Child Neurology
Seventh Edition

{There was} . . . a time when theses in medicine could still be beautifully literary, since ignorance about diseases and the human body still required that medicine be an art.
—Kurt Vonnegut, Jr.

Be kind to my mistakes, and live happy!
—Anonymous translator of Robinson Crusoe into Italian; cited by Walter De La Mare

All I have produced before the age of seventy is not worth taking into account.
—Hokusai, Katsushika

Child Neurology

Seventh Edition

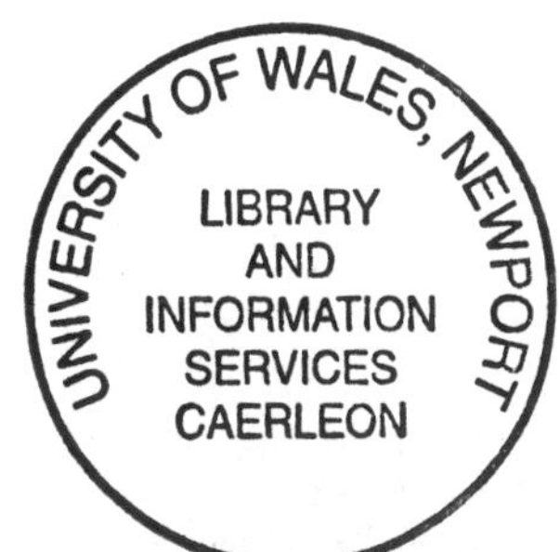

EDITED BY

JOHN H. MENKES, M.D.

Professor Emeritus
Departments of Neurology and Pediatrics
David Geffen School of Medicine at University of California Los Angeles
Los Angeles, California

HARVEY B. SARNAT, M.D., F.R.C.P.C.

Professor of Pediatrics, Pathology (Neuropathology), and Clinical Neurosciences
University of Calgary Faculty of Medicine
Chief, Division of Pediatric Neurology
Alberta Children's Hospital
Calgary, Alberta, Canada

BERNARD L. MARIA, M.D., M.B.A.

Jeffrey Edwin Gilliam Chair and Professor of Pediatrics and Neurosciences
Executive Director of the Charles P. Darby Children's Research Institute
Medical University of South Carolina
Charleston, South Carolina

Wolters Kluwer | Lippincott Williams & Wilkins
Health
Philadelphia • Baltimore • New York • London
Buenos Aires • Hong Kong • Sydney • Tokyo

Acquisitions Editor: Frances Destefano
Managing Editor: Joyce Murphy
Project Manager: Alicia Jackson
Senior Manufacturing Manager: Benjamin Rivera
Associate Marketing Director: Adam Glazer
Cover Designer: Joseph DePinho
Production Service: TechBooks
Printer: Quebecor World-Bogota

530 Walnut Street
Philadelphia, PA 19106 USA
LWW.com

Printed in Colombia

Library of Congress Cataloging-in-Publication Data

Child neurology / edited by John H. Menkes, Harvey B. Sarnat, Bernard L. Maria. — 7th ed.
p. ; cm.
Includes bibliographical references and index.
ISBN-13: 978-0-7817-5104-9
ISBN-10: 0-7817-5104-7
1. Pediatric neurology. I. Menkes, John H., 1928– II. Sarnat, Harvey B. III. Maria, Bernard L.
[DNLM: 1. Child. 2. Nervous System Diseases—Infant. WS 340 C5356 2005]
RJ486.C455 2005
618.92′8—dc22

2005021542

Care has been taken to confirm the accuracy of the information presented and to describe generally accepted practices. However, the authors, editors, and publisher are not responsible for errors or omissions or for any consequences from application of the information in this book and make no warranty, expressed or implied, with respect to the currency, completeness, or accuracy of the contents of the publication. Application of the information in a particular situation remains the professional responsibility of the practitioner.

The authors, editors, and publisher have exerted every effort to ensure that drug selection and dosage set forth in this text are in accordance with current recommendations and practice at the time of publication. However, in view of ongoing research, changes in government regulations, and the constant flow of information relating to drug therapy and drug reactions, the reader is urged to check the package insert for each drug for any change in indications and dosage and for added warnings and precautions. This is particularly important when the recommended agent is a new or infrequently employed drug.

Some drugs and medical devices presented in the publication have Food and Drug Administration (FDA) clearance for limited use in restricted research settings. It is the responsibility of the health care provider to ascertain the FDA status of each drug or device planned for use in their clinical practice.

To purchase additional copies of this book, call our customer service department at (800) 639-3030 or fax orders to (301) 824-7390. International customers should call (301) 714-2324.

Visit Lippincott Williams & Wilkins on the Internet: at LWW.com. Lippincott Williams & Wilkins customer service representatives are available from 8:30 am to 6 pm, EST.

10 9 8 7 6 5 4 3

To the teachers who have preceded me:
Blanche Bobbitt (1901-1988), who foresaw the importance of chemistry in the practice of medicine.

Sydney S. Gellis (1914–2002), who taught me that anything worth doing is worth doing well.

Alexander S. Nadas (1913–2000), who found humor in the most exasperating situations.

Sidney Carter (1912–2005), who showed me the value of a careful history and neurological examination.

David B. Clark (1913-1992), who demonstrated to me the humanity and intellectual rigor of nineteenth century British neurology.

J.H.M.

To my professors who, either as formal or indirect teachers, have been enlightening and inspiring influences in my career: Drs. LJ Thomas (zoologist), LMH Larramendi (neuroanatomist), FE Dreifuss (neurologist), MG Netsky (neuropathologist), EC Alvord Jr. (neuropathologist) and JH Menkes (neurologist).

And to my dear wife, Dr. Laura Flores-Sarnat, who has been enlightening, inspiring, loving and patient in both my professional and personal lives.

H.B.S

To my wife Barbara for her great love of children, To my son Alex for fueling a passion to make a difference, and To John Menkes, through the first (1974) and subsequent editions of this textbook, for igniting my development and that of so many others as child neurologists.

B.L.M.

To the teachers who have preceded me:

[illegible] (1907–1973), who first saw the importance of chemistry in the practice of medicine

[illegible] (1914–2003), who taught me that anything worth doing is worth doing well

[illegible] (1918–2000), who found humor in the most exasperating situations

[illegible]

[illegible] century [illegible]

J.H.M.

To my professors who, either as formal or indirect teachers, have been enlightening and standing influences in my career: [illegible]

And to my dear wife, Dr. [illegible], who has been a continuous, inspiring, loving and patient [illegible] professional and personal lives.

[illegible]

To my wife [illegible] for her [illegible] through the [illegible] and subsequent editions of this text and for [illegible]

[illegible]

CONTENTS

CONTRIBUTORS

James F. Bale, Jr., M.D.
Department of Pediatrics
University of Utah School of Medicine
Salt Lake City, Utah

Richard C. Ellenbogen, M.D.
Chairman
Department of Neurological Surgery
University of Washington
Seattle, Washington

Rena Ellen Falk, M.D.
Professor
Department of Pediatrics
University of California
Medical Director, Cytogenetics Laboratory
Steven Spielberg Pediatric Research Center
Cedars-Sinai Medical Center
Los Angeles, California

Christos D. Katsetos, M.D., Ph.D., M.R.C. Path
Research Professor
Department of Pediatrics
Drexel University College of Medicine
Director, Neurology Research Laboratory and
Department of Pathology and Laboratory Medicine
St. Chrisopher's Hospital for Children
Philadelphia, Pennsylvania

Marcel Kinsbourne, M.D.
Professor
Cognitive Studies
Tufts University
Medford, Massachusetts

Susan Koh, M.D.
Clinical Assistant Professor
Department of Pediatrics
David Geffen School of Medicine at UCLA
Director, Pediatric Epilepsy Monitoring Unit
Mattel Children's Hospital at UCLA
Los Angeles, California

Augustin Legido, M.D., Ph.D. M.B.A.
Professor
Departments of Pediatrics and Neurology
Drexel University College of Medicine
Chief
Section of Neurology
St. Christopher's Hospital for Children
Philadelphia, Pennsylvania

Laura Flores-Sarnat, M.D.
Pediatric Neurologist and Research Associate
Division of Pediatric Neurology
Alberta Children's Hospital
Calgary, Alberta, Canada

Bernard L. Maria, M.D., M.B.A.
Jeffrey Edwin Gilliam Chair and Professor of Pediatrics and Neurosciences
Executive Director of the Charles P. Darby Children's Research Institute
Medical University of South Carolina
Charleston, South Carolina

John H. Menkes, M.D.
Professor Emeritus
Departments of Neurology and Pediatrics
David Geffen School of Medicine at University of California Los Angeles
Los Angeles, California

Franklin G. Moser, M.D., FACR
Director of Clinical and Interventional Neuroradiology
Department of Imaging
Cedars-Sinai Medical Center
Los Angeles, California

E. Steve Roach, M.D.
Professor of Neurology
Department of Neurology
Wake Forest University School of Medicine
WFU-Baptist Medical Center
Winston-Salem, North Carolina

A. David Rothner, M.D.
Director of Patient Education
The Cleveland Clinic Foundation
Cleveland, Ohio

Raman Sankar, M.D., Ph.D.
Associate Professor of Neurology and Pediatrics
Department of Pediatrics
David Geffen School of Medicine at UCLA
Director of Training in Child Neurology
Mattel Children's Hospital at UCLA
Los Angeles, California

Cesar C. Santos, M.D.
Associate Professor
Department of Neurology
Wake Forest University School of Medicine
Chief
Division of Pediatric Neurology
WFU-Baptist Medical Center
Winston Salem, North Carolina

Harvey B. Sarnat, M.D.
Professor of Pediatrics, Pathology, and Clinical Neurosciences
University of Calgary
Alberta Children's Hospital
Calgary, Alberta, Canada

Samuel Robert Snodgrass, M.D.
Professor of Neurology
University of California
Los Angeles, California
Professor of Pediatrics and Neurology
Harbor UCLA Medical Center
Torrance, California

Silvia N. Tenembaum, M.D.
Pediatric Neurologist
Department of Neurology
Children's Hospital Dr. J.P. Garrahan
Buenos Aires, Argentina

William R.Wilcox, M.D., Ph.D.
Associate Professor
Department of Pediatrics
UCLA School of Medicine
Medical Geneticist
Cedars-Sinai Medical Center
Los Angeles, California

Frank Wood, Ph.D.
Professor and Section Head of Neuropsychology
Department of Neurology
Wake Forest University School of Medicine
Winston Salem, North Carolina

Joyce Wu, M.D.
Clinical Assistant Professor
Department of Pediatrics
David Geffen School of Medicine at UCLA
Clinical Attending Child Neurologist
Mattel Children's Hospital at UCLA
Los Angeles, California

PREFACE TO THE SEVENTH EDITION

It would be redundant to state that the world of Pediatric Neurology has changed considerably since the first edition of this work was published in 1974. At that time molecular genetics was in its infancy—Neil Holtzman and his group at Johns Hopkins had just reported on a mass screening program for phenylketonuria, and gene sequencing lay three years in the future—and neuroimaging was confined to pneumoencephalography, ventriculography and arteriography—Ambrose and Hounsfield's seminal paper on computerized tomography had been published in 1973, and the new technique was gaining acceptance at clinical centers. Since publication of the sixth edition in 2000, molecular genetics has made its impact felt on all aspects of the neurosciences. Not only has it affected neuropharmacology and our understanding of the heredodegenerative diseases of the nervous system, but it has also provided important insights into the processes that underlie the embryology of the nervous system, and allowed a transition from the traditional descriptive morphogenesis to concepts based on genetic programming. With these advances has come the first clarification of some of the common developmental defects and malformations. Another byproduct of the unraveling of molecular pathogenesis is a better understanding of mitochondrial diseases, which are being more frequently recognized, and which are now known to "cause any symptom in any tissue at any age by any inheritance."

The seventh edition pays tribute to these advances. They required a new chapter on mitochondrial encephalomyopathies, and an enlarged chapter on the New Neuroembryology. Another chapter that is new to this edition deals with Headaches and Non-epileptic Episodic Disorders. It was written in response to the increasing importance of these conditions in the general practice of pediatric neurology. The number of contributors to the book continues to increase, and now stands at 22, as compared with the five contributors to the first edition. Dr. Sarnat and I have called upon Bernard L. Maria to serve as co-editor of the seventh edition. Dr. Maria chose a career in pediatric neurology after reading the first 1974 edition of the book handed to him by his first mentor Bernard Lemieux in 1977. Now, nearly 30 years later, he contributes his expertise as co-editor in addition to having authored several chapters in child neurology and neuro-oncology.

As before, my co-editors and I have attempted to provide the reader with the most recent advances in the neurosciences, and to integrate these into the clinical practice of pediatric neurology. As before, we have not cast aside the classic contributions to neurology that form the essence of our discipline and that the younger practitioners may not have had the opportunity to absorb.

Finally, our thanks go out to Joyce Murphy and Adam Glazer at Lippincott, Williams and Wilkins, and to Stephanie Lentz at Techbooks without whose help this book would not have become a reality.

John H. Menkes, M.D.

PREFACE TO THE FIRST EDITION

Even in a textbook, prefaces are written not to be read but rather to blunt inevitable criticisms. One must therefore first ask, why, in view of the existence of several first-rate pediatric neurology texts, was this book ever written. The main excuse for becoming involved in such an undertaking, and for imposing another book upon an already overwhelmed medical audience, is the hope of being able to offer a new viewpoint of the field. More than any other branch of clinical neurology, pediatric neurology has felt the impact of the many recent advances in the neurosciences. Their magnitude becomes evident when the neurologic literature of the last century is read. At that time, clinical descriptions achieved a degree of clarity and conciseness, which has not been improved upon, and which at present is only rarely equaled. Yet the reader who finds the explanation of Tay-Sachs disease* offered during the last years of the nineteenth century must experience a sense of achievement at the great strides made during a relatively brief historical period. However, at the same time, one cannot but wonder how many of our "explanations" accepted and taught today, will make as little sense fifty years hence.

It is the aim of this text to incorporate some of the knowledge derived from the basic neurologic sciences into the clinical evaluation and management of the child with neurologic disease. Obviously, this can only be done to a limited extent. For some conditions the basic sciences have not yet offered any help, while for others, available experimental data only provide tangential information. Even when biochemical or physiologic information is pertinent to the conditions under discussion, their full presentation has been avoided, for to do so with any degree of completeness would require an extensive review of several scientific disciplines, which would go far beyond the intent of the text. The author and his colleagues have therefore chosen to review only aspects of the neurologic sciences with immediate clinical impact, and to refer the reader to the literature for some of the remaining information. They have also deemed it appropriate *not* to include a section on the neurologic examination of children. This subject is extremely well presented by R. S. Paine and T. E. Oppe, in *The Neurologic Examination of Children*,** a work everyone seriously interested in pediatric neurology should read.

In covering the field, extensive use of literature references has been made. These generally serve one or more of the following purposes:

(1) A classic or early description of the condition.
(2) Background information pertaining to the relevant neurologic sciences.
(3) A current review of the condition.
(4) In the case of some of the rarer clinical entities, the presentation of several key references was preferred to a brief and obviously inadequate summary.

It is hoped that this approach will serve to keep the text reasonably compact, yet allow it to be used as a guide for further reading.

John H. Menkes, M.D.
Los Angeles, California

*Namely, "an inherited weakness of the central nervous system, especially of the ganglion cells, and a premature degeneration due to exhaustion caused by this."

**London, Wm. Heinemann, 1966.

Neurologic Examination of the Child and Infant

John H. Menkes and Franklin G. Moser

The ever-increasing sophistication and accuracy of neurodiagnostic procedures might cause younger physicians to view the neurologic examination of the pediatric patient as obsolete and, like cardiac auscultation, a nostalgic ceremony engaged in by physicians trained before magnetic resonance imaging (MRI) and DNA hybridization (1). This is not how we view it. Excessive reliance on diagnostic procedures at the expense of an organized plan of approach, the "let's order an MRI and an electroencephalogram and then take a look at the kid" attitude, not only has been responsible for the depersonalization of neurologic care and the escalation of its costs, but also has made the analysis of neurologic problems unduly complex for the pediatrician or general practitioner. For these reasons, a presentation of some of the techniques of neurologic examination is still in order.

The pediatric neurologist who, through experience, has individualized the examination will find little new in this section, which was written with the pediatrician and general neurologist in mind. The pediatrician will find the section on the neurologic examination helpful; the general neurologist, who at times is called on to consult on an infant not much larger than the palm of the hand, may benefit from the section on the neurologic examination of the infant.

At its best, the neurologic evaluation is a challenge in logical deduction. It requires a clear plan at each step with the goal of answering the following questions:

1. Does the child have a neurologic disorder?
2. If so, where is the site of the lesion, or, as so often is the case in pediatric neurology, does it involve all parts of the brain to an equal degree?
3. What pathologic lesions are most likely to produce lesions at these sites?

The course of the illness, whether acute, subacute, static, or remitting, may provide a clue to the nature of the disease process.

It is at this point, and only at this point, that the physician draws up a differential diagnosis and calls on neurodiagnostic procedures to help decide which of the suspected conditions is the most likely.

If this systematic approach is followed, useless diagnostic procedures are avoided. For instance, an assay for arylsulfatase to exclude metachromatic leukodystrophy is inappropriate in a neurologic disorder that is clearly static. Similarly, neither computed tomography (CT) scans nor MRI of the brain assist materially in the differential diagnosis of a lower motor neuron disease.

NEUROLOGIC HISTORY

An accurate history, obtained from one or more members of the family, is often the most vital part of the neurologic evaluation. Additionally, if properly questioned, a child older than 3 to 5 years might provide information that not only is valuable, but also may be more reliable than that related by his or her parents. In taking a history from a youngster, the physician must learn not to ask leading questions and not to phrase them to obtain yes or no answers. The physician also must be responsive to the youngster's mood and cease taking a history as soon as fatigue or restlessness becomes evident. In a younger child or one with a limited attention span, the salient points of the history are best secured at the onset of the evaluation. The history is followed by the neurologic examination and, finally, by a second, more extensive review of the history.

In the assessment of a neurologic problem, an accurate review of the presenting illness is important. This is particularly the case in the youngster with headaches, seizures, or other types of recurrent disease and for the youngster with a learning disability or an attention-deficit disorder. In such patients, the history, particularly its social and environmental aspects, can be extensive enough to require more than one appointment.

A review of the developmental history necessitates a survey of antenatal, perinatal, and postnatal development.

This includes questioning the mother about the length of the pregnancy, any complications, including intercurrent infections, and drug intake. The mother who is concerned about her youngster may already have reviewed her pregnancy many times and may well provide much irrelevant information. For instance, an accident occurring during the second trimester is hardly the explanation for a meningomyelocele. The physician might well interrupt the questioning to reassure the mother that this event was not responsible for the child's neurologic defect.

A review of the perinatal events is always in order. As a rule, the youngster who has had an uncomplicated neonatal period and was discharged with the mother will not have sustained perinatal asphyxia, even though the infant might have had low Apgar scores or passage of meconium. The physician should not forget to obtain some information about the feeding history. Many children who later present with delayed development have had feeding problems, notably regurgitation, excessive colic, or frequent formula changes. A history of abnormal sleeping habits is also not unusual in the brain-damaged youngster.

The developmental milestones must always be recorded. Most mothers recall these and can compare one youngster with the siblings. Failure to remember any of the milestones is unusual, even in those of lower socioeconomic status; it suggests a postpartum depression.

A system review focuses on the major childhood illnesses, immunizations, and injuries. Recurrent injuries suggest hyperactivity, impaired coordination, or poor impulse control.

The family history is relevant in some of the neurologic disorders. The physician should remember that most neurodegenerative disorders are transmitted as a recessive gene and that questions about the health of siblings and the presence of consanguinity are in order. On the other hand, some of the epilepsies or migraine headaches tend to be transmitted as dominant traits; in fact, in children experiencing migraine headaches, a history of migraine in a first-degree relative can almost always be elicited.

GENERAL PHYSICAL EXAMINATION

The child's height, weight, blood pressure, and head circumference must always be measured and recorded. The youngster should be undressed by the parents, with the physician absent.

The physician should note the general appearance of the child, in particular the facial configuration and the presence of any dysmorphic features. Cutaneous lesions such as café au lait spots, angiomas, or areas of depigmentation are clues to the presence of phakomatoses. The condition of the teeth provides information about antenatal defects or kernicterus. The location of the hair whorl and the appearance of the palmar creases should always be noted. Abnormalities of whorl patterns can indicate the presence of cerebral malformations (2). The quality of the scalp hair, eyebrows, and nails also should be taken into account. It is important to inspect the midline of the neck, back, and pilonidal area for any defects, particularly for small dimples that might indicate the presence of a dermoid sinus tract. Comparison of the size of the thumbnails and their convexity might disclose a growth disturbance, a frequent accompaniment to a hemiparesis. Examination of chest, heart, and abdomen and palpation of the femoral pulses should always be part of the general physical examination. Finally, the presence of an unusual body odor may offer a clue to a metabolic disorder.

NEUROLOGIC EXAMINATION OF THE CHILD

In addition to the standard instruments used in neurologic examination, the following have been found useful: a tennis ball; a few small toys, including a toy car that can be used to assess fine motor coordination; a bell; and some object that attracts the child's attention (e.g., a pinwheel). A flashlight with a rubber adapter for transillumination is still used by some pediatric neurologists; it is cheaper and quicker than a CT scan or an ultrasound and often provides the same information. Most pediatric neurologists do not wear white coats.

In most intellectually healthy school-aged children, the general physical and neurologic examinations can be performed in the same manner as for adults, except that their more uncomfortable aspects, such as funduscopic examination, corneal and gag reflexes, and sensory testing, should be postponed until the end.

In younger children, the neurologic examination is a catch-as-catch-can procedure, with a considerable amount of information revealed by the youngster's play activities, including the child's dominant handedness and the presence of cerebellar deficits, a hemiparesis, and perhaps even a visual field defect.

The toddler is more difficult to examine. The toddler is best approached by seating the child in the mother's or father's lap and talking to the child. Because toddlers are fearful of strangers, the physician must first observe the youngster and defer touching him or her until some degree of rapport has been established. Offering a small, interesting toy may bridge the gap. In any case, the physician must be patient and wait for the youngster to make the first approach. Once frightened, most toddlers are difficult to reassure and are lost for the remainder of the examination.

Skull

The general appearance of the skull can suggest the presence of macrocephaly, microcephaly, or craniosynostosis. Prominence of the venous pattern might accompany increased intracranial pressure. Flattening of the occiput is seen in many developmentally delayed youngsters. Conversely, occipital prominence can indicate the Dandy-Walker malformation complex. Biparietal enlargement suggests the presence of subdural hematomas and should raise the suspicion of child abuse. Palpation of the skull can disclose ridging of the sutures, as occurs in craniosynostosis. Biparietal foramina are usually benign and are often transmitted as a dominant trait (3). Some are due to mutations in the *MSX2* gene, whereas in other families it is part of the 11p11.2 deletion syndrome (4). Prominence of the metopic suture is seen in some youngsters with developmental malformations. Percussion of the skull can reveal areas of tenderness resulting from localized osteomyelitis, an indication of an underlying brain abscess. Macewen (*cracked pot*) sign accompanies the separation of sutures and reflects increased intracranial pressure.

If accurately measured, serial head circumferences continue to be one of the most valuable parameters for assessing the presence of hydrocephalus or microcephaly. After multiple measurements are made with a good cloth or steel tape to ensure that the maximum circumference has been obtained, the value should be recorded on a head growth chart (Fig. I.1). Delayed head growth, particularly with evidence of arrest or slowing of head growth, reflects impaired brain growth from a variety of causes. Scalloping of the temporal fossae frequently accompanies microcephaly and suggests underdeveloped frontal and temporal lobes. Occasionally, one encounters a youngster, usually a girl, with a head circumference at or below the third percentile whose somatic measurements are commensurate and whose intellectual development is normal.

Palpation of the anterior fontanelle provides a simple way of estimating intracranial pressure. Normally, the fontanelle is slightly depressed and the pulsations are hardly felt. Auscultation of the skull using a bell stethoscope with the child in the erect position is performed over six standard listening points: globes, the temporal fossae, and the retroauricular or mastoid regions. In all cases, conduction of a cardiac murmur should be excluded. Spontaneous intracranial bruits are common in children. These are augmented by contralateral carotid compression. Wadia and Monckton (5) heard unilateral or bilateral bruits in 60% of 4- to 5-year-old children, 10% of 10-year-old children, and 45% of 15- to 16-year-old adolescents. Intracranial bruits are heard in more than 80% of patients with angiomas. Unlike benign bruits, they are accompanied by a thrill and are much louder and harsher. Intracranial bruits are heard in a variety of other conditions characterized by increased cerebral blood flow. These include anemia, thyrotoxicosis, and meningitis. Bruits also accompany hydrocephalus and some (not necessarily vascular) intracranial tumors. The technique and the history of auscultation for intracranial bruits are reviewed by Mackenzie (6).

Cranial Nerves

Olfactory Nerve

The olfactory nerve is only rarely assessed. Loss of olfactory nerve function can follow a head injury with fracture of the cribriform plate. Nerve function also can be lost when a tumor involves the olfactory bulbs. Olfactory sensation as transmitted by the olfactory nerve is not functional in the newborn, but is present by 5 to 7 months of age. By contrast, newborns do respond to inhalation of irritants, such as ammonia or vinegar, because the reflex is transmitted by the trigeminal nerve; hence, this reflex is preserved in the infant with arhinencephaly (7).

Optic Nerve

Much can be learned from a funduscopic examination, and more time is often spent with this than with any other part of the neurologic examination. With assistance from the parent or nurse, it is possible to examine even the most uncooperative youngster. If necessary, a mydriatic such as 2.5% or 10.0% phenylephrine (Neo-Synephrine) or 1% cyclopentolate (Cyclogyl) is used. Particular attention is paid to the optic discs, maculae, and appearance of the retina. In infants, the optic disc is normally pale and gray, an appearance similar to optic atrophy in later life. Optic nerve hypoplasia can be diagnosed if the discs are less than one-half normal size. The macular light reflex is absent until approximately 4 months of age. Premature and newborn infants have incompletely developed uveal pigment, resulting in a pale appearance of the fundus and a clear view of the choroidal blood vessels. Hyperemia of the disk, obliteration of the disc margins and absent pulsations of the central veins are the earliest and most important indications for papilledema. The differential diagnosis of papilledema is reviewed in Chapter 11.

Retinal hemorrhages are seen in one-third of vaginally delivered newborns. They are usually small and multiple, and their presence does not necessarily indicate intracranial bleeding. Persistence of the hyaloid artery is common in premature infants and is seen in approximately 3% of full-term infants. Chorioretinitis suggests an intrauterine infection. Less extensive and grouped pigmentation resembling the footprints of an animal (*bear tracks*) represents a harmless and common anomaly. This condition must be distinguished from the more extensive pigmentation seen in retinitis pigmentosa.

Visual acuity can be tested in the older child by standard means. In the toddler, an approximation can be obtained by observing him or her at play or by offering objects of varying sizes. Optokinetic nystagmus can be elicited by rotating a striped drum or by drawing a strip of cloth with black and white squares in front of the child's eyes. The presence of optokinetic nystagmus confirms cortical vision; its absence, however, is inconclusive. Unilateral

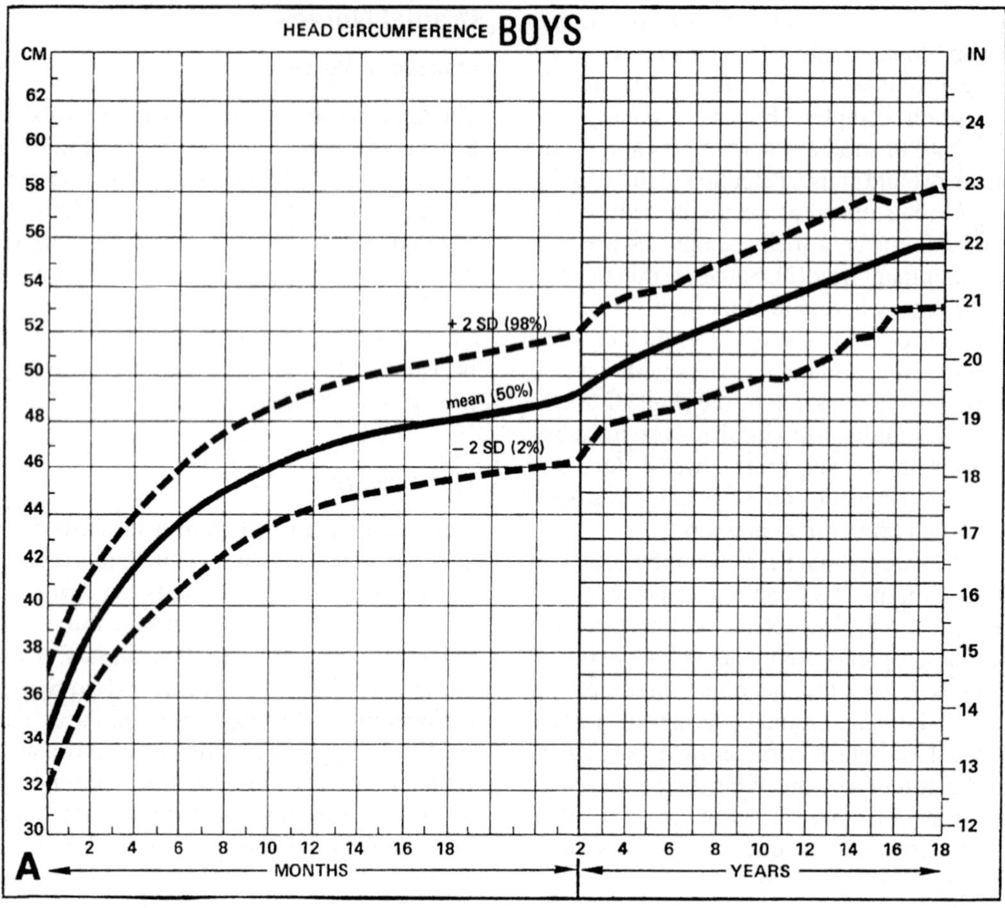

FIGURE I.1. Composite international and interracial head circumference graph. **A:** Boys. (*continued*)

optokinetic nystagmus suggests the presence of hemianopia. The visual fields can be assessed in toddlers and in infants younger than 12 months of age. The baby is placed in the mother's lap and the physician is seated in front of them, using a small toy to attract the baby's attention. An assistant standing in back of the infant brings another object into the field of vision, and the point at which the infant's eyes or head turns toward the object is noted.

The blink reflex, closure of the eyelids when an object is suddenly moved toward the eyes, is often used to determine the presence of functional vision in small infants. The reflex is absent in the newborn and does not appear until 3 or 4 months of age. It is present in approximately one-half of healthy 5-month-old infants and should be present in all infants by 1 year of age (8).

Oculomotor, Trochlear, and Abducens Nerves: Extraocular Movements

The physician notes the position of the eyes at rest. Noting the points of reflection of a flashlight assists in detecting a nonparallel alignment of the eyes. Paralysis of the oculomotor nerve results in lateral and slightly downward deviation of the affected eye. Paralysis of the abducens nerve produces a medial deviation of the affected eye, whereas paralysis of the trochlear nerve produces little change at rest. The *setting sun* sign, a forced downward deviation of the eyes at rest with paresis of upward gaze, is an indication of increased intracranial pressure, in particular pressure on the quadrigeminal plate causing impairment of the vertical gaze centers. This phenomenon also can be elicited in healthy infants younger than 4 weeks of age by suddenly changing the position of the head and in infants up to 20, or even 40, weeks of age by removing a bright light that had been placed in front of their eyes (9). Downward deviation of the eyes, skew deviation, and intermittent opsoclonus (irregular, chaotic oscillations of the eyes in horizontal, vertical, or oblique directions) may be noted transiently in healthy newborns (10).

Ocular bobbing refers to abnormal spontaneous vertical eye movements. In its most typical appearance, it consists of intermittent, often conjugate, fast downward movement of the eyes followed by, after a brief tonic interval, a slower return to the primary position (11). It is generally seen with pontine pathology, but also can be encountered

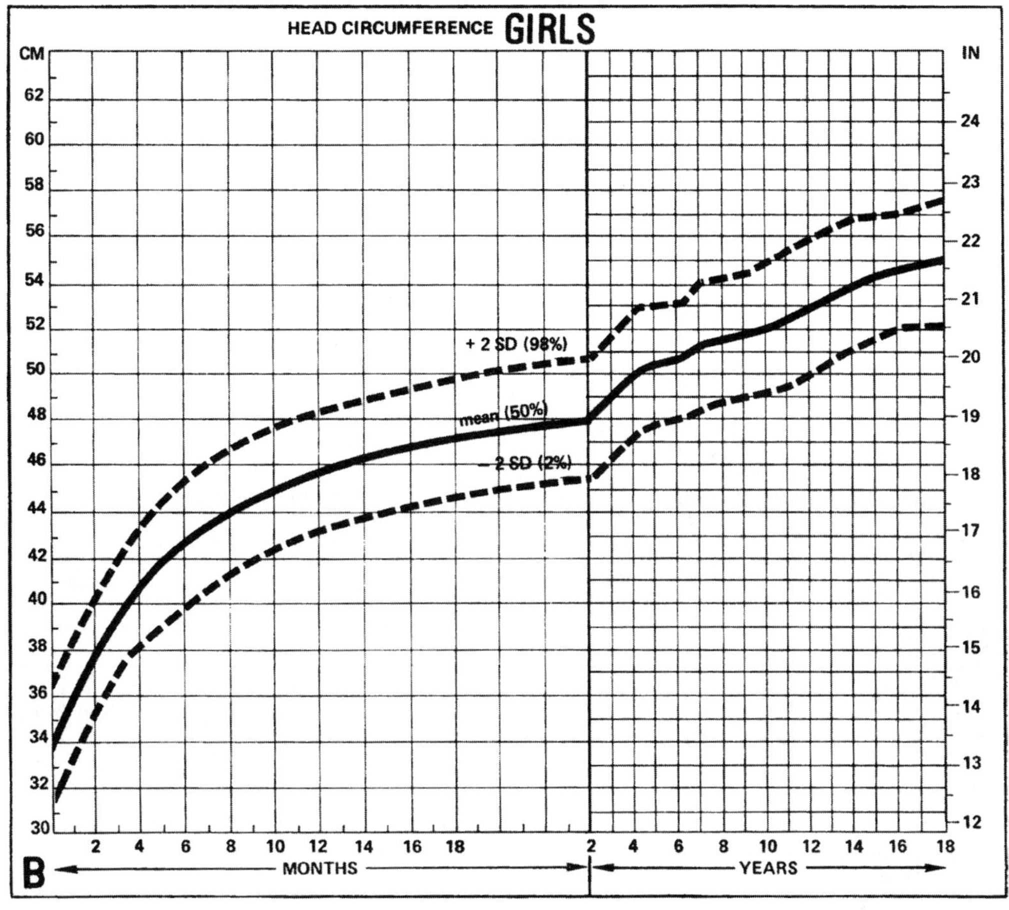

FIGURE I.1. *Continued.* **B:** Girls. SD, standard deviation. (Courtesy of the late Dr. G. Nellhaus, Napa VA Hospital, Napa, CA.)

in encephalitis and in some metabolic encephalopathies. It probably reflects residual eye movements of patients who have severe limitations of horizontal and vertical eye movements.

The doll's-eye phenomenon refers to the apparent turning of the eyes to the opposite direction in response to rotation of the head. It is seen in healthy newborns, in coma, and whenever optic fixation is impaired.

The size of the pupils, their reactivity to light, and accommodation and convergence are noted. In infants younger than 30 weeks' gestation, pupils are large and no response to light occurs. After 32 weeks' gestation, an absent light response is abnormal (12).

The association of meiosis, enophthalmos, ptosis, and lack of sweating on the ipsilateral side of the face was first described in 1869 and is known as Horner syndrome (13). The condition can result from damage to the cervical sympathetic nerves when it accompanies brachial plexus injuries or can be congenital, being transmitted as an autosomal dominant condition (14). A slight degree of anisocoria is not unusual, particularly in infants and small children. Fatigue-induced anisocoria also has been noted to be transmitted as an autosomal dominant trait (15).

Eye movements are examined by having the child follow an object while the mother holds the child's head. If the child permits it, the movement of each eye is examined separately while the other one is kept covered. The actions of the extraocular muscles are depicted in Fig. I.2. At birth, doll's-eye movements are normally elicitable, but little or no conjugation occurs. Shortly after birth, the eyes become conjugated, and by 2 weeks of age, the infant moves the eyes toward light and fixates. Following movements are complete in all directions by approximately 4 months of age, and acoustically elicited eye movements appear at 5 months of age (16). Depth perception using solely binocular cues appears by 24 months of age along with stable binocular alignment and optokinetic nystagmus.

Strabismus owing to muscular imbalance can be differentiated from a paralytic strabismus. In the former, the ocular movements are concomitant and full. In the latter, the disassociation of the eyes increases when the eyes enter the field of action of the paralyzed muscle. In abducens nerve palsies, failure of abduction is readily demonstrable. The combination of defective adduction and elevation with outward and downward displacement of the eye suggests a third-nerve palsy. Internuclear ophthalmoplegia

RIGHT UPWARD GAZE

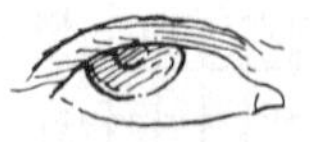

Rt. sup. rectus III

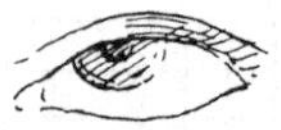

Lt. inf. oblique III

LEFT UPWARD GAZE

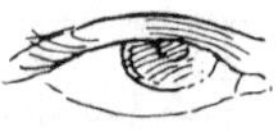

Rt. inf. oblique III

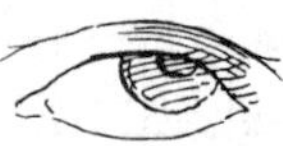

Lt. sup. rectus III

RIGHT LATERAL GAZE

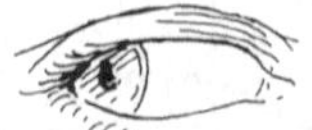

Rt. ext. rectus VI

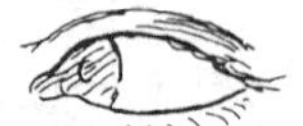

Lt. medial. rectus III

LEFT LATERAL GAZE

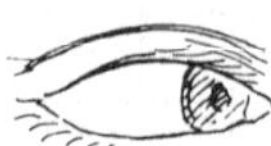

Rt. medial rectus III

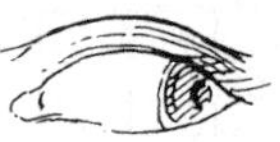

Lt. ext. rectus VI

RIGHT DOWNWARD GAZE

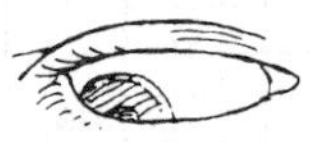

Rt. inf. rectus III

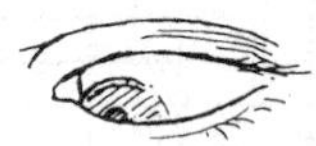

Lt. sup. oblique IV

LEFT DOWNWARD GAZE

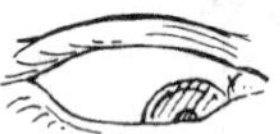

Rt. sup. oblique IV

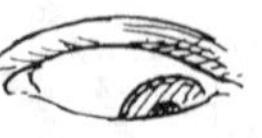

Lt. inf. rectus III

FIGURE I.2. Extraocular muscles involved in the various eye movements. Ext., exterior; inf., inferior; Lt., left; Rt., right; sup., superior. (Adapted from Farmer TW. *Pediatric neurology*, 3rd ed. New York: Harper & Row, 1983. With permission.)

(syndrome of the median longitudinal fasciculus) in its classical appearance consists of paralysis of adduction of the contralateral eye on lateral gaze, with nystagmus of the abducting eye and preservation of convergence. Ptosis and a large pupil with impaired constriction to light also can be present. Unilateral or bilateral congenital ptosis is relatively common, being transmitted as a dominant trait in some instance, and as X-linked in others (17). In some subjects with ptosis, reflex elevation or closure of the ptotic lid occurs in response to swallowing or movements of the jaw. Elevation has been termed the *Marcus Gunn sign* and closure the *reverse Marcus Gunn sign*. In instances of trochlear nerve palsy, the eye fails to move down when adducted. This defect is often accompanied by a head tilt.

In describing the presence of nystagmus, the physician should note the position of the eyes that produces the greatest amplitude of the nystagmus, the direction of the fast movement, and the quality or speed of the nystagmus. When the nystagmus is of small amplitude, it might be noted only on funduscopic examination.

Trigeminal Nerve

The action of the temporalis and masseter muscles is noted. Unilateral lesions of the trigeminal nerve result in a deviation of the jaw to the paralytic side and atrophy of the temporalis muscle. The jaw jerk can be elicited by placing one's finger below the lower lip of the slightly open mouth and tapping downward. An absent jaw jerk is rarely significant; upper motor neuron lesions above the level of the pons exaggerate the reflex.

The corneal reflex tests the intactness of the ophthalmic branch of the trigeminal nerve. A defect should be suspected when spontaneous blinking on one side is slower and less complete. The frequency of blinking increases with maturation and decreases in toxic illnesses.

Facial Nerve

Impaired motor function is indicated by facial asymmetry. Involvement of the facial nucleus or the nerve produces a lower motor neuron weakness in which upper and lower parts of the face are paralyzed. Normal wrinkling of the forehead is impaired, and the eye either cannot be closed or can be opened readily by the examiner. Weakness of the face can be obvious at rest and is accentuated when the child laughs or cries. When facial weakness is caused by corticobulbar involvement (upper motor neuron facial weakness), the musculature of the upper part of the face is spared. Although this sparing was believed to reflect bilateral enervation of the upper facial motor neurons, it now appears that upper facial motor neurons receive little direct cortical input, whereas lower facial neurons do (18).

Weakness is accentuated with volitional movements but disappears when the child laughs or cries. The converse, upper motor facial weakness associated with emotion and not evident on volitional movements, can be seen in thalamic lesions (19). The McCarthy reflex, ipsilateral blinking produced by tapping the supraorbital region, is diminished or absent in lower motor neuron facial weakness. Like the palpebral reflex, bilateral blinking induced by tapping the root of the nose, it can be exaggerated by upper motor neuron lesions. In hemiparesis or peripheral facial nerve weakness, the contraction of the platysma muscle is less vigorous on the affected side. This sign also carries Babinski's name.

An isolated weakness of the depressor of the corner of the mouth (depressor anguli oris) is relatively common in children. It results in a failure to pull the affected side of the mouth backward and downward when crying.

The sense of taste from the anterior two-thirds of the tongue is conveyed by the chorda tympani. Taste can be tested in children by applying solutions of sugar or salt to the previously dried and protruded tongue by cotton-tipped applicator sticks, making certain that the child does not withdraw the tongue into the mouth.

Cochlear and Vestibular Nerves

Hearing can be tested in the younger child by observing the child's response to a bell. Small infants become alert to sound; the ability to turn the eyes to the direction of the sound becomes evident by 7 to 8 weeks of age, and turning with eyes and head appears by approximately 3 to 4 months of age. Hearing is tested in older children by asking them to repeat a whispered word or number. For more accurate evaluation of hearing, audiometry or brainstem auditory-evoked potentials are necessary.

Vestibular function can be assessed easily in infants or small children by holding the youngster vertically so he or she is facing the examiner, then turning the child several times in a full circle. Clockwise and counterclockwise rotations are performed. The direction and amplitude of the quick and slow movements of the eye are noted. The healthy infant demonstrates full deviation of the eyes in the direction that he or she is being rotated with the quick phase of the nystagmus backward. When rotation ceases, these directions are reversed. This test has been found to be valuable in a newborn suspected of perinatal asphyxia, with an abnormal response suggesting impaired brainstem function between the vestibular and the oculomotor nuclei.

Glossopharyngeal and Vagus Nerves

Asymmetry of the resting uvula and palate and failure to elevate the palate during phonation indicate impaired vagal motor function. When upper or lower motor neuron involvement of the vagus nerve exists, the uvula deviates toward the unaffected side, and with movement, the palate is drawn away from the affected side.

The gag reflex tests the afferent and efferent portions of the vagus. This reflex is absent in approximately one-third of healthy individuals (20). Testing taste over the posterior part of the tongue is extremely difficult and, according to some opinions, generally not worth the effort.

Spinal Accessory Nerve

Testing the sternocleidomastoid muscle can be done readily by having the child rotate his or her head against resistance.

Hypoglossal Nerve

The position of the tongue at rest should be noted with the mouth open. The tongue deviates toward the paretic side. Fasciculations are seen as small depressions that appear and disappear quickly at irregular intervals. They are most readily distinguished on the underside of the tongue. Their presence cannot be determined with any reliability if the youngster is crying.

Motor System

The child's station (i.e., posture while standing) can usually be discerned before the start of the examination. Similarly, the walking and running gaits can be seen by playing with the youngster and asking him or her to retrieve a ball and run outside of the examining room. In the course of such an informal examination, sufficient information can be obtained so that the formal testing of muscle strength is only confirmatory.

Evaluation of the motor system in a school-aged child can be done in a formal manner. Examination of selected proximal and distal muscles of the upper and lower extremities is usually sufficient. A book published by the Medical Research Council is invaluable for this purpose (21): Muscle strength is graded from 0 to 5. The following grading system has been suggested:

0. No muscle contraction
1. Flicker or trace of contraction
2. Active movement with gravity eliminated
3. Active movement against gravity
4. Active movement against gravity and resistance
5. Normal power

Muscle tone is examined by manipulating the major joints and determining the degree of resistance. In toddlers or infants, inequalities of tone to pronation and supination of the wrist, flexion and extension of the elbow, and dorsi and plantar flexion of the ankle have been found to provide more information than assessment of muscle strength or reflexes.

A sensitive test for weakness of the upper extremities is the pronator sign, in which the hand on the hypotonic side hyperpronates to palm outward as the arms are raised over the head. Additionally, the elbow may flex (Fig. I.3). In the lower extremities, weakness of the flexors of the knee can readily be demonstrated by having the child lie prone and asking the child to maintain his or her legs in flexion at right angles at the knee (Barré sign).

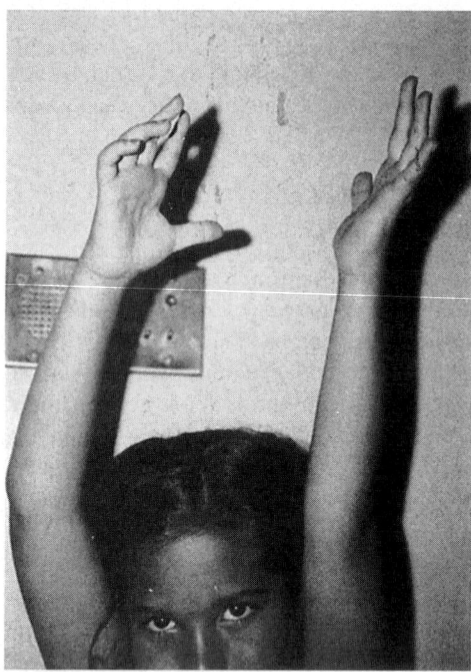

FIGURE I.3. The pronator sign. Weakness of the right upper extremity in a girl with a Brown-Séquard syndrome after spinal cord trauma.

Coordination

Coordination can be tested by applying specific tests for cerebellar function, such as having the youngster reach for and manipulate toys. One may be reluctant to use marbles for this purpose for fear that a small child might swallow them. Ataxia with tremor of the extremities can be demonstrated in the older child on finger-to-nose and heel-to-shin testing. Accentuation of the tremor as the extremity approaches the target is characteristic of cerebellar dysfunction (intention tremor). In the finger-to-nose test, the arm must be maintained abducted at the shoulder. The examiner can discover minor abnormalities by moving the finger to a different place each time. The ability to perform rapidly alternating movements can be assessed by having the child repeatedly pat the examiner's hand, or by having the child perform rapid pronation and supination of the hands. In the lower extremities, rapid tapping of the foot serves a similar purpose. Pyramidal and extrapyramidal lesions slow rapid succession movements but leave intact the execution of each stage of the movement so that no true dissociation occurs. The heel-to-shin test is not an easy task for many youngsters to comprehend, and performance must be interpreted with regard to the child's age and level of intelligence.

A variety of involuntary movements can be noted in the course of the examination. They may be seen when the child walks or is engaged in various purposeful acts.

Athetosis indicates an instability of posture, with slow swings of movement most marked in the distal portions of the limbs. The movements fluctuate between two extremes of posture in the hand, one of hyperextension of the fingers with pronation and flexion of the wrist and supination of the forearm and the other of intense flexion and adduction of the fingers and wrist and pronation of the forearm.

Choreiform movements refer to more rapid and jerky movements similar in their range to the athetoid movements but so fluid and continuous that the two extremes of posture are no longer evident (22). They commonly involve the muscles of the face, tongue, and proximal portions of the limbs. In children, athetosis and choreiform movements occur far more frequently as associated, rather than as isolated, phenomena.

Dystonia is characterized by fixation or relative fixation in one of the athetotic postures. When dystonia results from perinatal asphyxia, it is nearly always accompanied by other involuntary movements. The other manifestations of basal ganglia disorder (tremors and myoclonus) are usually less apparent. Tremors are rhythmic alterations in movement, whereas myoclonus is a relatively unpredictable contraction of one or more muscle groups. It can be precipitated by a variety of stimuli, particularly sudden changes in position, or by the start of voluntary movements. In addition to these movement disorders, children with dystonic cerebral palsy also exhibit sudden increases in muscle tone, often precipitated by attempts at voluntary movement (*tension*). These movements must be distinguished from seizures.

Small, choreiform-like movements are common in the healthy infant. They are transient; emerging at approximately 6 weeks of age, they become maximal between 9 and 12 weeks of age and taper off between 14 and 20 weeks of age. According to Prechtl and coworkers, their absence is highly predictive of neurologic abnormalities (23).

Sensory Examination

A proper sensory examination is difficult at any age, and almost impossible in an infant or toddler. Sensory modalities can be tested in the older child using a pin or preferably a tracing wheel. In infants or toddlers, abnormalities in skin temperature or in the amount of perspiration indicate the level of sensory deficit. The ulnar surface of the examiner's hand has been found to be the most sensitive, and by moving the hand slowly up the child's body, one can verify changes that one marks on the skin and rechecks on repeat testing.

Object discrimination can be determined in the healthy school-aged child by the use of coin, or small, familiar items such as paperclips or rubber bands.

Reflexes

The younger the child, the less informative are the deep tendon reflexes. Reflex inequalities are common and less reliable than inequalities of muscle tone in terms of

TABLE I.1 Segmental Levels of Major Deep Tendon Reflexes

Reflex	Segmental Level
Jaw jerk	V-trigeminal nerve
Biceps	C5–6
Triceps	C6–8
Radial periosteal	C5–6
Patellar	L2–4
Ankle	S1–2
Hamstrings	L4–S2

ascertaining the presence of an upper motor neuron lesion. The segmental levels of the major deep tendon reflexes are presented in Table I.1.

Little doubt exists that the Babinski response is the best-known sign of disturbed pyramidal tract function. To elicit it, the plantar surface of the foot is stimulated with a sharp object, such as the tip of a key, from the heel forward along the lateral border of the sole, crossing over the distal ends of the metatarsals toward the base of the great toe. Immediate dorsiflexion of the great toe and subsequent separation (fanning) of the other toes constitutes a positive response. Stimulation of the outer side of the foot is less objectionable and can be used in children who cannot tolerate the sensation of having their soles stimulated. The response is identical. An extensor plantar response must be distinguished from voluntary withdrawal, which, unlike the true Babinski response, is seen after a moment's delay. It also must be distinguished from athetosis of the foot (*striatal toe*). According to Paine and Oppe, a positive response to Babinski sign is seen normally in the majority of 1-year-old children and in many up to 2 1/2 years of age (24). In the sequential examination of infants conducted by Gingold and her group, the plantar response becomes consistently flexor between 4 and 6 months of age (25).

Many eponyms, 20 according to Wartenberg (26), have been attached to the reflexes elicitable from the sole of the foot. Some, such as Rossolimo reflex, which is elicited by tapping the plantar surface of the toe and producing a stretching of the plantar flexors, are muscle stretch reflexes. Others, such as Oppenheim reflex (a firm stroke with finger and thumb down the anterior border of the tibia) or Gordon reflex (a hard squeeze of the calf muscle), are variants of Babinski response.

In the upper extremity, Hoffmann reflex is elicited by flicking the terminal phalanx of the patient's middle finger downward between the examiner's finger and thumb. In hyperreflexia, the thumb flexes and adducts, and the tips of the other fingers flex. Wartenberg sign is elicited by having the patient supinate the hand, slightly flexing the fingers. The examiner pronates his or her own hand and links his or her own flexed finger with the patient's. Both flex their fingers against each other's resistance. In pyramidal tract disease, the thumb adducts and flexes strongly, a reemergence of the forced grasp reflex.

Clonus is a regular repetitive movement of a joint elicited by a sudden stretching of the muscle and maintaining the stretch. It is most easily demonstrable at the ankle by dorsiflexion of the foot. Clonus represents increased reflex excitability. Several beats of ankle clonus can be demonstrated in some healthy newborns and in some tense older children. A sustained ankle clonus is abnormal at any age and suggests a lesion of the pyramidal tract.

Chvostek sign, a contraction of the facial muscles after percussion of the pes anserinus of the facial nerve (just anterior to the external auditory meatus), is evidence of increased irritability of the motor fibers to mechanical stimulation such as occurs in hypocalcemia (27).

Children with developmental disabilities, such as minimal brain dysfunction and attention-deficit disorders, are often found to have *soft signs* on neurologic examination (see Chapter 18). These represent persistence of findings considered normal at a younger age. Of the various tests designed to elicit soft signs, tandem walking, hopping on one foot, and the ability of the child to suppress overflow movements when asked to repetitively touch the index finger to the thumb have been found to be the most useful. Forward tandem gait is performed successfully by 90% of 5-year-old children; 90% of 7-year-old children also can hop in one place, and synkinesis becomes progressively suppressed between 7 and 9 years of age (28).

Cognitive Function

Evaluation for the presence of cognitive limitations is an important part of the neurologic examination of developmentally delayed youngsters and of children with ostensibly normal intelligence who are referred because of school failure. Such an examination is extremely time consuming and might require a return visit. An outline of an evaluation of intelligence, speech, and disorders of cognitive function is presented in Chapter 18. Also provided are suggestions on how to interpret psychological data.

NEUROLOGIC EXAMINATION OF THE INFANT

The neurologic examination of an infant younger than 1 year of age can be divided into three parts: evaluation of posture and tone, evaluation of primitive reflexes, and examination of items that are relatively age invariable.

Posture and Muscle Tone

Evaluation of posture and muscle tone is a fundamental part of the neurologic examination of infants. It involves examination of the resting posture, passive tone, and active tone. Posture is appreciated by inspecting the undressed

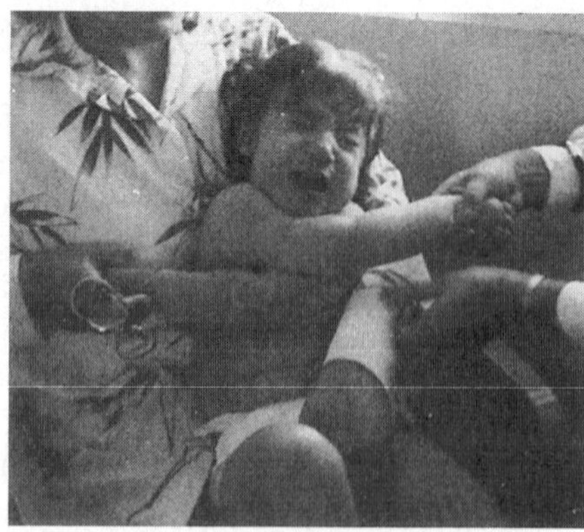

FIGURE I.4. Scarf sign in an infant with upper extremity hypotonia on a cerebral basis.

infant as the infant lies undisturbed. During the first few months of life, normal hypertonia of the flexors of the elbows, hips, and knees occurs. The hypertonia decreases markedly during the third month of life, first in the upper extremities and later in the lower extremities. At the same time, tone in neck and trunk increases. Between 8 and 12 months of age, a further decrease occurs in the flexor tone of the extremities together with increased extensor tone (29).

Evaluation of passive tone is accomplished by determining the resistance to passive movements of the various joints with the infant awake and not crying. Because limb tone is influenced by tonic neck reflexes, it is important to keep the child's head straight during this part of the examination. Passive flapping of the hands and the feet provides a simple means of ascertaining muscle tone. In the upper extremity, the scarf sign is a valuable maneuver. With the infant sustained in a semireclining position, the examiner takes the infant's hand and pulls the arm across the infant's chest toward the opposite shoulder (Fig. I.4). The position of the elbow in relationship to the midline is noted. Hypotonia is present if the elbow passes the midline. In the lower extremity, the fall-away response serves a similar purpose. The infant is suspended by the feet, upside down, and each lower extremity is released in turn. The rapidity with which the lower extremity drops when released is noted. Normally, the extremity maintains its position for a few moments, then drops. In hypotonia, the drop occurs immediately; in hypertonia, the released lower extremity remains up.

The traction response is an excellent means of ascertaining active tone. The examiner, who should be sitting down and facing the child, places his or her thumbs in the infant's palms and fingers around the wrists and gently pulls the infant from the supine position. In the healthy infant younger than 3 months of age, the palmar grasp reflex becomes operative, the elbows tend to flex, and the flexor muscles of the neck are stimulated to raise the head so that even in the full-term neonate the extensor and flexor tone are balanced and the head is maintained briefly in the axis of the trunk. The test is abnormal if the head is pulled passively and drops forward or if the head is maintained backward. In the former case, abnormal hypotonia of the neck and trunk muscles exists; in the latter case, abnormal hypertonia of the neck extensors exists. With abnormal hypertonia, one also might note the infant's head to be rotated laterally and extended when the infant is in the resting prone position.

Primitive Reflexes

The evaluation of various primitive reflexes is an integral part of the neurologic examination of the infant. Many of the reflexes exhibited by the newborn infant also are observed in a *spinal animal*, one in which the spinal cord has been permanently transected. With progressive maturation, some of these reflexes disappear (Tables I.2 and I.3). This disappearance should not be construed as meaning that they are actually lost, for a reflex once acquired in the course of development is retained permanently. Rather, these reflexes, which develop during intrauterine life, are gradually suppressed as the higher cortical centers become functional.

Segmental Medullary Reflexes

A number of segmental medullary reflexes become functional during the last trimester of gestation. They include (a) respiratory activity, (b) cardiovascular reflexes, (c) coughing reflex mediated by the vagus nerve, (d) sneezing reflex evoked by afferent fibers of the trigeminal nerve, (e) swallowing reflex mediated by the trigeminal and glossopharyngeal nerves, and (f) sucking reflex evoked by the afferent fibers of the trigeminal and glossopharyngeal nerves and executed by the efferent fibers of the facial, glossopharyngeal, and hypoglossal nerves.

Flexion Reflex

Another reflex demonstrable in the isolated spinal cord is the flexion reflex. This response is elicited by the unpleasant stimulation of the skin of the lower extremity, most consistently the dorsum of the foot, and consists of dorsiflexion of the great toe and flexion of the ankle, knee, and hip. This reflex has been elicited in immature fetuses and can persist as a fragment, the extensor plantar response, for the first 2 years of life. It is seen also in infants whose higher cortical centers have been profoundly damaged. Reflex stepping, which is at least partly a function of the flexion response, is present in the healthy newborn when the infant is supported in the standing position; it disappears in the fourth or fifth month of life.

TABLE I.2 Postural Reactions

Postural Reflex	*Stimulus*	*Origin of Afferent Impulses*	*Age Reflex Appears*	*Age Reflex Disappears*
Local static reactions				
Stretch reflex	Gravitation	Muscles	Any age	
Positive supporting action			Well developed in 50% of newborns	Indistinguishable from normal standing
Placing reaction			37 weeks	Covered up by voluntary action
Segmental static reactions	Movement	Contralateral muscles		
Crossed extensor reflex			Newborn	7–12 mo
Crossed adductor reflex to quadriceps jerk			3 mo	8 mo
General static reactions	Position of head in space	Otolith Neck muscles Trunk muscles		
Tonic neck reflex			Never complete and obligatory	
Neck-righting reflex			4–8 mo	Covered up by voluntary action
Grasp reflex				
Palmar			28 weeks	4–5 mo
Plantar			Newborn	9–12 mo
Moro reflex			28–32 weeks	4–5 mo
Labyrinthine accelerating reactions	Change in rate of movement	Semicircular canals		
Linear acceleration			4–9 mo	Covered up by voluntary action
Parachute reaction				
Angular acceleration			Any age	
Postrotational nystagmus				

From Menkes JH. The neuromotor mechanism. In: Cooke RE, ed. *The biologic basis of pediatric practice.* New York: McGraw-Hill, 1968. With permission.

Moro Reflex

The Moro reflex is best elicited by a sudden dropping of the baby's head in relation to its trunk. Moro, however, elicited this reflex by hitting the infant's pillow with both hands (30). The infant opens the hands, extends and abducts the upper extremities, and then draws them together. The reflex first appears between 28 and 32 weeks' gestation and is present in all newborns. It fades out between 3 to 5 months of age (25) (Table I.3). Its persistence beyond 6 months of age or its absence or diminution during the first few weeks of life indicates neurologic dysfunction.

Tonic Neck Response

The tonic neck response is obtained by rotating the infant's head to the side while maintaining the chest in a flat position. A positive response is extension of the arm and leg on the side toward which the face is rotated and flexion of the limbs on the opposite side (Fig. I.5). An asymmetric tonic neck response is abnormal, as is an obligatory and sustained pattern (i.e., one from which the infant is unable to extricate himself- or herself). Inconstant tonic neck responses can be elicited for as long as 6 to 7 months of age and can even be momentarily present during sleep in the healthy 2- to 3-year-old child (25) (Table I.3).

Righting Reflex

With the infant in the supine position, the examiner turns the head to one side. The healthy infant rotates the shoulder in the same direction, followed by the trunk, and finally the pelvis. An obligate neck-righting reflex in which the shoulders, trunk, and pelvis rotate simultaneously and in which the infant can be rolled over and over like a log is always abnormal. Normally, the reflex can be imposed briefly in newborns, but the infant is soon able to break through it.

Palmar and Plantar Grasp Reflexes

The palmar and plantar grasp reflexes are elicited by pressure on the palm or sole. Generally, the plantar grasp reflex is weaker than the palmar reflex. The palmar grasp reflex

TABLE I.3 Percentage of Healthy Babies Showing Various Infantile Reflexes with Increasing Age

	Signs that Disappear with Age			*Signs that Appear with Age*				
	Moro	*Tonic Neck Reflex*	*Crossed Adduction to Knee Jerk*	*Neck-Righting Reflex*	*Supporting Reaction*	*Landau*	*Parachute*	*Hand Grasp*
Age (mo)	*Extension Even Without Flexor Phase*	*Imposable Even for 30 secs or Inconstant*	*Strong or Slight*	*Imposable But Transient*	*Fair or Good*	*Head Above Horizontal and Back Arched*	*Complete*	*Thumb to Forefinger Alone*
1	93	67	?[a]	13	50	0	0	0
2	89	90	?[a]	23	43	0	0	0
3	70	50	41	25	52	0	0	0
4	59	34	41	26	40	0	0	0
5	22	31	41	38	61	29	0	0
6	0	11	21	40	66	42	3	0
7	0	0	12	43	74	42	29	16
8	0	0	15	54	81	44	40	53
9	0	0	6	67	96	97	76	63
10	0	0	3	100	100	100	79	84
11	0	0	3	100	100	100	90	95
12	0	0	2	100	100	100	100	100

[a] Divergence of experience and opinion between different examiners.

From Paine RS, Oppe TE. Neurological examination of children. *Clinics in Dev. Med.* 1996;20/21. London, William Heinemann.

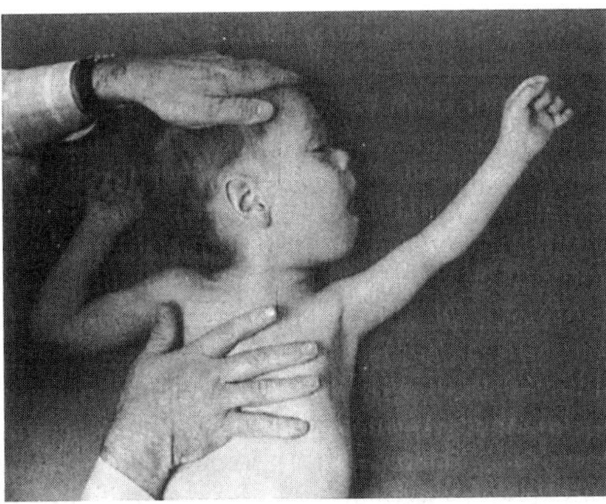

FIGURE I.5. Obligatory tonic neck response in a 6-year-old boy with severe spastic quadriplegia and extrapyramidal symptoms secondary to perinatal asphyxia.

appears at 28 weeks' gestation, is well established by 32 weeks, and becomes weak and inconsistent between 2 and 3 months of age, when it is covered up by voluntary activity. Absence of the reflex before 2 or 3 months of age, persistence beyond that age, or a consistent asymmetry is abnormal. The reappearance of the grasp reflex in frontal lobe lesions reflects the unopposed parietal lobe activity.

Vertical Suspension

The examiner suspends the child with his or her hand under its axillae and notes the position of the lower extremities. Marked extension or scissoring is an indication of spasticity (Fig. I.6).

Landau Reflex

To elicit the Landau response, the examiner lifts the infant with one hand under the trunk, face downward. Normally, a reflex extension of the vertebral column occurs, causing the newborn infant to lift the head to slightly below the horizontal, which results in a slightly convex upward curvature of the spine. With hypotonia, the infant's body tends to collapse into an inverted U shape.

Buttress Response

To elicit the buttress response, the examiner places the infant in the sitting position and displaces the center of gravity with a gentle push on one shoulder. The infant extends the contralateral arm and spreads the fingers. The reflex normally appears at approximately 5 months of age. Delay in its appearance and asymmetries are significant.

Parachute Response

The parachute reflex is tested with the child suspended horizontally about the waist, face down. The infant is then suddenly projected toward the floor, with a consequent extension of the arms and spreading of the fingers. Between 4 and 9 months of age, this reflex depends on visual and vestibular sensory input and is proportional to the size of the optic stimulus pattern on the floor (31) (Fig. I.7).

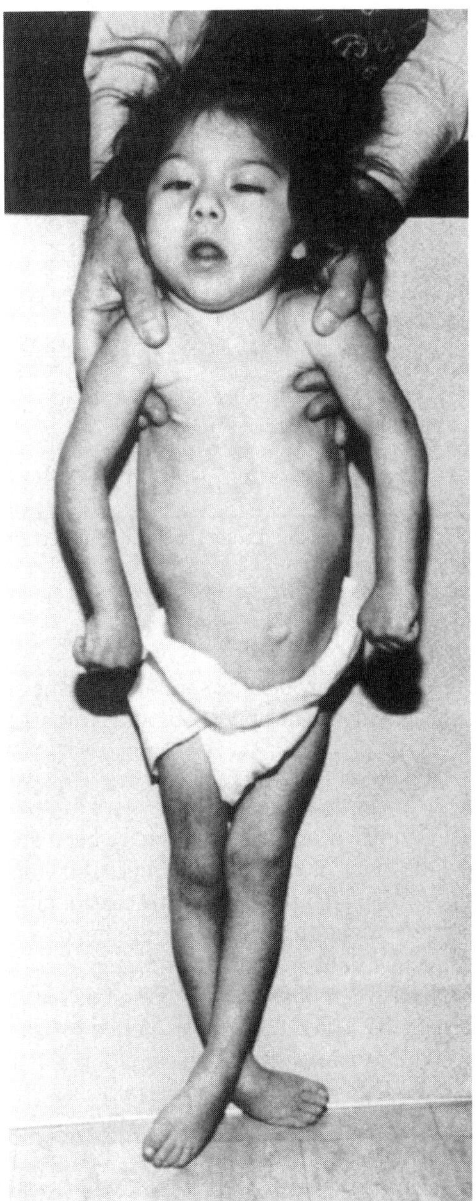

FIGURE I.6. Infant with upper motor neuron lesion demonstrates scissoring of the lower extremities when held in vertical suspension. Spastic quadriparesis followed perinatal asphyxia.

Reflex Placing and Stepping Responses

Reflex placing and stepping responses are of lesser value. Reflex placing is elicited by stimulating the dorsum of the foot against the edge of the examining table. Reflex stepping, which is at least partly a function of the flexion response to noxious stimuli, is present in the healthy

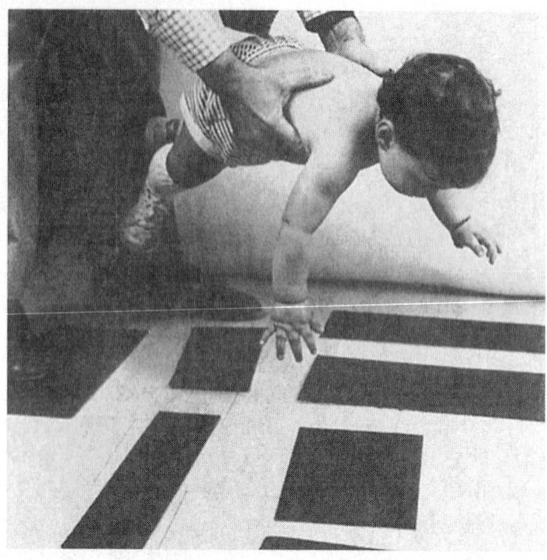

FIGURE I.7. Infant demonstrating the parachute reaction. Note the extended arms and spreading of the fingers. The minimal asymmetry in the response may be the consequence of an antecedent meningitis.

newborn when the newborn is supported in the standing position. The response disappears by 4 to 5 months of age.

Other Reflexes

A number of other primitive reflexes have been described. They include the curious bowing reflex first described by Gamper (31). This reflex, which occasionally can be demonstrated in healthy premature infants of 7 months' gestation, is invariably present in anencephalics. It sometimes can also be demonstrated in infants with severe spastic quadriparesis. The reflex can be elicited by placing the infant into the supine position and extending the thighs at the hip joints. The head then lifts itself slowly, followed by the trunk, so that the infant ultimately achieves the sitting position.

Other primitive reflexes add little to the neurologic examination of the infant. The physician should gather experience in a few selected tests rather than try to elicit the entire gamut of responses.

Age-Invariable Tests

The last part of the neurologic examination involves tests similar to those performed in older children or adults, such as the funduscopic examination and the deep tendon reflexes. These have been discussed already in the Cranial Nerves section and the Reflexes section. Though a variety of deep tendon reflexes can be elicited in the infant, they are of limited value except when they are clearly asymmetric. The triceps and brachioradialis reflexes are usually difficult to elicit during the period of neonatal flexion hypertonia. The patellar reflex is accompanied by adduction of the opposite thigh, the crossed adductor reflex. This reflex disappears by 9 to 12 months of age (24). An unsustained ankle clonus is common in the healthy neonate.

The ready availability of head ultrasound has for most practitioners relegated transillumination of the infant's skull to the scrap heap of history. Nevertheless, when performed correctly, it remains a quick and useful test for detecting the presence of hydrocephalus, subdural effusions, porencephalic cysts, and posterior fossa cysts (32).

It is not always possible to summarize the neurologic examination result of the infant as being normal or abnormal. Instead, an intermediate group of infants exists whose examination results are suspect. The examination should be recorded as such, with the ultimate decision being left to subsequent examinations. Only some 1% of these suspect infants turn out to have gross neurologic deficits (33).

NEURODIAGNOSTIC PROCEDURES

At the conclusion of history taking and physical examination, the physician sets up a differential diagnosis and calls on a variety of diagnostic procedures to ascertain the cause of the neurologic illness.

Some of the more commonly used procedures are commented on briefly to describe their applicability to various diagnostic problems and to direct the reader to more extensive sources.

Examination of the Cerebrospinal Fluid

In most cases, a sample of the cerebrospinal fluid (CSF) is obtained by lumbar puncture, a procedure introduced in 1891 by Quincke as a means of reducing the increased intracranial pressure in children with hydrocephalus (34). To perform a spinal tap, the child is held in the lateral recumbent position with the spine maintained maximally flexed. In the newborn or small infant, the tap is best performed with the baby in the sitting position. A small pillow placed against the abdomen keeps the spine flexed while an assistant maintains the head in a perfect anteroposterior alignment. After cleaning the back with an antibacterial solution, the tap is performed. One may omit local anesthesia because it entails twice as much struggling than a tap performed without it. A controlled clinical trial has come to a similar conclusion (35). In one medical center, eutectic mixture of local anesthetics (EMLA) cream, a topical anesthetic of mixture of 2.5% lidocaine and 2.5% prilocaine, applied as a thick layer over the puncture site approximately 1 hour before the tap has made the procedure easier for the child and doctor. For a small child or toddler, a 22-gauge needle is preferable, whereas for the newborn, a 23-gauge needle without a stylet is optimal. Several authors have suggested the use of an atraumatic needle that has a blunt tip rather than the beveled cutting edge of the Quincke needle. Based on experience derived from adult subjects, such a needle would reduce the incidence of post–lumbar puncture headaches in older children and adolescents (36). The needle is inserted into the L3–4 or, for a newborn, whose spinal cord terminates at a lower level than the older child's, into the L4–5 interspace, with the bevel being maintained parallel to the longitudinal dural fibers to decrease the size of the dural tear. The needle is then pushed forward as slowly as possible. Entry into the subarachnoid space can be felt by a sudden pop. A bloody tap usually results from the needle's going too deep and penetrating the dorsal epidural venous plexus overlying the vertebral bodies. Less often it is caused by injury to the vessels along the cauda equina. The person who holds the child in a perfect position is more important to the success of a lumbar puncture than the person who inserts the needle. Bonadio and coworkers constructed a graph relating the depth to which the needle must go to obtain clear CSF with body surface area (37).

If an opening pressure is essential, the stylet is replaced with a manometer, taking care to lose as little spinal fluid as possible. Because examination of the CSF for cells is more important than a pressure reading in most cases, a few drops of CSF should be collected at this point. An accurate recording of CSF pressure requires total relaxation of the child, a difficult and at times impossible task. The cooperative child may be released and the legs extended because falsely high pressures result when the knees are pressed against the abdomen. When the needle has been placed correctly, the fluid can be seen to move up and down the manometer with respirations. In older children, normal CSF pressure is less than 180 mm H_2O; usually it is between 110 and 150 mm H_2O. Pressure is approximately 100 mm H_2O in the newborn. Ellis and coworkers proposed that CSF pressure can be estimated by counting the number of drops that are collected through the needle during a fixed period of time, ranging from 12 to 39 seconds, depending on the temperature of the child and the gauge and the length of the needle. Their paper presents the counting period for which the number of drops counted equals the CSF pressure in centimeters of water (38). This method is not useful in cases in which the CSF viscosity is significantly increased. Queckenstedt test, compression of the jugular veins to determine the presence of a spinal subarachnoid block, has lost its usefulness. After the spinal tap is completed, the stylet, if such is used, is replaced, and the needle is given half a turn before being removed to prevent extensive spinal fluid leakage (39). This manipulation is believed to reduce the likelihood for a post–lumbar puncture headache (40).

The normal CSF is crystal clear. A cloudy fluid indicates the presence of cells. Fluid that contains more than 500 red blood cells/μL appears grossly bloody. If so, the possibility of a traumatic tap should be excluded by performing cell counts on three sequential samples of fluid. In the presence of an intracranial hemorrhage, little difference exists in the counts obtained from the first and last specimens. Performing sequential cell counts is a more reliable method of demonstrating intracranial bleeding than observing the presence of a xanthochromic fluid or crenated red cells (41). In the United States xanthochromia is generally assessed by visual inspection, spectrophotometry for the detection of CSF pigments is used almost universally in the United Kingdom (41a).

Crenation of red cells in CSF occurs promptly, whereas xanthochromia can be noted whenever contamination by red cells is heavy. In the term neonate, the mean protein concentration is 84 with a stardard deviation of $\pm$45 mg/dL (42); in the premature neonate, it is 115 mg/dL (43). The presence of blood from any source raises the total protein by 1.5 mg/dL of fluid for every 1,000 fresh red blood cells/μL (44). The number of white cells in normal CSF is higher in infants than in children. In the study conducted by Ahmed and colleagues, the mean white cell count in normal, noninfected neonates was 7/μL with a range of 0 to 130/μL (45).

In children older than 12 months of age, normal values range up to 3 cells/μL. Whereas polymorphonuclear cells can be present in the newborn, they are not found in CSF taken from healthy children older than 12 months of age (46). Blood-contaminated CSF complicates the determination of pleocytosis. Although it is frequently stated that the ratio of white blood cells to red blood cells does not differ from that present in peripheral blood (1:300), actual determinations by several groups of workers indicate that only approximately 20% of the predicted number of white blood cells are present in CSF; consequently, recalculation is necessary (47).

The normal immunoglobulin G (IgG) values for pediatric patients were compiled by Rust and coworkers (48). In tuberculous meningitis, a cobweb can form at the bottom of the tube; staining of this material can reveal the presence of acid-fast organisms. It is appropriate to consider the complications of lumbar puncture performed under these and other circumstances.

The possibility of herniation in the presence of increased intracranial pressure must be considered not only in cases of brain tumor, but also in purulent meningitis. The incidence of this complication was 4.3% in the series of Rennick et al. of 445 infants and children with bacterial meningitis (49). Obtaining a CT scan prior to a lumbar puncture in patients with meningitis to determine whether there is increased intracranial pressure is in our opinion unwarranted and only results in delayed appropriate treatment. As Oliver and coworkers (50) and Rennick and coworkers (49) also pointed out, the CT is generally normal in children with meningitis and increased intracranial pressure and does not disclose incipient cerebral herniation. This subject is also covered in Chapter 7.

The most common complication of lumbar puncture is headache. In the experience of Raskin it was encountered in 10% of subjects younger than 19 years of age (51). Its onset is between 15 minutes and 12 days after the tap, and it persists for an average of 4 days but as long as several weeks or months (51). It is most severe with the patient upright and subsides in the recumbent position. Nausea, vomiting, and, less often, vertigo can accompany the headache. It is generally accepted, although not proven conclusively, that the headache results from persistent leakage of CSF through a hole in the dura and arachnoid, with cerebral hypotension and a consequent stretching and displacement of pain-sensitive structures (51). In adults, but not in the pediatric population, the major factor in headache induction is the diameter of the hole made in the dura by the needle (52,53). Neither the amount of fluid removed nor the position of the patient during the puncture is important in terms of the incidence of post–lumbar puncture headache (53). If a small-gauge needle is used and CSF pressures are to be measured, the physician should allow sufficient time for equilibration.

The best current treatment of post–lumbar puncture headache is strict bed rest and the use of analgesics. Epidural injections of saline or intravenous caffeine have their advocates, but in the pediatric population these measures are generally unnecessary. Backache as a result of the trauma of the lumbar puncture is relatively common, but in children is generally not sufficiently severe to represent a major problem.

Less common complications of lumbar puncture include diplopia caused by unilateral or bilateral abducens palsy or combined fourth- and sixth-nerve palsies (54). This usually clears within a few days or weeks.

Trauma to the arachnoid and to dural vessels at the base of the vertebrae is fairly common, particularly in small infants, but unless the patient is suffering from a bleeding disorder, it is asymptomatic. An epidural hematoma and, even less likely, a subdural hematoma, and a subarachnoid hemorrhage after a lumbar puncture are extremely unusual complications (55). Frequent lumbar punctures, particularly when performed for the introduction of intrathecal medications, may result in the implantation of an epidermal tumor. Other, rarer complications, together with 789 references on complications of lumbar puncture, can be found in a review by Fredericks (56).

Cytologic studies can be performed on CSF after centrifugation and can assist in determining whether tumors have spread to the meninges or to the spinal subarachnoid space, as may occur in a medulloblastoma (57). Occasionally, the CSF contains choroid plexus and ependymal cells. These are particularly prominent in hydrocephalic infants (58).

Electroencephalography

Electroencephalography (EEG) remains the central tool for the clinical investigation of seizures and other paroxysmal disorders. The increasing importance of neuroimaging studies has circumscribed its usefulness, and many physicians call on EEG in clinical situations in which the procedure has little to offer (59).

EEG does not exclude the presence of epilepsy or organic disease, and its role in diagnosing the neuropsychiatric disorders is limited. A single normal tracing is of little value in excluding the diagnosis of epilepsy, and conversely, insignificant EEG abnormalities can accompany gross structural brain disease. Neither the technique of EEG nor the interpretation of normal and abnormal tracings are covered at this point. Instead, the reader is referred to Chapter 14.

EEG is indicated in transient alterations in cerebral function or behavior, central nervous system degenerative disorders (with photic stimulation), unexplained coma, prognosis after anoxic episodes and other acute cerebral problems, and the determination of brain death. It is of little help in developmental retardation, static encephalopathies unaccompanied by seizures, minimal brain dysfunction, attention-deficit disorders, and neuropsychiatric disorders (59).

Quantitative methods for data analysis of brain electrical activity (BEAM) can be used to compare signals from the various electrodes and so construct multicolor contour maps of brain activity. BEAM has found relatively little applicability in pediatric neurology. Even though this technique facilitates the detection of asymmetries, it remains investigational in mild to moderate head injuries, learning disabilities, and the attention-deficit disorders. No clinical application exists for quantitative EEG analysis without analysis of an accompanying routine EEG, and quantitative EEG by itself has not been proven useful in either the diagnosis or the treatment of children with learning or attention deficits (60,61,62). The issues involved in this procedure are discussed more extensively in Chapter 18.

Polysomnography

As interest in sleep disorders has increased, the polysomnogram has become more readily available, not only in university centers, but also in clinical sleep laboratories. The procedure consists in the simultaneous recording of multiple physiologic variables during sleep. These include an EEG, electromyogram, electrocardiogram, and electro-oculogram. Additionally, respiration is recorded. The procedure is invaluable in the evaluation of sleep apnea of infancy and the diagnosis of suspected nocturnal seizures, narcolepsy, periodic movement disorders, and parasomnias. It is discussed more extensively in books by Guilleminault (63) and Ferber and Kryger (64).

Electromyography

A concentric needle electrode inserted into muscle records the action potentials generated by muscle activity. These are amplified and displayed on a cathode ray oscilloscope. The amplified input also can be fed into a loudspeaker.

Normal resting muscle is electrically silent except for a small amount of electrical activity produced by insertion of the needle that rapidly dies away. This is termed the *insertion potential*. With slight voluntary activity, single action potentials become evident. With increasing volitional activity, motor unit discharges increase in number, and the frequency of discharge increases until an interference pattern of continuous motor activity is achieved.

The number or rate of motor unit discharge as well as the amplitude or shape of the individual discharges, can be abnormal. In establishing the diagnosis of myopathy, the duration of the discharge is more important than the amplitude inasmuch as the latter varies with age and with the muscle tested. Spontaneous discharges may be elicited from resting muscle or the insertion potential may be increased. After denervation of muscle, fibrillation potentials appear. They result from the periodic rhythmic twitching of single muscle fibers resulting from their hyperexcitability consequent to denervation. Fibrillation potentials appear on the average between 10 and 20 days after nerve section, and, as a rule, the greater the distance between the site of injury and the muscle, the longer it takes for the abnormality to develop. Spontaneous fibrillations also can be seen in hyperkalemic period paralysis, botulinus intoxication, muscular dystrophy, and some myopathies. They can be recorded in the proximal musculature of some term babies younger than 1 month of age and in some preterm infants (65).

Electromyography (EMG) is an integral part of the investigation of the patient with lower motor neuron disease. It is nonspecifically abnormal in upper motor neuron disease and in extrapyramidal disorders, and, therefore, has only limited use in these entities. High-spatial-resolution EMG, a noninvasive surface EMG technique, has been proposed for the diagnosis of pediatric neuromuscular disorders. As used in various European centers, its diagnostic validity appears to be similar to that of needle EMG (66). For a more extensive coverage of this procedure, the reader is referred to texts by Kimura (67) and Aminoff (68).

Nerve Conduction Studies

The conduction rates of motor nerves can be measured by stimulating the nerve at two points and recording the latency between each stimulus and the ensuing muscle contraction. The conduction rate depends on the patient's age and on the nerve tested. Normal values for pediatric patients were presented by Gamstorp (69).

Nerve conduction velocities can be used to distinguish demyelination from axonal degeneration of the peripheral nerve and also from muscular disorders. In peripheral nerve demyelination, nerve conduction velocities are generally reduced, whereas they are normal in axonal degenerations and in muscular diseases (see also Chapters 3 and 16). The procedure also provides information about the distribution of peripheral nerve lesions.

Sensory nerve conduction velocity can be determined in infants and children but is a more difficult procedure. It is useful in the study of the hereditary sensory and autonomic neuropathies and some of the heredodegenerative disorders.

Evoked Potentials

Evoked potentials are the brain's response to an external stimulus. Most evoked potentials, being of low amplitude (0.120 μV), cannot be seen on routine EEG, but must be extracted from background activity by computed signal averaging after repeated stimuli. The presence or absence of one or more evoked potential waves and their latencies (the time from stimulus to wave peaks) are used in clinical interpretations.

In pediatric neurology, visual-evoked responses (VERs), brainstem auditory-evoked responses (BAERs), and somatosensory-evoked potentials (SSEPs) are the most commonly used tests.

Visual-Evoked Responses

Flash and pattern shift VERs are in use. In one institution, pattern shift stimuli are preferred for older children in that they are more reliable and also can provide some information about visual acuity. Flash stimuli are used for infants and older but uncooperative youngsters. The amplitude and latencies of the VER as recorded from both occipital lobes are used for clinical purposes, with the former being less valuable in pediatrics because it is contingent on attention span and visual acuity.

VERs have found their place in the diagnosis of a variety of leukodystrophies, demyelinating diseases, and lipidoses. They can demonstrate clinically silent optic neuritis such as is present in spinocerebellar ataxia and various other system degenerations. VERs can be recorded reliably from neonates and have been used to measure visual acuity in infants and follow the development of the visual system (70,71).

Brainstem Auditory-Evoked Responses

A series of clicks delivered to one ear sequentially activates cranial nerve VIII, cochlear nucleus, superior olivary nucleus, nuclei of the lateral lemniscus, and inferior colliculus. In the neonate, the waves representing cranial nerve VIII (I), the superior olivary nucleus (III), and the inferior colliculus (V) are the most readily detectable. The BAER can be elicited in premature infants after 26 weeks' gestation, with amplitude increasing and latency decreasing as a function of increasing gestational age. Clinical interpretation of the BAER is based on the time interval between the waves and the interpeak latencies. These reflect the intactness of the brainstem auditory tract.

Diseases of the peripheral auditory nerve affect the latencies of all waves but do not alter interpeak latencies. The BAER is abnormal in various leukodystrophies, with most patients having central abnormalities. Clinically inapparent abnormalities of the auditory nerve can be demonstrated by BAER in Friedreich ataxia and the various hereditary motor and sensory neuropathies. The BAER is also abnormal in brainstem disease, such as occurs in neonates as a consequence of perinatal asphyxia or hyperbilirubinemia. It is also abnormal in bacterial meningitis and in the various viral encephalitides.

Indicative of brainstem damage, the BAER has been used for prognostic purposes in patients who are comatose subsequent to head trauma, cardiorespiratory arrest, or increased intracranial pressure.

Somatosensory-Evoked Potentials

SSEPs are recorded after stimulation of peripheral sensory nerves. Like BAERs, the waveforms and the anatomy of the sensory tracts are closely correlated. The cell bodies of the large-fiber sensory system lie in the dorsal root ganglia; their central processes travel rostrally in the posterior columns of the spinal cord to synapse in the dorsal column nuclei at the cervicomedullary junction. Second-order fibers cross the midline to the thalamus, whence third-order fibers continue to the frontoparietal sensorimotor cortex. Painless electrical stimuli at 4 to 5/sec are delivered to the skin overlying the median nerve at the wrist, the tibial nerve at the ankle, or the common peroneal nerve at the knee. Their intensity is adjusted to excite the largest myelinated fibers in the peripheral nerve. Waveforms are recorded along the somatosensory pathway: above the clavicle overlying the brachial plexus, at the posterior midline at the C2 vertebra to record the dorsal column nuclei, and on the scalp overlying the sensory cortex contralateral to the stimulated limb. When the lower extremities are stimulated, a recording electrode is placed over L1–3.

Clinical interpretation is based on interpeak latency, with particular attention paid to differences between the two sides. SSEPs can provide information on the integrity of the brachial plexus, and on spinal cord lesions if these involve the posterior columns. SSEPs can be used to evaluate children with myelodysplasia and provide useful information in patients with Friedreich ataxia and in the hereditary motor and sensory neuropathies. The role of multimodality-evoked potential recordings in the diagnosis of brain death is covered in Chapter 17.

The SSEP appears in the fetus at approximately 29 weeks of gestation, with a progressive decrease of response latency with increasing gestational age.

Electronystagmography

This procedure measures the rate and amplitude of eye movements at rest and after caloric or rotational stimulation. It is useful in the evaluation of children with vertigo and in the postconcussion syndrome (72,73).

NEUROIMAGING

Skull Radiography

Radiographs of the skull are hardly as valuable as they were before the advent of CT scan and MRI. Currently, they are used occasionally to detect and interpret localized lytic lesions, such as are seen in histiocytosis X, and to evaluate various congenital anomalies of the cranium, such as occur in achondroplasia, cleidocranial dysostosis, wormian bones, or hyperostosis. Plain skull radiography is clearly inferior to CT in the assessment of the child who has suffered a head injury, although, on occasion, radiography is better than CT in demonstrating a horizontal skull fracture.

In children, particularly in those between 4 and 8 years of age, prominence of convolutional markings is not a reliable indication of increased intracranial pressure. Separation of sutures is rare in children older than 10 years of age and is practically nonexistent beyond the age of 20 years.

Computed Tomography

The advent of CT and MRI revolutionized the diagnostic evaluation of the neurologic patients and eliminated the need for invasive studies such as pneumoencephalography and ventriculography.

The technique of CT was introduced by Ambrose and Hounsfield (74), who developed a scanning instrument based on theoretical work of Oldendorf (75). It permits visualization of even slight differences in the density of the intracranial contents without the need for and the complications of an invasive procedure. In essence, scattering of radiation is eliminated by the use of a thin x-ray beam so that the photon absorption by tissues can be calculated accurately using a sodium iodide crystal or solid-state detector. The x-ray tube and the detector move across the head and obtain readings of photon transmission through the head. The exact matrix depends on the particular scanning instrument used. After completion of the scan, the unit is rotated 1 degree and the process is repeated. In this fashion, the tube and the detector are rotated 180 degrees around the head. The resulting readings are fed into a computer that calculates the x-ray absorption coefficients of each of the voxels. The most recent machines are capable of acquiring multiple images at once using an array of thin x-ray detectors. These scanners are designed for spiral or helical scanning. With this technique the gantry rotates continuously as the table moves. The helical data set is then reconstructed into artificial slices for viewing. This technique shortens the scan time considerably. Scanners with the ability to acquire 64 slices are now available. This is beyond the technical need of most neuroimaging. Most scans are acquired as standard serial cuts of the head 2.5 or 5 mm thick. Multislice spiral imaging is used more commonly in the spine or with special techniques. The thin sections of 1 mm or less required for examination of the posterior fossa, the orbit, or the perisellar region are easily performed by the new generations of scanners. The total radiation dose for a complete scan of the head is approximately 6 rads, somewhat less than that produced by a routine skull series.

The CT scanning procedure takes some 5 to 30 minutes, and because even a slight degree of motion results in an artifact, the normally active child younger than 5 years of age requires sedation to prevent movement of the head. Oral chloral hydrate, rectal sodium pentothal (3 to 6 mg/kg for children younger than 4 years of age; 1.5 to 3 mg/kg for children older than 4 years), and meperidine (Demerol; 2 mg/kg up to 50 mg) are reliable and safe agents for this purpose. Chloral hydrate is administered orally as an initial dose of 60 to 75 mg/kg, with a subsequent dose of 45 to 50 mg/kg for those children in whom the initial dose was ineffective, with the maximum 2 g or 100 mg/kg, whichever is less (76,77). Newborns may not require sedation because simple bundling might hold the child still enough during the short scan times commonplace with newer machines.

Nonionic contrast media of the iodide type (e.g., iohexol) can be used to facilitate recognition of structure and vascularity. They have for the greater part replaced ionic contrast media because of their lower incidence of anaphylactoid reactions and other complications (78). Enhancement of tumors and surrounding abnormal tissue results from a breakdown of the blood–brain barrier. Rapid scanning in combination with iodinated contrast allows the acquisition of CT perfusion scans (79). By measuring the change in hounsifield units in each voxel while a bolus of contrast passes through, one can calculate blood flow transit time and blood volume. In addition to being most useful for rapid assessment of strokes, this technique has an array of other potential uses (79). Unlike MRI perfusion, it provides actual values as opposed to relative ones and is more anatomic than single photon emission computed tomography (SPECT) studies.

A CT scan is the procedure of choice for the emergency evaluation of the child who has suffered head trauma or who is suspected of having a subarachnoid hemorrhage. The CT scan is also preferable to MRI for the detection of intracranial calcifications such as are seen in intrauterine infections, the phakomatoses, and brain tumors. It also can be used to localize and define a brain abscess and to follow its course under therapy.

Although catheter angiography is still the procedure of choice for the ultimate delineation of vascular lesions, these are readily detected by CT scans, MRI, and MR angiography. The latter procedures also provide information not obtainable by catheter angiography, such as the presence and extent of an associated hematoma, subarachnoid blood, or edema. CT angiography is a noninvasive technique that uses a rapid intravenous contrast bolus and thin spiral scans of a defined area of vascular anatomy. It is most useful in evaluating complex circle of Willis aneurysms (80). CT angiography is best performed as a dedicated study with submillimeter spiral acquisitions (81) (Fig. I.8).

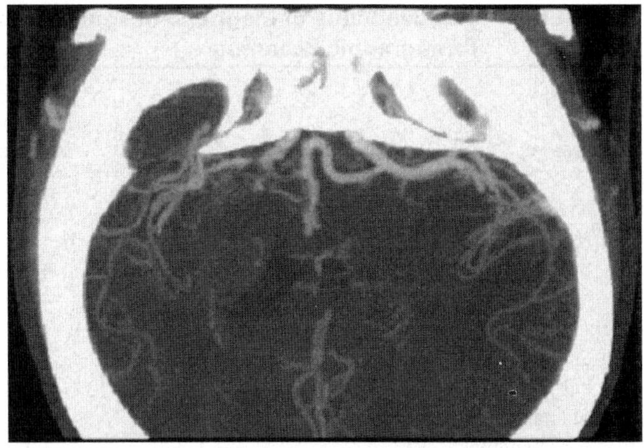

FIGURE I.8. Computed tomography angiography. The study demonstrates a variety of vascular abnormalities on the left side in a child with an early stage of moya-moya disease.

A CT scan is inferior to ultrasonography for the diagnosis of many of the early intracranial complications of prematurity and for the evaluation of an infant with hydrocephalus. The CT scan is also inferior to MRI in the detection of minor central nervous system malformations, the evaluation of structural epileptogenic lesions, and demyelinating processes.

Magnetic Resonance Imaging

Magnetic resonance imaging is a versatile and noninvasive procedure, whose clinical use was first described in 1977 (82). It provides information on brain structure without exposure to ionizing radiation. For a discussion of the fundamental physical principles of MRI and an explanation of its terminology, subjects far beyond the scope of this text, and for a more extensive presentation of its application the reader is referred to books such as those by Lee et al. (83). This section reviews the applications of MRI of the brain and compares them with those for CT scanning. Table I.4 shows the relative efficacy of the two procedures. Generally, T1-weighted images can provide a higher resolution view of structural anatomy, especially with thin-section techniques or three-dimensional acquisitions. T2-weighted images are preferred for the detection of various other abnormalities. Fluid-attenuated inversion recovery (FLAIR) is a T2-weighted technique that suppresses the background water signal that makes abnormal findings even more conspicuous.

As is the case for CT scanning, MR imaging necessitates sedation of infants and of children who cannot be expected to remain still for the duration of the procedure. In our institution this requires placement of an intravenous line, using intramuscular ketamine for children who are

TABLE I.4 Relative Value of Magnetic Resonance Imaging and Computed Tomographic Scanning

Disease	*Magnetic Resonance Imaging*	*Computed Tomographic Scanning*	*Metrizamide-Enhanced Computed Tomographic Scanning*
Tumors			
Low grade			
Supratentorial	+++	++	
Infratentorial	++++	++	
High grade			
Supratentorial	++++	++++	
Infratentorial	++++	++	
Metastases			
Supratentorial	+++	++	
Infratentorial	+++	+	
Demyelinating diseases	++++	++	
Trauma			
Craniocerebral	++	+++	
Spinal	+++[a]	+++	+++
Vasculitis (systemic lupus erythematosus)	+++	±	
Cervicomedullary junction and cervical spinal cord			
Congenital anomalies	++++	+	++
Tumors (intraaxial)			
Brainstem	++++	+	++
Cerebellopontine angle	+++	++	+++
Cervical spine	++++	±	++
Tumors (extraaxial)			
Brainstem	++++	+	++
Cervical spine	++++	±	+++

++++, preferred initial approach; +++, of definite value; ++, of value, but should not be considered as the initial diagnostic approach; +, of some value, but other procedures are superior; ±, of questionable value.

[a] Radiographic computed tomographic scanning is superior in visualizing bone abnormalities, whereas magnetic resonance imaging may be superior in demonstrating blood and spinal cord injury.

Adapted from Council of Scientific Affairs, Report of the Panel on Magnetic Resonance Imaging. Magnetic resonance imaging of the central nervous system. *JAMA* 1988;259:1211. With permission.

difficult to control, followed by intravenous midazolam and intravenous propofol or sevoflurane.

In the evaluation of tumors, MRI is generally superior to CT scanning for the detection and characterization of posterior fossa lesions, particularly when these are isodense and thus require contrast infusion for their delineation. It is also superior for the detection and delineation of low-grade tumors and provides a more precise definition of associated features, such as mass effects, hemorrhage, and edema. In a brainstem glioma, for instance, sagittal scans demonstrate the rostrocaudal extent of tumor, and tumors involving the sella or the chiasmatic cistern are more readily delineated by MRI than CT scanning because interference from surrounding bone limits the accuracy of CT scanning. The infusion of chelated gadolinium (i.e., gadopentetate dimeglumine) provides contrast enhancement for intracranial lesions with abnormal vascularity, such as the more malignant tumors, and detects lesions that disrupt the blood–brain barrier. These are best seen on T1-weighted images (84). Enhanced MRI facilitates the distinction between tumor and edema and between viable tissue and necrotic tissue. It also delineates any leptomeningeal spread of metastases and the spinal cord metastases so common in medulloblastomas. Gadolinium-contrast infusions also have been used to delineate the cerebral lesions of neurofibromatosis and tuberous sclerosis. Gadolinium contrast has proven to be an exceedingly safe material, with a complication rate of less than 1 in 10,000. The use of neuroimaging in the diagnosis of central nervous system tumors is discussed more extensively in Chapter 11.

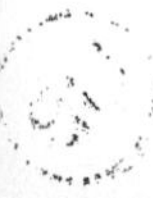

In spinal cord tumors, MRI is the procedure of choice. It is far superior in examination of inherent bone disease and in evaluation of the bone marrow.

In addition, MRI, by providing good gray–white differentiation, offers valuable information on the status of myelin in demyelinating diseases and during normal and abnormal development. When T2-weighted images are viewed, white matter appears lighter (higher signal intensity) than gray matter for the first 6 to 7 months of life. Between 8 and 12 months of age, the signal intensities from white and gray matter are approximately equal (Fig. I.9).

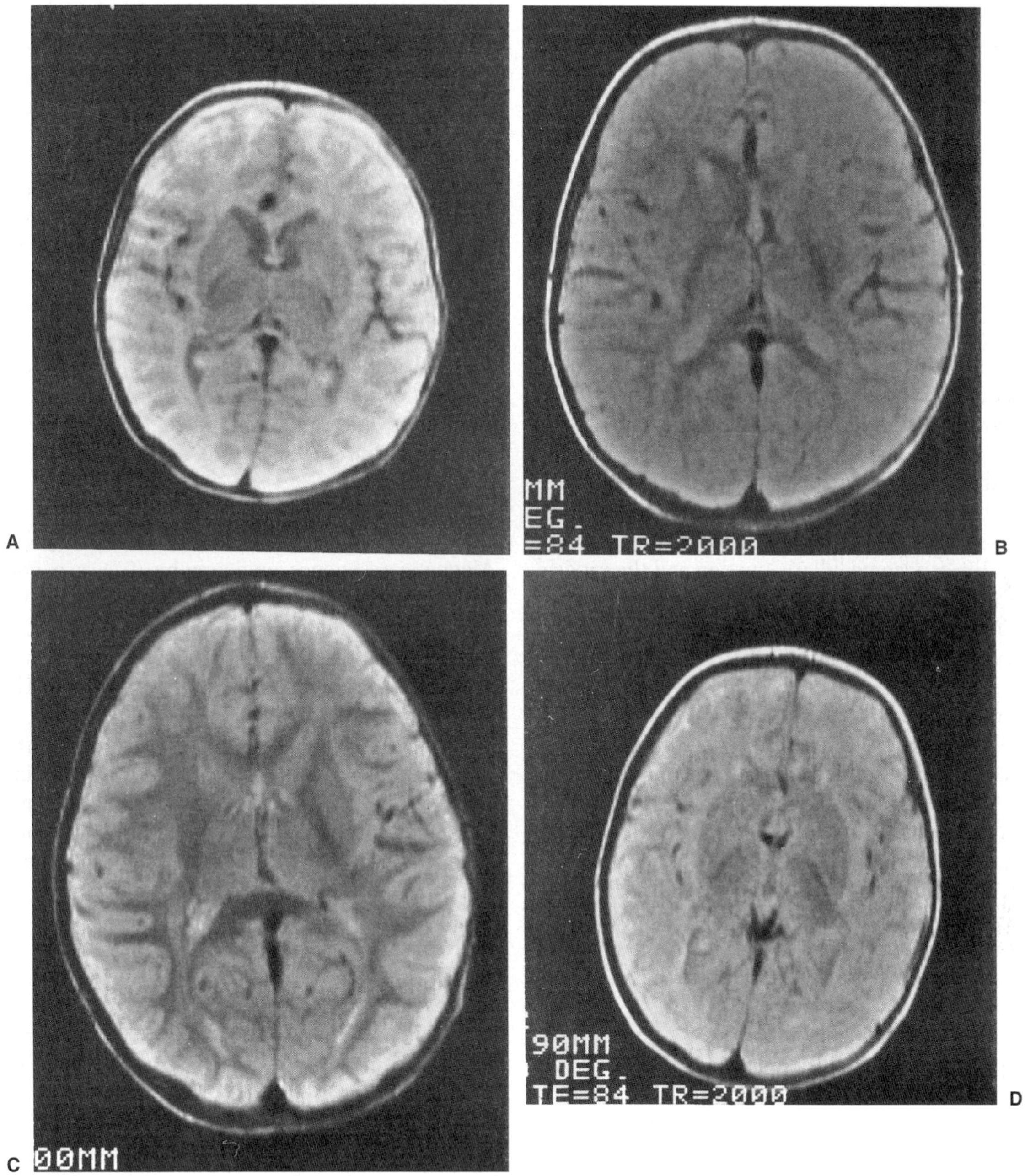

FIGURE I.9. Magnetic resonance imaging studies in normal and abnormal development. **A:** Normal development, age 3 months. Axial spin-echo (SE) (2,000/84). White matter has higher signal intensity than adjacent gray matter. Myelin is already present in the region of the thalamus and the posterior limbs of the internal capsule. A small amount of myelin is present in the occipital white matter. **B:** Normal development, age 10 months. Axial SE (2,000/84). The gray and white matter are isointense. Myelin is now present also in the anterior limbs of the internal capsule. **C:** Normal development, age 18 months. Axial SE (2,000/84). The white matter is hypointense relative to the gray matter. The area of myelinated white matter has now extended peripherally. **D:** Delayed development, age 18 months. Axial SE (2,000/84). White matter is transitional between having higher signal intensity than the adjacent gray matter and being isointense with gray matter. Myelin is present in the thalamus and the posterior limbs of the internal capsule. This picture is consistent with a normal development of between 3 and 6 months of age. (Courtesy of Dr. Rosalind B. Dietrich, Department of Radiology, Univ. of California, San Diego Medical Center, San Diego, CA.)

Thereafter, the brain has the adult appearance with gray matter lighter than white matter (85,86). This progression is delayed frequently in developmentally retarded youngsters (see Fig. I.9). MRI of the brain in preterm infants younger than 30 weeks' gestation demonstrates the presence of the germinal matrix at the margins of the lateral ventricles as small areas of high signal intensity on T1-weighted images and low signal intensity on T2-weighted images (87,88). The MRI also can be used to demonstrate the maturation of the cortical sulci (see Chapter 5).

For the evaluation of developmentally delayed children, particularly when anomalies of cortical architecture are suspected, MRI is far superior to CT scanning in that it can depict areas of micropolygyria, lissencephaly, or heterotopic gray matter. Additionally, the quality of images is superior to that offered by CT scans.

MRI is the procedure of choice for the evaluation of patients with refractory complex or simple partial seizures and is preferred to CT scanning in demonstrating abnormalities at the cervicomedullary junction and the cervical spinal cord. The procedure is, therefore, used as a follow-up study for the patient who has sustained cervical trauma or who is suspected of having an Arnold-Chiari malformation.

MRI has been used to map the distribution of brain iron. In the healthy brain, the concentration of iron is maximal in the globus pallidus, caudate nucleus, and putamen. It increases in the Hallervorden-Spatz syndrome, making MRI useful in its diagnosis.

Finally, in choosing between CT scanning and MRI, the physician should not forget that the critically ill patient with a variety of infusions and requiring respiratory support cannot be managed properly in many MRI units and that the procedure costs 20% to 300% more than CT scans (88).

The frequency of incidental findings on MR imaging in a normal population is significant. In a study conducted on 1,000 healthy volunteers, 18% of brain MRI demonstrated abnormal findings, the vast majority of which did not require follow-up evaluation (89).

Diffusion-Weighted Magnetic Resonance Imaging

In images obtained with diffusion-weighted MRI, contrast depends on differences in the molecular motion of water. Acute strokes, such as occur in sickle cell disease, and hypoxic-ischemic changes in mature brain are detected earlier by this technique than by conventional MRI (90,91). The advantages of this technique in neonatal hypoxic-ischemic encephalopathy are not as clear (92). Several methods, notably FLAIR pulse sequences, have been used to reduce CSF signal and produce heavy T2 weighting and thus provide additional anatomic detail. These are discussed in detail by Oatridge and colleagues (93). In our institution, a combination of FLAIR and diffusion-weighted images is used to evaluate the patient with hyperacute infarction (within 3 hours of onset).

Diffusion Tensor Imaging (DTI)

Whereas diffusion-weighted MRI examinations use the directionally random motion of water molecules that normally occurs, DTI takes advantage of the directional (anisotropic) motion of water molecules in white matter tracts (94). The tensor is the mathematical expression of the directional movement. DTI allows the plotting of white matter tracts throughout the brain. This technique is finding application in a wide array of situations, including abnormalities in brain development, hypoxic ischemic disease, and trauma (95,96) (Fig. I.10).

Magnetic Resonance Angiography

Magnetic resonance angiography (97) is a noninvasive technique that allows visualization of blood vessels. In those in the pediatric age group, who have a higher cerebral blood flow than adults, the large cerebral arteries and their major branches are routinely visualized. This procedure has replaced traditional angiography for most purposes and has proved helpful in evaluating dural sinuses and cerebral aneurysms and in studying arterial and venous components of an arteriovenous malformation. In particular, it is a noninvasive diagnostic tool for the evaluation of children with vascular accidents. Some centers use gadolinium enhancement to visualize veins and arteries with slower blood flow (98,99) (see Chapter 13).

Magnetic Resonance Spectroscopy

Magnetic resonance spectroscopy (MRS) is performed using the same magnets and computers as conventional MRI. Proton MRS is used more widely than ^{31}P-MRS. Unlike MRI, MRS provides information on the cerebral metabolites and some neurotransmitters in one or more small regions of interest (voxels). The major metabolites that can be detected by proton MRS include *N*-acetyl compounds, primarily *N*-acetylaspartate (NAA); creatine (including phosphocreatine and its precursor, creatine); and choline-containing compounds, including free choline, phosphoryl, and glycerophosphoryl choline. NAA is a neuronal marker, whereas the choline compounds are released in the course of membrane disruption. Proton MRS also can be used to determine the concentration of lactate, which accumulates as a result of tissue damage and consequent anaerobic metabolism (100–102). It is the most reliable procedure for diagnosinge defects in creatine transport (103). Neurotransmitters, such as gamma-aminobutyric acid and glutamate, also can be estimated using proton MRS. In neonates, the dominant peaks are

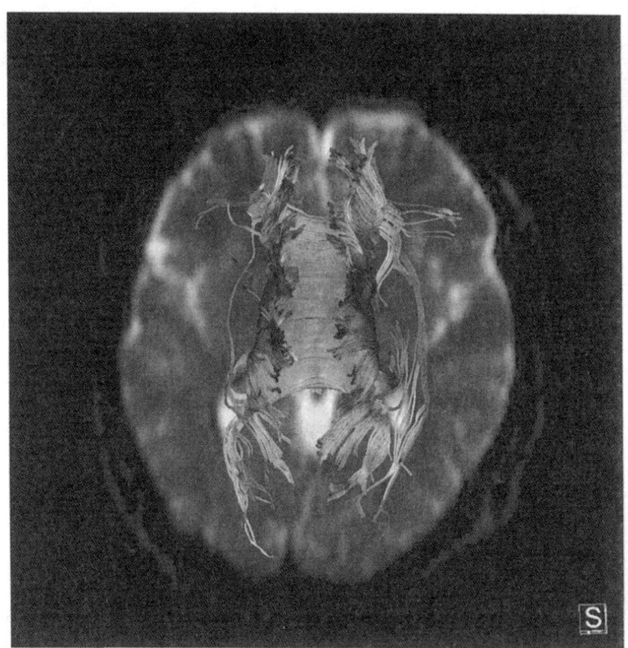

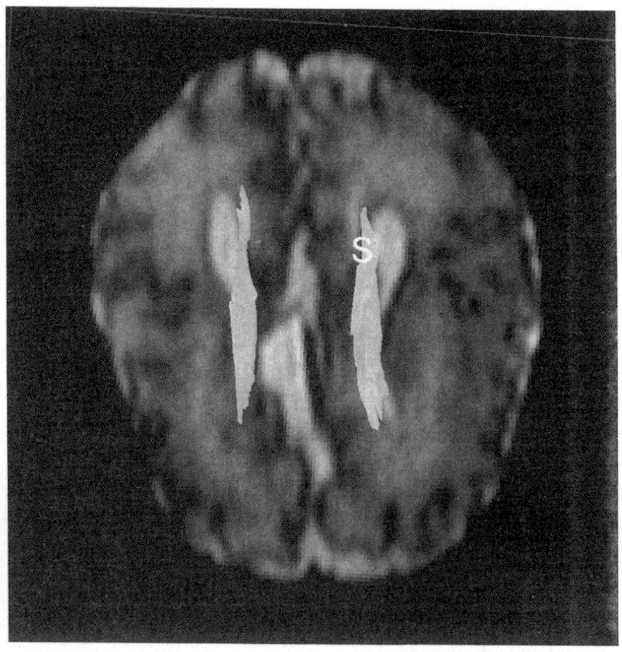

FIGURE I.10. Diffusion tensor imaging. **A:** Normal study demonstrating white matter tracts crossing the midline through the corpus callosum. **B:** Agenesis of the corpus callosum. Note the absence of fiber tracts crossing the midline.

the choline-containing compounds and myo-inositol. With maturation, NAA increases, so that by 4 months of age it becomes the major metabolic peak. As a consequence, the NAA/choline and NAA/creatine ratios increase rapidly with maturation, whereas the choline/creatine ratio decreases (100).

Concentrations of adenosine triphosphate, phosphocreatine, and some of the other high-energy phosphates involved in cellular energetics can be assessed using ^{31}P-MRS.

Spectra can be acquired within 1 hour, and changes in intracellular pH and metabolites can be followed. Proton and phosphorus MRS has been used in the evaluation of muscle diseases, localization of epileptic foci, evaluation of the extent of post-traumatic lesions, classification of brain tumors, and diagnosis of the various mitochondrial disorders, leukodystrophies, and other demyelinating disorders. These techniques also have been used to determine the extent, timing, and prognosis of perinatal asphyxia (101,104).

Perfusion MRI

Whereas CT perfusion uses the x-ray absorption of iodine to map perfusion, a bolus of gadolinium is used for MRI perfusion. The most frequently used technique involves signal loss caused by the influx of contrast and rapid sequences. Perfusion MRI can be used to assess the hemodynamic component in childhood CNS disease related to neoplasms and complications from their therapy, cerebrovascular occlusive disease, childhood CNS arteriopathies, and trauma. It has advantage over CT in that the entire brain can be scanned. As with CT perfusion, blood flow timing and blood volumes can be mapped (105).

Ultrasonography

As is more extensively discussed in Chapter 6, ultrasonography is widely used for the recognition of intracranial hemorrhage in the newborn and for the detection of a variety of nonhemorrhagic lesions, notably intracranial tumors, hydrocephalus, periventricular leukomalacia, and polycystic encephalomalacia (106). Additionally, ultrasonography detects areas of calcification, such as those caused by cytomegalovirus or *Toxoplasma* infections. Because the procedure is performed through the open anterior fontanelle, its accuracy decreases with the decreasing size of the fontanelle.

Positron Emission Tomography

Positron emission tomography (PET) enables one to detect localized functional abnormalities of the brain. It is based on the emission by certain unstable isotopes of positrons (positively charged electrons), which, after brief passage through tissue, collide with negatively charged electrons and emit energy that can be localized by tomography. Isotopes of carbon, nitrogen, oxygen, and fluorine have been used for PET scanning. All have short half-lives and are generally prepared by an on-site or nearby cyclotron. ^{18}F-labeled 2-fluorodeoxyglucose is particularly useful for measuring transport and phosphorylation of glucose in that it is not metabolized beyond deoxyglucose-6-phosphate and, therefore, remains within the brain. ^{18}F-labeled 2-fluorodeoxyglucose allows accurate measurements of cerebral blood flow and of local oxygen and glucose metabolism. Because the hallmark of an epileptic focus is an interictal area of reduced cerebral glucose metabolism, the PET scan has become invaluable in the assessment of candidates for surgical therapy of epilepsy (107). The PET scan is being used also for the early diagnosis of Huntington disease, the differential diagnoses of dementias, and the differentiation between radiation necrosis and tumor recurrence. Specific ligands have been used to investigate dopamine, opiate, and benzodiazepine receptor binding in various movement disorders. For the most part, these studies have not had any clinical applicability in pediatric cases. Finally, the PET scan has shown considerable promise in the study of the functional development of the normal and diseased human brain (108).

Single Photon Emission Computed Tomography (SPECT)

The so-called poor man's PET scan, SPECT depends on the gamma-ray emission of certain neutral lipophilic isotopes, notably ^{99}Tc, to measure regional cerebral blood flow. In the pediatric population, SPECT finds considerable use for the study of refractory epilepsies. In essence, the results with SPECT parallel those with PET scanning; generalized hyperperfusion is seen during a seizure in the generalized epilepsies, and regional hyperperfusion is seen for a few minutes before and during a seizure in an area that corresponds to the epileptic focus in partial seizures (109). Ictal hyperperfusion extends for approximately 10 minutes into the postictal period with hyperperfused surround that often is extensive (110). Interictally, a large proportion of patients show areas of hypoperfusion corresponding to the epileptic focus. For the purpose of localizing an epileptic focus, interictal hypoperfusion is less reliable than the data obtained by a combination of SPECT and MRI (109).

The simplicity and economy of SPECT are its biggest advantages. However, several drawbacks to this technique exist. For one, SPECT tracers are not natural biological molecules, and their physiologic behavior is not fully understood. Spatial resolution of SPECT is poorer than resolution by PET, and SPECT gives no information with respect to brain metabolism, nor does it permit quantitation of blood flow. Because in most instances brain metabolism and cerebral blood flow are closely linked and the isotopes used in SPECT do not require on-site production, this procedure has an important role in the evaluation of the difficult seizure patient (111). At present, no isotopes of carbon, oxygen, or nitrogen with usable half-lives and energies exist; this procedure has been therefore mainly limited to the study of cerebral perfusion (112). Newer pharmaceuticals, notably ^{99m}Tc-methoxyisobutylisonitrile, have been used to detect the metabolic activity of tumors (113).

Functional Magnetic Resonance Imaging

In our institution, the clinical applications of functional MRI are principally in the preoperative localization of the sensorimotor, visual, and language cortex in patients with intracranial tumors (114,115). Functional MRI allows the identification of cortical activation by examination of the oxygen level of the cortical veins. Oxygenated hemoglobin has different signal characteristics than hemoglobin. Blood flow to an actively functioning cortex provides more oxygen to neurons than is consumed by them, and as a result, the oxygen level in the corresponding veins increases.

Cerebral Arteriography

The visualization of cerebral blood vessels by the injection of radiopaque dyes was introduced by Moniz in 1927 (116). Various techniques are used for arteriography in children, most commonly cannulation of the brachial or femoral arteries under direct visualization. The exact amount injected depends on the size of the child, but, generally, nonionic contrast medium is injected directly. With the small catheters that are now available, selective angiography of the cerebral vessels can be performed on even the smallest infant (117). Lateral and anteroposterior views of the skull are taken simultaneously or with successive injections. The principal indication for the procedure is in the evaluation of vascular abnormalities, including arteriovenous malformations, aneurysms, and occlusive vascular disease (see Chapter 13). Tumors of the cerebral hemispheres are localized by the distortion of the normal vascular patterns of the carotid arterial or venous system or by the presence of abnormal vasculature. Although CT and MRI provide first-line evidence of the size and location of a brain tumor, arteriography using digital subtraction techniques offers excellent confirmatory data in terms of blood supply to the mass lesion.

Current angiographic techniques have permitted the development of interventional neuroradiology. Percutaneous endovascular procedures have become the major mode of treatment for a wide array of vascular lesions, including malformations of the vein of Galen, arteriovenous malformations, fistulas, and intracerebral aneurysms (see Chapter 13).

Radiography of the Spine and Myelography

Spinal radiographs and CT are important in the management of the youngster who has been subjected to craniocerebral or spinal trauma. In interpreting spine films, the pediatric neurologist must consider a number of relatively common normal variations. These include the forward subluxation of C2 on C3, a variety of anomalies of the odontoid process, including the presence of an accessory ossicle, and the occipitalization of C1 (118).

MRI is the optimal study for the delineation of spinal cord tumors, diastematomyelia, the tethered cord, and various spinal cord anomalies that are reviewed in Chapter 5.

Pneumoencephalography and Ventriculography

Because these procedures are of purely historical interest, a brief review suffices. In 1918, Dandy introduced the technique of visualizing the cerebral ventricles and subarachnoid spaces by the injection of air into the lumbar spinal canal (119).

When this technique was used, localization of intracranial neoplasms relied on the presence of abnormalities in ventricular size and location. The morbidity of the procedure was considerable. When air was used as the contrast medium, its introduction into the ventricular system almost invariably resulted in headache and vomiting. Less often, hypotensive episodes and focal or generalized seizures and CSF pleocytosis occurred.

REFERENCES

1. Craige E. Should auscultation be rehabilitated? *N Engl J Med* 1988;318:1611–1613.
2. Tirosh E, Jaffe M, Dar H. The clinical significance of multiple hair whorls and their association with unusual dermatoglyphics and dysmorphic features in mentally retarded Israeli children. *Eur J Pediatr* 1987;146:568–570.
3. Goldsmith WM. "The catlin mark": the inheritance of an unusual opening in the parietal bones. *J Hered* 1922;13:69–71.
4. Wuyts W, Cleiren E, Homfray T, et al. The *AlX4* homeobox gene is mutated in patients with ossification defect of the skull (foramina parietalia permagna, OMIM 168500). *J Med Genet* 2000;37:916–920.
5. Wadia NH, Monckton G. Intracranial bruits in health and disease. *Brain* 1957;80:492–509.
6. Mackenzie I. The intracranial bruit. *Brain* 1955;78:350–367.
7. Peiper A. *Cerebral function in infancy and childhood*. New York: Consultants Bureau, 1963:49–53.
8. Kasahara M, Inamatsu S. Der Blinzelreflex im Säuglingsalter. *Arch Kinderheilk* 1931;92:302.
9. Cernerud L. The setting-sun eye phenomenon in infancy. *Dev Med Child Neurol* 1975;17:447–455.
10. Hoyt CS, Mousel DK, Weber AA. Transient supranuclear disturbances of gaze in healthy neonates. *Am J Ophthalmol* 1980;89:708–713.
11. Mehler MF. The clinical spectrum of ocular bobbing and ocular dipping. *J Neurol Neurosurg Psychiatry* 1988;51:725–727.
12. Isenberg SJ. Clinical application of the pupil examination in neonates. *J Pediatr* 1991;118:650–652.
13. Horner JF. Ueber eine Form von Ptosis. *Klin Monatsbl Augenheilkd* 1869;7:193.
14. Hageman G, Ippel PF, te Nijenhuis FC. Autosomal dominant congenital Horner's syndrome in a Dutch family. *J Neurol Neurosurg Psychiatry* 1992;55:28–30.
15. Cheng MMP, Catalano RA. Fatigue-induced familial anisoria. *Am J Ophthal* 1990;109:480–481.
16. Jampel RS, Quaglio ND. Eye movements in Tay-Sachs disease. *Neurology* 1964;14:1013–1019.
17. McMullan TW, Crolla JA, Gregory SG. A candidate gene for congenital bilateral isolated ptosis identified by molecular analysis of a *de novo* balanced translocation. *Hum Genet* 2000;110:244–250.
18. Jenny AB, Saper CB. Organization of the facial nucleus and corticofacial projection in the monkey: a reconsideration of the upper motor neuron facial palsy. *Neurology* 1987;37:930–939.
19. Ross RT, Mathiesen R. Volitional and emotional supranuclear facial weakness. *N Engl J Med* 1998;338:1515.
20. Davies AE, Kidd D, Stone SP, et al. Pharyngeal sensation and gag reflex in healthy subjects. *Lancet* 1995;345:487–488.
21. Medical Research Council. *Aids to the examination of peripheral nerve injuries*. London: Balliere Tindall, 1986.
22. Denny-Brown D. *The basal ganglia*. Oxford: Oxford University Press, 1962.
23. Prechtl HFR, Einspieler C, Gioni G, et al. An early marker for neurological deficits after perinatal brain lesions. *Lancet* 1997;349:1361–1363.
24. Paine RS, Oppe TE. *Neurological examination of children: clinics in developmental medicine*, Vol. 20/21. London: William Heinemann, 1966.
25. Gingold MK, Jaynes ME, Bodensteiner JB, et al. The rise and fall of the plantar response in infancy. *J Pediatr* 1998;133:568–570.
26. Wartenberg R. *The examination of reflexes*, Chicago: Yearbook Publishers, 1945.
27. Chvostek F. Weitere Beiträge zur Tetanie. *Wiener Mediz Presse* 1879;20:1201, 1233, 1268, 1301.
28. Denckla MB. Development of motor coordination in normal children. *Dev Med Child Neurol* 1974;16:729–741.
29. Arniel-Tison C. A method for neurologic evaluation within the first year of life. *Curr Probl Pediatr* 1976;7:1.
30. Moro E. Das erste Trimenon. *Munch Med Wochenschr* 1918:1147.
31. Wenzel D. The development of the parachute reaction: a visuovestibular response. *Neuropädiatrie* 1978;9:351–359.

31a. Gamper, E. Refluxuntersuchungen an einem Anecephalus. *Z ges Neurol. Psychiat*. 1926;104:47–73.

32. Dodge PR, Porter P. Demonstration of intracranial pathology by transillumination. *Arch Neurol* 1961;5:594–605.
33. Nelson KB, Ellenberg JH. Neonatal signs as predictors of cerebral palsy. *Pediatrics* 1979;64:225–232.
34. Quincke H. Die Lumbarpunktion des Hydrocephalus. *Klin Wochenschr* 1891;28:929–933, 965–968.
35. Porter FL, Miller JP, Cole FS, et al. A controlled clinical trial of local anesthesia for lumbar punctures in newborns. *Pediatrics* 1991;88:663–669.
36. Birnbach DJ, Kuroda MM, Sternman D, et al. Use of atraumatic spinal needles among neurologists in the United States. *Headache* 2001;41:385–390.
37. Bonadio WA, Smith DS, Metrou M, et al. Estimating lumbar puncture depth in children. *N Engl J Med* 1988; 319:952–953.
38. Ellis RW, Strauss LC, Wiley JM, et al. A simple method of estimating cerebrospinal fluid pressure during lumbar puncture. *Pediatrics* 1992;89:895–897.
39. Nelson DA. Dangers of lumbar spinal needle placement. *Ann Neurol* 1989;25:310.
40. Strupp M, Brandt T. Should one reinsert the stylet during lumbar puncture? *N Engl J Med* 1997;336:1190.
41. Sha KH, Edlow JA. Distinguishing traumatic lumbar puncture from true subarachnoid hemorrhage. *J Emerg Med* 2002;23:67–74.

41a. Petzold A, Keit G, Sharpe LT. Spectophotometry for xanthochromia. *N Engl J Med* 2004;351:1695–1696.

42. Bonadio WA, Stanco L, Bruce R, et al. Reference values of normal cerebrospinal fluid composition in infants ages 0 to 8 weeks. *Pediatr Infect Dis J* 1992;11:589–591.

43. Volpe JJ. Neonatal intracranial hemorrhage. Pathophysiology, neuropathology, and clinical features. *Clin Perinatol* 1977;4:77–102.
44. Tourtellotte WW, Somers JF, Parker JA, et al. A study on traumatic lumbar punctures. *Neurology* 1958;8:129–134.
45. Ahmed A, Hickey SM, Ehrett S, et al. Cerebrospinal fluid values in the term neonate. *Pediatr Infec Dis J* 1996;15:298–303.
46. Portnoy JM, Olson LC. Normal cerebrospinal fluid values in children: another look. *Pediatrics* 1985; 75:484–487.
47. Rubenstein J, Yogev R. What represents pleocytosis in blood-contaminated ("traumatic tap") cerebrospinal fluid in children? *J Pediatr* 1985;107:249–251.
48. Rust RS, Dodson WE, Trotter JL. Cerebrospinal fluid IgG in childhood: the establishment of reference values. *Ann Neurol* 1988;23:406–410.
49. Rennick G, Shann F, de Campo J. Cerebral herniation during bacterial meningitis in children. *Brit Med J* 1993;306:953–955.
50. Oliver WJ, Shope TC, Kuhns LR. Fatal lumbar puncture: Fact versus fiction–an approach to a clinical dilemma. *Pediatrics* 2003;112:eI74–eI76.
51. Raskin NH. Lumbar puncture headache: a review. *Headache* 1990;30:197–200.
52. Tourtellotte WW, Henderson WG, Tucker RP. A randomized, double-blind clinical trial comparing the 22 versus 26 gauge needle in the production of the postlumbar puncture syndrome in normal individuals. *Headache* 1972;12:73–78.
53. Ebinger F, Kosel C, Pietz J, et al. Headache and backache after lumbar puncture in children and adolescents: a prospective study. *Pediatrics* 2004;113:1588–1592.
54. Niedermuller U, Trinka E, Bauer G. Abducens palsy after lumbar puncture. *Clin Neurol Neurosurg* 2002;104:61–63.
55. Kirkpatrick D, Goodman SJ. Combined subarachnoid and subdural spinal hematoma following spinal puncture. *Surg Neurol* 1975;3:109–111.
56. Fredericks JAM. Spinal puncture complications: complications of diagnostic lumbar puncture, myelography, spinal anesthesia and intrathecal drug anesthesia. In: Vinken PJ, Bruyn GW, Klawans HL, et al, eds. *Handbook of clinical neurology, Vol. 17 (61): Spinal cord trauma.* Amsterdam: Elsevier Science, 1992:147–189.
57. Glass JP, Melamed M, Chernick NL, et al. Malignant cells in cerebrospinal fluid (CSF): the meaning of a positive CSF cytology. *Neurology* 1979;29:1369–1375.
58. de Reuck J, Vanderdonckt P. Choroid plexus and ependymal cells in CSF cytology. *Clin Neurol Neurosurg* 1986;88:177–179.
59. Matoth I, Taustein I, Kay BS, et al. Overuse of EEG in the evaluation of common neurologic conditions. *Pedatr Neurol* 2002;27:378–383.
60. Binnie CD, Macgillivray BB. Brain mapping—a useful tool or a dangerous toy? *J Neurol Neurosurg Psychiatry* 1992;55:527–529.
61. Nuwer M. Assessment of digital EEG, quantitative EEG, and brain mapping: report of the American Academy of Neurology and the American Clinical Neurophysiology Society. *Neurology* 1997;49:277–292.
62. Barry RJ, Clarke AR, Johnstone SJ. A review of electrophysiology in attention-deficit/hyperactivity disorder: I. Qualitative and quantitative electroencephalography. *Clin Neurophysiol* 2003;114:171–183.
63. Guilleminault C. *Sleep and its disorders in children.* New York: Raven Press, 1987.
64. Ferber R, Kryger M, eds. *Principles and practice of sleep medicine in the child.* Philadelphia: Saunders, 1995.
65. Gamstorp I. *Pediatric neurology*, 2nd ed. London: Butterworth–Heinemann, 1985:45–47.
66. Huppertz HJ, Disselhorst-Klug C, Silny J, et al. Diagnostic yield of noninvasive high spatial resolution electromyography in neuromuscular diseases. *Muscle Nerve* 1997;20:1360–1370.
67. Kimura J. *Electrodiagnosis in diseases of nerve and muscle. Principles and practice*, 3rd ed. Oxford: Oxford University Press, 2001.
68. Aminoff MJ. *Electromyography in clinical practice: clinical and electrodiagnostic aspects of neuromuscular disease* 3rd ed. New York: Churchill Livingstone, 1997.
69. Gamstorp I. Normal conduction velocity of ulnar, median and peroneal nerves in infancy, childhood and adolescence. *Acta Paediatr Stockholm* 1963; 146(Suppl):68–77.
70. Moskowitz A, Sokol S. Developmental changes in the human visual system as reflected by the latency of the pattern reversal VEP. *Electroencephalogr Clin Neurophysiol* 1983;56:115.
71. Kos-Pietro S, Towle VL, Cakmur R, et al. Maturation of human visual evoked potentials: 27 weeks conceptional age to 2 years. *Neuropediatrics* 1997;28:318–323.
72. Taylor MJ, Boor R, Ekert PG. Preterm maturation of the somatosensory evoked potential. *Electroencephalogr Clin Neurophysiol* 1996;100:448–452.
73. Baloh RW, Honrubia V, eds. *Clinical neurophysiology of the vestibularsystem*, 3rd ed. Oxford: Oxford University Press, 2001.
74. Ambrose J, Hounsfield GN. Computerized transverse axial tomography. *Br J Radiol* 1973; 46:148–149.
75. Oldendorf W. Isolated flying spot detection of radiodensity discontinuities displaying the internal structural pattern of a complex object: IRE Trans Biomed Electronics . *Biomed Mater Eng* 1961;8:68–72.
76. Krauss B, Green SM. Sedation and analgesia for procedures in children. *N Engl J Med* 2000;342:938–945.
77. Olson DM, Sheehan MG, Thompson W, et al. Sedation of children for electroencephalograms. *Pediatrics* 2001;108:163–165.
78. Federle MP, Willis LL, Swanson DP. Ionic versus nonionic contrast media: a prospective study of the effect of rapid bolus injection on nausea and anaphylactoid reactions. *J Comput Assist Tomogr* 1998;22:341–345.
79. Eastwood JD, Lev MH, Provenzale JM. Perfusion CT with iodinated contrast material. *Am J Roentgenol* 2003;180:3–12.
80. Vieco PT. CT angiography of the intracranial circulation. *Neuroimaging Clin North Am* 1998;8:577–592.
81. Rankin SC. CT angiography. *Eur Radiol* 1999;9:297–310.
82. Hinshaw WS, Bottomley PA, Holland GN. Radiographic thin-section image of the human wrist by nuclear magnetic resonance. *Nature* 1977;270:722–723.
83. Lee SH, Rao KCVG, Zimmerman RA. *Cranial and spinal MRI and CT*, 4th ed. New York: McGraw-Hill, 1999.
84. Edelman RR, Warach S. Magnetic resonance imaging. *N Engl J Med* 1993;328:708–716.
85. Dietrich RB, Bradley WB, Zaragoza EJ, et al. MR evaluation of early myelination patterns in normal and developmentally delayed infants. *Am J Neuroradiol* 1988;9:69–76.
86. Byrd SE, Darling CF, Wilczynski MA. White matter of the brain: maturation and myelination on magnetic resonance in infants and children. *Neuroimag Clin North Am* 1993;3:247–266.
87. Battin MR, Maalouf EF, Counsell SJ, et al. Magnetic resonance imaging of the brain in very preterm infants: visualization of the germinal matrix, early myelination and cortical folding. *Pediatrics* 1998;101:957–962.
88. van Wezel-Meijler G, van der Knaap MS, Sie LT, et al. Magnetic resonance imaging of the brain in premature infants during the neonatal period: normal phenomena and reflection of mild ultrasound abnormalities. *Neuropediatrics* 1998;29:89–96.
89. Katzman GI, Dagher AP, Patronas NJ. Incidental findings on brain magnetic resonance imaging from 1000 asymptomatic volunteers. *JAMA* 1999;282:36–39.
90. Baird AE, Warach S. Magnetic resonance imaging of acute stroke. *J Cereb Blood Flow Metab* 1998;18:583–609.
91. Cowan FM, Pennock JM, Hanrahan JD, et al. Early detection of cerebral infarction and hypoxic ischemic encephalopathy in neonates using diffusion-weighted magnetic resonance imaging. *Neuropediatrics* 1994;25:172–175.
92. Tuor UI, Koslowski P, Del Bigio MR, et al. Diffusion- and T2-weighted increases in magnetic resonance images of immature brain during hypoxia-ischemia: transient reversal posthypoxia. *Exp Neurol* 1998;150:321–328.
93. Oatridge A, Hajnal JV, Cowan FM, et al. MRI diffusion-weighted imaging of the brain: contributions to image contrast from CSF signal reduction, use of a long echo time and diffusion effects. *Clin Radiol* 1993;47:82–90.
94. Jellison BJ, Field AS, Medow J, et al. Diffusion tensor imaging of white matter: a pictorial review of physics, fiber tract anatomy, and tumor imaging patterns. *Am J Neuroradiol* 2004;25:356–369.
95. Glenn OA, Henry RG, Berman J, et al. DTI-based three-dimensional tractography detects differences in the pyramidal tracts of infants

and children with congenital hemiparesis. *J Magnet Res Imaging* 2003;18:641–648.

96. Huisman TA, Schwamm LH, Schaefer PW, et al. Diffusion tensor imagaing as potential biomarker of white matter injury in diffuse axonal injury. *Am J Neuroradiol* 2004;25:370–376.
97. Zimmerman RA, Bilaniuk LT. Pediatric brain, head and neck, and spine magnetic resonance angiography. *Magn Reson Q* 1992;8:264–290.
98. Zimmerman RA, Bogdan AR, Gusnard DA. Pediatric magnetic resonance angiography: assessment of stroke. *Cardiovasc Intervent Radiol* 1992;15:60–64.
99. Brant-Zawadzki M, Heiserman JE. The roles of MR angiography, CT angiography and sonography in vascular imaging of the head and neck. *Am J Neuroradiol* 1997;18:1820–1825.
100. Holshouser BA, Ashwal S, Luh GY, et al. Proton MR spectroscopy after acute central nervous system injury: outcome prediction in neonates, infants and children. *Radiology* 1997;202:487–496.
101. Groenendaal F, Veenhoven RH, van der Grond J, et al. Cerebral lactate and *N*-acetyl-aspartate/choline ratios in asphyxiated full-term neonates demonstrated *in vivo* using proton magnetic resonance spectroscopy. *Pediatr Res* 1994;35:148–151.
102. Novotny E, Ashwal S, Shevell M. Proton magnetic resonance spectroscopy: an emerging technology in pediatric neurology research. *Pediatr Res* 1998;44:1–10.
103. Salomons GS, van Dooren SJ, Verhoeven NM, et al. X-linked creatine transporter defect: an overview. *J Inherit Metab Dis* 2003;26:309–318.
104. Wang Z, Zimmerman RA, Sauter R. Proton MR spectroscopy of the brain: clinically useful information obtained in assessing CNS diseases in children. *Am J Radiol* 1996;167:191–199.
105. Keston P, Murray AD, Jackson A. Cerebral perfusion imaging using contrast-enhanced MRI. *Clin Radiol* 2003;58:505–513.
106. Rennie JM. *Neonatal cerebral ultrasound*. Cambridge, Cambridge University Press, 1997.
107. Duncan JS. Imaging and epilepsy. *Brain* 1997;120:339–377.
108. Chugani HT. Functional brain imaging in pediatrics. *Pediatr Clin North Am* 1992;39:777–799.
109. Baumgartner C, Serles W, Leutmezer F, et al. Preictal SPECT in temporal lobe epilepsy: regional cerebral blood flow is increased prior to electroencephalography-seizure onset. *J Nucl Med* 1998;39:978–982.
110. Uvebrant P, Bjure J, Hedstrom A, Ekholm S. Brain single photon emission computed tomography (SPECT) in neuropediatrics. *Neuropediatrics* 1991;22:3–9.
111. Schulder M, Madjian JA, Liu WC, et al. Functional image-guided surgery of intracranial tumors located in or near the sensorimotor cortex. *J Neurosurg* 1998;89:412–418.
112. Prichard JW, Brass LM. New anatomical and functional imaging methods. *Ann Neurol* 1992;32:395–400.
113. O'Tuama LA, Treves ST, Larar JN, et al. Thallium-201 versus technicium-99m-MIBI SPECT in evaluation of childhood brain tumors: a within-subject comparison. *J Nucl Med* 1993;34:1045–1051.
114. Turner R. Magnetic resonance imaging of brain function. *Ann Neurol* 1994;35:637–638.
115. Ugrubil K, Toth L, Kim DS. How accurate is magnetic resonance imaging of brain function? *Trends Neurosci* 2003;26:108–114.
116. Moniz E. L'encephalographie arterielle, son importance dans la localization des tumeurs cerebrales. *Rev Neurol (Paris)* 1927;2:72–90.
117. Burrows PE, Robertson RI. Neonatal central nervous system vascular disorders. *Neurosurg Clin North Am* 1998;9:155–180.
118. Cattel HS, Filtzer DL. Pseudosubluxation and other normal variations in the cervical spine in children. *J Bone Joint Surg* 1965;47A:1295–1309.
119. Dandy WE. Ventriculography following the injection of air into the cerebral ventricles. *Ann Surg* 1918;68:5.

Chapter 1

Inherited Metabolic Diseases of the Nervous System

John H. Menkes and William R. Wilcox

The diseases considered in this chapter result from a single mutant gene that codes for an enzymatic protein that in most instances is involved in a catabolic pathway. The consequent homeostatic disturbances produce a neurologic or developmental abnormality. The separation between conditions considered in this chapter and those in Chapter 3 is admittedly arbitrary. Both chapters deal with single-gene defects, except that for diseases covered in this chapter, the defective gene is normally expressed in one or more organs, not necessarily in the nervous system, and chemical analyses of tissues are frequently diagnostic. Conditions considered in Chapter 3 are also the result of a single defective gene, but one that is mainly or exclusively expressed in the nervous system. Consequently, these entities lack characteristic chemical abnormalities of tissues or body fluids.

Since 1975, almost all of the nearly 500 neurologic and neuromuscular diseases caused by known enzymatic or protein defects have been mapped to a specific chromosome region, and a large proportion of them have been cloned. In the course of these advances, a considerable amount of metabolic, molecular, and genetic detail has become available, the full discussion of which is outside the domain of this text. Instead, the emphasis of this chapter is on the clinical presentation of the diseases, their diagnosis and treatment, and, when known, the mechanisms that induce the neurologic deficits. For a more extensive discussion of the genetic and molecular basis of the neurologic disorders, the reader is referred to a text by Rosenberg and coworkers (1) and the compendium edited by Scriver and coworkers (2). In addition, we recommend two small paperback handbooks written by Clarke (3) and Hoffman and coworkers (3a) that are intended to make inborn errors of metabolism accessible to physicians who do not have an in-depth knowledge of biochemistry and molecular biology. For readers who are computer minded there is a helpful Web site at http://www.geneclinics.org.

Screening of newborns by tandem mass spectroscopy of amino acids and acylcarnitines has found an incidence of inborn errors of metabolism (excluding phenylketonuria) of approximately 15.7 in 100,000 live births (3b). These disorders are therefore individually relatively uncommon in the practice of pediatric neurology. Their importance rests, however, on the insight these disorders offer into the relationship between a genetic mutation, the resultant disturbance in homeostasis, and a disorder of the nervous system.

The mechanisms by which inborn errors of metabolism produce brain dysfunction remain largely uncertain, although, for some conditions, a plausible theory of pathogenesis has been proposed. Not all enzyme defects lead to disease; a large number of harmless metabolic variants exist. They include pentosuria, one of the original four inborn errors of metabolism described by Garrod (4), and several others listed in Table 1.1. Many of these variants were discovered when individuals in institutions for the mentally retarded were screened for metabolic defects at a time when their incidence in normal populations had not been determined. Over the last decade the imperfect relationship between the gene defect and its phenotypic expression has become evident. A single gene defect can result in a variety of phenotypic expressions, and, conversely, what has been assumed to be a single neurologic phenotype can have multiple genetic etiologies. Even for phenylketonuria, long considered to be the epitome of a metabolic disorder, the relationship between the mutation in the gene for phenylalanine hydroxylase, blood phenylalanine levels, and the ultimate result, impairment in cognitive function, is complex and unpredictable (5,5a).

An introduction to the fundamentals of molecular genetics is far beyond the scope of this text. The reader interested in this subject is referred to books by Strachan and Read (6), Lodish and colleagues (7), and Lewin (8).

For practical purposes, we will divide metabolic disorders into the following groups:

Disorders of amino acid metabolism
Disorders of renal amino acid transport

TABLE 1.1 Inborn Errors of Amino Acid Metabolism Without Known Clinical Consequences

Histidinemia (OMIM 235800)
Cystathioninemia (OMIM 219500)
Hyperprolinemia I (OMIM 239500)
Hyperprolinemia II (OMIM 239510)
Hydroxyprolinemia (OMIM 237000)
Hyperlysinemia (OMIM 238700)
Saccharopinuria (OMIM 247900)
Dibasic aminoaciduria I (OMIM 222690)
Alpha-aminoadipic aciduria (OMIM 204750)
Alpha-ketoadipic aciduria (OMIM 245130)
Sarcosinemia (OMIM 268900)

Disorders of carbohydrate metabolism and transport
Organic acidurias
Disorders of fatty acid oxidation
Lysosomal disorders
Disorders of lipid and lipoprotein metabolism
Peroxisomal disorders
Carbohydrate-deficient protein syndromes
Familial myoclonus epilepsies
Ceroid lipofuscinosis and other lipidoses
Disorders of serum lipoproteins
Disorders of metal metabolism
Disorders of purine and pyrimidine metabolism
Porphyrias

EVALUATION OF THE PATIENT SUSPECTED OF HAVING A METABOLIC DISORDER

The spectacular advances of molecular biology have facilitated the diagnosis and prevention of genetic diseases and have brought humanity to the threshold of gene therapy. The clinician must, therefore, strive for an early diagnosis of inborn errors of metabolism to offer treatment whenever possible, provide appropriate genetic counseling, and, in many instances, give parents an opportunity for an antenatal diagnosis on the occasion of a subsequent pregnancy (9,10).

Since the initial descriptions of phenylketonuria and maple syrup urine disease, the protean clinical picture of the various inborn metabolic errors has become apparent. As a consequence, these disorders must be included in the differential diagnosis of neurologic problems whenever other causes are not evident from the child medical history and physical examination.

Two questions should be considered: What type of patient should be suspected of having an inborn error of metabolism, and what tests should be included in the diagnostic evaluation? It is clear that the greater the suspicion of a metabolic disorder, the more intense the investigative process must be.

TABLE 1.2 Clinical Syndromes Suggestive of An Underlying Metabolic Cause

Neurologic disorder, including mental retardation, replicated in sibling or close relative
Recurrent episodes of altered consciousness or unexplained vomiting in an infant
Recurrent unexplained ataxia or spasticity
Progressive central nervous system degeneration
Mental retardation without obvious cause

Table 1.2 lists some clinical syndromes (ranked by frequency) suggestive of an underlying metabolic cause.

A carefully obtained history and physical examination provide important clues to the presence of a metabolic disorder and its specific etiology (Table 1.3).

Metabolic investigations are less imperative for children who have focal neurologic disorders or who suffer from mental retardation in conjunction with major congenital anomalies. Dysmorphic features, however, have been found in some of the peroxisomal disorders, including Zellweger syndrome, in pyruvate dehydrogenase deficiency, in glutaric acidemia type II, and in Smith-Lemli-Opitz syndrome (11). These are given in Table 1.4.

When embarking on a metabolic investigation, procedures should be performed in ascending order of complexity and discomfort to patient and family.

Metabolic Screening

Routine screening of plasma and urine detects the overwhelming majority of disorders of amino acid metabolism and disorders manifested by an abnormality of organic acids as well as the common disorders of carbohydrate metabolism. Amino acid analysis can be performed by ion exchange chromatography, high-performance liquid chromatography, gas chromatography-mass spectrometry, or tandem mass spectrometry–mass spectrometry (TMS-MS). Analysis of organic acids is generally performed by gas–liquid chromatography with or without mass spectrometry. At our institution, metabolic screening usually includes plasma amino acids and urinary organic acids. The yield on these tests is low, and a high frequency of nonspecific or nondiagnostic abnormalities occurs. Urea cycle disorders are characterized by elevated concentrations of blood ammonia with the patient in the fasting state or on a high-protein intake (4 g/kg per day).

A number of genetic disorders are characterized by intermittent acidosis. Elevated lactic and pyruvic acid levels in serum or cerebrospinal fluid (CSF) are found in a number of the mitochondrial disorders. The lactate/pyruvate ratio may suggest the type of disorder. A normal ratio in

TABLE 1.3 Clinical Clues to the Diagnosis of Metabolic Diseases of the Nervous System

Clue	Diagnosis
Cutaneous abnormalities	
Increased pigmentation	Adrenoleukodystrophy
Telangiectases (conjunctiva, ears, popliteal areas)	Ataxia-telangiectasia
Perioral eruption	Multiple carboxylase deficiency
Abnormal fat distribution	Congenital disorders of glycosylation
Angiokeratoma (red macules or maculopapules) of hips, buttocks, scrotum	Fabry disease, sialidosis, fucosidosis type II
Oculocutaneous albinism	Chédiak-Higashi syndrome
Xanthomas	Cerebrotendinous xanthomatosis
Subcutaneous nodules	Ceramidosis (Farber disease)
Ichthyosis	Sjögren-Larsson syndrome (spasticity, seizures)
	Refsum disease (neuropathy, ataxia, phylanic acid)
	Dorfman-Chanarin syndrome (lipid storage in muscle, granulocytes, and so forth)
Inverted nipples	Congenital disorders of glycosylation
Abnormal urinary or body odor	
Musty	Phenylketonuria
Maple syrup or caramel	Maple syrup urine disease
Sweaty feet or ripe cheese	Isovaleric acidemia
Sweaty feet	Glutaric acidemia type II
Cat urine	3-Methylcrotonyl-CoA carboxylase deficiency
Cat urine	Multiple carboxylase deficiency
Hair abnormalities	
Alopecia	Multiple carboxylase deficiency
Kinky hair	Kinky hair disease
	Argininosuccinic aciduria
	Multiple carboxylase deficiency
	Giant axonal neuropathy
	Trichothiodystrophy (Pollitt syndrome; mental retardation, seizures)
Unusual facies	
Coarse	Mucopolysaccharidoses (Hunter-Hurler syndrome)
	I-cell disease (mucolipidosis II)
	GM, gangliosidosis (infantile)
	Sanfilippo syndrome
Slight coarsening (difficult to notice without comparing other family members)	Mucolipidosis III (pseudo-Hurler dystrophy)
	Fucosidosis II
	Mannosidosis
	Sialidosis II
	Aspartylglucosaminuria
High nasal bridge, prominent jaw, large pinnae	Congenital disorders of glycosylation
Ocular abnormalities	
Cataracts	Galactosemia
	Cerebrotendinous xanthomatosis
	Homocystinuria
Corneal clouding	Hurler syndrome
	Hunter syndrome (late in severe cases)
	Morquio syndrome
	Maroteaux-Lamy syndrome
Cherry-red spot	Tay-Sachs, Sandhoff diseases (GM_2 gangliosidosis)
	GM_1 gangliosidosis (infantile)
	Niemann-Pick disease (types A and C)
	Infantile Gaucher disease (type II)
	Sialidosis

TABLE 1.4 Abnormal Brain Development in Inborn Errors of Metabolism

Inborn Error of Metabolism	*Neural Tube Defect*	*Holoprosencephaly*	*Cerebellar Malformations*	*Hypoplastic Temporal Lobes*	*Migration Disorders*	*Dysgenetic Corpus Callosum*
Respiratory chain defect			+		±	±
Glutaric acidemia II			+	+	+	+
MTHFR deficiency	?					
Glutaric aciduria I				+		
Smith-Lemli-Opitz		+			+	+
CDG 1a			+			+
Menkes disease			+		+	+
Zellweger syndrome					+	+
Infantile Refsum					+	+
Bifunctional enzyme deficiency					+	
Pyruvate dehydrogenase deficiency					+	+
Fumarase deficiency					+	+
CPT 2 deficiency					+	
Nonketotic hyperglycinemia					+	+
3-Hydroxyisobutyric aciduria						+

MTHFR, methylene tetrahydrofoiate reductase; CDG, congenital disorders of glycosylation; CPT, carnitine palmitoyl transferase.

Adapted from Nissenkorn A, Michaelson M, Ben-Zeev B, et al. Inborn errors of metabolism: a cause of abnormal brain development. *Neurology* 2000;56:1265–1272. With permission of the authors.

the face of an elevated lactate points to a disorder of pyruvate metabolism, whereas an elevated lactate/pyruvate ratio suggests a defect in nicotinamide adenine dinucleotide (NADH) oxidation, such as occurs in genetic defects of the mitochondrial electron transport chain. Measurements of lactate and pyruvate are prone to errors due to poor venipuncture technique and delayed sample handling, and lactate/pyruvate ratios should therefore be interpreted with caution. As a rule, measurements of arterial blood or CSF lactate and pyruvate are more reliable. In some mitochondrial disorders elevation of lactate cannot be documented from assays of body fluids but only by finding an elevation of lactate in brain by magnetic resonance spectroscopy (MRS).

Determination of fasting blood sugar is also indicated as part of a metabolic workup. Should the suspicion for a metabolic disorder be high, any of these assays should be repeated when the child is ill with an intercurrent illness. For many disorders this is a safer approach than challenging the child with a protein or carbohydrate load. Other biochemical analyses required in the evaluation of a patient with a suspected metabolic defect include serum and urine uric acid, serum cholesterol, serum carnitine levels (including total, acyl, and free carnitine), immunoglobulins, thyroxine (T4), triiodothyronine (T3), serum copper, ceruloplasmin, magnesium, transferrin isoelectric focusing, and CSF glucose, protein, lactate, and amino acids. The assay of very long chain fatty acids is helpful in the diagnoses of adrenoleukodystrophy and other peroxisomal disorders.

Radiography

Radiographic examination of the vertebrae and long bones is helpful in the diagnosis of mucopolysaccharidoses, Gaucher diseases, Niemann-Pick diseases, and G_{M1} gangliosidosis. Neuroimaging studies, including magnetic resonance imaging (MRI), have been less helpful in pointing to any inborn metabolic error. Abnormalities such as agenesis of the corpus callosum and a large operculum seen in a few of the conditions covered in this chapter are nonspecific. The diagnostic yield of MRI is much higher in a child with mental retardation with or without seizures. As a rule, the more severe the mental retardation, the higher is the yield. Computed tomographic (CT) scanning contributes to the diagnosis of developmental delay in about 30% of children, whereas MRI shows a significant abnormality in 48% to 65% of patients presenting with global developmental delay (10). As is noted in Chapter 3 in the section entitled Diseases with Degeneration Primarily Affecting White Matter, MRI is also useful in the diagnosis of the various leukodystrophies. MRS is finding utility in diagnosing mitochondrial disorders and disorders of creatine synthesis.

TABLE 1.5 Inherited Metabolic Diseases Best Diagnosed from Analysis of Cerebrospinal Fluid

Disorder	Relevant CSF Assay
Glucose transport protein	Ratio of CSF/blood glucose
Mitochondrial encephalopathies	Lactate, pyruvate
Nonketotic hyperglycinemia	Ratio of CSF/plasma glycine
Serine synthesis defect	Amino acids
Defects in pathways of biogenic monoamines	Biogenic amines and metabolites
GTP cyclohydrolase deficiency	Biogenic amines and pterins
Cerebral dihydropteridine reductase deficiency	Biogenic amines and pterins
GABA transaminase deficiency	GABA
Defect of folate transport protein	5-Methyl tetrahydrofolate
Aromatic L-amino acid decarboxylase deficiency	Dopa, 5-HTP, HVA, HIAA

CSF, cerebrospinal fluid; GABA, gamma-aminobutyric acid; 5-HTP, 5-hydroxytryptophan; HVA, homovanillic acid; HIAA, hydroxyindoleaatic acid.

Adapted from Hoffmann GF, Surtees RAH, Weavers RA. Investigations of cerebrospinal fluid for neurometabolic disorders. *Neuropediatrics* 1998;29:59–71.

Serum Lysosomal Enzyme Screen

Should the clinical presentation suggest a lysosomal disorder, a leukocyte lysosomal enzyme screen should be performed. In particular, assays for α-galactosidase, arylsulfatase, and the hexosaminidases can be run accurately in a number of centers. Occasionally, healthy individuals have been found with marked deficiency in one or another of the lysosomal enzymes. This "pseudodeficiency" is due to a mutation that alters the ability of the enzyme to degrade the artificial substrate used for the enzyme assay but does not impair enzymatic activity toward the natural substrate.

Cerebrospinal Fluid Analyses

In addition to the mitochondrial disorders, several other inherited metabolic diseases require analyses of cerebrospinal fluid for diagnosis. These are listed in Table 1.5.

Structural and Biochemical Alterations

In a number of metabolic disorders, notably the lipidoses and white matter degenerations, diagnosis requires clinical evaluation and combined microscopic, ultrastructural, and biochemical studies on biopsied tissue. In the past, a brain biopsy was required for this purpose, but neuroimaging studies have made this procedure unnecessary in almost all instances. It has become clear that, if adequately sought for structural and biochemical alterations can be detected outside the central nervous system (CNS) in almost every leukodystrophy or lipidosis. Table 1.6 shows what diseases (discussed in this chapter and Chapter 3) are likely to be diagnosed by examination of various tissues.

TABLE 1.6 Common Diseases Diagnosed by Study of Tissues

Tissue Studied	Disease
Peripheral nerve	Metachromatic leukodystrophy
	Globoid cell leukodystrophy
	Infantile neuroaxonal dystrophy
	Fabry disease
	Refsum disease
	Tangier disease
Skin, conjunctivae, lymphocytes	Most lipidoses, particularly late infantile and juvenile neuronal ceroid lipofuscinosis
	Lafora disease
	Neuroaxonal dystrophy[a]
	Mucolipidosis
	Sanfilippo syndromes
	Fabry disease
Muscle	Late infantile and juvenile neuronal ceroid lipofuscinosis
	Familial myoclonus epilepsy
	Mitochondrial disorders
Bone marrow	Lysosomal storage diseases
	Niemann-Pick diseases
	Gaucher diseases
	G_{M1} gangliosidosis
	Mucopolysaccharidoses
	Mucolipidoses
Liver	Glycogen storage diseases
	Fructose 1,6-diphosphatase deficiency
	Nonketotic hyperglycinemia
	Lysinuric protein intolerance
	Primary hyperoxaluria type 1 (alanine-glyoxylate amino transferase deficiency)
	Wilson disease
	Menkes disease
	Niemann-Pick diseases

[a]When storage is confined to nerve fibers (e.g., neuroaxonal dystrophy), conjunctival biopsy is not diagnostic.

At this time, rectal biopsy and biopsies of other tissues such as kidney or tonsils are indicated only rarely. A liver biopsy is occasionally required to verify the actual enzymatic defect and is used to measure copper content in the diagnosis of Wilson disease, Menkes disease, and their variants. A conjunctival biopsy can be performed under local anesthetic and can be useful for excluding a lysosomal storage disease. When tissue biopsy suggests a specific metabolic disorder, highly sophisticated enzyme assays are required to confirm the diagnosis. Web sites that direct physicians to the various clinics that perform a given genetic test are maintained at http://www.genetests.org/ and http://biochemgen.ucsd.edu.

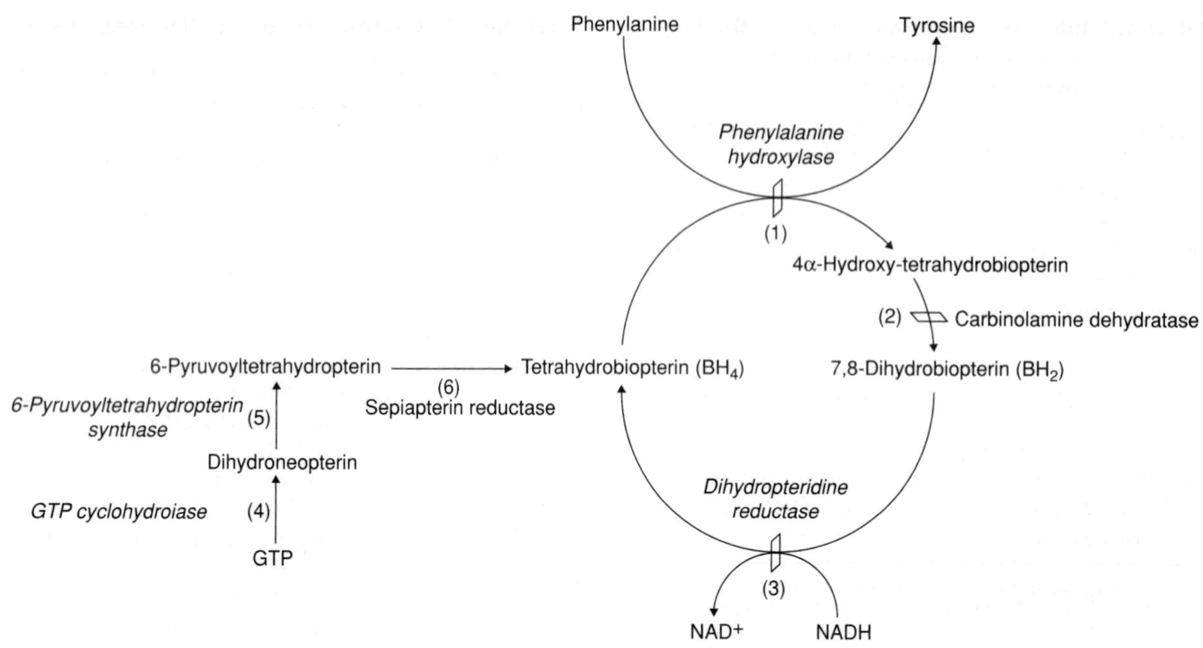

FIGURE 1.1. Phenylalanine metabolism. Phenylalanine is converted to tyrosine by the holoenzyme, phenylalanine hydroxylase (PAH). Phenylalanine hydroxylase requires tetrahydrobiopterin (BH4) as an active cofactor. BH4 is recycled by the sequential actions of (2) carbinolamine dehydratase and (3) dihydropteridine reductase. BH4 is synthesized *in vivo* from guanosine triphosphate (GTP) by a series of steps that involve (4) GTP cyclohydrolase and (5) 6-pyruvoyltetrahydropteridin (6-PT) synthase and (6) sepiatpterin reductase. Genetic defects in all these steps can result in hyperphenylalaninemia. A defect in GTP cyclohydrolase is seen also in dopa-responsive dystonia (see Chapter 3). (From Wilcox WR, Cedarbaum S. Amino acid metabolism. In: Rimoin DL, Connor JM, Pyeritz RE, et al., eds. *Principles and practice of medical genetics*, 4th ed. New York: Churchill Livingstone, 2002;2405–2440.)

DISORDERS OF AMINO ACID METABOLISM

Phenylketonuria (Online Mendelian Inheritance in Man [OMIM] Database, Number 261600)

Phenylketonuria (PKU) has long been the prototype for an inborn metabolic error that produces serious neurologic symptoms. We will therefore consider it in more detail than its frequency would warrant. Fölling, in 1934, first called attention to the condition in a report of 10 mentally defective patients who excreted large amounts of phenylpyruvic acid (12). The disease has since been found in all parts of the world, although it is rare in blacks and Ashkenazi Jews. Its incidence in the general population of the United States, as determined by screening programs, is approximately 1 in 14,000 (13).

Molecular Genetics and Biochemical Pathology

Phenylketonuria is an autosomal recessive disorder that results from a mutation in the gene that codes for phenylalanine hydroxylase (PAH), the enzyme that hydroxylates phenylalanine to tyrosine. The complete hydroxylation system consists in part of PAH, a PAH stabilizer, the tetrahydrobiopterin cofactor (BH4), dihydropteridine reductase (DHPR), which is required to recycle BH4, and a BH4-synthesizing system. This system involves guanosine triphosphate (GTP) cyclohydrolase and 6-pyruvoyl tetrahydropteridine synthetase (Fig. 1.1) (14).

PAH is normally found in liver, kidney, and pancreas but not in brain or skin fibroblasts. The enzyme is an iron-containing metalloprotein dimer of identical subunits with a molecular weight of approximately 100,000. The gene coding for the enzyme has been cloned and localized to the long arm of chromosome 12 (12q22–q24). The gene is approximately 90 kilobases (kb) long with 13 exons, and codes for a mature RNA of approximately 2,400 bases. Availability of this clone has facilitated the molecular genetic analysis of patients with PKU and has confirmed that PKU is the consequence of numerous mutant alleles arising in various ethnic groups. The majority of these mutations result in deficient enzyme activity and cause hyperphenylalaninemia. Mutations occur in all 13 exons of the gene and flanking sequence. Some cause phenylketonuria; others cause non-PKU hyperphenylalaninemia, whereas still others are silent polymorphisms present on both normal and mutant chromosomes (15,16). Some PAH alleles are more prevalent; five account for approximately 60% of European mutations and they tend to cluster in regions or are on only one of a few haplotypes. More than 495 mutations have been recorded. They are catalogued at http://www.pahdb.mcgill.ca.

Most mutations are missense mutations, although splice, nonsense, and silent mutations as well as single-base-pair frameshifts and larger deletions and insertions have been found. Most patients with PKU are compound heterozygotes rather than homozygotes in the precise meaning of the term (17). As a rule, the biochemical phenotype (i.e., the degree of phenylalanine elevation) does not correlate with the activity of PAH as predicted from the genetic mutation. In addition, no good correlation exists between PAH activity and intellectual function of untreated patients (18). Scriver (3,5) and others have pointed out that various environmental factors and modifying genes, such as the blood–brain barrier phenylalanine transporters, and variations in brain phenylalanine consumption rate may affect intellectual function in phenylketonuric patients (19,20).

The infant with classic PKU is born with only slightly elevated phenylalanine blood levels, but because of the absence of PAH activity, the amino acid derived from food proteins and postnatal catabolism accumulates in serum, CSF, and brain and is excreted in large quantities. In lieu of the normal degradative pathway, phenylalanine is converted to phenylpyruvic acid, phenylacetic acid, and phenylacetylglutamine.

The transamination of phenylalanine to phenylpyruvic acid is sometimes deficient for the first few days of life, and the age at which phenylpyruvic acid can be first detected varies from 2 to 34 days. From the first week of life, *o*-hydroxyphenylacetic acid also is excreted in large amounts.

In addition to the disruption of phenylalanine metabolism, tryptophan and tyrosine are handled abnormally. Normally, transport across the blood–brain barrier of a large neutral amino acid such as phenylalanine is determined by its plasma concentration and its affinity to the stereo-specific L-type amino acid carrier system (20). Supraphysiologic levels of phenylalanine competitively inhibit transport of tryptophan and tyrosine across the blood–brain barrier (21). Intestinal transport of L-tryptophan and tyrosine is also impaired in PKU, and fecal content of tryptophan and tyrosine is increased. These abnormalities are reversed by dietary correction of the plasma phenylalanine levels (22). Miyamoto and Fitzpatrick suggested that a similar interference might occur in the oxidation of tyrosine to 3-(3,4-dihydroxyphenyl) alanine (dopa), a melanin precursor, and might be responsible for the deficiency of hair and skin pigment in phenylketonuric individuals (23). The biochemical pathology of PKU is reviewed to a greater extent by Scriver and Kaufman (14).

Pathologic Anatomy

Alterations within the brain are nonspecific and diffuse. They involve gray and white matter, and they probably progress with age. Three types of alterations exist.

Interference with the Normal Maturation of the Brain

Brain growth is reduced, and microscopic examination shows impaired cortical layering, delayed outward migration of neuroblasts, and heterotopic gray matter (24). Additionally, the amount of Nissl granules is markedly deficient. This is particularly evident in those areas of the brain that are not fully developed at birth. Dendritic arborization and the number of synaptic spikes are reduced within the cortex (25). These changes point to a period of abnormal brain development extending from the last trimester of gestation into postnatal life (Fig. 1.2).

Defective Myelination

Defective myelination may be generalized or limited to areas where one would expect postnatal myelin deposition. Except for adult patients with PKU with neurologic deterioration, products of myelin degeneration are unusual (26). Myelin is usually relatively pale, and a mild degree of gliosis (Fig. 1.3) and irregular areas of vacuolation (status spongiosus) can be present. Areas of vacuolation usually are seen in central white matter of the cerebral hemispheres and in the cerebellum.

Diminished or Absent Pigmentation of the Substantia Nigra and Locus Ceruleus

Because substantia nigra and locus ceruleus are normally pigmented in albinos and tyrosinase activity cannot be demonstrated in normal neurons within the substantia nigra, diminished or absent pigmentation is not a result of tyrosinase inhibition by phenylalanine or its derivatives (27). Instead, neuromelanogenesis in the phenylketonuric patient must be interrupted at some other metabolic point, such as the metal-catalyzed pseudoperoxidation of dopamine derivatives probably responsible for the melanization of lipofuscin in the substantia nigra (26).

Clinical Manifestations

Phenylketonuric infants appear healthy at birth. In untreated infants, vomiting, which at times is projectile, and irritability are frequent during the first 2 months of life. By 4 to 9 months, delayed intellectual development becomes apparent (28). In the untreated classic case, mental retardation is severe, precluding speech and toilet training. Children in this category have an IQ below 50. Seizures, common in the more severely retarded, usually start before 18 months of age and can cease spontaneously. During

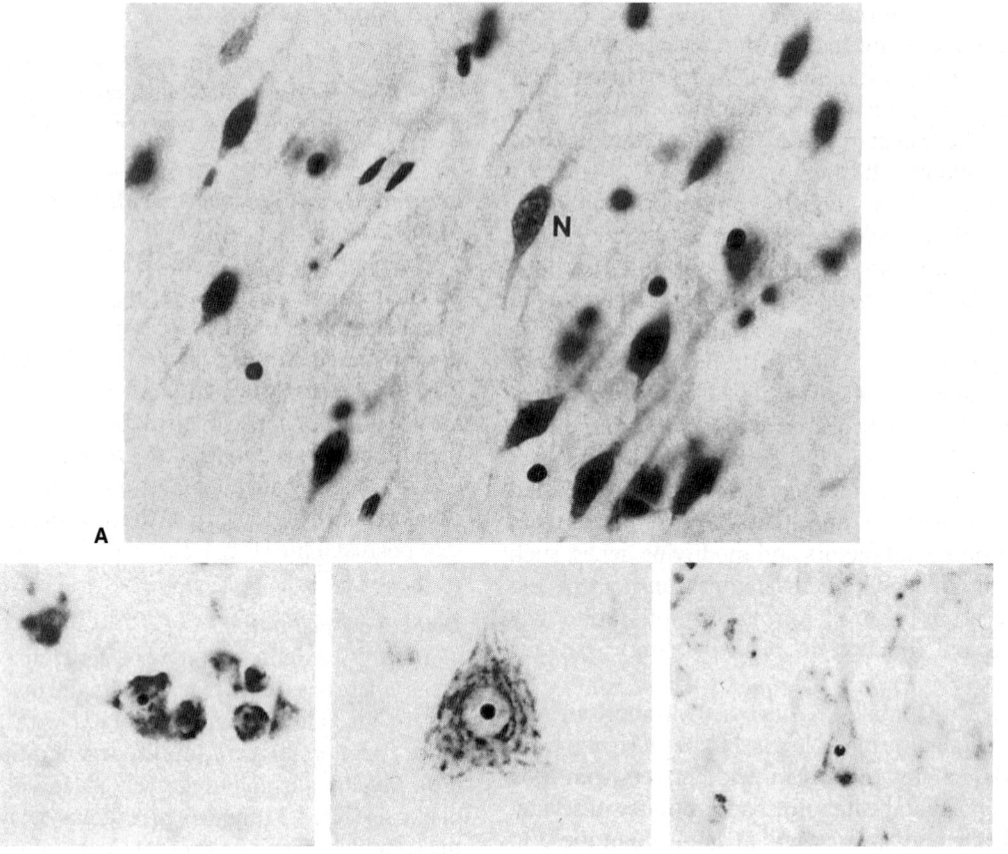

FIGURE 1.2. Phenylketonuria. **A:** Cresyl-violet-stained section showing spindle-shaped immature neuron (*N*) (×350). (Courtesy of Dr. Nathan Malamud, Langley Porter Neuropsychiatric Institute, San Francisco, CA.) **B:** Photomicrograph of Nissl-stained giant Betz cell from a healthy 4-month-old child. **C:** Photomicrograph of Nissl-stained Betz cells from a healthy 14-year-old child. **D:** Photomicrograph of Nissl-stained Betz cell from a 19-year-old with untreated phenylketonuria. Patient's developmental level was 4.6 months at age 5 years and 10 months; he was microcephalic and had seizures commencing at 10 years of age. Note that the Betz cells are reduced in size, with a pale cytoplasm and few well-formed Nissl granules. These cytoarchitectural abnormalities are nonspecific. (**B, C,** and **D** from Bauman ML, Kemper TL. Morphologic and histoanatomic observations of the brain in untreated human phenylketonuria. *Acta Neuropathol* 1982;58:55–63. With permission.)

infancy, they often take the form of infantile spasms, later changing into tonic-clonic attacks.

The untreated phenylketonuric child is blond and blue-eyed, with normal and often pleasant features. The skin is rough and dry, sometimes with eczema. A peculiar musty odor, attributable to phenylacetic acid, can suggest the diagnosis. Significant neurologic abnormalities are rare, although hyperactivity and autistic features are not unusual. Microcephaly may be present as well as a mild increase in muscle tone, particularly in the lower extremities. A fine, irregular tremor of the outstretched hands is seen in approximately 30% of the patients. Parkinsonian-like extrapyramidal symptoms also have been encountered (29). The plantar response is often extensor.

A variety of electroencephalographic (EEG) abnormalities has been found, but hypsarrhythmic patterns, recorded even in the absence of seizures, and single and multiple foci of spike and polyspike discharges are the most common (30).

MRI is abnormal in almost every patient, regardless of when treatment was initiated. On T2-weighted imaging, one sees increased signal in the periventricular and subcortical white matter of the posterior hemispheres. Increased signal can extend to involve the deep white matter of the posterior hemispheres and the anterior hemispheres. No signal abnormalities are seen in brainstem, cerebellum, or cortex, although cortical atrophy may be present (Fig. 1.4) (31,32). The severity of the abnormality is unrelated to the patient's IQ but is significantly associated with the phenylalanine level at the time of imaging. In adult patients with PKU who had come off their diets, resumption of dietary treatment can improve MRI abnormalities within

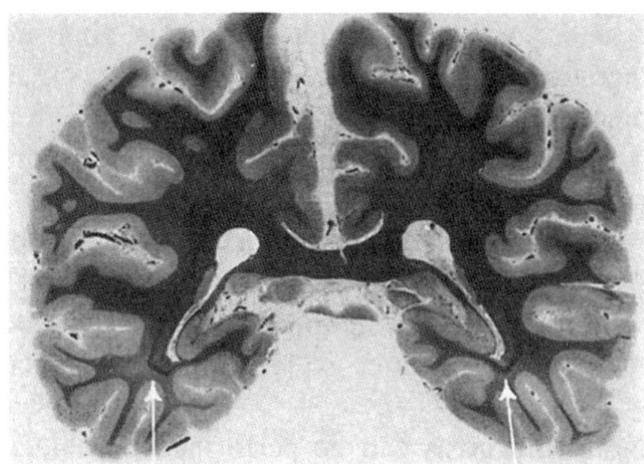

FIGURE 1.3. Phenylketonuria. Cerebrum of a 35-year-old man stained for myelin by the Loyez method. The individual was never treated. He sat at 1 year and walked at 3 years. He was microcephalic and spastic and never developed speech. Death was caused by pulmonary tuberculosis and dehydration. The visual radiations (*arrows*) stand out against the background of persisting pallor of the association tracts and nonspecific thalamic radiations. In a healthy brain of that age, the visual radiations are not distinguishable by tonality of staining from the completely myelinated white matter. (From Bauman ML, Kemper TL. Morphologic and histoanatomic observations of the brain in untreated human phenylketonuria. *Acta Neuropathol* 1982;58:55–63. With permission.)

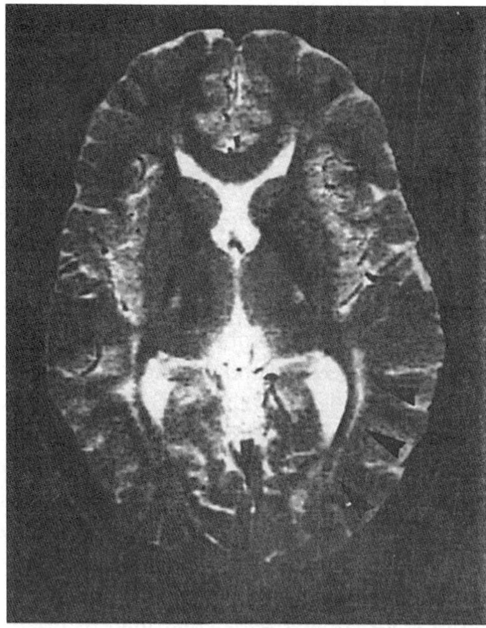

FIGURE 1.4. T2-weighted magnetic resonance imaging of a 16-year-old girl with phenylketonuria. The girl was treated from early infancy, and the diet was stopped at 12 years of age. At the time of the scan, her neurologic examination was normal, but her phenylalanine level was 27.0 mg/dL (1,639 μmol/L). The scan shows areas of high signal, particularly in the parieto-occipital areas, but also at the tips of the anterior horns of the lateral ventricles. (Courtesy of Dr. Alan J. Thompson, Neurorehabilitation Section, Institute of Neurology, University of London.)

a few weeks or months, an observation that strongly suggests that at least some of the MRI changes are the result of edema (32).

Heterozygous mothers tend to have elevated plasma phenylalanine levels and somewhat reduced tyrosine values during the latter part of pregnancy and after delivery. Mothers suffering from PKU have a high incidence of spontaneous abortions. It is now clear that when maternal blood phenylalanine levels are greater than 20 mg/dL (1,212 μmol/L) during pregnancy, fetal brain damage is almost inevitable, with mental retardation encountered in 92% of offspring and microcephaly in 73%. Offspring have an unusual facies: upturned nose, underdeveloped philtrum, and a thin upper lip (33). Additionally, a significant incidence of congenital heart disease and prenatal and postnatal growth retardation occurs (34). MRI in these children shows hypoplasia or partial agenesis of the corpus callosum and delayed myelination (35). These observations are best explained by a deleterious effect of elevated phenylalanine on the myelinating ability of oligodendrocytes.

Much, if not all, of the fetal damage appears to be preventable by placing phenylketonuric mothers on a phenylalanine-restricted diet before conception and maintaining blood phenylalanine levels below 6 mg/dL (360 μmol/L) throughout pregnancy (36). In the data compiled by Koch and coworkers the optimal outcome, as measured by the Wechsler Intelligence Scale for Children (WISC) score of offspring obtained at 7 years of age, was obtained when maternal blood phenylalanine levels of 120 to 360 μmol/L (2 to 6 mg/dL) were obtained by 8 to 10 weeks' gestation and maintained at those levels throughout pregnancy. However, there was considerable scatter in IQ even when the phenylalanine levels were maintained below 5 mg/dL (37). Birth weight and head circumference in infants of mothers so managed were normal, and no evidence existed for fetal nutritional deficiency. Offspring of mothers who experience mild PKU as defined by phenylalanine levels of less than 400 μmol/L (6.6 mg/dL) appear to be normal, and mothers do not require dietary intervention (38).

The pathogenesis of mental retardation in PKU is not completely understood (39). No evidence exists that phenylpyruvic acid or any of the other phenylalanine metabolites are neurotoxic at concentrations in which they are seen in PKU (40). Probably no single factor is responsible; instead, impairment of amino acid transport across the blood–brain barrier; disruption of the brain amino acid pool; with consequent defective proteolipid protein synthesis, impaired myelination, and low levels of neurotransmitters, such as serotonin, are responsible to varying degrees (41,42).

Diagnosis

With the worldwide practice of neonatal screening for phenylketonuria, the diagnosis is usually made during the first week of life, and it is now rare to encounter an older infant or child with undiagnosed PKU. As mentioned in the section on Molecular Genetics and Biochemical Pathology, plasma phenylalanine levels are elevated in the cord blood of phenylketonuric infants and increase rapidly within a few hours of birth. A screening program that involves spectrofluorometric or microbiologic estimation of blood phenylalanine is used commonly. Tandem mass spectrometric analysis of phenylalanine and other amino acids as well as of the acylcarnitines of the various organic acids is being used in some laboratories (43), and trials of this method for newborn screening are being instituted in several states. Whatever the method, the screening test requires a drop of whole blood placed on a filter paper. If the test is positive [a value greater than 2 to 4 mg/dL (120 to 240 μmol/L)], the diagnosis is confirmed by quantitative analysis of phenylalanine and tyrosine in blood. Although most infants whose blood phenylalanine levels are above the threshold value do not have PKU, such patients require prompt reevaluation by an appropriate laboratory to determine whether hyperphenylalaninemia is persistent and whether it is caused by PAH deficiency.

Of considerably greater concern are the false-negative test results. It is now clear that routine screening tests, when correctly performed after 12 hours of life, detect all infants with classic PKU. In a group of such infants studied by Koch and Friedman the lowest phenylalanine value recorded at 24 hours was 5.6 mg/dL (339 μmol/L); at 48 hours, 7.5 mg/dL (454 μmol/L); and at 72 hours, 8.4 mg/dL (509 μmol/L). Thus, even at 24 hours, none of the infants with classic PKU would have escaped detection (44). The Canadian experience of Hanley and coworkers is similar (45). As a rule, breast-fed PKU infants have higher phenylalanine levels than those who are formula fed. In some infants with mild hyperphenylalaninemia, the increase in blood phenylalanine is sufficiently slow to allow them to escape detection unless an assay is used, such as tandem mass spectroscopy, that can measure both phenylalanine and tyrosine, which decreases false-positive results. Some screening agencies obtain a second screening blood specimen from all infants whose first blood specimen was drawn during the first 24 hours of life (46,47).

Most infants with elevated blood phenylalanine detected by means of the newborn screening program do not have classic PKU; instead they have a transient or mild form of hyperphenylalaninemia that is usually benign. Patients with mild PKU have phenylalanine levels between 600 and 1200 μmol/L (10 to 20 mg/dL) on an unrestricted diet, and patients with mild hyperphenylalaninemia have levels below 600 μmol/L (10 mg/dl) on an unrestricted diet (48). A large proportion of these patients represent compound heterozygotes for a mutation that abolishes catalytic activity of PAH and one that reduces it (16,49–51). With normal protein intakes, the majority of such infants appear to have unimpaired intelligence, even when untreated (48).

Elevated blood phenylalanine levels also are observed in 25% of premature infants and occasionally in full-term newborns. In all of these patients, tyrosine levels are increased to a much greater extent than are phenylalanine levels.

Prenatal diagnosis can be performed by detection of the specific mutations in PAH identified in the family or by genetic linkage analysis (52,53). Modifier genes have not been identified.

Treatment

Two treatment strategies could be employed in PKU: modification of the phenotypic expression of the defective gene and definitive treatment by correcting the gene defect. Only the first approach has been used in clinical practice.

On referral of an infant with a confirmed positive screening test result, the first step is quantitative determination of serum phenylalanine and tyrosine levels. All infants whose blood phenylalanine concentration is greater than 10 mg/dL (600 μmol/L) and whose tyrosine concentration is low or normal (1 to 4 mg/dL) should be started on a low-phenylalanine diet immediately. Infants whose blood phenylalanine concentrations remain below 10 mg/dL (600 μmol/L) on an unrestricted diet are generally considered not to require a diet (54).

The accepted therapy for classic PKU is restriction of the dietary intake of phenylalanine by placing the infant on one of several low-phenylalanine formulas. The diet should be managed by a team consisting of a nutritionist, a physician with expertise in metabolic disorders, and a person to ensure dietary compliance. To avoid symptoms of phenylalanine deficiency, regular formula is added to the diet in amounts sufficient to maintain blood levels of the amino acid between 2 and 6 mg/dL (120 and 360 μmol/L). Generally, patients tolerate this diet quite well, and within 1 to 2 weeks, the serum concentration of phenylalanine becomes normal. Serum phenylalanine determinations are essential to ensure adequate regulation of diet. These are performed twice weekly during the first 6 months of life and twice monthly thereafter.

Strict dietary control should be maintained for as long as possible, and most centers strive to keep levels below 6.0 mg/dL (360 μmol/L), even in patients with moderate and mild PKU. Samples of low-phenylalanine menus are given by Buist and colleagues (55), and the nutritional problems inherent in prolonged use of a restricted diet are discussed by Acosta and colleagues (56). Dietary lapses are common, particularly in patients 15 years or older (57). They frequently are accompanied by progressive white matter abnormalities on MRI. Some workers have suggested supplementation of the low-phenylalanine diet with tyrosine, but no statistical evidence exists that this regimen results in a better intellectual outcome. This possibly could be due to failure to achieve adequate tyrosine levels in the brain even with tyrosine supplementation of 300 mg/kg (58). Failure to treat patients with mild hyperphenylalaninemias does not appear to produce either intellectual deficits or MRI abnormalities.

Patients with mild PKU or mild hyperphenylalaninemia have been treated successfully with tetrahydrobiopterin (BH4; 10 to 20 mg/kg per day) (59,59a). Most of these individuals have at least one missense mutation in the gene for phenylalanine hydroxylase, leading to some residual enzyme activity (60). The mechanism for this effect is unknown, as is the question of how to best select patients responsive to the cofactor. BH4 is being tested, but it is not yet approved for therapy in the United States.

Dietary therapy has for the greater part been effective in preventing mental retardation in patients with severe PKU. It has become apparent that the outcome depends on several factors. Most important is the age at which the diet was initiated. Smith and coworkers found that patients' IQ fell approximately 4 points for each month between birth and start of treatment (61). The average phenylalanine concentration while receiving treatment also affects outcome, with optimal average phenylalanine levels in the most recent cohorts being 5.0 to 6.6 mg/dL (300 to 400 μmol/L). Additionally, hypophenylalaninemia during the first 2 years of life [i.e., the length of time that phenylalanine concentration was below 2.0 mg/dL (120 μmol/L)] also affected outcome adversely. Even patients with normal IQ scores and with the most favorable diagnostic and treatment characteristics have lower IQs than other members of their families and suffer from cognitive deficits, educational difficulties, and behavioral problems, notably hyperactivity (61–63). As was already noted, dietary supplementation with tyrosine, although used in several centers, does not appear to improve performance on neuropsychologic tests (64). The most likely explanations for these deficits are inadequate dietary control and unavoidable prenatal brain damage from elevated phenylalanine (see Fig. 1.2) (24).

When patients who already have developed symptoms caused by classic PKU are placed and maintained on a low-phenylalanine diet, the epilepsy comes under control and their EEGs normalize. Microcephaly, if present, can correct itself, and abnormally blond hair regains its natural color.

Considerable uncertainty exists about when, if ever, to terminate the diet (65). In the series of Waisbren and coworkers (66), one-third of youngsters whose diet was discontinued at 5 years of age had a reduction in IQ of 10 points or more during the ensuing 5 years. The blood phenylalanine level when the children were off the restrictive diet predicted the change in IQ. Of the children whose IQs dropped 20 or more points, 90% had blood phenylalanine levels of 18 mg/dL (1,090 μmol/L) or higher, and 40% of those whose IQs rose 10 points or more had a phenylalanine level of less than 18 mg/dL (1,090 μmol/L). In young adult patients with PKU, discontinuation of the diet was accompanied by progressive spasticity and worsening white matter abnormalities (67). Reinstitution of the diet results in clear clinical improvement and resolution of new MRI abnormalities. Reports such as these speak against early relaxation of the restrictions on phenylalanine intake and indicate that dietary therapy for patients with classical PKU should be life-long (68,69).

The relative inadequacies of dietary therapy underscore the need for a more definitive approach to the treatment of PKU. Allogeneic or autologous bone marrow transplants are being used for the treatment of a variety of genetic diseases (Table 1.7). The likelihood that this procedure will cure or at least stabilize a genetic disease depends on the tissue-specific expression of the normal gene product, the patient's clinical symptoms, and the cellular transport of the normal gene product. In PKU, the defective enzyme is not normally expressed in bone marrow–derived cells, and bone marrow transplantation has no therapeutic value (see Table 1.7).

Another approach to treating the patient with PKU is the introduction of PAH gene into affected hepatic cells. Recombinant viruses containing human PAH have been introduced into mouse hepatoma cells, where they are able to continue expressing the human enzyme, lowering the phenylalanine level and normalizing coat color (70). The next step would be to find a virus that can infect human liver, maintain itself there without inducing damage to the organ, and allow the human gene to continue functioning in the new host. Ding and colleagues reviewed various approaches for nonviral gene transfer (71).

Other Conditions Characterized by Hyperphenylalaninemia

About 1% of infants with persistent hyperphenylalaninemia do not have PKU but lack adequate levels of BH4, the cofactor in the hydroxylation of phenylalanine to tyrosine. This can be due to a defect in BH4 biosynthesis or to a deficiency of dihydropteridine reductase (DHPR), one of the enzymes involved in the regeneration of BH4. These conditions are depicted in Table 1.8.

Dihydropteridine Reductase Deficiency (OMIM 231630)

The first and most common of these conditions to be recognized is characterized by undetectable DHPR activity in liver, brain, and cultured fibroblasts but normal hepatic PAH activity (72). DHPR is responsible for the regeneration

TABLE 1.7 Some Neurogenetic Diseases that can be Treated with Bone Marrow Transplantation (BMT) or Enzyme Replacement Therapy (ERT)

Disease	*Results of Treatment*
Gaucher disease (adult form)	Correctable by BMT, ERT; generalized genetic defect, symptoms restricted to lymphohematopoietic cells
Adrenoleukodystrophy	Correctable in early stages by BMT
Metachromatic leukodystrophy	Adult form can be stabilized by BMT in early stages
Globoid cell leukodystrophy	BMT may stabilize late-onset, slowly progressive form; generalized genetic defect
Hurler disease	Visceral symptoms improve with BMT, ERT, neurologic symptoms stabilize
Hunter disease	Visceral symptoms improve with BMT, ERT, neurologic symptoms progress
Sanfilippo diseases	No effect of BMT or ERT
Phenylketonuria	Not correctable by BMT; lymphohematopoietic cells do not express normal gene product
Chédiak-Higashi syndrome	Correctable by BMT; expression of genetic defect restricted to lymphoid and hematopoietic cells
Pompe disease	Cardiomyopathy responds to ERT; response of skeletal muscle is variable
Maroteaux-Lamy (MPS VI)	Visceral symptoms treated by ERT, BMT

of BH4 from quinoid dihydrobiopterin (see Fig. 1.1). BH4 levels are low in blood, urine, CSF, and a number of tissues. Because BH4 is an essential coenzyme for hydroxylation of not only phenylalanine, but also tyrosine and tryptophan, affected children show a defect in the synthesis of dopamine, norepinephrine, epinephrine, and serotonin.

The clinical picture of DHPR deficiency is one of developmental delay associated with the evolution of marked hypotonia, involuntary movements, oculogyric crises, and tonic-clonic and myoclonic seizures. None of these symptoms resolve with restriction of phenylalanine intake (73,74). Progressive intracranial calcifications can be demonstrated by CT scanning. These might be the consequence of reduced intracranial tetrahydrofolate (75) because folate deficiency, whether it is caused by inadequate intake or defective absorption, can induce intracranial calcifications. MRI demonstrates white matter abnormalities and cystic loss of parenchyma (76).

TABLE 1.8 Disorders of Phenylalanine Metabolism—the Hyperphenylalaninemias

Disorder	*Enzyme Deficiency*	*Inheritance Pattern and Chromosomal Locus*	*Gene Cloned*	*Heterozygote Detection*[a]	*Prenatal Diagnosis*[a]
Phenylketonuria (classic and mild forms)	Phenylalanine hydroxylase	AR (12q22–q24)	Yes	Yes	Possible
Dihydropteridine reductase deficiency	Dihydropteridine reductase	AR (4p 15.3)	Yes	Yes	Yes
Carbinolamine dehydratase deficiency	Carbinolamine dehydratase	AR (10q22)	Yes	Possible	Possible
Biopterin synthesis deficiency	GTP-cyclohydrolase	AR (14q22)	Yes	Possible	Yes
Biopterin synthesis deficiency	6-Pyruvoyl-tetrahydropterin synthase	AR (11q22–q23)	Yes	Possible	Yes
Biopterin synthesis deficiency	Sepiapterin reductase	AR (2p14–p12)	Yes	Possible	Possible

[a] "Yes" for heterozygote detection or prenatal diagnosis means that testing is clinically available by enzyme analysis, metabolite testing, linkage analysis, or mutation detection. Heterozygote testing or prenatal diagnosis is "Possible" by mutation detection or linkage analysis when the gene has been cloned or the chromosomal location is known. Such testing may only be available in research laboratories, if at all.

AR, autosomal recessive.

From Wilcox WR, Cedarbaum S. Amino acid metabolism. In: Rimoin DL, Connor JM, Pyeritz RE, et al., eds. *Principles and practice of medical genetics,* 4th ed. New York: Churchill Livingstone, 2002;2405–2440. With permission.

Treatment for patients with DHPR deficiency requires restriction of phenylalanine intake and administration of catechol and serotonin precursors. The former is given as levodopa-carbidopa (Sinemet) and the latter as 5-hydroxytryptophan (8 to 10 mg/kg per day). Additionally, folinic acid (12.5 mg per day) is added to the diet (77). Treatment of the other variants is discussed by Shintaku (78).

6-Pyruvoyl-Tetrahydropterin (6-PT) Synthase Deficiency (OMIM 261640)

Increased phenylalanine levels can result from inadequate biopterin synthesis. In 6-pyruvoyl-tetrahydropterin (6-PT) synthase deficiency the defect is localized to the synthetic pathway of BH4 at the point of the formation of 6-PT (see Fig. 1.1). The enzyme deficiency can be complete, partial, or transient or might affect only nonneural tissue (73,79,80).

The clinical picture of this entity is much like that of DHPR deficiency: progressive neurologic deterioration highlighted by hypotonia, involuntary movements, and seizures. Diagnosis of this variant depends on normal assays for PAH and dihydropteridine reductase and on determination of urinary or CSF pterins (81). MRI in this disorder is similar to that seen in classical PKU (82).

GTP Cyclohydrolase Deficiency (OMIM 233910)

Another rare cause for persistent hyperphenylalaninemia is a defect of GTP-cyclohydrolase, needed for the first step of BH4 biosynthesis (see Fig. 1.1) (83,84). Symptoms include hypotonia, seizures, and hyperthermia. Mutations in GTP-cyclohydrolase are also responsible for dopa-responsive dystonia, a condition covered in Chapter 3 in the section on Primary Dystonia. Symptoms in this condition differ considerably from those seen in hyperphenylalaninemia. The best explanation for the phenotypic diversity is that the mutant enzyme has a dominant negative effect on the normal enzyme (85).

Sepiapterin Reductase Deficiency (OMIM 182125)

The clinical picture in this condition does not differ significantly from that of DHPR deficiency, namely dystonia, spasticity, and progressive mental retardation. Blood phenylalanine levels are normal, and the diagnosis depends on demonstrating elevated CSF sepiapterin, biopterin, and dihydrobiopterin levels (86,87).

Carbinol Dehydratase Deficiency (OMIM 126090)

Children with this condition present with mild hyperphenylalaninemia, and the diagnosis is made by finding elevated urinary 7-biopterin (88).

Tyrosinosis and Tyrosinemia

Several clinically and biochemically distinct disorders are characterized by an elevation in serum tyrosine and the excretion of large amounts of tyrosine and its metabolites (89). Their clinical and biochemical characteristics are outlined in Table 1.9.

TABLE 1.9 Clinical and Genetic Features of the Tyrosinemias

Condition	*Clinical Manifestations*	*Enzyme Defect*	*Reference*
Tyrosinemia type I	Acute episodes of weakness, pain, self-mutilation, porphyria-like axonopathic process; seizures and extensor hypertonia; hepatic necrosis, renal tubular damage; carrier rate 1 in 20 in French Canadian isolates	Fumarylacetoacetase	90,91
Tyrosinemia type II	Mental retardation, herpetiform corneal ulcers, palmoplantar keratoses	Tyrosine transaminase soluble form	92,93
Tyrosinemia type III	Mild mental retardation	HPPA oxidase	94–96
Tyrosinosis	Only one reported case, asymptomatic	?	97
Tyrosinemia of prematurity	No clinical abnormalities, follow-up suggests impaired visual-perceptual function	Inactivation of HPPA oxidase by its substrate	98,99
Hawkinsinuria	Metabolic acidosis, failure to thrive, dominant inheritance, unusual, swimming pool odor	Excretion of a cysteine or glutathione-conjugated intermediate in conversion of HPPA to homogentisic acid (Hawkinsin[a])	100

HPPA, 4-hydroxyphenyl pyruvic acid.
[a]The name *Hawkinsin* is derived from the family in whom the disease was first described (100a).

Maple Syrup Urine Disease (OMIM 248600)

Maple syrup urine disease (MSUD) is a familial cerebral degenerative disease caused by a defect in branched-chain amino acid metabolism and characterized by the passage of urine that has a sweet, maple syrup–like odor. It was first described in 1954 by Menkes and coworkers (101). Since then, numerous other cases have been diagnosed throughout the world, and its incidence is estimated at 1 in 220,000 births (102). In some inbred populations, such as the Mennonites, the incidence is as high as 1 in 176 births (103). The disease occurs in all races and is transmitted in an autosomal recessive manner.

Molecular Genetics and Biochemical Pathology

MSUD is characterized by the accumulation of three branched-chain ketoacids: α-ketoisocaproic acid, α-ketoisovaleric acid, and α-keto-β-methylvaleric acid, the derivatives of leucine, valine, and isoleucine, respectively (104,105). Their accumulation is the consequence of a defect in oxidative decarboxylation of branched-chain ketoacids (Fig. 1.5).

The branched-chain α-ketoacid dehydrogenase complex is located within the mitochondrial inner membrane matrix compartment. It is a multienzyme complex comprising six proteins: $E_{1\alpha}$ and $E_{1\beta}$. which form the decarboxylase; E_2; E_3; and a branched-chain–specific kinase and phosphatase. The last two enzymes regulate the activity of the complex by phosphorylating and dephosphorylating the dehydrogenase. E_1 is a thiamin pyrophosphate-dependent enzyme. The second enzyme (E_2), dihydrolipoyltransacylase, transfers the acyl group from the first enzyme to coenzyme A. The third enzyme (E_3), dihydrolipoyldehydrogenase, a flavoprotein, reoxidizes the disulfhydryl form of lipoamide. The same enzyme is common to other α-ketoacid dehydrogenases, such as pyruvate and α-ketoglutarate dehydrogenase (106). The complex removes carboxyl groups from all three branched-chain ketoacids and converts those ketoacids to their respective coenzyme A derivatives (see Fig. 1.5, step 2). Chuang and coworkers reviewed the crystal structure of the various enzyme components and the structural basis for the various MSUD mutations (103).

With six genes involved in the function of the branched-chain ketoacid dehydrogenase complex, considerable room for heterogeneity exists. Mutations in the genes for $E_{1\alpha}$, $E_{1\beta}$, E_2, and E_3 have been described, with many MSUD patients being compound heterozygotes. These induce a continuum of disease severity that ranges from the severe, classic form of MSUD to mild and intermittent forms.

As a consequence of the enzymatic defect, the branched-chain ketoacids accumulate in serum and CSF and are excreted in large quantities in urine (105). Plasma levels of the respective amino acids (e.g., leucine, isoleucine, and valine) are elevated secondary to the increase in ketoacid concentrations. Alloisoleucine, which is formed by transamination of α-keto-β-methylvaleric acid, also has been found in serum (107). In some cases, the branched-chain hydroxyacids, most prominently α-hydroxyisovaleric acid (108), are excreted also. Sotolone, a derivative of α–ketobutyric acid, the decarboxylation of which is impaired by accumulation of α-keto-β-methylvaleric acid, is responsible for the characteristic odor of the patient's urine and perspiration (109).

Pathologic Anatomy

Structural alterations in the nervous system in untreated infants with MSUD are similar to, but more severe than, those seen in PKU. In infants dying during the acute phase of the disease, diffuse edema occurs (101). The cytoarchitecture of the cortex is generally immature, with fewer cortical layers and the persistence of ectopic foci of neuroblasts, an indication of disturbed neuronal migration. Dendritic development is abnormal, and the number of oligodendrocytes and the amount of myelin are less than would be seen in a healthy brain of comparable age (110). Marked astrocytic gliosis and generalized cystic degeneration occur (111). Little clinical or pathologic evidence exists for demyelination in patients who are treated early (112,113). On chemical examination, the concentration of myelin lipids is markedly reduced, with cerebrosides, sulfatides, and proteolipid protein almost completely absent. These abnormalities are not found in infants dying of the disease within the first days of life or in patients treated by restriction of branched-chain amino acid intake (113).

Clinical Manifestations

Various mutations result in five fairly distinct clinical phenotypes of MSUD. Patients can be homozygotes for the same allele or compound heterozygotes for different alleles. The classic form of MSUD accounts for approximately 75% of patients (103). Mutations in the E_1 decarboxylase component of the enzyme are associated with this phenotype (114). In the original four patients reported by Menkes and coworkers (101) as well as in subsequent cases, dystonia, opisthotonos, intermittent increase in muscle tone, and respiratory irregularities appeared within the first week of life in babies apparently healthy at birth (115). Subsequently, rapid deterioration of the nervous system occurred, and all but one died within 1 month. In some patients, cerebral edema is marked and can be fatal (116). Other patients, spastic and intellectually retarded, survived without treatment for several years. A fluctuating ophthalmoplegia correlates in intensity with serum leucine levels (117). Presentation with pseudotumor cerebri also has

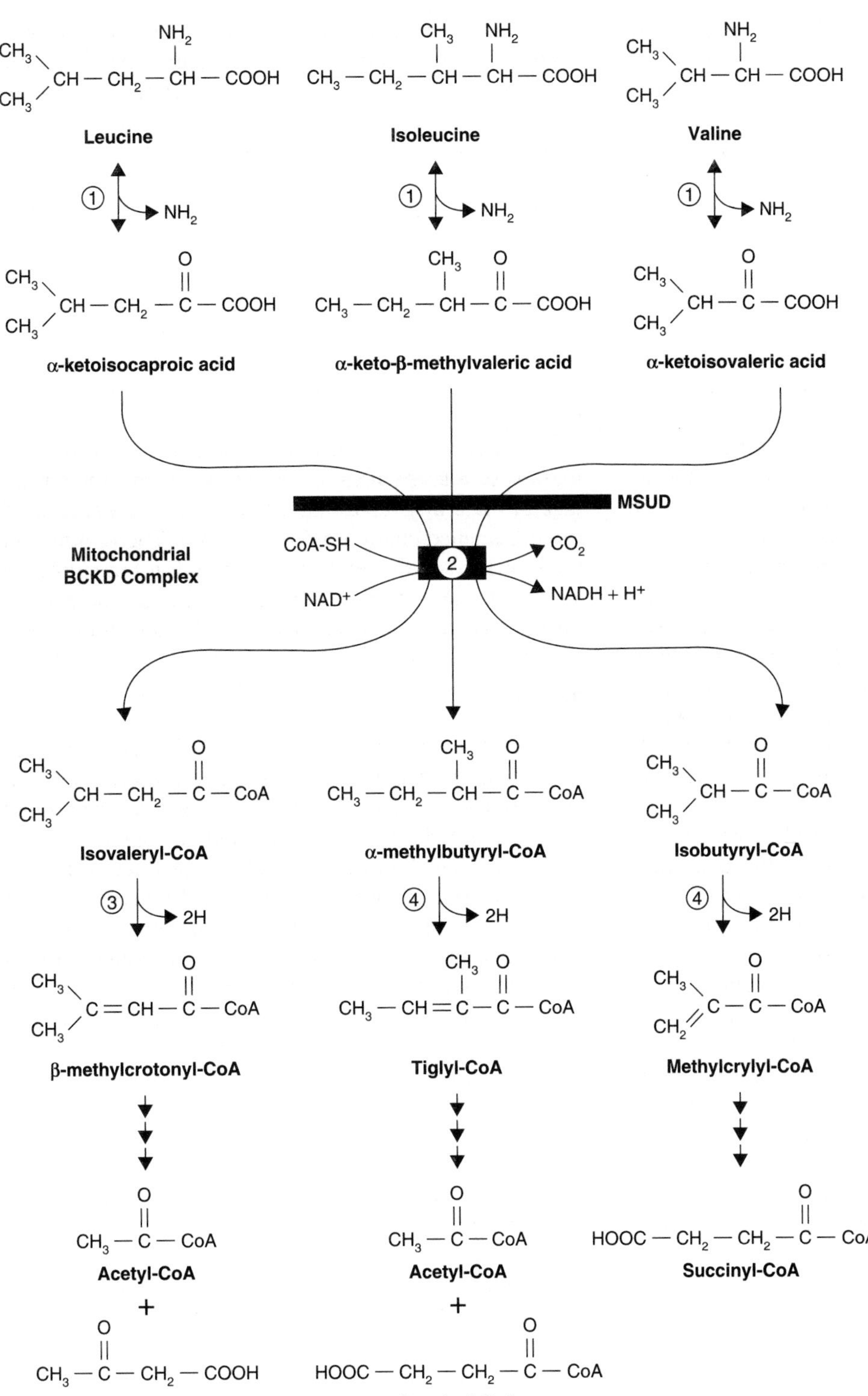

FIGURE 1.5. Degradation of leucine in mammalian tissues. In maple syrup urine disease, the metabolic block is located at step 2. In isovaleric acidemia, the block is confined to step 3. A rare entity with a possible metabolic block at step 4 also has been reported

been reported. Approximately 50% of patients with the classic form of MSUD develop severe hypoglycemia; this is probably the consequence of a defective gluconeogenesis from amino acids, particularly alanine (118).

MRI during the acute stage of the disease before treatment is characteristic. It demonstrates edema that is maximal in cerebellar deep white matter, the posterior portion of the brainstem, and the posterior limb of the internal capsule. Edema also is seen in the cortical U fibers, the head of the caudate, and the putamen (119,120). These findings are consistent with the location of status spongiosus noted on pathologic examination. The cause of the acute cerebral edema and its unique localization are unknown. Diffusion MRI suggests that in the myelinated areas of the brain there is an intramyelinic cytotoxic edema, whereas in the unmyelinated areas there is vasogenic interstitial edema (121,122). Because neurologic symptoms become apparent with relatively mild increases in plasma leucine concentrations, whereas there is little apparent toxicity associated with increased levels of isoleucine or valine, damage probably results from leucine accumulation or from accumulation of its ketoacid metabolite. As is the case in PKU, chronic brain damage is probably caused by interference with amino acid transport into the brain, a deranged amino acid environment, and, consequently, failure in biosynthesis of proteolipids, myelin, and neurotransmitters (123). In treated patients, the MRI discloses symmetric bilateral periventricular high signal intensity on T2-weighted images. This picture is similar to that seen in PKU and suggests focal dysmyelination (112).

The intermittent form of MSUD results from a variety of mutations in the gene for E_2, and branched-chain dehydrogenase activity is higher than in the classic form, usually 5% to 20% of normal (124). The clinical picture is that of intermittent periods of ataxia, drowsiness, behavior disturbances, and seizures that make their first appearance between ages 6 and 9 months. Attacks are generally triggered by infections, immunizations, or other forms of stress (125).

In the intermediate form, the clinical picture is one of mild to moderate mental retardation (126). Branched-chain dehydrogenase activity ranges from 5% to 20% of normal, and the defect is usually in the gene coding for E_1 (106).

A thiamin-responsive variant represents an entity in which, in some cases at least, a mutant exists in the gene for E_2 (103). Chuang and coworkers proposed that binding of the mutated, inactive E_2 component to the wild-type E_1 component enhances wild-type E_1 activity, and that the augmented E_1 activity is responsible for the response to thiamine (114).

Mutants defective in the gene for E_3 present with hypotonia, rapid neurologic deterioration, and severe lactic acidosis. This entity is discussed with the various other organic acidemias.

Diagnosis

The most common presentation of MSUD is that of a term infant who initially seems to be well for a few days and then deteriorates. The rate of deterioration varies, and most infants initially are believed to be septic. The neurologist called in to consult on such an infant should always consider the diagnosis of an inborn error of metabolism. Basic investigations at this point include blood or plasma pH, blood gases, glucose, electrolytes, liver function tests, ammonia, and plasma for amino acids and acyl carnitines. Urine for sugars, ketones, and organic acids is also indicated (127). In addition to MSUD, neurologic deterioration during the neonatal period is seen in various organic acidurias, urea cycle defects, fatty acid oxidation defects, and the congenital lactic acidoses. Clinically, MSUD is distinguished by the characteristic odor of the patient, a positive urine 2,4-dinitrophenylhydrazine test, and an elevation of the plasma branched-chain amino acids. The characteristic increase in plasma leucine, isoleucine, and valine is seen by the time the infant is 24 hours old, even in those infants who have not yet been given protein (128). Routine newborn screening for the condition using a bacterial inhibition assay analogous to that used for the neonatal diagnosis of PKU is performed in many states in the United States and in many other countries (129). Tandem mass spectroscopy also can be used and has the advantage of obtaining rapid quantitative measurements of all three branched-chain amino acids (43). The presence of the branched-chain ketoacid decarboxylases in cultivated amniocytes and chorionic villi allows the antenatal diagnosis of the disease as early as 10 weeks' gestation (130).

Treatment

Treatment consists in inhibiting endogenous protein catabolism, sustaining protein synthesis, preventing deficiencies of essential amino acids, and maintaining normal serum osmolarity (131). Morton and coworkers stressed that restriction of the dietary intake of the branched-chain amino acids through the use of one of several commercially available formulas is secondary in importance to inhibition of protein catabolism and enhancement of protein synthesis (131). For optimal results, infants should be placed on the diet during the first few days of life and should receive frequent measurements of serum amino acids. Prompt and vigorous treatment of even mild infections is mandatory; a number of children on this synthetic diet have died of septicemia (115,131).

Peritoneal dialysis or hemodialysis has been used to correct coma or other acute neurologic symptoms in the newly diagnosed infant (132). Another, simpler approach is to provide intravenously or by nasogastric tube an amino acid mixture devoid of leucine but containing large amounts of tyrosine, glutamine, and alanine (133). Morton and coworkers believe that the brain edema that is frequently seen in the acutely ill neonate results from hyponatremia and responds promptly to addition of oral and intravenous saline (131). Most of the children in whom long-term dietary therapy was initiated during the first 2 weeks of life and whose dietary control was meticulously maintained achieved normal or nearly normal IQs (131,134). In the experience of Hilliges and coworkers, the mean IQ of MSUD patients at 3 to 16 years of age was 74 $\pm$ 14, as compared with 101 $\pm$ 12 for early-treated patients with PKU. The length of time after birth that plasma leucine concentrations remain elevated appears to affect the IQ, as does the amount, if any, of residual branched-chain ketoacid dehydrogenase activity (135). The thiamin-responsive child is treated with 10 to 1,000 mg of thiamin per day (103).

Nonketotic Hyperglycinemia (OMIM 238300)

This relatively common family of diseases is marked by genetic and phenotypic heterogeneity, and considerable variation occurs in the severity of neurologic symptoms (136).

Five forms have been recognized:

1. In the most common, infantile form, neurologic symptoms begin during the neonatal period. They are highlighted by profound hypotonia, intractable generalized, reflex, or myoclonic seizures, apnea, and progressive obtundation with coma and respiratory arrest. The EEG demonstrates a burst-suppression pattern or, later, hypsarrhythmia (137). Nystagmus and a marked abnormality of the electroretinogram (ERG) also are seen (138). The majority of affected infants die during the neonatal period; those who survive are profoundly retarded. In some infants acute hydrocephalus develops between 2 and 6 months. In all instances this has been associated with a large retrocerebellar cyst (139).
2. A transient neonatal form has been recognized that initially is clinically indistinguishable from the permanent form of nonketotic hyperglycinemia. However, symptoms remit abruptly after a few days or months, and youngsters are left unimpaired (140). The condition appears to develop in some heterozygous carriers for nonketotic hyperglycinemia (141), and subsequent development is normal (142).
3. A less severe form becomes apparent during the latter part of the first year of life after several months of normal development. It is marked by progressive dementia leading to decerebrate rigidity. Extrapyramidal signs are not uncommon (143).
4. A juvenile form with mild mental retardation, hyperactivity, and language deficits also has been reported. They may represent survival to adulthood of individuals with the mild infantile form (144).
5. Bank and Morrow reported adults with a clinical picture of weakness and spasticity resembling spinocerebellar ataxia (145).

Pathologic examination of the brain in the infantile form of the disease discloses a reduction in white matter with an extensive spongy degeneration accompanied by marked gliosis (146). Partial or complete agenesis of the corpus callosum has been described, an indication of a significant intrauterine insult (137).

The marked increase in plasma and CSF glycine and the markedly elevated ratio of CSF glycine to blood glycine are diagnostic of the condition (137). It is important to note that one cannot rely on the plasma glycine alone to arrive at a diagnosis. The MRI shows decreased or absent supratentorial white matter, with thinning of the corpus callosum and cortical atrophy (147). On diffusion-weighted MRI symmetric lesions in the dorsal brainstem, cerebral peduncles, and posterior limbs of the internal capsule are noted, a picture compatible with a vacuolating myelopathy (148).

The basic defect in this condition is localized to the mitochondrial glycine cleavage system, which converts glycine to serine and is expressed in liver and brain. This complex reaction requires four protein components, and defects in one or another of three of these components have been documented (137). Some correlation exists between the clinical expression of the disease and the genetic defect. The classic neonatal form of the disease usually is associated with virtual absence of the pyridoxal-containing decarboxylase (P protein) and the milder atypical forms with a defect in the tetrahydrofolate-requiring transfer protein (T protein) (137,149).

The pathophysiology of the neurologic abnormalities has not been established fully. Glycine is an inhibitory neurotransmitter that acts mainly at spinal cord and brainstem levels. It also acts as a coagonist for the *N*-methyl-D-aspartate glutamate receptor, modulating its activity and probably producing seizures by an excitotoxic mechanism (137). The inhibitory effects of glycine are blocked by strychnine, but the effectiveness of strychnine on the basic course of the illness is questionable. Blockers of the *N*-methyl-D-aspartate receptor, such as dextromorphan or ketamine, have been used in conjunction with sodium benzoate, which is intended to couple with glycine. Despite these interventions the outcome for the neonatal form of nonketotic hyperglycinemia is dismal (150,151). If the patients survive the first 2 weeks of intubation, the apnea often resolves.

Defects in Urea Cycle Metabolism

Six inborn errors in the urea cycle have been described. Five of these represent a lesion at each of the five steps in the conversion of ammonia to urea (Fig. 1.6). These include argininosuccinic aciduria, citrullinuria, hyperargininemia, and two conditions termed hyperammonemia, the more common one attributable to a defect of ornithine transcarbamylase (OTC) and the other the result of a defect in mitochondrial carbamyl phosphate synthetase (CPS). The genes for all components of the urea cycle have been cloned. Additionally, a deficiency of *N*-acetylglutamate synthetase has been reported (152). This enzyme is responsible for the formation of *N*-acetylglutamate, a required activator for mitochondrial CPS. More recently two genetic defects affecting the citrulline and ornithine transporters have also been documented. The various deficits are summarized in Table 1.10.

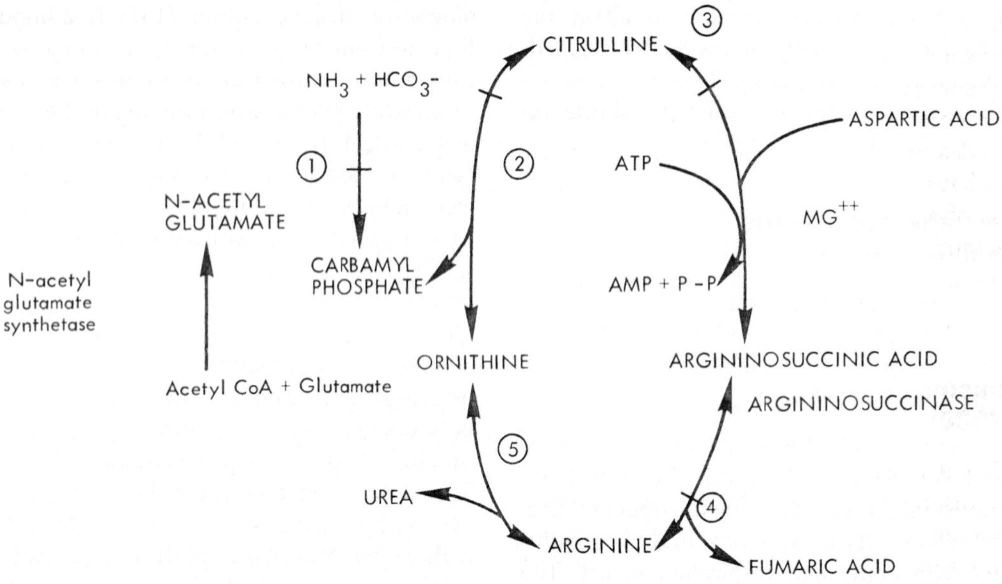

FIGURE 1.6. Normal urea cycle. In argininosuccinic aciduria, the cycle is blocked at step 4. In citrullinuria, the block occurs at step 3. In ornithine transcarbamylase deficiency, the block is at step 2. In carbamoylphosphate synthetase deficiency, the block is at step 1. A defect in *N*-acetylglutamate synthetase results in hyperammonemia by depriving step 1 of its activator, *N*-acetylglutamate. The enzyme is inhibited by a variety of organic thioesters, notably propionyl-CoA and isovaleryl-CoA. In hyperargininemia, the defect is one of arginase, step 5.

The biochemical aspects of the urea cycle were reviewed by Batshaw (153).

Because most systemic and neurologic symptoms in these diseases are the consequences of hyperammonemia or the accumulation of urea cycle intermediates, clinical manifestations of the urea cycle defects are nonspecific and overlap considerably. In their classic presentation, which occurs in some 60% of cases (154), the conditions become apparent between 24 and 72 hours of life. Initial symptoms include vomiting, lethargy, hyperpnea, and

TABLE 1.10 Disorders of Urea Cycle and of Ornithine

Disorder	*Enzyme Defect*	*Inheritance Pattern and Chromosomal Locus*	*Gene Cloned*	*Heterozygote Detection*[a]	*Prenatal Diagnosis*[a]
N-Acetylglutamate synthetase deficiency	*N*-Acetylglutamate synthetase	AR (17q21.31)	Yes	Possible	Possible
Carbamoylphosphate synthetase deficiency	Carbamoylphosphate synthetase I	AR (2q35)	Yes	Possible	Yes
Ornithine transcarbamylase deficiency	Ornithine transcarbamylase	XL (Xp21.1)	Yes	Yes	Yes
Citrullinemia, type I	Argininosuccinate synthetase	AR (9q34)	Yes	Possible	Yes
Citrullinemia, type II	Citrulline transporter	AR (7q21.3)	Yes	Possible	Possible
Argininosuccinic aciduria	Argininosuccinate lyase	AR (7cen-q11.2)	Yes	Yes	Yes
Arginase deficiency	Arginase I	AR (6q23)	Yes	Yes	Yes
Hyperornithinemia-hyperammonemia-homocitrullinuria syndrome	Ornithine transporter	AR (13q14)	Yes	Possible	Yes
Gyrate atrophy	Ornithine aminotransferase	AR (10q26)	Yes	Yes	Yes

AR, autosomal recessive; XL, X-linked.
[a]"Yes" for heterozygote detection or prenatal diagnosis means that testing is clinically available by enzyme analysis, metabolite testing, linkage analysis, or mutation detection. Heterozygote testing or prenatal diagnosis is "Possible" by mutation detection or linkage analysis when the gene has been cloned or the chromosomal location is known. Such testing may only be available in research laboratories, if at all.
From Wilcox WR, Cedarbaum S. Amino acid metabolism. In: Rimoin DL, Connor JM, Pyeritz RE, et al., eds. *Principles and practice of medical genetics,* 4th ed. New York: Churchill Livingstone, 2002;2405–2440. With permission.

hypotonia. These progress rapidly to seizures and coma. The EEG often shows burst suppression, and neuroimaging indicates the presence of cerebral edema.

When the enzyme deficiency is less severe, hyperammonemic episodes are delayed to late infancy or childhood. Patients have recurrent episodes of lethargy, vomiting, and, less often, seizures. Hyperactivity, behavioral abnormalities, and moderate to severe mental retardation are common, as is intolerance of protein-containing foods (155).

Argininosuccinic Aciduria (OMIM 207900)

Argininosuccinic aciduria is one of the more common of the urea cycle disorders. The condition is characterized by mental retardation, poorly formed hair, and accumulation of argininosuccinic acid in body fluids. It was first described in 1958 by Allan and coworkers (156).

Molecular Genetics and Biochemical Pathology

Argininosuccinic acid is a normal intermediary metabolite in the synthesis of urea (see Fig. 1.6). A deficiency in argininosuccinate lyase, an enzyme whose gene has been mapped to chromosome 7cn–q11.2, has been demonstrated in liver and skin fibroblast cultures (157).

The synthesis of urea is only slightly depressed, but a large proportion of labeled ammonium lactate administered to affected individuals is converted to glutamine (158). The manner in which children synthesize urea is not clear. It appears likely that in argininosuccinic aciduria, as well as in the other defects of urea cycle, substrate accumulates to a concentration at which the decreased substrate-binding capacity of the mutant enzyme is overcome by the accumulation of precursor to levels greater than the K_M for the mutated enzyme (159).

Pathologic Anatomy

The liver architecture is abnormal, with increased fat deposition. The brain of a neonate who succumbed to the disease was edematous, with poor demarcation of gray and white matter. The cortical layers were poorly developed, and myelination was defective with vacuolated myelin sheaths and cystic degeneration of white matter (160). An older patient had atypical astrocytes similar to the Alzheimer II cells seen in Wilson disease and in severe chronic liver disease (161).

Clinical Manifestations

As ascertained by newborn screening, the incidence of argininosuccinic aciduria is 1 in 70,000 in Massachusetts and 1 in 91,000 in Austria (162). Three distinct clinical forms have been recognized, each resulting from a different genetic mutation (163).

The most severe entity is the neonatal form. Infants feed poorly, become lethargic, develop seizures, and generally die within 2 weeks (160,164). In a second form, progression is less rapid, but similar symptoms appear in early infancy. In the majority of patients, including those described by Allan and coworkers (156), the presenting symptoms are mental retardation, recurrent generalized convulsions, poorly pigmented, brittle hair (trichorrhexis nodosa), ataxia, and hepatomegaly (165). Some patients have been seizure free, however, and have presented with little more than learning difficulties, and others (approximately 20% of all affected children) have normal intelligence without treatment (166).

Diagnosis

The presence of elevated blood ammonia should suggest a disorder in the urea cycle. Initial evaluation of such a child should include routine blood chemistries, plasma lactate levels, liver function tests, quantitative assay of plasma amino acids, and assay of urine for organic acids and orotic acid (153). The specific diagnosis of argininosuccinic aciduria can be made by a significant elevation of plasma citrulline and the presence of large quantities of plasma, urinary, and CSF argininosuccinic acid. In some instances, fasting blood ammonia level can be normal or only slightly elevated, but marked elevations occur after protein loading. Increased excretion of orotic acid is seen in all urea cycle defects, with the exception of CPS deficiency (167).

Treatment

Hyperammonemic coma in the neonate caused by any of the urea cycle defects requires prompt intervention. In essence, treatment consists of detoxification and removal of the excess ammonia and reduction in the formation of ammonia. Quantitative amino acid chromatography should be performed on an emergency basis, and the infant should be given a high dose of intravenous glucose with insulin to suppress protein catabolism. The elevated ammonia levels can be reduced by hemodialysis if available or by peritoneal dialysis (168). Details of treatment are presented by Brusilow and Horwich (166) and Batshaw and colleagues (169). Treatment for increased intracranial pressure, which frequently accompanies neonatal hyperammonemia, is symptomatic.

The long-term management of an infant who suffers a urea cycle defect is directed toward lowering blood ammonia levels and maintaining them as close to normal as possible. This is accomplished by providing the infant with alternative pathways for waste nitrogen synthesis and excretion. Infants with argininosuccinic aciduria are placed on a protein-restricted diet (1.2 to 2.0 g/kg per day), which is supplemented with L-arginine (0.4 to 0.7 g/kg per day), which promotes the synthesis of citrulline and argininosuccinate as waste nitrogen products, and citrate, which improves weight gain and reduces hepatomegaly (166,169). Sodium phenylbutyrate is added to divert ammonia from the urea cycle. A number of centers are now recommending the use of liver transplantation for argininosuccinic aciduria (170).

Episodes of hyperammonemia are generally triggered by intercurrent infections. Prevention of a rapid progression to death requires hospitalization and the use of intravenous therapy (166).

On this regimen, some children with argininosuccinic aciduria do well. Reduction of blood ammonia levels is accompanied by improved growth, reduction in liver size, cessation of seizures, and, in some patients, normal hair. Intellectual function is significantly impaired, however. In the experience of Batshaw and coworkers, all infants with the severe, neonatal form of the disease survived, although those who have been followed the longest have shown a significant lowering of their IQ (169). In the French long-term follow-up of 15 patients with argininosuccinic aciduria, none were doing well (171). Children with the late-onset variant fare much better, and, with therapy, achieve normal development (165). As a rule, the individual's ultimate IQ is a function of the severity and duration of hyperammonemic coma, and children who have not recovered from coma within 5 days do poorly (172). Valproic acid cannot be used in the treatment of seizures associated with this and with the other urea cycle defects because it induces severe hyperammonemia at even low doses (173).

Citrullinemia

In 1963, McMurray and associates reported a mentally retarded infant who had a metabolic block in the conversion of citrulline to argininosuccinic acid (see Fig. 1.6, step 3) (174). Since then, it has become clear that this condition, like many of the other inborn metabolic errors, is heterogeneous. Two genotypically and phenotypically distinct conditions have been recognized.

Argininosuccinic Acid Synthetase Deficiency (CTLI) (OMIM 215700)

The gene coding for argininosuccinic acid synthetase has been cloned. It is carried on chromosome 9 (175). At least 50 different genetic mutations have been recorded for infants with neonatal citrullinemia (176).

As a result of the enzymatic defect, the concentration of citrulline in urine, serum, and CSF is markedly increased, and administration of a protein meal results in a dramatic increase of blood ammonia and urinary orotic acid. Blood and urinary urea values are normal, indicating that urea production is not completely blocked. CT and MRI studies performed on patients with the neonatal form of citrullinemia show lesions in the thalami, basal ganglia, cortex, and subcortical white matter. Diffusion-weighted MR images indicate the presence of cytotoxic edema. Follow-up studies reveal subcortical cysts, ulegyria, and atrophy (177,178).

In Western countries, the most common presentation is in the neonatal period with lethargy, hypotonia, and seizures (179). In other instances, the disease is less severe, even though recurrent bouts of vomiting, ataxia, and seizures can start in infancy. A third form presents with mental retardation. Completely asymptomatic individuals also have been encountered (174,179).

Treatment for citrullinemia is similar to treatment for argininosuccinic aciduria, except that for long-term therapy, the low-protein diet is supplemented with arginine and sodium phenylbutyrate (166,169).

Citrullinuria in the absence of citrullinemia has been seen in patients with cystinuria. In this instance, citrulline is derived from arginine, which is poorly absorbed from the intestine (180).

Adult-Onset Type II Citrullinemia

Late-onset citrullinemia with loss of enzymatic activity in liver, but not in kidney or fibroblasts, is seen predominantly in Japan, where it constitutes the most common form of citrullinemia (181). It presents with cyclical changes in behavior, dysarthria, and motor weakness. It is due to mutations in citrin, a mitochondrial aspartate glutamate carrier (182,183).

Ornithine Transcarbamylase (OTC) Deficiency (OMIM 311250)

OTC is an enzyme coded by an X-linked gene and located in the mitochondrial matrix. Deficiency of OTC in the male infant is characterized biochemically by a catastrophic elevation of blood ammonia. This is accompanied by an increased excretion of orotic acid and a generalized elevation of plasma and urine amino acids. The disease was first reported in 1962 by Russell and coworkers (184) and is the most common of the urea cycle defects. The gene coding for the enzyme has been cloned and localized to the short arm of the X chromosome (Xp21.1), close to the Duchenne muscular dystrophy locus, and most families have their own unique mutation (185). The enzyme defect can be complete or, as occurs in some 10% to 20% of hemizygous male patients, it can be partial (186). As a consequence, blood ammonia levels are strikingly and consistently elevated (0.4 to 1.0 mg/dl, or 230 to 580 μmol/L, contrasted with normal values of less than 0.1 mg/dL, or 50 μmol/L), and CSF ammonia is at least 10 times normal. Additionally, there is an accumulation of glutamine, glutamate, and alanine. This is accompanied by a striking reduction in plasma citrulline and an increased excretion of orotic acid. The last is the consequence of a diffusion of excess carbamyl phosphate from mitochondria into cytosol, where it is converted into orotic acid (187).

As is the case in argininosuccinic aciduria, the neuropathologic picture is highlighted by the presence of Alzheimer II astrocytes throughout the brain (188). Unlike hepatic encephalopathy, a striking degree of neuronal necrosis also exists. Electron microscopic examination of liver can reveal striking abnormalities of the mitochondria (189).

As a rule, the magnitude of the enzymatic defect correlates with the severity of clinical symptoms. In male patients, the clinical picture is marked by severe hyperammonemia. When the condition presents during the neonatal period it is rapidly progressive, with a high incidence of mortality or profound neurologic residua. Symptoms usually are delayed until the second day of life and are highlighted by feeding difficulties, lethargy, and respiratory distress. The plasma ammonia level is at least five times normal, thus distinguishing the condition from sepsis (190). MRI demonstrates injury to the lentiform nuclei and the deep sulci of the insular and perirolandic region (191).

Less severe cases present with failure to thrive and with episodic attacks of headache and vomiting followed by periods of lethargy and stupor. These attacks are often the consequence of protein ingestion and are accompanied by high blood ammonia levels (192). Although hyperammonemia is probably responsible for a considerable proportion of the neurologic symptoms, alterations in neurotransmitters, notably quinolinic acid, a known excitotoxin that accumulates as a result of increased tryptophan transport across the blood–brain barrier, also could be involved (193).

The disease is expressed more variably in the heterozygous female patient, with manifestations ranging from apparent normalcy to profound neurologic deficits (187). In symptomatic female patients, behavioral abnormalities are almost invariable. In the series of Rowe and coworkers, irritability, temper tantrums, inconsolable crying, and hyperactivity were seen in every patient (187). Episodic vomiting and lethargy were also invariable. Ataxia was seen in 77% of female patients, reduced physical growth in 38%, and developmental delay in 35%. Seizures, generalized or focal, were seen in 23% (187). Blood ammonia and urinary orotic acid levels were elevated consistently when girls were symptomatic. Other girls are asymptomatic except for an aversion to protein-rich foods and possible subtle cognitive deficits (193). In some women the first hyperammonemic episode may occur in the postpartum period (194). Valproate therapy can induce fatal hepatotoxicity in male patients with OTC deficiency and in heterozygous female patients (195).

Treatment of OTC deficiency in the male or female patient is similar to treatment for argininosuccinic aciduria. It is directed at decreasing protein intake by means of a low-protein diet and increasing waste nitrogen excretion by the addition of sodium phenylbutyrate and arginine or citrulline to the diet (196). Liver transplant or isolated hepatocyte transplant has been suggested for the severe neonatal form, but the outcome for infants with no significant OTC activity is poor (171,197). Prospective treatment of infants at risk for neonatal OTC deficiency has been attempted with some success in that such infants appear to have a better neurologic outcome than those who have to be rescued from hyperammonemic coma (198).

In some hemizygous male patients, OTC deficiency is not complete, and the clinical course is not as severe. It can consist of several months of normal development followed by progressive cerebral degeneration or by the acute onset of cerebral and hepatic symptoms resembling those of Reye syndrome (199).

OTC is expressed only in liver and in the small intestine; prenatal diagnosis therefore depends on mutation detection or linkage analysis. Because some cases represent new mutations, linkage analysis is of limited use, except for offspring of obligate gene carriers (200). Of course one cannot predict whether a female patient will be asymptomatic or severely affected (186).

Carbamyl Phosphate Synthetase (CPS) Deficiency (OMIM 237300)

Carbamyl phosphate synthetase deficiency is a disorder of the urea cycle manifested by a reduction in hepatic mitochondrial CPS activity (see Fig. 1.6, step 1). This condition was reported first by Freeman and coworkers (201).

Symptoms of CPS deficiency are the most severe of any of the urea cycle defects, and the neonatal form of the condition, which is associated with complete absence of the enzyme, is usually fatal. In partial CPS deficiency, symptoms appear in infancy and consist of recurrent episodes of vomiting and lethargy, convulsions, hypotonia or hypertonia, and irregular eye movements (202). Imaging studies show changes that are almost identical to those seen in OTC deficiency. During the acute state there is cerebral edema (191,202).

Autopsy reveals ulegyria of cerebral and cerebellar cortex and hypomyelination of the centrum semiovale and the central part of the brainstem. In contrast to argininosuccinic aciduria, no Alzheimer cells are seen, probably because these cells take some time to develop and CPS deficiency is usually rapidly fatal (186,203).

Carbamyl phosphate synthetase deficiency is diagnosed by the presence of hyperammonemia in the absence of an elevation of plasma citrulline, argininosuccinic acids, or arginine. In contrast to OTC deficiency, orotic acid excretion is low or normal. Treatment for the neonatal and the less severe older-onset forms of CPS deficiency is similar to that for OTC deficiency, but the outcome in the neonatal form is uniformly poor (166,172).

Hyperargininemia (OMIM 207800)

Hyperargininemia, the least common of urea cycle disorders, has a clinical picture that differs from that of the other urea cycle disorders in that there is infrequent hyperammonemia. In the acute form cerebral edema and seizures begin during the neonatal period (204). In other instances, mental retardation, microcephaly, spastic diplegia, or quadriparesis becomes apparent during the first few months or years (205). The concentration of glutamine and arginine in plasma and CSF is elevated, and excretion of arginine, cystine, and lysine is increased, a urinary amino acid pattern resembling that of cystinuria. Blood ammonia levels are normal or slightly elevated. This is probably due to the presence of a second unaffected arginase gene locus expressed primarily in kidney mitochondria. A deficiency of arginase has been documented in red cells and liver (206).

Patients are treated with a diet consisting of a mixture of essential amino acids, exclusive of arginine, and supplemented by a commercial formula that furnishes fats, carbohydrates, vitamins, and minerals. Phenylbutyrate can also be added to the regimen. Replacement of arginase by means of periodic exchange transfusions has been suggested as a supplementary means of controlling blood and CSF arginine concentrations (207). In spite of therapy, spasticity often progresses. The effectiveness of liver transplants is unknown.

N-Acetylglutamate Synthetase Deficiency (OMIM 237310)

In the absence of the enzyme, a deficiency of *N*-acetylglutamate exists, an activator of mitochondrial CPS (185). Clinical manifestations range from fatal neonatal hyperammonemia to protein intolerance with recurrent episodes of hyperammonemia (208,209a). Treatment with carbamylglutamate has been successful.

Other Genetic Causes of Hyperammonemia

Hyperammonemia is seen in several other genetic disorders. Hyperammonemia, with increased excretion of orotic acid, is seen in periodic hyperlysinemia. For reasons as yet unknown, hyperammonemia can be induced by administration of large amounts of lysine and the condition diagnosed by the excretion of large amounts of lysine. It is considered with the other defects of lysine metabolism.

Ornithinemias

Another cause for intermittent hyperammonemia is ornithinemia. Clinically and biochemically this is a heterogeneous entity, At least two conditions have been delineated.

HHH Syndrome (OMIM 238970)

This condition is caused by a mutation in a gene encoding a mitochondrial ornithine transporter (210). As the name indicates, elevated plasma ornithine levels (hyperornithinemia) are accompanied by hyperammonemia and homocitrullinuria. In the neonatal form the clinical picture is of prolonged neonatal jaundice, mental retardation, infantile spasms, and intermittent ataxia (211,212). When the condition becomes apparent later in life, it is marked by spastic gait, myoclonic seizures, and ataxia (200).

Ornithine Aminotransferase Deficiency (OMIM 258870)

In this entity, ornithinemia is accompanied by gyrate atrophy of the choroid and retina, leading to night blindness. There is no hyperammonemia. The condition is most commonly encountered in the Finnish population, in which there is an incidence of 1 in 50,000. Intelligence is preserved, and no obvious neurologic or muscular symptoms occur, although type 2 muscle fiber atrophy is seen on biopsy (213) and peripheral nerve involvement can be shown electrically (214). Early white matter degenerative changes and premature cerebral atrophy can be documented on MRI, and MRS demonstrates reduced creatine in muscle and brain (215,216). The creatine deficiency can be partially corrected by creatine supplementation (216). Ocular symptoms seem to be ameliorated by a low-arginine diet or creatine supplementation.

Other Causes for Hyperammonemia

Transient hyperammonemia with consequent profound neurologic depression can be encountered in asphyxiated infants or with significant dehydration (217,218). This state should be differentiated not only from the various urea cycle defects, but also from the various organic acidemias, notably methylmalonic acidemia and propionic acidemia, which can induce hyperammonemia (219). In these conditions, the accumulation of organic acids inhibits the formation of *N*-acetylglutamine, the activator of mitochondrial CPS, and the activities of all five enzymes of the urea cycle are depressed. On a clinical basis, the organic acidemias can be distinguished from urea cycle defects in that infants with a urea cycle defect are asymptomatic for the first 24 hours of life and only rarely develop coma before 72 hours. Additionally, they demonstrate tachypnea rather than a respiratory distress syndrome. In contrast to the distressed neonates with hyperammonemia, infants with the various organic acidemias demonstrate ketonuria or ketonemia as well as acidosis (220).

Asymptomatic hyperammonemia is relatively common in low-birth-weight neonates. It probably is caused by shunting of blood away from the portal circulation of the liver into the systemic circulation.

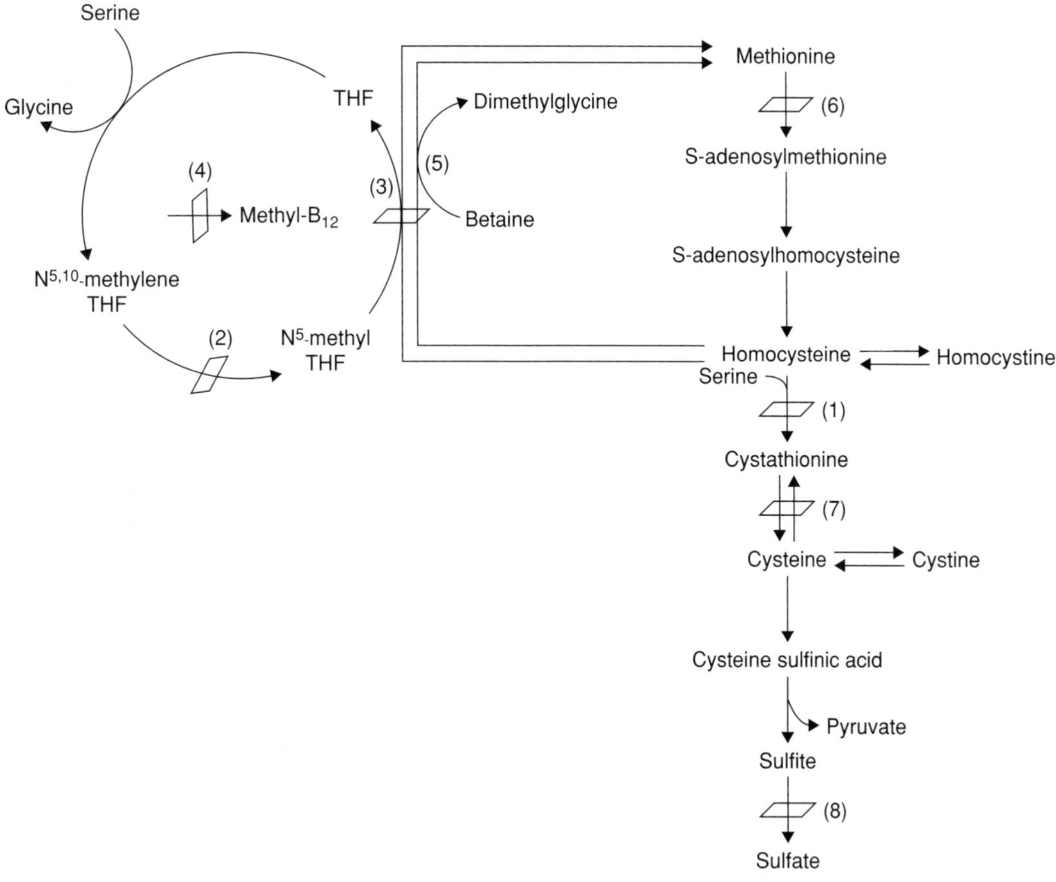

FIGURE 1.7. Normal metabolism of sulfur amino acids. THF, tetrahydrofolate. The known genetic defects that cause homocystinuria are a deficiency of cystathionine-β-synthase (1), $N^{5,10}$-methylenetetrahydrofolate reductase (2), methionine synthase or methionine synthase reductase (3), or deficient synthesis of methylcobalamine (4). Other defects in the pathway result in cystathioninuria due to γ-cystathionase deficiency (7), sulfite oxidase and molybdenum cofactor synthesis deficiencies (8), and hyperammonemia due to methionine adenosyltransferase deficiency (6). Betaine can be given therapeutically to treat homocystinuria by increasing remethylation of homocysteine via betaine-homocysteine methyltransferase (5). (From Wilcox WR, Cedarbaum S. Amino acid metabolism. In: Rimoin DL, Connor JM, Pyeritz RE, et al., eds. *Principles and practice of medical genetics*, 4th ed. New York: Churchill Livingstone, 2002;2405–2440.)

Mild hyperammonemia can also be seen in associated with hypoglycemia and hyperinsulinism due to mutations in the glutamate dehydrogenase gene (221).

Defects in the Metabolism of Sulfur Amino Acids

Homocystinuria (OMIM 236200)

The increased excretion of homocystine is a manifestation of several inborn errors of methionine metabolism. The most common of these errors is marked by multiple thromboembolic episodes, ectopia lentis, and mental retardation. Although discovered as late as 1962 by Field and reported subsequently by Carson and coworkers (222), the prevalence of homocystinuria varies considerably from one country to another, ranging from 1 in 65,000 in Ireland to approximately 1 in 335,000 worldwide (223). The gene for this autosomal recessive condition has been cloned; it is localized to the long arm of chromosome 21 (21q22.3).

Molecular Genetics and Biochemical Pathology

In the most common genetic form of homocystinuria, the mutation involves the gene for cystathionine synthase, the enzyme that catalyzes the formation of cystathionine from homocysteine and serine (Fig. 1.7) (224). The enzyme as purified from human liver has two identical subunits and contains bound pyridoxal phosphate (225). Considerable genetic heterogeneity exists among various cystathionine synthase–deficient families, but in the majority, the lesion resides in a structural gene for the enzyme (226). In most homocystinuric patients, the mutation does not cause dysfunction of the catalytic domain of this enzyme, but instead interferes with its activation by pyridoxine (227). As a result, enzyme activity is either

TABLE 1.11 Disorders of Sulfur Amino Acids

Disorder	Enzyme Deficiency	Inheritance Pattern and Chromosomal Locus	Gene Cloned	Heterozygote Detection[a]	Prenatal Diagnosis[a]
Hypermethioninemia	Methionine adenosyltransferase	AD (10q22) AR (10q22)	Yes	Possible	Possible
Cystathioninuria	γ-Cystathionase	AR (16)	Yes	Not indicated	Not indicated
Homocystinuria					
Pyridoxine-responsive and -nonresponsive homocystinuria	Cystathionine β-synthase	AR (21q22.3)	Yes	Yes	Yes
Homocystinuria and mild homocysteinemia	$N^{5,10}$-Methylenetetrahydrofolate reductase	AR (1p36.3)	Yes	Yes	Yes
Homocystinuria with megaloblastic anemia					
cbl E	Methionine synthase reductase	AR (5p15.3–p15.2)	Yes	Possible	Yes
cbl G	Methionine synthase	AR (1q43)	Yes	Possible	Possible
Homocystinuria with methylmalonic acidemia and megaloblastic anemia					
Intrinsic factor deficiency	Intrinsic factor	AR (11q13)	Yes	Possible	Possible
Ineerslund-Grasbeck syndrome	Cubilin (intrinsic factor receptor)	AR (10p12.1)	Yes	Possible	Possible
Transcobalamin II deficiency	Transcobalamin II	AR (22q11.2–qter)	Yes	Possible	Possible
cbl C	Synthesis of methyl and adenosylcobalamin	AR (?)	No	No	Possible
cbl D	Synthesis of methyl and adenosylcobalamin	AR (?)	No	No	Possible
cbl F	Cobalamin lysosomal release	AR (?)	No	No	?
Sulfite oxidase deficiency	Sulfite oxidase	AR (12q13.2–q13.3)	Yes	Possible	Possible
Molybdenum cofactor deficiency	Molybdenum cofactor synthesis	AR (6p21.3) (5q21)	 Yes Yes	Possible	Possible

[a]"Yes" for heterozygote detection or prenatal diagnosis means that testing is clinically available by enzyme analysis, metabolite testing, linkage analysis, or mutation detection. Heterozygote testing or prenatal diagnosis is "Possible" by mutation detection or linkage analysis when the gene has been cloned or the chromosomal location is known. Such testing may only be available in research laboratories, if at all.
AD, autosomal dominant; AR, autosomal recessive.
From Wilcox WR, Cedarbaum S. Amino acid metabolism. In: Rimoin DL, Connor JM, Pyeritz RE, et al., eds. *Principles and practice of medical genetics*, 4th ed. New York: Churchill Livingstone, 2002;2405–2440.

completely absent or, as is the case in a significant proportion of affected families (in the Australian series of Gaustadnes and coworkers approximately 38% of patients with homocystinuria), residual activity occurs (228). In the latter group, addition of pyridoxine (500 mg/day or more) stimulates enzyme activity and partially or completely abolishes the excretion of homocystine, the oxidized derivative of homocysteine. Pyridoxine-responsive patients tend to have a milder phenotype of the disease.

As a result of the block, increased amounts of homocystine, the oxidized derivative of homocysteine, and its precursor, methionine, are found in urine, plasma, and CSF. Administration of a methionine load to affected individuals produces a striking and prolonged increase in plasma methionine, but little alteration in the homocystine levels. In part, this reflects the low renal threshold for homocystine.

The various other genetic defects that result in an increased excretion of homocystinuria are depicted in Table 1.11. Homocystinuria also can result from an impaired methylation of homocysteine to methionine (see Fig. 1.7). When the metabolic block is at this point, plasma methionine concentrations are normal rather than increased, as is the case in the more common form of homocystinuria owing to cystathionine synthase deficiency. Methylation uses N^5-methyltetrahydrofolate as a methyl donor and a vitamin B_{12} derivative (methylcobalamin) as a cofactor. Methylation can be impaired as a result of lack of the cofactor methylcobalamin, or the enzyme. When synthesis of the vitamin B_{12} cofactor is defective, the biochemical picture is characterized by increased excretion of methylmalonic acid and homocystine. This condition is distinct from methylmalonic aciduria (MMA), which is the result of a reduced activity of methylmalonyl-CoA mutase, a cobalamin-dependent enzyme. Several errors in cobalamin metabolism have been recognized; the clinical picture includes mental retardation, seizures, failure to thrive, hypotonia, ataxia, and megaloblastic anemia. The conditions are covered in the section on Organic Acidurias, later in this chapter.

Another cause for homocystinuria is a defect in the methylation enzyme, methylene tetrahydrofolate reductase (MHTFR). The clinical picture in these patients is protean. Some are retarded or have been diagnosed as schizophrenic; others have recurrent episodes of vomiting and lethargy or muscular weakness and seizures. Vascular thromboses also have been encountered, but the skeletal and ocular changes of homocystinuria are absent (229,230). Folic acid has reduced the biochemical abnormalities in some patients with this condition but has been ineffectual in others. This severe disorder due to marked deficiency in MHTFR should be distinguished from the common "thermolabile" variant that mildly increases plasma homocysteine levels.

Pathologic Anatomy

The primary structural alterations in homocystinuria are noted in blood vessels of all calibers (231). Most of these show intimal thickening and fibrosis; in the aorta and its major branches, fraying of elastic fibers might be observed. Arterial and venous thromboses are common in a number of organs. Within the brain are usually multiple infarcted areas of varying age. The existence of dural sinus thrombosis has been recorded.

How the metabolic defect induces a propensity to vascular thrombosis has been reviewed by Welch and Loscalzo (232). It has also become evident that an increased plasma homocysteine concentration is an independent risk factor for atherosclerotic vascular disease.

Clinical Manifestations

The pyridoxine-unresponsive form of homocystinuria is more severe in its manifestations than the pyridoxine-responsive form.

Homocystinuric infants appear healthy at birth, and their early development is unremarkable until seizures, developmental slowing, or cerebrovascular accidents occur between 5 and 9 months of age. Ectopia lentis is seen in more than 90% of affected individuals. Lenticular dislocation has been recognized as early as age 18 months, but it generally occurs between 3 and 10 years of age. The typical older homocystinuric child's hair is sparse, blond, and brittle, and multiple erythematous blotches are seen over the skin, particularly across the maxillary areas and cheeks. The gait is shuffling, the extremities and digits are long, and genu valgum is present in most instances. Secondary glaucoma and cataracts are common (233).

In approximately 50% of the patients reported, major thromboembolic episodes have occurred on one or more occasions. These include fatal thromboses of the pulmonary artery, coronary arteries, and renal artery and vein. Multiple major cerebrovascular accidents also result in hemiplegia, and ultimately in a picture that closely resembles pseudobulbar palsy. Thromboembolic events are particularly common after even minor surgical procedures. It is likely that minor and unrecognized cerebral thrombi are the cause of the mental retardation that occurs in 50% of the patients (234,235). Routine laboratory study results are normal, but in a high proportion of patients, electromyography suggests myopathy (235).

Radiography reveals a biconcavity of the posterior aspects of the vertebrae (codfish vertebrae) (236). Additionally, scoliosis and osteoporosis become apparent in late childhood. Abnormalities of the hands and feet are noted also. These include metaphyseal spicules, enlargement of carpal bones, and selective retardation of the development of the lunate bone (237). Neuroimaging studies tend to show lesions due to vascular ischemia.

Diagnosis

The diagnosis of homocystinuria suggested by the appearance of the patient can be confirmed by the increased urinary excretion of homocystine, by elevated plasma methionine and homocystine, and by a positive urinary cyanide-nitroprusside reaction. Enzyme activity can be determined in cultured skin fibroblasts or in liver biopsy specimens.

Although ectopia lentis, arachnodactyly, and cardiovascular symptoms are seen also in Marfan syndrome, homocystinuria can be distinguished by its autosomal recessive transmission (in contrast to the dominant transmission of Marfan syndrome), the thromboembolic phenomena, the early appearance of osteoporosis, the biconcave vertebrae, and the peculiar facial appearance (238). The relatively long fingers seen in Marfan syndrome are present at birth, and the skeletal disproportion remains constant. In homocystinuria, the skeleton is normal for the first few years of life, but the limbs grow disproportionately long. Ectopia lentis is seen not only in homocystinuria but also as an isolated congenital defect in the Weill-Marchesani syndrome and in sulfite oxidase deficiency. In the latter condition, it occurs in conjunction with profound mental retardation, seizures commencing shortly after birth, acute hemiplegia, opisthotonos, and hyperacusis. Because the majority of cases are the result of a deficiency of the molybdenum cofactor rather than of the apoenzyme, this condition is covered more fully in the section dealing with disorders of metal metabolism.

Cystathionine synthase has been found in cultivated amniotic fluid cells, and the condition, therefore, can be diagnosed prenatally (239).

Treatment

Restriction of methionine intake lowers plasma methionine and eliminates the abnormally high urinary excretion of homocystine. Commercially available diets that are methionine free and are supplemented by carbohydrates, fats, and fat-soluble vitamins generally lower plasma methionine levels to the normal range (235). The diets are supplemented with cystine.

Other dietary measures include the addition of folic acid, based on the assumption that the mental defect is in part related to low serum folate levels (240). Dietary supplementation with betaine hydrochloride (*N,N,N*-trimethylglycine), a methyl donor, is generally used in pyridoxine-nonresponsive patients (241). However, several instances of progressive cerebral edema have been encountered in patients whose serum methionine levels had not been well controlled (242). Antithrombotic agents, such as aspirin or dipyridamole, are also given, although their effectiveness has not been proven.

Early therapy with good biochemical control results in a normal IQ and significantly reduces the incidence of thromboembolic episodes and other vascular complications in pyridoxine-nonresponsive patients (243,244).

In pyridoxine-responsive patients, large doses of the vitamin (250 to 1,200 mg/day) reduce or eliminate biochemical abnormalities. In the series of Mudd and coworkers, pyridoxine-responsive patients treated from the neonatal period on had an IQ ranging from 82 to 110. Virtually all patients with IQs greater than 90 were found to be responsive to pyridoxine (245).

Hypermethioninemia

Several other conditions are marked by elevated plasma methionine levels. The most common of these is a transitory methioninemia, seen in infants, many of who are premature and receiving a high-protein diet (at least 7 g/kg per day). It is likely that the biochemical abnormality is caused by delayed maturation of one or more of the enzymes of methionine metabolism.

Methioninemia, with or without tyrosinemia, accompanied by hepatorenal disease (tyrosinemia I) is considered in the section on tyrosinosis and tyrosinemia (see Table 1.9).

Persistent methioninemia associated with a deficiency of hepatic methionine adenosyltransferase is a benign metabolic variant unaccompanied by neurologic symptoms or impairment of cognition (246).

Other Rare Metabolic Defects

A few other extremely rare defects of amino acid metabolism associated with neurologic symptoms are presented in Table 1.12. Experience with disorders such as the iminoacidemias, cystathioninuria, and histidinemia should caution the reader against accepting a causal relationship between metabolic and neurologic defects.

DISORDERS OF RENAL AMINO ACID TRANSPORT

Renal amino acid transport is handled by five specific systems that have nonoverlapping substrate preferences. The disorders that result from genetic defects in each of these systems are listed in Table 1.13.

Hartnup Disease (OMIM 234500)

Hartnup disease is a rare familial condition characterized by photosensitive dermatitis, intermittent cerebellar ataxia, mental disturbances, and renal aminoaciduria. The name is that of the family in which it was first detected (262). The first gene to be identified was that for SLC6A19, a sodium-dependent amino acid transporter, on chromosome 5p15. Not all families are linked to chromosome 5p15, and there remains at least one other causative gene to be identified (263,264).

Molecular Genetics and Biochemical Pathology

The symptoms are the result of an extensive disturbance in sodium-dependent transport of neutral amino acids across the membrane of the brush border of the small intestine and the proximal renal tubular epithelium. Four main biochemical abnormalities exist: a renal aminoaciduria, increased excretion of indican, an abnormally high output of nonhydroxylated indole metabolites, and increased fecal amino acids. These deficits are discussed in detail by Milne and colleagues (265) and Scriver (266).

Pathologic Anatomy

Pathologic changes in the brain are nonspecific and are limited to neuronal degeneration and dysmyelination (267).

Clinical Manifestations

The incidence of the biochemical lesion responsible for Hartnup disease is 1 in 18,000 in Massachusetts, 1 in 70,000 in Vienna, and 1 in 33,000 in New South Wales, Australia (268). Clinical manifestations of Hartnup disease are the consequence of several factors. Polygenic inheritance is the major determinant for plasma amino acid levels, and symptoms are seen only in patients with the lowest amino acid concentrations. Because protein malnutrition further lowers amino acid levels, the disease

TABLE 1.12 Some Rarely Encountered Defects of Amino Acid Metabolism Associated with Neurologic Symptoms

Disease (Reference)	*Enzymatic Defect*	*Clinical Features*	*Diagnosis*
Hypervalinemia (247)[a]	Valine transaminase	Vomiting, failure to thrive, nystagmus, mental retardation	Increased blood and urine valine; no increased excretion of ketoacid
Hyper-β-alaninemia (248)	β-Alanine-α-keto-glutarate transaminase	Seizures commencing at birth, somnolence	Plasma urine β-alanine and β-aminoisobutyric acid elevated; urinary γ-aminobutyric acid elevated
Carnosinemia (249)	Carnosinase	Grand mal and myoclonic seizures, progressive mental retardation; most subjects are asymptomatic	Increased serum and urine carnosine; increased CSF homocarnosine
α-Methylacetoacetic aciduria (250,251)	3-Ketothiolase	Recurrent severe acidosis	α-Methyl acetoacetate and α-methyl-β-hydroxy butyric acid in urine
Hypertryptophanemia (252,253)	Tryptophan transaminase	Ataxia, spasticity, mental retardation, pellagra-like skin rash, cataracts	Elevated serum tryptophan, diminished or normal kynurenine, massive excretion of indole-acetic, -lactic, -pyruvic acids
Aspartylglycosaminuria (254,255)	Aspartylglucosaminidase	Progressive mental retardation, coarse facial features, changes in tubular bones of hand, vacuolated lymphocytes, mitral valve insufficiency	Elevated urine aspartylglucosamine
Glutamyl ribose-5-phosphate storage disease (256)	Deficiency of ADP-ribose protein hydrolase	Mental deterioration, seizures, microcephaly, proteinuria, coarse facies	Accumulation of glutamyl ribose-5-phosphate in brain and kidney
Glutamyl cysteine synthetase deficiency (257)	γ-Glutamylcysteine synthetase	Hemolytic anemia, spinocerebellar degeneration, peripheral neuropathy	Reduced erythrocyte glutathione, generalized aminoaciduria
Hyperoxaluria (258,259)	Type I: excessive oxalate synthesis; type II: defective hydroxypyruvate metabolism	Progressive renal insufficiency, dementia, peripheral neuropathy; type II milder than type I	Increased urinary oxalic acid with glycolic acid (type I) or L-glyceric acid
Aromatic L-aminoacid decarboxylase deficiency (261a,261b)	Aromatic L-aminoacid decarboxylase, DOPA decarboxylase	Hypotonia, paroxysmal dyskinesia, autonomic dysfunction	CSF homovanillic, 5-hydroxyindoleacetic acid reduced

ADP, adenosine 5′-diphosphate; CSF, cerebrospinal fluid.
[a]Hypervalinemia has not been seen since the original report in 1963.

itself, as distinguished from its biochemical defect, is seen mainly in malnourished children. Whenever dietary intake is satisfactory, neither neurologic nor dermatologic signs appear (268). In addition, no difference exists in rate of growth or IQ scores between groups with Hartnup disease and control groups. In the series of Scriver and coworkers, 90% of Hartnup patients had normal development (269). However, low academic performance and impaired growth were seen in those patients with Hartnup disease who, for genetic reasons, tended to have the lowest plasma amino acid levels (269).

When present, symptoms are intermittent and variable, and tend to improve with increasing age. A characteristic red, scaly rash appears on the exposed areas of the face, neck, and extensor surfaces of the extremities. This rash resembles the dermatitis of pellagra and, like it, is aggravated by sunlight. Cerebral symptoms can precede the rash for several years. They include intermittent personality changes, psychoses, migraine-like headaches, photophobia, and bouts of cerebellar ataxia. Changes in hair texture also have been observed. The four children of the original Hartnup family underwent progressive mental retardation, but this is not invariable. Renal and intestinal transport is impaired in 80% of patients and renal transport alone in 20% (269). The MRI is nonspecific; it demonstrates delayed myelination (270).

Diagnosis

Hartnup disease should be considered in patients with intermittent cerebral symptoms, even without skin involvement.

TABLE 1.13 Defects in Amino Acid Transport

Transport System	Condition	Biochemical Features	Clinical Features
Basic amino acids	Cystinuria (three types)	Impaired renal clearance and defective intestinal transport of lysine, arginine, ornithine, and cystine	Renal stones, no neurologic disease; ? increased prevalence in subjects with mental disease
Generalized	Lowe syndrome[a]	? Impaired intestinal transport of lysine and arginine; ? impaired tubular transport of lysine	Severe mental retardation, glaucoma, cataracts, myopathy; gender-linked transmission
Acidic amino acids	Dicarboxylic amino-aciduria	Increased excretion of glutamic, aspartic acids	Harmless variant
Neutral amino acids	Hartnup disease[b]	Defective intestinal and renal tubular transport of tryptophan and other neutral amino acids	Intermittent cerebellar ataxia; photosensitive rash
Proline, hydroxyproline, glycine	Iminoglycinuria	Impaired tubular transport of proline, hydroxyproline, and glycine	Harmless variant; transient iminoglycinuria normal in early infancy
β-Amino acids	None known	Excretion of β-aminoisobutyric acid and taurine in β-alaninemia is increased owing to competition at the tubular level	—
Lysinuric protein intolerance	Amino acid transporter	Mental retardation, vomiting diarrhea, failure to thrive; many patients from Finland	Increased excretion of ornithine, arginine, lysine (260,260a,260b,261,980)

[a] In Lowe syndrome, defects of amino acid transport are secondary to the defect in phosphatidyl inositol phosphatase.
[b] In Hartnup disease, amino acid transport is usually normal.

Numerous metabolic disorders with a partial enzymatic defect produce intermittent cerebellar ataxia. These include MSUD, lactic acidosis, pyruvate dehydrogenase deficiency, and some of the diseases caused by defects in the urea cycle. Additionally, episodic ataxia should be considered. This condition is caused by mutations in the calcium-channel voltage-dependent, P/Q type, alpha 1A subunit gene (*CACNA1A*), which is highly expressed in the cerebellum. Another rare condition to be considered in the differential diagnosis of Hartnup disease is hypertryptophanemia (see Table 1.12) and a disorder in kynurenine hydroxylation (271). Chromatography of urine for amino acids and indolic substances in the presence of a normal serum pattern is diagnostic for Hartnup disease. The absence of increased proline and hydroxyproline in the urine distinguishes Hartnup from generalized aminoaciduria that can be the result of many other disorders.

Treatment

The similarity of Hartnup disease to pellagra has prompted treatment with nicotinic acid (25 mg/day). Tryptophan ethylester also has been effective (272). However, the tendency for symptoms to remit spontaneously and for general improvement to occur with improved dietary intake and advancing age makes such therapy difficult to evaluate.

Lowe Syndrome (Oculocerebrorenal Syndrome) (OMIM 30900)

Lowe syndrome is an X-linked recessive disorder whose gene has been localized to the long arm of the X chromosome (Xq25–q26) and is characterized by severe mental retardation, myopathy, and congenital glaucoma or cataract. Biochemically, it is marked by a generalized aminoaciduria of the Fanconi type, renal tubular acidosis, and hypophosphatemic rickets (273,274). The gene responsible for the disorder has been cloned (275). It encodes a phosphatidyl inositol phosphatase located on the *trans*-Golgi network. The substrate for this phosphatase is a phospholipid with an important role in several basic cell processes, including cellular signaling, protein trafficking, and polymerization of the actin skeleton. Abnormalities in the structure of the actin skeleton of fibroblasts derived from patients with Lowe syndrome have been demonstrated (276). It is not clear how this lesion relates to the basic phenotypic defect, which is believed to be a defect in membrane transport (277).

Neuropathologic examination has disclosed rarefaction of the molecular layer of the cerebral cortex and parenchymal vacuolation or little more than ventricular dilation (278,279). The urinary levels of lysine are more elevated than those of the other amino acids, and defective uptake of lysine and arginine by the intestinal mucosa has been demonstrated in two patients (277).

The neurologic picture is that of a developmental delay or of progressive loss of acquired skills (280). This is accompanied by hypotonia, areflexia, and evidence of peripheral neuropathy with loss of myelinated fibers (281,282). CT scans reveal reduced density of periventricular white matter and marked scalloping of the calvarial bones, especially in the occipital region (283). T2-weighted MRI shows patchy, irregular areas of increased signal intensity

(283,285). Additionally, multiple periventricular cystic lesions have been observed (284).

Heterozygous female patients are neurologically healthy, with normal renal function, but have micropunctate cortical lens opacities (285).

Creatine Transporter Defect (OMIM 300036)

This X-linked disorder was first described in 2001 by Salomons and coworkers (286). It is marked by mental retardation and hypotonia. Some patients demonstrate an extrapyramidal disorder and have a drug-resistant seizure disorder (287). The condition is not rare. Screening of European X-linked mental retardation patients identified an incidence of at least 2.1%, making it almost as common as the fragile X syndrome (*FMR1* gene) (288). The defect has been localized to the creatine transporter gene (*SLC6A8*). Diagnosis is made by MRS, which demonstrates complete absence of the creatine peak. Urine and blood creatine levels are increased, and oral supplementation with creatine is ineffective in changing the MRS.

Creatine transporter defect should be distinguished from defects in guanidinoacetate *N*-methyl transferase (OMIM 601240), in which plasma guanidinoacetate levels are increased and urinary creatine levels are reduced (289). This condition is characterized by developmental arrest and deterioration, severe, early-onset seizures, and a variety of movement disorders (287,289). It should also be distinguished from arginine:glycine amidinotransferase deficiency (OMIM 602360), which presents with mental retardation, seizures, and autistic behavior and in which creatine supplementation not only normalizes the MRS, but also controls seizures and behavior (290).

DISORDERS OF CARBOHYDRATE METABOLISM AND TRANSPORT

Galactosemia (OMIM 230400)

Hepatomegaly, splenomegaly, and failure to thrive associated with the excretion of galactose were first pointed out by von Reuss in 1908 (291). Galactosemia is transmitted in an autosomal recessive manner. In the United States, it is seen with a frequency of 1 in 62,000; in Austria, 1 in 40,000 to 46,000; and in England, 1 in 72,000 (292).

Molecular Genetics and Biochemical Pathology

In 1917, Göppert demonstrated that galactosemic children excreted galactose after the ingestion of lactose (milk) and galactose (293). In 1956, Schwarz and associates found that administration of galactose to affected children gave rise to an accumulation of galactose-1-phosphate (294).

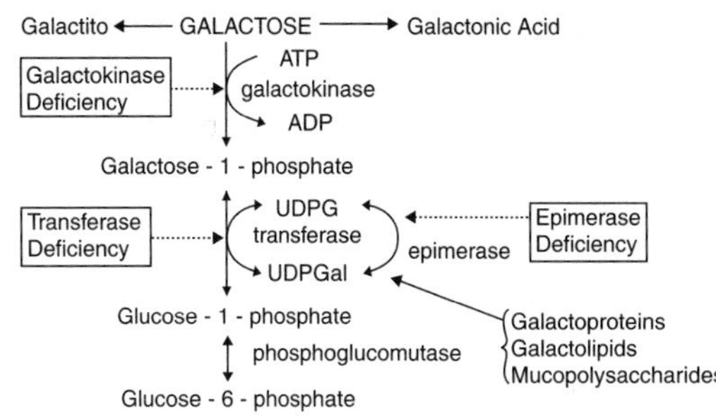

FIGURE 1.8. Pathways of galactose metabolism. In galactosemia, galactose-1-phosphate uridyltransferase is defective. (From Ng WG, Roe TF. Disorders of carbohydrate metabolism. In: Rimoin DL, Connor JM, Pyeritz RE, et al., eds. *Principles and practice of medical genetics*, 4th ed. New York: Churchill Livingstone, 2002.)

This was confirmed by Kalckar and his group, who were able to demonstrate a deficiency in galactose-1-phosphate uridyltransferase (GALT), the enzyme that catalyzes the conversion of galactose-1-phosphate into galactose uridine diphosphate (UDP-galactose) (Fig. 1.8) (295). The gene for galactosemia has been mapped to the small arm of chromosome 9 (9p13). It has been cloned and sequenced, and numerous mutations have been identified (296,297). Two point mutations (Q188R and K285N) account for 69% to 80% of galactosemia in whites and result in a complete enzyme deficiency; most of the remaining mutations result in detectable amounts of enzyme activity (296,297). In African-American patients, the most common mutation (S135L) accounts for 45% of the mutant alleles. Patients homozygous for the S135L allele have residual red cell GALT activity and a milder clinical course (298). Compound heterozygotes of a classic galactosemia allele and the Los Angeles or Duarte variant are asymptomatic.

In classic galactosemia, the metabolic block is essentially complete. Lactose of human or cow's milk is hydrolyzed to galactose and glucose, the latter being handled in a normal manner. The metabolism of galactose, however, stops after the sugar is phosphorylated to galactose-1-phosphate. This phosphate ester accumulates in erythrocytes, lens, liver, and kidney (299). Galactitol, the alcohol of galactose, also is found in the lens, brain, and urine of galactosemic individuals (300), and can be demonstrated in brain by MRS (303). Berry and coworkers postulated that galactitol induces cerebral edema that is occasionally present in neonates (301). Factors responsible for mental retardation can include a deficiency of uridine diphosphate galactose, a reduction of glycolytic intermediates, and a loss of adenosine triphosphate (ATP) (300).

Administration of galactose to affected infants results in marked hypoglycemia. This has been explained by an increased insulin release, prompted by the large amounts of circulating reducing substance, or by assuming interference by galactose-1-phosphate with normal glycogen breakdown. The peripheral hypoglycemia is enhanced by competition between glucose and galactose at the level of the hexose transport across the blood–brain barrier. As a consequence, the brain in galactosemic patients is in a constant hypoglycemic environment.

Intolerance to galactose decreases with increasing age. In part, this intolerance might be a result of the decreasing importance of milk as a food item. In patients with classic galactosemia who have been tested repeatedly, no increase in erythrocyte transferase activity has been found (302).

Pathologic Anatomy

The main pathologic lesions are found in the liver and brain. In the liver, several stages are recognized. Initially one sees a severe, diffuse, fatty metamorphosis. The hepatic cells are filled with large, pale, fat-containing vacuoles (303). If the disease remains untreated, the liver cell cords are transformed into pseudoglandular structures. The final stage is pseudolobular cirrhosis. Cerebral alterations are nonspecific. Edema, fibrous gliosis of white matter and marked loss of cortical neurons and Purkinje cells are the most prominent findings (304).

Clinical Manifestations

Infants with galactosemia appear healthy at birth, although their cord blood can already contain abnormally high concentrations of galactose-1-phosphate, and a few already have cataracts and hepatic cirrhosis, probably as a consequence of intrauterine galactosemia (305). In severe cases, symptoms develop during the first week of life. These include vomiting, diarrhea, listlessness, and failure to gain weight. Increased intracranial pressure due to cytotoxic cerebral edema can be a presenting sign (306). Infants are jaundiced. This may represent a persistence of neonatal jaundice or can appear at age 3 to 5 days (307). On a normal diet, hypoglycemia is not common. By age 2 weeks, hepatosplenomegaly and lenticular opacifications are easily detectable. The cataracts can be cortical or nuclear and can be present at birth (300). The most frequently observed opacity is a central refractile ring (308). The infants are hypotonic and often have lost the Moro reflex. Sepsis caused by *Escherichia coli* occurs with high frequency and is responsible for the majority of deaths during the neonatal period (309). Other secondary effects of deranged galactose metabolism include ovarian failure or atrophy and testicular atrophy (310). The MRI commonly shows multiple areas of increased signal in white matter, predominantly in the periventricular region (311).

If galactosemia goes untreated, growth failure becomes severe and the infant develops the usual signs of progressive hepatic cirrhosis. In some infants, the disease can be less severe and does not manifest until age 3 to 6 months, at which time the presenting symptoms are delayed physical and mental development. By then, cataracts can be well established and the cirrhosis far advanced.

In another group of galactosemic individuals, the diagnosis is not made until patients are several years old, often on evaluation for mental retardation. They might not have cataracts or albuminuria. Intellectual retardation is not consistent in untreated galactosemic children. When present, it is moderate; IQs range between 50 and 70. Asymptomatic homozygotes also have been detected. Most of these have some residual transferase activity.

Diagnosis

The enzyme defect is best documented by measuring the erythrocyte GALT activity. Several methods are available and have been be used for statewide and nationwide screening. In the Austrian screening program reviewed by Item and coworkers, only 1 in 190 infants who tested positive initially actually had galactosemia (297). Some of these were galactosemia carriers or Duarte/galactosemia compound heterozygotes.

Galactosuria, usually in combination with glucosuria or fructosuria, is seen in severe hepatic disorders of the neonatal period (e.g., neonatal hepatitis, tyrosinosis, congenital atresia of the bile ducts). Families in which several members are mentally defective and have congenital cataracts without an abnormality in galactose metabolism have been described by Franceschetti and others (312).

The antenatal diagnosis of galactosemia can be made by assay of GALT activity on cultured amniocytes or chorionic villi (315).

Treatment

When milk is withdrawn and lactose-free products such as Nutramigen or Prosobee are substituted, gastrointestinal symptoms are rapidly relieved and normal growth resumes. The progression of cirrhosis is arrested, and in 35% of patients, the cataracts disappear (307). Because infants have developed hypoglycemia when first placed on a galactose-free diet, it might be useful to add some glucose to the formula.

The propensity of galactosemic neonates for *E. coli* sepsis requires securing cultures of blood, urine, and CSF and treating against this organism until the test results are negative (309). In the larger series of Waggoner and coworkers, sepsis was suspected in 30% of neonates and confirmed in 10% (314).

Recommendations for the management of infants and children with galactosemia have been published by Walter and coworkers (315). Maintenance of the galactose-free diet and avoidance of milk and milk products is recommended until at least after puberty. In several children who returned to a milk-containing diet before puberty, cataracts flared up. Even after that age, some continue to be sensitive to milk products and prefer to avoid them. Intermittent monitoring of erythrocyte galactose-1-phosphate levels has been suggested. Even children with well-controlled galactosemia have elevated galactose-1-phosphate levels. Endogenous formation of galactose-1-phosphate from glucose-1-phosphate by way of the epimerase reaction (see Fig. 1.8) is believed to be responsible.

The long-term outlook for galactosemic patients is not as good as was initially believed, even when the diet is carefully monitored. A number of cases of progressive cerebellar ataxia and extrapyramidal movement disorders have been reported (316,317). In the series of Waggoner and colleagues, cerebellar deficits were seen in 18% (314); in the series of Kaufman and colleagues, the incidence was 27% (317). The cause for this syndrome is unclear, and MRI studies on patients with this syndrome do not differ from those without it (317). Rogers and Segal postulated that the syndrome results from an endogenous product of galactose-1-phosphate from UDP-glucose via the epimerase reaction (318). Another possibility is that a deficiency of UDP-galactose could limit the formation of cerebral glycoproteins and galactolipids. Administration of uridine, which has been suggested to prevent these complications, has not been effective (319).

Cognitive deficits are common. In 70% of galactosemic children treated from birth, the IQ was 90 or higher; however, approximately 50% of the youngsters had significant visual and perceptual deficits, and 33% had EEG abnormalities (320). Studies confirm that most patients have cognitive deficits in one or more areas. Verbal dyspraxia occurs in some 62%. Patients are unable to program their speech musculature and also show frequent disturbances in speech rhythm. Receptive language is normal (317,321). In addition, there appears to be a progressive decline in IQ with age (314,317). Neither IQ scores nor the presence of the dyspractic speech disorder are highly related with the age at which therapy is initiated or quality of control (314). Instead, cognitive and language deficits are likely to result from the *in utero* formation of potentially neurotoxic galactose-1-phosphate and the continued generation of galactose from glucose via UDP-galactose-4-epimerase (see Fig. 1.8) (300,322).

Two other defects of galactose metabolism have been recognized. A deficiency of galactokinase (see Fig. 1.8) is the more common (OMIM 230200). Cataracts are present in most patients and pseudotumor cerebri has been seen occasionally. The outlook in terms of mental function is better than for patients with galactosemia, and most appear to be normal (323). A very rare disorder, generalized deficiency of epimerase (OMIM 230350), the enzyme that converts UDP-glucose to UDP-galactose (see Fig. 1.8), can result in galactosuria, failure to thrive, sensorineural deafness, dysmorphic features, and mental retardation (324).

Fructose Intolerance (OMIM 229600)

Fructose intolerance, as distinguished from benign fructosuria, was first described by Chambers and Pratt in 1956 (325). The condition is transmitted as an autosomal recessive trait and is the consequence of a deficiency in the principal hepatic aldolase, aldolase B (326). The gene coding for aldolase B is located on the long arm of chromosome 9 (9q21.3–q22.2), and more than 25 mutations have been documented (327).

As a consequence of the metabolic defect, ingested fructose (or sucrose, which is split into fructose and glucose) is converted to fructose-1-phosphate, which accumulates in tissues and is responsible for renal and hepatic damage. Additionally, plasma lactate and urate levels increase (328). A glucagon-unresponsive hypoglycemia results from the blockage of glycogenolysis by fructose-1-phosphate at the point of phosphorylase and from the interruption of gluconeogenesis by the phosphate ester at the level of the mutant fructose-1,6-diphosphate aldolase.

The main pathologic abnormality is hepatic cirrhosis similar to that seen in galactosemia. The brain shows retarded myelination and neuronal shrinkage attributable to hypoglycemia (329). An associated coagulation defect can induce intracerebral hemorrhage.

Hereditary fructose intolerance is relatively rare in the United States and far more common in Europe. In Switzerland, the gene frequency is 1 in 80, and in Great Britain, 1 in 250 (328). The condition manifests by intestinal disturbances, poor weight gain, and attacks of hypoglycemia after fructose ingestion. Transient icterus, hepatic enlargement, fructosuria, albuminuria, and aminoaciduria follow intake of large quantities of fructose. Mild mental deficiency is frequent, and there may be a flaccid quadriparesis (330). Heterozygotes are predisposed to gout (328).

Diagnosis is based in part on the patient's clinical history, on the presence of a urinary reducing substance, and on the results of an intravenous fructose tolerance test (0.25 g/kg), a procedure that should be performed carefully under monitored conditions. An oral tolerance test is contraindicated in view of the ensuing severe gastrointestinal and systemic symptoms (331). For confirmation, a jejunal or liver biopsy with determination of fructose-1-phosphate aldolase levels is necessary (332). MRS has been used to confirm the diagnosis and to determine heterozygosity (328).

Other causes of increased fructose excretion include impaired liver function and fructosuria, which is an asymptomatic metabolic variant caused by a deficiency of fructokinase (OMIM 299800).

Treatment of hereditary fructose intolerance is relatively simple but is needed lifelong. It involves avoiding the intake of fruits and cane or beet sugar (sucrose).

Other Disorders of Carbohydrate Metabolism

Fructose-1,6-diphosphatase deficiency (OMIM 229700) is a rare disorder that manifests during the neonatal period with hyperventilation, hyperbilirubinemia, seizures, coma, and laboratory evidence of ketosis, hypoglycemia, and lactic acidosis (333). The diagnosis is difficult, and a variety of other causes for intermittent neonatal hypoglycemia must be excluded. The enzyme defect can be demonstrated by liver biopsy (334).

Of the various forms of mellituria seen in infancy and childhood, the most common are caused by the increased excretion of a single sugar, predominantly glucose. Isolated lactosuria and fructosuria are encountered also. Lactosuria usually is explained on the basis of congenital lactose intolerance or secondary lactose intolerance associated with enteritis, celiac disease, and cystic fibrosis. Essential pentosuria, one of the original inborn errors of metabolism described by Garrod, is a result of the excretion of L-xylulose. Ribosuria occurs in Duchenne muscular dystrophy, probably as the result of tissue breakdown. Sucrosuria has been reported in association with hiatal hernia and other intestinal disturbances.

A mixed-sugar excretion also can be seen in acute infections, liver disease, and gastroenteritis.

Glucose Transporter 1 Deficiency Syndrome (De Vivo Disease) (OMIM 606777)

This condition was first described in 1991 by De Vivo and coworkers (335). It is transmitted as an autosomal dominant trait, and, as the name indicates, results from a mutation in the gene for the glucose 1 transporter (GLUT 1). De Vivo and coworkers reviewed the molecular genetics of this condition (336).

The clinical picture is marked by the early onset of a seizure disorder accompanied by delayed development, the acquisition of microcephaly, incoordination, and spasticity. Other paroxysmal events have been observed. These include intermittent ataxia, confusion, or somnolence. Patients with intermittent ataxia and mental retardation in the absence of seizures have been reported, as have opsoclonic eye movements and a complex motor disorder with elements of ataxia, dystonia, and spasticity (336,337).

The presence of hypoglycorrhachia in the presence of normal blood sugar is diagnostic. Neuroimaging studies are generally unremarkable. In about 50% of patients the EEG demonstrates generalized spike or polyspike and wave discharges. Diffuse or focal slowing has also been observed. An erythrocyte glucose uptake study will confirm the diagnosis (338).

Treatment by means of the ketogenic diet or medium-chain triglycerides has been fairly effective. Ketone bodies are transported across the blood–brain barrier by monocarboxylic transporters and can be used as an alternative brain fuel. Barbiturates and caffeine, which inhibit glucose transport across the blood–brain barrier, should be avoided. α-Lipoic acid supplementation may be beneficial (336).

ORGANIC ACIDURIAS

A number of disorders of intermediary metabolism are manifested by intermittent episodes of vomiting, lethargy, acidosis, and the excretion of large amounts of organic acids. Even though the enzymatic lesions responsible are not related, they are grouped together because they are detected by analysis of urinary organic acids.

Propionic Acidemia (Ketotic Hyperglycinemia) (OMIM 232000; 232050)

Propionic acidemia, the first of the organic acidurias to be described, is characterized by intermittent episodes of vomiting, lethargy, and ketosis. Hsia and coworkers demonstrated a defect in propionyl-CoA carboxylase, a biotin-dependent enzyme that converts propionyl-CoA to methylmalonyl-CoA (339). The enzyme consists of two polypeptides, α and β, coded by genes (*PCCA* and *PCCB*) that are located on chromosomes 13 and 3, respectively. Considerable genetic heterogeneity exists, with defects in each of the two structural genes encoding the two subunits of propionyl-CoA carboxylase. Most of these are single-base substitutions (340). The clinical presentation of the two forms appears to be comparable; the original family had the *PCCA* type of propionic acidemia.

As a consequence of the metabolic block, not only is serum propionate elevated, but also several propionate derivatives accumulate (341). Hyperammonemia is frequent, probably as a consequence of an inhibition by the accumulating organic acids of *N*-acetylglutamate synthetase, the enzyme that forms *N*-acetylglutamate, a stimulator of carbamoyl-phosphate synthetase (see Fig. 1.6) (342). The severity of hyperammonemia appears to be proportional to the serum propionate levels (343). The mechanism for hyperglycinemia in this and in several of the other organic acidurias has not been fully elucidated. It appears likely, however, that propionate interferes with one of the components of the mitochondrial glycine-cleavage system.

In the classic form of the disease, symptoms start shortly after birth (344). In other cases, they might not become apparent until late infancy or childhood and are precipitated by upper respiratory or gastrointestinal infections. Marked intellectual retardation and a neurologic picture of a mixed pyramidal and extrapyramidal lesion ultimately become apparent (345). A less severe form of the disease is fairly common in Japan. It presents with mild mental retardation and extrapyramidal symptoms. It results from a mutation in *PCCB* (346). As a rule, attacks are precipitated by ingestion of proteins and various amino acids, notably leucine. In addition to ketoacidosis, hyperammonemia, persistent neutropenia, and thrombocytopenia occur. Propionic acidemia is seen in all patients, and plasma and urinary glycine levels are increased

(347). In some patients, MRI shows increased signal in the caudate nucleus and putamen on T2-weighted images (348).

Structural abnormalities in the brain are similar to those seen in PKU and other diseases of amino acid metabolism, namely retarded myelination and a spongy degeneration of gray and white matter (349,350).

Treatment involves a diet low in valine, isoleucine, threonine, and methionine, with carnitine supplementation (60 to 200 mg/kg per day). A commercial formula is available. A few patients have responded to biotin. Patients generally require a gastrostomy tube because of poor feeding. Courses of metronidazole have been used to decrease the amount of propionate produced by anaerobic intestinal bacteria. Cardiomyopathy and arrhythmias can further complicate the disease.

Propionic acidemia is biochemically and clinically distinct from familial glycinuria (OMIM 138500), a condition in which serum glycine levels are normal and the nervous system is unaffected (351). It also should be distinguished from iminoglycinuria and from nonketotic hyperglycinemia. Isovaleric acidemia and α-ketothiolase deficiency also can present with episodes of ketoacidosis and hyperglycinemia.

Methylmalonic Aciduria (OMIM 251000)

The classic presentation of MMA is one of acute neonatal ketoacidosis, with lethargy, vomiting, and profound hypotonia. Several genetic entities have been recognized. In all, the conversion of methylmalonyl-CoA to succinyl-CoA is impaired, a result either of a defect in the mitochondrial apoenzyme, methylmalonyl-CoA mutase, or in the biosynthesis, transport, or absorption of its adenosylcobalamin cofactor (352). The gene for methylmalonyl-CoA mutase has been cloned, and more than two dozen mutations have been recognized (353).

Approximately one-third of patients with MMA have the classic form of the disease (352). In this condition, the defect is localized to the apoenzyme methylmalonyl-CoA mutase. In the majority of patients, the enzyme is totally inactive, whereas in other patients with MMA, the apoenzyme defect is partial (354). In the remaining patients with MMA, constituting approximately 50% of a series of 45 patients assembled by Matsui and her group (352), dramatic biochemical improvement occurs with the administration of adenosylcobalamin, the cofactor for the mutase. In most of the responders, synthesis of adenosylcobalamin is blocked at the formation of the cofactor from cobalamin (cobalamin adenosyltransferase deficiency) or at one of the mitochondrial cobalamin reductases. In a small proportion of patients, the defect appears to involve adenosylcobalamin and methylcobalamin. Because the latter serves as cofactor for the conversion of homocysteine to methionine, children with this particular defect demonstrate homocystinuria and MMA (355). The various disorders in cobalamin absorption, transport, and use were reviewed by Shevell and Rosenblatt (356).

As ascertained by routine screening of newborns, a large proportion of infants with persistent MMA are asymptomatic and experience normal growth and mental development (357). These children may represent the mildest form of partial mutase deficiency. Small elevations in MMA and homocystine are also seen with maternal vitamin B_{12} deficiency, particularly common in vegans.

Infants suffering from the classic form of the disease (absence of the apoenzyme methylmalonyl-CoA mutase) become symptomatic during the first week of life, usually after the onset of protein feedings. The clinical picture is highlighted by hypotonia, lethargy, recurrent vomiting, and profound metabolic acidosis (352). Survivors of the initial crisis have recurrent episodes with intercurrent illnesses and often have spastic quadriparesis, dystonia, and severe developmental delay. When the apoenzyme defect is partial, patients generally become symptomatic in late infancy or childhood and are not as severely affected (354). MRI studies of the brain resemble those obtained on patients with propionic acidemia with delayed myelination and changes in the basal ganglia (358).

Pathologic changes within the brain also involve the basal ganglia predominantly, with neuronal loss and gliosis, or spongy changes in the globus pallidus and putamen. Abnormal laboratory findings in the classic form of MMA include ketoacidosis and an increased amount of methylmalonic acid in blood and urine. Hyperglycinemia is seen in 70% of classic cases, and hyperammonemia is seen in 75% (352). Hematologic abnormalities, notably leukopenia, anemia, and thrombocytopenia, are encountered in approximately 50% of the cases. These abnormalities result from the growth inhibition of marrow stem cells by methylmalonic acid (359).

Almost all of the survivors have some degree of neurologic impairment. This is in part the consequence of diminished protein tolerance and frequent bouts of metabolic decompensation. MMA is nephrotoxic leading to renal failure in the second decade of life (360). Late-onset patients fare better, and some have relatively minor neuromotor and mental handicaps (361).

At least four disorders of cobalamin absorption and transport and seven disorders of cobalamin utilization exist. In two of the cobalamin utilization defects, the output of methylmalonic acid is increased (cblA, cblB); in three, MMA and homocystinuria occur (cblC, cblD, and cblF); and in two, there is an increased excretion of homocystine (cblE and cblG) (356).

The clinical course of children experiencing a cofactor deficiency is not as severe as that of children with an apoenzyme deficiency, and nearly 60% of patients with the most common cobalamin utilization defect, cobalamin reductase deficiency (cblC), do not become symptomatic until after age 1 month (352). The clinical picture is variable (362). The majority of children present in infancy or during the first year of life with failure to thrive, developmental delay, and megaloblastic anemia. In others, the disease develops during adolescence, with dementia and a myelopathy (363,364). A progressive retinal degeneration has been observed (365). Pathologic findings in the cblC defect include a subacute combined degeneration of the spinal cord and a thrombotic microangiopathy (366).

The diagnosis of MMA can be suspected when urine treated with diazotized *p*-nitroaniline turns emerald green. MMA also is seen in pernicious anemia and vitamin B_{12} deficiency and in the infantile form of mitochondrial depletion syndrome (see Chapter 2). Cultured fibroblasts are used for the further delineation of the various metabolic defects responsible for MMA.

Infants with MMA should first be tested for vitamin B_{12} responsiveness (1 to 2 mg of cyanocobalamin or preferably hydroxycobalamin intramuscularly daily for several days). In those who fail to respond, a low-protein diet (0.75 to 1.2 g protein/kg per day) with the addition of L-carnitine is required (367). Vitamin B_{12}-responsive patients are treated with oral (1 mg/day) or intramuscular cobalamin (1 mg every 3 weeks), supplemented with L-carnitine (50 to 200 mg/kg per day) (369). In the child who does not respond to hydroxycobalamin, a trial of deoxyadenosylcobalamin is indicated, but the substance is hard to obtain (367). In children with the various cofactor deficiencies, the biochemical and clinical response to therapy is gratifying (362,368). Even an occasional patient with the apoenzyme deficiency can improve with therapy. Hepatic transplantation has been used in some of the more severe cases of vitamin B_{12}-nonresponsive methylmalonic aciduria. It appears that the procedure does not prevent neurologic dysfunction or progressive renal failure (369).

Isovaleric Aciduria (OMIM 243500)

A striking odor of urine, perspiration, and exhaled air, resembling stale perspiration, is characteristic of patients with isovaleric aciduria. The enzymatic lesion in this condition has been localized to isovaleryl-CoA dehydrogenase (see Fig. 1.5, step 3), a mitochondrial enzyme (370). The gene for this enzyme has been mapped to the long arm of chromosome 15 (15q12–q15) and has been cloned (371). As a consequence of the enzymatic defect, serum isovaleric acid concentrations are several hundred times normal, and the administration of L-leucine produces a sustained increase in isovaleric acid levels.

In addition to abnormally elevated concentrations of isovaleric acid in blood and urine, moderate hyperammonemia occurs. This is particularly evident during the neonatal period. Large quantities of isovaleryl glycine are excreted during acute episodes of acidosis and while the patient is in remission. During attacks, 3-hydroxyisovaleric acid, 4-hydroxyisovaleric acid and its oxidation products (methylsuccinic acid and methaconic acids), and isovaleryl glucuronide are excreted also (372). The acidosis seen during an attack appears to result from an accumulation of ketone bodies rather than from the presence of isovaleric acid.

Two clinical phenotypes are seen: an acute and commonly fatal neonatal form in which infants develop recurrent acidosis and coma during the first week of life, and a chronic form with recurrent attacks of vomiting, lethargy, ataxia, and ketoacidosis (373). Acute and chronic forms can be present in the same family. No correlation exists between the amount of residual enzyme activity and the clinical form of the disease. Instead, the severity of the disease appears to be a function of the effectiveness with which isovaleryl-CoA is detoxified to its glycine derivative (374). Attacks are triggered by infections or excessive protein intake. Pancytopenia is not uncommon; it is caused by arrested maturation of hematopoietic precursors (375).

Treatment involves a low-protein diet (1.5 to 2 g/kg per day) with L-carnitine (50 to 100 mg/kg per day). Glycine (250 mg/kg per day) has been used instead of carnitine. Glycine and carnitine aid in the mitochondrial detoxification of isovaleryl-CoA (374). For infants who survive the neonatal period, the outlook for normal intellectual development is fairly good, and 4 of 9 patients treated by Berry and coworkers at Children's Hospital of Philadelphia had IQs of greater than 95 (374).

A clinical picture resembling isovaleric aciduria develops after intoxication with achee, the fruit that induces Jamaican vomiting sickness and that contains hypoglycin, an inhibitor of several acyl-CoA dehydrogenases, including isovaleryl-CoA dehydrogenase (376).

Glutaric Acidurias

Several completely different genetic defects have been grouped under the term glutaric aciduria.

Glutaric Aciduria Type I (OMIM 231670)

This is a recessive disorder with an incidence of approximately 1 in 30,000. It is caused by a defect in the gene for glutaryl-CoA dehydrogenase. Biochemically, the condition is marked by the excretion of large amounts of glutaric, 3-hydroxyglutaric, and glutaconic acids. The clinical picture is protean, and the disorder is frequently undiagnosed or misdiagnosed. In approximately 20% of patients, glutaric aciduria I takes the form of a neurodegenerative condition commencing during the latter part of the first year of life and characterized by hypotonia, dystonia, choreoathetosis, and seizures (377). In most of the remaining patients, development is normal for as long as 2 years of age, and then, after what appears to be an infectious, an encephalitic, or a Reye syndrome–like illness or following routine immunization, neurologic deterioration occurs (378,379). In yet other cases, the clinical picture

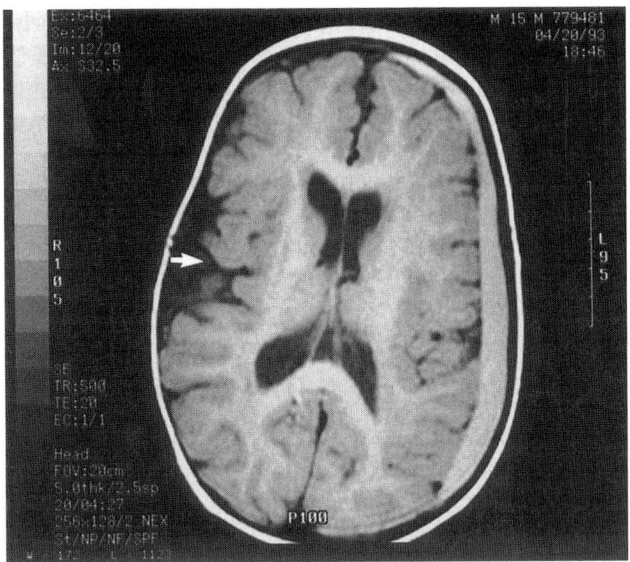

FIGURE 1.9. Glutaric aciduria I. Magnetic resonance imaging study. This T1-weighted image demonstrates an enlarged operculum on the right (*arrow*) and an extensive left subdural hematoma.

resembles extrapyramidal cerebral palsy (380). Rare cases remain asymptomatic. Macrocephaly is noted in 70% of cases (381). Lack of appetite, sleeplessness, and profuse sweating also is noted, as is hypoglycemia (382,383). No molecular basis for the clinical variability exists, and the severity of the clinical phenotype seems to be closely linked to the development of encephalopathic crises rather than to residual enzyme activity or genotype (384).

Neuroimaging shows frontotemporal cortical atrophy giving what has been termed a bat wing appearance. This is often accompanied by increased signal in the basal ganglia on T2-weighted images and caudate atrophy. Bilateral subdural hematomas have also been described (Fig. 1.9). When these are accompanied by retinal hemorrhages, an erroneous diagnosis of child abuse frequently is made (390).

Neuropathology shows temporal and frontal lobe hypoplasia, degeneration of the putamen and globus pallidus, mild status spongiosus of white matter, and heterotopic neurons in cerebellum (385). It is not clear why so much of the damage is localized to the basal ganglia. Kolker and coworkers postulated that 3-hydroxyglutaric acid, which is structurally related to glutamic acid, induces excitotoxic cell damage, and that in addition 3-hydroxyglutaric acid and glutaric acid modulate glutamatergic and gamma-aminobutyric acid (GABA)-ergic neurotransmission. Secondary amplification loops could also potentiate the neurotoxic properties of these organic acids (386).

A low-protein, high-calorie diet supplemented with a formula lacking lysine and tryptophan and containing carnitine has sometimes prevented further deterioration, but in the Scandinavian series of Kyllerman and colleagues almost all patients were left with a severe dystonic-dyskinetic disorder (387). The experience of Hoffmann and coworkers was similar (381). Strauss and colleagues, who worked with the disease in the Pennsylvania Amish population, however, found that good dietary care can reduce the incidence of basal ganglia injury to 35% (388).

Glutaric Aciduria Type II (Multiple Acyl-CoA Dehydrogenase Deficiency) (MADD) (OMIM 231680)

In this condition the defect has been localized to one of three genes involved in the mitochondrial β-oxidation of fatty acids: those coding for the α and β subunits of the electron transfer flavoprotein (ETF) and that coding for the electron transfer flavoprotein dehydrogenase (389,390). The clinical picture of GA II due to the different defects appears to be nondistinguishable; each defect can lead to a range of mild or severe cases, depending presumably on the location and nature of the intragenic lesion, that is, mutation, in each case. As a consequence of the enzyme deficiency there is increased excretion not only of glutaric acid, but also of other organic acids, including lactic, ethylmalonic, isobutyric, and isovaleric acids.

The heterogeneous clinical features of patients with MADD fall into three classes (391): a neonatal-onset form with congenital anomalies (type I), a neonatal-onset form without congenital anomalies (type II), and a late-onset form (type III).

Glutaric aciduria II can present in the neonatal period with an overwhelming and generally fatal metabolic acidosis coupled with hypoglycemia, acidemia, and a cardiomyopathy. Affected infants can have an odor of sweaty feet. As a rule, there is good correlation between the severity of the metabolic block, rather than its location and the severity of the disease, with null mutations producing the development of congenital anomalies and the presence of a minute amount of enzymatic activity allowing the development of type II disease (392).

Dysmorphic features are prominent in approximately one-half of cases (393). They include macrocephaly, a large anterior fontanel, a high forehead, a flat nasal bridge, and malformed ears. This appearance is reminiscent of Zellweger syndrome (Fig. 1.10). Neuroimaging discloses agenesis of the cerebellar vermis and hypoplastic temporal lobes (394). The neonatal-onset forms are usually fatal and are characterized by severe nonketotic hypoglycemia, metabolic acidosis, multisystem involvement, and excretion of large amounts of fatty acid- and amino acid-derived metabolites.

Standard treatment consists of a high-carbohydrate, low-fat and protein diet supplemented with carnitine. Van Hove and coworkers suggested that this condition be treated with D,L-3-hydroxybutyrate (430 to 700 mg/kg

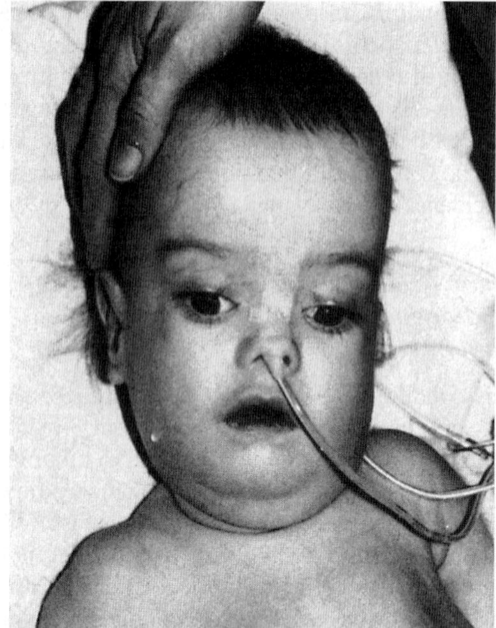

A

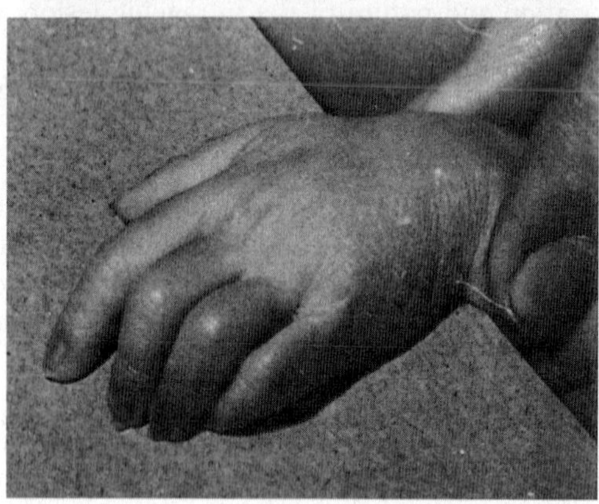

B

FIGURE 1.10. Zellweger syndrome. **A:** Typical facies with high forehead and flat facies. Redundant skin of the neck is seen. (Courtesy of the late Dr. H. Zellweger, University of Iowa, Iowa City, IA.) **B:** Hand, demonstrating camptodactyly of third, fourth, and fifth fingers. (Courtesy of Dr. J. M. Opitz, Shodair Children's Hospital, Helena, MT.)

per day). In their experience this treatment resulted in improvement of neurologic function and cardiac contractility (395).

Symptoms and age at presentation of late-onset MADD (type III) are highly variable and characterized by recurrent episodes of lethargy, vomiting, hypoglycemia, metabolic acidosis, and hepatomegaly often preceded by metabolic stress. Muscle involvement in the form of pain, weakness, and lipid storage myopathy also occurs. The organic aciduria in patients with the late-onset form of MADD is often intermittent and only evident during periods of illness or catabolic stress. Other cases present in early childhood with progressive spastic ataxia and high signal intensity on T2-weighted MRI in supratentorial white matter, a picture mimicking a leukodystrophy (398).

The neuropathologic picture is marked by diffuse gliosis of cerebrum, brainstem, and cerebellum, with foci of leukomalacia and striatal degeneration (393,397).

Some infants with glutaric aciduria II respond dramatically to riboflavin (100 mg three times a day). This riboflavin-responsive multiple acyl-CoA dehydrogenase deficiency may be identical to ethylmalonic-adipic aciduria (396,398,399).

Glutaric Aciduria Type III (OMIM 231690)

This condition is the result of a defect of peroxisomal glutaryl CoA oxidase. It results in a persistent isolated glutaric acid excretion, but the phenotype of this disorder is unknown, and it may well represent a benign inborn error (400).

The other, rarer organic acidurias are summarized in Table 1.15.

DISORDERS OF FATTY ACID OXIDATION

Up to 18 defects of hepatic mitochondrial fatty acid oxidation have been recognized, including eight defects of the β-oxidation cycle (401,402). Affected patients are unable to use fatty acids derived from adipose tissue or diet for energy production or hepatic ketone synthesis. Because fatty acids are the principal energy source during fasting, infants rapidly decompensate in the neonatal period or during a febrile illness. In addition to the acute metabolic decompensation that results when infants are fasted, resulting in a rapid evolution of seizures and coma, the clinical presentation of most of these conditions is marked by episodes of a nonketotic or hypoketotic hypoglycemia. The esterified-to-free-carnitine ratio is increased, and generally there is hypocarnitinemia. When the enzyme defect is limited to muscle, it can present with cardiomyopathy, muscle weakness, and myoglobinuria. These symptoms are features of defects in the transport of fatty acids into mitochondria and are covered in Chapter 2. Disorders of fatty acid oxidation are uncommon, and collectively, their incidence in Great Britain has been estimated at 1 in 5,000 live births (403).

Medium-Chain Acyl-CoA Dehydrogenase (MCAD) Deficiency (OMIM 201450)

The most common of the disorders of fatty acid oxidation is a defect involving medium-chain acyl-CoA dehydrogenase (MCAD). The incidence of this entity varies among

TABLE 1.14 Fatty Acid Oxidation Disorders

Disorder	Reference
Carnitine Cycle	
Carnitine transport defect	Stanley et al. (410)
Carnitine palmitoyl transferase I	Haworth et al. (411)
Carnitine acylcarnitine translocase	Stanley et al. (412)
Carnitine palmitoyl transferase II	Land et al. (413)
Mitochondrial β-Oxidation	
Medium-chain CoA acyldehydrogenase deficiency	Iafolla et al. (404)
Long-chain CoA acyldehydrogenase deficiency	Treem et al. (414)
Short-chain CoA acyldehydrogenase deficiency	Bhala et al. (415)
Very long chain CoA acyldehydrogenase deficiency	Souri et al. (416), Andresen et al. (417)
Short-chain 3-hydroxyacyl CoA dehydrogenase deficiency	Bennett et al. (418)
Long-chain hydroxy acyl Co-A deficiency	Spiekerkoetter et al. (419)

population groups. In whites, it has been estimated to be between 1 in 6,400 and 1 in 23,000 live births; thus, it appears to be almost as common as PKU (404–406).

Because MCAD is active over the range of C4 to C12 carbons, its deficiency permits fatty acid oxidation to progress only up to the point at which the carbon chain has been reduced to 12 (402). A single point mutation in the gene is responsible for the condition in more than 90% of symptomatic white patients. This mutation results in the substitution of glutamine for lysine in the MCAD precursor. This disrupts folding of the mature form and its assembly in mitochondria, with subsequent disappearance of the mutant MCAD.

Clinical symptoms usually develop during the first year of life and are characterized by episodes of hypoketotic hypoglycemia triggered by fasting or infections. These episodes result in lethargy, vomiting, and altered consciousness. In the experience of Rinaldo and colleagues, mortality of the first such episode of metabolic decompensation is 59% (407). In the series of Iafolla and coworkers, 36% of patients had sudden cardiorespiratory arrest (404). Although the last presentation resembles that of sudden infant death syndrome (SIDS), Miller and colleagues were unable to find any homozygotes for the glutamine-to-lysine mutation leading to MCAD deficiency in 67 SIDS babies (408), and Boles and colleagues found an incidence of only 0.6% among cases diagnosed as SIDS (409). In the latter study, another 0.6% of SIDS cases were believed to have glutaric aciduria II (409). The general practice of most coroners is to evaluate all cases of SIDS for an underlying metabolic disorder using blood, bile, vitreous humor, or tissue.

The MCAD deficiency is treated by supplemental L-carnitine, a low-fat diet, and avoidance of fasting, which rapidly initiates a potentially fatal hypoglycemia, which must be corrected by the prompt institution of glucose. The efficacy of supplemental L-carnitine is unclear. On follow-up of symptomatic patients, a significant proportion of survivors have global developmental delays, attention deficit disorder, and language deficits (404). Detection by tandem mass spectrometry newborn screening and early treatment can prevent this outcome.

Other Disorders of Fatty Acid Oxidation

Very Long Chain Acyl-CoA Deficiency (VLCAD) (OMIM 201475)

The other disorders of fatty acid β-oxidation are much less common. They are summarized in Table 1.14. In VLCAD the defect is at the first step of the fatty acid β-oxidation cycle. Clinically, failure of long-chain fatty acid β-oxidation leads to hypoketotic hypoglycemia associated with coma, liver dysfunction, skeletal myopathy, and hypertrophic cardiomyopathy. Patients are unable to metabolize fatty acids with 12 to 18 carbons (420–423). Three clinical forms have been recognized: a severe form with early onset and a high incidence of cardiomyopathy; a milder, childhood-onset form; and an adult form with rhabdomyolysis and myoglobinuria (422–424). The clinical picture appears to correlate with the amount of residual enzyme activity (417). VLCAD can be effectively treated with avoidance of fasting and a diet low in long-chain fats supplemented with medium-chain triglyceride oil and carnitine. Uncooked cornstarch at night can be added to the regimen (425).

Short-Chain Acyl-CoA Dehydrogenase Deficiency (SCAD) (OMIM 201470)

The short-chain acyl dehydrogenase is active from four to six carbons, and SCAD infants excrete large amounts of butyrate, ethylmalonate, methylmalonate, and methylsuccinate (426,427). The clinical picture is complex. Some patients develop acute acidosis and muscle weakness early in life; others develop a multicore myopathy in adolescence or in their adult years, and yet others remain clinically well (427,428). Whereas patients with MCAD and long-chain acyl-CoA deficiency tend to develop hypoketotic hypoglycemia, patients with short-chain acyl-CoA dehydrogenase deficiency may not have hypoglycemia. Most symptomatic patients have hypotonia, hyperactivity, and developmental delay. The condition can be intermittently symptomatic. In cases detected by newborn screening, care must be taken to determine whether the child is truly deficient and thus potentially at risk or merely harbors a common polymorphism in SCAD (429,430).

Long-Chain Hydroxy Acyl Co-A Deficiency (LCHAD) (OMIM 143450)

The mitochondrial trifunctional protein (MTP) is a multienzyme complex that catalyzes three of the four chain-shortening reactions in the β-oxidation of long-chain fatty acids. It is composed of four alpha subunits harboring long-chain enoyl-CoA hydratase and long-chain L-3-hydroxyacyl-CoA dehydrogenase and four beta subunits carrying the long-chain 3-ketoacyl-CoA dehydrogenase. Mutation in either subunit can result in reduced activity of all three enzymes.

Different phenotypes have been reported. There is a severe and generally fatal neonatal presentation with cardiomyopathy, Reye-like symptoms; a hepatic form with recurrent hypoketotic hypoglycemia; and a late-onset myopathic form with recurrent myoglobinuria (419,430a).

Defects in branched-chain acyl-CoA dehydrogenation also have been recognized. They are listed in Table 1.15.

The diagnosis of these disorders depends on the presence of the various dicarboxylic acids in urine, and more recently by the application of tandem mass spectrometry. The pros and cons of expanded neonatal screening to include the disorders of fatty acid oxidation are discussed by Dezateux (431).

Disorders of Biotin Metabolism

Four biotin-dependent enzymes have been described. All are carboxylases: propionyl-CoA carboxylase, 3-methylcrontonyl-CoA carboxylase, pyruvate carboxylase, and acetyl-CoA carboxylase. The covalent binding of biotin to these enzymes is catalyzed by holocarboxylase synthetase. A significant proportion of infants with organic aciduria are found to have impaired function of all four of these biotin-containing carboxylases (multiple carboxylase deficiency, holocarboxylase synthetase deficiency, OMIM 253270) (432). Most patients diagnosed with this condition became symptomatic in early infancy with metabolic acidosis, ketosis, and an erythematous rash. High concentrations of the metabolites α-hydroxyisovalerate, α-methylcrotonylglycine, α-hydroxypropionate, methyl citrate, and lactate are excreted in urine, which acquires a distinctive odor. The condition is caused by a deficiency in biotin holocarboxylase synthetase that is never complete (433). Symptoms are usually reversed by biotin, given in doses between 10 and 80 mg/day (434), but any permanent damage remains.

A second, more common disorder of biotin metabolism results from a deficiency of biotinidase (biotinidase deficiency, OMIM 253260). This condition is characterized by the onset of symptoms after the neonatal period, usually between ages 2 and 3 months. Biotinidase hydrolyzes the bond between biotin and lysine, the bound form in which biotin exists in the diet, and thus recycles biotin in the body (435). The enzyme deficiency can be complete or partial, with patients who have a partial deficiency tending to be asymptomatic unless stressed by prolonged infections (436). Considerable heterogeneity exists in profound biotinidase deficiency, and numerous mutations have been recognized (437). As ascertained by a screening program, the incidence of complete biotinidase deficiency in the United States is 1 in 166,000. The condition is rare in Asians (438).

Symptoms in complete biotinidase deficiency include lactic acidosis, alopecia, ataxia, spastic paraparesis, seizures, and an erythematous rash. Developmental delay soon becomes apparent. Hearing loss, acute vision loss, optic atrophy, and respiratory irregularities are seen in a significant proportion of cases (432,434). Plasma and urinary biotin levels are subnormal, and clinical and biochemical findings are rapidly reversed by the administration of oral biotin (5 to 10 mg/kg per day) (434). Children treated presymptomatically remain normal; those treated after becoming symptomatic are left with residual deficits, hearing impairment, optic atrophy, and developmental delay (439).

A unique familial syndrome of acute encephalopathy appearing between 1 and 14 years of age and marked by confusion and lethargy progressing to coma has been reported (440). The condition is associated with dystonia, chorea, rigidity, and, at times, opisthotonus and external ophthalmoplegia. It is completely reversible by the administration of biotin (5 to 10 mg/kg per day). MRI shows increased signal on T2-weighted images within the central part of the caudate and in parts or all of the putamen. Its cause is unknown, and all enzyme assay results have been normal.

Some of the other, even less commonly encountered organic acidurias are summarized in Table 1.15, together with any distinguishing clinical features. In most conditions, however, symptoms are indistinguishable; they consist mainly of episodic vomiting, lethargy, convulsions, and coma. Laboratory features include acidosis, hypoglycemia, hyperammonemia, and hyperglycinemia. The organic acidurias can be diagnosed during an acute episode by subjecting serum or, preferably, urine to organic acid chromatography. In addition, a marked reduction in plasma-free carnitine exists, accompanied by an increased ratio of esterified carnitine to free carnitine. These assays should be performed on any child with neurologic symptoms who has an associated metabolic acidosis or who is

TABLE 1.15 Some of the Rarer Organic Acidurias of Infancy and Childhood

Condition	Manifestations	Reference
2-Hydroxyglutaric aciduria	Mental deficiency, cerebellar dysfunction, brainstem and cerebellar atrophy, extrapyramidal signs, progressive macrocephaly	(441–443)
Glutathione synthetase deficiency (oxyprolinuria)	Neonatal acidosis, hemolytic anemia, retardation, seizures,	(444,445)
Succinic semialdehyde dehydrogenase deficiency (4-hydroxybutyric aciduria)	Severe, nonprogressive ataxia, hypotonia, mild mental retardation	(446–448)
3-Hydroxyisobutyric aciduria	Intracerebral calcifications, lissencephaly, polymicrogyria	(449,450)
3-Methylglutaconic aciduria (4 types)	Delayed speech, mental retardation, choreoathetosis, optic atrophy, cardiomyopathy	(451,452)
Ethylmalonic encephalopathy (also seen in SCAD deficiency, and multiple acyl CoA deficiency)	Encephalopathy, petechial lesions, CNS malformations, acrocyanosis, chronic diarrhea, excretion of ethylmalonic and methyl succinic acids	(453,454)
3-Hydroxy-3-methylglutaric aciduria	Fasting hypoglycemic coma	(455,456)
3-Hydroxy-2-methylbutyryl-CoA deficiency	Mental retardation, progressive deterioration in some, excretion of 3-hydroxy-2-methylbutyric acid, 2-ethylhydracrylic acid, tiglylglycine	(457,458)
Fumaric aciduria	Hypotonia, developmental delay, relative macrocephaly on MRI: large ventricles, open operculum, small brainstem structures	(459)

SCAD, short-chain acyl-CoA dehydrogenase deficiency; CNS, central nervous system; MRI, magnetic resonance imaging.

noted to have hyperglycinemia or hyperammonemia on routine biochemical analyses.

LYSOSOMAL DISORDERS

Lysosomes are subcellular organelles containing hydrolases with a low optimal pH (acid hydrolases) that catalyze the degradation of macromolecules. The lysosomal storage diseases, as first delineated by Hers (460), are characterized by an accumulation of undegraded macromolecules within lysosomes. The various groups are named according to the nature of the storage product. They include the glycogen storage diseases (glycogenoses), the mucopolysaccharidoses, the mucolipidoses, the glycoproteinoses, the sphingolipidoses, and the acid lipase deficiency diseases. The combined prevalence of all lysosomal storage diseases is 1 in 6,600 to 1 in 7,700 live births (461). The disease entities result from various single-gene mutations, with each of the enzyme defects induced by one of several different abnormalities on the genomic level (Table 1.16). The heterogeneity of the disorders is overwhelmingly complex (462). The enzyme itself can be defective, the result of a variety of single-base mutations or deletions that produce immunologically responsive or unresponsive enzyme proteins. The defect can impair glycosylation of the enzyme protein or cause a failure to generate a recognition marker that permits the enzyme to attach itself to the lysosomal membrane. Other mutations result in a lack of enzyme activator or substrate activator proteins or disrupt transport of the substrate across the lysosomal membrane. The various molecular lesions that lead to lysosomal storage are reviewed in a book edited by Platt and Walkley (463).

Glycogen Storage Diseases (Glycogenoses)

Of the various glycogenoses, only type II (Pompe disease) is a lysosomal disorder. For convenience, however, all the other glycogenoses are considered here as well.

Neuromuscular symptoms are seen in all but one of the eight types of glycogenoses (Table 1.17). Hypoglycemia is seen in types I, II, III, and VI and in the condition characterized by a defect in glycogen synthesis (type I_0). In type Ia, hypoglycemia is frequently severe enough to induce

TABLE 1.16 Molecular Lesions in the Lysosomal Storage Diseases

No immunologically detectable enzyme; includes conditions with grossly abnormal structural genes
Immunologically detectable, but catalytically inactive polypeptide; stability or transport of polypeptide abnormal
Enzyme catalytically active, but not segregated into lysosomes
Enzyme catalytically active, unstable in prelysosomal or lysosomal compartments
Lysosomal enzyme synthesized normally and transported into lysosomes; activator protein missing
Lysosomal enzyme deficiency results from intoxication with inhibitor of lysosomal enzyme[a]

[a]Not yet determined in humans, but inhibition of α-mannosidase by an alkaloid has been demonstrated.

Data from Kornfeld S. Trafficking of lysosomal enzymes in normal and disease states. *J Clin Invest* 1986;77:1–6. With permission.

TABLE 1.17 Enzymatically Defined Glycogenoses

Type	Defect	Structure of Glycogen	Involvement	Neuromuscular Symptoms
0	UDPG-glycogen transferase	Normal	Liver, muscle	Hypoglycemic seizures
Ia	Glucose-6-phosphatase complex (G6Pase)	Normal	Liver, kidney, intestinal mucosa	Hypoglycemic seizures, growth retardation, lactic acidemia
IaSP	Regulatory protein for glucose-6-phosphatase	Normal	Liver	Hypoglycemic seizures
Ib	Hepatic microsomal glucose-6-phosphate transport system	Normal	Liver	As Ia, but also impaired neutrophil function
Ic	Transporter of microsomal phosphate	Normal	Liver	Hypoglycemic seizures
Id	Defective microsomal glucose transport	Normal	Liver	As Ia
II	Lysosomal acid-α-1,4-glucosidase	Normal	Generalized	Progressive weakness
IIIa	Glycogen debrancher deficiency	Limit dextrin-like (short outer chains)	Muscle	Hypoglycemia, muscle weakness becomes more marked with age
IIIb	Glycogen debrancher deficiency	Limit dextrin-like	Liver	Hepatomegaly, hypoglycemia
IV	Brancher deficiency (amylo-1, 4–1,6-transglucosylase)	Amylopectin-like (long outer chains)	Generalized	Hypotonia, failure to thrive
V	Muscle phosphorylase	Normal	Muscle	Muscular cramps, weakness, atrophy (see Chapter 14)
VI	Liver phosphorylase	Normal	Liver, leukocytes	Hypoglycemia
VII	Phosphofructokinase	Normal	Muscle, erythrocytes	Muscular cramps, weakness (see Chapter 14)
VIII	Phosphorylase kinase	Normal	Liver	None
Danon disease	Lysosomal-associated membrane protein (LAMP-2)	Normal	Muscle, heart	Mild mental retardation

UDPG, uridine diphosphoglucose.

convulsions; indeed neuroimaging studies, EEGs, and psychometric tests indicate that many patients with glycogen storage disease type I have brain damage, probably the consequence of recurrent severe hypoglycemia (464).

A myopathy presenting with muscular stiffness and easy fatigability has been recognized in type IIIa glycogenosis. Undoubtedly, it is related to the accumulation of glycogen within muscle (465).

Hypotonia has been seen in the various type I glycogenoses and also has been the presenting symptom in type IV glycogenosis (466). Types V and VII glycogenoses are discussed in Chapter 15.

Type II Glycogenosis (Pompe Disease) (OMIM 232300)

Type II glycogenosis, first described by Pompe (467) in 1932, is a rare autosomal recessive disorder characterized by glycogen accumulation in the lysosomes of skeletal muscles, heart, liver, and CNS.

Molecular Genetics and Biochemical Pathology

Two groups of enzymes are involved in the degradation of glycogen. Phosphorylase initiates one set of breakdown reactions, cleaving glycogen to limit dextrin, which then is acted on by a debrancher enzyme (oligo-1,4-glucanotransferase and amyl-1,6-glucosidase) to yield a straight-chain polyglucosan, which is cleaved to the individual glucose units by phosphorylase. A second set of enzymes includes α-amylase, which cleaves glycogen to a series of oligosaccharides, and two α-1,4-glucosidases, which cleave the α-1,4 bonds of glycogen. There are two of these terminal glucosidases. One, located in the microsomal fraction, has a neutral pH optimum (neutral maltase); the other, found in lysosomes, has its maximum activity at an acid pH (3.5) (acid α-glucosidase). The gene for the latter enzyme has been mapped to the long arm of chromosome 17 (17q23) and has been cloned.

In type II glycogenosis, deficiency of lysosomal acid α-glucosidase leads to accumulation of lysosomal glycogen predominantly in liver, heart, and skeletal muscle (468). Like every other lysosomal protein, α-glucosidase is synthesized in a precursor form on membrane-bound polysomes and is sequestered in the lumen of the rough endoplasmic reticulum as a larger glycosylated precursor. Whereas the primary translational product of α-glucosidase mRNA is 100 kd, it becomes glycosylated to yield a 110-kd precursor, which in turn undergoes a posttranslational modification by phosphorylation to yield the mannose-6-phosphate recognition marker (469). Phosphorylation is an important step because formation of the marker distinguishes the lysosomal enzymes from

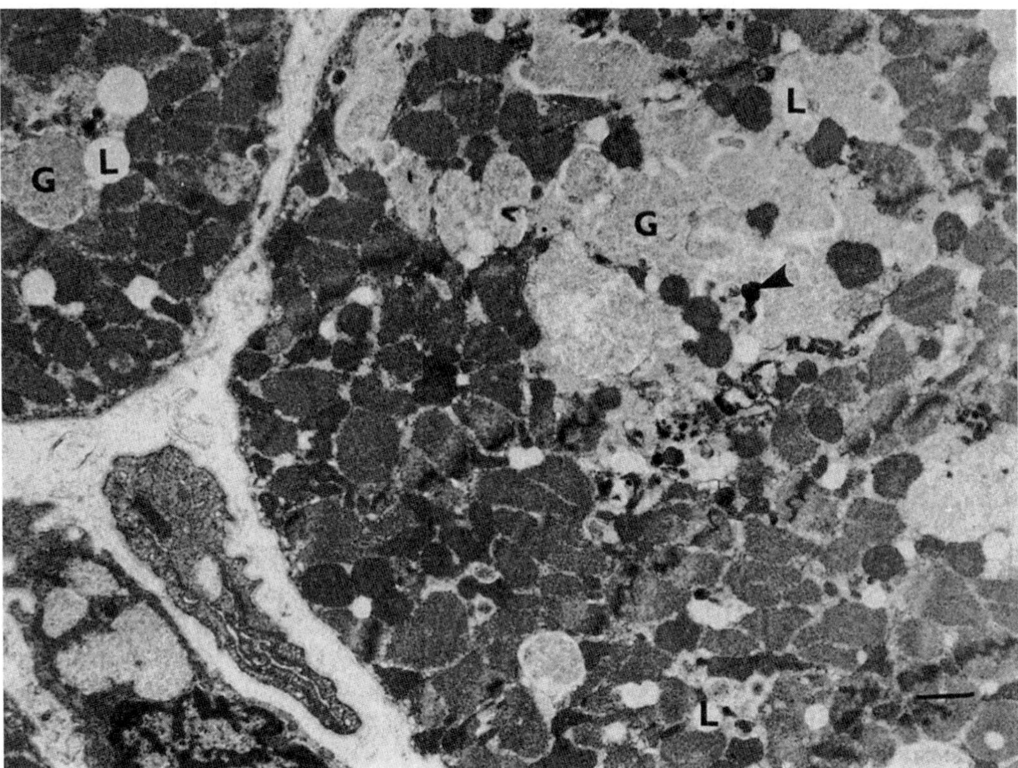

FIGURE 1.11. Glycogen storage disease type II (Pompe disease). Electron micrograph of several myofibers of various sizes demonstrating varying degrees of glycogen accumulations in sarcoplasm (***G***). Also seen are irregular electron-dense accumulations suggestive of lysosomes or autophagosomes (*arrowhead*). Large lipid droplets (***L***) appear between myofibrils (uranyl acetate and lead citrate, original magnification 9,600). (From Sarnat H. Lipid storage myopathy in infantile Pompe disease. *Arch Neurol* 1982;39:180. Copyright 1982, American Medical Association. With permission.)

secretory proteins and allows the lysosomal enzymes to be channeled to the lysosomes, to which they become attached by a membrane-bound mannose-phosphate–specific receptor. Additionally, the 110-kd precursor undergoes proteolytic processing to yield the two 76-kd and one 70-kd mature lysosomal enzyme polypeptides. With such a complex processing system, it is not surprising to encounter extensive clinical heterogeneity in glycogenosis II. Considerable genetic heterogeneity exists, and a variety of nonsense, frameshift, and missense mutations have been described. These result in partial or complete loss of enzyme activity. As a rule, the amount of residual enzyme activity correlates fairly well with the severity of the disease. Two relatively common mutations are responsible for a large proportion of the infantile form of Pompe disease. In whites, one of the more common mutations is a deletion of exon 18, which results in total loss of enzyme activity and the clinical manifestations of infantile glycogen storage disease (470,471).

Pathologic Anatomy

Glycogen can be deposited in virtually every tissue. The heart is globular, the enlargement being symmetric and primarily ventricular. In the infantile form, massive glycogen deposition occurs within the muscle fibers. In cross section, these appear with a central, clear area, giving a lacunate appearance. Glycogen also is deposited in striated muscle (particularly the tongue), in smooth muscle, and in the Schwann cells of peripheral nerves, kidney, and liver (Fig. 1.11). Ultrastructural studies of muscle show glycogen to be present in lysosomal sacs, where it occurs in conjunction with cytoplasmic degradation products. Additionally, it occurs free in cytoplasm (472). In the CNS, glycogen accumulates within neurons and in the extracellular substance (473). The anterior horn cells are affected predominantly, although deposits are seen in all parts of the neuraxis, including the cerebral cortex (474). Chemical analysis indicates an excess of glycogen in cerebral cortex and white matter and a deficiency in total phospholipid, cholesterol, and cerebroside. No evidence exists for primary demyelination.

Clinical Manifestations

Pompe disease can take one of three forms. In the classic, infantile form, the first symptoms usually appear by the second month of life. They include difficulty in feeding, with dyspnea and exhaustion interfering with sucking. Gradually, muscular weakness and impaired cardiac function become apparent. Marked cardiac enlargement is present at an early age. The heart appears globular on radiographic examination; murmurs are usually absent, but the heart tones have a poor quality and a gallop rhythm is often audible. The electrocardiogram shows characteristic high-voltage QRS complexes. Affected infants have poor muscle tone and few spontaneous movements, although the deep tendon reflexes are often intact. Skeletal muscles are often enlarged and gradually acquire a peculiar rubbery consistency. Electromyography shows lower motor neuron degeneration (475). Convulsions, intellectual impairment, and coma also have been observed. The liver, although usually not enlarged, is abnormally firm and easily palpable. Splenomegaly is rare. Infants are prone to intercurrent infections, particularly pneumonia, and usually die of these or bulbar paralysis by 1 year of age. In most patients having this clinical form, lysosomal α-glucosidase is catalytically inactive, although the protein is present in some families. The most common form of this variant, termed Antopol disease, is marked by severe cardiomyopathy, a mild myopathy, and mental retardation (476). Untreated, only 8% of all reported patients have survived beyond the first year of life (477).

α-Glucosidase deficiency also has been seen in older children and adults (juvenile and adult forms, respectively) (478). In these patients, organomegaly is absent, and muscle weakness is often slowly progressive or nonprogressive with maximum involvement of the proximal musculature of the lower extremities (479). Pharyngeal muscles can be involved as a consequence of glycogen storage in brainstem neurons (480). In most of the slowly progressive cases, residual lysosomal α-glucosidase activity is more than 10%. In others, the enzyme activity is undetectable, but the 110-kd precursor is present. Other individuals appear to be compound heterozygotes for different mutant alleles (478).

Diagnosis

When cardiac symptoms predominate, a differentiation from other causes of cardiomegaly and congestive failure in the absence of significant murmurs is required. These other causes include endocardial fibroelastosis, acute interstitial myocarditis, and aberrant coronary artery. When muscular weakness predominates, infantile spinal muscular atrophy (Werdnig-Hoffmann disease), the muscular dystrophies, myasthenia gravis, and hypotonic cerebral palsy must be considered (see Chapter 16). Cardiac involvement is generally late in Werdnig-Hoffmann disease and in the muscular dystrophies. In contrast to glycogen storage disease, the intellectual deficit in hypotonic cerebral palsy is usually severe and begins early. A muscle biopsy may be required to confirm the diagnosis. Blood chemistry, including fasting blood sugars and glucose tolerance tests, is normal.

α-Glucosidase activity of muscle and cultured fibroblasts is markedly diminished, and this assay serves as an excellent diagnostic aid (481). Examination of lymphocytes by electron microscopy frequently is successful in demonstrating and identifying the storage material. α-Glucosidase activity also can be shown in fibroblasts grown from normal amniotic fluid cells. This method can also be used for the antepartum diagnosis of Pompe disease and for the detection of heterozygotes.

Treatment

Several approaches to the treatment of glycogenosis II, as well as the other lysosomal defects, have been proposed. Enzyme replacement therapy, using twice-weekly infusions of recombinant human enzyme from rabbit milk or from genetically engineered Chinese hamster ovary cells overproducing acid α-glucosidase, has been used for the infantile and the late-onset forms of Pompe disease (482–484). The results have been encouraging in a few cases with the infantile form when treatment is started before irreversible damage has occurred (482). The cardiac muscle universally responds, whereas the response of skeletal muscle is variable. Because the enzyme does not cross the blood–brain barrier, it remains to be seen whether there will be late-onset complications in treated infantile Pompe patients. In the juvenile form of the disease enzyme replacement therapy has also resulted in some improvement (483). Adenovirus-mediated gene transfer holds some promise in delivering α-glucosidase to muscle (485). The problems inherent in gene delivery in Pompe disease are discussed by Ding and coworkers (486), and gene delivery to the brain is discussed by Kennedy (487).

Allogeneic bone marrow transplantation offers more promise for the treatment of some lysosomal storage diseases. In glycogenosis II, however, no beneficial result has been reported, despite successful engraftment. Liver transplantation has been used with some effect in types I, III, and IV glycogen storage disease (488). After transplant, the cells of the host organs become mixed with cells of the donor genome that migrate from the allograft into the tissues of the recipient and serve as enzyme carriers. This observation explains why some patients with such lysosomal storage diseases as type I Gaucher disease, Niemann-Pick disease, and Wolman disease receive more benefit from liver transplants than simply improved hepatic functions.

Danon Disease Glycogen Storage Disease IIa (OMIM 300257)

This condition is marked by the lysosomal storage of glycogen in the presence of normal acid maltase. It results from a mutation in the gene that codes for the lysosomal membrane protein 2 (LAMP-2) (489). The clinical picture is one of hypertrophic cardiomyopathy and myopathy, with mental retardation in about 70% of patients. Muscle biopsy discloses the presence of tiny vacuoles that resemble basophilic granules. Immunostaining for LAMP-2 shows complete absence of the protein. The brain MRI is generally normal. About 70% of female carriers are affected with cardiomyopathy. Myopathy is present in about one-third of carriers, and creatine kinase (CK) levels are increased (490).

Mucopolysaccharidoses

A syndrome consisting of mental and physical retardation, multiple skeletal deformities, hepatosplenomegaly, and clouding of the cornea was described by Hunter in 1917 (491), by Hurler in 1919 (492), and by von Pfaundler in 1920 (493). To Ellis and associates in 1936, the "large head, inhuman facies, and deformed limbs" suggested the appearance of a gargoyle (494). The syndrome is now known to represent six major entities, some with two or more subgroups that are distinguishable by their clinical picture, genetic transmission, enzyme defect, and urinary mucopolysaccharide (MPS) pattern (Table 1.18).

Molecular Genetics and Biochemical Pathology

The principal biochemical disturbance in the various mucopolysaccharidoses involves the catabolism of MPS. The chemistry of the MPS, also known as glycosaminoglycans, has been reviewed by Alberts and colleagues (495) and more extensively by Kjellen and Lindahl (496). These substances occur as large polymers having a protein core and multiple carbohydrate branches. Chondroitin-4-sulfate is found in cornea, bone, and cartilage. It consists of alternating units of D-glucuronic acid and sulfated *N*-acetylgalactosamine (Fig. 1.12).

Dermatan sulfate is a normal minor constituent of connective tissue and a major component of skin. It differs structurally from chondroitin-4-sulfate in that the uronic acid is principally L-iduronic rather than glucuronic acid (Fig. 1.12).

Heparan sulfate consists of alternating units of uronic acid and glucosamine. The former may be L-iduronic or D-glucuronic acid. Glucosamine can be acetylated on the amino nitrogen as well as sulfated on the amino nitrogen and hydroxyl group (Fig. 1.12). Generally, the MPS chains are linked to the serine of the protein core by means of a xylose-galactose-galactose-glucuronic acid-*N*-acetylhexosamine bridge.

The pathways of MPS biosynthesis are well established. The first step is the formation of a protein acceptor. Hexosamine and uronic acid moieties are then attached to the protein, one sugar at a time, starting with xylose. Sulfation occurs after completion of polymerization. The sulfate groups are introduced through the intermediary of an active sulfate. This is a labile nucleotide, identified as adenosine-3′-phosphate-5′-sulfatophosphate.

In the mucopolysaccharidoses, degradation of MPS is impaired because of a defect in one of several lysosomal hydrolases. This results in the accumulation of incompletely degraded molecules within lysosomes and the excretion of MPS fragments. The initial steps of MPS degradation (cleavage from the protein core) are intact in the mucopolysaccharidoses. In tissue where amounts of MPS are pathologic, such as liver, spleen, and urine, the protein core is completely lacking or represented only by a few amino acids.

In all of these diseases, therefore, the metabolic defect is located along the further degradation of the MPS, and in all but one, it involves the breakdown of dermatan sulfate and heparan sulfate (Fig. 1.12). As a result, large amounts (75 to 100 mg per 24 hours) of fragmented chains of these MPSs are excreted by individuals afflicted with the two major genetic entities: the autosomally transmitted Hurler syndrome (MPS IH; see Table 1.18) and the rarer X-linked Hunter syndrome (MPS II). These values compare with a normal excretion of 5 to 25 mg per 24 hours for all MPSs. Normal MPS excretion is distributed between chondroitin-4-sulfate (31%), chondroitin-6-sulfate (34%), chondroitin (25%), and heparan sulfate (8%) (497).

The biochemical lesions in the various mucopolysaccharidoses have been reviewed by Neufeld and Muenzer (498).

In the Hurler syndromes (MPS I), the activity of α-L-iduronidase is deficient (Fig. 1.12, step 1) (434). The iduronic acid moiety is found in dermatan and heparan sulfates (Fig. 1.12); therefore, the metabolism of both MPSs is defective. The gene for α-L-iduronidase has been mapped to chromosome 4 and has been cloned. Several hundred mutations have been described, with the frequency of each mutation differing from one genetic stock to the next. As a consequence of the genetic variability, a wide range of clinical phenotypes exists, from the most severe form, Hurler syndrome (IH), through an intermediate form (I H/S), to the mildest form, Scheie syndrome or MPS IS (499). Among patients of European origin, two mutations account for more than 50% of alleles (499).

In Hunter syndrome (MPS II), iduronate sulfatase activity is lost (Fig. 1.12, step 5) (500). Like L-iduronidase, this enzyme also is involved in the metabolism of dermatan and heparan sulfates. The gene for the enzyme is located on the distal portion of the long arm of the X chromosome (Xq28) in close proximity to the fragile X site. It has been cloned, and considerable genetic heterogeneity exists; in contrast to Hurler syndrome, there is a high incidence of gene deletions or rearrangements, and most families have their private mutation (500). Several phenotypic

TABLE 1.18 Classification of the Mucopolysaccharidoses

		Clinical Features				*Urinary Mucopolysaccharides*					
Type	***Eponym***	***Corneal Clouding***	***Dwarfism***	***Neurologic Signs***	***Cardiovascular Involvement***	***Heparan Sulfate***	***Dermatan Sulfate***	***Keratan Sulfate***	***Chondroitin-4-Sulfate***	***Chondroitin-6-Sulfate***	***Enzyme Defect***
I H	Hurler	Severe	Marked	Marked	Marked	+	+	–	–	–	α-L-IDURONIDASE
I S	Scheie	Severe	Mild	None	Late	+	+	–	–	–	α-L-IDURONIDASE
I H/S	Hurler-Scheie	Severe	Mild	None or mild	Late	+	+	–	–	–	α-L-IDURONIDASE
II A	Hunter (severe)	None	Marked	Mental retardation	Late	+	+	–	–	–	Iduronate sulfatase
II B	Hunter (mild)	None	Mild	Normal intellect, hearing deficits	Mild	+	+	–	–	–	Iduronate sulfatase
III A	Sanfilippo A	Absent	Moderate	Profound mental deterioration	Rare	+	–	–	–	–	Heparan-*N*-sulfatase
III B	Sanfilippo B	Absent	Moderate	Profound mental deterioration	Rare	+	–	–	–	–	α-*N*-acetylglucosaminidase
III C	Sanfilippo C	Absent	Moderate	Slow mental deterioration	Rare	+	–	–	–	–	Acetyl CoA: α-glucosaminide acetyltransferase
III D	Sanfilippo D	Absent	Moderate	Mild mental retardation	Rare	+	–	–	–	–	*N*-acetylglucosaminide 6-sulfate sulfatase
IV A	Morquio A	Late	Marked	None	Late	–	–	+	–	+	Galactose 6-sulfate sulfatase
IV B	Morquio B	Late	Marked	None	Late	–	–	+	–	–	β-Galactosidase
VI	Maroteaux-Lamy	Severe	Marked	None	Present	–	+	–	–	–	*N*-acetylgalactosamine 4-sulfate sulfatase
VII	Sly	Variable	Marked to severe	Variable; none	Present	±	±	–	+	+	β-Glucuronidase

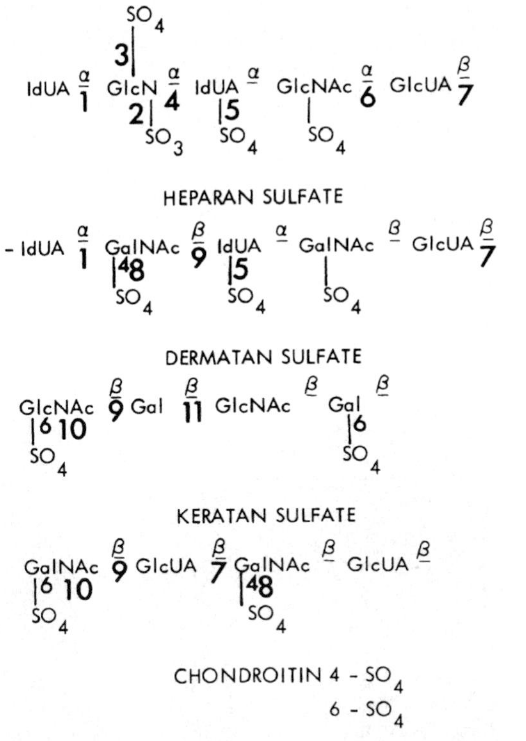

IdUA α 1 GlcN (3 SO4) α 4 (2 SO3) IdUA α (5 SO4) GlcNAc α 6 (SO4) GlcUA β 7

HEPARAN SULFATE

- IdUA α 1 GalNAc (4 8 SO4) β 9 IdUA (5 SO4) α GalNAc (SO4) β GlcUA β 7

DERMATAN SULFATE

GlcNAc (6 10 SO4) β 9 Gal β 11 GlcNAc β Gal (6 SO4) β

KERATAN SULFATE

GalNAc (6 10 SO4) β 9 GlcUA β 7 GalNAc (4 8 SO4) β GlcUA β

CHONDROITIN 4 - SO_4
6 - SO_4

FIGURE 1.12. Pathway of degeneration of mucopolysaccharides stored in the various mucopolysaccharidoses. The defects in the various entities as indicated by numbers: (1) Hurler and Scheie syndromes; (2) Sanfilippo syndrome type A; (5) Hunter syndrome; (6) Sanfilippo syndrome type B; (7) β-glucuronidase deficiency (MPS VII); (8) Maroteaux-Lamy syndrome; (9) Tay-Sachs and Sandhoff diseases (G_{M2} gangliosidoses); (10) Morquio syndrome; and (11) G_{M1} gangliosidosis. Step 3 is blocked by Sanfilippo syndrome type D. In Sanfilippo syndrome type C, acetylation of the free amino group of glucosamine (4) is defective. Gal, galactose; GalNAc, *N*-acetylgalactosamine; GlcN, glucosamine; GlcNAc, *N*-acetylglucosamine; GlcUA, glucuronic acid; IdUA, iduronic acid. (Courtesy of Dr. R. Matalon, Research Institute, Miami Children's Hospital, Miami, FL.)

forms of Hunter syndrome have been distinguished, and, as a rule, gene deletions result in a more severe clinical picture than point mutations. Hunter syndrome can rarely occur in female patients; in these circumstances, it results from X:autosome translocation or the unbalanced inactivation of the nonmutant chromosome (501).

In the four types of Sanfilippo syndrome (MPSs IIIA, B, C, and D), the basic defect involves the enzymes required for the specific degradation of heparan sulfate. In the A form of the disease, a lack of heparan-*N*-sulfatase (heparan sulfate sulfatase) occurs (Fig. 1.12, step 2), which is the enzyme that cleaves the nitrogen-bound sulfate moiety (498). In the B form, the defective enzyme is *N*-acetyl-α-D-glucosaminidase (Fig. 1.12, step 6) (498). In Sanfilippo syndrome, type C, the defect is localized to the transfer of an acetyl moiety from acetyl-CoA to the free amino group of glucosamine (Fig. 1.12, step 4) (498). In type D, the sulfatase for *N*-acetyl-glucosamine-6-sulfate is defective (Fig. 1.12, step 3) (498). The gene has been mapped to the long arm of chromosome 6 and has been cloned. Because all four of these enzymes are specific for the degradation of heparan sulfate, dermatan sulfate metabolism proceeds normally.

In Morquio syndrome (MPS IV) type A, the enzymatic lesion involves the metabolism of the structurally dissimilar keratan sulfate and chondroitin-6-sulfate. It is located at *N*-acetyl-galactosamine-6-sulfate sulfatase (Fig. 1.12, step 10) (498). Morquio syndrome type B, a clinically milder form, is characterized by a defect in β-galactosidase. The gene for this condition has been cloned. As a consequence of its defect, the removal of galactose residues from keratan sulfate is impaired. The defect is allelic with G_{M1} gangliosidosis, a condition in which a deficiency of β-galactosidase interrupts the degeneration of keratan sulfate and G_{M1} ganglioside (502). As a consequence of these defects, the urinary MPS in both forms of Morquio syndrome consists of approximately 50% keratan sulfate and lesser amounts of chondroitin-6-sulfate (see Table 1.18).

In Maroteaux-Lamy syndrome (MPS VI), the abnormality is an inability to hydrolyze the sulfate group from *N*-acetyl-galactosamine-4-sulfate (Fig. 1.12, step 8) (498). This reaction is involved in the metabolism of dermatan sulfate and chondroitin-4-sulfate (Fig. 1.12). The gene has been mapped to the long arm of chromosome 5 and has been cloned. Numerous mutations have been documented, and the phenotype of the condition is quite variable.

In MPS VII (Sly syndrome), a lack of β-glucuronidase (Fig. 1.12, step 7) has been demonstrated in a variety of tissues (498). The gene for this enzyme has been mapped to the long arm of chromosome 7 (7q21.11) and has been cloned. Numerous mutations have been described. As is the case for the other MPSs, these allelic forms have been postulated to explain differences in clinical manifestations in patients having the same enzymatic lesion.

Hurler Syndrome (Mucopolysaccharide I and IH) (OMIM 252800)

Pathologic Anatomy

Visceral alterations in Hurler syndrome are widespread and involve almost every organ. Large, vacuolated cells containing MPS can be seen in cartilage, tendons, periosteum, endocardium, and vascular walls, particularly the intima of the coronary arteries (503). Abnormalities occur in the cartilage of the bronchial tree, and the alveoli are filled with lipid-laden cells. The bone marrow is replaced in part by connective tissue that contains many vacuolated fibroblasts. The liver is unusually large, most parenchymal cells being at least double their normal size. On electron microscopy, MPSs are noted to accumulate in the lysosomes of most hepatic parenchymatous cells (504). The

Kupffer cells are swollen and contain abnormal amounts of MPS. In the spleen, the reticulum cells are larger than normal and contain the same storage material.

Changes within the CNS are widespread. The leptomeninges are edematous and thickened. The Virchow-Robin spaces are filled with MPS, and the periadventitial space in white matter is dilated and filled with viscous fluid and mononuclear cells containing MPS-positive vacuoles. The meningeal alterations produce partial obstruction of the subarachnoid spaces, which, in association with a narrowed foramen magnum, is responsible for the hydrocephalus that is often observed. The neurons are swollen and vacuolated, and their nuclei are peripherally displaced. Neuronal distention is most conspicuous in the cerebral cortex, but cells in the thalamus, brainstem, and particularly in the anterior horns of the spinal cord are involved also. In the cerebellum, the Purkinje cells contain abnormal lipid material and demonstrate a fusiform swelling of their dendrites. On electron microscopy, the storage material is in the form of membranes, zebra bodies, and, least common, lipofuscin material (505). The relationship of the pathologic appearance of neurons to the neurologic defects has been studied extensively. Because it has been best delineated in G_{M2} gangliosidosis, it is discussed under that section.

From a chemical viewpoint, the material stored in the brain is of two types. Within neurons are large amounts of two gangliosides: the G_{M2} ganglioside, which also is stored in the various G_{M2} gangliosidoses (Tay-Sachs disease), and the hexosamine-free hematocyte (G_{M3} ganglioside). The greater proportion of the stored material is within mesenchymal tissue and is in the form of dermatan and heparan sulfates (505).

Clinical Manifestations

A detailed review of the clinical manifestations of the various mucopolysaccharidoses can be found in the book by Beighton and McKusick (506). Hurler syndrome is inherited as an autosomal recessive disorder with an estimated incidence of 1 in 144,000 births (507). Affected children usually appear healthy at birth and, except for repeated infections, otitis in particular, remain healthy for the greater part of their first year of life. Slowed development can be the first evidence of the disorder. Bony abnormalities (dysostosis multiplex) of the upper extremities can be observed by 12 years of age and worsen thereafter. These changes are much more marked there than in the lower extremities, with the most striking being swelling of the central portion of the humeral shaft and widening of the medial end of the clavicle (Fig. 1.13), alterations that result from a thickening of the cortex and dilation of the medullary canal (508).

The typical patient is small with a large head and coarse facial features (Fig. 1.14). The eyes are widely spaced. The bridge of the nose is flat and the lips are large.

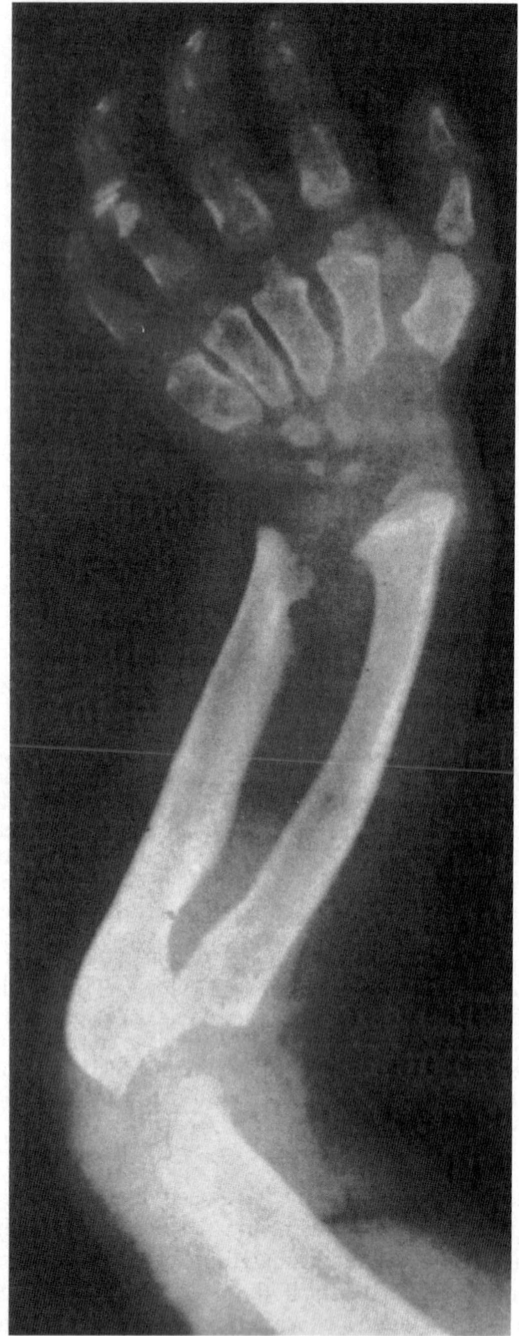

FIGURE 1.13. Hurler syndrome. Roentgenogram of upper extremity. The ulna and radius are short and wide and their epiphyseal ends are irregular. There is a Madelung deformity of the wrist (Madelung deformity is characterized by anatomic changes in the radius, ulna, and carpal bones, leading to palmar and ulnar wrist subluxation). The metacarpal bones and phalanges are also thickened and irregular and there is proximal pointing of the metacarpals.

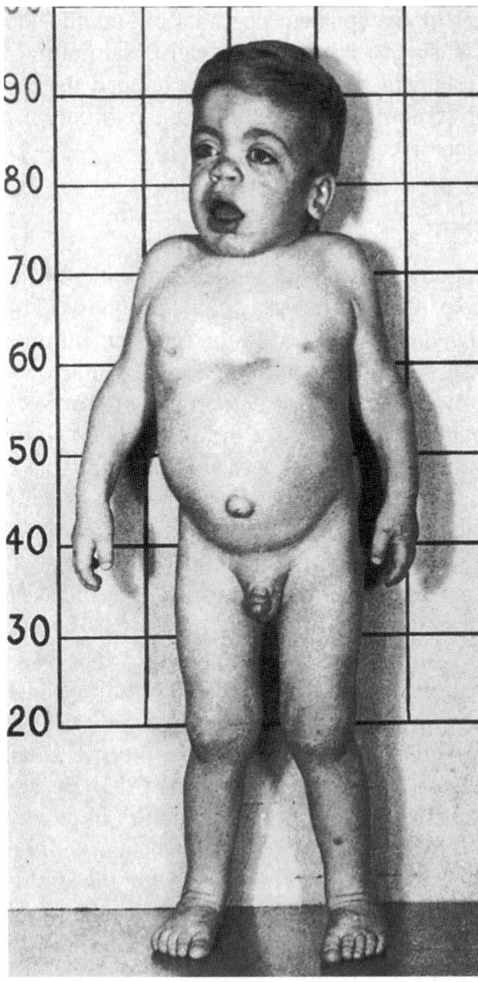

FIGURE 1.14. Hurler syndrome in a 4-year-old boy. The patient demonstrates the unusual, coarse facies, depressed bridge of the nose, open mouth, and large tongue. The hands are spadelike, the abdomen protrudes, and an umbilical hernia is present. (Courtesy of Dr. V. A. McKusick, Johns Hopkins Hospital, Baltimore, MD.)

The mouth is open and an almost constant nasal obstruction or upper respiratory infection exists. Kyphosis is marked and appears early. The hands are wide and the fingers are short and stubby, with contractures that produce a claw-hand deformity. A carpal tunnel syndrome caused by entrapment of the median nerve is common, as is odontoid hypoplasia, which can lead to C1–2 vertebral displacement and quadriplegia. The abdomen protrudes, an umbilical hernia is often present, and gross hepatosplenomegaly occurs. The hair is profuse and coarse. In older children, a unique skin lesion is observed occasionally (509). It consists of an aggregation of white, nontender papules of varying size, found symmetrically around the thorax and upper extremities. Corneal opacities are invariable. In most cases, progressive spasticity and mental deterioration occur. Blindness results from a combination of corneal clouding, retinal pigmentary degeneration, and optic atrophy. Optic atrophy is the consequence of prolonged increased intracranial pressure, meningeal infiltration constricting the optic nerve, and infiltration of the optic nerve itself. Cortical blindness caused by MPS storage in neurons of the optic system also has been observed. A mixed conductive and sensorineural deafness occurs (510).

Untreated, the disease worsens relentlessly, progressing more slowly in those children whose symptoms have a somewhat later onset. Many of the slower-progressing patients suffer from the intermediate Hurler-Scheie syndrome (MPS I H/S). A curious and unique feature of this particular variant is the presence of arachnoid cysts. Spinal cord compression is not unusual; in Hurler syndrome, it generally results from dural thickening.

Radiographic abnormalities in Hurler syndrome are extensive and have been reviewed by Caffey (see Fig. 1.13) (508). They are the prototype for the other mucopolysaccharidoses. The CSF is normal. When blood smears are studied carefully, granulocytes can be seen to contain darkly azurophilic granules (Reilly granules). Some 20% to 40% of lymphocytes contain metachromatically staining cytoplasmic inclusions. These are also seen in Hunter and Sanfilippo syndromes and in the GM1 gangliosidoses. MRI not only in Hurler but also in Hunter and Sanfilippo diseases shows five types of changes: (a) Cystic, "cribriform" changes due to abnormal enlargement of the perivascular spaces with MPS-laden cells. (b) Cystic lesions of the corona radiata, periventricular white matter, corpus callosum, and. less frequently, basal ganglia. These lesions have low signal intensity of T1-weighted images and high signal intensity on T2-weighted images. They reflect MPS deposition in the perivascular spaces. In the more advanced cases, increased patchy or diffuse signal is seen in periventricular white matter on T2-weighted images. (c) Ventricular enlargement and cerebral atrophy. (d) Spinal cord compression. (e) Mega cisterna magna or posterior fossa cysts (511,512).

Death is usually a result of airway obstruction or bronchopneumonia secondary to the previously described pulmonary and bronchial alterations. Coronary artery disease and congestive heart failure caused by MPS infiltration of the heart valves also can prove fatal, even as early as 7 years of age (513).

Diagnosis

Although classic Hurler syndrome offers little in the way of diagnostic difficulty, in many children, particularly in infants, some of the cardinal signs, such as hepatosplenomegaly, mental deficiency, bony abnormalities, or a typical facial configuration, are minimal or completely lacking (Fig. 1.15) (514). A qualitative screening test for increased output of urinary MPS usually confirms the diagnosis, whereas quantitative determinations of the various MPSs indicate the specific disorder. False-negative and false-positive test results are encountered, with the

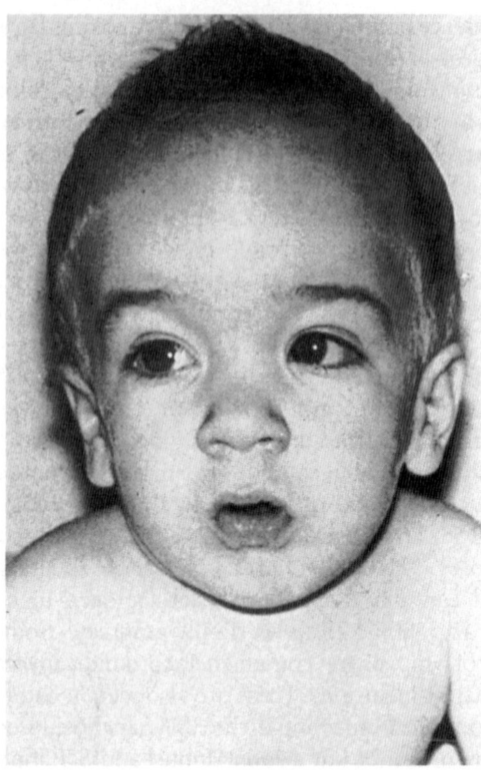

FIGURE 1.15. Infant with Hurler disease showing mild coarse features, presence of metopic suture, mild corneal clouding, and chronic rhinorrhea. (From Matalon R, Kaul R, Michals K. The mucopolysaccharidoses and the mucolipidoses. In: Rosenberg RN, Prusiner SB, DiMauro S, Barchi RL, eds. *The molecular and genetic basis of neurological disease*. Stoneham, MA: Butterworth–Heinemann, 2nd ed., 1997;340. With permission.)

latter being fairly common in newborns. A more definitive diagnosis requires an assay for α-L-iduronidase. If Hurler disease is suspected, the assay can be performed on lymphocytes or cultured fibroblasts (498). These assays also can serve for carrier detection or prenatal diagnosis (498).

In a number of conditions, the facial configuration seen in Hurler syndrome, the body abnormalities, and hepatosplenomegaly are unaccompanied by an abnormal MPS excretion. The first of these entities to have been defined was generalized G_{M1} gangliosidosis, formerly known as pseudo-Hurler syndrome. This condition is characterized by hepatosplenomegaly, mental retardation, and bony abnormalities but a normal MPS output. The basic defect is one of ganglioside degradation (see the section on sphingolipidoses later in this chapter).

Patients presenting with dwarfism, early psychomotor retardation, unusual facies, a clear or only faintly hazy cornea, and normal MPS excretion manifest the syndrome termed mucolipidosis II, or I-cell disease. This entity is discussed with the mucolipidoses.

Other conditions to be considered in the differential diagnosis are mucolipidoses III and IV and the various disorders of glycoprotein degradation: mannosidosis, fucosidosis, sialidosis, and aspartylglycosaminuria. Finally, hypothyroidism must always be excluded in the youngster with small stature, developmental retardation, and unusual facies (see Chapter 17).

Treatment

Bone marrow transplantation has dramatically improved the course of Hurler disease and its prognosis (514a). The beneficial effects result from the replacement of enzyme-deficient macrophages and microglia by marrow-derived macrophages that provide a continuous source of normal enzyme, which can enter the brain and digest stored MPS. Several hundred patients with Hurler disease have undergone bone marrow transplantation with considerable improvement of their dysmorphic features, cardiac defects, hepatosplenomegaly, and hearing. Macrocephaly tends to resolve, as does odontoid hypoplasia, but the skeletal abnormalities progress (515). In the British series of Vellodi and colleagues, the intelligence of 60% of children improved or showed no further deterioration after bone marrow transplant (516). In the American series of Guffon and colleagues, 46% of patients had normal intelligence and 15% had borderline intelligence (517). Because little improvement occurs in mental function in children who are severely retarded, Vellodi and colleagues did not recommend bone marrow transplants for those older than 2 years of age (516). Guffon and colleagues considered an initial IQ of lower than 70 to be the main criterion for excluding a patient from consideration for transplant (517). As a rule, no improvement occurs in corneal clouding, and orthopedic problems tend to persist (518). Bone marrow transplant has not improved the CNS manifestations of Hunter or Sanfillipo diseases, and the procedure is no longer performed for those conditions.

Enzyme replacement therapy is being used extensively for patients with Hurler disease as well as for some of the other MPSs. In the placebo-controlled series of Wraith and coworkers weekly infusions of 100 U/kg of α-L-iduronidase (Laronidase) significantly reduced hepatomegaly, MPS excretion, respiratory function, and sleep apnea. Growth rate and weight gain improved, and there was an increase in the range of motion of shoulder and elbow (519). Although nearly all patients developed immunoglobulin G (IgG) antibodies, these tended to fall after continued therapy as patients developed immune tolerance (520). Neurologic symptoms are not reversible with enzyme replacement therapy. Prior enzyme replacement therapy may help to improve engraftment and survival for those undergoing bone marrow transplantation (521). There is hope that intrathecal therapy may be useful for treating the brain in the future.

MPS I is frequently accompanied by hydrocephalus that can escape detection by neuroimaging until it is advanced. It is important to also monitor the opening pressure on lumbar puncture and perform an early shunt to preserve intellectual function. Older patients may develop cord compression from meningeal involvement and benefit from laminectomy.

Scheie Syndrome (Mucopolysaccharide IS)

Scheie syndrome is due to mutations in the gene for α-L-iduronidase that induce a less severe phenotype than is seen in Hurler disease. The major manifestations are corneal clouding, organ enlargement, and joint stiffness (522). Intelligence is unaffected until late in life, and, until then, neurologic symptoms are limited to a high incidence of carpal tunnel syndrome (compression of the median nerve as it transverses the carpal tunnel of the wrist).

On autopsy, relatively little MPS storage is found within the leptomeninges, and the neurons appear normal (505).

Scheie syndrome is diagnosed in patients who have the biochemical and enzymatic defects of Hurler syndrome but lack skeletal and severe neurologic involvement. Hurler-Scheie genetic compounds also have been reported (MPS I H/S). This disorder is characterized by hepatosplenomegaly, corneal clouding, slow mental deterioration, and, ultimately, the evolution of increased intracranial pressure resulting from obstruction at the basilar cisterns (506). Winters and associates described neuronal storage in this entity (523).

Hunter Syndrome (Mucopolysaccharide II) (OMIM 309900)

This condition is transmitted as an X-linked recessive disorder, with a variety of alleles believed responsible for differences in severity of clinical manifestations. Its frequency in British Columbia is 1 in 111,000 births (524).

Depending on whether mental deterioration is present, the syndrome is separated into mild and severe forms (IIA and IIB, respectively). In the mild form, the abnormal facial configuration is first noted during early childhood. Dwarfism, hepatosplenomegaly, umbilical hernia, and frequent respiratory infections are almost invariable. Cardiac disease, particularly with valvular abnormalities, was seen in more than 90% of patients in the series of Young and Harper and was the most common cause of death (525). Additionally, joints are involved widely, with a particular predilection for the hands. Neurologic symptoms in the mild form of Hunter syndrome are limited to progressive head growth (generally unaccompanied by ventricular enlargement or hydrocephalus), sensorineural deafness, and retinitis pigmentosa with impaired visual-evoked responses. The latter two symptoms are explained by the autopsy finding of vacuolated ganglion cells in the eighth nerve nucleus and retina (526). Papilledema is common; seen in the presence of normal CSF pressure and normal-sized ventricles, it probably results from local infiltrative processes around the retinal veins. It can be present for 8 years or longer without apparent loss of vision (527).

In the severe form of the disease, the clinical picture is highlighted by the insidious onset of mental retardation, first noted between ages 2 and 3 years. Seizures are seen in 62% and a persistent, unexplained diarrhea in 65% of patients (528). Upper airway obstruction is common and difficult to correct because tracheostomy presents major anesthetic risks (527). Corneal clouding is unusual but its presence does not speak against the diagnosis of Hunter syndrome (529). In the series of Young and Harper, death occurred at an average age of 12 years (530). Multiple nerve entrapments can occur in Hunter as well as in Hurler syndrome as the consequence of connective tissue thickening through MPS deposition (530).

Alterations within the brain are similar to those seen in Hurler syndrome. Considerable leptomeningeal MPS storage occurs, mainly in the form of dermatan and heparan sulfates. The neuronal cytoplasm is distended with lipid-staining material, probably of ganglioside nature (531). Electron microscopy reveals the presence of lamellar figures in cortical neurons (532). The storage process commences during early intrauterine development (533).

The enzyme deficiency can be ascertained in serum, lymphocytes, and fibroblasts. Prenatal diagnosis of Hunter syndrome can be performed by examining amniotic fluid cells and by assaying for idurono-sulfate-sulfatase in cell-free amniotic fluid (498). Approximately one-fourth of mothers are noncarriers (i.e., their affected male offspring represent a new mutation).

Unlike MPS I, bone marrow transplantation, for unclear reasons, does not preserve intellectual function in MPS II. Enzyme replacement therapy is being tested.

Sanfilippo Syndrome (Mucopolysaccharides IIIA, B, C, and D) (OMIM 252900; 252920; 252930; 252940)

This heterogeneous syndrome, first described in 1963 by Sanfilippo and coworkers, is characterized by mental deterioration that commences during the first few years of life. It is accompanied by subtle somatic features of a mucopolysaccharidosis (534). With an incidence of at least 1 in 24,000, it is the most common of the mucopolysaccharidoses (498), and in the experience of Verity and coworkers it is the most common condition that causes progressive neurologic and intellectual deterioration (535).

Four genetically and biochemically, but not clinically, distinct forms have been recognized. In all, delayed development is the usual presenting symptom. It is first noted between ages 2 and 5 years and is gradually superseded by evidence of neurologic regression. This is most rapid in type A. Abnormally coarse facial features are usually

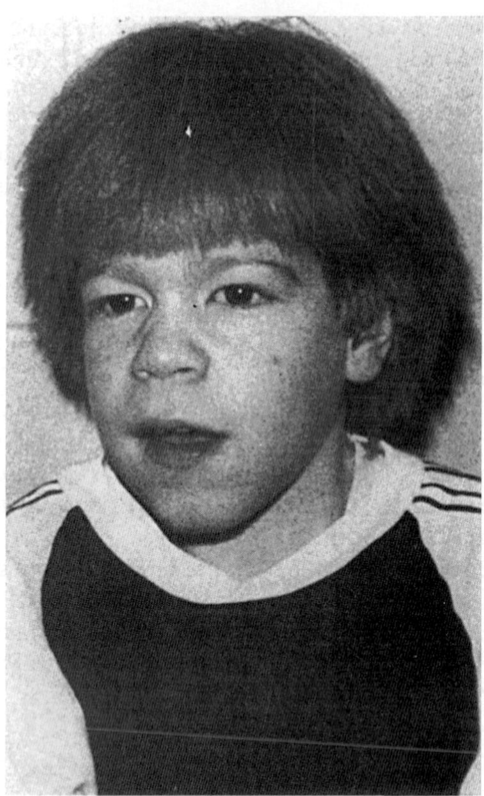

FIGURE 1.16. Patient with Sanfilippo A syndrome, showing the relatively mild coarsening of facial features. (From Matalon R, Kaul R, Michals K. The mucopolysaccharidoses and the mucolipidoses. In: Rosenberg RN, Prusiner SB, DiMauro S, Barchi RL, eds. *The molecular and genetic basis of neurological disease*. Stoneham, MA: Butterworth–Heinemann, 2nd ed., 1997;344. With permission.)

evident even earlier but generally go unnoticed because they are never as prominent as in the other mucopolysaccharidoses (Fig. 1.16). No growth retardation, no corneal opacification, and only mild hepatosplenomegaly occur. Diarrhea is seen in more than 50% of patients (536). Loss of extension of the interphalangeal joints was present in all patients in the series of Danks and coworkers, whereas limitation of elbow extension was characteristic for the rare type D (536,537). In addition to mental deterioration, the neurologic examination can disclose ataxia, coarse tremor, progressive spasticity, and, as the illness advances, bulbar palsy. The changes seen on MRI are similar to those for Hurler and Hunter syndromes (512). Although hydrocephalus can be caused by meningeal thickening, it is more often the result of malformations of the foramen magnum or of an underdeveloped dens, with increased thickness of the ligaments surrounding it (538).

Other common radiographic features are widening of the anterior two-thirds of the ribs and elongation of the radius. Peripheral blood smears can reveal cytoplasmic inclusions in lymphocytes or polymorphs, and bone marrow aspirates can be positive for storage material.

The disease is inexorably progressive, and most patients die before 20 years of age. Generally, the downhill course is most rapid in the type A variant (539).

Morphologic alterations within the CNS are similar to those seen in Hurler syndrome, but heparan sulfate is the major MPS stored in the leptomeninges and brain (505,531).

The clinical diagnosis of Sanfilippo syndrome is difficult to establish and also can be missed on random MPS screening. It must be considered in any mentally retarded child who has only minor physical stigmata (see Fig. 1.16). Examination of a 24-hour urine collection discloses the excretion of heparan sulfate (see Table 1.18). Enzyme assays on serum, skin fibroblasts, and lymphocytes confirm the diagnosis and identify the specific type. Treatment of type A disease with bone marrow transplantation does not appear to be of benefit (540). Sleep and behavioral disturbances are the most distressing to parents and difficult to manage, although shunting may improve behavior in some cases (541,542).

Morquio Syndrome (Mucopolysaccharides IVA and B) (OMIM 253000; 253010)

The clinical manifestations of Morquio syndrome involve the skeleton primarily and the nervous system only secondarily. Skeletal manifestations include growth retardation and deformities of the vertebral bodies and epiphyseal zones of the long bones. Generally, type A is more severe than type B. However, type A shows considerable clinical heterogeneity. Absence or severe hypoplasia of the odontoid process or atlantoaxial instability is invariable (543), and neurologic symptoms result from chronic or acute compression of the spinal cord. This compression can be the result of atlantoaxial subluxation, the presence of a gibbus, or dural thickening as a consequence of MPS deposition. These complications are best visualized by MRI. The mild form of Morquio syndrome (MPS IVB) presents with growth retardation, bony abnormalities (dysostosis multiplex), and corneal opacities. Mental functioning generally remains normal. Corneal opacities, sensorineural hearing loss, and mental retardation are encountered occasionally (544). Neuroimaging studies can show ventricular dilation and progressive white matter disease.

It is not clear why the nervous system is generally spared in Morquio syndrome B, whereas an equally severe defect of β-galactosidase results in G_{M1} gangliosidosis. The best explanation is that in Morquio syndrome type B, the mutation affects the activity of β-galactosidase for keratan sulfate, whereas in G_{M1} gangliosidosis, the mutation affects the enzyme's ability to degrade ganglioside. β-Galactosidase deficiency also can be caused by a lack of a protective protein. This is the case in mucolipidosis I, in which a deficiency of β-galactosidase and sialidase occurs.

Pathologic examination of the brain reveals leptomeningeal thickening and neuronal storage. Neuronal storage tends to be localized; Koto and coworkers found it primarily within the thalamus and hippocampus. On ultrastructural examination, the material appears similar to that stored in Hurler syndrome (544).

The diagnosis of Morquio syndrome can be made by the presence of keratan sulfate in urine (see Table 1.18) and by assaying for enzyme activity in leukocytes or fibroblasts.

Maroteaux-Lamy Syndrome (Mucopolysaccharide VI) (OMIM 253200)

In this condition, first described in 1963 by Maroteaux, Lamy, and colleagues (545), neurologic complications result from compression myelopathy and hydrocephalus (506,546). Several clinical variants with differing severity of expression have been recognized. The severe form resembles Hurler syndrome, except that the intellect remains normal. Skeletal and corneal involvement is generally severe in this form, and the facial appearance is characteristic for MPS. The milder forms of the disease show some of the clinical manifestations, but to a lesser extent.

The excretion of dermatan sulfate in the absence of urinary heparan sulfate is strongly suggestive of the diagnosis (see Table 1.18). The enzyme implicated in the disease (*N*-acetylgalactosamine-4-sulfate sulfatase, or arylsulfatase B) is readily assayed in a variety of tissues, and antenatal diagnosis has been possible.

The initial results from enzyme replacement therapy using human recombinant *N*-acetylgalactosamine 4-sulfatase appear to be promising (547).

Sly Syndrome (Mucopolysaccharide VII) (OMIM 253220)

The clinical appearance of patients with Sly syndrome varies considerably. Some are of normal intelligence or only mildly retarded, whereas others present with hydrops fetalis, severe retardation, and macrocephaly (548). Hepatomegaly is generally present, and the facial and skeletal abnormalities are characteristic for a mucopolysaccharidosis. The increased excretion of heparan sulfate and dermatan sulfate is shared with MPSs I, II, and V, but a deficiency of β-glucuronidase (see Table 1.18) is readily detected in serum, leukocytes, and fibroblasts (549).

Enzyme replacement therapy initiated at birth improved the behavioral performance and reduced hearing loss in the murine model of MPS VII (550), suggesting that early enzyme replacement therapy might be effective in the human as well.

Mucolipidoses

Mucolipidoses have the clinical features of both the mucopolysaccharidoses and the lipidoses. At least four mucolipidoses have been distinguished, characterized by MPS storage despite normal excretion of MPS. All of them are rare.

The most likely to be encountered is mucolipidosis II [ML II, or inclusion cell (I-cell) disease (OMIM 252500)]; its prevalence in a French Canadian isolate is 1 in 6,000 (551). This condition is the consequence of a defect in UDP-*N*-acetylglucosamine:*N*-acetylglucosaminyl-1-phosphotransferase, the enzyme responsible for attaching a phosphate group to mannose and synthesizing mannose-6-phosphate, which acts as a recognition marker for lysosomal enzymes. In the absence of this recognition marker, lysosomal enzymes are prevented from reaching lysosomes and instead are routed into the extracellular space and excreted (552).

As in all other lysosomal disorders, considerable clinical and biochemical heterogeneity exists. The clinical and radiologic features of this autosomal recessive disorder are reminiscent of Hurler syndrome, although in distinction, I-cell disease is apparent at birth. Features seen in the affected newborn include hypotonia, coarse facial appearance, striking gingival hyperplasia, congenital dislocation of the hips, restricted joint mobility, and tight, thickened skin (552). Radiographic changes of dysostosis multiplex develop between 6 and 10 months of age, although periosteal cloaking can occur even prenatally. Subsequently, growth failure, microcephaly, and progressive mental deterioration become apparent. Hepatomegaly and corneal clouding are inconstant. Most patients die during childhood (552). Nonimmune hydrops fetalis can be seen in some pregnancies. Bone marrow transplantation has shown some promise (553).

Cultured fibroblasts and bone marrow cells contain numerous inclusions. Visible by phase-contrast microscopy, these inclusions represent enlarged lysosomes filled with MPS and membranous material. The brain has no significant neuronal or glial storage, and the clinically evident mental deterioration cannot, as yet, be explained on a morphologic basis (554).

In ML II and ML III, a number of lysosomal enzymes (e.g., α-L-iduronidase, β-glucuronidase, and β-galactosidase) are elevated markedly in plasma and deficient in fibroblasts. Enzyme levels in liver and brain are normal (555).

ML III is a milder form of ML II. In this condition, the defect in the phosphorylation of mannose is also defective, although to a lesser degree than in ML II, and the activity of *N*-acetylglucosaminyl-1-phosphotransferase is considerably reduced.

Symptoms of ML III do not become apparent until after age 2 years, and learning disabilities or mental retardation are mild. Restricted mobility of joints and growth retardation occur. Radiographic examination shows a pattern of dysostosis multiplex with severe pelvic and vertebral abnormalities. Fine corneal opacities and valvular heart disease are occasionally present (556). The disease can be diagnosed by the presence of elevated lysosomal enzymes in plasma. Prolonged survival is possible but complicated by osteopenia, which may respond to bisphosphonates.

ML IV (OMIM 252650) is a relatively common disease in Ashkenazi Jews (557), with the estimated heterozygote frequency being 1/100 (558). Two mutations account for 95% of the cases in this population group (558). Symptoms are nonspecific, and probably many cases go undiagnosed. Developmental delay and impaired vision become apparent during the first year of life. Corneal opacities are almost invariable, as is strabismus and an ERG with markedly reduced amplitude. Photophobia was noted in 25% of the children in the Israeli series of Amir and coworkers (557). A striking hypotonia and extrapyramidal signs also have been encountered, and some patients have been evaluated for a congenital myopathy. Seizures are not part of the clinical picture. Skeletal deformities and visceromegaly are absent (559). Curiously, patients with ML IV are constitutionally achlorhydric with a secondary elevation of serum gastrin (559). Although visual function deteriorates, Amir and coworkers found no intellectual deterioration (557). MRI consistently demonstrates a hypoplastic corpus callosum; additionally, there can be delayed myelination (560). MPS excretion is normal, but the urine contains large quantities of G_{M3} gangliosides, phospholipids, and neutral glycolipids. The diagnosis is made by visualizing the polysaccharide and lipid-containing inclusion organelles using electron microscopy of a conjunctival or skin biopsy. In contrast to ML II, ML IV shows a variety of inclusions in neurons, glia, and the perivascular cells of brain (561).

The gene for ML IV encodes a transmembrane protein, mucolipin 1, a member of the transient receptor potential gene family that is involved in endosomal transport within the cell (562).

Mucolipidosis I (sialidosis) is considered with the glycoproteinoses.

Glycoproteinoses: Disorders of Glycoprotein Degradation

In four storage diseases, the primary enzymatic defect involves the degradation of glycoproteins. These substances, which in essence are peptides linked to oligosaccharides, are widely distributed within cells, the cell membrane, and outside the cells; they are particularly abundant in nervous tissue (563). Because some of the same oligosaccharide linkages also are found in glycolipids, a single enzymatic lesion affects the degradation of more than one macromolecule. For this reason, some of the sphingolipid storage diseases and the mucolipidoses have an impaired glycoprotein breakdown, and, conversely, the glycoproteinoses also can have a defective sphingolipid catabolism.

Fucosidosis (OMIM 230000)

Although a severe and a mild form of this autosomal recessive disorder have been distinguished on clinical grounds, both forms have been identified within the same family, and there appears to be a clinical continuum (564). A deficiency of α-L-fucosidase can be documented. Fucosidase is responsible for cleavage of the fucose moieties linked to *N*-acetylglucosamine (Fig. 1.17). The gene for the enzyme has been mapped to the distal portion of the short arm of chromosome 1 (1p34.1-p36.1). It has been cloned and sequenced. Considerable genetic heterozygosity exists, and numerous mutations have been recognized (565).

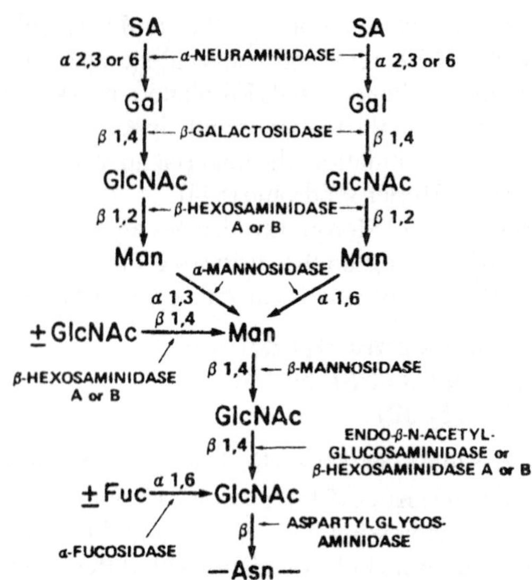

FIGURE 1.17. Probable steps for the degradation of a complex type oligosaccharide structure. Asn, asparigine; Fuc, fucose; Gal, galactose; GlcNAc, *N*-acetylglucosamine; Man, mannose; SA, sialic acid. (From Thomas GH. Disorders of glycoprotein degradation: α-mannosidosis, β-mannosidosis, β-fucosidosos, sialidosis and aspartylglycosaminuria. In: Scriver CR, Beaudet AL, Sly WS, Valle D. eds. *The metabolic basis of inherited diseases*, 5th ed. New York: McGraw–Hill, 2001:3510. With permission.)

In approximately 60% of patients, the condition has a rapidly progressive course, with intellectual deterioration and spasticity commencing at approximately 1 year of age. This is accompanied by growth retardation. In the series of Willems and coworkers, facial features were coarse in 79% of patients, and skeletal abnormalities (dysostosis multiplex) were seen in 58% (565). MR imaging studies are unusual. Aside from showing increased signal in white matter the globus pallidus shows increased intensity on T1-weighted images and decreased intensity on T2-weighted and fluid attenuation inversion recovery (FLAIR) images. The putamen shows increased intensity on T2-weighted images (566). The chloride content of sweat is increased markedly. In the same series seizures were noted in 36% of cases. The patient usually dies by age 35 years. When the condition is more protracted, the clinical picture is similar, except that angiokeratoma of the skin, particularly of the gingiva and genitalia, is invariable. These skin manifestations are indistinguishable from those seen in

Fabry disease and sialidosis and are not seen when the disease progresses rapidly (567). Treatment with bone marrow transplantation has shown promise in arresting the progress of the illness (568), as has infusion of recombinant alpha-L-fucosidase (569).

Pathologic examination discloses cytoplasmic vacuolization in most organs, notably in liver. Vacuolization also occurs in neurons and glial cells within brain and spinal cord (570).

Biochemical analysis reveals fucose-rich glycolipids in a variety of organs. In brain, the storage material is of two types: One is a fucose-containing decasaccharide, the other a fucose-containing disaccharide (563). Because α-L-fucoside residues are components of the blood group antigens, Lewis activity in red cells and saliva is expressed to an unusually high degree.

α- and β-Mannosidosis

α-Mannosidosis (OMIM 248500), first described in 1967, is characterized by a Hurler-like facial appearance, mental retardation, skeletal abnormalities, hearing loss, and hepatosplenomegaly (571). Considerable clinical heterogeneity exists, with a severe infantile form (type I) and a more common, milder, juvenile-adult form (type II) having been distinguished (563). Deficiency of both cellular and humoral immunity has been observed and may account for the frequent infections seen in patients with this condition (563).

Neuronal storage of mannose-rich oligosaccharides is widespread within the brain and spinal cord (572). The basic lesion is a mutation of the α-mannosidase gene, which leads to deficiency of α-mannosidoses A and B in liver, brain, peripheral leukocytes, serum, and skin fibroblasts. α-Mannosidase normally hydrolyses the trisaccharide mannose-mannose-*N*-acetylglucosamine (see Fig. 1.17), which consequently is excreted in large amounts (573). Bone marrow or hematopoietic stem cell transplantation has been effective in slowing or arresting the progression of the disease, including the cognitive loss (568,574).

A defect in β-mannosidase (OMIM 248510) also has been reported (575). It is marked by developmental regression and coarse facial features and, occasionally, a peripheral neuropathy, but neither organomegaly nor corneal clouding (575,576).

Sialidosis (OMIM 256550)

Lysosomal neuraminidase initiates the hydrolysis of sialylated glycoconjugates by removing their terminal sialic acid residues. In humans,primary or secondary deficiency of this enzyme leads to twoclinically similar neurodegenerative lysosomal storage disorders:sialidosis and galactosialidosis (see Fig. 1.17) (577). The gene that codes for sialidase has been mapped to the short arm of chromosome 6p21.3. It has been cloned, and three types of mutations have been documented. Patients with the most severe form of the disease have a catalytically inactive enzyme that is not localized to the lysosome. Patients with intermediate severity have a catalytically inactive enzyme that is localized to the lysosome, and patients with a mild form of the disease have a catalytically active enzyme that is localized to the lysosome (578).

Two clinical forms of sialidosis are recognized. In type I sialidosis (cherry-red spot myoclonus syndrome), the milder form of the disease, neurologic symptoms begin after age 10 years. Initially, these include diminished visual acuity (notably night blindness), a macular cherry-red spot, ataxia with gait abnormalities, nystagmus, and myoclonic seizures. Neuropathy and punctate lenticular opacities also can be present (579). Patients do not have dysmorphic features or deterioration of intelligence and have a normal life span.

Type II, the severe, congenital form of primary neuraminidase deficiency with dysmorphic features, is characterized by hepatosplenomegaly, corneal opacifications, dysostosis multiplex, hydrops fetalis, ascites, and a pericardial effusion. The condition is rapidly fatal. Pathologic examination of the brain discloses membrane-bound vacuoles in cortical neurons and Purkinje cells and zebra bodies in spinal cord neurons. Vacuoles are also seen in the glomerulus and tubular epithelial cells of the kidney and in hepatocytes, endothelial cells, and Kupffer cells of the liver (582).

Sialidosis should be distinguished from a galactosialidosis (OMIM 256540), a condition in which both neuraminidase and β-galactosidase (G_{M1} ganglioside β-galactosidase) are deficient. This deficiency is the consequence of a primary deficiency of a protective protein/cathepsin A. This protein forms a high-molecular-weight multienzyme complex containing both neuraminidase and β-galactosidase. As a result of this association both enzymes are correctly compartmentalized in lysosomes and are protected from rapid proteolipid degradation (581). In the absence of this protective protein, both protein complexes are reduced and endothelin-1 accumulates in neurons and glial cells of cerebellum, hippocampus and the anterior horns of the spinal cord. Its storage may be responsible for some of the neurologic deficits (582).

Two forms of galactosialidosis have been recognized. The infantile form has its onset early in life, with hydrops, coarse facies, and skeletal changes (583). The other form, which is more common among Japanese, has a juvenile onset, with coarse facies, dysostosis multiplex, conjunctival telangiectases, angiokeratoma, corneal clouding, a macular cherry-red spot, hearing loss, mental retardation, and seizures (583,584).

Sialic Acid Storage Diseases (OMIM 269920)

Several clinical disorders of sialic acid metabolism are marked by lysosomal storage and an abnormally increased urinary excretion of sialic acid. The most common of these entities has been termed Salla disease, after a small town in northern Finland close to the Russian border where this disease is particularly prevalent and where the vast majority of patients share the same founder mutation (585). It is characterized by growth retardation, coarse facies, early delay in mental development, and the evolution of ataxia, spasticity, and extrapyramidal movements. The peripheral nervous system is also affected with demonstrable dysmyelination (586). The disease is slowly progressive and is compatible with a normal life span. Free sialic acid is elevated in urine, blood, and fibroblasts. The combination of early-onset psychomotor retardation and a normal life span without any evidence for deterioration throughout childhood makes this entity unique among lysosomal storage diseases.

This condition is allelic with infantile sialic acid storage disease. This condition is marked by hypotonia, congenital ascites, progressive organomegaly, and delayed development. In some instances there is hydrops fetalis and a prominent telangiectatic skin rash.

The basic defect for both Salla disease and infantile sialic acid storage disease involves a gene that codes for sialin, a lysosomal membrane protein that transports sialic acid out of lysosomes (587).

A third, rare, sialic acid storage disease is sialuria. These patients have coarse facies and static mental retardation. Sialuria is due to mutations in uridinediphosphate-*N*-acetylglucosamine (UDP-GlcNAc) 2-epimerase that interrupt feedback inhibition, resulting in massive excess production of sialic acid (588,589).

The sialic acid storage diseases are probably more common than has been appreciated up to now. The diagnosis can be suspected from the presence of cytoplasmic vacuoles in lymphocytes and from the presence of membrane-bound vacuoles in a conjunctival biopsy (590). Unfortunately, none of the screening tests for oligosaccharides can detect free sialic acid, and all lysosomal enzymes are normal.

Aspartylglycosaminuria (OMIM 208400)

This condition is caused by a defect in the enzyme that cleaves the *N*-acetylglucosamine–asparagine bond (Fig. 1.17, Table 1.12). Like Salla disease, aspartylglycosaminuria is common in Finland (591). The clinical picture is one of mental deterioration commencing between ages 6 and 15 years, coarse facial features, lenticular opacities, bony changes (dysostosis multiplex), and mitral insufficiency. Vacuolated lymphocytes are noted in the majority of patients. The disease is identified by the excretion of aspartylglucosamine and is detected by routine amino acid chromatography (255).

Sphingolipidoses

This group of disorders includes a number of hereditary diseases characterized by an abnormal sphingolipid metabolism, which in most instances leads to the intralysosomal deposition of lipid material within the CNS. Clinically, these conditions assume a progressive course that varies only in the rate of intellectual and visual deterioration.

With the rapid advances in the knowledge of the composition, structure, and metabolism of cerebral lipids, these disorders are best classified according to the chemical nature of the storage material or, if known, according to the underlying enzymatic block. Although such an arrangement is adhered to in this section, the chemistry and metabolism of sphingolipids often prove too complex for the clinician who is not continuously involved in this field. To make matters more difficult, diseases with a similar phenotypic expression can be caused by completely different enzymatic blocks; conversely, an apparently identical genetic and biochemical defect can produce completely different clinical pictures.

Gangliosidoses

In choosing the name gangliosides, Klenk emphasized the localization of these lipids within the ganglion cells of the neuraxis (592). His finding has since been amply confirmed by work indicating that gangliosides are found mainly in nuclear areas of gray matter and are present in myelin in only small amounts.

Gangliosides are components of the plasma membranes. They are composed of sphingosine, fatty acids, hexose, hexosamine, and neuraminic acid (Fig. 1.18). The sphingosine–fatty acid moiety (ceramide) is hydrophobic and acts as a membrane anchor, whereas the hexose, hexosamine, and neuraminic moieties are hydrophilic and extracellular. The pattern of gangliosides is cell-type specific and changes with growth and differentiation. Gangliosides interact at the cell surface with membrane-bound receptors and enzymes; they are involved in cellular adhesion processes and signal transduction events. In addition, they are believed to play a role in the binding of neurotransmitters and other extracellular molecules. They also have a neuronotropic function, which is discussed in connection with the pathogenesis of neurologic deficits in some of the gangliosidoses. Gangliosides are degraded in the cellular lysosomal compartment. The plasma membranes containing gangliosides that are destined for degradation are endocytosed and are transported through the endosomal compartments to the lysosome. There, a series of hydrolytic enzymes cleaves the sugar moieties sequentially to yield ceramide, which is further degraded to sphingosine and fatty acids.

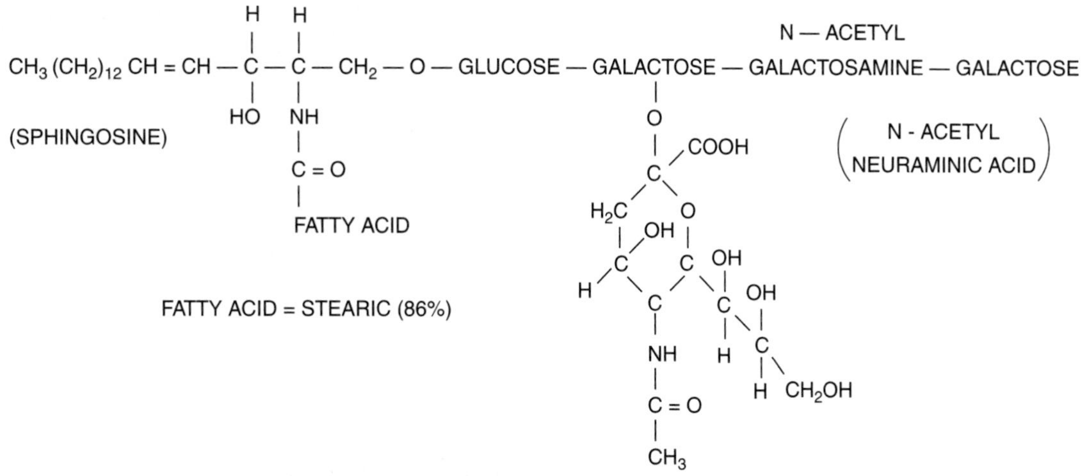

$CH_3(CH_2)_{12}CH = CH - C(H)(HO) - C(H)(NH) - CH_2 - O -$ GLUCOSE — GALACTOSE — N—ACETYL GALACTOSAMINE — GALACTOSE

(SPHINGOSINE)

NH — C = O — FATTY ACID

FATTY ACID = STEARIC (86%)

(N - ACETYL NEURAMINIC ACID)

COOH, H_2C, O, OH, OH, OH, NH, C = O, CH_3, CH_2OH

FIGURE 1.18. Structure of a monosialoganglioside.

At least 10 different gangliosides have been isolated from brain. Of these, 4 are major components and account for more than 90% of the total ganglioside fraction of brain.

As is depicted in Fig. 1.18, the major gangliosides contain the skeleton ceramide-glucose-galactose-galactosamine-galactose. *N*-Acetylneuraminic acid (NANA) is attached to the proximal galactose in the monosialoganglioside, whereas in the two major disialo species, an additional NANA unit is attached either to the terminal galactose or to the first NANA.

G_{M2} Gangliosidoses (Tay-Sachs Disease) (OMIM 272800)

Tay-Sachs disease, the prototype of this group of diseases, was first described by Tay, who noted the retinal changes in 1881 (593), and by Sachs in 1887 (594).

Molecular Genetics and Biochemical Pathology

On chemical analysis of brain tissue, the most striking abnormality is the accumulation of G_{M2} ganglioside in cerebral gray matter and cerebellum 100 to 300 times the normal level. The structure of G_{M2} ganglioside that accumulates in Tay-Sachs disease is depicted in Fig. 1.19. It consists of ceramide to which 1 mol each of glucose, galactose, *N*-acetylgalactosamine, and *N*-acetylneuraminic acid has been attached. Cerebral white matter, liver, spleen, and serum also contain increased amounts of G_{M2} ganglioside. The ganglioside content of viscera is not increased. Several other glycosphingolipids are found in lesser amounts.

In most instances, storage of G_{M2} ganglioside is the result of a defect in hexosaminidase. Two isozymes of hexosaminidase have been recognized. Hexosaminidases A and B are the two major tissue isozymes; hexosaminidase A is composed of one α subunit and one β subunit, whereas hexosaminidase B is composed of two slightly different β subunits. The gene locus for the α subunit has been mapped to chromosome 15 (15q23–q24); for the β subunit, it is on the long arm of chromosome 5 (5q11.2–q13.3) (595). Both genes have been cloned, and numerous mutations have been described. These are being catalogued on the G_{M2} database (http://www.hexdb.mcgill.ca/).

In the classic form of Tay-Sachs disease, the disorder affects the α chain, and hexosaminidase A is inoperative (Fig. 1.19, step A II) in brain, blood, and viscera (596).

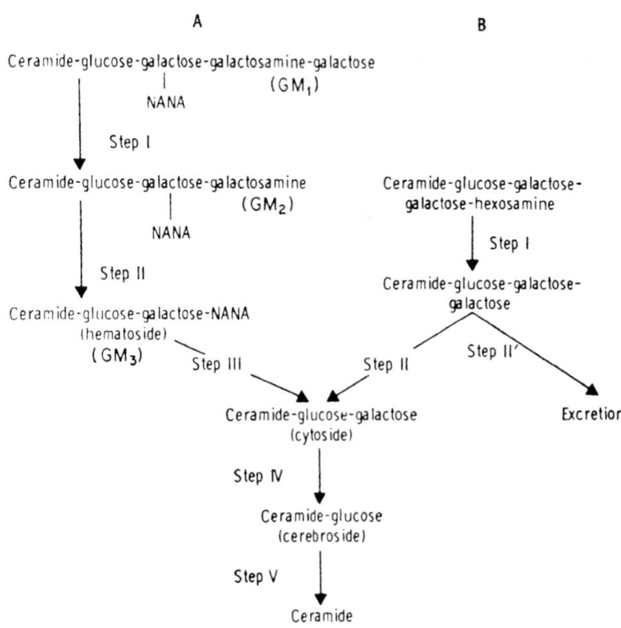

FIGURE 1.19. Degradative pathways for sphingolipids. Metabolic defects are located at the following points: generalized gangliosidosis G_{M1} at step A I; Tay-Sachs disease and variants of generalized gangliosidosis G_{M2} at step A II; adult Gaucher disease at step A V; and Fabry disease at step B II. Enzymes for these reactions have been demonstrated in mammalian brain. NANA, *N*-acetylneuraminic acid.

Total hexosaminidase activity is usually normal, but the hexosaminidase B component in the CNS acting on its own is unable to hydrolyze G_{M2} ganglioside *in vivo*.

In the Jewish form of generalized G_{M2} gangliosidoses three molecular lesions have been found in what had once been considered a pure genetic entity, and a large proportion of patients are compound heterozygotes. The most common mutation, accounting for 73% of Ashkenazi Jews carrying the gene for Tay-Sachs disease in the series of Grebner and Tomczak (597), is a four-base-pair insertion in exon 11 (595). In 18% of cases, there was a single base substitution in intron 12 resulting in defective splicing of the messenger RNA, whereas in 3.3% there was a point mutation on exon 7 (595). In French Canadian patients, an ethnic group in whom the gene frequency for Tay-Sachs disease is equal to that in Ashkenazi Jews, a large deletion in the gene coding for the α chain has been recognized in about 80% of the mutant alleles. The deletion involves part of intron 1, all of exon 1, and probably also the promoter region for the gene. As a consequence, neither mRNA nor immunoprecipitable hexosaminidase A protein is produced. Clinically, this variant is indistinguishable from the Jewish form of Tay-Sachs disease (598).

Mutations in the gene that codes for the gene for the β subunit result in a deficiency of hexosaminidase A and hexosaminidase B, a condition that is termed Sandhoff disease. The most common genetic defect producing this condition is a large deletion in the gene coding for the β subunit (595). Infants with this disorder are non-Jewish, have a mild visceromegaly, and accumulate much larger amounts of globoside (ceramide-glucose-galactose-galactose-galactosamine) in viscera than infants with Tay-Sachs disease (601). Sandhoff disease accounts for approximately 7% of the G_{M2} gangliosidoses (600).

A defect at a third gene locus that codes for the G_{M2} activator protein produces the AB variant. The action of the activator is to extract a single G_{M2} molecule from its micelles to form a water-soluble protein–lipid complex that acts as the true substrate for hexosaminidase A (601). In this entity, accounting for less than 4% of the G_{M2} gangliosidoses in the United Kingdom (600), both hexosaminidase components are present but are inactive with respect to hydrolyzing G_{M2}. The clinical picture of this condition resembles that of classical Tay-Sachs disease. Aside from the G_{M2} activator, four other sphingolipid activator proteins (saposins) have been recognized. They are derived from a single precursor protein (prosaposin); their genetically inherited defects lead to other lysosomal storage diseases (602).

Some children who show the clinical picture of late infantile or juvenile amaurotic idiocy (see the section on generalized G_{M1} gangliosidosis later in this chapter) have been found to have G_{M2} gangliosidosis and a partial defect of hexosaminidase A (603). They account for approximately 25% of English patients with G_{M2} gangliosidosis (600). Patients with the adult or chronic form of G_{M2} gangliosidosis are compound heterozygotes between one of the infantile mutations and a point mutation at exon 7 in the gene for the α chain (595). The clinical picture is one of a child with learning disability who, over the years, develops a gradually progressive muscular weakness. At times, this picture is complicated by ataxia, at other times by dystonia (604). Finally, there are asymptomatic individuals with little more than 10% residual hexosaminidase A activity (602).

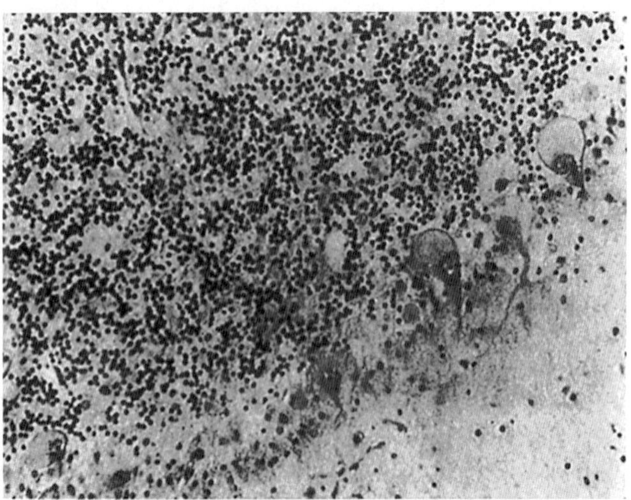

FIGURE 1.20. Tay-Sachs disease. Purkinje cells, showing swollen cell bodies and an occasional antler-like dendrite. In general, lipid storage in the cerebellum is less extensive than in the cerebral cortex (cresyl violet, ×150). (Courtesy of the late Dr. D. B. Clark, University of Kentucky, Lexington, KY.)

Pathologic Anatomy

The pathologic changes in Tay-Sachs disease are confined to the nervous system and represent the most fulminant of all the cerebroretinal degenerations. Almost every neuron in the cerebral cortex is distended markedly, its nucleus is displaced to the periphery, and the cytoplasm is filled with lipid-soluble material (Fig. 1.20). A similar substance is stored in the apical dendrites of the pyramidal cells. As the disease progresses, the number of cortical neurons diminishes, with only a few pyknotic cells remaining. The gliotic reaction is often extensive. In the white matter, myelination can be arrested, and in the terminal stages, demyelination, accumulation of lipid breakdown products, and widespread status spongiosus are observed commonly. Similar alterations affect the cerebellar Purkinje cells and, to a somewhat lesser degree, the larger neurons of the brainstem and spinal cord. In the retina, the ganglion cells are distended with lipid. At the margin of the fovea, considerable reduction in the number of ganglion cells and an accumulation of large phagocytic cells occurs.

On electron microscopic examination of the involved neurons, the lipid is found in the membranous cytoplasmic bodies, which are round, oval, and 0.5 to 2.0 μm

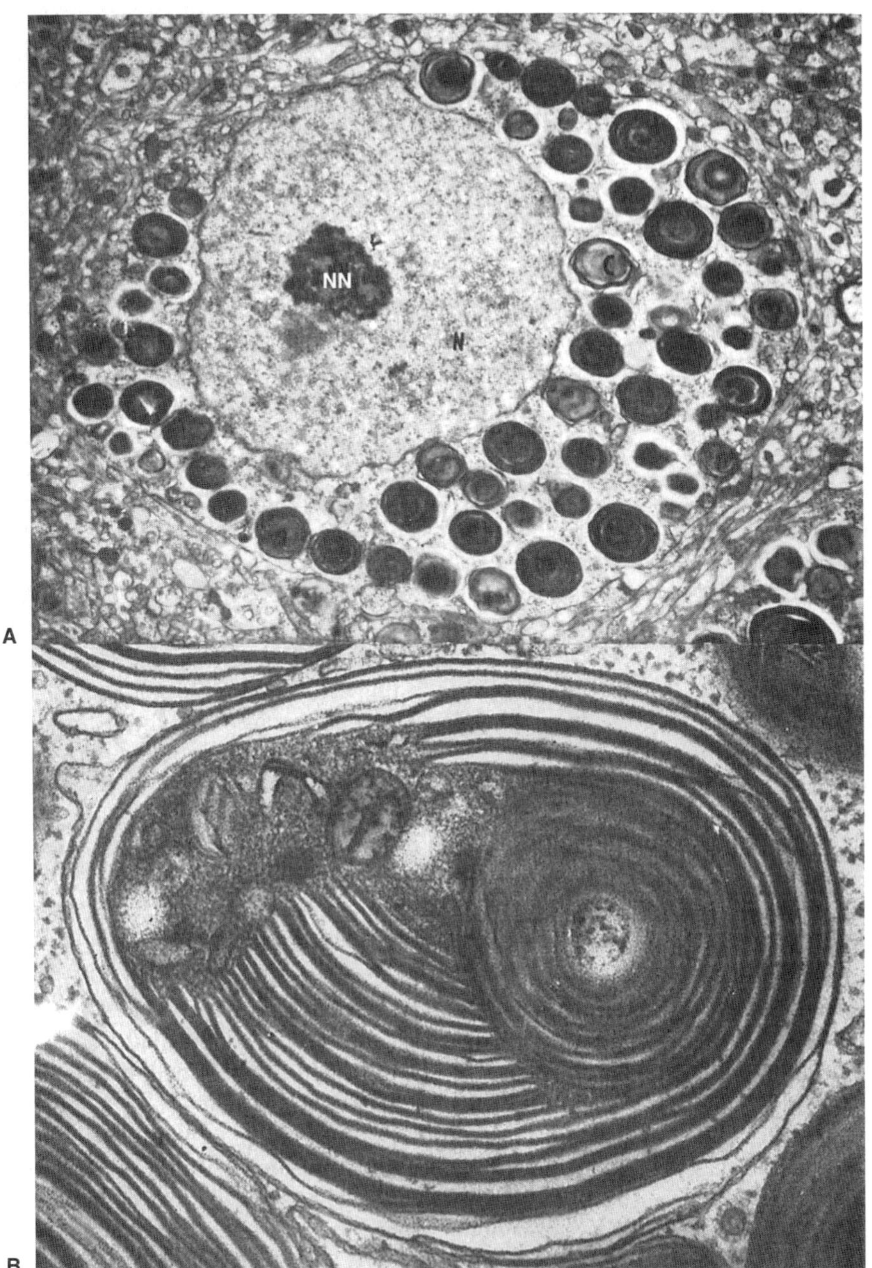

FIGURE 1.21. Tay-Sachs disease, cortical biopsy. **A:** Neuron showing cytoplasmic granules. These are ganglioside in nature. Electron microscopic examination (×10,000). NN, nucleolus; N, nucleus; C, cytoplasmic granule. **B:** Cytoplasmic granule showing lamellar arrangement. Lamellae are approximately 25 Å thick. Electron microscopic examination (×10,000). (From Terry RD, Weiss M. Studies in Tay-Sachs disease: ultrastructure of cerebrum. *J Neuropathol Exp Neurol* 1963;22:18–55. With permission.)

in diameter. They occupy a considerable portion of the ganglion cell cytoplasm (Fig. 1.21). The membranous bodies also can be located in axis cylinders, glial cells, and perivascular cells (605). Membranous cytoplasmic bodies consist of aggregates of lipids (90%) and protein (10%). The composition of lipids is approximately one-third to one-half gangliosides (mainly G_{M2}), approximately 20% phospholipids, and 40% cholesterol. *In vitro* experiments show membranous cytoplasmic bodies to be formed in neurons as a consequence of high ganglioside concentrations in the presence of phospholipids and cholesterol.

By means of Golgi stains and electron microscopy, massively expanded neuronal processes can be demonstrated even in the earliest stages of Tay-Sachs disease. These meganeurites are found specifically at the axon hillock of the cell and displace distally the initial segment of the axon. With progressive enlargement, they become interspersed between the neuronal soma and the axon. Growth of new neurites is increased, probably as a response to excessive amounts of gangliosides, and dendritic spines are lost (606). Abnormal synapses are formed. As a consequence, GABA-ergic connections are enhanced, and the cholinergic connections are altered. The synaptic alterations can be seen early in the disease, much before ganglioside storage has produced a mechanical disruption of cell cytoplasm and organelles (607). Their presence readily explains the neuronal dysfunction and the early onset of neurologic deficits. Similar but less prominent meganeurites have been observed in Hurler syndrome, Sanfilippo syndrome, and in some of the other gangliosidoses.

Clinical Manifestations

Before the 1970s, when carrier screening became available, the classic form of Tay-Sachs disease was usually confined to Jewish families, particularly those of Eastern European background. Since then the condition has been encountered in a variety of ethnic groups. It is transmitted as an autosomal recessive trait. In the United States, the gene frequency is 1 in 27 among Ashkenazi Jews and 1 in 380 among non-Jews.

Infants appear healthy at birth. Until 3 to 10 months of age, growth and development are essentially unremarkable. Listlessness and irritability are usually the first indications of the illness, as well as hyperacusis in approximately one-half of the infants. Soon thereafter, an arrest in intellectual development and a loss of acquired abilities are observed. Examination at this time shows a generalized hypotonia and what is termed a cherry-red spot in both macular areas. The cherry-red spot at the fovea is due to the red of the choroids being visible through an area of the retina that is relatively free of the white, lipid-swollen ganglion cells. The cherry-red spot is characteristic of Tay-Sachs disease, although it is also seen in the other forms of G_{M2} and occasionally is observed in Niemann-Pick disease (types A and C), generalized G_{M1} gangliosidosis, Farber lipogranulomatosis, infantile Gaucher disease, metachromatic leukodystrophy, and sialidosis (608). In Tay-Sachs disease, it is invariably present by the time neurologic symptoms have developed.

No significant enlargement of liver or spleen occurs. The neurologic symptoms progress rapidly to complete blindness and loss of all voluntary movements. Pupillary light reflexes remain intact, however. The hypotonia is replaced by spasticity and opisthotonus. Convulsions appear at this time and can be generalized, focal, myoclonic, or gelastic. In the final stages, a progressive enlargement of the head has been observed; it is invariably present if the disease has lasted more than 18 months (609). The condition terminates fatally by the second or third year of life.

The CSF is normal. In the early stages of the disease, neuroimaging shows low density on CT scans in caudate, thalamus and putamen, and cerebral white matter, with increased signal on T2-weighted MRI in these areas (610). The caudate nuclei appear swollen and protrude into the lateral ventricles.

The clinical pictures of Sandhoff disease and the AB form of G_{M2} gangliosidosis are similar to that of classic Tay-Sachs disease, except for the presence of organomegaly. Juvenile variants of Sandhoff disease have been described. As a rule, these children have late infantile or juvenile progressive ataxia (611).

Other clinical variants of G_{M2} gangliosidosis have been recognized in which the picture is highlighted by motor neuron disease (612) or by a movement disorder (615). As a rule, such patients have traces of hexosaminidase A activity.

Diagnosis

The diagnosis of Tay-Sachs disease is made easily on clinical grounds in an infant with a progressive degenerative disease of the nervous system when the infant has the characteristic retinal cherry-red spot and lacks significant visceromegaly. Hexosaminidase assay of serum confirms the clinical impression and also can be used to detect the heterozygote. Prenatal diagnosis by assaying the hexosaminidase A content of amniotic fluid or of fibroblasts cultured from amniotic fluid is possible during the second trimester of gestation (595).

The serum hexosaminidase assay has been automated and used in mass screening surveys. For the Ashkenazi Jewish population, in whom DNA testing identifies 99.9% of carriers, DNA testing is the preferred method for ascertaining carriers (614). For non-Jewish individuals the enzyme assay can be performed initially and, if necessary, followed up by DNA mutation analysis (614). The apparent deficiency of the enzyme in clinically healthy individuals has already been discussed in this section; see Molecular Genetics and Biochemical Pathology.

Treatment

No effective treatment is known for this condition. The process of G_{M2} ganglioside accumulation and subsequent degeneration of brain structure and function is already well established by the second trimester of fetal development, so that postnatal enzyme replacement therapy and bone marrow transplantation cannot be expected to be effective. In fact, trials of bone marrow transplants have only slowed but not halted the progression of Tay-Sachs disease (595). Prevention of lysosomal storage by administration of *N*-butyldeoxynojirimycin (NB-DNJ), an inhibitor of glycosphingolipid synthesis, has been found to prevent G_{M2} in the brain of mice with Tay-Sachs disease and Sandhoff disease. This approach has been used in the treatment of non-neuropathic Gaucher disease and might be of help in a few patients with some residual hexosaminidase activity (615,616).

Generalized G_{M1} Gangliosidosis (OMIM 230500)

Although it is customary to classify G_{M1} gangliosidosis into infantile, late infantile or juvenile, and adult forms according to the age of onset, a continuum of onset occurs, and this classification is merely one of convenience.

G_{M1} gangliosidosis is not a rare condition; the infantile form was once known as a variant of Tay-Sachs disease with visceral involvement or as pseudo-Hurler syndrome. It was delineated in 1964 by Landing and coworkers (617). The basic enzymatic lesion, a defect in lysosomal β-galactosidase and storage of a monosialoganglioside G_{M1} (see Fig. 1.19, step A I), was discovered in 1965 by O'Brien and coworkers (618).

The clinical picture of the late infantile and juvenile forms of generalized G_{M1} gangliosidosis resembles the Batten-Bielschowsky or Spielmeyer-Vogt types of late infantile and juvenile amaurotic idiocies, whereas the adult form of G_{M1} gangliosidosis is a slowly progressive disease characterized by focal neurologic signs, such as ataxia and movement disorders.

Molecular Genetics and Biochemical Pathology

Total ganglioside content of brain and viscera is increased, and the stored G_{M1} ganglioside constitutes up to 90% of total gray matter gangliosides. Additionally, the asialo derivative of G_{M1} (G_{A1}) is present in large amounts. The ganglioside also is stored in liver and spleen. The ultrastructure of the stored material in the liver, however, is entirely different from the membranous cytoplasmic bodies found in neurons. This difference has been attributed to the accumulation of numerous mannose-containing oligosaccharides, which probably result from defective glycoprotein catabolism (619). It is the storage of these compounds that accounts for the hepatomegaly seen in generalized G_{M1} gangliosidosis but not in G_{M2} gangliosidosis. A profound deficiency (less than 0.1% of normal) of β-galactosidase, the enzyme that catalyzes the cleavage of the terminal galactose of G_{M1} (see Fig. 1.19, step A I), has been demonstrated in several tissues of all patients with G_{M1} gangliosidoses regardless of their clinical course (620).

The β-galactosidase is synthesized in a precursor form, which is processed via an intermediate form to the mature enzyme that aggregates in lysosomes as a high-molecular-weight complex of β-galactosidase, a protective protein, and a lysosomal neuraminidase. The β-galactosidase precursor is encoded on the short arm of chromosome 3, and numerous mutations have been recognized, with most patients being compound heterozygotes and the degree of residual β-galactosidase activity determining the clinical course of the disease. In type B Morquio disease, several other mutations of the β-galactosidase gene have been identified (621). It is of note that the same mutation can result in type B Morquio disease and G_{M1} gangliosidosis, with the phenotypic expression being dependent on the nature of the second allele with which it is paired (622). Type B Morquio disease is considered in the section on the mucopolysaccharidoses. A combined defect in β-galactosidase and neuraminidase produces a clinical picture of cherry-red spots and myoclonus. It is the consequence of a defective protective protein and considered in the section on sialidase deficiency.

Pathologic Anatomy

The pathologic picture shows neuronal storage resembling that of G_{M2} gangliosidosis (Tay-Sachs disease). The neurons are distended with *p*-aminosalicylic acid (PAS)–positive lipid material; electron microscopy shows that they contain a large number of membranous cytoplasmic bodies similar to those seen in Tay-Sachs disease (623). Myelin is defective, probably the consequence of oligodendroglial loss and impaired axoplasmic transport (624). Additionally, many unusual membrane-bound organelles appear to be derived from lysosomes. Abnormalities also are seen in the extraneural tissues. In the kidneys, a striking vacuolization of the glomerular epithelial cells and the cells of the proximal convoluted tubules occurs. In the liver, a marked histiocytosis is associated with vacuolization of the parenchymal cells. Visceral storage of G_{M1} is less prominent in the slower progressive forms.

Clinical Manifestations

For clinical purposes, it is preferable to adhere to the traditional classification of the disease and to divide generalized gangliosidosis into three types. The infantile form of G_{M1} is a severe cerebral degenerative disease that can be clinically evident at birth. The infant is hypotonic with a poor sucking reflex and poor psychomotor development. Characteristic facial abnormalities include frontal bossing, depressed nasal bridge, macroglossia, large, low-set ears, and marked hirsutism. Dermal melanocytosis is seen in about one-fourth of patients. This is a condition characterized by persistent or progressive extensive, blue cutaneous pigmentation and indistinct borders in a dorsal and ventral distribution. This skin lesion is characteristic for lysosomal storage disease. The most common lysosomal storage disease associated with dermal melanocytosis is Hurler syndrome (625). Hepatosplenomegaly usually is present after age 6 months. Approximately 50% of patients have cherry-red spots. The skeletal deformities (dysostosis multiplex) are similar to those seen in Hurler syndrome (508,626). Patients with hepatosplenomegaly and rapid neurologic deterioration that begins during the first few months of life, but without facial coarsening or many skeletal deformities, also have been recognized (627).

In the late infantile and juvenile forms of generalized G_{M1} gangliosidosis, neurologic symptoms usually become manifest after 1 year of age. Hyperacusis can be striking; seizures, frequently taking the form of myoclonic epilepsy, occur in approximately 50% of the patients, and a slowly progressive mental deterioration develops. Bony abnormalities and hepatosplenomegaly are absent, and optic atrophy, when present, is usually unaccompanied by a cherry-red spot (628).

In the chronic adult form, progressive intellectual deterioration becomes apparent between 6 and 20 years of age. It is accompanied by ataxia, a variety of involuntary movements, and spasticity. In other cases, the condition is marked by progressive athetosis or dystonia but no dementia (629). Pathologic studies reveal that in this, as well as in other sphingolipidoses, the storage material in the more chronically progressive disorders is localized predominantly to the basal ganglia, notably the caudate and lenticular nuclei (630). In this region, axonal and dendritic changes analogous to those seen in G_{M2} gangliosidosis are maximal. The cause for the regional predilection is utterly obscure.

Diagnosis

The diagnosis of G_{M1} gangliosidosis is suggested by the early onset of clinical manifestations and rapid neurologic deterioration in a patient who has features and radiologic bone changes reminiscent of Hurler syndrome and by the absence of β-galactosidase in conjunctiva, leukocytes, skin, urine, or viscera. Because so many phenotypic variants of this disorder exist, it is advisable to perform a conjunctival biopsy or to assay for β-galactosidase in any patient with an unexplained progressive neurologic disorder. Enzyme assays on fibroblasts cultured from amniotic fluid allow an antenatal diagnosis in offspring of affected families (631).

Treatment

No treatment is available. G_{M1} gangliosidosis has not been treated successfully by bone marrow transplantation or enzyme infusions.

Gaucher Disease (OMIM 230800; 230900; 23100)

Under the name of Gaucher disease are grouped three fairly distinct clinical conditions (chronic, infantile, and juvenile Gaucher disease) that are characterized by storage of cerebrosides in the reticuloendothelial system. The entity was first described by Gaucher in 1882 (632). It is the most prevalent of the hereditary storage diseases (633).

Three forms have been delineated, with a considerable phenotypic continuum between the two neuropathic forms, and it is likely that nonhereditary factors modify disease expression (634). The most common form is chronic non-neuronopathic (type 1) Gaucher disease, a slowly progressive condition with marked visceral involvement but no nervous system involvement, except in a few instances in which it develops late in life. Occasionally, this form can appear at birth or during early childhood.

The acute neuronopathic form (type 2) is a rare disorder, with a rapid downhill course and marked cerebral involvement. The subacute or juvenile neuronopathic form (type 3) is characterized by splenomegaly, anemia, and neurologic deterioration that develop in the first decade of life. A high incidence of this condition has been reported from the northern part of Sweden, and it therefore is also known as Norbottnian Gaucher disease.

Molecular Genetics and Biochemical Pathology

The enzymatic defect in the various forms of Gaucher disease is an inactivity of a lysosomal ceramide glucoside-cleaving enzyme, glycosyl ceramide β-glucosidase (glucocerebrosidase) (635). The gene for this enzyme has been mapped to the long arm of chromosome 1. It has been isolated and sequenced. Numerous mutations have been identified, with two point mutations accounting for some 80% of mutant alleles. As yet, poor correlation exists between the genetic mutation and the ensuing clinical picture, and an individual's genotype predicts neither the severity nor the course of the illness, although, as a rule, the clinical picture is similar in siblings (636).

As a consequence of the genetic lesion, glucocerebrosidase is defective, and glucocerebroside is the principal sphingolipid stored within the reticuloendothelial system in adult Gaucher disease (637). In affected individuals, the spleen contains greatly increased amounts of ceramide glucoside, ceramide dihexosides, and hematosides (ceramide-glucose-galactose-NANA) (638).

Pathologic Anatomy

The outstanding feature of all types of Gaucher disease is the widespread presence of large numbers of Gaucher cells in spleen, liver, lymph nodes, and bone marrow (Fig. 1.22). These are modified macrophages, appearing as spherical or oval cells between 20 and 50 μm in diameter with a lacy, striated cytoplasm that contrasts with the vacuolated foam cells of Niemann-Pick disease. Electron microscopy reveals irregular inclusion bodies containing tubular elements (639).

In the neuronopathic form (type 2) of Gaucher disease, the cerebral alterations are of five types. These are foci of acute cell loss with neuronophagia, microglial nodules, and chronic neuronal dropout accompanied by gliosis. Additionally, perivascular Gaucher cells can be seen in white matter, particularly in the subcortical area. They are derived from vascular adventitial histiocytes. Finally, a subtle neuronal cytoplasmic accumulation of a PAS-positive material occurs, which on electron microscopy appears as tubular and fibrillar inclusions, similar to the tubules of isolated glucocerebrosides (640). These are detected principally in the large nerve cells outside the cerebral cortex. A marked degree of cytoplasmic storage is not characteristic of infantile Gaucher disease.

The interrelation between the lipid storage and neuronal cell death is not clear. The selective neuronal loss

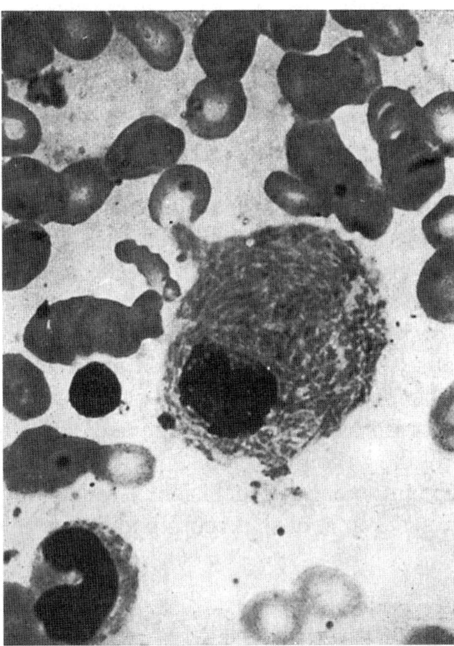

FIGURE 1.22. Typical Gaucher cell together with a lymphocyte and a juvenile neutrophil from the sternal bone marrow in a patient with Gaucher disease. (McGovern MM, Desnick RJ. Abnormalities in the monocyte-microphage system; Lysomal storage diseases. In Green JP, Foerster J, Lukens JN, et al. *Wintrobe's Clinical Hematology,* 11th ed., Philadelphia, Lippincott Williams & Wilkins, 2004;1821. With permission.)

in cerebral cortical layers 3 and 5 and hippocampal layers CA2–4 and 4b points to cytotoxic action (641). Lloyd-Evans and coworkers found that elevation of intracellular glucosylceramide results in increased functional calcium stores in cultured neurons. Glucosylceramide as well as glucosylsphingosine and galactosylsphingosine (psychosine), stimulate calcium release from brain microsomes. In the case of glucosylceramide and galactosylsphingosine the calcium release was mediated through the ryanodine receptors (642). This phenomenon may explain some of the neuropathology.

Clinical Manifestations

In the neuronopathic (type 2 infantile) form of Gaucher disease, the onset of symptoms is generally noted at age 4 or 5 months with anemia, apathy, and loss of intellectual achievements (643,644). These are followed by a gradually progressive spasticity. Neck retraction and bulbar signs are observed frequently, and the infant can have considerable difficulty in swallowing. An acquired oculomotor apraxia also has been noted in this form as well as in the subacute neuronopathic (type 3) form (645). Splenomegaly is usually quite marked, but liver and lymph nodes might not be enlarged. Pulmonary infiltration owing to aspiration or alveolar consolidation by Gaucher cells can be noted. Occasionally, retinal cherry-red spots are present. Radiographic examination reveals rarefaction at the lower ends of the femora. Laboratory studies show only anemia and thrombocytopenia. A neonatal form of Gaucher disease with complete deficiency of glucocerebrosidase is associated with congenital ichthyosis, hepatosplenomegaly, hydrops fetalis, and a rapidly progressive downhill course. This condition has been noted to have a prenatal onset (646).

The subacute neuronopathic form (type 3) becomes apparent during the first decade of life, manifesting by a slowly progressive hepatosplenomegaly, intellectual deterioration, cerebellar ataxia, and spasticity (647). Myoclonic seizures are common (648). They are accompanied by giant potentials on the somatosensory-evoked potentials (SEP), an indication of abnormal cortical inhibition (649). A horizontal supranuclear gaze palsy can develop early in the disease and was found in almost all patients in the series of Harris and colleagues (645). Neuroimaging studies are generally unremarkable. A disproportionately large number of patients have been encountered in Norrbotten in northern Sweden (650). The condition is caused by a single mutation that has been seen in other parts of the world (651).

The chronic non-neuronopathic (type 1) form of Gaucher disease, which is much more common than the other two forms and which occasionally is clinically evident during infancy, rarely involves the CNS, although some patients can develop an atypical form of parkinsonism and dementia during their adult years (633).

Diagnosis

The diagnosis of neuronopathic Gaucher disease must be considered in a child with anemia, splenomegaly, and intellectual deterioration. The presence of Gaucher cells in bone marrow aspirates supports the diagnosis, although Gaucher cells also can be seen in chronic myelocytic leukemia or, occasionally, in thalassemia major. The main difficulty, from a clinical standpoint, is excluding Niemann-Pick disease type A. Assay of glucocerebrosidase in leukocytes and fibroblast cultures, using synthetic or labeled natural substrates, provides a definitive diagnosis and can be used to identify the heterozygote for intrauterine diagnosis of the disease (633).

Treatment

Two forms of therapy are being used in Gaucher disease: enzyme replacement therapy and substrate reduction therapy. Intravenous infusions of glucocerebrosidase purified from human placenta have been effective in reversing most of the systemic manifestations in the non-neuronopathic and the neuronopathic forms. The neurologic symptoms are less amenable to treatment, and in a series of 21 patients with type 3 disease cognitive function decreased in 8 patients while under therapy, with 3 of these patients developing myoclonic seizures (652). This lack of effectiveness results from the inability of intravenous administered glucocerebrosidase to cross the blood-brain barrier in significant amounts. Convection-enhanced delivery of the enzyme to the brain has been effective in experimental animals, and could provide a better treatment option (645a). In substrate reduction therapy an inhibitor of glucosylceramide synthase (Miglustat) is used to reduce the rate of substrate formation to a level that can be metabolized by the residual glucocerebrosidase (653).

Bone marrow transplantation has been attempted in the subacute form (type 3) of the disease with an encouraging response in some cases (568). As is the case for the other lysosomal storage diseases, gene therapy using retroviral vectors to transfer the cDNA for the human glucocerebrosidase gene into hematopoietic stem cells is still in the experimental phase.

Fabry Disease (OMIM 301500)

This rare metabolic disorder is characterized by the storage of ceramide trihexoside and dihexoside and is transmitted as an X-linked recessive condition with unusually frequent penetrance into the heterozygous female patient (654–659).

Molecular Genetics and Biochemical Pathology

The basic defect involves α-galactosidase A, an enzyme that is specific for cleavage of the terminal galactose moiety of globotriaosylceramide (ceramide trihexoside), which has an α configuration (see Fig. 1.19, step B II) (659a). The gene for α-galactosidase A is localized to the long arm of the X chromosome (Xq21.33–q22). It has been completely sequenced, and more than 200 mutations have been documented, with almost every family having its own private mutation, making phenotype difficult to predict from genotype (660). Examination of the synthesis and processing of the enzyme indicates that Fabry disease, like most other lysosomal storage diseases, represents a heterogeneous group of mutations affecting enzyme synthesis, processing, and stability. In some patients, deficiency of α-galactosidase A is the result of a complete absence of the protein; in others, the α-galactosidase A polypeptides are synthesized but are rapidly degraded after their transport to lysosomes (661). Yet other patients, with a milder clinical form of the disease, have residual enzyme activity. As a consequence of the enzymatic defect, large amounts of globotriaosylceramide (ceramide-glucose-galactose-galactose), normally present in minute amounts in plasma and kidneys, have been isolated from affected tissues, and lesser quantities of a ceramide dihexoside (ceramide-galactose-galactose) are found in kidney (662).

Pathologic Anatomy

On pathologic examination, foam cells with vacuolated cytoplasm are found in smooth, striated, and heart musculature; bone marrow; reticuloendothelial system; and renal glomeruli. Much of the pathology of the disorder can be explained by storage within the vascular endothelium.

In the CNS, lipid storage is highly selective and is primarily confined to the lysosomes of vascular endothelium, including that of the choroid plexus. The accumulation of the glycolipid leads to degenerative and proliferative changes and tissue ischemia and infarctions. In some cases, glycolipid also occurs in neurons of the autonomic nervous system, such as the intermediolateral cell columns of the thoracic cord, the dorsal autonomic nuclei of the vagus, hypothalamus, amygdala, and anterior nuclei of the thalamus (663). In these areas, the permeability of the blood–brain barrier can be sufficiently great to allow entrance of the glycolipid (664). On ultrastructural examination, the intraneuronal inclusions resemble those seen in Hurler syndrome, in that zebra bodies are prominent (663).

Clinical Manifestations

Fabry disease was first described in 1898 on the basis of its dermatologic lesions (665). It is a rare condition with an incidence of approximately 1 in 40,000 (654). Manifestations usually begin in childhood, but can be delayed into the second or third decade of life. The clinical picture is believed to result from direct involvement of various tissues by lipid deposits or by vascular disease involving the small arteries and arterioles, predominantly in the posterior circulation (666). The disease is a systemic disorder. The first manifestations are usually acroparesthesias, fatigue with exercise, and cold and heat intolerance first appearing in early childhood (657,667). The punctate, angiectatic skin rash, which gave the condition its original name, angiokeratoma corpus diffusum, is commonly the next manifestation, and usually, as in Fabry's original case, appears in late childhood (668). It is most frequently seen about the hips, umbilicus, and genitalia, but can sometimes assume a butterfly distribution over the face. Diarrhea and postprandial pain are common, and many patients are underweight. Most male patients sweat poorly. The most debilitating symptoms are the acroparesthesial crises in the hands and feet, which become progressively more frequent and can be generalized, lasting for days to weeks, and are accompanied by fever and an elevated sedimentation rate. It is likely that these episodes of acroparesthesia result from peripheral nerve involvement (654). Corneal opacifications, best seen by slit-lamp examination, are common. They have been seen in infancy (669). A peripheral neuropathy affecting the small myelinated and unmyelinated fibers commonly develops as the disease progresses (670). In older patients, hypertension, recurrent cerebral infarction, and hemorrhage are the usual neurologic complications. Neuroimaging studies can be used to delineate the early cerebrovascular alterations consisting of small white matter hyperintense lesions on T2-weighted images and

T1 hyperintensity in the pulvinar (671–673). Untreated, the illness is progressive; death is usually caused by renal failure or cardiac dysfunction. Variants atypical through lack of cutaneous manifestations or isolated renal, cardiac, and corneal involvement (cornea verticillata) are fairly common (576).

Heterozygous female patients can be totally asymptomatic or be as severely affected as male patients. Acroparesthesias, exercise intolerance, and cardiac involvement are particularly common (655).

Diagnosis

Fabry disease should be considered in children who have intermittent burning pain in their feet, legs, and fingertips, aggravated by warm weather or exercise. In the early stages of the disease, angiomas must be sought with care. The umbilicus and scrotum are the most likely sites (654). In male patients, the diagnosis also can be made by finding lipid-like inclusions in the endothelium and smooth muscle of skin biopsies. Biopsy of the peripheral nerve can reveal swelling and disruption of unmyelinated axons and zebra bodies in perineural fibroblasts (670). The diagnosis in male patients is confirmed by finding a marked deficiency of α-galactosidase A in plasma or serum leukocytes or in cultured skin fibroblasts (670). Female patients must be diagnosed by mutation testing. The disease severity does not correlate with blood enzyme levels in female patients.

Treatment

Phenytoin, carbamazepine, gabapentin, or a combination of these drugs can be of considerable benefit in relieving the intermittent pain if nonsteroidal antiinflammatory agents are insufficient. Avoidance of extremes of heat and cold, reduction of fevers, and spraying of water on the body (to substitute for sweating) can be helpful measures. Enzyme replacement therapy using 1 mg/kg of α-galactosidase A (Fabrazyme) every 2 weeks reverses systemic manifestations of the disease, stabilizes renal function, and decreases the episodes of acroparesthesia, although improvement in pain may take over a year. These infusions, although very expensive, are well tolerated and are free of major side reactions (674–676). In Europe, α-galactosidase B (Replagal), an enzyme functionally identical to α-galactosidase A, is available and infused at the lower dose of 0.2 mg/kg every other week (677). Enzyme replacement therapy improves peripheral nerve function (678) and cardiac function (679) and reduces cerebral hyperperfusion (680,681).

Schindler Disease

Schindler disease, a very rare disorder first recognized in 1988, is believed to be the consequence of a defect in lysosomal α-*N*-acetylgalactosaminidase (α-NAGA) (α-galactosidase B). The condition is marked by storage of glycopeptides and oligosaccharides with termination α-*N*-acetylgalactosaminyl moieties. The neuropathologic picture resembles that of infantile neuroaxonal dystrophy (Seitelberger disease), a condition covered in Chapter 3, in that axonal spheroids are seen throughout the neocortex.

Clinical heterogeneity is marked; the same genotype can present with a progressive disease leading to the vegetative state or be totally asymptomatic (682). In many of the reported cases the illness becomes apparent during the second year of life and manifests itself by developmental deterioration, myoclonic seizures, and cortical blindness. Angiokeratoma and tortuous conjunctival vessels are seen in the older patients (683). No organomegaly occurs and there is no vacuolization of peripheral lymphocytes or granulocytes. The diagnosis is made by analysis of plasma or leukocyte lysosomal enzymes and analysis of oligosaccharides in nondesalted urine (683,684).

Niemann-Pick Diseases (OMIM 257200)

The prototype of these conditions was first described in 1914 by Niemann (685). Their traditional nomenclature as proposed in 1958 by Crocker and Farber (686) implies that these conditions are biochemically and enzymatically related. Actually, this is not the case. Niemann-Pick disease types A (NPA) and B (NPB) are recessively inherited lysosomal storage diseases that feature a deficiency in sphingomyelinase activity and an accumulation of sphingomyelin in the reticuloendothelial system. They are allelic and result from mutations in the gene that codes for sphingomyelinase. Types C (NPC) and D (NPD) are characterized by an accumulation of cholesterol and sphingomyelin. They result from an abnormal intracellular translocation of cholesterol derived from low-density lipoproteins with NPD being an allelic variant of NPC. Callahan proposed a classification by which the various conditions are grouped into type I (formerly types A and B) and type II (formerly types C and D) (687). From a clinical point of view, it is still preferable, however, to retain the older classification.

Niemann-Pick Disease Type A

Clinically, NPA is characterized by autosomal recessive transmission with a predilection for Ashkenazi Jewish families [approximately 30% of patients in the series of Crocker and Farber (686)]. Symptoms become apparent during the first year of life with hepatosplenomegaly, which can lead to massive abdominal distention, and with poor physical and mental development. Other systemic symptoms include persistent neonatal jaundice, diarrhea, generalized lymphadenopathy, and pulmonary infiltrates.

In approximately one-third of patients, neurologic symptoms predominate initially, and few children survive

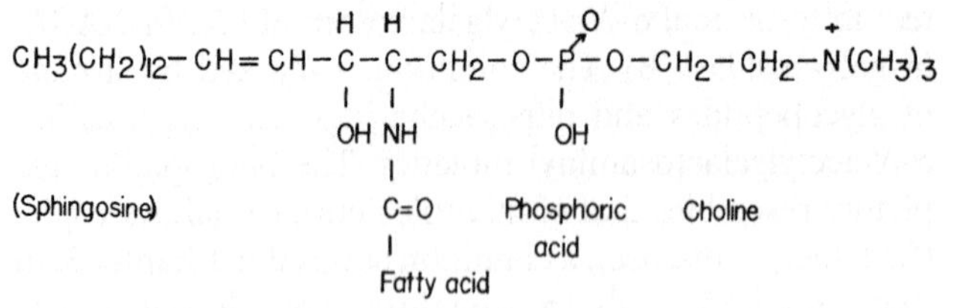

$$CH_3(CH_2)_{12}-CH=CH-\underset{OH}{\overset{H}{C}}-\underset{NH-C(=O)-\text{Fatty acid}}{\overset{H}{C}}-CH_2-O-\underset{OH}{\overset{O}{P}}-O-CH_2-CH_2-\overset{+}{N}(CH_3)_3$$

(Sphingosine) Fatty acid Phosphoric acid Choline

FIGURE 1.23. Structure of a sphingomyelin.

beyond infancy without apparent involvement of the nervous system. Seizures, particularly myoclonic jerks, are common, and marked spasticity can develop before death. Approximately one-half of the infants have hypotonia; with progression of the disease, the nerve conduction velocities slow. On biopsy of the peripheral nerves, the Schwann cells are filled with inclusion bodies (688). Retinal cherry-red spots are found in approximately 25% of patients and can antedate neurologic abnormalities (686). Corneal and lenticular opacifications are common (673a). The progression of the disease is variable, but death usually occurs before age 5 years.

The pathologic hallmark of NPA is the presence of large, lipid-laden cells in the reticuloendothelial system, mostly in spleen, bone marrow, liver, lungs, and lymph nodes. In the brain, massive, generalized deposition of foam cells and ballooned ganglion cells occurs, primarily in the cerebellum, brainstem, and spinal cord (690). Lipid storage also occurs in the endothelium of cerebral blood vessels, in arachnoid cells, and in the connective tissue of the choroid plexus.

Biochemical examination documents the storage of sphingomyelin in affected organs. This compound was first described in 1884 by Thudichum, the father of neurochemistry (691), and was found to have the structure depicted in Fig. 1.23.

Chemical and histochemical studies have shown sphingomyelin to be a major myelin constituent. It is also a normal component of spleen. Sphingomyelinase, which cleaves sphingomyelin into phosphatidylcholine and ceramide, is normally present in liver, kidney, spleen, and brain. Two forms of this enzyme have been distinguished. The lysosomal form has an acidic pH optimum, which distinguishes it from the microsomal form, which has a basic pH optimum. In NPA, the lysosomal enzyme is defective. The gene for lysosomal sphingomyelinase has been mapped to the short arm of chromosome 11p15.1–p15.4. It has been cloned and sequenced, and a variety of mutations have been described. Mutations lacking catalytically active sphingomyelinase result in NPA, whereas mutations that produce a defective enzyme with some residual catalytic activity result in NPB (692). Two common mutations are responsible for more than 50% of Ashkenazi Jewish patients with NPA (693).

Niemann-Pick Disease Type B

Classic NPB is very rare, and the majority of NPB patients develop neurologic symptoms later in life (694). The absence of any childhood neurologic manifestations in NPB precludes its extensive discussion. Suffice it to say that the clinical picture is one of hepatosplenomegaly, hyperlipidemia, and interstitial pulmonary infiltrates. In some cases, sphingomyelin storage occurs in retinal neurons, peripheral nerves, and the endothelium of the cerebral vasculature (695).

Niemann-Pick Disease Type C (OMIM 257220)

Niemann-Pick disease type C (NPC) is more common than NPA and NPB combined and is seen in a variety of ethnic groups. Its prevalence in Western Europe has been estimated at 1 in 150,000, but it is much higher in certain geographic isolates such as in the French Acadians of Nova Scotia. It has been described under several terms, notably Niemann-Pick types E and F, a condition in which vertical supranuclear ophthalmoplegia and sea-blue histiocytes were accompanied by hepatic cirrhosis and juvenile dystonic lipidosis. As can be surmised from the multitude of eponyms, the clinical picture is extremely heterogeneous, even within the same family, and reports describe a continuum of severity, with neurologic symptoms appearing any time from infancy to late adult life. Two genotypes have been recognized. About 95% of patients with NPC have mutations in the NPC1 gene that has been mapped to 18q11; the remainder have mutations in the NPC2 gene mapped to 14q24.3 (696).

NPC1

Clinically, the disorder is heterogeneous, but three phenotypes have been described with considerable overlap among them:

1. An early-onset, rapidly progressive form is seen in about 20% of cases. It is marked by severe liver dysfunction and developmental delay in infancy, followed by supranuclear gaze palsy, ataxia, increasing spasticity, and seizures in those who survive the neonatal period. In its most severe form, comprising another 10% of patients with NPC1, the disease presents in infancy with prolonged neonatal jaundice, often associated with cholestasis and giant cell hepatitis, hepatosplenomegaly, and a rapid progression (697) Neurologic signs or symptoms may not be apparent (698).
2. A late infantile/juvenile form is seen in 50% of patients. In this entity, the disease makes its first appearance between ages 2 and 4 years. Neurologic symptoms predominate, and in children younger than 5 years cerebellar ataxia is the presenting feature. Older children present with learning difficulties. Dystonia and other basal ganglia symptoms are common, as are

myoclonic or akinetic seizures, ataxia, and macular cherry-red spots. A supranuclear paralysis of vertical gaze is characteristic for this condition. Some degree of hepatosplenomegaly is found in some 90% of patients, but is not as striking as in NPA and can become less marked as the illness progresses (699). Sea-blue histiocytes and foam cells are seen in the bone marrow in virtually every instance (700).

3. A late-onset variant with a clinical picture similar to the juvenile-onset variant can appear during adolescence or adult life.
4. A non-neuronopathic form of NPC1 has also been described.

On pathologic examination of the brain, the condition is marked by a massive loss of nerve cells and the lysosomal accumulation of unesterified cholesterol and sphingolipids within neurons. Lysosomal accumulation of unesterified cholesterol and sphingolipids is also seen in liver and spleen (701). Cytoskeletal abnormalities are seen within neurons. These consist of Alzheimer Disease (AD)-type neurofibrillary tangles (NFTs) composed of hyperphosphorylated tau proteins. Tau proteins are low-molecular-weight, microtubule-associated proteins that are normally found predominantly in axons of the central nervous system (702). In the most severely affected patients there is also a deposition amyloid beta protein such as is seen in Alzheimer disease. This deposition is particularly marked in patients who are homozygous for ApoE4 (703).

The gene that is defective in NPC1 encodes a transmembrane protein that is involved in mobilization of endosomal cholesterol to the plasma membrane. Cholesterol is delivered to cells by the low-density-lipoprotein (LDL) pathway. In the cell, after LDL receptor-mediated endocytosis, the LDL particles are transported to lysosomes, where cholesterol esters are hydrolyzed by acid lipase. Unesterified cholesterol is used for synthesis of membranes and sterol derivatives and regulates *de novo* cholesterol biosynthesis and LDL uptake. In NPC1 cholesterol biosynthesis is not suppressed despite high levels of free intracellular cholesterol (704). The relation between the disorder of cholesterol metabolism and the development of Alzheimer-like pathology is an area of intense investigation (705).

NPC2

Although genetically distinct, NPC2 is phenotypically similar to NPC1. The rate of disease progression is variable, and death may occur by 6 months of age or not until adult life. In the small number of patients surveyed, pulmonary symptoms including pulmonary fibrosis was common (706). The condition results from mutations in HE1, a ubiquitously expressed soluble lysosomal protein that binds cholesterol (707).

Niemann-Pick Disease Type D

The clinical presentation of NPD, now known to be allelic with NPC, is indistinguishable from the slowly progressive form of NPC, except that patients are from southwestern Nova Scotia, a geographic isolate where the heterozygote frequency for this condition ranges between 1 in 4 and 1 in 10 (708,709).

Diagnosis

Hepatosplenomegaly, anemia, and failure to thrive in children who show intellectual deterioration can suggest one of the forms of Niemann-Pick disease with neurologic involvement. Leukocytes and skin fibroblasts of patients with NPA are deficient in sphingomyelinase. Sphingomyelinase activity has been found in cultured amniotic fibroblasts, allowing an intrauterine diagnosis of NPA and NPB (695).

Diagnosis of both NPC1 and NPC2 can be made by demonstrating delayed LDL-derived cholesterol esterification and increased amounts of unesterified cholesterol in fibroblasts. Staining with filipin demonstrates the intracellular accumulation of cholesterol (701). A small percentage of patients with NPC show near-normal results of the biochemical tests. Fibroblasts derived from these NPC-variant patients act as in a sphingolipid storage disease and accumulate a fluorescent sphingolipid in their lysosomes rather than in the Golgi complex as is the case in normal cells (710).

The presence of sea-blue histiocytes in the bone marrow also serves to diagnose NPC.

Treatment

Liver or bone marrow transplantation has been unsuccessful in the treatment of NPA and NPC. Enzyme replacement therapy is being developed for patients with NPB who have no neurologic symptoms. No evidence indicates that dimethylsulfoxide or cholesterol-lowering agents improve neurologic symptoms in NPC.

Wolman Disease (Acid Lipase Deficiency Disease) (OMIM 278000)

This condition was first described by Wolman and his group in 1956 (711). The clinical manifestations resemble those of NPA and include failure in weight gain, a malabsorption syndrome, and adrenal insufficiency. Lipoproteins and plasma cholesterol are reduced and acanthocytes are evident (712). A massive hepatosplenomegaly occurs, and radiographic examination reveals the adrenals to be calcified. Neurologic symptoms are usually limited to delayed intellectual development. Pathologic examination shows xanthomatosis of the viscera. Sudanophilic material is stored in the leptomeninges, retinal ganglion cells, and nerve cells of the myenteric plexus. Sudanophilic granules outline the cortical capillaries, and sudanophilic demyelination occurs (713).

A striking accumulation of cholesterol esters and triglycerides occurs in affected tissues. Lipid accumulation is greatest in tissues that synthesize the most cholesterol esters. These tissues include the adrenal cortex, liver, intestine, spleen, and lymph nodes. Relatively little lipid storage occurs in the brain. The basic enzymatic defect is a deficiency in lysosomal acid lipase, an enzyme that normally hydrolyzes cholesterol esters and medium- and long-chain triglycerides (714). The gene coding for this enzyme has been mapped to chromosome 10q23.2 and has been cloned. Acid lipase deficiency has been demonstrated in fibroblasts, which lack the ability to hydrolyze cholesterol esters entering the cells bound to low-density lipoproteins. Because free low-density lipoproteins are not present in the cell, the suppression of 3-hydroxy-3-methylglutaryl-CoA reductase, which normally regulates endogenous cholesterol synthesis, also is impaired (715).

Deficiency of lysosomal acid lipase is responsible for two clinically distinguishable phenotypes: Wolman disease and cholesterol ester storage disease (CESD). Wolman disease is a severe infantile-onset variant, whereas CESD is a milder condition and often remains unrecognized until adult life. Lipid deposition is widespread, but hepatomegaly may be the only clinical manifestation. Most but not all patients with CESD have genetic mutations that result in residual acid lipase activity, whereas the mutations resulting in Wolman disease produce a nonfunctioning enzyme (716,717). Wolman disease also should be distinguished from triglyceride storage disease type I, in which only the hydrolysis of triglycerides is impaired and in which infants are developmentally retarded (718).

Bone marrow transplant has produced a long-term remission with normalization of peripheral lysosomal acid lipase activity and improved developmental milestones (719). 3-Hydroxy-3-methylglutaryl coenzyme A (HMG CoA) reductase inhibitors have only been minimally beneficial.

Ceramidosis (Farber Lipogranulomatosis) (OMIM 228000)

Ceramidosis, which is probably the rarest of the lysosomal storage diseases, was first described by Farber and associates (720). The clinical features are unique and manifest during the first few weeks of life. The infant becomes irritable, has a hoarse cry, and develops nodular erythematous swelling of the wrists. Over subsequent months, nodules develop in numerous sites, particularly in areas subject to trauma, such as joints and the subcutaneous tissue of the buttocks. Severe motor and mental retardation occur. Hepatosplenomegaly has been seen in approximately 70% of reported cases (721). In approximately two-thirds of cases, the disease progresses rapidly, and death usually occurs by 2 years of age. As a rule, the earlier the dermal nodules appear, the more malignant is the illness. Variants that resemble a malignant form of histiocytosis X have been reported (722).

The basic pathologic lesion is a granuloma formed by the proliferation and ballooning of mesenchymal cells that ultimately become enmeshed in dense hyaline fibrous tissue. Within the CNS, neurons and glial cells are swollen and contain stored material (723).

The enzymatic defect responsible has been localized to lysosomal acid ceramidase, which is absent from brain, kidney, and skin fibroblasts (724). The gene coding for the enzyme has been cloned, and numerous pathogenic mutations have been defined (725). A consequence of the defect is a striking increase in ceramides in affected tissues. Gangliosides also are increased, particularly in the subcutaneous nodules, which have the ganglioside concentration of normal gray matter. Mildly affected patients in whom mental function is unimpaired also have been encountered (697). Bone marrow transplantation has been unsuccessful in correcting the neurologic deficits, and no treatment exists for this disorder (721).

Cystinosis (OMIM 219800)

Neurologic symptoms are not commonly part of the clinical picture of early-onset or infantile nephropathic cystinosis. However, with the successful management of end-stage renal disease and longer survival of patients, neurologic complications are becoming apparent (725). Cystine accumulates in the form of cystine crystals in lysosomes of a variety of organs. In the brain, they are seen in the interstitial macrophages of choroid plexus (726). Two forms of neurologic disorder have been recognized. One form is marked by progressive cerebellar signs, spasticity, pseudobulbar palsy, and dementia. The second form presents with the sudden onset of changes in consciousness and hemiparesis (727). A myopathy caused by accumulation of cystine in and around muscle fibers, and oral motor dysfunction also has been recorded (728). Computed tomography (CT) scans have revealed progressive ventricular dilation and calcifications in the periventricular white matter (729). A young man with a progressive parkinsonian movement disorder has been seen at our hospital. Treatment with cysteamine can be effective in some cases with encephalopathy (727).

DISORDERS OF LIPID AND LIPOPROTEIN METABOLISM

Globoid cell leukodystrophy and metachromatic leukodystrophy have been shown to result from a disorder in lipid metabolism. These conditions are discussed in Chapter 3 with the other leukodystrophies.

Cerebrotendinous Xanthomatosis (OMIM 213700)

Although cerebrotendinous xanthomatosis, a rare but well-defined familial disease, was first described by van Bogaert and associates in 1937 (730), its unique chemical feature, deposition of cholestanol (dihydrocholesterol) within the nervous system, was uncovered only in 1968 by Menkes and associates (731). The disease is characterized by xanthomas of tendons and lungs, cataracts, slowly progressive cerebellar ataxia, spasticity, and dementia. It has a predilection for Sephardic Jews of Moroccan ancestry.

Although, as a rule, the disease is not apparent until late childhood, some 35% of patients in the series of Berginer and colleagues were symptomatic before age 10 years (732). Progression is generally slow, and in many instances, the illness does not interfere with a normal life span. The triad of progressive spinocerebellar ataxia, pyramidal signs, and mental retardation is seen in the large majority of patients with cerebrotendinous xanthomatosis, and mental retardation is seen in more than 90% (732). Cataracts are present in 76% of patients and generally are seen as early as 56 years of age. Seizures are encountered in 40% to 50% of patients and can be the presenting symptom (733). Intractable diarrhea can be a major manifestation during childhood (chologenic diarrhea) (734). A sensory and motor neuropathy also has been documented (703). Tendon xanthomas can be apparent in childhood, most commonly over the Achilles and triceps tendons. Serum cholesterol levels tend to be low, and cholestanol concentrations in serum and erythrocytes are elevated (732). CT reveals the presence of hyperdense nodules in the cerebellum and diffuse white matter hypodensity. MRI demonstrates atrophy of cerebrum and cerebellum, with occasional atrophy of the brainstem and corpus callosum. Increased signal is seen on T2-weighted images in the dentate nucleus, globus pallidus, substantia nigra, and inferior olive, extending into the white matter as the disease progresses. Occasionally hypodensity on T2-weighted images is present in the dentate nucleus, related to deposition of hemosiderin and calcifications (735).

On pathologic examination, the brainstem and cerebellum are the two areas within the nervous system most affected. Myelin destruction, a variable degree of gliosis, and xanthoma cells are visible (736).

On chemical examination, large amounts of free and esterified cholestanol are found stored in the nervous system. The sterol is located not only in such affected areas as the cerebellum, but also in histologically normal myelin. The content of cholestanol in the tendon xanthomas is increased, but here the predominant sterol is cholesterol (731).

The defect in cerebrotendinous xanthomatosis has been localized to the mitochondrial sterol 27-hydroxylase (737). The gene has been cloned, and numerous mutations have been documented (738,739). As a consequence of the enzymatic defect, chenodeoxycholic acid is absent from bile, and cholic acid biosynthesis proceeds via the 25-hydroxylated intermediates. Large amounts of C-27 bile alcohols in the form of glucuronides are present in bile, plasma, and urine. Batta and coworkers explained the deposition of cholestanol within the CNS, where it can comprise as much as 50% of the total sterols, by a disorder in the blood–brain barrier induced by the presence of large amounts of bile alcohol glucuronides (740).

Treatment with chenodeoxycholic acid (15 mg/kg per day) reverses the elevated CSF cholestanol levels and induces a 50% reduction of plasma cholestanol, an increase in IQ, and a reversal of neurologic symptoms (741). Additionally, improvement occurs in the EEG, somatosensory-evoked potentials, and the MRI (732,741).

Smith-Lemli-Opitz Syndrome (OMIM 270400)

Smith-Lemli-Opitz syndrome, an autosomal recessive condition, is marked by the combination of mental retardation, hypotonia, midface hypoplasia, congenital or postnatal cataracts, and ptosis. Anomalies of the external male genitalia and the upper urinary tract are common (742). The prevalence of Smith-Lemli-Opitz syndrome has been estimated at 1 in 20,000, making it one of the more common metabolic causes for mental retardation (743,744). The basic biochemical defect involves the gene coding for sterol delta-7-reductase, the enzyme that converts 7-dehydrocholesterol to cholesterol, the last step of cholesterol biosynthesis (744). The gene has been mapped to chromosome 11q12–q13 and has been cloned. A number of mutations have been documented that result in reduced expression of the enzyme (745,746). As a consequence of the enzymatic defect, the concentration of plasma 7-dehydrocholesterol is markedly increased and plasma cholesterol is significantly reduced.

The clinical picture of Smith-Lemli-Opitz syndrome ranges in severity from little more than syndactyly of the second and third toes to holoprosencephaly with profound mental retardation (746). As a rule, the lower the plasma cholesterol, the more severe is the clinical picture. Although the disease has been divided into two types, with type II being more severe than type I, there is a continuum of clinical severity. A low plasma cholesterol level should suggest the diagnosis, which can be confirmed by finding an elevated 7-dehydrocholesterol level on gas–liquid chromatography/mass spectroscopy (747). In 10% of patients, plasma cholesterol levels are normal, and the diagnosis depends on quantitation of 7-dehydrocholesterol (747). Some patients excrete large amounts of 3-methylglutaconic acid, and this can be detected on screening of urinary organic acids (748).

Several other disorders of cholesterol biosynthesis are associated with dysmorphogenesis of the brain and other organs, notably the limbs (748a). Cholesterol can modulate

TABLE 1.19 Genetic Disorders of Cholesterol Biosynthesis

Disorder	*Clinical Picture*	*Reference*
Smith-Lemli-Opitz syndrome	Microcephaly, holoprosencephaly, facial and limb anomalies	
Desmosterolosis	Macrocephaly, rhizomelic limb shortening, facial anomalies	
Lathosterolosis	Dysmorphic features, microcephaly, facial anomalies	Brunetti-Pieri et al. (753)
Mevalonic acidemia	Growth failure, developmental delay, hypotonia, ataxia, facial anomalies	
Conradi-Hünermann syndrome	Lethal in males; asymmetric limb shortening, scoliosis, cataracts, facial anomalies, patchy alopecia, skin defects, occasional mental retardation	
CHILD syndrome	Lethal in males; unilateral erythematous exfoliative dermatitis, punctate calcifications of epitheses	
Antley-Bixler syndrome	Craniosynostosis, severe midface hypoplasia, proptosis, choanal atresia/stenosis, frontal bossing, dysplastic ears, depressed nasal bridge, radiohumeral synostosis, long-bone fractures and femoral bowing, urogenital abnormalities	Hassell and Butler (753)

CHILD, congenital hemidysplasia, ichthyosiform erythroderma, and limb defects.
These conditions are reviewed by Haas and coworkers (750), Herman (753), Porter (754), and Krakowiak and coworkers (755).

the activity of the Hedgehog proteins (see Chapter 5), which control the embryonic development of forebrain and limbs (749,750). The various other genetic disorders of cholesterol biosynthesis are listed in Table 1.19.

Smith-Lemli-Opitz syndrome has been treated with dietary cholesterol supplementation, which unfortunately does not improve the development of affected children (756).

PEROXISOMAL DISORDERS

Peroxisomes are ubiquitous organelles containing more than 50 enzymes involved in anabolic and catabolic reactions, including plasmalogen and bile acid biosynthesis, gluconeogenesis, the removal of excess peroxides, purine catabolism, and β-oxidation of very long chain fatty acids. Peroxisomes do not contain DNA, and peroxisomal matrix and membrane proteins, therefore, must be imported from the cytosol where they are synthesized. Peroxisomal structure and function and peroxisomal biogenesis have been reviewed by Moser (757), Gould and colleagues (758), and Wanders (759). At least 20 disorders of peroxisomal function have been identified. They can be classified into two groups.

In group 1, a disorder of peroxisome biogenesis, the number of peroxisomes is reduced and the activities of many peroxisomal enzymes are deficient. Zellweger cerebrohepatorenal syndrome, neonatal adrenoleukodystrophy, and infantile Refsum disease belong to this group.

In group 2, peroxisomal structure and function are normal, and the defect is limited to a single peroxisomal enzyme. At least 13 disorders exist in which a single peroxisomal enzyme is defective (757). X-linked adrenoleukodystrophy, in which peroxisomal fatty acid β-oxidation is defective, and adult Refsum disease, in which phytanic acid α-oxidation is deficient, belong to this group. X-linked adrenoleukodystrophy is covered in Chapter 3 with the other leukodystrophies.

The major clinical features of the disorders of peroxisomal assembly are outlined in Table 1.20.

Disorders of Peroxisomal Biogenesis

The basic defect in disorders of peroxisomal biogenesis involves the incorporation of the peroxisomal proteins into peroxisomes. The proteins of peroxisomal matrix and membranes are encoded by nuclear genes and are synthesized on cytoplasmic polyribosomes. They are then targeted to the peroxisomes. Protein targeting is achieved through the interaction of specific peroxisomal-targeting signals on these proteins with their cognate cytoplasmic receptors. The major targeting signal is a C-terminal tripeptide (PTS1). Less commonly, a nine-amino acid signal is used (PTS2). These receptors, bound to their cargo, interact with specific docking proteins in the peroxisomal membrane. Finally, by a process not fully understood, the peroxisomal proteins enter the peroxisome (758). As ascertained from the results of complementation analyses, at least 15 different groups of defects affect peroxisomal biogenesis, implying that at least 15 genes are involved in the formation of normal peroxisomes and in the transport of peroxisomal enzymes (757). No correlation exists between the complementation group and the phenotypic features, and Zellweger syndrome is represented in 13 of the 15 complementation groups (757).

As a consequence of the defect of peroxisomal membrane proteins, enzymes normally found within the peroxisomal matrix are absent or located in the cytosol, and cultured fibroblasts derived from patients with Zellweger syndrome contain empty membranous sacs, designated as peroxisomal ghosts (760).

Zellweger Syndrome

The differentiation of the disorders of peroxisomal biogenesis into Zellweger syndrome, neonatal adrenoleukodystrophy, and infantile Refsum disease is not based on a

TABLE 1.20 Major Clinical Features of Disorders of Peroxisomal Assembly and Their Occurrence in Various Peroxisomal Disorders

Feature	*ZS*	*NALD*	*IRD*	*Oxidase Deficiency*	*Bifunctional Enzyme Deficiency*	*RCDP*	*DHAP Synthase Deficiency*	*DHAP Alkyl Transferase Deficiency*
Average age at death or last follow-up (years)	0.76	2.2	6.4	4.0	0.75	1.0	0.5	?
Facial dysmorphism	++	+	+	0	73%	++	++	++
Cataract	80%	45%	7%	0	0	72%	+	+
Retinopathy	71%	82%	100%	2+	+	0	0	0
Impaired hearing	100%	100%	93%	2+	?	71%	33%	100%
Psychomotor delay	4+	3–4+	3+	2+	4+	4+	4+	?
Hypotonia	99%	82%	52%	+	4+	±	±	?
Neonatal seizures	80%	82%	20%	50%	93%	±	?	?
Large liver	100%	79%	83%	0	+	0	?	0
Renal cysts	93%	0	0	0	0	0	0	0
Rhizomelia	3%	0	0	0	0	93%	+	+
Chondrodysplasia punctata	69%	0	0	0	0	100%	+	+
Neuronal migration defect	67%	20%	±	?	88%	±	?	?
Coronal vertebral cleft	0	0	0	0	0	+	+	+
Demyelination	22%	50%	0	60%	75%	0	0	0

Percentages indicate the percentage of patients in whom the abnormality is present; 0, abnormality is absent; ± to 4+, degree to which an abnormality is present.
DHAP, dihydroacetone phosphate; IRD, infantile Refsum disease; NALD, neonatal adrenoleukodystrophy; RCDP, rhizomelic chondrodysplasia punctata; ZS, Zellweger syndrome.
From Moser HW. Peroxisomal disorders, In: Rosenberg RN, Prusiner SB, DiMauro S, et al., eds. *The molecular and genetic basis of neurologic and psychiatric disease,* 3rd ed. Philadelphia: Butterworth–Heinemann, 2003:214.
With permission of Dr. Hugo Moser, Director, Neurogenetics Research Center, Kennedy Krieger Institute, Johns Hopkins University, Baltimore, MD.

fundamental genetic difference but on the severity of the disease, with Zellweger syndrome the most severe and infantile Refsum disease the least severe. All three entities are autosomal recessive disorders, with the Zellweger form having a frequency of 1 in 100,000 births. Several genetic defects cause the disorders of peroxisomal biogenesis. Mutations in either one of two adenosinetriphosphatases (ATPases), peroxin 1 (PEX1) and peroxin 6 (PEX6), are common causes of these disorders (761). The gene for PEX1, which is responsible for about two-thirds of patients with Zellweger syndrome (762), encodes a 147-kd member of the AAA protein family (ATPases associated with diverse cellular activities), and at least 30 mutations of this gene have been recorded (762). PEX1 is believed to interact with PEX6, a different member of the AAA protein family, and the two proteins are active in the import of protein into the peroxisomal matrix. At least seven other genetic mutations have been delineated (758). The phenotypic severity of Zellweger syndrome appears to correlate well with the gene defect, in that mutations with the most significant loss of protein function result in the most severe clinical symptoms (762).

In its classic form, Zellweger syndrome is marked by intrauterine growth retardation, hypotonia, profound developmental delay, hepatomegaly, variable contractures in the limbs, and renal glomerular cysts. Impaired hearing and nystagmus are common, as are irregular calcifications of the patellae. Facies are unusual with a large fontanel, a high forehead with shallow supraorbital ridges, a low or broad nasal bridge, and a variety of eye and ear anomalies (763) (see Fig. 1.10). A number of migrational disorders of the brain have been documented, including macrogyria, polymicrogyria, and heterotopic gray matter in the cerebral hemispheres and cerebellum (764–766). Based on experimental studies, Janssen and coworkers suggested that peroxisomal metabolism in the brain and in extraneural tissue affects the normal neocortical development (767). MRI discloses impaired myelination and diffusely abnormal gyral patterns with areas of pachygyria and micropolygyria. These abnormalities are most severe in the perisylvian and perirolandic regions (768).

The plasma fatty acid pattern in Zellweger syndrome is abnormal, with large amounts of very long chain fatty acids. Most patients also have elevations in plasma or urinary pipecolic acid. Additionally, phytanic levels are elevated, and the urinary excretion of dicarboxylic acids is increased (769).

Neonatal Adrenoleukodystrophy and Infantile Refsum Disease

These two entities represent less severe expressions of disordered peroxisomal biogenesis. Neonatal adrenoleukodystrophy is an autosomal recessive disease, in contrast to the X-linked adrenoleukodystrophy of later onset, with symptoms becoming apparent during the first 3 months of life. It is marked by dysmorphic features, hearing deficit, hypotonia, hepatomegaly, seizures, and retinal degeneration (770).

The clinical features of infantile Refsum disease are similar. They include a sensorineural hearing loss, retinitis pigmentosa, and mental retardation. Facial dysmorphism and hypotonia are less marked, and neonatal seizures are less common than in Zellweger syndrome (770). As in Zellweger syndrome, serum phytanic acid, pipecolic acid, and very long chain fatty acids are present in increased amounts in plasma, and urinary pipecolic acid is elevated (757).

The diagnosis of these conditions is best made by assay of plasma very long chain fatty acids and can be confirmed by phytanic acid and pipecolic acid determinations in plasma or urine (757). Morphologic examination of established fibroblast cultures or tissue obtained by liver biopsy is also of diagnostic assistance (757).

Rhizomelic Chondrodysplasia Punctata (RCDP)

RCDP, an autosomal recessive disorder, is marked by severe proximal shortening of humeri and femora and mental retardation with or without spasticity. Patients have flat facies and a low nasal bridge; cataracts are seen in 72% and ichthyosis in 28% (757). Radiography shows punctate epiphyseal and extraepiphyseal mineralization. Similar calcifications are seen in warfarin embryopathy, maternal lupus, and Conradi-Hünermann syndrome. The last is an X-linked, dominant, male lethal disorder in which intelligence is relatively preserved (771).

Neuropathologic examination in RCDP shows little more than cortical atrophy; no abnormality in myelination or disorders of cortical migration occur. A defect in the gene for PEX7, a gene involved in the import of protein to the peroxisomal matrix, has been demonstrated in most instances of this condition (757).

RCDP can also result from defects in alkyl-dihydroxyacetonephosphosphate synthase (OMIM 600121) and dihydroxyacetonephosphate acyltransferase (OMIM 222765), two enzymes required for ether lipid synthesis. In neither of these latter genetic defects is there an elevation of serum phytanic acid.

Single-Peroxisomal-Enzyme Defects

Refsum Disease (Heredopathia Atactica Polyneuritiformis) (OMIM 266500)

Although Refsum disease has been known since 1944, when Refsum (772) described two families with polyneuritis, muscular atrophy, ataxia, retinitis pigmentosa, diminution of hearing, and ichthyosis, an underlying disorder in lipid metabolism was uncovered only some 20 years later (773).

The disease usually makes its appearance between ages 4 and 7 years, most commonly with partial, intermittent peripheral neuropathy. This neuropathy can be accompanied by sensorineural deafness, ichthyosis, and cardiomyopathy. The CSF shows albuminocytologic dissociation with a protein level between 100 and 600 mg/dL.

In brain, lipids are deposited in swollen nerve cells and in areas of demyelination with the formation of fatty macrophages (774). The characteristic alterations in peripheral nerve are hypertrophy, sometimes with onion bulb formation, and a loss of myelinated fibers. Electron microscopy reveals Schwann cells to contain paracrystalline inclusions. In all organs, including the brain, quantities of lipids are increased. The lipids contain, as one of their major fatty acids, a branched-chain compound, 3,7,11,15-tetramethylhexadecanoic acid (phytanic acid). Blood levels of phytanic acid are increased. In contrast to normal levels of 0.2 mg/dL or less, they range between 10 and 50 mg/dL. Very long chain fatty acids are normal.

These changes result from a defect in the gene that codes for phytanoyl-coenzyme A hydroxylase. As a consequence, there is a block in the peroxisomal α-oxidation of phytanic to prostanoic acid (Fig. 1.24) (775). Phytanic acid is almost exclusively of exogenous origin and derived mainly from dietary phytol ingested in the form of nuts, spinach, or coffee. When patients are placed on a phytol-free diet, blood phytanic acid levels decrease slowly, and within 1 year reach levels of approximately one-fourth of the original values (776). This change is accompanied by increased nerve conduction velocities, return of reflexes, and improvement in sensation and objective coordination. Periodic plasma exchanges have been used to reduce body

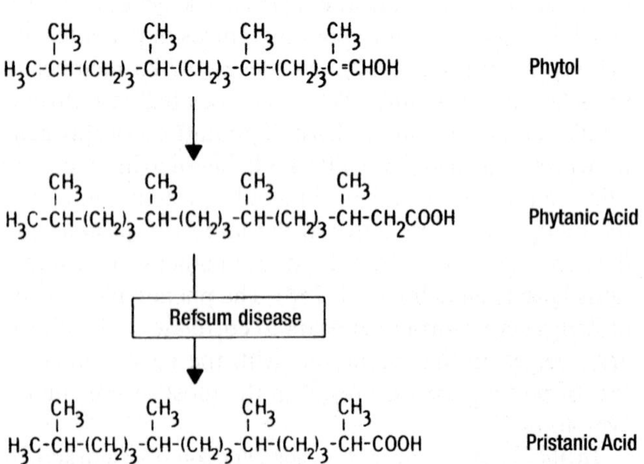

FIGURE 1.24. Phytol metabolism. In Refsum disease, the metabolic block is located at the conversion of phytanic to pristanic acid.

stores of phytanic acid and appear to be particularly effective during the early phases of therapy (776).

The mechanism by which phytanic acid produces the variety of clinical manifestations is not clear. One attractive hypothesis is that its structural similarity to the farnesol and the geranyl-geranyl groups permits phytanic acid to interfere with the formation of cytosolic prenylated proteins and prevents anchoring of cytosolic proteins to membranes.

The differential diagnosis of Refsum disease includes other causes of chronic and intermittent polyneuritis, such as α-lipoprotein deficiency (Tangier disease), which can be diagnosed by examination of the plasma lipoproteins and by the low serum cholesterol levels. Other similar clinical entities are relapsing infectious polyneuritis, the mitochondrial myopathies (ophthalmoplegia plus), acute intermittent porphyria, recurrent exposures to toxins, particularly alcohol or lead, and the various hereditary sensory motor neuropathies described in Chapter 3.

TABLE 1.21 Single-Peroxisomal-Enzyme Defects

Disorder	Enzyme
X-linked adrenoleukodystrophy	ALDP–ATP binding transporter protein
Acyl-CoA oxidase deficiency	Acyl-CoA oxidase
Bifunctional protein deficiency	Bifunctional protein
Racemase deficiency	Racemase
Rhizomelic chondrodysplasia punctata	Dihydroxyacetone phosphate acyl transferase Alkyldihydroxyacetone phosphate synthase
Refsum disease	Phytanoyl-CoA hydroxylase
Mevalonate kinase deficiency	Mevalonate kinase
Glutaric aciduria type 3	Glutaryl CoA oxidase
Acatalasemia	Catalase
Primary hyperoxaluria, type 1	Alanine:glyoxylate aminotransferase

ALDP, adrenoleukodystrophy protein.

Mevalonic Aciduria (OMIM 251170)

Mevalonic aciduria is an inborn error of cholesterol biosynthesis whose clinical picture is heterogeneous (777). Most often it is highlighted by neonatal acidosis, the evolution of cataracts, and seizures (778). Recurrent attacks of fever, profound diarrhea and a malabsorption syndrome are accompanied by hyperimmunoglobulin D and an increased excretion of leukotriene E4 during the febrile episodes (779). Hepatomegaly, lymphadenopathy, and anemia can suggest a congenital infection. Affected infants have a triangular face with down-slanted eyes and large, posteriorly rotated, low-set ears. The diagnosis can be suspected by a markedly reduced blood cholesterol level and confirmed by analysis of urinary organic acids. However, blood cholesterol may be normal, and mevalonic acid may only be present when the child is ill, and even then in only low quantities (779a). The defect is localized to mevalonate kinase, a peroxisomal enzyme, which is virtually absent in fibroblasts. The pathogenesis of the clinical manifestations is unknown (780).

Some of the other conditions resulting from defects of single peroxisomal enzymes are summarized in Table 1.21.

CARBOHYDRATE-DEFICIENT GLYCOPROTEIN SYNDROMES (CONGENITAL DISORDERS OF GLYCOSYLATION, CDG)

Carbohydrate-deficient glycoprotein syndromes (CDGS) were first described in 1987 by Jacken and coworkers (781). They represent a group of heterogeneous genetic neurologic disorders with multisystem involvement that result from the abnormal synthesis of N-linked and, less commonly, so far, of O-linked oligosaccharides (782,782a). CDG has been reported throughout the world; all entities are transmitted as autosomal recessive traits and all, except for CDG Ib, result in primary dysfunction of the nervous system. The phenotypic extent of these disorders is still being delineated, with the most severe disorders having been the first to be defined.

Almost all proteins that are secreted or membrane-bound have carbohydrate side chains. N-Linked oligosaccharides are a prominent structural feature of cell surfaces and are essential to the function of cell surface receptors, protein targeting and turnover, and cell-to-cell interaction. The synthesis of the oligosaccharides, their transfer to the nascent polypeptide chain, and their subsequent modifications require a pathway of more than 100 steps. The disorders in this section all have a defect in this pathway, with the characteristic biochemical abnormality in CDG being the hypoglycosylation of glycoproteins. As a result, the carbohydrate side chain of glycoproteins is either truncated or completely absent. At least 17 subtypes have been recognized (Table 1.22). Those in group I are due to defects in the assembly and transfer of the carbohydrate chain, whereas those in group II result from defects in processing of the carbohydrate chains.

Type Ia is the most common form of CDG, with a frequency of 1 in 80,000 births (783). Patterson recognizes four phases (784). Initially the typical presentation is that of a hypotonic and hyporeflexic infant with failure to thrive and numerous dysmorphic features. Most frequently one observes inverted nipples and an abnormal distribution of fat in the suprapubic area and buttocks. Facies are unusual, with a high nasal bridge, prominent jaw, and large pinnae. Mortality during infancy may be up to 20% (785). The second phase, up to the end of the

TABLE 1.22 Carbohydrate-Deficient Glycoprotein Syndromes

Type	Central Nervous System Symptoms	Systemic Symptoms	Enzyme Defect
Ia	Hypotonia, hyporeflexia, seizures, strokelike episodes, retinitis pigmentosa	Failure to thrive, dysmorphic facies, inverted nipples, fat pads in public and gluteal areas, pericardial effusion	Phosphomannomutase 2
Ib	None	Protein-losing enteropathy, recurrent thrombotic events, hepatic fibrosis	Phosphomannose isomerase
Ic	Moderate mental retardation, seizures, less severe than Ia	—	α-1,3-Glucosyltransferase
Id	Profound delay, optic atrophy, seizures with hypsarrhymia	Iris colobomas	α-1,3-Mannosyltransferase
Ie	Same as Ia	Same as Ia	Dolicholphosphate mannose synthase
If	Short stature, psychomotor retardation	Retinitis pigmentosa, ichthyosis	Mannose-P-dolichol untilization defect
Ig	Hypotonia, retardation, microcephaly	Facial dysmorphism, frequent infections	Dolichol-P-mannose:dolichol mannosyltransferase
Ih	Normal development	Intrauterine growth retardation, protein-losing enteropathy	Dolichol-P-glucose:dolichol glucosyltransferase
Ii	Mental retardation, seizures, hypomyelination	Coloboma of iris, hepatomegaly, coagulation disorders	GDP-Mannose:mannosedolichol mannosyltransferase
Ij	Hypotonia, intractable seizures, mental retardation, microcephaly	Micrognathia, single flexion creases of hands, skin dimples on upper thighs	UDP-GlcNAc:Dolichol phosphate *N*-acetylglycosamine-phosphate transferase
Ik	Multifocal seizures, contractures	Fetal hydrops, multiple dysmorphic features, large fontanel, hypertelorism	GDP-Mannose:GlcNAc2-dolichol mannosyltransferase
Il	Developmental delay, hypotonia, seizures	Hepatomegaly	α-1,2-Mannosyltransferase
IIa	Severe delay, hypotonia, handwashing movements	Coarse facies, low-set ears	*N*-Acetylglucosamine transferase II
IIb	Hypotonia, seizures	Dysmorphic features	α-1,2-Glucosidase
IIc	Mental retardation, microcephaly	Recurrent infections, persistent neutrophilia	GDP-fucose transporter 1
IId	Hypotonia, Dandy-Walker malformation	Spontaneous hemorrhages	β-1,4-Galactosyltransferase
IIe	Hypotonia, seizures	Dysmorphic features	Defect of oligomeric Golgi complex
Unknown	Hypotonia progressing to spastic quadriparesis, infantile spasms	—	Unknown

first decade, is marked by afebrile seizures and strokelike episodes, the latter possibly the consequence of a transient coagulopathy induced by intercurrent infections. Later in childhood there is a slowly progressive cerebellar ataxia, wasting of the lower extremities, and retinitis pigmentosa. Symptoms during adult life include mental retardation, severe ataxia, and hypogonadism. MRI studies show cerebellar hypoplasia, brainstem atrophy, and occasionally Dandy-Walker malformation (786). Microcephaly can develop or can be present at birth.

CDG Ib has no neurologic manifestations (787), and CDG Ic has a milder phenotype than CDG Ia. It is marked by moderate mental retardation, hypotonia, seizures, and ataxia (788). Children with CDG I and CDG Ie have severe mental retardation, cortical blindness, and intractable seizures. Some have dysmorphic features.

CDG should be considered in any child with mental retardation, hypotonia, and seizures, particularly when there is evidence of unexplained multisystem disease (784). Diagnosis of the N-linked forms of CDG is best and most quickly made by demonstrating the presence of abnormal transferrin and by its pattern as shown on immunoaffinity and mass spectrometry (782,789). The condition cannot be diagnosed prenatally until at least 36 weeks' gestation (790). Therapy with intravenous mannose or fucose has been suggested and may be effective in specific types (784).

FAMILIAL MYOCLONUS EPILEPSIES

The various metabolic diseases that produce progressive myoclonus epilepsy are listed in Table 1.23. Of these various entities, Lafora disease and Unverricht-Lundborg disease are covered in this section.

Lafora Disease

Lafora disease, first described by Lafora in 1911 (791), is marked by generalized, myoclonic, and focal occipital seizures commencing between 11 and 18 years of age

TABLE 1.23 Metabolic Causes for Progressive Myoclonic Epilepsy

Myoclonus epilepsy with ragged-red fibers (MERRF)
Unverricht Lundborg disease
Neuronal ceroid lipofuscinosis (Batten-Spielmeyer-Vogt disease; CLN 3)
Lafora disease
Late-onset GM_2 gangliosidosis
G_{M1} gangliosidosis, juvenile type
Niemann-Pick disease
Galactosialidosis
Arylsulfatase A deficiency

and accompanied by a fairly rapidly progressive dementia. It is clinically and genetically distinct from Unverricht-Lundborg disease, first described by Unverricht in 1891 (792).

Although clinically the disease is fairly homogeneous, at least two genes are responsible. In about 80% of patients, the gene (*EPM2A*) has been mapped to 6q24. It encodes a protein, named laforin, that functions as a tyrosine phosphatase that associates with polyribosomes and binds to polyglucosans, the storage material in Lafora disease (793). A variety of mutations in the gene have been described and cosegregate with Lafora disease.

A second gene (*EPM2B*) responsible for Lafora disease maps to chromosome 6p22 and encodes malin, believed to function as a ubiquitin ligase (794). Both laforin and malin colocalize to the endoplasmic reticulum, suggesting that they operate in a related pathway that protects against polyglucosan accumulation.

The pathologic picture of Lafora disease is unique. Many concentric amyloid (Lafora) bodies are found within the cytoplasm of ganglion cells throughout the neuraxis, particularly in the dentate nucleus, substantia nigra, reticular substance, and hippocampus (Fig. 1.25). Histochemically, these inclusions react as a protein-bound MPS. Similar amyloid material has been found in heart and liver (795). In the liver, the material causes cells to acquire a ground-glass appearance with eccentric nuclei and clear halos at their periphery. The cytoplasm contains PAS-positive basophilic material. Electron microscopy reveals short, branching filaments (796). Inclusions also are seen in eccrine sweat glands and muscle (797). Isolation and hydrolysis of organelles from the brain has shown them to consist of polyglucosan, a glucose polymer (linked in the 1:4 and 1:6 positions) chemically related to glycogen.

Clinical Manifestations

Lafora disease appears between ages 11 and 18 years with the onset of grand mal and myoclonic seizures. At first, the myoclonic seizures are triggered by photic stimulation or proprioceptive impulses and are much more frequent when formal tests of coordination are attempted, simulating the intention tremor of cerebellar ataxia. The EEG is usually abnormal, with generalized and focal and multifocal posterior epileptiform discharges (797). The interval between the bilateral sharp waves and the

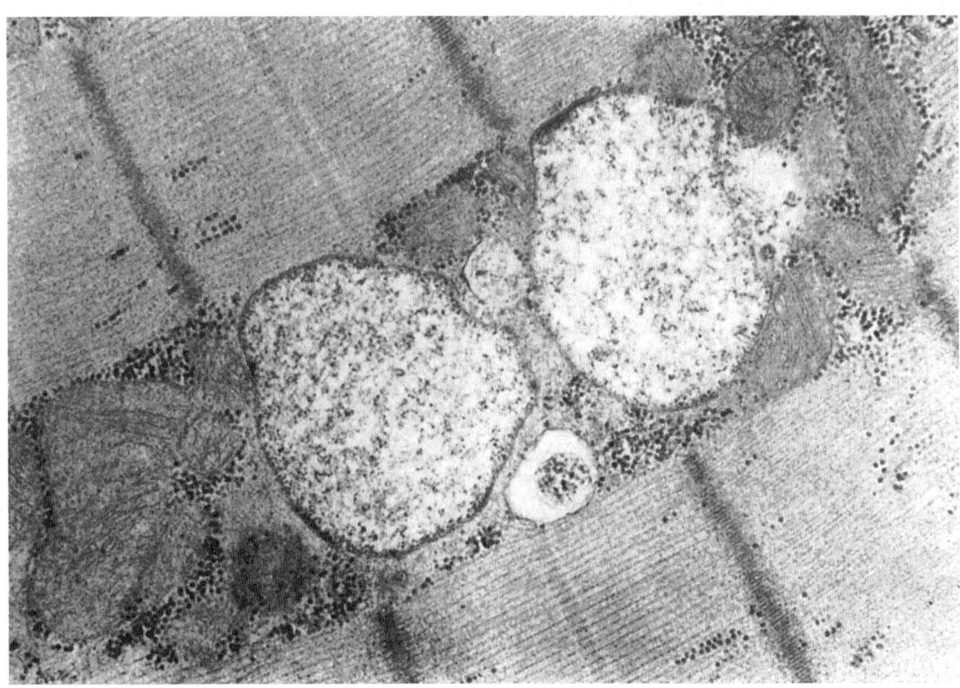

FIGURE 1.25. Myoclonus epilepsy. Electron micrograph showing inclusion bodies in muscle. (Courtesy of Dr. M. Anthony Verity, Department of Pathology, University of California, Los Angeles, Los Angeles, CA.)

myoclonus is 15 ms in the upper extremities and 25 ms in the lower extremities, suggesting that cortical discharges and myoclonic seizures are secondary to a brainstem focus.

With progression of the disease, the major seizures become less frequent, myoclonus increases in intensity, and intellectual deterioration occurs. A terminal stage of dementia, spastic quadriparesis, and almost constant myoclonic seizures is reached within 4 to 10 years of the first symptoms.

The diagnosis of Lafora disease is confirmed by the characteristic polyglucosan storage material in muscle and in the sweat glands (obtained by skin biopsy). In liver, PAS-positive material is found in the extracellular spaces (798). Electron microscopy reveals a disrupted endoplasmic reticulum and large vacuoles containing electron-dense material (799). Storage material can be detected in liver before the appearance of neurologic symptoms (800).

No therapy has been found to arrest the progression of neurologic symptoms. The seizures are generally difficult if not impossible to control with anticonvulsants.

Unverricht-Lundborg Disease (OMIM 254800)

Unverricht-Lundborg disease is an autosomal recessive disorder that tends to start somewhat earlier than Lafora disease. It is manifested by myoclonic and generalized seizures and a slowly progressive intellectual deterioration. The condition is common in North Africa and in the Baltic region; in Finland, its incidence is 1 in 20,000 (797). The gene responsible for both the Baltic and Mediterranean forms of Unverricht-Lundborg disease has been mapped to chromosome 21q22.3 and has been named *EPM1*. It encodes cystatin B, one of several cysteine protein inhibitors whose function is to inactivate proteases that leak out of lysosomes, and has a role in the programming of cell apoptosis. In the majority of patients, the mutation is an unstable minisatellite repeat expansion in the promoter region of the cystatin B gene which results in loss of expression of cystatin B, inducing uncontrolled cell apoptosis (801). There is no apparent correlation between the mutant repeat length and the disease phenotype (802). A defect in another cysteine protein inhibitor, cystatin C, is responsible for hereditary cerebral amyloid angiopathy.

The pathologic picture of Unverricht-Lundborg disease is marked by neuronal loss and gliosis, particularly affecting the Purkinje cells in the cerebellum and cells in the medial thalamus and spinal cord.

The disorder becomes manifest between 6 and 16 years of age, with the mean age of onset 10 years of age. Stimulus-sensitive myoclonus initiates the disease in approximately one-half of the children, and tonic-clonic seizures initiate it in the remainder. Myoclonus is induced by maintenance of posture or initiation of movements indicating a pathological hyperexcitability of the sensorimotor cortex (803). Myoclonus and seizures are difficult to control, and a slow and interfamily variable progression to ataxia and dementia occurs. The EEG shows progressive background slowing and 3- to 5-Hz spike wave or multiple spike wave activity. The temporal relationship between the electrical discharges and the myoclonus is variable. Marked photosensitivity and giant somatosensory-evoked potentials occur (803).

Treatment of myoclonus is difficult, and of the many anticonvulsants used, levetiracetam appears to be the most promising. Vagal nerve stimulation also offers promise in controlling the myoclonic seizures and ataxia. Tonic-clonic seizures tend to respond to the usual anticonvulsant therapy, notably valproate, clonazepam, and lamotrigine. The response to *N*-acetylcysteine has been variable (804).

Myoclonic seizures also occur in idiopathic epilepsy and in a variety of degenerative diseases, most commonly the infantile and juvenile lipofuscinoses. They also are found in the mitochondrial myopathies, sialidosis, and subacute sclerosing panencephalitis. Finally, dentatorubral atrophy (Ramsay Hunt syndrome) must be considered in the differential diagnosis of myoclonic seizures. As depicted by Hunt in 1921, the last is a progressive cerebellar ataxia accompanied by myoclonic seizures and atrophy of the dentate nucleus and superior cerebellar peduncles without the presence of amyloid bodies (see Chapter 3).

CEROID LIPOFUSCINOSIS AND OTHER LIPIDOSES

Neuronal Ceroid Lipofuscinoses

The neuronal ceroid lipofuscinoses (NCLs) are characterized by the accumulation of autofluorescent neuronal storage material within neuronal lysosomes, leading to neuronal death and cerebral atrophy. Traditionally the various NCLs were differentiated according to the age at which neurologic symptoms first become evident and the ultrastructural morphology of the inclusions. This classification has now been supplemented by genetic analysis.

The major subtypes are the infantile form, first reported from Finland in 1973 by Santavuori and her associates (805), the late infantile form first described by Jansky in 1909 (806) and subsequently by Bielschowsky (807) and Batten (808), the juvenile form described by Spielmeyer (809), and the adult form first described by Kufs (810). At least four other disease gene loci have been mapped, bringing the current total number of NCLs to nine subtypes. All are transmitted in an autosomal recessive manner. In addition, an autosomal dominant form of NCL has been delineated and is one cause for early onset of dementia (811). The relative frequencies of autosomal recessive forms in the clinical and pathologic series of Wisniewski and colleagues are as follows: infantile NCL, 11.3%; late

TABLE 1.24 Molecular Genetics of the Neuronal Ceroid Lipofuscinoses (NCLs)

Clinical Description	*Ultrastructural Characteristics*	*Location of Gene*	*Gene Defect*	*Reference*
Infantile NCL (Santavuori)	Granular osmiophilic deposits	1p32	Palmitoyl-protein thioesterase 1 (CLN1)	Das et al. (813)
Late-infantile NCL (Jansky-Bielschowsky)	Curvilinear bodies	11p15.5	Tripeptidyl-peptidase 1 (CLN2)	Sleat (814)
Juvenile NCL (Spielmeyer-Vogt)	Fingerprint bodies, curvilinear bodies, granular osmiophilic deposits	16p12.1	Transmembrane protein (CLN3)	Munroe et al. (815)
Adult NCL (Kufs)	Ceroid lipofuscin, curvilinear bodies	?	CLN4	International Batten Disease Consortium (816)
Finnish variant of late infantile NCL	Subunit c of mitochondrial adenosine triphosphate synthase	13q22	Soluble lysosomal protein (CLN5)	Tyynela et al. (817); Isosomppi et al. (818)
Indian variant of late infantile NCL	Curvilinear bodies, fingerprint profiles	15q21–q23	Transmembrane protein (CLN6)	Sharp et al. (819)
Northern epilepsy/Turkish variant	Autofluorescent material	8p23	CLN8 allelic with CLN7 transmembrane protein	Ranta et al. (820)
Serbian-German variant	Autofluorescent curvilinear material	?	(CLN9)	Schulz et al. (821)

infantile NCL (LINCL), 36.3%; juvenile NCL, 51.1%; and adult NCL, 1.3% (812). The molecular genetics of the various NCLs is outlined in Table 1.24. A mutation database can be accessed at http://www.ucl.ac.uk/ncl.

Infantile Neuronal Ceroid Lipofuscinosis (Santavuori Disease, CLN1) (OMIM 256730)

This condition was first reported in Finland in 1973 by Santavuori and associates (805). Its incidence in that country is 1 in 13,000, but the disease has been reported worldwide. The gene for infantile NCL has been mapped to chromosome 1p32. It encodes a lysosomal enzyme, palmitoyl-protein thioesterase (PPT1), which hydrolyzes fatty acids from cysteine residues in lipid-modified proteins undergoing degradation in the lysosome (813,822). PPT1 has been localized to synaptosomes and synaptic vesicles.

The principal features of the illness include intellectual deterioration that becomes apparent between 9 and 19 months of age (later than the generalized G_{M2} gangliosidoses), ataxia, myoclonic seizures, and visual failure, with a brownish pigmentation of the macula, hypopigmentation of the fundi, and optic atrophy (823). A retinal cherry-red spot is absent, but a pigmentary retinal degeneration is not unusual (824). Head growth ceases early, and in contrast to G_{M2} gangliosidosis, most infants become microcephalic before age 24 months.

The EEG shows a progressive decrease in amplitude and an increased proportion of slow waves. Concurrently, a progressive loss of the ERG and the visual-evoked responses occur (823,825). The MRI can be abnormal before the development of neurologic symptoms (826).

Pathologic examination shows the brain to be small with diffuse cortical atrophy. Microscopic examinations performed during the early stages of the illness show the neuronal cytoplasm to be slightly distended by granular, PAS-, and Sudan black–positive autofluorescent material. On ultrastructural examination, this material consists of granular osmiophilic deposits (Fig. 1.26). It resembles ordinary lipofuscin, except that the granules are far more uniform and no associated lipid droplet component exists. Similar storage material can be found in approximately 20% of lymphocytes (827). Chemically, the storage material consists mainly of sphingosine activator proteins A and D (saposins A and D). These are small lysosomal proteins that activate the various hydrolases required for the degradation of sphingolipids (602). The relationship between the defect in the gene coding for PPT1 and the accumulation of the sphingosine activator proteins is unclear (817). As the disease progresses, a gradual and ultimately near total loss of cortical neurons occurs (823).

Late Infantile Neuronal Ceroid Lipofuscinosis (Late Infantile Amaurotic Idiocy, Jansky-Bielschowsky Disease, CLN2) (OMIM 204500)

The onset of the clinical syndrome occurs later than that of the classic form of G_{M2} gangliosidosis. The condition does not affect Jewish children predominantly, its progression

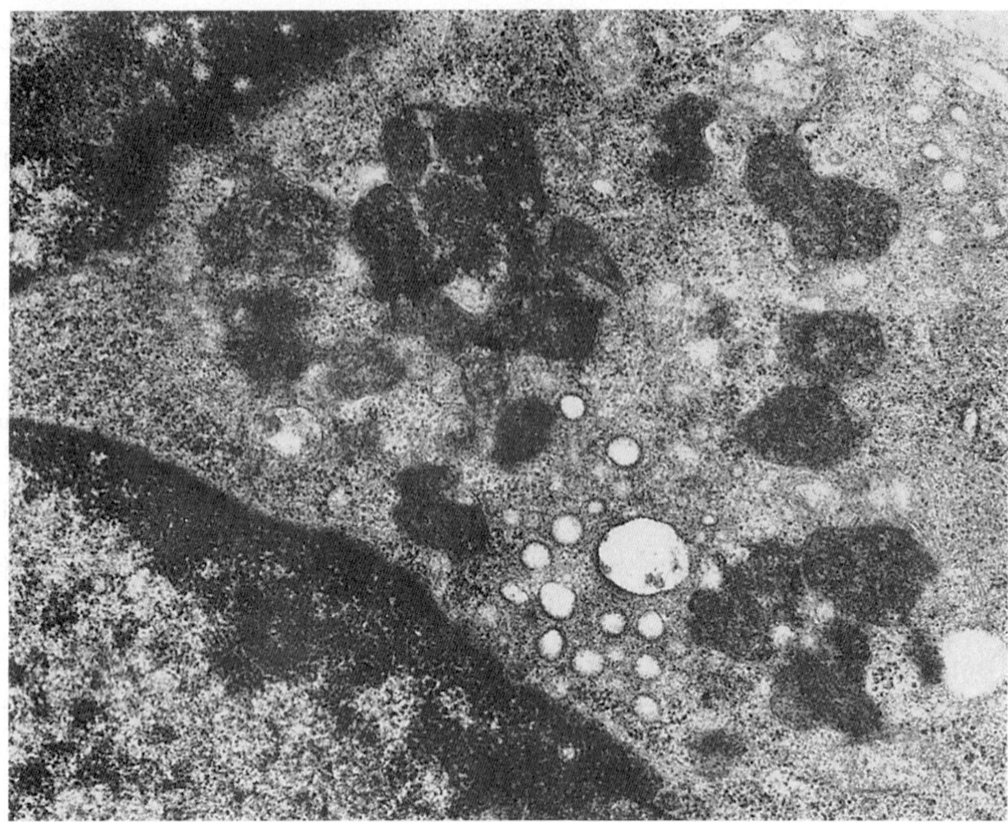

FIGURE 1.26. Electron micrograph showing granular osmiophilic deposits in the cytoplasm of an eccrine clear cell. Biopsy of a 3-year-old child with blindness, dementia, and spastic quadriparesis, who began having seizures and myoclonus at age 15 months (×25,000). (Courtesy of Dr. Stirling Carpenter, Montreal Neurological Institute, Montreal, Canada.)

is slower, and patients lack the usual retinal cherry-red spot. In the experience of Verity and coworkers CLN2 was the second most common cause of progressive neurologic and intellectual deterioration, only eclipsed by Sanfilippo disease (535).

The gene for the condition has been mapped to chromosome 11p15.5. It encodes a lysosomal tripeptidyl-peptidase 1 (816,830). Many of the CLN2 mutations induce major misfolding of the precursor peptidase, and as a result post-translational processing and lysosomal targeting of tripeptidyl peptidase is disrupted (829).

CLN2 is characterized by normal mental and motor development for the first 24 months of life, although in many instances, slight clumsiness or a slowing in the acquisition of speech can be recalled retrospectively. The usual presenting manifestations are myoclonic or major motor seizures. Ataxia develops subsequently and is accompanied by a slowly progressive retinal degeneration, which is generally not obvious until the other neurologic symptoms have become well established. Visual acuity is decreased, and a florid degeneration occurs in the macular and perimacular areas. The macular light reflex is defective, and a fine brown pigment is deposited. The optic disc is pale. Photic stimulation at two or three flashes per second elicits high-amplitude polyphasic discharges at the time of the child's first seizure or within a few months thereafter (832). These abnormalities have been noted even before the onset of neurologic symptoms.

The ERG is abnormal and is lost early in the course of the disease as a consequence of storage material in the rod and cone layer of the retina. This finding is in marked contrast to the preservation of the ERG in the G_{M2} gangliosidoses, in which retinal lipid storage is limited to the ganglion layer. The visual-evoked responses are also abnormal, in that the early components are grossly enlarged (825). Marked spasticity, as well as a parkinsonian picture, can develop terminally. The condition progresses fairly slowly, and death does not occur until late childhood.

Laboratory studies have rarely shown an increase in CSF protein. Neuroimaging studies show nonspecific changes with generalized atrophy most evident in the cerebellum (830). However, these studies distinguish the lipofuscinoses from the various leukodystrophies, in which there are striking alterations of white matter.

Microscopic examination of the affected brain reveals generalized neuronal swelling of lesser amplitude than in

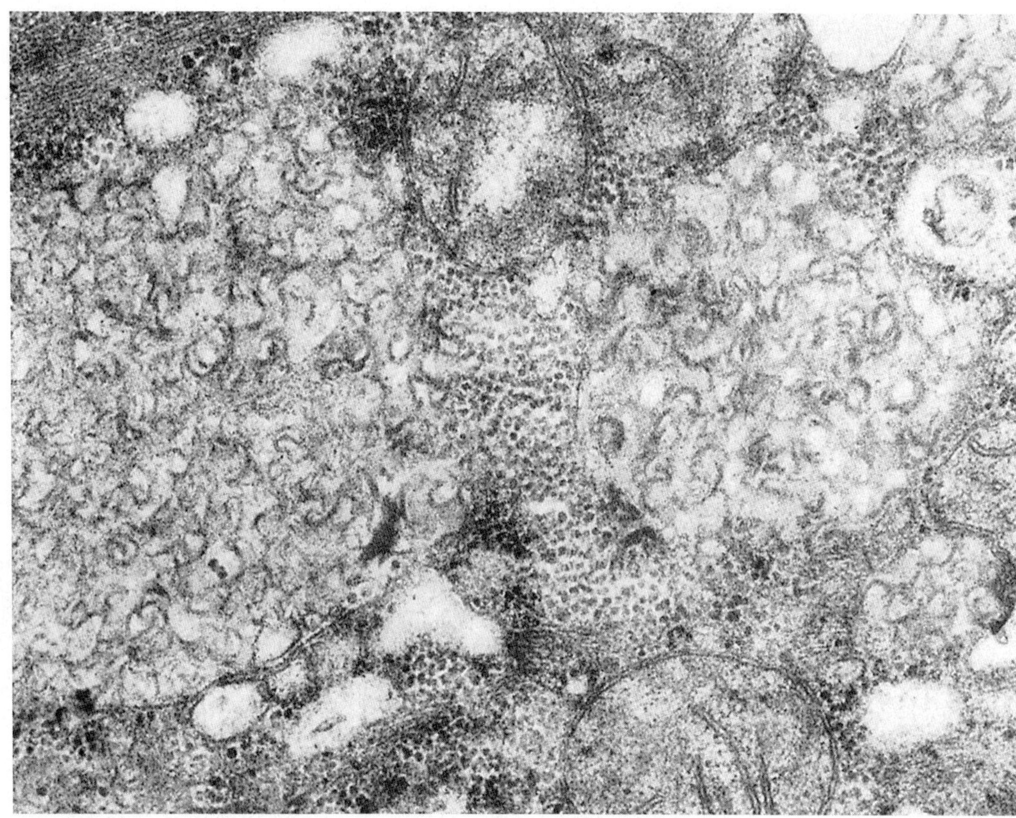

FIGURE 1.27. Curvilinear body storage disease. Electron micrograph showing curvilinear bodies in an eccrine clear cell. Skin biopsy of a 4-year-old boy with seizures, myoclonus, and visual impairment, whose symptoms started at age 3 years (×50,000). (Courtesy of Dr. Stirling Carpenter, Montreal Neurological Institute, Montreal, Canada.)

generalized G_{M2} gangliosidosis. The intraneuronal material stains with PAS and Sudan black, but, unlike the lipid stored in G_{M2} gangliosidosis, it is nearly insoluble in lipid solvents and is invariably autofluorescent. The material is principally the hydrophobic mitochondrial ATP synthase subunit c, a normal component of the inner mitochondrial membrane (831). Sleat and coworkers postulated this protein to be a substrate for the defective carboxypeptidase (814).

On ultrastructural examination, the storage material most commonly seen consists of curved stacks of lamellae with alternating dark and pale lines, the so-called curvilinear bodies (Fig. 1.27) (832). In a few cases, the storage material has a "fingerprint" configuration (Fig. 1.28), which is more typical of juvenile NCL. This designation is based on its appearance in groups of parallel lines, each pair separated by a thin lucent space. Some cases have only granular osmiophilic material (see Fig. 1.26). These different appearances of the storage material probably reflect differences in the genetic lesions in phenotypically similar patients, and mutations in CLN1 gene have been documented in some of these cases (833).

The stored material is distributed widely and is seen not only in neurons and astrocytes, but also in Schwann cells, smooth and skeletal muscle, fibroblasts, and secretory cells in such organs as thyroid, pancreas, and eccrine sweat glands (834).

By electron microscopy, the material can be identified in biopsies of skin, skeletal muscle and conjunctivae, and peripheral lymphocytes as well as in urinary sediment (834). Kurachi and colleagues suggested a new method for the rapid diagnosis of CLN2 using specific polyclonal antibodies against the CLN2 gene product. They found a marked reduction in CLN2 immunoreactivity in lymphocytes and fibroblasts (835).

CLN5 (Finnish-Variant Late Infantile Neuronal Ceroid Lipofuscinosis) (OMIM 256731)

This variant of LINCL has been encountered in Finland, where it is a relatively common disease, with an incidence of 1 in 21,000 (836). The gene for this entity has been mapped to chromosome 13q21.1–q 32. It encodes a transmembrane protein of unknown function (823). Vesa and coworkers found that the wild-type CLN5 protein interacts with the proteins of CNL2 and CLN3, whereas the mutant

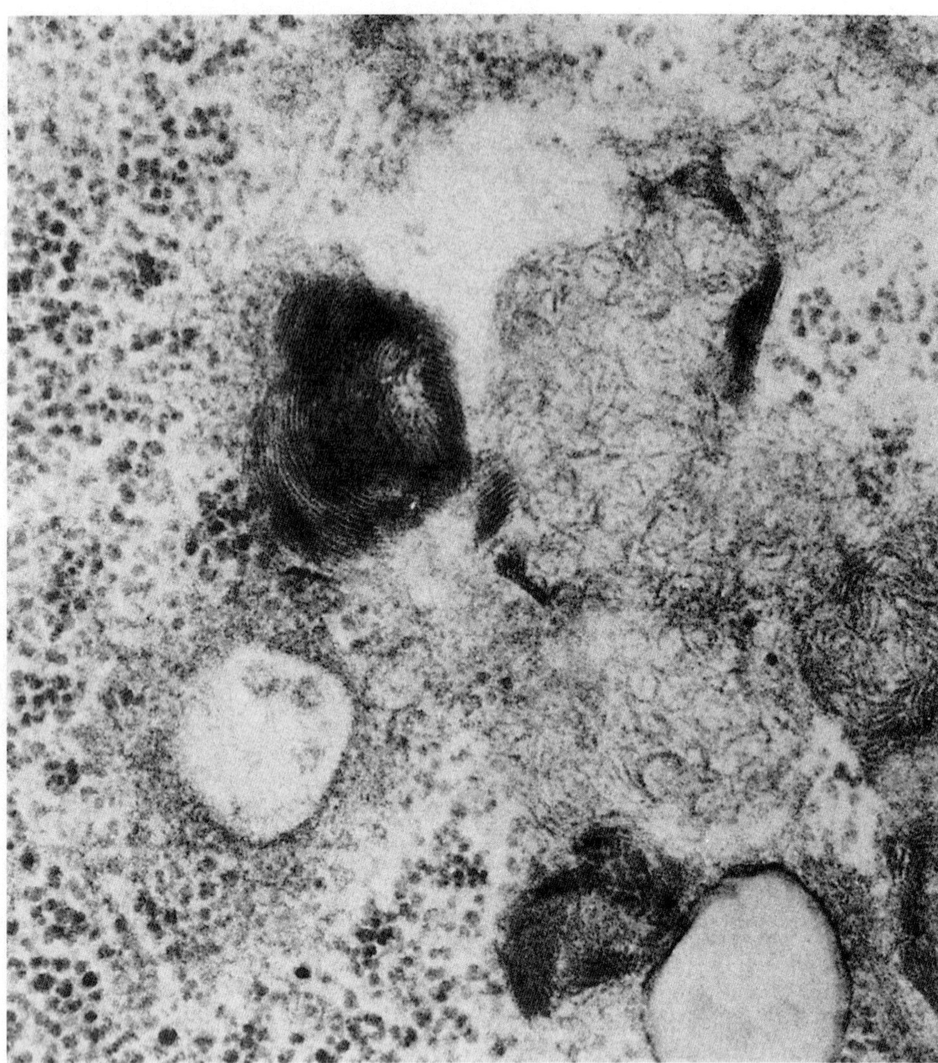

FIGURE 1.28. "Fingerprint" profiles. Skin biopsy from a 5-year-old boy with a 6-month history of akinetic and myoclonic seizures and pigmentary retinal degeneration. Fingerprint profiles are present in sweat glands (×115,000). (Courtesy of Dr. Stirling Carpenter, Montreal Neurological Institute, Montreal, Canada.)

CLN5 protein lost its ability to interact with the CLN2 protein (837).

The disease is marked by the onset of symptoms between 4 and 7 years of age, early visual failure, a somewhat slower progression, and the presence of curvilinear and "fingerprint" storage material in all tissues but lymphocytes (see Table 1.25).

Juvenile Neuronal Ceroid Lipofuscinosis (Juvenile Amaurotic Idiocy; Spielmeyer-Vogt Disease, CLN3) (OMIM 204200)

Juvenile neuronal ceroid lipofuscinosis was mentioned first in 1893 by Freud (838) and subsequently by Spielmeyer (809) and Vogt (839). The gene for this condition has been localized to chromosome 16p12.1 (819). It encodes a lysosomal transmembrane protein (battenin) of unknown function (815,840). The most common genomic mutation involves a 1.02-kb deletion.

As described in the classic monographs, visual and intellectual deterioration first becomes apparent between 4 and 10 years of age. Fundoscopic examination at that time reveals abnormal amounts of peripheral retinal pigmentation and early optic atrophy. In the majority of patients, seizures develop between the ages of 8 and 13 years (841). Loss of motor function becomes apparent subsequently. Ataxia and seizures are usually not seen; in the series of Järvelä and colleagues, extrapyramidal signs, notably parkinsonism, were seen during the second to third decade of life in approximately one-third of patients homozygous for the 1.02-kb deletion (841). A reduced striatal dopamine transporter density as measured by single-photon emission computed tomography (SPECT) is commensurate with this clinical finding (842). Although many patients whose illness commences during the early school years follow this clinical pattern, variations do occur.

The EEG is generally abnormal, in that it demonstrates large-amplitude slow wave and spike complexes, often without the photosensitivity noted in CLN1. The ERG is

TABLE 1.25 Clinical Differentiation of the Neuronal Ceroid Lipofuscinoses

	Infantile (Santavuori) CLN1	*Late Infantile (Jansky-Bielschowsky) CLN2*	*Variant Late Infantile CLN5*	*Juvenile (Spielmeyer-Vogt) CLN3*
Age at onset	9–19 mo	2–4 yr	5–7 yr	4–10 yr
Visual failure	Early	Late	Early	Early
Ataxia	Marked	Marked	Marked	Mild and late
Myoclonic seizures	Present	Present	Present	Occasional
Retinal pigment aggregation	Not seen	Rarely seen	Not seen	Invariable after 11–13 yr
Abnormal photic stimulation	Not seen	Positive early and persists	Develops late, disappears	Not seen
Visual-evoked potentials	Abolished early	Abnormal early and persists	Abnormal early, abolished later	Abolished early
Lymphocyte-electron microscopy	Granular amorphous inclusions	Inclusions with curvilinear bodies, fingerprint bodies	Negative	Vacuoles containing fingerprint bodies

Adapted from Santavuori P, Rapola J, Sainio K, et al. A variant of Jansky-Bielschowski disease. *Neuropediatrics* 1982;13:135–141. With permission.

absent, even in the early stages of the illness, and the visual-evoked potentials lose their amplitude as the disease progresses. Large complexes such as are present in CNL1 are not noted. The MRI shows mild to moderate atrophy (841).

Light microscopy reveals mild ballooning of cortical neurons, often with storage apparent in the initial segment of the axon. The cell is packed with PAS- and Sudan black–positive autofluorescent material that is resistant to lipid solvents. Electron microscopy reveals inclusions consisting of prominent "fingerprint" formations (see Fig. 1.28). These also are seen in some cases of CNL1. They may be interspersed with poorly organized lamellar material, sometimes referred to as rectilinear profiles. These inclusions are thin stacks of lamellae with the same periodicity as curvilinear bodies, but more likely to be straight than curved (841a). "Fingerprint" profiles also can be seen in a variety of other cell types throughout the body, but the extent of storage is considerably less than in CNL1, and much more variability is present from case to case and organ to organ. The "fingerprint" profiles are found regularly within eccrine sweat gland secretory cells and in some lymphocytes (843). In rare instances, clinically indistinguishable from the majority of CNL3 cases, the cytoplasmic inclusions are composed of granular osmiophilic material (see Fig. 1.26). Granular osmiophilic and fingerprint inclusions also have been seen in Kufs disease (CLN4), the adult form of NCL (843).

As is the case for CLN5, biochemical studies on the storage material show the presence of the subunit c of the mitochondrial ATP synthase (817,844). The pathogenetic mechanisms in this disorder remain unclear, as does the role of autoantibodies against the 65 kD form of glutamic acid decarboxylase found in sera of patients with Batten disease. These antibodies are distinct from those seen in stiff-man syndrome (846a). What has been amply demonstrated is that cell death in CNL3 is the result of apoptosis, and that two segments in the CNL3 protein are vital in regulating normal cell growth and apoptosis (846b). Furthermore, whereas wild-type CLN3 localizes to both the Golgi network and the plasma membrane, mutant CNL3 protein is retained within the Golgi network and is mislocalized to lysosomes (846c).

Several other NCLs (CLNs 6, 7, 8, and 9) have been described, and the heterogeneity of the various clinical entities has become fully apparent. They are summarized in Table 1.24.

Diagnosis of the Ceroid Lipofuscinoses

The ceroid lipofuscinoses should be considered in the differential diagnosis of the infant or child who presents with seizures and loss of acquired milestones coupled with progressive visual impairment. The first step in the diagnostic process is an EEG, with emphasis on photic stimulation at 2 to 3 Hz. CNL3 generally gives an exaggerated photic response. The visual-evoked potentials and ERGs also tend to be abnormal in this disorder. A lysosomal enzyme screen must be performed to exclude the majority of the other lysosomal storage diseases. Imaging studies exclude the various white matter degenerations. The definitive diagnosis usually can be arrived at by an enzymatic assay and/or morphologic examination of readily available tissue, such as skin, conjunctiva, muscle, peripheral nerves, or lymphocytes. In all instances, electron microscopy and histochemical examinations are necessary for a diagnosis (see Table 1.25). On skin biopsy in children with CNL3, the curvilinear storage material is best seen in histiocytes and smooth muscle cells, but it can be found in virtually any cell type. In the other ceroid lipofuscinoses, examination of sweat glands is mandatory because other cell types are involved inconsistently (831); in the hands of some investigators, electron microscopic examination of muscle obtained on biopsy is equally reliable (845).

Human immunodeficiency virus encephalopathy is becoming an important cause for progressive intellectual deterioration. Although in most instances CNS involvement is preceded by bouts of systemic infection, this is not invariable. The condition is covered more fully in Chapter 7. Finally, despite its present rarity, juvenile paresis, caused by congenital syphilitic infection, which is often accompanied by retinal degeneration, must always be included in the differential diagnosis.

Rectal biopsy with its attendant discomfort and morbidity is no longer indicated. When skin, conjunctiva, and muscle have failed to yield a diagnosis, and MRI and MRS have been uninformative, a brain biopsy has to be considered.

DISORDERS OF SERUM LIPOPROTEINS

Abetalipoproteinemia (OMIM 200100)

Abetalipoproteinemia, an unusual disorder, was first described by Bassen and Kornzweig in 1950 (846). The main clinical manifestations include acanthocytosis (large numbers of burr-shaped erythrocytes) (Fig. 1.29, which may account for more than one-half of the circulating erythrocytes, hypocholesterolemia, progressive combined posterior column degeneration, peripheral neuritis, mental retardation, retinitis pigmentosa, and steatorrhea. The disorder is transmitted in an autosomal recessive manner.

In the first year of life, infants develop a typical celiac syndrome with abdominal distention, diarrhea, foul-smelling stools, decreased fat absorption, and, occasionally, osteomalacia. The majority of affected infants are below the third percentile for height and weight. Neurologic symptoms are first noted between ages 2 and 17 years, and 33% of patients are symptomatic before age 10 years.

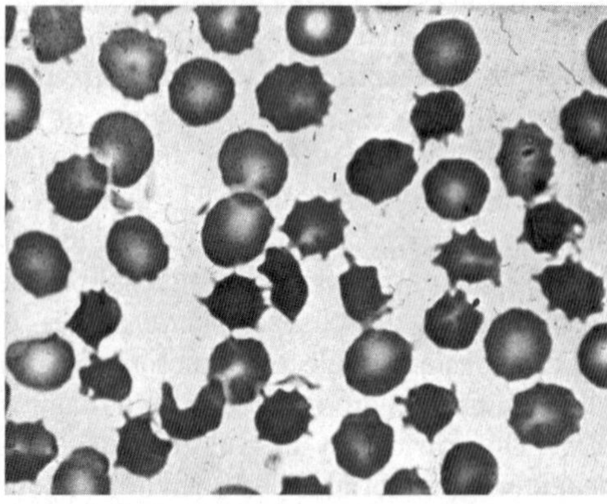

FIGURE 1.29. Acanthocytes from a patient with abetalipoproteinemia. (From Wintrobe MM, et al. *Clinical hematology*, 8th ed. Philadelphia: Lea & Febiger, 1981.)

Commonly, the initial symptom is unsteadiness of gait. This is caused by a combination of ataxia, proprioceptive loss, and muscle weakness. Deep tendon reflexes are generally absent, and cutaneous sensory loss is often demonstrable (847). Extensor plantar responses are noted occasionally. Mental retardation has been seen in approximately 33% of patients (848). The retinal degeneration is accompanied by decreased visual acuity and night blindness. The ERG and the visual-evoked potentials are often abnormal even in the early stages of the disease. Somatosensory-evoked potentials were abnormal in some 40% of patients in the series of Brin and coworkers (849). Cardiac abnormalities, including irregularities of rhythm, are common.

Autopsy reveals extensive demyelination of the posterior columns and spinocerebellar tracts and neuronal loss in the anterior horns, cerebellar molecular layer, and cerebral cortex (850). Ceroid and lipofuscin deposits are seen in muscle. They are similar to the inclusions in cystic fibrosis patients and probably reflect vitamin E deficiency (851).

Characteristic laboratory findings include low serum cholesterol (usually in the range of 20 to 50 mg/dL), low serum triglycerides (2 to 13 mg/dL), depressed total serum lipids (80 to 285 mg/dL), and vitamin E levels below 1.3 μg/mL, as contrasted with a normal range of 5 to 15 μg/mL (849,852).

As indicated by its name, the hallmark of the disease is the complete absence of serum β-lipoproteins. This in turn leads to an absence of all apolipoprotein β-containing lipoproteins (i.e., chylomicrons, very low density lipoproteins, and low-density lipoproteins).

In the majority of cases, the disease is caused by a defect in the gene that codes for the microsomal triglyceride transfer protein (853). This protein mediates the transfer of lipid molecules from their site of synthesis in the membranes of the endoplasmic reticulum to the nascent lipoprotein particles in the endoplasmic reticulum. In some cases, the lack of microsomal transfer protein could reflect its downregulation in response to another, more proximate defect or could result from a mutation in the gene that controls the formation of microsomal transfer protein (854).

As a consequence of the absence of β-lipoproteins, fat absorption is deficient. Normally, ingestion of fat is followed by absorption of lipids by the mucosal cells, from which the lipids are released in the form of chylomicrons and discharged into the lymphatic system. In abetalipoproteinemia, no fat is detectable in the lymphatic spaces of the small bowel and no chylomicrons appear in the plasma after fat loading. This defect is consequent to a defect in lipid transport from the mucosal cells into the lymphatic system, β-lipoproteins apparently being necessary to the formation of chylomicrons. Fat-soluble vitamins transported in chylomicrons are also poorly absorbed, resulting in the low serum levels of vitamins E and A.

Neurologic symptoms are probably the result of inadequate body stores of vitamin E, with resulting peroxidation of the unsaturated myelin phospholipids. In support of this hypothesis is the finding of a nearly identical neurologic picture when vitamin E deficiency results from chronic fat malabsorption, as is seen in cystic fibrosis and cholestatic liver disease (see Chapter 17), or when it is due to mutations in the gene for the alpha-tocopherol transfer protein (855).

Supplementation of the diet with vitamin E (100 mg/kg per day given orally) appears to prevent the development or progression of neurologic and retinal lesions. All children started on such high doses of vitamin E before age 16 months have remained normal neurologically and developmentally up to at least 27 years of age (853,856). No evidence exists that intramuscular vitamin E is superior. In addition to vitamin E, current therapeutic regimens suggest administration of vitamin A (200 to 400 IU/kg per day) and vitamin K_1 (5 mg/day). Fagan and Taylor suggested that improvement of patients can best be followed by repeated somatosensory-evoked potentials (857).

The presence of low blood cholesterol should alert the clinician to abetalipoproteinemia. Low cholesterol also is seen in hypobetalipoproteinemia, malnutrition, and a variety of absorption defects.

The occurrence of acanthocytes in peripheral blood is not limited to abetalipoproteinemia. Acanthocytes are mature erythrocytes with many irregularly arranged spiny projections (see Fig. 1.29). They are best detected on a fresh blood smear using conventional light microscopy. A 1:1 saline dilution may reveal their presence when undiluted blood fails to show the cells. Acanthocytes occasionally have been seen in patients with anemia or advanced cirrhosis. They also have been present in patients with triglyceride hyperlipemia and in families with extrapyramidal movement disorders resembling Hallervorden-Spatz disease. Several other families have been reported in whom an extrapyramidal disorder (parkinsonism, chorea, vocal tics), motor neuron disease, areflexia, and mental retardation were associated with the presence of acanthocytes but in whom serum lipids were normal (neuroacanthocytosis) (858,859). In most instances, the disease has its onset between 25 and 45 years of age. The gene for this autosomal recessive condition has been mapped to chromosome 9q2. It codes for chorein, a protein that has been implicated in protein sorting (860).

Several forms of hypobetalipoproteinemia have been recognized. The majority of affected children or adolescents are heterozygotes for the gene coding for apoprotein B. Neurologic symptoms are absent or are limited to a loss of deep tendon reflexes; rarely, there is progressive demyelination,with ataxia and mental deterioration (853). Homozygotes for the condition resemble clinically patients with abetalipoproteinemia. Treatment with large doses of vitamin E (1,000 to 2,000 mg/day for infants, up to 10,000 to 20,000 mg/day for older children and adults) appears to arrest the progressive neurologic symptoms (853).

Tangier Disease (Hypoalphalipoproteinemia) (OMIM 205400)

Tangier disease is a hereditary disorder of lipid metabolism distinguished by almost complete absence of high-density plasma lipoproteins, reduction of low-density plasma lipoproteins, cholesterol, and phospholipids, normal or elevated triglyceride levels, and storage of cholesterol esters in the reticuloendothelial system of the liver, spleen, lymph nodes, tonsils, and cornea. The name of the disease refers to an island in Chesapeake Bay where the first two patients were found.

Symptoms usually are limited to enlargement of the affected organs, notably the tonsils. Retinitis pigmentosa and peripheral neuropathy have been observed (863). Peripheral neuropathy was noted in nearly 50% of the reported patients. Nerve biopsy reveals three different types of changes. One group had a multifocal demyelination with large amounts of neutral lipids within Schwann cells, particularly those associated with unmyelinated fibers. In another group (whose clinical manifestations include facial weakness, weakness of the small hand muscles, spontaneous pain, and loss of pain and temperature sensations), no demyelination occurs, but lipid is deposited in Schwann cells. A third type is a distal sensory neuropathy (862). A syringomyelia-like phenotype has also been encountered (863).

The gene has been mapped to chromosome 9q22–q31. It codes for ATP-binding cassette transporter 1 (ABCA1), whose function is to bind and promote cellular cholesterol and phospholipid efflux to apolipoprotein I (apoA-I) (864).

DISORDERS OF METAL METABOLISM

Wilson Disease (Hepatolenticular Degeneration) (OMIM 277900)

Wilson disease is an autosomal recessive disorder of copper metabolism that is associated with cirrhosis of the liver and degenerative changes in the basal ganglia. The fact that, once diagnosed, Wilson disease is eminently treatable prompts a more extensive discussion than would otherwise be justified by the frequency of the disease.

During the second half of the nineteenth century, a condition termed pseudosclerosis was distinguished from multiple sclerosis by the lack of ocular signs. In 1902, Kayser observed green corneal pigmentation in one such patient (865); in 1903, Fleischer, who had also noted the green pigmentation of the cornea in 1903, commented on the association of the corneal rings with pseudosclerosis (866). In 1912, Wilson gave the classic description of the disease and its pathologic anatomy (867).

Because the derangement of copper metabolism is one of the important features of this condition, it is pertinent to review briefly the present knowledge of the field (868).

Copper homeostasis is an important biological process. By balancing intake and excretion, the body avoids copper toxicity on the one hand, and on the other hand ensures the availability of adequate amounts of the metal for a variety of vital enzymes, such as cytochrome oxidase and lysyl hydroxylase. The daily dietary intake of copper ranges between 1 and 5 mg. Healthy children consuming a free diet absorb 150 to 900 μg/day, or approximately 40% of dietary copper (869). Cellular copper transport consists of three processes: copper uptake, intracellular distribution and use, and copper excretion (870).

The site of copper absorption is probably in the proximal portion of the gastrointestinal tract. The metallothioneines (MTs), a family of low-molecular-weight metal-binding proteins containing large amounts of reduced cysteine, are involved in regulating copper absorption at high copper intakes. In addition to playing a role in the intestinal transport of the metal, MTs are probably also involved in the initial hepatic uptake of copper.

After its intestinal uptake, copper enters plasma, where it is bound to albumin in the form of cupric ion. Within 2 hours, the absorbed copper is incorporated into a liver protein. Cellular copper uptake is facilitated by Ctr1, a membrane protein that transports the metal in a high-affinity, metal-specific manner. The concentration of copper in normal liver ranges from 20 to 50 μg/g dry weight. Once within the hepatocyte, copper is bound to metallochaperones, a family of proteins that deliver it to various specific sites. The chaperone Atox1, through direct interaction with the Wilson disease P-type ATPase (ATP7b), delivers copper to the hepatic secretory pathway for excretion into bile. ATP7b is predominantly located in the *trans*-Golgi network and functions to transfer copper for incorporation into apoceruloplasmin or excretion into bile. Within hepatocyte cytoplasm copper is complexed to what is probably a polymeric form of MT. Lastly, copper can combine with apoceruloplasmin to form ceruloplasmin, which then reenters the circulation (871). More than 95% of serum copper is in this form (870).

Ceruloplasmin is an alpha-globulin with a single continuous polypeptide chain and a molecular weight of 132 kd; it has six copper atoms per molecule. The protein is a ferroxidase that has an essential role in iron metabolism. Although it is not involved in copper transport from the intestine, it is considered to be the major vehicle for the transport of copper from the liver and to function as a copper donor in the formation of a variety of copper-containing enzymes. Ceruloplasmin controls the release of iron into plasma from cells, in which the metal is stored in the form of ferritin. It is also the most prominent serum antioxidant, and as such, it catalyzes the oxidation of ferrous ion to ferric ion and prevents the oxidation of polyunsaturated fatty acids and similar substances. Finally, it modulates the inflammatory response and can regulate the concentration of various serum biogenic amines.

The concentration of ceruloplasmin in plasma is normally between 20 and 40 mg/dL. It is elevated in a variety of circumstances, including pregnancy and other conditions with high estrogen concentrations, infections, cirrhosis, malignancies, hyperthyroidism, and myocardial infarction. The concentration of ceruloplasmin is low in healthy infants up to approximately 2 months of age and in children experiencing a combined iron and copper deficiency anemia. In the nephrotic syndrome, low levels are caused by the vast renal losses of ceruloplasmin. Ceruloplasmin also is reduced in kinky hair disease (KHD; Menkes disease), a condition discussed in the next section.

Several other copper-containing proteins have been isolated from mammalian tissues. Most prominently, these include the enzymes cytochrome *c* oxidase, dopamine β-hydroxylase, superoxide dismutase, and tyrosinase. None of these is altered in Wilson disease.

Molecular Genetics and Biochemical Pathology

Knowledge of disturbed copper metabolism in Wilson disease did not progress for more than three decades. In 1913, 1 year after Wilson's report, Rumpel found unusually large amounts of copper in the liver of a patient with hepatolenticular degeneration (872). Although this finding was confirmed and an elevated copper concentration also was detected in the basal ganglia by Lüthy (873), the implication of these reports went unrecognized until 1945 when Glazebrook demonstrated abnormally high copper levels in serum, liver, and brain in a patient with Wilson disease (874). In 1952, 5 years after the discovery of ceruloplasmin, several groups of workers simultaneously found it to be low or absent in patients with Wilson disease. Although for many years it was believed that Wilson disease was caused by ceruloplasmin deficiency, it has become evident that the absence of ceruloplasmin (aceruloplasminemia) results in a severe disorder of iron metabolism (875,876).

The gene for Wilson disease has been mapped to chromosome 13q14.3–q21.1. It has been cloned and encodes a copper-transporting P-type ATPase that is expressed in many tissues, including the brain (877). The ATPase is present in two forms. One is probably localized to the late endosomes where it is involved in the delivery of copper to apoceruloplasmin (877a). The other form, probably representing a cleavage product, is found in mitochondria (878,879). More than 300 mutations have been described. Some mutations are population specific, others are common in many nationalities. The majority are missense mutations or small insertions or deletions (880). Most patients are compound heterozygotes (881).

The genetic mutation induces extensive changes in copper homeostasis. Normally, the amount of copper in the body is kept constant through excretion of copper from the liver into bile. The two fundamental defects in Wilson disease are a reduced biliary transport and excretion of copper and an impaired formation of plasma ceruloplasmin (880). Biliary excretion of copper is between 20% and 40% of normal, and fecal output of copper is reduced also (882). Apoceruloplasmin is present in the liver of patients with Wilson disease, but due to a lack of copper available for incorporation, apoceruloplasmin is rapidly degraded.

Most important, copper accumulates within liver. At first, it is firmly bound to copper proteins, such as ceruloplasmin and superoxide dismutase, or is in the cupric form complexed with MT. When the copper load overwhelms the binding capacity of MT, cytotoxic cupric copper is released, causing damage to hepatocyte mitochondria and peroxisomes (883,884). Ultimately, copper leaks from liver into blood, where it is taken up by other tissues, including brain, which in turn are damaged by copper.

Pathologic Anatomy

The abnormalities in copper metabolism result in a deposition of the metal in several tissues. In the brain, the largest proportion of copper is located in the subcellular soluble fraction, where it is bound not only to cerebrocuprein, but also to a number of other normal cerebral proteins. Anatomically, the liver shows a focal necrosis that leads to a coarsely nodular, postnecrotic cirrhosis. The nodules vary in size and are separated by bands of fibrous tissues of different widths. Some hepatic cells are enlarged and contain fat droplets, intranuclear glycogen, and clumped pigment granules; other cells are necrotic with regenerative changes in the surrounding parenchyma (885).

Electron microscopic studies indicate that copper is initially spread diffusely within cytoplasm, probably as the monomeric MT complex. Later in the course of the disease, the metal is sequestered within lysosomes, which become increasingly sensitive to rupture. Copper probably initiates and catalyzes oxidation of the lysosomal membrane lipids, resulting in lipofuscin accumulation. Within the kidneys, the tubular epithelial cells can degenerate, and their cytoplasm can contain copper deposits.

In the brain, particularly in patients whose symptoms commenced before the onset of puberty, the basal ganglia show the most striking alterations. They have a brick-red pigmentation; spongy degeneration of the putamen frequently leads to the formation of small cavities (867). Microscopic studies reveal a loss of neurons, axonal degeneration, and large numbers of protoplasmic astrocytes, including giant forms termed Alzheimer cells. These cells are not specific for Wilson disease; they also can be seen in the brains of patients dying in hepatic coma or as a result of argininosuccinic aciduria or other disorders of the ammonia cycle. Opalski cells, also seen in Wilson disease, are generally found in gray matter. They are large cells with a rounded contour and finely granular cytoplasm. They probably represent degenerating astrocytes. In approximately 10% of patients, cortical gray matter and white matter are more affected than the basal ganglia. Here, too, extensive spongy degeneration and proliferation of astrocytes is seen (886). Copper is deposited in the pericapillary area and within astrocytes, but it is uniformly absent from neurons and ground substance.

Lesser degenerative changes are seen in the brainstem, dentate nucleus, substantia nigra, and convolutional white matter. Copper also is found throughout the cornea, particularly the substantia propria, where it is deposited in an alcohol-soluble, and probably chelated, form. In the periphery, the metal appears in granular clumps close to the endothelial surface of Descemet membrane. Here, the deposits are responsible for the appearance of the Kayser-Fleischer ring. The color of the Kayser-Fleischer ring varies from yellow to green to brown. Copper deposition in this area occurs in two or more layers, with particle size and distance between layers influencing the ultimate appearance of the ring (887).

Clinical Manifestations

Wilson disease is a progressive condition with a tendency toward temporary clinical improvement and arrest. Its prevalence is about 1 in 30,000 (870). The condition occurs in all races, with a particularly high incidence in Eastern European Jews, in Italians from southern Italy and Sicily, and in people from some of the smaller islands of Japan—groups with a high rate of inbreeding.

In a fair number of cases, primarily in young children, initial symptoms can be hepatic, such as jaundice or portal hypertension, and the disease can assume a rapidly fatal course without any detectable neurologic abnormalities (888,889). In many of these patients, an attack of what appears to be an acute viral hepatitis heralds the onset of the illness (890). The presentation of Wilson disease with hepatic symptoms is common among affected children in the United States. In the series of Werlin and associates, who surveyed patients in the Boston area, the primary mode of presentation was hepatic in 61% of patients younger than age 21 years (891). In approximately 10% of affected children in the United States, Wilson disease presents as an acute or intermittent, Coombs-test-negative, nonspherocytic anemia that is accompanied by leukopenia and thrombocytopenia (891).

When neurologic symptoms predominate, the appearance of the illness is delayed until 10 to 20 years of age, and the disease progresses at a slower rate than in the hepatic form. The youngest reported child with cerebral manifestations of Wilson disease was 4 years old. The first signs are usually bulbar; these can include indistinct speech and difficulty in swallowing. A rapidly progressive dystonic syndrome is not unusual when the disease presents in childhood. Such patients can present with acute dystonia, rigidity, and fever, with an occasional elevation of serum creatine phosphokinase (892). Rarely, hemiparesis can be the initial presentation (893).

In the experience of Arima and his group, 33% of children presented with hepatic symptoms, mainly jaundice or ascites (888). They were 4 to 12 years old at the time of medical attention. Cerebral symptoms, notably dystonia, drooling, or gait disturbances, were the presenting symptoms in 30% of children. These patients were 9 to 13 years of age. The remainder had a mixed hepatocerebral picture and were 6 to 12 years old at the time of medical attention. Minor intellectual impairment or emotional disturbances also can be observed, but seizures or mental deterioration are not prominent features of the disease.

Before long, the patient has a characteristic appearance. A fixed smile is a result of retraction of the upper lip; the mouth hangs open and drools. Speech is often severely impaired. Tremors are usually quite marked. Though they often are unilateral during the early stages of the disease, sooner or later they become generalized. The tremors are present at rest, but become exaggerated with movements and emotional disturbance. Initially fine, they gradually become coarse as the illness progresses until they assume a characteristic "wing-beating" appearance. Rigidity, contractures, and tonic spasms advance steadily and can involve the extremities. Dementia can be severe in some patients, whereas other patients are merely emotionally labile. A nearly pure Parkinson-like syndrome and progressive choreoathetosis or hemiplegia also have been described. In essence, Wilson disease is a disorder of motor function; despite often widespread cerebral atrophy, no sensory symptoms or reflex alterations occur.

Without treatment, death ensues within 1 to 3 years of the onset of neurologic symptoms and is usually a result of hepatic insufficiency.

The intracorneal, ring-shaped pigmentation first noted by Kayser and Fleischer might be evident to the naked eye or might appear only with slit-lamp examination. The ring can be complete or incomplete and is present in 75% of children who present with hepatic symptoms and in all children who present with cerebral or a combination of cerebral and hepatic symptoms (888). The Kayser-Fleischer ring can antedate overt symptoms of the disease and has been detected even in the presence of normal liver functions. In the large clinical series of Arima, it was never present before 7 years of age (888). "Sunflower" cataracts are less commonly encountered.

CT scans usually reveal ventricular dilation and diffuse atrophy of the cortex, cerebellum, and brainstem. Approximately one-half of the patients have hypodense areas in the thalamus and basal ganglia. Increased density owing to copper deposition is not observed. Generally, MRI correlates better with clinical symptoms than CT. A diagnostic appearance of the MRI has been termed the "face of the giant Panda" (894). This is due to an accentuation of the

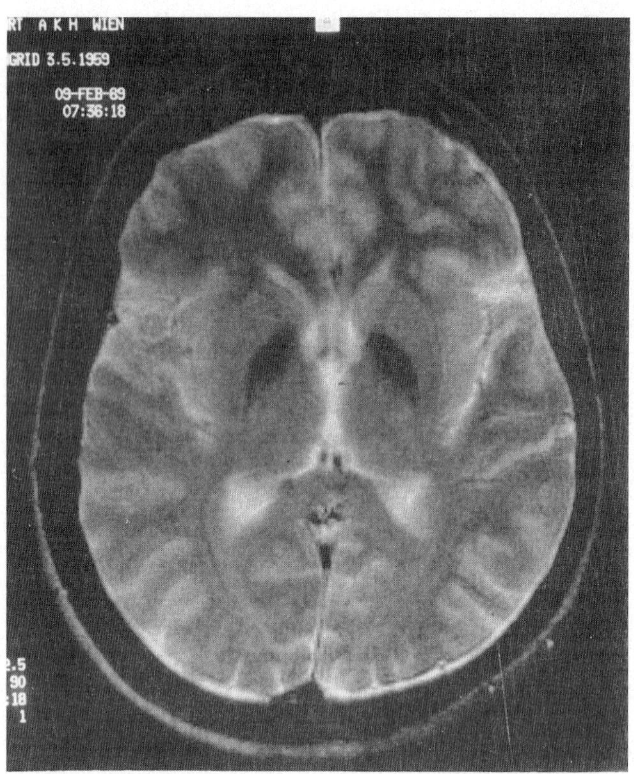

FIGURE 1.30. Wilson disease. Coronal T2-weighted magnetic resonance images of a 22-year-old woman with Wilson disease. There are bilateral hyperintense thalamic lesions that are hypointense on T1-weighted images. (Courtesy of Dr. I. Prayer, Zentral Institut für Radiodiagnose und Ludwig Boltzmann Institut, University of Vienna, Austria.)

normal low intensity of the red nucleus and substantia nigra by the surrounding increased intensity of the midbrain and tegmentum. MRI also demonstrates abnormal signals (hypointense on T1-weighted images and hyperintense on T2-weighted images) most commonly in the putamen, thalami, and the head of the caudate nucleus (Fig. 1.30). The midbrain is also abnormal, as are the pons and the cerebellum. Cortical atrophy and focal lesions in cortical white matter also are noted. Correlation with clinical symptoms is not good, in that patients with neurologic symptoms can have normal MRI results and other individuals with no neurologic symptoms can have abnormal MRI results (895,896). Positron emission tomography (PET) demonstrates a widespread depression of glucose metabolism, with the greatest focal hypometabolism in the lenticular nucleus. This abnormality precedes any alteration seen on CT scan (897).

Diagnosis

When Wilson disease presents with neurologic manifestations, some of the diagnostic features are the progressive extrapyramidal symptoms commencing after the first decade of life, abnormal liver function, aminoaciduria, cupriuria, and absent or decreased ceruloplasmin. The presence of a Kayser-Fleischer ring is the most important diagnostic feature; its absence in a child with neurologic symptoms rules out the diagnosis of Wilson disease. The ring is not seen in the majority of presymptomatic patients, nor is it seen in 15% of children in whom Wilson disease presents with hepatic symptoms (890).

An absent or low serum ceruloplasmin level is of lesser diagnostic importance; some 5% to 20% of patients with Wilson disease have normal levels of the copper protein. In affected families, the differential diagnosis between heterozygotes and presymptomatic homozygotes is of utmost importance because it is generally accepted that presymptomatic homozygotes should be treated preventively (898).

The presymptomatic child with Wilson disease can have a Kayser-Fleischer ring (seen in 33% of presymptomatic patients in Walshe series), an increased 24-hour urine copper level (greater than 100 μg/24 hours), hepatosplenomegaly (seen in 38% of cases), and abnormal neuroimaging (seen in approximately one-fourth of cases). Approximately one-half of the patients with presymptomatic Wilson disease had no physical findings, and urinary copper excretion can be normal in children younger than the age of 15 years. Should the diagnosis in a child at risk still be in doubt, an assay of liver copper is indicated (898). Low ceruloplasmin levels in an asymptomatic family member only suggest the presymptomatic stage of the disease; some 10% of heterozygotes have ceruloplasmin levels below 15 mg/dL. Because gene carriers account for approximately 1% of the population, gene carriers with low ceruloplasmin values are seen 40 times more frequently than patients with Wilson disease and low ceruloplasmin values. Therefore, when low ceruloplasmin levels are found on routine screening and are unaccompanied by any abnormality of hepatic function or copper excretion, the individual is most likely a heterozygote for Wilson disease.

When a liver biopsy has been decided on, histologic studies with stains for copper and copper-associated proteins and chemical quantitation for copper are performed. In all confirmed cases of Wilson disease, hepatic copper is greater than 3.9 μmol/g dry weight (237.6 μg/g) as compared with a normal range of 0.2 to 0.6 μmol/g (Fig. 1.31). The finding of normal hepatic copper concentration excludes the diagnosis of Wilson disease (871). Because of the large number of mutations causing the disease, a combination of mutation and linkage analysis is required for prenatal diagnosis. As a rule, this technique is not useful in the diagnosis of an individual patient. However, about one-third of North American Wilson disease patients have a point mutation (His1069Glu), and screening for this mutation can be performed readily (899).

Wilson disease is one of a number of metabolic diseases that can present with extrapyramidal signs and symptoms. These conditions and the best means of diagnosing them are listed in Table 1.26.

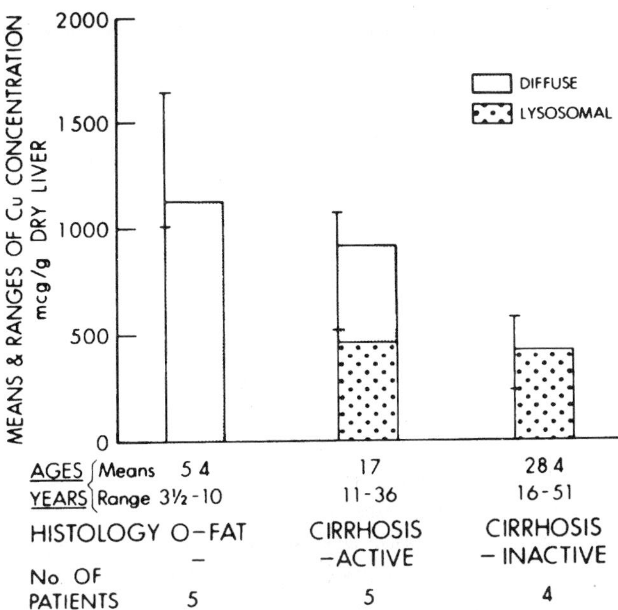

FIGURE 1.31. Mean values and ranges of hepatic copper concentrations in patients with Wilson disease, grouped according to age and stage of disease (mean age, 5.4 years). Asymptomatic children with minimal histologic abnormalities (mean age, 17 years). Adolescents and young adults with active liver disease (mean age, 28.4 years). Adults with neurologic symptoms of Wilson disease and inactive cirrhosis. The height of the bar graph indicates the concentration of copper in each group. A striking decrease is seen with advancing age and progression of the disease, and the intracellular distribution of copper changes from its diffuse cytoplasmic distribution in the hepatocytes of children to its lysosomal concentration in the hepatocytes of patients with advanced disease. (From Scheinberg IH, Sternlieb I. *Wilson disease*. Philadelphia: Saunders, 1984. With permission.)

Treatment

All patients with Wilson disease, whether symptomatic or asymptomatic, require treatment. The aims of treatment are initially to remove the toxic amounts of copper and secondarily to prevent tissue reaccumulation of the metal (900,901).

Treatment can be divided into two phases: the initial phase, when toxic copper levels are brought under control, and maintenance therapy. There is no agreed-on regimen for treatment of the new patient with neurologic or psychiatric symptoms. In the past, most centers recommended starting patients on d-penicillamine (600 to 3,000 mg/day). Although this drug is effective in promoting urinary excretion of copper, adverse reactions during the initial and maintenance phases of treatment are seen in approximately 25% of patients. These include worsening of neurologic symptoms during the initial phases of treatment, which frequently is irreversible. Skin rashes, gastrointestinal discomfort, and hair loss are encountered also. During maintenance therapy, one may see polyneuropathy,

TABLE 1.26 Genetic Metabolic Diseases Presenting with Basal Ganglia Signs

Disease	*Diagnostic Tests*
Dihydropteridine reductase deficiency	Blood phenylalanine, CSP biopterin metabolites
Dihydrobiopterine synthetase deficiency	Blood phenylalanine, CSF biopterin metabolites
Propionic acidemia	Urinary organic acids
Nonketotic hyperglycinemia	Blood amino acids
Glutaric aciduria type I	Urine organic acids
Mucolipidosis type IV	Conjunctival biopsy
Salla disease	Urinary sialic acid
GM_1 gangliosidosis, juvenile	Conjunctival biopsy
GM_2 gangliosidosis	Conjunctival biopsy
Niemann-Pick disease type C (juvenile dystonic lipidosis)	Bone marrow aspirate
Neuroacanthocytosis	Blood smear
Wilson disease	Ceruloplasmin, slit-lamp, urinary Cu
Menkes variant	Serum copper, ceruloplasmin
Lesch-Nyhan disease	Urinary uric acid
Creatine deficiency syndrome	Magnetic resonance marrow spectroscopy of brain
Cystinosis	Bone marrow aspiration
Mitochondrial disorders	See Chapter 2

CSF, cerebrospinal fluid.

polymyositis, and nephropathy. Some of these adverse effects can be prevented by giving pyridoxine (25 mg/day).

Because of these side effects, many institutions now advocate initial therapy with ammonium tetrathiomolybdate (60 to 300 mg/day, administered in six divided doses, three with meals and three between meals). Tetrathiomolybdate forms a complex with protein and copper and when given with food blocks the absorption of copper. The major drawback to using this drug is that it has not been approved for general use in this country.

Triethylene tetramine dihydrochloride (trientine) (250 mg four times a day, given at least 1 hour before or 2 hours after meals) is also a chelator that increases urinary excretion of copper. Its effectiveness is less than that of penicillamine, but the incidence of toxicity and hypersensitivity reactions is lower.

Zinc acetate (50 mg of elemental zinc acetate three times a day) acts by inducing intestinal MT, which has a high affinity for copper and prevents its entrance into blood. Zinc is far less toxic than penicillamine but is much slower acting. Diet does not play an important role in the management of Wilson disease, although Brewer recommends restriction of liver and shellfish during the first year of treatment (901).

Zinc is the optimal drug for maintenance therapy and for the treatment of the presymptomatic patient. Trientine in combination with zinc acetate has been suggested for patients who present in hepatic failure. Liver transplantation can be helpful in the patient who presents in end-stage liver disease. The procedure appears to correct the metabolic defect and can reverse neurologic symptoms (902). Schumacher and colleagues (904a) have also recommended its use for patients with normal liver function, but whose neurological symptoms have not responded to the various chelating agents.

With these regimens, gradual improvement in neurologic symptoms occurs. As a rule, brainstem auditory-evoked potentials improve within 1 month of the onset of therapy, with the somatosensory-evoked responses being somewhat slower to return to normal (903). The Kayser-Fleischer ring begins to fade within 6 to 10 weeks of the onset of therapy and disappears completely in a couple of years (904). Improvement of neurologic symptoms starts 5 to 6 months after therapy has begun and is generally complete in 24 months. As shown by serial neuroimaging studies, a significant regression of lesions occurs within thalamus and basal ganglia (895). Successive biopsies show a reduction in the amount of hepatic copper. Total serum copper and ceruloplasmin levels decrease, and the aminoaciduria and phosphaturia diminish.

As a rule, patients who are started on therapy before the evolution of symptoms remain healthy. Children who have had hepatic disease exclusively do well, and in 80%, hepatic functions return to normal. Approximately 40% of children who present with neurologic symptoms become completely asymptomatic and remain so for 10 or more years. Children with the mixed hepatocerebral picture do poorly. Fewer than 25% recover completely, and approximately 25% continue to deteriorate, often with the appearance of seizures. In all forms of the disease, the earlier the start of therapy, the better is the outlook (888).

When symptom-free patients with Wilson disease discontinue chelation therapy, their hepatic function deteriorates in 9 months to 3 years, a rate that is far more rapid than deterioration after birth (905). Scheinberg and coworkers postulate that penicillamine not only removes copper from tissue, but also detoxifies the metal by inducing MT synthesis (906).

Aceruloplasminemia (OMIM 604290)

The clinical picture of aceruloplasminemia is one of dementia, diabetes, ataxia, and extrapyramidal movements. MRI and neuropathologic examinations demonstrate iron deposition in the basal ganglia. The condition has its onset in middle age, and to our knowledge has not been reported in the pediatric population. It is due to a mutation in the gene that codes for ceruloplasmin, which acts as a ferroxidase, mediating oxidation of ferrous to ferric iron (907).

Menkes Disease (Kinky Hair Disease, KHD) (OMIM 309400)

This focal degenerative disorder of gray matter was described in 1962 by Menkes and associates (908). It is transmitted as an X-linked disorder.

Molecular Genetics and Biochemical Pathology

The characteristic feature of KHD, as expressed in the human infant, is a maldistribution of body copper so that it accumulates to abnormal levels in a form or location that renders it inaccessible for the synthesis of various copper enzymes (909,910). Most of the clinical manifestations can be explained by the low activities of the various copper-containing enzymes. Patients absorb little or no orally administered copper; when the metal is given intravenously, they experience a prompt increase in serum copper and ceruloplasmin (911). Copper levels are low in liver and brain but are elevated in several other tissues, notably intestinal mucosa, muscle, spleen, and kidney. The copper content of cultured fibroblasts, myotubes, or lymphocytes derived from patients with KHD is several times greater than of control cells; however, the kinetics of copper uptake in these cells is normal (912).

ATP7A, the gene for KHD, has been mapped to Xq13.3. It encodes an energy-dependent, copper-transporting P-type membrane ATPase (MNK) (913,914). The ATPase is one of a family of membrane proteins that transports cations across plasma and endoplasmic reticulum membranes. The structural homology between *ATP7A* and the *ATP7B*, the gene for Wilson disease, is considerable in the 3′ two-thirds of the genes, but there is much divergence between them in the 5′ one-third (914). *ATP7A* is expressed in most tissues, including brain, but not in liver. At basal copper levels, the protein (MNK) is located in the *trans*-Golgi network, the sorting station for proteins exiting from the Golgi apparatus, where it is involved in copper uptake into its lumen (915). At increased intra- and extracellular copper concentrations the MNK protein shifts toward the plasma membrane, presumably to enhance removal of excess copper from the cell (916,917). Numerous mutations have been recognized, and it appears as if almost every family has its own private mutation (918).

As a consequence of the defect in the transport protein, copper becomes inaccessible for the synthesis of ceruloplasmin, superoxide dismutase, and a variety of other copper-containing enzymes, notably ascorbic acid oxidase, cytochrome oxidase, dopamine β-hydroxylase, and lysyl hydroxylase.

Because of the defective activity of these metalloenzymes, a variety of pathologic changes are set into motion. Arteries are tortuous, with irregular lumens and a frayed and split intimal lining (Fig. 1.32A). These abnormalities reflect a failure in elastin and collagen cross-linking caused by dysfunction of the key enzyme for this process, copper-dependent lysyl hydroxylase.

Changes within the brain result from vascular lesions, copper deficiency, or a combination of the two. Extensive focal degeneration of gray matter occurs, with neuronal loss and gliosis and an associated axonal degeneration in white matter. Cellular loss is prominent in the cerebellum. Here, Purkinje cells are hard hit; many are lost, and others show abnormal dendritic arborization (weeping willow) and perisomatic processes. Focal axonal swellings (torpedoes) are observed also (908,919). Electron microscopy often shows a marked increase in the number of mitochondria in the perikaryon of Purkinje cells and to a lesser degree in the neurons of cerebral cortex and the basal ganglia (919). Mitochondria are enlarged, and intramitochondrial electron-dense bodies are present. The pathogenesis of these changes is a matter of controversy.

Clinical Manifestations

KHD is a rare disorder; its frequency has been estimated at 1 in 114,000 to 1 in 250,000 live births (920). Baerlocher and Nadal provided a comprehensive review of the clinical features (921). In the classic form of the illness symptoms appear during the neonatal period. Most commonly, one observes hypothermia, poor feeding, and impaired weight gain. Seizures soon become apparent. Marked hypotonia, poor head control, and progressive deterioration of all neurologic functions are seen. The facies has a cherubic appearance with a depressed nasal bridge and reduced movements (922) (Fig. 1.32B). There also is gingival enlargement and delayed eruption of primary teeth. The optic discs are pale, and microcysts of the pigment epithelium are seen (923). The most striking finding is the appearance of the scalp hair; it is colorless and friable. Examination under the microscope reveals a variety of abnormalities, most often pili torti (twisted hair), monilethrix (varying

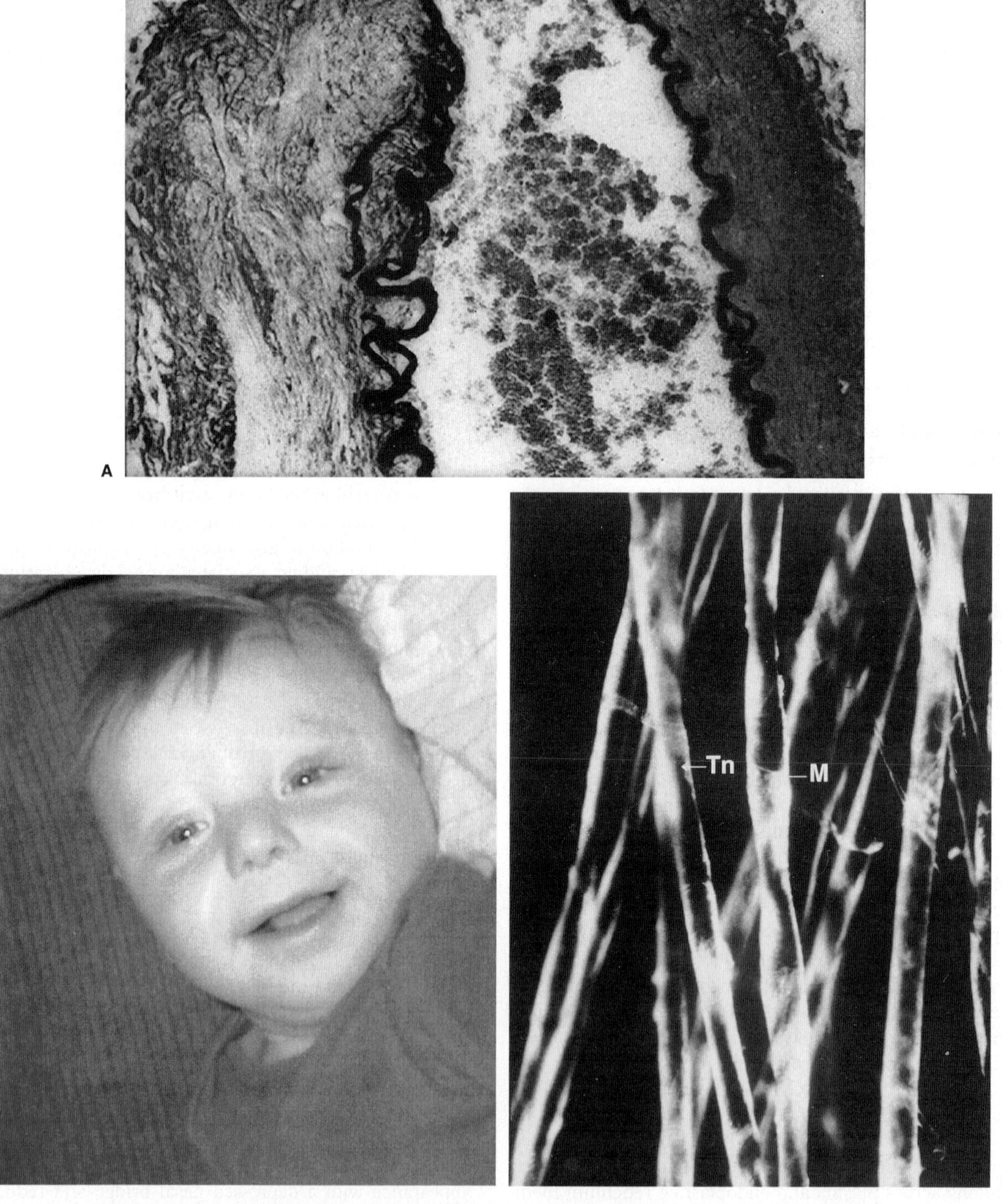

FIGURE 1.32. Menkes disease. **A:** Section of a large artery from a patient with Menkes disease. Note frayed and split internal elastic lamina. **B:** Typical "cherubic" facies of a boy with Menkes disease. **C:** Abnormalities of hair shaft. M, monilethrix; Tn, trichorrhexis nodosa.

diameter of hair shafts), and trichorrhexis nodosa (fractures of the hair shaft at regular intervals) (Fig. 1. 32C) (923).

Radiography of long bones reveals metaphyseal spurring and a diaphyseal periosteal reaction reminiscent of scurvy (924). The urinary tract is not spared. Hydronephrosis, hydroureter, and bladder diverticula are common (925).

Neuroimaging discloses cerebral atrophy and bilateral ischemic lesions in deep gray matter or in the cortical areas, the consequence of vascular infarctions (926). A progressive tortuosity and enlargement of intracranial vessels also can be shown by MRI angiography. Similar changes are seen in the systemic vasculature (927). Asymptomatic subdural hematomas are almost invariable, and when these occur in conjunction with a skull fracture, the diagnosis of nonaccidental trauma is frequently considered (928,929). EEGs show multifocal paroxysmal discharges or hypsarrhythmia. Visual-evoked potentials are of low amplitude or completely absent (930).

The course is usually inexorably downhill, but the rate of neurologic deterioration varies considerably. There are recurrent infections of the respiratory and urinary tracts, and sepsis and meningitis are fairly common. I have seen a patient in his 20s, and numerous patients have been reported whose clinical manifestations are less severe than those seen in the classic form of KHD, and it appears likely that a continuum in disease severity exists. The correlation between the severity of phenotype and the type of mutation is not good, and variable clinical expressions for identical mutations have been observed (931,932).

One of the most important clinical variants is occipital horn syndrome. As originally described, this condition is characterized by occipital exostoses, which appear as bony horns on each side of the foramen magnum, cutis laxa, and bladder diverticula (933). Mental retardation is frequent but not invariable. The neuropathology of this disease is similar to that seen in the classic forms of KHD (934). Serum copper and ceruloplasmin are usually but not invariably low. A variety of mutations of *ATP7A* have been described, and in some there is complete absence of the normal gene product (935).

Diagnosis

The clinical history and the appearance of the infant should suggest the diagnosis. Serum ceruloplasmin and copper levels are normally low in the neonatal period and do not reach adult levels until 1 month of age. Therefore, these determinations must be performed serially to demonstrate a failure of the expected increase. The diagnosis can best be confirmed by demonstrating the intracellular accumulation of copper and decreased efflux of ^{64}Cu from cultured fibroblasts (936). The increased copper content of chorionic villi has been used for first-trimester diagnosis of the disease (936). These analyses require considerable expertise, and only few centers can perform them reliably.

In heterozygotes, areas of pili torti constitute between 30% and 50% of the hair. Less commonly, skin depigmentation is present. Carrier detection by measuring the accumulation of radioactive copper in fibroblasts is possible but is not very reliable (936). The full neurodegenerative disease, accompanied by chromosome X/2 translocation, has been encountered in girls (937).

Trichorrhexis nodosa also can be seen not only in argininosuccinic aciduria and giant axonal neuropathy, but also in a number of other conditions that result in a structural abnormality of the hair shaft. A condition characterized by short stature, ataxia, physical and mental retardation, ichthyotic skin, and brittle hair and nails with reduced content of cysteine-rich matrix proteins has been termed trichothiodystrophy (TTD) (938). Approximately one-half of the patients have photosensitivity. Several genetically distinct entities are included in this group, with DNA repair-deficient TTD resulting from mutations in the DNA repair and transcription factor (939). Other disorders in the hair shaft are reviewed in conjunction with photographs of their microscopic appearance in an article by Whiting (940).

Treatment

Copper supplementation, using daily injections of copper-histidine, appears to be the most promising treatment. Parenterally administered copper corrects the hepatic copper deficiency and restores serum copper and ceruloplasmin levels to normal. The effectiveness of treatment in arresting or reversing neurologic symptoms probably depends on whether some activity of the copper-transporting enzyme MNK has been preserved and whether copper supplementation has been initiated promptly (936,941). Therefore, it is advisable to commence copper therapy as soon as the diagnosis is established if the child has good neurologic function and to continue therapy until it becomes evident that cerebral degeneration cannot be arrested.

Molybdenum Cofactor Deficiency (OMIM 252150)

Three enzymes require molybdenum for their function: sulfite oxidase, xanthine dehydrogenase, and aldehyde oxidase. Three genetically distinct disorders result in a defect of the molybdenum cofactor. Each of these represents a defect in one of the four genes involved in the biosynthesis of the molybdenum cofactor.

Most commonly, one encounters a defect in *MOCS1*, the gene that codes for the enzyme involved in the formation of the cofactor precursor (942). MOCS2 prevents the conversion of the precursor into molybdopterin. A third genetically distinct disorder affects the formation of gephyrin, a molecule that assists with the insertion of molybdenum into molybdopterin (943).

About 100 cases of the various molybdenum cofactor deficiencies have been described worldwide. Clinically, all three disorders are autosomal recessive and are marked by intractable seizures, often starting in the neonatal period, severe developmental delay, and multiple cerebral infarcts producing a neuroimaging picture that resembles severe perinatal asphyxia (944). Molybdenum cofactor deficiency can be suspected by elevated serum lactate levels, low serum and urinary uric acid, and increased urinary sulfite. A dipstick test (Merckoquant; Merck, Darmstadt, Germany) applied to fresh urine detects the increased presence of sulfites (3a,945). Treatment with dietary restriction of methionine has been attempted (946).

Isolated sulfite oxidase deficiency produces a clinical picture similar to molybdenum cofactor deficiency, namely a profound developmental delay, hypotonia, and seizures, which generally start in the neonatal period. Dislocated lenses are apparent in some cases (947,948). Neuroimaging studies show initial cerebral edema followed by dramatic multicystic leukoencephalopathy. We emphasize that neonatal isolated sulfite oxidase deficiency should be included in the differential diagnosis of neonates with unexplained hypoxic-ischemic changes on neuroimaging studies (949). Dietary therapy of this condition with reduced methionine intake and a synthetic amino acid mixture lacking cystine and methionine has resulted in normal growth and apparently normal psychomotor development (950).

DISORDERS OF PURINE AND PYRIMIDINE METABOLISM

Lesch-Nyhan Syndrome (OMIM 308000)

The occurrence of hyperuricemia in association with spasticity and severe choreoathetosis was first reported by Catel and Schmidt in 1959 (951). Since then, the disease has been observed in all parts of the world. It is transmitted as an X-linked disorder, with the gene mapped to Xq26–q27.2 (952).

Molecular Genetics and Biochemical Pathology

The structure of the gene whose defect is responsible for Lesch-Nyhan syndrome has been elucidated. It codes for the enzyme hypoxanthine-guanine phosphoribosyltransferase (HGPRT), which is defective in this condition. More than 200 mutations have been recorded; most families studied have their private mutation, and the same mutation is encountered rarely in unrelated individuals (953). Some 85% of these are point mutations or small deletions, and patients produce detectable amounts of normal-sized HGPRT (954). As a consequence of the genetic mutation, HGPRT activity is reduced to less than 0.5% of normal in a number of tissues, including erythrocytes and fibroblast cultures.

Because of HGPRT deficiency, hypoxanthine cannot be reused, and whatever hypoxanthine is formed is either excreted or catabolized to xanthine and uric acid. Additionally, phosphoribosylpyrophosphate, a known regulator of *de novo* purine synthesis, is increased. For these reasons, *de novo* uric acid production is increased markedly, and serum urine and CSF uric acid levels are elevated. The excretion of other purines, such as xanthine and hypoxanthine, is increased also (954).

The mechanism by which HGPRT deficiency induces the neurologic disorder is unclear. An abnormality in the dopaminergic system has been well documented. In basal ganglia, notably in the terminal-rich regions of the caudate, putamen, and nucleus accumbens septi, the dopamine concentration is reduced, as are the activities of dopa decarboxylase and tyrosine hydroxylase. Such findings point to a functional loss of a significant proportion of nigrostriatal and mesolimbic dopamine tracts. Using a ligand that binds to dopamine transporters, Wong and coworkers showed a reduction in the density of dopamine-containing neurons (955). A reduction in norepinephrine turnover and a diminution in the function of the striatal cholinergic neurons also have been documented. These alterations of the normal neurotransmitter balance within basal ganglia could account for the movement disorder characteristic of Lesch-Nyhan syndrome (956). Based on animal data, it has been postulated that the self-injurious behavior that is so characteristic of the condition is the consequence of destruction of dopaminergic fibers early in development and subsequent exposure to dopamine agonists (953). Impaired adenosine transport and apoptosis induced by the accumulation of 5′-aminoimidazole-4-carboxamide riboside have also been proposed as contributing to the neurologic manifestations (957,958).

As would be expected from the Lyon hypothesis, the heterozygote female patient has two cell populations, one with full enzymatic activity and the other enzyme deficient. Heterozygotes can be ascertained by determining HGPRT activity in hair follicles.

Pathologic Anatomy

The morphologic alterations seen in the brain are sparse and can be explained by the uremia, which is often present terminally (959). The dopamine-producing cells in the substantia nigra appear grossly unaffected.

Clinical Manifestations

Clinically, patients with HPRT deficiency fall into three groups. The most severely affected have all the features of classic Lesch-Nyhan disease, another group has neurologic manifestations and hyperuricemia, and yet a third group has isolated hyperuricemia without neurologic deficits (953).

In the classic form of Lesch-Nyhan disease children appear healthy at birth, and initial gross motor milestones are achieved appropriately. During the first year of life, psychomotor retardation becomes evident. Extrapyramidal movements appear between 8 and 24 months of age and persist until obliterated by progressive spasticity. Seizures occur in approximately 50% of the patients. A curious and unexplained feature of the disease is the involuntary self-destructive biting of fingers, arms, and lips, which becomes apparent by 4 years of age. Children are disturbed by their compulsion to self-mutilation and are happier when maintained in restraints. The teeth may have to be removed to prevent damage to the lips and tongue. Hematuria and renal calculi are seen in the majority of individuals, and ultimately renal failure develops. Gouty arthritis and urate tophi are also late complications. A megaloblastic anemia is common. Intellectual levels range from moderate mental retardation to low average (960). In later years, a large proportion of patients develop vocal tics reminiscent of those seen in Tourette disease.

In the second group of patients there is excessive uric acid production, gouty arthritis, and mild neurologic symptoms, most commonly a spinocerebellar syndrome or mild mental retardation, or mild mental retardation, short stature, and spasticity (953,961,962).

The least severely affected group has defective HGPRT with hyperuricemia and renal symptoms but no neurologic deficits (953).

Diagnosis

The features of the illness, in particular self-mutilation and extrapyramidal movements, make a diagnosis possible on clinical grounds. Although serum uric acid is usually elevated, diagnosis is best confirmed from the urinary uric acid content, a urinary uric acid to creatine ratio of 3 to 1 or higher being almost diagnostic (953). Enzymatic analyses of lysed erythrocytes, cultured skin fibroblasts, cultured amniotic fluid cells, or other tissue are easily carried out and confirm the diagnosis and can be used for antenatal diagnosis (953,963). Routine MRI studies reveal mild cerebral atrophy. Volumetric MRI shows a one-third reduction in caudate volume (964).

Other Disorders of Purine and Pyrimidine Metabolism

A variety of other disorders of purine and pyrimidine metabolism are summarized in Table 1.27.

An X-linked syndrome marked by developmental delay, ataxia, and sensorineural deafness in which hyperuricemia is caused by superactivity of phosphoribosyl pyrophosphate synthetase and excessive purine production has been reported (965) (OMIM 311850). Another disorder of purine metabolism, adenylosuccinate lyase deficiency (OMIM 103050), is manifested by the presence of large amounts of succinyladenosine and succinylaminoimidazole carboxamide riboside and succinyl adenosine in body fluids. The clinical picture is one of severe mental retardation, seizures, and autistic features, or exclusively austistic features (966,967). These disorders can be identified by subjecting urine to the Bratton-Marshall reaction. This test is described by Laikind and coworkers (968). Castro and coworkers stress the need to subject the urine of children with unexplained neurologic disease and autism to this simple test (970).

Treatment

Allopurinol (20 mg/kg per day), a xanthine oxidase inhibitor that blocks the last steps of uric acid synthesis, has been used in treating the renal and arthritic manifestations of the disease. The decrease in uric acid excretion induced by this drug is accompanied by an increase of hypoxanthine and xanthine but does not alter the neurologic manifestations of the disease (953). A variety of drugs such as serotonin agonists or antagonists have been used in an attempt to suppress self-mutilation, none with any clear effect. Chronic stimulation of the globus pallidus has been effective in at least one patient (969). Bone marrow transplantation has been ineffective (953).

Disorders of Pyrimidine Metabolism

A condition termed thymine-uraciluria in which increased excretion of uracil, thymine, and 5-hydroxymethyluracil are accompanied by seizures and mental retardation has been reported (970,971). The defect is one of dihydropyrimidine dehydrogenase (OMIM 274270). Patients develop severe reactions to 5-fluorouracil, with cerebellar ataxia and progressive obtundation (970).

Creatine Deficiency Syndrome (OMIM 601240)

Creatine deficiency syndrome, a disorder of creatine biosynthesis, is caused by a deficiency in hepatic guanidinoacetate methyltransferase. The condition is marked by a progressive extrapyramidal movement disorder, seizures,

TABLE 1.27 Disorders of Purine and Pyrimidine Metabolism with Neurologic Phenotypes

Disorder	*Biochemical Abnormality*	*Clinical Manifestations*
Lesch-Nyhan (HGPTR deficiency)	Elevated urine uric acid	Extrapyramidal disorder, self-mutilation
Phosphoribosylpyrophosphate synthase superactivity	Elevated urine uric acid	Developmental delay, ataxia, sensorineural deafness
Adenosine monophosphate deaminase deficiency 1 (myoadenylate deaminase)	Decreased lactate formation on ischemic forearm test	Hypotonia, exertional myalgia, poor exercise tolerance or no symptoms
Purine nucleotide phosphorylase deficiency	Elevated urine/plasma inosine, guanosine	T-cell immunodeficiency, cerebral vasculopathy, strokes
Adenylosuccinate lyase (adenyl succinase) deficiency	Succinyl adenosine, succinylaminoimidazole carboxamide ribotide elevated in plasma, urine, CSF	Severe mental retardation, seizures, autistic features
Uridine monophosphate synthase deficiency	Orotic acid elevation in urine	Mental retardation
Dihydropyrimidine dehydrogenase deficiency	Increased excretion of uracil, thymine, 5-hydroxymethyluracil	Mental retardation, adverse reaction to 5-fluorouracil
Dihydropyrimidinase deficiency	Increased excretion of uracil, thymine	Dysmorphic features, intractable seizures, severe developmental delay

CSF, cerebrospinal fluid; HGPTR, hypoxanthine guanine phosphoribosyl transferase.

and microcephaly. On MRI, delayed myelination is seen, and on MRS, the creatine and creatine phosphate peaks are virtually absent. Treatment with oral creatine (400 to 500 mg/kg per day) results in gradual improvement in some of the symptoms (972). Defects in creatine transport are covered in another part of this chapter.

Porphyrias

Of the various inherited disorders of the heme biosynthetic pathway that result in the accumulation of porphyrin or porphyrin precursors, only congenital erythropoietic porphyria is observed with any frequency during childhood. It results in cutaneous photosensitivity and hemolytic anemia but it is not accompanied by neurologic symptoms.

Acute intermittent porphyria is transmitted as an autosomal dominant trait with variable, but generally low, penetrance. Symptoms usually begin at puberty or shortly thereafter, and are most pronounced in young adults. Prior to that symptoms are vague and of short duration (973). Manifestations consist of recurrent attacks of autonomic dysfunction, intermittent colicky abdominal pain, convulsions, and a polyneuritis, which usually predominantly affects the motor nerves. The upper limbs are generally more involved, and the paralysis progresses until it reaches its maximum within several weeks. Seizures are relatively rare. Mental disturbances, notably anxiety, insomnia, and confusion, are common, but no skin lesions develop (974,975). Attacks can be precipitated by a variety of drugs, notably anticonvulsants.

Decreased activity of porphobilinogen deaminase to 50% of normal has been demonstrated in several tissues, notably in erythrocytes, where the enzyme can be assayed most readily. The gene for the enzyme is located on the long arm of chromosome 11 (11q23–qter), and more than 100 allelic variants have been documented (976). This heterogeneity is in part responsible for the variable expression of the disease.

The pathogenesis of the neurologic symptoms is poorly understood (975). The various hypotheses are reviewed by Bissell (975). The most likely explanation is that multiple

TABLE 1.28 Neurologic Symptoms in the Hereditary Porphyrias

Disease	*Neurologic Signs and Symptoms*
Acute intermittent porphyria	Recurrent attacks of autonomic dysfunction, abdominal pain, seizures, motor polyneuropathy
δ-Aminolevulinic acid dehydratase deficiency	Motor polyneuropathy
Congenital erythropoietic porphyria	No neurologic symptoms, severe cutaneous photosensitivity
Porphyria cutanea tarda	No neurologic symptoms, cutaneous photosensitivity
Hereditary coproporphyria	As in acute intermittent porphyria, cutaneous photosensitivity
Variegate porphyria	Acute neurovisceral crises, photosensitive skin; rarely starts before third decade of life
Protoporphyria	Cutaneous photosensitivity, no neurologic symptoms except in endstage liver disease

factors, notably δ-aminolevulinic acid (ALA), which has structural resemblance to GABA, act on the nervous system concomitantly or sequentially.

The diagnosis is arrived at by demonstrating increased urinary porphobilinogen and urinary ALA during an attack. Between attacks, the excretion of both metabolites decreases but is rarely normal. Clinically silent carriers do not excrete increased amounts of these metabolites (977).

The neurologic signs and symptoms of the various porphyrias are summarized in Table 1.28. We should point out that increased excretion of ALA without increased porphobilinogen excretion is seen in lead poisoning and hereditary tyrosinemia.

REFERENCES

1. Rosenberg RN, Prusiner SB, DiMauro S, et al., eds. *The molecular and genetic basis of neurologic and psychiatric disease,* 3rd ed. Philadelphia: Butterworth–Heinemann, 2003.
2. Scriver CR, Beaudet AL, Sly WS, et al., eds. *The metabolic and molecular bases of inherited disease,* 8th ed. New York: McGraw-Hill, 2001.
3. Clarke JTR. *A clinical guide to inherited metabolic diseases,* 2nd ed. Cambridge: Cambridge University Press, 2002.
3a. Hoffmann GF, Nyhan WL, Zschocke J, et al. *Inherited metabolic diseases.* Philadelphia: Lippincott Williams & Wilkins, 2002.
3b. Wilcken B, Wiley V, Hammond J, et al. Screening newborns for inborn errors of metabolism by tandem mass spectrometry. *N Engl J Med* 2003;348:2304–2312.
4. Garrod AE. The Croonian lectures on inborn errors of metabolism. Lecture IV. *Lancet* 1908;2:214–220.
5. Scriver CR. Why mutation analysis does not always predict clinical consequences: explanation in the era of genomics. *J Pediatr* 2002;140:502–506.
5a. Enns GM, Martinez DR, Kuzmin AI, et al. Molecular correlations in phenylketonuria: mutation patterns and corresponding biochemical and clinical phenotypes in a heterogeneous California population. *Pediatr Res* 1999;46:594–602.
6. Strachan T, Read AP. *Human molecular genetics,* 3rd ed. New York: Garland, 2004.
7. Lodish H, Berk A, Matsudaine P, et al., eds. *Molecular cell biology,* 5th ed. New York: Scientific American Books, 2003.
8. Lewin B. *Genes VIII.* New York: Oxford University Press, 2003.
9. Burton BK. Inborn errors of metabolism. The clinical diagnosis in early infancy. *Pediatrics* 1987;79:359–369.
10. Shevell M, Ashwal S, Donley D, et al. Practice parameter: evaluation of the child with global developmental delay. *Neurology* 2003;60:367–380.
11. Nissenkorn A, Michelson M, Ben-Zeev B, et al. Inborn errors of metabolism: a cause of abnormal brain development. *Neurology* 2001;56:1265–1272.
12. Fölling A. Uber Ausscheidung von Phenylbrenztraubensäure in den Harn als Stoffwechselanomalie in Verbindung mit Imbezillität. *Z Physiol Chem* 1934;227:169–176.
13. Berman JL, Cunningham GC, Day RW, et al. Causes of high phenylalanine with normal tyrosine. *Am J Dis Child* 1969;117:654–656.
14. Scriver CR, Kaufman S. Phenylalanine hydroxylase deficiency. In: Scriver CR, Sly WS, Childs B, et al., eds. *The metabolic and molecular bases of inherited disease,* 8th ed. New York: McGraw-Hill, 2001:1667–1724.
15. Eisensmith RC, Martinez DR, Kuzmin AI, et al. Molecular basis of phenylketonuria and a correlation between genotype and phenotype in a heterogeneous southeastern US population. *Pediatrics* 1996;97:512–516.
16. Guldberg P, Ray F, Zschocke J, et al. A European multicenter study of phenylalanine hydroxylase deficiency: classification of 105 mutations and a general system for genotype-based prediction of metabolic phenotype. *Am J Hum Genet* 1998;63:71–79.
17. Okano Y, Eisensmith EC, Guttler F, et al. Molecular basis of phenotypic heterogeneity in phenylketonuria. *N Engl J Med* 1991;324:1232–1238.
18. Ramus SJ, Forrest SM, Pitt DD, et al. Genotype and intellectual phenotype in untreated phenylketonuria patients. *Pediatr Res* 1999;45:474–481.
19. Moller HE, Weglage J, Bick U, et al. Brain imaging and proton magnetic resonance spectroscopy in patients with phenylketonuria. *Pediatrics* 2003;112:1580–1583.
20. Pietz J, Kreis R, Rupp A, et al. Large neutral amino acids block phenylalanine transport into brain tissue in patients with phenylketonuria. *J Clin Invest* 1999;103:1169–1178.
21. Hanley WB, Lee AW, Hanley AJ, et al. "Hypotyrosinemia" in phenylketonuria. *Mol Genet Metab* 2000;69:286–294.
22. Yarbro MT, Anderson JA. L-Tryptophan metabolism in phenylketonuria. *J Pediatr* 1966;68:895–904.
23. Miyamoto M, Fitzpatrick TB. Competitive inhibition of mammalian tyrosinase by phenylalanine and its relationship to hair pigmentation in phenylketonuria. *Nature* 1957;179:199–200.
24. Malamud N. Neuropathy of phenylketonuria. *J Neuropathol Exp Neurol* 1966;25:254–269.
25. Bauman ML, Kemper TL. Morphologic and histoanatomic observations of the brain in untreated human phenylketonuria. *Acta Neuropathol* 1982;58:55–63.
26. Crome L. The association of phenylketonuria with leucodystrophy. *J Neurol Neurosurg Psychiatr* 1962;25:149–153.
27. Barden H. The histochemical relationship of neuro-melanin and lipofuscin. *J Neuropathol Exp Neurol* 1969;28:419–441.
28. Partington MW. The early symptoms of phenylketonuria. *Pediatrics* 1961;27:465–473.
29. MacLeod MD, Monroe JF, Ledingham JG, et al. Management of the extrapyramidal manifestations of phenylketonuria with L-dopa. *Arch Dis Child* 1983;58:457–458.
30. Gross PT, Berlow S, Schuett VE, et al. EEG in phenylketonuria. Attempt to establish clinical importance of EEG changes. *Arch Neurol* 1981;38:122–126.
31. Pearsen KD, Gean-Marton AD, Levy HL, et al. Phenylketonuria: MR imaging of the brain with clinical correlation. *Radiology* 1990;177:437–440.
32. Cleary MA, Walter JH, Wraith JE, et al. Magnetic resonance imaging in phenylketonuria: reversal of cerebral white matter changes. *J Pediatr* 1995;127:251–255.
33. Kang E, Paine RS. Elevation of plasma phenylalanine levels during pregnancies of women heterozygous for phenylketonuria. *J Pediatr* 1963;63:282–289.
34. Levy HL, Gulberg P, Guttler F, et al. Congenital heart disease in maternal phenylketonuria: report from the Maternal PKU Collaborative Study. *Pediat Res* 2001;49:636–642.
35. Levy HL, Lobbregt D, Barnes PD, et al. Maternal phenylketonuria: magnetic resonance imaging of the brain in offspring. *J Pediatr* 1996;128:770–775.
36. Widaman KF, Azen C. Relation of prenatal phenylalanine exposure to infant and childhood cognitive outcomes: results from the International Maternal PKU Collaborative Study. *Pediatrics* 2003;112:1537–1543.
37. Koch R, Hanley W, Levy H, et al. The Maternal Phenylketonuria International Study: 1984–2002. *Pediatrics* 2003;112:1523–1529.
38. Levy HL, Weisbren SE, Guttler F, et al. Pregnancy experiences in the woman with mild hyperphenylalaninemia. *Pediatrics* 2003;112:1548–1552.
39. Scriver CR, Clow CL. Phenylketonuria: epitome of human biochemical genetics. *N Engl J Med* 1980;303:1336–1342.
40. Kaufman S. An evaluation of the possible neurotoxicity of metabolites of phenylalanine. *J Pediatr* 1989;114:895–900.
41. Menkes JH, Koch R. Phenylketonuria. In: Vinken PJ, Bruyn GW, eds. *Handbook of clinical neurology, Vol. 29.* Amsterdam: North-Holland, 1977:29–51.
42. Hommes FA. On the mechanism of permanent brain dysfunction in hyperphenylalaninemia. *Biochem Med Metabol Biol* 1991;46:277–287.

43. Bartlett K, Eaton SJ, Pourfarzam M. New developments in neonatal screening. *Arch Dis Child Fetal Neonatal Ed* 1997;77:F151–F154.
44. Koch R, Friedman EG. Accuracy of newborn screening programs for phenylketonuria. *J Pediatr* 1981;98:267–270.
45. Henley WR, Demshar H, Preston MA, et al. Newborn phenylketonuria (PKU) Guthrie (BIA) screening and early hospital discharge. *Early Hum Dev* 1997;47:87–96.
46. Doherty LB, Rohr FJ, Levy HL. Detection of phenylketonuria in the very early newborn population. *Pediatrics* 1991;87:240–244.
47. Sinai LN, Kim SC, Casey R, et al. Phenylketonuria screening: effect of early newborn discharge. *Pediatrics* 1995;96:605–608.
48. Weglage J, Pietsch M, Feldmann R, et al. Normal clinical outcome in untreated subjects with mild hyperphenylalaninemia. *Pediatr Res* 2001;49:532–536.
49. Economou-Petersen E, Henriksen KF, Guldberg P, et al. Molecular basis for nonphenylketonuria hyperphenylalanemia. *Genomics* 1992;14:1–5.
50. Guttler F, Ledley FD, Lidsky AS, et al. Correlation between polymorphic DNA haplotypes at phenylalanine hydroxylase locus and clinical phenotypes of phenylketonuria. *J Pediatr* 1987;110:68–71.
51. National Institutes of Health Consensus Development Panel/ National Institutes of Health Consensus Development Statement: Phenylketonuria screening and management, October 16–18, 2000. *Pediatrics* 2001;108:972–982.
52. DiLella AG, Huang WM, Woo SLC. Screening for phenylketonuria mutations by DNA amplifications with the polymerase chain reaction. *Lancet* 1988;1:497–499.
53. Ledley FD. Clinical application of genotypic diagnosis for phenylketonuria: theoretical considerations. *Eur J Pediatr* 1991; 150:752–756.
54. Cedarbaum S. Phenylketonuria: an update. *Curr Opin Pediatr* 2002;14:702–706.
55. Buist NR, Prince AP, Huntington KL, et al. A new amino acid mixture permits new approaches to the treatment of phenylketonuria. *Acta Paediatr Suppl* 1994;407:75–77.
56. Acosta PB, Yanicelli S, Marriage B, et al. Nutrient intake and growth of infants with phenylketonuria undergoing therapy. *J Pediatr Gastroenterol Nutr* 1998;27:297–291.
57. Walter JH, White FJ, Hall SK, et al. How practical are recommendations for dietary control in phenylketonuria? *Lancet* 2002; 360:55–57.
58. Kalsner LR, Rohr FJ, Strauss KA, et al. Tyrosine supplementation in phenylketonuria: diurnal blood tyrosine levels and presumptive brain influx of tyrosine and other large neutral amino acids. *J Pediatr* 2001;139:421–427.
59. Muntau AC, Röschinger W, Habich M, et al. Tetrahydrobiopterin as an alternative treatment for mild phenylketonuria. *N Engl J Med* 2002;347:2122–2132.
59a. Shintaku H, Kure S, Ohura T, et al. Long-term treatment and diagnosis of tetrahydrobiopterin responsive hyperphenylalaninemia with a mutant phenylalanine hydroxylase gene. *Pediatr Res* 2004;55:425–430.
60. Spaapen LJ, Rubio-Gonzalbo ME. Tetrahydrobiopterin-responsive phenylalanine hydroxylase deficiency. *Mol Genet Metab* 2003;78:93–99.
61. Smith I, Beasley MG, Ades AE. Intelligence and quality of dietary treatment in phenylketonuria. *Arch Dis Child* 1990;65:472–478.
62. Brunner RL, Jordan MK, Berry HK. Early treated phenylketonuria: neuropsychologic consequences. *J Pediatr* 1983;102:831–835.
63. Smith I, Beasley MG, Wolff OH, et al. Behavior disturbance in 8-year-old children with early treated phenylketonuria. *J Pediatr* 1988;112:403–408.
64. Smith ML, Hanley WB, Clarke JT, et al. Randomised controlled trial of tyrosine supplementation on neuropsychological performance in phenylketonuria. *Arch Dis Child* 1998;78:116–121.
65. Holtzman NA, Kronmal RA, van Doorminck W, et al. Effect of age at loss of dietary control on intellectual performance and behavior of children with phenylketonuria. *N Engl J Med* 1986;314:593–598.
66. Waisbren SE, Mahon BE, Schnell RR, et al. Predictors of intelligence quotients and intelligence quotient change in persons treated for phenylketonuria early in life. *Pediatrics* 1987;79:351–355.
67. Thompson AJ, Smith I, Brenton D, et al. Neurological deterioration in young adults with phenylketonuria. *Lancet* 1990;336:602–605.
68. Villasana D, Butler IJ, Williams JC, et al. Neurological deterioration in adult phenylketonuria. *J Inherit Metab Dis* 1989;12:451–457.
69. Endres W. Diet in phenylketonuria: how long? Policies under discussion. *Ann Nutr Metab* 1998;4:221–227.
70. Oh HJ, Park ES, Kong S, et al. Long-term enzymatic and phenotypic correction in the phenylketonuria mouse model by adeno-associated virus vector-mediated gene transfer. *Pediatr Res* 2004;56:278–284.
71. Ding Z, Harding CO, Thony B. State-of-the-art 2003 on PKU gene therapy. *Mol Genet Metab* 2004;81:3–8.
72. Gröbe H, Bartholome K, Milstien S, et al. Hyperphenylalaninemia due to dihydropteridine reductase deficiency. *Eur J Pediatr* 1978;129:93–98.
73. Dhondt JL. Tetrahydrobiopterin deficiencies: preliminary analysis from an international survey. *J Pediatr* 1984;104:501–508.
74. Smith I, Leeming RJ, Cavanagh MP, et al. Neurological aspects of biopterin metabolism. *Arch Dis Child* 1986;61:130–137.
75. Woody RC, Brewster MA, Glasier C. Progressive intracranial calcification in dihydropteridine reductase deficiency prior to folinic acid therapy. *Neurology* 1989;39:673–675.
76. Sugita R, Takahashi S, Ishii K, et al. Brain CT and MR findings in hyperphenylalaninemia due to dihydropteridine reductase deficiency (variant of phenylketonuria). *J Comput Assist Tomogr* 1990;14:699–703.
77. Irons M, Levy HL, O'Flynn ME, et al. Folic acid therapy in treatment of dihydropteridine reductase deficiency. *J Pediatr* 1987;110:61–67.
78. Shintaku H. Disorders of tetrahydrobiopterin metabolism and their treatment. *Curr Drug Metab* 2002;3:123–131.
79. Dhondt JL, Guibaud P, Rolland MO, et al. Neonatal hyperphenylalaninaemia presumably caused by a new variant of biopterin synthetase deficiency. *Eur J Pediatr* 1988;147:153–157.
80. Thony B, Leimbacher W, Blau N, et al. Hyperphenylalaninemia due to defects in tetrahydrobiopterin metabolism: molecular characterization of mutations in 6-pyruvoyl-tetrahydropterin synthase. *Am J Hum Genet* 1994;54:782–792.
81. Hoganson G, Berlow S, Kaufman S, et al. Biopterin synthesis defects: problems in diagnosis. *Pediatrics* 1984;74:1004–1011.
82. Brismar J, Aqueel A, Gascon G, et al. Malignant hyperphenylalaninemia: CT and MR of the brain. *Am J Neuroradiol* 1990;11:135–138.
83. Niederwieser A, Blau N, Wang M, et al. GTP cyclohydrolase I deficiency, a new enzyme defect causing hyperphenylalaninemia with neopterin, biopterin, dopamine and serotonin deficiencies and muscular hypotonia. *Eur J Pediatr* 1984;141:208–214.
84. Blau N, Ochinose H, Nagatsu T, et al. A missense mutation in a patient with guanosine triphosphate cyclohydrolase I deficiency missed in the newborn screening program. *J Pediatr* 1995;126:401–405.
85. Hirano M, Yanagihara T, Ueno S. Dominant negative effect of GTP cyclohydrolase I mutations in dopa-responsive hereditary progressive dystonia. *Ann Neurol* 1998;44:365–371.
86. Blau N, Bonafé L, Thöny B. Tetrahydrobiopterin deficiencies without hyperphenylalaninemia: Diagnosis and genetics of DOPA-responsive dystonia and sepiapterin reductase deficiency. *Mol Genet Metab* 2001;74:172–185.
87. Zorzi G, Redweik U, Trippe H, et al. Detection of sepiapterin in CSF of patients with sepiapterin reductase deficiency. *Mol Genet Metab* 2002;75:174–177.
88. Thony B, Neuheiser F, Kierat L, et al. Mutations in the pterin-4-alpha-carbinolamine dehydratase (PCBD) gene cause a benign form of hyperphenylalaninemia. *Hum Genet* 1998;103:182–187.
89. Scriver CR, Larochelle J, Silverberg M. Hereditary tyrosinemia and tyrosyluria in a French-Canadian geographic isolate. *Am J Dis Child* 1967;113:41–46.
90. Grompe M. The pathophysiology and treatment of hereditary tyrosinemia type I. *Semin Liver Dis* 2001;20:563–571.
91. Laine J, Salo MK, Krogerus L, et al. The nephropathy of type I tyrosinemia after liver transplantation. *Pediatr Res* 1995;37:640–645.

92. Westphal EM, Natt E, Grimm T, et al. The human tyrosine aminotransferase gene: characterization of restriction fragment length polymorphisms and haplotype analysis in a family with tyrosinemia type II. *Hum Genet* 1988;79:260–264.
93. Andersson S, Nemeth A, Ohisalo J, et al. Persistent tyrosinemia associated with low activity of tyrosine aminotransferase. *Pediatr Res* 1984;18:675–678.
94. Menkes JH, Jervis GA. Developmental retardation associated with an abnormality in tyrosine metabolism. *Pediatrics* 1961;28:399–409.
95. Ellaway CJ, Holme E, Standing S, et al. Outcome of tyrosinaemia type III. *J Inherit Metab Dis* 2001;24:824–832.
96. Ruetschi U, Rymo L, Lindstedt S. Human 4-hydroxyphenylpyruvate dioxygenase gene (HPD). *Genomics* 1997;44:292–299.
97. Medes G. A new error of tyrosine metabolism: tyrosinosis. The intermediary metabolism of tyrosine and phenylalanine. *Biochem J* 1932;26:917–940.
98. Menkes JH, Welcher SW, Levi HS, et al. Relationship of elevated blood tyrosine to the ultimate intellectual performance of premature infants. *Pediatrics* 1972;49:218–224.
99. Mamunes P, Prince PE, Thornton NH, et al. Intellectual deficits after transient tyrosinemia in the term neonate. *Pediatrics* 1976;57:675–680.
100. Lehnert W, Stogmann W, Engelke U, et al. Long-term follow up of a new case of hawkinsuria. *Eur J Pediatr* 1999;158:578–582.
100a. Niederweiser A, Matasovic A. Tippett P, et al. A new sulfur aminoacid, named hawkensin, identified in a baby with transient tyrosinemia and her mother. *Clin Chim Acta* 1977;76:345–356.
101. Menkes JH, Hurst PL, Craig JM. A new syndrome: progressive familial infantile cerebral dysfunction associated with unusual urinary substance. *Pediatrics* 1954;14:462–467.
102. Roth KS. Newborn metabolic screening: a search for "nature's experiments." *South Med J* 1986;79:47–54.
103. Chuang DT, Chuang JL, Cox RP. Maple syrup urine disease: clinical and biochemical perspectives. In: Rosenberg RN, Prusiner SB, DiMauro S, et al., eds. *The molecular and genetic basis of neurological disease,* 3rd ed. Philadelphia: Butterworth–Heinemann, 2003:635–642.
104. Menkes JH. Maple syrup disease: investigations into the metabolic defect. *Neurology* 1959;9:826–835.
105. Menkes JH. Maple syrup disease: isolation and identification of organic acids in the urine. *Pediatrics* 1959;23:348–353.
106. Chuang DT. Maple syrup urine disease: it has come a long way. *J Pediatr* 1998;132:S17–S23.
107. Mamer OA, Reimer ML. On the mechanisms of the formation of L-alloisoleucine and the 2-hydroxy-3-methylvaleric acid stereoisomers from L-isoleucine in maple syrup urine disease patients and in normal humans. *J Biol Chem* 1992;267:22141–22147.
108. Lancaster G, Mamer OA, Scriver CR. Branched-chain α-keto acids isolated as oxime derivatives. Relationship to the corresponding hydroxy acids and amino acids in maple syrup urine disease. *Metabolism* 1974;23:257–265.
109. Podebrad F, Heil M, Reichert S, et al. 4,5-Dimethyl-3-hydroxy-2[5H]-furanone (sotolone)—the odor of maple syrup urine disease. *J Inherit Metab Dis* 1999;22:107–114.
110. Kamei A, Takashima S, Chan F, et al. Abnormal dendritic development in maple syrup urine disease. *Pediatr Neurol* 1992;8:145–147.
111. Martin JJ, Schlote W. Central nervous system lesions in disorders of amino-acid metabolism: a neuropathological study. *J Neurol Sci* 1972;15:49–76.
112. Müller K, Kahn T, Wendel U. Is demyelination a feature of maple syrup disease? *Pediatr Neurol* 1993;9:375–382.
113. Menkes JH, Solcher H. Effect of dietary therapy on cerebral morphology and chemistry in maple syrup disease. *Arch Neurol* 1967;16:486–491.
114. Chuang H, Wynn RM, Moss CC, et al. Structural and biochemical basis of novel mutations in homozygous Israeli maple syrup urine disease patients: a proposed mechanism for thiamin-responsive phenotypes. *J Biol Chem* 2004;279:17792–17800.
115. Dickinson JP, Holton JB, Lewis GM, et al. Maple syrup urine disease. Four years' experience with dietary treatment of a case. *Acta Paediat Scand* 1969;58:341–351.
116. Riviello JJ, Rezvani I, Di George AM, et al. Cerebral edema causing death in children with maple syrup urine disease. *J Pediatr* 1991;119:42–45.
117. MacDonald JT, Sher PK. Ophthalmoplegia as a sign of metabolic disease in the newborn. *Neurology* 1977;27:971–973.
118. Haymond MW, Ben-Galim E, Strobel KE. Glucose and alanine metabolism in children with maple syrup urine disease. *J Clin Invest* 1978;62:398–405.
119. Felber SR, Sperl W, Chemelli A, et al. Maple syrup urine disease: metabolic decompensation monitored by proton magnetic resonance imaging and spectroscopy. *Ann Neurol* 1993;33:396–401.
120. Brismar J, Aqeel A, Brismar G, et al. Maple syrup urine disease: findings on CT and MRI scans of the brain in 10 infants. *Am J Neuroradiol* 1990;11:1219–1228.
121. Righini A, Ramenghi LA, Purini R, et al. Water apparent diffusion coefficient and T2 changes in the acute stage of maple syrup urine disease: evidence of intramyelinic and vasogenic-interstitial edema. *J Neuroimaging* 2003;13:162–165.
122. Ha JS, Kim TK, Eun BL, et al. Maple syrup urine disease encephalopathy: a follow-up study in the acute stage using diffusion-weighted MRI. *Pedatr Radiol* 2004;34:163–166.
123. Menkes JH. The pathogenesis of mental retardation in phenylketonuria and other inborn errors of amino-acid metabolism. *Pediatrics* 1967;39:297–308.
124. Tsuruta M, Mitsubichi H, Mardy S, et al. Molecular basis of intermittent maple syrup urine disease: novel mutations in the E2 gene of the branched-chain alpha-keto acid dehydrogenase complex. *J Hum Genet* 1998;43:91–100.
125. Goedde HW, Langenbeck U, Brackertz D. Clinical and biochemical-genetic aspects of intermittent branched-chain ketoaciduria. *Acta Paediatr Scand* 1970;59:83–87.
126. Schulman JD, Lustberg TJ, Kennedy JL, et al. A new variant of maple syrup urine disease (branched chain ketoaciduria): clinical and biochemical evaluation. *Am J Med* 1970;49:118–124.
127. Leonard JV, Morris AAM. Inborn errors of metabolism around time of birth. *Lancet* 2000;358:583–587.
128. Wendel U, Lombeck I, Bremer HJ. Maple-syrup-urine disease. *N Engl J Med* 1983;308:1100–1101.
129. Naylo EW, Guthrie R. Newborn screening for maple syrup urine disease (branched-chain ketoaciduria). *Pediatrics* 1978;61:262–266.
130. Elsas LJ, Priest JH, Wheeler FB, et al. Maple syrup urine disease: coenzyme function and prenatal monitoring. *Metabolism* 1974;23:569–579.
131. Morton DH, Strauss KA, Robinson DL, et al. Diagnosis and treatment of maple syrup disease: a study of 36 patients. *Pediatrics* 2002;109:999–1008.
132. Puliyanda DP, Harmon WE, Peterschmitt MJ, et al. Utility of hemodialysis in maple syrup urine disease. *Pediatr Nephrol* 2002;17:239–242.
133. Nyhan WL, Rice-Kelts M, Klein J, et al. Treatment of the acute crisis in maple syrup urine disease. *Arch Pediatr Adolesc Med* 1998;152:593–598.
134. Clow CL, Reade TM, Scriver CR. Outcome of early and long-term management of classical maple syrup urine disease. *Pediatrics* 1981;68:856–862.
135. Hilliges C, Awiszus D, Wendel U. Intellectual performance of children with maple syrup urine disease. *Eur J Pediatr* 1993;152:144–147.
136. Tada K. Nonketotic hyperglycinemia: clinical metabolic aspects. *Enzyme* 1987;38:27–35.
137. Hamosh A, Johnston MV. Nonketotic hyperglycinemia. In: Scriver CR, Sly WS, Childs B, et al., eds. *The metabolic and molecular bases of inherited disease,* 8th ed. New York: McGraw-Hill, 2001:2065–2078.
138. Hayasaka S, Setogawa T, Hara S, et al. Nystagmus and subnormal electroretinographic response in nonketotic hyperglycinemia. *Graefes Arch Clin Exp Ophthalmol* 1987;225:277–278.
139. van Hove JLK, Kishnani PS, Demaerel P, et al. Acute hydrocephalus in nonketotic hyperglycinemia. *Neurology* 2000;54:754–756.
140. Luder AS, Davidson A, Goodman SI, et al. Transient nonketotic hyperglycinemia in neonates. *J Pediatr* 1989;114:1013–1015.

141. Kure S, Kojima K, Ichinohe A, et al. Heterozygous GLDC and GCSH mutations in transient neonatal hyperglycinemia. *Ann Neurol* 2002;52:643–646.
142. Zammarchi E, Donati MA, Ciani F. Transient neonatal nonketotic hyperglyceinemia: a 13-year-follow-up. *Neuropediatrics* 1995;26: 328–330.
143. Frazier DM, Summer GK, Chamberlin HR. Hyperglycinuria and hyperglycinemia in two siblings with mild developmental delays. *Am J Dis Child* 1978;132:777–781.
144. Flannery DB, Pellock J, Bousonis D, et al. Nonketotic hyperglycinemia in two retarded adults: a mild form of infantile nonketotic hyperglycinemia. *Neurology* 1983;33:1064–1066.
145. Bank WJ, Morrow G. A familial spinal cord disorder with hyperglycinemia. *Arch Neurol* 1972;27:136–144.
146. Trauner DA, Page T, Greco C, et al. Progressive neurodegenerative disorder in a patient with nonketotic hyperglycinemia. *J Pediatr* 1981;98:272–275.
147. Press GA, Barshop BA, Haas RH, et al. Abnormalities of the brain in nonketotic hyperglycinemia: MR manifestations. *Am J Neuroradiol* 1989;10:315–321.
148. Khong PL, Lam BC, Chung BH, et al. Diffusion-weighted MR imaging in neonatal nonketotic hyperglycenemia. *Am J Neuroradiol* 2003;24:1181–1183.
149. Tada K, Kure S, Kume A, et al. Genomic analysis of nonketotic hyperglycinemia: a partial deletion of P-protein gene. *J Inherit Metab Dis* 1990;13:766–770.
150. Deutsch SI, Rosse RB, Mastropaolo J. Current status of NMDA antagonist interventions in the treatment of nonketotic hyperglycinemia. *Clin Neuropharmacol* 1998;21:71–79.
151. Chien YH, Hsu CC, Huang A, et al. Poor outcome for neonatal-type nonketotic hyperglycinemia treated with dose sodium benzoate and dextromorphan. *J Child Neurol* 2004;19:39–42.
152. Elpeleg ON, Colombo JP, Amir N, et al. Late-onset form of partial *N*-acetylglutamate synthetase deficiency. *Eur J Pediatr* 1990;149:634–636.
153. Batshaw ML. Inborn errors of urea synthesis. *Ann Neurol* 1994;35:133–141.
154. Matsuda I, Nagata N, Matsuura T, et al. Retrospective survey of urea cycle disorders: Part I. Clinical and laboratory observations of thirty-two Japanese male patients with ornithine transcarbamylase deficiency. *Am J Med Genet* 1991;38:85–89.
155. Rowe PC, Newman SL, Brusilow SW. Natural history of symptomatic partial ornithine transcarbamylase deficiency. *N Engl J Med* 1986;314:541–547.
156. Allan JD, Cusworth DC, Dent CE, et al. A disease, probably hereditary, characterized by severe mental deficiency and a constant gross abnormality of amino acid metabolism. *Lancet* 1958;1:182–187.
157. O'Brien WE, Barr RH. Argininosuccinate lyase: purification and characterization from human liver. *Biochemistry* 1981;20:2056–2060.
158. Crane CW, Gay WMB, Jenner FA. Urea production from labeled ammonia in argininosuccinic aciduria. *Clin Chim Acta* 1969;24: 445–448.
159. Kay JD, Oberholzer VG, Seakins JW, et al. Effect of partial ornithine carbamoyltransferase deficiency on urea synthesis and related biochemical events. *Clin Sci* 1987;72:187–193.
160. Carton, D, De Schrijver F, Kint J, et al. Argininosuccinic aciduria: neonatal variant with rapid fatal course. *Acta Paediatr Scand* 1969;58:528–534.
161. Lewis PD, Miller AL. Argininosuccinic aciduria: case report with neuropathological findings. *Brain* 1970;93:413–422.
162. Levy HL, Coulombe JT, Shih VE. Newborn urine screening. In: Bickel H, Augustin AV, et al. eds. *Neonatal screening for inborn errors of metabolism*. Berlin: Springer-Verlag, 1980:89.
163. Walker DC, McCloskey DA, Simard LR, et al. Molecular analysis of human argininosuccinate lyase: mutant characterization and alternative splicing of the coding region. *Proc Natl Acad Sci USA* 1990;87:9625–9629.
164. Glick NR, Snodgrass PJ, Schafer IA. Neonatal argininosuccinicaciduria with normal brain and kidney but absent liver argininosuccinate lyase activity. *Am J Hum Genet* 1976;28:22–30.
165. Widhalm K, Koch S, Scheibenreiter S, et al. Long-term follow-up of 12 patients with the late-onset variant of argininosuccinic acid lyase deficiency: no impairment of intellectual and psychomotor development during therapy. *Pediatrics* 1992;87:1182–1184.
166. Brusilow SW, Horwich AL. Urea cycle enzymes. In: Scriver CR, Beaudet AL, Sly WS, et al., eds. *The metabolic and molecular bases of inherited disease,* 8th ed. New York: McGraw-Hill, 2001:1909–1964.
167. Bachmann C, Colombo JP. Diagnostic value of orotic acid excretion in heritable disorders of the urea cycle and in hyperammonemia due to organic acidurias. *Eur J Pediatr* 1980;134:109–113.
168. Rutledge SL, Havens PL, Haymond MW, et al. Neonatal hemodialysis: effective therapy for the encephalopathy of inborn errors of metabolism. *J Pediatr* 1990;116:125–128.
169. Batshaw ML, MacArthur RB, Tuchman M. Alternative pathway therapy for urea cycle disorders: twenty years later. *J Pediatr* 2001;138:546–555.
170. Lee B, Goss J. Long-term correction of urea cycle disorders. *J Pediatr* 2001;138(1 Suppl):S62–S71.
171. Saudubray JM, Touati G, Delonlay P, et al. Liver transplantation in urea cycle disorders. *Eur J Pediatr* 1999;158(Suppl 2):S55–S59.
172. Msall M, Batshaw ML, Suss R, et al. Neurologic outcome in children with inborn errors of urea synthesis: outcome of urea-cycle enzymopathies. *N Engl J Med* 1984;310:1500–1505.
173. Morgan HB, Swaiman KF, Johnson BD. Diagnosis of argininosuccinic aciduria after valproic acid-induced hyperammonemia. *Neurology* 1987;37:886–887.
174. McMurray WC, Rathbun JC, Mohyuddin F, et al. Citrullinuria. *Pediatrics* 1963;32:347–357.
175. Beaudet AL, O'Brien WE, Bock HG, et al. The human argininosuccinate locus and citrullinemia. *Adv Hum Genet* 1986;15:161–196.
176. Gao HZ, Kobayashi K, Tabeta A, et al. Identification of 16 novel mutations in the argininosuccinate synthetase gene and genotype–phenotype correlation in 38 classical citrullinemia patients. *Hum Mutat* 2003;22:24–34.
177. Albayram S, Murphy KJ, Gailloud P, et al. CT findings in the infantile form of citrullinemia. *Am J Neuroradiol* 2002;23:334–336.
178. Majoie CB, Mourmans JM, Akkerman EM, et al. Neonatal citrullinemia: comparison of conventional MR, diffusion-weighted, and diffusion tensor findings. *Am J Neuroradiol* 2004;25: 32–35.
179. Wick H, Bachmann C, Baumgartner R, et al. Variants of citrullinaemia. *Arch Dis Child* 1973;48:63–64.
180. Milne MD, London DR, Asatoor AM. Citrullinuria in cases of cystinuria. *Lancet* 1962;2:49–50.
181. Oyanagi K, Hakura Y, Tsuchiyama A, et al. Citrullinemia: quantitative deficiency of argininosuccinate synthetase in the liver. *Tohoku J Exp Med* 1986;148:385–391.
182. Saheki T, Kobayashi K, Iijima M, et al. Adult-onset type II citrullinemia and idiopathic neonatal hepatitis caused by citrin deficiency: involvement of the aspartate glutamate carrier for urea synthesis and maintenance of the urea cycle. *Mol Genet Metab* 2004;81(Suppl 1):S20–S26.
183. Palmieri F. The mitochondrial transporter family (SLC25): physiological and pathological implications. *Pflugers Arch* 2004;447:689–709.
184. Russell A, Levin B, Oberholzer VG, et al. Hyperammonaemia: a new instance of an inborn enzymatic defect of the biosynthesis of urea. *Lancet* 1962;2:699–700.
185. Tuchman M, Morizono H, Rajagopal BS, et al. The biochemical and molecular spectrum of ornithine transcarbamylase deficiency. *J Inherit Metab Dis* 1998;21(Suppl 1):40–58.
186. Wendel U, Wilchowski E, Schmidke J, et al. DNA analysis of ornithine transcarbamylase deficiency. *Eur J Pediatr* 1988;147:368–371.
187. Rowe PC, Newman SL, Brusilow SW. Natural history of symptomatic partial ornithine transcarbamylase deficiency. *N Engl J Med* 1986;314:541–546.
188. Dolman CL, Clasen RA, Dorovini-Zis K. Severe cerebral damage in ornithine transcarbamylase deficiency. *Clin Neuropathol* 1988;7: 10–15.
189. Shapiro JM, Schaffner F, Tallan HH, et al. Mitochondrial abnormalities of liver in primary ornithine transcarbamylase deficiency. *Pediatr Res* 1980;14:735–739.

190. Maestri NE, Clissold D, Brusilow SW. Neonatal onset ornithine transcarbamylase deficiency: a retrospective analysis. *J Pediatr* 1999;134:268–272.
191. Takanashi J, Barkovich AJ, Cheng SF, et al. Brain MR imaging in neonatal hyperammonemic encephalopathy resulting from proximal urea cycle disorders. *Am J Neuroradiol* 2003;24:1184–1187.
192. Bachmann C. Ornithine transcarbamoyl transferase deficiency: findings, models and problems. *J Inherit Metab Dis* 1992;15:578–591.
193. Batshaw ML, Roan J, Jung AL, et al. Cerebral dysfunction in asymptomatic carriers of ornithine transcarbamylase deficiency. *N Engl J Med* 1980;302:482–485.
194. Arn PH, Hauser ER, Thomas GH, et al. Hyperammonemia in women with a mutation at the ornithine carbamoyltransferase locus. A cause of postpartum coma. *N Engl J Med* 1990;322:1652–1655.
195. Hjelm M, de Silva LV, Seakins JW, et al. Evidence of inherited urea cycle defect in a case of fatal valproate toxicity. *Br Med J* 1986;292:23–24.
196. Maestri NE, Brusilow SW, Clissold DB, et al. Long-term treatment of girls with ornithine transcarbamylase deficiency. *N Engl J Med* 1996;335:855–859.
197. Horslen SP, McCowan TC, Goertzen TC, et al. Isolated hepatocyte transplantation in an infant with a severe urea cycle disorder. *Pediatrics* 2003;111:1262–1267.
198. Maestri NE, Hauser ER, Bartholomew D, et al. Prospective treatment of urea cycle disorders. *J Pediatr* 1991;119:923–928.
199. Yudkoff M, Yang W, Snodgrass PJ, et al. Ornithine transcarbamylase deficiency in a boy with normal development. *J Pediatr* 1980;96:441–443.
200. Tuchman M, Morizono H, Rajagopal BS, et al. Identification of "private" mutations in patients with ornithine transcarbamylase deficiency. *J Inherit Metab Dis* 1997;20:525–527.
201. Freeman JM, Nicholson JF, Schimke RT, et al. Congenital hyperammonemia. *Arch Neurol* 1970;23:430–437.
202. Takeoka M, Soman TR, Shih VE, et al. Carbamyl phosphate synthetase I deficiency: a destructive encephalopathy. *Pediatr Neurol* 2001;24:193–199.
203. Ebels EJ. Neuropathological observations in a patient with carbamylphosphate synthetase deficiency and in two sibs. *Arch Dis Child* 1972;47:47–51.
204. Picker JD, Puga AC, Levy HL, et al. Arginase deficiency with lethal neonatal expression: evidence for the glutamine hypothesis of cerebral edema. *J Pediatr* 2003;142:349–352.
205. Snyderman SE, Sansaricq C, Norton PM, et al. Argininemia treated from birth. *J Pediatr* 1979;95:61–63.
206. Iyer R, Jenkinson CP, Vockley JG, et al. The human arginases and arginase deficiency. *J Inherit Metab Dis* 1998;21(Suppl 1):86–100.
207. Mizutani N, Hayakawa C, Maehara M, et al. Enzyme replacement therapy in a patient with hyperargininemia. *Tohoku J Exp Med* 1987;151:301–307.
208. Guffon N, Vianey-Saban C, Bourgeois J, et al. A new neonatal case of *N*-acetylglutamate synthase deficiency treated by carbamylglutamate. *J Inherit Metab Dis* 1995;18:61–65.
209. Plecko B, Erwa W, Wermuth B. Partial *N*-acetylglutamate synthetase deficiency in a 13-year-old girl: diagnosis and response to treatment with *N*-carbamylglutamate. *Eur J Pediatr* 1998;157:996–998.
209a. Caldovic L, Morizono H, Panglao MG, et al. Null mutations in the N-acetylglutamate synthase gene associated with acute neonatal disease and hyperammonenua. *Hum Genet* 2003;112:364–368.
210. Camacho JA, Obie C, Biery B, et al. Hyperornithinaemia-hyprammonaemia-homocitrullinuria syndrome is caused by mutation in a gene encoding a mitochondrial ornithine transporter. *Nat Genet* 1999;22:151–158.
211. Zammarchi E, Ciani F, Pasquini E, et al. Neonatal onset of hyperornithemia-hyperammonemia-homocitrullinuria syndrome with favorable outcome. *J Pediatr* 1997;131:440–443.
212. Salvi S, Santorelli FM, Bertini E, et al. Clinical and molecular findings in hyperornithinemia-hyperammonemia-homocitrullinuria syndrome. *Neurology* 2001;57:911–914.
213. Valtonen M, Nanto-Salonen K, Heinanen K, et al. Skeletal muscle of patients with gyrate atrophy of the choroid and retina and hyperornithinaemia in ultra-low-field magnetic resonance imaging and computed tomography. *J Inherit Metab Dis* 1996; 19:729–734.
214. Peltola KE, Jaaskelainen S, Heinonen OJ, et al. Peripheral nervous system in gyrate atrophy of the choroids and retina with hyperornithinemia. *Neurology* 2002;59:735–740.
215. Valtonen M, Nanto-Salonen K, Jaaskelainen S., et al. Central nervous system involvement in gyrate atrophy of the choroids and retina with hyperornithinaemia. *J Inherit Metab Dis* 1999;22:855–866.
216. Nanto-Salonen K, Komu M, Lundbom N, et al. Reduced brain creatine in gyrate atrophy of the choroid and retina with hyperornithinemia. *Neurology* 1999;53:249–250.
217. Van Geet C, Vandenboesche L, Eggermont E, et al. Possible platelet contribution to pathogenesis of transient neonatal hyperammonemia syndrome. *Lancet* 1991;337:73–75.
218. Ellison PH, Cowger ML. Transient hyperammonemia in the preterm infant: neurologic aspects. *Neurology* 1981;31:67–770.
219. Ogier de Baulny H, Slama A, Touati G, et al. Neonatal hyperammonemia caused by a defect of carnitine-acylcarnitine translocase. *J Pediatr* 1995;127:723–728.
220. Hudak ML, Jones MD, Brusilow SW. Differentiation of transient hyperammonemia of the newborn and urea cycle enzyme defects by clinical presentation. *J Pediatr* 1985;107:712–719.
221. Stanley CA, Lieu YK, Hsu BYL, et al. Hyperinsulinism and hyperammonemia in infants with regulatory mutations of the glutamate dehydrogenase gene. *N Engl J Med* 1998;338:1352–1357.
222. Carson NAJ, Cusworth DC, Dent CE. Homocystinuria: a new inborn error of metabolism associated with mental deficiency. *Arch Dis Child* 1963;38:425–436.
223. Naughten ER, Yap S, Mayne PD. Newborn screening for homocystinuria: Irish and world experience. *Eur J Pediatr* 1998; 157(Suppl 2):S84–S87.
224. Mudd SH, Finkelstein JD, Irrevere F, et al. Homocystinuria: an enzymatic defect. *Science* 1964;143:1443–1445.
225. Kraus J, Packman S, Fowler B, et al. Purification and properties of cystathionine-β-synthase from human liver. *J Biol Chem* 1978;253:6523–6528.
226. Fowler B, Kraus J, Packman S, et al. Homocystinuria: evidence for three distinct classes of cystathionine-β-synthase mutants in cultured fibroblasts. *J Clin Invest* 1978;61:645–653.
227. Shan X, Kruger WD. Correction of disease-causing CBS mutations in yeast. *Nat Genet* 1998;19:91–93.
228. Gaustadnes M, Wilcken B, Oliveriusova J, et al. The molecular basis of cystathionine beta-synthase deficiency in Australian patients: genotype–phenotype correlations and response to treatment. *Hum Mutat* 2002;20:117–126.
229. Haworth JC, Dilling LA, Surtees RA, et al. Symptomatic and asymptomatic methylene tetrahydrofolate reductase deficiency in two adult brothers. *Am J Med Genet* 1993;45:572–576.
230. Freeman JM, Finkelstein JD, Mudd SH. Folate-responsive homocystinuria and "schizophrenia": a defect in methylation due to deficient 5,10-methylene tetrahydrofolate reductase activity. *N Engl J Med* 1975;292:491–496.
231. Gibson JB, Carson NA, Neill DW. Pathological findings in homocystinuria. *J Clin Pathol* 1964;17:427–437.
232. Welch GN, Loscalzo J. Homocysteine and atherosclerosis. *N Engl J Med* 1998;338:1042–1050.
233. Presley GD, Sidbury JB. Homocystinuria and ocular defects. *Am J Ophthalmol* 1967;63:1723–1727.
234. Wilcken B, Turner G. Homocystinuria in New South Wales. *Arch Dis Child* 1978;53:242–245.
235. Mudd SH, Levy HL, Skovby F. Disorders of transsulfuration. In: Scriver CR, Beaudet AL, Sly WS, et al., eds. *The metabolic and molecular bases of inherited disease*, 8th ed. New York: McGraw-Hill, 2001:2007–2056.
236. Thomas PS, Carson NA. Homocystinuria: the evolution of skeletal changes in relation to treatment. *Ann Radiol* 1978;21:95–104.
237. Schedewie H, Willich E, Grobe H, et al. Skeletal findings in homocystinuria: a collaborative study. *Pediatr Radiol* 1973;1:12–23.
238. Brenton DP, Dow CJ, James JI, et al. Homocystinuria and Marfan's syndrome: a comparison. *J Bone Joint Surg* 1972;54B:277–298.

239. Kurczynski TW, Muir WA, Fleisher LD, et al. Maternal homocystinuria: studies of an untreated mother and fetus. *Arch Dis Child* 1980;55:721–723.
240. Morrow G, Barness LA. Combined vitamin responsiveness in homocystinuria. *J Pediatr* 1972;81:946–954.
241. Singh RH, Kruger WD, Wang L, et al. Cystathione beta-synthase deficiency: effects of betaine supplementation after methionine restriction in B6-nonresponsive homocystinuria. *Genet Med* 2004;6:90–95.
242. Yaghmai R, Kashani AH, Geraghty MT, et al. Progressive cerebral edema associated with high methionine levels and betaine therapy in a patient with cystathione beta-synthase (CBS) deficiency. *Am J Med Genet* 2002;108:57–63.
243. Yap S, Naughten ER, Wilcken B, et al. Vascular complications of severe hyperhomocysteinemia in patients with homocysteinuria due to cystathionine beta-synthase deficiency: effects of homocysteine-lowering therapy. *Semin Thromb Hemost* 2000;26:335–340.
244. Yap S, Rushe H, Howard PM, et al. The intellectual abilities of early-treated individuals with pyridoxine-nonresponsive homocystinuria due to cystathionine-beta-synthase deficiency. *J Inherit Metab Dis* 2001;24:437–447.
245. Mudd SH, Shouby F, Levy HL, et al. The natural history of homocystinuria due to cystathionine-β-synthase deficiency. *Am J Hum Genet* 1985;37:1–31.
246. Mudd SH, Levy HL, Tangerman A, et al. Isolated persistent hypermethioninemia. *Am J Hum Genet* 1995;57:882–892.
247. Wada Y, Tada K, Minagawa A. Idiopathic hypervalinemia: probably a new entity of inborn error of valine metabolism. *Tohoku J Exp Med* 1963;81:46–55.
248. Higgins JJ, Kaneski CR, Bernardini I, et al. Pyridoxine-responsive hyper-β-alaninemia associated with Cohen's syndrome. *Neurology* 1994;44:1728–1732.
249. Willi SM, Zhang Y, Hill JB, et al. A deletion in the long arm of chromosome 18 in a child with serum carnosinase deficiency. *Pediatr Res* 1997;41:210–213.
250. Yamaguchi S, Orii T, Sakura N, et al. Defect in biosynthesis of mitochondrial acetoacetyl-coenzyme A thiolase in cultured fibroblasts from a boy with 3-ketothiolase deficiency. *J Clin Invest* 1988;81:813–817.
251. Fukao T, Yamaguchi S, Wakazono A, et al. Identification of a novel exonic mutation at -13 from 5′ splice site causing exon skipping in a girl with mitochondrial acetoacetyl-coenzyme A thiolase deficiency. *J Clin Invest* 1994;93:1035–1041.
252. Salih MA, Bender DA, McCreanor GM. Lethal familial pellagra-like skin lesions associated with neurologic and developmental impairment and the development of cataracts. *Pediatrics* 1985;76:787–793.
253. Martin JR, Mellor CS, Fraser FC. Familial hypertryptophanemia in two siblings. *Clin Genet* 1995;47:180–183.
254. Isenberg JN, Sharp HL. Aspartylglucosaminuria: psychomotor retardation masquerading as a mucopolysaccharidosis. *J Pediatr* 1975;86:713–717.
255. Tollersrud OK, Nilssen O, Tranebjaerg L, et al. Aspartylglucosaminuria in northern Norway: a molecular and genealogical study. *J Med Genet* 1994;31:360–363.
256. Williams JC, Butler IJ, Rosenberg HS, et al. Progressive neurologic deterioration and renal failure due to storage of glutamyl ribose-5-phosphate. *N Engl J Med* 1984;311:152–155.
257. Konrad PN, Richards F 2nd, Valentine WN, et al. γ-Glutamylcysteine synthetase deficiency. A cause of hereditary hemolytic anemia. *N Engl J Med* 1972;286:557–561.
258. Small KW, Letson R, Scheinman J. Ocular findings in primary hyperoxaluria. *Arch Ophthalmol* 1990;108:89–93.
259. Seargeant LE, de Groot GW, Dilling LA, et al. Primary oxaluria type 2 (l-glyceric aciduria): a rare cause of nephrolithiasis in children. *J Pediatr* 1991;118:912–914.
260. Simell O. Lysinuric protein intolerance and other cationic aminoacidurias. In: Scriver CR, Sly WS, Childs B, et al., eds. *The metabolic and molecular bases of inherited disease,* 8th ed. New York: McGraw-Hill, 2001:4933–4956.
260a. Simell O, Perheentupa J, Rapola J, et al. Lysinuric protein intolerance. *Am J Med* 1975;59:229–240.
260b. Lauteala T, Sistonen P, Savontaus ML, et al. Lysinuric protein intolerance (LPI) gene maps to the long arm of chromosome 14. *Am J Hum Genet* 1997;60:1479–1486.
261. Borsani G, Bassi MT, Sperandeo MP, et al. SLC7A7, encoding a putative permease-related protein, is mutated in patients with lysinuric protein intolerance. *Nat Genet* 1999;21:297–301.
261a. Swoboda KJ, Saul JP, McKenna CE, et al. Aromatic L-amino acid decarboxylase deficiency: overview of clinical features and outcomes. *Ann Neurol* 2003;54(Suppl 6):S49–S55.
261b. Fiumara A, Bräutigam C, Hyland K, et al. Aromatic L-aminoacid decarboxylase deficiency with hyperdopaminuria. Clinical and laboratory findings in response to different therapies. *Neuropediatrics* 2002;33:203–208.
262. Baron DN, Dent CE, Harris H, et al. Hereditary pellagra-like skin rash with temporary cerebellar ataxia, constant renal aminoaciduria, and other bizarre biochemical features. *Lancet* 1956;2:421–426.
263. Nozaki J, Dakeishi M, Ohura T, et al. Homozygosity mapping to chromosome 5p15 of a gene responsible for Hartnup disorder. *Biochem Biophys Res Commun* 2001;284:255–260.
264. Kleta R, Romeo E, Ristic Z, et al. Mutations in SLC6A19, encoding B0AT1, cause Hartnup disorder. *Nat Genet* 2004;36:999–1002.
265. Milne MD, Crawford MA, Girao CB, et al. The metabolic disorder in Hartnup disease. *Q J Med* 1960;29:407–421.
266. Scriver CR. Hartnup disease: a genetic modification of intestinal and renal transport of certain neutral α-amino acids. *N Engl J Med* 1965;273:530–532.
267. Schmidtke K, Endres W, Roscher A, et al. Hartnup syndrome, progressive encephalopathy and alfa-albuminaemia. A clinicopathologic case study. *Eur J Pediatr* 1992;151:899–903.
268. Wilcken B, Yu JS, Brown DA. Natural history of Hartnup disease. *Arch Dis Child* 1977;52:38–40.
269. Scriver CR, Mahon B, Levy HL, et al. The Hartnup phenotype: mendelian transport disorder multifactorial disease. *Am J Hum Genet* 1987;40:401–412.
270. Erly W, Castillo M, Foosaner D, et al. Hartnup disease: MR findings. *Am J Neuroradiol* 1991;12:1026–1027.
271. Clayton PT, Bridges NA, Atherton DJ, et al. Pellagra with colitis due to a defect in tryptophan metabolism. *Eur J Pediatr* 1991;150:498–502.
272. Jonas AJ, Butler IJ. Circumvention of defective neutral amino acid transport in Hartnup disease using tryptophan ethyl ester. *J Clin Invest* 1989;84:200–204.
273. Lowe CU, Terry M, MacLachlan EA. Organic aciduria, decreased renal ammonia production, hydrophthalmos and mental retardation: a clinical entity. *Am J Dis Child* 1952;83:164–184.
274. Charnas LR, Bernardini I, Rader D, et al. Clinical and laboratory findings in the oculocerebrorenal syndrome of Lowe, with special reference to growth and renal function. *N Engl J Med* 1991;324:1318–1325.
275. Lin T, Orrison BM, Leahey AM, et al. Spectrum of mutations in the OCR1 gene in the Lowe oculocerebrorenal syndrome. *Am J Hum Genet* 1997;60:1384–1388.
276. Suchy SF, Nussbaum RL. The deficiency of PIP2 5-phosphatase in Lowe syndrome affects actin polymerization. *Am J Hum Genet* 2002;71:1420–1427.
277. Bartsocas CS, Levy HL, Crawford JD, et al. A defect in intestinal amino acid transport in Lowe's syndrome. *Am J Dis Child* 1969;117:93–95.
278. Richards W, Donnell GN, Wilson WA, et al. The oculo-cerebro-renal syndrome of Lowe. *Am J Dis Child* 1965;109:185–203.
279. Matin MA, Sylvester PE. Clinicopathological studies of oculocerebrorenal syndrome of Lowe, Terrey and MacLachlan. *J Ment Defic Res* 1980;24:1–17.
280. Kenworthy L, Park T, Charnas LR. Cognitive and behavioral profile of the oculocerebrorenal syndrome of Lowe. *Am J Med Genet* 1993;46:297–303.
281. Charnas L, Bernar J, Pezeshkpour GH, et al. MRI findings and peripheral neuropathy in Lowe's syndrome. *Neuropediatrics* 1988;19:7–9.
282. Charnas LR, Gahl WA. The oculocerebrorenal syndrome of Lowe. *Adv Pediatr* 1991;38:75–101.
283. O'Tuama LA, Laster DW. Oculocerebrorenal syndrome: case report with CT and MR correlates. *Am J Neuroradiol* 1987;8:555–557.

284. Demmer LA, Wippold FJ, Dowton SB. Periventricular white matter cystic lesions in Lowe (oculocerebrorenal) syndrome. A new MR finding. *Pediatr Radiol* 1992;22:76–77.
285. Cibis GW, Waeltermann JM, Whitcraft CT, et al. Lenticular opacities in carriers of Lowe's syndrome. *Ophthalmology* 1986;93:1041–1045.
286. Salomons GS, van Dooren SJ, Verhoeven NM, et al. X-linked creatine-transporter gene (SLC6A8) defect: a new creatine-deficiency. *Am J Hum Genet* 2001;68:1497–1500.
287. Bizzi A, Bugiani M, Salomons GS, et al. X-linked creatine deficiency syndrome: a novel mutation in creatine transporter gene SLC6A8. *Ann Neurol* 2002;52:227–231.
288. Rosenberg RH, Almeida LS, Kleefstra T, et al. High prevalence of SLC6A8 deficiency in X-linked mental retardation. *Am J Hum Genet* 2004;75:97–105.
289. Leuzzi V. Inborn errors of creatine metabolism and epilepsy: clinical features, diagnosis, and treatment. *J Child Neurol* 2002;17(Suppl 3):3S89–3S97.
290. Battini R, Leuzzi V, Carducci C, et al. Creatine depletion in a new case with AGAT deficiency: clinical and genetic study in a large pedigree. *Med Genet Metab* 2002;77:326–331.
291. von Reuss A. Zuckerausscheidung im Säuglingsalter. *Wien Med Wochenschr* 1908;58:799–803.
292. Shih V, Levy HI, Karolkewicz V, et al. Galactosemia screening of newborns in Massachusetts. *N Engl J Med* 1971;284:753–757.
293. Göppert F. Galaktosurie nach Milchzuckergabe bei angeborenem, familiärem chronischem Leberleiden. *Berl Klin Wochenschr* 1917;54:473–477.
294. Schwarz V, Golberg L, Komrower GM, et al. Some disturbances of erythrocyte metabolism in galactosaemia. *Biochem J* 1956;62:34–40.
295. Kalckar HM, Anderson EP, Isselbacher KJ. Galactosemia, a congenital defect in a nucleotide transferase. *Biochim Biophys Acta* 1956;62:262–268.
296. Elsas LJ, Lai K. The molecular biology of galactosemia. *Genet Med* 1998;1:40–48.
297. Item C, Hagerty BP, Muhl A, et al. Mutations at the galactose-1-*p*-uridyltransferase gene in infants with a positive galactosemia newborn screening test. *Pediatr Res* 2002;51:511–516.
298. Wang BB, Xu YK, Ng WG, et al. Molecular and biochemical basis of galactosemia. *Mol Genet Med* 1998;63:263–269.
299. Schwarz V, Golberg L. Galactose-1-phosphate in galactose cataract. *Biochim Biophys Acta* 1955;18:310–311.
300. Holton JB. Galactosaemia: pathogenesis and treatment. *J Inherit Metab Dis* 1996;19:3–7.
301. Berry GT, Hunter JV, Wang Z, et al. *In vivo* evidence of brain galactitol accumulation in an infant with galactosemia and encephalopathy. *J Pediatr* 2001;138:260–262.
302. Holton JB, Walter JH, Tyfield LA. Galactosemia. In: Scriver CR, Beaudet AL, Sly WS, et al, eds. *The metabolic and molecular bases of inherited disease,* 8th ed. New York: McGraw-Hill, 2001:1553–1578.
303. Smetana HF, Olen E. Hereditary galactose disease. *Am J Clin Pathol* 1962;38:3–25.
304. Haberland C, Perou M, Brunngraber EG, et al. The neuropathology of galactosemia. *J Neuropathol Exp Neurol* 1971;30:431–447.
305. Allen JT, Gillett M, Holton JB, et al. Evidence of galactosemia *in utero* [Letter]. *Lancet* 1980;1:603.
306. Huttenlocher PR, Hillman RE, Hsia YE. Pseudotumor cerebri in galactosemia. *J Pediatr* 1970;76:902–905.
307. Hsia DY, Walker FA. Variability in the clinical manifestations of galactosemia. *J Pediatr* 1961;59:872–883.
308. Walsh FB, Hoyt WF. *Clinical neuro-ophthalmology,* 3rd ed. Baltimore: Williams & Wilkins, 1969:802.
309. Levy HL, Sepe SJ, Shih VE, et al. Sepsis due to *Escherichia coli* in neonates with galactosemia. *N Engl J Med* 1977;297:823–825.
310. Kaufman FR, Xu YK, Ng WG, et al. Correlation of ovarian function with galactose-1-phosphate uridyl transferase levels in galactosemia. *J Pediatr* 1988;112:754–756.
311. Nelson MD Jr, Wolff JA, Cross CA, et al. Galactosemia: evaluation with MR imaging. *Radiology* 1992;184:255–261.
312. Franceschetti A, Marty F, Klein D. Un syndrome rare: heredoataxie avec cataracte congenitale et retard mental. *Confin Neurol* 1956;16:271–275.
313. Jakobs C, Kleijer WJ, Allen J, et al. Prenatal diagnosis of galactosemia. *Eur J Pediatr* 1995;154(Suppl 2):S33–S36.
314. Waggoner DD, Buist NRM, Donnell GN. Long-term prognosis in galactosemia: results of a survey of 350 cases. *J Inherit Metab Dis* 1990;13:802–818.
315. Walter JH, Collins JE, Leonard JV. Recommendations for the management of galactosaemia: UK Galactosaemia Steering Group. *Arch Dis Child* 1999;80:93–96.
316. Böhles H, Wenzel D, Shin YS. Progressive cerebellar and extrapyramidal motor disturbances in galactosemic twins. *Eur J Pediatr* 1986;145:413–417.
317. Kaufman FR, McBride-Chang C, Manis FR, et al. Cognitive functioning, neurologic status and brain imaging in classical galactosemia. *Eur J Pediatr* 1995;154(Suppl 2):S2–S5.
318. Rogers S, Segal S. Modulation of rat tissue galactose-1-phosphate uridyltransferase by uridine and uridinetriphosphate. *Pediatr Res* 1991;30:222–226.
319. Manis FR, Cohn LB, McBride-Chang C, et al. A longitudinal study of cognitive functioning in patients with classical galactosemia, including a cohort treated with oral uridine. *J Inherit Metab Dis* 1997;20:535–549.
320. Fishler K, Koch R, Donnell GN, Wenz E. Developmental aspects of galactosemia from infancy to childhood. *Clin Pediatr* 1980;19:38–44.
321. Nelson CD, Waggoner DD, Donnell GN, et al. Verbal dyspraxia in treated galactosemia. *Pediatrics* 1991;88:346–350.
322. Gitzelmann R, Steinmann B. Galactosemia: how does long-term treatment change the outcome? *Enzyme* 1984;32:37–46.
323. Bosch AM, Bakker HD, van Gennip AH, et al. Clinical features of galactokinase deficiency: a review of the literature. *J Inherit Metab Dis* 2002;25:629–634.
324. Walter JH, Roberts RE, Besley GT, et al. Generalised uridine diphosphate galactose-4-epimerase deficiency. *Arch Dis Child* 1999;80:374–376.
325. Chambers RA, Pratt RTC. Idiosyncrasy to fructose. *Lancet* 1956;2:340.
326. Nikkila EA, Somersalo O, Pitkanen E, et al. Hereditary fructose intolerance: an inborn deficiency of liver aldolase complex. *Metabolism* 1962;11:727–731.
327. Esposito G, Vitagliano L, Santamaria R, et al. Structural and functional analysis of aldolase B mutants related to hereditary fructose intolerance. *FEBS Lett* 2002;531:152–156.
328. Oberhaensli RD, Rajagopalan B, Taylor DJ, et al. Study of hereditary fructose intolerance by use of ^{31}P magnetic resonance spectroscopy. *Lancet* 1987;2:931–934.
329. Lindemann R, Gjessing LR, Merton B, et al. Amino acid metabolism in hereditary fructosemia. *Acta Paediat Scand* 1970;59:141–147.
330. Rennert OM, Greer M. Hereditary fructosemia. *Neurology* 1970;20:421–425.
331. Steinmann B, Gitzelmann R. The diagnosis of hereditary fructose intolerance. *Helv Paediatr Acta* 1981;36:297–316.
332. Steinmann B, Gitzelmann R, Van den Berghe G. Disorders of fructose metabolism. In: Scriver CR, Sly WS, Childs B, et al., eds. *The metabolic and molecular bases of inherited disease,* 8th ed. New York: McGraw-Hill, 2001:1489–1520.
333. Moses SW, Bashan N, Flasterstein BF, et al. Fructose-1,6-diphosphatase deficiency in Israel. *Isr J Med Sci* 1991;27:1–4.
334. Buhrdel P, Bohme HJ, Didt L. Biochemical and clinical observations in four patients with fructose-1,6-diphosphatase deficiency. *Eur J Pediatr* 1990;149:574–576.
335. De Vivo DC, Trifiletti RR, Jacobson RI, et al. Defective glucose transport across the blood–brain barrier as a cause of persistent hypoglycorrhachia, seizures, and developmental delay. *N Engl J Med* 1991;325:703–709.
336. De Vivo DC, Wang D, Pascual JM. Disorders of glucose transport. In: Rosenberg RN, Prusiner SB, DiMauro S, et al.,eds. *The molecular and genetic basis of neurological disease,* 3rd ed. Philadelphia: Butterworth–Heinemann, 2003:625–634.

337. Overweg-Plandsoen WC, Groener JE, Wang D, et al. GLUT-1 deficiency without epilepsy—an exceptional case. *J Inherit Metab Dis* 2003;26:559–563.
338. Klepper J, Garcia-Alvarez M, O'Driscoll KR, et al. Erythrocyte 3-*o*-methyl-D-glucose uptake assay for diagnosis of glucose-transporter-protein syndrome. *J Clin Lab Anal* 1999;13:116–121.
339. Hsia YE, Scully KL, Rosenberg LE. Inherited propionyl-CoA deficiency in "ketotic hyperglycinemia." *J Clin Invest* 1971;50:127–130.
340. Perez B, Desviat LR, Rodriguez-Pombo R, et al. Propionic acidemia: identification of twenty-four novel mutations in Europe and North America. *Mol Genet Metab* 2003;78:59–67.
341. Menkes JH. Idiopathic hyperglycinemia: isolation and identification of three previously undescribed urinary ketones. *J Pediatr* 1966;69:413–421.
342. Coude FX, Sweetman L, Nyhan WL. Inhibition by propionyl CoA of *N*-acetylglutamate synthetase in rat liver mitochondria. *J Clin Invest* 1979;64:1544–1551.
343. Wolf B, Hsia YE, Tanaka K, et al. Correlation between serum propionate and blood ammonia concentration in propionic acidemia. *J Pediatr* 1978;93:471–473.
344. Childs B, Nyhan WL, Borden M, et al. Idiopathic hyperglycinemia and hyperglycinuria. A new disorder of amino acid metabolism. *Pediatrics* 1961;27:522–538.
345. Surtees RAH, Matthews EE, Leonard JV. Neurologic outcome of propionic acidemia. *Pediatr Neurol* 1992;8:333–337.
346. Yorifuji T, Kawai M, Muroi J, et al. Unexpectedly high prevalence of the mild form of propionic acidemia in Japan: presence of a common mutation and possible clinical implications. *Hum Genet* 2002;111:161–165.
347. Ando T, Rasmussen K, Nyhan WL, et al. Propionic acidemia in patients with ketotic hyperglycinemia. *J Pediatr* 1971;78:827–832.
348. Bergman AJ, Van der Knaap MS, Smeitink JA, et al. Magnetic resonance imaging and spectroscopy of the brain in propionic acidemia: clinical and biochemical considerations. *Pediatr Res* 1996;40:404–409.
349. Shuman RM, Leech RW, Scott CR. The neuropathology of the non-ketotic and ketotic hyperglycinemias: three cases. *Neurology* 1978;28:139–146.
350. Feliz B, Witt DR, Harris BT. Propionic academia: a neuropathology case report and review of prior cases. *Arch Pathol Lab Med* 2003;127:e325–e328.
351. de Vries A, Kochwa S, Lazebnik J, et al. Glycinuria: a hereditary disorder associated with nephrolithiasis. *Am J Med* 1957;23:408–415.
352. Matsui SM, Mahoney MJ, Rosenberg LE. The natural history of the inherited methylmalonic acidemias. *N Engl J Med* 1983;308:857–861.
353. Peters HL, Nefedov M, Lee LW, et al. Molecular studies in mutase-deficient (MUT) methylmalonic aciduria: identification of five novel mutations. *Hum Mutat* 2002;20:406.
354. Shevell MI, Matiaszuk N, Ledley FD, Rosenblatt DS. Varying neurologic phenotypes among mut0 and mut- patients with methylmalonylCoA mutase deficiency. *Am J Med Genet* 1993;45:619–624.
355. Mitchell GA, Watkins D, Melancon SB, et al. Clinical heterogeneity in cobalamin C variant of combined homocystinuria and methylmalonic aciduria. *J Pediatr* 1986;108:410–415.
356. Shevell MI, Rosenblatt DS. Vitamins: Cobalamin and folate. In: Rosenberg RN, Prusiner SB, DiMauro S, et al., eds. *The molecular and genetic basis of neurological disease,* 3rd ed. Philadelphia: Butterworth-Heinemann, 2003:699–704.
357. Ledley FD, Levy HL, Shih VE, et al. Benign methylmalonic aciduria. *N Engl J Med* 1984;311:1015–1018.
358. Brismar J, Ozand PT. CT and MR of the brain in disorders of the propionate and methylmalonate metabolism. *Am J Neuroradiol* 1994;15:1459–1473.
359. Inoue S, Krieger I, Sarnaik A, et al. Inhibition of bone marrow stem cell growth *in vitro* by methylmalonic acid: a mechanism for pancytopenia in a patient with methylmalonic acidemia. *Pediatr Res* 1981;15:95–98.
360. Rutledge SL, Geraghty M, Mroczek E, et al. Tubulointerstitial nephritis in methylmalonic acidemia. *Pediatr Nephrol* 1993;7:81–82.
361. Van der Meer SB, Poggi F, Spada M, et al. Clinical outcome of long-term management of patients with vitamin B12-unresponsive methylmalonic acidemia. *J Pediatr* 1994;125:903–908.
362. Rosenblatt DS, Laframboise R, Pichette J, et al. New disorder of vitamin B12 metabolism (cobalamin F) presenting as methylmalonic aciduria. *Pediatrics* 1986;78:51–54.
363. Shinnar S, Singer HS. Cobalamin C mutation (methylmalonic aciduria and homocystinuria) in adolescence: a treatable cause of dementia and myelopathy. *N Engl J Med* 1984;311:451–454.
364. Mitchell GA, Watkins D, Melancon SB, et al. Clinical heterogeneity in cobalamin C variant of combined homocystinuria and methylmalonic aciduria. *J Pediatr* 1986;108:410–415.
365. Robb RM, Dowton SB, Fulton AB, Levy HL. Retinal degeneration in vitamin B12 disorder associated with methylmalonic aciduria and sulfur amino-acid abnormalities. *Am J Ophthalmol* 1981;97:691–696.
366. Russo P, Doyon J, Sonsino E, et al. A congenital anomaly of vitamin B12 metabolism: a study of three cases. *Hum Pathol* 1992;23:504–512.
367. Fenton WA, Gravel RA, Rosenblatt DS. Disorders of propionate and methylmalonate metabolism. In: Scriver CR, Beaudet AL, Sly WS, et al., eds. *The metabolic and molecular bases of inherited disease,* 8th ed. New York: McGraw-Hill, 2001:2165–2194.
368. Chalmers RA, Bain MD, Mistry J, et al. Enzymological studies on patients with methylmalonic aciduria: basis for a clinical trial of deoxyadenosylcobalamin in a hydroxocobalamin-unresponsive patient. *Pediatr Res* 1991;30:560–563.
369. Nyhan WL, Gargus JJ, Boyle K, et al. Progressive neurologic disability in methylmalonic academia despite transplantation of the liver. *Eur J Pediatr* 2002;161:377–379.
370. Tanaka K, Budd MA, Efron ML, et al. Isovaleric acidemia; new genetic defect of leucine metabolism. *Proc Natl Acad Sci USA* 1966;56:236–242.
371. Mohsen AW, Anderson BD, Volchenboum SL, et al. Characterization of molecular defects in isovaleryl-CoA dehydrogenase in patients with isovaleric acidemia. *Biochemistry* 1998;37:10325–10335.
372. Hine DG, Tanaka K. The identification and the excretion pattern of isovaleryl glucuronide in the urine of patients with isovaleric acidemia. *Pediatr Res* 1984;18:508–512.
373. Ando T, Nyhan WL, Bachmann C, et al. Isovaleric acidemia: identification of isovalerate, isovalerylglycine, and 3-hydroxyisovalerate in urine of a patient previously reported as butyric and hexanoic acidemia. *J Pediatr* 1973;82:243–248.
374. Berry GT, Yudkoff M, Segal S. Isovaleric acidemia: medical and neurodevelopmental effects of long-term therapy. *J Pediatr* 1988;113:58–64.
375. Kelleher JF Jr, Yudkoff M, Hutchinson R, et al. The pancytopenia of isovaleric acidemia. *Pediatrics* 1980;65:1023–1027.
376. Tanaka K, Isselbacher KT, Shih V. Isovaleric and methylbutyric acidemias induced by hypoglycin A: mechanism of Jamaican vomiting sickness. *Science* 1972;175:69–71.
377. Goodman SI, Markey SP, Moe PG, et al. Glutaric aciduria: a "new" disorder of amino acid metabolism. *Biochem Med* 1975;12:12–21.
378. Haworth JC, Booth FA, Chudley AE, et al. Phenotypic variability in glutaric aciduria type I: report of fourteen cases in five Canadian Indian kindreds. *J Pediatr* 1991;118:52–58.
379. Goodman SI, Norenberg MD, Shikes RH, et al. Glutaric aciduria: biochemical and morphologic considerations. *J Pediatr* 1977;90:746–750.
380. Hauser SE, Peters H. Glutaric aciduria type I: an underdiagnosed cause of encephalopathy and dystonia-dyskinesia syndrome in children. *J Paediatr Child Health* 1998;34:302–304.
381. Hoffmann GF, Athanassopoulos S, Burlina AB, et al. Clinical course, early diagnosis, treatment, and prevention of disease in glutaryl-CoA dehydrogenase deficiency. *Neuropediatrics* 1996;27:115–123.
382. Dunger DB, Snodgrass GJ. Glutaric aciduria type I presenting with hypoglycaemia. *J Inherit Metab Dis* 1984;7:122–124.
383. Busquets C, Merinero B, Christensen E, et al. Glutary-CoA dehydrogenase deficiency in Spain: evidence of two groups of patients, genetically, and biochemically distinct. *Pediatr Res* 2000;48:315–322.

384. Twomey EL, Naughton ER, Donoghue VB, et al. Neuroimaging findings in glutaric aciduria type 1. *Pediatr Radiol* 2003;33:823–830.
385. Kimura S, Hara M, Nezu A, et al. Two cases of glutaric aciduria type 1: clinical and neuropathological findings. *J Neurol Sci* 1994;123: 38–43.
386. Kolker S, Koeller DM, Okun JG, et al. Pathomechanisms of neurodegeneration in glutaryl-CoA dehydrogenase deficiency. *Ann Neurol* 2004;55:7–12.
387. Kyllerman M, Skjeldal O, Christensen E, et al. Long-term follow-up, neurological outcome and survival rate in 28 Nordic patients with glutaric aciduria type 1. *Eur J Paediatr Neurol* 2004;8:121–129.
388. Strauss KA, Puffenberger RG, Robinson DL, et al. Type I glutaric aciduria, part 1: natural history of 77 patients. *Am J Med Genet* 2003;121C:38–52.
389. Amendt BA, Rhead WJ. The multiple acyl-coenzyme A dehydrogenation disorders, glutaric aciduria type II and ethylmalonic-adipic aciduria: mitochondrial fatty acid oxidation, acyl-coenzyme A dehydrogenase, and electron transfer flavoprotein activities in fibroblasts. *J Clin Invest* 1986;78:205–213.
390. Loehr JP, Goodman SI, Frerman FE. Glutaric acidemia type II: heterogeneity of clinical and biochemical phenotypes. *Pediatr Res* 1990;27:311–315.
391. Frerman FE, Goodman SI. Defects of electron transfer flavoprotein and electron transfer flavoprotein-ubiquinone oxidoreductase: glutaric aciduria type II. In: Scriver CR, Beaudet AL, Sly WS, et al., eds. *The metabolic and molecular bases of inherited disease*. New York: McGraw-Hill, 2001:2357–2365.
392. Olsen RKJ, Andresen BS, Christensen E, et al. Clear relationship between ETF/ETFDH genotype and phenotype in patients with multiple acyl-CoA dehydrogenation deficiency. *Hum Mutat* 2003;22:12–23.
393. Wilson GN, de Chadarevian JP, Kaplan P, et al. Glutaric aciduria type II: review of the phenotype and report of an unusual glomerulopathy. *Am J Med Genet* 1989;32:395–401.
394. Takanashi J, Fujii K, Sugita K, et al. Neuroradiologic findings in glutaric aciduria type II. *Pediatr Neurol* 1999;20:142–145.
395. Van Hove, Grunewald S, Jaeken J, et al. D, L-3-hydroxybutyrate treatment of multiple acyl-CoA dehydrogenase deficiency (MADD). *Lancet* 2003;361:1433–1435.
396. Uziel G, Garavaglia B, Ciceri E, et al. Riboflavin-responsive glutaric aciduria type II presenting as a leukodystrophy. *Pediatr Neurol* 1995;13:333–335.
397. Chow CW, Frerman FE, Goodman SI, et al. Striatal degeneration in glutaric acidaemia type II. *Acta Neuropathol* 1989;77:554–556.
398. Gregersen N, Christensen MF, Christensen E, et al. Riboflavin responsive multiple acyl-CoA dehydrogenation deficiency. Assessment of 3 years of riboflavin treatment. *Acta Paediatr Scand* 1986;75:676–681.
399. Green A, Marshall TG, Bennett MJ, et al. Riboflavin-responsive ethylmalonic-adipic aciduria. *J Inherit Metab Dis* 1985;8: 67–70.
400. Knerr I, Zschocke J, Trautment U, et al. Glutaric aciduria type III: a distinctive non-disease. *J Inherit Metab Dis* 2002;25:483–490.
401. Hale DE, Bennett MJ. Fatty acid oxidation disorders: a new class of metabolic diseases. *J Pediatr* 1992;121:1–11.
402. Eaton S, Bartlett K, Pourfarzam M. Mammalian mitochondrial β-oxidation. *Biochem J* 1996;320:345–357.
403. Bennett MJ, Worthy E, Pollitt RJ. The incidence and presentation of dicarboxylic aciduria. *J Inherit Metab Dis* 1987;10:322–323.
404. Iafolla AK, Thompson RJ Jr, Roe CR. Medium-chain acyl-coenzyme A dehydrogenase deficiency: clinical course in 120 affected children. *J Pediatr* 1994;124:409–415.
405. Tanaka K, Gregersen N, Ribes A, et al. A survey of the newborn populations in Belgium, Germany, Poland, Czech Republic, Hungary, Bulgaria, Spain, Turkey, and Japan for the G985 variant allele with haplotype analysis at the medium-chain acyl-CoA dehydrogenase gene locus: clinical and evolutionary considerations. *Pediatr Res* 1997;41:201–209.
406. Andresen BS, Dobrowolski SF, O'Reilly L, et al. Medium-chain acyl-CoA dehydrogenase (MCAD) mutations identified by MS/MS-based prospective screening of newborns differ from those observed in patients with clinical symptoms: identification and characterization of a new, prevalent mutation that results in mild MCAD deficiency. *Am J Hum Genet* 2001;68:1408–1418.
407. Rinaldo P, O'Shea JJ, Coates PM, et al. Medium-chain acyl-CoA dehydrogenase deficiency: diagnosis by stable isotope dilution analysis of urinary *n*-hexanoylglycine and 3-phenylpropionylglycine. *N Engl J Med* 1988;319:1308–1313.
408. Miller ME, Brooks JG, Forbes N, et al. Frequency of medium-chain acyl-CoA dehydrogenase deficiency G-985 mutation in sudden infant death syndrome. *Pediatr Res* 1992;31:305–307.
409. Boles RG, Buck EA, Blitzer MG, et al. Retrospective biochemical screening of fatty acid oxidation disorders in postmortem livers of 418 cases of sudden death in the first year of life. *J Pediatr* 1998;132:924–933.
410. Stanley CA, DeLeeuw S, Coates PM, et al. Chronic cardiomyopathy and weakness or acute coma in children with a defect in carnitine uptake. *Ann Neurol* 1991;30:709–716.
411. Haworth JC, Demaugre F, Booth FA, et al. Atypical features of the hepatic form of carnitine palmitoyltransferase deficiency in a Hutterite family. *J Pediatr* 1992;121:553–557.
412. Stanley CA, Hale DE, Berry GT, et al. Brief report: a deficiency of carnitine-acylcarnitine translocase in the inner mitochondrial membrane. *N Engl J Med* 1992;327:19–23.
413. Land JM, Mistry S, Squier M, et al. Neonatal carnitine palmitoyltransferase-2-deficiency: a case presenting with myopathy. *Neuromusc Disord* 1995;5:129–137.
414. Treem WR, Stanley CA, Hale DE, et al. Hypoglycemia, hypotonia, and cardiomyopathy: the evolving clinical picture of long-chain acyl-CoA dehydrogenase deficiency. *Pediatrics* 1991;87:328–333.
415. Bhala A, Willi SM, Rinaldo P, et al. Clinical and biochemical characterization of short-chain acyl-coenzyme A dehydrogenase deficiency. *J Pediatr* 1995;126:910–915.
416. Souri M, Aoyama T, Orii K, et al. Mutation analysis of very-long-chain acyl-coenzyme A dehydrogenase (VLCAD) deficiency: identification and characterization of mutant VLCADF cDNAs from four patients. *Am J Hum Genet* 1996;58:97–106.
417. Andresen BS, Olpin S, Poorthuis BJ, et al. Clear correlation of genotype with disease phenotype in very-long-chain acyl-CoA dehydrogenase deficiency. *Am J Hum Genet* 1999;64:479–494.
418. Bennett MJ, Weinberger MJ, Kobori JA, et al. Mitochondrial short-chain l-3-hydroxyacyl coenzyme A dehydrogenase deficiency: a new defect of fatty acid oxidation. *Pediatr Res* 1996;39:185–188.
419. Spiekerkoetter U, Sun B, Khuchua Z, et al. Molecular and phenotypic heterogeneity in mitochondrial trifunctional protein deficiency due to beta-subunit mutations. *Hum Mutat* 2003;21:598–607.
420. Hale DE, Batshaw ML, Coates PM, et al. Long-chain acyl coenzyme A dehydrogenase deficiency: an inherited cause of nonketotic hypoglycemia. *Pediatr Res* 1985;19:666–671.
421. Amendt BA, Moon A, Teel L, et al. Long-chain acyl-coenzyme A dehydrogenase deficiency. Biochemical studies in fibroblasts from three patients. *Pediatr Res* 1988;23:603–605.
422. Aoyama T, Souri M, Ueno I, et al. Cloning of human very-long-chain acyl-coenzyme A dehydrogenase and molecular characterization of its deficiency in two patients. *Am J Hum Genet* 1995;57:273–283.
423. Aoyama T, Souri M, Ushikubo S, et al. Purification of human very-long-chain acyl-coenzyme A dehydrogenase and characterization of its deficiency in seven patients. *J Clin Invest* 1995;95:2465–2473.
424. Mathur A, Sims HF, Gopalakrishnan D, et al. Molecular heterogeneity in very-long-chain acyl-CoA dehydrogenase deficiency causing pediatric cardiomyopathy and sudden death. *Circulation* 1999;99:1337–1343.
425. Cox GF, Souri M, Aoyama T, et al. Reversal of severe hypertrophic cardiomyopathy and excellent neuropsychologic outcome in very-long-chain acyl-coenzyme A dehydrogenase deficiency. *J Pediatr* 1998;133:247–253.
426. Bhala A, Willi SM, Rinaldo P, et al. Clinical and biochemical characterization of short-chain acyl-coenzyme A dehydrogenase deficiency. *J Pediatr* 1995;126:910–915.
427. Bok LA, Vreken P, Wijburg FA, et al. Short-chain acyl-CoA dehydrogenase deficiency: studies in a large family adding to the complexity of the disorder. *Pediatrics* 2003;112:1152–1155.

428. Tein I, Haslam RH, Rhead WJ, et al. Short-chain acyl-CoA dehydrogenase deficiency: a cause of ophthalmoplegia and multicore myopathy. *Neurology* 1999;52:366–372.
429. Nagan N, Kruckeberg KE, Tauscher AL, et al. The frequency of short-chain acyl-CoA dehydrogenase gene variants in the US population and correlation with the C(4)-acylcarnitine concentration in newborn blood spots. *Mol Genet Metab* 2003;78:239–246.
430. Gregersen N, Andresen BS, Corydon MJ, et al. Mutation analysis in mitochondrial fatty acid oxidation defects: Exemplified by acyl-CoA dehydrogenase deficiencies, with special focus on genotype-phenotype relationship. *Hum Mutat* 2001;18:169–289.
430a. Schwab KO, Ensenauer R, Matern D, et al. Complete deficiency of mitochondrial trifunctional protein due to a novel mutation within the beta-subunit of the mitochondrial trifunctional protein gene leads to failure of long-chain fatty acid beta-oxidation with fatal outcome. *Eur J Pediatr* 2003;162:90–95.
431. Dezateux C: Newborn screening for medium chain acyl-CoA dehydrogenase deficiency: evaluating the effects on outcome. *Eur J Pediatr* 2003;162(Suppl 1):S25–S28.
432. Wolf B, Heard SG. Screening for biotinidase deficiency in newborns: worldwide experience. *Pediatrics* 1990;85:512–517.
433. Yang X, Aoki Y, Li X, et al. Structure of human holocarboxylase synthetase gene and mutation spectrum of holocarboxylase synthetase deficiency. *Hum Genet* 2001;109:526–534.
434. Wolf B. Disorders of biotin metabolism: treatable neurologic syndromes. In: Rosenberg RN, Prusiner SB, DiMauro S, et al., eds. *The molecular and genetic basis of neurological disease,* 3rd ed. Philadelphia: Butterworth–Heinemann, 2003:705–710.
435. Wolf B, Heard GS, Jefferson LG, et al. Clinical findings in four children with biotinidase deficiency detected through a statewide neonatal screening program. *N Engl J Med* 1985;313:16–19.
436. Pomponio RJ, Hymes J, Reynolds TR, et al. Mutations in the human biotinidase gene that cause profound biotinidase deficiency in symptomatic children: molecular, biochemical, and clinical analysis. *Pediatr Res* 1997;42:840–848.
437. Hymes J, Stanley CM, Wolf B. Mutations in BTD causing biotinidase deficiency. *Hum Mutat* 2001;200:375–381.
438. Hart PS, Hymes J, Wolf B. Biochemical and immunological characterization of serum biotinidase in profound biotinidase deficiency. *Am J Hum Genet* 1992;50:126–136.
439. Weber P, Scholl S, Baumgartner ER. Outcome in patients with profound biotinidase deficiency: relevance of newborn screening. *Dev Med Child Neurol* 2004;46:481–484.
440. Ozand PT, Gascon GG, Al Essa M, et al. Biotin-responsive basal ganglia disease: a novel entity. *Brain* 1998;121:1267–1279.
441. Chen E, Nyhan WL, Jakobs C, et al. L-2-Hydroxyglutaric aciduria: neuropathological correlations and first report of severe neurodegenerative disease and neonatal death. *J Inherit Metab Dis* 1996;19:335–343.
442. Barbot C, Fineza I, Diogo L, et al. L-2-Hydroxyglutaric aciduria: clinical, biochemical and magnetic resonance imaging in six Portuguese pediatric patients. *Brain Dev* 1997;19:268–272.
443. van der Knaap MS, Jakobs C, Hoffman GF, et al. D-2-Hydroxyglutaric aciduria: biochemical marker or clinical disease entity? *Ann Neurol* 1999;45:111–119.
444. Spielberg SP, Kramer LI, Goodman SI, et al. 5-Oxoprolinuria: biochemical observations and case report. *J Pediatr* 1977;91:237–241.
445. Ristoff E, Mayatepek E, Larsson A. Long-term clinical outcome in patients with glutathione synthetase deficiency. *J Pediatr* 2001;139:79–84.
446. Pearl PL, Gibson KM, Acosta MT, et al. Clinical spectrum of succinic semialdehyde dehydrogenase deficiency. *Neurology* 2003;60: 1413–1417.
447. Gibson KM, Christensen E, Jakobs C, et al. The clinical phenotype of succinic semialdehyde dehydrogenase deficiency (4-hydroxybutyric aciduria): case reports of 23 new patients. *Pediatrics* 1997;99:567–574.
448. Chambliss KL, Hinson DD, Trettel F, et al. Two exon-skipping mutations as the molecular basis of succinic semialdehyde dehydrogenase deficiency (4-hydroxybutyric aciduria). *Am J Hum Genet* 1998;63:399–408.
449. Ko FJ, Nyhan WL, Wolff J, et al. 3-Hydroxyisobutyric aciduria: an inborn error of valine metabolism. *Pediatr Res* 1991;30:322–326.
450. Chitayat D, Meagher-Villemure K, Mamer OA, et al. Brain dysgenesis and congenital intracerebral calcification associated with 3-hydroxyisobutyric aciduria. *J Pediatr* 1992;121:86–89.
451. Gibson KM, Elpeleg ON, Jakobs C, et al. Multiple syndromes of 3-methylglutaconic aciduria. *Pediatr Neurol* 1993;9:120–123.
452. Zeharia A, Elpeleg ON, Mukamel M, et al. 3-Methylglutaconic aciduria: a new variant. *Pediatrics* 1992;89:1080–1082.
453. Nowaczyk MJ, Lehotay DC, Platt BA, et al. Ethylmalonic and methylsuccinic aciduria in ethylmalonic encephalopathy arise from abnormal isoleucine metabolism. *Metabolism* 1998;47:836–839.
454. McGowan KA, Nyhan WL, Barshop BA, et al. The role of methionine in ethylmalonic encephalopathy with petechiae. *Arch Neurol* 2004;61:570–574.
455. Robinson BH, Oei J, Sherwood WG, et al. Hydroxymethylglutaryl CoA lyase deficiency: features resembling Reye syndrome. *Neurology* 1980;30:714–718.
456. Thompson GN, Hsu BY, Pitt JJ, et al. Fasting hypoketotic coma in a child with deficiency of mitochondrial 3-hydroxy-3-methylglutaryl-CoA synthase. *N Engl J Med* 1997;337:1203–1207.
457. Ensenauer R, Niederhoff H, Ruiter JP, et al. Clinical variability in 3-hydroxy-2-methylbutyryl-CoA dehydrogenase deficiency. *Ann Neurol* 2002;51:656–659.
458. Offman R, Ruiter JP, Feenstra M, et al. 2-Methyl-3-hydroxybutyryl-CoA dehydrogenase deficiency is caused by mutations in the *HADH2* gene. *Am J Hum Genet* 2003;72:1300–1307.
459. Kerrigan JF, Aleck KA, Tarby TJ, et al. Fumaric aciduria: clinical and imaging features. *Ann Neurol* 2000;47:583–588.
460. Hers HG. Inborn lysosomal diseases. *Gastroenterology* 1965;48: 625–633.
461. Meikle PJ, Hopwood JJ, Clagne AE, et al. Prevalence of lysosomal storage disorders. *J Am Med Assoc* 1999;281:249–254.
462. Kornfeld S. Trafficking of lysosomal enzymes in normal and disease states. *J Clin Invest* 1986;77:1–6.
463. Platt FM, Walkley SU, eds. *Lysosomal disorders of the brain*. Oxford: Oxford University Press, 2004.
464. Melis D, Parenti G, Della Casa R, et al. Brain damage in glycogen storage disease type I. *J Pediatr* 2004;144:637–642.
465. Murase T, Ikeda H, Muro T, et al. Myopathy associated with type III glycogenosis. *J Neurol Sci* 1973;20:287–295.
466. Zellweger H, Mueller S, Ionasescu V, et al. Glycogenosis IV, a new cause of infantile hypotonia. *J Pediatr* 1972;80:842–844.
467. Pompe JC. Over idiopathische hypertrophie van het hart. *Ned Tijdschr Geneeskd* 1932;76:304–307.
468. Kishnani PS, Howell RR. Pompe disease in infants and children. *J Pediatr* 2004;144(Suppl 5):S35–S43.
469. Kroos MA, Van der Kraan M, Van Diggelen OP, et al. Two extremes of the clinical spectrum of glycogen storage disease type II in one family: a matter of genotype. *Hum Mutat* 1997;9:17–22.
470. Kleijer WJ, Van der Kraan M, Kroos MA, et al. Prenatal diagnosis of glycogen storage disease type II. Enzyme assay or mutation analysis? *Pediatr Res* 1995;38:103–106.
471. Hirschhorn R, Reuser AJJ. Glycogen storage disease type II: Acid α-glucosidase (acid maltase) deficiency. In: Scriver CR, Beaudet AL, Sly WS, et al., eds. *The metabolic and molecular bases of inherited disease*. 8th ed. New York: McGraw-Hill, 2001:3389–3420.
472. Engel AG, Hirschhorn R. Acid maltase deficiency. In: Engel AG, Franzini-Armstrong C, eds. *Myology. Basic and clinical,* 2nd ed. New York,McGraw-Hill, 1994;2:1533–1553.
473. Gambetti T, DiMauro S, Baker L. Nervous system in Pompe's disease: ultrastructure and biochemistry. *J Neuropathol Exp Neurol* 1971;30:412–430.
474. Martin JJ, de Barsy T, van Hoof F, et al. Pompe's disease: an inborn lysosomal disorder with storage of glycogen. *Acta Neuropathol* 1973;23:229–244.
475. Lenard HG, Schaub J, Keutel J, et al. Electromyography in type II glycogenosis. *Neuropädiatrie* 1974;5:410–424.
476. Verloes A, Massin M, Lombet J, et al. Nosology of lysosomal glycogen storage diseases without *in vitro* maltase deficiency. Delineation of a neonatal form. *Am J Med Genet* 1997;72:135–142.
477. van den Hout HM, Hop W, van Diggelen OP, et al. The natural course of infantile Pompe disease: 20 original cases compared with 133 cases from the literature. *Pediatrics* 2003;112:332–340.

478. Lam CW, Yuen YP, Chan KY, et al. Juvenile-onset glycogen storage disease type II with novel mutations in acid alpha-glucosidase gene. *Neurology* 2003;60:715–717.
479. Swaiman KF, Kennedy WR, Sauls HS. Late infantile acid maltase deficiency. *Arch Neurol* 1968;18:642–648.
480. Matsuishi T, Yoshino M, Terasawa K, Nonaka I. Childhood acid maltase deficiency: a clinical, biochemical, and morphologic study of three patients. *Arch Neurol* 1984;41:47–52.
481. Broadhead DM, Butterworth J. α-Glucosidase in Pompe's disease. *J Inherit Metab Dis* 1978;1:153–154.
482. Winkel LP, Kamphoven JH, van den Hout HJ, et al. Morphological changes in muscle tissue of patients with infantile Pompe's disease receiving enzyme replacement therapy. *Muscle Nerve* 2003;27:743–751.
483. Winkel LP, van den Hout HJ, Kamphoven JH, et al. Enzyme replacement therapy in late-onset Pompe's disease: a three-year follow-up. *Ann Neurol* 2004;55:495–502.
484. Amalfitano A, Bengur AR, Morse RP, et al. Recombinant human acid alpha-glucosidase enzyme therapy for infantile glycogen storage disease type II: results of a phase I/II trial. *Genet Med* 2001;3:132–138.
485. Sun B, Chen YT, Bird A, et al. Packaging of an AAV vector encoding human acid alpha-glucosidase for gene therapy in glycogen storage disease type II with a modified hybrid adenovirus-AAV vector. *Mol Ther* 2003;7:467–477.
486. Ding E, Hu H, Hodges BI, et al. Efficacy of gene therapy for a prototypical lysosomal storage disease (GSD-II) is critically dependent on vector dose, transgene promoter, and the tissues targeted for vector transduction. *Mol Ther* 2002;5:436–446.
487. Kennedy PG. Potential use of herpes simplex virus (HSV) vectors for gene therapy of neurological disorders. *Brain* 1997;120:1245–1259.
488. Matern D, Starzl TE, Arnaout W, et al. Liver transplantation for glycogen storage disease types I, III, and IV. *Eur J Pediatr* 1999;158(Suppl 2):S43–S48.
489. Nishino I. Lysosomal membrane disorders. In: Rosenberg RN, Prusiner SB, DiMauro S, et al., eds. *The molecular and genetic basis of neurological disease,* 3rd ed. Philadelphia: Butterworth–Heinemann, 2003:309–314.
490. Sugie K, Yamamoto A, Murayama K, et al. Clinicopathological features of genetically confirmed Danon disease. *Neurology* 2002;58:1773–1778.
491. Hunter C. A rare disease in two brothers. *Proc R Soc Med* 1917;10: 104–116.
492. Hurler G. Uber einen Typ multipler Abartungen, vorwiegend am Skelett-system. *Z Kinderheilk* 1919;24:220–234.
493. von Pfaundler M. Demonstrationen über einen Typus kindlicher Dysostose. *Jahrb Kinderheilk* 1920;92:420–421.
494. Ellis RWB, Sheldon W, Capon NB. Gargoylism (chondro-osteo-dystrophy, corneal opacities, hepatosplenomegaly, and mental deficiency). *Q J Med* 1936;5:119–139.
495. Alberts B, Johnson A, Lewis J, et al. Cell junctions, cell adhesion and the extracellular matrix. In: Alberts B, Johnson, Lewis J, et al., eds. *The molecular biology of the cell,* 4th ed. New York: Garland, 2002;1065–1126.
496. Kjellen L, Lindahl V. The proteoglycans structures and functions. *Annu Rev Biochem* 1991;60:443–475.
497. Varadi DP, Cifonelli JA, Dorfman A. The acid mucopolysaccharides in normal urine. *Biochem Biophys Acta* 1967;141:117.
498. Neufeld EF, Muenzer J. The mucopolysaccharidoses. In: Scriver CR, Sly WS, Childs B, et al., eds. *The metabolic and molecular bases of inherited disease,* 8th ed. New York: McGraw-Hill, 2001:3421–3452.
499. Scott HS, Bunge S, Gal A, et al. Molecular genetics of mucopolysaccharidosis type I: diagnostic, clinical and biological implications. *Hum Mutat* 1995;6:288–302.
500. Froissart R, Maire I, Millat G, et al. Identification of iduronate sulfatase gene alterations in 70 unrelated Hunter patients. *Clin Genet* 1998;53:362–368.
501. Clarke JT, et al. Hunter disease (mucopolysaccharidosis type II) associated with unbalanced inactivation of the X-chromosomes in a karyotypically normal girl. *Am J Hum Genet* 1991;49:289–297.
502. Groebe H, Krins M, Schmidberger H, et al. Morquio syndrome (mucopolysaccharidosis IV B) associated with β-galactosidase deficiency: report of two cases. *Am J Hum Genet* 1980;32:258–272.
503. Renteria VG, Ferrans VJ, Roberts WC. The heart in Hurler syndrome: gross histologic and ultrastructural observations in five necropsy cases. *Am J Cardiol* 1976;38:487–501.
504. Van Hoof F, Hers HG. L'ultrastructure des cellules hepatiques dans la maladie de Hurler (gargoylisme). *C R Acad Sci Paris* 1964;259:1281–1283.
505. Dekaban AS, Constantopoulos G. Mucopolysaccharidosis types I, II, III A and V. Pathological and biochemical abnormalities in the neural and mesenchymal elements of the brain. *Acta Neuropathol* 1977;39:1–7.
506. Beighton P, McKusick VA. *Heritable disorders of connective tissue,* 5th ed. St. Louis: Mosby, 1993.
507. Lowry RB, Applegarth DA, Toone JR, et al. An update on the frequency of mucopolysaccharide syndromes in British Columbia. *Hum Genet* 1990;85:389–390.
508. Caffey J. Gargoylism (Hunter-Hurler disease, dysostosis multiplex, lipochondrodystrophy): prenatal and postnatal bone lesions and their early postnatal evolution. *AJR Am J Roentgenol* 1952;67:715–731.
509. Levin S. A specific skin lesion in gargoylism. *Am J Dis Child* 1960;99:444–450.
510. Friedmann I, Spellacy E, Crow J, et al. Histopathological studies of the temporal bones in Hurler's disease [mucopolysaccharidosis (MPS) IH]. *J Laryngol Otol* 1985;99:29–41.
511. Seto T, Kono K, Morimoto K, et al. Brain magnetic resonance imaging in 23 patients with mucopolysaccharidoses and the effect of bone marrow transplantation. *Ann Neurol* 2001;50:79–92.
512. Lee C, Dineen TE, Brack M, et al. The mucopolysaccharidoses: characterization by cranial MR imaging. *Am J Neuroradiol* 1993;14:1285–1292.
513. Gross DM, Williams JC, Caprioli C, et al. Echocardiographic abnormalities in the mucopolysaccharide storage diseases. *Am J Cardiol* 1988;61:170–176.
514. Roubicek M, Gehler J, Spranger J. The cliniical spectrum of α-L-iduronidase deficiency. *Am J Med Genet* 1985;20:471–481.
514a. Meunzer J, Fisher A. Advances in the treatment of mucopolysaccharidosis type I. *N Engl J Med* 2004;350:1932–1934.
515. Peters C, Shapiro EG, Krivit W. Hurler syndrome: past, present, and future. *J Pediatr* 1998;133:7–9.
516. Vellodi A, Young EP, Cooper A, et al. Bone marrow transplantation for mucopolysaccharidosis type I: experience of two British centres. *Arch Dis Child* 1997;76:92–99.
517. Guffon N, Souillet G, Maire I, et al. Follow-up on nine patients with Hurler syndrome after bone marrow transplantation. *J Pediatr* 1998;133:119–125.
518. Weisstein JS, Delgado E, Steinbach LS, et al. Musculoskeletal manifestations of Hurler syndrome: long-term follow-up after bone marrow transplantation. *J Pediatr Orthop* 2004;24:97–101.
519. Wraith JE, Clarke LA, Beck M, et al. Enzyme replacement therapy for mucopolysaccharidoses I: a randomized, double-blinded, placebo-controlled, multinational study of recombinant human alpha-L-iduronidase (laronidase). *J Pediatr* 2004;144:581–588.
520. Kakavanos R, Turner CT, Hopwood JJ, et al. Immune tolerance after long-term enzyme-replacement therapy among patients who have mucopolysaccharidoses I. *Lancet* 2003;361:1608–1613.
521. Kakkis ED, Muenzer J, Tiller GE, et al. Enzyme-replacement therapy in mucopolysaccharidoses I. *N Engl J Med* 2001;344:182–188.
522. Scheie HG, Hambrick GW, Barness LA Jr. A newly recognized forme fruste of Hurler's disease (gargoylism). *Am J Ophthalmol* 1962;53:753–769.
523. Winters PR, Harrod MJ, Molenich-Heetred SA, et al. α-L-iduronidase deficiency and possible Hurler-Scheie genetic compound. Clinical, pathologic, and biochemical findings. *Neurology* 1976;26:1003–1007.
524. Lowry RB, Applegarth DA, Toone JR, et al. An update on the frequence of mucopolysaccharide syndromes in British Columbia. *Hum Genet* 1990;85:389–390.
525. Young IS, Harper PS. Mild form of Hunter's syndrome: clinical delineation based on 31 cases. *Arch Dis Child* 1982;57:828–836.

526. Topping TM, Kenyon KR, Goldberg MF, et al. Ultrastructural ocular pathology of Hunter's syndrome. Systemic mucopolysaccharidosis type II. *Arch Ophthalmol* 1971;86:164–177.
527. Young ID, Harper PS. Long-term complications in Hunter's syndrome. *Clin Genet* 1979;16:125–132.
528. Young ID, Harper PS. The natural history of the severe form of Hunter's syndrome: a study based on 52 cases. *Dev Med Child Neurol* 1983;25:481–489.
529. Spranger J, Cantz M, Gehler J, et al. Mucopolysaccharidosis II (Hunter disease) with corneal opacities: report of two patients at the extremes of a wide clinical spectrum. *Eur J Pediatr* 1978;129:11–16.
530. Karpati G, Carpenter S, Eisen AA, et al. Multiple peripheral nerve entrapments: an unusual phenotypic variant of the Hunter syndrome (mucopolysaccharidosis II) in a family. *Arch Neurol* 1974;31:418–422.
531. Constantopoulos G, McComb RD, Dekaban AS. Neurochemistry of the mucopolysaccharidoses: brain glycosaminoglycans in normals and four types of mucopolysaccharidoses. *J Neurochem* 1976;26:901–908.
532. Murphy JV, Hodach AE, Gilbert EF, et al. Hunter's syndrome: ultrastructural features in young children. *Arch Pathol Lab Med* 1983;107:495–499.
533. Meier C, Wismann U, Herschkowitz N, et al. Morphological observations in the nervous system of prenatal mucopolysaccharidosis II (M. Hunter). *Acta Neuropathol* 1979;48:139–143.
534. Sanfilippo SJ, Podosin R, Langer LO, et al. Mental retardation associated with acid mucopolysaccharidúria (heparitin sulfate type). *J Pediatr* 1963;63:837–838.
535. Verity CM, Nicoll A, Will RG, et al. Variant Creutzfeld-Jakob disease in UK children: a national surveillance study. *Lancet* 2000;356:1224–1227.
536. Danks DM, Campbell PE, Cartwright E, et al. The Sanfilippo syndrome: clinical, biochemical, radiological, haematological and pathological features of nine cases. *Austr Paediat J* 1972;8:174–186.
537. Kaplan P, Wolfe LS. Sanfilippo syndrome type D. *J Pediatr* 1987;110:267–271.
538. Federico A, Capece G, Cecio A, et al. Sanfilippo B syndrome (MPS III B): case report with analysis of CSF mucopolysaccharides and conjunctival biopsy. *J Neurol* 1981;225:77–83.
539. van de Kamp JJP, Niermeijer MF, von Figura K, et al. Genetic heterogeneity and clinical variability in the Sanfilippo syndrome (types A, B, and C). *Clin Genet* 1981;20:152–160.
540. Shapiro EG, Lockman LA, Balthazor M, Krivit W. Neuropsychological outcomes of several storage diseases with and without bone marrow transplantation. *J Inherit Metab Dis* 1995;18:413–429.
541. Fraser J, Wraith JE, Delatycki MB. Sleep disturbance in mucopolysaccharidosis type III (Sanfilippo syndrome): a survey of managing clinicians. *Clin Genet* 2002;62:418–421.
542. Robertson SP, Klug GL, Rogers JG. Cerebrospinal fluid shunts in the management of behavioural problems in Sanfilippo syndrome (MPS III). *Eur J Pediatr* 1998;157:653–655.
543. Nelson J, Thomas PS. Clinical findings in 12 patients with MPS IV A (Morquio's disease). Further evidence for heterogeneity. Part III: odontoid dysplasia. *Clin Genet* 1988;33:126–130.
544. Koto A, Horwitz AL, Suzuki K, et al. The Morquio syndrome: neuropathology and biochemistry. *Ann Neurol* 1978;4:26–36.
545. Maroteaux P, Leveque B, Marie J, et al. Une nouvelle dysostose avec elimination urinaire de chondroitine-sulfate B. *Presse Med* 1963;71:1849–1852.
546. Peterson DI, Bacchus H, Seaich L, et al. Myelopathy associated with Maroteaux-Lamy syndrome. *Arch Neurol* 1975;32:127–129.
547. Harmatz P, Whitley CB, Waber L, et al. Enzyme replacement therapy in mucopolysaccharidosis VI (Maroteaux-Lamy syndrome). *J Pediatr* 2004;144:547–580.
548. Lee JE, Falk RE, Ng WG, et al. Beta-glucoronidase deficiency. A heterogeneous mucopolysaccharidosis. *Am J Dis Child* 1985;139:57–59.
549. Beaudet AL, DiFerrante NM, Ferry GD, et al. Variation in the phenotypic expression of β-glucuronidase deficiency. *J Pediatr* 1978;86:388–394.
550. O'Connor LH, Erway LC, Vogler CA, et al. Enzyme replacement therapy for murine mucopolysaccharidosis type VII leads to improvements in behavior and auditory function. *J Clin Invest* 1998;101:1394–1400.
551. De Braekeleer M. Hereditary disorders in Saguenay-Lac-St. Jean (Quebec, Canada). *Hum Hered* 1991;41:141–146.
552. Beck M, Barone R, Hoffmann R, et al. Inter- and intrafamilial variability in mucolipidosis II (I-cell disease). *Clin Genet* 1995;47:191–199.
553. Greval S, Shapiro E, Braunlin E, et al. Continued neurocognitive development and prevention of cardiopulmonary complications after successful BMT for I-cell disease: a long-term follow-up report. *Bone Marrow Transplant* 2003;32:957–960.
554. Martin JJ, Leroy JG, Farriaux JP, et al. I-cell disease (mucolipidosis II). A report on its pathology. *Acta Neuropathol* 1975;33:285–305.
555. Leroy JG, Ho MW, MacBrinn MC, et al. I-cell disease; biochemical studies. *Pediatr Res* 1972;6:752–757.
556. Kelly TE, Thomas GH, Taylor HA Jr, et al. Mucolipidosis III (pseudo-Hurler polydystrophy). Clinical and laboratory studies in a series of 12 patients. *Johns Hopkins Med J* 1975;137:156–175.
557. Amir N, Zlotogora J, Bach G. Mucolipidosis type IV: clinical spectrum and natural history. *Pediatrics* 1987;79:953–959.
558. Bach G. Mucolipidosis type IV. *Mol Genet Metab* 2001;73:197–203.
559. Schiffmann R, Dwyer NK, Lubensky IA, et al. Constitutive achlorhydria in mucolipidosis type IV. *Proc Natl Acad Sci USA* 1998;95:1207–1212.
560. Frei KP, Patronas MJ, Crutchfield KE, et al. Mucolipidosis type IV. Characteristic MRI findings. *Neurology* 1998;51:565–569.
561. Tellez-Nagel I, Rapin I, Iwamoto T, et al. Mucolipidosis IV. *Arch Neurol* 1976;33:828–835.
562. LaPlante JM, Falardeau J, Sun M, et al. Identification and characterization of the single channel function of human mucolipin-1 implicated in mucolipidosis type IV, a disorder affecting the lysosomal pathway. *FEBS Lett* 2002;532:183–187.
563. Johnson WG. Disorders of glycoprotein degradation: sialidosis, fucosidosis, alpha-mannosidosis, beta-mannosidosis, and aspartylglycosaminuria In:Rosenberg RN, Prusiner SB, DiMauro S, et al., eds. *The molecular and genetic basis of neurologic and psychiatric disease*. Philadelphia: Butterworth–Heinemann, 2003:279–290.
564. Willems PJ, Gatti R, Darby JK, et al. Fucosidosis revisited: a review of 77 patients. *Am J Med Genet* 1991;38:111–131.
565. Willems PJ, Seo HC, Coucke P, et al. Spectrum of mutations in fucosidosis. *Eur J Hum Genet* 1999;7:60–67.
566. Galluzzi P, Rufa A, Balestri P, et al. MR brain imaging of fucosidosis type I. *Am J Neuroradiol* 2001;22:777–770.
567. Troost J, Staal GE, Willemse J, et al. Fucosidosis I. Clinical and enzymological studies. *Neuropaediatrie* 1977;8:155–162.
568. Krivit W, Peters C, Shapiro EG. Bone marrow transplantation as effective treatment of central nervous sytem disease in globoid cell leukodystrophy, metachromatic leukokystrophy, adenoleukodystrophy, mannosidosis, fucosidosis, aspartylglucosaminuria, Hurler, Maroteaux-Lamy, and Sly syndromes, and Gaucher disease type III. *Curr Opin Neurol* 1999;12:167–176.
569. Bielicki J, Muller V, Fuller M, et al. Recombinant canine alpha-l-fucosidase: expression, purification, and characterization. *Mol Genet Metab* 2000;69:24–32.
570. Larbrisseau A, Brouchu P, Jasmin G. Fucosidose de type 1 Etude anatomique. *Arch Fr Pediatr* 1979;36:1013–1023.
571. Kistler JP, Lott IT, Kolodny EH, et al. Mannosidosis. New clinical presentation, enzyme studies and carbohydrate analysis. *Arch Neurol* 1977;34:45–51.
572. Sung JH, Hayano M, Desnick RJ. Mannosidosis: pathology of the nervous system. *J Neuropathol Exp Neurol* 1977;36:807–820.
573. Norden NE, Lundblad A, Svensson S, et al. Characterization of two mannose-containing oligosaccharides from the urine of patients with mannosidosis. *Biochemistry* 1974;13:871–874.
574. Grewal SS, Shapiro EG, Krivit W, et al. Effective treatment of alpha-mannosidosis by allogeneic hematopoietic stem cell transplantation. *J Pediatr* 2004;144:569–573.
575. Wenger DA, Sujansky E, Fennessey PV, et al. Human β-mannosidase deficiency. *N Engl J Med* 1986;315:1201–1205.

576. Kleijer WJ, Hu P, Thoomes R, et al. β-Mannosidase deficiency: heterogenous manifestation in the first female patient and her brother. *J Inherit Metab Dis* 1990;13:867–872.
577. Young ID, Young EP, Mossman J, et al. Neuraminidase deficiency: case report and review of the phenotype. *J Med Genet* 1987;24:283–290.
578. Bonten EJ, Arts WF, Beck M, et al. Novel mutations in lysosomal neuraminidase identify functional domains and determine clinical severity in sialidosis. *Hum Mol Genet* 2000;9:275–2725.
579. Steinman L, Tharp BR, Dorfman LJ, et al. Peripheral neuropathy in the cherry-red spot-myoclonus syndrome (sialidosis type I). *Ann Neurol* 1980;7:450–456.
580. Yamano T, Shimada M, Matsuzaki K, et al. Pathological study on a severe sialidosis (α-neuraminidase deficiency). *Acta Neuropathol* 1986;71:278–284.
581. Malvagia S, Morrone A, Caciotti A, et al. New mutations in the PPBG gene lead to loss of PPCA protein which affects the level of the beta-galactosidase/neuraminidase complex and the EBP-receptor. *Mol Genet Metab* 2004;82:48–55.
582. Itoh K, Oyanagi K, Takahashi H, et al. Endothelin-1 in the brain of patients with galactosialidosis: its abnormal increase and distribution pattern. *Ann Neurol* 2000;47:122–126.
583. Kleijer WJ, Geilen GC, Janse HC, et al. Cathepsin A deficiency in galactosialidosis: studies of patients and carriers in 16 families. *Pediatr Res* 1996;39:1067–1071.
584. Okada S, Yutaka T, Kato T, et al. A case of neuraminidase deficiency associated with a partial β-galactosidase defect. *Eur J Pediatr* 1979;130:239–249.
585. Renlund M, Aula P, Raivio KO, et al. Salla disease: a new lysosomal storage disorder with disturbed sialic acid metabolism. *Neurology* 1983;33:57–66.
586. Varho TT, Alajoki LE, Posti KM, et al. Phenotypic spectrum of Salla disease, a free sialic acid storage disorder. *Pediatr Neurol* 2002;26:267–273.
587. Kleta R, Morse RP, Orvisky E, et al. Clinical, biochemical, and molecular diagnosis of a free sialic acid storage disease patient of moderate severity. *Mol Genet Metab* 2004;82:137–143.
588. Robinson RO, Fensom AH, Lake BD. Salla disease—rare or underdiagnosed. *Dev Med Child Neurol* 1997;39:153–157.
589. Enns GM, Seppala R, Musci TJ, et al. Clinical course and biochemistry of sialuria. *J Inherit Metab Dis* 2001;24:328–336.
590. Leroy JG, Seppala R, Huizing M, et al. Dominant inheritance of sialuria, an inborn error of feedback inhibition. *Am J Hum Genet* 2001;68:1419–1427.
591. Matilainen R, Airaksinen E, Mononen T, et al. A population-based study on the causes of mild and severe mental retardation. *Acta Paediatr* 1995;84:261–266.
592. Klenk E. Beiträge zur Chemie der Lipoidosen: Niemann-Picksche Krankheit und amaurotische Idiotie. *Z Physiol Chem* 1939; 262:128–143.
593. Tay W. Symmetrical changes in the region of the yellow spot in each eye of an infant. *Trans Ophthalmol Soc UK* 1880–1881;1:55–57.
594. Sachs B. On arrested cerebral development, with special reference to its cortical pathology. *J Nerv Ment Dis* 1887;14:541–553.
595. Kolodny EH, Neudorfer O. The GM2 gangliosidoses. In: Rosenberg RN, Prusiner SB, DiMauro S, et al., eds. *The molecular and genetic basis of neurological and psychiatric disease*, 3rd ed. Boston: Butterworth–Heinemann, 2003:239–246.
596. Mahuran DJ. The biochemistry of *HEXA* and *HEXB* gene mutations causing GM2 gangliosidosis. *Biochim Biophys Acta* 1991;1096:87–94.
597. Grebner EE, Tomczak J. Distribution of three α-chain β-hexosaminidase A mutations among Tay-Sachs carriers. *Am J Hum Genet* 1991;48:604–607.
598. Myerowitz R, Hogikyan ND. A deletion involving Alu sequences in the β-hexosaminidase α-chain gene of French Canadians with Tay-Sachs disease. *J Biol Chem* 1987;263:15396–15397.
599. Sandhoff K, Andreae U, Jatzkewitz H. Deficient hexosaminidase activity in an exceptional case of Tay-Sachs disease with additional storage of kidney globoside in visceral organs. *Life Sci* 1968;7:283–288.
600. Ellis RB, Ikonne JU, Patrick AD, et al. Prenatal diagnosis of Tay-Sachs disease [Letter]. *Lancet* 1973;2:1144–1145.
601. Hama Y, Li YT, Li SC. Interaction of GM2 activator protein with glycosphingolipids. *J Biol Chem* 1997;272:2828–2833.
602. Sandhoff K, Kolter T. Biochemistry of glycosphingolipid degradation. *Clin Chim Acta* 1997;266:51–61.
603. Menkes JH, O'Brien JS, Okada S, et al. Juvenile GM2 gangliosidosis. Biochemical and ultrastructural studies on a new variant of Tay-Sachs diseases. *Arch Neurol* 1971;25:14–22.
604. Navon R, Kolodny EH, Mitsumoto H, et al. Ashkenazi-Jewish and non-Jewish adult GM2 gangliosidosis patients share a common genetic defect. *Am J Hum Genet* 1990;46:817–821.
605. Terry RD, Weiss M. Studies in Tay-Sachs disease: ultrastructure of cerebrum. *J Neuropathol Exp Neurol* 1963;22:18–55.
606. Walkley SU, Siegel DA, Dobrenis K, Zervas M. GM2 ganglioside as a regulator of pyramidal neuron dendritogenesis. *Ann N Y Acad Sci* 1998;845:188–199.
607. Walkley SU. Pathobiology of neuronal storage disease. *Int Rev Neurobiol* 1988;29:191–244.
608. Kivlin JD, Sanborn GE, Myers GG. The cherry-red spot in Tay-Sachs and other storage diseases. *Ann Neurol* 1985;17:356–360.
609. Aronson SM, Lewitan A, Rabiner AM, et al. The megaloencephalic phase of infantile amaurotic familial idiocy: cephalometric and pneumoencephalographic studies. *Arch Neurol Psychiatr* 1958;79:151–163.
610. Yoshikawa H, Yamada KN. Sakuragawa MRI in the early stage of Tay-Sachs disease. *Neuroradiology* 1992;34:394–395.
611. Johnson WG. Genetic heterogeneity of hexosaminidase-deficiency diseases. *Res Publ Assoc Res Nerv Ment Dis* 1983;60:215–237.
612. Cashman NR, Antel JP, Hancock LW, et al. *N*-acetyl-β-hexosaminidase β locus defect and juvenile motor neuron disease: a case study. *Ann Neurol* 1986;19:568–572.
613. Oates CE, Bosch EP, Hart EN. Movement disorders associated with chronic GM2 gangliosidoses. *Eur Neurol* 1986;25:154–159.
614. Sutton VR. Tay-Sachs disease screening and counseling familes at risk for metabolic disease. *Obstet Gynecol Clin North Am* 2002;29:287–296.
615. Platt FM, Neises GR, Reinkensmeier G, et al. Prevention of lysosomal storage in Tay-Sachs mice treated with *N*-butyldeoxynojirimycin. *Science* 1997;276:428–431.
616. Butters TD, Dwe RA, Platt FM. New therapeutics for the treatment of glycosphingolipid lysosomal storage diseases. *Adv Exp Med Biol* 2003;535:219–226.
617. Landing BH, Silverman FN, Craig JM, et al. Familial neurovisceral lipidosis. An analysis of eight cases of a syndrome previously reported as "Hurler-variant, pseudo-Hurler disease" and "Tay-Sachs disease" with visceral involvement. *Am J Dis Child* 1964;108:503–522.
618. O'Brien JS, Stern MB, Landing BH, et al. Generalized gangliosidosis: another inborn error of ganglioside metabolism? *Am J Dis Child* 1965;109:338–346.
619. Wolfe LS, Senior RG, Ng-Ying-Kin NM. The structures of oligosaccharides accumulating in the liver of GM1-gangliosidosis, type I. *J Biol Chem* 1974;249:1828–1838.
620. Okada S, O'Brien JS. Generalized gangliosidosis: β-galactosidase deficiency. *Science* 1968;160:1002–1004.
621. Callahan JW. Molecular basis of GM1 gangliosidosis and Morquio disease, type B. Structure-function studies of lysosomal beta-galactosidase and the non-lysosomal beta-galactosidase-like protein. *Biochim Biophys Acta* 1999;1455:85–103.
622. Paschke E, Milos I, Keimer-Erlacher H, et al. Mutation analyses in 17 patients with deficiency in acid beta-galactosidase: three novel point mutations and high correlation of mutation W273L with Morquio disease type B. *Hum Genet* 2001;109:159–166.
623. Suzuki K, Suzuki K, Chen GC. Morphological, histochemical and biochemical studies on a case of systemic late infantile lipidosis (generalized gangliosidosis). *J Neuropathol Exp Neurol* 1968;27:15–38.
624. Van Der Voorn JP, Kamphorst W, Van Der Knaap MS, et al. The leukoencephalopathy of infantile GM1 gangliosidosis: oligodendrocytic leoss and axonal dysfunction. *Acta Neuropathol* 2004;107:539–545.
625. Hanson M, Lupski JR, Hicks J, et al. Association of dermal melanocytosis with lysosomal storage disease: clinical features and

hypotheses regarding pathogenesis. *Arch Dermatol* 2003;139:916–920.

626. O'Brien JS. Generalized gangliosidosis. *J Pediatr* 1969;75:167–186.
627. Farrell DF, MacMartin MP. GM1-gangliosidosis: enzymatic variation in a single family. *Ann Neurol* 1981;9:232–236.
628. Wolfe LS, Callahan J, Fawcett JS, et al. GM1-gangliosidosis without chondrodystrophy or visceromegaly. *Neurology* 1970;20:23–44.
629. Guazzi GC, D'Amore I, van Hoof F, et al. Type 3 (chronic) GM1 gangliosidosis presenting as infanto-choreo-athetotic dementia, without epilepsy, in three sisters. *Neurology* 1988;38:1124–1127.
630. Goldman JE, Katz D, Rapin I, et al. Chronic GM1-gangliosidosis presenting as dystonia. I. Clinical and pathologic features. *Ann Neurol* 1981;9:465–475.
631. Lowden JA, Cutz E, Conen PE, et al. Prenatal diagnosis of GM1-gangliosidosis. *N Engl J Med* 1973;288:225–228.
632. Gaucher PCE. De l'épithélioma primitif de la rate.Thèse,Université de Paris, 1882.
633. Brady RO, Schiffmann R. Gaucher disease. In: Rosenberg RN, Prusiner SB, DiMauro S, et al., eds. *The molecular and genetic basis of neurological disease,* 3rd ed. Philadelphia: Butterworth–Heinemann, 2003:229–234.
634. Goker-alpan O, Schiffman R, Park JK, et al. Phenotypic continuum in neuronopathic Gaucher disease: an intermediate phenotype between type 2 and type 3. *J Pediatr* 2003;143:273–276.
635. Brady RO, Kanfer JN, Bradley RM, Shapiro D. Demonstration of a deficiency of glucocerebroside-cleaving enzyme in Gaucher's disease. *J Clin Invest* 1966;45:1112–1115.
636. Masuno M, Tomatsu S, Sukegawa K, et al. Non-existence of a tight association between a 444-leucine to proline mutation and phenotypes of Gaucher disease: high frequency of a NciI polymorphism in the non-neuronopathic form. *Hum Genet* 1990;84:203–206.
637. Lieb H. Cerebrosidspeicherung bei Splenomegalie Typus-Gaucher. *Z Physiol Chem* 1924;140:305–315.
638. Philippart M, Rosenstein B, Menkes JH. Isolation and characterization of the main splenic glycolipids in the normal organ and in Gaucher's disease: evidence for the site of metabolic block. *J Neuropathol Exp Neurol* 1965;24:290–303.
639. Lee RE. The fine structure of the cerebroside occurring in Gaucher's disease. *Proc Natl Acad Sci USA* 1968;61:484–489.
640. Grafe M, Thomas C, Schneider J, et al. Infantile Gaucher's disease: a case with neuronal storage. *Ann Neurol* 1988;23:300–303.
641. Wong K, Sidransky E, Verma A, et al. Neuropathology provides clues to the pathophysiology of Gaucher disease. *Mol Genet Metab* 2004;82:192–207.
642. Lloyd-Evans E, Pelled D, Riebeling C, et al. Glucosylceramide and glucosylsphingosine modulate calcium mobilization from brain microsomes via different mechanisms. *J Biol Chem* 2003;278:23594–23599.
643. Rodgers CL, Jackson SH. Acute infantile Gaucher's disease: case report. *Pediatrics* 1951;7:53–59.
644. Sidransky E. New perspectives in type 2 Gaucher disease. *Adv Pediatr* 1997;44:73–107.
645. Harris CM, Taylor DS, Vellodi A. Ocular motor abnormalities in Gaucher disease. *Neuropediatrics* 1999;30:289–293.
646. Sidransky E, Sherer D, Ginns EI. Gaucher disease in the neonate: a distinct Gaucher phenotype is analogous to a mouse model created by targeted disruption of the glucocerebrosidase gene. *Pediatr Res* 1992;32:494–498.
647. Nishimura RN, Barranger JA. Neurologic complications of Gaucher's disease, type 3. *Arch Neurol* 1980;37:92–93.
648. Park JK, Orvisky E, Tayebi N, et al. Myoclonic epilepsy in Gaucher disease: genotype–phenotype insights from a rare patient subgroup. *Pediatr Res* 2003;53:387–395.
649. Garvey MA, Toro C, Goldstein S, et al. Somatosensory evoked potentials as a marker of disease burden in type 3 Gaucher disease. *Neurology* 2001;56:391–394.
650. Erikson A. Gaucher disease-Norrbottnian type (III). Neuropaediatric and neurobiological aspects of clinical patterns and treatment. *Acta Paediatr Scand Suppl* 1986;326:1–42.
651. Dahl N, Lagerstrom M, Erikson A, et al. Gaucher disease type III (Norrbottnian type) is caused by a single mutation in exon 10 of the glucocerebrosidase gene. *Am J Hum Genet* 1990;47:275–278.
652. Altarescu G, Hill S, Wiggs E, et al. The efficacy of enzyme replacement therapy in patients with chronic neuronopathic Gaucher's disease. *J Pediatr* 2001;138:539–547.

652a. Lonser RR, Walbridge S, Murray GJ, et al. Convection perfusion of glucocerebrosidase for neuronopathic Gaucher's disease. *Ann Neurol* 2005;57:542–548.

653. Moyses C. Substrate reduction therapy: clinical evaluation in type 1 Gaucher disease. *Phil Trans R Soc Lond B Biol Sci* 2003;358:955–960.
654. Desnick RJ. Fabry disease: α-galactosidase A deficiency. In: Rosenberg RN, Prusiner SB, DiMauro S, et al., eds. *The molecular and genetic basis of neurological disease,* 3rd ed. Philadelphia: Butterworth–Heinemann, 2003:315–322.
655. MacDermot KD, Holmes A, Miners AH. Anderson-Fabry disease: clinical manifestations and impact of disease in a cohort of 60 obligate carrier females. *J Med Genet* 2001;38:769–775.
656. Mehta A, Ricci R, Widmer U, et al. Fabry disease defined: baseline clinical manifestations of 366 patients in the Fabry Outcome Survey. *Eur J Clin Invest* 2004;34:236–242.
657. Reis M, Ramaswami U, Parini R, et al. The early clinical phenotype of Fabry disease: a study on 35 European children and adolescents. *Eur J Pediatr* 2003;162:767–772.
658. Desnick RJ, Brady R, Barranger J, et al. Fabry disease, an under-recognized multisystemic disorder: expert recommendations for diagnosis, management, and enzyme replacement therapy. *Ann Intern Med* 2003;138:338–346.
659. Branton MH, Schiffmann R, Sabnis SG, et al. Natural history of Fabry renal disease: influence of alpha-galactosidase A activity and genetic mutations on clinical course. *Medicine* 2002;81:122–138.

659a. Schram AW, Hamers MN, Brouwer-Kelder B, et al. Enzymological properties and immunological characterization of α-galactosidase isoenzymes from normal and Fabry human liver. *Biochim Biophys Acta* 1997;482:125–137.

660. Eng CM, Ashley GA, Burgert TS, et al. Fabry disease: thirty-five mutations in the alpha-galactosidase A gene in patients with classic and variant phenotypes. *Mol Med* 1997;3:174–182.
661. Lemansky P, Bishop DF, Desnick RJ, et al. Synthesis and processing of α-galactosidase A in human fibroblasts. Evidence for different mutations in Fabry disease. *J Biol Chem* 1987;262:2062–2065.
662. Sweeley CC, Klionsky B. Fabry's disease: classification as a sphingolipidosis and partial characterization of a novel glycolipid. *J Biol Chem* 1963;238:3148–3150.
663. Grunnet ML, Spilsbury PR. The central nervous system in Fabry's disease. *Arch Neurol* 1973;28:231–234.
664. Kaye EM, Kolodny EH, Logigian EL, et al. Nervous system involvement in Fabry's disease: clinicopathological and biochemical correlation. *Ann Neurol* 1988;23:505–509.
665. Fabry J. Ein Beitrag zur Kenntnis der Purpura haemorrhagica nodularis (Purpura papulosa hemorrhagica Hebrae). *Arch Dermatol Syph* 1898;43:187–200.
666. Mitsias P, Levine SR. Cerebrovascular complications of Fabry's disease. *Ann Neurol* 1996;40:8–17.
667. Desnick RJ, Brady RO. Fabry disease in childhood. *J Pediatr* 2004;144(5 Suppl):S20–S26.
668. deGroot WP. Fabry's disease in children. *Br J Dermatol* 1970;82:329–332.
669. Sher NA, Letson RD, Desnick RJ. The ocular manifestations of Fabry's disease. *Arch Ophthalmol* 1979;97:671–676.
670. Cable WJL, Dvorak AM, Osage JE, et al. Fabry disease: significance of ultrastructural localization of lipid inclusions in dermal nerves. *Neurology* 1982;32:347–353.
671. Crutchfield KE, Patronas NJ, Dambrosia JM, et al. Quantitative analysis of cerebral vasculopathy in patients with Fabry disease. *Neurology* 1998;50:1746–1749.
672. Takanashi J, Barkovich AJ, Dillon WP, et al. T1 hyperintensity in the pulvinar: key imaging feature for diagnosis of Fabry disease. *Am J Neuroradiol* 2003;24:916–921.
673. Moore DF, Ye F, Schiffmann R, et al. Increased signal intensity in the pulvinar on T1 weighted images: a pathognomonic MR imaging sign of Fabry disease. *Am J Neuroradiol.* 2003;24:1096–1101.

673a. Franceschetti AT, Philippart M, Franceschetti A. A study of Fabry's disease: I. Clinical examination of a family with cornea verticillata. *Dermatologica* 1969;138:209–221.

674. Desnick RJ. Enzyme replacement and enhancement therapies for lysosomal disease. *J Inherit Metab Dis* 2004;27:385–310.
675. Eng CM, Guffon N, Wilcox WR, et al. International Collaborative Fabry Disease Study Group. Safety and efficacy of recombinant human alpha-galactosidase A—replacement therapy in Fabry's disease. *N Engl J Med* 2001;345:9–16.
676. Wilcox WR, Banikazemi M, Guffon N, et al. International Fabry Disease Study Group. Long-term safety and efficacy of enzyme replacement therapy for Fabry disease. *Am J Hum Genet* 2004;75:65–74.
677. Schiffmann R, Kopp JB, Austin HA et al. Enzyme replacement therapy in Fabry disease: a randomized controlled trial. *JAMA* 2001;285:2743–2749.
678. Hilz MJ, Brys M, Marthol H, et al. Enzyme replacement therapy improves function of C-, Adelta-, and Abeta-nerve fibers in Fabry neuropathy. *Neurology*. 2004;62:1066–1072.
679. Baehner F, Kampmann C, Whybra C, et al. Enzyme replacement therapy in heterozygous females with Fabry disease: results of a phase IIIB study. *J Inherit Metab Dis* 2003;26:617–627.
680. Moore DF, Scott LT, Gladwin MT, et al. Regional cerebral hyperperfusion and nitric oxide pathway dysregulation in Fabry disease: reversal by enzyme replacement therapy. *Circulation* 2001;104:1506–1512.
681. Moore DF, Altarescu G, Ling GS, et al. Elevated cerebral blood flow velocities in Fabry disease with reversal after enzyme replacement. *Stroke* 2002;33:525–531.
682. Bakker HD, de Sonnaville ML, Vreken P, et al. Human alpha-*N*-acetylgalactosaminidase (alpha-NAGA) deficiency: no association with neuroaxonal dystrophy? *Eur J Hum Genet* 2001;9:91–96.
683. Desnick RJ, Schindler D. Schindler disease: Deficient α-*N*-acetylgalactosaminidase activity. In: Rosenberg RN, Prusiner SB, DiMauro S, et al., eds. *The molecular and genetic basis of neurological disease,* 3rd ed. Philadelphia: Butterworth–Heinemann, 2003:323–330.
684. De Jong J, van den Berg C, Wijburg H, et al. Alpha-*N*-acetylgalactosaminidase deficiency with mild clinical manifestations and difficult biochemical diagnosis. *J Pediatr* 1994;125:385–391.
685. Niemann A. Ein unbekanntes Krankheitsbild. *Jahrb Kinderheilk* 1914;79:1–10.
686. Crocker AC, Farber S. Niemann-Pick disease: a review of 18 patients. *Medicine* 1958;37:1–95.
687. Callahan JW. The cerebral defect in Tay-Sachs disease and Nie mann-Pick disease. *J Neurochem* 1961;7:69–80.
688. Gumbinas M, Larsen M, Liu HM. Peripheral neuropathy in classic Niemann-Pick disease: ultrastructure of nerves and skeletal muscles. *Neurology* 1975;25:107–113.
689. Walton DS, Robb RM, Crocker AC. Ocular manifestations of Group A Niemann-Pick disease. *Am J Ophthalmol* 1978;85:174–180.
690. Ivemark BI, Svennerholm L, Thoren C, et al. Niemann-Pick disease in infancy: report of two siblings with clinical, histologic, and chemical studies. *Acta Paediatr* 1963;52:391–401.
691. Thudichum JLW. *A treatise on the chemical constitution of the brain, based throughout upon original researches*. London: Bailliere, Tindall and Cox, 1884.
692. Takahashi T, Suchi M, Desnick RJ, et al. Identification and expression of five mutations in the human acid sphingomyelinase gene causing types A and B Niemann-Pick disease. Molecular evidence for genetic heterogeneity in the neuronopathic and non-neuronopathic forms. *J Biol Chem* 1992;267:12552–12558.
693. Levran O, Desnick RJ, Schuchman EH. Identification and expression of a common missense mutation (L302P) in the acid sphingomyelinase gene of Ashkenazi Jewish type A Niemann-Pick disease patients. *Blood* 1992;80:2081–2087.
694. Harzer K, Rolfs A, Bauer P. et al. Niemann-Pick disease type A and B are clinically but also enzymatically heterogenous: pitfall in the laboratory diagnosis of sphingomyelinase deficiency associated with the mutation Q292K. *Neuropediatrics* 2003;34:301–306.
695. Wenger DA, Kudoh T, Sattler M, et al. Niemann-Pick disease type B: prenatal diagnosis and enzymatic and chemical studies on fetal brain and liver. *Am J Hum Genet* 1981;33:337–344.
696. Vanier MT, Millat G. Niemann-Pick disease type C. *Clin Genet* 2003;64:269–281.
697. Guibaud P, Vanier MT, Malpuech G, et al. Forme infantile précoce, cholestatique, rapidement mortelle, de la sphingomyélinose type C. *Pediatrie* 1979;34:103–114.
698. Kelly DA, Pormann B, Mowat AP, et al. Niemann-Pick disease type C. Diagnosis and outcome in children, with particular reference to liver disease. *J Pediatr* 1993;123:242–247.
699. Philippart M, Martin L, Martin JJ, et al. Niemann-Pick disease: morphologic and biochemical studies in the visceral form with late central nervous system involvement (Crocker's group C). *Arch Neurol* 1969;20:227–238.
700. Vanier MT, Wenger DA, Comly ME, et al. Niemann-Pick disease group C: clinical variability and diagnosis based on defective cholesterol esterification. A collaborative study on 70 patients. *Clin Genet* 1988;33:331–348.
701. Patterson MC. A riddle wrapped in a mystery: understanding Niemann-Pick disease, type C. *Neurologist* 2003;9:301–310.
702. Lee VMY, Gioedert M, Trojanowski JQ. Neurodegenerative tauopathies. *Annu Rev Neurosci* 2001;24:1121–1159.
703. Saito Y, Suzuki K, Hulette CM, Murayama S. Aberrant phosphorylation of alpha-synuclein in human Niemann-Pick type C1 disease. *J Neuropathol Exp Neurol* 2004;63:323–328.
704. Frolov A, Zielinski SE, Crowley JP, et al. NPC1 and NPC2 regulate cellular cholesterol homeostasis through generation of low density lipoprotein cholesterol–derived oxysterols. *J Biol Chem* 2003;278:25517–25525.
705. Nixon RA. Niemann-Pick Type C disease and Alzheimer's disease: the APP-endosome connection fattens up. *Am J Pathol* 2004;164:757–761.
706. Millat G, Chikh K, Naureckiene S, et al. Niemann-Pick disease type C: spectrum of HE1 mutations and genotype/phenotype correlations in the NPC2 group. *Am J Hum Genet* 2001;69:1013–1021.
707. Naureckiene S, Sleat DE, Lackland H, et al. Identification of HE1 as the second gene of Niemann-Pick C disease. *Science* 2000;290:2298–2301.
708. Jan MM, Camfield PR. Nova Scotia Niemann-Pick disease (type D): clinical study of 20 cases. *J Child Neurol* 1998;13:75–78.
709. Greer WL, Riddell DC, Gillan TL, et al. The Nova Scotia (type D) form of Niemann-Pick disease is caused by a G3097T transversion in NPC1. *Am J Hum Genet* 1998;63:52–54.
710. Sun X, Marks DL, Park WD, et al. Niemann-Pick C variant detection by altered sphingolipid trafficking and correlation with mutations within a specific domain of NPC1. *Am J Hum Genet* 2001;68:1361–1372.
711. Abramov A, Schorr S, Wolman M. Generalized xanthomatosis with calcified adrenals. *Am J Dis Child* 1956;91:282–286.
712. Eto Y, Kitagawa T. Wolman's disease with hypolipoproteinemia and acanthocytosis: clinical and biochemical observations. *J Pediatr* 1970;77:862–867.
713. Wolman M. Involvement of nervous tissue in primary familial xanthomatosis with adrenal calcification. *Pathol Eur* 1968;3:259–265.
714. Patrick AD, Lake BD. Deficiency of an acid lipase in Wolman's disease. *Nature* 1969;222:1067–1068.
715. Brown MS, Sobhani MK, Brunschede GY, et al. Restoration of a regulatory response to low density lipoprotein in acid lipase-deficient human fibroblasts. *J Biol Chem* 1976;251:3277–3286.
716. Pagani F, Pariyarath R, Garcia R, et al. New lysosomal acid lipase gene mutants explain the phenotype of Wolman disease and cholesteryl ester storage disease. *J Lipid Res* 1998;39:1382–1388.
717. Zschenker O, Jung N, Rethmeier J, et al. Characterization of lysosomal acid lipase mutations in the signal peptide and mature polypeptide region causing Wolman disease. *J Lipid Res* 2001;42:1033–1140.
718. Galton DJ, Gilbert C, Reckless JP, et al. Triglyceride storage disease. *Q J Med* 1974;43:63–71.
719. Krivit W, Peters C, Dusenbery K, et al. Wolman disease successfully treated by bone marrow transplantation. *Bone Marrow Transplant* 2000;26:567–570.
720. Farber S, Cohen J, Uzman LL. Lipogranulomatosis: a new lipoglycoprotein storage disease. *J Mount Sinai Hosp N Y* 1957;24:816–837.
721. Moser HW. Farber disease: Acid ceramidase deficiency, Farber lipogranulomatosis. In: Rosenberg RN, Prusiner SB, DiMauro S,

et al., eds. *The molecular and genetic basis of neurological disease,* 3rd ed. Philadelphia: Butterworth–Heinemann, 2003:299–304.
722. Antonarakis SE, Valle D, Moser HW, et al. Phenotypic variability in siblings with Farber disease. *J Pediatr* 1984;104:406–409.
723. Burck U, Moser HW, Goebel HH, et al. A case of lipogranulomatosis Farber: some clinical and ultrastructural aspects. *Eur J Pediatr* 1985;143:203–208.
724. Chen WW, Moser AB, Moser HW. Role of lysosomal acid ceramidase in the metabolism of ceramide in human skin fibroblasts. *Arch Biochem* 1981;208:444–455.
725. Jonas AJ, Conley SB, Marshall R, et al. Nephropathic cystinosis with central nervous system involvement. *Am J Med* 1987;83:966–970.
726. Levine S, Paparo G. Brain lesions in a case of cystinosis. *Acta Neuropathol* 1982;57:217–220.
727. Broyer M, Tete MJ, Guest G, et al. Clinical polymorphism of cystinosis encephalopathy. Results of treatment with cysteamine. *J Inherit Metab Dis* 1996;19:65–75.
728. Gahl WA, Delakas MC, Charnas L, et al. Myopathy and cystine storage in muscles in a patient with nephropathic cystinosis. *N Engl J Med* 1988;319:1461–1464.
729. Cochat P, Drachman R, Gagnadoux MF, et al. Cerebral atrophy and nephropathic cystinosis. *Arch Dis Child* 1986;61:401–403.
730. van Bogaert L, Scherer HJ, Epstein E. *Une forme cérébrale de la cholestérinose généralisée.* Paris: Masson, 1937.
731. Menkes JH, Schimschock JR, Swanson PD. Cerebrotendinous xanthomatosis: the storage of cholestanol within the nervous system. *Arch Neurol* 1968;19:47–53.
732. Berginer VM, Salen G, Patel S. Cerebrotendinous xanthomatosis. In: Rosenberg RN, Prusiner SB, DiMauro S, et al. *The molecular and genetic basis of neurologic and psychiatric disease.* 3rd ed. Philadelphia: Butterworth–Heinemann, 2003:575–582.
733. Arlazoroff A, Roitberg B, Werber E, et al. Epileptic seizures as a presenting symptom of cerebrotendinous xanthomatosis. *Epilepsia* 1991;32:657–661.
734. Kuriyama M, Fujiyama J, Yoshidome H, et al. Cerebrotendinous xanthomatosis: clinical and biochemical evaluation of eight patients and review of the literature. *J Neurol Sci* 1991;102: 225–232.
735. Barkhof F, Verrips A, Wesseling P, et al. Cerebrotendinous xanthomatosis: the spectrum of imaging findings and the correlation with neuropathologic findings. *Radiology* 2000;217:869–876.
736. Schimschock JR, Alvord EC, Swanson PD. Cerebrotendinous xanthomatosis: clinical and pathological studies. *Arch Neurol* 1968;18:688–698.
737. Cali JJ, Russell DW. Characterization of human sterol 27-hydroxylase: a mitochondrial cytochrome P-450 that catalizes multiple oxidation reactions in bile acid biosynthesis. *J Biol Chem* 1991;266:7774–7778.
738. Chen W, Kubota S, Teramoto T, et al. Genetic analysis enables definite and rapid diagnosis of cerebrotendinous xanthomatosis. *Neurology* 1998;51:865–867.
739. Verrips A, Hoefsloot LH, Steenbergen GC, et al. Clinical and molecular genetic characteristics of patients with cerebrotendinous xanthomatosis. *Brain* 2000;123:908–919.
740. Batta AK, Salen G, Shefer S, et al. Increased plasma bile alcohol glucuronides in patients with cerebrotendinous xanthomatosis: effect of chenodeoxycholic acid. *J Lipid Res* 1987;28:1006–1012.
741. Van Heijst AF, Verrips A, Weners RA, et al. Treatment and follow-up of children with cerebrotendinous xanthomatosis. *Eur J Pediatr* 1998;157:313–316.
742. Johnson VP. Smith-Lemli-Opitz syndrome: review and report of two affected siblings. *Z Kinderheilk* 1975;119:221–234.
743. Smith DW, Lemli L, Opitz JM. A newly recognized syndrome of multiple congenital anomalies. *J Pediatr* 1964;64:210–217.
744. Tint GS, Irons M, Elias ER, et al. Defective cholesterol biosynthesis associated with the Smith-Lemli-Opitz syndrome. *N Engl J Med* 1994;330:107–113.
745. Wassif CA, Maslen C, Kachilele-Linjewile S, et al. Mutations in the human sterol delta7-reductase gene at 11q12–13 cause Smith-Lemli-Opitz syndrome. *Am J Hum Genet* 1998;63:55–62.
746. Fitzky BU, Witsch-Baumgarner M, Erdel M, et al. Mutations in the delta7-sterol reductase gene in patients with the Smith-Lemli-Opitz syndrome. *Proc Natl Acad Sci USA* 1998;95:8181–8186.
747. Cunniff C, Kratz LE, Moser A, et al. Clinical and biochemical spectrum of patients with RSH/Smith-Lemli-Opitz syndrome and abnormal cholesterol metabolism. *Am J Med Genet* 1997;68: 263–269.
748. Kelley RI, Kratz L. 3-Methylglutaconic acidemia in Smith-Lemli-Opitz syndrome. *Pediatr Res* 1995;37:671–674.
748a. Rossi M, Vajro P, Iorio R, et al. Characterization of liver involvement in defects of cholesterol biosynthesis: long-term follow-up and review. *Am J Med Genet A* 2005;132:144–151.
749. Gofflot F, Hers C, Illien F, et al. Molecular mechanisms underlying limb anomalies associated with cholesterol deficiency during gestation: implications of Hedgehog signaling. *Hum Mol Genet* 2003;12:1187–1198.
750. Haas D, Kelley RI, Hoffman GF. Inherited disorders of cholesterol biosynthesis. *Neuropediatrics* 2001;32:113–122.
751. Brunetti-Pierri N, Corso G, Rossi M, et al. Lathosterolosis, a novel multiple-malformation/mental retardation syndrome due to deficiency of 3beta-hydroxysteroid-delta5-desaturase. *Am J Hum Genet* 2002;71:952–958.
752. Hassell S, Butler MG. Antley-Bixler syndrome: report of a patient and review of the literature. *Clin Genet* 1994;46:372–376.
753. Herman GE. Disorders of cholesterol biosynthesis: prototypic metabolic malformation syndromes. *Hum Mol Genet* 2003;12(Spec Issue No 1):R75–R88.
754. Porter FD. Human malformation syndromes due to inborn errors of cholesterol synthesis. *Curr Opin Pediatr* 2003;15:607–613.
755. Krakowiak PA, Wassif CA, Kratz L, et al. Lathosterolosis: an inborn error of human and murine cholesterol synthesis due to lathosterol 5-desaturase deficiency. *Hum Mol Genet* 2003;12:1631–1641.
756. Sikora DM, Ruggiero M, Petit-Kekel K, et al. Cholesterol supplementation does not improve developmental progress in Smith-Lemli-Opitz syndrome. *J Pediatr* 2004;144:783–791.
757. Moser HW. Peroxisomal disorders. In: Rosenberg RN, Prusiner SB, DiMauro S, et al. *The molecular and genetic basis of neurologic and psychiatric disease.* 3rd ed. Philadelphia: Butterworth–Heinemann, 2003:213–228.
758. Gould SJ, Raymond GV, Valle D. The peroxisomal biogenesis disorders. In: Scriver CR, Beaudet AL, Sly WS, et al., eds. *The metabolic and molecular bases of inherited diseases.* New York, McGraw Hill, 2001:3185–3218.
759. Wanders RJ. Metabolic and molecular basis of peroxisomal disorders: a review. *Am J Med Genet* 2004;126A:355–375.
760. Santos MJ, Imanaka T, Shio H, et al. Peroxisomal membrane ghosts in Zellweger syndrome—aberrant organelle assembly. *Science* 1988;239:1536–1538.
761. Geisbrecht BV, Collins CS, Reuber BE, et al. Disruption of a PEX1-PEX6 interaction is the most common cause of the neurologic disorders Zellweger syndrome, neonatal adrenoleukodystrophy, and infantile Refsum disease. *Proc Natl Acad Sci USA* 1998;95:8630–8635.
762. Preuss N, Brosius U. Biermanns M, et al. PEX1 mutations in complementation group 1 of Zellweger spectrum patients. *Pediatr Res* 2002;51:706–714.
763. Opitz JM, et al. The Zellweger syndrome (cerebrohepatorenal syndrome). *Birth Defects Orig Artic Ser* 1969;5:144–160.
764. Kamei A, Houdou S, Takashima S, et al. Peroxisomal disorders in children: immunohistochemistry and neuropathology. *J Pediatr* 1993;122:573–579.
765. Volpe JJ, Adams RD. Cerebrohepatorenal syndrome of Zellweger: an inherited disorder of neuronal migration. *Acta Neuropathol* 1972;20:175–198.
766. Gressens P, Baes M, Leroux P, et al. Neuronal migration disorder in Zellweger mice is secondary to glutamate receptor dysfunction. *Ann Neurol* 2000;48:336–343.
767. Janssen A, Gressens P, Grabenbauer M, et al. Neuronal migration depends on intact peroxisomal function in brain and in extraneuronal tissues. *J Neurosci* 2003;23:9732–9741.
768. Barkovich AJ, Peck WW. MR of Zellweger syndrome. *Am J Neuroradiol* 1997;18:1163–1170.

769. Rocchiccioli F, Aubourg P, Bougnères PF. Medium- and long-chain dicarboxylic aciduria in patients with Zellweger syndrome and neonatal adrenoleukodystrophy. *Pediatr Res* 1986;20:62–66.
770. Moser AB, Rasmussen M, Naidu S, et al. Phenotype of patients with peroxisomal disorders subdivided into sixteen complementation groups. *J Pediatr* 1995;127:13–22.
771. Happle R. X-linked chondrodysplasia punctata. Review of literature and report of a case. *Hum Genet* 1979;53:65–73.
772. Refsum S. Heredopathia atactica polyneuritiformis. *Acta Psychiatr Scand* 1946;38(Suppl):93–103.
773. Richterich R, Van Mechelen P, Rossi E. Refsum's disease (heredopathia atactica polyneuritiformis): an inborn error of lipid metabolism with storage of 3,7,11,15-tetramethyl hexadecanoic acid. *Am J Med* 1965;39:230–236.
774. Cammermeyer J. Neuropathologic changes in hereditary neuropathies: manifestation of the syndrome heredopathia atactica polyneuritiformis in the presence of interstitial hypertrophic polyneuropathy. *J Neuropathol Exp Neurol* 1956;15:340–361.
775. Jansen GA, Wanders RJ, Watkins PA, et al. Phytanoyl-coenzyme A hydroxylase deficiency—the enzyme defect in Refsum's disease. *N Engl J Med* 1997;337:133–134.
776. Gibberd FB, Billimoria JD, Page NG, et al. Heredopathia atactica polyneuritiformis (Refsum's disease) treated by diet and plasma-exchange. *Lancet* 1979;1:575–578.
777. Prietsch V, Mayatepek K, Krastel H, et al. Mevalonate kinase deficiency: enlarging the clinical and biochemical spectrum. *Pediatrics* 2003;111:258–261.
778. Simon A, Kremer HP, Wevers RA, et al. Mevalonate kinase deficiency: Evidence for a phenotypic continuum. *Neurology* 2004;62:994–997.
779. Frenkel J, Willemsen MA, Weemaes CM, et al. Increased urinary leukotriene E(4) during febrile attcks in the hyperimmunoglobulinaemia D and periodic fever syndrome. *Arch Dis Child* 2001;85:158–159.
779a. Simon A, Kremer HPH, Wevers RA, et al. Mevalinate kinase deficiency. Evidence for a phenotypic continuum. *Neurology* 2004; 62:994–997.
780. Hoffmann GF, Charpentier C, Mayatepek E, et al. Clinical and biochemical phenotype in 11 patients with mevalonic aciduria. *Pediatrics* 1993;91:915–921.
781. Jacken J, Eggermont E, Stibler H. An apparent homozygous X-linked disorder with carbohydrate-deficient serum glycoproteins. *Lancet* 1987;2:1398.
782. Leonard J, Grünewald S, Clayton P. Diversity of congenital disorders of glycosylation. *Lancet* 2001;357:1382–1383.
782a. Marquardt T, Denecke J. Congenital disorders of glycosylation: review of their molecular bases, clinical presentations, and specific therapies. *Eur J Pediatr* 2003;162:359–379.
783. Miossec-Chauvet E, Mikaeloff Y, Heron D, et al. Neurological presentation in pediatric patients with congenital disorders of glycosylation type 1a. *Neuropediatrics* 2003;34:1–6.
784. Patterson MC. Metabolic disorders—congenital disorders of glycosylation. In: Rosenberg RN, Prusiner SB, DiMauro S, et al. *The molecular and genetic basis of neurologic and psychiatric disease*. 3rd ed. Philadelphia: Butterworth–Heinemann, 2003:643–650.
785. Krasnewich D, Gahl WA. Carbohydrate-deficient glycoprotein syndrome. *Adv Pediatr* 1997;44:109–140.
786. Peters V, Penzien JM, Reiter G, et al. Congenital disorders of glycosylation IId (CDG-IId)—a new entity. Clinical presentation with Dandy-Walker malformation and myopathy. *Neuropediatrics* 2002;33:27–32.
787. Babovic-Vuksanovic D, Patterson MC, Schwenk WF, et al. Severe hypoglycemia as a presenting symptom of carbohydrate-deficient glycoprotein syndrome. *J Pediatr* 1999;135:775–781.
788. Grünewald S, Imbach T, Huijben K, et al. Clinical and biochemical characteristics of congenital disorder of glycosylation type Ic, the first recognized endoplasmic reticulum defect in *N*-glycan synthesis. *Ann Neurol* 2000;47:776–781.
789. Bergen HR, Lacey JM, O'Brien JF, et al. Online single-step analysis of blood proteins: the transferrin story. *Anal Biochem* 2001;296:122–129.
790. Stibler H, Skovby F. Failure to diagnose carbohydrate-deficient glycoprotein syndrome prenatally. *Pediatr Neurol* 1994;11:71.
791. Lafora GR. Über das Vorkommen amyloider Körperchen in Innern der Ganglienzell. *Virchows Arch Pathol Anat* 1911;205:295–303.
792. Unverricht H. *Die Myoklonie*. Leipzig: Franz Deuticke, 1891.
793. Chan EM, Ackerley CA, Lohi H, et al. Laforin preferentially binds the neurotoxic starch-like polyglucosans, which form in its absence in progressive myoclonus epilepsy. *Hum Mol Genet* 2004;13:1117–1129.
794. Chan EM, Young EJ, Ianzano L. Mutations in NHLRC1 cause progressive myoclonus epilepsy. *Nat Genet* 2003;35:125–127.
795. Harriman DGF, Millar JHD. Progressive familial myoclonic epilepsy in three families: its clinical features and pathological basis. *Brain* 1955;78:325–349.
796. Nishimura RN, Ishak KG, Reddick R, et al. Lafora disease: diagnosis by liver biopsy. *Ann Neurol* 1980;8:409–415.
797. Berkovic SF, Andermann F, Carpenter S, et al. Progressive myoclonus epilepsies: specific causes and diagnosis. *N Engl J Med* 1986;315:296–304.
798. Janeway R, Ravens JR, Pearce LA, et al. Progressive myoclonus epilepsy with Lafora inclusion bodies. I. Clinical, genetic, histopathologic and biochemical aspects. *Arch Neurol* 1967;16: 565–582.
799. Odor DL, Janeway R, Pearce LA, et al. Progressive myoclonus epilepsy with Lafora inclusion bodies. II. Studies of ultrastructure. *Arch Neurol* 1967;16:583–594.
800. Baumann RJ, Kocoshis SA, Wilson D. Lafora disease: liver histopathology in presymptomatic children. *Ann Neurol* 1983; 14:86–89.
801. Virtaneva K, D'Amato E, Miao J, et al. Unstable minisatellite expansion causing recessively inherited myoclonus epilepsy, EPM1. *Nat Genet* 1997;15:393–396.
802. Lalioti MD, Antonarakis SE, Scott HS. The epilepsy, the protease inhibitor and the dodecamer: progressive myoclonus epilepsy, cystatatin b and a 12-mer repeat expansion. *Cytogenet Genom Res* 2003;100:213–223.
803. Forss N, Silen T, Karjalaeinen T. Lack of activation of human secondary somatosensory cortex in Unverricht-Lundborg type of progressive myoclonus epilepsy. *Ann Neurol* 2001;49: 90–97.
804. Edwards MJ, Hargreaves IP, Heales SJ, et al. *N*-Acetylcysteine and Unverricht-Lundborg disease: variable response and possible side effects. *Neurology* 2002;59:1447–1449.
805. Santavuori P, Haltia M, Rapola J, et al. Infantile type of so-called neuronal ceroid lipofuscinosis. Part I. A clinical study of 15 patients. *J Neurol Sci* 1973;18:257–267.
806. Jansky J. Über einen noch nicht beschriebenen Fall der familiären amaurotischen Idiotie mit Hypoplasie des Kleinhirns. *Z Erforsch Behandl Jugendlich Schwachsinns* 1909;3:86–88.
807. Bielschowsky M. Über spätinfantile familiäre amaurotische Idiotie mit Kleinhirn Symptomen. *Dtsch Z Nervenheilk* 1914;50:7–29.
808. Batten FE. Family cerebral degeneration with macular change (so-called juvenile form of family amaurotic idiocy). *Q J Med* 1914;7:444–454.
809. Spielmeyer W. Weitere Mitteilung ueber eine besondere Form von familiärer amaurotischer Idiotie. *Neurol Zbl* 1905;24:1131–1132.
810. Kufs M. Über eine Spätform der amaurotischen Idiotie und ihre heredofamiliären Grundlagen. *Z Ges Neurol Psychiat* 1925;95:169–188.
811. Josephson SA, Schmidt RE, Millsap P, et al. Autosomal dominant Kufs' disease: a cause of early dementia. *J Neurol Sci* 2001;188:51–60.
812. Wisniewski KE, Kida E, Patxot OF, et al. Variability in the clinical and pathological findings in the neuronal ceroid lipofuscinoses: review of data and observations. *Am J Med Genet* 1992;42:525–532.
813. Das AK, Becerra CH, Yi W, et al. Molecular genetics of palmitoyl-protein thioesterase deficiency in the U.S. *J Clin Invest* 1998;102:361–370.
814. Sleat DE, Donnelly RJ, Lackland H, et al. Association of mutations in a lysosomal protein with classical late-infantile neuronal ceroid lipofuscinosis. *Science* 1997;277:1802–1805.
815. Munroe PB, Mitchison HM, O'Rawe AM, et al. Spectrum of mutations in the Batten disease gene, CLN3. *Am J Hum Genet* 1997;61:310–316.

816. International Batten Disease Consortium. Isolation of a novel gene underlying Batten disease (CLN3). *Cell* 1995;82:949–957.
817. Tyynela J, Suopanki J, Baumann M, et al. Sphingolipid activator proteins (SAPs) in neuronal ceroid lipofuscinosis. *Neuropediatrics* 1997;28:49–52.
818. Isosomppi, J. Vesa J, Jalanko A, et al. Lysosomal localization of the neuronal ceroid lipofuscinosis CLN5 protein. *Hum Mol Genet* 2002;11:885–891.
819. Sharp JD, Wheeler RB, Lake BD, et al. Loci for classical and a variant late infantile neuronal ceroid lipofuscinosis map to chromosomes 11p15 and 15q21–23. *Hum Mol Genet* 1997;6:591–595.
820. Ranta S, Topcu M, Tegelberg S, et al. Variant late infantile neuronal ceroid lipofuscinosis in a subset of Turkish patients is allelic to Northern epilepsy. *Hum Mutat* 2004;3:300–303.
821. Schulz A, Dhar S, Rylova S, et al. Impaired cell adhesion and apoptosis in a novel CLN9 Batten disease variant. *Ann Neurol* 2004;56:342–350.
822. Mole S, Gardener M. Molecular genetics of the neuronal ceroid lipofuscinoses. *Epilepsia* 1999;40(Suppl 3):29–32.
823. Santavuori P, Haltia M, Rapola J. Infantile type of so-called neuronal ceroid-lipofuscinosis. *Dev Med Child Neurol* 1974;16:644–653.
824. Bateman JB, Philippart M. Ocular features of the Hagberg-Santavuori syndrome. *Am J Ophthalmol* 1986;102:262–271.
825. Harden A, Pampiglione G, Picton-Robinson N. Electroretinogram and visual evoked response in a form of "neuronal lipidosis" with diagnostic EEG features. *J Neurol Neurosurg Psychiatry* 1973;36:61–67.
826. Vanhanen SL, Puranen J, Autti T, et al. Neuroradiological findings (MRS, MRI, SPECT) in infantile neuronal ceroid-lipofuscinosis (infantile CLN1) at different stages of the disease. *Neuropediatrics* 2004;35:27–35.
827. Baumann RJ, Markesbery WR. Santavuori disease: diagnosis by leukocyte ultrastructure. *Neurology* 1982;32:1277–1281.
828. Zhong N, Wisniewski KE, Hartikainen J, et al. Two common mutations in the CLN2 gene underlie late infantile neuronal ceroid lipofuscinosis. *Clin Genet* 1998;54:234–238.
829. Steinfeld R, Steinke HB, Isbrandt D, et al. Mutations in classical late infantile neuronal ceroid lipofuscinosis disrupt transport of tripeptidyl-peptidase I to lysosomes. *Hum Mol Genet* 2004;13:2483–2491.
830. Pampiglione G, Harden A. So-called neuronal ceroid lipofuscinosis: neurophysiological studies in 60 children. *J Neurol Neurosurg Psychiat* 1977;40:323–330.
831. Seitz D, Grodd W, Schwab A, et al. MR imaging and localized proton MR spectroscopy in late infantile neuronal ceroid lipofuscinosis. *Am J Neuroradiol* 1998;19:1373–1377.
832. Palmer DN, Jolly RD, van Mil HC, et al. Different patterns of hydrophobic protein storage in different forms of neuronal ceroid lipofuscinosis (NCL, Batten disease). *Neuropediatrics* 1997;28:45–48.
833. Carpenter S, Karpati G, Andermann F, et al. The ultrastructural characteristics of the abnormal cytosomes in Batten-Kufs' disease. *Brain* 1977;100:137–156.
834. Farrell DF, Sumi SM. Skin punch biopsy in the diagnosis of juvenile neuronal ceroid-lipofuscinosis. *Arch Neurol* 1977;34:39–44.
835. Kurachi Y, Oka A, Mizuguchi M, et al. Rapid immunologic diagnosis of classic late infantile neuronal ceroid lipofuscinosis. *Neurology* 2000;54:1676–1680.
836. Santavuori P, Rapola J, Sainio K, et al. A variant of Jansky-Bielschowski disease. *Neuropediatrics* 1982;13:135–141.
837. Vesa J, Chin MH, Oelgeschlager K, et al. Neuronal ceroid lipofuscinoses are connected at molecular level: interaction of CLN5 protein with CLN2 and CLN3. *Mol Biol Cell* 2002;13:2410–2420.
838. Freud S. Ueber familiaere Formen von cerebralen Diplegien. *Neurol Zentralbl* 1893;12:512–515, 542–547.
839. Vogt H. Ueber familiaere amaurotische Idiotie und verwandte Krankheitsbilder. Monatsschr *Psychiat Neurol* 1905;18:161–171, 310–357.
840. Mole S, Gardner M. Molecular genetics of palmitoyl-proteinthioesterase deficiency in the U.S. *J Clin Invest* 1998;102: 361–370.
841. Järvelä I, Autti T, Lamminranta S, et al. Clinical and magnetic resonance imaging findings in Batten disease: analysis of the major mutation (1.02-kb deletion). *Ann Neurol* 1997;42:799–802.
841a. Goebel HH. The neuronal ceroid lipofuscinoses. *Semin Pediatr Neurol* 1996;3:270–278.
842. Aberg L, Liewendahl K, Nikkinen P, et al. Decreased striatal dopamine transporter density in JNCL patients with parkinsonian symptoms. *Neurology* 2000;14:1069–1074.
843. Ikeda K, Goebel HH. Ultrastructural pathology of human lymphocytes in lysosomal disorders: a contribution to their morphological diagnosis. *Eur J Pediatr* 1982;138:179–185.
843a. Kornfeld M. Generalized lipofuscinosis (generalized Kufs' disease). *J Neuropathol Exp Neurol* 1972;31:668–682.
844. Vesa J, Peltonen L. Mutated genes in juvenile and variant late infantile neuronal ceroid lipofuscinoses encode lysosomal proteins. *Curr Mol Med* 2002;2:439–444.
844a. Ramirez-Montealegre D, Chattopadhyah S, Churran T, et al. Autoimmunity to glutamic acid decarboxylase in the neurodegenerative disorder Batten disease. *Neurology* 2005;64:743–745.
844b. Lane SC, Jolly RD, Schmechel DE, et al. Apoptosis as the mechanism of neurodegeneration in Batten's disease. *J Neurochem* 1996;67:677–683.
844c. Persaud-Sawin D, McNamara JO, Rylova S, et al. A galactosylceramide binding domain is involved in trafficking of CLN3 from Golgi to rafts via recycling endosomes. *Pediatr Res* 2004;56:449–463.
845. Goebel HH, Zeman W, Pilz H. Significance of muscle biopsies in neuronal ceroid-lipofuscinoses. *J Neurol Neurosurg Psychiatry* 1975;38:985–993.
846. Bassen FA, Kornzweig AL. Malformation of erythrocytes in cases of atypical retinitis pigmentosa. *Blood* 1950;5:381–387.
847. Schwarz JF, et al. Bassen-Kornzweig syndrome: deficiency of serum β-lipoprotein. *Arch Neurol* 1963;8:438–454.
848. Kane JP, Havel RJ. Disorders in the biogenesis and secretion of lipoproteins containing the B apolipoproteins. In: Scriver CR, Beaudet AL, Sly WS, et al., eds. *The metabolic and molecular bases of inherited disease,* 8th ed. McGraw-Hill,New York, 2001:2717–2753.
849. Brin MF, Pedley TA, Lovelace RE, et al. Electrophysiologic features of abeta-lipoproteinemia: functional consequences of vitamin E deficiency. *Neurology* 1986;36:669–673.
850. Sobrevilla LA, Goodman ML, Kane CA. Demyelinating central nervous system disease, macular atrophy, and acanthocytosis (Bassen-Kornzweig syndrome). *Am J Med* 1964;37:821–832.
851. Lazaro RP, Dentinger MP, Rodichok LD, et al. Muscle pathology in Bassen-Kornzweig syndrome and vitamin E deficiency. *Am J Clin Pathol* 1986;86:378–387.
852. Blum CB, Deckelbaum RJ, Witte LD, et al. Role of apolipoprotein E-containing lipoproteins in abetalipoproteinemia. *J Clin Invest* 1982;70:1157–1169.
853. Malloy MJ, Kane JP. Lipoprotein disorders. In: Rosenberg RN, Prusiner SB, DiMauro S, et al., eds. *The molecular and genetic basis of neurologic and psychiatric disease,* 3rd ed. Philadelphia: Butterworth-Heinemann, 2003:555–564.
854. Ohashi K, Ishibashi S, Osuga J, et al. Novel mutations in the microscomal triglyceride transfer protein gene causing abetalipoproteinemia. *J Lipid Res* 2000;41:1199–1204.
855. Cellini E, Piacentini S, Nacmias B, et al. A family with spinocerebellar ataxia type 8 expansion and vitamin E deficiency ataxia. *Arch Neurol* 2002;59:1952–1953.
856. Muller DPR, Lloyd JK. Effect of large oral doses of vitamin E on the neurologic sequelae of patients with abeta-lipoproteinemia. *Ann N Y Acad Sci* 1982;393:133–144.
857. Fagan ER, Taylor MJ. Longitudinal multimodal evoked potential studies in abetalipoproteinemia. *Can J Neurol Sci* 1987;14:617–621.
858. Hardie RJ, Pullon HW, Harding AE, et al. Neuroacanthocytosis: a clinical, haematological and pathological study of 19 cases. *Brain* 1991;114:13–49.
859. Bird TD, Cederbaum S, Valey RW, et al. Familial degeneration of the basal ganglia with acanthocytosis: a clinical, neuropathological, and neurochemical study. *Ann Neurol* 1978;3:253–258.

860. Dobson-Stone C, Danek A, Rampoldi L, et al. Mutational spectrum of the CJAC gene in patients with chorea-acanthocytosis. *Eur J Hum Genet* 2002;10:773–781.
861. Engel WK, Dorman JD, Levy RI, et al. Neuropathy in Tangier disease. α-Lipoprotein deficiency manifesting as familial recurrent neuropathy and intestinal lipid storage. *Arch Neurol* 1967;17:19.
862. Thomas PK. Inherited neuropathies related to disorders of lipid metabolism. *Adv Neurol* 1988;48:133–144.
863. Zuchner S, Sperfeld AD, Senderek J, et al. A novel nonsense mutation in the ABC1 gene causes a severe syringomyelia-like phenotype of Tangier disease. *Brain* 2003;126:920–927.
864. Stefkova J, Poledne R, Hubacek JA. ATP-binding cassette (ABC) transporters in human metabolism and diseases. *Physiol Res* 2004;53:235–243.
865. Kayser B. Ueber einen Fall von angeborener grünlicher Verfärbung der Cornea. *Klin Monatsbl Augenheilkd* 1902;40:22–25.
866. Fleischer B. Über einer der "Pseudosklerose" nahestehende bisher unbekannte Krankheit (gekennzeichnet durch Tremor psychische Störungen, bräunliche Pigmentierung bestimmter Gewebe, insbesondere auch der Hornhautperipherie, Lebercirrhose). *Dtsch Z Nervenheilk* 1912;44:179–201.
867. Wilson SAK. Progressive lenticular degeneration: a familial nervous disease associated with cirrhosis of the liver. *Brain* 1912;34:295–509.
868. Menkes JH. Disorders of copper metabolism: Wilson disease and Menkes disease.Rosenberg RN, Prusiner SB, DiMauro S, et al., eds. *The molecular and genetic basis of neurologic and psychiatric disease,* 3rd ed. Philadelphia: Butterworth–Heinemann, 2003:687–692.
869. Vulpe CD, Packman S. Cellular copper transport. *Ann Rev Nutr* 1995;15:293–322.
870. Gitlin JD. Wilson disease. *Gastroenterology* 2003;125:1868–1877.
871. Tapia L, Gonzalez-Aguerre M, Cisternas MF, et al. Metallothionein is crucial for safe intracellular copper storage and cell survival at normal and supra-physiological exposure levels. *Biochem J* 2004;378:617–624.
872. Rumpel A. Über das Wesen und die Bedeutung der Leberveränderungen und der Pigmentierungen bei den damit verbundenen Fällen von Pseudosklerose, zugleich ein Beitrag zur Lehre der Pseudosklerose (Westphal-Strümpell). *Dtsch Z Nervenheilk* 1913;49:54–73.
873. Lüthy F. Über die hepato-lentikuläre Degeneration (Wilson-Westphal-Strümpell). *Dtsch Z Nervenheilk* 1931;123:101–181.
874. Glazebrook AJ. Wilson's disease. *Edinburgh Med J* 1945;52:83–87.
875. Mukhopadhyay CK, Attieh ZK, Fox PL. Role of ceruloplasmin in cellular iron uptake. *Science* 1998;279:714–716.
876. Gitlin JD. Aceruloplasminemia. *Pediatr Res* 1998;44:271–276.
877. Tanzi RE, Petrukhin K, Chernov I, et al. The Wilson's disease gene is a copper-transporting ATPase with homology to the Menkes disease gene. *Nat Genet* 1993;5:344–350.
877a. Harada M, Kawaguchi T, Kumemura H, et al. The Wilson disease protein ATPTB resides in the late endosomes with Rab7 and the Niemann-Pick C1 protein. *Am J Pathol* 2005;166:499–570.
878. Lutsenko S, Cooper MJ. Localization of the Wilson's disease protein product to mitochondria. *Proc Natl Acad Sci USA* 1998;95: 6004–6009.
879. Schaefer M, Hopkins RG, Failla ML, et al. Hepatocyte-specific localization and copper-dependant trafficking of the Wilson's disease protein in the liver. *Am J Physiol* 1999;276:G639–G646.
880. His G, Cox DW. A comparison of the mutation spectra of Menkes disease and Wilson disease. *Hum Genet* 2004;114:165–172.
881. Thomas GR, Forbes JR, Roberts EA, et al. The Wilson disease gene: spectrum of mutations and their consequence. *Nat Genet* 1995;9:210–217.
882. Frommer DJ. Defective biliary excretion of copper in Wilson's disease. *Gut* 1974;15:125–129.
883. Gu M, Cooper JM, Butler P, et al. Oxidative-phosphorylation defects in liver of patients with Wilson's disease. *Lancet* 2000; 356:469–474.
884. Sheline CT, Choi DW. Cu2+ toxicity inhibition of mitochondrial dehydrogenases *in vitro* and *in vivo*. *Ann Neurol* 2004;55:645–653.
885. Strohmeyer FW, Ishak, KG. Histology of the liver in Wilson's disease: a study of 34 cases. *Am J Clin Pathol* 1980;73:12–24.
886. Richter R. The pallial component in hepatolenticular degeneration. *J Neuropathol Exp Neurol* 1948;7:1–18.
887. Uzman LL, Jakus MA. The Kayser-Fleischer ring: a histochemical and electron microscope study. *Neurology* 1957;7:341–355.
888. Arima M, Takeshita K, Yoshino K, et al. Prognosis of Wilson's disease in childhood. *Eur J Pediatr* 1977;126:147–154.
889. Slovis TL, Dubois RS, Rodgerson DO, et al. The varied manifestations of Wilson's disease. *J Pediatr* 1971;78:578–584.
890. Scott J, Golan JL, Samourian S, et al. Wilson's disease, presenting as chronic active hepatitis. *Gastroenterology* 1978;74:645–651.
891. Werlin SL, Grand RJ, Perman JA, et al. Diagnostic dilemmas of Wilson's disease: diagnosis and treatment. *Pediatrics* 1978;62:47–51.
892. Kontaxakis V, Stefanis C, Markidis M, et al. Neuroleptic malignant syndrome in a patient with Wilson's disease [Letter]. *J Neurol Neurosurg Psychiatr* 1988;51:1001–1002.
893. Carlson MD, Al-Mateen M, Brewer GJ. Atypical childhood Wilson's disease. *Pediatr Neurol* 2004;30:57–60.
894. Hitoshi S, Iwata M, Yoshikawa K. Mid-brain pathology of Wilson's disease: MRI analysis of three cases. *J Neurol Neurosurg Psychiatr* 1991;54:624–626.
895. Prayer L, Wimberger D, Kramer J, et al. Cranial MRI in Wilson's disease. *Neuroradiology* 1990;32:211–214.
896. King AD, Walshe JM, Kendall BE, et al. Cranial MR imaging in Wilson's disease. *Am J Roentgenol* 1996;167:1579–1584.
897. Hawkins RA, Mazziotta JC, Phelps ME. Wilson's disease studied with FDG and positron emission tomography. *Neurology* 1987;37:1707–1711.
898. Walshe JM. Diagnosis and treatment of presymptomatic Wilson's disease. *Lancet* 1988;2:435–437.
899. Shah AB, Chernov I, Zhang HT, et al. Identification and analysis of mutation in the Wilson disease gene (ATP7B): population frequencies, genotype–phenotype correlation, and functional analyses. *Am J Hum Genet* 1997;61:317–328.
900. Brewer GJ, Yuzbasiyan-Gurkan V. Wilson's disease. *Am J Med* 1992; 71:139–164.
901. Brewer GJ. Practical recommendations and new therapies for Wilson's disease. *Drugs* 1995;50:240–249.
902. Emre S, Atillasoy EO, Ozdemir S, et al. Orthotopic liver transplantation for Wilson's disease: a single-center experience. *Transplantation* 2001;72:1232–1236.
902a. Schumacher G, Platz KP, Mueller AR, et al. Liver transplantation: treatment of choice for hepatic and neurological manifestations of Wilson's disease. *Clin Transplant* 1997;11:217–224.
903. Grimm G, Oder W, Prayer L, et al. Evoked potentials in assessment and follow-up of patients with Wilson's disease. *Lancet* 1990;336:963–964.
904. Mitchell AM, Heller GL. Changes in Kayser-Fleischer ring during treatment of hepatolenticular degeneration. *Arch Ophthalmol* 1968;80:622–631.
905. Walshe JM, Dixon AK. Dangers of non-compliance in Wilson's disease. *Lancet* 1986;1:845–847.
906. Scheinberg IH, Sternlieb I, Schilsky M, et al. Penicillamine may detoxify copper in Wilson's disease. *Lancet* 1987;2:95.
907. Miyajima M. Aceruloplasminemia, an iron metabolic disorder. *Neuropathology* 2003;23:345–350.
908. Menkes JH, Alter M, Weakley D, et al. A sex-linked recessive disorder with growth retardation, peculiar hair, and focal cerebral and cerebellar degeneration. *Pediatrics* 1962;29:764–779.
909. Danks DM, Campbell PE, Stevens BJ, et al. Menkes' kinky hair syndrome: an inherited defect in copper absorption with widespread effects. *Pediatrics* 1972;50:188–201.
910. Cox DW. Disorders of copper transport. *Br Med Bull* 1999;55:544–555.
911. Bucknall WE, Haslam RH, Holtzman NA. Kinky hair syndrome: response to copper therapy. *Pediatrics* 1973;52:653–657.
912. van den Berg GJ, Kroon JJ, Wijburg FA, et al. Muscle cell cultures in Menkes' disease: copper accumulation in myotubes. *J Inherit Metab Dis* 1990;13:207–211.
913. Vulpe C, Levinson B, Whitney S, et al. Isolation of a candidate gene for Menkes disease and evidence that it encodes a copper-transporting ATPase. *Nat Genet* 1993;3:7–13.

914. Harrison MD, Dameron CT. Molecular mechanisms of copper metabolism and the role of the Menkes disease protein. *J Biochem Mol Toxicol* 1999;13:93–106.
915. Andrews NC. Mining copper transport genes. *Proc Natl Acad Sci USA* 2001;98:6543–6545.
916. Goodyer ID, Jones EE, Monaco AP, et al. Characterization of the Menkes protein copper-binding domains and their role in copper-induced protein relocalization. *Hum Mol Genet* 1999;8:1473–1478.
917. Cobbold C, Coventry J, Ponnambalam S, et al. The Menkes disease ATPase (ATP7A) is internalized via a Rac-1 regulated, clathrin and caveolae-independent pathway. *Hum Mol Genet* 2003;12:1523–1533.
918. Moller LB, Tumer Z, Lund C, et al. Similar splice-site mutations of the ATP7A gene lead to different phenotypes: classical Menkes disease or occipital horn syndrome. *Am J Hum Genet* 2000;66:1211–1220.
919. Hirano A, Liena JF, French JH, et al. Fine structure of the cerebellar cortex in Menkes kinky-hair disease X-chromosome-linked copper malabsorption. *Arch Neurol* 1977;34:52–56.
920. Tnnesen T, Kleijer WJ, Horn N. Incidence of Menkes disease. *Hum Genet* 1991;86:408–410.
921. Baerlocher K, Nadal D. Das Menkes-Syndrom. *Ergeb Inn Mediz* 1988;57:79–144.
922. Grover WD, Johnson WC, Henkin RI. Clinical and biochemical aspects of trichopoliodystrophy. *Ann Neurol* 1979;5:65–71.
923. Seelenfreund MH, Gartner S, Vinger PE. The ocular pathology of Menkes' disease. *Arch Ophthalmol* 1968;80:718–720.
924. Wesenberg RL, Gwinn JL, Barnes GR. Radiologic findings in the kinky hair syndrome. *Radiology* 1968;92:500–506.
925. Wheeler EM, Roberts PF. Menke's steely hair syndrome. *Arch Dis Child* 1976;51:269–274.
926. Hsich GE, Robertson RL, Irons M, et al. Cerebral infarction in Menkes' disease. *Pediatr Neurol* 2000;23:425–428.
927. Kim OH, Suh JH. Intracranial and extracranial MR angiography in Menkes disease. *Pediatr Radiol* 1997;27:782–784.
928. Ubhi T, Reece A, Craig A. Congenital skull fracture as a presentation of Menkes disease. *Dev Med Child Neurol* 2000;42:347–348.
929. Menkes, JH. Subdural haematoma, non-accidental head injury or...? *Eur J Paediatr Neurol* 2001;5:175–176.
930. Ferreira RC, Heckenlively JR, Menkes JH, et al. Menkes disease. New ocular and electroretinographic findings. *Ophthalmology* 1998;105:1076–1078.
931. Borm B, Moller LB, Hausser I, et al. Variable clinical expression of an identical mutation in the ATP7A gene for Menkes disease/occipital horn syndrome in three affected males in a single family. *J Pediatr* 2004;145:119–121.
932. Tumer Z, Bir Moller L, Horn N. Screening of 383 unrelated patients affected with Menkes disease and finding of 57 gross deletions in *ATP7A*. *Hum Mutat* 2003;22:457–464.
933. Proud VK, Mussell HG, Kaler SG, et al. Distinctive Menkes disease variant with occipital horns: delineation of natural history and clinical phenotypes. *Am J Med Genet* 1996;65:44–51.
934. Palmer CA, Percy AK. Neuropathology of occipital horn syndrome. *J Child Neurol* 2001;16:764–766.
935. Dagenais SL, Adam AN, Innis JW, et al. A novel frameshift mutation in exon 23 of *ATP7A* (MNK) results in occipital horn syndrome and not in Menkes disease. *Am J Hum Genet* 2001;69:420–427.
936. Tümer Z, Horn N. Menkes disease: recent advance and new aspects. *J Med Genet* 1997;34:265–274.
937. Kapur S, Higgins JV, Delp K, et al. Menkes' syndrome in a girl with X-autosome translocation. *Am J Hum Genet* 1987;26:503–510.
938. Stefanini M, Vermeulen W, Weeda G, et al. A new nucleotide-excision-repair gene associated with the disorder trichothiodystrophy. *Am J Hum Genet* 1993;3:817–821.
939. Giglia-Mari G, Coin F, Ranish JA, et al. A new, tenth subunit of TFIIH is responsible for the DNA repair syndrome trichothiodystrophy group A. *Nat Genet* 2004;36:714–719.
940. Whiting DA. Structural abnormalities of the hair shaft. *J Am Acad Dermatol* 1987;16:1–25.
941. Christodoulou J, Danks DM, Sarkar B, et al. Early treatment of Menkes disease with parenteral copper-histidine: long-term follow-up of four treated patients. *Am J Med Genet* 1998;76:154–164.
942. Reis J, Johnson JL. Mutations in the molybdenum cofactor biosynthetic genes *MOCS1*, *MOCS2*, and *GEPH*. *Hum Mutat* 2003;21:569–576.
943. Reiss J, Gross-Hardt S, Christensen E, et al. A mutation in the gene for the neurotransmitter receptor-clustering protein gephyrin causes a novel form of molybdenum cofactor deficiency. *Am J Hum Genet* 2001;68:208–213.
944. Slot HMJ, Overweg-Plandsoen WC, Bakker HD, et al. Molybdenumcofactor deficiency: an easily missed cause of neonatal convulsions. *Neuropediatrics* 1993;24:139–142.
945. Koch H. Dipsticks and convulsions. *Lancet* 1998;352:1824.
946. Boles RG, Ment LR, Meyn MS, et al. Short-term response to dietary therapy in molybdenum cofactor deficiency. *Ann Neurol* 1993;34:742–744.
947. Rupar CA, Gillett J, Gordon BA, et al. Isolated sulfite oxidase deficiency. *Neuropediatrics* 1996;27:299–304.
948. Garrett RM, Johnson JL, Graf TN, et al. Human sulfite oxidase R160Q; identification of the mutation in a sulfite oxidase-deficient patient and expression and characterization of the mutant enzyme. *Proc Natl Acad Sci USA* 1998;95:6394–6398.
949. Topcu M, Coskun T, Haliloglu G, et al. Molybdenum cofactor deficiency: report of three cases presenting as hypoxic-ischemic encephalopathy. *J Child Neurol* 2001;16:264–270.
950. Touati G, Rusthoven E, Depondt E, et al. Dietary therapy in two patients with a mild form of sulphite oxidase defieincy. Evidence for clinical and biological improvement. *J Inherit Metab Dis* 2000;23:45–53.
951. Catel W, Schmidt J. Über familiäre gichtische Diathese in Verbindung mit zerebralen und renalen Symptomen bei einem Kleinkind. *Dtsch Med Wochenschr* 1959;84:2145–2147.
952. Lesch M, Nyhan WL. A familial disorder of uric acid metabolism and central nervous system function. *Am J Med* 1964;36:561–570.
953. Nyhan WL.Purines In: Rosenberg RN,Prusiner SB,DiMauro S, et al., eds. *The molecular and genetic basis of neurologic and psychiatric disease,* 3rd ed. Philadelphia: Butterworth–Heinemann, 2003:657–662.
954. Seegmiller JE. Contributions of Lesch-Nyhan syndrome to the understanding of purine metabolism. *J Inherit Metab Dis* 1989;12:184–196.
955. Wong DF, Harris JC, Naidu S, et al. Dopamine transporters are markedly reduced in Lesch-Nyhan disease *in vivo*. *Proc Natl Acad Sci USA* 1996;93:5539–5543.
956. Jankovic J, Caskey TC, Stout JT, et al. Lesch-Nyhan syndrome: a study of motor behavior and cerebrospinal fluid neurotransmitters. *Ann Neurol* 1988;23:466–469.
957. Torres RJ, Deantonio I, Prior C, et al. Adenosine transport in peripheral blood lymphocytes from Lesch-Nyhan patients. *Biochem J* 2004;377:733–739.
958. Garcia-Gil M, Pesi R, Perna S, et al. 5′-Aminoimidazole-4-carboxamide riboside induces apoptosis in human neuroblastoma cells. *Neuroscience* 2003;117:811–820.
959. Watts RW, Spellacy E, Gibbs DA, et al. Clinical, postmortem, biochemical and therapeutic observations on the Lesch-Nyhan syndrome with particular reference to the neurological manifestations. *Q J Med* 1982;201:43–78.
960. Matthews WS, Solan A, Barabas G. Cognitive functioning in Lesch-Nyhan syndrome. *Dev Med Child Neurol* 1995;37:715–722.
961. Kelley WN, Greene ML, Rosenbloom FM, et al. Hypoxanthine-guanine phosphoribosyl transferase deficiency in gout. *Ann Intern Med* 1969;70:155–206.
962. Page T, Nyhan WL, Morena de Vega V. Syndrome of mild mental retardation, spastic gait, and skeletal malformations in a family with partial deficiency of hypoxanthine-guanine phosphoribosyl transferase. *Pediatrics* 1987;79:713–717.
963. Page T, Broock RL, Nyhan WL, et al. Use of selective media for distinguishing variant forms of hypoxanthine phosphoribosyl transferase. *Clin Chim Acta* 1986;154:195–201.
964. Harris JC, Lee RR, Jinnah HA, et al. Craniocerebral magnetic resonance imaging measurement and findings in Lesch-Nyhan syndrome. *Arch Neurol* 1998;55:547–553.

965. Becker MA, Puig JG, Mateos FA, et al. Inherited superactivity of phosphoribosylpyrophosphate synthetase: association of uric acid overproduction and sensorineural deafness. *Am J Med* 1988;85:383–390.
966. Castro M, Perez-Cerda C, Merinero B, et al. Screening for adenylsuccinate lyase deficiency: clinical, biochemical and molecular findings in four patients. *Neuropediatrics* 2002;33:186–189.
967. Edery P, Chabrier S, Caballos-Picot I, et al. Intrafamilial variability in the phenotypic expression of adenylosuccinate lyase deficiency: a report on three patients. *Am J Med Genet* 2003;120A:185–190.
968. Laikind PK, Seegmiller JE, Grober HE. Detection of 5′-phosphoribosyl-4-(*N*-succinylcarboxamide)-5-aminoimidazole in urine by use of the Bratton-Marshall reaction: identification of patients deficient in adenylosuccinate lyase activity. *Anal Biochem* 1986;156:81–90.
969. Taira T, Kobayashi T, Hori T. Disappearance of self-mutilating behavior in a patient with Lesh-Nyhan syndrome after bilateral chronic stimulation of the globus pallidus internus. Case report. *J Neurosurg* 2003;98:414–416.
970. Diasio RB, Beavers TL, Carpenter JT. Familial deficiency of dihydropyrimidine dehydrogenase: biochemical basis for familial pyrimidinemia and severe 5-fluorouracil–induced toxicity. *J Clin Invest* 1988;81:47–51.
971. Van Kuilenburg AB, Vreken P, Abeling NG, et al. Genotype and phenotype in patients with dihydropyrimidine dehydrogenase deficiency. *Hum Genet* 1999;104:1–9.
972. Schulze A, Hess T, Wevers R, et al. Creatine deficiency syndrome caused by guanidinoacetate methyltransferase deficiency: diagnostic tools for a new inborn error of metabolism. *J Pediatr* 1997;131:626–631.
973. Hultdin J, Schnauch A, Wikberg A, et al. Acute intermittent porphyria in childhood: a population based study. *Acta Paediatr* 2003;92:562–568.
973a. Kauppinen R. Porphyrias. *Lancet* 2005;365:241–252.
974. Barclay N. Acute intermittent porphyria in childhood. A neglected diagnosis? *Arch Dis Child* 1974;49:404–406.
975. Bissell DM. The porphyrias. In: Rosenberg RN, Prusiner SB, DiMauro S, et al., eds. *The molecular and genetic basis of neurologic and psychiatric disease,* 3rd ed. Philadelphia: Butterworth–Heinemann, 2003:663–678.
976. McDonagh AF, Bissell DM. Porphyria and porphyrinology—the past fifteen years. *Semin Liver Dis* 1998;18:3–15.
977. Kushner JP. Laboratory diagnosis of the porphyrias. *N Engl J Med* 1991;324:1432–1434.
978. Palacin M, Bertran J, Chillaron J, et al. Lysinuric protein intolerance: mechanisms of pathophysiology. *Mol Genet Metab* 2004;81(Suppl 1):S27–S37.

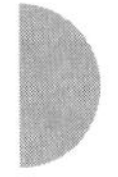

Chapter 2

Mitochondrial Encephalomyopathies

Harvey B. Sarnat and John H. Menkes

> Mitochondrial disease may cause
> any symptom
> in any tissue
> at any age
> by any inheritance.
> *A. Munnich*

The above definition of mitochondrial diseases summarizes the clinician's dilemma in diagnosing this most ubiquitous of metabolic disorders, with pathogenic mitochondrial DNA mutations being found in at least 1 in 8,000 individuals (1). Nevertheless, there are some patterns of specific mitochondrial syndromes that can be recognized at least enough to justify the extensive laboratory investigations required for confirmation. Because mitochondria are essential organelles of nearly all cells, with the exception of mature erythrocytes, mitochondrial diseases may affect any organ system and for this reason are now termed *mitochondrial cytopathies*. The most frequently affected organs are striated muscle, central nervous system, and heart. Diagnostic changes may be demonstrated in striated muscle even in patients who do not overtly manifest myopathic symptoms and signs; hence the muscle biopsy can be valuable diagnostic procedure.

ORIGIN OF MITOCHONDRIA

Mitochondria were free-living independent organisms with their own unique DNA and membranes about 2 billion years ago, when they developed a symbiotic relationship with the evolving proeukaryocytes, and the two have lived more or less harmoniously as eukaryotic cells ever since. The cell depends on its mitochondria for the generation of oxidative enzymes of aerobic energy production, and the mitochondria depend upon the cell's nuclear DNA to provide the majority of the subunits for its respiratory chain complexes.

HISTORY OF DISCOVERY OF MITOCHONDRIA AND DISEASES OF THE ORGANELLE

The first probable human visualization of mitochondria was in 1841, when intracellular granules were described using the crude optics of early microscopes. In 1890 Altmann (2) recognized the ubiquitous nature of "bioblasts" as elementary organs living in cells, and in 1898 Benda named the organelle the "mitochondrion" (3). The ultrastructure of mitochondria was described in 1952 by Palade (4), and mitochondrial DNA (mtDNA) was defined by Nass and Nass in 1963 (5). Luft was the first to describe a mitochondrial disease in 1962, deciphering a deficit in oxidative phosphorylation in a patient with a now rare disease (6). Ragged-red fibers were described in the muscle biopsy and recognized as associated with mitochondrial disorders in 1963 by Engel and Cunningham (7). In the early 1970s, several disorders of brain and muscle involving deficiencies in respiratory chain enzymes were described, and in 1973, DiMauro and DiMauro provided the first examples of myopathies due to isolated deficiencies of muscle carnitine and carnitine palmitoyltransferase (8). By 1981, the complete genomic sequence of human mtDNA was documented (9). In 1984 phenotype–genotype correlations were being made by Pavlakis et al. (10), and the concept of mitochondrial syndromes was founded. In 1988, major advances occurred with the description by Holt et al. (11) of human encephalomyopathies associated with large deletions of mtDNA and the description by Wallace et al. (12) of Leber hereditary optic neuritis as due to a point mutation at nucleoprotein (np)11778 in mtDNA, a clinical disorder subsequently shown to be a syndrome associated with several additional mtDNA point mutations in other patients, as is the case with most mitochondrial disorders. Hundreds of point mutations or deletions of mtDNA have been described since 1990, and new genetic varieties are continuously being discovered. Mitochondrial diseases also can result from mutations in the nDNA that encodes respiratory chain subunits or parts of mitochondrial membranes, even with a normal mtDNA genome. In 2003, Servidei showed that large-scale mtDNA rearrangements, rather than mtDNA deletions or point mutations, are the basis of some mitochondrial diseases (13). Nearly all of the distinctive clinical and pathologic patterns of mitochondrial diseases were initially thought to be singular diseases but now are recognized as syndromes in which the same phenotype can be produced by multiple mitochondrial genotypes.

FUNCTIONS OF MITOCHONDRIA

The biochemical aspects of mitochondrial structure and function are reviewed more extensively by Lodish et al. (14) and Schapira (15). The primary function of mitochondria is to generate the high-energy phosphate bond in ATP by phosphorylation of adenosine diphosphate (ADP). The energy required for this reaction is derived from oxidation of the metabolic products of carbohydrates, fatty acids, and proteins. These processes of energy generation are collectively referred to as *oxidative phosphorylation*. Energy production is the only function of mitochondrial DNA; unlike the nuclear DNA of the cell, mtDNA does not determine any features of anatomic structure of the body, growth, or tissue differentiation.

Mitochondrial oxidative phosphorylation involves electron transport among five respiratory chains of enzymes, termed *respiratory complexes*. Complex I is nicotinamide adenine dinucleotide diaphorase; complex II is succinate dehydrogenase; complex III is ubiquinone or cytochrome *b* oxidase; complex IV is cytochrome *c* oxidase; complex V is ATP synthase. Coenzyme Q10 helps to mediate transport from complex I to complexes III and IV.

Pyruvate dehydrogenase is one of the most complex enzymes known, with a molecular weight of greater than 7 million. It contains multiple subunits of three catalytic enzymes (E_1, E_2, and E_3), two regulatory polypeptides, and five different coenzymes. The pyruvate dehydrogenase complex mediates the oxidation of pyruvate to acetyl coenzyme A to carbon dioxide, to generate reduced electron carriers through a series of nine reactions, carried out within the mitochondrial matrix by the citric acid cycle of Krebs. These reactions are carried out on the inner mitochondrial membrane by the electron transport chain, a set of electron carriers grouped into five multienzyme complexes. The free energy released during oxidation is stored in an electrochemical proton gradient across the inner mitochondrial membrane. The movement of protons back across the mitochondrial membrane is then coupled with the synthesis of ATP from ADP and phosphate. Coenzyme Q10 subserves the transport of electrons from complex I to complexes III and IV.

Transport of free fatty acids into mitochondria as fuel is mediated by carnitine. Within the mitochondria, the fatty acids are uncoupled from carnitine, a carrier molecule, and react with coenzyme A (CoA) to form an acyl-CoA. By a series of four sequential reactions (beta-oxidation), each molecule of acyl-CoA is oxidized to form one molecule of acetyl-CoA and an acyl-CoA shortened by two carbon atoms. Because most defects of beta-oxidation present with organicaciduria, these conditions are considered in Chapter 1 in the section dealing with organic acidurias. Amino acids are oxidized within the mitochondria; after transamination to their respective ketoacids, the amino acids alanine, aspartic acid, and glutamic acid enter the citric acid cycle.

In addition to its principal function in energy metabolism, mtDNA has additional functions during development. It is important for neuroblast polarity by modulating calcium homeostasis in microtubules and also regulates the *bcl2* gene for apoptosis. Damage to mtDNA and loss of the mitochondrial membrane potential are demonstrated in apoptotic cell death (16).

GENETICS OF MITOCHONDRIAL STRUCTURE AND DISEASES

The genetics of mitochondrial cytopathies is complex. The mitochondrion has its own DNA (mtDNA) on a single, circular chromosome of about 16.5 kilobases (kb). The mtDNA has an intimate relation with the cell's nuclear DNA (nDNA), and for each of the five respiratory complexes, the majority of the subunits are encoded by nDNA, not mtDNA. Complex I consists of 41 subunits, of which only 7 are encoded in the mtDNA; the other 34 are encoded in the nDNA. Complex II has only 4 subunits, all of which are encoded in nDNA. Complex III has 10 subunits, 1 encoded by mtDNA and 9 by nDNA. Complex IV has 13 subunits, 3 encoded by mtDNA and 10 by nDNA. Complex V has 12 subunits, 2 encoded by mtDNA and 10 by nDNA. The nDNA encodes the vast majority of the mitochondrial proteins, including all proteins present in the outer membrane and the matrix. The respiratory complexes are located on the inner membrane.

Because in the formation of the zygote, almost all mitochondria are contributed by the ovum, mtDNA is maternally inherited (17). Maternal inheritance appears to be operative in a small but significant proportion of inherited mitochondrial diseases; in the remainder transmission is as an autosomal recessive trait or is sporadic or unpredictable (18). Because the nuclear genome contributes subunits to the respiratory complexes, some mitochondrial diseases may follow a Mendelian pattern of inheritance, in which the metabolic defect is due to defective subunits encoded by mutation in nDNA, with preservation of normal mtDNA. Inheritance in these mutations is nearly always autosomal recessive. Some cases of Leigh encephalopathy provide a good example of this phenomenon. Nine different genetic defects have been documented in this syndrome, five of which involve mtDNA and four of which involve nDNA. If a point mutation in mtDNA is involved, the obligatory transmission is maternal, though not involving the X chromosome of nDNA.

Homoplasmy refers to the situation in which all mtDNA molecules within the cell are identical, the normal condition. If mutations in mtDNA occur, two populations of mtDNA then coexist, the *heteroplasmic* condition. Most pathogenic mtDNA mutations are *heteroplasmic*. In this situation the ratio of normal to abnormal mtDNA determines the clinical expression as well as the severity of the mitochondrial disease. A 100% abnormal mtDNA is incompatible with life. Differences in this ratio of heteroplasmy among cells in different organs determine the clinical expression in each organ system. Heteroplasmy may occur not only at the level of the cell, but also at the level of the individual mitochondrion, *intramitochondrial heteroplasmy*.

At the time of cell division, mitochondria and mtDNA are randomly partitioned into the two daughter cells, *mitotic segregation*. The proportion of normal and abnormal mtDNA inherited by each daughter cell is not necessarily equal, and a *threshold effect* of mtDNA mutation may influence clinical expression including age of onset of symptoms (19).

As an example of heteroplasmy, in the nucleotide (nt)-8993 T→C mutation that substitutes leucine for arginine, if less than 70% of the mtDNA shows this point mutation, the patient has the NARP (nystagmus, ataxia, and retinitis pigmentosa) syndrome; if the mutation involves 90% or more, the patient presents with Leigh encephalopathy. Between 70% and 90% mutated mtDNA produces mixed or variable clinical expression.

Another class of mtDNA abnormalities is large-scale mtDNA rearrangements, such as kilobase deletions of the mitochondrial chromosome. Patients may harbor a 5- or 7.5-kb mtDNA deletion (the most common varieties), with striking differences in the proportion of deleted mtDNA molecules within the total mtDNA population. Sometimes as little as 2% mitochondria with significant deletions may be enough to render the individual symptomatic. High levels of these large-scale mtDNA deletions frequently occur in patients with Kearns-Sayre and PEO (progressive external ophthalmoplegia) syndromes (20). Approximately one-third of Kearns-Sayre patients harbor the same kind of mtDNA deletion, often designated *the common 5-kb deletion*, but occasional patients with Kearns-Sayre syndrome have larger, 11-kb deletions, with correspondingly more severe neurologic, muscular, and cardiac manifestations (21,22).

Many of the common point mutations are now known, particularly in mitochondrial myopathies with ragged-red fibers, in mitochondrial cardiomyopathies, and in some mitochondrial encephalopathies, especially Leigh encephalopathy, but new mutations are published weekly in this rapidly expanding field of genetics. A table summarizing the known mtDNA point mutations and deletions in mitochondrial encephalomyopathies is updated quarterly in the journal *Neuromuscular Disorders* (23). Many mitochondrial point mutations are expressed in both striated muscle and central nervous system (CNS). For example, Kearns-Sayre syndrome is clinically mainly a myopathy but also involves the visual system of the brain, demonstrated during life by abnormally slow visual-evoked potentials.

Most genetic laboratories that study mtDNA employ batteries of several point mutations that they screen for the common, well-documented mutations, but cannot test the entire mitochondrial genome. At times, point mutations are found in nucleotide sequences that are not evolutionarily conserved, do not specify highly conserved amino acid residues, and/or are not associated with an amino acid substitution. The interpretation of such defects or polymorphic variants, in the context of clinical and pathologic presentation, often is problematic and uncertain.

CLINICAL SYNDROMES OF MITOCHONDRIAL CYTOPATHIES

Because mitochondria are present in almost every cell, the wide variety of clinical presentations is not surprising. Mitochondrial disorders can be initially classified by clinical criteria in accordance with the organ systems most affected. One principle of mitochondrial diseases in general is that rarely is only one organ affected, and the clinical involvement of multiple organ systems is an important feature that allows the clinician to suspect a mitochondrial disease. The combination of symptoms and signs referable to the central and/or peripheral nervous system and striated muscle is the most frequent. Clinical manifestations are extremely variable, even with a known pathogenic point mutation and even among affected members of the same family. Phenotype–genotype correlations often are poor for the clinical identification of specific mtDNA point mutations or at times for specific mitochondrial syndromes (24–26). Multiple genotypes of both mtDNA and nDNA defects may produce similar clinical and pathologic presentations, hence the common patterns of mitochondrial disorders and syndromes.

Each of the mitochondrial syndromes has some constant clinical features that raise suspicion of the diagnosis and justify investigations to confirm or refute this provisional diagnosis. For instance, some patients fit a classical clinical and pathologic phenotype for MELAS (mitochondrial encephalopathy with lactic acidosis and strokelike episodes) but have an mtDNA point mutation that is more typical for MERRF (myoclonic epilepsy with ragged-red fibers), or they show a mixed MELAS/MERRF phenotype (27,28) or MERRF/Kearns-Sayre phenotype (29). Many mitochondrial cytopathies cannot be classified under a single clinical eponym.

Because each of the mitochondrial syndromes may be a similar clinical expression of multiple genetic defects, and the ratio of normal to abnormal mitochondria is variable between different patients even in the same family and between different organs, the phenotype–genotype correlations often are poor. Myopathology–genotype correlations are somewhat more reliable, but even the muscle biopsy does not always predict the precise genetic mutation.

The neurologic manifestations of mitochondrial diseases are many, but the most common in infancy are seizures, including infantile spasms and myoclonic epilepsy, visual impairment, deafness, central dysphagia, apnea and respiratory failure, diffuse muscular hypotonia, and global developmental delay. In older children and young adults, neurologic deficits include dystonia, cerebellar deficits, spastic diplegia, memory loss, cognitive deficits, progressive hearing loss, dementia, and autism. Regression and loss of skills may be seen as with any neurodegenerative disease. Peripheral neuropathy also occurs in mitochondrial disease and may contribute to the hypotonia and weakness. Because extraocular muscles have more mitochondria per unit volume of tissue than do most other muscles, they often are involved and produce progressive external ophthalmoplegia of all six muscles. Respiratory insufficiency may result from myopathic involvement or from central respiratory failure or a combination.

Lactic acidosis is a prominent feature of many mitochondrial diseases but not all. It is universally present in MELAS syndrome and helps to define this entity but is not present in MERRF and Kearns-Sayre syndromes. It is present in most cases of Leigh encephalopathy but not all; lactic acidosis is more likely in those cases with mtDNA mutations than in cases with nDNA defects. In some patients, the serum lactate may be normal but cerebrospinal fluid (CSF) lactate is elevated. When drawing serum lactate levels, it is important to also measure pyruvate. The most common cause of high serum lactate is that the tourniquet has been left on the arm too long while searching for a good vein; the resulting acute anaerobic state causes pyruvate to become converted to lactate; hence the lactate is high but the pyruvate is very low. In mitochondrial cytopathies, by contrast, if the lactate is elevated, the pyruvate is normal or also high (30). Simultaneous measurement of serum pyruvate will thus remove all doubt about whether an elevated lactate is merely a biological artifact. Other differential diagnoses of high serum lactate are shown in Table 2.1.

Imaging of the brain is an important diagnostic study in patients with mitochondrial cytopathy involving encephalopathy. Characteristic lesions may be seen with both computed tomography (CT) and magnetic resonance imaging (MRI) in the regions of the basal ganglia in particular (Fig. 2.1).

TABLE 2.1 Conditions Producing Lactic Acidosis in Infancy and Childhood

Pyruvate Dehydrogenase Complex
Pyruvate decarboxylase (E_1)
Dihydrolipoamide acetyltransferase (E_2)
Dihydrolipoamide dehydrogenase (E_3)
Pyruvate Dehydrogenase Phosphatase
Pyruvate decarboxylase activator
Gluconeogenesis
Glucose-6-phosphatase (glycogen storage disease type I)
Fructose-1,6-diphosphatase
Pyruvate carboxylase
Carboxylase Defects
Propionyl-CoA carboxylase
3-Methylcrotonyl-CoA carboxylase
Multiple carboxylase deficiency
Organic Acidurias
Glutaric aciduria I
Glutaric aciduria II
Phosphoenolpyruvate carboxykinase deficiency
Nongenetic Causes
Sepsis
Circulatory failure, shock, hypoxia
Short-bowel syndrome
Urinary tract infection caused by *Enterobacter cloacae* (a lactic acid–producing organism)
Seizures
Reye syndrome
Salicylate poisoning
Liver failure
Administration of intravenous glucose in newborns
Bacterial meningitis (cerebrospinal fluid lactic acid)

Mitochondrial syndromes can be broadly divided into two large categories: those in which the muscle biopsy exhibits ragged-red fibers and those that show many other features of mitochondrial myopathy but not ragged-red fibers. Ragged-red fibers are muscle fibers seen in frozen section and stained with modified Gomori trichrome stain that show irregularly shaped, bright red deposits in the subsarcolemmal and intermyofibrillar sarcoplasm, contrasting with the green myofibrils. The red color with this histochemical stain is derived from the strongly lipophilic chromotrope-2R in the stain, which has a particularly strong affinity for phospholipids; mitochondrial membranes contain a large amount of the phospholipid *sphingomyelin*. Electron microscopic examination of the ragged-red zone reveals large numbers of closely packed normal and abnormal mitochondria.

A majority of adults presenting clinically with mitochondrial cytopathy have a ragged-red fiber syndrome with combined complex I and IV deficiencies, whereas most infants and children symptomatic with mitochondrial

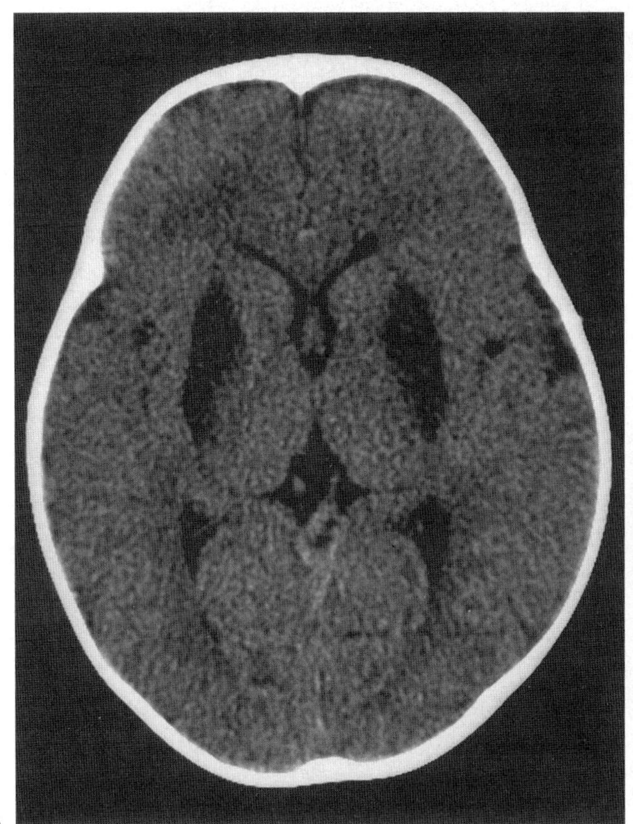

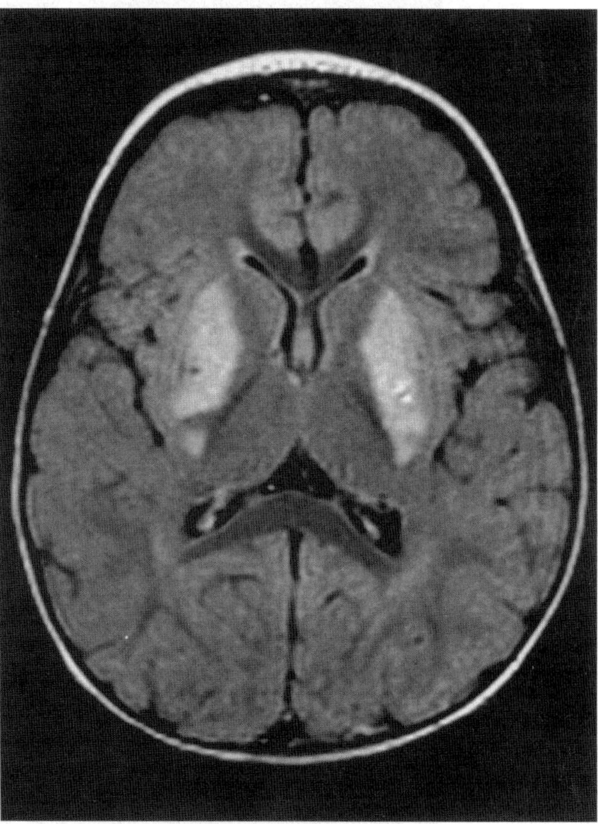

FIGURE 2.1. Imaging of a 21-month-old girl with Leigh encephalopathy. **A:** Computed axial tomography shows symmetric hypodense areas in the region of basal ganglia. **B:** Magnetic resonance imaging-T2 FLAIR (fluid attenuation inversion recovery) reveals high signal intensity in the same region. This is a characteristic finding in many mitochondrial diseases with many types of mutations in mtDNA. The muscle biopsy of this child showed no ragged-red fibers but many fibers deficient in cytochrome *c* oxidase and subsarcolemmal crescents of intense oxidative activity. She had quantitative defects in respiratory chains I, III, and V, but known mtDNA mutations could not be demonstrated.

disease do not have this combination, hence the designation non–ragged-red fiber syndromes. A common combination defect in early childhood is one of complexes III and V, which is unusual in adults (31). Infants with complex I and IV defects may not show ragged-red fibers histologically by trichrome stain until 3 years of age or older; hence this marker is not entirely reliable in infant muscle biopsies.

RAGGED-RED FIBER MITOCHONDRIAL SYNDROMES

MELAS (Mitochondrial Encephalopathy with Lactic Acidosis and Strokelike Episodes)

First described by Pavlakis et al. (10), the clinical onset of this disorder usually is in late childhood or early adult life, but it can present even in infancy. In more than 60% of patients symptoms appear before 15 years of age (32,33). Neurologic deficits are transient ischemic episodes and permanent cerebral infarcts and are referable to vessels as large as the middle cerebral artery or as small as arterioles producing multiple microinfarcts in the brain. The cerebral cortex and subcortical white matter is most frequently involved, particularly in the parieto-occipital region, but the thalamus, corpus striatum, globus pallidus, brainstem, and cerebellum also may be affected with similar lesions. Though all patients with MELAS have strokes, they are not always the initial symptoms. Migrainous headaches, vomiting, seizures, deafness, and focal neurologic deficits are frequent presentations, and some patients suffer progressive dementia (34). The occipital lesions may lead to hemianopia or to cortical blindness. Though muscle is involved pathologically with ragged-red fibers, weakness, myalgias, and other neuromuscular symptoms and signs rarely are evident. Retinitis pigmentosa and cardiomyopathy occur rarely.

The reason for the strokes is the high mutation load of the mtDNA in endothelial cells of cerebral vessels, which leads to deficient pinocytotic vesicles, endothelial swelling, and vascular occlusion.

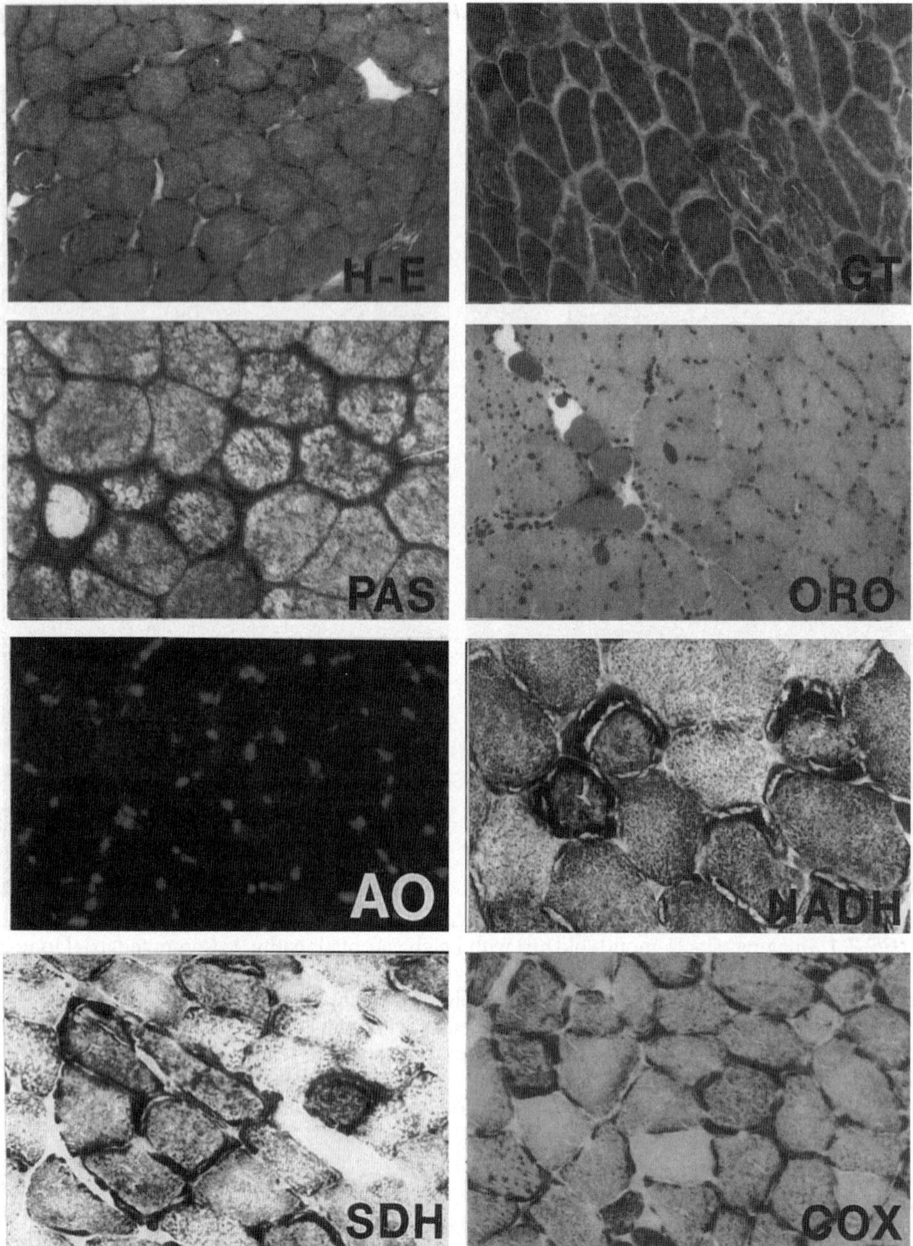

FIGURE 2.2. Quadriceps femoris muscle biopsy of a young woman with right spastic hemiplegia since infancy due to a large left middle cerebral artery infarct and porencephaly. She also has several smaller cerebral infarcts bilaterally, demonstrated by magnetic resonance imaging. She has acquired microcephaly, persistent lactic acidosis, and generalized weakness that has progressed over the last 2 years, hence the muscle biopsy at this time. The clinical diagnosis is MELAS (mitochondrial encephalopathy with lactic acidosis and strokelike episodes) syndrome. Hematoxylin-eosin (H-E) stain shows variation in myofiber diameter and several fibers with basophilic sarcoplasmic masses, corresponding to ragged-red fibers clearly identified with modified Gomori trichrome (GT) stain because these subsarcolemmal zones are irregular in shape and intensely red in color, whereas the normal myofibrils are green. Glycogen is abundantly stained (p-aminosalicylic acid, PAS) in these subsarcolemmal masses and is digested by diastase (not shown); one fiber shows loss of PAS staining except for its ragged-red margins. Neutral lipid, demonstrated by oil red O (ORO), is not increased within myofibers but is globular in the perimysium. Acridine orange (AO) fluorochrome shows no orange-red fluorescence in the ragged-red zones or within myofibrils. The oxidative enzymatic stains nicotinamide adenine dinucleotide (NADH), succinate dehydrogenase (SDH), and cytochrome *c* oxidase (COX) all exhibit intense mitochondrial enzymatic activity in the subsarcolemmal zones corresponding to ragged-red fibers. Two myofibers show no COX activity and a few others show weak activity, strong evidence of a mitochondrial defect, though nonspecific for which mitochondrial disease. Frozen sections. ×250 (H-E, GT, ORO, AO), ×400 (PAS, NADH, SDH, COX). From a color plate in Sarnat HB, Marín-García J. Pathology of mitochondrial encephalomyopathies. *Can J Neurol Sci* 2005;32:152–166. With permission of the *Canadian Journal of Neurological Sciences*.

Point mutations in mtDNA are the cause of this syndrome; hence the transmission is maternal but not X linked. The most frequent mutation, accounting for about 80% of cases, is an A→G point mutation at the nt-3243 locus, involving the $tRNA_{Leu(UUR)}$ gene (35). In another 10% of cases, the locus is T→C at nt 3271 of the same gene. The remaining cases are due to mtDNA point mutations at other loci, and new genetic mutations are being identified continuously; hence MELAS is a true syndrome. The genetic mutation may be identified in blood in most patients; if this approach is not diagnostic, muscle biopsy will identify the ragged-red fiber histopathology and provide tissue for quantitative mitochondrial studies of respiratory chain enzymes, showing a defect in respiratory complexes I and IV and sometimes others as well, and identify known mtDNA point mutations that are screened.

Calcifications in the globus pallidus and other parts of the basal ganglia can sometimes be demonstrated by CT. The MRI appearance and distribution of infarcts large enough to be seen is characteristic (36). Serum creatine kinase (CK) is usually normal, but may be mildly elevated due to an increase in either the BB (brain) or MM (striated muscle) isozyme. Serum lactate is consistently elevated in this disorder, regardless of the specific point mutation and even during asymptomatic phases; pyruvate remains normal or also is elevated. The muscle biopsy is characteristic, as shown in Fig. 2.2 and Table 2.2.

TABLE 2.2 Mitochondrial Respiratory Chain Enzymes of The Patient Whose Muscle Biopsy Is Shown in Fig. 2.2

	Specific Level	*Range of Eight Controls*
Complex I (NADH)	<0.003	0.014–0.055
Complex II (SDH)	0.022	0.003–0.035
Complex III (cytochrome *b*)	0.005	0.013–0.060
Complex IV (COX)	0.039	0.075–0.225
Complex V (ATP synthase)	0.020	0.060–0.300
Citrate synthase	0.235	0.090–0.262

NADH, nicotinamide adenine dinucleotide; SDH, succinate dehydrogenase; COX, cytochrome *c* oxidase; ATP, adenosine triphosphate.
There is significantly decreased activity in complexes I, III, IV, and V. The defects in complexes I and IV correlate well with ragged-red fibers. Citrate synthase is normal, an internal control demonstrating that the number of functional mitochondria is satisfactory to render the values valid, and the specific deficiencies demonstrated were each confirmed when calculated as a ratio of citrate synthase. All units are expressed as μmol of substrate/min per mg of protein. None of the described mitochondrial DNA mutations or deletions were identified, hence the patient must have a novel mutation, but clinical, pathologic, and biochemical profile clearly are consistent with the MELAS (mitochondrial encephalopathy with latic acid and strokelike episodes) syndrome.

MERRF (Myoclonic Epilepsy with Ragged-Red Fibers)

This condition was first described by Fukuhara and colleagues (37). Clinical onset is during childhood or young adult life, and as the name suggests, the syndrome is highlighted by myoclonus and myoclonic epilepsy, progressive ataxia, and myopathy. Seizures are the usual presenting symptom in childhood and may take mixed forms. Cerebellar ataxia and dementia leading to mental retardation follow and are progressive (38). In contrast to MELAS, cerebral infarcts are uncommon, but some patients have a mixed MELAS/MERRF phenotype. Other, less constant clinical features include small stature, deafness, optic atrophy, progressive external ophthalmoplegia, peripheral neuropathy, and cutaneous lipomas.

About 80% of MERRF patients harbor an mtDNA point mutation at the nt-8344 locus of the $tRNA_{Lys}$ gene (34,39,40), but numerous other mutations in this gene are being recognized (41). If the genetic defect is not confirmed in a blood sample, muscle biopsy is diagnostic.

Kearns-Sayre Syndrome

First described by Kearns and Sayre in 1958, this ragged-red fiber mitochondrial cytopathy involves brain and muscle (42). It is the most frequent and best studied from both clinical and molecular aspects. The known genetic bases are all different point mutations of mtDNA; hence it is a syndrome, not a single disease.

As defined by DiMauro and coworkers (43), the condition is characterized by its onset before 15 years but rarely before 5 years of age, the presence of progressive external ophthalmoplegia involving all extraocular muscles, pigmentary degeneration of the retina (retinitis pigmentosa) and one or more of the following: cardiac conduction block, cerebellar deficits, CSF protein greater than 100 mg/dL, or myopathy affecting facial cervical and limb girdle muscles (43). A common additional finding is growth retardation. It can be present before age 5 years and thus precede neurologic and myopathic signs. Peripheral neuropathy occurs in some cases, and altered mitochondria may be demonstrated in axons in sural nerve biopsies (44). Cataracts, neurosensory hearing loss, ichthyosis, a variety of endocrinopathies, and proximal renal tubular acidosis also have been recorded (45,46). The disease is progressive because with time, the fraction of mtDNA containing the deletion increases. This could reflect the fact that mitochondria containing deletions replicate preferentially and accumulate in the ragged-red fibers (47)

Investigations nearly always show a normal serum lactate but elevated CSF lactate. The serum CK is normal or mildly elevated to about 600 IU/L. Visual-evoked potentials often show slow conduction in central visual pathways (geniculocalcarine projections) that is not explained by the retinitis pigmentosa, though visual function usually remains normal except for diplopia resulting from ophthalmoplegia. The muscle biopsy exhibits multiple ragged-red fibers and also increased lipid within myofibers, a feature that helps to distinguish this disorder from

MELAS and MERRF ragged-red syndromes (48). Cardiac investigations should be performed in all patients to detect potentially treatable heart block.

Neuropathologic findings in Kearns-Sayre syndrome include spongiform encephalopathy involving both gray and white matter of the cerebrum and cerebellum and primarily gray matter of the brainstem. Extensive neuronal loss is seen throughout the brainstem and cerebellum, and demyelination of white matter possibly secondary to axonal degeneration. Calcium deposits occur in the thalamus and globus pallidus, involving individual mineralized neurons, and also in the parenchyma. Mitochondrial ultrastructural abnormalities are not consistently shown in the brain despite the neuropathologic lesions (48,49).

PEO (Progressive External Ophthalmoplegia)

This disorder tends to affect adults and rarely has an onset in childhood or adolescence. It is closely related to Kearns-Sayre syndrome both clinically and genetically, and the muscle biopsy also appears virtually identical, including the increased lipid in myofibers, both ragged-red and others (50).

Pearson Syndrome

This ragged-red fiber disorder is marked by refractory sideroblastic anemia, exocrine pancreatic dysfunction, insulin-dependent diabetes mellitus, lactic acidosis, and 3-methylglutaconic aciduria. It is usually fatal during infancy and early childhood, but after age 5 years, survivors develop symptoms and signs typical of Kearns-Sayre syndrome (51). It is clinically distinguishable by the infantile features of endocrinopathies and anemia, the early onset, and the presence of lactic acidosis. The genetic basis is mtDNA deletions similar to those of Kearns-Sayre syndrome, demonstrable in many tissues.

NON–RAGGED-RED FIBER MITOCHONDRIAL SYNDROMES

Leigh Encephalopathy (Subacute Periventricular Necrotizing Encephalopathy)

This syndrome, first described by Leigh in 1951 (52), has many genetic mutations of both mtDNA and nDNA and is the most frequent mitochondrial disease of the perinatal period and early infancy. Transmission may be maternal if the principal mutation affects mtDNA, or it may present as a Mendelian autosomal recessive trait if the principal mutation affects nDNA. X-linked recessive inheritance is a rarer genetic pattern, when a mutation involves the pyruvate dehydrogenase E_1 gene on the X chromosome. Autosomal recessive cases often involve pyruvate carboxylase deficiency, *SURF1* (a nonencoding "housekeeping" gene of uncertain function) mutation with complex IV deficiency, or isolated complex I deficiency (53,54). A combination of complex III and V deficiency is common, with or without other respiratory chain complexes also being deficient.

Leigh disease can commence at birth. The clinical presentation in the newborn is one of diffuse encephalopathy, but neonatal seizures are infrequent. Infants usually feed poorly or are unable to swallow and may aspirate. Central respiratory insufficiency is sometimes a serious complication in the absence of pulmonary disease and is evidence of brainstem tegmental lesions in the floor of the fourth ventricle involving the fasciculus solitarius. Though the pupils generally remain reactive, the infants do not fixate visually and do not respond reflexively to bright lights shown in the eyes. Reactions to olfactory and auditory stimuli similarly are less than expected. Muscle tone may be hypotonic, or, occasionally, early spastic diplegia may become evident, associated with clonus.

Often infants appear normal at birth, but within the first 3 months of life develop progressive lethargy, visual impairment, dysphagia, and hypotonia with weakness and paucity of movement. Older infants and toddlers may exhibit dyskinesias and progressive cerebellar deficits in addition. In the New York series of Macaya and colleagues, movement disorders, notably dystonia and myoclonus, formed a prominent part of the neurologic picture in 86% of patients (55); in some they were the presenting signs (56). Seizures are uncommon, even in later infancy and early childhood. A male predominance occurs; 66% of patients in the series of DiMauro and colleagues were male (57).

The neurologic deficits are progressive, and most patients die within days to weeks if already symptomatic as neonates or within months to a few years if onset is later in infancy.

In the majority of patients, including neonates, serum lactate is elevated, with normal or mildly high pyruvate. CSF lactate may be elevated despite normal serum lactate. Serum CK is normal. Imaging studies, CT and MRI, show characteristic findings of periventricular leukomalacia and a hyperintense T2 signal in the basal ganglia and thalami. The electroencephalogram (EEG) is usually nonparoxysmal but shows diffuse, poorly regulated, and excessively slow background rhythms in both wakefulness and sleep.

The muscle biopsy is diagnostic even in the neonate (48). Ragged-red fibers are not found (because complexes I and IV are not usually involved together in Leigh encephalopathy and also because these fibers are rare in infancy even in ragged-red fiber diseases); neutral lipid is increased in some cases. Ultrastructural studies of muscle show many abnormal mitochondria with altered cristae. Paracrystalline structures are rare in muscle but are sometimes seen in the periventricular region of the lateral ventricles at autopsy. Quantitative studies of respiratory chain enzymes in muscle are invariably abnormal. The exact pattern depends on the mtDNA or nDNA defect, which may or may not be evident on screening the common point mutations and deletions. Isolated complex IV (cytochrome *c* oxidase) deficiency is common, but isolated complex I and isolated complex V or combined complexes III and V as well as pyruvate dehydrogenase deficiencies have also been documented (58,59).

Neuropathologic examination shows encephalomalacia and necrosis of periventricular tissue around the lateral ventricles, sometimes the third and floor of the fourth ventricles, and even around the central canal of the spinal cord. Calcified neurons are seen in the thalamus and basal ganglia. Minor developmental malformations are found in the cerebellum, the bases of some cerebellar folia show pan-neuronal loss and gliosis, and convolutions of the inferior olivary nuclei are abnormally formed. Myelination of the white matter of the cerebrum and cerebellum is deficient; small cryptic angiomas of the choroid plexuses may be present (48).

When Leigh encephalopathy is the result of a pyruvate dehydrogenase deficiency, treatment with a ketogenic diet may be beneficial, not only in improving the lactic acidosis and MRI lesions, but in preventing irreversible brain damage (58,59).

NARP (Neuropathy, Ataxia, Retinitis Pigmentosa)

This mitochondrial syndrome is closely related to Leigh encephalopathy and, in effect, is the same disease with a quantitative difference in the ratio of normal versus abnormal mtDNA. A point mutation at the nt-8993 locus of the mitochondrial ATPase-6 gene inhibits oxidative phosphorylation and results in enhanced free radical production (60). When the mutation involves 90% or more of mtDNA, Leigh encephalopathy results; when it involves 70% or less of mtDNA, NARP is expressed; patients with between 70% and 90% mutated mtDNA have a mixed syndrome. The onset of NARP is not as early as it is in Leigh disease and usually occurs during childhood. Progressive cerebellar ataxia and motor and sensory polyneuropathy with weakness and paresthesias are the presenting symptoms. Visual loss, particularly for night vision, and the development of tunnel vision are noted later, and funduscopic examination reveals retinitis pigmentosa, most prominently in the periphery of the retina.

Mitochondrial Depletion Syndrome of Early Infancy

Mitochondrial disease may present in the neonatal period or even be clinically evident in fetal life. The two most frequent mitochondrial syndromes of early infancy are Leigh encephalopathy and the mitochondrial depletion syndrome.

The mitochondrial depletion syndrome is an autosomally recessive condition that generally takes two forms. The hepatocerebral form is marked by an early onset of hepatic failure, encephalopathy, and renal tubulopathy. The gastrointestinal encephalomyopathy form is defined clinically by severe gastrointestinal dysmotility, cachexia, ptosis, peripheral neuropathy and leukoencephalopathy (20,61–70). Epidermolysis of the skin may occur in some neonates (64).

The syndrome is associated with at least two genetic mutations: the nuclear-encoded mitochondrial deoxyguanosine kinase gene (*DGUOK*) and the nuclear-encoded mitochondrial thymidine kinase gene (*TK2*) (71). Although many of the patients with the gastrointestinal encephalopathy form have a defect in *TK2*, the genotype–phenotype correlations are far from exact. As is the case in Leigh encephalopathy, most infants have persistent lactic acidosis. CSF lactate might be elevated in some cases with normal serum lactate. Infants can die in the neonatal period or occasionally survive several weeks or even months. Clinical suspicion of the syndrome is raised by unexplained multisystem metabolic disease in the absence of a history of hypoxia or ischemia or other metabolic diseases. Confirmation is by muscle biopsy, but the histopathologic and histochemical findings can be normal or subtle, and quantitative analysis of respiratory chain enzymes is required. Ultrastructural alterations of mitochondria usually are demonstrated but also may be subtle.

The diagnostic findings of this condition are supported by the quantitative studies of mitochondrial respiratory chain enzymes. The four respiratory complexes with subunits encoded by mtDNA (i.e., complexes I, III, IV, and V) exhibit abnormally low activities, but point mutations of mtDNA are not demonstrated, whereas the level of mtDNA is markedly reduced. Citrate synthase is low or normal. Normal levels of complex II (succinate ubiquinone reductase) activity in conjunction with reduced complex I, III, and IV activities is suggestive of the mtDNA depletion syndrome (67). It has been demonstrated in rats that mtDNA can be totally depleted by the administration of drugs and toxins, such as zidovine (AZT). In these cases the number of mitochondria and their replication are not affected, though the ultrastructure is abnormal (70).

Alpers syndrome is an autosomal recessive neurodegenerative disease of childhood characterized by seizures, hypotonia, loss of mental function, impaired hearing and vision, and hepatic insufficiency, as described by Alpers in 1931 (72). CSF lactate and pyruvate are elevated in the presence of normal serum lactate. This disorder is now known to be another mtDNA depletion syndrome, and mutations in DNA polymerase gamma have been demonstrated in some patients with the syndrome (73,74).

LHON (Leber Hereditary Optic Neuropathy)

The clinical deficit usually is an isolated bilateral optic neuropathy, with insidious onset in late adolescence and early adult life, between 15 and 35 years of age.

Several defects in mtDNA have been recognized. The three most frequent defects are at np 11778 (69%), nt 14484 (14%), and np 3460, all encoding regions for complex I subunits. Although other mutations have been reported, these three account for 80% to 95% of cases of LHON in all ethnic groups.

Relatively little difference in the clinical picture of Leber disease exists among patients harboring the three major mutations (75). As a rule, the younger the patient at the onset of symptoms, the better is the ultimate outcome, and some 80% of patients with onset of vision loss before 20 years of age recover sufficiently to be able to drive a car (75).

The onset of symptoms is insidious, usually occurring between 18 and 24 years of age and without any obvious precipitating cause. Visual loss progresses rapidly until it reaches a static phase. The initial complaint is a sudden blurring of central vision that progresses to dense central scotomas. In many patients, vision loss is at first unilateral. Examination of the fundi in the earliest states of the illness can reveal hyperemia and edema of the optic nerve head, dilation and tortuosity of peripapillary arteries but not veins, circumpapillary telangiectasia, and sometimes focal microhemorrhages. Visual-evoked potentials are delayed and of low amplitude early in the course of the disease and later are totally extinguished (76). Female (50%) and also male (33%) descendents of affected patients also have abnormal visual-evoked responses despite lack of visual loss.

Visual loss is irreversible, but a few patients have shown spontaneous dramatic reversal of visual loss with restoration, and as many as half of patients with LHON experience some improvement of vision; the mutation at bp 3460 has a better prognosis than other mutations (75).

Inconstant associated features in LHOH include cardiac conduction defects, movement disorders, minor skeletal anomalies, and a slowly progressive myopathy.

An association of LHON with small stature, generalized childhood-onset severe dystonia, progressive dementia and corticospinal tract and bulbar deficits results from a mutation in the *ND6* gene for complex I (77).

MRI often shows bilateral abnormalities in the putamen and caudate nuclei in T2-weighted images but these changes are common to many other non-LHON mitochondrial encephalomyopathies.

Neuropathologic examination reveals a loss of ganglion cells from the fovea centralis, marked atrophy of the optic nerves, and demyelination of the papillomacular bundle of the retina, optic nerves, chiasm, and tracts. Despite severe neuronal loss and gliosis of the lateral geniculate bodies, the visual cortex remains histologically normal (78). The muscle biopsy shows enlargement in mitochondrial size, aggregation in the subsarcolemmal region, and abnormal cristae. Myofilaments of the muscle fiber itself may be disrupted and nemaline rods are occasionally seen (79).

There is a greater susceptibility of male patients to visual loss than of female patients, despite the maternally transmitted mtDNA point mutations; this male predominance is unexplained (75).

The genetic defect can usually be confirmed from a blood sample, or from muscle biopsy tissue if the blood results are inconclusive. Electrocardiogram should be performed because the conduction defects are a potentially treatable complication.

DEFECTS OF MITOCHONDRIAL TRANSPORT (LIPID STORAGE MYOPATHIES)

Since their first description by Engel and coworkers in 1970 on the basis of a pathologic picture of lipid droplets within type 1 fibers (80), a number of distinct biochemical entities have been recognized, all sharing a defect in the use of long-chain fatty acids by skeletal muscle.

Carnitine (L-3-hydroxy-4-trimethylammonium butyrate) is present in large amounts in skeletal muscle, where it stimulates mitochondrial oxidation of the coenzyme A derivatives of long-chain fatty acids (acyl-CoA), notably palmitate, by facilitating their transport from cytoplasm into the inner mitochondrial compartment (Fig. 2.3). The transfer of palmitoyl acyl-CoA is accomplished by its transesterification to form a long-chain fatty acylcarnitine. This reaction is catalyzed by carnitine palmitoyl transferase I, an enzyme located on the outer surface of the inner mitochondrial membrane. Carnitine is supplied for this reaction by a sodium-dependent carnitine transporter (OCTN2). A translocase then carries the acylcarnitine across the barrier of the inner mitochondrial membrane. There the acylcarnitine complex is cleaved by a second carnitine palmitoyl transferase (II) to form acyl-CoA, which then enters the β-oxidation pathway (81).

Carnitine occurs naturally in food, notably in meat and fish, but the amounts ingested in a normal diet are insufficient to meet body requirements. Carnitine is also synthesized in several tissues, including liver, according to the pathway outlined in Fig. 2.3. Aside from functioning in the transport of fatty acids into mitochondria, carnitine is used to detoxify the acyl-CoA compounds. Large amounts of acyl-CoA derivatives, such as are seen in the various organic acidurias (see Chapter 1), can inhibit a variety of enzymes, notably the pyruvate dehydrogenase complex and

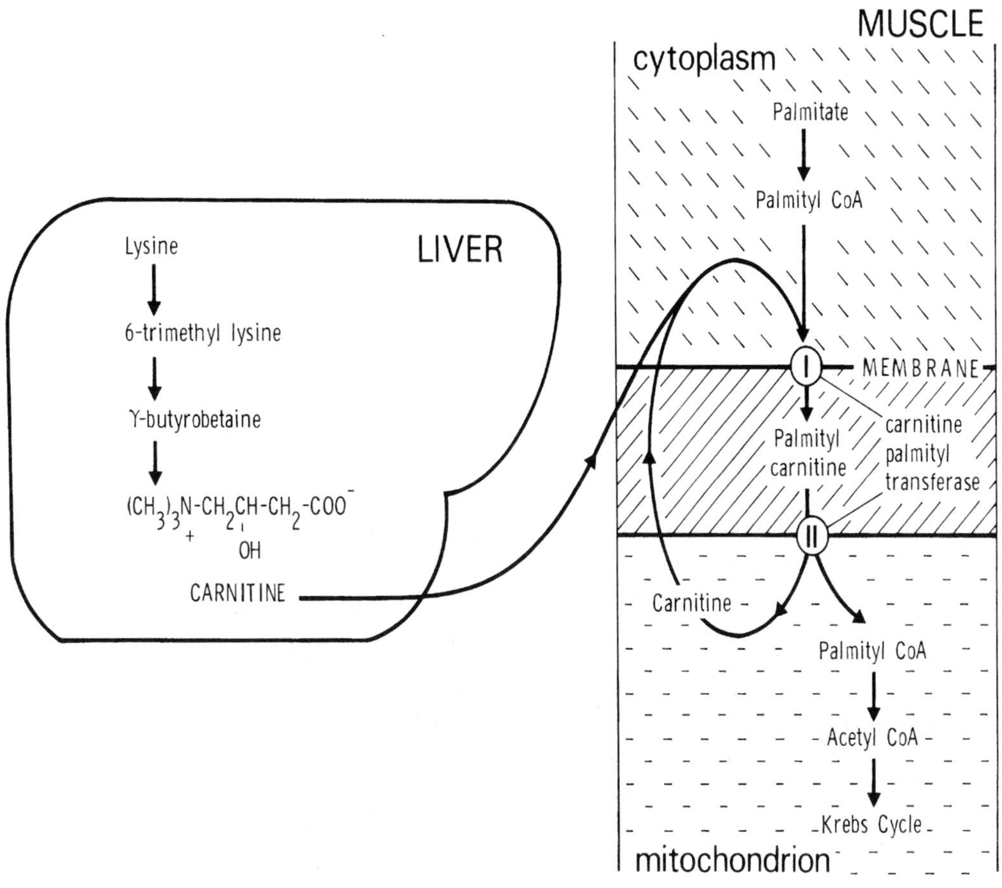

FIGURE 2.3. Muscle carnitine metabolism. Not shown in this figure is a carnitine transporter that carries carnitine to the inner aspect of the outer mitochondrial membrane, where carnitine palmityl transferase I (CPT I) catalyzes its reaction with palmityl-CoA to form palmitylcarnitine. After the formation of palmitylcarnitine, a translocase carries the acylcarnitine to the inner aspect of the inner mitochondrial membrane, where CPT II converts palmitylcarnitine to free carnitine and palmityl-CoA.

glutamate dehydrogenase, which in turn aggravates the basic enzymatic defect and sets into motion a vicious circle. When the amount of carnitine is insufficient to buffer the toxic acyl-CoA compounds, a carnitine deficiency is said to exist (82).

Normal total plasma carnitine concentrations run between 40 and 60 μmol/L, with between 70% and 90% of carnitine in the free (unesterified) state (83,84). Patients with secondary carnitine deficiency generally have a high ratio of plasma acylcarnitine (esterified carnitine) to free carnitine. The causes for secondary carnitine deficiency are many (85). Aside from its presence in the various acyl-CoA dehydrogenase deficiencies and the organic acidemias, it is seen in disorders of mitochondrial function, in several other inborn errors of metabolism, including maple syrup urine disease, in infants having an inadequate dietary intake, in Reye syndrome, in renal failure, and in patients receiving valproate or salicylates (82).

Most workers distinguish between a primary or systemic and a secondary carnitine deficiency, with secondary deficiency being encountered far more commonly. Primary carnitine deficiency encompasses some of the previously reported cases of muscle carnitine deficiency. Several infants who initially were thought to have a primary systemic carnitine deficiency were subsequently found to have a defect in medium-chain acyl-CoA dehydrogenase, another infant was found to have a defect in short-chain acyl-CoA dehydrogenase, and another patient with muscle carnitine deficiency was shown to have a defect in short-chain acyl-CoA dehydrogenase that for unknown reasons was restricted to muscle (83,86). The primary carnitine deficiencies have been divided into systemic and muscle forms, a distinction that will likely turn out to be artificial. Systemic forms have low levels of carnitine in plasma, liver, and muscle, whereas muscle forms have low carnitine levels in muscle only.

The most clearly defined primary carnitine deficiency syndrome is an autosomal recessive disorder characterized by a defect in intracellular uptake of carnitine (87). Primary carnitine deficiency is caused by mutations in the gene that encodes a plasmalemmal, sodium ion-dependent, high-affinity carnitine transporter, OCTN2 (88,89). The gene has been mapped to 5q33.1.

The clinical picture is highlighted by a progressive cardiomyopathy, skeletal myopathy, hypoketotic hypoglycemia, and hyperammonemia that develops in late infancy or early childhood. This was the clinical presentation in 70% of cases compiled by Stanley and coworkers (87). In 45%, the initial manifestation was an episode of hypoglycemic coma. Rarely, the presentation resembles a sudden infant death syndrome–like episode (88,90). Plasma and muscle carnitine levels are markedly reduced, and a defect in carnitine uptake has been shown in fibroblasts and leukocytes. The renal transport system for carnitine is believed to be impaired also, resulting in defective renal conservation of carnitine. Skeletal muscle contains lipid inclusions that are mainly seen in type 1 fibers. Electron microscopy shows the mitochondria to appear abnormal, with increased number and size, and intramitochondrial inclusions (91). There is an associated metabolic acidosis, probably secondary to an accumulation of lactic acid, and urinary organic acids are normal or show only slight elevations of medium-chain dicarboxylic acids.

Response to treatment with oral carnitine (50 mg/kg per day of L-carnitine) corrects the clinical signs of myopathy, although skeletal muscle carnitine levels remain markedly reduced (92).

Carnitine Palmitoyl Transferase Deficiencies

Cases with documented carnitine palmitoyl transferase II deficiency are more common than those with carnitine palmitoyl transferase I deficiency, of which there are only a few adequately documented cases. In these, children present with recurrent Reye syndrome–like episodes, marked by nonketotic hypoglycemic coma, mild hyperammonemia, renal tubular acidosis, and elevated plasma free fatty acids (93). Treatment with medium-chain triglycerides that are transported into mitochondria without the need of the carnitine palmitoyl transferase system has been effective. The gene for carnitine palmitoyl transferase I deficiency has been mapped to chromosome 11q13, whereas the gene for carnitine palmitoyl transferase II deficiency has been mapped to chromosome 1p32.

Carnitine palmitoyl transferase II deficiency has two modes of presentation. In older children or adults the disorder is characterized by exercise intolerance and attacks of rhabdomyolysis with myoglobinuria precipitated by fasting, cold stress, prolonged but not necessarily strenuous physical activity, or high fat intake (94–96). In newborns, carnitine palmitoyl transferase II deficiency is a generally lethal disease, marked by hypoglycemia, cardiac arrhythmia, or severe myopathy (97–99). Serum and muscle carnitine levels are generally reduced, and palmitoyl transferase activity is decreased in muscle and in various other tissues, including liver and fibroblasts (100). Although there is some lipid accumulation in muscle, this disorder is not a lipid myopathy, in that there is little or no lipid storage in muscle. Probably, this enzymatic defect precludes the use of fatty acids required to maintain muscle energy when glycogen stores are depleted by prolonged exercise. A high carbohydrate intake before exercise usually prevents symptoms, and treatment with medium-chain triglycerides appears also to be effective.

Another disorder in mitochondrial oxidation of fatty acids affects the carnitine-acylcarnitine translocase. This is an autosomal recessive disorder has been mapped to 3p21–p31. Symptoms develop in infancy and are marked by seizures, apnea, and bradycardia. Generalized muscle weakness becomes apparent in survivors (101). Dietary supplementation with carnitine appears to be ineffective in this condition (102).

Lipid Myopathy with Normal Carnitine Levels

In several instances, the pathologic picture of lipid inclusions within type 1 muscle fibers has been unaccompanied by any discernible disorder in the metabolism of fatty acids (103,104). The clinical picture of these conditions is variable; most patients have a congenital, nonprogressive myopathy. Because most of the clinical descriptions lack biochemical and enzymatic studies, their nature is unclear. One form, Dorfman-Chanarin disease, is characterized by congenital ichthyosis, cardiomyopathy, and neutral lipid storage in muscles, hepatocytes, granulocytes, and the gastrointestinal endothelium. It is accompanied by impaired oxidation of long-chain fatty acids (105,106). The various lipid storage myopathies have been reviewed by Cwik (107).

PATHOLOGY OF MITOCHONDRIAL CYTOPATHIES

Alterations in mitochondrial structure and function are most commonly sought for in muscle, blood, skin, or brain.

Muscle Biopsy

If the specific genetic defect is not known, muscle is the best tissue to investigate for mitochondrial disease even in the absence of clinical signs pointing to a myopathy. If the defect is known, genetic confirmation can be feasible from a blood sample. Several previous parallel pathologic studies of muscle and brain including our personal experience confirm the reliability of histopathologic observations performed on muscle tissue (15,108–115).

Whereas all muscles show similar findings, the quadriceps femoris muscle (vastus lateralis) is generally most

TABLE 2.3 Microscopic Features in the Muscle Biopsy of Mitochondrial Cytopathies

Feature	*Comment*
Ragged-red fibers	Uncommon in children younger than 5 years of age
Neutral lipids	Increased lipid is a constant finding in Kearns-Sayre syndrome, not in MELAS or MERRF; found in some genetic forms of Leigh encephalopathy
Glycogen	Can be abundant, suggesting glycogenosis
Oxidative enzymes[a]	
NADH-TR (complex I)	
SDH (complex II)	Reduction or absence shows a defect in complex II
COX (complex IV)	Scattered absence of COX is not specific for complex IV deficiency, but is strong evidence of mitochondrial cytopathy
Ribosomal RNA (48)	Not increased, unlike regenerating myofibers
Fiber-type ratios and distribution	Quadriceps normally shows type I predominance (116)
Denervation–reinnervation (neurogenic atrophy) of muscle (48,117,118)	
Features not characteristic of mitochondrial cytopathies	But seen in myopathies where mitochondrial function is impaired
Extensive myofiber degeneration or necrosis	Mutation in subunit II of COX (complex IV) is a rare cause of rhabdomyolysis (119)
Regeneration	
Inflammatory cell infiltrates	

NADH-TR, nicotinamide adenine dinucleotide-tetrazolium reductase; SDH, succinate dehydrogenase; COX, cytochrome *c* oxidase; MELAS, mitochondrial encephalopathy with lactic acidosis and strokelike episodes; MERRF, myoclonic epilepsy with ragged-red fibers.
[a]Specific and reliable histochemical stains are not available to demonstrate complex III (ubiquinol; cytochrome *b* oxidase) and complex V (ATP synthase).

suitable for study. Samples are set aside for microscopy, histochemical studies, and electron microscopy. The microscopic features in a muscle biopsy of mitochondrial cytopathy are summarized in Table 2.3.

Table 2.4 summarizes the histochemical differences among the various mitochondrial myopathies that offer clues to a specific diagnosis.

Electron Microscopy

After histochemical studies, electron microscopy (EM) is regarded as the next level of complexity in investigating a muscle biopsy for mitochondrial disease. EM demonstrates characteristic ultrastructural alterations in mitochondria in the majority of cases of mitochondrial cytopathy. These are summarized in Table 2.5.

An abnormality in the mitochondrial ultrastructure provides valid justification to proceed with the third, and most expensive, aspect of the workup, the quantitative analysis of respiratory chain enzymes and screening of mtDNA for deletions and point mutations.

Quantitative Determination of Respiratory Chain Complexes

The respiratory complexes located on the inner mitochondrial membrane and each consisting structurally of several subunits encoded in either mtDNA and nDNA can be biochemically measured in a quantitative fashion and compared with normal control muscle. Citrate synthase, a Krebs cycle enzyme located in the mitochondrial matrix and present in all mitochondria, serves as an internal

TABLE 2.4 Correlation of Histochemical Findings with Specific Defects in Mitochondrial Respiratory Complexes

Ragged-red fibers	Combination defects in complexes I and IV
Increased lipid in ragged-red fibers	Kearns-Sayre, PEO (not MELAS, MERRF)
Increased lipid in non–ragged-red myopathy	Some, but not all, mitochondrial myopathies; specific, constant correlations not determined
Absent SDH in all fibers	Severe complex II defect
Absent COX in all fibers	Severe complex IV defect; defective CoQ10
Absent COX in scattered myofibers (often associated with increased SDH in those fibers)	Nonspecific for complexes, but reliable finding indicating mitochondrial myopathy
Increased glycogen in ragged-red fibers	Nonspecific for complexes

PEO, progressive external ophthalmoplegia; MELAS, mitochondrial encephalopathy with lactic acid and strokelike episodes; MERRF, myoclonic epilepsy with ragged-red fibers; SDH, succinate dehydrogenase; COX, cytochrome *c* oxidase.

TABLE 2.5 Electron Microscopic Changes in Mitochondrial Cytopathies

Excessive numbers of mitochondria in subsarcolemmal and intermyofibrillar spaces
Excessively bizarre shapes of mitochondria
Excessively large size or length of mitochondria
Irregularities of cristae, stacking, and whorling
Multiple small, electron-dense spherical granules
Paracrystalline structures with a regular geometric periodicity; these are the most pathognomonic of the various ultrastructural alterations (48,120); also seen in liver, brain (121, 122)

control of whether the number of functional mitochondria is sufficient to validate the results of the respiratory chain enzymes.

Some respiratory chain deficiencies are potentially reversible or produce only mild, benign clinical manifestations, particularly in children (123–125). At each stage of the investigation, the total data collected must be reassessed to decide whether to proceed further.

Skin Biopsy

Punch biopsy of the skin seems an attractive alternative to muscle biopsy because it is simple, less invasive, and can be performed by any nonsurgical clinician. Epidermal cells are a poor source of mitochondria, but the smooth muscle of the pili erecti muscles and the axoplasm of cutaneous nerves have mitochondria suitable for ultrastructural examination (48,126). Fibroblasts also sometimes show good mitochondria but they are not as large as those in smooth muscle. Fibroblasts are more easily cultured than myocytes.

Correlations of Clinical and Pathologic Phenotype with Genotype

Attempts to correlate the clinical picture with specific respiratory complex deficiencies have yielded only limited success. Muscle pathology offers a better correlation, though it also is not definitive. Some biochemical deficiencies in respiratory enzymatic activities are secondary to nonmitochondrial conditions (127), and defects in the respiratory chain can be nonspecific in children (128,129).

CLINICAL INVESTIGATIONS OF MITOCHONDRIAL ENCEPHALOMYOPATHIES

The clinical investigation of a child in whom mitochondrial disease is suspected from clinical presentation should begin with serum lactate and pyruvate and possibly CSF lactate. Neuroimaging often provides useful clues, with particularly characteristic changes seen on MRI (Fig. 2.1). The serum CK usually is normal or mildly elevated. If mitochondrial cardiomyopathy is suspected, electrocardiogram (ECG) and echocardiogram are useful, and sometimes a small myocardial biopsy can be taken during cardiac catherization.

If a specific category of mitochondrial cytopathies is suspected, such as the syndromes of MELAS, Kearns-Sayre, LHON, or Leigh encephalopathy, mtDNA deletions may sometimes be demonstrated in blood to confirm the diagnosis. Muscle biopsy is the ultimate gold standard for studying mitochondria and performing all of the studies outlined previously. Skin biopsy may sometimes supplement the workup.

Detection of mtDNA Deletions in Blood

Southern blot hybridization analysis can demonstrate mtDNA deletions in muscle tissue but not always in blood in a subgroup of patients with myopathic signs (130,131). The highly sensitive polymerase chain reaction (PCR) can be used in blood for the detection of mtDNA deletions in several mitochondrial myopathies, and panels have been developed for screening the common mutations in categories, such as for MELAS, Kearns-Sayre, PEO, or LHON.

PATHOLOGIC FINDINGS IN BRAIN

The mitochondria of neurons, glial cells, and endothelial cells all can be affected in the various mitochondrial cytopathies, and endothelial cells sometimes show the greatest alterations, leading to cytoplasmic swelling, decreased pinocytotic vesicles, and impaired blood flow. This is the basis of both strokelike episodes (i.e., transient ischemia) and true microinfarcts and macroinfarcts in the brain in MELAS syndrome and sometimes in other mitochondrial encephalopathies as well. Additional characteristic alterations demonstrated at postmortem examination in patients with mitochondrial cytopathies, particularly in infants and children, include (a) individual mineralized neurons in the thalamus, hypothalamus, and sometimes the basal ganglia (i.e., neuronal calcinosis); (b) white matter gliosis, particularly in the brainstem and cerebellum; (c) dysmyelination or demyelination of white matter in the cerebral hemispheres; (d) focal dysplasias and neuronal loss in the inferior olivary (Fig. 2.4), red and dentate nuclei, and the cerebellar cortex; (e) periventricular necrosis or spongiform changes in Leigh encephalopathy; and (f) alterations in ependymal cells (48,132–134).

Whereas the changes in brain just described are consistent with and may be strongly suggestive of mitochondrial disease, none of these alterations individually is pathognomonic and all may be seen at times in other diseases.

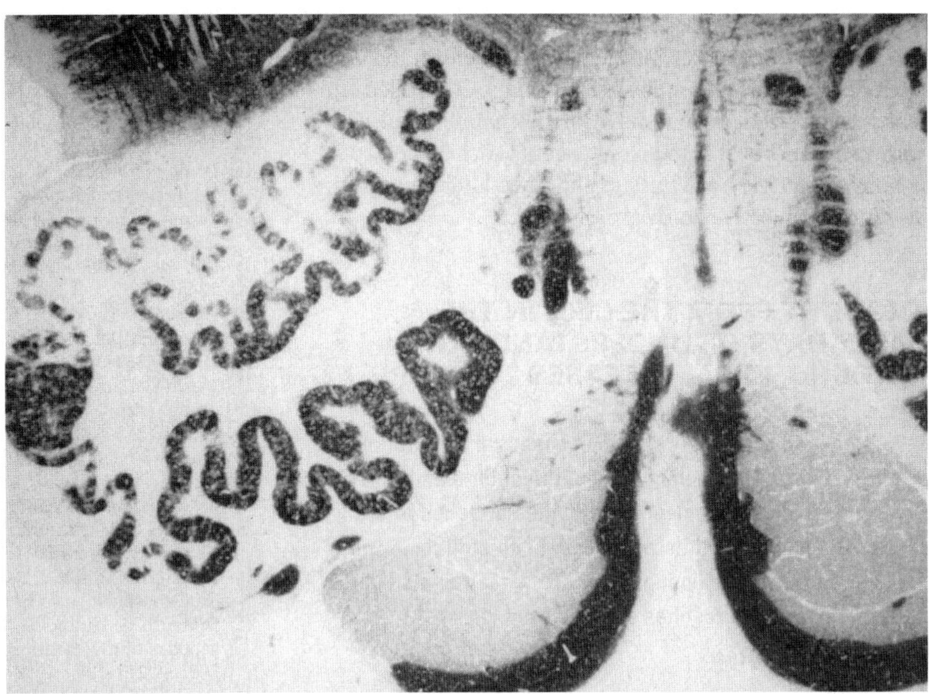

FIGURE 2.4. Characteristic lesions of inferior olivary nucleus in mitochondrial cytopathy of a 3-month-old infant girl, born at term, with Leigh encephalopathy. Olivary convolutions are preserved but the superior lip shows irregular loss of synaptic vesicle immunoreactivity, whereas normal activity is preserved in the inferior lip, in the dorsal and medial accessory olives, and in the arcuate nucleus at the medial and inferior margins of the pyramids. This finding is characteristic and almost pathognomonic of mitochondrial encephalopathies of infancy and is not typical in other cerebral malformations. It may be difficult to detect, however, in sections stained with hematoxylin-eosin. Paraffin section. Synaptophysin immunocytochemistry. ×40.

It is becoming increasingly evident that mitochondrial disorders are associated with a large number of diseases that are not primary mitochondrial cytopathies but in which a disturbance in mitochondrial function may contribute to pathogenesis or clinical manifestations. The involved disorders fall into nearly all categories of disease: metabolic and degenerative, inflammatory, developmental malformations, and neoplastic. They are listed in Table 2.6.

TREATMENT OF MITOCHONDRIAL CYTOPATHIES

There is no definitive treatment of mitochondrial diseases as this time. Pharmacologic substances that provide an improved substrate for mitochondrial function are used and include a "cocktail" of mainly coenzyme-Q10 (CoQ10), L-carnitine, the antioxidant α-tocopherol (vitamin E) (154), and creatine monohydrate (155). Alpha-tocopherol is theoretically more effective than ascorbic acid (vitamin C) because it helps to regulate superoxide generation in mitochondria (156), but some authors find it ineffective (157). Alpha-tocopherol, crucial for mitochondrial integrity, is localized in the outer mitochondrial membrane, unlike the respiratory chain complexes, which are localized in the inner membrane (158). CoQ10 not only serves an important function in electron transport, but subserves membrane polarity of many subcellular organelles and is a gene regulator that upregulates some genes and downregulates others (159–161). Other substances suggested as useful treatment in mitochondrial defects, but of less well established value, include quinones as substitutive electron carriers or antioxidants (160), niacin, thiamin, and the B-complex of vitamins in general, but good evidence of the efficacy of water-soluble vitamins is lacking (157).

TABLE 2.6 Mitochondrial Alterations in Diseases of Central Nervous System and Muscle That Are Not Primary Mitochondrial Cytopathies

Glycogenosis (type II, and adult-onset acid maltase deficiency) (48,135)
Spinal muscular atrophy (136,137)
Infantile-onset spinocerebellar ataxia (*SCA8*) (138,139)
Some cerebellar ataxias are associated with coenzyme Q10 deficiency (140)
Congenital myopathy (120)
Inflammatory necrotizing myositis (polymyositis) (141,142)
Septo-optic-pituitary dysplasia–associated respiratory complex III dysfunction (cytochrome *b*) (143)
Cerebro-hepato-renal disease (Zellweger syndrome) (144,145)
Neoplastic cells (146)
Antiepileptic medications administered to pregnant women can impair fetal mitochondrial function (147)
Toxic and drug-induced mitochondrial cytopathies
Immunosuppressive drugs
Antimetabolic drugs
Antibacterial and antiviral agents (148,149)
Statins (150, 151)
Antiepileptic drugs (valproate) (152)
Steroid therapy, chronic (153)

No longitudinal pathologic studies are available that prospectively compare muscle biopsies before and after treatment, either in humans or in animals. Controlled clinical trials of the various advocated treatments also are wanting. Reports of responses to agents such as CoQ10 are encouraging (161,162) but are still anecdotal and require systematic objective study (163).

THOUGHT FROM THE CELL IN THE EARLY DAYS OF UNDERSTANDING MITOCHONDRIAL DISEASES

> I am obliged to do a great deal of essential work for my mitochondria. My nuclei code out the outer membranes of each, and a good many of the enzymes attached to the cristae must be synthesized by me. Each of them, by all accounts, makes only enough of its own materials to get along on, and the rest has to come from me.
>
> *L. Thomas, 1974 (164)*

REFERENCES

1. Chinnery PF, DiMauro S, Shanske S, et al. Risk of developing a mitochondrial DNA deletion disorder. *Lancet* 2004;364:592–596.
2. Altmann R. *Die Elementarorganismen und ihre Beziehungen zu den Zellen*. Leipzig: Veit Co., 1890.
3. Benda, C. Ueber die Spermatogenese der Vertebraten und hoeherer Evertebraten. II. Theil. Die Histiogenese der Spermien. *Arch. Anat. Physiol. [Physiol.]* 1898;393–398.
4. Palade GE. The fine structure of mitochondria. *Anat Rec* 1952;114: 427–451.
5. Nass MM, Nass S. Intramitochondrial fibers with DNA characteristics. I. Fixation and electron staining reactions. *J Cell Biol* 1963;19: 593–611.
6. Luft R., Ikkos D, Palmieri G, et al. A case of severe hypermetabolism of nonthyroid origin with a defect in the maintenance of mitochondrial respiratory control: a correlated clinical, biochemical, and morphological study. *J Clin Invest*. 1962;41:1776–1804.
7. Engel WK, Cunningham GG. Rapid examination of muscle tissue. An improved trichrome method for fresh-frozen biopsy sections. *Neurology* 1963;13:919–923.
8. DiMauro S, DiMauro PM. Muscle carnitine palmityltransferase deficiency and myoglobinuria. *Science* 1973;182:929–931.
9. Anderson S, Bankier AT, Barrell BG, et al. Sequence and organization of the human mitochondrial genome. *Nature* 1981;290:457–465.
10. Pavlakis SG, Phillips PC, DiMauro S, et al. Mitochondrial myopathy, encephalopathy, lactic acidosis, and strokelike episodes: a distinctive clinical syndrome. *Ann Neurol*. 1984;16:481–488.
11. Holt IJ, Harding AE, Morgan-Hughes JA. Deletions of muscle mitochondrial DNA in patients with mitochondrial myopathies. *Nature* 1988;331:717–719.
12. Wallace DC, Singh G, Lott MT, et al. Mitochondrial DNA mutation associated with Leber's hereditary optic neuropathy. *Science* 1998;242:1427–1430.
13. Servidei S. Mitochondrial encephalopathies: gene mutation. *Neuromusc Disord* 2003;13:848–853.
14. Lodish H, Berk A, Matsodaira P, et al. Cellular energetics. In: *Molecular cell biology*, 5th ed. New York: Freeman, 2004: 301–350.
15. Schapira AHV. *Mitochondrial function and dysfunction*. New York: Academic Press, 2003.
16. Santos JH, Hunakova L, Chen Y, et al. Cell-sorting experiments link persistent mitochondrial DNA damage with loss of mitochondrial membrane potential and apoptotic cell death. *J Biol Chem* 2003;278:1728–1734.
17. Chinnery PF, Turnbull DM. Mitochondrial medicine. *Q J Med* 1997;90:657–667.
18. Poulton J, Macaulay V, Marchington DR. Mitochondrial genetics '98. Is the bottleneck cracked? *Am J Hum Genet* 1998;62:752–757.
19. Verma A, Moraes CT. Mitochondrial disorders. In: Bradley WG, Daroff RB, Fenichel GM, et al., eds. *Neurology in clinical practice*, 4th ed. Philadelphia: Butterworth–Heinemann, 2004;II:1833–1845.
20. Elpeleg O, Mandel H, Saada A. Depletion of the other genome—mitochondrial DNA depletion syndromes in humans. *J Mol Med* 2002;80:389–396.
21. Marín-García J, Goldenthal MJ, Sarnat HB. Kearns-Sayre syndrome with a novel mitochondrial DNA deletion. *J Child Neurol* 2000;15:555–558.
22. Marín-García J, Goldenthal MJ, Flores-Sarnat L, et al. Severe mitochondrial cytopathy with complete A-V block, PEO and mtDNA deletions. *Pediatr Neurol* 2002;27:213–216.
23. Servidei S. Mitochondrial encephalomyopathies: gene mutations. *Neuromusc Disord* 2004;14:107–116.
24. DiMauro S, Bonilla E, DeVivo DC. Does the patient have a mitochondrial encephalopathy? *J Child Neurol* 1999;14(Suppl 1):S23–S35.
25. DiMauro S, Hirano M, Kaufmann P, et al. Clinical features and genetics of myoclonic epilepsy with ragged red fibers. *Adv Neurol* 2002;89:217–229.
26. Darin N, Oldfors A, Moslemi AR, et al. Genotypes and clinical phenotypes in children with cytochrome-*c*-oxidase deficiency. *Neuropediatrics* 2003;34:311–317.
27. Sakuta R, Honzawa S, Murakami N, et al. Atypical MELAS associated with mitochondrial tRNALys gene A8296G mutation. *Pediatr Neurol* 2002;27:397–400.
28. Melone MAB, Tessa A, Petrini S, et al. Revelation of a new mitochondrial DNA mutation (G121147A) in a MELAS/MERRF phenotype. *Arch Neurol* 2004;61:269–272.
29. Nishigaki Y, Tadesse S, Bonilla E, et al. A novel mitochondrial $tRNA_{Leu(UUR)}$ mutation in a patient with features of MERRF and Kearns-Sayre syndrome. *Neuromusc Disord* 2003;13:334–340.
30. Kaufmann P, Shungu PC, Sano MC, et al. Cerebral lactic acidosis correlates with neurological impairment in MELAS. *Neurology* 2004;62:1297–1302.
31. Marín-García J, Goldenthal MJ, Sarnat HB. Probing striated muscle mitochondrial pheonotype in neuromuscular disorders. *Pediatr Neurol* 2003;29:26–33.
32. Taylor RW, Chinnery PF, Haldane F, et al. MELAS associated with a mutation in the valine transfer RNA gene of mitochondrial DNA. *Ann Neurol* 1996;40:459–462.
33. Ciafaloni E, Ricci E, Servidei S, et al. MELAS: Clinical features, biochemistry, and molecular genetics. *Ann Neurol* 1992;31:391–398.
34. Zeviani M, Tiranti V, Piantadosi C. Mitochondrial disorders. *Medicine* 1998;77:59–72.
35. Okhuijsen-Kroes EJ, Trijbels JM, Sengers RC, et al. Infantile presentation of the mtDNA A3243G tRNA(Leu(UUR)) mutation. *Neuropediatrics* 2001;32:183–190.
36. Kim IO, Kim JH, Kim WS, et al. Mitochondrial myopathy-encephalopathy-lactic acidosis-and strokelike episodes (MELAS) syndrome: CT and MR findings in seven children. *Am J Roentgenol.* 1996;166:641–645.
37. Fukuhara N, Tokiguchi S, Shirakawa K, et al. Myoclonus epilepsy associated with ragged-red fibres (mitochondrial abnormalities): disease entity or a syndrome? Light-and electron-microscopic studies of two cases and review of literature. *J Neurol Sci* 1980;47:117–133.
38. Tulinius MH, Holme E, Kristiansson B, et al. Mitochondrial encephalomyopathies in childhood. II. Clinical manifestations and syndromes. *J Pediatr* 1991;119:251–259.
39. Zeviani M, Tiranti V, Piantadosi C. Mitochondrial disorders. *Medicine* 1998;77:59–72.
40. Shoffner JM, Lott MT, Lezza AM, et al. Myoclonic epilepsy and ragged-red fiber disease (MERRF) is associated with a mitochondrial DNA tRNA(Lys) mutation. *Cell*. 1990;61:931–937.

41. Rossmanith W, Raffelsberger T, Roka J, et al. The expanding mutational spectrum of MERRF substitution G8361A in mitochondrial tRNA Lys gene. *Ann Neurol* 2003;54:820–823.
42. Kearns TP, Sayre GP. Retinitis pigmentosa, external ophthalmoplegia and complete heart block: unusual syndrome with histologic study in one of two cases. *Arch Ophthalmol* 1958;60:280–289.
43. DiMauro S, Bonilla E, Zeviani M, et al. Mitochondrial myopathies. *Ann Neurol* 1985;17:521–538.
44. Yiannikas C, McLeod JG, Pollard JD, et al. Peripheral neuropathy associated with mitochondrial myopathy. *Ann Neurol* 1986;20:249–257.
45. Danta G, Hilton RC, Lynch PG. Chronic progressive external ophthalmoplegia. *Brain* 1975;98:473–492.
46. Karpati G, Carpenter S, Larbrisseau A, et al. The Kearns-Shy syndrome. A multisystem disease with mitochondrial abnormality demonstrated in skeletal muscle and skin. *J Neurol Sci*. 1973;19:133–151.
47. Shoubridge EA, Karpati G, Hastings KEM. Deletion mutants are functionally dominant over wild-type mitochondrial genomes in skeletal muscle fiber segments in mitochondrial diseases. *Cell* 1990; 62:43–49.
48. Sarnat HB, Marín-García J. Pathology of mitochondrial encephalomyopathies. *Can J Neurol Sci* 2005;32:152–166.
49. Sparaco M, Bonilla E, DiMauro S, Powers JM. Neuropathology of mitochondrial encephalomyopathies due to mitochondrial DNA defects. *J Neuropathol Exp Neurol* 1993;52:1–10.
50. Agostino A, Valletta L, Chinnery PF, et al. Mutations of ANT1, Twinkle, and POLG1 in sporadic progressive external ophthalmoplegia (PEO). *Neurology* 2003;60:1354–1356.
51. McShane MA, Hammans SR, Sweeney M, et al. Pearson syndrome and mitochondrial encephalopathy in a patient with a deletion of mtDNA. *Am J Hum Genet* 1991;48:39–42.
52. Leigh D. Subacute necrotizing encephalomyelopathy in an infant. *J Neurol Neurosurg Psych* 1951;14:216–222.
53. Zhu Z, Yao J, Johns T, et al. *SURF1*, encoding a factor involved in the biogenesis of cytochrome c oxidase, is mutated in Leigh syndrome. *Nat Genet* 1998;20:337–343.
54. Tiranti V, Jaksch M, Hofmann S, et al. Loss-of-function mutations of *SURF-1* are specifically associated with Leigh syndrome with cytochrome *c* oxidase deficiency. *Ann Neurol* 1999;46:161–166.
55. Macaya A, Munell F, Burke RE, et al. Disorders of movement in Leigh syndrome. *Neuropediatrics* 1993;24:60–67.
56. Campistol J, Cusi V, Vernet A, et al. Dystonia as a presenting sign of subacute necrotizing encephalomyelopathy in infancy. *Eur J Pediatr* 1986;144:589–591.
57. DiMauro S, Lombes A, Nakase H, et al. Cytochrome *c* oxidase deficiency. *Pediatr Res* 1990;28:536–541.
58. Wijburg FA, Barth PG, Bindoff LA, et al. Leigh syndrome associated with a deficiency of the pyruvate dehydrogenase complex: results of treatment with a ketogenic diet. *Neuropediatrics* 1992;23:147–152.
59. Wexler ID, Hemalatha SG, McConnell J, et al. Outcome of pyruvate dehydrogenase deficiency treated with ketogenic diets. Studies in patients with identical mutations. *Neurology* 1997;49:655–1661.
60. Mattiazzi M, Vijayvergiya C, Gajewski CD, et al. The mtDNA T8993G (NARP) mutation results in an impairment of oxidative phosphorylation that can be improved by antioxidants. *Hum Mol Gene* 2004;13:869–879.
61. Ricci E, Moraes CT, Servidei S, et al. Disorders associated with depletion of mitochondrial DNA. *Brain Pathol* 1992;2:141–147.
62. Saada A, Shaaag A, Mandel H, et al. Mutant mitochondrial thymidine kinase in mitochondrial DNA depletion myopathy. *Nat Genet* 2001;29:342–344.
63. Wang L, Eriksson S. Mitochondrial deoxyguanosine kinase mutations and mitochondrial DNA depletion syndrome. *FEBS Lett* 2003;554:319–322.
64. Arnon S, Avram R, Dolfin T, et al. Mitochondrial DNA depletion presenting prenatally with skin edema and multisystem disease immediately after birth. *Prenat Diagn* 2002;22:34–37.
65. Salviati L, Sacconi S, Mancuso M, et al. Mitochondrial DNA depletion and dGK gene mutations. *Ann Neurol* 2002;52:311–317.
66. Mancuso M, Salviati L, Sacconi S, et al. Mitochondrial DNA depletion: mutations in thymidine kinase gene with myopathy and SMA. *Neurology* 2002;59:1197–1202.
67. Hargreaves P, Rahman S, Guthrie P, et al. Diagnostic value of succinate ubiquinone reductase activity in the identification of patients with mitochondrial DNA depletion. *J Inherit Metab Dis* 2002;25: 7–16.
68. Mancuso M, Filosto M, Bonilla E, et al. Mitochondrial myopathy of childhood associated with mitochondrial DNA depletion and a monozygous mutation (T77M) in the TK2 gene. *Arch Neurol* 2003;60:1007–1009.
69. Marín-García J, Ananthakrishnan R, Goldenthal MJ, et al. Cardiac mitochondrial dysfunction and DNA depletion in children with hypertrophic cardiomyopathy. *J Inherit Metab Dis* 1997;20:674–680.
70. Holmuhamedov E, Jahangir A, Bienengraeber M, et al. Deletion of mtDNA disrupts mitochondrial function and structure, but not biogenesis. *Mitochondrion* 2003;3:13–19.
71. Hirano M, Nishigaki Y, Marti R. Mitochondrial neurogastrointestinal encephalomyopathy (MNGIE): a disease of two genomes. *Neurologist* 2004;10:8–17.
72. Alpers BJ. Diffuse progressive degeneration of the gray matter of the cerebrum. *Arch Neurol Psychiatr* 1931;25:469–505.
73. Naviaux RK, Nguyen KV. *POLG* mutations associated with Alpers' syndrome and mitochondrial DNA depletion. *Ann Neurol* 2004;55:706–712.
74. Tesarova M, Mayr JA, Wenchich L, et al. Mitochondrial DNA depletion in Alpers syndrome. *Neuropediatrics* 2004;35:215–223.
75. Riordan-Eva P, Harding AE. Leber's hereditary optic neuropathy: the clinical relevance of different mitochondrial DNA mutations. *J Med Genet* 1995;32:81–87.
76. Nikoskelainen E, Savontaus ML, Wanne OP, et al. Leber's hereditary optic neuroretinopathy, a maternally inherited disease. *Arch Ophthalmol* 1987;105:665–671.
77. Jun AS, Brown MD, Wallace DC. A mitochondrial DNA mutation at nucleotide pair 14459 of the NADH dehydrogenase subunit 6 gene associated with maternally inherited Leber hereditary optic neuropathy and dystonia. *Proc Natl Acad Sci USA* 1994;91:6206–6210.
78. Adams JH, Blackwood W, Wilson J. Further clinical and pathological observations on Leber's optic atrophy. *Brain* 1966;89:15–26.
79. Uemura A, Osame M, Nakagawa M, et al. Leber's hereditary optic neuropathy: mitochondrial and biochemical studies on muscle biopsies. *Br J Ophthalmol* 1987;71:531–536.
80. Engel WK, Vick NA, Glueck CJ, Levy RI. A skeletal muscle disorder associated with intermittent symptoms and a possible defect of lipid metabolism. *N Engl J Med* 1970;282:697–704.
81. Murthy MS, Pande SV. Characterization of a solubilized malonyl-CoA-sensitive carnitine palmitoyltransferase from the mitochondrial outer membrane as a protein distinct from the malonyl-CoA-insensitive carnitine palmitoyltransferase of the inner membrane. *Biochem J* 1990;268:599–604.
82. Stumpf DA, Parker WD, Angelini C. Carnitine deficiency, organic acidemias, and Reye's syndrome. *Neurology* 1985;35:1041–1045.
83. Coates PM, Hale DE, Finocchiaro G, et al. Genetic deficiency of short-chain acyl-coenzyme A dehydrogenase in cultured fibroblasts from a patient with muscle carnitine deficiency and severe skeletal muscle weakness. *J Clin Invest* 1988;81:171–175.
84. Winter SC, Szabo-Aczel S, Curry CJ, et al. Plasma carnitine deficiency. Clinical observations in 51 pediatric patients. *Am J Dis Child* 1987;141:660–665.
85. Breningstall GN. Carnitine deficiency syndromes. *Pediatr Neurol* 1990;6:75–81.
86. Turnbull DM, Bartlett K, Stevens DL, et al. Short-chain acyl CoA dehydrogenase deficiency associated with a lipid-storage myopathy and secondary carnitine deficiency. *N Engl J Med* 1984;311:1232–1236.
87. Stanley CA, DeLeeuw S, Coates PM, et al. Chronic cardiomyopathy and weakness or acute coma in children with a defect in carnitine uptake. *Ann Neurol* 1991;30:709–716.
88. Treem WR, Stanley CA, Finegold DN, et al. Primary carnitine deficiency due to a failure of carnitine transport in kidney, muscle, and fibroblasts. *N Engl J Med* 1988;319:1331–1336.
89. Nezu J, Tamai I, Oku A, et al. Primary systemic carnitine deficiency is caused by mutations in a gene encoding sodium-ion dependent carnitine transporter. *Nat Genet* 1999;21:91–94.

90. Bonnet D, Martin D, Pascale De Lonlay, et al. Arrhythmias and conduction defects as presenting symptoms of fatty acid oxidation disorders in children. *Circulation* 1999;100:2248–2253.
91. Di Donato S. Disorders of lipid metabolism affecting skeletal muscle: carnitine deficiency syndromes, defects in the catabolic pathway, and Chanarin disease. In: Engel AG, Franzini-Armstrong C, eds. *Myology*, 2nd ed. New York: McGraw-Hill, 1994;1587–1609.
92. Lamhonwah AM, Olpin SE, Pollitt RJ, et al. Novel OCTN2 mutations: no genotype-phenotype correlations: early carnitine therapy prevents cardiomyopathy. *Am J Med Genet* 2002;111:271–284.
93. Falik-Borenstein ZC, Jordan SC, Saudubray JM, et al. Brief report: renal tubular acidosis in carnitine palmitoyltransferase type 1 deficiency. *N Engl J Med* 1992;327:24–27.
94. Kelly KJ, Garland JS, Tang TT, et al. Fatal rhabdomyolysis following influenza infection in a girl with familial carnitine palmityl transferase deficiency. *Pediatrics* 1989;84:312–316.
95. Vladutin G.D. Biochemical and molecular correlations in carnitine palmitoyltransferase II deficiency. *Muscle Nerve* 1999;22:949–951.
96. Thullier L, Rostave H, Droin V, et al. Correlation between genotype, metabolic data, and clinical presentation in carnintine palmitoyl transferase 2 (CPT2) deficiency. *Hum Mut* 2003;21:493–500.
97. Hug G, Bove KE, Soukup S. Lethal neonatal multiorgan deficiency of carnitine palmitoyl transferase II. *N Engl J Med* 1991;325:1862–1864.
98. Demaugre F, Bonnefont JP, Colonna M, et al. Infantile form of carnitine palmitoyltransferase II deficiency with hepatomuscular symptoms and sudden death: physiopathological approach to carnitine palmitoyltransferase II deficiencies. *J Clin Invest* 1991;87:859–864.
99. Land JM, Mistry S, Squier W, et al. Neonatal carnitine palmitoyltransferase-2 deficiency: a case presenting with myopathy. *Neuromuscul Disord* 1995;5:129–137.
100. Meola G, Bresolin N, Rimoldi M, et al. Recessive carnitine palmityl transferase deficiency: biochemical studies in tissue cultures and platelets. *J Neurol* 1987;235:74–79.
101. Stanley CA, Hale DE, Berry GT, et al. Brief report: a deficiency of carnitine-acylcarnitine translocase in the inner mitochondrial membrane. *N Engl J Med* 1992;327:19–23.
102. Iacobazzi V, Pasquali M, Singh R, et al. Respopnse to therapy in carnitine/actyl carnitine translocase (CACT) deficiency due to a novel missense mutation. *Am J Med Genet* 2004;126A:150–155.
103. Jerusalem F, Spiess H, Baumgartner G. Lipid storage myopathy with normal carnitine levels. *J Neurol Sci* 1975;24:273–283.
104. Sengers RC, Stadhouders AM, Jaspar HH, et al. Cardiomyopathy and short stature associated with mitochondrial and/or lipid storage myopathy of skeletal muscle. *Neuropaediatrie* 1976;7:196–208.
105. Williams ML, Koch TK, O'Donnell JJ, et al. Ichthyosis and neutral lipid storage disease. *Am J Med Genet* 1985;20:711–726.
106. Lefevre C, Jobard F, Caux F, et al. Mutations in *CGI-58*, the gene encoding a new protein of the esterase/lipase/thioesterase subfamily, in Chanarin-Dorfman syndrome. *Am J Hum Genet* 2001;69:1002–1012.
107. Cwik VA. Disorders of lipid metabolism in skeletal muscle. *Neurol Clin* 2000;18:167–180.
108. Schröder R, Vielhaber S, Wiedemann FR, et al. New insights into the metabolic consequences of large-scale mtDNA deletions: a quantitative analysis of biochemical, morphological and genetic findings in human skeletal muscle. *J Neuropathol Exp Neurol* 2000;59:353–360.
109. Vogel H. Mitochondrial myopathies and the role of the pathologist in the molecular era. *J Neuropathol Exp Neurol* 2001;60:217–227.
110. Rollins S, Prayson RA, McMahon JT, et al. Diagnostic yield muscle biopsy in patients with clinical evidence of mitochondrial cytopathy. *Am J Clin Pathol* 2001;116:326–330.
111. Carpenter S, Karpati G. *Pathology of skeletal muscle*, 2nd ed. New York: Oxford University Press, 2001: 453–459.
112. Vielhaber S, Varlamov DA, Kudina TA, et al. Expression pattern of mitochondrial respiratory chain enzymes in skeletal muscle of patients harboring the A3243G point mutation or large-scale deletions of mitochondrial DNA. *J Neuropathol Exp Neurol* 2002;61:885–895.
113. Oldfors A, Tulinius M. Mitochondrial encephalomyopathies. *J Neuropathol Exp Neurol* 2003;62:217–227.
114. Ricoy-Campo JR, Cabello A. Mitocondriopatías. *Rev Neurol* (Barcelona) 2003;37:775–779.
115. Kyriakides T, Drousiotou A, Panasopoulou A, et al. A comparative morphological study in 33 cases of respiratory chain encephalomyopathies. *Acta Myol* 2003;22:48–52.
116. Fardeau M, Tomé FMS, Rolland JC. Congenital neuromuscular disorder with predominant mitochondrial changes in type II muscle fibers. *Acta Neuropathol* 1981;(Suppl 7):279–282.
117. Peyronnard JM, Charron L, Bellavance A, et al. Neuropathy and mitochondrial myopathy. *Ann Neurol* 1980;7:262–268.
118. Yiannikas C, McLeod JG, Pollard JD, Baverstock J. Peripheral neuropathy associated with mitochondrial myopathy. *Ann Neurol* 1986;20:249–257.
119. McFarland R, Taylor RW, Chinnery PF, et al. A novel sporadic mutation in cytochrome-*c*-oxidase subunit II as a cause of rhabdomyolysis. *Neuromusc Disord* 2004;14:162–166.
120. Bonilla E, Schotland DL, DiMauro S, et al. Electron cytochemistry of crystalline inclusions in human skeletal muscle mitochondria. *J Ultrastruct Res* 1975;51:404–408.
121. Nishino I, Kobayashi O, Goto YI, et al. A new congenital muscular dystrophy with mitochondrial structural abnormalities. *Muscle Nerve* 1998;21:40–47.
122. Bhawat AG, Ross RC. Hepatic intramitochondrial crystalloids. *Arch Pathol* 1971;91:70–77.
123. DiMauro S, Nicholson JF, Hays AP, et al. Benign infantile mitochondrial myopathy due to reversible cytochrome-*c*-oxidase deficiency. *Ann Neurol* 1983;14:226–234.
124. Wada H, Woo M, Nishio H, et al. Vascular involvement in benign infantile mitochondrial myopathy caused by reversible cytochrome-*c*-oxidase deficiency. *Brain Dev* 1996;18:263–268.
125. Castro-Gago M, Eirís J, Pintos E, et al. Miopatía congénita benigna asociada a deficiencia parcial de los complejos I y III de la cadena respiratoria mitocondrial. *Rev Neurol* (Barcelona) 2000;31:838–841.
126. Kubota Y, Ishii T, Sugihara H, et al. Skin manifestations of a patient with mitochondrial encephalomyopathy with lactic acidosis and strokelike episodes (MELAS syndrome). *J Am Acad Dermatol* 1999;41:469–473.
127. Schapira AHV. Primary and secondary defects of the mitochondrial respiratory chain. *J Inherit Metab Dis* 2002;25:207–214.
128. Marín-García J, Goldenthal MJ, Sarnat HB. Probing striated muscle mitochondrial phenotype in neuromuscular disorders. *Pediatr Neurol* 2003;29:26–33.
129. Tsao CY, Mendell JR, Lo WD, et al. Mitochondrial respiratory-chain defects presenting as nonspecific features in children. *J Child Neurol* 2000;15:445–448.
130. Poulton J, Deadman ME, Turnbull DM, et al. Detection of mitochondrial DNA deletions in blood using the polymerase chain reaction: noninvasive diagnosis of mitochondrial myopathy. *Clin Genet* 1991;39:33–38.
131. De Coo IF, Gussinklo T, Arts PJ, et al. A PCR test for progressive external ophthalmoplegia and Kearns-Sayre syndrome on DNA from blood samples. *J Neurol Sci* 1997;149:37–40.
132. Sparaco M, Bonilla E, DiMauro S, et al. Neuropathology of mitochondrial encephalomyopathies due to mitochondrial DNA defects. *J Neuropathol Exp Neurol* 1993;52:1–10.
133. Powers JM, De Vivo DC. Peroxisomal and mitochondrial disorders. In: Graham DI, Lantos PL, eds. *Greenfield's Neuropathology*, 7th ed. London: Arnold Press; 2002;1:737–798.
134. Tanji K, Hays AP, Bonilla E. Mitochondrial alterations in ependymal cells of Kearns- Sayre syndrome [Abstract]. *J Neuropathol Exp Neurol* 2003;62:567.
135. Fernández R, Fernández JM, Cervera C, et al. Adult glycogenosis II with paracrystalline mitochondrial inclusions and Hirano bodies in skeletal muscle. *Neuromusc Disord* 1999;9:136–143.
136. Pons R, Andreetta F, Wa CH, et al. Mitochondrial myopathy simulating spinal muscular atrophy. *Pediatr Neurol* 1996;15:153–158.
137. Berger A, Mayr JA, Meierhofer D, et al. Severe depletion of mitochondrial DNA in spinal muscular atrophy. *Acta Neuropathol* 2003;105:245–251.
138. Nikali K, Isosomppi J, Lonnqvist T, et al. Toward cloning of a novel ataxia gene: refined assignment and physical map of the IOSCA locus (*SCA8*) on 10q24. *Genomics* 1997;39:185–191.
139. Nikali K, Lönnqvist T, Suomalainen A, et al. Infantile onset spinocerebellar ataxia is caused by recessive mutations in a gene encoding a mitochondrial protein [Abstract]. *Eur J Paediatr Neurol* 2003;7:285.

140. Lamperti C, Naini A, Hirano M, et al. Cerebellar ataxia and coenzyme Q10 deficiency. *Neurology* 2003;60:1206–1208.
141. Rifai Z, Welle S, Kamp C, et al. Ragged-red fibers in normal aging and inflammatory myopathy. *Ann Neurol* 1995;37:24–29.
142. Carpenter S, Karpati G, Johnston W, et al. Coexistence of polymyositis (PM) with mitochondrial myopathy [Abstract]. *Neurology* 1992;42(Suppl 3):388.
143. Schuelke M, Krude H, Finckh B, et al. Septo-optic dysplasia associated with a new mitochondrial cytochrome *b* mutation. *Ann Neurol* 2002;51:388–392.
144. Sarnat HB, Machin G, Darwish HZ, et al. Mitochondrial myopathy of cerebro-hepato-renal (Zellweger) syndrome. *Can J Neurol Sci* 1983;10:170–177.
145. Kelley RI. The cerebrohepatorenal syndrome of Zellweger. Morphological and metabolic aspects. *Am J Med Genet* 1983;16:503–517.
146. Lorenc A, Bryk J, Golik P, et al. Homoplasmic MELAS A3243G mtDNA mutation in a colon cancer sample. *Mitochondrion* 2003;3:119–124.
147. Wu SP, Shuy MK, Liou HH, et al. Interaction between anticonvulsants and human placental carnitine transporter. *Epilepsia* 2004;45:204–210.
148. Yerroum M, Pham-Dang C, Authier FJ, et al. Cytochrome *c* oxidase deficiency in the muscle of patients with zidovudine myopathy is segmental and affects both mitochondrial DNA- and nuclear DNA-encoded subunits. *Acta Neuropathol* 2000;100:82–86.
149. Luca CC, Lam BL, Moraes CT. Erythromycin as a potential precipitating agent in the onset of Leber's hereditary optic neuropathy. *Mitochondrion* 2004;4:31–36.
150. Phillips PS, Haas RH, Bannykh S, et al. Statin-associated myopathy with normal creatine kinase levels. *Ann Intern Med* 2002;137:581–585.
151. Silver MA, Langsjoen PH, Szabo S, et al. Statin cardiomyopathy? A potential role for co-enzyme Q10 therapy for statin-induced changes in diastolic LV performance: description of a clinical protocol. *Biofactors* 2003;18:125–127.
152. Melegh B, Trombitás K. Valproate treatment induces lipid globule accumulation with ultrastructural abnormalities of mitochondria in skeletal muscles. *Neuropediatrics* 1997;28:257–261.
153. Mitsui T, Umaki Y, Nagasawa M, et al. Mitochondrial damage in patients with long-term corticosteroid therapy: development of oculoskeletal symptoms similar to mitochondrial disease. *Acta Neuropathol* 2002;104:260–266.
154. Chow CK. Vitamin E regulation of mitochondrial superoxide generation. *Biol Signals Recept* 2001;10:112–124.
155. Komura K, Hobbiebrunken E, Ekkehard KG, et al. Effectiveness of creatine monohydrate in mitochondrial encephalomyopathies. *Pediatr Neurol* 2003;28:53–58.
156. Brierley EJ, Johnson MA, Bowman A, et al. Mitochondrial function in muscle from elderly athletes. *Ann Neurol* 1997;41:114–116.
157. Matthews PM, Ford B, Dandurand RJ, et al. Coenzyme Q10 with multiple vitamins is generally ineffective in treatment of mitochondrial disease. *Neurology* 1993;43:884–890.
158. Li X, May MM. Location and recycling of mitochondrial α-tocopherol. *Mitochondrion* 2003;3:29–38.
159. Linnane AW, Kopsidas G, Zhang C, et al. Cellular redox activity of coenzyme Q10: effect of CoQ10 supplementation on human skeletal muscle. *Free Radic Res* 2002;36:445–453.
160. Geromel V, Darin N, Chrétien D, et al. Coenzyme Q(10) and idebenone in the therapy of respiratory chain diseases: rationale and comparative benefits. *Mol Genet Metabol* 2002;77:21–30.
161. Van Maldergem L, Trijbels F, DiMauro S, et al. Coenzyme Q-responsive Leigh's encephalopathy in two sisters. *Ann Neurol* 2002;52:750–754.
162. Huang CC, Kuo HC, Chu CC, et al. Rapid visual recovery after coenzyme Q10 treatment of Leber hereditary optic neuropathy [Comment]. *J Neuro-Ophthalmol* 2002;22:66.
163. Berbel-García A, Barabara-Farre JR, Etessam JP, et al. Coenzyme Q 10 improves lactic acidosis, strokelike episodes, and epilepsy in a patient with MELAS (mitochondrial myopathy, encephalopathy, lactic acidosis and strokelike episodes). *Clin Neuropharmacol* 2004;27:187–191.
164. Thomas L. Organelles as organisms. In: *The Life of a Cell*. New York: Viking Press, 1974:72.

Chapter 3

Heredodegenerative Diseases

John H. Menkes

Advances in molecular biology have pointed to a basic similarity between diseases of metabolic origin (see Chapter 1) and heredodegenerative diseases. Nevertheless, essential differences remain. In metabolic disorders, the biochemical derangement of tissue or body fluids has led, in enzymopathies such as phenylketonuria or maple syrup urine disease, to the identification of the basic biochemical defect. Subsequent purification of the normal protein has permitted isolation of the gene that codes for it and has led to the determination of the molecular abnormality or abnormalities in the gene in patients with the disease. This process has been termed *functional cloning*.

Many of the conditions covered in this chapter do not yet have a biochemical explanation. This lack has prompted the application of positional cloning (*reverse genetics*, a process in which the gene responsible for the disorder is isolated without its protein product being known). Theoretically, the process is simple; the approximate map position of the gene is established by linkage studies on extended families experiencing the disease. In many instances, cytogenetics and the use of a large number of polymorphic markers allow assignment of the gene to a specific chromosome with a resolution of roughly several million base pairs. This first step has been accomplished for quite a few of the conditions covered in this chapter. The second step involves a more exact localization of the gene site and subsequent isolation and cloning of the gene. Although this has been a complicated and labor-intensive process, it has been achieved for a significant proportion of the heredodegenerative diseases covered in this chapter.

A shortcut to this process, which is also applicable to the rarer diseases, has been the use of *candidate genes*. A number of genes coding for proteins and enzymes vital to brain function have been mapped, cloned, and sequenced. When a new disease locus is assigned to a chromosomal region using linkage analysis, candidate genes from the same region are surveyed and features of these candidate genes are compared with the features of the particular disease. Conversely, when a new gene is assigned to a chromosomal region, candidate diseases are analyzed by an analogous process. This approach has led to the observation that abnormalities in the gene for myelin proteolipid protein (PLP) are responsible for Pelizaeus-Merzbacher disease (PMD), with the gene for both PLP and the disease localized to the q22 segment of the X chromosome. One of the genes for Charcot-Marie-Tooth (CMT) disease [hereditary motor sensory neuropathy (HMSN) type IA] was isolated by this combined approach.

The interested reader is referred to reviews of this constantly evolving field in Chapters 14 (Identifying Human Disease Genes) and 16 (Molecular Pathology) in the text by Strachan and Reed (1) and Chapter 1 (Introduction to Medical Genetics and Methods of DNA Testing) in the book edited by Pulst (2).

For the clinician, it is still best that the heredodegenerative diseases are grouped according to their clinical presentation and according to the site in the brain that incurs the major anatomic or functional insult. The categories are (a) heredodegenerative diseases of the basal ganglia, (b) heredodegenerative diseases of the cerebellum, brainstem, and spinal cord, (c) heredodegenerative diseases of the peripheral and cranial nerves, and (d) diffuse cerebral degenerative diseases. A variety of intermediate forms have been well documented.

As our knowledge of the interrelation between genotype and phenotype expands it has become evident that many common neurologic phenotypes have multiple genetic etiologies and, conversely, that there are many examples of mutations in single genes that produce distinct phenotypes. This chapter will provide examples of both phenomena. Thus there are at least 21 genetic forms of autosomal dominant cerebellar ataxias, and the Charcot-Marie-Tooth phenotype results from mutations in more than a dozen different genes. On the other hand, different mutations in the voltage-dependent calcium-channel gene (*CACNA1A*) can produce one of the dominant spinocerebellar ataxias (SCA6), episodic ataxia (EA2), or familial hemiplegic migraine. Even when there appears to be a clear relationship between a mutated gene and its phenotype, the correlation between genotype and phenotype is far from complete, and there are often known or unknown genetic or environmental phenotypic modifiers that affect penetrance and expression. One example of this perplexing situation is the situation in DYT1 dystonia, one of the primary torsion dystonias, in which the question of why dystonia is only present in some 30% of gene carriers is completely unresolved. Another such example is the recently uncovered effect of genetic modifiers on the splicing machinery that can result in changes in the levels of normal transcripts or in the relative ratios of wild type to mutant transcripts such as has been documented for familial dysautonomia.

HEREDODEGENERATIVE DISEASES OF THE BASAL GANGLIA

Huntington Disease

Huntington disease (HD) is a chronic progressive degenerative disease characterized by involuntary movements, mental deterioration, and an autosomal dominant transmission. Although its essential features were first described by Waters (3) in 1841, Huntington provided its most accurate and graphic description in residents of East Hampton, Long Island (4).

The prevalence of HD in the general population has been estimated at between 5 and 10 per 100,000 (5). Although all patients early in the history of the United States were descendants of two English brothers, the disease has since been found in all races and nationalities.

Morphologic abnormalities are limited to the brain. Grossly, patients have gyral atrophy affecting primarily the frontal lobes and generalized and symmetric dilatation of the lateral ventricles. The striatum (caudate nucleus and putamen) is markedly shrunken, with the tail of the caudate nucleus being the area that is most affected (Fig. 3.1). Light microscopic examination demonstrates three processes: neuronal loss, which is associated with the presence of brain macrophages and neuronal satellitosis; lipopigment deposition in neurons and astroglia in excess of that expected for the patient's age; and a relative astrocytic proliferation (6). In adults, these changes are found in the caudate nucleus, putamen, and, to a lesser extent, the cortex, notably the frontal lobes (7). The ventrolateral thalamic nucleus, subthalamic nucleus, and, in some cases, spinal cord also may be involved. As a rule, the caudate nucleus, particularly its periventricular portion, is more affected than the putamen, whereas the nucleus accumbens generally is spared until late in the disease process.

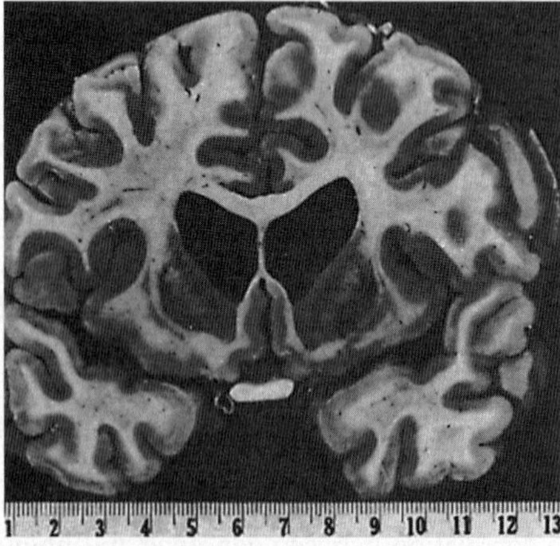

FIGURE 3.1. Huntington disease. Gross atrophy of the caudate nucleus gives the lateral ventricles a butterfly appearance. (Courtesy of Dr. J. A. N. Corsellis, The Maudsley Hospital, London.)

The pathology of juvenile HD is somewhat similar. Children presenting with the rigid form of the disease appear to have a marked destruction of the putamen (8,9). Severe astrogliosis of the globus pallidus may occur without neuronal loss, and hyperpigmentation of the substantia nigra has been noted in some juvenile patients (10).

Electron microscopy of frontal lobe biopsies reveals a generalized, nonspecific derangement of all membrane structures, a consequence of cell death.

Cell death within the striatum does not affect all neurons equally. The medium-sized gamma-aminobutyric acid (GABA)-ergic spiny projection neurons, which make up approximately 95% of human striatal neurons and contain a variety of neuropeptides, notably enkephalins and substance P, are the first to be affected (11). They are the source of the striatal output projections to the external globus pallidus and to the substantia nigra pars reticulata. By contrast, medium-sized aspiny interneurons containing somatostatin and staining with the histochemical marker nicotinamide adenine dinucleotide phosphate (NADPH)–diaphorase are relatively spared, as are the large, aspiny, cholinergic neurons and neurons immunoreactive for neuropeptide Y.

Selective cell loss also is observed in the cortex, where a depletion of the large pyramidal neurons in cortical layers III, V, and VI and sparing of the GABA-ergic local circuit neurons occur (12). During the initial phases of the disease, cell loss is at least partially compensated by augmentation of the dendritic trees of the surviving pyramidal cells. This observation could explain the normal cortical metabolic activity that is observed in the early phase of the illness (13).

Pathogenesis and Molecular Genetics

The gene for HD has been mapped to the short arm of chromosome 4 (4p16.3) (14). This work represented the first successful linkage analysis in humans using polymorphic DNA markers. The gene whose mutation causes HD is widely expressed in all regions of normal and HD brain and in various other organs. It encodes a large cytoplasmic protein named huntingtin (15). Wild-type huntingtin is essential for normal embryogenesis and the formation of forebrain (16).

HD is an autosomal dominant condition; therefore one mutated gene suffices to cause the disease. Because hemizygous loss of one of the two Huntington genes—as occurs in Wolf-Hirschhorn syndrome—does not produce an HD phenotype, it is evident that the mutation confers a deleterious function on the mutant huntingtin. The disease is now known to result from an expansion of a trinucleotide repeat in the coding region of the gene (17). Trinucleotide repeats are repeated units of three nucleotides in genomic DNA. In the case of HD, it is the trinucleotide (triplet) cytosine-adenine-guanine (CAG) that is repeated. Whereas in the normal population this trinucleotide repeat ranges from 9 to 34 copies, the length of this repeat is expanded in HD to a mean of 42 to 46 copies. This long run of CAGs in the HD gene encodes a polyglutamine tract near the amino terminus of huntingtin. In HD the length of the repeat is highly unstable. Whereas during maternal transmission it changes by only a few repeats and on rare occasions has been shown to contract, in paternal transmission the length of the repeat increases dramatically in approximately one-third of cases. Of patients with repeats of 55 or more, 90% have an onset of the disease by age 30 years, and a good negative correlation exists between the length of the repeat and the age of onset of neurologic symptoms, with the longest repeats resulting in juvenile HD (18).

When HD appears sporadically, it is often the result of an expansion from an already large repeat. Such an expansion is more likely to occur on the paternally derived allele and has been correlated with advanced paternal age (19). The basic processes responsible for the instability of some repeat trinucleotide DNA sequences, a process termed *dynamic mutation*, are unclear (20).

A similar expansion of genes with triplet repeats is seen in a number of neurologic conditions (Table 3.1). It would now appear that whenever a dominantly transmitted heredodegenerative disease manifests genetic anticipation (i.e., whenever a progressively earlier onset of neurologic symptoms occurs in successive generations), a repeat expansion of trinucleotide repeats is suspected (21) (see Chapter 4, Fig. 4.5). However, Fraser stressed that ascertainment bias, that is, that the younger generation has not yet reached the age when the disease becomes manifest, and truncation bias, meaning that parents with an early onset of disease do not have offspring, also should be considered as a cause for anticipation in neurologic conditions (22). In addition, a high incidence of repeat expansions occurs in the normal population, and between 30% and 35% of humans have CAG repeat lengths in their genomes that exceed 40 repeats, an indication that trinucleotide expansion is not invariably associated with a disease process.

It is not fully understood how the expanded triplet repeat on the Huntington gene causes the disease. Several investigators have observed neuronal intranuclear inclusions immunoreactive for huntingtin epitopes in cortical and striatal neurons of HD brain (23). These inclusions comprise truncated derivatives of the mutated huntingtin and are also found in presymptomatic HD (24). It is likely that the expanded polyglutamine tract alters the physical properties of huntingtin in such a manner as to induce its accumulation within the cell nucleus. This contrasts with the cytoplasmic location of wild-type huntingtin (24a). Nuclear accumulation of mutant huntingtin induces cell dysfunction and ultimately neuronal death. Of note is the presence of ubiquitin in these inclusions. Ubiquitin is a small protein that is crucial for the degradation of many cytosolic nuclear and endoplasmic reticulum proteins (25). Because binding of ubiquitin to proteins marks them for subsequent degradation, this finding suggests that mutant huntingtin has been targeted for proteolysis but that the degradation was somehow incomplete.

TABLE 3.1 Triplet-Repeat Diseases

Very Large Expansions of Repeats Outside Coding Sequences
Fragile X syndrome A (FRAXA)
Fragile X syndrome E (FRAXE)
Myotonic dystrophy (DM1)
Spinocerebellar ataxia 8 (SCA8)
Juvenile myoclonus epilepsy (JME)
Intronic Expansions
Friedreich ataxia (FA)
Spinocerebellar ataxia 11 (SCA11)
Myotonic dystrophy (DM2)
CAG Expansions in Translated Regions
Spinobulbar atrophy, X-linked (Kennedy disease)
Spinocerebellar ataxia 1 (SCA1)
Spinocerebellar ataxia 2 (SCA2)
Spinocerebellar ataxia 3 (SCA3, Machado-Joseph disease)
Spinocerebellar ataxia 6 (SCA6) ? Pathogenic
Spinocerebellar ataxia 7 (SCA7)
Spinocerebellar ataxia 17 (SCA17)
Dentatorubral-pallidoluysian atrophy (DPRLA)
Huntington disease (HD)

How mutant huntingtin induces a selective cell death is the subject of much research. More than a dozen proteins interact with the amino terminal of huntingtin. Some are involved in intracellular signaling; others are involved in transcriptional events, and the function of yet others is poorly characterized (26,27). Experimental work suggests that polyglutamine-expanded huntingtin acts within the nucleus to induce apoptotic cell death (28). Antiapoptotic compounds protect neurons against the mutant huntingtin, as does blocking nuclear localization of mutant huntingtin (29).

The mechanisms for selective vulnerability that is so characteristic for HD are unclear. Current thinking is that overactivity of the *N*-methyl-D-aspartate (NMDA)-type glutamate receptors, particularly the NR2B subtype, is at least contributory in that it can result in excitotoxicity-induced cell death in the medium-sized spiny GABA-ergic projection neurons that are enriched in the NR2B receptors (30). In support of this hypothesis is the marked reduction in NMDA-receptor binding in the putamen of brains in patients with HD as compared with normal brains (31).

It is not clear whether mitochondrial dysfunction and consequent oxidative stress represent primary abnormalities or are secondary to early neuronal dysfunction (32). Respiratory complex II/III is deficient in putamen derived from patients with HD but is normal in their cerebral cortex, cerebellum, and cultured fibroblasts. This observation suggests that mitochondrial dysfunction parallels the severity of neuronal loss and could be secondary to cell damage induced by excitotoxicity and the ensuing generation of free radicals and superoxide (33).

Clinical Manifestations

Although symptoms usually begin between ages 35 and 40 years, approximately 5% of patients are younger than 14 years (34). In general, the age when symptoms have their onset is inversely related to the CAG repeat number (35). However, the age of onset is also a function of genes other than the HD gene and is partially environmentally determined (36). Age of onset also decreases as the number of affected male ancestors increases. This finding is most striking when both the affected parent and grandparent are men. In a large series of patients with juvenile HD (patients whose symptoms become apparent before 20 years of age), Myers and coworkers found that 83% inherited the disease from their fathers (34). The onset of neurologic symptoms in siblings of patients with juvenile HD is approximately 27 years. This timing is significantly earlier than in the general population of patients with HD (37). The best explanation for the phenomenon of paternal inheritance of juvenile HD is that an expansion of the triplet repeat occurs during spermatogenesis.

The clinical picture of HD as it presents in children differs from that of affected adults (Table 3.2).

TABLE 3.2 Clinical Features of Huntington Disease of Childhood (28 Cases)

Features	Number of Patients
Age of onset	
Younger than 5 years of age	7
5 to 10 years of age	21
Hyperkinesia or choreoathetosis	13
Rigidity	19
Seizures	13
Mental deterioration	22
Cerebellar symptoms	5

Data from Jervis GA. Huntington's chorea in childhood. *Arch Neurol* 1963;9:244–257; and Markham CH, Knox JW. Observations in Huntington's chorea. *J Pediatr* 1965;67:46–57. With permission.

As surveyed by Cotton and colleagues (38), the initial stages of the illness are marked by mental deterioration or behavioral abnormalities (20 of 40 patients), gait disturbances, usually the consequence of rigidity (18 of 40 cases), cerebellar signs (15 of 40 cases), and, less commonly, seizures. In the Dutch series of Siesling and coworkers, behavioral disorders were the first feature of juvenile HD in 70% and chorea was seen in 48% (39). Some 70% of children in this series who presented with chorea developed rigidity in the course of the disease. Mental deterioration can commence before 2 years of age (40). It is not clear whether the intellectual decline results from striatal or cortical dysfunction.

The clinical onset of rigid cases is earlier than in patients who have chorea as the predominant movement disorder (39). Additionally, in almost 90% of rigid juvenile HD cases, the disease is paternally inherited. This contrasts with approximately 70% for juvenile HD with chorea (39,41).

When present, choreoathetosis resembles that seen in Sydenham chorea, but the movements have a greater affinity for the trunk and proximal musculature and, unlike those in Sydenham chorea, are rarely asymmetric. They are increased by voluntary physical activity and excitement and cease during sleep. Seizures are rare in adults with HD but affect approximately 50% of children. In some cases, they are the most prominent symptom and herald the onset of neurologic deterioration. Grand mal attacks are the most common; minor motor and myoclonic seizures and action myoclonus also have been observed (40). Spasticity, although rare in adults, can be prominent in juvenile HD (42). Cerebellar signs occasionally can be a major feature. Although optic nerve atrophy is not seen, impairment of ocular motility is an early sign and resembles oculomotor apraxia (9). In such instances, requesting the patient to look from side to side elicits closure of the eyelids or a rapid, jerking movement of the head with an attendant delay in the movement of the eyeballs. Unlike in oculomotor apraxia, random and vertical eye movements also are affected.

The disease progresses more rapidly in children than in adults, with an average duration of illness in the reported juvenile cases of 8 years, as contrasted with a range of 10 to 25 years for adults (43). Rate of progression of the disease has also been shown to be directly proportional to the number of CAG repeats.

Homozygotes for HD have been identified in a large Venezuelan kindred (44). Their neurologic picture and the age when symptoms became apparent did not differ from those of the heterozygotes, an indication that the HD gene is phenotypically completely penetrant in the heterozygous state.

Laboratory studies are normal, although the electroencephalogram result is often abnormal, and the cerebrospinal fluid (CSF) protein concentration is sometimes elevated. Computed tomography (CT) scanning and magnetic resonance imaging (MRI) are equally reliable in demonstrating caudate atrophy, but can show normal results even when there are significant neurologic symptoms. The appearance of images on these scans is often not specific, but there can be abnormal T2 prolongation in the putamen (45). A more sensitive and more specific study involves positron emission tomography (PET) scanning after the infusion of radiolabeled fluorodeoxyglucose. A marked reduction in caudate glucose metabolism is observed in all symptomatic patients, regardless of whether atrophy is evident on CT or MRI scans, and in approximately one-third of presymptomatic individuals at risk for the disease (46). A reduced glucose metabolism is accompanied by a reduction in dopamine D_1- and D_2-receptor binding in caudate and putamen. A good correlation exists between intellectual deterioration and the reduction in D_2-receptor binding (47).

Diagnosis

The capacity to monitor the size of the trinucleotide repeat in individuals at risk for HD has revolutionized preclinical and prenatal testing for the disorder. The following diagnostic guidelines have been established: (a) Allele sizes of 26 or fewer CAG repeats have never been associated with the HD phenotype or with mutations to longer repeats. (b) Allele sizes of 27 to 35 repeats have not been associated with the HD phenotype but have been associated with mutability when transmitted paternally. It is likely that some patients with sporadic HD represent the occasional expansion of high-normal paternal alleles into the affected range. (c) Allele sizes of 36 to 39 have been associated with HD phenotype but also have been seen in apparently unaffected individuals. (d) Allele sizes of 40 or more CAG repeats have always been accompanied by HD pathology (48). In the experience of Kremer and colleagues, who obtained molecular data from 1,007 individuals, 1.2% of patients with a clinical diagnosis of HD possessed repeats that fell into the normal range (49). It is not known whether these patients have a phenocopy of HD or whether they were misdiagnosed. Until effective treatment becomes available, the World Federation of Neurology does not advise that patients under 18 years of age be tested for the disease (50). I believe this is a complex issue and that the decision to administer or not to administer the test to children must be evaluated on a case-by-case basis.

The clinical diagnosis of HD rests on the neurologic examination, a positive family history, and neuroimaging studies. HD should be differentiated from the various conditions in which a movement disorder arises during childhood or adolescence. These include idiopathic torsion dystonia (dystonia musculorum deformans), Hallervorden-Spatz syndrome, Wilson disease, and juvenile Parkinson's disease. When intellectual deterioration is the chief feature, the various lipidoses should also be considered. Since 1980 there has been a resurgence of Sydenham chorea in the United States. Even though an antecedent streptococcal infection usually cannot be elicited, the distribution of the involuntary movements assists in the diagnosis, as does immune evidence of a streptococcal infection.

Treatment

No treatment has been effective in reversing or arresting the progressive dementia. Choline, reserpine, and various phenothiazines, however, can alleviate the choreiform movements, and levodopa, bromocriptine, and amantadine can provide some benefit in the rigid form of the disease.

Huntington Disease–Like Disorders

There are several disorders that present with symptoms commensurate with HD but in which genetic analysis shows neither a pathologic CAG triplet expansion nor a linkage to 4p16.3. The best studied of these has been termed HD-like 2. It has been mapped to chromosome 16q24.4 and represents a CAG/CTG expansion in the gene that codes for junctophilin-3, a protein that is involved in the formation of junctional membrane structures (51). The clinical picture in this condition resembles that of HD.

In HD-like 3, a condition that has been mapped to chromosome 4p15.3, the clinical picture resembles that of juvenile HD, but transmission appears to be autosomal recessive (52). The condition manifests itself at about 3 to 4 years of age and is characterized by both pyramidal and extrapyramidal abnormalities. The MRI shows caudate atrophy.

HD-like 1 disease is linked to chromosome 20p12. This condition is a familial prion disease with a large insertion in the prior protein gene (53).

Hereditary benign chorea is a syndrome that is not too rarely encountered by a pediatric neurologist interested in movement disorders. This autosomal dominant condition, first described by Pincus and Chutorian (54), has its onset in infancy or early childhood and is nonprogressive, with peak severity in the second decade of life and movement diminishing during the adult years (55,56). Mild mental retardation is seen in a few patients, but there is no mental deterioration. PET scans in patients with this condition also demonstrate caudate hypometabolism. In some families the condition has been mapped to the long arm of chromosome 14, but there is significant genetic heterogeneity (57). Mutations in the thyroid transcription factor 1 gene, a homeodomain-containing transcription factor essential for the organogenesis of the lung, the thyroid, and the basal ganglia, have been documented in some patients carrying this disease (58).

Several conditions are now recognized in which an extrapyramidal disorder is accompanied by the presence of acanthocytes. These are red blood cells with an irregular body and spicules of variable length that are irregularly distributed over the surface of the cell (see Chapter 1,

Fig. 1.32). The differentiation between acanthocytes and red cells with rounded projections (echinocytes) and their visualization is discussed by Feinberg and coworkers (59). Acanthocytes are seen in more than 50% of all red cells derived from patients with abetalipoproteinemia but also have been observed in an occasional patient with Hallervorden-Spatz disease, HD-like 2 disease, hypobetalipoproteinemia, acanthocytosis, retinitis pigmentosa, pallidal degeneration syndrome (HARP syndrome: hypoprebetalipoproteinemia, acanthocytosis, and retinitis pigmentosa), and a condition termed *chorea-acanthocytosis*.

Symptoms of HARP syndrome generally appear during the first decade of life and are marked by dystonia, dysarthria, and impaired gait (60).

Typically, chorea-acanthocytosis is characterized by chorea, orofacial dyskinesia with dysarthria, and depressed or absent reflexes. Seizures, dementia, and self-mutilation also have been observed. The age of onset is usually during the second decade or later (61). This condition is not rare in the south of Japan and can be transmitted in both a recessive and a dominant manner (62). The diagnosis of neuroacanthocytosis rests on the demonstration of acanthocytes in a dried blood smear or in saline-diluted wet preparations. Serum lipoprotein electrophoresis and vitamin E levels are normal. Neuroimaging demonstrates caudate atrophy, and MRI reveals increased signal in the caudate and lentiform nuclei. PET scans indicate a severe loss of striatal dopamine D_2-receptor-binding sites and a marked reduction in the [^{18}F]dopa uptake in the posterior putamen. These point to a selective degeneration of dopaminergic projections from the substantia nigra compacta to the posterior putamen (63). Further discussion of the various neurologic syndromes associated with peripheral acanthocytosis is given in Chapter 1.

Primary Dystonia (Dystonia Musculorum Deformans, Torsion Dystonia, DYT1)

Primary dystonia (dystonia musculorum deformans, torsion dystonia) is characterized by sustained muscle contraction frequently causing twisting and repetitive movements or abnormal postures. It was first described by Schwalbe in 1908 as a variant of hysteria (64) and more definitively by Oppenheim in 1911 (65). It is now evident that this condition represents several genetically distinct entities distinguishable from the various acquired dystonias that result from perinatal asphyxia, trauma, toxins, or vascular disease.

Pathogenesis and Molecular Genetics

Several genes have been implicated in the various hereditary dystonias. The disorders are summarized in Table 3.3. The clinical entity that most commonly manifests during childhood has been termed *early-onset dystonia* (DYT1). The gene for this condition has been mapped to chromosome 9q34. A single mutation, a 3-base pair (bp) deletion, in the coding sequence of the gene is found in almost all cases seen in Ashkenazi Jewish families (66). Identical gene mutations also have been documented in patients with completely different ethnicities. This suggests that DYT1 is an example of a recurrent mutation causing a dominantly inherited condition (85,86). The DYT1 gene codes for a protein termed torsin A, an adenosine triphosphate (ATP)-binding protein, which is a member of the AAA protein family. These proteins participate in a variety of biological functions including membrane trafficking, organelle biosynthesis, and protein chaperone activities. They achieve these tasks by unfolding proteins or disassembling protein complexes. The mutation causes torsin A to relocalize from the endoplasmic reticulum, where it is normally located, to the nuclear envelope, recruiting the wild-type torsin A to the nuclear envelope with it (87–89,89a).

The pathophysiology of primary dystonia (dystonia musculorum deformans) is unknown. Clinical and electrophysiologic observations indicate that dystonic movements and postures result from a functional disturbance of the basal ganglia. In particular, the striatal control of the globus pallidus and the substantia nigra pas reticulata is impaired. Microelectrode recording conducted in the course of pallidotomy shows a decreased discharge rate from both the internal and external segments of the globus pallidus, probably as a consequence of an increased inhibitory output from the striatum. In addition, the pattern of spontaneous neuronal activity is highly irregular (90). As a result, there is an alteration of thalamic control of cortical motor planning and execution of movements, reducing the brainstem and spinal cord inhibitory mechanisms (91,92). As a consequence, prolonged abnormal cocontractions of agonist and antagonist muscles occur, with abnormal recruitment (overflow) to the more distant musculature. Marsden postulated that a defect in the presynaptic inhibitory mechanisms in the spinal cord causes the failure in reciprocal inhibition (93).

Even though primary dystonia is believed to be a functional disorder of the basal ganglia, no consistent anatomic abnormalities are seen in this region. Neuropathologic examination of patients with dystonia musculorum deformans has been negative or has revealed nonspecific changes (94). However, McNaught and coworkers recently demonstrated the presence of perinuclear inclusions in cholinergic and other neurons of the midbrain reticular formation, an indication of altered protein handling such as is seen in several other neurodegenerative disorders (94a). Dopamine levels are slightly reduced in the rostral striatum, but not enough to explain the symptoms. This is in contrast to autopsy specimen from patients with

TABLE 3.3 Hereditary Dystonias

Disease	Gene Locus	Inheritance	Mutated Gene Product	Ethnic Predilection	Symptoms	Reference
DYT1	9q34	AD	Torsin A ATPase	Ashkenazi Jewish	Childhood limb onset dystonia becoming generalized	66
DYT2		AR		Gypsy, Sephardic Jews	Early onset of dystonia in extremities, torticollis, blepharospasm	67,68
DYT3	Xq13.1	XR		Filipino	Adult onset, blepharospasm, torticollis, parkinsonism	69
DYT4		AD		Australian	Adolescence to adult, torticollis, dysphonia	70
DYT5a	14q22.1	AD	GTP cyclohydrolase	Japan	Childhood onset, generalized dystonia, diurnal fluctuations, dopa-responsive	71
DYT5b	11p15.5	AR	Tyrosine hydroxylase	None	Childhood onset, generalized dystonia, diurnal fluctuations, dopa-responsive	72
DYT6	8p21–q22	AD		Mennonites	Indistinguishable from DYT1, but later onset	73
DYT7	18p	AD		German	Onset in sixth decade, torticollis, tremor, dysphonia	74
DYT8	2q34	AD		None	Paroxysmal nonkinesigenic dyskinesia	75
DYT9	1p21–p13.3	AD		None	Paroxysmal choreoathetosis with episodic ataxia	76
DYT10	16p11.2–q12.1	AD		None	Paroxysmal kinisigenic choreoathetosis	77
DYT11a	7q21	AD	ε-Sarcoglycan	None	Myoclonic jerks, dystonia, relieved with alcohol, onset childhood, adolescence	78
DYT11b	11q23	AD	Dopamine receptor D_2	None	Same as DYT11a	79
DYT12	19q13	AD			Rapid onset of dystonia and parkinsonism in childhood, adolescence	80
DYT13	1p36.13–36.32	AD			Onset childhood to adult life, benign, slow progression	81
DYT14	14q13	AD			Dopa-responsive dystonia	82
DYT15	18p11	AD		Canada	Like DYT11a	82a
Deafness-dystonia syndrome	Xq22	XR	DDP1/TIMM8a	None	Deafness, rapidly progressive dystonia, some with mental retardation, cortical blindness	83,84

AD, autosomal dominant; AR, autosomal recessive; XR, X-linked recessive; DPP1/TIMM8a, deafness-dystonia protein 1/ translocase of mitochondrial inner membrane 8a.

dopa-responsive dystonia, in whom dopamine levels range between 3% and 20% of normal (95). When discrete lesions result in a secondary focal or hemidystonia, these lesions are localized to the thalamus, caudate nucleus, putamen, or globus pallidus (93).

Clinical Manifestations

Dystonia has been classified according to the body distribution of the abnormal movements. Generalized dystonia (dystonia musculorum deformans) is the most common form seen in children. In this condition, one or both legs and some other region of the body are affected (96). Focal dystonia refers to involvement of a single region. It includes the eyelids (blepharospasm), mouth (oromandibular dystonia), larynx (spastic dysphonia), neck (torticollis), and hand (writer's cramp). In segmental dystonia, two or more contiguous regions are involved. Focal and segmental dystonias are seen rarely during the first two decades of life. Torticollis, when seen in infants and children, is a relatively common condition but is unrelated to primary dystonia. It is considered in Chapter 6.

DYT 1

Generalized DYT1 dystonia is transmitted as an autosomal dominant condition with a low penetrance, probably between 30% and 40% (97). The factors that control penetrance, be they genetic or environmental, are unknown (98). The degree of penetrance is not dependent on the gender of the transmitting parent.

Primary dystonia caused by a defect in the DYT1 gene is the most common type of childhood dystonia. It has a relatively high incidence among Ashkenazi Jews. This entity begins between the ages of 4 and 16 years and is characterized by an initially rapid deterioration. The first symptoms in both the childhood and late-onset forms of hereditary dystonia are involuntary movements or posturing of one portion of the body (99). Most commonly, the initial movement consists of a plantar, flexion-inversion movement of the foot that can first appear when walking (Fig. 3.2). Initially, symptoms are intermittent and, because they are more severe under stress, they frequently are misdiagnosed as representing a hysterical reaction. In due time, however, they become constant. As the disease progresses, involuntary flexion or extension appears at the wrist, and, finally, torsion spasms of the neck and trunk become evident. These movements can be triggered by motion of any other part of the body or ultimately they can appear spontaneously. Eventually, the affected limbs assume a fixed, continuously maintained, abnormal attitude on which athetotic fluctuations in time are superimposed. On examination, the muscles resist passive movements and after forcible deflection, tend to return to their original position.

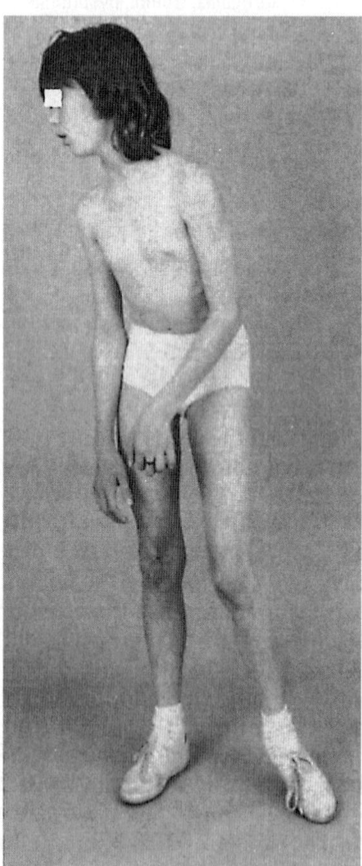

FIGURE 3.2. Dystonia musculorum deformans. Dystonic posturing of left arm and left lower extremity. Flexion at the knee and equinovarus positioning of the foot are typical for this condition. Additionally, this $11^1/_2$-year-old girl has torticollis. Symptoms started at age 9 years with a change in voice, followed by torsion of the distal portion of her left lower extremity at age 10 years.

In some cases, the involuntary movements affect the face and interfere with speech and swallowing. Dystonia of the visceral musculature, particularly paroxysmal dyspnea, has been described. As a rule, all movements cease during sleep. The intellect remains normal in all instances. The childhood-onset form of the disease tends to progress relentlessly, and, in general, the earlier the onset of symptoms, the more rapid is their advance. In the experience of Marsden and Harrison (100), 79% of children whose involuntary movements appeared before 11 years of age progressed to generalized dystonia. Individuals whose sole symptom is a mixed resting and intention tremor, writer's cramp, or torticollis frequently are seen in affected families and probably represent a partial expression of the disease (99,101).

Neuroimaging in primary dystonia is usually unremarkable. On PET scan of a movement-free patient, a significant increase is seen in the cerebral glucose metabolism in the caudate and lentiform nuclei, cerebellum, and those areas of the frontal lobes that receive projections from the mediodorsal thalamic nucleus (92,102). In clinically nonpenetrant individuals, resting glucose utilization in putamen, anterior cingulate, and cerebellar hemispheres is also increased (103).

In contrast to the generalized forms of hereditary dystonia, segmental and focal forms are rarely encountered in children. The most common of these conditions is spasmodic torticollis, which can appear in isolation or as part of a segmental dystonia, with muscle spasms also affecting the upper extremity. Focal dystonias also include writer's cramp, blepharospasm, spasmodic dysphonia, and oromandibular dystonia. Although these entities tend to remain restricted, they progress in some instances to generalized dystonia (104). In most instances these forms represent a partial expression of primary dystonia (DYT1) (101).

DYT5

A hereditary progressive form of dystonia with marked diurnal fluctuations and a striking response to low doses of dopaminergic drugs has been seen in Japan and accounts for approximately 5% to 10% of all dystonias seen in the West (71,105). Both autosomal dominant and autosomal recessive forms have been described (see Table 3.3). The autosomal dominant form is the result of a defect in the gene that codes for guanosine triphosphate (GTP) cyclohydrolase I; the recessive form is caused by a defect in the gene for tyrosine hydroxylase (71,72). GTP cyclohydrolase I deficiency also is seen in hyperphenylalaninemia (see Chapter 1). The clinical picture for both forms is similar to early-onset generalized dystonia, with onset during the first decade of life. It generally startes with a postural dystonia in one extremity, and within a few years becomes generalized. A postural tremor of the hands is often present. In approximately one-fourth of children, the diurnal fluctuations are not apparent (71).

Patients with generalized dystonia and severe developmental delay and failure to achieve normal motor milestones also have been described. These patients are compound heterozygotes for mutations in the gene coding for GTP cyclohydrolase, but unlike patients with autosomal recessive GTP cyclohydrolase I deficiency, these patients do not demonstrate a marked elevation of plasma phenylalanine. These individuals respond dramatically to therapy with a combination of levodopa and tetrahydrobiopterin (BH_4) (106). Diagnosis of this condition and related conditions such as the recently described infantile parkinsonism-dystonia depends on reliable quantification of the abnormal metabolites in the CSF (107,108).

DYT11

Myoclonic dystonia, a dominantly transmitted form in which torsion dystonia is accompanied by myoclonic jerks, can develop during childhood. Both myoclonus and dystonia improve dramatically with ingestion of alcohol or with a combination of trihexyphenidyl hydrochloride and valproic acid (109). The two genetically distinct forms appear to have similar phenotypes (Table 3.3).

Diagnosis

Primary dystonia (dystonia musculorum deformans) must be differentiated from dystonia arising as a consequence of a known central nervous system (CNS) insult (symptomatic or secondary dystonia) or because of other hereditary neurologic disorders. In children, dystonic symptoms are most often the result of perinatal asphyxia (see Chapter 6). Under such circumstances, the movement disorder generally appears before the third year of life, although, exceptionally, the involuntary movements do not begin until 5 to 15 years of age or even later, with the child having exhibited minimal or no neurologic abnormalities before that time (110,111). In a number of these patients, dystonic symptoms are not static but continue to progress throughout life.

Dystonic movements also can develop after acute viral encephalitis, carbon monoxide poisoning, and the ingestion of various drugs, notably phenytoin, carbamazepine, phenothiazines, butyrophenones, benzamides (e.g., Tigan), tricyclic antidepressants, chloroquine, antihistamines (e.g., Benadryl), ketamine, and lithium (112). Many children who develop drug-induced dystonia suffered from preexisting brain damage. Dystonia also can follow craniocerebral trauma. Under these circumstances, it is typically unilateral (hemidystonia). Typical dystonia also can follow peripheral trauma, with the traumatized limb being the one initially affected by the movement disorder (113,114). It is unclear what role trauma plays in the clinical expression that otherwise would have been asymptomatic for the DYT1 gene.

Dystonic movements also are seen in Leigh syndrome and Wilson disease. In Wilson disease, Kayser-Fleischer rings are invariable, the serum ceruloplasmin is generally depressed, and speech or the facial musculature is often preferentially affected. Other heredodegenerative diseases in which dystonia can be a prominent clinical feature include various lipidoses (G_{M1} and G_{M2} gangliosidosis, juvenile neuronal ceroid lipofuscinosis, and Niemann-Pick disease type C), metachromatic leukodystrophy (MLD), and glutaric acidemia type I.

Treatment

Two modes of treatment, pharmacologic agents and neurosurgery, have been used to alleviate the symptoms of dystonia. The effectiveness of drug treatment is unpredictable and inconsistent, but approximately one-half of the patients experience significant improvement. Trihexyphenidyl (Artane) is probably best used for DYT1 patients with this disease, whereas levodopa, given alone or with a decarboxylase inhibitor (Sinemet), appears to be most beneficial in patients with late-onset dystonia. Trihexyphenidyl is administered to children in extremely large doses (60 to 80 mg/day or even more). Doses begin at 2 to 4 mg/day, and the drug is gradually increased until maximum benefit or intolerable side effects are encountered (115). Tetrabenazine, a dopamine-depleting drug, can be given in doses of 50 to 200 mg/day. Its effect is potentiated by combining it with lithium (approximately 900 mg/day) (116). In some patients, a combination of trihexyphenidyl, dextroamphetamine, and tetrabenazine appears to be fairly effective, as is the cocktail of trihexyphenidyl, pimozide, and tetrabenazine used in the United Kingdom (117). The concomitant administration of baclofen (40 to 120 mg/day) can enhance the effectiveness of drug therapy (118). Other drugs that can be beneficial to an occasional patient include carbamazepine (Tegretol), bromocriptine, and diazepam (Valium).

Botulinum toxin (Botox) has been effective in the treatment of blepharospasm and other craniocervical dystonias, but it is used only rarely in generalized dystonia because of the number of large muscles affected. It can be used, however, for the most disabling or painful muscles in conjunction with the other medications (96).

Unilateral or bilateral pallidotomy and pallidal stimulation are options for patients who have been unresponsive to pharmacologic treatment. The latter procedure is preferred in our institution. Results from several centers indicate that this procedure induces a marked but gradual improvement over the course of several months (118a). Patients with secondary dystonia derive neither functional nor objective improvement (119,120). Pallidotomy appears to be equally effective (120). Because of a high incidence of relapses and the development of dysarthria in more than half of the patients who undergo bilateral procedures, cryothalamectomy is no longer used for amelioration of dystonia.

In general, it appears that not severely affected patients with the early onset form of hereditary dystonia (DYT1) respond more favorably to drugs, whereas patients with severe generalized DYT1 dystonia, and focal or segmental dystonia are likely to be more amenable to the use of botulinum toxin or surgery.

In light of the empirical and often not very successful treatment of patients with DYT1 dystonia, inhibiting the expression of the mutant torsin with the aid of mutant-specific small interfering RNA (siRNA) appears to be a new and potentially exciting approach (121).

Tardive Dyskinesia

Tardive dyskinesia is encountered in the pediatric population in association with the use of neuroleptic medications, notably phenothiazines, butyrophenones, and diphenylbutylpiperidine (Pimozide) (122). Its prevalence is much higher in children treated with conventional antipsychotics than in those given atypical antipsychotics. The condition is not one entity, but a number of different syndromes. Its incidence is not known. Studies on an inpatient population of psychotic children and adolescents receiving neuroleptics suggest that extrapyramidal movement disorders are seen during drug therapy or on drug withdrawal in as many as 50% (123). In most instances, the movement disorder is transient. It is more common in children who have had prenatal and perinatal complications or those who have received high doses of the medication for months or years or after an increase in the dose (124). However, low doses given over brief periods also have induced the movement disorder.

The severity of movements varies considerably. Characteristically, they consist of orofacial dyskinesias, notably stereotyped involuntary protrusion of the tongue, lip smacking, and chewing. A variety of other involuntary movements also can be present. After the medication is discontinued, these can improve in the course of several months or they can persist. Withdrawal dyskinesias generally disappear after a few weeks or months. Persistent dystonia has been associated with the use of neuroleptics. The clinical appearance of this movement disorder differs from tardive dyskinesia by the absence of orofacial dyskinesias.

Tardive dyskinesia is believed to result from a hypersensitivity of the dopamine receptors induced by the neuroleptic medications. A full review of the pathophysiology of this disorder is beyond the scope of this text.

Why this condition appears in some patients and not in others is unclear. The concomitant administration of anticholinergic drugs does not predispose to the appearance of tardive dyskinesia nor do drug holidays prevent it. In my experience, several patients with tardive dyskinesia have had a family history of a movement disorder (such as writer's cramp or tremor), suggesting a genetic predisposition.

In making the diagnosis of tardive dyskinesia, one should bear in mind that a number of movement disorders, notably HD and Wilson disease, are preceded by behavior problems, personality changes, or psychoses that could require the use of neuroleptic agents. It is also necessary to differentiate tardive dyskinesia from the choreiform movements of hyperkinetic children, the peculiar movements of institutionalized youngsters exhibiting mental retardation, and the choreoathetosis of children with cerebral palsy that can be suppressed by neuroleptics.

A variety of drugs has been used for the treatment of persistent tardive dyskinesia. Jankovic and his group favor tetrabenazine given solely or in combination with lithium (116). In their series, which mainly comprised adults, a persistent excellent response was seen in 85% of patients. A variety of other drugs (reserpine, clonidine, and clozapine) also has been used. In many instances; however, if the movement disorder has established itself and has failed to subside with withdrawal of the responsible neuroleptic, the outlook for remission is not good. The effectiveness of branched-chain amino acids in the treatment of tardive dyskinesia is under investigation (125).

The neuroleptic malignant syndrome is another neurologic disorder believed to result from the administration of dopamine receptor–blocking neuroleptics. The principal clinical features of this condition are hyperthermia, muscular rigidity, tremors, rhabdomyolysis, and disorientation. Tachycardia and hypertension also can develop (126,127). The condition can be life-threatening, and prompt treatment is required. Anticholinergics, bromocriptine, and dantrolene have been used to treat this condition. Although the last drug is favored by many authors (128) it was not useful in the series of patients reported by Silva and coworkers (129).

Hallervorden-Spatz Disease (Pantothenate Kinase–Associated Neurodegeneration; PKAN)

In 1922, Hallervorden and Spatz described Hallervorden-Spatz disease, a rare familial disorder that began before age 10 years and was characterized by clubfoot deformity, gradually increasing stiffness of all limbs, impaired speech, and dementia (130).

Pathogenesis and Molecular Genetics

PKAN is an autosomal recessive disorder, with the gene mapped to chromosome 20p13. It encodes pantothenate kinase 2 (PANK2), the first enzyme in the biosynthesis of coenzyme A (131). Normally, PANK2 localizes to mitochondria and phosphorylates pantothenate, *N*-pantothenoyl-cysteine, and pantetheine (132). The mutated sequence leads to skipping of the mitochondrial targeting signal and causes PANK2 to be localized to the cytosol (133). It is not clear how this leads to the deposition of iron. One likelihood is that *N*-pantothenoyl-cysteine and pantetheine induce free radical damage to cells and that, additionally, iron is chelated by the cysteine-containing compounds that accumulate as the result of the enzyme defect.

Pathology

Three pathologic abnormalities occur in Hallervorden-Spatz disease. These are (a) intracellular and extracellular iron deposition in the globus pallidus, substantia nigra, and, less often, cerebral cortex; (b) a variable degree of neuronal loss and gliosis in the globus pallidus and the pars reticularis of the substantia nigra; and (c) widely disseminated rounded structures, identified as axonal spheroids and seen with particular frequency in the basal ganglia (134).

Microscopically, the pigment is located within neurons and glial cells and in the neuropil, particularly around large blood vessels of affected areas. Histochemical and chemical analyses indicate that it contains iron and is related to neuromelanin. The cytoplasm of the renal tubules contains a brown granular pigment similar in composition to that deposited in nerve tissues (135).

Clinical Manifestations

Considerable variability occurs in time of onset of symptoms and in the major manifestations of Hallervorden-Spatz disease (136). In the classic form of the disease, symptoms become apparent during early childhood (137). These include a progressive impairment of gait caused by a dystonic equinovarus pes deformity of the feet and rigidity of the legs, slowing and diminution of all voluntary movements, dysarthria, and in some children mental deterioration (138). Approximately 50% of patients, however, exhibit a choreiform and athetotic movement disorder. Spasticity has been evident in some cases and atrophy of distal musculature or seizures in others. Retinitis pigmentosa was seen in 20% of patients compiled by Dooling and colleagues (136) and in 68% of patients in the series of Hayflick and her group (137). Optic atrophy is seen in only about 3% of patients (137).

A form of PKAN that has a later onset and is more slowly progressive has also been delineated. Symptoms tend to be first noted in the second decade and are marked by speech difficulties and extrapyramidal dysfunction, the latter resembling parkinsonism (137).

Neuroimaging studies are of considerable assistance in the diagnosis of the disease. The CT scan shows bilateral high-density lesions within the globus pallidus (139). The presence of iron within the basal ganglia is best detected by MRI using a T2-weighted spin-echo pulse sequence at high field strength (1.5 Tesla). Marked hypointensity of the globus pallidus is seen, and the low-signal area surrounds a circumscribed region of high signal, the *eye-of-the-tiger sign* (140).

No effective treatment exists for the condition. In view of the enzymatic defect, high doses of pantothenic acid (up to 10 g/day) have been recommended in the hope of driving any residual enzyme activity by substrate overload (137). In my experience, neither pantothenic acid supplementation nor iron chelation has been effective. Movement disorders, notably dystonia, can sometimes be controlled by pallidal stimulation (140a). Pallidotomy has not been effective at our institution.

Several variants of Hallervorden-Spatz disease have been reported (134). Of these the most likely to be encountered is marked by hypoprebetalipoproteinemia, acanthocytosis, and retinitis pigmentosa. It has been termed the HARP syndrome (134,141). This condition is allelic with PKAN (141,141a).

Familial Idiopathic Calcification of Basal Ganglia (Fahr Disease)

Fahr disease is not a single entity but several genetically and clinically distinct disorders that share the characteristic of calcific deposits within the basal ganglia (Fig. 3.3). A brain that demonstrated calcification within the basal ganglia was first described by Bamberger in 1855 (142). In 1930, Fahr reported a case of idiopathic calcification of the cerebral blood vessels in an adult with progressive neurologic symptoms (143). Since then, several genetic disorders subsumed under the term *Fahr disease* have been delineated (144).

One form of familial calcification of the basal ganglia is best exemplified by two sets of siblings reported by Melchior and coworkers (145). In these children, the disease was marked by mental deterioration, which became apparent within the first 2 years of life, and a choreoathetotic movement disorder. Microcephaly and seizures also can be present, and in one patient, calcification could be seen on ophthalmoscopic examination of the fundi. An autosomal recessive transmission is likely.

Another group has been designated as Aicardi-Goutiéres syndrome. It is an autosomal recessive progressive encephalopathy, with its onset in infancy, first described in 1984 (146). Initial symptoms include feeding difficulties and irritability. In some patients, previously acquired skills are lost and spasticity develops. Microcephaly is common (147). The diagnostic features include basal

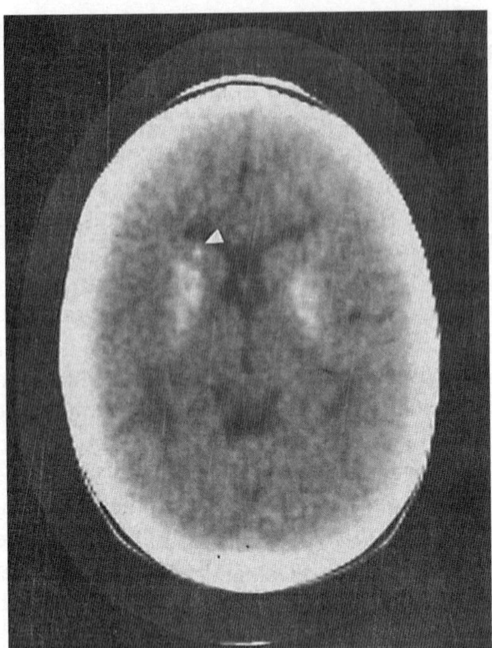

FIGURE 3.3. Calcified basal ganglia in a 10-year-old girl. Computed tomographic scan without contrast. The calcification is principally in the putamen and globus pallidus. Additionally, a focus of calcification in the caudate nucleus appears on the left (*arrowhead*). (Courtesy of Dr. Robert Sedgwick, and the late Dr. Lawrence S. Fishman, Children's Hospital, Los Angeles, CA.)

ganglia calcifications, a mild but persistent CSF lymphocytosis, CSF protein elevation, and a high level of interferon-α in CSF and serum (147). MRI studies show increased signal in central white matter (148). In one variant of Aicardi-Goutiéres syndrome CSF interferon-α is normal but CSF neopterin and biopterin are elevated (149).

An autosomal dominant type of calcification of the basal ganglia is represented by the family reported by Boller and coworkers (150). Affected members developed chorea and dementia in the third or fourth decade. The family reported by Moskowitz and coworkers was clinically similar, and its members excreted greater-than-normal amounts of 3′,5′-AMP in response to administration of purified parathormone (151). In another family, calcification of the basal ganglia transmitted as an autosomal dominant trait was linked to chromosome 14q (152).

On pathologic examination, calcium deposits are found within capillaries and the media of the small and medium-sized arteries and less often the veins. Free calcium also is seen within brain tissue in the basal ganglia, cortex, and dentate nucleus of the cerebellum. There might be an accompanying demyelination (153).

Calcification of the basal ganglia also can be seen secondary to a number of well-delineated conditions. Most often, the picture is encountered in disorders of calcium metabolism, including hypoparathyroidism, pseudohypoparathyroidism, and hyperparathyroidism. Additionally, calcification of the basal ganglia, accompanied by deposition of the mineral in other parts of the brain, is seen in tuberous sclerosis, toxoplasmosis, cytomegalic inclusion disease, AIDS, chronic Epstein-Barr infection, Cockayne syndrome, Wilson disease, and Down syndrome (154). Calcification of the basal ganglia has variously been reported as a consequence of perinatal asphyxia, but in my experience, this situation is extremely unusual. A differential diagnosis of basal ganglia calcification as detected by CT scans was presented by Harrington and coworkers (155).

Hereditary (Familial) Tremor

Hereditary (familial) tremor represents the most common yet the most benign movement disorder seen in childhood. Symptoms usually become evident around puberty, although patients aged 5 years or younger have been observed.

The condition is polygenic, and in most families it is transmitted as an autosomal dominant trait. Two genetic loci have been established. One, obtained from an Icelandic family, is on chromosome 3q13 (*FET1*) (156). The other locus was obtained from a large American family and is on chromosome 2p22–p25 (*FET2*) (157). The presence of clinical anticipation suggests that an expanded CAG trinucleotide sequence will turn out to be responsible for the disease in some families. Without doubt, other gene loci will be found in the course of the next few years.

The pathophysiology of familial tremor is in dispute. Autopsy has shown no significant abnormality (157a). Marsden distinguished two forms. The first he termed an exaggerated physiologic essential tremor with a frequency of 8 to 12 Hz, which depends on a peripheral reflex. The second form represents a pathologic essential tremor having a frequency of 4 to 7 Hz, which is largely dependent on an interaction between an overactive central generator, which does not arise in the cerebellum, but is transmitted through the cerebellothalamocortical pathway. It arises by abnormal cerebellar afferent input from areas such as the inferior olive (158,159). On PET, overactivity of this loop is confirmed by the observed hypermetabolism of the medulla, presumably reflecting inferior olivary activity, and abnormal bilateral cerebellar blood flow during tremor and at rest (160).

Essential tremor in childhood is seen predominantly in boys (161). On examination, there is a rhythmic tremor, with the frequency of oscillation usually being between 4 and 8 Hz (158). The tremor increases with movement, becoming accentuated as the limb approaches its target, and, except in the most severe cases, is absent when the limb is at rest. It disappears with sleep. The tremor initially affects one or both of the upper extremities but usually does not interfere with fine coordination. With tremor progression, the patient can develop head nodding. The lower extremities are affected less often, and intelligence, gait, and strength remain normal (162,163). Speech and eyelids are rarely affected during childhood, and head tremor is unusual. Brief episodes of shuddering or stiffening of the body, usually associated with excitement, might be observed in infancy or early childhood. They are believed to represent an antecedent to familial tremor (164).

Although the disease is progressive during its early stages, it arrests during much of adult life and interferes little with the patient's daily activity. In later life, however, the condition can suddenly become aggravated, and senile tremor can be a late manifestation of essential tremor.

The diagnosis of essential tremor rests on the exclusion of other disorders of the basal ganglia. Tremors can accompany DYT1 (162), spasmodic torticollis, and writer's cramp. They probably represent a partial expression of primary dystonia. Tremors also are seen in Wilson disease and HD. A family history of the disorder and examination of the parents and other family members are helpful.

Treatment

In most cases of familial tremor, the tremor is not sufficiently severe to require treatment during childhood and adolescence. Propranolol, a nonselective β-adrenoreceptor antagonist, relieves familial tremor. It also has been used to treat shuddering attacks (165). For adults, doses range from 120 to 240 mg/day, given in divided doses. No correlation exists between plasma levels of propranolol and tremorolytic action (166). Small doses of primidone (50 mg/day) or of topiramate (50 mg/day) are equally and in some patients even more effective (167,168).

Restless Legs Syndrome

Restless legs syndrome is a common disorder. It affects between 2% and 5% of the population. It is characterized by a creeping-crawling or aching sense of discomfort in both legs that creates an irresistable need to move them. Symptoms are most common at night before going to sleep. In addition, brief involuntary flexion of the lower extremities can be noted during sleep. Occasionally, the movements also affect the upper extremities. In approximately one-third of patients, there is a family history, and an autosomal dominant transmission appears likely. The cause for the movements is not clear. Trenkwalder and colleagues suggested the presence of brainstem disinhibition that activates a spinal generator for the involuntary limb movements (169). CSF orexin-A levels are increased in patients, most strikingly in those with an early onset of the condition (169a). In the experience of Walters and colleagues, approximately 20% of adult patients with restless legs syndrome had an age of onset before 10 years. Diagnosis was usually not made at that time; instead, the condition was considered as growing pains or attention-deficit/hyperactivity disorder (ADHD) (170). The association of ADHD and restless legs syndrome has also been made prospectively. In the series of Picchietti and Walters, 15 of 16 children with severe restless legs syndrome also had ADHD (171). The diagnosis of restless legs syndrome is best made by polysomnography or videotaping, which discloses the periodic limb movements during sleep. Treatment with clonazepam or adopaminergic agent such as levodopa or bromocriptine has been quite effective (172).

Juvenile Parkinson's Disease

As is commonly defined, juvenile Parkinson's disease refers to a condition in which symptoms of Parkinson's disease make their appearance before age 20 years. This is in distinction to early-onset Parkinson's disease, a condition that becomes apparent between the ages of 20 and 40 years. Our concepts of juvenile Parkinson's disease have undergone marked changes. Although it had been known for many years that when Parkinson's disease develops during the first two decades of life, the familial occurrence can be as high as 40%, the genetic transmission had not been clarified until recently.

The initial report of juvenile Parkinson's disease by Hunt in 1917 probably described four unrelated adolescent patients with dopa-responsive dystonia (173). Since then, genetic analysis has confirmed the clinical impression that juvenile Parkinson's disease is a heterogeneous condition, and at least three autosomal dominant and at least three autosomal recessive forms have been delineated.

One of the genes for an autosomal dominant form has been mapped to chromosome 4q21–q23 (PARK1) (174). This gene encodes α-synuclein, a neuron-specific presynaptic membrane protein, which is a component of Lewy bodies, the fibrous cytoplasmic inclusions seen in dopaminergic neurons of the substantia nigra in adult-onset Parkinson's disease (175). Two mutations in the gene for synuclein have been described (176).

Other loci for autosomal dominant early-onset Parkinson's disease (PARK3) have been mapped to chromosome 2p13 (177), and chromosome 12q12 (177a). The genes for the autosomal recessive forms of juvenile Parkinson's disease (PARK2, PARK6, PARK7) have been mapped to chromosomes 6q15.2–q27, 1p35–p36, and 1p36, respectively (178). The gene for PARK2 encodes a protein, named parkin, which is abundant in all parts of the brain, including the substantia nigra (179). A variety of mutations in the gene, including deletions and point mutations, can lead to clinical picture of juvenile Parkinson's disease (180,181).

The clinical picture of PARK1 and PARK3 is similar, and in most instances symptoms do not become apparent until the third or fourth decade. Autosomal recessive PARK2 is encountered frequently in Japan (182). Symptoms appear as early as the second half of the first decade of life. Initial signs are a gait disturbance with retropulsion, a fine tremor, hyperreflexia, and dystonic posturing of the foot. Parkinsonian symptoms improve with sleep. Good response occurs with levodopa, although dopa-induced dyskinesia can appear within a few months of starting the medication. No intellectual deterioration occurs. MRI study results are normal (182). Neuropathologic studies show neuronal loss and gliosis in the pars compacta of the substantia nigra. In the median portion of the substantia nigra and in the locus ceruleus, neuronal loss and poor melanization of the nigral neurons occur. No Lewy bodies are detectable in either the autosomal recessive or the autosomal dominant forms (183,184).

The pathophysiology of Parkinson disease is a topic that should be relegated to a text on adult disorders.

Juvenile Parkinson's disease should be distinguished from Wilson disease, dopa-responsive dystonia, and spinocerebellar ataxia 2 (SCA2) or other spinocerebellar ataxias that can manifest with prominent parkinsonism. We have encountered identical twins with a clinical picture of the dystonic, dopa-responsive form of juvenile Parkinson's disease who were found to have neuronal intranuclear inclusion disease (185). Another condition to be considered is rapid-onset dystonia-parkinsonism (DYT12), which can have its onset as early as the second decade of life (80,186).

Familial Infantile Bilateral Striatal Necrosis

This rare entity, first described by Paterson and Carmichael (187), is probably an autosomal recessive condition and has been mapped to chromosome 19q (188). It is marked by developmental arrest, dysphagia, choreoathetosis, pendular nystagmus, and optic atrophy. MR imaging studies demonstrate marked atrophy of the basal ganglia. On autopsy there is severe atrophy of the lenticular nuclei with neuronal loss and gliosis (189). Most often the condition develops gradually, but there have been instances in which it appeared acutely following an infectious illness. It is not clear whether this acute form and another form that develops later in life are expressions of the same genetic defect.

Gilles de la Tourette Syndrome

Gilles de la Tourette syndrome, which straddles the fields of neurology and psychiatry, was first described in 1885 by Georges Gilles de la Tourette (190). It is characterized by multiple, uncontrollable muscular and vocal tics and, in the classic cases, obscene utterances. Although in the past the condition was considered to be rare and caused by emotional and psychiatric factors, it is now clear that it represents a continuum from mild and transient tics at one end to the complete Tourette syndrome (TS) at the other.

Pathogenesis and Pathology

The pathogenesis of TS is unknown. Although the current working hypothesis proposes an autosomal dominant transmission of the disease, this has not been fully documented. Family studies have shown that the increase of TS in first-degree relatives of TS patients is at least beween 10% and 15%, a value that is about 10 times that seen in the general population (191). There also is a significant difference in concordance for monozygotic and dizygotic twins (191). A systematic genome scan has shown that four regions (4q, 7q, 8p, and 11q) may contain TS-related genes (192). Specifically, no confirmed linkage has been documented to the various dopamine-receptor genes or to the dopamine-transporter gene. Failure to establish such a linkage could reflect diagnostic uncertainties, including an unclear definition of TS, the variable clinical expression of the disorder, and genetic heterogeneity. Walkup and coworkers suggested that the susceptibility for TS is inherited by a major locus in combination with a multifactorial background (193). Because cases of secondary TS, such as after carbon monoxide poisoning, have shown lesions in the basal ganglia (194), a disorder in the circuitry of the basal ganglia has been postulated, with a working hypothesis being that TS is a developmental disorder of synaptic transmission that results in the disinhibition of the cortico-striatal-thalamic-cortical circuitry (192,195).

Neuropathologic studies have failed to find any consistent structural alterations within basal ganglia. Volumetric MRI suggests that the left-sided predominance of the putamen visualized in healthy right-handed boys is absent in TS and that there is a tendency to right-sided predominance (196). Neurochemical examinations indicate low levels of serotonin in brainstem, low levels of glutamate in globus pallidus, and low levels of cyclic AMP in the cortex (192). Using single-photon emission computed tomography or PET, some but not all studies have found an increase in the density of the presynaptic dopamine transporter and the postsynpatic D_2 dopamine receptor, a suggestion that there is abnormal regulation of dopamine release and uptake. These findings have been partly confirmed by postmortem studies that demonstrate increased prefrontal (but not striatal) D_2 protein in TS brain (197).

The observation that children with TS have significantly increased antineuronal antibodies against human putamen suggests an autoimmune mechanism. A number of studies have found a relationship between a prior streptococcal infection and various movement disorders aside from Sydenham chorea, but such a link has not been proven for TS (197a). This topic is covered more fully in Chapter 8 in the section on pediatric autoimmune neuropsychiatric disorders associated with streptococcal infection (PANDAS).

Clinical Manifestations

A variety of estimates have been presented for the prevalence of TS in the United States. These range from 5 in 10,000, as determined in North Dakota children (198), to as high as 4.2% when all types of tic disorders are included (192). Boys are affected more frequently than girls by a ratio of between 3:1 and 5:1. The syndrome is rare in blacks; in Cleveland, 97% of TS patients were white (199). In approximately 33%, the condition is familial, and relatives can have multiple tics, an obsessive–compulsive disorder, or the complete TS (200,201).

Symptoms generally appear between ages 5 and 10 years. Although periods of remission occur and TS tends to become less severe after adolescence, the condition usually persists for life, and only 8% of children have complete and permanent remission. In the survey of Pappert and colleagues more than one-fourth of adults with TS were disabled due to alcohol abuse, criminality, and unemployment. Tic severity was not, however, a primary factor for disability. It was of note that early life dysfunction correlated with dysfunction during adult life (202).

The initial clinical picture is usually one of multifocal tics affecting the face and head. These progress to vocal tics, such as grunting, coughing, sneezing, and barking and, in the most severe cases, to coprolalia or compulsive echolalia. Tics can be voluntarily suppressed for variable periods, but an accompanying increase in internal tension ultimately results in a symptomatic discharge. Compulsive self-mutilation has been noted in a significant number of cases. In patients in the Cleveland series, an attention-deficit disorder was documented in 35%, learning disabilities in another 22%, and serious psychiatric disorders in 9% (197a). Coprolalia was encountered in only 8%, an indication that even mild cases of the syndrome are coming to physicians' attention. An increased incidence in TS during the winter months has been observed, and the role of group A streptococcal infection as a trigger for tics has been suggested by several workers (203,204). As observed in the genetic studies, obsessive–compulsive traits also are characteristic; in contrast to TS they tend to occur more frequently in girls (200).

Clinical findings suggest that brain function is abnormal in a high proportion of these children. On neurologic examination, a large number of patients exhibit "soft" signs. Approximately 15% of cases are precipitated by stimulant medications, such as methylphenidate hydrochloride (Ritalin), pemoline (Cylert), and dextroamphetamine sulfate (Dexedrine) (205).

Electroencephalogram results have been reported to be abnormal in as many as 55% of affected patients, sometimes even revealing frank paroxysmal discharges. Sleep is disturbed. The amount of stages 3 and 4 sleep is increased, the number of awakenings is increased, and the amount of rapid eye movement sleep is decreased. Sleep electroencephalography (EEG) shows high-voltage slow waves with awakening and immature arousal pattern (206).

Treatment

The goal of treatment is to achieve a satisfactory balance between maximal control of tics and a minimum of side effects. Several medications are being used, but few have been tested in placebo-controlled studies (191). Postsynaptic D_2-receptor antagonists are generally the most reliable drugs for the treatment of TS. Although a recent publication lists 20 drugs that have been advocated for treatment, most clinicians favor haloperidol or pimozide (206a). Haloperidol (0.5 to 2.0 mg/day) improves symptoms in up to 80% of affected children, although side effects prevent the drug from being used for long-term therapy in more than one-third of patients (207), and Robertson and Stern no longer consider it as the first-line drug (208). Because of the marked sedation and alterations in personality induced by the drug, I agree with them. Pimozide appears to be at least as effective as haloperidol, producing significant improvement in 70% of patients with fewer side effects (209). As recommended by Shapiro and coworkers, the starting dose for children is 1 mg given at bedtime, with the dose increased 1 mg every 5 to 7 days until at least a 70% reduction of symptoms occurs or until adverse side effects appear (209). Regeur and coworkers used a dose range of 0.5 to 9.0 mg/day (210). Pergolide, a mixed D_1, D_2, D_3 agonist, was used by Gilbert and coworkers at Cincinnati Children's Hospital with good results in a randomized, double-blind crossover trial, but other centers have not found it to be as efficacious (211). Kurlan considers α-adrenergic agonists, such as clonidine or guanfacine, to be the first-line medications for the treatment of tics, with second-line agents being the atypical antipsychotics such as resperidone and olanzapine (212).

Other drugs that have been advocated for the treatment of TS include tetrabenazine, clonidine, and fluphenazine. The variety of medications that have been proposed indicates that none are of exceptional value and that all have their drawbacks.

A large proportion of children with TS (21% to 90%) develop symptoms of ADHD at some time in their life. Because many of the medications used in the treatment of TS are sedative, they tend to worsen ADHD, and generally ADHD needs to be treated as well. In my practice I find that given the choice, it is more important for the emotional adjustment of the child and the family to treat the ADHD than the TS. Kurlan and colleagues found that methylphenidate and clonidine particularly when given in combination are effective for children with ADHD who have comorbid tics or TS. In their series of children with combined TS and ADHD, methylphenidate used in the same dose as in children without tics was quite effective, and tics worsened in only 20% of patients, a figure that was no greater than in placebo-treated children (213). I should point out that Leckman and coworkers found that clonidine might not become effective until it has been given for some 3 months. They also noted that even after brief discontinuation, its reinstitution does not result in an improvement until after 2 weeks to 4 months (214).

Side effects are similar for all drugs but are least common with pimozide. Acute dystonia is seen in some 5% to 9% of patients receiving pimozide; akathisia is seen in some 25%, but usually disappears within the first 3 months of therapy. Tardive dyskinesia is seen with haloperidol and pimozide; it is more common with haloperidol (215). Other side effects include weight gain, gynecomastia, and, rarely, nonspecific alterations of the electrocardiogram.

Paroxysmal Dyskinesias

The first entity of this rare set of disorders, which straddle the boundary between seizures and basal ganglia diseases, was described by Mount and Reback in 1940 (216). In its classic form, it is characterized by paroxysmal attacks of choreiform, athetoid, dystonic, or tonic movements lasting from a few seconds to several minutes. Consciousness remains unimpaired. Goodenough and coworkers (217) classified the reported cases into familial and acquired (sporadic), with the majority falling into the latter group (218).

Lance distinguished two types of familial dyskinesias (219). In one group, termed *kinesigenic paroxysmal dyskinesias* (PKDs, DYT10), attacks are regularly precipitated by movement, especially movement occurring after prolonged immobility. Paroxysms begin almost always in childhood, usually between ages 6 and 16 years. The movements most often resemble dystonia, although some patients can exhibit a choreiform or even a ballistic component (77). About one-fourth of patients in the series of Houser and coworkers had other affected family members (220). Attacks usually last less than 5 minutes. In the familial cases, the condition appears to be transmitted as an autosomal dominant trait. Attacks respond promptly to anticonvulsants, notably carbamazepine or phenytoin (220). Curiously, blood levels required to control attacks (4 to 5 μg/mL) are well below the range considered to be therapeutic for seizure disorders (221).

The condition has been mapped to 16p11.2–q12.1 (222). In several families there is an association between PKD and benign infantile convulsions (224).

The pathophysiology of this disorder is unclear. Mir and coworkers have recently found characteristic abnormalities in cortical and spinal inhibitory circuits, in particular a reduced short intracortical inhibition (223). In my experience *paroxysmal nonkinesigenic dykinesia* (PNKD, DYT8) is a more common entity. Attacks arise spontaneously or are triggered by fatigue. They first appear before 5 years of age and most often take the form of dystonia, although a mixed movement disorder also can be seen (220). The family history is consistent with an autosomal dominant transmission, and the gene has been mapped to chromosome 2q34 (225). In the experience of Demirkiran and Jankovic, attacks usually last longer than 5 minutes in 65% of instances, but the duration of attacks cannot be used to classify the various paroxysmal dyskinesias (220). The response to anticonvulsants is not as good as in the kinesigenic cases. Between attacks, the child is usually in excellent health, although some children have shown mild choreiform movements or a seizure disorder and some have been developmentally delayed (226,227).

Another autosomal dominant PNKD has been mapped to chromosome 1p (228). In this condition, a spastic paraplegia occurs during and between episodes of dyskinesia. Less often one encounters exertion-induced dyskinesias or sleep-induced dyskinesias (220).

Acquired paroxysmal dyskinesias are often seen in children who had previously experienced perinatal asphyxia or other static encephalopathies as well as in patients with reflex epilepsy and metabolic disorders, notably idiopathic hyperparathyroidism. The condition also is seen in multiple sclerosis. In some cases of acquired paroxysmal dyskinesia, attacks have responded to diphenhydramine (227). Other patients respond to clonazepam or acetazolamide. Bressman and coworkers distinguished a psychogenic form of paroxysmal dystonia. Patients belonging to this group respond to placebo, hypnotherapy, or faith healing (218).

A transient form of dystonia arising during infancy is marked by periods of opisthotonos and dystonic posturing of the upper limbs occurring during the waking state and generally lasting no more than a few minutes. The attacks resolve within a few months. No family history exists, and this entity is distinct from Sandifer syndrome, which accompanies hiatus hernia (see Chapter 6), and from paroxysmal torticollis, a precursor to migraine (229).

The essence of the paroxysmal dyskinesias is unknown. Stevens (230) and Homan and associates (222) postulated that they represent a convulsive disorder akin to the reflex epilepsies. During an attack, however, the EEG does not disclose any paroxysmal features and differs little from the interictal tracing. Most likely, in analogy with paroxysmal ataxia, a condition covered in a subsequent section, the paroxysmal dyskinesias will turn out to represent different types of channelopathies.

Hyperekplexia

Familial startle disease or hyperekplexia is characterized by transient, generalized rigidity in response to unexpected loud noises or sudden tactile stimulation. A large number of patients exhibit severe muscle stiffness at birth (*stiff baby syndrome*) (231). Infants present with marked irritability and recurrent startles in response to handling or sounds, or tapping on the face or the bridge of the nose. This can be accompanied by rhythmic, jerky movements and occasionally by episodes of breath holding (232). The condition is misdiagnosed frequently as spastic quadriparesis. Muscle tone returns to normal in early childhood, but patients continue to have sudden falls in response to startle and they can suppress the startle reaction if they are able to anticipate the stimulus (233). The "jumping Frenchmen of Maine" probably represent an extensive family with such a condition (234). The EEG and electromyography (EMG) results are generally normal.

The condition has been mapped to chromosome 5q33–q35 (235), and in most instances it is caused by mutations in the alpha1 subunit (GLRA1) of the inhibitory glycine receptor. This receptor facilitates fast-response, inhibitory glycinergic neurotransmission in the brainstem and spinal cord leading to a reduction of the excitatory startle response. Both autosomal dominant and recessive forms have been described, arising from different mutations of GLRA1 (236–238). Mutations in the beta subunit of the inhibitory glycine receptor have also been found (239). Symptoms improve markedly with administration of clonazepam or valproate.

Another rare entity that borders between seizures and movement disorders is one of hereditary chin trembling, which can be associated with nocturnal myoclonus (240). The condition responds to administration of botulinum toxin (241).

HEREDODEGENERATIVE DISEASES OF THE CEREBELLUM, BRAINSTEM, AND SPINAL CORD

Heredodegenerative diseases of the cerebellum, brainstem, and spinal cord involve a slow, progressive deterioration of one or more of the functions subserved by the cerebellum, brainstem, or spinal cord. This deterioration is caused by neuronal atrophy within the affected tract or tracts, commencing at the axonal periphery and advancing in a centripetal manner. Familial distribution is the usual pattern. In the past, classification of these disorders based on clinical and pathologic data led to numerous debates, which are now being resolved with the increasing availability of genetic data. Two groups can be distinguished: the autosomal recessive ataxias and the autosomal dominant ataxias. In this chapter, emphasis is placed on those conditions that are more prevalent during childhood and adolescence.

Friedreich Ataxia

Friedreich ataxia (FRDA) was first distinguished from syphilitic locomotor ataxia by Friedreich in 1863, who reported all the essential clinical and pathologic features of the condition (242). Characterized by ataxia, nystagmus, kyphoscoliosis, and pes cavus, it occurs throughout the world as an autosomal recessive trait.

Molecular Genetics, Pathology, and Pathogenesis

The gene for FRDA has been mapped to chromosome 9q13. It has been cloned and codes for a protein termed frataxin (243). Some 94% of FRDA patients are homozygous for an expanded GAA repeat in an intron of the gene. The remaining individuals, some 5%, are compound heterozygotes with an expanded repeat on one allele and a point mutation or deletion on the other (244). Compound heterozygotes have a somewhat earlier onset of symptoms and are more likely to show optic atrophy (245). The number of GAA repeats ranges from 6 to 29 in healthy individuals and from 120 to 1,700 in FRDA patients, with the size of the expanded repeat correlating fairly well wth age of onset and disease severity (244,246,247). The expression of frataxin is markedly reduced in FRDA, and the pattern of frataxin expression in normal tissues approximates the sites of pathologic changes in the disease (243). Frataxin is normally localized to mitochondria, where it plays a critical role in iron homeostasis (248). In yeast and mouse models of FRDA frataxin deficit results in reduced activity of numerous mitochondrial enzymes, notable complexes I, II, and III of the mitochondrial respiratory chain (249), and aconitase (250). Impaired mitochondrial function is probably the result of iron overload in mitochondria and tissue damage from free radical toxicity and abnormal antioxidant responses (251,252). In patients with FRDA there is an accumulation of iron in myocardial cells and in the dentate nucleus (244). The mechanism by which frataxin regulates iron metabolism is uncertain, but it is likely that the protein acts as an iron chaperone or an iron store (248,250). How the GAA triplet-repeat expansion results in a reduced expression of frataxin in mitochondria is not clear. The most likely possibility is that the unusual DNA structure interferes with transcription (253). Interestingly, the at one time discredited finding of abnormalities in the pyruvate dehydrogenase complex and in the activity of the mitochondrial malic enzyme can now be explained (254).

The essential pathologic process in FRDA as well as in the other cerebellar degenerations is a dying back of neurons in certain systems from the periphery to the center with eventual disappearance of the cell body (255). The principal lesions are found in the long ascending and descending tracts of the spinal cord (Fig. 3.4). The peripheral nerves also can be affected, as can the brainstem and, less often, the cerebellum. All these areas show axonal degeneration, demyelination, and a compensatory gliosis. Degenerative cellular changes are most striking in Clarke column and the dentate nucleus. They occur to a lesser extent in a variety of other nuclei of the lower brainstem and in the Purkinje cells. Cell loss and gliosis also are seen in the vestibular and auditory systems (256). Other areas of gray matter are usually unaffected.

Abnormalities of the viscera are limited to the heart and the pancreas. There is cardiomegaly, with myocytic hypertrophy and chronic interstitial fibrosis, and an inflammatory infiltrate (257). In the pancreas there is a loss of islet cells.

Clinical Manifestations

Friedreich ataxia accounts for about three-fourth of cases in whites with hereditary ataxia having their onset before age 25 years. The prevalence in Great Britain is

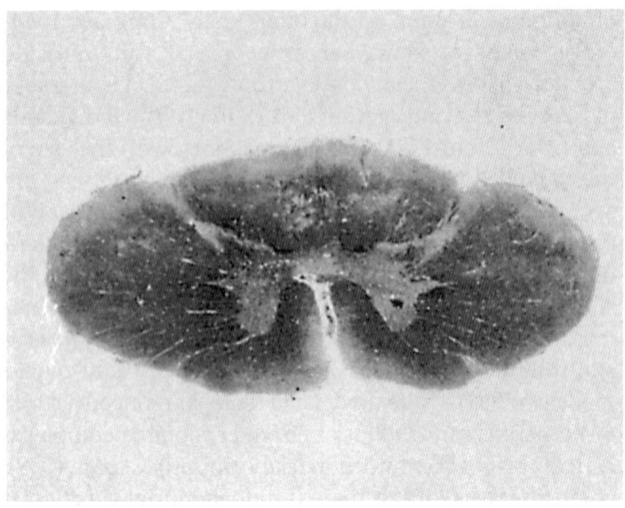

FIGURE 3.4. Friedreich ataxia. Section of spinal cord stained for myelin. The area of myelination involves the posterior columns and the lateral and ventral spinocerebellar tracts. The corticospinal tracts are relatively spared, although demyelination is more extensive than would be expected from the clinical picture at the time of demise. (Courtesy of Dr. K. E. Earle, Armed Forces Institute of Pathology, Washington, DC.)

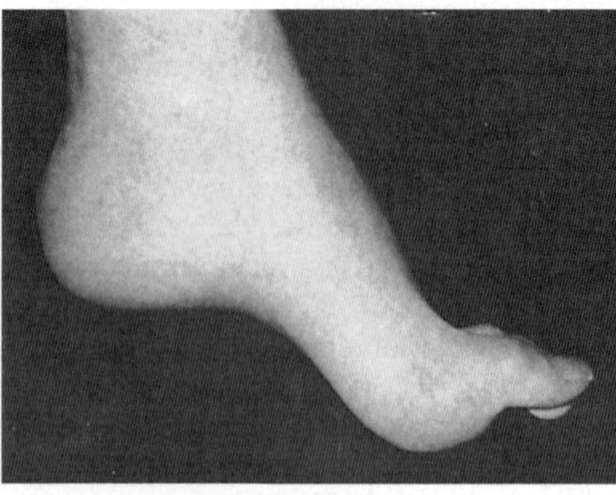

FIGURE 3.5. Typical pes cavus foot deformity seen in Friedreich ataxia. The patient is a 12-year-old girl.

approximately 1 in 48,000 (257). In western Norway, it is 1 in 100,000. Although considerable variability occurs in age of onset, in most families the disease begins at the same period of time in each affected individual. The first symptoms can be seen as early as age 2 years, and the mean age of onset is 10 years of age (258). The clinical manifestations are outlined in Table 3.4 (259). Children can be slow in learning to walk or can begin to stumble frequently. Less commonly, abnormal speech or incoordination of hand movements is the initial complaint.

TABLE 3.4 Frequency of Neurologic Symptoms in 72 Patients with Friedreich Ataxia

Symptom	*Percent Incidence*
Truncal ataxia	100
Dysarthria	82
Nystagmus	33
Dysmetria of upper extremities	89
Decreased vibration sense in lower extremities	72
Areflexia of lower extremities	100
Weakness of lower extremities	69
Atrophy of lower extremities	46
Extensor plantar reflex	83
Pes cavus	83
Scoliosis	78
Diabetes	15
Abnormal electrocardiographic results	79

Data from Klockgether T, Evert B. Genes involved in hereditary ataxias. *Trends Neurosci* 1998;21:413–418. With permission.

Neurologic symptoms advance relentlessly. Although the disease evolves rapidly in a few children, progression is slow in the vast majority, and, occasionally, long static periods occur. Intercurrent infections frequently aggravate existing symptoms and bring new ones to light. The patient with fully developed FRDA has an immature, dysmorphic appearance with a number of skeletal deformities, some of which can exist from birth. In approximately three-fourths of the patients, the feet have a high arch (pes cavus), hammer toes, and wasting of the small muscles of the sole (Fig. 3.5). This abnormality, present at birth, might for many years represent the only sign of FRDA. Kyphoscoliosis is present in 75% to 90% of patients (257,259).

The most prominent sign, however, is ataxia. As might be expected from the pathologic lesions, ataxia is caused by a combination of cerebellar asynergia and loss of posterior column sensation. Ataxia is usually more marked in the legs than in the arms and is most evident when the child's gait or station is examined. Speech is invariably involved and acquires a staccato or explosive character, which is the result of an incoordination of respiration and phonation. Nystagmus is seen in 20% to 40% of cases (257–259). It is usually bilateral and is present only on lateral movements of the eyes. Additionally, one frequently observes broken-up, jerky pursuit movements. Nystagmus on upward gaze is rare, as is optic atrophy (255). In the series of Pandolfo (260) the latter was seen in 13% of cases. Optic atrophy can be congenital or can have its onset during early infancy, progressing rapidly after its inception.

Carroll and coworkers found color vision to be impaired in 40% of patients, and abnormalities in the visual-evoked potentials were seen in two-thirds of the patients (261). The two principal abnormalities were a generalized reduction in amplitude of the potentials and a prolongation in their latency. The reduction in amplitude is probably the consequence of a loss of functional fibers in the visual pathway. Electroretinogram results are usually normal. Vestibular involvement, including loss of caloric reactions and attacks of vertigo, was already described by Friedreich (242). Attacks of vertigo often appear early and ultimately are seen in approximately 50% of the patients. Sensorineural hearing loss was seen in about 20% of Pandolfo's series; it is caused by degeneration of the cochlear neurons (256,260,262).

Weakness of the distal musculature of the lower limbs and wasting of the small muscles of the hands and feet are common and are out of proportion to the degree of disuse. A loss of vibratory and proprioceptive sensation occurs, and in the advanced cases, the other sensory modalities also are likely to be affected, notably in the distal portions of the extremities (255,257). Pains, cramps, and paresthesias are common.

In the experience of Harding, reported before the discovery of frataxin, deep tendon reflexes were absent in 74% of patients, with the patellar reflex being lost in 99%. An extensor plantar response could be elicited in 89% (257,258). In the series of Pandolfo, controlled by determination of genotype, areflexia in the lower extremities was seen in 75% of cases and an extensor plantar response was seen in only 62% of cases (260).

MRI studies can show enlargement of the fourth ventricle and atrophy of the superior vermis, brainstem, and spinal cord (259). The somatosensory-evoked potentials recorded over the clavicles are abnormal even in the earliest stages of the disease (263). They are unaccompanied, however, by a delay in peripheral nerve conduction. Sphincter disturbance is rare except for occasional urgency of micturition (257). Neither mental retardation nor dementia was encountered in Harding's large series (257,258). Electrocardiographic and echocardiographic evidence of myocarditis has been found in 80% to 90% of patients (259,260). T-wave abnormalities and congenital heart block are particularly common (264). Echocardiographic abnormalities are seen early; most commonly interventricular septal hypertrophy is seen (257). About 10% of patients develop diabetes mellitus and about 20% have carbohydrate intolerance (260).

The patient with an advanced case of FRDA is bedridden with dysphagia and other bulbar signs. Death is caused by inanition or, more commonly, myocarditis with intractable congestive failure.

Heterozygotes for FRDA are neurologically normal. According to Harding, they demonstrate neither pes cavus nor scoliosis (257).

When patients with clinically typical FRDA are examined for GAA trinucleotide expansion, a small proportion do not show an expanded allele. It is possible that these patients have point mutations or deletions in the gene for FRDA on both chromosomes (265) or have a genetically different disease with an FRDA phenotype. Conversely, triplet expansions have been seen in a number of patients with atypical ataxia and in patients presenting with generalized chorea (266).

Diagnosis

In the typical patient, the clinical diagnosis is suggested by the presence of childhood-onset progressive ataxia, skeletal deformities, an abnormal visual-evoked potential, and an abnormal echocardiogram result. The diagnosis is confirmed by determination of the size of GAA repeats, which can now be performed commercially. Ataxia-telangiectasia (see Chapter 12) is the second-most-common cause of childhood-onset progressive ataxia. It is distinguished clinically by cutaneous telangiectases, a history of frequent serious respiratory infections, absent or marked reduction of immunoglobulin A (IgA) globulins, an elevated α-fetoprotein, and a lack of skeletal deformities and sensory signs.

Harding described an autosomal recessive form of cerebellar ataxia in which deep tendon reflexes are preserved and in which optic atrophy, diabetes, and cardiac abnormalities cannot be demonstrated (257). Symptoms appear between 18 months and 20 years of age, and the progression of the illness is slower than in the classic form of FRDA. Most of these patients are now known to have the same mutation as is seen in typical FRDA (244).

Several other forms of ataxia having their onset in childhood and having an autosomal recessive inheritances have been recognized. They are summarized in Table 3.5.

An autosomal recessive infantile-onset spinocerebellar ataxia (IOSCA) is seen not infrequently in Finland and is probably identical with an entity once termed *Behr disease*. Symptoms develop during the second year of life and are highlighted by cerebellar ataxia, a peripheral sensory neuropathy, deafness, optic atrophy, athetosis, and seizures. Hypogonadism can be documented in female patients (269,270). Pathologic examination shows atrophy in the spinal cord: the dorsal roots, posterior columns, and posterior spinocerebellar tracts. There is a severe neuronal loss in the dorsal nucleus. The dentate nuclei and inferior olives are also atrophic (279).The gene for this condition has been mapped to chromosome 10q24 (280).

A recessively inherited ataxia caused by a mutation of the α-tocopherol transfer protein has a clinical picture that resembles FRDA (268). Age of onset is younger than 20 years in patients who stem from the Mediterranean region but is later in Japanese cases.

The other recessively inherited ataxias are even rarer. These include an entity characterized by cerebellar ataxia, mental deficiency, congenital cataracts, impaired physical growth, and various skeletal anomalies. It was first described by Marinesco and Sjögren, Garland, and others (275,276). The brain shows marked cerebellar atrophy, especially affecting the vermis, with almost complete loss of Purkinje and granule cells and with gliosis of the dentate

TABLE 3.5 Recessively Inherited Ataxias

Name	Locus	Clinical Manifestations	Reference
Friedreich ataxia (FRDA)	9q	Ataxia, dysarthria, position-sense loss, cardiomyopathy	244
Ataxia-telangiectasia	11q22–q23	Ataxia, choreoathetosis, ocular apraxia, telangiectasia of conjunctivae	Chapter 12
Charlevoix-Saguenay	13q11	Spasticity, gait ataxia, abnormal eye movements	267
Vitamin E deficiency	8q13.1–q13.3	Variable age of onset, FRDA phenotype	268
Infantile-onset SCA	10q24	Ataxia, sensory neuropathy, optic atrophy, seizures, athetosis	269,270
Ataxia-ocular motor apraxia (AOA1)	9p13	Onset 3–12 years, ocular motor apraxia, chorea, mental deterioration, hypoalbuminemia	271,272
AOA2	9q34	Onset in childhood, ocular apraxia, ataxia, senataxin mutation	273,273a
Ataxia with hearing impairment	6p21–p23	Ataxia, hearing impairment, optic atrophy	274
Marinesco-Sjogren	5q31	Ataxia, mental retardation, congenital cataracts, skeletal abnormalities	275,276
Cayman	19p13.3	Nonprogressive ataxia, mental retardation	277
Ataxia and hypogonadism		Mental retardation, seizures, muscle CoQ deficiency	278

SCA, spinocerebellar ataxia; CoQ, coenzyme Q.

nucleus. The presence of a myopathy is suggested by EMG and by the presence of fiber-type disproportion, fibrosis, and lipid deposition on biopsy (276). Electron microscopic studies on sural nerve biopsies demonstrate numerous abnormally enlarged lysosomes. Lysosomal enzyme study results, however, have been normal. The condition has been mapped to chromosome 5q31 (281).

A recessively inherited form of spastic ataxia has been described in an isolated French Canadian community of Quebec (Charlevoix-Saguenay syndrome) (267). The condition has been mapped to chromosome 13q11, and the gene (*SACS*) codes for a protein that is believed to be involved in chaperone-mediated protein folding (282).

Treatment

Children with FRDA should remain active for as long as possible and participate in physical therapy and programmed remedial exercises. These should focus on balance training and muscle strengthening. In my experience, the cardiomyopathy does not interfere with such an exercise program. Orthopedic surgery for skeletal deformities, particularly progressive scoliosis, which is a major cause for morbidity, might be necessary if bracing does not arrest the progression of the scoliosis (283). The antioxidant idebenone, a synthetic analogue of coenzyme Q10, has induced a significant reduction of cardiac hypertrophy at doses as low as 5 mg/kg and improved cardiac function, but in the experience of Buyse and coleagues did not arrest the progression of ataxia (284). The effectiveness of much higher doses (60 to 70 mg/kg) on the neurologic manifestations is under trial (285).The use of mitochondrially targeted antioxidants (mitoquinone–ubiquinone conjugated to a lipophilic cation that enchances its mitochondrial uptake) is also under investigation. Nontargeted antioxidants such as coenzyme Q10 stabilize or reverse the cardiomyopathy but at the doses used have no effect on the ataxia (285). In the experience of the Ataxia Clinic at the University of California, Los Angeles, patients feel better when their carbohydrate intake is restricted. Children with FRDA should be seen by cardiologists and orthopedic surgeons at regular intervals (once or twice a year). With good supportive care, patients can expect to live into their 40s or 50s.

Dominant Spinocerebellar Ataxias (SCAs) (Olivopontocerebellar Atrophies)

The SCAs represent some 25 genetically distinct autosomal dominant conditions, some of which were in the past designated as olivopontocerebellar atrophies and whose prototypes were first described by Menzel in 1890, Déjérine and Thomas in 1900, and Holmes in 1907 (286–288). Clinically, they manifest by progressive cerebellar ataxia, tremor, speech impairment, and, in some instances, marked extrapyramidal signs, cranial nerve palsies, and peripheral neuropathy (see Table 3.6). Approximately one-third of cases with autosomal dominant ataxia do not correspond to any of the mapped conditions, so that, over time, further genetic subtypes will undoubtedly be delineated.

SCA1, SCA2, SCA3, SCA6, SCA7, and SCA17 are caused by the inheritance of an expansion of CAG repeats coding for an extended polyglutamine tract. This expansion is located in the coding region of the respective genes. The genes *SCA8*, *SCA10*, and *SCA12* have expansions of CTG, ATTCT, and CAG repeats, respectively, in their noncoding region. Although the mean age of onset of these disorders is during the fourth decade of life, the conditions have sometimes been encountered in children. The length

TABLE 3.6 Dominantly Inherited Ataxias

Name	Locus	Clinical Manifestations	Reference
SCA1	6p22–p23 with CAG repeats	Ataxia, dysarthria, bulbar dysfunction	289
SCA2	12q23–q24.1 with CAG repeats	Ataxic gait, slow sacchadic eye movements, dystonia, chorea, myoclonus, dementia	290
SCA3	14q24.3–q32 with CAG repeats	Ataxia, diconjugate eye movements, extrapyramidal signs, peripheral neuropathy	291
SCA4	16q24–qter	Rare, ataxia, peripheral neuropathy, pyramidal tract involvement	292
SCA5	11q13	Slowly progressive ataxia does not shorten life span	293
SCA6	19p13.2 with CAG repeats in *CACNA 1A*	Slowly progressive ataxia, dysphagia, vertigo; not seen in children	294
SCA7	3p14.1–p21.1 with CAG repeats	Ataxia with progressive macular degeneration, dysarthria, pyramidal tract signs	295
SCA8	13q21 with CTG repeats in noncoding region	Seen in adolescence; predominantly cerebellar disease; no relation between expansion size and disease severity	296,297
SCA10	22q13–qter with ATTCT repeats	Seen in adolescence; ataxia and seizures, polyneuropathy	298
SCA11	15q14–q21.3	Rare, slowly progressive, mild ataxia	299
SCA12	15q31–q33 with CAG repeats in protein phosphatase 2A	Not seen before third decade; hand tremor, bradykinesia; no relation between repeat size and age of onset	300
SCA13	19q13.3–q14.4	Rare; can start in childhood with mental deterioration	301
SCA14	19q13.4–qter	Rare; can start in second decade with myoclonus	302,302a
SCA16	8q22.1–q24.1	Starts after third decade; ataxia, head tremor, dysarthria	303
SCA17	6q27 with CAG repeats of TATA-binding protein	Ataxia, dementia, parkinsonism; can start in second decade	304
SCA18	7q22–q32	Juvenile patients with progressive myoclonus epilepsy, ataxia, dementia	305
SCA19	1p21–q21	Ataxia, tremor, myoclonus, dementia	306
SCA21	7p21.3–p15.1	Ataxia, extrapyramidal signs, dementia	307
SCA22	1p21–q23	Gait ataxia; onset as early as first decade; may be identical with SCA 19	308
SCA25	2p	Ataxia and sensory neuropathy; can start as early as 17 mo	309
SCA26	19p13.3	Slowly progressive pure cerebellar ataxia, adult onset	309a

SCA, spinocerebellar ataxia.

of the expanded repeat tends to increase from generation to generation, and there is an inverse correlation between the size of the repeat and the age when symptoms become apparent. As a result, a progressively earlier onset of symptoms occurs in successive generations, a phenomenon termed *anticipation*.

SCA1

In the series of Benton and colleagues, some 6% of families with autosomal dominant SCA have a defect in *SCA1* (310). In the Italian series of Brusco and coworkers, *SCA1* accounted for 21% of patients with hereditary ataxia (310a). *SCA1* codes for a protein termed ataxin 1. It is found ubiquitously and is a nuclear protein in all cells with the exception of the cerebellar Purkinje cells, where it is cytoplasmic as well as nuclear. As is the case for HD, the extended polyglutamine tract is believed to induce neuronal degeneration in an as-yet-undefined manner. Lin and coworkers attributed the toxic effects of the expanded polyglutamine tracts to downregulation of a number of neuronal genes (311).

Expanded repeats tend to increase in length more with paternal than with maternal transmission; as a consequence, the majority of patients with juvenile onset are offspring of affected men. In the series of Pandolfo and Montermini, 16% of SCA1 patients developed symptoms before 15 years of age (289). Characteristic symptoms include ataxia, ophthalmoplegia, and pyramidal and extrapyramidal signs. Neuropathologically, patients with SCA1 show gross atrophy of the cerebellum, cerebellar peduncles, and basis ponti. The Purkinje cells appear most affected. A marked reduction in the number of granule cells and neuronal loss in the dentate nucleus are seen. Pathologic changes can also involve the basal ganglia, spinal cord, retina, and peripheral nervous system.

SCA2

SCA2 is phenotypically similar to SCA1, but movement disorders and a neuropathy are common. The gene for the disease codes for a highly basic protein, ataxin 2, having no similarity with any other proteins. Ataxin 2 is found in all parts of the brain, but an ataxin 2–binding protein is predominantly expressed in the cerebellum (312). In the series of Benton and colleagues, SCA2 was encountered in 21% of families with autosomal dominant cerebellar ataxia (310). In the Italian series of Busco and coworkers, SCA2 accounted for 24% of cases of dominant cerebellar ataxia (310a). SCA2 is the most common dominant cerebellar ataxia in India. SCA2 is also the most common dominant cerebellar ataxia in children seen in the Ataxia Clinic at the University of California, Los Angeles (S. Perlman, personal communication, 2004). The onset of neurologic symptoms is before 10 years of age in some 3% of patients. In these children, the disease is nearly always paternally transmitted.

SCA3

SCA3, also known as Machado-Joseph disease, is also phenotypically similar. In the series of Pandolfo and Montermini, the onset of neurologic symptoms was before 15 years of age in 7% of patients (289). In Germany, this condition is the most common of the autosomal dominant cerebellar ataxias, being found in 42% of the families with autosomal dominant ataxia (313). In the series of Benton and colleagues, this condition was seen in only 8% of families (310). SCA3 accounted for only 1% of cases in the Italian series of Brusco and coworkers (310a). The mechanism of neuronal damage in this condition is not yet clarified. Schmidt and coworkers found the polyglutamine-expanded protein displayed an increased propensity to misfold and aggregate and that the nuclear aggregates of the mutant protein form the ubiquinated neuronal intranuclear inclusions seen in the pons and substantia nigra (314).

SCA6

SCA6 was seen in 11% of the families compiled by Benton and colleagues (310). It differs from the other autosomal dominant cerebellar ataxias in that the mutation affects a gene with a known function, the gene for the α_{1A} voltage-dependent calcium-channel subunit, *CACNA1A*, which has its strongest expression in Purkinje cells (251). Two other neurologic disorders are caused by mutations in the same gene: hereditary paroxysmal (episodic) ataxia (EA2), considered in another part of this section, and familial hemiplegic migraine, considered in Chapter 15. It is not completely clear how mutations on the same gene can cause such markedly different syndromes. However, studies have shown that patients with familial hemiplegic migraine tend to have missense mutations, whereas patients with episodic ataxia tend to have missense mutations and other mutations that lead to a truncated protein. SCA6 is a slowly progressive disorder and does not develop during childhood (294). MRI shows little more than cerebellar and brainstem atrophy.

SCA7

SCA7 is clinically distinct in that ataxia is almost always associated with early retinal degeneration (310,315). The condition can manifest as early as the first year of life, usually with ataxia and progressive vision loss (310). After SCA2, SCA7 is the most common dominant cerebellar ataxia in the pediatric age group (S. Perlman, personal communication, 2004). SCA7 appears to be phenotypically similar but genetically distinct from hereditary dentatorubral-pallidoluysian atrophy (DRPLA; Haw River syndrome). The latter entity has a predilection to Japanese families and results from a CAG trinucleotide expansion on chromosome 12p13.1–p12.3 (316,317). The clinical picture of DRPLA varies even within the same family. It may present with learning disabilities, followed by progressive cerebellar signs, choreoathetosis, myoclonus, and dementia. As implied by the name, degenerative changes are seen in the globus pallidus, dentate and red nuclei, and Purkinje cells (305).

The various other dominant SCAs are summarized in Table 3.6. Because in some families the onset of symptoms is in the first or second decade of life, these conditions must be kept in mind when evaluating children with progressive ataxia.

Diagnosis

The diagnosis of autosomal dominant cerebellar ataxia is based on the underlying genetic mutation. Molecular genetic analyses for SCA1, SCA2, SCA3, SCA6, SCA 7, SCA8, SCA10, SCA17, and DRPLA can now be performed commercially.

In the child who presents with progressive ataxia, the differential diagnosis depends on the rapidity with which the symptoms have appeared. When they are of short duration, ataxia is most likely to be neoplastic, toxic, autoimmune, or infectious. If the ataxia is slowly progressive, posterior fossa tumors must be excluded. Structural anomalies of the upper cervical spine and foramen magnum (e.g., platybasia) can present with ataxia, as does hydrocephalus caused by partial obstruction at the aqueduct of Sylvius (see Chapter 5). The lipidoses, particularly the group of late-infantile amaurotic idiocies, also can present a primarily cerebellar picture (see Chapter 1).

Of the familial cerebellar degenerations presenting during childhood, ataxia-telangiectasia and FRDA are the most common. Several conditions, collectively termed *Ramsay Hunt syndrome*, present with progressive cerebellar ataxia, myoclonus, and seizures. Refsum disease is characterized by cerebellar ataxia, deafness, retinitis pigmentosa, and polyneuritis. It is produced by a defect in the oxidation of branched-chain fatty acids (see Chapter 1). Sporadic cerebellar degenerations of childhood also can be caused by toxins such as lead or organic mercury compounds (see Chapter 10).

Familial Episodic (Paroxysmal) Ataxia

Four genetically distinct forms of familial episodic (paroxysmal) ataxia (EA) have been recognized. Episodic ataxia 1 (EA1) is characterized by brief bouts of ataxia or dysarthria lasting seconds to minutes, with interictal myokymia, usually involving the muscles about the eyes and the hands. Attacks are usually triggered by startle or exercise (317a). In some families, acetazolamide is of marked benefit; in others anticonvulsants are helpful. Other findings are joint contractures and paroxysmal choreoathetosis. No progressive cerebellar degeneration occurs. The episodes of ataxia become less frequent as the child matures and often completely disappear by the end of the second decade. This condition is linked to chromosome 12q13 and is the consequence of a mutation in the gene that codes for a brain potassium channel (*KCNA1*) (318).

A second form of episodic ataxia (EA2) is marked by attacks that last for up to several days. Attacks are triggered by emotional upset, physical exertion, or fevers (319). The condition can have its onset as early as 3 years of age (320). In some patients, migraine-like headaches, vertigo, and nausea accompany the attacks, a clinical picture that suggests a diagnosis of basilar migraine (see Chapter 15) (321). Interictal downbeat and rebound nystagmus is common. Progressive cerebellar ataxia can be present in some. In about two-thirds of patients attacks respond to acetazolamide (321). The mutation for EA2 has been mapped to chromosome 19p and, like *SCA6*, affects the gene for the α_{1A} voltage-dependent calcium-channel subunit, *CACNA1A* (322). The same gene also is affected in familial hemiplegic migraine (see Chapter 15).

Two other genetically distinct forms of EA have been encountered, termed EA3 and EA4 (323,324). These conditions differ clinically in that attacks are triggered by fatigue. Attacks are frequently accompanied by tinnitus and do not respond to acetazolamide (323).

Ramsay Hunt Syndrome (Dentatorubral Atrophy)

This condition was first described by J. Ramsay Hunt in 1921 in a family with myoclonus epilepsy and cerebellar ataxia (325). Autopsy showed well-marked degeneration of the spinocerebellar tracts, atrophy of the dentate nucleus, and pallor of the superior cerebellar peduncle, including the dentatorubral tract. It probably represented a mitochondrial disorder, and Andermann and coworkers suggested that the name Ramsay Hunt syndrome no longer served a useful purpose (326).

Familial Spastic Paraplegia (FSP)

Characterized by progressive spastic paraplegia and first described by Seeligmüller in 1876 (327), the familial spastic paraplegias (FSPs) appear to be the most common system degenerations of childhood, with Charcot-Marie-Tooth disease and Friedreich ataxia being far less common (328). Harding subdivided this condition into *pure* and *complicated* forms (257). Both forms exhibit various modes of inheritance. Autosomal dominant transmission is found in about 70% of pure FSP. Less often, FSP is transmitted in an X-linked or an autosomal recessive manner.

Pathogenesis and Molecular Genetics

Some 20 gene loci responsible for pure or complicated FSP have been found, and the genes for 8 of these have been identified. Some of these are outlined in Table 3.7. Spastic paraplegia 4 (SPG4) is the most common of the FSPs. The condition has been mapped to chromosome 2p21–p24 (329), and the gene codes for spastin, an ATPase belonging to the AAA family (ATPases associated with diverse cellular activities), believed to be involved in the energy-dependent rearrangement of protein complexes. The normal function of spastin and the mechanism by which mutations in the spastin gene cause axonal degeneration are not fully understood. The current hypothesis is that mutant spastic is bound to microtubules and directly or indirectly blocks the action of wild-type spastin or some other critical microtubule-associated protein. This would disrupt microtubule dynamics and impair organelle transport on the microtubule network, leading in a manner not yet explained to axonal degeneration (330–332). Several hundred spastin mutations have been described, and it appears as if almost every family has its private mutation (332).

Mutations in the gene for atlastin (leading to the condition SPG3A) are responsible for approximately 10% of autosomal dominant pure FSPs (333). The gene codes for a widely expressed GTPase that is most abundant in brain and spinal cord. Mutations in the neuronal-specific kinesin gene (*KIF5A*) are responsible for SPG10, another pure FSP. Mutations in spartin are associated with Troyer syndrome, a condition in which spastic paraparesis is complicated by dysarthria, distal amyotrophy, and mental retardation (334). The proteins encoded by all four of these genes are believed to bind to microtubules and could be involved in intracellular trafficking (332).

The other genetic mutations result in disordered cell recognition (*L1-CAM* gene, defective in X-linked SPG1), abnormalities in myelination (the proteolipid protein gene *PLP1*, responsible for X-linked SPG2), and abnormalities in mitochondrial molecular chaperones [paraplegin gene, responsible for SPG7, and heat-shock protein (HSP) 60 gene, responsible for SPG13] (332).

Pathology

The major changes occur in the spinal cord. Axonal degeneration of the pyramidal tracts is always present and is maximal in the terminal portions. In affected tracts, the

TABLE 3.7 Molecular Genetics of the Familial Spastic Paraplegias (FSP)

Disease	Locus	Gene Product	Clinical Manifestations	Reference
SPG1	Xq28	L1-CAM, cell adhesion molecule	SP, MR, absent extensor pollicis longus muscle, or MR, or X-linked hydrocephalus	Chapter 5 337
SPG2	Xq22	Proteolipid protein, DM20	Pure, complicated FSP, Pelizaeus Merzbacher disease, X-linked	338
SPG3A	14q12–q21	Atlastin	Pure SP, AD	333
SPG4	2q21–q24	Spastin	Pure SP, AD	339,340
SPG5	8q11–q13		Pure SP, AR	332
SPG6	15q11.2–q12	NIPA1	Pure SP, AD	341
SPG7	16q24.3	Paraplegin	Pure SP, complicated SP, AR	342
SPG8	8q24		Pure SP, AD	332
SPG9	10q23.3–q24.2		Complicated SP, bilateral cataracts, GE reflux, AD	343
SPG10	12q13	KIF5A	Pure SP, AD	344
SPG11	15q13–q15		Pure SP, complicated SP, AR	345
SPG12	19q13		Pure SP, AD	332
SPG13	2q24–q34	HSP60	Pure SP, AD	346
SPG14	3q27–q28		Complicated SP, MR, distal motor neuropathy, AR	347
SPG15	14q22–q24		Kjellin syndrome, SP, pigmented maculopathy, distal amyotrophy, MR, AR	348
SPG16	Xq11.2		Pure or complicated SP, X-linked	332
SPG17	11q12–q14		Mild SP, amyotrophy of hands, AD	349
SPG19	9q33–q34		Pure SP, AD	332
SPG20	13q12.3	Spartin	Troyer syndrome, SP, distal muscle wasting, AR	350
SPG23	1q24–q32		Vitiligo, hyperpigmentation, premature graying, AR	350a
SPG25	6q23–q24.1		AR disc herniation	350b
SPG27	10q22.1–q24.1		AR	350c

SP, spastic paraplegia; MR, mental retardation; AD, autosomal dominant; AR, autosomal recessive; GE, gastroesophageal; HSP, heat-shock protein.

myelin sheath is lost and the axis cylinder disappears. Ascending tracts also can be involved, in particular the posterior columns, spinocerebellar fibers, and cells of the dorsal root ganglion, which can degenerate and show satellitosis (335,336). No signs of primary demyelination are seen. It is of note that in the autosomal recessive form linked to chromosome 16q24.3 (SPG7) (see Table 3.7), the gene defect involves a protein (paraplegin), a nuclear-encoded mitochondrial metalloprotease, and that muscle biopsy discloses ragged-red fibers (351).

Clinical Manifestations

The Hereditary Spastic Paraplegia Working Group found that families in which the disease is transmitted by an autosomal dominant gene far outnumber those in whom an autosomal recessive gene has been implicated (352). The clinical picture of the various genetic forms of FSP appears to be unrelated to the gene defect. In all forms, a marked intrafamilial variability in age of onset exists, and even in genetically homogeneous kindreds the distinction between early- and late-onset FSP proposed by Harding (353) does not hold true (354).

In the recessive variants of FSP, the average age at onset of symptoms is 11.5 years; in the dominant forms, it is 20 years (353). However, 40% of patients develop symptoms before 5 years of age (257,353). Children can be slow in learning to walk, and once they do walk, their gait is stiff and awkward and their legs are scissored. Muscle tone is increased, the deep tendon reflexes are hyperactive, and the plantar responses are extensor. No muscular atrophy occurs, and, despite the pathologic involvement of the posterior columns, usually no impairment of position or vibratory sensation can be demonstrated by clinical examination. Bladder and bowel control is retained during the early stages of the illness. As a rule, the rate of progress of the illness is extremely slow; it is faster in children affected with the recessive forms. When children suffer from one of the dominant forms, the condition often remains static until they are in their 30s, and in the experience of Harding, only one patient became unable to walk before 50 years of age (257). The upper extremities often remain virtually unaffected until the terminal stage of the disease.

At least three forms of X-linked spastic paraplegia have been recognized. Like the dominant types of FSP, these have been divided into pure and complicated forms. One of the genes for the pure form has been localized to Xq28 (SPG1) (337) (see Table 3.7). Another gene is on Xq21 and codes for proteolipid protein, which is defective in Pelizaeus-Merzbacher disease (PMD). Several different missense mutations in the gene for PLP protein result in X-linked FSP (SPG2) (see Table 3.7), whereas other missense mutations or a deletion of the gene result in PMD. This indicates that these two conditions are allelic disorders (355).

Harding distinguished the pure form of FSP from the complicated type, which is marked by a variety of associated neurologic features (257,353). The range of additional clinical features is enormous, and overlaps exist among the various groups. Grouped together, the complicated forms of FSPs are at least as common as the pure form. The most commonly encountered complicated forms comprise a combination of mild paraparesis with moderate to severe amyotrophy of the small hand muscles and the distal portion of the lower extremities. In other families, spastic paraplegia is associated with dementia, seizures, optic neuritis, movement disorders, cardiac abnormalities, and hypopigmentation of the skin. In several families, ataxia, nystagmus, and dysarthria accompany spastic paraplegia. This mixed picture has been termed *spastic ataxia.* These syndromes have been seen in Amish families (Troyer syndrome) and in French Canadian isolates (Charlevoix-Saguenay syndrome). Most of the cases are dominantly inherited, but autosomal recessive and X-linked complicated FSP have been reported.

Diagnosis

In the absence of a family history, the diagnosis of FSP is determined by exclusion. Motor and sensory nerve conduction times are normal, but somatosensory-evoked potentials are absent or reduced, not only in affected patients, but also in clinically healthy family members at risk for the disease. Progression of symptoms speaks against spastic diplegia of perinatal origin (see Chapter 6). Sensory deficits and sphincter disturbances, which usually accompany spinal cord tumors, are rarely seen in the early stages of FSP (353). Nevertheless, in the absence of a convincing family history, MRI studies of the spinal cord are required to exclude a spinal cord neoplasm.

Treatment

In view of the slow progression of symptoms, an active physiotherapy program should be designed. Orthopedic surgery, unless essential to relieve contractures, should be discouraged.

Fazio-Londe Disease

Fazio-Londe disease, a rare condition, also termed *progressive bulbar paralysis of childhood*, is probably heterogeneous and distinct from spinal muscular atrophy (Werdnig-Hoffmann disease) (see Chapter 16) and from amyotrophic lateral sclerosis, which is a sporadic degeneration of the anterior horn cells and pyramidal fibers occurring in adult life.

The clinical picture reflects a progressive deterioration of the anterior horn cells, particularly those of the bulbar musculature and pyramidal tracts. Symptoms begin at a variable age. In a family I have encountered, symptoms began during early childhood. They progress fairly rapidly and lead to death in approximately one decade (356).

McShane and colleagues distinguished two forms of progressive bulbar palsy presenting in the first two decades (357). In bulbar hereditary motor neuropathy I, bilateral nerve deafness is prominent and accompanies involvement of the motor components of the cranial nerves. This condition is inherited as an autosomal recessive disorder. Bulbar hereditary motor neuropathy II is usually recessive. In some patients, the degree of pyramidal tract involvement is minimal and can be limited to extensor plantar responses; the clinical picture is, therefore, essentially that of the late-onset form of Werdnig-Hoffmann disease. In other families, clinical or pathologic evidence of posterior column deficit relates this particular form of heredodegenerative disease to the spinocerebellar group (258). When anterior horn cell involvement is exclusively distal and is accompanied by significant spasticity and slow progression, the condition can be related to the complicated form of FSP (257). This variant can be transmitted rarely as a dominant trait.

In a few families, progressive degeneration of the anterior horn cells and pyramidal tracts appears before age 20 years. Those families include a large series of cases among the Chamorro tribe of Guam, in whom anterior horn cell degeneration is associated frequently with parkinsonism and dementia. This condition has been linked to a plant-excitant neurotoxin (see Chapter 10). In the other families transmission is either autosomal dominant or autosomal recessive. The dominant form is clinical and pathologically indistinguishable from sporadic amyotrophic lateral sclerosis (ALS), and like sporadic ALS is a disease of adult life. Recessive forms of ALS usually have a juvenile onset. The most prevalent form has been mapped to chromosome 2q33 and has been designated as ALS2. The various forms of familial ALS are summarized in Table 3.8.

The most likely form to be encountered in the pediatric population is ALS2. The clinical picture is heterogeneous. In some patients the disease may take the form of a motor neuron disease that commences as early as 3 years of age. In other families, the disease resembles familial spastic paraparesis with stiffness and spasticity commencing in the lower extremities (359,361). The condition has been mapped to chromosome 2q33, and the mutated gene codes for alsin, a large cytosolic protein (366). The function of alsin is not clear; it seems to belong to the family of the guanine nucleotide exchanging factor (GEF) for small GTPases.

TABLE 3.8 Familial Amyotrophic Lateral Sclerosis (ALS)

Name	Gene Locus	Inheritance	Clinical Manifestations	Reference
ALS1	21q22.1–q22.2	AD; defect in SOD1	Adult onset; indistinguishable from sporadic ALS; about 20% of familial cases	358
ALS2	2q33	AR; defect in alsin	Distal muscular atrophy, increased reflexes, fasciculations; onset in first decade	359–361
ALS3	18q21	AD	Adult onset	362
ALS4	9p34	AD; DNA/RNA helicase	Onset second decade; impaired gait, weakness wasting hand muscles; normal life expectancy	363,364
ALS5	15q15.1–q21.1	AR	Early age; slowly progression	365

AD, autosomal dominant; AR, autosomal recessive; SOD, superoxide dismutase.
See also Swash M. How many ALS syndromes? *Neurology* 2002;59:967.

The diagnosis of juvenile ALS rests on the presence of a pure motor neuronopathy with or without the presence of long tract signs. Tumors of the brainstem must be excluded. When pyramidal tract signs are not striking, myasthenia gravis or an ocular muscle dystrophy should be excluded.

Treatment

No treatment is available.

HEREDODEGENERATIVE DISEASES OF THE PERIPHERAL AND CRANIAL NERVES

In the past, heredodegenerative diseases of the peripheral and cranial nerves were grouped according to their clinical presentation and the histopathology and electrophysiology of the peripheral nerves. Advances in molecular biology have permitted a classification to be made in terms of genetic characteristics (367). The clinical characteristics of the various hereditary peripheral neuropathies in a pediatric population are depicted in Table 3.9 and their relative frequencies in Table 3.10 (398).

The classification of the various hereditary peripheral neuropathies presents the physician who is not completely immersed into this field with an almost unsurveyable complexity. Several considerations can facilitate navigation. The first point is whether the peripheral neuropathy is axonal or demyelinating. In an axonal neuropathy the axon or the neuron suffers the primary injury; if myelin sheath degenerate subsequently, this represents Wallerian degeneration. In a demyelinating neuropathy the myelinating Schwann cells are affected first, and axons may degenerate subsequently. As simple as this distinction appears, in a given patient it is sometimes difficult to decide whether demyelination or axonal degeneration was the primary event. The demyelinating neuropathies are characterized by severely reduced motor nerve conduction velocities (NCV) (less than 38 m/sec) and segmental demyelination and remyelination with onion bulb formations on nerve biopsy. The axonal neuropathies are characterized by normal or mildly reduced NCVs and chronic axonal degeneration and regeneration on nerve biopsy. CMT1 represents the group of CMT patients in whom demyelination is the primary event and the disease is transmitted in a dominant manner, whereas CMT2 represents patients in whom axonal degeneration is the primary event and the disease is transmitted in a dominant manner. There are some families in whom the distinction between a dominantly inherited axonal and demyelinating neuropathy is unclear. These have been placed into the I-CMT group. Patients assigned CMT3 were once classified Déjérine-Sottas syndrome. Patients who have been classified as CMT4 have an autosomal recessive demyelinating neuropathy, whereas patients with an autosomal recessive axonal neuropathy are classified as AR-CMT2. Based on the gene locus, the various CMT groups are further subdivided into CMT1A through (presently) K, CMT2A through G, and, for the X-linked conditions, CMT1X1 through CMT1X3.

Further complicating this classification is the fact that mutations in the same gene can cause widely different clinical manifestations. Thus mutations in peripheral myelin protein 22 kd (PMP-22) can cause Déjérine-Sottas syndrome, CMT1A, and hereditary neuropathy with pressure palsies, and mutations in protein P_0 (MPZ) can cause Déjérine-Sottas disease, congenital hypomyelinating neuropathy, CMT1B, and CMT2.

Charcot-Marie-Tooth Disease (CMT)

Charcot-Marie-Tooth disease, also called peroneal muscular atrophy, was described by Virchow in 1855 (399), Charcot and Marie in France in 1886 (400), and Tooth in England in 1886 (401), who considered it as a peroneal type of familial progressive muscular atrophy. As already indicated, CMT1 is characterized pathologically by extensive segmental demyelination and remyelination and by a consequential thickening of peripheral nerves to the point

TABLE 3.9 Heredodegenerative Diseases of the Peripheral Nerves

Name	Locus	Gene Product	Clinical Picture	Pathology	Reference
Autosomal Dominant Conditions					
CMT1A	17p11	PMP-22	Weakness, wasting of lower, than upper limbs, sensory loss, delayed NCV, pes cavus, onset first decade of life	Segmental demyelination, onion bulbs, hypertrophy	368
CMT1B	1q22–23	P_0			369,370
CMT1C	16p13.3–p12				371
CMT1D	10q21.1–q22.1	EGR2			372
CMT2A	1p36.2	KIF1Bs	Similar to CMT1 but onset in second decade, slower progress, normal NCV	Axonal degeneration	373,374
CMT2B	3q13–q22				
CMT2C			Similar to CMT1 but with paresis of diaphragm and vocal cord		375
CMT2D	7p14		Similar to CMT2A but upper extremities more involved		376
CMT2E	8p21	NFL			377
CMT2F	7q11–q21	HSP27			378
CMT2G	12q12–q13.3				379
X-linked Conditions					
CMTX1	Xq13.1	Connexin 32	Variable depending on type of mutation	Axonal neuropathy and demyelinating	380,381
CMTX2	Xp22.2		Infantile onset, pes cavus, some have MR		382
CMTX3	Xq26		Late onset, distal weakness, normal intelligence, may have spastic paraparesis		382
Autosomal Recessive Conditions					
CMT3 (Déjérine-Sottas)	Various	PMP-22, P_0, connexin 32, EGR2, periaxin	Early hypotonia, MR, slowed NCV	Hypomyellnation, demyelination, onion bulb formation	383,368
CMT 4A	8q13–q21.1	GDAP1	Early onset rapidly progressive distal weakness and atrophy	Loss of large myelinated fibers, hypomyelination, onion bulb formation	384
CMT 4B1	11q22	MTMR2		Focally folded myelin	385
CMT 4B2	11p15				386
CMT 4C	5q23–33		As CMT, but early onset severe scoliosis	Demyelination	387
CMT 4D	8q24	NDRG1	Much like CMT1		388
AR CMT 2A	1q21.2	LMNA	Onset in first or second decade, weakness, atrophy, posterior anterior tibial muscles, mild sensory disturbance	Loss of large myelinated fibers	389
AR CMT 2B	19q13.3				
Hereditary Sensory and Autonomic Neuropathies (HSANs)					
HSAN I	9q22.1–q22.3	LCB1	AD, onset in second to fourth decade, sensory loss over feet, pain > touch, ulcers on feet, NCV normal	Loss of unmyelinated fibers, reduced small myelinated fibers, large myelinated fibers preserved	390,391
HSAN II	12p13.33	HSN2 protein	AR, congenital; light touch, pain affected most, limbs more than trunk, unrecognized injuries	Total loss myelinated fibers, reduced unmyelinated fibers	392,393
HSAN III (FD)	9q31	IKBKAP	See Table 3.11	Decrease number of neurons in autonomic, spinal ganglia, absence of gamma-moter neurons	394,395
HSAN IV	1q21–q22	TRKA	AR; bouts of high fever, anhidrosis, normal sensory nerve action potential	Absence of unmyelinated fibers	396,397

(continued)

TABLE 3.9 (Continued) Heredodegenerative Diseases of the Peripheral Nerves

Name	Locus	Gene Product	Clinical Picture	Pathology	Reference
HSAN V			Congenital insensitivity to pain, anhidrosis	Absence of small myelinated fibers	392
Hereditary Motor Neuropathies (HMNs)					
HMN 1	Same as HSAN I				
HMN 2	12q24		AD, distal muscle weakness, childhood or adult onset		
HMN 5	7p15; 11q13	GARS	Distal UE atrophy, no sensory signs, very slow progression		397a
HMN 7	2q14		AD, distal spinal muscular atrophy, vocal cord paralysis, sensory neural hearing loss		397b

AD, autosomal dominant; AR, autosomal recessive; CMT, Charcot-Marie-Tooth disease; EGR2, a zinc-finger protein; FD, familial dysautonomia; GARS, glycyl tRNA synthetase; GDAP1, ganglioside-induced differentiation-associated protein 1; HSP27, heat-shock protein 27; IKBKAB, inhibitor of kappa light polypeptide gene enhancer in B-cell kinase complex-associated protein; KIF1Bβ, kinesin family 1B, long isoform; LCB1, subunit of palmitoyl transferase; LMNA, lamin A; MR, mental retardation; MTMR2, myotubularin gene-related protein; NCV, nerve conduction velocity; NDRG, Nmyc downstream-regulated gene; NFL, neurofilament protein, light polypeptide; PMP-22, peripheral myelin protein 22 kD; TRKA, tyrosine kinase receptor for nerve growth factor; UE, upper extremity.

at which they become palpably enlarged (367). By contrast, in CMT2, which is a far less common entity, there is no pathologic evidence for demyelination; instead, axonal degeneration occurs. The pathologic features of demyelination and remyelination are shared by an entity formerly termed Lévy-Roussy syndrome (hereditary areflexic dystasia) and by most cases of Déjérine-Sottas syndrome (CMT3).

CMT1 is a relatively common condition and constitutes 51% of pooled pediatric cases of hereditary peripheral neuropathies (401a). The prevalence of all forms of CMT1 is 3.8 per 10,000 population, and by definition they are transmitted as autosomal dominant disorders with a high degree of penetrance (401b).

TABLE 3.10 Specific Diagnostic Entities in 103 Children with Peripheral Neuropathies

Conditions	Number of Patients
HMSN	63
CMT1 (HMSN1)	31
Autosomal dominant (CMT1A, B, C)	21
Sporadic or recessive (CMT4A A, B)	10
CMT2 (HMSN2)	32
Autosomal dominant (CMT2 A, B)	27
Parents unknown	4
Sporadic or recessive (CMT2D)	1
Hereditary sensory neuropathies	3
Heredodegenerative CNS disorders with peripheral neuropathies	37
Spastic paraplegias	9
Heredoataxias	6
Friedreich ataxia	3
Abetalipoproteinemia	2
Lysosomal disorders	9
Globold cell leukodystrophy (Krabbe disease)	5
Other neurometabolic disorders	7
Unknown or undiagnosed	6

CMT, Charcot-Marie-Tooth disease; CNS, central nervous system; HMSN, hereditary motor and sensory neuropathies.

Adapted from Hagberg B, Westerberg B. The nosology of genetic peripheral neuropathies in Swedish children. *Dev Med Child Neurol* 1983;25:3–18. With permission.

Pathology, Pathogenesis, and Molecular Genetics

Because only a few complete postmortem examinations are available, the changes within the CNS have not been well documented. Most commonly, the patient has degeneration of the posterior columns, loss of anterior horn cells, and degeneration of the spinocerebellar tracts and the anterior and posterior nerve roots (401c). Biopsy of the peripheral nerves reveals a diminution in fascicle size and a reduction in the number of myelinated fibers, with the greatest loss among those of large diameter. Unmyelinated fibers appear normal (367). As a consequence of repeated demyelination and remyelination, greater-than-normal variation exists in the distance between nodes.

Depending on the duration and severity of the disease, gross enlargement of the proximal portions of the peripheral nerves, plexi, and roots are seen, with lesser involvement of the distal peripheral nerves and cranial nerves. Microscopic examination shows increased thickness of the myelin sheath and endoneurium and an increase in collagen around the individual fibers. Because of their appearance on transverse section, the concentric lamellae

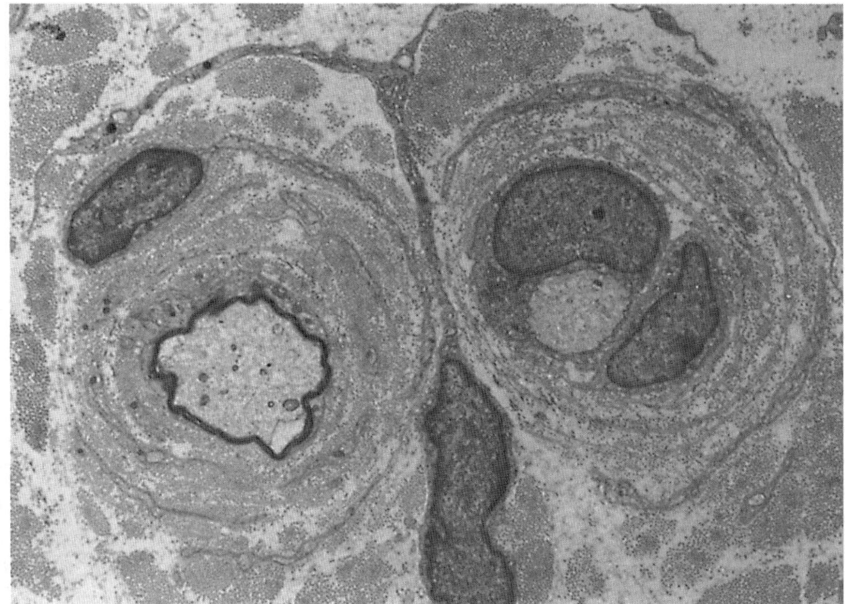

FIGURE 3.6. Sural nerve biopsy in a 2-year-old girl. Electron micrograph, hereditary motor sensory neuropathy type III (Déjérine-Sottas disease). Large *onion bulbs* are seen containing small fibers with absent or thin myelin sheaths. Symptoms of proximal weakness became apparent prior to 1 year of age, and the girl did not walk until $2^1/_2$ years of age. Ataxia was seen, and the peripheral nerves were enlarged on clinical examination. Pupils were normal, and no cranial nerve deficits were seen. (Courtesy of Dr. Robert Ouvrier, The Children's Hospital, Camperdown, Sydney, Australia.)

surrounding the nerve fibers were first termed *onion bulbs* by Déjérine and Sottas (402) (Fig. 3.6). Electron microscopy shows these to contain only Schwann cells and their processes, and they probably reflect a nonspecific regenerative Schwann cell response to injury (383,403). The lamellae can be seen in even the youngest patients (368). Some demyelination occurs, particularly in younger patients (369). Degenerative changes in the skeletal muscles are secondary to damage of the peripheral nerves.

CMT1 is genetically heterogeneous (404). In the most common form, type CMT1A, the genetic defect is a large (1.5 megabase [Mb]) submicroscopic duplication of the proximal portion of the short arm of chromosome 17 (17p11.2), a region that contains the gene for PMP-22 (405), thus producing a segmental trisomy. This duplication arises as a spontaneous mutation in some 10% to 20% of patients, and nearly 90% of sporadic cases of CMT demonstrate this abnormality. It has been conjectured, but is still unproven, that PMP-22 is an important structural component of peripheral myelin (406). How overexpression of PMP-22 results in the clinical manifestations of CMT1A has not been fully clarified. In animals, overexpression of PMP-22 interferes with the growth and differentiation of Schwann cells. This, however, does not appear to be the case in patients with CMT1A (405). Approximately 30% of patients with CMT1A show a point mutation in the gene for PMP-22 (407). Patients who have only one copy of the gene for PMP-22 develop the condition known as hereditary neuropathy with liability to pressure palsies, whereas patients with four copies of the gene have the clinical picture of Déjérine-Sottas disease. These entities are covered later in this chapter.

The gene for the less common entity CMT1B has been localized to the long arm of chromosome 1 (1q22–q23). The major structural protein of peripheral myelin, P_0, a glycoprotein involved in the compaction of the multilamellar myelin sheaths, has been localized to this site, and both deletions and point mutations in this gene can cause CMT1B (370).

At least three X-linked forms of CMT1 also have been described (Table 3.10). Collectively these account for approximately 10% of all CMT cases (408). The gene for one form is on the short arm of the chromosome (Xp22.2); for the other, the gene is on the long arm (Xq13.1) and codes for connexin 32. At least 240 mutations in the gene sequence of connexin have been documented (409). Connexins are membrane-spanning proteins that are localized adjacent to the nodes of Ranvier and in the Schmidt-Lantermann incisures of peripheral nerve. They assemble to form gap junctions, channels that facilitate the transfer of ions and small molecules between cells (373).

In addition to these X-linked conditions, at least two other forms of CMT1 have been delineated. They have been designated as CMT1C, an autosomal dominant condition whose gene is located on chromosome 16p13.1–p12.3 (371), and CMT1D, whose gene is located on chromosome 1q21.1–q22.1 (see Table 3.10). The gene for CMT1D has been characterized as an early growth response 2 (EGR2) gene and is believed to play a role in the regulation of cellular proliferation (410).

The recessive demyelinating neuropathies are less common and have been grouped as CMT4A to 4F. Mutations in the ganglioside-induced differentiation-associated protein 1 (GDAP1) gene have been shown to be responsible for CMT4A (411,412). CMT4C is a childhood-onset demyelinating form with early onset of scoliosis. The gene for this condition has been mapped to chromosome 5q23–q33 and codes for a protein of unknown function (413).

Clinical Manifestations

The various genetic subtypes of CMT1 can manifest at any age, but in general, a bimodal distribution can be distinguished, with onset in the first two decades or after the fifth decade of life. Only the patients with the earlier onset are discussed here.

Symptoms can become apparent before 1 year of age (368). As a rule, the phenotype for CMT1B is more severe than for CMT1A, with somewhat earlier onset of symptoms (370). Patients with point mutations in the gene for PMP-22 tend to have a more severe expression of the disease than those who have a duplication, and onion bulbs can be detected in abundance on nerve biopsies at an early age (369). In general, the peroneal muscles are involved first, and delay in walking or a slapping, storklike gait might motivate the parents to bring the child to the physician. In the upper extremities, weakness and atrophy are at first limited to the small muscles of the hand but later spread to the forearm. The face, trunk, and proximal muscles usually are spared, although nystagmus or facial weakness is not uncommon.

In the fully developed condition, examination reveals a pes cavus deformity (368,414), scoliosis, and contractures of the wrist and fingers that have produced a claw hand. The patient has striking atrophy and weakness of the distal musculature, which contrasts with the preservation of the bulk and strength of the proximal parts. Sensation, particularly vibratory and position sense, is reduced over the distal portions of the extremities. Vasomotor signs are common and include flushing and cyanosis or marbling of the skin. The ankle reflexes are generally lost; other deep tendon reflexes are preserved. The plantar responses can be difficult to elicit.

Progression of the disease is slow, and spontaneous arrests are common. The CSF protein level is elevated in one-half of the cases, but no other abnormalities exist. Median nerve sensory action potentials are generally absent, and motor nerve conduction velocities along the peroneal nerve are slowed. Slowed nerve conduction velocities are characteristic for the various forms of CMT1 and can be recorded before any clinical manifestations or in cranial nerves that remain uninvolved (415). This feature distinguishes the various forms of CMT1 from the forms of CMT2 in which nerve conduction velocities are normal or only slightly decreased. Sensory neural deafness with or without mental retardation has accompanied CMT1 in several families (416,417) The gene for this condition has been mapped to 17p11. It is therefore allelic with CMT1A, and it is the result of a four-amino acid deletion in the PMP-22 gene (416).

Diagnosis

The demyelinating forms of CMT are diagnosed on the basis of the characteristic distal distribution of the slowly progressive muscular wasting and weakness and the presence of sensory deficits. In approximately 10% to 20% of patients, the duplication of the PMP-22 gene is *de novo* and is usually of paternal origin. Sensory deficits distinguish the various forms of CMT1 from the slowly progressive distal myopathies. Nerve conduction velocities are reduced markedly and, as a rule, also are abnormal in one of the parents (368,401a,415). Conduction of visual-evoked potentials is slowed in approximately one-half of the patients, including those who deny visual symptoms. Although histologic abnormalities are noted on biopsy of the peripheral nerves, they are not pathognomonic.

A dominantly inherited syndrome considered to be an intermediate between peroneal muscular atrophy and FRDA was described by Roussy and Lévy (418) and by Symonds and Shaw in 1926 (418a). This condition is now considered to be CMT1 (257).

Several syndromic motor sensory neuropathies have been delineated (419). One form is accompanied by sensory neural deafness, but its gene has been mapped to chromosome 8q24, distinguishing it from the form that results from a deletion in the PMP-22 gene. Another form is associated with mental retardation, facial dysmorphism, and hypogonadism. It has been mapped to the terminal portion of the long arm of chromosome 18. A third form has been mapped to chromosome 10q23. It is marked by limb weakness starting in the latter part of the first decade. It is accompanied by a foot deformity, distal sensory loss, and occasional cranial nerve involvement (419).

A commercial diagnostic service that tests for PMP22, Connexin 32, P_0, early growth response gene 2 (EGR2), neurofilament light (NFL), Periaxin, ganglioside-induced differentiation associated protein 1 (GDAP1), liposaccaride-induced tumor necrosis factor-alpha-factor (LITAF) and mitofusin-2 (MFN-2) by DNA sequencing is now available.

Treatment

Aside from orthopedic measures designed to prevent the disabling deformities and intensive physical therapy, no specific therapy is available. Prenatal diagnosis for CMT1A is available and is based on demonstrating the duplication of the PMP-22 gene.

Charcot-Marie-Tooth Disease (Peroneal Muscular Atrophy), Axonal Type (CMT2)

CMT2 is also genetically heterogeneous, with 11 genetic loci having been delineated. Mutations in genes for a small heat-shock protein, a light neurofilament protein, and a mitochondrial GTPase have been documented (420–422).

Pathologically, the condition is characterized by axonal degeneration of the peripheral nerves, with demyelination being secondary. The clinical picture is similar to that of the CMT1 neuropathies, except that the progression of the disability is generally slower. Because a significant proportion of axons are spared, nerve conduction velocities are often normal or near normal. EMG reveals denervation. Patients satisfying clinical and pathologic criteria for CMT2 made up 5% of the pooled pediatric series of hereditary peripheral neuropathies compiled by Hagberg and Lyon (401a). The various forms of CMT2 are transmitted as a dominant trait (see Table 3.9), and one parent can show abnormalities on EMG but no other clinical abnormalities (423).

Déjérine-Sottas Disease (Hypertrophic Interstitial Neuropathy of Infancy, CMT3)

The prototype of a severe form of hereditary demyelinating neuropathy was described by Déjérine and Sottas (402). Déjérine-Sottas disease (hypertrophic interstitial neuropathy of infancy, hereditary motor sensory neuropathy type III) has been shown to consist of several genetically distinct entities, all of them marked by onset of symptoms in infancy or childhood and progressing to severe disability. In the pooled series of Hagberg and Lyon published in 1981, patients corresponding to CMT3 accounted for 12% of children with hereditary peripheral neuropathies (401a). Several autosomal dominant and autosomal recessive conditions result in this clinical picture. They include mutations in the gene for PMP-22, various mutations in the gene for P_0, tandem duplications of the gene for P_0, mutations for connexin 32, mutations for a zinc finger protein (EGR2), and mutations for periaxin. EGR2 is essential for the normal development of myelinating Schwann cells, and periaxin is believed to be required for the maintenance of a normal peripheral myelin sheath. Periaxin gene mutations are also associated with CMT4F, one of the autosomal recessive demyelinating neuropathies (424). In the majority of patients with CMT3, a *de novo* mutation or autosomal dominant transmission has been demonstrated (425), whereas in other cases it appears to be autosomal recessive (426).

The pathologic picture of Déjérine-Sottas disease is highlighted by hypomyelination of the peripheral nerves, with hypertrophic changes and the presence of onion bulbs (426). In some patients with the clinical picture of Déjérine-Sottas disease, a unique pathologic picture of focally folded myelin sheaths is seen (426).

Clinical Manifestations

As first described in two siblings by Déjérine and Sottas in 1893 (402), the clinical picture is marked by hypotonia, muscular atrophy, and weakness, accompanied by ataxia and sensory disturbances. Facial weakness and an unusual thick-lipped, pouting (*tapir mouth*) appearance are characteristic. The disease begins early in life, prior to 1 year of age in the majority of patients (368). The rate of progression varies considerably, even within the same family (383). In approximately 10% of patients, the neuropathy is evident at birth (401a).

Initial symptoms also include a delay in motor milestones or, in children with later onset of the illness, a disturbance of gait or weakness of the hands. Nerve conduction times are extremely slow, usually less than 10 per second. As the disease progresses, distal weakness and atrophy become evident. Distal sensory impairment is usual and tends particularly to affect vibration sense. In contrast to the initially reported cases, pupillary abnormalities are seen rarely. Kyphoscoliosis or pes cavus is common [occurring in two-thirds of cases in the series of Ouvrier and coworkers (368)]. Intelligence is unaffected.

Laboratory findings include an elevated CSF protein content (seen in 75% of patients) and abnormal sensory and motor nerve conduction velocities (427). EMG shows widespread evidence of peripheral denervation with frequent fibrillation potentials at rest.

Diagnosis

The diagnosis of Déjérine-Sottas disease (CMT3) should be considered in any chronic progressive peripheral neuropathy of childhood. Clinical enlargement of the nerves was seen in all children in the series of Ouvrier and coworkers (368). This finding, however, was only seen in a small percentage of cases examined by Tyson and colleagues (426). Even when present, it is not specific for CMT3, and is also encountered in one-fourth of patients with CMT1. Clinical enlargement also should be distinguished from nerves made easily visible by muscular atrophy.

Congenital hypomyelinating neuropathy can be due to a variety of gene mutations (428). This condition has its onset early in infancy, or even prenatally, with arthrogryposis, hypotonia, and areflexia. The weakness has a distal to proximal gradient. Nerve conduction velocities are severely slowed or absent.

Other conditions that produce a chronic demyelinating polyneuropathy with its onset in infancy include metachromatic leukodystrophy (MLD), Niemann-Pick disease type C, and chronic polyneuropathy secondary to nonspecific infections.

Several entities present as hereditary motor sensory neuropathies. These include Refsum disease, which is considered in Chapter 1, and hereditary motor neuropathies associated with spastic paraplegia (429), optic atrophy (430,431), retinitis pigmentosa (432), and agenesis of the corpus callosum (Andermann syndrome) (433).

Treatment

Aside from orthopedic measures and consistent, active physiotherapy, no specific treatment exists. Corticosteroids have been ineffective.

Hereditary Neuropathy with Liability to Pressure Palsies (Tomaculous Neuropathy)

Hereditary neuropathy with liability to pressure palsies (HNPP) is a dominantly transmitted condition characterized by recurrent peripheral nerve palsies, often precipitated by only slight trauma (434). Distal nerves are affected more commonly, and both patients and asymptomatic carriers show slowed motor and sensory conduction velocities even in childhood. Psychomotor development is unaffected. On nerve biopsy one almost always sees focal myelin thickenings, termed tomacula, which result from redundant loop formation within the myelin sheaths and are seen in both motor and sensory nerves (435–437). HNPP can be accompanied by nerve deafness or scoliosis (438). In approximately 70% of patients, HNPP results from a 1.5-Mb deletion on chromosome 17 p11.2, the site that spans the gene for PMP-22 (434), with a consequent underexpression of PMP-22 (439).

The relationship between HNPP and Smith-Magenis syndrome is unclear. The latter condition is a contiguous-gene–deletion syndrome of chromosome 17p11.2. Smith-Magenis syndrome is characterized by brachycephaly, midface hypoplasia, broad nasal bridge, brachydactyly, speech delay, and a hoarse, deep voice. Signs suggestive of peripheral neuropathy (e.g., decreased or absent deep tendon reflexes, pes planus or pes cavus, decreased sensitivity to pain, and decreased leg muscle mass) were found in 55% of patients (440). However, unlike patients with Charcot-Marie-Tooth disease type 1A, these patients demonstrated normal nerve conduction velocities, and there was no susceptibility to pressure palsies. Two-thirds of the patients demonstrated self-destructive behavior or mental retardation.

Hereditary Brachial Plexus Neuropathy (Hereditary Neuralgic Amyotrophy)

A dominantly transmitted form of brachial plexus neuropathy has been known for nearly 100 years. One gene for this condition has been mapped to chromosome 17q25, but there is considerable genetic heterogeneity (441). Brachial plexus neuropathy is characterized by recurrent attacks of pain affecting the neck and shoulders followed within hours or days by a weakness of muscles enervated by the brachial plexus. Attacks tend to be precipitated by infection or mild trauma. In addition to muscles enervated by the brachial plexus, the lower extremities are affected in approximately 20% of cases. Cranial nerves, notably X, VII, and VIII, also can be involved, resulting in hoarseness owing to paralysis of the vocal cords, impaired swallowing, facial weakness, and sensorineural deafness. Functional recovery takes place within a few months but atrophy and weakness can persist. Associated anomalies are not unusual. Affected children have closely spaced eyes or other dysmorphic features (442,443). Ring-shaped creases on the arms, resembling those of the Michelin tire man, are frequent. Unusual skin folds are also seen on the neck (442). Although the condition usually presents during the second to third decade of life, it also can affect neonates, producing what appears to be a traumatic brachial plexus injury.

Nerve conduction velocities are normal during both the attack and the recovery period, but EMG can reveal evidence of denervation. Biopsy of the peripheral nerves reveals regions of tomaculous (sausage-like) thickening of the myelin sheath. Perivascular inflammation with disruption of the vessel walls has also been noted (444). Corticosteroid therapy does not appear to affect the course of the attacks. In at least one instance there was a favorable response to high-dose intravenous globulin. The gene for this condition has been mapped to chromosome 17q24–q25 (445).

Hereditary brachial plexus neuropathy can be distinguished on clinical grounds from HNPP. In the latter condition, attacks are not preceded by pain and generally affect the distal nerves. Nerve biopsy is characteristic. Hereditary brachial plexus neuropathy also should be distinguished from acute brachial plexus neuropathy. This condition mainly affects adults, is bilateral in 25% to 33% of cases, and is triggered by infections and immunizations, notably by tetanus toxoid. Epidemics or clusters of brachial plexus neuropathy have been observed (446).

Hereditary Sensory and Autonomic Neuropathies (HSAN)

At least five clinical entities exist under hereditary sensory and autonomic neuropathies, all characterized by a progressive loss of function that predominantly affects the peripheral sensory nerves (447). These conditions are less common than the hereditary motor sensory neuropathies; their incidence has been estimated at 1 in 25,000, approximately 1/10 that of CMT1 (448), and collectively these conditions accounted for 3% of the hereditary peripheral neuropathies of infants and children pooled by Hagberg and Lyon (401a).

The clinical presentation depends on the population of affected neurons or axons. When degeneration of the large-diameter afferent fibers occurs, as in Friedreich ataxia, position sense is involved primarily. When the small afferent and autonomic fibers are affected, an increased threshold to nociception and thermal discrimination occurs accompanied by autonomic and trophic changes.

Type I (Hereditary Sensory Radicular Neuropathy; HSAN I)

Hereditary sensory radicular neuropathy is the most common of the hereditary sensory and autonomic neuropathies. It is transmitted as an autosomal dominant

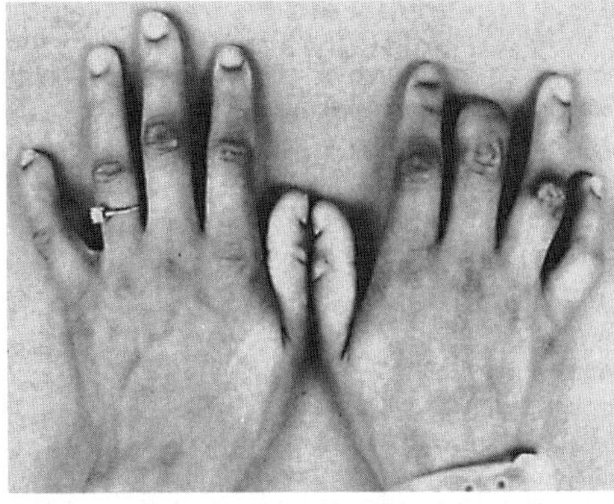

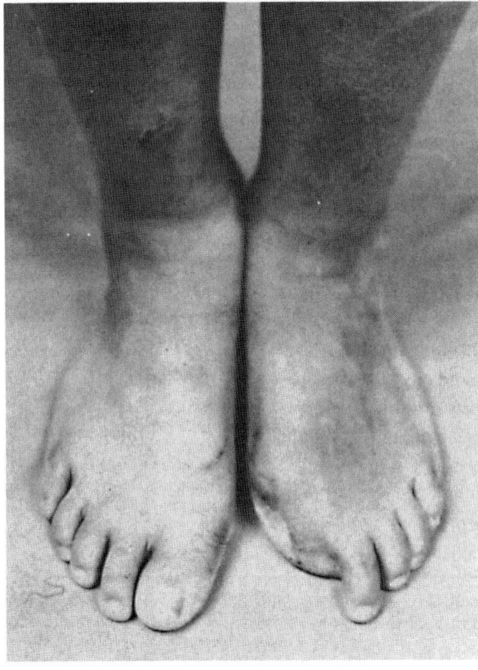

FIGURE 3.7. Hereditary sensory radicular neuropathy. Trophic changes in digits of upper and lower extremities. (Courtesy of Dr. K. E. Astrom, Massachusetts General Hospital, Boston, MA.)

trait and is characterized by a sensory deficit in the distal portion of the lower extremities, chronic perforating ulcerations of the feet, and progressive destruction of the underlying bones. It is identical to familial lumbosacral syringomyelia. Pathologic examination discloses degeneration of the dorsal root ganglia and of the dorsal roots of the spinal cord segments supplying the lower limbs (390).

Symptoms appear in late childhood or early adolescence. Initially, patients have episodes of cellulitis of the feet accompanied by a progressive loss of sensation in the lower extremities, which is associated with painless lacerations and trophic ulcers (Fig. 3.7). On examination, perception of pain is affected more than touch or deep pressure perception. Sweating is impaired. The distal portions of the upper extremities also can be affected. Sharp, brief pains can occur in the legs and resemble the lightning pains of tabes dorsalis. Many of the cases have accompanying nerve deafness and atrophy of the peroneal muscles (390).

The gene for this disorder has been mapped to 9q22.1–q22.3 (448). The gene (*SPTLC1*) encodes a subunit of serine palmitoyl transferase (LCB1), the enzyme that catalyzes the first step of sphingolipid biosynthesis (391). It is not clear how this defect induces the neuropathy, but experimental studies have shown that mutant LCB1 can confer a dominant negative effect on serine palmitoyl transferase (449).

Histopathologic examination shows a marked reduction in the number of unmyelinated fibers. Small myelinated fibers are decreased to a lesser degree and large myelinated fibers are affected least (447). Motor nerve conduction velocities are normal but the sensory nerve action potentials are absent.

Type II (Congenital Sensory Neuropathy; HSAN II)

Congenital sensory neuropathy is characterized by its autosomal recessive inheritance and by an onset of symptoms in early infancy or childhood. The gene for this condition has been mapped to chromosome 12p13.33. The functions of the gene, named *HSN2*, are not known (450).

The upper and lower extremities are affected with chronic ulcerations and multiple injuries to fingers and feet. Pain sensation is involved most, with temperature and touch sensations affected to a lesser extent. Deep pain is impaired and the deep tendon reflexes are reduced (392). Autoamputation of the distal phalanges is common, as is a neuropathic joint degeneration (451). The condition progresses slowly, if at all (393). Sensory nerve action potentials are reduced or absent. Nerve biopsy shows a total loss of myelinated fibers and reduced numbers of unmyelinated fibers.

Type III (Familial Dysautonomia, Riley-Day Syndrome; HSAN III)

Although the name *familial dysautonomia* suggests that the disease is exclusively a disorder of the autonomic nervous system, peripheral sensory neurons, peripheral motor neurons, and other neuronal populations also are affected.

In the first description of the disease in 1949, Riley and coworkers pointed out excessive sweating, poor temperature control, skin blotching, defective lacrimation, indifference to pain, absent deep tendon reflexes, and motor incoordination (452). The condition is transmitted as an autosomal recessive trait and is confined to Jews of Eastern European descent. In the United States, the frequency of the carrier state as determined by screening for the splice-site mutation in this ethnic group is 1 in 32 (453).

The gene for dysautonomia (*IKBKAP*) has been localized to chromosome 9q31. It codes for a protein named I Kappa 3 Kinase-associated protein (IKAP), which is the largest member of a three-subunit protein complex called core elogator. Core elongator has been localized to cytoplasm, but its function has not been clarified (454). In dysautonomia the mutation that accounts for more than 99.5% of all cases is a single-base change at base pair 6 of the donor splice site of intron 20. This mutation causes a tissue-specific decreased splicing efficiency with sporadic skipping of exon 20 (454,455). Cells from patients retain some capacity to produce the normal protein; thus the wild-type:mutant ratio is highest in lymphoblasts cultured from patients and lowest in postmortem central and peripheral nervous system (454). Nissim-Raffinia and Kerem reviewed the role of splicing regulation in determining the severity and the tissue-specific expression of genetic diseases (456).

Pathology

No consistent structural abnormality has been found within the CNS. The sympathetic ganglia are hypoplastic and the number of neurons in the spinal ganglia is reduced, with hypoplasia of the dorsal root entry zones and Lissauer tract (457). Substance P immune reactivity in the substantia gelatinosa of the spinal cord and the medulla is depleted, a finding consistent with a supposition that this undecapeptide is involved in the transmission of pain impulses (458).

Some patients have shown degenerative changes in the reticular substance of the pons and medulla with focal lack of myelination and neuronal depletion (459). Additionally, fibers are lost from the lateral and ventral spinothalamic tracts, the posterior columns, and the spinocerebellar tracts, and myelin sheaths are lacking in the mesencephalic roots of the trigeminal nerve. These changes are slowly progressive without neuronophagia or evidence of myelin breakdown.

In peripheral nerves, the number of myelinated and nonmyelinated axons is reduced and the transverse fascicular area is diminished. Most important, the catecholamine endings appear to be absent (460).

Clinical Manifestations

Familial dysautonomia is characterized by symptoms referable to the sensory and autonomic nervous system (394). No single feature, but rather the association of several, points to the diagnosis.

Nervous system dysfunction is usually evident from birth as a poor or absent suck reflex, hypotonia, and hypothermia. Nursing difficulties result in frequent regurgitation (394). A high incidence of breech presentation (31%) is unrelated to the birth weight but reflects intrauterine hypotonia. Retarded physical development, poor temperature control, and motor incoordination become prominent during early childhood, and subsequently other clinical features are detected (Table 3.11) (395). These include inability to produce overflow tears with the usual stimuli, absent or hypoactive deep tendon reflexes, absent corneal reflexes, postural hypotension, relative indifference to pain, and absence of the fungiform papillae on the tongue in association with a marked diminution in taste sensation (Fig. 3.8) (461). Many patients have serious feeding difficulties, including cyclic vomiting and recurrent pneumonia. In part, these problems can be attributed to absent or decreased lower esophageal peristalsis, a dilated esophagus, and impaired gastric motility (462). Taste and smell are significantly impaired (463). Scoliosis is frequent and becomes more marked with age. Intelligence remains normal. Many patients die from the disease during infancy or childhood. In some 40%, death is a consequence of pulmonary failure or cardiorespiratory arrest, usually during sleep or precipitated by hypotension (394). A prolongation of the QT interval seen in approximately one-third of patients could predispose them to sudden death from ventricular arrhythmia (464). Aspiration or

TABLE 3.11 Clinical Features of Familial Dysautonomia

Disturbances of Autonomic Nervous System	
Reduced or absent tears	+++
Peripheral Vascular Disturbances	
Hypertension with excitement	++
Postural hypotension	+++
Skin blotching with excitement or with eating	++
Cold hands and feet	+++
Excessive perspiration	+++
Erratic temperature control	++
Disturbed swallowing reflex	+++
Drooling beyond usual age	++
Cyclic vomiting	++
Disturbances of Voluntary Neuromuscular System	
Absent or hypoactive deep tendon reflexes	+++
Poor motor coordination	+++
Dysarthria	+++
Convulsions	+
Abnormal electroencephalographic results	++
Sensory Disturbances	
Relative indifference to pain	+++
Corneal anesthesia	++
Psychological Disturbances	
Apparent mental retardation	++
Breath-holding spells in infancy	++
Emotional lability	+++
Other Disturbances	
Absence of fungiform papillae	+++
Corneal ulcerations	++
Frequent bronchopneumonia	++
Retardation of body growth	++
Scoliosis	++

+, common; ++, occurs frequently but not required for the diagnosis; +++, probably present in all cases.

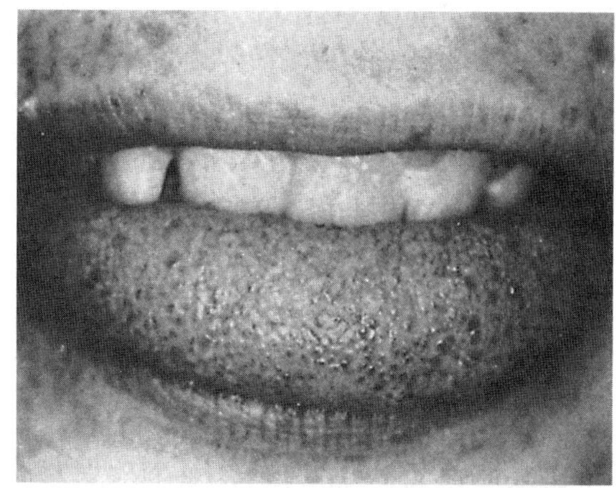

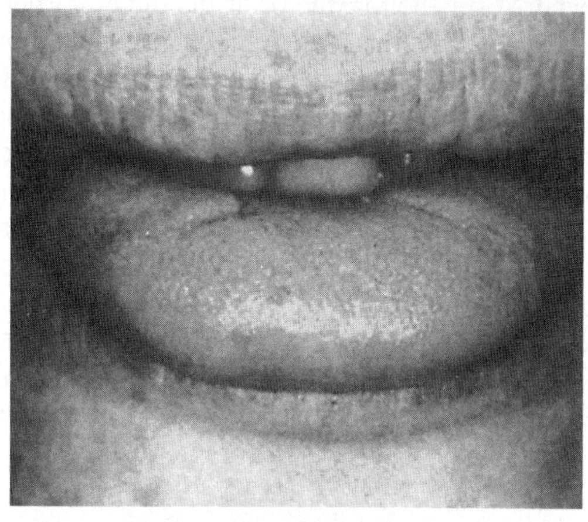

FIGURE 3.8. Familial dysautonomia. **A:** Tip of the tongue of a healthy child. The dark spots are blood cells seen through the clear epithelium of the fungiform papillae. **B:** In familial dysautonomia, no fungiform papillae exist, and the tongue appears smooth. (Courtesy of Dr. Felicia Axelrod, Department of Pediatrics, New York University, New York, NY.)

infectious pneumonia is another common cause for demise. Still, approximately 40% of living patients are 20 years of age or older (394). Some symptoms, notably cyclic vomiting, become less marked with age; others, in particular the sensory loss, are slowly progressive (465).

The brainstem auditory-evoked potentials are abnormally prolonged in most patients (466). Neuroimaging studies have been unremarkable.

Other clinical aspects of this systemic disease, including ophthalmologic abnormalities, anesthetic hazards, and various emotional problems, are discussed by Goldberg and associates (467) and Axelrod (394).

Diagnosis

The clinical diagnosis of dysautonomia rests on the patient's history, genetic background, and clinical features of the condition, in particular the absence of fungiform papillae, absent corneal reflexes, decreased or absent deep tendon reflexes, and decreased response to pain. I have found the intradermal histamine test to be the most reliable. In healthy individuals, intradermal injection of histamine phosphate (0.03 to 0.05 mL of a 1:1,000 solution) produces a local wheal and a red erythematous flare extending 1 to 3 cm beyond the wheal. In dysautonomic patients beyond the newborn period, the flare response is absent. A similar lack of response can be seen in atopic dermatitis and in some disorders of the spinal cord or peripheral nerves (e.g., other progressive sensory neuropathies). A commercial genetic test is available.

Treatment

Treatment is symptomatic (394). Impaired swallowing is best managed by experimenting with nipples of different sizes and with thickened feedings. If these methods fail, gavage feedings are necessary. When gastroesophageal reflux results in intractable pulmonary problems, gastrostomy feeding and fundal plication are required (468). Vomiting is managed by correcting the dehydration, which generally is isotonic. Gastric distention is relieved by using bethanechol chloride. Oral doses range from 1 to 2 mg/kg per day, given in several divided doses, although the amount required varies from one child to the next. Cessation of vomiting is promoted by the use of diazepam (0.1 to 0.2 mg/kg per dose) given intravenously. Diazepam is also the most effective treatment for hypertension and is given intramuscularly in doses of 0.5 to 1.0 mg/kg. Crises are best handled with diazepam or with the combination of diazepam and chlorpromazine (0.5 to 1.0 mg/kg given intramuscularly) (394). Aspiration pneumonia is prevented by maintaining the head in an elevated position. Feeding and swallowing difficulties in the infant might necessitate gavage. Hypertensive crises are treated with sedation and chlorpromazine.

Type IV (Congenital Insensitivity to Pain and Anhidrosis; HSAN IV)

Congenital insensitivity to pain and anhidrosis is a recessive condition that becomes apparent in early life. The gene for this condition has been mapped to chromosome 1q21–q22. It codes for a high-affinity tyrosine kinase receptor for nerve growth factor (396).

Affected infants present with episodes of high fever often related to the environmental temperature, anhidrosis, and insensitivity to pain. Palmar skin is dry, thickened, and hyperkeratotic, and Charcot joints (sensory arthropathy) are commonly present. Painless heel ulcerations are frequent and are slow to heal. Children respond to tactile stimulation, and deep tendon reflexes are often preserved. Self-mutilatory behavior is common, as are corneal ulcers. About 20% of infants succumb to hyperpyrexia within the first 3 years of life (397). Peripheral nerve biopsy shows the small unmyelinated fibers to be almost totally absent (469). Axonal microtubules are reduced and the mitochondria are abnormally enlarged. Muscle biopsy discloses an accumulation of lipid droplets and reduced cytochrome *c* oxidase (470). In contrast to the other sensory neuropathies, motor and sensory nerve action potentials are normal.

An autosomal recessive neuropathy seen in Navajo children is similar pathologically. Clinically, the Navajo children do not experience bouts of hyperpyrexia and are developmentally normal (471).

Type V (Hereditary Sensory and Autonomic Neuropathy; HSAN V)

Hereditary sensory and autonomic neuropathy also manifests with congenital insensitivity to pain and anhidrosis. It is distinct from congenital insensitivity to pain and anhidrosis (HSAN IV) by a selective absence of the small myelinated fibers (392). This condition, in association with neurotrophic keratitis, has been seen in Kashmir (472).

Other Hereditary Sensory Neuropathies

Several other, probably distinct, forms of hereditary sensory neuropathies have been reported. In addition, an entity exists termed *asymbolia to pain*, or congenital indifference to pain, in which pain sensation is appreciated but its unpleasant quality is lost. It is an autosomal recessive disorder that is often accompanied by auditory imperception (473).

Giant Axonal Neuropathy (GAN)

Giant axonal neuropathy, an autosomal recessive disorder, was described in 1972 by Berg and colleagues (474). The gene for GAN has been mapped to chromosome 16q24.1. It encodes a protein named gigaxonin, which is one of the BTB/kelch superfamily of cytoskeletal proteins that have been termed the "propellers of cell function"(475). The condition probably represents a generalized disorder of cytoplasmic microfilament formation.

The condition is characterized clinically by a chronically progressive, peripherally mixed neuropathy having its onset in early childhood. Most of those affected have pale or slightly reddish hair, which is unusually tight and curly. Scanning electron microscopy of the hair shafts shows an irregular cuticle and longitudinal grooves (476). Ataxia and nystagmus are not unusual. Biopsy of the motor and sensory nerves reveals decreased numbers of myelinated and unmyelinated fibers and the presence of focal axonal enlargements that are more common distally and adjacent to a node of Ranvier. Ultrastructurally, these swellings are replete with aggregates of neurofilaments (477). Swollen axons also have been found within the CNS (478). Similar axonal enlargements have been seen in neuroaxonal dystrophy and in glue-sniffing neuropathy.

Progressive Facial Hemiatrophy (Parry-Romberg Syndrome)

Although evidence for a mendelian basis for this condition is lacking, it is presented in this chapter for the sake of convenience.

Progressive facial hemiatrophy is characterized by progressive wasting of the face, including the subcutaneous tissue, fat, cartilage, and bone. The disease makes its appearance in early childhood and occasionally is present at birth. Approximately 75% of patients with progressive facial hemiatrophy are affected before 20 years of age. In approximately 25%, local trauma appears to predispose to the condition. Initially, shrinkage of the subcutaneous tissue occurs over the maxilla or at the upper corner of the nasolabial fold. As the disease progresses slowly over the course of several years, the remainder of the facial half becomes involved (Fig. 3.9). Patients experience no muscular weakness, loss of trigeminal nerve function, or atrophy of the skin. The hair, including the eyelashes and eyebrows, is affected commonly, and alopecia and blanching, particularly along the paramedian area, can precede all other manifestations of the condition.

Cerebral symptoms include seizures that can be generalized or focal (particularly sensory focal) and minimal pyramidal tract signs (479,480). Seizures can take

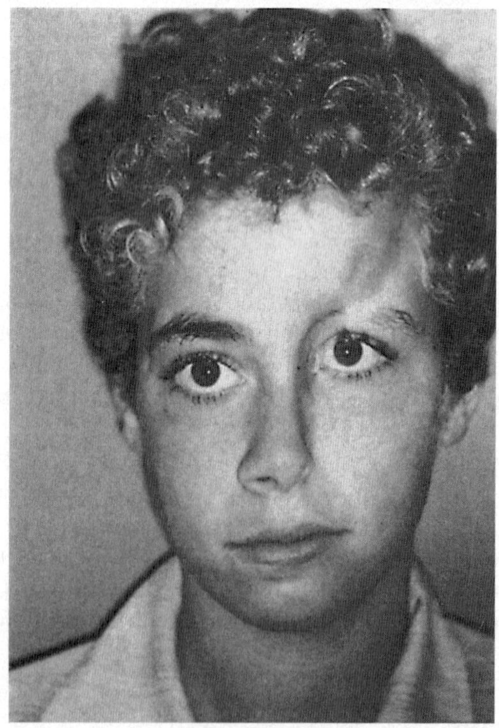

FIGURE 3.9. Progressive facial hemiatrophy in a 16-year-old boy. The scarlike coup de sabre is characteristic for this condition but also may be seen in scleroderma. (Courtesy of Dr. Creighton G. Bellinger, Glendale, CA.)

a course that is suggestive of Rasmussen encephalitis, an indication, perhaps, that the two conditions share a similar underlying etiology (481) (see Chapter 7). However, in Parry-Romberg syndrome, seizures can often be controlled with anticonvulsants, which is rarely so in Rasmussen encephalitis. No definite pathologic changes have been found in the few brains examined, although some have shown nonspecific inflammatory processes (479,482). The CT scan can be normal or show intracerebral calcifications or atrophy. The calcification is generally ipsilateral to the facial hemiatrophy (480). MRI demonstrates areas of ipsilateral cortical dysgenesis or increased signal in the ipsilateral white matter on T2-weighted images (483).

Although the appearance of the patient with progressive hemiatrophy is characteristic, lipodystrophy and scleroderma should be considered in the differential diagnosis. In lipodystrophy, the involvement is bilateral and spares cartilage and bone; in scleroderma, the skin becomes cold, waxy, and inelastic and adheres to the subcutaneous tissue. In familial hemiatrophy, the skin usually remains normal.

Aside from cosmetic surgery, no appropriate therapy for this condition is available. The atrophy progresses for several years but never becomes complete.

Progressive Hereditary Nerve Deafness

Various heredodegenerative diseases of the CNS are accompanied by a progressive sensory neural hearing loss. These include such heredodegenerations as CMT disease, FRDA, and the hereditary sensory neuropathies. Progressive nerve deafness also is seen in association with retinitis pigmentosa (Usher syndromes), recessive conditions with a variable degree of penetrance. In Refsum disease, nerve deafness accompanies retinitis pigmentosa, ataxia, and polyneuropathy.

A number of syndromes in which progressive nerve deafness accompanies lesions of the visual system have been summarized by Fischel-Ghodsian and Falk (484) and Fraser (485). In all of these, deafness begins insidiously and progresses slowly; the ability to hear high tones is usually lost first. A differential diagnosis of profound hearing loss in childhood is presented in Chapter 5 (see Table 5.15). Ménière disease, a condition characterized by progressive deafness, tinnitus, and paroxysms of vertigo, is essentially a disorder of middle life.

Retinitis Pigmentosa

Retinitis pigmentosa represents a common cause of hereditary visual impairment. It is a component of the more than 400 hereditary diseases that affect the retina, macula, and choroids. Retinitis pigmentosa can be subdivided into a group in which the disease process is confined to the eye and a group in which it accompanies a systemic or heredodegenerative disorder. A list of the various mapped or cloned human genes that cause retinal degenerations is provided by Heckenlively and Daiger (486).

DIFFUSE CEREBRAL DEGENERATIVE DISEASES

Various hereditary diseases that affect the CNS in a nonselective manner are included in diffuse cerebral degenerative diseases. Although in some the evidence indicates a defect in cerebral metabolism, the relationship between the enzymatic defect and the neurologic abnormalities has not always been defined completely.

Diseases with Degeneration Primarily Affecting White Matter (Leukodystrophies)

Traditionally the leukodystrophies have been grouped by the histochemical characteristics of the myelin breakdown products. The following major entities can be distinguished: adrenoleukodystrophy (ALD), Pelizaeus-Merzbacher disease (PMD), Canavan disease (spongy degeneration of white matter), Alexander disease, MLD, and Krabbe disease (globoid cell leukodystrophy).

Adrenoleukodystrophy

Adrenoleukodystrophy is the most common and clearly defined form of sudanophilic cerebral sclerosis, with an incidence of 1 in 10,000 male individuals. It is also the most common inherited peroxisomal disorder. The condition can take one of three forms: (a) rapidly progressive, inflammatory cerebral form, which is characterized by visual and intellectual impairment, seizures, spasticity, and a more or less rapid progression to death, (b) adrenomyeloneuropathy (AMN), which has its onset in the third or fourth decade with slowly progressive paraparesis, and (c) Addison's disease without neurologic symptoms.

Pathology, Molecular Genetics, and Pathogenesis

ALD is an X-linked condition, and the gene *ABCD1*, whose mutation causes the disease, has been mapped to chromosome Xq28. The gene encodes a protein, ALDP, that is a member of the family of ATP-binding-cassette transport systems (called *cassette* because the ATP fits into the molecule like a cassette into a tape player). These proteins use the energy derived from the hydrolysis of ATP to transport substrates, including very long chain fatty acid (VLCFA)-CoA synthetase, across a membrane such as that of the peroxisome against a concentration gradient (487). As a result of the transporter defect, the first step in the β-oxidation of the VLCFA, namely the synthesis of

VLCFA-CoA, becomes inoperative. The biological functions of the transporters have been reviewed by Stefkova and coworkers (488). More than 500 different mutations in the gene that codes for the VLCFA-CoA transporter, including missense and frameshift mutations, have been documented in patients with different phenotypes of ALD, and no correlation between genotype and phenotype can be demonstrated (499).

The pathogenesis of the CNS lesion in ALD is poorly understood (490). The presence of the slowly progressive adult form and the severe childhood form of ALD in the same nuclear family, the observation of different phenotypes in identical twins (491), and the rapid progression of the disease after years of dormancy all suggest that nongenetic factors, modifier genes, or both are important in the expression of the disease. The increased expression of proinflammatory cytokines, such as tumor necrosis factor-α and interleukin-1β in astrocytes and microglia in demyelinating lesions of patients with the childhood form of ALD, suggests an important role of cytokines in the pathogenesis of the disease (492).

Pathologic features include widespread demyelination and gliosis of cerebral white matter. The demyelination generally spares subcortical fibers and exhibits a rostrocaudal progression, with the earliest abnormalities evident in the occipital and posterior parietal lobes. Inflammatory cells are common and are seen in a perivascular distribution. Macrophages are filled with material that has positive results for periodic acid–Schiff and oil red O, and probably consist of VLCFA esters. In the zona fasciculata and reticularis of the adrenal gland, ballooned cells are evident. Many of these have striated cytoplasm and vacuolations. Similar lipid inclusions are found in Schwann cells of the peripheral nerves and in testes (493). The structure of peroxisomes is morphologically normal.

Chemical analysis demonstrates the accumulation of VLCFAs with carbon chain lengths of 22 to 30 (C_{22} to C_{30}), notably C_{26}, in white matter cholesterol esters, cerebrosides, and gangliosides. VLCFAs, particularly C_{26}, also are increased in cultured fibroblasts and serum (494). These VLCFAs are partly of exogenous origin, and their β-oxidation normally occurs within peroxisomes (495). The biochemical defect, however, does not directly involve the oxidation of VLCFAs, as was originally surmised.

Clinical Manifestations

Of the three phenotypes the cerebral form of ALD is the most common; it represented 48% of the collected patients in Moser's group (496). In the Australian series of Kirk and colleagues, it comprised 54% (497). Adrenomyeloneuropathy was found in 25% of ALD hemizygotes and Addison disease without neurologic involvement was found in 10% of Moser's cases (476), and these were found in 25% and 16%, respectively, in the series of Kirk and colleagues (497). The various phenotypes frequently occur within the same family, and the manifestations of the disease can differ significantly in closely related family members (498). In some individuals progression is fairly rapid, whereas in others the course can be relapsing and remitting (499).

Onset of the cerebral form of ALD is usually between ages 5 and 8 years, with a gradual disturbance in gait and slight intellectual impairment. Abnormal pigmentation or classic adrenal insufficiency sometimes precedes neurologic abnormalities by several years. In other cases, adrenocortical atrophy is asymptomatic throughout life (493). Early seizures of several types are common, as are attacks of crying and screaming. Visual complaints are initially rare, whereas swallowing is disturbed in approximately one-third of the children. Spastic contractures of the lower extremities appear, and frequently the child becomes ataxic. Extrapyramidal symptoms also can be observed. Cutaneous melanosis or evidence of Addison disease can often be detected.

The CSF protein content can be elevated, and a mild lymphocytosis can develop. MRI is more sensitive than the CT scan in terms of showing the extent of abnormal white matter. Abnormalities that are seen as high signal on T2-weighted sequences are first noted in the periventricular posterior parietal and occipital regions and extend anteriorly with progression of the disease. Demyelination can be accompanied by a contrast-enhancing area at the margins of the lesion that probably represents an inflammatory reaction. Calcification is not unusual (500,501). The MRI and MR spectroscopy also are abnormal in the preclinical stage of the disease (502). Because patients may remain asymptomatic in the face of an abnormal MRI until as long as their seventh decade of life, there is little predictive significance to these neuroimaging abnormalities. Evoked potentials are normal when neurologic symptoms first make their appearance; they become abnormal as the demyelinating lesions extend into the brainstem and into the parieto-occipital lobes. The auditory-evoked potential, one of the most sensitive indices of brainstem demyelination, is abnormal in obligatory carriers (503). The urinary excretion of adrenal androgens and corticosteroids is decreased, and adrenocorticotropic hormone stimulation fails to produce an increase in the 17-hydroxycorticoid excretion.

Adrenomyeloneuropathy generally has its onset in adult life, with only 8% of cases developing before 21 years of age (496,504). The condition is characterized by spastic paraparesis, distal neuropathy, adrenal insufficiency, and hypogonadism. At times the condition can mimic a hereditary form of spastic paraparesis (504a). MRI of the brain is abnormal in approximately one-half of patients, and cognitive function is reduced in approximately 40% (496).

Between 15% and 20% of female carriers develop a spastic paraparesis or a mild peripheral neuropathy. In 16% of these patients the MRI is abnormal (496).

Diagnosis

The diagnosis is suspected on the basis of the clinical picture. It can be confirmed by finding abnormally high levels of plasma VLCFAs, in particular a significantly elevated level of C_{26} saturated fatty acid and abnormally high ratios of C_{26} to C_{22} and C_{24} to C_{22} fatty acids. Some 85% of obligatory heterozygotes also can be diagnosed by their increased VLCFA levels in plasma and cultured fibroblasts (505). Mutation analysis is probably the most reliable method for the diagnosis of the heterozygote (505). Plasma VLCFA levels are unaffected by the usual food intake or by storage at room temperature for up to 2 weeks. Elevated levels of VLCFAs also are seen in some of the other peroxisomal disorders (see Chapter 1).

Treatment

Two forms of therapy can be considered: dietary therapy and bone marrow transplantation. Although the VLCFAs are, in part, of dietary origin, restriction of their intake does not affect the progressive worsening of the condition. A diet containing 20% erucic acid, a monounsaturated 22-carbon fatty acid (22:1), in addition to 80% oleic acid normalizes the levels of plasma C_{26} within a month. This diet, which goes under the name *Lorenzo oil*, has been tested in various centers, but in view of the variability of the clinical course of ALD it is difficult to evaluate its effectiveness. In the experience of van Geel and coworkers, dietary therapy with Lorenzo oil failed to improve the abnormal visual-evoked responses (506). It is the opinion of Gartner and colleagues that no scientific evidence exists to recommend this diet for patients with neurologic symptoms (500). Thrombocytopenia is a fairly common complication of treatment with Lorenzo oil (507).

Bone marrow transplantation has been used widely over the last few years. The outcome is encouraging in boys who are in the early stages of the disease, with an overall 5-year survival in this group of 92% (508). In this series, there was a 95% 5-year survival in boys who were treated when their performance IQ was above 80, and who showed only mild MRI abnormalities (508). In the experience of Shapiro and coworkers, the procedure did not arrest peripheral nerve demyelination (509).

Other therapeutic approaches include the use of lovastatin, which normalizes plasma VLCFAs, and 4-phenylbutyrate, which normalizes brain VLCFAs in mice by enhancing an alternative pathway for VLCFA oxidation (510) and increasing peroxisomal oxidation of VLCFA in fibroblast cultures (511).

In addition to the adrenoleukodystrophies, two other forms of sudanophilic diffuse sclerosis have been documented. The sporadic form is probably related to multiple sclerosis and is considered in Chapter 8. The other form is a sudanophilic diffuse sclerosis occurring as an autosomal recessive disorder, which in some families is accompanied by meningeal angiomatosis (512). It is not well substantiated as a discrete entity, and the white matter lesions are now believed to be hypoxic in nature.

Pelizaeus-Merzbacher Disease

Pelizaeus-Merzbacher disease (PMD) is a rare, slowly progressive disorder of myelin formation first described by Pelizaeus (513) in 1885 and Merzbacher in 1910 (514). The classic form of the condition has its onset in infancy and is transmitted in a gender-linked manner with the gene localized to the long arm of the X chromosome (Xq21.2–q22). The families described by Pelizaeus and Merzbacher fall into this category, as do the cases reported by Seitelberger (515) and Boulloche and Aicardi (516).

Pathology, Pathogenesis, and Molecular Genetics

The pathologic picture demonstrates widespread lack of myelin, although islands of myelination, particularly around small blood vessels, are preserved. Little sudanophilic material is present, and chemical examination of the brain reveals the white matter lipids to be normal or reduced. As expected from the absence of sudanophilic material, and in contrast to ALD, no increase in cholesterol esters is seen (516a). The axons in demyelinated areas are covered by their lipid sleeves, which give histochemical reactions for sphingolipids. Oligodendrocytes contain spherical lamellated cytoplasmic inclusions and numerous myelin balls at their periphery (516b). This pathologic picture suggests that the basic defect is impaired formation of myelin, a situation reminiscent of that observed in *jimpy* mice. This animal model suffers from a defect in PLP, one of the two major myelin membrane proteins. Indeed, the gene that encodes PLP, the *PLP* gene, has been found to be defective in PMD. In addition to PLP, the *PLP* gene also encodes another myelin protein, DM20. PLP and DM20 are two isoforms. They are hydrophobic membrane proteins that account for approximately one-half of the protein content of adult brain. The mRNAs that encode them are synthesized by alternative splicing of the primary transcript of the *PLP* gene.

A number of mutations in this gene have been described in patients with PMD. The most common of these is a duplication of the *PLP1* gene (518). Other mutations in order of frequency include missense mutations, insertions, and deletions (517). Missense mutations account for some 10% to 25% of families with PMD (518). Mutations in the noncoding region of the gene have also been described. The phenotype associated with this mutation is severe, with onset of symptoms between birth and 16 months (519). Mutations that truncate *PLP1* expression or result in a null mutation produce a clinical picture that combines demyelination and a peripheral neuropathy (520). Otherwise, the phenotype for the various mutations and duplications appears to be fairly comparable (518).

One of the intriguing questions that now is becoming unraveled is how the gene mutation in PMD results in dysfunction of oligodendrocytes and failure of myelination. Total absence of PLP due to gene deletion or a null mutation is associated with a more benign form than is seen in patients who have a gene duplication (517). It has recently become apparent that PMD is only one of many diseases in which mutant proteins aggregate in various subcellular departments and cause cell death. In PMD it appears that accumulation of the mutant protein in oligodendrocytes perturbs the viability of the cells by activating what has been termed the unfolded protein response (521). This is a stress response mediated by the endoplasmic reticulum leading ultimately to programmed cell death and apoptosis of the oligodendrocytes (522). For a review of this dynamic and exciting field see Gow and Sharma (523) and Kaufman (524).

The gene defect associated with PMD is allelic with that causing SPG2, one of the X-linked forms of hereditary spastic paraplegia (355) (see Table 3.7).

Clinical Manifestations

The clinical course differs from the other leukodystrophies only by the presence, before 3 months of age, of arrhythmically trembling and roving eye movements. Head control is poor, and cerebellar ataxia, including intention tremor and scanning speech, is frequent. Over the years, optic atrophy, involuntary movements, and spasticity become apparent, whereas the nystagmus can disappear. The disease progresses slowly, with many plateaus. The CSF is normal, as are other laboratory studies (525). Abnormalities of myelin are disclosed by MRI. Nezu and colleagues distinguished three patterns: diffuse alterations in hemispheric white matter and the corticospinal tracts, diffuse alterations in hemispheric white matter with a normal corticospinal tract, and least often, patchy changes in the white matter of the cerebral hemispheres (526). Little correlation exists between the type of MRI abnormality and the gene defect, and these changes do not appear to progress (526).

A connatal form of PMD that has an early, possibly prenatal onset and progresses rapidly also has been reported. It appears to be allelic with the classic form of PMD (527).

Diagnosis

In the absence of other affected members of the family, the diagnosis cannot be made with certainty solely on clinical grounds or by neuroimaging. However, ocular and cerebellar symptoms of extremely slow progression and the gender-linked recessive transmission tend to differentiate PMD from other degenerative conditions. The absence of remissions and early onset distinguish it from multiple sclerosis. Gene duplications can be detected by fluorescence *in situ* hybridization, using a PLP probe (528). This assay can also be utilized for the prenatal diagnosis of the condition (529). Considerable doubt exists over whether MRI can be used for carrier detection.

An X-linked disease has been reported that clinically resembles PMD in which there were capillary calcifications in the basal ganglia and dentate nucleus and in which the gene locus was on the long arm of the X chromosome but outside the region for the *PLP* gene (530).

Treatment

No effective treatment is available.

Spongy Degeneration of the Cerebral White Matter (Canavan Disease)

Spongy degeneration of the cerebral white matter (Canavan disease) is a rare familial degenerative disease of cerebral white matter first described by Canavan in 1931 (531). The condition is inherited as an autosomal recessive trait, with the gene having been mapped to chromosome 17 pter–p13 and cloned. It codes for an enzyme, aspartoacylase, that hydrolyzes *N*-acetylaspartic acid to L-aspartic acid. A point mutation in the gene for aspartoacylase is a common finding in Canavan disease. In the series of Kaul and coworkers, 12 of 17 patients with this condition had this abnormality, the remainder were compound heterozygotes with one allele having the point mutation (532).

The condition is fairly rare worldwide, but the carrier rate has been found to be as high as 1 in 40 to 1 in 57 in the Ashkenazi Jewish population, with two point mutations accounting for more than 99% of patients (533,534). In the most common clinical variant, symptoms appear between the second and fourth months of life and include failure of intellectual development, optic atrophy, and hypotonia. Subsequently, seizures appear and a progressive increase occurs in muscular tone. Choreoathetotic movements are noted occasionally. A relative or absolute macrocephaly is often evident by age 6 months. It was seen in all Arab cases reported by Gascon and colleagues (535) and was seen in 92% of children in the series of Traeger and Rapin (536). In almost all, it could be documented by 1 year of age. The visual-evoked responses are frequently absent or delayed; they were normal in only 1 of 8 children reported by Gascon and colleagues (535). Nystagmus was seen in 88% of children and seizures in 63% (536). Death usually ensues before 5 years of age (537), although survival into the second or third decade of life is not uncommon (536).

Variants in which the onset of neurologic symptoms occurs within the first few days of life or after age 15 years also have been recognized (537).

The main pathologic findings are in white matter, particularly that of the convolutional areas, which is replaced by a fine network of fluid-containing cystic spaces that give the characteristic spongy appearance. The central portions and the internal capsule remain relatively spared. Edema fluid collects in the cytoplasm of astrocytes and intramyelinic vacuoles that result from splitting of the myelin sheath at the intraperiod lines (537,538). Products of myelin degradation cannot be found (539). In addition, axonal degeneration of the peripheral nerves is present, with clumping and granular disintegration of axonal material (540).

The most striking finding in patients with Canavan disease is the increased amount of *N*-acetylaspartic acid (NAA) in plasma, urine, and brain (533), the consequence of aspartoacylase deficiency. In brain, NAA is localized within neurons. Its function is not known; presumably it serves as a source of acetyl groups for the synthesis of myelin lipids (541). The cause for the neurologic deterioration is unknown; it is possible that the accumulation of NAA causes an osmoregulatory disturbance.

The clinical diagnosis of Canavan disease rests on the progressive neurologic deterioration in a child with megalocephaly, optic atrophy, and seizures. It is confirmed by assay of urine for NAA. On nuclear magnetic resonance spectroscopy (MRS), the ratio of NAA to creatine and choline is strikingly increased; the actual concentration of NAA is not increased (542). On MRI, diffuse white matter degeneration is seen, with abnormally high signal throughout cerebral white matter on T2-weighted images (543) (Fig. 3.10). As the disease progresses, cerebral atrophy becomes marked.

In many cases the course of the disease is slowly progressive. I have seen children who were relatively intact neurologically even in the face of striking MRI abnormalities.

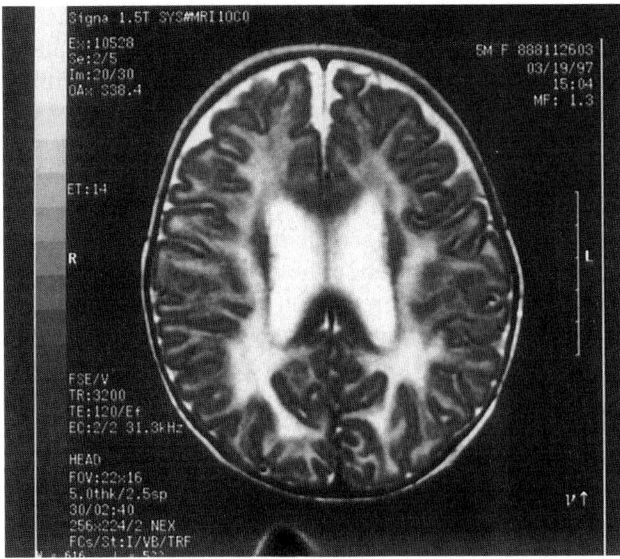

FIGURE 3.10. Spongy de eneration of cerebral white matter (Canavan disease). Magnetic resonance imaging study. T2-weighted axial views show a marked increase in signal in the white matter that is most evident in the posterior portions of the hemispheres. (Courtesy of Dr. Franklin G. Moser, Division of Neuroradiology, Cedars-Sinai Medical Center, Los Angeles, CA.)

Alexander Disease

First described by Alexander in 1949 (544), this condition most commonly begins within the first year of life with intellectual deterioration, macrocephaly, spasticity, and seizures. The gene has been mapped to chromosome 17q21 and codes for glial fibrillary acidic protein (GFAP) (545). Four clinical forms of Alexander disease have been recognized; all have mutations in the gene that codes for GFAP. The infantile form is the most common; it accounted for 26 of 44 genetically confirmed cases in the series of Li and coworkers (546). The juvenile form, with onset between 5 and 9 years of age, accounted for 15 patients, and the adult form was seen in 3 subjects. Bulbar signs are almost invariable additional symptoms in the juvenile form (547). A neonatal form has its onset in the first month of life followed by rapid progression. All children in this group develop hydrocephalus and increased intracranial pressure as a consequence of aqueductal stenosis caused by astroglial proliferation (548). Macrocephaly is less common in the juvenile form; it was only seen in 27% of cases in the series of Li and coworkers (546). The adult form appears to have an autosomal dominant transmission (549), and macrocephaly is not seen in this group (546).

Microscopic examination of the brain reveals diffuse demyelination. The distinctive feature is the presence of innumerable Rosenthal fibers that are particularly dense around blood vessels. Rosenthal fibers are rounded, oval, or club-shaped, densely osmiophilic bodies in the cytoplasm of enlarged astrocytes. It is believed that their formation is initiated by oxidative stress (550). The cells contain stress proteins, such as α-B-crystallin and HSP27. Crystallins are enormously large proteins normally secreted in the lens of the eye and in normal astrocytes. In Alexander disease, they form insoluble astrocytic aggregates (551). Both HSP27, and α-B-crystallin are increased in the CSF.

Diagnosis usually depends on a combination of neuroimaging and gene analysis. MRI results show extensive cerebral white matter changes with frontal predominance, a periventricular rim with increased signal on T1-weighted images and decreased signal on T2-weighted images, and abnormalities of the basal ganglia, thalamus, and brainstem (552,552a). The location of the abnormal signal correlates with areas where there is an accumulation of Rosenthal fibers (553). Although their appearance on neuroimaging studies has been claimed to be diagnostic for one or another of the leukodystrophies, their appearance is rarely specific. Instead, they show an evolution in the course of the disease from a normally appearing brain, to one in which white matter is diffusely abnormal, to an ultimate picture of generalized gray and white matter atrophy. Because, as a rule, the lesions are more extensive when visualized by MRI than by CT scans, MRI is the imaging study of choice in any infant or child with suspected leukodystrophy. Gene analysis is available commercially and should be performed when the MRI suggests the diagnosis.

Metachromatic Leukodystrophy (MLD)

Metachromatic leukodystrophy is a lysosomal storage disease marked by the accumulation of cerebroside sulfate (sulfatide) within the nervous system and other tissue. Although first described in 1910 by Alzheimer (554), the condition was not fully delineated until 1933 when Greenfield noted it to be a form of diffuse sclerosis in which oligodendroglial degeneration was characteristic (555).

Pathology and Molecular Genetics

Diffuse demyelination and accumulation of metachromatically staining granules are the outstanding pathologic features. (Metachromatic staining implies that the tissue–dye complex has an absorption spectrum sufficiently different from the original dye to produce an obvious contrast in color. The spectral shift is caused by the polymerization of the dye, which is induced by negative charges such as RSO_3 present in close proximity to one another within the tissue.) Metachromatically staining granules are either free in the tissues or stored within glial cells and macrophages. Metachromatic material is almost always found in neuronal cytoplasm, distending the cell body as in G_{M2} gangliosidosis but to a lesser extent. Electron microscopy demonstrates cytoplasmic inclusions and alteration in the lamellar structure of myelin (Fig. 3.11). Demyelination is diffuse but especially affects those tracts that myelinate during the latter part of infancy. All the involved areas have loss of oligodendroglia. Metachromatic granules also are found in the renal tubules, bile duct epithelium, gallbladder, islet cell and ductal epithelium of pancreas, reticular zone of adrenal cortex, and liver.

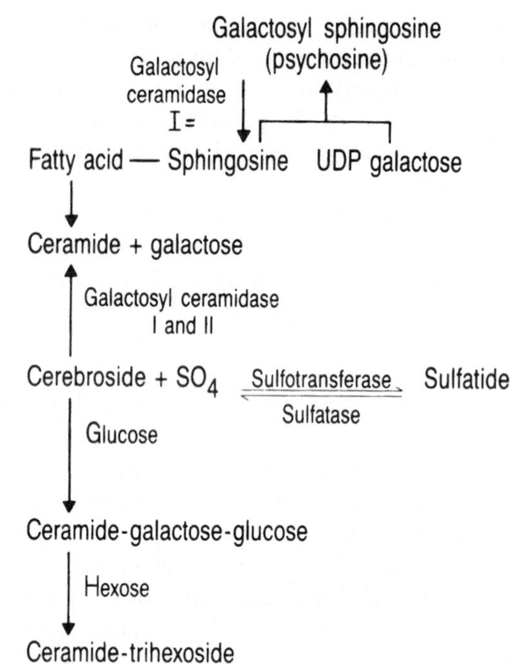

FIGURE 3.12. Glycolipid metabolism in brain. In metachromatic leukodystrophy, sulfatase is defective. In globoid cell leukodystrophy, galactosylceramidase I is deficient. As a consequence, galactosyl sphingosine (psychosine) accumulates. In addition, a secondary increase exists in ceramide dihexoside and trihexoside. UDP, uridine diphosphate.

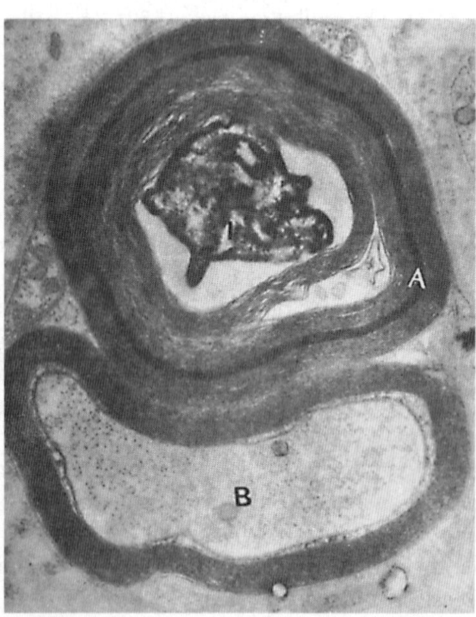

FIGURE 3.11. Metachromatic leukodystrophy. Electron microscopic examination. Sural nerve biopsy (×18,400). Within the myelin loop is a circular band of increased density (*A*). Large cytoplasmic inclusions (*I*) corresponding in size and distribution to metachromatic material observed in frozen sections of the same nerve can be seen. The adjacent axon and myelin are normal (*B*). (Courtesy of Dr. H. De F. Webster, National Institutes of Health, Bethesda, MD.)

In 1959, Austin showed the metachromatic material to be a sulfatide (i.e., a sulfuric acid ester of cerebroside) and a major constituent of myelin glycolipids (556). Subsequently, Austin and associates (557) and Jatzkewitz and Mehl (558) found the basic enzymatic defect in late infantile MLD to be an inactivity of a heat-labile cerebroside sulfatase (arylsulfatase-A). This defect results in the blocked hydrolysis of sulfatides to cerebrosides (Fig. 3.12). A marked reduction but not complete absence of arylsulfatase-A activity has been found in gray and white matter, kidney, liver, urine, leukocytes, and cultured skin fibroblasts (559). The gene coding for arylsulfatase-A has been mapped to chromosome 22q13.31–qter. It has been cloned and characterized, and nearly 100 mutations have been identified (560). Two mutations are particularly common in whites. In one [termed *allele I* by Polten and colleagues (561)], a G-to-A transition eliminates the splice donor site at the start of intron 2, with the resultant total loss of enzyme activity. Another common mutation (termed *allele A*) is characterized by a C-to-T transition that results in the substitution of leucine for proline at amino acid 426. This produces an enzyme with 3% residual activity. In the experience of Barth and colleagues, who

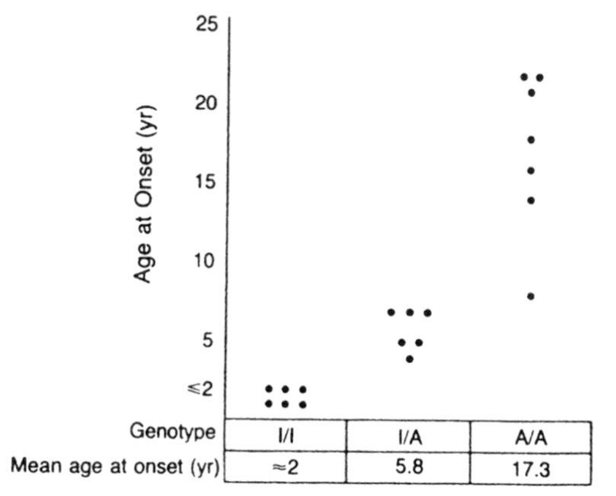

FIGURE 3.13. Arylsulfatase-A genotype and age at onset of symptoms for metachromatic leukodystrophy. The arylsulfatase-A genotype was plotted against the age at onset of clinical symptoms in 19 patients for whom such data were available. (From Polten A, Fluharty AL, Fluhart CB, et al. Molecular basis of different forms of metachromatic leukodystrophy. *N Engl J Med* 1991;324:18–22. With permission.)

studied mainly families from the United Kingdom, these two mutations accounted for 59% of the genetic lesions causing MLD (562). Numerous other, less common mutations in the gene have been demonstrated. These include both point mutations and gene deletions (560).

As a rule, the phenotype of each mutation can be inferred from their clinical expression in combination with other MLD mutations. In the series of Polten and colleagues, 21% of patients with the late infantile form of MLD were homozygous for the I/I genotype and another 48% had an I haplotype. Compound heterozygosity I/A was seen in 27% of juvenile cases (561) (Fig. 3.13). Homozygosity for allele A was seen in 45% of patients with the adult form of MLD, and another 27% had the A haplotype. A significant proportion of individuals with the A/A haplotype demonstrated the juvenile form of MLD. Thus, a considerable degree of phenotypic variation exists among patients with identical A/A genotypes, suggesting that nonallelic or environmental factors affect the age when neurologic symptoms make their appearance.

A reduction in arylsulfatase-A activity to 5% to 10% of control values is seen in up to 20% of the healthy population. This nonpathogenic reduction in enzyme activity is caused by homozygosity for a pseudodeficiency allele (562a). Individuals who are homozygous for this allele are asymptomatic, although in some, MRI shows lesions of white matter (563).

Less commonly, MLD is caused by a deficient cerebroside sulfatase activator protein, saposin B. The saposins are small glycoproteins that are required for sphingolipid hydrolysis by lysosomal hydrolases. Four saposins arise through hydrolytic cleavage from one gene product, prosaposin; other saposins arise from different genes. At least four different mutations in the gene for saposin B have been recognized (564). Patients with cerebroside activator protein deficiency present as the late infantile or juvenile form of MLD (560). The role of saposins in the various lysosomal storage diseases was reviewed by O'Brien and Kishimoto (565).

The mechanism by which sulfatide accumulation results in brain damage is not completely clear. Sulfatides are stored in oligodendrocytes and Schwann cells, and isolated myelin contains excess amounts of sulfatides. These are believed to result in an unstable molecular structure of myelin and myelin's consequent breakdown. Additionally, sulfatide accumulation might be responsible for the destruction of oligodendroglia and possibly for damage to neurons as well (566).

Clinical Manifestations

The incidence of the several forms of MLD is approximately 1 in 40,000 births. Symptoms can appear at any age. In the late infantile variant, a gait disorder, caused by either poor balance or a gradual stiffening, and strabismus occur by age 2 years. Impairment of speech, spasticity, and intellectual deterioration appear gradually, and, occasionally, coarse tremors or athetoid movements of the extremities develop. Deep tendon reflexes in the legs are reduced or even absent. Unexplained bouts of fever or severe abdominal pain can develop as the disease advances. Optic atrophy becomes apparent. Seizures are never prominent, although they can appear as the disease progresses (567). Progression is inexorable, with death occurring within 6 months to 4 years after the onset of symptoms. The CSF protein is elevated, the conduction velocity in the peripheral nerves is decreased, and the electroretinograms, in contrast to the various juvenile amaurotic idiocies, is normal. Auditory-evoked potentials can be abnormal even in presymptomatic patients (568). On MRI, the areas of demyelination are marked by high signal intensity on T2-weighted images. These are first seen in the periventricular regions and the centrum semiovale. The splenium and the genu of the corpus callosum also are affected (569), as are the internal capsule and the pyramidal tracts. Characteristically, the subcortical white matter, including the arcuate fibers, tends to be spared until late in the disease (569).

The juvenile form of MLD is somewhat rarer. It was first described by Scholz (570) and subsequently by others (571). Neurologic symptoms become evident at between 5 years of age and adulthood and progress slowly. Older patients develop an organic mental syndrome and progressive corticospinal, corticobulbar, cerebellar, or, rarely, extrapyramidal signs (572). The adult form of MLD, which has been seen as early as 15 years of age, generally begins with a change in personality and psychiatric problems (573). Rarely, the disease begins as a peripheral neuropathy.

The variant forms with arylsulfatase-activator deficiency present a clinical picture of late infantile or juvenile MLD (560).

Multiple sulfatase deficiency (mucosulfatidosis) is characterized by mental deterioration, coarse facial features, hepatosplenomegaly, skeletal anomalies, and ichthyosis. The clinical severity of this condition is variable; it ranges from a severe neonatal form to phenotypes that have only mild neurologic involvement (574). The gene for this disease (*SUMF1*) has been mapped to chromosome 3p26. It encodes a protein that is involved in a post-translational modification at the catalytic site of all sulfatases and is necessary for their function (574). At least 13 different sulfatases are defective. Patients accumulate sulfatides, acid mucopolysaccharides (heparan sulfate), and cholesterol sulfate in brain, liver, and kidney. Urinary excretion of mucopolysaccharides, notably heparan sulfate, is increased (575). The CSF protein content is elevated, and nerve conduction is slowed.

Diagnosis

The time of onset of neurologic symptoms and the presence of ataxia, spasticity, and particularly depressed deep tendon reflexes with elevated CSF protein content should suggest the diagnosis, which is confirmed by a marked reduction in urinary or leukocyte arylsulfatase-A activity. Other abnormal laboratory test results include slowed motor nerve conduction velocities, a reduced auditory-evoked brainstem response, and a nonfunctioning gallbladder. Brown metachromatic bodies can be found on biopsy of various peripheral nerves as early as 15 months after the onset of symptoms (Fig. 3.14). Segmental demyelination of peripheral nerves is encountered in other leukodystrophies, including globoid cell leukodystrophy, Canavan disease (540), and, rarely, GM_2 gangliosidosis and Spielmeyer-Vogt disease.

The assay of fibroblast arylsulfatase-A activity can be used for the biochemical identification of heterozygotes for MLD and for the diagnosis of multiple sulfatase deficiency. Cultured amniotic fluid cells can serve for the antenatal diagnosis of the disorder. Asymptomatic individuals with pseudodeficiency of arylsulfatase are distinguished from presymptomatic individuals with MLD by the presence of normal levels of urinary sulfatides and normal nerve conduction velocities.

Treatment

As is the case for several of the other lysosomal disorders, bone marrow transplantation is being used to treat the late infantile and the juvenile forms of MLD. Long-term results in patients with the juvenile form of MLD have been particularly encouraging when performed prior to the onset of neurologic deficits, in that engraftment develops with normalization of leukocyte arylsulfatase-A activity and a decrease in the sulfatide content of peripheral nerves, with a frequent but not invariable consequent arrest of neurologic deterioration (560,576). Retroviral or adenovirus-mediated gene transfer has been successful under experimental conditions, but these techniques have not been applied to the patient population.

Globoid Cell Leukodystrophy (Krabbe Disease)

Globoid cell leukodystrophy (GLD; Krabbe disease) was first described in 1908 by Beneke (577) and, more definitively, in 1916 by Krabbe (578), who noted the characteristic globoid cells in affected white matter.

Pathology

The white matter of the cerebrum, cerebellum, spinal cord, and cortical projection fibers is extensively demyelinated, with only minimal sparing of the subcortical arcuate fibers (579). Additionally, there is an almost total loss of oligodendroglia. In areas of recent demyelination,

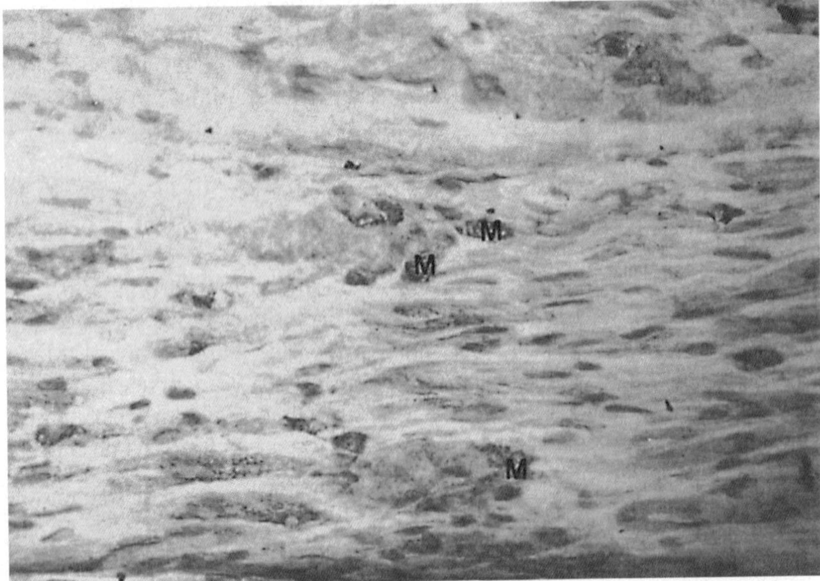

FIGURE 3.14. Metachromatic leukodystrophy. Peripheral nerve biopsy, longitudinal section, stained with acetic cresyl violet (acid pH). Innumerable coarse and fine clumps of golden brown crystalline granules (*M*). The 5-year-old girl had onset of intellectual deterioration at $3^1/_2$ years of age. This was accompanied by seizures and impaired coordination. Nerve conduction times were markedly prolonged and cerebrospinal fluid protein was elevated.

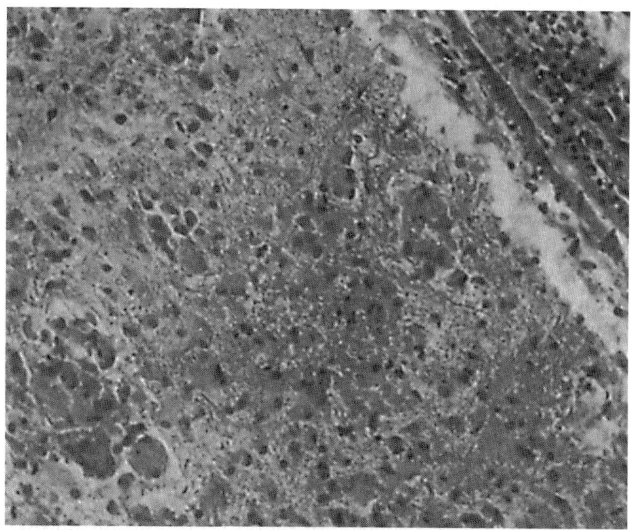

FIGURE 3.15. Globoid cell leukodystrophy. Cerebral white matter. Aggregates of globoid cells are seen in the vicinity of a blood vessel in the lower left corner. A considerable increase in cellularity occurs in the demyelinated area (hematoxylin and eosin, ×280).

mononuclear epithelioid cells and large (20 to 50 μm) multinucleated globoid cells are seen around the smaller blood vessels (Fig. 3.15). The globoid cells are believed to arise from vascular adventitia. Histochemical reactions and chemical analyses on globoid cell–rich fractions prepared by differential centrifugation show that a protein-bound cerebroside is stored within them. The appearance of globoid cells is believed to be stimulated by the release of cerebrosides from myelin because a similar cellular response can be produced in experimental animals through intracerebral injection of natural and synthetic cerebrosides (580).

Small clusters of globoid cells occur in a number of degenerative diseases of myelin, and the distinguishing feature of GLD is not the mere presence of these cellular elements, but their vast number. Ultrastructural examination reveals intracellular and extracellular crystalline inclusions, most commonly seen within the globoid cells, which correspond to the periodic acid-Schiff–positive material (581). The peripheral nerves show segmental demyelination and marked endoneurial fibrosis. Electron microscopy reveals curved or straight tubular structures in the cytoplasm of Schwann cells, around small blood vessels, or in the proliferated endoneurial collagenous tissue (582). Globoid cells also have been noted in lungs, spleen, and lymph nodes (583).

Biochemical Pathology and Molecular Genetics

The basic biochemical defect in GLD is a deficiency of a galactosylceramidase (galactocerebroside β-galactosidase) (see Fig. 3.12). Galactosylceramidase activity is reduced in a number of tissues, including leukocytes, brain, liver, spleen, and cultured skin fibroblasts (584). Because galactosylsphingosine (psychosine) is broken down only by galactosylceramidase, the substance accumulates in brain, peripheral nerve, liver, and kidney. Galactosylsphingosine has profound cytotoxic effects, inhibiting mitochondrial functions and inducing a globoid cell response and the destruction of oligodendrocytes by apoptosis (585,586). With the disappearance of oligodendrocytes, cerebroside biosynthesis ceases and the formation of myelin is arrested.

The gene coding for galactocerebrosidase (GALC) has been mapped to chromosome 14q31. The gene has been cloned, and more than 70 mutations have been documented. These include deletions of varying sizes and numerous point mutations. In general terms, a fair inverse correlation exists between the amount of residual galactocerebrosidase activity and the severity of the clinical manifestations. However, as is the case for ALD and some of the disorders of lysosomal function, intrafamilial variability of clinical manifestations has been described (587), including symptomatic and asymptomatic siblings harboring the same genetic mutation (588). The factors responsible for this variability are unknown.

Clinical Manifestations

Three clinical forms of GLD have been distinguished: the classic infantile form, the late infantile or juvenile form, and the adult form. In the infantile form, the disease begins acutely at 46 months of age with restlessness, irritability, and progressive stiffness. Convulsions can develop later. Frequently, these are tonic spasms induced by light, noise, or touch. Infants show increased muscular tone, with few spontaneous movements. Optic atrophy and hyperacusis are seen often. The deep tendon reflexes are characteristically difficult to elicit and can be absent in the legs. Terminally, infants are flaccid and develop bulbar signs (589).

A small proportion of patients have a later onset and slower evolution of their illness. Their neurologic symptoms include most commonly a slowly evolving spastic paraparesis. Less often the predominant symptoms include a motor and sensory neuropathy, hemiparesis, cerebellar ataxia, or cortical blindness (588).

Laboratory studies in the infantile form reveal a consistent elevation of CSF protein content. Conduction velocity of motor nerves is reduced. In the late-onset forms, both CSF protein and nerve conduction time can be normal (590). The MRI shows increased signal on T2-weighted images in the affected white matter, notably in the parietal lobes (590a). A curious MRI finding seen in GLD as well as in MLD are radially oriented hypointense stripes in the abnormally hyperintense white matter. Postmortem studies have shown that, in GLD, these stripes represent perivenular clusters of lipid-containing globoid cells (590b). In the late-onset Krabbe disease, the white matter lesions are more restricted and mainly affect the periventricular region, corpus callosum, or occipital lobes (588).

Diagnosis

The salient clinical diagnostic feature for the infantile form of GLD is peripheral nerve involvement: depressed deep tendon reflexes, elevated CSF protein, and delayed nerve conduction in a deteriorating infant. Various other degenerative conditions present a clinical picture akin to GLD. In general, G_{M2} gangliosidosis (Tay-Sachs disease) can be distinguished by the characteristic retinal changes. Juvenile amaurotic idiocy and MLD have a somewhat later onset. In the rare progressive degenerations of the gray matter, seizures tend to appear earlier and more frequently. The marked white matter involvement as seen on MRI and the near absence of serum, leukocyte, or skin fibroblast galactosylceramidase are the most definitive tests. An antenatal diagnosis can be made by means of this enzymatic assay (585).

Treatment

Allogeneic bone marrow transplantation has arrested the anticipated evolution of neurologic signs in a number of patients with GLD, notably those with a late onset and slower progression. In these instances nerve conduction studies improved and the CSF protein levels decreased following hematopoietic stem cell transplantation (591). Entrance of donor-derived mononuclear cells into the CNS occurs over the course of several months to years. As a consequence, the procedure is much less effective in the rapidly progressive infantile form than in the more slowly developing late-onset forms, and early-onset GLD patients do not appear to benefit (592).

Other Hereditary Demyelinating Conditions

Several entities in which demyelination is part of the pathologic picture are mentioned here.

Cockayne Syndrome

Cockayne syndrome is one of several known disorders of DNA repair (593). This rare condition, transmitted as an autosomal recessive trait, was first described by Cockayne in 1936 (594). Several different genotypes have been documented. The most common of these (seen in about 80% of patients) is a gene that has been mapped to chromosome 5 and encodes the Cockayne syndrome B protein. This protein is essential for transcription-coupled DNA repair (TCR), which is dependent on RNA polymerase II elongation (595). It is also involved in several other processes, including transcription by RNA polymerase I, transcription-coupled nucleotide excision repair, and base excision repair of some types of oxidative damage in nuclei and mitochondria (596). The nucleotide excision repair pathway is responsible for the removal from DNA of a variety of lesions, including those induced by ultraviolet light.

Nucleotide excision repair is a six-step process requiring a large number of gene products. It recognizes and removes lesions from DNA by a dual incision around the lesion in the damaged strand along with flanking nucleotides. Excision is followed by repair synthesis using the undamaged strand as template and by ligation. As determined by hybridization in culture using cell fusion agents, seven excision-deficient complementation groups have been identified, of which at least two have the clinical picture of Cockayne syndrome (597). Skin fibroblasts derived from patients with Cockayne syndrome show marked sensitivity to ultraviolet light. This is the consequence of a specific defect in the repair of lesions in strands of actively transcribed genes (598). It is not clear why the nervous system is singled out for defects in conditions in which impaired DNA repair exists. This extremely complex area is covered in a review by Wood (599) and in the text by Strachan and Reed (1).

Yet other patients with Cockayne syndrome have mutations in the Cockayne syndrome A protein, and a large variety of mutations are seen in the xeroderma pigmentosum-Cockayne syndrome (XP-CS) (600).

Cockayne syndrome is a progressive disorder, characterized by an unusual progeroid facies (large ears and sunken eyes), failure of growth first manifested after the second year of life, slowly progressive intellectual deterioration, lack of subcutaneous fat, pigmentary retinal degeneration, nerve deafness, and hypersensitivity of skin to sunlight. There is an associated leukodystrophy (600–602). In the Turkish patients of Özdirim and colleagues, ocular abnormalities including cataracts, retinitis pigmentosa, optic atrophy, and miosis unresponsive to mydriatics was recorded in 88% of children (601). A peripheral neuropathy also has been demonstrated, and nerve conduction and brainstem auditory-evoked responses are abnormal (601,603). Radiographic examinations reveal thickening of the skull bones and kyphoscoliosis. Calcifications, particularly involving the basal ganglia are common. MRI reveals loss of white matter and white matter hyperintensity on T2-weighted images (601,603).

On pathologic examination, generally patchy demyelination and atrophy of white matter and cerebellum are seen. The brain can undergo perivascular calcification in the basal ganglia and cerebellum, changes termed a *calcifying vasopathy* (604).

Except in the classic case, diagnosis of Cockayne syndrome is difficult. Not all patients have a photosensitive dermatitis, intracranial calcifications are seen only in some 40% to 50% of patients, and optic atrophy is seen in approximately one-half. Even fibroblast ultraviolet sensitivity is not present invariably (605).

Cockayne syndrome is one of three neurologic disorders in which an abnormality in DNA repair has been documented. Ataxia-telangiectasia is considered in Chapter 12. Xeroderma pigmentosum is also a markedly heterogeneous condition, with seven complementation groups (596). In this condition, there is also a defect in the nucleotide excision pathway (598). Xeroderma pigmentosum is characterized by extreme photosensitivity of the skin, resulting in a variety of cutaneous abnormalities in the areas of skin exposed to sunlight and a 1,000-fold increase in the incidence of melanoma and cutaneous basal and squamous cell carcinomas (600). Additionally, neurologic symptoms develop in 20% of patients (606). These include progressive mental deterioration, microcephaly, ataxia, choreoathetosis, a sensorineural hearing loss, and a peripheral neuropathy (607,608). Some patients with xeroderma pigmentosum can present with physical and mental retardation, optic atrophy, retinitis pigmentosa, premature senility, and other clinical features of Cockayne syndrome (598,600).

A related condition is the MICRO syndrome. This is an autosomal recessive condition, manifested by congenital microcephaly, microcornea, cortical dysplasias, cataracts, optic atrophy, and profound mental retardation. Unlike Cockayne syndrome, cultured cells do not show hypersensitivity to ultraviolet radiation (609).

Vanishing White Matter Disease

This condition was first described by van der Knaap and colleagues in 1997 (610). It is an autosomal recessive disorder that can be caused by a mutation in any of the five genes that encode subunits of the translation initiation factor eIF2B (611). The gene that is most commonly affected has been mapped to chromosome 3q27. It encodes the ε subunit. The factor eIF2B plays an important role in initiation of mRNA translation in that it activates eIF2, another initiation factor (611).

The onset of neurologic signs is usually in infancy or early childhood. There is often a rapid deterioration following an infection or minor head trauma (611). Abnormalities consist mainly of cerebellar ataxia and spasticity; epilepsy and optic atrophy may develop, but are not obligatory. Mental abilities may also be affected, but not to the same degree as the motor functions. MR imaging studies are diagnostic. They demonstrate cavitation and vacuolation of the cerebral hemispheric white matter; with time, part or all of the white matter has a signal intensity close to or the same as CSF on proton-density, T2-weighted, T1-weighted, and fluid attenuation inversion recovery (FLAIR) images. The U fibers, the corpus callosum, and the internal capsule tend to be spared (611,612). Cerebellar atrophy varies from mild to severe and primarily involves the vermis. On MRS there is a reduction of all metabolites and a relative increase of lactate and glucose in white matter (612).

The clinical severity of the condition is related to age of onset but not to the genotype. It can range from a rapidly fatal infantile to an asymptomatic adult form (613). Cree leukoencephalopathy also has a homozygous mutation in the ε subunit of eIF2B (613).

Other Diseases of Cerebral White Matter

The widespread use of MRI in the evaluation of children with neurologic disorders, particularly those with intellectual deterioration, has resulted in the description of several other groups of patients who demonstrate white matter changes compatible with a leukodystrophy but whose clinical picture does not fall into any of the previously described categories (Table 3.12). These conditions are not rare. In the series of Kristjánsdóttir and colleagues reported in 1996, of 78 patients with MRI abnormalities that primarily involved white matter, only 32 could be given a specific diagnosis. In the remaining 46 children, the cause of the white matter abnormalities could not be ascertained. Of these children, 17 (37%) had a clearly progressive course and 13 (28%) were stationary over the course of at least 3 years (614).

Neuroaxonal Dystrophies (Seitelberger Disease)

Neuroaxonal dystrophies (Seitelberger disease) are rare degenerative disorders of the nervous system that share a pathologic picture of focal axonal swelling in myelinated and nonmyelinated central and peripheral nervous system axons. Several entities have been described; the most likely of which to be encountered is the late infantile form. As first documented by Seitelberger (625), it has its onset between 1 and 2 years of age. The clinical picture is marked by mixed upper and lower motor neuron signs; the pathologic picture is one of focal axonal swelling throughout the neuraxis (626). Loss of microtubules and abnormalities of neurofilaments with resulting failure of axonal transport may result in focal axonal swelling and could represent the fundamental disorder in this condition (626a).

Affected individuals develop neurologic abnormalities within the first 2 years of life. These include progressive weakness, hypotonia, and muscular atrophy accompanied by evidence of corticospinal tract involvement and anterior horn cell disease. Tendon reflexes are usually hyperactive and urinary retention is common, as are disturbances of ocular mobility and optic atrophy (626). Convulsions are rare. The most characteristic finding on neuroimaging is a diffuse and prominent hyperintensity of the cerebellar cortex, the dentate nucleus, and the pyramidal tracts seen on T2-weighted MRI (627,628). This is accompanied by diffuse cerebellar atrophy. The diagnosis can best be made by biopsy of the peripheral nerves, which demonstrates globular swellings (neuroaxonal spheroids) along the course of the axons, particularly at the neuromuscular junction. Similar changes are seen in the peripheral nerve endings

TABLE 3.12 Newly Recognized Forms of Leukodystrophy

Name	Clinical Picture	Magnetic Resonance Imaging Result	Reference
Megalencephalic leukodystrophy	High incidence in Asian Indians, megalencaphaly, slowly progressive spasticity, MLC1 gene mutation, chromosome 22qter	Extensive white matter changes out of proportion to clinical picture, subcortical cystlike spaces in frontoparietal anterior temporal areas	615,616,616a
Hypomyelination and increased *N*-acetylaspartyl glutamate	Early-onset nystagmus, seizures, resembling connatal form of PMD	Almost complete absence of myelin	617
Hypomyelination with atrophy of basal ganglia and cerebellum (HABC)	Onset 2 mo to 3 yr; delayed motor development followed by deterioration; spasticity, rigidity, ataxia, choreoathetosis, dystonia	Diffuse myelin deficiency increased signal on T2, progressive atrophy putamen, head of caudate, cerebellum	618,619
Leukoencephalopathy with brainstem and spinal cord involvement	Onset in childhood, slowly progressive, variable mental deficits, pyramidal, cerebellar dysfunction	Extensive diffuse or spotty WM abnormalities, selective involvement pyramidal tract, sensory tracts, cerebellar peduncles, MRS shows increased lactate	619,620
	Autosomal dominant, macrocephaly, nystagmus, spasticity, nonprogressive	Obstructive hydrocphalus caused by cerebellar enlargement, abnormal cerebellar WM, progresses to atrophy	621
Leukoencephalopathy with bilateral anterior temporalobe cysts	Delayed initial development, spasticity, normal HC, or microcephaly, no obvious progression	Cystic lesions in anterior temporal lobes, periventricular demyelination	622,623
LCC syndrome (leukoencephalopathy, brain calcifications, cysts)	Onset early childhood, progressive dystonia, spasticity, ataxia	Diffuse leukodystrophy, sparing U fibers, CC; calcifications in basal ganglia, thalamus, subcortical WM, interhemispheric cyst	624

CC, corpus callosum; HC, head circumference; MLC1, megalencephalic leukoencephalopathy with subcortical cysts; MRS, magnetic resonance spectroscopy; PMD, Pelizaeus-Merzbacher disease; WM, white matter.

of conjunctivae and on skin biopsy (629). These are best seen by electron microscopy. In some cases, biopsy results of peripheral tissue were negative and the diagnosis rested on brain biopsy (630).

The presence of neuroaxonal spheroids is, however, nonspecific. They also are seen in a juvenile form of neuroaxonal dystrophy that becomes symptomatic between 9 and 17 years of age (631).

Axonal swelling also is encountered in numerous other conditions. These include vitamin E deficiency, the olivopontocerebellar atrophies, FRDA, human T-cell lymphotropic virus 1 tropic myeloneuropathy, GM_1 and GM_2 gangliosidoses, α-*N*-acetylgalactosaminidase deficiency (Schindler disease), and the amyotrophic lateral sclerosis-Parkinson's-dementia complex seen on Guam. Hallervorden-Spatz disease (PKAN) and infantile neuroaxonal dystrophy share several pathologic features, but haplotype analysis in several families affected with neuroaxonal dystrophy has not revealed any mutations in *PANK2* or in other genes of coenzyme A biogenesis (631a).

Rett Syndrome

Rett syndrome is a unique and relatively common condition, with an incidence of 1 in 10,000 to 1 in 15,000 girls, which places it second as a cause for mental retardation in female patients. Inasmuch as progressive dementia is one of its main features, it is considered in this chapter.

A syndrome of cerebral atrophy and hyperammonemia occurring exclusively in girls was first described by Rett in 1966 (632). Since then, it has become evident that hyperammonemia is present only rarely in these children, and that in fact characteristic laboratory abnormalities are absent.

Molecular Genetics and Pathogenesis

The gene for Rett syndrome has been mapped to Xq28 (633). The gene, *MeCP2*, encodes methylated CpG-binding protein 2 (634). This protein is one of four known proteins that selectively bind methylated DNA and mediate transcriptional repression (635,636). It interacts with the Sin3A/histone co-repressor complex and histone deacetylases. Deacetylation of histones converts chromatin structure from an active into an inactive state. *MeCP2* is widely expressed and is abundant in brain. Amir and coworkers showed that mutations in *MeCP2* account for about 70% to 80% of Rett patients (634). More than 200 such mutations have been recorded; they are distributed along the whole gene and include all types of mutations. The majority of these mutations are *de novo* on the paternal chromosome (637). The condition is almost exclusively seen in girls because of the predominance of the mutation on the paternal X chromosome and also because of the early postnatal lethal effects of the disease-causing mutations in hemizygous boys (638). Approximately 99.5% of cases of Rett syndrome are sporadic (639). However, the incidence of familial cases is higher than is expected by chance. Villard proposed that in these familial cases the unaffected carrier mothers have a completely biased X-chromosome inactivation favoring expression of the normal allele (640).

The manner in which the abnormality of the *MeCP2* protein and the consequent overexpression of genes result in neurologic deficits is not understood. One likely hypothesis is that loss of function of *MeCP2* protein leads to overexpression of genes that could interfere with the later stages of cerebral maturation and result in disruption of genetic programs that establish and refine synaptic connections (634). Because olfactory receptor neurons are replaced throughout life by ongoing postnatal neurogenesis, Ronnett and coworkers biopsied nasal epithelium from patients with Rett syndrome (641). They found an increased ratio of immature to mature neurons and dysmorphic and shrunken cell bodies and processes of the olfactory receptor neurons.

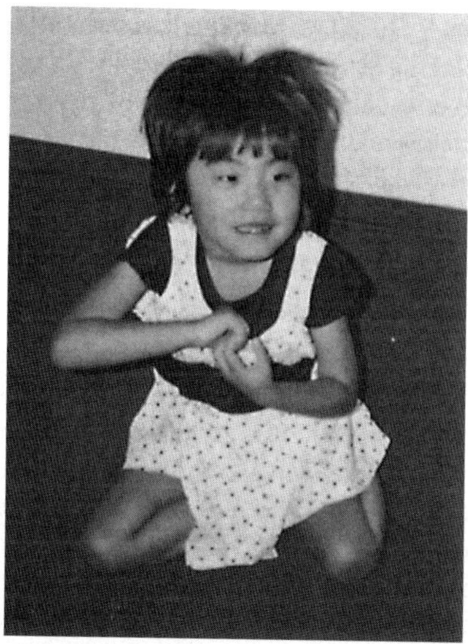

FIGURE 3.16. Rett syndrome. The girl demonstrates the typical hand-washing posture of the upper extremities.

Pathology

Pathologic examination of the brain obtained from Rett patients discloses diffuse cerebral atrophy with increased amounts of neuronal lipofuscin and an underpigmentation of the substantia nigra. Neuronal size is reduced and cell-packing density is increased throughout the brain. These changes are most evident in the medial temporal lobe (642). Decreased length and complexity of dendritic branching in premotor, frontal, motor, and limbic cortex is seen (643). Abnormalities also are seen in the cerebellum with reduced numbers of Purkinje cells (642). These pathologic changes are most consistent with a curtailment of brain maturation early in development (642). Immunochemical studies of microtubule-associated proteins, which are expressed during dendritic formation in embryonic mammalian brain, also suggest a disturbance in the early stages of neocortical maturation (639). Neurochemical studies and evaluation of patients with PET point to abnormalities in the cholinergic and the dopaminergic pathways (639). It is not known whether these changes are primary or secondary to abnormalities in neurotrophins.

Clinical Manifestations

There is a wide range of phenotypic expression. At this point it would appear that patients with missense mutations present with milder phenotypes than those with nonsense mutations (644). In typical cases the clinical picture is fairly characteristic and suggests the diagnosis (639,645). Although hypotonia is often noted, girls develop normally until 6 to 12 months of age. Thereafter, a deceleration in head growth and a clear developmental regression occur. Microcephaly develops, as do pyramidal tract signs and an autistic-like behavior. One-third of children experience seizures and almost all have abnormal EEG results. Purposive hand use is lost between 6 and 30 months; it is replaced by hand wringing or hand-to-mouth (hand-washing) movements (Fig. 3.16) (646). Gait apraxia and truncal ataxia develop subsequently. Intermittent hyperventilation with a disorganized breathing pattern during the waking state is characteristic and is seen as early as 2 years of age (647). Neuroimaging shows little more than progressive cortical atrophy and hypoplasia of the corpus callosum, the latter probably secondary to neuronal reduction (648).

In some 25% of patients who have a typical clinical picture of Rett syndrome there have been no obvious mutations of the *MeCP2* gene. Conversely, *MeCP2* mutations have been found in children without the classical Rett phenotype (649). Although most *MeCP2* mutations are lethal for boys, Dotti and coworkers found six men with mental retardation and spastic paraparesis who had a point mutation in the *MeCP2* gene. Other male patients have a clinical picture of autism, mental retardation, and an Angelman syndrome–like presentation (650). Most of these cases are probably due to mosaicism.

Rett syndrome allows prolonged survival. By the second decade of life, patients become stable. Seizures may subside, children may regain their ability to walk, their hand use improves, and they often have improved social interaction (639). Supportive care and active physical therapy have been fairly effective in preventing contractures. In our experience, treatment with carbamazepine, even in the absence of overt seizures, appears to improve alertness.

In the differential diagnosis of Rett syndrome, other conditions that induce a developmental regression coupled with seizures, cerebellar signs, or autistic behavior have to be considered. These include some of the lipofuscinoses, Angelman syndrome, and the spinocerebellar degenerations. The characteristic loss of hand use and the negative imaging studies assist in arriving at the diagnosis. This can be confirmed by genetic testing. A commercial testing service is available that detects mutations in exons 1 to 4 of the *MeCP2* gene.

Diseases with Degeneration Primarily Affecting Gray Matter

Degenerative conditions that primarily affect cerebral gray matter are less common than those affecting white matter. Although clearly these entities do not represent a single genetic condition, they have in the past been referred to as *Alpers syndrome* (651). The nature of the entities such as those described by Alpers in 1931 and Ford and coworkers in 1951 (652) cannot now be determined, but in retrospect one suspects that many were instances of metabolic defects, such as the mitochondrial encephalopathies.

In several forms of gray matter degeneration, the pathologic picture is unique. One of these conditions, which has aroused some interest, is intranuclear hyaline inclusion disease. This disorder is marked by slowly progressive pyramidal or extrapyramidal signs and mental deterioration. First symptoms appear between the ages of 3 and 12 years. Brainstem signs such as blepharospasm or cranial nerve palsies are common, as are oculogyric crises. Eosinophilic neuronal intranuclear inclusions are seen in neurons of the central and autonomic nervous system (185,653). The similarity in this pathologic picture between this condition and the polyglutamine diseases suggest that the inclusions are formed during a proteolysis-related process and that the condition is due to accumulation of an as-yet-unidentified abnormal protein or dysfunction of the intranuclear ubiquitin-proteosome pathway (654). Several centers have suggested a rectal biopsy as a means of making a diagnosis during the patient's lifetime (655,656).

An autosomal recessive progressive neuronal degeneration with liver disease presents during the first year of life with developmental delay and failure to thrive. Seizures are prominent, and clinical and pathologic evidence of liver failure occurs (657,658). The condition goes under the name of Alpers-Huttenlocher disease. One such patient had a marked depletion of mitochondria in skeletal muscle and no detectable activity of liver and muscle mitochondrial DNA polymerase γ (659). Because many children suffering from this condition have been placed on valproate for control of their seizures, this degenerative disease can mimic valproate-induced hepatic encephalopathy.

REFERENCES

1. Strachan T, Read AP. *Human molecular genetics*, 3rd ed. London: Garland Science, 2004:416–433, 462–485.
2. Pulst SM. Introduction to medical genetics and methods of DNA testing. In: Pulst SM, ed. *Genetics of movement disorders*. Amsterdam: Academic Press, 2003:1–18.
3. Bruyn GW. Huntington's chorea—historical, clinical and laboratory synopsis. In: Vinken PJ, Bruyn GW, eds. *Handbook of neurology: diseases of the basal ganglia*. Amsterdam: North-Holland, 1968;298–378.
4. Huntington G. On chorea. *Med Surg Rep* 1872;26:317–321.
5. Conneally PM. Huntington's disease: genetics and epidemiology. *Am J Hum Genet* 1984;36:506–526.
6. Tellez-Nagel I, Johnson AB, Terry RB. Studies on brain biopsies of patients with Huntington's chorea. *J Neuropathol Exp Neurol* 1974;33:308–332.
7. Vonsattel JP, DiFiglia. Huntington's disease. *J Neuropath Exp Neurol* 1998;57:369–384.
8. Jervis GA. Huntington's chorea in childhood. *Arch Neurol* 1963; 9:244–257.
9. Markham CH, Knox JW. Observations in Huntington's chorea. *J Pediatr* 1965;67:46–57.
10. Carlier G, Reznik M, Franck G, et al. Etude anatomo-clinique d'une forme infantile de la maladie de Huntington. *Acta Neurol Belg* 1974;74:36–63.
11. Richfield EK, Maguire-Zeiss KA, Voukeman HE, et al. Preferential loss of preproenkephalin versus preprotachykinin neurons from the striatum of Huntington's disease patients. *Ann Neurol* 1995;38:852–861.
12. Storey E, Kowall NW, Finn SF, et al. The cortical lesion of Huntington's disease: further neurochemical characterization and reproduction of some of the histological and neurochemical features by *N*-methyl-D-aspartate lesions of rat cortex. *Ann Neurol* 1992;32:526–534.
13. Sotrel A, Williams RS, Kaufmann WE, et al. Evidence for neuronal degeneration and dendritic plasticity in cortical pyramidal neurons of Huntington's disease: a quantitative Golgi study. *Neurology* 1993;43:2088–2096.
14. Gusella JF, Wexler NS, Connealy PM, et al. A polymorphic DNA marker genetically linked to Huntington's disease. *Nature* 1983;306:234–238.
15. Sapp E, Schwartz C, Chase K, et al. Huntington localization in brains of normal and Huntington's disease patients. *Ann Neurol* 1997;42:604–612.
16. Reiner A, Dragatsis I, Zeitlin S, et al. Wild-type huntingtin plays a role in brain development and neuronal survival. *Mol Neurobiol* 2003;28:259–276.
17. The Huntington's Disease Collaborative Research Group. A novel gene containing a trinucleotide repeat that is expanded and unstable on Huntington's disease chromosomes. *Cell* 1993;72:971–983.
18. Duyao MP, Ambrose C, Myers R, et al. Trinucleotide repeat length instability and age of onset in Huntington's disease. *Nat Genet* 1993;4:387–392.
19. Myers RH, MacDonald ME, Koroshetz WJ, et al. *De novo* expansion of a $(CAG)_n$ repeat in sporadic Huntington's disease. *Nat Genet* 1993;5:168–173.
20. Sinden RR, Potaman VN, Oussatcheva E, et al. Triplet DNA structures and human genetic disease: dynamic mutations from dynamic DNA. *J Biosci* 2002;27:53–65.
21. La Spada AR, Paulson HL, Fischbeck KH. Trinucleotide repeat expansion in neurological disease. *Ann Neurol* 1994;36:814–822.
22. Fraser FC. Trinucleotide repeats not the only cause of anticipation. *Lancet* 1997;350:459–460.
23. Gourfinkel-An I, Cancel G, Trottier Y, et al. Differential distribution of the normal and mutated forms of Huntington in the human brain. *Ann Neurol* 1997;42:712–719.
24. Gomez-Tortosa E, MacDonald ME, Friend JC, et al. Quantitative neuropathological changes in presymptomatic Huntington's disease. *Ann Neurol* 2001;49:29–34.

24a. Cornett J, Cao F, Wang CE, et al. Polyglutamine expansion of huntingtin impairs its nuclear export. *Nat Genet* 2005;37:198–204.

25. Alves-Rodrigues A, Gregori L, Figueiredo-Pereira ME. Ubiquitin, cellular inclusions and their role in neurodegeneration. *Trends Neurosci* 1998;21:516–520.
26. Faber PW, Barnes GT, Srinidhi J, et al. Huntington interacts with a family of WW domain proteins. *Hum Mol Genet* 1998;7:1463–1474.
27. Sieradran KA, Mann DM. The selective vulnerability of nerve cells in Huntington's disease. *Neuropathol Appl Neurobiol* 2001;27: 1–21.

28. Lin YF. Expression of polyglutamine-expanded Huntington activates the SEK1-JNK pathway and induces apoptosis in a hippocampal neuronal line. *J Biol Chem* 1998;273:28873–28877.
29. Saudou F, Finkbeiner S, Devys D, et al. Huntingtin acts in the nucleus to induce apoptosis but death does not correlate with the formation of intranuclear inclusions. *Cell* 1998;95:55–66.
30. Li L, Murphy TH, Hayden MR, et al. Enhanced striatal NR2B-containing *N*-methyl-D-aspartate receptor mediated synaptic currents in a mouse model of Huntington disease. *J Neurophysiol* 2004;92:2738–2746.
31. Young AB, Greenamyre JT, Hollingsworth Z, et al. NMDA receptor losses in putamen from patients with Huntington's disease. *Science* 1988;241:981–983.
32. Guidetti P, Charles V, Chen EY, et al. Early degenerative changes in transgenic mice expressing mutant huntingtin involve dendritic abnormalities but no impairment of mitochondrial energy production. *Exp Neurol* 2001;169:340–350.
33. Tabrizi SJ, Cleeter MW, Xuereb J, et al. Biochemical abnormalities and excitotoxicity in Huntington's disease brain. *Ann Neurol* 1999;45:25–32.
34. Myers RH, Cupples LA, Schoenfeld M, et al. Maternal factors in onset of Huntington's disease. *Am J Hum Genet* 1985;37:511–523.
35. Rubinstein DC. Molecular biology of Huntington's disease (HD) and HD-like disorders. In: Pulst SM, ed. *Genetics of movement disorders*. Amsterdam: Academic Press, 2003:365–383.
36. Wexler NS, Lorimer J, Porter J, et al. Venezuelan kindreds reveal that genetic and environmental factors modulate Huntington's disease age of onset. *Proc Natl Acad Sci USA* 2004;101:3498–3503.
37. Hayden MR, Soles JA, Ward RH. Age of onset in siblings of persons with juvenile Huntington's disease. *Clin Genet* 1985;28:100–105.
38. Cotton JB, Grenier JL, Ladreyt JP, et al. La maladie de Huntington chez l'enfant: a propos d'une observation anatomo-clinique. *Pediatrie* 1975;30:609–619.
39. Siesling S, Vegter-van der Vlis M, Roos RA. Juvenile Huntington's disease in the Netherlands. *Pediatr Neurol* 1997;17:37–43.
40. Haslam RHA, Curry B, Johns R. Infantile Huntington's disease. *Can J Neurol Sci* 1983;10:200–203.
41. van Dijk JG, van der Velde EA, Roos RA, et al. Juvenile Huntington's disease. *Hum Genet* 1986;73:235–239.
42. Katafuchi Y, Fujimoto T, Ono E, et al. A childhood form of Huntington's disease associated with marked pyramidal signs. *Eur Neurol* 1984;23:296–299.
43. Myers RH, Vonsattel JP, Stevens TJ, et al. Clinical and neuropathologic assessment of severity in Huntington's disease. *Neurology* 1988;38:341–347.
44. Young AB, Shoulson I, Penney JB, et al. Huntington's disease in Venezuela: neurologic features and functional decline. *Neurology* 1986;36:244–249.
45. Schapiro M, Cecil KM, Doescher J, et al. MR imaging and spectroscopy in juvenile Huntington disease. *Pediatr Radiol* 2004;34:640–643.
46. Mazziotta JC, Phelps ME, Pahl JJ, et al. Reduced cerebral glucose metabolism in asymptomatic subjects at risk for Huntington's disease. *N Engl J Med* 1987;316:357–362.
47. Laurence AD, Weeks RA, Brooks DJ, et al. The relationship between striatal dopamine receptor binding and cognitive performance in Huntington's disease. *Brain* 1998;121:1343–1355.
48. ACMG/ASHG Statement. Laboratory guidelines for Huntington disease genetic testing. The American College of Medical Genetics/American Society of Human Genetics Huntington Disease Genetic Testing Working Group. *Am J Hum Genet* 1998;62:1243–1247.
49. Kremer B, Goldberg P, Andrew SE, et al. A worldwide study of the Huntington's disease mutation. The sensitivity and specificity of measuring CAG repeats. *N Engl J Med* 1994;330:1401–1406.
50. World Federation of Neurology—Committee of the International Huntington's Association and the World Federation of Neurology. Ethical issues policy statement on Huntington's disease molecular genetics predictive test. *J Med Genet* 1990;27:34–38.
51. Stevanin G, Camuzat A, Holmes SE, et al. CAG/CTG expansion at the Huntington's disease-like 2 locus are rare in Huntington's disease patients. *Neurology* 2002;58:965–967.
52. Kambouris M, Bohlega S, Al-Tahan A, et al. Localization of the gene for a novel autosomal recesssive neurodegenerative Huntington-like disorder to 4p15.3. *Am J Hum Genet* 2000;67:262–263.
53. Moore RC, Xiang F, Monaghan J, et al. Huntington disease phenocopy is a familial prion disease. *Am J Hum Genet* 2001;69:1385–1388.
54. Pincus JH, Chutorian A. Familial benign chorea with intention tremor: a clinical entity. *J Pediatr* 1967;70:724–729.
55. Kleiner-Fisman G, Rogaeva E, Halliday W, et al. Benign hereditary chorea: clinical, genetic and pathological findings. *Ann Neurol* 2003;54:244–247.
56. Stapert JLRH, Busard BL, Gabreels FJ, et al. Benign (nonparoxysmal) familial chorea of early onset: an electroneurophysiological examination of two families. *Brain Dev* 1985;7:38–42.
57. Breedveld GJ, Percy AK, MacDonald ME, et al. Clinical and genetic heterogeneity in benign hereditary chorea. *Neurology* 2002;59:579–584.
58. Breedveld GJ, van Dongen JW, Danesino C, et al. Mutations in TITF-1 are associated with benign hereditary chorea. *Hum Mol Genet* 2002;11:971–979.
59. Feinberg TE, Cianci CD, Morrow JS, et al. Diagnostic tests for choreoacanthocytosis. *Neurology* 1991;41:100–106.
60. Orrell RW, Amrolia PJ, Heald A, et al. Acanthocytosis, retinitis pigmentosa, and pallidal degeneration: a report of three patients, including the second reported case with hypoprebetalipoproteinemia (HARP syndrome). *Neurology* 1995;45:487–492.
61. Hardie RJ, Pullon HW, Harding AE, et al. Neuroacanthocytosis: a clinical, haematological and pathological study of 19 cases. *Brain* 1991;114:13–49.
62. Shibasaki H, Sakai T, Nishimura H, et al. Involuntary movements in chorea-acanthocytosis: a comparison with Huntington's chorea. *Ann Neurol* 1982;12:311–314.
63. Brooks DJ, Ibanez V, Playford ED, et al. Presynaptic and postsynaptic striatal dopaminergic function in neuroacanthocytosis: a positron emission tomographic study. *Ann Neurol* 1991;30:166–171.
64. Schwalbe MW. *Eine eigentuehmliche, tonische Krampfform mit hysterischen Symptomen*. Berlin: G. Schade, 1908.
65. Oppenheim H. Ueber eine eigenartige Krampfkrankheit des kindlichen und jugentlichen Alters (dysbasia lordotica progressiva, dystonia musculorum deformans). *Neurol Centralbl* 1911;30:1090–1107.
66. Ozelius LJ, Hewett JW, Page CE, et al. The early-onset torsion dystonia gene (*DYT1*) encodes an ATP-binding protein. *Nat Genet* 1997;17:40–48.
67. Gimenez-Roldan S, Delgado G, Marin M, et al. Hereditary torsion dystonia in gypsies. *Adv Neurol* 1988;50:73–91.
68. Khan NL, Wood NW, Bhatia KP. Autosomal recessive, DYT2-like primary torsion dystonia: a new family. *Neurology* 2003;61:1801–1803.
69. Lee LV, Kupke KG, Caballar-Gonzaga F, et al. The phenotype of the X-linked dystonia-parkinsonism syndrome: an assessment of 42 cases in the Philippines. *Medicine* 1991;70:179–187.
70. Ahmad F, Davis MB, Waddy HM, et al. Evidence for locus heterogeneity in autosomal dominant torsion dystonia. *Genomics* 1993;15:9–12.
71. Nygaard TG, Marsden CD, Fahn S. Dopa-responsive dystonia: long-term treatment response and prognosis. *Neurology* 1991;41:174–181.
72. Hoffman GF, Assmann B, Bräutigam C, et al. Tyrosine hyroxylase deficiency causes progressive encephalopathy and Dopa-responsive dystonia. *Ann Neurol* 2003;54(Suppl 6):S56–S65.
73. Almasy L, Bressman SB, Raymond D, et al. Idiopathic torsion dystonia linked to chromosome 8 in two Mennonite families. *Ann Neurol* 1997;42:670–673.
74. Leube B, Rudnicki D, Ratzlaff T, et al. Idiopathic torsion dystonia: assignment of a gene to chromosome 18p in a German family with adult onset, autosomal dominant inheritance and purely focal distribution. *Hum Mol Genet* 1996;5:1673–1677.
75. Mount LA, Reback S. Familial paroxysmal choreo-athetosis. *Arch Neurol Psychiatr* 1940;44:841–847.
76. Muller U, Steinberger D, Nemeth AH. Clinical and molecular genetics of primary dystonia. *Neurogenetics* 1998;1:165–177.
77. Demirkiran M, Jankovic J. Paroxysmal dyskinesias: clinical features and classification. *Ann Neurol* 1995;38:571–579.

78. Hjermind LE, Werdelin LM, Eiberg H, et al. A novel mutation in the ε-sarcoglycan gene causing myoclonus-dystonia syndrome. *Neurology* 2003;60:1536–1539.
79. Doheny DO, Brin MF, Morrison CE, et al. Phenotypic features of myoclonus-dystonia in three kindreds. *Neurology* 2002;59:1187–1196.
80. Pittock SJ, Joyce C, O'Keane V, et al. Rapid-onset dystonia-parkinsonism: a clinical and genetic analysis of a new kindred. *Neurology* 2000;55:991–995.
81. Bentivoglio AR, Ialongo T, Contarino MF, et al. Phenotypic characterization of DYT13 primary torsion dystonia. *Mov Disord* 2004:19:200–206.
82. Grötzsch H, Pizzolato GP, Ghika J, et al. Neuropathology of a case of dopa-responsive dystonia associated with a new genetic locus, *DYT14*. *Neurology* 2002;58:1839–1843.
82a. Grimes DA, Han F, Lang AE, et al. A novel locus for inherited myoclonus-dystonia on 18p11. *Neurology* 2002;59:1183–1186.
83. Tranebjaerg L, Schwartz C, Eriksen H, et al. A new X linked recessive deafness syndrome with blindness, dystonia, fractures, and mental deficeincy is linked to Xq22. *J Med Genet* 1995;32:257–263.
84. Roesch K, Hynds PJ, Varge R, et al. The calcium-binding aspartate/glutamate carriers, citrin and aralar1, are new substrates for the DDP1/TIMM8a-TIMM13 complex. *Hum Mol Genet* 2004;13:2101–2111.
85. Klein C, Brin MF, de Leon D, et al. *De novo* mutations (GAG deletion) in the *DYT1* gene in two non-Jewish patients with early-onset dystonia. *Hum Mol Genet* 1998;7:1133–1136.
86. Lebre AS, Durr A, Jedynak P, et al. *DYT1* mutation in French families with idiopathic torsion dystonia. *Brain* 1999;122:41–45.
87. Goodchild RE, Dauer WT. Mislocalization to the nuclear envelope: an effect of the dystonia causing torsinA mutation. *Proc Natl Acad Sci USA* 2004;101:847–852.
88. Kamm C, Boston H, Hewett J, et al. The early onset dystonia protein torsinA interacts with kinesin light chain 1. *J Biol Chem* 2004;279:19882–19992.
89. Gonzalez-Alegre P, Paulson HL. Aberrant cellular behavior of mutant torsinA implicates nuclear envelope dysfunction in DYT1 dystonia. *J Neurosci* 2004;24:2593–2601.
89a. Goodchild RE, Dauer WT. The AAA+ protein torsin A interacts with a conserved domain present in LAP1 and a novel ER protein. *J Cell Biol* 2005;168:855–862.
90. Vitek JL, Chockkan V, Zhang JY, et al. Neuronal activity in the basal ganglia in patients with generalized dystonia and hemiballismus. *Ann Neurol* 1999;46:22–35.
91. Berardelli A, Rothwell JC, Hallett M, et al. The pathophysiology of primary dystonia. *Brain* 1998;121:1195–1212.
92. Eidelberg D, Moeller JR, Antonini A, et al. Functional brain networks in DYT1 dystonia. *Ann Neurol* 1998;44:303–312.
93. Marsden CD, Obeso JA, Zarranz JJ, et al. The anatomical basis of symptomatic hemidystonia. *Brain* 1985;108:463–483.
94. Zeman W. Dystonia: an overview. *Adv Neurol* 1976;14:91–103.
94a. McNaught KSP, Kapustin A, Jackson T, et al. Brainstem pathology in DYT1 primary torsion dystonia. *Ann Neurol* 2004;56:540–547.
95. Furukawa H, Hornykiewicz O, Fahn S, et al. Striatal dopamine in early-onset primary torsion dystonia with the *DYT1* mutation. *Neurology* 2000;54:193–1195.
96. Ozelius LJ, Bressman SB. DYT1 dystonia. In: Pulst SM, ed. *Genetics of movement disorders*. Amsterdam: Academic Press, 2003:407–418.
97. Gasser T, Fahn S, Breakefield XO. The autosomal dominant dystonias. *Brain Pathol* 1992;2:297–308.
98. Bird TD. Penetrating observations of dystonia. *Ann Neurol* 1998;44:299–300.
99. Marsden CD, Harrison MJG, Bundey S. Natural history of idiopathic torsion dystonia. *Adv Neurol* 1976;14:177–187.
100. Marsden CD, Harrison MJG. Idiopathic torsion dystonia: a review of 42 patients. *Brain* 1974;97:93–810.
101. Bressman SB, de Leon D, Raymond D, et al. Clinical-genetic spectrum of primary dystonia. *Adv Neurol* 1998;78:79–91.
102. Karbe H, Holthoff VA, Rudolf J, et al. Positron emission tomography demonstrates frontal cortex and basal ganglia hypometabolism in dystonia. *Neurology* 1992;42:1540–1544.
103. Carbon M, Su S, Dhawan V, et al. Regional metabolism in primary torsion dystonia: effects of penetrances and genotype. *Neurology* 2004;62:1384–1390.
104. Sheehy MP, Marsden CD. Writer's cramp—a focal dystonia. *Brain* 1982;105:461–480.
105. Segawa M, Nomura Y, Nishiyama N. Autosomal dominant guanosine triphosphate cyclohydrolase I deficiency (Segawa disease). *Ann Neurol* 2003;54(Suppl 6):S32–S45.
106. Furukawa Y, Kish SJ, Bebin EM, et al. Dystonia with motor delay in compound heterozygotes for GTP-cyclohydrolase I gene mutations. *Ann Neurol* 1998;44:10–16.
107. Assmann B, Surtees R, Hoffmann GF. Approach to the diagnosis of neurotransmitter diseases exemplified by the differential diagnosis of childhood-onset dystonia. *Ann Neurol* 2003;54(Suppl 6):S18–S24.
108. Assman BE, Robinson RO, Surtees RA, et al. Infantile parkinsonism-dystonia and elevated dopamine metabolites in CSF. *Neurology* 2004;62:1872–1874.
109. Pueschel SM, Friedman JH, Shetty T. Myoclonic dystonia. *Childs Nerv Syst* 1992;8:61–66.
110. Hansen RA, Berenberg W, Byers RK. Changing motor patterns in cerebral palsy. *Dev Med Child Neurol* 1970;12:309–314.
111. Burke RE, Fahn S, Gold AP. Delayed onset dystonia in patients with "static" encephalopathy. *J Neurol Neurosurg Psychiatry* 1980;43:789–797.
112. Goetting MG. Acute lithium poisoning in a child with dystonia. *Pediatrics* 1985;76:978–980.
113. Schott GD. Induction of involuntary movements by peripheral trauma: an analogy with causalgia. *Lancet* 1986;2:712–716.
114. Trauma and dystonia [Editorial]. *Lancet* 1989;1:759–760.
115. Burke RE, Fahn S, Marsden CD. Torsion dystonia: a double-blind, prospective trial of high-dosage trihexyphenidyl. *Neurology* 1986;36:160–164.
116. Jankovic J, Beach J. Long-term effects of tetrabenazine in hyperkinetic movement disorders. *Neurology* 1997;48:358–362.
117. Marsden CD, Marion MH, Quinn N. The treatment of severe dystonia in children and adults. *J Neurol Neurosurg Psychiatry* 1984;47:1166–1173.
118. Greene PE, Fahn S. Baclofen in the treatment of idiopathic dystonia in children. *Mov Disord* 1992;7:48–752.
118a. Vidailhet M, Vercueil L, Houeto JL, et al. Bilateral deep-brain stimulation of the globus pallidus in primary generalized dystonia. *N Engl J Med* 2005;352:459–467.
119. Coubes P, Roubertie A, Vayssiere N, et al. Treatment of DYT1-generalised dystonia by stimulation of the internal globus pallidus. *Lancet* 2000;355:2220–2221.
120. Eltahaway HA, Saint-Cyr J, Giladi N, et al. Primary dystonia is more responsive than secondary dystonia to pallidal interventions: outcome after pallidotomy or pallidal deep brain stimulation. *Neurosurgery* 2004;54:613–619.
121. Gonzalez-Alegre P, Miller VM, Davidson BL, et al. Toward therapy for DYT1 dystonia: allele-specific silencing of mutant torsinA. *Ann Neurol* 2003;53:781–787.
122. Singer HS. Tardive dyskinesia: a concern for the pediatrician. *Pediatrics* 1986;77:553–556.
123. Kumra S, Jacobsen LK, Lenane M, et al. Case series: spectrum of neuroleptic-induced movement disorders and extrapyramidal side effects in childhood-onset schizophrenia. *J Am Acad Child Adolesc Psychiatry* 1998;37:221–227.
124. Campbell M, Armenteros JL, Malone RP, et al. Neuroleptic-related dyskinesias in autistic children: a prospective, longitudinal study. *J Am Acad Child Adolesc Psychiatry* 1997;36:835–843.
125. Richardson MA, Small AM, Read LL, et al. Branched chain amino acid treatment of tardive dyskinesia in children and adolescents. *J Clin Psychiatry* 2004;65:92–96.
126. Joshi PT, Capozzoli JA, Coyle JT. Neuroleptic malignant syndrome: life-threatening complication of neuroleptic treatment in adolescents with affective disorders. *Pediatrics* 1991;87:235–239.
127. Rodnitzky RL. Drug-induced movement disorders in children. *Semin Pediatr Neurol* 2003;10:80–87.
128. Goulon M, de Rohan-Chabot P, Elkharrat D, et al. Beneficial effects of dantrolene in the treatment of neuroleptic malignant syndrome. *Neurology* 1988;33:516–518.

129. Silva RR, Munoz DM, Alpert M, et al. Neuroleptic malignant syndrome in children and adolescents. *J Am Acad Child Adolesc Psychiatry* 1999;38:187–194.
130. Hallervorden J, Spatz H. Erkrankung im System mit besonderer Beteilung des Globus Pallidus und der Substantia Nigra. *Z Ges Neurol Psychiat* 1922;79:254–302.
131. Zhou B, Westway SK, Levinson B, et al. A novel pantothenate kinase gene (*PANK2*) is defective in Hallervorden-Spatz syndrome. *Nat Genet* 2001;28:345–349.
132. Hortnagel K, Prokisch H, Meitinger T. An isoform of hPANK2 deficient in pantothenate kinase-associated neurodegeneration localizes to mitochondria. *Hum Mol Genet* 2003;12:321–327.
133. Johnson MA, Kao YM, Westaway SK, et al. Mitochondrial localization of human PANK2 and hypotheses of secondary iron accumulation in pantothenate kinase-associated neurodegeneration. *Ann N Y Acad Sci* 2004;1012:282–298.
134. Halliday W. The nosology of Hallervorden-Spatz disease. *J Neurol Sci* 1995;134[Suppl]:84–91.
135. Nakai H, Landing BH, Schubert WK. Seitelberger's spastic amaurotic axonal idiocy: report of a case in a 9 year old boy with comment on visceral manifestations. *Pediatrics* 1960;25: 441–449.
136. Dooling EC, Schoene WC, Richardson EP Jr. Hallervorden-Spatz syndrome. *Arch Neurol* 1974;30:70–83.
137. Hayflick SJ, Westaway SK, Levinson B, et al. Genetic, clinical, and radiographic delineation of Hallervorden-Spatz syndrome. *N Engl J Med* 2003;348:33–40.
138. Swaiman KF. Hallervorden-Spatz syndrome and brain iron metabolism. *Arch Neurol* 1991;48:1285–1293.
139. Savoiardo M, Halliday WC, Nardocci N, et al. Hallervorden-Spatz disease: MR and pathologic findings. *Am J Neuroradiol* 1993;14:155–162.
140. Sehti KD, Adams RJ, Loring DW, et al. Hallervorden-Spatz syndrome: clinical and magnetic resonance imaging correlations. *Ann Neurol* 1988;24:692–694.
140a. Castelnau P, Cif L, Valente EM, et al. Pallidal stimulation improves pantothenate kinase-associated neurodegeneration. *Ann Neurol* 2005;57:738–741.
141. Ching KH, Westaway SK, Glitschier J, et al. HARP syndrome is allelic with pantothenate kinase-associated neurodegeneration. *Neurology* 2002;58:1673–1674.
141a. Houlden H, Lincoln S, Farrer M, et al. Compund heterozygous *PANK2* mutations confirm HARP and Hallervorden-Spatz syndromes are allelic. *Neurology* 2003;61:1423–1426.
142. Bamberger H. Beobachtungen und Bemerkungen über Hirnkrankheiten. *Verh Phys Med Ges* (Würzburg)1855;6:325–328.
143. Fahr T. Idiopatische Verkalkung der Hirngefässe. *Zentralbl Allg Pathol Pathol Anat* 1930;50:129–133.
144. Billard C, Dulac O, Bouloche J, et al. Encephalopathy with calcifications of the basal ganglia in children: a reappraisal of Fahr's syndrome with respect to 14 new cases. *Neuropediatrics* 1989;20:12–19.
145. Melchior JC, Benda CE, Yakovlev PI. Familial idiopathic cerebral calcifications in childhood. *Am J Dis Child* 1960;99:787–803.
146. Aicardi J, Goutières F. A progressive encephalopathy in infancy with calcifications of the basal ganglia and chronic cerebrospinal fluid lymphocytosis. *Ann Neurol* 1984;15:49–54.
147. Goutières F, Aicardi J, Barth PG, et al. Aicardi-Goutières syndrome: an update and results of interferon-α studies. *Ann Neurol* 1998;44:900–907.
148. McEntagart M, Kamel H, Lebon P, et al. Aicardi-Goutières syndrome: an expanding phenotype. *Neuropediatrics* 1998;29:163–167.
149. Blau N, Bonafe L, Krageloh-Mann I, et al. Cerebrospinal fluid pterins and folates in Aicardi-Goutières syndrome: a new phenotype. *Neurology* 2003;61:642–647.
150. Boller F, Boller M, Gilbert J. Familial idiopathic cerebral calcifications. *J Neurol Neurosurg Psychiatry* 1977;40:280–285.
151. Moskowitz MA, Winickoff RN, Heinz ER. Familial calcification of the basal ganglions: a metabolic and genetic study. *N Engl J Med* 1971;285:72–77.
152. Geschwind DH, Loginov M, Stern JM. Identification of a locus on chromosome 14q for idiopathic basal ganglia calcification (Fahr disease). *Am J Hum Genet* 1999;63:764–772.
153. Jervis GA. Microcephaly with extensive calcium deposits and demyelination. *J Neuropathol Exp Neurol* 1954;13:318–329.
154. Marasco JA, Feczko WA. Basal ganglia calcification in Down's syndrome. *Comput Tomogr* 1979;3:111–113.
155. Harrington MG, MacPherson P, McIntosh WB, et al. The significance of the incidental finding of basal ganglia calcification on computed tomography. *J Neurol Neurosurg Psychiatry* 1981;44:1168–1170.
156. Gulcher JR, Jonsson P, Kong A, et al. Mapping of a familial esssential tremor gene, *FET1*, to chromosome 3q13. *Nat Genet* 1997;17:84–87.
157. Higgins JJ, Pho LT, Nee LE. A gene (*ETM*) for essential tremor maps to chromosome 2p22–p25. *Mov Disord* 1997;12:859–864.
157a. Rajput A, Robinson CA, Rajput AH. Essential tremor course and disability: A clinicopathologic study of 20 cases. *Neurology* 2004;62:932–936.
158. Marsden CD, Obeso J, Rothwell JC. Benign essential tremor is not a single entity. In: Yahr MD, ed. *Current concepts in Parkinson's disease*. Amsterdam: Excerpta Medica, 1983:31–46.
159. Pinto AD, Lang AE, Chen R. The cerebellothalamocortical pathway in essential tremor. *Neurology* 2003;60:1985–1987.
160. Deuschl G, Elble RJ. The pathophysiology of essential tremor. *Neurology* 2000;54(Suppl 4):S14–S20.
161. Louis ED, Dure LS, Pullman S. Essential tremor in childhood: a series of nineteen cases. *Mov Disord* 2001;16:921–923.
162. Koller WC, Busenbark K, Miner K. The relationship of essential tremor to other movement disorders: report on 678 patients. *Ann Neurol* 1994;35:717–723.
163. Critchley M. Observation on essential (heredofamilial) tremor. *Brain* 1949;72:113–139.
164. Vanasse M, Bedard P, Andermann F. Shuddering attacks in children: an early clinical manifestation of essential tremor. *Neurology* 1976;26:1027–1030.
165. Barron TF, Younkin DP. Propanolol therapy for shuddering attacks. *Neurology* 1992;42:258–259.
166. Calzetti S, Findley LJ, Perucca E, et al. Controlled study of metopronol and propanolol during prolonged administration in patients with essential tremor. *J Neurol Neurosurg Psychiatry* 1983;45:893–897.
167. Koller WC, Royse VL. Efficacy of primidone in essential tremor. *Neurology* 1986;36:121–124.
168. Gatto EM, Roca MC, Raina G, et al. Low doses of topiramate are effective in essential tremor: a report of three cases. *Clin Neuropharmacol* 2003;26:294–296.
169. Trenkwalder C, Bucher SF, Oertel WH. Electrophysiological pattern of involuntary limb movements in the restless legs syndrome. *Muscle Nerve* 1996;19:155–162.
169a. Allen RP, Mignot E, Ripley B, et al. Increased CSF hypocretin-1 (orexin-A) in restless legs syndrome. *Neurology* 2002;59:639–641.
170. Walters AS, Picchietti DL, Ehrenberg BL, et al. Restless legs syndrome in childhood and adolescence. *Pediatr Neurol* 1994;11:241–245.
171. Picchietti DL, Walters AS. Moderate to severe periodic limb movement disorder in childhood and adolescence. *Sleep* 1999;22:297–300.
172. Early CJ. Restless legs syndrome. *N Engl J Med* 2003;348:2103–2109.
173. Hunt JR. Progressive atrophy of the globus pallidus. (Primary atrophy of the pallidal system.) A system disease of the paralysis agitans type, characterized by atrophy of the motor cells of the corpus striatum: a contribution to the functions of the corpus striatum. *Brain* 1917;40:58–148.
174. Polymeropoulos MH, Higgins JJ, Golbe LI, et al. Mapping of a gene for Parkinson's disease to chromosome 4q21–q23. *Science* 1996;274:1197–1199.
175. Nussbaum RL, Polymeropoulos MH. Genetics of Parkinson's disease. *Hum Mol Genet* 1997;6:1687–1691.
176. Langston JW, Golbe LI, Lee SJ. Park 1 and α-synuclein: A new era in Parkinson's research. In: Pulst SM, ed. *Genetics of movement disorders*. Amsterdam: Academic Press, 2003:287–304.

177. Gasser T, Muller-Myhsok B, Wszolek ZK, et al. A susceptibility locus for Parkinson's disease maps to chromosome 2p13. *Nat Genet* 1998;18:262–265.
177a. Di Fonzo A, Rohé CF, Ferreira J, et al. A frequent LRRK2 gene mutation associated with autosomal dominant Parkinson's disease. *Lancet* 2005;365:412–415.
178. Krüger R, Riess O. Park3, ubiquitin hydrolase-L1 and other PD loci. In: Pulst SM, ed. *Genetics of movement disorders*. Amsterdam: Academic Press, 2003:315–323.
179. Kitada T, Asakawa S, Hattori N, et al. Mutations in the Parkin gene cause autosomal recessive juvenile parkinsonism. *Nature* 1998;392:605–608.
180. Hattori N, Kitada T, Matsumine H, et al. Molecular genetic analysis of a novel Parkin gene in Japanese families with autosomal recessive juvenile parkinsonism: evidence for variable homozygous deletions in the parkin gene in affected individuals. *Ann Neurol* 1998;44:935–941.
181. Abbas N, Lucking CB, Ricard S, et al. A wide variety of mutations in the Parkin gene are responsible for autosomal recessive parkinsonism in Europe. *Hum Mol Genet* 1999;8:567–574.
182. Ishikawa A, Tsuji S. Clinical analysis of 17 patients in 12 Japanese families with autosomal-recessive type juvenile parkinsonism. *Neurology* 1996;47:160–166.
183. Takahashi H, Ohama E, Suzuki S, et al. Familial juvenile parkinsonism: clinical and pathologic study in a family. *Neurology* 1994;44:437–441.
184. Dwork AJ, Balmaceda C, Fazzini EA, et al. Dominantly inherited, early-onset parkinsonism: neuropathology of a new form. *Neurology* 1993;43:69–74.
185. Haltia M, Somer H, Palo J, et al. Neuronal intranuclear inclusion disease in identical twins. *Ann Neurol* 1984;15:316–321.
186. Dobyns WB, Ozelius LJ, Kramer PL, et al. Rapid-onset dystonia-parkinsonism. *Neurology* 1993;43:2596–2602.
187. Paterson D, Carmichael EA. Form of familial cerebral degeneration chiefly affecting the lenticular nucleus. *Brain* 1924;47:207–231.
188. Basel-Vanagaite L, Straussberg R, Ovadia H, et al. Infantile bilateral strial necrosis maps to chromosome 19p. *Neurology* 2004;62:87–90.
189. Straussberg R, Shorer Z, Weitz R, et al. Familial infantile bilateral striatal necrosis: clinical features and response to biotin treatment. *Neurology* 2002;59:983–989.
190. de la Tourette G. Etude sur une affection nerveuse, characterisée par de l'incoordination motrice, accompagnée d'echolalie et de coprolalie. *Arch Neurol* (Paris) 1885;9:158–200.
191. Lombroso PJ, Mercadante MT, Scahill L. Obsessive-compulsive disorder and Tourette syndrome. In: Rosenberg RN, Prusiner SB, DiMauro S, et al., eds. *The molecular basis of neurologic and psychiatric disease*, 3rd ed. Philadelphia: Butterworth–Heinemann, 2003:767–778.
192. Jancovic J. Tourette's syndrome. *N Engl J Med* 2001;345:1184–1192.
193. Walkup JT, LaBuda MC, Singer HS, et al. Family study and segregation analysis of Tourette's syndrome: evidence for a mixed model of inheritance. *Am J Hum Genet* 1996;59:684–693.
194. Pulst S, Walshe TM, Romero JA. Carbon monoxide poisoning with features of Gilles de la Tourette's syndrome. *Arch Neurol* 1983;40:443–444.
195. Numura Y, Segawa M. Neurology of Tourette's syndrome (TS). TS as a developmental dopamine disorder: a hypothesis. *Brain Dev* 2003;25(Suppl 1):S37–S42.
196. Singer HS, Reiss AL, Brown JE, et al. Volumetric MRI changes in basal ganglia of children with Tourette's syndrome. *Neurology* 1993;43:950–956.
197. Minzer K, Lee O, Hong JJ, et al. Increased prefrontal D2 protein in Tourette syndrome: a postmortem analysis of frontal cortex and striatum. *J Neurol Sci* 2004;219:55–61.
197a. Singer HS, Giuliano JD, Hansen BH, et al. Antibodies against human putamen in children with Tourette's syndrome. *Neurology* 1998;50:1618–1624.
198. Burd L, Kerbeshian J, Wikenheiser M, et al. A prevalence study of Gilles de la Tourette's syndrome in North Dakota school-age children. *J Am Acad Child Adolesc Psychiatry* 1980;25:552–553.
199. Ehrenberg G, Cruse RP, Rothner AD. Tourette's syndrome: an analysis of 200 pediatric and adolescent cases. *Clev Clin Q* 1986;53:127–131.
200. Golden GS. Tics and Tourette's: a continuum of symptoms? *Ann Neurol* 1978;4:145–148.
201. Chase TN, Friedhoff AJ, Cohen DJ, eds. *Tourette syndrome: genetics, neurobiology, and treatment*. New York: Raven Press, 1992.
202. Pappert EJ, Goetz CG, Louis ED, et al. Objective assessments of longitudonal outcome in Gilles de la Tourette's syndrome. *Neurology* 2003;61:936–940.
203. Snider LA, Seligman LD, Letchen BR, et al. Tics and problem behaviors in school children: prevalence, characterization, and associations. *Pediatrics* 2002;110:331–336.
204. Cardona F, Orefici G. Group A streptococcal infections and tic disorders in an Italian pediatric population. *J Pediatr* 2001;138:71–75.
205. Lowe TL, Cohen DJ, Detlor J, et al. Stimulant medications precipitate Tourette's syndrome. *JAMA* 1982;247:1729–1731.
206. Glaze DG, Frost JD, Jankovic J. Sleep in Gilles de la Tourette's syndrome: disorder of arousal. *Neurology* 1983;33:586–592.
206a. Jimenez-Jimenez FJ, Garcia-Ruiz PJ. Pharmacologic options for the treatment of Tourette's disorder. *Drugs* 2001;61:2207–2220.
207. Leckman JF, Detlor J, Harcherik DF, et al. Short-and long-term treatment of Tourette's syndrome with clonidine: a clinical perspective. *Neurology* 1985;35:343–351.
208. Robertson MM, Stern JS. Gilles de la Tourette syndrome: symptomatic treatment based on evidence. *Eur Child Adolesc Psychiatry* 2000;9(Suppl 1):160–175.
209. Shapiro AK, Shapiro E, Fulop G. Pimozide treatment of tic and Tourette disorders. *Pediatrics* 1987;79:1032–1039.
210. Regeur L, Pakkenberg B, Fog R, et al. Clinical features and long-term treatment with pimozide in 65 patients with Gilles de la Tourette's syndrome. *J Neurol Neurosurg Psychiatry* 1986;49:791–795.
211. Gilbert DL, Dure L, Sethuraman G, et al. Tic reduction with pergolide in a randomized controlled trial in children. *Neurology* 2003;60:606–611.
212. Kurlan R. New treatment for tics? *Neurology* 2001;56:580–581.
213. Kurlan R, Goetz CG, McDermott MP, et al. Treatment of ADHD in children with tics. A randomized controlled trial. *Neurology* 2002;58:527–536.
214. Leckman JF, Ort S, Caruso KA, et al. Rebound phenomenon in Tourette's syndrome after abrupt withdrawal of clonidine. *Arch Gen Psychiatry* 1986;43:1168–1176.
215. Sallee FR, Nesbitt L, Jackson C, et al. Relative efficacy of haloperidol and pimozide in children and adolescents with Tourette's disorder. *Am J Psychiatr* 1997;154:1057–1062.
216. Mount LA, Reback S. Familial paroxysmal choreoathetosis. *Arch Neurol Psychiatry* 1940;44:841–847.
217. Goodenough DJ, Fariello RG, Annis BL, et al. Familial and acquired paroxysmal dyskinesias. *Arch Neurol* 1978;35:827–831.
218. Bressman SB, Fahn S, Burke RE. Paroxysmal nonkinesigenic dystonia. *Adv Neurol* 1988;50:403–413.
219. Lance JW. Familial paroxysmal dystonic choreo-athetosis and its differentiation from related syndromes. *Ann Neurol* 1977;2:285–293.
220. Houser MK, Soland VL, Bhatia KP, et al. Paroxysmal kinesigenic choreoathetosis: a report of 26 cases. *J Neurol* 1999;246:120–126.
221. Homan RW, Vasko MR, Blaw M. Phenytoin concentrations in paroxysmal kinesigenic choreoathetosis. *Neurology* 1980;30:673–676.
222. Bennett LB, Roach ES, Bowcock AM. A locus for paroxysmal kinesigenic dyskinesia maps to human chromosome 16. *Neurology* 2000;54:125–130.
223. Mir P, Huang YZ, Gilio F, et al. Abnormal cortical and spinal inhibition in paroxysmal kinesigenic dyskinesia. *Brain* 2005;128:291–299.
224. Cuenca-Leon E, Cormand B, Thomson T, et al. Paroxysmal kinesigenic dyskinesia and generalized seizures: clinical and genetic analysis in a Spanish pedigree. *Neuropediatrics* 2002;33:288–293.
225. Raskind WH, Bolin T, Wolff J, et al. Further localization of a gene for paroxysmal dystonic choreoathetosis to a 5-cM region on chromosome 2q34. *Hum Genet* 1998;102:93–97.

226. Pryles CV, Livingston S, Ford FR. Familial paroxysmal choreoathetosis of Mount and Reback: study of a second family in which this condition is found in association with epilepsy. *Pediatrics* 1952;9:44–47.
227. Rosen JA. Paroxysmal choreoathetosis. *Arch Neurol* 1964;11:385–387.
228. Auburger G, Ratzlaff T, Lunkes A, et al. A gene for autosomal dominant paroxysmal choreoathetosis/spasticity (CSE) maps to the vicinity of a potassium channel gene cluster on chromosome 1p, probably within 2 cM between D1S443 and D1S197. *Genomics* 1996;31:90–94.
229. Angelini L, Rumi V, Lamperti E, et al. Transient paroxysmal dystonia in infancy. *Neuropediatrics* 1988;19:171–174.
230. Stevens H. Paroxysmal choreoathetosis. *Arch Neurol* 1966;14:415–420.
231. Lingam S, Wilson J, Hart EW. Hereditary stiff-baby syndrome. *Ann Neurol* 1980;8:195–197.
232. Shahar E, Raviv R. Sporadic major hyperekplexia in neonates and infants: clinical manifestations and outcome. *Pediatr Neurol* 2004;31:30–34.
233. Stevens H. Jumping Frenchmen of Maine. *Arch Neurol* 1965;12:311–314.
234. Wilkins DE, Hallet M, Wess MM. Audiogenic startle reflex of man and its relationship to startle syndromes. *Brain* 1986;109:561–573.
235. Ryan SG, Sherman SL, Terry JC, et al. Startle disease or hyperexplexia: response to clonazepam and assignment of the gene (*STHE*) to chromosome 5q by linkage analysis. *Ann Neurol* 1992;31:663–668.
236. Rees MI, Andrew M, Jawad S, et al. Evidence for recessive as well as dominant forms of startle disease (hyperekplexia) caused by mutations in the alpha 1 subunit of the inhibitory glycine receptor. *Hum Mol Genet* 1994;3:2175–2179.
237. Humeny A, Bonk T, Becker K, et al. A novel recessive hyperekplexia allele *GLRA1* (S231R): genotyping by MALDI-TOF mass spectrometry and functional characterisation as a determinant of cellular glycine receptor trafficking. *Eur J Hum Genet* 2002;10:188–196.
238. Vergouwe MN, Tijssen MA, Peters AC, et al. Hyperekplexia phenotype due to compound heterozygosity for *GLRA1* gene mutations. *Ann Neurol* 1999;46:634–638.
239. Rees MI, Lewis TM, Kwok JB, et al. Hyperekplexia associated with compound heterozygote mutations in the beta-subunit of the human inhibitory glycine receptor (GLRB). *Hum Mol Genet* 2002;11:853–860.
240. Johnson LF, Kinsbourne M, Renuart AW. Hereditary chin-trembling with nocturnal myoclonus and tongue-biting in dizygous twins. *Dev Med Child Neurol* 1971:13:726–729.
241. Gordon K, Cadera W, Hinton G. Successful treatment of hereditary trembling chin with botulinum toxin. *J Child Neurol* 1993;8:154–156.
242. Friedreich N. Ueber degenerative Atrophie der spinalen Hinterstränge. *Virchows Arch Path Anat* 1863;26:391–419.
243. Campuzano V, Montermini L, Molto MD, et al. Friedreich's ataxia: autosomal recessive disease caused by an intronic GAA triplet repeat expansion. *Science* 1996;271:1423–1427.
244. Pandolfo M. Friedreich Ataxia. In: Pulst SM, ed. *Genetics of movement disorders*, Amsterdam: Academic Press, 2003:166–178.
245. Cossée M, Durr A, Schmitt M, et al. Friedreich's ataxia: point mutations and clinical presentation of compound heterozygotes. *Ann Neurol* 1999;45:200–206.
246. Dürr A, Cossee M, Agid Y, et al. Clinical and genetic abnormalities in patients with Friedreich's ataxia. *N Engl J Med* 1996;335:1169–1175.
247. Montermini L, Richter A, Morgan K, et al. Phenotypic variability in Friedreich's ataxia: role of the associated GAA triplet repeat expansion. *Ann Neurol* 1997;41:675–682.
248. Isaya G, O'Neill HA, Gakh O, et al. Functional studies of frataxin. *Acta Paediatr* 2004:93(Suppl 455):68–71.
249. Rotig A, de Lonley P, Chretien D, et al. Aconitase and mitochondrial iron-sulphur protein deficiency in Friedreich's ataxia. *Nat Genet* 1997;17:215–217.
250. Bulteau AL, O'Neill HA, Kennedy MC, et al. Frataxin acts as an iron chaperone protein to modulate mitochondrial aconitase activity. *Science* 2004;305:242–245.
251. Klockgether T, Evert B. Genes involved in hereditary ataxias. *Trends Neurosci* 1998;21:413–418.
252. Pandolfo M. Molecular pathogenesis of Friedreich Ataxia. *Arch Neurol* 1999;56:1201–1208.
253. Bidchandani SI, Ashikawa T, Patel PI. The GAA triplet-repeat expansion Friedreich's ataxia interferes with transcription and may be associated with an unusual DNA structure. *Am J Hum Genet* 1998;62:111–121.
254. Blass JP, Kark RAP, Menon NK. Low activities of the pyruvate and oxoglutarate dehydrogenase complexes in five patients with Friedreich's ataxia. *N Engl J Med* 1976;295:62–67.
255. Greenfield JG. *The spino-cerebellar degenerations*. Oxford: Blackwell, 1954.
256. Oppenheimer DR. Brain lesions in Friedreich's ataxia. *Can J Neurol Sci* 1979;6:173–176.
257. Harding AE. *The hereditary ataxias and related disorders*. Edinburgh: Churchill Livingstone, 1984.
258. Harding AE. Friedreich's ataxia: a clinical and genetic study of 90 families with an analysis of early diagnostic criteria and intrafamilial clustering of clinical features. *Brain* 1981;104:589–620.
259. De Michele G, Di Maio L, Filla A, et al. Childhood onset of Friedreich's ataxia: a clinical and genetic study of 36 cases. *Neuropediatrics* 1996;27:3–7.
260. Pandolfo M. Friedreich's ataxia and iron metabolism. In: Rosenberg RN, Prusiner SB, DiMauro S, et al., eds. *The molecular basis of neurologic and psychiatric disease*, 3rd ed. Philadelphia: Butterworth–Heinemann, 2003:679–686.
261. Carroll WM, Kriss A, Baraitser M, et al. The incidence and nature of visual pathway involvement in Friedreich's ataxia. *Brain* 1980;103:413–434.
262. van Bogaert L, Martin L. Optic cochleovestibular degeneration in the hereditary ataxias. I. Clinico-pathological and genetic aspects. *Brain* 1974;97:15–40.
263. Jones SJ, Baraitser M, Halliday AM. Peripheral and central somatosensory nerve conduction defects in Friedreich's ataxia. *J Neurol Neurosurg Psychiatry* 1980;43:495–503.
264. Boyer SH, Chisholm AW, McKusick VA. Cardiac aspects of Friedreich's ataxia. *Circulation* 1962;25:493–505.
265. Schols L, Amoiridis G, Przuntek H, et al. Friedreich's ataxia: revision of the phenotype according to molecular genetics. *Brain* 1997;120:2131–2140.
266. Hanna MG, Davis MB, Sweeney MG, et al. Generalized chorea in two patients harboring the Friedreich's ataxia gene trinucleotide repeat expansion. *Mov Disord* 1998;13:339–340.
267. Bouchard JP, Barbeau A, Bouchard R, et al. Autosomal recessive spastic ataxia of Charlevoix-Saguenay. *Can J Neurol Sci* 1978;5:61–69.
268. Hentati F, Amouri R, Peki M, et al. Familial ataxia with isolated vitamin E deficiency (AVED). In: Pulst SM, ed. *Genetics of movement disorders*. Amsterdam: Academic Press, 2003:179–187.
269. Koskinen TP, Santavuori P, Sainio K, et al. Infantile onset spinocerebellar ataxia with sensory neuropathy—a new inherited disease. *J Neurol Sci* 1994;121:50–56.
270. Koskinen TP, Pihko H, Voutilainen R. Primary hypogonadism in females with infantile onset spinocerebellar ataxia. *Neuropediatrics* 1995;26:263–266.
271. Shimazaki H, Takiyama Y, Sakoe K, et al. Early-onset ataxia with ocular motor apraxia and hypoalbuminemia. The aprataxin gene mutation. *Neurology* 2002;59:590–595.
272. Sano Y, Date H, Igarashi S, et al. Aprataxin, the causative protein for EAOH is a nuclear protein with a potential role as a DNA repair protein. *Ann Neurol* 2004;55:241–249.
273. Nemeth AH, Bochukova E, Dunne E, et al. Autosomal recessive cerebellar ataxia with ocular motor apraxia (ataxia-telangiectasia-like syndrome) is linked to chromosome 9q34. *Am J Hum Genet* 2000;67:1320–1326.
273a. Moreira MC, Klur S, Watanabe M, et al. Senataxin, the ortholog of a yeast RNA helicase, is mutant in ataxia-ocular apraxia. *Nat Genet* 2004;36:225–227.
274. Bomont P, Watanabe M, Gershoni-Barush R, et al. Homozygosity mapping of spinocerebellar ataxia with cerebellar atrophy and peripheral neuropathy to 9q33–34, and with hearing impairment and optic atrophy to 6p21–23. *Eur J Hum Genet* 2000;8:986–990.

275. Garland H, Moorhouse D. An extremely rare recessive hereditary syndrome including cerebellar ataxia, oligophrenia, cataract, and other features. *J Neurol Neurosurg Psychiatry* 1953;16:110–116.
276. McLaughlin JF, Pagon RA, Weinberger E, et al. Marinesco-Sjögren syndrome: clinical and magnetic resonance imaging features in three children. *Dev Med Child Neurol* 1996;38:356–370.
277. Nystuen A, Benke PJ, Merren J, et al. A cerebellar ataxia locus identified by DNA pooling to search for linkage disequilibrium in an isolated population from the Cayman Islands. *Hum Mol Genet* 1996;5:525–530.
278. Gironi M, Lamperti C, Nemni R, et al. Late-onset cerebellar ataxia with hypogonadism and muscle coenzyme Q10 deficiency. *Neurology* 2004;62:818–820.
279. Lonnqvist T, Paetau A, Nikali K, et al. Infantile onset spinocerebellar ataxia with sensory neuropathy (IOSCA): neuropathological features. *J Neurol Sci* 1998;161:57–63.
280. Nikali K, Saharinen J, Peltonen L. cDNA cloning, expression profile and genomic structure of a novel human transcript on chromosome 10q24, and its analyses as a candidate gene for infantile onset spinocerebellar ataxia. *Gene* 2002;299:111–115.
281. Lagier-Tourenne C, Tranebaerg L, Chaigne D, et al. Homozygosity mapping of Marinesco-Sjogren syndrome to 5q31. *Eur J Hum Genet* 2003;11:770–778.
282. Engert JC, Berube P, Mercier J, et al. ARSACS, a spastic ataxia common in northeastern Quebec, is caused by mutations in a new gene encoding an 11.5 kb ORF. *Nat Genet* 2000;24:120–125.
283. Shapiro F, Specht L. The diagnosis and orthopaedic treatment of childhood spinal muscular atrophy, peripheral neuropathy, Friedreich ataxia, and arthrogryposis. *J Bone Joint Surg Am* 1993;75:1699–1714.
284. Buyse G, Mertens L, Di Salvo G, et al. Idebenone treatment in Friedreich's ataxia: neurological, cardiac, and biochemical monitoring. *Neurology* 2003;60:1679–1681.
285. Perlman S. Symptomatic and disease-modifying therapy for the progressive ataxias. *Neurologist* 2004;10:275–289.
286. Menzel P. Beitrag zur Kentniss der hereditären Ataxie und Kleinhirnatrophie. *Arch Psychiatr Nervenkr* 1890:22:160–190.
287. Dejerine J, André-Thomas A. L'atrophie olivoponto-cérébelleuse. *Nouv Iconog Salpètr* 1900;13:330–370.
288. Holmes GM. A form of familial degeneration of the cerebellum. *Brain* 1907;30:466–489.
289. Pandolfo M, Montermini L. Molecular genetics of the hereditary ataxias. *Adv Genet* 1998;38:31–68.
290. Babovic-Vuksanovic D, Snow K, Patgterson MC, et al. Spinocerebellar ataxia type 2 (SCA2) in an infant with extreme CAG repeat expansion. *Am J Med Genet* 1998;79:383–387.
291. Zhou XY, Fan MZ, Yang BX, et al. Machado-Joseph disease in four Chinese pedigrees: molecular analysis of 15 patients including two juvenile cases and clinical correlations. *Neurology* 1997;48:482–485.
292. Mizusawa H. Spinocerebellar ataxia type 4 (SCA4). In: Pulst SM, ed. *Genetics of movement disorders*. Amsterdam: Academic Press, 2003:71–73.
293. Ranum RPW, Dick KA, Day JW. Spinocerebellar ataxia 5 (SCA5). In: Pulst SM, ed. *Genetics of movement disorders*. Amsterdam: Academic Press, 2003:75–80.
294. Ikeuchi T, Takano H, Koide R, et al. Spinocerebellar ataxia type 6: CAG repeat expansion in α_{1a} voltage-dependent calcium channel gene and clinical variations in Japanese populations. *Ann Neurol* 1997;42:879–884.
295. Lebre AS, Stevann G, Brice A. Spinocerebellar ataxia 7 (SCA7). In: Pulst SM, ed. *Genetics of movement disorders*. Amsterdam: Academic Press, 2003:85–94.
296. Day JW, Schut LJ, Moseley ML, et al. Spinocerebellar ataxia type 8. Clinical features in a large family. *Neurology* 2000;55:649–657.
297. Schöls L, Bauer I, Zühlke C, et al. Do CTG expansions at the SCA8 locus cause ataxia? *Ann Neurol* 2003;54:110–115.
298. Rasmussen A, Matsuura T, Ruano L, et al. Clinical and genetic analysis of four Mexican families with spinocerebellar ataxia type 10. *Ann Neurol* 2001;50:234–239.
299. Vakharia H, Oh MK, Pulst SM. Spinocerebellar ataxia 11 (SCA11). In: Pulst SM, ed. *Genetics of movement disorders*. Amsterdam: Academic Press, 2003:117–119.
300. Srivastava A, Choudhry S, Gopinath MS, et al. Molecular and clinical correlation in five Indian families with spinocerebellar ataxia 12. *Ann Neurol* 2001;50:796–800.
301. Fujigasaki H, Dürr A, Stevanin G, et al. Spinocerebellar ataxia 13, 14, and 16. In: Pulst SM, ed. *Genetics of movement disorders*. Amsterdam: Academic Press, 2003:133–138.
302. Yamashita I, Sasaki H, Yabe I, et al. A novel locus for dominant cerebellar ataxia (SCA14) maps to a 10.2 cM interval flanked by D19S206 and D19S605 on chromosome 19q13.4–qter. *Ann Neurol* 2000;48:156–163.
302a. Chen DH, Cimino PJ, Ranum LPW, et al. The clinical and genetic spectrum of spinocerebellar ataxia 14. *Neurology* 2005;64:1258–1260.
303. Miyoshi Y, Yamada T, Tanimura M, et al. A novel autosomal dominant spinocerebellar ataxia (SCA16) linked to chromosome 8q22.1–24.1. *Neurology* 2001;57:96–100.
304. Tsuji S. Spinocerebellar ataxia 17 (SCA17). In: Pulst SM, ed. *Genetics of movement disorders*. Amsterdam: Academic Press, 2003:139–141.
305. Oyanagi S. Hereditary dentatorubral-pallidoluysian atrophy. *Neuropathology* 2000;20(Suppl):S42–S46.
306. Verbeek DS, Schelhaas JH, Ippel EF, et al. Identification of a novel SCA locus (*SCA19*) in a Dutch autosomal dominant cerebellar ataxia family on chromosome region 1p21–q21. *Hum Genet* 2002;111:388–393.
307. Vuillaume L, Devos D, Schraein-Maschke S, et al. A new locus for spinocerebellar ataxia (*SCA21*) maps to chromosome 7p21.3–p15.1. *Ann Neurol* 2002;52:666–670.
308. Chung MY, Lu YC, Cheng NC, et al. A novel autosomal dominant spinocerebellar ataxia (SCA22) linked to chromosome 1p21–q23. *Brain* 2003;126:1293–1299.
309. Stevanin G, Bouslam N, Thobois S, et al. Spinocerebellar ataxia with sensory neuropathy (SCA25) maps to chromosome 2p. *Ann Neurol* 2004;55:97–104.
309a. Yu GY, Howell MJ, Roller MJ, et al. Spinocerebellar ataxia type 26 maps to chromosome 19p13.3 adjacent to SCA6. *Ann Neurol* 2005;57:349–354.
310. Benton CS, de Silva R, Rutledge SL, et al. Molecular and clinical studies in SCA-7 define a broad clinical spectrum and the infantile phenotype. *Neurology* 1998;51:1081–1086.
310a. Brusco A, Gellera C, Cagnoli C, et al. Molecular genetics of hereditary spinocerebellar ataxia: mutation analysis of spinocerebellar ataxia genes and CAG/CTG repeat expansion detection in 225 Italian families. *Arch Neurol* 2004;61:727–733.
311. Lin X, Antalffy B, Kang D, et al. Polyglutamine expansion downregulates specific neuronal genes before pathologic changes in SCA1. *Nat Neurosci* 2000;3:157–163.
312. Huynh DP, Del Bigio MR, Ho DH, et al. Expression of ataxin-2 in brains from normal individuals and patients with Alzheimer's disease and spinocerebellar ataxia 2. *Ann Neurol* 1999;45:232–241.
313. Schöls L, Amoiridis G, Buttner T, et al. Autosomal dominant cerebellar ataxia: phenotypic differences in genetically defined subtypes? *Ann Neurol* 1997;42:924–932.
314. Schmidt T, Lindenberg KS, Krebs A, et al. Protein surveillance machinery in brains with spinocerebellar ataxia type 3: redistribution and differential recruitment of 26S proteasome subunits and chaperones to neuronal intranuclear inclusions. *Ann Neurol* 2002;51:302–310.
315. Gouw LG, Digre KB, Harris CP, et al. Autosomal dominant cerebellar ataxia with retinal degeneration: clinical, neuropathologic, and genetic analysis of a large kindred. *Neurology* 1994;44:1441–1447.
316. Van Leeuwen MA, van Bogaert L. Hereditary ataxia with optic atrophy of the retrobulbar neuritis type, and latent pallido-Luysian degeneration. *Brain* 1949;72:340–363.
317. Warner TT, Williams LD, Walker RW, et al. A clinical and molecular genetic study of dentatorubral-pallidoluysian atrophy in four European families. *Ann Neurol* 1995;37:452–459.
317a. Brunt ER, van Weerden TW. Familial paroxysmal kinesigenic ataxia and continuous myokymia. *Brain* 1990;113:1361–1382.
318. Browne DL, Gancher ST, Nutt JG, et al. Episodic ataxia/myokymia syndrome is associated with point mutations in the human potassium channel gene *KCNA1*. *Nat Genet* 1994;8:136–140.

319. Subramony SH, Schott K, Raike RS, et al. Novel *CACNA1A* mutation causes febrile episodic ataxia with interictal cerebellar deficits. *Ann Neurol* 2003;54:725–731.
320. Baloh RW, Yue Q, Furman JM, et al. Familial episodic ataxia: clinical heterogeneity in four families linked to chromosome 19p. *Ann Neurol* 1997;41:8–16.
321. Jen J, Kim GW, Baloh RW. Clinical spectrum of episodic ataxia type 2. *Neurology* 2004;62:17–22.
322. Ophoff RA, Terwindt GM, Vergouwe MN, et al. Familial hemiplegic migraine and episodic ataxia type-2 are caused by mutations in the Ca^{2+} channel gene *CACNL1A4*. *Cell* 1996;87:543–552.
323. Jen JC, Baloh RW. Episodic and intermittent ataxias. In: Pulst SM, ed. *Genetics of movement disorders*. Amsterdam: Academic Press, 2003:205–212.
324. Steckley JL, Ebers GC, Cader MZ, et al. An autosomal dominant disorder with episodic ataxia, vertigo, and tinnitus. *Neurology* 2001;57:1499–1502.
325. Hunt JR. Dyssynergia cerebellaris myoclonica—primary atrophy of the dentate system. *Brain* 1921;44:490–538.
326. Andermann, Berkovic S, Carpenter S, et al. The Ramsay Hunt syndrome is no longer a useful diagnostic category. *Mov Disord* 1989;4:13–17.
327. Seeligmüller A. Sklerose der Seitenstränge des Rückenmarks bei 4 Kindern derselben Familie. *Dtsch Med Wochenschr* 1876;2:185–186.
328. Dyken P, Krawiecki N. Neurodegenerative diseases of infancy and childhood. *Ann Neurol* 1983;13:351–364.
329. Hedera P, Rainier S, Alvarado D, et al. Novel locus for autosomal dominant hereditary spastic paraplegia, on chromosome 8q. *Am J Hum Genet* 1999;64:563–569.
330. McDermott CJ, Grierson AJ, Wood JD, et al. Hereditary spastic paraparesis:disrupted intracellular transport associated with spastin mutation. *Ann Neurol* 2003;54:748–755.
331. Errico A, Claudiani P, D'Addio M, et al. Spastin interacts with the centrosomal protein NA14, and is enriched in the spindle pole, the midbody, and the distal axon. *Hum Mol Genet* 2004;13:2121–2132.
332. Reid E. Science in motion: common molecular pathological themes emerge in the hereditary spastic paraplegias. *J Med Genet* 2003;40:81–86.
333. Zhao X, Alvarado D, Rainier S, et al. Mutations in a newly identified GTPase cause autosomal dominant hereditary spastic paraparesis. *Nat Genet* 2001;29:326–331.
334. Patel H, Cross H, Proukakis C, et al. *SPG20* is mutated in Troyer syndrome, an hereditary spastic paraplegia. *Nat Genet* 2002;31:347–348.
335. Behan WMH, Maia M. Strumpell's familial paraplegia: genetics and neuropathology. *J Neurol Neurosurg Psychiatry* 1974;37: 8–20.
336. Schwarz GA, Liu C. Hereditary spastic paraplegia. *Arch Neurol Psychiatry* 1956;75:144–162.
337. Jouet M, Rosenthal A, Armstrong G, et al. X-linked spastic paraplegia (SPG1), MASA syndrome and X-linked hydrocephalus result from mutations in the *L1* gene. *Nat Genet* 1994;7:402–406.
338. Saugier-Veber P, Munnich A, Bonneau D, et al. X-linked spastic paraplegia (SPG1) and Pelizaeus-Merzbacher disease are allelic disorders at the proteolipid protein locus. *Nat Genet* 1994;6:257–262.
339. Fink JK, Rainir S. Hereditary spastic paraplegia: spastin phenotype and function. *Arch Neurol* 2004;61:830–833.
340. Hentati A, Deng HX, Zhai H, et al. Novel mutations in spastin gene and absence of correlation with age at onset of symptoms. *Neurology* 2000;55:1388–1390.
341. Rainier S, Chai JH, Tokarz D, et al. *NIPA1* gene mutations cause autosomal dominant hereditary spastic paraplegia (SPG6). *Am J Hum Genet* 2003;73:967–971.
342. De Michele G, De Fusco M, Cavalcanti F, et al. A new locus for autosomal recessive hereditary spastic paraplegia maps to chromosome 16q24.3. *Am J Hum Genet* 1998;63:135–139.
343. Seri M, Cusano R, Forabosco P, et al. Genetic mapping to 10q23.2–q24.2, in a large Italian pedigree, of a new syndrome showing bilateral cataracts, gastroesophageal reflux, and spastic paraparesis with amyotrophy. *Am J Hum Genet* 1999;64:586–593.
344. Reid E, Kloos M, Ashley-Koch A, et al. A kinesin heavy chain (KIF5A) mutation in hereditary spastic paraplegia (SPG10). *Am J Hum Genet* 2002;71:1189–1194.
345. Shibasaki Y, Tanaka H, Iwabuchi K, et al. Linkage of autosomal recessive hereditary spastic paraplegia with mental impairment and thin corpus callosum to chromosome 15q13–15. *Ann Neurol* 2000;48:108–112.
346. Hansen JJ, Durr A, Cournu-Rebeix I, et al. Hereditary spastic paraplegia SPG13 is associated with a mutation in the gene encoding the mitochondrial chaperonin Hsp60. *Am J Hum Genet* 2002;70:1328–1332.
347. Vazza G, Zortea M, Boaretto F, et al. A new locus for autosomal recessive spastic paraplegia associated with mental retardation and distal motor neuropathy, *SPG14*, maps to chromosome 3q27–q28. *Am J Hum Genet* 2000;67:504–509.
348. Hughes CA, Byrne PC, Webb S, et al. *SPG15*, a new locus for autosomal recessive complicated HSP on chromosome 14q. *Neurology* 2001;56:1230–1233.
349. Windpassinger C, Wagner K, Petek E, et al. Refinement of the Silver syndrome locus on chromosome 11q12–q14 in four families and exclusion of eight candidate genes. *Hum Genet* 2003;114:99–109.
350. Cross HE, McKusick VA. The Troyer syndrome. A recesssive form of spastic paraplegia with distal muscle wasting. *Arch Neurol* 1967;16:473–485.
350a. Lison M, Kornbrut B, Feinstein A, et al. Progressive spastic paraparesis, vitiligo, premature graying, and distinct facial appearance: a new genetic syndrome in 3 sibs. *Am J Med Genet* 1981;9:351–357.
350b. Zortea M, Vettori A, Trevisan CP, et al. Genetic mapping of a susceptibility locus for disc herniation and spastic paraplegia on 6q23.3–q24.1. *J Med Genet* 2002;39:387–390.
350c. Meijer I, Cossette P, Roussel J, et al. A novel locus for pure recessive hereditary spastic paraplegia maps to 10q22.1–10q24.1. *Ann Neurol* 2004;56:579–582.
351. Casari G, De Fusco M, Ciarmatori S, et al. Spastic paraplegia and OXPHOS impairment caused by mutations in paraplegin, a nuclear-encoded mitochondrial metalloprotease. *Cell* 1998;93:973–983.
352. Fink JK, Heiman-Patterson T, Bird T, et al. Hereditary spastic paraplegia: advances in genetic research. *Neurology* 1996;46:1507–1514.
353. Harding AE. Hereditary "pure" spastic paraplegia: a clinical and genetic study of 22 families. *J Neurol Neurosurg Psychiatry* 1981;44: 871–883.
354. Dürr A, Davoine CS, Paternotte C, et al. Phenotype of autosomal dominant spastic paraplegia linked to chromosome 2. *Brain* 1996;119:1487–1496.
355. Saugier-Veber P, Monnich A, Bonneau D, et al. X-linked spastic paraplegia and Pelizaeus-Merzbacher disease are allelic disorders at the proteolipid protein locus. *Nat Genet* 1994;6:257–262.
356. Huang S, Zhuyu, Li H, et al. Another pedigree with pure autosomal dominant spastic paraplegia (AD-FSP) from Tibet mapping to 14q11.2–q24.3. *Hum Genet* 1997;100:620–623.
357. McShane MA, Boyd S, Harding R, et al. Progresive bulbar paralysis of childhood. A reappraisal of Fazio-Londe disease. *Brain* 1992;115:1889–1900.
358. Veltema AN, Roos RA, Bruyn GW. Autosomal dominant adult amyotrophic lateral sclerosis. A six generation Dutch family. *J Neurol Sci* 1990;97:93–115.
359. Yamanaka K, Van de VeldeC, Eymard-Pierre E, et al. Unstable mutants in the peripheral endosomal membrane component ALS2 cause early-onset motor neuron disease. *Proc Natl Acad Sci USA* 2003;100:16041–16046.
360. Yang Y, Hentati A, Deng HX, et al. The gene encoding alsin, a protein with three guanine-nucleotide exchange factor domains, is mutated in a form of recessive amyotrophic lateral sclerosis. *Nat Genet* 2001;29:160–165.
361. Lesca G, Eymard-Pierre E, Santorelli FM, et al. Infantile ascending hereditary spastic paralysis (IAHSP): clinical features in 11 families. *Neurology* 2003;60:674–682.
362. Hand CK, Khonis J, Salachas F, et al. A novel locus for familial amyotrophic lateral sclerosis, on chromosome 18q. *Am J Hum Genet* 2002;70:251–256.

363. De Jonghe P, Auer-Grumbach M, Irobi J, et al. Autosomal dominant juvenile amyotrophic lateral sclerosis and distal hereditary motor neuropathy with pyramidal tract signs: synonyms for the same disorder? *Brain* 2002;125:1320–1325.
364. Chen YZ, Bennett CL, Huynh HM, et al. DNA/RNA helicase gene mutations in a form of juvenile amyotrophic lateral sclerosis. *Am J Hum Genet* 2004;74:1128–1135.
365. Hentati A, Ouahchi K, Pericak-Vance MA, et al. Linkages of a commoner form of recessive amyotrophic lateral sclerosis to chromosome 15q15-q22 markers. *Neurogenetics* 1998;2:55–60.
366. Topp JD, Gray NW, Gerard RD, et al. Alsin is a Rac1 guanine-nucleotide exchange factor. *J Biol Chem* 2004;279:24612–24623.
367. Dyck PJ, Chance P, Lebo R, et al. Hereditary motor and sensory neuropathies. In: Dyck PJ, Thomas PK, eds. *Peripheral neuropathy*, 3rd ed. Philadelphia: Saunders, 1993:1094–1136.
368. Ouvrier RA, McLeod JG, Conchin TE. The hypertrophic forms of hereditary motor and sensory neuropathy. *Brain* 1987;110:121–148.
369. Gabreels-Festen AA, Bolhuis PA, Hoogendijk JE, et al. Charcot-Marie-Tooth disease type 1A: morphological phenotype of the 17p duplication versus PMP point mutations. *Acta Neuropathol* 1995;90:645–649.
370. Bird TD, Kraft GH, Lipe HP, et al. Clinical and pathological phenotype of the original family with Charcot-Marie-Tooth type 1B: a 20-year study. *Ann Neurol* 1997;41:4663–4669.
371. Street VA, Goldy JD, Golden AS, et al. Mapping of Charcot-Marie-Tooth disease type 1C to chromosome 16p identifies a novel locus for demyelinating neuropathies. *Am J Hum Genet* 2002;70:244–250.
372. Warner LE, Mancias P, Butler IJ, et al. Mutations in the early growth response (EGR2) gene are associated with hereditary myelinopathies. *Nat Genet* 1998;18:382–384.
373. Suter U, Snipes GJ. Biology and genetics of hereditary motor and sensory neuropathies. *Annu Rev Neurosci* 1995;18:45–75.
374. Muglia M, Zappiea M, Timmerman V, et al. Clinical and genetic study of a large Charcot-Marie-Tooth type 2A family from southern Italy. *Neurology* 2001;56:100–103.
375. Kok C, Kennerson ML, Spring PJ, et al. A locus for hereditary sensory neuropathy with cough and gastroesophageal reflux on chromosome 3p22–p24. *Am J Hum Genet* 2003;73:632–637.
376. Ionasescu V, Searby C, Sheffield VC, et al. Autosomal dominant Charcot-Marie-Tooth axonal neuropathy mapped on chromosome 7p (CMT2D). *Hum Mol Genet* 1996;5:1373–1375.
377. Georgiou DM, Zidar J, Korosec M, et al. A novel *NF-L* mutation Pro22Ser is associated with CMT2 in a large Slovenian family. *Neurogenetics* 2002;4:93–96.
378. Ismailov SM, Fedotov VP, Dadali EL, et al. A new locus for autosomal dominant Charcot-Marie-Tooth disease type 2 (CMT2F) maps to chromosome 7q11–q21. *Eur J Hum Genet* 2001;9:646–650.
379. Nelis E, Berciano J, Verpoorten N, et al. Autosomal dominant axonal Charcot-Marie-Tooth disease type 2 (CMT2G) maps to chromosome 12q12–q13.3. *J Med Genet* 2004;41:193–197.
380. Bergoffen J, Scherer SS, Wang S, et al. Connexin mutations in X-linked Charcot-Marie-Tooth disease. *Science* 1993;262:2039–2042.
381. Birouk N, LeGuern E, Maisonobe T, et al. X-linked Charcot-Marie-Tooth disease with connexin 32 mutations: clinical and electrophysiologic study. *Neurology* 1998;50:1074–1082.
382. Ionasescu VV, Trofatter J, Haines JL, et al. X-linked recessive Charcot-Marie-Tooth neuropathy: clinical and genetic study. *Muscle Nerve* 1992;15:368–373.
383. Webster H deF, Schroder JM, Asbury AK, et al. The role of Schwann cells in formation of "onion bulbs" found in chronic neuropathies. *J Neuropathol Exp Neurol* 1967;26:276–299.
384. Ben Othmane K, Hentati F, Lennon F, et al. Linkage of a locus (*CMT4A*) for autosomal recessive Charcot-Marie-Tooth disease to chromosome 8q. *Hum Mol Genet* 1993;2:1625–1628.
385. Bolino A, Brancolini V, Bono F, et al. Localization of a gene responsible for autosomal recessive demyelinating neuropathy with focally folded myelin sheaths to chromosome 11q23 by homozygosity mapping and haplotype sharing. *Hum Mol Genet* 1996;5:1051–1054.
386. Gambardella A, Bolino A, Muglia M, et al. Genetic heterogeneity in autosomal recessive hereditary motor and sensory neuropathy with focally folded myelin sheaths (CMT4B). *Neurology* 1998;50:799–801.
387. Gabreels-Festen A, van Beersum S, Eshuis L, et al. Study on the gene and phenotypic characterisation of autosomal recessive demyelinating motor and sensory neuropathy (Charcot-Marie-Tooth disease) with gene locus on chromosome 5q23–q33. *J Neurol Neurosurg Psychiatry* 1999;66:569–574.
388. Hunter M, Bernard R, Freitas E, et al. Mutation screening of the N-myc downstream-regulated gene 1 (*NDRG1*) in patients with Charcot-Marie-Tooth disease. *Hum Mutat* 2003;22:129–135.
389. Bouhouche A, Benomar A, Birouk N, et al. A locus for an axonal form of autosomal recessive Charcot-Marie-Tooth disease maps to chromosome 1q21.2–q21.3. *Am J Hum Genet* 1999;65:722–727.
390. Denny-Brown D. Hereditary sensory radicular neuropathy. *J Neurol Neurosurg Psychiatry* 1951;14:237–252.
391. Dawkins JL, Hulme DJ, Brahmbhatt SB, et al. Mutations in *SPTLC1*, encoding serine palmitoyltransferase, long chain base subunit-1, cause hereditary sensory neuropathy type I. *Nat Genet* 2001;27:309–312.
392. Dyck PJ, Mellinger JF, Reagan TJ, et al. Not "indifference to pain" but varieties of hereditary sensory and autonomic neuropathy. *Brain* 1983;106:373–390.
393. Verity CM, Dunn HG, Berry K. Children with reduced sensitivity to pain: assessment of hereditary sensory neuropathy types II and IV. *Dev Med Child Neurol* 1982;24:785–797.
394. Axelrod FB. Familial dysautonomia. *Muscle Nerve* 2004;29:352–363.
395. Yatsu F, Zussman W. Familial dysautonomia (Riley-Day syndrome): case report with postmortem findings of a patient at age thirty-one. *Arch Neurol* 1964;10:459–463.
396. Mardy S, Miura Y, Endo F, et al. Congenital insensitivity to pain with anhydrosis: novel mutations in the *TRKA* (*NTRK1*) gene encoding a high-affinity receptor for nerve growth factor. *Am J Hum Genet* 1999;64:1570–1579.
397. Rosemberg S, Marie SK, Kliemann S. Congenital insensitivity to pain with anhidrosis (hereditary sensory and autonomic neuropathy tyhpe IV). *Pediatr Neurol* 1994;11:50–56.
397a. Christodoulou K, Kyriakides T, Hristova AH, et al. Mapping of a distal form of spinal muscular atrophy with upper limb predominance to chromosome 7p. *Hum Mol Genet* 1995;4:1629–1632.
397b. Pridmore C, Baraitser M, Brett EM, et al. Distal spinal muscular atrophy with vocal cord paralysis. *J Med Genet* 1992;29:197–199.
398. Hagberg B, Westerberg B. The nosology of genetic peripheral neuropathies in Swedish children. *Dev Med Child Neurol* 1983;25:3–18.
399. Virchow R. Ein Fall von progressiver Muskelatrophie. *Virchows Arch Pathol Anat* 1855;8:537–540.
400. Charcot JM, Marie P. Sur une forme particulière d'atrophie musculaire progressive, souvent familiales débutant par les pieds et les jambes, et atteignant plus tard les mains. *Rev Med* (Paris) 1885;6:97–138.
401. Tooth HH. *The peroneal type of progressive muscular atrophy*. London: H. K. Lewis, 1886.
401a. Hagberg B, Lyon G. Pooled European series of hereditary peripheral neuropathies in infancy and childhood. *Neuropaediatrie* 1981;12:9–17.
401b. Dyck PJ, Lambert EH. Lower motor and primary sensory neuron diseases with peroneal muscular atrophy. II. Neurologic, genetic, and electrophysiologic findings in various neuronal degenerations. *Arch Neurol* 1968;18:619–625.
401c. de Recondo J. Hereditary neurogenic muscular atrophies. In: Vinken PJ, Bruyn GW, eds. *Handbook of clinical neurology: system disorders and atrophies, Part I, Vol 21*. New York: Elsevier North-Holland, 1975:271–317.
402. Dejerine J, Sottas J. Sur la nevrite interstitielle hypertrophique et progressive de l'enfance. *C R Soc Biol* (Paris) 1893;45:63–96.
403. Behse F, Buchthal F. Peroneal muscular atrophy (PMA) and related disorders. II. Histological findings in sural nerves. *Brain* 1977;100:67–85.
404. Lupski JR. Charcot-Marie-Tooth polyneuropathy: duplication, gene dosage, and genetic heterogeneity. *Pediatr Res* 1999;45:159–165.

405. Hanemann CO, Muller HW. Pathogenesis of Charcot-Marie-Tooth 1A (CMT 1A) neuropathy. *Trends Neurosci* 1998;21:282–286.
406. Berger P, Young P, Suter U. Molecular cell biology of Charcot-Marie-Tooth disease. *Neurogenetics* 2002;4:1–15.
407. Roa BB, Garcia CA, Suter U, et al. Charcot-Marie-Tooth disease type1A: association with a spontaneous point mutation in the *PMP22* gene. *N Engl J Med* 1993;329:96–101.
408. Ionasescu VV, Trofatter J, Haines JL, et al. Heterogeneity in X-linked recessive Charcot–Marie-Tooth neuropathy. *Am J Hum Genet* 1991;48:1075–1083.
409. Menichella DM, Goodenough DA, Sirkowski E, et al. Connexins are critical for normal myelination in the CNS. *J Neurosci* 2003;23:5963–5973.
410. Warner LE, Mancias P, Butler IJ, et al. Mutations in the early growth response 2 (EGR2) gene are associated with hereditary myelinopathies. *Nat Genet* 1998;18:382–384.
411. Nelis E, Erdem S, Van Den Bergh PY, et al. Mutations in GDAP1: autosomal recessive CMT with demyelination and axonopathy. *Neurology* 2002;59:1865–1872.
412. Senderek J, Bergmann C, Ramaekers VT, et al. Mutations in the ganglioside-induced differentiation-associated protein-1 (GDAP1) gene in intermediate type autosomal recessive Charcot-Marie-Tooth neuropathy. *Brain* 2003;126:642–649.
413. Senderek J, Bergmann C, Stendel C, et al. Mutations in a gene encoding a novel SH3/TPR domain protein cause autosomal recessive Charcot-Marie-Tooth type 4C neuropathy. *Am J Hum Genet* 2003;73:1106–1119.
414. Tyrer JH, Sutherland JM. The primary spinocerebellar atrophies and their associated defects, with a study of the foot deformity. *Brain* 1961;84:289–300.
415. Nicholson GA. Penetrance of the hereditary motor and sensory neuropathy Ia mutation: assessment by nerve conduction studies. *Neurology* 1991;41:547–552.
416. Sambuughin N, de Bantel A, McWilliams S, et al. Deafness and CMT disease associated with a novel four amino acid deletion in the *PMP22* gene. *Neurology* 2003;60:506–508.
417. Sabatelli M, Mignogna T, Lippi G, et al. Hereditary motor and sensory neuropathy with deafness, mental retardation, and absence of sensory large myelinated fibers: confirmation of a new entity. *Am J Med Genet* 1998;75:309–313.
418. Roussy G, Lévy G. Sept cas d'une maladie familiale particuliere: troubles de la marche, pieds bots, et areflexie tendineuse generalisée, avec, accessoirement, legere maladresse des mains. *Rev Neurol* (Paris) 1926;1:427–450.
418a. Symonds CP, Shaw ME. Familial claw foot with absent tendon jerks: a "forme fruste" of the Charcot-Marie-Tooth disease. *Brain* 1926;44:387–403.
419. Thomas PK, Kalaydjieva L, Youl B, et al. Hereditary motor and sensory neuropathy–Russe: new autosomal recessive neuropathy in Balkan gypsies. *Ann Neurol* 2001;50:452–457.
420. Mersiyanova IV, Perepelov AV, Polyakov AV, et al. A new variant of Charcot-Marie-Tooth disease type 2 is probably the result of a mutation in the neurofilament-light gene. *Am J Hum Genet* 2000;67:37–46.
421. Zuchner S, Mersiyanova IV, Muglia M, et al. Mutations in the mitochondrial GTPase mitofusin 2 cause Charcot-Marie-Tooth neuropathy type 2A. *Nat Genet* 2004;36:449–451.
422. Evgrafov OV, Mersiyanova I, Irobi J, et al. Mutant small heat-shock protein 27 causes axonal Charcot-Marie-Tooth disease and distal hereditary motor neuropathy. *Nat Genet* 2004;36:602–606.
423. Hagberg B, Westerberg B, Conradi N, et al. Peripheral neuropathies in childhood: Gothenburg 1973–78. *Neuropaediatrie* 1979;10(Suppl):426.
424. Takashima H, Boerkoel CF, De Jonghe P, et al. Periaxin mutations cause a broad spectrum of demyelinating neuropathies. *Ann Neurol* 2002;51:709–715.
425. Lynch DR, Hara H, Yum SW, et al. Autosomal dominant transmission of Dejerine-Sottas disease (HMSN III). *Neurology* 1997;49:601–603.
426. Tyson J, Ellis D, Fairbrother U, et al. Hereditary demyelinating neuropathy of infancy: a genetically complex syndrome. *Brain* 1997;120:47–63.
427. Bradley WG, Aguayo A. Hereditary chronic polyneuropathy: electrophysiologic and pathologic studies in affected family. *J Neurol Sci* 1969;9:131–154.
428. Szigeti K, Saifa GM, Armstrong D, et al. Disturbance of muscle fiber differentiation in congenital hypomyelinating neuropathy caused by a novel myelin protein zero mutation. *Ann Neurol* 2003;54:398–402.
429. Vucic S, Kennerson M, Zhu D, et al. CMT with pyramidal features. Charcot-Marie-Tooth. *Neurology* 2003;60:696–699.
430. MacDermot KD, Walker RWH. Autosomal recessive hereditary motor and sensory neuropathy with mental retardation, optic atrophy and pyramidal tract signs. *J Neurol Neurosurg Psychiatry* 1987;50:1342–1347.
431. Ippel EF, Wittebol-Post D, Jennekens FGI, et al. Genetic herogeneity of hereditary motor and sensory neuropathy type VI. *J Child Neurol* 1995;10:459–463.
432. Massion-Verniory L, Dumont D, et al. Rétinite pigmentaire familiale compliquée d'une amyotrophie neurale. *Rev Neurol (Paris)* 1946;78:561–571.
433. Dupre N, Howard HC, Mathieu J, et al. Hereditary motor and sensory neuropathy with agenesis of the corpus callosum. *Ann Neurol* 2003;54:9–18.
434. Mariman ECM, Gabreels-Festen AA, van Beersum SE, et al. Prevalence of the 1.5-Mb 17p deletion in families with hereditary neuropathy with liability to pressure palsies. *Ann Neurol* 1994;36:650–655.
435. Behse F, Buchthal F, Carlsen F, et al. Hereditary neuropathy with liability to pressure palsies: electrophysiological and histopathological aspects. *Brain* 1972;95:777–794.
436. Sellman MS, Mayer RF. Conduction block in hereditary neuropathy with susceptibility to pressure palsies. *Muscle Nerve* 1987;10:621–625.
437. Andersson PB, Yuen H, Parko K, So YT. Electrodiagnostic features of hereditary neuropathy with liability to pressure palsies. *Neurology* 2000;54:40–44.
438. Gabreels-Festen AAWM, Gabreels FA, Joosten EM, et al. Hereditary neuropathy with liability to pressure palsies in childhood. *Neuropediatrics* 1992;23:138–143.
439. Nicholson GA, Valentijn LJ, Cheryson AK, et al. A frame shift mutation in the *PMP22* gene in hereditary neuropathy with liability to pressure palsies. *Nat Genet* 1994;6:263–266.
440. Greenberg F, Lewis RA, Potocki L, et al. Multi-disciplinary clinical study of Smith-Magenis syndrome. *Am J Med Genet* 1996;62:247–254.
441. Jeannet PV, Watts GDJ, Bird TD, et al. Craniofacial and cutaneous findings expand the phenotype of hereditary neuralgic amyotrophy. *Neurology* 2001;57:1963–1968.
442. Thomas PK, Ormerod IE. Hereditary neuralgic amyotrophy associated with a relapsing multifocal sensory neuropathy. *J Neurol Neurosurg Psychiatry* 1993;56:107–109.
443. Airaksinen EM, Iivanainen M, Karli P, et al. Hereditary recurrent brachial plexus neuropathy with dysmorphic features. *Acta Neurol Scand* 1985;71:309–316.
444. Klein CJ, Dyck PJ, Friedenberg SM, et al. Inflammation and neuropathic attacks in hereditary brachial plexus neuropathy. *J Neurol Neurosurg Psychiatry* 2002;73:45–50.
445. Stogbauer F, Young P, Timmerman V, et al. Refinement of the hereditary neuralgic amyotrophy (HNA) locus to chromosome 17 q24–q25. *Hum Genet* 1997;99:685–687.
446. Zeharia A, Mukamel M, Frishberg Y, et al. Benign plexus neuropathy in children. *J Pediatr* 1990;116:276–278.
447. Dyck PJ. Neuronal atrophy and degeneration predominantly affecting peripheral sensory and autonomic neurons. In: Dyck PJ, Thomas PK, Griffin JW, eds. *Peripheral neuropathy*, 3rd ed. Philadelphia: Saunders, 1993:1065–1093.
448. Nicholson GA, Dawkins JL, Blair IP, et al. The gene for hereditary sensory neuropathy type I (HSN-I) maps to chromosome 9q22.1–q22.3 *Nat Genet* 1996;13:101–104.
449. Bejaoui K, Uchida Y, Yasuda S, et al. Hereditary sensory neuropathy type 1 mutations confer dominant negative effects on serine palmitoyltransferase, critical for sphingolipid synthesis. *J Clin Invest* 2002;110:1301–1308.
450. Lafreniere RG, MacDonald ML, Dube MP, et al. Identification of a novel gene (*HSN2*) causing hereditary sensory and autonomic

neuropathy type II through the Study of Canadian Genetic Isolates. *Am J Hum Genet* 2004;74:1064–1073.
451. Davar G, Shalish C, Blumenfeld A, et al. Exclusion of p75NGFR and other candidate genes in a family with hereditary sensory neuropathy type II. *Pain* 1996;67:135–139.
452. Riley CM, Day RL, Greeley DM, et al. Central autonomic dysfunction with defective lacrimation. I. Report of five cases. *Pediatrics* 1949;3:468–478.
453. Dong J, Edelmann L, Bajwa AM, et al. Familial dysautonomia: detection of the IKBKAP IVS20(+6T→C) and R696P mutations and frequencies among Ashkenazi Jews. *Am J Med Genet* 2002;110:253–257.
454. Cuajungco MP, Leyne M, Mull J, et al. Tissue-specific reduction in splicing efficiency of IKBKAP due to the major mutation associated with familial dysautonomia. *Am J Hum Genet* 2003;72:749–758.
455. Mezey E, Parmalee A, Szalayova I, et al. Of splice and men: what does the distribution of IKAP mRNA in the rat tell us about the pathogenesis of familial dysautonomia? *Brain Res* 2003;983:209–214.
456. Nissim-Rafinia M, Kerem B. Splicing regulation as a potential genetic modifier. *Trends Genet* 2002;18:123–127.
457. Pearson J. Familial dysautonomia (a brief review). *J Auton Nerv Syst* 1979;1:119–126.
458. Pearson J, Brandeis L, Cuello AC. Depletion of substance-P-containing axons in substantia gelatinosa of patients with diminished pain sensitivity. *Nature* 1982;295:61–63.
459. Brown WJ, Beauchemin JA, Linde LM. A neuropathological study of familial dysautonomia (Riley-Day syndrome) in siblings. *J Neurol Neurosurg Psychiatry* 1964;27:131–139.
460. Pearson J, Dancis J, Axelrod F, Grover N. The sural nerve in familial dysautonomia. *J Neuropathol Exp Neurol* 1975;34:413–424.
461. Axelrod FB, Pearson J. Familial dysautonomia. In: Gomez MR, ed. *Neurocutaneous diseases: a practical approach*. Boston: Butterworth–Heinemann, 1987:200–208.
462. Linde LM, Westover JL. Esophageal and gastric abnormalities in dysautonomia. *Pediatrics* 1962;29:303–306.
463. Gadoth N, Mass E, Gordon CR, et al. Taste and smell in familial dysautonomia. *Dev Med Child Neurol* 1997;39:393–397.
464. Glickstein JS, Schwartzman D, Friedman D, et al. Abnormalities of the corrected QT interval in familial dysautonomia: an indicator of autonomic dysfunction. *J Pediatr* 1993;122:925–928.
465. Axelrod FB, Iyer K, Fish I, et al. Progressive sensory loss in familial dysautonomia. *Pediatrics* 1981;67:517–522.
466. Lahat E, Aladjem M, Mor A, et al. Brainstem auditory evoked potentials in familial dysautonomia. *Dev Med Child Neurol* 1992;34:690–693.
467. Goldberg MF, Payne JW, Brunt PW. Ophthalmologic studies of familial dysautonomia: the Riley-Day syndrome. *Arch Ophthalmol* 1968;80:732–743.
468. Udassin R, Seror D, Vinograd I, et al. Nissen fundoplication in the treatment of children with familial dysautonomia. *Am J Surg* 1992;164:332–336.
469. Goebel HH, Veit S, Dyck PJ. Confirmation of virtual unmyelinated fiber absence in hereditary sensory neuropathy type IV. *J Neuropathol Exp Neurol* 1980;39:670–674.
470. Edwards-Lee TA, Cornford ME, Yu KT. Congenital insensitivity to pain and anhidrosis with mitochondrial and axonal abnormalities. *Pediatr Neurol* 1997;17:356–361.
471. Johnsen SD, Johnson PC, Stein SR. Familial sensory autonomic neuropathy with arthropathy in Navajo children. *Neurology* 1993;43:1120–1125.
472. Donaghy M, Hakin RN, Bamford JM, et al. Hereditary sensory neuropathy with neurotrophic keratitis. *Brain* 1987;110:561–583.
473. Nagasako EM, Oaklander AL, Dworkin RH. Congenital insensitivity to pain: an update. *Pain* 2003;101:213–219.
474. Berg BO, Rosenberg SH, Asbury AK. Giant axonal neuropathy. *Pediatrics* 1972;49:894–899.
475. Bomont P, Cavalier L, Blondeau F, et al. The gene encoding gigaxonin, a new member of the cytoskeletal BTB/kelch repeat family, is mutated in giant axonal neuropathy. *Nat Genet* 2000;26:370–374.
476. Treiber-Held S, Budjarjo-Welim H, Riemann D, et al. Giant axonal neuropathy: a generalized disorder of intermediate filaments with longitudinal grooves in the hair. *Neuropediatrics* 1994;25:89–93.
477. Bruno C, Bertini E, Federico A, et al. Clinical and molecular findings in patients with giant axonal neuropathy (GAN). *Neurology* 2004;62:13–16.
478. Carpenter S, Karpati G, Andermann F, et al. Giant axonal neuropathy: a clinically and morphologically distinct neurological disease. *Arch Neurol* 1974;31:312–316.
479. Wolf SM, Verity MA. Neurological complications of progressive facial hemiatrophy. *J Neurol Neurosurg Psychiatry* 1974;37:997–1004.
480. Asher SW, Berg BO. Progressive hemifacial atrophy. *Arch Neurol* 1982;39:44–46.
481. Shah JR, Juhasz C, Kupsky WJ, et al. Rasmussen encephalitis associated with Parry-Romberg syndrome. *Neurology* 2003;61:395–397.
482. Wartenberg R. Progressive facial hemiatrophy. *Arch Neurol Psychiatr* 1945;54:75–97.
483. Dupont S, Catala M, Hasboun D, et al. Progressive facial hemiatrophy and epilepsy: a common underlying dysgenetic mechanism. *Neurology* 1997;48:1013–1018.
484. Fischel-Ghodsian N, Falk RE. Hereditary hearing impairment. In: Rimoin DL, Connor JM, Pyeritz RE, et al, eds. *Principles and practice of medical genetics*, 4th ed. New York: Churchill Livingstone, 2002:3637–3670.
485. Fraser GR. The causes of profound deafness in childhood. In: Wolstenholme GEW, Knight J, eds. *Sensorineural hearing loss*. London: Churchill, 1970:5–40.
486. Heckenlively JR, Daiger SP. Hereditary retinal and choroidal degenerations. In: Rimoin DL, Connor JM, Pyeritz RE, et al., eds. *Principles and practice of medical genetics*, 4th ed. New York: Churchill Livingstone, 2002:3555–3593.
487. Mosser J, Lutz Y, Stoeckel ME, et al. The gene responsible for adrenoleukodystrophy encodes a peroxisomal membrane protein. *Hum Mol Genet* 1994;3:265–171.
488. Stefkova J, Poledne R, Hubacek JA. ATP-binding casette (ABC) transporters in human metabolism and diseases. *Physiol Res* 2004;53:235–243.
489. Kemp J, Pujol A, Waterham HR, et al. *ABCD1* mutations and the X-linked adrenoleukodystrophy mutation database: role in diagnosis and clinical correlations. *Hum Mutat* 2001;18:499–515.
490. Dubois-Dalcq M, Feigenbaum V, Aubourg P. The neurobiology of X-linked adrenoleukodystrophy: a demyelinating peroxisomal disorder. *Trends Neurosci* 1999;22:4–12.
491. Korenke GC, Fuchs S, Krasemann E, et al. Cerebral adrenoleukodystrophy (ALD) in only one of monozygotic twins with an identical ALD genotype. *Ann Neurol* 1996;40:254–257.
492. Pahan K, Khan M, Singh I. Therapy for X-adrenoleukodystrophy: normalization of very-long-chain fatty acids and inhibition of induction of cytokines by cAMP. *J Lipid Res* 1998;39:1091–1100.
493. Schaumburg HH, Powers JM, Raine CS, et al. Adrenoleukodystrophy: a clinical and pathological study of 17 cases. *Arch Neurol* 1975;33:577–591.
494. Menkes JH, Corbo LM. Adrenoleukodystrophy: accumulation of cholesterol esters with very-long-chain fatty acids. *Neurology* 1977;27:928–932.
495. Kishimoto Y, Moser HW, Kawamura N, et al. Adrenoleukodystrophy: evidence that abnormal very-long-chain fatty acids of brain cholesterol tests are of exogenous origin. *Biochem Biophys Res Commun* 1980;96:69–76.
496. Moser HW, Moser AB, Smith KD, et al. Adrenoleukodystrophy: phenotypic variability and implications for therapy. *J Inherit Metab Dis* 1992;15:645–664.
497. Kirk EP, Fletcher JM, Sharp P, et al. X-linked adrenoleukodystrophy: the Australasian experience. *Am J Med Genet* 1998;76:420–423.
498. Wichers M, Kohler W, Brennemann W, et al. X-linked adrenomyeloneuropathy associated with 14 novel ALD-gene mutations: no correlation between type of mutation and age of onset. *Hum Genet* 1999;105:116–119.
499. Walsh PJ. Adrenoleukodystrophy: report of two cases with relapsing and remitting courses. *Arch Neurol* 1980;37:448–450.

500. Gartner J, Braun A, Holzinger A, et al. Clinical and genetic aspects of X-linked adrenoleukodystrophy. *Neuropediatrics* 1998;29:3–13.
501. Kumar AJ, Rosenbaum AE, Naidu S, et al. Adrenoleukodystrophy: correlating MR imaging with CT. *Radiology* 1987;165:497–504.
502. Rajanayagam V, Balthazor M, Shapiro EG, et al. Proton MR spectroscopy and neuropsychological testing in adrenoleukodystrophy. *Am J Neuroradiol* 1997;18:1909–1914.
503. Moloney JBM, Masterson JG. Detection of adrenoleukodystrophy carriers by means of evoked potentials. *Lancet* 1982;2:852–853.
504. O'Neill BP, Marmion LC, Feringa ER. The adrenoleukomyeloneuropathy complex: expression in four generations. *Neurology* 1981;31:151–156.
504a. Shaw-Smith CJ, Lewis SJ, Reid E. X-linked adrenoleukodystrophy presenting as autosomal dominant pure hereditary spastic paraparesis. *J Neurol Neurosurg Psychiatry* 2004;75:686–688.
505. Boehm CD, Cutting GR, Lachtermacher MB, et al. Accurate DNA-based diagnostic and carrier testing for X-linked adrenoleukodystrophy. *Mol Genet Metab* 1999;66:128–136.
506. van Geel BM, Assies J, Haverkort EB, et al. Progression of abnormalities in adrenomyeloneuropathy and neurologically asymptomatic X-linked adrenoleukodystrophy despite treatment with "Lorenzo's oil." *J Neurol Neurosurg Psychiatry* 1999;67:290–299.
507. Zinkham WH, Kickler T, Borel J, et al. Lorenzo's oil and thrombocytopenia in patients with adrenoleukodystrophy. *N Engl J Med* 1993;328:1126–1127.
508. Peters C, Charnas LR, Tan Y, et al. Cerebral X-linked adrenoleukodystrophy: the international hematopoietic cell transplantation experience from 1982 to 1999. *Blood* 2004;104:881–888.
509. Shapiro E, Krivit W, Lockman L, et al. Long-term effect of bone-marrow transplantation for childhood-onset cerebral X-linked adrenoleukodystrophy. *Lancet* 2000;356:713–718.
510. Kemp S, Wei HM, Lu JF, et al. Gene redundancy and pharmacological gene therapy: implications for X-linked adrenoleukodystrophy. *Nat Med* 1998;4:1261–1268.
511. McGuiness MC, Zhang HP, Smith KD. Evaluation of pharmacological induction of fatty acid beta-oxidation in X-linked adrenoleukodystrophy. *Mol Genet Metab* 2001;74:256–263.
512. Hooft DG, van Bogaert L, Guazzi GC. Sudanophilic leukodystrophy with meningeal angiomatosis in two brothers: infantile form of diffuse sclerosis with meningeal angiomatosis. *J Neurol Sci* 1965;2:30–51.
513. Pelizaeus F. Ueber eine eigentümliche Form spastischer Lähmung mit Cerebralerscheinungen auf hereditärer Grundlage. *Arch Psychiatr Nervenkr* 1885;16:698–710.
514. Merzbacher L. Eine eigenartige familiär-hereditäre Erkrankungsform. *Z Ges Neurol Psychiatry* 1910;3:1–138.
515. Seitelberger F. Pelizaeus-Merzbacher disease. In: Vinken PJ, Bruyn GW, eds. *Handbook of clinical neurology*, Vol. 10. New York: Elsevier North-Holland, 1970:150–202.
516. Boulloche J, Aicardi J. Pelizaeus-Merzbacher disease: clinical and nosological study. *J Child Neurol* 1986;1:233–239.
516a. Watanabe I, Patel V, Goebel HH, et al. Early lesion of Pelizaeus-Merzbacher disease: electron microscopic and biochemical study. *J Neuropathol Exp Neurol* 1973;32:313–333.
516b. Golomb MR. Walsh LE, Carvalho KS, et al. Clinical findings in Pelizaeus-Merzbacher disease. *J Child Neurol* 2004;19:328–331.
517. Koeppen AH, Robitaille Y. Peilizaeus-Merzbacher disease. *J Neuropathol Exp Neurol* 2002;61:747–759.
518. Sistermans EA, de Coo RF, De Wijs IJ, et al. Duplication of the proteolipid protein gene is the major cause of Pelizaeus-Merzbacher disease. *Neurology* 1998;50:1749–1754.
519. Hobson GM, Davis AP, Stowell NC, et al. Mutations in noncoding regions of the proteolipid protein gene in Pelizaeus-Merzbacher disease. *Neurology* 2000;55:1089–1096.
520. Shy ME, Hobson G, Jain M, et al. Schwann cell expression of PLP1 but not DM20 is necessary to prevent neuropathy. *Ann Neurol* 2003;53:354–365.
521. Southwood CM, Garbern J, Jiang W, et al. The unfolded protein response modulates disease severity in Pelizaeus-Merzbacher disease. *Neuron* 2002;36:585–596.
522. Forman MS, Lee VM, Trojanowski JQ. "Unfolding" pathways in neurodegenerative disease. *Trends Neurosci* 2003;26:407–410.
523. Gow A, Sharma R. The unfolded protein response in protein aggregating diseases. *Neuromolecular Med* 2003;4:73–94.
524. Kaufman RJ. Orchestrating the unfolded protein response in health and disease. *J Clin Invest* 2002;110:1389–1398.
525. Tyler HR. Pelizaeus-Merzbacher disease: a clinical study. *Arch Neurol Psychiatry* 1958;80:162–169.
526. Nezu A, Kimura S, Takeshita S, et al. An MRI and MRS study of Pelizaeus-Merzbacher disease. *Pediatr Neurol* 1998;18:334–337.
527. Iwaki A, Muramoto T, Iwaki I, et al. A missense mutation in the proteolipid protein gene responsible for Pelizaeus-Merzbacher disease in a Japanese family. *Hum Mol Genet* 1993;2:19–22.
528. Woodward K,Kendall E, Vetrie D, Malcolm S. Pelizaeus-Merzbacher disease: identification of Xq22 proteolipid-protein duplications and characterization of breakpoints by interphase FISH. *Am J Hum Genet* 1998;63:207–217.
529. Inoue K, Kanai M, Tanabe Y, et al. Prenatal interphase FISH diagnosis of *PLP1* duplication associated with Pelizaeus-Merzbacher disease. *Prenat Diagn* 2001;21:1133–136.
530. Lazzarini A, Schwarz KO, Jiang S, et al. Pelizaeus-Merzbacher-like disease: exclusion of the proteolipid protein locus and documentation of a new locus on Xq. *Neurology* 1997;49:824–832.
531. Canavan MM. Schilder's encephalitis periaxialis diffusa. *Arch Neurol Psychiatry* 1931;25:299–308.
532. Kaul R, Gao GP, Balamuragan K, et al. Cloning of the human aspartoacylase cDNA and a common missense mutation in Canavan's disease. *Nat Genet* 1993;5:118–123.
533. Matalon R, Matalon KM. Canavan disease. In: Rosenberg RN, Prusiner SB, DiMauro S, et al., eds. *The molecular basis of neurologic and psychiatric disease*, 3rd ed. Butterworth-Heinemann, Philadelphia, 2003:383–387.
534. Feigenbaum A, Moore R, Clarke J, et al. Canavan disease: carrier frequency determination in the Ashkenazi Jewish population and development of a novel molecular diagnostic assay. *Am J Med Genet* 2004;124:142–147.
535. Gascon GG, Ozand PT, Mahdi A, et al. Infantile CNS spongy degeneration—14 cases: clinical update. *Neurology* 1990;40:1876–1882.
536. Traeger EC, Rapin I. The clinical course of Canavan disease. *Pediatr Neurol* 1998;18:207–212.
537. Adachi M, Schneck L, Cara J, Volk BW. Spongy degeneration of the central nervous system (van Bogaert and Bertrand type; Canavan's disease): a review. *Hum Pathol* 1973;4:331–447.
538. Gambetti P, Mellman WJ, Gonatas NK. Familial spongy degeneration of the central nervous system (van Bogaert-Bertrand Disease). *Acta Neuropathol* 1969;12:103–115.
539. Banker BQ, Robertson JT, Victor M. Spongy degenerations of the central nervous system in infancy. *Neurology* 1964;14:981–1001.
540. Suzuki K. Peripheral nerve lesion in spongy degeneration of the central nervous system. *Acta Neuropathol* 1968;10:95–98.
541. Birken DL, Oldendorf WH. *N*-acetyl-L-aspartic acid: a literature review of a compound prominent in 1H NMR spectroscopic studies of brain. *Neurosci Biobehav Rev* 1989;13:23–31.
542. Barker PB, Bryan RN, Kumar AJ, Naidu S. Proton NMR spectroscopy of Canavan's disease. *Neuropediatrics* 1992;23:263–267.
543. Patel PJ, Kolawole TM, Mahdi AH, et al. Sonographic and computed tomographic findings in Canavan's disease. *Br J Radiol* 1986;59:1226–1228.
544. Alexander WS. Progressive fibrinoid degeneration of fibrillary astrocytes associated with mental retardation in hydrocephalic infant. *Brain* 1949;72:373–381.
545. Brenner M, Johnson AB, Boespflug-Tanguy O, et al. Mutations in *GFAP*, encoding glial fibrillary acidic protein, are associated with Alexander disease. *Nat Genet* 2001;27:117–124.
546. Li R, Johnson AB, Salomons GS, et al. Glial fibrillary acidic protein mutations in infantile, juvenile, and adult forms of Alexander disease. *Ann Neurol* 2005;57:310–326.
547. Pridmore CL, Baraitser M, Harding B, et al. Alexander's disease: clues to diagnosis. *J Child Neurol* 1993;8:134–144.
548. Springers, Erlewein R, Naegele T, et al. Alexander disease—classification revisited and isolation of a neonatal form. *Neuropediatrics* 2000;31:86–92.
549. Stumpf E, Masson H, Duquette A, et al. Adult Alexander disease with autosomal dominant transmission: a distinct entity

caused by mutation in the glial fibrillary protein gene. *Arch Neurol* 2003;60:1307–1312.
550. Castellani RJ, Perry G, Harris PL, et al. Advanced lipid peroxidation end-products in Alexander's disease. *Brain Res* 1998;787:15–18.
551. Iwaki T, Kume-Iwaki A, Liem RK, et al. α B-crystallin expressed in non-lenticular tissues and accumulates in Alexander's disease brains. *Cell* 1989;57:71–78.
552. van der Knaap MS, Naidu S, Breiter SN, et al. Alexander disease: diagnosis with MR imaging. *Am J Neuroradiol* 2001;22:541–552.
552a. van der Knaap MS, Salomons GS, Li R, et al. Unusual variants of Alexander disease. *Ann Neurol* 2005;57:327–338.
553. Shah M, Ross JS. Infantile Alexander disease: MR appearance of a biopsy-proven case. *Am J Neuroradiol* 1990;11:1105–1106.
554. Alzheimer A. Beiträge zur Kenntnis der pathologischen Neuroglia und ihrer Beziehungen zu den Abbauvorgängen im Nervengewebe. In: Nissl F, Alzheimer A, eds. *Histologische und histopathologische Arbeiten über die Grosshirnrinde*. Jena, Germany: Gustav Fischer, 1910;3:401–562.
555. Greenfield JG. A form of progressive cerebral sclerosis in infants associated with primary degeneration of the interfascicular glia. *J Neurol Psychopathol* 1933;13:289–302.
556. Austin J. Metachromatic sulfatides in cerebral white matter and kidney. *Proc Soc Exp Biol Med* 1959;100:361–364.
557. Austin JH, Balasubramanian AS, Pattabiraman TN, et al. A controlled study of enzymatic activities in three human disorders of glycolipid metabolism. *J Neurochem* 1963;10:805–816.
558. Jatzkewitz H, Mehl EL. Cerebrosidesulphatase and arylsulphatase: a deficiency in metachromatic leukodystrophy (ML). *J Neurochem* 1969;16:19–28.
559. Austin JH. Studies in metachromatic leukodystrophy. *Arch Neurol* 1973;28:258–264.
560. Kolodny EH, Neudorfer O. Metachromatic leukodystrophy and multiple sulfatase deficiency: sulfatide lipidosis. In: Rosenberg RN, Prusiner SB, DiMauro S, et al., eds. *The molecular basis of neurologic and psychiatric disease*, 3 rd ed. Butterworth–Heinemann, Philadelphia, 2003:247–253.
561. Polten A, Fluharty AL, Fluhart CB, et al. Molecular basis of different forms of metachromatic leukodystrophy. *N Engl J Med* 1991;324:18–22.
562. Barth ML, Fensom A, Harris A. Prevalence of common mutations in the arylsulphatase: a gene in metachromatic leukodystrophy patients diagnosed in Britain. *Hum Genet* 1993;91:73–77.
562a. Harvey JS, Carey WF, Morris CP. Importance of the glycosylation and polyadenylation variants in metachromatic leukodystrophy pseudodeficiency phenotype. *Hum Mol Genet* 1998;7:1215–1219.
563. Penzien JM, Kappler J, Herschkowitz N, et al. Compound heterozygosity for metachromatic leukodystrophy and arylsulfatase: a pseudodeficiency allele is not associated with progressive neurological disease. *Am J Hum Genet* 1993;52:557–564.
564. Zhang XL, Rafi MA, De Gala G, et al. The mechanism for a 33 nucleotide insertion in mRNA causing sphingolipid activator protein (SAP1) deficient metachromatic leukodystrophy. *Hum Genet* 1991;87:211–215.
565. O'Brien JS, Kishimoto Y. Saposin proteins: structure, function, and role in human lysosomal storage disorders. *FASEB J* 1991;5:301–308.
566. Gieselmann V. Metachromatic leukodystrophy: recent research developments. *J Child Neurol* 2003;18:591–594.
567. McFaul R. Metachromatic leucodystrophy: review of 38 cases. *Arch Dis Child* 1982;57:168–175.
568. Brown FR 3rd, Shimizu H, McDonald JM, et al. Auditory evoked brain stem response and high-performance liquid chromatography sulfatide assay as early indices of metachromatic leukodystrophy. *Neurology* 1981;31:980–985.
569. Kim TS, Kim IO, Kim WS, et al. MR of childhood metachromatic leukodystrophy. *Am J Neuroradiol* 1997;18:733–738.
570. Scholz W. Klinische, pathologische anatomische und erbiologische Untersuchungen bei familiärer diffuser Hirnsklerose im Kindesalter. *Z Ges Neurol Psychiat* 1925;99:651–717.
571. Menkes JH. Chemical studies of two cerebral biopsies in juvenile metachromatic leukodystrophy: the molecular composition of cerebroside and sulfatides. *J Pediatr* 1966;69:422–431.
572. Austin JH, Armstrong D, Fouch S, et al. Metachromatic leukodystrophy (MLD): VIII. MLD in adults: diagnosis and pathogenesis. *Arch Neurol* 1968;18:225–240.
573. Alves D, Pires MM, Guimaraes A, et al. Four cases of late onset metachromatic leucodystrophy in a family: clinical, biochemical and neuropathological studies. *J Neurol Neurosurg Psychiatry* 1986;49:1417–1422.
574. Cosma MP, Pepe S, Parenti G, et al. Molecular and functional analysis of *SUMF1* mutations in multiple sulfatase deficiency. *Hum Mutat* 2004;23:576–581.
575. Eto Y, Tahara T, Tokoro T, et al. Various sulfatase activities in leukocytes and cultured skin fibroblasts from heterozygotes for the multiple sulfatase deficiency (mukosulfatidosis). *Pediatr Res* 1983;17:97–100.
576. Kidd D, Nelson J, Jones F, et al. Long-term stabilization after bone marrow transplantation in juvenile metachromatic leukodystrophy. *Arch Neurol* 1998;55:98–99.
577. Beneke R. Ein Fall hochgradigster ausgedehnter Sklerose des Zentralnervensystem. *Arch Kinderheilk* 1908;47:420–422.
578. Krabbe K. A new familial infantile form of diffuse brain sclerosis. *Brain* 1996;39:74–114.
579. Norman RM, Oppenheimer DR, Tingey AH. Histological and chemical findings in Krabbe's leucodystrophy. *J Neurol Neurosurg Psychiatry* 1961;24:223–232.
580. Austin JH, Lehfeldt D. Studies in globoid (Krabbe) leukodystrophy: III. Significance of experimentally produced globoidlike elements in rat white matter and spleen. *J Neuropathol Exp Neurol* 1965;24:265–289.
581. Andrews JM, Cancilla PA, Grippo J, et al. Globoid cell leukodystrophy (Krabbe's disease): morphological and biochemical studies. *Neurology* 1971;21:337–352.
582. Martin JJ, Ceuterick C, Martin L, et al. Leucodystrophie à cellules globoïdes (maladie de Krabbe) lésions nerveuses périphériques. *Acta Neurol Belg* 1974;74:356–375.
583. Hager H, Oehlert W. Ist die diffuse Hirnsklerose des Typ Krabbe eine entzündliche Allgemeinerkrankung? *Z Kinderheilk* 1957;80: 82–96.
584. Kobayashi T, Shinoda H, Goto I, et al. Globoid cell leukodystrophy is a generalized galactosylsphingosine (psychosine) storage disease. *Biochem Biophys Res* 1987;144:41–46.
585. Wenger DA, Suzuki K, Suzuki Y, et al. Galactosylceramide lipidosis: globoid cell leukodystrophy (Krabbe's disease). In: Scriver CR, Beaudet AL, Sly WS, et al., eds. *The metabolic basis of inherited disease*, 8th ed. New York: McGraw-Hill, 2001:3669–3694.
586. Haq E, Giri S, Singh I, et al. Molecular mechanism of psychosine-induced cell death in human oligodendrocyte cell line. *J Neurochem* 2003;86:1428–1440.
587. De Gasperi R, Gama Sosa MA, Sartorato EL, et al. Molecular heterogeneity of late-onset forms of globoid cell leukodystrophy. *Am J Hum Genet* 1996;59:1233–1242.
588. Satoh JI, Tokumoto H, Kurohara K, et al. Adult-onset Krabbe disease with homozygous T1853C mutation in the galactocerebrosidase gene: unusual MRI findings of corticospinal tract demyelination. *Neurology* 1997;49:1392–1399.
589. Wenger DA. Krabbe disease: Globoid cell leukodystrophy. In: Rosenberg RN, Prusiner SB, DiMauro S, et al., eds. *The molecular basis of neurologic and psychiatric disease*, 3rd ed. Butterworth–Heinemann, Philadelphia, 2003:255–261.
590. Loonen MCB, Van Diggelen OP, Janse HC, et al. Late-onset of globoid cell leucodystrophy (Krabbe's disease): clinical and genetic delineation of two forms and their relation to the early-infantile form. *Neuropediatrics* 1985;16:137–142.
590a. Zarifi MK, Tzika AA, Astrakas LG, et al. Magnetic resonance spectroscopy and magnetic resonance imaging findings in Krabbe's disease. *J Child Neurol* 2001;16:522–526.
590b. van der Voorn JP, Pouwels PJ, Kamphorst W, et al. Histopathologic correlates of radial stripes on MR images in lysosomal storage disorders. *AJNR Am J Neuroradiol* 2005;26:442–446.
591. Krivit W, Shapiro EG, Peters C, et al. Hematopoietic stem-cell transplantation in globoid-cell leukodystrophy. *N Engl J Med* 1998;338:1119–1126.
592. Caniglia M, Rana I, Pinto RM, et al. Allogeneic bone marrow

transplantation for infantile globoid-cell leukodystrophy (Krabbe's disease). *Pediatr Transplant* 2002;6:427–431.
593. Woods CG. DNA repair disorders. *Arch Dis Child* 1998;78:178–184.
594. Cockayne EA. Dwarfism with retinal atrophy and deafness. *Arch Dis Child* 1936;11:1–8.
595. Van Den Boom V, Ciutterio K, Hoogstraten D, et al. DNA damage stabilizes interaction of CSB with the transcription elongation machinery. *J Cell Biol* 2004;166:27–36.
596. Licht CL, Stevsner T, Bohr VA. Cockayne syndrome group B cellular and biochemical function. *Am J Hum Genet* 2003;73:1217–1239.
597. Citterio E, Rademakers S, van der Horst GT, et al. Biochemical and biological characterization of wild-type and ATPase-deficient Cockayne syndrome B repair protein. *J Biol Chem* 1998;273:11844–11851.
598. Vermeulen W, Jaeken J, Jaspers NG, et al. Xeroderma pigmentosum complementation group G associated with Cockayne syndrome. *Am J Hum Genet* 1993;53:185–192.
599. Wood RD. DNA repair in eukaryotes. *Annu Rev Biochem* 1996;65: 135–167.
600. Rapin I, Lindenbaum Y, Dickson DW, et al. Cockayne syndrome and xeroderma pigmentosum. *Neurology* 2000;55:1442–1449.
601. Özdirim E, Topku M, Ozon A, et al. Cockayne syndrome: review of 25 cases. *Pediatr Neurol* 1996;15:312–316.
602. Nance MA, Berry SA. Cockayne syndrome: review of 140 cases. *Am J Med Genet* 1992;42:68–84.
603. Sugita K, Takanashi J, Ishii M, et al. Comparison of MRI white matter changes with neuropsychologic impairment in Cockayne syndrome. *Pediatr Neurol* 1992;8:295–298.
604. Moossy J. The neuropathology of Cockayne's syndrome. *J Neuropathol Exp Neurol* 1967;26:654–660.
605. Sugita K, Suzuki N, Kojima T, et al. Cockayne syndrome with delayed recovery of RNA synthesis after ultraviolet irradiation but normal ultraviolet survival. *Pediatr Res* 1987;21:34–37.
606. Butler IJ. Xeroderma pigmentosum. In: Rosenberg RN, Prusiner JB, DiMauro S, et al. *The molecular and genetic basis of neurological disease*, 2 nd ed. Boston: Butterworth–Heinemann, 1997:959–967.
607. Kanda T, Oda M, Yonezawa M, et al. Peripheral neuropathy in xeroderma pigmentosum. *Brain* 1990;113:1025–1044.
608. Mimaki T, Itoh N, Abe J, et al. Neurological manifestations in xeroderma pigmentosum. *Ann Neurol* 1986;20:70–75.
609. Graham JM, Hennekam R, Dobyns WB, et al. MICRO syndrome: an entity distinct from COFS syndrome. *Am J Med Genet* 2004;128:235–245.
610. van der Knaap MS, Barth PG, Gabreels FJ, et al. A new leukoencephalopathy with vanishing white matter. *Neurology* 1997;48:845–855.
611. van der Knaap MS, Leegwater PAJ, Könst AAM, et al. Mutations in each of the five subunits of translation initiation factor eIF2B can cause leukoencephalopathy with vanishing white matter. *Ann Neurol* 2002;51:264–270.
612. Brück W, Herms J. Brockmann K, et al. Myelinopathia centralis diffusa (vanishing white matter disease): evidence of apoptotic oligodendrocyte degeneration in early lesion development. *Ann Neurol* 2001;50:532–536.
613. Fogli A, Schiffmann R, Bertini E, et al. The effect of genotype on the natural history of eIF2B-related leukodystrophies. *Neurology* 2004;62:1509–1517.
614. Kristjansdottir R, Uvebrant P, Hagberg B, et al. Disorders of the cerebral white matter in children: the spectrum of lesions. *Neuropediatrics* 1996;27:295–298.
615. Singhal BS, Gursahani RD, Udani VP, et al. Megalencephalic leukodystrophy in an Asian Indian ethnic group. *Pediatr Neurol* 1996;14:291–296.
616. Gorospe JR, Singhal BS, Kainu T, et al. Indian Agarwal megalencephalic leukodystrophy with cysts is caused by a common *MLC1* mutation. *Neurology* 2004;62:878–882.
616a. Henneke M, Preuss N, Engelbrecht V, et al. Cystic leukoencephalopathy with megalencephaly. A distinct disease entity in 15 children. *Neurology* 2005;64:1411–1416.
617. Woolf NI, Willemsen MA, Engelke UF, et al. Severe hypomyelination associated with increased levels of *N*-acetylaspartylglutamate in CSF. *Neurology* 2004;62:1503–1508.
618. van der Knaap MS, Naidu S, Pouwels PJ, et al. New syndrome characterized by hypomyelination with atrophy of the basal ganglia. *Am J Neuroradiol* 2002;23:1466–1474.
619. Schiffmann R, van der Knaap MS. The latest on leukodystrophies. *Curr Opin Neurol* 2004;17:187–192.
620. Serkov SV, Pronin IN, Bykova OV, et al. Five patients with a recently described novel leukoencephalopathy with brainstem and spinal cord involvement and elevated lactate. *Neuropediatrics* 2004;35:1–5.
621. Gripp KW, Zimmerman RA, Wang CJ, et al. Imaging studies in a unique familial dysmyelinating disorder. *Am J Neuroradiol* 1998;19:1368–1372.
622. Olivier M, Lenard HG, Aksu F, et al. A new leukoencephalopathy with bilateral anterior temporal lobe cysts. *Neuropediatrics* 1998;29:225–228.
623. Battini R, Bianchi MC, Tosetti M, et al. Leukoencephalopathy with bilateral anterior temporal lobe cysts: a further case of this new entity. *J Child Neurol* 2002;17:773–776.
624. Nagae-Poetscher LM, Bibat G, Philippart M, et al. Leukoencephalopathy, cerebral calcifications, and cysts: new observations. *Neurology* 2004;62:1206–1209.
625. Seitelberger F, Gross H. Ueber eine spätinfantile Form der Hallervorden-Spatzschen Krankheit. II. Histochemische Befunde, Erörterung der Nosologie. *Dtsch Z Nervenheilk* 1957;176:104–125.
626. Aicardi J, Castelein P. Infantile neuroaxonal dystrophy. *Brain* 1979;102:727–748.
626a. Gordon N. Infantile neuroaxonal dystrophy (Seitelberger's disease). *Dev Med Child Neurol* 2002;44:849–851.
627. Tanabe Y, Iai M, Ishii M, et al. The use of magnetic resonance imaging in diagnosing infantile neuroaxonal dystrophy. *Neurology* 1993;43:110–113.
628. Sener RN. Diffusion magnetic resonance imaging in infantile neuroaxonal dystrophy. *J Comput Assist Tomogr* 2003;27:34–37.
629. Ferreira RC, Mierau GW, Bateman JB. Conjunctival biopsy in infantile neuroaxonal dystrophy. *Am J Ophthalmol* 1997;123:264–266.
630. Ramaekers VT, Lake BD, Harding B, et al. Diagnostic difficulties in infantile neuroaxonal dystrophy. *Neuropediatrics* 1987;18:170–175.
631. Williamson K, Sima AA, Curry B, et al. Neuroaxonal dystrophy in young adults: a clinicopathological study of two unrelated cases. *Ann Neurol* 1982;11:335–343.
631a. Hörtnagel K, Nardocci N, Zorzi G, et al. Infantile neuroaxonal dystrophy and pantothenate kinase–associated neurodegeneration. Locus heterogeneity. *Neurology* 2004;63:922–924.
632. Rett A. Ueber ein eigenartiges hirnatrophisches Syndrom bei Hyperammonamie im Kindesalter. *Wien Med Wochenschr* 1966;116:723–726.
633. Sirianni N, Naidu S, Pereira J, et al. Rett syndrome: confirmation of X-l inked dominant inheritance and localization of the gene to Xq28. *Am J Hum Genet* 1998;63:1552–1558.
634. Amir RE, Van den Veyver IB, Wan M, et al. Rett syndrome is caused by mutations in X-linked *MECP2*, encoding methyl-CpG-binding protein 2. *Nat Genet* 1999;23:185–188.
635. Fuks F, Hurd PJ, Wolff D, et al. The methyl-CpG-binding protein MeCP2 links DNA methylation to histone methylation. *J Biol Chem* 2002;278:4035–4040.
636. Hendrich B, Bird A. Identification and characterization of a family of methyl-pG-binding proteins. *Mol Cell Biol* 1998;18:6538–6547.
637. Mittenberger-Miltenyi G, Laccone F. Mutations and polymorphisms in the human methyl CpG-binding protein MECP2. *Hum Mutat* 2003;22:107–115.
638. Topcu M, Akyerli C, Sayi A., et al. Somatic mosaicism of a *MECP2* mutation associated with classic Rett syndrome in a boy. *Eur J Hum Genet* 2002;77–81.
639. Naidu S. Rett syndrome: a disorder affecting early brain growth. *Ann Neurol* 1997;42:3–10.
640. Villard L, Levy N, Xiang F, et al. Segregation of a totally skewed pattern of X chromosome inactivation in four familial cases of Rett syndrome without *MECP2* mutation: implications for the disease. *J Med Genet* 2001;38:435–442.
641. Ronnett GV, Leopold D, Cai X, et al. Olfactory biopsies demonstrate a defect in neuronal development in Rett's syndrome. *Ann Neurol* 2003;54:206–218.

642. Baumann ML, Kemper TL, Arin DM. Pervasive neuroanatomic abnormalities of the brain in three cases of Rett syndrome. *Neurology* 1995;45:1581–1586.
643. Armstrong DD, Dunn K, Antalffy B. Decreased dendritic branching in frontal, motor and limbic cortex in Rett syndrome compared with trisomy 21. *J Neuropathol Exp Neurol* 1998;57:1013–1017.
644. Schanen C, Houwink EJ, Dorrani N, et al. Phenotypic manifestations of *MECP2* mutations in classical and atypical Rett syndrome. *Am J Med Genet* 2004;126A:129–140.
645. The Rett Syndrome Diagnostic Criteria Work Group. Diagnostic criteria for Rett syndrome. *Ann Neurol* 1988;23:425–428.
646. Hagberg B, Aicardi J, Dias K, et al. A progressive syndrome of autism, dementia, ataxia, and loss of purposeful hand use in girls: Rett's syndrome—report of 35 cases. *Ann Neurol* 1983;14:471–479.
647. Glaze DG, Frost JD Jr, Zoghbi HY, et al. Rett's syndrome: characterization of respiratory patterns and sleep. *Ann Neurol* 1987;21:377–382.
648. Nihei K, Naitoh H. Cranial computed tomographic and magnetic resonance imaging studies on the Rett syndrome. *Brain Dev* 1990;12:101–105.
649. Hoffbuhr K, Devaney JM, LaFleur B, et al. *MeCP2* mutations in children with and without the phenotype of Rett syndrome. *Neurology* 2001;56:1486–1495.
650. Dotti MT, Orrico A, De Stefano N, et al. A Rett syndrome *MECP2* mutation that causes mental retardation in men. *Neurology* 2002;58:226–230.
651. Alpers BJ. Diffuse progressive degeneration of the cerebral gray matter. *Arch Neurol Psychiatry* 1931;25:469–505.
652. Ford FR, Livingston S, Pryles CV. Familial degeneration of the cerebral gray matter in childhood, with convulsions, myoclonus, spasticity, cerebellar ataxia, choreoathetosis, dementia, and death in status epilepticus: differentiation of infantile and juvenile types. *J Pediatr* 1951;39:33–43.
653. Sung JH, Ramirez-Lassepas M, Mastri AR, et al. An unusual degenerative disorder of neurons associated with a novel intranuclear hyaline inclusion (neuronal intranuclear hyaline inclusion disease). *J Neuropathol Exp Neurol* 1980;39:107–130.
654. Takahashi-Fujigasaki J. Neuronal intranuclear hyaline inclusion disease. *Neuropathology* 2003;23:351–359.
655. Goutières F, Mikol J, Aicardi J. Neuronal intranuclear inclusion disease in a child: diagnosis by rectal biopsy. *Ann Neurol* 1990;27:103–106.
656. Kulikova-Schupak R, Knupp KG, Pascual JM, et al. Rectal biopsy in the diagnosis of neuronal intranuclear hyaline inclusion disease. *J Child Neurol* 2004;19:59–62.
657. Wilson DC, McGibben D, Hicks EM, et al. Progressive neuronal degeneration of childhood (Alpers syndrome) with hepatic cirrhosis. *Eur J Pediatr* 1993;152:260–262.
658. Harding BN. Progressive neuronal degeneration of childhood with liver disease (Alpers-Huttenlocher syndrome): a personal review. *J Child Neurol* 1990;5:273–287.
659. Naviaux RK. Mitochondrial DNA polymerase α-deficiency and mtDNA depletion in a child with Alpers' syndrome. *Ann Neurol* 1999;45:54–58.

Chapter 4

Chromosomal Anomalies and Contiguous-Gene Syndromes

John H. Menkes and Rena E. Falk

This chapter considers conditions that develop as a result of chromosomal abnormalities. Abnormalities of chromosomes are either constitutional or acquired. Acquired chromosomal abnormalities develop postnatally, affect only one clone of cells, and are implicated in the evolution of neoplasia. Constitutional abnormalities, on the other hand, develop during gametogenesis or early embryogenesis and affect a significant portion of an individual's cells. Until recently, detection of constitutional abnormalities was limited to disorders that resulted in gains or losses of an entire chromosome or large portions thereof—abnormalities readily visible by standard cytogenetics. The smallest loss or gain visible with standard cytogenetic preparations is about 4 megabases (Mb) of DNA (1). The introduction of chromosomal banding techniques with increasing degrees of resolution, the widespread use of fluorescence *in situ* hybridization (FISH), and supplemental molecular analyses have refined cytogenetic analysis and have permitted detection of uniparental disomies and innumerable subtle, often submicroscopic (cryptogenic), deletions, duplications, or translocations. This has removed any clear dividing line between changes considered to be chromosomal abnormalities and those considered to be molecular defects (1). Because in humans more than 30,000 genes are expressed in brain, it comes as no surprise that impaired brain function is the most common symptom of chromosomal anomalies.

In considering the significance of some of the subtle chromosomal abnormalities, one must keep in mind that many of the abnormal chromosomal constitutions have been ascertained by searching the genome of mentally or neurologically handicapped individuals with multiple congenital abnormalities, thus introducing an obvious sampling bias. To complicate matters, chromosomal abnormalities are seen in only a fraction of handicapped individuals, whereas a sizable proportion of healthy adults have been found to have chromosomal variants. These include variations in Y chromosomal length, variations in satellite size or location, and variations in size of secondary constrictions as well as some forms of mosaicism, balanced translocations, and differences in the intensity and appearance of bands revealed by staining techniques. Small supernumerary chromosomes (*marker chromosomes*) may serve as a case in point. This abnormality is seen in 0.3 to 1.2 of 1,000 newborns and in 0.7 to 1.5 of 1,000 fetuses on amniocentesis. Even though the origin of the marker chromosome may be ascertained by FISH, for the purpose of genetic counseling, the prognosis of the marker is still uncertain in many cases (2).

An evaluation of the relationship of chromosomal abnormalities to neurologic deficits can be achieved by controlled, blind-coded cytogenetic surveys in groups of unclassifiable individuals with mental retardation and control individuals. One such study published in 1977 and using routine cytogenetics detected chromosomal abnormalities in 6.2% of patients with mental retardation and 0.7% of controls (3). Using banding techniques, Jacobs and colleagues found a 0.92% prevalence of structural chromosomal abnormalities in unselected newborns (4). Small chromosomal rearrangements affecting the telomeres (the specialized structure at the tips of chromosomes) have been detected in some 5% of individuals with mental retardation and in up to 7.4% of individuals with moderate to severe mental retardation (5,6). This relatively high yield prompts the use of such techniques in the investigation of children with global developmental delay, even in the absence of dysmorphic features (7). However, the cost of a systematic surveillance of the newborn population using high-resolution chromosomal banding, DNA polymorphisms, and subtelomeric FISH panels remains prohibitive.

The limitations of prenatal and neonatal surveillance programs are discussed more fully by Hook and colleagues (8). Studies in other species, as well as in humans, have shown that major duplications or deficiencies in autosomes tend to be lethal (9), with death occurring either *in utero* or in the immediate postnatal period (10). Few of the autosomal trisomies are compatible with survival.

Thus, the most common trisomy, that of chromosome 16, accounts for 7.5% of all spontaneous abortions but is not compatible with live birth, and only 2.8% of trisomy 13, 5.4% of trisomy 18, and 23.8% of trisomy 21 cases are live born (8).

This chapter is confined to the neurologic sequelae of chromosomal abnormalities. For the basic principles of cytogenetics and more detailed phenotypes of chromosomal disorders consult one of several excellent monographs (11–14).

AUTOSOMAL ABNORMALITIES

Down Syndrome (Trisomy 21)

Down syndrome (trisomy 21), the most common autosomal anomaly in live births and the most common single cause of mental retardation, was first differentiated from other forms of mental retardation in 1866 by Down (15) and Seguin (16). Demographic factors, notably the higher proportion of older women bearing children, has caused an increase in the incidence of this condition. However, prenatal diagnosis programs also have affected the incidence. The most recent figures in the United States (1997) indicate an incidence of 9.9 per 10,000 live births, and 43% occur in births to women aged 35 years and older (17). This is significantly less than the incidence of 1 in 500 recorded in 1950, and reflects the effectiveness of prenatal screening programs (18).

Etiology and Pathogenesis

Down syndrome is associated with either an extra chromosome 21 or an effective trisomy for chromosome 21 by its translocation to another chromosome, usually chromosome 14, or, less often, to another acrocentric chromosome, especially chromosome 21 or 22 (19).

A few terms require definition. In the general population about 1 couple in 500 carries a reciprocal translocation. A *reciprocal translocation* is a structural alteration of chromosomes that usually results from breakage of two chromosomes with the subsequent exchange of the resultant chromosomal segments. In general, this event occurs most frequently at prophase of the first meiotic cell division. The segments exchanged are nearly always from nonhomologous chromosomes and are usually not the same size. Such an rearrangement is said to be *balanced* when none of the chromosomal material appears to be duplicated or deleted on standard or high-resolution analysis.

Robertsonian translocation results from centromeric fusion of two acrocentric chromosomes. A larger chromosome is formed, with the resultant loss of the short-arm regions of the participating chromosomes, resulting in a complement of 45 chromosomes in the *balanced carrier.* In a survey that was based on prenatal genetic studies performed with banding the frequency of balanced chromosomal rearrangements was 1 in 250 or 0.4%. Reciprocal translocations were seen in 0.17%, inversions in 0.12%, and Robertsonian translocations in 0.11% (19a). On a clinical basis, it is impossible to distinguish between patients with Down syndrome caused by ordinary trisomy 21 and those caused by translocation. The frequency of trisomy 21 increases with maternal age and reaches an incidence of 1 in 54 births in mothers aged 45 years or older (20). In contrast to ordinary trisomy, the incidence of translocation Down syndrome is independent of maternal age. Most translocations producing Down syndrome arise *de novo* in the affected child and are not associated with familial Down syndrome. Data obtained between 1989 and 1993 on prenatal and postnatal diagnoses of 1,811 Down syndrome children born to mothers aged 29 years or younger show regular trisomy 21 in 90.8% (19). Of a group of 235 translocation Down syndrome individuals, 42% of cases involved a translocation between chromosome 21 and chromosome 14, whereas 38% showed a translocation involving two 21 chromosomes. In translocation patients for whom cytogenetic results were available from both parents, 21;21 translocations were almost invariably *de novo*, whereas 37% of 14;21 translocations were inherited from the mother and 4% derived from the father (19). Of 51 cases of 21;21 translocation investigated, 50 were *de novo* and one was of maternal origin (19).

Approximately 1% of couples experience the recurrence of Down syndrome as a result of regular trisomy 21. In most instances, this is caused by previously unrecognized mosaicism in one parent (21). In families in whom Down syndrome results from a translocation, the risk for subsequent affected children is significantly higher; it is 15% if the mother is the carrier, but less than 5% if the father is the translocation carrier (22).

By the use of polymorphic DNA markers, several studies have concluded that the extra chromosome is maternally derived and mainly is the consequence of errors in the first meiotic division in more than 90% of cases (23). The mean maternal age associated with errors in meiosis is approximately 33 years, significantly higher than the mean reproductive age in the United States. In 4.3%, there were errors in paternal meiosis. In these cases, and in the remainder, caused by errors in mitosis, maternal age is not increased (24). Several explanations have been put forth to account for the maternal age effect. With increasing age there are a decreasing number of chiasmata, that is, crossovers, sites where recombination occurs because of breakage and reunion between homologous chromosomes (25). The most likely hypothesis is that the decrease in chiasmata contributes to nondisjunction by disrupting the process of separation of the chromosomal homologues.

To understand the molecular pathogenesis of Down syndrome, two questions must be answered: (a) How does

TABLE 4.1 Genes Localized to Chromosome 21 Believed to Affect Brain Development, Neuronal Loss, and Alzheimer's Type Pathology

Symbol	Name	Possible Effect in Down Syndrome
SIM2	Single-minded homologue 2 (*Drosophila*)	Brain development: required for synchronized cell division and establishment of proper cell lineage
DYRK1A	Dual-specificity tyrosine-(Y)-phosphorylation–regulated kinase 1A	Brain development: expressed during neuroblast proliferation and believed to be an important homologue in regulation of cell-cycle kinetics during cell division
GART	Phosphoribosylglycinamide formyltransferase Phosphoribosylglycinamide synthetase Phosphoribosylaminoimidazole synthetase	Brain development: expressed during prenatal development of the cerebellum
PCP4	Purkinje cell protein 4	Brain development: function unknown but found exclusively in the brain and most abundantly in the cerebellum
DSCAM	Down syndrome cell adhesion molecule	Brain development and possible candidate gene for congenital heart disease: expressed in all regions of the brain and believed to have a role in axonal outgrowth during development of the nervous system
GRIK1	Glutamate receptor, Ionotropic, kainite 1	Neuronal loss: function unknown, found in the cortex in fetal and early postnatal life and in adult primates, most concentrated in pyramidal cells in the cortex
APP	Amyloid beta (A4) precursor protein (protease nexin-II, Alzhelmer disease)	Alzheimer type neuropathy: seems to be involved in plasticity, neurite outgrowth, and neuroprotection
S100B	S100 calcium-binding protein, beta (neural)	Alzheimer type neuropathy: stimulates glial proliferation
SOD1	Superoxide dismutase 1, soluble (amyotrophic lateral sclerosis, adult)	Accelerated aging? Scavenges free superoxide molecules in the cell and might, accelerate aging by producing hydrogen peroxide and oxygen

From Roizen NJ, Patterson D. Down syndrome. *Lancet* 2003;361:1281–1289. With permission of the authors.

the presence of a small acrocentric chromosome in triplicate and the increased expression of genes on this chromosome produce the anatomic and functional abnormalities of the Down syndrome phenotype, and (b) are we able to identify specific regions of chromosome 21 whose duplication is responsible for each of the phenotypic features of Down syndrome?

The sequencing of chromosome 21 has resulted in the identification of more than 300 genes, of which at least 165 have been confirmed experimentally (26). Of these at least 9 are believed to affect brain development and function (Table 4.1). Studies on individuals with partial trisomy 21 have suggested that overexpression and subsequent interactions of genes on chromosome 21q22 contribute significantly to the phenotype of Down syndrome (25,27). Two genes in this region have received particular attention. The gene for a Down syndrome cell adhesion molecule (DSCAM) is expressed in the developing nervous system, and, like other cell adhesion molecules, this molecule is critical for cellular migration, axon guidance, and the formation of neural connections (see Chapter 5) (25). Another gene localized to the 21q22 region is that for DYRK1A, a serine/threonine protein kinase, required for postembryonic proliferation of neuronal cell types. The overexpression of this gene is believed to interfere with postembryonic neurogenesis (27). However, the 21q22 region can hardly be considered "critical" for the production of the clinical syndrome, and duplication of genes in regions distinct from 21q22 are believed to be responsible for many of the typical Down syndrome features (28).

It also is not known how the presence of extra copies of genes and their regulatory sequences produces the Down syndrome phenotype. Although, on a theoretical basis, one would expect gene product levels 1.5 times normal, this is not always the case. For example, expression of the amyloid precursor protein (APP) is approximately four times normal in the brains of patients with Down syndrome (29). Its role in the development of early-onset Alzheimer disease in patients with Down syndrome is considered in the subsequent section.

Pathology

Malformations affect principally the heart and the great vessels. Approximately 20% to 60% of Down syndrome individuals have congenital heart disease. Defects in the atrioventricular septum were the most common abnormalities encountered by Rowe and Uchida in 36% of their patients, most of whom were younger than 2 years of age (30). A ventricular septal defect was present in 33% and a patent ductus arteriosus was present in 10% of patients. Among the other malformations, gastrointestinal anomalies were the most common. These included duodenal stenosis or atresia, anal atresia, and megacolon. Hirschsprung disease was seen in approximately 6% of patients (31).

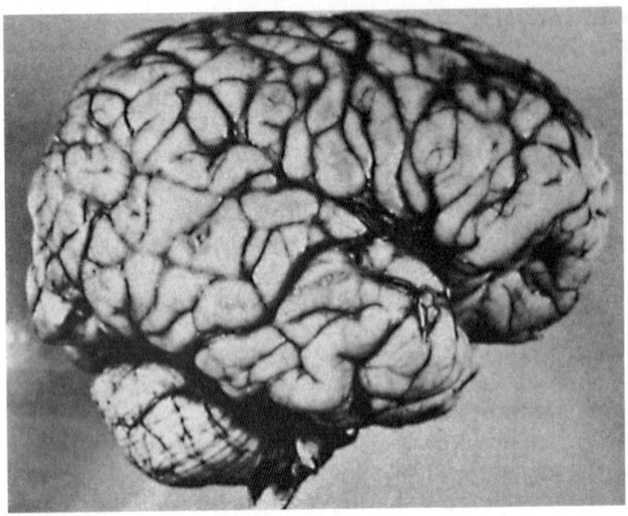

FIGURE 4.1. Lateral view of the brain of a 10-year-old boy with Down syndrome showing the typical small superior temporal gyrus and the large operculum. (From Lemire RJ, Loeser JD, Alvord C. *Normal and abnormal development of the human nervous system*. Hagerstown, MD: Harper & Row, 1975. With permission.)

Malformations of the spine, particularly of the upper cervical region, can occasionally produce neurologic symptoms. These are considered at another point of this chapter.

Grossly, the brain is small and spherical, and the frontal lobes, brainstem, and cerebellum are smaller than normal. The number of secondary sulci is generally reduced, the tuber flocculi persist, and the superior temporal gyrus is poorly developed (Fig. 4.1). A number of microscopic abnormalities also have been described (32,33). In essence, these involve reduction of neuronal density in various areas of the cortex, a loss of cortical interneurons, an accumulation of undifferentiated fetal cells in the cerebellum, and a reduction in the number of spines along the apical dendrites of pyramidal neurons, believed to indicate a reduction in the number of synaptic contacts (34). Interestingly, the dendritic tree is greater than normal in early infancy, but the excessive early outgrowth is followed by atrophy (35). Becker and colleagues explained these observations as an abortive attempt by neurons to compensate for the decreased number of spines and synapses on their receptive surfaces (35).

Abnormalities of the basal nucleus have received particular attention because an early and significant loss of cholinergic neurons in this area is a feature of both Down syndrome and Alzheimer disease. In Down syndrome the cell count is one-third normal, even before the onset of dementia, and it decreases progressively with age (36).

The most intriguing neuropathologic observation is the premature development of changes within the brain compatible with a morphologic diagnosis of Alzheimer disease. The spatial pattern of involvement of the brain by senile plaques and tangles follows that seen in Alzheimer disease. Thus, the amygdala, hippocampus, and the association areas of the frontal, temporal, and parietal cortex are particularly vulnerable to these changes (37). They are found in 15% of patients with Down syndrome aged 11 to 20 years, in 36% of patients aged 21 to 30 years, and in all patients who died aged 31 years or older (38). Microscopic alterations include pigmentary degeneration of neurons, senile plaques, and calcium deposits within the hippocampus, basal ganglia, and cerebellar folia. The calcium deposits in the cerebellar folia can be extensive enough to be seen on neuroimaging studies. As in Alzheimer disease, the brains of individuals with Down syndrome have reduced choline acetyltransferase activity, not only in areas that contain plaques, but also in those that appear microscopically normal (39,40).

Underlying the evolution of Alzheimer disease in children with Down syndrome is an excessive buildup of amyloid β-protein (AβP). This buildup is believed to be the consequence of an overexpression of the gene for amyloid β precursor protein (AβPP), mapped to chromosome 21q21. AβPP is cleaved to form AβP through the sequential action of beta-secretase and gamma-secretase. The gene for beta-secretase is also located on chromosome 21q22, and levels of this enzyme are significantly higher in Down syndrome fetal tissue than in controls, an indication that this gene is also overexpressed in Down syndrome (41). Cleavage of AβP by beta-secretase produces Aβ40, a soluble intracellular form, and plasma and tissue levels of soluble Aβ40 are higher in individuals with Down syndrome than in controls (42,43). Longer, less soluble forms, Aβ42 and Aβ43, are produced by the action of gamma-secretase, and Aβ42 is present in the brain of fetuses affected with Down syndrome as early as 21 weeks' gestation (44,45). These insoluble aggregates of AβP readily form fibrils and are responsible for the ultimate appearance of both senile plaques and amyloid deposits in cerebral blood vessels (46). Why the appearance of plaques and amyloid deposits is delayed for decades after the appearance of Aβ42 remains unclear. Also unclear is the role played by mitochondrial dysfunction in the abnormal processing of AβPP (47).

Clinical Manifestations

The clinical picture of Down syndrome is protean and consists of an unusual combination of anomalies rather than a combination of unusual anomalies (22). The condition is seen more frequently in male individuals, with one study showing a male-to-female ratio of 1.23 to 1, but in mosaic individuals the male-to-female ratio is 0.8 to 1 (19).

The birth weight of Down syndrome infants is less than normal, and 20% weigh 2.5 kg or less (48). Neonatal complications are more common than normal, a consequence of fetal hypotonia and a high incidence of breech presentations. Physical growth is consistently delayed, and the

TABLE 4.2 Intellectual Functioning of Children with Down Syndrome

Age (Yr)		Mean	Standard Deviation	Range
0–1	Developmental quotient	65	±15	27–100
1–2	Developmental quotient	51	±11	23–73
2–3	Developmental quotient	46	±8	32–55
3–4	Intelligence quotient	43	±16	10–55
4–9	Intelligence quotient	43	±7	10–61

Modified from Smith GF, Berg JM. *Down's anomaly,* 2nd ed. Edinburgh: Churchill Livingstone, 1976. With permission.

adult Down syndrome individual has a significantly short statue (49). The mental age that is ultimately achieved varies considerably. It is related in part to environmental factors, including the age at institutionalization for non–home-reared individuals, the degree of intellectual stimulation, and the evolution of presenile dementia even before puberty. As a rule, the developmental quotient (DQ) is higher than the IQ and decreases with age (Table 4.2) (50). Most older patients with Down syndrome have IQs between 25 and 49, with the average approximately 43. The social adjustment tends to be approximately 3 years ahead of that expected for the mental age (50). Del Bo and coworkers found that the decline in full-scale IQ with age was faster in those individuals who carry the apolipoprotein E4 allele, an important risk factor for both sporadic and familial late-onset Alzheimer disease (51).

Mosaicism can be found in approximately 2% to 3% of patients with Down syndrome. In these instances, the patient exhibits a mixture of trisomic and normal cell lines. As a group, these individuals tend to achieve somewhat higher intellectual development than nonmosaic individuals, and, in particular, they possess better verbal and visual-perceptual skills (52).

Aside from mental retardation, specific neurologic signs are rare and are limited to generalized muscular hypotonia and hyperextensibility of the joints. This is particularly evident during infancy and occurs to a significant degree in 44% of patients younger than 9 years of age (53).

Whereas major motor seizures are seen no more frequently in Down syndrome infants than in the general population, the association between infantile spasms and Down syndrome is greater than chance (54). Attacks can occur spontaneously or, less often, follow insults such as perinatal hypoxia. The electroencephalogram (EEG) demonstrates hypsarrhythmia or modified hypsarrhythmia (55). In the experience of Nabbout and coworkers a 6-month course of vigabatrin monotherapy has been effective, and with prompt treatment the prognosis for seizure control and preservation of intelligence is relatively good (54,56). In the experience of Stafstrom and Konkol, only 3 of 16 patients with Down syndrome with infantile spasms had persistent seizures, and the degree of cognitive impairment did not exceed that expected for the general Down syndrome population (55). A progressive disorganization of the EEG accompanies the evolution of Alzheimer dementia (57). Neuroimaging characteristically reveals large opercula, an indication of the underdeveloped superior temporal gyrus, and, in older patients, evidence exists of premature aging (58). Symmetric calcifications in basal ganglia, notably in the globus pallidus, are common, particularly in adults (59,60).

Numerous case reports and series have associated atlantoaxial instability and dislocation with Down syndrome. The instability, seen in some 15% to 40% of patients, results from laxity of the transverse ligaments that hold the odontoid process close to the anterior arch of the atlas (61). The instability is usually asymptomatic, but neck pain, hyperreflexia, progressive impairment of gait, and urinary retention have been encountered (62). Other patients have experienced an acute traumatic dislocation. In view of this catastrophic complication, children with Down syndrome should undergo a complete neurologic examination, including neuroimaging with lateral views of the cervical spine in flexion and extension, if they plan to participate in competitive sports (e.g., Special Olympics) or in sports that could result in trauma to the head or neck. Children who have this abnormality should be excluded from these activities. Children with atlantoaxial instability who develop neurologic signs require surgical stabilization of the joint (62,63).

In addition to these neurologic abnormalities, patients with Down syndrome exhibit a number of dysmorphic features. None of these is present invariably, nor are any consistently absent in the healthy population, but their conjunction contributes to the characteristic appearance of the patient.

The eyes show numerous abnormalities, almost all of which have been encountered in other chromosomal anomalies (64). The palpebral fissures are oblique (upslanting) and narrow laterally. Patients have a persistence of a complete median epicanthal fold, a fetal characteristic rarely present in healthy children older than age 10 years but observed in 47% of trisomy 21 patients aged 5 to 10 years and in 30% of older patients (65). Brushfield spots are an accumulation of fibrous tissue in the superficial layer of the iris. They appear as slightly elevated light spots encircling the periphery of the iris (Fig. 4.2). According to Donaldson, Brushfield spots are present in 85% of Down syndrome individuals, as compared with 24% of controls (66). Blepharitis and conjunctivitis are common, as are lenticular opacifications and keratoconus, particularly in older patients. Many children with Down syndrome benefit from spectacles to correct refractive errors and astigmatism.

Anomalies of the external ear are also frequent. The ear is small, low set, and often C-shaped, with a simple helix

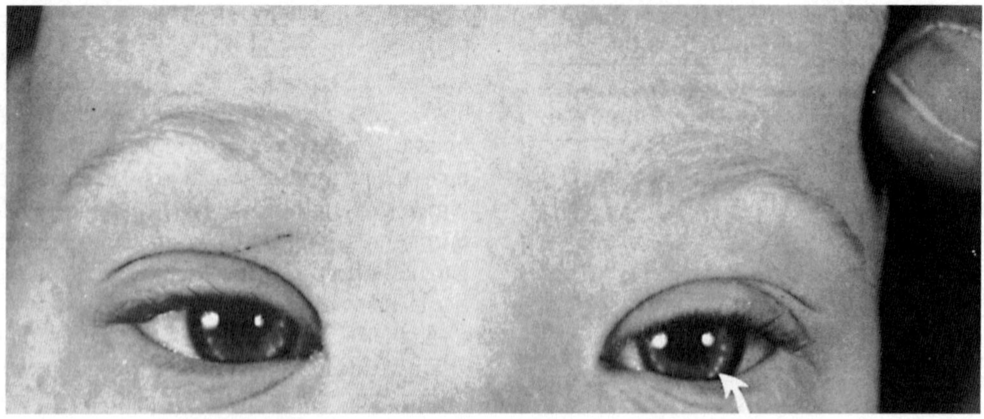

FIGURE 4.2. Five-year-old child with Down syndrome demonstrating Brushfield spots (*arrow*). (Courtesy of the late Dr. H. Zellweger, Department of Pediatrics, University of Iowa, Iowa City, IA.)

and hypoplastic tragus. The cartilage is often deficient. Additionally, the diameter of the external auditory meatus is abnormally narrow, which precludes good visualization of the tympanic membrane.

Structural anomalies of the middle and inner ear might contribute significantly to the language delay commonly encountered in children with Down syndrome. Congenital malformations of the bones of the middle ear, permanent fixation of the stapes, and shortening of the cochlear spiral are encountered frequently (67). Additionally, children, particularly infants, are prone to acute and chronic otitis, middle ear effusions, and endolymphatic hydrops with subsequent conductive and neurosensory hearing loss.

According to Balkany and colleagues (68), 64% of patients with Down syndrome have binaural hearing loss. In 83%, the hearing loss is conductive, and in the remainder, sensorineural. Brainstem auditory-evoked potentials can be used to determine the type and severity of hearing loss in young or uncooperative children (69). Because of the frequency of impaired hearing, a comprehensive hearing evaluation is indicated during the first 6 to 12 months of life.

The lips of the patient with Down syndrome have radial furrows, and, as a consequence of the generalized hypotonia, the tongue, often fissured, tends to protrude because the maxilla is too small and the palate is too narrow to accommodate it. A typical finding, particularly evident in infants, is a roll of fat and redundant skin in the nape of the neck, which, combined with the short neck and low hairline, gives the impression of webbing.

The extremities are short. The fifth digit is incurved, and the middle phalanx is hypoplastic (clinodactyly). As a consequence, its distal interphalangeal crease is usually proximal to the proximal interphalangeal crease of the ring finger. Additionally, the distal and proximal interphalangeal creases are closely spaced, and there might be a single flexion crease on the fifth digits. The simian line, a single transverse palmar crease, is present bilaterally in 45% of patients (Fig. 4.3). In the feet, a diastasis between the first and second toes (sandal gap) is the most characteristic anatomic abnormality.

A juvenile rheumatoid arthritis–like progressive polyarthritis has been seen with some frequency. A number of other autoimmune disorders, notably diabetes mellitus type 1, also have a greater-than-chance association with Down syndrome, as do a variety of endocrine abnormalities (70). Down syndrome is associated with several autoimmune conditions and with a variety of endocrine abnormalities (71). An elevation of antithyroid antibody is common, and nearly 50% of trisomy 21 patients, mostly male patients, have reduced thyroid function in later life (72). Congenital hypothyroidism and primary gonadal deficiency are fairly common, but hypothyroidism can appear at any age. Gonadal deficiency progresses from birth to adolescence and becomes manifest in adult life with resultant infertility in virtually all nonmosaic male patients (73).

The dermatoglyphic pattern of the patient with Down syndrome shows several abnormalities. Of these, a distally displaced triradius, the palmar meeting point of three differently aligned fine creases, is seen in 88% of patients but in only 10% of controls (50). Dermatoglyphic abnormalities of the fingerprint patterns are equally characteristic (see Fig. 4.3) (50,74).

Abnormalities of the skin are common. Xeroderma and localized chronic hyperkeratotic lichenification are seen in 90% and 75% of patients, respectively. Vitamin A levels are reduced in 15% to 20% of patients.

As of 1997, the median age at death of Down patients was 49 years (75). Several factors contribute to the reduced life expectancy. The most important of these is the high incidence of major cardiovascular malformations; these account for 80% of deaths. In one study, 92.2% of Down syndrome patients without congenital heart disease survived to age 24 years, as contrasted with 74.6% of patients with congenital heart disease (76). As expected, mortality

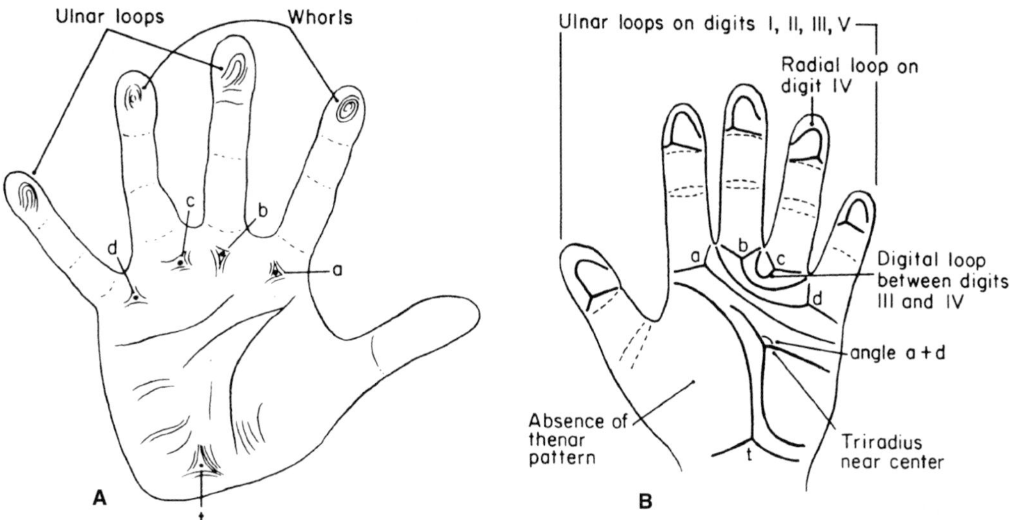

FIGURE 4.3. Outlines of the digital, palmar, and plantar configurations. **A:** Healthy child. The triradii are *a*, *b*, *c*, *d*, and *t*—the meeting point of sets of parallel ridges; *t* is located near the base of the fourth metacarpal bone at some point on its axis. **B:** Child with Down syndrome. A transverse palmar crease occurs, fingers tend to have a loop pattern, and the triradius subtends an angle of approximately 80 degrees with points *a* and *d* instead of the normal 45 degrees. (Modified from Penrose LS. Fingerprints, palms and chromosomes. *Nature* 1963;197:933.)

in those with congenital heart disease is the greatest during the first year of life (77). Of less significance in terms of influencing life expectancy is a 10- to 20-fold increase in lymphoblastic leukemia (78). As a rule, acute myeloid leukemia predominates in children with Down syndrome younger than age 4 years, whereas acute lymphoblastic leukemia predominates in older children (78). Also shortening the life expectancy of children with Down syndrome is an unexplained high susceptibility to infectious illnesses and the early appearance of Alzheimer disease, which results in a marked decrease in survival after 35 years of age (75,79). The clinical picture of Alzheimer disease in patients with Down syndrome corresponds to that in patients without Down syndrome. Deterioration of speech and gait are early findings. Epileptic seizures and myoclonus are common and were seen in 78% and 85% of patients, respectively, in the Dutch series of Evenhuis (80). Loss of cognitive function, including memory loss, generally remains unrecognized until the later stages of the disease.

Diagnosis

The diagnosis of Down syndrome is made by the presence of the characteristic physical anomalies and is confirmed by cytogenetic analysis. Karyotyping of all cases of Down syndrome is indicated to identify those that result from chromosomal translocation. When translocation is present, the karyotype of both parents must be ascertained to determine whether one of them carries a balanced translocation.

First-trimester screening is indicated for mothers ages 35 or older at term as well as in the young mother who has had a previous child with Down syndrome. Low maternal serum α-fetoprotein, reduction of unconjugated estriol, and elevated chorionic gonadotropins are independent predictors of Down syndrome, as is an ultrasonic measurement of the fetal nuchal translucency (81). Serum inhibin, a glycoprotein of placental origin, is elevated in maternal serum in women with Down syndrome fetuses and has been suggested as another useful screening marker (82), as is pregnancy-associated protein A (83). Biggio and coworkers discussed the cost-effectiveness, reliability, and complications of the various current screening strategies (84).

The diagnosis of a mosaic Down syndrome does not present any difficulty except when the frequency of the abnormal karyotype is low (85). However, accurate prediction of the phenotype in mosaic cases is problematic. Eventually, routine screening of all mothers for Down syndrome will be possible. One approach is the implementation of a polymerase chain reaction (PCR)–based technique that uses chromosome 21 markers to detect abnormal gene copy numbers in fetal cells (86,87).

Treatment

Despite the number of vigorously and fervently advocated regimens, none has proved to be successful in improving the mental deficit of the child with Down syndrome. Medical intervention is directed toward treatment and prophylaxis of infections, treatment of hearing and visual deficits, early recognition and treatment of hypothyroidism, and, if possible, correction of congenital heart disease or any other significant malformation. Although not proven statistically, early intervention appears to be of benefit in enhancing communication and self-help skills.

The early administration of 5-hydroxytryptophan, a serotonin precursor, appears to reverse the muscular hypotonia characteristically present in the infant with Down syndrome (88), and in some instances can accelerate motor milestones. Unfortunately, this has no effect on the ultimate level of intelligence (89).

The treatment of the Down syndrome child with mental retardation is similar to that of children with mental retardation from any cause and having the same potential of intellectual and social function. The topic, particularly the role of early intervention and total communication programs, is discussed in Chapter 18.

Other Abnormalities of Autosomes

Autosomal trisomies, and even double autosomal trisomies, are seen in some 20% of spontaneously aborted fetuses, and only a small minority of trisomic conceptuses are live born. Aside from trisomy 21, trisomies involving the other, larger chromosomes are associated with multiple severe malformations of the brain and viscera, and affected children usually do not survive infancy. The two entities most commonly encountered by the pediatric neurologist are trisomies of chromosomes 13 and 18. The incidence of these and other chromosomal abnormalities is presented in Table 4.3 (90).

TABLE 4.3 Incidence of Chromosomal Anomalies Among 3,658 Newborns in a Danish Population Between 1980 and 1982

Chromosomal Anomalies	*Total*	*Rate Per 1,000*
Autosomal Chromosomes		
+ 13	0	
+ 18	1	0.27
+ 21	5	1.37
+ 8	1	0.27
+ ring	2	0.55
13/14 translocation	2	0.55
14/21 translocation	1	0.27
Reciprocal translocations	7	1.91
Inversion chromosomes 2 and 6	2	0.55
Inversion chromosome 9[a]	35	9.57
Duplications	2	0.55
Others	1	0.27
Total autosomal anomalies	59	16.13
Sex Chromosome Anomalies		
47,XXY	3	1.60
47,XYY	2	1.07
47,XXX	3	1.68
45,XO (including mosaics)	4	2.24
Others	3	1.63
Total sex chromosome anomalies	15	4.10
Total chromosome anomalies	74	20.23

[a] No physical abnormalities accompany balanced translocations or inversion of chromosome 9.

Data from Nielsen J, Wohlert M, Faaborg-Andersen J, et al. Incidence of chromosome abnormalities in newborn children. Comparison between incidences in 1969–1974 and 1980–1982 in the same area. *Hum Genet* 1982;61:98–101. With permission.

Trisomy 13 (Patau Syndrome)

Trisomy 13 (Patau syndrome) occurs in fewer than 1 in 5,000 births (91). Approximately one-half of cases are diagnosed prenatally through a combination of routine ultrasound and serum screening (92). The clinical picture is characterized by feeding difficulties, apneic spells during early infancy, and striking developmental retardation (93–95). Patients have varying degrees of median facial anomalies, including cleft lip and/or palate, premaxillary agenesis, and micrognathia. The ears are low set and malformed, and many infants are deaf. Polydactyly, flexion deformities of the fingers, and a horizontal palmar crease are common. The dermatoglyphics are abnormal (Fig. 4.4). Cardiovascular anomalies are present in 80% of patients, most commonly in the form of a patent ductus arteriosus or a ventricular septal defect. Approximately 33% of patients have polycystic kidneys. An increased frequency of omphalocele and neural tube defects also exists. Microcephaly is present in 83% and microphthalmus in 74% of cases (94).

The major neuropathologic abnormality is holoprosencephaly (arrhinencephaly), a complex group of malformations that have in common absence of the olfactory bulbs

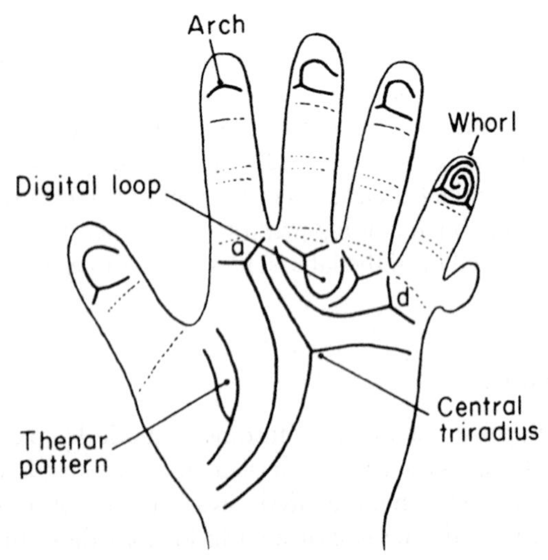

FIGURE 4.4. Dermatoglyphics in trisomy 13. Polydactyly is present. The angle subtended by points *a*, *d*, and the central triradius is almost 90 degrees. Unlike in Down syndrome, both arches and whorls can be present. (Modified from Penrose LS. Fingerprints, palms and chromosomes. *Nature* 1963;197:933.)

and tracts and other cerebral anomalies, notably only one ventricle and absence of the interhemispheric fissure (see Chapter 5). On autopsy, a number of microscopic malformations are observed, including heterotopic nerve cells in the cerebellum and in the subcortical white matter (96–98).

Absence of the olfactory apparatus is not specific for trisomy 13. In the series of Gullotta and coworkers (99), this malformation was encountered at autopsy in 40% of trisomy 13 patients. It also occurs with deletion of the short arm of chromosome 18 (18p), in the trisomy 18 syndrome, and with deletion of the long arm of chromosome 13 (13q). A condition termed *pseudotrisomy 13 syndrome* is fairly common. This entity is characterized by alobar holoprosencephaly, cardiac anomalies, and postaxial polydactyly, accompanied by apparently normal cytogenetics (100). Cardiac, pulmonary, genital, or other skeletal malformations also can be present (101). The condition is transmitted as an autosomal recessive trait (102).

The prognosis for children with chromosome 13 trisomy is poor. Approximately 50% die during the first month of life, and only 20% survive into the second year.

Trisomy 18 (Edwards Syndrome)

Trisomy 18 (Edwards syndrome) was first described in 1960 by Edwards (103). Its incidence appears to be on the increase; with the most recently recorded prevalence in Hawaii being 4.7 in 10,000 (91). The incidence in conceptuses is much higher, and only 2.5% of trisomy 18 conceptuses are live born. The anomaly is seen much more frequently in girls, the most recent male:female ratio being 0.65 (104). This suggests that a high proportion of affected male fetuses succumb during gestation. Like other autosomal trisomies, trisomy 18 results from an error in maternal meiosis, with the additional chromosome demonstrating maternal origin in 96% of cases (105).

The clinical picture is highlighted by a long, narrow skull with prominent occiput, characteristic facies, low-set, malformed ears, a mildly webbed neck, and marked physical and mental retardation (94,99). A typical picture of camptodactyly (flexion contractures of the fingers) and abnormal palmar flexion creases occurs. The second and fourth fingers characteristically overlie the third, and the fifth finger overlies the fourth. Distally implanted, retroflexible thumbs are encountered frequently. As in trisomy 13, omphalocele, polycystic kidneys, and congenital heart disease are common. A striking dermatoglyphic pattern, relatively less common in other autosomal anomalies, is the presence of simple arches on all fingers.

No consistent central nervous system malformation is associated with the trisomy 18 syndrome. The most common anomaly is agenesis of the corpus callosum, occasionally associated with nerve cell heterotopias of the cerebellum or white matter (97,99). In more than 50% of patients, the brain is small, but normal on gross and routine microscopic examination (99). The prognosis for children with trisomy 18 is poor, and 90% die by 1 year of age. The mean survival time is 10 months for girls and 23 months for boys (106). The natural history of trisomy 18 and trisomy 13 in long-term survivors has been well characterized (106,107).

Other trisomies are much less common (see Table 4.3) but have been found with relatively high frequency in spontaneous human abortions (9). Mosaic trisomy syndromes have been recognized for chromosomes 8, 9, 16, and 20. Mosaicisms for other autosomal trisomies have been reported very rarely (108). Their clinical appearance is reviewed by Schinzel (12) and Tolmie (109).

STRUCTURAL AUTOSOMAL ANOMALIES

The best described of the numerous classical deletion syndromes are the 5p- (cri du chat), and the 4p- (Wolf-Hirschhorn) syndromes.

Cri du Chat Syndrome

A number of cytogenetically visible structural anomalies of the autosomal chromosomes have been reported and have been accompanied by neurologic defects, notably mental retardation and microcephaly. The most common of these entities is a deletion of the short arm of chromosome 5 (5p), which causes the cri du chat syndrome (110). Through the combined phenotypic and molecular analysis of affected individuals the genes responsible for this condition have been mapped to 5p15.2 and 5p15.3. Deletion of a critical region in 5p15.2 results in the characteristic facial features and the severe mental retardation, whereas deletion of 5p15.3 is associated only with the meowing cry (111). The telomerase reverse transcriptase gene is localized to the region that is lost in cri du chat syndrome. The phenotypic effects of haploinsufficiency for this gene are unknown (112).

Cri du chat syndrome is seen with a frequency of 1 in 20,000 to 50,000 births (22,110). A low birth weight and failure in physical growth are associated with a characteristic cry likened to that of a meowing kitten. Infants have microcephaly, large corneas, moon-shaped facies, ocular hypertelorism, epicanthal folds, transverse palmar (simian) creases, and generalized muscular hypotonia. The brain, although small, is grossly and microscopically normal, representing a rare example of true microcephaly (113).

Wolf-Hirschhorn Syndrome

The Wolf-Hirschhorn syndrome is caused by partial monosomy of the short arm of chromosome 4, with the region

TABLE 4.4 Some Structural Autosomal Anomalies Associated With Neurologic Symptoms

Chromosomal Anomaly[a]	*Clinical Picture*[b]	*Reference*
Trisomy short arm of 4	Microcephaly, growth retardation, prominent glabella, rounded nose, low-set ears	Patel et al. (117)
Trisomy long arm of 7	Low birth weight, fuzzy hair, small palpebral fissures, micrognathia, abnormal low-set ears	Vogel et al. (118)
Trisomy of 8 (mosaic)	Long, slender trunk, restricted articular function of large and small joints, thickened skin with deep furrows, absent patella	Riccardi (119)
Trisomy of 9 (mosaic)	Upward-slanted eyes, small palpebral fissures, broad base and prominent tip of nose	Qazi et al. (120)
Trisomy short arm of 9	Microcephaly, enophthalmos, antimongoloid slant, bulbous nose with inverted nostrils, protruding ears	Hacihanefioglu et al. (121)
Trisomy long arm of 10	Microcephaly, wide forehead, arched and widely spaced eyebrows, small palpebral fissures, carp mouth, microphthalmia	Aalfs et al. (122)
Trisomy long arm 11 (partial)	Short nose, long philtrum, micrognathia, retracted lower lip, micropenis	Pihko et al. (123)
Deletion 11q2 (Jacobsen syndrome)	Trigonocephaly, growth retardation, ptosis, congenital heart disease, pancytopenia	Wardinsky et al. (124)
Deletion long arm 12 (partial)	Hypertonia, mental retardation, congenital anomalies	Tengstrom et al. (125)
Trisomy distal portion long arm of 13	Microcephaly, narrow temples, long incurved eyelashes, abnormal dentition, low-set or malformed ears	Schinzel et al. (126)
Ring 14	Mixed major and minor motor seizures; no major congenital anomalies and few facial stigmata	Lippe and Sparkes (127)
Deletion short arm of 18	Holoprosencephaly, congenital ptosis, microcephaly, hypertension, epicanthal folds	Tsukahara et al. (128), Tezzon (129)
Deletion long arm of 18	Hypoplasia first metacarpals, hypoplasia nasomaxiliary region, microcephaly, carp mouth	Mahr et al. (130)
Deletion long arm of 21	Microcephaly, downward slant of palpebral fissures, low-set ears, high-arched or cleft palate	Mikkelsen and Vestermark (131)
Trisomy of 22	Microcephaly, large, deep-set eyes, growth retardation, micrognathia, low-set malformed ears, preauricular skin tags, finger-like thumbs, small penis, undescended testis	Bacino et al. (132)
Trisomy long arm of 22	Coloboma of iris (cat's-eye syndrome), microcephaly, micrognathia, low-set ears	Hirschhorn et al. (133)

[a] p denotes the short arm and q denotes the long arm of the chromosome.
[b] Mental retardation is common to all of these chromosomes.

critical for the development of this disorder being 4p16.3 (114,115). The syndrome is characterized by a facies that has been likened to that of a helmet of a Greek warrior. Frontal bossing, a high frontal hairline, a broad, beaked nose, prominent glabella, and ocular hypertelorism are seen. Major malformations occur commonly, especially cleft lip and palate, and mental retardation is usually severe. Deletions in the region responsible for Wolf-Hirschhorn syndrome overlap those seen in Pitt-Rogers-Danks syndrome. The latter entity has a somewhat different phenotype. It is marked by prenatal and postnatal growth retardation, microcephaly, prominent eyes, a large mouth, and maxillary hypoplasia. Mental retardation is somewhat less severe than is seen in the Wolf-Hirschhorn syndrome. Wright and coworkers proposed that the two conditions result from the absence of similar, if not identical genetic segments, and that the clinical differences between the two syndromes result from allelic variation in the remaining homologue (116).

Other structural autosomal anomalies associated with neurologic symptoms are summarized in Table 4.4.

Partial deletions and partial trisomies have been described for almost every chromosome, but few of these entities are sufficiently characteristic to allow the practitioner to suspect the diagnosis without cytogenetic analysis. In particular, the phenotypic expressions of ring chromosomes overlap those of partial deletions, showing so much variability that one cannot arrive at any conclusions with respect to their clinical pictures. Furthermore, certain features, especially microcephaly, are common to many of the chromosomal anomalies, and they also are encountered in the absence of any discernible chromosomal defect. Therefore, only those anomalies that occur with sufficient frequency to establish a fairly definite clinical

TABLE 4.5 Subtelomeric Deletions

1p
1q
2q
3p
5q
6p
6q
14q
18p
22q

In all of these subtelomeric deletions the clinical picture is that of mild to moderate developmental delay, hypotonia, microcephaly, minor facial anomalies, and growth retardation (135) The 2q subtelomeric deletion may be associated with autistic features (139).

picture are discussed here. The most complete review of the various neurologic deficits seen in chromosomal disorders is that by Kunze (134).

SUBTELOMERIC ABNORMALITIES

Deletions, duplications, and cryptic imbalance rearrangements of the telomeres—the terminal segments of chromosomes—have received an increasing amount of attention in the last few years. It has become apparent that abnormalities in these regions are responsible for at least 5% to 10% of nonsyndromic mental retardation as well as for cases of mental retardation associated with multiple congenital anomalies. Several techniques have been used to screen for these abnormalities. Fluorescence *in situ* hybridization (FISH) is being replaced by comparative genomic hybridization (CGH). In this method an abnormal and a control genome are compared for DNA copy differences. This technique is being adapted for rapid and sensitive automation (135–138). The recognized subtelomeric deletions are listed in Table 4.5.

SEX CHROMOSOME ABNORMALITIES

Sex chromosome abnormalities consist of various aneuploidies involving the sex chromosomes. As determined by most surveys of the newborn population (139a) or of cells obtained at amniocentesis (140), the incidence of sex chromosome abnormalities is approximately 2.5 in 1,000 phenotypic male infants and 1.4 in 1,000 phenotypic female infants (139a). Although considerable geographic variation occurs, the two most common abnormalities in phenotypic male patients are the XYY and the XXY (Klinefelter) syndromes (139a). Because monosomy X (45,X) is highly lethal, a significantly lower incidence of sex chromosome abnormalities is found in newborns than is found at amniocentesis, and in a large proportion of individuals with sex chromosome abnormalities, particularly phenotypic male individuals, the condition remains undiagnosed throughout life (140,141). The great majority of the abnormalities in female individuals (75%) involve the XXX syndrome, with less than 25% being monosomy X (Turner syndrome) or variants thereof (142).

Klinefelter Syndrome

Klinefelter syndrome was first described by Klinefelter in 1942 in male patients who suffered from increased breast development, lack of spermatogenesis, and increased excretion of follicle-stimulating hormone. The chromosome constitution of XXY, present in most patients, was elucidated in 1959 (143).

The condition occurs in 1 in 500 to 1,000 male births (142). Although affected persons are relatively tall with an eunichoid habitus, the diagnosis is usually not made until adult life, and hormone assays are normal before the onset of puberty (144). Neurologic examination shows decreased muscle tone and some dysmetria or tremor; the major deficits encountered in unselected patients are cognitive disorders. In the Denver series, IQs were 10 points lower than in controls (145), whereas in the Edinburgh series of Ratcliffe, the mean IQ of XXY patients was 96, as contrasted with a mean IQ of 105 for controls (146). A high incidence of impaired auditory sequential memory occurs, which results in delayed language development and a variety of learning disorders, notably dyslexia (147). An increase in the incidence of behavioral abnormalities also has been observed (146). EEG abnormalities, including spike and spike-wave discharges, are said to be common (148). On high-resolution magnetic resonance imaging (MRI) left temporal lobe gray matter is significantly reduced and brain volume is less than that of controls (149,150). A greater-than-chance association exists between Klinefelter syndrome and midline suprasellar or pineal germinomas (151), male breast cancer, and insulin-resistant diabetes.

XYY Karyotype

The XYY karyotype is another common chromosomal anomaly encountered in the phenotypic male individual, with a frequency as high as 4 in 1,000 male newborns (152).

In the past, the XYY karyotype was thought to be associated with unusually tall stature, a predisposition to criminality, and dull normal intelligence. Controlled studies have indeed shown a small, statistically significant deficit in the Webster Intelligence Test for Children Verbal and Full Scale IQs, but none in the Performance scores (153). Boys with XYY syndrome can exhibit minor neurologic abnormalities, including intention tremor, mild motor incoordination, and limitation of motion at the elbows secondary to radioulnar synostoses (154,155). The last defect is also seen in Klinefelter syndrome.

The initial impression that a high proportion of XYY individuals exhibit antisocial behavior aroused much controversy because in some surveys individuals were ascertained by screening of psychiatric wards, prisons, and maximum-security hospitals (156). Careful behavioral studies have confirmed, however, that XYY patients tend to have a higher incidence of temper tantrums than controls and exhibit other forms of overt impulsive behavior, poor long-term planning, and an inability to handle aggression in a socially acceptable manner (153,157). In addition there is an increased incidence of criminal convictions during adolescence and adulthood, which is thought to reflect reduced cognitive functioning of XYY individuals (158).

Other Sex Chromosonal Polysomies

In a phenotypically male patient, the greater the number of X chromosomes, the more severe is the mental retardation. XYYY individuals, such as the one reported by Townes and associates, exhibit only mild retardation (159), whereas all of the 12 XXXYY male patients reviewed by Schlegel had major intellectual deficit, with IQs varying from 35 to 74 (160). Patients with the XXXY syndrome have severe mental retardation, small testes, microcephaly, and a variety of minor deformities (161). The XXXXY chromosomal anomaly is characterized by mental retardation, hypotonia, and a facial appearance reminiscent of Down syndrome. The palpebral fissures are upslanted, and the individual has epicanthal folds, excess posterior cervical skin, and widely spaced eyes. The fifth digits are usually shorter and curved inward (162,163).

In the phenotypic female patient, the presence of more than two X chromosomes also is associated with mental retardation. The most common of these disorders is the XXX syndrome, which is seen in 1 in 1,000 newborn female infants (164). Although no specific clinical pattern exists for female individuals with the XXX sex chromosome complement and there is considerable variability in their cognitive abilities, the majority have an IQ less than that of their siblings and are at risk for language problems, learning disabilities, and impaired social adaptation (145). Additionally, the girls are clumsy and poorly coordinated, with hypotonia of their musculature. Tetrasomy and pentasomy X female patients usually show mental retardation, with the observed degree of retardation increasing with the number of supernumerary X chromosomes (165).

Turner Syndrome (Ullrich-Turner Syndrome)

In 1938, Turner described a syndrome of sexual infantilism, cubitus valgus, and webbed neck in women of short stature (166). Ford and colleagues in 1959, found this condition to be generally associated with the 45,X chromosomal complement (167). In actuality, when cytogenetic techniques are combined with DNA analysis, the large majority, probably more than 75% of liveborn individuals, are 45,X mosaics who have a normal XX cell line, another abnormal cell line, or both. In the experience of Alvarez-Nava and colleagues and Lopez and colleagues 7.7% and 12%, respectively, of patients whose karyotype was 45,X had some Y chromosome material (168,169). Other Turner patients could have mosaicisms that are present in low frequencies (micromosaicism), which cannot be detected by the relatively insensitive techniques of conventional cytogenetics, but which can be demonstrated by FISH or, in the case of the Y chromosome, by PCR for the sex-determining region (SRY) or for various other sequences found on the Y chromosome (170–172).

Turner syndrome is seen in approximately 0.2 per 1,000 female individuals (173). The clinical and endocrinologic picture of Turner syndrome is complex; this discussion is confined to the neurologic symptoms (174). As a rule, the apparent absence of the X chromosome is not associated with a gross intellectual deficit (175). However, severe mental retardation and a variety of gross congenital malformations are seen in some Turner syndrome patients with a tiny ring X chromosome (176). In these individuals, the *XIST* locus on their ring X chromosome is not present or is not expressed. This results in defective X inactivation of the ring X chromosome and leads to functional disomy of the genes on the ring X chromosome (177, 178). The role of *XIST* in X chromosome inactivation was discussed by Lyon (179) and Kuroda and Meller (180).

Although the incidence of Turner syndrome is no greater in institutionalized individuals with retardation than in the newborn (181), the majority of patients have a right–left disorientation and a defect in perceptual organization (*space-form blindness*) (182–184). This is particularly true for those individuals who have an apparent 45,X karyotype and is less marked in children with obvious mosaicism (185). Patients in whom the X chromosome is paternally derived have better verbal skills and social adjustment than those in whom the X chromosome is maternally derived (186). The defects in perceptual organization correlate with magnetic resonance imaging evidence of reduced volume of cerebral hemisphere and parieto-occipital brain matter, including hippocampus, lenticular, and thalamic nuclei, being more marked on the right (187). Treatment with growth hormone starting at an early age and before induction of puberty increases the final height of patients (188). Estrogen treatment was discussed by Bouthelier and coworkers (189).

An autosomal dominant condition that is phenotypically similar to Turner syndrome but occurs in karyotypically normal female and male patients (Noonan syndrome) is associated commonly with short stature, congenital heart disease—generally pulmonic stenosis—hypertelorism, a triangular, high, broad forehead, hypotonia, auditory nerve deafness, and mild mental retardation (190,191). Patients have a wide range in their IQ and a variable pattern of verbal–performance discrepancies (190). As in Turner syndrome, lymphedema is a frequent occurrence; it results from dysplasia of the lymphatic vessels (192). Some patients have cortical dysplasia (193). The condition has an incidence of 1 in 1,000 to 1 in 1,250 (190). One causal gene has been mapped to 12q24.1; it encodes a nonreceptor protein tyrosine phosphatase (PTPN11) that is involved in several intracellular signal transduction pathways (194).

The association of Noonan syndrome with neurofibromatosis has been reported by several authors, and accounts for as much as 10% of patients with neurofibromatosis 1 (NF1) (195). Most patients with this syndrome have mutations in the NF1 gene, and it is not clear what distinguishes this variant form of NF1.

Three other syndromes clinically resemble Noonan syndrome. The LEOPARD syndrome is an autosomal dominantly inherited condition. LEOPARD is an acronym for its clinical manifestations: multiple lentigines, electrocardiographic conduction abnormalities, ocular hypertelorism, pulmonic stenosis, abnormal genitalia, retardation of growth, and sensorineural deafness. The condition is allelic to Noonan syndrome (196). Costello syndrome is an autosomal recessive condition that has been mapped to 22q13.1. It is marked by mental retardation, cutis laxa, and, in many instances, papillomata of mouth and nares (197). Cardio-facial-cutaneous syndrome is characterized by mild to moderate mental retardation, microcephaly, various cardiac abnormalities, and sparse, friable, and slow-growing hair. The facies show bitemporal narrowing, a prominent forehead, hypoplastic supraorbital ridges, a bulbous nose with a low nasal bridge, hypoplastic philtrum, an antimongoloid slant of the palpebral fissures, and posteriorly rotated auricles. Neuroimaging studies have been normal (198,199).

CHROMOSOMAL ANOMALIES IN VARIOUS DYSMORPHIC SYNDROMES (CONTIGUOUS-GENE SYNDROMES, MICRODELETION SYNDROMES)

In addition to deletions that are readily detected cytogenetically, combined molecular and cytogenetic analysis has led to the identification of small deletions in a number of clinically well-defined syndromes. These are outlined in Table 4.6. The term *contiguous-gene syndrome*, coined by Schmickel (215), refers to the patterns of phenotypic expression resulting from the inactivation or overexpression, as a result of deletion, duplication, or other means, of a set of adjacent genes in a specific chromosome region.

These conditions are distinct from the various syndromes that result from gross chromosomal deletion or duplication in that they are not readily demonstrable by classic cytogenetic techniques (216). The use of improved techniques for the examination of chromosomal structure has revealed that chromosomal anomalies are encountered in some syndromes with a far greater frequency than can be explained by chance. The number of recognizable syndromes has continued to multiply over the last few decades, and their clinical diagnosis has become

TABLE 4.6 Microdeletion Syndromes With Prominent Neurologic Symptoms

Chromosome	Syndrome	FISH Probe	Reference
4p16	Wolf-Hirschhorn	+	114
5p16	Cri du chat	+	111
7p13	Cephalopolysyndactyly	+	200
7q11.23	Williams	+	See text
7q34	Holoprosencephaly	−	201
8q24	Langer-Giedion	−	202,203
11p15[a]	Beckwith-Wiedemann	+	204–206
11q13	Wilms tumor, aniridia, mental retardation, genitourinary anomalies hemihypertrophy (WAGR syndrome)	+	207
15q12	Prader-Willi/Angelman	+	See text
16p13.3	α-Thalassemia, mental retardation	+	208
16p13.3	Rubinstein-Taybi	+	209, 210
17p11.2	Smith-Magenis	+	211
17p13	Miller-Dieker	+	212,213
22q11.2	Velocardiofacial syndrome; Di George syndrome	+	See text
Xp21.2	Duchenne muscular dystrophy	+	See Chapter 16
Xq21.1	Choroideremia, mental retardation	+	214

FISH, fluorescence *in situ* hybridization.
[a]Developmental dysregulation rather than deletion of a cluster of imprinted genes.

increasingly difficult. Books by Jones (13) and Buyse (217) are invaluable assistants for that task, but even with their aid, diagnosis is often in dispute. An online database for the diagnosis of genetic and dysmorphic syndromes (Online Mendelian Inheritance in Man, OMIM) has been prepared by McKusick and his group and is continuously updated by the National Center for Biotechnology Information. It can be accessed at http://www.ncbi.nlm.nih.gov/entrez.

Two disorders with a marked difference in clinical expression are associated with interstitial deletions of chromosome 15q11–q13, Prader-Willi, and Angelman syndromes.

The observation that the clinical picture of deletion 15q11–q13 depended on whether the deleted chromosome is derived from mother or father provided the first clear example of genomic imprinting in the human. Certain regions of the human genome normally exhibit gene expression from only one of the two inherited genes. This monoallelic expression of biallelic genes is regulated by a variety of mechanisms. The decision of which of the two alleles is expressed can be on a random basis or it can be according to the parent of origin. The term *genomic imprinting* refers to the differential expression of genetic material depending on whether it is inherited from the male or female parent. The absence of biparental contributions to the genome, which cannot be detected by routine cytogenetic examination, may be responsible for a large proportion of syndromes for which no chromosomal anomaly has been demonstrated. Hall also suggested that the phenotypic differences in any given chromosomal syndrome may reflect the parental origin of the affected chromosome (218). Some children with a cytogenetically normal karyotype have uniparental disomy (UPD) rather than biparental inheritance of a specific chromosome pair. In some instances, UPD has no effect on the phenotype; in other instances it exerts a profound effect. The latter occurs for several reasons. In some cases (isodisomy), UPD results in homozygosity for one or more deleterious genes. When imprinted regions are involved, UPD may result in loss of expression or overexpression of a critical imprinted gene or genes. In addition, Lalande suggested that genomic imprinting perturbs the timing of normal chromosomal replication (219). The molecular mechanisms for imprinting are not fully understood, but allele-specific DNA methylation has been demonstrated to play a vital part. A more extensive discussion of imprinting in Prader-Willi and Angelman syndromes is provided by Nicholls and Knepper (220), Strachan and Read (221), and Perk and coworkers (222).

Prader-Willi Syndrome

Prader-Willi syndrome, marked by obesity, small stature, hyperphagia, and mental retardation, was first described by Prader and coworkers (223). It is not an uncommon condition, and its prevalence has been estimated at 1 in 10,000 to 25,000 births (224).

When chromosomes are examined by FISH analysis, approximately 70% of patients with Prader-Willi syndrome demonstrate a deletion of the proximal part of the long arm of chromosome 15 (15q11–q13) (225). These deletions, which are occasionally visible by high-resolution banding techniques, occur exclusively on the paternally derived chromosome. Some of the remaining patients with Prader-Willi syndrome have other abnormalities in the same region of chromosome 15, including molecular deletions, translocation, duplication, or inverted, repeated DNA elements (226). In about 20% of patients karyotype appears normal, but restriction fragment length polymorphism analyses show the presence of two maternally derived chromosomes 15 and no paternal chromosome 15, consistent with maternal UPD for chromosome 15 (227). Thus, in at least 95% of patients, partial or complete absence of the paternal chromosome 15 occurs. In the remainder of the patients, the condition results from mutations in the imprinting center (216,228,229). Point mutations have not been encountered. Although monozygotic twins concordant for Prader-Willi syndrome have been reported and familial cases are known (230), the vast majority of cases occurs sporadically.

The clinical picture is fairly uniform (231). Breech presentation is common. Characteristically, the face is long, the forehead narrow, and the eyes almond shaped. Symptoms of hypothermia, hypotonia, and feeding difficulties become evident in infancy. Hypotonia is occasionally so striking that infants are evaluated for muscle disorders (232). Small hands and feet are noted in early childhood. Over the years, hyperphagia and excessive weight gain develop. Overeating is believed to reflect reduced satiation rather than increased hunger (233). Hypotonia tends to improve, but short stature, hypogonadism, and mild to moderately severe mental retardation become evident (13,230,231). Several endocrine abnormalities have been documented, but many of these reflect the severe obesity rather than an underlying disorder (224,231). Most patients have hypersomnolence; daytime hypoventilation also has been observed (234). Approximately one-half of Prader-Willi patients are hypopigmented, a finding that is associated frequently with cytogenetic deletions and may be related to deletion of the *P* gene, which maps to the Prader-Willi syndrome region. The gene codes for a transmembrane polypeptide that may transport small molecules such as tyrosine, the precursor of melanin. A defect in this gene is associated with one form of oculocutaneous albinism (235). Many patients have strabismus, and, curiously, as is the case in albinos, visual-evoked potentials have demonstrated that optic fibers from the temporal retina cross at the chiasm rather than project to the ipsilateral occipital lobe (236).

Anatomic examinations of the brain and of muscle biopsies and neuroimaging studies have not been helpful in providing insight into the cause of the mental retardation and hypotonia, but MRI has suggested abnormalities

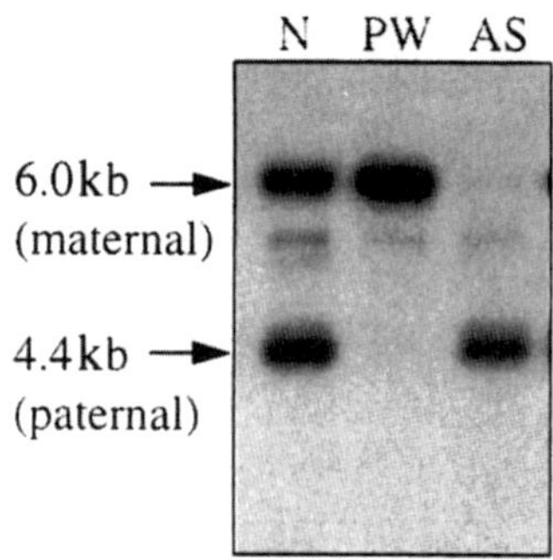

FIGURE 4.5. Southern blot analysis exhibiting a maternal 6.0-kb fragment and a paternal 4.4-kb fragment in a healthy person **(lane N)**. In the patient with Prader-Willi syndrome **(lane PW)**, the 4.4-kb fragment is lacking because of either deletion on paternal chromosome 15 or maternal uniparental disomy. In the patient with Angelman syndrome **(lane AS)**, lack of the maternal 6.0-kb fragment indicates either deletion on maternal chromosome 15 or paternal uniparental disomy. (From Schad CR, Jalal SM, Thibodeau SN. Genetic testing for Prader-Willi and Angelman syndromes. *Mayo Clin Proc* 1995;70:1195–1196. With permission.)

in cortical development (237). Electron microscopy of skin biopsies has revealed a reduction in the number of melanin-containing cells.

The diagnosis of Prader-Willi syndrome is prompted by historic and clinical features and is confirmed by methylation PCR analysis of the promoter region of the gene for small nuclear ribonucleoprotein polypeptide N (SNRPN), which is part of the imprinted gene cluster at 15q11–q13 (238). Whereas healthy individuals have biparental and always different methylation patterns, patients with Prader-Willi or Angelman syndromes caused by either deletions or UPD show a uniform methylation pattern, reflecting the absence of the paternal allele (238). This procedure is available commercially and is less costly than FISH or microsatellite polymorphism typing (Fig. 4.5) (239). Only patients with abnormal methylation will require further diagnostic investigation with FISH using probes from the 15q11–q13 region to confirm deletions. Cytogenetic studies are less revealing but can be useful in the rare instances of inherited rearrangements or markers.

Angelman Syndrome

A deletion of the maternally derived chromosome 15q11–q13 is seen in approximately 75% of children with the Angelman "happy puppet" syndrome. Some 2% of patients with this condition have paternal UPD, 5% have a defect in the imprinting center, and 8% of cases result from a defect in a gene involved in the ubiquitin-mediated protein degradation pathway (*UBE3A*) (216,240). The cause of the condition in the remaining patients is unexplained (241).

The incidence of Angelman syndrome is less than 1 in 10,000. The clinical picture is marked by severe mental retardation, microcephaly, and puppet-like, jerky, but not truly ataxic, movements. Frequent paroxysms of unprovoked laughter lend the syndrome its name. Several authors have noted that the lack of expressive speech in these children is disproportionate to the degree of retardation. Seizures are common and include almost every seizure type (242), most commonly atypical absences and myoclonic seizures (243). The interictal EEG is said to be characteristic. It shows bifrontally dominant rhythmic runs of notched slow waves or slow and sharp waves, especially during sleep, when they can become continuous. At times, patients exhibit a rhythmic myoclonus involving hands and face that is accompanied by rhythmic, 5- to 10-Hz EEG activity (244). With maturation, prolonged runs of 23-Hz, high-amplitude (200 to 500 μV) spike and wave discharges make their appearance. This EEG result abnormality can be seen in the absence of seizures, and no correlation exists with electrical paroxysms and outbursts of 0laughter (245). As a rule, intellectual deficits and the seizure disorder is more severe in patients with a chromosome 15q11–q13 deletion than in those with UPD or mutations of the *UBE3A* gene (240,243). The seizure disorder is believed to be the consequence of reduced expression of the gene for GABRB3, of one of the three gamma-aminobutyric acid $(GABA)_A$-receptor subunits, which has been mapped to the imprinted Angelman deletion region (246,247). Although a number of familial cases of Angelman syndrome have been reported, the recurrence risk for the condition is low except for those cases in which neither a deletion nor paternal UPD can be demonstrated. The latter cases may represent an autosomal recessive disorder caused by mutation in the *UBE3A* gene.

Examination of the brain shows mild cerebral atrophy but normal gyral development. Marked cerebellar atrophy is seen, with loss of Purkinje and granule cells, and a marked decrease in dendritic arborizations (248).

Diagnosis may be made by FISH analysis in the case of deletions of 15q, but methylation studies detect a higher proportion of cases. Mutation analysis for *UBE3A* is not available commercially.

Other conditions with uniparental disomy have now been recognized. They are summarized in Table 4.7.

TABLE 4.7 Symptomatic Uniparental Disomies

Chromosome	*Clinical Manifestations*	*Reference*
pUPD6	Transient neonatal diabetes mellitus	249
mUPD7	Russell-Silver syndrome	
pUPD11	Beckwith-Wiedemann syndrome	204–206
mUPD14	Prader-Willi–like appearance, short stature, mental retardation	250
pUPD14	Skeletal anomalies, unusual facies, mental retardation	251
mUPD15	Prader-Willi syndrome	See text
pUPD15	Angelman syndrome	See text

Uniparental disomies (UPDs) of the other chromosomes have no apparent phenotypic effect (249).

Miller-Dieker Syndrome

Miller-Dieker syndrome is characterized by lissencephaly, microcephaly, severe to profound mental retardation, and an unusual facies marked by a high forehead, vertical soft tissue furrowing, and a small, anteverted nose (13,212). More than 90% of patients with this condition have visible or submicroscopic deletions of 17p13.3 (216). The chromosomal abnormality results in a deletion of one copy of *LIS-1*, a gene in this region. This gene encodes a protein that is a subunit of a brain platelet-activating factor acetylhydrolase. During early development, this protein is localized predominantly to the Cajal-Retzius cells, bipolar neurons of the preneuronal migration stage, and developing ventricular neuroepithelium (252).

The Miller-Dieker syndrome is a major cause for lissencephaly. This condition, which is discussed more extensively in Chapter 5, results from the arrest of migrating neurons in the formation of the cortical plate (253). In the experience of Lo Nigro and coworkers about one-third of patients with isolated lissencephaly have deletions in 17p13.3 (213). In addition, molecular analyses can reveal point mutations in the *LIS-1* gene (213). For a more extensive discussion of lissencephaly, see Chapter 5.

Rubinstein-Taybi Syndrome

Rubinstein-Taybi syndrome was first described by Rubinstein and Taybi (254). It is marked by microcephaly, a hypoplastic maxilla with a narrow palate, a prominent, beaked nose, the presence of broad thumbs and great toes, and a moderate degree of mental retardation. Postnatal growth retardation occurs, and other facial abnormalities are common. These include downward-slanting palpebral fissures, low-set ears, heavy, highly arched eyebrows, and long eyelashes (209). Although familial cases have been reported, the recurrence risk is on the order of 0.1%.

Many patients with the Rubinstein-Taybi syndrome have breakpoints or deletions of chromosome 16p13.3, and a gene for a nuclear protein that is involved in cyclic-AMP–regulated gene expression appears to be responsible for the clinical manifestations of the syndrome (210,216,255). There is a significant amount of genetic heterogeneity, and mutations in the EP300 gene have also been found (255a). This gene codes for a histone acetyltransferase that regulates transcription via chromatin remodeling and is important in the processes of cell proliferation and differentiation.

Kabuki Syndrome

This syndrome, first reported from Japan, is so named because the facies of patients resembles the makeup used by actors in the Kabuki theatre. The condition is marked by mild to moderate mental retardation, brachydactyly, long palpebral fissures, eversion of the lateral portion of the lower eyelid, and arching of the eyebrows. There is postnatal growth retardation, and, in about one-third of patients, there are cardiac defects (256). Duplication of chromosome 8p22–p23.1 is believed to be responsible for the condition (257).

Cornelia de Lange Syndrome (Brachmann-de Lange Syndrome)

Cornelia de Lange syndrome (Brachmann-de Lange syndrome) is characterized by marked growth retardation, severe mental retardation, a low-pitched, growling cry, bushy eyebrows, hirsutism, and various malformations of the hands and feet (13,258). Although this condition is usually sporadic, it has a low recurrence rate, and an autosomal dominant inheritance has been proposed. The condition is believed to result from mutations of a gene mapped to chromosome 5p13.1 and named *NIPBL* because it is the human homologue of *Nipped-B*, a *Drosophila* fly gene involved in Notch signaling, a process that regulates cell proliferation and neuronal plasticity (259; also see Chapter 5).

Williams Syndrome

Williams syndrome is a disorder marked by an unusual, elfin-like facies (Fig. 4.6A), supravalvular aortic stenosis, hypercalcemia, and significant physical and mental retardation. The incidence of the condition has been estimated at 1 in 10,000 (216). The condition is caused by a heterozygous deletion in chromosome 7q11.23. The deleted interval is believed to contain some 25 to 30 genes, notably *ELN*, the gene that encodes elastin. The other genes that are deleted commonly include *LIMK1*, which encodes a protein tyrosine kinase; *CLIP-115* which is involved in the regulation of the dynamic aspects of the cell cytoskeleton; *STX1A*, which encodes a component of the synaptic apparatus; *FZD3*, which also is expressed in brain (260,261); and *GTF2IRD*, *GTF21*, and *TFII-I* (262). Deletion of *LIMK*, *TFII-I*, *GTF2IRD1*, and *GTF2I* are believed to be responsible for the cognitive impairment, notably the defects in visuospatial construction (261–264).

Mental retardation is usually not severe, and language ability may be quite good, with some children having an extraordinary talent for music. Hypersociability ("Everybody in the world is my friend") is a striking characteristic and is evident in very young children (265). This contrasts with severe deficits in a number of nonverbal tasks, notably spatial cognition, planning, and problem solving (266,267). An aortic systolic murmur, most commonly caused by supravalvular aortic stenosis, is present in a large proportion of children. In addition, diffuse or segmental stenoses of a variety of arteries occur, including the carotid, which can result in cerebrovascular accidents (268,269). Patients can die from azotemia or can become normocalcemic spontaneously. Early feeding difficulties, a hoarse cry, and small, widely spaced teeth are other frequent manifestations. Hypertension is fairly

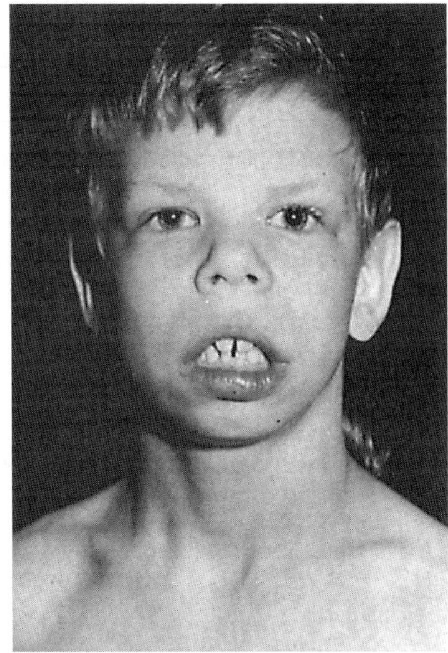
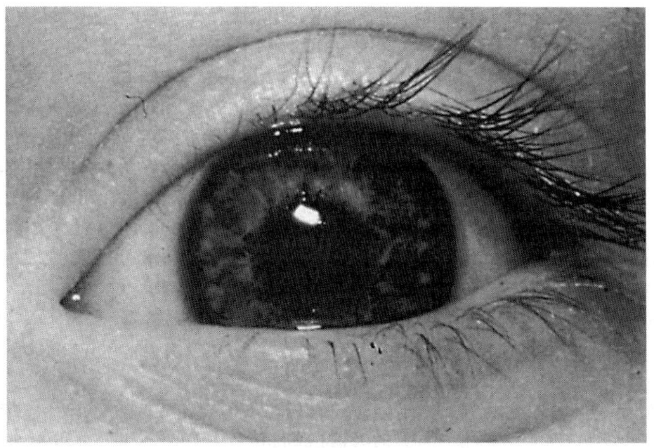

A B

FIGURE 4.6. **A:** Williams syndrome. The facial appearance in patients is remarkably uniform. This boy's eyebrows flare medially, his nasal bridge is depressed, the epicanthal folds are prominent, and the nares are anteverted. Note prominent lips and full cheeks. (Courtesy of Prof. K. Kruse, Medizinische Universität zu Lübeck, Germany, and Dr. R. Pankau, Universitäts Kinderklinik, Kiel, Germany.) **B:** Williams syndrome. A stellate pattern exists in the iris. (Courtesy Dr. G. Holmström, Department of Ophthalmology, Hospital for Sick Children, Great Ormond Street, London.)

common. More than one-half of children have a stellate pattern in their irises, which is uncommon in control individuals (Fig. 4.6B). The abnormality is believed to result from hypoplasia of the stroma of the iris (270). Magnetic resonance imaging shows cerebral hypoplasia and alterations in the relative size of paleocerebellar to neocerebellar portions of the vermis. There is a significant reduction in white matter in the posterior half of the brain, and the size of the posterior portion of the corpus callosum is reduced (271). The cardiac murmur, characteristic facies, and mental retardation or borderline intellectual functioning persist into adult life (272). On pathologic examination, the brain is microcephalic, with paucity of gray matter neurons, foci of ectopic gray matter, and a variety of cytoarchitectural abnormalities (273).

Hypercalcemia is relatively infrequent (274) and is not commonly documented by the time the diagnosis is made, although normocalcemic children can still have difficulty handling an intravenous load of calcium (275). No significant disturbance in vitamin D metabolism occurs, and the cause for the tendency to hypercalcemia is unexplained.

Velocardiofacial Syndrome; Di George Syndrome (Catch-22 Syndrome)

Velocardiofacial syndrome is the most frequent microdeletion syndrome, with an incidence that approximates 2 in 10,000 (276). It is characterized by an overt or submucous cleft palate, velopharyngeal insufficiency resulting in a distinctive hypernasal speech, cardiac malformations that are often conotruncal defects, and parathyroid deficiency with hypocalcemia. The face is marked by a prominent, bulbous nose, ocular hypertelorism, a squared nasal root, and micrognathia. The majority of children have learning disabilities or suffer from mild mental retardation (277). Approximately 25% of patients develop a variety of psychiatric disorders in late adolescence or adult life, and there appears to be an increased susceptibility to schizophrenia (278). Hypocalcemia has been documented in approximately 20% of patients (277). The term DiGeorge syndrome has generally been reserved for children who present as neonates with thymic hypoplasia and hypocalcemia.

Cytogenetic analysis using FISH probes has shown deletions within 22q11.21. At least 30 genes have been mapped to this area. Deletions or mutations of *TBX1,* a gene that has been mapped to 22q11.2, have been found in nearly all patients with this syndrome (279). Rarely, the DiGeorge phenotype is associated with deletions on chromosome 10p14 (280).

Other microdeletion syndromes are presented in Table 4.6.

Numerous other malformation syndromes are encountered frequently in the practice of child neurology. Most are characterized by mental retardation and small stature. Some of these conditions are outlined in Table 4.8. In due time and with a better understanding of molecular pathogenesis, all of these entities will undoubtedly be found to represent contiguous-gene syndromes or single-gene defects.

TABLE 4.8 Some of the Rare Malformation Syndromes Affecting the Nervous System

Condition	Manifestations	Reference
Bird-headed dwarf (Seckel)	Low birth weight, microcephaly, craniosynostosis, dislocation of joints, numerous bony defects, unusual facies, autosomal recessive inheritance	Seckel (281), Shanske et al. (282), Kilinc et al. (283)
Börjeson syndrome	Seizures, hypogonadism, obesity, swelling of subcutaneous tissue of face, narrow palpebral fissures, large ears	Börjeson et al. (284), Turner et al. (285)
Cockayne syndromes	Impaired hearing, retinal degeneration, aged appearance, cataracts, intracranial calcifications, peripheral neuropathy	Chapter 2
Coffin-Siris syndrome	Mental retardation, coarse facial appearance, short fifth finger with absence of nail, Dandy-Walker deformity	Tunneson et al. (286), Fleck et al. (287)
De Sanctis-Cacchione syndrome (mutation identical to Cockayne syndromes)	Xeroderma pigmentosum, microcephaly: autosomal recessive transmission, defect in DNA repair	Reed et al. (288), Colella et al. (289)
Hallermann-Streiff syndrome	Microphthalmia, hypotrichosis, malar hypoplasia, small nose, microcephaly	Hoefnagel and Bernirschke (290), Cohen (291)
Laurence-Moon syndrome	Obesity, mental retardation, polydactyly, retinitis pigmentosa, hypogonadism	Chapter 17
Leprechaunism	Large nares, low-set ears, sunken eyes, absent subcutaneous adipose tissue, short limbs, insulin receptor gene mutation	Longo et al. (292), Kosztolanyi (293)
Lowe syndrome	Cataracts, glaucoma, hypotonia, aminoaciduria, organic aciduria, choreoathetosis, X-linked transmission	Chapter 1
Schwartz-Jampel syndrome	Congenital blepharophimosis, continuous muscle contractions	Chapter 16
Sjögren-Larsson syndrome	Slowly progressive oligophrenia, spasticity, ichthyosis, deficiency of fatty alcohol:nicotinamide-adenine dinucleotide oxidoreductase	Chapter 1
Sotos syndrome	Large-for-gestational-age infant, large hands and feet, macrocephaly, advanced bone age, wide range in IQ	Chapter 17
Zellweger syndrome (cerebrohepatorenal)	Hypotonia, high forehead with flat facies, poor suck, seizures, absent deep tendon reflexes, camptodactyly, peroxisomal disorder	Chapter 1

Fragile X Syndrome

Even though the diagnosis of fragile X syndrome is now made by DNA analysis rather than cytogenetic analysis, for traditional reasons this condition is best considered in this chapter.

The fact that a preponderance of patients in institutions for those with mental retardation are boys or men has long been recognized, and various pedigrees corresponding to a sex-linked inheritance of mental retardation were recorded by Martin and Bell (294) and Renpenning and colleagues (295), among many others. No cytogenetic abnormality could be found consistently in these persons until 1977, when Harvey and associates (296) and Sutherland (297) demonstrated a fragile site within the terminal region of the long arm of the X chromosome (Xq27) when cells were cultured in folic acid–deficient media.

Etiology, Pathogenesis, and Molecular Genetics

The progressive unraveling of the nontraditional inheritance pattern of the fragile X syndrome was chronicled by Tarleton and Saul (298). The fragile X gene (*FMR-1*) has been isolated, cloned, and characterized. It contains a trinucleotide sequence (CGG) that in the normal genome is repeated from 6 to 55 times (299). In persons with the fragile X syndrome, this repeat is expanded (amplified) to several hundred copies (full mutation), whereas asymptomatic carriers for fragile X carry between 50 and 230 copies (premutation) (Fig. 4.7). The premutation tends to remain stable during spermatogenesis, but frequently expands to a full mutation during oogenesis. All male individuals with a full mutation but only 53% of female individuals with a full mutation are mentally impaired (300). The marked expansion of the CGG repeat sequence is accompanied by inactivation through methylation of a sequence (CpG island) adjacent to, but outside of, the *FMR-1* gene, believed to represent the promoter region for gene transcription. As a consequence, the *FMR-1* gene is not expressed in the majority of fragile X patients, and its gene product, the fragile X mental retardation protein (FMRP), is reduced or completely absent. FMRP is an RNA-binding protein that shuttles between the nucleus and the cytoplasm. It is believed to act as a translational repression and regulates translation of dendritic RNAs and normal maturation of synaptic connections (301, 301a). This is confirmed by the rapid

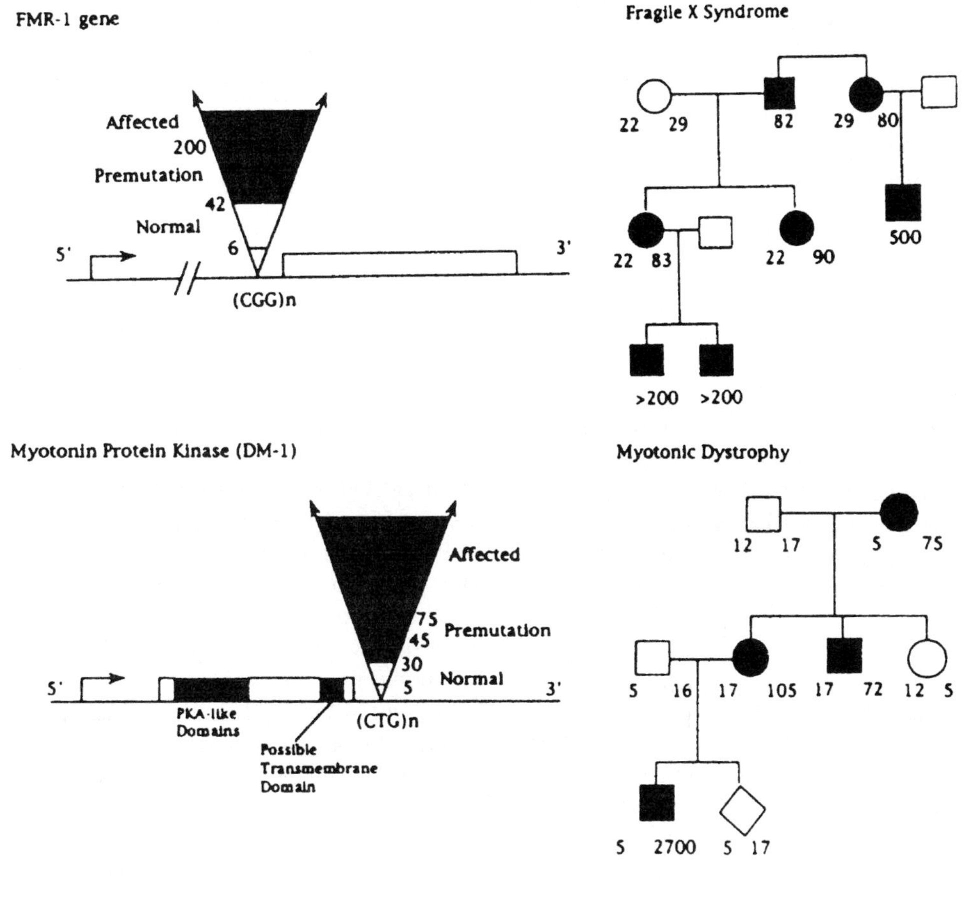

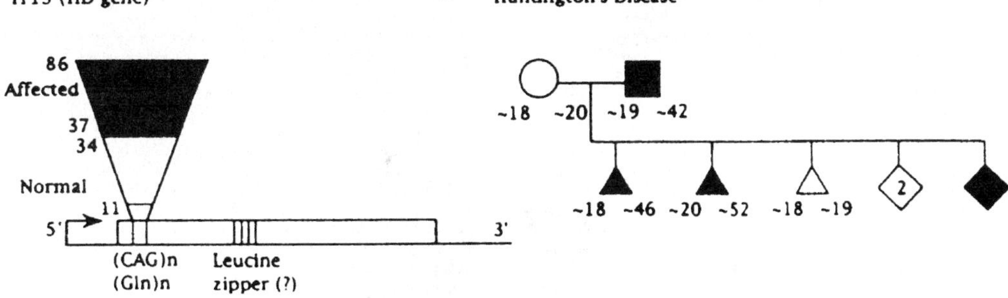

FIGURE 4.7. Diseases caused by expansion of trinucleotide repeats. On the left, a schematic diagram of each gene, with the repeat region depicted as an inverted pyramid and the numbers of repeats beside it. Open regions represent the normal variation of repeat numbers. A representative pedigree for each disorder is depicted on the right, with the number of repeats in each allele displayed below the symbols. Open symbols represent unaffected individuals. Circles represent female individuals, squares represent male individuals, diamonds or triangles represent individuals whose sex is not identified, with a number inside to indicate more than one person. (Adapted from Ross CA, McInnis MG, Margolis RL, et al. Genes with triplet repeats: candidate mediators of neuropsychiatric disorders. *Trends Neurosci* 1993;16:254. With permission of Dr. C. A. Ross, Laboratory of Molecular Neurobiology, Departments of Psychiatry and Neuroscience, Johns Hopkins University School of Medicine, Baltimore, MD.)

production of FMRP in response to stimulation of the glutamate receptor function (302,303). Good correlation exists between the degree of methylation at the *FMR-1* locus and phenotypic expression (304). However, some fragile X male patients continue to express the mRNA for FMRP despite the expectation that in view of its hypermethylation the *FMR-1* gene should be silent. Neither this phenomenon nor the reasons for hyperexpansion of the *FMR-1* gene are truly understood (305). It is becoming apparent that any mutation in the *FMR-1* gene, including deletions or point mutations such as the one described by Hammond and colleagues, that results in the failure to form FMRP can give rise to the fragile X phenotype (306).

Normally, the *FMR-1* gene is expressed in many tissues, including brain, where expression is particularly high in the lateral geniculate nucleus (307). There it is expressed in high levels in the neuronal perikarya, where it is concentrated in ribosome-rich regions. The protein also has been localized to large- and small-caliber dendrites.

Pathology

No specific neuropathology has been recognized. On gross examination, the posterior vermis is reduced in size, with a compensatory increase in the size of the fourth ventricle. Magnetic resonance imaging studies have confirmed that the volume of the posterior vermis and the volume of the superior temporal gyrus are significantly reduced, whereas the volume of the hippocampus is increased (308,309). Ultramicroscopy shows abnormal synapses, suggesting defective neuronal maturation or arborization (310).

Clinical Manifestations

The condition is relatively common, second only to Down syndrome as a genetic cause for mental retardation. It was seen with a frequency of 0.92 in 1,000 male individuals in British Columbia (311). In Coventry, England, the prevalence was 1 in 1,370 male individuals and 1 in 2,083 female individuals (312). Some 9% of male patients with IQs between 35 and 60 and no neurologic signs have the fragile X syndrome (313). On screening using DNA analysis, 0.4% of unselected women have been found to carry premutations of 55 to 101 repeats (314).

Fragile X is a clinically subtle dysmorphic syndrome. The male patient has a long face, prominent brow, somewhat square chin, large, floppy ears, and macro-orchidism without any obvious evidence of endocrine dysfunction (Fig. 4.8A) (315). Although macro-orchidism can be present at birth (315), it is difficult to recognize in the prepubertal boy, as are most of the other physical features (316). Approximately 10% of patients have a head circumference greater than the 97th percentile, and the fragile X syndrome may mimic the features of cerebral gigantism

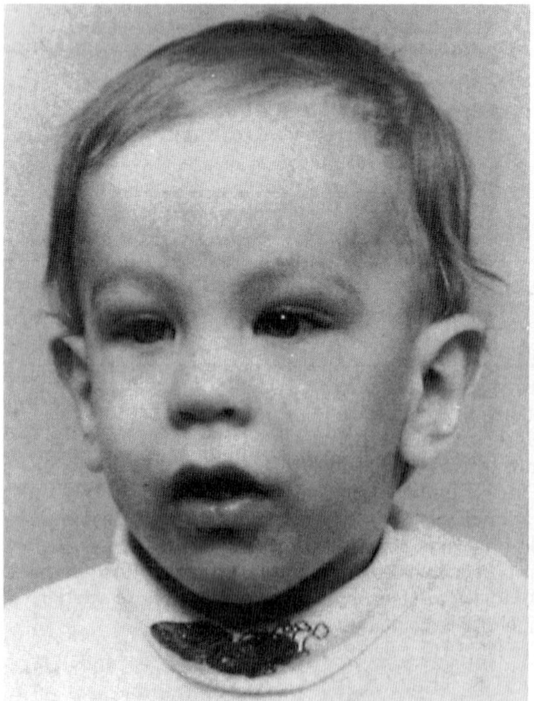
A

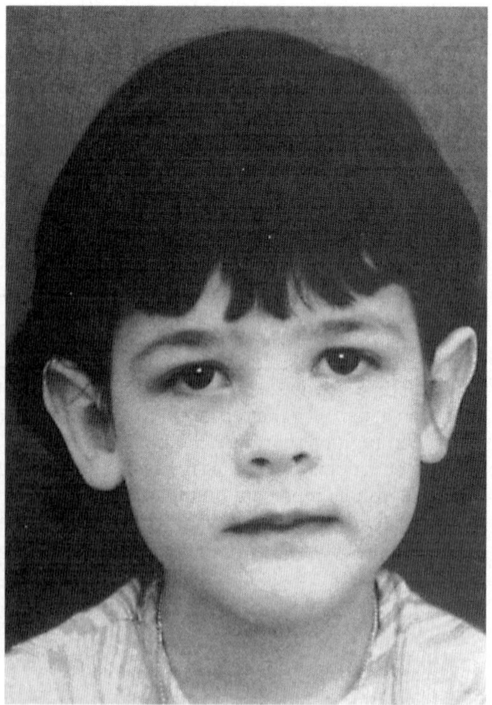
B

FIGURE 4.8. **A:** Fragile X syndrome in a 2.5-year-old boy. Note the long hypotonic face, high forehead, epicanthal folds, and prominent ears. **B:** Five-year-old fragile X–positive girl, referred because of behavior problems. Note the prominent ears. (From Chudley AE, Hagerman RJ. Fragile X syndrome. *J Pediatr* 1987;110:821–831. With permission.)

(317,318). A number of clinical features reflect connective tissue dysplasia (316). These include hyperextensible finger joints, flat feet, aortic root dilatation, and mitral valve prolapse. A Prader-Willi phenotype has also been encountered (319).

The neurologic picture is highlighted by retarded language development and hyperactivity. Delayed motor development is seen in some 20% of male patients, and seizures have been experienced by 25% to 40% of male patients. These are major motor or partial complex seizures, and as a rule they respond well to anticonvulsant therapy (317). They do not correlate with the severity of the mental retardation. Gross neurologic deficits are the exception, although some patients have been considered to be hypotonic (317). The severity of mental retardation varies considerably. Most male patients exhibit mental retardation in the moderate to severe range; in the experience of Hagerman and her group, 13% of boys have an IQ of 70 or higher but experience significant learning disabilities (320). The majority of male individuals who carry a premutation are clinically unaffected, but some have significant learning disabilities (321). A neurologic syndrome marked by ataxia, progressive dementia, peripheral neuropathy, and mild parkinsonian features is seen in some premutation carriers (321a). Pathologic examination of the brain discloses a striking loss of Purkinje cells and eosinophilic intranuclear inclusions in neurons and astrocytes throughout the cerebrum and brainstem (322,323).

The prevalence of autistic symptoms among male patients with the fragile X syndrome has been noted as considerable. Hagerman and coworkers found that 16% of male patients with the fragile X syndrome experienced infantile autism and a large proportion of the remainder had some autistic features, including poor eye contact, fascination with spinning objects, and impaired relatedness (324). However, Einfeld and Hall could not detect any difference in the incidence of autistic behavior between individuals with fragile X and matched control individuals with mental retardation (325), and the association of fragile X with autism probably reflects the association with mental retardation and autism (326). Rogers and coworkers proposed that about one-third of individuals with fragile X meet the criteria for autism, whereas the remainder do not (327).

In the affected female individual, clinical features are extremely variable. Typical physical features are generally absent or are relatively unremarkable (Fig. 4.8B). In the experience of Hagerman and coworkers, 25% of girls had an IQ below 70 and another 28% had IQs between 70 and 84 (328). Of those girls who had a normal IQ, approximately one-half had learning difficulties. Conversely, in the experience of Turner and coworkers, approximately 5% of schoolgirls with mild mental retardation had the "marker" X chromosome (329). No evidence exists for any deterioration in intelligence in female patients, although the IQ of most boys with the full expansion decreases over time (322).

Female carriers of the premutation are subject to ovarian failure. As already mentioned, they are also prone to develop the tremor/ataxia syndrome, but unlike their male counterparts, they do not demonstrate any dementia (321a,323,330).

Diagnosis

Diagnosis of the fragile X syndrome in affected individuals and carriers can be made readily by means of molecular DNA techniques (Fig. 4.9). This procedure has replaced cytogenetic fragile X testing as the diagnostic method of choice because the latter technique can result in false-negative results (331) (Fig. 4.10).

Four other fragile sites have been found cytogenetically on the long arm of chromosome X. *FRAXE*, located on band Xq28, is often associated with a mild form of mental retardation. In this disorder, a GCC repeat occurs on Xq28 (332,333). Healthy individuals have up to 25 copies of the repeat; those with mental retardation have more than 200 copies. In contrast to the fragile X syndrome (*FRAXA*), the repeat is equally unstable when inherited from father or mother. The frequent presence of normal intelligence in this variant reflects a relatively high incidence of mosaicism, with coexistent small and large amplifications (334). The function of *FRAXE* is unknown (335).

FRAXF and *FRAXD* are less common. Patients with *FRAXF* suffer mental retardation with seizures (336), whereas *FRAXD*, located on band Xq27.2, is a common fragile site inducible in most healthy people and of no clinical significance (299).

The fragile X syndrome accounts for one-third to one-half of X-linked mental retardation. Additionally, more than 90 X-linked disorders exist, more than 40 of which have been mapped, in which mental retardation is a prominent clinical feature (299), and at least 10 nonsyndromic mental retardation genes have been mapped (337). One common entity, exemplified by the family originally reported by Renpenning and coworkers (295), is characterized by fairly severe mental retardation, microcephaly, short stature, and a normal karyotype (338). Patients belonging to the family reported by Martin and Bell (294) have subsequently been found to have the fragile X syndrome (299). Another entity, initially described as nonsyndromic mental retardation is accompanied by a mutation in *ARX*, a homeobox gene, which is known to have a variable expression leading to seizures, notably infantile spasms, lissencephaly, focal dystonia, and autism (339).

Treatment

No specific treatment exists for youngsters with the fragile X syndrome. Instead, management involves a multidisciplinary approach with early speech and language therapy and behavior modification (316).

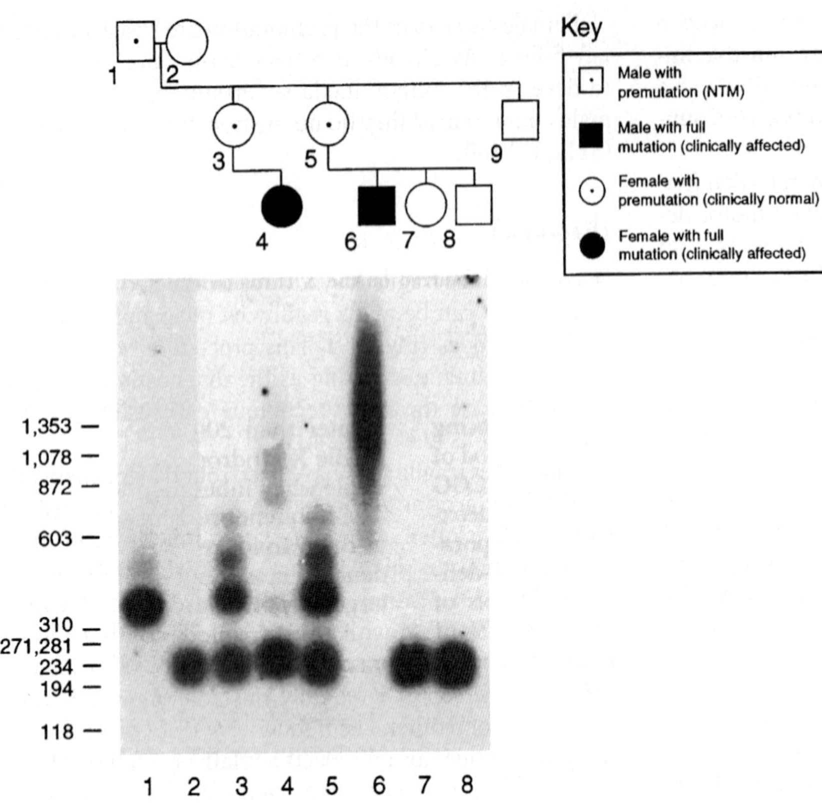

FIGURE 4.9. Pedigree and polymerase chain reaction blot of fragile X family. **Lane 1:** Male individual with premutation (phenotypically normal transmitting male individual). The polymerase chain reaction blot shows only one band with a slightly greater molecular weight than normal. **Lanes 2 and 7:** Healthy female individuals. On polymerase chain reaction a single band occurs, with approximately 234 base pairs. **Lanes 3 and 5:** Female individuals with premutation. Their polymerase chain reaction blots show two groups of bands, one single band representing the normal X chromosome and the other showing a series of bands with amplification up to approximately 700 base pairs. **Lane 4:** Phenotypically affected female patient with full mutation. The polymerase chain reaction blot shows a band representing the normal X chromosome and a smear of bands demonstrating the expansion. **Lane 6:** Male patient with full mutation. His polymerase chain reaction blot shows a smear of bands, which extends to over several thousand base pairs. **Lane 8:** Healthy male individual. (Courtesy of Genica Pharmaceuticals Corporation, Worcester, MA.)

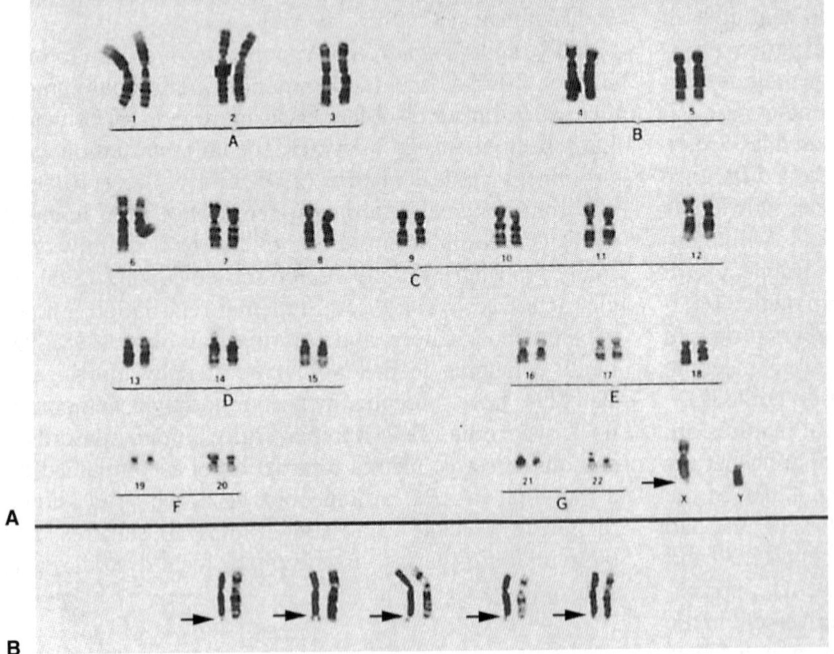

FIGURE 4.10. X-linked mental retardation associated with the fragile X chromosome. **A:** Representative Giemsa (GTG) banded karyotype of a 12-year-old boy with mental retardation with relative macrocephaly, prominent brows, deep-set eyes, large ears, and megalotestes. The fragile site (*arrow*) was demonstrated in 28% of cells cultured in folic acid–deficient media. **B:** Fragile X chromosomes from the same patient. Each pair represents the single X chromosome from a cell that was first analyzed unbanded **(left)**, for easier recognition of the fragile site (*arrows*), then banded **(right)** to confirm that the fragile site occurred on the X chromosome. (Courtesy of Dr. Rena Falk, Cedars-Sinai Medical Center, Los Angeles, CA.)

ROLE OF CYTOGENETICS IN NEUROLOGIC DIAGNOSIS

Because chromosomal anomalies are seen in up to 10% of developmentally delayed children, cytogenetic examination is an essential part of the evaluation of any youngster with a substantial mental handicap for which no obvious cause has been uncovered even in the absence of dysmorphic features or features suggestive of a specific syndrome. This yield contrasts with a yield of about 1% for routine metabolic screening (7).

In most laboratories, phytohemagglutinin-stimulated lymphocytes serve for the analysis. However, in at least one entity, the Pallister-Killian syndrome, a condition marked by profound mental retardation, streaks of hypopigmentation and hyperpigmentation, and facial dysmorphism, isochromosome 12p has been detected in buccal smears and fibroblasts but not in lymphocytes (340). Some children with hypomelanosis of Ito have chromosomal mosaicism that may be demonstrated in skin and blood or only in fibroblast cultures. This condition is considered in Chapter 12.

Chromosomal banding is always indicated, and chromosomal analysis using only a conventional solid stain no longer has any role in pediatric neurology. The most popular banding technique in North America is Giemsa-trypsin banding (G banding). Quinacrine fluorescent banding (Q banding) and reverse banding (R banding) are additional techniques that are useful adjuncts in some cases. When an anomaly is identified, more than one technique might be needed to delineate its location and the size of any deletion or extra chromosomal fragment. When the location for the abnormality is suspected (e.g., chromosome 15q for Prader-Willi syndrome), molecular cytogenetic analyses using FISH techniques or high-resolution studies focusing on that site are indicated. FISH probes are available for the known microdeletion syndromes (Table 4.6) (341).

Chromosome-specific subtelomeric probes are available commercially, and if financially feasible should form part of an evaluation for nonsyndromic mental retardation.

DNA studies are routine in the evaluation of the fragile X syndrome in the assessment of nonspecific mental retardation in both male and female patients. When these study results are negative and the phenotype is highly suggestive of the fragile X syndrome, mutation analysis for the *FMR-1* gene should be performed. Subtle chromosomal deletions or other anomalies are best detected by examining cells in late prophase or early metaphase using high-resolution analysis, a technique more laborious and expensive than standard analysis. A newer alternative is the use of comparative genomic hybridization (CGH) (342). CGH and array CGH will detect not only subtelomeric deletions, but also deletions and duplications along the lengths of the chromosomes, assuming that the deletion or duplication is not so small as to be spaced between two adjacent probes in the set (343).

Unstable DNA sequences, as are seen in fragile X syndrome, myotonic dystrophy, and several of the heredodegenerative conditions, can be diagnosed by molecular techniques to quantify repeat expansions. Such procedures are available for clinical problems (342).

Because applying all the available cytogenetic techniques to the diagnosis of every child with mental retardation is not feasible, patients with the greatest likelihood of chromosomal anomalies should be selected.

1. Chromosomal analysis is indicated in several circumstances: in the presence of clinically suspected autosomal syndromes (e.g., Down syndrome, cri du chat syndrome). In Down syndrome and in other trisomies, chromosomal analysis distinguishes nondisjunction trisomy from clinically identical translocation syndromes and mosaics.
2. In the presence of clinically suspected sex chromosome syndromes (e.g., Klinefelter syndrome, Turner syndrome).
3. Whenever mental retardation is accompanied by two or more major congenital anomalies, particularly when these involve the mesodermal or endodermal germ layers.
4. Whenever mental retardation is accompanied by minor congenital anomalies, particularly when these involve the face, hands, feet, or ears. In this respect, the frequency of minor anomalies of the face, mouth, ears, and extremities in a healthy population must be kept in mind. In a survey of 74 healthy children, Walker demonstrated between two and three such stigmata per child (343). Their incidence in the healthy pediatric population is depicted in Table 4.9.

TABLE 4.9 Incidence of Stigmata in 74 Healthy Children

Anomaly	*Percentage*
High palate	16.7
Head circumference >1 standard deviation outside normal range	15.3
Adherent ear lobes	14.0
Gap between first and second toe	11.7
Stubbed fifth finger	8.1
Curved fifth finger	7.7
Hypertelorism	6.8
Low-seated ears	4.5
Epicanthal folds	3.2
Syndactyly toes	2.7

From Walker HA. Incidence of minor physical anomalies in autistic patients. In: Coleman M, ed. *autistic Syndrome.* New York: Elsevier Science, 1976: 95–115. With permission.

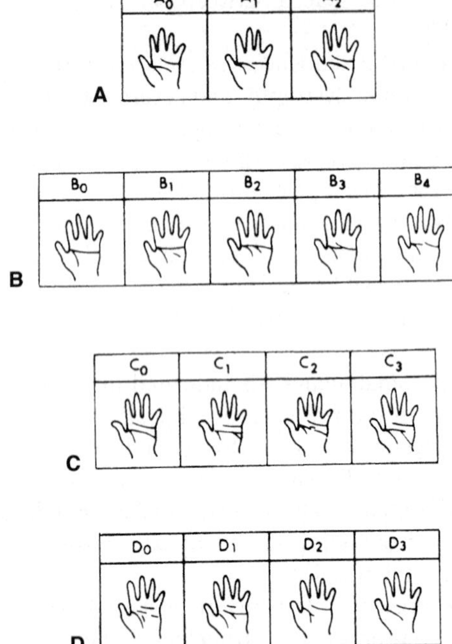

FIGURE 4.11. Palmar crease variants. **A:** Normal palmar creases. Variant A_0 is found in 94% of healthy children. **B:** Simian crease and its variants. **C:** Sydney line and its variants (301). The Sydney line is a proximal transverse crease that extends from beyond the hypothenar eminence to the ulnar margin of the palm. In contrast to the simian crease, a distal palmar crease also occurs (see Fig. 4.3) (303). **D:** Other unusual palmar creases. (Adapted from Dar H, Schmidt R, Nitowsky HM. Palmar crease variants and their clinical significance: a study of newborns at risk. *Pediatr Res* 1977;11:103–108. With permission. Further subvariants are depicted in the original publication.)

5. Whenever mental retardation is accompanied by small stature, physical underdevelopment, or dysmorphic features, including abnormalities of palmar creases (Fig. 4.11) or dermal ridge patterns (dermatoglyphics), or by abnormalities in the scalp hair whorl pattern (344,345). Because skin creases form at 11 to 12 weeks' gestation, these abnormalities point to an insult in early intrauterine life (345,346). Facial abnormalities are a particularly sensitive indicator of developmental anomalies of the brain. The explanation for this rests on the fact that facial development is dependent on prosencephalic and rhombencephalic organizing centers. Thus, any major defect in forebrain development can be reflected in the development of the face (139). This topic is covered more extensively in Chapter 5.
6. In the absence of a history of perinatal trauma, we obtain a cytogenetic survey in children who have microcephaly or the syndrome of muscular hypotonia with brisk deep tendon reflexes (atonic cerebral palsy). In addition, methylation studies or FISH for del(15q11.2) should be considered in the latter situation.
7. Whenever a family history exists of frequent unexplained stillbirths, neonatal deaths, or mental retardation.
8. In the presence of any new dominantly inherited syndrome (e.g., retinoblastoma) in addition to mental retardation.

Present cytogenetic techniques are so sensitive that they have uncovered minor chromosomal anomalies in unselected newborn populations (see Table 4.3). It is unclear how many of the rarer chromosomal variations are consistently responsible for neurologic symptoms and how many are the consequences of the same environmental event (e.g., exposure to virus, drugs, irradiation) that induced the abnormal offspring. The coming availability of multicolor FISH and array CGH to screen children with nonspecific mental retardation for cryptic subtelomeric deletions could well result in detection of abnormalities in a further 6% of children with mental retardation (4,347,348).

REFERENCES

1. Strachan T, Read AP. *Human molecular genetics*, 3rd ed. London: Garland Science, 2004.
2. Blennow E, Nielsen KB, Telenius H, et al. Fifty probands with extra structurally abnormal chromosomes characterized by fluorescence *in situ* hybridization. *Am J Med Genet* 1995;55:85–94.
3. Tharapel AT, Summit RL. A cytogenetic survey of 200 unclassifiable mentally retarded children with congenital anomalies and 200 normal subjects. *Hum Genet* 1977;37:329–338.
4. Jacobs PA, Browne C, Gregson N, et al. Estimates of the frequency of chromosome abnormalities detectable in unselected newborns using moderate levels of banding. *J Med Genet* 1992;29:103–108.
5. Flint J, Knight S. The use of telomere probes to investigate submicroscopic rearrangements associated with mental retardation. *Curr Opin Genet Dev* 2003;13:310–316.
6. Baralle D. Chromosomal aberrations, subtelomeric defects, and mental retardation. *Lancet* 2001;358:7–8.
7. Shevell M, Ashwal S, Donley D, et al. Practice parameter: evaluation of the child with global developmental delay: report of the Quality Standards Subcommittee of the American Academy of Neurology and the Practice Committee of the Child Neurology Society. *Neurology* 2003;60:367–380.
8. Hook EB, Healy N, Willey A. How much difference does chromosome banding make? *Ann Hum Genet* 1989;54:237–242.
9. Griffin DK. The incidence, origin and etiology of aneuploidy. *Int Rev Cytol* 1996;167:263–296.
10. Kuleshov NP. Chromosome anomalies of infants dying during the perinatal period and premature newborn. *Hum Genet* 1976;31:151–160.
11. Ferguson-Smith M, Smith K. Cytogenetic analysis. In: Rimoin DL, Connor JM, Pyeritz RE, et al., eds. *Principles and practice of medical genetics*, 4th ed. New York: Churchill Livingstone, 2002:690–722.
12. Schinzel A. *Catalogue of unbalanced chromosome aberrations in man*, 2nd ed. Berlin: de Gruyter, 2001.
13. Jones KL. *Smith's Recognizable patterns of human malformation*, 5th ed. Philadelphia: Saunders, 1997.
14. Pai GS, Lewandowski RC, Borgaonkar DS. *Handbook of chromosomal syndromes*. New York: Wiley-Liss, 2001.
15. Down JLH. Observation on an ethnic classification of idiots. *Clin Lect Rep Lond Hosp* 1866;3:259–262.
16. Seguin E. *Idiocy: its treatment by the physiological method*. New York: William Wood, 1866.

17. Olsen CL, Cross PK, Gensburg IJ. Down syndrome: interaction between culture, demography, and biology in determining the prevalence of a genetic trait. *Hum Biol* 2003;75:503–520.
18. Böök JA, Reed SC. Empiric risk figures in mongolism. *J Am Med Assoc.* 1950;143:730–732.
19. Mutton D, Alberman E, Hook EB. Cytogenetic and epidemiological findings in Down syndrome, England and Wales 1989 to 1993. *J Med Genet* 1996;33:387–394.
19a. Van Dyke DL, Weiss L, Roberson JR, et al. The frequency and mutation rate of balanced autosomal rearrangements in man estimated from prenatal genetic studies for advanced maternal age. *Am J Hum Genet* 1983;35:301–308.
20. Pueschel M, ed. *New perspectives on Down syndrome*. Baltimore: Paul Brookes, 1987.
21. Sachs ES, Jahoda MG, Los FJ, et al. Trisomy 21 mosaicism in gonads with unexpectedly high recurrence risks. *Am J Med Genet* 1990;(Suppl 7):186–188.
22. Tolmie JL. Down syndrome and other autosomal trisomies. In: Rimoin DL, Connor JM, Pyeritz RE, eds. *Principles and practice of medical genetics*, 4th ed. New York: Churchill Livingstone, 2002:1129–1183.
23. Hassold T., Sherman S. Down syndrome: genetic recombination and the origin of the extra chromosome 21. *Clin Genet* 2000;57:95–100.
24. Antonarakis SE. Human chromosome 21: genome mapping and exploration, circa 1993. *Trends Genet* 1993;9:142–148.
25. Yamakawa K, Huot YK, Haendelt MA, et al. DSCAM: a novel member of the immunoglobulin superfamily maps in a Down syndrome region and is involved in the development of the nervous system. *Hum Mol Genet* 1998;7:227–237.
26. Roizen NJ, Patterson D. Down syndrome. *Lancet* 2003;361:1281–1289.
27. Wegiel J, Kuchna I, Nowicki K, et al. Cell type- and brain structure-specific patterns of distribution of minibrain kinase in human brain. *Brain Res* 2004;1010:69–80.
28. Korenberg JR, Chen XN, Schipper R, et al. Down syndrome phenotypes: the consequences of chromosomal imbalance. *Proc Natl Acad Sci USA* 1994;91:4997–5001.
29. Neve RL, Finch EA, Dawes LP. Expression of the Alzheimer amyloid precursor gene transcripts in human brain. *Neuron* 1988;1:669–677.
30. Rowe DR, Uchida IA. Cardiac malformation in mongolism. A prospective study of 184 mongoloid children. *Am J Med* 1961;31:726–735.
31. Garver KL, Law JC. Garver B. Hirschsprung disease: a genetic study. *Clin Genet* 1985;28:503–508.
32. Ross MH, Galaburda AM, Kemper TL. Down's syndrome: is there a decreased population of neurons? *Neurology* 1984;34:909–916.
33. Epstein CJ, Down syndrome. In: Rosenberg RN, Prusiner SB, DiMaura S, et al. *The molecular and genetic basis of neurologic and psychiatric disease*, 3rd ed. Philadelphia: Butterworth–Heineman, 2003:125–134.
34. Suetsugu M, Mehraein P. Spine distribution along the apical dendrites of the pyramidal neurons in Down syndrome. *Acta Neuropathol* 1980;50:207–210.
35. Becker LE, Armstrong DL, Chan F. Dendritic atrophy in children with Down's syndrome. *Ann Neurol* 1986;20:520–526.
36. Casanova MF, Walker LC, Whitehouse PJ, et al. Abnormalities of the nucleus basalis in Down syndrome. *Ann Neurol* 1985;18:310–313.
37. Hyman BT, West HL, Rebeck GW, et al. Neuropathological changes in Down's syndrome hippocampal formation. Effect of age and apolipoprotein E genotype. *Arch Neurol* 1995;52:373–378.
38. Wisniewski KE, Wisniewski HM, Wen GY. Occurrence of neuropathological changes and dementia of Alzheimer disease in Down syndrome. *Ann Neurol* 1985;17:278–282.
39. Yates CM, Simpson J, Mahoney AF, et al. Alzheimer-like cholinergic deficiency in Down syndrome [Letter]. *Lancet* 1980;2:979.
40. Hayn M, Kremser K, Singewarld N, et al. Evidence against the involvement of reactive oxygen species in the pathogenesis of neuronal death in Down syndrome and Alzheimer's disease. *Life Sci* 1996;59:537–544.
41. Barbiero L, Benussi L, Ghidoni R, et al. BACE-2 is overexpressed in Down syndrome. *Exp Neurol* 2003:182:335–345.
42. Tokuda T, Fujushima T, Ikeda S, et al. Plasma levels of amyloid β proteins Aβ1-40 and Aβ1-42(43) are elevated in Down syndrome. *Ann Neurol* 1997;41:271–273.
43. Head E, Lott IT. Down syndrome and beta-amyloid deposition. *Curr Opin Neurol* 2004;17:95–100.
44. Schupf N, Patel B, Silverman W, et al. Elevated plasma amyloid beta-peptide 1-42 and onset of dementia in adults with Down syndrome. *Neurosci Lett* 2001;301:199–203.
45. Teller JK, Russo C, DeBusk LM, et al. Presence of soluble amyloid β peptide precedes amyloid plaque formation in Down syndrome. *Nature Med* 1996;2:93–95.
46. Iwatsubo T, Mann DM, Odaka K, et al. Amyloid β protein (Aβ) deposition: Aβ42(43) precedes Aβ40 in Down syndrome. *Ann Neurol* 1995;37:294–299.
47. Busciglio J, Pelsman A, Wong C, et al. Altered metabolism of the amyloid beta precursor protein is associated with mitochondrial dysfunction in Down syndrome. *Neuron* 2002;28:677–688.
48. Levinson A, Friedman A, Stamps F. Variability of mongolism. *Pediatrics* 1955;16:43–54.
49. Cowie VA. *A study of the early development of mongols*. Oxford: Pergamon Press, 1970.
50. Smith GF, Berg JM. *Down's anomaly*, 2nd ed. Edinburgh: Churchill Livingstone, 1976.
51. Del Bo R, Comi GP, Bresolin N, et al. The apolipoprotein E epsilon4 allele causes a faster decline of cognitive performances in Down's syndrome subjects. *J Neurol Sci* 1997;145:87–91.
52. Fishler K, Koch R. Mental development in Down syndrome mosaiciscm. *Am J Ment Retard* 1991;96:345–351.
53. Loesch-Mdzewska D. Some aspects of the neurology of Down syndrome. *J Ment Defic Res* 1968;12:237–246.
54. Nabbout R, Melki I, Gerbaka B, et al. Infantile spasms in Down syndrome: good response to a short course of vigabatrin. *Epilepsia* 2001;42:1580–1583.
55. Stafstrom CE, Konkol RJ. Infantile spasms in children with Down syndrome. *Dev Med Child Neurol* 1994;36:576–585.
56. Eisermann MM, DeLaRaillere A, Dellatolas G, et al. Infantile spasms in Down syndrome—effects of delayed anticonvulsive treatment. *Epilepsy Res* 2003;55:21–27.
57. Crapper DR, Dalton AJ, Skoptiz N, et al. Alzheimer degeneration in Down syndrome. Electrophysiologic alterations and histopathologic findings. *Arch Neurol* 1975;32:618–623.
58. Roth GM, Sun B, Greensite FS, et al. Premature aging in persons with Down syndrome: MR findings. *Am J Neuroradiol* 1996;17:1283–1289.
59. Okaro S, Takeuchi Y, Kohmura E, et al. Globus pallidus calcification in Down syndrome with progressive neural deficits. *Pediatr Neurol* 1992;8:72–74.
60. Wisniewski KE, French JH, Rose JF, et al. Basal ganglia calcification (BGC) in Down syndrome (DS)—another manifestation of premature aging. *Ann N Y Acad Sci* 1982;396:179–189.
61. Pueschel SM, Scola FH. Atlantoaxial instability in individuals with Down syndrome: epidemiologic, radiographic, and clinical studies. *Pediatrics* 1987;80:555–560.
62. Taggard DA, Menezes AH, Ryken TC. Treatment of Down syndrome–associated craniovertebral junction abnormalities. *J Neurosurg* 2000;93:205–213.
63. Lowry DW, Pollack IF, Clyde B, et al. Upper cervical spine fusion in the pediatric population. *J Neurosurg* 1997;87:671–676.
64. Ginsberg J, Bofinger MK, Roush JR. Pathologic features of the eye in Down syndrome with relationship to other chromosomal anomalies. *Am J Ophthalmol* 1977;83:874–880.
65. Eissler R, Longenecker LP. The common eye findings in mongolism. *Am J Ophthalmol* 1962;54:398–406.
66. Donaldson DD. The significance of spotting of the iris in mongoloids: Bruschfield's spots. *Arch Ophthalmol* 1961;65:26–31.
67. Balkany TJ, Mischke RE, Downs MP, et al. Ossicular abnormalities in Down's syndrome. *Otolaryngol Head Neck Surg* 1979;87:372–384.
68. Balkany TJ, Downs MP, Jafek BW, et al. Hearing loss in Down's syndrome: a treatable handicap more common than generally recognized. *Clin Pediatr* 1979;18:116–118.

69. Roizen NJ, Wolters C, Nichol T, et al. Hearing loss in children with Down syndrome. *J Pediatr* 1993;123:S9–S12.
70. Olson JC, Bender JC, Levinson JE, et al. Arthropathy of Down syndrome. *Pediatrics* 1990;86:931–936.
71. Carlsson A, Axelsson I, Borulf S, et al. Prevalence of IgA-antigliadin antibodies and IgA-antiendomysium antibodies related to celiac disease in children with Down syndrome. *Pediatrics* 1998;101:272–275.
72. Loudon MM, Day RE, Duke EM. Thyroid dysfunction in Down syndrome. *Arch Dis Child* 1985;60:1149–1151.
73. Hsiang YH, Berkovitz GD, Bland GL, et al. Gonadal function in patients with Down syndrome. *Am J Med Genet* 1987;27:449–458.
74. Reed TE, Borgaonkar JC, Conneally PM, et al. Dermatoglyphic nomogram for the diagnosis of Down syndrome. *J Pediatr* 1970; 77:1024–1032.
75. Yang Q, Rasmussen SA, Friedman JM. Mortality associated with Down syndrome in the USA from 1983 to 1997: a population-based study. *Lancet* 2002;359:1019–1025.
76. Hijii T, Fukushige J, Igarashi H, et al. Life expectancy and social adaptation in individuals with Down syndrome with and without surgery for congenital heart disease. *Clin Pediatr* 1997;36:327–332.
77. Hayes C, Johnson Z, Thornton L, et al. Ten-year survival of Down syndrome births. *Int J Epidemiol* 1997;26:822–829.
78. Lange BJ, Kobrinksy N, Barnard DR, et al. Distinctive demography, biology, and outcome of acute myeloid leukemia and myelodysplastic syndrome in children with Down syndrome: Children's Cancer Group Studies 2861 and 2891. *Blood* 1998;91:608–615.
79. Strauss D, Eyman RK. Mortality of people with mental retardation in California with and without Down syndrome, 1986–1991. *Am J Ment Retard* 1996;100:643–653.
80. Evenhuis HM. The natural history of dementia in Down syndrome. *Arch Neurol* 1990;47:263–267.
81. Wapner R, Thom E, Simpson JL, et al. First-trimester screening for trisomies 21 and 18. *N Engl J Med* 2003;349:1405–1413.
82. Aitken DA, Wallace EM, Crossley JA, et al. Dimeric inhibin as a marker for Down's syndrome in early pregnancy. *N Engl J Med* 1996;334:1231–1236.
83. Brambati B, Tului L, Bonacci I, et al. Serum PAPP-A and free β-HCG are first trimester screening markers for Down syndrome. *Prenat Diagn* 1994;14:1043–1047.
84. Biggio JR, Morris TC, Owen J, Stringer JS. An outcomes analysis of five prenatal screening strategies for trisomy 21 in women younger than 35 years. *Am J Obstet Gynecol* 2004;190:721–729.
85. Kardon NB, Chernay PR, Hsu LY, et al. Pitfalls in prenatal diagnosis resulting from chromosomal mosaicism. *J Pediatr* 1972;80:297–299.
86. Mansfield ES. Diagnosis of Down syndrome and other aneuploidies using quantitative polymerase chain reaction and small tandem repeat polymorphisms. *Hum Mol Genet* 1993;2:43–50.
87. Pertl B, Kopp S, Kroisel PM, et al. Rapid detection of chromosome aneuploidies by quantitative fluorescence PCR: first appplication on 247 chorionic villus samples. *J Med Genet* 1999;36:300–303.
88. Bazelon M, Paine RS, Cowie VA, et al. Reversal of hypotonia in infants with Down syndrome by administration of 5-hydroxytryptophan. *Lancet* 1967;1:1130–1133.
89. Weise P, Koch R, Shaw KN, et al. The use of 5-HTP in the treatment of Down syndrome. *Pediatrics* 1974;54:165–168.
90. Nielsen J, Wohlert M, Faaborg-Andersen J, et al. Incidence of chromosome abnormalities in newborn children. Comparison between incidences in 1969–1974 and 1980–1982 in the same area. *Hum Genet* 1982;61:98–101.
91. Forrester MB, Merz RD. Trisomies 13 and 18: prenatal diagnosis and epidemiologic studies in Hawaii, 1986–1997. *Genet Test* 1999:3:335–340.
92. Abramsky L, Chapple J. Room for improvement? Detecting autosomal trisomies without serum screening. *Publ Health* 1993;107:349–354.
93. Patau K, Smith DW, Therman E, et al. Multiple congenital anomaly caused by an extra autosome. *Lancet* 1960;1:790–793.
94. Taylor AI. Autosomal trisomy syndromes: A detailed study of 27 cases of Edwards' syndrome and 27 cases of Patau's syndrome. *J Med Genet* 1968;5:227–252.
95. Zoll B, Wolf J, Lensing-Hebben D, et al. Trisomy 13 (Patau syndrome) with an 11-year survival. *Clin Genet* 1993;43:46–50.
96. Norman RM. Neuropathological findings in trisomies 13–15 and 17–18 with special reference to the cerebellum. *Dev Med Child Neurol* 1966;8:170–177.
97. Inagaki M, Ando Y, Mito T, et al. Comparison of brain imaging and neuropathology in cases of trisomy 18 and 13. *Neuroradiology* 1987;29:474–479.
98. Moerman P, Fryns JP, vasn der Steen K, et al. The pathology of trisomy 13 syndrome. A study of 12 cases. *Hum Genet* 1988;80:349–356.
99. Gullotta F, Rehder H, Gropp A. Descriptive neuropathology of chromosomal disorders in man. *Hum Genet* 1981;57:337–344.
100. Boles RG, Teebi AS, Neilson KA, et al. Pseudo-trisomy 13 syndrome with upper limb shortness and radial hypoplasia. *Am J Med Genet* 1992;44:638–640.
101. Cohen MM, Gorlin RJ. Pseudo-trisomy 13 syndrome. *Am J Med Genet* 1991;39:332–335.
102. Amor DJ, Woods CG. Pseudotrisomy 13 syndrome in siblings. *Clin Dysmorphol* 2000;9:115–118.
103. Edwards JH, Harnden DG, Cameron AH, et al. A new trisomic syndrome. *Lancet* 1960;1:787–789.
104. Carothers AD, Boyd E, Lowther G, et al. Trends in prenatal diagnosis of Down syndrome and othrautosomal trisomies in Scotland 1990 to 1994, with associated cytogenetic and epidemiological findings. *Genet Epidemiol* 1999:179–190.
105. Fisher JM, Harvey JF, Morton NE, et al. Molecular studies of trisomy 18. *Am J Hum Genet* 1993;52:1139–1140.
106. Baty BJ, Blackburn BL, Carey JC. Natural history of trisomy 18 and trisomy 13: I. Growth, physical assessment, medical histories, survival, and recurrence risk. *Am J Med Genet* 1994;49:175–188.
107. Baty BJ, Jorde LB, Blackburn BL, et al. Natural history of trisomy 18 and trisomy 13: II. Psychomotor development. *Am J Med Genet* 1994;49:189–194.
108. Basaran N, Berkil H, Ay N, et al. A rare case: mosaic trisomy 22. *Ann Genet* 2001;44:183–186.
109. Tolmie JL. Down syndrome and other autosomal trisomies. In: Rimoin DL, Connor JM, Pyeritz RE, et al., eds. *Principles and practice of medical genetics*, 4th ed. New York: Churchill Livingstone, 2002:1129–1183.
110. Lejeune J, LaFourcade J, Berger R, et al. Three cases of partial deletion of the short arm of chromosome 5. *C R Hebd Seances Acad Sci* (Paris) 1964;257:3098–3102.
111. Gersh M, Grady D, Rojas K, et al. Development of diagnostic tools for the analysis of 5p deletions using interphase FISH. *Cytogenet Cell Genet* 1997;77:246–251.
112. Zhang A, Zheng C, Hou M, et al. Deletion of the telomerase reverse transcriptase gene and haploinsufficiency of telomere maintenance in Cri du chat syndrome. *Am J Hum Genet* 2003;72:940–948.
113. Solitare GB. The cri-du-chat syndrome: Neuropathologic observations. *J Ment Defic Res* 1967;11:267–277.
114. Fang YY, Bain S, Haan EA, et al. High resolution characterization of an interstitial deletion of less than 1.9 Mb at 4p16.3 associated with Wolf-Hirschhorn syndrome. *Am J Med Genet* 1997;71:453–457.
115. Gandelman KY, Gibson L, Meyn MS, et al. Molecular definition of the smallest region of deletion in the Wolf-Hirschhorn syndrome. *Am J Hum Genet* 1992;51:571–578.
116. Wright TJ, Clemens M, Quarrell O, et al. Wolf-Hirschhorn and Pitt-Rogers-Danks syndromes caused by overlapping 4p deletions. *Am J Med Genet* 1998;75:345–350.
117. Patel SV, Dagnew H, Parekh AJ, et al. Clinical manifestations of trisomy 4p syndrome. *Eur J Pediatr* 1995;154:425–431.
118. Vogel W, Siebers JW, Reinwein H. Partial trisomy 7q. *Ann Genet* 1973;16:227–280.
119. Riccardi VM. Trisomy 8: An international study of 70 patients. *Birth Defects* 1977;13:171–184.
120. Qazi QH, Masakaw A, Madahar C, et al. Trisomy 9 syndrome. *Clin Genet* 1977;12:221–226.
121. Hacihanefioglu S, Guven GS, Deviren A, et al. Trisomy 9p syndrome in two brothers: with new clinical findings and review of the literature. *Genet Couns* 2002;13:41–48.

122. Aalfs CM, Hoovers JM, Nieste-Otter MA, et al. Further delineation of the partial proximal trisomy 10q syndrome. *J Med Genet* 1995;32:968–971.
123. Pihko H, Therman E, Uchida IA. Partial 11q trisomy syndrome. *Hum Genet* 1981;58:129–134.
124. Wardinsky TD, Weinberger E, Pagon RA, et al. Partial deletion of the long arm of chromosome 11 [del(11)q23.3–qter)] with abnormal white matter. *Am J Med Genet* 1990;35:60–63.
125. Tengstrom C, Wilska M, Kahkonen M, et al. Partial trisomy 12q: clinical and cytogenetic observations. *Clin Genet* 1985;28:112–117.
126. Schinzel A, Schmid W, Mursett G. Different forms of incomplete trisomy 13: Mosaicism and partial trisomy for the proximal and distal long arm. *Humangenetik* 1974;22:287–298.
127. Lippe BM, Sparkes RS. Ring 14 chromosome: association with seizures. *Am J Med Genet* 1981;9:301–305.
128. Tsukahara M, Imaizumi K, Fujita K, et al. Familial del (18p) syndrome. *Am J Med Genet* 2001;99:67–69.
129. Tezzon F, Zanoni T, Passarin MG, et al. Dystonia in a patient with deletion of 18p. *Ital J Neurol Sci* 1998;19:90–93.
130. Mahr RN, Moberg PJ, Overhauser J, et al. Neuropsychiatry of 18q-syndrome. *Am J Med Genet* 1996;67:172–178.
131. Mikkelsen M, Vestermark S. Karyotype 45, XX,-21/46, XX, 21q- in an infant with symptoms of the G-d eletion syndrome. *J Med Genet* 1974;11:389–393.
132. Bacino CA, Schreck R, Fischel-Ghodsian N, Clinical and molecular studies in full trisomy 22: further delineation of the literature. *Am J Med Genet* 1995;56:359–365.
133. Hirschhorn K, Lucas M, Wallace I. Precise identification of various chromosome abnormalities. *Ann Hum Genet* 1973;36:375–379.
134. Kunze J. Neurological disorders in patients with chromosomal anomalies. *Neuropädiatrie* 1980;11:203–249.
135. Irons M. Use of subtelomeric fluorescence in situ hybridization in cytogenetic diagnosis. *Curr Opin Pediatr* 2003;15:594–597.
136. Yu W, Ballif BC, Kashork CD, et al. Development of a comparative genomic hybridization microarray and demonstration of its utility with 25 well-characterized 1p36 deletions. *Hum Mol Genet* 2003;12:2145–2152.
137. Albertson DG, Pinkel D. Genomic microarrays in human genetic disease and cancer. *Hum Molec Genet* 2003;12(Rev Issue 2):R145–R152.
138. Veltman JA, Schoenmakers EFPM, Eussen BH, et al. High-output analysis of subtelomeric chromosome rearrangements by use of array-based comparative genomic hybridization. *Am J Hum Genet* 2002;70:1269–1276.
139. Winter RM. What's in a face? *Nat Genet* 1996;12:124–129.
139a. Hamerton JL, Canning N, Ray M, et al. Cytogenetic survey of 14,069 newborn infants: I. Incidence of chromosome abnormalities. *Clin Genet* 1975;8:223–243.
140. Ferguson-Smith MA, Yates JRW. Maternal age specific rates for chromosome aberration and factors influencing them: report of a collaborative study on 52,965 amniocenteses. *Prenat Diagn* 1984;4:5–44.
141. Abramsky L, Chapple J. 47, XXY (Klinefelter syndrome) and 47,XYY: estimated rates of and indication for postnatal diagnosis with implications for prenatal counselling. *Prenat Diagn* 1997;17:363–368.
142. Allanson JE, Graham GE. Sex chromosome abnormalities. In: Rimoin DL, Connor JM, Pyeritz RE, et al., eds. *Principles and practice of medical genetics*, 4th ed. New York: Churchill Livingstone, 2002:1184–1201.
143. Jacobs PA, Strong JA. A case of human intersexuality having a possible XXY sex-determining mechanism. *Nature* 1959;183:302–303.
144. Salbenblatt JA, Bender BG, Puck MH, et al. Pituitary-gonadal function in Klinefelter syndrome before and during puberty. *Pediatr Res* 1985;19:82–86.
145. Robinson A, Bender BG, Linden MG, et al. Sex chromosome aneuploidy: The Denver Prospective Study. *Birth Defects* 1990; 26:59–115.
146. Ratcliffe SG, Bancroft J, Axworthy D, et al. Klinefelter's syndrome in adolescence. *Arch Dis Child* 1982;57:6–12.
147. Bender B, Fry E, Pennington B, et al. Speech and language development in 41 children with sex chromosome anomalies. *Pediatrics* 1983;71:262–267.
148. Dumermuth G. EEG Untersuchungen beim jugendlichen Klinefelter-syndrom. *Helv Paediatr Acta* 1961;16:702–710.
149. Patwardhan AJ, Eliez S, Bender B, et al. Brain morphology in Klinefelter syndrome: extra X chromosome and testosterone supplementation. *Neurology* 2000;54:2218–2223.
150. Warwick MM, Doody GA, Lawrie SM, et al. Volumetric magnetic resonance imaging study of the brain in subjects with sex chromosome aneuploidies. *J Neurol Neurosurg Psychiatry* 1999;66:628–632.
151. Hashimoto M, Hatasa M, Shinoda S, et al. Medulla oblongata germinoma in association with Klinefelter syndrome. *Surg Neurol* 1992;37:384–387.
152. Sergovich F, Valentine GH, Chen AT, et al. Chromosome aberrations in 2159 consecutive newborn babies. *N Engl J Med* 1969;280:851–855.
153. Radcliffe SG, Butler GE, Jones M. Edinburgh study of growth and development of children with sex chromosome abnormalities. IV. *Birth Defects Orig Articles Ser* 1990;26:1–48.
154. Daly DF. Neurological abnormalities in XYY males. *Nature* 1969;221:472–473.
155. Cleveland WW, Arias D, Smith GF. Radio-ulnar synostosis, behavioral disturbance and XYY chromosomes. *J Pediatr* 1969;74:103–106.
156. Jacobs PA, Price WH, Court Brown WM, et al. Chromosome studies on men in a maximum security hospital. *Ann Hum Genet* 1968;31:339–358.
157. Money J, Annecillo C, Van Orman B, et al. Cytogenetics, hormones and behavior disability: comparison of XYY and XXY syndromes. *Clin Genet* 1974;6:170–182.
158. Gotz MJ, Johnstone EC, Radcliffe SG. Criminality and antisocial behaviour in unselected men with sex chromosome abnormalities. *Psychol Med* 1999;29:953–962.
159. Townes PL, Ziegler NA, Lenhard LW. A patient with 48 chromosomes (XYYY). *Lancet* 1965;1:1041–1043.
160. Schlegel RJ, Aspillaga MJ, Neu R, et al. Studies on a boy with XXYY chromosome constitution. *Pediatrics* 1965;36:113–119.
161. Zollinger H. XXXY syndrome: two new observations at early age and review of literature. *Helv Paediatr Acta* 1969;24:589–599.
162. Zaleski WA, Houston CS, Pozsonyi J, et al. The XXXXY chromosome anomaly: report of three new cases and review of 30 cases from the literature. *Can Med Assoc J* 1966;94:1143–1154.
163. Peet J, Weaver DD, Vance GB. 49, XXXXY: a distinct phenotype. Three new cases and review. *J Med Genet* 1998;35:420–424.
164. Linden MG, Bender BG, Harmon RJ, et al. 47, XXX: what is the prognosis? *Pediatrics* 1988;82:619–630.
165. Brody J, Fitzgerald MG, Spiers ASD. A female child with five X chromosomes. *J Pediatr* 1967;70:105–109.
166. Turner HH. A syndrome of infantilism, congenital webbed neck and cubitus valgus. *Endocrinology* 1938;23:566–574.
167. Ford CE, Jones KW, Polani PE, et al. A sex chromosome anomaly in case of gonadal dysgenesis (Turner's syndrome). *Lancet* 1959;1:711–713.
168. Alvarez-Nava F, Soto M, Sanchez MA, et al. Molecular analysis in Turner syndrome. *J Pediatr* 2003;142:336–340.
169. Lopez N, Canto P, Aguinaga M, et al. Frequency of Y chromosomal material in Mexican patients with Ullrich-Turner syndrome. *Am J Med Genet* 1998;76:120–124.
170. Held KR, Kerber S, Kaminsy E, et al. Mosaicism in 45, X Turner syndrome: does survival in early pregnancy depend on the presence of two sex chromosomes? *Hum Genet* 1992;88:288–294.
171. Henn W, Zang KD. Mosaicism in Turner's syndrome. *Nature* 1997;390:569.
172. Mancilla EE, Poggi H, Repetto G, et al. Y chromosome sequences in Turner's syndrome: association with virilization and gonadoblastoma. *J Pediatr Endocrinol Metab* 2003;16:1157–1163.
173. Gravholt CH, Juul S, Naeraa RW, et al. Morbidity in Turner syndrome. *J Clin Epidemiol* 1998;51:147–158.
174. Saenger P. Turner's syndrome. *N Engl J Med* 1996;335:1749–1754.
175. Money J. Two cytogenetic syndromes: Psychologic comparisons. I. Intelligence and specific factor quotients. *J Psychiatr Res* 1964;2:223–231.

176. Van Dyke DL, Wiktor A, Palmer CG, et al. Ullrich-Turner syndrome with a small ring X chromosome and presence of mental retardation. *Am J Med Genet* 1992;43:996–1005.
177. Migeon BR, Luo S, Jani M, Jeppesen P. The severe phenotype of females with tiny ring X chromosomes is associated with inability of these chromosomes to undergo X inactivation. *Am J Hum Genet* 1994;55:497–504.
178. Herzing LBK, Romer JT, Horn JM, et al. Xist has properties of the X-chromosome inactivation centre. *Nature* 1997;386:272–275.
179. Lyon MF. X-chromosome inactivation and human genetic disease. *Acta Paediatr Suppl* 2002;91:107–112.
180. Kuroda MI, Meller VH. Transient Xist-ence. *Cell* 1997;91:9–11.
181. Miller OJ. The sex chromosome anomalies. *Am J Obstet Gynecol* 1964;90:1078–1139.
182. Alexander D, Walker HT, Money J. Studies in direction sense. I. Turner's syndrome. *Arch Gen Psychiatry* (Chicago) 1964;10:337–339.
183. Waber DP. Neuropsychological aspects of Turner's syndrome. *Dev Med Child Neurol* 1979;21:58–70.
184. Bender B, Puck M, Salbenblatt J, et al. Cognitive development of unselected girls with complete and partial X monosomy. *Pediatrics* 1984;73:175–182.
185. Temple CM, Carney RA. Intellectual functioning of children with Turner syndrome: a comparison of behavioural phenotypes. *Dev Med Child Neurol* 1993;35:691–698.
186. Skuse DH, James RS, Biship DV, et al. Evidence from Turner's syndrome of an imprinted X-l inked locus affecting cognitive function. *Nature* 1997;387:705–708.
187. Murphy DGM, De Carli C, Daly E, et al. X-chromosome effects on female brain: A magnetic resonance imaging study of Turner's syndrome. *Lancet* 1993;342:1197–2000.
188. Gault EJ, Paterson WF, Young D, et al. Improved final height in Turner's syndrome following growth-promoting treatment at a single centre. *Acta Paediatr* 2003;92:1033–1038.
189. Gracia Bouthelier R, Oliver Iguacel A, Gonzalez Casado I, et al. Optimization of treatment in Turner's syndrome. *J Pediatr Endocrinol Metab* 2004;17(Suppl 3):427–434.
190. Noonan JA. Noonan syndrome revisited. *J Pediatr* 1999;135:667–668.
191. Sharland M. Burch M, McKenna WM, et al. A clinical study of Noonan syndrome. *Arch Dis Child* 1992;67:178–183.
192. Witt DR, Hoyme HE, Zonana J, et al. Lymphedema in Noonan syndrome: clues to pathogenesis and prenatal diagnosis and review of the literature. *Am J Med Genet* 1987;27:841–856.
193. Saito Y, Sasaki M, Hanoaka S, et al. A case of Noonan syndrome with cortical dysplasia. *Pediatr Neurol* 1997;17:266–269.
194. Musante L, Kehl HG, Majewski F, et al. Spectrum of mutations in PTPN11 and genotype–phenotype correlation in 96 patients with Noonan syndrome and five patients with cardio-facio-cutaneous syndrome. *Eur J Hum Genet* 2003;11:201–206.
195. Baralle D. Mattocks C, Kalidas K, et al. Different mutations in the NF1 gene are associated with neurofibromatosis-Noonan syndrome (NFNS). *Am J Med Genet* 2003;119A:1–8.
196. Digilio MC, Conti E, Sarkozy A., et al. Grouping of multiple-lentigines/LEOPARD and Noonan syndromes on the PTPN11 gene. *Am J Hum Genet* 2002;71:389–394.
197. Hennekam RCM. Costello syndrome: an overview. *Am J Med Genet* 2003;117C:42–48.
198. Reynolds JF, Neri G, Hermann JP, et al. New multiple congenital anomalies/mental retardation syndrome with cardio-facial-cutaneous involvement—the CFC syndrome. *Am J Med Genet* 1986:25:413–427.
199. Gross-Tsur V, Grosss-Kieselstein E, Amir N. Cardio-facio-cutaneous syndrome: neurological manifestations. *Clin Genet* 1990;38:382–386.
200. Debeer R, Peeters H, Driess S, et al. Variable phenotype in Greig cephalopolysyndactyly syndrome: clinical and radiological findings in 4 independent families and 3 sporadic cases with identified GLI3 mutations. *Am J Med Genet* 2003;120A:49–58.
201. Frints SG, Schrander-Stumpel CT, Schoenmakers EF, et al. Strong variable cllinical presentation in 3 patients with 7q terminal deletion. *Genet Couns* 1998;9:5–14.
202. Langer LO, Krassikoff N, Laxova R, et al. The tricho-rhino-phalangeal syndrome with exostoses (Langer-Giedion syndrome): four additional patients without mental retardation and review of the literature. *Am J Med* 1984;19:81–111.
203. Ludecke HJ, Wagner MJ, Nardmann J, et al. Molecular dissection of a contiguous gene syndrome: localization of the genes involved in the Langer-Giedion syndrome. *Hum Mol Genet* 1995;4:31–36.
204. Hatada I, Nebetani A, Morisaki H, et al. New p57KIP2 mutations in Beckwith-Wiedemann syndrome. *Hum Genet* 1997;100:681–683.
205. Weksberg R, Smith AC, Squire J, et al. Beckwith-Wiedemann syndrome demonstrates a role for epigenetic control of normal development. *Hum Mol Genet* 2003;12(Spec Issue No 1):R61–R68.
206. Pettenati MJ, Haines JL, Higgins RR, et al. Wiedemann-Beckwith syndrome: presentation of clinical and cytogenetic data on 22 new cases and review of the literature. *Hum Genet* 1986;74:143–154.
207. Crolla JA, Cawdery JE, Oley CA, et al. A FISH approach to defining the extent and possible clinical significance of deletions at the WAGR locus. *J Med Genet* 1997;34:207–212.
208. Borgione E, Sturnio M, Spalletta A., et al. Mutational analysis of the ATRX gene by DGGE: a powerful diagnostic approach for the ATRX syndrome. *Hum Mutat* 2003;21:529–534.
209. Hennekam RCM, Stevens CA, van de Kamp JJP. Etiology and recurrence risk in Rubinstein-Taybi syndrome. *Am J Med Genet Suppl* 1990;6:17–29.
210. Petrij F, Giles RH, Dauwerse HG, et al. Rubinstein-Taybi syndrome caused by mutations in the transcriptional co-activator CBP. *Nature* 1995;376:348–351.
211. Spadoni E, Colapietro P, Bozzola M, et al. Smith-Magenis syndrome and growth hormone deficiency. *Eur J Pediatr* 2004;163:353–358.
212. Jones KL, Gilbert EF, Kaveggia EG, et al. The Miller-Dieker syndrome. *Pediatrics* 1980;66:277–281.
213. Lo Nigro C, Chong CS, Smith AC. Point mutations and an intragenic deletion in LIS1, the lissencephaly causative gene in isolated lissencephaly sequence and Miller-Dieker syndrome. *Hum Mol Genet* 1997;6:157–164.
214. Yatema HG, van den Helm B, Kissing J, et al. A novel ribosomal S6-kinase (RSK4; RPS6KA6) is commonly deleted in patients with complex X-linked mental retardation. *Genomics* 1999;62:332–343.
215. Schmickel RD. Contiguous gene syndromes: A component of recognizable syndromes. *J Pediatr* 1986;109:231–241.
216. Budarf ML, Emanuel BS. Progress in the autosomal segmental aneusomy syndromes (SASs): single or multi-locus disorders. *Hum Mol Genet* 1997;6:1657–1665.
217. Buyse ML. *Birth defects encyclopedia*. Cambridge, MA: Blackwell Science, 1990.
218. Hall JG. Genomic imprinting: Nature and clinical relevance. *Annu Rev Med* 1997;48:35–44.
219. Lalande M. Parental imprinting and human disease. *Annu Rev Genet* 1996;30:173–195.
220. Nicholls RD, Knepper JL. Genome organization, function, and imprinting in Prader-Willi and Angelman syndromes. *Annu Rev Genom Hum Genet* 2001;2:153–175.
221. Davies W, Isles AR, Wilkinson LS. Imprinted gene expression in the brain. *Neurosci Biobehav Rev* 2005;29:421–430.
222. Perk J, Makedonski K, Lande L, et al. The imprinting mechanism of the Prader-Willi/Angelman regional control center. *EMBO J* 2002;21:5807–5814.
223. Prader A, Labhart A, Willi H. Ein Syndrom von adipositas, Kleinwuchs, Kryptorchismus, und Oligophrenie nach myotonieartigen Zustand im Neugeborenenalter. *Schweiz Med Wschr* 1956;86:1260–1261.
224. Bray GA, Dahms WM, Swerdloff RS, et al. The Prader-Willi syndrome: a study of 40 patients and a review of the literature. *Medicine* 1983;62:59–80.
225. Mascari MJ, Gottlieb W, Rogan PK, et al. The frequency of uniparental disomy in Prader-Willi syndrome: implications for molecular diagnosis. *N Engl J Med* 1992;326:1599–1607.
226. Donlon TA, Lalande M, Wyman A, et al. Isolation of molecular probes associated with the chromosome 15 instability in the Prader-Willi syndrome. *Proc Natl Acad Sci USA* 1986;83:4408–4412.

227. Nicholls RD, Kroll JH, Butler MG, et al. Genetic imprinting suggested by maternal heterodisomy in non-deletion Prader-Willi syndrome. *Nature* 1989;342:281–285.
228. Glenn CC, Driscoll DJ, Yang TP, et al. Genomic imprinting: potential function and mechanisms revealed by the Prader-Willi and Angelman syndromes. *Mol Hum Reprod* 1997;3:321–332.
229. Ohta T, Gray TA, Rogan PK, et al. Imprinting-mutation mechanisms in Prader-Willi syndrome. *Am J Hum Genet* 1999;64:397–413.
230. Hall BD, Smith DW. Prader-Willi syndrome. A resume of 32 cases including an instance of affected first cousins, one of whom is of normal stature and intelligence. *J Pediatr* 1972;81:286–293.
231. Holm VA, Cassidy SB, Butler MG, et al. Prader-Willi syndrome: Consensus diagnostic criteria. *Pediatrics* 1993;91:398–402.
232. Miller SP, Riley P, Shevell MI. The neonatal presentation of Prader-Willi syndrome revisited. *J Pediatr* 1999;134:226–228.
233. Lindgren AC, Barkeling B, Hagg A, et al. Eating behavior in Prader-Willi syndrome, normal weight, and obese control groups. *J Pediatr* 2000;137:50–55.
234. Kaplan J, Fredrickson PA, Richardson JW. Sleep and breathing in patients with the Prader-Willi syndrome. *Mayo Clin Proc* 1991;66:1124–1126.
235. Spritz RA, Bailin T, Nicholls RD, et al. Hypopigmentation in the Prader-Willi syndrome correlates with *P* gene deletion but not with haplotype of the hemizygous *P* allele. *Am J Med Genet* 1997;71:57–62.
236. Creel DJ, Bendel CM, Wiesner Gl, et al. Abnormalities of the central visual pathways in Prader-Willi syndrome associated with hypopigmentation. *N Engl J Med* 1986;314:1606–1609.
237. Yoshii A, Krishnamoorthy KS, Grant PE. Abnormal cortical development shown by 3D MRI in Prader-Willi syndrome. *Neurology* 2002;59:644–645.
238. Klein O, Cotter P, Albertson D, et al. Prader-Willi syndrome resulting from an unbalanced translocation: characterization by array comparative genomic hybridization. *Clin Genet* 2004;65:477–482.
239. Schad CR, Jalal SM, Thibodeau SN. Genetic testing for Prader-Willi and Angelman syndromes. *Mayo Clin Proc* 1995;70:1195–1196.
240. Lossie AC, Whitney MM, Amidon D, et al. Distinct phenotypes distinguish the molecular classes of Angelman syndrome. *J Med Genet* 2001;38:834–845.
241. Hitchins MP, Dhalla RS, de Vries F, et al. Investigations of UBE3A and MECP2 in Angelman syndrome (AS) and patients with features of AS. *Am J Med Genet* 2004;125A:167–172.
242. Matsumoto A, Kumagai T, Miura K, et al. Epilepsy in Angelman syndrome associated with chromosome 15q deletion. *Epilepsia* 1992;33:1083–1090.
243. Minassian BA, De Lorey TM, Olsen RW, et al. Angelman syndrome: Correlations between epilepsy phenotypes and genotypes. *Ann Neurol* 1998;43:485–493.
244. Guerrini R, De Lorey TM, Bonanni P, et al. Cortical myoclonus in Angelman syndrome. *Ann Neurol* 1996;40:39–48.
245. Boyd SG, Harden A, Patton MA. The EEG in early diagnosis of the Angelman (happy puppet) syndrome. *Eur J Pediatr* 1988;147:508–513.
246. Dan B, Boyd SG. Angelman syndrome reviewed from a neurophysiological perspective. The UBE3A-GABRB3 hypothesis. *Neuropediatrics* 2003;34:169–176.
247. Holopainen IE, Metsähonkala EL, Kokkonen H, et al. Decreased binding of [^{11}C] flumazenil in Angelman syndrome patients with $GABA_A$ receptor β_3 subunit deletions. *Ann Neurol* 2001;49:110–113.
248. Jay V, Becker LE, Chan FW, et al. Puppet-like syndrome of Angelman: a pathologic and neurochemical study. *Neurology* 1991;41:416–422.
249. Eggermann T, Zerres K, Eggermann K, et al. Uniparental disomy: clinical indications for testing in growth retardation. *Eur J Pediatr* 2002;161:305–312.
250. Cox H, Bullman H, Temple IKJ. Maternal UPD(14) in the patient with a normal karyotype: clinical report and a systemic search for cases in samples sent for testing for Prader-Willi syndrome. *Am J Med Genet A* 2004;127:21–25.
251. Chu C, Schwartz S, McPherson E. Paternal uniparental isodisomy for chromosome 14 in a patient with a normal 46, XY karyotype. *Am J Med Genet* 2004;127A:167–171.
252. Clark GD, Mizuguchi M, Antalffy B, et al. Predominant localization of the LIS family of gene products to Cajal-Retzius cells and ventricular neuroepithelium in the developing human cortex. *J Neuropath Exp Neurol* 1997;56:1044–1052.
253. Sarnat HB, Flores-Sarnat L. Etiological classification of CNS malformations: integration of molecular, genetic and morphological criteria. *Epileptic Disord* 2003;(5 Suppl 2):S35–S43.
254. Rubinstein JH, Taybi H. Broad thumbs and toes and facial abnormalities. *Am J Dis Child* 1963;105:588–608.
255. Coupry I, Monnet L, Attia AA, et al. Analysis of CBP (CREBBP) gene deletions in Rubinstein-Taybi syndrome patients using real-time quantitative PCR. *Hum Mutat* 2004;23:278–284.
255a. Roelfsema JH, White SJ, Ariyurek Y, et al. Genetic heterogeneity in Rubinstein-Taybi syndrome: mutations in both the CBP and EP300 genes cause disease. *Am J Hum Genet* 2005;76:572–580.
256. Niikawa N, Kuroki Y, Kajii T., et al. Kabuki make-up (Niikawa-Kuroki) syndrome: a study of 62 patients. *Am J Med Genet* 1988;31:565–589.
257. Milunski JM, Huang XL. Unmasking Kabuki syndrome: chromosome 8p22–8p23.1 duplication revealed by comparative genomic hybridization and BAC-FISH. *Clin Genet* 2003;64:509–516.
258. Ptacek LJ, Opitz JM, Smith DW, et al. The Cornelia de Lange syndrome. *J Pediatr* 1963;63:1000–1020.
259. Krantz ID, McCallum J, DeScipio C, et al. Cornelia de Lange syndrome caused by mutations in *NIPBL*, the human homolog of *Drosophila melanogaster Nipped-B*. *Nat Genet* 2004;36:631–635.
260. Rossen ML, Sarnat HB. Why should neurologists be interested in Williams syndrome? *Neurology* 1998;51:8–9.
261. Tassabehji M, Metcalve E, Karmiloff-Smith A, et al. Williams syndrome: use of chromosomal microdeletions as a tool to dissect cognitive and physical phenotypes. *Am J Hum Genet* 1999;64:118–125.
262. Hirota H, Matsuoka R, Chen XN, et al. Williams syndrome deficits in visual spatial processing linked to GTF2IRD1 and GTF2I on chromosome 7q11.23. *Genet Med* 2003;5:311–321.
263. Meng X, Lu X, Li Z, et al. Complete physical map of the common deletion region in Williams syndrome and identification and characterization of three novel genes. *Hum Genet* 1998;103:590–599.
264. Danoff SK, Taylor He, Blackshow S, et al. TFII-I, a candidate gene for Williams syndrome cognitive profile: parallels between regional expression in mouse brain and human phenotype. *Neuroscience* 2004:123:931–938.
265. Doyle TF, Bellugi U, Korenberg JR, et al. "Everybody in the world is my friend" hypersociability in young children with Williams syndrome. *Am J Med Genet* 2004;124A:263–273.
266. Korenberg JR, Chen XN, Hirota H, et al. VI. Genome structure and cognitive map of Williams syndrome. *J Cogn Neurosci* 2000;12(Suppl 1):89–107.
267. Karmiloff-Smith A, Grant J, Berthout I, et al. Language and Williams syndrome: how intact is "intact"? *Child Dev* 1997;68:246–262.
268. Wollack JB, Kaifer M, La Monte MP, et al. Stroke in Williams syndrome. *Stroke* 1996;27:143–146.
269. Sadler LS, Gingell R, Martin DJ. Carotid ultrasound examination in Williams syndrome. *J Pediatr* 1998;132:354–356.
270. Holmström G, Almond G, Temple K, et al. The iris in Williams syndrome. *Arch Dis Child* 1990;65:987–989.
271. Schmitt JE, Eliez S, Warsofsky IS, et al. Corpus callosum morphology of Williams syndrome: relation to genetics and behavior. *Dev Med Child Neurol* 2001;43:155–159.
272. Morris CA, Demsey SA, Leonard CO, et al. Natural history of Williams syndrome: physical characteristics. *J Pediatr* 1988;113:318–326.
273. Crome L, Sylvester PE. A case of severe hypercalcaemia of infancy with an account of the neuropathological findings. *Arch Dis Child* 1960;35:620–625.
274. Sforzini C, Milani D, Fossali E, et al. Renal tract ultrasonography and calcium homeostasis in Williams-Beuren syndrome. *Pediatr Nephrol* 2002:17:899–902.

275. Jones KL, Smith DW. The Williams elfin facies syndrome. *J Pediatr* 1975;86:718–723.
276. Oskarsdottir S, Vujic M, Fasth A. Incidence and prevalence of the 22q11 deletion syndrome: a population-based study in western Sweden. *Arch Dis Chid* 2004;89:148–151.
277. Goldberg R, Motzkin B, Marion R, et al. Velo-cardio-facial syndrome: a review of 120 patients. *Am J Med Genet* 1993;45:313–319.
278. Murphy KC. Schizophenia and velo-cardio-facial syndrome. *Lancet* 2002;359:426–430.
279. Yagi H, Furutani Y, Hamada H, et al. Role of TBX1 in human del 22q11.2 syndrome. *Lancet* 2003;362:1366–1373.
280. Bartsch O, Nemeckova M, Kocarek E, et al. DiGeorge/velocardiofacial syndrome: FISH studies of chromosomes 22q11 and 10p14, and clinical reports on the proximal 22q11 deletion. *Am J Med Genet* 2003;117A:1–5.
281. Seckel HP. *Bird-headed dwarfs*. Springfield, IL: Charles C. Thomas, 1960.
282. Shanske A, Caride DE, Menasse-Palmer L, et al. Central nervous system anomalies in Seckel syndrome: report of a new family and review of the literature. *Am J Med Genet* 1997;70:155–158.
283. Kilinc MO, Ninis VN, Ugur SA, et al. Is the novel SCKL3 at 14q23 the predominant Seckel locus? *Eur J Hum Genet* 2003;11:851–857.
284. Borjeson M, Forssman H, Lehmann O. An X-linked, recessively inherited syndrome characterized by grave mental deficiency, epilepsy, and endocrine disorder. *Acta Med Scand* 1962;171:13–21.
285. Turner G, Lower KM, White SM, et al. The clinical picture of the Borjeson-Forssman-Lehmann syndrome in males and heterozygous females with PHF6 mutations. *Clin Genet* 2004:65:226–232.
286. Tunneson WW, McMillan JA, Levin MA. The Coffin–Siris syndrome. *Am J Dis Child* 1978;132:393–395.
287. Fleck BJ, Pandya A, Vanner L, et al. Coffin-Siris syndrome: review and presentation of new cases from a questionnaire study. *Am J Med Genet* 2001;99:1–7.
288. Reed W, May SB, Nickel WR. Xeroderma pigmentosum with neurological complications: The de Sanctis–Cacchione syndrome. *Arch Dermatol* (Chicago) 1965;91:224–226.
289. Colella S, Nardo T, Botta E., et al. Identical mutations in the CSB gene associated with either Cockayne syndrome or the DeSanctis-Caccione variant of xeroderma pigmentosum. *Hum Mol Genet* 2000;9:1171–1175.
290. Hoefnagel D, Bernirschke K. Dyscephalia and mandibulo-oculo-cephalis (Hallermann-Streiff syndrome). *Arch Dis Child* 1965;40:57–61.
291. Cohen MM. Hallermann-Streiff syndrome. A review. *Am J Med Genet* 1991;41:488–499.
292. Longo N., Wang Y, Smith SA, et al. Genotype–phenotype correlation in inherited severe insulin resistance. *Hum Mol Genet* 2002;11:1465–1475.
293. Kosztolanyi G. Leprechaunism/Donohue syndrome/insulin receptor gene mutations: a syndrome delineation story from clinicopathological description to molecular understanding. *Eur J Pediatr* 1997;156:253–255.
294. Martin JP, Bell J. Pedigree of mental defect showing sex-linkage. *J Neurol Psychiatry* 1943;6:154–157.
295. Renpenning H, Gerrard JW, Zaleski WA, et al. Familial sex-linked mental retardation. *Can Med Assoc J* 1967;87:954–956.
296. Harvey J, Judge C, Wiener S. Familial X-linked retardation with an X chromosome abnormality. *J Med Genet* 1977;14:46–50.
297. Sutherland GR. Heritable fragile sites on human chromosomes. Demonstration of their dependence on the type of tissue culture medium. *Science* 1977;197:265.
298. Tarleton JC, Saul RA. Molecular genetic advances in fragile X syndrome. *J Pediatr* 1993;122:169–185.
299. Sutherland GR, Gecz J, Mulley JC. Fragile X syndrome and other causes of X-linked mental handicap. In: Rimoin DL, Connor JM, Pyeritz RE, et al. eds. *Principles and practice of medical genetics*, 4th ed. New York: Churchill Livingstone, 2002:2801–2826.
300. Rousseau F, Heitz D, Biancalana V, et al. Direct diagnosis by DNA analysis of the fragile X syndrome of mental retardation. *N Engl J Med* 1991;325:1673–1681.
301. Zalfa F, Bagni C. Molecular insights into mental retardation: multiple functions for the fragile X mental retardation protein? *Curr Issues Mol Biol* 2004;6:73–88.
301a. Bagni C, Greenough WT. From mRNP trafficking to spine dysmorphogenesis: the roots of fragile X syndrome. *Nat Rev Neurosci* 2005;6:376–387.
302. Feng Y, Gutekunst CA, Eberhart DE, et al. Fragile X mental retardation protein: nucleocytoplasmic shuttling and association with somatodendritic ribosomes. *J Neurosci* 1997;17:1539–1547.
303. Weiler IJ, Irwin SA, Klintsova AY, et al. Fragile X mental retardation protein is translated near synapses in response to neurotransmitter activation. *Proc Natl Acad Sci USA* 1997;94:5395–5400.
304. McConkie-Rosell A, Lackiewticz AM, Spiridigliozzi GA, et al. Evidence that methylation of the *FMR-1* locus is responsible for variable phenotypic expression of the fragile X syndrome. *Am J Hum Genet* 1993;53:800–809.
305. Tassone F, Hagerman PJ. Expression of the *FMR1* gene. *Cytogenet Genome Res* 2003;100:124–128.
306. Hammond LS, Macias MM, Tarleton JC, et al. Fragile X syndrome and deletions in *FMR1*: new case and review of the literature. *Am J Med Genet* 1997;72:430–434.
307. Kogan CS, Boutet I, Cornish K, et al. Differential impact of the *RMR1* gene on visual processing in fragile X syndrome. *Brain* 2003:127:591–601.
308. Reiss AL. Lee J, Freund L. Neuroanatomy of fragile X syndrome: the temporal lobe. *Neurology* 1994;44:1317–1324.
309. Mostofsky SH, Mazzocco MM, Aakalu G, et al. Decreased cerebellar posterior vermis size in fragile X syndrome: correlation with neurocognitive performance. *Neurology* 1998;50:121–130.
310. Rudelli RD, Brown WT, Wisniewski K, et al. Adult fragile X syndrome. Clinico-neuropathologic findings. *Acta Neuropathol* 1985; 67:289–295.
311. Herbst DS. Non-specific X-linked mental retardation. I. A review with information from 24 new families. *Am J Med Genet* 1980; 7:443–460.
312. Webb TP, Bundey SE, Thake AI, et al. Population incidence and segregation ratios in the Martin-Bell syndrome. *Am J Med Genet* 1986;23:573–580.
313. Webb TP, Bundey SE, Thake AI, et al. The frequency of the fragile X chromosome among school children in Coventry. *J Med Genet* 1987;29:711–719.
314. Rousseau F, Rouillard P, Morel ML, et al. Prevalence of carriers of premutation-size alleles of the *FMR1* gene and implications for the population genetics of the fragile X syndrome. *Am J Hum Genet* 1993;57:1006–1018.
315. De Arce MA, Kearns A. The fragile X syndrome: The patients and their chromosomes. *J Med Genet* 1984;21:84–91.
316. Chudley AE, Hagerman RJ. Fragile X syndrome. *J Pediatr* 1987;110:821–831.
317. Wisniewski KE, French JH, Fernando S, et al. Fragile X syndrome: associated neurological abnormalities and developmental disabilities. *Ann Neurol* 1985;18:665–669.
318. Beemer FA, Veenema H, de Pater JM. Cerebral gigantism (Sotos syndrome) in two patients with Fra (X) chromosomes. *Am J Med Genet* 1986;23:221–226.
319. Stalker HJ, Keller KL, Gray BA, et al. Concurrence of fragile X syndrome and 47, XYY in an individual with a Prader-Willi–like phenotype. *Am J Med Genet* 2003;116A:176 178.
320. Hagerman RJ, Hull CE, Safanda JF, et al. High functioning fragile X males: demonstration of an unmethylated, fully expanded *FMR1* mutation associated with protein expression. *Am J Med Genet* 1994;51:298–308.
321. Hagerman RJ, Staley LW, O'Conner R, et al. Learning-disabled males with a fragile X CGG expansion in the upper premutation size range. *Pediatrics* 1996;97:122–126.
321a. Berry-Kravis E, Potanos K, Weinberg D, et al. Fragile X-associated tremor/ataxia syndrome in sisters related to X-inactivation. *Ann Neurol* 2005;57: 144–147.
322. Greco CM, Hagerman RJ, Tassone F, et al. Neuronal intranuclear inclusions in a new cerebellar tremor/ataxia syndrome among fragile X carriers. *Brain* 125:1760–1771.
323. Hagerman RA, Leavitt BR, Farzin F., et al. Fragile-X-associated tremor/ataxia syndrome (FXTAS) in females with the *FMR1* premutation. *Am J Hum Genet* 2004;74:1051–1056.

324. Hagerman RJ, Jackson AW, Levitas A, et al. An analysis of autism in 50 males with the fragile X syndrome. *Am J Med Genet* 1986;23:359–374.
325. Einfeld S, Hall W. Behavior phenotype of the fragile X syndrome. *Am J Med Genet* 1992;43:56–60.
326. Fisch GS. Is autism associated with the fragile X syndrome? *Am J Med Genet* 1992;43:47–55.
327. Rogers SJ, Wehner DK, Hagerman R. The behavioral phenotype in fragile X: symptoms of autism in very young children with fragile X syndrome, idiopathic autism, and other developmental disorders. *J Dev Behav Pediat* 2001;22:409–417.
328. Hagerman RJ, Jackson C, Amiri K, et al. Girls with fragile X syndrome: Physical and neurocognitive status and outcome. *Pediatrics* 1992;89:395–400.
329. Turner G, Brookwell R, Daniel A, et al. Heterozygous expression of X-linked mental retardation and X-chromosome marker fra(X) q27. *N Engl J Med* 1980;303:662–664.
330. Barry-Kravis E, Lewin F, Wuu J, et al. Tremor and ataxia in fragile X premutation carriers: blinded videotape study. *Ann Neurol* 2003;53:616–623.
331. Gringras P, Barnicoat A. Retesting for fragile X syndrome in cytogenetically normal males. *Dev Med Child Neurol* 1998;40:62–64.
332. Gu Y, Shen Y, Gibbs RA, et al. Identification of *FMR2*, a novel gene associated with the FRAXE CCG repeat and CpG island. *Nat Genet* 1996;13:109–113.
333. Barnicoat AJ, Wang O, Turk J, et al. Clinical, cytogenetic, and molecular analysis of three families with FRAXE. *J Med Genet* 1997;34:13–17.
334. Knight SJ, Flannery AV, Hirst MC, et al. Trinucleotide repeat amplification and hypermethylation of a CpG island in FRAXE mental retardation. *Cell* 1993;74:127–134.
335. Gecz J. The *FMR2* gene, FRAXE and non-specific X-linked mental retardation: clinical and molecular aspects. *Ann Hum Genet* 2000;64:95–106.
336. Hirst MC, Barnicoat A, Flynn G, et al. The identification of a third fragile site, FRAXF, in Xq27–q28 distal to both FRAXA and FRAXE. *Hum Mol Genet* 1993;2:197–200.
337. Molinari F, Rio M, Meskenaite V, et al. Truncating neurotrypsin mutation in autosomic recessive nonsyndromic mental retardation. *Science* 2002;298:1779–1781.
338. Fox P, Fox D, Gerrard JW. X-linked mental retardation: Renpenning revisited. *Am J Med Genet* 1980;7:491–495.
339. Kato M,. Das S, Petras K., et al. Mutations of ARX are associated with striking pleiotropy and consistent genotype–phenotype correlation. *Hum Mutat* 2004;23:147–159.
340. Velagaleti GV, Tapper JH, Rampy BA, et al. A rapid and noninvasive method for detecting tissue-limited mosaicism: detection of i(12)(p10) in buccal smear from a child with Pallister-Killian syndrome. *Genet Test* 2003;7:219–223.
341. Ferguson-Smith MA, Smith K. Cytogenetic analysis. In: Rimoin DL, Connor JM, Pyeritz RE, et al., eds. *Principles and practice of medical genetics*, 4th ed. New York: Churchill Livingstone, 2002:690–722.
342. Carvalho B, Ouwerkerk E, Meijer GA, et al. High resolution microarray comparative genomic hybridization analysis using spotted oligonucleotides. *J Clin Pathol* 2004:57:644–646.
343. Walker HA. Incidence of minor physical anomalies in autistic patients. In: Coleman M, ed. *Autistic syndrome*. New York: Elsevier Science, 1976:95–115.
344. Smith DW, Gong BT. Scalp hair patterning as a clue to early fetal development. *J Pediatr* 1973;83:374–380.
345. Purvis-Smith SG. The Sydney line: a significant sign in Down's syndrome. *Aust Paediatr J* 1972;8:198–200.
346. Shiono H, Azumi J. The Sydney line and the simian line: the incidence in Down's syndrome patients with mental retardation and Japanese controls. *J Ment Defic Res* 1982;26:3–10.
347. Shaffer LG, Bejjani BA. A cytogeneticist's perspective on genomic microarrays. *Hum Reprod Update* 2004;10:221–226.
348. Wolff DJ, Clifton K, Karr C, et al. Pilot assessment of the subtelomeric regions of children with autism: detection of a 2q deletion. *Genet Med* 2002;4:10–12.

Chapter 5

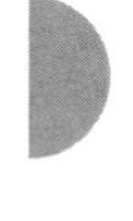

Neuroembryology, Genetic Programming, and Malformations of the Nervous System

PART 1
The New Neuroembryology

Harvey B. Sarnat

> Preformation is represented by DNA, not by . . . a tiny adult in every sperm.
>
> *Antonio García-Bellido, 1998* (1)

Traditional embryology is descriptive morphogenesis: detailed observations of gross and microscopic changes in organs and tissues in the developing embryo and fetus. The *new neuroembryology* is an integration of classic embryology with the insight into molecular genetic programs that direct cellular and regional differentiation to provide an explanation for the precise spatial and temporal sequences of these anatomic changes. Traditional embryology recognizes a series of developmental processes that are not entirely sequential because of a great deal of temporal overlap as the various processes proceed simultaneously. Several excellent recent textbooks effectively integrate descriptive morphogenesis and genetic programming (2–4). In human neuropathology, the gross and microscopic changes seen postmortem are temporally sequenced so precisely that they allow a precise correlation of brain maturation with gestational age and provide evidence of developmental delay in some cases (5).

By means of molecular genetics, the focus on the concepts of normal and abnormal development of the nervous system has shifted from traditional categories of structural change, such as neuronogenesis, cell migration, axonal projection, and synaptogenesis, to an understanding of preprogrammed mechanisms that allow these overlapping processes to proceed. Interactions of genes or their transcription products specify differentiation; developmental genes may be expressed only transiently in the embryo or continuously throughout life. After development appears complete, they conserve the identity of individual cellular types even in the adult and perhaps provide clues to degenerative processes that begin after the nervous system is mature.

The relevance of the new neuroembryology to clinical pediatric neurology, apart from new insights, is in its promise of new approaches for the prevention, and perhaps even potential treatment, of malformations of the nervous system. As a result of these new concepts, one must consider an entirely new and still largely unfamiliar classification of cerebral malformations. Such a classification is to be based on the defective expression or coexpression of transcription products of various developmental genes that determine and coordinate every aspect of neuroembryonic development, from gastrulation and the creation of a neuroepithelium to the last detail of postnatal synaptogenesis and myelination. Of additional importance is the understanding that the development of the nervous system no longer can be isolated from the rest of the embryonic and fetal body, because it is influenced by surrounding structures and also influences them: Segmentation of spinal nerve roots by mesodermal somites is an example of the former, and craniofacial development induced by neural crest migrating from the neural tube exemplifies the latter.

GASTRULATION

> It is not birth, marriage, or death, but gastrulation which is truly the most important time in your life.
>
> *Lewis Wolpert, 1978* (2)

Gastrulation is the birth of the nervous system. It is the time when a neuroepithelium may first be recognized as distinctive from other cells or tissues. In simple chordates, such as amphioxus and amphibians, gastrulation is the invagination of a spherical blastula. In birds and mammals, the blastula is collapsed as a flattened, bilayered disc, and gastrulation appears not as an invagination, but as a groove between two ridges on one surface of this disc, the primitive streak on the epiblast. The primitive streak establishes, in each embryo, the basic body plan of all vertebrates: a midline axis, bilateral symmetry, rostral and caudal ends, and dorsal and ventral surfaces.

As the primitive streak extends forward, an aggregate of cells at one end is designated the primitive node or Hensen's node. Hensen's node defines the rostral direction. Cells of the epiblast on either side move toward the primitive streak, stream through it, and emerge beneath it to pass into the narrow cavity between the two sheets of cells, the epiblast above and the hypoblast below. These migratory cells give rise to the mesoderm and endoderm internally, and some then replace the hypoblast (2).

After extending approximately halfway across the blastoderm (epiblast), the primitive streak with Hensen's node reverses the direction of its growth to retreat, moving posteriorly as the head fold and neural plate form anterior to Hensen's node. As the node regresses, a notochordal process develops in the area rostral to it and somites begin to form on either side of the notochord, the more caudal somites differentiating first and successive ones anterior to somites already formed. The notochord induces epiblast cells to form neuroectoderm (see the following Induction section).

INDUCTION

> Experimental studies of the formation of the neural plate have yielded extraordinarily interesting information as the way one part of a developing embryo may influence the differentiation of other parts.
>
> *B. M. Patten, 1951* (6)

Induction is a term denoting the influence of one embryonic tissue on another so that both the inducer and the induced differentiate as different mature tissues. In the case of the nervous system, the creation and subsequent development of the neural tube may be defined in terms of gradients of inductive influences.

Induction usually occurs between germ layers, as with the notochord (mesoderm) inducing the floor plate of the neural tube (ectoderm). Induction also may occur within a single germ layer, however. An example is the optic cup (neuroectoderm) inducing the formation of a lens and cornea from the overlying epithelium (surface ectoderm) that otherwise would have simply differentiated as more epidermis. Neural induction is the differentiation or maturation of structures of the nervous system from undifferentiated ectodermal cells because of the influence of surrounding embryonic tissues not of ectodermal origin. *Neural induction* is a term also used to describe the opposite: the effects of primitive neural tissues on the development of non-neural structures. An example is craniofacial development, in which neural crest cells migrating from the prosencephalon and mesencephalon of the neural tube induce the formation of membranous cranial and facial bone, cartilage, connective tissue, blood vessels, nerve sheaths, ocular globes, and many other tissues of the face and head (see the Neural Crest section later in this chapter).

Induction was discovered in 1924 by Hans Spemann and Hilde Mangold, who demonstrated that the dorsal lip of the newt gastrula was capable of inducing the formation of an ectopic second nervous system when transplanted to another site in a host embryo, in another individual of the same species, or in a ventral site of the same embryo (7). This dorsal lip of the amphibian gastrula (also known as the *Spemann organizer*) is homologous with Hensen's node of embryonic birds and mammals. The transplantation of the primitive node in a similar manner as in the Spemann and Mangold experiments in amphibians yields similar results.

The first gene isolated from the Spemann organizer was *Goosecoid* (*Gsc*), a homeodomain protein (for definition, see Patterning of the Neural Tube: Axes and Gradients of Growth and Differentiation section) able to recapitulate the transplantation of the dorsal lip tissue. When injected into an ectopic site, *Gsc* also normally induces the prechordal mesoderm and contributes to prosencephalic differentiation (8–10). Another gene also expressed in Hensen's node and even before the primitive streak is fully formed, *Wnt-8C*, also is essential for the regulation of axis formation and later for hindbrain patterning in the region of the future rhombomere 4 (see Segmentation section) (11). The regulatory gene *Cnot*, with major domains in the primitive node, notochord, and prenodal and postnodal neural plate, is another important molecular genetic factor responsible for the induction of prechordal mesoderm and for the formation of the notochord in particular (12). The gene (transcription factor) *Gooseberry* (*Gox*) is unique in being the only identified gene to be expressed in the primitive streak that loses expression at the onset of notochord formation. The *Gox* gene probably regulates the primitive streak either positively, by promoting its elongation, or negatively, by suppressing formation of the notochordal process. Another possible function is to promote a mesodermal lineage of epiblast cells as they ingress through the primitive streak. Several other genes essential in creating the fundamental architecture of the embryo and its nervous system are already expressed in the primitive node (10), and many reappear later to influence more advanced stages of ontogenesis.

The specificity of induction is not the inductive molecule, but rather the receptor in the induced cell. This distinction is important because foreign molecules similar in structure to the natural inductor molecule may at times be recognized erroneously by the receptor as identical; such foreign molecules thus can behave as teratogens if the embryo is exposed to such a toxin. Induction occurs during a precise temporal window; the time of responsiveness of the induced cell is designated its competence, and it is incapable of responding either before that precise time or thereafter (13).

Induction receptors are not necessarily in or on the plasma membrane of the cell, but also can be in the cytoplasm or in the nucleoplasm. Retinoic acid (see Retinoic Acid section) is an example of a nuclear inducer. In some cases, the stimulus acts exclusively at the plasma membrane of target cells and does not require actual penetration of the cell (13,14). The receptors that represent the specificity of induction also are genetically programmed: A gene known as *Notch* is particularly important in regulating the competence of a cell to respond to inductive cues from within the neural tube and in surrounding embryonic tissues (15). Some mesodermal tissues, such as smooth muscle of the fetal gut, can act as mitogens on the neuroepithelium by increasing the rate of cellular proliferation (16,17), but this phenomenon is not true neural induction because the proliferating cells do not differentiate or mature. Some organizer and regulatory genes of the nervous system, such as *Wnt-1*, also exhibit mitogenic effects (18), and both insulin-like and basic fibroblast growth factors (bFGF) act as mitogens as well (19–21).

The early formation of the neural plate is not accomplished exclusively by mitotic proliferation of neuroepithelial cells, but also by a conversion of surrounding cells to a neural fate. In amphibians, a gene known as *Achaete-scute* (*Xash-3*) is expressed early in the dorsal part of the embryo from the time of gastrulation and acts as a molecular switch to change the fate of undifferentiated cells to become neuroepithelium rather than surface ectodermal or mesodermal tissues (22). Some cells differentiate as specific types because they are actively inhibited from differentiating as other cell types. All ectodermal cells are preprogrammed to form neuroepithelium, and neuroepithelial cells are preprogrammed to become neurons if not inhibited by genes that direct their differentiation along a different lineage, such as epidermal, glial, or ependymal (23–25).

SEGMENTATION

> The primitive segmentation of the vertebrate brain is a problem which has probably attracted as much of the attention of morphologists as any one of the great, unsettled questions of the day, and many views have been advanced.
>
> *C. F. W. McClure, 1890* (26)

Over a century ago, the concept of segmentation was already an issue actively debated by biologists who were intrigued by the repeating units along the rostrocaudal axis of many worms and insects as well as by the somites of embryonic vertebrates. Segmentation of the neural tube creates intrinsic compartments that restrict the movement of cells by physical and chemical boundaries between adjacent compartments. These embryonic compartments are known as *neuromeres*.

The spinal cord has the appearance of a highly segmented structure but is not intrinsically segmented in the embryo, fetus, or adult. Instead it corresponds in its entirety to the caudalmost of the eight neuromeres that create the hindbrain. The apparent segmentation of the spinal cord is caused by clustering of nerve roots imposed by true segmentation of surrounding tissues derived from mesoderm, tissues that form the neural arches of the vertebrae, the somites, and associated structures. Neuromeres of the hindbrain are designated rhombomeres (27–30). The entire cerebellar cortex, vermis, flocculonodular lobe, and lateral hemispheres, develops from rhombomere 1 with a small contribution from the mesencephalic neuromere, but the dentate and other deep cerebellar nuclei are formed in rhombomere 2 (31,32). The rostral end of the neural tube forms a mesencephalic neuromere and probably six forebrain neuromeres, as three diencephalic and three telencephalic prosomeres (33–36). The segmentation of the human embryonic brain into neuromeres is summarized in Table 5.1.

The segments of the embryonic neural tube are distinguished by physical barriers formed by processes of early-specializing cells that resemble the radial glial cells that appear later in development (37,38) and also by chemical barriers from secreted molecules that repel migratory cells. Cell adhesion is increased in the boundary zones between rhombomeres, which also contributes to the creation of barriers against cellular migration in the longitudinal axis (38). Limited mitotic proliferation of the neuroepithelium occurs in the boundary zones between rhombomeres. Although cells still divide in this zone, their nuclei remain near the ventricle during the mitotic cycle and do not move as far centrifugally within the elongated cell cytoplasm during the interkinetic gap phases as they do in general (38). The rhombomeres of the brainstem

TABLE 5.1 Segmentation of the Neural Tube

Neuromere[a]	*Derived Structures in Mature Central Nervous System*
Rhombomere 8	Entire spinal cord; caudal medulla oblongata; cranial nerves XI, XII
Rhombomere 7	Medulla oblongata; cranial nerves IX, X; neural crest
Rhombomere 6	Medulla oblongata; cranial nerves VIII, IX
Rhombomere 5	Medulla oblongata; cranial nerves VI, VII; no neural crest
Rhombomere 4	Medulla oblongata; cranial nerves VI, VII; neural crest
Rhombomere 3	Caudal pons; cranial nerve V; no neural crest
Rhombomere 2	Caudal pons; cranial nerves IV, V; cerebellar nuclei
Rhombomere 1	Rostral pons; cerebellar cortex
Mesencephalic neuromere	Midbrain; cranial nerve III; neural crest
Diencephalic prosomere 2	Dorsal diencephalon
Diencephalic prosomere 1	Ventral diencephalon
Prosencephalic prosomere 2	Telencephalic nuclei; olfactory bulb
Prosencephalic prosomere 1	Cerebral cortex; hippocampus; corpus callosum

[a]Rhombomere 3 is associated with the first branchial arch; rhombomeres 4 and 5 are associated with the second branchial arch; rhombomere 7 is associated with the third branchial arch.

also may be visualized as a series of transverse ridges and grooves on the dorsal surface, the future floor of the fourth ventricle; these ridges are gross morphologic markers of the hindbrain compartments (26,30).

The first evidence of segmentation is a boundary that separates the future mesencephalic neuromere from rhombomere 1 of the hindbrain. More genes play a role in this initial segmentation of the neural tube than in the subsequent formation of other boundaries that develop to separate other neuromeres. Furthermore, the mesencephalic–metencephalic region appears to develop early as a single independent unit or *organizer* for other neuromeres rostral and caudal to that zone (39,40). The organizer genes recognized at the mesencephalic–metencephalic boundary for this earliest segmentation of the neural tube include *Pax-2*, *Wnt-1*, *En-1*, *En-2*, *Pax-5*, *Pax-8*, *Otx-1*, *Otx-2*, *Gbx-2*, *Nkx-2.2*, and *FGF-8*.

The earliest gene known with regional expression in the mouse is *Pax-2*, which is expressed even before the neural plate forms. It is the earliest gene recognized in the presumptive region of the midbrain–hindbrain boundary (41,42). In invertebrates, *Pax-2* is important for the activation of *Wingless* (*Wg*) genes; this relationship is relevant because the first gene definitely associated with an identified midbrain–hindbrain boundary in vertebrates is *Wnt-1*, a homologue of *Wg*. The regulation of *Wnt-1* may be divided into two phases: In the early phase (1 to 2 somites), the mesencephalon broadly expresses the gene throughout. In the later phase (15 to 20 somites), expression is restricted to dorsal regions, the roof plate of the caudal diencephalon, mesencephalon and myelencephalon, and spinal cord. It also is expressed in a ring that extends ventrally just rostral to the midbrain–hindbrain boundary and in the ventral midline of the caudal diencephalon and mesencephalon (43–45). *Wnt-1* is essential in activating and preserving the function of the *Engrailed* genes *En-1* and *En-2*. *En-1* is coexpressed with *Wnt-1* at the one-somite stage, in a domain only slightly caudal to *Wnt-1*, which includes the midbrain and rhombomere 1, the rostral half of the pons, and the cerebellar cortex but excludes the diencephalon (46). The activation of *En-2* begins at the four-somite stage, and its function in mesencephalic and rhombomere 1 development is similar, with differences in some details, particularly their roles in cerebellar development (47,48). Finally, the homeobox gene *Otx-2* appears early in the initial boundary zone of the midbrain–hindbrain, and, as with *Wnt-1*, it appears to be essential for the later expression of *En-1* and *En-2* and also of *Wnt-1* (49,50).

The creation of neuromeres allows the development of structures within regions of the brain without the neuroblasts that form these nuclei wandering to other parts of the neuraxis where they would not be able to later establish their required synaptic relations. The interaction of genes with one another is a complexity that makes analysis of single-gene expression more difficult in interpreting programmed malformations of the brain.

PATTERNING OF THE NEURAL TUBE: AXES AND GRADIENTS OF GROWTH AND DIFFERENTIATION

Basic characteristics of the body plan are called *patterning* (27). They are the anatomic expression of the genetic code within the nuclear DNA of every cell, but they also may result from signals from neighboring cells, carried by molecules that are secretory translation products of various families of organizer genes, each in a highly precise and predictable temporal and spatial distribution.

The early development of the central nervous system (CNS) of all vertebrates, even before the closure of the neural placode or plate to form the neural tube, requires the establishment of a fundamental body plan of bilateral symmetry, cephalization, or the identity of head and tail ends, and dorsal and ventral surfaces. This fundamental architecture of the body and of the neural tube requires the establishment of definite axes of growth and gradients of genetic expression and differentiation: (a) a *longitudinal axis* with rostrocaudal and caudorostral gradients, (b) a *vertical axis* with dorsoventral and ventrodorsal gradients, and (c) a *horizontal axis* with mediolateral and lateromedial gradients. Both normal ontogenesis and abnormal development of the embryonic nervous system involve these axes and gradients and should be put into this perspective (51).

These axes of the body itself, and of the CNS, require the expression of genes that impose the gradients of differentiation and growth. The genes that determine the polarity and gradients of the anatomic axes are called *organizer genes*. Many express themselves not only in the CNS but in other organs and tissues as well (2,45). The bilateral symmetry of many organs and programmed asymmetries, probably including such neural structures as the different targets of the left and right vagal nerves and left–right asymmetries in the cerebral cortex, is determined in large part by *Pitx-2*, a gene expressed as early as in the primitive node (52).

The RNA that represents a transcript of the DNA translates a peptide, a glycoprotein, or some other molecule that acts to induce or at times to serve as a growth factor. Some genes also function to stimulate or inhibit the expression of others, or an antagonism or equilibrium can exist between certain families of genes, exemplified by those that exert a dorsoventral gradient and those that cause a ventrodorsal gradient.

The difference between an *organizer gene* and a *regulator gene* really lies in its function, and often the same gene subserves both roles at different stages of development. The definitions and programs of these two groups are summarized in Tables 5.2 and 5.3.

Evolutionary Conservation of Genes

The sequences of nucleotides of DNA are so primordial to animal life that identical or nearly identical base pairs exist not only in all vertebrates, but in all invertebrates as well, from the simplest worms to the most complex primates (53). The evolutionary biologists of the nineteenth century, such as Charles Darwin and Thomas Huxley, were constantly searching for "the missing links" between mammals and other vertebrates, between humans and other primates, and, most of all, between invertebrates and vertebrates because comparative anatomy did not provide a sufficiently satisfactory answer. They never found the missing link because the technology of their day could not elucidate this fundamental and profound question. The missing link sought by the nineteenth-century evolutionary biologists lies in the identical sequences of nucleic acid residues that form the same organizer genes in all animals, from the simplest worms to humans.

Despite evolutionary conservation of genes, there may be some variability among species in the compartmental site within the embryonic neural tube of structures programmed by these genes. For example, the abducens motor nucleus forms in rhombomere 6 in elasmobranchs (sharks) but in rhombomere 5 in mammals; the trigeminal/facial boundary shifts from rhombomere 4 in lampreys to rhombomere 3 in birds and mammals.

TABLE 5.2 Programs of Developmental Genes

- I. **Organizer Genes**
  - A. Cell proliferation
  - B. Identity of organs or tissues (e.g., neural, renal)
  - C. Axes of polarity and growth
    1. Ventrodorsal
    2. Dorsoventral
    3. Rostrocaudal
    4. Caudorostral
    5. Mediolateral
    6. Lateromedial
  - D. Segmentation
  - E. Left–right symmetry or asymmetry
- II. **Regulator Genes**
  - A. Differentiation of structures and specialization within organ
  - B. Cell lineage: differentiation and specialization of individual cells
  - C. Inhibition of other genetic programs in order to change a cell lineage

Transcription Factors and Homeoboxes

The genes that program the development of the nervous system are specific series of DNA base pairs linked to small proteins called *transcription factors*. These transcription factors are essential for the functional expression of these genes. A frequent transcription factor is the basic helix-loop-helix structure. It is so fundamental to the evolution of life that it appears for the first time in certain bacteria, even before a cell nucleus evolved to concentrate the DNA (53).

The zinc finger is another DNA-binding, gene-specific transcription factor. It consists of 28 amino acid repeats with pairs of cysteine and histidine residues, each sequence folded around a zinc ion (54). *Krox-20* (this gene name is applied to the mouse; in the human it is redesignated *EGR2*) is a zinc finger gene expressed in alternating rhombomeres, especially rhombomere 3 and rhombomere 5; neural crest tissue does not migrate from those two rhombomeres (see Neural Crest section). *Krox-20* also

TABLE 5.3 Organizer and Regulator Genes of the Embryonic and Fetal Nervous System

Gene	Region	Functions	References
Achaete-scute	Epiblast	Changes the fate of undifferentiated cells to form neuroepithelium	22
BMP4 (bone morphogenic protein)	Hensen's node; neural plate	Inhibits cells from forming neural tissue; dorsalizing to neural tube; of transforming growth factor β family	24,25
Cart1	Head mesenchyme	Organizes head mesoderm before neural crest arrival	94
Cnot	Hensen's node	Induces the primitive node to form notochordal process; induces neural placode	12
Delta	—	Antagonizes *Notch;* inhibits neural differentiation	—
Dab-1 (*Disabled-1*)	Laminated cortices	Acts downstream of *rein* for terminal neuroblast migration and cortical lamination	—
Dix1, Dix2 (*Distal-less*)	Prosomeres; ventral thalamus; anterior hypothalamus; corpus striatum	Subcortical neuroblast migration; interneuron migration from basal forebrain to neocortex	23
Dorsalin1	Neural tube	Dorsalizing; of transforming growth factor β family	95
Doublecortin	Telencephalon	Neuroblast migration; Xq22.3–q23 locus; defective in subcortical laminar heterotopia (band heterotopia; double-cortex syndrome)	96,97
EMX2	Telencephalon	Neuroblast migration; defective in schizencephaly	98
En-1, En-2 (*engralled*)	Mesencephalon, r1	Formation of mesencephalon and metenoephalon, including entire cerebellar cortex	31,32,39,43,45–48, 99–101
FLM-A (*Filamin A*)	Telencephalon	Neuroblast migration; defective in X-linked dominant periventricular heterotopia	102
Gbx-2 (unplugged)	r1–r3	Specification of anterior hindbrain; contributes to formation of the cerebellum, motor trigeminal nerve	40
Gox (*Gooseberry*)	Primitive streak	Regulates elongation of primitive streak; disappears at onset of notochord formation; related to *Otx* homeobox; promotes epiblast cells to become mesoderm	—
Gsc (*Goosecoid*)	Hensen's node, neural plate	Induces prechordal mesoderm and prosencephalon; ectopically duplicates neural tube	8–10
Hex3	Prosencephalon	Folate-dependent gene; defective in septo-optic dysplasia	—
HNF3β (*winged helix*)	Notochord	Regulates floor plate development; suppresses dorsalizing influence of *Pax-3*	72
Hox-1.5	r3; r5	Segmentation; formation of parathyroid, thymus (ref. *Hox* family)	—
Hox-1.6 (*Hoxa-1*)	r4–r7	Rostrocaudal gradient and segmentation	28–30,80,82–84
Hox-2.1	r8	Rostrocaudal gradient of spinal cord	—
Hox-2.6	Border r6/7–r8	Rostrocaudal gradient and segmentation	—
Hox-2.8	Border r2/3–r8	Rostrocaudal gradient and segmentation; regulates axonal projections from r3	—
Hox-2.9 (*Hoxb-1*)	r4	Formation of neural crest	59,80
HNF (*forkhead*)	Neural plate	Patterning of the midline of the neural tube	—
Islet-1	Ventral neural tube	Motor neuroblast differentiation	103
Islet-3	Neural plate	Floor plate differentiation; suppresses *Pax-3*	104
Krox-20 (*EGR2*)	r3; r5	Zinc finger; regulates expression of *Hox* genes; regulates myelination of Schwann cells	55–57
L1CAM	Mesencephalon; telencephalon	Formation of aqueduct; cerebral neuroblast migration defective in X-linked hydrocephalus with aqueductal stenosis and also reported in hemimegalencephaly	105,106
Lhx2	Prosomeres	*LIM*-family homeobox; development of hippocampus and cellular proliferation for neocortex; development of eye before formation of optic cup	107

(*continued*)

TABLE 5.3 (Continued) Organizer and Regulator Genes of the Embryonic and Fetal Nervous System

Gene	Region	Functions	References
LIM	Neural plate; prechordal mesenchyme	Organizer of cephalic mesenchyme before migration of neural crest; organizer of neural placode	104,108
LIS1	Cortical plate	Neuroblast migration; 17p13.3 locus; defective in lissencephaly type I	109–112
Math1	r1, cerebellum	Differentiation of cerebellar granule cells	113
Math5	Optic cup	Retinal differentiation	93
MNR	Motor neuroblasts	Motor neuron identity	114
Neuro-D	Ectodermal cells	Neuronal differentiation; three subtypes on human chromosomes 2, 5, 17; related to gene regulating transcription of insulin; retinal development	85–88,89–92
Neurogenin (*Ngn*)	Ectodermal cells	Neuronal differentiation in central nervous system and peripheral nervous system; expressed earlier than *neuro-D;* interacts with *Delta* and *Notch;* family of subtypes	115–117
Nkx2.1	Prosomeres	Differentiation of hypothalamus; induced by *Shh*	118
Nkx2.2	All neuromeres	Specifies diencephalic neuromeric boundaries; interacts with *Dlx1* and transcription factor TTF1 for prosencephalic differentiation	118,119
Nkx6.1	Diencephalon-r8; motor neurons	Induced by *Shh* and repressed by *BMP7;* coexpressed with *Istet-1* in motor neurons	118
Nkx6.2	Diencephalon-r8	Same as *gtx;* glial cell differentiation	118
Noggin	Hensen's node	Inhibits *BMP4* to allow neural plate differentiation	24,25,120
Notch	Neural plate; neuroepithelium	Regulates the competence of cells to respond to inductive signals; differentiation of neural placode; asymmetric distribution in cytoplasm during mitotic cycle	121,122
Numb	Neural plate; fetal neuroepithelium	Antagonizes *Notch* by preventing neural differentiation	121,123
Otx-1 (orthodenticle)	Mesencephalon/r1 boundary; telencephalon; sensory nerves	Onset of neuromere formation; corticogenesis; sense organ development	—
Otx-2 (orthodenticle)	Prestreak blastomere; neural plate	Gastrulation; specification and maintenance of anterior neural plate	49,50
Pit1 (pituitary-specific)	Adenohypophysis	Differentiation of anterior pituitary	—
ptc (patched)	Cerebellar cortex	Regulates granule cell proliferation; tumor-suppressor gene	124–128
Pax-2 (paired)	Primitive streak; r2–r8; prosomeres	Dorsalizing polarity gradient; segmentation regulated by notochord and floor plate; formation of ventral half of optic cup, retina, and optic nerve; overlaps and partially redundant with *Pax-5*	39,43,77,129
Pax-3 (paired)	r1; r8	Identity of Bergmann glia; active spinal cord dorsalizing gradient	77
Pax-5 (paired)	r1	Partially redundant with *Pax-2* for differentiation of cerebellar cortex; dorsalizing gradient	77,129
Pax-6 (paired)	r1; r8; prosomeres	Identity of cerebellar granule cells; active in spinal cord as dorsalizing gradient; neuroblast migration to cerebral cortex and deep telencephalic nuclei	76,77
Pitx	Primitive streak	Determines right–left asymmetries of internal organs	52
Reelin (*reln*)	Laminar cortices	Extracellular matrix glycoprotein product secreted by Cajal-Retzius neurons and cerebellar granule cells, essential for terminal neuroblast migration and laminar architecture	95,130–132

(*continued*)

TABLE 5.3 (Continued) Organizer and Regulator Genes of the Embryonic and Fetal Nervous System

Gene	Region	Functions	References
RhoB	Dorsal neural tube	Delamination of neural crest cells; *BMP* gene	133
Shh (*Sonic hedgehog*)	Notochord; floor plate; prechordal mesoderm	Induces floor plate; ventralizing influence of neural tube; ventral midline of prosencephalon; induction of motor neurons; mitogen to cerebellar granule cells	66–70,74,75,124, 127,134
Slug	Neural crest	Neural crest differentiation; homologue of *Snail* in invertebrates	—
SMN (survival motor neuron)	Motor neuroblasts	Arrests apoptosis of motor neuroblasts	135,136
TSC1, TSC2	Neuraxis	Encodes proteins hamartin and tuberin; *TSC1* at 9q34 locus; *TSC2* at 16p13.3 locus; both defective in tuberous sclerosis	137–142
Twist	Hensen's node	Organizer of cephalic mesenchyme before migration of neural crest; cranial neural tube morphogenesis	143
TOAD-64 (*uno-33*)	Growth cones	Promotes axonal outgrowth	144
Wnt-1 (*wingless*)	r1; r3–r8	Formation of mesencephalic–metencephalic boundary; formation of mesencephalon, rostral pons, and cerebellum; essential for expression of *En-1*; weak dorsal polarizing influence in r3–r8; mitogen	31,39,43,46,78,95, 145,146
Wnt-3 (*wingless*)	Mesencephalon; r1; r3–r8	Overlaps and redundant with *Wnt-1* in mesencephalic neuromere and r1; strong dorsal polarizing influence in r3–r8 including spinal cord; differentiation of brainstem nuclei; identity of Purkinje cells	78,147
Wnt-7 (*wingless*)	Prosomeres	Differentiation of structures of diencephalon and telencephalon	34
Wnt-8 (*wingless*)	Epiblast; primitive streak; r1–r8	Primitive streak formation; segmentation	11
Zic1	Cerebellum	Zinc finger; differentiation of granule cells	148,149

An *organizer gene* is defined as one that programs the differentiation of the neural placode, neural axes, and gradients and segmentation of the neural plate and neural tube; a *regulator gene* is defined as one that programs the differentiation of specific structures and cellular types in the developing nervous system and conserves their identity and mediates developmental processes such as neuroblast migration or synaptogenesis. The genes are listed alphabetically rather than by function because many of the same genes serve various functions at different stages, as organizer genes in early ontogenesis and as regulator genes at later periods. This is a partial list of some of the most important in the nervous system of the more than 80,000 genes that have already been identified in the human genome. Developmental genes recognized in invertebrate such as *Drosophila*, but for which the vertebrate homologue has not yet been identified, are excluded.

r1, rhombomere 1; r2, rhombomere 2, and so forth.

serves an additional function in the peripheral nervous system, where it regulates myelination by Schwann cells (55). Finally, *Krox-20* regulates the expression of some other genes, most notably those of the *Hox* family (56–60). Examples of other zinc fingers include *Zic*, *TFIIIA*, *cSnR* (snail related), and *PLZF* (human promyelocytic leukemia zinc finger) (61).

Complexes of retinoic acid with its intranuclear receptor form still other transcription factors important in nervous system development, both normal and abnormal (see Retinoic Acid section). A unique transcription factor with coactivation domain requirements, *Pit*, programs anterior pituitary differentiation (62,63).

Growth factors, which also are molecules created by DNA sequences, are other influences on the establishment of the plan of the neural tube. Biologically, they act as transcription factors: bFGF behaves as an auxiliary inductor of the longitudinal axis with a rostrocaudal gradient during the formation of the neural tube (64).

Some transcription factors include homeoboxes. These are restricted DNA sequences of 183 base pairs of nucleotides that encode a class of proteins sharing a common or similar 60-amino acid motif termed the *homeodomain* (27). Homeodomains contain sequence-specific DNA-binding activities and are integral parts of the larger regulatory proteins, the transcription factors. Homeoboxes or homeotic genes are classified into various families with common molecular structure and similar general expression in ontogenesis. Homeoboxes are associated especially with genes that program segmentation and rostrocaudal gradients of the neural tube. Some of the important families of homeobox genes in the development of the vertebrate nervous system are *Gsc*, *Hox*, *En*, *Wnt*, *Shh*, *Nkx*, *LIM*, and *Otx*.

Families of Developmental Genes of the Central Nervous System

The genes that program the axes and gradients of the neural tube may be classified as families by their similar nucleic acid sequences and also by their similar general functions, although important differences occur within a family in the site or neuromere where each gene is expressed and in the anatomic structures they form. A dorsalizing gene not only has a dorsal territory of expression, but also causes the ventral parts of the neural tube to differentiate as dorsal structures if influences from ventralizing genes do not antagonize them with sufficient strength, and vice versa. A good example is the development of the somite. The sclerotome, which forms cartilage and bone of the vertebral body, normally is situated ventral to the myotome, which forms muscle cells, and the dermatome. Ectopic cells of the floor plate or of the notochord implanted next to the somite of the chick embryo cause a ventralization of the somite, so that excess cartilage and bone are formed and a deficiency of muscle and dermis occurs (65,66). The floor plate or notochord, in this instance, is the ventralizing inductor of the mesodermal somite, and it is now known that the genetic factor responsible is the transcription product of the gene *Sonic hedgehog* (*Shh*), which also serves as a strong ventralizing gradient force in the neural tube (25,67–70). If a section of notochord is implanted ectopically dorsal or lateral to the neural tube, a second floor plate forms opposite the notochord and motor neurons differentiate on either side of it, despite the presence of a normal floor plate and motor neurons in the normal position (71,72). *Shh*, a strong gene of the ventrodorsal gradient that becomes expressed as early as in the primitive node, has induced the ventralization of a dorsal region of the neural tube or duplicates the neural tube. Such an influence in the human fetus, the so-called split notochord, could be an explanation of the rare cases of diplomyelia or diastematomyelia (73). Excessive *Shh*, particularly its N-terminus cleavage product, upregulates floor plate differentiation at the expense of motor neuron formation (68) and might even induce duplication of the neuraxis. Furthermore, *Shh* also exerts a strong influence on the differentiation of ventral and medial structures of the prosencephalon (74), and the defective expression resulting from a mutation of this gene is thought to be the molecular basis of the human malformation holoprosencephaly (75).

To establish an equilibrium with genes with a ventralizing influence, other families of genes exercise a dorsalizing influence, causing the differentiation of dorsal structures of the neural tube; the *PAX* family is an example (74,77). The *WNT* family also is dorsalizing in the hindbrain; *in situ* hybridization shows its transcription products expressed diffusely only in the early neuroepithelium and restricted to dorsal regions as the neural tube develops (78). The zinc finger gene *Zic2* has a dorsalizing gradient in the forebrain. The rostrocaudal axis of the neural tube and segmentation, or the formation of neuromeres, are directed in large part by a family of 38 genes called *Hox* genes, which are divided into four groups (28,29,79–83). Each of 13 *HOX* genes is expressed in certain rhombomeres and not in others (see Table 5.3). In addition to their functions in establishing the compartments or rhombomeres of the brainstem and effecting the differentiation of certain anatomic structures, *Hox* genes also serve as guides of growth cones that are forming the long descending and ascending pathways between the brain and spinal cord (84).

Another important organizer gene expressed early in ontogenesis is *Neuro-D*, which appears in primitive neuroepithelium just after gastrulation and continues to be expressed throughout fetal life and at maturity, even appearing in cultured cortical neurons (85,86). *Neuro-D* converts ectoderm from an epidermal to a neural lineage and thus is important in the early differentiation of the neuroepithelium (87). Transcription products of *Neuro-D* may be cloned from neuroblastoma cell lines expressed in fetal brain and adult cerebellum (88). *Neuro-D* also serves as a regulator gene for the differentiation of retinal neurons, including photoreceptor cells (89,90). The multiple functions of human *Neuro-D* are related to at least three subtypes that map to human chromosomes 2q32, 5q23–q31, and 17q12 (91,92). *Math*5 also is expressed during the earliest stages of retinal neurogenesis (93) and probably has a close interaction with *Neuro-D*.

Genes that direct the specific differentiation of structures are called regulatory genes, and frequently are the same genes that served as organizer genes in an earlier period. The most important families for the development of the brainstem and midbrain are *Engrailed* (*EN*), *Wingless* (*WNT*), *HOX*, *EGR*, and *Paired* (*PAX*). Table 5.3 summarizes the sites of expression and functions of the most important organizer and regulator genes. Genes have peculiar names that do not correspond to their function. At times the same gene is given a slightly different name in vertebrates and invertebrates, despite an identical nucleotide sequence. For example, *Sonic hedgehog* in vertebrates is simply *Hedgehog* in invertebrates. Other *hedgehog* genes in vertebrates are *Desert hedgehog* and *Indian hedgehog*, but these do not appear to be involved in the ontogenesis of the neural tube.

Many genes exert influences on the expression of others and some serve redundant functions with others. The gene *En-1* has a strong domain in the mesencephalic neuromere and also in rhombomere 1, the rhombomere that forms the rostral half of the pons and the cerebellar cortex. This same territory corresponds to the neuromeric expressions of *Wnt-1* and *Wnt-3*. One of the *Wnt* genes is necessary to augment the expression of *En-1*; if a loss of *Wnt-1* or *Wnt-3* occurs by mutation, the other *Wnt* gene is able to compensate alone, and no malformation of the brain is observed in homozygotes. The overlapping and redundant expression of these two *Wnt* genes provides a kind of plasticity at the molecular level for the developing nervous system. If *Wnt-1* expression is lost, however, the expression of *Wnt-3* is insufficient to compensate in the rostral regions of the future brainstem, and the result is a defective midbrain and pons and cerebellar hypoplasia (39,46,99,150). The genes *En-1* and *En-2* have similar functions with differences in some details and are demonstrated in the human fetus as well as in the mouse (100).

Another complexity in gene interrelationships is that many regulatory genes change their territories of expression in different stages of development, increasing to include more rhombomeres or broader expression early in development and being more restricted in domain later. At times, the expression of a gene in the wrong neuromere, called *ectopic expression*, interferes with normal development.

Retinoic Acid

Retinoic acid, the alcohol of which is vitamin A, is a hydrophobic molecule secreted by the notochord and ependymal floor plate cells (151). Retinoid-binding proteins and receptors are already strongly expressed in mesenchymal cells of the primitive streak and in the preotic region of the early-developing hindbrain (152). Ependymal cells other than those of the floor plate and neuroepithelial cells have retinoic acid receptors but do not secrete this compound.

Retinoic acid diffuses across the plasma membrane without requiring active transport and binds to intracellular receptors. It enters the cell nucleus, where it binds to a specific nuclear receptor protein and changes the structural configuration of that protein, enabling it to attach to a specific receptor on a target gene, where the complexes formed by retinoic acid and its receptor then function as a transcription factor for neural induction (153,154). Other transcription factors of developmental genes already mentioned are the basic helix-loop-helix and zinc fingers.

Retinoic acid functions as a polarity molecule for determining the anterior and posterior surfaces of limb buds and, in the nervous system, is important in segmentation polarity and is a strong rostrocaudal polarity gradient (2,155,156). Excessive retinoic acid acts on the neural tube of amphibian tadpoles to transform anterior neural tissue to a posterior morphogenesis, resulting in extreme microcephaly and suppression of optic cup formation (154). Failure of optic cup formation may be caused by retinoic acid suppression by genes of the *LIM* family, such as *Islet-3* and *Lim-1* (104,107). Retinoic acid upregulates homeobox genes, those of the *HOX* family and *Krox-20* in particular, and causes ectopic expression of these genes in rhombomeres where normally they are not expressed (157). An excess of retinoic acid, whether endogenous or exogenous as in mothers who take an excess of vitamin A during early gestation, results in severe malformations of the hindbrain and spinal cord. A single dose of retinoic acid administered intraperitoneally to maternal hamsters on embryonic day 9.5 results in the Chiari type II malformation and often meningomyelocele in the fetuses (158–160). In cell cultures of cloned CNS stem cells from the mouse, retinoic acid enhances neuronal proliferation and astroglial differentiation (161).

SUMMARIZED PRINCIPLES OF GENETIC PROGRAMMING

The molecular genetic regulation of neural tube development may be summarized as a series of principles of genetic programming (51).

Principle 1: *Developmental genes are reused repeatedly*. Nature recognizes useful genes and uses them over and over again during embryonic development, but developmental genes play different roles at different stages. An organizer gene of the neural axis or of segmentation may later serve as a regulator gene for the differentiation and maintenance of specific cells of the CNS. Genes of growth factors also are reused at different stages; the fibroblast growth factor gene *EGF8* is active during gastrulation but later contributes to cardiac, craniofacial, midbrain, cerebellar, and forebrain development (162). The classification of a gene as an *organizer* or a *regulator*, therefore, depends on the specific embryonic stage and its function at that stage of development.

Principle 2: *Domains of organizer genes change in successive stages*. The domains, or territories of expression, of organizer genes generally are diffuse initially and become more localized or confined to certain neuromeres as the neural tube develops.

Principle 3: *Relative gene domains may differ in various neuromeres*. The domain of one gene may be dorsal to another in rostral neuromeres and ventral to it in caudal neuromeres at any given stage of development. An example is the case of *Nkx2.2* and *Nkx6.1*, both of which are coexpressed throughout most of the length of the neural tube. The domain of *Nkx2.2* is dorsal to that of *Nkx6.1* in the diencephalic and mesencephalic neuromeres but shifts to a position ventral to that of *Nkx6.1* in the hindbrain and spinal cord (118,119).

Principle 4: *Some genes activate, regulate, or suppress the expression of others*. Some organizer genes act sequentially, so that one already-expressed gene initiates the expression of another that follows or that becomes coexpressed. A failure of the first gene thus may result in a lack of expression of others, producing a more extensive developmental defect than might be anticipated from the loss of the first gene alone. An example is the normal cascade of *Pax-2* activating *Wnt-1* at the mesencephalic–metencephalic boundary at the beginning of neuromere formation; *Wnt-1* then activates *En-1* and *En-2*. Another example is the activation by *Shh* of *Nkx-2.1* in the rostral neural plate and *Nkx-6.1* in the caudal neural plate (118).

Some genes act by inhibiting or antagonizing the genetic programs of others. *Notch* and *Achaete-scute* change the fate of undifferentiated cells so that they form neuroepithelium and signal the formation of the neural plate; *Numb* and *Delta* antagonize these genes and inhibit neural differentiation. Bone morphogenic protein 4 (*BMP4*), expressed in Hensen's node, inhibits ectodermal germ cells from forming neural tissue and promotes epidermal differentiation, but *Noggin* inhibits *BMP4*, thus allowing neural plate formation to proceed (24,25). The formation of dorsal structures including the neural plate in the early embryo depends on the absence of *BMP4* expression. *Wnt-1* and *Wnt-3* cause neural crest cells to form melanocytes instead of proceeding with neuronal fates (163).

All neuroepithelial cells are preprogrammed to form neurons; glial and ependymal cells can form only when this program is inhibited (24,101,164).

Principle 5: *Defective homeoboxes usually have reduced domains*. A defective homeobox gene, especially one of segmentation, usually is expressed in fewer neuromeres than normal, a reduction in its domain; it may even lose all of its expression. These changes occur in the homozygous and not the heterozygous state of genetic animal models.

Principle 6: *Some genes may compensate for the loss of others if their domains overlap: redundancy and synergy*. Some genes coexpressed in the same neuromeres may compensate, in part or in full, for the loss of expression of one of the pair, so that anatomic development, maturation, and function of the nervous system all proceed normally. An example is the coexpression of *Wnt-1* and *Wnt-3* in the myelencephalic rhombomeres. If *Wnt-1* is defective in rhombomeres 4 to 9 of the mouse but *Wnt-3* continues to be normally expressed, the hindbrain develops normally. This principle is known as *redundancy*. In the continued expression in adult life of some regulator genes to conserve cell identity, oculomotor, trochlear, and abducens neurons, but not hypoglossal or spinal motor neurons, are conserved by *Wnt-1*– and *LIM*-family genes. These genes can compensate for loss of expression of other genes expressed in all motor neurons to preserve normal extraocular muscle innervation in spinal muscular atrophy. Specification of specific motor neuron identity also is provided by the *MNR2* gene product (114). *Neurogenin* is another gene that, after its organizer function of directing neuronal lineage, has a regulator function in determining the type of neuron in both the central and peripheral nervous systems (115–117).

A variation of the principle of redundancy is synergy, cooperation of two or more genes to produce effects that none is capable of achieving alone. An example is the synergy between *Pax-2* and *Pax-5* in midbrain and cerebellar development (129). If one of this pair is lost, partial but not total compensation may occur.

Principle 7: *An organizer gene may be upregulated to be expressed in ectopic domains*. Certain molecules may act as teratogens in the developing nervous system if the embryo is exposed to an excess, whether the excess is exogenous or endogenous in origin. The inductive mechanism is the upregulation of organizer genes so that they become expressed in ectopic domains such as in neuromeres where they do not normally play a role in development. An example is retinoic acid, which induces ectopic expression of *Hox* genes.

Upregulation of some genes may suppress the expression of others, also contributing to dysgenesis. The overexpression of *LIM* proteins containing only *Islet-3* homeodomains in the zebrafish causes an early termination of expression of *Wnt-1*, *En-2*, and *Pax-2* in the midbrain neuromere and rhombomere 1. This results in severe mesencephalic and metencephalic defects and prevents the formation of optic vesicles. These defects can be rescued by the simultaneous overexpression of *Islet-3* (165).

Principle 8: *Developmental genes regulate cell proliferation to conserve constant ratios of synaptically related neurons*. An example of this principle is the constant, fixed ratio maintained between Purkinje cells and granule cells in the cerebellar cortex (147). This ratio is lower in less complex mammals than in humans. The ratio was 1:778 in the mouse and 1:2,991 in the human in one study (166) and 1:449 in the rat and 1:3,300 in the human in another (167). To regulate granule cell proliferation, *Shh* and its receptor *Patched* (*Ptc*) are important genes. *Ptc* protein is localized to granule cells and *Shh* protein to Purkinje cells, thus providing a molecular substrate for signaling between these synaptically related neurons to establish the needed amount of granule cell production (124–126). *Shh* protein in Purkinje cells acts as a mitogen on external granule cells (127). To make the system even more complex, *Ptc* also interacts through activation of another gene, *Smoothened*. A hemizygous deletion of *ptc* in mice results in uncontrolled, excessive proliferation of granule cells and often also leads to neoplastic transformation to medulloblastoma (124). Mutations in the human *PTC* gene are associated with sporadic basal cell carcinomas of the skin and also primitive neuroectodermal tumors of the cerebellum, so that this gene is involved in at least a subset of human medulloblastomas (128). Theoretically, the focal loss of *PTC* expression also might be a basis for dysplastic gangliocytoma of the cerebellum, also known as

Lhermitte-Duclos disease, a focal hamartoma, rather than a neoplasm (73).

NEURULATION

Neurulation is the bending of the neural placode to form the neural tube. This process requires both extrinsic and intrinsic mechanical forces in addition to the dorsalizing and ventralizing genetic effects described in the Patterning of the Neural Tube: Axes and Gradients of Growth and Differentiation section (Table 5.4). This bending of the neural placode to form a closed tube is called *primary neurulation*. The term *secondary neurulation* refers only to the most caudal part of the spinal cord (i.e., conus medullaris) that develops from the neuroepithelium caudal to the site of posterior neuropore closure. This part of the spinal cord forms not as a tube, but rather as a solid cord of neural cells in which ependymal cells differentiate in its core and *canalize* the cord, often giving rise to minor aberrations (168). It was previously believed that this is the manner in which the entire spinal cord of fishes is formed, but dorsal folding of the neural plate actually occurs as in other vertebrates (169).

These forces arise in part from the growth of the surrounding mesodermal tissues on either side of the neural tube, the future somites (170). After surgical removal of mesoderm and endoderm from one side of the neuroepithelium in the experimental animal, the neural tube still closes but is rotated and becomes asymmetric (171). The mesoderm appears to be important for orientation but not for closure of the neural tube. The expansion of the surface epithelium of the embryo is the principal extrinsic force for the folding of the neuroepithelium to form the neural tube (172). Cells of the neural placode are mobile and migrate beneath the surface ectoderm, raising the lateral margins of the placode toward the dorsal midline. The growth of the whole embryo itself does not appear to be an important factor because neurulation proceeds equally well in anamniotes (e.g., amphibians), which do not grow during this period, and in amniotes (e.g., mammals), which grow rapidly at this time (173).

TABLE 5.4 Factors Involved in Closure of Neuroepithelium to form the Neural Tube

- **I. Extrinsic Mechanical Forces**
  - A. Surrounding mesodermal tissues
  - B. Surface epithelium
- **II. Intrinsic Mechanical Forces**
  - A. Wedge shape of floor plate cells
  - B. Differential growth in dorsal and ventral zones
  - C. Adhesion molecules
  - D. Orientation of mitotic spindles of neuroepithelium
  - E. Large fetal central canal
- **III. Molecular Genetic Programming**
  - A. Induction of floor plate by *Sonic hedgehog*
  - B. Ventralizing gene transcription products
  - C. Dorsalizing gene transcription products
  - D. Genetic transcription products that regulate axonal guidance, both attraction and repulsion, across midline and in longitudinal axis
- **IV. Separation of Neural Crest**

Among the intrinsic forces of the neuroepithelium, the cells of the floor plate have a wedge shape, narrow at the apex and broad at the base, which facilitates bending (174). Although the width of the floor plate is small, its site in the ventral midline is crucial and sufficient to allow it to have a significant influence. It represents yet another aspect of floor plate induction by the notochord, besides its influence on the differentiation of neural cells (175). Ependymal cells that form the floor plate are the first neural cells to differentiate, and they induce a growth of the parenchyma of the ventral zone more than in the dorsal regions (73,176); this mechanical effect also may facilitate the curving of the neural placode. The direction of proliferation of new cells in the mitotic cycle, determined in part by the orientation of the mitotic spindle, becomes another mechanical force shaping the neural tube (173,174). Adhesion molecules are probably yet another important mechanical factor for neurulation. In later stages, the ependymal-lined central canal, which is much larger in the fetus than in the newborn, may have a role in exerting a centrifugal force for the tubular shape. In early spinal cord development, the central canal is a tall, narrow, midline slit, and only later in fetal life does it assume a rounded contour as seen in transverse sections (73).

Neuroepithelial cells of the neural placode or plate downregulate the polarity of their plasma membrane, so that apical and basilar surfaces are not as distinct, before neural tube closure; cell differentiation in general involves such changes in cell polarity (177). Finally, the rostrocaudal orientation of the majority of mitotic spindles of the neuroepithelium and the direction in which they push by the mass of daughter cells they form also influence the shape of the neural tube (178).

The neural tube closes in the dorsal midline first in the cervical region, with the closure then extending rostrally and caudally, so that the anterior neuropore of the human embryo closes at 24 days and the posterior neuropore closes at 28 days, the distances from the cervical region being unequal. This traditional view of a continuous, zipper-like closure is an oversimplification. In the mouse embryo, the neural tube closes in the cranial region at four distinct sites, with the closure proceeding bidirectionally or unidirectionally and in general synchrony with somite formation (179,180). An intermittent pattern of anterior neural tube closure involving multiple sites also has been described in human embryos (181). In this closure, the principal rostral neuropore closes bidirectionally (182) to form the lamina terminalis, an essential primordium of the forebrain (73). A rare anomaly of a human tail may occur. A true vestigial tail is the most distal remnant of the embryonic tail and contains adipose and connective tissue, central bundles of striated muscle, blood vessels, and nerves and is covered by skin, but bone, cartilage, and spinal cord are lacking. Pseudotails are usually an anomalous elongation of the coccygeal vertebrae. In many instances, they contain lipomas, gliomas, teratomas, or even a thin, elongated parasitic fetus (183). Pseudotails often cause tethering of the spinal cord or may even be associated with spinal dysraphism (184,185).

EXPRESSION OF REGULATOR GENES AFTER THE FETAL PERIOD: CONSERVATION OF CELL IDENTITY

Many developmental genes continue to be expressed after the period of ontogenesis and into adult life. In particular, those that direct the differentiation of particular types of cells also may preserve the unique identity of these distinct cells in the mature state. In the cerebellar cortex, *Wnt-3* preserves the identity of Purkinje cells (147); *Pax-3* is responsible for the preservation of Bergmann glia (77); and granule cells are supported by several genes, the most important being *Pax-6*, *Zic-1*, and *Math-1* (77,113,148,149). If one of these genes fails to be expressed, there may be compensation because of the principle of redundancy, but if this phenomenon is incomplete or fails to occur, the motor neurons may never differentiate or may later die by apoptosis and disappear. Theoretically, although not yet proved, such a mechanism might explain human cases of granuloprival cerebellar hypoplasia in which a sparse number or total absence of granule cells is seen in the presence of a normal complement of Purkinje cells and other cellular elements of the cerebellar cortex (73). On the other hand, the preservation of *Wnt-3* expression in Purkinje cells also depends in part on its relations with granule cells (147), so that synaptic contacts probably also impart genetic information between mature neurons.

Another example of genetic expression to preserve cell identity is in motor neurons. The earliest stimulus of motor neuron differentiation is *Shh*, induced by the notochord and floor plate (67,68,70,174). Despite the similar morphologic appearance and function of ocular and spinal motor neurons, differences exist in the genes that program their development and maintenance. *Wnt-1*–knockout mice fail to develop oculomotor and trochlear nuclei and their extraocular muscles are altered or deficient, but spinal and hypoglossal motor neurons are not altered (65,145,146). Even among the three pairs of motor nuclei subserving the various extraocular muscles, abducens motor neurons may be selectively involved or spared in relation to motor neurons of the trochlear and oculomotor nuclei (145). Genes of the large *LIM* family, particularly *Lim-1*, *Lim-2*, *Islet-1*, and *Islet-2*, also are expressed in motor neurons, and each individual gene in this family defines a subclass of motor neurons for the topographic projection of axonal projections (103,108,186). Insulin-like growth factor also has been identified as a regulator of apoptosis of developing motor neurons and may express a differential effect (180). These differences in genetic programming of motor neurons in various neuromeres perhaps explain oculomotor sparing with progressive degeneration of spinal and hypoglossal motor neurons in spinal muscular atrophy (Werdnig-Hoffmann disease).

ANATOMIC AND PHYSIOLOGIC PROCESSES OF CENTRAL NERVOUS SYSTEM DEVELOPMENT

Redundancy

One of the most important general principles of neuroembryology is that of redundancy. The redundancy of some genes with overlapping domains and their ability to compensate for lack of expression of others has already been mentioned in the Patterning of the Neural Tube: Axes and Gradients of Growth and Differentiation section. Another redundancy is the production of neuroblasts. An overproduction by 30% to 50% of neuroblasts occurs in all regions of the nervous system, depending on the number of symmetric mitotic cycles, followed by apoptosis of the surplus cells that are not needed to be matched to targets. Immature axonal projections are redundant because many collaterals form diffuse projections, followed during maturation by retraction of many to leave fewer but more specific connections. Synapses also are overly produced, followed by synaptic pruning to provide greater precision.

Embryologic Zones of the Neural Tube

After neurulation, the closed neural tube has an architecture of two concentric rings as viewed in transverse section: The inner ring is the ventricular zone, consisting of the proliferative, pseudostratified columnar neuroepithelium; the outer ring is the marginal zone, a cell-sparse region of fibers and extracellular matrix proteins (73). Details of the mitotic patterns in the ventricular zone are discussed later (see Neuroepithelial Cell Proliferation section).

With further development, four concentric zones appear. A subventricular zone outside the proliferative ventricular zone is composed of postmitotic, premigratory neuroblasts and glioblasts and radial glial cells. After radial migration of neuroblasts begins, an intermediate zone is formed by the radial glial processes and the migratory neuroblasts adherent to them; this intermediate zone eventually becomes the deep subcortical white matter of the cerebral hemispheres. In the cerebrum, migratory neuroblasts destined to form the cerebral cortex begin to form an unlaminated cortical plate within the marginal zone. This event divides that zone into an outermost, cell-sparse region, thereafter known as the *molecular layer* (eventually layer 1 of the mature cerebral cortex), and the innermost portion of the marginal zone isolated by the intervening cortical plate, known as the *subplate zone*. This region contains many neurons that form transitory pioneer axons to establish the corticospinal and other long projection pathways, but eventually the subplate zone becomes incorporated into layer 6 of the maturing cortex and disappears as a distinct anatomic region.

In the brainstem and spinal cord, the two and later four concentric zones clearly identified in the cerebrum are similar, although in modified form. They become even further altered in the cerebellum with an apparent inversion, the granule cells migrating from the surface inward rather than from the periventricular region outward. An ependymal epithelium eventually forms at the ventricular surface of the ventricular zone, creating an additional, innermost zone not present in the embryo except for the floor plate in the ventral midline (see Role of the Fetal Ependyma section).

Neuroepithelial Cell Proliferation

Early cleavages in the fertilized ovum to form the blastula and the blastomere (gastrula) involve a simple proliferation of cells cycling between the mitotic (M-phase) and resting (S-phase) states, a process similar to DNA replication in bacteria. As the neuroectoderm forms in the epiblast at postovulatory week 3 in the human embryo, it becomes organized as a pseudostratified columnar epithelium, a sheet of bipolar cells all oriented so that one cytoplasmic process extends to the dorsal (future ventricular) surface and the other process extends to the ventral (future pial) surface. The nucleus of each of these spindle-shaped cells moves to and fro within its own cytoplasmic extensions. M-phase occurs at or near the ventricular surface and S-phase occurs at the other end. Transitional periods between these two states are known as gap phases: G1 when the nucleus moves distally toward the pial surface and G2 when the nucleus approaches the ventricular surface (187). The introduction of gap phases in the mitotic cycle allows for adjustments to be made in the replication of DNA during G1, and the sequence ensures that G2 cells do not undergo an extra round of S-phase, which might lead to a change in ploidy as the chromosomes segregate in the dividing cell (188). In this way, errors may be corrected before the next mitosis, thus allowing for more plasticity than the all-or-none principle of simple cell division.

TABLE 5.5 Generation of Motor Neurons in the Lumbar Spinal Cord of the Chick Embryo

Progenitor stem cells	60
Motor neuroblasts generated	24,000
Mature motor neurons required	12,000
Motor neurons generated in seven symmetric mitotic cycles	7,680
Motor neurons generated in eight symmetric mitotic cycles	15,360

From Burek MJ, Oppenheim RW. Programmed cell death in the developing nervous system. *Brain Pathol* 1996;6:427–446. With permission.

Mitoses continue to occur at the ventricular surface as the neural plate folds and becomes a neural tube. The differentiation of an ependyma at the ventricular surface signals the termination of mitotic activity and indeed of the ventricular zone because the remaining cells in the periventricular region all are postmitotic, premigratory neuroblasts and glioblasts, hence, of the subventricular zone (73,174).

Because mitoses increase cell populations exponentially, a finite number of mitotic cycles is needed to produce the requisite number of neurons needed in a given part of the nervous system. In the cerebrum of the rat, 10 mitotic cycles in the ventricular zone generate all the neurons of the cerebral cortex; in the human, 33 mitotic cycles generate a much larger number of neurons than simply three times the number in the rat cortex (190). Eight symmetric mitotic cycles are required to produce the minimum essential number of motor neuroblasts in the spinal cord of the chick (Table 5.5) (123).

The orientation of the mitotic spindle at the ventricular surface is important in the fate of the daughter cells after each mitosis because certain gene products are distributed asymmetrically within the mother cell and because with some orientations both daughter cells do not retain their attachments to the ventricular wall (122,190,191). *Notch* and *Numb* are genes with antagonistic functions, situated at opposite poles of the neuroepithelial cell. If the cleavage plane of the mitotic spindle is perpendicular to the ventricular surface, the daughter cells each retain an attachment to that surface and inherit equal amounts of *Notch* and *Numb*. This situation is called *symmetric cleavage* and both daughter cells reenter the mitotic cycle in the same manner as their common precursor cell. If, however, the mitotic spindle is parallel to the ventricular surface, the two daughter cells are unequal because only one can retain an attachment to the ventricle, and one inherits most of the *Notch* and the other inherits most of the *Numb* gene product. This situation is asymmetric cleavage. Only one of the cells, the one at the ventricular surface, reenters the mitotic cycle, and the other, more distal cell has completed its final mitosis and rapidly moves away from its sister to begin differentiation as a neuroblast and prepare for radial migration from the subventricular zone. *Notch* and *Numb* have additional distinctive functions later in cortical neuronogenesis (121).

Neuronal polarity, establishing from which side of the cell the axon will sprout and from which cell surfaces the dendrites will form, is determined at least in part at the time of the final mitosis. Microtubule arrays are the most fundamental components of the mitotic spindle, forming during prophase as the centrosome replicates; the *minus* ends of the microtubules remain associated with the centrosome, whereas the *plus* ends emanate outward, with the duplicated centrosomes driven to opposite poles of the cell as a direct result of microtubule organization. The mitotic spindle consists of regions in which microtubules are uniformly oriented in tandem and in parallel and other regions where the microtubules are more haphazardly oriented; the former becomes the axonal end of the cell and the latter, the opposite pole or the dendritic end (192).

In the postnatal human infant, mitotic activity of neuronal precursors continues to be seen, although sparse, in the outer half of the external granule cell layer of the cerebellum; external granule cells do not complete their migration until after 1 year of age; hence, the potential for regeneration after prenatal and even postnatal loss of some of these cells still exists. Another well-documented region of continued neuronal turnover in the human nervous system is the primary olfactory neurons (193).

A few neuroblasts appear to undergo division even during migration, which are exceptions to the general rule (194). A population of quiescent neuroepithelial stem cells in the subventricular zone of the mammalian forebrain retains a proliferative potential even in the adult (195). Great interest has been shown in this inconspicuous and sparse cell population because of its potential in neuronal regeneration and repair of the damaged brain and spinal cord.

Apoptosis

In every region of the nervous system, an overgeneration of neuroblasts occurs, more than are required at maturity by 30% to 70%. Surplus cells survive for a period of days or weeks and then spontaneously undergo a cascade of degenerative changes and disappear without inflammatory responses to cell death or the proliferation of glial scars. This physiologic process of programmed cell death, or apoptosis, was discovered in 1949 by Hamburger and Levi-Montalcini, who demonstrated its occurrence in the spinal dorsal root ganglion of the chick embryo (196). The phenomenon subsequently has been confirmed by numerous other investigators, and indeed it is a general principle of development in all animals, from the simplest worms to humans, and involves all organ systems, not just the nervous system (197–200). Examples of apoptosis that continues throughout life are found in any tissue that has a constant turnover of cells, such as the 120-day half-life of erythrocytes and the continuous replacement of intestinal mucosal epithelial cells (of mesodermal origin) and of epidermal cells of the skin (of ectodermal origin).

Apoptosis differs from cell death by necrosis (e.g., from ischemia, hypoxia, toxins, infections) in several important morphologic details in addition to the absence of tissue response to the loss, except for the removal of the cellular debris by phagocytic microglial cells (i.e., modified macrophages). In neural cell apoptosis, the sequence begins with shrinkage of the nucleus, condensation of chromatin, and increased electron opacity of the cell. These events are followed by disappearance of the Golgi apparatus, loss of endoplasmic reticulum, and disaggregation of polyribosomes; final steps are the formation of ribosomal crystals and the breakdown of the nuclear membrane (196). Mitochondria are preserved until late stages of apoptosis, whereas they swell and disintegrate early in cellular necrosis.

Apoptosis is genetically patterned, as with other events in nervous system development. The process is programmed into every cell, but its expression is blocked by the inhibitory influence of certain genes, such as *bcl-2* and the immediate early proto-oncogene c-*fos*, and this genetic regulation also is modulated by trophic factors of other cells in the vicinity that preserve metabolic integrity. For example, nerve growth factor and bFGF block cell death and preserve the identity of various cell lineages in the nervous system (201–204). The apoptotic process also may be accelerated or retarded by metabolic factors, such as plasma concentrations of thyroid hormone, serum ammonia, local neurotoxins, including excitatory amino acids such as aspartate (204), lactic acidosis, and imbalances of calcium and electrolytes. Insulin-like growth factor regulates apoptosis in avian motor neuroblasts (186a).

Synaptic relations are another *environmental factor* within the brain that affects apoptosis: An inverse relationship exists between the rate of apoptosis of spinal motor neurons and synaptogenesis. On the afferent side, neurons degenerate if they fail to be innervated or if they lose their entire afferent supply because of the loss of presynaptic neurons. This phenomenon is called *transsynaptic degeneration* and is exemplified in the lateral geniculate body after optic nerve lesions and in the inferior olivary nucleus after destruction of the central tegmental tract. On the efferent side, motor neurons degenerate if they fail to match with target muscle fibers or if their muscle targets are removed, as after amputation of a limb bud of an embryo or even the amputation of an extremity in the adult.

Proteins programmed from exons 7 and 8 of the *survival motor neuron* (*SMN*) gene at the 5q11–q13 locus are defective in spinal muscular atrophy (Werdnig-Hoffmann and Kugelberg-Welander diseases); this is an example of a gene that normally arrests apoptosis in spinal motor neurons after all muscular targets are matched (135,136), as earlier predicted by Sarnat (205; see Chapter 16). This degenerative disease thus occurs because a physiologic process in the early fetus becomes pathologic in late fetal life and the postnatal period because of its failure to stop, with continued progressive death of motor neurons.

Apoptosis occurs in two phases. The first is the programmed death of incompletely differentiated cells and represents the numerically most important phase of this process; even completely undifferentiated neuroepithelial cells undergo apoptosis, but the factors that select these short life cycles are poorly understood (206). The second phase is the cell death of mature, well-differentiated neurons. This process continues in the early postnatal period in the rat cervical spinal cord (207).

"Transitory" Neurons of the Fetal Brain

Certain populations of cells of the fetal brain serve an important function in development but are not required after maturity. An example is the radial glial cell of the fetal cerebrum that guides migratory neuroblasts from the subventricular zone to the cerebral cortical plate. After all neuroblasts and glioblasts have migrated, these radial glia retract their long processs, which spans almost the entire cerebral mantle, to become fibrillary astrocytes of the subcortical white matter of the mature brain. External granule cells of the cerebellum migrate to the mature internal granular layer until the external layer no longer exists after 18 months of age. Subplate pyramidal neurons of the early fetal cerebral cortex, deep to the cortical plate, project pioneer axons to initially form the internal capsule and corticospinal tract. They later become incorporated into layer 6 so that the subplate zone no longer is microscopically recognizable (208,209). These examples identify cells that appear to be transient but do not really disappear or degenerate; they only change their site and shape.

The Cajal-Retzius neurons of the molecular layer of the immature cerebral cortex are another important population that appears to be present only in the fetus, begins to decrease in density at about 32 weeks' gestation, and is sparse in the term neonate and rare in the adult brain. It was previously thought to disappear by apoptosis (210), but it is now known that these neurons persist but are so "diluted" during late fetal and postnatal life by the growth of the brain that they become extremely sparse (209,211,212).

The Cajal-Retzius neuron already is present and mature in the marginal layer of the telencephalon before the first wave of radial migration from the subventricular zone as a part of the plexus that exists before formation of the cortical plate (73,213–216). The cells may migrate rostrally from the midbrain neuromere at the time of neural tube formation (209). Other authors contend that they arise in the ganglionic eminence and travel tangentially, because they synthesize gamma-aminobutyric acid and express the *LIM* gene *Lhx6* (217,218). They are bipolar neurons that form axons and dendritic trunks running parallel to the pial surface of the brain. With formation of the cortical plate, axonal collaterals of Cajal-Retzius neurons plunge into the cortical plate to create the first intrinsic cortical synaptic circuits by forming synapses on neurons of layer 6 from the earliest waves of radial migration.

Cajal-Retzius neurons also appear to play an important role in radial neuroblast migration and in the developing laminar architecture of the cerebral cortex. The *Reelin* gene–associated antigen in the reeler mouse model is expressed strongly in Cajal-Retzius neurons and is crucial to the laminar organization of cortical neurons (130,131,219). Lack of Cajal-Retzius cells in embryonic mice results in disruption of radial glial fibers and cortical dysgenesis (220). These neurons also are probably important for the organization of inhibitory hippocampal commisural connections (221,222). This gene programs an extracellular glycoprotein of the same name that is secreted by Cajal-Retzius cells in the cerebrum and by external granule cells in the cerebellum and without which the laminar architecture of the cortex is disrupted severely. Cajal-Retzius cells also strongly express the *LIS* family of genes, which have been shown to be defective in lissencephaly type I (Miller-Dieker syndrome) (109). An excess of persistent Cajal-Retzius neurons in the mature brain, by contrast, is associated with polymicrogyria (223). Cajal-Retzius cells synthesize gamma-aminobutyric acid as their principal neurotransmitter and probably acetylcholine as well; immunocytochemical reactivity to calcium-binding proteins suggests that they represent a heterogeneous population (209,211,224).

The subpial granular layer of Brun over the cerebral cortex is composed of astrocytes, by contrast with the neuronal external granular layer in the cerebellar cortex. These subpial astrocytes are prominent at 26 to 32 weeks' gestation in the human fetus or preterm neonate and are nearly gone by 40 weeks, having migrated into the cortex to become protoplasmic astrocytes (5,73).

In summary, the apparent populations of "transitory" cells of the brain are really not transitory at all.

Role of the Fetal Ependyma

The ependyma of the mature brain is little more than a decorative lining of the ventricular system, serving minor functions in the transport of ions and small molecules between the ventricles and the cerebral parenchyma and perhaps having a small immunoprotective role. The fetal ependyma, by contrast, is an essential and dynamic structure that contributes to a number of developmental processes (73,176,225).

The floor plate is the first region of the neuroepithelium to differentiate as specific cells. It forms the ventral midline of the ependyma in the spinal cord and brainstem as far rostrally as the midbrain, but a floor plate is not recognized in the prosencephalon, perhaps not in diencephalic neuromeres because of the infundibulum in the ventral midline, or in the telencephalon. The floor plate has an active expression of *Shh* and contributes to the differentiation of motor neurons and of other parts of the ependyma. It also secretes retinoic acid, unlike other ependymal cells that merely have retinoid receptors.

The ependyma develops in a precise temporal and spatial pattern. The last surfaces of the ventricular system to be completely covered by ependyma are in the lateral ventricles at 22 weeks' gestation (225). In some parts of the neuraxis, it is advantageous for ependymal differentiation to be delayed as long as possible to permit the requisite numbers of neuroblasts to be produced in the ventricular zone because once the ependyma forms in a particular region, all mitotic activity ceases at the ventricular surface (176,225–227). One function of the fetal ependyma, therefore, is to regulate the arrest of mitotic proliferation of neuroepithelial cells.

The fetal ependyma is structurally different from the adult version. Rather than a simple cuboidal epithelium as in the adult, it is a pseudostratified columnar epithelium, each cell having at least a slender cytoplasmic process contacting the ventricular surface even though its nucleus may be at some distance. This arrangement is needed so that ependymal cells do not divide after differentiation, and a provision is required for enough cells to cover the entire expanding ventricular surface. With growth of the fetus, the extra layers of ependymal cells become thinned as the ependyma spreads to cover the expanding ventricular surface. At the basal surface of fetal ependymal cells is a process that radiates into the parenchyma. This process may reach the pial surface of the spinal cord and brainstem but never spans the entire cerebral hemisphere and only extends into the subventricular zone (i.e., germinal matrix) and into the deeper portions of the intermediate zone. The fetal ependyma also differs from the adult version in expressing certain intermediate filament proteins, such as vimentin and glial fibrillary acidic protein, and some other molecules such as S-100β protein (225). As in the adult, the fetal ependyma is ciliated at its apical (i.e., ventricular) surface.

Ependymal cells are important elements in guiding the intermediate trajectories of axonal growth cones (227,228). In some places, the basal processes of fetal ependymal cells actually form mechanical tunnels to guide axonal growth in developing long tracts. Ependymal cells and their processes also secrete molecules that attract or repel axons and may be specific for some and not for other axons. Floor plate ependymal cells synthesize netrin, a diffusible neurotrophic factor, permitting the passage of commissural axons but repelling fibers of longitudinal tracts (229–231). Netrin may be bifunctional, acting as attractants of decussating axons at some sites, such as the floor plate in the spinal cord, but as repellants in other sites, such as trochlear axons (230). In the developing dorsal columns of the spinal cord, the dorsal median raphé formed by ependymal cells of the roof plate prevents the wandering to the wrong side of the spinal cord of rostrally growing axons by secreting a proteoglycan, keratan sulfate, that strongly repels axonal growth cones (227). Ependymal processes do not guide migratory neuroblasts, despite their appearance resembling radial glial fibers.

The loss of S-100β protein from ependymal cells of the lateral ventricles appears to coincide with the end of cell migration from the subventricular zone and the beginning conversion of radial glial cells into mature astrocytes (176). Whether the ependyma is inducing this conversion is uncertain, but circumstantial evidence suggests such a function.

Neuroblast Migration

Almost no neurons occupy sites in the mature human brain that are the sites where these cells underwent their terminal mitosis and began differentiation. In some simple vertebrates, such as the salamander, mature neurons often are situated in the periventricular zone where they originated (232), but in humans, such periventricular maturation is regarded as heterotopic and pathologic. Neuroblasts thus migrate to sites often distant from their birthplace to establish the needed synaptic relations with both similar and different types of neurons and to send axonal projections grouped with similar fibers to form tracts or fascicles to distant sites along the neuraxis. The synaptic architecture of the cerebral or cerebellar cortices would not be possible without such neuroblast migration.

Several mechanisms subserve neuroblast migration. The most important from the standpoint of transporting the majority of neuroblasts, whether into cortical or nuclear structures, is the use of radial glial fiber guides. In the cerebrum, glial cells of the subventricular zone develop a long, slender process that spans the entire cerebral mantle to terminate as an end-foot on the pial membrane at the surface of the brain (73,233). These specialized radial glial cells are transitory and, after all migration is complete, they retract their radial process and mature to become fibrillary astrocytes of the subcortical white matter. The radial glial process of these cells serves a unique function during fetal life of guiding migratory cells, both neuroblasts and glioblasts, from the subventricular zone or germinal matrix to their destination in the cerebral cortex or in other forebrain structures. They perform this function as a *monorail*, with migratory cells actually gliding along their surface. Fetal ependymal cells also have basal processes that extend into the germinal matrix, but they do not reach as far as the cortex or even into the deep white matter, differ morphologically, and serve entirely different functions that do not include the guidance of migratory cells (73,176). In the cerebellum, the specialized Bergmann glial cells, which occupy the Purkinje cell layer and have radiating processes that extend to the surface of the cerebellar cortex, provide a similar function for the migration inward of granule cells from the fetal external granular layer to the mature internal site within the folia (73). Bergmann cells and their processes persist into adult life, unlike the change that occurs before birth in the radial glial cells of the cerebrum. In addition to the radial migration of neuroblasts into the cortical plate along radial glial fibers, a tangential migration along axons also occurs, so that the columns of neurons in the cortex are not the sole progeny of one or a few progenitor neuroepithelial cells, but are mixed with cells arising at some distance away (see later discussion).

The transport of migratory neuroepithelial cells along the radial glial fiber requires a number of adhesion molecules to prevent the cell from detaching too early. Adhesion molecules also lubricate their path of travel and perhaps provide nutrition to the cells as they move and continuously change their position in relation to capillaries within the white matter parenchyma (234). These molecules are secreted either by (a) the migratory neuroblast itself, (b) the radial glial cell, or (c) others already present in the extracellular matrix. Astrotactin is an example of a protein molecule produced by the neuroblast during migration that helps adhere the cell to the radial glial fiber and is essential in the establishment of the laminar architecture of the neocortex, hippocampus, olfactory bulb, and cerebellar cortex (235). The gene that encodes astrotactin is also related to the synthesis of epidermal growth factor and fibronectin (235). Examples of molecules synthesized by the radial glial cell for purposes of neuroblast adhesion are S-100β protein (174) and L1-neural cell adhesion molecule (L1-NCAM) (215); the defective expression of the gene that regulates the L1-NCAM protein results in polymicrogyria, pachygyria, and X-linked recessive fetal hydrocephalus (105). Other molecules synthesized by the radial glial cell also have been identified (236).

Some molecules contributing to cell adhesion, such as fibronectin, laminins, and collagen type IV, needed for the formation of extracellular basement membranes, are found in the extracellular matrix (237). In addition to providing a substrate for normal neuroblast and glioblast migration, the motility and infiltration of brain parenchyma by neoplastic cells of neural origin depends largely on extracellular matrix proteins.

Reelin (*Reln*) is a gene and glycoprotein transcription product secreted by Cajal-Retzius neurons in the cerebrum and by external granule cells in the cerebellum that is essential to terminal migration and the laminal architecture of cortices. The reeler mouse is a model that lacks expression of the *reln* gene and exhibits severe disruption of laminated structures of the brain (130,131). Another gene and its protein, *Disabled-1* (*Dab-1*), act downstream of *Reln* in a signaling pathway of laminar organization, functioning in phosphorylation-dependent intracellular signal transduction (95).

Not all cells migrating within the developing brain use radial glial fibers. Some migrations proceed along the axons of earlier and now established cells in the spinal cord, brainstem, olfactory bulb, and cerebellum, using the axon in the same manner as a radial glial fiber. Tangential migrations perpendicular to the radial glial fibers also occur in the cerebral cortex and contribute to a mixture of clones in any given region so that all neurons are not from the same neuroepithelial stem cells originating in the same zone of the germinal matrix (238–242). These neuroblasts migrate not on glial processes, but along axons of other, more mature neurons (242). The site of origin of these cells migrating tangentially is not well documented, but they begin their tangential course outside the proliferative ventricular zone (240). Some may arise in the ganglionic eminence and provide some Cajal-Retzius neurons (217,218). They might even represent the persistent stem cells that have since the 1990s been recognized in the adult brain and become of great interest because of their potential value in regeneration of the damaged nervous system if they can be stimulated and mobilized. How these tangential migrations occur, skipping from one radial glial fiber to another or traveling between radial glia, is incompletely resolved. The migration of interneurons from the basal forebrain to the neocortex is mediated by the *Distalless* (*Dlx*) family of genes (243), but little more is known about the genetic basis of tangential migration.

At the surface of the cerebrum, the migratory neuroblasts reverse direction so that the earlier migrations are displaced into deeper layers of the cortical plate by the more recent arrivals. Layer 6 therefore represents the earliest wave of radial neuroblast migration from the subventricular zone, and layer 2 consists of the last neurons to migrate.

The Cajal-Retzius cells of the molecular zone, which were in place before the first radial migrations occurred (214–216), are important to the architectural integrity of the developing cortex and appear to influence cell placement within the cortical plate, even before distinct lamination occurs. The pial membrane and the subpial granular layer of Brun (which in the human fetal cerebrum is a transitory layer of glial cells, unlike the cerebellar cortex, in which the external granule cell layer is neuroblasts) are important in reversing the direction of migration as cells arrive at the surface. Deficiency of these components in certain malformations, such as holoprosencephaly and lissencephaly, results in extensive overmigration with neuronal ectopia in the leptomeninges (73).

Several genes are now recognized to be defective in disorders of neuroblast migration in humans, although the precise mechanisms by which these genes mediate migration in the healthy fetus are incompletely understood. The *LIS1* gene at the 17p13.3 locus is responsible for lissencephaly type I in Miller-Dieker syndrome and also in isolated lissencephaly (110–112). *Doublecortin* is a gene (this is also the name of the gene product or signaling protein) that is defective or unexpressed in X-linked dominant subcortical laminar heterotopia, also known as band heterotopia or double cortex (96,97). Bilateral periventricular heterotopia, another X-linked dominant trait, is associated with deficiency of expression of *filamin A* (102,244). The neural cell adhesion molecule L1-CAM is implicated in hemimegalencephaly (106) and also in X-linked recessive hydrocephalus with pachygyria and often with aqueductal stenosis (245).

Axonal Pathfinding

The outgrowth of a single axon precedes the formation of the multiple dendrites and is one of the first morphologic events marking the maturation of a neuroblast in becoming a neuron. It occurs at times even during the course of migration before the cell has arrived at its final destination, and, in some cases, such as the external granule cells of the cerebellum, even occurs before migration starts. The tip of the growing axon, termed the *growth cone* by Ramón y Cajal (246), is neither pointed nor blunt, but instead is a constantly changing complex of cytoplasmic fingers or extensions, the *filopodia*, enclosed by a membrane that extends between filopodia to form veils or webs. The cytoplasm of the filopodia is filled with microtubules, filaments, and mitochondria. Filopodia extend and retract with amoeboid movements.

To develop polarity, by which an axon emerges at one site and not at others, neuroblasts share membrane protein–sorting mechanisms with epithelial cells, the other important polarized type of cell. The axonal cell surface is analogous to the apical plasma membrane of epithelial cells, such as ependymal cells or intestinal mucosal cells, and the somatodendritic plasma membrane is analogous to the basolateral epithelial surface (247–249). A complex interaction of sorting signals from glycolipid proteins within the plasma membrane and soluble attachment protein receptors that promote the docking of vesicles with target membranes results in intracellular membrane fusions that differ in various parts of the neuroblast plasma membrane and are required for membrane assembly during axonal growth (248).

Three fundamental mechanisms guide axons to their destination, which may be at a great distance from the cell body (250,251). A fourth mechanism, proposed a century ago, has been resurrected as plausible. (a) *Cell–cell interactions*: Molecular signals generated by the target cell induce the growth cone to form a synapse. This mechanism is effective only as the axon approaches within 1 to 2 mm of the target. (b) *Cell–substrate interactions*: Molecules known as integrins bind the cell to an extracellular protein matrix, such as fibronectin or laminin. Such substrates serve as adhesive surfaces for growth cones, allowing them to pull themselves along, but also might provide directional cues as attractants or repellants. (c) *Chemotactic interactions*: Secretory molecules may release powerful attractants or repellants to keep the axon aligned along an intended course in its intermediate trajectory; growth cones are exquisitely sensitive to certain chemicals and grow toward or away from these molecules. (d) It was once thought that electric or electromagnetic fields were important influences in orienting the growing axon; this discarded theory is being reconsidered in a more modern context, although its importance is still poorly substantiated. Local electric fields might change the course of growing axons by altering receptive properties of their membrane to neurotransmitters and attractant and repellent molecules (252).

The glycosaminoglycans and proteoglycan molecules are important examples of growth cone repellants in the developing CNS. An example is keratan sulfate (unrelated biochemically to the epidermal protein keratin). This compound is secreted in many tissues of the fetal body at sites where nerves are not needed or desired: the epiphyseal plates of growing bones; the epidermis (to prevent nerves from growing through the skin); the notochordal sheath; and the developing neural arches of the vertebrae (to segment and guide nerve roots from the spinal cord between rather than through the somites) (251). The highly segmented somites are important early guides of neural crest cellular migration as well as of axonal projections peripherally (253). Within the CNS, fetal ependymal cells synthesize keratan sulfate, in part to prevent axons from growing into the ventricles of the brain and in part to prevent aberrant decussation of developing long tracts and the wandering of axons toward wrong targets (176,227). The dorsal median raphé that separates the dorsal columns of the two sides of the spinal cord in the dorsal midline, probably programmed by dorsalizing genes such as those of the *PAX* family, is composed of ependymal roof plate processes that secrete keratan sulfate at the time when the axons of the dorsal columns are growing rostrally. The raphé serves to repel growth cones that might otherwise decussate prematurely before reaching the gracile and cuneate nuclei of the medulla oblongata (227,228). The effects of such repellent molecules are selective, however. Keratan sulfate secreted by the floor plate and the dorsal median septum of the midbrain collicular plate does not prevent the passage of commissural fibers at those sites, although the substance repulses axons of descending and ascending long tracts. Perhaps the passage of commissural fibers is mediated by attractants of such fibers, such as netrin, that overcome a negative influence of keratan sulfate. The floor plate also repulses axons of developing motor neurons so that they extend into the spinal roots only on the side of their soma (254). Another family of proteins, the semaphorins/collapsins, acts mainly as growth cone repellants both in neural tissue, including the floor plate, and throughout the body in non-neural tissues (255). Thus, the midline septa composed of floor and roof plate basal processes act as chemical barriers to some axons but are not physical barriers despite their appearance in histologic stained sections because commissural axons easily pass through them. Other examples of growth cone attractants are nerve growth factor and S-100β protein.

The cytoskeleton plays a central role in axonal guidance. The internal organization of actin filaments and microtubules changes rapidly within the growth cone before large-scale changes in growth cone shape are seen. These changes are evoked by local environmental molecules that stabilize local changes of cytoskeletal polymers in the growth cone (256). Although microtubule assembly in the growing axon is required for the axon to extend along its pathway, drugs that disrupt microtubule assembly do not impede the assembly and growth at the axonal tip (257). Growth cone collapse is a part of the normal process of axonal growth and may become pathologic if excessive; it is induced by a platelet-activation factor (258).

Finally, or perhaps first of all, homeobox-containing genes are involved in the regulation of axonal growth. A gene expressed early in neuronal differentiation, *TOAD-64* ("turned on after division"; with an identical nucleotide sequence to *unc-33* in nematodes) is strongly expressed by its protein transcription product in growth cones and is downregulated after axonal projection is complete. Mutations in this gene result in aberrations in axonal outgrowth in the mouse (144). The overexpression of *Hox-2* reverses axonal pathways from rhombomere 3 (84). Boundary regions between adjacent domains of regulatory gene expression influence where the first axons extend (249). Initial tract formation is associated with the selective expression of certain cell adhesion molecules and their regulatory gene transcripts (259).

Some long tracts are preceded by pioneer axons formed by transitory neurons that appear to serve as guides for the growth cones of permanent axons and without which the permanent axons detour to heterotopic sites. An example is the pioneer axons from subplate neurons as the cortical plate is beginning to form; these pioneer axons establish the internal capsule and precede the passage of axons from pyramidal cells of the future layers 5 and 6 of the cortex. After the pyramidal cell axons are guided into the internal capsule, the pioneer axons and their cells of origin disappear, probably by apoptosis. An epidermal growth factor is expressed by pioneer neurons and by Cajal-Retzius cells in the reeler mouse, a model of migrational disorders and cortical dysgenesis (132,260).

Dendritic Proliferation and Synaptogenesis

Dendrites sprout only after the axon begins its projection from the same neuron. The branching pattern of dendrites and the formation of spines on these dendritic arborizations, on which synapses form, are varied and characteristic for each type of neuron. In the cerebral cortex, synaptogenesis occurs after migration of the neuron to its mature site is complete. In the cerebellar cortex, external granule cells project bipolar axons as parallel fibers in the molecular zone and form synapses with Purkinje cell dendrites before migrating to their mature site in the interior of the folium.

An excessive number of synapses generally forms, and many are later deleted with the retraction of redundant collateral axons (261). In addition, transitory neurons, such as the Cajal-Retzius neurons of the fetal cerebral cortex, form temporary synapses. As with other aspects of neural development, a critical period of synapse elimination occurs (262). Class 1 major histocompatibility complex glycoproteins may be involved in synaptic remodeling during fetal development and infancy. In the optic system, considerable amounts of these surface-expressed proteins are demonstrated on neurons of the lateral geniculate body in the late fetal and early postnatal periods, a period when synaptogenesis and especially synaptic retraction are most active (263).

Most of the dendritic arborization and synapatogenesis in the cerebral cortex occur during late gestation and early infancy, a circumstance that renders this developmental process particularly vulnerable to toxic, hypoxic, ischemic, and metabolic insults in the postnatal period, especially in neonates born prematurely. Synapses increase in the human visual striate (occipital) cortex to reach a maximum at 2 to 4 months postnatally; they then remain at a plateau until about 8 months, thereafter steadily decreasing until about 11 years of age, when they are at the stable mature number (264). This "pruning" of synapses allows for greater precision and specificity than more diffuse connections can provide.

When an axonal terminal reaches a dendritic spine and cell–cell contact is achieved, a chemical synapse usually forms rapidly. Some *promiscuous* neurons may even secrete transmitter before contacting their targets, inducing an overabundance of synapses that then undergo additional electrical activity–dependent refinement (265). Dendritic spines determine the dynamics of intracellular second-messenger ions, such as calcium, and probably provide for synaptic plasticity by establishing compartmentalization of afferent input based on biochemical rather than electrical signals (266).

Neurotropins play an important role in the modulation of synaptogenesis as selective retrograde messengers (267). Trans-synaptic signaling by neurotropins and neurotransmitters also may influence neuronal architecture such as neurite sprouting and dendritic pruning (268,269). The effects of neurotrophic factors may be lamina specific within the cortex and have opposite effects in different layers. Brain-derived neurotrophic factor stimulates dendritic growth in layer 4 neurons, whereas neurotropin-3 inhibits this growth; brain-derived neurotrophic factor is inhibitory and neurotropin-3 is stimulatory, by contrast, for neuroblasts in layer 6 (270).

Prostaglandins and their inducible synthetase enzymes (e.g., cyclo-oxygenase 2) are expressed by excitatory neurons at postsynaptic sites in the cerebral cortex and hippocampus. They modulate *N*-methyl-D-aspartate–dependent responses, such as long-term potentiation, and show a spatial and temporal sequence of expression that may be demonstrated in the fetal brain by immunocytochemistry. This expression is highly localized to dendritic spines and reflects functional rather than structural features of synapse formation (271–274). Prostaglandin signaling of cortical development and synaptogenesis in particular thus are mediated through dendrites, and the same is likely for neurotropin signaling (275).

Glial cells are important in promoting dendritic development (276). In addition to the axodendritic and axosomatic synapses, a few specialized sites in the developing brain show dendrodendritic contacts. An example is the spines of olfactory granule cells (259).

The electroencephalogram (EEG) is the most reliable and accessible noninvasive clinical measure of functional synaptogenesis in the cerebral cortex of the preterm infant. The maturation of EEG patterns involves a precise and predictable temporal progression of changes with conceptional age, including the development of sleep–wake cycles.

Neuronal and Glial Cell Maturation

Neuronal and epithelial cells are the most polarized cells of the body: epithelial cells must have apical and basal surfaces, and neurons must form an axon at one end and dendrites at other cell surfaces (260,261,277,278). The development of cell polarity is one of the first events in neuronogenesis. The structural and molecular differences that distinguish axonal and dendritic domains play an integral role in every aspect of neuronal function (278). Neuronal polarity begins with the final mitosis of the neuroepithelial cell and is determined by the orientation of microtubules in the mitotic spindle (192).

Two other combined features distinguish neurons from all other cells in the body: an electrically polarizing and excitable plasma membrane and secretory function. Muscle cells have excitable membranes but do not secrete; endocrine and exocrine cells are secretory but do not have polarized membranes. Only neurons have both.

The development of electrical polarity of the cell membrane is an important maturational feature that denotes when a neuroblast becomes a neuron. This process depends on the development of ion channels as well as a means of delivering continuous energy production necessary to maintain a resting membrane potential. This membrane potential is mediated by voltage-gated ion channels and does not require another energy-generating mechanism such as the adenosine triphosphatase (ATPase) pumps mediated by Na^+/K^+, Ca^{2+}, or Mg^{2+}. The importance of glial cells for ion transport in this regard may be greater than once believed, and astrocytes play an important role in regulating the cerebral microenvironment in addition to their nutritive functions and their contribution to the blood–brain barrier (276).

The onset of synthesis of neurotransmitter substances, their transport down the axon, and the formation of terminal axonal storage vesicles for these compounds are other features that denote the transition from neuroblast to neuron. Transmitter biosynthesis may begin before neuroblast migration is completed, although the secretion of these substances is delayed until synapses are formed with target cells. Some substances that later serve as neurotransmitters, including most of the neuropeptides, acetylcholine, and γ-aminobutyric acid, may be synthesized early in embryonic or fetal life before they could possibly function as transmitters and may serve a neurotrophic function.

A number of proteins are produced by mature neurons and not by immature nerve cells. Antibodies against such proteins may be used to demonstrate the maturation of neuroblasts in the human fetal brain (at autopsy) by immunocytochemistry. One such example is neuronal nuclear antigen (NeuN) (279). By coupling such studies with immunocytochemical markers of axonal maturation, such as the use of antibodies against synaptic vesicle proteins, it is possible to demonstrate the temporal relation of terminal axonal maturation and the maturation of their target neuron (280). This sequence may be altered in some cerebral malformations and may explain why some infants with severe malformations such as holoprosencephaly have intractable epilepsy whereas others with similar anatomic lesions, by imaging and even by histopathologic examination, have few or no seizures.

Some genes appear to be essential for the regulation of trophic factors or differentiation and growth of the individual neural cell. *TSC1* and *TSC2* are genes that produce products, respectively termed hamartin and tuberin, that are defective in tissues, both neural and non-neural, in patients with tuberous sclerosis (137–142) (see Chapter 12). *TSC1* is localized on chromosome 9q34 (139). It accounts for only the minority of patients with this autosomal dominant disease (140). *TSC2* has its locus at 16p13.3.

Myelination

As with other aspects of nervous system development, myelination cycles (i.e., the time between onset and termination of myelination in a given pathway) are specific for each tract and precisely time linked. Some pathways myelinate in a rostrocaudal progression. The human corticospinal tract at birth is myelinated in the corona radiata, internal capsule, middle third of the cerebral peduncle, upper pons; very lightly myelinated in the pyramids; and unmyelinated in the spinal cord. Other pathways myelinate

TABLE 5.6 Myelination Cycles in the Human Central Nervous System Based on Myelin Tissue Stains

Pathway	Begins	Completed
Spinal motor roots	16 wk	42 wk
Spinal sensory roots	20 wk	5 mo
Cranial motor nerves III, IV, V, VI	20 wk	28 wk
Ventral commissure, spinal cord	24 wk	4 mo
Dorsal columns, spinal cord	28 wk	36 wk
Medial longitudinal fasciculus	24 wk	28 wk
Habenulopeduncular tract	28 wk	34 wk
Acoustic nerve	24 wk	36 wk
Trapezoid body and lateral lemniscus	25 wk	36 wk
Acoustic radiations (thalamocortical)	40 wk	3 yr
Inferior cerebellar peduncle (inner part)	26 wk	36 wk
Inferior cerebellar peduncle (outer parts)	32 wk	4 mo
Middle cerebellar peduncle (pontocerebellar)	42 wk	3 yr
Superior cerebellar peduncle	28 wk	6 mo
Medial lemniscus	32 wk	12 mo
Optic nerve	38 wk	6 mo
Optic radiations (geniculocalcarine)	40 wk	6 mo
Ansa reticularis	28 wk	8 mo
Fornix	2 mo	2 yr
Mammillothalamic tract	8 mo	6 yr
Thalamocortical radiations	2 mo	7 yr
Corticospinal (pyramidal) tract	38 wk	2 yr
Corpus callosum	2 mo	14 yr
Ipsilateral intracortical association fibers, frontotemporal and frontoparietal	3 mo	32 yr

Myelination determined by light microscopy using luxol fast blue and other myelin stains; composite from various authors. Gestational age stated in weeks; postnatal age stated in months and years.

From Sarnat HB. *Cerebral dysgenesis: embryology and clinical expression.* New York: Oxford University Press, 1992. With permission.

in their proximal and distal portions at the same time. Some pathways myelinate early and others late, but no axons myelinate during the growth of the axonal growth cone, before it reaches its target. The medial longitudinal fasciculus acquires myelin at 24 weeks' gestation and is fully myelinated within 2 weeks. The corticospinal tract begins myelinating at approximately 38 weeks and is not complete until 2 years of age. The corpus callosum begins myelination at approximately 4 months postnatally and is not complete until late adolescence. The last tract to complete myelination is the ipsilateral association bundle that interconnects the anterior frontal and the temporal lobes, which is not complete until 32 years of age (281). Myelination cycles as determined by special myelin stains of sections of fetal and postnatal CNS tissue at autopsy are summarized in Table 5.6. The traditional stain is luxol fast blue, but newer methods using gallocyanin stains (e.g., Lapham stain) and immunocytochemical demonstration of myelin basic protein provide earlier detection of myelin formation at the light microscopic level; electron microscopy remains the most sensitive morphologic method for documenting the onset of myelination in brain tissue. The sequences of proteins and lipids incorporated into myelin also may be studied biochemically at autopsy in immature brains.

Myelination also may be determined in living patients by magnetic resonance imaging (MRI). T1-weighted images are more sensitive than T2 sequences early, and T2 is more sensitive as myelination advances with maturation, but the present generation of imaging does not show the earliest onset of myelination that can be demonstrated histologically. This difference in sensitivity accounts for somewhat different tables of myelination used by neuroradiologists and neuropathologists (Table 5.7).

Myelination depends on the normal differentiation and integrity of oligodendrocytes in the CNS and Schwann cells in the peripheral nervous system (282–284). As with other developmental processes in the nervous system, the programming of differentiation of these myelin-producing cells and of myelin formation is under genetic regulation (276,277). The *Krox-20* mouse gene (*EGR2* in humans), previously discussed as a zinc finger homeobox gene expressed in rhombomeres 3 and 5, also plays an important role in myelination by Schwann cells (55). It is a paradox that *Krox-20*/*EGR2* is expressed only in rhombomeres 3 and 5, rhombomeres that do not form neural crest tissue

TABLE 5.7 First Appearance of Myelination in the Human Brain Based on Magnetic Resonance Imaging

Anatomic Region	*T1-Weighted*	*T2-Weighted*
Middle cerebellar peduncle	Birth	Birth to 2 mo
Cerebral white matter	Birth to 4 mo	3–5 mo
Internal capsule, posterior limb		
Anterior portion	Birth	4–7 mo
Posterior portion	Birth	Birth to 2 mo
Internal capsule, anterior limb	2–3 mo	7–11 mo
Corpus callosum, genu	4–6 mo	5–8 mo
Corpus callosum, splenium	3–4 mo	4–6 mo
Occipital white matter		
Central	3–5 mo	9–14 mo
Peripheral	4–7 mo	11–15 mo
Frontal white matter		
Central	3–6 mo	11–16 mo
Peripheral	7–11 mo	14–18 mo
Centrum semiovale	2–6 mo	7–11 mo

From Barkovich AJ. *Pediatric neuroimaging*, 2nd ed. New York: Raven, 1995. With permission.

although adjacent and intervening rhombomeres do (61,62), and Schwann cells are derived from neural crest. The *PMP-22* gene, which is defective in several hereditary motor sensory neuropathies, programs proteolipid protein by encoding an axonally regulated Schwann cell protein incorporated into peripheral myelin (285), but whether it serves a function in the CNS is uncertain.

In addition to their role in generating myelin sheaths around some axons, oligodendrocytes express nerve growth factor and may secrete other molecules that stimulate the growth of axons (286). Insulin-like growth factor also may play a role in central myelination and conserving axonal integrity (287). The embryonic expression of myelin genes in the brain provides evidence of the focal source of oligodendroglial precursors in the ventricular zone of the neural tube (284a). Gangliosides are complex lipids that form part of the myelinating membranes of oligodendrocytes and Schwann cells, and their composition is important in the development of myelin (288).

Oligodendrocytes may ensheath several axons in the CNS, but in the peripheral nervous system each Schwann cell myelinates only a single axon, though some Schwann cells may enclose one to four unmyelinated axons. At midgestation, a single Schwann cell may enclose as many as 25 axons, but this ratio becomes smaller with progressive maturation (289).

Myelination is an important parameter of the maturation of the brain in a clinically measurable index. Delayed myelination occurs in many metabolic diseases involving the nervous system, in fetal and postnatal malnutrition if the lipids and proteins are not available to be incorporated, and at times as a nonspecific feature of global developmental delay (73). Late progenitors of oligodendrocytes are vulnerable to hypoxic/ischemic injury in the human fetus and premature infant, and their damage results in white matter injury, periventricular leukomalacia, a common cause of spastic diplegia (290).

Neural Crest

Ontogenesis of Neural Crest Tissue

The neural crest is a transient population of embryonic cells derived from ectoderm and defined by their migratory behavior and ability to form numerous derivatives (291–294). Primordial neural crest cells first appear at the lateral margins of the neural placode shortly after gastrulation. As neurulation proceeds, the curling of the neural placode shifts these cells to the dorsomedial neural groove. With closure of the dorsal midline, the neural crest cells separate from the newly formed neural tube and begin migrating along prescribed routes throughout the embryo, initiating the peripheral nervous system, including dorsal root and autonomic ganglia, Schwann cells of peripheral nerves, and chromaffin tissue in the adrenal medulla, carotid body, and other sites. Neural crest also differentiates as mesodermal cells, including melanocytes, endothelial cells, smooth muscle of blood vessels, interstitial connective tissue, the ocular sclera, cartilage, and membranous (but not endochondral) bone, especially in the craniofacial skeleton (291–296). When neural crest meets an epithelium, cartilage forms; when it meets mesodermal tissue, membranous bone forms. This explains why we have cartilage in our ears and bone forms our orbits. Neural crest cells terminally differentiate only after reaching their final destination.

Neural crest is so pervasive that some authors have suggested its status be promoted as a fourth germ layer (297), but this is not a correct or useful reclassification because, though incipient neural crest cells first appear at the lateral margins of the neuroepithelial placode on the day of gastrulation, these cells are not yet "committed" to a specific fate. Lineage analyses have demonstrated that individual neural fold cells can form either epidermis or neural crest cells, hence they are not truly neural crest until after gastrulation. Moreover, to create another germ layer, other germ layers would have to yield tissues previously assigned as ectoderm and mesoderm. The whole concept of embryonic germ layers may soon be regarded as a relic of the pre–molecular genetic era, hence this is a moot point.

Neural crest arises segmentally in all three primitive cerebral vesicles: rhombencephalon, mesencephalon, and prosencephalon. Neural crest cells migrate in a somewhat different manner from each part of the embryonic neural tube after segmentation and the formation of neuromeres at 4 to 8 weeks' gestation. The neural crest may be divided into three groups on this basis. The prosencephalic neural crest migrates rostrally into the head as a midline *vertical sheet* of cells (36). The mesencephalic neural crest, which arises not only from the mesencephalic neuromere (i.e., r0, future midbrain), but also from the first two hindbrain rhombomeres (neuromeres r1 and r2' (the rostral half of r2), migrates as *streams* of cells into the face and cranium. The rhombencephalic neural crest, arising from the hindbrain, migrates as *segmental blocks* of cells, mainly caudal to the head (293,294).

Neural crest is thus responsible for much of craniofacial development (292–294). For this reason, many developmental malformations of the brain are associated with dysmorphic facies or cranial bone defects (298–300). Neuroembryology involves the study of more than the central and peripheral nervous systems.

Though patterns of genetic expression in the hindbrain contribute to the segmental arrangement of neural crest cells, cellular migratory pathways also are guided by attractant and repulsant paracrine molecules secreted by surrounding tissues such as the otic capsule, the somites, and the vertebral neural arches. The "delamination" of neural crest cells, their separation from the dorsal midline of the neural tube, is probably mediated by several genes and molecules; rhoB appears to be one of these factors (133).

In addition, neural crest cells possess *integrin* receptors for interacting with extracellular matrix molecules (301). Changes in the distribution of *extracellular matrix* components during neural crest migration impose migratory guidance limits as well (302). The extracellular matrix glycoprotein tenascin is required for proper cranial neural crest migration, and its absence in the chick embryo leads to neural tube defects and aggregates of ectopic neural crest cells (303).

As with other parts of the neural tube, neural crest tissue has a rostrocaudal gradient of differentiation. The fate of neural crest cells is not entirely predetermined; environmental factors may induce differentiation of different cells than were originally intended. For example, although early-migrating neural crest cells generally form dorsal root ganglion cells, when these early-migrating cells are ablated, the late-migrating neural crest cells that ordinarily form mesodermal structures change their fate to become primary sensory neurons. Transplanted early-migrating neural crest cells do not always differentiate as neurons under all conditions (304,305).

Neurotrophic factors, such as neurotrophin-3 (NT3), also influence the fate of neural crest cells and are essential for survival of sympathetic neuroblasts and innervation of specific organs (305–309). NT3 is the principal, and perhaps the only, neurotrophin needed by neurons of the myenteric plexus (307–309), but other neural crest derivatives require other factors. Gene products of *BMP2* and *BMP4* regulate the onset of NT3 during fetal gut development, and *BMP4* and NT3 (with its receptor TrkC) are needed to preserve the integrity of the submucosal and myenteric plexuses. Nerve growth factor (NGF), the first neurotrophin identified, was first demonstrated in dorsal root ganglia. Brain-derived neurotrophic factor (BDNF), ciliary neurotrophic factor (CNTF), and glial-derived neurotrophic factor (GNTF) all are associated with neural crest migration or differentiation.

The origin of neural crest is topographically unequal in the neuraxis. The streams of cells arising in the midbrain contribute to craniofacial structure. In the hindbrain, migratory mesencephalic neural crest cells from rl and r2 populate the trigeminal ganglion, and streams of rhombencephalic neural crest form the mandibular arch; cells from r4 form the hyoid arch and the geniculate and vestibular ganglia; those from r6 populate the third and fourth branchial arches and associated peripheral ganglia (293,294). Rhombomeres 3 and 5 do not appear to have neural crest cells, but actually neural crest cells of r3 and r5 are generated and mix with neural crest cells of the adjacent rostral and caudal rhombomeres to migrate together (294,310). This explains the fusion of the proximal maxillary and mandibular branches of the trigeminal nerve.

Genetic Programs of Neural Crest

Many genes are involved in the formation, migration, and terminal differentiation of neural crest into its various cellular types. These cells do not differentiate until arriving in their target zone. Recent molecular genetic data diminish the conceptual importance of embryonic germ layers, long believed to be fundamental in cellular lineage, because it is now recognized that the same organizer and regulator genes program development and cytologic differentiation in various tissues and that genes do not respect embryonic germ layers. Examples are the *HOX* and *PAX* families, both primordial in the embryonic segmentation of the neural tube, but also in the ontogenesis of bone, kidney, gut, and many other tissues. Even single-gene deletions or mutations may downregulate other downstream genes in a cascade, permit the overexpression of antagonistic genes, or otherwise alter complex multigenetic interactions. Trophic factors important in neural crest migration and maturation also might be defective in some syndromes. Neural crest induction occurs continuously over a long period starting at gastrulation and persisting well past the time of neural tube closure (295). Neural crest can be induced to form in early neuroectoderm by the proximity of non-neural surface ectoderm (311–313).

Many genes are essential to the formation of neural crest, but the most important are those having a strong *dorsalizing* effect in the vertical axis of the neural tube: *Zic2*, *Bmp4*, *Bmp7*, and *Pax3*. The transforming growth factor-beta (TGFβ) superfamily, and in particular *Bmp4* and *Bmp7*, promote neural crest differentiation at the time of neural tube closure; these two genes can even substitute for non-neural ectoderm in inducing neural crest cells (312,314). Ventralizing genes of the vertical axis, such as *Shh*, expressed by both notochord and floor plate cells of the neural tube, inhibit neural crest formation (314). Experimentally, either notochordal tissue or *Shh*-expressing cells grafted adjacent to the neural folds prevent neural crest formation (120). The gene *Noggin*, a strong antagonist of *Bmp* genes, also inhibits neural crest formation (120,315).

At a later stage in neural tube development, the segmentation genes that program the formation of neuromeres also can promote neural crest, especially those with a dorsalizing effect in the vertical axis. The segmentation homeobox *Wingless* family, particularly *Wnt-1* and *Wnt-3a*, not only are important for the formation of neuromeric compartments and their boundaries in the hindbrain, but also promote neural crest formation (316–318). Outside the neural tube, however, these same *Wnt* genes cause neural crest to become melanocytes rather than neurons such as autonomic ganglion cells (163).

The human gene *EGR2* (known as *Krox-20* in the mouse), another homeobox gene of segmentation and a zinc finger gene (see the Transcription Factors and Homeoboxes section for definition), limits its expression to rhombomeres r3 and r5. *EGR2* inhibits neural crest formation, but the incipient neural crest cells of these two rhombomeres shift to the immediately adjacent anterior and posterior rhombomeres where *EGR2* is not expressed (56). This shifted neural crest cells mix with the neural crest being generated in those rhombomeres, so that neural crest cells that migrate caudally around the otic vesicle are from both r5 and r6 (56,294). *Hox-1.5* and *Hox-2.9* regulate the premigratory and migratory neural crest cells from r4 (318).

The gene *Slug* (*Snail* in invertebrates) is essential for later stages of neural crest differentiation. Though also detected in early stages of the neural placode prior to neural crest migration and in early migratory cells to the periphery, its transcript is later downregulated during later migration and also *in vitro* in the absence of tissue interactions (295,319,320). *Slug* then is later re-expressed in stronger form. *Slug* is a "zinc finger" (for definition, see the Transcription Factors and Homeoboxes section) (321). In the amphibian embryo, *Slug* expression does not itself induce neural crest, but in the presence of *Wnt* signals, abundant neural crest is generated (322). *Bmp4* is upregulated in the isolated neural folds just prior to the upregulation of *Slug*.

Other genes implicated in neural crest development include *Otx* (*Emx1, 2*), *Phox*, *Dlx*, *Mash1*, and *Twist*. The *PAX* and *MSX* families are of particular importance in craniofacial development associated with prosencephalic and mesencephalic neural crest migration (320). *Twist* in head mesenchyme is obligatory for cranial neural tube morphogenesis and for cranial neural crest formation and migration (143). The proto-oncogene c-*myc* is another essential regulator of neural crest formation (323).

WHAT IS A BRAIN AND HOW DOES IT DIFFER FROM A GANGLION?

After reviewing the many aspects of neuroembryology, one can address a fundamental question of when does the differentiating tissue at the rostral end of the neural tube become a brain. Does it begin as a "cerebral ganglion" or "cephalic ganglion" and only later meet the criteria of being a "brain" or is it a brain from the beginning? What are these criteria? The definition of *brain* is primordial to embryologic understanding. A brain, in the most universal terms as applies to all vertebrates and invertebrates, has the following characteristics: (a) It is located in the head or rostral end of the organism; (b) it subserves the entire body, not just restricted segments; (c) it has functionally specialized parts; (d) it is bilobar; (e) neurons form the surface with their axons in the central core; (f) interneurons are more numerous than primary sensory or primary motor neurons that project neurites into the periphery; and (g) multisynaptic rather than monosynaptic circuits predominate (324). The definition specifically excludes functional aspects, including cognition, which may differ at various stages of maturation and between species. Ganglia, such as autonomic and dorsal root ganglia, fail to fulfill any of these criteria and, from the time that neuroepithelium begins to differentiate in the rostral end of the neural tube, it is a true brain. A "cephalic ganglion" does not exist at any time during ontogenesis in any animal that aggregates neurons to be a central nervous system, including in the simplest flatworms, and probably never existed in evolution (324).

PART 2

Malformations of the Central Nervous System

John H. Menkes, Harvey B. Sarnat, and Laura Flores-Sarnat

Malformations of the brain and spinal cord may be genetically determined or acquired. The great majority of dysgeneses that occur early in gestation have a genetic basis, whereas those that begin late in gestation are more likely to be secondary to destructive lesions such as infarcts that interfere with development of particular structures. The distinction between atrophy, the shrinkage of a previously well-formed structure, and hypoplasia, the deficient development of a structure that never achieves normal size, is not always clear in degenerative processes or in those acquired lesions of fetal life in which an insult is imposed on a structure that is not yet fully formed. Examples are ischemic lesions in fetal brain associated with congenital cytomegalovirus infections and fetal degenerative diseases such as pontocerebellar hypoplasia and polymicrogyria, which develop in zones of relative ischemia that surround porencephalic cysts resulting from an occlusion of the middle cerebral artery incurred in fetal life. White matter infarcts in the cerebrum may destroy radial glial fibers and prevent normal migration of neuroblasts and glioblasts from the subventricular zone or germinal matrix (see Chapter 6).

Regardless of their cause, malformations are traditionally classified as disturbances in developmental processes. These are outlined in Table 5.8.

Whereas this type of classification retains validity for understanding the type of developmental process most disturbed, such as cellular proliferation or neuroblast migration, the new understanding of developmental genes and their role in the ontogenesis of the nervous system provides a new, complementary molecular genetic classification of early neurogenesis that recognizes the genetic regulation of development. An example of an attempt to use these new data to organize the thinking about developmental malformations of the brain is proposed in Table 5.9, a table that will undoubtedly undergo considerable revision in the coming years as more data become available.

Because the nervous system develops in a precise temporal as well as spatial sequence, it is often possible to assign a precise timing of a malformation, or at least to date the earliest time when the insult was first expressed. In most cases, an insult, whether caused by overexpression or underexpression of a developmental gene or caused by an ongoing acquired process such as a congenital viral infection or repeated episodes of ischemia, affects nervous system development over an extended period of time. Thereby, the insult involves processes that occur at various stages of development, not just at a single precise moment. As discussed in the Patterning of the Neural Tube:

TABLE 5.8 Traditional Classification of Central Nervous System Malformations as Disorders of . . .

1. Neurulation
2. Cell proliferation: neurogenesis and gliogenesis
3. Apoptosis
4. Migration of neuroblasts and glioblasts
5. Axonal projection and pathfinding
6. Dendritic sprouting and synaptogenesis
7. Myelination

TABLE 5.9 Proposed Molecular Genetic Classification of Malformations of Early Central Nervous System Development

I. **Disorders of the Primitive Streak and Node**
   A. Overexpression of genes
   B. Underexpression of genes

II. **Disorders of Ventralization of the Neural Tube**
   A. Overexpression of the ventrodorsal gradient
      1. Duplication of spinal central canal
      2. Duplication of ventral horns of spinal cord
      3. Diplomyelia (and diastematomyelia?)
      4. Duplication of entire neuraxis
      5. Ventralizing induction of somite
         a. Segmental amyoplasia
   B. Underexpression of ventrodorsal gradient
      1. Fusion of ventral horns of spinal cord
      2. Sacral (thoracolumbosacral) agenesis
      3. Arhinencephaly
      4. Holoprosencephaly

III. **Disorders of Dorsalization of the Neural Tube**
   A. Overexpression of dorsoventral gradient
      1. Duplication of dorsal horns of spinal cord
      2. Duplication of dorsal brainstem structures
   B. Underexpression of dorsalization of the neural tube
      1. Fusion of dorsal horns of spinal cord
      2. Septo-optic dysplasia (?)

IV. **Disorder of the Rostrocaudal Gradient, Segmentation, or Both**
   A. Decreased domains of homeoboxes
      1. Agenesis of mesencephalon and metencephalon
      2. Global cerebellar aplasia or hypoplasia
      3. Aplasia of basal telencephalic nuclei
   B. Increased domains of homeoboxes or ectopic expression
      1. Chiari II malformation

Axes and Gradients of Growth and Differentiation section, developmental genes may serve as organizer genes early in ontogenesis and as regulator genes later on, thus involving various processes. Defective expression of *SHH*, for example, may result in holoprosencephaly because of its early effects on midline ventralization in the prosencephalon but may affect granule cell proliferation in the cerebellum as well; the timing of these two events is quite different.

The accounts that follow are traditional descriptions of major malformations of the human nervous system, but the new perspective of molecular genetic programming will be an integral part of the understanding of these disorders of development. Finally, it must always be recognized that just as no two adults, even monozygotic twins, are identical, no two fetuses are identical and no two cerebral malformations are identical. Individual biological variations occur in abnormal as well as in normal development, and allowance must be made for small differences while recognizing the principal patterns that denote pathogenesis.

The importance of disordered nervous system maturation in causing chronic abnormalities of brain function only recently has become fully apparent. Estimates suggest that 3% of neonates have major CNS or multisystem malformations (325), and 75% of fetal deaths and 40% of deaths within the first year of life are secondary to CNS malformations (326). Furthermore, 5% to 15% of pediatric neurology hospital admissions appear to be primarily related to cerebral and spinal cord anomalies (327). Genetic and nongenetic interactions are responsible for 20% of CNS malformations; monogenic malformations, whether autosomal or X-linked, account for 7.5% of malformations; chromosomal factors account for 6%; and well-delineated environmental factors, including maternal infections, maternal diabetes, irradiation, and drugs (e.g., thalidomide, valproic acid, methylmercury, excessive vitamin A or retinoic acid) account for at least another 3.5%. In the remainder, more than 60% of cases, the cause of the CNS malformation is uncertain (328–330). As more associations with specific genes and their defective expression become known, this number will undoubtedly become smaller.

EMBRYONIC INDUCTION DISORDERS (0 TO 4 WEEKS' GESTATION)

Embryogenic induction disorders represent a failure in the mutual induction of mesoderm and neuroectoderm. The primary defect is a failure of the neural folds to fuse and form the neural tube (ectoderm), with secondary maldevelopment of skeletal structures enclosing the CNS (mesoderm). This process is called *neurulation*. In addition to the mesodermal notochord inducing the floor plate of the neural tube, the neural tube induces many non-neural structures of mesodermal origin. Craniofacial development is induced by the anterior neural tube and mediated by the migration of mesencephalic and prosencephalic neural crest tissue (293,294). This relation explains the midfacial hypoplasia in holoprosencephaly, the absence of calvarial bones and hypotelorism in anencephaly, and hypertelorism in agenesis of the corpus callosum and in many genetic syndromes such as Noonan syndrome (298,300).

Defects range from anencephaly to sacral meningomyelocele in the cephalic to caudal direction of the neural tube, and from holoprosencephaly to craniospinal rachischisis (midline posterior splitting of skull and vertebral column) in the anterior to posterior direction. For convenience, they are divided into dorsal (posterior) and ventral (anterior) midline defects. The former is named *dysraphism* to indicate the persistent continuity between posterior neuroectoderm and cutaneous ectoderm. Midline cerebral malformations with dysmorphic facies, such as holoprosencephaly, are not in this category. Some dorsalizing genes, expressed in the dorsal part of the neural tube (e.g. , *ZIC2*, several *PAX* genes, the *BMP* family), may cause CNS malformations without dysraphism, however, when mutations occur. Ventral midline defects that involve more structures than just the neural tube are called *facio-telencephalopathy* to connote the noncleavage of the ventral neural tube, cephalic mesoderm, and adjacent foregut entoderm.

Dorsal Midline Central Nervous System–Axial Skeletal Defects: Dysraphism

A large number of midline anomalies occur, and the chance of several midline defects occurring conjointly is greater than the product of their individual occurrence.

Anencephaly

Anencephaly is the paradigm of the various dysraphic disorders. Although affected infants rarely survive early infancy, insight into the mechanics of neural ontogenesis provided by this disorder is enormous.

Pathogenesis and Pathology

Both genetic predisposition and environmental insults are responsible for the condition. The defect is time specific in that the insult probably occurs after the onset of neural fold development (16 days) but before closure of the anterior neuropore (24 to 26 days). The stimulus is nonspecific because a variety of insults have been implicated. These include drugs (330), infections (331), chemical disorders such as maternal diabetes or folic acid deficiency (332), and irradiation (333). Whatever the actual teratogenic stimulus might be, it induces four basic defects: (a) A defective notochord and prechordal mesoderm (the notochord proper extends rostrally only to the midbrain) causes failure of the cephalic neural folds to fuse into a neural tube. (b) Failure of development of the meninges and cranial bones exposes the brain to amniotic fluid, with subsequent encephaloclastic degeneration of forebrain germinal cells. (c) Paraxial mesoderm fails to differentiate into well-formed somites and hence into sclerotomes, the latter being the primordium for the base of the skull and vertebrae. (d) A failure of prosencephalic and mesencephalic neural crest formation and migration results in midfacial hypoplasia with hypotelorism resembling that of holoprosencephaly and failure of formation of the meninges over the forebrain and membranous bone of the cranial vault (298,300). Thus, mutual induction between the germ layers fails at time-specific stages, resulting in deformities of both nervous tissue and supporting axial and membranous bone (300,334). Genetic factors are suspected in many cases, but no specific gene or its locus has yet been identified.

Studies of human embryos suggest that the splitting of an already closed neural tube might account for anencephaly and other dysraphic conditions (335). Gardner and Breuer argued not only that dysraphic states are a consequence of neural tube rupture after closure, but also that a number of associated non-neural anomalies, including asplenia, renal agenesis, and tracheoesophageal fistula, result from the damage of primordia of other organs by the overdistended neural tube (336). Osaka and coworkers discounted these theories on the basis that in human embryos dysraphism can be observed before completion of neural tube closure (337,338). Muscle differentiates normally in anencephaly despite disruption of motor innervation, suggesting that motor innervation occurs after muscle development and, therefore, after embryogenesis and neural tube closure (339). A primary defect of neural crest could explain many of the non-neurologic features of anencephaly (300).

Examination of the nervous system shows the spinal cord, brainstem, and cerebellum to be small. Descending tracts within the spinal cord, particularly the corticospinal tract, are absent. Above the midbrain, glial and vascular tissue with remnants of midbrain and diencephalon exist. Sometimes the basal telencephalic nuclei are partially or even fully formed (73). The pituitary is absent, with secondary adrenal hypoplasia. The optic nerves are absent but the eyes are normal, indicating that the anterior cephalic end of the neural tube, whence the optic vesicles spring, closed and diverticulated properly.

In addition to the primary defect of development, anencephaly involves an important encephaloclastic component (73,300). Because neural tissue is directly exposed to amniotic fluid, which is caustic, a progressive destruction of neural tissue and a compensatory proliferation of small blood vessels occurs to create the area cerebrovasculosa in the nubbin of tissue representing the residual prosencephalon. A poorly organized network of thin-walled vascular channels of variable size that are not mature capillaries, arterioles, or venules is enmeshed with glial processes and scattered (haphazardly oriented neurons and neuroblasts, lacking recognizable architecture as either nuclei or laminated cortex). Anencephaly is therefore difficult to analyze histopathologically because of the simultaneous presence of both primary dysplastic and secondary destructive processes.

The calvarium fails to develop, and the frontal and parietal bones are partially absent; the rostral half of the occipital bone is membranous and also is deficient, but the posterior part, not of neural crest origin, is preserved. Malformations of the foramen magnum and cervical vertebrae are frequent. The reduced forehead and relatively large ears and eyes lend a froglike appearance to the face; facial structures are developed, but midfacial hypoplasia with hypotelorism occurs in some cases (300), and there is an occasional lateral cleft lip or palate.

Some authors use the term *aprosencephaly* for cases in which the calvarium is intact, in distinction from *atelencephaly*, in which the cranium is open (340,341). In *exencephaly*, a rare condition, the membranous bones of the cranial vault are absent and the preserved but disorganized brain is covered by vascular epithelium. The condition is believed to be a stage in the development of anencephaly, with more complete destruction of the exposed brain being a matter of time (342).

Epidemiology

Anencephaly is the most common major CNS malformation in the West (343). The incidence of this malformation differs in various parts of the world. It is high in Ireland, Scotland, and Wales and low in Japan. The incidence of anencephaly and of neural tube defects in general is very high in northern but not southern China (344). It is high also in Mexico near the Texas border (345). Other areas of high incidence include Egypt, the Arabian subcontinent, and New Zealand. As a rule, the incidence increases with increasing maternal age and decreasing socioeconomic status.

The rate of anencephaly as well as that of the other neural tube defects has declined. In the 1960s, the incidence ranged from 0.65 per 1,000 births in Japan to more than 3 in 1,000 in the British Isles, with a maximum incidence of 8 in 1,000 occurring in Ireland in 1960. Prior peaks in incidence had been recorded during the years of 1929 through 1932 and 1938 through 1941. Since then, there has been a steady decline in both the United States and the United Kingdom. Between 1971 and 1989, the annual rate of various forms of spina bifida fell from 2 in 1,000 to 0.6 in 1,000 (346), with a relative increase in the proportion of spina bifida to anencephaly (347). In part, this decline reflects the widespread use of antenatal screening, but other factors, notably the correction of maternal vitamin deficiency, also might be responsible (346,348).

Anencephaly is seen 37 times more frequently in female than in male newborns (349). The recurrence rate in families with an affected child is 35%, although almost 10% of siblings of anencephalics have major anomalies of neural tube closure: anencephaly, spina bifida cystica, and encephalocele (350). The transmission appears to be matrilineal. No relationship to consanguinity is evident, nor to concordance in monozygotic twins, and the recurrence rate for a maternal half-sibling is the same as for a full sibling. These factors weigh against a simple polygenetic inheritance pattern and are more consistent with the interaction of genetic and environmental factors (351).

Clinical Manifestations

Anencephalic patients do not survive infancy. During their few weeks of life, they exhibit slow, stereotyped movements and frequent decerebrate posturing. Head, facial, and limb movements can be spontaneous or pain induced. The Moro reflex and some brainstem functions and automatisms, such as sucking, rooting, and righting responses, are present and are more readily and more reproducibly elicited than in healthy infants. The *bowing reflex*, which occasionally can be demonstrated in healthy premature infants of 7 months' gestation, is invariably present in anencephalics (352) (see Introduction chapter). Seizures have been observed in anencephalic infants, an indication that some types of neonatal seizures originate in the deeper structures of the brain (353).

The presence of anencephaly and other open neural tube defects can be predicted by measuring α-fetoprotein (AFP) in amniotic fluid or maternal serum. AFP is the major serum protein in early embryonic life, representing 90% of total serum globulin. It is a fetus-specific α_1-globulin that is probably involved in preventing fetal immune rejection; it is produced first by the yolk sac and later by the fetal liver and gastrointestinal tract. It normally passes from fetal serum into fetal urine and then into amniotic fluid. Because of a substantial leak of fetal blood components directly into amniotic fluid, AFP concentrations in amniotic fluid and maternal serum AFP levels are elevated in anencephaly and in open spina bifida or cranium bifidum (354).

Normal AFP in adult serum is less than 10 ng/mL. In normal maternal serum and amniotic fluid, it ranges from 15 to 500 ng/mL. At 15 to 20 weeks' gestation, an AFP concentration of 1,000 ng/mL or greater strongly suggests an open neural tube defect, and the current screening of serum detects 79% of cases of open spina bifida at 16 to 18 weeks (355). Determining gestational age is critical, however, because normal AFP concentration varies considerably with fetal age, peaking between 12 and 15 weeks' gestation. Amniotic fluid AFP screening is more reliable, detecting 98% of open spina bifida cases (356). The amniotic fluid must be assessed for contamination by fetal hemoglobin, which complicates amniocentesis, because a 200:1 AFP gradient exists between fetal serum and amniotic fluid. The reliability of ultrasonography depends on the experience of the operators; in good hands, the procedure is more than 99% specific (355). False-positive results are obtained in a variety of unrelated conditions, principally in the presence of multiple pregnancies, threatened abortion or fetal death, or when an error is made in dating the pregnancy. Amniotic fluid AFP obtained between 15 and 20 weeks' gestation is most specific (356); however, closed neural tube defects such as skin-covered lipomyelomeningoceles, encephaloceles, and meningoceles go undetected. These lesions constitute between 5% and 10% of total neural tube defects (357,358).

Mothers who have borne one or more children with neural tube defects, spinal dysraphism, or multiple vertebral anomalies; who have a family history of any of these disorders; or who are surviving patients with spina bifida are at risk for bearing children with neural tube defects and should undergo screening.

Supplementation of the maternal diet with folic acid or with a multivitamin preparation that contains folic acid even before conception has been proposed to prevent neural tube defects. An extensive, controlled British study indicated that the recurrence rate of neural tube defects can be reduced sharply by folic acid supplementation (359). A multivitamin cocktail including folic acid, ascorbic acid, and riboflavin, given from at least 28 days before conception up to the second missed menstrual period, reduced the recurrence rates for neural tube defects from 4.2% to 0.5% in mothers with a previous neural tube defect pregnancy and from 9.6% to 2.3% in mothers who had given birth to two or more offspring with neural tube defects (360,361). These findings were duplicated in an American study, which showed that a vitamin supplement including 0.8 mg of folic acid, started 1 month before conception reduced significantly the incidence of neural tube defects (362,363). The reason for the apparent effect of folic acid is unclear, and the significance of these findings must be evaluated in the light of the declining incidence of neural tube defects in areas where no vitamin supplementation is used (346,364,365). Mice with a mutation of the *Cart1* gene develop acrania and meroanencephaly, and this can be prevented by prenatal folic acid treatment (94).

Meningomyelocele (Spina Bifida) and Encephalocele (Cranium Bifidum)

As the older names imply, *spina bifida* and *cranium bifidum* share a failure of bone fusion in the posterior midline of the skull (cranium bifidum) or the vertebral column (spina bifida). The result is a bony cleft through which the meninges and varying quantities of brain or spinal cord tissue protrude. In cranium bifidum, the neural herniation is termed *encephalocele* and can consist of brain parenchyma and meninges or only of meninges. These form the wall of a saclike cyst filled with cerebrospinal fluid (CSF). Posterior encephaloceles may contain only supratentorial structures, only posterior fossa structures, or both. In spina bifida, the herniation is called *meningocele* or *meningomyelocele*, depending on whether the meninges herniate alone or together with spinal cord parenchyma and nerve roots. The traditional names *spina bifida* and *cranium bifidum* are now less frequently used than in the older literature because of the recognition that the bony cleft may not be the primary defect in all cases, but instead that the pathogenesis may involve neural induction of mesodermal tissues in the dorsal midline, including leptomeninges, dura mater, and bone.

Spina bifida occulta is a minor fusion failure of the posterior vertebral arches unaccompanied by herniation of meninges or neural tissue. Spina bifida cystica collectively designates meningocele, meningomyelocele, and other cystic lesions (Fig. 5.1). Similarly, in the head, cranium bifidum comprises meningocele, a herniation of meninges containing only CSF, and the more commonly occurring encephalocele, in which the sac contains neural and glial tissue. *Rachischisis* refers to a severe condition with an extensive defect of the craniovertebral bone with exposure of the brain, spinal cord, and meninges. *Myeloschisis* is another defect in the tissues over the lower spinal cord. Neural tissue is exposed at the surface as a flat, red lesion with a velvety appearance over the sacral region, without protruding as a myelomeningocele sac.

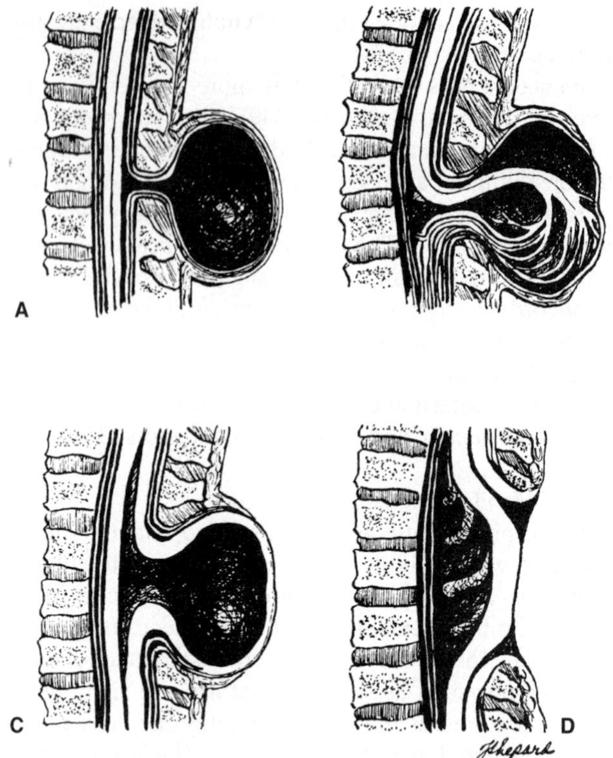

FIGURE 5.1. Drawings of various forms of spinal dysraphic lesions (spina bifida cystica). **A:** Meningocele. Through the bony defect (spina bifida), the meninges herniate and form a cystic sac filled with spinal fluid. The spinal cord does not participate in the herniation and might or might not be abnormal. **B:** Myelomeningocele. The spinal cord is herniated into the sac and ends there or can continue in an abnormal way further downward. **C:** Myelocystocele or syringomyelocele. The spinal cord shows hydromyelia; the posterior wall of the spinal cord is attached to the ectoderm and is undifferentiated. **D:** Myelocele. The spinal cord is araphic; a cystic cavity is in front of the anterior wall of the spinal cord. (From Benda CE. *Developmental disorders of mentation and cerebral palsies.* New York: Grune and Stratton, 1952. With permission.)

Pathogenesis

Spina bifida and cranium bifidum are not only disorders of induction; they also are associated with major abnormalities of cellular migration and secondary mechanical deformities of the nervous system. The continuity between neural and cutaneous ectodermal derivates is regarded as evidence that the primary defect is in the neural tube closure (366,367). Based on studies with embryos of mutant mice with genetically abnormal neurulation and a sacral neural tube defect, McLone and Naiditch (368) proposed a unified theory for the development of the associated anomalies that incorporates some of the prior observations of Padget (334).

According to these authors, the initial event is a failure of the neural folds to close completely, leaving a dorsal myeloschisis. This is followed by a failure of the normal, transient occlusion of the central cavity of the spinal cord. These two events result in the escape of CSF into the amniotic cavity and a collapse of the primitive ventricular system. The failure of the primitive cranial ventricular system to distend results in a posterior fossa that is too small to accommodate the growing cerebellum and leads to upward and downward herniation of the structures within the posterior fossa. Additionally, the failure of the normal distention of the ventricular system leads to inadequate support for the normal outward migration of neuroblasts and a failure to maintain the normal pattern of ossification in the calvarium.

Marín-Padilla proposed that the primary defect is a limited injury to the primitive streak and primitive node, which impairs local growth of skeletal elements, which in turn interferes with closure of the neural tube (369). Although the specific genes involved have not been identified, this hypothesis may be expanded to invoke a mechanism of failed expression of one or more organizer genes during the primitive streak and neural placode stages of early ontogenesis.

These defects are time specific, which is why the most common sites for the lesion in surviving children are either lumbosacral or occipital, these being the last levels at which neural tube closure normally occurs. The initiation

TABLE 5.10 Timetable of Human Central Nervous System Ontogenesis

Days of Gestation	*Event*	*Effect of Toxic Stimulus*
0–18	Three germ layers elaborate and early neural plate forms	No effect or death
18	Neural plate and groove develop	Anterior midline defects (18–23 days)
22–23	Optic vesicles appear	Induction hydrocephalus (18–60 days)
24–26	Anterior neuropore closed	Anencephaly (after 23 days to ?)
26–28	Posterior neuropore closed, ventral horns form	Cranium bifidum, spina bifida cystica, spina bifida occulta (after 26 days to ?)
28–32	Anterior and posterior nerve roots form	—
32	Cerebellar primordium, vascular circulation	Microcephaly (30–130 days), cellular proliferation syndromes (30–175 days), migration anomalies (30 days to complete development of each brain subdivision)
33–35	Prosencephalon cleaves to form palred telencephalon; five cerebral vesicles, choroid plexi, dorsal root ganglion develop	Holoprosencephaly
41	Region of olfactory bulb appears in forebrain	Arhinencephaly
56	Differentiation of cerebral cortex, meningitis, ventricular foramina, central nervous system circulation	Dandy-Walker malformation
70–100	Corpus callosum	Agenesis of corpus callosum
70–150	Primary fissures of cerebral cortex, spinal cord ends at L3 level	Lissencephaly, pachygyria
140–175	Neuronal proliferation in cerebral cortex ends	Defects of cellular architectonics, myelin defects (175 days to 4 yr postnatally)
7–9 mo	Secondary and tertiary sulci	Destructive pathologic changes first noted
175 days to 4 yr postnatally	Neuron blast migration, glial cell production, myelin formation, axosomatic and axodendritic synaptic connections, spinal cord ends L1–2 level	—

of a defect at an earlier stage leads to a more extensive defect, which is incompatible with survival. In the same way, a simple meningocele results when the insult occurs after the spinal cord has formed, whereas a myelomeningocele arises from an earlier insult, which must occur before closure of the posterior neuropore (i.e., before 26 to 28 days' gestation) (Table 5.10) (370).

The cause of these anomalies is unknown. As is the case for anencephaly, it is likely that genetic defects, probably at more than one locus, interact with environmental factors to produce the varying dysraphic conditions. Spinal dysraphic lesions are among the most common anomalies of the nervous system. As with anencephaly, the incidence is highest in Ireland and lowest in Japan and also is influenced by season, socioeconomic status, gender, ethnicity, and such maternal factors as parity, age, prior offspring with neural tube defects, and maternal heat exposure (371). Recurrence rates for mothers who have previously given birth to a child with an open neural tube defect are 1.5% to 2.0%, and for mothers with two affected children, the recurrence rate is 6% (372). The recurrence risk is also higher than normal if close relatives are affected. Less is known about the epidemiology of cranium bifidum, the incidence of which is approximately 1/10 that of spina bifida cystica (341,373).

Pathology

Meningomyelocele (Spina Bifida Cystica). Of the defects collectively termed spina bifida cystica, 95% are myelomeningoceles and 5% are meningoceles. Locations of the defect in liveborn infants are depicted in Table 5.11.

TABLE 5.11 Site of Lesion of Spina Bifida Cystica

Level[a]	*Number of Patients*
Cervical	51
Thoracic	103
Thoracolumbar	137
Lumbar	583
Lumbosacral	382
Sacral	119
Anterior	6
Thoracic	3
Pelvic	3
Undesignated	9
Total	1,396

[a]Level of the meningeal sac in 1,396 consecutive patients treated for spina bifida cystica in the Boston Children's Medical Center.
From Matson DD. *Neurosurgery of infancy and childhood,* 2nd ed. Springfield, IL: Charles C. Thomas, 1969. With permission.

A lumbar or lumbosacral defect is most common; it corresponds to the site of the posterior neuropore closure. Cervical lesions are the least frequent posterior defects. Anterior midline defects of the vertebral arches are uncommon and constituted less than 0.5% of cases in the experience of Matson (373). Approximately 100 anterior sacral meningoceles have been reported, the majority in female patients (374). These conditions should be differentiated from spinal meningeal malformations, which can occur in isolation or in association with systemic malformations (375). Spinal meningeal malformations are relatively common in patients with the various mucopolysaccharidoses and in neurofibromatosis.

Cervical and thoracic meningoceles have narrow bases and are usually not associated with hydrocephalus. By contrast, 90% or more of lumbosacral myelomeningoceles are accompanied by Chiari type II malformations and hydrocephalus. As originally described by Chiari, type I malformations consist of heterotopic, downwardly displaced cerebellar tissue in the absence of space-occupying lesions other than hydrocephalus. Type III malformations consist of cervical spina bifida accompanied by a cerebellar encephalocele. Type IV is a heterogeneous variant in which the cerebellum and brainstem remain in their entirety within the posterior fossa but the cerebellum is small (376,377). Type IV is now an obsolete term of historical interest and is redesignated *cerebellar hypoplasia*.

In 88% of children with lumbar or lumbosacral meningomyeloceles, the spinal cord demonstrates abnormalities in the cervical region (Table 5.12) (366). The majority of instances involve hydrosyringomyelia; less often, diplomyelia or winged and dorsally slit cords are present (378,379). In greater than 70% of cases, the medulla overrides the cervical cord dorsally, in association with type II Chiari malformation (Figs. 5.2 and 5.3). Chiari II malformation is the most constant accompanying feature of lumbosacral meningomyeloceles and is present in nearly all cases. Of patients with spina bifida cystica, 70% show defects in the posterior arch of the atlas, which is bridged by a firm fibrous band, suggesting that congenital atlantoaxial dislocation is a mild expression of an induction disorder (380). Examination of the parenchyma of the spinal cord reveals atrophic or poorly developed ventral horn cells, absent or abnormal corticospinal and ascending sensory tracts, incomplete posterior horns, and exceedingly small and deranged ventral and dorsal root fibers. These changes result in muscle denervation during fetal life and ultimately produce limb deformities and joint contractures.

Defects of cellular migration in the cerebral hemispheres are extremely common (see Table 5.12). These include gray matter heterotopia, schizencephaly, gyral anomalies, agenesis of the corpus callosum, and mesodermal ectopia (366,381,382).

A number of mesodermal lesions accompany the ectodermal defects. In addition to the spinal canal being widened and the posterior arches being malformed, the vertebral bodies can be misshapen with resulting kyphosis or scoliosis. Rib anomalies are common. Mesodermal dysplasia of the skull produces defects in the membranous bones of the calvarium, a condition termed *lacunar skull* or *craniolacunia* (*Lückenschadel*). This peculiar, honeycombed appearance of the skull is seen in some 85% of patients with the Chiari type II malformation. The skull changes are transient and disappear in the first few months after birth. They are probably the result of a defect in membranous bone formation and are not secondary to *in utero* intracranial hypertension, as is often stated (383). The lattice pattern in the inner table of the cranium does not correspond to cerebral convolutions. Lacunar skull also can be seen, rarely, in neonates with normal brains, no midline defects over the spine or head, and no neurologic symptoms (384).

TABLE 5.12 Central Nervous System Anomalies Associated with Meningomyelocele, Hydrocephalus, and Chiari Malformation

	Percentage of Cases
Spinal Cord Malformation	88
Hydromyelia	68
Syringomyelia	36
Diplomyelia (complete duplication over several segments)	36
Diastematomyelia (splitting without duplication)	8
Brainstem Malformation	76
Hypoplasia of cranial nerve nuclei	20
Hypoplasia/aplasia of olives	20
Hypoplasia/aplasia of basal pontile nuclei	16
Malformations of Ventricular System	92
Aqueductal stenosis	52
Aqueductal forking	48
Aqueductal atresia	8
Cerebellar Malformations	72
Heterotaxias (disordered combination of mature neurons and germinal cells)	48
Heterotopias	40
Cerebral Malformations	92
Heterotopias	44
Polymicrogyria	40
Disordered lamination	24
Polymicrogyria	12
Agenesis of the Corpus Callosum	12

Data are based on 25 autopsied patients with meningomyeloceie and hydrocephalus.

Modified from Gilbert JN, Jones KL, Rorke LB, et al. Central nervous system anomalies associated with meningomyelocele, hydrocephalus, and the Chiari malformation: reappraisal of theories regarding the pathogenesis of posterior neural tube closure defects. *Neurosurgery* 1986;18:559–564. With permission.

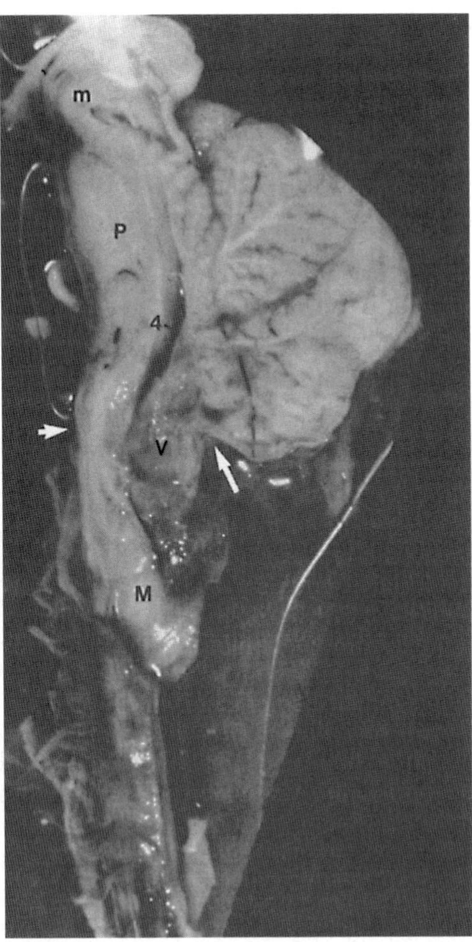

FIGURE 5.2. Chiari type II malformation. Sagittal section through the cerebellum and brainstem in a newborn boy. Anterior is to the reader's left. Arrows mark the location of the foramen magnum. The medulla (*M*) protrudes below the foramen magnum into the cervical spinal cord canal to overlap the cervical spinal cord. The medulla buckles dorsally to form a kink. The cerebellar vermis (*V*) is indented by the posterior lip of the foramen magnum. The fourth ventricle (*4*) is elongated, and the midbrain (*m*) is beaked. The pons (*P*) is demonstrated also. (From Naidich TP, McLone DG, Fulling KH. The Chiari II malformation: part IV. The hind-brain deformity. *Neuroradiology* 1983;25:179–197. With permission.)

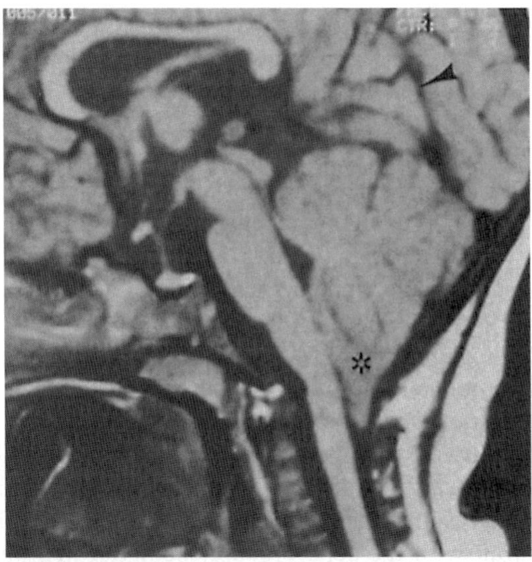

FIGURE 5.3. Chiari type II malformation. Magnetic resonance imaging study. The fourth ventricle and aqueduct are stretched only slightly. Cerebellar heterotopia includes both the inferior vermis and tonsil (*asterisk*). The tentorial opening is wide, and vertical orientation is seen at line of attachment along the straight sinus (*black arrowhead*). (Courtesy of Dr. Taher El Gammal, Department of Radiology, Medical College of Georgia, Augusta, GA, and the American Society of Neuroradiology.)

Deformities of the lower extremities are common and are of two types. In the first type, the various clubfoot and rocker-bottom foot deformities result from the unopposed action of the intrinsic foot muscles or the muscles at the ankle joint. In the second type, the deformities are positional; they result from intrauterine pressure on the paralytic limbs.

Other anomalies accompany myelodysplasia with a greater-than-normal incidence. These include intestinal malformations (e.g., duodenal atresia, pyloric stenosis, anal stenosis), renal anomalies, notably renal agenesis, urogenital defects, cardiac malformations, and tracheoesophageal fistulas.

Spina Bifida Occulta. In spina bifida occulta, no herniation of the meninges is present and the skin of the back is completely epithelialized, although always showing some abnormality such as a nevus, dermal sinus, and dimple (35%), an underlying lipoma (29%), or a hirsute area (372). Radiography reveals a variety of deformities, the most common of which are widening of the spinal canal, fusion of the vertebral bodies, fused and malformed laminae, spina bifida, and, sometimes, a midline bone mass within the spinal canal. These skin and bone abnormalities are indications that the cord and nerve roots are malformed also. There may be a localized doubling of the cord (diplomyelia), a sagittal splitting of the cord (diastematomyelia), absent or adherent nerve roots, or an intradural lipoma attached to the cord. Abnormalities of the filum terminale, notably a shortening, which gives the appearance of a lengthening of the cord but actually results from a failure of the cord to dedifferentiate during early embryonic life, were seen in 24% of patients in Anderson's series (383). Duplication of the spinal cord or portions of it, such as the central canal, is associated, as discussed in the Families of Developmental Genes of the Central Nervous System section, with upregulation of an early ventralizing influence of a gene such as *Sonic hedgehog*.

These lesions must be recognized because they can cause progressive loss of neural functioning during the childhood growth spurt. In many cases, operative intervention to free the cord or nerves is indicated to prevent further damage or prophylactically to avoid such damage. One distinction of occult dysraphism is that it never seems to be accompanied by a Chiari II malformation. However, its genetic origins in familial cases are the same as those of spina bifida cystica, so that both types of spina bifida can occur in the same family. The chances that parents of a child with spina bifida occulta could have another offspring with spina bifida cystica are the same as when the proband has spina bifida cystica (385).

Cranium Bifidum. Several types of simple midline or paired paramedian skull defects are grouped under the term *cranium bifidum occultum*. These include the persistence of wide fontanelles and parietal foramina (386). Persistently large foramina are seen in families, and the condition is sometimes transmitted as an autosomal dominant trait with the gene probably being located on the short arm of chromosome 11 (387). The condition has been termed Caitlin marks, named after the family in which it was described. Excessively large anterior and posterior fontanelles as hypomineralization of the cranium also occurs in hypophosphatasia; serum calcium and phosphate should be measures in such patients. Parietal foramina are generally asymptomatic, although they have been reported to be accompanied by a seizure disorder. The radiographic changes in the various congenital anomalies of the skull are reviewed by Kaplan and colleagues (388). Persistence of the fontanelle is sometimes accompanied by cleidocranial dysostosis, Marden-Walker syndrome, Schinzel-Giedion syndrome, and several other malformation syndromes (389).

Cranium bifidum (cephalocele, encephalocele) is a much more serious condition. Like anencephaly, it has been postulated to represent a defect in the closure of the anterior neuropore. Hoving and coworkers, however, proposed that the underlying defect is a disturbance in the separation of neural and surface ectoderm (390). Marín-Padilla suggested that it results from a deficiency in local growth of the basicranium, with the timing of the insult and the amount of damage to mesodermal cells determining whether the result is anencephaly, Chiari II malformation, or cranium bifidum (369).

The incidence of cranium bifidum is approximately 1/10 that of spina bifida cystica. In the Western world, approximately 85% of these lesions are dorsal defects involving the occipital bone. Parietal, frontal, or nasal encephaloceles are far less common. In Asia, the majority of encephaloceles are anterior and involve the frontal, nasal, and orbital bones (373,391,392). The lesions of cranium bifidum, regardless of whether they are a meningocele or contain neural tissue, and consequently are an encephalomeningocele, are usually classified together as encephaloceles. As with myelomeningoceles, the sac can be covered by partially transparent abnormal meninges, but in most lesions, the herniation is fully epithelialized with either dysplastic or normal skin. Cutaneous abnormalities are frequent and consist of port wine stains, abnormal patterning of scalp hair, a hairy nevus over the posterior lumbosacral region, and, occasionally, excessive amounts of subcutaneous lipomatous tissue.

In the series of Simpson and coworkers, 34% of occipital meningoencephaloceles contained only cerebral tissue, 21% had cerebral and cerebellar tissue, and 37% had nodules of glial cells and dysplastic neural tissue (393). In 5% the sac contained cerebellar tissue only. Some of these infants would represent the Chiari III malformation. MRI is invaluable in determining the contents of the encephalocele (341).

Lorber and Schofield reported 147 cases of posteriorly located encephaloceles (392). Of this group, one-fifth were cranial meningoceles and the remainder were encephalomeningoceles. Of those patients who survived into childhood, 25% of those who harbored a meningocele and 75% of those with an encephalomeningocele exhibited mental retardation. All patients with microcephaly had neural tissue within the sac, and all exhibited mental retardation. The presence of neural tissue in the sac usually was associated with malformations of the hindbrain or, less often, with holoprosencephaly or agenesis of the corpus callosum (394). In the series of Lorber and Schofield, 16% of patients with encephaloceles had other anomalies, including myelomeningocele, cleft palate, congenital malformations of the heart, and Klippel-Feil syndrome (392). Hydrocephalus was present in more than 59% of patients and was more common in those with encephalomeningoceles. In a small proportion of patients with encephaloceles, the condition is part of a known syndrome. These were listed by Cohen and Lemire (395). Meckel-Grüber syndrome is probably the most common of these. It is an autosomal recessive condition with its gene mapped to chromosome 17q21–q24. It is characterized by an occipital encephalocele, holoprosencephaly, the Dandy-Walker syndrome, orofacial clefts, microphthalmia, polydactyly, polycystic kidneys, and cardiac anomalies (396).

In Western countries, only a small fraction of encephaloceles are located anteriorly. Most of these patients are otherwise completely healthy neurologically, and hydrocephalus is rare. The only associated CNS malformations are agenesis or lipomas of the corpus callosum (397). Midline frontal encephaloceles may be due to defective migration of the vertical sheet of prosencephalic neural crest (300). Anterior encephaloceles located at the cranial base often cause no external physical abnormalities, or they might be accompanied by such midline defects as hypertelorism, cleft lip, and cleft palate. An encephalocele presenting a mass that obstructs the nares can be mistaken for a nasal polyp. Its removal can result in a persistent CSF leak and meningitis.

On examination, the encephalocele is usually fully epithelialized, although the skin can be dysplastic. Its size ranges from the insignificant to a sac that can rival the calvarium in size. Pedunculate lesions are less likely to contain neural tissue than sessile lesions. Transillumination can provide an indication of neural tissue in the sac; however, neuroimaging studies are definitive and detect associated CNS abnormalities.

Meningocele. A meningocele, by definition, represents the herniation of only the meninges through the defective posterior arches; the sac does not contain neural elements. Meningoceles account for less than 5% of patients with spina bifida cystica (398). *Meningomyelocele* must be differentiated from meningocele because the prognoses are vastly different. The meningomyelocele sac contains, in addition to cutaneous and subcutaneous tissues, meninges, fragments of bone, cartilage, and fibrous tissue, and neural elements. The neural tissue includes nerve roots and sometimes dysplastic spinal cord fragments and poorly differentiated neuroepithelium. An infant with a meningocele has little or no associated CNS malformation, rarely develops hydrocephalus, and usually has a normal neurologic examination. The anatomic distribution of meningoceles is the same as for myelomeningoceles. In general, meningoceles are fully epithelialized and tend to be more pedunculated than sessile lesions. Occasionally, a myelomeningocele is differentiated from a meningocele only at the time of operative repair. Some meningoceles contain a significant component of adipose tissue and are designated lipomeningoceles. These have a poorer long-term prognosis because the lipomatous portion often envelops nerve roots of the cauda equina and is not easily dissected from the roots at the time of surgery without sacrificing roots and creating a major neurologic deficit in the lower limbs and some visceral organs such as the urinary bladder.

Clinical Manifestations

Meningomyelocele (Spina Bifida Cystica). At birth, spina bifida cystica can assume a variety of appearances. These range from complete exposure of neural tissue to a partially epithelialized membrane. Most often, a saclike structure is located at any point along the spinal column. Usually, the sac is covered by a thin membrane that is prone to tears, through which the CSF leaks. Of defects, 95% are myelomeningoceles and produce neurologic dysfunction corresponding to their anatomic level (399).

The lumbosacral region is the site of 80% of meningomyeloceles (see Table 5.11). These produce a variety of conus, epiconus, and cauda equina syndromes (Table 5.13). When the lesion is below L2, the cauda equina bears the brunt of the damage. Children exhibit varying degrees of flaccid, areflexic paraparesis and sensory deficits distal from the dermatome of L3 or L4. The sphincter and detrusor functions of the bladder are compromised and dribbling incontinence occurs. An absent or unilateral anal skin reflex and poor tone of the rectal sphincter are often apparent and can result in rectal prolapse. If the lesion is located at the thoracolumbar level or higher, the anal tone is often normal and the bladder is hypertonic. Lesions below S3 cause no motor impairment but can result in bladder and anal sphincter paralysis and saddle anesthesia involving the dermatomes of S3 through S5. Electromyographic studies and nerve conduction velocities obtained in the lower extremities of affected newborns suggest that the paralysis is the outcome of a combined upper and lower motor neuron lesion (400). Upper motor neuron lesions that result from involvement of the corticospinal tracts, however, usually are obscured by the more severe involvement of the nerve roots, cauda equina, and ventral horn cells.

TABLE 5.13 Neurologic Syndromes with Myelomeningoceles

Lesion Level	Spinal-Related Disability
Above L3	Complete paraplegia and dermatomal para-anesthesia Bladder and rectal incontinence Nonambulatory
L4 and below	Same as for above L3 except preservation of hip flexors, hip adductors, knee extensors Ambulatory with aids, bracing, orthopedic surgery
S1 and below	Same as for L4 and below except preservation of feet dorsiflexors and partial preservation of hip extensors and knee flexors Ambulatory with minimal aids
S3 and below	Normal lower extremity motor function Saddle anesthesia Variable bladder–rectal incontinence

Cauda equina lesions produce muscular denervation *in utero*, resulting in joint deformities of the lower limbs. These are most commonly flexion or extension contractures, valgus or varus contractures, hip dislocations, and lumbosacral scoliosis. The expression of the contracture depends on the extent and severity of dermatome involvement.

Hydrocephalus associated with type II Chiari malformation complicates more than 90% of lumbosacral myelomeningoceles (401). It is manifest at birth in 50% to 75% of cases. In approximately 25% of infants with this condition, the head circumference is below the fifth percentile (373). In these infants and in the group whose head circumference is normal at birth, the ventricles are dilated at birth. This finding suggests that hydrocephalus almost always precedes operative closure of the myelomeningocele sac (402). Hammock and coworkers proposed that some of the infants with large ventricles but normal head circumference have normal-pressure hydrocephalus, and that these patients, like adults with this syndrome, might benefit from shunting procedures (403).

Clinical signs of progressive hydrocephalus accompanying a myelomeningocele include an abnormal increase in head circumference, full fontanelle, spreading of sutures, hyper-resonant calvarial percussion note, dilated scalp veins, deviation of the eyes below the horizontal (*setting sun sign*), strabismus, and irritability. MRI studies have become the definitive diagnostic procedure for the evaluation of spina bifida cystica and the various other dysraphic conditions (381). They reveal the downward displacement of the stretched brainstem, with a kink between the medulla and the cervical spinal cord, and herniation of the cerebellar vermis. These findings are best seen on sagittal views. As a consequence of these malformations, CSF circulation is blocked at the level of the foramen magnum. Additionally, a significant incidence of hydromyelia of the cervical or thoracic spinal cord occurs (404). MRI and cine-MRI also can be used to display the patency of the aqueduct (405). Using MRI, El Gammal and coworkers found aqueductal stenosis in 40% of patients with myelomeningocele (404).

Other cerebral anomalies also have been described (366). These include microgyria and other types of cortical dysgenesis. These are frequently visualized by MRI studies but may be difficult to see if a deficit in cortical lamination is at the microscopic level, below the limit of resolution of imaging.

In the first few weeks or months of life, a small percentage of infants develop lower cranial nerve palsies and impaired brainstem function. This dysfunction is characterized by vocal cord paralysis with inspiratory stridor, retrocollis, apneic episodes, difficulty with feeding, and inability to handle secretions (406,407). Additionally, progressive spasticity of the upper extremities can develop (406). The reason for this progressive neurologic deficit is unclear. It might relate to compression of the cranial nerves and brainstem in the shallow posterior fossa. Downward pressure from inadequately controlled hydrocephalus has been suggested as an explanation for infants whose symptoms resolve with surgery. In others, brainstem hemorrhage, brainstem ischemia, or an underlying neuronal agenesis is present (406,408). Anterior sacral meningoceles are characterized by unremitting and unexplained constipation and a smooth pelvic mass. Their presence can be diagnosed by MRI studies.

Radiography of the spine reveals the extent of the nonfused vertebrae. The relationship between the cord segment and the vertebral bodies is abnormal. Although at birth the terminal segments of the normal cord lie between the vertebral bodies of T11 and L1, in infants with myelomeningocele the cord can extend as far down as L5 or even lower. The position of the spinal cord segments remains normal in the lower cervical and upper thoracic levels (409).

A dysraphic lesion that straddles the categories of occult and cystic spina bifida is the *subcutaneous lipoma* extending intradurally through a posterior vertebral arch defect to end within the substance of a low-lying conus medullaris. A more extreme example of this type of lesion is the *lipomeningomyelocele* (Fig. 5.4). This lesion can be included in either the cystic or the occult dysraphic category because a huge mass is evident with some lesions, whereas others are only a minimal deformity of the back. The mass is invariably located in the lumbosacral region. It can be midline or eccentric, is fully epithelialized, and frequently is associated with a cutaneous angioma, a hair patch, one or more dimples, or a sinus tract. In addition to the fatty tissue, the mass can be cystic or occasionally it can contain cartilage. These lesions are usually not associated with the Chiari malformations, hydrocephalus, or other CNS anomalies.

Though some infants with lumbosacral lipoma have no neurologic deficit, it is more common to find the lower lumbar or sacral segments affected, with resultant motor or sensory loss in the feet and bladder and bowel dysfunction. The quantity of subcutaneous lipomatous material varies. It extends through the defective posterior arches to become intimate with the low-lying and tethered conus medullaris. The dura is dysplastic and blends into the fatty tissue or forms cystic cavities filled with CSF.

Surgical intervention is advised at approximately age 3 months, not simply for cosmetic reasons, but, more important, to decompress and untether as far as possible the spinal cord, thus preventing progressive neurologic dysfunction. These patients require full orthopedic and urologic evaluation. A considerable proportion present with urologic symptoms, notably incontinence, soiling, and recurrent urinary tract infections (410).

Occasionally, a *sacrococcygeal teratoma* is mistaken for spina bifida cystica. Sacrococcygeal teratomas are only approximately 1/40 as frequent as spina bifida cystica, with a marked female preponderance. As the name implies, a sacrococcygeal teratoma is located in the sacrococcygeal region, whereas the lesion of spina bifida cystica is above the coccyx. Other than the breakdown of skin owing to tumor necrosis, no cutaneous abnormalities are seen. Deformities of the lower extremities and neurologic deficits are unusual, and radiography of the vertebral column is normal. Calcium deposits within the teratoma are seen in approximately one-third of patients. Imaging studies of the region confirm the diagnosis. A sacrococcygeal teratoma must be surgically removed in the first few days of life because the incidence of malignancy increases from 10% at birth to more than 50% by 2 months of age (411).

Malformations and infections of the genitourinary tract occur in up to 90% of newborns with spina bifida cystica, and renal disease is the most common cause of morbidity and mortality after age 3 years (412). Most commonly, a disturbance in bladder function is evident. One group, representing 33% of patients, shows more or less constant dribbling, and the bladder content is easily expressed manually. Direct cystometry reveals absent detrusor activity (413). In another, larger group of patients,

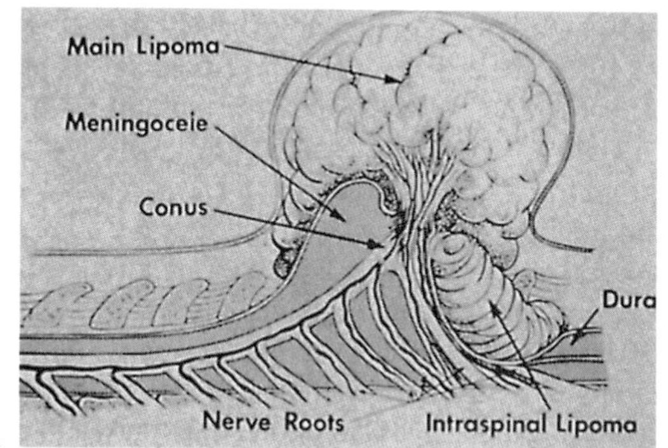

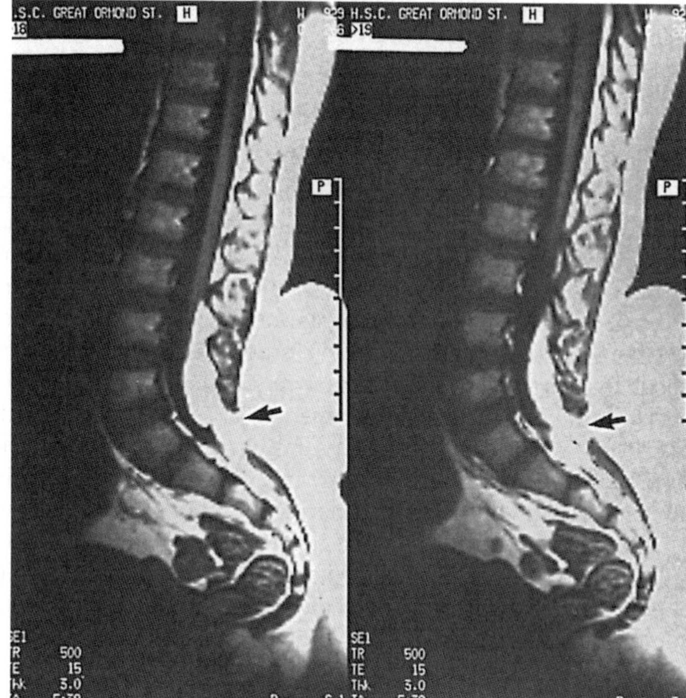

FIGURE 5.4. **A:** Diagrammatic sagittal view of a lumbosacral lipomyelomeningocele. The subcutaneous lipoma extends through the defect in the posterior arches to end in the low-lying conus medullaris. The skin over the lesion is fully epithelialized, and it had been covered by a large tuft of hair. (From Milhorat TH. *Pediatric neurosurgery*. Philadelphia: Davis, 1978. With permission.) **B:** Lipomyelomeningocele. T1-weighted magnetic resonance imaging shows the subcutaneous lipoma extending through the defect in the posterior arches (*arrow*) into the low-lying conus. (Courtesy of Dr. Brian Kendall, Institute of Neurology, London.)

detrusor contractions are weak, but bladder emptying is inefficient, and outlet obstruction at the level of the external sphincter occurs. This obstruction is believed to result from impaired coordination between the detrusor and sphincter functions and reflects a lesion of the spinal cord between the pontine-mesencephalic center regulating the vesicourethral unit and the sacral area. Bladder sensation is intact in some children. This latter type of upper motor neuron defect results in a high incidence of bladder trabeculation, an elevated resting bladder pressure, and dilatation of the upper urinary tract, often reaching enormous proportions (414). Continence appears to depend more on preservation of detrusor activity than of sphincter function. Serial neurologic evaluations indicate that these abnormalities are not static, but tend to change, particularly during the first year of life. Some children with complete or nearly complete denervation of the external sphincter improve, whereas others deteriorate (415). When deterioration occurs in childhood, it most likely occurs in patients with dyssynergia with a small, trabeculated, noncompliant bladder (416). Persistent bacteriuria is seen in 50% of 2-year-old children, with hydronephrosis being found in 25% (417).

The three fundamental urologic problems are infection, incontinence, and retrograde high pressure on the upper urinary tract, producing hydronephrosis and hydroureter. Therefore, early and constant monitoring of the urinary tract with intravenous pyelograms, cultures with colony counts, and voiding cystography is an essential part of any therapeutic program (418). To assess the efficacy of clean intermittent catheterization and to time appropriate surgical intervention for the prevention or arrest of upper urinary tract damage, more complex urodynamic studies are available.

Spina Bifida Occulta. Spina bifida occulta, referring to a simple bony anomaly in which there has not been complete fusion of the laminae in the midline, is extremely common. It is found in 25% of children hospitalized for any reason and in 10% of the general pediatric population. It generally involves the posterior arches of L5 and S1. Although it is usually asymptomatic and is found incidentally on radiographic examination, the skin of the low midback region can manifest a hairy tuft, dimple, dermal sinus, or mass caused by a subcutaneous lipoma or teratoma. In the child who has a neurogenic bladder; foot deformities, particularly a broad, shortened, or elevated arch of the foot; or a variety of neurologic deficits of the lower limbs, spina bifida occulta can suggest an underlying malformation of the spinal cord (383,391). In these patients, neurologic deficits, even in the absence of urinary tract or cutaneous abnormalities, are an indication for neuroimaging studies.

Cranium Bifidum Occultum. The degree of neurologic and developmental damage in this condition depends on the quantity of protruded tissue, the degree of hydrocephalus, and the extent of hindbrain lesions or cerebral hemisphere dysplasias that result from the associated disorder of cellular migration and organization (331,382).

Often, no functional impairment is noted until childhood, by which time mild mental retardation, spastic diplegia, and impaired cognitive function or seizures can be evident. In the newborn, the mass must be distinguished from cephalhematoma, inclusion cysts of the scalp, cystic hygromas, caput succedaneum, and, in the case of anterior defects, nasal polyps. Its location along the midline, with pulsations synchronous with the heart rate, and absence of periosteal new bone formation distinguish cranium bifidum from these other conditions. Skull radiography reveals the bony defect, and neuroimaging studies define the ventricular system and quantity of neural tissue within the sac.

Treatment

Spina Bifida Cystica. The management of spina bifida cystica was given new energy by English orthopedic surgeons in the early 1960s (419,420). Their studies suggested that skin closure within 24 hours of birth reduces mortality and morbidity from meningitis and ventriculitis. They argued that early closure not only prevents local infection and trauma to the exposed neural tissue, but also avoids stretching additional nerve roots, which is likely to occur as the cystic sac expands during the first 24 hours. As a consequence, further deterioration of lower limb function and sphincter control is prevented, and motor power of the legs is maintained (421).

In 1971, Lorber (422) proposed the principle of selective surgery and suggested four adverse criteria: a high level of paraplegia, clinically evident hydrocephalus present at birth, congenital lumbar kyphosis, and other major malformations. Other workers, however, have obtained a relatively good outcome in approximately one-half of infants who would have fared badly according to Lorber criteria (423). A further hindrance to the prediction of the future neurologic status of an infant with myelomeningocele is the subsequent progressive cavitation of the cervical and thoracic spinal cord that produces increasing weakness and spasticity of the upper extremities and causes progressive scoliosis (424).

The questions as to whether and when to operate on neonates with spina bifida cystica have perhaps generated more concern and anxiety than any others in pediatric neurosurgery. Many clinicians have refrained from operating on children who had one or more of Lorber adverse criteria. In a paper published in 1974, these selected infants were found to have a 2-year survival rate of 0% to 4% (425).

The reluctance of many American clinicians to follow Lorber criteria in carefully selecting children to treat surgically has been justified by the observation that two or more of the contraindications to operation are commonly compatible with survival and with a quality of life more acceptable than had been expected. In addition, with modern methods of management the purported selection criteria advocated in the past have been shown to have little prognostic value, and in terms of mortality, the ultimate outcome for patients in unselected series compares favorably with that of patients managed according to selection criteria. The effect of early treatment on disability is far less, however. As a rule, the higher the sensory level, the lower is the survival rate, the lower is the IQ, and the lower is the likelihood of employability (426). For a review of the present position, see the papers by McLone (427) and Hobbins (428). A survey published in 1990 found that in an unselected adult population of myelomeningocele patients, some 50% of survivors were ambulatory and 25% were continent. Of the survivors, 50% were able to live without supervision in adapted accommodations and 70% were employable, 25% being able to manage competitive employment (426). McLone concluded that "nearly all children born with a meningomyelocele should have the lesion repaired surgically within 24 hours of birth and should have hydrocephalus treated by shunt diversion . . . and other appropriate management" (429).

Almost all workers agree that when a patient has been selected for surgical treatment, the procedure should be undertaken within 24 hours of birth and no later than 1 week of age. The claim that delivery by cesarean section before the onset of labor results in better motor function requires confirmation (430), as do the benefits of an *in utero* repair of the myelomeningocele (431). Early surgery undoubtedly prevents further loss of functioning neural tissue as a result of trauma and infection. Additionally, prompt closure results in shorter hospitalization, easier care of the infant, and psychological benefit to the family and nursing staff. It is important to emphasize to the family that closing the defect does not reverse the neurologic impairment already present, and that often much additional treatment will be necessary. It is our view that if major malformations of other organ systems are present or if MRI demonstrates major abnormalities of cortical architecture, parents should be advised of these malformations and of the likelihood of a poor intellectual and functional outcome. As a rule, intelligence is related to the thickness of the cortex at the time of shunt insertion and to the sensory level present at birth, with infants who had a lesion in the thoracic region faring worse than those who had a lumbar or sacral lesion (432,433). Children who required a shunt because of hydrocephalus did not perform as well intellectually as those who did not. In particular, those children whose shunt required one or more revisions showed a significant reduction in their cognitive score (433). Bier and colleagues also stressed the importance of socioeconomic factors in the ultimate outcome, particularly in the verbal scores of affected children (433).

If the neonate is to be treated, as is usually the case, the sac is kept clean and moist before surgery by an undercover of gauze sponges wet with a povidone-iodine solution. To prevent colonization of the gastrointestinal tract and to keep the meconium sterile, the infant is not fed. Systemic broad-spectrum antibiotics, especially against *Staphylococcus* and coliform organisms, are started when the infant arrives at the hospital and are continued for several days after closure of the sac. Postoperatively, the infant is kept prone for the first week to diminish the risk of urine or feces contaminating the wound. If fluid is present beneath the skin at the repair site, it can be aspirated and a pressure dressing can be applied. Persistent fluid buildup indicates an accumulation of CSF at this location and requires the insertion of a ventriculoperitoneal shunt, even though the ventricles can still be only mildly dilated. Preventing the accumulation of CSF at the repair site allows the wound to heal completely, and rarely is any additional surgery needed at this site. Bladder emptying is assured either with Credé maneuver or with intermittent catheterization. If Credé maneuver is used, occasionally catheterizing the infant is advisable to confirm that the residuals are low.

In the course of follow-up examinations, the head circumference and the appearance of the fontanelle are monitored, and imaging is used whenever the findings suggest increased intracranial pressure. As judged by imaging studies, more than 90% of infants with spina bifida cystica ultimately develop progressive hydrocephalus. Of these, 80% do so within the first 6 months of life and require a shunting procedure (434,435). Approximately 20% of children with myelomeningocele develop symptoms of hindbrain, cranial nerve, or spinal cord compression (436,437). In the majority of cases, manifestations develop before the age of 3 months (408). If the infant develops progressive lower cranial nerve palsies and brainstem signs, it often becomes necessary to decompress the posterior fossa and upper cervical spine, assuming that the hydrocephalus is under good control (437).

Contracture deformities of the lower limbs require physical therapy, leg braces, and stabilization of dislocated hips. Muscle or tendon transplants and joint arthrodeses might be necessary in the ambulating child. Postoperatively, neuropathic fractures resulting from paralysis and prolonged immobility are common. They are best prevented by early active and passive range-of-motion exercises (438).

Kyphosis is an occasional serious and sometimes life-threatening development as the child assumes the sitting posture. It occurs in the more severe cases of extensive lumbosacral myelomeningocele as a result of the paralysis of trunk muscles and from the bone deformity associated with the primary lesion. The spinal deformity poses a threat to respiratory function, to the health of the skin overlying the repaired lesion, and sometimes to the function of surviving cord and nerves. An early decision with respect to reducing the deformity must be made in these circumstances. The deformity is best reduced by the difficult procedure of excision of the vertebral bodies at the level of the kyphosis. In some severe cases, it is possible to perform bony excision at the time of the primary operation. Not providing such treatment can cause a marked reduction in life expectancy.

Spinal cord tethering, of the type found in spina bifida occulta, is present in a small proportion of patients with myelomeningocele. This tethering occurs in addition to the obvious union of the neural elements with the superficial tissues, which is the essential feature of a myelomeningocele. Thus, diastematomyelia, other forms of tethering, and hydromyelia can be present. These additional lesions can be detected by MRI. In the series of Caldarelli and colleagues, routine MRI screening disclosed cavitation of the spinal cord in 22.5% of spina bifida patients. Approximately one-half of the lesions were clinically asymptomatic (439). Deciding whether and when to intervene surgically when such a lesion is found is difficult and requires considerable neurosurgical judgment.

Disorders of the excretory system are the most common cause of morbidity and mortality in patients who survive longer than 2 years. Fernandez and colleagues outlined five points that are invaluable in the management of the child with neurogenic bladder. These are (a) achieving urinary continence, (b) achieving good bladder emptying, (c) lowering intravesical pressure, (d) preventing urinary tract infections, and (e) treating vesicoureteral reflux (440).

In lumbosacral spina bifida cystica, few children attain urinary continence, although McLone and his group believe that bladder and bowel control can be achieved by school age in almost 90% of surviving children (429). The mechanism for urinary incontinence cannot be predicted by the neurologic examination; instead it requires urodynamic testing, including cystometrography, uroflometry, and electromyography of the urinary sphincter (441). When these studies show the bladder to be atonic but with adequate urethral resistance, treatment is by intermittent catheterization, often in conjunction with cholinergic agents such as bethanechol, which can reduce the residual volume of the bladder. When the bladder is atonic and urethral resistance is inadequate, treatment should be directed to increasing outlet resistance. One way this can be accomplished is by creating an artificial urinary sphincter. Ephedrine, an α-adrenergic agent that acts on the bladder neck, or imipramine can improve continence in the denervated bladder by increasing muscle tone, thereby increasing resistance to bladder outflow. Conversely, this resistance can be diminished by phenoxybenzamine or diazepam.

When incontinence results from a spastic bladder and decreased bladder capacity and urethral resistance is adequate, the high intravesical pressure is managed with anticholinergic drugs. For this purpose, Fernandez and colleagues recommend oxybutynin chloride (0.2 mg/kg per day given in two divided doses), which inhibits the muscarinic action of acetylcholine on smooth muscle (440). Other drugs that have been suggested include propantheline bromide and imipramine hydrochloride. Serial cystometrograms are indicated to monitor drug response. When intermittent catheterization and anticholinergic drugs are insufficient, urinary diversion or bladder augmentation should be considered, with the latter procedure being used more frequently in children (440).

When incontinence is of mixed origin, a combination of medication, intermittent catheterization, and implantation of an artificial urinary sphincter should be tried. In all instances, however, an associated malformation of the urinary tract, such as double ureter or single kidney, must be kept in mind and must be diagnosed to provide comprehensive care.

In the absence of vesicoureteral reflux and in the presence of normal upper tracts, urine cultures taken every 6 months and urograms or imaging studies done every 13 years should suffice. Acute urinary tract infection demands prompt and appropriate antibiotics because infection inevitably leads to persistent vesicoureteral reflux. Such reflux, together with residual urine, produces trigonal hypertrophy and results in retrograde high pressure and eventual hydronephrosis.

Vesicoureteral reflux should be monitored by isotope cystography and requires long-term treatment with low doses of antibiotics such as nitrofurantoin or trimethoprim sulfa. Urinary acidification can be useful in inhibiting calculus formation.

Bowel incontinence owing to a flaccid external sphincter, although not as serious a medical problem as bladder incontinence, poses a much greater social disability. Constipation and impaction of stool are major problems after the first few years of life. Routine enemas or suppositories and biofeedback training have been used with some degree of success, especially when anorectal manometric data demonstrate some rectal sensation and when the patient is able to effect some contraction of skeletal muscle (442,443). Another approach to alleviating the fecal incontinence can be achieved in carefully selected and motivated children who have failed to respond to the other approach and wish to avoid a colostomy. By means of an appendicostomy, a relatively simple operation, the appendix is inserted into the anterior aspect of the cecum, and retrograde colonic enemas can be performed. The slow washing out of the colonic contents by injection of water through the appendicostomy may be needed only every 24 to 48 hours, leaving the child free to take part in normal activities for the remainder of the time. The procedure can be carried out by itself or in combination with surgery for urinary incontinence (444).

The long-term care of the patient with spina bifida cystica requires a multidisciplinary effort. In addition to continuing neurologic and neurosurgical evaluations, the infant also should be seen at regular intervals by orthopedic surgeons, urologists, physiotherapists, and nursing and social services. Details of ongoing care are covered more extensively in a multiauthored book edited by Rekate (445).

Spina Bifida Occulta. The availability of neuroimaging has allowed a more complete diagnosis of occult dysraphism. Diagnosis is particularly important because the lesions are frequently multiple and surgical intervention at more than one level is indicated.

Clear indications for surgery include the finding of progressive neurologic defects, the presence of an associated tumor or a dermal sinus that carries the risk of meningitis or deep abscess, or a history of meningitis. Considerable debate exists about the need to operate when a malformation has been discovered in the absence of a progressive neural loss. It is our opinion that a child with a lower limb malformation (a small and deformed foot is the most common manifestation) or with a skin stigmata should have plain radiography of the entire spine or MRI studies whenever these are available. When vertebral column malformation is disclosed on the radiographic films, follow-up imaging studies are necessary. Should these reveal an abnormal attachment of the cord or nerve roots, operative intervention to remove that attachment is required as a prophylactic measure, even when no history of progressive damage exists.

Meningocele. If the meningocele is fully epithelialized and not draining CSF and if the skin over the sac is not ulcerated, immediate repair is not needed and surgery can be deferred for several months. As is the case with spina bifida cystica, the possibility of an additional dysraphic anomaly such as a tethered cord or diastematomyelia requires complete imaging studies. Lesions that protrude minimally do not necessarily require surgical intervention. Imaging studies of the brain are suggested to assess ventricular size and to detect those few infants who develop hydrocephalus. A small proportion of meningoceles present ventrally as a pelvic mass, or, even more uncommonly, as a posterior mediastinal mass. These lesions are usually not detected in the newborn period.

Cranium Bifidum Cysticum. Cranium bifidum cysticum requires immediate repair if CSF is leaking or if the defect is not covered by skin. If the defect is completely epithelialized, it should be closed before the infant's discharge from the hospital; if the lesion is small and less unsightly, closure can be postponed until later in the first year of life. When the lesion is tender and a source of distress to the infant, early surgical repair is indicated. Posterior encephaloceles are often associated with posterior fossa malformations leading to hydrocephalus. MRI should be done before surgical operation in all cases. Anterior encephaloceles should be repaired by a neurosurgeon working with a cosmetic surgeon.

Prognosis

Follow-up studies have been performed to compare the survival and quality of life among patients treated without surgery, patients who were operated on selectively (i.e., if they lacked the adverse criteria), and patients who received routine early operation (446). Some 45% of infants with myelomeningoceles who are not treated surgically die within the first year of life, most often as a consequence of hydrocephalus or CNS infections (447). Of the survivors, approximately 50% are minimally handicapped (448). The rest are severely handicapped. With operation, approximately 90% survive into their teens, but less than 33% of these are minimally handicapped (449).

Nonselective surgical intervention results in a large number of survivors with major disabilities. By adolescence, 66% of this group are wheelchair dependent because many will have given up assisted walking as they gained weight. Furthermore, 40% have IQs below 80; 66% have no continence of bladder and bowel; 66% have visual defects, including strabismus, corneal scarring, and blindness; 25% have a seizure disorder; and 25% develop precocious puberty. Approximately 90% experience pressure sores, burns, and fractures (450). Incontinence becomes the dominant issue in the surviving adolescent; some undergo urinary diversion and others respond to intermittent catheterization. In most cases, incontinence adversely affects their academic and social life, and more than 90% can be expected to have some degree of personal, social, and economic dependence (451). Long-term studies on patients who had selective surgical intervention have not been completed.

When death occurs after early childhood, it is usually the result of urinary tract infection with sepsis and renal failure. Less often, it is the consequence of increased intracranial pressure resulting from poorly treated or intractable hydrocephalus. In some cases, death is the consequence of pulmonary disease caused by progressive kyphoscoliosis.

Even though surgical and medical advances have improved the prognosis for children with spina bifida cystica, the essence of treatment is prevention of the condition by correction of any maternal nutritional deficiency and prenatal screening programs not only of the high-risk population but also of the general population (452).

Chiari Malformations

The third major expression of dysraphism was first observed by Cleland in 1883 (453), but was more definitively described in Vienna by Chiari in 1891 and 1896 (376,377).[1] Chiari malformations are characterized by cerebellar elongation and protrusion through the foramen magnum into the cervical spinal cord. Primary anomalies of the hindbrain and skeletal structures with consequent mechanical deformities produce four different positions of the cerebellum and brainstem relative to the foramen magnum and upper cervical canal (455) (Figures 5.2 and 5.3).

Pathogenesis

Traditional theories of the pathogenesis of the Chiari malformations have been mechanical in nature, but a molecular genetic mechanism of pathogenesis has recently been proposed (456).

1. The *traction theory* suggests that tethering of the spinal cord pulls the caudal medulla oblongata and posterior cerebellum through the foramen magnum as the spinal column grows faster than the spinal cord (457). This theory has been totally discredited both experimentally in animals and in humans; traction on the lower spinal cord distorts only the most caudal few segments (458).
2. The *pulsion theory* suggests fetal hydrocephalus causes pressure and displacement downward of the brainstem and cerebellum during development (459,460).
3. The *hydrodynamic* or *oligo-CSF* or so-called *unified theory* of Chiari malformations attributes a paucity of sufficient fluid to distend the cerebral vesicles early in cerebral development because the open neural tube allows leakage and prevents the accumulation of fluid within

[1] Although Chiari described this condition with meticulous neuropathologic examinations. Arnold, who later published a single case of a sacral teratoma with a downward herniation of "a ribbon of cerebellum" through the foramen magnum (454), had his name subsequently added ahead of Chiari's by two of Arnold's students in honor of their professor. The former widely used term "Arnold-Chiari malformation" no longer is employed, as a correction of this historical error.

the ventricular system (461). Hydrodynamics may indeed play a minor role, but does not explain the entire malformation or its early pathogenesis.

4. The *crowding theory* asserts that the posterior fossa itself is too small and the confined neural structures within it are forced through the foramen magnum as they grow.

   None of these theories fully accounts for all of the manifestations of Chiari malformations, such as the primary intramedullary dysplasia that usually is found in the brainstem and cerebellum, the accompanying aqueductal stenosis and hydromyelia in many cases, and the inconstant forebrain anomalies in some, such as absence of the corpus callosum. This crowding theory of Marín-Padilla (462) could play a role late in gestation, as the posterior fossa is indeed pathologically reduced in volume, but it cannot explain the pathogenesis of the malformation earlier than 30 weeks, before the cerebellum has grown so that its volume no longer is accommodated in the posterior fossa, and also fails to explain the reason for the small posterior fossa.

5. The *birth trauma theory* is wholly without merit, and cases are well documented, both in the literature and in our neuropathologic experience, of fetuses of less than 20 weeks' gestation with well-formed Chiari malformations (73).

6. The hypothesis that appears to have the greatest consistency with all aspects of Chiari malformations, particularly types II and III, is a *molecular genetic hypothesis* that the malformation is caused by ectopic expression of homeobox genes of rhombomere segmentation. The *HOX* family is implicated in particular because not only do they program segmentation of the hindbrain, but they also are important for the development of the basioccipital, exoccipital, and supraoccipital bones of paraxial mesodermal origin that are hypoplastic in Chiari malformations and result in the abnormally low placement of the torcula and tentorium that causes the posterior fossa to be reduced in volume; *HOX* genes play no role, by contrast, in the development of membranous bones of most of the cranial vault, which are of neural crest origin (456). Experimentally, Chiari II malformations and often meningomyeloceles may be created in fetal rodents by administering a single dose of retinoic acid (vitamin A) to the maternal animal on embryonic day 9.5 (462). Retinoic acid is known to cause ectopic expression of genes of the *Hox* and *Krox* (human *EGR2*) families in mice, resulting in brainstem and cerebellar malformations. The ependyma shows upregulation of vimentin only in the regions of dysgenesis in Chiari malformations, unlike other cerebral malformations and congenital hydrocephalus of other causes; vimentin expression may be upregulated by genetic mutation of *HOX* genes (463).

Types of Chiari Malformations

Type I. In type I malformation, clinically the least severe, the medulla is displaced caudally to the spinal canal and the inferior pole of the cerebellar hemispheres is protruded through the foramen magnum in the form of two parallel, tonguelike processes. This cerebellar displacement can extend as far down as the third cervical vertebra. Though sometimes called a "herniation," this term is incorrect because it implies that it is being squeezed down, which is not the pathogenesis. Malformations at the base of the skull and the upper cervical spine are sometimes present. These include basilar impression, atlas assimilation, atlantoaxial dislocation, asymmetric small foramen magnum, and Klippel-Feil syndrome. Hydromyelia, syringomyelia, syringobulbia, and diastematomyelia are frequently present (464).

The Chiari malformation type I is generally asymptomatic in childhood, becoming clinically apparent only in adolescence or adult life. The ready availability of MRI studies that demonstrate the malformation has led to a more complete understanding of the clinical spectrum of this condition. Symptoms result from direct medullary compression, compromise of the vasculature supplying the medulla, or, less frequently, from hydrocephalus that develops from aqueductal stenosis or obstruction of the fourth ventricle at its outlet foramina or at the foramen magnum. With obstruction at the foramen magnum, torticollis, opisthotonus, and signs of cervical cord compression are evident. Headache, vertigo, laryngeal paralysis, and progressive cerebellar signs can be accompanied by lower cranial nerve deficits that are often asymmetric (465). Other symptoms of this condition include recurrent apneic attacks and pain in the neck and the occipital region that is exacerbated by laughing or straining. In the series of 43 patients reported by Nohria and Oakes, the mean age at presentation was 17.5 years (466). Hydrosyringomyelia was seen in 65% and scoliosis in 30%. Hydrocephalus was only seen in 12%.

Type II. In type II, the most common of the Chiari malformations to be diagnosed in childhood, any combination of features of type I malformation can be associated with noncommunicating hydrocephalus and lumbosacral spina bifida. Additionally, the medulla and cerebellum, together with part or all of the fourth ventricle, are displaced into the spinal canal (325,407). The medulla and pons are ventrally linked and juxtaposed (see Figs. 5.2 and 5.3). The pons and cranial nerves are elongated and the cervical roots are compressed and forced to course upward, rather than downward, to exit through their respective foramina. Cervicothoracic hydromyelia and syringomyelia also can be present, and both the foramina of Luschka and Magendie and the basal cisterns are occluded as a result of impaction of the foramen magnum or atresia of the foramina outlets (467).

These anatomic features can be demonstrated readily by MRI studies. Additionally, one can observe that the posterior fossa is smaller than normal and that the tentorium has a low attachment to the occipital bone (407). In 75% of patients, the underdeveloped tentorium allows inferior displacement of the medial posterior cerebrum (444).

In addition to these gross abnormalities, developmental arrests of the cerebellar and brainstem structures, heterotopia of cerebral gray matter, and polymicrogyria also occur. The cortical defects point to an additional defect in cerebral cellular migration and are not explained by obstructive hydrocephalus alone (366,468).

In more than 90% of patients, type II Chiari malformation is seen in conjunction with spina bifida cystica, hydrocephalus, and any combination of the assorted defects already cited for type I (469). Conversely, all patients with spina bifida cystica and hydrocephalus exhibit the type II defect. The clinical presentation of this condition was first noted in 1941 by Adams and colleagues, who demonstrated the lesion by intraspinal injection of lipiodol (470). In the more recent experience of Vandertop and colleagues, 21% of patients develop signs of Chiari II malformation despite good control of their hydrocephalus (437). Symptoms usually develop in infants. They include swallowing difficulties, seen in 71% of the series of Vandertop and coworkers; stridor, seen in 59%; arm weakness, seen in 53%; apneic spells, seen in 29%; and aspiration, seen in 12%. Surgical decompression and sectioning a tight and dense fibrotic band that is often present at the C1 level produces significant improvement in the majority of infants.

Type III. Type III variant can have any of the features of types I or II. Additionally, the entire cerebellum is herniated through the foramen magnum with a cervical spina bifida cystica. Hydrocephalus is seen regularly and is the result of differing degrees of atresia of the fourth ventricle foramina, aqueductal stenosis, or impaction at the foramen magnum. Rhombencephalosynapsis can rarely be part of type III (471).

Management

The clinical condition and therapeutic regimen for the various Chiari syndromes are described in other sections (see Spina Bifida Cystica, Cranium Bifidum, and Hydrocephalus).

Other Spinal Cord Dysraphic States

The vast majority of other dysraphic states are confined to the spinal cord and its vertebral and cutaneous environment. Like anencephaly and spina bifida, they result from a combination of environmental and genetic components (472). They are of subtle expression and usually are associated with spina bifida occulta along with a tethered cord, a mass lesion, or both (473). A tethered conus medullaris is diagnosed by its position below L2 and by a filum terminale that is wider than 2 mm and is located in the posterior portion of the spinal cord. Tethering results in traction and damage to neural tissue. If a mass lesion is present (e.g., lipoma, syrinx), compression of neural tissue occurs (473).

Neurologic dysfunction can be present already in the neonate with an occult dysraphic lesion. If so, it most frequently involves the lower lumbar and sacral segments and produces motor and sensory loss or sphincter impairment. Musculoskeletal deformities primarily involve the foot, but scoliosis can develop. With somatic growth, the neurologic deficit can worsen or can become apparent if not already present. The progression and development of neurologic symptoms is believed to result from the differential growth between the spinal column and the spinal cord, compression of neural elements, or damage from repeated local trauma (397). Normally, the conus medullaris ascends from the lower lumbar to the upper lumbar level during growth. If tethered by a lipomatous mass, a hypertrophic filum terminale, or a bony spur such as is associated with diastematomyelia, spinal cord ascent is impaired, causing neural damage.

Dysraphisms are often heralded by cutaneous or subcutaneous lesions, such as a hairy tuft, hemangioma, lipoma, sinus, or dimple. We advise imaging studies of the spine and the spinal cord in any neonate with these cutaneous abnormalities. If a patient has neurologic abnormalities and a bony defect in addition to the cutaneous lesions, imaging and surgical exploration are indicated.

In some cases, successful intrauterine surgery of the fetus to repair the meningomyelocele has resulted in dramatic correction of anatomic defects including hydrocephalus and lessening or correction of the Chiari malformation, and this evidence has been cited in support of the hydrodynamic theory of pathogenesis (474,475), but the relief of some anatomic defects to lessen clinical manifestations does not detract from a molecular theory of pathogenesis.

Diplomyelia and Diastematomyelia

Diplomyelia is a complete duplication of a region of spinal cord; *diastematomyelia* is a vertical division of the spinal cord into two separate halves, usually by an abnormal bony, cartilaginous or fibrous septum over several segments. These two conditions are traditionally discussed together, but they actually are quite different with distinct mechanisms of formation, though not all of the details of pathogenesis are known.

Based on neuroimaging, Pang and coworkers used the term *split cord malformation* (SCM) and distinguished two types (476), but both really correspond to diastematomyelia. In the first, each of two hemicords is each contained within its own dural tubes and they are separated by a rigid osseocartilaginous median septum. This condition generally corresponds to diastematomyelia. In the second, the two hemicords are housed in a single dural tube and are separated by a nonrigid fibrous median septum. The state of the dural tube and the nature of the median septum can be demonstrated by imaging studies (476). For this purpose, high-resolution, thin-cut, axial computed tomographic (CT) myelography using bone algorithms is more sensitive than MRI (477).

According to Pang and colleagues, both types of SCM result from adhesions between ectoderm and endoderm, which lead to an accessory neuroenteric canal around which an endomesenchymal tract condenses, which bisects the developing notochord and causes the formation of two hemineural plates (476). A true vertical bisection of the notochord would yield two complete spinal cords, not two hemicords, because two floor plates would be induced, though the resulting two spinal cords may have imperfect architecture (73).

Diplomyelia represents a complete duplication of the spinal cord, usually in the lumbar region, 79% in the series of Pang, in which they mistakenly assumed that diplomyelia was a form of diastematomyelia, and occasionally extending for 10 segments or more (477). Because it is a true duplication, each affected spinal segment has four dorsal roots and four anterior horns. The lesion can be associated with extensive spina bifida cystica or with tumors of the spinal cord or it can occur in the absence of other neurologic lesions (478). Diplomyelia could be caused by upregulation of an early gene, expressed in the primitive streak stage, that could also cause conjoined twinning in animals, such as *Wnt-8c*, or diplomyelia could result from upregulation in the caudal part of the neural tube of a ventralizing gene from the notochord, such as *SHH*, that causes duplication of the neuraxis; defective *SHH* expression conversely causes sacral agenesis with severe dysplasia of the spinal cord in those segments (479).

The term *diastematomyelia* is derived from the Greek *diastema*, meaning cleft. The condition is marked by a cleft in the spinal cord, which becomes divided longitudinally by a septum of bone and cartilage emanating from the posterior vertebral arch and extending anteriorly. Each half of the cord has its own dural covering. The cord or cauda equina becomes impaled by the bony spur, and differential growth between vertebral column and spinal cord results in stretching of the cord above its point of fixation. An alternative, pathogenetic hypothesis postulates that progressive cord or cauda equina damage results from minor trauma and traction at the spur during head and neck flexion in the growing child. In the majority of patients, diastematomyelia is confined to the low thoracolumbar region, usually extending for 1 to 2 segments, rarely for as many as 10 segments (480). Diplomyelia and diastematomyelia no longer should be regarded as variants of the same process because the pathogenesis is different and the neuropathologic lesions are certainly quite different.

Some 80% to 95% of patients with diastematomyelia are female (481). A variety of skin lesions mark the site of the defect. Most commonly [56% of cases in the series of Pang (477)], these are tufts of hair or dimples, but subcutaneous lipomas, vascular malformations, or dermal sinuses also can be present. Additionally, anomalies of the craniobasal bones may occur as well as syringomyelia and hydromyelia (see Fig. 5.1C). A *neurenteric cyst* (a persistent embryonic communication with the gut) can be located in the cleft portions of the spinal cord (482).

Progressive sensorimotor deficits represent the most common clinical manifestation for both diplomyelia and diastematomyelia (477,483). They were seen in 87% of symptomatic children and are commonly asymmetric. Pain was seen in 37% of children. Sensorimotor deficits may take two forms. The first is a predominantly unilateral, nonprogressive hypotonia and weakness. The second syndrome is seen in approximately two-thirds of cases. In this entity, the patient experiences weakness and spasticity of the lower extremities with awkward gait, incontinence of bladder and rectum, and, less commonly, posterior root pain. Symptoms either appear *de novo* or are superimposed on the first syndrome. A combination of upper and lower motor neuron signs in the lower extremities is associated with atrophy of the leg muscles and skeletal deformities of the feet (484). The difference in shape and dimensions of the lower limbs is often quite striking and is believed to result from a combination of prenatal and postnatal asymmetry of growth stimulus secondary to differences in nerve supply. Spinothalamic and posterior column sensory deficits correspond with the level of the lesion. With suspicion aroused by cutaneous anomalies and neurologic dysfunction of the lower limbs and sphincters, diagnosis can best be made by means of MRI of the spinal cord. Because sagittal images may be difficult to interpret in patients with severe scoliosis, coronal images should always be obtained.

Surgery for SCM type I cases (diastematomyelia) has a higher risk of morbidity than is seen for SCM type II cases (diplomyelia), particularly when one hemicord is markedly smaller and, therefore, more delicate (477). Surgical removal of the bony spur allows the cord to become freely movable. Although this does not alter the nonprogressive hypoplastic syndrome, it prevents the onset or arrests and even improves the progressive *de novo* syndrome (482,485). The more recent the neurologic deficit, the more likely it is to be reversible; hence, prophylactic surgery for the infant or young child without neurologic deficit is indicated. Periodic postoperative follow-up is necessary because regrowth of bone spurs has been reported (486).

Syringomyelia and Hydromyelia

Hydromyelia is an enlargement or dilatation of the central canal of the spinal cord. *Syringomyelia* involves extension of an enlarged central canal into the cord parenchyma, usually one or both dorsal horns and dorsal columns. Syringomyelia and hydromyelia are traditionally believed to represent different expressions of the same pathologic process because hydromyelia at times can progress to syringomyelia. However, hydromyelia can occur as a developmental anomaly, associated with Chiari malformations in particular, whereas syringomyelia can be an acquired lesion of the spinal cord secondary to trauma, infarction, or intramedullary tumors. The two terms thus are not synonymous and interchangeable.

As originally defined, syringomyelia is a condition of tubular cavitation within the spinal cord. When the cystic lesion extends into the medulla and pons, the condition is termed *syringobulbia*. When hydromyelia is a developmental defect from early fetal life, the large central canal is fully lined by ependyma, though it overexpresses vimentin (463). By contrast, the hydromyelia that results from acquired injuries postnatally usually leaves a central canal with ependymal discontinuities and large gaps.

When syringomyelia is associated with Chiari type I or II malformation, as it often is, it is accompanied by tonsillar herniation and an apparent occlusion of the outlet foramina of the fourth ventricle. The diameter of the cervical spinal canal is enlarged, and extensive scoliosis or kyphoscoliosis can be present. Some cases of syringomyelia are post-traumatic, a condition more fully covered in Chapter 9 (Fig. 5.5). Others, nearly 20%, are associated with a spinal cord tumor (487). Rarely, spinal cord gray and white matter is disorganized, a microscopic picture analogous to schizencephaly of the cerebral cortex. In the majority of cases, however, the cause of syringomyelia remains essentially unknown despite numerous theories and many clinical and experimental studies intended to explain the condition (488). One theory, as proposed by Oldfield and colleagues, is based on their observations, supported by MRI and cine-MRI, that in patients with syringomyelia associated with the Chiari I malformation the subarachnoid space is partially occluded at the level of the foramen magnum by the displaced brainstem and cerebellar tonsils (489). This displacement impedes the rapid upward and downward movement of CSF during the cardiac cycle and produces a systolic pressure wave in the spinal CSF that forces CSF into the spinal cord through the perivascular and interstitial spaces.

Hydromyelia, a dilated central canal without extension into the spinal cord parenchyma, resembles the healthy fetal condition at midgestation, although often in a more extreme form. At 6 to 12 weeks' gestation, the central canal is a tall, vertical slit extending almost the entire vertical axis of the neural tube. It is initially lined by undifferentiated neuroepithelium with mitotic activity at the surface of the central canal; a pseudostratified columnar ependymal epithelium then develops and stops all mitotic activity, first at the basal plate and later at the alar plate. The slit becomes round in transverse sectional views and progressively narrows as the fetus and infant mature. In early adult life the canal ceases to exist altogether and its site is identified by clusters and rosettes of residual ependymal cells, but the lumen is obliterated. Hydromyelia of the cervical and often of the thoracic and lumbosacral spinal cord usually accompanies Chiari II malformations, and the ependyma lining it overexpresses vimentin as a persistent fetal feature that normally disappears by 34 weeks' gestation. Vimentin expression continues into adult life in patients with Chiari malformations, but does so only in the regions of dysgenesis of the ventricles, not in the normal lateral or third ventricles or in normal segments of the spinal cord (463).

Though sometimes recognized during childhood, syringomyelia usually does not become symptomatic until adult life (489). The vast majority of lesions involve the

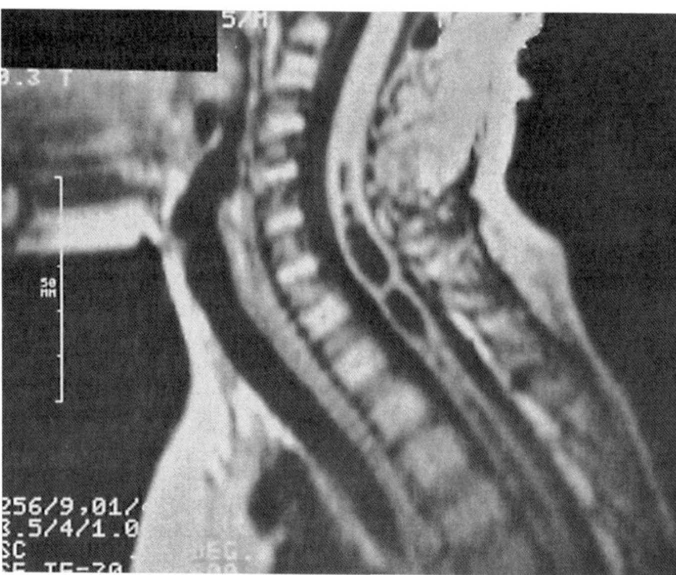

FIGURE 5.5. Cervical syringomyelia. Magnetic resonance imaging study. The syrinx was essentially asymptomatic in this 4-year-old boy. It was discovered when imaging studies were done as part of an evaluation for a hemiplegia, which was found to be caused by a parietal porencephaly.

cervical cord, and, therefore, the upper extremities are preferentially involved. However, a syrinx is sometimes encountered in spinal dysraphism of the lower spine, when it is usually associated with other malformations in this region. Because the cavities tend to be more central than eccentric, they damage fibers crossing through the central white matter of the cord and thus compromise temperature and pain sensation, sparing sensory modalities mediated by the posterior columns. This disassociated anesthesia is responsible for cutaneous trophic, sudomotor, and vasomotor disorders, including painless ulcerations, coldness, cyanosis, and hyperhidrosis. It also causes the painless arthropathies, the Charcot joints similar to those seen in tabes dorsalis, but involving joints of the upper rather than the lower extremities.

As the syrinx enlarges, involvement of anterior horn cells, pyramidal tracts, and posterior columns in the cervical region leads to segmental asymmetric lower motor neuron signs in the upper and lower extremities. Spasticity, hyper-reflexia, and loss of position and vibratory sense occur. In children, the first sign can be a rapidly progressive scoliosis (490). In syringobulbia, asymmetric lower cranial nerve palsies occur, and the condition is almost always associated with anomalies of the craniobasal bones. Brainstem tumors are occasionally present. Syrinxes in the child or adult can impinge on dorsal motor nuclei of the vagus nerve, producing episodic stridor with laryngospasm, or they can compromise the nucleus ambiguous, causing chronic stridor and vocal cord paralysis (491).

Diagnosis is best made by MRI studies. Sagittal views provide excellent visualization of the cystic cavity and of the anatomy at the level of the foramen magnum. Gadolinium enhancement can be used to verify the presence of an adjoining tumor (492). Considerable dispute exists about the best means of managing the lesion (487,493). Posterior fossa and upper cervical decompression is the recommended treatment for the most common form of syringomyelia seen in the pediatric population (i.e., that associated with Chiari type II malformation and downward displacement of the cerebellar tonsils and outlet obstruction of the fourth ventricle) (487,494). In patients in whom such decompression fails to stabilize the neurologic deterioration and in whom persistence of a dilated cyst can be demonstrated, shunting of the CSF from the cystic cavity into the neighboring subarachnoid space is recommended (487,492). The value of occluding the opening from the fourth ventricle into the syringomyelic cavity has come under question, but is still recommended when syringomyelia is associated with the Dandy-Walker syndrome (487,495,496). Follow-up examinations by MRI are required.

Sacral Agenesis

Sacral agenesis is marked by total absence of the coccyx and the lower two or three sacral vertebrae and hypoplasia of the vertebrae just above the aplastic segments. An associated anomalous development of the lumbosacral cord and other major or minor dysraphisms occur. Lipoma of the conus medullaris and filum terminale often accompany the defect (497). Sacral agenesis is associated in animals and humans with underexpression of *Sonic hedgehog* at the caudal end of the neural tube. The same molecular defect when expressed only at the rostral end of the neural tube is associated with holoprosencephaly. The gene for sacral agenesis has been mapped to chromosome 7q36, the same region that contains a gene for holoprosencephaly (498). Sacral agenesis, therefore, represents a genetic disorder of neural induction and of failure in induction of the sclerotome in the ventral half of the paired somites. In severe cases, the entire somite may fail to develop at the sacral and lumbar levels, hence the myotome is affected as well and fails to generate myocytes, resulting in segmental amyoplasia. Sensory innervation from the dorsal horns and dorsal roots remains well preserved, by contrast, and autonomic neural structure and function are variably involved (499).

Neurologic signs are those of a flaccid neurogenic bladder with dribbling incontinence, motor deficits, to a lesser extent sensory deficits of the lower extremities, lower extremity muscle hypoplasia, and skeletal arthrogryposis (499). Recurrent urinary tract infection and hydronephrosis, aggravated by delay in diagnosing the primary process, are major sources of morbidity (500). The defect has been associated with imperforate anus, malrotation of the bowel, and genital anomalies. All malformations can be dated to the first 7 weeks of gestation (501). Sacral agenesis is seen in approximately 1% of offspring of diabetic mothers, and Passarge and Lenz postulated that insulin interferes with the differentiation of caudal chordamesoderm (502). The *caudal regression syndrome* refers to severe sacral agenesis associated with *syringomelia* or lack of separation of the two legs, as with manatees or seals.

Neurodermal Sinus

The majority of dermal sinuses (e.g., the pilonidal sinus) do not connect with the CNS and are therefore of limited neurologic importance.

Neurodermal sinuses are relatively frequent among cases of occult spinal dysraphism (383). They represent a communication lined by stratified squamous epithelium between skin and any portion of the neuraxis. Most commonly, the defects are in the lumbosacral region and the occiput, defects in the lumbosacral region occurring approximately nine times as frequently as those in the occiput. These two levels are at the terminal closure sites of the neural tube.

The sinus is often surrounded by a small mound of skin, the dimple, or other cutaneous lesions such as tufts of hair or angiomas. It often overlies a spina bifida occulta. It can expand into an epidermoid or dermoid cyst at its proximal end, causing segmental neurologic deficits, either through mass effect or by traction on the neuraxis. Cerebellar and brainstem signs or, on occasion, hydrocephalus can be produced by a neurodermal sinus in the occipital region. The presence of an open sinus tract can provide a portal of entry for bacterial infections, and a neurodermal sinus is an important cause for recurrent meningitis. In other cases, the dermoid cyst enlarges rapidly through infection of its contents, becoming an intraspinal abscess. When the lesion is in the lumbosacral region, coliform bacteria and staphylococci are the most common invaders; a sinus tract in the occiput is more likely to produce recurrent staphylococcal meningitis. Such defects must be scrupulously sought in any case of CNS infection (503). Any dermal sinus ending that is above the level of the lower sacrum should be traced with neuroimaging studies.

These lesions require surgical exploration and complete excision of the sinus before the development of symptoms. An occipital sinus is treated by primary excision of the entire sinus tract, and of the proximal cyst if it is present. In Matson's experience, surgical results were poorer when performed after the development of infection, with death resulting from chronic meningitis or hydrocephalus (373).

Congenital Scalp Defect

A congenital defect of the scalp, also known as *aplasia cutis congenita*, is a relatively rare anomaly seen in either sex. It can occur in isolation or in combination with a wide variety of other cerebral or extracranial anomalies (504). Rarely, congenital scalp defects are associated with similar cutaneous lesions elsewhere on the body. In 80% of instances the defect is sporadic; in the remainder it is inherited as autosomal dominant or autosomal recessive traits (331). The defect can vary from one that is small to one that includes most of the calvarial surface. Although in two-thirds of cases the underlying skull is intact, other cases involve underlying defects of periosteum, skull, and dura that often close spontaneously during the first few months after birth. The defect is generally at the vertex, although some lesions occur off the midline. The brain is usually normal, but imaging is justified to verify this assumption. Posterior midline scalp defects can be accompanied by mental retardation, congenital deafness, and hypothyroidism, the Johanson-Blizzard syndrome, and are seen in infants with deletion of the short arm of chromosome 4 (505). A small skin defect can be closed, but if it is large, grafting might be required. It is important to keep the lesion clean and moist before surgical repair. A dermoid or epidermoid cyst may occur in the site of the anterior fontanelle as a benign lesion.

Congenital Defects of the Cranial Bones

Congenital defects of the skull bones without loss of overlying skin or underlying dura result from a failure of ossification that usually occurs at the vertex either as enlarged persistent biparietal foramina or as an absence of the sphenoid wing. The latter can result in a pulsating exophthalmos that can damage the globe or optic nerve. In approximately 50% of the cases, this defect is associated with neurofibromatosis. Diagnosis is made by radiography or CT.

DEVELOPMENTAL ANOMALIES OF THE CEREBELLUM

In the Chiari malformation, the cerebellar hemispheres that remain in the posterior fossa are frequently hypoplastic. On microscopic examination, the cerebellum often shows disorganization of the normal lamination with the Purkinje cells being heterotopic or focally absent.

Complete cerebellar aplasia is a rare condition. It is attributed to destruction of the cerebellum rather than representing a true aplasia (506). However, molecular genetic manipulations in mice demonstrate that global cerebellar aplasia results from homozygous deletion of *Wnt-1*, *En-1*, or both genes, and *En-2*–defective expression results in cerebellar hypoplasia (46). In all three of these genetic mutations, agenesis of the mesencephalon and metencephalon (rostral pons) also is present in the mouse. Each of these genes is essential for the development of the midbrain neuromere (r0) and rhombomere 1 (r1). Nearly identical lesions can occur in humans, and it seems likely that an *EN2* mutation accounts for this combination of focal malformations of derivatives of r0 and r1 that cannot be explained as infarction or on any other basis (507).

Cerebellar Hypoplasias

Under *cerebellar hypoplasias* are grouped several entities in which the cerebellum does not achieve its full developmental potential. Cerebellar hypoplasia can be categorized as global or as selective for the vermis or the lateral hemispheres.

Global hypoplasia of the cerebellum can be caused by a variety of endogenous or exogenous factors. It is seen as an autosomal recessive trait, in a variety of chromosomal disorders, and as a result of intrauterine exposure to drugs or irradiation. Patients with the autosomal recessive condition demonstrate a small cerebellum with an atrophic cerebellar cortex. Granule cells are markedly reduced or absent. Purkinje cells can be normal or can demonstrate a variety of abnormalities. Clinically, children present with delayed development, generalized muscular hypotonia, fixation nystagmus, esotropia, and, in the more severe cases, microcephaly and a seizure disorder (508). Ataxia and intention tremor were seen in all older children reported by Sarnat and Alcalá, but the common presentation in infancy was hypotonia and gross motor developmental delay; phasic nystagmus was variably expressed at any age (509). Migratory disorders of the cerebral cortex frequently accompany this condition (510).

Two syndromes of an autosomal recessive form of pontocerebellar hypoplasia have been reported. One type is accompanied by ventral horn cell degeneration similar to that seen in infantile spinal muscular atrophy; the other is marked by progressive microcephaly and extrapyramidal movements appearing during the first year of life (511). However, pontocerebellar hypoplasias may not be simple developmental malformations, but progresssive degenerative diseases beginning in fetal life, and hence combine hypoplasia with atrophy of incompletely developed structures of the brain and involve supratentorial as well as posterior fossa structures.

Aplasia of the Vermis

Selective aplasia of the vermis can be genetic or acquired. Acquired vermal aplasia or hypoplasia results from a variety of teratogens acting on the brain during the seventh to eighth weeks of gestation, a time when the neural folds of the developing cerebellum meet in the midline to enclose the fourth ventricle and form the vermis (512). Hypoplasia of the cerebellar vermis occurs sporadically, as an autosomal dominant trait (513) or as *Joubert syndrome*, an autosomal recessive condition. Since its first description in 1969 by Joubert and coworkers (514), this disorder has been reported from all parts of the world. Patients usually present in infancy with respiratory irregularities, notably hyperpnea alternating with apnea. These were seen in 44% of patients in the series of Kendall and colleagues (515). Abnormal eye movements, notably nystagmus and impaired supranuclear control, were seen in 67%. Reduced visual acuity or retinal dystrophy were seen in 44%. Cyclic conjugate lateral deviation of the eyes accompanied by head turning also has been described (516). Hypotonia and mental retardation are common, as are polycystic kidneys and congenital anomalies of the extremities. Variants of Joubert syndrome also are described; in one form, supratentorial white matter shows delayed myelination as a probable autosomal recessive trait in siblings (517). Hypoplasia of the cerebellar vermis also is well documented in many cases of infantile autism, but the genetics is uncertain (518).

Selective aplasia of the vermis may leave a CSF-filled extension of the subarachnoid space that separates the medial borders of the preserved lateral hemispheres, as in Joubert syndrome or associated with Dandy-Walker malformation, or it may be associated with fusion of the medial wall of the hemispheres and of the dentate nuclei that obliterates this space and also causes the fourth ventricle to be shallow, tall, and distorted. This latter condition is termed *rhombencephalosynapsis* and is most often a cerebellar component of the forebrain malformation septo-optic-pituitary dysplasia, but not of holoprosencephaly (512). The condition occasionally is associated with the Chiari III malformation (471). Children present with cerebellar deficits and mental retardation of variable severity (506,510).

Partial or complete absence of the vermis can be visualized by neuroimaging or on pathologic examination. In some cases the cerebellar folia are normal; in others the hemispheres are hypoplastic with hypomyelination of cerebellar white matter. The brainstem is often hypoplastic with absence of the pyramidal decussations and a variety of abnormalities at the cervicomedullary junction (515). Commonly, an associated atrophy of the cerebral hemispheres occurs. Diagnosis of the condition is best made by MRI. In some cases the secondary enlargement of the cisterna magna bears some resemblance to the Dandy-Walker syndrome (519).

A rare, sporadic malformation in which hypoplasia of the vermis is associated with an occipital encephalocele and ventrolateral dislocation of the hypoplastic cerebellar hemispheres has been termed *inverse cerebellum* or *tectocerebellar dysraphia*. Hydrocephalus, microcephaly, agyria, and dysplasia of the corpus callosum are associated findings (520). The Dandy-Walker syndrome, which, in part, is characterized by complete or partial agenesis of the vermis, is covered in another section of this chapter.

Aplasia of the Cerebellar Hemispheres

Selective agenesis of the cerebellar hemispheres with preservation of the vermis is associated with secondary degeneration of cerebellofugal and cerebellopetal tracts, abnormalities in the basal ganglia, microcephaly, and mental retardation (521). Generalized disorganization of the cerebellar cortex usually is accompanied by such major cerebral malformations as holoprosencephaly. Because migration of the external granular layer of the cerebellum continues into the second year of postnatal life, focal dysplasias of the cerebellum can result from either prenatal or perinatal insults. When the dysplasias are prenatal, they are marked by heterotopia of undifferentiated neuroepithelial cells and hypertrophy and proliferation of the cells of the cerebellar cortex.

The condition known as *cerebellar hypertrophy*, *dysplastic gangliocytoma of the cerebellum*, or *Lhermitte-Duclos syndrome* manifests as a cerebellar tumor. It is covered in Chapter 11, although it is really a malformation and not a true neoplasm.

DEVELOPMENTAL ANOMALIES OF THE BASE OF THE SKULL AND UPPER CERVICAL VERTEBRAE

Platybasia

The terms *platybasia* and *basilar impression* frequently are used interchangeably, but they are not the same. *Platybasia* refers to a condition in which the angle formed by a line connecting the nasion, tuberculum sellae, and anterior margin of the foramen magnum is greater than 143 degrees.[2] The diagnosis of platybasia in young infants should be made cautiously because it also represents a normal transitory developmental stage. Basilar impression, by contrast, refers to a pathologic upward displacement of the occipital bone and cervical spine with protrusion of the odontoid process into the foramen magnum. It is a common complication of conditions in which the bones are vulnerable to deformity or easy fracture, as in osteogenesis imperfecta.

Platybasia also is sometimes applied to a familial disorder characterized by a deformity of the osseous structures at the base of the skull that produces an upward displacement of the floor of the posterior fossa and a narrowing of the foramen magnum. Basilar impression, with which platybasia often is confused, may be transmitted as an autosomal dominant trait with occasional lack of penetrance (522). As a rule, neurologic symptoms do not appear until the second or third decade of life. When they do, they are progressive and are caused by compression of the cervical spinal cord. Commonly, they include progressive spasticity, incoordination, and nystagmus with lower cranial nerve palsies. Platybasia after 2 years of age can be associated with other malformations of the CNS, including the Chiari malformations and aqueductal stenosis.

The diagnosis is suggested by a short neck and a low hairline. It is confirmed by radiography of the skull and upper cervical spine. These reveal an odontoid process that extends above a line drawn from the dorsal lip of the foramen magnum to the dorsal margin of the hard palate.

Treatment is by surgical decompression of the posterior fossa and upper cervical cord (510).

Klippel-Feil Syndrome

Klippel-Feil syndrome, first described in 1912 by Klippel and Feil (523), is characterized by a fusion or reduction in the number of cervical vertebrae. The embryonic defect is a failure of segmentation of the chordamesoderm and its derivative sclerotomes that ultimately go on to form the cervical vertebrae. It is probably a disorder of segmentation of embryonic somitosomes into distinct segmental somites, including the sclerotomes that form the vertebrae. The most likely, though not yet proved, etiology of Klippel-Feil malformation of the cervical spine is defective expression of a *HOX*-family gene that programs segmentation not only of the hindbrain, but also of somites, including sclerotomes that form vertebral bodies. In most cases the syndrome appears sporadically; in isolated families an autosomal dominant transmission has been recorded.

On examination, affected children have a short neck and a low hairline. Passive and active movements of the neck are limited. Neurologic symptoms are variable. Progressive paraplegia owing to compression of the cervical cord can appear early in life. Some children exhibit retardation or show learning deficits. An association with mirror movements has been reported. It could reflect the *soft signs* seen in children with mild intellectual deficits, or result from an inadequate decussation of the pyramidal tracts or dorsal closure of the cord (524). Associated malformations are common and include spina bifida, syringomyelia, and fibrosis of the lateral rectus muscle of the eye (Duane syndrome) (Table 5.14). The constellation of Klippel-Feil syndrome, congenital sensorineural hearing loss, and abducens palsy is known as the Wildervanck syndrome (Table 5.15). Wildervanck syndrome is limited to female patients, suggesting that the condition is lethal in the hemizygous male individual. Klippel-Feil syndrome also can be accompanied by congenital heart disease (538,539).

The diagnosis of Klippel-Feil syndrome rests on radiographic demonstration of fused cervical or cervicothoracic vertebrae, hemivertebrae, or atlanto-occipital fusion. MRI can demonstrate compression of the cervical cord, syringomyelia, and other CNS anomalies.

With clinical evidence for compression of the cervical cord, laminectomy is indicated.

Cleidocranial Dysostosis

Cleidocranial dysostosis is transmitted as an autosomal dominant trait and is characterized by rudimentary clavicles, a broad head, delayed or defective closure of the anterior fontanelle, mental deficiency, and a variety of cerebral malformations (540). Other skeletal malformations are common. These include spina bifida, short and wide fingers, and delayed ossification of the pelvis.

ANTERIOR MIDLINE DEFECTS

Holoprosencephaly

Holoprosencephaly is a disorder of forebrain cleavage of the early prosencephalon to form two distinct telencephalic hemispheres. Six different genes have been identified in various patients with holoprosencephaly, yet all six together represent only about 20% of total cases studied, hence there are likely many more yet to be discovered. Of the six known genes, five follow a ventrodorsal gradient or have a ventralizing effect and one (*ZIC2*) is a dorsalizing gene. A defective expression of the transcription product of the gene *Sonic hedgehog* (*SHH*) has been shown to be the responsible molecular event in some cases, both in

[2] Platybasia is actually more of an anthropological term than a medical one, which anthropologists use, for example, to help distinguish Neanderthals from Cro-Magnons or *Homo sapiens*.

TABLE 5.14 Unusual Congenital Defects of the Cranial Nerves and Related Structures

Condition	Effects	Reference
Marcus Gunn syndrome	Eyelid lifts when jaw is opened and closes when jaw is closed, or vice versa	Falls et al. (525)
Duane syndrome	Fibrosis of one or both laferal rectus muscles results in retraction of the globe on adduction of the eye	Duane (526)
Congenital optic nerve hypoplasia	Congenitally small and atrophic discs; poor vision, diminished pupillary light response; occasionally accompanied by hypopituitarism	Margalith et al. (527), Skarf and Hoyt (528)
Congenital nystagmus	Rapid and fine nystagmus, often pendular; head often turned so that eyes are in the position of least nystagmus, may be dominant or sex-linked recessive trait	
Congenital anomaly of facial nerve	Weakness associated with deformities of ipsilateral ear	Dickinson et al. (529)
Congenital hypoplasia of depressor of anguli oris	Asymmetric face when crying; may have associated congenital heart disease, genitourinary or skeletal anomalies	Nelson and Eng (530)
CHARGE syndrome	Congenital anomaly of facial nerve, arhinencephaly, coupled with coloboma of iris, congenital heart disease, choanal atresia, mental retardation, genital hypoplasia, ear anomalies	Pagon et al. (531)

animal models and in humans (541,542); defective expression of this gene at the caudal end of the neural tube causes sacral agenesis (see later discussion), but both malformations never occur in the same individual. As a consequence of downregulation of *SHH* (human locus 7q36qter), the formation of a median (interhemispheric) fissure and the development of paired telencephalic hemispheres from the prosencephalon fail (543). The defect in cleavage continues to influence the development of other cerebral structures that occur at a later time in ontogenesis. For example, the corpus callosum fails to form and, unlike cases of isolated callosal agenesis, a bundle of Probst composed of misdirected callosal axons within the same hemisphere where they arose also is absent. Various migrational abnormalities occur. As with anencephaly, the dysplasia is time specific and the stimulus is nonspecific. Normally, cleavage of the hemispheres occurs at 33 days' gestation. Thus, of the major induction malformations, holoprosencephaly has the shortest vulnerable period and one of the earliest onsets.

Holoprosencephaly may result from multiple genetic defects. *SHH* expression can be altered in inborn metabolic diseases of cholesterol synthesis, notably in the Smith-Lemli-Opitz syndrome in which the conversion of the cholesterol precursor 7-dehydrocholesterol to cholesterol is defective. In this condition, which is frequently accompanied by holoprosencephaly, the *SHH* protein product undergoes autoproteolysis to form a cholesterol-modified active product (544) (see Chapter 1). Other ventralizing genes identified in human holoprosencephaly include *SIX3* at 2q21 (545), *TGIF* at 18p11.3 (546), *PTCH*, which is an *SHH* receptor, at 9q22.3 (547), and the head inducer *DKK* at 10q11.2 (548). In still other cases of holoprosencephaly, a mutation of the zinc-finger dorsalizing gene *ZIC2* at 13q32 occurs (549). Because this genetic defect is associated with 13q deletions, it may be the cause of holoprosencephaly in infants with 13 trisomy (550).

Holoprosencephaly generally is sporadic. In Japan, the incidence is 0.4% of aborted fetuses and 6 in 10,000 liveborn babies (550). A variety of chromosomal abnormalities are linked with holoprosencephaly. Besides trisomy of chromosome 13, these include a partial deletion of the long arm of chromosome 13, ring chromosome 13, trisomy of chromosome 18, partial deletion of the short arm of chromosome 18, ring chromosome 18, and partial trisomy of chromosome 7 (551,552) (see Chapter 4). The malformation also is associated with such maternal disorders as diabetes mellitus, syphilis, cytomegalic inclusion disease, and toxoplasmosis (553). The risk of recurrence in siblings of affected patients is 6%. If a chromosomal anomaly is identified, the risk for recurrence is 2%, but is higher if mother is older than 35 years of age (554). After chromosomal disorders, maternal diabetes mellitus, including gestational diabetes, is the most common condition associated with holoprosencephaly.

An autosomal dominant form of holoprosencephaly has been well described. The gene for this disorder has been localized to the telomeric region of the long arm of chromosome 7 (7q36.2) and has been shown to be associated with defective expression of *SHH* (542,555). In several reported families with this disorder, penetrance has been 88%, with mental retardation representing a mild expression of the defect (556). In a minority of cases, holoprosencephaly has been transmitted as an autosomal recessive condition, and this trait is described in each of the identified genetic mutations (545–549,557,558).

TABLE 5.15 Common Causes for Profound Hearing Loss in Childhood

Condition	Associated Anomalies	Incidence (% of Total Deaf Children)	Reference
Genetically Determined			
Clinically undifferentiated			
Autosomal recessive	None	25.4	Fraser (532)
Autosomal dominant	None	12.2	
Sex-linked	None	1.7	Parker (533)
Autosomal recessive syndromes			
Pendred syndrome	Sporadic goiter	5.6	
Usher syndrome	Retinitis pigmentosa, impaired vestibular function, ataxia	1.2	Konigsmark (534)
Surdocardiac syndrome	Syncopal attacks, impaired cardiac conduction	0.7	Jervell and Lange-Nielson (535)
Autosomal dominant syndromes			
Waardenburg syndrome	Widely spaced median canthi, flat nasal root, white forelock, heterochromia iridis	<1	Waardenburg (536)
Wildervanck syndrome	Klippel-Feil anomalies, osseous malformations of labyrinth, cleft palate, abducens palsy, female/male ratio 10:1	<1	Wildervanck (537)
Malformations			
Malformations of middle ear	Defective embryogenesis of first and second branchial arches, conductive and sensorineural hearing loss	1.8	
	Ear pits, preaurical tubercle, malformed ears; conductive and sensorineural hearing loss		
Prenatally Acquired			
Rubella	Cataracts, congenital heart disease, microcephaly	8.0	
Syphilis		Rare	
Toxoplasmosis			
Drug ingestion (streptomycin, quinine)			
Perinatally Acquired	Associated cerebral palsy, rarely associated kernicterus	16.0	
Postnatally Acquired			
Head injury	Variable	22.9	
Meningitis	Variable		
"Mild" virus infections	Often unilateral		

Adapted from Fraser GR. The causes of profound deafness in childhood. In: Worstenholme GE, Knight J, eds. *Sensorineural hearing loss. A CIBA Foundation Symposium.* London: Churchill, 1970:5–40. With permission.

Holoprosencephaly has been recognized in various degrees of severity, but these morphologic variants are only degrees of severity and do not refer to the genetic defect because all three anatomic forms have been described in association with each of the six known genetic mutations (559–562). In its most complete expression (alobar holoprosencephaly), the brain is characterized by a single midline ventricular cavity encompassed within an undivided prosencephalic vesicle (Fig. 5.6). The thalamus remains undivided, the inferior frontal and temporal regions are often absent, and the remainder of the isocortex is rudimentary, with only the primary motor and sensory cortex present. The olfactory bulbs and tracts are absent, and indeed the original descriptive name applied to this malformation was *arhinencephaly*, but poorly differentiated primordial olfactory bulbs may be adherent to the entorhinal cortex as seen by careful microscopic examination; hence this may be a problem of growth and migration of the olfactory bulbs rather than total agenesis (298). Many other neuropathologic details are well described in holoprosencephaly (298,563,564). The brainstem and cerebellum are present and fully differentiated. Minor focal dysplasias of the cerebellar cortex may be present, however. Gray matter heterotopia and agenesis of the septum

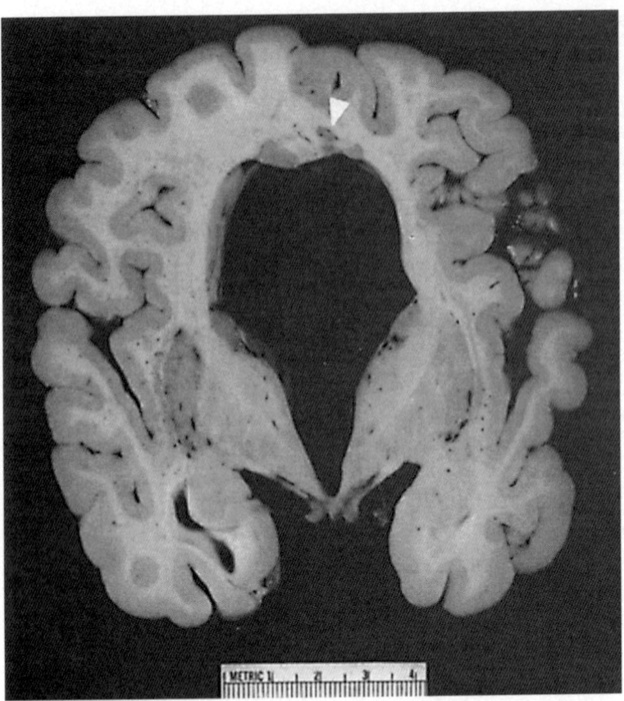

FIGURE 5.6. Holoprosencephaly. In this coronal section, note the common lateral and third ventricles. Midline fusion of the frontal lobes is seen in the absence of the interhemispheric fissure. Note the subependymal heterotopia at the usual location of the corpus callosum (*arrowhead*). These may give rise to seizure foci. (Courtesy of Dr. Hideo H. Itabashi, Department of Pathology, Los Angeles County Harbor Medical Center, Torrance, CA.)

pellucidum result from abnormal cellular migration (565). The lamination and general architecture of the cortex is abnormal, and extensive sites of overmigration occur beyond the limits of the pia mater into the leptomeninges. Some of these overmigrated nodules become isolated from the brain as ectopia and others remain attached to the cerebral surface or connected by a stalk. These nodules are sometimes known by the ignoble term *brain warts*. In holoprosencephaly, absence or severe deficiency occurs of the external granular layer of Brun, a transient layer of glial cells at the cerebral cortical surface during the stage of radial migrations. Its absence could account for the failure to limit overmigration (298).

One of the most important aspects of brain development in holoprosencephaly is the extent of gradients of genetic expression, regardless of which gene is mutated (298). Most genes affecting the embryonic nervous system have a maximal expression in one part of the neural tube and their effects become lessened or disappear in progressively more distal regions. In holoprosencephaly, the most severe defect in the lateral gradient is in the midline, and more-lateral structures of the cerebral cortex are less affected, so that the most lateral regions of frontal, parietal and temporal and occipital lobes may show histologically normally laminated neocortex, whereas severely disorganized cortical architecture is seen in midline and parasagittal sections, and less severely dysplastic cortex is found in intermediate regions (298). The extent of the mediolateral gradient may determine such clinical expression of cerebral cortical function as epilepsy, degree of mental retardation, and various cognitive defects. The rostrocaudal gradient in the longitudinal axis may extend from the telencephalon to involve the diencephalon, with noncleavage of the thalamus, and may extend further into the midbrain, with noncleavage of the superior colliculi and atresia of the cerebral aqueduct. Involvement of the midbrain neuromere also affects the mesencephalic neural crest formation that determines the extent of the midfacial hypoplasia, and this rostrocaudal gradient is unrelated to the severity of malformation of the forebrain; hence a normal face can be seen in alobar holoprosencephaly if the midbrain is normal, and severe midfacial hypoplasia can occur in the mild lobar form if the midbrain is involved (298).

The clinical picture of this condition is highlighted by midline facial abnormalities, which are seen in the large majority of children with alobar holoprosencephaly and in many cases with milder forms of holoprosencephaly. The clinical and imaging classification of holoprosencephaly into alobar, semilobar, and lobar forms reflects the degree of genetic deficiency and how far caudally in the neural tube the underexpression extends rather than fundamental differences in pathogenesis. In alobar holoprosencephaly, the neurologic picture is characterized by severe to profound mental retardation, seizures, rigidity, apnea, and temperature imbalance. Hydrocephalus can develop as a consequence of aqueductal obstruction, and associated hypothalamic or pituitary malformation can induce endocrine disorders; epilepsy is variable and only a minority of infants with holoprosencephaly have seizures in the neonatal period or later, though infantile spasms and other severe forms of epilepsy can occur (561,562).

The anatomic forms of holoprosencephaly can be defined by CT, MRI, and neuropathologic examination. The most extreme form, *alobar holoprosencephaly*, is characterized by a monoventricle continuous with the third ventricle, so that foramina of Monro cannot be recognized. This single midline ventricle is large, and the cerebral cortex and hippocampi are continuous across the frontal midline; none of the horns of the lateral ventricles are differentiated. The third ventricle may be atretic because of nonfusion of the thalamus or many be large and incorporated into the forebrain monoventricle. Hydrocephalus may be present because of aqueductal atresia, especially in cases with midfacial hypoplasia. In alobar holoprosencephaly, there is always a large dorsal cyst. This is a fluid-filled cavity that fills the posterior half of the cranial cavity, so that the holoprosencephalic brain actually only occupies the rostral half of the cranium. At times, the dorsal cyst herniates through the anterior fontanelle to form a special type of encephalocele found only in holoprosencephaly. This cephalocele has ependymal remnants in its wall to indicate that it arose within the ventricular system and is not an arachnoidal cyst. The origin of the dorsal cyst may be the large suprapineal recess of the third ventricle (298). A single midline, meandering anterior cerebral artery is present, but both middle cerebral arteries are present (566). The deep venous system of the brain also is malformed (567).

In semilobar holoprosencephaly, the intermediate degree of severity, an incomplete hemispheric fissure is seen posteriorly, and the occipital lobes and the occipital horns of the lateral ventricles are well differentiated, indicating that the rostrocaudal gradient of genetic expression in the cerebral cortex is less extensive than in the alobar form. In lobar holoprosencephaly, the mildest form, partial fusion of the hemispheres or sometimes only of the hippocampus, occurs frontally, with complete separation occipitally. The olfactory bulbs may be differentiated but are hypoplastic.

The type of midfacial hypoplasia ranges from mild hypotelorism and hypoplasia of the bridge of the nose to the most extreme form, cyclopia with a single median eye and a proboscis above the median eye instead of a nose (559,568,569). The two most frequent severe variants are related to which wave of mesencephalic neural crest tissue has been affected (293,298,300). If the first streams of mesencephalic neural crest are defective, there is a midline cleft of the lip and palate because of agenesis of the premaxilla and vomer bones, and hypotelorism, but both eyes and both nostrils are differentiated. If the second streams of mesencephalic neural crest are preferentially impaired, cebocephaly results. In this case, the premaxilla is present, but there is a single nare in the midline of the nose because the lateral haves of the nose on each side fuse because of lack of development of the medial halves of each heminare. A single central incisor has been observed in approximately 25% of cases of the autosomal dominant form of holoprosencephaly (544), and this finding also indicates a disruption of the second of the three main waves of mesencephalic neural crest migration. The severity of facial anomalies often reflects the severity of the cerebral malformations ("the face predicts the brain") but there are many exceptions, and this often-quoted statement by DeMyer et al. (570) was modified by Sarnat and Flores-Sarnat to "the face predicts the neural crest migration" (298) and reversed by Carstens to indicate the importance of neural tube induction of facial mesoderm: "the brain predicts the face" (294).

In cyclopia, the face is marked by a single median orbital fossa and eye with a protruding, noselike appendage above the orbit. Because the medial side of the globe of the eye is formed from the second mesencephalic neural crest migration and the lateral side by the third, the pathogenesis of the median eye is the same principle as the single nare in cebocephaly. Other dysplastic features include polydactyly and cardiac and digestive tract anomalies. Hypotelorism, a median cleft lip, and a nose that lacks its bridge, columella, or septum almost always denote some degree of holoprosencephaly, even if not associated with any of the aforementioned major anomalies (551,568). The diagnosis of hypotelorism should be based on formal measurements of the interpupillary, interorbital, and intercanthal distances (571). The most severe craniofacial malformations are usually associated with the most severe cerebral form, alobar holoprosencephaly, but this is not always the case, and cyclopia and cebocephaly can be seen in semilobar and even in lobar holoprosencephalies.

The term *arhinencephaly* has been used to describe a variety malformations ranging from isolated absence or hypoplasia of the olfactory bulbs and tracts to the association of this anomaly with the various forms of holoprosencephaly (551,572). Arhinencephaly can be unilateral and associated with hemifacial microsomia and oculoauriculovertebral dysplasia (Goldenhar syndrome) (573). It also can be accompanied by hypogonadotropic hypogonadism (Kallmann syndrome) (574).

Diagnostic studies in holoprosencephaly should include facial radiography to show deformed anterior craniobasal bones, cytogenetics, and MRI for definitive evaluation of the CNS abnormalities. The EEG, visual-evoked potentials, and auditory-evoked potentials are generally abnormal. When the patient has many extracephalic abnormalities, a chromosomal anomaly is likely, whereas in their absence, the karyotype is usually normal. Neuroendocrine studies should be performed to study the function of the hypothalamic–pituitary axis. A simple but often neglected part of the neurologic examination of young infants is a test for olfactory reflexes using a nonirritating substance such as peppermint (not alcohol or ammonia): In most neonates a sucking response is elicited, and in about one-third there is arousal withdrawal; a good and reproducible response indicates that arinencephaly is not present (575).

Septo-Optic-Pituitary Dysplasia

Septo-optic-pituitary dysplasia, first described in 1956 by DeMorsier (576), bears some similarities to holoprosencephaly in being another disorder of midline cleavage and hypoplasia of median diencephalic and telencephalic structures. Some cases are associated with mutations or deletions in the *HESX1* gene (577,578), and in others the *PAX3* gene has been shown to be defective (579). Septo-optic-pituitary dysplasia includes agenesis of the septum pellucidum, hypoplasia of the optic nerves and chiasm with resultant blindness or severe visual impairment, hypoplasia of the infundibulum with growth hormone deficiency and short stature, and, in approximately one-third of children, diabetes insipidus (580,581). Although growth hormone deficiency is the most common isolated posterior pituitary insufficiency in septo-optic-pituitary dysplasia, some patients have panhypopituitarism. Endocrine function, therefore, should be evaluated in all children in whom the diagnosis is confirmed by imaging. Psychomotor function can be preserved (582). Optic nerve hypoplasia can occur in the absence of any other developmental anomaly, and as such it is a relatively common congenital anomaly (583). The condition is reviewed by Zeki and Dutton (584).

The insult responsible for septo-optic-pituitary dysplasia probably begins at approximately 37 days' gestation, though underexpression of an organizer gene would begin even earlier. A variety of causes have been recorded, including maternal diabetes, maternal anticonvulsant intake, and cytomegalic inclusion disease (585). Additionally, optic nerve hypoplasia is seen in conjunction with the Klippel-Trenaunay-Weber syndrome, chondrodysplasia punctata, and Kallmann syndrome (hypogonadotropic hypogonadism) (585,586).

Noncleft Median Face Syndrome

Noncleft median face syndrome includes several syndromes familiar to pediatricians, such as Treacher Collins syndrome, Crouzon disease, and Apert syndrome. It also embraces the chromosomal trisomies 18 and 21. The facial deformities are mild but stereotyped, characterized by mongoloid and antimongoloid slants and abnormally spaced eyes (hypertelorism or hypotelorism). In a significant proportion of cases, pathologic examination or neuroimaging studies of the brain reveal maldevelopment of the neocortex with frequent migration anomalies causing defective cortical lamination, and occasional failure of inductive diverticulation.

DISORDERS OF CELLULAR PROLIFERATION

Rarely, severely hypoplastic brains are found that appear to be developmental arrests at early embryonic or fetal stages. Two examples are illustrated in Fig. 5.7. These maturational arrests appear to be a failure of adequate cellular proliferation in the neural tube, and the etiology is probably multiple. One mechanism may be if the ependyma is induced to differentiate too early, so that all of the mitotic cycles at the ventricular wall are not completed (73,587). Whether accelerated apoptosis may be destroying cells as they are formed at an excessive rate is speculative as another mechanism. Congenital viral infections often produce brains that are excessively small and lack the number of neurons and glial cells expected, but this is often the result of microinfarcts due to endothelial cell and vascular involvement. Vaccines in the first trimester of pregnancy also are implicated in some cases, but this is difficult to prove (588).

DISORDERS OF CELLULAR MIGRATION (1 TO 7 MONTHS' GESTATION)

Although disorders of organ induction are known to produce secondary histogenic migratory anomalies, this section is confined to those disorders of cellular migration that are unassociated with defects of embryogenesis. Over the last few years, MRI has permitted diagnosis of these

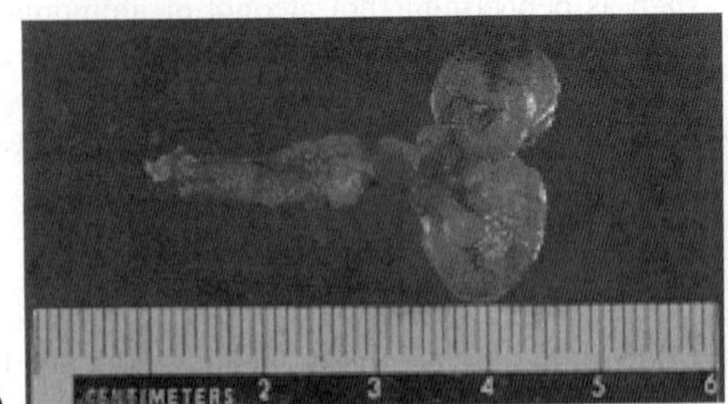

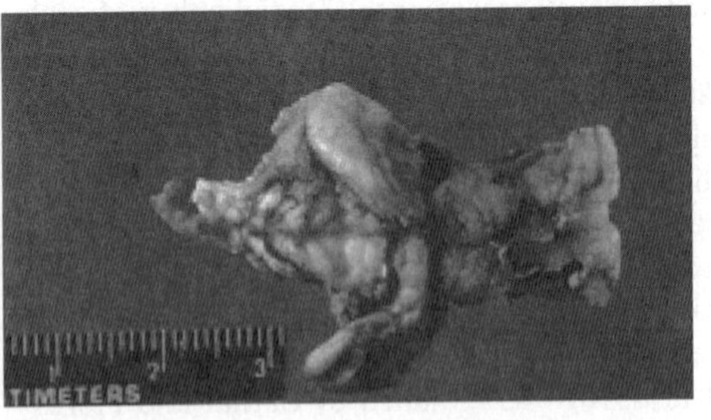

FIGURE 5.7. **A.** Global cerebral hypoplasia in a 21-week fetus, a maturational arrest probably due to deficient neuronogenesis. The cerebral hemispheres, brainstem and cerebellum are all very small and underdeveloped even for this gestational age. The brain weighed 2.3 g (normal mean for age is 58.0 g). (From Sarnat HB. *Cerebral dysgenesis. Embryology and clinical expression*. New York: Oxford University Press, 1992. With permission.) **B.** Dorsal view of brainstem and cerebellum of a full-term neonate, showing an exposed fourth ventricle because the cerebellum is arrested in development while still at the rhombic lip stage or a little beyond. The mother had received a swine influenza vaccine in the first trimester, but whether this was the cause is uncertain. (From Sarnat HB, Rybak G, Kotagal S, et al. Cerebral embryopathy in late first trimester: possible association with swine influenza vaccine. *Teratology* 1979;20:93–100. With permission.)

conditions during the lifetime of the affected child, and it is becoming apparent that their incidence is much greater than had previously been estimated. Sarnat, Barth, and Barkovich and their coworkers have published reviews of these various disorders (73,589,590). Nevertheless, many microdysplasias of the cerebral cortex that are focal migratory disturbances are beneath the limits of resolution of imaging studies and are only seen microscopically. In the past these were poorly understood because autopsy confirmation of the clinical suspicion was rarely available, but it is now with the advent of epilepsy surgery and the availability of surgical brain tissue; these malformations are now being well studied.

The various conditions associated with migration defects are listed in Table 5.16. They include the phakomatoses; a variety of metabolic, genetic, and chromosomal syndromes; and maternal and environmental causes.

Migratory disorders develop when neuroblasts of the subventricular zone (i.e., the germinal matrix), which forms the wall of the lateral ventricles, fail to reach their intended destination in the cerebral cortex. This results in focal or generalized structural deformities of the cerebral hemispheres. These are discussed in sequence of their ontogenetic chronology.

TABLE 5.16 Conditions Associated With Neuroblast Migratory Disorders

Metabolic Diseases
Zellweger disease
Neonatal adrenoleukodystrophy
Glutaric aciduria, type II
Kinky hair disease
G_{M2} gangliosidosis
Chromosomal Anomalies
Trisomy 13
Trisomy 18
Trisomy 21
Deletion 4p
Deletion 17p13 (Miller-Dieker syndrome)
Neuromuscular Disease
Walker-Warburg syndrome
Fukuyama muscular dystrophy
Myotonic dystrophy
Anterior horn arthrogryposis
Neurocutaneous Syndromes
Incontinentia pigmenti
Neurofibromatosis
Hypermelanosis of Ito
Encephalocraniocutanous lipomatosis (590a)
Tuberous sclerosis
Epidermal nevus syndrome (590b)
Multiple Congenital Anomalies Syndromes
Smith-Lemli-Opitz syndrome
Potter syndrome (590c)
Cornelia de Lange syndrome
Meckel-Gruber syndrome
Orofacial-digital syndrome
Coffin-Siris syndrome
Other Syndromes
Thanatophoric dysplasia (590d)
Pachygyria and congenital nephrosis (590e)
Aicardi syndrome
Joubert syndrome
Hemimegalencephaly
Maternal and Environmental Causes
Infection
Cytomegalovirus
Intoxication
Carbon monoxide
Isoretinoic acid (590f)
Fetal alcohol syndrome
Methylmercury
Ionizing radiation

[a]Reference citations are given for syndromes not covered in this text.
Adapted from Barth P. Disorders of neuronal migration. *Can J Neurol Sci* 1987;14:1–16. With permission.

Schizencephaly

Schizencephaly is characterized by clefts placed symmetrically within the cerebral hemispheres and extending from the cortical surface to the underlying ventricular cavity (Figs. 5.8 and 5.9) (73,589–591). The walls of the cleft may be in apposition or separated. The cerebral cortex that surrounds the cleft may be normal or show areas of polymicrogyria. This suggests that in many instances schizencephaly results from pathogenetic processes similar to those that cause polymicrogyria, but are more extensive and involve the entire thickness of the developing cerebral hemispheres (592).

A mutation of the homeobox gene *EMX2* has been identified in schizencephaly (98,593). This mutation does not account for all cases, however, and some are not really primary developmental malformations at all, but occur secondary to porencephaly or other encephaloclastic lesions acquired during midfetal life (73).

Schizencephaly should be distinguished from porencephaly caused by a variety of vascular or infectious insults to the brain during late fetal or early infantile life. A porencephalic cyst results from the dissolution of necrotic regions of brain, with cavitation and cyst formation within the parenchyma of the cerebral hemispheres. Porencephalic cysts communicate with the ventricular system or may extend to the cerebral cortical surface but do not destroy the thin pial membrane. Occasionally, they act as a space-occupying lesion, causing symptoms of increased intracranial pressure (594). Most important, they are asymmetric, not aligned with the primary fissures, and unassociated with major cerebral migration defects.

The clinical picture of schizencephaly is characterized by a wide range of neurologic and developmental defects. Epilepsy may be the most serious complication, and seizures often are the presenting symptom. Hypotonia,

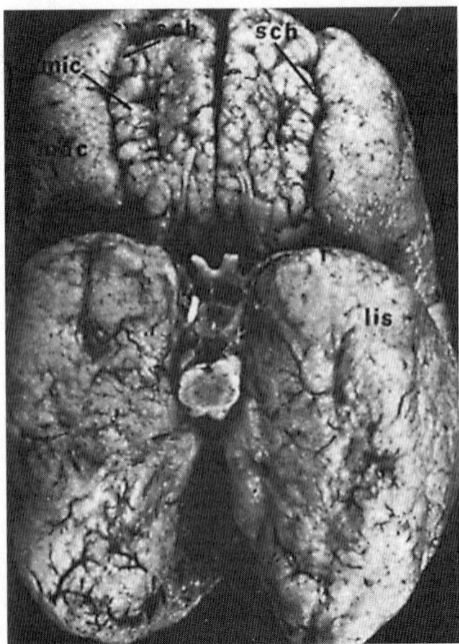

FIGURE 5.8. Schizencephaly (*sch*). Ventral view of the brain in a severely retarded 10-year-old boy. In addition to the symmetric clefts in the orbital walls of the frontal lobes, the brain also shows failure of sulcation (lissencephaly, *lis*) and microgyria (*mic*) of the frontal lobes. (From Yakovlev PI, Wadsworth RC. Schizencephalies. A study of the congenital clefts in the cerebral mantle. *J Neuropathol Exp Neurol* 1946;5:116, 169. With permission.)

hemiparesis, or spastic quadriparesis can be accompanied by a seizure disorder and microcephaly. Imaging studies usually show bilateral, symmetric, or asymmetric clefts (594,595). On clinical grounds porencephaly differs from schizencephaly in that the patient frequently has a well-documented history of a destructive insult to the brain, and neurologic deficits are often focal, asymmetric, or silent and compatible with relatively normal development. Unlike schizencephaly, a porencephalic cyst can occur as a one-way ball valve–type communication with the ventricular system. It can enlarge progressively and behave like an expanding lesion impinging on the ventricular system to produce hydrocephalus (372).

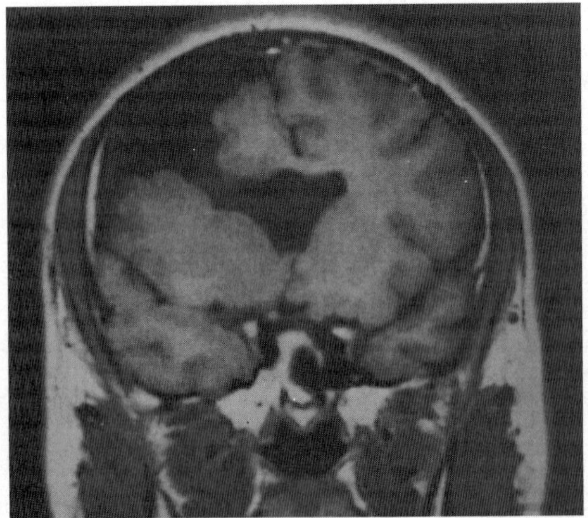

FIGURE 5.9. Schizencephaly. T1-weighted magnetic resonance imaging study of a 17-year-old patient with seizures and mild developmental delay. Coronal images reveal a large unilateral cleft lined with cortex. (Courtesy of Dr. A. J. Barkovich, Department of Radiology, University of California, San Francisco, CA.)

Lissencephaly (Agyria-Pachygyria, Macrogyria)

Lissencephaly, a term coined by Owen in 1868, literally means *smooth brain*. The term is used synonymously with agyria. In pachygyria (macrogyria), the pathology is less

A

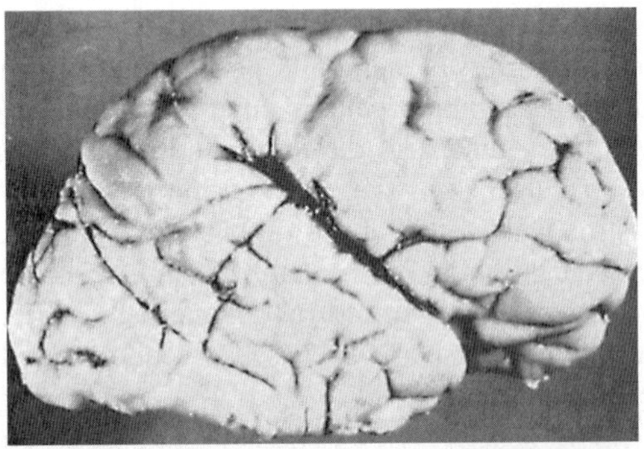

B

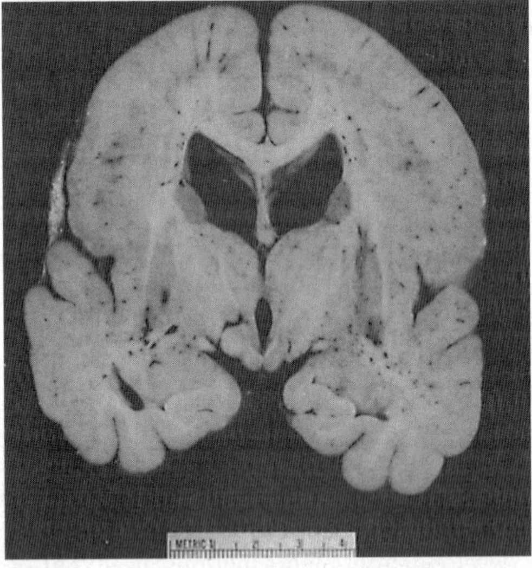

FIGURE 5.10. Lissencephaly (agyria). **A:** External view of the brain. Note the severe degree of diffuse pachygyria with a large area of frontoparietal agyria from a $6\frac{1}{2}$-year-old with marked hypotonia, profound retardation, and minor motor seizures. Microscopic examination of the brain showed an abnormally laminated cortex in the temporoparietal and occipital regions, abnormally formed neurons, almost complete loss of Purkinje cells, and loss of granule cells in cerebellum. (From Druckman R, Chad D, Alvord EC. A case of atonic cerebral diplegia with lissencephaly. *Neurology* 1959;9:806. With permission.) **B:** Coronal section of another brain showing the typical deep cortical mantle and sparse central white matter. The mediotemporal areas show a cortical ribbon of normal appearance. The deep nuclei are grossly intact. (Courtesy Dr. Hideo H. Itabashi, Department of Pathology, Los Angeles County Harbor Medical Center, Torrance, CA.)

severe than that in lissencephaly, and areas of normal laminar organization are seen. Lissencephaly and pachygyria may occur together in the same brain and are not mutually exclusive, but represent degrees of the same fundamental disorder in cell migration and cortical organization.

In lissencephaly the cerebral hemispheres approximate the smooth 20-week fetal cerebral cortex, with absence of secondary sulci. The condition results from a migratory defect believed to occur between 12 and 16 weeks' gestation. The insult, whatever it may have been, prevents succeeding waves of migrating neurons from reaching their destined positions in the cerebral cortex. Thus, gray matter heterotopia, macrogyria, polymicrogyria, and schizencephaly, together with defective cortical lamination, often accompany this condition (Fig. 5.10) (596).

Two major types of lissencephaly have been defined by neuropathologic examination and MRI (73,597,598). In the Miller-Dieker syndrome, classical or type I lissencephaly (Fig. 5.11), a point mutation and microdeletion of the *LIS1* gene occurs at the 17p13.3 locus (598–600). The *LIS1* gene is strongly expressed in Cajal-Retzius neurons and periventricular neuroepithelium and is essential for the normal course of radial migration (601). Cajal-Retzius cells also express the *Reelin* gene, which is essential for cortical laminar architecture (211). Intracellular levels of the *LIS1* protein correlate well with clinical and imaging findings (602). Several genetic defects in lissencephaly

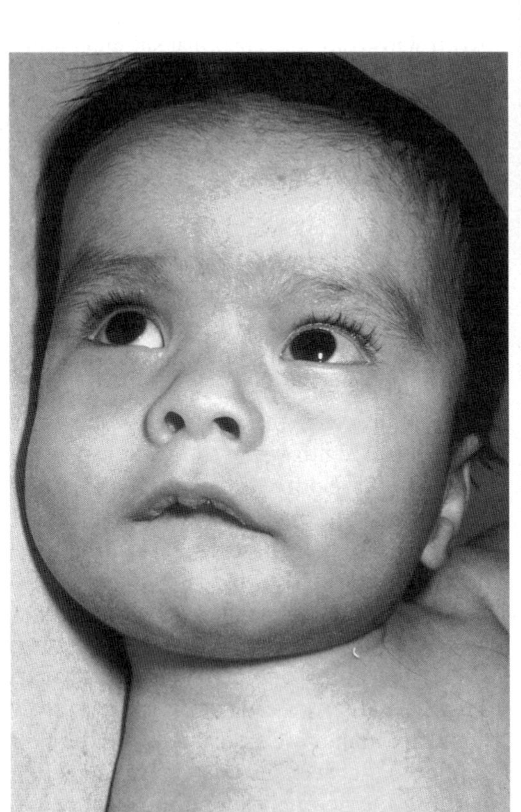

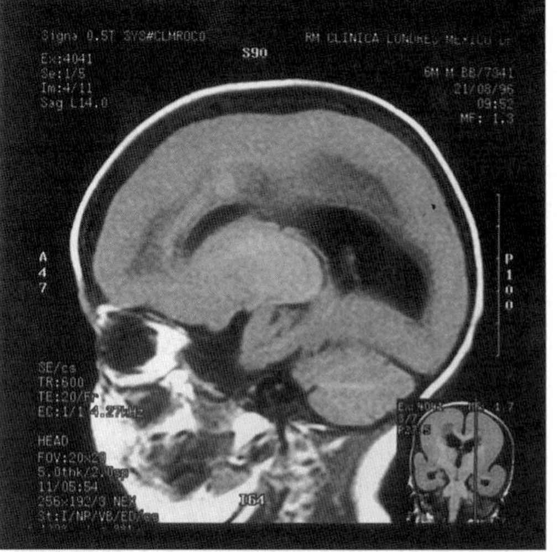

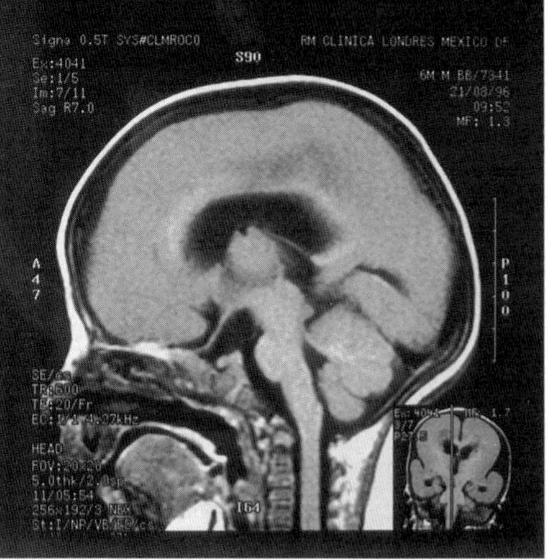

FIGURE 5.11. A 7-month-old boy with Miller-Dieker syndrome. **A:** The face shows characteristic features of a high forehead, long philtrum of the upper lip, and upturned nares. The (**B**) midsagittal and (**C**) parasagittal T1-weighted magnetic resonance imaging shows total lissencephaly with grossly well-formed brainstem and cerebellum. The corpus callosum is thin. Lateral ventricles are mildly dilated, and the subarachnoid spaces over the cerebral hemispheres and brainstem cisternae are wide. (Courtesy of Dr. Laura Flores-Sarnat, Alberta Children's Hospital, Calgary, Canada and Bernardo Boleaga Durán, Clínica Londres, Mexico City.)

type II have been identified recently and include *POMT1* in Walker-Warburg syndrome and *Fukutin* in Fukuyama congenital muscular dystrophy (603,604).

Pathologic examination of the brain in lissencephaly type I reveals that the cortex is four-layered. Layer 1 corresponds to the molecular layer; layer 2 contains neurons of the normal layers III, V, and VI; layer 3 is cell sparse, possibly representing persistence of the fetal subplate zone; and layer 4 is thick and extends almost to the ependyma, from which it is separated by a band of white matter (73,592). This layer contains heterotopic, incompletely migrated neurons (596).

Lissencephaly type II is characterized by an almost complete absence of cortical layering. Cortical neurons are randomly displaced and disoriented, so that pyramidal neurons normally confined to layers 3, 5, and 6 are found throughout the cortex, including its most superficial parts, and their dendritic trunks often are horizonal, rather than perpendicular, to the cortical surface. In other instances the entire neuron may be inverted, and many heterotopic neurons occur in the subcortical white matter (73). Vascular bundles and fibroglia tissue are seen perpendicular to the surface. These penetrate the brain from the thickened meninges and separate the cortex into glomerulus-like nests of neurons. Hydrocephalus often accompanies lissencephaly type II. It results from meningeal thickening that obliterates the subarachnoid space around the brainstem and at the base of the brain (519). The glioneuronal heterotopia extend into the leptomeninges and represent overmigration because of gaps or breaches in the pia mater or in the basal lamina that normally would limit the extent of radial migration. This mechanism has been well demonstrated in the mouse with mutation of the *Fukutin* gene, the gene that is responsible for Fukuyama muscular dystrophy in Japan. This condition is associated with lissencephaly type II and with dysplasias of many other organs; the molecular basis of this genetic mutation, and also of mutations of the *POMT1* gene in Walker-Warburg syndrome, is hypoglycosylation of α-dystroglycan, a membrane component that helps to link the basal lamina to the plasma membrane in both brain and muscle, hence the association with congenital muscular dystrophy (603,604).

Though the lissencephalies were previously considered to be rare, they are now more readily diagnosable with MRI studies (Fig. 5.12). Lissencephaly type I is the most common and accounted for 43% of the lissencephalies in the series of Aicardi; pachygyria was seen in 26% and lissencephaly type II in 14% of all lissencephalies (605). The clinical picture of complete lissencephaly type I is homogeneous. All patients have profound mental retardation, marked hypotonia (hypotonic cerebral palsy), and seizures. These may include massive myoclonus and tonic seizures, which often are preceded by infantile spasms. In 76% of cases, the EEG shows high-amplitude (300 μV) 10- to 16-Hz rhythms (605). Microcephaly was present in approximately one-half of patients in the series of Gastaut and coworkers (606). The high frequency of seizures, particularly infantile spasms, was also noted by Alvarez and his group (607).

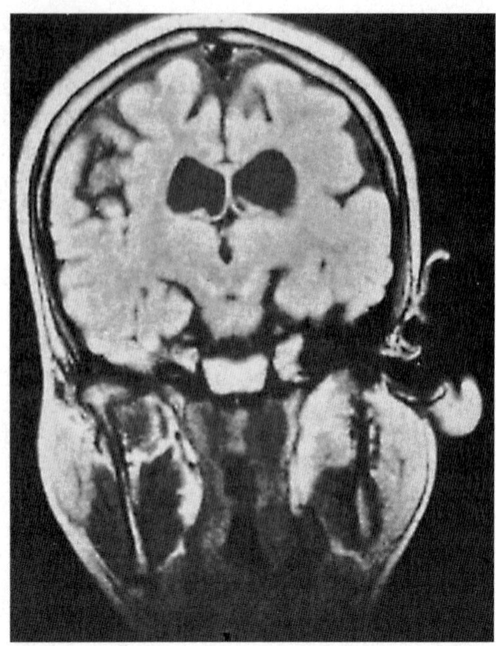

FIGURE 5.12. Pachygyria. T1-weighted magnetic resonance imaging study shows a number of anomalies. These include areas of total absence of gyri (lissencephaly), areas of large, broad gyri (pachygyria), and abnormal sulcation of the right parietal operculum. The left parietal operculum is also abnormal in that the sylvian fissure is enlarged. This 19-year-old man has a long-standing seizure disorder, characterized by generalized tonic-clonic and atonic seizures, partly resistant to anticonvulsant therapy. He is functioning in the borderline range.

In pachygyria, the MRI study shows an abnormally thick cortex, with white matter not penetrating into the convolutions. Both entire hemispheres are involved. Cases described with only one hemisphere being abnormal or restricted to the opercular area (Fig. 5.13) are really hemimegalencephaly (see later in this section). The toxic stimuli that induce macrogyria can occur up to the fifth month of gestation, by which time the primary sulci have already become elaborated. Thus, secondary sulcation is aborted and tertiary sulcation is prevented. Other migrational anomalies are associated, and the clinical picture is similar to that seen in lissencephaly type I, but less severe. Because the anomalies tend to be more asymmetric, the neurologic deficits are often lateralized. Areas of focal cortical dysplasia frequently act as an epileptic focus giving rise to focal clonic seizures or focal myoclonus. These architectonic abnormalities can now be visualized by MRI (Fig. 5.14) (608).

Lissencephaly type II is most often seen in the Walker-Warburg syndrome but also occurs in Fukuyama

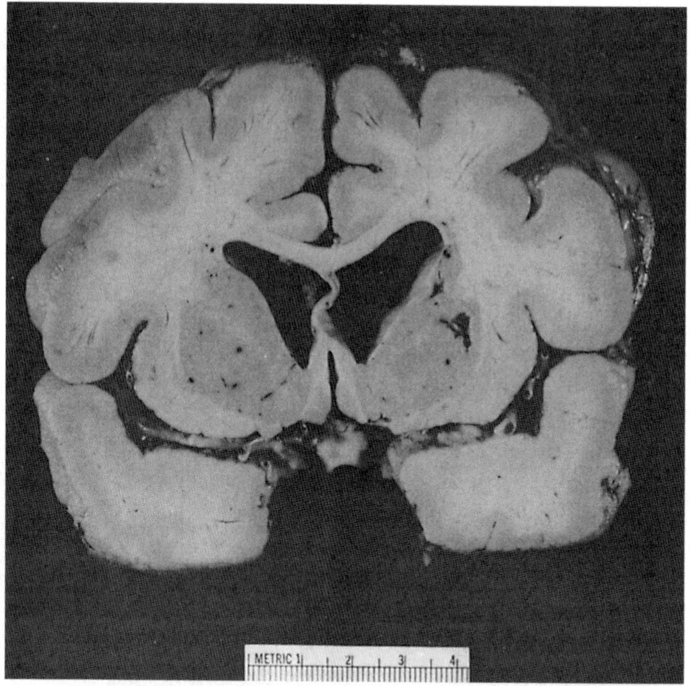

FIGURE 5.13. Pachygyria (macrogyria). This developmental disturbance of the convolutional pattern has thickened and irregular convolutions. Note the scarcity of sulci, especially in the temporal lobes. This patient survived for many years. (Courtesy of Dr. Hideo H. Itabashi, Department of Pathology, Los Angeles County Harbor Medical Center, Torrance, CA.)

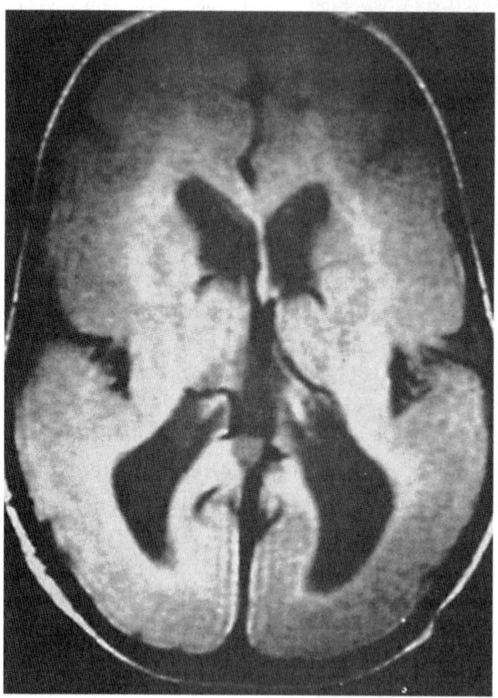

FIGURE 5.14. Pachygyria. T1-weighted magnetic resonance imaging study of a 4-month-old infant presenting with seizures. Axial image demonstrates thickening of gray matter and thinning of white matter in this patient with lissencephaly. Pachygyria is present in the frontal lobes with agyria in the temporoparieto-occipital region. The distribution of the more severely affected regions posteriorly and the less severely affected regions anteriorly suggests a vascular component to this anomaly. (Courtesy of Dr. A. J. Barkovich, Department of Radiology, University of California, San Francisco, CA.)

congenital muscular dystrophy and in muscle-eye-brain disease of Santavuori. Walker-Warburg syndrome is an autosomal recessive disorder characterized by the additional features of hydrocephalus, retinal or other ocular malformations, and the occasional presence of an occipital encephalocele. Most patients with this condition die before 2 years of age. Of the other syndromes associated with lissencephaly type II, muscle-eye-brain disease of Santavuori is mainly found in Finland, and Fukuyama muscular dystrophy is almost exclusively limited to the Japanese population.

Although lissencephaly is seen in the Miller-Dieker syndrome (see Chapter 4), only 5% of infants demonstrated this chromosomal anomaly in Aicardi's series (605). The malformation also can be seen after cytomegalovirus infection and in a variety of other, rarer syndromes. These are listed in Table 5.16 and are reviewed by Dobyns and coworkers (609).

Polymicrogyria

Polymicrogyria results from an insult to the nervous system sustained before the fifth month of gestation. The affected brain resembles a chestnut kernel and is characterized by an excess of secondary and tertiary sulci, resulting in gyri that are too small and too numerous (Fig. 5.15). In addition to the gyral anomalies, polymicrogyria is characterized by other migrational defects, gray matter heterotopia, defective cortical cell polarization, and abnormal cellular lamination. Microscopically, the brain resembles that of a 4- to 6-month-old fetus. Layering abnormalities are generally present and tend to be of two types. In one

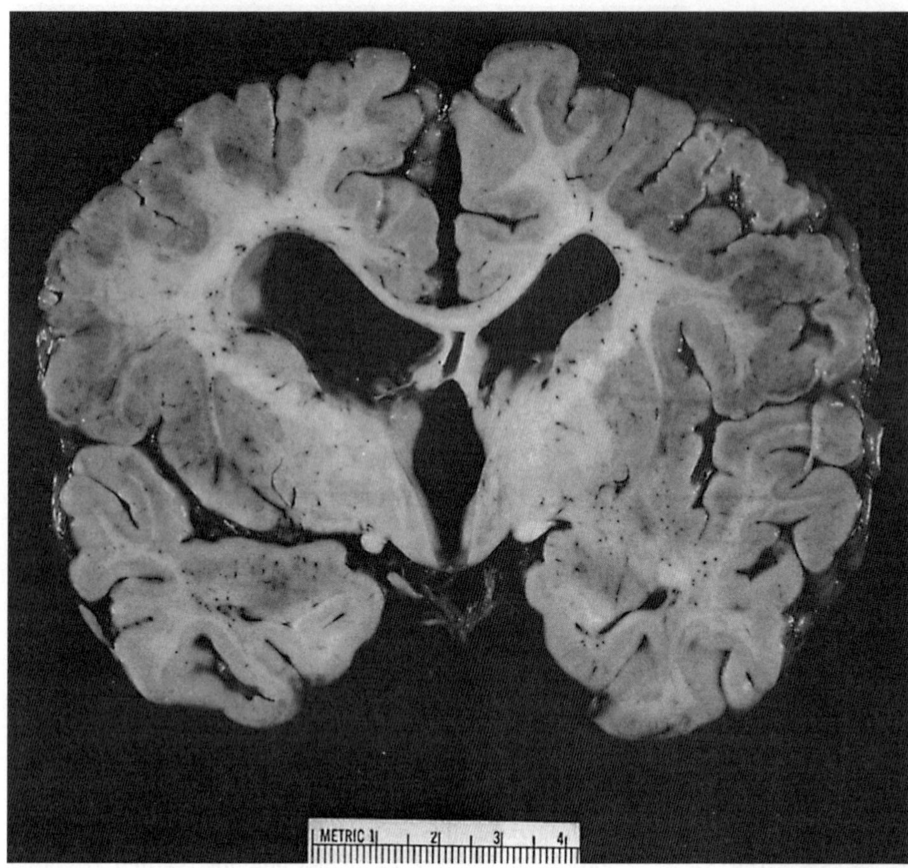

FIGURE 5.15. Polymicrogyria. Coronal section of frontal lobe. Excessive secondary and tertiary sulci are present, resulting in gyri that are too small and too numerous. (Courtesy of Dr. Hideo H. Itabashi, Department of Pathology, Los Angeles County Harbor Medical Center, Torrance, CA.)

type, four cellular layers of cerebral cortex occur, compared with the normal six, and the layering is irregular and more columnar than laminar. The reduced number of migrating cells results in a decreased amount of white matter and in hypoplastic pyramidal tracts. In the other form, no layers can be discerned (589). The anomaly can be generalized or affect only focal areas of the cerebral cortex. The cerebellum also shows deformities, with a failure in the development of a normal folial pattern. Gray matter heterotopia occurs along the brainstem and cerebellar axis. The abnormal cellular architecture serves to distinguish this anomaly from microgyria seen as a consequence of perinatal destructive lesions.

The mechanism causing polymicrogyria is under dispute (589). Barth suggested that early fetal accidents, possibly ischemic cortical damage, at 13 to 16 weeks' gestation cause the unlayered form of polymicrogyria, whereas late fetal accidents occurring between 20 and 24 weeks cause four-layered polymicrogyria. Other cases clearly are primary malformations. Polymicrogyria is reported in brains with persistent large numbers of fetal Reelin-secreting Cajal-Retzius cells in the molecular zone of the cerebral cortex (223), but the significance in pathogenesis is uncertain.

The clinical picture in polymicrogyria is generally one of mental retardation and spasticity or hypotonia with active deep tendon reflexes (hypotonic cerebral palsy; see Chapter 6). The important role of focal polymicrogyria in producing an intractable seizure disorder has become evident by neuroimaging studies. In particular, a syndrome of opercular polymicrogyria, or *congenital bilateral perisylvian syndrome*, has been delineated. In addition to seizures, patients present with mental retardation, dysarthria, abnormal tongue movements, and dysphagia (610). Polymicrogyria is seen in the insular and opercular region, and at times the malformation extends to involve the parietal and the superior temporal region. Guerrini and colleagues described a syndrome of symmetric parasagittal parieto-occipital polymicrogyria. The condition manifests by seizures and mild developmental delay. The lesion is located in the watershed vascular territory between the anterior cerebral artery and the posterior cerebral artery, and the authors suggested that it is the consequence of perfusion failure occurring between the 20th and 24th weeks of gestation (611). The predisposition of the opercular region to polymicrogyria has been confirmed by other groups and by our clinical experience (612,613).

MRI sometimes diagnoses polymicrogyria during the patient's lifetime (Fig. 5.16) (614), but in other cases the abnormal pattern of gyration is difficult to detect by MRI and nearly impossible by CT scan. In some cases, the abnormality can be detected by demonstrating a focal area

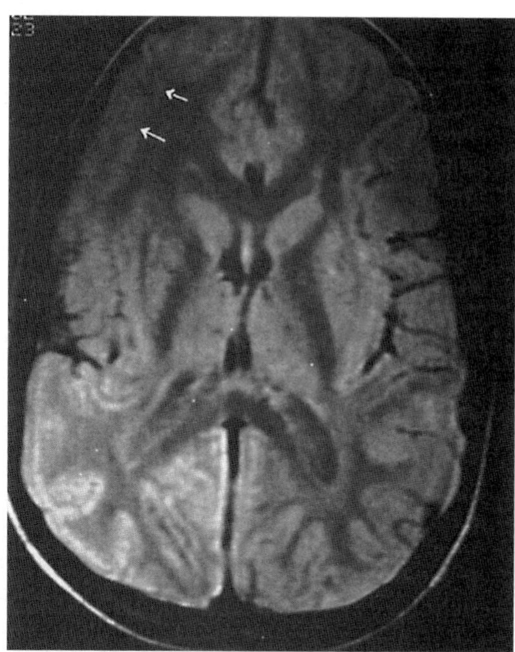

FIGURE 5.16. Polymicrogyria. T2-weighted magnetic resonance imaging study of an 8-year-old child presenting with developmental delay. Axial images reveal thickening of the right posterior frontal cortex (*arrows*). This region has no gyri; instead, paradoxically smooth cortex is seen, as in all cases of polymicrogyria. The normal finger-like projections of white matter are absent. (Courtesy of Dr. A. J. Barkovich, Department of Radiology, University of California, San Francisco, CA.)

of delayed maturation of subcortical white matter (615). The distinction between polymicrogyria and macrogyria cannot always be made by MRI. In both conditions one can see a thickened cortex with absence of detectable gyri, and the irregularities on the surface of what is believed to be a macrogyric cortex actually represent polymicrogyria. Approximately 25% of patients with polymicrogyria have abnormally prolonged T2 relaxation of the underlying white matter (614). Polymicrogyria may coexist with pachygyria and lissencephaly.

Subcortical Laminar Heterotopia (Band Heterotopia, Double Cortex)

Subcortical laminar heterotopia is a rare genetic disorder that is transmitted as an X-linked dominant trait, so that nearly all patients are female (616). A few male patients have survived spontaneous fetal loss and been born live; these boys have a particularly severe form of the disorder with lissencephaly in addition (617). The defective gene, called *doublecortin*, and its transcription product have been identified (618–620).

On pathologic examination, arrested radial neuroblast migration in the cerebrum is seen, so that a layer of gray matter heterotopia forms beneath the normal surface cortex and the periventricular zone, separated from both the cortex and the subependymal region by white matter (Fig. 5.17). Because of the distinctive appearance by MRI, the condition has sometimes been termed the *double cortex syndrome*, but the internal architecture of the subcortical heterotopia is not laminar as in normal cortex, though the overlying cerebral cortex has normal structure. Synaptic connections between the disorganized subcortical heterotopia and the overlying cortex probably account for

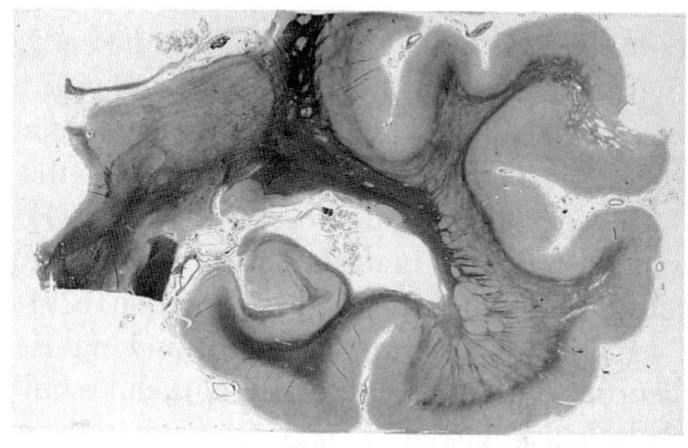

A

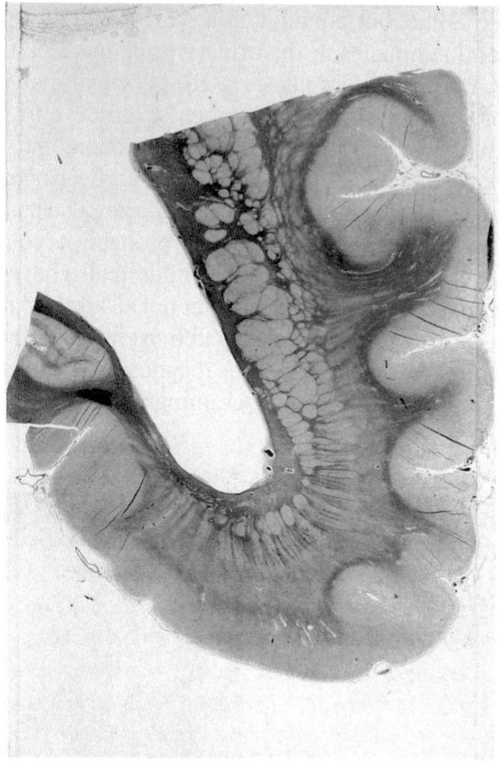

B

FIGURE 5.17. Subcortical laminar heterotopia in a young adult woman with intractable epilepsy who died in status epilepticus. This is an X-linked dominant trait. Islands of nonlaminated and disorganized gray matter are found in the subcortical white matter of the **(A)** temporal and **(B)** occipital lobes, forming a *double cortex* as a second layer of gray matter beneath the "normal" cortex at the surface and separated from it and from the ventricular wall by white matter (Luxol fast blue/periodic acid–Schiff reaction). (Courtesy of Dr. Ellsworth C. Alvord, Jr., University of Washington, Seattle, WA.)

the severe seizure disorder. Positron emission tomography demonstrates that the subcortical heterotopia has the same degree of glucose metabolism as the overlying true cortex (621).

Bilateral Periventricular Nodular Heterotopia

Bilateral periventricular nodular heterotopia is an arrest of neuroblast migration before such migration even is initiated, so that neurons mature in the subventricular zone without migrating along radial glia. It is another X-linked dominant trait that occurs almost exclusively in girls and is expressed clinically with epilepsy and mental retardation (622–626). Most girls, but also some boys, with this condition have a genetic mutation of *filamin A* (*FLNA*), a gene that is expressed early in the initiation of radial migration of neuroblasts from the subventricular zone (627), so that these cells fail to even begin migrating and mature *in situ* into neurons that form subventricular nodules but cannot establish their intended synaptic relations in the cerebral cortex. Some, but not all, families exhibit dysmorphic facies and anomalies in the urinary tract and rectal polyps (625). Maturing neuroblasts of the germinal matrix form nodules of gray matter that often protrude into the lateral ventricle and form internal connections but cannot establish the synaptic relations with cortical neurons at the surface of the brain. The surface cortex also has abnormal architecture, however, which probably accounts for the severe epilepsy (626). Some children also have hydrocephalus for uncertain reason, but not all affected families have the *FLNA* genetic defect and must have another gene defect not yet found (628). The diagnosis is established by MRI or by neuropathologic examination. It should not be confused with subependymal glial nodules that occur as a reactive change to periventricular leukomalacia, infantile hydrocephalus, ventriculitis, congenital infections, or acquired complications of prematurity.

The occasional boy with periventricular nodular heterotopia has a gene defect that has not yet been delineated.

Agenesis of the Corpus Callosum

The corpus callosum is the largest interhemispheric commissure. The failure of this commissure to form is traditionally regarded as a "midline defect" because normal callosal fibers cross the midline, but it should be reclassified as a disorder of axonal projection. The callosal axons are not absent, but rather are diverted to form an abnormal *bundle of Probst* in the dorsalmedial part of the hemisphere ipsilateral to their origin. The small pyramidal neurons of layer 3 are the cells of origin of the majority of callosal axons, and this layer is normal in microscopic examination of the cerebral cortex. The anterior commissure often is enlarged to three to four times its normal size, suggesting that some callosal axons find another route to reach the other hemisphere and many other aberrant crossings also occur, though not necessarily as an easily recognized, compact bundle of fibers. In some cases, the internal capsules and the rest of the corticospinal tracts are greatly enlarged and form thick axonal bundles in the ventral funiculi of the spinal cord, probably representing both aberrant callosal axons and normal corticospinal axons.

Agenesis of the corpus callosum is a relatively common condition in the developmentally disabled population, with an incidence as detected by CT of 2.3% (629) (Fig. 5.18). Sarnat postulated that agenesis of the corpus callosum results from the failure of the programmed cell death;

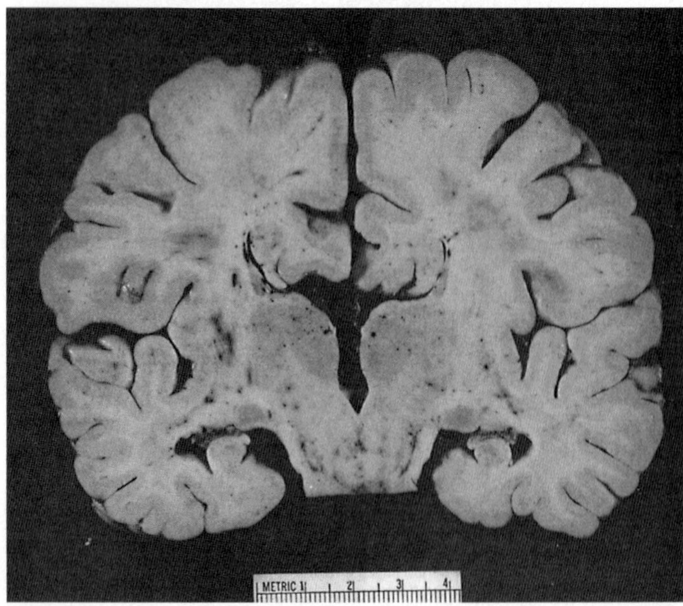

FIGURE 5.18. Agenesis of corpus callosum. Coronal section of brain. In this instance, the anomaly was not accompanied by abnormalities of cellular proliferation. (Courtesy of Dr. Hideo H. Itabashi, Department of Pathology, Los Angeles County Harbor Medical Center, Torrance, CA.)

in this instance glial cells of the lamina terminalis that form the initial septum do not degenerate in time to permit the passage of callosal axons (73). Experimental evidence of this mechanism is demonstrated in a murine model (630). The normally formed callosal fibers, being unable to cross the midline, are diverted to follow a path of least resistance, forming the bundle of Probst in the dorsomedial wall of the ipsilateral hemisphere, from which some fibers eventually make aberrant decussations. The bundle of Probst is interposed between the medial hemispheric wall and the lateral ventricle, splaying the lateral ventricles apart and giving a characteristic appearance in imaging studies and in coronal sections of the brain at autopsy.

The presence of heterotopic callosal axons that cannot cross the midline distinguishes agenesis of the corpus callosum with formation of the bundle of Probst from agenesis of the corpus callosum such as is seen in holoprosencephaly, in which callosal axons usually do not form. Most callosal axons in normal brains arise from the pyramidal cells of layer 3 of the cerebral cortex, unlike the corticospinal axons, which originate mainly from pyramidal cells of layers 5 and 6.

Agenesis of the corpus callosum takes one of two forms. In one type, partial or complete agenesis of the corpus callosum is accompanied solely by defects of contiguous and phylogenetically related structures. Abnormalities include a disturbance in the convolutional pattern of the medial wall of the hemisphere, which assumes a radiate arrangement. A complete or partial absence of the cingulate gyrus and of the septum pellucidum also can be observed. The most striking feature in these brains is the presence of the bundle of Probst. In this type of agenesis of the corpus callosum, significant neurologic abnormalities can be absent. If present and nonspecific, they can include seizures or mild to moderate mental retardation and impaired visual, motor, and bimanual coordination (see Fig. 5.1) (631,632).

As the corpus callosum forms from anterior to posterior, partial agenesis generally manifests by the presence of the anterior portions, the genu and body, and absence of the posterior portions, the splenium and rostrum (633). Myelination starts in the posterior portion of the corpus callosum, which begins to show increased signal on T1-weighted images at 3 to 4 months of age; the genu shows increased signal at 6 months of age (634).

In the second form, agenesis of the corpus callosum is accompanied by numerous abnormalities of cellular proliferation, including polymicrogyria and heterotopia of gray matter. In these patients and in families in which the trait is transmitted by one of at least two X-linked genes, severe intellectual retardation and seizures are present (635–637). The cortical anomalies are demonstrable by MRI or by positron emission tomography (636).

Agenesis of the corpus callosum accompanies a variety of chromosomal defects and the Dandy-Walker syndrome. It also was seen in 17% of patients with inherited metabolic disorders in the series of Bamforth and coworkers (638). These conditions include nonketotic hyperglycinemia, Zellweger syndrome, neonatal adrenoleukodystrophy, Menkes disease, glutaric aciduria type II, and pyruvate dehydrogenase deficiency, especially when the $E_1\alpha$ subunit is affected (639). Thus, the possibility of an inborn metabolic error should be considered in patients with agenesis of the corpus callosum.

A diminished width (hypoplasia) of the corpus callosum can be secondary to a reduced number of cortical neurons that give rise to callosal axons. This is not a developmental malformation. It may result from a variety of acquired insults and is a common consequence of supratentorial atrophy (640).

Agenesis of the corpus callosum is an integral part of Aicardi syndrome. This condition, which has been described in female patients only, is characterized by severe mental retardation, generalized tonic-clonic and myoclonic seizures that have their onset between birth and age 4 months, and chorioretinal lacunae. Hemivertebrae and costovertebral anomalies are common. In most instances, no other siblings are affected, and the syndrome is believed to result from an intrauterine insult between 4 and 12 weeks' gestation (641,642). The question as to whether an increased lethality of male fetuses occurs and the role of nonrandom inactivation of the X chromosome in the phenotypic expression of this condition remain unclarified.

Agenesis of the corpus callosum is also seen in the FG syndrome (FG stands for the initials of one of the families in which the syndrome was described). This syndrome is transmitted as an X-linked condition and is marked by the additional presence of constipation, imperforate anus, and a facial configuration highlighted by epicanthal folds and a fish-shaped (inverted-V) mouth (637,643). Other associated gastrointestinal (GI) anomalies in some cases of callosal agenesis are hypertrophic pyloric stenosis and aganglionic megacolon or Hirschsprung disease (644). Some patients have feeding difficulties without these lesions of the GI tract (645).

Agenesis of the corpus callosum is sometimes associated with interhemispheric lipomas or arachnoidal cysts that replace a portion of the commissure (646–648). These are developmental defects in which primitive meninx becomes mixed with neural tissue. Partial agenesis of the corpus callosum may selectively involve the rostrum, the middle, or the splenium, with or without the additional imposition of a lipoma or an arachnoidal cyst.

In isolated callosal agenesis, the clinical symptoms and signs can be subtle and often are unrecognized, though the incidence of epilepsy, usually complex partial seizures, is higher than in the normal population. Because of difficulty with interhemispheric transfer, objects placed in the left hand and perceived in the right parietal cortex are difficult to name because the data must be transferred back to the left hemisphere where speech is localized, but stereognosis and graphesthesia are normal in the right hand; this provides a useful clinical test during neurologic examination in older children if callosal agenesis is known or is suspected. The EEG shows lack of synchrony of sleep spindles after 18 months of age, when spindles of the two hemispheres normally occur together.

Colpocephaly

In colpocephaly the occipital horns of the lateral ventricles are disproportionately enlarged. Colpocephaly can occur in association with agenesis of the posterior fibers of the corpus callosum, as a primary developmental malformation, or as an acquired lesion, a consequence of severe periventricular leukomalacia, or intrauterine infections (73). This acquired form is probably the most common cause of colpocephaly. The clinical picture is nonspecific. As a rule, mental retardation of variable severity and seizures occur (649). Hypertelorism can be present. Visual function is usually normal. The diagnosis is made by neuroimaging. This condition should be distinguished from obstructive hydrocephalus; developmental colpocephaly does not require surgical treatment (650).

Cavum Septi Pellucidi

The development of the cavum septi pellucidi depends on and follows the evolution of the corpus callosum (651). The cavum is present in healthy fetal brain, in 97% of preterm infants, and in 56% of term infants (652). Its incidence diminishes further with increasing age. Persistence of its posterior extension, the cavum vergae, is less common; it is seen in only 7% of term neonates. The presence of a cavum septi pellucidi or both the cavi septi pellucidi and the cavum vergae generally represents incidental findings in healthy individuals. Less commonly, these defects occur in association with induction or migratory disorders, particularly if a cavum vergae is present (653). A large cavum septi pellucidi more frequently occurs in brains with other dysgeneses, with generalized atrophy, or in metabolic encephalopathies; hence it should alert the clinician to investigate further (654,655). Neuroimaging studies establish the diagnosis and also may reveal associated defects of cellular proliferation and migration. Although in agenesis of the corpus callosum the cavum appears to be absent by neuroimaging, careful neuropathologic studies disclose that the leaves of the septum pellucidum are actually displaced laterally and adhere to the widely separated medial walls of the lateral ventricles.

MICROCEPHALY

Microcephaly was defined by a head circumference, as measured around the forehead and the occipital protuberance, that is more than two standard deviations below the mean for age, sex, and race (see Introduction chapter, Fig. I.1) (656). This definition was challenged because 1.9% of healthy school children were found to have a head circumference less than two standard deviations below the mean (657) and because in some families with normal intelligence, microcephaly and short stature are inherited as dominant or recessive traits (658,659). When children with a head circumference less than two standard deviations but greater than three standard deviations below the mean were examined, 10.5% had an IQ below 70, 28.1% had a borderline IQ (71 to 80), and 14.0% had an IQ above 100. Of children with both height and head circumference less than two standard deviations below the mean, 13.3% had an IQ below 70. When children with a head circumference of less than three standard deviations below the mean were tested at 7 years of age, 51.2% had an IQ below 70 and 17.1% were borderline. None had an IQ above 100 (660).

Head circumference should always be compared with other concurrent growth parameters: If the child has a weight and a length or a height also at or below the 2nd centile, the apparent microcephaly may be less significant than if these other measures of growth are at or above the 50th centile. Head circumference also should be compared with previous measurements of the same child, ideally from birth, to determine whether microcephaly is congenital or acquired.

Except in cases of premature closure of the sutures (craniosynostosis), the small size of the skull reflects a small brain, but it is not the size of the brain that determines the presence of mental retardation, but the underlying structural pathology of the brain. An abnormally small brain results either from anomalous development during the first 7 months of gestation (primary microcephaly) or from an insult incurred during the last 2 months of gestation or during the perinatal period (secondary microcephaly).

Primary Microcephaly

Primary microcephaly results from a variety of genetic and environmental insults that cause anomalies of induction and migration. *Micrencephaly*, by contrast with *microcephaly*, denotes a small brain or cerebral hypoplasia rather than a small head, and is an imaging or neuropathologic diagnosis. Micrencephaly and coexist with microcephaly or with a normal-sized head.

Genetic Defects

Primary microcephaly can be transmitted as an autosomal recessive or as an autosomal dominant disorder (658,661,662). The brain can weigh as little as 500 g and resemble that of a 3- to 5-month-old fetus (663). Numerous migrational anomalies are seen, including schizencephaly, lissencephaly, pachygyria, polymicrogyria, and agenesis of

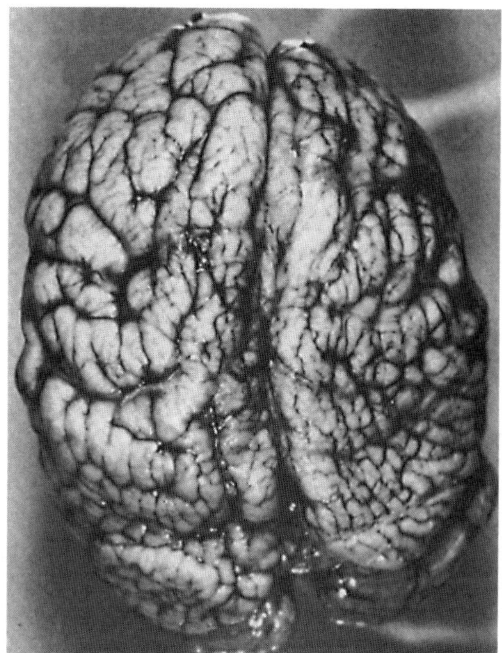

FIGURE 5.19. Primary microcephaly. Dorsal view of the brain of a 9-year-old boy with severe microcephaly (brain weight was 700 g) and polymicrogyria. Note the regional differences, with the parieto-occipital regions being more severely involved, and a gradation to a more normal pattern frontally, especially in the larger hemisphere. Other malformations are not unusual. (From Lemire RJ, Loeser JD, Leech RW. *Normal and abnormal development of the human nervous system.* Hagerstown, MD: Harper & Row, 1975. With permission.)

the corpus callosum (Figs. 5.19 and 5.20). Gray matter heterotopia occur, and neurons are reduced in number and abnormal in configuration (Figs. 5.20 and 5.21). Cortical lamination is defective, with grouping of cortical neurons in columnar blocks.

Numerous families with primary microcephaly have been recorded. In at least one, the gene has been mapped to the short arm of chromosome 8 (8pter–p22). Tolmie and colleagues distinguished two forms of autosomal recessive microcephaly, both of them characterized by a head circumference at birth that was more than five standard deviations below the mean. In one form, affected individuals were in the mildly retarded range with a normal facial appearance. In the other, more frequently encountered form, microcephaly was complicated by spasticity and seizures. Patients with this genetically transmitted microcephaly exhibited a receding forehead, and profound retardation was seen (664). Ocular abnormalities, including chorioretinopathy and cataracts, also have accompanied primary microcephaly (665,666). We have seen two siblings, brother and sister, with associated insulin-dependent diabetes mellitus (see Chapter 17).

In some patients, microcephaly results from an arrest in neuronogenesis before the requisite number of mitotic cycles is completed in the telencephalic neuroepithelium. One factor known to arrest mitotic activity is precocious differentiation of the ependyma, perhaps induced by fetal exposure to some toxin or virus that acts as a teratogen by imitating an inductive gene or molecule that normally initiates ependymal differentiation in a preprogrammed temporal sequence (663).

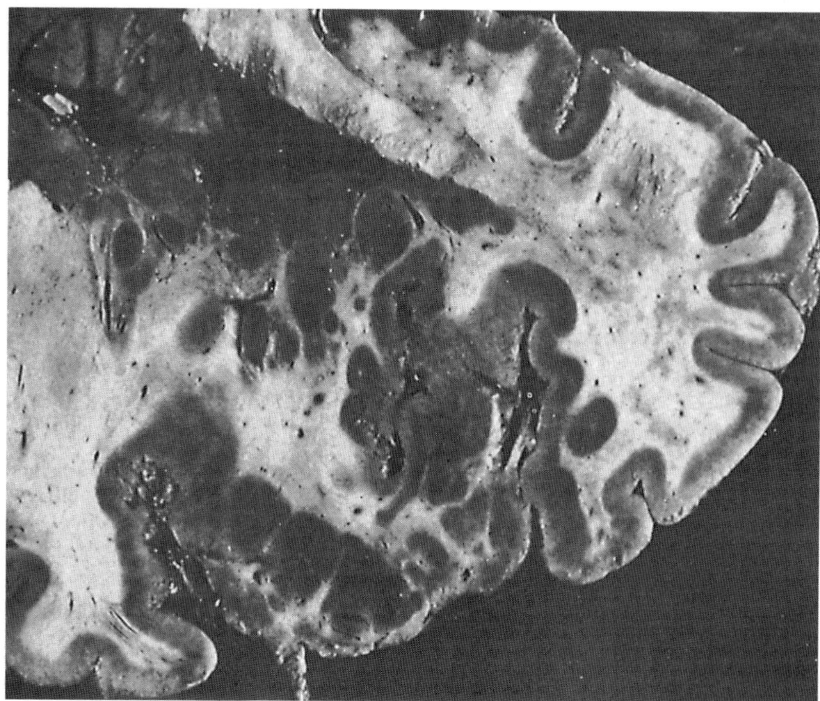

FIGURE 5.20. Heterotopia of gray matter. Disruption of the cortex is present, with islands of heterotopic gray matter extending between the ependyma of the lateral ventricle and the surface. (From Layton DD. Heterotopic cerebral gray matter as an epileptogenic focus. *J Neuropathol Exp Neurol* 1962;21:244. With permission.)

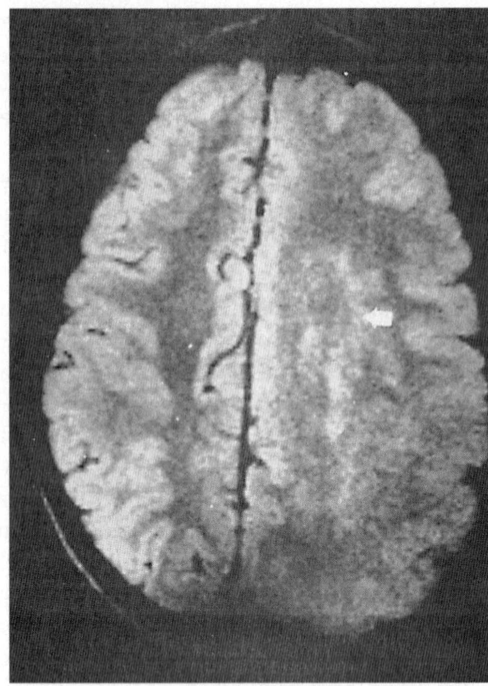

FIGURE 5.21. Gray matter heterotopia. T2-weighted magnetic resonance imaging study of a 7-year-old child presenting with seizures reveals foci that are isointense with gray matter lying within the centrum semiovale (*arrow*). (Courtesy of Dr. A. J. Barkovich, Department of Radiology, University of California, San Francisco, CA.)

The recurrence of microcephaly after one affected child is relatively high, the exact frequency in each of the reported series depending on the incidence of autosomal recessive microcephaly. It was 19% in the series of Tolmie and colleagues (664). Prenatal diagnosis by ultrasound has been attempted by serial biparietal diameter measurements. This procedure discriminates poorly between affected and unaffected fetuses until the third trimester of gestation (664).

Disorders of Karyotype

Numerous chromosomal disorders, including trisomies, deletions, and translocation syndromes, are associated with primary microcephaly (see Chapter 4, Table 4.3). In addition, at least 20 well-defined dysmorphic syndromes with normal karyotypes, inherited or not inherited (e.g., Cornelia de Lange, Hallermann-Streiff, and Seckel syndromes), are associated with microcephaly (see Chapter 4, Table 4.8).

Irradiation

Microcephaly can result from exposure to ionizing radiation during the first two trimesters, particularly between 4 and 20 weeks' gestation (667,668). The earlier the insult, the smaller is the brain and the more disabling are the resulting neurologic abnormalities. Maternal exposure within 1,500 m of the epicenter of the Hiroshima atomic bomb resulted in microcephaly when the gestational age at the time of exposure was 15 weeks or less (669). During the first 4 months of gestation, diagnostic irradiation of 1 cGy or less appears to pose little or no risk (670).

Infections in Utero

A variety of infectious agents, notably cytomegalovirus, *Toxoplasma*, and the rubella virus, are responsible for microcephaly. These disorders are discussed in Chapter 7.

Chemical Agents

In experimental animals, a wide variety of chemical agents has been found to produce microcephaly associated with induction and migration anomalies. Drugs implicated include cortisone, sulfhydryl enzyme inhibitors, aminopterin, triethylenemelamine, and nitrogen mustard. Additionally, mothers who suffer from untreated phenylketonuria have a high risk of bearing microcephalic offspring. This problem is considered in Chapter 1.

All causes of primary microcephaly, genetic, irradiation, chromosomal, infectious, or chemical, are time specific in that the toxic stimulus must occur during the period of induction and major cellular migration.

Secondary Microcephaly

A variety of insults, infectious, traumatic, metabolic, and anoxic, occurring during the last part of the third trimester, the perinatal period, and early infancy cause destruction of brain with multiple areas of cystic degeneration, encephalomalacia, and porencephaly, accompanied by inflammatory gliotic scarring and shrinkage. As a consequence, little postnatal growth occurs and sutures close early. In secondary microcephaly, brain anomalies such as those in primary microcephaly are absent except for instances of cerebellar gray matter heterotopia and hypoplasia.

Clinical Manifestations

It is clear that both primary and secondary microcephaly display a broad spectrum of neurologic disorders. These disorders range from decerebration to a mild impairment of fine motor coordination, from complete nonresponsiveness to educable mental retardation, and from severe autistic behavior to mild hyperkinesis.

Diagnosis

In the diagnostic evaluation of the microcephalic child, various possible causes must be considered. Serologic studies for intrauterine infections, cytogenetics, amino acid screening, and CT for intracranial calcifications should be considered. MRI demonstrates abnormalities in cortical architecture (671). Craniosynostosis can be distinguished from microcephaly by an abnormally shaped skull and by the presence at birth of bony union between sutures. In the experience of Matson, in no patient with craniosynostosis was the affected suture open at birth (373).

The prognosis for relative microcephaly (i.e., a head circumference within the normal range, above the 10th percentile for gestational age, but proportionately small compared with length or weight) was examined by Brennan and coworkers, who used data collected as part of the Collaborative Perinatal Project. In their series, such infants do not show any developmental delay when tested at 7 years of age (672). It is otherwise for infants whose head circumference at birth is below the 10th percentile for gestational age. Both term infants and those small for gestational age having small head circumferences fare poorly, and according to Lipper and coworkers, head circumference at birth appears to be the most important variable for future neurodevelopmental outcome (673).

Microcephaly on rare occasions can be reversed with treatment of the underlying cause. This has been reported for phenylketonuria, chronic hypoglycemia, and diet-induced hypochloremic metabolic alkalosis (see Chapter 17).

CRANIOSYNOSTOSIS

Craniosynostosis is defined as the premature closure at birth of one or more cranial sutures.[3] It is termed *simple* when only one suture is fused and *compound* when two or more sutures are affected. Primary craniosynostosis results from an abnormality of the mesenchymal matrix and is not the consequence of impaired brain growth. Secondary craniosynostosis is the consequence of one of various mechanical, metabolic, or hematologic disorders. Craniosynostosis can be an isolated phenomenon or can form part of a generalized dysmorphologic, chromosomal, or genetic syndrome (675). Several well-defined genetic diseases are known to associated with craniosynostosis and for which the specific genetic mutation is demonstrated; these include Apert, Crouzon, Pfeiffer, Muenke, Saethre-Chotzen, and Shprintzen-Goldberg syndromes as the best recognized (676). Disturbances of fibroblast growth factor receptors (FGFRs) 1, 2, and 3 and causative genes such as *TWIST* have been proved (677).

In the healthy newborn, all sutures are separated by several millimeters, except the metopic suture, which closes antenatally. Metopic craniosynostosis, which manifests itself by a midfrontal ridge, is relatively common in small infants but is of little or no clinical significance. No known neurologic consequences exist, and surgery is contraindicated.

By age 3 months, the posterior fontanelle is closed. By age 6 months, fibrous union of suture lines occurs and serrated edges interlock. By age 20 months, the anterior fontanelle is closed. At age 8 years, ossification of craniobasal bones is complete. By age 12 years, the sutures cannot be separated by raised intracranial pressure; they continue to be visible on radiography until age 20 years. Solid bony union of all sutures is complete by the eighth decade of life.

Etiology

No histologic abnormality of the prematurely fused sutures exists, and the pathogenesis is heterogeneous, with more than 100 syndromes of developmental defects having been described. These syndromes, which taken together constitute approximately 10% of craniosynostoses, are listed in monographs by David and coworkers (675) and Cohen (677). It appears likely therefore that calvarial involvement represents but one expression of a more widespread fundamental germ layer disturbance (678). The molecular basis of several craniosynostosis syndromes has been identified. Dominant mutations in three fibroblast growth factor receptor genes have been shown to be responsible for Crouzon, Jackson-Weiss, Pfeiffer, and Apert syndromes (679,680). Undoubtedly, other genetic mutations will be uncovered. Although animal experiments have shown that immobilization of a suture can lead to its fusion, the importance of intrauterine constraint in producing craniosynostosis has been questioned (681,682).

Secondary synostosis can be caused by a variety of metabolic disorders, including hyperthyroidism (683), Hurler syndrome, Conradi syndrome (684), and various forms of rickets, notably vitamin D deficiency, hypophosphatemia, hypophosphatasia, and azotemic osteodystrophy (685). It also is associated with such hematologic disorders as thalassemia and sickle cell anemia (686). In microcephaly and after reduction of increased intracranial pressure (as occurs with surgical treatment of hydrocephalus), a secondary premature fusion of the sutures occurs. In general, the deformities produced by secondary synostosis are much less pronounced than those with the primary form and rarely, if ever, appear to impair brain growth. Hence, corrective surgery for secondary synostosis is not indicated.

[3] Craniosynostosis was first described by Homer in the person of Thersites, "whose skull went up to a point ... [He was a] fluent orator though ... the ugliest man who came beneath Ilion." Virchow, in 1851, provided a more complete clinical characterization (674).

TABLE 5.17 Distribution of Suture Involvements in 136 Patients With Craniosynostosis

Suture Affected	Term	Male	Female	Total	Percentage
Sagittal	Scaphocephaly (dollchocephaly)	45	10	55	40
Both coronals	Acrocephaly	12	16	28	20.5
One coronal	Plagiocephaly	10	12	22	16
All in vault	Oxycephaly	7	5	12	9
Sagittal and coronal	—	4	8	12	9
Metopic	Trigonocephaly	4	2	6	4.5
Sagittal and lambdoid	—	1	0	1	1
Total		**83**	**53**	**136**	**100**

From Till K. *Paediatric neurosurgery.* Oxford: Blackwell, 1975. With permission.

Clinical Manifestations

Craniosynostosis occurs in fewer than 5 in 10,000 births. The anatomic classification of craniosynostosis depends on the description of head contour or on the suture or sutures involved. The final skull shape depends on which sutures close, the duration and order of the closure process, and the success or failure of other sutures to compensate by expansion. As a rule, skull growth is inhibited in a direction at right angles to the closed sutures. The frequency of the various types of craniosynostosis is given in Table 5.17 (687).

Premature closure of the sagittal suture, the most common form of craniosynostosis, results in elongation of the skull in the anteroposterior direction. Associated anomalies are seen in 26% of patients, and between 5% and 40% of affected children exhibit mental retardation (688,689). When the coronal suture fuses prematurely, the brain expands in a lateral direction. In this condition, the incidence of associated anomalies is higher: 33% with involvement of one coronal suture and 59% with involvement of both coronal sutures (363). Approximately 50% of affected children with synostosis of both coronal sutures exhibit mental retardation (688).

Of all types of craniosynostosis, oxycephaly can produce the most severe CNS involvement. Increased intracranial pressure, divergent strabismus, optic atrophy, anosmia, and bilateral pyramidal tract signs can either occur as associated CNS anomalies or because nonfused sutures are not sufficient to allow for expansion of the brain.

Psychomotor retardation can result from prolonged increased intracranial pressure, but more often it is caused by associated cerebral malformations or concurrent hydrocephalus (689,690). Retardation is noticeably absent in the majority of children with sagittal craniosynostosis, however, so that the need to treat is at times debatable.

In Crouzon syndrome (craniofacial dysostosis), premature closure of multiple sutures is associated with an abnormally high forehead, hypertelorism, shallow orbits with resultant exophthalmos, micrognathia, choanal atresia, prognathism, beaked nose, and high arched palate, but is usually associated with normal intellect. Chronic tonsillar herniation accompanies Crouzon syndrome and was seen in 73% of patients studied by Cinalli and coworkers (691). Hydrocephalus develops in a large proportion of patients. It is believed to result from intracranial venous hypertension (692) or from the early closure of the lambdoid sutures (693). Crouzon syndrome tends to be hereditary or familial, and its gene has been mapped to the long arm of chromosome 10 (10q26). It codes for fibroblast growth factor receptor 2. Numerous mutations of fibroblast growth factor receptor 2 have been described and have been found to cause various craniosynostotic syndromes aside from Crouzon syndrome (679,693,694).

In Apert syndrome (acrocephalosyndactyly), the head and facial configuration are similar to that seen in Crouzon syndrome, but syndactyly or polydactyly is present as well. Most cases are sporadic. In the majority, the condition results from one of two mutations in the gene for fibroblast growth factor receptor 2 (695). Nonprogressive ventriculomegaly, hydrocephalus, and megalencephaly are often demonstrated (691). When measured, intracranial pressure is increased in some 80% of patients. The most likely cause of this phenomenon is impaired flow of CSF through the basilar cisterns. Only a small proportion of patients with Apert syndrome have normal intelligence, and malformations of the imbic structures, corpus callosum, and gyral abnormalities are common (696,697).

A variety of other genetic or sporadically occurring constitutional dysplastic features are associated with craniosynostosis (674,677,698).

Diagnosis

In the small infant, the diagnosis can be suspected in the presence of an abnormally shaped head or face. CT is usually definitive. It reveals the extent of premature fusion and frequently shows an increased density of the fused suture. The early radiologic change is a loss of the pattern of interdigitations of the bone, until the suture becomes a simple line of separation of the bones. Bridging of this gap then begins, followed by a thickening of the bone along the line of the former suture. If the sagittal suture is involved, the anterior fontanelle is obliterated. With increased intracranial pressure, imaging studies performed after age 6 months can show demineralization and thinning of bone with increased digital impressions. MRI is necessary if hydrocephalus or abnormalities of cortical architecture are suspected.

One important differential diagnosis is that of microcephaly. Oxycephaly in particular, characterized by deformity of skull contour, closure of sutures at birth or during the neonatal period, and increased intracranial pressure, can mimic primary microcephaly. The differentiation of infants with unilambdoid synostosis (plagiocephaly) from those with positional flattening (deformational occipital plagiocephaly) can be difficult. In the experience of Menard and David, only 1% of children with unilateral occipital plagiocephaly were found to have true lambdoid synostosis (698).

The shape of the skull of a newborn who has been in the breech position *in utero* can suggest sagittal synostosis. In the breech baby, however, the biparietal diameter is normal, and no ridging is present at the sagittal suture, which appears normal on radiography. With time, the misshapen head can be expected to improve spontaneously (699).

Treatment

Craniosynostosis is treated surgically in children with multiple suture closure to prevent any brain damage that could result from chronic increased intracranial pressure and in children with synostosis of only one suture to affect a good cosmetic result.

A consensus exists regarding the need for a surgical procedure in the presence of increased intracranial pressure (700). There has been considerable debate, however, regarding the need for surgery in children with synostosis of only one suture, particularly in plagiocephaly and scaphocephaly (premature closure to the sagittal suture). Some clinicians believe that scaphocephaly is rarely complicated by intellectual or neurologic dysfunction and that skull surgery is not justified for cosmetic reasons alone (688). Considerable debate exists concerning the optimal management of plagiocephaly. Rekate reviewed the literature and found no prospective, randomized, controlled trials. The various recommended treatment options include observation only, mechanical correction of the deformity by wrapping of the head, and various types of surgical interventions. It is not known whether children whose plagiocephaly has gone uncorrected have suffered from failure in intervention (701).

We believe that surgery for craniosynostosis should be viewed as a corrective rather than a cosmetic procedure and that a child with uncorrected synostosis and a significant skull deformity is fated to a lifetime of being considered and treated as abnormal.

It is fortunate that scaphocephaly is the disorder in most of the patients with synostosis; the technical procedure to correct this condition is easy, and, if properly performed, it produces uniformly excellent results. The most common method of treating sagittal synostosis is to remove the midline strip of bone several centimeters in width from anterior to the coronal suture, to posterior to the lambdoidal sutures. Interpositional material is placed on the bony edges to prevent early refusion. Removal of a much wider strip of bone without interpositional material can serve the same purpose. The application of a fixative solution, such as Zenker, to the dura mater for this or any form of synostosis with the intent to retard reossification is definitely not recommended because the solution can penetrate the dura and injure the brain (702) or can destroy the ossifying potential of the dura, necessitating subsequent cranioplasty (703).

Several techniques are advocated for the correction of the other synostoses (704). These are necessarily complex in most cases, particularly if surgical treatment has been delayed until later in childhood and when multiple sutures are involved, as in Crouzon disease. Surgery during the first 6 months of life is far more successful, having the advantage of using brain growth to assist in achieving a more normal skull shape as well as removing any impediment to brain development.

Morbidity consists of local hematoma, wound infection, or, rarely, the development of a leptomeningeal cyst. The more complex procedures should be performed only at centers with frequent experience with them, where the operative mortality is virtually nil and prolonged morbidity is less than 1% (705).

MACROCEPHALY

Macrocephaly is defined as a head circumference that is more than two standard deviations more than the mean for age, sex, race, and gestation (see Introduction chapter, Fig. I.1). It is not a disease, but a syndrome of diverse causes. Table 5.18 outlines the most important diagnostic considerations appropriate for each age group. We stress that evaluation of a child is necessary whenever a single head circumference measurement is outside the range of normal or when graphing of serial measurements documents a progressive, relative enlargement of the head as evidenced by the crossing of one or more percentile lines.

The differential diagnosis of macrocephaly takes into account the various conditions most likely for the age of the patient. The history must answer three important questions: Was the patient abnormal from birth or was there a period of normal growth and development before

TABLE 5.18 Common Causes of Macrocephaly and Time of Clinical Presentation

Early Infantile (Birth to 6 mo of age)	Hydrocephalus (progressive or "arrested")	
	Induction disorders	Spina bifida cystica, cranium bifidum, Chiari malformations (types I, II, and III), aqueductal stenosis, holoprosencephaly
	Mass lesions	Neoplasms, atrioventricular malformations, congenital cysts
	Intrauterine infections	Toxoplasmosis, cytomegalic inclusion disease, syphilis, rubella
	Perinatal or postnatal infections	Bacterial, granulomatous, parasitic
	Perinatal or postnatal hemorrhage	Hypoxia, vascular malformation, trauma
	Hydranencephaly	
	Subdural effusion	
	Hemorrhagic, infectious, cystic hygroma	
	Normal variant (often familial)	
Late Infantile (6 mo to 2 yr of age)	Hydrocephalus (progressive or "arrested")	
	Space-occupying lesions	Tumors, cysts, abscess
	Postbacterial or granulomatous meningitis	
	Posthemorrhagic	Trauma or vascular malformation
	Dandy-Walker syndrome	
	Subdural effusion	
	Increased intracranial pressure syndrome	
	Pseudotumor cerebri	Lead, tetracycline, hypoparathyroidism, corticosteroids, excess or deficiency of vitamin A, cyanotic congenital heart disease
	Primary skeletal cranial dysplasias (thickened or enlarged skull)	
	Osteogenesis imperfecta, hyperphosphatemia, osteopetrosis, rickets	
	Megalencephaly (increase in brain substance)	
	Metabolic central nervous system diseases	Leukodystrophies (e.g., Canavan, Alexander), lipidoses (Tay-Sachs), histiocytosis, mucopolysaccharidoses
	Proliferative neurocutaneous syndromes	von Recklinghausen tuberous sclerosis, hemanglomatosis, Sturge-Weber
	Cerebral gigantism	Sotos syndrome
	Achondroplasia	
	Primary megalencephaly	May be familial and unassociated with abnormalities of cellular architecture, or associated with abnormalities or cellular architecture
Early to Late Childhood (older than 2 yr of age)	Hydrocephalus (progressive or "arrested")	
	Space-occupying lesions	
	Preexisting induction disorder	Aqueductal stenosis
	Postinfectious	
	Hemorrhagic	
	Chiari type I malformation	
	Megalencephaly	
	Proliferative neurocutaneous syndromes	
	Familial	
	Pseudotumor cerebri	
	Normal variant	

deterioration set in? Is there a family history of neurologic or cutaneous abnormalities? Is there a history of CNS trauma or infection?

The patient and family should be examined for cutaneous lesions such as angiomas, café-au-lait spots, vitiligo, shagreen patches, telangiectasia, and subcutaneous nodules. Measurement of the head circumference of both parents provides valuable information. We stress that we have seen children with proven hydrocephalus with parents who have exceptionally large heads. The fundi must be evaluated for papilledema, macular degeneration such as is seen in lipidoses, chorioretinitis and cataracts produced by intrauterine infections, and optic nerve tumors caused by phakomatoses. The fontanelle, if open, is palpated for increased intracranial pressure and its size is measured. The ranges of normal size were recorded by Popich and Smith (706).

In 90% of healthy infants, the anterior fontanelle closes between 7 and 19 months of age, and in the remainder, by 26 months. The average time of closure is 16.3 months for boys and 18.8 months for girls (707). Persistent enlargement of the fontanelle is seen not only in hydrocephalus, but also in athyrotic hypothyroidism, achondroplasia, cleidocranial dysostosis, Down syndrome, trisomies 13 and 18, osteogenesis imperfecta, and the rubella syndrome. In addition to examination of the fontanelle, the skull should be auscultated for intracranial bruits.

Should ultrasonography demonstrate ventricular enlargement, the next question to be answered is whether ventriculomegaly is atrophic or is caused by obstruction and increased intracranial pressure. Routine MRI or cine-MRI is useful to ascertain the presence of CSF flow through the foramen of Monro, aqueduct of Sylvius, and foramen of Magendie. MRI provides evidence for a mass lesion such as a neoplasm, a vascular malformation, subdural fluid collections, or porencephalic cysts. CT scans are essential to assess the presence of intracranial calcifications produced by prenatal infections, hypoparathyroidism, or parasitic cysts. Long-bone radiographs can be used to determine the presence of spinal dysraphism. Increased cortical thickness of long bones suggests primary skeletal disturbances; fractures in different stages of healing suggest the diagnosis of a battered infant and a subdural hematoma.

Additional studies depend on diagnostic expectations for each age group (see Table 5.18).

Megalencephaly

Megalencephaly results from excessive amounts of normal brain constituents, cellular proliferation, inadequate physiologic apoptosis, or storage of metabolites. This condition is reviewed in a monograph by Gooskens (708). Some genes are now identified, such as *FoxG1*, that cause overgrowth of the neural tube in animals (709); whether these are involved in human megalencephaly is unknown.

In true megalencephaly, the increase in all neural elements is usually accompanied by overgrowth, abnormal migration, abnormal organization of some or all cellular and fiber elements of gray and white matter, giant neurons, gray matter heterotopia, and defective cortical lamination. The brain, which normally weighs 350 g at term (1,250 to 1,400 g at maturity), can be twice as heavy as expected for the age. True megalencephaly is primarily a proliferation disorder of embryonic origin, hamartomatous in nature with occasional malignant transformation, and, therefore, related to such phakomatoses as tuberous sclerosis and neurofibromatosis. In lissencephaly, the brain usually is small because of inadequate neuroepithelial cell proliferation, but if the proliferation is normal, the brain is excessively large because the lack of convolutions require a larger tissue volume to accommodate the cortex.

The classical clinical picture of true megalencephaly is one of mental retardation, seizures, hypotonia or mild pyramidal tract, and cerebellar deficits. These symptoms are occasionally progressive. The skull bones are thin, the anterior fontanelle is large, and sutures are slow in closing. The head reveals neither frontal bossing suggestive of hydrocephalus nor lateral bulging seen so often with infantile subdural fluid collections. Multiple minor congenital anomalies are frequently present, including hypertelorism, abnormal dermatoglyphics, and high arched palate. These stigmata also are seen in cerebral gigantism (Sotos syndrome) (see Chapter 17). Megalencephaly accompanies cutaneous and subcutaneous abnormalities in a variety of syndromes, notably disseminated hemangiomatosis, neurofibromatosis, multiple hemangiomas and pseudopapilledema, angiomatosis and lipomatosis, Bannayan syndrome (710), Beckwith-Wiedemann syndrome (see Chapter 17), and Klippel-Trenaunay-Weber syndrome (see Chapter 13). A dominantly inherited syndrome of megalencephaly, hypotonia, proximal muscle weakness, and increased intercellular muscle lipids has been described (711). A number of patients also have café-au-lait lesions and pigmented lesions of the penis; thus this condition may be identical to the Ruvalcaba-Myhre-Smith and Bannayan syndromes (712).

Although the prevalence of megalencephaly is increased in children with learning disabilities (713), the majority of children with this condition have normal to superior intelligence, and a large brain has been seen in many geniuses. In the large series of Lorber and Priestley, 88% of children with megalencephaly had normal to superior intelligence and 5% were in the borderline range (714). Sandler and coworkers found that when children with macrocephaly were compared with unaffected siblings, the former group had delayed motor milestones, speech and articulation problems, and difficulties with visuomotor integration (714a). In the series of Lorber and Priestley, the male-to-female ratio was 4:1, height and weight were within the normal range in 90% and 91%, respectively, and at least 39% had a family history of an enlarged head, most commonly in the child's father (715). In such families, transmission of the condition is most likely to be as an autosomal dominant trait.

Benign enlargement of the subarachnoid space over the cerebral hemispheres may result in a macrocephaly with a normal-sized brain (716). Such children have a normal head circumference at birth, and reach a maximal size at the 90th centile or above at age 5 to 12 months, thereafter stabilizing or showing a relative slow decrease in head size until age 5 years. Psychomotor development is normal, but the children usually are hypotonic without weakness.

The occurrence in siblings suggests an autosomal recessive trait. Diagnosis is by CT or MR imaging of the brain.

Hemimegalencephaly

This is a unique cerebral malformation that does not correspond to any normal stage of development. It is an asymmetric hamartomatous dysgenesis limited to one cerebral hemisphere and causing that side of the brain to be larger than the other. Hemimegalencephaly may be classified as isolated, not associated with other abnormalities, or syndromic, associated in particular with several neurocutaneous syndromes: most frequently epidermal nevus syndrome, Klippel-Trenaunay syndrome, and Proteus syndrome (717). A rare variant, called *total hemimegalencephaly*, involves the ipsilateral cerebellar hemisphere and hemibrainstem, which also are enlarged. There is no difference between isolated and syndromic forms (717).

Three grades of severity may be recognized, both anatomically and in clinical expression, and these correlate with prognosis. The imaging characteristics are distinctive and identify the grade of the malformation. The hemisphere is variably enlarged, totally or in part, the midline is shifted, the distinction between gray and white matter is poor, lissencephaly or pachygyria may be seen focally in parts of the cerebral cortex, and the corpus callosum is asymmetric. A shift of the occipital pole across the midline, the *occipital sign*, is a characteristic finding (717). In severe cases, epilepsy may be intractable and require surgical treatment (718).

The pathologic lesions are hamartomatous because of abnormal cell morphology as well as disorganized histologic architecture (719–721). Though frequently classified as a disorder of neuroblast migration because of the abnormalities of cortical gyration and lamination, the migratory disorder is secondary (720). Hemimegalencephaly is more likely a disturbance of cellular lineage, similar to tuberous sclerosis (720). Histopathologically, many hypertrophic cells, including "balloon cells," are found with abnormal processes that have immunocytochemical markers of neuronal, glial, or mixed lineage (720,721). Several genes of body symmetry are known, such as *Pitx-2* (52) and *Lefty-1* and *Lefty-2* (722), but it is uncertain which specific genes play a role in pathogenesis (717).

Hydrocephalus

Hydrocephalus is commonly defined as a pathologic increase in the cerebral ventricular volume. Although this increase can occur from a reduction in the volume of cerebral tissue resulting from either malformation or atrophy (hydrocephalus *ex vacuo*), the type of hydrocephalus considered here is that which results from an imbalance between the formation of CSF and its absorption. With the possible exception of choroid plexus papilloma, in which CSF overproduction has been postulated to occur, hydrocephalus results from blockage of CSF pathways or impaired absorption. An impairment to the normal flow or to the return of CSF into the blood leads to an increase in ventricular pressure because no mechanism exists for homeostasis and reduction of CSF formation. The increased pressure and the ventricular enlargement that follows account for the clinical findings. The timing, site of the obstruction, and cause of hydrocephalus, particularly the presence or absence of associated cerebral malformations, determine the type of hydrocephalus, the extent of any brain damage, and the outcome.

Ontogenesis and Physiology of the Cerebrospinal Fluid

Excellent books reviewing the embryology, anatomy, and physiology of the CSF dynamics and of the ventricular and subarachnoid spaces are those by Fishman, who also discusses the alterations of CSF in various disease processes (723), and Davson and colleagues (724). As noted in Table 5.10, closure of the neural tube and primordial cephalization occur by 28 days' gestation. In humans, the cerebral vesicles with a central lumen develop from the cephalic end of the neural tube. These represent the major brain subdivisions and the tentatively defined ventricles, both of which become further elaborated as certain regions constrict and others expand to form the basic pattern of the ventricular system.

During the second month of gestation, choroid plexi primordia develop, first as a mesenchymal invagination of the roof of the fourth ventricle, then by a similar invagination of the lateral and third ventricles (725). By the third month, the plexi fill 75% of the lateral ventricle and then begin to decrease in relative size. During the third trimester, the plexi become cellular and glycogen rich. After birth, glycogen is lost as the cells begin aerobic oxidation (726). Changes occur during fetal life in the intermediate filament protein content of ependyma and choroid plexus epithelial cells (727).

As the plexi develop in the second month, the fetal ventricles are large relative to the thickness of the cortical wall, and this relative dilatation disappears with further development of white and gray matter. It is not clear when CSF secretion is initiated, but complete circulation from ventricle to the subarachnoid spaces does not occur until after 2 months' gestation (728).

At this time, the fourth ventricle exit foramina develop. These are the foramina of Luschka, two lateral apical roof apertures leading to the pontine cistern, and the foramen of Magendie, a single median posterior roof aperture leading to the cisterna magna (729). Initially, the outlets from the fourth ventricle are covered with a membrane, which does not impair CSF outflow because drainage occurs via intercellular pores in the membrane. The membrane develops progressively larger pores and becomes progressively thinner until it no longer is present (729). The fully developed choroid plexi are outpouchings into the ventricular cavity of ependyma-lined blood vessels of the pia mater. Most of the CSF is produced within the ventricular system by the choroid plexi; however, a sizable proportion, some 10% to 20%, evidently is formed by the parenchyma of cerebrum and spinal cord (730).

The accepted view is that CSF bulk flow occurs from the site of its production in the ventricles to its absorption in the arachnoid (pacchionian) granulations. In the adult human, CSF is secreted at a rate of 500 mL per 24 hours, or between 0.2% and 0.5% of the total volume per minute (723,731). The rate of CSF formation ranges from 0.3 to 0.4 mL/min in children (732) and adults (724). Total CSF volume in the newborn is 50 mL and increases with age to an adult volume of 150 mL. At CSF pressures below 200 mm H_2O, production of CSF is independent of pressure (733); however, a prolonged and marked increase in intraventricular pressure owing to hydrocephalus can slightly reduce the rate of CSF formation (733).

The mechanisms responsible for the formation of CSF are primarily active and specific transport, simple diffusion, and carrier-mediated diffusion. The choroid plexus has the morphologic characteristics associated with secretory function. It has been compared with the proximal renal tubules in that it can both secrete and absorb a number of substances (734). Unlike parenchymal capillaries, in which the tight junctions between endothelial cells constitute the blood–brain barrier, the capillaries of the choroid plexus are fenestrated and devoid of tight junctions. Tight junctions are found on the astrocytic side of the choroid epithelium, however, and these constitute the blood–CSF barrier (734).

CSF is not quite an ultrafiltrate of plasma. Its concentrations of potassium, calcium, bicarbonate, and glucose are lower than in an ultrafiltrate, whereas those of sodium, chloride, and magnesium are higher. These small differences are important because they affect the excitability of neurons.

CSF appears to be formed in a two-step process. The first step is the formation by hydrostatic pressure of a plasma ultrafiltrate through the nontight-junctioned choroidal capillary endothelium into the connective tissue stroma beneath the epithelium of the villus. The passage is driven by hydrostatic pressure. The ultrafiltrate is transformed subsequently into a secretion by an active metabolic process within the choroidal epithelium. Although the exact mechanism for this process is unknown, one model suggests that sodium-and-potassium–activated adenosine triphosphatase pumps sodium into the basal side of the cell with water passively following the osmotic gradient thus created.

Carbonic anhydrase catalyzes the formation of bicarbonate inside the cell, with the hydrogen ion being fed back to the sodium pump as a counter-ion to potassium (723). In a manner analogous to that on the basal side of the epithelium, sodium-potassium adenosine triphosphatase located in the microvilli on the astrocytic surface extrudes sodium into the ventricle, followed by osmotically drawn water. Because the cells do not swell or shrink, the sum of the two processes must be in balance. Carbonic anhydrase is not specific to choroid plexus epithelial cells, however, and, in fact, is found in all secretory and ion-exchanging cells of the body, including kidney, intestinal mucosa, and endocrine glands.

The absorption of CSF depends in the main on bulk flow. Pulsatile movements of the CSF, as generated by the systolic expansion of the vasculature of the cerebral and basilar arterial systems, can be demonstrated by cine-MRI. No evidence exists, however, that they contribute significantly to the circulation of the CSF. Based on his data obtained by radiocisternography and gated MRI, Greitz argued that CSF flow is primarily pulsatile and that no significant bulk flow occurs except within the ventricles, notably in the aqueduct (735). He suggested that CSF absorption is not limited to the arachnoid granulations, but can occur anywhere in the CNS via the brain extracellular space, which communicates with the subarachnoid space.

Whatever the actual forces involved in CSF absorption, 80% enters directly into the cisternal system with subsequent drainage from the cerebral subarachnoid space into the cortical venous system; 20% circulates into the subarachnoid space of the spinal cord, but eventually is drained to a great extent from cerebral subarachnoid space, with lesser drainage from the spinal subarachnoid space into the spinal venous system. Spinal descent of CSF, however, might prove to be an important alternative pathway in pathologic conditions.

CSF drainage occurs in part by way of the arachnoidal villi and granulations. These are essentially microtubular envaginations of the subarachnoid space into the lumen of large dural and venous sinuses (736). The distinction between arachnoid villi and granulations is one of size, and arachnoid granulations probably develop from villi with increasing age. Arachnoid villi are present in the fetus and newborn infant; arachnoid granulations become evident by 18 months of age and are visible to the naked eye by 3 years of age (737). They are located principally in the parieto-occipital region of the superior sagittal sinus, in the lateral sinuses of the posterior fossa, and at dural reflections over cranial nerves.

Three factors control CSF drainage: CSF pressure, pressure within the dural sinuses and the cortical venous system, and resistance of the arachnoidal villi to CSF flow (738). Changes in any of these variables significantly affect CSF flow. Normally, pressure is greater in the subarachnoid CSF than in the sagittal sinus, whether the body is recumbent or erect. The normal lumbar CSF pressure is 150 mm H_2O in the laterally recumbent adult and up to

180 mm H_2O in the child, substantially greater than the mean pressure of 90 mm H_2O in the superior sagittal sinus. The capacity for drainage is two to four times the normal rate of CSF production (732).

The labyrinth of small tubules in the villi can behave as one-way valves, in that they are closed by high pressure in the venous sinus and opened by high CSF pressure (736). The factors that control CSF drainage in the human are uncertain, and the only proven force is that of a hydrostatic gradient. Increased CSF pressure does not facilitate the flow of macromolecules through the villi from the CSF, which suggests that the *valves* do not enlarge in response to increased pressure (739). Furthermore, it appears that drainage does not depend on the colloid osmotic pressure difference between CSF and sinus blood because the tubules are permeable to protein (736). Ultrastructural analysis of human specimens has failed to demonstrate the one-way valves of the villi seen in animals (740).

Experimental work with animals, including primates, suggests that a significant amount, perhaps as much as one-half, of the CSF drains through the lymphatics (741,742). To what extent this process exists in humans is unknown, but support for the concept comes from the clinical observation that children with an obstructed CSF-diverting shunt occasionally develop nasal congestion and periorbital or facial swelling. The lymphatic drainage of CSF might play a role in the pathophysiology of hydrocephalus, either as an alternative pathway for drainage or, in cases of impaired access to the lymphatic system, as a cause of hydrocephalus.

The question of whether CSF can be absorbed by the brain is unresolved. The penetration of substances into the periventricular region of hydrocephalic animals has been well documented (743). CT scans demonstrate periventricular hypodensity in the presence of hydrocephalus, the result of CSF migrating into the area surrounding the ventricles in the presence of increased intraventricular pressure (744). This hypodensity is confirmed by MRI studies that show increased signal intensity in the periventricular regions. The presence of CSF in brain parenchyma, however, does not necessarily equate with absorption of CSF, and experimental evidence supports the contention that the brain, rather than absorbing CSF, acts as a conduit for fluid to move from the ventricles into the subarachnoid spaces or into the prelymphatic channels of the blood vessels (745).

CSF also can drain from the subarachnoid spaces surrounding the cranial and spinal nerve root sleeves, with entry into the lymphatic system. Studies by Nabeshima and colleagues (746) showed that an outer arachnoid layer between the subarachnoid spaces and the dura functions as the blood–CSF barrier at this location. At higher-than-normal intraventricular pressures, this barrier can be disrupted with resultant penetration of macromolecules into the extracellular space of the dura mater and the dural lymphatic channels. It is possible that at high pressures, disruption of this arachnoid barrier permits significant absorption of CSF.

Pathogenesis

Any block in the CSF pathway from the site of formation to that of absorption results in increased CSF pressure. By convention, hydrocephalus is divided into noncommunicating and communicating forms. In noncommunicating hydrocephalus, the subarachnoid space is usually compressed; in communicating hydrocephalus it is enlarged. With one possible exception (discussed later), all hydrocephalic conditions are obstructive.

In noncommunicating hydrocephalus, the obstructive site is within the ventricular system, including the outlet foramina of the fourth ventricle. In communicating hydrocephalus, the obstruction occurs distal to the fourth ventricle foramina, in the cisterns or cerebral subarachnoid space itself.

A condition termed *external hydrocephalus* has been identified with increasing frequency by means of neuroimaging studies. It is seen in infants with enlarged heads or rapid head growth. In all instances, subarachnoid spaces are widened bilaterally in the frontal and sometimes in the frontoparietal regions. The ventricles are of normal size or only slightly enlarged. The condition gradually resolves during the second year of life, and the large majority of infants, 89% in the series of Alvarez and coworkers (747) and 100% in the series of Andersson and coworkers (748), are developmentally normal. External hydrocephalus is more common in premature infants, and in 88% of cases a family history of enlarged head exists (747). It probably results from a developmental delay in arachnoidal function, but could also be acquired residually on trauma, spontaneous subarachnoid hemorrhage, or infection.

CSF formation in hydrocephalus is normal or nearly normal (749). In compensated hydrocephalus, the rate of absorption equals the rate of formation, whereas in uncompensated hydrocephalus only a small fraction of the total amount formed is not absorbed. Because CSF formation is relatively constant, CSF pressure depends on the change in resistance to flow or absorption, the resistance to ventricular enlargement by brain elasticity, and the meninges, skull, and scalp. Thus, the intracranial pressure in an infant with hydrocephalus whose head can enlarge fairly easily can be just a little above normal, whereas the same impairment of flow in an older child or adult with more rigid sutures causes a greater and more rapid increase in pressure.

Impaired CSF absorption in communicating hydrocephalus can occur at some or all of the following sites: the arachnoid villi, lymphatic channels associated with the cranial and spinal nerves, lymphatic channels in the adventitia of the cerebral vessels, and arachnoid membrane. If

CSF outflow from the ventricles is blocked, as occurs in noncommunicating hydrocephalus, absorption could still occur through the adventitia of the blood vessels, through the stroma of the choroid plexus, and by passage of CSF through the extracellular space of the cortical mantle to reach the brain surface. Additional ways for CSF to exit the ventricles would be through the dilated spinal cord central canal (750) or through a fistulous opening created by a rupture of the ventricular system into the subarachnoid space at the lamina terminalis or the suprapineal recess (398).

The rate of ventricular enlargement depends on the degree to which the resistance to absorption has increased and on the distensibility of the ventricular system.

Regardless of the site of obstruction, it is the arterial pulse thrust, not only of the choroid plexus, but also of the cerebral arteries, that is believed to be responsible for compressing the ventricular wall, enlarging the ventricular cavity (751), and producing parenchymal disruption (752). This pulse thrust increases with increasing mean CSF pressure and splits the ventricular ependymal lining, as demonstrated in the experimental animal (752,753). Splitting of the ependymal lining, in turn, produces transependymal flow of CSF into white matter, resulting in spongy and edematous white matter, dissolution of nerve fibers, and a significant degree of neuronal and astrocytic swelling in the deep areas of gray matter (754). This transependymal flow, if it continues for long, is a likely cause of the loss of neural and glial tissue (cerebral atrophy), contributing to the thinning of the cerebral mantle. The more immediate cause of cerebral thinning, however, is the loss of extracellular water absorbed into the blood. A reversal of this process allows the remarkably rapid reduction in ventricular size that can be observed when the ventricular pressure is relieved by drainage or shunting.

Additionally, the cilia that normally cover the ependymal surfaces of the ventricular walls disappear (755). The impact of their loss on CSF dynamics and metabolism is unknown. Also unclear is the extent to which normally nonfunctioning drainage routes, including the choroid plexi and the periventricular capillaries, become operative with increased CSF pressure and contribute to equalizing the rates of CSF formation and absorption in the human hydrocephalic patient. However, in both hydrocephalic animals (756,757) and humans (758), stabilization of ventricular pressure and the cessation of growth of the ventricular cavity appear to result from the availability of these other drainage pathways. In hydrocephalic children, ventricular pressure varies greatly with respiration, cardiovascular changes, and activity (759). Because ventricular pressure is increased by sucking and crying, normal pressure and high-pressure hydrocephalus might be the same phenomenon, differing only in time and rate of development, degree of obstruction, and parenchymal integrity (748).

Additionally, the combination of ventriculomegaly and increased intracranial pressure can produce brain damage by reducing cerebral blood flow, in particular through the anterior cerebral arteries, and thus lead to ischemic injury of the cerebral cortex adjacent to the interhemispheric fissure and the basal forebrain (760).

Pathology

The three general causes of hydrocephalus are excess secretion caused by choroid plexus papilloma, obstruction within the ventricular cavity (noncommunicating hydrocephalus), and absorptive block within the subarachnoid space (communicating hydrocephalus).

Excess Secretion Caused by Choroid Plexus Papilloma

The papilloma is a large aggregate of choroidal fronds that are microscopically similar to normal choroid plexi and produce great quantities of CSF. Accounting for 1% to 4% of childhood intracranial tumors, they usually occur after infancy and are associated with signs of increased intracranial pressure, although some of the more than 400 reported cases were found incidentally at postmortem examination. Whereas in a number of instances the mass effect of the tumor or the presence of proteinaceous and xanthochromic CSF, most likely the result of bleeding stemming from the neoplasm, suggested that obstruction of CSF flow is responsible for hydrocephalus, preoperative and postoperative studies of CSF production substantiated earlier suggestions that, in at least some cases, the tumor produces hydrocephalus by CSF oversecretion (761,762).

Obstruction within the Ventricular Cavity

Any obstruction from the foramina of Monro or to the foramina of Magendie and Luschka produces noncommunicating hydrocephalus. Space-occupying lesions in the cerebral hemispheres tend to compress the ventricular system, whereas tumors in the posterior fossa or arteriovenous malformations involving the vein of Galen can produce kinking or obstruction of the aqueduct or obstruction at the fourth ventricular outflow. These conditions are discussed in Chapter 11. The other, more complex causes of aqueductal obstruction are discussed here.

Aqueductal Stenosis. Aqueductal stenosis is responsible for 20% of cases of hydrocephalus. Its incidence ranges from 0.5 to 1.0 in 1,000 births, with a recurrence risk in siblings of 1.0% to 4.5% (763). Normally, the aqueduct, lined by ependyma, is 3 mm in length at birth and its mean cross section is 0.5 mm^2 (764), with the cross-sectional area ranging from 0.2 to 1.8 mm^2 (765). The cross section is somewhat larger in the fetus, but after birth does not change significantly with age. In aqueductal stenosis, the aqueduct is smaller but remains histologically normal. In particular, no gliosis is present. Constrictions of the aqueduct to less than 0.14 mm^2 can occur at two points: The first is beneath the midline of the superior quadrigeminal bodies and the second is at the intercollicular sulcus (766).

The onset of symptoms is usually insidious and can occur at any time from birth to adulthood. In many instances, aqueductal stenosis is accompanied by aqueductal forking or marked branching of the channels. Associated malformations in neighboring structures are common. These include fusion of the quadrigeminal bodies, fusion of the third nerve nuclei, and more-caudal defects of neural tube closure such as spina bifida cystica or occulta. These associated anomalies raise the possibility that aqueductal stenosis itself probably represents a mild expression of a neural tube defect (767).

A small percentage of the anomalies (approximately 2%) are caused by one or more sex-linked recessive genes (768). This entity, more correctly known as X-linked hydrocephalus because not all cases actually have aqueductal stenosis as the only basis, has been shown to be caused by a mutation in the *L1* gene, the product of which is a member of the superfamily of cell adhesion molecules (768,769). Numerous such mutations have been documented (769). Yamasaki and colleagues divided them into three groups. Mutations that disrupt only the cytoplasmic domain of *L1* result in the mildest phenotype. Point mutations and truncations of the *L1* extracellular domain produce a more severe phenotype with pronounced hydrocephalus and profound mental retardation (769). This disorder also results in pachygyria and polymicrogyria, and the acronym of CRASH syndrome has been proposed to account for the major features of the disorders: corpus callosum hypoplasia, retardation, adducted thumbs, spastic paraplegia, and hydrocephalus (769). The presence of these malformations helps to explain the intellectual, cognitive, and motor handicaps even after the hydrocephalus is compensated by shunting (770).

In at least some instances, noninflammatory aqueductal stenosis is the consequence of inapparent viral infections (see Chapter 7).

Aqueductal Gliosis. Aqueductal gliosis, a postinfectious noninflammatory process, is usually secondary to a perinatal infection or hemorrhage. With the increasing survival of newborns affected with bacterial meningitis or intracranial hemorrhage, this condition has assumed greater importance. The ependymal lining is permanently destroyed because it is highly vulnerable to insult and cannot regenerate; the aqueduct is replaced by multiple ependymal cell clusters and rosettes of blind tubules (771). Marked fibrillary gliosis of adjacent tissue is evident, and the occlusion is progressive. As with aqueductal stenosis, its onset is insidious. No foreign inflammatory cells are found in the region of the cerebral aqueduct either during the period of active fetal infection or afterward (772).

Aqueductal gliosis occasionally accompanies neurofibromatosis. A variant, also postinflammatory, appears as a septal obstruction at the caudal end of the aqueduct. This obstruction is the result of a membrane of neuroglial overgrowth associated with "granular ependymitis," though this term is not acccurate because it is not an inflammatory condition (506). Aqueductal stenosis and gliosis have been produced in experimental animals by intrauterine viral infections, and a patient has been reported with aqueductal stenosis after mumps encephalitis (see Chapter 7).

Descending from the ventricular system, the next major area of obstruction is at the fourth ventricle. This is the site of obstruction in approximately one-half of hydrocephalic children.

Chiari Malformations. Chiari malformations, congenital malformations involving the fourth ventricle, which alone or combined with other anomalies account for 40% of all hydrocephalic children, are discussed in the prior Chiari Malformation section.

Dandy-Walker Malformation. Dandy-Walker malformation, described in 1914 by Dandy and Blackfan (773), is characterized by a triad of complete or partial agenesis of the cerebellar vermis, cystic dilatation of the fourth ventricle, and an enlarged posterior fossa with upward displacement of the transverse sinuses, tentorium, and torcular (774). The basic embryonic failure in this malformation is controversial. It is unrelated to occlusion of the foramina of Luschka and Magendie for three reasons. First, the foramina are open in as many as 80% of patients. Second, the associated malformations of vermis and fourth ventricle occur before development of the foramina, which is after the fourth month of gestation in the case of the foramen of Magendie and even later for the foramina of Luschka (73). Third, the lack of massive hydrocephalus at birth in most infants suggests that CSF circulation is present at that time. The best explanation is that of Benda and others, who consider the Dandy-Walker syndrome to be a defect of neural tube closure at the cerebellar level occurring at approximately 4 weeks' gestation (774,775). Of uncertain relevance to humans is a phylogenetic perspective that many birds normally have an expanded posterior membrane of the fourth ventricle without apertures, resembling a Dandy-Walker malformation, and the large membrane permits sufficient transudate of fluid between the fourth ventricle and subarachnoid space to provide adequate CSF flow.

The most striking abnormality is the presence of a hugely dilated fourth ventricle that acts as a cyst and is roofed by a neuroglial-vascular membrane lined with ependyma. This cyst herniates caudally and separates the cerebellar hemispheres posteriorly, displacing them anteriorly and laterally (Fig. 5.22). The vermis and choroid plexi are rudimentary. The foramina of the fourth ventricle

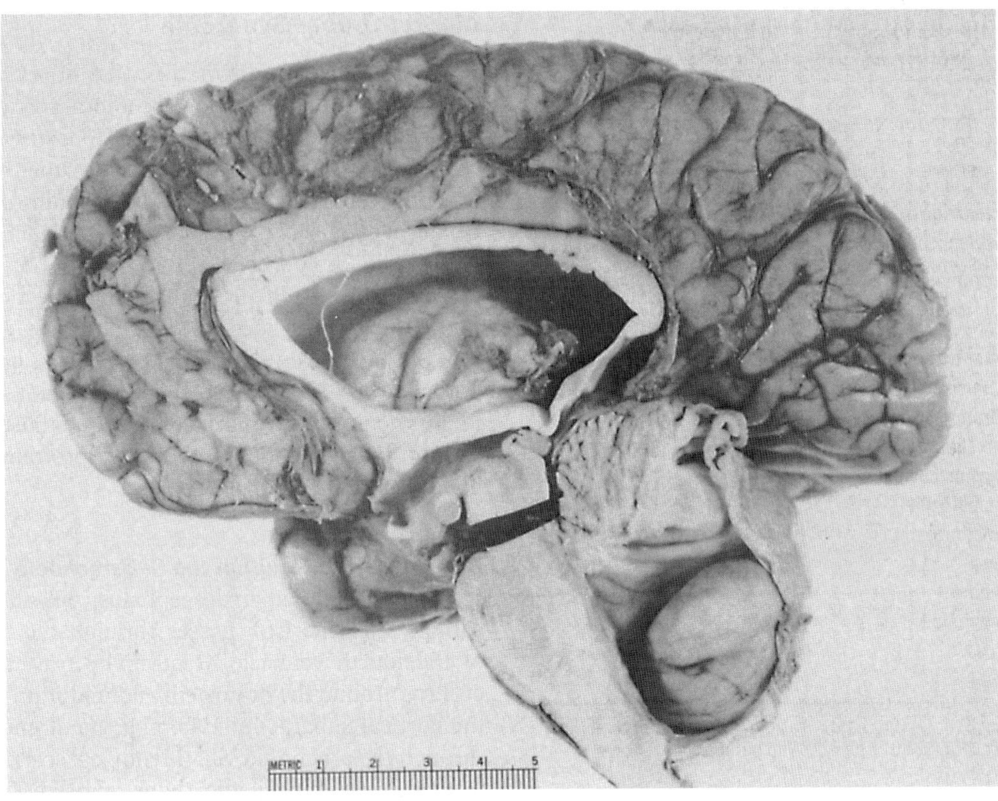

FIGURE 5.22. Dandy-Walker syndrome with obstruction of the foramina of Magendie and Luschka. Midsagittal section showing the absence of posterior cerebellar tissue. A dilatation of the fourth ventricle and a huge cyst within the posterior fossa confluent with the fourth ventricle are seen. The tentorium is displaced upward, and the lateral ventricle is markedly enlarged. (Courtesy of Dr. Hideo H. Itabashi, Department of Pathology, Los Angeles County Harbor Medical Center, Torrance, CA.)

are often occluded by membranes or are atretic. Hart and coworkers, however, were able to demonstrate patency of the foramen of Magendie in 7% of their cases (774).

Other associated neural and systemic anomalies include agenesis of the corpus callosum, aqueductal stenosis, occipital encephalocele, polymicrogyria, syringomyelia, heterotopias, facial angiomas, midline cleft palate, cardiovascular malformations, and polycystic kidneys (775,776).

A variant in which cystic dilatation of the fourth ventricle and hypoplasia of the cerebellar vermis exists without enlargement of the posterior fossa is more common than the classic Dandy-Walker malformation and accounts for one-third of posterior fossa malformations. A number of supratentorial malformations accompany this condition (506). The diagnosis of "Dandy-Walker variant" is frequently made by both radiologists and clinicians but often is meaningless because there are no firm imaging criteria. Some of these cases represent nothing more than megacisterna magna, a normal variant, some are arachnoidal cysts of the posterior fossa, and some are Joubert syndrome or other cerebellar hypoplasias. This "diagnosis" should, therefore, be critically reviewed and not accepted at face value.

The Dandy-Walker syndrome also must be distinguished from retrocerebellar arachnoidal cysts (mega cisterna magna) and posterior fossa arachnoid cysts (777). In mega cisterna magna the vermis is intact, the cisterna magna is markedly enlarged, and the posterior fossa is enlarged. Mental retardation caused by associated supratentorial anomalies is common. In posterior fossa arachnoid cysts, symptoms arise from hydrocephalus, which occasionally is accompanied by cerebellar deficits (506).

The incidence of Dandy-Walker syndrome is 1 per 25,000 to 30,000 births, with the condition having a slight predilection for girls (776). Hydrocephalus is not present at birth; it appears by 3 months of age in some 75% of infants, and the diagnosis is established by 1 year of age in 80%. In some instances, hydrocephalus fails to develop and the condition remains asymptomatic throughout life (775). In addition to the clinical features outlined in Table 5.19, infants can have a large occiput, with an inion that is higher than normal. They can experience recurrent attacks of pallor, ataxia, and abnormal respirations. In the series of Tal and coworkers, 7 of 10 infants died of sudden respiratory arrest (775). Because in 5 of those 7 infants

TABLE 5.19 Clinical Features in 40 Cases of Dandy-Walker Syndrome

Disorder	*Number of Cases*
Macrocrania	29
Hypotonia	10
Headache and vomiting	6
Downwardly displaced eyeballs	6
Spasticity	3
Hemiparesis	1
Seizures	6
Enlarged posterior fossa	6
Seventh-nerve palsy	1
Cerebellar syndrome	1
Associated anomalies	
Agenesis of corpus callosum	3
Occipital encephalocele	7
Hemispheric malformation	1
Facial angiomas	4
Malformed fingers	2
Onset of hydrocephalus	
At birth	6
By 1 yr of age	31

Adapted from Hirsh JF, et al. The Dandy-Walker malformation: a review of 40 cases. *J Neurosurg* 1984;61:515–522. With permission.

previously placed ventricular shunts were patent, pressure of the cyst on the pontine respiratory center appears likely. Mental retardation is common and is probably the consequence of cortical malformations. In the series of Maria and coworkers 47% of children had normal intelligence, another 26% had learning disabilities, and the remainder had moderate or severe delay (778). The syndrome also is associated with a number of other conditions, including the Klippel-Feil syndrome, Cornelia de Lange syndrome, Rubinstein-Taybi syndrome, and hypertelorism.

Correction of hydrocephalus involves cystoperitoneal, ventriculoperitoneal, or both kinds of shunts (775,776). Cystoperitoneal shunting, because it avoids the risk of an entrapped fourth ventricle, is considered by many to be the best procedure for this condition (776). Fewer shunt malfunctions occur in part because the cyst does not collapse (779). Curless and coworkers suggested that cine-MRI be used to determine the presence of aqueductal flow and that if normal flow is present, a single posterior ventricular shunt can safely be placed (780). McLaurin and Crone stated that the incidence of aqueductal stenosis is sufficiently high to warrant Y shunting of the cyst and the lateral ventricles or shunting of the cyst (779).

Other conditions that frequently obstruct fourth ventricular outflow are space-occupying lesions, particularly those involving the posterior fossa. Less often, a retrocerebellar subdural hematoma or bacterial or granulomatous meningitis occludes the foramina of Magendie and Luschka (781).

Meckel-Grüber Syndrome

This syndrome is a distinctive triad of severe malformations of the brain, consisting of cerebral cortical dysgenesis reminiscent of lissencephaly type II, posterior encephalocele, and rhombic roof dysgenesis. Other, less constant features reported include Chiari malformation, cerebellar hypoplasia, micrencephaly, arhinencephaly, polymicrogyria, holoprosencephaly, and even anencephaly (782). Obstructive hydrocephalus may be a complication. The pathogenesis is probably a defective ventral induction of the neural tube by the prechordal mesoderm and notochord. A specific genetic basis is not known. Most infants do not survive early infancy, and those who do with extraordinary supportive care have profound neurologic handicaps and a poor prognosis.

Absorptive Block within the Subarachnoid Space

Of all childhood hydrocephalus, 30% are communicating. After the CSF passes through the exit foramina of the fourth ventricle, it normally traverses the basal cisterns around the brainstem and midbrain on the way to the cortical subarachnoid compartment and is absorbed through the arachnoid villi. Meningeal scarring can result from subarachnoid hemorrhage or bacterial meningitis. When this scarring occludes the exits from the cisterns or involves the arachnoid villi, the CSF circulation is impeded. The resulting increase in intracranial pressure then enlarges not only the four ventricles, but also the subarachnoid compartment over the cerebral hemispheres.

Intraventricular hemorrhage is common in premature infants, particularly in babies weighing less than 1,500 g. Subarachnoid hemorrhage is usually seen in both premature and full-term infants. The pathogenesis and pathology of these conditions are discussed in Chapter 6. The fibrosis of the pacchionian granulations is so slow that decompensation and hydrocephalus often do not present clinically until 6 to 12 months after the perinatal hemorrhagic event.

Meningitis can produce communicating hydrocephalus in the acute phase by the clumping of purulent fluid in the drainage channels and in the chronic phase by the organizing of exudate and blood, resulting in fibrosis of the subarachnoid spaces (see Chapter 7). As a rule, bacterial meningitis tends to produce cerebral cortical arachnoiditis, whereas granulomatous or parasitic meningitis produces cisternal obstruction. Rarely, viral meningitis can result in obstruction at either point. Intrauterine infections are discussed in Chapter 7.

Two causes of communicating hydrocephalus, although uncommon, deserve mention. The first is a diffuse meningeal malignant tumor caused by lymphoma or leukemia. This condition is discussed in Chapter 17. The second is an extra-axial arachnoid cyst that can be located in the basal cistern, over the cerebral cortex, or in the paramesencephalic region (783). This condition is considered later in this chapter.

Finally, chronic obstruction of the vein of Galen or the major sinuses has been held responsible for communicating hydrocephalus. Rosman and Shands postulated that increased intracranial venous pressure produces hydrocephalus if the patient is under 18 months of age. If increased venous pressure develops in a child older than 3 years of age, pseudotumor cerebri is more likely to result. The difference in response to venous obstruction might relate to an expansile calvarium and softer, less myelinated periventricular parenchyma in the infant, which permit greater ventricular dilatation under high pressure (784). Little experimental evidence supports this clinical impression (785). Occasionally, however, large space-occupying lesions within the posterior fossa can cause hydrocephalus without impinging on the fourth ventricle, perhaps as the result of venous obstruction.

Other Types of Hydrocephalus

Normal-Pressure Hydrocephalus (Hakim Syndrome) and Arrested (Compensated) Hydrocephalus

With advancing diagnostic and surgical technology, these conditions, which can be seen with any of the various types of hydrocephalus, have assumed increased importance (786). Normal-pressure hydrocephalus, conceptually and clinically defined primarily by Hakim, is an instance of indolently progressive hydrocephalus in which CSF pressure is within the physiologic range but in which a marked increase in CSF pulse pressure results in slow ventricular expansion and progressive white matter damage (787). The cause and pathophysiology of the condition are poorly understood, and the condition may represent a primary disorder in the cerebral parenchyma rather than a compromise of CSF compensatory pressure mechanisms (788). The pathogenesis of normal-pressure hydrocephalus, as it is seen in the elderly, undoubtedly differs from that in infants and children, in whom the most common cause is communicating hydrocephalus with incomplete arachnoidal obstruction to CSF drainage. Primary events include neonatal intraventricular hemorrhage, spontaneous subarachnoid hemorrhage, intracranial trauma, infections, and surgery (788,789). The clinical presentation in childhood resembles that seen in adult life. In the series of Bret and Chazal, psychomotor retardation, psychotic-like behavior, gait abnormalities, and sphincter disturbances were seen in a large proportion of children (789).

Arrested hydrocephalus occurs when CSF formation and absorption are in balance and no more CSF accumulates. Milhorat (790) defined arrested hydrocephalus as the surgical or spontaneous termination of a hydrocephalic condition, with subsequent return to normal of the pressure gradient across the cerebral mantle. Others regard this condition as hydrocephalus that has been treated or resolved rather than arrested, and they are skeptical about whether hydrocephalus can ever be truly arrested. Indeed, in some patients, hydrocephalus can progress so slowly that the advancing neurologic dysfunction becomes evident only over the course of several years. In other cases, hydrocephalus becomes reactivated after a seemingly insignificant head trauma or viral illness. Even if no further net accumulation of CSF occurs, the increased resistance to CSF absorption establishes a new equilibrium at an increased intracranial pressure.

As a consequence, the head circumference is usually near or above the 97th percentile, and if above the 97th percentile, it generally parallels it. On neuroimaging studies, the ventricles are moderately to markedly dilated. The larger the ventricles, the less likely it is that ventricular size will further increase. On clinical evaluation, these children tend to be clumsy and uncoordinated, with verbal IQ better than performance IQ. Tone and deep tendon reflexes are often increased, and optic atrophy, papilledema, and visual field defects can be present.

Fetal Hydrocephalus

The advent and refinement of high-resolution ultrasonography and CT has allowed the prenatal diagnosis of much fetal pathology. In particular, the diagnosis of hydrocephalus has made it possible to consider intrauterine shunting of ventricular fluid into the amniotic sac (791,792). More recently, a rapid technique of fetal MRI that allows good-resolution images without the requirement for sedation to abolish fetal movements has become the best modality for the demonstration of fetal brain pathology (793). The majority of fetuses that have undergone such shunting have had aqueductal stenosis or communicating hydrocephalus. Treatment at present must be regarded as experimental in view of the inability to be sure that intraventricular pressure is high relative to the intrauterine pressure together with our imperfect knowledge of the natural history of fetal hydrocephalus. A number of factors need to be considered before surgery is selected. These include the presence of other CNS malformations such as spina bifida cystica and the Chiari deformity. It is usually considered wrong to attempt amelioration of hydrocephalus in such cases. Karyotyping and screening of the family for X-linked hydrocephalus are also necessary. Renier and coworkers stressed that antenatal ventriculomegaly is not synonymous with hydrocephalus, and a significant proportion of infants with ventriculomegaly are found to have normal CSF pressures after birth (794). It is also difficult to determine from ultrasonography alone whether hydrocephalus is so severe that treatment is contraindicated or whether it is sufficiently mild to allow the pregnancy to go to term (795).

In approximately one-half of the cases collected by Glick and coworkers, hydrocephalus was accompanied by other major anomalies that precluded treatment (795). Even when treatment is selected, the outlook is poor. In Renier's series of 106 infants with hydrocephalus at birth, 62% survived to 10 years of age. Of the survivors, 28% had IQs above 80 and 50% had IQs below 50 (794). Although grim, this prognosis is still better than that for infants who develop hydrocephalus secondary to a perinatal intraventricular hemorrhage.

If intrauterine surgery is elected, the shunt should be inserted before 32 weeks' gestation. If at ventriculostomy the pressure is less than 60 mm H_2O, the insertion of a shunting tube might not be justified. The current mortality for this procedure is 15% to 20%. Follow-up ultrasonographic studies may document an arrest of progressive ventricular enlargement or decompression. At birth, the shunt is converted to a ventriculoperitoneal bypass.

Clinical Manifestations

Four major factors influence the clinical course in hydrocephalus: the time of onset, the duration of increased intracranial pressure, the rate at which intracranial pressure increases, and any preexisting structural lesions. The time when hydrocephalus develops in relation to closure of the cranial sutures determines whether enlargement of the head is the presenting sign. Before 2 years of age, progressive enlargement of the head is almost invariably a presenting complaint. When hydrocephalus develops after 2 years of age, any changes in head circumference are overshadowed by other neurologic manifestations. In older infants and children, the space-occupying lesions responsible for hydrocephalus often produce focal neurologic signs before causing CSF obstruction.

Neonatal Period through Infancy (0 to 2 Years)

Hydrocephalus causing an abnormally large head or abnormally accelerating head growth during this time is usually caused by a major defect in embryogenesis. Chiari malformations with or without spina bifida cystica, aqueductal stenosis, and aqueductal gliosis account for 80% of all hydrocephalus in this period and represent 60% of all hydrocephalus regardless of age (796). The remainder of cases are a consequence of intrauterine infection, anoxic or traumatic perinatal hemorrhage, and neonatal bacterial or viral meningoencephalitis. Rare causes include congenital midline tumor, choroid plexus papilloma, and arteriovenous malformation of the vein of Galen or straight sinus. Apart from the features unique to each disease, they all produce a stereotyped clinical picture.

The etiology, presenting signs, management, and sequels of perinatal intracranial hemorrhage are described in Chapter 6.

The head grows at an abnormal rate and is macrocephalic within 12 months, if not at birth. The forehead is disproportionately large, giving an inverted triangular appearance to the head. The skull is thin, hair can be sparse, and the sutures are excessively separated. This results in an accentuated *cracked-pot* sound on percussion of the skull. The anterior fontanelle is tense and the scalp veins are dilated, strikingly so when the infant cries. A divergent strabismus with the eyeballs rotated downward is often noted. This *setting-sun sign* is caused by pressure of the third ventricle's suprapineal recess on the mesencephalic tectum, causing impairment of the vertical gaze centers. The sign, however, also can be elicited in healthy infants (see Introduction chapter). Other ocular disturbances include unilateral or bilateral abducens nerve paresis, nystagmus, ptosis, and a diminished pupillary light response. Optic atrophy caused by compression of the chiasm and optic nerves by a dilated anterior portion of the third ventricle can occur. Papilledema is rare, perhaps because of the presence of open sutures.

Early infantile automatisms persist, indicating a failure in the development of normal cortical inhibition. Responses such as the parachute reflex, which is expected to appear later in infancy, fail to develop. Opisthotonus can be striking. A common finding is spasticity of the lower extremities, resulting from proportionately more stretching and distortion of myelinated paracentral corticospinal fibers arising from the leg area of the motor cortex. These fibers have a longer distance to travel around the dilated ventricle than do the corticospinal and corticobulbar fibers supplying the upper extremities and face. Mild spasticity and weakness, however, occur in the upper limbs. Clinical signs are caused more by myelin disruption than by cellular loss (797).

Of great importance is the development of deranged lower brainstem function caused by bilateral corticobulbar disruption, a condition termed *pseudobulbar palsy*. This is manifested by difficulty in sucking, feeding, and phonation, and results in regurgitation, drooling, and aspiration. Laryngeal stridor, although not common, is distressing. Some of these symptoms also can be the consequence of an associated Chiari II malformation, causing vagal nerve traction or perhaps infarction of the vagal nuclei in the medulla. Corticobulbar deficits together with a change in acoustic properties of brain and calvarium are believed to account for the characteristic shrill, brief, and high-pitched cry.

Other features of early infantile hydrocephalus relate more to specific causes. The clinical picture of Dandy-Walker syndrome is fairly characteristic and is covered in another section of this chapter (see Dandy-Walker Malformation section).

The Chiari malformation type II is almost always associated with meningomyelocele and, occasionally, with a short, malformed neck that results from basilar impression or the Klippel-Feil anomaly.

If hydrocephalus is rapidly progressive, as in acute bacterial meningitis or diffuse cortical thrombophlebitis, then emesis, somnolence, irritability, seizures, and cardiopulmonary embarrassment occur despite open sutures. Neonates with severe hydrocephalus associated with congenital anomalies usually do not survive the neonatal period.

Early to Late Childhood (2 to 10 Years)

In this age group, neurologic symptoms caused by increased intracranial pressure or by focal deficits referable to the primary lesion tend to appear before any significant changes in head size.

The most common causes for hydrocephalus during this period of life are posterior fossa neoplasms and obstructions at the aqueduct. The Chiari type I malformation, with abnormalities of the craniobasal bones and cervical vertebrae, also can be encountered in this age group.

The clinical picture of the various space-occupying lesions is discussed in Chapter 11. A unique hydrocephalic syndrome (the bobble-head doll syndrome) is characterized by two to four head oscillations per second, psychomotor retardation, and obstructive lesions in or around the third ventricle or aqueduct (798). It is important to recognize that head bobbing can be a sign of obstructive hydrocephalus in which, it is postulated, a dilated third ventricle impinges on the medial aspect of the dorsomedial nucleus of the thalamus.

Between 2 and 10 years of age, the infections most likely to cause hydrocephalus are tuberculosis and fungal or parasitic infections. Hydrocephalus resulting from any one of these agents has its special features; however, in almost all instances, increased intracranial pressure produces papilledema, strabismus, and headache on awakening in the morning that improves after emesis or upright posture. The cracked-pot sound is prominent on skull percussion. Pyramidal tract signs are more marked in the lower limbs for reasons noted previously.

Additional features seen in this late-onset group are encountered also in the early-onset group in whom hydrocephalus has become arrested or marginally compensated, either spontaneously or because of surgical intervention. These features include endocrine changes resulting in small stature with growth hormone deficiency (799), obesity, gigantism, delayed or precocious puberty, primary amenorrhea or menstrual irregularities, absent secondary sexual characteristics, hypothyroidism, and diabetes insipidus (800,801). They are probably caused by abnormal hypothalamic–pituitary axis function, which is a consequence of compression of this axis by an enlarged third ventricle, a particular risk in aqueductal stenosis. Spastic diplegia is prominent, and both upper limbs exhibit mild pyramidal tract signs resulting in fine motor incoordination. Perceptual motor deficits and visual–spatial disorganization ensue as a consequence of stretched corticospinal fibers of parietal and occipital cortex owing to dilated posterior horns of the lateral ventricles. Performance intelligence is considerably worse than verbal intelligence and learning problems are common (802). Some children are sociable and conversationally bright and exhibit relatively good memory, but they are often hyperkinetic, emotionally labile, and unable to conceptualize (803).

Diagnosis

In infants, the initial diagnosis of hydrocephalus is based on a head circumference that, regardless of absolute size, crosses one or more grid lines (1 cm on the chart; see Introduction chapter, Fig. I.1, and Fig. 5.23). Such infants require prompt diagnostic evaluation, even when overt neurologic signs are absent.

An evaluation of a premature infant for possible hydrocephalus must take into account its normal postnatal head growth (804). In preterm infants whose weight is appropriate for gestational age, head growth velocity increases progressively after birth, with maximum velocity occurring between 30 and 40 days (805). The less mature the infant, the smaller are the initial increments of head growth and the later is the time of maximal growth. The initial delay of head growth and probably of brain growth is related, in part, to the presence of respiratory distress and possibly also to exposure to oxygen (806). It does not correlate with caloric intake. A special head circumference chart applicable to preterm infants was compiled by Babson and Benda (Fig. 5.23) (807).

Because acceleration of skull growth occurs later than increase in ventricular size, skull circumference measurements poorly reflect the increase in ventricular size. This is particularly the case for children older than age 18 months, in whom head circumference might not be abnormally large in the presence of hydrocephalus.

Various diagnostic studies of different complexities are used for the diagnosis of hydrocephalus and increased ventricular size. Transillumination of the skull is the least complex diagnostic study; nowadays, unfortunately, it is only rarely used (808).

Ultrasonography has proven to be invaluable in monitoring the ventricular system in infants with hydrocephalus (Fig. 5.24). Because the technique does not delineate intracranial anatomy as well as CT scans or MRI, its value lies not so much in establishing the diagnosis of hydrocephalus as in permitting sequential assessment of the adequacy of medical and surgical therapy (809,810). Fetal ultrasonography also has been useful in the diagnosis of hydrocephalus and Dandy-Walker syndrome (811).

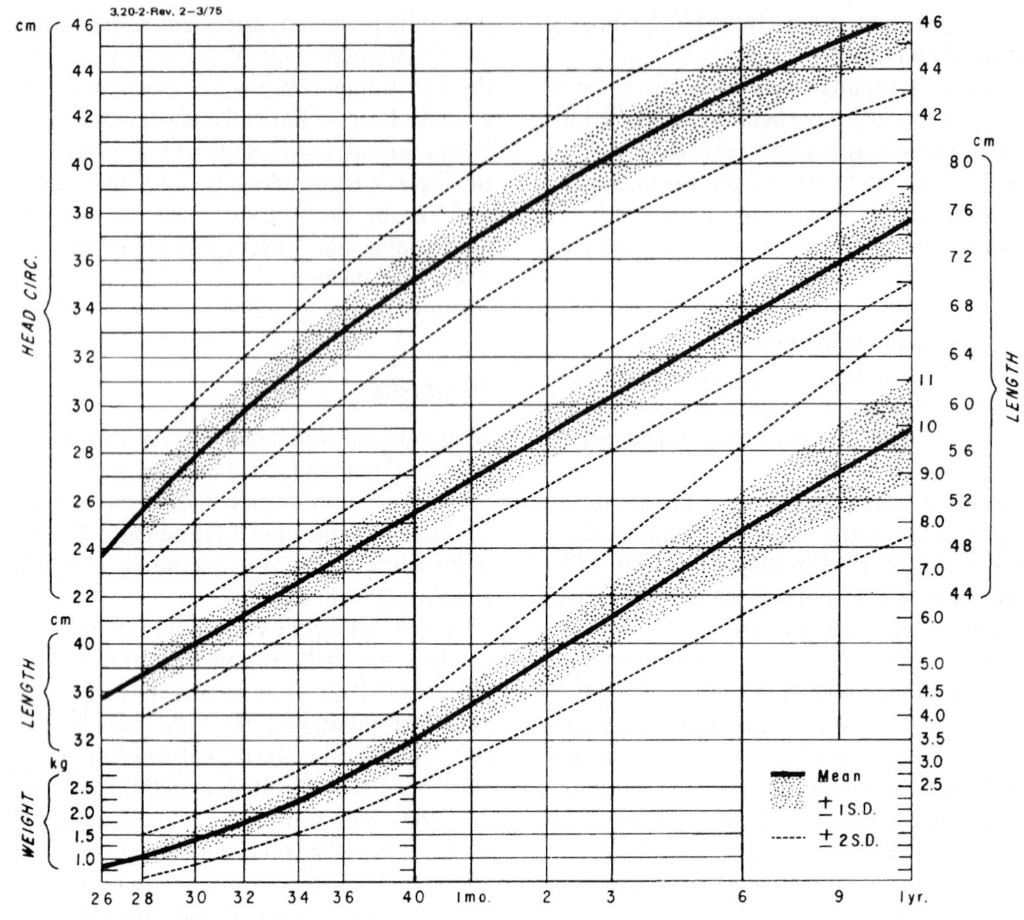

FIGURE 5.23. A fetal–infant growth graph for infants of varying gestational ages. (Courtesy of Dr. S. G. Babson, Department of Pediatrics, University of Oregon School of Medicine, Portland, OR.)

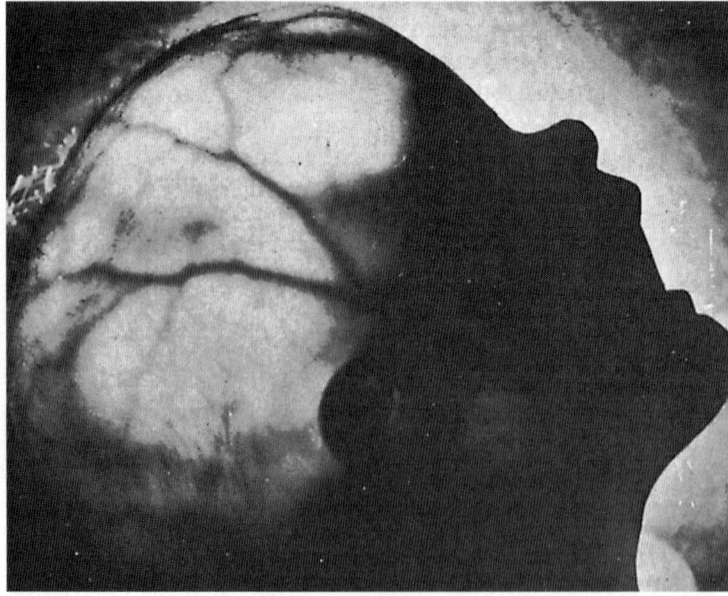

FIGURE 5.24. Hydrocephalus in a neonate. Coronal ultrasonographic scan of hydrocephalus in a 2-day-old child with lumbosacral myelomeningocele. Marked dilatation of the bodies of the lateral ventricles (*LV*) and their temporal horns (*LVt*) is present. The third ventricle (*V3*) is enlarged also, but to a lesser degree. (From Babcock DS, Han BK. The accuracy of high-resolution, real-time, ultrasonography of the head in infancy. *Radiology* 1981;139:665. With permission.)

Although in the past CT scans have proven of value in the diagnostic evaluation of the infant or child with hydrocephalus, we believe that MRI is the preferred procedure. It demonstrates not only the size and position of the ventricles, but also the width of the subarachnoid spaces at the base of the brain and over its convexity. It is also the preferred means for measuring changes in ventricular size after a shunting procedure.

MRI is also the optimal method for determining the cause of the hydrocephalus. The Dandy-Walker syndrome can be diagnosed by observing an enlarged fourth ventricle and a large posterior fossa cyst on sagittal views. Communicating hydrocephalus manifests by dilatation of the entire ventricular system and the subarachnoid spaces at the base of the brain and over the lower portion of the convexity. Aqueductal stenosis can be demonstrated by the dilatation of the lateral and third ventricles, the presence of a normal-sized or small fourth ventricle, and absence of the normal flow-related signal void in the aqueduct (812,813).

It is sometimes difficult to distinguish between ventricular enlargement secondary to hydrocephalus and that resulting from white matter atrophy. Some findings that point to hydrocephalus include dilatation of the temporal horns commensurate with dilatation of the lateral ventricles, enlargement of the anterior and posterior recesses of the third ventricle, and effacement of the cortical sulci (814).

A high-resolution axial technique can be used to quantitate CSF flow through the aqueduct and is a useful adjunct to MRI (815). Additionally, MRI can delineate a variety of cerebral anomalies and readily excludes the presence of tumors or larger arteriovenous malformations. Differentiation of normal and increased pressure hydrocephalus by MRI studies is under investigation (816,817). Cine-MRI also holds great promise in the evaluation of CSF dynamics in obstructive and communicative hydrocephalus (818,819).

Information concerning CSF clearance, particularly in patients with normal-pressure hydrocephalus, is provided by radioisotope cisternography. This procedure consists of the injection into the lumbar sac or cisterna of ^{131}I-labeled serum albumin, technetium, or indium (820). Emission of gamma radiation is measured by an external scanner. In communicating hydrocephalus, the radioisotope collects entirely within the ventricular system and persists there for 24 to 48 hours (821). In noncommunicating hydrocephalus and in healthy individuals, no retrograde filling is present. In the healthy individual, all the supratentorial cisterns are well visualized within 4 hours. By 12 to 24 hours, the radioisotope is concentrated over the cerebral convexities toward the parasagittal area. By 48 hours, the CSF is clear.

When hydrocephalus develops after infancy, children show symptoms and signs of increased intracranial pressure. Their diagnostic evaluation is similar to that suggested for tumor suspects (see Chapter 11).

Treatment

The general principles of treatment are surgical correction of CSF obstruction, reduction of CSF production by drugs or surgical therapy, ventricular bypass into a normal intracranial channel in noncommunicating hydrocephalus, and ventricular bypass into an extracranial compartment in either noncommunicating or communicating hydrocephalus.

In the child with rapidly progressive hydrocephalus of whatever cause, the need for therapy is obvious. However, the patient in whom hydrocephalus progresses slowly or who is suspected of having an arrested process presents a difficult therapeutic problem (822). Ultimately, clinical findings and serial imaging studies will determine whether treatment is indicated. At present, we believe that the diagnosis of arrested hydrocephalus cannot be made in a patient with macrocephaly despite a normal head growth curve and normal CSF pressures unless ventricular size stabilizes as ascertained by imaging studies (786,790). We concur with the suggestion of McLone and Aronyk that children older than 3 years of age with stable ventricular size be monitored if their intellectual performance is within the normal range and appears stable (822). Children younger than 3 years of age with large ventricles should be shunted if doubt exists, because the outcome of nontreatment is uncertain.

Ventriculomegaly after meningitis or in conjunction with spina bifida cystica does not require a shunting procedure unless serial imaging studies demonstrate it to be progressive. Once progression has become evident, needless procrastination or failure to treat can result in further compromise of both cognitive function and fine and gross motor coordination. The underlying cause of hydrocephalus and serial developmental examinations can provide clues to the ultimate prognosis and contribute to the criteria for the decision to perform surgery.

Medical Treatment

As a rule, medical management of hydrocephalus has failed because in most cases hydrocephalus is the result of impaired CSF absorption and the available pharmacologic agents have little or no effect on this process. Most agents known to decrease CSF formation under experimental conditions cannot be tolerated by humans when given in sufficiently high doses to diminish CSF production. Notable exceptions are acetazolamide and furosemide. These agents, given singly or in conjunction (e.g., 100 mg/kg per day of acetazol-amide and 1 mg/kg per day of furosemide), decrease CSF production, acetazolamide by inhibiting choroid plexus carbonic anhydrase and furosemide probably by inhibiting chloride transport. Each agent reduces CSF formation by approximately 50%, and the combined effect of the two drugs appears to be greater than the additive effect. Reduction of normal CSF production by one-third reduces intracranial pressure by only 1.5 cm H_2O. This differential explains the clinical limitations of agents that reduce CSF formation (823,824). These drugs are used as a temporizing measure or are used preoperatively in patients with acute hydrocephalus in whom immediate surgery is not possible. Nephrocalcinosis is a potentially serious complication.

Surgical Treatment

Several methods of surgical treatment have been used.

Direct Approach. The best treatment for hydrocephalus is to remove the obstruction. This is possible only in the small proportion of patients in whom a tumor or cyst within or beyond the ventricular system can be resected. Surgical attempts to eliminate the obstruction in aqueductal stenosis, Dandy-Walker malformation, and Chiari malformation type II associated with myelodysplasia have been abandoned because the failure rate has been high and the associated morbidity and mortality are considerable.

Indirect Approach. Two techniques of indirect approach are of great historical interest: endoscopic choroid plexus extirpation (plexectomy or electric coagulation) and third or fourth ventriculostomy. Choroid plexus extirpation had been used successfully in communicating hydrocephalus since 1934, with an arrest rate of 65% (825). Although complicated by intracerebral hemorrhage and, potentially, cystic dilatations of the endoscopic tracts as well as an operative mortality of 10%, the elimination of the choroid plexus pulse effect, one of the reasons for ventricular dilatation, provided a pathophysiologic rationale for this approach.

Ventricular Bypass. Therapeutically, the distinction between communicating (extraventricular) and noncommunicating (intraventricular) hydrocephalus has been rendered less important by modern shunt technology. In both types, the lateral ventricle is used as the drained reservoir. The CSF is bypassed from the ventricle, the site of its production, around the obstruction, and into a freely draining compartment of the body.

Surgical fenestration of the third ventricle into the basal cisterns and placement of a tube between a lateral ventricle and the cervical subarachnoid space (ventriculocisternostomy or Torkildsen procedure) are ways of bypassing the obstruction in noncommunicating hydrocephalus. Use of these methods depends on the patency of the basal cisterns and subarachnoid spaces, a condition that is not always present and must be verified before surgery. In general, these shunts are restricted to older children with noncommunicating hydrocephalus or to children with hydrocephalus caused by posterior fossa mass lesions obstructing outflow (819). In the experience of Cinalli and colleagues, when this procedure was performed using endoscopic guidance, good results were obtained in some 70% of infants or children with primary aqueductal stenosis, and they considered this procedure to be preferable to shunt placement (826).

Extracranial Shunts

Ventriculoperitoneal Shunts. The modern era of extracranial shunts began in 1949 when Matson introduced diversion of CSF into the ureter (827). Subsequent development of pressure-regulated one-way flow valves made this procedure unnecessary and avoided the sacrifice of a kidney. Additionally, ureteral shunts were associated with such major complications as gram-negative ventriculitis and life-threatening electrolyte imbalances (705). Steady improvement in shunting hardware and a progressive decline in shunt-related complications have made extracranial shunting the procedure of choice whenever the direct surgical removal of the obstruction is not possible.

Extracranial shunts currently used include the ventriculoperitoneal, ventriculoatrial, ventriculopleural, and lumboperitoneal varieties. Although the ventriculoatrial shunt was the first to enjoy widespread success, it has largely been supplanted by the ventriculoperitoneal shunt because the latter is technically easier to insert and is associated with less severe complications. Ventriculoperitoneal shunts were not widely used until the last three decades because the peritoneal end frequently became obstructed. The development of newer silicone elastomers and the insertion of sufficient tubing to allow the abdominal end to move freely about the peritoneal cavity have largely eliminated this problem.

Several types of valves are used. The Holter valve consists of two stainless steel check valves connected by silicone tubing. The Pudenz-Heyer-Schulte valve is a plastic bubble pump placed under the scalp with its distal end connected to the slit valve. Both apparatuses can be pumped. The Holter valve can be attached to many types of reservoirs placed in the burr hole to measure ventricular pressure and to instill antibiotics. Other, increasingly sophisticated devices are used. Of note are the programmable valves (i.e., valves whose flow characteristics can be altered by application of a magnetic field external to the head) and the Delta valve (Medtronic, Minneapolis, MN). The Delta valve incorporates an antisiphon device and adjusts the flow automatically to maintain intraventricular pressure within a narrow range in the face of the significant changes in CSF pressure that result from changes in posture or altered intracranial conditions. Many shunt valves can be preset to open at high or low CSF pressures, depending on the individual needs of the patient, such as the size of the lateral ventricles and thickness of the cerebral mantle. The various available shunting devices are discussed by Post (828).

Ventriculovascular Shunts. The ventriculovascular shunt was the preferred pathway before improvement of the peritoneal shunt and it still is preferred in some adult patients. A medium- or high-pressure valve is required. The slit one-way valve opens at a predetermined intraventricular pressure and closes once the pressure decreases below that level, thus preventing retrograde flow of venous blood into the ventricular cavity.

Lumboperitoneal and Other Shunts. Lumboperitoneal and other shunts are used infrequently in the pediatric age group because they are limited to the treatment of communicating hydrocephalus and pseudotumor cerebri. In pseudotumor cerebri, the narrower ventricles can make the insertion of a ventricular catheter technically difficult. Insertion of a lumboperitoneal shunt and its subsequent revision require a greater amount of operative manipulation than with other shunts and can be associated with scoliosis and nerve root irritation. Although the CSF can be diverted into the pleural cavity, frequent and progressive pleural effusions that require subsequent removal of the shunt in infants and small children restrict use of this type of a procedure to the older child or adult.

Complications of Shunts. The best way to avoid shunt complications is not to insert an unnecessary shunt. Shunt complications can be divided into those that are common to all types of shunts and those that are unique to one particular type (829). All shunts are subject to obstruction, disconnection, and infection, and revisions are often required periodically with somatic growth. The frequency and location of obstruction and disconnection depend to a degree on the shunting hardware. In general, the most frequent malfunction is that of occlusion of the ventricular catheter by choroid plexus or glial tissue that actually grows into the lumen of the catheter. Disconnection can occur at any point within the system, but most commonly it occurs where the various components are joined. Pressure-regulated valves in the shunting system can cause obstruction, drain CSF at higher or lower pressures than intended, and, rarely, allow retrograde flow. The last is of concern only in ventriculovascular shunts.

Use of a shunt valve that opens at too low a CSF pressure in an infant with a thin cerebral mantle and greatly enlarged lateral ventricle might result in collapse of the brain and massive subdural hematoma formation.

Though considerable apprehension has been expressed that an elevated CSF protein content can obstruct the valves, this has not been confirmed (830). We have noted, however, that increased CSF protein is commonly associated with a higher incidence of ventricular catheter obstruction. We advocate the use of radiopaque material to visualize the entire length of the shunt and thus determine the continuity of the shunting system on plain radiography. We also recommend that a reservoir be placed in the system to allow access to the CSF. By tapping the reservoir, pressures can be measured, functioning of the system can be ascertained, and CSF can be obtained for examination as necessary.

Imaging techniques that use contrast agents or radioisotopes can be used to determine the patency of the shunt. Each type of shunting system has its own peculiarities that determine how best to ascertain the adequacy of its function. That most shunting systems contain a pumping mechanism, in either the valve or the reservoir, that is designed to test whether the shunt is functioning properly is unfortunate because the correlation between the response to pumping and functioning of the shunt is poor. Many functioning shunts do not pump normally, whereas other shunts that pump well are malfunctioning. We therefore strongly advocate that the response to pumping of the shunt not be used to establish its adequacy. In a shunt-dependent child, malfunction results in a progressive increase in intracranial pressure, which can be acute or chronic, depending on the rate at which intracranial pressure becomes elevated. The symptoms differ little from those seen before the insertion of the shunt.

The implantation of foreign material, even when it is completely tissue compatible, carries the risk of infection in the neighboring areas (831). Prevention of infection, clearly of primary importance, can be achieved only by meticulous attention to aseptic technique during insertion, revision, or tapping. The value of antibiotic prophylaxis in preventing shunt infections has been established (831). In our hospitals, coverage for gram-positive organisms is given preoperatively and for the first 24 hours after operation, using first-generation cephalosporins, such as cephalothin or cefazolin. To prevent emergence of vancomycin-resistant organisms, vancomycin is not used for bacterial prophylaxis. Reduction of operating time and the use of experienced neurosurgeons also has a beneficial effect on the occurrence of infection, which now occurs in 1% to 5% of procedures in many pediatric neurosurgical centers. Superficial sepsis in the area of the wound usually responds to antibiotic treatment, whereas deeper infection is uncommon when proper operative technique has been used.

More frequent is the development of infection secondary to colonization of the valve or catheters, which leads to peritonitis with a ventriculoperitoneal shunt or bacteremia with a ventriculoatrial shunt. Although insidious in onset and sometimes difficult to diagnose, infection secondary to colonization usually develops within 6 months of shunt insertion. In the experience of Meirovitch and his group, reporting from Israel on patients collected between 1972 and 1984, 44% of infections developed during the first postoperative week and more than one-half developed during the first postoperative month (833). As a rule, the infection rate is higher in neonates and small infants (834). In the experience of one center, the incidence is 15.7% when shunts are performed in infants younger than 6 months of age, as contrasted to 5.6% when patients older than 6 months are shunted. As a rule, the incidence of infection is inversely proportional to the experience of the neurosurgeon. Some centers propose the use of prophylactic antibiotics to reduce the incidence of infections.

The most common organisms encountered are coagulase-positive or coagulase-negative staphylococci (835,836). These accounted for 67% of infections in the 1992 series of Pople and colleagues (834). The remainder represents a variety of pathogens. Nearly all the organisms that have been responsible for shunt infections are normal skin commensals, and intensive typing procedures have shown that the invading organism is usually indistinguishable from the patient's skin flora. Most infections occur within 4 months of the placement of an initial shunt and within 2 months of the placement of a revised shunt (836). Shunt infection can manifest by fever, shunt malfunction, irritability, vomiting, meningism, and swelling or redness over a portion or all of the shunting tract (833,836). Less commonly, one sees generalized symptoms such as meningitis or peritonitis with a ventriculoperitoneal shunt or septicemia with a ventriculoatrial shunt. Peripheral leukocytosis is seen in approximately one-half of instances. In the case of a ventriculoperitoneal shunt, obstruction owing to infection usually occurs at the distal end.

Infections also can occur as a result of breakdown of the skin over the hardware. In some instances, the infection is confined to the ventricular system and the shunt, without any external evidence of infection. Initial and recurrent infection rates are similar in all types of shunts (833).

The most reliable way to confirm a shunt infection is to identify organisms on a Gram-stained smear or obtain multiple CSF cultures from the shunting system (835). A less time-consuming test is to measure serum C-reactive protein, supplemented by coagulase-negative staphylococcus antibody testing in the CSF (830). Increased CSF eosinophilia is seen in approximately 28% of shunt infections. In approximately 80% of these it is accompanied by blood eosinophilia. The distribution of infectious agents in shunt infections with eosinophilia is no different than in those without it (837).

The management of shunt infections remains a matter of debate. All authorities advocate the use of appropriate intraventricular and systemic antibiotics combined with one of four approaches: removal of the infected shunt and placement of an external ventricular drainage system; removal of the infected shunt without replacement until a short course of antibiotics is completed, with the hydrocephalus being controlled by an external ventricular drain or repeated CSF aspirations; removal of the infected shunt with immediate insertion of a new shunt; or clearing of the infection without replacement of the shunting system (830,831,835,836). We advocate complete removal of the entire infected shunt, placement of a ventricular drain, and replacement of the shunt at a subsequent time. In the experience of Ronan and colleagues, this approach had a better outcome, with a relapse rate of only 4.5% (836). The appropriate antibiotic, chosen, if possible, according to the sensitivity of the organisms, is injected into the ventricles; at the same time, a broad-spectrum antibiotic is given systemically. The infection is usually overcome in 4 days, and on the seventh day the shunt can be reinserted.

Complications unique to peritoneal shunts include ascites, pseudocyst formation, perforation of a viscus or of the abdominal wall, and intestinal obstruction (838). The use of a coiled spring inside the peritoneal catheter to prevent its kinking (Raimondi catheter) is responsible for the majority of abdominal complications (839). The length of the tube in the peritoneal cavity does not appear to be a factor in subsequent complications (839).

The older the shunted patient is and the bigger the ventricles are at the time of surgery, the greater is the likelihood of a significant subdural fluid collection. Fluid collection can occur spontaneously or after seemingly minor head trauma. Its incidence can be reduced by the use of a higher-pressure valve. If it is asymptomatic, treatment is not indicated, but if it is accompanied by clinical symptoms, the fluid should be drained, usually by insertion of a subdural peritoneal shunt.

The incidence of seizures in patients with shunted hydrocephalus is higher than in unshunted patients (828,840). That the shunting procedure contributes to a seizure disorder is substantiated by EEG abnormalities localized to the site of shunt insertion (841). We do not believe that anticonvulsants should be given prophylactically.

Another, rarer complication of the shunting procedure is the *slit ventricle syndrome*. This condition refers to symptoms and signs of intermittent intracranial hypertension in a child who has been treated for hydrocephalus by the insertion of a shunt and whose ventricular system is found to be much smaller than normal. The patient, whose condition has usually been stable for months or years after the initial shunt placement, develops headache, vomiting, or impaired consciousness. A large proportion of patients, 27% in the series of Baskin and colleagues, develop Parinaud syndrome (842). The cause for this potentially fatal syndrome has not been satisfactorily explained; it might represent several different entities (843). Rekate suggested that chronic monitoring of intracranial pressure will uncover the cause of the syndrome (844). In a significant proportion of patients with small ventricles, intracranial pressure monitoring has revealed paroxysms of high pressure, even though the shunt appears to function normally. This may be the result of intermittent occlusion of the ventricular catheter in a shunt-dependent patient. In others, intracranial pressure is extremely low. This could result from an acquired rigidity of the periventricular tissue. In either case, the failure for ventriculomegaly to develop is unexplained. Epstein suggested that the diminished CSF volume is insufficient to buffer the normally occurring fluctuations in intracranial blood pressure and blood volume (819). Small ventricles revealed by neuroimaging studies, however, are often seen in patients who are clinically asymptomatic.

Regular monitoring by neuroimaging studies to monitor ventricle size should prevent the development of slit ventricle syndrome. Additionally, the appearance of a seizure disorder or the deterioration of the EEG should suggest this condition (845).

Treatment of the established condition is difficult and often ineffective. Baskin and colleagues suggested that patients undergo fiberoptic intracranial pressure monitoring after removal or externalization of their shunts. They found that a significant number of patients tolerated removal of their shunts. Those who demonstrated a need for CSF drainage underwent endoscopic third ventriculostomy with improvement or resolution of complaints in 73% of cases (842). No attempt should be made to insert a new ventricular catheter, because its failure and consequent hemorrhage are likely. Another approach would be to insert a valve that opens at a moderately higher pressure than the one already present or to use an antisiphoning device (844). The newer, self-adjustable or externally adjustable valves might also prove to be capable of avoiding the syndrome.

Prognosis

Based on studies of the natural course of untreated (846) and spontaneously arrested hydrocephalus (803,846), it is clear that surgery reduces mortality and limits morbidity. Untreated, hydrocephalus has a 50% mortality. In one study, 50% of the survivors were exhibited mental retardation in the illiterate range or worse, and fewer than 10% were intellectually normal. More than two-thirds of survivors had major physical handicaps (846,847). Other studies of spontaneously arrested hydrocephalus revealed an IQ of greater than 90 in one-third of survivors and disabling neurologic defects in two-thirds (7803). These defects included ataxia, spastic diplegia, compromised fine motor coordination, and perceptual deficits.

In surgically treated hydrocephalus, survival rate is at least 90%, and the IQ is normal or nearly normal in approximately two-thirds of patients. As a rule, verbal IQ is higher than performance IQ, and the classic *cocktail chatter* of a hydrocephalic child is a common occurrence (848). Neither site of obstruction nor number of shunt revisions or infections has an adverse effect on IQ. No evidence exists that prompt shunting enhances the ultimate IQ. Instead, IQ is a function of the etiology of the hydrocephalus, in particular, the presence or absence of concurrent cerebral malformations (849). Posterior fossa malformations do not affect IQ (848). In general, the narrower the cortical mantle and the smaller the brain mass, the worse is the eventual outcome. The outcome for normal cognitive function in preterm infants with shunted posthemorrhagic hydrocephalus is poor. This topic is covered in greater detail in Chapter 6.

The question of whether a shunt, once placed, can ever be removed was considered by Hemmer and Böhm (850). In their series, only 9% of shunts could be removed in children with communicating hydrocephalus or hydrocephalus associated with myelomeningoceles. We believe that no asymptomatic shunting device should ever be removed because, in many instances, it is impossible to establish beyond doubt whether the shunt is totally nonfunctional (851,852). In this respect, it is reassuring to remember that a nonfunctioning shunt rarely, if ever, becomes infected.

Hydranencephaly

Pathology

In hydranencephaly, the greater portions of both the cerebral hemispheres and the corpus striatum are reduced to membranous sacs composed of glial tissue covered by intact meninges and encompassing a cavity filled with clear CSF. Occasionally, the CSF is opaque and protein rich. Basal portions of frontal, temporal, and occipital lobe are preserved together with scattered islands of cortex elsewhere. The diencephalon, midbrain, and brainstem are usually normal except for rudimentary descending corticobulbar and corticospinal tracts. The cerebellum can be normal, hypoplastic, or damaged (853,854). In some cases, the ependyma lining the covering membrane is intact, the choroid plexus is preserved, and the aqueduct is stenotic. Other patients have large bilateral schizencephalic clefts in which pia and ependyma are joined, and they demonstrate other migration anomalies of fetal morphogenesis. In still other brains, bilateral porencephalic cysts replace the parenchyma normally perfused by the middle and anterior cerebral arteries. The latter instances show pathologic evidence of a destructive lesion.

Pathogenesis

The pathology suggests at least four different pathogenetic mechanisms. Some authorities, citing the presence of preserved ependyma and aqueductal stenosis in some cases, have argued that hydranencephaly is a type of hydrocephalus that has run its course *in utero*. In other instances, hydranencephaly can be the consequence of intrauterine infections or other gestational insults (854,855). In other cases, the condition can represent a genetically determined defect in vascular ontogenesis or can be the outcome of vascular occlusion of both internal carotid arteries or their main branches (853,856). A proliferative vasculopathy with an autosomal recessive inheritance also has been described (857). A few cases appear to be caused by defects in embryogenesis and subsequent cellular migration, resulting in schizencephaly and cortical agenesis (382).

Clinical Manifestations

Infants appear healthy at birth or have a somewhat large head that enlarges progressively. Spontaneous and reflex activity is often normal. However, failure in the development of cerebrocortical inhibition results in the persistence and exaggeration of reflexes, which becomes apparent by the second or third postnatal week. Over the subsequent weeks, hyper-reflexia, hypertonia, quadriparesis, and decerebration develop, together with irritability, infantile spasms, and dysconjugate extraocular movements. Generalized or minor motor seizures also become apparent. EEG can be normal at first, but later becomes abnormal, varying from a diffusely slow to an isoelectric pattern. The visual-evoked responses are absent, but brainstem auditory-evoked responses are preserved (858). Environmentally related behavioral automatisms can occur in those surviving early infancy (859).

Diagnosis

In an infant with an enlarged head or abnormally accelerating head growth, ultrasonography is mandatory to exclude severe hydrocephalus and expanding bilateral porencephalic cysts under increased pressure. Neuroimaging studies exclude massive bilateral subdural effusions that can mimic hydranencephaly on ultrasonography. MRI, in addition to defining the anatomic limits of the fluid-filled intracranial cavity and demonstrating residual structures in the basal telencephalic nuclei, diencephalon, and of the posterior fossa, also can demonstrate absence of flow in the internal carotid arteries (860). Most infants with hydranencephaly do not survive beyond the second year of life; they succumb to intercurrent infections or to an unexplained deficit of vital function. Survival for several years has been reported, however (859).

Treatment

No treatment is available for hydranencephaly.

Arachnoidal Cysts

Arachnoidal cysts are fluid-filled cavities situated within the arachnoid membrane and lined with collagen and cells arising from the arachnoid. They are believed to result from an anomalous splitting of the arachnoid membrane and to date from the sixth to the eighth fetal week. Some communicate freely with the subarachnoid space; in other patients contrast material introduced into the subarachnoid space does not enter the cyst or only does so slowly. Approximately one-half of the cysts are located in the middle cranial fossa (861), one-third are in the posterior fossa, and 10% are found in the suprasellar region (Fig. 5.25). Approximately one-fourth of the middle cranial fossa cysts are bilateral and some are accompanied by hypogenesis or compression of the temporal lobe (862). Additionally, they can cause a diffuse expansion and thinning of the bones of the vault and an elevation of the lesser wing of the sphenoid (687).

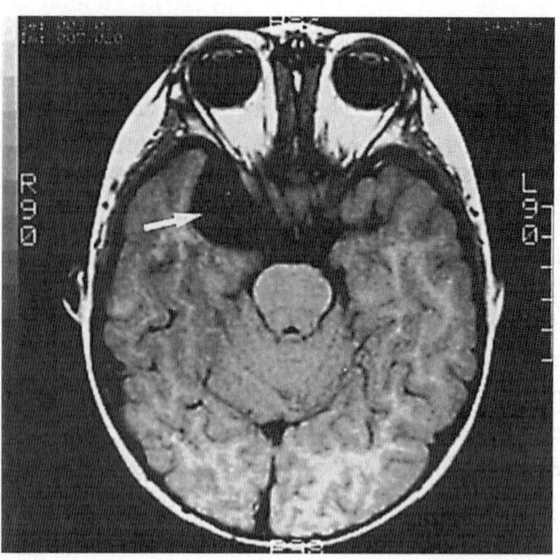

FIGURE 5.25. Arachnoid cyst. The T1-weighted (466/16/1) axial magnetic resonance imaging demonstrates the presence of a discrete low-intensity structure (*arrow*) in the right middle fossa that displaces the anterior temporal lobe laterally. The lesion had high intensity on T2-weighted images, consistent with CSF signal characteristics. The patient was a 3.5-year-old boy who presented with headaches and whose neurologic examination was benign. No evidence exists of a pressure effect on the imaging study.

Though in many instances a small cyst is clinically silent, larger cysts or cysts located in the posterior fossa can produce signs and symptoms of increased intracranial pressure. The cyst has the potential of producing hydrocephalus by increasing the resistance to CSF flow in the subarachnoid space. As the cyst enlarges, it eventually produces extrinsic compression of the ventricular system or of the subarachnoid channels. Symptoms can begin at any time during life. Aside from hydrocephalus, they include headaches and seizures. The relationship between headaches or seizures and the presence of an arachnoid cyst is often difficult to establish. Hemorrhage into an arachnoid cyst can cause the sudden onset of focal neurologic signs. A subdural hematoma has been reported to originate from a preexisting arachnoid cyst (863). Spinal cord arachnoid cysts can be intradural or, less frequently, extradural. They may present as space-occupying lesions with radicular pain, progressive weakness and spasticity, scoliosis, recurrent urinary tract infections, and constipation (864). An accompanying neural tube defect is common (865).

With the increased use of imaging studies, many cysts are discovered accidentally, particularly in the course of evaluating a seizure patient. Gandy and Heier believe that removal of the cyst does not improve seizure control (783). In other instances, removal of the cyst has been associated with complete or improved seizure control (866). Because the large majority of cysts remain constant in size and only large cysts tend to expand, we suggest only those cysts that present as space-occupying lesions should require surgical removal.

Achondroplasia

Achondroplasia is an abnormality of endochondral bone development transmitted as an autosomal dominant trait. It occurs in approximately 1 in 25,000 births, and 80% occur sporadically as new mutations. The gene for achondroplasia has been mapped to the tip of the short arm of chromosome 4 (4p16.3) in close proximity to the gene for Huntington disease (867). The gene (*FGFR3*) codes for a tyrosine kinase transmembrane receptor for fibroblast growth factor (867). FGRFs are members of a superfamily that bind fibroblast growth factors and initiate an intracellular signaling cascade. Remarkable genetic homogeneity exists, and almost all achondroplastic patients have the same point mutation.

Clinically, a decrease in the rate of endochondral bone formation is seen with normal membranous bone formation. The condition is characterized by dwarfism and a variety of skeletal abnormalities. Neurologic symptoms are the result of macrocephaly, which might or might not be accompanied by hydrocephalus, and cervicomedullary compression.

Because the cranial base is the only portion of the skull that is preformed in cartilage, its growth is selectively impaired, and a compensatory growth of the calvaria and an increase in the vertical diameter of the skull occur. The skull base is narrowed and the petrous pyramids tower. This results in an abnormal orientation of inner and middle ear structures (868). These growth changes produce a characteristic brachycephalic configuration and narrowing of all foramina that pass through the base of the skull.

As Dandy (869) demonstrated in 1921 using pneumoencephalography, the ventricular system is enlarged in approximately 50% of achondroplastic individuals (870). The cause for ventricular dilatation is under debate. Some authorities have suggested that it results from a mechanical block to the flow of CSF in the area of the foramen magnum, which is abnormally small in almost all patients with achondroplasia. This is confirmed by invasive monitoring, which has demonstrated an elevation of intracranial pressure (870). In addition, venography of the jugular veins demonstrates stenosis at the level of the jugular foramen and a pressure gradient across the foramen. Flodmark suggested that this phenomenon is responsible for venous hypertension and impaired CSF absorption (863). Yamada and colleagues confirmed the presence of both causes for hydrocephalus (859). Venous decompression at the jugular foramen and construction of a venous bypass from the transverse sinus to the jugular vein have reduced ventriculomegaly, as has venous decompression at the jugular foramen (871,872).

Cervicomedullary compression resulting from stenosis of the foramen magnum is a serious complication, presenting at any time from infancy to adult life. In the series of Ryken and Menezes, 3.2% of patients with achondroplasia demonstrated symptoms or signs of progressive compression of neural structures at the level of the foramen magnum (873). These included a variety of respiratory complications that are frequent in achondroplasia, notably apnea and respiratory irregularities. In the series of Nelson and coworkers, the incidence of apnea was 28% (874). Other signs include ataxia and spastic quadriparesis. In some instances brainstem compression can be insidious and can lead to syringobulbia, quadriparesis, and sudden infant death syndrome (875). Rarely, other neurologic signs are seen, including weak cry, failure to thrive, hypersomnia, and persistent papilledema (875,876). Paraplegia can develop as a result of compression of the spinal cord in the thoracic area (877). Mental retardation and seizures are not common features of achondroplasia (878). Although sensorineural hearing loss is common and subtle cognitive deficits have been uniformly demonstrated, general intelligence is within normal limits in most patients.

Considerable controversy exists as to on whom and when to perform suboccipital decompressive surgery (875,879,880). On the one hand, surgery is not without risk, and almost all achondroplastic infants who present with spasticity ultimately attain normal motor development if left alone (879). In addition, because the foramen magnum grows faster than the spinal cord, the impingement of the posterior rim of the foramen magnum on the cord decreases with maturation. On the other hand, MRI and pathologic evidence suggests deformational and traumatic changes to the spinal cord as a result of foramen magnum stenosis (880). We believe MRI evidence of notching or indentation of the spinal cord at the level of the foramen magnum has little clinical significance, and that unless evidence exists of spasticity or increased signal within the spinal cord on T2-weighted images, decompressive surgery can be deferred.

Osteopetrosis

The *osteopetroses* are a rare and heterogeneous group of disorders characterized by generalized bone sclerosis with thickening and increased fragility of cortical and spongy bone. Both autosomal dominant and autosomal recessive forms have been encountered, with the former being more common. As a result of a defect in osteoclast function, bone resorption is reduced, and the skull base is thickened and the foramina are narrowed. The autosomal dominant form has a benign prognosis, and individuals may remain asymptomatic. The recessive form is characterized by delayed psychomotor development, optic atrophy, conductive hearing loss, and facial nerve palsy (881,882). Other neurologic complications include hydrocephalus and intracranial hemorrhage (882). The earlier the onset of symptoms, the more malignant is the course.

Cerebral atrophy with secondary ventricular dilatation is frequently evident. A combination of calvarial thickening and hydrocephalus explains the degree of macrocephaly only in part. The process involves all skeletal bone and results in hematologic and bleeding disorders and in frequent fractures.

Computed tomographic scans are diagnostic. MRI often reveals delayed myelination and cerebral atrophy. Calcifications can be seen in the periventricular area and the falx (883). The only curative treatment is early allogeneic bone marrow transplantation. Surgical decompression can stabilize cranial nerve deficits, especially optic nerve entrapments. Visual-evoked potentials and electroretinography can be used to show the first indications of visual impairment (884).

A syndrome of osteopetrosis, renal tubular acidosis, and cerebral calcification is inherited as an autosomal recessive trait. Mental retardation is common, and patients have unusual facies. The primary defect in this entity appears to be one of carbonic anhydrase II, one of two enzymes catalyzing the association of water and carbon dioxide to form bicarbonate (885,886). Osteopetrosis also has been associated with infantile neuroaxonal dystrophy (887).

Möbius Syndrome

Möbius syndrome, first described by Harlan in 1880 (888), Chisholm in 1882 (889), and more extensively Möbius in 1888 and 1892 (890,891), is characterized by congenital paralysis of the facial muscles and impairment of lateral gaze.

Möbius syndrome results from diverse causes. The most frequent cause is symmetric tegmental infarcts in the fetal or neonatal brainstem associated with an episode of hypoperfusion from the basilar artery. The tegmentum is a watershed zone in the brainstem, with end-arterial perfusion from the paramedian penetrating and long circumferential arteries from the basilar artery (892). This pathogenesis is discussed more fully in Chapter 6 on neonatal asphyxia. Möbius syndrome often is accompanied by central respiratory insufficiency, central dysphagia, and other cranial neuropathies extending even as far caudally as to involve the hypoglossal nucleus, all explicable by the bilateral columnar tegmental watershed infarcts (892). Other pathologic lesions include complete or partial absence of the facial nuclei, dysplasia of the facial musculature, and hypoplasia of the facial nerve. The entity also has been seen in a variety of conditions involving progressive disease of muscle, ventral horn cells, or peripheral neurons. In some instances, there is absence, faulty attachment, or fibrosis of the extraocular muscles, whereas in other cases, the brainstem nuclei show multiple areas of calcification and necrosis, suggesting a prenatal vascular etiology (893–895). The symmetric calcified lesions with chronic gliosis, including gemistocytes, are in the tegmentum of the pons and medulla oblongata, a watershed zone of the brainstem between the territories of the paramedian penetrating arteries and the long circumferential arteries, both branches of the basilar artery. The vascular anatomy and the histopathologic findings at birth indicate a period of systemic hypotension in fetal life at least 4 to 6 weeks before birth (892). In a few cases, the electromyography points to the presence of a supranuclear lesion (896,897).

Most patients with Möbius syndrome have a variable degree of unilateral, asymmetric, or symmetric bilateral facial paralysis, with an inability to abduct the eyes beyond the midline (898). Occasionally, the weakness is restricted to portions or quadrants of the face (Fig. 5.26). Atrophy of the tongue, paralysis of the soft palate or masseters, congenital clubfoot, deafness, or a mild spastic diplegia also can be present. Because of bulbar deficits, the language and communication disorder is far greater than general intelligence would predict (899). Möbius syndrome is nonprogressive. In some instances, however, myotonic dystrophy or muscular dystrophy can accompany Möbius syndrome (900).

Congenital Sensorineural Deafness

Congenital deafness resulting from a lesion of the acoustic nerve can occur in isolation or in combination with a variety of anomalies. The conditions can appear sporadically or be transmitted in a dominant, recessive, or sex-linked manner (534,901). In the experience of Das, a family history of deafness was elicited in 23% of children assessed for bilateral sensorineural hearing loss. Perinatal asphyxia was believed to be responsible for 13%, congenital infections for 8.2%, bacterial meningitis for 6.5%, chromosomal anomalies for 5.3%, and a variety of syndromes, notably Waardenburg syndrome, for 5.3%. In 34%, the cause was unknown (902). Mutations in the *connexin 26* gene are the most common cause of genetic hearing loss (903). Other causes for profound hearing loss occurring in childhood are outlined in Table 5.15.

In a significant proportion of patients, dermatologic manifestations accompany the hearing loss. Waardenburg syndrome, probably the most common entity of this group, is characterized by dystopia of the medial canthi, an

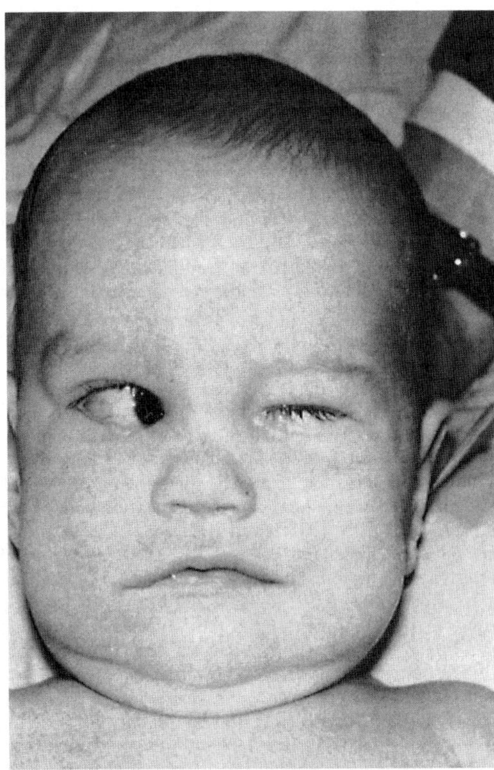

FIGURE 5.26. Möbius syndrome. As the infant cries, she demonstrates the bilateral weakness of the lower facial musculature and the marked weakness of the right upper facial muscles. Additionally, a palsy of both external recti, tongue, and palatal musculature occurred, requiring gastrostomy feeding.

elevated nasal root, a white forelock, and heterochromia iridis. Four genetic and clinical forms are known and are transmitted as an autosomal dominant trait (536), though sporadic cases also appear. The genetic mutation in Waardenburg syndrome types I and III is *PAX3*, which is located on the long arm of chromosome 2 (2q35–2q37) and normally encodes a protein termed HuP2. HuP2 protein binds DNA, and the gene that codes for it is suspected to belong to a family of genes, the homeobox genes, that regulate mammalian development; in animals, mutations in these genes result in major developmental abnormalities (904,905). Type II is the only one that is not associated with dystopia of the ocular canthi. It is due to a mutation in the microphthalmia transcription factor, human microophthalmia (MITF) (906). Many features of Waardenburg syndrome can be explained as a disorder of neural crest migration, and indeed some authors classify it as a neurocristopathy, but it also has many features of neurocutaneous syndromes and shares their embryologic etiology (907). The deafness that is part of most forms of Waardenburg syndrome is probably due to degeneration of the stria vascularis, a neural crest derivative that covers and protects the cochlear hair cells and without which the hair cells degenerate. In type III, variable musculoskeletal abnormalities and occasionally meningomyelocele and mental retardation are additional features. Type IV includes aganglionic megacolon (Hirschsprung disease), congenital hypomyelinating neuropathy, and CNS hypomyelination due to a mutation in the *SOX10* gene (908,909); both peripheral features can be directly ascribed to defective rhombencephalic neural crest.

In another group of syndromes, congenital sensorineural deafness is associated with visual symptoms. In Usher syndrome, a condition transmitted in an autosomal recessive manner, congenital neural hearing loss is seen in conjunction with progressive visual impairment and retinitis pigmentosa (534,910). Usher syndrome is the most common of a number of conditions in which retinitis pigmentosa is combined with deafness. These are reviewed by Mills and Calver (910). When a sensorineural hearing loss accompanies a neurologic disorder, it is usually in the framework of a peripheral neuropathy, and the hearing loss is progressive rather than congenital (534).

A distinct syndrome of congenital weakness of the musculature of the face, tongue, and palate unassociated with atrophy was termed *congenital suprabulbar paresis* by Worster-Drought (911). This condition is related to the perisylvian syndrome, in which facio-lingual-masticatory diplegia results from bilaterally anterior opercular infarctions. In the congenital form of this condition, marked feeding difficulties are accompanied by dysarthria, restricted tongue movements, and an absent gag reflex. Intellect is relatively preserved. In the series of Kuzniecky and coworkers, seizures were documented in 87% (912). These tend to have their onset after the age of 5 years, and most commonly are atonic and tonic drop attacks. Neuroimaging studies frequently disclose polymicrogyria, which has a predilection for the opercular areas. Associated malformations, notably arthrogryposis, clubfeet, and spastic quadriparesis, are not uncommon (911,912).

Other congenital disorders of the cranial nerves and the musculature innervated by them are presented in Table 5.14 (525–533,535,537).

REFERENCES

1. García-Bellido A. The development of concepts on development: a dialogue with Antonio García-Bellido (Interview by Enrique Cerda-Olmedo). *Int J Dev Biol* 1998;42:233–236.
2. Wolpert L, Beddington R, Brocken J, et al. *Principles of development*. Oxford: Oxford University Press, 1998.
3. Gilbert SF. *Developmental biology*, 7th ed. Sunderland, MA: Sinauer, 2003.
4. Blechschmidt E. *The ontogenetic basis of human anatomy*. Berkeley, CA: North Atlantic Books, 2004.
5. Sarnat HB. Microscopic criteria to determine gestational age of the fetal and neonatal brain. In: García JH, ed. *Neuropathology: the diagnostic approach*. St. Louis, MO: Mosby, 1997:529–540.
6. Patten BM. *Early embryology of the chick*, 4th ed. New York: McGraw-Hill, 1951.
7. Spemann H, Mangold H. Über Induktion von Embryonalanlagen

durch Implantation arfremder Organisatoren. *Wilhelm Roux Arch Entwicklungsmech* 1924;100:599–638.
8. Cho KWY, Blumberg B, Steinbeisser H, et al. Molecular nature of Spemann's organizer: the role of the *Xenopus* homeobox gene *goosecoid*. *Cell* 1991;67:1111–1120.
9. Wakamiya M, Rivera-Pérez JA, Baldini A, et al. *Goosecoid* and *goosecoid*-related genes in mouse embryogenesis. *Cold Springs Harbor Symp Quant Biol* 1997;62:145–149.
10. De Robertis EM, Kim S, Leyns L, et al. Patterning by genes expressed in Spemann's organizer. *Cold Springs Harbor Symp Quant Biol* 1997;62:169–175.
11. Hume CR, Dodd J. Cwnt-8C: a novel *Wnt* gene with a potential role in primitive streak formation and hindbrain organization. *Development* 1993;119:1147–1160.
12. Stein S, Kessel M. A homeobox gene involved in node, notochord and neural plate formation of chick embryos. *Mech Dev* 1995;49:37–48.
13. Duprat AM, Gualandris L, Kan P, et al. Review: neural induction. *Arch Anat Microsc Morphol Exp* 1987;75:211–227.
14. Tiedemann H. The molecular mechanism of neural induction: neural differentiation of *Triturus* ectoderm exposed to Hepes buffer. *Roux's Arch Dev Biol* 1986;195:399–402.
15. Fortini ME, Artavanis-Tsakonas S. Notch: neurogenesis is only part of the picture. *Cell* 1993;75:1245–1247.
16. Fontaine-Pérus JC, Chanconie M, Le Douarin NM, et al. Mitogenic effect of muscle on the neuroepithelium of the developing spinal cord. *Development* 1989;107:413–422.
17. Fontain-Pérus J. Migration of crest-derived cells from gut: gut influences on spinal cord development. *Brain Res Bull* 1993;30:251–255.
18. Dickson ME, Krumlauf R, McMahon AP. Evidence for a mitogenic effect of *Wnt-1* in the developing mammalian central nervous system. *Development* 1994;120:1453–1471.
19. DiCicco-Bloom E, Black IB. Insulin growth factors regulate the mitotic cycle in cultured rat sympathetic neuroblasts. *Proc Natl Acad Sci USA* 1988;85:4066–4070.
20. Tao Y, Black LB, DiCicco-Bloom E. Neurogenesis in neonatal rat brain is regulated by peripheral injection of basic fibroblast growth factor (bFGF). *J Comp Neurol* 1996;376:653–663.
21. Tao Y, Black IB, DiCicco-Bloom E. *In vivo* neurogenesis is inhibited by neutralizing antibody to basic fibroblast growth factor. *J Neurobiol* 1997;33:289–296.
22. Turner DL. Weintraub H. Expression of *Achaete-scute* homolog 3 in *Xenopus* embryos converts ectodermal cells to a neural fate. *Genes Dev* 1994;8:1434–1447.
23. Anderson DJ. A molecular switch for the neuron-glia developmental decision. *Neuron* 1995;15:1219–1222.
24. Hemmati-Brivantou A, Melton D. Vertebrate embryonic cells will become nerve cells unless told otherwise. *Cell* 1997;88:13–17.
25. Tanabe Y, Jessell TM. Diversity and pattern in the developing spinal cord. *Science* 1996;274:1115–11123.
26. McClure CFW. The segmentation of the primitive vertebrate brain. *J Morphol* 1890;4:35–56.
27. Keynes R, Lumsden A. Segmentation and the origin of regional diversity in the vertebrate central nervous system. *Neuron* 1990;2:1–9.
28. McGinnis W, Krumlauf R. Homeobox genes and axial patterning. *Cell* 1992;68:283–302.
29. Keynes R, Krumlauf R. *Hox* genes and regionalization of the nervous system. *Annu Rev Neurosci* 1994;17:109–132.
30. Guthrie S. Patterning the hindbrain. *Curr Opin Neurobiol* 1996;6:41–48.
31. Wassef M, Joyner AL. Early mesencephalon/metencephalon patterning and development of the cerebellum. *Perspect Dev Neurobiol* 1997;5:3–16.
32. Goldowitz D, Hamre K. The cells and molecules that make a cerebellum. *Trends Neurosci* 1998;21:375–382.
33. Figdor MC, Stem CD. Segmental organization of embryonic diencephalon. *Nature* 1993;363:630–634.
34. Rubenstein JLR, Shimamura K, Martínez S. Regionalization of the prosencephalic neural plate. *Annu Rev Neurosci* 1998;21:445–477.
35. Rubenstein JLR, Beachy PA. Patterning of the embryonic forebrain. *Curr Opin Neurobiol* 1998;8:18–26.
36. Puelles L, Rubinstein JL. Forebrain gene expression domains and the evolving prosomeric model. *Trends Neurosci* 2003;26:469–476.
37. Mai JK, Andrressen C, Ashwell KWS. Demarcation of prosencephalic regions by CD15-positive radial glia. *Eur J Neurosci* 1998;10:746–751.
38. Guthrie S, Butcher M, Lumsden A. Patterns of cell division and interkinetic nuclear migration in the chick embryo hindbrain. *J Neurobiol* 1991;22:742–754.
39. Joyner AL. *Engrailed, Wnt* and *Pax* genes regulate midbrain-hindbrain development. *Trends Genet* 1996;12:15–20.
40. Wassarman KM, Lewandoski M, Campbell K., et al. Specification of the anterior hindbrain organizer is dependent on *Gbx2* gene function. *Development* 1997;124:2923–2934.
41. Nomes HO, Dressler GR, Knapik EW, et al. Spatially and temporally restricted expression of *Pax-2* during neurogenesis. *Development* 1990;109:797–809.
42. Puschel AW, Westerfeld M, Dressler G. Comparative analysis of *Pax-2* protein distributions during neurulation in mice and zebrafish. *Mech Dev* 1992;38:197–208.
43. Rowitch DH, McMahon AP. *Pax-2* expression in the murine neural plate precedes and encompasses the expression domains of *Wnt-1* and *En-1*. *Mech Dev* 1995;52:3–8.
44. Rowitch DH, Danielian PS, Lee SMK, et al. Cell interactions in patterning the mammalian midbrain. *Cold Springs Harbor Symp Quant Biol* 1997;62:535–544.
45. Wurst W, Auerback AB, Joyner AL. Multiple developmental defects in *Engrailed-1* mutant mice: an early mid-hindbrain deletion and patterning defects in forelimbs and sternum. *Development* 1994;120:2065–2075.
46. McMahon AP, Joyner AL, Bradley A, et al. The midbrain-hindbrain phenotype of *Wnt-1-/Wnt-1*-mice results from stepwise deletion of *engrailed*-expressing cells by 9.5 days postcoitum. *Cell* 1992;69:581–595.
47. Millen KJ, Hui C-C, Joyner AL. A role for *En-2* and other murine homologues of *Drosophila* segment polarity genes in regulating position information in the developing cerebellum. *Development* 1995;121:3935–3945.
48. Kuemerle B, Zanjani H, Joyner A, et al. Pattern deformities and cell loss in *Engrailed-2* mutant mice suggest two separate patterning events during cerebellar development. *J Neurosci* 1997;17:7881–7889.
49. Rhinn M, Dierich A, Shawlot W, et al. Sequential roles for *Otx2* in visceral endoderm and neuroectoderm for forebrain and midbrain induction and specification. *Development* 1989;125:845–856.
50. Acampora D, Simeone A. Understanding the roles of *Otx1* and *Otx2* in the control of brain mophogenesis. *Trends Neurosci* 1999;22:116–122.
51. Sarnat HB, Menkes JH. How to construct a neural tube. *J Child Neurol* 2000;15:110–124.
52. Ryan AK, Blumberg B, Rodríguez-Estaban C, et al. *Pitx2* determines left-right asymmetry of internal organs in vertebrates. *Nature* 1998;394:545–551.
53. De Pomerai D. *From gene to animal: an introduction to the molecular biology of animal development*, 2nd ed. Cambridge: Cambridge University Press, 1990.
54. El-Baradi T, Pieler T. Zinc finger proteins: what we know and what we would like to know. *Mech Dev* 1991;35:155–169.
55. Topilko P, Schneider-Maunoury S, Levi G, et al. *Krox-20* controls myelination in the peripheral nervous system. *Nature* 1994;371:796–799.
56. Schneider-Maunoury S, Topilko P, Seitanidou T, et al. Disruption of *Krox-20* results in alteration of rhombomeres 3 and 5 in the developing hindbrain. *Cell* 1993;75:1199–1214.
57. Nieto MA, Sechrist J, Wilkinson DG, et al. Relationship between spatially restricted *Krox-20* gene expression in branchial neural crest and segmentation in the chick embryo hindbrain. *EMBO J* 1995;14:1697–1710.
58. Wilkinson DG, Krumlauf R. Molecular approaches to the segmentation of the hindbrain. *Trends Neurosci* 1990;13:335–339.
59. Morriss-Kay GM, Murphy P, Hill RE, et al. Effects of retinoic acid excess on expression of *Hox-2.9* and *Krox-20* and on morphological segmentation in the hindbrain of mouse embryos. *EMBO J* 1991;10:2985–2995.

60. Nonchev S, Maconochie M, Vesque C, et al. The conserved role of *Krox-20* in directing *Hox* gene expression during vertebrate hindbrain segmentation. *Proc Natl Acad Sci USA* 1996;93:9339–9345.
61. Cook M, Gould A, Brand N, et al. Expression of the zinc-finger gene *PLZF* at rhombomere boundaries in the vertebrate hindbrain. *Proc Natl Acad Sci USA* 1995;92:2249–2253.
62. Ingraham HA, Chen PRP, Mangalan HJ, et al. A tissue-specific transcription factor containing a homeodomain specifies a pituitary phenotype. *Cell* 1988;55:519–529.
63. Xu L, Lavinsky RM, Dasen JS. Signal-specific co-activator domain requirements for *Pit-1* activation. *Nature* 1998;395:301–306.
64. Doniach T. Basic FGF as an inducer of anteroposterior neural pattern. *Cell* 1995;83:1067–1070.
65. Brand-Saberi B, Ebensperger C, Wilting J, et al. The ventralizing effect of the notochord on somite differentiation in chick embryos. *Anat Embryol* 1993;188:239–245.
66. Pourquié O, Coltey M, Teillet MA, et al. Control of dorsoventral patterning of somite derivatives by notochord and floor plate. *Proc Natl Acad Sci USA* 1993;90:5242–5246.
67. Martí E, Bumcrot DA, Takada R, et al. Requirement of 19K form of Sonic hedgehog for induction of distinct ventral cell types in CNS explants. *Nature* 1995;375:322–325.
68. Roelink H, Porter JA, Chiang C, et al. Floor plate and motor neuron induction by different concentrations of the amino-terminal cleavage product of Sonic hedgehog autoproteolysis. *Cell* 1995;81:445–455.
69. Tabin CJ, McMahon AP. Recent advances in hedgehog signalling. *Trends Cell Biol* 1997;7:442–446.
70. Goulding M. Specifying motor neurons and their connections. *Neuron* 1998;21:943–946.
71. van Straaten HWM, Hekking JWM, Wiertz-Hoessels EJLM, et al. Effect of the notochord on the differentiation of the floor plate area in the neural tube of the chick embryo. *Anat Embryol* 1988;177:317–324.
72. Sasaki H, Hogan BLM. HNF-3β as a regulator of floor plate development. *Cell* 1994;76:103–115.
73. Sarnat HB. *Cerebral dysgenesis: embryology and clinical expression*. New York: Oxford University Press, 1992.
74. Ericson J, Muhr J, Placzek M, et al. Sonic hedgehog induces the differentiation of ventral forebrain neurons: a common signal for ventral patterning within the neural tube. *Cell* 1995;81:747–756.
75. Roessler E, Belloni E, Gaudenz K, et al. Mutations in the human *Sonic hedgehog* gene cause holoprosencephaly. *Nat Genet* 1996;14:357–360.
76. Callaerts P, Halder G, Gehring WJ. *Pax-6* in development and evolution. *Annu Rev Neurosci* 1997;20:483–532.
77. Stoykova A, Gruss P. Roles for *Pax* genes in developing and adult brain as suggested by expression patterns. *J Neurosci* 1994;14:1395–1412.
78. Saint-Jeannet JP, He X, Varmus HE, et al. Regulation of dorsal fate in the neuraxis by *Wnt-1* and *Wnt-3a*. *Proc Natl Acad Sci USA* 1997;94:13713–13718.
79. Briscoe J, Wilkinson DG. Establishing neuronal circuitry: *Hox* genes make the connection. *Genes Dev* 2004;18:1643–1648.
80. Murphy P, Hill RE. Expression of the mouse labial-like homebox-containing genes, *Hox-2.9* and *Hox-1.6*, during segmentation of the hindbrain. *Development* 1991;111:61–74.
81. Boncinelli E, Somma R, Acampora D, et al. Organization of human homeobox genes. *Hum Reprod* 1988;3:880–886.
82. Capecchi MR. *Hox* genes and mammalian development. *Cold Springs Harbor Symp Quant Biol* 1997;62:273–281.
83. Stern CD, Foley AC. Molecular dissection of *Hox* gene induction and maintenance in the hindbrain. *Cell* 1998;94:143–145.
84. Kessel M. Reversal of axonal pathways from rhombomere 3 correlates with extra *Hox* expression domains. *Neuron* 1993;10:379–393.
85. Lee JE. *NeuroD* and neurogenesis. *Dev Neurosci* 1997;19:27–32.
86. Katayama M, Mizuta I, Sakayama Y, et al. Differential expression of *neuroD* in primary cultures of cerebral cortical neurons. *Exp Cell Res* 1997;236:412–417.
87. Lee JE, Hollenberg SM, Snider I, et al. Conversion of *Xenopus* ectoderm into neurons by *NeuroD*: a basic helix-loop-helix protein. *Science* 1995;268:836–844.
88. Yokoyama M, Nishi Y, Miyamoto Y, et al. Molecular cloning of a human *neuroD* from a neuroblastoma cell line specifically expressed in the fetal brain and adult cerebellum. *Brain Res Mol Brain Res* 1996;42:135–139.
89. Morrow EM, Furukawa T, Lee JE, et al. *NeuroD* regulates multiple functions in the developing neural retina in rodent. *Development* 1998;126:23–36.
90. Yan RT, Wang SZ. *NeuroD* induces photoreceptor cell overproduction *in vivo* and *de novo* generation *in vitro*. *J Neurobiol* 1998;15:485–496.
91. Tamimi R, Steingrimsson E, Copeland NG, et al. The *NEUROD* gene maps to human chromosome 2q32 and mouse chromosome 2. *Genomics* 1996;34:418–421.
92. Tamimi RM, Steingrimsson E, Montgomery-Dyer K, et al. *NEUROD2* and *NEUROD3* genes map to human chromosomes 17q12 and 5q23-q31 and mouse chromosomes 11 and 13, respectively. *Genomics* 1997;40:355–357.
93. Brown NL, Kanekar S, Vetter ML, et al. *Math5* encodes a murine basic helix-loop-helix transcription factor expressed during early stages of retinal neurogenesis. *Development* 1998;125:4621–4633.
94. Zhao Q, Behringer RR, de Crombrugghe B. Prenatal folic acid treatment suppresses acrania and meroanencephaly in mice mutant for the *Cart1* homeobox gene. *Nat Genet* 1996;13:275–283.
95. Rice DS, Sheldon M, D'Arcangelo G, et al. *Disabled-1* acts downstream of *Reelin* in a signaling pathway that controls laminar organization in the mammalian brain. *Development* 1998;125:3719–3729.
96. Gleeson JG, Allen KM, Fox JW, et al. *Doublecortin*, a brain-specific gene mutated in human X-linked lissencephaly and double cortex syndrome, encodes a putative signaling protein. *Cell* 1998;92:63–72.
97. des Portes V, Pinard JM, Billuart P, et al. A novel CNS gene required for neuronal migration and involved in X-linked subcortical laminar heterotopia and lissencephaly syndrome. *Cell* 1998;92:51–61.
98. Faina GT, Cardini FA, D'Incerti L, et al. Familial schizencephaly associated with *EMX2* mutation. *Neurology* 1997;48:1403–1406.
99. Millen KJ, Wurst W, Herrup K, et al. Abnormal embryonic cerebellar development and patterning of postnatal foliation in two mouse *Engrailed-2* mutants. *Development* 1994;120:695–706.
100. Zec N, Rowitch DH, Bitgood MJ, et al. Expression of the homeobox-containing genes *EN1* and *EN2* in human fetal midgestational medulla and cerebellum. *J Neuropathol Exp Neurol* 1997;56:236–242.
101. Condron BG, Patel NH, Zinn K. *Engrailed* controls glial/neuronal cell fate decisions at the midline of the central nervous system. *Neuron* 1994;13:541–554.
102. Fox JW, Lamperti ED, Eksioglu YZ, et al. Mutations in *filamin 1* prevent migration of cerebral cortical neurons in human periventricular heterotopia. *Neuron* 1998;21:1315–1325.
103. Pfaff SL, Mendelsohn M, Stewart CL, et al. Requirement of *LIM* homeobox gene *Isl1* in motor neuron generation reveals a motor neuron-dependent step in interneuron differentiation. *Cell* 1996;84:309–320.
104. Kikuchi Y, Segawa H, Tokumoto M, et al. Ocular and cerebellar defects in zebrafish induced by overexpression of the LIM domains of the *Islet-3 LIM*/homeo-domain protein. *Neuron* 1997;18:369–382.
105. Jouet M, Kenwrick S. Gene analysis of L1 neural cell adhesion molecule in prenatal diagnosis of hydrocephalus. *Lancet* 1995;345:161–162.
106. Tsuru A, Mizuguchi M, Uyemura K, et al. Immunohistochemical expression of cell adhesion molecule L1 in hemimegalencephaly. *Pediatr Neurol* 1997;16:45–49.
107. Porter FD, Drago J, Xu Y, et al. *Lhx2*, a *LIM* homeobox gene, is required for eye, forebrain, and definitive erythrocyte development. *Development* 1997;124:2935–2944.
108. Tsuchida T, Ensini M, Morton SB, et al. Topographic organization of embryonic motor neurons defined by expression of *LIM* homeobox genes. *Cell* 1994;79:957–970.
109. Clark DC, Mizuguchi M, Antalffy B, et al. Predominant localization of the LIS family of gene products to Cajal-Retzius cells and ventricular neuroepithelium in the developing human cortex. *J Neuropathol Exp Neurol* 1997;56:1044–1052.

110. Dobyns WB, Reiner O, Carrozzo R, et al. Lissencephaly: a human brain malformation associated with deletion of the *LIS1* gene located at chromosome 17p13. *JAMA* 1993;270:2838–2842.
111. Lo Nigro C, Chong SS, Smith ACM, et al. Point mutations and an intragenic deletion in *LIS1*: the lissencephaly causitive gene in isolated lissencephaly sequence and Miller-Dieker syndrome. *Hum Mol Genet* 1997;6:157–164.
112. Chong SS, Pack SD, Roschke AV, et al. A revision of the lissencephaly and Miller-Dieker syndrome critical regions in chromosome 17p13.3. *Hum Mol Genet* 1997;6:147–155.
113. Ben-Arie N, Bellen HJ, Armstrong DL, et al. *Math1* is essential for genesis of cerebellar granule neurons. *Nature* 1997;390:169–172.
114. Tanabe Y, William C, Jessell JM. Specification of motor neuron identity by the *MNR2* homeodomain protein. *Cell* 1998;95:67–80.
115. Ma Q, Kinter C, Anderson DJ. Identification of *neurogenin*—a vertebrate neuronal determination gene. *Cell* 1996;87:43–52.
116. Sommer I, Ma Q, Anderson DJ. Neurogenins: a novel family of atonal-related bHLH transcription factors are putative mammalian neuronal determination genes that reveal progenitor cell heterogeneity in the developing CNS and PNS. *Mol Cell Neurosci* 1996;8:221–241.
117. Ma Q, Chen Z, del Barco Barrantes I, et al. *Neurogenin1* is essential for the determination of neuronal precursors for proximal cranial sensory ganglia. *Neuron* 1998;20:469–482.
118. Qiu M, Shimamuira K, Sussel L, et al. Control of anteroposterior and dorsoventral domains of *Nkx-6.1* gene expression relative to other *Nkx* genes during vertebrate CNS development. *Mech Dev* 1998;72:77–88.
119. Price M, Lazzaro D, Pohl T, et al. Regional expression of the homeobox gene *Nkx-2.2* in the developing mammalian forebrain. *Neuron* 1992;8:241–255.
120. McMahon JA, Takada S, Zimmerman LB, et al. *Noggin*-mediated antagonism of *BMP* signaling is required for growth and patterning of the neural tube and somite. *Genes Dev* 1998;12:1438–1452.
121. Zhong W, Jiang MM, Weinmaster G, et al. Differential expression of mammalian *Numb*, *Numblike* and *Notch1* suggests distinct roles during mouse cortical neurogenesis. *Development* 1997;124:1887–1897.
122. Chenn A, McConnell SK. Cleavage orientation and the asymmetric inheritance of Notch1 immunoreactivity in mammalian neurogenesis. *Cell* 1995;82:631–641.
123. Burek MJ, Oppenheim RW. Programmed cell death in the developing nervous system. *Brain Pathol* 1996;6:427–446.
124. Goodrich LV, Mienkovi L, Higgins KM, et al. Altered neural cell fates and medulloblastoma in mouse *patched* mutants. *Science* 1997;277:1109–1113.
125. Traiffort E, Charaytoniuk DA, Faure H, et al. Regional distribution of *Sonic hedgehog, Patched* and *Smoothened* mRNA in the adult rat brain. *J Neurochem* 1998;70:1327–1330.
126. Goodrich LV, Scott MP. *Hedgehog* and *Patched* in neural development. *Neuron* 1998;21:1243–1257.
127. Wechsler-Reya, Scott MP. Control of neuronal precursor proliferation in the cerebellum by *Sonic hedgehog*. *Neuron* 1999;22:103–114.
128. Walter M, Reifenberger J, Summer C, et al. Mutations in the human homologue of the *Drosophila* segment polarity gene *patched* (*PTCH*) in sporadic basal cell carcinomas of the skin and primitive neuroectodermal tumors of the central nervous system. *Cancer Res* 1997;57:2581–2585.
129. Urbnek P, Fetka I, Meisler MH, et al. Cooperation of *Pax2* and *Pax5* in midbrain and cerebellum development. *Proc Natl Acad Sci USA* 1997;94:5703–5708.
130. Ogawa M, Miyata T, Nakajima K, et al. The *reeler* gene-associated antigen on Cajal-Retzius neurons is a crucial molecule for laminar organization of cortical neurons. *Neuron* 1995;14:899–912.
131. Curran T, D'Arcangelo G. Role of reelin in the control of brain development. *Brain Res Rev* 1998;26:285–294.
132. Hirotsune S, Takahara T, Sasaki N, et al. The *reeler* gene encodes a protein with an EGF-like motif expressed by pioneer neurons. *Nat Genet* 1995;10:77–83.
133. Jeh-Ping L, Jessell TM. A role for rhoB in the delamination of neural crest cells from the dorsal neural tube. *Development* 1998;125:5055–5067.
134. Ericson J, Briscoe J, Rashbass P, et al. Graded Sonic hedgehog signaling and the specification of cell fate in the ventral neural tube. *Cold Springs Harbor Symp Quant Biol* 1997;62:451–466.
135. Lefebvre S, Burglen L, Reboullet S, et al. Identification and characterization of a spinal muscular atrophy determining gene. *Cell* 1995;80:155–165.
136. Roy N, Mahadevan MS, McLean M, et al. The gene for neuronal apoptosis inhibitory protein is partially deleted in individuals with spinal muscular atrophy. *Cell* 1995;80:167–178.
137. Menchine M, Emeline JK, Mischel PS, et al. Tissue and cell-type specific expression of the tuberous sclerosis gene, *TSC2*, in human tissues. *Modern Pathol* 1996;9:1071–1080.
138. Wienecke R, Maize JC Jr, Reed JA, et al. Expression of the *TSC2* product tuberin and its target Rap1 in normal human tissues. *Am J Pathol* 1997;150:43–50.
139. van Slegtenhorst M, de Hoogt R, Hermans C, et al. Identification of the tuberous sclerosis gene *TSC1* on chromosome 9q34. *Science* 1997;277:805–808.
140. Ali JB, Sepp T, Ward S, et al. Mutations in the *TSC1* gene account for a minority of patients with tuberous sclerosis. *J Med Genet* 1998;35:969–972.
141. Au KS, Rodriguez JA, Finch JL, et al. Germ-line mutational analysis of the *TSC2* gene in 90 tuberous sclerosis patients. *Am J Hum Genet* 1998;62:286–294.
142. Kwiatkowska J, Jozwiak S, Hall F, et al. Comprehensive mutational analysis of the *TSC1* gene: observations on frequency of mutation, associated features, and non-penetrance. *Ann Hum Genet* 1998;18:9365–9375.
143. Chen ZF, Behringer RR. *Twist* is required in head mesenchyme for cranial neural tube morphogenesis. *Genes Dev* 1995;9:686–699.
144. Minturn JE, Fryer HJL, Geschwing DH, et al. *TOAD-64P*: a gene expressed early in neuronal differentiation in the rat is related to *unc-33*, a *C. elegans* gene involved in axon outgrowth. *J Neurosci* 1995;15:6757–6766.
145. Fritzsch B, Nichols DH, Echelard Y, et al. Development of midbrain and anterior hindbrain ocular motoneurons in normal and *Wnt-1* knockout mice. *J Neurobiol* 1995;27:457–469.
146. Porter JD, Baker RS. Absence of oculomotor and trochlear motorneurons leads to altered extraocular muscle development in the *Wnt-1* null mutant mouse. *Dev Brain Res* 1997;100:121–126.
147. Salinas PC, Fletcher C, Copeland NG, et al. Maintenance of *Wnt-3* expression in Purkinje cells of the mouse cerebellum depends on interaction with granule cells. *Development* 1994;120:1277–1286.
148. Aruga J, Yokota N, Hashimoto M, et al. A novel zinc finger protein, Zic, is involved in neuronogenesis, especially in the cell lineage of cerebellar granule cells. *J Neurochem* 1994;63:1880–1890.
149. Aruga J, Minowa O, Yaginuma H, et al. Mouse Zic1 is involved in cerebellar development. *J Neurosci* 1998;18:284–293.
150. Mastick GS, Fan CM, Tessier-Lavigne M, et al. Early deletion of neuromeres in *Wnt-1-/-* mutant mice: evaluation by morphological and molecular markers. *J Comp Neurol* 1996;374:246–258.
151. Wagner M, Thaller C, Jessell T, et al. Polarizing activity and retinoid synthesis in the floor plate of the neural tube. *Nature* 1990;345:819–822.
152. Ruberte E, Dolle P, Chambon P, et al. Retinoid acid receptors and cellular retinoid binding proteins. II. Their differential pattern of transcription during early morphogenesis in mouse. *Development* 1991;111:45–60.
153. Summerbell D, Maden M. Retinoic acid, a developmental signalling molecule. *Trends Neurosci* 1990;13:142–147.
154. Momoi M, Yamagata T, Ichihashi K, et al. Expression of cellular retinoic-acid binding protein in the developing nervous system of mouse embryos. *Dev Brain Res* 1990;54:161–167.
155. Thaller C, Eichele G. Isolation of 3,4-didehydroretinoic acid: a novel morphogenetic signal in the chick wing bud. *Nature* 1990;345:815–819.
156. Brockes J. Reading the retinoid signals. *Nature* 1990;345:766–768.
157. Durston AJ, Timmermans JPM, Hage WJ, et al. Retinoic acid causes an anteroposterior transformation in the developing central nervous system. *Nature* 1989;340:140–144.
158. Marín-Padilla M, Marin-Padilla MT. Mophogenesis of experimentally induced Arnold-Chiari malformation. *J Neurol Sci* 1981;50:29–55.

159. Marín-Padilla M. Embryology and pathology of the axial skeleton and neural dysraphic disorders. *Can J Neurol Sci* 1991;18:153–169.
160. Alles AJ, Sulik KK. Retinoic acid-induced spina bifida: evidence for a pathogenetic mechanism. *Development* 1990;108:73–81.
161. Wohl CA, Weiss S. Retinoic acid enhances neuronal proliferation and astroglial differentiation in cultures of CNS stem cell-derived precursors. *J Neurobiol* 1998;37:281–290.
162. Meyers EN, Lewandoski M, Martin GR. An Fgf8 mutant allelic series generated by Cre- and Flp-mediated recombination. *Nat Genet* 1998;18:136–141.
163. Dorsky RI, Moon RT, Raible DW. Control of neural crest cell fate by the *Wnt* signaling pathway. *Nature* 1998;396:370–373.
164. Shah NM, Marchionni MA, Isaacs I, et al. Glial growth factor restricts mammalian neural crest stem cells to a glial fate. *Cell* 1994;77:349–360.
165. Hirate Y, Mieda M, Harada T, et al. Identification of ephrin-A3 and novel genes specific to the midbrain-MHB in embryonic zebrafish by ordered differential display. *Mech Dev* 2001;107:83–96.
166. Lange W. Regional differences in the cytoarchitecture of the cerebellar cortex. In: Palay SL, Chan-Palay V, eds. *The cerebellum: new vistas*. Berlin: Springer-Verlag, 1982:93–107.
167. Korbo L, Andersen BB, Ladefoged O, et al. Total numbers of various cell types in rat cerebellar cortex using an unbiased stereological method. *Brain Res* 1993;609:262–268.
168. Lemire RJ. Variations in development of the caudal neural tube in human embryos (Horizons XIV-XXI). *Teratology* 1969;2:361–370.
169. Papan C, Campos-Ortega JA. On the formation of the neural keel and neural tube in the zebrafish *Danio* (*Brachydanio*) *rerio*. *Roux's Arch Dev Biol* 1994;203:178–186.
170. Smith JL, Schoenwolf GC. Neurulation: coming to closure. *Trends Neurosci* 1997;20:510–517.
171. Schoenwolf GC, Smith JL. Mechanisms of neurulation: traditional viewpoint and recent advances. *Development* 1990;109:243–270.
172. Alvarez I, Schoenwolf GC. Expansion of surface epithelium provides the major extrinsic force for bending of the neural plate. *J Exp Zool* 1992;261:340–348.
173. Jacobson AG. Experimental analysis of the shaping of the neural plate and tube. *Am Zool* 1991;31:628–643.
174. Schoenwolf GC, Franks MV. Quantitative analyses of changes in cell shapes during bending of the avial neural plate. *Dev Biol* 1984;105:257–272.
175. Smith J, Schoenwolf GC. Notochordal induction of cell wedging in the chick neural plate and its role in neural tube formation. *J Exp Zool* 1989;25:49–62.
176. Sarnat HB. Role of the human fetal ependyma. *Pediatr Neurol* 1992;8:163–178.
177. Aaku-Saraste E, Oback B, Hellwig A, et al. Neuro-epithelial cells downregulate their plasma membrane polarity prior to neural tube closure and neurogenesis. *Mech Dev* 1997;69:71–81.
178. Sausedo RA, Smith JL, Schoenwolf GC. Role of randomly oriented cell division in shaping and bending of the neural plate. *J Comp Neurol* 1997;381:473–488.
179. Juriloff DM, Harris JM, Tom C, et al. Normal mouse strains differ in the site of initiation of closure of the cranial neural tube. *Teratology* 1991;44:225–233.
180. Golden JA, Chernoff GF. Intermittent pattern of neural tube closure in two strains of mice. *Teratology* 1993;47:73–80.
181. Busam KJ, Roberts DJ, Golden JA. Clinical teratology counseling and consultation. Case report: two distinct anterior neural tube defects in a human fetus: evidence for an intermittent pattern of neural tube closure. *Teratology* 1993;48:399–403.
182. O'Rahilly R, Müller F. Bidirectional closure of the rostal neuropore in the human embryo. *Am J Anat* 1989;184:259–268.
183. Dao AH, Netsky MG. Human tails and pseudotails. *Hum Pathol* 1984;15:449–453.
184. Lu FL, Wang PJ, Teng RJ, et al. The human tail. *Pediatr Neurol* 1998;19:230–233.
185. James HE, Canty TG. Human tail and associated spinal anomalies. *Clin Pediatr* 1995;34:386–388.
186. Appel B, Korzh V, Glasgow E, et al. Motoneuron fate specification revealed by patterned *LIM* homeobox gene expression in embryonic zebrafish. *Development* 1995;121:4117–4125.
186a. D'Costa AP, Prevette DM, Houenou LJ, et al. Mechanisms of insulin-like growth factor regulation of programmed cell death of developing avian motoneurons. *J Neurobiol* 1998;36:379–394.
187. Sauer FC. Mitosis in the neural tube. *J Comp Neurol* 1935;62:377–405.
188. Nurse P. Ordering S-phase and M-phase in the cell cycle. *Cell* 1994; 79:547–550.
189. Caviness VS Jr, Pinto-Lord MC, Evrard P. The development of laminated patterns in the mammalian neocortex. In: Connelly TG, ed. *Morphogenesis and pattern formation*. New York: Raven Press, 1981:103–126.
190. Zhong W, Feder JN, Jiang MM, et al. Asymmetrical localization of a mammalian numb homolog during mouse cortical neuronogenesis. *Neuron* 1996;17:43–53.
191. Mione MC, Cavanaugh JFR, Harris B, et al. Cell fate specification and symmetrical/asymmetrical divisions in the developing cerebral cortex. *J Neurosci* 1997;17:2018–2029.
192. Bass PW. Microtubules and neuronal polarity: lessons from mitosis. *Neuron* 1999;22:23–31.
193. Crews L, Hunter D. Neurogenesis in the olfactory epithelium. *Perspect Dev Neurobiol* 1994;2:151–161.
194. Menezes JRL, Smith CM, Nelson KC, et al. The division of neuronal progenitor cells during migration in the neonatal mammalian forebrain. *Mol Cell Neurosci* 1995;6:496–508.
195. Kendler A, Golden JA. Progenitor cell proliferation outside the ventricular and subventricular zones during human brain development. *J Neuropathol Exp Neurol* 1996;55:1253–1258.
196. Hamburger V, Levi-Montalcini R. Proliferation, differentiation and degeneration in the spinal ganglia of the chick embryo under normal and experimental conditions. *J Exp Zool* 1949;111:457–502.
197. O'Connor TM, Wyttenback CR. Cell death in the embryonic chick spinal cord. *J Cell Biol* 1974;60:448–459.
198. Okado N, Oppenheim RW. Cell death of motorneurons in the chick embryo spinal cord. *J Neurosci* 1984;4:1639–1652.
199. Harris AJ, McCaig CD. Motorneuron death and motor unit size during embryonic development of the rat. *J Neurosci* 1984;4:13–24.
200. Ferrer I, Serrano T, Soriano E. Naturally occurring cell death in the subicular complex and hippocampus in the rat during development. *Neurosci Res* 1990;8:60–66.
201. Diener PS, Bregman BS. Neurotrophic factors prevent the death of CNS neurons after spinal cord lesions in newborn rats. *NeuroReport* 1994;5:1913–1917.
202. Pittman RN, Wang S, DiBenedetto AJ, et al. A system for characterizing cellular and molecular events in programmed neuronal cell death. *J Neurosci* 1993;13:3669–3680.
203. Gómez-Pinilla F, Lee JWK, Cotman CW. Distribution of brain fibroblast growth factor in the developing brain. *Neuroscience* 1994;61:911–923.
204. Page KJ, Saha A, Everitt BJ. Differential activation and survival of basal forebrain neurons following infusions of excitatory amino acids: studies with the intermediate early gene c-*fos*. *Exp Brain Res* 1993;93:412–422.
205. Sarnat HB. Commentary: Pathology of spinal muscular atrophy. In: Gamstorp I, Sarnat HB. *Progressive spinal muscular atrophies*. New York: Raven Press, 1984:91–110.
206. Homma S, Yaginuma H, Oppenheim RW. Programmed cell death during the earliest stages of spinal cord development in the chick embryo: a possible means of early phenotypic selection. *J Comp Neurol* 1994;345:377–395.
207. Nurcombe V, McGrath PA, Bennett MR. Postnatal death of motor neurons during the development of the brachial spinal cord of the rat. *Neurosci Lett* 1981;27:249–254.
208. Allendoerfer KL, Shatz CJ. The subplate, a transient neocortical structure: its role in the development of connections between thalamus and cortex. *Annu Rev Neurosci* 1994;17:185–218.
209. Sarnat HB, Flores-Sarnat L. Cajal-Retzius and subplate neurons: their role in cortical development. *Eur J Paediatr Neurol* 2002;6: 91–97.
210. Derer P, Derer M. Cajal-Retzius cell ontogenesis and death in mouse brain visualized with horseradish peroxidase and electron microscopy. *Neuroscience* 1990;32:707–717.
211. Belichennko PV, Vogt Weisenhorn DM, Myklóssy J, et al.

Calretinin-positive Cajal-Retzius cells persist in the adult human neocortex. *NeuroReport* 1995;6:1869–1874.
212. Martin R, Gutiérrez A, Marín-Padilla M, et al. Persistence of Cajal-Retzius cells in the adult human cerebral cortex. An immunohistochemical study. *Histol Histopathol* 1999;14:487–490.
213. Duckett S, Pearse AGE. The cells of Cajal-Retzius in the developing human brain. *J Anat* 1968;102:183–187.
214. Marín-Padilla M. Dual origin of the mammalian neocortex and evolution of the cortical plate. *Anat Embryol* 1978;152:109–126.
215. Bayer SA, Altman J. Development of layer 1 and the subplate in the rat neocortex. *Exp Neurol* 1990;107:48–62.
216. Marín-Padilla M. Cajal-Retzius cells and the development of the neocortex. *Trends Neurosci* 1998;21:64–71.
217. Lavdas AA, Girgoriou M, Pachnis V, et al. The medial ganglionic eminence gives rise to a population of early neurons in the developing cerebral cortex. *J Neurosci* 1999;19:7881–7888.
218. Maricich SM, Gilmore ED, Herrup K. The role of tangential migration in the establishment of the mammalian cortex. *Neuron* 2001;31:175–178.
219. Deguchi K, Inoue K, Avila WE, et al. *Reelin* and *disabled-1* expression in developing and mature human cortical neurons. *J Neuropathol Exp Neurol* 2003;62:676–684.
220. Noctor SC, Palmer SL, Hasling T, et al. Interference with the development of early generated neocortex results in disruption of radial glia and abnormal formation of neocortical layers. *Cerebr Cortex* 1999;9:121–136.
221. Borrell V, Ruiz M, Del Río J, et al. Development of commissural connections in the hippocampus of Reeler mice: evidence of an inhibitory influence of Cajal-Retzius cells. *Exp Neurol* 1999;156:268–282.
222. Del Río J, Heimrich B, Borrell V, et al. A role for Cajal-Retzius cells and reelin in the development of hippocampal connections. *Nature* 1997;385:70–74.
223. Eriksson SH, Thom M, Heffernan J, et al. Persistent *Reelin*-expressing Cajal-Retzius cells in polymicrogyria. *Brain* 2001;124:1350–1361.
224. Huntley GW, Jones EG. Cajal-Retzius neurons in developing monkey neocortex show immunoreactivity to calcium binding proteins. *J Neurocytol* 1990;19:200–219.
225. Sarnat HB. Regional differentiation of the human fetal ependyma: immunocytochemical markers. *J Neuropathol Exp Neurol* 1992;51:58–75.
226. Smart IHM. Proliferative characteristics of the ependymal layer during the early development of the spinal cord in the mouse. *J Anat* 1972;111:365–380.
227. Snow DM, Steindler DA, Silver J. Molecular and cellular characterization of the glial roof plate of the spinal cord and optic tectum: a posible role for a proteoglycan in the development of an axon barrier. *Dev Biol* 1990;138:359–376.
228. Bovolentá P, Dodd J. Guidance of commissural growth cones at the floor plate in embryonic rat spinal cord. *Development* 1990;109:435–447.
229. Kennedy TE, Serafini T, de la Torre J, et al. Netrins are diffusible chemotropic factors for commissural axons in the embryonic spinal cord. *Cell* 1994;78:425–435.
230. Colamarino SA, Tessier-Lavigne M. The axonal chemoattractant netrin-1 is also a chemorepellant for trochlear motor neurons. *Cell* 1995;81:621–629.
231. Keynes R, Cook GMW. Axonal guidance molecules. *Cell* 1995;83:161–169.
232. Sarnat HB, Netsky MG. *Evolution of the nervous system*, 2 nd ed. New York: Oxford University Press, 1981.
233. Roessmann U, Gambetti P. Astrocytes in the developing human brain: an immunohistochemical study. *Acta Neuropathol* 1986;70:308–313.
234. Anton ES, Cameron RS, Rakic P. Role of neuron-glial junctional domain proteins in the maintenance and termination of neuronal migration across the embryonic cerebral wall. *J Neurosci* 1996;16:1193–2283.
235. Zheng C, Heintz N, Hatten ME. CNS gene encoding astrotactin which supports neuronal migration along glial fibers. *Science* 1996;272:417–419.
236. Herman JP, Victor JC, Sanes JR. Developmentally regulated and spatially restricted antigens of radial glial cells. *Dev Dyn* 1993;197:307–318.
237. Thomas LB, Gates MA, Steindler DA. Young neurons from the adult subependymal zone proliferate and migrate along an astrocyte, extracellular matrix-rich pathway. *Glia* 1996;17:1–14.
238. O'Rourke NA, Dailey ME, Smith SJ, et al. Diverse migratory pathways in the developing cerebral cortex. *Science* 1992;258:299–302.
239. Rakic P. Radial versus tangential migration of neuronal clones in the developoing cerebral cortex. *Proc Natl Acad Sci USA* 1995;92:11323–11327.
240. O'Rourke NA, Sullivan DP, Kaznowski CE, et al. Tangential migration of neurons in the developing cerebral cortex. *Development* 1995;121:2165–2176.
241. Wichterle H, García-Verdugo JM, Alvarez-Buylla A. Direct evidence for homotypic glia-independent neuronal migration. *Neuron* 1997;18:779–791.
242. McManus MF, Nasrallah IM, Gopal PP, et al. Axon mediated interneuron migration. *J Neuropathol Exp Neurol* 2004;63:932–941.
243. Anderson SA, Eisenstat DD, Shi L, et al. Interneuron migration from basal forebrain to neocortex: dependence on *Dlx* genes. *Science* 1997;278:474–476.
244. Eksioglu YZ, Scheffer IE, Cardena P, et al. Periventricular heterotopia: an X-linked dominant epilepsy locus causing aberrant cerebral cortical development. *Neuron* 1996;16:77–87.
245. Graf WD, Born DE, Sarnat HB. The pachygyria-polymicrogyria spectrum of cortical dysplasia in X-linked hydrocephalus. *Eur J Pediatr Surg* 1998;8(Suppl 1):1–14.
246. Ramón y Cajal, S de. *Histologie du systéme nerveux central de l'homme et des vértébrés*. Paris: Maloine, 1909–1911.
247. Dotti CG, Simons K. Polarizing sorting of viral glycoproteins to at the axon and dendrites of hippocampal neurons in culture. *Cell* 1990;62:63–72.
248. Higgins D, Burack M, Lein P, et al. Mechanisms of neuronal polarity. *Curr Opin Neurobiol* 1997;7:599–604.
249. Bredt DS. Sorting out genes that regulate epithelial and neuronal polarity. *Cell* 1998;94:691–694.
250. Tessier-Lavigne M, Placzek M, Lumsden AGS, et al. Chemotropic guidance of developing axons in the mammalian central nervous system. *Nature* 1988;336:775–778.
251. Oakley RA, Tosney KW. Contact-mediated mechanisms of motor axon segmentation. *J Neurosci* 1993;13:3773–3792.
252. Erskine L, McCaig CD. Growth cone neurotransmitter receptor activation modulates electric field-guided nerve growth. *Dev Biol* 1995;171:330–339.
253. Tosney KW. Somites and axon guidance. *Scan Electron Microsc* 1988;2:427–442.
254. Guthrie S, Pini A. Chemopulsion of developing motor axons by the floor plate. *Neuron* 1995;14:1117–1130.
255. Dodd J, Schuchardt A. Axon guidance: a compelling case for repelling growth cones. *Cell* 1995;81:471–474.
256. Tanaka E, Sabry J. Making the connection: cytoskeletal rearrangements during growth cone guidance. *Cell* 1995;83:171–176.
257. Yu W, Baas PW. The growth of the axon is not dependent upon net microtubule assembly at its distal tip. *J Neurosci* 1995;15:6827–6833.
258. Clark GD, McNeil RS, Bix GL, et al. Platelet-activating factor produces neuronal growth cone collapse. *NeuroReport* 1995;6:2569–2575.
259. Wilson SW, Placzek M, Furley AJ. Border disputes: do boundaries play a role in growth-cone guidance? *Trends Neurosci* 1993;16:316–323.
260. Chédodtal A, Pourquié O, Sotelo C. Initial tract formation in the brain of the chick embryo: selective expression of the BEN/SCI/DM-GRASP cell adhesion molecule. *Eur J Neurosci* 1995;7:193–212.
261. Purves D, Lichtman JW. Elimination of synapses in the developing nervous system. *Science* 1980;210:153–157.
262. Van Huizen F, Romijn HJ, Corner MA. Indications for a critical period for synapse elimination in developing rat cerebral cortex cultures. *Dev Brain Res* 1987;31:1-6.
263. Corriveau RA, Huh GS, Shatz CJ. Regulation of class I MHC gene expression in the developing and mature CNS by neural activity. *Neuron* 1998;21:506–520.

264. Huttenlocher PR, de Courten C. The development of synapses in striate cortex of man. *Hum Neurobiol* 1987;6:1–9.
265. Haydon PG, Drapeau P. From contact to connection: early events during synaptogenesis. *Trends Neurosci* 1995;18:196–201.
266. Koch C, Zador A. The function of dendritic spines: devices subserving biochemical rather than electrical compartmentalization. *J Neurosci* 1993;13:413–422.
267. Thoenen H. Neurotrophins and neuronal plasticity. *Science* 1995; 270:593–598.
268. Greenough WT. Structural correlates of information storage in the mammalian brain: a review and hypothesis. *Trends Neurosci* 1984;7:229–233.
269. Lipton SA, Kater SB. Neurotransmitter regulation of neuronal outgrowth, plasticity and survival. *Trends Neurosci* 1989;12:265–270.
270. McAllister AK, Katz LC, Lo DC. Opposing roles for endogenous BDNF and NT-3 in regulating cortical dendritic growth. *Neuron* 1997;18:767–778.
271. Breder CD, Dewitt D, Kraig RP. Characterization of inducible cyclooxygenase in rat brain. *J Comp Neurol* 1995;355:296–315.
272. Kaufmann WE, Worley PF, Pegg J, et al. Cox-2: a synapatically induced enzyme is expressed by excitatory neurons at postsynaptic sites in rat cerebral cortex. *Proc Natl Acad Sci USA* 1996;93:2317–2321.
273. Lerea LS, McNamara JO. Ionotropic glutamate receptor subtypes activate c-*fos* transcription by distinct calcium-requiring intracellular signaling pathways. *Neuron* 1993;10:31–41.
274. Williams JH, Errington ML, Lynch MA, et al. Arachidonic acid induces a long-term activity-dependent enhancement of synaptic transmission in the hippocampus. *Nature* 1989;341:739–742.
275. Shepherd GM, Greer CA. The dendritic spine: adaptations of structure and function for different types of synaptic integrations. In: Lesek R, Black M, eds. *Intrinsic determinants of neuronal form and function*. New York: Liss, 1989:245–314.
276. Walz W. Role of glial cells in the regulation of the brain microenvironment. *Progr Neurobiol* 1989;33:309–333.
277. Prochianz A. Neuronal polarity: giving neurons heads and tails. *Neuron* 1995;15:743–746.
278. Craig AM, Banker G. Neuronal polarity. *Annu Rev Neurosci* 1994; 17:267–310.
279. Sarnat HB, Nochlin D, Born DE. Neuronal nuclear antigen (NeuN): a marker of neuronal maturation in the early human fetal nervous system. *Brain Dev* 1998;20:88–94.
280. Sarnat HB, Born DE. Synaptophysin immunocytochemistry with thermal intensification: a marker of terminal axonal maturation in the human fetal nervous system. *Brain Dev* 1999;21:41–50.
281. Yakovlev PI, Lecours AR. The myelination cycles of regional maturation of the brain. In: Minkowsky A, ed. *Regional development of the brain in early life*. Philadelphia: Davis. 1967:3–70.
282. Hasegawa M, Houdou S, Mito T, et al. Development of myelination in the human fetal and infant cerebrum: a myelin basic protein immunohistochemical study. *Brain Dev* 1992;14:1–6.
283. Colello RJ, Pott U. Signals that initiate myelination in the developing mammalian nervous system. *Mol Neurobiol* 1997;15:83–100.
284. Compston A, Zajicek J, Sussman J, et al. Glial lineages and myelination in the central nervous system. *J Anat* 1997;190:161–200.
284a. Yu WP, Collarini EJ, Pringle NP, et al. Embryonic expression of myelin genes: evidence for a focal source of oligodendrocyte precursors in the ventricular zone of the neural tube. *Neuron* 1994;12:1353–1362.
285. Lemke G. The molecular genetics of myelination: an update. *Glia* 1993;7:263–271.
286. Byravan S, Foster LM, Phan T, et al. Murine oligodendroglial cells express nerve growth factor. *Proc Natl Acad Sci USA* 1994;91:8812–8816.
287. Zumkeller W. The effect of insulin-like growth factors on brain myelination and their potential therapeutic application in myelination disorders. *Eur J Paediatr Neurol* 1997;4:91–101.
288. Ogawa-Goto K, Abe T. Gangliosides and glycosphingolipids of peripheral nervous system myelins: a minireview. *Neurochem Res* 1998;23:305–310.
289. Hasan SU, Sarnat HB, Auer RN. Vagal nerve maturation in the fetal lamb: an ultrastructural and morphometric study. *Anat Rec* 1993;237:527–537.
290. Back SA, Luo NL, Borenstein NS, et al. Late oligodendrocyte progenitors coincide with the developmental window of vulnerability for human perinatal white matter injury. *J Neurosci* 2001;21:1302–1312.
291. Le Douarin N, Kalcheim C. *The neural crest*, 2nd ed. Cambridge: Cambridge University Press, 1999.
292. Hall BK. *The neural crest in development and evolution*. New York: Springer-Verlag, 1999.
293. Carstens MH. Development of the facial midline. *J Craniofac Surg* 2002;13:129–187.
294. Carstens MH. Neural tube programming and craniofacial cleft formation. *Eur J Paediatr Neurol* 2004;8:160–178.
295. Basch ML, Selleck MAJ, Bronner-Fraser M. Timing and competence of neural crest formation. *Devel Neurosci* 2000;22:217–227.
296. Tan SS, Morriss-Kay GM: The development and distribution of the cranial neural crest in the rat embryo. *Cell Tiss Res* 1985;240:403–416.
297. Hall BK. The neural crest as a fourth germ layer and vertebrates as quadroblastic not triploblastic. *Evol Dev* 2000;2:3–5.
298. Sarnat HB, Flores-Sarnat L. Neuropathologic research stategies in holoprosencephaly. *J Child Neurol* 2001;16:918–931.
299. Dambska M, Schmidt-Sidor B, Maslinska D, et al. Anomalies of cerebral structures in acranial neonates. *Clin Neuropathol* 2003;22:291–295.
300. Sarnat HB, Flores-Sarnat L, Carstens MH. Hypotelorism and hypertelorism: neural crest induction of craniofacial development. *J Child Neurol* 2005;20:*in press*.
301. Bronner-Fraser M: Neural crest formation and migration in the developing embryo. *FASEB J* 1994;8:699–706.
302. Sadaghiani B, Crawford BJ, Vielkind JR: Changes in the distribution of extracellular matrix components during neural crest development in *Xipbophorus* spp. embryos. *Can J Zool* 1994;72:1340–1353.
303. Bronner-Fraser M. Distribution and function of tenascin during cranial neural crest development in the chick. *J Neurosci Res* 1988;21:135–147.
304. Raible DW, Eisen JS: Regulative interactions in zebrafish neural crest. *Development* 1996;122:501–507.
305. El Shamy WM, Linnarsson S, Lee KF, et al. Prenatal and postnatal requirements of NT-3 for sympathetic neuroblast survival and innervation of specific targets. *Development* 1996;122:491–500.
306. Gershon MD. Neurotrophins in enteric nervous system development. In: Sieber-Blum M, ed. *Neurotrophins and the neural crest*. Boca Raton, FL: CRC Press, 1999:173–202.
307. Chalazonitis A. Neurotrophin-3 as an essential signal for the developing nervous system. *Mol Neurobiol* 1996;12:39–53.
308. Chalazonitis A. Neurotrophin-3 in the development of the enteric nervous system. *Progr Brain Res* 2004;146:243–263.
309. Sieber-Blum M, ed. *Neurotrophins and the neural crest*. Boca Raton, FL: CRC Press, 1999.
310. Lumsden A, Sprawson N, Graham A: Segmental origin and migration of neural crest cells in the hindbrain region of the chick embryo. *Development* 1991;113:1281–1291.
311. Selleck MAJ, García-Castro M, Artinger KB, et al. Dorsalization of the neural tube by the non-neural ectoderm. *Development* 1995;121:2099–2106.
312. Liem KF Jr, Tremmi G, Roelink H, et al. Dorsal differentiation of neural plate cells induced by *BMP*-mediated signals from epidermal ectoderm. *Cell* 1995;82:969–979.
313. Bronner-Fraser M. Origins and developmental potential of the neural crest. *Exp Cell Res* 1995;218:405–417.
314. Selleck MAJ, García-Castro M, Artinger KB, et al. Effects of *Shh* and *noggin* on neural crest formation demonstrate that *BMP* is required in the neural tube but not ectoderm. *Development* 1998;125:4919–4930.
315. Dickinson M, Selleck M, McMahon A, et al. Dorsalization of the neural tube by the non-neural ectoderm. *Development* 1995; 121:2099–2106.
316. LaBonne C. Vertebrate development: *wnt* signals at the crest. *Curr Biol* 2002;12:R743–R744.
317. Chisaka O, Capecchi MR. Regionally restricted developmental defects resulting from targeted disruption of the mouse homeobox gene *Hox 1.5*. *Nature* 1991;350:473–479.

318. Hunt P, Wilkinson DG, Krumlauf R. Patterning of the vertebrate head: murine *Hox-2* genes mark distinct subpopulations of premigratory and migrating neural crest. *Development* 1991;112: 43–51.
319. LaBonne C, Bronner-Fraser M. *Snail*-related transcriptional repressors are required in *Xenopus* for both the induction of the neural crest and its subsequent migration. *Dev Biol* 2000;221:195–205.
320. Nieto MA, Sargent MG, Wilkinson DG, et al. Control of cell behaviour during vertebrate development by *Slug*, a zinc finger gene. *Science* 1994;264:835–839.
321. LaBonne C, Bronner-Fraser M. Neural crest induction in *Xenopus*: evidence for a two-signal model. *Development* 1998;125:2403–2414.
322. Bei M, Peters H, Maas RL. The role of *PAX* and *MSX* genes in craniofacial development. In: *Craniofacial surgery*. Lin KY, Ogle RC, Jane JA, eds. Philadelphia: Saunders, 2002:101–112.
323. Bellmeyer A, Krase J, Lindgren J, et al. The protooncogene *c-myc* is an essential regulator of neural crest formation in *Xenopus*. *Dev Cell* 2003;4:827–839.
324. Sarnat HB, Netsky MG. When does a ganglion become a brain? Evolutionary origin of the central nervous system. *Semin Pediatr Neurol* 2002;9:240–253.
325. Kalter H, Warkany J. Medical progress. Congenital malformations: etiologic factors and their role in prevention. *N Engl J Med* 1983;308:424–431.
326. Adams RD, Sidman RL. *Introduction to neuropathology*, New York: McGraw-Hill, 1968.
327. Bird TD, Hall JG. Clinical neurogenetics: a survey of the relationship of medical genetics to clinical neurology. *Neurology* 1977;27:1057–1060.
328. Opitz JM, Gilbert EF. CNS anomalies and the midline as a "developmental field." *Am J Med Genet* 1982;12:443–455.
329. Nance WE. Anencephaly and spina bifida: an etiologic hypothesis. *Birth Defects Orig Artic Ser* 1971;7:97–102.
330. Robert E, Guibaud P. Maternal valproic acid and congenital tube defects. *Lancet* 1982;2:937.
331. Johnson RT. Effects of viral infection on the developing nervous system. *N Engl J Med* 1972;287:599–604.
332. Navarrete VN, Rojas CE, Alger CR, et al. Subsequent diabetes in mothers delivered of a malformed infant. *Lancet* 1970;2:993–994.
333. Giroud A. Causes and morphogenesis of anencephaly. In: Wolstenholme GE, O'Connor CM, eds. *CIBA Foundation symposium on congenital malformations*. London: Churchill Livingstone, 1960.
334. Müller F, O'Rahilly R. Development of anencephaly and its variants. *Am J Anat* 1991;190:193–218.
335. Padget DH. Development of so-called dysraphism with embryologic evidence of clinical Arnold-Chiari and Dandy-Walker malformations. *Johns Hopkins Med J* 1972;130:127–165.
336. Gardner WJ, Breuer AC. Anomalies of heart, spleen, kidneys, gut and limbs may result from an overdistended neural tube: a hypothesis. *Pediatrics* 1980;65:508–514.
337. Osaka K, Matsumoto S, Tanimura T. Myeloschisis in early human embryos. *Childs Brain* 1978;4:347–359.
338. Osaka K, Tanimura T, Hirayama A, et al. Myelomeningocele before birth. *J Neurosurg* 1978;49:711–724.
339. Toop J, Webb JN, Emery AE. Muscle differentiation in anencephaly. *Dev Med Child Neurol* 1973;15:164–170.
340. García CA, Duncan C. Atelencephalic microcephaly. *Dev Med Child Neurol* 1977;19:227–232.
341. Iivanainen M, Haltia M, Lydecken K. Atelencephaly. *Dev Med Child Neurol* 1977;19:663–668.
342. Naidich TP, Altman NR, Braffman BH, et al. Cephaloceles and related malformations. *Am J Neuroradiol* 1992;13:655–690.
343. Naggan L, Macmahon B. Ethnic differences in the prevalence of anencephaly and spina bifida in Boston, Massachusetts. *N Engl J Med* 1967;277:1119–1123.
344. Pei LJ, Li Z, Li S, et al. The epidemiology of neural tube defects in high-prevalence and low-prevalence areas of China. *Chin J Epidemiol* 2003;24:465–470 [in Chinese].
345. Ramírez-Espitia JA, Benavides FG, Lacasana-Navarro M, et al. Mortality from neural tube defects in Mexico. *Salud Pública Méx* 2003;45:356–364 [in Spanish].
346. Stone DH. The declining prevalence of anencephalus and spina bifida: its nature, causes and implications. *Dev Med Child Neurol* 1987;29:541–546.
347. Yen IH, Khoury MJ, Erickson JD, et al. The changing epidemiology of neural tube defects: United States 1968–1989. *Am J Dis Child* 1992;146:857–861.
348. Carstairs V, Cole S. Spina bifida and anencephaly in Scotland. *Br Med J* 1984;289:1182–1184.
349. Nakano KK. Anencephaly: a review. *Dev Med Child Neurol* 1973; 15:383–400.
350. Fedrick J. Anencephalus in the Oxford Record Linkage Study area. *Dev Med Child Neurol* 1976;18:643–656.
351. James WH. The sex ratios of anencephalics born to anencephalic-prone women. *Dev Med Child Neurol* 1980;22:618–622.
352. Peiper A, Hempel HC, Wunscher W. Der gampersche verbeugungsreflex. *Monatsschr Kinderheilkd* 1959;107:393–622.
353. Danner R, Shewman A, Sherman MP. Seizures in an atelencephalic infant: is the cortex essential for neonatal seizures? *Arch Neurol* 1985;42:1014–1016.
354. Brock DJ. Biochemical and cytological methods in the diagnosis of neural tube defects. *Progr Med Genet* 1977;2:1–37.
355. Nicolaides KH, Campbell S, Gabbe SG, et al. Ultrasound screening for spina bifida: cranial and cerebellar signs. *Lancet* 1986;2: 72–74.
356. Brock DJ. α-Fetoprotein and the prenatal diagnosis of central nervous system disorders: a review. *Childs Brain* 1976;2:1–23.
357. Laurence KM. Fetal malformations and abnormalities. *Lancet* 1974;2:939–942.
358. Milunsky A. Prenatal detection of neural tube defects: false positive and negative results. *Pediatrics* 1977;59:782–783.
359. MRC Vitamin Study Research Group. Prevention of neural tube defects: result of the Medical Research Council Vitamin Study. *Lancet* 1991;338:131–137.
360. Smithells RW, Nevin NC, Seller MJ, et al. Further experience of vitamin supplementation for prevention of neural tube defect recurrences. *Lancet* 1983;1:1027–1031.
361. Rhoads GG, Mills JL. Can vitamin supplements prevent neural-tube defects? Current evidence and ongoing investigations. *Clin Obstet Gynecol* 1986;29:569–1986.
362. Czeizel AE, Dudas I. Prevention of the first occurrence of neural-tube defects by preconceptional vitamin supplementation. *N Engl J Med* 1992;327:1832–1835.
363. Centers for Disease Control and Prevention Bulletin. Spina bifida and anencephaly before and after folic acid mandate–United States, 1995–1996 and 1999–2000. *MMWR Morb Mortal Wkly Rep* 2004;53(17):362–365.
364. Lemire RJ. Neural tube defects. *JAMA* 1988;259:558–562.
365. Morrison K, Papapetrou C, Hol FA, et al. Susceptibility to spina bifida: an association study of five candidate genes. *Ann Hum Genet* 1998;62:379–396.
366. Gilbert JN, Jones KL, Rorke LB, et al. Central nervous system anomalies associated with meningomyelocele, hydrocephalus, and the Arnold-Chiari malformation: reappraisal of theories regarding the pathogenesis of posterior neural tube closure defects. *Neurosurgery* 1986;18:559–564.
367. Dekaban AS. Anencephaly in early human embryos. *J Neuropathol Exp Neurol* 1963;22:533–548.
368. McLone DG, Naidich TP. Developmental morphology of the subarachnoid space, brain vasculature, and contiguous structures, and the cause of the Chiari II malformation. *Am J Neuroradiol* 1992;13:463–482.
369. Marín-Padilla M. Embryology and pathology of axial skeletal and neural dysraphic disorders. *Can J Neurol Sci* 1991;18:153–169.
370. Dryden R. The fine structure of spina bifida in an untreated three-day chick embryo. *Dev Med Child Neurol* 1971;25(Suppl):116–124.
371. Milunsky A, Ulcickas M, Rothman KJ, et al. Maternal heat exposure and neural tube defects. *JAMA* 1992;268:882–885.
372. Milunsky A. Prenatal detection of neural tube defects. VI. Experience with 20,000 pregnancies. *JAMA* 1980;244:2731–2735.
373. Matson DD. *Neurosurgery of infancy and childhood*, 2nd ed. Springfield, IL: Charles C. Thomas, 1969.
374. Anderson FM, Burke BL. Anterior sacral meningocele. *JAMA* 1977;237:39–42.

375. Richaud J. Spinal meningeal malformations in children (without meningoceles or meningomyeloceles). *Childs Nerv Syst* 1988;4:79–87.
376. Chiari H. Ueber Veränderungen des Kleinhirns infolge von Hydrocephalie des Grosshirns. *Dtsch Med Wochenschr* 1891;17:1172–1175.
377. Chiari H. Über die Veränderungen des Kleinhirns, des Pons und der Medulla Oblongata in Folge von congenitaler Hydrocephalie des Grosshirns. *Denkschrift Akad Wiss Wien* 1895;63:71–116.
378. Mackenzie NG, Emery JL. Deformities of the cervical cord in children with neurospinal dysraphism. *Dev Med Child Neurol* 1971;25(Suppl)):58–67.
379. Emery JL, Lendon RG. Clinical implications of cord lesions in neurospinal dysraphism. *Dev Med Child Neurol* 1972;27(Suppl):45–51.
380. Blaauw G. Defect in posterior arch of atlas in myelomeningocele. *Dev Med Child Neurol* 1971;25(Suppl):113–115.
381. Brunberg JA, Latchaw RE, Kanal E, et al. Magnetic resonance imaging of spinal dysraphism. *Radiol Clin North Am* 1988;26:181–205.
382. Yakovlev PI, Wadsworth RC. Schizencephalies: a study of the congenital clefts in the cerebral mantle. *J Neuropathol Exp Neurol* 1946;5:116–130, 169–206.
383. Anderson FM. Occult spinal dysraphism: a series of 73 cases. *Pediatrics* 1975;55:826–835.
384. Taylor B, Sarnat HB, Seibert JJ. Neonatal lacunar skull without neurologic disease. Report of 3 cases. *South Med J* 1982;75:875–877.
385. Carter CO, Evans KA, Till K. Spinal dysraphism: genetic relation to neural tube malformations. *J Med Genet* 1976;13:343–350.
386. Little BB, Knoll KA, Klein VR, et al. Hereditary cranial bifidum and symmetric parietal foramina are the same entity. *Am J Med Genet* 1990;35:453–458.
387. Bartsch O, Wuyts W, Van Hul W, et al. Delineation of a contiguous gene syndrome with multiple exostoses, enlarged parietal foramina, craniofacial dysostosis, and mental retardation caused by deletions in the short arm of chromosome 11. *Am J Hum Genet* 1996;58:734–742.
388. Kaplan SB, Kemp SS, Oh KS. Radiographic manifestations of congenital anomalies of the skull. *Radiol Clin North Am* 1991;29:195–218.
389. Jones KL. *Smith's Recognizable patterns of human malformation*, 5th ed. Philadelphia: Saunders, 1997:778–779.
390. Hoving EW, Vermeij-Keers C, Mommaas-Kienhuis AM. Separation of neural and surface ectoderm after closure of the rostral neuropore. *Anat Embryol* 1990;182:455–463.
391. Suwanwela C, Suwanwela N. A morphological classification of sincipital encephalomeningoceles. *J Neurosurg* 1972;36:201–211.
392. Lorber J, Schofield JK. The prognosis of occipital encephalocele. *Z Kinderchir* 1979;28:347–351.
393. Simpson DA, David DJ, White J. Cephaloceles: treatment, outcome and antenatal diagnosis. *Neurosurgery* 1984;15:14–21.
394. Smith MT, Huntington HW. Inverse cerebellum and occipital encephalocele: a dorsal fusion uniting the Arnold-Chiari and Dandy-Walker spectrum. *Neurology* 1977;27:246–251.
395. Cohen MM, Lemire RM. Syndromes with cephaloceles. *Teratology* 1982;25:161–172.
396. Summers MC, Donnenfeld AE. Dandy-Walker malformation in the Meckel syndrome. *Am J Med Genet* 1995;55:57–61.
397. Zee CS, McComb JG, Segall HD, et al. Lipomas of the corpus callosum associated with frontal dysraphism. *J Comput Assist Tomogr* 1981;5:201–205.
398. French BN. Midline fusion defects and defects of formation. In: Youmans JR, ed. *Neurological surgery*, 3rd ed. Philadelphia: Saunders, 1990:1081–1235.
399. Stark GD. Neonatal assessment of the child with a meningomyelocele. *Arch Dis Child* 1971;46:539–548.
400. Mortier W, von Bernuth H. The neural influence on muscle development in myelomeningocele: histochemical and electrodiagnostic studies. *Dev Med Child Neurol* 1971;25(Suppl):82–89.
401. Laurence KM. The natural history of spina bifida cystica: detailed analysis of 407 cases. *Arch Dis Child* 1964;39:41–57.
402. Lorber J. Ventriculo-cardiac shunts in the first week of life. *Dev Med Child Neurol* 1969;20(Suppl):13–22.
403. Hammock MK, Milhorat TH, Baron IS. Normal pressure hydrocephalus in patients with myelomeningocele. *Dev Med Child Neurol* 1976;37(Suppl):55–68.
404. El Gammal T, Mark EK, Brooks BS. MR imaging of Chiari II malformation. *Am J Roentgenol* 1988;150:163–170.
405. Quencer RM. Intracranial CSF flow in pediatric hydrocephalus: evaluation with cine MR imaging. *Am J Neuroradiol* 1992;13:601–608.
406. Charney EB, Rorke LB, Sutton LN, et al. Management of Chiari II complications in infants with myelomeningocele. *J Pediatr* 1987;111:364–371.
407. Venes JL, Black KL, Latack JT. Preoperative evaluation and surgical management of the Arnold-Chiari II malformation. *J Neurosurg* 1986;64:363–370.
408. Bell WO, Charney EB, Bruce DA, et al. Symptomatic Arnold-Chiari malformation: review of experience with 22 cases. *J Neurosurg* 1987;66:812–816.
409. Naik DR, Emery JL. The position of the spinal cord segments related to the vertebral bodies in children with meningomyelocele and hydrocephalus. *Dev Med Child Neurol* 1968;16(Suppl):62–88.
410. Kaplan WE, McLone DG, Richards I. The urological manifestations of the tethered spinal cord. *Z Kinderchir* 1987;42(Suppl 1): 27–31.
411. Altman RP, Randolph JG, Lilly JR. Sacrococcygeal teratoma: American Academy of Pediatrics, Surgical Section Survey-1973. *J Pediatr Surg* 1974;9:389–398.
412. Smith ED. *Spina bifida and the total care of spinal meningomyelocele*, Springfield, IL: Charles C. Thomas, 1965.
413. Stark G. Prediction of urinary continence in myelomeningocele. *Dev Med Child Neurol* 1971;13:388–389.
414. Stark G. The pathophysiology of the bladder in myelomeningocele and its correlation with the neurological picture. *Dev Med Child Neurol* 1968;16(Suppl):76–86.
415. Spindel MR, Bauer SB, Dyro FM, et al. The changing neurourologic lesion in myelodysplasia. *JAMA* 1987;258:1630–1633.
416. Brem AS, Martin D, Callaghan J, et al. Long-term renal risk factors in children with meningomyelocele. *J Pediatr* 1987;110:51–55.
417. Thomas M, Hopkins JM. A study of the renal tract from birth in children with myelomeningocele. *Dev Med Child Neurol* 1971;25(Suppl):96–100.
418. Guthkelch AN. Aspects of the surgical management of myelomeningocele: a review. *Dev Med Child Neurol* 1986;28:525–532.
419. Sharrard WJ, Zachary RB, Lorber J. Survival and paralysis in open myelomeningocele with special reference to the time of repair of the spinal lesion. *Dev Med Child Neurol* 1967;11(Suppl):35–50.
420. Sharrard WJ, et al. A controlled trial of immediate and delayed closure of spina bifida cystica. *Arch Dis Child* 1963;38:18–22.
421. Brocklehurst G. *Spina bifida for the clinician*. London: Heinemann, 1976.
422. Lorber J. Spina bifida cystica: results of treatment of 270 consecutive cases with criteria for selection for the future. *Arch Dis Child* 1972;47:8548–8573.
423. Soare PL, Raimondi AJ. Intellectual and perceptual motor characteristics of treated myelomeningocele children. *Am J Dis Child* 1977;131:199–204.
424. Park TS, Cail WS, Maggio WM, et al. Progressive spasticity and scoliosis in children with myelomeningocele. *J Neurosurg* 1985;62:367–375.
425. Lorber J. Selective treatment of myelomeningocele: to treat or not to treat? *Pediatrics* 1974;53:307–308.
426. Hunt GM. Open spina bifida: outcome for a complete cohort treated unselectively and followed into adulthood. *Dev Med Child Neurol* 1990;32:108–118.
427. McLone DG. Care of the neonate with a myelomeningocele. *Neurosurg Clin N Am* 1998;9:111–120.
428. Hobbins JC. Diagnosis and management of neural tube defects today. *N Engl J Med* 1991;324:690–691.
429. McLone DG. Continuing concepts in the management of spina bifida. *Pediatr Neurosurg* 1992;18:254–256.
430. Luthy DA, Wardinsky T, Shurtleff DB, et al. Cesarean section before the onset of labor and subsequent motor function in infants with meningomyelocele diagnosed antenatally. *N Engl J Med* 1991;324:662–666.

431. Tulipan N, Bruner JP. Myelomeningocele repair *in utero*: a report of three cases. *Pediatr Neurosurg* 1998;28:177–180.
432. Hunt GM, Holmes AE. Some factors relating to intelligence in treated children with spina bifida cystica. *Am J Dis Child* 1976;130:823–827.
433. Bier JB, Morales Y, Liebling J, et al. Medical and social factors associated with cognitive outcome in individuals with myelomeningocele. *Dev Med Child Neurol* 1997;39:263–266.
434. Carmel PW. Management of the Chiari malformation in childhood. *Clin Neurosurg* 1983;30:385–406.
435. Laurence KM, Tew BJ. Follow-up of 65 survivors from 425 cases of spina bifida born in South Wales between 1956 and 1962. *Dev Med Child Neurol* 1967;119(Suppl):13.
436. Paul KS, Lye RH, Strang FA, et al. Arnold-Chiari malformation: review of 71 cases. *J Neurosurg* 1983;58:183–187.
437. Vandertop WP, Asai A, Hoffman HJ, et al. Surgical decompression for symptomatic Chiari II malformation in neonates with myelomeningocele. *J Neurosurg* 1992;77:541–544.
438. Drummond DS, Moreau M, Cruess RL. Postoperative neuropathic fractures in patients with myelomeningocele. *Dev Med Child Neurol* 1981;23:147–150.
439. Caldarelli M, Di Rocco C, La Marca F. Treatment of hydromyelia in spina bifida. *Surg Neurol* 1998;50:411–420.
440. Fernandes ET, Reinberg Y, Vernier R, et al. Neurogenic bladder dysfunction in children: review of pathophysiology and current management. *J Pediatr* 1994;124:1–7.
441. González R. Urinary incontinence. In: Kelalis PK, Panayotis P, King LR, et al., eds. *Clinical pediatric urology*. Philadelphia: Saunders, 1992:384–398.
442. Whitehead WE, Parker LH, Masek BJ, et al. Biofeedback treatment of fecal incontinence in patients with meningomyelocele. *Dev Med Child Neurol* 1981;23:313–320.
443. Wald A. Use of biofeedback in treatment of fecal incontinence in patients with meningomyelocele. *Pediatrics* 1981;68:45–49.
444. Malone PS, Ransley PG, Kiely EM. Preliminary report: the antegrade continence enema. *Lancet* 1990;336:1217–1218.
445. Rekate HL. *Comprehensive management of spina bifida*. Boca Raton, FL: CRC Press, 1991.
446. Laurence KM. Effect of early surgery for spina bifida cystica on survival and quality of life. *Lancet* 1974;1:301–304.
447. Menzies RG, Parkin JM, Hey EN. Prognosis for babies with meningomyelocele and higher lumbar paraplegia at birth. *Lancet* 1985;2:993–997.
448. Hide DW, Williams HP, Ellis HL. The outlook for the child with a myelomeningocele for whom early surgery was considered inadvisable. *Dev Med Child Neurol* 1972;14:304–307.
449. McLaughlin JF, Parker LH, Masek BJ, et al. Influence of prognosis on decisions regarding the care of newborns with myelodysplasia. *N Engl J Med* 1985;312:1589–1594.
450. Hunt GM. Spina bifida: implications for 100 children at school. *Dev Med Child Neurol* 1981;23:160–172.
451. Gilbertson M, Newman B, Tomlinson J, et al. ASBAH-independence. *Z Kinderchir Grenzgeb* 1979;28:425–432.
452. Leonard CO, Freeman JM. Spina bifida: a new disease. *Pediatrics* 1981;68:136–137.
453. Cleland J. Contribution to the study of spina bifida, encephalocele, and anencephalus. *J Anat Physiol* 1883;17:257–292.
454. Arnold J. Myelocyste. Transposition von Gewebskeimen und Symposodie. *Beitr Pathol Anat* 1894;16:1–28.
455. Harding B, Copp AJ. Malformations. In: Graham DI, Lantos PL, eds. *Greenfield's Neuropathology*, 6 th ed. New York: Oxford University Press, 1997:417–422.
456. Sarnat HB. Pathogenesis of Chiari malformations: mechanical, hydrodynamic and molecular genetic theories. *J Neuropathol Exp Neurol* 2005;*in press*.
457. Lichtenstein BW. 'Spinal dysraphism': spina bifida and myelodysplasia. *Arch Neurol Psychiatr* 1940;44:792–818.
458. Goldstein F, Kepes JJ. The role of traction in the development of the Arnold-Chiari malformation. An experimental study. *J Neuropathol Exp Neurol* 1966;25:654–666.
459. Gardner WJ. Hydrodynamic factors in Dandy-Walker and Arnold-Chiari malformtions. *Childs Brain* 1977;3:200–212.
460. Masters CL. Pathogenesis of Arnold-Chiari malformation: the significance of hydrocephalus and aqueductal stenosis. *J Neuropathol Exp Neurol* 1978;37:56–74.
461. McClone DG, Knepper PA. The cause of Chiari II malformation: a unified theory. *Pediatr Neurol* 1989;15:1–12.
462. Marin-Padilla M, Marin-Padilla MT. Morphogenesis of experimentally induced Arnold-Chiari malformation. *J Neurol Sci* 1981;50: 29–55.
463. Sarnat HB. Regional ependymal upregulation of vimentin in Chiari II malformation, aqueductal stenosis and hydromyelia. *Pediatr Dev Pathol* 2004;7:48–60.
464. Elster AD, Chen MY. Chiari I malformations: clinical and radiological reappraisal. *Radiology* 1992;183:347–353.
465. Pascual J, Oterino A, Berciano J. Headache in type I Chiari malformation. *Neurology* 1992;42:1519–1521.
466. Nohria V, Oakes WJ. Chiari I malformation: a review of 43 patients. *Pediatr Neurosurg* 1990–1991;16:222–227.
467. Gardner WJ. Anatomic features common to the Arnold-Chiari and the Dandy-Walker malformations suggests a common origin. *Cleve Clin Q* 1959;26:206–222.
468. Peach B. Arnold-Chiari malformation: anatomic features of 20 cases. *Arch Neurol* 1965;12:613–621.
469. Emery JL, MacKenzie NG. Medullocervical dislocation deformity (Chiari II deformity) related to neurospinal dysraphism (meningomeylocele). *Brain* 1973;96:155–162.
470. Adams RD, Schatzki R, Scoville WB. The Arnold-Chiari malformation diagnosis: demonstration by intraspinal lipiodol and successful surgical treatment. *N Engl J Med* 1941;225:125–131.
471. Schachenmayr W, Friede RL. Rhombencephalosynapsis: a Viennese malformation? *Dev Med Child Neurol* 1982;24:178–182.
472. Carter CO, Evans KA, Till K. Spinal dysraphism: genetic relation to neural tube malformations. *J Med Genet* 1976;13:343–350.
473. James CC, Lassman LP. *Spinal dysraphism: spina bifida occulta*. London: Butterworth, 1972.
474. Bruner JP, Tulipan N, Paschall RI, et al. Fetal surgery for myelomeningocele and the incidence of shunt-dependent hydrocephalus. *JAMA* 1999;282:1819–1825.
475. Olutoye OO, Adzick NS. Fetal surgery for myelomeningocele. *Sem Perinatol* 1999;23:462–473.
476. Pang D, Dias MS, Ahab-Barmada M. Split cord malformation. Part I: a unified theory of embryogenesis for double spinal cord malformations. *Neurosurgery* 1992;31:451–480.
477. Pang D. Split cord malformation. Part II: clinical syndrome. *Neurosurgery* 1992;31:481–500.
478. Yamada S, Zinke DE, Sanders D. Pathophysiology of "the tethered cord syndrome." *J Neurosurg* 1981;54:494–503.
479. Sarnat HB. Molecular genetic classification of central nervous system malformations. *J Child Neurol* 2000;15:675–687.
480. Dryden RJ. Duplication of the spinal cord: a discussion of the possible embryogenesis of diplomyelia. *Devel Med Child Neurol* 1980;22:234–243.
481. Naidich TP, Zimmerman RA, McLone DG, et al. Congenital anomalies of the spine and spinal cord. In: Atlas SW, ed. *Magnetic resonance imaging of the brain and spine*. New York: Raven Press, 1991:902–907.
482. Bremer JL. Dorsal intestinal fistula; accessory neurenteric canal; diastematomyelia. *Arch Pathol Lab Med* 1952;54:132–138.
483. Guthkelch AN. Diastematomyelia with median septum. *Brain* 1974;97:729–742.
484. Sheptak PE, Susen AF. Diastematomyelia. *Am J Dis Child* 1967;113: 210–213.
485. Hendrick EB. On diastematomyelia. *Prog Neurol Surg* 1971;4:277–288.
486. Pang D, Parrish RG. Regrowth of diastematomyelic bone spur after extradural resection: case report. *J Neurosurg* 1983;59:887–890.
487. Batzdorf U. *Syringomyelia: concepts in diagnosis and treatment*. Baltimore: Williams & Wilkins, 1990.
488. Williams B. Pathogenesis of syringomyelia. In: Batzdorf U, ed. *Syringomyelia: current concepts in diagnosis and treatment*. Baltimore: Williams & Wilkins, 1991:59–90.
489. Oldfield EH, Muraszko K, Shawker TH, et al. Pathophysiology of syringomyelia associated with Chiari I malformation of the cerebellar tonsils: implications for diagnosis and treatment. *J Neurosurg* 1994;80:3–15.

490. Williams B. Syringomyelia. *Neurosurg Clin N Am* 1990;1:653–685.
491. Hall PV, Lindseth RE, Campbell RI. Myelodysplasia and developmental scoliosis: a manifestation of syringomyelia. *Spine* 1976;1:48–56.
492. Alcalá H, Dodson WE. Syringobulbia as a cause of laryngeal stridor in childhood. *Neurology* 1975;25:875–878.
493. Powell M. Syringomyelia: how MRI aids diagnosis and management. *Acta Neurochir* 1988;43(Suppl):17–21.
494. Wisoff JH. Hydromyelia: a critical review. *Childs Nerv Syst* 1988;4:1–8.
495. Filizzolo F, Versari P, D'Aliberti G, et al. Foramen magnum decompression versus terminal ventriculostomy for the treatment of syringomyelia. *Acta Neurochir* 1988;96:96–99.
496. Logue V, Edwards MR. Syringomyelia and its surgical treatment—an analysis of 75 patients. *J Neurol Neurosurg Psychiatry* 1981;44:273–284.
497. Towfighi J, Housman C. Spinal cord abnormalities in caudal regression syndrome. *Acta Neuropathol* 1991;81:458–466.
498. Lynch SA, Bond PM, Copp AJ, et al. A gene for autosomal dominant sacral agenesis maps to the holoprosencephaly region at 7q36. *Nat Genet* 1995;11:93–95.
499. Sarnat HB, Case ME, Graviss R. Sacral agenesis: neurologic and neuropathologic features. *Neurology* 1976;26:1124–1129.
500. Thompson IM, Kirk RM, Dale M. Sacral agenesis. *Pediatrics* 1974;54:236–238.
501. Mills JL, Baker L, Goldman AS. Malformations in infants of diabetic mothers occur before the seventh gestational week: implications for treatment. *Diabetes* 1979;28:292–293.
502. Passarge E, Lenz W. Syndrome of caudal regression in infants of diabetic mothers: observation of further cases. *Pediatrics* 1966;37:672–675.
503. Matson DD, Jerva MJ. Recurrent meningitis associated with congenital lumbo-sacral dermal sinus tract. *J Neurosurg* 1966;25:288–297.
504. Frieden IJ. Aplasia cutis congenita: a clinical review and proposal for classification. *J Am Acad Dermatol* 1986;14:646–660.
505. Hurst JA, Baraitser M. Johanson-Blizzard syndrome. *J Med Genet* 1989;26:45–48.
506. Altman NR, Naidich TP, Braffman BH. Posterior fossa malformations. *Am J Neuroradiol* 1992;13:691–724.
507. Sarnat HB, Benjamin DR, Siebert JR, et al. Agenesis of the mesencephalon and metencephalon with cerebellar hypoplasia: putative mutation in the *EN2* gene. Report of 2 cases in early infancy. *Pediatr Dev Pathol* 2002;5:54–68.
508. Pascual-Castroviejo I, Gutierrez M, Morales C, et al. Primary degeneration of the granular layer of the cerebellum: a study of 14 patients and review of the literature. *Neuropediatrics* 1994;25:183–190.
509. Sarnat HB, Alcalá H. Human cerebellar hypoplasia: a syndrome of diverse causes. *Arch Neurol* 1980;37:300–305.
510. Friede RL. *Developmental neuropathology*, 2nd ed. Berlin: Springer-Verlag, 1989:361–371.
511. Barth PG, Blennow G, Lenard HG, et al. The syndrome of autosomal recessive pontocerebellar hypoplasia, microcephaly, and extrapyramidal dyskinesia (pontocerebellar hypoplasia type 2): compiled data from 10 pedigrees. *Neurology* 1995;45:311–317.
512. Isaac M, Best P. Two cases of agenesis of the vermis of the cerebellum with fusion of the dentate nuclei and cerebellar hemispheres. *Acta Neuropathol* 1987;74:278–280.
513. Tomiwa K, Baraitser M, Wilson J. Dominantly inherited congenital ataxia with atrophy of the vermis. *Pediatr Neurol* 1987;3:360–362.
514. Joubert M, Eisenring JJ, Andermann F. Familial agenesis of the cerebellar vermis. *Neurology* 1969;19:813–825.
515. Kendall B, Kingsley D, Lambert SR, et al. Joubert syndrome: a clinico-radiological study. *Neuroradiology* 1990;31:502–506.
516. Legge RH, Weiss HS, Hedges TR 3rd, et al. Periodic alternating gaze deviation in infancy. *Neurology* 1992;42:1740–1743.
517. DeMyer W, Espay A, Walsh L, et al. Vermian hypoplasia and arrested cerebral myelination in two sisters: variant of Joubert syndrome or new syndrome? *J Child Neurol* 2003;18:755–762.
518. Kaufmann WE, Cooper KL, Mostoffsky SH, et al. Specificity of cerebellar vermian abnormalities in autism: a quantitative magnetic resonance imaging study. *J Child Neurol* 2003;8:463–470.
519. Bordarier C, Aicardi J, Goutières F. Congenital hydrocephalus and eye abnormalities with severe developmental brain defects: Warburg's syndrome. *Ann Neurol* 1984;16:60–65.
520. Dehdashti AR, Abouzeid H, Momjian S, et al. Occipital extra- and intracranial lipoencephalocele associated with tectocerebellar dysraphia. *Childs Nerv Syst* 2004;20:225–228.
521. Robain O, Dulac O, Lejeune J. Cerebellar hemispheric agenesis. *Acta Neuropathol* 1987;60:137–141.
522. Bull JS, Nixon WLP, Pratt RTC. Radiological criteria and familial occurrence of primary basilar impression. *Brain* 1955;78:229–247.
523. Klippel M, Feil A. Anomalie de la colonne vertebrale par d'absence des vertèbres cervicales. *Bull Mém Soc Anat Paris* 1912;87:185–188.
524. Gunderson CH, Solitare GB. Mirror movements in patients with Klippel-Feil syndrome. *Arch Neurol* 1968;18:675–679.
525. Falls HF, Kruse WT, Cotterman CW. Three cases of Marcus Gunn phenomenon in two generations. *Am J Ophthalmol* 1949; 32(Part 2):53–59.
526. Duane A. Congenital deficiency of abduction, associated with impairment of abduction retraction movements, contractions of the palpebral fissure and oblique movements of the eye. *Arch Ophthalmol* 1905;34:133–159.
527. Margalith D, Jan JE, McCormick AQ, et al. Clinical spectrum of congenital optic nerve hypoplasia: review of 51 patients. *Dev Med Child Neurol* 1984;26:311–322.
528. Skarf B, Hoyt CS. Optic nerve hypoplasia in children: association with anomalies of the endocrine and CNS. *Arch Ophthalmol* 1984;102:62–67.
529. Dickinson JT, Srisomboon P, Kamerer DB. Congenital anomaly of the facial nerve. *Arch Otolaryngol* 1968;88:357–359.
530. Nelson KB, Eng GD. Congenital hypoplasia of the depressor anguli oris muscle: differentiation from congenital facial palsy. *J Pediatr* 1972;81:16–20.
531. Pagon RA, Graham JM Jr, Zonana J, et al. Coloboma, congenital heart disease, and choanal atresia with multiple anomalies: CHARGE association. *J Pediatr* 1981;99:223–227.
532. Fraser GR. The causes of profound deafness in childhood. In: Worstenholme GE, Knight J, eds. *Sensorineural hearing loss. A CIBA Foundation symposium*. London: Churchill, 1970:5–40.
533. Parker N. Congenital deafness due to a sex-linked recessive gene. *Ann Hum Genet* 1958;10:196–200.
534. Konigsmark BW. Hereditary deafness in man. *N Engl J Med* 1969;281:713–720, 774–778, 827–832.
535. Jervell A, Lange-Nielsen F. Congenital deaf-mutism, functional heart disease with prolongation of the Q-T interval and sudden death. *Am Heart J* 1957;54:59–68.
536. Waardenburg PJ. A new syndrome combining developmental anomalies of the eyelids, eyebrows and nose root with pigmentary defects of the iris and head hair and with congenital deafness. *Am J Hum Genet* 1951;3:195–253.
537. Wildervanck LS. Hereditary malformations of the ear in three generations. Marginal pits, preauricular appendages, malformations of the auricle and conductive deafness. *Acta Otolaryngol* 1962;54:553–560.
538. Morrison SG, Perry LW, Scott LP. Congenital brevicollis (Klippel-Feil syndrome) and cardiovascular anomalies. *Am J Dis Child* 1968;115:614–620.
539. Foster JB, Hudgson P, Pearce GW. The association of syringomyelia and congenital cervico-medullary anomalies: pathological evidence. *Brain* 1969;92:25–34.
540. Bach C, Faure C, Schaefer P, et al. La dysostose cléido-cranienne étude de six observations: association à des manifestations neurologiques. *Ann Pediatr* (Paris) 1966;13:67–77.
541. Belloni E, Muenke M, Roessler E, et al. Identification of *Sonic hedgehog* as a candidate gene responsible for holoprosencephaly. *Nat Genet* 1996;14:353–356.
542. Roessler E, Belloni E, Gaudenz K, et al. Mutations in the human *Sonic hedgehog* gene cause holoprosencephaly. *Nat Genet* 1996;14:357–360.
543. Müller F, O'Rahilly R. Mediobasal prosencephalic defects, including holoprosencephaly and cyclopia, in relation to the development of the human forebrain. *Am J Anat* 1989;185:391–414.
544. Kelley RL, Roessler E, Hennekam RC, et al. Holoprosencephaly in RSH/Smith-Lemli-Opitz syndrome: does abnormal cholesterol

metabolism affect the function of *Sonic hedgehog*? *Am J Med Genet* 1996;66:78–84.

545. Wallis DE, Roessler E, Hehr U, et al. Mutations in the homeodomain of the human *SIX3* gene cause holoprosencephaly. *Nat Genet* 1999;22:196–198.
546. Gripp KW, Wotton D, Edwards MC, et al. Mutation in *TGIF* cause holoprosencephaly and link *NODAL* signalling to human neural axis determination. *Nat Genet* 2000;25:205–208.
547. Ming JE, Kaupas ME, Roessler E, et al. Mutations in *PATCHED-1*, the receptor for *SONIC HEDGEHOG*, are associated with holoprosencephaly. *Hum Genet* 2002;110:297–301.
548. Roessler E, Du Y, Glinka A, et al. The genomic structure, chromosome location, and analysis of the human *DKK1* head inducer gene as a candidate for holoprosencephaly. *Cytogenet Cell Genet* 2000;89:220–224.
549. Brown SA, Warburton D, Brown LY, et al. Holoprosencephaly due to mutations in *ZIC2*, a homologue of *Drosophila odd-paired*. *Nat Genet* 1998;20:180–183.
550. Matsunaga E, Shiota K. Holoprosencephaly in human embryos: epidemiologic study of 150 cases. *Teratology* 1977;16:261–272.
551. Kobori JA, Herrick MK, Urich H. Arhinencephaly: the spectrum of associated malformations. *Brain* 1987;110:237–260.
552. Ming PL, Goodner DM, Park TS. Cytogenetic variants in holoprosencephaly. Report of a case and review of the literature. *Am J Dis Child* 1976;130:864–867.
553. Barr M, Hanson JW, Currey K. Holoprosencephaly in infants of diabetic mothers. *J Pediatr* 1983;102:565–568.
554. Burck U. Genetic counselling in holoprosencephaly. *Helv Paediatr Acta* 1982;37:231–237.
555. Gurrieri F, Trask BJ, van den Engh G, et al. Physical mapping of the holoprosencephaly critical region on chromosome 7q36. *Nat Genet* 1993;3:247–251.
556. Ardinger HH, Bartley JA. Microcephaly in familial holoprosencephaly. *J Craniofac Genet Dev Biol* 1988;8:53–61.
557. McKusick VA. Holoprosencephaly. In: *Mendelian inheritance in man. Catalogs of autosomal dominant, autosomal recessive, and X-linked phenotypes*, 10th ed. Baltimore: Johns Hopkins University Press 1992:1443–1444.
558. Sarnat HB. CNS malformations: gene locations of known human mutations. *Eur J Paediatr Neurol* 2004;8:105–108.
559. DeMyer W. The median cleft face syndrome. *Neurology* 1967;17: 961–972.
560. DeMyer W. Classification of cerebral malformations. *Birth Defects Orig Artic Ser* 1971;7:78–93.
561. Plawner LL, Delgado MR, Miller VS, et al. Neuroanatomy of holoprosencephaly as predictors of function: beyond the face predicting the brain. *Neurology* 2002;59:1058–1066.
562. Hahn JS, Pinter JD. Holoprosencephaly: genetic, neuroradiological and clinical advances. *Semin Pediatr Neurol* 2002;9:309–319.
563. Golden JA. Holoprosencephaly: a defect in brain patterning. *J Neuropathol Exp Neurol* 1998;57:991–999.
564. Golden JA. Towards a greater understanding of the pathogenesis of holoprosencephaly. *Brain Dev* 1999;21:513–521.
565. Dekaban AS. Arhinencephaly. *Am J Ment Defic* 1948;63:428–432.
566. Maki Y, Kumagai K. Angiographic features of alobar holoprosencephaly. *Neuroradiology* 1974;6:270–276.
567. Osaka K, Sato M, Yamasaki S, et al. Dysgenesis of the deep venous system as a diagnostic criterion for holoprosencephaly. *Neuroradiology* 1977;13:231–238.
568. DeMyer W. Median facial malformations and their implications for brain malformations. *Birth Defects Orig Artic Ser* 1975;7:155–181.
569. Winter RM. What's in a face? *Nat Genet* 1996;12:124–129.
570. DeMyer W, Zeman W, Palmer CG. The face predicts the brain: diagnostic significance of median facial anomalies for holoprosencephaly (arhinencephaly). *Pediatrics* 1864;34:256–263.
571. DeMyer W. Orbital hypertelorism. In: Vinken PJ, Bruyn GW, eds. *Handbook of clinical neurology. Vol. 30. Congenital malformations of the brain and skull*. Part I. New York: Elsevier North-Holland, 1977:235–255.
572. DeMyer W, Zeman W, Palmer CG. Familial alobar holoprosencephaly (arhinencephaly) with median cleft lip and palate. *Neurology* 1963;13:913–918.
573. Aleksic S, Budzilovich G, Reuben R, et al. Unilateral arhinencephaly in Goldenhar Gorlin syndrome. *Dev Med Child Neurol* 1975;17:498–504.
574. Merriam GR, Beitins IZ, Bode HH. Father-to-son transmission of hypogonadism with anosmia. *Am J Dis Child* 1977;131:1216–1219.
575. Sarnat HB. Olfactory reflexes in the newborn infant. *J Pediatr* 1978;92:624–626.
576. DeMorsier G. Études sur les dysgraphies cranioencéphaliques. II. Agénesie du septum lucidum avec malformation du tractus optique. La dysplasie septo-optique. *Schweiz Arch Neurol Psychiat* 1956;77:267–292.
577. Dattani MT, Martínez-Barbera JP, Thomas PQ, et al. Mutations in the homeobox gene *HESX1/Hesx1* associated with septo-optic dysplasia in human and mouse. *Nat Genet* 1998;19:125–133.
578. Tajima T, Hattorri T, Nakajima T, et al. Sporadic heterozygous frameshift mutation of *HESX1* causing pituitary and optic nerve hypoplasia and combined pituitary hormone deficiency in a Japanese patient. *J Clin Endocrinol Metab* 2003;88:45–50.
579. Carey ML, Friedman TB, Asher JH Jr, et al. Septo-optic dysplasia and WS1 in the proband of a WS1 family segregating for a novel mutation in *PAX3* exon 7. *J Med Genet* 1998;35:248–250.
580. Roessmann U, Velasco ME, Small EJ, et al. Neuropathology of "septo-optic dysplasia" (de Morsier's syndrome) with immunohistochemical studies of the hypothalamus and pituitary gland. *J Neuropath Exp Neurol* 1987;46:597–608.
581. Masera N, Grant DB, Stanhope R, et al. Diabetes insipidus with impaired osmotic regulation in septo-optic dysplasia and agenesis of the corpus callosum. *Arch Dis Child* 1994;70:51–53.
582. Michaud J, Mizrahi EM, Urich H. Agenesis of the vermis with fusion of the cerebellar hemispheres, septo-optic dysplasia and associated anomalies. *Acta Neuropathol* 1982;56:161–166.
583. Fielder AR, Levene MI, Trounce JQ. Optic nerve hypoplasia in infancy. *J R Soc Med* 1986;79:25–29.
584. Zeki SM, Dutton GN. Optic nerve hypoplasia in children. *Br J Ophthalmol* 1990;74:300–304.
585. Nelson M, Lessell S, Sadun AA. Optic nerve hypoplasia and maternal diabetes mellitus. *Arch Neurol* 1986;43:20–25.
586. Parr JH. Midline cerebral defect and Kallmann's syndrome. *J R Soc Med* 1988;81:355–356.
587. Sarnat HB. Role of human fetal ependyma. *Pediatr Neurol* 1992;8:163–178.
588. Sarnat HB, Rybak G, Kotagal S, et al. Cerebral embryopathy in late first trimester: possible association with swine influenza vaccine. *Teratology* 1979;20:93–100.
589. Barth P. Disorders of neuronal migration. *Can J Neurol Sci* 1987;14:1–16.
590. Barkovich AJ, Gressens P, Evrard P. Formation, maturation, and disorders of brain neocortex. *Am J Neuroradiol* 1992;13:423–446.
590a. Haberland C, Perou M. Encephalocraniocutaneous lipomatosis. *Arch Neurol* 1970;22:144–155.
590b. Choic BH, Kudo M. Abnormal neuronal migration and gliomatosis cerebri in epidermal nevus syndrome. *Acta Neuropathol* 1981;53:318–325.
590c. Grunnet ML, Bale JF. Brain abnormalities in infants with Potter syndrome (oligohydramnios tetrad). *Neurology* 1981;31:1571–1574.
590d. Shigematsu H, Takashima S, Otani K, et al. Neuropathological and Golgi study on a case of thanatophoric dysplasia. *Brain Dev* 1985;7:628–632.
590e. Robain O, Deonna T. Pachygyria and congenital nephrosis: disorder of migration and neuronal orientation. *Acta Neuropathol* 1983;60:137–140.
590f. Hansen LA, Pearl GS. Isoretinoin teratogenicity: case report with neuropathogical findings. *Acta Neuropathol* 1985;65:335–337.
591. Dekaban A. Large defects in cerebral hemispheres associated with cortical dysgenesis. *J Neuropathol Exp Neurol* 1965;24:512–530.
592. Barkovich AJ, Kjos B. Schizencephaly: correlation of clinical findings with MR characteristics. *Am J Neuroradiol* 1992;13:85–94.
593. Granata T, Farina L, Faiella A, et al. Familial schizencephaly associated with *EMX2* mutation. *Neurology* 1997;48:1403–1406.
594. Tardieu M, Evrard P, Lyon G. Progressive expanding congenital porencephalies: a treatable cause of progressive encephalopathy. *Pediatrics* 1981;68:198–202.

595. Miller GM, Stears JC, Guggenheim MA, et al. Schizencephaly: a clinical and CT study. *Neurology* 1984;34:997–1001.
596. Steward RM, Richman DP, Caviness VS. Lissencephaly and pachygyria: an architectonic and topographical analysis. *Acta Neuropathol* 1975;31:1–12.
597. Barkovich AJ, Koch TK, Carrol CL. The spectrum of lissencephaly: report of 10 patients analyzed by magnetic resonance imaging. *Ann Neurol* 1991;30:139–146.
598. Dobyns WB, Stears JC, Guggenheim MA, et al. Lissencephaly: a human brain malformation associated with deletion of the *LIS1* gene located at chromosome 17p13. *JAMA* 1993;270:2838–2842.
599. Lo Nigro C, Chong CS, Smith AC, et al. Point mutations and an intragenic deletion in *LIS1*: the lissencephaly causative gene in isolated lissencephaly sequence and Miller-Dieker syndrome. *Hum Mol Genet* 1997;6:157–164.
600. Chong SS, Pack SD, Roschke AV, et al. A revision of the lissencephaly and Miller-Dieker syndrome critical regions in chromosome 17p13.3. *Hum Mol Genet* 1997;6:147–155.
601. Clark DC, Mizuguchi M, Antalffy B, et al. Predominant localization of the *LIS* family of gene products to Cajal-Retzius cells and ventricular neuroepithelium in the developing human cortex. *J Neuropathol Exp Neurol* 1997;56:1044–1052.
602. Fogli A, Guerrini R, Moro F, et al. Intracellular levels of the LIS1 protein correlate with clinical and neuroradiological findings in patients with classical lissencephaly. *Ann Neurol* 1999;45:154–161.
603. Beltran-Valero de Barnabé D, Currier S, Steinbrecher A, et al. Mutations in the *O*-mannosyltransferase gene *POMT1* give rise to the severe neuronal migration disorder Walker-Warburg syndrome. *Am J Hum Genet* 2002;71:1033–1043.
604. Yamamoto T, Kato Y, Karita M, et al. Expression of genes related to muscular dystrophy with lissencephaly. *Pediatr Neurol* 2004;31:183–190.
605. Aicardi J. The agyria-pachygyria complex: a spectrum of cortical malformations. *Brain Dev* 1991;13:1–8.
606. Gastaut H, Pinsard N, Raybaud C, et al. Lissencephaly (agyria-pachygyria): clinical findings and serial EEG studies. *Dev Med Child Neurol* 1987;29:167–180.
607. Alvarez LA, Yamamoto T, Wong B, et al. Miller-Dieker syndrome: a disorder affecting specific pathways of neuronal migration. *Neurology* 1986;36:489–493.
608. Kuzniecky R, Berkovic S, Andermann F. Focal cortical myoclonus and rolandic cortical dysplasia: clarification by magnetic resonance imaging. *Ann Neurol* 1988;23:317–325.
609. Dobyns WB, Stratton RF, Greenberg F. Syndromes with lissencephaly. Miller-Dieker and Norman-Roberts syndrome and isolated lissencephaly. *Am J Med Genet* 1984;18:509–526.
610. Kuzniecky R, Andermann F, Guerrini R. Congenital bilateral perisylvian syndrome: study of 31 patients. *Lancet* 1993;341:608–612.
611. Guerrini R, Dubeau F, Dulac O, et al. Bilateral parasagittal parietooccipital polymicrogyria and epilepsy. *Ann Neurol* 1997;41:65–73.
612. Gropman AL, Barkovich AJ, Vezina LG, et al. Pediatric congenital bilateral perisylvian syndrome: clinical and MRI features in 12 patients. *Neuropediatrics* 1997;28:198–203.
613. Becker PS, Dixon AM, Troncoso JC. Bilateral opercular polymicrogyria. *Ann Neurol* 1989;25:90–92.
614. Palmini A, Andermann F, Olivier A, et al. Focal neuronal migration disorders and intractible partial epilepsy: a study of 30 patients. *Ann Neurol* 1991;30:741–749.
615. Sankar R, Curran JG, Kevill JW, et al. Microscopic cortical dysplasia in infantile spasms: evolution of white matter abnormalities. *Am J Neuroradiol* 1995;16:1265–1272.
616. Palmini A, Andermann F, Aicardi J, et al. Diffuse cortical dysplasia or the "double cortex" syndrome. *Neurology* 1991;41:1656–1662.
617. Pinard J-M, Motte J, Chiron C, et al. Subcortical laminar heterotopia and lissencephaly in two families: a single X-l inked dominant gene. *J Neurol Neurosurg Psychiatry* 1994;57:914–920.
618. Gleeson JG, Allen KM, Fox JW. *Doublecortin*, a brain-specific gene mutated in human X-l inked lissencephaly and double cortex syndrome, encodes a putative signaling protein. *Cell* 1998;92:63–72.
619. Gleeson JG, Minnerath SR, Fox JW, et al. Characterization of mutations in the gene *doublecortin* in patients with double cortex syndrome. *Ann Neurol* 1999;45:146–153.
620. des Portes V, Pinard JM, Billuart P, et al. A novel CNS gene required for neuronal migration and involved in X-l inked subcortical laminar heterotopia and lissencephaly syndrome. *Cell* 1998;92:51–61.
621. Miura K, Watanabe K, Maeda N, et al. Magnetic resonance imaging and positron emission tomography of band heterotopia. *Brain Dev* 1993;15:288–290.
622. Huttenlocher PR, Taravath S, Mojtahedi S. Periventricular heterotopia and epilepsy. *Neurology* 1994;44:51–55.
623. Dubeau F, Tampieri D, Lee N. Periventricular and subcortical nodular heterotopia: a study of 33 patients. *Brain* 1995;118:1273–1287.
624. Li LM, Dubeau F, Andermann F, et al. Periventricular nodular heterotopia and intractable temporal lobe epilepsy: poor outcome after temporal lobe resection. *Ann Neurol* 1997;41:662–668.
625. Musumeci SA, Ferri R, Elia M, et al. A new family with periventricular nodular heterotopia and peculiar dysmorphic features. *Arch Neurol* 1997;54:61–64.
626. Eksioglu YZ, Scheffer IE, Cardenas P, et al. Periventricular heterotopia: an X-l inked dominant epilepsy locus causing aberrant cerebral cortical development. *Neuron* 1996;16:77–87.
627. Sheen VL, Dixon PH, Fox JW, et al. Mutations in the X-linked *filamin1* gene cause periventricular nodular heterotopia in males as well as in females. *Hum Mol Genet* 2001;10:1165–1783.
628. Sheen VL, Basel-Vanagaite L, Goodman JR, et al. Etiological heterogeneity of familial periventricular heterotopia and hydrocephalus. *Brain Dev* 2004;26:326–334.
629. Jeret JS, Serur D, Wisniewski K, et al. Frequency of agenesis of the corpus callosum in the developmentally disabled population as determined by computerized tomography. *Pediatr Neurosci* 1986;12:101–103.
630. Zaki W. Le processus dégénératif au cours du développement du corps colleux. *Arch Anat Microscp Morphol Exp* 1985;74:133–149.
631. Ettlinger G, Blakemore CB, Milner AD, et al. Agenesis of the corpus callosum: a behavioral investigation. *Brain* 1972;95:327–346.
632. Serur D, Jeret JS, Wisniewski K. Agenesis of the corpus callosum: clinical, neuroradiological and cytogenetic studies. *Neuropediatrics* 1988;19:87–91.
633. Barkovich AJ, Lyon G, Evrard P. Formation, maturation, and disorders of white matter. *Am J Neuroradiol* 1992;13:447–461.
634. Barkovich AJ, Kjos B. Normal postnatal development of the corpus callosum as demonstrated by MR imaging. *Am J Neuroradiol* 1988;9:487–491.
635. Menkes JH, Philippart M, Clark DB. Hereditary partial agenesis of the corpus callosum. *Arch Neurol* 1964;11:198–208.
636. Khanna S, Chugani HT, Messa C, et al. Corpus callosum agenesis and epilepsy: PET findings. *Pediatr Neurol* 1994;10:221–227.
637. Graham JM, Tackels D, Dibbern K, et al. FG syndrome: report of three new families with linkage to Xq12-q22.1. *Am J Med Genet* 1998;80:145–156.
638. Bamforth F, Bamforth S, Poskitt K, et al. Abnormalities of corpus callosum in patients with inherited metabolic diseases. *Lancet* 1988;2:451.
639. Dobyns WB. Agenesis of the corpus callosum and gyral malformations are frequent manifestations of nonketotic hyperglycinemia. *Neurology* 1989;39:817–820.
640. Njiokiktjien C, Valk J, Ramaekers G. Malformation or damage of the corpus callosum? A clinical and MRI study. *Brain Dev* 1988;10:92–99.
641. deJong JG, Delleman JW, Houben M, et al. Agenesis of the corpus callosum, infantile spasms, ocular anomalies (Aicardi's syndrome). *Neurology* 1976;26:1152–1158.
642. Bertoni JM, von Loh S, Allen RJ. The Aicardi syndrome: report of 4 cases and review of the literature. *Ann Neurol* 1979;5:475–482.
643. Burn J, Martin N. Two retarded male cousins with odd facies, hypotonia, and severe constipation: possible examples of the X-linked FG syndrome. *J Med Genet* 1983;20:97–99.
644. Sayed M, Al-Alaiyan S. Agenesis of corpus callosum. Hypertrophic pyloric stenosis and Hirschsprung disease: coincidence or common etiology? *Neuropediatrics* 1996;27:204–206.
645. Ng Y, McCarthy CM, Tarby T, et al. Agenesis of the corpus callosum is associated with feeding difficulties. *J Child Neurol* 2004;19:443–446.

646. Barkovich AJ, Simon EM, Walsh CA. Callosal agenesis with cyst. A better understanding and new classification. *Neurology* 2001;56:220–227.
647. Dávila-Gutiérrez G. Agenesis and dysgenesis of the corpus callosum. *Semin Pediatr Neurol* 2002;9:292–301.
648. Sherr EH, Barkovich AJ, Hetts S, et al. Agenesis of the corpus callosum: analysis of the phenotypic spectrum [Abstract]. *Ann Neurol* 2003;54(Suppl 7):S108–S109.
649. Landman J, Weitz R, Dulitzki F, et al. Radiological colpocephaly: a congenital malformation or the result of intrauterine and perinatal brain damage. *Brain Dev* 1989;11:313–316.
650. Flores-Sarnat L. *Colpocephaly*. San Diego, CA: MedLink, 2004.
651. Rakic P, Yakovlev P. Development of the corpus callosum and cavum septi in man. *J Comp Neurol* 1968;132:45–72.
652. Nakajima Y, Yano S, Kuramatsu T, et al. Ultrasonographic evaluation of cavum septi pellucidi and cavum vergae. *Brain Dev* 1986;8:505–508.
653. Miller ME, Kido D, Horner F. Cavum vergae: association with neurologic abnormality and diagnosis by magnetic resonance imaging. *Arch Neurol* 1986;43:821–823.
654. Bodensteiner JB. The saga of the septum pellucidum: a tale of unfunded clinical investigations. *J Child Neurol* 1995;10:227–231.
655. Pauling KJ, Bodensteiner JB, Hogg JP, et al. Does selection bias determine the prevalence of the cavum septi pellucidi? *Pediatr Neurol* 1998;19:195–198.
656. Nellhaus G. Head circumference from birth to 18 years. *Pediatrics* 1968;41:106–114.
657. Sells CJ. Microcephaly in a normal school population. *Pediatrics* 1977;59:262–265.
658. Burton BK. Dominant inheritance of microcephaly with short stature. *Clin Genet* 1981;20:25–27.
659. Dorman C. Microcephaly and intelligence. *Dev Med Child Neurol* 1991;33:267–269.
660. Dolk H. The predictive value of microcephaly during the first year of life for mental retardation at 7 years. *Dev Med Child Neurol* 1991;33:974–983.
661. Book JA, Schut JW, Reed AC. A clinical and genetical study of microcephaly. *Am J Ment Defic* 1953;57:637–660.
662. Merlob P, Steier D, Reisner SH. Autosomal dominant isolated ("uncomplicated") microcephaly. *J Med Genet* 1988;25:750–753.
663. Connolly CJ. The fissural pattern of primate brain. *Am J Phys Anthropol* 1936;21:301–422.
664. Tolmie JL, McNay M, Stephenson JB, et al. Microcephaly: genetic counselling and antenatal diagnosis after the birth of an affected child. *Am J Med Genet* 1987;27:583–594.
665. McKusick VA, Stauffer M, Knox DL, et al. Chorioretinopathy with hereditary microcephaly. *Arch Ophthalmol* 1966;75:597–600.
666. Scott-Emuakpor A, Heffelfinger J, Higgins JV. A syndrome of microcephaly and cataracts in four siblings: a new genetic syndrome? *Am J Dis Child* 1977;131:167–169.
667. Miller RW, Blot WJ. Small head after *in utero* exposure to atomic radiation. *Lancet* 1972;2:784–787.
668. Dekaban A. Abnormalities in children exposed to x-radiation during various stages of gestation: tentative timetable of radiation injury to the human fetus, Part I. *J Nucl Med* 1968;9:471–477.
669. Wood JW, Johnson KG, Omori Y. *In utero* exposure to the Hiroshima atomic bomb: an evaluation of head size and mental retardation 20 years later. *Pediatrics* 1967;39:385–392.
670. Amatuzzi R. Hazards to the human fetus from ionizing radiation at diagnostic dose levels: review of the literature. *Perinatol Neonatal* 1980;4:23–30.
671. Steinlin M, Zurrer M, Martin E, et al. Contribution of magnetic resonance imaging on the evaluation of microcephaly. *Neuropediatrics* 1991;22:184–189.
672. Brennan TL, Funk SG, Frothinghom TE. Disproportionate intrauterine head growth and developmental outcome. *Dev Med Child Neurol* 1985;27:746–750.
673. Lipper E, Lee K, Gartner LM, et al. Determinants of neurobehavioral outcome in low-birth-weight infants. *Pediatrics* 1981;67:502–505.
674. Virchow R. Ueber den Cretinismus, namentlich in Franken, and über pathologische Schädelformen. *Verh Phys Med Ges* (Würzburg) 1851;2:230–271.
675. David JD, Poswillo D, Simpson D. *The craniosynostoses*. Berlin: Springer-Verlag, 1982.
676. Flores-Sarnat L. New insights into craniosynostosis. *Semin Pediatr Neurol* 2002;9:274–291.
677. Cohen MM Jr. Craniosynostosis update 1987. *Am J Med Genet* 1988;4(Suppl):99–148.
678. Park EA, Powers GF. Acrocephaly and scaphocephaly with symmetrically distributed malformations of the extremities: A study of the so-called acrocephalosyndactylism. *Am J Dis Child* 1920;20:235–315.
679. Moloney DM, Wall SA, Ashworth GJ, et al. Prevalence of Pro250Arg mutation of fibroblast growth factor receptor 3 in coronal craniosynostosis. *Lancet* 1997;349:1059–1062.
680. Passos-Bueno MR, Sertie AL, Richieri-Costa A, et al. Description of a new mutation and characterization of FGFR1, FGFR2, and FGFR3 mutations among Brazilian patients with syndromic craniosynostoses. *Am J Med Genet* 1998;78:237–241.
681. Graham JM, Badura RJ, Smith DW. Coronal cranio-stenosis: fetal head constraint as one possible cause. *Pediatrics* 1980;65:995–999.
682. Babler WJ, Persing JA, Persson KM, et al. Skull growth after coronal suturectomy, periostectomy, and dural transection. *J Neurosurg* 1982;56:529–535.
683. Menking M, Wiebel J, Schmid WU, et al. Premature craniosynostosis associated with hyperthyroidism in 4 children with reference to 5 further cases in the literature. *Monatsschr Kinderheilkd* 1972;120:106–110.
684. Comings DE, Papazian C, Schoene HR. Conradi's disease: Chondrodystrophia calcificans congenita, congenital stippled epiphyses. *J Pediatr* 1968;72:63–69.
685. Reilly BJ, Leeming JM, Fraser D. Craniosynostosis in the rachitic spectrum. *J Pediatr* 1964;64:396–405.
686. Cohen MM Jr. Perspectives on craniosynostosis. *West J Med* 1980;132:507–513.
687. Till K. *Paediatric neurosurgery*. Oxford: Blackwell, 1975.
688. Freeman JM, Borkowf S. Craniostenosis: review of the literature and report of 34 cases. *Pediatrics* 1962;30:57–70.
689. Müke R. Neue Gesichtspunkte zur Pathogenese und Therapie der Kraniosynostose. *Acta Neurochir* 1972;26:191–250, 293–326.
690. Fishman MA, Hogan GR, Dodge PR. The concurrence of hydrocephalus and craniosynostosis. *J Neurosurg* 1971;34:621–629.
691. Cinalli G, Renier D, Sebag G, et al. Chronic tonsillar herniation in Crouzon's and Apert's syndromes: the role of premature synostosis of the lambdoid suture. *J Neurosurg* 1995;83:575–582.
692. Francis PM, Beals S, Rekate HL, et al. Chronic tonsillar herniation and Crouzon's syndrome. *Pediatr Neurosurg* 1992;18:202–206.
693. Steinberger D, Vriend G, Mulliken JB, et al. The mutations of FGFR2-associated craniosynostoses are clustered in five structural elements of immunoglobulin-like domain III of the receptor. *Hum Genet* 1998;102:145–150.
694. Schaefer F, Anderson C, Can B, et al. Novel mutation in the FGFR2 gene at the same codon as the Crouzon syndrome mutations in a severe Pfeiffer syndrome type 2 case. *Am J Med Genet* 1998;75:252–255.
695. Park WJ, Theda C, Maestri NE, et al. Analysis of phenotypic features and FGFR2 mutations in Apert syndrome. *Am J Hum Genet* 1995;57:321–328.
696. Cohen MM, Kreiborg S. The central nervous system in the Apert syndrome. *Am J Med Genet* 1990;35:36–45.
697. Ladda RL, Stoltzfus E, Gordon SL, et al. Craniosynostosis associated with limb reduction malformations and cleft lip/palate: a distinct syndrome. *Pediatrics* 1978;61:12–15.
698. Menard RM, David DJ. Unilateral lambdoid synostosis: morphological characteristics. *J Craniofac Surg* 1998;9:240–246.
699. Lee FA, McComb JG. The breech head. Personal communication.
700. Dohn DF. Surgical treatment of unilateral coronal craniosynostosis (plagiocephaly): report of three cases. *Clev Clin Q* 1963;30:47–54.
701. Rekate HL. Occipital plagiocephaly: a critical review of the literature. *J Neurosurg* 1998;89:24–30.
702. McComb JG, Withers GJ, Davis RL. Cortical damage from Zenker's solution applied to the dura mater. *Neurosurgery* 1981;6:68–71.
703. Anderson FM. Treatment of coronal and metopic synostosis: 107 cases. *Neurosurgery* 1981;8:143–149.

704. Marsh JL, Schwartz HG. The surgical correction of coronal and metopic craniosynostoses. *J Neurosurg* 1983;59:245–251.
705. Shillito J, Matson DD. Craniosynostosis: a review of 519 surgical patients. *Pediatrics* 1968;41:829–853.
706. Popich GA, Smith DW. Fontanels: range of normal size. *J Pediatr* 1972;80:749–752.
707. Aisenson MR. Closing of the anterior fontanelle. *Pediatrics* 1950;6:223–226.
708. Gooskens RHJM. *Megalencephaly: a subtype of macrocephaly*. Wijk bij Duurstede, Netherlands: Drukwerkverzorging ADDIX, 1987.
709. Ahlgren S, Vogt P, Bronner-Fraser M. Excess *FoxG1* causes overgrowth of the neural tube. *J Neurobiol* 2003;57:337–349.
710. Saul RA, Stevenson RE, Bley R. Mental retardation in the Bannayan syndrome. *Pediatrics* 1982;69:642–644.
711. Powell BR, Budden SS, Buist NRM. Dominantly inherited megalencephaly, muscle weakness, and myoliposis: a carnitine-deficient myopathy within the spectrum of the Ruvalcaba-Myhre-Smith syndrome. *J Pediatr* 1993;123:70–75.
712. Cohen MM. Bannayan-Riley-Ruvalcaba syndrome: renaming three formerly recognized syndromes as one etiologic entity. *Am J Med Genet* 1990;35:291.
713. Smith RD. Abnormal head circumference in learning-disabled children. *Dev Med Child Neurol* 1981;23:626–632.
714. Lorber J, Priestley BL. Children with large heads: a practical approach to diagnosis in 557 children with special reference to 109 children with megalencephaly. *Dev Med Child Neurol* 1981;23:494–504.
714a. Sandler AD, Knudsen MW, Brown TT, et al.. Neurodevelopmental dysfunction among nonreferred children with idiopathic megalencephaly. *J Pediatr* 1997;31:320–324.
715. Wilson SAK. Megalencephaly. *J Neurol Psychopathol* 1934;14:173–186.
716. Pascual-Castroviejo I, Pascual-Pascual SI, Velásquez-Fragua R. Ensanchamieneto benigno de los espaacios subaracnoideos. Estudios y seguimiento de diez casos. [Benign enlargement of the subarachnoid spaces. A study and follow-up of ten cases]. *Rev Neurol* (Barcelona) 2004;39:701–706.
717. Flores-Sarnat L. Hemimegalencephaly. Part 1. Genetic, clinical and imaging aspects. *J Child Neurol* 2002;17:373–384.
718. Di Rocco C, Iannelli A. Hemimegalencephaly and intractable epilepsy: complications of hemispherectomy and their correlations with the surgical technique. A report of 15 cases. *Pediatr Neurosurg* 2000;33:198–207.
719. Robain O, Floquet C, Heldt N, et al. Hemimegalencephaly: a clinicopathological study of four cases. *Neuropathol Appl Neurobiol* 1988;14:125–135.
720. Takashima S, Chan F, Becker LE, et al. Aberrant neuronal development in hemimegalencephaly: immunocytochemical and Golgi studies. *Pediatr Neurol* 1991;7:275–280.
721. Flores-Sarnat L, Sarnat HB, Dávila-Gutiérrez G, et al. Hemimegalencephaly. Part 2. Neuropathology suggests a disorder of cellular lineage. *J Child Neurol* 2003;18:776–785.
722. Saijoh Y, Adachi H, Mochida K, et al. Distinct transcriptional regulatory mechanisms underlie left-right asymmetric expression of *lefty-1* and *lefty-2*. *Genes Dev* 1999;13:259–269.
723. Fishman RA. *Cerebrospinal fluid in diseases of the nervous system*, 2nd ed. Philadelphia: Saunders, 1992.
724. Davson H, Welch K, Segal MB. *Physiology and pathophysiology of the cerebrospinal fluid*. Edinburgh: Churchill Livingstone, 1987.
725. Müller F, O'Rahilly R. The human brain at stages 18–20, including the choroid plexuses and the amygdaloid and septal nuclei. *Anat Embryol* 1990;182:285–306.
726. Shuangshoti S, Netsky MG. Histogenesis of choroid plexus in man. *Am J Anat* 1966;118:283–316.
727. Sarnat HB. Histochemistry and immunocytochemistry of the developing ependyma and choroid plexus. *Microsc Res Tech* 1998;41:14–28.
728. Dooling EC, Chi Je G, Gilles FH. Ependymal changes in the human fetal brain. *Ann Neurol* 1977;1:535–541.
729. McComb JG. Cerebrospinal fluid physiology of the developing fetus. *Am J Neuroradiol* 1992;13:595–599.
730. Rottenberg DA, Howieson J, Deck MDF. The rate of CSF formation in man: preliminary observations on metrizamide washout as a measure of CSF bulk flow. *Ann Neurol* 1977;2:503–510.
731. Masserman JH. Cerebrospinal hydrodynamics. IV. Clinical experimental studies. *Arch Neurol Psychiatr* 1934;32:523–553.
732. Cutler RWP, Page L, Galicich J, et al. Formation and absorption of cerebrospinal fluid in man. *Brain* 1968;91:707–720.
733. Lorenzo AV, Page LK, Watters GV. Relationship between cerebrospinal fluid formation, absorption and pressure in human hydrocephalus. *Brain* 1970;93:679–692.
734. Rubin LL, Staddon JM. The cell biology of the blood–brain barrier. *Annu Rev Neurosci* 1999;22:11–28.
735. Greitz D. Cerebrospinal fluid circulation and associated intracranial dynamics: a radiologic investigation using MR imaging and radionuclide cisternography. *Acta Radiol* 1993;34(Suppl 386):1 23.
736. Welch K, Friedman V. The cerebrospinal fluid valves. *Brain* 1960;83:454–469.
737. Upton ML, Weller RO. The morphology of cerebrospinal fluid drainage pathways in human arachnoid granulations. *J Neurosurg* 1985;63:867–875.
738. Mann JD, Butler AB, Rosenthal JE, et al. Regulation of intracranial pressure in rat, dog, and man. *Ann Neurol* 1978;3:156–165.
739. James AE, McComb JG, Christian J, et al. The effect of cerebrospinal fluid pressure on the size of the drainage pathways. *Neurology* 1976;26:659–663.
740. Shabo AL, Maxwell DS. The morphology of the arachnoid villi: a light and electronmicroscopic study in the monkey. *J Neurosurg* 1968;29:451–463.
741. McComb JG, Davson H, Hyman S, et al. Cerebrospinal fluid drainage as influenced by ventricular pressure in the rabbit. *J Neurosurg* 1982;56:790–797.
742. McComb JG. Recent research into the nature of cerebrospinal fluid formation and absorption. *J Neurosurg* 1983;59:369–383.
743. James AE Jr, Strecker EP, Sperber E, et al. An alternative pathway of cerebrospinal fluid absorption in communicating hydrocephalus: transependymal movement. *Radiology* 1974;111:143–146.
744. Hiratsuka H, Tabata H, Tsuruoka S, et al. Evaluation of periventricular hypodensity in experimental hydrocephalus by metrizamide CT ventriculography. *J Neurosurg* 1982;56:235–240.
745. Zervas NT, Liszczak TM, Mayberg MR, et al. Cerebrospinal fluid may nourish cerebral vessels through pathways in the adventitia that may be analogous to systemic vasa vasorum. *J Neurosurg* 1982;56:475–481.
746. Nabeshima S, Reese TS, Landis DM, et al. Junctions in the meninges and marginal glia. *J Comp Neurol* 1975;164:127–170.
747. Alvarez LA, Maytal J, Shinnar S. Idiopathic external hydrocephalus: natural history and relationship to benign familial macrocephaly. *Pediatrics* 1986;77:901–907.
748. Andersson H, Elfverson J, Svendson P. External hydrocephalus in infants. *Childs Brain* 1984;11:398–402.
749. Lorenzo AV, Bresnan MJ, Barlow CF. Cerebrospinal fluid absorption deficit in normal pressure hydrocephalus. *Arch Neurol* 1974;30:387–393.
750. Murthy VS, Deshpande DH. The central canal of the filum terminale in communicating hydrocephalus. *J Neurosurg* 1980;53:528–532.
751. Bering EA. Circulation of the cerebrospinal fluid: demonstration of the choroid plexuses as the generator of the force of flow of fluid and ventricular enlargement. *J Neurosurg* 1962;19:405–413.
752. Weller RO, Wisniewski H. Histological and ultrastructural changes with experimental hydrocephalus in adult rabbits. *Brain* 1969;92:819–828.
753. Milhorat TH, Clark RG, Hammock MK, et al. Structural, ultrastructural and permeability changes in the ependyma and surrounding brain favoring equilibration in progressive hydrocephalus. *Arch Neurol* 1970;22:397–407.
754. Weller RO, Shulman K. Infantile hydrocephalus: clinical, histological, and ultrastructural study of brain damage. *J Neurosurg* 1972;36:255–267.
755. Bannister CM, Chapman SA. Ventricular ependyma of normal and hydrocephalic subjects: a scanning electronmicroscopic study. *Dev Med Child Neurol* 1980;22:725–735.
756. Levin VA, Milhorat TH, Fenstermacher JD, et al. Physiological

studies on the development of obstructive hydrocephalus in the monkey. *Neurology* 1971;21:238–246.
757. Hochwald GM, Lux WE Jr, Sahar A, et al. Experimental hydrocephalus: changes in cerebrospinal fluid dynamics as a function of time. *Arch Neurol* 1972;26:120–129.
758. Shulman K, Marmarou A. Pressure-volume considerations in infantile hydrocephalus. *Dev Med Child Neurol* 1971;25(Suppl):90 95.
759. Hayden PW, Shurtleff DB, Foltz EL. Ventricular fluid pressure recordings in hydrocephalic patients. *Arch Neurol* 1970;23:147–154.
760. Hill A, Volpe JJ. Decrease in pulsatile flow in the anterior cerebral arteries in infantile hydrocephalus. *Pediatrics* 1982;69:4–7.
761. Milhorat TH, Hammock MK, Davis DA, et al. Choroid plexus papilloma. I. Proof of cerebral spinal fluid overproduction. *Childs Brain* 1976;2:273–289.
762. Eisenberg HM, McComb JG, Lorenzo AV. Cerebrospinal fluid overproduction and hydrocephalus associated with choroid plexus papilloma. *J Neurosurg* 1974;40:381–385.
763. Adams C, Johnston WP, Nevin NC. Family study of congenital hydrocephalus. *Dev Med Child Neurol* 1982;24:493–498.
764. Emery JL, Staschak MC. The size and form of the cerebral aqueduct in children. *Brain* 1972;95:591–598.
765. Woollam DHM, Millen JW. Anatomical considerations in the pathology of stenosis of the cerebral aqueduct. *Brain* 1953;76:104–112.
766. Russell DS. Observations on the pathology of hydrocephalus. *Medical Research Council special report series, no*. 265. London: His Majesty's Stationery Office, 1949:138.
767. McMillan JJ, Williams B. Aqueduct stenosis: case review and discussion. *J Neurol Neurosurg Psychiatry* 1977;40:521–532.
768. Parisi MA, Dobyns WB. Human malformations of the midbrain and hindbrain: review and proposed classification scheme. *Mol Genet Metab* 2003;80:36–53.
769. Yamasaki M, Thompson P, Lemmon V. CRASH syndrome: Mutations in L1CAM correlate with severity of the disease. *Neuropediatrics* 1997;28:175–178.
770. Graf WD, Born DE, Sarnat HB. The pachygyria-polymicrogyria spectrum of cortical dysplasia in X-linked hydrocephalus. *Eur J Pediatr Surg* 1998;8(Suppl 1):10–14.
771. Sarnat HB. Ependymal reactions to injury: a review. *J Neuropathol Exp Neurol* 1995;54:1–15.
772. Benda C. *Developmental disorders of mentation and cerebral palsies*. New York: Grune and Stratton, 1952.
773. Dandy WE, Blackfan KD. Internal hydrocephalus: an experimental, clinical and pathological study. *Am J Dis Child* 1914;8:406–482.
774. Hart NM, Malamud N, Ellis WG. The Dandy-Walker syndrome: a clinicopathological study based on 28 cases. *Neurology* 1972;22:771–780.
775. Tal Y, Freigang B, Dunn HG, et al. Dandy-Walker syndrome: analysis of 21 cases. *Dev Med Child Neurol* 1980;22:189–201.
776. Hirsch JF, Pierre-Kahn A, Renier D, et al. The Dandy-Walker malformation: a review of 40 cases. *J Neurosurg* 1984;61:515–522.
777. Cartwright MJ, Eisenberg MB, Page LK. Posterior fossa arachnoid cyst presenting with an isolated twelfth nerve paresis: case report and review of the literature. *Clin Neurol Neurosurg* 1991;93: 69–72.
778. Maria BL, Zinreich SJ, Carson BC, et al. Dandy-Walker syndrome revisited. *Pedatr Neurosci* 1987;13:45–51.
779. McLaurin RL, Crone KR. Dandy-Walker malformation. In: Wilkins RH, Rengachary SS, eds. *Neurosurgery*, 2nd ed. New York: McGraw-Hill, 1996:3669–3672.
780. Curless RG, Quencer RM, Katz DA, et al. Magnetic resonance demonstration of intracranial CSF flow in children. *Neurology* 1992;42:377–381.
781. Gilles FH, Shillito J. Infantile hydrocephalus: retrocerebellar subdural hematoma. *J Pediatr* 1970;76:529–537.
782. Ahdab-Barmada M, Claassen D. A distinctive triad of malformations of the central nervous system in the Meckel-Grüber syndrome. *J Neuropathol Exp Neurol* 1990;49:610–620.
783. Gandy SE, Heier LA. Clinical and magnetic resonance features of primary intracranial arachnoid cysts. *Ann Neurol* 1987;21:342–348.
784. Rosman NP, Shands KN. Hydrocephalus caused by increased intracranial venous pressure: a clinicopathological study. *Ann Neurol* 1978;3:445–450.
785. Beck DJK, Russell DS. Experiments on thrombosis of the superior longitudinal sinus. *J Neurosurg* 1946;3:337–347.
786. Gordon N. Normal pressure hydrocephalus and arrested hydrocephalus. *Dev Med Child Neurol* 1977;19:540–543.
787. Hakim S, Venegas JG, Burton JD. The physics of the cranial cavity, hydrocephalus and normal pressure hydrocephalus: mechanical interpretation and mathematical model. *Surg Neurol* 1976;5:187–210.
788. Mori K, Mima T. To what extent has the pathophysiology of normal pressure hydrocephalus been clarified? *Crit Rev Neurosurg* 1998;8:232–243.
789. Bret P, Chazal J. Chronic ("normal pressure") hydrocephalus in childhood and adolescence: a review of 16 cases and reappraisal of the syndrome. *Childs Nerv Syst* 1995;11:687–691.
790. Milhorat TH. *Hydrocephalus and the cerebrospinal fluid*. Baltimore: Williams & Wilkins, 1972:137, 170.
791. Rogers M, Kaplan AM, Ben-Ora A. Fetal hydrocephalus. Use of ultrasound in diagnosis and management. *Perinatol Neonatol* 1980;4(6):31–34.
792. Johnson ML, Pretorius D, Clewell WH, et al. Fetal hydrocephalus: diagnosis and management. *Semin Perinatol* 1983;7:83–89.
793. Huisman TA, Wiser J, Martin E, et al. Fetal magnetic resonance imaging of the central nervous system: a pictorial essay. *Eur Radiol* 2002;12:1952–1961.
794. Renier D, Sainte-Rose C, Pierre-Kahn A, et al. Prenatal hydrocephalus: outcome and prognosis. *Childs Nerv Syst* 1988;4:213–222.
795. Glick PL, Harrison MR, Nakayama DK, et al. Management of ventriculomegaly in the fetus. *J Pediatr* 1984;105:97–105.
796. Laurence KM. The pathology of hydrocephalus. *Ann R Coll Surg Engl* 1959;24:388–401.
797. Rubin RC. The effect of the severe hydrocephalus on size and number of brain cells. *Dev Med Child Neurol* 1972;27(Suppl):117 120.
798. Tomasovic JA, Nellhaus G, Moe PG. The bobble-head doll syndrome: an early sign of hydrocephalus. Two new cases and review of the literature. *Dev Med Child Neurol* 1975;17:777–783.
799. Hier DB, Wiehl AC. Chronic hydrocephalus associated with short stature and growth hormone deficiency: case report. *Ann Neurol* 1977;2:246–248.
800. Kim CS, Bennett DR, Roberts TS. Primary amenorrhea secondary to noncommunicating hydrocephalus. *Neurology* 1969;19:533–535.
801. Fiedler R, Krieger DT. Endocrine disturbances in patients with congenital aqueductal stenosis. *Acta Endocrinol* 1975;80:1–13.
802. Miller E, Sethi L. The effect of hydrocephalus on perception. *Dev Med Child Neurol* 1971;25(Suppl):77 81.
803. Hagberg B, Sjörgen I. The chronic brain syndrome of infantile hydrocephalus: a follow-up study of 63 spontaneously arrested cases. *Am J Dis Child* 1966;112:189–196.
804. Sher PK, Brown SB. A longitudinal study of head growth in preterm infants. I. Normal rates of head growth. *Dev Med Child Neurol* 1975;17:705–710.
805. Fujimura M, Seryu J. Velocity of head growth during the perinatal period. *Arch Dis Child* 1977;52:105–112.
806. Fujimura M. Factors which influence the timing of maximum growth rate of the head in low birthweight infants. *Arch Dis Child* 1977;52:113–117.
807. Babson SG, Benda GI. Growth graphs for the clinical assessment of infants of varying gestational age. *J Pediatr* 1976;89:814–820.
808. Dodge PR, Porter P. Demonstration of intracranial pathology by transillumination. *Arch Neurol* 1961;5:594–605.
809. Horbar JD, Walters CL, Philip AG, et al. Ultrasound detection of changing ventricular size in posthemorrhagic hydrocephalus. *Pediatrics* 1980;66:674–678.
810. Afschrift M, Jeannin P, de Praeter C, et al. Ventricular taps in the neonate under ultrasonic guidance: technical note. *J Neurosurg* 1983;59:1100–1101.
811. Newman GC, Buschi AI, Sugg NK, et al. Dandy-Walker syndrome diagnosed *in utero* by ultrasonography. *Neurology* 1982;32:180–184.

812. Britton J, Marsh H, Kendall B, et al. MRI and hydrocephalus in childhood. *Neuroradiology* 1988;30:310–314.
813. Atlas SW, Mark AS, Fram EK. Aqueductal stenosis: evaluation with gradient-echo rapid MR imaging. *Radiology* 1988;169:449–453.
814. Barkovich AJ, Edwards MSB. Applications of neuroimaging in hydrocephalus. *Pediatr Neurosurg* 1992;18:65–83.
815. Nitz WR, Bradley WG Jr, Watanabe AS, et al. Flow dynamics of cerebrospinal fluid: assessment with phase-contrast velocity MR imaging performed with retrospective cardiac gating. *Radiology* 1992;183:395–405.
816. Ohara S, Nagai H, Matsumoto T, et al. MR imaging of CSF pulsatory flow and its relation to intracranial pressure. *J Neurosurg* 1988;69:675–682.
817. Schroth G, Klose U. Cerebrospinal fluid flow. III. Pathological cerebrospinal fluid pulsations. *Neuroradiology* 1992;35:16–24.
818. Quencer RM. Intracranial CSF flow in pediatric hydrocephalus: evaluation with cine-MR imaging. *Am J Neuroradiol* 1992;13:601–608.
819. Goumnerova LC, Frim DM. Treatment of hydrocephalus with third ventriculocisternostomy: outcome and CSF flow patterns. *Pediatr Neurosurg* 1997;27:149–152.
820. DiChiro G, Ashburn WL, Briner WH. Technetium Tc 99m serum albumin for cisternography. *Arch Neurol* 1968;19:218–227.
821. McCullough DC, Harbert JC, Di Chiro G, et al. Prognostic criteria for cerebrospinal fluid shunting from isotope cisternography in communicating hydrocephalus. *Neurology* 1970;20:594–598.
822. McLone DG, Aronyk KE. An approach to the management of arrested and compensated hydrocephalus. *Pedatr Neurosurg* 1993;19:101–103.
823. Schain RJ. Carbonic anhydrase inhibitors in chronic infantile hydrocephalus. *Am J Dis Child* 1969;117:621–625.
824. Mealey J Jr, Barker DT. Failure of oral acetazolamide to advert hydrocephalus in infants with myelomeningocele. *J Pediatr* 1968;72:257–259.
825. Putnam TJ. Treatment of hydrocephalus by endoscopic coagulation of choroid plexuses: description of a new instrument and preliminary report of results. *N Engl J Med* 1934;210:1373–1376.
826. Cinalli G, Sainte-Rose C, Chumas P, et al. Failure of third ventriculostomy in the treatment of aqueductal stenosis in children. *J Neurosurg* 1999;90:448–454.
827. Matson DD. A new operation for the treatment of communicating hydrocephalus: report of a case secondary to generalized meningitis. *J Neurosurg* 1949;6:238–247.
828. Post EM. Shunt systems. In: Wilkins RH, Rengachary SS, eds. *Neurosurgery*, 2nd ed. New York: McGraw-Hill, 1996:3645–3653.
829. McLaurin RL. Ventricular shunts: complications and results. In: Section of Pediatric Neurosurgery, American Association of Neurological Surgeons, eds. *Pediatric neurosurgery. Surgery of the developing nervous system*, 2nd ed. New York: Grune and Stratton, 1989:219–229.
830. Forslund M, Bjerre I, Jeppson JO. Cerebrospinal fluid protein in shunt-treated hydrocephalic children. *Dev Med Child Neurol* 1976;18:784–790.
831. Bayston R. *Hydrocephalus shunt infections*. London: Chapman and Hall, 1989.
832. Haines SJ, Walters BC. Antibiotic prophylaxis for cerebrospinal fluid shunts: a metanalysis. *Neurosurgery* 1994;34:87–92.
833. Meirovitch J, Kitai-Cohen Y, Keren G, et al. Cerebrospinal fluid shunt infections in children. *Pediatr Infect Dis J* 1987;6:921–924.
834. Pople IK, Bayston R, Hayward RD. Infection of cerebrospinal fluid shunts in infants: a study of etiologic factors. *J Neurosurg* 1992;77:29–36.
835. Forward KR, Fewer HD, Stiver HG. Cerebrospinal fluid shunt infections: a review of 35 infections in 32 patients. *J Neurosurg* 1983;59:389–394.
836. Ronan A, Hogg GG, King GL. Cerebrospinal fluid shunt infections in children. *Pediatr Infect Dis J* 1995;14:782–786.
837. Vinchon M, Vallee L, Prin L, et al. Cerebrospinal fluid eosinophilia in shunt infections. *Neuropediatrics* 1992;23:235–240.
838. Davidson RI. Peritoneal bypass in the treatment of hydrocephalus: historical review and abdominal complications. *J Neurol Neurosurg Psychiatry* 1976;39:640–646.
839. McComb JG. Comments. In: Abu-Dulu K, Pode D, Hadani M, et al. Colonic complications of ventriculo-peritoneal shunts. *Neurosurgery* 1983;13:167–169.
840. Copeland GP, Foy PM, Shaw MD. The incidence of epilepsy after ventricular shunting operations. *Surg Neurol* 1982;17:279–281.
841. Laws ER, Niedermeyer E. EEG findings in hydrocephalic patients with shunt procedures. *Electroenceph Clin Neurophysiol* 1970;29:325.
842. Baskin JJ, Manwaring KH, Rekate HL. Ventricular shunt removal: the ultimate treatment of the slit ventricle syndrome. *J Neurosurg* 1998;88:478–484.
843. Epstein FJ. Increased intracranial pressure in hydrocephalic children with functioning shunts: a complication of shunt dependency. *Concepts Pediatr Neurosurg* 1983;4:119–130.
844. Rekate HL. Classification of slit-ventricle syndromes using intracranial pressure monitoring. *Pediatr Neurosurg* 1993;19:15–20.
845. Saukkonen A, Serlo W, von Wendt L. Electroencephalographic findings and epilepsy in the slit ventricle syndrome of shunt treated hydrocephalic children. *Childs Nerv Syst* 1988;4:344–347.
846. Laurence KM, Coates S. Natural history of hydrocephalus: detailed analysis of 182 unoperated cases. *Arch Dis Child* 1962;37:345–362.
847. Laurence KM. Neurologic and intellectual sequelae of hydrocephalus. *Arch Neurol* 1969;20:73–81.
848. Riva D, Milani N, Giorgi C, et al. Intelligence outcome in children with shunted hydrocephalus. *Childs Nerv Syst* 1994;10:70–73.
849. Hirsch JF. Consensus: long-term outcome in hydrocephalus. *Childs Nerv Syst* 1994;10:64–69.
850. Hemmer R, Böhm B. Once a shunt, always a shunt. *Dev Med Child Neurol* 1976;18(Suppl):69 73.
851. Hayden PW, Shurtleff DB, Stuntz TJ. A longitudinal study of shunt function in 360 patients with hydrocephalus. *Dev Med Child Neurol* 1983;25:334–337.
852. Lorber J, Pucholt V. When is a shunt no longer necessary? An investigation of 300 patients with hydrocephalus and myelomeningocele: 11–22-year follow-up. *Z Kinderchir* 1981;34:327–329.
853. Lindenberg R, Swanson PD. "Infantile hydrancephaly." A report of five cases of infarction of both cerebral hemispheres in infancy. *Brain* 1967;90:839–850.
854. Fowler M, Dow R, White TA, et al. Congenital hydrocephalus-hydrancephaly in five siblings with autopsy studies: a new disease. *Dev Med Child Neurol* 1972;14:173–188.
855. McElfresh AE, Arey JB. Generalized cytomegalic inclusion disease. *J Pediatr* 1957;51:146–156.
856. Myers RE. Brain pathology following fetal vascular occlusion: an experimental study. *Invest Ophthalmol* 1969;8:41–50.
857. Hockey A. Proliferative vasculopathy and an hydrancephalic-hydrocephalic syndrome: a neuropathological study of two siblings. *Dev Med Child Neurol* 1983;25:232–239.
858. Lott IT, McPherson DL, Starr A. Cerebral cortical contributions to sensory evoked potentials: hydran-encephaly. *Electroenceph Clin Neurophysiol* 1986;64:218–223.
859. Hoffman J, Liss L. "Hydranencephaly." A case report with autopsy findings in a 7-year-old girl. *Acta Paediatr Scand* 1969;58:297–300.
860. García-Íñigo P, Paniagua-Escudero JC, de Castro-García FJ, et al. Hidranencefalia. Hallazgos en tomografía axial computerizada y resonancia magnética [Hydranencephaly. Findings in computed axial tomography and magnetic resonance]. *Rev Neurol* (Barcelona) 2004;39:398–399.
861. Wang PJ, Lin HC, Liu HM, et al. Intracranial arachnoid cysts in children: related signs and associated anomalies. *Pediatr Neurol* 1998;19:100–104.
862. Robertson SJ, Wolpert SM, Runge VM. MR imaging of middle cranial fossa arachnoid cysts: temporal lobe agenesis syndrome revisited. *Am J Neuroradiol* 1989;10:1007–1010.
863. Flodmark O. Neuroradiology of selected disorders of the meninges, calvarium and venous sinuses. *Am J Neuroradiol* 1992;13:483–491.
864. Aithala GJ, Sztriha L, Amirlak I, et al. Spinal arachnoid cyst with weakness in the limbs and abdominal pain. *Pediatr Neurol* 1999;20:155–156.
865. Rabb CH, McComb JG, Raffel C, et al. Spinal arachnoid cysts in the pediatric age group: an association with neural tube defects. *J Neurosurg* 1992;77:369–372.
866. Sato K, Shimoji T, Yaguchi K, et al. Middle fossa arachnoid

cyst: clinical, neuroradiological and surgical features. *Childs Brain* 1983;10:301–316.
867. Horton WA. Molecular genetic basis of the human chondrodysplasias. *Endocrinol Metab Clin North Am* 1996;25:683–697.
868. Shohat M, Flaum E, Cobb SR, et al. Hearing loss and temporal bone structure in achondroplasia. *Am J Med Genet* 1993;45:548–551.
869. Dandy WE. Hydrocephalus in chondrodystrophy. *Bull Johns Hopkins Hosp* 1921;32:5–10.
870. Reid CS, Pyeritz RE, Kopits SE, et al. Cervicomedullary compression in young patients with achondroplasia: value of comprehensive neurologic and respiratory evaluation. *J Pediatr* 1987;110:522–530.
871. Yamada Y, Ito H, Otsubo Y, et al. Surgical management of cervicomedullary compression in achondroplasia. *Childs Nerv Syst* 1996;12:737–741.
872. Lundar T, Bakke SJ, Nornes H. Hydrocephalus in an achondroplastic child treated by venous decompression at the jugular foramen: case report. *J Neurosurg* 1990;73:138–140.
873. Ryken TC, Menezes AH. Cervicomedullary compression in achondroplasia. *J Neurosurg* 1994;81:43–48.
874. Nelson FW, Hecht JT, Horton WA, et al. Neurological basis of respiratory complications in achondroplasia. *Ann Neurol* 1988;24:89–93.
875. Pauli RM, Horton VK, Glinski LP, et al. Prospective assessment of risks for cervicomedullary-junction compression in infants with achondroplasia. *Am J Hum Genet* 1995;56:732–744.
876. Landau K, Gloor BP. Therapy-resistant papilledema in achondroplasia. *J Neuroopthalmol* 1994;14:24–28.
877. Hahn YS, Engelhard HH 3rd, Naidich T, et al. Paraplegia resulting from thoracolumbar stenosis in a 7-month-old achondroplastic dwarf. *Pediatr Neurosci* 1989;15:39–43.
878. Rogers JG, Perry MA, Rosenberg LA. I.Q. measurements in children with skeletal dysplasia. *Pediatrics* 1979;63:894–897.
879. Rimoin DL. Cervicomedullary junction compression in infants with achondroplasia: when to perform neurosurgical decompression. *Am J Hum Genet* 1995;56:824–827.
880. Pauli RM. Surgical intervention in achondroplasia. *Am J Hum Genet* 1995;56:1501–1502.
881. Elster AD, Theros EG, Key LL, et al. Cranial imaging in autosomal recessive osteopetrosis. Part II. Skull base and brain. *Radiology* 1992;183:137–144.
882. Lehman RAW, Reeves JD, Wilson WB, Wesenberg RL. Neurological complications of infantile osteopetrosis. *Ann Neurol* 1977;2:378–384.
883. Patel PJ, Kolawole TM, al-Mofada S, et al. Osteopetrosis: brain ultrasound and computed tomography findings. *Eur J Pediatr* 1992;151:827–828.
884. Thompson DA, Kriss A, Taylor D, et al. Early VEP and ERG evidence of visual dysfunction in autosomal recessive osteopetrosis. *Neuropediatrics* 1998;29:137–144.
885. Ohlsson A, Cumming WA, Paul A, et al. Carbonic anhydrase II deficiency syndrome: recessive osteopetrosis with renal tubular acidosis and cerebral calcification. *Pediatrics* 1986;77:371–381.
886. Al Rajeh S, Mouzan MI, Ahlberg A, et al. The syndromes of osteopetrosis, renal acidosis and cerebral calcification in two sisters. *Neuropediatrics* 1988;19:162–165.
887. Rees H, Ang LC, Casey R, et al. Association of infantile neuroaxonal dystrophy and osteopetrosis: a rare autosomal recessive disorder. *Pediatr Neurosurg* 1995;22:321–327.
888. Harlan GC. Congenital paralysis of both abducens and both facial neres. *Trans Am Ophthalmol Soc* 1880;3:216–218.
889. Chisholm JJ. Congenital paralysis of the sixth and seventh pairs of cranial nerves in an adult. *Arch Opthalmol* 1882;11:323–325.
890. Möbius PJ. Uber angeborene doppelseitige Abducens-Facialis-Lähmung. *München Med Wochenschr* 1888;35:91, 108.
891. Möbius PJ. Ueber infantilen Kernschwund. *München Med Wochenschr* 1892;39:17, 41, 55.
892. Sarnat HB. Watershed infarcts in the fetal and neonatal brainstem. An aetiology of central hypoventilation, dysphagia, Möbius syndrome and micrognathia. *Eur J Paediatr Neurol* 2004;8:71–87.
893. Thakkar N, O'Neil W, Duvally J, et al. Möbius syndrome due to brain stem tegmental necrosis. *Arch Neurol* 1977;34:124–126.
894. Singh B, Shahwan SA, Singh P, et al. Möbius syndrome with basal ganglia calcification. *Acta Neurol Scand* 1992;85:436–438.
895. D'Cruz O'NF, Swisher CN, Jaradeh S, et al. Möbius syndrome: evidence for a vascular etiology. *J Child Neurol* 1993;8:260–265.
896. Richter RB. Unilateral congenital hypoplasia of the facial nucleus. *J Neuropathol Exp Neurol* 1960;19:33–41.
897. Pitner SE, Edwards JE, McCormick WF. Observations of pathology of Möbius syndrome. *J Neurol Neurosurg Psychiatry* 1965;28:362–374.
898. Henderson JL. The congenital facial diplegia syndrome: clinical features, pathology and etiology—a review. *Brain* 1939;62:381–403.
899. Meyerson MD, Foushee DR. Speech, language and hearing in Möbius syndrome. *Dev Med Child Neurol* 1978;20:357–365.
900. Sudarshan A, Goldie WD. The spectrum of congenital facial diplegia (Möbius syndrome). *Pediatr Neurol* 1985;1:180–185.
901. Steele MW. Genetics of congenital deafness. *Pediatr Clin North Am* 1981;28:973–980.
902. Das VK. Aetiology of bilateral sensorineural hearing impairment in children: a 10 year study. *Arch Dis Child* 1996;74:8–12.
903. Cohn ES, Kelley PM, Fowler TW, et al. Clinical studies of families with hearing loss attributable to mutations in the connexin 26 gene (GJB2/DFNB1). *Pediatrics* 1999;103:546–550.
904. Baldwin CT, Hoth CF, Amos JA, et al. An exonic mutation in the HuP2 paired domain gene causes Waardenburg's syndrome. *Nature* 1992;355:637–638.
905. DeStefano AL, Cupples LA, Arnos KS, et al. Correlation between Waardenburg syndrome phenotype and genotype in a population of individuals with identified *PAX3* mutations. *Hum Genet* 1998;102:499–506.
906. Tassabehji M, Newton VE, Read AP. Waardenburg syndrome type 2 caused by mutations in the *human microphthalmia* (*MITF*) gene. *Nat Genet* 1994;8:251–255.
907. Sarnat HB, Flores-Sarnat L. Embryology of the neural crest: its inductive role in the neurocutaneous syndromes. *J Child Neurol* 2005;20: *in press*.
908. Chan KK, Wong CK, Lui VC, et al. Analysis of *SOX10* mutations identified in Waardenburg-Hirschsprung patients: differential effects on target gene regulation. *J Cell Biochem* 2003;90:573–583.
909. Inoue K, Shilo K, Boerkoel CF, et al. Congenital hypomyelinating neuropathy, central demyelination and Waardenburg-Hirschsprung disease: phenotypes linked by *SOX10* mutation. *Ann Neurol* 2002;52:836–842.
910. Mills RP, Calver DM. Retinitis pigmentosa and deafness. *J R Soc Med* 1987;80:17–20.
911. Worster-Drought C. Suprabulbar paresis and its differential diagnosis, with special reference to acquired suprabulbar paresis. *Dev Med Child Neurol* 1974;(Suppl 30):1–33.
912. Kuzniecky R, Andermann F, Guerrini R. The epileptic spectrum in the congenital bilateral perisylvian syndrome. CBPS Multicenter Collaborative Study. *Neurology* 1994;44:379–385.

Chapter 6

Perinatal Asphyxia and Trauma

John H. Menkes and Harvey B. Sarnat

> The name "cerebral palsy" is thus nothing other than an invented word, the product of our nosographic classification, a label which we attach to a group of clinical cases: it should not be defined, rather it should be explained by reference to these clinical cases.
>
> *Sigmund Freud (1, p. 3)*

Although more than 160 years has elapsed since the publication of Little's classic paper linking abnormal parturition, difficult labor, premature birth, and asphyxia neonatorum with a "spastic rigidity of the limbs" (2), the pathogenesis of cerebral birth injuries is far from completely understood. This is not because of lack of interest. The evolution and ultimate neurologic picture of cerebral palsy (i.e., the various syndromes of a persistent but not necessarily unchanging disorder of movement and posture resulting from a nonprogressive lesion of the brain acquired during development) have been recorded in innumerable papers. These include Little's 1843 paper on spastic diplegia (2) and Cazauvielh's 1827 monograph on congenital hemiplegia (2a), both also containing descriptions of childhood dyskinesia.

Investigations into the causes of cerebral palsy have taken various approaches. Prospective and retrospective studies have attempted to link the various neurologic abnormalities to specific disorders of gestation or the perinatal period. Pathologic studies of the brain have produced careful descriptions of various cerebral abnormalities in patients with nonprogressive neurologic disorders and have led to attempts, often highly speculative, to formulate their causes. A third line of investigation has been to induce perinatal injuries in experimental animals and to correlate the subsequent pathologic and clinical pictures with those observed in children. These approaches have been supplemented by neuroimaging studies conducted during the perinatal period and in later life. Images have been correlated with neurologic or developmental outcome or with the pathologic examination of the brain.

The various investigations have demonstrated that a given clinical neurologic deficit can be caused by a cerebral malformation of gestational origin, by destructive processes of antenatal, perinatal, or early postnatal onset affecting a previously healthy brain, or by the various processes acting in concert. Developmental anomalies are discussed in Chapter 5 and intrauterine infections in Chapter 7. This chapter considers perinatal trauma, perinatal asphyxia, and the neurologic complications of prematurity.

The reader is referred to the classic texts by Friede (3) on developmental neuropathology, and by Volpe (4) on neonatal neurology.

CRANIOCEREBRAL TRAUMA

Mechanical trauma to the central or peripheral nervous system is probably the insult that is understood best. Trauma to the fetal head can produce extracerebral lesions, notably molding of the head, caput succedaneum, subgaleal hemorrhage, and cephalhematoma.

The fetal head is often asymmetric owing to intrauterine or intravaginal pressure. The sutures override one another, the fontanelles are small or obliterated, and the tissues overlying the skull can be soft because of caput succedaneum. A caput usually appears at the vertex and is commonly accompanied by marked molding of the head. The hemorrhage and edema are situated between the skin and the aponeurosis. When the hemorrhage is beneath the aponeurosis, it is termed a *subgaleal hemorrhage*. As it does in a caput, blood crosses suture lines, but bleeding can continue after birth, and at times the blood loss is quite extensive.

Cephalhematoma and Subgaleal Hematoma

Cephalhematoma is a usually benign hemorrhage between the periosteum of the skull (pericranium) and the calvarium. It results from direct physical trauma or from the differential between intrauterine and extrauterine pressure. Vaginal delivery is not necessarily a prerequisite for its occurrence; it has been encountered in infants born by cesarean section. Neonatal cephalhematoma occurs in from 1.5% to 2.5% of deliveries. Approximately 15% occur bilaterally. A linear skull fracture is seen in 5% of unilateral and in 18% of bilateral cephalhematoma (5). A depressed skull fracture may underlie a minority of cephalhematomas and cannot be detected with certainty by palpation on physical examination, so that a computed tomography (CT) scan or skull radiography may be indicated in infants with cephalhematoma and neurologic symptoms or signs. Routine ultrasound examination does not detect this lesion. Less commonly, a hematoma lies between the galea of the scalp and the periosteum. The subperiosteal hematoma is sharply delineated by the suture lines, whereas the subgaleal hematoma is not so limited and, therefore, is more diffuse. The hematoma is usually absorbed within 3 to 4 weeks, and aspiration, which can allow the introduction of infection, is contraindicated. On rare occasions, the scalp swelling is caused not by a hematoma, but by cerebrospinal fluid (CSF) that leaked from the subarachnoid compartment via a dural tear and a skull fracture. Swelling from CSF does not usually disappear in 4 weeks, and diagnosis by aspiration becomes necessary, followed by operative repair, to avoid a *growing fracture* (6). Although occasionally a subperiosteal hematoma calcifies (Fig. 6.1), it should cause little concern because calcium deposits are usually reabsorbed before the end of the first year, leaving no residual asymmetry.

Management of a cephalhematoma is fundamentally nonoperative. Underlying skull fractures do not create a therapeutic problem and need no specific therapy unless a significant depression of bone fragments occurs.

Large cephalhematomas can result in anemia or, more often, in hyperbilirubinemia owing to absorption of hemoglobin breakdown products (7). With the advent of the vacuum extractors, there has been an increased occurrence of subgaleal hematomas. In the experience of Chadwick and his group, 89% of neonates who had experienced a subgaleal hematoma had a vacuum extractor applied to their head at some time in the course of delivery (8). Intracranial hemorrhage, skull fracture, and cerebral edema (9) can complicate a subgaleal hematoma, as can hypovolemia, coagulopathy, and jaundice, the latter consequences of extensive blood loss (8).

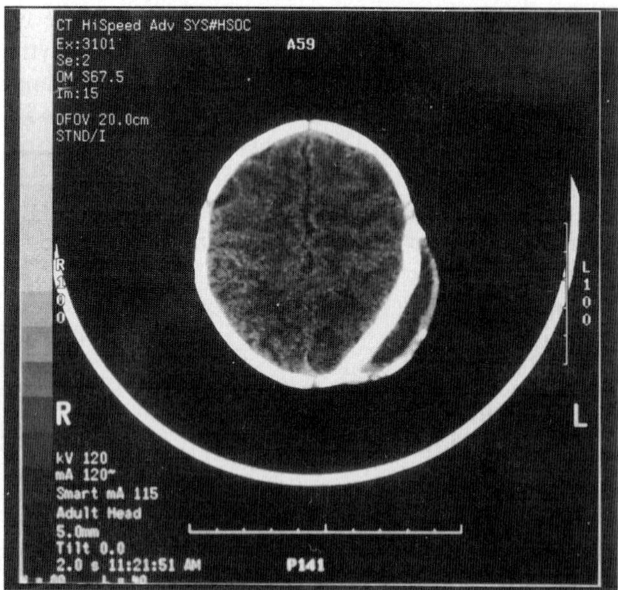

FIGURE 6.1. CT scan of a calcified cephalhematoma. (Courtesy of Dr. Franklin G. Moser, Division of Neuroradiology, Cedars-Sinai Medical Center, Los Angeles, CA.)

Skull Fracture

The skull of the newborn is poorly mineralized and extremely pliable. These factors permit considerable distortion of the head without injury to the skull. Nevertheless, a variety of skull fractures can be seen in the newborn. These can be incurred *in utero*, during labor, or secondary to the application of forceps.

The most common fracture is linear and is localized to the parietal or frontal regions. When no displacement is present, the fracture should heal spontaneously, and no treatment is indicated.

A depressed skull fracture can result from pressure of the head against the pelvis. In addition, incorrect application of the obstetric forceps is often held responsible for the small, *ping-pong ball* depression.

Traumatic Intracranial Hemorrhage

Mechanical trauma to the infant's brain during delivery can induce lacerations in the tentorium or cerebral falx with subsequent subdural hemorrhage. With improved obstetric techniques, large subdural hemorrhages have become relatively uncommon, generally occurring only in large full-term infants delivered through an inadequate birth canal. In the series of Gröntoft published in 1953 (10), two-thirds of infants with tentorial lacerations weighed more than 4,500 g. Similar lesions can be seen in the premature infant (11). In the more recent study of Whitby and coworkers, who subjected normal asymptomatic neonates to magnetic resonance imaging (MRI), 6.1% of infants delivered vaginally without instrumentation had subdural hemorrhages. The incidence of subdural hemorrhages was markedly increased when delivery required instrumentation. In all instances, the hemorrhage had completely resolved by 4 weeks of age, without any apparent sequelae (11a).

Small arachnoid hemorrhages are frequent with moulding of the head because of the rupture of small arachnoid bridging veins. They often are too sparce to be detected by CT, but CSF examination discloses red blood cells and increased protein. If extensive, subarachnoid hemorrhage in the neonate may provoke seizures. Only rarely are there permanent neurological sequelae to perinatal subarachnoid hemorrhage, but slowly progressive late hydrocephalus may occur in the second half of the first year.

Compression of the head along its occipitofrontal diameter, resulting in vertical molding, can occur with vertex presentations, whereas compression of the skull between the vault and the base, resulting in an anteroposterior elongation, is likely to be the outcome of face and brow presentations. Tears of the falx and tentorium can be caused by both forms of overstretch. In particular, the use of vacuum extraction can produce vertical stress on the cranium, with tentorial tears (12). Such hemorrhages are extremely common; in the series of Avrahami and colleagues published in 1993, they could be demonstrated by CT in all of 10 infants delivered by vacuum extraction (13). Most of these are minor and inconsequential. In stretch injuries, damage usually occurs where the falx joins the anterior edge of the tentorium and the hemorrhage is usually infratentorial. Tears and thromboses of the dural sinuses and of the larger cerebral veins, including the vein of Galen, are accompanied commonly by subdural hemorrhages. These can be major and potentially fatal or minor and clinically unrecognizable. The hemorrhages are mainly localized to the base of the brain; when the tears extend to involve the straight sinus and the vein of Galen, hemorrhages expand into the posterior fossa. The latter are poorly tolerated and can be rapidly fatal (14). Rarely, they can develop *in utero*, the consequence of motor vehicle accidents or other nonpenetrating trauma. *In utero* intracranial hemorrhage caused by unknown causes has been seen in infants born to Pacific Island mothers, probably the consequence of abdominal massage by traditional Pacific Island healers (15,16).

Overriding of the parietal bones occasionally produces a laceration of the superior sagittal sinus and a major fatal hemorrhage. Tearing of the superficial cerebral veins is probably relatively common. The subsequent hemorrhage results in a thin layer of blood over the cerebral convexity. Bleeding is often unilateral and usually is accompanied by a subarachnoid hemorrhage. This form of hemorrhage usually results in minimal or no clinical signs. Because the superficial cerebral veins of the premature infant are underdeveloped, this hemorrhage is limited to full-term infants (17).

Subdural hemorrhage within the posterior fossa is being increasingly recognized by neuroimaging studies. The hemorrhage can be the result of a tentorial laceration or a traumatic separation of the cartilagenous joint between the squamous and lateral portions of the occiput in the course of delivery (11). Symptoms typically appear after a lag period of 12 hours to 4 days (18). They are relatively nonspecific and differ little from those seen with intracranial hemorrhage or hypoxic-ischemic encephalopathy (HIE). They include decreased responsiveness, apnea, bradycardia, opisthotonus, and seizures (19). As the subdural hematoma enlarges, the fourth ventricle is displaced forward and soon becomes obstructed, producing signs of increased intracranial pressure. Posterior fossa hemorrhage can be accompanied by intraventricular hemorrhage (IVH) or an intracerebellar hematoma (20). An intracerebral hemorrhage is a less common result of craniocerebral trauma. It is usually seen in conjunction with a major subdural or epidural hemorrhage (4).

Gross traumatic lesions to the brainstem are uncommon. Like spinal cord injuries, they are most likely to occur in the course of breech deliveries. Injury results from traction on the fetal neck during labor or delivery, with the force of excessive flexion, hyperextension, or torsion of the spine being transmitted upward. A compression injury can ensue, with the medulla being drawn into the foramen magnum. Other instances involve laceration of the cerebellar peduncles accompanied by local brainstem hemorrhage. Generally, death occurs during the course of labor or soon after birth as a consequence of damage to the vital medullary centers (21).

Spinal cord injuries are discussed in the section dealing with perinatal injuries to the spinal cord.

HYPOXIC ISCHEMIC ENCEPHALOPATHY (HIE)

Whereas in the past mechanical damage to the brain contributed significantly to mortality during the neonatal period and to subsequent persistent neurologic deficits, mortality and neurologic deficits are now more commonly the consequences of developmental anomalies and HIE, acting singly or in concert.

HIE is the consequence of a deficit of oxygen supply to the brain. This can result from a reduced amount of oxygen in the blood (hypoxia) or a reduced supply of blood to the brain (ischemia). Hypoxia and ischemia singly or conjointly can occur during the perinatal period as a consequence of asphyxia. Many definitions exist for the term *perinatal*. In the context of this chapter, we restrict it to the period extending from the onset of labor to the end of the first week of postnatal life.

No generally accepted definition exists for *asphyxia* (22). It can be inferred on the basis of indirect clinical markers: depressed Apgar scores, cord blood acidosis, or clinical signs in the neonate caused by HIE. From the physiologic viewpoint, asphyxia is a condition in which the brain is subjected not only to hypoxia, but also to ischemia and hypercarbia, which, in turn, can lead to cerebral edema and various circulatory disturbances (4). The incidence of postasphyxial encephalopathy in Leicester, England, from 1980 to 1984 was 6 in 1,000 full-term infants, with 1 in 1,000 infants dying or experiencing severe neurologic deficits as a consequence of the asphyxial insult (23,24). More recent data compiled from Goteborg, Sweden, for the period of 1985 to 1991 showed an incidence of neonatal HIE of 1.8 per 1,000 (25).

Asphyxia can occur at one or more times during intrauterine and extrauterine life. The relative frequency of antepartum, intrapartum, and postpartum asphyxia is a matter of considerable dispute. In the large clinical series of asphyxiated infants published by Brown and associates in 1974, the insult was believed to have occurred primarily antepartum in 51%, intrapartum in 40%, and postpartum in 9% (26). Low and coworkers, who published autopsies on perinatal deaths of full-term and premature infants in 1989, found the insult to be antepartum in 10%, antepartum and intrapartum in 40%, intrapartum in 16%, and in the neonatal period in 34% (27).

Antepartum abnormalities can either be sufficient cause for neonatal encephalopathies or risk factors that render the fetus more susceptible to asphyxia during the birth process. Volpe (4) estimated that some 70% of neonatal encephalopathy is related to intrapartum insults. Half of these infants have additional antepartum risk factors for asphyxial injury. The injury is primarily antepartum in 20% and postpartum in 10%. Based on retrospective case evaluations, Badawi and colleagues estimated that as few as 4% of term infants with neonatal encephalopathy had an insult limited to the intrapartum period without any evidence of an antepartum insult (28,29). In another 25% of infants with neonatal encephalopathy intrapartum hypoxia was superimposed on preconceptional or antepartum risk factors. These findings are in sharp contrast to those of Cowan and coworkers, who examined a stringently defined sample of neonates with neonatal encephalopathy using MRI studies and/or autopsy. Cowen and coworkers found an acute intrapartum insult in 80%, and a preexisting injury in less than 1% (30). The discrepancies between these two studies are difficult to resolve. In part they could be due to the less restricted criteria for neonatal encephalopathy used by Badawi and coworkers, who included infants with obvious chromosomal and neurodevelopmental abnormalities and those who presented with neonatal encephalopathy late in the first week of life.

A related question deals with the importance of perinatal asphyxia as a cause for cerebral palsy. Here a consensus finds that the majority of cases of cerebral palsy did not have neonatal encephalopathy. Based on retrospective MRI studies of children with cerebral palsy, Truwit and coworkers found that in 17% of patients born at term cerebral palsy was related to intrapartum asphyxia. In another 7% it was associated with intrauterine and perinatal insults (31). A Swedish population-based study compiled by Hagberg and coworkers for the period of 1991 to 1994 found that in term births intrapartum asphyxia considered severe enough to cause cerebral palsy was recorded and documented in 28% of cases. More than half of the children in this group showed extrapyramidal symptoms (31a). Using retrospective clinical analysis but excluding children with extrapyramidal cerebral palsy, Blair and Stanley estimated that in 8% of cases intrapartum asphyxia was the possible cause of brain damage (32). Nelson and Grether, who also limited themselves to children with spastic cerebral palsy, found that 6% of cases were attributable to a potentially asphyxiating complication during birth (33). In another retrospective study Gaffney and coworkers found that only 12% of all children with cerebral palsy had evidence of neonatal encephalopathy (34).

From these studies we can conclude that whereas intrapartum asphyxia is a common cause for neonatal encephalopathy, it is a not the major cause for cerebral palsy. Cerebral palsy is a heterogeneous symptom complex that in most instances is the consequence of genetic and antenatal factors and in the majority of instances is not preceded by neonatal encephalopathy (35–37).

Pathogenesis and Pathology

There are two facets to the pathogenesis of asphyxial brain damage: cerebrovascular physiologic factors ensuing from asphyxia, and the subsequent cascade of cellular and molecular events triggered by hypoxia-ischemia leading to cell damage and death within the central nervous system (CNS). These two aspects were reviewed by Volpe (38), Johnston and colleagues (39), and McLean and Ferriero (39a).

Cerebrovascular Physiologic Factors

Because of its relatively low energy demands, the neonatal brain has a considerable resistance to hypoxia, and most hypoxic injuries to neonates result from a combination of hypoxia and ischemia. Alterations in cerebral blood flow induced by asphyxia are therefore of primary importance in understanding the genesis of birth injuries (Fig. 6.2). Following the onset of asphyxia, cardiac output is redistributed so that a larger proportion enters the brain. This results in a 30% to 175% increase in cerebral blood flow. The increase in cerebral blood flow is induced locally by a reduction in cerebrovascular resistance and systemically by hypertension. The severity and the speed of onset of the asphyxial insult determine the cerebrovascular response (40). When asphyxia is severe and develops rapidly, cerebral blood flow decreases rather than increases, probably due to increased cerebrovascular resistance. When the hypoxic-ischemic insult is prolonged, these homeostatic mechanisms fail, cerebral vascular autoregulation is lost, cardiac output decreases, and systemic hypotension develops with reduced cerebral blood flow (41) (see Fig. 6.2).

Normal brain vasculature can compensate for the decreased cerebral perfusion by rapid dilatation of the smaller vessels, so that cerebral blood flow is maintained relatively constant as long as blood pressure is kept within the normal range. The constancy of cerebral blood flow in the face of fluctuations in systemic blood pressure is termed *autoregulation*. The large cerebral blood vessels are believed to be more important for cerebral autoregulation in the neonate than the arterioles, with the response to changes in blood pressure being endothelium dependent (42). A number of chemicals have been implicated in the control of cerebral arterial tone (43). Nitric oxide, by

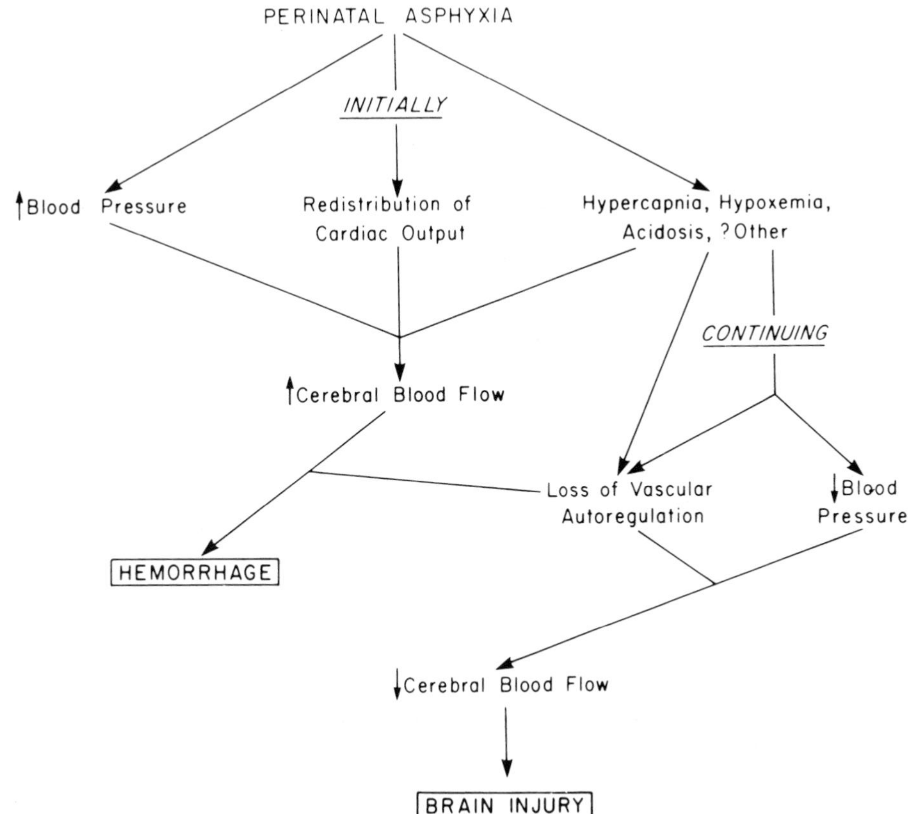

FIGURE 6.2. Interrelationships between perinatal asphyxia, alterations in cerebral blood flow, and brain damage. In addition to the mechanisms depicted, acidosis can induce focal or generalized cerebral edema, which reduces cerebral blood flow. (From Volpe JJ. *Neurology of the newborn*, 3rd ed. Philadelphia: Saunders, 1995. With permission.)

acting on the calcium-activated potassium channel of vascular endothelium, induces vascular dilatation. Adenosine also mediates vasodilatation, whereas endothelin-1 and prostanoids mediate vasoconstriction (42,44). Hypoxia, hypercarbia, and hypoglycemia all impair cerebral autoregulation. When autoregulation becomes defective as a result of hypoxia, cerebral arterioles fail to respond to changes in perfusion pressure and carbon dioxide concentrations, resulting in a pressure-passive cerebral blood flow.

It is clear that in a clinical setting multiple factors can act in concert to cause cerebral vessels to become unresponsive to systemic blood pressure (45,46). Although in the preterm infant the lower limits of autoregulation are very close to the mean systemic arterial pressure, adequate cerebral perfusion can be maintained as long as the mean arterial blood pressure ranges between 24 and 39 mm Hg (47). When hypotension exceeds these lower limits, the preterm infant is unable to compensate for the drop in blood pressure. With the arteriolar system unable to respond to decreased perfusion pressure by vasodilatation, there is a striking reduction in cerebral blood flow (47).

After termination of the ischemic insult there is a marked increase in cerebral blood flow, probably the result of the various vasodilating factors already cited. This early increase in cerebral perfusion is followed by a decline and a second, delayed increase in cerebral blood flow, probably the consequence of an increased synthesis of nitric oxide. It is during this second phase that most of the deleterious events occur that lead to cell death within the brain.

Asphyxial brain injury is similar regardless of whether the brain has incurred a global asphyxial insult as occurs in perinatal asphyxia, hypoperfusion as after cardiac arrest (see Chapter 17), or focal ischemia as after a vascular occlusion (see Chapter 13). Some authors (and lawyers) attribute great significance to meconium as a cause of intrapartum or neonatal asphyxia, but the expulsion of meconium into the amniotic fluid in the first place often is due to a generalized parasympathetic discharge with increased peristalsis that results from fetal distress or an hypoxic-ischemic insult *in utero*. Aspirated meconium at delivery can complicate the problem further by obstructing the infant's airway, but meconium per se is not a cause of asphyxia.

The mechanisms for brain damage in asphyxial brain injury are not completely clear. Volpe, in reviewing the physiologic aspects of asphyxial injury, suggested that the loss of vascular autoregulation coupled with hypotension reduces cerebral blood flow to the point of producing tissue necrosis and subsequent cerebral edema (4). Combined clinical and imaging studies by Lupton and associates in which intracranial pressure of asphyxiated term infants was correlated with their CT scan corroborate Volpe's view that tissue necrosis precedes cerebral edema rather than vice versa, with maximum abnormalities being seen between 36 and 72 hours after the insult (48). Nevertheless, it is still likely that tissue swelling can to some extent further restrict cerebral blood flow and cause secondary edema. The earliest phase of cerebral edema probably reflects a cytotoxic component, whereas a vasogenic component characterizes the edema that accompanies extensive tissue injury (49). In asphyxiated newborns, increased intracranial pressure after perinatal asphyxia is a relatively uncommon complication; in the series of Lupton and coworkers it was encountered in only 22% of asphyxiated infants (48). It is important that the clinician recognize that a bulging fontanelle and split sutures in the neonate after an asphyxiating or severe ischemic insult does not signify potentially reversible cerebral edema after obstructive hydrocephalus, mass lesions such as subdural hematomas, and meningitis have been excluded, but rather irreversible encephalomalacia with massive necrosis in both gray and white matter, and hence is a very bad prognostic sign.

Cellular and Molecular Events Triggered by Hypoxia-Ischemia

Over the last few years increasing attention has been paid to the molecular and cellular aspects of cell death within the nervous system. Gluckman et al. distinguished two phases (50). The first phase occurs during the insult and the immediate period of reperfusion and reoxygenation. The second phase evolves after a period of some hours and extends for at least 72 hours. During the first phase, asphyxia rapidly results in the conversion of nicotinamide adenine dinucleotide (NAD) to reduced NADH. As the energy demands fail to be met, there is a shift from aerobic to anaerobic metabolism, causing acceleration of glycolysis and increased lactate production. In experimental animals, brain lactate increases within 3 minutes of induction of asphyxia (51). At the same time, the concentration of tricarboxylic acid cycle intermediates decreases and the production of high-energy phosphates diminishes. These changes result in a rapid fall in phosphocreatine and a slower reduction in brain adenosine triphosphate (ATP) concentrations. With reduction of ATP levels the various ion pumps, notably the Na^+–K^+ pump, the most important transporter for maintaining high intracellular concentrations of potassium and low intracellular concentrations of sodium, becomes inoperative. As ion pump function is lost, the neuronal membrane begins to change. Some neurons, such as the CA1 and the CA3 hippocampal neurons, hyperpolarize, whereas others, such as the dentate granule cells, depolarize. If anoxia persists, all cells undergo a rapid and marked depolarization with complete loss of membrane potential.

The aforementioned changes in lactate and high-energy phosphates can be documented in the asphyxiated infant by proton and ^{31}P magnetic resonance spectroscopy. These studies show an early increase in lactate (52). A decrease in phosphocreatine during the initial insult is reversed on resuscitation but is followed by a slow, secondary decline some 24 hours later. Intracellular pH and other indices of cellular energy status frequently remain normal for the first day of life (53,54).

Decreases in intracellular and extracellular pH precede changes in membrane potential as hypoxia induces production of lactate and intracellular acidosis. The decrease in extracellular pH is believed to be the consequence of extrusion of intracellular hydrogen ions, intracellular lactate, or both. At the time when the neuronal membrane potential is abolished, there are a number of striking ionic changes. They include an efflux of potassium and an influx into cells of sodium, chloride, and calcium. The increase in intracellular calcium appears to play a critical role in cellular injury. It results from a failure of energy-dependent calcium pumping mechanisms and an opening of voltage-dependent calcium channels. The accumulation of intracellular calcium in turn initiates a cascade of deleterious events:

1. Activation of phospholipases. These induce membrane injury and the release of arachidonic acid, which in turn produces large amounts of oxygen radicals.
2. Activation of proteases. These disrupt the microtubules and cytoskeleton.
3. Activation of nucleases. These cause an injury to the nucleus.
4. Activation of nitric oxide synthetase. This results in an overproduction of nitric oxide, which has neuronal toxicity on its own or when converted to peroxynitrite. One target of nitric oxide and peroxynitrite is mitochondria, and with severe hypoxic-ischemic insults there can be complete mitochondrial failure.
5. Glutamate release. Among the numerous factors responsible for asphyxial neuronal damage, glutamate release and the resultant excitotoxicity have received the most attention and are probably the most important determinants for neuronal death. Increased glutamate is the consequence of increased release of the neurotransmitter and impaired reuptake (55). The mechanism for increased glutamate release is controversial, and there is evidence that it may not be entirely calcium dependent, but may also be due to a reversal of the neuronal glutamate transporters, which instead of removing extracellular glutamate, release glutamate (56). Whatever the mechanism, the result is an excessive stimulation of the neuronal excitatory receptors. This is evidenced by focal elevations in the regional cerebral glucose metabolism in basal ganglia and cerebral cortex in infants who sustained asphyxial brain damage (57).

Glutamate also binds to postsynaptically located glutamate receptors that regulate calcium channels, and its release results in a further increase in intracellular calcium. Several other mechanisms also have been implicated in the increase of excitatory amino acids. These reactions were reviewed by Berger and coworkers (58) and Johnston and coworkers (39,59).

How excitotoxins induce cell death is not completely clear. Rothman and Olney proposed that prolonged neuronal depolarization induces both a rapid and a slowly evolving cell death (60). Rapid cell death is caused by an excessive influx of sodium through glutamate-gated ion channels. This leads to the entry of chloride into neurons. The increased intracellular chloride induces further cation influx to maintain electroneutrality, and the chloride and cation entry draws water into cells with ultimate osmotic lysis. Most important, calcium influx occurs. A sustained increase in intracellular calcium induces the "toxic cascade," outlined above whose end result is cell death by necrosis (61,62).

6. Release of neuron-specific enolase (NSE). NSE is a glycolytic enzyme present in all classes of neurons, and concentrations in blood and CSF of normal infants and children can be measured and are reliable (62a). NSE becomes markedly elevated in the serum and CSF following cardiac arrest, stroke, or other lesions that cause necrosis of neurons (62b). In neonatal rats, NSE elevation after hypoxia is attenuated by lactate (62c), and in adult mice, *Bcl-2* is under the control of NSE and is becomes overexpressed in hippocampal CA1 and dentate gyrus neurons after hypoxic-ischemic insults; the importance of this is that *Bcl-2* suppresses apoptosis and delays cell death, and hence may play a protective role (62d). NSE levels in CSF also may provide a useful clinical marker of cerebral infarction or other irreversible brain damage in neonates. NSE immunoreactivity can be readily detected in neurons in tissue sections and has been used for years by pathologists as a neuronal marker.

Inflammatory reactions involving a variety of cytokines may also contribute to hypoxic-ischemic cell death. The increase in cytokines could stem from an infection, notably a chorioamnionitis that predates the hypoxic-ischemic insult, or it could result from the activation of microglia by asphyxia (63,64).

The late phase of asphyxial injury and cell death is marked by an inappropriate induction of apoptosis. Apoptosis refers to the activation of genetically determined cell-suicide programs. Choi proposed that a single insult might trigger both excitotoxic necrosis and apoptosis, with the severity and duration of the insult determining which death pathway predominates (61). In regions containing large amounts of apoptosis inhibitors, necrosis predominates; conversely, in the absence of endogenous apoptosis inhibitors, hypoxia-ischemia induces apoptosis (39a). Nakajima and coworkers found that apoptosis is more prevalent than necrosis in the hypoxic-ischemic newborn brain (65), suggesting that the impact of apoptosis-executing caspases, key effectors of apoptotic death, is much greater in the immature than in the mature brain (66). The factors that promote postasphyxial apoptosis are under intense investigation. They are believed to include free radicals, increased expression and enhanced concentrations of inflammatory cytokines, and alterations in the concentrations or the response to endogenous growth factors (67). The observation that neurotropins, such as brain-derived neurotrophic factor, act as neuroprotectors after a hypoxic insult provides evidence for the importance of neurotropins in mediating postasphyxial brain injury (68). Asphyxia also induces both rapid and delayed changes in the transcription of several genes, notably *c-fos*, *c-jun*, and some of the heat-shock proteins (69, 70,71). These substances are believed to have a significant influence on the extent of apoptosis (70). The contributions of hypoglycemia and intracellular acidosis, whether caused by accumulation of lactic acid or products of ATP hydrolysis, to the extent and severity of asphyxial brain damage have not been resolved (72).

A large number of strategies aimed at blocking the postasphyxial events that lead to neuronal damage have been proposed. These involve inhibition of glutamate release, blockade of glutamate receptors, inhibition of the cytokine effects, and blockade of apoptotic cell death. None has had any significant clinical application (39,73,74). They are reviewed by Berger and coworkers (58). More recently, the effectiveness of growth factors such as erythropoietin and brain-derived neurotrophic factor in improving outcome after an asphyxial insult has been encouraging (39a).

Imaging of the Neonatal Brain after Hypoxic-Ischemic Encephalopathy

The findings in imaging studies of the neonatal brain after hypoxic-ischemic injury depend on several factors, most of them temporal: the gestational age of the infant; the time since the insult; and whether there was a single temporal event or repeated or chronic hypoxic or ischemic periods. Ultrasound studies are the most accessible because they can be performed noninvasively at the bedside in even the sickest infants, through the anterior fontanelle, and can be compared with prenatal ultrasound studies of the fetal head and also performed serially postnatally. They are excellent for demonstrating ventricular size, and often can detect cerebral edema, periventricular lesions and hemorrhages and infarcts. Ultrasound is not very precise for structures far from the midline, such as the cerebral cortex, nor for posterior fossa structures.

Computed tomography offers better resolution than ultrasound and is very good for detecting intracerebral hemorrhages, calcifications, ventricular size, and periventricular leukomalacia, but it lacks the detail provided by MRI as well as the versatility of different MRI modalities. CT can be performed easily in neonates, even those on ventilators, and does not require anesthesia, but the infant must be transported to the radiology suite.

Magnetic resonance imaging provides the most information but has the limitation of not being accessible to very sick infants on life support who cannot be moved and are connected to a ventilator. In chronic states, when the infant is more stable, three distinctive patterns are demonstrated by MRI following hypoxic-ischemic injuries: periventricular leukomalacia occurs mainly in preterm infants with subacute or chronic hypoxia-ischemia; basal ganglionic and thalamic infarcts occur in term neonates with profound asphyxia; multicystic encephalomalacia occurs in a minority of infants with severe encephalopathy following relatively mild hypoxic-ischemic events (74a). Diffusion-weighted MRI of the neonate can identify early injury after an insult because of its ability to detect subtle alterations in brain water content (39a,74b–74c). Magnetic resonance spectroscopy (MRS), especially if done as a three-dimensional study in the neonatal brain, can detect metabolites such as lactate, *N*-acetyl aspartate, choline, and creatine that provide functional data regarding metabolic integrity in specific regions of the brain (74c,74e).

Selective Vulnerability

Whatever the biochemical and physiologic mechanisms for brain damage, the relative resistance of the neonate's brain to hypoxia has been known for some time. Probably this phenomenon reflects a slower overall cerebral metabolism and smaller energy demands by the brain of the neonate compared with that of the adult. Total metabolism of the brain of a newborn mouse is approximately 10% that of the adult mouse's brain, and glycolysis also proceeds at a much slower rate (75). In that respect the relative resistance of the cardiovascular system to hypoxic injury also can be operative.

The factors that determine the selective vulnerability of certain neuronal populations are incompletely understood. In part, regional distribution of injury reflects the vascular supply to the brain, with the injury being maximal in the border zones between the major cerebral arteries. In the striatum, the topography of neuronal death is probably related to the density of excitatory receptors and the expression of the various receptor subtypes (76). The Myers model of "partial" versus "total" asphyxia, resulting in different sites of the principal lesions in neonatal monkeys, cannot be extrapolated to the human condition. This is because the monkey brain is more mature at birth, in terms not only of structure, synaptic organization, and myelination, but also in terms of better autoregulation of cerebral blood flow. In addition, the monkey brain is considerably smaller than the human brain, with a shorter distance for blood flow to reach terminal perfusion, and blood vessels are narrower than in the human neonate. Human cerebral arterioles do not acquire their muscular walls until near term, an anatomic prerequisite for autoregulatory function in cerebral blood flow, whereas the monkey already has mature cerebral vasculature for several weeks before birth.

It is this combination of vascular and metabolic factors that results in the various distinct pathologic lesions that have been well described by classic pathologists over the course of the last century.

Multicystic Encephalomalacia

The neonatal brain responds to infarction differently than the mature brain. Rather than dense gliotic scars, pseudocysts are the usual long-term residual lesions. The reasons for the formation of cysts in the newborn brain are that areas of infarction tend to be relatively larger than in the adult because collateral circulation is less well developed and because the ability of neonatal brain to mobilize reactive gliosis is limited. The number of astrocytes per volume of neonatal brain is approximately one-sixth that of the adult brain in both gray and white matter; hence the response to injury is not nearly as effective and the glial cells present are only able to form thin septa without neurons, compartmentalizing the empty space after macrophages have cleared away the necrotic tissue. These glial septa create the multiple pseudocysts of multicystic encephalomalacia. They are pseudocysts rather than true cysts because they are not lined by an epithelium, as are ependymal cysts. Multicystic encephalomalacia is therefore the end result of extensive cerebral infarcts.

When the primate fetus is subjected to acute total asphyxia, a reproducible pattern of brain disorders ensues (77,78). This pattern includes bilaterally symmetric lesions in the thalamus and in a number of brainstem nuclei, notably the nuclei of the inferior colliculi, superior olive, and lateral lemniscus. The neurons of the cerebral cortex, particularly the hippocampus, are especially vulnerable, as are the Purkinje cells of the cerebellum (4,79).

Soon after the initial insult, the first changes observed using electron microscopy are in the neuronal mitochondria, the internal structure of which becomes swollen and disrupted (80). Gradual widespread transneuronal degeneration follows. With progressively longer periods of total asphyxia, the destructive changes in the thalamus become more extensive, and damage begins to appear in the putamen and in the deeper layers of the cortex. (Fig. 6.3). In its extreme form, asphyxiated animals show an extensive cystic degeneration of both cortex and white matter. Connective tissue replaces the damaged areas in the forebrain, but a relative lack of cellular reaction occurs in the central nuclear areas (78).

This experimentally produced picture resembles cystic encephalomalacia (central porencephaly, cystic degeneration) of the human brain, a condition characterized by the formation of cystic cavities in white matter (Fig. 6.4). When small, the cysts are trabeculated and do not communicate with the ventricular system. In their most extensive

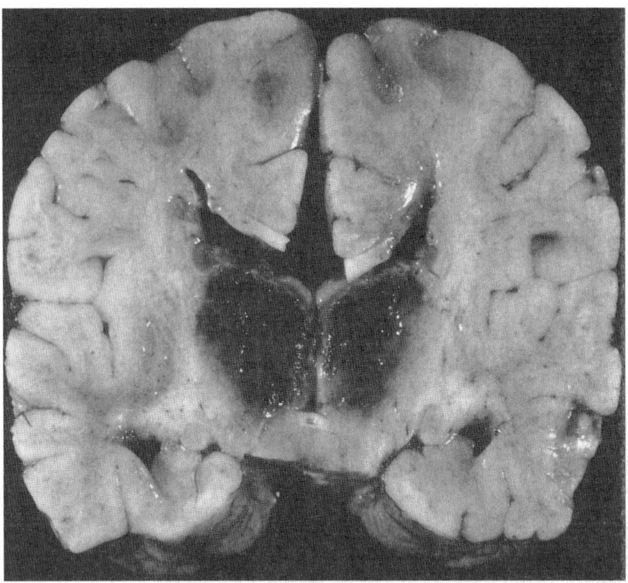

FIGURE 6.3. Coronal section of cerebral hemispheres at autopsy of a 9-month-old boy with bilateral thalamic hemorrhages. This is part of the pattern of deep infarction due to severe and prolonged perfusion failure of the brain secondary to shock. Hemorrhagic infarcts are more common than ischemic infarcts in the thalamus of fetuses and young infants. The hemorrhages do not extend into the lateral or third ventricles, and the cerebrum is otherwise normally developed and without other lesions, though microscopically it showed extensive neuronal changes of hypoxic-ischemic encephalopathy (not shown).

form they can involve both hemispheres, leaving only small remnants of cortical tissue. The cavities are generally believed to be the products of insufficient glial reaction, perhaps the result of cerebral immaturity, or to reflect the sudden and massive tissue damage caused by the aforementioned circulatory or anoxic events. This pathologic picture is seen not only as a consequence of severe perinatal asphyxia, as first established by Little (2), but also in twin pregnancies after intrauterine fetal death and in fetal viral encephalitides such as herpes simplex (81–83). Infants surviving this type of insult usually develop a severe form of spastic quadriparesis.

The pathologic differentiation between cystic degeneration and hydranencephaly is discussed in Chapter 5.

Selective Neuronal Necrosis and Laminar Necrosis of the Cortex

The distribution of cerebral lesions induced by acute total asphyxia rarely reproduces the distribution of lesions found in infants who have survived partial but prolonged asphyxia. When prolonged partial asphyxia is induced experimentally, primates develop high carbon dioxide partial pressure (pCO_2) levels and mixed metabolic and respiratory acidosis (78,84). These are usually accompanied by marked brain swelling, which compresses the small blood vessels of the cerebral parenchyma. The resultant increase in vascular resistance superimposed on the systemic alterations leads to various focal cerebral circulatory lesions whose location is governed in part by vascular patterns and in part by the gestational age of the fetus at the time of the asphyxial insult (85,86). Selective necrosis of neurons may be followed by mineralization of those cells.

The neonatal cerebral cortex is vulnerable to *laminar necrosis* after a severe ischemic insult. This selective neuronal necrosis involves some layers more than others. In preterm and term infants, layers 3 and 5, which contain pyramidal cells, are most vulnerable, but in later infancy and childhood, layer 4 is most severely affected. This layer contains granule cells that are sensory, rather than motor, in function. Layer 4 is largest in the striate (occipital) cortex, where it is the principal visual receptive zone. Laminar necrosis is extensive degeneration of neurons in the affected layers, with relatively better preservation in other layers, though pyknosis and karyorrhexis indicating dying neurons are seen in neurons in all layers. These changes may be expressed in infants who survive as cortical blindness and spastic diplegia, though damage in other parts of the brain, such as the lateral geniculate body and periventricular leukomalacia also contribute to the clinical deficits. Laminar necrosis may be identified in MRI, particularly in fluid-attenuated inversion recovery (FLAIR) sequences, as a bright line of increased signal within the cortex and parallel to the surface of the brain (Fig. 6.5).

Periventricular Leukomalacia

One lesion that occurs with particular frequency in the premature infant is periventricular leukomalacia (PVL) (Figs. 6.6 and 6.7). First delineated by Banker and Larroche (87), this condition consists of a bilateral, fairly symmetric necrosis having a periventricular distribution. The two most common sites are at the level of the occipital radiation and in the white matter around the foramen of Monro (88,89). In addition, there can be diffuse cerebral white matter necrosis that usually spares the gyral cores (90). Preterm infants of 22 to 30 weeks' gestation tend to experience more widespread and confluent periventricular necrosis, whereas older premature infants exhibit more-focal necrosis (91).

The evolution of PVL has been studied by neuropathologic and neuroimaging methods. Within 6 to 12 hours of the suspected insult, coagulation necrosis occurs in the affected areas, accompanied by proliferation of astrocytes and microglia, loss of ependyma, and, in some cases, subcortical degeneration. Focal axonal disruption and death of oligodendroglia are some of the earliest signs of injury, with the developing oligodendroglia being especially vulnerable (4).

The pathogenesis of PVL is uncertain and is most likely to be multifactorial. Five major factors are believed to be operative.

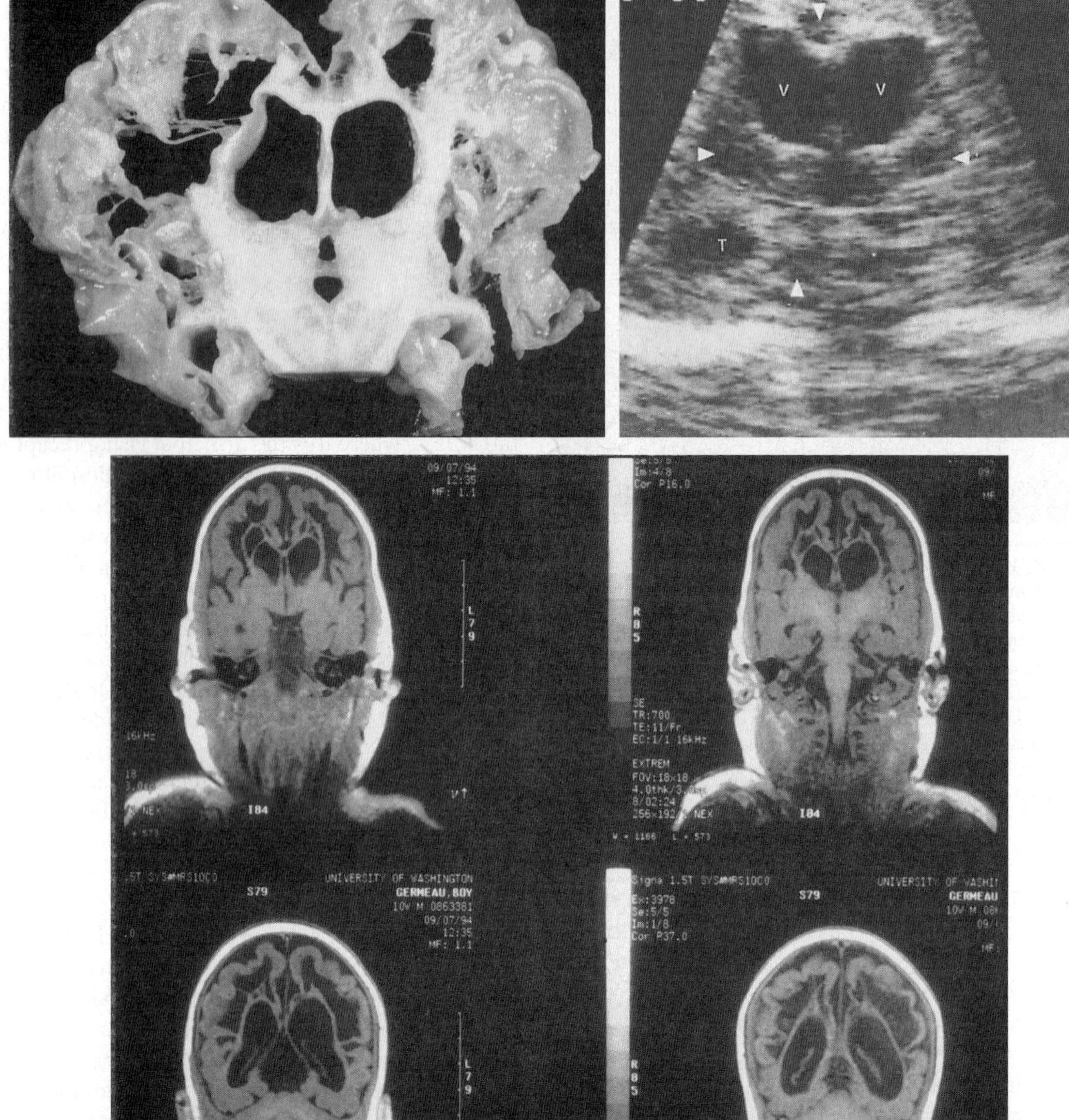

FIGURE 6.4. Cystic encephalomalacia. **A:** Coronal section of cerebral hemispheres of a 14-month-old boy with multicystic encephalomalacia. This is the gross pathologic appearance of lesions similar to those seen in panel C by MRI. The architecture of the cerebral white matter and cerebral cortex, including the gyri, is severely disrupted by these extensive infarcts and cerebral atrophy. The lateral and third ventricles are dilated to compensate for the atrophy. Deep structures appear better preserved, but microscopically also showed extensive neuronal loss and microinfarcts. **B:** Coronal sonogram of the same infant. Moderate ventriculomegaly and numerous poorly defined anechoic areas in periventricular parenchyma and in basal ganglia are visible (*arrowheads*) (*V*, lateral ventricles; *T*, temporal horn of lateral ventricle). Ultrasonography was performed at 7 months of age, autopsy at 16 months. The infant had a history of seizures and profound developmental retardation. In this instance, the most likely cause for the condition appeared to have been a cytomegalovirus infection. **C:** Coronal T1-weighted MRI of a 9-week-old boy, born at 31 weeks' gestation, showing multicystic encephalomalacia throughout the white matter. The ventricles are large because of the atrophy of cerebral parenchyma, both gray and white matter. This is the result of severe hypoxic/ischemic encephalopathy in the perinatal period. (Panel B, from Stannard MW, Jimenez JF. Sonographic recognition of multiple cystic encephalomalacia. *Am J Neuroradiol* 1983; 4:11. With permission.)

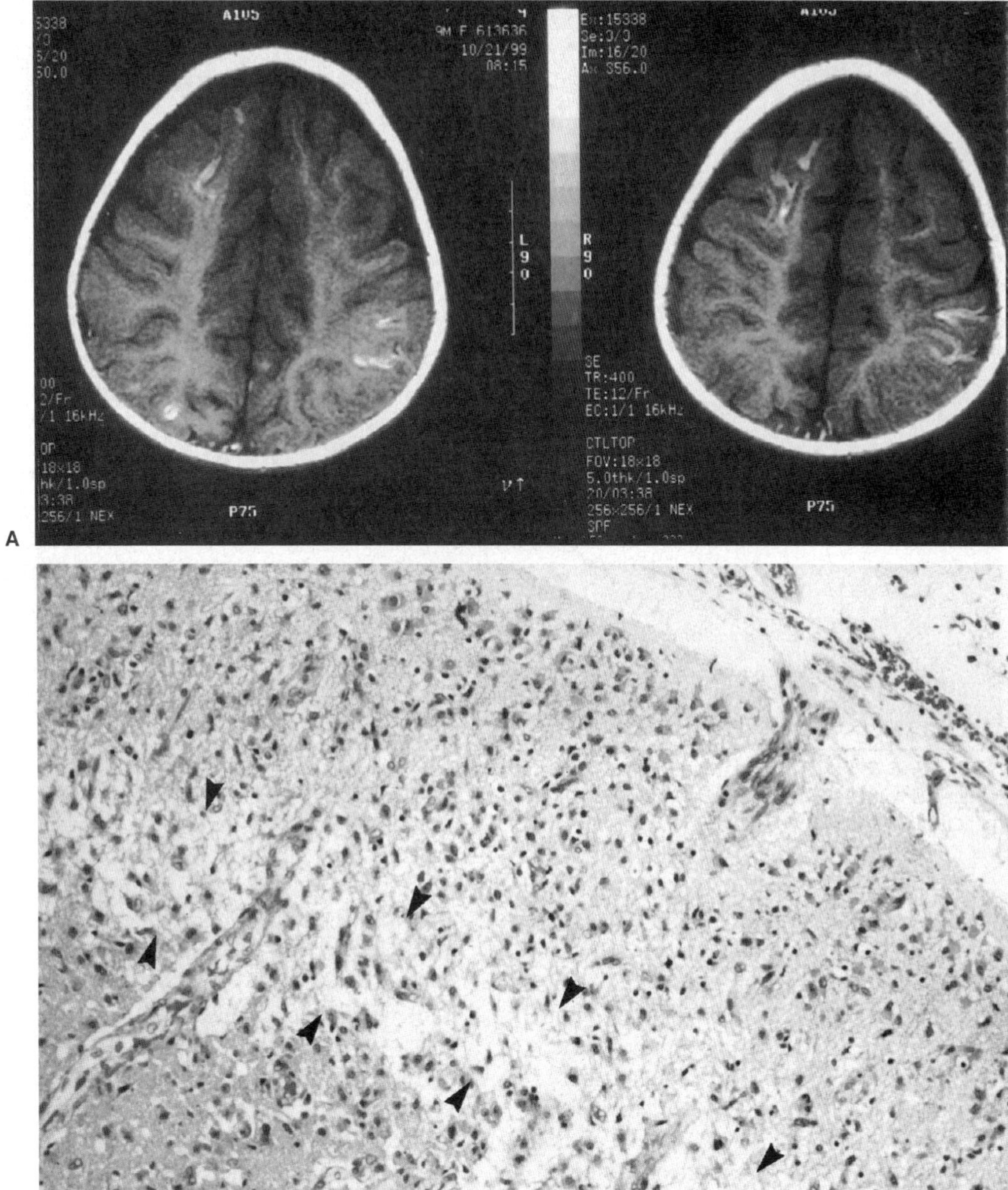

FIGURE 6.5. **A:** MRI-T2 fluid-attenuated inversion recovery (FLAIR) sequence of a term neonate with laminar necrosis of the cerebral cortex. The bright signal within the cortex corresponds to necrosis in layer 4. **B:** Section of occipital lobe of a 5-year-old girl who suffered severe perinatal asphyxia and also had congenital hydrocephalus, successfully shunted in the neonatal period. She had an additional hypoxic event 3 weeks prior to death. Dark, shrunken nuclei of dying and dead neurons are seen in all layers (arrows), but layer 4 is undergoing actual necrosis of the entire layer, known as laminar necrosis of the cortex.

1. A failure in perfusion of the periventricular region. The distribution of the focal necrotic changes of PVL suggests inadequate circulatory perfusion and infarction in the arterial end zones, areas that are most susceptible to a fall in cerebral blood flow and reduced perfusion (92). The anatomic picture indicating a low blood flow to cerebral white matter has been confirmed by cerebral blood studies (93).
2. A second factor in the pathogenesis of PVL is derived from the observation by Doppler ultrasound studies that cerebral vascular autoregulation is impaired in a substantial proportion of premature infants, with a

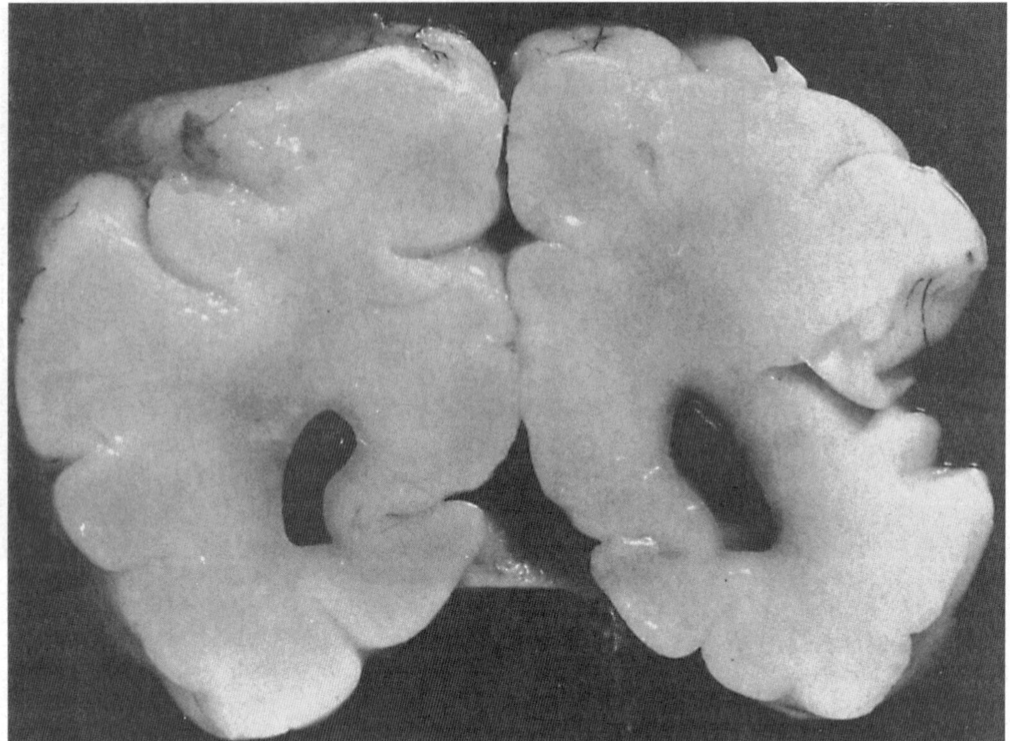

FIGURE 6.6. Periventricular leukomalacia. Semicircular areas of malacia surround both lateral ventricles. (From Cooke RE. *The biologic basis of pediatric practice*. New York: McGraw-Hill, 1968. With permission.)

propensity for pressure-passive circulation (94). Loss of autoregulation is particularly common in preterm infants who have experienced hypoxic-ischemic events (94). Because even in healthy preterm infants white matter has an extremely low perfusion, the vulnerability of the periventricular region to ischemia becomes readily explicable (45,93). Experimental work has demonstrated that hypotension induced by exsanguination or by administration of endotoxin results in reduced perfusion of periventricular white matter and occipital white matter. By contrast, these measures do not induce any significant reduction in blood flow to the cerebral cortex or to the deep gray matter nuclei (95). In substantiation of the clinical importance of impaired autoregulation in the induction of PVL, Volpe demonstrated that the subset of premature infants with pressure-passive cerebral circulation have an extremely high incidence of PVL (96).

3. A third factor in the pathogenesis of PVL pertains to the intrinsic vulnerability of the early-differentiating oligodendroglia (preoligodendroglia, i.e., cells at a developmental stage before the acquisition of myelin) to excitatory neurotransmitters, such as glutamate, and to attack by free radicals (97–99). This vulnerability may be the consequence of a lack of such antioxidant enzymes as catalase and glutathione peroxidase during a period when oligodendroglia undergo rapid iron acquisition (96,100). Elevated levels of lipid peroxidation products have been found in the CSF of premature infants who had evidence of white matter injury by MRI (99).
4. An increasing amount of clinical and experimental evidence shows that cytokines play an important role in the induction of white matter damage (98,101). The administration of interferon-alpha 2a to term infants as treatment for hemangiomas has resulted in spastic diplegia and delayed myelination. In some instances, diplegia did not resolve with discontinuation of cytokine therapy (102). Retrospective assays of neonatal blood have shown that preterm and term children with spastic diplegia had higher blood levels of various cytokines, including interferon-alpha, interferon-gamma, interleukin 6 (IL-6), IL-8, and tumor necrosis factor (TNF)-alpha, than did control children (103) It is of note that the association between elevated cord blood levels of cytokines and the development of white matter damage is weaker in premature than in term infants (104). In the study of Grether and colleagues, serum interferon levels were elevated in 78% of children with spastic diplegia but only in 20% of children with hemiparesis and in 42% of children who developed quadriparesis (103). Cytokines can also be demonstrated

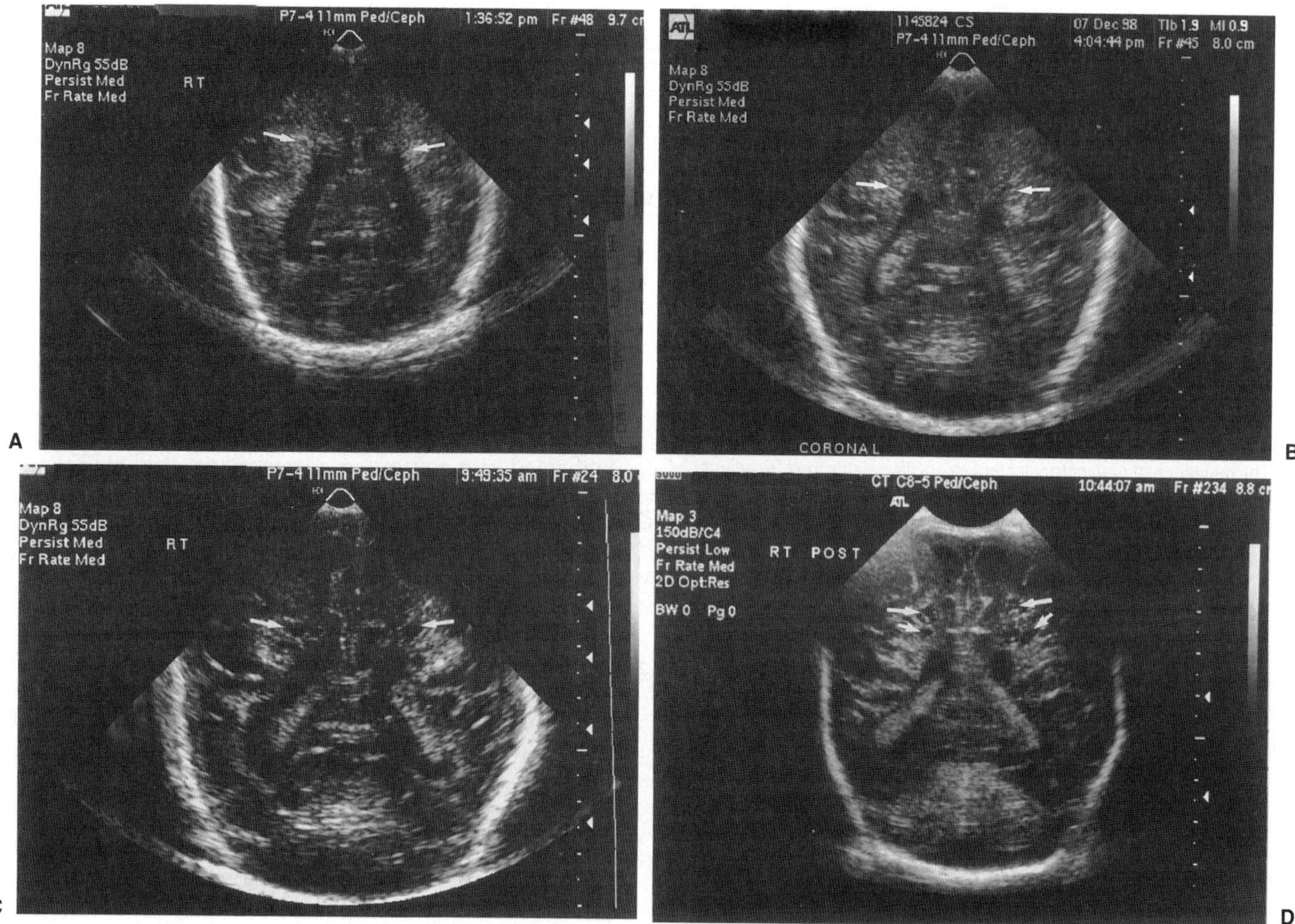

FIGURE 6.7. Evolution of cystic periventricular encephalomalacia. Ultrasound, coronal views. **A:** At 4 days of age, there are focal echodense areas bilaterally in the periventricular white matter (*arrows*). **B:** At 9 days of age, the bilateral periventricular echogenicity is more clearly evident (*arrows*). **C:** At 23 days of age, early cystic changes are seen bilaterally in the periventricular region (*arrows*). These are more severe on the right. **D:** At 1 month of age, multiple periventricular cystic changes are seen (*arrows*). This boy was the 1,445-g product of a 30-week twin pregnancy. His neonatal course was complicated by recurrent apnea and bradycardia. A septic work-up was negative. Neurologic examination was unremarkable but for jerky movements of the extremities. At 5 months of age, this youngster had spastic diplegia most severe in the trunk and lower extremities. (Courtesy of Dr. Nancy Niparko, Cedars-Sinai Medical Center, Los Angeles, CA.)

by *in situ* immunohistochemical methods in neurons in the neocortex, hippocampus, basal ganglia, and thalamus of infants with PVL (105). It appears likely that cytokines such as interferon-alpha, interferon-gamma, tumor necrosis factor-alpha, IL-6, or IL-8 might damage white matter by leading to hypotension or by inducing ischemia through intravascular coagulation. Cytokines also could have a direct adverse effect on developing oligodendroglia or induce the product of other cytokines such as platelet-activating factor, which can further damage cells (106).

5. The role of hypocarbia during the first days of life in mechanically ventilated premature infants in predisposing them to PVL has been suggested by several studies (107). Fritz and coworkers proposed that hypocarbia reduces cerebral blood flow and decreases tissue oxidative metabolism, with increased intracellular calcium and the various secondary events already described (108).

From a clinical point of view, spastic diplegia is the most common and most consistent sequela of PVL. It is nearly always bilateral, although often asymmetric in severity. Because of the propensity of the periventricular necrotizing lesions to appear earliest and most prominently around the occipital horns of the lateral ventricles, optic radiation fibers may be involved and sometimes also result in cortical visual impairment.

A number of adverse perinatal events correlate with the development of PVL. Most important, PVL tends to occur

TABLE 6.1 Incidence of Periventricular Leukomalacia According to Gestational Age

Gestational Age (weeks)	*Ultrasound Incidence of Cystic Periventricular Leukomalacia (%)*[a]
<27	7.2
27	12.9
28	15.7
29	10.5
30	12.4
31	6.5
32	4.3
Total	9.2

[a]The incidence of periventricular leukomalacia is calculated for infants surviving at least 7 days.
From Zupan V, Gonzalez P, Lacaze-Masmonteil T, et al. Periventricular leukomalacia: risk factors revisited. *Dev Med Child Neurol* 1996;38:1061. With permission.

in the larger premature infant, with the highest incidence by both neuropathologic and ultrasound criteria being between 27 and 30 weeks' gestational age (109,110) (Table 6.1). In the more recent French series of Baud and coworkers, published in 1999, the highest incidence (12.9%) was, however, seen in infants whose gestational age was 24 to 26 weeks (111). Other notable risk factors include prenatal factors such as premature, prolonged, or both premature and prolonged rupture of membranes, chorioamnionitis, and intrauterine infections (109,110,112). Several perinatal and postnatal factors also appear to be of importance. These are listed in Table 6.2 (4,113,114). In many instances, however, infants in whom PVL evolved had a relatively benign postnatal course (110). Although systemic hypotension has been suggested as an important pathogenetic factor, several studies failed to show an association between hypotension and PVL (115,116). In part, this lack of documentation reflects the lack of direct and continuous blood pressure recordings, or it might indicate that PVL results from a discrepancy between the metabolic requirements of periventricular white matter and its perfusion (117). We also stress that in infants of less than 31 weeks' gestation, relatively small reductions in systemic blood pressure (less than 30 mm Hg) for 1 hour or longer suffice to induce cerebral infarcts (118). This is particularly true in those in whom autoregulation is defective or has been disrupted by asphyxia. As a rule, the less mature the periventricular vasculature, the less significant are the clinical complications that accompany the evolution of PVL.

TABLE 6.2 Factors Predisposing to the Evolution of White Matter Damage in Premature Infants

Low Apgar score
Prolonged need for ventilatory assistance
Need for extracorporeal membrane oxygenation (ECMO)
Recurrent episodes of apnea and bradycardia
Hypercarbia
Hypocarbia
Patent ductus arteriosus
Hypoplastic left heart syndrome
Administration of indomethacin

Several observational studies have reported that both maternal preeclampsia and the prenatal administration of magnesium resulted in a lower incidence of spastic diplegia, and by inference of PVL, in very low birth weight infants (119,120,121). These observations could not be confirmed in a controlled, retrospective study (122), and randomized clinical trials will be necessary to determine the effectiveness of magnesium. In addition, there are large and still unexplained differences among centers in the outcomes of extremely low birth weight infants, which also will require controlled clinical trials (123).

Newer imaging techniques such as ultrasonography and magnetic resonance imaging (MRI) permit the following of the evolution of PVL. In the series of infants autopsied by Iida and colleagues (90), the prenatal onset of PVL was observed in 20% of stillborn infants and in 16.4% of infants who died by 3 days of age. These findings have been confirmed by ultrasound studies showing the presence of cystic PVL as early as the third day of life (90,124). The evolution of PVL can be followed by ultrasonography. During the first week of life, transient hyperechoic periventricular areas are frequent and probably represent a persistent germinal matrix (125). Persistent echogenic foci are pathologic, however. They too are seen during the first week of postnatal life. Within 1 to 3 weeks they are replaced with echolucent, cystic foci (cystic leukomalacia) (see Fig. 6.7C and D). As the intracystic fluid becomes resorbed, these cysts disappear and are replaced by gliosis (126). PVL can be accompanied by cystic lesions in the subcortical white matter and by delayed myelination (127). In some instances, gliosis becomes interspersed with areas of microcalcification (128). Calcification is more likely when lesions are not extensive. Premature infants with PVL have a marked reduction in cerebral cortical gray matter volume at term as compared to premature infants without PVL. This may reflect destruction of corticopedal, corticofugal, and associative fibers with secondary impairment of neuronal differentiation (129).

Periventricular echodensities can reflect several neuropathologic entities aside from PVL. They also are observed in hemorrhagic infarctions such as are seen in association with IVH and in ischemic edema (130). PVL becomes hemorrhagic in up to 25% of infants (131), mostly a consequence of a hemorrhage into the ischemic area, the outcome of subsequent reperfusion (4).

Parasagittal Cerebral Injury

The most common site of brain damage in the term newborn is the cortex. Experimental studies have confirmed that the parasagittal cortex is the earliest and most severely damaged on prolonged asphyxia, with the amount of damage increasing geometrically with increasing duration of asphyxia (132). The lesions characteristically involve the territory supplied by the most peripheral branches of the three large cerebral arteries (Fig. 6.8) (133). Infarctions in this area are secondary to arterial or venous stasis and thromboses. One common pattern for the distribution of lesions, termed arterial "border zone" or "watershed lesions," usually results from a sudden decrease in systolic blood pressure and cerebral perfusion. *Watershed* is a term first used in the early nineteenth century in England to describe the strip of land between two more or less parallel rivers or streams. This strip was protected from damming of one stream because it had an alternative water supply from the other, but it also was the most vulnerable and the first land to become parched during periods of general drought because it received the last water from both streams. Extrapolated to the cerebrovascular circulation, a watershed thus is the territory between two major arterial supplies, protected from occlusion of one of the arteries but vulnerable to an even transient period of systemic hypotension or hypoperfusion. The best-known watershed zones in the brain are between the anterior and middle cerebral artery circulations and between the middle and posterior cerebral circulations. Watershed zone infarcts are not infrequent in the neonate in these same regions that are affected in adults (Fig. 6.9), and usually denote a previous episode of systemic hypotension associated with fetal distress during late gestation or just prior to birth. Watershed zone infarcts in the full-term neonatal cerebrum are usually ischemic infarcts, but in about 30% of cases they are hemorrhagic. In preterm infants, hemorrhagic watershed infarcts are more frequent than ischemic infarcts.

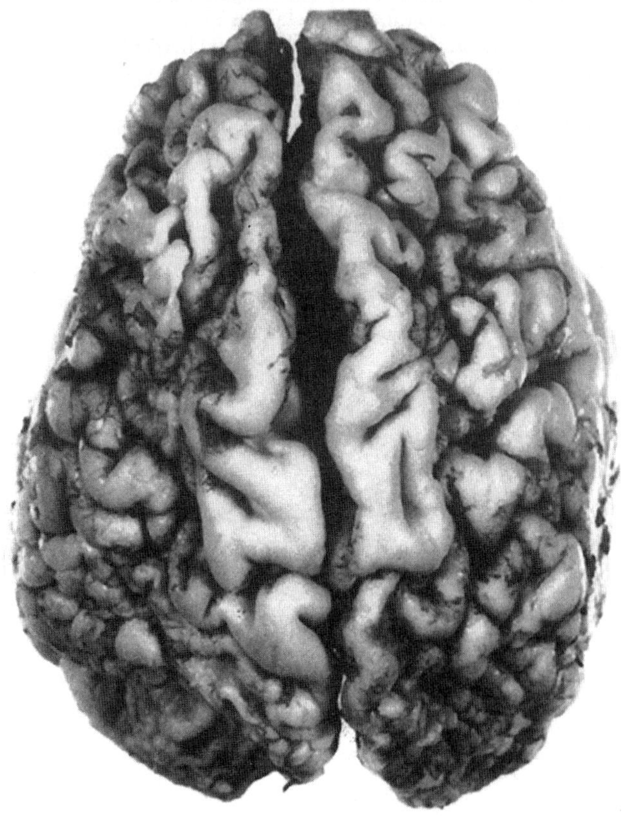

FIGURE 6.8. Watershed pattern in a 10-year-old child with history of prolonged labor and spastic quadriparesis. Symmetric atrophy is seen in border zones of anterior, middle, and posterior cerebral arteries. (From Lindenberg R. Compression of brain arteries as pathogenetic factor for tissue necrosis and their areas of predilection. *J Neuropathol Exp Neurol* 1955;14:223. With permission.)

Another watershed zone occurs in the tegmentum of the brainstem. A series of 25 to 30 paired triads of vessels arise from the basilar artery; this series extends from the upper midbrain to the lower medulla oblongata. The three vessels of the triad on each side of the brainstem are (a) the paramedian penetrating artery, which extends dorsally next to the midline from the basilar artery to the floor of the fourth ventricle; (b) the short branches of the circumferential artery, which travels from the basilar artery around the outside of the brainstem to penetrate and supply the ventrolateral brainstem; and (c) the long branches of the circumferential artery, which encircles the brainstem and then penetrates dorsolaterally. The tegmentum of the pons and medulla is a watershed zone between the territories of the paramedian penetrating and the long circumferential arteries (Fig. 6.10) (133a).

Damage is maximal in the posterior parietal-occipital region, becoming less marked in the more anterior portions of the cortex. The lesions in the affected area can be located in the cortex or in the white matter. When gray matter is affected, damage usually involves the portions around the depth of the sulci. In part, this distribution can reflect the effect of cerebral edema on the drainage of the cortical veins, and, in part, it can be the consequence of the impoverished vascular supply of this area in the healthy human newborn. Bilateral parasagittal infarction also may result from sagittal sinus thrombosis, an event usually associated with infections (sepsis and meningitis) or with dehydration in young infants.

Lesions involving damage to the deeper portions of gray matter have been termed *ulegyria* (mantle sclerosis, lobar sclerosis, nodular cortical sclerosis) (3). A common abnormality, ulegyria accounts for approximately one-third of clinical defects caused by circulatory disorders during the neonatal period (133). Its characteristic feature is the localized destruction of the lower parts of the wall of the convolution, with relative sparing of the crown. This produces

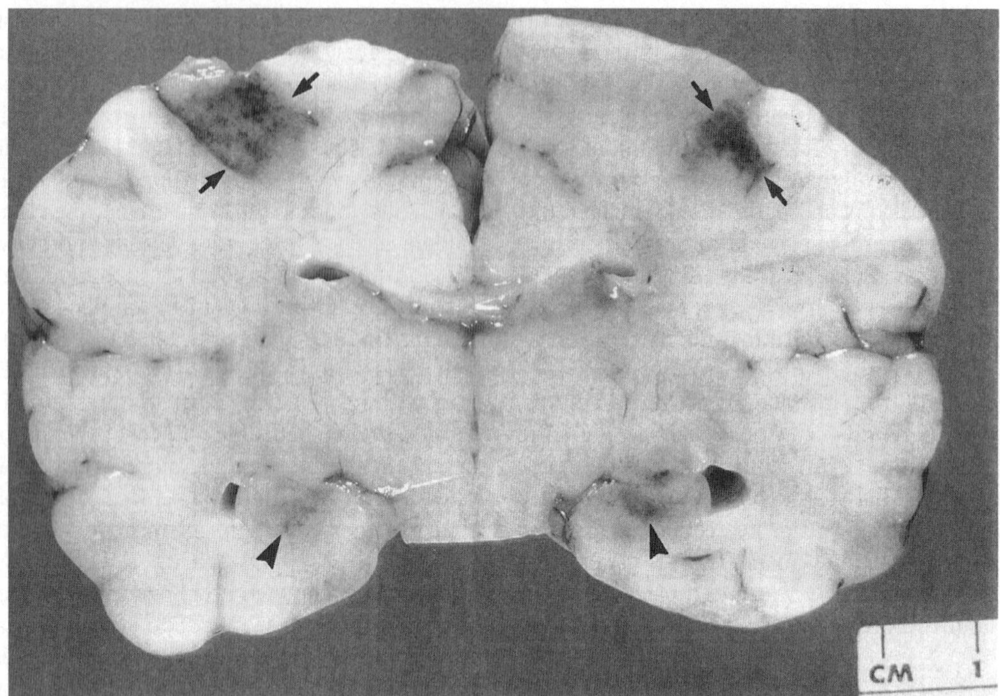

FIGURE 6.9. Coronal section of cerebrum, at the level of the thalamus and third ventricle, of a 35-week preterm infant who suffered multiple episodes of severe bradycardia during prolonged labor and lived only a few hours after birth. Bilateral watershed hemorrhagic infarcts are seen at the junctions between anterior cerebral and middle cerebral artery territories (*arrows*) and between the middle cerebral and posterior cerebral artery territories (*arrowheads*). The ventricles are normal and no periventricular hemorrhages are seen.

a "mushroom" gyrus (Fig. 6.11). The margins of affected gray matter often contain abnormally dense aggregates of myelinated fibers, whereas adjacent white matter shows a considerable amount of myelin loss and compensatory gliosis (134). Later, coarse bundles of abnormally oriented, heavily myelinated fibers traverse the gliotic tissue, and the myelin sheaths enclose astrocytic processes as well as axons, similar to status marmoratus of the basal ganglia (135). Laminar necrosis of layer 3 often accompanies ulegyria.

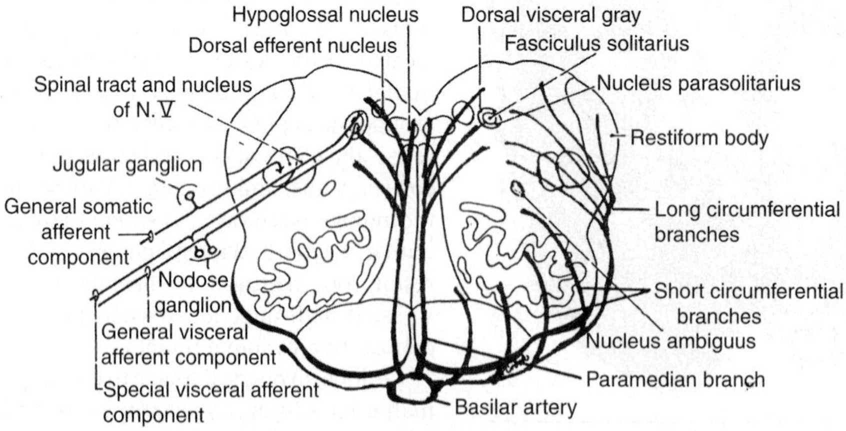

FIGURE 6.10. Drawing of a transverse section of the medulla oblongata to demonstrate the tegmental watershed zone, where the end-perfusions overlap from the parasagittal penetrating artery and the long circumferential artery, both arising from the basilar artery. Within this tegmental zone are the nucleus/tractus solitarius (respiratory center) and nucleus ambiguus (deglutition center) as well as several cranial nerve nuclei. (From Sarnat HB. Watershed infarcts in the fetal and neonatal brainstem. An aetiology of central hypoventilation, dysphagia, Möbius syndrome and micrognathia. *Eur J Paediatr Neurol* 2004;8:71–87. With permission.)

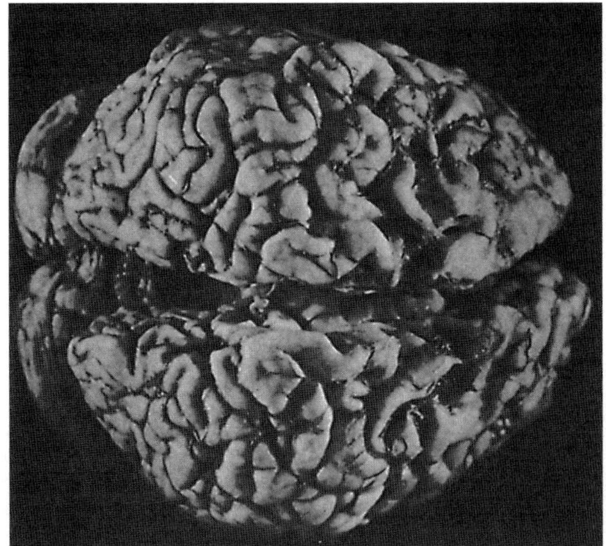

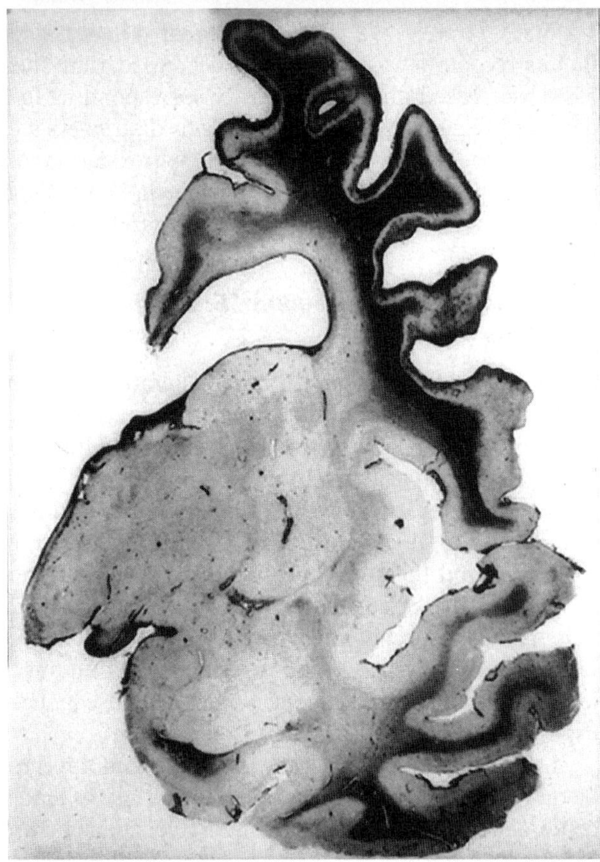

FIGURE 6.11. **A:** Lobar sclerosis (ulegyria) in a 5-year-old child with mental retardation and spastic since infancy. Sclerosis and distortion of the frontoparietal convolutions of the cerebrum are present. **B:** Coronal section of same brain showing shrunken and gliotic convolutions. The sulci are deepened and widened (Holzer's stain for myelin fibers). (From Towbin A. *The pathology of cerebral palsy*. Springfield, IL: Charles C Thomas, 1960. With permission.)

Ulegyria can be extensive or so restricted that the gross appearance of the brain is normal. It most commonly occurs in major arterial watershed border zones, in a parasagittal distribution in the venous drainage territory of the superior sagittal sinus, or within the territory of a major cerebral artery with partial occlusion (136). The perisulcal topography of the necrosis is related to reduced perfusion as a consequence of impaired sulcal venous drainage resulting from the compression of the stems of veins that ascend between gyri that have become edematous from previous hypoxic episodes (137). When ulegyria is widespread, an associated cystic defect in the subcortical white matter (porencephalic cyst) and dilatation of the lateral ventricles often occur. The meninges overlying the affected area are thickened and the small arteries occasionally can show calcifications in the elastica. Less often, ulegyria involves the cerebellum.

Marin-Padilla studied the postinjury gray matter alterations in ulegyria and found that the surviving cortex acquires a cortical dysplasia that affects the structural and functional differentiation of neurons, glial elements, and synaptic organization. Marin-Padilla proposed that the consequences of the acquired cortical dysplasia represent the main pathogenetic mechanism for epilepsy and other neurologic sequelae to perinatal brain damage (138).

Abnormalities of Basal Ganglia

Abnormalities within the basal ganglia are seen in the majority of patients subjected to perinatal asphyxia [84% in the series of Christensen and Melchior (139)]. One common lesion seen in this area has been termed *status marmoratus*. This picture was described first by Anton (140) in 1893 and later by the Vogt and Vogt (141). Fundamentally, the pathologic picture is one of glial scarring corresponding to the areas of tissue destruction. It is characterized by a gross shrinkage of the striatum, particularly the globus pallidus, associated with defects in myelination. Although in some cases myelinated nerve fibers, probably of astrocytic origin (135), are found in coarse networks resembling the veining of marble (hence the name of the condition, status marmoratus) (Fig. 6.12), in other cases the principal pattern is one of a symmetric demyelination (status dysmyelinatus) (142). Hypermyelination and demyelination probably represent different responses to the same insult. Hypermyelination probably results from oligodendrocytes becoming activated to produce excessive myelin, and, lacking enough axons to ensheath, they envelop astrocytic processes. The number of nerve cells in the affected areas is usually conspicuously reduced, with the smaller neurons in the putamen and caudate nucleus appearing more vulnerable. Cystic changes within the basal ganglia were stressed by Denny-Brown but are rarely extensive (143). Although the abnormalities within the basal ganglia are often the most striking, a variety of associated cortical lesions can be detected in most instances.

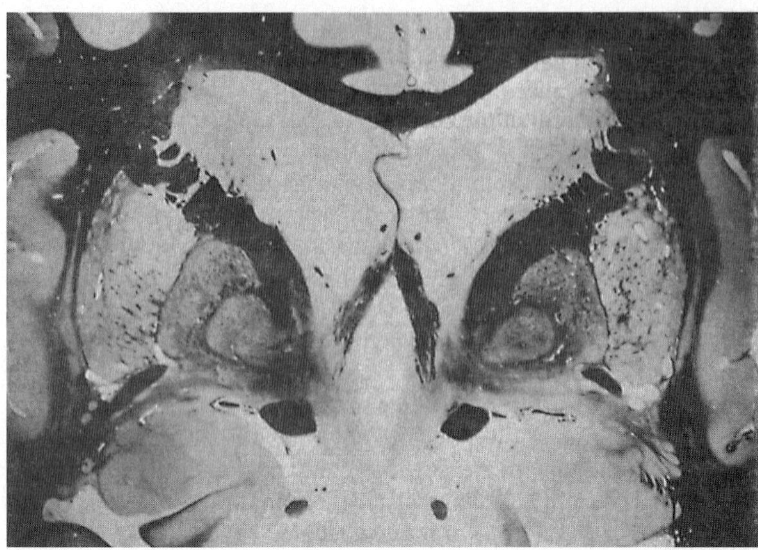

FIGURE 6.12. Status marmoratus of basal ganglia. (From Merritt HH. *A textbook of neurology*, 6th ed. Philadelphia: Lea & Febiger, 1979. With permission.)

It has been our experience, as well as that of others, that this condition is the result of an acute, severe hypoxic insult (144). As a rule, the asphyxia is not as prolonged as that which results in multicystic encephalomalacia, a condition in which there is also extensive damage to the cerebral cortex and white matter. The reason for the selective vulnerability of the basal ganglia to asphyxia is alluded to in another section of this chapter.

Given that these regions have a higher baseline oxygen consumption than other regions of the brain, as has been evidenced by positron emission tomography (PET) (145), other factors also must be operative to account for the particular vulnerability of the putamen and anterior thalamus (146). The most recent thinking is that the topography of neuronal death points to a primary role of glutamate excitotoxicity in basal ganglia neuronal damage, with the type of cell death induced by asphyxia (necrosis or apoptosis) being determined by neuronal maturity and the severity and duration of asphyxia (147). Also playing a role is the density of excitatory receptors, the differential expression of ionotropic and metabotropic glutamate receptors, their differential sensitivities, and the expression of the various receptor subtypes (76,147). Variations in the subunit composition of the receptor and changes in the expression of glutamate receptors with maturation may also influence the sensitivity of neurons to perinatal asphyxia (147a). Because astrocytes and oligodendroglia also express glutamate receptors, these cells may participate in basal ganglia injury (147). The striatal gamma-aminobutyric acid (GABA)-ergic, medium-sized inhibitory neurons also are sensitive to asphyxia, whereas the striatal cholinergic interneurons are resistant to asphyxia (76). Basal ganglionic neurons expressing nitric oxide synthase participate in oxidative stress and excitotoxicity, which often lead to the death of neighboring cells (147b,148).

In infants who suffer basal ganglia necrosis secondary to asphyxia, neuronal immunoreactivity to the various glutamate receptors was consistently decreased, with the areas of decreased immune reactivity corresponding to the damaged regions (149). Neonatal asphyxia triggers a cascade of gene expressins for tyrosine hydroxylase and D_1 and D_2 dopamine receptors in experimental animals, but the importance of this finding is unclear (150).

Abnormalities of Cerebellum, Brainstem, and Pons

Occasionally, the major structural alterations resulting from perinatal injury are localized to the cerebellum. In the majority of instances, the involvement is diffuse, with widespread disappearance of the cellular elements of the cerebellar cortex, notably the Purkinje cells, and the dentate nucleus (3,151). As with the periventricular germinal matrix around the lateral ventricles, the external granular layer of the cerebellum is vulnerable to spontaneous hemorrhage, especially in preterm infants of young gestational age. However, in the vast majority of infants, selective cerebellar involvement is not the consequence of asphyxia (152).

In general, the human neonatal brainstem appears to be more resistant to ischemic and hypoxic insults than the cerebral cortex, but it is not invulnerable, and sometimes lesions are more prominent in the brainstem than in supratentorial structures. The lesions are usually symmetric and involve both gray matter nuclei and adjacent white matter tracts, but the gray matter is more focally involved, perhaps because of its higher metabolic rate. Lesions may involve the inferior or superior colliculi almost selectively (3), or infarction may occur in the central core of the brainstem or selectively in the periaqueductal gray matter (3,136,153,154). Such multiple deep microinfarcts at times extend rostrally to involve deep supratentorial structures such as the thalamus and corpus striatum (155). Bilateral tegmental infarcts of the pons and medulla oblongata in particular are frequent sequelae of transient fetal hypotension because the tegmentum is a watershed zone, futher discussed later (133a). Because of the microscopic size of many of the deep infarcts, particularly those of the brainstem, they are difficult to identify on neuroimaging. Nevertheless, some older lesions that occurred in fetal life several weeks before delivery may be visualized in CT by their calcification in the floor of the fourth ventricle (133a,155a). MRI occasionally demonstrates infarcts in the tegmentum or floor of the fourth ventricle if they are large enough (155b).

Infarction in the nuclei of the brainstem and thalami, induced in experimental animals by total asphyxia of 10 to 25 minutes' duration, also can be seen in asphyxiated human infants with a history of acute profound asphyxial damage (156). Additionally, transient compression of the vertebral arteries in the course of rotation or hyperextension of the infant's head during delivery can be a cause for circulatory lesions of the brainstem (157,158).

Involvement of the nucleus ambiguous, just ventrolateral to the tractus solitarius, can result in dysphagia because this nucleus provides motor neurons for the muscles of deglutition. Involvement of the trigeminal motor nucleus by tegmental infarcts may damage motor neurons to the masticatory muscles, such as the masseter and pterygoids, and, in late gestation, the lack of function of these muscles leads to a lack of stimulus to growth of the mandible, so that micrognathia and even ankylosis of the temporomandibular joint is present by the time of birth (133a). Because the paired triads of vessels from the basial artery are 25 to 30 in number, from the midbrain to the caudal end of the medulla oblongata, the watershed tegmental infarcts are columnar and may extend posteriorly to even involve the hypoglossal nucleus so that the infant has atrophy and fasciculations of the tongue that may be mistaken for spinal muscular atrophy (133a,155c).

Neurosensory hearing loss after basilar artery insufficiency has both central and peripheral bases: The lateral lemniscus is at the margin of the tegmental watershed zone and the inferior colliculus is one of the most constant regions infarcted; the stria vascularis and hair cells of the cochlea receive their arterial supply from the basilar artery via the inferior anterior cerebellar artery (IACA). The labyrinth (semicircular canals) also receives arterial blood from the IACA, but its cells seem more resistant to irreversible injury from ischemia.

Table 6.3 lists the lesions and clinical expression seen with tegmental infarcts, but only rarely does an infant exhibit all deficits. Though much more frequent in fetuses and neonates than at any other time in life, tegmental watershed infarcts also can occur in older children and adults.

Unilateral tegmental infarcts also can involve the fetal and neonatal brainstem but are rare; such asymmetric lesions are more likely the result of a vascular anomaly of the basilar artery or birth trauma to the veretebral arteries than of generalized hypoperfusion of the brainstem due to transient shock in the fetus or neonate (133a,158).

TABLE 6.3 Clinical Sequelae of Tegmental Watershed Infarcts

Clinical Presentation	*Brainstem Structures Damaged*
Möbius syndrome	Nucleus VI, loop of VII, and more (155a,155b)
Micrognathia, ankylosis of jaw	Trigeminal motor V nucleus
Central respiratory failure	Nucleus/tractus solitarius IX, X
Dysphagia	Nucleus ambiguus X
Poor peristalsis, bradycardia	Dorsal motor nucleus X
Atrophy, fasciculations of tongue	Hypoglossal nucleus XII
Neurosensory hearing loss	Lateral lemniscus, inferior colliculus VIII

See also Sugama et al. (155c).

Pontosubicular Degeneration

Pontosubicular degeneration in isolation or accompanied by widespread cerebral damage has been described in premature and term infants (3,156,157). It is not a rare entity. It has been demonstrated in up to 59% of infants born before 38 weeks' gestation who died in the first month of postnatal life, which suggests that it is the most common cerebral lesion of preterm neonates, exceeding even germinal matrix hemorrhages (4,159–161).

The condition represents a unique topology of pathologic neuronal apoptosis in the fetal and neonatal brain following hypoxia or ischemia. As its descriptive name implies, it selectively involves relay nuclei of the corticopontocerebellar pathway in the basis pontis and the subiculum, a transitional cortex between the three-layered hippocampus and the six-layered hippocampal gyrus. Although it may coexist with other hypoxic lesions in the cortex, thalamus, and cerebellum, these other regions are disproportionately less severely involved than the pontine nuclei and subiculum (136,159,162). Usually, there are no lesions in the tegmentum of the pons, although in rare instances symmetric microinfarcts have been described (163,164). Focal white matter infarcts also occur occasionally.

This distribution of infarcts is generally seen in infants older than 29 weeks' gestation, most commonly in infants of 32 to 36 weeks' gestation. The pattern can also occur in stillborns (165) and term infants and has occasionally been encountered in adult brains (166). The reason that pontosubicular degeneration is not better recognized by clinicians is that it is difficult to demonstrate during life and remains essentially a postmortem neuropathologic diagnosis.

The combination of infarcts in the basis pontis and the subiculum is difficult to explain because these regions do not share common afferent or efferent fiber connections, use different neurotransmitters, have morphologically different types of neurons, arise from different embryologic primordia, and belong to different functional systems of the brain.

The pathogenesis of pontosubicular degeneration is poorly understood. Hyperoxemia in the presence of acidosis and hypoxia is described in some infants, suggesting that oxygen toxicity plays a role (160), but these cases represent only a small minority. Pontine neurons exhibiting karyorrhexis are immunoreactive to ferritin if accompanied by spongy changes and gliosis, suggesting that iron may be released to the damaged pontine neurons (167). *In situ* DNA fragmentation studies indicate apoptosis rather than frank necrosis as the mechanism of cellular death (168,169).

Pontosubicular degeneration has been described in stillborn fetuses, indicating that the lesions may result from intrauterine fetal distress and are not necessarily acquired intrapartum or postpartum (165,170,171). Sarnat provided details of the histologic progression of changes in the degenerating neurons (136).

Spinal Cord Lesions

The spinal cord is also vulnerable to hypoxic-ischemic injuries, and damage to anterior horn cells results from hypoperfusion of the watershed area between the vascular distribution of the anterior spinal and the dorsal spinal arteries (172). The resultant hypotonia is generally attributed to cerebral injury, but electromyography (EMG) can demonstrate a lower motor neuron injury.

Infarcts

An infarct, the consequence of a focal or generalized disorder of cerebral circulation that occurs during the antenatal or early postnatal period and acts in isolation, is a relatively rare cause of brain damage. In the series of autopsies studied by Barmada and colleagues, arterial infarcts were seen in 5.4%, and infarcts of venous origin were found in 2.4% (173). Almost 90% are unilateral, and in 83% the infarct is in the distribution of the middle cerebral artery (4). It is presumed to be the result of embolization arising from placental infarcts or of thrombosis caused by vascular maldevelopment, sepsis, or, as in the case of a twin to a macerated fetus, the exchange of thromboplastic material from the dead infant (3). In the series of Fujimoto and colleagues, 22% followed perinatal asphyxia; their onset was in the first 3 days of life (174). Infarcts can be asymptomatic or present with convulsions. Of 90 term infants presenting with seizures solely within 72 hours of birth, Cowan et al. found that 35 (39%) had focal cerebral infarction in arterial or parasagital distribution (30). Such infarctions are generally thought to be unrelated to intrapartum difficulties or the presence of neonatal encephalopathy, although the incidence of antenatal and intrapartum problems is higher in this group of infants than in a control population (175). Sreenan and coworkers had a different experience (176). In their series neonatal encephalopathy was encountered in 56% of infants who developed cerebral infarctions, and various adverse perinatal events occurred in about 75%. The presence of an inherited thrombophilic abnormality increased the risk of focal infarction. In the same population Mercuri and coworkers found that 30% of infants with focal infarction had a thrombophilic abnormality, usually heterozygosity for factor V Leiden or a high factor VIII concentration (177). In the series of Golumb and coworkers (178), 70% of infants with ischemic stroke who did not suffer from neonatal encephalopathy had anticardiolipin antibodies. Golumb reviewed the various prothrombotic disorders that contribute to the development of neonatal thrombotic infarcts (179).

Focal infarctions are less common in the premature than the term infant, and compared with the term infant the premature infant has a better prognosis with regard to neurologic residua (180).

With increased use of neuroimaging studies, dural sinus thrombosis can be demonstrated as a consequence of severe perinatal asphyxia (181). The condition is also seen in a variety of other conditions that predispose the infant to a hypercoagulable state (182,183).

Porencephaly

A porencephalic cyst is a large intraparenchymal cyst that always communicates with the ventricular system. Loculated cysts entirely within the subcortical white matter are not porencephalic and are pseudocysts rather than true cysts because they lack an epithelial lining. Porencephalic cysts are partly, though usually sparsely, covered by ependyma. Porencephaly results from infarction in the territory of a major artery, usually the middle cerebral artery, although at times it may be a sequel to a grade 4 intraventricular hemorrhage (IVH) that extends the ventricle lumen into the empty parenchymal space left by the reabsorption of the hematoma. It is not a watershed infarct.

Porencephalic cysts often appear to communicate also with the overlying subarachnoid space, and such a communication may be reported by radiologists, but careful neuropathologic examination demonstrates that a thin pial membrane and sometimes arachnoidal tissue separate the porencephalic and subarachnoid compartments. (Fig. 6.13). The pia derives its vascular supply from meningeal rather than cerebral vessels. This membrane is too thin to resolve by CT or MRI, but is important during life in terms of fluid shifts and CSF flow.

The cerebral cortex immediately surrounding a porencephalic cyst often appears to be polymicrogyric. This is secondary to ischemia and atrophy of immature gyri and should not be misconstrued as a primary dysgenesis. These small gyri are gliotic and have extensive neuronal loss.

Porencephaly is usually limited to one hemisphere, and the clinical correlates are spastic hemiplegia, hemisensory deficits, and often hemianopia. Porencephalic cysts following grade 4 IVH are visualized in survivors 10 days to 8 weeks after the event (184). Although it is not a

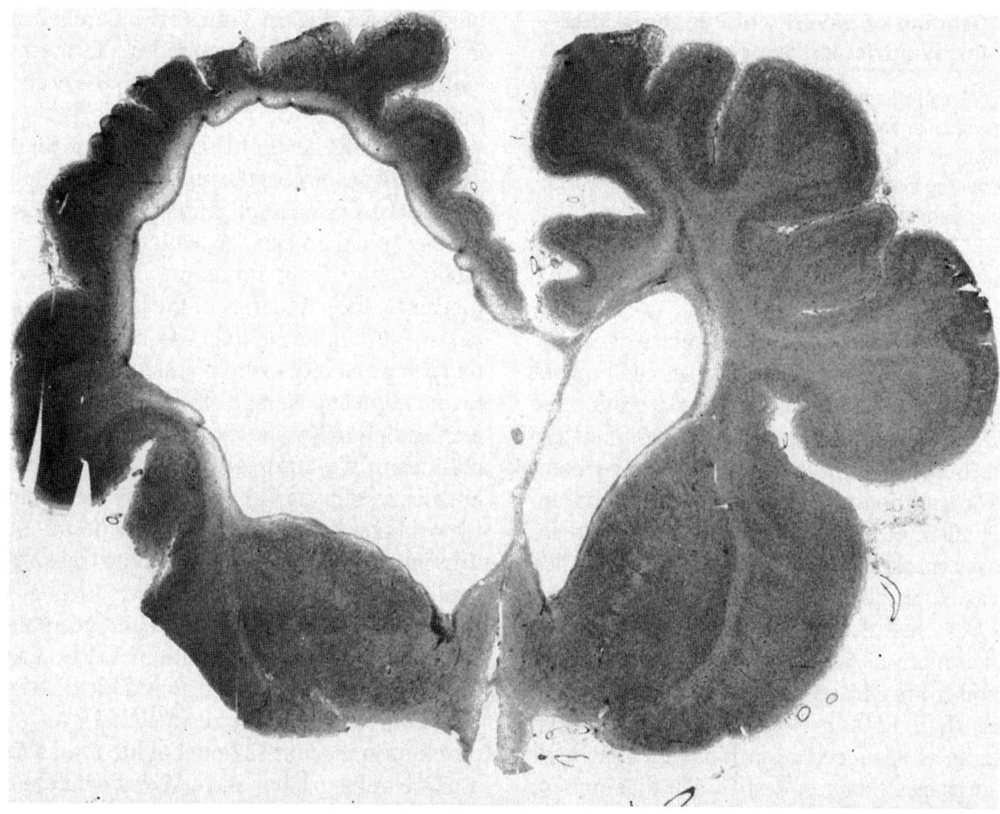

FIGURE 6.13. Porencephaly in middle cerebral artery distribution of a 4-month-old boy born at 30 weeks' gestation and who suffered fetal distress for more than a week before delivery. This coronal section of the brain at autopsy shows a large cavity replacing most of the right cerebral hemisphere and continuous with the lateral ventricle on that side. A thin ribbon of white matter and a thin cortex remain, but there is polymicrogyria of the right hemisphere in response to the atrophy. The left, "good" hemisphere shows pachygyria because the convolutional development of the brain became arrested at the time of onset of the fetal distress. Hematoxylin-eosin. ×1.5 (original magnification).

progressive lesion and does not obstruct the flow of CSF in the chronic phase, the porencephalic cyst occasionally enlarges and causes symptoms of intracranial hypertension. The reason for this phenomenon is the pulsation of the choroid plexus, which may induce a "waterhammer effect" because the force of the pulsations is transmitted to a larger surface area and the resistance to stretch is therefore less. The choroid plexus does not derive its blood supply from the middle cerebral artery; hence it usually survives the infarct. In some cases, a ventriculoperitoneal shunt may be required to prevent further enlargement of the porencephalic cyst, encroachment on functional brain, and midline shift.

Rarely, porencephaly is transmitted as an autosomal dominant disorder with incomplete penetrance. The presentation is with variable degrees of hemiparesis, seizures, and mental retardation (185). A thrombotic event during late pregnancy is believed to be responsible. The gene has been mapped to chromosome 13qter (186).

Intracranial Hemorrhage

Whereas mechanical trauma can be responsible for a subdural hemorrhage and, less commonly, a primary subarachnoid hemorrhage, it plays a relatively unimportant role in the evolution of periventricular-intraventricular hemorrhage (IVH), the most common form of neonatal intracranial hemorrhage (Table 6.4) (4,187,188). The various grades of hemorrhage are defined in Table 6.5 and depicted in Figs. 6.14, 6.15, and 6.16.

The site of the bleeding that results in an IVH is determined by the maturity of the infant. In the premature

TABLE 6.4 Major Types of Neonatal Intracranial Hemorrhage and Usual Clinical Setting

Type of Hemorrhage	*Usual Clinical Setting*
Subdural	Full-term >premature; trauma
Primary subarachnoid	Premature > full-term; trauma or "hypoxic" event(s)
Intracerebellar	Premature; "hypoxic" event(s); trauma (?)
Periventricular-intraventricular	Premature > full-term; "hypoxic" event(s)

From Volpe JJ. *Neurology of the newborn,* 3rd ed. Philadelphia: Saunders, 1995. With permission.

TABLE 6.5 Grading of Severity of Periventricular-Intraventricular Hemorrhage

Grade	Description
Grade I:	Germinal matrix hemorrhage with no or minimal intraventricular hemorrhage (IVH)
Grade II:	IVH involving less than 50% of ventricular area
Grade III:	IVH involving more than 50% of ventricular area
Grade IV:	IVH plus periventricular hemorrhagic infarction

Determination of the amount of blood in the ventricular system is best made on the parasagittal scan on ultrasonography.

infant, bleeding originates in the capillaries of the subependymal germinal matrix, usually over the body of the caudate nucleus (188). With increasing maturation the germinal matrix involutes, so that in the term infant the choroid plexus becomes the principal site of the hemorrhage (114,188). Although Hayden and coworkers encountered IVH in 4.6% of term neonates (189), its incidence increases markedly with decreasing maturity, so that when ultrasonography is performed on infants with birth weights less than 1,500 g, a hemorrhage can be documented in as many as 50%. A high-grade hemorrhage is more common in this group than in infants with birth weights greater than 1,500 g (190–192). At times, even premature infants of advanced gestational age may have extensive hemorrhages that can destroy the thalamus or basal ganglia (Figs. 6.3 and 6.15). Cerebellar hemorrhages in prematures usually arise in the external granular layer, a neuroepithelium corresponding to the periventricular germinal matrix.

The pathogenesis of IVH is not completely understood. The predisposition of the premature infant to IVH is in part due to the presence of a highly vascularized subependymal germinal matrix, to which a major portion of the blood supply of the immature cerebrum is directed. Furthermore, the capillaries of the premature infant have less basement membrane than those of the mature brain, and there is a paucity of tight junctions that is compounded by incomplete coverage of blood vessels by astrocytic end feet leading to fragility of the blood vessels. Finally, abnormalities in the autoregulation of arterioles in premature and distressed term infants impair the infants' response to hypoxia and hypercarbia and thus permit transmission of arterial pressure fluctuations to the fragile periventricular capillary bed.

Prenatal as well as perinatal and postnatal factors have been implicated in the evolution of IVH . Lack of adequate matching for gestational age and birth weight have, however, confounded many results (193). As a rule, IVH that develops in the first 12 hours of life is associated with variables relating to labor and delivery, whereas IVH that starts

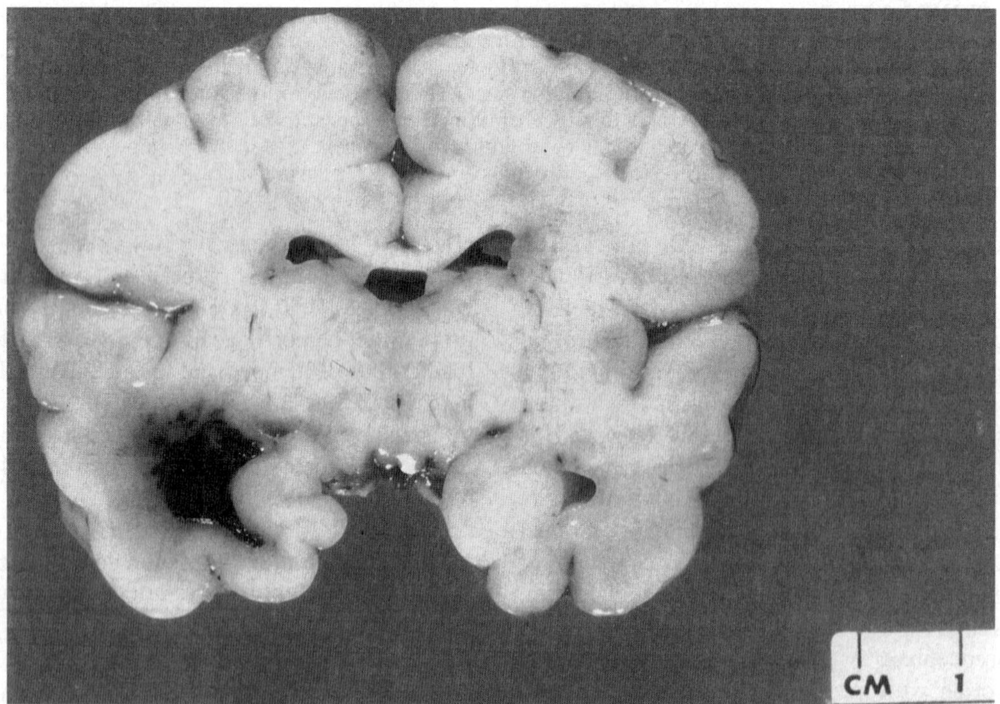

FIGURE 6.14. Intraventricular hemorrhage, grade 2. Focal hemorrhage of the germinal matrix breaking through the ependyma and causing focal intraventricular hemorrhage that does not extend throughout or dilate the ventricular system. The coronal section of this brain of a 32-week premature infant shows hemorrhage into the left temporal horn and local dilatation of that horn, but blood does not extend into the frontal horn or across the midline, and the rest of the ventricular system is not dilated. In the dorsolateral periventricular region of the involved temporal horn, hemorrhage is seen in the parenchyma, but confined to that zone.

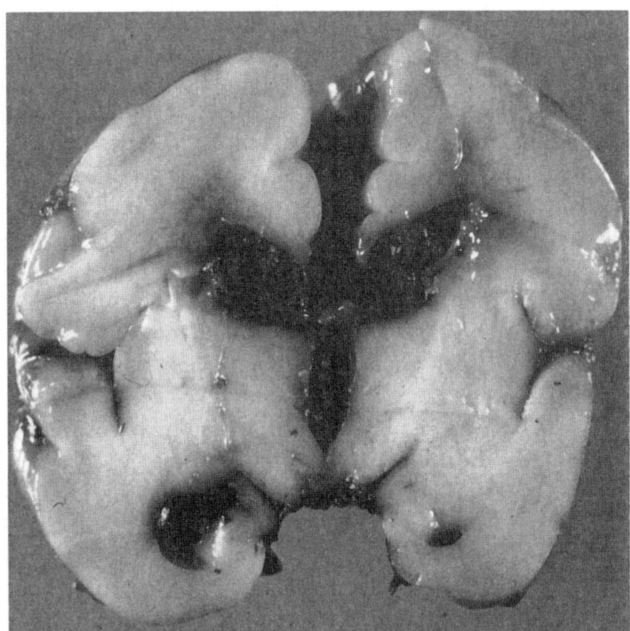

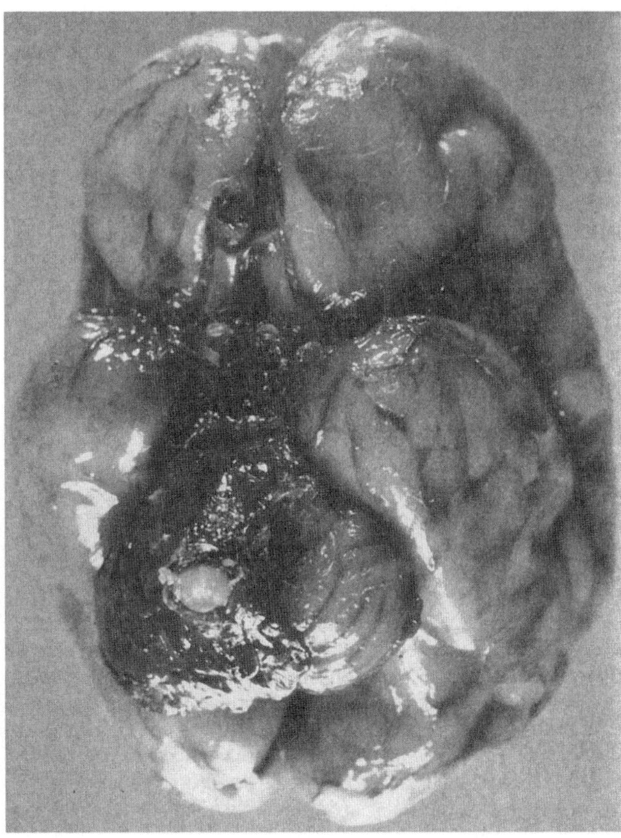

FIGURE 6.15. **A:** Intraventricular hemorrhage, grade 3. More extensive intraventricular hemorrhage than in Fig. 5.2, in a 28-week premature infant. Hemorrhage extends throughout the ventricular system and causes dilatation of the lateral ventricles bilaterally and the third ventricle; the original site of origin of the hemorrhage may be difficult to identify, but periventricular leukomalacia is seen around both frontal horns and the left side of the third ventricle. **B:** Blood from the lateral and third ventricles is seen in the subarachnoid space at the base of the brain, having exuded through the aqueduct and fourth ventricle and out the foramina of Luschka and Magendie during the course of cerebrospinal fluid flow.

later is associated with postpartum variables. Premature rupture of membranes and maternal chorioamnionitis increase the risk for the condition, suggesting that cytokines play a role in its evolution (192,194,195).

In most infants, acute fluctuations in cerebral blood flow and an impaired cerebral vascular autoregulation are more important than prenatal factors in the evolution of an IVH. Clinical studies have shown that infants with intact cerebrovascular autoregulation are at low risk for IVH. In contrast, a variety of adverse factors that disrupt autoregulation are associated with a high risk of IVH. These include low Apgar scores, respiratory distress, artificial ventilation, the presence of a patent ductus arteriosus, and the various complications of perinatal and postnatal asphyxia (192,194,196). An elevation of venous pressure also has been implicated. Such an elevation can occur in the course of labor and delivery, or it can accompany positive-pressure ventilation, pneumothorax, hypoxic-ischemic myocardial failure, or hyperosmolality induced by administration of excess sodium bicarbonate (4).

The importance of pneumothorax caused by positive-pressure ventilation in producing IVH was stressed by McCord and coworkers, who were able to reduce the incidence of respiratory distress syndrome and with it the incidence of IVH by treatment with surfactant (197). In addition to surfactant, maternal tocolysis using ritrodrine, early low-dose indomethacin, and antenatal steroid treatment also reduce the incidence of IVH in very low birth weight premature infants (193,198–200). Neonatal risk factors that predispose to the evolution of IVH include clotting disorders, reduced hemoglobin, hypercarbia, and hypoglycemia (4).

In the premature infant, the hemorrhage does not occur at the time of delivery but tends to commence later, most commonly 24 to 48 hours after a major asphyxial insult, whether at the time of birth or subsequently (192,201). In the experience of Ment and associates, 74% of hemorrhages were detected by ultrasonography within 30 hours after birth (202) (Fig. 6.16). In the series of Trounce and colleagues, 15% of infants developed an IVH after 2 weeks

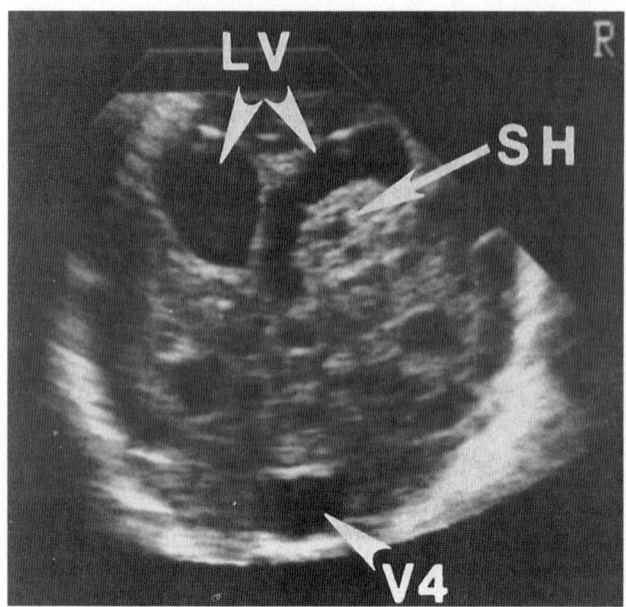

FIGURE 6.16. Intraventricular hemorrhage in a 1,400-g infant of 30 weeks' gestation who suffered birth asphyxia. Coronal ultrasonographic scan reveals moderate hydrocephalus and a large subependymal hemorrhage (*SH*) in the wall of the right lateral ventricle (*LV*, lateral ventricles; *V4*, fourth ventricle). (From Babcock DS, Han BK. The accuracy of high-resolution, real-time ultrasonography of the head in infancy. *Radiology* 1981;139:665. With permission.)

of age (191). In some infants bleeding can be a slow process rather than a sudden event (203). The extent of the hemorrhage can range from a slight oozing to a massive intraventricular bleed with an associated asymmetric periventricular hemorrhagic infarction and an extension of the blood into the subarachnoid space of the posterior fossa (see Figs. 6.14 and 6.15) (204).

Blood usually clears rapidly from the intraventricular and subarachnoid spaces. In fact, hemosiderin deposition, a reliable and permanent neuropathologic marker of old hemorrhage in the adult brain, is found rarely in children's brains after an IVH. Despite the resolution of the fresh blood, brain injury is a relatively common result of IVH. Several mechanisms are believed to play a role (4).

1. The injury can be the result of an antecedent asphyxial injury that predisposed the infant to the bleeding.
2. In the presence of a large IVH, intracranial pressure will increase, which, in turn, will reduce cerebral perfusion.
3. The IVH can induce arterial vasospasm. As demonstrated by PET, cerebral blood flow becomes abolished in the area of an intraparenchymal hematoma and is reduced twofold to threefold over the entire affected hemisphere (205). How a hemorrhage induces such widespread vasospasm is unclear. Like the vasospasm encountered in older children and adults after a subarachnoid hemorrhage induced by the rupture of an aneurysm (see Chapter 13), the vasospasm could be related to the presence of high concentrations of blood in the CSF (206). Vasospasm may well have its major effect on the middle cerebral artery; as judged from the pulsatility index in the anterior cerebral artery, Perlman and Volpe found no consistent effect of an IVH on flow in the anterior cerebral artery (207).
4. Metabolic alterations are responsible for subsequent neurologic abnormalities. Cerebral glucose metabolism is markedly reduced (208), and, as determined by MR spectroscopy, the brain phosphocreatine concentration is reduced for several weeks after the hemorrhage (209).
5. Unilateral or grossly asymmetric destruction of periventricular white matter can be the result of an ischemic reperfusion injury. A fan-shaped hemorrhagic infarct, visualized by ultrasonography as an intracerebral periventricular, echodense lesion, is not unusual and can be demonstrated in approximately 15% of infants with IVH and in approximately one-third of those who harbor a severe hemorrhage (4,210) (Fig. 6.17). It is marked by a large region of hemorrhagic necrosis in the periventricular white matter at the point where the medullary veins become confluent and join the terminal vein in the subependymal region. The necrosis is usually markedly asymmetric; it is unilateral in the majority of instances (96). Approximately 80% of cases are accompanied by a large IVH, and, in the past, the

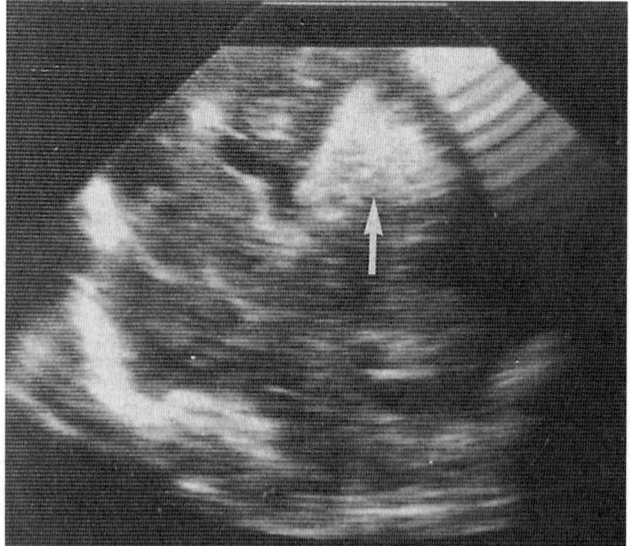

FIGURE 6.17. Intracerebral hemorrhage in a neonate. Coronal ultrasonographic scan. The arrow indicates the presence of the hematoma. Displacement of the ventricular system occurred. (Courtesy of Dr. Eric E. Sauerbrei, Kingston General Hospital, Kingston, Ontario, Canada.)

infarction was mistakenly described as a parenchymal extension of the IVH. Periventricular hemorrhagic infarction is believed to result from the IVH compressing and obstructing the terminal veins and interfering with their drainage (211). The periventricular hemorrhagic infarct produces tissue destruction and formation of cystic cavities and is associated with a poor functional outcome. Porencephalic cysts can develop in survivors and are visualized in 10 days to 8 weeks after the event (212).

6. White matter injury can also result from the toxic effects of proinflammatory cytokines or the release of a variety of reactive oxygen species (213). Iron released during heme catabolism has the potential of generating hydroxyl radicals and inducing oxidative damage on immature oligodendroglia.

Progressive ventricular dilatation is a common sequel to IVH (Fig. 6.18). Evolving 1 to 3 weeks after the hemorrhage, it is caused by a fibrotic reaction that obliterates the subarachnoid spaces and induces ventricular dilatation with or without increased intracranial pressure (normal-pressure hydrocephalus) (4). The factors responsible for normal-pressure hydrocephalus in the neonate are poorly understood.

When an IVH occurs in term infants, it generally emanates from the choroid plexus, less frequently from the subependymal germinal matrix. The major causes are trauma and perinatal asphyxia (4). In the experience of Volpe, approximately one-half of term newborns with IVH experienced difficult deliveries. The experience of Palmer and Donn is similar (214). In approximately 25% of cases, the IVH is of unknown etiology. One cause that probably accounts for a large number of these cases is a cryptic hemangioma of the choroid plexus, well demonstrated at autopsy (215,216). The lesions range in size from thin-walled cavernous angiomas to fully formed arteriovenous malformations. They are sometimes difficult to show by imaging, in part because the hemorrhage may destroy the original vascular malformation or obscure its remains (216). Unruptured angiomas of the choroid villi are not uncommon as incidental findings at autopsy and must be distinguished from simple vascular congestion. It is a relatively common complication of Sturge-Weber syndrome (see Chapter 12). One of us (H.S.) has found them to be more frequent in patients with cerebral malformations or chromosomal abnormalities.

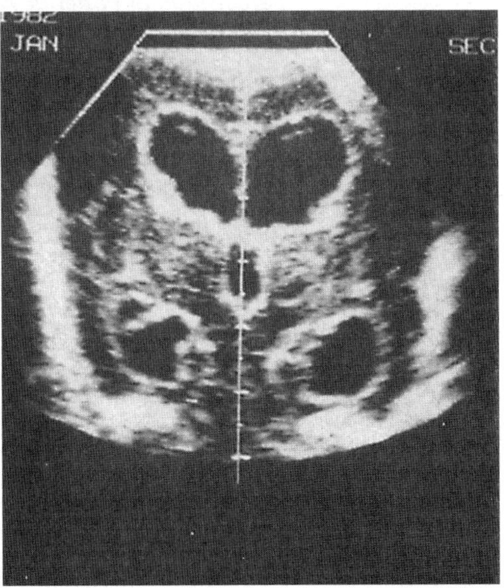

FIGURE 6.18. Posthemorrhagic hydrocephalus in a 2-week-old premature infant. The lateral ventricles and the third ventricle are dilated; the fourth ventricle is not visualized. The increased echogenicity of the ventricular wall indicates posthemorrhagic hydrocephalus, as distinct from hydrocephalus resulting from a malformation, in which the hyperecho ring is absent. (Courtesy of Dr. W. Donald Shields, Division of Pediatric Neurology, University of California, Los Angeles, CA.)

Term infants with IVH tend to become symptomatic at a later age, often not until the fourth week of life. Irritability, changes in alertness, and seizures are common presenting symptoms. In the series of Palmer and Donn, seizures were the first symptom in 69% of cases; 23% of infants presented with apnea (214).

Extension of intracranial hemorrhage to the spinal canal is more frequent than is recognized. Both epidural and subdural bleeding have been encountered, the former being far more common. Epidural bleeding is associated not only with intracranial hemorrhage owing to asphyxia, but also with traumatic birth injuries (217,218). Although these hemorrhages either are asymptomatic or induce deficits that are obscured by the more obvious symptoms of an intracranial hemorrhage, diagnosis by MRI of the spinal cord is now possible.

Primary and Secondary Malformations of the Central Nervous System

In addition to direct trauma, asphyxia, and circulatory disturbances, malformations of the CNS play an important part in the genesis of the lesions of perinatal asphyxia and trauma. Little doubt exists that in the premature infant, for instance, both faulty maturation of the nervous system and a greater vulnerability to perinatal trauma and asphyxia are responsible for the high incidence of neurologic deficits (Table 6.6) (219). The relative frequency of prenatal and perinatal brain lesions in individuals with moderate or severe mental retardation can be determined from autopsy studies such as those by Freytag and Lindenberg (133) (Table 6.7) or from MRI evaluation of children with mental retardation and/or cerebral palsy (31).

Ischemic, hypoxic, and traumatic insults of the fetal brain in the second and third trimesters can induce malformations that are not primary defects of genetic

TABLE 6.6 Neuropathology in Premature and Full-Term Infants with Cerebral Palsy

	Pathology	
Birth Weight (g)	*Birth Injury (Number of Cases)*	*Central Nervous System Malformation (Number of Cases)*
Less than 2,000	3	3
2,000–2,500	2	1
2,501–3,000	0	6
3,001–3,500	10	4
Greater than 3,500	7	7
Total known	22	21

From Malamud N, Itabashi HH, Castor-Messinger HB. An etiologic and diagnostic study of cerebral palsy. *J Pediatr,* 1964;66:270. With permission.

programming. Because development is incomplete, lesions that interrupt or alter radial glial fibers, for example, can prevent further neuroblast and glioblast migration before the process is complete and may result in focal dysplasias of cortical lamination and in deep heterotopia of neurons arrested in migration (Fig. 6.19). The abnormal synaptic relations that result from the abnormal anatomic positions of neurons may become a basis for later epilepsy (138).

Clinical Manifestations of Cerebral Perinatal Injuries

This section describes the clinical appearance of the neonate who has been subjected to perinatal asphyxia or trauma. It also traces the evolution of the spastic and extrapyramidal deficits and concludes with a discussion of the various syndromes of cerebral palsy, acknowledging that in many instances cerebral malformations play an etiologic role equaling or surpassing that of perinatal asphyxia and trauma.

The interested reader is referred to the pioneering studies by Paine on the evolution of tone and postural reflexes in neurologically damaged neonates (220,221).

Neonatal Period

The degree of a newborn's functional abnormality secondary to asphyxia incurred during labor and delivery depends on the severity, timing, and duration of the insult. (See the Introduction chapter for a description of the essentials of a neurologic examination of the infant or small child.)

After birth, the infant subjected to perinatal asphyxia shows certain alterations in alertness, muscle tone, and respiration. These important clinical features of HIE were first graded by Sarnat and Sarnat (222) (Table 6.8). Several

TABLE 6.7 Frequency of Brain Lesions

Type of Lesion	*Number of Patients with Lesion*[a]			*Percentage of Patients With Demonstrable Lesions*	
Prenatal	150			50.5	
Malformations		93			31.3
Chiari malformation			23		
Microgyria, pachygyria, agyria			18		
Primary microcephaly			9		
Agenesis of corpus callosum			8		
Heterotopic gray matter			6		
Abnormal convolutional pattern			6		
Other malformations			23		
Down syndrome		31			10.4
Hydrocephalus		23			7.7
Prenatal Infections		2			0.7
Unclassified		1			0.3
Perinatal	47			15.8	
Circulatory lesions			42		14.1
Mechanical birth trauma			5		1.7
[genetic disorders (e.g., leukodystrophies, lipidoses, tuberose sclerosis)]	27			9.1	
Postnatal					
Postnatal owing to exogenous causes (meningitis, encephalitis)	44			14.8	
Unknown whether perinatal or prenatal	29			9.8	

[a] No morphologic lesions were detectable in another 62 autopsies.

Adapted from Freytag E, Lindenberg R. Neuropathological findings in patients of a hospital for the mentally deficient: a survey of 359 cases. *Johns Hopkins Med J* 1967;121:379. With permission.

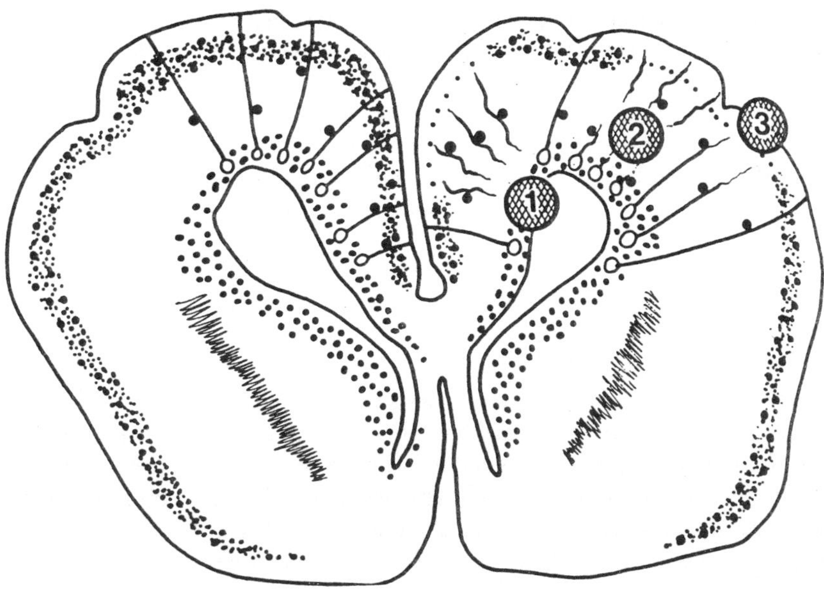

FIGURE 6.19. Drawing of a coronal section of the cerebral hemisphere of a preterm infant to illustrate three possible sites where ischemic-hypoxic lesions might disrupt radial glial cells or their fibers to interfere with neuroblast and glioblast migration and thus cause secondary, acquired malformations as focal cortical dysplasias and subcortical heterotopia of incompletely migrated cells: (*1*) In the periventricular region, periventricular leukomalacia or grade 1 or 2 germinal matrix hemorrhage; (*2*) in the deep subcortical white matter, as either ischemic or hemorrhagic infarction; and (*3*) at the pial surface, where injury might cause retraction of radial glial end-feet. Examples of insults at the pial surface include contusions of the brain at delivery, subarachnoid hemorrhage, and neonatal meningitis. (From Sarnat HB. *Cerebral dysgenesis. Embryology and clinical expression*. New York: Oxford University Press, 1992. With permission.)

other grading schemes have been devised. In essence, they are similar to that of Sarnat and Sarnat; however, some schemes place infants with repetitive or prolonged seizures into grade 3 rather than grade 2 (22). Sarnat and Sarnat specifically excluded seizures as a criterion for grading acute encephalopathy because of poor correlation with outcome in their experience and because some of the most severely involved infants in stage 3 do not have seizures because the cerebral cortex is so severely impaired that it can no longer generate epileptic activity. They did include electroencephalographic (EEG) criteria, however, as a measure of cerebral function rather than of paroxysmal activity. They also emphasized the importance of autonomic features, with sympathomimetic effects in stage 1 and strong parasympathetic (i.e., vagal) effects in stage 2.

TABLE 6.8 Clinical Features of Hypoxic-Ischemic Encephalopathy

Stage 1
Hyperalert
Normal muscle tone
Weak suck
Low threshold Moro
Mydriasis
No seizures
Stage 2
Lethargic or obtunded
Mild hypotonia
Weak or absent suck
Weak Moro
Miosis
Focal or multifocal seizures
Stage 3
Stuporous, responds to strong stimuli only
Flaccid
Intermittent decerebration
Absent suck
Absent Moro
Poor pupillary light response

Adapted from Sarnat HB, Sarnat MS. Neonatal encephalopathy following fetal distress. *Arch Neurol* 1976;33:696.

In the experience of Levene and coworkers, 3.9 in 1,000 newborn term infants develop grade 1 HIE, 1.1 in 1,000 develop grade 2 HIE, and 1.0 in 1,000 develop grade 3 HIE (223).

Infants with grade 1 HIE are irritable with some degree of feeding difficulty and are in a hyperalert state in which their eyes are open with a "worried" facial appearance and a decreased frequency of blinking. They seem hungry and respond excessively to stimulation. Tremulousness, especially when provoked by abrupt changes of limb position or tactile stimulation, can resemble seizures. Mild degrees of hypotonia can be documented by a head lag and a lack of the normal biceps flexor tone in the traction response from the supine position. The Landau reflex is often abnormal, in that the infant's body tends to collapse into an inverted U shape.

A greater hypoxic insult results in the evolution of grade 2 HIE. Infants are lethargic or obtunded with delayed or incomplete responses to stimuli. Focal or multifocal seizures are common. Severely asphyxiated infants develop clinical signs of grade 3 HIE. The infant is markedly hypotonic. The sucking and swallowing reflexes are absent, producing difficulties in feeding. Palmar and plantar grasps are weak, the Moro reflex can be absent, and the placing and stepping reactions are impossible to elicit.

A variety of respiratory abnormalities can be encountered. These include a failure to initiate breathing after birth, which suggests a hypoxic depression of the respiratory reflex within the brainstem. Tachypnea or dyspnea in the absence of pulmonary or cardiac disease also suggests a neurologic abnormality. Periodic bouts of apnea are normal in the smaller premature infant. In larger infants, periodic apnea can result from a depression of the respiratory reflex or can indicate a seizure disorder (see Chapter 14).

The Apgar score has been used to measure the severity of the initial insult. Although in the past the score was used to determine the presence of a hypoxic insult, to do so is a misapplication. For instance, in the experience of Sykes and coworkers, only 20% of infants with a 5-minute Apgar score of less than 7 had an umbilical artery pH below 7.10 (224). Conversely, virtually all of the infants of 35 to 36 weeks' gestation with a cord pH below 7.25 had a 5-minute Apgar score of 7 or more. In preterm infants the Apgar score is of even less value, and the more premature the infant, the more likely it is that the Apgar score will be low in the presence of a normal cord pH (225). Instead, the value of the Apgar score lies in being a simple and valuable predictor for survival during the neonatal period and for the ultimate outcome. In the series of Casey and coworkers, the neonatal mortality for term infants with a 5-minute Apgar score of 0 to 3 was 244 per 1,000, as contrasted with a mortality of 0.2 per 1,000 for intants with a 5-minute Apgar score of 7 to 10 (226). The extended Apgar scores (Apgar scores taken at 10 and 20 minutes of life), however, are even more valuable in predicting neurologic outcome, in that the likelihood of ensuing cerebral palsy increases significantly once the Apgar score remains under 3 for 10 minutes or longer (227). Moster and colleagues (228) noted that infants with 5-minute Apgar scores of 0 to 3 had an 81-fold increased risk for cerebral palsy compared with infants who had scores of 7 to 10. Term infants who had 5-minute Apgar scores of 0 to 3 and who also had signs consistent with neonatal encephalopathy had a significantly increased risk for impaired minor motor skills, reduced performances in reading and mathematics, and a variety of behavioral problems (229).

After 12 to 48 hours, the clinical picture of the previously hypotonic or flaccid infant (grade 3) can change to that of grade 2 or 1.5 (26). The infant becomes jittery, the cry is shrill and monotonous, the Moro reflex becomes exaggerated, and the infant has an increased startle response to sound. The deep tendon reflexes become hyperactive, and an increased extensor tone develops. Seizures can appear at this time. These signs of cerebral irritation also are noted in an infant who has experienced a major intracranial hemorrhage. In the series of Brown and associates (26), 24% of infants who were judged to have been subjected to perinatal hypoxia demonstrated hypotonia progressing to extensor hypertonus. In the experience of DeSouza and Richards, this clinical course has an ominous prognosis, for none of the infants following it were ultimately free of neurologic deficits (230). In our experience, the greater the delay in emerging from grade 3 HIE, the worse is the ultimate prognosis.

In other instances [24% in the series of Brown and associates (26)], an infant who was judged to have sustained perinatal asphyxia exhibits hypertonia and rigidity during the neonatal period. The clinical picture of spasticity in the neonate is modified by the immaturity of some of the higher centers. In the spastic infant, the deep tendon reflexes are not exaggerated but can be depressed as a result of muscular rigidity. Hyperreflexia becomes evident only during the second half of the first year of life. A more reliable physical sign indicating spasticity is the presence of a sustained tonic neck response, which indicates a tonic neck pattern that can be imposed on the infant for an almost indefinite time and that the infant cannot break down. Such a response is never normal (see Introduction chapter, Fig. I.5). Spastic hemiparesis is manifest during the neonatal period in only 10% of infants (231), usually by a reduction of spontaneous movements or by excessive fisting in the upper extremity. Obvious paralyses during the neonatal period are rarely caused by cerebral damage; instead, they suggest a peripheral nerve or spinal cord lesion.

The evolution of IVH can go unrecognized clinically in more than 50% of infants (232,233). The remainder can have a sudden, sometimes catastrophic deterioration highlighted by alterations in consciousness, abnormalities of eye movements, and respiratory irregularities. Deterioration can continue over several hours, then stop, only to resume hours or days later (4). The presence of a full fontanelle is noted in approximately one-third of asphyxiated infants (26). It can be the consequence of a massive intracranial hemorrhage, cerebral edema, or, less often, an acute subdural hemorrhage, the result of concomitant cerebral trauma (234).

Seizures secondary to perinatal asphyxia usually occur after 12 hours of age. However, when asphyxia is acute and profound, as can happen when a cord prolapse occurs, or when there is significant perinatal trauma, seizures can begin much earlier, and as a rule their onset cannot be used to time the asphyxial episode. The characterization and classification of seizures has been facilitated by the development of time-synchronized video and EEG/polygraphic monitoring. Generalized tonic-clonic convulsions are rare in the newborn. More often, one observes unifocal or multifocal clonic movements that tend to move from one part of the body to another. Generalized slow myoclonic jerks are another common neonatal seizure. EEG abnormalities do not accompany some behaviors previously considered to be neonatal seizures. These include a high percentage of tonic seizures, particularly those manifest by transient opisthotonos, and the various unusual forms of seizure activity ("subtle seizures"). Subtle seizures include paroxysmal blinking, changes in vasomotor tone, nystagmus, chewing, swallowing, or pedaling or swimming movements. These seizures probably represent primitive brainstem and spinal motor patterns released from the normal tonic inhibition of forebrain structures (235). Apnea is not observed as the sole seizure manifestation. Seizures resulting from birth trauma or perinatal asphyxia often cease spontaneously within a few days or weeks or become relatively easy to control with adequate doses of anticonvulsants. The topic of neonatal seizures is taken up in greater detail in Chapter 14.

Evolution of Motor Patterns

Infants who have suffered perinatal asphyxia experience various sequential changes of muscle tone and an abnormal evolution of postural reflexes.

Most often, there is a gradual change from the generalized hypotonia in the newborn period to spasticity in later life. In these patients, the earliest sign of spasticity is the presence of increased resistance on passive supination of the forearm or on flexion and extension of the ankle or knee. In spastic diplegia, this abnormal stretch reflex is first evident in the lower extremities and is often accompanied by the appearance of extension and scissoring in vertical suspension (see Introduction chapter, Fig. I.6), the late appearance or asymmetry of the placing response, a crossed adductor reflex that persists beyond 8 months of age, and the increased mobilization of extensor tone in the supporting reaction (221). In spastic hemiplegia, abnormalities first become apparent in the upper extremity. When five infants with unilateral hemispheric lesions detected by routine imaging studies during the first week of life were subjected to regular neurologic examinations, no abnormalities could be detected until 3 months of age, when one of the infants showed an asymmetric popliteal angle. Between 3 and 6 months of age the signs were subtle and usually consisted of asymmetric kicking in vertical suspension, which was seen in three infants by 6 months of age. Hand preference became apparent between 3 and 9 months of age (236). In some instances asymmetries of generalized movements and "fidgety" movements can be detected as early as 3 weeks of age (237). The absence of "fidgety" movements is also a good predictor for the development of dyskinetic and spastic quadriparetic cerebral palsy (238). As a rule, the more severe the hemiplegia, the earlier do the abnormalities make their appearance. Other signs of hemiparesis include inequalities of muscle tone, asymmetry of fisting, and inequalities of the parachute reaction (see Introduction chapter, Fig. I.7). In many instances, parents also note poor feeding and frequent regurgitation.

Ingram observed a remarkably constant sequence of neurologic manifestations in the progression from hypotonia to spasticity (239). The hypotonic stage lasts from 6 weeks to 17 months or longer. In general, the longer its duration, the more severely handicapped is the child.

In a significant percentage of children, 1.3% in the series of Skatvedt (240), but 20% of the group with cerebral palsy at the Southbury Training School, Southbury, Connecticut (241), the hypotonic state persists beyond the second or third year of life, and, accordingly, the condition is designated as hypotonic (atonic) cerebral palsy, a term first proposed by Förster in 1910 (242). The differential diagnosis between hypotonic cerebral palsy and abnormalities in muscle function is discussed more fully in Chapter 16.

A stage of intermittent dystonia often becomes apparent when the infant is first able to hold up his or her head. At that time, abrupt changes in position, particularly extension of the head, elicit a response that is similar to extensor decerebrate rigidity. The frequency with which this intermediate dystonic stage is observed is probably a function of the care with which neurologic observations are performed. In the majority of children, dystonic episodes are present from 2 to 12 months of age. Ultimately, as rigidity appears, episodes become less frequent and more difficult to elicit. Transient dystonic posturing, notably torticollis or opisthotonos, has been associated with maternal use of cocaine (243).

In a smaller number of children with cerebral palsy, a transition occurs from the diffuse hypotonia seen in the neonatal period to an extrapyramidal form of cerebral palsy. Although a characteristic feature of the motor activity of the healthy premature and full-term infant is the presence of choreoathetoid movements of the hands and feet, the fully developed clinical picture of dyskinesia is not usually apparent until the second year of life (Table 6.9) (221). Until then, the neurologic picture is marked

TABLE 6.9 Evolution of Athetosis in Infants with Extrapyramidal Cerebral Palsy

Age (Months)	*Cumulative Percentage of Patients Showing Athetosis in Reaching for Objects*
6	0
9	12
12	36
15	56
18	64
21	64
24	72
27	76
30	84
33	88
36	92

From Paine RS, Brazelton TE, Donovan DE, et al. Evolution of postural reflexes in normal infants and in the presence of chronic brain syndromes. *Neurology* 1964;14:1036. With permission.

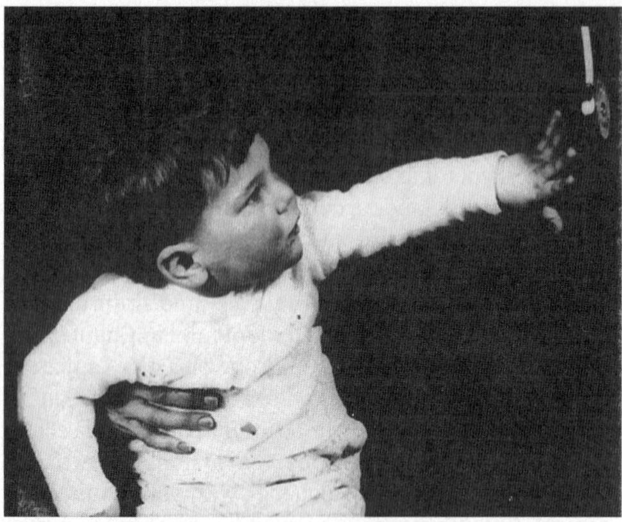

FIGURE 6.20. Athetotic posture of the hand in an infant. The child is attempting to reach a proffered object. (From Cooke RE. *The biologic basis of pediatric practice*. New York: McGraw-Hill, 1968. With permission.)

by persistent hypotonia accompanied by retention of the immature postural reflexes. In particular, the tonic neck reflex, the righting response, and the Moro reflex are retained for longer periods in infants with extrapyramidal cerebral palsy than in those in whom a spastic picture predominates (221). In general, the earliest specific evidence for extrapyramidal disease is observed in the posturing of the fingers when the infant reaches for an object (Fig. 6.20). This can be noted as early as 9 months of age, and, as a rule, the early appearance of extrapyramidal movements indicates that the ultimate disability will be mild. In the child with dyskinesia, dystonic posturing can be elicited by sudden changes in the position of the trunk or limbs, particularly by extension of the head. Characteristically, when an infant with early extrapyramidal disease is placed with support in the sitting position, the infant resists passive flexion of the neck and tends to retroflex the back and shoulders. The assessment of the general movement patterns was used by Prechtl to accurately predict the ultimate evolution of cerebral palsy (244).

Every physician examining infants suspected of having sustained a cerebral birth injury has encountered a group of patients who appear to have clear-cut neurologic signs in early infancy but who, on subsequent examinations, have lost all of their motor dysfunction (245). Many of these have not escaped brain damage; follow-up studies show them to have delayed milestones, a high incidence of mental retardation (22%), abnormalities of extraocular movements (22%), and afebrile seizures (4.4%) (245). Still, approximately one-third appear normal, or, at worst, demonstrate mild perceptual handicaps or hyperkinetic behavior patterns (246).

Childhood

With the decline in neonatal mortality and improved documentation, the prevalence of cerebral palsy rose significantly in most countries during the 1970s and 1980s but has remained fairly stable in the last 10 years. A recent estimate is 2.4 per 1,000 children (247). This contrasts with in prevalence of 1.23 in 1,000 3-year-old children born in Northern California between 1983 and 1985 (248). In this group of children, 53% of children with cerebral palsy had birth weights of 2,500 g or less and 28% had birth weights less than 1,500 g. In Sweden, 2.12 in 1,000 children born between 1991 and 1994 were diagnosed as suffering from cerebral palsy; 38% of these children were preterm (31a). The increase in the incidence of cerebral palsy as a consequence of a decrease in neonatal mortality and the increased frequency of multiple births also has been reported from Australia, England, and Ireland (249).

In older children, the manifestations of cerebral birth injuries are so varied that it is difficult to devise an adequate scheme of classification. Yet the differences in cause, clinical picture, and prognosis require that cerebral palsy be subdivided into various entities based on the clinical picture. In this chapter, the following system is used:

Spastic cerebral palsy
Spastic quadriparesis
Spastic diplegia
Spastic hemiparesis
Extrapyramidal cerebral palsies
Hypotonic (atonic) cerebral palsy
Cerebellar cerebral palsy
Mixed and atypical forms

Table 6.10 shows the incidence of some of these forms of cerebral palsy. As many as one-seventh of children show a mixture of clear-cut pyramidal and extrapyramidal signs, and almost every child with spastic diplegia is found to

TABLE 6.10 Incidence of Various Forms of Cerebral Palsy

Classification[a]	*Crothers and Paine (N = 161) (%)*	*Grether et al. (N = 176) (%)*
Spastic	64.6	82
Quadriplegia	19.0	22
Diplegia	2.8	41
Hemiplegia	40.5	19
Monoplegia	0.4	—
Triplegia	1.9	—
Extrapyramidal	22.0	5[b]
Mixed Types	13.1	13

[a]Category of cerebral palsy as diagnosed by examining physician.
[b]Includes cases of ataxic cerebral palsy.

TABLE 6.11 Incidence of Abnormalities of Pregnancy and Delivery in Patients with Hemiparetic Cerebral Palsy

Abnormality	Number of Patients
Pregnancy	5
Delivery	20
Neither	27
Total	52

From Cohen ME, Duffner PK. Prognostic indicators in hemiparetic cerebral palsy. *Ann Neurol* 1981;9:353. With permission.

have spastic quadriparesis on careful examination of the upper extremities. A number of authors have distinguished an ataxic form of cerebral palsy (239,240). In Skatvedt's series, published in 1958, this condition accounted for approximately 7% of children with cerebral palsy (240). Subsequent series do not distinguish this form of cerebral palsy. In most instances, neuropathologic studies on patients with cerebellar signs have revealed malformations of the cerebellum, often accompanied by even more conspicuous malformations of the cerebral hemispheres (151,152,157). Conversely, most patients with histologically verified lesions of the cerebellum attributable to perinatal trauma or asphyxia did not show cerebellar signs during their lifetime (139). Although Crothers and Paine (231) distinguished a condition termed *spastic monoplegia* (Table 6.11), this entity is probably rare. Most children fitting this designation have spastic hemiparesis revealed on subsequent examinations (231).

Spastic Quadriparesis

The category spastic quadriparesis includes a group of children whose appearance corresponds to the description of spastic rigidity as given by Little (2) and contains some of the most severely damaged patients. *Quadriplegia* is a poor term grammatically because it links a Latin prefix with a Greek root, but it is deeply entrenched in the literature and tradition. In the Northern California series, spastic quadriparesis accounted for 22% of all children with cerebral palsy who were examined (250). This form of cerebral palsy was seen in 6% of Swedish children with cerebral palsy (31a).

Although a mixed etiology exists for this form of cerebral palsy, abnormalities in delivery, particularly a prolonged second stage of labor, precipitate delivery, or fetal distress, are common causes. These abnormalities accounted for some 30% of cases in a 1989 Swedish series, whereas prenatal factors were thought to be responsible for 55% (251). In the Australian series, intrapartum events were believed to be responsible in some 20% of children. It was higher in those children who had an associated athetosis (252).

In his classic pathologic studies, Benda noted the frequent occurrence of an extensive cystic degeneration of the brain (multicystic encephalomalacia, polyporencephaly) (see Fig. 6.4) (253). Other cerebral abnormalities included destructive cortical and subcortical lesions, PVL, and a variety of developmental malformations or residua of intrauterine infections.

Neuroimaging studies support the clinical and pathologic impressions of a multiplicity of causes for this form of cerebral palsy. MRI studies on term infants with spastic quadriparesis demonstrate a mixture of multicystic encephalomalacia, parasagittal cortical lesions, and a variety of developmental abnormalities such as polymicrogyria and schizencephaly. It is of note that in a series of 26 term infants with spastic quadriparesis subjected to MRI, 12 (46%) demonstrated PVL (254). In term infants with spastic quadriparesis who suffered perinatal asphyxia, parasagittal cortical lesions, multicystic encephalomalacia, and basal ganglia lesions were the most common lesions (254). Several other studies as well as our own clinical experience corroborate these findings (31a,255).

Patients with spastic quadriparesis demonstrate a generalized increase in muscle tone and rigidity of the limbs on both flexion and extension. In the experience of one of us (J.H.M.), the right side is more severely affected in the majority of children. In the most extreme form of spastic quadriparesis, the child is stiff and assumes a posture of decerebrate rigidity. Generally, impairment of motor function is more severe in the upper extremities. Few voluntary movements are present, and vasomotor changes in the extremities are common. Most children have pseudobulbar signs, with difficulties in swallowing and recurrent aspiration of food material. Optic atrophy and grand mal seizures are noted in approximately one-half of patients (239).

Intellectual impairment is severe in nearly all instances, and no child in Ingram's series was considered to be educable (239).

Spastic Diplegia

As defined by Freud, who coined the term *diplegia*, this condition is characterized by bilateral spasticity, with greater involvement of the legs than arms (256). Although the term *diplegia* inaccurately describes the clinical findings, we continue to use it for the sake of convenience. In the experience of Ford, spastic diplegia was the most common form of cerebral palsy encountered at Johns Hopkins Hospital (257). As is evident from Table 6.10, the incidence of spastic diplegia increased between the 1950s and the 1990s. In Sweden, this form of cerebral palsy accounts for 25% of cerebral palsy in term infants, 83% in infants with a gestational age of less than 28 weeks, 76% in infants with a gestational age of 28 to 31 weeks, and 56% in infants with a gestational age of 32 to 36 weeks (31a). The experience in Northern California is somewhat similar. Spastic diplegia is seen in 48% of those with birth weights less

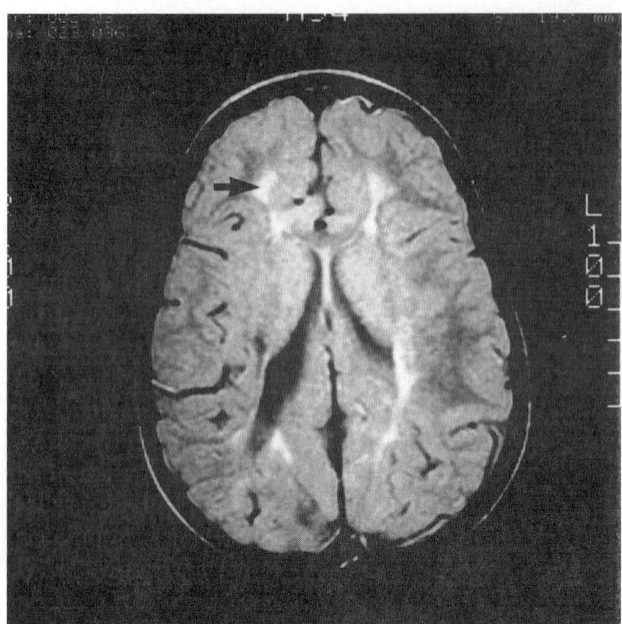

FIGURE 6.21. Magnetic resonance imaging of spastic diplegia. Axial T2-weighted images show marked widening of occipital horns and markedly reduced occipitoparietal white matter, which is nearly absent on the right. Increased signal is seen in a periventricular distribution, particularly at the tips of the frontal horns (*arrow*), and in the occipital white matter. On sagittal views the corpus callosum was markedly thinned. This 7-year-old girl was the product of a 27-week twin pregnancy, with a birth weight of 1,022 g. Neonatal course was complicated by respiratory distress syndrome, which required ventilation for the first 2 months of life, and sepsis. The child now shows spastic quadriparesis that is more marked in the lower extremities, a seizure disorder, and severe mental retardation. The other twin died of sepsis during the first month of life.

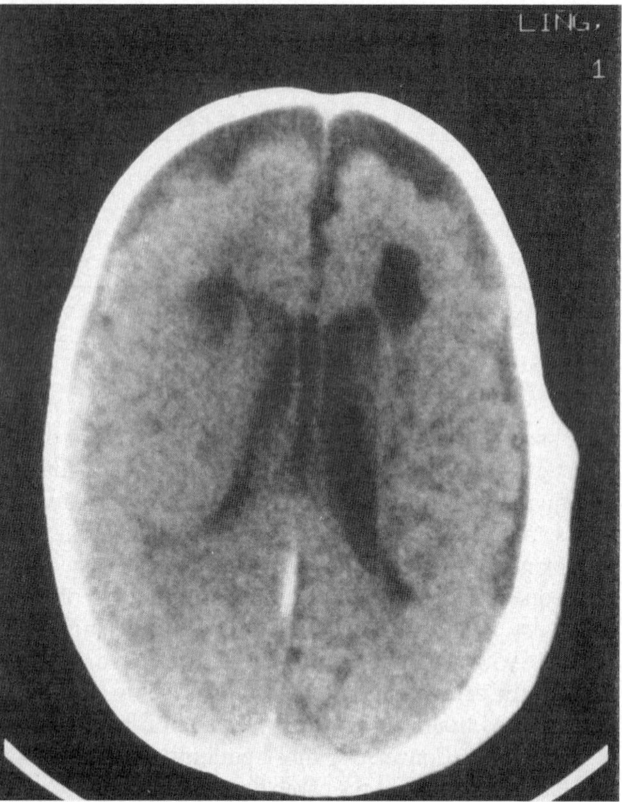

FIGURE 6.22. Axial CT of a 4-month-old boy, born at 32 weeks' gestation, with bilateral cystic infarcts of the periventricular white matter at the angles of the frontal horns of the lateral ventricles. Low-density lesions extend posteriorly from these cysts in the periventricular region as *periventricular leukomalacia*. A smaller cystic infarct is seen at the angle of the right occipital horn as well. Patchy, small, low-density infarcts are seen throughout the subcortical white matter.

than 1,500 g, as contrasted with an incidence of 23% in children with cerebral palsy with birth weights of 1,500 to 2,499 g and 28% of those with birth weights greater than 2,500 g (250). In other studies, the frequency of prematurity is equally striking. In the classic series of Ingram, 44% of children with spastic diplegia had a birth weight of 2,500 g or less (239).

Full-term and premature infants appear to differ with respect to the cause of this condition as determined by pathologic examination or neuroimaging studies. In premature infants, the most common finding is PVL. It was present in nearly all premature infants with spastic diplegia subjected to MRI (254,255,258). Most commonly, periventricular high-intensity areas are seen on T2-weighted images (Fig. 6.21). These are most marked in the white matter adjacent to the trigones and the bodies of the ventricles, and at times can be asymmetric. Additionally, a marked loss of periventricular white matter is seen; it is most striking in the trigonal region with compensatory ventricular dilatation (259). Cystic lesions at the angles of the frontal horns are characteristic (Fig. 6.22). The distribution of the periventricular high-intensity areas corresponds to the anatomic distribution of PVL. The location of the white matter lesions produces an interruption of the downward course of the pyramidal fibers from the cortical leg area as they traverse the internal capsule, which explains the predominant involvement of the lower extremities. Lesions of the internal capsule and the thalamus also are noted on MRI. These usually are seen in the more severely affected children (260). Yokochi observed a paroxysmal downward deviation of the eyes in a large proportion of children with thalamic lesions (260).

In term infants with spastic diplegia, PVL as well as cortical abnormalities, porencephaly, and various congenital malformations of the gyri such as micropolygyria also have been seen (139) (see Chapter 5).

The most striking physical finding in children with spastic diplegia is the increased muscle tone in the lower extremities. The severity of the spasticity varies from case to case. In the most involved patients, Ingram was able to distinguish a state in which rigidity predominates and the limbs tend to be maintained in extension (239). Thus, when a child is held vertically, the rigidity of the lower extremities becomes most evident, whereas the adductor spasm of the hips maintains the lower extremities in a scissored position (see Fig. I.6).

This stage is succeeded by the spastic phase, when flexion of the hips, knees, and, to a lesser extent, elbows becomes predominant. When the diplegia is less severe, patients show only impaired dorsiflexion of the feet, with increased tone at the ankles, which causes them to walk with the feet in the equinus position (toe walking). In such instances, the tone in the upper extremities is often normal to passive movement, but the child maintains the elbows flexed when walking (teddy-bear gait). Toe walking is not always due to cerebral palsy. Other causes include various myopathies and neuropathies and spinal dysraphism; most commonly, toe walking is habitual, and some of these individuals have a short Achilles tendon. The differential diagnosis of toe walking is reviewed by Sala and coworkers (261).

In other instances, spasticity of the lower extremities is accompanied by impaired coordination of fine and rapid finger movements and by a slight weakness of the wrist extensors. Sensory impairment is rare. The deep tendon reflexes are hyperactive in all extremities, unless muscular rigidity makes them difficult to elicit. An ankle clonus and an extensor plantar response usually can be obtained. Dystonia, athetosis, and mixed types of involuntary movements occasionally are seen in more severe cases and can interfere considerably with muscular control.

After a variable period, usually more than 2 years, contractures appear. These tend to be more severe in the distal musculature, particularly at the ankles. As a consequence, feet tend to become fixed in plantar flexion, knees in flexion, and hips in flexion and adduction. Vasomotor changes and dwarfing of the pelvis and lower extremities are often striking and, in general, parallel the severity of the paresis. Optic atrophy, field defects, and involvement of the cranial nerves are relatively rare. A convergent strabismus is common, however, and was seen in 43% of Ingram's diplegic patients (239). Of the children in Ingram's series, 44% had a speech defect; most often, this was a matter of retarded speech development and an inability to pronounce consonants.

Seizures are a common accompaniment of spastic diplegia and were seen in 27% in Ingram's series (239) and in 16% of the patients reported by Veelken and colleagues (262). Most often these are grand mal seizures, and their incidence is unrelated to the severity of the motor handicap, although the presence of minor motor seizures is usually limited to patients with significant involvement of the upper extremities.

As a rule, the more severe the motor deficit, the more severe is the retardation in the patient. Of 29 children with little impairment of the upper extremities (spastic paraplegia), 6 had IQs above 100, but all of 27 children with major involvement of the upper extremities had an IQ below 100 (239). In the more recent series of Olsén and coworkers, 25% of infants with birth weights less than 1,750 g who had minor neurodevelopmental dysfunction at 8 years of age demonstrated PVL. Furthermore, 25% neurologically and developmentally normal ex-premature infants also demonstrated PVL that was generally considered mild (258). The majority of preterm infants with MRI changes indicative of PVL tend to have visual motor and visuoperceptual deficits (263), although a significant proportion have grossly normal intelligence (254).

The cognitive functions of premature infants are covered in the Prematurity with Neurologic Complications section later in this chapter.

Spastic Hemiparesis

Spastic hemiparesis is characterized by a unilateral paresis that nearly always affects the upper extremity to a greater extent than the lower and ultimately is associated with some spasticity and flexion contractures of the affected limbs. Its incidence ranges from 0.41 to 0.79 per 1,000 live births (264), and it accounted for 19% of children with cerebral palsy in the series of Grether and coworkers (250). In the Swedish series of Hagberg and coworkers, spastic hemiparesis accounted for 44% of term infants with cerebral palsy and 9% of cerebral palsy in infants with a gestational age of less than 28 weeks, 10% in infants with a gestational age of 28 to 31 weeks, and 32% in infants with a gestational age of 32 to 36 weeks (31a).

The correlation of congenital hemiparesis with cerebral abnormalities was established by Cazauvielh in 1827 (2a); an antecedent history of abnormalities of labor and delivery was proposed by McNutt (265), Freud and Rie (266), and Ford (267). Since then it has become clear that the pathogenesis is multifactorial and that both morphogenetic and clastic lesions are responsible, with the relatively low incidence of abnormalities of pregnancy and delivery in this form of cerebral palsy being quite striking (Table 6.11). In the series of 91 cases reported by Cioni and coworkers, first-trimester lesions were seen in 14% of cases. These included focal cortical dysplasias, migration disorders, and schizencephaly (264). Other causes for hemiparesis include pachygyria and unilateral hemimegalencephaly (268,269). On the basis of fetal ultrasound studies coupled with pathologic examination of the brain, Larroche postulated that intrauterine arterial ischemic lesions are a frequent cause for congenital hemiparesis. These can be induced by maternal hemodynamic disturbances, emboli arising from the placenta, anomalies in the fetal circulation, or, in twin pregnancies, from the fetal transfusion syndrome (270). The role of these various intrauterine insults in the pathogenesis of hemiparetic cerebral palsy also was stressed by Nelson (271).

Third-trimester lesions were seen in 45% of patients in the series of Cioni and coworkers (264). These were mainly periventricular white matter lesions resulting from periventricular leukodystrophy. In a large proportion of patients in this group, the lesions were bilateral, and 58% of these patients were born preterm. Periventricular venous infarctions have also been reported. These are due to venous ischemia caused by impaired drainage of veins that drain blood from periventricular white matter (272). Perinatal lesions were seen in 30% of cases. These mainly involved an infarction of a major artery, usually the main branch or a cortical branch of the middle cerebral artery (264).

As implied from these clinical and neuroimaging data, the pathologic picture in congenital hemiparesis is varied. Benda emphasized the frequency with which mantle sclerosis (ulegyria) can be found (253) (see Fig. 6.11), but a number of other abnormalities of the cerebral hemispheres also are encountered. These are often bilateral (255).

As already noted, of the various unilateral lesions seen in term infants with congenital hemiparesis, vascular infarcts are prominent. These are usually seen in the territory of the middle cerebral artery, with the left artery being more frequently affected than the right (273). As a rule, middle cerebral artery infarctions are more commonly seen in infants older than 37 weeks' gestation (273,274). A variety of causes have been implicated in the focal infarction. These include perinatal asphyxia, thromboembolism, polycythemia, dehydration, cocaine abuse, extracorporeal membrane oxygenation, and a coagulopathy, notably a mutation in factor V Leiden (273,275).

For unknown reasons, the hemiparesis is only rarely documented at birth, although some subsequently hemiparetic infants present with focal seizures during the first few days of life (276). As already stated in the section that deals with the evolution of motor patterns, even the most careful neurologic examination frequently does not detect the hemiparesis for several months (236). The right side is more commonly affected. The incidence of right-sided involvement in three major series is 55% (277), 59% (239), and 66% (231).

The evolution of the hemiparesis from its appearance in the neonate to the spasticity seen in the older child was traced by Byers (278). In older children, the extent of impaired voluntary function varies considerably from one patient to another. In the series of Cioni and coworkers, 54% of patients whose hemiparesis resulted from first-trimester insults and 70% of patients who experienced a perinatal insult were more affected in their upper limb. This contrasted with the group that experienced a third-trimester insult, in whom the lower extremity was more affected in 54% (264). The reorganizational potential of the brain after the various lesions that cause hemiparesis has been studied by means of transcranial magnetic stimulation and functional magnetic resonance imaging during hand movements (278a). As a rule, the earlier the lesion is acquired, the better the prognosis with respect to hand movements, and the efficacy of sensorimotor reorganization decreases markedly towards the end of gestation. When a lesion destroys the normal contralateral corticospinal control over the paretic hand, the contralesional hemisphere develops ipsilateral corticospinal tracts to the paretic hand. These ipsilateral corticospinal tracts can mediate a useful hand function, but normal hand function is only possible when crossed corticospinal tracts are preserved.

In the upper extremity, fine movements of the hand are generally the most affected, notably the pincer grasp of thumb and forefinger, extension of the wrist, and supination of the forearm. Proximal muscle power is well preserved, and function in the upper extremity relates to speed of movement and power in the distal musculature. In the lower extremity, dorsiflexion and eversion of the foot are impaired most frequently, with power in the proximal muscles being preserved. Increased flexor tone is invariable, leading to a hemiparetic posture, with flexion at the elbow, wrist, and knees and an equinus position of the foot. Despite these abnormalities, most children with pure hemiparetic cerebral palsy walk by 20 months of age (279). Deep tendon reflexes are increased, and Babinski and, less often Hoffmann, reflexes can be elicited. In most children, the palmar grasp reflex persists for many years.

A large proportion of hemiparetic children have involuntary movements of the affected limbs. Goutières and coworkers found dystonia in 12% and choreoathetosis in 9% of hemiparetic children (280). These disorders are seen most clearly in the hand, where the patient demonstrates an avoidance response and athetotic posturing of the hand, producing overextension of the fingers and occasionally of the wrist as the child attempts to hold an object (281). This type of posture is similar to that of patients with parietal lobe lesions. Just as the grasp reflex in frontal lobe lesions reflects unopposed parietal lobe activity, this avoidance response reflects the unopposed frontal lobe activity (282). The affected side of the brain also participates in overflow movements, which are involuntary changes in position of the affected side associated with voluntary movements of the unaffected side. Before 10 years of age these movements are more evident in the unaffected hand; thereafter, they occur in both affected and unaffected hands (283). These changes are believed to reflect callosal inhibition of the uncrossed motor pathways and the organizational changes of the pyramidal motor system (284) and Staudt and coworkers have found that mirror movements in the paretic hand during voluntary movements of the nonparetic hand indicate the presence of ipsilateral corticospinal tract enervation of the paretic hand (278a).

Sensory abnormalities of the affected limbs are common and were documented by Tizard and associates in 68% of patients with hemiparesis (285). Stereognosis is impaired most frequently; less often, two-point discrimination and position sense is defective. In addition to sensory impairment, frequently a neglect and unawareness of the affected side deficits aggravates considerably the handicap induced by the hemiparesis. In general, the severity of the sensory defect does not correlate with the severity of the hemiparesis.

Growth disturbances of the affected limbs are extremely common and, like the sensory defects, probably reflect damage to the parietal lobes. Failure of growth, most evident in the upper extremities and particularly in the terminal phalanges and in the size of the nail beds, is a result of underdevelopment of muscle and bone. Growth arrest is not always accompanied by sensory changes.

Between 17% and 27% of hemiparetic patients have homonymous hemianopia. When adequate testing of the visual fields is possible, sparing of the macula can often be demonstrated (231). Abnormalities in cranial nerve function are frequent and usually the result of a supranuclear involvement of the muscles enervated by the lower cranial nerves. Facial weakness is probably the most common abnormality, being noted in approximately three-fourths of the patients (239,278). Deviation of the tongue and convergent strabismus are seen less often.

More than one-half of hemiparetic patients develop seizures, with the actual incidence probably being a function of the duration of follow-up (278,283,286). In 52%, seizures first appear before 18 months of age, and only 8% of hemiparetic children suffer their first attack after age 10 years. For those who had experienced seizures during the neonatal period, the likelihood of recurrence is high, being 100% in the series of Cohen and Duffner (283).

Seizures are usually in the form of major or focal motor attacks. A considerable proportion of children who for months or even years have only focal seizures can develop generalized convulsions (267). As a rule, anticonvulsant therapy is effective in reducing the frequency of attacks, but only a small proportion of children have remission of seizures for longer than 2 years. In these patients, anticonvulsant withdrawal after 2 seizure-free years results in a high rate of relapse, 62% in the series of Delgado and coworkers (286). We would be most reluctant to ever discontinue anticonvulsant therapy in a seizure-free child with hemiparetic cerebral palsy. In a small group of seizure patients, attacks persist despite medication. These patients should be considered for surgical removal of the portion of the cerebral cortex from which the seizure originates or for hemispherectomy, should there be more than one focus. The presurgical evaluation of such a patient is covered in Chapter 14.

The EEG and neuroimaging studies are of considerable prognostic value for a patient with hemiparetic cerebral palsy. A paroxysmal EEG almost invariably indicates the presence of a seizure disorder. Approximately one-half of hemiparetic children have average IQs, and 18% score above 100 (245). In the series of Cioni and coworkers mental retardation was documented in 30% of hemiparetic patients who sustained a first-trimester insult and in 18% of patients with a perinatal injury (264). Nearly all of hemiparetic patients are educationally competitive and ultimately become at least partially independent economically (287). Neither the IQ nor the type of deficit, be it delayed language development or perceptual handicaps, depends on which hemisphere has sustained the major damage or the extent of structural damage, a reflection on hemispheric equipotentiality in the small infant. Neither is there a consistent relationship between the extent of the lesion, the severity of the hemiparesis, and the functional outcome (274). In our opinion, other developmental malformations of the brain undetectable by imaging studies probably determine the ultimate outcome.

Extrapyramidal Cerebral Palsies

Extrapyramidal cerebral palsies are characterized by the predominant presence of a variety of abnormal motor patterns and postures secondary to a defective regulation of muscle tone and coordination (288–290). Spasticity frequently accompanies the involuntary movements, and primitive reflex patterns can often be demonstrated.

This form of cerebral palsy is considered to be the result of damage to the extrapyramidal system. In contrast to spastic hemiparesis, whose cause is manifold, it appears to be caused by several fairly well-delineated insults acting singly, successively, or in concert. In the series reported from Hagberg's unit, 58% of children with extrapyramidal cerebral palsy had experienced perinatal asphyxia. A further 34% were of low birth weight, and many of these were small for gestational age, with placental infarction and maternal toxemia being the most frequent prenatal risk factors (291). Kyllerman's group, studying a different Swedish population, came to similar conclusions (292,293). They distinguished two groups of extrapyramidal cerebral palsies: the hyperkinetic form, characterized by choreiform and choreoathetoid movements, and the more severely involved dystonic form, characterized by abnormal postures. The hyperkinetic group consisted of premature infants with asphyxia and hyperbilirubinemia; the dystonic group consisted of small-for-gestational-age infants who experienced asphyxia in the perinatal period or during the last trimester of their gestations. When extrapyramidal cerebral palsy affects term infants who are appropriate for gestational age, the characteristic antecedent event is a severe but brief hypoxic stress late in labor, with a relatively mild degree of subsequent HIE (294).

An extrapyramidal syndrome caused exclusively by kernicterus was not encountered in the large series of dyskinetic children reported in 1975 by Hagberg and colleagues (291). Kernicterus is discussed more fully in Chapter 10.

The clinical picture of extrapyramidal cerebral palsy evolves gradually from diffuse hypotonia with lively reflexes in infancy to choreoathetosis during childhood (295).

The onset of choreoathetosis usually occurs between the second and third years of life (see Table 6.9), with the most severely affected children continuing to manifest hypotonia for the longest time (221). Bobath observed that hypotonic infants destined to develop extrapyramidal movements demonstrate a head lag when pulled into the sitting position. However, when pushed into the sitting position, their arms and shoulders press back. This resistance persists when the infant's body is pushed forward into flexion (296). One of us (J.H.M.) termed this phenomenon the *Bobath response*. The onset of involuntary movements, almost invariably in the form of generalized or focal dystonia, can occur as late as the third decade of life (297). This delay in the clinical expression of a static cerebral lesion probably reflects changes with maturation in function and distribution of the various neurotransmitters.

A syndrome of transient dystonia characterized by hyperextension of the neck, hyperpronation of the forearm, and palmar transient flexion of the wrists has been reported (298). We have seen such children; as a rule, the dystonia subsides before the third year of life.

In the final stage of dyskinesia, a number of involuntary movements are recognized. Although collectively these have been termed *choreoathetosis*, the clinical picture is more complex. In most patients, a variety of involuntary movements, appearing discretely or in transitional forms, can be recognized. Their appearance and definition are discussed in the Introduction chapter. These various dyskinesias combine with spasticity, which is seen in a large proportion of children, to interfere markedly with all types of voluntary movements.

Development of motor function is usually far more delayed than would be expected from the child's intelligence. Approximately one-half walk before the fourth year. In Ingram's series, the average age at which children walked unsupported was 2 years and 5 months (239). The delay in gait correlates well with delays in the other motor milestones. Crothers and Paine showed that persistence of the obligatory tonic neck reflex (see Introduction chapter, Fig. I.5) suggests a bad prognosis in terms of the ability to walk without assistance and, to a lesser extent, the severity of athetosis (231). In their experience, walking is highly improbable as long as an obligatory tonic neck response can be elicited. Correlation of obligatory tonic neck response with intelligence was not uniform, and the persistence of the reflex does not necessarily indicate intellectual incompetence.

Skilled hand movements, such as those required for self-feeding, dressing, and writing, are equally impaired, and the disability in hand function can be severe enough to render a child virtually helpless. An occasional patient learns to perform these movements with the mouth or feet. Speech defects occur frequently in children with extrapyramidal cerebral palsy. In many, development of speech is retarded because of the uncoordinated movements of lips, tongue, palate, and respiratory muscles. In approximately two-thirds of children, incoordination of the muscles of respiration and speech is responsible for delayed speech (240); however, approximately one-half of patients begin to say intelligible words before 2 years of age (231), and almost all children who do not exhibit severe retardation are able to speak by 4 years of age.

A number of patients with moderately severe dyskinesia have impaired swallowing and control of saliva; drooling can persist for as long as 6 years of age. Cranial nerve involvement is less common than in the other forms of cerebral palsy. Strabismus is seen in approximately one-third of patients, however, and one-third have nystagmus (239). Seizures are encountered in approximately 25% to 40% of patients (246,299). Optic atrophy is rare. A sensorineural hearing loss can be documented in approximately one-half of children whose intelligence level permits adequate testing (292).

In a considerable proportion of children with extrapyramidal involvement, delayed language skills and gross motor handicaps can cause an erroneous underestimation of intelligence (Table 6.12) (231). In the experience of Crothers and Paine, 65% had IQs over 70 and 45% had IQs of 90 or better (231). The series of Kyllerman and associates, compiled in 1982, indicated that 78% of

TABLE 6.12 Validity of Early Estimate of Intelligence in Two Types of Cerebral Palsy

	Original Estimate		*Estimate at Follow-Up*		
Type of Cerebral Palsy	***Range***	***Number of Patients***	***Same***	***Higher***	***Lower***
Hemiplegia	Superior	4	2	—	2
	Average	17	13	1	3
	Below average	19	11	1	7
	Inadequate or defective	27	25	2	—
Extrapyramidal	Superior	5	5	—	0
	Average	13	10	0	3
	Below average	6	6	0	0
	Inadequate or defective	27	16	11	—

From Crothers B, Paine RS. *The natural history of cerebral palsy.* Cambridge, MA: Harvard University Press, 1959. With permission.

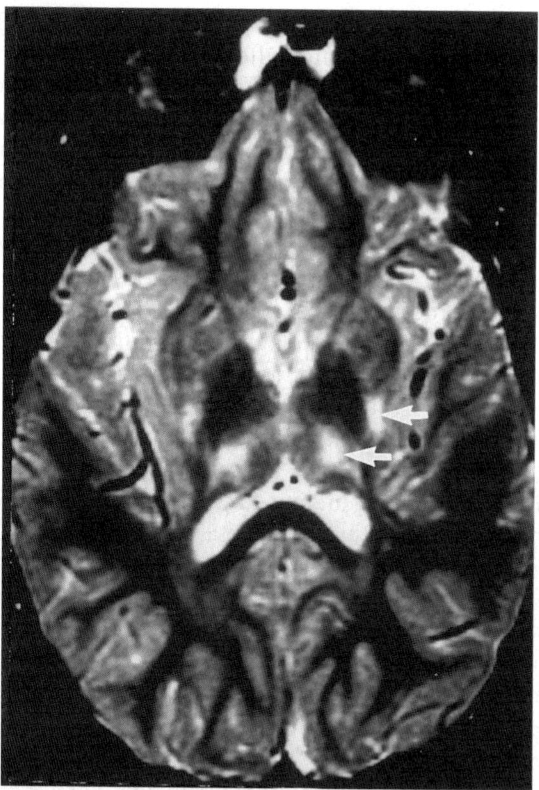

FIGURE 6.23. Axial T2-weighted image (3,000/150/1) illustrating bilateral symmetric focal hyperintensities in the posterior putamen and the ventrolateral nucleus of the thalamus (*arrows*). The patient was a 6 1/2-year-old boy who experienced severe shoulder dystocia. Birth weight was 4,230 g. Apgar scores were 1 and 0 at 1 and 5 minutes, respectively. Arterial pH was 6.84 at 4 hours and 20 minutes of age. The child demonstrated a mixed, but mainly extrapyramidal, form of cerebral palsy. He had low-normal intelligence.

children with the choreoathetotic movement disorder demonstrated IQs of 90 or higher (293). Children with the dystonic form of cerebral palsy do not fare as well. A large proportion of children with normal or near-normal intelligence, however, have an educational disability sufficiently severe to require their attendance at special schools.

On MRI, we have found a uniform picture of bilateral high-intensity signals in the anterior lateral thalamus, posterior thalamus, and posterior putamen in children with pure postasphyxial extrapyramidal cerebral palsy (146) (Fig. 6.23). The location of the changes corresponds with the location of glial scarring seen by Hayashi and colleagues in autopsied individuals who had experienced perinatal asphyxia (300). MRI abnormalities within the basal ganglia are seen in a variety of metabolic, genetic, and toxic disorders (301). These are summarized in Table 6.13.

Hypotonic (Atonic) Cerebral Palsy

Hypotonic (atonic) cerebral palsy, a relatively common condition, is characterized by generalized muscular hypotonia that persists beyond 2 to 3 years of age and that does not result from a primary disorder of muscle or peripheral nerve. Characteristically, the deep tendon reflexes are normal or even hyperactive, and the electrical reactions of muscle and nerve are normal. Over the years, more than one-half of these children develop frank cerebellar deficits with incoordination, ataxia, and impaired rapid succession movements. Another one-third have profound retardation; the remainder develop minimal cerebral dysfunction syndrome (302). Hypotonic cerebral palsy also can be a forerunner to extrapyramidal cerebral palsy, but in the majority of children, the involuntary movements are apparent before 3 years of age (see Table 6.9).

The cause of hypotonia in this form of cerebral palsy is still a matter of considerable speculation. In many instances, muscle biopsy discloses a pattern termed *fiber type disproportion*, in which the type 1 muscle fibers are significantly smaller than type 2 fibers. Additionally, the number of type 1 fibers often is increased. This pathologic picture is nonspecific and is a manifestation of a delay in muscle maturation (303). In the fetus, type 1 fibers, which are rich in oxidative enzymes, form only a small proportion of total muscle fibers, whereas the type 2 fibers, which are rich in glycolytic enzymes, are predominant at 25 weeks'

TABLE 6.13 Basal Ganglia Abnormalities on Magnetic Resonance Imaging in Children with Extrapyramidal Movement Disorders

Condition	*Caudate*	*Putamen*	*Globus Pallidus*	*Thalamus*
Perinatal asphyxia	+	+		+
Maple syrup disease	+	+		
Propionic acidemia	+	+		
Glutaric aciduria I	+	+		
Lesch-Nyhan disease	±			
Leigh syndrome	±	+	+	
Wilson disease	±	+		+
Methylmalonic acidemia		+	+	
Kernicterus			+	
Carbon monoxide			+	
3-Nitropropionic acid		+	+	

gestation, but not at term (303,304). Lesny suggested that the condition is a syndrome of extremely delayed brain development, with the generalized hypotonia representing the earliest sign of a cerebellar disorder (302). In the majority of his patients, prenatal factors, acting singly or in concert with other noxious influences, were presumably responsible. By contrast, perinatal asphyxia was believed responsible in less than 5% of children. Our own experiences are identical. We have found neuroimaging studies of little help in arriving at an anatomic diagnosis; some patients have a small cerebellum with a prominent fourth ventricle; a significant proportion of these children merely show ventriculomegaly and gyral atrophy (152).

Cerebellar Cerebral Palsy

A small number of children experience a static neurologic disorder in which cerebellar signs predominate. The majority of these have a developmental anomaly of the cerebellum. In others, generally children of normal intelligence, the symptoms appear to be the consequence of perinatal trauma or perinatal asphyxia.

Mixed Forms of Cerebral Palsy

In the experience of most physicians, a considerable proportion of children with cerebral palsy exhibit a mixture of spasticity and extrapyramidal movements (see Table 6.10). This combination can be manifested by minor amounts of athetotic posturing, as observed in a high percentage of children with spastic hemiparesis, or by the presence of extensor plantar responses in patients with predominantly extrapyramidal disease. When the mixed form is most obvious, the clinical picture is one of hyperreflexia, spasticity, and contractures in a child with frank dystonia or other extrapyramidal movements.

Diagnosis

The diagnosis of a neurologic disorder incurred in a term infant that has resulted from perinatal asphyxia is surrounded by much discussion and controversy. The issue was reviewed from a predominantly obstetric point of view by MacLennan, heading an International Cerebral Palsy Task Force (305). The conclusions of the task force evoked criticisms from pediatric neurologists, neonatologists, and others (306,307). From our point of view, diagnosis of asphyxia of sufficient severity to induce a permanent neurologic disorder in a term infant is based on a history of intrauterine distress, a history of an abnormal neonatal course, and laboratory studies and/or imaging studies that point to perinatal asphyxia.

Prenatal and Intrauterine Factors

Evidence of intrauterine distress includes an alteration of fetal heart rate pattern, the passage of meconium, and abnormalities in fetal acid–base status as determined by scalp or cord blood sampling. Although beat-to-beat variability and deceleration beginning after the start of a contraction and peaking well after the peak of the uterine contraction (late decelerations) are ominous in terms of fetal well-being, they do not seem to predict ultimate neurologic or intellectual deficits (308). In the experience of Valentin and coworkers, infants who demonstrated a pattern of reduced variability, reduced variability with late decelerations, or bradycardia with late decelerations had the most abnormal cord arterial pHs (309) and would therefore be at greatest risk for neurologic abnormalities. However, Nelson and coworkers in a retrospective study found that 37% of children with cerebral palsy showed none of the risk factors on prenatal fetal heart monitoring (310). In view of the heterogeneity of the cerebral palsy population this is not a surprising finding. Passage of large amounts of meconium after rupture of the fetal membranes also correlates with the subsequent presence of neurologic deficits (311). However, infants with developmental abnormalities as well as those who have sustained neurologic injuries before the onset of labor are likely to demonstrate abnormal fetal heart rate patterns during labor (308). Mothers of infants whose neurologic handicaps were secondary to cerebral malformations have a statistically higher incidence of vaginal bleeding during pregnancy and a suggestively higher incidence of prenatal infections. Additionally, a breech presentation and the application of midforceps are significantly associated with both mechanical and asphyxial birth injury.

The relationship between arterial cord blood values and ultimate neurologic deficits has been the subject of several investigations. Infants with a complicated neonatal course tend to have a lower cord arterial pH and a significantly greater mean base deficit than those with an uncomplicated neonatal course (312,313). However, fewer than one-half of infants with an arterial cord pH of 7.00 or less have neonatal complications (314), and, conversly, infants born with acute birth asphyxia do not invariably demonstrate umbilical artery acidemia at birth (315). Hermansen pointed out that an infant may produce acid in the tissues without developing acidemia, with different mechanisms being responsible for a lack of acidosis in the presence of acidemia. Thus in the presence of complete circulatory arrest, acid may accumulate in fetal tissues but not enter the bloodstream until after resuscitation and after circulation has been restored (315). Concomitant hypoglycemia could result in an inability to produce lactate. Because lactate is a crucial energy substrate in the brain during recovery from ischemia, a reduction in lactate would put the neonate at an increased risk for neurologic damage (316,317). Sehdev and coworkers found the combined presence of a high arterial base deficit and a low 5-minute Apgar score to be good predictors for neonatal morbidity (314). An arteriovenous pCO_2 difference of greater than 25 torr has been found to be a highly specific parameter for identifying asphyxiated infants who go on to develop HIE (318). Hypoglycemia (blood sugar of less than 40 mg/dL on the initial specimen) is another important risk factor for perinatal brain injury, particularly in infants who require resuscitation and have severe fetal acidemia (318a).

An infant small for gestational age (SGA) (i.e., one whose birth weight is more than two standard deviations below the mean for any given week of gestation) is at an increased risk for perinatal asphyxia, the meconium aspiration syndrome, hypoglycemia, and the complications of polycythemia. In a survey of children with spastic cerebral palsy, 30.4% were below the 10th percentile for birth weight and 15.5% were below the 3rd percentile for birth weight. SGA infants between 34 and 37 weeks' gestational age were at highest risk of developing spastic cerebral palsy (319). Amiel-Tison and Pettigrew suggested that intrauterine growth retardation is an adaptive response to placental insufficiency and that as judged from their physical examinations and their brainstem-evoked responses, SGA infants are neurologically more mature than infants whose birth weights are appropriate for their gestational age (AGA) (320). Generally, the infant who is both underweight and short experienced an insult in early fetal life, whereas the infant who is underweight but of normal growth suffered an insult that was briefer and occurred later during gestation. Under both circumstances, brain growth, as inferred from head circumference, is less affected than body weight or length.

Whether SGA infants ultimately develop learning disorders and minor cognitive and behavioral abnormalities beyond those caused by socioeconomic factors has not been fully resolved. Long-term follow-up studies indicate that SGA infants have a slightly increased risk for developmental delay when compared to AGA infants (321). Although verbal IQ was not confounded by parental demographic and child-rearing factors, these variables accounted for much of the deficits in nonverbal IQ (322). Sommerfelt and coworkers found maternal smoking to be associated with birth of a SGA infant and a reduction of 5 points in performance IQ at 5 years of age (322). They were, however, unable to determine whether the effect of maternal smoking was due to maternal socioeconomic or child-rearing factors (322).

History of an Abnormal Neonatal Course

An abnormal neonatal course is the most important diagnostic feature of perinatal asphyxia that has been sufficiently severe to cause neurologic deficits. This includes delayed or impaired respiration requiring resuscitative measures such as endotracheal intubation and assisted ventilation. Additionally, depressed Apgar scores, particularly when the score is 3 or less for more than 10 minutes, correlate with subsequent development of neurologic complications, including neonatal seizures, and the ultimate evolution of cerebral palsy (227,314). It must be remembered, however, that a low Apgar score does not by itself indicate perinatal asphyxia because other causes, notably brain malformations, maternal drugs, or anesthesia, can be responsible for the low score (323). Watershed infarcts in the fetal brainstem can be expressed as failure of the central respiratory drive (324). Some of the other structural CNS lesions responsible for apnea at birth include a variety of CNS malformations and degenerative disorders (325). It therefore comes as no surprise that in the classic study of Sykes et al. published in 1982, 73% of neonates with severe acidosis had a 1-minute Apgar score of 7 or higher, and only 21% of infants with a 1-minute Apgar score of less than 7 had severe acidosis (224). Other studies confirm this work. Thus, Socol and coworkers found that 60% of infants with a 5-minute Apgar score of 3 or less had an umbilical artery pH of greater than 7.0 and 54% had an arterial pH of greater than 7.10 (312). The results of Goldenberg and colleagues are similar (225). Thus, neither scalp pH nor umbilical artery pH can provide more than inferential evidence for perinatal asphyxia and its severity.

Other abnormalities observed during the neonatal period include seizures, hypotonia, and a bulging fontanel; less obvious abnormalities are irritability, feeding difficulties, excessive jitters, or an abnormal cry. In addition, there may be clinical or laboratory evidence for asphyxial damage to organs other than the brain. The multiple-organ-dysfunction phenomenon is mechanistically related to the diving reflex. The reflex, activated by asphyxia, consists in shunting blood from the skin and splanchnic area to the heart, adrenals, and brain, ostensibly to protect these vital organs from hypoxic-ischemic injury (326). In the experience of Shah and coworkers all infants who had experienced asphyxial injury to the brain showed evidence of at least one organ dysfunction in addition to brain (327). Renal, cardiovascular, pulmonary, and hepatic dysfunction was present in 91 (70%), 80 (62%), 112 (86%), and 110 (85%) infants, respectively.

The infant whose birth was complicated but whose neonatal period was uneventful (i.e., activity after the first day of life was normal, incubator care was not required beyond 3 days of age, and the infant did not have feeding problems, impaired sucking, respiratory difficulties, or neonatal seizures) is not at increased risk for neurologic damage, and the absence of these symptoms and signs in a youngster who subsequently presents with cerebral palsy points to a cause other than intrapartum hypoxia (328).

Laboratory Studies Suggesting Perinatal Asphyxia

Increased amounts of nucleated red blood cells (nRBC) are frequently seen in the infant who presents with acute, subacute, or chronic asphyxia. However, despite previous reports to the contrary (329), there is a large overlap between nRBC values after acute and chronic asphyxia.

Furthermore, asphyxia of any duration dues not always cause an increased nRBC count, and extreme increases can be found without asphyxia (330).

Examination of the CSF can provide some evidence for perinatal asphyxia in that the concentration of CSF protein can be elevated after perinatal asphyxia. In the term neonate, the mean protein concentration is 90 mg/dL; values higher than 150 mg/dL are considered abnormal. In the premature neonate, the mean CSF protein is 115 mg/dL (331). The presence of blood from any source raises the total protein by 1.5 mg/dL of fluid for every 1,000 fresh red blood cells/μL (332). An elevation in the ratio of CSF lactate to pyruvate has been found to persist in asphyxiated infants for several hours after normal oxygenation has been reestablished (333), as does a striking elevation of blood creatine kinase-BB isozyme (334). A normal CSF does not exclude the possibility of perinatal asphyxia.

EEG has been used not only for the recognition of seizures, but also as a reliable predictor of neurodevelopmental outcome. In particular, the background activity recorded 72 hours after birth best predicts the outcome (335,336), whereas the prognostic significance of paroxysmal abnormalities is less certain (337). The amplitude-integrated EEG obtained 3 and 6 hours after birth is also a good predictor of outcome (338). All infants with a discontinuous EEG had an abnormal outcome, and those with an extremely discontinuous EEG or low voltage died or had severely abnormal outcome (338).

Several groups of French and Dutch workers have found the presence of positive rolandic sharp waves to be a specific and sensitive marker for PVL and white matter damage. In their experience EEG abnormalities can be detected before the appearance of ultrasound abnormalities of cystic PVL (339,340).

Neuroimaging studies are invaluable in diagnosing the presence and the extent of tissue damage in the asphyxiated neonate and in determining the extent of an intracranial hemorrhage. Ultrasonography scans are most commonly used. Their advantage is that examinations can be performed at the bedside and serially without harmful effects to the infant. In general, the brain is examined in two planes: coronal and sagittal. This technique provides excellent visualization of the ventricular system, basal ganglia, choroid plexus, and corpus callosum (204,341).

The location, extent, and course of an IVH can readily be followed by ultrasonography. IVHs produce strong echoes in the normally echo-free ventricles. Subependymal and intracerebral hemorrhages also are identified readily. Partridge and associates suggested that for their optimal detection, the scan be performed routinely at 4 to 7 days of age in all infants with birth weights less than 1,500 g (342). Follow-up scans for ventricular size should be done at 14 days of age and, in infants who demonstrate ventricular dilatation, at least weekly thereafter until ventricular size is stabilized, with a final examination being conducted at 3 months of age.

The various grades of IVHs are defined in Table 6.5. As already mentioned in the section that deals with intracranial hemorrhage, parenchymal hemorrhagic necrotic lesions, the so-called grade IV hemorrhage seen in 15% of infants with IVH, probably result from a clot-induced impairment of venous flow and consequent venous infarction of brain tissue rather than representing an extension of an IVH (211).

Ultrasonography also has been used to demonstrate PVL, which initially presents as persistent periventricular echodense areas, and as echolucent cystic areas after the second week of life. These lesions are seen most commonly near the lateral ventricles, in front of the anterior horns, in the corona radiata, or posterior to the occipital horns (343,344).

Ultrasonography is of somewhat more limited value in the evaluation of the asphyxiated neonate. In the hands of Eken and coworkers, the use of a high-resolution transducer led to the detection of echogenicity in the cortex, which correlated well with the location of pathologic changes on autopsy (345). Although ultrasonography is inferior to CT scans in revealing details of brain anatomy, the procedure can be used to detect porencephalic cysts and other major structural lesions of the cerebrum.

The CT scan has wide diagnostic application to the newborn with neurologic disease. It is useful in diagnosing not only an intracranial hemorrhage, but also a variety of congenital malformations. For the first 48 to 72 hours after an asphyxial insult, the CT is more sensitive than MRI in demonstrating cortical changes because on MRI the edematous cortex is isodense with white matter. CT scans performed on asphyxiated infants 1 to 2 weeks after birth demonstrate local areas of hyperperfusion, with a dense network of proliferating capillaries that almost completely replaces the parenchyma. This alteration is most often observed in the basal ganglia, but it also can occur in the brainstem and cerebellum, the periventricular area, the depth of the cortical sulci, and the hippocampus. The bright thalamus syndrome probably represents an example of hyperperfusion as documented by cranial ultrasound (346). Shewmon and coworkers considered this hypervascularity a response to the antecedent hypoxia and reduced cerebral blood flow (347).

Whereas certain pathologic appearances (e.g., hemorrhage) are readily interpreted, difficulties are encountered in the CT analysis of parenchymal changes. These difficulties occur because of the frequent presence of alternating areas of high and low densities within the cerebral substance that lack adult equivalents. Both gray and white matter, however, have lower attenuation coefficients in neonates than in older children, and the difference in density between gray and white matter is greater than that in adults. Sulci and subarachnoid spaces are often prominent and should not be interpreted as cerebral atrophy (348,349).

In the preterm infant, interpretation of the CT scan is further complicated by the poor visualization of the ventricular system owing to its small volume in relation to brain parenchyma. Localized areas of low density in the periventricular region and hypodense parenchymal areas have little significance. In most instances, these changes are transient and can reflect a developmental stage (350). In most instances ultrasound is more useful than CT in providing prognostic information in the preterm infant during the neonatal period.

In the clinically stable term infant MRI is the preferred neuroimaging study for delineating the extent and nature of asphyxial damage. Diffusion-weighted MRI, in which the image contrast depends on differences in the molecular motion of water, allows detection of changes within minutes of the injury and therefore much earlier than conventional MRI (351). FLAIR sequences are complementary to conventional MRI imaging in detecting early evidence of hypoxic-ischemic damage, but are not suitable for assessing myelination of the neonatal brain (352).

MRI performed within the first 10 days of life on asphyxiated infants demonstrates three patterns of damage (353,354). In term infants, abnormalities are most commonly confined to the thalamus and basal ganglia. Almost all of these infants suffered an acute profound asphyxial insult (146,354). Mercuri and coworkers noted that there was a better association between basal ganglia lesions and Apgar scores than with cord pH (355). In a second group, abnormalities are predominantly in the cerebral cortex and subcortical white matter. Periventricular white matter abnormalities are generally seen in preterm infants or in infants believed to have sustained *in utero* asphyxial damage before 34 to 35 weeks' gestation (296) (Fig. 6.21). In the series of Sie and coworkers 26% of infants who demonstrated PVL on MRI were born at term (354). In some infants, imaging discloses a mixed pattern of abnormalities (353). Brainstem and cerebellar abnormalities are less common (356). Contrast enhancement of abnormalities in the thalamus and basal ganglia, in particular, correlates with tissue necrosis, and thus predicts a poor outcome (357). Focal parenchymal hemorrhages, mainly in a parietal or parieto-occipital distribution, were common in the series of Keeney and coworkers (358). These were unilateral or bilateral and generally resolved to be replaced by atrophy, thinning of myelin, or hemosiderin deposition. Basal ganglia hemorrhage occurred in 5% of asphyxiated infants; it was seen in 63% of term infants who had developed an IVH (359). On follow-up MRI studies, basal ganglia hemorrhage can resolve or the hemorrhage can be replaced by cysts or a calcification. For reasons as yet unknown, calcification can appear as early as 2 weeks after the asphyxial insult (360).

MRI also assists in determining the extent and progress of myelination and can be used to follow the loss of water from white matter with maturation (361). When diffusion tensor magnetic resonance imaging is used, the abnormal postinjury white matter development seen on pathologic examination can be demonstrated (362,363). In preterm infants these abnormalities can persist for many years and generally involve the posterior portion of the corpus callosum and the anterior and posterior parts of the internal capsule. These changes are present even in the absence of any demonstrable periventricular leukodystrophy (364). In the normal newborn, white matter is lighter than gray matter when T2-weighted spin-echo pulse sequences are used (365,366). Areas of myelination are seen in the cerebellum and thalami, which, therefore, have a lower signal intensity. After perinatal asphyxia, there is a delay in myelination. This is best identified after 7 to 8 months of age. In the premature infant, PVL is accompanied by delayed myelination; IVH, as a rule, is not (367).

Positron emission tomography has been used to measure regional cerebral blood flow in infants who have sustained perinatal asphyxia. Discrepant results have been obtained. In the series of Lou and coworkers performed during the first few hours after birth, a low cerebral blood flow was associated with a poor outcome (368). Rosenbaum and coworkers, who performed the study during the first and second weeks of life, found that an abnormally high cerebral blood flow was followed by a poor outcome (369). The difference between the two studies probably reflects the timing of when these were performed. Because there is no definition of a threshold below which there is invariable brain damage, measurement of cerebral blood flow is of little clinical assistance.

Total and regional cerebral glucose metabolism have been measured by PET. When determined 4 to 24 days after birth the total cerebral metabolic rate for glucose decreased with increasing severity of hypoxic-ischemic encephalopathy. As was noted in normal infants, the deep subcortical parts, thalamus, basal ganglia, and sensorimotor cortex were the most metabolically active, with the total metabolic rate increasing with maturation (370). PET also has been used to study the functional anatomic correlations in children with long-standing cerebral palsy. In the latter group, abnormalities in glucose metabolism generally correspond to abnormalities of brain structure demonstrable by other neuroimaging studies, although metabolic impairment is usually more extensive than anatomic involvement (371).

Proton MR spectroscopy, which determines the relative amounts of various brain metabolites, is a noninvasive procedure that can provide information on the severity of asphyxial brain damage, its evolution, and, by inference, its prognosis. The physical and chemical principles that form the basis of this technique were presented by Novotny and colleagues (372). When infants subjected to perinatal asphyxia are studied, there is an initial increase in the concentration of inorganic phosphate and a reduction of phosphocreatine. The ratio of inorganic phosphate to phosphocreatine is a surrogate measure of adenosine diphosphate (ADP) concentration, which accumulates as adenosine triphosphate (ATP) concentration falls, and thus it reflects the phosphorylation potential within brain. After resuscitation these values normalize, but a second period of delayed energy failure begins 8 to 24 hours later. This period is marked by a second reduction of phosphorylation potential, an increase in lactate as is evidenced by the ratio of lactate to creatine and lactate to *N*-acetylaspartate (373), and the development of an alkaline intracellular pH (374). The magnitude of change appears to correlate with the severity of injury and the neurodevelopmental outcome at 1 year of age (373). When MR spectroscopy is performed 1 to 2 weeks after birth, the ratio of *N*-acetylaspartate to creatine is generally reduced and the lactate is normal. However, a persistent basal ganglia lactic alkalosis has been seen in some infants who had a poor outcome from their asphyxial injuries (374–376). The reason for persistently elevated basal ganglia lactate in infants with asphyxial damage is unclear (374,375,377). Robertson and coworkers postulated that brain alkalosis is induced by an altered buffering mechanism due to upregulation of the Na^+/H^+ transporter by focal areas of ischemia or by proinflammatory cytokines (374,378). Such brain alkalosis may be detrimental to cell survival and may increase the glycolytic rate in astrocytes, leading to an increased production of lactate (378,379).

On ^{31}P MR spectroscopy a reduction in the ratio of phosphocreatine MR signals to inorganic phosphate MR signals is considered an excellent indication of cerebral asphyxia, as is a decrease in brain intracellular pH (53,380). Techniques for spatial localization of these metabolic changes have been developed (381). These show that the metabolic derangement is most marked in the deeper layers of the cerebral cortex, an observation consistent with the known vulnerability of subcortical regions to hypoxic-ischemic injury (382).

Abnormalities in the brainstem auditory-evoked response and the visual-evoked response correlate well with the severity of the asphyxial insult. In infants who experienced perinatal asphyxia, the brainstem auditory-evoked response can be completely abolished or the interval between the auditory nerve action potential and the nerve action potential arising from the inferior colliculi can be prolonged (383). In the experience of Muttitt and her group, a visual-evoked response that is absent or remains abnormal throughout the first week of life invariably predicts an abnormal neurologic outcome (384).

Cerebral Doppler studies have been used in some centers to evaluate infants with perinatal asphyxia and intracranial hemorrhage. Technical aspects, methodology, and clinical applications of this technique are reviewed by Raju (385). Ilves and coworkers concluded that cerebral blood-flow velocities are of little predictive value when performed 2 to 6 hours after asphyxia. Studies conducted 12 hours after asphyxia showed infants with severe HIE to have increased cerebral blood flow velocities in the anterior, medial cerebral, and basilar arteries as compared to a control group (386).

In evaluating an older child with cerebral palsy, the best diagnostic tool is an MRI, which can demonstrate abnormalities of myelination, areas of atrophy, cystic degeneration, and any anomalies in cortical architecture. Other diagnostic studies, notably CT, are of less help.

Treatment

Perinatal Asphyxia and Its Complications

The prevention of perinatal trauma and asphyxia is largely the task of the obstetrician and is, therefore, outside the scope of this text. Treatment of the asphyxiated neonate is largely outside the domain of the neurologist who will be called on to assist in the management of cerebral edema and neonatal seizures.

Neither fluid restriction nor corticosteroids are effective in the management of postasphyxial cerebral edema. Mannitol will reduce brain edema but does not affect the clinical outcome. The value of hyperventilation or osmotic agents in improving the outcome of infants with cerebral edema is probably also minimal (223). Mild head cooling and mild systemic hypothermia have also been suggested for treating the infant with severe HIE (387). Although two small randomized, controlled trials demonstrated no evidence of harm, evidence is inadequate to assess its efficacy. The treatment of neonatal seizures is considered in Chapter 14.

Experimental work suggests that there is a therapeutic window of some 1 to 2 hours between the time an infant has been resuscitated successfully from perinatal asphyxia and the onset of the cascade of secondary changes that lead to apoptotic and necrotic neuronal death. Several pharmaceutical agents have been proposed that could intervene in the production of secondary brain injury.

N-methyl-D-aspartate (NMDA) antagonists, notably MK-801, have been found to protect the brain from experimentally induced asphyxial injuries, even when administered up to 1 hour after the insult. None of them has been used in the human neonate. Calcium-channel blockers, inhibitors of nitric oxide production, and oxygen-free radical inhibitors and scavengers such as allopurinol and indomethacin also have been suggested but have not received any clinical trials (388). Under experimental conditions, antisense oligodeoxynucleotides to one of the NMDA-receptor channel complexes inhibit synthesis of the protein component of the channel and selectively reduce the expression of NMDA receptors and the extent of focal ischemic infarctions. Although the use of antisense nucleotides represents a novel and exciting approach to the treatment of asphyxia, it has undergone no clinical trials (389).

Intraventricular Hemorrhage and Ventricular Enlargement

Several regimens have been suggested to prevent IVH or to reduce its severity. Antenatal administration of glucocorticoids, usually betamethasone or dexamethasone, clearly reduces the incidence of IVH in premature infants. Our nurseries at Cedars-Sinai Medical Center use prenatal treatment of the fetus with corticosteroids to prevent respiratory distress syndrome and thereby lessen the likelihood for IVH. Antenatal treatment with betamethasone is also associated with a decreased incidence of cystic PVL in very small premature infants (111).

Infants with birth weights lower than 1,250 g are given prophylactic indomethacin. Indomethacin (0.1 mg/kg) given at 6 to 12 hours and every 24 hours for two further doses lowered the incidence of the most extensive hemorrhages (grades III and IV) (390,391). Indomethacin reduces cerebral blood flow velocity and increases cerebral vascular resistance and thus attenuates the adaptive vasodilatory response to asphyxia (392). It also reduces the formation of free radicals and accelerates maturation of the microvasculature in the germinal matrix (393). Ethamsylate administration also is associated with a lowered incidence of IVH, particularly the more extensive hemorrhages (394).

We believe that maintaining a good airway with a good cardiovascular support system and trying to prevent excessive swings in blood pressure and cardiac output reduce the likelihood of a large IVH. Additionally, allowing the pCO_2 to increase, but maintaining it below 55 mm Hg, appears to reduce the incidence of pneumothorax, which contributes to the evolution of IVH. Such factors as hypoxemia, acidemia, and rapid volume expansion all can lead to extension of the hemorrhage and should therefore be avoided.

Other therapeutic modalities that have been investigated include the prenatal administration of phenobarbital, which in combination with vitamin K does not appear to reduce the incidence of severe IVH (395).

Vitamin E supplementation in preterm infants reduced the risk of IVH but increased the risk of sepsis. In very low birth weight infants it increased the risk of sepsis, and reduced the risk of severe retinopathy and blindness among those examined. This evidence does not support the routine use of vitamin E supplementation by intravenous route at high doses (396).

Antenatal treatment with magnesium has not resulted in a statistically significant reduction of IVH or cerebral palsies in very preterm births (397).

In treating progressive ventricular enlargement, many centers suggest that lumbar punctures should be performed first unless ultrasound or CT evidence exists of noncommunication between the ventricles and the spinal subarachnoid space. Acetazolamide or furosemide can be used as an adjunct to lumbar punctures. If these interventions fail to arrest the progressive ventricular enlargement, external ventricular drainage is indicated (398). A ventricular reservoir is inserted, and serial reservoir taps are performed until the ventricular fluid protein falls below 2,000 mg/dL and there has been no resolution of the hydrocephalus, as indicated by serial ultrasounds. At that time, a ventriculo-peritoneal shunt replaces the reservoir. Serial monitoring with ultrasonography is recommended in all infants who have had an IVH, whatever treatment has been adopted. Randomized, controlled trials have found that neither acetazolamide nor furosemide can control posthemorrhagic ventricular dilatation (399).

Only a small proportion of patients undergoing a shunting procedure become neurologically and developmentally healthy adults. Several studies have demonstrated that in these patients nonverbal skills are more impaired than verbal skills. The outlook for infants whose hydrocephalus responds to medical treatment with repeated lumbar punctures, osmotic diuretics, or acetazolamide is significantly better than it is for those who require a shunt (400). It is equally evident that the extent of parenchymal damage that attends IVH determines the ultimate prognosis (4,400).

Cerebral Palsy

The treatment of children with cerebral palsy has been the subject of innumerable publications, most of them surprisingly uncritical and devoid of controls. Although cerebral palsy is, by definition, a "static encephalopathy," the associated musculoskeletal pathology is progressive Tizard proposed that before treatment is initiated, the following points should be considered (401): (a) Does the child need treatment? (b) What are the aims of treatment? (c) Do the family and child have the time required for treatment? (d) Will treatment disrupt family life?

Various means are available for the treatment of spasticity, which represents the most important disorder of motor control in children with cerebral palsy (247). Management involves the use of a continuity of modalities, and most patients require a combination of modalities. Thus, Graham and coworkers found that the combination of physiotherapy and orthotics increased the benefits from intramuscular botulinum toxin (402).

Nonsurgical Therapy

Physiotherapy is the most traditional and principal nonsurgical form of treatment. Its aims are to prevent additional deformities and to promote functionally useful posture and movements. From the studies of Crothers and Paine (231) and Paine (403), it seems clear that to be most effective, the program must be determined by the nature of the handicap. Fixsen divided orthopedic management into two aspects: the management of the child who will ultimately become ambulatory and hat of the nonambulatory child (404).

Intensive physical therapy (1 hour a day, 5 days a week) has been considered to be helpful for children with spastic hemiparesis and spastic diplegia. If possible, effectiveness of management should be monitored by gait analysis (404). Most children with these forms of cerebral palsy require regular physiotherapy as soon as they begin to walk, with special attention to the presence of contractures in the lower extremity. There is little evidence-based data supporting the effectiveness of physiotherapy. In evaluating effectiveness of the physiotherapy for spastic children, Wright and Nicholson found no evidence that it improved the range of dorsiflexion of the ankle or abduction of the hip or that it affected the retention or loss of reflex automatisms (405). A controlled study of infants with spastic diplegia found that the routine use of physical therapy offered no short-term advantages over an infant stimulation program (406). A randomized, controlled trial also found no statistical difference between intensive and routine physiotherapy (2 to 15 hours per 3 months) when measured by changes in gross motor function or performance (407). Bracing often is necessary. According to Tardieu and his group, bracing for 6 hours a day prevents contractures at the ankle (408). It is difficult to state categorically at what age treatment should be initiated. The controlled studies by Paine indicate that the eventual gait is better and contractures are fewer when physical therapy is begun before the age of 2 years (403).

Much controversy surrounds the management of the hemiplegic hand. No differences in hand function, quality of upper extremity movement, or parents' perception of the child's hand function were noted when children received intensive neurodevelopmental therapy plus casting or regular occupational therapy. However, casting appears to be more effective in older children (409). Ultimate hand function is usually not improved by physical therapy or surgery, and when the hemiplegia is complicated by a hemisensory deficit, the affected hand will probably never do more than assist the good hand (410). Forced-use treatment of the hemiparetic upper extremity has shown some benefit, but growth of the affected side is not improved by any mode of treatment (411). When the hemiplegia is mild, children achieve a good gait whether treated or not.

Few objective data indicate that either physiotherapy or orthopedic measures improve the disabilities of the child with a predominantly extrapyramidal disorder. In these patients, hand function and the quality of the ultimate gait depend principally on the original severity of the disorder, and most children with extrapyramidal movements, particularly those with unimpaired intelligence, are able to teach themselves to assume certain positions and perform substitute movements by which involuntary movements are avoided. The substitute movements are often so complex that they could not possibly be invented by therapists. In all instances, coordination and function tend to improve with age. Various drugs have been tried for relief of the extrapyramidal movements. None of these has resulted in long-term benefit sufficient to outweigh the side effects (401).

Various pharmacologic approaches have been tried for relief of spasticity. The most commonly used medications are baclofen, diazepam, and dantrolene. Doses are started at low levels and are increased until spasticity improves or side effects, notably drowsiness, occur. As a rule, these medications only have a small effect. The intrathecal administration of baclofen by continuous infusion is proving to be an effective means for treating spasticity in the lower extremities in a selected group of patients who have responded favorably to a trial dose of intrathecal baclofen (412–414). Complications of this procedure are seen in about one-fourth of patients. In the experience of Gooch and coworkers, they mainly involved mechanical failures of the pump or the catheter (415). Side effects from the drug are usually temporary and can be managed by reducing the rate of infusion.

The injection of botulinum toxin A (Botox) into the gastrosoleus and hamstring group of muscles appears to improve gait for up to 6 months and may help to delay or obviate the need for serial casting or orthopedic surgery (416). The effect of the toxin becomes evident within 12 hours to 7 days, and the effect can last between 2 and 10 months (416,417). Graham and coworkers presented a consensus statement with respect to patient selection and assessment, drug dosage, injection technique, and outcome measurements (418). Forssberg and Tedroff believed that treatment should be initiated at a time when children are still developing their motor control apparatus. This might prevent them from entering a vicious cycle in which CNS lesions affect the musculoskeletal system, thereby preventing the development of motor functions (419). Graham confirmed their experience (420). In addition, experimental data on the formation of a cortical somatotopic map during early life indicate that the periphery plays an instructional role on the formation of central neuronal structures (421). The economics and effectiveness of this type of treatment also require further study.

No evidence indicates that treatment programs that attempt to modify sensory input, inhibit primitive reflexes, or modify or inhibit abnormal movement patterns are ever successfully incorporated into the maturing nervous system with resulting improvement in motor function. Several authorities and parent groups have expressed their enthusiasm for infant stimulation programs. Even lacking objective evidence of their usefulness, they are apparently beneficial in controlling behavior and are here to stay (422,423).

Surgical Therapy

Despite physical therapy, approximately one-half of the patients with spastic diplegia, spastic quadriparesis, or hemiparesis ultimately require some form of orthopedic procedure. Nonambulatory children, in particular, have a high incidence of spinal deformities, and more than 50% develop progressive displacement and dysplasia of the hips, and up to 20% ultimately develop frank dislocation (404). Children with spastic quadriparesis who are unable to walk at most at risk. Graham recommended a hip surveillance program for such children and stressed the benefits of reconstructive surgery (424,425).

Park and Owen divided surgical procedures into two categories: lengthening or release of muscles and tendons and procedures involving bones (426). The former procedures include tenotomy of the hip adductors, hamstring lengthening, and lengthening of the heel cords or the posterior tibial tendons. The majority of such operations are performed between 4 and 8 years of age. Surgery on bones is generally carried out in older individuals with the aim of correcting fixed deformities (427,428). The outcome of these procedures is not related to the age at surgery; instead, the more severe the deficit, the greater is the improvement. Long-term follow-ups, however, indicate that the greatest gains are seen 1 year after surgery; thereafter, function tends to return to preoperative levels (429).

Another type of surgical approach has been directed to correcting the pathophysiology underlying the spastic muscle. Normally, muscle tone results from a stream of impulses from the muscle spindles activating the motoneurons (the large motor neurons of the anterior horns). In spasticity, increased activity of the two types of small, gamma-motoneurons results from an imbalance of two opposing influences, facilitation and inhibition. Facilitation is brought about by afferent fibers from the muscle spindles and inhibition is mediated by the descending pyramidal tract fibers. When the descending pyramidal tract fibers have been damaged, inhibition is reduced. Stimulation of the cerebellum has been offered as a means of enhancing inhibition. However, neither chronic cerebellar stimulation nor the implantation of a subcutaneous dorsal column stimulator in the high cervical region of the spinal cord has been effective. Peacock and his group suggested a compensatory reduction of facilitation by selective sectioning of the posterior roots of the spinal cord (430). This procedure requires sectioning of those rootlets between the levels of L2 to S1 or S2 involved in spasticity-producing circuits, whose electrical stimulation induces either a tetanic muscle contraction or a diffusion of muscle contraction to muscle groups other than those being stimulated. This procedure is relatively free of complications, and any sensory loss induced by it appears to be minor and transient. Although the efficacy of the procedure and its neurophysiologic rationale have been questioned, several series have reported good results on patients who have severe spasticity in the lower extremities but near-normal intelligence, no major contractures, and no movement disorder. With good patient selection, significant improvement occurs in muscle tone, range of motion, and speed of walking, and in some studies the outcome is better than in children who are treated with intensive physiotherapy alone (431). Other studies failed to show an additional functional benefit of dorsal rhizotomy to a physical therapy program, but in some instances upper limb function also improves (432, 433). Rhizotomy should not be performed on patients whose spasticity enables them to maintain the erect position (434).

Because an effective treatment program requires considerable time and effort by the child's family and a large number of skilled personnel, deciding whether to advise treatment for the child with retardation with cerebral palsy is difficult. Obviously, the goals for the cerebral palsy child and the time spent achieving them must be realistic. It is beyond the scope of this book to explore the emotional and social factors that need to be considered in the evaluation of each case.

From time to time a number of methods have been proposed for the treatment of cerebral palsy. Some of these, such as the use of hyperbaric oxygen, are based on unproven or even false concepts of neuromuscular function, and claims for effectiveness are more a matter of bias than objective evaluation. Reviews by Koman and coworkers (247), Dormans (435), Tilton (436), and Bobath and Bobath (437) can be consulted for further information on treatment programs, particularly with respect to orthopedic therapy, speech therapy, and handling of social and educational problems.

Non-neurological Complication of Cerebral Palsy

A high incidence of ocular abnormalities is found in children with cerebral palsy. The most common abnormality encountered is strabismus, mainly caused by esotropia, which is found in approximately one-half of the patients with ocular problems (438). The condition is most common in children with spastic diplegia and least common in those with extrapyramidal cerebral palsy. Strabismus that fluctuates from esotropia to exotropia, apparently unrelated to accommodative effort, is particularly common in children with extrapyramidal cerebral palsy and can be the first sign of this disorder (439). The cause for convergent strabismus is unknown, but because the alignment of the eye is often correctable under anesthesia, probably overactivity of the convergence center is at fault. Approximately one-third of patients have defects of horizontal conjugate gaze. Generally, surgical treatment of the eye muscles is deferred until the child has reached an age at which the degree of deviation is stable. Surgery is indicated when binocular vision is evident on sensory testing. If a surgical procedure is performed too early, the child, who has not yet achieved a fusion potential, does not maintain the correct alignment, and strabismus recurs. Only 10% to 15% of children with cerebral palsy ever achieve binocular vision. In the remainder, surgery serves only cosmetic purposes.

Asphyxiated infants can be cortically blind or can have delayed visual maturation. As a rule the presence and severity of visual impairment is proportional to the severity of brain lesions. Moderate or severe basal ganglia lesions and severe white matter changes are always associated with abnormal visual function (440). Delayed visual maturation can reflect delayed myelination and dendritic and synapse formation. The visual-evoked response in these children is usually abnormal, whereas the electroretinogram (ERG) is normal (441). As a rule, visual assessment at 5 months of age is predictive of visual outcome at school age (440). However, many cortically blind infants make a remarkable recovery, although often a residue of visual perceptual handicaps remains (441–443).

Impaired feeding and swallowing are relatively common. Symptoms result in part from an increased bite reflex and tongue thrust and in part from incoordination of the swallowing mechanism (gastroesophageal reflux) (444). Dysfunctional problems can include drooling, coughing or aspiration, abnormal breathing patterns, uncoordinated swallowing, an absence of bilabial close on the spoon or cup, prolonged bottle feeding or impaired sucking, inadequate jaw or tongue movements, and rejection of textured foods. Additionally, dystonic hyperextension of the head allows liquids and foods to move into the trachea by gravity and causes aspiration and upper respiratory dysfunction.

Treatment for these problems is practical, but tedious. A major component in the treatment process is positioning (i.e., breaking up abnormal patterns such as hyperextension of the head by means of a hands-on technique in addition to the wheelchair headrest) (445).

The sequential steps for successful oral feeding intake are (a) tactile desensitization to allow oral intake of textured foods; (b) active feeding techniques to retrain lip and tongue movements, bilabial closure on the spoon and cup, and reduction of the tongue thrust; (c) active feeding techniques to encourage normal chewing skills; and (d) active feeding techniques to encourage automatic jaw closure, decrease drooling, and encourage normal breathing and swallowing patterns (446). Small amounts of benztropine (Cogentin) (0.5 to 6 mg/day) and other anticholinergics have been used successfully to reduce drooling (447). The neural control of swallowing was reviewed by Jean (448).

Approximately one-third of children with cerebral palsy develop significant lower urinary tract symptoms, notably daytime urinary incontinence, urgency, and frequency. Videourodynamic studies disclose that the most common finding, seen in 74%, is hyper-reflexia of the detrusor muscle of the bladder with reduced bladder capacity. Less often, 19% in the experience of Reid and Borzyskowski, detrusor sphincter dyssynergia occurs, which is a contraction of the detrusor concurrent with involuntary contraction of the external urethral sphincter. Treatment includes anticholinergic drugs, intermittent catheterization, antibiotic prophylaxis, and surgery. Reid and Borzyskowski reviewed evaluation and management of these conditions (449).

In a large proportion of children with cerebral palsy, learning is impaired by defects in visual or auditory perception. The procedures by which these defects can be evaluated and the educational aspects of perceptual and spatial handicaps are discussed in Chapter 18.

Prognosis

Perinatal Asphyxia

Underlying the prognosis of the asphyxiated infant is the unanswered question about whether asphyxia produces a continuum of brain damage (i.e., whether mild asphyxia causes a small amount of damage and more severe asphyxia causes more severe damage) or a threshold exists beyond which the brain is damaged in an all-or-none manner. It is our opinion that there is a threshold of asphyxia beyond which there is a continuum of brain injury, and below this threshold there is no damage.

It is clear that most infants who experience perinatal asphyxia do not exhibit abnormal neurologic signs or subsequent evidence of brain injury. It is also clear that unless clinical signs of neurologic abnormality are present during the neonatal period, the outcome of perinatal asphyxia is entirely favorable. In the experience of Dubowitz and Dubowitz, all term infants who were healthy on neonatal examination were healthy at 1 year of age (450). The best predictor of outcome from a perinatal asphyxia is the clinical status of the infant during the neonatal period as assessed by the Sarnat scale (see Table 6.8). Numerous studies have confirmed the prognostic value of such an assessment (222,451). In terms of outcome, staging is best done according to the most severe signs and according to the most severe stage of encephalopathy between 1 hour and 7 days of life (451). In the experience of Robertson and

Finer, all infants with stage 1 encephalopathy had a normal outcome, and their cognitive performance at 8 years of age did not differ from that of controls. The results of Handley-Derry and coworkers are similar (452). Infants with stage 3 encephalopathy fare poorly. Robertson and Finer found that 82% died by school age and 18% were severely handicapped (451). The outcome of infants with moderate (stage 2) HIE is less certain. Robertson and Finer found that 80% were neurologically normal, 15% were neurologically disabled, and 5% died (451). Of the nondisabled survivors in this series as well as in several others a large proportion had significant cognitive dysfunction and poor school performance (451). In the study of Robertson and Finer, the presence of neonatal seizures did not appear to affect the prognosis. Temple and coworkers, however, found that infants who developed neonatal seizures after an asphyxial injury demonstrated significant cognitive deficits, even when the neurologic examination was normal (453). Infants with subtle seizures and infants who demonstrate more than two seizure types tend to have a worse outcome in terms of continued epileptic manifestations and mental retardation (454). Renal injury, particularly prolonged oliguria, when associated with asphyxia also presages a poor neurologic outcome (455).

Other factors that influence the infant's response to an asphyxial insult, and thus his or her outcome, include preexisting cerebral anomalies, fetal maturity, cerebral energy stores at the time of asphyxia, the adequacy of uteroplacental blood flow, and the fetal adaptive response to asphyxia. This adaptive response involves a redistribution of cardiac output so that blood flow to brain and heart is maintained at the expense of blood flow to kidney, the gastrointestinal tract, and the musculoskeletal system. Finally, experimental data indicate that not only can asphyxial injury cause neuronal loss, but it also can interfere with the normal developmental processes including cortical reorganization, formation of synaptic connections, and programmed cell death that may have been in progress at the time of injury (138,363,456).

In view of the interaction of these several factors, it should come as no surprise that many infants with severe and prolonged asphyxia recover without any neurodevelopmental deficits, and an arterial cord pH as low as 6.60 is compatible with normal neurologic and cognitive examinations at a mean age of 47 months (313). Nevertheless, aggressive resuscitation of the newborn infant is not in order. Levene recommends that if an infant has no cardiac output after 10 minutes of effective resuscitation, treatment should be abandoned (223). The outcome of infants with good cardiac output who do not breathe spontaneously by 20 minutes is poor, and only 25% were left without significant neurologic deficits (457). These considerations are important in a time of medical cost control.

Several other methods have been used in an attempt to identify infants with a poor prognosis. The most traditional of these has been the Apgar score, even though it is now evident that a low Apgar score does not indicate the presence of asphyxia in either term or premature infants (225,227). Whereas the predictive value of the 1- and 5-minute Apgar scores in terms of subsequent neurologic deficits is limited, term infants with 5-minute Apgar scores of 6 or less are three times as likely to be neurologically abnormal at 1 year of age as those with scores of 6 to 10 (458). The likelihood of permanent brain damage increases even more significantly when depressed Apgar scores persist. Of infants with scores of 3 or less at 10 minutes of age, 68% die during the first year of life, and 12.5% of survivors are neurologically damaged. The prognosis is even worse when an Apgar score of 3 or less persists for 20 minutes. Of those infants, 87% die, and 36% of survivors have cerebral palsy (227). A poor outcome was seen in 30% of infants with a low Apgar score but no significant acidosis (459). In some instances, this is due to acidosis paradox, discussed in another portion of this chapter (315,316).

Fetal blood sampling can provide somewhat better prognostic information, although there still are no absolute values of blood pO_2, pCO_2, or pH beyond which irreparable brain damage is certain to ensue. Studies designed to correlate the severity of acidosis in term infants at birth with outcome have failed to show any consistent relationship (460,461). When infants with umbilical cord pH of 7.0 or less are selected to be followed, the outcome is still unpredictable; however, when severe acidemia is associated with persistent bradycardia or seizures, the outcome is poor in 85% of cases (210). Because most of the asphyxial insults were believed to occur *in utero* during labor, electronic monitoring of the fetal heart rate was considered to be of prognostic value. Prospective studies have indicated otherwise. Although one-fourth of high-risk infants whose fetal heart rate patterns showed severe variable decelerations or late decelerations were neurologically abnormal at 1 year of age, these abnormalities did not persist into later childhood (308,462). Ekert and coworkers presented a model that can predict within 4 hours of birth a poor outcome from perinatal asphyxia (463). The three major adverse factors singled out by them were onset of spontaneous respirations after 10 minutes of life, administration of chest compression, and onset of seizures before 4 hours of age.

Because a significant proportion of infants with a neurologic examination consistent with Sarnat stage 2 fare well, prognosis in this group should be influenced by the results of neurodiagnostic tests (464).

The EEG is one of the commonly used means of evaluating the neonate with a history of perinatal asphyxia and clinical evidence for moderate or severe HIE. Recovery is more likely to occur if the tracing is normal or if it demonstrates a single focus rather than showing multifocal paroxysmal discharges or a burst-suppression pattern (465,466). Serial EEGs first obtained between 12 and

36 hours of life and then between 7 and 9 days postpartum provide a better indication of ultimate outcome (467).

CT scanning and MRI, particularly when coupled with EEG, provide the best prognostic tools. The presence of areas of decreased density in brain parenchyma seen on CT predicts a major neurologic handicap. This likelihood is particularly true when two or more focal areas of hypodensity exist or when the density of the basal ganglia is reduced (468). Asphyxiated infants with normal CT rarely exhibit major neurologic residua.

MRI provides more detail about the anatomic localization and severity of asphyxial injury and is a better means of predicting the ultimate outcome than the Apgar score or staging the severity of neonatal encephalopathy (469,470). Lesions of the basal ganglia are generally predictive of a poor outcome. Parasagittal lesions, focal areas of necrosis, have a better outlook. Asphyxiated infants with a normal MRI do well developmentally and neurologically.

MR spectroscopy is a potentially valuable prognostic tool. Neonates with poor outcomes had significantly lower *N*-acetyl aspartate (NAA)/choline ratios and significantly higher choline/creatine ratios in the occipital region compared with patients with good to moderate outcomes. In addition, the persistence of lactic acids predicts a poor outcome (471,472). The practical problems associated with obtaining such a study preclude it from being widely used in the early evaluation of asphyxiated infants.

The question of whether asphyxia resulting in mild to moderate neonatal encephalopathy can result in mild mental retardation or learning disabilities in the absence of gross neurologic deficits has not been resolved. Nelson and Ellenberg failed to find a statistically significant increase in mental retardation in children with low Apgar scores who did not also have cerebral palsy (227). They concluded that when mental retardation is a consequence of perinatal asphyxia, it is usually severe and accompanied by evidence of neurologic damage, notably spastic quadriparesis, athetosis, or both. Recent work by Hopkins-Golightly and colleagues however argues against the presence of an all-or-none threshold phenomenon for development of brain injury and cognitive impairment, and suggests that there is a continuum of brain injury in asphyxia (472a). This issue is further discussed in Chapter 18.

TABLE 6.14 Survival and Incidence of Early Childhood Disability in Infants with Birth Weights of 500 to 1,250 g

	Birth Year (%)			
	1978 to 1979		1988 to 1989	
One-Year Survival				
500–749 g	3		41	
750–999 g	21		64	
1,000–1,250 g	67		86	
Specific Disabilities				
Cerebral palsy	17		10	
500–749 g		0		15
750–999 g		13		10
1,000–1,250 g		18		9
Mental Retardation	11		7	
500–749 g		0		15
750–999 g		20		4
1,000–1,250 g		9		6

Adapted from Robertson CMT, Hrynchyshyn GJ, Etches PC, et al. Population-based study of the incidence, complexity, and severity of neurologic disability among survivors weighing 500–1,250 grams at birth: a comparison of two birth cohorts. *Pediatrics* 1992;90:750.

Prematurity with Neurologic Complications

Modern methods of perinatal care have brightened the outlook in terms of survival of even the smallest premature infant. However, concurrent with a decrease in neonatal mortality, there has been an increase in the incidence of neurologic handicaps in the smallest group of preterm infants (249). The incidence of neurologic disabilities in infants born from 1978 to 1979 as compared with infants born from 1988 to 1989 is depicted in Table 6.14 (473).

Four factors contribute to the increased incidence of neurologic disability in the smallest preterm infants: the presence and severity of PVL, the presence and severity of periventricular and intraventricular hemorrhages, the effects of premature delivery and neonatal complications on cerebral cortical and white matter organization, and the likelihood that a significant proportion of premature infants are neurologically compromised prior to birth.

The presence of PVL as detected on ultrasound or by neuroimaging studies predicts the evolution of spastic diplegia over the ensuing months. In addition, children with PVL have a significantly curtailed intellect. In the study by Pharoah and colleagues, 68% of children with spastic diplegia had an IQ of 70 or higher, 15% had moderate mental retardation, and 17% had severe mental retardation (474). Visual perceptual deficits and other cognitive disorders are common in the group of children with PVL who appear to have grossly normal intelligence.

Several studies indicate that children who had sustained an uncomplicated IVH (grades I or II) have subtle neurologic deficits. Most of these are not apparent during the first few years of life but can be documented when follow-up examinations are performed between 5 and 7 years of age or later (475,476,477). The risk of developing neurologic deficits is significantly increased for infants who have sustained a major IVH. In the series of Fazzi and colleagues, only 20% of infants who sustained this lesion were considered to have developed normally at 2 years of age. By 5 to 7 years of age, this figure had declined to 8% (477). Other follow-up studies have yielded similar results (475,478).

The cause of the cognitive and attention deficits of premature infants who are grossly normal neurologically is not clear. Based on experimental work of Ghosh and Shatz (479), Volpe postulated that neurons in the subependymal germinative zone, the subplate neurons, which are involved in cerebral cortical organization, are disrupted by the presence of even minor germinal matrix hemorrhages or PVL (480). Their injury could lead to the variety of cortical deficits that are so common in small premature infants. One should also remember that most of the growth of cortical connections and complexity occurs after 25 weeks' gestation. Whereas neuronal migration is largely complete by 25 weeks, glial migration continues, as does cortical connectivity. The cerebral cortex of extremely premature infants when imaged at gestational age 38 to 42 weeks has less cortical surface area and is less complex than that of the normal term newborn (481). It is likely that these deficits acquired during a critical period of brain development are permanent.

Numerous follow-up studies have been done on small preterm infants. The earlier reports were relatively optimistic; more recent series have noted a significant incidence of cognitive and behavioral abnormalities that lead to learning disabilities. In the United Kingdom series of infants with gestational age of 25 weeks or less, collected in 1995 by Wood and coworkers, 49% of the surviving children had significant disability detected at 30 months of postconceptual age. About half of these infants (23% of surviving infants) had severe disability (482). This study is probably more reliable than those that report outcome according to birth weight categories, which can be confounded by the inclusion of infants that are more gestationally mature but were growth restricted. Using the latter methodology, Hirata and colleagues found that in a group of infants with birth weights between 501 and 750 g, of the 40% who survived, 66% appeared normal, some 20% had borderline or low-average IQs, and approximately 10% had significant neurologic sequelae (483). Kitchen and coworkers examined infants with birth weights between 500 and 999 g at 2 years of age. Their results were similar, with 68% of surviving infants born between 1985 and 1987 having no apparent functional handicap (484). However, as a rule, a large proportion of neurodevelopmental deficits are not apparent during the first 2 to 3 years of life. The experience of Collin and coworkers, who followed infants into their preschool years, underlines this fact. They observed a downward drift in performance between infancy and preschool, with only approximately one-third of children who were deemed developmentally normal when seen between 12 and 25 months of age performing in the normal range when reassessed at approximately 4 years of age (485). The negative effect of extreme prematurity on cognitive and language function appears to be modified in infants from families with a high socioeconomic status (485a). Hack and coworkers believed that perinatal growth failure, as reflected in a subnormal head circumference at 8 months of age, predicts impaired cognitive function and academic achievement. Because most very low birth weight infants had a normal head circumference at birth, postnatal events are responsible for impairment in head growth and, by inference, brain maturation (486). More recently published studies show similar results (487,488).

Child with Cerebral Palsy as an Adult

The ultimate social adjustment of the patient with cerebral palsy is determined primarily by the severity of the physical and mental handicap. Individuals who can be predicted to be unable to work are those with an IQ under 50, are nonambulatory and without communication skills, and need assistance in using their hands. Those predicted for sheltered work are those with IQs between 50 and 79 who walk and have some communication skills (489). Generally, mental handicap is less of a barrier to useful employment than physical handicap. In the series of Sala and Grant, all children with spastic hemiparesis became ambulatory. Children with spastic diplegia became ambulatory in 86% to 91% of cases, with those who were able to sit independently by 2 years of age having the best prognosis for ambulation (490). Patients with hemiplegia are most often able to become competitive, approximately one-third of them being economically productive. One-fourth of patients with extrapyramidal disorders are ultimately able to work competitively (287). The outlook for patients with spastic quadriparesis is far worse. In the series of Crothers and Paine, published in 1959, none of the adult patients with spastic quadriparesis was gainfully employed (231). Also important in the ultimate prognosis is the presence or absence of associated disabilities, including seizures, and impairment of vision or hearing.

Adults with cerebral palsy develop a variety of new functional disabilities. These include lower extremity contractures, scoliosis, cervical pain, and back pain (491). For those who are mobile when they become adults there is a marked decline in ambulation in late adulthood, and few of the 60-year-olds who walked well preserved this skill over the following 15 years (492). Speech and self-feeding appear to be well preserved over the years. Survival rates of ambulatory older adults are only moderately worse than those of the general population (492).

Finally, and most difficult to evaluate when first seeing a patient, is the attitude of the patient and his or her family to the disability and the stability of the home in view of the severe and chronic emotional trauma caused by cerebral palsy (489).

Various estimates of life expectancy of children with cerebral palsy have been published. As a rule, life expectancy in mildly to moderately disabled children is only slightly curtailed (493), and 98% of persons without severe disabilities live to age 35 years (473). Life expectancy for the profoundly handicapped and immobile child, however, is severely curtailed (494), and more than one-third of those with severe disability l die before age 30 years (495).

PERINATAL INJURY TO THE SPINAL CORD

Because of the relative resistance of the spinal cord to asphyxia, perinatal spinal cord injuries are almost invariably the consequence of trauma. Although spinal birth injuries were first described during the nineteenth century, much of the understanding of them can be attributed to the classic papers of Crothers (496), Ford (497), and Crothers and Putnam (498). Relatively common in the early 1900s, this type of birth injury has become less common with improved obstetric practice, and by 1959 it constituted only 0.6% of the series of children with cerebral palsy encountered by Crothers and Paine (231).

Pathogenesis and Pathology

Perinatal traumatic lesions of the spinal cord result more commonly from stretching of the cord than from compression or transection (499). Longitudinal or lateral traction to the infant's neck or excessive torsion, particularly in the course of a difficult breech delivery, stretches the cord, its covering meninges, the surface vessels, and the nerve roots. Lesions are most frequent in the lower cervical and upper thoracic regions (500). The most common gross pathologic findings are epidural hemorrhage, dural laceration with subdural hemorrhage, tears of the nerve roots, laceration and distortion of the cord, and focal hemorrhage and malacia within the cord (499). Ischemic lesions of the cord are less common. Gross or petechial hemorrhages also can be seen within the substance of the cord, and myelination of the tracts can be impaired above the transection (501).

Clinical Manifestations

Three-fourths of infants who suffer a spinal birth injury had a difficult breech delivery, with arrest of the aftercoming head. As a rule, children with cephalic presentation develop upper cervical lesions, whereas cervical cord damage resulting from breech delivery involves the lower cervical cord (502,503). In the series of Mills and coworkers, upper cervical cord injury was accompanied by hypoxic-ischemic encephalopathy in 64% of instances (504). When damage to the cord is severe, the neonate dies during labor or soon after. With a less extensive injury, infants show respiratory depression and generalized hypotonia or flaccid paraplegia (505). Associated urinary retention and abdominal distention with paradoxical respirations occur (506). In addition to impaired motor function, sensation and perspiration are absent below the level of injury. The deep tendon reflexes usually cannot be elicited during the neonatal period, and mass reflex movements do not become apparent until later.

In approximately 20% of cases, damage to the brachial plexus also can be documented. In other cases, the lower brainstem is involved as well, with consequent bulbar signs.

The clinical picture after complete transection of the spinal cord is discussed in Chapter 9. A high percentage of survivors have normal intelligence.

Diagnosis

The presence of poor muscle tone and flaccid weakness involving all extremities or only the legs after a breech extraction should suggest a cord injury. Although not easy to demonstrate, loss of sensory function should always be sought.

Neuromuscular disorders, notably infantile spinal muscular atrophy (Werdnig-Hoffmann disease), are not associated with loss of sensory function or loss of sphincter control. Of the other neuromuscular disorders, congenital myasthenia gravis is diagnosed by reversibility of symptoms after injection of anticholinesterase drugs (see Chapter 16).

Occasionally, an infant with a congenital tumor of the cervical or lumbar cord presents a clinical picture akin to that of a spinal cord injury. Abnormalities of the skin along the posterior lumbosacral midline, including dimpling, hemangiomas, or tufts of hair, are commonly seen in congenital tumor of the lumbar cord (507). Neuroimaging studies are diagnostic, and an MRI can demonstrate the pathologic findings and predict the long-term neurologic outcome. As a rule, hemorrhage within the spinal cord predicts poor outcome. The use of gradient echo acquisition sequences increases the sensitivity of the MRI and can show the hemorrhage within 3 hours of its occurrence (504).

Treatment and Prognosis

In most infants, fractures or fracture dislocations of the spine are absent, and the treatment is that outlined in Chapter 9 for spinal cord injuries of older children. Although the majority of clinically apparent spinal birth injuries are severe and irreversible, milder degrees of injury are potentially reversible.

PERINATAL INJURIES OF CRANIAL NERVES

Facial Nerve

The most common cranial nerve to be involved in birth trauma is the facial nerve. According to Hepner (508), some facial nerve injury is evident in 6% of neonates. The injury results from pressure of the sacral prominence of the maternal pelvis against the facial nerve distal to its emergence from the stylomastoid foramen (pes anserinus). Less often, compression results from forceps application. These insults are more likely to produce swelling of tissue around the nerve than complete or partial anatomic interruption of the fibers.

The degree of facial paresis ranges from complete loss of function in all three main branches to weakness limited to a small group of muscles. One common picture is a mild paresis of the lower portion of the face, particularly the depressor muscle of the lower lip and the depressor muscle of the angle of the mouth, which is manifested most clearly when the infant cries by a failure in downward movement of the affected corner of the mouth. Because the mentalis muscle, innervated by the same nerve fibers as the depressor anguli oris, usually is unaffected, the condition probably reflects a maldevelopment rather than perinatal trauma (see Table 5.14) (509).

In most instances, the facial nerve palsy is mild, and some improvement becomes evident within a week. In the more severe cases, the start of recovery can be delayed for several months. Electrodiagnostic studies can be used to provide information on the extent and cause of nerve damage. The ability to produce contraction of the muscle by stimulating the nerve implies that the conductivity of the nerve is only partially interrupted and suggests a favorable prognosis. Good recovery is possible, however, even when electrical reactions are completely absent (510). In traumatic facial nerve palsy, electrical studies performed within 48 hours of birth are normal and do not become abnormal until 72 or more hours. By contrast, the initial electrical study results are abnormal in congenital developmental weakness (511). Another less common traumatic cause for facial nerve palsy present at birth is a basilar skull fracture.

Acquired facial nerve palsy should be distinguished from the various developmental facial nerve palsies. The most common of these is seen with Möbius syndrome (see Chapter 5). This condition generally involves a bilateral facial palsy, often accompanied by weakness of one or both abducens nerves or of other cranial nerves. Occasionally, Möbius syndrome is limited to one side of the face, or even one part of the face, and can be associated with the Poland syndrome (hypoplasia of the pectoralis major, and nipple and syndactyly of the hand). In Goldenhar syndrome, hypoplasia of the facial musculature is associated with anomalies of the ear and vertebral anomalies. Unilateral facial nerve palsy can also accompany Catch-22 syndrome (velocardiofacial syndrome, microdeletion of chromosome 22q11) (512,513) (Chapter 4).

Treatment of the facial nerve palsy is limited to protection of the eye by application of methylcellulose drops and by taping the paralytic lid. Electrical stimulation of the nerve does not hasten recovery. Neurosurgical repair of the nerve should be considered only when evidence suggests that the nerve is severed. Recovery is complete in about 90% of acquired facial nerve palsy. Facial nerve palsy accompanying the various developmental disorders has a poorer prognosis (512).

Other Cranial Nerves

Conjunctival and retinal hemorrhages are common in the newborn infant, but birth injury involving the optic nerve exclusively is relatively rare. Unilateral and bilateral optic atrophy result from direct injury to the nerve through fracture of the orbit or, less often, through the base of the skull (514,515).

A transient postnatal paralysis of the abducens and oculomotor nerves is occasionally encountered. Paralysis of the oculomotor nerve can take the form of a transient postnatal ptosis (516). Congenital suprabulbar paresis, as first delineated by Worster-Drought (517), is considered in Chapter 5. Symmetric tegmental infarcts of the brainstem sometimes extend as far caudally as the lower medulla and may involve the hypoglossal nuclei or the intramedullary course of their axons, causing atrophy and fasciculation of the tongue that may suggest spinal muscular atrophy (Werdnig-Hoffmann disease) (163).

Hearing is impaired in approximately one-fourth of children with cerebral palsy. Perinatal asphyxia is accompanied by hemorrhages in the inner ear and damage to the auditory pathway within the brainstem (518,519). These injuries can be documented by the brainstem auditory-evoked potentials. An injury to the peripheral portion of the auditory pathway results in a heightened threshold and a prolonged latency of all responses, whereas an injury to the brainstem results in a prolonged latency of waves, which represents activity beyond the point of injury. Both types of abnormalities have been encountered in asphyxiated neonates (520,521). Hecox and Cone stressed the prognostic value of a diminished amplitude of wave V, which reflects midbrain function, relative to wave I, which reflects the activity of the VIII nerve. They found that an abnormal amplitude ratio is an excellent predictor of a poor outcome of asphyxial injury to both premature and term infants (522).

PERINATAL INJURIES OF PERIPHERAL NERVES

Brachial Plexus

Although perinatal injuries of the peripheral nerves were first described by Smellie (523), the present-day understanding of the interrelationship between palsies of the upper extremity and injuries of the brachial plexus comes from a group of nineteenth-century French neurologists. This includes Danyau (524) and Duchenne (525), who were the first to describe obstetric injuries to the fifth and sixth cervical roots (Erb-Duchenne palsy), and Klumpke (526), who described the lesion of the lower trunk of the cervical plexus that now bears her name.

Pathogenesis and Pathology

As a rule, brachial plexus injuries result from stretching of the plexus owing to turning the head away from the shoulder in a difficult cephalic presentation of a large infant. An injury also can be consequent to stretching of the brachial plexus owing to traction on the shoulder in the course of delivering the aftercoming head in a breech presentation (527,528). The condition has been reported in a few instances after delivery by cesarean section (529). However, whatever scant evidence exists for a classical brachial plexus injury resulting from intrauterine maladaptation is principally based on faulty interpretation of EMG (530,531). When intrauterine palsies do occur, they are characterized by limb atrophy and abnormal dermatoglyphics at birth (532).

In most instances, the brachial plexus is compressed by hemorrhage and edema within the nerve sheath. Less often, there is an actual tear of the nerves, or avulsion of the roots from the spinal cord occurs, with segmental damage to the gray matter of the spinal cord (443). With traction, the fifth cervical root gives way first, then the sixth, and so on down the plexus. Thus, the mildest plexus injuries involve only C5 and C6, and the more severe involve the entire plexus (528).

Clinical Manifestations

The incidence of brachial plexus injury in 2000 was 4.6 per 1,000 births (533). This figure should be contrasted with an incidence of 2.2 per 1,000 births in 1994 as determined from the Swedish Medical Birth Registry (534) and an incidence of 1.3 per 1,000 births in 1980, a significant increase over the course of the last 20 years. The incidence of brachial plexus palsy is 45 times greater in infants with birth weights greater than 4,500 g than in those that weigh less than 3,500 g (534). In approximately 80% of infants, Erb-Duchenne paralysis is confined to the upper brachial plexus (535). Involvement was unilateral in approximately 95% of instances in the series of Eng and coworkers (532). One of us (J.H.M.) has seen an infant with what appeared to be bilateral brachial plexus injury who had agenesis of the biceps muscles. The right side is more frequently affected than the left, with the ratio in the series of Eng and coworkers being 55:45 (535). The weakness is recognized soon after delivery, with the involved arm assuming a characteristic posture. The shoulder is adducted and internally rotated, the elbow extended, the forearm pronated, and the wrist occasionally flexed. This position results from paralysis of the deltoid, the supraspinatus and infraspinatus, biceps, and brachioradialis muscles. The Moro reflex is absent or diminished on the affected side, but the grasp reflex remains intact. Unlike in the healthy neonate, the biceps reflex is abolished or is less active than the triceps reflex. In most infants, a sensory loss cannot be demonstrated, although occasionally cutaneous sensation is lost over the deltoid region and the adjacent radial surface of the upper arm.

Fractures of the clavicle or humerus, slippage of the capital head of the radius, and subluxation of the shoulder and the cervical spine often accompany a brachial plexus injury (528). When a significant degree of injury to the fourth cervical root is present, phrenic nerve paralysis can accompany injury to the upper brachial plexus (536). An affected infant can show signs of respiratory distress, including tachypnea, cyanosis, and decreased movement of the affected hemithorax. When the phrenic nerve palsy is unaccompanied by injury to the brachial plexus, as occurs occasionally, the condition can mimic congenital pulmonary or heart disease (537,538).

In the more severely involved infants, 12% in the series of Eng and colleagues (532), the entire brachial plexus is damaged and the arm is completely paralyzed. The limb is flaccid, the Moro and grasp reflexes are unelicitable, deep tendon reflexes are absent, and sensory loss occurs over a portion of the extremity.

Isolated paralysis of the lower part of the brachial plexus (Klumpke paralysis) is relatively uncommon. It constituted only 2.5% of brachial plexus birth palsies in the experience of Ford (257), and a spinal cord lesion should be suspected whenever the paralysis involves the intrinsic muscles of the hand (532). The clinical picture of a lower plexus injury includes weakness of the flexors of the wrist and fingers, an absent grasp reflex, and a unilateral Horner syndrome caused by involvement of the cervical sympathetic nerves. Loss of sensation and sudomotor function over the hand can sometimes be demonstrated. Interference with the sympathetic innervation of the eye results in a delay or failure in pigmentation of the iris, and it is one of several causes for heterochromia iridis (539).

Diagnosis

The diagnosis of brachial plexus injury is usually readily apparent from the posture of the affected arm and from the absence of voluntary and reflex movements. Radiographic examinations can detect associated fractures, usually of the clavicle, humerus, or both, whereas fluoroscopy can be used to ascertain any limitation of diaphragmatic movement. In severe injuries causing avulsion of the spinal roots and bleeding into the subarachnoid space, the CSF can be bloody. MRI can be used to visualize the brachial plexus and to demonstrate root evulsions (540,541). The presence of pseudomeningoceles is a bad prognostic sign (540). EMG performed 2 to 3 weeks after the injury can confirm the extent of denervation. Because fibrillation potentials are seen in the proximal musculature of some healthy newborns during the first month of life and in the distal musculature during the first 3 months of life, an indication that the muscles are not completely innervated, both sides should always be studied (542). Repeated EMG examinations at 6-week intervals indicate the degree of recovery (532).

Congenital Horner syndrome can occur in the absence of trauma and can be associated with anomalies of the cervical vertebrae, enterogenous cysts, or congenital nerve deafness (543,544). The association of heterochromia iridis, congenital nerve deafness, white forelock, broad root of the nose, and lateral displacement of the medial canthi of the eyes and inferior lacrimal puncta is well recognized under the term *Waardenburg syndrome* (see Chapter 5) (543,544).

Treatment and Prognosis

Treatment and prognosis is a function of the severity of the injury. Hoeksma and coworkers distinguished five grades of injury (533):

1. Loss of conduction in affected axons
2. Loss of axon continuity
3. Loss of continuity of nerve fibers
4. Loss of continuity of fasciculi
5. Tearing or evulsion of the entire nerve trunk

In grades 1 and 2, complete recovery can be expected. In grade 1, this occurs within days to 2 to 3 weeks; in grade 2, recovery can take up to several months. In grade 3, axonal regeneration is complicated by intrafascicular scarring and the regeneration of axons in foreign endoneural tubes. In grades 4 and 5, axon regeneration can take several months or never. As a rule, external rotation and supination are the most affected movements and the last to show recovery.

Gentle passive exercises of the affected arm should be instituted at approximately 1 week after birth. The infant's sleeve should be pinned in a natural position rather than in abduction and external rotation as many texts suggest (257). Follow-up studies indicate that overimmobilization of the affected arm is conducive to contractures and deformities that can persist despite spontaneous recovery of nerve function (545).

There is no consensus with respect to selection criteria for surgical intervention. Grossman reviewed the criteria for early surgical repair and stressed that whether surgery is performed at 3 months of age, as recommended by some surgeons, or at at 6 to 8 months of age makes little difference in terms of ultimate functional outcome (546). His group also has found that even when surgery is performed after one year of age, there can be significant functional improvement in selected cases (546a). Hoeksma and colleagues stated that when there is no sign of biceps by 3 months of age, the outlook is poor (533). Many surgeons use the absence of biceps contraction at 3 months of age as the criterion for placing an infant into the surgical group (546). The good surgical results with early intervention should be tempered by reflecting on the high incidence of improvement with conservative management (547,548). In the series of Michelow and colleagues, 92% of infants recovered spontaneously (549). Hoeksma and coworkers, however, reported only 66% complete recovery. In half of these children recovery was delayed up to 16 months of age (533). The presence of elbow flexion and elbow, wrist, and finger extension at 3 months of age is predictive of a good recovery (533,546). Eng and colleagues believed that if contraction occurs in the biceps and deltoid muscles by 2 months of age, shoulder function will recover almost completely. Mild sequelae, such as winging of the scapula and limited shoulder flexion and abduction, are common, however (532). We believe that if no improvement is noted in 3 to 6 months, surgical exploration of the brachial plexus should be considered, with repair of the damaged segment. In most instances in which poor recovery occurs, nerve damage is caused by avulsion of the spinal roots and surgical repair would, therefore, not be expected to result in any improvement.

In most cases, most of the recovery occurs between 2 and 14 months of age, with the condition becoming essentially stationary thereafter (534). Rossi and colleagues, however, believed that significant improvement is still possible up to the start of school (550).

As a rule, when the entire plexus is involved and an associated Horner syndrome exists, the outlook for full recovery is poor. Almost all children are left with hypoplasia of the limb and well-defined motor deficits, usually more marked in the proximal musculature. Contractures at the shoulder and elbow are common; approximately one-third have a clear-cut sensory deficit, whose location is variable. Trophic changes involving the fingers are unusual (535,550). They were seen in 2% of children in the series of Eng and colleagues (532).

Some infants have an apparently good return of neuromuscular function and sensation yet are unable to use the affected arm (535). Probably, transitory sensory motor deprivation in early life impairs the development of normal movement patterns and the organization of cortical body image (551). This would be in line with what has been observed with respect to the organization of the visual system after early deafferentation (552).

Other Peripheral Nerves

Birth injuries to the other peripheral nerves are relatively uncommon. Injury to the lumbosacral plexus can occur rarely after a frank breech delivery. Sciatic nerve palsy has been observed after injection of hypertonic glucose into the umbilical artery. It is caused by thrombosis of the inferior gluteal artery and is accompanied by circulatory changes in the buttock (553,554).

Palsies of the radial nerve (555) and obturator nerve (556) also have been recorded. The former is generally the consequence of intrauterine nerve compression.

Idiopathic Torticollis

Because idiopathic torticollis, a relatively common condition, is in some instances believed to be related to perinatal trauma, it is considered in this chapter.

Torticollis, meaning *twisted neck*, is a syndrome characterized by contracture of the sternocleidomastoid muscle accompanied by a tilt of the head to the affected side and a rotation of the neck so that the chin points to the opposite shoulder. Asymmetry of the skull and facial bones can be present.

The condition can be congenital, acquired, spasmodic, or intermittent.

Congenital muscular torticollis is encountered most frequently. It is characterized by the presence of a tumor in the affected sternocleidomastoid muscle. In the majority of cases, the tumor develops during the first few weeks of life, gradually disappearing by age 46 months. In the experience of Coventry and Harris (557), the tumor disappeared at a mean age of 14 weeks.

Considerable debate surrounds the cause of this condition. Although some instances are associated with congenital malformations of the cervical spine, abnormalities in the function of the extraocular muscles, and tumors of the brainstem or spinal cord, the majority of cases are truly idiopathic. The two most likely etiologic factors are restricted movement of the head owing to an unusual fetal posture or amniotic adhesions, and perinatal trauma to the sternocleidomastoid muscle (558). A relatively high incidence of breech deliveries (28% to 40%) is compatible with either cause.

Pathologic examination of the muscle usually reveals extensive fibrosis and nonspecific myopathic changes. When the condition is chronic, evidence exists for denervation and reinnervation, probably secondary to repeated episodes of minor trauma to the muscle, which results in an entrapment neuropathy of the accessory nerve. The innervation of the sternocleidomastoid is unique in the body because the accessory nerve to the clavicular head passes through the sternal head and may become entrapped or compressed by fibrosis, producing denervation of the clavicular head (558). Separate arterial supplies predispose to ischemia in the sternal head, resulting in focal myopathy with fibrosis (558). The sternocleidomastoid tumor is not a neoplasm, either benign or malignant; it is composed of actively proliferating fibroblastic tissue that surrounds fragments of atrophic or degenerating muscle fibers (559,560). The initial tumor is usually a hematoma.

Caputo and coworkers noted that when torticollis is the consequence of disturbed function of the extraocular muscles it disappears when the infant is placed into the supine position or when one eye is occluded (561).

Considerable debate surrounds the treatment of congenital torticollis. However, the majority of clinicians opts for early physical therapy measures such as stretching and massage rather than surgical sectioning of the sternocleidomastoid muscle, removal of the tumor, or a combination of the two procedures (562). With physical therapy, the torticollis resolves in 70% of children by 12 months of age regardless of its severity or the presence or absence of focal fibrosis (563).

Acquired torticollis most commonly is associated with an infratentorial tumor. It also can be seen with colloid cysts of the third ventricle, syringomyelia, and spinal cord tumors. On rare occasions, it develops in the course of a progressive muscular disease.

The association of torticollis with hiatus hernia and gastroesophageal reflux (Sandifer syndrome) was first reported by Kinsbourne (564). Torticollis can be present at birth; generally, no shortening of the sternocleidomastoid muscle occurs.

Spasmodic torticollis, occurring in isolation or progressing to a focal, segmental, or generalized dystonia, is rare during childhood. This condition is discussed to a greater extent in Chapter 3.

Paroxysmal torticollis is characterized by recurrent episodes of head tilting starting in infancy. These episodes are sometimes accompanied by vomiting and ataxia. The EEG and caloric tests during an attack are usually normal. Generally, symptoms subside within a few hours or days. Attacks occur at monthly intervals, and the condition remits spontaneously within a few years or is replaced by vertigo or migraine (565,566). A family history of similar attacks is not uncommon, and in some families there is a linkage to a calcium-channel gene (*CACNA1A*) (566).

REFERENCES

1. Freud S. *Die infantile cerebrallähmung*. Vienna: Alfred Hoelder, 1897.
2. Little WJ. Course of lectures on the deformities of human frame. *Lancet* 1843;1:318–322.

2a. Cazauvielh JB. *Recherches sur l'agénése cérèbrale et la paralysie congéniale*. Paris: Migneret, 1827.

3. Friede RL. *Developmental neuropathology*, 2nd ed. Berlin: Springer-Verlag, 1989.
4. Volpe JJ. *Neurology of the newborn*, 4th ed. Philadelphia: Saunders, 2001.
5. Zelson C, Lee SJ, Pearl M. The incidence of skull fractures underlying cephalhematomas in newborn infants. *J Pediatr* 1974;85:371–373.
6. Papaefthymiou G, Oberbauer R, Pendl G. Craniocerebral birth trauma caused by vacuum extraction: a case of growing skull fracture as a perinatal complication. *Childs Nerv Syst* 1996;12:117–120.
7. Kozinn PJ, Ritz ND, Moss AH, et al. Massive hemorrhage—scalps of newborn infants. *Am J Dis Child* 1964;108:413–417.
8. Chadwick LM, Pemberton PJ, Kurinczuk JJ. Neonatal subgaleal haematoma: associated risk factors, complications and outcome. *J Paediatr Child Health* 1996;32:228–232.
9. Amar AP, Aryan HE, Meltzer HS, et al. Neonatal subgaleal hematoma causing brain compression: report of two cases and review of the literature. *Neurosurgery* 2003;52:1470–1474.
10. Gröntoft O. Intracerebral and meningeal haemorrhages in perinatally deceased infants. II. Intracerebral haemorrhages: a pathologico-anatomical and obstetrical study. *Acta Obstet Gynecol Scand* 1953;32:308–334.

11. Wigglesworth JS, Husemeyer RP. Intracranial birth trauma in vaginal breech delivery: the continued importance of injury to the occipital bone. *Br J Obstet Gynecol* 1977;84:684–691.
11a. Whitby EH, Griffiths PD, Rutter S, et al. Frequency and natural history of subdural haemorrhages in babies and relation to obstetric factors. *Lancet* 2004;363:846–851.
12. Hanigan WC, Morgasn AM, Stahlberg LK, et al. Tentorial hemorrhage associated with vacuum extraction. *Pediatrics* 1990;85:534–539.
13. Avrahami E, Frishman E, Minz M. CT demonstration of intracranial haemorrhage in term newborn following vacuum extractor delivery. *Neuroradiology* 1993;35:107–108.
14. Menezes AH, Smith DE, Bell WE. Posterior fossa hemorrhage in the term neonate. *Neurosurgery* 1983;13:452–456.
15. Gunn TR, Mok PM, Becroft DMO. Subdural hemorrhage *in utero*. *Pediatrics* 1985;76:605–610.
16. Akman CI, Cracco J. Intrauterine subdural hemorrhage. *Dev Med Child Neurol* 2000;42:843–846.
17. Gröntoft O. Intracranial haemorrhage and bloodbrain barrier problems in the newborn: pathologico-anatomical and experimental investigation. *Acta Pathol Microbiol Scand Suppl* 1954;100:1–109.
18. Blank NK, Strand R, Gilles FH. Posterior fossa subdural hematomas in neonates. *Arch Neurol* 1978;35:108–111.
19. Fishman MA, Percy AK, Cheek WR, et al. Successful conservative management of cerebellar hematomas in term neonates. *J Pediatr* 1981;98:466–468.
20. Ravenel SD. Posterior fossa hemorrhage in the newborn. *Pediatrics* 1979;64:39–42.
21. Towbin A. Latent spinal cord and brain stem injury in newborn infants. *Dev Med Child Neurol* 1969;11:54–68.
22. Leviton A, Nelson KB. Problems with definitions and classifications of newborn encephalopathy. *Pediatr Neurol* 1992;8:85–90.
23. Levene MI, Kornberg J, Williams THC. The incidence and severity of post-asphyxial encephalopathy in fullterm infants. *Early Hum Dev* 1985;11:21–26.
24. Levene MI, Fenton AC, Evans DH, et al. Severe birth asphyxia and abnormal cerebral blood-flow velocity. *Dev Med Child Neurol* 1989;31:427–434.
25. Thornberg K, Thiringer K, Odeback A, et al. Birth asphyxia: incidence, clinical course and outcome in a Swedish population. *Acta Paediatr* 1995;84:927–932.
26. Brown JK, Purvis RJ, Forfar JO, et al. Neurological aspects of perinatal asphyxia. *Dev Med Child Neurol* 1974;16:567–580.
27. Low JA, Robertson DM, Simpson LL. Temporal relationships of neuropathologic conditions caused by perinatal asphyxia. *Am J Obstet Gynecol* 1989;160:608–614.
28. Badawi N, Kurinczuk JJ, Keogh JM, et al. Antepartum risk factors for newborn encephalopathy: the Western Australian case–control study. *Br Med J* 1998;317:1549–1553.
29. Badawi N, Kurinczuk JJ, Keogh JM, et al. Antepartum risk factors for newborn encephalopathy: the Western Australian case–control study. *Br Med J* 1998;317:1554–1558.
30. Cowen F, Rutherford M, Groenendaal F, et al. Origin and timing of brain lesions in term infants with neonatal encephalopathy. *Lancet* 2003;361:736–742.
31. Truwit CL, Barkovich AJ, Koch TK, et al. Cerebral palsy: MR findings in 40 patients. *Am J Neuroradiol* 1992;13:67–78.
31a. Hagberg B, Hagberg R, Beckung E, et al. Changing panorama of cerebral palsy in Sweden. VIII. Prevalence and origin in the birth year period 1991–1994. *Acta Paediat* 2001;90:271–277.
32. Blair E, Stanley FJ. Intrapartum asphyxia: A rare cause of cerebral palsy. *J Pediatr* 1988: 112:515–519.
33. Nelson KB, Grether JK. Potentially asphyxiating conditions and spastic cerebral palsy in infants of normal birth weight. *Am J Obstet Gynecol* 1998;179:507–513.
34. Gaffney G, Flavell V, Johnson A, et al. Cerebral palsy and neonatal encephalopathy. *Arch Dis Child* 1994;70:F195–F200.
35. Croen LA, Grether JK, Curry CJ, et al. Congenital abnormalities among children with cerebral palsy: more evidence for prenatal antecedents. *J Pediatr* 2001;138:804–810.
36. Nelson KB. Can we prevent cerebral palsy? *N Engl J Med.* 2003;349:1765–1770.
37. Hankins GDV, Speer M. Defining the pathogenesis and pathophysiology of neonatal encephalopathy and cerebral palsy. *Obstet Gynecol* 2003;102:628–636.
38. Volpe JJ. Hypoxic-ischemic encephalopathy: biochemical and physiologic aspects. In: Volpe JJ. *Neurology of the newborn*, 4th ed. Philadelphia: Saunders, 2001: 217–304.
39. Johnston MV, Trescher WH, Ishida A, et al. Neurobiology of hypoxic-ischemic injury in the developing brain. *Pediatr Res* 2001;49:735–741.
39a. McLean C, Ferriero D. Mechanisms of hypoxic-ischemic injury in the term infant. *Semin Perinatol* 2004;28:425–432.
40. Bennet L, Peebles DM, Edwards AD, et al. The cerebral hemodynamic response to asphyxia and hypoxia in the near-term fetal sheep as measured by near infrared spectroscopy. *Pediatr Res* 1998;44:951–957.
41. van Bel F, Dorrepaal CA, Benders MJ, et al. Changes in cerebral hemodynamics and oxygenation in the first 24 hours after birth asphyxia. *Pediatrics* 1993;92:365–372.
42. Martínez-Orgado J, Gonzalez R, Alonso MJ, et al. Endothelial factors and autoregulation during pressure changes in isolated newborn piglet cerebral arteries. *Pediatr Res* 1998;44:161–167.
43. Del Toro J, Louis PT, Goddard-Finegold J. Cerebrovascular regulation and neonatal brain injury. *Pediatr Neurol* 1991;7:3–12.
44. Blood AB, Hunter CJ, Power GG. Adenosine mediates decreased-cerebral metabolic rate and increased cerebral blood flow during acute moderate hypoxia in the near-term fetal sheep. *J Physiol* 2003;553:935–945.
45. Pryds O. Control of cerebral circulation in the high-risk neonate. *Ann Neurol* 1991;30:321–329.
46. Boylan GB, Young K, Paneral RB, et al. Dynamic cerebral autoregulation in sick newborn infants. *Pediatr Res* 2000;48:12–17.
47. Tyszczuk L, Meek J, Elwell C, et al. Cerebral blood flow is independent of mean arterial blood pressure in preterm infants undergoing intensive care. *Pediatrics* 1998;102:337–341.
48. Lupton BA, Hill A, Roland EH, et al. Brain swelling in the asphyxiated term newborn: pathogenesis and outcome. *Pediatrics* 1988;82:139–146.
49. Vannucci RC, Christensen MA, Yager JY. Nature, time-course, and extent of cerebral edema in perinatal hypoxic-ischemic brain damage. *Pediatr Neurol* 1993;9:29–34.
50. Gluckman PD, Pinal CS, Gunn AJ. Hypoxic-ischemic brain injury in the newborn: pathophysiology and potential strategies for intervention. *Semin Neonatol* 2001;6:109–120.
51. Vannucci RC, Duffy TE. Cerebral metabolism in newborn dogs during reversible asphyxia. *Ann Neurol* 1977;1:528–534.
52. Barkovich AJ, Westmark KD, Bedi HS, et al. Proton spectroscopy and diffusion imaging on the first day of life after perinatal asphyxia: preliminary report. *Am J Neuroradiol* 2001;22:1786–1794.
53. Hope PL, Costello AM, Cady EB, et al. Cerebral energy metabolism studied with phosphorus NMR spectroscopy in normal and birth-asphyxiated infants. *Lancet* 1984;2:366–370.
54. Azzopardi D, Wyatt JS, Cady EB, et al. Prognosis of newborn infants with hypoxic-ischemic brain injury assessed by phosphorus magnetic resonance spectroscopy. *Pediatr Res* 1989;25:441–451.
55. Szatkowski M, Attwell D. Triggering and execution of neuronal death in brain ischemia: two phases of glutamate release by different mechanisms. *Trends Neurosci* 1994;17:359–365.
56. Rossi DJ, Oshima T, Attwell D. Glutamate release in severe brain ischaemia is mainly by reversed uptake. *Nature* 2000;403:316–321.
57. Blennow M, Ingvar M, Lagercrantz H, et al. Early [^{18}F]FDG positron emission tomography in infants with hypoxic-ischemic encephalopathy shows hypermetabolism during the postasphyctic period. *Acta Paediatr* 1995;84:1289–1295.
58. Berger R, Garnier Y, Jensen A. Perinatal brain damage: underlying mechanisms and neuroprotective strategies. *J Soc Gynecol Invest* 2002;9:319–328.
59. Johnston MV, Nakajima W, Hagberg H. Mechanisms of hypoxic neurodegeneration in the developing brain. *Neuroscientist* 2002;8:212–220.
60. Rothman SM, Olney JW. Excitotoxicity and the NMDA receptor. *Trends Neurosci* 1987;10:299–302.
61. Choi DW. Calcium still center-stage in hypoxic-ischemic neuronal death. *Trends Neurosci* 1995;18:58–60.

62. Sattler R, Tymianski M. Molecular mechanisms of glutamate receptor-mediated excitotoxic neuronal cell death. *Mol Neurobiol* 2001;24:107–129.

62a. Rodríguez-Nuñez A, Eiris CE, Rodríguez-García J, et al. Neuron-specific enolase levels in the cerebrospinal fluid of neurologically healthy children. *Brain Dev* 1999;21:16–19.

62b. Schoerkhuber W, Kittler H, Sterz F, et al. Time course of serum neuron-specific enolase. A predictor of neurological outcome in patients resuscitated from cardiac arrest. *Stroke* 1999;30:1598–1603.

62c. Ohki S, Togari H, Sobajima H, et al. Lactate attenuates neuron specific enolase elevation in newborn rats. *Pediatr Neurol* 1999;21:543–547.

62d. Wang HD, Fukuda T, Suzuki T, et al. Differential effects of *Bcl-2* overexpression on hippocampal CA1 neurons and dentate granule cells following hypoxic ischemia in adult mice. *J Neurosci Res* 1999;57:1–12.

63. Ivacko JA, Sun R, Silverstein FS. Hypoxic-ischemic brain injury induces an acute microglial reaction in perinatal rats. *Pediatr Res* 1996;339:39–47.

64. Shalak, LF, Laptook AR, Jafri HS. Clinical chorionamnionitis, elevated cytokines, and brain injury in term infants. *Pediatrics* 2002;110:673–680.

64a. Graham EM, Sheldon RA, Flock DL, et al. Neonatal mice lacking functional Fas death receptors are resistant to hypoxic-ischemic brain injury. *Neurolbiol Dis* 2004;17:89–98.

65. Nakajima W, Ishida A, Lange MS, et al. Apoptosis has a prolonged role in the neurodegeneration after hypoxic ischemia in the newborn rat. *J Neurosci* 2000;20:7994–8004.

66. Hu BR, Liu CL, Ouyang Y, et al. Involvement of caspase-3 in cell death after hypoxia-ischemia declines during brain maturation. *Cereb Blood Flow Metab* 2000;20:1294–1300.

67. Lindvall O, Kokaia Z, Bengzon J, et al. Neurotrophins and brain insults. *Trends Neurosci* 1994;17:490–496.

68. Cheng Y, Gidday JM, Yan Q, et al. Marked age-dependent neuroprotection by brain-derived neurotrophic factor against neonatal hypoxic-ischemic brain injury. *Ann Neurol* 1997;41:521–529.

69. Blumenfeld KS, Welsh FA, Harris VA, Pesenson, MA. Regional expression of *cfos* and heat shock protein-70 mRNA following hypoxia-ischemia in immature rat brain. *J Cereb Blood Flow Metab* 1992;12:987–995.

70. Fellman V, Raivio KO. Reperfusion injury as the mechanism of brain damage after perinatal asphyxia. *Pediatr Res* 1997;41:599–606.

71. Ringstedt T, Tang LQ, Persson H, et al. Expression of c-*fos*, tyrosine hydroxylase, and neuropeptide mRNA in the rat brain around birth: effects of hypoxia and hypothermia. *Pediatr Res* 1994;37:15–20.

72. Vannucci RC, Yager JY. Glucose, lactic acid, and perinatal hypoxic-ischemic brain damage. *Pediatr Neurol* 1992;8:3–12.

73. Delivoria-Papadopoulos M, Misbra OP. Mechanisms of cerebral injury in perinatal asphyxia and strategies for prevention. *J Pedatr* 1998;132:S30–S34.

74. Arvin KL, Han BH, Du Y, et al. Minocycline markedly protects the neonatal brain against hypoxic-ischemic injury. *Ann Neurol* 2002;52:54–61.

74a. Sie LT, van der Knaap MS, Osting J, et al. MR patterns of hypoxic-ischemic brain damage after prenatal, perinatal or postnatal asphyxia. *Neuropediatrics* 2000;31:128–136.

74b. Westmark KD, Barkovich AJ, Sola A, et al. Patterns and implications of MR contrast enhancement in perinatal asphyxia: a preliminary report. *Am J Neuroradiol* 1995;16:685–692.

74c. Ferriero DM. Neonatal brain injury. *N Engl J Med* 2004;351:1985–1995.

74d. Roelants-van Rijn AM, Nikkels PG, Groenendaal F, et al. Neonatal diffusion-weighted MR imaging: relation with histopathology or follow-up MR examination. *Neuropediatrics* 2001;32:286–294.

74e. Vigneron DB, Barkovich AJ, Noworolski SM, et al. Three-dimensional proton MR spectroscopy imaging of premature and term neonates. *Am J Neuroradiol* 2001;22:1424–1433.

75. Thurston JH, McDougal DB. Effect of ischemia on metabolism of the brain of the newborn mouse. *Am J Physiol* 1969;216:348–352.

76. Calabresi P, Centonze D, Bernardi G. Cellular factors controlling neuronal vulnerability in the brain: a lesson from the striatum. *Neurology* 2000;55:1249–1255.

77. Ranck JB, Windle WF. Brain damage in the monkey, *Macaca mulatta*, by asphyxia neonatorum. *Exp Neurol* 1959;1:130–154.

78. Myers RE. Experimental models of perinatal brain damage: relevance to human pathology. In: Gluck L, ed. *Intrauterine asphyxia and developing fetal brain*. Chicago: Year Book, 1977: 37–97.

79. Norman MG. Perinatal brain damage. *Perspect Pediatr Pathol* 1978;4:41–92.

80. Brown AW, Brierley JB. The earliest alterations in rat neurones and astrocytes after anoxia-ischaemia. *Acta Neuropathol* 1973;23:9–22.

81. Lyen KR, Lingam S, Butterfill AM, et al. Multicystic encephalomalacia due to fetal viral encephalitis. *Eur J Pediatr* 1981;137:11–16.

82. Weiss JL, Cleary-Goldman J, Tanji K, et al. Multicystic encephalomalacia after first-trimester intrauterine fetal death in monochorionic twins. *Am J Obstet Gynecol* 2004;190:563–656.

83. Vasileiadis GT, Roukema HW, Romano W, et al. Intrauterine herpes simplex infection. *Am J Perinatol* 2003;20:55–58.

84. Brann AW, Myers RE. Central nervous system findings in the newborn monkey following severe *in utero* partial asphyxia. *Neurology* 1975;25:327–338.

85. Towbin A. Cerebral hypoxic damage in fetus and newborn: basic patterns and their clinical significance. *Arch Neurol* 1969;20:35–43.

86. Skov H, Lou H, Pederson H. Perinatal brain ischaemia: impact at four years of age. *Dev Med Child Neurol* 1984;26:353–357.

87. Banker BQ, Larroche JC. Periventricular leukomalacia of infancy. *Arch Neurol* 1962;7:386–410.

88. de Reuck J, Chatta AS, Richardson EP. Pathogenesis and evolution of periventricular leukomalacia in infancy. *Arch Neurol* 1972;27:229–236.

89. Shuman RM, Selednik LL. Periventricular leukomalacia: a one-year autopsy study. *Arch Neurol* 1980;37:231–235.

90. Iida K, Takashima S, Takeuchi Y, et al. Neuropathologic study of newborns with prenatal-onset leukomalacia. *Pediatr Neurol* 1993;9:45–48.

91. Deguchi K, Oguchi K, Matsuura N, et al. Periventricular leukomalacia: relation to gestational age and axonal injury. *Pediatr Neurol* 1999;20:370–374.

92. Nelson MD, Gonzalez-Gomez I, Gilles FH. Search for human telencephalic ventriculofugal arteries. *AJNR Am J Neuroradiol* 1991;12:215–222.

93. Börch K, Greisen G. Blood flow distribution in the normal human preterm brain. *Pediatr Res* 1998;43:28–33.

94. Blankenberg FG, Loh NN, Norbash AM, et al. Impaired cerebrovascular autoregulation after hypoxic-ischemic injury in extremely low-birth-weight neonates: detection with power and pulsed wave Doppler US. *Radiology* 1997;205:563–568.

95. Young RS, Hernandez MJ, Yagel SK. Selective reduction of blood flow to white matter during hypotension in newborn dogs: a possible mechanism of periventricular leukomalacia. *Ann Neurol* 1982;12:445–448.

96. Volpe JJ. Neurologic outcome of prematurity. *Arch Neurol* 1998;55:297–300.

97. Yonezawa M, Back SA, Gan X, et al. Cystine deprivation induces oligodendroglial death: rescue by free radical scavengers and by a diffusible glial factor. *J Neurochem* 1996;67:566–573.

98. Rezaie P, Dean A. Periventricular leukomalacia, inflammation and white matter lesions within the developing nervous system. *Neuropathology* 2002;22:106–132.

99. Inder T, Mocatta T, Darlow B, et al. Elevated free radical products in the cerebrospinal fluid of VLBW infants with cerebral white matter injury. *Pediatr Res* 2002;52:213–218.

100. Baud O, Greene AE, Li J, et al. Glutathione peroxidase-catalase cooperativity is required for resistance to hydrogen peroxide by mature rat oligodendrocytes. *J Neurosci* 2004;24:1531–1540.

101. Dammann O, Durum S, Leviton A. Do white cells matter in white matter damage? *Trends Neurosci* 2002;25:20–21.

102. Barlow CF, Priebe CJ, Mulliken JB, et al. Spastic diplegia as a complication of interferon alfa-2a treatment of hemangiomas of infancy. *J Pediatr* 1998;132:527–530.

103. Grether JK, Nelson KB, Dambrosia JM, et al. Interferons and cerebral palsy. *J Pediatr* 1999;134:324–332.

104. Hagberg H. No correlation between cerebral palsy and cytokines in postnatal blood of preterms. *Pediatr Res* 2003;53:544–545.
105. Kadhim H, Tabarki B, De Prez C, et al. Cytokine immunoreactivity in cortical and subcortical neurons in periventricular leukomalacia: are cytokines implicated in neuronal dysfunction in cerebral palsy *Acta Neuropathol* 2003;105:209–216.
106. Damman O, Leviton A. Maternal intrauterine infection, cytokines, and brain damage in the preterm infant. *Pediatr Res* 1997;42:1–8.
107. Giannakopoulou C, Korakaki E, Manoura A, et al. Significance of hypocarbia in the development of periventricular leukomalacia in preterm infants. *Pediatr Int* 2004;46:268–273.
108. Fritz KI, Ashraf QM, Mishra OP, et al. Effect of moderate hypocapnic ventilation on nuclear DNA fragmentation and energy metabolism in the cerebral cortex of newborn piglets. *Pediatr Res* 2001;50:586–589.
109. Zupan V, Gonzalez P, Lacaze-Masmonteil T, et al. Periventricular leukomalacia: risk factors revisited. *Dev Med Child Neurol* 1996;38:1061–1067.
110. Perlman JM, Risser R, Broyles RS. Bilateral cystic periventricular leukomalacia in the premature infant: associated risk factors. *Pediatrics* 1996;97:822–827.
111. Baud O, Foix-L'Helias L, Kaminski M, et al. Antenatal glucocorticoid treatment and cystic periventricular leukomalacia in very premature infants. *N Engl J Med* 1999;341:1190–1196.
112. Murphy DJ, Sellers S, MacKenzie IZ, et al. Case–control study of antenatal and intrapartum risk factors for cerebral palsy in very preterm singleton babies. *Lancet* 1995;346:1449–1454.
113. Hesser U, Katz-Salamon M, Mortensson W, et al. Diagnosis of intracranial lesions in very low-birth-weight infants by ultrasound: incidence and association with potential risk factors. *Acta Paediatr Suppl* 1997;419:16–26.
114. Trounce JQ, Shaw DE, Levene MI, et al. Clinical risk factors and periventricular leucomalacia. *Arch Dis Child* 1988;63:17–22.
115. Koppelman AE. Blood pressure and cerebral ischemia in very low-birth-weight infants. *J Pediatr* 1990;116:1000–1002.
116. Perlman JM, Risser R, Broyles RS. Bilateral cystic periventricular leukomalacia in the premature infant: associated risk factors. *Pediatrics* 1996;97:822–827.
117. Ment LR, Stewart WB, Duncan CC, et al. Beagle puppy model of perinatal infarction: acute changes in cerebral blood flow and metabolism during hemorrhagic hypotension. *J Neurosurg* 1985;63:441–447.
118. Miall-Allen VM, DeVries LS, Whitelaw AGL. Mean arterial blood pressure and neonatal cerebral lesions. *Arch Dis Child* 1987;62:1068–1069.
119. Gray PH, O'Callaghan MJ, Mohay HA, et al. Maternal hypertension and neurodevelopmental outcome in very preterm infants. *Arch Dis Child Fetal Neonatal Ed* 1998;79:F88–F93.
120. Spinillo A, Capuzzo E, Cavallini A, et al. Preeclampsia, preterm delivery, and infant cerebral palsy. *Eur J Obstet Gynecol Reprod Biol* 1998;77:151–155.
121. Hirtz DG, Nelson K. Magnesium sulfate and cerebral palsy in premature infants. *Curr Opin Pediatr* 1998;10:131–137.
122. Wilson-Costello D, Borawski E, Friedman H, et al. Perinatal correlates of cerebral palsy and other neurologic impairment among very-low-birth-weight children. *Pediatrics* 1998;102:315–322.
123. Vohr BR, Wright LL, Dusick AM, et al. Center differences and outcomes of extremely low birth weight infants. *Pediatrics* 2004;113:781–789.
124. Pidcock FS, Graziani LJ, Stanley C, et al. Neurosonographic features of periventricular echodensities associated with cerebral palsy in preterm infants. *J Pediatr* 1990;116:417–422.
125. Van Wezel-Meijler G, van der Knaap MS, Sie LT, et al. Magnetic resonance imaging of the brain in premature infants during the neonatal period: normal phenomena and reflection of mild ultrasound abnormalities. *Neuropediatrics* 1998;29:89–96.
126. Rodriguez J, Claus P, Verellen G, et al. Periventricular leukomalacia: ultrasonic and neuropathological correlations. *Dev Med Child Neurol* 1990;32:347–355.
127. DeVries LS, Connell JA, Dubowitz LM, et al. Neurological, electrophysiological and MRI abnormalities in infants with extensive cystic leukomalacia. *Neuropediatrics* 1987;18:61–66.
128. Fawer CL, Calame A, Perentes E, et al. Periventricular leukomalacia: a correlative study between real-time ultrasound and autopsy findings. *Neuroradiology* 1985;27:292–300.
129. Inder TE, Huppi PS, Warfield S, et al. Periventricular white matter injury in the premature infant is followed by reduced cerebral cortical gray matter volume at term. *Ann Neurol* 1999;46:755–760.
130. Perlman JM, Rollins N, Burns D, et al. Relationship between periventricular intraparenchymal echodensities and germinal matrix-intraventricular hemorrhage in the very-low-birth-weight neonate. *Pediatrics* 1993;91:474–480.
131. Armstrong D, Norman MG. Periventricular leucomalacia in neonates: complications and sequelae. *Arch Dis Child* 1974;49:367–375.
132. Williams CE, Gunn AJ, Mallard C, et al. Outcome after ischemia in the developing sheep brain: an electroencephalographic and histological study. *Ann Neurol* 1992;31:14–21.
133. Freytag E, Lindenberg R. Neuropathological findings in patients of a hospital for the mentally deficient: a survey of 359 cases. *Johns Hopkins Med J* 1967;121:379–392.
133a. Sarnat HB. Watershed infarcts in the fetal and neonatal brainstem. An aetiology of central hypoventilation, dysphagia, Möbius syndrome and micrognathia. *Eur J Paediatr Neurol* 2004;8: 71–87.
134. Norman RM, Urich H, McMenemey WH. Vascular mechanisms of birth injury. *Brain* 1957;80:49–58.
135. Borit A, Herndon RM. The fine structure of plaques fibromyeliniques in ulegyria and in status marmoratus. *Acta Neuropathol* 1970;14:304–311.
136. Sarnat HB. Perinatal hypoxic/ischemic encephalopathy: neuropathological features. In: García JH, ed. *Neuropathology: the diagnostic approach*. St. Louis, MO: Mosby, 1997: 541–580.
137. Norman MG. On the morphogenesis of ulegyria. *Acta Neuropathol* 1981;53:331–332.
138. Marin-Padilla M. Developmental neuropathology and impact of perinatal brain damage. III. Gray matter lesions of the neocortex. *J Neuropathol Exp Neurol* 1999;58:407–429.
139. Christensen E, Melchior J. Cerebral palsy: a clinical and neuropathologic study. Clinics in Developmental Medicine #25. Heinemann Medical Books, London, 1967.
140. Anton G. Ueber die Betheiligung der grossen basalen Gehirnganglien bei Bewegungsstörungen und insbesondere bei Chorea: Mit Demonstrationen von Gehirnschnitten. *Wien Klin Wochenschr* 1893;6:859–861.
141. Vogt C, Vogt O. Zur Lehre der Erkrankungen des striären Systems. *J Psychol Neurol* 1919–1920;25:627–846.
142. Malamud N. Status marmoratus: a form of cerebral palsy following either birth injury or inflammation of the central nervous system. *J Pediatr* 1950;37:610–619.
143. Denny-Brown D. *The basal ganglia*. Oxford: Oxford University Press, 1962.
144. Pasternak JF, Gorey MT. The syndrome of acute near-total intrauterine asphyxia in the term infant. *Pediatr Neurol* 1998;18:391–398.
145. Chugani HT, Phelps ME, Mazziotta JC. Positron emission tomography study of human brain functional development. *Ann Neurol* 1987;22:487–497.
146. Menkes JH, Curran J. Clinical and magnetic resonance imaging correlates in children with extrapyramidal cerebral palsy. *AJNR Am J Neuroradiol* 1994;15:451–457.
147. Martin LJ, Brambrink AM, Lehmann C, et al. Hypoxia-ischemia causes abnormalities in glutamate transporters and death of astroglia and neurons in newborn striatum. *Ann Neurol* 1997;42:335–348.
147a. Silverstein FS, Torke L, Barks J, Johnston MV. Hypoxia-ischemia produces focal disruption of glutamate receptors in developing brain. *Brain Res* 1987;431:33–39.
147b. Ferriero DM, Holtzman DM, Black SM, et al. Neonatal mice lacking neuronal nitric oxide synthase are less vulnerable to hypoxic-ischemic injury. *Neurobiol Dis* 1996;3:64–71.
148. Back SA, Luo NI, Borenstein NS, et al. Late oligodendrocyte progenitors coincide with the developmental window of vulnerability for human perinatal white matter injury. *J Neurosci* 2001;21:11302–1312.
149. Meng SZ, Ohyu J, Takashima S. Changes in AMPA glutamate and

dopamine D_2 receptors in hypoxic-ischemic basal ganglia necrosis. *Pediatr Neurol* 1997;17:139–143.
150. Gross J, Muller I, Chen Y, et al. Perinatal asphyxia induces region-specific long-term changes in mRNA levels of tyrosine hydroxylase and dopamine D(1) and D(2) receptors in rat brain. *Brain Res Mol Brain Res* 2000;79:110–117.
151. Courville CB. Structural alterations in the cerebellum in cases of cerebral palsy: their relation to residual symptomatology in the ataxic-atonic group. *Bull Los Angeles Neurol Soc* 1959;24:148–165.
152. Sarnat HB, Alcala H. Human cerebellar hypoplasia: a syndrome of diverse causes. *Arch Neurol* 1980;37:300–305.
153. Adams RD, Prodhom LS, Rabinowicz T. Intrauterine brain death: neuroaxial reticular core necrosis. *Acta Neuropathol* 1977;40:41–49.
154. Azzarellli B, Caldemeyer KS, Phillips JP, et al. Hypoxic-ischemic encephalopathy in areas of primary myelination: a neuroimaging and PET study. *Pediatr Neurol* 1996;14:108–116.
155. Natsume J, Watanabe K, Kuno K, et al. Clinical, neurophysiologic, and neuropathological features of an infant with brain damage of total asphyxia type (Myers). *Pediatr Neurol* 1995;13:61–64.
155a. Dooley JM, Stewart WA, Hayden JD, et al. Brainstem calcification in Möbius syndrome. *Pediatr Neurol* 2004;30:39–41.
155b. Pedraza S, Gamez J, Rovira A, et al. MRI findings in Möbius syndrome: correlation with clinical features. *Neurology* 2000;55:1058–1060.
155c. Sugama S, Ariga M, Hoashi E, et al. Brainstem cranial nerve lesions in an infant with hypoxic cerebral injury. *Pediatr Neurol* 2003;29:256–259.
156. Roland EH, Hill AG, Norman MG, et al. Selective brainstem injury in an asphyxiated newborn. *Ann Neurol* 1988;23:89–92.
157. Friede RL. Ponto-subicular lesions in perinatal anoxia. *Arch Pathol* 1972;94:343–354.
158. Yates PO. Birth trauma to vertebral arteries. *Arch Dis Child* 1959;34:436–441.
159. Skullerud K, Westre B. Frequency and prognostic significance of germinal matrix hemorrhage, periventricular leukomalacia, and pontosubicular necrosis in preterm infants. *Acta Neuropathol* 1986;70:257–261.
160. Ahdab-Barmada M, Moosey J, Painter M. Pontosubicular necrosis and hyperoxemia. *Pediatrics* 1989;66:840–847.
161. Paneth N, Rudelli R, Kazan E, et al. *Brain damage in the preterm infant*. London: MacKeith Press and Cambridge University Press, 1994.
162. Skullerud K, Torvik A, Skaare-Botner L. Progressive degeneration of the cerebral cortex in infancy. *Acta Neuropathol* 1973;24:153–160.
163. Leech RW, Alvord CE Jr. Anoxic-ischemic encephalopathy in the human neonatal period: the significance of brainstem involvement. *Arch Neurol* 1977;34:109–113.
164. Schneider H, Ballowitz L, Schachinger H, et al. Anoxic encephalopathy with predominant involvement of basal ganglia, brainstem, and spinal cord in the perinatal period. *Acta Neuropathol* 1975;32:2878–2980.
165. Grafe MR, Kinney HC. Neuropathology associated with stillbirth. *Semin Perinatol* 2002;26:83–88.
166. Pullicino P, Ostrow P, Miller L, et al. Pontine ischemic rarefaction. *Ann Neurol* 1995;37:460–466.
167. Ozawa H, Nishida A, Mito T, et al. Ferritin immunohistochemical study on pontine nuclei from infants with pontosubicular neuron necrosis. *Brain Dev* 1995;17:20–23.
168. Brück Y, Bruck W, Kretzschmar HA, et al. Evidence for neuronal apoptosis in pontosubicular neuronal necrosis. *Neuropathol Appl Neurobiol* 1996;22:23–29.
169. van Landeghem FK, Felderhoff-Mueser U, Moysich A, et al. Fas (CD95/Apo-1)/Fas ligand expression in neonates with pontosubicular neuron necrosis. *Pediatr Res* 2002;51:129–135.
170. Skullerud K, Skjaeraasen J. Clinicopathological study of germinal matrix hemorrhage, pontosubicular necrosis, and periventricular leukomalacia in stillborn. *Childs Nerv Syst* 1988;4:88–91.
171. Mito T, Kamei A, Takashima S, et al. Clinicopathological study of pontosubicular necrosis. *Neuropediatrics* 1993;24:204–207.
172. Clancy RR, Sladky JT, Rorke LB. Hypoxic-ischemic spinal cord injury following perinatal asphyxia. *Ann Neurol* 1989;25:185–189.
173. Barmada MA, Moosey J, Shuman RM. Cerebral infarction with arterial occlusion in neonates. *Ann Neurol* 1979;6:495–502.
174. Fujimoto S, Yokochi K, Togari H, et al. Neonatal cerebral infarction: symptoms, CT findings, and prognosis. *Brain Dev* 1992;14:48–52.
175. Mercuri E, Rutherford M, Cowan F, et al. Early prognostic indicators in infants with neonatal cerebral infarction: a clinical, EEG and MRI study. *Pediatrics* 1999;108:39–46.
176. Sreenan C, Bhargava R, Robertson CMT. Cerebral infarction in the term newborn: Clinical presentation and long-term outcome. *J Pediatr* 2000;137:351–355.
177. Mercuri E, Cowan F, Gupte G, et al. Prothrombotic disorders and abnormal neurodevelopmental outcome in infants with neonatal cerebral infarction. *Pediatrics* 2001;107:1400–1404.
178. Golomb MR, MacGregor DL, Domi L, et al. Presumed pre- or perinatal arterial ischemic stroke: risk factors and outcomes. *Ann Neurol* 2001;50:163–168.
179. Golomb MR. The contribution of prothrombotic disorders to peri- and neonatal ischemic stroke. *Semin Thromb Hemost* 2003;29:415–424.
180. De Vries LS, Regev R, Connell JA, et al. Localized cerebral infarction in the premature infant: an ultrasound diagnosis correlated with computed tomography and magnetic resonance imaging. *Pediatrics* 1988;81:36–40.
181. Battin MR, Teele RL. Abnormal sagittal sinus blood flow in term infants following a perinatal hypoxic ischaemic insult. *Pediatr Radiol* 2003;33:559–562.
182. Shevell MI, Silver K, O'Gorman AM, et al. Neonatal dural sinus thrombosis. *Pediatr Neurol* 1989;5:161–165.
183. Voorhies TM, Lipper EG, Lee BC, et al. Occlusive vascular disease in asphyxiated newborn infants. *J Pediatr* 1984;105:92–96.
184. Dykes FD, Lazzarra A, Ahmann P, et al. Intraventricular hemorrhage: a prospective evaluation of etiopathogenesis. *Pediatrics* 1980;66:42–49.
185. Mancini CM, de Coo IF, Lequin MH, et al. Hereditary porencephaly: clinical and MRI findings in two Dutch families. *Eur J Paediatr Neurol* 2004;8:45–54.
186. Aguglia U, Gambardella A, Breedveld GI, et al. Suggestive evidence for linkage to chromosome 13qter for autosomal dominant type I porencephaly. *Neurology* 2004;62:1613–1615.
187. Wigglesworth JS. Current problems in brain pathology in the perinatal period. In: Pape KE, Wigglesworth JS. *Perinatal brain lesions*. Boston: Blackwell, 1989: 1–23.
188. Mitchell W, O'Tuama L. Cerebral intraventricular hemorrhages in infants: a widening age spectrum. *Pediatrics* 1980;65:35–39.
189. Hayden CK, Shatturck KE, Richardson CJ, et al. Subependymal germinal matrix hemorrhage in full-term neonates. *Pediatrics* 1985;75:714–718.
190. Bergman I, Bauer RE, Barmada MA, et al. Intracerebral hemorrhage in the fullterm neonatal infant. *Pediatrics* 1985;75:488–496.
191. Trounce JQ, Rutter N, Levene MI. Periventricular leucomalacia and intraventricular haemorrhage in the preterm neonate. *Arch Dis Child* 1986;61:1196–1202.
192. Investigators DEN. The correlation between placental pathology and intraventricular hemorrhage in the preterm infant. *Pediatr Res* 1998;43:15–19.
193. Linder N, Haskin O, Levit O, et al. Risk factors for intraventricular hemorrhage in very low birth weight premature infants: A retrospective case–control study. *Pediatrics* 2003;111:e608–e615.
194. Vohr B, Ment LR. Intraventricular hemorrhage in the preterm infant. *Early Hum Dev* 1996: 44:1–16.
195. De Felice C, Toti P, Laurinu RN, et al. Early neonatal brain injury in histologic chorioamnionitis. *J Pediatr* 2001;138:101–104.
196. Perlman JM, Goodman S, Kreusser KL, et al. Reduction in intraventricular hemorrhage by elimination of fluctuating cerebral blood-flow velocity in preterm infants with respiratory distress syndrome. *N Engl J Med* 1985;312:1353–1357.
197. McCord FB, Curstedt T, Halliday HL, et al. Surfactant treatment and incidence of intraventricular haemorrhage in severe respiratory distress syndrome. *Arch Dis Child* 1988;63:10–16.
198. Weintraub Z, Solovechick M, Reichman B, et al. Effect of maternal tocolysis on the incidence of severe periventricular/

intraventricular haemorrhage in very low birthweight infants. *Arch Dis Child Fetal Neonatal Ed* 2001;85:F13–F17.
199. Salhab WA, Hynan LS, Perlman JM. Partial or complete antenatal steroids treatment and neonatal outcome in extremely low birth weight infants < or = 1000 g: is there a dose-dependent effect? *J Perinatol* 2003;23:668–672.
200. Ment LR, Vohr B, Westerveld M, et al. Outcome of children in the indomethacin intraventricular hemorrhage prevention trial. *Pediatrics* 2000;105:485–491.
201. Tsiantos A, Victorin L, Relier JP, et al. Intracranial hemorrhage in the prematurely born infant: timing of clots and evaluation of clinical signs and symptoms. *J Pediatr* 1974;85:854–859.
202. Ment LR, Duncan CC, Ehrenkranz RA, et al. Intraventricular hemorrhage in preterm neonate: timing and cerebral blood flow changes. *J Pediatr* 1984;104:419–425.
203. Levene MI, de Vries LS. Extension of neonatal intraventricular haemorrhage. *Arch Dis Child* 1984;59:631–636.
204. Babcock DS, Han BK. The accuracy of high-resolution: real-time ultrasonography of the head in infancy. *Radiology* 1981;139:665–676.
205. Volpe JJ, Herscovitch P, Perlman JM, et al. Positron emission tomography in the newborn: extensive impairment of regional cerebral blood flow with intraventricular hemorrhage and hemorrhagic intracerebral involvement. *Pediatrics* 1983;72:589–601.
206. Edvinsson L, Lou HC, Tvede K. On the pathogenesis of regional cerebral ischemia in intracranial hemorrhage: a causal influence of potassium? *Pediatr Res* 1986;20:478–480.
207. Perlman JM, Volpe JJ. Cerebral blood flow velocity in relation to intraventricular hemorrhage in the premature newborn infant. *J Pediatr* 1982;100:956–959.
208. Altman DI, Volpe JJ. Cerebral blood flow in the newborn infant: measurement and role in the pathogenesis of periventricular and intraventricular hemorrhage. *Adv Pediatr* 1987;34:111–138.
209. Younkin D. *In vivo* ^{31}P nuclear magnetic resonance measurement of chronic changes in cerebral metabolites following neonatal intraventricular hemorrhage. *Pediatrics* 1988;82:331–336.
210. Perlman JM, Risser R. Severe fetal acidemia: neonatal neurologic features and short-term outcome. *Pediatr Neurol* 1993;9:277–282.
211. Taylor GA. Effect of germinal matrix hemorrhage on terminal vein position and patency. *Pediatr Radiol* 1995;25:S37–S40.
212. Grant EG, Kerner M, Schellinger D, et al. Evolution of porencephalic cysts from intraparenchymal hemorrhage in neonates: sonographic evidence. *Am J Roentgenol* 1982;138:467–470.
213. Savman K, Nilsson UA, Blennow M, et al. Non–protein-bound iron is elevated in cerebrospinal fluid from preterm infants with posthemorrhagic ventricular dilatation. *Pediatr Res* 2001;208–212.
214. Palmer TW, Donn SM. Symptomatic subarachnoid hemorrhage in the term newborn. *J Perinatol* 1991;11:112–116.
215. Doe FD, Shuangshoti S, Netsky MG. Cryptic hemangioma of the choroid plexus. *Neurology* 1972;22:1233–1239.
216. Wakai S, Andoh Y, Nagai M, et al. Choroid plexus arteriovenous malformations in a full-term neonate. *J Neurosurg* 1990;72:127–129.
217. Volbert H, Schweitzer H. Ueber Häufigkeit, Lokalization und Aetiologie von Blutungen im Wirbelkanal bei unreifen Früchten und Frühgeburten. *Geburtshilfe Frauenheilkd* 1954;11:1041–1048.
218. Coutelle C. Ueber epidurale Blutungen in den Wirbelkanal bei Neugeborenen und Säuglingen und ihre Beziehung zu anderen perinatalen Blutungen. *Z Geburtshilfe Gynaekol* 1960;156:19–52.
219. Drillien CM. Aetiology and outcome in low-birth-weight infants. *Dev Med Child Neurol* 1972;14:563–574.
220. Paine RS, Brazelton TE, Donovan DE, et al. Evolution of postural reflexes in normal infants and in the presence of chronic brain syndromes. *Neurology* 1964;14:1036–1048.
221. Paine RS. The evolution of infantile postural reflexes in the presence of chronic brain syndromes. *Dev Med Child Neurol* 1964;6:345–361.
222. Sarnat HB, Sarnat MS. Neonatal encephalopathy following fetal distress: a clinical and electroencephalographic study. *Arch Neurol* 1976;33:696–705.
223. Levene M. Management of the asphyxiated full-term infant. *Arch Dis Child* 1993;68:612–616.
224. Sykes GS, Molloy PM, Johnson P, et al. Do Apgar scores indicate asphyxia? *Lancet* 1982;1:494–496.
225. Goldenberg RL, Huddleston JF, Nelson KG. Apgar scores and umbilical arterial pH in preterm newborn infants. *Am J Obstet Gynecol* 1984;149:651–654.
226. Casey BM, McIntire DD, Leveno KJ. The continuing value of the Apgar score for the assessment of newborn infants. *N Engl J Med.* 2001;344:467–471.
227. Nelson KB, Ellenberg J. Neonatal signs as predictors of cerebral palsy. *Pediatrics* 1979;64:225–232.
228. Moster D, Lie RT, Irgens LM, et al. The association of Apgar score with subsequent death and cerebral palsy: a population-based study in term infants. *J Pediatr* 2001;138:798–803.
229. Moster D, Lie RT, Markestad T. Joint association of Apgar scores and early neonatal symptoms with minor disabilities at school age. *Arch Dis Child Fetal Neonatal Ed* 2002;86:F16–F21.
230. DeSouza SW, Richards B. Neurological sequelae in newborn babies after perinatal asphyxia. *Arch Dis Child* 1978;53:564–569.
231. Crothers B, Paine RS. *The natural history of cerebral palsy*. Cambridge, MA: Harvard University Press, 1959.
232. Lazzara A, Ahmann P, Dykes F, et al. Clinical predictability of intraventricular hemorrhage in preterm infants. *Pediatrics* 1980;65:30–34.
233. Dubowitz LMS, Levene MI, Morante A, et al. Neurologic signs in neonatal intraventricular hemorrhage: a correlation with real-time ultrasound. *J Pediatr* 1981;99:127–133.
234. Chamnanvanakij S, Rollins N, Perlman JM. Subdural hematoma in term infants. *Pediatr Neurol* 2002;26:301–304.
235. Mizrahi EM, Kellaway P. Characterization and classification of neonatal seizures. *Neurology* 1987;37:1837–1844.
236. Bouza H, Rutherford M, Acolet D, et al. Evolution of early hemiplegic signs in full-term infants with unilateral brain lesions in the neonatal period: a prospective study. *Neuropediatrics* 1994;25:201–207.
237. Guzzetta A, Mercuri E, Rapisardi G, et al. General movements detect early signs of hemiplegia in term infants with neonatal cerebral infarction. *Neuropediatrics* 2003;34:61–66.
238. Einspieler C, Cioni G, Paolicelli PB, et al. The early markers for later dyskinetic cerebral palsy are different from those for spastic cerebral palsy. *Neuropediatrics* 2002:33:73–78.
239. Ingram TT. *Paediatric aspects of cerebral palsy*. Edinburgh: Livingstone, 1964.
240. Skatvedt M. Cerebral palsy: a clinical study of 370 cases. *Acta Paediatr Scand* 1958;46(Suppl):3.
241. Yannet H, Horton F. Hypotonic cerebral palsy in mental defectives. *Pediatrics* 1952;9:204–211.
242. Förster O. Der atonische-astatische Typus der infantilen Cerebrallähmung. *Dtsch Arch Klin Med* 1910;98:216–244.
243. Beltran RS, Coker SB. Transient dystonia of infancy: a result of intrauterine cocaine exposure? *Pediatr Neurol* 1995;12:354–356.
244. Prechtl HFR. General movement assessment as a method of developmental neurology: new paradigms and their consequences. *Dev Med Child Neurol* 2001;43:836–842.
245. Nelson KB, Ellenberg JH. Children who "outgrew" cerebral palsy. *Pediatrics* 1982;69:529–536.
246. Taudorf K, Hansen EJ, Melchior JC, et al. Spontaneous remission of cerebral palsy. *Neuropediatrics* 1986;17:19–22.
247. Koman LA, Smith BP, Shilt JS. Cerebral palsy. *Lancet* 2004;363:1619–1631.
248. Cummins SK, Nelson KB, Grether JK, et al. Cerebral palsy in four Northern California counties: births 1983 through 1985. *J Pediatr* 1993;123:230–237.
249. Stanley FJ. Survival and cerebral palsy in low-birth-weight infants: implications for perinatal care. *Paediatr Perinat Epidemiol* 1992;6:298–310.
250. Grether JK, Cummins SK, Nelson KB. The California Cerebral Palsy Project. *Pediatr Perinat Epidemiol* 1992;6:339–351.
251. Edebol-Tysk K, Hagberg B, Hagberg G. Epidemiology of spastic tetraplegic cerebral palsy in Sweden. II. Prevalence, birth data and origin. *Neuropediatrics* 1989;20:46–52.
252. Stanley FJ, Blair E, Hockey A, et al. Spastic quadriplegia in Western Australia: a genetic and epidemiological study. I: Case population and perinatal risk factors. *Dev Med Child Neurol* 1993;35:191–201.

253. Benda CE. *Developmental disorders of mentation and cerebral palsies*. New York: Grune & Stratton, 1952.
254. Krageloh-Mann I, Petrsen D, Hagberg G, et al. Bilateral spastic cerebral palsy—MRI pathology and origin. Analysis from a representative series of 56 cases. *Dev Med Child Neurol* 1995;37:379–397.
255. Okumura A, Kato T, Kuno K, et al. MRI findings in patients with spastic cerebral palsy. II. Correlation with type of cerebral palsy. *Dev Med Child Neurol* 1997;39:369–372.
256. Freud S. *Zur Kenntnis der cerebralen Diplegien des Kindesalters*. Leipzig: Deuticke, 1893.
257. Ford FR. *Diseases of the nervous system in infancy, childhood and adolescence*, 5th ed. Springfield, IL: Charles C. Thomas, 1966.
258. Olsén P, Paakko E, Vainionpaa L, et al. Magnetic resonance imaging of periventricular leukomalacia and its clinical correlation in children. *Ann Neurol* 1997;41:754–761.
259. Yokochi K, Aiba K, Horie M, et al. Magnetic resonance imaging in children with spastic diplegia: correlation with the severity of their motor and mental abnormality. *Dev Med Child Neurol* 1991;33: 18–25.
260. Yokochi K. Thalamic lesions revealed by MR associated with periventricular leukomalacia and clinical profiles of subjects. *Acta Paediatr* 1997;86:493–496.
261. Sala DA, Shulman LH, Kennedy RF, et al. Idiopathic toe-walking: a review. *Dev Med Child Neurol* 1999;41:846–848.
262. Veelken N, Hagberg B, Hagberg G, et al. Diplegic cerebral palsy in Swedish term and preterm children: differences in reduced optimality, relations to neurology and pathogenetic factors. *Neuropediatrics* 1983;14:20–28.
263. Olsén P, Vainionpaa L, Paakko E, et al. Psychological findings in preterm children related to neurologic status and magnetic resonance imaging. *Pediatrics* 1998;102:329–336.
264. Cioni G, Sales B, Paolicelli PB, et al. MRI and clinical characteristics of children with hemiplegic cerebral palsy. *Neuropediatrics* 1999;30:249–255.
265. McNutt SJ. Apoplexia neonatorum. *Am J Obstet* 1885;18:73–81.
266. Freud S, Rie O. *Klinische Studie ueber die halbseitige Cerebrallähmung der Kinder*. Vienna: M. Perles, 1891.
267. Ford FR. Cerebral birth injuries and their results. *Medicine* 1926;5:121–194.
268. Wiklund LM, Uvebrant P, Flodmark O. Morphology of cerebral lesions in children with congenital hemiplegia. *Neuroradiology* 1990;32:179–186.
269. Barkovich AJ, Chuang SH. Unilateral megalencephaly: correlation of MR imaging and pathologic characteristics. *AJNR Am J Neuroradiol* 1990;11:523–531.
270. Larroche JC. Fetal encephalopathies of circulatory origin. *Biol Neonate* 1986;50:61–74.
271. Nelson KB. Prenatal origin of hemiparetic cerebral palsy: how often and why? *Pediatrics* 1991;88:1058–1062.
272. Takanashi J, Barkovich AJ, Ferriero DM, et al. Widening spectrum of congenital hemiplegia. Periventricular venous infarction in term neonates. *Neurology* 2003;61:531–533.
273. De Vries LS, Groenendaal F, Eken P, et al. Infarcts in the vascular distribution of the middle cerebral artery in preterm and full-term infants. *Neuopediatrics* 1997;28:88–96.
274. Bouza H, Dubowitz LM, Rutherford M, et al. Late magnetic resonance imaging and clinical findings in neonates with unilateral lesions on cranial ultrasound. *Dev Med Child Neurol* 1994;36:951–964.
275. Thorarensen O, Ryan S, Hunter J, et al. Factor V Leiden mutation: an unrecognized cause of hemiplegic cerebral palsy, neonatal stroke, and placental thrombosis. *Ann Neurol* 1997;42:372–375.
276. Lanska MJ, Lanska DJ, Horwitz SJ, et al. Presentation, clinical course, and outcome of childhood stroke. *Pediatr Neurol* 1991;7:333–341.
277. Perlstein MA, Hood PN. Infantile spastic hemiplegia: incidence. *Pediatrics* 1954;14:436–441.
278. Byers RK. Evolution of hemiplegias in infancy. *Am J Dis Child* 1941;61:915–927.
278a. Staudt M, Gerloff C, Grodd W, et al. Reorganization in congenital hemiparesis acquired at different gestational ages. *Ann Neurol* 2004;56:854–863.
279. Brown JK, Rodda J, Walsh EG, et al. Neurophysiology of lower-limb function in hemiplegic children. *Dev Med Child Neurol* 1991;33:1037–1047.
280. Goutières F, Challamel MJ, Aicardi J, et al. Les hémiplégies congénitales: sémiologie, étiologie et prognostic. *Arch Fr Pediatr* 1972;29:839–851.
281. Twitchell TE. The grasping deficit in infantile hemiparesis. *Neurology* 1958;8:13–21.
282. Denny-Brown D, Chambers RA. The parietal lobe and behaviour. *Assoc Res Nerv Ment Dis Proc* 1958;36:35–117.
283. Cohen ME, Duffner PK. Prognostic indicators in hemiparetic cerebral palsy. *Ann Neurol* 1981;9:353–357.
284. Nass R. Mirror movement asymmetries in congenital hemiparesis: the inhibition hypothesis revisited. *Neurology* 1985;35:1059–1062.
285. Tizard JP, Paine RS, Crothers B. Disturbances of sensation in children with hemiplegia. *JAMA* 1954;155:628–632.
286. Delgado MR, Riela AR, Mills J, et al. Discontinuation of antiepileptic drug treatment after two seizure-free years in children with cerebral palsy. *Pediatrics* 1996;97:192–197.
287. Cohen P, Kohn JG. Follow-up study of patients with cerebral palsy. *West J Med* 1979;130:6–11.
288. Kyllerman M. *Dyskinetic cerebral palsy*. London: Allen and Unwin, 1981.
289. Brun A, Kyllerman M. Clinical, pathogenetic and neuropathologic correlates in dystonic cerebral palsy. *Eur J Pediatr* 1979;131: 93–104.
290. Audry J. *Étude de pathologie nerveuse. L'athétose double et les chorées chroniques de l'enfance*. Paris: J.B. Baillière, 1892.
291. Hagberg B, Hagberg G, Olow I. The changing panorama of cerebral palsy in Sweden, 1954–1970. II. Analysis of the various syndromes. *Acta Paediatr Scand* 1975;64:187–200.
292. Kyllerman M, Bager B, Bensch J, et al. Dyskinetic cerebral palsy. I. Clinical categories, associated neurologic abnormalities and incidences. *Acta Paediatr Scand* 1982;71:543–550.
293. Kyllerman M. Dyskinetic cerebral palsy. II. Pathogenetic risk factors and intrauterine growth. *Acta Paediatr Scand* 1982;71: 551–558.
294. Rosenbloom L. Dyskinetic cerebral palsy and birth asphyxia. *Dev Med Child Neurol* 1994;36:285–289.
295. Polani PE. The clinical natural history of choreoathetoid cerebral palsy. *Guy Hosp Rep* 1959;108:32–45.
296. Bobath KA. Neurophysiological basis for the treatment of cerebral palsy. *Clin Dev Med* 1991;75:73.
297. Saint Hilaire MH, Burke RE, Bressman SB, et al. Delayed-onset dystonia due to perinatal or early childhood asphyxia. *Neurology* 1991;41:216–222.
298. Deonna TW, Ziegler AL, Nielsen J. Transient idiopathic dystonia in infancy. *Neuropediatrics* 1991;22:220–224.
299. Carlsson M, Hagberg G, Olsson I. Clinical and aetiological aspects of epilepsy in children with cerebral palsy. *Dev Med Child Neurol* 2003;45:371–376.
300. Hayashi M, Satoh J, Sakamoto K, et al. Clinical and neuropathological findings in severe athetoid cerebral palsy: a comparative study of globo-luysian and thalamo-putaminal groups. *Brain Dev* 1991;13:47–51.
301. Malamud N, Itabashi HH, Castor-Messinger HB. An etiologic and diagnostic study of cerebral palsy. *J Pediatr* 1964;66:270–293.
302. Lesny IA. Follow-up study of hypotonic forms of cerebral palsy. *Brain Dev* 1979;1:87–90.
303. Fenichel GM. Cerebral influence on muscle fiber typing: the effect of fetal immobilization. *Arch Neurol* 1969;20:644–649.
304. Iannaccone ST, Bove KE, Vogler CA, et al. Type 1 fiber size disproportion: morphometric data from 37 children with myopathic, neuropathic, or idiopathic hypotonia. *Pediatr Pathol* 1987;7:395–419.
305. MacLennan A. A template for defining a causal relation between acute intrapartum events and cerebral palsy: international consensus statement. *Br Med J* 1999;319:1054–1059.
306. Rosenbloom, L, Rennie JM. Birth asphyxia and cerebral palsy. *Br Med J*. 2000;320:1076.
307. Dear P, Newell S. Establishing probable cause in cerebral palsy. *Br Med J* 2000;320:1075–1076.
308. Painter MJ. Fetal heart rate patterns, perinatal asphyxia, and brain injury. *Pediatr Neurol* 1989;5:137–144.

309. Valentin L, Ekman G, Isberg PE, et al. Clinical evaluation of the fetus and neonate: relation between intra-partum cardiotocography, Apgar score, cord blood acid-base status and neonatal morbidity. *Arch Gynecol Obstet* 1993;253:103–115.
310. Nelson KB, Dambrosia JM, Ting TY, et al. Uncertain value of electronic fetal monitoring in predicting cerebral palsy. *N Engl J Med* 1996;334:613–618.
311. Meis PJ, Hall M, Marshall JR, et al. Meconium passage: a new classification for risk assessment during labor. *Am J Obstet Gynecol* 1978;131:509–513.
312. Socol ML, Garcia PM, Riter S. Depressed Apgar scores, acid-base status, and neurologic outcome. *Am J Obstet Gynecol* 1994;170:991–998.
313. Perlman JM, Risser R. Can asphyxiated infants at risk for neonatal seizures be rapidly identified by current high-risk markers? *Pediatrics* 1996;97:456–462.
314. Sehdev HM, Stamilio DM, Macones GA, et al. Predictive factors for neonatal morbidity in neonates with an umbilical arterial cord pH less than 7.00. *Am J Obstet Gynecol* 1997;177:1030–1034.
315. Hermansen MC. The acidosis paradox: asphyxial brain injury without coincident acidemia. *Dev Med Child Neurol* 2003;45:353–356.
316. Lin JP. The acidosis paradox: asphyxial brain injury without coincident acidemia. *Dev Med Child Neurol* 2003;45:431.
317. Schurr A. Bench-to-bedside review: A possible resolution of the glucose paradox of cerebral ischemia. *Crit Care* 2002;6:330–334.
318. Belai Y, Goodwin TM, Durand M, et al. Umbilical arteriovenous pO_2 and pCO_2 differences and neonatal morbidity in term infants with severe acidosis. *Am J Obstet Gynecol* 1998;178:13–19.
318a. Salhab WA, Wyckoff MH, Laptook AR, Perlman JM. Initial hypoglycemia and neonatal brain injury in term infants with severe fetal acidemia. *Pediatrics* 2004;114:361–366.
319. Blair E, Stanley F. Intrauterine growth and spastic cerebral palsy. I. Association with birth weight for gestational age. *Am J Obstet Gynecol* 1990;162:229–237.
320. Amiel-Tison C, Pettigrew AG. Adaptive changes in the developing brain during intrauterine stress. *Brain Dev* 1991;13:67–76.
321. Sommerfelt K, Sonnander K, Skranes J, et al. Neuropsychologic and motor function in small-for-gestation preschoolers. *Pediatr Neurol* 2002;26:186–191.
322. Sommerfelt K, Andersson HW, Sonnadner K, et al. Cognitive development of term small for gestational age children at five years of age. *Arch Dis Child* 2000;83:25–30.
323. Committee on Fetus and Newborn, American Academy of Pediatrics. Use and abuse of the Apgar score. *Pediatrics* 1996;98:141–142.
324. Sarnat HB. Watershed infarcts in the fetal and neonatal brainstem. An aetiology of central hypoventilation, dysphagia, Möbius syndrome and micrognathia. *Eur J Paediatr Neurol* 2004;8:71–87.
325. Brazy JE, Kinney HC, Oakes WJ. Central nervous system structural lesions causing apnea at birth. *J Pediatr* 1987;111:163–175.
326. Jensen A, Garnier Y, Berger R. Dynamics of fetal circulatory responses to hypoxia and asphyxia. *Eur J Obstet Gynecol Reprod Biol* 1999;84:155–172.
327. Shah P, Riphagen S, Beyene J, et al. Multiorgan dysfunction in infants with post-asphyxial hypoxic-ischemic encephalopathy. *Arch Dis Child Fetal Neonatal Ed* 2004;89:F152–F155.
328. Freeman JM, Nelson KB. Intrapartum asphyxia and cerebral palsy. *Pediatrics* 1988;82:240–249.
329. Naeye RL, Localio AR. Determining the time before birth when ischemia and hypoxemia initiate ceebral palsy. *Obstet Gynecol* 1995;86:713–719.
330. Hermanson MC. Nucleated red blood cells in the fetus and newborn. *Arch Dis Child Fetal Neonatal Ed* 2001;84:F211–F215.
331. Volpe JJ. Neonatal intracranial hemorrhage. *Clin Perinatol* 1977;4:77–102.
332. Tourtellotte WW, Somers JF, Parker JA, et al. et al. A study on traumatic lumbar punctures. *Neurology* 1958;8:159–160.
333. Svenningsen NW, Siesjö BK. Cerebrospinal fluid lactate/pyruvate ratio in normal and asphyxiated neonates. *Acta Paediatr Scand* 1972;61:117–124.
334. Walsh P, Jedeikin R, Ellis G, et al. Assessment of neurologic outcome in asphyxiated term infants by use of serial CK-BB isoenzyme measurement. *J Pediatr* 1982;101:988–992.
335. Biagioni E, Mercuri E, Rutherford M, et al. Combined use of electroencephalogram and magnetic resonance imaging in full-term neonates with acute encephalopathy. *Pediatrics* 2001;107:461–466.
336. Holmes GL, Lombroso CT. Prognostic value of background patterns in the neonatal EEG. *J Clin Neurophysiol.* 1993;10:323–352.
337. Biagioni E, Boldrini A, Bottone U, et al. Prognostic value of abnormal EEG transients in preterm and full-term neonates. *Electroencephalogr Clin Neurophysiol.* 1996;99:1–9.
338. Toet MC, Hellstrom-Westas L, Groenendaal F, et al. Amplitude integrated EEG 3 and 6 hours after birth in full term neonates with hypoxic-ischemic encephalopathy. *Arch Dis Child Fetal Neonatal Ed* 1999;81:F19–F23.
339. Baud O, d'Allest AM, Lacaze-Marmonteil T, et al. The early diagnosis of periventricular leukomalacia in premature infants with positive rolandic sharp waves on serial electroencephalography. *J Pediatr* 1998;132:813–817.
340. Vermeulen RJ, Sie LT, Jonkman EJ, et al. Predictive value of EEG in neonates with periventricular leukomalacia. *Dev Med Child Neurol* 2003;45:586–590.
341. Levene MI, Williams JL, Fawer CL. *Ultrasound of the infant brain*. Oxford: Blackwell, 1985.
342. Partridge JC, Babcock DS, Steichen JJ, et al. Optimal timing for diagnostic cranial ultrasound in low-birth-weight infants: detection of intracranial hemorrhage and ventricular dilation. *J Pediatr* 1983;102:281–287.
343. Graham M, Leven ML, Trounce JO, et al. Prediction of cerebral palsy in very low-birth-weight infants: prospective ultrasound study. *Lancet* 1987;2:593–596.
344. Fawer CL, Deibold P, Calame A. Periventricular leucomalacia and neurodevelopmental outcome in preterm infants. *Arch Dis Child* 1987;62:30–36.
345. Eken P, Jansen GH, Groenendaal F, et al. Intracranial lesions in the full-term infant with hypoxic ischaemic encephalopathy: ultrasound and autopsy correlation. *Neuropediatrics* 1994;25:301–307.
346. Shen EY, Huang CC, Chyou SC, et al. Sonographic finding of the bright thalamus. *Arch Dis Child* 1986;61:1096–1099.
347. Shewmon DA, Fine M, Masden JC, Palacios E. Postischemic hypervascularity of infancy: a stage in the evolution of ischemic brain damage with characteristic CT scan. *Ann Neurol* 1981;9:358–365.
348. Hope PL, Gould SJ, Howard S, et al. Precision of ultrasound diagnosis of pathologically verified lesions in the brains of very preterm infants. *Dev Med Child Neurol* 1988;30:457–471.
349. Fitzhardinge PM, Flodmark O, Fitz CR, et al. The prognostic value of computed tomography of the brain in asphyxiated premature infants. *J Pediatr* 1982;100:476–481.
350. Picard L, Claudon M, Roland J, et al. Cerebral computed tomography in premature infants with an attempt at staging developmental features. *J Comput Assist Tomogr* 1980;4:435–444.
351. Cowan FM, Pennock JM, Hanrahan JD, et al. Early detection of cerebral infarction and hypoxic ischemic encephalopathy in neonates using diffusion-weighted magnetic resonance imaging. *Neuropediatrics* 1994;25:172–175.
352. Sie LT, Barkhof F, Lafeber HN, et al. Value of fluid-attenuated recovery sequences in early MRI of the brain in neonates with a perinatal hypoxic-ischemic encephalopathy. *Eur Radiol* 2000;10:1594–1601.
353. Barkovich AJ. Perinatal asphyxia: MR findings in the first 10 days. *AJNR Am J Neuroradiol* 1995;16:427–438.
354. Sie LT, van der Knaap MS, Oosting J, et al. MR patterns of hypoxic-ischemic damage after prenatal, perinatal or postnatal asphyxia. *Neuropediatrics* 2000;31:128–136.
355. Mercuri E, Rutherford M, Barnett A, et al. MRI lesions in infants with neonatal encephalopathy. Is the Apgar score predictive? *Neuropediatris* 2002;35:150–156.
356. Sugama S, Eto Y. Brainstem lesions in children with perinatal brain injury. *Pediatr Neurol* 2003;28:212–215.
357. Barkovich AJ, Truwit CL. Brain damage from perinatal asphyxia: correlation of MR findings with gestational age. *AJNR Am J Neuroradiol* 1990;11:1087–1096.
358. Keeney SE, Adcock EW, McArdle CB. Prospective observations of 100 high-risk neonates by high field (1.5 Tesla) magnetic resonance imaging of the central nervous system. II. Lesions associated with hypoxic-ischemic encephalopathy. *Pediatrics* 1991;87:431–438.

359. Roland EH, Flodmark O, Hill A. Thalamic hemorrhage with intraventricular hemorrhage in the full-term newborn. *Pediatrics* 1990;85:737–742.
360. Michoni G, Willinsky R. Rapid postanoxic calcification of the basal ganglia. *Neurology* 1992;42:2144–2146.
361. Byrne P, Welch R, Johnson MA, et al. Serial magnetic resonance imaging in neonatal hypoxic-ischemic encephalopathy. *J Pediatr* 1990;117:694–700.
362. Huppi PS, Murphy B, Maier SE, et al. Microstructural brain development after perinatal cerebral white matter injury assessed by diffusion tensor magnetic resonance imaging. *Pediatrics* 2001;107:455–460.
363. Marin-Padilla M. Developmental neuropathology and impact of perinatal brain damage. II. White matter lesions of the neocortex. *J Neuropathol Exp Neurol* 1997;56:219–235.
364. Nagy Z, Westerberg H, Skare S, et al. Preterm children have disturbances of white matter at 11 years of age as shown by diffusion tensor imaging. *Pediatr Res* 2003;54:672–679.
365. Holland BA, Haas DK, Norman D, et al. MRI of normal brain maturation. *AJNR Am J Neuroradiol* 1986;7:201–208.
366. Johnson MA, Pennock JM, Bydder GM, et al. Serial imaging in neonatal cerebral injury. *AJNR Am J Neuroradiol* 1987;8:83–92.
367. van de Bor M, Guit GL, Schreuder AM, et al. Early detection of delayed myelination in preterm infants. *Pediatrics* 1989;84:407–411.
368. Lou HC, Skov H, Henricksen L. Intellectual impairment with regional cerebral dysfunction after low neonatal cerebral blood flow. *Acta Paediatr Scand* 1989;36(Suppl):72–82.
369. Rosenbaum JL, Almli CR, Yundt KD, et al. Higher neonatal cerebral blood flow correlates with worse childhood neurologic outcome. *Neurology* 1997;49:1035–1041.
370. Thorngren-Jerneck K, Ohlsson T, Sandell A, et al. Cerebral glucose metabolism measured by positron emission tomography in term newborn infants with hypoxic ischemic encephalopathy. *Pediatr Res* 2001;49:495–501.
371. Kerrigan JF, Chugani HT, Phelps ME. Regional cerebral glucose metabolism in clinical subtypes of cerebral palsy. *Pediatr Neurol* 1991;7:415–425.
372. Novotny E, Ashwal S, Shevell M. Proton magnetic resonance spectroscopy: an emerging technology in pediatric neurology research. *Pediatr Res* 1998;44:1–10.
373. Hanrahan JD, Cox IJ, Azzopardi D, et al. Relation between proton magnetic resonance spectroscopy within 18 hours of birth asphyxia and neurodevelopment at 1 year of age. *Dev Med Child Neurol* 1999;41:76–82.
374. Robertson NJ, Cox IJ, Cowan FM, et al. Cerebral intracellular lactic alkalosis persisting months after neonatal encephalopathy measured by magnetic resonance spectroscopy. *Pediatr Res* 1999;46:287–296.
375. Hanrahan JD, Cox IJ, Edwards AD, et al. Persistent increases in cerebral lactate concentration after birth asphyxia. *Pediatr Res* 1998;44:304–311.
376. Miller SP, Newton N, Ferreiro DM, et al. Prediction of 30-month outcome after perinatal depression: role of proton MRS and socioeconomic factors. *Pediatr Res* 2002;52:71–77.
377. Robertson NJ, Cowan FM, Cox IJ, et al. Brain alkaline intracellular pH after neonatal encephalopathy. *Ann Neurol* 2002;52:732–742.
378. Robertson NJ, Stafler P, Battini R, et al. Brain lactic alkalosis in Aicardi-Goutieres syndrome. *Neuropediatrics* 2004;35:20–26.
379. Penrice J, Cady EB, Lorek A, et al. Proton magnetic resonance spectroscopy of the brain in normal preterm and term infants, and early changes after perinatal hypoxia-ischemia. *Pediatr Res* 1996;40:6–14.
380. Hamilton PA, Hope PL, Cady EB, et al. Impaired energy metabolism in brains of newborn infants with increased cerebral echo-densities. *Lancet* 1986;1:1242–1246.
381. Gadian DG, Williams SR, Bates TE, et al. NMR spectroscopy: current status and future possibilities. *Acta Neurochir* 1993;57(Suppl):18.
382. Moorcraft J, Bolas NM, Ives NK, et al. Spatially localized magnetic resonance spectroscopy of the brains of normal and asphyxiated newborns. *Pediatrics* 1991;87:273–282.
383. Despland PA, Galambos R. The auditory brain stem response (ABR) is a useful diagnostic tool in the intensive care nursery. *Pediatr Res* 1980;14:154–158.
384. Muttitt SC, Taylor MJ, Kobayashi JS, et al. Serial visual evoked potentials and outcome in term birth asphyxia. *Pediatr Neurol* 1991;7:86–90.
385. Raju TNK. Cerebral Doppler studies in the fetus and newborn infant. *J Pediatr* 1991;119:165–174.
386. Ilves P, Lintrop M, Metsvaht T, et al. Cerebral blood-flow velocities in predicting outcome of asphyxiated newborn infants. *Acta Paediatr* 2004;93:523–528.
387. Batten MR, Penrice J, Gunn TR, et al. Treatment of term infants with head cooling and mild systemic hypothermia (35.0°C and 34.5°C) after perinatal asphyxia. *Pediatrics* 2003;111:244–251.
388. Vanucci RC, Perlman JM. Interventions for perinatal hypoxic-ischemic encephalopathy. *Pediatrics* 1997;100:1004–1014.
389. Wahlestedt C, Golanov E, Yamamoto S, et al. Antisense oligodeoxynucleotides to NMDA-R1 receptor channel protect cortical neurons from excitotoxicity and reduce focal ischaemic infarctions. *Nature* 1993;363:260–263.
390. Ment LR, Oh W, Ehrenkranz RA, et al. Low-dose indomethacin and prevention of intraventricular hemorrhage: a multicenter randomized trial. *Pediatrics* 1994;93:543–550.
391. Yanowitz TD, Baker RW, Sobchak Brozanski B. Prophylactic indomethacin reduces grades III and IV intraventricular hemorrhages when compared to early indomethacin treatment of a patent ductus arteriosus. *J Perinatol* 2003;23:317–322.
392. Yanowitz TD, Yao AC, Werner JC, et al. Effects of prophylactic low-dose indomethacin on hemodynamics in very low-birth-weight infants. *J Pediatr* 1998;132:28–34.
393. Volpe J. Brain injury caused by intraventricular hemorrhage: is indomethacin the silver bullet for prevention? *Pediatrics* 1994;93:673–677.
394. Benson JWT, Drayton MR, Hayward C, et al. Multicentre trial of ethamsylate for prevention of periventricular hemorrhage in very low-birth-weight infants. *Lancet* 1986;2:1297–1300.
395. Shankaran S, Papile LA, Wright LL, et al. The effects of antenatal phenobarbital therapy on neonatal intracranial hemorrhage in preterm infants. *N Engl J Med* 1997;337:466–471.
396. Brion LP, Bell EF, Raghuveer TS. Vitamin E supplementation for prevention of morbidity and mortality in preterm infants. *Cochrane Database Syst Rev* 2003;CD003665.
397. Crowther CA, Hiller JE, Doyle LW, et al. Effect of magnesium sulfate given for neuroprotection before preterm birth: a randomized, controlled trial. *Obstet Gynecol Surv* 2004;59:330–332.
398. Engelhard HH, Andrews CO, Slavin KV, et al. Current management of intraventricular hemorrhage. *Surg Neurol* 2003;60:15–21.
399. Kennedy CR, Ayers S, Campbell MJ, et al. Randomized, controlled trial of acetazolamide and furosemide in posthemorrhagic ventricular dilatation in infancy: follow-up at 1 year. *Pediatrics* 2001;108:597–607.
400. Fletcher JM, Landry SH, Bohan TP, et al. Effects of intraventricular hemorrhage and hydrocephalus on the long-term neurobehavioral development of preterm very-low-birth-weight infants. *Dev Med Child Neurol* 1997;39:596–606.
401. Tizard JPM. Cerebral palsies: treatment and prevention. The Croonian lecture 1978. *J R Coll Physicians Lond* 1980;14:72–77.
402. Graham HK, Aoki KR, Autti-Rämö I, et al. Recommendations for the use of botulinum toxin type A in the management of cerebral palsy. *Gait Posture* 2000;11:67–79.
403. Paine RS. On the treatment of cerebral palsy: the outcome of 177 patients, 74 totally untreated. *Pediatrics* 1962;29:605–616.
404. Fixsen JA. Orthopedic management of cerebral palsy. *Arch Dis Child* 1994;71:396–397.
405. Wright T, Nicholson J. Physiotherapy for the spastic child: an evaluation. *Dev Med Child Neurol* 1973;15:146–163.
406. Palmer FB, Shapiro BK, Wachtel RC, et al. The effects of physical therapy on cerebral palsy: a controlled trial in infants with spastic diplegia. *N Engl J Med* 1988;318:803–808.
407. Bower E, Michell D, Burnett M, et al. Randomized controlled trial of physiotherapy in 56 children with cerebral palsy followed for 18 months. *Dev Med Child Neurol* 2001;43:4–15.

408. Tardieu C, Lespargot A, Tabary C, et al. For how long must the soleus muscle be stretched each day to prevent contracture? *Dev Med Child Neurol* 1988;30:3–10.
409. Law M, Russell D, Pollock N, et al. A comparison of intensive neurodevelopmental therapy plus casting and a regular occupational therapy program for children with cerebral palsy. *Dev Med Child Neurol* 1997;39:664–670.
410. Goldner JL. The upper extremity in cerebral palsy. In: Samilson RL, ed. *Orthopaedic aspects of cerebral palsy*. Philadelphia: Lippincott, 1975.
411. Willis JK, Morello A, Davie A, et al. Forced use treatment of childhood hemiparesis. *Pediatrics* 2002;110:94–96.
412. Gerszten PC, Albright AL, Johnstone GF. Intrathecal baclofen infusion and subsequent orthopedic surgery in patients with spastic cerebral palsy. *J Neurosurg* 1998;88:1099–1013.
413. Awaad Y, Tayem H, Munoz S, et al. Functional assessment following intrathecal baclofen therapy in children with spastic cerebral palsy. *J Child Neurol* 2003: 18:26–34.
414. Sussman MD, Aionna MD. Treatment of spastic diplegia in patients with cerebral palsy. *J Pediatr Orthop B* 2004:13:S1–S12.
415. Gooch JL, Oberg WA, Grams B, et al. Complications of intrathecal baclofen pumps in children. *Pediatr Neurosurg* 2003:39:1–6.
416. Jefferson RJ. Botulin toxin in the management of cerebral palsy. *Dev Med Child Neurol* 2004;46:491–499.
417. Wong V. Use of botulinum toxin injection in 17 children with spastic cerebral palsy. *Pediatr Neurol* 1998;18:124–131.
418. Graham HK, Aoki KR, Autti-Ramo I, et al. Recommendations for the use of botulinum toxin type A in the management of cerebral palsy. *Gait Posture* 2000:11:67–79.
419. Forssberg H, Tedroff KB. Botulinum toxin treatment in cerebral palsy: intervention with poor evaluation. *Dev Med Child Neurol* 1997;39:635–640.
420. Graham HK. Botulinum toxin A in cerebral palsy. Functional outcomes. *J Pediatr* 2000;137:300–303.
421. Killackey HP, Rhades RW, Bennett-Clarke CA. The formation of a cortical somatotopic map. *Trends Neurosci* 1995;18:402–407.
422. Ferry PC. Infant stimulation programs: a neurologic shell game? *Arch Neurol* 1986;43:281–282.
423. Russman BS. Are infant stimulation programs useful? *Arch Neurol* 1986;43:282–283.
424. Graham HK. Painful hip dislocation in cerebral palsy. *Lancet* 2002;359:907–908.
425. Owens KL, Pyman J, Gargan MF, et al. Bilateral hip surgery in severe cererebral palsy. *J Bone Joint Surg* 2001;83B:1161–1167.
426. Park TS, Owen JH. Surgical management of spastic diplegia in cerebral palsy. *N Engl J Med* 1992;326:745–749.
427. Banks HH. The foot and ankle in cerebral palsy. In: Samilson RL, ed. *Orthopaedic aspects of cerebral palsy*. Philadelphia: Lippincott, 1975.
428. Ruda R, Frost HM. Cerebral palsy: spastic varus and forefoot adductus treated by intramuscular posterior tibial tendon lengthening. *Clin Orthop* 1971;79:61–70.
429. Damron T, Breen AL, Roecker E. Hamstring tenotomies in cerebral palsy: long-term analysis. *J Pediatr Orthop* 1991;514–519.
430. Peacock WJ, Arens LJ, Berman B. Cerebral palsy spasticity: selective posterior rhizotomy. *Pediatr Neurosci* 1987;13:61–66.
431. Steinbok P, Reiner AM, Beauchamp R, et al. A randomized clinical trial to compare selective posterior rhizotomy plus physiotherapy with physiotherapy alone in children with spastic diplegic cerebral palsy. *Dev Med Child Neurol* 1997;39:178–184.
432. McLaughlin JF, Bjornson KF, Astley SJ, et al. Selective dorsal rhizotomy: efficacy and safety in an investigator-masked randomized clinical trial. *Dev Med Child Neurol* 1998;40:220–232.
433. Peacock WJ, Staudt LA. Spasticity in cerebral palsy and the selective posterior rhizotomy procedure. *J Child Neurol* 1990;5:179–185.
434. Bleck EE. Posterior rootlet rhizotomy in cerebral palsy. *Arch Dis Child* 1993;68:717–719.
435. Dormans JP. Orthopedic management of children with cerebral palsy. *Pediatr Clin North Am* 1993;40:645–657.
436. Tilton AD. Approach to the rehabilitation of spasticity and neuromuscular disorder in children. *Neurol Clin* 2003;21:853–881.
437. Bobath B, Bobath K. *Motor development in the different types of cerebral palsy*. London: Heineman, 1975.
438. Black P. Visual disorders associated with cerebral palsy. *Br J Ophthalmol* 1982;66:46–52.
439. Buckley E, Seaber JH. Dyskinetic strabismus as: a sign of cerebral palsy. *Am J Ophthalmol* 1981;91:652–657.
440. Mercuri E, Anker S, Guzzetta A, et al. Visual function at school age in children with neonatal encephalopathy and low Apgar scores. *Arch Dis Child Fetal Neonatal Ed* 2004;89:F258–F262.
441. Cocker KD, Moseley MJ, Stirling HF, et al. Delayed visual maturation: pupillary responses implicate subcortical and cortical visual systems. *Dev Med Child Neurol* 1998;40:160–162.
442. Huo R, Burden SK, Hoyt CS, et al. Chronic cortical visual impairment in children: aetiology, prognosis, and associated neurological deficits. *Br J Ophthalmol* 1999;83:670–675.
443. Foley J, Gordon N. Recovery from cortical blindness. *Dev Med Child Neurol* 1985;27:383–387.
444. Menkes JH, Ament ME. Neurologic disorders of gastroesophageal function. *Adv Neurol* 1988;49:409–416.
445. Reilly S, Skuse D. Characteristics and management of feeding problems of young children with cerebral palsy. *Dev Med Child Neurol* 1992;34:379–388.
446. Yossen F. Personal communication, 1989.
447. Jongerius PH, van Tiel P, van Limbeek J, et al. A systematic review for evidence of efficacy of anticholinergic drugs to treat drooling. *Arch Dis Child* 2003;88:911–914.
448. Jean A. Brain stem control of swallowing: neuronal network and cellular mechanisms. *Physiol Rev* 2001;81:929–969.
449. Reid CJD, Borzyskowski M. Lower urinary tract dysfunction in cerebral palsy. *Arch Dis Child* 1993;68:739–742.
450. Dubowitz L, Dubowitz V. The neurological assessment of the preterm and full-term newborn infant. *Clinics in Developmental Medicine* Vol 79, 1981.
451. Robertson CMT, Finer NN. Long-term follow-up of term neonates with perinatal asphyxia. *Clin Perinatol* 1993;20:483–500.
452. Handley-Derry M, Low JA, Burke SO, et al. Intrapartum fetal asphyxia and the occurrence of minor deficits in 4- to 8-year-old children. *Dev Med Child Neurol* 1997: 39:508–514.
453. Temple CM, Dennis J, Carney R, et al. Neonatal seizures: long-term outcome and cognitive development among "normal" survivors. *Dev Med Child Neurol* 1995;37:109–118.
454. Brunquell PJ, Glennon CM, DiMario FJ, et al. Prediction of outcome based in clinical seizure type in newborn infants. *J Pediatr* 2002;140:707–712.
455. Perlman JM, Tack ED. Renal injury in the asphyxiated newborn: relationship to neurologic outcome. *J Pediatr* 1988;113:875–879.
456. Janowsky JS, Finlay BL. The outcome of perinatal brain damage: the role of normal neuron loss and axon retraction. *Dev Med Child Neurol* 1986;28:375–389.
457. Ergander U, Eriksson M, Zetterstrom R. Severe neonatal asphyxia: incidence and prediction of outcome in the Stockholm area. *Acta Paediatr Scand* 1983;72:321–325.
458. Drage JS, Kennedy C, Berendes H, et al. The Apgar score as an index of infant morbidity: a report from the collaborative study of cerebral palsy. *Dev Med Child Neurol* 1966;8:141–148.
459. Dennis J, Johnson A, Mutch L, et al. Acid-base status at birth and neurodevelopmental outcome at four-and-one-half years. *Am J Obstet Gynecol* 1989;161:213–220.
460. Dijxhoorn MJ, Visser GH, Fidler VJ, et al. Apgar score, meconium, and acidaemia at birth in relation to neonatal neurological morbidity in term infants. *Br J Obstet Gynaecol* 1986;93:217–222.
461. Fee SC, Malee K, Deddish R, et al. Severe acidosis and subsequent neurologic status. *Am J Obstet Gynecol* 1990;162:802–806.
462. Painter MJ, Depp R, O'Donoghue MN. Fetal heart rate patterns and development in the first year of life. *Am J Obstet Gynecol* 1978;132:271–277.
463. Ekert P, Perlman M, Steinlin M, et al. Predicting the outcome of postasphyxial hypoxic-ischemic encephalopathy within 4 hours of birth. *J Pediatr* 1997;131:613–617.
464. Majnemer A, Mazer B. Neurologic evaluation of the newborn infant: definition and psychometric properties. *Dev Med Child Neurol* 1998;40:708–715.
465. Holmes G, Lombroso CT. Prognostic value of background patterns in the neonatal EEG. *J Clin Neurophysiol* 1993;10:323–352.

466. Sinclair DB, Campbell M, Byrne P, et al. EEG and long-term outcome of term infants with neonatal hypoxic-ischemic encephalopathy. *Clin Neurophysiol* 1999;110:655–659.
467. Zeinstra E, Fock JM, Begeer JH, et al. The prognostic value of serial EEG recordings following acute neonatal asphyxia in full-term infants. *Eur J Paediatr Neurol* 2001;5:155–160.
468. Roland EH, Poskitt K, Rodriguez E, et al. Perinatal hypoxic-ischemic thalamic injury: clinical features and neuroimaging. *Ann Neurol* 1998;44:161–166.
469. Rutherford MA, Pennock JM, Counsell SJ, et al. Abnormal magnetic resonance signal in the internal capsule predicts poor neurodevelopmental outcome in infants with hypoxic-ischemic encephalopathy. *Pediatrics* 1998;102:323–328.
470. Barnett A, Mercuri E, Rutherford M, et al. Neurological and perceptual-motor outcome at 5–6 years of age in children with neonatal encephalopathy: relationship with neonatal brain MRI. *Neuropediatrics* 2002;33:242–248.
471. Martin E, Buchli R, Ritter S, et al. Diagnostic and prognostic value of cerebral 31P magnetic resonance spectroscopy in neonates with perinatal asphyxia. *Pediatr Res* 1996;40:749–758.
472. Shu SK, Ashwal S, Holshouser BA, et al. Prognostic value of 1H-MRS in perinatal CNS insults. *Pediatr Neurol* 1997;17:309–318.
472a. Hopkins-Golightly T, Razs, Sander CJ. Influence of slight to moderate risk for birth anoxia on acquisition of cognitive and language function in the pretern infant: A cross-sectional comparison with preterm-birth controls. *Neuropsychology* 2003;17: 3–13.
473. Robertson CMT, Hrynchyshyn GJ, Etches PC, et al. Population-based study of the incidence, complexity, and severity of neurologic disability among survivors weighing 500–1,250 grams at birth: a comparison of two birth cohorts. *Pediatrics* 1992;90:750–755.
474. Pharoah PO, Cooke T, Rosenbloom L, et al. Effects of birth weight, gestational age, and maternal obstetrical history on birth prevalence of cerebral palsy. *Arch Dis Child* 1987;62:1035–1040.
475. Lowe J, Papile LA. Neurodevelopmental performance of very-low-birth-weight infants with mild periventricular, intraventricular hemorrhage: outcome at 5–6 years of age. *Am J Dis Child* 1990;144:1242–1245.
476. van de Bor M, Verloove-Vanhorick SP, Baerts W, et al. Outcome of periventricular-intraventricular haemorrhage at 5 years of age. *Dev Med Child Neurol* 1993;35:33–41.
477. Fazzi E, Orcesi S, Telesca C, et al. Neurodevelopmental outcome in very low-birth-weight infants at 24 months and 5 to 7 years of age: changing diagnosis. *Pediatr Neurol* 1997;17:240–248.
478. Jongmans M, Henderson S, de Vries L, et al. Duration of periventricular densities in preterm infants and neurological outcome at 6 years of age. *Arch Dis Child* 1993;69(Spec Issue 1):9–13.
479. Ghosh A, Shatz CJ. A role for subplate neurons in the patterning of connections from thalamus to neocortex. *Development* 1993;117:1031–1047.
480. Volpe JJ. Subplate neurons—missing link in brain injury of the premature infant? *Pediatrics* 1996;97:112–113.
481. Ajayi-Obe M, Saeed N, Cowan FM, et al. Reduced development of cerebral cortex in extremely preterm infants. *Lancet* 2000;356:1162–1163.
482. Wood NS, Marlow N, Costeloe K, et al. Neurologic and developmental disability after extremely preterm birth. *N Engl J Med* 2000;343:378–384.
483. Hirata T, Epcar JT, Walsh A, et al. Survival and outcome of infants 501 to 750 gm: a six-year experience. *J Pediatr* 1983;102:741–748.
484. Kitchen WH, Doyle LW, Ford GW, et al. Changing two-year outcome in infants weighing 500–999 grams at birth: a hospital study. *J Pediatr* 1991;118:938–943.
485. Collin MF, Halsey CL, Anderson CL. Emerging developmental sequelae in the "normal" extremely low-birth-weight infant. *Pediatrics* 1991;88:115–120.
485a. Kilbride HW, Thorstad K, Daily DK. Preschool outcome of less than 801 gram preterm infants compared with full-term siblings. *Pediatrics* 2004;113:742–747.
486. Hack M, Breslau N, Aram D, et al. Effect of very low-birth-weight and subnormal head size on cognitive abilities at school age. *N Engl J Med* 1991;325:231–237.
487. Piecuch RE, Leonard CH, Cooper BA, et al. Outcome of extremely low-birth-weight infants (500 to 999 grams) over a 12-year period. *Pediatrics* 1997;100:633–639.
488. Hack M, Taylor HG, Klein N, et al. School-age outcomes in children with birth weights under 750 g. *N Engl J Med* 1994;331:753–759.
489. O'Grady RS, Crain LS, Kohn J. The prediction on long-term functional outcomes of children with cerebral palsy. *Dev Med Child Neurol* 1995;37:997–1005.
490. Sala DA, Grant AD. Prognosis for ambulation in cerebral palsy. *Dev Med Child Neurol* 1995;37:1020–1026.
491. Murphy KP, Molnar GE, Lankasky K. Medical and functional status of adults with cerebral palsy. *Dev Med Child Neurol* 1995;37:1075–1084.
492. Strauss D, Ojdana K, Shavelle R, et al. Decline in function and life expectancy of older persons with cerebral palsy. *Neuro Rehabilitation* 2004;19:69–78.
493. Hutton JL, Cooke T, Pharoah POD. Life expectancy in children with cerebral palsy. *Br Med J* 1994;309:431–435.
494. Crichton JU, Mackinnon M, White CP. The life expectancy of persons with cerebral palsy. *Dev Med Child Neurol* 1995;37:567–576.
495. Hutton JL, Culver AF, Mackie PC. Effect of severity of disability on survival in north east England cerebral palsy cohort. *Arch Dis Child* 2000;83:468–474.
496. Crothers B. Injuries of the spinal cord in breech extractions as an important cause of fetal death and paraplegia in childhood. *Am J Med Sci* 1923;165:94–110.
497. Ford FR. Breech delivery in its possible relations to injury of the spinal cord with special reference to infantile paraplegia. *Arch Neurol Psychiatr* 1925;14:742–750.
498. Crothers B, Putnam MC. Obstetrical injuries of spinal cord. *Medicine* 1927;6:4–126.
499. Towbin A. Latent spinal cord and brain stem injury in newborn infants. *Dev Med Child Neurol* 1969;11:54–68.
500. Byers RK. Spinal cord injuries during birth. *Dev Med Child Neurol* 1975;17:103–110.
501. Hedley-Whyte ET, Gilles FH. Observations on myelination of human spinal cord and some effects of parturitional transection. *J Neuropathol Exp Neurol* 1974;33:436–445.
502. Rossitch E, Oakes WJ. Perinatal spinal cord injury: clinical, radiographic, and pathologic features. *Pediatr Neurosurg* 1992;18:149–152.
503. MacKinnon JA, Perlman M, Kirpalani H, et al. Spinal cord injury at birth: diagnostic and prognostic data in twenty-two patients. *J Pediatr* 1993;122:431–437.
504. Mills JF, Dargaville PA, Coleman LT, et al. Upper cervical spinal cord injury in neonates: the use of magnetic resonance imaging. *J Pediatr* 2001;138:105–108.
505. Bucher HU, Boltshauser E, Friderich J, et al. Birth injury to the spinal cord. *Helv Paediatr Acta* 1979;34:517–527.
506. Melchior JC, Tygstrup I. Development of paraplegia after breech presentation. *Acta Paediatr Scand* 1963;52:171–176.
507. Schwartz HG. Congenital tumors of spinal cord in infants. *Ann Surg* 1952;136:183–192.
508. Hepner WR Jr. Some observations on facial paresis in the newborn infant: etiology and incidence. *Pediatrics* 1951;8:494–497.
509. Nelson KB, Eng GD. Congenital hypoplasia of the depressor anguli oris muscle: differentiation from congenital facial palsy. *J Pediatr* 1972;81:16–20.
510. Douglas DB, Kessler RE. Significance of electrical reactions in facial palsy of newborn: a case report. *Behav Neuropsychiatry* 1971;2:67.
511. Shapiro NL, Cunningham MJ, Parikh SR, et al. Congenital unilateral facial paralysis. *Pediatrics* 1996;97:261–265.
512. Toelle SP, Boltshauser E. Long-term outcome in children with congenital unilateral facial nerve palsy. *Neuropediatrics* 2001;32:130–135.
513. Ehara H, Hara H, Takeshita K. Catch 22: a possible cause of congenital unilateral facial nerve palsy. *Eur J Pediatr* 1997;156:739.
514. Vannas M. Zur Sehnervenatrophie nach Geburtsverletzung. *Acta Ophthalmol* 1933;11:514–525.
515. Gifford H. Congenital defects of abduction and other ocular movements and their relation to birth injuries. *Am J Ophthalmol* 1926;9:3–22.

516. Cogan DG. *Neurology of the ocular muscles*, 2nd ed. Springfield, IL: Charles C. Thomas, 1975.
517. Worster-Drought C. Suprabulbar paresis. *Dev Med Child Neurol* 1974;16 (Suppl):1–33.
518. Spector GJ, Pettit WJ, Davis G, et al. Fetal respiratory distress causing CNS and inner ear hemorrhage. *Laryngoscope* 1978;88:764–784.
519. Orita Y, Sando I, Miura M, et al. Cochleosaccular pathology after perinatal and postnatal asphyxia: histopathologic findings. *Otol Neurotol* 2002;23:4–38.
520. Galambos R, Despland PA. The auditory brain stem response (ABR) evaluates risk factors for hearing loss in the newborn. *Pediatr Res* 1980;14:159–163.
521. Henderson-Smart DJ, Pettigrew AG, Campbell DJ. Clinical apnea and brain-stem neural function in preterm infants. *N Engl J Med* 1983;308:353–357.
522. Hecox KE, Cone B. Prognostic importance of brain-stem auditory evoked responses after asphyxia. *Neurology* 1981;31:1429–1434.
523. Smellie WA. *Treatise on the theory and practice of midwifery: a collection of preternatural cases and observations in midwifery*, Vol 3, 3rd ed. London: D. Wilson & T. Durham, 1766.
524. Danyau N. Un cas de paralysie du bras, chez un enfant nouveau né. *Bull Soc Chir Paris* 1851;2:148–151.
525. Duchenne GB. *De l'Electrisation Localisée*. Paris: Bailliere, 1872.
526. Klumpke A. Contribution a l'étude des paralysies radiculaires du plexus brachial; paralysies radiculaires totales; paralysies radiculaires inférieres; de la participation des filets sympathiques oculopupillaries dans ces paralysies. *Rev Méd Paris* 1885;5:591–596.
527. Shoemaker J. Ueber die Aetiologie der Entbindungslähmungen, speziell der Oberarmparalysen. *Z Geburtshilfe Gynaekol* 1899;41:33–53.
528. Clark LP, Taylor AS, Prout FP. A study on brachial birth palsy. *Am J Med Sci* 1905;130:670–707.
529. Gherman RB, Goodwin TM, Ouzounian JG, et al. Brachial plexus palsy associated with cesarean section: an *in utero* injury? *Am J Obstet Gynecol* 1997;177:1162–1164.
530. Jennet RJ, Tarby TJ, Kreinick CJ. Brachial plexus palsy: an old problem revisited. *Am J Obstet Gynecol* 1992;166:1673–1677.
531. Dunn DW, Engle WA. Brachial plexus palsy: intrauterine onset. *Pediatr Neurol* 1985;1:367–369.
532. Eng GD, Binder H, Getson P, et al. Obstetrical brachial plexus palsy (OBPP) outcome with conservative management. *Muscle Nerve* 1996;19:884–891.
533. Hoeksma AF, ter Steeg AM, Nelissen RG, et al. Neurological recovery in obstetric brachial plexus injuries: an historical cohort study. *Dev Med Child Neurol* 2004;46:76–83.
534. Bager B. Perinatally acquired brachial plexus palsy—a persisting challenge. *Acta Paediatr* 1997;86:1214–1219.
535. Eng GD. Brachial plexus palsy in newborn infants. *Pediatrics* 1971;48:18–28.
536. Schifrin N. Unilateral paralysis of the diaphragm in the newborn infant due to phrenic nerve injury: with and without associated brachial palsy. *Pediatrics* 1952;9:69–121.
537. Adams FH, Gyepes MT. Diaphragmatic paralysis in the newborn infant simulating cyanotic heart disease. *J Pediatr* 1971;78:119–121.
538. Smith BT. Isolated phrenic nerve palsy in the newborn. *Pediatrics* 1972;49:449–451.
539. Robinson GC, Dikranian DA, Roseborough GF. Congenital Horner's syndrome and heterochromia iridium: their association with congenital foregut and vertebral anomalies. *Pediatrics* 1965;35:103–107.
540. Yilmaz K, Caliskan M, Oge E, et al. Clinical assessment, MRI, and EMG in congenital brachial plexus palsy. *Pediatr Neurol* 1999;21:705–710.
541. Posniak HV, Olson MC, Dudiak CM, et al. MR imaging of the brachial plexus. *Am J Roentgenol* 1993;161:373–379.
542. Eng GD. Spontaneous potentials in premature and full-term infants. *Arch Phys Med Rehabil* 1976;57:120–121.
543. DiGeorge AM, Olmsted RW, Harley RD. Waardenburg's syndrome: syndrome of heterochromia of irides, lateral displacement of medial canthi and lacrimal puncta, congenital deafness and other characteristic associated defects. *J Pediatr* 1960;57:649–669.
544. Pardono E, van Bever Y, can den Ende J, et al. Waardenburg syndrome: clinical differentiation between types I and II. *Am J Med Genet* 2003;117A:223–235.
545. Adler JB, Patterson RL. Erb's palsy: long-term results of treatment in eighty-eight cases. *J Bone Joint Surg* 1967;49A:1052–1064.
546. Grossman JAI. Early operative intervention for birth injuries to the brachial plexus. *Sem Pediat Neurol* 2000;7:36–43.
546a. Grossman JAI, DiTaranto P, Price AE, et al. Multidisciplinary management of brachial plexus birth injuries: the Miami experience. *Semin Plastic Surg* 2004; 18:319–326.
547. Laurent JP, Lee R, Shenaq S, et al. Neurosurgical correction of upper brachial plexus birth injuries. *J Neurosurg* 1993;79:197–203.
548. Greenwald AG, Shute P, Shively J. Brachial plexus birth palsy: a 10-year report on the incidence and prognosis. *J Pediatr Orthop* 1984;4:689–692.
549. Michelow BJ, Clarke HM, Curtis CG, et al. The natural history of obstetrical brachial plexus palsy. *Plast Reconstruct Surg* 1994;93:675–680.
550. Rossi LN, Vassella F, Mumenthaler M. Obstetrical lesions of the brachial plexus: natural history in 34 personal cases. *Eur Neurol* 1982;21:1–7.
551. Schlaggar BL, Fox K, O'Leary DDM. Postsynaptic control of plasticity in developing somatosensory cortex. *Nature* 1993;364:623–626.
552. Brown T, Cupido C, Scarfone H, et al. Developmental apraxia arising from neonatal brachial plexus palsy. *Neurology* 2000;55:24–30.
553. Penn A, Ross WT. Sciatic nerve palsy in newborn infants: report of case. *S Afr Med J* 1955;29:553–554.
554. San Agustin M, Nitowsky HM, Borden JN. Neonatal sciatic palsy after umbilical vessel injection. *J Pediatr* 1962;60:408–413.
555. Escolar DM, Jones HR. Pediatric radial mononeuropathies: a clinical and electromyographic study of sixteen children with review of the literature. *Muscle Nerve* 1996;19:878–883.
556. Craig WS, Clark JMP. Obturator palsy in the newly born. *Arch Dis Child* 1962;37:661–662.
557. Coventry MB, Harris LE. Congenital muscular torticollis in infancy: some observations regarding treatment. *J Bone Joint Surg Am* 1959;41:815–817.
558. Sarnat HB, Morrissy RT. Idiopathic torticollis: sternocleidomastoid myopathy and accessory neuropathy. *Muscle Nerve* 1981;4:374–380.
559. Sanerkin NG, Edwards P. Birth injury to the sternomastoid muscle. *J Bone Joint Surg Br* 1966;48:441–447.
560. Lidge RT, Bechtol RC, Lambert CN. Congenital muscular torticollis: etiology and pathology. *J Bone Joint Surg Am* 1957;39:1165–1182.
561. Caputo AR, Mickey KJ, Guo S, et al. The sit-up test: an alternative clinical test for evaluating pediatric torticollis. *Pediatrics* 1990;90:612–615.
562. Morrison DL, MacEwen GD. Congenital muscular torticollis: observations regarding clinical findings, associated conditions and results of treatment. *J Pediatr Orthop* 1982;2:500–505.
563. Binder H, Eng GD, Gaiser JF, Koch B. Congenital muscular torticollis: results of conservative management with long-term follow-up in 85 cases. *Arch Phys Med Rehabil* 1987;68:222–225.
564. Kinsbourne M. Hiatus hernia with contortions of the neck. *Lancet* 1964;1:1058–1061.
565. Deonna T, Martin D. Benign paroxysmal torticollis in infancy. *Arch Dis Child* 1981;56:956–959.
566. Giffin NJ, Benton S, Goadsby PJ. Benign paroxysmal torticollis of infancy: four new cases and linkage to *CACNA1A*. *Dev Med Child Neurol* 2002;44:490–493.

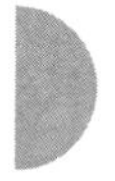

Chapter 7

Infections of the Nervous System

Bernard L. Maria and James F. Bale, Jr.

Many different pathogens can invade and damage the developing or mature central nervous system (CNS). These infectious disorders share several clinical and pathologic features, with unique signs or symptoms attributable to the pathogen, tropism, virulence, or variations in the host immune responses. In general terms, CNS infections can be categorized according to the nature of the infectious pathogen—viral, bacterial, protozoan, or fungal—and by the location of the infection—parenchymal, meningeal, or vascular. The diagnosis of infectious disorders of the CNS requires laboratory studies, including isolation or molecular detection of the specific pathogen and the identification of organism-specific serologic or pathologic abnormalities.

MENINGITIS

Menigitis refers to inflammation of the leptomeninges, the connective tissue layers in closest proximity to the surface of the brain. Meningitis can be caused by bacteria, viruses, parasites, and fungi as well as by noninfectious conditions including inflammatory disorders (e.g., systemic lupus erythematosis or Kawasaki disease) and neoplasia (e.g., leukemic meningitis) (1). Historically, meningitis due to viruses and certain other nonbacterial pathogens has been designated "aseptic meningitis."

Bacterial Meningitis

In the United States, approximately 25,000 cases of meningitis occur annually among children and adults (1). The pathogens causing pediatric bacterial meningitis vary considerably according to the age of the child. In newborns *Streptococcus agalactiae* (group B streptococcus), *Escherichia coli, Staphylococcus* species, *Listeria monocytogenes,* and *Pseudomonas aeruginosa* are the most frequent causes of bacterial meningitis. *Citrobacter* species, other potential causes of neonatal meningitis, account for less than 5% of cases but produce brain abscesses in approximately 75% of the infected infants. By contrast, two organisms, *Streptococcus pneumoniae,* a gram-positive diplococcus, and *Neisseria meningitides,* a gram-negative diplococcus, cause most cases of bacterial meningitis among children and adolescents living in regions with compulsory immunization for *Haemophilus influenzae* type b (Hib). Prior to the development and marketing of an effective Hib vaccine, however, as many as 1 in every 400 children between 1 and 4 years of age experienced bacterial meningitis due to this organism.

Among unimmunized children, *H. influenzae* meningitis remains a potential threat and occurs more commonly among African Americans and Native Americans and in children with asplenia, sickle cell anemia, and HIV infection. Risk factors for *S. pneumoniae* meningitis include the foregoing as well as nephritic syndrome, cochlear implantation, and cerebrospinal fluid (CSF) leaks. College students and persons with inherited complement deficiencies have increased risks of *N. meningitides* infection.

Pathology and Pathophysiology

Anatomic and Immunologic Features

Bacteria reach the leptomeninges by hematogenous spread, passage through the choroid plexus, rupture of superficial cortical abscesses, or contiguous spread from an adjacent infection (2). Hematogenous spread occurs during bacteremia and can result from passive transfer of organisms by infected leukocytes. Organisms can also enter the CNS from damaged blood vessels, via neurosurgical procedures, or via compound (open) fractures of the skull. In rare instances, bacterial meningitis can complicate congenital defects such as myelomeningoceles or dermal sinuses that allow direct bacterial invasion of CSF or by spread of bacteria from adjacent infections, such as parameningeal abscess, or osteomyelitis of the cranial bones.

In most instances, meningitis begins with bacterial colonization of the nasopharynx and bacteremia (2). The probability of meningitis correlates with the magnitude and duration of the bacteremia, which relate directly to the size of the intranasal inoculum. *S. pneumoniae, H. influenzae,* and *N. meningitidis* secrete proteases that neutralize

TABLE 7.1 Frequency of the Common Forms of Acute Meningitis in Infancy and Childhood[a]

	<1 Month	1–23 Months	2–18 Years	19–59 Years	>60 Years
Haemophilus influenzae[b]	—	5	10	15	5
Streptococcus pneumoniae	10	45	30	60	60
Neisseria meningitidis	—	30	60	20	5
β-Hemolytic *Streptococcus*	70	20	5	5	5
Listeria monocytogenes	20	—	—	10	15

[a]Figures are percentage of total cases within a given age group.
[b]Immunization against *Haemophilus influenzae* has significantly reduced the proportion of this type of meningitis in selected regions of the world.
Modified from Schuchat A, et al., for the Active Surveillance Team. Bacterial meningitis in the United States in 1995. *N Engl J Med* 1997;337:970.

secretory IgA and impair the mucosal cilia. Invasion of *N. meningitidis* and *S. pneumoniae* across the nasopharyngeal mucosal epithelium can occur by endocytosis and transport across the cell in membrane-bound vacuoles. *H. influenzae* invades directly through tight junctions between columnar epithelial cells (3). Once in the bloodstream, organisms can avoid lysis by circulating complement (3).

The blood–brain barrier, composed of the arachnoid membrane, the choroid plexus epithelium, and the endothelial cells of the cerebral microvasculature, separates the intravascular compartment from the brain and CSF. This barrier effectively prevents ingress of many molecules and particles, including many infectious agents; it is unclear how most organisms causing meningitis breach this barrier (4). Pneumococci use a surface protein to bind to the receptor for platelet activating factor on cytokine-activated cerebral endothelial cells. By corrupting host chemokine receptor pathways, bacteria enter the cell, and the receptor is recycled for subsequent reuse (5). In meningitis, the blood–brain barrier can be disrupted by separation of intercellular tight junctions, primarily in the endothelial cells of the cerebral microvasculature and, to a lesser degree, in the endothelium of the choroid plexus (4–6). Matrix metalloproteinases, nitric oxide, reactive oxygen species, and metabolites of the arachidonic pathway participate in the disruption of the blood–brain barrier (7). Upon entering the CSF, bacteria encounter few host defenses because the CSF generally lacks antibody, complement, and opsonic activity.

Unique bacterial antigens, often capsular polysaccharides, contribute to the virulence and neurotropisms of certain bacteria (1,2,8). *E. coli* K1 strains cause the majority of cases of neonatal *E. coli* meningitis, emphasizing the importance of this antigen in the organism's virulence. Mortality and morbidity in *E. coli* meningitis are greater when it is caused by K1 strains as compared with non-K1 strains. The clinical and pathologic aspects of meningitis are summarized in works by Schuchat and coworkers (9), Saez-Llorens and coworkers (10), Smith (11), and Tunkel and Scheld (12,13). Table 7.1 summarizes the frequency of several bacterial pathogens (9).

The fundamental pathologic process in bacterial meningitis is inflammation of the leptomeninges. This begins with hyperemia of the meningeal vessels, and soon thereafter, neutrophils migrate into the subarachnoid space (Fig. 7.1). The subarachnoid exudate increases rapidly and within a few hours extends into the sheaths of blood vessels and along cranial and spinal nerves. Phagocytic polymorphonuclear leukocytes predominate during the initial stages, and lymphocytes and histiocytes increase over the subsequent days. Fibrinogen and other blood proteins contribute to the inflammatory exudates, and plasma

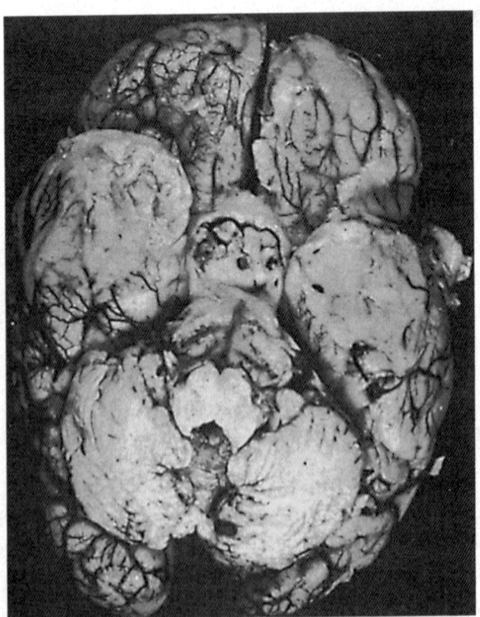

FIGURE 7.1. *Haemophilus influenzae* meningitis. The brain is swollen with flattening of the gyri. The meninges are thickened, and purulent material lies along the bases and over the temporal and frontal poles. (Courtesy of Dr. P. Cancella, Department of Pathology, University of California, Los Angeles, CA.)

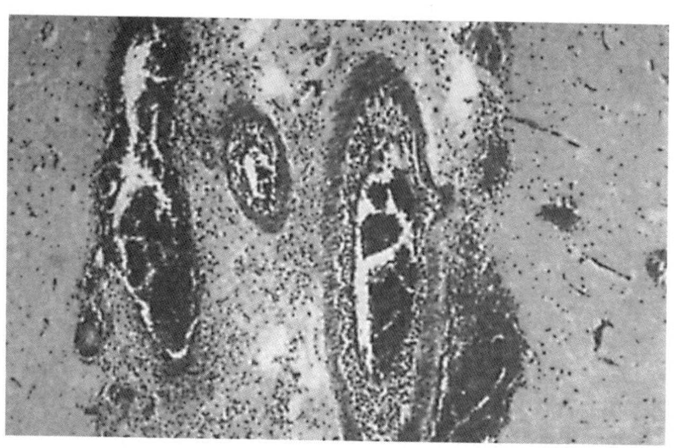

FIGURE 7.2. *Haemophilus influenzae* meningitis. A purulent exudate is seen in the subarachnoid space surrounding the venules, which are partially or completely thrombosed (hematoxylin and eosin stain, ×25). (Courtesy of Dr. P. Cancella, Department of Pathology, University of California, Los Angeles, CA.)

cells appear. Fibroblasts participate in the organization of exudate and fibrosis of the arachnoid.

The meningeal infection spreads along the penetrating cortical vessels in the Virchow-Robin spaces. The adventitia of these vessels, formed by an investment of the arachnoid membrane, is invariably involved, even in the initial stages of meningitis. Subarachnoid arteries also are affected. Endothelial cells swell, proliferate, and constrict the vessel lumen in 48 to 72 hours. Adventitial connective tissue becomes infiltrated by neutrophils, and a layer of inflammatory cells also appears beneath the arterial intima. Foci of necrosis of the arterial walls can develop and occasionally cause arterial thrombosis and infarction. Stroke and other vascular phenomena can be demonstrated in children with meningitis (14). A similar process occurs in the veins (15) with foci of necrosis and thrombi that can occlude the vascular lumen. Venous thrombosis is thought to occur more frequently than arterial thrombosis during bacterial meningitis (Fig. 7.2).

With resolution of meningitis, cells disappear in the order in which they appeared. The number of neutrophils diminishes after a few weeks, whereas lymphocytes, plasma cells, and macrophages can persist for months. The extent of resolution depends on the stage at which infection is arrested. If infection is controlled early, residua can be minimal, but an infection lasting several weeks produces permanent fibrosis of the meninges, resulting in a cloudy arachnoid membrane and adhesions between the arachnoid and dura.

The inflammatory response elicited by bacteria and bacterial cell wall fragments contributes to meningitis-induced tissue injury (16,17). Bacterial lipopolysaccharide elicits a monocytic response in the parenchyma (18). Thus, therapy with bacterial drugs that lyse bacteria can transiently exacerbate inflammatory responses and potentially increase the severity of tissue injury. Corticosteroids, when given immediately prior to antibiotic therapy, can minimize the inflammatory response (19) and reduce the likelihood of certain complications, especially sensorineural hearing loss in children with *H. influenzae* meningitis.

Cytokines, soluble proteins released by host cells in response to bacterial products, participate in the pathogenesis of meningeal inflammation (20–23). Cytokines can increase blood–brain barrier permeability, decrease autoregulation of cerebral blood flow, and induce cytotoxic edema. Cytokines can recruit leukocytes into an infected compartment. Proinflammatory cytokines include tumor necrosis factor-alpha (TNF-α), interleukin (IL)-1β (IL-1β), IL-6, IL-8, IL-10, and transforming growth factor β(TGF-β) (23) (Table 7.2). TNF-α, a major contributor to the pathogenesis of bacterial meningitis and its complications, is a low-molecular-weight protein secreted by activated macrophages, leukocytes, endothelial cells, microglia, and astrocytes. TNF-α increases the permeability of the blood–brain barrier (23,34), induces cell lysis, and mediates myelin and oligodendrocyte damage (35). Levels of TNF-α are transiently elevated to more than 200 pg/mL

TABLE 7.2 Cytokines that Increase in Response to Meningitis

Cytokine	Serum	Cerebrospinal Fluid		Reference
		Viral	Bacterial	
IL-1	+	+	++	22,24,25
IL-6	++	++	++	26–28
IL-8		+	++	24
IL-9	–	+		29
Tumor necrosis factor	+	+	+	30–32
Tumor growth factor-β			+	33
Platelet-activating factor	–	–	+	30
C-reactive protein	+	+	++	27
Alpha-2 microglobulin		–	+	27

IL, interleukin.

in CSF in the majority of patients in the first 24 to 48 hours of purulent meningitis (24). By contrast, CSF concentrations of TNF-α usually remain normal in patients with viral meningitis (36,37).

IL-1β, a highly potent inducer of neutrophil accumulation and procoagulant, stimulates the release of other cytokines such as TNF and IL-6 and of hypothalamic corticotrophin-releasing factor. The latter increases systemic levels of adrenocorticotrophic hormone (ACTH) (38). ACTH can increase blood–brain barrier permeability for albumin with augmentation of edema. Peak concentrations of CSF IL-1b more than 100 pg/100 mL correlate with poor outcome for neonatal gram-negative meningitis and childhood pyogenic meningitis (24,39). IL-1 and TNF-α act synergistically to disrupt the blood–brain barrier and can stimulate human vascular endothelial cells to promote transendothelial passage of neutrophils (40).

IL-6, which is also a pyrogen, plays a role in the induction and propagation of inflammatory responses. Increased levels of IL-6 are detected in CSF of patients with bacterial meningitis (30), and serum concentrations are also elevated, in contrast to the compartmentalization of the responses of other cytokines in meningitis (30,31,41). Levels of IL-8, a leukocyte chemotactic agent that promotes leukocyte adherence, are increased in CSF of patients with meningococcal meningitis but not aseptic meningitis (42). IL-10 is not present in serum but is elevated in CSF in the first 48 to 72 hours of viral meningitis. It is believed to downregulate inflammation and may contribute to chronicity of disease.

Cytokines released from damaged cells stimulate leukocyte chemotaxis from blood into CSF, a response more pronounced in the juvenile than in the adult brain (43). Chemokines include diverse agents such as platelet-activating factor, IL-b, families of cysteine-containing chemokines, and the macrophage inhibitory proteins (MIPs). Ectopic expression of chemokines in the CNS leads to dramatic accumulation of circulating leukocytes in brain parenchyma and CSF with accompanying pathology (44). Conversely, inhibition of leukocyte trafficking to the brain attenuates inflammation and tissue damage, indicating that leukocytes are an important mediator of neuronal injury. This inhibition can occur at the level of the leukocyte integrins that serve as adhesion molecules or at the level of the endothelial adhesion receptors, such as selectins and intercellular adhesion molecules (45).

Reactive oxygen and nitrogen species, potent antimicrobial factors, can also damage host cells. Microglia, when activated with interferon-beta and bacterial lipopolysaccharide, cause neuronal cell injury by a nitric oxide mechanism (46,47). Nitric oxide, a gas with a half-life of seconds, regulates vascular tone and perfusion pressure. In excess amounts, as generated in the CSF during infection, nitric oxide enhances blood–brain barrier permeability and leukocytosis (48). Administration of inhibitors of inducible nitric oxide synthase decreases the bystander damage to host cells during meningitis. The mean concentration of nitric oxide is significantly elevated in CSF during the early stages of bacterial but not aseptic meningitis (49).

When the fibrinopurulent exudate accumulates in large quantities, hydrocephalus can be produced by obstruction of the foramina of Luschka and Magendie or the aqueduct of Sylvius. Communicating hydrocephalus can result from inflammation or exudate in the subarachnoid space around brainstem and over the cerebral convexity. The exudate can interfere with CSF flow from the cisterna magna and lateral recesses to the basal cisterns or with absorption of CSF by arachnoid granules (Fig. 7.2).

Brain perfusion can be impeded by acute increases in intracranial pressure (50), changes in the vascular bed, or acute ventricular dilatation. Brain metabolism changes to glycolysis with increased glucose oxidation and lactate production and the depletion of high-energy compounds, such as phosphocreatine and adenosine triphosphate (ATP). Brain edema in bacterial meningitis can be vasogenic, the result of increased permeability of the blood–brain barrier, or cytotoxic. Both vasogenic and cytotoxic edema can be induced by components of the neutrophil membrane (51). Cytotoxic brain edema is marked by increased brain water, cellular swelling, increased intracellular sodium, and loss of intracellular potassium (51). Brain edema can depolarize neuronal membranes and lead to seizure activity. These changes are mediated in part by polyunsaturated fatty acids released from leukocytes and possibly brain cell membranes (52). Vasogenic edema, caused by the opening of tight junctions between cerebral capillary endothelial cells and increased micropinocytosis across endothelial cells, can result from the presence of bacteria as well as inflammation. Additionally, there are concomitant increases in superoxide and lipid peroxidation, believed to result from inhibition of superoxide dismutase activity. Arachidonic acid, formed in part by cleavage of phospholipids by phospholipase A2, accumulates not only in meningitis, but also in other pathologic insults such as ischemia, hypoxia, and trauma. Dexamethasone, which inhibits phospholipase A2 and stabilizes cell membranes, reduces arachidonic acid–induced brain edema *in vivo* but not *in vitro* (see Table 7.3) (52). Bacterial cells or cell fragments also induce cerebral arteriolar vasodilatation by formation of oxygen free radicals.

Gram-negative endotoxin in the CSF can induce respiratory and circulatory failure (53). Symptoms include pulmonary edema, which develops from an intense systemic vasoconstriction; subendocardial hemorrhages; myocardial necrosis; hemorrhagic lesions in the adrenal corticomedullary junction; and ulcerations of the intestinal mucosa. McCracken observed that the endotoxin concentrations in CSF correlate with clinical severity and neurologic outcome of *H. influenzae* type B meningitis (54).

TABLE 7.3 Therapeutic Interventions Against the Inflammatory Response

Intervention	Action
Anti-CD-18 monoclonal antibodies to adhesion glycoproteins	Inhibit cytokine-Induced leukocytosis and brain edema (21)
Pentoxifylline	Inhibits release from microglia of tumor necrosis factor, interleukin-1
Transforming growth factor-β	Inhibits cytokine production, adhesion of granulocytes to endothelium
Dexamethasone	Inhibits cytokine-induced exudation of neutrophils in cerebrospinal fluid (21)
	Inhibits secretion of interleukin-1β
	Inhibits secretion of tumor necrosis factor-α
	Inhibits phospholipase A_2, decreases release of free arachidonic acid, decreases production of prostanoids, leukotrienes (14)
Dexamethasone and nifedipine	Inhibit production of nitric oxide synthetase
Anticytokine antibody, interleukin-1, receptor antagonist soluble tumor necrosis factor receptor	Block cytokine action
Nonsteroidal anti-inflammatory drug	Inhibits production of variety of cytokines (34)
Thalidomide	Inhibits tumor necrosis factor production
Interleukin-10	Downregulation of macrophage activation
Fucoidin	Competitive inhibition of selectin, mediated leukocyte adhesion

During the early stages of meningitis, regional cerebral blood flow is increased; however, in severe meningitis cerebral blood flow is reduced (55). Paulson and colleagues observed that cerebral blood flow was reduced to 72% of normal in meningitis and the cerebral arteriovenous oxygen difference to 63% of normal, with a consequent decrease in oxygen consumption to 42% of the normal levels (56). Although autoregulation is lost in experimental meningitis, its role in the pathogenesis of childhood meningitis is less clear. Ashwal and colleagues observed that autoregulation of cerebral blood flow was preserved in children with bacterial meningitis (57). The changes in cerebral blood flow secondary to changes in carbon dioxide partial pressure (pCO_2) indicate that hyperventilation can reduce cerebral blood flow below ischemic thresholds. For this reason hyperventilation to reduce intracranial pressure in meningitis may potentiate neuronal injury. Mortality in bacterial meningitis and other serious CNS infections correlates, in part, with decreased cerebral perfusion pressure (58).

Clinical Manifestations

The early signs of neonatal bacterial meningitis may consist only of low-grade fever, poor feeding, somnolence, "fussy" behavior, or irritability (Table 7.4). Later, vomiting, lethargy, and seizures ensue. The physical examination in infants with meningitis can be equally nonspecific, showing somnolence, irritability, hyper-reflexia, and a full or bulging fontanel. Meningeal signs are present infrequently. Systemic signs can include hypotension and features of disseminated intravascular coagulopathy (DIC).

The signs and symptoms of meningitis in older children include fever, headache, nausea and vomiting, nuchal rigidity, alterations of sensorium, convulsions, cranial

TABLE 7.4 Signs and Symptoms in 39 Infants with Neonatal Meningitis

	Premature Infants		Full-Term Infants	
	Initial	Overall	Initial	Overall
Anorexia or vomiting	4	10	4	15
Lethargy	3	12	1	13
Irritability	0	0	4	15
Jaundice	3	10	2	3
Respiratory distress	5	11	1	5
Diarrhea	1	3	1	4
Bulging fontanelle	0	0	0	13
Convulsions	0	2	1	9
Nuchal rigidity	0	1	0	6
Fever	0	2	8	19
Pyoderma	0	0	1	6
Total	16		23	

From Groover RV, Sutherland JM, Landing BH. Purulent meningitis of newborn infants: eleven year experience in the antibiotic era. *N Engl J Med* 1961;264:1115. With permission.

nerve palsies, disturbances in vision, and occasionally papilledema (59). Headache, often accompanied by photophobia, results from inflammation of the meningeal vessels and from increased intracranial pressure. Head retraction, neck stiffness, and spinal rigidity are caused by irritation of the meninges and spinal roots, which elicits protective reflexes intended to shorten the spinal axis and immobilize the irritated tissue (60). With lengthening of the spine, nerve roots are stretched, and the resulting pain and reflex spasm is the basis of Kernig and Brudzinski signs. Spinal rigidity is a more sensitive sign of meningeal irritation than nuchal rigidity, especially in young children. Nuchal stiffness is most readily demonstrated with the child in the sitting position with the legs extended (61). Systemic signs can include pneumonia in children with pneumococcal or *H. influenzae* meningitis and petechiae, purpura, or signs of DIC in children with meningococcal meningitis. Rash, purpura, and DIC can also be observed occasionally in children with *H. influenzae* meningitis.

Seizures can be generalized or partial in infants or children with bacterial meningitis. Dodge and Swartz reported seizures in 44% of patients with *H. influenzae* meningitis, 25% of those with *S. pneumoniae* infections, 10% of those with meningococcal infections, and 78% of those with streptococcal meningitis (62). Focal seizures can be the result of localized involvement of the cerebral hemispheres by bacteria, cytokines, or vascular lesions. In a study by Samson and associates (63), 18% of patients had their first febrile convulsion in the course of meningitis. A lumbar puncture, therefore, is advised in children with their first febrile convulsion, especially in infants or unimmunized children. Lumbar puncture also deserves consideration when febrile convulsions recur and meningitis is suspected (64) or the seizure has atypical features (65). Focal neurologic signs in infants or children with bacterial meningitis can indicate Todds paralysis, ischemic stroke, or sinovenous thrombosis.

Abnormalities of cranial nerves III, IV, and VI can result from local inflammation of the perineurium or impaired vascular supply to the nerves. Transient opsoclonus can occur (66). Cochlear and vestibular deficits occur owing to septic involvement of the endolymphatic and perilymphatic systems of the scala tympani (67) or are caused by cytolytic toxins elaborated by bacteria (68). Conductive hearing loss can result from middle ear dysfunction following meningitis (69). Sensorineural hearing loss, the most common sequela of bacterial meningitis, is more likely in children younger than 1 month or older than 5 years of age, children with hydrocephalus, and those with a decreased CSF glucose (70). Jiang and coworkers suggested that a slightly depressed amplitude of the brainstem auditory potential wave V is a sensitive indicator of brainstem dysfunction in children recovering from meningitis (71). Otoacoustic emissions can detect meningitis-induced sensorineural hearing loss in young infants (72). Selective paralysis of downward gaze can occur (73). In a few rare instances, acute cerebellar ataxia can be the presenting symptom in *H. influenzae* or *N. meningitidis* infection (74). Cortical blindness also has been encountered (75).

In young infants, widened sutures can be observed within 2 days after onset of meningitis (76); however, progressive ventricular enlargement can develop without excessive head growth during or after acute bacterial meningitis (77). This enlargement results from cerebral destruction (passive ventriculomegaly) or from the effects of increased intraventricular pressure on already compromised brain parenchyma. In young infants, the low water content of brain parenchyma, lack of myelin, and relatively large subarachnoid spaces permit ventricular enlargement without corresponding increases in head circumference. Cranial bruits over the anterior fontanel and the posterior temporal areas are more common in children with bacterial meningitis than in febrile or healthy controls (72).

Complications

Ventriculitis

Ventriculitis commonly accompanies bacterial meningitis in young infants; in one series, 92% of neonates with fatal meningitis had ventriculitis (79,80). When ventriculitis is accompanied by an obstruction of the aqueduct of Sylvius, the infection can behave like a brain abscess. Rapid increase in intraventricular pressure can induce brainstem herniation and impair perfusion of the periventricular structures. Ventriculitis, treated with high doses of parenteral antibiotics, occasionally requires neurosurgical drainage (80).

Subdural Effusion and Subdural Empyema

Subdural effusions, a complication observed in the majority of young infants with bacterial meningitis, usually occur bilaterally over the frontoparietal region, although localized collections can develop over the occipital region. Effusions are most common when meningitis results from *H. influenzae* (45% of all effusions); less often, pneumococcus (30% of all effusions) and meningococcus (9% of all effusions) are the responsible pathogens. Subdural effusions result from efflux of intravascular fluids as a consequence of thrombophlebitis of the veins bridging the subdural space, abnormal vascular permeability at the arachnoid–dura interface, or arachnoiditis. Most effusions occur in children younger than 2 years of age. Other factors that favor the evolution of a subdural effusion include a rapid onset of illness, low peripheral white blood count, and high levels of CSF protein and bacterial antigen. Although children with effusions are more likely to have acute neurologic abnormalities or seizures, their outcome is similar to that of children without effusions (81).

Subdural empyema represents infection of the subdural space. In contrast to subdural effusions, subdural empyema rarely complicates bacterial meningitis (82). Indications for suspecting a subdural effusion or subdural

TABLE 7.5 Indications for Suspecting a Subdural Effusion in Infants with Purulent Meningitis

1. Failure of temperature curve to show progressive decline after 72 hours of adequate antibiotic and supportive treatment
2. Persistent positive spinal culture results after 72 hours of appropriate antibiotic therapy
3. Occurrence of focal or persistent convulsions
4. Persistence or recurrence of vomiting
5. Development of focal neurologic signs
6. An unsatisfactory clinical course, particularly evidence of increased intracranial pressure after 72 hours of antibiotic therapy

From Matson DD. *Neurosurgery of infancy and childhood,* 2nd ed. Springfield, IL: Charles C. Thomas, 1969. With permission.

empyema in the presence of meningitis are summarized in Table 7.5 (83). The criteria set forth by Matson more than 30 years ago are still applicable; in particular, the presence of fever that lasts more than 3 to 5 days after the start of antibiotic therapy should prompt initiation of diagnostic studies for these complications. The conditions can be diagnosed best by using gadolinium-enhanced magnetic resonance imaging (MRI).

In a subdural effusion, the fluid is xanthochromic or blood-tinged initially and can become less yellow with repeated taps. The protein content ranges between 50 and 1,000 mg/dL and is always higher than the CSF protein obtained simultaneously. Compared with serum, subdural fluid has a disproportionately high albumin-to-globulin ratio. MRI generally shows the fluid to be isointense relative to CSF on both T1- and T2-weighted images. In subdural empyema, the fluid shows a markedly elevated white count and protein concentration, with the glucose concentration being generally less than in CSF (84). On MRI the subdural empyema is hyperintense relative to CSF on proton density-weighted and T2-weighted images. Gadolinium enhancement of the adjacent leptomeninges can be observed in either empyema or effusion.

Subdural effusions can be managed conservatively, and aspiration or surgical intervention is no longer recommended unless empyema is strongly suspected. Most subdural fluid collections resorb spontaneously (81). Surgical intervention can be indicated if the effusion becomes hemorrhagic or causes significant midline shift. The technique for a subdural tap is described by Matson (77). Persistence of subdural effusions can indicate underlying cortical damage (85).

Fluid and Electrolyte Disturbances

Hyponatremia occurs in approximately 20% of patients with meningitis (86). Hyponatremia can be the result of an intracellular shift of sodium with an extracellular shift of potassium as a consequence of the inflammation, the syndrome of inappropriately high secretion of antidiuretic hormone (SIADH), or increased release of atrial natriuretic peptide. Inappropriate ADH release, which can occur with or without clinical hyponatremia, occurs in almost every case of bacterial meningitis and in approximately 60% of cases of viral meningitis (87). Hyponatremia leads to hypervolemia, oliguria, and increased urinary osmolality, despite low serum osmolality. When hyponatremia becomes severe, symptoms can include restlessness, irritability, and convulsions. The diagnosis can be established by measuring serum electrolytes and osmolality and urine output, specific gravity, and osmolality. The condition is treated by restricting free water intake; hypertonic saline solutions can be considered cautiously in children with seizures (88).

Recurrent Meningitis

Recurrent bacterial meningitis can be caused by acquired or congenital anatomic defects, foci of infection, or immunologic disorders. Skull fractures, especially those affecting the base of the brain and extending to the sinuses and petrous pyramids, are the most common cause of recurrent meningitis. They are discussed in Chapter 9. Congenital defects include myelomeningoceles, neurenteric cysts, midline or spinal dermal sinuses, and anomalies of the labyrinthine capsule and stapes foot plate. These conditions are covered in Chapter 5. Neuroschisis that allows entry of bacteria in the CSF can occur as an anterior encephalocele in the nasopharynx or as a small defect in the cribriform or orbital plate. Meningitis caused by these defects can occur in late childhood (89).

Splenectomy, congenital immunodeficiencies such as agammaglobulinemia, or acquired immune disorders such as HIV infection can predispose children or adults to bacterial meningitis. Children with leukemia and lymphoma have a particularly high incidence of recurrent purulent and fungal meningitis (see Chapter 17). Recurrence caused by the same organism can also occur if the initial therapy was inadequate or the organism was resistant to antibiotics (90). The incidence of chronic complications of meningitis is listed in Table 7.6.

TABLE 7.6 Major Complications Seen in 71 Children after Recovery from Meningitis

Complication	*Number of Cases*
Mental retardation	3
Seizures	3
Hemiparesis or quadriparesis	1
Bilateral deafness	4
Vestibular disturbance	1
Hydrocephalus	1
Total	13 (18%)

Modified from Dodge PR, Swartz MN. Bacterial meningitis: a review of selected aspects. I. Special neurologic problems, postmeningitic complications and clinicopathological correlations. *N Engl J Med* 1965;272:954.

Diagnosis

The diagnosis of meningitis requires prompt lumbar puncture and analysis of the CSF (91,92). The technique of lumbar puncture and the interpretation of CSF findings are discussed in the Introduction chapter. Children with focal neurologic deficits, coma, or papilledema require head computed tomography (CT) prior to performing a lumbar puncture (93). When a CT is indicated, a blood culture should be obtained (94) and empiric therapy should be initiated as rapidly as possible while awaiting the imaging study. A brief delay between lumbar puncture and antibiotic treatment may not interfere with isolation of the causative organism.

The gold standard for the diagnosis of bacterial meningitis is identification by culture and Gram stain of CSF. Most bacteria responsible for meningitis can be readily detected by all microbiology laboratories. Culture also provides clinically useful information regarding antibiotic sensitivity. Several bacteria can also be detected by CSF analysis using the polymerase chain reaction (PCR), including the nucleic acids of *N. meningitidis* (95), *H. influenzae,* and *Mycobacterium tuberculosis* (96). PCR can be useful in the diagnosis of meningitis caused by spirochetes (97) and several viruses (98,99) and has considerable promise for detecting bacteria in children with meningitis that is partially treated or due to nonculturable organisms. Partial treatment of bacterial meningitis reduces the sensitivity of culture and Gram stain from 97% to 73% (100) but does not substantially alter the protein or glucose content of the CSF (101).

The CSF in bacterial meningites is usually cloudy and under increased pressure. During the acute stage, polymorphonuclear leukocytes predominate, whereas mononuclear cells appear in the later stages. The cell counts generally range between 1,000 and 10,000 cells/μL, but as many as 6% of cases have few or no cells during the earliest stage of the infection (102). Organisms can be seen intracellularly and extracellularly in smears and can be visualized or cultured in the absence of pleocytosis on rare occasions (103). Eosinophilic leukocytes can be seen in the CSF of patients with parasitic infestations of the CNS, including cysticercosis, trichinosis, toxocariasis, toxoplasmosis, ascariasis, angiostrongyliasis, echinococcosis, gnathostomiasis, or coccidiomycosis (104).

The cerebrospinal fluid typically has a low glucose content in children with bacterial meningitis, often to undetectable levels. In bacterial meningitis, the CSF-to-blood glucose ratio is usually below 0.40 (105). First observed by Lichtheim (106), the decrease was attributed initially to consumption of glucose by bacteria growing in the CSF. Although there remains controversy regarding the cause of hypoglycorrhachia in bacterial meningitis, the finding likely represents a combination of altered transport into the CSF compartment and alterations in glycolysis and the blood–brain barrier (107). Prockop and Fishman observed that the facilitated diffusion of glucose from blood to CSF and from CSF to blood is impaired in bacterial meningitis, although the increase in nonspecific bulk transport of glucose can compensate for the deficit (108). Low CSF glucose also occurs in sarcoidosis, mumps meningitis, herpes zoster meningitis, CNS leukemia, and meningeal carcinomatosis (109).

CSF protein is elevated in 80% to 92% of patients (59), commonly to levels of 100 mg/dL and higher, and some studies show correlations between mortality and increased CSF protein. CSF lactate concentrations can also be increased in bacterial meningitis (110), whereas CSF lactate is normal in aseptic meningitis unless cerebral hypoxia or edema has activated glycolytic pathways (111,112). The slow decrease of CSF lactate to normal with a 3-day course of antibiotic therapy can be useful in the diagnosis of partially treated bacterial meningitis (113) and can aid in differentiating bacterial meningitis from aseptic meningitis (114). The decrease in CSF pH, which also occurs in bacterial meningitis, is more transient than the elevation of CSF lactate and has less diagnostic utility (113).

Neuroimaging studies have important adjunctive roles in identifying the complications of bacterial meningitis, such as hydrocephalus, subdural effusions, or subdural empyema, and in detecting parameningeal abscesses or CSF leaks. Indications for neuroimaging in acute bacterial meningitis include depressed level of consciousness, prolonged, partial, or late seizures, focal neurologic deficits, enlarging head circumference, persistent or recurrent fever during the later stages of treatment, and recurrent meningitis (91–93,115). Neuroimaging studies can also improve clinicians' ability to predict sequelae in children who survive bacterial meningitis. Imaging should be considered strongly in neonates with bacterial meningitis, especially when gram-negative organisms are identified.

In the series of Rennick and colleagues, cerebral herniation occurred in 4.3% of children with meningitis (116). When ventricular dilatation or other imaging signs of increased pressure are present, lumbar puncture should be deferred to diminish the risk of herniation. This is particularly true if the child has a Glasgow Coma Score of 7 or less (117). Severe cerebral edema complicating neonatal meningitis can be associated with uncal herniation (118).

Treatment

Because of the life-threatening nature of bacterial meningitis and the potential for permanent neurodevelopmental sequelae, antibiotic therapy should be instituted as soon as the diagnosis is suspected. The management of the pediatric patients with meningitis is reviewed by Saez-Lorens and McCracken (1), Quagliarello and Scheld (3), Feigin and Pearlman (119), and Wubbel and McCracken (120).

Empiric antibiotic therapy for meningitis in infants younger than 1 month of age consists of therapy with ampicillin, 150 to 300 mg/kg per day in divided doses every 6 to

TABLE 7.7 General Recommendations Regarding Treatment of Meningitis

Known Organisms	*Primary Treatment for Susceptible Organisms*	*Alternative Treatment*
Streptococcus pneumoniae	Third-generation cephalosporin	Vancomycin
Neisseria meningitidis	Penicillin	Cefotaxime
Haemophilus influenzae	Ceftriaxone	Cefotaxime
Staphylococci	Nafcillin, oxacillin	Vancomycin (if methicillin resistance is suspected)
Listeria monocytogenes	Ampicillin and aminoglycoside	Trimethoprim-sulfa
Usual gram-negative rods	Cefotaxime, ceftizoxime, ceftriaxone	Ampicillin and aminoglycoside
Resistant gram-negative rods (especially *Pseudomonas*)	Ceftazidime and aminoglycoside (intravenous, intrathecal)	Ticarcillin, mezlocillin, and aminoglycoside
Anaerobes (including *Bacteroides fragilis*)	Penicillin and metronidazole	Chloramphenicol
Unknown pyogenic organism in neonates (younger than 2 months of age)	Ampicillin and aminoglycoside	Ampicillin and third-generation cephalosporin (e.g., cefotraxime)
Unknown pyogenic organism in children	Ampicillin and chloromycetin	Third-generation cephalosporin and penicillin

Adapted from Wubbel L, McCracken GH Jr. Management of bacterial meningitis. *Pediatr Rev* 1998;19:78; and Kennedy SS, Zacharski LR, Beck JR. Thrombotic thrombocytopenic purpura: analysis of 48 unselected cases. *Semin Thromb Hemost* 1980;6:341.

8 hours, and gentamicin, 2.5 to 7.5 mg/kg per day in one to three divided doses, or cefotaxime, 150 to 300 mg/kg per day divided every 6 to 8 hours, depending on the gestational and postnatal age of the infant (121). Antibiotic therapy should be modified once the identity and sensitivity profile of the pathogen have been determined (Table 7.7). Therapy for group B streptococcal meningitis can consist of ampicillin, as just described, or penicillin G, 250,000 to 450,000 U/kg per day intravenously in three divided doses for infants less than 1 week old and 450,000 U/kg per day in four divided doses for infants older than 1 week. Some add gentamicin, 2.5 to 7.5 mg/kg per day in one to three divided doses. *E. coli* meningitis can be treated with ampicillin or an expanded-spectrum cephalosporin and gentamicin, as just described. Listeria are not sensitive to cephalosporins, including the expanded-spectrum formulations, so therapy consists of 14 to 21 days of intravenous ampicillin, 150 to 300 mg/kg per day in three to four divided doses, and gentamicin, 2.5 to 7.5 mg/kg per day in one to three divided doses, depending on the infant's gestational and postnatal age (121). Infants with uncomplicated cases of meningitis require 14 to 21 days of intravenous antibiotic therapy, and complicated cases may require more prolonged treatment.

Empiric antibiotic therapy for suspected bacterial meningitis in children older than 1 month of age consists of cefotaxime, 300 mg/kg per day in three or four divided doses, or ceftriaxone, 100 mg/kg per day intravenously divided every 12 hours, and vancomycin, 60 mg/kg per day in four divided doses (121). Vancomycin, used because of potential resistance of *S. pneumoniae* to penicillin and cephalosporins, should be discontinued as soon as the causative organism is shown to be susceptible to penicillin, cefotaxime, or ceftriaxone. Resistance of *S. pneumoniae* to penicillin and cephalosporins remains a potential problem in most regions. The prevalence of strains with decreased susceptibility to penicillin approaches 50% in some areas of the United States (122). Penicillin G, 250,000 units/kg per day (maximum dose 12 million units/day), can be used in children or adolescents with meningococcal meningitis.

Children or adolescents with suspected meningitis require droplet and standard precautions for the first 24 hours of appropriate antibiotic therapy. Repeat lumbar puncture should be considered after 24 to 48 hours of therapy to confirm sterilization of the CSF in infants and in children with pneumococcal meningitis who received dexamethasone or have infections with strains that are nonsusceptible to penicillin or cephalosporins. Infants older than 1 month of age, children, and adolescents with bacterial meningitis should receive 7 to 14 days of therapy, depending on the organism and the presence of any complications.

Adjunctive management of infants and children with suspected or proven bacterial meningitis includes control of increased intracranial pressure, treatment of seizures, correction of electrolyte disturbances, treatment of fever, and close monitoring for subdural effusions and severe systemic complications such as DIC, hemorrhagic purpura, or renal failure (123,124). Strategies for the management of childhood bacterial meningitis can be found in the 2003 *Red Book* of the American Academy of Pediatrics (121).

Dexamethasone therapy, an adjunct in meningitis therapy in infants and children with *H. influenzae* meningitis and perhaps also in adults with bacterial meningitis, is controversial in children with *S. pneumoniae* or *N. meningitidis* meningitis. Clinical trials with dexamethasone in children with *H. influenzae* meningitis demonstrated a significantly lower incidence of profound hearing loss in the dexamethasone-treated group (125–128). Recommendations regarding dexamethasone therapy can be found in the most recent edition of the *Red Book* (121).

Increased intracranial pressure can cause significant alterations in consciousness and can contribute to the morbidity of bacterial meningitis. Intracranial pressure can be reduced by cautious removal of CSF, as might occur with an extraventricular drainage device, or by the use of hyperosmolar agents. These agents can sometimes improve the child's sensorium promptly. Mannitol is effective for the cytotoxic edema but not for the vasogenic edema of meningitis. Intracranial pressure can be reduced by elevating the head of the patient's bed by 30 degrees, and pressure spikes associated with suctioning can be minimized by careful sedation. Hyperventilation as a means to lower intracranial pressure by reducing Pco_2 may be detrimental (57).

Seizures require prompt treatment using lorazepam, 0.05 to 0.1 mg/kg as needed, followed by loading doses of either phenobarbital, 10 to 20 mg/kg, or fosphenytoin, 15 to 20 mg/kg. Maintenance doses of either phenobarbital or fosphenytoin may be necessary thereafter. Sedation can accompany anticonvulsant therapy. The potential for SIADH in children with bacterial meningitis necessitates close monitoring of fluid therapy, serum electrolytes, and urine output.

Prognosis

The outcome of bacterial meningitis is influenced by the age of the child, the species of the bacterial pathogen, and the duration of disease before the initiation of appropriate antibiotic therapy. In general, the prognosis is less favorable in neonates, regardless of the pathogen, and in older children with pneumococcal meningitis. In some but not all studies (118,129,130), sequelae are more likely in children whose diagnosis and treatment are delayed. Kresky and colleagues observed sequelae in 12% of children whose treatment was begun within 24 hours of the onset of symptoms versus 59% in children who began treatment 3 or more days after the onset of symptoms (131).

In the experience of Thomas, sensorineural hearing loss, the most common sequela of bacterial meningitis, was observed in 8.5% of the surviving children (132); hearing loss was bilateral and severe in 5.6%. Children who survive bacterial meningitis also have learning disabilities, motor problems, speech delay, hyperactivity, blindness, obstructive hydrocephalus, and recurrent seizures. Grimwood and colleagues observed that approximately one in four school-aged meningitis survivors had serious and disabling sequelae, a functionally important behavior disorder, or neuropsychological or auditory dysfunction that adversely affected academic performance (133). Children who have meningitis in the first year of life and survive are at greatest risk for neurodevelopmental sequelae (134).

Hearing loss develops during the first 48 hours of the illness (135) and results from infectious and immune-mediated injury to the cochlea and, occasionally, the semicircular canals. Less often, deafness is caused by an arachnoiditis of the eighth nerve or damage to the auditory projection areas. Recovery of hearing can begin during the first 2 weeks, but hearing can continue to improve for as long as 6 months. However, because hearing loss can be permanent, audiometry is required in all infants, children, and adolescents who recover from bacterial meningitis (136,137).

The 20-year risk for subsequent unprovoked seizures is 13% for patients with early seizures and 2.4% for those without early seizures. When seizures develop, their incidence is highest during the first 5 years after meningitis, but the risk remains elevated during the subsequent 15 years (138). Patients who develop intractable seizures after meningitis incurred before 4 years of age have a high incidence of neocortical seizure foci or mesial temporal sclerosis. The latter group of patients can respond to surgical intervention should seizures remain unresponsive to anticonvulsant therapy (139).

In a meta-analysis of reports of meningitis in children 2 months to 19 years of age published between 1955 and 1993, Baraff and colleagues found that children from developed countries had a lower mortality (4.8% vs. 8.1%) and a lower likelihood of sequelae (17.5% vs. 26.1%) than those from underdeveloped countries (140). Mortality was highest for meningitis caused by *S. pneumoniae* (15.3%) and lowest for that caused by *N. meningitis* (7.5%) and *H. influenzae* (3.8%) (140).

Common Forms of Meningitis

Meningococcal Meningitis

N. meningitidis causes three distinct clinical entities: meningitis, as discussed previously; septicemia, which can precede invasion of the CNS or be an isolated but fulminant form with petechiae and purpura (Waterhouse-Friderichsen syndrome); and chronic meningococcemia, in which an equilibrium between bacteria and host has become established (141). Genetic factors determine, in part, the susceptibility to meningococcal disease. Families with low TNF production have a 10-fold increased risk for fatal outcome, whereas high IL-10 production, a potent inhibitor of TNF (142), increases the risk 20-fold. Children with complement deficiency are also at risk (143), suggesting that screening for complement disorders should be considered in children or adolescents with meningococcal infections.

The meningococcus produces petechial, maculopapular, or morbilliform skin lesions in approximately 75% of patients. Petechiae also are occasionally seen in patients with *H. influenzae*, pneumococcal, or streptococcal meningitis. Septicemia with *N. meningitidis* can lead to tissue sensitization and purpura fulminans as a consequence of disseminated intravascular coagulation. Purpura fulminans also has been observed during infections with other *Neisseria* species, including *N. catarrhalis* (144), *N. subflava* (145), and *N. gonorrhoeae* (146).

Meningococcal septicemia can cause a rapidly evolving fulminant illness with high rates of morbidity and mortality. The pathogenesis of this disorder reflects bacterial embolization and endotoxin-induced shock (147–149). Pulmonary microvascular thromboses, composed of platelets and leukocytes, can lead to severe cor pulmonale. Meningococcal endotoxin activates the cascades of procoagulation, anticoagulation, and fibrinolysis as well as the cytokine network and the complement system. Meningococcal endotoxin also produces disseminated intravascular coagulation with rapid consumption of fibrinogen and formation of fibrin thrombi in adrenal glands and renal glomeruli. The fibrin thrombi cause hemorrhagic infarction of the adrenal glands and renal cortical necrosis. Bilateral adrenal hemorrhages occur in two-thirds of fatal cases.

Chronic meningococcemia produces intermittent chills or fever, evanescent rash, joint pain or swelling, or joint effusions. Symptoms can regress without specific therapy or recur over several days or weeks. The rash can assume the form of petechiae, erythema nodosum, papulonecrotic tuberculids, macules, or maculopapules. Recurrent neisserial infections of the nervous system are rare, but they occur with increased frequency in patients with deficiencies of immunoglobulin G (IgG) subclass (150) or complement (151). Complications of meningococcal bacteremia include pericarditis, arthritis, hypopyon, and panophthalmitis (152). Autopsy of 200 fatal cases of meningococcal infection revealed acute interstitial myocarditis with focal necrosis and hemorrhage in 78% (153). Deafness after meningococcal meningitis is more frequent with infections by the uncommon serogroups (W135, X, Y, 29E) than with meningitis caused by serogroup B (154).

Chemoprophylaxis of family members and other intimate contacts is recommended; current information can be found in the *Red Book* (121,155). Rifampin is the drug of choice in children, whereas rifampin, ceftriaxone, or ciprofloxacine can be used in adults. A quadrivalent vaccine (groups A, C, Y, and W135) is available in the United States for children 2 years of age and older (121). Vaccination of college students who live in dormatories is recommended, given the potential for epidemic meningococcal disease on college campuses (121).

Haemophilus Meningitis

Before the availability of *H. influenzae* (Hib) vaccine, *H. influenzae* was the leading cause of meningitis in the United States, causing 8,000 to 11,000 cases annually (1,3,9). Between the years 1985 and 1991 the incidence of *H. influenzae* meningitis in the United States decreased by 82% (156,157) after the widespread introduction of the vaccine (Table 7.1). *H. influenzae* vaccines consist of capsular polysaccharides covalently linked to a carrier protein. They are not effective against unencapsulated organisms that are also potential causes of CNS disease (158). *Haemophilus* meningitis is occasionally caused by types A through F or nontypable species (159,160). Although *H. influenzae* meningitis occurs almost exclusively in unimmunized children younger than 6 years of age (121), cases have been described in neonates or apparently healthy adults (161).

Hearing loss, the most common neurologic sequela of *H. influenzae* meningitis, affects approximately 11% of surviving children. Hearing deficits range from mild to profound hearing loss and are more common in children who began treatment 24 hours or more after the onset of symptoms (162). In approximately one-half of the affected children the hearing loss is bilateral. Approximately 15% of survivors have neurologic defects, such as a learning disability, focal neurologic deficits, epilepsy, cortical blindness, or mental retardation (163,164). Mortality rates range from 3% to 5%. Factors associated with poor prognosis include age less than 1 year, illness duration of more than 3 days before therapy, and onset or persistence of seizures after 3 days of treatment (162). Rarely, carotid artery occlusion (165,166), pericarditis, myocarditis, atrioventricular block (167), epiglottitis, cellulitis, and septic arthritis can accompany *H. influenzae* meningitis (168).

The risk of disease in household contacts is increased considerably during the month after exposure to the index case. Clusters of cases have also been encountered in day care centers. Rifampin prophylaxis has been recommended for index cases during their hospitalization, usually just before discharge, and for adults and children in households of an unvaccinated child younger than 4 years of age, households with an unimmunized child under 1 year of age, and households with an immunocompromised child. Prophylaxis should be given as soon as possible because 54% of secondary cases occur in the first week after hospitalization of the index case (121).

Pneumococcal Meningitis

Predisposing factors for childhood meningitis with *S. pneumoniae*, the most common cause of meningitis after the neonatal period in populations with compulsory immunization for *H. influenzae*, include an upper respiratory infection, acute or chronic otitis media, purulent conjunctivitis, and CSF rhinorrhea secondary to developmental abnormalities or trauma (59). Splenectomy, congenital or acquired immunodeficiencies, and disorders that alter splenic function (e.g., sickle cell disease) increase substantially the risk of pneumococcal disease, including meningitis (169–171).

The pathogenesis of pneumococcal meningitis differs because the gram-positive organism does not contain endotoxin. Pneumococci adhere to cerebral capillaries using a surface protein, CbpA, that recognizes carbohydrates.

Once attached, invasion involves bacterial recognition of the receptor for platelet-activating factor (PAF) (172). Once in the CSF, a variety of pneumococcal components, including the cell wall, lipoteichoic acid, and several cytotoxins, incite the inflammatory response (173). The cytotoxin pneumolysin contributes to loss of cochlear cells in meningitic hearing loss but does not contribute to cell damage or inflammation in the brain itself (174).

Approximately one-third of children who survive pneumococcal meningitis have sequelae, 19% with hearing loss and 25% with neurologic complications (175). Overall mortality in the series reported by Kornelisse and coworkers was 17%. Coma at admission, respiratory distress, shock, CSF protein level of 250 mg/dL or greater, peripheral white count of less than 5,000 cells/μL, and a serum sodium of less than 135 mEq/L are associated with increased risks of mortality. Of the surviving children described by Arditi and colleagues, 25% had neurologic sequelae, and 32% had unilateral or bilateral hearing loss. In this study the incidence of hearing loss was higher in those who had received dexamethasone (176), illustrating further the controversy associated with dexamethasone therapy in childhood bacterial meningitis.

Staphylococcal Meningitis

Staphylococcus aureus accounts for 0.8% to 8.8% of bacterial meningitis cases in patients of all ages. Approximately 20% of cases occurred in neonates, 10% in children, and 70% in adults (177). As many as 90% of cases occur in association with predisposing factors, such as recent neurosurgical procedures or head trauma. *S. aureus* causes 12% to 36% of CSF shunt infections, and *S. epidermidis* causes the majority of the remainder. Meningitis can develop from staphylococcal abscesses within the brain parenchyma or from spinal epidural abscesses. More distant staphylococcal infections, such as oral or abdominal abscesses, sinusitis, osteomyelitis, pneumonia, cellulitis, infected shunts or intravascular grafts, decubitus ulcers, and even abdominal abscesses, have been implicated in occasional cases of *S. aureus* meningitis. *S. aureus* is the most likely cause of meningitis in persons with infective endocarditis. Other predisposing factors include immunodeficiency disorders, diabetes mellitus, renal failure, and malignancy (178–180). Coagulase-negative staphylococci, especially slime-producing variants (181), can cause indolent infections of ventriculoatrial and ventriculoperitoneal shunts (182,183) (see Chapter 5 for a further discussion of shunt-related infections).

Acute Purulent Meningitis in the Neonate

Neonatal meningitis has an overall incidence of 0.2 to 0.32 cases per 1,000 live births (184). Meningitis occurs more often in male infants (68% to 76%) (185), except for group B streptococcal meningitis, which has a female preponderance (186). Other potential neonatal pathogens include *E. coli, Listeria monocytogenes, Citrobacter* species, *Klebsiella-Enterobacter* species, *Pasteurella multocida* (187), *Flavobacterium, Pseudomonas cepacia* (188), *Salmonella* species (189), *N. meningitidis* (190), and, rarely, *H. influenzae.* The median age of infants with neonatal meningitis is 10 days (191). Predisposing factors include maternal infections chorioamnionitis, premature rupture of membranes, neonatal urinary anomalies, neural tube defects, and immune dysfunction common among newborns (192–194). Infections of the respiratory tract and skin can also predispose to meningitis; bacterial meningitis complicates 20% to 30% of infants with septicemia.

CSF findings can be confusing in neonatal meningitis, given the broad ranges of normal values for cell count and protein content (194–199). White blood counts of less than 32 cells/μL occur in 29% of group B streptococcal and 4% of gram-negative neonatal meningitis; protein concentrations of less than 170 mg/dL occur in 47% and 23%, and CSF-to-blood glucose ratios of grerater than 0.44 occur in 45% and 15%, respectively (198). CSF values for healthy term and preterm infants are presented in the Introduction chapter.

Since the late 1970s group B *Streptococcus* (*S. agalactiae*) has been an extremely important pathogen in the neonate (200–202). The two clinically and epidemiologically distinct forms of group B streptococcal disease are now recognized as a paradigm for several bacterial pathogens that infect the neonate. In the first, termed "early-onset disease," symptoms begin within 10 days of birth. The infants are often seriously ill with respiratory distress, shock, or DIC at the time of diagnosis, and the mortality is quite high (58%). In this form of infection, bacteria can be isolated often from CSF, blood, and other fluids or tissues. In the second clinical pattern, termed "late-onset disease," symptoms begin after 10 days of age. The infants are less severely ill, and death or permanent neurologic sequelae are less frequent (19%). Organisms are usually isolated from the CSF or blood only. However, infants with late-onset disease with several bacteria, including group B *Streptococcus,* can have osteomyelitis, which can cause pseudoparalysis of the upper or lower extremities.

The diagnosis of group B neonatal meningitis can be confirmed by lumbar puncture. Blood cultures are positive in 50% to 90% of infants with early-onset meningitis (203,204), and cultures of the nasopharynx may yield the causative organism in as many as 40% of cases. Antigen detection systems for analysis of CSF or urine have variable sensitivity and specificity and are generally not recommended. The prognosis of neonatal meningitis remains discouraging despite 21 to 28 days of therapy with the available antimicrobials (Table 7.7). In the series of Hristeva and coworkers the mortality was 26% with neurologic sequelae in 27% of survivors (204). Most experts recommend repeat CSF analysis after 48 hours of therapy to ensure eradication of bacteria from the CSF of infants with neonatal meningitis (121).

Chronic and Granulomatous Bacterial Meningitis

Tuberculous Meningitis

Despite advances in chemotherapy, meningitis caused by *Mycobacterium tuberculosis* remains a serious worldwide pediatric problem, and even in the United States, tuberculous meningitis causes more deaths than any other form of tuberculosis. In England and Wales, tuberculous meningitis occurred in 4.4% of children reported during 1983 to have tuberculosis (205).

Pathology and Pathophysiology. In children, tuberculous meningitis almost always accompanies generalized miliary tuberculosis. In an older clinical series published in 1997 (206), 68% of children with meningitis had miliary tuberculosis, and conversely, 81% of children with miliary disease developed tuberculous meningitis. In a Turkish series published in 1998, miliary tuberculosis was seen by chest radiography in 20% (207).

In the majority of cases in the United States, infection is caused by the human type of mycobacteria. Bovine tuberculosis has become uncommon because of the widespread pasteurization of milk. The human form also is more common in tropical countries because of the relative inaccessibility of nonhuman milk and milk products.

Involvement of the meninges is probably secondary to a small tuberculoma in the cortex or the leptomeninges (1), and the brains of most patients who die of tuberculous meningitis demonstrate older superficial foci. Tuberculomas of the choroid plexus are a less common site for the infection.

At autopsy, the meninges look gray and opaque, and a gelatinous exudate fills the basal cisterns, particularly the anterior portion of the pons. Small tubercles can appear over the convexity of the brain or the periventricular area. The basal ganglia and thalamus in the region of the lenticulostriate and thalamo-perforating arteries are involved in 46% of cases (208).

Microscopic examination shows the exudate to consist of lymphocytes, plasma cells, and large histiocytes with typical caseation. Langhans giant cells are rare. The meningeal arteries are inflamed and thrombosed, and secondary infarctions of the superficial cortex are common. Tuberculomas are now relatively rare in Western countries, but were at one time one of the most common causes for a posterior fossa mass in children (209). They occur most commonly in the cerebellum and less often within the brainstem.

Clinical Manifestations. The most common form of tuberculous meningitis, constituting approximately 70% of all cases, is a caseous meningitis that results from direct invasion of the meninges. In approximately 75% of children, this invasion occurs while the primary focus is fresh (i.e., less than 6 months old). The illness is often precipitated by an acute infectious disease, commonly measles. Before 1955, its incidence in the United States was highest in the spring. When tuberculous meningitis is part of the initial attack, its incidence is highest among children between the ages of 1 and 2 years. When it is a complication of systemic tuberculosis, it is more likely to affect older children.

Untreated, tuberculous meningitis rapidly progresses to death, with an average duration of only 3 weeks. Lincoln distinguished three stages of the illness, each lasting approximately 1 week (210).

In the initial stage (stage 1), gastrointestinal symptoms predominate, and no definite neurologic manifestations are seen. The child can be apathetic or irritable with intermittent headache, but the results of the neurologic examination are negative. In approximately 10% of patients, commonly in infants, a febrile convulsion is the most significant symptom of this stage.

During stage 2, the child develops drowsiness and disorientation, with signs of meningeal irritation. The deep tendon reflexes are hyperactive, abdominal reflexes disappear, and ankle and patellar clonus can be present. Cranial nerve signs are evident, with involvement of cranial nerves VII, VI, and III, in that order of frequency (207). Choroid tubercles are present in 10% of patients.

During stage 3, the patient is comatose, although periods of intermittent wakefulness can occur. The pupils are fixed, and recurrent clonic spasm of the extremities, irregular respiration, and a rising fever are present. Hydrocephalus develops in approximately two-thirds of patients whose illness lasts longer than 3 weeks. It was apparent at presentation in 80% of patients in the Turkish series of Yaramis and coworkers (207). It is particularly common when treatment is delayed or inadequate.

A serous form of tuberculous meningitis is encountered less commonly. In children known to have active primary tuberculosis, the presenting symptom is meningeal irritation. Unlike in tuberculous meningitis, the CSF is normal.

A third form of tuberculous meningitis, seen in 17% of instances, consists of cases with primary spinal cord infection. These children can have major problems with blockage of the spinal canal that can be associated with Pott disease. Spinal tuberculosis can be differentiated from the other types by its history and laboratory findings. The symptoms usually last longer, often existing for 6 months before meningitis is considered. A fall often produces back pain and staggering or clumsy gait. Abdominal pain, presumably of root origin, is common. Nuchal or spinal rigidity can develop while the sensorium remains clear. CSF can be scant and show marked elevation in protein.

Recognition of tuberculous meningitis can be difficult because the characteristic signs and symptoms of meningitis can be absent during the early stages of the illness. In the series of Idriss and coauthors, nuchal rigidity occurred in 77%, apathy in 72%, fever in 47%, vomiting in 30%, drowsiness in 23%, headache in 21%, coma in 14%, convulsions, sweating, facial palsy, optic atrophy, and abducens and oculomotor palsies each in 9%, hemiparesis in 5%, and eighth-nerve palsy and diabetes insipidus each in 2% (211).

Metabolic disturbances during tuberculous meningitis include metabolic alkalosis, hyponatremia, hypochloremia, and hypotonic expansion of extracellular fluid. Intracellular potassium concentration is normal or decreased, whereas sodium concentration within red cells and skeletal muscle generally increases. No evidence exists for a salt-losing renal lesion in tuberculous meningitis, although hypervolemia can result in secondary hypoaldosteronism and increased secretion of atrial natriuretic peptide factor (212). The hyponatremic syndrome in tuberculous meningitis is associated with elevations in atrial naturietic peptide more often (65%) than elevation of vasopressin (3%) (212). Vomiting often tends to aggravate electrolyte disturbances.

The presence of focal neurologic signs in a patient with tuberculous meningitis and with hypoglycorrhachia persisting beyond 12 weeks should suggest a tuberculous brain abscess or tuberculoma (213,214). Tuberculomas or vascular occlusions can develop weeks or months after active therapy is instituted (215). However, they were seen in only 2% of patients in the series of Yaramis and colleagues (207). The presence of these complications indicates the need for revision of chemotherapy. Paradoxic expansion of intracranial tuberculomas can occur during therapy (216).

Tuberculous spinal arachnoiditis, which occurs in 7% to 42% of cases, can cause paraplegia or quadriplegia (217). Sensory loss can occur with a sensory level, root distribution pattern, bladder or bowel involvement, or root pain (218).

Diagnosis. The diagnosis of tuberculous meningitis depends on the clinical picture of a subacute meningitis, a history of exposure to the disease, often from an otherwise asymptomatic older relative, a positive skin test result, and the CSF changes.

Anergy to tuberculosis can occur in up to 36% of patients (218). In the experience at Bellevue Hospital, New York City, 85% of patients had positive reactions. Another 10% were inadequately tested or died before tuberculin tests could be completed (210,219). In the Turkish series, only 30% had a positive skin test result (207). In the series of Kent and coworkers, which included both children and adults, 75% of patients reacted positively to 100 U or less of purified protein derivative (220). A decreased humoral immune response can occur in the presence of intact cell-mediated immunity (221). The chest radiograph is not always reliable; in the series of Zarabi and colleagues, children with tuberculous meningitis had normal chest radiograph results in 43% of cases, signs of disseminated miliary tuberculosis in 23%, and calcifying primary intrathoracic tuberculosis in 10% (222). In the more recent series of Yaramis and colleagues, the chest radiograph result was abnormal in 87%; a hilar adenopathy was the most common abnormality, being present in 34% (207).

The CSF findings are characteristic. The fluid has a ground glass appearance and when spun down forms a pellicle in which the organisms can occasionally be visualized. In 85% of cases the total CSF cell count was less than 500 cells/μL (207). The cells are composed of reactive mononuclear and ependymal cells with few polymorphonuclear cells. CSF protein is invariably increased (207,220). Of tuberculous meningitis patients reported from Turkey, 83% showed a sugar of 40 mg/dL or less (207). In the Australian series of Kent and colleagues, the initial CSF glucose was normal in 60%, but in the majority of patients (74%) who initially had a normal CSF glucose level, subsequent values fell below normal (220). Tuberculous meningitis can be diagnosed rapidly by means of the polymerase chain reaction (PCR), enzyme-linked immunosorbent assay (ELISA), and latex particle agglutination detection of mycobacterial antigen (159,223,224). ELISA detection of IgG and IgM antibodies and identification of tuberculostearic acid in CSF with gas chromatography and mass spectrometry also can assist in arriving at a diagnosis of tuberculous meningitis (225). CSF culture results for mycobacteria are positive in less than one-half of instances (207). Performing repeated lumbar punctures and obtaining large volumes of CSF markedly enhance the likelihood of obtaining a positive culture result (226). The PCR for early detection of *M. tuberculosis* in CSF has a sensitivity of only 48%; microscopy has a sensitivity of 9% (159). Fatal *Mycobacterium avium* meningitis has been confused with meningitis caused by *M. tuberculosis* in immunocompetent children (227).

Diffuse or focal electroencephalographic (EEG) abnormalities occur in approximately 80% of cases (228). Neuroimaging is of relatively little assistance in the diagnosis of tuberculous meningitis. Cranial CT within 1 week of initial symptoms can reveal basilar enhancement, ventricular dilatation, or infarction (207,229). MRI with gadolinium enhancement also can demonstrate meningeal inflammation. Mild to marked third ventricular enlargement is extremely common and was invariably present in one study (230). Severe hydrocephalus was demonstrable by CT scans in 87% of children with tuberculous meningitis but in only 12% of adults. Visible infarcts are present in 28% to 40% of cases, usually involving the territory of the middle cerebral artery. Patients with nonenhancing lesions have a good prognosis, whereas those with enhancing lesions are likely to die or have irreversible sequelae despite medical therapy or shunting (205,230).

The appearance of tuberculomas revealed by neuroimaging studies differs from that of abscesses, metastases, and gliomas. MRI of tuberculomas shows large, ring-enhancing lesions with low intensity on T2-weighted images and intermediate intensity on T1-weighted images. Small lesions with ring enhancement on CT scan show a central bright signal on T2-weighted images with a peripheral low-intensity rim, surrounded by high-intensity edema (231).

Treatment. Therapy for tuberculous meningitis must be prompt and adequate (232). It includes appropriate chemotherapy, correction of fluid and electrolyte disturbances, and relief of increased intracranial pressure.

Treatment of tuberculous meningitis, as recommended by the Committee on Infectious Diseases of the American Academy of Pediatrics (233), should include daily doses of four drugs for 2 months: isoniazid (INH), rifampin, pyrazinamide, and streptomycin. This is followed by INH and rifampin administered daily or twice weekly under direct observation for 10 months. For patients who may have acquired tuberculosis in geographic locales where resistance to streptomycin is common, capreomycin (15 to 30 mg/kg per day) or kanamycin (15 to 30 mg/kg per day) may be used instead of streptomycin. Treatment of tuberculomas should be similar to that for tuberculous meningitis. CSF penetration of INH (89%) and pyrazinamide (91%) changes little during the course of therapy for tuberculous meningitis; penetration of rifampin (5%) and streptomycin (20%) can decline to result in subtherapeutic levels. Corticosteroids have little effect on the penetration of these drugs (234).

INH (10 to 15 mg/kg per day up to a maximum dose of 300 mg/day, 20 to 40 mg/kg per dose twice weekly up to a maximum of 900 mg per dose) is a bactericidal and bacteriostatic drug that interacts with nucleic acid synthesis and inhibits production of cell wall mycolic acid (235). Peak serum concentrations usually range from 6 to 20 μg/mL. The optimal duration of treatment with INH is not known, but therapy should be continued for at least 1 year. Peripheral neuritis can complicate the use of INH in some patients. This complication can be prevented or relieved by pyridoxine (25 to 50 mg/day). Adding pyridoxine is probably not necessary for infants or children unless they are malnourished, but it is recommended for adolescents (232). Other adverse reactions can include gastrointestinal and hematologic hypersensitivity and lupus-like reactions. Hepatitis is rare in children younger than 11 years of age. When INH is used together with rifampin, the incidence of hepatotoxicity increases if the INH dose exceeds 10 mg/kg per day.

Rifampin (10 to 20 mg/kg up to 600 mg daily or twice weekly) is a bactericidal drug that inhibits RNA synthesis by binding to bacterial DNA-dependent RNA polymerase. Rifampin is recommended for children with resistant organisms. Adverse reactions include gastrointestinal and hematologic hypersensitivity, most often thrombocytopenia, flulike symptoms, and hepatitis. Birth control pills may be rendered ineffective.

Pyrazinamide (20 to 40 mg/kg per day or 50 to 70 mg/kg twice weekly up to 2,000 mg/day) is a bacteriostatic drug used for drug-resistant organisms. It can cause hepatotoxicity, hyperuricemia, arthritis, skin rash, and gastrointestinal upset.

Streptomycin (20 mg/kg intramuscularly daily or twice weekly up to 1,000 mg/day) is a bactericidal drug that blocks protein synthesis. Adverse reactions include ototoxicity with greater incidence of vestibular than auditory involvement, hypersensitivity, and, rarely, nephrotoxicity. Streptomycin toxicity usually develops after 12 weeks of therapy.

Ethambutol (15 to 25 mg/kg per day or 50 mg/kg per dose twice weekly up to 2,500 mg/day) is a bacteriostatic drug that has replaced para-aminosalicylic acid in older individuals. It is usually reserved for children older than 5 years of age because of the risk of optic neuritis or optic atrophy in younger children. These complications are rare if the recommended dose is not exceeded. Impairment of visual acuity or color vision may occur, as well as rashes, gastrointestinal symptoms, and fever.

Para-aminosalicylic acid (200 mg/kg per day in three divided doses up to 12 g/day) reduces the emergence of drug-resistant strains. Gastrointestinal side effects can be intolerable.

In the United States, the incidence of drug-resistant strains has been low, but is becoming an increasing problem, and in some regions of the world resistance to INH can be as high as 30%. This percentage makes a laboratory evaluation of drug susceptibility imperative. Ethionamide, cycloserine, kanamycin, amikacin, ofloxacin, ciprofloxacin, and capreomycin should be considered in multidrug-resistant tuberculosis (236).

Spinal arachnoiditis is a common complication of tuberculous meningitis. Intrathecal hyaluronidase has been reported in a nonrandomized trial to reduce the mortality and disability of patients with tuberculous meningitis when compared with a control group (217).

Adjuvant treatment with corticosteroids such as prednisone remains controversial. In the study of Schoeman and coworkers (237), prednisone improved the survival rate and intellectual outcome of patients with tuberculous meningitis; it did not affect the incidence of motor deficits, blindness, deafness, increased intracranial pressure, or basal ganglia infarction (237). Its use has been recommended for seriously ill patients (233,238). In other studies, corticosteroids reduced intracranial pressure, basal exudate, and cerebral edema without altering morbidity or mortality (234,239) and relieved pulmonary symptoms in miliary tuberculosis (232). The neurologic state of patients sometimes deteriorates shortly after the initiation of therapy. Corticosteroid treatment can benefit this condition and can favorably influence mortality if started before the onset of coma (238,240). Most experts consider 1 to 2 mg/kg per day of prednisone or its equivalent given for 6 to 8 weeks to be appropriate (233).

Intracranial pressure above 400 mm of CSF significantly impairs perfusion of cerebral tissue, and patients who have consistent severe elevations of intracranial pressure require short courses of dexamethasone (6 mg/m^2 every 4 to 6 hours) to reduce edema or neurosurgical intervention with ventriculo-external or ventriculoperitoneal shunts to relieve acute hydrocephalus (241,242). Hydrocephalus becomes more marked at pressures up to 600 mm CSF, by which point hemoperfusion has fallen to approximately 40% of normal. Peacock and Deenny observed that ventriculoperitoneal shunting of patients with tuberculous meningitis resulted in a better outcome than was seen in matched nonshunted children (243).

The treatment of tuberculoma has been considered by Bhagwati and Parulekar. In their experience, some 60% of the patients responded to drugs alone and 23% required surgical intervention for failure to respond or mass effect (244). Infratentorial tuberculomas associated with hydrocephalus should receive ventriculoperitoneal shunts.

Prognosis. Untreated tuberculous meningitis was invariably fatal. With the newer treatment regimens, fewer survivors have major sequelae than were observed several decades ago (245). Even so, in the experience of Deeny and coworkers, reported in 1985, only 18% of survivors were neurologically and intellectually normal (246). As a rule, the prognosis is good for patients presenting with stage 1 disease and generally poor for those presenting with stage 3 disease. In the series of Kent and colleagues 25% of patients presenting with stage 2 disease died or were left with sequelae (220). With treatment, CSF glucose returns to normal within 1 to 2 months and CSF protein becomes normal within 4 to 26 months (220).

Major neurologic sequelae include hydrocephalus, spastic pareses, seizures, paraplegia, and sensory disturbances of the extremities. Late ophthalmologic complications include optic atrophy and blindness. Hearing and vestibular residua can occur as a consequence of both streptomycin therapy and the disease process itself. Minor neurologic sequelae include cranial nerve palsies, nystagmus, ataxia, mild disturbances of coordination, and spasticity.

Intellectual defects occur in approximately two-thirds of survivors (246). These patients have a high incidence of encephalographic abnormalities, which correlate with the persistence of sequelae such as convulsions and mental subnormality. Intracranial calcifications develop in approximately one-third of children who recover from tuberculous meningitis (247). Panhypopituitarism has been reported after cured tuberculous meningitis (248). One-fifth of survivors have such selective pituitary hypothalamic disturbances as sexual precocity, hyperprolactemia, and deficiencies in ADH, growth hormone, corticotropin, and gonadotropin (249).

Children younger than 3 years of age have a poorer prognosis for survival than do older children, a fact that might relate to the easier recognition of the disorder in older children (246,250).

Meningitis Caused by Unusual Organisms

Table 7.8 summarizes the essential clinical features of the various meningeal infections produced by some of the less common organisms and indicates the recommended forms of treatment (251–263).

BRAIN ABSCESSES

Brain abscess is a relatively uncommon but life-threatening infection in children (264). A brain abscess consists of localized free or encapsulated pus within the brain substance. Although the condition has been known for more than 200 years and its association with cyanotic congenital heart disease was described more than 100 years ago, the absence of classic signs and symptoms hinders its early clinical diagnosis and treatment.

Etiology and Pathogenesis

Predisposing contiguous site or distant pathologic states are always present. In the experience of Ersahin and coworkers, reported in 1994, the cause of the abscess was meningitis in 36% of cases, otitis in 27%, head injury in 16%, and congenital heart disease in 9%. Multiple abscesses occurred in 29% of the children (265). However, congenital heart disease was the most common predisposing factor between 1981 and 2000 and from 1945 to1980 at Children's Hospital Boston (266). Pyogenic organisms gain access to the brain substance by one of three routes. The first is through the bloodstream either from a remote infection, as a consequence of sepsis, or in association with a cardiopulmonary malfunction, most commonly cyanotic congenital heart disease with a right-to-left shunt. The second is by extension of contiguous infections such as leptomeningitis, infections of the middle ear, or infections of the paranasal sinuses either directly or as a result of septic thrombophlebitis of bridging veins. The third is as a complication of a penetrating wound. Children with chronic bacterial infection are more prone to this complication, in that they can develop an infected infarct (267).

The most common causative organisms in order of frequency are anaerobic and microaerophilic streptococci, *Fusobacterium* species, β-hemolytic streptococci,

TABLE 7.8 Some Rarer Organisms Responsible for Meningitis

Organism (Reference)	Clinical Features	Treatment of Choice
Listeria monocytogenes (253–255)	Primary meningitis in newborn infants or later in first month of life, rhombencephalitis	Ampicillin (150–250 mg/kg/day) IV, alone or in combination with trimethoprim-sulfamethoxazole or aminoglycosides
Proteus spp. (256)	Neonatal meningitis or secondary to otitis media, genitourinary tract infection; hydrocephalus, hemorrhagic necrosis of brain are common complications; cerebrospinal fluid culture results may be negative with ventricular culture results positive	Variable sensitivities: usually penicillin, kanamycin, ampicillin, chloramphenicol
Mima polymorpha (257)	Neonatal meningitis	Variable: sensitivities necessary (usually sensitive to ampicillin or gentamicin)
Salmonella	Neonatal meningitis	Third-generation cephalosporins, chloramphenicol
Klebsiella pneumoniae	Secondary to middle ear or respiratory tract, wound infections; usually younger than age 1 year, high mortality	Variable: sensitivities necessary
Bacillus anthracis (258)	Secondary to septicemia from primary cutaneous or visceral lesion; fulminant course, trismus common; meningitis often hemorrhagic	Penicillin, corticosteroids
Yersinia pestis (252)	Regional adenopathy, meningitis; may have primary cutaneous lesion	Chloramphenicol, gentamicin IV and IT, streptomycin, tetracycline
Pasteurella ureae (259)	Basal skull fracture with otorrhea	Ampicillin
Pasteurella pneumotropica	Seizures, contact with animals	Sensitivities necessary
Citrobacter (260)	Meningitis in newborn infant; abscesses form in most patients	Sensitivities necessary
Brucella spp. (261–264)	Chronic meningitis with increased intracranial pressure, prolonged indolent course; encephalitis, meningoencephalitis; parenchymatous dysfunction without direct evidence of infection (e.g., cerebellum)	Tetracyclines, sulfonamides, (trimethoprim-sulfamethoxazole), streptomycin, rifampin in some combination
Yersinia enterocolitica (264)	Enterocolitis, meningitis	Trimethoprim-sulfamethoxazole, cefotaximes, aminoglycoside, doxicillin (in children older than 9 years of age)

IV, intravenous; IT, intrathecal.

S. aureus, and pneumococci. *Actinomyces* (gram positive) as well as *Bacteroides* and other gram-negative rods, particularly *Haemophilus* species, are seen less often (268,269). Abscesses caused by *Aspergillus* and *Nocardia* (270) or protozoa such as *Toxoplasma* (271) are even rarer in the nonimmunocompromised host. Anaerobic organisms alone cause approximately 56% of brain abscesses, aerobic bacteria alone cause approximately 18%, and mixed aerobic and anaerobic bacteria cause approximately 26% (272,273). Frequently, the organism cannot be identified, often owing to failure to perform the appropriate cultures or the use of antibiotics before securing cultures.

Pathology

The earliest stage of an abscess is cerebritis (septic encephalitis). This is usually localized in the white matter even when infection has to pass through the cortex. It is an edematous area with softening and congestion of brain tissue, often with numerous petechial hemorrhages. The center becomes liquefied, thus forming the abscess cavity (Fig. 7.3). Initially, its wall is poorly defined and irregular. Gradually, a firmer, thicker wall develops, which ultimately can become a thick, firm, concentric capsule of fibrous tissue. The adjacent brain tissue is infiltrated with polymorphonuclear leukocytes and plasma cells near the abscess, with lymphocytes in the more peripheral zones, and heavy lymphocytic cuffing of vessels in the area. In more chronic abscesses, a border of granulation tissue merges gradually into a collagenous capsule. Abscesses enlarge within the softer and less vascular white matter and extend toward the ventricles, rupturing into this space, rather than into the subarachnoid fluid. Seeding of the leptomeninges and subsequent meningitis results from local thrombophlebitis more often than from actual rupture.

Abscesses resulting from hematogenous spread can be localized within any part of the brain, but most commonly occur in the distribution of the middle cerebral artery at the junction of gray and white matter of the cerebral

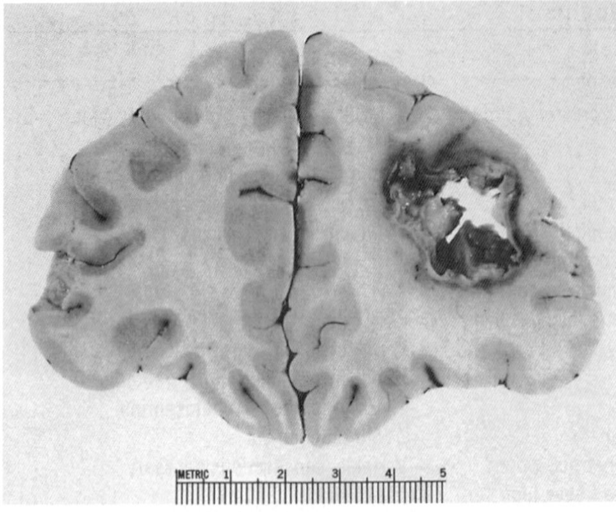

FIGURE 7.3. Anterior frontal lobe abscess in a child with cyanotic congenital heart disease. The brain is edematous and flattening of the gyri is seen. Gross representation of coronal section. (Courtesy of Dr. Hideo H. Itabashi, Departments of Pathology and Neurology, Los Angeles County Harbor Medical Center, Torrance, CA.)

TABLE 7.9 Incidence of Symptoms and Neurologic Findings in 19 Cases of Brain Abscess with Congenital Heart Disease

Symptoms	*Number of Patients*
Headache, vomiting, or both	15
Seizures	7
Fever (101°F or more)	6
Listlessness	4
Disorientation	4
Neck pain	4
Neurologic sign	
Lateralizing signs	15
Papilledema	13
Hemiparesis	12
Increased deep tendon reflexes	12
Extensor plantar responses	9
Pupillary changes	7
Stupor	6
Neck stiffness	5
Aphasia	5
Homonymous hemianopia	4
Localized percussion tenderness of skull	[a]

[a] Although not cited, this is a common neurologic sign and is valuable in localizing the abscess.
Adapted from Raimondi AJ, Matsumoto S, Miller RA. Brain abscess in children with congenital heart disease. I. *J Neurosurg* 1965;23:588.

hemispheres. By contrast, abscesses derived from contiguous sources tend to be superficial and close to the infected bone or dura. Multiple abscesses occur in 6% of patients, usually when sepsis or congenital heart disease is the predisposing cause.

Clinical Manifestations

During initial stages of the brain abscess, the clinical picture can be nonspecific. The patient, who can have cyanotic congenital heart disease or a primary infection, develops the complex of headache, vomiting, and convulsions, either partially or in its entirety. As the abscess progresses, the neurologic signs, which initially were minimal or completely absent, become readily apparent. As indicated in Table 7.9 (274), they include papilledema, lateralizing signs, notably hemiparesis or homonymous hemianopia, and more obvious indications of increased intracranial pressure. Focal percussion tenderness often aids in the localization of the lesion. Untreated, the condition is usually fatal, either as a consequence of decompensated increased intracranial pressure or from sudden rupture of the abscess into the ventricular system. Sudden rupture is marked by a sudden high fever, meningeal signs, and deterioration of consciousness (275).

Cerebellar abscesses are most commonly seen in association with mastoid infections and occur most frequently during the second and third decades of life. Symptoms and neurologic signs are those associated with any posterior fossa mass lesion. Mastoid infections also give rise to abscesses of the temporal lobe. Abscesses of the pituitary fossa can have a prolonged course that simulates a slow-growing tumor (276).

Intramedullary abscesses of the spinal cord have been observed in infants as young as 8 days of age. In a review of 73 cases, 17% were found to have occurred before the age of 5 years (277).

Diagnosis

Peripheral blood counts are usually of little value in establishing the diagnosis of brain abscess. Peripheral white blood cell counts of greater than 11,000 cells/μL occur in only one-third of patients (278). The erythrocyte sedimentation rate is normal in 11% of patients. The CSF leukocyte count in patients without congenital heart disease is greater than 5 cells/μL in 80% of cases. In patients with congenital heart disease, the CSF cell count is normal in 47% and the CSF protein is normal in 67% (278). Generally, the more striking the CSF pleocytosis, the closer the abscess is to the ventricular lining. Hypoglycorrhachia of less than 45 mg/dL occurs in approximately 30% of cases. Bacterial culture results of CSF are usually negative unless the abscess is leaking into the ventricular system (278). As a rule, a lumbar puncture should be avoided in children with brain abscess because the procedure results in neurologic deterioration in 15% to 33% of cases and the information is of little use in management (278).

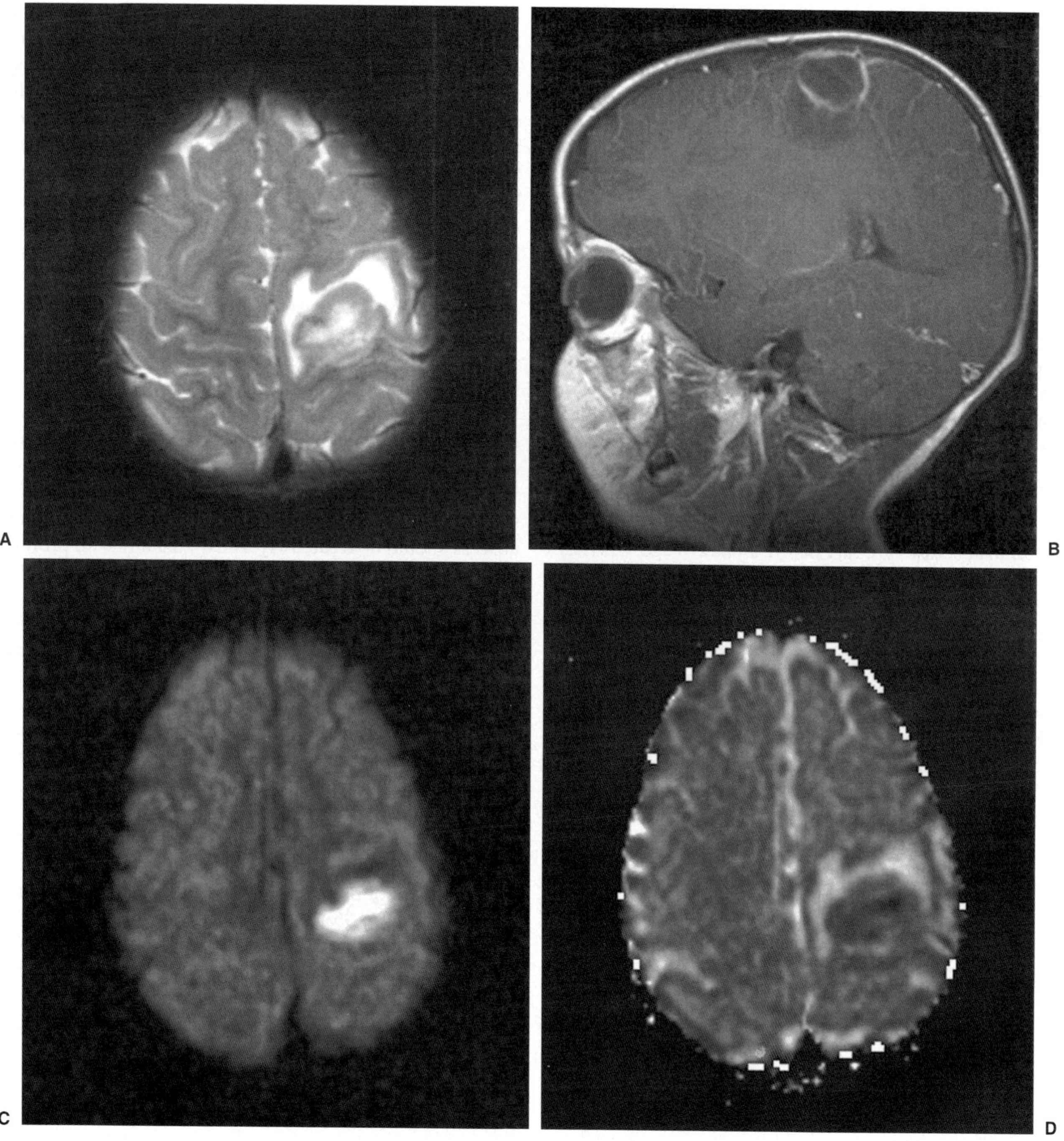

FIGURE 7.4. Brain abscess. **A:** Axial T2-weighted image showing a hyperintense lesion with hypointense rim and surrounding vasogenic edema in the posterior left frontal lobe. **B:** Sagittal post-contrast T1-weighted image demonstrating hypointense central portion and rim enhancement of the mass. **C:** The lesion is very bright on the axial diffusion-weighted image. **D:** Corresponding apparent diffusion coefficient map revealing the low signal intensity of the mass, consistent with restricted diffusion of water molecules. Surrounding vasogenic edema is hyperintense due to increased diffusion.

The EEG almost always shows a focal slowing, which corresponds closely to the location of the abscess. Neuroimaging studies (CT and MRI) are essential diagnostic tools for making an accurate diagnosis (279) (Fig. 7.4). These reveal a focal process that rapidly assumes the character of a mass lesion with a contrast-enhancing margin (279). If MRI is not available, CT or cerebral arteriography is the preferred procedure when the abscess requires further delineation (280). Focal arterial displacement and the presence of the ripple sign, a concentric, curvilinear displacement of opacified sulci in the late arterial phase caused by perifocal edema, are helpful arteriographic findings (281). Hyperintensity on diffusion-weighted imaging (DWI) with a reduced apparent diffusion coefficient (ADC) is characteristic of brain abscess (Fig. 7.4); in the absence of restricted diffusion on DWI, *in vivo* proton magnetic resonance spectroscopy can distinguish brain abscesses from cystic tumors (282–285).

In patients with cyanotic congenital heart disease, a brain abscess must be differentiated from intracranial vascular accidents and hypoxic attacks. Thromboses of arteries, veins, and dural sinuses are particularly common in severely cyanotic infants. Although dehydration and stasis play a minor role in the evolution of cerebral vascular thromboses, in the series of Tyler and Clark virtually every infant who experienced a thrombosis had an arterial oxygen saturation of 10 volumes percent or less (286). Except for a more abrupt onset of symptoms, the clinical picture can mimic that of an abscess; however, the patient's age is of considerable importance in the differential diagnosis. Brain abscesses are rare before 2 years of age, whereas vascular thromboses are rare in patients older than 2 years (286). Emboli in patients with congenital heart disease are highly unusual, and when present they are precipitated by cardiac or other surgery. The differential diagnosis of these two entities and their distinction from hypoxic attacks, which are often accompanied by headaches, is further covered in the section on neurologic complications of cardiac disease in Chapter 17.

A partially treated meningitis also should be considered in the differential diagnosis of a brain abscess. It lacks the neurologic and EEG evidence of focal central involvement, and, of course, neuroimaging studies are diagnostic.

Clark pointed out that old focal neurologic signs, which are often present in the patient with cyanotic congenital heart disease, are aggravated by stress, including a recent infection (287). The ensuing picture simulates a progressive lesion.

Treatment

Treatment of any brain abscess should include a diligent search for the source of infection (288,289). In a child without congenital heart disease, the presence of multiple brain abscesses should raise the question of immunodeficiency. Fungal brain abscesses in immunocompromised patients have death rates in excess of 95% (290). Once the diagnosis has been made, proper selection of antimicrobial agents with good penetration of the CNS should follow. Initial therapy should include coverage for anaerobic as well as aerobic organisms. The antibiotics of choice are generally intravenous penicillin G, chloramphenicol, and metronidazole. Oxacillin or methicillin also should be started until it is established that a β-lactamase–producing organism is not involved. Ampicillin can be used, but is not as effective as penicillin against anaerobic organisms. Surgical drainage should be performed without delay, and antibiotic therapy should be withheld until immediately after cultures have been obtained (278,291–293). In the early phase of cerebritis, however, infection can respond to antibiotic therapy alone. Subsequent therapy is guided by laboratory determination of antibiotic sensitivity and by neuroimaging studies (294). It is continued for a minimum of 3 weeks and often for 4 to 6 weeks. Intravenous fluid is usually limited to 1,500 mL/m^2 to minimize cerebral edema.

Controversy surrounds the indications for surgical therapy and the various surgical methods. These methods include tapping of the abscess, with or without excision of the shrunken abscess capsule, and operative removal of the acute abscess (295). Generally, surgical therapy is indicated when the patient does not improve after 24 hours of antibiotic therapy, when clinical status deteriorates, or when there is life-threatening displacement of cerebral structures. Sinusitis or mastoiditis contiguous to a brain abscess should be treated vigorously, usually with prompt surgery. A short course of corticosteroids to reduce life-threatening edema can be used safely.

When an abscess is fully established, surgical treatment is usually necessary. Mampalam and Rosenblum compared treatment by surgical excision with treatment by aspiration (278). Excision resulted in a shorter course of antibiotic therapy, but there was no difference in morbidity or mortality. Wright and Ballantine recommended total excision of brain abscesses, having had no deaths with this approach (296), whereas significant mortality was associated with drainage or medical treatment alone. Berlit and coworkers recommended burr hole aspiration plus antibiotic treatment of brain abscesses. In their study, mortality for this group was 9%, as opposed to 62% for the subgroup treated with antibiotics alone (297). The affected region is aspirated and the aspirate examined for aerobic and anaerobic bacteria, mycobacteria, fungi, and parasites, notably *Toxoplasma*. Patients with increased intracranial pressure should not receive halothane, trichloroethylene, or methoxyflurane because these agents can cause considerable increase in intracranial pressure (298). Because seizures can occur owing to the cortical injury produced by the brain abscess or its surgical therapy, anticonvulsant medication should be used during the acute phase.

Brain abscess in the early phase of cerebritis may respond to antimicrobial therapy without surgical drainage (299,300).

Complications

Residual defects include seizure activity, localized neurologic abnormalities, mental retardation, and hydrocephalus. Intracranial complications of frontal sinusitis (Pott's puffy tumor) include hemiparesis, obtundation, and aphasia (301). Seizures can appear at any time between 1 month and 15 years after a supratentorial abscess, with the latent period being somewhat shorter when the abscess occurs in the temporal lobe. In 40% of patients, seizures develop within 1 year, and the mean time of onset is 3.3 years. No relationship exists between the development of seizures and the age of the patient or the mode of surgical therapy (302).

The overall mortality has declined from 30% in the pre-CT era to almost none in the past few years. The prognosis remains poor in infants with brain abscesses, with mortality approaching 50% (303).

Subdural Abscesses

Subdural abscesses or subdural empyema result from sepsis, from a direct extension of an infection such as an osteomyelitis, or from bacterial contamination of a subdural effusion in meningitis or a post-traumatic subdural hematoma. Approximately two-thirds occur subsequent to a prior craniotomy. Otitis media and pneumococcal meningitis are other sources of organisms for subdural abscesses in children, whereas sinusitis is a more common antecedent in adults. Approximately 9% of children with brain abscesses develop subdural empyemas. These lesions generally occur over the convexity of the brain, but 12% are found interhemispherically.

Signs and symptoms are those of a space-occupying lesion in association with evidence of infection. Increased intracranial pressure and focal neurologic findings, notably focal seizures, are common (304,305).

The presence of subdural abscesses is demonstrated by neuroimaging (18). Sinusitis-induced subdural empyemas may not become apparent on CT scan until 1 or 2 weeks after symptoms develop, hence they may be missed on initial CT scans (306). Enhancement of membranes with gadolinium on MRI can occur when no enhancement is seen on CT (307). Diffusion MR imaging can be valuable in distinguishing subdural empyema from effusion and in the follow-up of subdural collections (308). Early diagnosis and prompt chemotherapy and surgical drainage are imperative (269). Craniotomy is the surgical procedure of choice, but more limited procedures (burr holes and craniectomies) should be performed in patients in septic shock, for patients with parafalcine empyemas, or for children with subdural empyemas secondary to meningitis (309,310). Subdural infections are caused by the same spectrum and distribution of bacteria as those causing brain abscesses (269).

Epidural Abscesses

Epidural abscesses can develop from contiguous infection of structures that surround the brain and spinal cord. They can arise from local infection or can be secondary to congenital anomalies such as dermal sinuses (311,312). Bacteremia and trauma also have been implicated. Approximately one-third of cases involve staphylococcal organisms (313). Epidural abscesses complicating sinus infections most commonly present with purulent nasal or aural discharge, fever, headache, scalp swelling, signs or symptoms of raised intracranial pressure, and, rarely, focal neurologic findings or seizures (314,315). Epidural abscesses can have a more indolent course than subdural empyemas (316).

Infection of the spinal epidural space, though extremely rare in childhood, produces a devastating neurologic picture. The main determinant of outcome for patients with spinal epidural abscess is neurologic status at the time of diagnosis (317). The infection is limited to the dorsal surface of the cord except in the cord's lower sacral portion, where the abscess completely surrounds the cord. The anatomy of the epidural space limits extension to vertical spread and produces extradural compression. Epidural infections can result from the use of epidural catheters for prolonged postoperative analgesia in children (318).

The clinical course can be acute and rapidly progressive or chronic. The acute form, more common in children, is usually the result of a metastatic infection, whereas chronic lesions are commonly caused by a direct extension of a spinal osteomyelitis. The classic case of spinal epidural abscess follows a fairly typical pattern of development. Within 1 to 2 weeks of an infection, backache develops; this backache is enhanced by jarring or straining and is accompanied by local spinal tenderness. Within a few days, tenderness progresses to radicular pain followed by symptoms of cord involvement, including weakness of voluntary movements and impaired sphincter control. Paraplegia can be complete within a few hours or days.

In many patients, the history and neurologic signs are impossible to differentiate from those of acute transverse myelitis. Intradural extramedullary tumors can produce a similar clinical picture.

A history compatible with infection, in association with focal pain in the region of the spine, especially when accompanied by neurologic symptoms of spinal cord or root involvement, should suggest the diagnosis, which can be confirmed by neuroimaging studies (18). Prompt blood cultures can reveal the causative organism. Lumbar puncture should not be performed because of the risk of spreading the infection to the subdural or subarachnoid space. Aspiration can be performed with a large-gauge needle, but only under radiographic guidance. If the CSF is examined, it shows pleocytosis and an elevated protein level.

An epidural abscess that has produced neurologic deficit is treated by laminectomy with decompression and drainage. In view of the rapid progression of potentially irreversible symptoms, this condition is a surgical emergency. Antibiotic therapy is secondary. If tuberculosis of the spine is suspected, antituberculous therapy should be

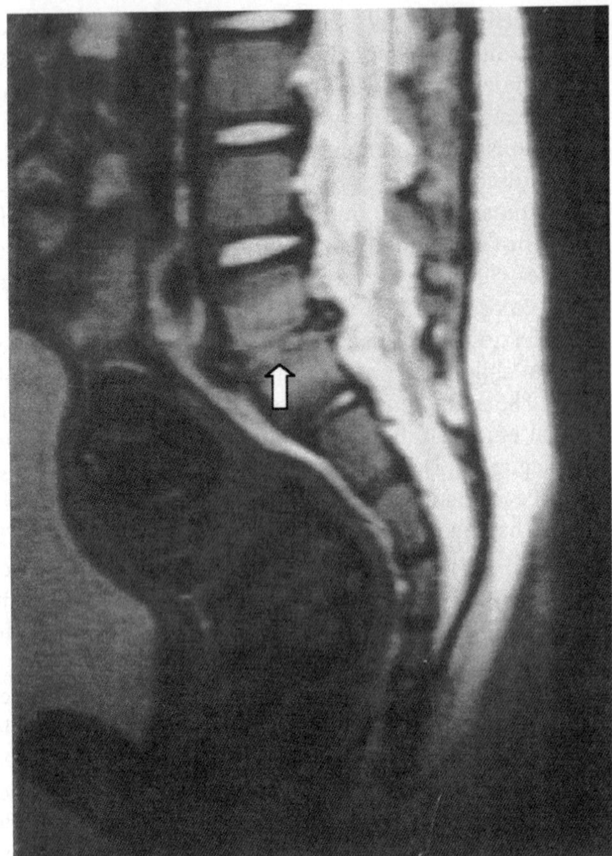

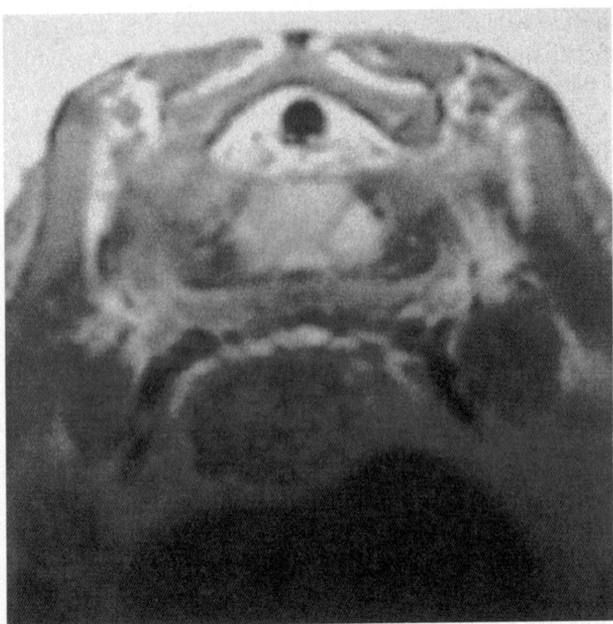

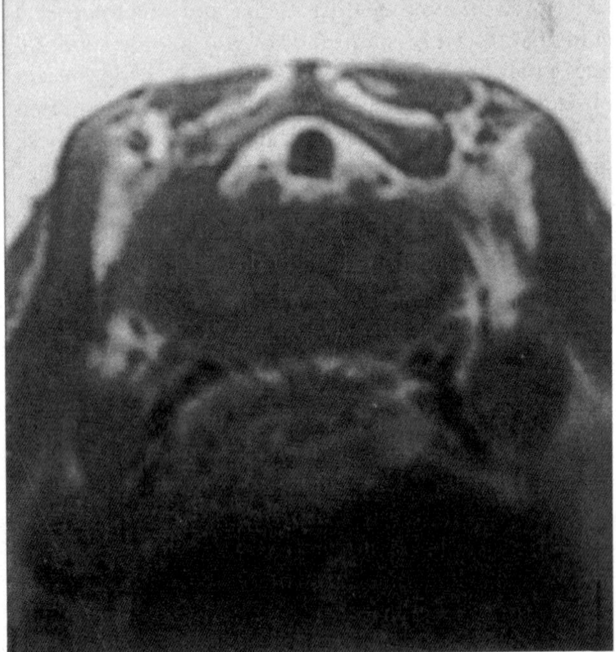

FIGURE 7.5. Septic discitis. Magnetic resonance imaging scan of the lumbar spine of a 14-month-old child who stopped cruising. **A:** Sagittal T2-weighted scan showing reduced signal in the L5/S1 intervertebral disc (*arrow*) and high signal in the end plate and adjacent medullary bone. **B:** Axial T1-weighted scan after contrast demonstrated intense contrast enhancement of the disc. **C:** Axial T1-weighted scan showing nerve roots surrounded by fat. (Courtesy of Dr. Philip Anslow, Department of Radiology, Radcliffe Infirmary, Oxford, England.)

instituted pending identification of the causative organisms. Sinus-related intracranial epidural abscesses in children may be managed without neurosurgical procedures in the setting of adequate sinus drainage, appropriate antibiotic therapy, and minimal extradural mass effect from the abscess (308).

Intramedullary Abscesses

Approximately 27% of intramedullary abscesses occur before age 10 years, and 40% occur during the first two decades of life (319). The abscess develops by spread from infected contiguous dermal sinuses or, less often, from suppurative foci at other sites. In some instances, particularly since the advent of antibiotics, the disease can be insidious, and in approximately one-fourth of cases, the infection has been present for at least 4 months before diagnosis. The thoracic cord is involved in most instances. Symptoms generally simulate an intramedullary tumor.

Infections of Intervertebral Disc Space

Self-limited intervertebral disc space infections can occur in children. These infections can be caused by *S. aureus* or diphtheroids, but often no organism can be isolated.

Infections of the disc space are characterized by back pain with or without fever, a variable incidence of hip pain or abdominal pain, radiographic evidence of narrowing of the intervertebral space, enhanced radionuclide uptake, and an elevated sedimentation rate (320). Cross-sectional MRI is probably the most useful diagnostic procedure (321) (Fig. 7.5). Treatment by immobilization relieves pain. Antibiotics have been used, but are not always needed. Scoliosis and complete interbody ankylosis can occur (322,323). In a follow-up of 35 children on average 17 years after discitis, flexion of the low back was normal in 90% but extension was markedly restricted in 86%, 80% had narrowing of the vertebral canal, 74% had a block vertebrae, and 43% still complained of backache (324). Nonspecific discitis without bacterial cause can occur in young children. It is characterized by restriction of spinal mobility and an elevated sedimentation rate. Biopsy usually reveals chronic or subacute inflammation, although approximately one-third of the biopsies yield normal tissue. The disease is usually self-limiting in most cases with only minor residual radiographic changes (325).

Intraventricular Shunt Infections

The management of infected cerebrospinal shunts is covered in Chapter 5.

CONGENITAL INFECTIONS

Introduction

Several pathogens, grouped traditionally as TORCH infections—an acronym designating toxoplasmosis, others, rubella, cytomegalovirus, and herpes (326)—are potential causes of deafness, vision loss, and behavioral or neurologic disorders among young children throughout the world (Table 7.10). Although the introduction of the rubella vaccine in the late 1960s led to a dramatic reduction in the incidence of the congenital rubella syndrome (CRS), the last several decades have brought only modest changes in the epidemiology of congenital infections. This section describes the major pathogens causing intrauterine infections and summarizes information on pathogenesis, clinical manifestations, treatment, and prevention.

TABLE 7.10 Infectious Agents Potentially Associated with Intrauterine Central Nervous System Infections

Viruses	Protozoa
Rubella	*Toxoplasma gondii*
Cytomegalovirus	*Trypanosoma cruzi*
Herpes simplex virus type 2	
Varicella-zoster virus	**Other**
Lymphocytic choriomeningitis virus	*Treponema pallidum*
Western equine encephalitis virus	

Pathogenesis and Pathology

Intrauterine infections reflect the complex interaction of the mother's immune status, the placenta, the fetus, and the infectious pathogen (327). Relatively few microorganisms can cross the placenta and damage the developing fetus. Women who possess antibodies to specific pathogens have reduced risks of transmitting the agents to their infants. By contrast, women who experience primary infections with these pathogens during their pregnancies have substantial risks of delivering infants with symptomatic congenital infections.

The agents causing intrauterine infections reach the placenta and the fetus during maternal viremia, parasitemia, or spirochetemia. There, the pathogens replicate, invade the fetal circulation, and disseminate hematogenously to the target organs of the developing fetus. For certain agents, such as rubella and varicella-zoster virus (VZV), the fetal consequences of infection reflect the timing of maternal infection (328,329). Maternal rubella during the initial 8 weeks, for example, produces cataracts and congenital heart lesions, whereas sensorineural hearing loss correlates with infection during the first 16 weeks. Stillbirth or spontaneous abortion can also occur during this time interval. The risk of the fetal varicella syndrome is restricted to first-trimester maternal varicella.

During maternal infections with *Toxoplasma gondii* the likelihood of transmission to the fetus increases during gestation, but maternal infections early in pregnancy are more likely to produce several fetal infections (330). For other agents, such as cytomegalovirus (CMV), the relationship between the timing of infection and the likelihood of fetal damage is less clear (331,332). CMV infection during critical stages of fetal development can produce severe CNS malformations, such as lissencephaly or schizencephaly (333,334), but damage to other tissues, including the retina, cochlea, liver, or spleen, can occur irrespective of the timing of maternal infection.

Intracranial calcifications, a hallmark of intrauterine infections, accompany infections with several pathogens, including CMV, rubella, herpes simplex virus (HSV), VZV, human immunodeficiency virus (HIV), lymphocytic choriomeningitis (LCM) virus, and *T. gondii*. Calcifications indicate tissue necrosis and dystrophic changes. The location of the calcifications provides a useful clue regarding the etiology of intrauterine infections. Periventricular calcifications commonly occur with CMV (Fig. 7.6), rubella, and LCM virus, whereas diffuse parenchymal as well as periventricular calcifications suggest congenital

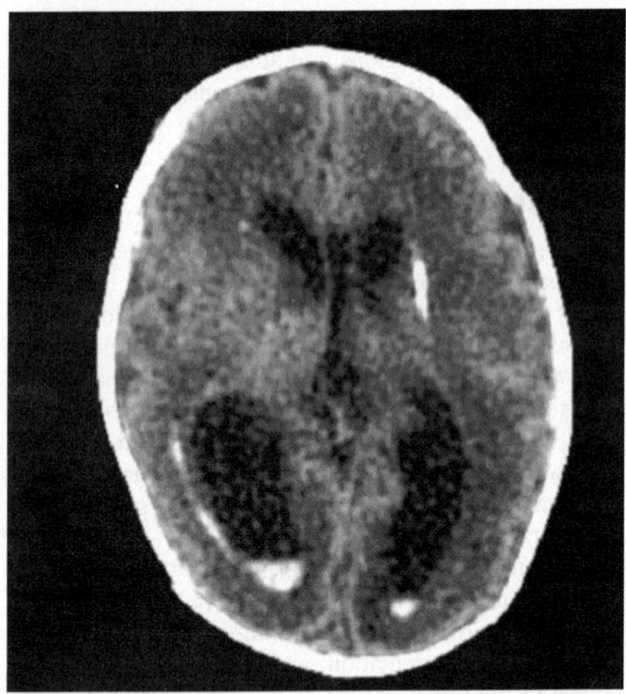

FIGURE 7.6. Unenhanced head CT of a premature infant with congenital cytomegalovirus infection showing a dense periventricular calcification as well as an intraventricular hemorrhage.

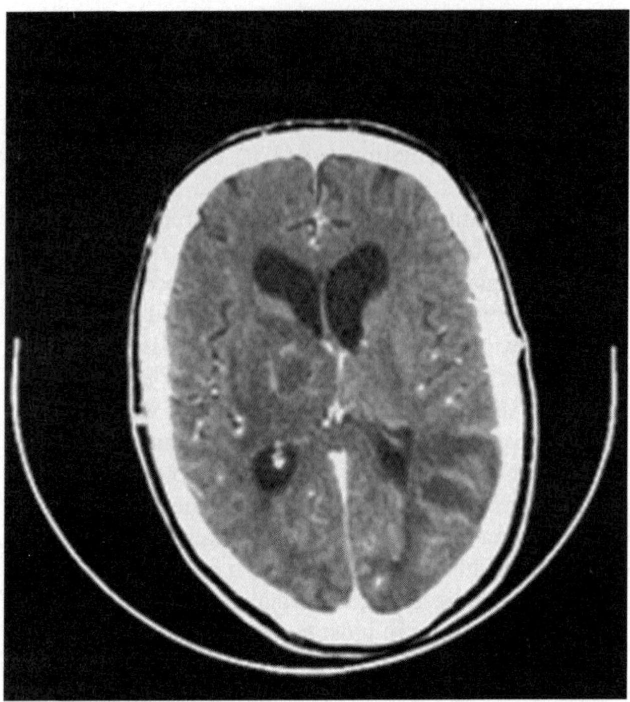

FIGURE 7.7. Unenhanced head CT of a child with congenital toxoplasmosis showing mild cerebral atrophy and scattered, parenchymal calcifications.

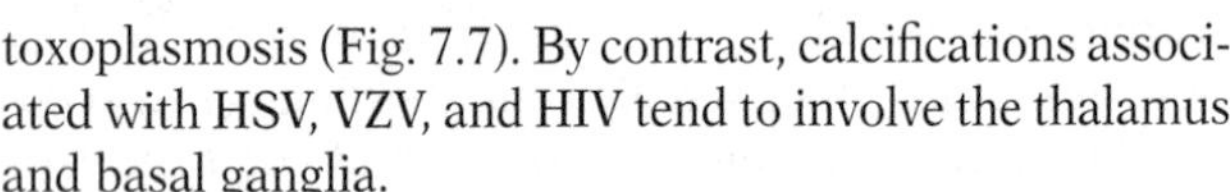

toxoplasmosis (Fig. 7.7). By contrast, calcifications associated with HSV, VZV, and HIV tend to involve the thalamus and basal ganglia.

Cystic necrosis occurs during intrauterine infections with HSV and VZV as well as with Venezuelan equine encephalitis virus, a pathogen endemic to Latin America and a rare cause of intrauterine infection. These pathologic abnormalities result from tissue invasion, virus replication, and immune-mediated tissue destruction. In severe cases, tissue destruction can lead to extensive encephalomalacia or hydranencephaly. Infectious vasculopathy contributes to the tissue changes associated with several intrauterine infections, including rubella, congenital syphilis, CMV, and VZV. The prevention and treatment of the various congenital infections are summarized in Table 7.11.

Cytomegalovirus (CMV)

Epidemiology

In the United States and many developed countries, 0.4% to 2.5% of newborns shed CMV at birth (331). The incidence of acquired CMV infection among children and adults, including women of childbearing age, averages 1% to 2% per year. By adulthood, 40% to 100% of the population has been infected with CMV. Infants acquire CMV postnatally from their breast-feeding mothers, and young children become infected through contact with CMV-excreting playmates (335). Adults acquire CMV via blood transfusion, sexual contact, organ transplantation, or contact with young children (336). Adults with multiple sexual partners have increased rates of CMV acquisition (332).

Pathogenesis and Pathology

Approximately 40% of women who acquire primary CMV infection during pregnancy transmit CMV to the fetuses, and 5% to 10% of the infected infants have CMV disease (337). Although seronegative women have the greatest risk of transmitting CMV to their unborn infants, fetal infections can occur in CMV-seropositive women who are reinfected with new CMV strains (338). CMV infection begins with replication of the virus in lymphoid tissues adjacent to the genital tract or oropharynx. Viremia then develops and leads to infection of systemic organs, including the placenta of pregnant women. Although most fetal tissues support CMV replication, major sites of infection are the liver, spleen, brain, and retina. The virus enters the brain via the choroid plexus and spreads centrifugally from the subependymal region. Pathologic changes within the brain include hemorrhage, cystic degeneration, dystrophic calcification, and perivascular mononuclear inflammation (332).

TABLE 7.11 Prevention and Treatment of Intrauterine Infections

Infectious Disorder or Organism	*Preventive Measures*	*Therapy*
Cytomegalovirus	Avoiding contact with young children during pregnancy; practicing monogamy	Ganciclovir[a]
Herpes simplex virus	None established	Acyclovir[b]
Varicella zoster virus	Avoiding contact with persons with chickenpox Immunization[c]	None
Rubella	Immunization in childhood	None
Lymphocytic choriomeningitis virus	Avoiding contact with mice and hamsters during pregnancy	None
Toxoplasma gondii	Avoiding contact with cats and modifying diet practices; prenatal therapy with spiramycin or sulfadiazine-pyrimethamine	Sulfadiazine and pyrimethamine
Syphilis	Avoiding contact with infected persons; maternal therapy	Penicillin

[a]Experimental; see text.
[b]Acyclovir therapy will diminish viral shedding but will not affect neurologic outcome in congenitally infected infants.
[c]Presumptive benefit of childhood immunization.

Clinical Manifestations

The majority of CMV-infected neonates have no signs of CMV infection at birth. Approximately 5% to 10% of the infected newborns have systemic signs (currently designated "congenital CMV disease") (Table 7.12) consisting of jaundice, hepatomegaly, splenomegaly, petechial or purpuric rash, intrauterine growth retardation, or respiratory distress (339–343). Neurologic features include microcephaly, chorioretinitis, seizures, sensorineural hearing loss, and alterations in muscle tone.

Diagnosis

The diagnosis of intrauterine infection is established by detecting CMV in clinical samples during the first 3 weeks of life (331,332). Because congenitally infected infants shed enormous quantities of CMV in their urine, culturing urine or saliva using the shell vial assay is the gold standard for the diagnosis of intrauterine CMV infection. Performing PCR or assaying CMV-specific IgG or IgM in the infant's serum has much lower sensitivity. CMV antigenemia assays have no role in the diagnosis of intrauterine CMV infections.

Approximately 50% of the infants with congenital CMV disease have periventricular calcifications (Fig. 7.6), and infants with calcifications have higher rates of permanent neurodevelopmental disabilities (344,345). Neuroimaging studies may also show periventricular leukomalacia, polymicrogyria, pachygyria, schizencephaly, or lissencephaly. Because CT detects small calcifications more effectively than MRI, CT is the preferable imaging study in the perinatal period. MRI provides more accurate

TABLE 7.12 Neonatal Clinical Features in Infants with Proven Intrauterine Infections with Cytomegalovirus and *Toxoplasma gondii*, the Most Frequent Pathogens Associated with Congenital Infections in Most Developed Nations

	Approximate Prevalence (%)	
Feature	*CMV*[a]	*T. gondii*[b]
Petechiae	50	20
Microcephaly	50	15
Hydrocephalus	5	40
Intrauterine growth retardation	50	10
Hepatomegaly	45	50
Splenomegaly	45	50
Jaundice at birth	40	65
Sensorineural hearing loss	40	—
Abnormal tone	25	30
Chorioretinitis	10	75
Seizures	10	15
Death	5	5
Pneumonitis	5	10
Congenital heart disease	—	—

[a]Modified from data of the National Congenital Cytomegalovirus Disease Registry (339).
[b]Modified from data of Koskiniemi M, Lappalainen M, Hedman K. Toxoplasmosis needs evaluation: An overview and proposals. *Am J Dis Child* 1989;143:724–728; Couvreur J, Desmonts G. Congenital and maternal toxoplasmosis. *Dev Med Child Neurol* 1962;4:519–530; and McAuley J, Boyer K, Patel D, et al. Early and longitudinal evaluations of treated infants and children and untreated historical patients with congenital toxoplasmosis. The Chicago Collaborative Treatment Trial. *Clin Infect Dis* 1994;18:38–72.

information regarding cortical dysplasia, polymicrogyria, and other disorders of neuronal migration associated with congenital CMV infection.

Prevention, Treatment, and Prognosis

There are no vaccines for preventing CMV infections. Pregnant women can reduce their risk of infection by avoiding direct contact with the urine and saliva of young, toddler-aged children (346). Should inadvertent skin contact occur, hand washing with soap and water eliminates the virus from the skin. Postnatal therapy with ganciclovir can reduce the severity of sensorineural hearing loss and can treat CMV-induced pneumonia in congenitally infected infants (341). In the treatment trial sponsored by the National Institute of Allergy and Infectious Diseases–Children's Antiviral Study Group (NIH-CASG), infants received 6 mg/kg per dose intravenously every 12 hours for 6 weeks (Table 7.11) (341,347).

The majority of infants with silent CMV infections escape neurodevelopmental sequelae, but 7% to 10% of these will later exhibit sensorineural hearing loss. Because of the high incidence of intrauterine CMV infection, this disorder represents the most common cause of nongenetic deafness in many regions (348). By contrast, infants with congenital CMV disease have high rates (greater than 90%) of neurodevelopmental sequelae, consisting of cerebral palsy, seizures, sensorineural hearing loss, mental retardation, behavioral disorders, and vision loss (331,332,349). Approximately 9,000 infants annually in the United States have audiologic or neurologic sequelae of intrauterine CMV infections (331).

Toxoplasma gondii

Epidemiology

Humans acquire *T. gondii* by ingesting undercooked meat that contains bradyzoites, the encysted form found in tissues, or by ingesting fruits, vegetables, and other foods contaminated by oocysts, the highly infectious form of the organism (350). Infected cats, major contributors to human infection, excrete vast quantities of oocysts (351). Approximately 0.1% to 2% of the adult population acquires *T. gondii* annually. Rates of congenital infection vary from 1 per 12,000 live births to as high as 1 per 1,000 (330,347,350–352).

Pathogenesis and Pathology

Fetal infections complicate approximately 40% of the *T. gondii* infections in pregnant women (330,350). Healthy women infected with *T. gondii* rarely have recognizable symptoms, although an acute mononucleosis-like illness develops occasionally. Infections during the first trimester, when transmission to the fetus is less likely, can produce spontaneous abortion, whereas infections during the third trimester, when transmission frequently occurs, usually cause subclinical fetal infection. Infections during the second trimester often produce severe fetal disease. Congenital toxoplasmosis produces a diffuse, granulomatous meningoencephalitis that can lead to aqueductal obstruction, fetal hydrocephalus, and dystrophic parenchymal calcification.

Clinical Manifestations

Approximately 85% of the infants with intrauterine *T. gondii* infections lack symptoms at birth, but many of these infants later have ophthalmologic or neurologic sequelae (330,342,350,353). Symptomatic neonates exhibit jaundice, splenomegaly, hepatomegaly, fever, anemia, chorioretinitis, hydrocephalus or microcephaly, and petechiae secondary to thrombocytopenia (Table 7.12; Fig. 7.8) (330). Intrauterine coinfections with *T. gondii* and HIV or CMV can occur.

Diagnosis

The diagnosis of intrauterine infection with *T. gondii* can be made postnatally by detecting anti-*Toxoplasma* antibodies of several classes—IgM, IgG, IgA, and IgE—in the newborn infant's serum (354,355). Serologic studies of infants

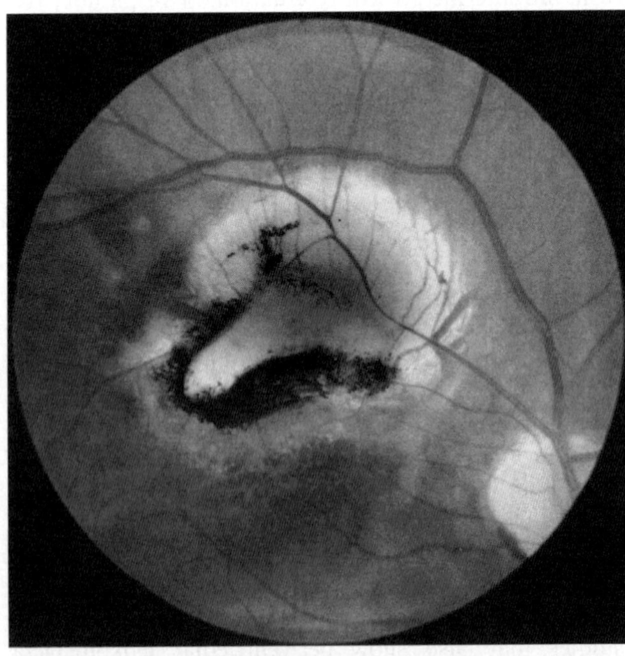

FIGURE 7.8. Chorioretinitis in toxoplasmosis. (Courtesy of Dr. John Chang, Department of Ophthalmology, University of California, Los Angeles, CA.)

and their mothers should be sent to an experienced laboratory, such as the Palo Alto Laboratories (phone number 650-853-4828), that performs a battery of serologic studies for *T. gondii*. As many as 25% of infected infants lack anti-*Toxoplasma* IgM. Inoculation of fresh placental tissues into laboratory mice can be used to confirm the diagnosis of congenital toxoplasmosis, and PCR can detect *T. gondii* in clinical specimens (356). Imaging studies in infants with congenital toxoplasmosis may show intracranial calcifications and ventriculomegaly, reflecting hydrocephalus or passive ventricular enlargement (330).

Prevention, Treatment, and Prognosis

Pregnant women can reduce their risk of exposure to *T. gondii* by avoiding cat excreta and modifying their dietary habits (357). Treating infected mothers with spiramycin or pyrimethamine-sulfadiazine has been advocated to reduce the risk of congenital toxoplasmosis, although the effectiveness of these strategies is unproven (358,359). Therapeutic abortion has been considered when the diagnosis of intrauterine toxoplasmosis is confirmed and CNS damage has been detected by fetal ultrasonography.

The neurologic prognosis of infants with congenital toxoplasmosis can be improved by early shunting of obstructive hydrocephalus and prolonged antitoxoplasma therapy postnatally (330,343,360). Infants should receive sulfadiazine, 100 mg/kg per day, and pyrimethamine, 1 mg/kg per day, for 6 months followed by the same dose three times per week for an additional 6 months. Infants require folinic acid, 5 to 10 mg three times weekly. Among infants who do not receive antitoxoplasma therapy, 80% have epilepsy, 70% have cerebral palsy, 60% have visual impairment, and nearly 60% have intelligence quotients less than 70 (330). Treated infants have considerably lower rates of neurodevelopmental complications (343,360).

Herpes Simplex Virus Type 2

Epidemiology

Intrauterine HSV disease, a rare disorder, nearly always results from HSV-2 infection. The incidence of HSV-2 infection is highest among young women, approximately 2% of whom acquire the virus each year (361); approximately 30% of 30-year-old women have serologic evidence of prior HSV-2 infection. The risk of HSV-2 infection among U.S. women is associated with several sociodemographic factors, including African-American race, lower income, greater number of lifetime sexual partners, earlier age of sexual intercourse, and drug use (362).

Pathogenesis and Pathology

As many as 2% of pregnant women become infected with HSV during pregnancy, but the majority of these infections do not produce fetal or neonatal disease (363). Primary maternal infection usually occurs without recognizable symptoms. The risk of intrauterine transmission of HSV-2 to the fetus appears to be very low. Fewer than 50 cases of intrauterine HSV infection have been described. HSV may reach the fetus during maternal viremia or through an ascending intrauterine infection. The virus replicates in several tissues, including the skin, liver, lung, eye, and brain, producing tissue necrosis, cystic degeneration, and dystrophic calcifications (364).

Clinical Manifestations

Infants with congenital HSV infections have skin vesicles or scarring, chorioretinitis, microcephaly, and microophthalmia (365–367). Intrauterine growth retardation can also be present. Of 13 infants identified by the NIH-CASG, 12 had skin lesions, 8 had chorioretinitis, 7 had microcephaly, and 5 had hydranencephaly, evidence of severe brain necrosis (366). Less severe congenital HSV-2 infections likely occur.

Diagnosis

The diagnosis of congenital HSV-2 infection can be made by detecting the virus in skin lesions or body fluids, using cell culture or PCR (368). Samples for virus isolation should include skin vesicle fluid, CSF, and swabs of the conjunctiva, rectum, and oropharynx. Ophthalmologic examination may reveal chorioretinitis and microphthalmia. Infants with intrauterine HSV infections frequently have dense calcifications of the basal ganglia and thalami, diffuse, hemispheric cystic lesions, and a lissencephalic-like cerebral cortex (369).

Prevention, Treatment, and Prognosis

Preventing neonatal HSV-2 infection, including intrauterine infection, remains problematic, and most women who give birth to infants with congenital HSV infection have no history of genital HSV infection (369). Although infants with neonatal HSV infections require prolonged high-dose therapy with acyclovir (60 mg/kg per day for 21 days) (369), acyclovir has little or no benefit for the severe CNS damage that accompanies intrauterine HSV-2 infection. Infants with congenital HSV-2 infections often die in infancy; survivors usually have cerebral palsy, epilepsy, and mental retardation (366).

Varicella-Zoster Virus

Epidemiology

Chickenpox affects approximately 0.05% of pregnant women (370). Women who acquire VZV before week 20 of gestation have a 2% risk of delivering an infant with the fetal varicella syndrome (371,372). By contrast, fetal varicella syndrome is highly unlikely in women who have chickenpox during the last half of pregnancy. Maternal VZV reactivation (zoster) poses little or no risk to the developing fetus.

Pathogenesis and Pathology

VZV displays tropism for the brain, retina, skin, and long tracts or neurons of the spinal cord. Lytic infection of neurons depletes neuronal populations, leading to the clinical manifestations described in the following paragraph. Pathologic changes include tissue necrosis, mononuclear inflammation, and cystic degeneration. CNS necrosis can manifest as severe cystic encephalomalacia or hydranencephaly (364).

Clinical Manifestations

The clinical manifestations of the congenital varicella syndrome consist of intrauterine growth retardation, limb hypoplasia, chorioretinitis, cataracts, microphthalmia, cutaneous scaring (cicatrix), and neurologic abnormalities (329,364,373,374). The latter can include microcephaly, hydrocephalus/hydranencephaly, seizures, Horner syndrome, and cranial neuropathies.

Diagnosis

Infection can be established by detecting the virus in fetal tissues using culture or PCR and by detecting VZV-specific IgM in fetal blood samples obtained by cordocentesis (376,376). At birth, infants with the fetal varicella virus syndrome no longer shed VZV, and VZV-specific IgM can be undetectable. Imaging studies may show intracranial calcifications, cortical dysplasia, or hydranencephaly (364,377).

Prevention, Treatment, and Prognosis

Although the efficacy of varicella-zoster immune globulin (VZIG) in preventing the fetal varicella syndrome is unproven, VZIG should be considered when susceptible pregnant women have been exposed to persons with chickenpox (378). VZIG should be given within 96 hours of the exposure. Postnatal therapy with acyclovir or other antiviral medications provides no benefit for infants with the congenital varicella syndrome. A substantial number of infants with the fetal varicella syndrome will die in infancy, and survivors usually have permanent sequelae affecting vision or neurologic development (329,364).

Lymphocytic Choriomeningitis Virus

Epidemiology

Lymphocytic choriomeningitis (LCM) virus, an arenavirus that naturally infects the feral house mouse, *Mus musculus,* can also infect humans (379). Seroprevalence rates of 0.3% to 5.0% have been observed among persons living in the United States, Canada, and Argentina (380–383). Intrauterine LCM virus infection is presumed to be a rare condition, but no surveillance studies have been performed to establish the incidence of the disorder.

Pathogenesis and Pathology

Human infection results from inhalation of infected aerosols, direct contact with LCM virus-shedding animals, or ingestion of material contaminated by infected excreta (384). Infected adults can experience an influenza-like illness with fever, malaise, and myalgia. Fetal infections are associated with periventricular calcifications, cortical dysplasia, and diffuse lymphocytic meningitis that can involve the ependyma of the aqueduct of Sylvius and cause hydrocephalus (385).

Clinical Manifestations

The clinical features of congenital LCM virus infection mimic those of intrauterine CMV disease and congenital toxoplasmosis (379,385,386). Among 26 reported cases reviewed by Wright and colleagues in 1997, 88% had chorioretinopathy, 43% had macrocephaly at birth, and 13% were microcephalic (385). Occasional infants had vesicular or bullous skin lesions. Virtually all infants were born at term and had normal birth weights. Approximately 50% of mothers who gave birth to the infants reviewed in this study recalled influenza-like illness during pregnancy, and one-fourth reported contact with rodents, usually mice, during their pregnancy.

Diagnosis

The diagnosis of congenital LCM virus infection is established by serologic studies of the mother and infant (379,385). Antibodies against LCM virus can be detected in the infant's serum or CSF. Because of the low seroprevalence of LCM virus infection in the general population, detecting LCM virus-specific antibodies, particularly LCM virus-specific IgM, strongly supports the diagnosis. The virus can be detected by PCR, but this method does not yet have diagnostic utility in human infections. Imaging studies in infants with congenital LCM virus infections may show hydrocephalus or cortical dysplasia (385).

Prevention, Treatment, and Prognosis

No vaccine is available for preventing LCM virus infections; pregnant women should avoid mice and pet hamsters during their pregnancy. Effective postnatal antiviral therapy of LCM virus infections has not been described. Approximately 35% of the reported infants died from complications of congenital LCM virus infection (379,385). Surviving infants commonly had cerebral palsy, epilepsy, vision loss, and mental retardation. LCM virus-infected infants with hydrocephalus may require shunt placement.

Rubella

Epidemiology

In the pre-vaccine era, epidemics of rubella caused thousands of cases of the congenital rubella syndrome (CRS), but after licensure of the rubella vaccine in 1969 and aggressive immunization programs in the 1980s, the incidence of the CRS in the United States and other nations declined dramatically (386). In the United States, only one to three cases of CRS were reported to the Centers for Disease Control and Prevention annually by the late 1980s, an incidence of less than 0.1 case of CRS per 100,000 live births (387). In recent years, CRS in the United States has virtually disappeared except among the offspring of immigrants from regions without compulsory immunization (388).

Pathogenesis and Pathology

Maternal rubella during the initial 8 weeks produces cataracts and congenital heart lesions, whereas hearing loss correlates with infection during the first 16 weeks (328). Infections after the week 16 of gestation usually leave no sequelae other than a risk of sensorineural hearing loss. Pathologic changes within the CNS consist of diffuse meningoencephalitis, cystic degeneration, and dystrophic calcification. Cardiac lesions include peripheral pulmonic stenosis, patent ductus arteriosus, and atrial or ventricular septal defects (389).

Clinical Manifestations

Infants with CRS can have cataracts, retinopathy, microphthalmia, microcephaly or sensorineural hearing loss, meningoencephalitis, osteopathy, pneumonitis, hepatitis, hepatosplenomegaly, thrombocytopenia, and jaundice (Table 7.12) (389–391). The propensity of the rubella virus to infect the heart causes myocarditis, patent ductus arteriosus, valvular stenosis, or septal defects at the atrial or ventricular level (389).

Diagnosis

CRS is diagnosed by isolating virus from nasal secretions, urine, or CSF or detecting rubella virus-specific IgM in the infant's serum (370,392). Postnatal persistence of rubella-specific IgG supports the diagnosis of CRS. Imaging studies can show periventricular calcifications, periventricular leukomalacia, or subependymal cysts.

Prevention, Treatment, and Prognosis

CRS cannot be treated effectively by postnatal antiviral therapy; infection must be prevented by vaccination. Maternal antibody prior to conception or at the time of maternal rubella exposure indicates that the fetus is not at risk. Termination of pregnancy is considered in confirmed primary rubella infections early in gestation (370). When termination is not an option, immune globulin can be considered, although the efficacy of this approach is unproven (370). Progressive sensorineural hearing loss can develop in children who survive CRS, and children with CRS also have an increased risk of growth failure or diabetes mellitus in the second or third decade of life (393–395). Neurologic sequelae include microcephaly, language delay, autistic features, and developmental or mental retardation.

Syphilis

Epidemiology

The overall incidence of congenital syphilis is low in the United States, but *Treponema pallidum* remains endemic in large urban areas and the rural South (396–399). In virtually all other developed countries syphilis rarely occurs. A transient resurgence of congenital syphilis in the United States in the late 1980s and early 1990s was attributed to maternal use of illicit drugs, especially cocaine (398).

Pathogenesis and Pathology

Untreated early maternal infection causes perinatal death, stillbirth, or miscarriage in approximately 40% of pregnancies (400). Although congenital syphilis can occur during all stages of maternal infection, fetal infection is most likely during secondary-stage maternal infections, when rates of transmission range from 60% to 100%. Maternal–fetal transmission complicates approximately 30% of latent maternal infections. Pathologic features in infants with congenital syphilis include periostitis, osteochondritis, leptomeningitis, endarteritis, periarteritis, and mixed inflammatory infiltration of multiple organs or tissues, including the liver, lungs, skin, eyes, inner ear, and central nervous system (401).

Clinical Manifestations

Early signs of congenital syphilis, present at birth or evident during the first 2 years of life (399–401), consist of intrauterine growth retardation, rash, hepatosplenomegaly, jaundice, lymphadenopathy, pseudoparalysis, and bony abnormalities. Hemolytic anemia, thrombocytopenia, leukocytosis, or leukopenia can be present, and long-bone radiographs in the perinatal period may show osteochondritis. The latter can mimic nonaccidental trauma. Late signs of congenital syphilis, features evident after 2 years of age, include sensorineural deafness, dental abnormalities, saddle nose, saber shins, hydrocephalus, and developmental delay (400,401).

Diagnosis

Infants with suspected congenital syphilis require (a) quantitative treponemal and nontreponemal assays of serum, (b) routine studies and nontreponemal and treponemal assays of CSF, and (c) long-bone radiographs. Definitive diagnosis is made by demonstrating spirochetes in exudates or tissues using dark-field or direct immunofluorescence microscopy (402). Serologic tests consist of nontreponemal tests, such as the Venereal Disease Research Laboratory (VDRL) slide test or rapid plasmin reagin (RPR), and treponemal tests, such as the fluorescent treponemal antibody absorption (FTA-ABS) test or the *T. pallidum* particle agglutination (TP-PA). Infants likely have congenital syphilis when spirochetes are present in tissues or when they have reactive CSF VDRL or FTA-ABS tests or serum quantitative treponemal tests four times higher than the mother (402).

Prevention and Treatment

Pregnant women with acquired syphilis require penicillin treatment, using one to three doses of penicillin G benzathine (2.4 million units intramuscularly), at 1-week intervals if more than one dose is given, irrespective of the timing of pregnancy (404). No effective alternatives exist for penicillin-allergic persons, so desensitization should be performed. Neonates with proven or highly suspected symptomatic congenital syphilis require aqueous crystalline penicillin G, 50,000 U/kg intravenously every 12 hours during the first week of life and every 8 hours thereafter for a total of 10 days (401). Alternatively, procaine penicillin G can be given intramuscularly at a dose of 50,000 U/kg once a day for 10 days. If penicillin G cannot be given, treatment recommendations can be found at www.cdc.gov/nchstp/dstd/penicillinG.htm. Infectious disease experts should be consulted regarding current treatment strategies for infants whose mothers received inadequate treatment, infants with asymptomatic infections, or infants older than 4 weeks with possible syphilis and neurologic involvement.

Congenital Chagas Disease

Infants with congenital Chagas disease, caused by intrauterine infection with *Trypanosoma cruzi,* resemble those with congenital toxoplasmosis (403,404). Hepatosplenomegaly, petechiae, jaundice, anemia, and seizures are potential complications. The diagnosis can be established by detecting serologic responses or parasitemia. Infected persons, including infants, can be treated with nifurtimox (405).

VIRAL INFECTIONS

Viral infections of the CNS are usually benign and self-limited with a good clinical outcome. A subset of viruses, however, can result in a severe clinical course with a high morbidity and mortality. Acute encephalitis is more common in children (more than 16 cases per 100,000 patient-years) than in adults (between 3.5 and 7.4 cases per 100,000 patient-years) (406). The number of annual cases of primary and postinfectious encephalitis reported to the Centers for Disease Control and Prevention from 1989 to 1994 ranged from 717 to 1,341 and from 82 to 170, respectively. Since 1995, these clinical entities are no longer nationally notifiable.

Pathogenesis

Viruses can cause CNS damage through direct invasion of central nervous tissues (primary or infectious encephalitis) or through the generation of an immune response to a systemic viral infection (postinfectious encephalomyelitis) (407).

In a naturally acquired infection, virus spreads to the CNS through two main mechanisms: hematogeneous and neuronal. These two mechanisms are not mutually exclusive and can occur concurrently to spread a virus.

Hematogenous Spread

The most common pathway for spread of virus to the CNS is by way of the bloodstream. Viral growth generally begins in extraneural tissue: poliomyelitis in the gut or regional lymphatics; herpes simplex in the respiratory tract or gastrointestinal mucosa; arbovirus in the vascular epithelium; and coxsackievirus, reovirus, rabies, and variola in brown fat. The viremia is maintained by shedding of the virus, absorption into red blood cells, or growth within leukocytes. Virus in blood can enter the CSF by either passing through or growing through the choroid plexus. Growth of virus in the choroid plexus might explain the ease with which echovirus and coxsackievirus can be isolated from the CSF. Migration of infected phagocytes through cerebral vessels and replication of virus in the endothelial cells with growth or passive transfer through the blood–brain barrier also can occur.

Once within the nervous system, the virus can spread by direct contiguity or through the limited extracellular space. Neurovirulent viruses that lack the neuroinvasive ability to cross the blood–brain barrier are able to produce infection once the barrier is breached by bacterial lipopolysaccharide (407).

Neuronal Spread

Less commonly, neuronal spread occurs from peripheral and cranial nerves. Viruses can enter the nervous system tissue by centripetal spread along the endoneurium, perineural Schwann cells, and fibrocytes of peripheral nerves. Once the virus has gained access to the spinal cord by this route, it can spread randomly along the endoneurium or the interstitial space within the nerve. Spread within the nerve is significant for rabies and for some herpes simplex infections. Penetration at sensory or motor nerve endings with transport to specific sensory ganglion cells or motor neurons by retrograde axoplasmic flow has been demonstrated for herpes simplex, polio viruses, and rabies virus.

Spread by way of the olfactory system has been demonstrated in herpes simplex, poliomyelitis, and arbovirus infections. These viruses spread along olfactory rods and nerve fibers to the mitral cell neurons of the olfactory bulb, or along the interstitial spaces, endoneurium, and perineurium of the olfactory nerves to the parenchymal cells of the olfactory bulb, and from there along the subarachnoid cuffs to the meninges (408).

Pathology

Cells of the CNS vary in their susceptibility to viral infection. Thus, herpes simplex seems to infect all cell types, whereas poliomyelitis has a predilection for the larger motor cells, Purkinje cells, and cells of the reticular formation. Susceptibility is determined by cell receptor sites and by the route of entry.

The reactions of brain tissue to viral invasion are similar in all forms of encephalitis. The most obvious histologic lesion is a cellular infiltration. Initially, this consists largely of polymorphoneutrophils; later, round cells predominate. Proliferation of microglial cells can be diffuse or focal. With diffuse proliferation, the cells accumulate around degenerated or dying nerve cells, a phenomenon associated with neuronophagia. Most commonly, alterations within nerve cells consist of a loss of Nissl granules and eosinophilia of the cytoplasm. Inclusion bodies within neurons and glial cells, such as the Negri bodies seen in rabies, can be typical of the disease or can represent nonspecific degeneration products.

Arteritis and other alterations of the vessel walls are observed in a number of conditions, notably in the equine encephalitides. Demyelination can result from the loss of cortical nerve cells or can occur independently, as in subacute sclerosing panencephalitis (SSPE) or other slow virus infections.

Viral infections are characterized by intrathecal production of oligoclonal immunoglobulin within the CNS. Viral-specific IgM is produced during the early stage of infection, with specific IgG and IgA produced slightly later.

The patient's humoral and cellular immune response to infection can contribute to the disease picture. For instance, in experimental lymphocytic choriomeningitis, the virus causes severe meningeal infiltrates only in immunologically mature and competent animals. TNF, the cytokine associated with inflammation in bacterial infections, is not demonstrable in many viral infections of the nervous system (409,410). Leukotriene B4, a potent chemotactic factor for leukocytes, and leukotriene C4, which increases vascular permeability and causes smooth muscle contraction, are increased in the CSF of children with aseptic meningitis and encephalitis (411). Suppression of the immune response with dexamethasone may have no benefit or can even be deleterious (412). For a review of T-cell activation, critical to activation of the immune response to viruses, see the publication by Reiser and Stadecker (413).

Apoptosis is a common pathway to virus-induced cell death. It can result from viral infection of cells or from the action of leukocytes and their products. This subject has been extensively reviewed by Razvi and Welsh (414).

Clinical Manifestations

Viruses can cause encephalitis (inflammation of the brain) and meningitis (inflammation of the meninges). These processes can be seen independently as well as concurrently.

Acute Encephalitis

The initial clinical picture can be protean, manifesting as a systemic infection without neurologic symptoms or findings. Fever, irritability, headaches, nausea, vomiting, poor appetite, and restlessness precede neurologic symptoms. In Finnish studies, the most characteristic neurologic symptoms of viral encephalitis during the acute phase were lowered consciousness manifested by disorientation, confusion, somnolence, or coma. These symptoms were recorded in 58% of patients. Ataxia was seen in 58%; an altered mental status, notable aggressiveness, and apathy were seen in 40%. Seizures, either generalized (32%), focal (5%), or both, were encountered less commonly.

Neurologic findings were generally nonspecific, and meningeal symptoms and signs were not always present (415,416). The incidence of CNS viral infections in association with neonatal seizures may be much higher than previously reported (417). The CSF examination was often frequently normal early in the disease (418). As a general rule, the initial CSF pleocytosis is characterized by a rapidly decreasing proportion of granulocytes. The transient elevation in CSF granulocyte colony-stimulating factor observed during the initial stages of aseptic meningitis is associated with this change (419). The development of PCR has greatly increased our ability to diagnose viral infections of the CNS, particularly for herpes and enteroviral infections (420). Young age, disorientation, and loss of consciousness are serious prognostic signs in encephalitis, especially if the encephalitis is caused by herpes simplex. In the study by Klein and coworkers, focal signs on neurologic examination and abnormal neuroimaging studies were the only two factors present at admission that predicted a poor short-term outcome (421). Unilateral hyperperfusion demonstrated by single photon emission CT (SPECT) also is associated with a poor prognosis in encephalitis (422).

Viral Meningitis (Aseptic Meningitis)

This is a clinical syndrome characterized in children by fever, abrupt onset of headaches, vomiting, irritability, and physical findings of meningeal irritation such as Kernig and Brudzinski signs. Infants present with a mild syndrome without the physical findings found in older children. The spinal fluid reveals less than 1,000 white blood cells with a mononuclear predominance, although early in the course of the illness, a polymorphonuclear predominance may be observed. CSF glucose is normal or slightly decreased, and CSF protein is slightly elevated. The Gram stain is universally negative, as are bacterial, mycobacterial, and fungal cultures.

Diagnosis

The diagnosis of a presumptive CNS viral infection starts with a thorough and meticulous history looking for significant exposures within the previous 2 to 3 weeks. The exposure of the patient to sick humans or animals (especially horses), travel history, and exposure to mosquitoes, rodents, and ticks helps to ascertain potential etiologies. The physical examination provides useful information about the extent of the disease and guides the choice of diagnostic studies required.

The analysis of the CSF is crucial in the search of the etiologic diagnosis. The cytochemical analysis combined with specific virologic (PCR and cultures) and serologic tests (specific IgM, IgG, or both) can assist in confirming the etiology. CSF also helps to rule out other treatable infectious or noninfectious causes, which could mimic a viral process. Thus, it is important in a child with a clinical picture of aseptic meningoencephalitis to rule out fungal, mycobacterial, and parasitic infections by performing appropriate stains and cultures. Bacterial infections of the CNS need to be ruled out by Gram stains, rapid antigen tests, and cultures. Viral cultures of blood, stool, and throat serve as a useful diagnostic tool. Blood obtained in the beginning of the clinical course as well as 2 to 3 weeks later can be used for the serologic confirmation of diseases through the observation of a fourfold increase in the specific antibody titer.

The value of neuroimaging studies lies not in determining the etiology of the viral encephalitis or meningitis, but in assessing the degree of CNS damage. For this purpose, MRI has been found to be more helpful than CT (423).

By the combined use of the various diagnostic studies, the etiology of viral meningitis or encephalitis can be determined in approximately 60% of patients (416).

This section considers the various types of viral infections according to etiology. A survey of their relative frequencies, as derived from data of Koskiniemi and Vaheri, is presented in Table 7.13 (424). Table 7.14 compiles the etiologic agents, type of disease, mechanism of acquisition,

TABLE 7.13 Known Reported Causes of Encephalitis in 412 Children 16 Years or Younger (1968 Through 1987)

Pathogen	*Percentage of Known Agents*
Measles, Mumps, Rubella Group[a]	30.4
Measles	12.8
Mumps	16.0
Rubella	1.6
Herpes Group	24.1
Varicella	15.4
Herpes simplex virus	6.4
Cytomegalovirus	1.3
Epstein-Barr virus	1.0
Respiratory Group	18.3
Adenovirus	8.7
Parainfluenza virus and respiratory syncytial virus	4.2
Influenza A and B viruses	5.4
Enterovirus Group	9.7
Enteroviruses	7.7
Rotavirus	1.0
Reovirus	1.0
Mycoplasmal Pneumonia	13.1
More Than One Virus	2.9
Postvaccination Encephalitis (Measles-Mumps-Rubella, Polio)	1.0
Agent Unknown	32.0

[a]No case of mumps, measles, or rubella encephalitis was encountered after 1982.

Adapted from Koskiniemi M, Vaheri A. Effect of measles, mumps, rubella vaccination on pattern of encephalitis in children. *Lancet* 1989;1:31.

TABLE 7.14 Common Viral Infections of the Central Nervous System

Viral Agent	*Disease*	*Transmission*	*Incidence*	*Fatality Rate*	*Laboratory Confirmation*
Herpesvirus					
Herpes simplex	Encephalitis	Human	Common	>70% if untreated	PCR has become method of choice
	Meningoencephalitis				
	Aseptic meningitis		Rare	<1%	Culture of CSF, brain biopsy
Varicella-zoster	Cerebellitis	Human	Uncommon	None	Clinical picture, culture of skin lesions, DFA of skin or brain tissue, serology
	Encephalitis		Rare		
	Aseptic meningitis		Rare		
	Transverse myelitis		Very rare		
	Reye syndrome		Very rare	>40%	
Cytomegalovirus	Encephalitis	Human	Uncommon	Rare	Culture of CSF, brain, PCR becoming gold standard, serology
	Meningitis		Rare		
Epstein-Barr virus	Encephalitis	Human	Uncommon	Rare	Serology is most useful, PCR of CSF
	Meningitis	Rare			
	Transverse myelitis				
	Guillain-Barré syndrome				
Human herpesvirus type 6	Encephalitis	Human	Uncommon	No	Culture PBMC, saliva, PCR on CSF, serology
	Meningitis				
	Encephalomyelitis				
Human herpesvirus type 7	Acute hemiplegia	Human	?	?	Culture PBMC, saliva, PCR on CSF, serology
	Seizures				
Enteroviruses					
Polio virus	Meningitis	Human	None in United States, clinical disease in developing countries	5%–50%	Culture, PCR
	Paralytic polio				
Coxsackievirus (C) and echovirus (E)	Meningitis	Human	Very common	None	Culture of stool, CSF, PCR of CSF very useful, serology
	Encephalitis		Rare (C), uncommon (E)		
	Paralytic disease		Common (C), rare (E)[a]		
	Guillain-Barré syndrome		Uncommon (C), rare (E)		
	Transverse myelitis		Rare		
	Cerebellitis		Rare		
	Peripheral neuritis		Rare		
Newer enteroviruses	Meningitis	Human	Uncommon	Rarely fatal	Viral culture, serology not useful
	Encephalitis				
	Paralytic disease				
	Encephalomyelitis				

(continued)

TABLE 7.14 (Continued). Common Viral Infections of the Central Nervous System

Viral Agent	*Disease*	*Transmission*	*Incidence*	*Fatality Rate*	*Laboratory Confirmation*
Arboviruses[b]					
Western equine encephalitis virus[c]	Meningitis Encephalitis	Mosquitoes/birds	Common	10% in infants	Serology, antigen detection in brain
Eastern equine encephalitis virus[d]	Meningitis Encephalitis	Mosquitoes/birds	Uncommon	50% in all ages	Serology, IgM, ELISA, culture and antigen in brain
Venezuelan equine encephalitis virus[e]	Meningitis Encephalitis	Mosquitoes/horses	Uncommon	$<1\%$	Serology, IgM, ELISA
Japanese encephalitis virus[f]	Meningitis Encephalitis	Mosquitoes/swine/birds	Very common	25%	ELISA, serology, CSF antigen
St. Louis encephalitis virus[g]	Meningitis Encephalitis Febrile headache	Mosquitoes/birds	Common	7%–20%	Serology, CSF IgM, ELISA
West Nile fever virus[h]	Meningitis Encephalitis Myelitis	Mosquitoes/birds	Common	10%	Serology, CSF IgM, ELISA
Murray Valley virus[i]	Encephalitis	Mosquitoes/birds	Uncommon	20%	Serology
Tick-borne encephalitis virus[j]	Meningitis Encephalitis Myelitis Radiculoneuritis	Ticks rodents	Uncommon	1%	Serology, CSF IgM, ELISA
California (La Crosse) encephalitis virus[k]	Meningitis Encephalitis	Mosquitoes/chipmunks Squirrels	Common	$<1\%$	Serology, culture, CSF IgM, ELISA
Paramyxoviruses					
Measles virus	Encephalitis	Human	Uncommon	$<5\%$	Serology
	Subacute sclerosing panencephalitis		Rare	100%	Elevated CSF globulin
Mumps virus	Meningitis Encephalitis	Human	Common in unvaccinated	$<1\%$	Serology, culture of CSF
Togaviruses					
Rubella virus	Encephalitis Guillain-Barré syndrome Optic neuritis Myelitis Progressive panencephalitis	Human	Rare	$<1\%$	Serology

Orthomyxoviruses					
Influenza virus	Encephalitis	Human	Uncommon	<1%	Culture of respiratory secretions, serology
	Transverse myelitis			<1%	
	Reye syndrome			>40%	
Rabdoviruses					
Rabies virus	Encephalitis	Bats, raccoons, skunks, dogs, squirrels, cats	Common	>99%	Antigen detection in brain, culture, serology
	Encephalomyelitis				
Adenoviruses					
Adenovirus	Meningitis	Human	Rare	<1%	Culture of CSF, brain
	Encephalitis				
Retroviruses					
Human immunodeficiency virus	Encephalitis	Human	Uncommon	100%	Serology, culture of CSF, PCR of CSF
	Transverse myelitis				
	Leukoencephalopathy				
Arenaviruses					
Lymphocylic choriomeningitis virus	Meningitis	Mice/hamsters	Rare	<2%	CSF, blood, urine cultures, serology
	Encephalitis				

CSF, cerebrospinal fluid; DFA, direct fluorescent antibody; ELISA, enzyme-linked immunosorbent assay; IgM, immunoglobulin M; PBMC, peripheral blood mononuclear cells; PCR, polymerase chain reaction.
[a] Incidence varies according to serotypes.
[b] Incidence depends on geographic region.
[c] Seen in United States west of Mississippi River.
[d] Seen in United States Atlantic and Gulf Coast states.
[e] Seen in southwestern United States, Florida, and Central and South America.
[f] Seen in Southeast Asia, India, and Nepal.
[g] Seen in all of United States.
[h] Seen in Africa, Middle East, Southeast Asia, India, Australia, areas of Europe, and the northeastern United States.
[i] Seen in Australia.
[j] Seen in Central Europe and Russia.
[k] More than 90% of cases seen in Midwest of United States.

TABLE 7.15 Viruses That have been Rarely Associated with Central Nervous System Disease

Virus	*Disease*
Parainfluenza	Aseptic meningitis
	Guillain-Barré syndrome
	Demyelinating disease
	Encephalomyocarditis
	Aseptic meningitis
Rotavirus	Aseptic meningitis
	Encephalitis
Coronavirus	Aseptic meningitis
	Polyradiculitis
	Multiple sclerosis?
Parvovirus B19	Aseptic meningitis
	Encephalitis
Rhinoviruses	Aseptic meningitis

frequency, fatality rates, and laboratory confirmation, as derived from data from Cassady and Whitley (425) and Johnson (426). Table 7.15 lists some of the more uncommon viral pathogens that have been associated with CNS disease.

Enterovirus Infections

Enterovirus (a group of RNA viruses) infections include poliomyelitis (3 types), coxsackie groups A (22 serotypes) and B (6 serotypes), and the echovirus group (31 serotypes). Viruses isolated after the original classification are simply assigned an enterovirus number (serotypes 68 to 72) (427).

Organisms enter the body through the oral or respiratory tracts, replicate, and extend to the regional lymphoid tissue, induce a minor viremia, and subsequently can invade multiple sites, including the nervous system. The clinical picture produced by these agents depends on factors such as type and virulence of the virus, the site of CNS invasion, and, as is the case for poliomyelitis, host factors such as degree of susceptibility and recent inoculations or trauma (428).

Enterovirus infection is transmitted principally by direct or indirect contamination through infected fecal material. Organisms can be isolated from the oropharynx, stool, blood, or CSF. Isolation of virus from CSF confirms the cause of a specific episode (428). Diagnosis by isolation of an enterovirus from stool can be misleading because virus can be excreted for 12 to 17 weeks after infection. In such a situation, only a definite increase in the titer of antibodies to the isolated agent can confirm a recent significant infection.

The clinical manifestations of an enterovirus infection of the nervous system can take several forms.

In aseptic meningitis, children usually have an infection associated with epidemic disease caused by coxsackieviruses A9 and B2, 4, and 5 or echoviruses 4, 6, 9, 11, 16, 30, and 33; other types, such as echoviruses 18, 7, and 13, have also emerged in outbreaks (429). Febrile infants infected with coxsackievirus group B and echoviruses 11 and 30 were more likely to have aseptic meningitis than those infected with other serotypes (430). Berlin and coworkers were able to identify the viral pathogen in 62% of children younger than 2 years of age with aseptic meningitis; group B coxsackievirus or echoviruses were implicated in 92% of the laboratory-diagnosed cases (431). In 63.5% of cases, the infection developed at 8 weeks of age or earlier (432). Fever, pharyngitis, or other respiratory symptoms are common. Abdominal pain can occur. Rash is common but its incidence depends on the specific viral agent; one-third to one-half of patients with echovirus 9 meningitis have exanthem. This rash is variable in appearance, but can be petechial and simulate the rash of meningococcemia. Herpangina, pleurodynia, or myocarditis are associated findings that suggest enterovirus infection (433). SIADH occurs in approximately 9% of children with enteroviral meningitis. It usually lasts less than 2 days (428,431). Multiple attacks of enteroviral aseptic meningitis occasionally have occurred in the same individual.

Enterovirus encephalitis is most commonly caused by echovirus type 9, less commonly by echoviruses 4, 6, 7, 11, and 30 and coxsackievirus B5. Outbreaks of encephalitis have been associated with enterovirus 71 (434) where systemic inflammatory responses may trigger cardiopulmonary collapse (435), especially in younger children (436–439). Three neurologic syndromes have been observed. Most commonly, there is a rhombencephalitis marked by myoclonic jerks, ataxia, and various brainstem signs; less often there is an aseptic meningitis or an acute flaccid paralysis (434,440). Enteroviruses account for approximately 10% to 20% of the cases of encephalitis of proven viral etiology. Neurologic symptoms can be diffuse or focal (441). Clinical manifestations of the diffuse form of encephalitis range from mild changes of mental status to coma, whereas focal neurologic symptoms include focal seizures, hemichorea, or ataxia. Although the general prognosis is favorable, fatal cases of enterovirus encephalitis involving coxsackieviruses B3 and B6, echoviruses 2, 9, 17, and 25, and enterovirus 70 have been reported (428,431). There is some evidence of efficacy of the antiviral agent pleconaril in enteroviral meningitis (438,442).

Coxsackieviruses and echoviruses can on rare occasions cause paralytic syndromes that are clinically indistinguishable from paralytic poliomyelitis. The course is less severe, however, and of shorter duration. Acute paralytic syndromes also can occur after acute epidemic conjunctivitis caused by enterovirus type 70 (443). The three patterns most commonly seen are limb involvement only (43%), involvement of nerves and limbs (33%), and involvement of one or more cranial nerves only (24%). Severe, diffuse pain that does not conform to root or nerve distribution and that is sometimes associated with muscle tenderness usually precedes the onset of paralysis (444). Approximately one-half of patients have fasciculations during the acute paralytic stage. In some instances, radiculitis, myelitis, or radiculomyelitis can occur (445).

Coxsackieviruses and echoviruses have been associated with a variety of other neurologic conditions, notably Guillain-Barré syndrome, transverse myelitis, dermatomyositis, polymyositis, cerebellar ataxia, and the syndrome of opsoclonus-myoclonus (431,446,447). Pulmonary edema, thought to be neurogenic in origin, has been associated with enterovirus 71 (448). Cardiopulmonary failure occurs in the absence of severe neurologic signs but is accompanied by severe, widespread inflammation of the brainstem and spinal cord (449).

Enterovirus infections of neonates are a serious and potentially fatal condition. Vertical transmission of enteroviruses can occur transplacentally, during delivery, and during the postpartum period. Whereas the presence of a primary maternal infection during late pregnancy can lead to stillbirth and severe neonatal disease manifested within the first 2 days of life, this is not a common occurrence. The majority of children manifest symptoms between the third and tenth days of life. This reflects the transmission of the virus by genital, respiratory, and gastrointestinal secretions during the immediate perinatal period. Enteroviruses reported to cause neonatal disease include coxsackieviruses B1 through B5 and echoviruses 5, 7, 9, 11, 17, 19, and 22 (450).

Signs and symptoms suggestive of severe CNS involvement include extreme lethargy, flaccid paralysis, and coma. These symptoms usually are associated with a multisystem organ involvement that includes liver, heart, and lungs with hypocoagulability and bleeding, a picture suggestive of neonatal sepsis (451). In the experience of Rorabaugh and associates, only 8.7% of infants younger than 16 weeks of age show meningeal irritation when first examined (432). A more benign picture of isolated aseptic meningitis also has been seen. Febrile seizures might be caused by enteroviral infection in the central nervous system, especially in summer months (452). Because of the decline in neonatal bacterial meningitis, enteroviruses have become the most common cause of meningitis in neonates older than 7 days and are responsible for one-third of all cases of neonatal meningitis (453). Repeat episodes of meningitis caused by different strains of enterovirus can occur within 1 month of each other (454).

A long-term follow-up study suggests that approximately 10% to 15% of infants who recover from enterovirus infections incurred during the first year of life have motor deficits or subnormal intelligence (455–457). Enterovirus infections in infants younger than 3 months of age can cause subtle deficits in language skills, particularly in receptive language. These children, therefore, should be monitored carefully for language development (458). When infection incurred after the first year of life, no residua are usually demonstrable.

Persistent and fatal enteroviral CNS infections can occur in patients with agammaglobulinemia (441,459).

The diagnosis of enteroviral infections is based in the recovery of the virus in feces, urine, blood, or CSF or from cultures obtained on biopsy specimen during the acute episode of the disease (460,461). The PCR technique is highly sensitive and specific for the detection of virus-specific DNA. Its speed, accuracy, and sensitivity make it superior to virus culture of CSF for the diagnosis of enterovirus meningitis (462,463).

Poliomyelitis

Although poliomyelitis caused by wild virus has been eradicated from the Western hemisphere since 1994, it remains a problem in developing countries. An extensive discussion is warranted because it serves as a prototype for viral infections of the nervous system.

Poliomyelitis is an acute infectious disease first described by Heine in 1840 (464). It affects the motor neurons of the spinal cord and brain and results in an asymmetric flaccid paralysis of the voluntary muscles. The severity of the illness varies; asymptomatic or mild cases are approximately 100 times more common than the classic paralytic disease. Poliomyelitis can occur throughout the world. It is contracted earlier in life and is less likely to be symptomatic in areas with inadequate sanitation because poor sanitation is conducive to exposure at an age when lingering transferred maternal immunity can attenuate the clinical picture.

With widespread immunization, poliomyelitis has become preventable, and recurrent major epidemics are no longer encountered. Approximately 8 to 10 cases per year have been reported in the United States. All of these have been associated with the use of the oral polio vaccine (OPV). These cases are more commonly associated with the administration of the first dose of vaccine (1 per 720,000 recipients of OPV) (465,466). Based on the lack of wild cases and the occurrence of vaccine-associated paralytic polio (VAPP), the Advisory Committee on Immunization Practices voted to recommend a sequential schedule of inactivated polio vaccine (IPV) and OPV for polio immunization, with either all OPV or all IPV as acceptable alternatives (467).

Pathology

Alterations found within the CNS depend on the stage of the disease at the time of death. In the early days of the illness, neurons undergo a variety of nonspecific microscopic

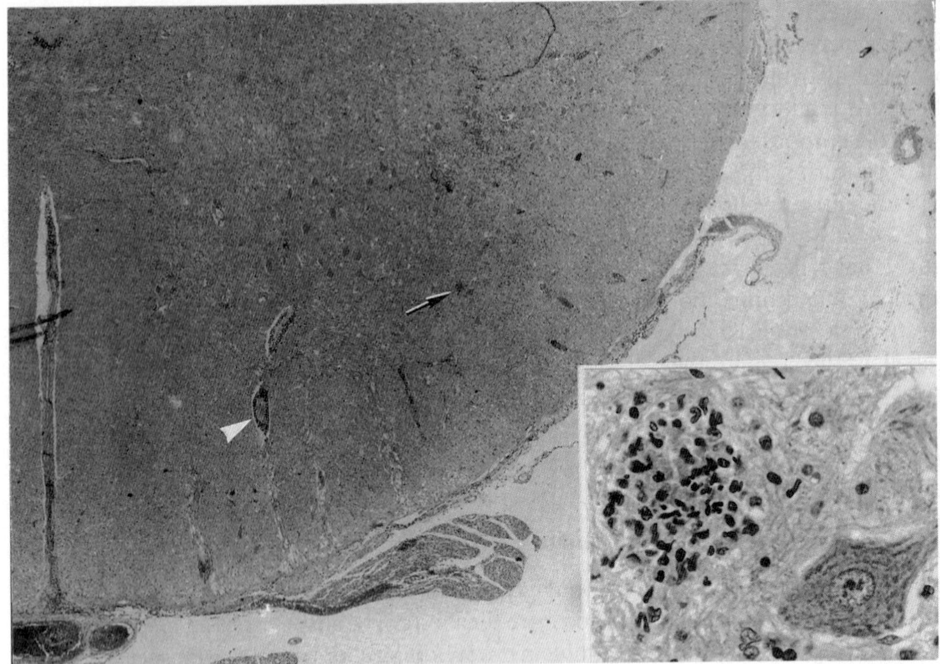

FIGURE 7.9. Poliomyelitis, acute stage. Anterolateral quadrant of the spinal cord at lumbrosacral enlargement shows widespread inflammation, mainly in the anterior horn. Perivascular cuff of chronic inflammatory cells (*white arrowhead*) and neuronophagia (*black arrow*) are apparent (H and E stain, ×22). Inset shows details of neuronophagia (hematoxylin and eosin stain, ×450). West Nile encephalitis shows a similar picture. (Courtesy of Dr. Hideo H. Itabashi, Departments of Pathology and Neurology, Los Angeles County Harbor Medical Center, Torrance, CA.)

changes that vary in severity and result directly from viral invasion. These changes are accompanied by an initial polymorphonuclear reaction, which later becomes mononuclear. As the illness progresses, motor neurons degenerate, become surrounded by inflammatory cells, and undergo neuronophagia. The distribution of lesions is characteristic of poliomyelitis. Lesions are usually mild and restricted to layers 3 and 5 in the precentral gyrus and adjacent cortex, thalamus, and globus pallidus (468). Neuronal necrosis can be caused by toxic levels of neurotransmitters such as quinolinic acid that occur in areas of the brain affected by the virus as well as from direct viral damage to neurons (469).

Cerebellar vermis and deep cerebellar nuclei are often severely involved, whereas the cerebellar hemispheres are usually free of lesions (470). In addition, marked involvement of motor and sensory cranial nuclei of the medulla occurs, especially the vestibular and ambiguous nuclei and throughout the reticular formation. The basis pontis and inferior olivary nuclei are usually spared.

In the spinal cord, lesions usually are restricted to the anterior horn cells, although some cases also show spotty involvement of the neurons in the intermediate, intermediolateral, and posterior gray columns (Fig. 7.9). Extension of lesions to the sensory spinal ganglia is the rule in more extensive cord involvement. The cervical and lumbar cords tend to be more affected than the thoracic region.

Clinical Manifestations

The clinical picture of poliomyelitis ranges from a nonspecific mild febrile illness to a severe and potentially fatal paralytic disease. An inapparent infection is estimated to occur in 90% to 95% of infected individuals, a minor nonparalytic illness in 4% to 8%, and paralytic poliomyelitis in 1% to 2% (Fig. 7.10). The incubation period ranges between 3 and 35 days, with an average of 17 days (471).

The minor illness coincides with the period of viremia and the appearance of virus in the stool. It lasts 24 to 48 hours and is manifested by nonspecific symptoms of headache, vomiting, sore throat, and gastrointestinal disturbances.

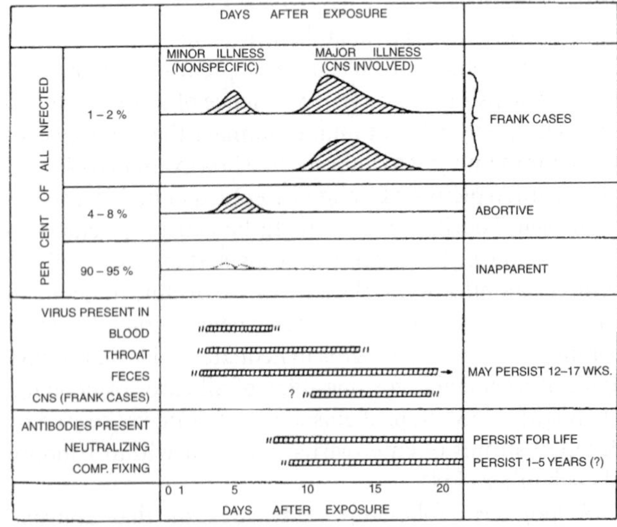

FIGURE 7.10. Schematic diagram of the clinical and subclinical forms of poliomyelitis, showing presence of virus and antibodies in relation to the development and subsidence of infection. (From Horsfall FL, Tamm I. *Viral and rickettsial infections of man*, 4th ed. Philadelphia: Lippincott, 1965. With permission.)

The major illness can follow in 2 to 5 days of recovery from the minor illness. When mild, it produces aseptic meningitis with fever, headache, vomiting, and meningeal irritation. The disease might not advance any further or it might progress to the paralytic stage.

The clinical course and picture of paralytic poliomyelitis varies with the age of the patient and the site of maximal involvement. The classic diphasic course is more common in children than in adults. It was noted in 37% of children aged 2 to 9 years but only in 11% of adolescents 15 years or older (472). In the remaining cases, the preparalytic stage is mild or inapparent. Infants show relatively little fever and lack meningeal signs despite extensive and often symmetric paralysis. Paralysis occurs in 90% of infants younger than 1 year of age who develop symptomatic infections with poliomyelitis virus (473).

The presenting symptom of paralytic poliomyelitis is pain, often severe and localized to the lower back. It usually is accompanied by hyperesthesia, drowsiness, or irritability. The initial indications of paralysis are localized muscular pain, fasciculation, twitching, and diminution or loss of the deep tendon reflexes. The paralysis appears during the first or second day of the major illness. Often it reaches its maximum within a few hours, and, less commonly, it can advance for 4 to 5 days. The fever that generally accompanies the paralysis falls by lysis.

Table 7.16 shows the distribution of paralysis, as encountered in an early epidemic (474). Curiously, when an infected child had received an injection before the onset of symptoms, the illness more likely involves the injected limb. A similar problem has been encountered when intramuscular injections are given within 30 days of immunization with oral poliovirus vaccine (475). These observations can be explained by the upregulation of the poliovirus receptor consequent to trauma. The poliovirus receptor is an integral membrane protein with structural characteristics of the immunoglobulin superfamily of proteins (476,477).

TABLE 7.16 Distribution of Paralysis in 5,784 Cases of Acute Anterior Poliomyelitis

Location	*Percentage of Cases*
Leg	78.6
Arm	41.4
Trunk	27.8
Throat and neck	5.8
Cranial nerves	13.8
Facial muscles	40.9
Pharyngeal	31.9
Ocular	30.1
Palatal	15.8
Glossal	5.6
Masticatory	2.9

Modified from Wernstedt W. Epidemiologische Studien über die zweite grosse Poliomyelitisepidemie in Schweden 1911–1913. *Ergebn Inn Med Kinderheilkd* 1924;26:248.

Spinal, bulbar, and encephalitic forms of poliomyelitis have been recognized. Spinal paralytic poliomyelitis is characterized by an asymmetric, scattered, flaccid paralysis that more frequently involves the lower extremities. On examination, the weakness is accompanied by muscle tenderness and spasm. Deep tendon reflexes in the affected area are usually absent. Autonomic involvement can be manifested by excessive sweating and vasomotor disturbances. Some 10% to 20% of patients have bladder involvement, notably sphincter spasm and overflow incontinence (478). Pyramidal tract and segmental sensory involvement are extremely rare.

The bulbar form of poliomyelitis generally evolves with explosive rapidity. Other areas of the neuraxis, most often the cervical cord, also are affected in 90% of cases.

The clinical picture of bulbar poliomyelitis reflects the site of involvement. Most commonly, the paralysis affects the facial, pharyngeal, and ocular muscles (see Table 7.16) (474,479). Involvement of the reticular formation can lead to respiratory and cardiovascular irregularities (480). Pulmonary edema is regarded as a manifestation of extensive damage to both the dorsal nuclei of the vagus and the medial reticular (vasomotor) nuclei of the medulla (481). When the tenth cranial nerve is involved, there is impairment of swallowing and faulty innervation of the larynx. This presents a serious threat to life by obstruction of the airway and is an indication for early elective tracheotomy. Fatal involvement of the respiratory center or the circulatory center may occur. Hypertension can develop secondary to medullary involvement or hypocapnia. Hypothalamic dysfunction is manifested by impaired temperature regulation and hypertension (482). Papilledema results from carbon dioxide retention caused by inadequate pulmonary ventilation. It also is associated with a high CSF protein, which interferes with normal CSF absorption.

In as many as one-third of cases, poliomyelitis is accompanied by symptoms and signs of encephalitis, including changes in consciousness, anxiety, irrationality, and restlessness or hyperactivity, muscular tremors, and twitching. These signs should first be considered as caused by hypoxia even in the absence of cyanosis. Only when these symptoms persist after adequate oxygenation can they be attributed to viral involvement of the cortex. Other complications of the acute stage of poliomyelitis include infections of the respiratory tract and atelectasis.

Paralytic ileus with gastric atony can result from viral damage to the vegetative centers or altered serum potassium concentrations.

Diagnosis

The blood is usually normal, although leukopenia can be found in the early stages of the illness. The CSF is almost always abnormal. CSF pressure is normal but can become elevated with carbon dioxide retention. The cell count is highest in the preparalytic stage, when polymorphonuclear cells predominate. The average count of 185 cells/μL decreases to 50 cells/μL at 1 week after the onset of paralysis. By then there is a predominantly monocytic response. The protein content is normal in the early stages of the illness. In the experience of Merritt and Fremont-Smith, it reached a maximum 25 days after the onset of paralysis (483). Thereafter, the protein content decreased gradually, remaining elevated long after the pleocytosis had disappeared. The sugar content is normal.

The virus is best isolated from the stool and oropharynx. Poliovirus has been isolated from the stool as early as 19 days before onset of illness and as late as 3 months after onset. The mean duration of virus excretion is approximately 5 weeks after onset of clinical illness. Poliovirus is rarely isolated from the CSF. The PCR technique performed on CSF (484), stool, blood, and throat specimens (485) is a sensitive, specific, and rapid technique for the diagnosis of enteroviral infections. It also has been used to differentiate wild poliovirus infections from vaccine strains and from other enteroviral infections (486). Serologic diagnosis is impractical but can be made by demonstrating an elevation in the specific complement fixation or neutralizing antibody titers. The etiologic diagnosis of inapparent, abortive, or nonparalytic poliomyelitis can be made only by laboratory studies.

Currently, poliomyelitis occurs rarely, and no confirmed case of wild-type polio virus infection has been reported in the United States since 1991 (487). Since then, all cases encountered in the United States have been associated with vaccination (488,489). All patients who develop poliomyelitis soon after oral vaccine administration should be evaluated for humoral and cellular immunosuppression (490). In the survey of Nkowane and coworkers, 33% of cases of poliomyelitis encountered between 1973 and 1984 were seen in recipients of OPV, 48% in contacts of such recipients, and 13% in immunodeficient patients (488). Virus reversion to the neurovirulent form involves point mutations at a single or several nucleotide positions (491).

On rare occasions, children who have been previously vaccinated with OPV present with an ascending paralysis simulating Guillain-Barré syndrome in association with a subsequent poliomyelitis type 1 infection (492,493).

Differential Diagnosis

In patients who are not immunodeficient and who have not been exposed to the vaccine, the diagnosis of poliomyelitis has become difficult. A number of other enteroviruses, notably coxsackieviruses and echoviruses, can produce a flaccid paralysis. When these conditions are unassociated with an exanthem, their diagnosis rests on PCR, viral isolation, or serologic confirmation. An illness resembling acute poliomyelitis also has been observed after infection with Epstein-Barr virus (494) as well as with an agent of the Russian spring-summer louping ill group of viruses (495).

Poliomyelitis must be differentiated from infectious polyneuritis, which has as presenting symptom a symmetric paralysis, usually progresses for more than 3 days, and is unaccompanied by fever. When sensory deficits can be documented, they confirm the diagnosis of polyneuritis. The absence of pleocytosis in the presence of a progressive paralysis also argues for polyneuritis.

A poliomyelitis-like paralysis (Hopkins syndrome) can occur during recovery from an asthma-like respiratory tract disease (496) (see Chapter 17). In some instances this syndrome can result from enterovirus or herpesvirus type 1 infections (497). Other conditions that mimic poliomyelitis include epidemic motor polyradiculoneuritis, insect and snake bites, schistosomiasis of the spinal cord, ingestion of chemicals such as arsenic and organic phosphates, trichinosis, and tetanus (498–500).

Prognosis

Recovery from nonparalytic forms of poliomyelitis is complete. The degree of disability that results from paralytic poliomyelitis depends on the extent of involvement. Function generally improves as pain and spasm recede after the acute phase. Overall mortality for the paralytic disease is approximately 4%. Spontaneous recovery of muscle function begins within a few weeks. Some involved neurons recover, but muscles totally paralyzed 1 month after the onset of the illness become completely normal only 1.4% of the time (501). Muscles severely paralyzed at the end of the acute period regain functional strength in 50% of cases and become normal in 20%. Moderately paralyzed muscles recover in 90% of cases. One-half the affected muscles continue to improve after 1 year. Three-fourths of functional recoveries occur in the first year, slightly less than one-fourth during the second year, and 5% during the third year. In general, prognosis is best for the proximal muscles in the lower extremities; it is poorest for the opponens pollicis and abdominal muscles (502).

Children with severe paralytic disease have developed a progressive neurologic disorder marked by increased weakness, fatigability, and pain some 30 to 40 years after the initial infection. Several explanations for this postpolio syndrome have been proposed. Sharief and colleagues suggested that it results from a chronic progression of the infection because there is intrathecal production of detectable IgM oligoclonal bands specific for poliovirus in the CSF and elevated CSF levels of IL-2 (503). Mononuclear perivascular cuffs occur in postpolio patients dying as long as 38 years after poliomyelitis (504). Late decompensation also could result from the combination of an abnormal enlargement of the motor units, resulting from the loss of the anterior horn cells, and the increased end-plate complexity seen with aging (504,505). Another factor that could cause postpolio syndrome is chronic muscle overuse because 40% of children with severe residual paralytic disease have elevated creatine kinase levels (505). Patients with residual leg weakness are twice as likely to report symptoms in those limbs as those with residual arm weakness (506). Sleep apnea can be a late complication of the postpolio syndrome (507). Relapses and second attacks of poliomyelitis are extremely rare. Other than a continued exercise program, there is no effective treatment for this condition (508).

Treatment

Control of poliomyelitis has been achieved by the use of orally administered live attenuated virus vaccine. Because of the vaccine-associated paralytic polio, changes in the poliovirus vaccine schedule occurred in 1997. Details of the advised vaccination schedules are presented in the 1997 Report of the Committee on Infectious Diseases, American Academy of Pediatrics (509).

Oral attenuated poliomyelitis vaccine should not be given to individuals with altered immunocompetence. Inactivated poliomyelitis vaccine is recommended for adults 18 years or older because of the increased risk of vaccine paralysis in that age group (488,489) and for immunization of HIV-positive children (509). For a detailed discussion of the response to vaccination, the characteristics of immunity, and the complications of vaccination, the reader is referred to Salk and Salk (510).

During the acute phase of the illness, treatment is solely symptomatic.

Coxsackievirus

An increasing number of coxsackievirus strains have been reported as causing infections of the human nervous system. The clinical pictures produced by the various strains of coxsackievirus are indistinguishable. Neurologic manifestations include aseptic meningitis, encephalitis, acute flaccid paralysis, Guillain-Barré syndrome, transverse myelitis, cerebellar ataxia, opsoclonus-myoclonus, and epidemic pleurodynia (511). These occur with both group A and B infections.

The clinical picture of aseptic meningitis caused by infection with coxsackievirus is nonspecific. The illness is preceded by a prodromal phase manifested by malaise and gastrointestinal disturbances, during which time viremia can be demonstrated. Neurologic symptoms can develop in association with pleurodynia, particularly in older children infected with B1 and B3 viruses. Exanthems are rare.

Coxsackieviruses B5, 1, 2, and 4 and A9 have been associated with the development of a clinical picture of encephalitis. The outcome is usually favorable. Serotypes A5, A9, and B2 have been associated with focal encephalitis (512).

Group A viruses also can cause acute lymphonodular pharyngitis, acute parotitis, hand-foot-and-mouth disease, polymyositis, chronic myopathies, and respiratory infections. Group B viruses have been associated with pleurodynia (Bornholm disease or epidemic pleurodynia) and diarrhea. Both types have been associated with pericarditis and myocarditis.

Anatomic alterations within the CNS are slight and nonspecific. They include meningeal inflammation and focal glial infiltration of gray and white matter of cerebrum, brainstem, and cerebellum (513).

A mild paralytic disease has been reported (514,515) as well as acute cerebellar ataxia, unilateral paralysis of the oculomotor nerve, palatal paralysis, and a postencephalitic parkinsonian picture (515,516). Focal necrotizing encephaloclastic lesions with subsequent porencephalic cyst formation also can occur.

Coxsackievirus infection is diagnosed by recovering the virus from blood or CSF, feces, and oropharyngeal swabbings, by detection of viral DNA by PCR in CSF or in brain biopsies, and by demonstrating an at least fourfold increase in neutralizing antibodies against the isolated virus.

The prognosis for recovery is usually excellent, and treatment is purely symptomatic.

Echovirus

Echoviruses are the most frequent cause of enterovirus infection of the nervous system. Sporadic infections have been described for 25 members of the group, whereas outbreaks usually occur with types 4, 6, 9, 11, 16, 18, and 30.

The clinical manifestations vary. Most common is an aseptic meningitis. All echovirus serotypes except 24, 26, 29, and 32 are associated with this entity (517). The illness is biphasic and generally self-limited. It presents a nonspecific picture of fever, headache, signs of meningeal irritation, sore throat, neck and back pain, and, occasionally, myalgia. In some cases, symptoms simulate basilar migraine (518). The illness usually resolves in 7 to 10 days. Certain viral strains can produce an illness associated with exanthematous or petechial rashes that can antecede or be associated with the period of central nervous involvement.

Although most patients have no paralytic residua, a few patients have been left with impaired strength in the anterior neck muscles. Rarely, a paralytic disease indistinguishable from poliomyelitis can occur with echovirus infections. Paralysis can be mild and transient or so severe as to be permanent or fatal. In the latter case, the virus has been isolated from CNS tissue.

Encephalitis manifested by focal or generalized seizures, disorders of sensorium, tremor, cranial nerve deficits, disorders of ocular movement, choreiform movements, paresthesias, and other signs of cerebral dysfunction have been associated with echovirus infections (519). Cerebellar ataxia of short duration (520) and acute ascending polyradiculomyelitis also have been described (521) as has muscular hypotonia in association with bilateral edema of the basal ganglia (522). Encephalitis with white matter necrosis can occur in the neonatal period (523). Persistent and fatal CNS infections with echoviruses can occur in patients with agammaglobulinemia (524). The course of these infections can be ameliorated by repeated administration of intravenous infusions of gamma globulin and intrathecal administration of gamma globulin prepared for intravenous use (524,525).

The diagnosis of echovirus infection usually rests on laboratory tests. IgG echovirus antibody elevation has been demonstrated in CSF of individuals with and without meningeal involvement. Because antibody titers to other viruses also are elevated, IgG echovirus antibody elevation reflects a nonspecific transport of IgG-associated viral antibodies from the serum to the CSF or reflects endogenous production of multiple antibodies within the CNS (526). PCR of CSF and a fourfold rise of specific antibodies confirm the etiologic agent.

Newer Enteroviruses

Four new enteroviruses (serotypes 68 through 71) have been recognized. These viruses can cause sporadic or epidemic infections of hand-foot-and-mouth disease and they have been recognized throughout the world. Serotypes 70 and 71 have been associated with CNS infections such as aseptic meningitis, encephalitis, and encephalomyelitis. Serotype 71 is responsible for more serious CNS disease, leading to acute paralytic manifestations indistinguishable from poliomyelitis and fatal encephalomyelitis (433,434,527).

The diagnosis is based on the virus isolation from skin vesicles, CSF, and brain tissue, using a monoclonal fluorescent antibody technique. No specific serologic diagnosis exists. Treatment of these infections is supportive.

Reovirus

Reovirus type 1 can cause meningitis in young infants (528).

Adenoviruses

Adenovirus infections usually cause an acute respiratory disease associated with conjunctivitis or keratoconjunctivitis. In a small percentage of cases, these symptoms are associated with involvement of the nervous system, notably a severe encephalitis or meningoencephalitis (529,530). A syndrome of reversible encephalopathy has also been reported (531). Neonatal infections usually are generalized. In fatal cases with neonatal encephalitis the CSF has been reported to be normal (532).

The diagnosis of these infections can be made through the isolation of the virus from the CSF or brain. A fourfold rise in adenoviral antibodies can provide a retrospective diagnosis. The prognosis of the CNS manifestations of adenoviruses is difficult to ascertain because of the few reported cases. No specific treatment for these infections is available.

Human Herpesvirus Types 6 and 7

Exanthem Subitum (Roseola Infantum)

Roseola, the most common exanthem of infancy, is characterized by the relative absence of prodromal symptoms, a rapid increase in body temperature, and conspicuously little listlessness or irritability. The temperature remains elevated for 3 to 5 days and subsides with the appearance of maculopapular rash. A bulging fontanel, the result of increased intracranial pressure, occurs during the second to fifth day of fever in about one-third of children (533). The condition occurs at a median age of 9 months when caused by human herpesvirus-6 (HHV-6), and at a median age of 26 months when caused by human herpesvirus-7 (HHV-7) (534). Other viral agents also are believed to be responsible for this condition (535).

CNS involvement can occur from 1 day before the onset of fever to day 2 of the illness (533). Neurologic complications include aseptic meningitis, acute disseminated encephalomyelitis (536,537), acute encephalitis (538), and acute cerebellitis.

The incidence of seizures varies considerably from one series of cases to the next (539). In the prospective study of Hall and coworkers, HHV-6 infection accounted for one-third of all febrile seizures younger than the age of 2 years (540). Persistent neurologic complications and death have been reported. The former include hemiparesis, recurrent seizures, and mental retardation. The cause of the residual encephalopathy is unknown (536).

HHV-6 DNA has been detected in the CSF of children who had three or more febrile seizures. This observation suggests that in some instances recurrence of febrile convulsions is associated with reactivation of the virus (540,541,542).

Approximately one-fifth of children have CSF with either a pleocytosis of more than 5 white blood cells/μL or a protein of more than 45 mg/dL; CSF glucose is normal. Approximately one-fourth of children have encephalopathy or encephalitis; all of these have an abnormal EEG. Transient periodic complexes can occur over the temporal lobes similar to those described for herpes simplex virus encephalitis (536). Unilateral or bilateral CT changes usually begin as hypodense areas that can progress to irregular cerebral atrophy or become hemorrhagic (536).

The association of HHV-6 with the neurologic complications is suggested by the concomitant isolation of virus, the identification of DNA by PCR in the CSF (543), and the fourfold increase in specific neutralizing antibodies. HHV-6 reactivations include a number of neurologic complications later in life (544).

HHV-7 has been associated with febrile seizures, a severe encephalopathy, and in two instances acute hemiplegia by the isolation of HHV-7 through viral culture and PCR (545,546). The diagnosis of HHV-7 is based on the methods described for HHV-6 (547).

Many strains of HHV-6 are sensitive *in vitro* to ganciclovir and foscarnet (548). Doses of 10 mg/kg per day in two divided doses of ganciclovir or 180 mg/kg per day in three divided doses of foscarnet can be given in cases of serious CNS infections caused by HHV-6.

Arboviruses

Arthropod-borne (arbo) viruses are RNA viral agents transmitted between susceptible vertebrate hosts by means of blood-sucking arthropods (549). Approximately 200 viruses have been tentatively classified into this group, and approximately 150 of these have been assigned to 21 groups that share common antigens. At least 51 have been associated with human disease. The epidemiology of these infections is largely determined by the nature and lifestyle of the vector. Most of the infections are sustained in sylvan hosts, with transmission through humans and domestic animals being usually incidental and insignificant in the natural history of the virus. Of greatest significance in the United States are the La Crosse (LAC) strain of the California encephalitis group, St. Louis encephalitis (SLE), western equine encephalitis (WEE), eastern equine encephalitis (EEE), Venezuelan equine encephalitis (VEE), Colorado tick fever, West Nile virus, and Powassan encephalitis. In this section we also include Dengue virus and Japanese encephalitis virus.

In humans, these viruses can be asymptomatic or can produce a mild generalized illness. The full-blown diseases, which are discussed in this section, are the least common manifestations of infection.

The nonspecificity of symptoms necessitates diagnosis by means of laboratory studies. Viral-specific IgM antibodies appear in serum in the first week of illness, and serologic tests on paired samples taken several weeks apart can suggest a recent infection (550). The detection of virus-specific IgM in the CSF is diagnostic. Virus can be isolated from blood or from nervous tissue by means of biopsies or autopsies.

La Crosse Encephalitis

LAC, a member of the California serogroup of *Bunyavirus*, is the most commonly reported cause of mosquito-borne disease in the United States (551). This disease, originally encountered most frequently in Midwestern states, also has become endemic in the mid-Atlantic region. Since 1993, West Virginia has had more reported cases that any other state (552). *Aedes triseriatus,* the principal mosquito vector, transmits the virus during the summer and early fall. Tree holes that contain water as well as discarded automobile tires that hold rainwater serve as the breeding habitat for the mosquito. Unlike St. Louis encephalitis virus and other arboviruses that cause epidemic disease, La Crosse virus infections exhibit an endemic pattern.

In 99% of instances, LAC virus infection is asymptomatic. The symptomatic disease can be mild or severe (553). LAC is the most prevalent and most pathogenic of the California serogroup of viruses (554,555).

Pathology

The alterations within the brain are largely microscopic. They are those of an acute encephalitis without distinctive findings (553).

Clinical Manifestations

The peak incidence of LAC is between July and October. There is a strong association between rural outdoor exposure and the presence of antibodies and clinical illness; the incidence of antibodies is 26.8% in rural populations and 15.3% in urban areas. Significant increases in antibody titer occur between ages 5 and 9 years among rural populations and between ages 10 and 19 years among urban populations living in endemic areas (556). Male individuals are affected three times as often as female individuals.

The clinical picture is that of a meningoencephalitis with fever, changes in consciousness, headache, and meningeal irritation (553,557,558). Balfour and associates defined two clinical patterns (559). A mild form begins with a 2- to 3-day prodromal stage characterized by fever, headache, malaise, and gastrointestinal symptoms. An increase in temperature on approximately the third day is associated with lethargy and evidence of meningeal irritation. Symptoms abate over 7 or 8 days without overt neurologic residua.

The severe form begins abruptly with fever and headache, followed in 12 to 24 hours by sudden onset of focal or generalized seizures. These have been reported in 40% to 50% of patients with neurologic symptoms (559). Hypernatremia and increased body temperature may be related to clinical deterioration (560).

The CSF shows pleocytosis, which in 85% of cases is mainly mononuclear. The protein content is mildly elevated in 20% of the patients and the glucose content is normal. The LAC PCR test for cerebrospinal fluid enables rapid diagnosis (554). Presence of the SIADH is common. The EEG is always abnormal, with abnormalities persisting for months or years in 55% of cases (561).

Diagnosis

In contrast to infections caused by enteroviruses, LAC is not biphasic and is not obviously associated with upper respiratory signs or symptoms. Familial outbreaks are extremely rare. EEG and neuroimaging demonstrate a focal process in 15% to 40% of patients (559). Such focal involvement also is observed in herpes simplex encephalitis; in both conditions, the CSF can be hemorrhagic. Specific

IgM and IgG serologies in CSF and serum confirm the viral etiology. A fourfold increase in these antibodies provides a retrospective diagnosis. If a brain biopsy is performed, infected brain cells can be detected by a monoclonal antibody technique (562).

Prognosis

LAC is a relatively mild illness, with a case fatality rate in symptomatic cases of less than 1% (551). Permanent neurologic residua are uncommon, but patients can have a variety of neurologic and behavioral residua (558,563). Older children and adolescents tend to show emotional lability, difficulty in learning, and personality problems. Later, difficulties in processing visual and auditory information become apparent, and some children develop behavior that resembles the organic hyperkinetic syndrome (564). However, a controlled assessment of 29 children who recovered from encephalitis failed to demonstrate significant personality changes when compared with the premorbid state (564).

Treatment

The treatment of neurologic manifestations of LAC has changed over the last few years. Ribavirin, which is active *in vitro* against LAC (565,566), was given for 10 days to a child for a severe, biopsy-proven case of LAC encephalitis, with a good outcome (565). Future studies will determine the need for its routine use.

St. Louis Encephalitis

SLE was first recognized in St. Louis in the summer of 1932 during an epidemic of encephalitis that originated in Paris, Illinois. Since then, sporadic outbreaks have occurred in the St. Louis area, California, the Rio Grande valley, Florida, and the central river valleys and western coastal regions of the United States. The vector for this virus is the *Culex* mosquito, and the virus has been isolated from overwintering mosquitoes (567,568).

Pathology

Diffuse vascular congestion and edema occur with meningeal and perivascular infiltration, petechiae, and glial nodules. Lesions predominate in the thalamus and substantia nigra. The cortex, anterior horns of the spinal cord, molecular and Purkinje cell layers, and dentate nucleus of the cerebellum also are involved (569).

Clinical Manifestations

Most commonly, this virus produces a clinically inapparent infection, and the ratio of asymptomatic to symptomatic cases has ranged from 19:1 to 427:1 in various outbreaks (570). Most cases occur in late summer and early fall; boys are affected three times more often than girls in some epidemics. Generally, the severity of the encephalitis and the extent of residua are greater in the older age groups (571).

The clinical manifestations of SLE range from a nonspecific flulike illness to fatal cases of encephalitis. In the 1964 Houston epidemic, most children had fever, headache, and meningeal irritation. Ataxia was noted in 27%, and fine tremors of the upper extremity in 19%. Cranial nerve palsies were encountered in 12% (570). Occasionally, the virus is responsible for transient parkinsonism (572), the syndrome of opsoclonus and myoclonus (573), and acute cerebellar ataxia (574). The latter two conditions are covered in Chapter 8.

Abnormalities in the CSF are those expected for a viral encephalitis, namely pleocytosis, which initially is predominantly polymorphonuclear, but later becomes mononuclear; a mild elevation of protein levels; and a normal sugar content (575). The EEG is often abnormal. Electromyographic studies have shown fasciculations in 59% of cases, fibrillations in 8%, and excessive insertional potentials in 54%. In some cases, these abnormalities have persisted for more than 1 month (570). The diagnosis is confirmed by specific IgM serology in the CSF or blood. When obtained within 4 days of the clinical onset of the disease, the serology has been positive in 75% of cases. Fourfold increases in specific IgG antibodies in blood can provide a retrospective diagnosis. Viral isolation should be pursued when a brain biopsy or autopsy is obtained.

Prognosis

SLE is intermediate in severity between California encephalitis and the equine encephalitides. The mortality in the 1964 St. Louis epidemic was 8% in children younger than 10 years of age. In more recent epidemics, it has ranged from 0% to 22%. Major sequelae occur less frequently than after EEE or WEE, but have been observed in 7.7% to 10.0% of survivors. Most commonly, they involve disturbances of gait and equilibrium, difficulties in speech and vision, and changes in personality (575,576). Children and young adults are much less prone to long-term motor disability than older adults (575).

Treatment

Treatment is symptomatic and supportive. No specific antiviral therapy or vaccines are available.

Western Equine Encephalitis

WEE is caused by a group A arbovirus from the family Togaviridae. It occurs in the western United States and in the central states west of the Mississippi Valley. The virus was first isolated in 1930 in California from horses with encephalitis. The chief vectors are several *Culex* mosquitoes, notably *Culex tarsalis* in the United States. The enzoonotic cycle is kept between mosquitoes, birds, and other vertebrate hosts. Horses and humans become dead-end hosts.

Pathology

The alterations within the nervous system in WEE are similar to those seen in the other encephalitides caused by arboviruses. The greatest damage is usually in the basal ganglia and cerebral white matter, with foci of demyelination and necrosis. The subcortical white matter is more extensively damaged than the cortex in the majority of fatal cases (577). White matter subjacent to cortex is more involved than deeper white matter in some children. Striking involvement of the substantia nigra might explain the relatively frequent appearance of parkinsonism as a late sequel of WEE (578,579). Extensive cystic degeneration of white matter can occur in infants.

A striking finding, noted as late as 5 years after onset of the acute illness, is the presence of both chronic inactive areas of destruction and active foci of glial proliferation and perivascular cuffing. This finding suggests that a slowly progressive form of the disease can continue for years (580).

Chronic cases can have a significant endothelial proliferation with a vasculitis producing almost complete occlusion of small vessels. Scattered areas of focal necrosis often contain phagocytic elements. In some cases, extensive cavities replace brain tissue (576,581).

Clinical Manifestations

Clinically inapparent infections far outnumber overt infections, although infants younger than 1 year of age have an equal incidence of apparent and inapparent infections (582).

In infants younger than 1 year of age, one common clinical picture is that of a sudden onset of high fever, seen in 92% of patients, accompanied by focal or generalized seizures, seen in 77% of patients (583). Older children have a severe encephalitis with fever, headache, vomiting, changes in consciousness, and meningeal signs. Convulsions develop in approximately 50% of children aged 1 to 4 years and in 9% of children aged 5 to 14 years.

Symptoms usually persist for approximately 10 days, then gradually subside. In fatal cases, the course is rapidly progressive. The CSF findings resemble those encountered in the other arbovirus infections (583).

The mortality in different epidemics has ranged from 9% to 23%. Sequelae are frequent and are most severe in very young infants; 56% of infants who contracted the illness when they were younger than 1 month of age had major sequelae (576). These include microcephaly, pyramidal or extrapyramidal motor impairment, seizures, and developmental retardation (580). Follow-up studies conducted on survivors reveal that the younger the patient is at the time of illness, the greater are the incidence and severity of sequelae (580,581). In older infants and in children, the sequelae are less severe. In Finley's series, no patient contracting the illness between ages 1 and 2 years developed motor or behavior problems; 25%, however, developed seizures (580). Such seizures represent persistence of convulsions that first appeared during the acute illness.

The diagnosis is based on the detection of specific IgM and IgG in CSF and blood. The virus can be isolated rarely from blood or CSF. When brain tissue is obtained, the virus can be easily cultured.

No vaccine or specific treatment is available.

Eastern Equine Encephalitis

EEE is a group A arbovirus from the family Togaviridae first isolated in 1933 from brain tissue of infected horses. It is distributed along the Atlantic coast from the northeastern United States to Argentina. Small epidemics have been encountered in Massachusetts, New Jersey, Florida, Texas, and, more recently, Jamaica. The virus is transmitted by a variety of mosquitoes, *Culiseta melanura* being the most common in the United States. Birds are the amplifying host and horses and humans are dead-end hosts (550).

Pathology

The outstanding feature of EEE is the predominance of neutrophilic leukocytes in the infiltrates, which undoubtedly reflects the rapid demise of most fatally infected patients. Focal or diffuse accumulations of neutrophils and histiocytes are prominent in the leptomeninges and in the cerebral cortex, particularly the occipital and frontal lobes and hippocampus (584).

Foci of tissue damage with rarefaction necrosis permeated by neutrophilic leukocytes and pleomorphic ameboid cells are often found. Neuronolysis, often with adjacent neutrophilic leukocytes and microglial cells, is common in fulminant cases. Large perivascular collections of neutrophils, histiocytes, and other ameboid cells are detected in the white matter in regions of cortical involvement. Other sites of predilection are the basal ganglia and brainstem. Edema and congestion are prevalent early. Vascular lesions characterized by numerous small thrombi in arterioles and venules can occur. Many vessels show complete involvement of their walls with neutrophilic infiltration and fibrin deposition. As the disease progresses, the dominant cell type changes to mononuclear lymphocytes and macrophages (576,584).

Clinical Manifestations

Infected children have a subclinical to clinical ratio of 2:1 to 8:1; adults have a ratio of 4:1 to 50:1 (585). For this reason, EEE is particularly common in infants, with two-thirds of the clinical cases being younger than 2 years old. It is usually fulminant with an abrupt onset, high fever, stupor or coma, convulsions, and signs of meningeal irritation. Patients can die within 48 hours of their initial symptoms or can survive for a few days, dying from damage of the vital medullary centers, dural sinus thrombosis, or subarachnoid hemorrhage. Survivors can remain comatose for several days or weeks before becoming responsive.

Laboratory studies are not diagnostic. The peripheral blood can show a prominent leukocytosis. The increase in CSF pressure can be striking. Initial CSF cell counts range between 250 and 2,000 white blood cells/μL, often containing almost 100% polymorphonuclear cells. The pleocytosis diminishes rapidly, and mononuclear cells predominate after 3 days in surviving patients (584). The EEG almost invariably shows generalized slowing and disorganization of the background activities, with the occasional patient demonstrating epileptiform discharges. The confirmation of the diagnosis is obtained through specific serology in CSF (IgM), a fourfold increase in the titer of serum antibodies, and/or the isolation of EEE virus from CSF or brain tissue (586).

Neuroimaging study results can be norma or show diffuse edema or a variety of focal lesions. In the review by Deresiewicz and coworkers, abnormal findings included focal lesions in the basal ganglia, thalami, and brainstem. Cortical lesions, meningeal enhancement, and periventricular white matter changes were less common. The presence of large radiographic lesions did not predict a poor outcome (586).

Prognosis

Infection with the virus of EEE has the most serious prognosis of all virus infections prevalent in the United States. The mortality in EEE in patients younger than 10 years is approximately 60% (585). The case fatality rate for all patients reported to the Centers for Disease Control and Prevention between 1988 and 1994 was 36%, with 35% of surviving patients showing moderate to severe sequelae. These include mental retardation, motor dysfunction, deafness, and seizures. Complete neurologic recovery is seen in only a small proportion of survivors. A high CSF white count or severe hyponatremia was predictive of a poor outcome (586).

Venezuelan Equine Encephalomyelitis

Although VEE, a group A arbovirus, is indigenous to Colombia, Venezuela, and Panama, it was responsible for the 1971 Texas encephalitis epidemic. The organism was also responsible for an outbreak of encephalitis in 1995 in Colombia and Venezuela that involved 75,000 to 100,000 cases (587). The organism has been isolated from many wild rodents as well as from *Aedes* and *Culex* mosquitoes (588).

VEE is much more benign than California (La Crosse) encephalitis, SLE, EEE, and WEE. It is marked by sudden onset of malaise, chills and fever, nausea and vomiting, headache, myalgia, and bone pain. The fever lasts from 24 to 96 hours, then abruptly drops. A period of 2 to 3 weeks of marked asthenia can follow. In contrast to other arboviruses, whose ratios of inapparent to apparent infections range from 23:1 to 500:1, in VEE a ratio of 11:1 has been reported.

The CSF findings are as in the other arbovirus infections. Virus can be isolated from serum during the first 3 days of the illness in 75% of confirmed cases (588).

PCR provides a fast, sensitive, and specific method for the detection of viral DNA in infected blood. The detection of specific IgM in CSF and serum and the observation of a fourfold increase in specific IgG in serum provide serologic confirmation of the disease.

Prognosis is good, and, with good care, fatalities are rare.

Japanese Encephalitis

Japanese encephalitis virus is transmitted by culicine mosquitoes between birds and humans. Histologic changes are most marked in the thalamus and brainstem. Patients who die rapidly can have no histologic signs of inflammation, yet have immunohistochemical evidence of viral antigen in morphologically normal neurons. Clinical features of this condition are much like those of the other encephalitides (589,590). Fever, headache, and vomiting are followed by meningism and coma. Convulsions have been reported in 85% of children. A characteristic mask-like facies with a vacant stare or grimacing or lip-smacking can occur, as can a paralytic disease that mimics acute poliomyelitis. Pyramidal tract signs, a rare complication in poliomyelitis, should suggest the diagnosis of Japanese encephalitis in endemic areas (591). In the 1986 Nepal epidemic, children accounted for the majority of hospitalized cases. The fatality rate in children was markedly less than that in adults (592). In the Indian epidemic studied by Kumar and colleagues, of children with proven Japanese encephalitis, the case fatality rate was 32%; major sequelae occurred in 45%; only 29% were healthy on follow-up (593). Sequelae of the disease were more severe when the initial illness was prolonged or was associated with focal neurologic deficits. Children are more likely to have dystonia as a sequela when compared to adults (594). A TNF concentration of greater than 50 pg/mL in serum correlated significantly with a fatal outcome, whereas high levels of Japanese encephalitis virus–IgM antibodies (more than 500 units) in the CSF were associated with a nonfatal outcome (595). Elevated levels of proinflammatory cytokines and chemokines are associated with a poor outcome (596).

The MRI in Japanese encephalitis patients shows lesions in the thalamus, cortex, midbrain, cerebellum, and spinal cord. Classically, the lesions are hyperintense in T2-weighted images and hypodense in T1-weighted images (597). In some 70% of cases these are hemorrhagic. According to Kumar and coworkers, bilateral thalamic involvement, especially hemorrhagic, can be considered to be characteristic of Japanese encephalitis in endemic areas (598). Diffusion-weighted MR imaging best demonstrates bilateral thalamic disease in Japanese encephalitis (599).

A specific diagnosis can be made by detecting a fourfold increase in specific IgG antibodies in acute and convalescent sera and by measuring Japanese encephalitis virus IgM in serum and CSF by ELISA. IgM can be detected 1 week after the onset of clinical symptoms. Virus isolation can be performed but needs to be done during the first 7 days of the disease prior to the mounting of an immune response.

No effective treatment exists, and high-dose dexamethasone treatment has been of no benefit. Interferon-alpha has been used in a small number of patients, and bigger trials are being awaited to assess its efficacy. The use of sedation has been shown to independently improve outcome (600). An inverse association between interferon-gamma levels and the severity of postencephalitic sequelae has been reported (601). Motor evoked potentials may be useful in predicting motor outcome (602). A Japanese encephalitis vaccine is available in the United States (550).

West Nile Virus

Since its introduction into the United States in 1999, West Nile virus has become a significant cause of arboviral infection of the central nervous system. The most recent data issued by the Centers for Disease Control and Prevention indicate that in 2004 the virus was reported from 40 states with more than 2,300 cases, of whom over 800 developed neurologic manifestations, resulting in 79 deaths. Reports of neurologic complications in children with West Nile virus infections have been rare (602a), and in 2002 only 4% of cases with neurologic manifestations occurred in patients younger than 18 years (602a).

The neurologic picture can be that of myalgia and lethargy, a viral meningitis, or, most seriously, an encephalitis with ataxia, extrapyramidal movements, cranial nerve abnormalities, optic neuritis, and a poliomyelitis. The last can take the form of a rapidly ascending quadriplegia that mimics Guillain-Barré syndrome or a picture whose clinical, pathologic and electrophysiologic features are indistinguishable from poliovirus-induced poliomyelitis (602b). This is marked by a focal, asymmetric weakness unaccompanied by sensory changes. Pathologic examination of the spinal cord discloses the ventral horn to bear the brunt of the infection. There one observes neuronophagia, perivascular inflammation, and microglial proliferation. The dorsal roots and sympathetic ganglia can also be affected (602c). Electrodiagnostic studies can demonstrate widespread fibrillation potentials and compound motor action potentials of normal or reduced amplitude. MR imaging of the spinal cord demonstrates hyperintensity in the anterior horns on T2-weighted images (602d).

In the milder cases recovery is complete (602a), but the severely paralyzed patient remains quadriplegic and ventilator dependent.

Powassan Encephalitis

Powassan encephalitis is a virus within the group of tick-borne flaviviruses. In North America it is transmitted by ticks to small mammals. Human infections are related to outdoor activities and tick bites. Canada and the northeastern, north central, and western United States are the geographic areas of distribution of this disease.

The incubation period ranges from 4 to 21 days, after which fevers, headache, lethargy, vomiting, and photophobia appear as early signs, followed by an increase in the intracranial pressure reflected by alterations of consciousness, seizures, ophthalmoplegia, and motor impairment (603). The disease tends to be similar to the CNS disease caused by the mosquito-borne viral meningoencephalitis. Mortality approximates 1%, and sequelae such as hemiplegia, quadriplegia, aphasia, and chronic convulsive disorders have been reported.

The diagnosis is based on the detection of specific IgM antibodies in serum, CSF, or both. Powassan encephalitis can be isolated from brain tissue in biopsies and autopsies. No specific therapy for Powassan encephalitis is available.

Dengue Fever

Dengue is unique among flaviviruses in that humans are the most important natural host and infections are frequently symptomatic. *Aedes aegypti* mosquitoes are the most common vectors. Neurologic complications referred to as dengue encephalopathy can occur secondary to the two forms of the disease, Dengue hemorrhagic fever or an acute febrile illness with facial flushing, headache, arthralgia, myalgia, retro-orbital pain, petechiae, and a fine maculopapular rash. Dengue fever is caused by four distinct viral species. Immunity to a heterologous Dengue serotype predisposes to Dengue hemorrhagic fever (604). In most cases neurologic manifestations are thought to be manifestations secondary to severe disease. Dengue-associated encephalopathy is seen in less than 1% of cases of Dengue fever (605). Intracranial hemorrhages and cerebral edema can occur. A Reye-like metabolic encephalopathy secondary to hepatic failure can occur. Occasionally, there can be direct invasion of the CNS. Lethargy, confusion, convulsions, and coma are the most common clinical features, but meningism, paresis, and cranial nerve palsies can occur (606). CSF can be normal or show mild pleocytosis (606).

TABLE 7.17 Distribution of Arbovirus-Caused Encephalitides

Condition	Distribution	Vector	Reference
Japanese encephalitis	Eastern Siberia, China, Korea, Taiwan	Mosquito	576,607,608
Toscana virus	Tuscany, Italy	Sandfly	609
Murray Valley encephalitis	Eastern Australia, Northern Territory, New Gulnea	Mosquito	609a–609c
Tick-borne encephalitides			
European	Europe	Tick *(Ixodes ricinus)*	576,610
Far Eastern (Russian spring-summer encephalitis)	Siberia, Far East	Tick *(Ixodes persulcatus)*	611
Kyasanur Forest disease	India	Tick	612
Powassan virus	Ontario, Canada	Tick	613
Colorado tick fever	Western United States	Wood tick	576,613a,614
Kumlinge disease		Tick	615
Louping Ill	Scotland	Tick *(Ixodes ricinus)*	610,616

Other Arboviruses

The distribution of encephalitides caused by other arboviruses is summarized in Table 7.17.

Rift Valley Fever

Rift Valley fever is caused by a virus of the phlebotomus fever serogroup. It has an ever-widening distribution in Africa and is capable of widespread epizootics and epidemics such as the Egyptian outbreak of 1977, which had an estimated morbidity of 200,000 and a mortality of 600. The disease is characterized by sudden onset of fever, occasionally with one early recurrence (saddleback fever), severe myalgia, especially in the lower back, headache, retro-orbital pain, conjunctival suffusion, vomiting, and anorexia. The disease usually lasts 4 to 7 days.

Three forms of complications occur. Retinal complications can develop 7 to 20 days after the onset of other symptoms, with decrease in visual acuity that can result in permanent loss of central vision in the more severe cases owing to edema, exudates, hemorrhage, and vasculitis. Meningoencephalitis can occur during convalescence from a febrile illness lasting 5 to 10 days, often beginning with hallucinations, disorientation, and vertigo. Residual neurologic deficits can occur, but fatalities are infrequent. Hemorrhagic Rift Valley fever with jaundice and hemorrhagic phenomena can develop in 2 to 4 days. This is the chief cause of mortality; in 3 to 6 days, the patient either dies or begins a slow convalescence (617).

Mumps

Mumps virus was the most common cause of CNS involvement by any of the contagious diseases of childhood before the widespread use of mumps immunization. It is now much less common in countries with effective vaccination programs. It remains a frequent complication in nonimmunized populations and vaccine failures can occur. The most common complication of mumps is an aseptic meningitis syndrome; meningoencephalitis is a much rarer manifestation. CNS involvement has been observed in up to 65% of cases, most with meningitis (618). Mumps virus involvement of the nervous system can occur with or without signs of clinical parotitis. The incidence of neurologic involvement is difficult to estimate, but CFS pleocytosis has been demonstrated in 56% of patients with parotitis. Meningoencephalitis is far less common, developing in 0.2% of cases (619). In approximately one-third of children, CNS symptoms occur in the absence of clinical parotitis, although subclinical parotitis usually can be documented by elevations in serum amylase. More commonly CNS symptoms accompany the swelling or develop from 8 days before to 20 days after the appearance of clinical parotitis (620). Male patients are three or four times more likely to have neurologic symptoms than female patients. Signs of meningeal irritation may or may not be present; headache, nausea, and vomiting are associated with the benign leptomeningeal form of the disease. In this entity recovery is complete. Brainstem encephalitis and acute disseminating encephalomyelitis are rare complications of mumps (618).

Mumps meningoencephalitis is a far more serious condition. Signs and symptoms in order of observed frequency include fever, vomiting, nuchal rigidity, lethargy, headache, convulsions, and delirium. Vertigo, ataxia, facial nerve palsy, and optic atrophy also have been reported (621,622). Sequelae are relatively common. They were seen in 25% of survivors in the Finnish series of Koskiniemi and coworkers (623) and were most common when children presented with seizures or altered consciousness. Interestingly, the prognosis was worse in those patients without salivary gland swelling. Behavioral disturbances and persistent headache are the most common sequelae. Other residua include ataxia, extrapyramidal disorders, optic neuritis and atrophy, facial palsy, impairment of extraocular muscles, neurogenic deafness, and a seizure disorder (624,625). Hydrocephalus related to ependymal changes in the aqueduct of Sylvius is a rare sequela (625).

Facial nerve paralysis can be caused by swollen parotid gland compression of the nerve or by cranial neuritis. Labyrinthine and vestibular nerve involvement can result in neurogenic vertigo. Transverse myelitis can occur. In rare instances, there is chronic progressive encephalitis (626).

Mumps infection also can result in muscle weakness, which is most marked in the neck flexors and becomes evident at the end of the acute phase. Muscle weakness can persist for as long as 5 months.

The CSF usually shows an early granulocytic pleocytosis that soon has a lymphocytic predominance and an elevated protein count. Hypoglycorrhachia is present in approximately 10% of cases (622,623,627). Serum amylase is elevated in patients with clinical as well as many with subclinical parotitis. After mumps meningitis, CSF pleocytosis may persist for months, and mumps virus-specific oligoclonal IgG can persist for more than a year (628). Rapid direct diagnosis of mumps meningitis is possible by demonstration of mumps virus antigen in CSF (629).

MRI is more reliable than CT in confirming involvement of the brain parenchyma in mumps encephalitis (630). The reactions to measles, mumps, and rubella immunization are described in Chapter 8.

Herpes Simplex

Herpes simplex viruses are widespread organisms that commonly infect humans. They produce a protean picture that only rarely results in neurologic manifestations. Prenatal herpes infection is referred to in the Congenital Infections section in this chapter.

Etiology

Herpes simplex viruses are members of the herpesvirus family, whose genomes consist of a single double-stranded DNA molecule. They occur in two distinct serotypes, which are distinguishable by serologic and cultural means (631,632). Individual strains can be characterized by restrictive endonucleases, so epidemiologic studies can identify sources of contact. Type 1 virus, generally associated with orofacial herpes infections, is identified in most cases of herpes simplex encephalitis in patients 6 months of age or older. Type 2 virus is identified in genital herpes and causes most of the congenital or perinatally acquired infections (633).

Pathology

Experimental virus invasion of the nervous system has been demonstrated after intranasal inoculation. The virus spreads by infection of mucosal and submucosal cells, ultimately crossing the cribriform plate, or by infection of endoneural and perineural cells of the olfactory fibers to involve the parenchymal cells of the olfactory bulb (634). The first neurons to be infected are usually constituents of the peripheral nervous system. Viral infection then spreads by continuity to other neurons through synaptic contact. Neuronal apoptosis accounts for acute CNS injury (635,636). For an extensive review of the biology of the herpes viruses in infections of the nervous system, see the review by Enquist and coauthors (637).

CNS infection by herpes simplex virus shows the usual microscopic picture of viral encephalitis: lymphocytic infiltration of the meninges, perivascular aggregates of lymphocytes and histiocytes in the cortex and subjacent white matter, and proliferation of microglia with formation of glial nodules.

Several pathologic features are distinctive, however. One feature is the severity of the process. Necrosis is unusually severe in the areas of greatest involvement, with gross softening, destruction of architecture, hemorrhage, and, in severe cases, loss of all nervous and glial elements. Another feature is the topography of lesions. Lesions are generally widespread, with many foci of hemorrhage and necrosis, but the mediotemporal and orbital regions are the most severely damaged. A final feature is inclusion bodies. Intranuclear Cowdry type A inclusion bodies are recognized in neurons, oligodendroglia, and astrocytes (638).

Persistence of herpesvirus type 1 in trigeminal ganglia (639) and type 2 in sacral ganglia (640) leads to recurrent cutaneous or mucosal infections by means of axonal spread. Latent herpes virus type 1 infection of the trigeminal ganglia occurs in 18% of individuals from newborn to 20 years of age (641).

Clinical Manifestations

Encephalitis can occur as part of a systemic herpes infection or as an isolated phenomenon. It can develop from a primary infection or from reactivation of a preexisting infection (642). Encephalitis also has developed after long-term corticosteroid therapy and experimentally after injection of epinephrine or induction of anaphylactic shock (643).

Cases of neonatal herpes meningoencephalitis caused by type 2 infection generally are associated with disseminated herpes infection. When the infection is contracted during the perinatal period, an event usually associated with primary infection of the mother, symptoms can begin as early as the first few days of life (644).

In another group of type 2 infections, infants become symptomatic at 4 months of age or later in association with serologic evidence of probable reinfection or reactivation. When first seen, these infants' IgG antibody to herpes simplex virus is already elevated, suggesting maternal transfer of considerable antibody or a prior infection.

Specific IgM and IgG responses occur in serum and CSF during the acute disease. Localization of the type 2 infection tends to be frontoparietal rather than temporal, as occurs in type 1 infection. The association of type 2 virus with diffuse meningoencephalitis rather than with a hemorrhagic or necrotizing focal disease can reflect in part its greater incidence in young infants (645).

The incidence of CNS involvement in herpes simplex infections is uncertain, but the virus probably accounts for approximately 10% of all viral infections of the CNS, and herpes simplex virus is the most common cause of sporadic, fatal meningoencephalitis in the United States. Of all herpes cases, 31% occur in patients younger than 20 years of age and 12% occur in patients between 6 months and 10 years of age (646). In general, the incidence of herpes is lowest between the ages of 5 and 15 years (647). Herpes encephalitis has no clear seasonal incidence (646).

Prodromal symptoms unrelated to CNS disease occur in approximately 60% of patients. Fever and malaise are most common; symptoms of respiratory infection are present in one-third of patients. This prodromal period usually lasts 1 to 7 days.

Neurologic involvement includes aseptic meningitis and a diffuse or focal encephalitis (647). Aseptic meningitis is relatively benign and is encountered in approximately 20% of cases. Patients experience an acute febrile illness with headache and stiff neck, occasionally with orchitis or pneumonitis, and recover uneventfully in 4 to 7 days. CSF pleocytosis is common, ranging from 300 to 1,000 cells with a protein concentration from 50 to approximately 200 mg/dL. In 12% of cases, the initial CSF examination is normal (648). Though the condition is asymptomatic, CSF changes can persist for months.

More often, herpes is associated with encephalitis. The clinical findings are of two kinds: nonspecific changes of encephalitis, including fever, papilledema, meningeal irritation, and global confusion; and changes referable to focal necrosis, usually of the orbital or temporal regions of the brain, including anosmia, memory loss, disordered behavior, and olfactory or gustatory hallucinations (638). Only 22% of patients have a history of recurrent herpes simplex lesions (646).

Focal symptoms and neurologic findings are not unusual. They include focal seizures, seen in 28% of patients, and hemiparesis, seen in 33%. In the series of Whitley and associates, ataxia was seen in 40% of patients, cranial nerve deficits in 32%, papilledema in 14%, and visual field loss in 14% (646).

Initial signs of herpes encephalitis are frequently referable to the CNS. The most common early symptoms are alterations in consciousness (97%), fever (90%), headache (81%), personality change (71%), generalized, but often partial, motor seizures (67%), vomiting (46%), and hemiparesis (33%). The most common neurologic findings include changes in personality (85%), dysphasia (76%), autonomic dysfunction (60%), ataxia (40%), hemiparesis (38%), seizures (38%, of which 74% are focal, 26% generalized, and 13% mixed), cranial nerve defects (32%), papilledema (14%), and visual field loss (14%). Essentially similar histories and neurologic findings were obtained from a group of patients who did not have biopsy evidence of herpes simplex encephalitis, and no signs are pathognomonic for herpes simplex encephalitis (646).

Herpes simplex encephalitis can occasionally present as apyrexial, with focal seizures and normal neuroimaging studies. Less commonly, it can present as an opercular syndrome with anarthria and impairment of mastication and swallowing. This is caused by focal, bilateral cortical involvement of the anterior opercular regions (649). In other cases, expressive aphasia or paresthesias precede the more severe CNS signs.

The mortality from herpes simplex encephalitis is considerable, and approximately one-half of the survivors aged 5 to 11 years have major residual deficits (642). These include severe disturbances in mental function, either diffuse cerebral damage or isolated damage to memory or speech areas. Selective cognitive deficits, mental retardation, personality changes, incoordination, hyperkinetic movement disorders, seizures, or hemiparesis also can persist (650).

Diagnosis

The clinical picture of herpes encephalitis or herpes aseptic meningitis can be indistinguishable from that produced by other viral organisms. However, localizing signs, mostly focal seizures and paralyses, are found in approximately three-fourths of patients. When present, focal temporal lobe or limbic symptoms suggest the diagnosis, as can the presence of a bloody or xanthochromic CSF. A history of preceding herpetic infection or the presence of mucocutaneous herpes is present in fewer than 50% of patients. In neonates, the differential diagnosis is principally between group B streptococcal meningitis and enteroviral meningoencephalitis.

The CSF can be normal in the first hours of encephalitis, but virtually all patients develop CSF abnormalities. The CSF is under increased pressure and shows pleocytosis. In 92% of cases, the cell count is less than 500 cells/μL, in 22% of cases there are fewer than 50 cells/μL. The CSF protein elevation can persist for months. In other cases, a hemorrhagic encephalitis produces a xanthochromic or bloody CSF, usually with fewer than 500 red cells/μL. Infants younger than 1 month of age tend to have a mild hypoglycorrhachia (651).

The EEG is of considerable diagnostic aid. The result is usually diffusely abnormal, although in some patients it demonstrates a focal temporal or frontal lesion or focal centrotemporal spike complexes recurring every 1 to 2 seconds against a slow-wave background (652,653). A

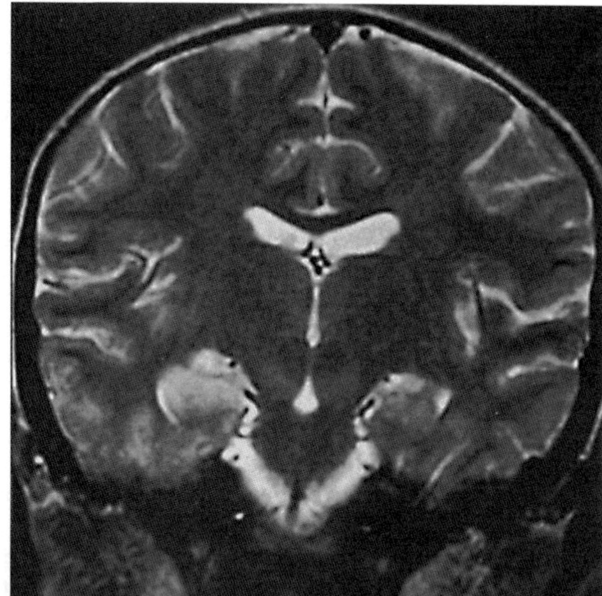

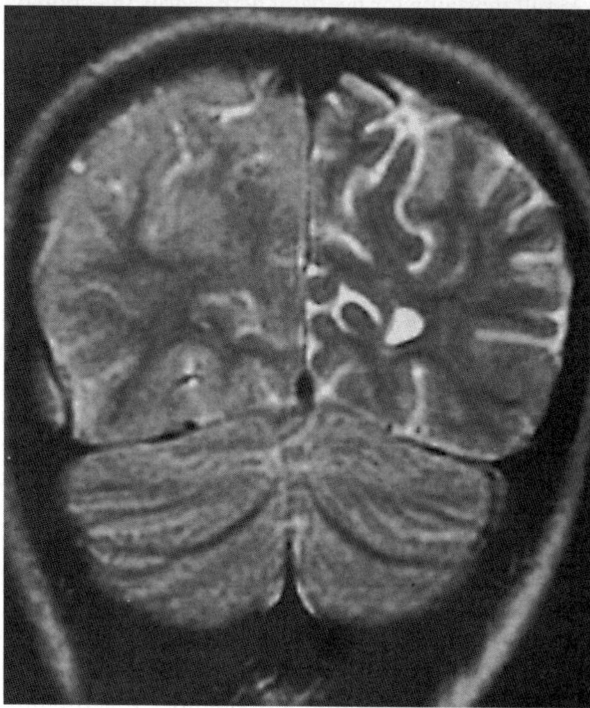

FIGURE 7.11. Herpes simplex encephalitis in an 8-year-old child. Coronal T2-weighted magnetic resonance images. **A:** Focal involvement of right hippocampus and inferior temporal region. **B:** Focal involvement of right parieto-occipital region. (Courtesy of Dr. Philip Anslow, Department of Radiology, Radcliffe Infirmary, Oxford, England.)

burst-suppression pattern is considered to be characteristic for this condition. Neuroimaging studies also are of considerable diagnostic assistance. The MRI can demonstrate unilateral or bilateral inflammation of the temporal lobe on T2-weighted images (Fig. 7.11). These abnormalities can be seen in the presence of a normal CSF (654,655). They also are noted before any detectable abnormality on CT scan, which does not become evident until days 3 to 11 of illness (655).

Rapid diagnosis of herpesvirus encephalitis can best be achieved by demonstration of viral DNA in the CSF by PCR (656,657). This test has largely replaced brain biopsy as the major diagnostic procedure. When DNA primers with sequences common to herpes simplex viruses 1 and 2 have been used, a sensitivity of greater than 95% and a specificity of 100% have been reported in patients with brain biopsy–proven herpes simplex encephalitis (658). Viral culture of CSF has a relatively high yield in neonates (30% to 50%); in older children the viral culture is positive in only 1% of the cases. No clear correlation exists between the viral load as measured from the number of infected cells in the CSF and the patient's morbidity (659). Viral DNA also can be detected in the serum in neonatal infections but not in the serum of older children (660). Serum serologic diagnosis has not been satisfactory for herpes encephalitis. Fourfold increases in titer can occur from herpes infection at other sites. A prior herpesvirus infection can cause elevations in titer that do not change significantly during neurologic involvement. However, a simultaneous serum–CSF herpes antibody titer ratio of 20 or less is diagnostic of herpes encephalitis (661). This change is usually found after the second week of illness (662). A rise in CSF or serum IgM herpes antibody correlates best with an active herpetic process (663). Some acute cases of herpes encephalitis can represent reactivation of latent infection or reinfection rather than new infection.

If the clinical picture and neurodiagnostic procedures are at all suggestive of herpes simplex encephalitis, treatment with acyclovir, as discussed later, should be instituted immediately. If the clinical picture and the neuroimaging studies are not diagnostic or if progress during treatment with acyclovir is unsatisfactory, a brain biopsy is recommended (664,665). For histologic confirmation or virus isolation, the biopsy should be obtained early in the course of the illness and must be taken from the involved area either by needle aspiration or direct surgical approach. Histopathologic changes can be missed if the biopsy is taken from the wrong site, or it can be misinterpreted because Cowdry type A inclusion bodies can be absent or can occur in other diseases such as subacute sclerosing panencephalitis. Even in proven cases, attempts at viral isolation from brain tissue can be unsuccessful. In their series published in 1982, Nahmias and coworkers correlated the histologic, serologic, and clinical findings on patients undergoing brain biopsy for suspected herpes encephalitis (666).

Of patients in their series with negative brain biopsy findings, 23% had diseases requiring other forms of therapy. Conditions that mimic focal encephalitis caused by herpes simplex include other forms of encephalitis, bacterial abscess, and tuberculosis (667). Mesenrhombоencephalitis, which can be established as caused by herpes simplex virus in approximately 30% of cases, also can be caused by agents such as Listeria monocytogenes (668). Focal EEG and CT findings during an acute episode of encephalomyelopathy caused by mitochondrial encephalopathy lactic acidosis stroke (MELAS) syndrome can lead to the erroneous presumptive diagnosis of herpes encephalitis (669).

Treatment

Untreated, the disease pursues an unremitting downhill course. Currently accepted treatment for herpes encephalitis involves acyclovir (664). Treatment should start as soon as possible after the onset of infection if permanent brain damage is to be minimized, although early therapy is not the only determinant of a satisfactory outcome. The quantity of virus produced and the extent and site of brain involvement also influence the outcome (667).

Acyclovir is given in a dose of 10 to 20 mg/kg (500 mg/m^2 of body surface area for children younger than 12 years of age) every 8 hours, in the form of a 20-mg/mL solution, administered over 1 hour for a 14- to 21-day course (670). Caution should be exercised because extravasation of the drug may cause a marked local bullous inflammatory reaction. Toxic side effects of acyclovir include renal tubular crystalluria with elevation of serum creatinine or, less commonly, an encephalopathy (671).

Strains of herpes simplex types 1 and 2 resistant to acyclovir have been isolated from patients treated with several courses of the drug (672). These resistant strains have evolved after 7 days of acyclovir therapy, and most have been isolated from immunocompromised individuals (673,674). Should acyclovir therapy fail to arrest the disease, a trial of intravenous foscarnet is recommended (674). The drug is given at a dose of 60 mg/kg every 8 hours intravenously for 14 days. PCR of the CSF should be considered at completion of therapy for encephalitis to monitor treatment response (675,676).

Generally, mortality and morbidity are less in younger patients, especially when treatment is initiated early in the course of the disease and before consciousness deteriorates (677). Approximately one-half of patients recover completely. Such recovery occurs more often when therapy is instituted before the onset of stupor. When encephalitis is accompanied by seizures and coma, the outcome is generally poor. Only 10% of patients in whom therapy is delayed to that stage recover (678). These results stress the need for early therapy whenever herpes simplex encephalitis is suspected. Surviving patients usually improve in 10 to 25 days. They do not experience persistent chronic encephalitis.

Some 5% to 26% of patients have relapses after a dramatic initial response to therapy, usually 1 to 3 months after treatment (667,675,679). Involuntary movement disorders such as choreoathetosis or chorea can occur 1 to 18 days after relapse (680). They are much more often associated with relapse than with the primary illness. In some instances of relapses, viral DNA can be demonstrated in CSF (681), although brain biopsy does not reveal any evidence of recrudescent infection or demyelination (667).

In neonatal herpes simplex encephalitis, the outcome generally depends on the type of virus responsible. Neonates have a low risk of herpes simplex virus infection if virus exposure occurs at the time of delivery to mothers with recurrent genital herpes simplex virus infection. This is because of placental transfer of maternal-specific neutralizing antibody. The risk is much greater if the mother has acute genital herpes and lacks neutralizing antibody at the time of delivery (681). In the experience of Corey and coworkers, all infants with type 1 virus had normal results on follow-up during the second year of life, compared with 28% of infants surviving type 2 herpesvirus infection (682). Even infants treated promptly for type 2 herpes have a poor outcome. In the various reported series the overall mortality for neonatal herpesvirus infection of the CNS ranges between 15% and 27% (683,684). Malm and associates found that, of the survivors, 48% were healthy, whereas 39% had severe disabilities such as severe mental retardation and quadriparesis (684). Of children surviving with severe or mild neurologic impairment, 94% had ophthalmologic abnormalities (684).

Influenza Virus

Influenza viruses are classified as orthomyxoviruses. They are RNA viruses of three major antigenic types: A, B, and C. Influenza viruses are responsible for an acute respiratory infection of worldwide distribution, but can attack any portion of the neuromuscular system.

Encephalomyelitis can be attended by changes in consciousness, opisthotonos, ataxia, or a transverse myelopathy. In etiologic studies of encephalitis or encephalopathy, influenza A and/or B have been identified in up to 10% of pediatric cases (685). Seizures are not infrequent, although in some cases they represent activation of a preexisting epileptic focus. Although neurovirulent influenza A virus demonstrates a predilection for the substantia nigra in experimental animals, no clear association with postencephalitic parkinsonism has been demonstrated (686). Two forms of influenza virus–induced acute infectious polyneuritis have been recognized. In the first, seen only in children, the course is mild and lasts 2 to 10 days. Weakness usually is limited to the lower extremities. The second form resembles classic Guillain-Barré syndrome (see Chapter 8).

Myositis caused by one of several strains of influenza viruses and involving primarily the gastrocnemius and soleus muscles also has been encountered. Symptoms appear as the respiratory phase of the illness wanes. They include muscle pain and tenderness that is exaggerated by bedrest. Symptoms last from a few days to several weeks.

An elevation of serum creatine phosphokinase levels is often noted (687,688).

The CSF in influenza meningoencephalitis can be normal or can reveal a mild pleocytosis. Mild pleocytosis has been noted also in patients with the respiratory form of influenza who lack overt CNS symptoms. Virus isolation has been successful only rarely (689).

MRI during acute influenza A encephalitis reveals multifocal areas of involvement in the cortex and subcortical white matter that can persist for long periods (688). Pontine lesions also may occur (689). Diffusion-weighted imaging may demonstrate lesions more clearly than conventional MRI (685). The clinical outcome is related to degree of CNS injury and neuronal apoptosis (690,691). The involved areas have decreased blood flow by SPECT. This is in distinction from the increased blood flow usually noted in the focal lesions of acute herpes simplex encephalitis (688). Symmetric hypodense lesions within the thalami and pons can be the major findings on CT (689).

Parainfluenza virus type 3 can cause encephalitis with periodic breathing, opsoclonus-myoclonus, or a clinical picture resembling herpes simplex encephalitis. These patients have recovered without neurologic residue (692,693). Parainfluenza virus type 4 can cause aseptic meningitis in children (694).

Varicella-Zoster Virus

Varicella-zoster virus (VZV) reaches the CNS through the bloodstream or by direct spread from sensory ganglia where it is harbored latently.

The virus causes two diseases: varicella (chickenpox) and herpes zoster (shingles). Varicella is the manifestation of the primary VZV infection, whereas herpes zoster, more commonly seen in adults, is the result of the reactivation of a VZV infection. Both may lead to neurologic infection and disease. VZV can lead to neurologic disease through direct viral invasion (infectious) or by the development of a specific immune response (postinfectious). The occurrence of neurologic symptoms in some chickenpox-infected children before the onset of the rash points to the former type of disease mechanism (695). In addition, some of the symptoms are the result of a vasculopathy that involves large and small cerebral vessels (696–701).

Herpes Zoster

The neurologic complications of varicella are rare (702). Clinical, epidemiologic, and virologic evidence has established that herpes zoster results from varicella virus that is localized to cranial sensory and dorsal root ganglia and their connections and to the skin area corresponding to the distribution of the involved sensory nerves (699). It is believed that the initial varicella exposure results in viral invasion of neuronal and glial tissue, and any subsequent reversion to generalized infection is suppressed by persistent immunity. During latency, the viral genomes are found in nonneuronal cells, only spreading to neuronal cells on reactivation of the virus (700). Gradual attenuation of the resistance, or immune suppression as a consequence of intrinsic or extrinsic factors, can lower cellular immunity to a level that permits the virus to activate. The observation that immune individuals show immunologic evidence of reinfection with VZV indicates that herpes zoster also can become symptomatic through reacquisition of virus (701). Serologic and viral studies do not distinguish between varicella virus and herpes zoster, although zoster patients carry a higher immune titer for varicella. Zoster vesicle fluid can produce typical varicella lesions in susceptible children, and in children with leukemia, live attenuated varicella vaccine can cause herpes zoster in immunized children (703).

Pathology

Pathologic changes in herpes zoster are usually limited to one dorsal root or sensory ganglion and the corresponding nerve (704). Infiltration with lymphocytes, plasma cells, and polymorphonuclear cells occurs around a central area of congestion and hemorrhage caused by intense inflammation and hemorrhagic necrosis. Nerve cells in the area demonstrate degeneration and neuronophagia. Involvement often extends to the spinal cord, where microglial cells abound in the dorsal horns, in Clarke's column, and in the lateral and ventral horns. Anterior horn cells can show chromatolysis and neuronophagy. Similar involvement in the brainstem accompanies infection of the trigeminal or glossopharyngeal nerves.

Pathologic lesions in varicella-zoster encephalomyelitis include focal areas of necrosis and perivascular demyelination. These are mainly seen in cortex and peripheral white matter. Gliosis and astrocytic proliferation also are present. Cowdry type A inclusion bodies with VZV particles are most abundant in oligodendroglia near the focus of necrosis, but can be found in ganglial cells, damaged nerve roots, vasa nervorum, peripheral nerve endoneurium, perineurium, and epineurium, and Schwann cells of peripheral nerves (705). In trigeminal herpes zoster, tissue damage in the brainstem can extend to the spinal and principal nucleus of the trigeminal nerve and mildly disseminate to the bulbo-ponto-mesencephalic region. The mesencephalic trigeminal nucleus is spared. Myositis with demonstrable VZV in the masseter muscle can complicate trigeminal herpes zoster (706).

Clinical Manifestations

The incidence of herpes zoster increases steadily with increasing age. The condition occurs in approximately 0.74 in 1,000 children up to 9 years of age, 1.38 in 1,000 children 10 to 19 years of age, and approximately 2.5 in 1,000 individuals through age 49 years (707). Neonatal cases have been described. Generally, children older than age 2 years who develop herpes zoster have had a previous attack of varicella; those younger than 2 years of age might have been exposed during gestation or infancy without clinical disease. Incidence of second attacks is 3 to 5 per 1,000 (707). Rarely, children develop segmental symptoms of herpes zoster during an attack of varicella.

Essential to the diagnosis of herpes zoster are grouped vesicular lesions distributed over one or more dermatomes. Systemic reactions, usually fever, nuchal rigidity, headache, and enlargement of the regional lymph nodes, are common in children. In 89% of patients younger than age 12 years, the lesion is localized to the thoracolumbar area (Fig. 7.12). Cervical herpes is seen in 8% and maxillary lesions in 3% of children. Ophthalmic herpes and geniculate herpes are extremely rare.

The skin lesions first appear as erythematous papules that progress to vesicles in 12 to 24 hours and to pustules in 72 hours. Lesions often appear in the proximal area of the dermatome and spread peripherally. When pustulation appears, the surrounding erythema begins to subside, and in 7 to 8 days pustules begin to dry up. Crusts form in 10 to 12 days and fall off in 2 or 3 weeks. Unilateral involvement is the rule, with bilateral involvement occurring in only 0.5% of cases.

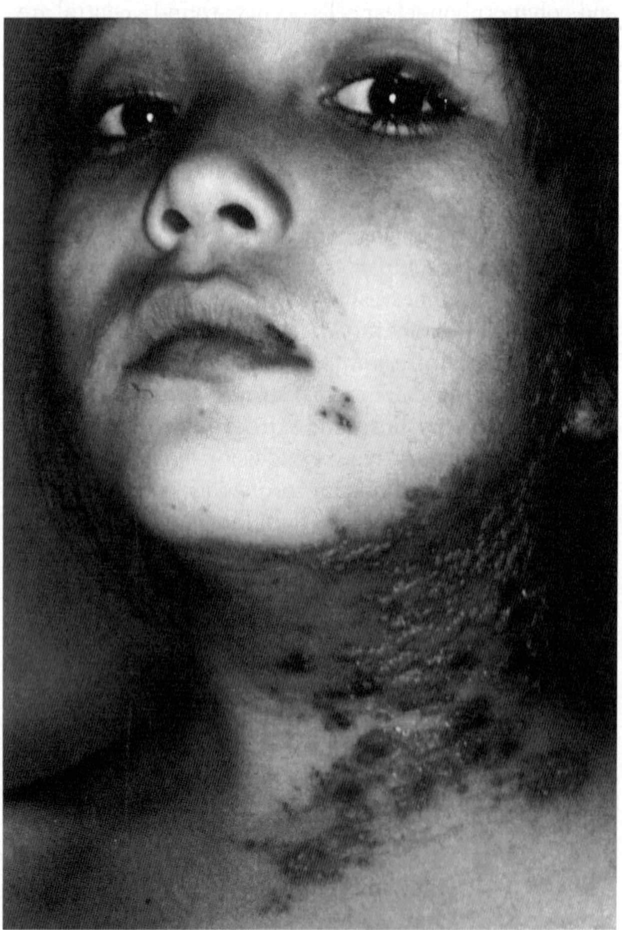

FIGURE 7.12. Herpes zoster showing the skin eruption over the third and fourth cervical dermatomes.

Pain, noted by approximately two-thirds of children, can be a prodrome, can occur during the acute infection, or can develop after the skin inflammation has subsided. The pain is evanescent in some and persistent in others; it bears no relationship to the severity of cutaneous lesions. Patients describe it as pruritic, aching, stabbing, or burning.

The most common adult complication of herpes zoster, postherpetic neuralgia, is unusual in children (708). Although in the series of Kost and Straus, 18% of patients younger than 19 years of age developed postherpetic neuralgia, the pain lasted less than 1 month in almost all of them and lasted longer than 1 year in only 4% (709). Sensory deficits and tactile allodynia coexist in the involved dermatomes.

There has been considerable interest in the cause of the persistent pain. The observation that the number of nerve endings in unilateral postherpetic neuralgia is reduced in both the ipsilateral and contralateral dermatomes suggests a central process (710). Kost and Straus postulated that after their injury peripheral nerves discharge spontaneously and have lower activation thresholds and an exaggerated response to stimuli (709). In addition, axonal regrowth after injury produces nerve sprouts that are prone to unprovoked discharges. The increased peripheral activity leads to hyperexcitability of the dorsal horns and an exaggerated central response to all input (711). The pain of postherpetic neuralgia can be intractable to treatment (712).

Localized paralysis and atrophy of muscles after an attack of herpes zoster are not unusual and in some instances are permanent. Ascending myelitis and diffuse encephalomyelitis have been reported also (713).

Hemiparesis, ipsilateral to ophthalmic herpes zoster, can occur after a delay of several weeks to 6 months. It usually involves a territory of the middle cerebral artery. VZV antigen has been demonstrated in the media of the middle cerebral artery ipsilateral to the site of the infection and contralateral to the hemiparesis (714,715). Hemiparesis also can develop some 3 weeks to 2 months after primary chickenpox. The vascular lesions are usually in the basal ganglia, internal capsule, or both, with occasional involvement of the cortex. Children usually recover without recurrences (716,717).

Disseminated herpes zoster occurs in 2% to 5% of cases. Widespread lesions involving the skin, mucous membranes, and lungs and a clinical syndrome with many characteristics of varicella can develop in 2 to 12 days, usually by 6 days after the onset of herpes zoster (718). Viremia has been documented just before dissemination of dermal lesions. The more severe cases of disseminated herpes zoster correlate positively with prolonged viremia (719).

Neurologic complications of herpes zoster can occur when the rash is present or months thereafter and are more common in immunocompromised hosts. They include encephalitis, leukoencephalitis, herpes zoster ophthalmicus with delayed contralateral hemiparesis, myelitis, and cranial and peripheral nerve palsies (557,702,720). The most common neurologic complication is postherpetic neuralgia, which fortunately is rare in children.

Herpes zoster encephalitis is diffuse and can occur from the start of the appearance of the rash to up to 1 year later. It is seen more frequently in immunocompromised hosts. The clinical symptoms are acute or subacute delirium with few or no focal findings. The presence of viral particles and the rapid clinical improvement when acyclovir is administered speak of the likely infectious pathogenesis.

Patients with acquired immunodeficiency syndrome (AIDS) and with other immunodeficiencies have been found to develop other VZV-induced neurologic disorders such as multifocal leukoencephalitis, ventriculitis, myelitis, and focal brainstem lesions (721,722). Because patients with AIDS have to be severely immunosuppressed to develop these entities, they have been reported mainly in adults. With the development of effective therapies and prolongation of life for pediatric HIV infections, these entities will probably begin to surface in the pediatric population.

An acute aseptic meningitis syndrome (723), acute polyneuritis, myelitis, and encephalitis (724) also have been described in serologically proven varicella-zoster infection, in some instances without demonstrable skin lesions (725,726).

The appearance of herpes zoster lesions in preadolescent children can be the first manifestation of HIV infection acquired in the neonatal period (727). Once established, this exacerbation of infection elicits an anamnestic immune response too late to abort the process (698).

The association of herpes zoster with leukemia and Hodgkin disease has been well documented. Treatment of the underlying malignancy with corticosteroids, antimetabolites, and alkylating agents does not appear to have an adverse effect on the course of herpes (728).

Herpes zoster of the geniculate ganglion is a rare cause of facial nerve palsy in the pediatric population. In some instances, herpetic lesions are seen on the tympanic membrane and in the auricular sensory distribution of the facial nerve (729). VZV DNA can be demonstrated by PCR in the auricular lesions (730). The diagnosis can best be made by gadolinium-enhanced MRI of the facial nerve. This demonstrates discrete or, in the more severe cases, diffuse enhancement of the facial and vestibulocochlear nerves in the internal auditory canal and labyrinth (731). Early treatment with acyclovir and prednisone has been recommended (732).

Diagnosis

VZV infections can cause CNS disease with or without the presence of characteristic skin eruptions. When present, the clinical characteristics of the skin rash in children with chickenpox and herpes zoster are cardinal in the diagnosis of these clinical entities (see Fig. 7.12). In the differential diagnosis of facial palsy, herpetic lesions of the tympanic membrane and external auditory canal should be sought. The isolation of VZV from skin lesions and the detection of specific antigens within epithelial cells by the use of fluorescent monoclonal antibodies by direct fluorescent antibody testing provide confirmation of the etiologic diagnosis. The direct fluorescent antibody monoclonal test is much more sensitive than Tzank smear in the diagnosis of VZV infections.

In the CSF, a mild pleocytosis occurs with mononuclear predominance and a protein elevation; hypoglycorrhachia can occur (138). IgG and IgA varicella-zoster antibodies are found in CSF when neurologic complications are present (723,733). Early diagnosis can be established by the detection of virus-specific DNA sequences in the CSF (734–736). Viral isolation in cell culture is considered the gold standard but is difficult to perform and usually too slow to be of diagnostic assistance.

Treatment

As a rule, antiviral treatment of children with uncomplicated chickenpox or shingles and normal immune status is not warranted. However, secondary skin lesions should be prevented. Oral acyclovir for 7 days reduces the duration of the acute phase of herpes zoster; a further 14 days of therapy is of only slight additional benefit (737). Maximum benefit is obtained when acyclovir is started within the first 24 hours of the disease, and treatment is ineffective if delayed beyond 72 hours after the onset of the illness (738). Acyclovir-resistant zoster myelitis has responded to famciclovir (739). The concurrent use of a short course of prednisolone can accelerate healing and reduce the severity of pain in herpes zoster during the first 2 weeks of therapy, but is associated with an increased incidence of adverse reactions. Neither drug seems to influence the incidence or severity of postherpetic neuralgia (737,738).

Treatment with intravenous acyclovir (500 mg/m^2 every 8 hours for a minimum of 7 days) is reserved for children with a normal immune status who develop CNS manifestations of varicella before the appearance of the rash or who develop severe encephalitis within the first week of the rash. Treatment also is indicated for children who develop shingles with neurologic or ophthalmologic complications and for immunocompromised children who develop either chickenpox or herpes zoster. Controlled studies have shown that intravenous acyclovir reduces the risk for cutaneous and visceral dissemination of VZV in immunocompromised hosts (740) and that it improves the clinical outcome of neurologic complications (741).

Little experience has accrued in the management of prolonged herpetic pain in the pediatric population. In adults, persistent pain has been treated with topical lidocaine preparations. Amitriptyline or desipramine give moderate to complete relief in approximately one-half of patients. Carbamazepine and gabapentin also have been recommended (710,742) as well as ketamine and a variety of antiviral agents, including acyclovir, famciclovir, and valacyclovir (710).

Rabies

Rabies is an acute infection of the nervous system caused by an RNA virus with a predilection for exocrine glands, kidneys, and the nervous system. The virus is present in the saliva of infected mammals and is transmitted by bite. The disease was well described by Greek and Roman clinicians. Pasteur's study of the disease led to his 1885 development of a modified virus vaccine, which is still the basis for immunization (743).

Etiology and Pathology

At least six antigenically distinct strains of rabies virus affect animals in the United States (744). Of these, four affect humans (745). Worldwide, the dog is the principal vector of human infection. The virus carried in saliva is transmitted when the dog bites or causes a skin abrasion. Of the 18 cases of rabies reported in the United States between 1980 and 1993, only 8 were acquired in the United States. Virus isolates suggest that 6 of these were acquired from the reservoir in bats, 1 from the reservoir in dogs, and 1 from the reservoir in skunks (744). A number of other mammals have been found to be responsible for human infections (744,746). The disease also has been contracted by indirect exposure, probably by inhalation of virus particles in a bat-infested cave or after corneal transplants. In one series, no history of animal bite was obtained in 39% of cases (747). A heavy inoculum accompanying considerable tissue damage, such as occurs with a wolf bite, is much more likely to cause fatality than a lesser bite. Bites around the face and neck are the most dangerous; a fatal clinical illness is 10 times more likely after a face bite than a bite on the upper extremity and 28 times more likely after a face bite than a bite on a lower extremity (748).

The virus enters the nervous system through the nicotinic acetylcholine receptor of the neuromuscular junction (744,749) and reaches the CNS along peripheral nerves (750). The essential pathology of rabies is that of a generalized encephalomyelitis. When the bite occurs on the extremities, the corresponding posterior horn of the spinal cord shows hyperemia, neuronophagia, and cellular infiltrations. Intracytoplasmic eosinophilic inclusions (Negri bodies) (Fig. 7.13), demonstrated in the neurons in most cases, consist of many aggregated viral particles and are pathognomonic for the disease (751). Negri bodies are most numerous in the forebrain, and their formation is likely influenced by factors that vary in different neuronal cell types (752). Usually, they abound in the pyramidal layer of the hippocampus, but they are common also in the cerebral cortex and the cerebellar Purkinje cells. These inclusions are seen after infection only with street or "wild" virus, not with fixed or adapted virus. Another eosinophilic cytoplasmic body, the lyssa body, is seen not only in rabies, but also in a variety of other degenerative conditions not related to virus infection. Van Gehuchten and Nelis lesions, in which ganglion cells are pushed further and further apart because of dense proliferation of capsular cells, occur in the cranial nerve and spinal ganglia.

Centrifugal spread of the virus from the CNS occurs and results in infection of acinar cells in the salivary and submaxillary glands with secretion of virus in the saliva. Spread of virus to muscles of the head and neck and to the cornea make these sites useful for diagnosis by biopsy of the nape of the neck or by corneal smear.

Microscopic lesions are distributed differently in the two clinical types of disease. In the classic form after a dog bite and characterized clinically by restlessness and dysphagia, the chief lesions are in the brainstem, notably in the jugular, gasserian, and dorsal root ganglia, and in the lower two-thirds of the medulla. Infiltrations can be seen also in the substantia nigra, hypothalamic nuclei, peripheral nerves, spinal cord, and cerebral and cerebellar hemispheres.

The paralytic form after bat bites results in congestion of the cord and a striking softening of the lower cord. Neuronal degeneration is marked in both anterior and posterior horns and extends up into the medulla. Microglial infiltration is marked, but Negri bodies are often sparse or absent. Paralytic rabies appears to correlate with absence of significant immune response to the infection (753).

Clinical Manifestations

The highest incidence of rabies in humans occurs in children younger than age 15 years. The incubation period usually ranges from 1 to 3 months, but it can be as short as 4 days (746) or as long as 4 years (754).

Rabies infection has three phases: the initial phase, the excitement phase, and the paralytic phase. Once symptoms develop, progression to death is usually relentless over the course of 7 to 14 days (744). The initial or premonitory phase, lasting 2 to 4 days, is characterized by fever, headache, anorexia, malaise, and sore throat. Gastrointestinal and upper respiratory symptoms and subtle changes in mental status can occur (755). The body temperature can be mildly elevated, but it is seldom higher than 102°F. The most striking symptom during this

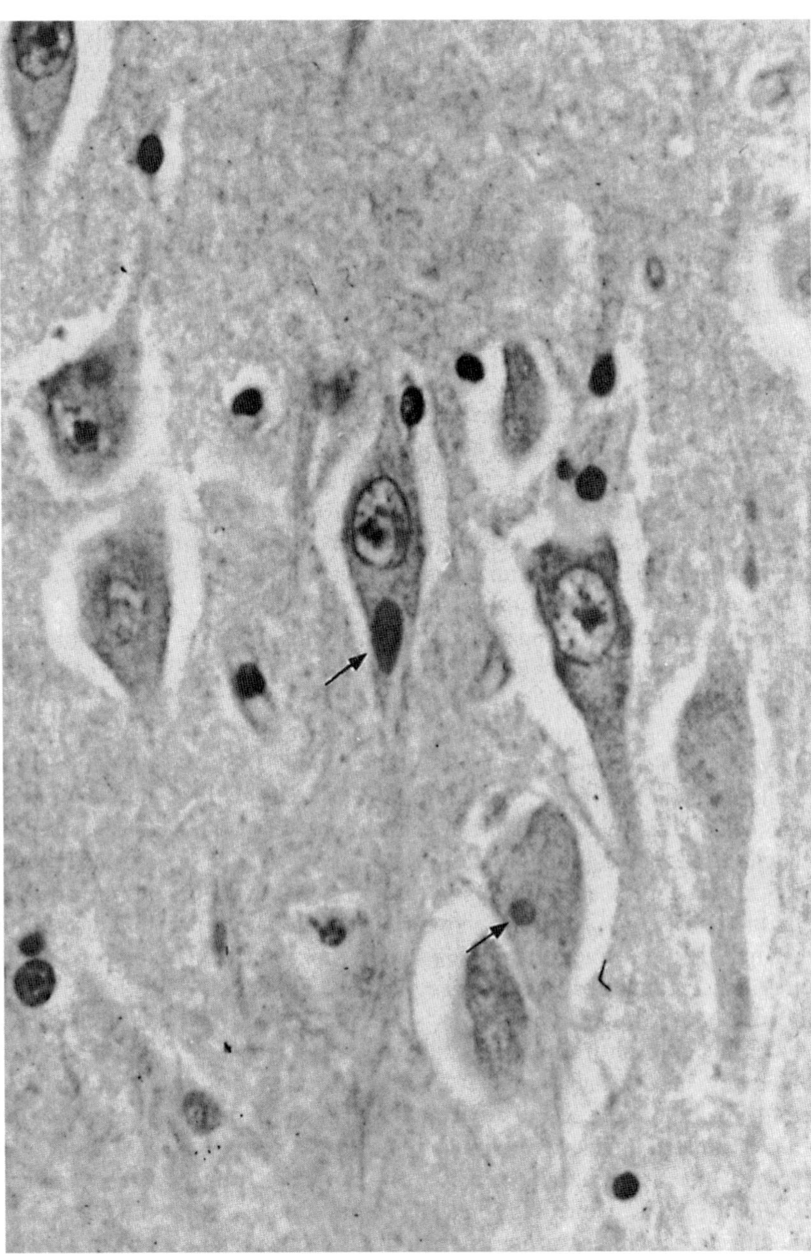

FIGURE 7.13. Rabies. Photomicrograph showing Negri bodies (*arrows*) in neuronal cytoplasm of the dorsal cell band of the hippocampus (original magnification ×160). (Courtesy of Dr. Hideo H. Itabashi, Departments of Pathology and Neurology, Los Angeles County Harbor Medical Center, Torrance, CA.)

period is numbness or paresthesia in the region of the bite. Numbness occurs in approximately 80% of cases and has been ascribed to the direct action of the virus on sensory neurons. Decreased sensitivity to local pain can be demonstrated, yet, paradoxically, patients complain of drafts and bedclothes that cause general stimulation of the skin.

Symptoms of the second or excitement phase usually have a gradual onset. Hyperacusis and photophobia can occur. Signs include hyperactive deep tendon reflexes, increased muscle tone, and tics. Facial expression becomes overactive. Signs referable to the autonomic system can be prominent; they include pupillary dilatation, lacrimation, excessive salivation, priapism, and increased perspiration. SIADH and diabetes insipidus have been reported, but the secretion of anterior pituitary hormones does not seem to be affected (756). A combination of hypoxia, hypocapnia, and respiratory alkalosis early in the disease gradually changes to hypoventilation and increasing periods of respiratory arrest (756).

As the excitement phase progresses, the patient becomes increasingly nervous, sleepless, anxious, and apprehensive. The outstanding clinical sign of rabies is related to the act of swallowing. When fluid comes in contact with the fauces, it is expelled with considerable violence. The patient experiences painful spasmodic contractions of the muscles of deglutition and of the accessory muscles of respiration. Subsequently, the sight, smell, or sound of liquids can precipitate spasm. Drooling of bloody saliva can be prominent at this time (757). Choking from attempts at swallowing can result in such severe spasm of the respiratory muscles that prolonged apnea develops with cyanosis and anoxia. The term *hydrophobia* was derived from this phenomenon.

Convulsions are common, as is maniacal behavior, such as tearing of clothes and bedding. Periods of intense excitement are interspersed with relative quiet, during which the patient is oriented and responds intelligently.

Patients can die in the acute excitement stage in the course of a convulsion, often before the paralytic phase becomes evident. Depressive or paralytic symptoms can dominate the disease picture from its onset or can supervene at any time. Weakness of muscle groups in the vicinity of the bite can become apparent early in the disease. If the patient survives the acute excitement stage, muscle spasms often cease within 1 to 3 days and the patient becomes quiet. The patient might be able to swallow with difficulty. The face becomes expressionless; anxiety and excitement are replaced by apathy, stupor, and coma. Bowel and bladder control can be lost. For a few hours the patient can seem to improve, but this apparent remission is rapidly followed by progressive paralysis. Silent or radiculomyelitis rabies, presenting with ascending paralysis like Guillain-Barré syndrome, constitutes 20% of cases with pathologic abnormalities involving spinal cord or dorsal ganglion cells (758).

In rare instances, ascending paralysis begins in the muscles of the legs and progresses without relationship to the original site of infection. Rabies in humans caused by the bite of the vampire bat, as described in Trinidad, is uniformly of the paralytic type (759).

Death can result from heart failure as well as hypoxia. Myocarditis has been reported (760). The disease has been uniformly fatal, but several survivors have been reported after prolonged intensive care unit support.

The white blood count is increased and can range from 20,000 to 30,000 white blood cell/μL with a polymorphonuclear preponderance. Proteinuria, glycosuria, and acetonuria are frequently minimal. CSF cell count usually is within normal limits, but mononuclear pleocytosis of more than 100 cells has been encountered (747,761).

Diagnosis

The diagnosis of rabies in humans is based on the history, clinical features, and laboratory tests. The long incubation periods often make the history of a bite unreliable, and laboratory test results, including serum antibodies, can be negative for long periods of time. Fluorescent antibody tests on saliva can be equally disappointing (762). The diagnosis is confirmed by fluorescence microscopy or virus isolation using corneal smears or skin or muscle biopsies from the nape of the neck, or by examination of saliva or CSF. Serologic diagnosis of rabies is possible by serum-virus neutralization tests, indirect fluorescent antibody titration, or the complement fixation test (763). Presence of rabies antibodies in the CSF, serum, or both is indicative of rabies. Examination of the brain of the animal involved also can be helpful. MR imaging may be helpful in distinguishing radiculomyelitic rabies from acute disseminated encephalomyelitis (758).

Prevention and Treatment

Once symptoms are present, rabies progresses inexorably and is generally fatal. Only three symptomatic persons have been known to survive; all received some form of rabies vaccine (764,765). The recommended procedure for preventing the disease in the exposed child has been summarized (744,766). Immediate and thorough washing with soap and water of all bite wounds and scratches markedly reduces the likelihood of rabies (744). Among infectious diseases, rabies is unique in that the long incubation period allows the induction of active as well as passive immunity before the onset of illness. Active immunity is achieved by use of one of several types of rabies vaccines. In the United States the most widely used of these is the human diploid cell culture vaccine. This provides better protection than other types of killed-virus vaccines and causes fewer adverse reactions (766). Deltoid injection is recommended because it produces a better immune response and fewer vaccine failures than gluteal injection (767). A combination of rabies immune serum (40 IU/kg body weight for equine antirabies serum or 20 IU/kg body weight for human rabies immune globulin) and human diploid cell vaccine has proved extremely effective in preventing the disease (766). Details of the immunization regimen are given in the *Red Book* of the American Academy of Pediatrics (746).

Passive immunization by means of hyperimmune antirabies serum should be administered concurrently with the first dose of rabies vaccine unless the child has been previously vaccinated against rabies. The recommended dose is 20 IU/kg of body weight. Approximately one-half of the dose is used to infiltrate the wound; the remainder is given intramuscularly. Human rabies immune globulin should be used whenever possible, and if it is not available, purified equine globulin at a dose of 40 IU/ kg is the recommended choice. Passive antibody can inhibit the response to vaccine; therefore, the recommended dose should not be exceeded. One case of complex partial seizures immediately after treatment with human diploid cell rabies vaccine and human rabies immune globulin was reported (768). Prophylactic immunization with human diploid cell vaccine or rhesus rabies vaccine (absorbed) should be considered for persons in high-risk groups, such as veterinarians, animal handlers, certain laboratory workers, children living in areas where rabies is a constant threat, and persons traveling to areas where rabies is common (744,746).

The complications of rabies vaccination are discussed in Chapter 8.

Lymphocytic Choriomeningitis Virus

Lymphocytic choriomeningitis virus (LCMV) is an arenavirus that causes human disease ranging from a mild flulike illness to meningitis. It also is associated with a congenital viral infection. LCMV is a chronic infection of mice and hamsters. Humans become infected through the inhalation or ingestion of dust or food contaminated by the virus in urine, feces, blood, or secretions of infected animals. No human-to-human transmission has been reported.

Etiology and Pathology

LCMV is a relatively common infection, with a frequency comparable with that of mumps. The overall prevalence in North America ranges from 3.5% (769) to 4.0% (770). The prevalence of antibody in persons younger than 30 years of age is 0.3%, whereas in those older than 30 years it is 5.4% (769). Female individuals were found to be more likely to be seropositive (770). In the United States, hamsters have been described as vectors in several reports, including those of outbreaks in families.

Although transmission has been postulated to occur through inhalation or ingestion of dried mouse urine or feces, the high prevalence of the disease suggests the existence of other infectious routes. The benign nature of the illness has precluded extensive pathologic studies. Meningeal reactions can be present, but the most constant lesion is a perivascular accumulation of glial cells, lymphocytes, and fat granules (771,772).

Clinical Manifestations

Infections by the LCMV virus can result in a number of clinical forms. The disease is often inapparent. Chorioretinal scars can be an isolated manifestation of LCMV (773). In other cases, a flulike picture develops after an incubation period of 1 to 3 weeks. The course can be biphasic, or symptoms of meningitis or meningoencephalomyelitis can begin abruptly without antecedent prodrome.

When evident, the initial phase can be influenza-like, with retro-orbital headache, photophobia, severe myalgia, malaise, chills, anorexia, and aching nonpleuritic chest pains. Fever ranges from 100°F to 104°F. This period lasts from 5 days to 3 weeks (774). In one reported case, parotitis with isolation of virus antedated the onset of symptoms of meningitis by 9 days (775). The initial phase can pass without signs of meningeal involvement.

Of cases with definite signs of meningeal involvement, 50% have a prodromal period as described previously. The remainder have an abrupt onset of meningeal signs similar to those seen in acute purulent meningitis (776). Moderately severe nuchal rigidity can be noted with presence of Kernig and Brudzinski signs in approximately 75% of patients. Consciousness is impaired in approximately two-thirds of cases, and patients occasionally complain of syncope, vertigo, abdominal pain, tremor, or insomnia (776). Recovery from the meningitic form of LCMV can be prompt or can take several weeks or as long as 4 months.

In a few children, encephalitic symptoms predominate. These include alterations of sensorium, seizures, hemiplegia, extrapyramidal signs, cranial nerve palsies, and cerebellar dysfunction (771). Cases simulating bulbar poliomyelitis or infectious polyneuritis also have been reported (777).

The CSF findings in LCMV are characteristic of the disease. The cell count is almost always elevated and can be as high as 6,000 cells/μL. Except for the first few days of the illness, the response is predominantly mononuclear. Cell counts and CSF protein tend to remain elevated for several weeks to months. The concentration of CSF glucose remains normal (777).

During the convalescent period, arthralgia of the hands and shoulders is common. In rare instances, arthralgia is associated with nonmigratory pain and swelling of the small joints of the fingers. Mild generalized alopecia 2 to 3 weeks after the onset of the illness and a delayed orchitis also have been described (774). Hydrocephalus caused by posterior fossa arachnoiditis, which produces headache and prolonged increased intracranial pressure, represents a more serious delayed complication of LCMV (776).

A congenital LCMV syndrome that resembles congenital toxoplasmosis has been reported. It is manifested by chorioretinitis, which was present in 88% of infants in the series of Wright and colleagues, macrocephaly, microcephaly, and intracranial calcifications, the last observed in 19% of infants (778). The disease had a 35% mortality, and 63% of survivors had severe neurologic residua. Approximately one-half of mothers experienced an illness compatible with LCMV during pregnancy.

Diagnosis

Although the clinical picture of LCMV is not characteristic, the diagnosis can be suspected from a history of exposure to rodents and the CSF findings, particularly from the persistent and marked monocytic pleocytosis. LCMV can be confirmed by virus isolation. Viremia can persist until approximately day 15 of the disease. Virus titers in CSF are lower and are present for a shorter period despite the prolonged abnormalities in cell and protein content. Pharyngeal secretions and urine also can yield the virus. Indirect fluorescent or complement fixation antibodies appear 2 to 3 weeks after the onset of the illness, reach their maximum titers 5 to 6 weeks after the onset of the illness, and decrease to low or undetectable levels in several months. Neutralizing antibodies appear later, 2 to 6 weeks after the onset of symptoms, but persist for 6 months to 5 years (769). Acute and convalescent sera can be tested for increases in antibody titers. An increase in the specific IgM in blood and CSF is diagnostic. A nested reverse transcription–PCR assay has been developed for the detection of LCMV RNA in CSF (779).

LCMV can be distinguished from bacterial infections, particularly from tuberculous meningitis, in that in the latter the CSF sugar is almost invariably depressed. Mycotic and spirochetal infections, when associated with normal CSF sugar, can be excluded by isolating the infecting organisms. In meningeal carcinomatosis, the CSF sugar is usually normal. Differential diagnosis rests on the microscopic examination of a cell block prepared from the centrifuged CSF.

Treatment

No specific treatment or vaccine is available.

Epstein-Barr Virus (Infectious Mononucleosis)

Epstein-Barr virus (EBV) is a herpesvirus responsible for infectious mononucleosis. In the United States infectious mononucleosis is seen mainly in adolescents and young adults, whereas in developing countries the primary infection with EBV occurs in the first 2 years of life. The younger the child, the more likely it is that the infection will be asymptomatic. The most common clinical findings include fevers, lymphadenopathy, pharyngitis, splenomegaly, and hepatomegaly. Rare complications include optic disc vasculitis (780). The laboratory hallmarks are a lymphocytosis with more than 10% of atypical lymphocytes, transaminitis, and neutropenia. Specific serologic diagnosis is easily made from serum.

Minor neurologic disturbances, such as headache and nuchal rigidity, are common in infectious mononucleosis, but serious neurologic complications occur in only 1% to 7% of cases (781,782). These include, in order of frequency, an aseptic, lymphocytic meningitis, polyneuritis, encephalomyelitis, and mononeuritis. Seizures, subtle corticospinal tract signs, vertical nystagmus, confusion, disorientation, or coma can occur (782). A poliomyelitis-like syndrome also has been reported (783). In some cases, neurologic symptoms are the first or the only clinical manifestations of the disease (782).

The pathogenesis of EBV-associated neurologic disease can be immune mediated, infectious, or both. Whereas some studies have found no traces of EBV in CSF or brain tissue (784), others have recovered EBV from the CSF (785).

Neurologic symptoms can occur as early as a week before the onset of systemic manifestations or they can be delayed until several weeks after recovery from systemic manifestations (644,786). The clinical features of acute EBV myeloradiculitis, encephaloradiculitis, encephalomyeloradiculitis, and subacute meningomyeloradiculitis are distinctive (787).

The presenting symptoms of lymphocytic meningitis and other aseptic meningitides are usually headache, malaise, and nuchal rigidity. Peripheral neuritis can be mild or severe. Motor and sensory functions are usually impaired, and CSF changes similar to those in acute infectious polyneuritis (Guillain-Barré syndrome) have been reported (493,788).

Presenting symptoms of encephalomyelitis involve the cerebrum, cerebellum, brainstem, or spinal cord, singly or in combination (786,789,790). Menigoencephalitis with a lymphoma-like response can occur in immunocompetent individuals (791). Generalized or myoclonic seizures or metamorphopsia "Alice in Wonderland syndrome" can be evident (792). Localized brainstem encephalitis and mononeuritis of a variety of nerves also have been reported (790). These mononeuritides include an olfactory and an optic neuritis, the latter with papillitis (793). Palsies of one or more cranial nerves have been encountered (794,795), as has that of the nerve to the serratus anterior muscle (796). An undulating course with exacerbations and remissions of encephalitic signs has been described (797). Because the manifestations of EBV infection of the nervous system can be protean, all acute neurologic diseases of undetermined origin should be screened for EBV (788).

Approximately 30% of patients with infectious mononucleosis have 5 or more cells/μL in the CSF (798). These alterations can persist for months, often after complete clinical recovery. EEG abnormalities have been noted in a large proportion of children (786,798).

The diagnosis of EBV encephalitis can be made by detecting the viral genome in CSF through PCR (799,800). EBV serology can be determined by virus-specific immunofluorescence or by a variety of spot tests (801). Patients usually recover from the neurologic sequelae within a few days to several months. In some cases, a poor correlation exists between the severity of the neurologic disorder and the clinical course, prognosis, and laboratory findings (802).

The role played by EBV in the development of nasopharyngeal carcinoma, Hodgkin disease, systemic lupus, and lymphoma in immunosuppressed patients is outside the scope of this text.

Treatment

No specific therapy or vaccine is available, and response to acyclovir therapy is variable.

Rotavirus Encephalitis

Afebrile benign convulsions can occur during the course of rotavirus gastroenteritis. CSF increases in leukocytes have been minimal (15 white blood cells/μL); protein and sugar are unchanged. Rotavirus genome and antivirus IgG in the CSF and changes in CT have been demonstrated. No sequelae have been reported (803). Rare fatal rotaviral infections have been reported in cases of diffuse endothelialitis and concomitant cardiac and CNS damage (804).

Cytomegalovirus

CMV involvement of the nervous system most often is a complication of the immunocompromised host, but it can also occur in immunocompetent young children and adolescents. CMV infections are common among young children. If the child is an immunocompetent host, CMV causes in the great majority of cases an asymptomatic infection and in a small minority a clinical picture that resembles infectious mononucleosis (805).

Neurologic complications are seen in 5% of normal hosts during CMV mononucleosis. They include encephalitis (806), acute idiopathic polyneuritis (807), Guillain-Barré syndrome (808,809), and a potential association with Rasmussen syndrome (810). Immunocompromised hosts, such as patients with AIDS and children who are receiving immunosuppressant drugs, have a much higher likelihood of developing disseminated CMV infections with neurologic compromise than immunocompetent patients. In some instances activation of a latent infection may be caused by enterovirus infection (493,811).

The diagnosis of CMV CNS infections is best made by PCR of CSF (812) or, if available, by tissue obtained at brain biopsy. The CSF reveals pleocytosis with high protein content and hypoglycorrhachia. Serologic studies have little diagnostic value in these patients.

Whereas the treatment of CMV chorioretinitis has been extensively studied and found to be efficacious, no double-blinded, placebo-controlled studies of anti-CMV therapy in patients with neurologic compromise have been reported. Treatment of adult patients with CMV neurologic disease with ganciclovir has given mixed results, ranging from lack of clinical response to clinical improvement. The most commonly used antivirotics are: ganciclovir, foscarnet, cidofovir, valganciclovir, and valaciclovir (813).

Cat-Scratch Disease

Cat-scratch disease is an infectious illness, first described by Debré in 1950 (814), and contracted by a scratch from a cat. It is characterized by fever, a primary cutaneous lesion with regional lymphadenitis, and occasional neurologic complications.

Etiology

Cat-scratch disease is a syndrome caused by members of the alpha-proteobacteria, most commonly *Bartonella henselae.* Less commonly, *Afipia felis* and *Bartonella quintana* have been implicated (815–817). These agents are small, gram-negative rods that can be visualized only with difficulty in lymph node sections (818). They have been successfully cultivated (819). *B. henselae,* although serologically cross-reactive with *A. felis,* differs from it in its genetic structure. It is responsible for the majority of cases seen in the United States (816).

Clinical Manifestations

Neurologic manifestations are encountered in approximately one-third of cases of cat-scratch fever (60). They follow the initial symptoms of the illness, usually by 1 to 5 weeks (815,820). In the series of Carithers and Margileth, encephalitis accounted for 80% of neurologic complications, whereas seizures were present in 46, and combative behavior in 40% of children. Twenty percent had cranial nerve palsies or peripheral nerve involvement. Optic neuritis was seen in 13% (821). Cerebral arteritis and a transverse myelitis also have been reported (820,822,823).

The onset of the encephalitic phase is usually precipitous, with convulsions, confusion, lethargy, stupor, and coma. Status epilepticus lasting up to several hours can occur (824). Despite the apparent severity of the picture, the patient improves rapidly and generally returns to consciousness in 2 to 10 days. Varieties of transient neurologic sequelae have been encountered, and an occasional patient has died from the encephalitis.

The CSF is usually normal. Rarely, a mild to moderate mononuclear pleocytosis occurs. The EEG is almost uniformly abnormal during the acute phase of the illness. Focal or generalized abnormalities can persist for several years, even after an apparently complete clinical recovery.

Diagnosis

A history of contact with cats, a cat scratch, or a primary dermal lesion is obtainable in 90% of cases (820). The diagnosis is suggested by positive serology against *B. henselae* or *B. quintana* or by lymph node biopsy with demonstration of necrotizing granulomatous lymphadenitis and visualization of *B. henselae* organisms. False-negative serologic diagnosis may occur because antigenic variability results in distinct serogroups that do not cross-react (825). The organism can be cultivated with difficulty. Eighty-eight percent of patients with suspected cat-scratch disease have serum antibodies that react with *B. henselae* antigen. This assay also can be useful for diagnosis of cat-scratch disease in the immunocompromised host (826,827). The most sensitive test available for detecting the presence of *B. henselae*

DNA sequences is the PCR. This test can be performed on sterile fluids and from tissues obtained at biopsy.

Treatment

No immunization is available. A variety of antibiotics, notably aprofloxacin and azithromycin, have been suggested but no controlled trials have been described (821). Corticosteroids may improve the encephalopathy in cat-scratch disease (828).

SLOW VIRUS INFECTIONS AND RELATED DISORDERS

Although scrapie, a chronic spongiform encephalopathy of sheep, was first described by Sigurdsson in 1954 (829), the concept that an infectious transmissible agent can modify normal gene products and continue to propagate within the host for several months to years and ultimately produce a progressive debilitative disease of the nervous system is relatively new (830). These agents, called *prions*, have been implicated in animal and human disease. Although they differ from all other conventional infectious agents, they are included in this section (831).

In humans, three forms of prion disease are manifest as transmissible, sporadic, and inherited disorders (830). Transmissible forms require B lymphocytes to become neuroinvasive (832). These include Creutzfeldt-Jakob disease (CJD), bovine spongiform encephalopathy, Gerstman-Strõussler-Scheinker syndrome, fatal familial insomnia, kuru, and iatrogenic CJD (830,833,834). New-variant CJD (nvCJD), described in Europe, is caused by the same prion strain as bovine spongiform encephalopathy (835). All entities involve the aberrant metabolism and resulting accumulation of the prion protein. The conversion of the normal cellular protein (PrP^{c}) to the abnormal disease-causing isoform (PrP^{Sc}) involves a conformational change in the protein. PrP^{c} and PrP^{Sc} are membrane-bound phosphatidylinositol sialoglycoproteins (836). The conformational change renders the protein more resistant to protease digestion and nondenaturing detergents. The mechanism whereby transmission of abnormal prion protein induces changes in normal prion protein of susceptible hosts is unknown (837). PrP^{Sc} is the source of plaques and amyloid found in the transmissible spongiform encephalopathies (832). Inherited prion diseases in humans are associated with at least 20 different mutations of the *PrP* gene. These different mutations account for the conformational changes that confer diversity to prion diseases (834). However, a few sporadic cases of CJD, and possibly a few cases of sporadic Gerstman-Strõussler-Scheinker syndrome, have no demonstrable mutation of the *PrP* gene. In scrapie, these glycosylated phosphatidylinositol prion proteins result in the production of protease-resistant filaments that differ from normal, protease-susceptible neurofilaments. In scrapie, PrP^{Sc} reaches concentrations 20 times that of PrP^{c}, which remains unchanged during scrapie. In normal animals PrP^{Sc} is distributed in the cell bodies and proximal dendrites of many neurons, with much less in the neuropil. In experimental scrapie, PrP is lost from most cell bodies, but high concentrations of PrP are found in the neuropil (838). The gene that encodes the precursor of an amyloid protein (*PrP*) involved in the pathogenesis of spongiform encephalopathies is located on the short arm of human chromosome 20. A different gene appears to control the incubation time for scrapie. The molecular basis of neurologic dysfunction is unknown, although cellular receptor-mediated responses are altered (839,840). For a more complete discussion of this rapidly evolving field, the reader is referred to reviews by Kovacs and coworkers (841) and Weisman (842).

Slowly progressive infections can also be caused by lentiviruses (e.g., AIDS, HIV), or by conventional agents. Examples of conventional agents include SSPE caused by measles virus, progressive rubella panencephalitis, progressive multifocal leukoencephalopathy (papovavirus), subacute encephalitis (herpes simplex), chronic mumps encephalitis (843), progressive bulbar palsy with epilepsy (Russian spring-summer encephalitis) (844), recurrent Japanese encephalitis virus (845), and CMV brain infection. Only slow infections that become clinically symptomatic during childhood are discussed here.

Human Immunodeficiency Virus/Acquired Immunodeficiency Syndrome

The acquired immunodeficiency syndrome (AIDS) virus (also called human immunodeficiency virus, HIV) has an affinity for the CD4 receptor, a membrane protein of T4 lymphocytes (846,847). When complexed with antibody the virus binds to Fc receptors. It also binds to galactosylceramide on brain and bowel cells and the chemokine receptors CXCR4 and CCR5 (848). Several mechanisms have been proposed to account for the effects of the virus on the CNS. These include a direct effect of the virus, the effects of viral products on neurons and other cells of the nervous system (849), macrophage expression of cytokines (847,850), and upregulation of unique monocyte subsets to induce neuronal apoptosis (851). In addition, neurologic symptoms can arise as a result of complications of an immunodeficient state or through a combination of these factors (849,852–854). Brain involvement can occur soon after infection because infected microglia have been identified in brain parenchyma as early as 7 days after transfusion with infected blood (855).

Neurologic disorders that result from primary infections of the nervous system include congenital or neonatal infections that can produce early signs of mental retardation and developmental delay (856) or produce mental deterioration of delayed onset (857,858). Metabolic changes demonstrable by MR spectroscopy can occur in newborn children of HIV-seropositive mothers (853). Postnatal infections in children or young adults result from parenteral injection of blood products or from sexual transmission or intravenous drug use.

Productive HIV-1 infection of the CNS is probably limited to macrophages, microglia, and astrocytes. High levels of plasma virus and low CD4 counts relatively early in HIV infection are associated with increased risk of neurologic disease (859). Most studies fail to localize HIV antigen to nerve cells (860,861). The HIV viral load of the nervous system is low in presymptomatic AIDS. With the onset of symptomatic HIV infection of the nervous system, the brain and spinal cord have high viral loads, which correlates with the presence of giant cell encephalitis or myelitis (861).

Inflammatory cell infiltrates, multinucleated cells, microglial nodules, white matter pallor, and calcification mainly in the vessels of the basal ganglia and deep cerebral white matter characterize the autopsy findings (860,862). Encephalitic changes are focally distributed in the brain, where in severe cases they are associated with multinucleated cell encephalitis. There is preferential involvement of the diencephalic structures, particularly the globus pallidus, but also the substantia nigra and deeper white matter, with less frequent infection of the cerebral cortex. Patients with only mild AIDS dementia have pathologic findings usually restricted to central gliosis and white matter pallor with limited inflammatory response (863,864). Brains from children have fewer HIV-1–infected macrophages, multinucleated giant cells, and microglia than brains from adults (865). Cellular changes are numerous in the globus pallidus and less so in the corpus striatum and thalamus. Infratentorial involvement is most prevalent in the ventral midbrain, especially the substantia nigra and the dentate nucleus. Lower levels of infection, often patchy, occur in the cerebral and cerebellar white matter and the pontine base. HIV-1–positive cells are usually less numerous in the cerebral cortex, medulla, and spinal cord (861,865). Although the cerebral cortex is relatively preserved in most cases, massive and diffuse destruction of the cerebral cortex with severe neuronal loss caused by HIV has been reported (866).

With primary brain involvement, oligoclonal antibody to HIV is synthesized within the blood–brain barrier. Viral particles, viral DNA, RNA, and other viral antigens can be demonstrated in CNS tissue or CSF. However, lack of correlation between the amount of viral antigen present and the extent of the lesion suggests that one or more additional factors such as cytokines or cytokine activation of nitric oxide, blood–brain barrier dysfunction, blockage of neurotrophic factors, disturbance of ion channels by viral proteins, or direct damage to neurons and glial cells play a role in the disease (867–869).

Clinical Manifestations

Maternal-to-infant transmission of HIV-1 occurs in 13% to 40% of pregnancies of infected mothers (870). Mothers who transmit infection to their offspring have higher mean concentrations of IgG_1 antibodies to a portion of the viral envelope (gp160) than nontransmitters (870). Infants born to mothers with more advanced disease before delivery have a greater risk of serious manifestations of disease or early death than those whose mothers have less advanced disease (871). In the experience of Sperling and coworkers, infants born to untreated mothers with HIV-1 infections have a 22% chance of acquiring HIV-1, whereas the risk was 7.6% for zidovudine-treated mothers (872). The rate of HIV transmission by untreated mothers to newborn infants is 25% when membranes are ruptured more than 4 hours before delivery and 14% when membranes are ruptured for less than 4 hours (873). Among infants with maternally transmitted HIV infection, approximately one-fifth have rapid progression to profound immunodeficiency, whereas the remainder have much slower progression (871). On rare occasions postnatal infection appears to have been acquired by way of breast milk (874). The incubation period is generally shorter in congenital infections than in acquired ones.

During the clinically latent period, DNA provirus is active and progressive in lymphoid tissue (875,876). After an intrauterine HIV-1 infection, neurologic signs can appear as early as 3 weeks of age. After a perinatal infection, approximately 50% of patients develop signs or symptoms by 12 months of age, 78% by 2 years of age, and 82% by 3 years of age (877). Belman and coworkers found neurologic problems in 90% of prenatally and perinatally infected infants followed for an average of 18 months (878). In a subsequent study, the same workers found that uninfected children with antibody passively transferred from infected mothers did not differ from controls in neurologic status or growth (879). Infected children who remain free from AIDS-defining illnesses for the first 2 years of life have only a slightly increased frequency of neurologic abnormalities, which, when these do develop, are often transient or mild. In the original study by Roy and coworkers, 71% of the affected children presented with progressive encephalopathy characterized by developmental delay with loss of acquisitions and cognitive decline, impaired growth, microcephaly, and corticospinal dysfunction (870). Cerebral atrophy was present in all cases, and basal ganglia calcification could be demonstrated in 29%. Cooper and coworkers (871) reported that encephalopathy represented the first AIDS-defining condition in 67% of HIV-infected children and was diagnosed in 21% of HIV-infected children by age 2 years. Encephalopathy was correlated with a high viral load in infancy and with a median survival of 14 months after the diagnosis was made.

An acute meningoencephalitis syndrome can present during acute HIV-1 infection. This syndrome must be considered in the differential diagnosis of aseptic meningitis (882). Childhood infection also can result in acute or subacute dementia, chronic aseptic meningitis, acute encephalopathy, or granulomatous angiitis involving the CNS. Pediatric HIV-1 infection frequently involves the corticospinal tract with involvement of myelin alone or both myelin and axons (877). Spinal cord involvement has been associated with vacuolar myelopathy in adults, but this is rare in children (877). Peripheral nerve involvement has been associated with distal symmetric sensorimotor neuropathy, mononeuritis multiplex, chronic inflammatory demyelinating polyradiculoneuropathy, and a polyneuritis mimicking the Guillain-Barré syndrome (493). Progressive multifocal leukoencephalopathy has been reported in HIV-infected children (883). Clinical deterioration can be acute, chronic, or characterized by intermittent decline. Intellectual deterioration is often accompanied by progressive corticospinal or corticobulbar signs, ataxia, or disturbance of tone. Microcephaly can result from involvement of the developing brain (862,884). Seizures or myoclonus are an uncommon occurrence (877).

Bale and coworkers found that on admission to a longitudinal study of HIV-positive hemophiliacs, 11% had cranial nerve dysfunction, 17% had abnormal deep tendon reflexes, 23% had abnormal strength, 25% had abnormal coordination, and 31% had abnormal tone bulk or range of motion. Fewer than than 2% demonstrated abnormal movements or had abnormalities of sensation or mental status (885). A subsequent follow-up of this group showed that there was a progressive increase in the incidence of behavior change, gait disturbance, and muscle atrophy (886). Major depression is significantly associated with neuroimaging or clinical neurologic abnormalities (877). The neurologic and developmental effects of HIV and AIDS in children and adolescents are reviewed elsewhere (888).

The EEG shows diffuse background slowing. CSF can be normal or have mild pleocytosis or an elevation in protein (862). Neuroimaging studies are relatively insensitive to the primary changes of HIV encephalitis during the early stages of the disease. In the series of DeCarli and associates, who used CT to study children with symptomatic but untreated AIDS who did not have cerebral complications from other causes, ventricular enlargement was seen in 78%, cortical atrophy in 69%, white matter attenuation in 26%, and cerebral calcification in 19% (889). All children with intracerebral calcifications were encephalopathic. CT abnormalities were present in some children during the presymptomatic stage before onset of encephalopathy. MRI demonstrates focal or multifocal areas of demyelination that appear as progressive, high-intensity T2-weighted images, usually in the periventricular white matter and centrum semiovale (890). Central atrophy, primarily affecting the subcortical white matter or the basal ganglia regions in MRI of children, can be suggestive of AIDS encephalopathy (891). A correlation between HIV RNA levels in the CSF and progressive neurologic disease has been found (892).

Other neuroimaging findings include cerebrovascular complications such as arterial ectasia and arterial fibrosing sclerosis (893). MR spectroscopy of the basal ganglia has been used before and after antiretroviral therapy to show a normalization of the N-acetylaspartate/creatinine and lactate levels, an indication of decreased inflammation (894). Salvan and coworkers (895) used in vivo proton MR spectroscopy to study the cerebral metabolism of HIV-infected children with and without encephalopathy. Children with progressive encephalopathy had an abnormal profile consisting of an increased proportion of lipid signals, decreased proportion of N-acetylaspartate, and increased proportion of the myo-inositol signal. None of the children without encephalopathy had these changes.

Secondary opportunistic infections of the brain accompanying HIV infection include CMV encephalitis, toxoplasmosis, CMV viral lymphoma, progressive multifocal leukoencephalopathy, and, less commonly, viral encephalitis owing to VZV or herpes simplex virus. Myelitis has resulted from VZV, herpes simplex, and CMV. Meningitis can result from typical and atypical mycobacteria, especially *Mycobacterium avium intracellulare*, cryptococcal, and other fungal meningitides. Cerebral infection with Bartonella henselae, the agent implicated in cat-scratch disease, has been associated with AIDS encephalopathy (826,896). Radiculitis has been caused by varicella-zoster or by CMV.

Diagnosis

Diagnosis of HIV infection in an infant relies on the performance of virologic assays. The HIV DNA PCR is the method of choice for the diagnosis of HIV infection during the first 6 months of life. This test result is positive in 38% of prenatally HIV-infected children within the first 48 hours of life (897). After 2 weeks of age, 93% of the HIV-infected neonates had a positive PCR assay result. The majority of HIV-infected infants has a positive DNA PCR by 1 month of age, and all infants are positive by 6 months of age. Whereas the HIV-1 culture is as sensitive as the HIV DNA PCR (898), it is more cumbersome to perform and more expensive. The initial testing ideally should be performed within the first 48 hours of life. A positive test result indicates an intrauterine acquisition of HIV and predicts rapid progression of the infection (899). Passively acquired maternal IgG antibody to HIV detectable by ELISA or Western blot declines slowly: Sixty percent of uninfected children have negative test results at 12 months of age, 80% at 15 months, and 100% by 18 months. Indications of neonatal infection include prolonged persistence of IgG antibody or a fourfold increase in titer, the presence of IgG subclasses that differ from that of the mother, appearance of new bands on Western blot, or specific anti-HIV IgM or IgA antibody (896,900). The serologic diagnosis of HIV infection by ELISA and Western blot analysis is reliable in infants 18 months and older. In neonates serologic detection of HIV infection is complicated by the presence of HIV antigens complexed to passively transferred maternal antibody. Early detection of HIV infection in neonates can be achieved by serologic testing with immune-complex–dissociated HIV p24 antigen (896). Detection of p24 antigen in the neonate predicts the development of early and severe HIV-related disease (900). Viral culture at birth can identify only approximately one-half of HIV-infected newborns, probably because infections acquired late in pregnancy or during delivery may be missed (900).

HIV DNA, HIV RNA, and HIV-1 culture have been performed on CSF and brain tissues from children with HIV infection and encephalopathy. Sei and coworkers (901) evaluated the levels of HIV RNA in CSF in children with HIV encephalopathy. They found that the levels were highest in children with severe encephalopathy, intermediate when the encephalopathy was moderate, and the lowest in nonencephalopathic children. These findings speak to the potential role of increased viral replication within the CNS in the progression of HIV encephalopathy. Cerebrospinal fluid concentration of proinflammatory mediators may be involved in the pathogenesis of CNS disease in HIV-infected children (902).

The diagnosis of an acute postnatally acquired HIV-1 infection cannot be made with standard serologic tests. Serologic tests first become positive 22 to 27 days after infection. Earlier diagnosis must rely on detection of p24 antigen in serum or plasma (882).

Treatment

Every HIV-infected infant younger than 12 months of age, independent of clinical, immunologic, and virologic status, should receive combination antiretroviral therapy. Most experts agree that the same criteria apply to children older than 1 year. Aggressive antiretroviral therapy using three drugs is preferred. The combination of two nucleoside reverse transcriptase inhibitors and a protease inhibitor is the combination of choice. This combination of drugs has led to a significant decrease in the mortality of patients with HIV infection and an accompanying significant improvement in quality of life.

Antiretroviral therapy improves and even reverses the course of the HIV encephalopathy in children. For CNS disease, zidovudine, stavudine, and lamivudine are preferred over didanosine because of their better CNS penetration. The protease inhibitors are highly bound to serum proteins with low penetration in the CNS. Ongoing trials will determine which is the best combination of drugs to fight HIV within the CNS, particularly in children with low blood CD8+ T lymphocytes at highest risk of developing progressive encephalopathy (903,904).

A more extensive discussion of treatment, complications of treatment, and control measures for AIDS is beyond the scope of this text.

HUMAN T-LYMPHOTROPIC VIRUS MYELONEUROPATHIES

Four different neurologic diseases are related to infection with human T-lymphotropic virus types I and II (HTLV-I and HTLV-II): tropical spastic paraparesis/HTLV-I–associated myelopathy (TSP/HAM), polymyositis, progressive neurologic abnormalities without immune reactivity against the virus, and tropical ataxic neuropathy (905–908).

TSP/HAM usually occurs in high-HTLV-I–endemic areas such as southern Japan, equatorial Africa, and the Seychelles as well as in high endemic foci in Central and South America, Melanesia, and South Africa. Sporadic cases have been described in the United States and Europe.

Neuropathologic changes in TSP/HAM consist most notably of chronic inflammatory changes in the spinal cord that are prominent as a meningomyelitis of the lower thoracic region. Radiculitis, leptomeningitis, and pial thickening can occur. With time the inflammatory changes predominate in the perivascular region and are accompanied by hyalinosis of blood vessels, meningeal fibrosis, glial scars, and progressive atrophy of the spinal cord. Early lesions usually demonstrate destruction of myelin; later, both myelin and axons are destroyed (906). Both immunologic response and viral load play a role in the development of symptoms. Symptomatic patients have an activated immune response and as much as 50 times more HTLV-I proviral DNA in peripheral blood lymphocytes than do seropositive asymptomatic persons. HTLV-I RNA is present in CD4+ lymphocytes and astrocytes (909). These lymphocytes are thought to enter the nervous system, where they evoke local expansion of virus-specific CD8+ cytotoxic T lymphocytes, which together with cytokines cause the pathologic lesions (910).

Symptoms may appear as early as 6 years of age, although onset before the age of 20 years is uncommon (906). The onset is insidious without prodromata or provocation. Symptoms include stiffness or weakness in one or both legs, often associated with lumbar pain, and various sensory symptoms in the legs including numbness, burning, and "pins and needles." Urinary frequency and urgency are common. The disease progresses at a variable rate, but usually reaches a plateau. After 10 years, 30% of patients are bedridden and 45% cannot walk unaided. Complete paralysis can occur within 2 years

(906). Early onset has been associated with more rapid progression.

The clinical presentation is one of spastic paraparesis or paraplegia. Minor sensory involvement of the posterior columns and spinothalamic tract are found in the lower extremities. Cerebellar signs limited to intention tremor have been reported in 20% of patients. Cranial nerves are usually spared, but optic neuropathy can develop occasionally. Cognitive functions remain normal (906).

MRI of the spinal cord can be normal or show atrophy of the thoracic spinal cord with a diffuse high signal on T2-weighted images. Approximately one-half of patients have nonspecific lesions of the brain, which consist of increased signal on T2-weighted images and decreased signal on T1-weighted images, either contiguous with the ventricles or scattered throughout deep cerebral white matter (906). EEGs are abnormal in up to 64% of patients, and visual-evoked responses are abnormal in approximately 30% of cases (906). Somatosensory-evoked potentials are abnormal in the legs in two-thirds of patients and in the arms in one-third of patients (906). Conduction velocities can be reduced in the spinothalamic tracts and posterior columns without clinical impairment of sensation (908).

The CSF usually demonstrates a mild pleocytosis, elevated IgG, and intrathecal production of oligoclonal antibodies against HTLV-I (906). Rarely, TSP/HAM coexists with adult T-cell leukemia.

The pathologic features of polymyositis associated with HTLV-I are indistinguishable from polymyositis in noninfected individuals. Specific diagnosis is made by demonstration of virus in inflammatory lymphocytes or HTLV-I–positive endomysial macrophages of the involved tissue by PCR (905). HTLV-I– and HTLV-I–positive lymphocytes do not infect muscle. Virus, which persists in tissues other than muscle, triggers T-cell–mediated and major histocompatibility complex I–restricted cytotoxicity (911).

Chronic progressive myelopathy without detectable HTLV-I antibodies is observed most frequently in HTLV-I–endemic areas. HTLV-I–related DNA sequences have been demonstrated in peripheral blood mononuclear cells of these patients by PCR. Patients have a clinical disease similar to TSP/HAM, except that the onset of disease is at a younger age and little or no sphincteric or sensory disturbance occurs (906).

Interferon-alpha is of benefit in HTLV-I–associated myelopathy, although the therapy has a considerable incidence of side effects (912).

HTLV-II causes a myelopathy similar to HTLV-I except that it is associated with more prominent ataxia and mental changes (tropical ataxic neuropathy) (907,908).

Creutzfeldt-Jakob Disease

Transmitted CJD has occurred after inoculation of prion protein by injection of human growth hormone (913–915), and the risk is raised if growth hormone administration occurred at ages 8 to 10 years in the United Kingdom from 1959 through 1985 (916). The disease also develops in older patients after corneal transplantation and after implantation of cerebral electrodes. Spontaneous CJD can develop in adolescence as early as 16 years of age, with dementia progressing to severe disability within 12 months and death within 28 months (917). Some 5% to 10% of spongiform encephalopathies are familial (918,919).

PrPCJD, an abnormal isoform of prion protein that accumulates in the brain in parallel with development of the disease, differs in location in iatrogenic and in spontaneous CJD. PrPCJD is found in high concentrations in the cerebellum of iatrogenic CJD cases in comparison with sporadic cases; conversely, PrPCJD amounts are greater in the forebrain of sporadic CJD than in iatrogenic cases (920).

The condition is marked by dementia, accompanied by pyramidal tract disease, extrapyramidal signs, and myoclonus, which is often stimulus sensitive. Initial symptoms also can be highlighted by cerebellar signs, which are followed by mental deterioration and myoclonus, with death ensuing within a few months (917). The EEG is characteristic: it demonstrates periodic complexes of spike or slow-wave activity at intervals of 0.5 to 2.0 seconds (921).

Conventional laboratory studies of CSF are usually unremarkable. Elevations in neuron-specific enolase and demonstration of 14-3-3 brain protein in CSF have been associated with early diagnosis of CJD (922,923).

Kuru

Kuru, first described by Berndt in 1954 (924), is a progressive degenerative disease of the CNS with predominantly cerebellar features. The disease is limited to the Fore tribe of the eastern highlands of central New Guinea, in a population that until recently practiced cannibalism (925).

Pathologic changes are seen only on microscopy (926). They include widespread neuronal degeneration that is most marked within the cerebellum, proliferation of astroglia and microglia, and minimal demyelination. The disease has been transmitted experimentally to the chimpanzee, in which it develops after incubation periods ranging from 18 to 30 months (927). It is now believed to have passed from human to human by cutaneous inoculation during the cannibalistic ingestion of infected human brain, although one well-documented case was seen in a visitor to the endemic area (928).

The clinical course is remarkably uniform. In boys, the mean age of onset is approximately 14 years of age. In female patients, the age of onset has a bimodal distribution, with one mode occurring at approximately 8 years of age and the other at 33 years of age. The earliest case of kuru occurred in a child 5 years of age. The initial symptom is ataxia, which is progressive and accompanied by a fine tremor of the trunk, extremities, and head. During the second to third month of illness, the tremor becomes more coarse and severe, and choreiform movements can appear (929). Intelligence is preserved, although alterations in mood are common. In most children, the disease is fatal within 6 to 9 months of onset (930).

Laboratory studies have been unremarkable and in particular have shown no abnormalities of the CSF (915).

Although no therapy has been effective once symptoms have become apparent, abolition of cannibalism among the Fore tribe has led to disappearance of the illness.

New-Variant Creutzfeldt-Jakob Disease

New-variant Creutzfeldt-Jakob disease or bovine spongiform encephalopathy has occurred in adolescents as young as 14 years of age. Involvement of lymphoid tissue as early as 8 months before the onset of symptoms (931), as well as early involvement of nervous tissue, has been demonstrated (932). This variant has clinical features that help distinguish it from other phenotypes. Psychiatric symptoms, most often depression, are common. Ataxia and involuntary movements occur in all cases, and akinetic mutism is often a late occurrence. One-third of patients develop persistent and often painful sensory symptoms (933,934). These symptoms, except for their early age of onset, may overlap with atypical cases of sporadic CJD. For epidemiologic aspects of this disorder, see the review by Collee and Bradley (935).

Fatal familial insomnia, a rare prion disease usually seen only in adults, has caused death in a 13-year-old child (936).

Subacute Sclerosing Panencephalitis

SSPE is a slow virus infection, first described in Tennessee children by Dawson in 1934 (937) and caused by measles virus, which presents a clinical picture of CNS degeneration characterized by myoclonic seizures, involuntary movements, and mental deterioration. Although SSPE was once a relatively common condition, its frequency has been decreased significantly by the widespread use of measles immunization. This topic is reviewed by Bergamini and coworkers (938).

Etiology and Pathology

The alterations within the brain are usually evident on both gross and microscopic examination. They consist of a subacute encephalitis that is accompanied by demyelination.

Lesions generally involve the cerebral cortex, hippocampus, thalamus, brainstem, and cerebellar cortex. In the cerebral cortex, the histologic picture is a nonspecific one of subacute encephalitis with cell loss that is sometimes accompanied by neuronophagia and meningeal and perivascular infiltration. Perivascular cells are predominantly CD4+ T cells, whereas the parenchymal inflammatory infiltrate are B cells (939). Inclusions are seen within both the nucleus and the cytoplasm of neurons and glial cells. Characteristically, they consist of homogeneous eosinophilic material (Cowdry type A); less often, the inclusions are small and multiple (Cowdry type B). They are almost always found in the brainstem (940). Older patients often show neurofibrillary tangles in neurons and fibrillary tangles in oligodendroglia (939).

The demyelination is particularly evident in the more chronic cases. It is sudanophilic with astrocytic and fibrillary gliosis and is independent of the loss of cortical neurons. In its early stages, SSPE affects the occipital areas primarily; subsequently, it spreads to the anterior portions of the cerebral hemispheres, subcortical structures, brainstem, and spinal cord (941). The presence of measles virus antigen has been convincingly demonstrated by several methods, including *in situ* hybridization to nucleic acid sequences from the measles virus matrix (M) protein (942).

The interplay between viral mutation and abnormal host response to the virus that results in SSPE is not clear. At one time it was thought that the pathogenesis of SSPE involved an abnormality in the host synthesis in brain of the M protein, one of the nonglycosylated polypeptides of the measles virus involved in the assembly of viral nucleocapsid with the viral glycoproteins in the cell membrane. It is now clear that multiple viral mutations rather than host factors cause defective measles virus gene expression in SSPE (943,944). Although strains of SSPE measles virus can code for M protein, the conformation of the protein is defective and it is unable to bind to nucleocapsids (945).

Host factors are probably also important. Patients with SSPE have low titers of antibody to the M protein, even though they have high titers of antibody to the other measles virus polypeptides (943). Oligoclonal IgG in the sera of patients with SSPE is only partially specific for measles antigens (946).

SSPE patients have an increased CSF-to-serum ratio of β_2-microglobulin and higher than normal levels of serum-soluble IL-2 receptor and CSF-soluble CD8. During clinical worsening of the disease, the level of CSF-soluble CD8 increases, whereas the level of serum β_2-microglobulin decreases (947).

Clinical Manifestations

SSPE is more common in rural than in urban populations. The age of onset ranges from 5 to 15 years, and boys are more frequently affected than girls by a factor of three to five. Occasional cases begin in adult life. Children with SSPE are more likely to have been infected with natural measles than with a live vaccine strain. The risk of SSPE after measles is 4.0 in 100,000 cases compared with a risk after measles vaccine of 0.14 in 100,000 cases. Children with early measles infection are more prone to the disease. When measles is contracted in children younger than

1 year of age, the risk for SSPE is 16 times greater than when measles is contracted in children older than 5 years of age. Receipt of measles vaccine subsequent to natural measles does not increase the incidence of SSPE. During the period 1970 through 1986, 36.6% of SSPE was vaccine associated, with SSPE developing after a latency of 7.7 years. The median interval between natural measles and the onset of SSPE is 8 years (948).

Initially, personality changes and an insidious deterioration of intellect occur. Seizures, usually appearing within 2 months, characteristically are myoclonic jerks, initially of the head and subsequently of the trunk and limbs. Muscular contraction is followed by 1 to 2 seconds of relaxation associated with a decrease in muscle action potentials or complete electrical silence. The myoclonic jerks do not interfere with consciousness but may be a troublesome cause of falling episodes. They are exaggerated by excitement and disappear during sleep. Although initially they are infrequent and might be regarded as stumbling, clumsiness, or possibly ataxia, later in the course of the illness they occur every 5 to 15 seconds. Patients can present with intractable simple partial seizures (949).

Spontaneous speech and movements decrease, although comprehension seems relatively well preserved.

With further progression of the illness, extrapyramidal dyskinesia and spasticity become more prominent. The former includes athetosis, chorea, ballismus, and dystonic movements with transient periods of opisthotonus. Swallowing difficulties can develop at this stage. Progressive vision loss associated with focal chorioretinitis, cortical blindness, and, occasionally, optic atrophy also has been noted (950,951).

In the terminal stages of the disease, a progressive unresponsiveness is associated with increasing extensor hypertonus and decerebrate rigidity. Respirations become irregular and stertorous, and the patient has a variety of signs of hypothalamic dysfunction. These include vasomotor instability, hyperthermia, profuse sweating, and disturbances of pulse and blood pressure.

Ocular involvement is present in 56% of patients with SSPE. When present, it is bilateral in approximately 80% of patients. Optic neuritis occurs in 72% of involved eyes, retinitis in 35%, and macular pigment disturbances in 9%. Visual agnosia can occur but is rare. Ophthalmologic involvement precedes the neurologic signs in approximately 10% of patients (952).

The clinical course is characterized by slowly progressive deterioration or variable periods of remission, with the mean duration of the disease being approximately 12 months (953). Patients have lived for as short as 6 weeks after the onset of symptoms or as long as 20 years. Patients with remissions that last up to 25 years have been encountered (954).

A fulminant disease that can be as brief as 1 month has been described after acquired measles (955). It is probably related to measles inclusion body encephalitis, which is encountered in immunocompromised children.

Cerebral metabolism during SSPE has been studied by positron emission tomography. During the initial active period of disease progression, inflammation in the basal ganglia appears to lead to neuronal excitation accompanied by hypermetabolism. This is followed by widespread functional inhibition of cortical metabolism. Striatal inflammation ends with necrosis and hypometabolism. Later, deep midbrain and brainstem structures become hypermetabolic. No such changes are found during clinical remission (956). CT scans obtained during the early stages of SSPE show small ventricles and obliteration of hemispheric sulci and interhemispheric fissures. Atrophy of white and gray matter can be seen after a prolonged course, but tomograms are normal, sometimes for as long as 5 years after onset of the disease (957).

MRI shows abnormal signal in gray and white matter, which reflects the inflammatory process and occasionally mimics a neoplasm. These abnormalities can resolve during progression of the disease (958). Two types of MRI abnormalities are observed: focal areas of increased signal intensity on T2-weighted images (hypointense or isointense on T1-weighted images) and atrophy (959). Although the cortical and subcortical lesions seen on MRI have some correlation with clinical findings, the extent of the periventricular white matter lesions and cortical atrophy generally does not correlate with the neurologic status (960). Typically, the CSF contains a normal or slightly elevated protein concentration, but the concentration of gamma globulin, predominantly oligoclonal IgG, is always increased to amounts that can vary from slightly above normal to 60% of the total protein concentration. Antibodies against measles virus can be demonstrated in both serum and CSF by a variety of techniques. Almost invariably, the ratio of the IgG and IgA antibody content in the CSF compared with that in serum is disproportionately high because of intrathecal production of antibody. CSF pleocytosis can be absent or minimal, with a variable proportion of mononuclear cells.

The EEG is characteristic. Paroxysmal bursts of high-voltage diphasic activity of 2 to 3 seconds' duration occur synchronously throughout the tracing and are often associated with spike discharges. They are followed by a short period of flattened activity. The entire pattern, termed a *suppression burst* (Fig. 7.14), occurs in approximately 80% of patients (961). These discharges are believed to arise from the mesencephalic activating system or the subcortical area adjacent to the thalamus (962). The background activity can be normal initially; later, it becomes disorganized. These EEG abnormalities can be seen as early as 4 years before the clinical appearance of myoclonus (963). Terminally, paroxysmal activity can decrease, or it can disappear completely with periods of hyperpyrexia. The myoclonic contractions can coincide with the paroxysmal

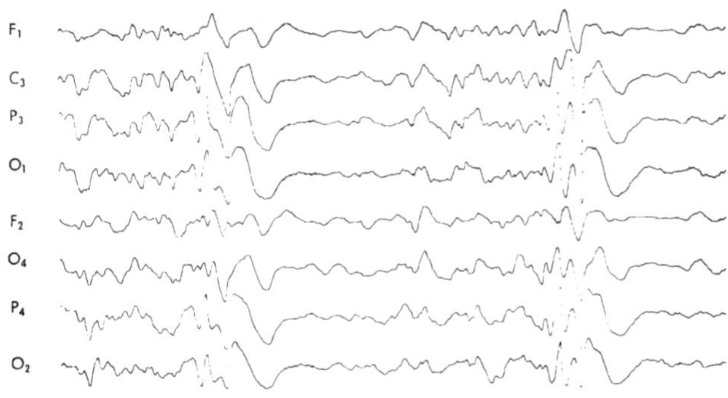

FIGURE 7.14. Subacute sclerosing panencephalitis. Electroencephalogram in a 5-year-old boy, showing characteristic suppression bursts. Unipolar leads, F1, C3, P3, O1, left frontal, central, parietal, and occipital leads; F2, C4, P4, O2, right frontal, central, parietal, and occipital leads.

bursts observed by EEG or they can be disassociated from them. During sleep, the myoclonic discharges disappear, but the paroxysmal EEG bursts continue.

Diagnosis

The clinical picture of intellectual deterioration associated with myoclonic seizures and the presence of suppression bursts suggests SSPE. The diagnosis is confirmed by the strikingly elevated levels of measles antibodies in the serum and CSF.

SSPE should be distinguished from subacute measles encephalitis with immunosuppression measles inclusion body encephalitis (MIBE), which occurs in children with immunocompromised cellular immunity. One to 6 months after exposure to measles virus, a neurologic disorder can develop with seizures, neurologic deficits, stupor, coma, and death over a period of a few days to a few weeks. Seizures, often severe, may take the form of epilepsia partialis continua. The CSF can have no abnormalities and no elevation in measles antibody titers, although measles virus can be demonstrated in the brain. Eosinophilic inclusions occur in the neurons and glia. Variable degrees of necrosis and a paucity of inflammation are found in the brain (964,965). Quantitative differences occur in the pattern of measles mRNA expression in brain tissue with restricted expression of envelope proteins (M, F, and H) (966).

SSPE also should be differentiated from the group of late infantile or juvenile lipidoses (see Chapter 1), progressive rubella panencephalitis, and the various degenerations of white matter. Affected children frequently have a history of recent falls, which suggests cerebral trauma or akinetic seizures. Occasionally, patients can demonstrate lateralizing neurologic signs or, less commonly, papilledema, findings that can lead to an erroneous diagnosis of an intracranial space-occupying lesion.

Treatment

No adequate therapy is available. Nonrandomized studies suggest, but by no means confirm, that isoprinosine can prolong life in patients with SSPE (967). Anlar and coworkers recommend intraventricular interferon and oral isoprinosine, especially for those with slowly progressive disease (968). Administration of human interferon alone to patients with SSPE has been of uncertain benefit in cases of mild progression and did not alter the course of patients with rapid deterioration (969). Carbamazepine is of some benefit for myoclonus-induced falling episodes (970).

Progressive Rubella Panencephalitis

A chronically progressive panencephalitis, appearing after congenital or acquired rubella, has been described in 12 children and young adults, all male (971,972). The brain shows diffuse destruction of white matter with perivascular mononuclear and plasma cells and with fibrillary astrocytosis. Moderate neuronal loss occurs, and microglial nodules are present. Inclusion bodies have not been found. Cerebellar involvement is prominent (973).

Symptoms appear 4 to 14 years after the rubella infection. Initially, an insidiously progressive dementia occurs, followed by progressive pyramidal and extrapyramidal deficits. Truncal ataxia and myoclonic seizures are often prominent. The condition progresses over several years and is ultimately fatal.

The EEG demonstrates high-voltage slow-wave activity without the periodicity characteristic of SSPE (971). Examination of the CSF reveals mononuclear pleocytosis and an elevation of protein. Oligoclonal IgG constitutes 30% to 52% of the total CSF protein, indicating considerable antibody production within the brain (851). Oligoclonal IgG antibodies to rubella virus also are present in serum (974).

Rubella virus has been isolated from brain and peripheral leukocytes (975). The persistence of circulating interferon and IgM antibody to rubella, the presence of circulating immune complexes in serum, and the presence in serum of a possible blocking factor of lymphocyte cytotoxicity for rubella-infected target cells imply that unusual immune responses play a role in this disorder (976). A serum inhibitor of interferon production by normal donor lymphocytes is present on stimulation with rubella antigen (977).

LEPROSY

More than 5.5 million patients suffer from leprosy worldwide, with an incidence of approximately 1 million new patients per year (978). A majority of affected patients live in underdeveloped countries, but increasing numbers of affected patients live in North America and Europe, largely because of increasing immigration and travel. There is a male predominance in leprosy patients after the age of puberty, with a male-to-female ratio of between 1.5 and 2.0 to 1 (979). Although drug treatment is effective in achieving microbiologic cure and reducing transmission, approximately 25% of survivors are left with chronic disability (980).

Infection with *Mycobacterium leprae* is probably only acquired from contact with infected individuals discharging viable organisms. Infection rates are highest in children living in close proximity to patients with lepromatous leprosy, who excrete large numbers of bacilli. A naturally occurring leprosy-like disease among wild armadillos and the detection of living *M. leprae* in mosquitoes suggest that nonhuman reservoirs of leprosy may exist and that in some instances an intermediate host is involved (981).

The spectrum of clinical disease is broad and depends on the individual's immune response to the bacillus. The disease can be classified clinically and histologically into five stages: full lepromatous, borderline lepromatous, borderline, borderline tuberculoid, and full tuberculoid (982). Patients with lepromatous leprosy have extensive disease that is often bilateral, with large numbers of bacilli present in the lesions and nasal secretions and associated with multiple erythematous macules, papules, or nodules. Nerve involvement in lepromatous disease is diffuse but less severe than in tuberculoid cases. Palpable nerve thickening is uncommon and sensory loss is patchy, typically a mononeuritis multiplex (983). In these lesions messenger RNAs coding for IL-4, IL-5, and IL-10 predominate (984).

Tuberculoid leprosy is characterized by isolated disease, with large erythematous plaques that have sharply demarcated outer edges. The center of the plaques is flattened and the area is anesthetic. Hypopigmented macules can be present. Peripheral nerves can be visibly swollen. In tuberculoid leprosy, bacilli are seldom seen within the lesions and are not present in the nasal secretions. In these lesions, messenger RNAs for IL-2 and interferon-gamma are most evident (984). Patients with borderline lepromatous and borderline tuberculoid disease have features between those of lepromatous and tuberculous forms. In all forms of the disease, T cells are Ia-positive, which is evidence for an activated state (985,986).

The histologic features of lepromatous and borderline lepromatous leprosy are poorly formed granulomata that are largely comprised of foamy macrophages (987). Epithelioid cell formation is poorly developed, only scanty lymphocytes are seen, and Langerhans-type giant cells are absent. Large numbers of mycobacteria are visible within the granuloma. Bacilli can be seen extensively proliferating within Schwann cells and perineural cells of nerve bundles, but structural preservation of axons is better than in tuberculoid disease (988). In tuberculoid leprosy, a well-developed granulomatous process has histologic features similar to the lesions of sarcoidosis. Epithelioid cells are prominent, as are Langerhans giant cells. Extensive lymphocyte infiltrates are seen, but bacilli are infrequently seen. Nerve bundles are grossly swollen and infiltrated with mononuclear inflammatory cells. In late cases, there is extensive fibrous replacement of the most distal segments of peripheral nerves, and fibrous plaques can prevent regenerating axons from reaching cutaneous nerves (988).

Immunologic mechanisms underlie the different clinical manifestations of the disease. Patients with lepromatous leprosy are anergic to *M. leprae* and have a generalized impairment of delayed T-cell hypersensitivity responses (989). Immunoglobulin levels are markedly increased, indicating a polyclonal proliferative response, and a variety of autoimmune phenomenon may be present including a false-positive VDRL test, autoantibodies to testicular germinal cells and thyroglobulin, and positive antinuclear factor or rheumatoid factor (989,990). Patients with tuberculoid leprosy have positive lepromin reactions and exhibit normal delayed T-cell hypersensitivity tests to other antigens (991).

Reversal reactions are seen when patients with borderline leprosy are treated and probably present an increasing inflammatory response caused by the acquisition of T-cell immunity to the mycobacteria (992). Lepromatous skin lesions may rapidly develop brawny, raised induration and in some cases ulceration. There is worsening of the neuritis, with swelling of the nerve and loss of motor function. Reversal reactions entail a reduction in the number of bacilli, extensive edema formation, and an increase in the number of lymphocytes in the inflammatory infiltrate.

The neurologic consequences of leprosy range from isolated anesthetic areas caused by denervation to severe peripheral neuropathy with loss of both sensory and motor functions (993). The neurologic lesions of leprosy are of three types (994,995). Purely sensory polyneuritis results in loss of light touch, light pain, and temperature sense in a glove-and-stocking distribution, whereas deep pressure and deep pain, vibration, and joint sense are preserved. Sensory polyneuritis can occur without characteristic skin lesions. A less common lesion is a mixed sensory polyneuritis and mononeuritis with paralysis in a peripheral nerve distribution and sensory loss more widely distributed than in sensory polyneuritis (996). Rarely, a myositis occurs or a pure mononeuritis, which results in a motor deficit with a peripheral nerve distribution (997,998).

Symptoms can begin abruptly or develop insidiously. Peripheral nerve trunks can become enlarged, hard, and tender. The most commonly involved nerves include the ulnar nerve just above the elbow, the lateral popliteal nerve at the neck of the fibula, the posterior tibial nerve behind the internal malleolus, and the great auricular nerve. Intense neuralgia or shooting pains can precede impairment of sensation (996). In addition to the sensory loss, sudomotor dysfunction with anhidrosis is commonly seen in the absence of evidence of vasomotor abnormality. Ocular complications are extremely common, and approximately 2% of infected patients are blind (999). Reversal reactions occurring in borderline leprosy, often during the initial months of treatment, may result in damage to trigeminal and facial nerves. Facial nerve dysfunction causes inability to close the eyes fully (1000). This causes exposure keratitis and progressive scarring over the lower half of the cornea, which may ultimately result in blindness. Involvement of the trigeminal nerve also may cause hypoanesthesia, and traumatic damage to the cornea may result. The eye may be directly involved by acute uveitis and episcleritis as a component of erythema nodosum leprosum or by the presence of ocular lepromas. Dysfunctional and anesthetic limbs are extremely susceptible to damage, and serious deformities with destruction to limbs and digits are often the result.

The diagnosis of leprosy should be considered in patients presenting with dermatologic, neurologic, or multisystem complaints who have come from parts of the world where the disease is endemic (1001). Hypoesthesic or anesthetic skin lesions, with or without associated nerve thickenings, are important diagnostic clues. Ultrasonography and magnetic resonance imaging can detect nerve abnormalities (1002). The diagnosis can be confirmed by skin biopsy, which should include both a central and a peripheral area of the lesion and should be examined histologically, including with mycobacterial stains.

The management of leprosy is difficult. The entire spectrum of leprosy can be seen in nerve aspirates (1003), and all patients should receive multidrug chemotherapy. The treatment regimen and the adverse reactions to treatment are beyond the scope of this text. The interested reader is referred to reviews by Jacobson and Krahenbuhl (982), Nations and colleagues (1004), Willcox (1005), and Manandhar et al. (1006).

Damage to nerves frequently progresses or worsens after the initiation of treatment, particularly in patients with lepromatous or borderline lepromatous disease. Patients undergoing reversal reactions are treated with corticosteroids to reduce the inflammatory response.

SPIROCHETAL INFECTIONS

Leptospirosis

Leptospirosis, caused by *Leptospira icterohaemorrhagiae, L. canicola, L. pomona,* or *L. grippotyphosa,* is an uncommon cause of meningitis. The state of Hawaii has the highest reported annual incidence in the United States (1007), although the disease is reemerging following recreational freshwater exposure in the continental United States (1008). It is characterized by sudden onset of fever, muscle pain, articular symptoms, epigastric pain, and headache. Hemorrhagic symptoms can occur. Conjunctival suffusion is present in 25% to 30% of patients with leptospirosis and may be pathognomonic for the infection (1007). Jaundice, hepatosplenomegaly, renal damage, and vascular involvement are common. Single or multiple relapses occur, but almost all patients recover. The death rate in icteric leptospirosis is highest (1009).

Signs of meningeal irritation occur in approximately 10% of patients (1010,1011). These commence between the days 5 and 14 of the illness, most often by the end of the first week. Symptoms are of variable severity and do not correlate with the severity of other manifestations of the infection. Symptoms subside in 1 to 14 days.

Thrombocytopenia and polymorphonuclear leukocytosis are common. Urinalysis frequently shows hematuria and albuminuria occuring during the early phase of the illness (1007). CSF pleocytosis is usually below 500 white blood cells/μL, with a progressive increase in the proportion of mononuclear cells. It can persist for several weeks. Protein can range from normal to 140 mg/dL. Leptospiral meningitis is regarded as an antigen–antibody reaction; this explains the absence of early CSF pleocytosis, the abrupt onset of meningeal symptoms toward the end of the first week of illness, the rapid disappearance of leptospires after the onset of meningitis, and the uniformly good prognosis (1012). A severe form of encephalitis, myelitis, and peripheral neuritis caused by leptospirosis has been seen on rare occasions (1013). CNS involvement can occur without evidence of renal dysfunction or jaundice (1013).

Leptospirosis is diagnosed by isolation of the organism or by antibody studies in blood (first 7 days), CSF (4 to 10 days), and urine (greater than 10 days) (1014). Penicillin is the drug of choice. It is given for 7 days and appears to be effective, even when started late in the course of the illness (1015). Doxycycline prophylaxis did not prevent leptospiral infection in an endemic area, but it had a significant protective effect in reducing the morbidity and mortality during outbreaks (1016).

Syphilis

The resurgence of syphilis throughout the world gives added importance to congenital and acquired cases of neurosyphilis seen in infancy or childhood. The incidence of both acquired and congenital syphilis has risen significantly in the last decade (1017). Meningovascular syphilis accounts for 35% to 40% of all cases of neurosyphilis (1018).

Pathology and Pathogenesis

The pathology of congenital neurosyphilis resembles that of the acquired forms (1019) and is described in more detail in the Congenital Infections section. Neurosyphilis takes either the meningovascular or the parenchymatous form. In both forms, the infectious process begins in the meninges as a widespread diffuse arachnoiditis with inflammation concentrated around the meningeal vessels and the branches that penetrate into the cortex. Small meningeal vessels can show thickening and infiltration of the adventitia as well as intimal proliferation; syphilitic phlebitis is less common, although both can result in infarction with localized lesions of the brain or spinal cord.

Obstructive or communicating hydrocephalus can result from meningeal fibrosis and obliteration of the subarachnoid spaces.

Diffuse meningeal inflammation of the secondary stage can be carried over into the tertiary stage with increased fibrosis of the meninges and the formation of small, often miliary gummas.

In parenchymatous congenital syphilis, as in juvenile paresis, diffuse degeneration occurs with cerebral and cerebellar atrophy. Microscopic changes include round cell meningeal and perivascular infiltration, loss and degenerative changes in the nerve cells with an increase in microglia and astroglia, a disturbance of normal cytoarchitecture, deposition of iron pigment, and presence of spirochetes.

Clinical Manifestations

The CNS becomes involved during the first few months or years of life. In 50% to 80% of cases of congenital neurosyphilis, one or more of the stigmata of congenital syphilis are present. These include interstitial keratitis, chorioretinitis, defective teeth, malformed or "saddle" nose, frontal bossing of the skull, saber shins, Clutton joints, and rhagades, either singly or in combination. Nerve deafness, which, when seen with dental deformities and interstitial keratitis, forms the classic Hutchinson triad, is infrequent. Painful bone involvement can cause pseudoparalysis. Syphilitic meningitis is more common during the first few months of postnatal life, whereas vascular syndromes are prevalent during the first 2 years of life.

Syphilitic meningitis usually appears between ages 3 and 12 months with a sudden onset of convulsions, listlessness, apathy, vomiting, feeding difficulties, or progressive enlargement of the head. Nuchal rigidity, a full fontanel, head retraction, various cranial nerve palsies with optic atrophy, or strabismus can develop in the course of the illness.

Chronic syphilitic meningitis can give rise to hydrocephalus. Rarely present at birth, hydrocephalus usually develops progressively at 9 to 12 months, sometimes accompanied by cranial nerve deficits. Congenital cerebrovascular syphilis can result in diverse vascular syndromes because of arteritis and thrombosis of cerebral vessels (1019, 1020).

Mental deficiency, mental subnormality, and behavior disorders are more common in patients with congenital syphilis than in the general population, not because of the infection itself, but because of other hereditary and environmental factors (1021).

Tertiary congenital syphilis begins after 5 to 25 years of infection, the same interval as for acquired syphilis. Juvenile paresis is the most common form of congenital tertiary neurosyphilis. It usually begins between ages 6 and 21 years, the average age of occurrence being 13 years. Male and female patients are affected equally often. The onset of juvenile paresis in children with marked mental retardation is vague and impossible to date. When the children exhibit moderate retardation or normal intelligence, onset of juvenile paresis is marked by loss of previous accomplishments.

Patients with juvenile paresis most commonly have simple mental deterioration characterized by regression, confusion, flattened affect, and restless, non-purposeful behavior. The neurologic syndromes of juvenile paresis are more diverse and advanced than those of acquired paresis, and in 25% of cases, cerebellar deficits are conspicuous. In 50% of children, one or more limbs are spastic. Seizures occur in 30% to 40%. Spinal cord involvement indicating taboparesis is present in 10% to 15% of cases. Optic atrophy with or without chorioretinitis is present in 12% to 18%, compared with an incidence of 5% in the acquired form of disease. The facial nerve is involved in 10% of cases, the auditory nerve in 2%, and the hypoglossal nerve in approximately 10% to 15%. Other deficits and multiple cranial nerve deficits can occur also. Untreated, the disease steadily progresses to death in 2 to 5 years.

Tabes dorsalis is rare in congenital syphilis and eventually develops in only 1.5% to 9.0% of those afflicted. Its age of onset corresponds to that of congenital paretic neurosyphilis. Often the first symptom is failing vision or urinary incontinence, which is often nocturnal. Approximately one-half of the cases have cranial nerve palsies; strabismus is common. Pupillary abnormalities are almost always present; the pupils are usually dilated and fixed, although Argyll Robertson pupils can occur. Lightning pains and gastric crises are relatively uncommon, and ataxia and arthropathies are rare.

The clinical course of tabes dorsalis is mild, and many of the cases are discovered during routine examination of syphilitic children.

Diagnosis

The diagnosis of active neurosyphilis is based on serologic evidence of treponemal infection, demonstration of *Treponema pallidum* DNA by PCR, or rabbit infectivity testing (1022). Serum and CSF treponema antibody tests provide evidence of past infection but give no information about CNS activity (1023). The CSF in paretic neurosyphilis shows a mononuclear pleocytosis ranging from 10 to 100 cells/μL, with the degree of pleocytosis being an indicator of disease activity. In 80% of cases, the protein content is elevated, with a disproportionate rise in gamma globulin and the presence of oligoclonal banding (1023). Contamination of CSF with as little as 0.008 μL/mL of fluorescent treponemal antibody absorption test (FTA-ABS)–reactive blood (equivalent to adding 43 red blood cells to 1 mL of CSF) can result in a false-positive FTA reaction (1024). The specificity of the CSF VDRL in diagnosing probably active neurosyphilis is 100%, but its sensitivity is only 27%. The insensitivity of the CSF VDRL limits its usefulness as a screening test for neurosyphilis. The CSF FTA-ABS is more sensitive for screening, but its lack of specificity in distinguishing active neurosyphilis from past syphilitic infections necessitates the use of clinical judgment based on clinical history, clinical findings, and CSF evaluation (1025). The presence of maternal reagin or immunoglobulins passively transferred to the newborn renders early diagnosis of congenital syphilis more difficult. The presence of elevated IgM levels in the newborn or PCR assay of serum or blood is indirect evidence of prenatal infection (1026). Assay for both specific neonatal IgM antibody and *T. pallidum* DNA in the serum and CSF is recommended for the diagnosis of asymptomatic infected neonates (1027). Demonstration of IgM FTA reactivity is specific for fetal infection (1028) but is positive in only approximately 40% of asymptomatic infected neonates (1022).

Inadvertent partial therapy can render the VDRL test result negative, whereas the serum FTA or *T. pallidum* immobilization (TPI) test result remains positive.

The differential diagnosis of juvenile paresis is that of any progressive degenerative disease of the nervous system with onset in childhood (see Chapter 1). Thus, leukodystrophies and the various lipid storage disorders should be among possible conditions to be considered.

Treatment

Penicillin G is the drug of choice for treatment of all stages of neurosyphilis (1023). Details of treatment are beyond the scope of this text. The reader is referred to the *Red Book* of the American Academy of Pediatrics (1029). The treatment of children with acquired syphilis must include an evaluation for sexual abuse and other sexually transmitted diseases (1030).

Recommended follow-up for children younger than age 2 years is clinical examination and quantitative VDRL titer at 2, 4, 6, 12, and 24 months. Quantitative VDRL titers should be followed until they become nonreactive. CSF should be rechecked 1 year after completion of treatment.

If CSF serologies are nonreactive in children with congenital syphilis older than 2 years, qualitative serologic tests for syphilis should be done at 6-month intervals for 2 years. If CSF serology is reactive, quantitative serologic tests for syphilis and CSF examinations should be done quarterly for 1 year, then semiannually for 2 additional years. The disease is regarded as inactive in the nervous system when the cell count and protein level have returned to normal. Serofast cases should be observed carefully. Persistence of serologic titer does not necessarily mean that previous therapy was inadequate or that additional treatment is indicated.

Lyme Disease

Lyme disease is caused by a spirochete, *Borrelia burgdorferi*. At least four genospecies are recognized throughout the world, each with its own degree of virulence (1031). Whereas in the United States only *B. burgdorferi* has been reported in humans, most of the illness in Europe is caused by *B. afzelii* and *B. garinii* (1032). There is evidence that the *Borrelia* genotype determines the severity of disease and disparities between Lyme disease in humans in the United States and Europe (1033). The organism can be isolated from blood, skin lesions, brain, or CSF of infected patients. It also has been isolated from the nymphal and adult forms of its vectors, *Ixodes scapularis* and *I. pacificus* (1031,1034,1035). In Europe, another common vector is *I. ricinus* (1036). A bimodal age of distribution of Lyme disease occurs in the United States, with the highest incidence rates in children aged 5 to 9 years and in adults older than 30 years (1031). Lyme neuroborreliosis occurs in 1 of every 620 infected children (1037). The presence of headache, fatigue, paresthesia, or stiff neck is not sufficient for diagnosis of neuroborreliosis (1032).

The pathology of neuroborreliosis is highlighted by an inflammatory thrombotic vasculopathy that can cause axonal sensorimotor degeneration of the peripheral nerves through involvement of vasa nervorum and causes ischemic lesions of the CNS (1037). Large areas of demyelination in periventricular white matter as well as lymphocytic vasculitis have been found in fatal cases (1038). Cellular and humoral autoimmune mechanisms also are important, and the serum of infected patients contains IgM antibodies that cross-react with an axonal component (1039).

Three stages of Lyme disease have been distinguished. The first stage is highlighted by the presence of a unique skin lesion, erythema chronicum migrans, which can be accompanied by fatigue (54%), myalgia (44%), arthralgia (44%), fever, chills, or both (39%), malaise, lymphadenopathy, and symptoms that suggest meningeal irritation: headache (42%) and neck stiffness (35%). The rash may not occur in some 10% to 20% of patients (1031,1035,1036,1040). The second stage features systemic involvement. A variety of neurologic complications develop during this stage in some 15% to 20% of patients. The third stage is seen in untreated patients 1 to 3 years after the initial infection. It is marked by chronic arthritis, but a variety of neurologic complications also can be encountered.

The neurologic symptoms and signs of neuroborreliosis are protean and can involve any portion of the neuraxis. In Europe, more than 80% of childhood neuroborreliosis manifests as facial palsy or an aseptic meningitis (161,1037). A predominantly mononuclear CSF pleocytosis occurs in 95% of children with neuroborreliosis (1037). Oligoclonal IgG antibodies are found in the CSF in only one-third of children (1037). Facial palsy usually occurs ipsilateral to a tick bite on the head or neck, but it can be bilateral (1041). It may develop during the first week of treatment, but this does not constitute treatment failure (1031). Additionally, one encounters a variety of cranial neuropathies other than that of the facial nerve (1037,1042,1043), a spastic or flaccid paralysis, chorea, cerebellar dysfunction, seizures, and a radiculoneuritis (1044,1045). A predominantly mononuclear CSF pleocytosis occurs in 95% of children with neuroborreliosis (1037). A chronic lymphocytic meningitis has been seen in approximately 6% of children. It can last up to 6 years. Meningeal signs are rare despite significant CSF changes (1046). A clinical picture similar to that of Guillain-Barré syndrome occurs in 1.8% of children (1028,1035). It is atypical in that it can have CSF pleocytosis in the range of 35 to 120 cells/μL, with 60% to 100% mononuclear cells (1047). Rarely, cases present with pseudotumor cerebri (1048,1049). Painful lymphocytic meningoradiculoneuritis (Bannwarth syndrome) has been associated serologically with Lyme disease (1050). This expression of the disease is much more common in Europe than in the United States, where headache, stiff neck, and subtle encephalitic signs with less radiculopathy are more likely (1036). On rare occasions, an acute focal meningoencephalitis (1051) or an acute psychosis (1052) can be the first signs of the disease. Lyme neuroborreliosis can be difficult to distinguish from viral meningitis. The presence of cranial neuropathies, papilledema, or erythema migrans is a characteristic that should suggest Lyme disease (1053).

A chronic course occurs in 6% of children. A wide spectrum of abnormalities also is seen during this, the third stage of Lyme disease. A subacute encephalopathy is the most common neurologic complication. It is characterized by cognitive deficits and disturbances of mood and sleep (1035,1054). A destructive chronic meningoencephalitis can progress over many years in untreated individuals (1055). A chronic lymphocytic meningitis or a subacute encephalitis also can accompany this stage of the disease (1052,1054). Chronic meningoradiculomyelitis has been associated with persistent intrathecal secretion of oligoclonal *B. burgdorferi*-specific IgG (1056,1057). However, radiculitis with pathologic changes of peripheral neuropathy can occur without intrathecal synthesis of specific antibody (1058). In addition to arthritis, an occasional case can present as Shulman syndrome (eosinophilic fasciitis) (1059).

In comparison with adults, children with neuroborreliosis have less common and milder radicular pain and less facial diplegia, but more often have headache, clinical signs of meningitis, and fever. Monosymptomatic paresis, usually facial paresis, without concomitant pain, fever, or neck stiffness occurs almost exclusively in children (1060).

EEG changes, usually in the form of moderate generalized slowing, occur in approximately one-third of children with Lyme neuroborreliosis. Children with facial palsy caused by Lyme disease have abnormal EEGs more often than those with idiopathic facial palsy or facial palsy caused by other causes. It also is of diagnostic significance that nearly all children with facial palsy caused by Lyme disease have CSF pleocytosis or intrathecal production of antibodies to *B. burgdorferi,* whereas only 11.7% of children with facial palsy caused by unknown causes have CSF pleocytosis (1061).

MRI scans can show punctate areas of increased signal in white matter of the cerebral hemispheres on both T1- and T2-weighted images (1045,1056,1062). Proton magnetic resonance spectroscopy is also nonspecific in neuroborreliosis (1063). In patients with Lyme disease radiculitis, enhancement of the roots may be noted on T1-weighted MR images (1064).

The diagnosis of acute childhood Lyme neuroborreliosis is most reliably made by demonstrating the presence of IgM antibodies to *B. burgdorferi* (1037) or by PCR, a more sensitive method. Tests on CSF may give false-negative results because of strain variation or false-positive results in the absence of active infection (1065). In some cases the comparison of antibody content for equal amounts of serum and CSF IgG confirms intrathecal *Borrelia* antibody production (1046). Oligoclonal IgG antibodies are found in the CSF in only one-third of children (1037). Serologic diagnosis is not always reliable because seronegative Lyme disease can occur in patients with vigorous T-cell proliferative responses to whole *B. burgdorferi* organisms (1056,1065). After effective therapy the presence of specific activated IgM class B cells, an indication of acute disease, is the earliest marker to disappear (1066). Although in some cases Western blot and ELISA may be discordant, positive results from both tests strongly support the diagnosis of Lyme disease (1067).

The paradox of the difficulty in demonstrating the causative agent within the neuraxis in the face of significant neurologic dysfunction can perhaps be explained by the presence of neuroactive kyurenines elicited by immune stimulation. Levels of quinolinic acid, an excitotoxin and an *N*-methyl-D-aspartate agonist, are substantially elevated in CSF of patients with CNS Lyme disease and correlate with CSF leukocytosis (1068). Direct invasion of the CNS has been confirmed by demonstration of *B. burgdorferi* DNA in areas with inflammatory changes (1038).

For early disease, doxycycline (100 mg twice daily) is the preferred drug for children 8 years of age or older; for younger children, penicillin V or amoxicillin (25 mg to 50 mg/kg per day in three divided doses, maximum 1 to 2 g/day) is recommended (1069). Treatment is recommended for 14 to 21 days (1069). Treatment for 21 to 28 days is recommended for isolated facial palsy (1069). In the later stages of the disease, high-dose intravenous penicillin is used. Ceftriaxone (75 to 100 mg/kg, intravenously or intramuscularly once daily, maximum 2 g/day), cefotaxime, and intravenous penicillin G (300,000 U/kg per day given in divided doses every 4 hours for 14 to 21 days, maximum 20 million U/day) are recommended for the treatment of meningitis or encephalitis (1070,1071). Treatment within the first year of infection results in a more favorable clinical response than later therapy, and probably reduces the incidence of neurologic complications attributable to the disease (1037,1072). Lyme radiculoneuritis has responded to intravenous gamma globulin (1073).

Lyme borreliosis can cause long-term residual cognitive deficits in verbal memory, mental flexibility, verbal associative functions, and articulation (1074). Thus, Lyme disease in children may be accompanied by long-term neuropsychiatric disturbances, resulting in psychosocial and academic difficulties (1075). However, outcomes of children with facial nerve palsy attributable to Lyme disease are comparable to those who did not have Lyme disease (1076).

Tick-Borne Relapsing Fever

Tick-borne relapsing fever is caused by spirochetes of the genus *Borrelia,* which can vary their surface antigens extensively (1077,1078). The most important agent in the western United States is *B. hermsii,* which is transmitted through the bite of the argasid tick (*Ornithodoros hermsii*) (1079). Neurologic involvement occurs in 5% to 10% of patients (1080).

Mycoplasma Infections

Although *Mycoplasma* species, usually *M. pneumoniae,* are generally implicated in pneumonia and other respiratory tract infections, the organisms also produce neurologic disease in up to 0.1% of infections and in 7% of *Mycoplasma*-infected patients treated in hospitals (1081). CNS disease can be caused by direct CNS invasion, microthromboembolism, or an immune-mediated disseminated encephalomyelitis (493,1082–1084).

Male patients are more commonly affected by a factor of four (1085). Neurologic complications of *M. pneumoniae* infections can be divided into seven categories: encephalitis, myelitis, meningitis or meningoencephalitis, encephalomyelitis, cranial neuritis or radiculitis, Guillain-Barré syndrome, and vascular problems. Meningeal, cerebral, brainstem, spinal cord, and nerve root involvement can occur singly or in combination (1086).

Cerebral involvement with an altered mental state and a nonfocal or focal encephalitis is the most common neurologic manifestation of a *Mycoplasma* infection (1087–1089). Symptoms include seizures, somnolence, and changes in consciousness. Encephalitis can be focal and involve principally the putamen and head of the caudate nucleus with symptoms of drowsiness, seizures, bradykinesia, dysarthria, ocular movement disorders, and dysphagia. Convulsions occur in 51% of children. Status epilepticus can develop with tonic-clonic seizures that often last for hours, sometimes for days. Ataxia was noted in 19% of children in a Finnish series (1081). An encephalitis lethargica–like illness also has been seen (1090). Other, less common manifestations of CNS involvement with *Mycoplasma* include cranial nerve dysfunction (1091), an ascending paralysis (Guillain-Barré syndrome) (493), and stroke resulting from occlusion of the internal carotid artery (1091). Myalgias and arthralgias are encountered in 15% to 45% of cases. Neonatal infections of the CNS can occur (1092,1093) and can complicate a severe intraventricular hemorrhage (1094).

An EEG obtained in the first week after onset of illness shows severe generalized disturbance in 58% of children. During the second to fourth weeks after onset, the EEG abnormality becomes worse in 25% of patients (1081). Serial EEGs initially may show bilateral periodic lateralized epileptiform discharges that subsequently are replaced by other abnormalities (1095).

Myelitis can be symptomatic (1096) or can be associated with clinically silent lesions demonstrable by MRI (1097).

In the meningitis-meningoencephalitis group the CSF can be normal or show a marked pleocytosis of up to 4,000 white blood cells/μL. In the Finnish series of pediatric patients with *Mycoplasma* encephalitis, the CSF was normal during the first week of illness in 70% of patients. CSF protein ranged from normal to 164 mg/dL (1081). The cranial neuritis-radiculitis group is characterized by a more modest CSF pleocytosis that decreases more slowly. Although symptoms usually remit in 4 to 10 weeks, pleocytosis of up to 60 white blood cells/μL can persist for 6 to 24 weeks, but rarely longer. CSF IgM elevation occurs in all patients except those with Guillain-Barré syndrome. Blood–brain barrier disruption, which is demonstrated by elevation in lipoprotein, albumin, or α_2-microglobulin, occurs in most cases (1098).

The diagnosis of a *Mycoplasma* infection rests on elevation of the *M. pneumoniae* complement fixation (1099) or specific IgG or IgM antibody titers (1100). The increase in titer commences 7 to 9 days after the onset of symptoms and peaks at 3 to 4 weeks. IgM antibody persists for approximately 15 months, whereas CF and IgG antibodies persist for approximately 3 years (1099,1100). A fourfold rise in titer is necessary for diagnosis. An increase in cold agglutinin titers is less reliable. CNS infection can be confirmed by demonstration of *M. pneumoniae* DNA in CSF using the method of nested PCR (1101). Isolation of organisms from CSF is rarely successful.

Antimicrobial therapy has been ineffective in modifying the course of neurologic complications (1099).

Recovery is often slow and can require many months of hospitalization. Patients having focal encephalitis or nerve root involvement run the greatest risk for residua. In the Finnish series, the mortality was 10%. Severe neurologic damage such as psychomotor retardation, movement disorders, choreoathetosis, or recurrent convulsions occurred in 24% of patients. Only 52% of patients recovered completely by 2 to 26 weeks after discharge (1081). One-third of patients who recovered had permanent or persistent defects.

MYCOTIC INFECTIONS OF THE NERVOUS SYSTEM

Mycotic infections of the nervous system lead to a chronic granulomatous meningitis or abscesses. The infection can be primary or, more commonly, secondary to diabetes or other chronic illnesses, immune deficiency, debilitation, or an infection elsewhere in the body that requires antibiotic therapy (1102).

Candidiasis

Candida albicans can produce candidemia and subsequent meningitis in infants born with major congenital anomalies such as intestinal malrotation and meconium ileus, and it can complicate ventriculoatrial shunt created for hydrocephalus (1103). *Candida* meningitis also is an uncommon complication of prolonged antibiotic or corticosteroid therapy, irradiation, immune suppression, total parenteral alimentation, surgery, or extensive burns (1104,1105). The most common symptoms are headache, photophobia, nuchal rigidity, and delerium. The CSF usually shows a pleocytosis dominated by neutrophils and mononuclear cells, an elevated protein concentration, and a normal or low glucose concentration (1106). When Candida is the primary invader of the nervous system, it usually progresses to gross abscess formation; patients in whom it is a secondary invader complicating antibiotic therapy can develop diffuse cerebritis with widespread microabscesses (1107). These microabscesses are found throughout the brain in association with other granuloma-like lesions containing epithelioid and giant cells. Meningeal inflammation also can occur. *Candida* can invade the walls of blood vessels, with granulomatous vasculitis and resulting thrombi formation producing necrosis and hemorrhages (1107). Children at risk for candidemia represent a heterogeneous population, and non-*albicans* species are a more prevalent cause of infections (1108). Because candidal infection cannot be reliably diagnosed from CSF changes, culture of the organism from the CSF or from biopsies is needed for diagnosis, and large volumes (greater than 5 mL) of CSF should be cultured (1106). The subacute course, lack of a characteristic clinical picture, variable CSF findings, difficulty in recovering the organism from the CNS and its slow *in vitro* growth, and misinterpretation of positive cultures as representing contaminants all contribute to a delay in diagnosis (1105). A *Candida* cell wall component, mannan, has been used in diagnosing CNS candidosis, but it has limited value in the diagnosis of invasive candidosis (1106).

The combination of amphotericin B and 5-flucytosine is the treatment of choice (1109). This combination takes advantage of a synergistic effect and permits lower and less toxic doses of amphotericin (1104,1109). Fluconazole, an oral antifungal drug, is better tolerated than 5-fluorocytosine and has been advocated as an alternative for amphotericin B in immunocompetent patients with candidemia (1110). Because amphotericin B–resistant *Candida* species have been reported, susceptibility testing of isolates is mandatory; the mortality of fungemia is still unacceptably high (1111).

Coccidioidomycosis

Coccidioides immitis can produce a chronic meningitis, usually by inhalation of the spore form. The disease is endemic to the southwestern United States. The infection rate is particularly high in California's southern San Joaquin Valley, southern Nevada, central and southern Arizona, southern New Mexico, and throughout western Texas along the Mexican border. Outside of the United States, a high infection rate exists in the northern states of Mexico, Honduras, Venezuela, and the Chaco region of Bolivia, Paraguay, and Argentina (1112).

Symptoms are mainly headache, low-grade fever, weight loss, progressive obtundation, and minimal meningeal signs (1113). Multiple sites of obstruction can develop, particularly at the outlets of the fourth ventricle and the upper parts of the spinal cord, leading to hydrocephalus and isolation of these regions from therapy (1114). Patients with active or untreated disease usually have hydrocephalus and intense enhancement of the cervical subarachnoid space and basilar, sylvian, and interhemispheric cisterns on postcontrast MRI scans. Focal areas of ischemia or infarction are common (1115). Spinal disease can be the first manifestation of disseminated coccidioidomycosis (1116).

The CSF is almost always abnormal. Mononuclear pleocytosis ranges up to more than 1,000 cells/μL. The protein is usually elevated, whereas the glucose concentration is reduced in approximately 75% of cases (1112). *Coccidioides* spherules can be recognized in the CSF by direct examination using lactophenol cotton blue or India ink preparations or after culture.

The diagnosis of coccidioidomycosis is suggested by the presence of pulmonary lesions. A skin test result is usually positive, but can be misleading because some disseminated cases are nonreactive. The complement fixation and precipitin tests assist in the diagnosis. The precipitin test result becomes negative after approximately 3 to 4 months, however, regardless of the progression of the disease (1117).

Amphotericin B has traditionally been the recommended antibiotic for the treatment of coccidioidal meningitis. Details of treatment are given in the *Red Book* of the American Academy of Pediatrics (1118). Fluconazole, one of a series of antifungal azoles, is an effective and well-tolerated drug, which is successful in arresting the progress of the disease (1110,1119). According to Kauffman, it has replaced amphotericin as the drug of choice (1120). In addition, several lipid formulations of amphotericin that are less nephrotoxic came on the market in the late 1990s (1121). In a randomized, double-blind trial, neither fluconazole nor itraconazole showed statistically superior efficacy in nonmeningeal coccidioidomycosis, although there was a trend toward slightly greater efficacy with itraconazole (1122). Most improvement occurs within 4 to 8 months after the start of therapy. Relapses can occur in up to 25% of patients after discontinuation of prolonged therapy (1110,1123,1124). Approximately half of children with disseminated disease require surgery for debridement, central venous access, or CSF access and shunting (1125).

Coccidioidomycosis meningitis is rarely completely eradicated. Intensive follow-up is necessary, and repeated courses of antifungal therapy are required to suppress the infection.

Histoplasmosis

Histoplasmosis, caused by *Histoplasma capsulatum*, is endemic to the northeastern, central, and south-central United States (1112). CNS involvement is seen only after disseminated involvement, although clinical signs of dissemination may be lacking. The highest incidence of CNS involvement is among HIV-infected individuals (1126). It occurs in approximately one-fourth of cases with signs of clinical dissemination and in 7.6% of all *Histoplasma* infections (1127). Not all patients with CNS histoplasmosis have symptomatic disease at other sites (1128).

Infants and children younger than age 3 years can have systemic signs, including fever, anemia, or hepatosplenomegaly and, less often, weight loss, adenopathy, or cough. Neurologic symptoms are usually absent. Older children can have tetany or pyramidal tract signs (1127). The CSF is abnormal in all age groups. Hyperactive T-suppressor cells in CSF can suppress proliferative responses to Histoplasma antigen, whereas T cells from blood do not. This difference can result in a selective lack of cellular and humoral response in some patients (1129). Serologic tests are positive in only 80% of patients with disseminated histoplasmosis (1128).

Brain changes include the formation of granulomas within the parenchyma or in the perivenous regions, a meningitis that most often involves the basilar regions, and the formation of isolated abscesses. Cerebral or spinal mass lesions may resemble neoplasms (1130).

Skin tests or complement fixation tests are generally used for the diagnosis of *Histoplasma* infections. The results are often negative in patients with CNS disease, however, and a bone marrow biopsy is probably the best diagnostic procedure (1127). Brain biopsy with appropriate stains and cultures is the gold standard for diagnosis of cerebral histoplasmosis (1128,1131).

Treatment with amphotericin B is similar to the treatment for coccidioidomycosis, but various reports underline the mostly fatal prognosis (1126). Fluconazole, itraconazole, and, to a lesser extent, other azoles have proven effective alternatives to amphotericin B for *Histoplasma* meningitis (1110,1120,1126,1132). There is some evidence that combination therapy of amphotericin B plus fluconazole is not more effective than monotherapy (1133,1134).

Cryptococcosis

Cryptococcosis is one of the most common fungal infections of the nervous system. It is caused by *Cryptococcus neoformans*, an organism that is widely distributed and is often isolated from soil, particularly in the vicinity of pigeon nests (1102).

The pathologic changes in the brain vary. Some areas have only minimal inflammation, whereas others have pseudotubercles composed of giant cells, epithelioid cells, and lymphocytes. Patients with cryptococcal meningitis have significantly lower natural killer cytotoxic activity of their peripheral blood mononuclear leukocytes. This can be fully reconstituted *in vitro* with IL-2, but not with interferon-gamma (1135).

The infection is rare in children, and most affected have underlying disease such as AIDS, leukemia, SLE, or other immunosuppressive disorders (1136–1139). Adults are more commonly involved because of greater exposure and because of the predilection of cryptococcal infection for debilitated or immunocompromised individuals. African Americans with AIDS are more likely than whites with AIDS to develop the disease (1136).

Symptoms usually reflect meningeal involvement, although, occasionally, neurologic signs or alterations in mental status predominate. Children are more likely than adults to have seizures (1140). Spinal arachnoiditis can occur without meningitis (1141).

The diagnosis is difficult. Approximately one-half of patients with active cryptococcal disease have a negative cryptococcal antigen skin test result. Complement fixation, latex agglutination, fluorescent antibody, and hemagglutination tests also have been employed (1142).

The CSF in patients with cryptococcal meningitis resembles the CSF of tuberculous meningitis, with a moderate lymphocytic pleocytosis, increased protein content [more in adults than children (1140)], and decreased sugar content. The diagnosis depends on culture of organisms from the fluid or demonstration in CSF of the cryptococcal polysaccharide by latex agglutination tests. Culture-negative meningitis occurs frequently, even in experienced laboratories, although the chance of obtaining a positive culture result is higher if the CSF is dripped directly into the culture medium (1143). India ink preparations are positive in 71% of cases (1144). A latex agglutination test result can be positive, even when organisms cannot be demonstrated by other methods (1145). Neuroimaging abnormalities are present in the basal ganglia and white matter in virtually all patients (1146).

Untreated cryptococcal meningitis is fatal within a few months. In immunocompetent patients, combined therapy with amphotericin B and 5-flucytosine is the treatment of choice (1147,1148). Amphotericin B nephrotoxicity can be minimized by use of amphotericin B lipid emulsion, although anaphylaxis has been reported (1449,1150). Plasma levels of 5-flucytosine should be monitored because of the potential for bone marrow suppression (1110). Fluconazole is as effective as amphotericin B for treatment of cryptococcal meningitis in the immunocompromised host (1110,1120,1148,1151,1152).

Some of the rarer fungal infections of the nervous system are summarized in Table 7.18.

RICKETTSIAL INFECTIONS AND SCRUB TYPHUS

A number of rickettsial organisms invade the nervous system and produce neurologic symptoms. Based on serologic and clinical characteristics, six major rickettsial entities have been recognized.

The epidemic louse-borne form of typhus fever is caused by *Rickettsia prowazekii;* the endemic murine type is caused by *R. typhi.* Rocky Mountain spotted fever is caused by *R. rickettsii* in the Western hemisphere. Scrub typhus is caused by *Orientia tsutsugamushi* (formerly *R. tsutsugamushi*) and is found in Australasia (Japan, India, and Australia) (1164). *Orientia tsutsugamushi* has been removed from the genus *Rickettsia,* and a bewildering array of new rickettsial pathogens is reviewed elsewhere (1165). Q fever is caused by *Coxiella burnetii.* Rickettsialpox is caused by *R. akari,* with the agent being transmitted to humans by the mouse mite. Trench fever is transmitted to humans by the louse and is caused by *R. quintana.* Finally, *R. felis* is maintained in cat fleas by transovarian transmission (1166).

Rocky Mountain Spotted Fever

In the United States, the most common rickettsial disease is Rocky Mountain spotted fever (1167). This condition has been reported from almost all parts of the United States, notably the Appalachian and the western Rocky Mountain areas (1168). The main vectors for humans are the Rocky Mountain wood tick (*Dermacentor andersoni*); the dog tick (*Dermacentor variabilis*), which is more prevalent in the eastern United States; and the Lone Star tick (*Amblyomma americanum*), which is prevalent in the Gulf states (1169).

The rickettsial organisms invade the human by way of a tick bite followed by contamination by tick feces. Thus, early removal of the tick can prevent the disease. One can

TABLE 7.18 Characteristics of Rarer Fungal Infections of the Nervous System

Organism (Disease)	*Major Central Nervous System Symptoms*	*Therapy*	*Reference*
Actinomyces bovis (actinomycosis)	Chronic low-grade meningitis, abscesses	Penicillin, tetracycline, surgical drainage	1153
Aspergillus niger (aspergillosis)	Multiple brain abscesses, vascular thromboses	Amphotericin B	1102,1154
Aspergillus fumigatus	Meningoencephalitis, single or multiple brain abscesses, granulomas, myelopathy	Amphotericin B	1155,1156
Blastomyces dermatitidis (blastomycosis)	Meningitis	Amphotericin B, ketoconazole	1157
Cephalosporium granulomatis	Meningitis	Amphotericin B	1158
Phycomycetes rhizopus (mucormycosis)	Thromboses of cerebral and meningeal arteries	Amphotericin B	1159,1160
Nocardia asteroides (nocardiosis)	Meningitis, multiple focal abscesses	Sulfadiazine or trimethoprim-sulfamethoxazole	1161–1163

best remove a tick by grasping its body with a pair of tweezers and applying gentle traction until it releases its hold in 30 to 60 seconds. This method also reduces the chance of leaving behind the head with biting mouth.

Rickettsia first enter the nuclei of the capillary endothelial cells, where they multiply and destroy the cells. The lesions extend along the blood vessels to the arterioles, where smooth muscle cells of the media are invaded and destroyed. Vascular lesions result in scattered thrombosis and extravasation of blood, producing microinfarcts. Alterations within the nervous system are more striking in Rocky Mountain spotted fever than in any of the other rickettsial diseases. The patient has areas of petechial hemorrhages, perivascular infiltration, glial nodules, and minute sites of focal necrosis. Patches of demyelination are seen throughout the brain (1170).

Clinical Manifestations

Neurologic symptoms are prominent in Rocky Mountain spotted fever. Meningoencephalitis, a major manifestation of the disease, evolves after an incubation period of 4 to 8 days (1171). The acute phase begins with headache, myalgia, fever, and shaking chills. Meningeal signs can be prominent (1172). Mental confusion, hallucination, or delirium can appear and progress to coma. Muscular twitchings, fibrillary tremors, fasciculations, and convulsions are common. Focal motor seizures can occur. A variety of neurologic signs, including diffuse hyper-reflexia, choreoathetosis, sixth-nerve palsies, alteration in pupillary size and reflexes, cerebellar signs, and neurogenic bladder, can develop (1173). Deafness often develops during the acute illness (1174). A variety of ophthalmologic signs have been noted, including retinal edema, papilledema, and choroiditis. Choked discs can be observed in the presence of normal intracranial pressure as a consequence of vasculitis (1175). Intracranial hemorrhage can result from thrombocytopenia and hypofibrinogenemia secondary to intravascular coagulation (1176).

After several days of fever, the rash usually begins over the extremities. Approximately 10% of patients do not develop a rash (1177). When present, it spreads centripetally, and in 2 to 3 days changes from a macular to a maculopapular petechial eruption. Hemorrhagic areas can coalesce to form ecchymotic lesions. At this point, myocardial involvement can lead to cardiac failure with hypotension, tachycardia, and shock. Renal and hepatic involvements result in oliguria and hypoproteinemia with generalized edema.

Residual neurologic deficits might not be immediately apparent. At reevaluation after 1 to 8 years, 16% of survivors showed definite neurologic abnormalities, although one-half of this group had no objective changes during the acute phase of the illness. A variety of neurologic residua were observed, including mental retardation, behavioral disturbances, impairment of coordination, and hypotonia. In one-third of patients, the EEG was persistently abnormal (1176). Perceptuomotor deficits also have been observed as a late sequela (1178).

Diagnosis

The diagnosis of Rocky Mountain spotted fever rests in part on a history of exposure and the development of the characteristic rash. Rocky Mountain spotted fever should be considered as a diagnosis in family members and contacts who have febrile illness and share environmental exposures with the patient (1179). The CSF is normal in 56% of cases. In the remainder, white blood cell count can range from 11 to 300 cells/μL; only one-fourth of these have more than 50% polymorphonuclear cells. Modest elevations in protein content occur in approximately 33% of cases; the sugar content remains normal. Laboratory diagnosis can be made by complement fixation, rickettsial agglutination, Felix-Weil reaction, or indirect fluorescent antibody studies (1180). It is noteworthy that the relatively high provalence of seropositivity among children living in the southern United States suggests that infection with *R. rickettsii* may be common and subclinical. Thus, we should be cautious in interpreting single immunofluorescence antibody assay titers in children with suspected Rocky Mountain spotted fever (1181).

Treatment

Chloramphenicol or a tetracycline is the preferred antibiotic. Doxycycline is the agent of choice in children 8 years of age and younger. They are continued until at least 1 week after the patient has become afebrile. Intravenous tetracycline should be avoided because it can cause hepatic necrosis (1182). High mortality rates in untreated patients and rapid progression of illness to death among fatal cases highlight the need for rapid treatment decisions. Understanding the appropriate time and place for empiric therapy is important both in limiting iatrogenic events stemming from ineffective antibiotic prophylaxis and also in minimizing morbidity and mortality from delayed diagnosis or undertreatment of Rocky Mountain spotted fever (1177).

For a discussion of the neurologic complications of typhus and the other rickettsial infections, the reader is referred to the classic papers by Noad and Haymaker on the complications of scrub typhus (tsutsugamushi fever) (1183) and by Herman on typhus fever (1184). Chloramphenicol-resistant and doxycycline-resistant strains of scrub typhus have been reported (1185).

Q Fever

Although Q fever usually presents as a febrile illness with mild to moderate pneumonia, headache is the most common neurologic manifestation of *Coxiella burnetii* infection. Children are less frequently symptomatic than adults following infection, and may have milder cases (1186). Lymphocytic meningitis and encephalitis can occur with minimal changes in the CSF (1187).

PROTOZOAL AND PARASITIC INFECTIONS OF THE NERVOUS SYSTEM

Aside from toxoplasmosis and cysticercosis, no protozoal and parasitic organisms commonly invade the nervous system of children in the United States and Western Europe (1188).

Generally, parasitic infestations of the CNS can produce diffuse symptoms of meningoencephalitis, a space-occupying lesion, or lesions caused by the migration of larvae through brain substance.

Cysticercosis

Cysticercosis of the CNS has become a relatively common entity in those areas of the United States settled by immigrants from various Latin American countries. The condition is not unusual in Chile, Mexico, Peru, India, and the Middle East. In Mexico, for instance, cysticercosis accounts for approximately 25% of intracranial tumors. The infection is almost always caused by the encysted form of *Taenia solium*. In the parenchymatous form of cysticercosis, the organisms encyst within the parenchyma of the brain. They also can seed into the ventricles or cisterns, producing chronic inflammation of the leptomeninges and ependyma. The inflammation becomes much worse after the death of the organisms (1189). Serial CT or MR scans demonstrate that cysts can disappear in a few months or can progress to residual calcified lesions (1190–1192).

The most common symptoms are focal or generalized seizures, found as the presenting feature in up to 90% of patients (1193,1194); increased intracranial pressure, found in 44% to 75% of cases (1193–1195); and cranial nerve palsies. Tumor and encephalitic and basilar meningitic forms of infestation also have been described (1189,1196).

Cysts, sometimes free floating, can occur in the CSF. These can cause acute neurologic symptoms by obstructing the aqueduct if they are in the third ventricle (1197). Cysts can cause spinal cord compression if they are in the spinal canal. CT visualization may require CSF contrast media.

The racemose form of cyst can invade the ventricular or subarachnoid spaces and persist there for many years. Intermittent rupture of cysts contiguous to CSF can cause a marked inflammatory response with transient high fevers. In approximately one-third to two-thirds of cases, CSF eosinophilia is present. Approximately one-half of patients show intracranial calcification by CT scan (1195). Kramer and associates documented the natural history of cerebral cysticercosis with serial CT scans. In the early acute stage, they found focal nonenhancing areas of edema that progress to homogeneously enhancing lesions. In the chronic phase, beginning a few months after infestation, nonenhancing cysts occur that later demonstrate ring enhancement. Lesions can completely resolve then, or they can resolve totally or partially before developing punctate calcifications (1190). Positive CSF serology results are diagnostic. For a detailed review of the neurologic aspects of cysticercosis, see the publication by Garg (1198).

Praziquantel is effective against the parenchymatous form of the disease but has limited usefulness against the racemose form. The treatment of cysticercosis with praziquantel and albendazole is reviewed by Liu and coworkers (1199) and Bale (1200). When cysts produce CSF obstruction, they must be removed surgically (1189).

In the United States, parenchymatous cerebral cysticercosis has a good prognosis. Seizures are usually easily controlled and the disease is self-limited and does not require therapy (1201). Albendazole is recommended for the treatment of persistent, solitary cysticercosis granulomas in patients with seizures (1202).

Trichinosis

Trichinosis is caused by a nematode, *Trichinella spiralis*, that most often infests live pigs and is ingested when pork is raw or poorly cooked. The encysted larvae escape to all parts of the body by the bloodstream but survive and grow only in skeletal muscle.

Microscopy reveals parasites within the muscle fibers, where they set up a focal inflammation and ultimately become calcified. Within the CNS, filiform larvae are found in the capillaries and in parenchyma, where they cause a focal inflammatory response (1203).

The clinical picture is highlighted by fever, myalgia, and abdominal pain. Muscles innervated by the cranial nerves, including the extraocular and masticatory muscles, can be involved. In 10% to 20% of infestations, the nervous system also is invaded within the first weeks of the onset of infection. CNS damage can be caused by larval migration, vascular obstruction, toxic parasite antigens, and inflammatory and eosinophile infiltration (1204). Encephalitis or meningeal signs can be present along with papilledema and focal neurologic abnormalities including bilateral facial palsies (1205,1206). Sagittal sinus thrombosis can occur (1207), and the disease can be fatal (1208).

The most striking laboratory findings include eosinophilia and occasional electrocardiographic abnormalities compatible with a myocarditis. The diagnosis rests on a history of potential exposure, persistent eosinophilia, increasing serum antibody titer, and positive muscle biopsy result. In approximately one-fourth of patients, larvae are seen in the CSF (1205).

Mebendazole is the recommended treatment (1209). Thiabendazole (25 mg/kg twice a day for 5 to 7 days) kills adult worms in the intestine but seems to be ineffective against encysted larvae. Corticosteroids are recommended for severe symptoms to reduce inflammation and edema, but improvement is generally not dramatic.

When the infection has not been extensive, the prognosis for survival is good, but weakness and electrocardiographic abnormalities can persist for long periods after apparent clinical recovery. In chronic infections, radiography of the muscles, particularly those of the gastrocnemius, reveals the calcified filarial cysts.

Cerebral Malaria

Malaria remains one of the most important causes of childhood mortality and morbidity worldwide. The World Health Organization estimated that at least 1 million children die of malaria annually in Africa (1210). The vast majority of deaths from malaria are caused by cerebral malaria, which is the most common, severe, and potentially fatal complication of *Plasmodium falciparum* infection. The clinical severity of malaria is highly dependent on the malaria-specific immune status of the infected individual.

In malaria-endemic countries, cerebral malaria most commonly affects young children. However, in nonendemic areas and in nonimmune travelers who acquire malaria, cerebral malaria can occur at any age (1211,1212). In the past, it was assumed that most patients who recover from acute cerebral malaria have no sequelae of the illness. However, increasingly it is recognized that a significant proportion of survivors are left with long-term neurologic sequelae (1213,1214). Cerebral malaria is, therefore, an important cause of long-term childhood neurologic disability in many countries.

Pathophysiology

A major impediment to improving the prognosis of cerebral malaria is the inadequate understanding of the pathophysiology of the disorder. Early neuropathologic studies indicated that cerebral malaria was associated with preferential sequestration of parasitized erythrocytes within the cerebral microvasculature (1215). These observations led to the hypothesis that sequestration of parasitized cells in the cerebral capillary bed is a key initial step in the pathogenesis of cerebral malaria (1216,1217). Although more recent studies in fatal cases have confirmed that there are indeed large numbers of parasitized red blood cells within capillaries, a number of features argue against simple mechanical occlusion of the vasculature by parasitized erythrocytes as the prime cause of the disorder (1211,1217). Diffuse encephalopathy, rather than focal neurologic abnormalities, is the usual manifestation of cerebral malaria. Furthermore, complete recovery of neurologic function occurs in a majority of patients, including those who have been in deep coma. Such a course would be unlikely if thrombotic occlusion of the vasculature had occurred.

Adherence of parasitized red cells to the endothelium occurs through a specific, receptor-mediated interaction. Many different endothelial receptors for infected red cells have been identified (1218). Some, notably CD 36 and thrombospondin, are used by all strains of malaria parasites, others, such as intercellular adhesion molecule-1 (ICAM-1), are specific for certain parasite strains (1219). Binding to ICAM-1 is highest in patients with cerebral malaria, with the degree of binding correlating with the severity of the illness (1219). Genetic factors also appear to play a role in the degree of binding of parasitized red cells in cerebral vascular endothelium. Individuals homozygous for certain mutations in the gene coding for ICAM-1 have an increased susceptibility to develop severe cerebral malaria (1220).

Intact parasitized red cells can modulate the immune system by adherence to dendritic cells, thereby inhibiting their maturation and their capacity to stimulate T cells (1221). Cytokines such as TNF, released during malaria infection, may increase expression of ICAM-1 and facilitate increased adherence of parasitized cells within the cerebral circulation (1222,1223). The mechanisms by which parasitized red cells within the cerebral circulation alter brain function are unclear. Candidate toxic mediators include malaria-derived cytokines such as TNF, and nitric oxide (1215,1223,1224). TNF levels are increased in children with severe malaria and are higher in those who die in comparison with survivors (1225). Increased IL-1 levels also correlate positively with outcome (1225–1227). It is unclear, however, whether TNF is a specific mediator of the inflammatory process in cerebral malaria or simply a marker of the severity of that process. Anti-TNF therapy, however, inhibits fever in cerebral malaria (1228).

Metabolic factors also have been implicated in the pathophysiology of cerebral malaria. Hypoglycemia is found in almost one-third of children with cerebral malaria, and children who are hypoglycemic on admission are at significantly greater risk of death from the development of neurologic sequelae (1229,1230). Hypoglycemia is accompanied by elevated plasma lactate levels, with acidosis and lactate concentrations in plasma and CSF being significantly higher in patients with a poor outcome than in those who make a full recovery (1229). Among the metabolic derangements, acidosis has emerged as a central feature of severe malaria and the major predictor of a fatal outcome (1231). Plasma insulin concentrations are appropriately low, suggesting that inhibition of gluconeogenesis is the most likely mechanism responsible for hypoglycemia (1229,1232). Competition between parasites and host cells for essential nutrients may contribute to the metabolic derangement. Release of toxic metabolites that impair brain cell metabolism also may occur (1211). An association between some cases of fatal cerebral malaria and inducible nitric oxide synthase polymorphism (*NOS2* locus) has been reported (1233).

Little evidence exists to suggest cerebral edema plays a significant role in the pathophysiology of cerebral malaria, even though MRI shows brain volume to be increased during the acute phase of cerebral malaria. Instead, this results from an increase in the volume of intracerebral blood, probably the consequence of the sequestration of parasitized erythrocytes (1234). Turner (1215) and Miller and coworkers (1235) reviewed the pathophysiology of cerebral malaria.

Clinical Manifestations

The clinical features of cerebral malaria are those of an acute encephalopathic illness, and overlap other infective and metabolic causes of childhood encephalopathy (1236,1237). In the series of Newton and Warrell, 82% of children with cerebral malaria developed seizures before hospitalization (1238). Another 15% were deeply unconscious, with a Glasgow Coma Score of less than 6. Hypoglycemia was seen in 23% and metabolic acidosis in 42%. Retinal hemorrhage was noted in 6% (1238). In children younger than 5 years of age, the disease typically presents with fever, headache, malaise, anorexia, and vomiting. Neurologic signs are those of a diffuse encephalopathy with symmetric upper motor neuron signs and brainstem disturbances, including dysconjugate gaze, palsies, hypotonicity or hypertonicity, extensor plantar responses, absent abdominal reflexes, and stertorous breathing. Retinal hemorrhages can be present, and decorticate and decerebrate posturing are seen in severe cases (1229,1239).

Diagnosis

In malaria-endemic areas, two difficulties exist in the diagnosis of cerebral malaria. First, malaria parasitemia in a child with neurologic abnormalities does not exclude the possibility of other diagnoses such as bacterial meningitis. Second is the converse: Occasionally, patients with cerebral malaria may not have detectable *P. falciparum* in the peripheral blood, either because of sequestration of the parasitized cells within the vasculature or due to previous antimalarial treatment. In such cases, treatment for cerebral malaria must always be commenced without awaiting definite confirmation of the diagnosis (1236,1237). PCR is used mainly to confirm positive blood smears and is valuable in identification of malaria species (1240). In children with malaria who have experienced febrile convulsions, the possibility of cerebral malaria must always be considered if neurologic abnormality persists or progresses 30 minutes after convulsions have stopped. Lumbar puncture is generally required to exclude the possibility of bacterial meningitis. The CSF in cerebral malaria contains normal numbers of white blood cells and normal or minimally elevated concentrations of protein. CSF glucose may be depressed and CSF lactate increased (1229,1241). All of the clinical features of cerebral malaria can be seen in other bacterial and viral infections of the CNS or in a variety of metabolic disorders (1236,1237,1241). Imaging studies may reveal nonspecific findings that are consistent with cerebral edema or ischemia (1240).

Treatment

In childhood malaria, death can occur within hours of the onset of illness. Antimalarial drugs are the only specific therapy known to arrest the infection, and children suspected of having cerebral malaria must receive the best available antimalarials by the parenteral route as quickly as possible. Specific therapy should not be delayed if cerebral malaria is suspected but cannot be ruled out by appropriate investigations. Parenteral quinine is recommended in most countries for patients with cerebral malaria because of the worldwide spread of chloroquine-resistant *P. falciparum*. In countries with low levels of chloroquine resistance, chloroquine is often given to patients with uncomplicated malaria, with quinine being reserved for those with severe malaria. Even with parenteral administration, quinine may take up to 48 hours to achieve desirable plasma concentrations, and a loading dose is frequently recommended (1242). Quinine dihydrochloride is given in a dose of 20 mg of salt (16.7 mg of base) per kg body weight by intravenous infusion over 4 hours as a loading dose, followed by 10 mg of salt (8.3 mg of base) per kg infused over 4 hours, every 12 hours until the patient regains consciousness. Quinidine gluconate is used as an alternative to quinine in some countries (1243). Quinine may be given by intramuscular route if intravenous access is difficult. Careful monitoring of blood glucose is required, although hyperinsulinemia has rarely been documented during treatment of children with cerebral malaria. Quinine does not result in rapid parasite clearance, and many regimes use additional antimalarial agents such as pyrimethamine sulfadoxine or mefloquine to ensure parasite killing once consciousness has been regained.

A number of new antimalarial agents have been evaluated for use in cerebral malaria, particularly in regions where multidrug-resistant parasites are increasingly found. The artemethrin derivative artemetha, developed in China from the traditional remedy Qinghausu, is among the most promising antimalarial drugs (1244). In studies in Malawi, artemetha was found to clear parasitemia more rapidly than quinine and was associated with more rapid recovery from coma (1245). Mortality for children treated with artemether (20.5%) is similar to that for children treated with quinine (21.5%) (1246). Further trials are required to establish whether this agent is associated with improved mortality. In areas of the world, such as the Thai–Burmese border, where an increasing resistance of organisms to quinine has occurred, combination regimes of quinine with tetracycline cotrimoxazole or artemisinin or its derivatives may be required. In some areas of Africa combined therapy of artemisinin or its derivatives and pyrimethamine-sulfadoxine has been recommended (1247). Some of the less prevalent antiparasitic drugs (1248) are available from the Parasitic Disease Drug Service of the Centers for Disease Control and Prevention in Atlanta. Artemisinin derivatives are suited for use in rural zones (1249–1253).

As in any comatose patients, successful outcome of patients with cerebral malaria also depends on control of convulsions, with particular attention to fluid and electrolyte balance, maintenance of the airway, and good nursing care. Disruption in axonal transport may represent a final common pathway leading to neurologic dysfunction in cerebral malaria (1254). The vast majority of patients with cerebral malaria are treated in hospitals with minimal facilities for intensive medical support. Patients with cerebral malaria in more-developed countries are treated with full intensive care support, including elective ventilation to optimize cerebral perfusion. A wide number of adjunctive agents have been suggested as being beneficial in the treatment of cerebral malaria. These include corticosteroids, heparin, mannitol, low-molecular-weight dextran, prostacyclin, TNF antibodies, and desferrioxamine. Most of these agents have not been subjected to controlled clinical trials or clinical trials have shown no benefit. However, a randomized, double-blind, placebo-controlled trial of iron chelation therapy with desferrioxamine documented more rapid resolution of coma and increased parasite clearance in patients receiving desferrioxamine (1255). Further trials of this and other experimental agents such as anti-TNF antibodies are required before any specific recommendations can be made. Parecetamol significantly delays the clearance time of *P. falciparum* in children; its role in the treatment of malaria is uncertain (1256).

Prognosis

The mortality for patients admitted with cerebral malaria ranges from 6% to 30% in different series. Some of the variation in mortality is explained by differences in the criteria for diagnosis (1229). A number of clinical and laboratory features that are present on admission of children with cerebral malaria are predictive of severe disease and a poor outcome. These include profound coma, signs of decerebration, absence of corneal reflex, and convulsions at the time of admission. Laboratory findings predictive of a poor outcome are hypoglycemia, leukocytosis, hyperparasitemia, elevated concentrations of alanine and 5-nucleotidase, elevated plasma or CSF lactate, and pigmented monocytes and neutrophils (1229,1257).

Although in the past, survivors of cerebral malaria were thought to have an excellent prognosis for full neurologic recovery, more recent studies from several countries have documented a significant rate of long-term neurologic sequelae (1213,1229). Approximately 10% to 30% of survivors experience neurologic deficits including hemiplegia, ataxia, and generalized motor deficits, with spasticity or hypotonia (1238,1258). The prevalence of epilepsy is more than twice that reported after complicated febrile seizures (1259). No detailed studies are available of long-term effects on intellect or later development. It is likely that an even greater proportion of survivors have experienced subtle long-term residua (1214). Persistence of neurologic abnormalities is associated with the same poor prognostic features that are predictive of increased mortality.

A postmalaria neurologic syndrome occurs rarely in patients who have recovered from *P. falciparum* malaria. It occurs more often after treatment with mefloquine, but also occurs in patients who have not received this drug. This syndrome usually occurs within 2 months after recovery from malaria and usually lasts 1 to 10 days. It is characterized by one or more of the following: psychosis or acute confusional episodes, generalized convulsions, tremors, or fever. At the time of this complication, blood smear results for malaria parasites are negative. CSF can show a mild pleocytosis (8 to 80 white blood cells) with lymphocyte predominance and a mild elevation in protein (1260).

Prophylaxis

Chloroquine can no longer be recommended for prophylaxis because of widespread resistance to the drug, especially in Africa. Resistance to sulfadoxine/pyrimethamine also has been reported in Africa. A combination of atovaquone plus proguanil prophylaxis has been recommended in children (1261).

Trypanosomiasis

The CNS can be involved in both African and American trypanosomiasis. African trypanosomiasis is caused by *Trypanosoma brucei,* of which there are two subspecies, *gambiense* and *rhodesiense.* CNS involvement is the major clinical complication of African trypanosomiasis and is fatal if untreated.

Pathogenesis and Pathology

African trypanosomiasis is transmitted to humans by the bite of blood-sucking flies of the genus *Glossina* (tsetse fly). The *gambiense* form occurs in West and central sub-Saharan Africa and the *rhodesiense* form occurs in east and south East Africa. Although 25 to 50 million people live in areas of Africa where the disease is endemic, the disease is distributed in patches in approximately 200 known hyperendemic foci. The official incidence figures of 20,000 to 25,000 cases annually are probably a substantial underestimate, considering that over 7,000 cases were diagnosed in 1987 alone in an epidemic in Uganda (1262,1263).

The pathogenesis of trypanosomiasis is not completely understood. Parasites enter the body after the bite of the infected fly. Active parasite replication and invasion of local tissues occurs, leading to an inflammatory nodule at the site of the bite. The trypanosomes enter the lymphatics, causing lymphadenopathy, and the bloodstream, causing parasitemia. During the hemolymphatic stage of the illness, recurrent episodes of fever and constitutional symptoms occur, which remit spontaneously and are followed by intervening periods of well-being (1264). The trypanosomes are coated with a glycoprotein called the variant surface glycoprotein, which shields underlying structures from host antibodies. Each parasite has more than 1,000 different genes for this protein, only one form of which is expressed on the surface of the parasite at a particular point in time (1264,1265). The production of host antibodies to this antigenic surface results in clearance of the parasite from the blood and cessation of symptoms. However, a new wave of parasitemia follows, resulting from the growth of a population of parasites with a new, antigenically distinct surface glycoprotein. This cycle of parasite proliferation and humeral immune response may be repeated for months or years and is associated with a marked elevation in immunoglobulins. Eventually, the parasite invades the brain, probably via the choroid plexus, and induces a lymphocytic/plasmacytic meningoencephalitis. An interaction of the parasite with the cytokine network of the host is believed to play a role in the proliferation of the parasite and in evoking the inflammation (1265,1266). Inflammatory lesions occur predominantly in a perivascular distribution with sparing of neuronal elements. In some fatal cases, demyelination and choroid plexus involvement occur. An acute hemorrhagic encephalopathy with discrete and confluent hemorrhages also can occur (1267,1268). The mechanisms by which trypanosomes damage the brain are unclear. It has been suggested that toxins produced by the trypanosomes induce vascular injury or induce a CNS metabolic derangement (1265,1266). Alternatively, brain injury may be caused by the host inflammatory response, and evidence of autoantibodies directed against brain myelin proteins can be detected in a high proportion of cases (1269). Immunofluorescence studies have shown deposition of complement and immunoglobulins in brain tissue, suggesting immune complex deposition as a mechanism of vascular injury (1270).

Clinical Manifestations

Clinical features of the East African and West African forms of trypanosomiasis differ, with *T. rhodesiense* causing a much more acute and fulminant disease. In *T. rhodesiense* infection, the CNS involvement occurs early, with death occurring within weeks to months in untreated cases. The *gambiense* form of the disease is indolent and is characterized by prominent lymphadenopathy, a gradual onset, and late CNS involvement. The illness may last months to years. The hemolymphatic stage of both diseases is associated with constitutional symptoms, such as weakness, joint pains, weight loss, and headache (1271). Major CNS symptoms include headache, alterations in mentation and behavior, abnormal sleep patterns, and progressive deterioration of consciousness. Psychological and behavioral changes, including personality disorder, psychosis, and major affective disorders, are common (1272). Excessive sleeping increases as the disease progresses. Extrapyramidal symptoms and signs, with cerebellar ataxia, parkinsonian rigidity, and convulsions, appear as the disease progresses, as does papilledema. Stupor and coma ultimately develop, and the mortality in untreated cases approaches 100% (1273).

Diagnosis

Diagnosis depends on the demonstration of parasites in fluid aspirates from chancre or lymph nodes or in blood, bone marrow, or CSF. Repeated examinations may be necessary because of the cyclic nature of parasitemia (1274). CSF abnormality is always present in severe disease, with pleocytosis and elevated protein. Microscopically visible trypanosomes are found in less than 20% of cases. CSF immunoglobulin, particularly IgM, is increased markedly. Serologic methods are available for detecting antibodies against the parasite in both the blood and CSF (1274). Trypanosomiasis-related immunoglobulin patterns are of value in differential diagnosis (1275).

Treatment

Treatment of cerebral trypanosomiasis is difficult. Intravenous suramin is effective in the lymphatic stage of the disease, but is ineffective once CNS invasion occurs (1264,1276). Pentamidine can be used in early cases of *T. gambiense* infection, but is ineffective against *T. rhodesiense* disease. The only agent that can penetrate the CNS and is effective in CNS disease is melarsoprol, which is given as a single daily intravenous injection of 3.6 mg/kg for 3 days and is repeated three times with a rest period of 7 days between courses (1276,1277). Patients with severe disease also should receive a short course of suramin before receiving melarsoprol. Of treated patients, 10% to 18% experience severe complications of treatment with symptoms of arsenical encephalopathy, which may be fatal (1266). A number of other agents are under investigation that may prove to be less toxic, including difluoromethyl ornithine (DFMO) (1278).

American Trypanosomiasis

CNS disease is extremely rare in adult Chagas disease, but is seen as a complication of congenital infection with *Trypanosoma cruzi* (1279). Transmission to the fetus occurs in 2% of pregnancies if the mother is seropositive.

The majority of cases of Chagas disease with CNS involvement are in children younger than 1 year of age. Parasites can be found in the CSF after acute infection at any age, but clinical or pathologic meningoencephalitis is rare. It is usually fatal when it does occur. Histologic findings are those of scattered granulomas in which amastigote forms of the parasite can be found (1280).

Acute chagasic encephalitis manifests with a range of signs from tremor to spasticity, coma, and convulsions (1281). Infants with congenital infection show delayed development or regression. Diagnosis can be established by finding parasites in the blood, tissues, or CSF. Serologic testing can be helpful. Treatment is with the trypanocides nifurtimox and benznidazole.

Echinococcosis (Hydatid Disease)

Hydatid cysts in the CNS produce symptoms of space-occupying lesions. In children, they are found in the brain (77%), spine (18%), and skull (8%) (1282,1283). The preferred management is surgical extirpation (1282,1284). Prolonged courses of mebendazole or albendazole have been used in inoperable cases (1284).

Amebic Infections of the Central Nervous System

Amebic infections of the CNS caused by both pathogenic and free-living amebas occur infrequently. Cerebral amebiasis occurs when *Entamoeba histolytica* spreads from its normal site of infection in the bowel to cause amebic abscesses within the CNS (1285). Considering that in any year more than 400 million people are infected with *E. histolytica,* CNS infection is remarkably rare. Most patients with amebic brain abscesses are young adults, and the disease affects male much more than female patients. The majority of reported patients died, possibly because the diagnosis is seldom made during life (1286). At necropsy, the brain is swollen with areas of focal meningitis. Multiple focal, hemorrhagic necrotic lesions are usually found, the walls of which are infiltrated by mononuclear cells. Amebas may be identified within these necrotic lesions. The presenting features are indistinguishable from those of brain abscesses or tumors (1287). Computed tomography and magnetic resonance imaging are helpful in the diagnosis of cerebral hydatid disease (1288). CSF may be normal or show nonspecific changes, and biopsy of the lesions may be required to establish the diagnosis. It is likely that prompt treatment with metronidazole coupled with surgical aspiration or excision of accessible lesions may improve the prognosis of what has been up to now a largely fatal illness (1289).

Primary amebic meningoencephalitis is caused by free-living amebas belonging to two genera, *Naegleria* and *Acanthamoeba.* The organisms flourish in warm, moist conditions, and infection in children is usually acquired while swimming in unchlorinated freshwater sources (1290). *N. fowleri* is the most common species associated with acute primary amebic meningoencephalitis, whereas *Acanthamoeba* may cause a more chronic granulomatous amebic encephalitis. The amebas enter the nasal cavity during swimming or diving and, in some patients, invade the roof of the nasal cavity, crossing the olfactory epithelium and ascending into the anterior cranial fossa through the cribriform plate. The amebas reach the meninges surrounding the frontal lobes, where they multiply, spread, and destroy the brain substance (1291). Less commonly, bloodstream invasion can occur. *Acanthamoeba* species also can invade the CNS from a primary corneal infection of the eye (1291).

The histologic findings are severe meningoencephalitis and necrosis (1292). An intense polymorphonuclear infiltrate occurs, with areas of hemorrhage and necrosis. In cases of *Acanthamoeba* infection, single or multiple brain abscesses can be found, and histologic findings of granulomatous meningitis can be present.

The acute form of primary amebic meningoencephalitis presents with sudden onset of high fever, photophobia, headache, and progression to coma (1293). The initial features are indistinguishable from those of acute bacterial meningitis. Subacute or chronic meningoencephalitis can present more insidiously with symptoms suggesting a brain tumor or abscess. Most cases are diagnosed initially as having bacterial meningitis. The CSF is consistent with findings of bacterial meningitis with pleocytosis, hypoglycorrhachia, and elevated protein concentration. The diagnosis can be made before death by examination of fresh, warm specimens of CSF to detect ameboid movements of the motile trophozoites. Identification of organisms by PCR is under investigation (1294). After death, the parasite can be visualized with light or electron microscopy within the brain. In the chronic form of the disorder, no trophozoites are found in the CSF and the diagnosis can only be made by biopsy of a necrotic lesion detected by neuroimaging.

The free-living amebas are sensitive to a variety of antimicrobial agents, including amphotericin B, pentamidine, tetracycline, and rifampicin. Most of the reported cases have been fatal, but treatment with intravenous pentamidine or with amphotericin and rifampicin may reduce the mortality if diagnosis is made early (1295,1296).

NEMATODE INFECTIONS

Angiostrongyliasis

The nematode *Angiostrongylus cantonensis* is a common cause of eosinophilic meningitis in many countries, including Thailand, Malaysia, Vietnam, and the Pacific Islands. Additional cases have been reported from the Middle East and Africa (1297). Rats are the definitive host of the parasite, and human infection follows ingestion of the larvae present in contaminated foods such as mollusks. The larvae migrate to the CNS, where they die and initiate an intense inflammatory process. Symptoms begin 6 to 30 days after ingesting raw mollusks and include headache, stiff neck, paresthesias, and vomiting. The CSF characteristically shows leukocytosis with a high proportion of eosinophils and elevated protein concentration. Immuno-PCR is a promising technique for diagnosis of *A. cantonensis* infection (1298).

The prognosis is generally good. Most patients recover within 1 or 2 weeks, but full resolution of symptoms may take considerably longer (1299). The treatment is symptomatic, although thiabendazole may hasten clearance of the parasite. The neurologic complications of strongyloidiasis were reviewed by Lowichik and Ruff (1300).

Gnathostomiasis

Gnathostoma spinigerum may cause a serious CNS infection acquired by ingestion of raw or partially cooked animal flesh. The parasite is widely distributed in the Far East, and although most cases have been reported from Thailand and Japan, the disease has now been recognized in various parts of Mexico (1301). The parasite causes a variety of neurologic syndromes including radiculomyelitis, encephalitis, and subarachnoid or intracerebral hemorrhage (1302). Highly motile larvae or worms invade nerve roots and migrate to the spinal canal or the spinal cord itself, from which they migrate to the brain. This explains the diverse clinical findings of radicular pain, radicular myelitis, eosinophilic meningitis, or encephalitis. In endemic areas, painless migratory subcutaneous edema is highly suggestive of the subcutaneous form of the disease. CNS involvement is suggested by sudden onset of severe radicular pain followed by CNS signs (1303). Typical CSF findings are a moderate leukocytosis with a high percentage of eosinophils, elevated protein, and elevated blood cells. Serology is the criterion standard for diagnosing gnathostomiasis, whereas MR imaging represents a complimentary tool for assessing severity and extent of disease (1304).

No specific drug treatment has been shown to be of benefit, and patients have to be treated symptomatically. Corticosteroids may be used to reduce inflammation and edema.

Toxocariasis

Nematodes of the genus *Toxocara* are common parasites of dogs and cats, and humans become infected through ingestion of soil containing ova, which hatch in the small intestine to produce larvae that pass through the intestinal wall and migrate into the tissues. Visceral larvae migrans refers to the disorder produced during migration of the larvae through the organs. The larvae elicit granulomatous inflammation associated with eosinophilia. When the larvae come to rest in the tissues, necrosis develops in the surrounding area, with infiltration of polymorphonuclear cells, eosinophils, and histiocytes. Focal granuloma with multinucleated giant cells may develop. Because toxocariasis is rarely fatal, only a few descriptions of CNS pathology in this disorder are found (1305).

Seroprevalence studies indicate that *Toxocara* infection is common in young children, with a majority of the infections being asymptomatic. The usual manifestations of visceral larvae migrans are abdominal pain, anorexia, nausea, vomiting, behavior disturbance, cough, wheeze, and fever. Striking eosinophilia is usually present and should suggest the diagnosis. The most common CNS symptom is headache, which is present in a high proportion of cases but may be unrelated to direct CNS invasion. Encephalitis, myelitis, and seizures are reported (1306–308). Children with idiopathic epilepsy have antitoxocaral antibodies more often than controls. This association has led to the suggestion that in some instances toxocariasis can be a precipitant of epilepsy (1309). Although people of all ages are at risk, the more severe symptoms occur mainly in children ages 1 to 7 years (1310).

CENTRAL NERVOUS SYSTEM DISEASE CAUSED BY TREMATODES

Schistosomiasis

Schistosomiasis is one of the most important parasitic diseases, occurring in more than 200 million people worldwide. Of the various *Schistosoma* species, *S. mansoni*, *S. haematobium*, and *S. japonicum* are the most common disease-causing organisms (1311). CNS schistosomiasis usually follows migration of adult worms to the CNS, with eggs being laid in the spinal cord or brain vasculature. In other cases, eggs are embolized from the portal mesenteric system to the brain and spinal cord (1312). The size of the eggs produced by the different species determines the site of CNS involvement (1313). *S. japonicum* eggs are more likely to reach the brain, whereas the larger eggs of *S. mansoni* cause mostly spinal lesions. *S. haematobium* also causes mainly spinal cord disease. The presence of eggs within the CNS can elicit an inflammatory reaction characterized by infiltration of lymphocytes, eosinophils, and macrophages and lead to a florid granulomatous reaction (1311).

Acute schistosomiasis occurs predominantly in children, adolescents, and young adults. Neurologic syndromes can occur in nonimmune individuals with Katayama fever, which probably results from an immunologic reaction to cercaria, schistosomula, and eggs (1312). Mental confusion, seizures, coma, visual defects, and signs of increased intracranial pressure can occur. Occasionally, hemiplegia or other focal neurologic signs can occur. Schistosomal myelopathy is more commonly symptomatic than cerebral schistosomiasis (1313,1314). Symptoms, which depend on the site of involvement, include paraplegia, sphincter dysfunction, areflexia, radiculopathy, and a rapidly progressive transverse myelitis usually affecting the lumbosacral segments of the spinal cord. These reflect the presence of single or multiple granulomata in the spinal cord with cord compression and necrosis (1311). Examination of the CSF in acute schistosomiasis can show an increase in protein concentration and lymphocytosis with eosinophilia (1315).

Neurologic symptoms occurring in chronic schistosomiasis include headache, confusion, seizures, and incoordination. Schistosomal myeloradiculopathy is less frequent than cerebral disease (1308).

The diagnosis of schistosomiasis depends on a history of potential exposure and a high index of suspicion. In some cases, blood and CSF eosinophilia are seen. *Schistosoma eggs* can be detected in feces or urine or by rectal snips, and serologic tests can indicate previous exposure. Intracerebral and spinal cord lesions can be demonstrated by neuroimaging studies (1316). The presence in CSF of an IgG specific for schistosome-soluble egg antigen is highly specific but not very sensitive for the diagnosis (1317).

Treatment of schistosomiasis depends on a combination of drug therapy with praziquantel to eradicate the infection and measures to reduce inflammation (1318). Neurologic disease during Katayama fever responds to corticosteroids. Surgical decompression may be required for lesions that compress the spinal cord. The effectiveness of a vaccine is under investigation (1319). It is interesting to note that schistosomiasis alters the progression of experimental autoimmune encephalomyelitis (1320) and that it may protect against human multiple sclerosis (1321).

Paragonimiasis

Infestation with paragonimiasis, a common condition in Southeast Asia and in certain parts of Africa and South America, generally causes pulmonary symptoms. Occasionally, the organism can cause serious neurologic disease. *Paragonimus westermani,* the oriental lung fluke, is the most common etiologic agent, although other species also can cause CNS infection. Infection is acquired through ingestion of seafood or contaminated water. The metacercaria excyst in the small intestine, penetrate the bowel wall, and migrate into the tissues. Larval flukes migrate to the lung and, occasionally, elsewhere in the body. Flukes can migrate from the lung through the jugular and carotid foramina at the base of the skull to reach the temporal and occipital lobes of the brain, where they cause necrosis and an eosinophilic, granulomatous reaction. The spinal cord can be invaded through the intervertebral disc. Adult flukes can invade muscle, usually the psoas.

Common symptoms include headache, nausea and vomiting, seizures, visual disturbance, focal motor defects, and other neurologic signs. These symptoms can have features suggestive of meningitis, meningoencephalitis, encephalopathy, brain tumor, or brain abscess (1322–1324). Diagnosis of cerebral paragonimiasis is based on an epidemiologic history of exposure. Eosinophilia may be present, but all other features overlap with those of other CNS disorders, including tuberculosis. CT scanning may show calcification and ventricular dilatation. Contrast-enhanced MRI can be used to assess the extent of the inflammatory activity (1325). Biopsy of a CNS lesion may be required to confirm the diagnosis. The disease is treated by praziquantel or bithionol to eradicate the parasite. Convulsion and coma can occur as complications of treatment for cerebral paragonimiasis. The dosage may require adjustment, and corticosteroids should be given as in cysticercosis. Surgery may be required for focal lesions.

OTHER NEUROLOGIC DISORDERS OF PRESUMED INFECTIOUS ETIOLOGY

Sarcoidosis

Nervous system sarcoidosis is unusual in children. The cause of the disease is problematic, but for convenience it is classified with infectious diseases. Although sarcoidosis occurs throughout the world, it is particularly common in the southeastern portions of the United States, where it predominates among blacks. Genetic factors have been implicated (1326). Most affected children are between 9 and 15 years old. Children are more likely to have seizures, less likely to have cranial nerve palsies, and perhaps more likely to have a space-occupying lesion (1327).

Pathologically, the disease is characterized by widely disseminated epithelioid cells, tubercles with little or no necrosis, and giant cells. The predominant lymphocyte at the site of disease is the T4-helper/inducer cell. Locally, the T4-to-T8 ratio is increased, whereas it is reduced in the peripheral circulation (1328). Tissues most frequently involved are the lymph nodes, lungs, skin, eyes, and bones. In adults, any part of the nervous system can be affected, in particular the cranial nerves, meninges, and musculature (1329,1330). In children, neurologic symptoms are most commonly associated with uveoparotid fever. This syndrome, first described by Heerfordt (1331), is characterized by ocular disturbances, most commonly uveitis and less commonly optic neuritis, swelling of the parotid gland, and facial nerve palsy. Facial nerve palsy usually follows a subacute course; it appears after the parotid swelling and subsides with it. It occurs in 4% of children with sarcoidosis (1332). Meningeal signs, peripheral neuritis, papilledema, and diabetes insipidus are other rare findings associated with childhood CNS sarcoidosis (1332). Intramedullary spinal cord involvement can occur (1333). The CSF protein content can show an elevation with evidence of intrathecal production of oligoclonal IgM and IgG (1334). Other cases demonstrate intrathecal production of polyclonal IgG. However, only 24% of cases have either an elevated IgG index or an increased synthesis rate (1335). Cranial MRI evaluation should be done on all children with systemic sarcoidosis because clinically inapparent neurosarcoidosis can occur (1336).

Sarcoidosis has a slowly progressive course, with a tendency to undergo partial or complete spontaneous remissions.

The diagnosis of sarcoidosis depends on the clinical and radiologic features along with histologic evidence of epithelioid cell granulomas on biopsy of the lung or other tissue. Because facial weakness is rare in mumps, the association of parotid swelling and facial palsy should suggest sarcoidosis. In the rare condition termed *Melkersson* syndrome, recurrent facial nerve palsy is accompanied by edema of the face or lips. This condition is covered in Chapter 8. The MRI is not characteristic in CNS sarcoidosis. It can resemble multiple sclerosis with periventricular and multifocal lesions in the white matter (1337). A fuller discussion of the diagnostic problems is beyond the scope of this text; the reader is referred to reviews by Scott (1338), Newman and colleagues (1326), and Baumann and Robertson (1327).

Treatment with corticosteroids tends to improve cerebral, ocular, and facial nerve involvement. Other immunosuppressive drugs can be of benefit should corticosteroid therapy fail. Surgical intervention may be required for hydrocephalus or expanding mass lesions (1326).

Encephalopathy and Fatty Degeneration of the Viscera (Reye Syndrome)

Reye syndrome, which was first described by Reye and coworkers in 1963 (1339), is an acute illness after a viral infection, characterized by a progressive encephalopathy, hypoglycemia, and disordered hepatic function (1340). The disease, once relatively common, has almost completely disappeared, and so most currently encountered cases are atypical (1341).

Etiology and Pathology

The cause of Reye syndrome is unknown; the essential pathophysiology consists of a generalized impairment of mitochondrial function (1342) from infectious, metabolic, toxic, or other causes (1343). Reye syndrome is associated with an upregulated isoprenoid pathway, elevated hypothalamic digoxin secretion, and right hemispheric chemical dominance (1344). The syndrome has accompanied a large number of viral illnesses, notably varicella, influenza, and parainfluenza (1339,1342,1345). In northern Thailand, a condition resembling Reye syndrome has been associated with a toxin from *Aspergillus flavus* (1346). Most importantly, the association between the disease and administration of salicylates used to treat the fever accompanying the antecedent illnesses has been established by epidemiologic studies (1347). The incidence of Reye syndrome has decreased dramatically with the decreased use of salicylates as an antipyretic in childhood infections. It is important to note, however, that there are no reported cases of Reye syndrome when aspirin was used in antiplatelet doses of 3 to 5 mg/kg per day. A significant proportion of cases are caused by a variety of inborn errors of metabolism.

The serum from patients with Reye syndrome contains an inhibitor of mitochondrial function capable of inducing in normal mitochondria morphologic changes similar to those seen in patients with Reye syndrome. The inhibitor's properties resemble those of a dicarboxylic acid, and analysis of serum from patients with Reye syndrome demonstrates a marked increase in both medium- and long-chain dicarboxylic acids. The clinical similarity of Reye syndrome to Jamaican vomiting sickness and the various inborn errors of fatty acid metabolism in which dicarboxylic acids accumulate suggests that dicarboxylic acids indeed play a crucial role in the disease. These conditions are more fully discussed in the section on organic acidurias in Chapter 1.

In fatal cases, the brain shows severe edema and brainstem herniation. The histopathologic changes are nonspecific. The cortical neurons are either swollen or shrunken and deeply staining. Astrocytes and oligodendroglia are swollen without microglial proliferation. Some cells are laden with sudanophilic granules. Brain mitochondria are usually grossly deformed and swollen. Their matrix is rarefied, and its materials are coarsely granular. Cristae are fragmentary, widely spaced, and few in number.

The liver is enlarged and yellow, with fatty infiltration observed in every cell. This extensive fatty change is unassociated with necrosis. Electron microscopy reveals the most striking abnormalities to be in mitochondria, which are swollen and pleomorphic (1338). Similar changes are seen in the kidney, occasionally the myocardium, and pancreatic acinar cells.

Clinical Manifestations

Reye syndrome is primarily a disease of childhood, and more than 90% of reported cases have been in persons younger than 15 years of age.

A variety of antecedent illnesses are associated with Reye syndrome. In order of their frequency, these are respiratory, varicella, and gastrointestinal illnesses, the last with diarrhea as the main symptom. Prodromal symptoms of Reye syndrome can be mild or can consist of nonspecific complaints such as malaise, cough, rhinorrhea, or sore throat. The child rapidly deteriorates, usually after 1 to 3 days, but sometimes as late as 2 to 3 weeks, with vomiting and the onset of stupor or coma, which is sometimes followed by convulsions. Wild delirium and unusual restlessness have been noted in approximately one-half of patients as the level of consciousness declines. Various types of seizures occur in approximately 85% of cases (1349).

With coma, the child develops changes in muscle tone, decorticate and decerebrate status, or opisthotonus. The pupils become dilated, unresponsive to light, or unequal. Central neurogenic hyperventilation or shallow breathing can occur. Symptoms often correlate with metabolic disturbances or brainstem herniation. The liver is frequently enlarged.

The clinical course of Reye syndrome is rapid, and in one series, 61% of deaths occurred within 24 hours of the onset of CNS manifestations. The cause of death in most cases is encephalopathy with cerebral edema leading to increased intracranial pressure and brainstem compression. Reye syndrome can stop progressing at any stage, with complete recovery in 5 to 10 days.

EEG changes correlate with the severity of Reye syndrome and with prognosis. Aoki and Lombroso characterized the EEG changes (1350).

Diagnosis

A bout of vomiting followed by the sudden onset of a profound disturbance of consciousness associated with hepatic dysfunction and hypoglycemia should suggest the diagnosis of Reye syndrome. This is supported by abnormal liver function test results, such as elevated serum transaminases, prolonged prothrombin times, and high arterial blood ammonia with or without hypoglycemia. Hypoglycemia and impaired gluconeogenesis are not the only signs of disturbed glucose metabolism; blood lactate, pyruvate, acetoacetate, glycerol, glucose, glucagon, insulin, and growth hormone can be elevated. The CSF is normal. Biopsy of the liver confirms the diagnosis (1351). A variety of toxic substances, notably ethanol, and salicylates can produce a similar picture.

Treatment

Reye syndrome can be a mild, self-limited disease or a rapidly progressive, relentless, fatal illness (1348). Control of intracranial hypertension is one of the most critical issues in the care of patients with Reye syndrome (1352). An important adjunct to therapy is the monitoring of intracranial pressure. If possible, all patients with Reye syndrome should receive care in a setting where intracranial pressure can be monitored if coma evolves. Careful attention to metabolic and physiologic disturbances can be life saving in severe cases.

Generally, the residual neurologic deficit is proportional to the severity of the disease (1353,1354). Among survivors of Reye syndrome, 30% of those developing decerebrate posturing or seizures during hospitalization had serious neurologic sequelae when discharged. Evidence of increased intracranial pressure and a blood ammonia level greater than 300 g/dL were associated with a significantly greater mortality, as were hyperkalemia, hyperpnea, and hematemesis (1342). Disorders of voice and speech can be the major disabling handicaps in survivors of Reye syndrome (1355). If the neurologic phase of Reye syndrome resolves, visceral function is expected to recover completely within a few days. However, the severity and duration of both metabolic and hydrostatic effects on the nervous system will determine prognosis (1356).

Hemorrhagic Shock and Encephalopathy Syndrome

This syndrome, first described by Levin and coworkers in 1983 (1357), affects previously healthy infants and young children. It manifests with a sudden onset of fever, watery diarrhea, shock, disseminated intravascular coagulation, and renal and hepatic dysfunction (1357,1358). The encephalopathy is characterized by seizures and coma. Neuroimaging studies demonstrate cerebral edema with relative sparing of cerebellum and basal ganglia (1359,1360). The differential diagnosis should include bacterial and viral septicemia, hemolytic uremic syndrome, toxic shock syndrome, Reye syndrome, and some inborn errors of metabolism (1361). The majority of survivors have significant neurologic deficits. Bacterial culture results have been uniformly negative, and the etiology of hemorrhagic shock and encephalopathy syndrome is unknown. Sofer and coworkers suggested that the condition is the result of hyperpyrexia in genetically susceptible infants (1362). However, not all cases of hemorrhagic shock and encephalopathy syndrome have factors conducive to overheating (1363).

Behçet Disease

Behçet disease is a chronic and relapsing condition characterized by keratitis, uveitis, recurrent ulcerations of the mouth and genitalia, and a variety of skin lesions (1364,1365). Although the disease largely affects adults, it may occur in children as young as 2 years of age, and transient ulcerative manifestations have been observed in newborns of mothers with Behçet disease (1366). The nervous system is involved in approximately one-fifth of patients (1367).

Although reports of viral isolation from affected patients have prompted classification of this disease with infectious illnesses, no convincing evidence exists for such an etiology, and bacterial, autoimmune, and environmental factors also have been suggested (1368). Allen proposed that an underlying genetic predisposition coupled with a triggering event leads to alterations in immune function and response (1369). Brain pathology is not specific. Multiple foci of necrotizing lymphocytic perivenular and pericapillary inflammatory cuffing are found in gray and white matter, and thrombosis of small vessels or of the large veins and dural sinuses occurs (1370). Endothelial damage and increased polymorphonuclear leukocyte activity in the active stage of Behçet's disease result in decreased antioxidant paraoxonase activity and increased lipid peroxidation (1371).

In most patients, neurologic manifestations of Behçet disease include aseptic meningitis or a recurrent meningoencephalitis (1372). Parenchymal involvement is associated with cognitive dysfunction (1373). Less often an episodic progressive brainstem syndrome occurs (1372,1374). Dural sinus thrombosis or pseudotumor cerebri also can develop with subsequent increase in intracranial pressure (1375). A mild CSF pleocytosis is common, with most patients having fewer than 60 white blood cells/μL. Latencies of cognitive evoked potentials (P300) are significantly longer in patients with attention and memory deficits (1373). As in adults with Behçet disease, single photon emission computed tomography studies can disclose areas of hypoperfusion that seem normal on MRI (1376). The MRI shows scattered areas of high signal intensity on T2-weighted images, with a predilection for central structures of the cerebrum, cerebral peduncles, and basis pontis during the acute illness. This evolves to atrophy of posterior fossa structures with signal attenuation suggestive of hemosiderin deposits (1377). The condition is rare in the United States but appears to be relatively common in Turkey and Japan (1378). Patients with an Asian heritage have been associated with HLA-B5 haplotype (1379). As with most inflammatory diseases that involve the CNS, the neurologic manifestations are not specific, and the diagnosis rests on the presence of systemic manifestations. These include a marked cutaneous sensitivity to trauma, recurrent aphthous stomatitis, recurrent genital aphthous ulcers, and ocular manifestations, notably anterior uveitis. Devlin and coworkers recommended performing contrast-enhanced MRI and CSF analysis in any patient who fulfills the criteria for systemic Behçet disease and who has a history of altered mental status, recurrent headache, or altered neurologic examination (1365).

The neurologic complications are generally treated with corticosteroids, although immunomodulators or chlorambucil also have been used (1379,1380). Interferon-α2b can benefit refractory ocular disease (1381). Colchicine is said to prevent relapses (1379).

Uveomeningoencephalitic Syndrome (Vogt-Koyanagi-Harada Syndrome)

Another cause for uveomeningitic disease in the pediatric population is Vogt-Koyanagi-Harada syndrome. This is an uncommon condition characterized by the association of uveitis, a meningoencephalitis of variable severity, occasional loss of skin and hair pigmentation, and auditory disturbances (1382).

The condition is presumed to be a class II major histocompatibility complex autoimmune inflammatory disease primarily directed at the antigens of melanocytes, with particular injury to pigmented structures of the eye (1383,1384). The condition is more frequently encountered in the Japanese population, in whom a strong association exists with HLA-DR4 (1383). A secondary association to HLA-DR1 also exists, involving a sequence that is linked with susceptibility to rheumatoid arthritis (1383). The incidence of keratoconjunctivitis sicca is higher in Vogt-Koyanagi-Harada patients and might be related to HLA-DR4 (1385). An inflammatory process similar to that found in the ocular choroid but directed at melanocytes of the inner ear may account for the frequent finding of auditory disturbance in Vogt-Koyanagi-Harada syndrome (1386). Melanin-laden macrophages may constitute a significant portion of the pleocytic cells found in CSF of patients with Vogt-Koyanagi-Harada syndrome (1387). It is unclear what provokes the autoimmune response in Vogt-Koyanagi-Harada syndrome. Autoreactive T cells against tyrosinase and/or tyrosinase-related-protein-1 may contribute to the development of the disease (1388).

The onset of Vogt-Koyanagi-Harada syndrome is typically one of a subacute onset of bilateral anterior, posterior, or both uveitis associated with ocular pain (1389). This may be followed by abrupt onset of aseptic meningitis or meningoencephalitis. Meningeal signs may be the first sign of disease and are found at some stage in approximately 60% of cases of Vogt-Koyanagi-Harada syndrome (1390). In the series of Beniz and coworkers, symptoms included meningismus, predominantly headache (67%), tinnitus (17%), dysacusis (13%), alopecia (13%), vitiligo (10%), and poliosis (6%) (1391). Ocular findings included iridocyclitis, vitreitis, diffuse swelling of the choroid, serous retinal detachment, or optic disc hyperemia (1391). Most cases occur during adult life, and in the series of Belfort and coworkers only 12% of patients were younger than 20 years of age (1392), the youngest being 4 years of age

(1393). Waxing and waning abnormalities of cranial nerve function may be noted, especially of the third, seventh, and eighth cranial nerves. Tonic pupils, dysfunction of ocular accommodation, and corneal anesthesia are additional possible features (1394). Development of areas of depigmentation (poliosis), involving eyebrows and eyelashes, alopecia, and dermal vitiligo are other common late manifestations.

A lymphocytic CSF pleocytosis is typical. Optical coherence tomography can be helpful in characterizing the patterns of retinal detachment (1395). MRI studies can show multiple focal lesions or increased T2 signal in the periventricular area (1396,1397).

Treatment with high doses of corticosteroids has been advocated. In patients whose neurologic symptoms do not respond, intravenous immune globulin can be of benefit (1397). Intravitreal triamcinolone acetonide provides short-term improvement in visual acuity and serous retinal detachments; systemic corticosteroid use may be spared, shortened, or even eliminated when intravitreal steroids are used (1398). Recovery takes place gradually over several months but is usually incomplete, with both visual and auditory system sequelae (1382). In children, the outcome for visual acuity is poor, and in the series of Tabbara and colleagues, 61% of children required cataract surgery and 61% had a final visual acuity of 20/200 or worse (1399). Final visual acuity is significantly better in younger patients and in those who have less extensive retinal detachment, no pigmentary change, and no complications (1400–1402).

Mollaret Meningitis

A recurrent, benign, lymphocytic meningitis, probably of diverse causes (1403,1404), but presumed to be infectious, was first described by Mollaret (1405). Mollaret meningitis's association with herpes simplex types 1 and 2 has been suggested by the demonstration of viral DNA in the CSF (1403,1406). Herpes simplex type 2 is the most commonly isolated agent (1407). Symptoms recur at intervals of weeks or months over the course of several years, and as many as five or more attacks can occur (1408). Seizures or coma have been reported, but focal neurologic signs are uncommon. Episodes are often associated with fever, but may not be associated with active herpetic lesions on the skin or mucous membranes. Large mononuclear cells can be found in the CSF early in the course of an exacerbation (1409), but a CSF protein elevation is not invariable. The EEG can be normal or can demonstrate focal accentuations without spikes (1410). The long-term prognosis is good, with spontaneous recovery and no residua.

Mollaret meningitis should be distinguished from chronic granulomatous infections of the nervous system, from an aseptic meningitis syndrome induced by trimethoprim therapy (1411), and from an intracranial epidermoid cyst (1404). Yamamoto and colleagues recommended acyclovir prophylaxis for those patients with detectable herpes simplex virus DNA in the CSF (1412).

Benign Paroxysmal Vertigo

The most common causes of vertigo in children are migraine and benign paroxysmal vertigo of childhood (1413). Benign paroxysmal vertigo is characterized by recurrent attacks of vertigo associated with vomiting, pallor, nystagmus, and profuse sweating. Although benign paroxysmal vertigo is unaccompanied by loss of consciousness, children are known to fall during an attack. Episodes can last a few minutes to several hours or can recur for many weeks or even months, gradually decreasing in severity (1414). The age occurrence is usually 1 to 5 years (1415). A similar condition, epidemic vertigo, has occurred in epidemics, with more than one case appearing in the same family (1416). The preservation of consciousness during an attack and abnormalities in labyrinthine function distinguish benign paroxysmal vertigo from complex partial seizures with a vertiginous component and from vestibulogenic epilepsy, in which an attack is triggered by labyrinthine stimulation (1417–1419). In some children, recurrent attacks of vertigo are ultimately replaced by typical migraine (see Chapter 15). Benign paroxysmal vertigo also should not be confused with vestibular neuronitis or Ménière vertigo, a condition that is almost exclusively limited to the adult years (1420). Comprehensive otologic and neurologic examinations are required for proper diagnosis (1413,1421).

Epidemic Encephalitis

Epidemic encephalitis, first described by von Economo in 1917, attained epidemic proportions throughout Europe and the United States over the subsequent few years (1422). Since then, it has become progressively less common, although sporadic cases still occur (1423). Al-Mateen and coworkers encountered one such case, confirmed by the presence of increased signal intensity on MRI from the basal ganglia and substantia nigra and associated with *Mycoplasma* encephalitis (1090).

Epidemic encephalitis presented as an acute encephalitis that was often marked by somnolence and oculomotor palsies. The encephalitis cleared completely or left a variety of residua, including mental disturbances and disorders of eye movements. After a quiescent interval of months or years, many of the survivors developed a chronic progressive extrapyramidal disorder marked by parkinsonism, oculogyric crises, tremors, and dystonia (1424).

A common residual finding in children was a postencephalitic behavior syndrome marked by hyperkinesia, shortened attention span, and impaired fine motor function (1425). This picture resembled attention-deficit hyperactivity disorder (ADHD). As a consequence, many children with this condition used to be regarded as postencephalitic without having any history of encephalitis (see Chapter 18).

Kawasaki Disease (Mucocutaneous Lymph Node Syndrome)

Kawasaki disease is a triphasic illness, possibly related to superantigen expansion and activation of T cells (1426) by bacterial (1427) or viral infection (1428,1429). T-cell autoreactivity for antibodies to antigenic determinants of human heat-shock protein that develop during the course of the disease has been related to susceptibility to this condition (1430). Serum levels of an array of cytokines are elevated in Kawasaki disease; cytokines may mediate endothelial damage and lead to coronary artery disease while also producing systemic signs of inflammation (1431–1433). There may be a genetic predisposition to Kawasaki disease (1434).

Kawasaki disease has an acute phase lasting approximately 2 weeks (1435). In typical cases, this phase is marked by a febrile period of more than 5 days, an erythematous rash, conjunctival injection, erythema and crusting of lips and mouth, a strawberry tongue, swelling of hands and feet, and lymph node enlargement. After approximately 10 days, the fever subsides and the subacute phase begins. Arthritic manifestations, cardiac disease with coronary obstruction or aneurysms, and thrombocytosis can occur during this period, as can desquamation of the fingers and toes. Sterile pyuria or proteinuria, diarrhea, abdominal distress, hepatitis, or hydrops of the gallbladder also is encountered. The convalescent phase can last for several months. If death occurs, it is usually caused by cardiac complications. Older age at onset (greater than 8 years of age) is associated with higher mortality rates (1436).

Nearly all patients with Kawasaki disease demonstrate some degree of CNS involvement. Irritability, mood lability, and sleep disturbances are common. Semicoma or coma can occur for several days. Approximately one-fourth of children have an aseptic meningitis with severe lethargy and nuchal rigidity. Severe myositis can occur (1437). Facial palsy is a rare complication (1438). In up to 40% of patients the CSF shows a mononuclear pleocytosis of up to 320 cells. Protein and glucose are usually normal (1439,1440).

Treatment with intravenous gamma globulin (2 g/kg as a single dose given over 10 to 12 hours; a second infusion may be needed of 400 mg/kg per day for 4 days) and aspirin decreases the cardiac sequelae and leads to rapid resolution of sequelae (1441–1443). Okada and colleagues showed in a randomized, prospective study that intravenous gamma globulin with corticosteroids was more effective than intravenous gamma globulin alone in reducing circulating levels of all inflammatory cytokines and IL-10 in patients with acute Kawasaki disease (1431). Plasma exchange also can be of benefit (1444).

Chronic Focal Encephalitis (Rasmussen Encephalitis)

Chronic focal encephalitis (Rasmussen syndrome), first described in 1958, is characterized by uncontrollable focal seizures associated with focal inflammation in cerebral tissue (1445). The current concept is that the condition represents a syndrome with a heterogeneous etiology (1446). Evidence exists for a viral etiology, in that in some cases CMV and herpes simplex virus genomes can be demonstrated in brain tissue (1447–1449). Although some studies have shown the presence of serum autoantibodies to glutamate receptor GluR3 (1450), Watson and coworkers were not able to duplicate this finding (1450a). Elevated serum antinuclear antibody titers, CSF evidence of endogenous production of IgG, and immunofluorescent staining of brain tissue for IgG, IgM, IgA, C3, and C1q also have been described (1451).

On pathologic examination of brain, the cortex of the affected side is thinned and scarred. Microscopically, perivascular lymphocytic infiltrates are seen with vascular injury and astrogliosis. Microglial nodules can occur; leptomeningeal infiltration is rare. Neuronal loss and cortical atrophy can be marked (1452). The contralateral side is generally normal.

Typically, patients develop simple partial seizures before age 10 years. An antecedent febrile illness is usually absent. In more than one-half of children, these seizures progress to epilepsia partialis continua. Complex partial seizures or secondary generalized seizures also can occur. As a result of the disease process, most patients experience a developmental arrest or regression. Neuropsychologic deficits or behavioral disturbances can result, in part from the persistent seizure activity or from large doses of anticonvulsants (1453).

Hart and coworkers described a form of chronic encephalitis with onset of seizures in adolescence without apparent cause and pathologic features of chronic encephalitis. These cases differ from classical Rasmussen encephalitis in that the course is more benign, an increased incidence of occipital involvement occurs, and the response to surgery is variable (1454).

EEG in Rasmussen encephalitis demonstrates broadly distributed but lateralized spike foci with underlying slow-wave disturbances, usually in the centrotemporal region (1453). CSF changes can include a mild pleocytosis or elevation of protein.

Neuroimaging studies generally show the progressive evolution of focal or hemispheric atrophy (1455,1456).

Regional hypoperfusion and interictal hypometabolism can be demonstrated by PET or SPECT scanning (1457,1458). Proton MR spectroscopy is more sensitive than MRI in that it provides evidence for progressive neuronal damage at a stage when the MRI shows normal results. Even this sensitive study fails to show any abnormalities on the contralateral side (1459).

The sudden onset in a previously healthy youngster of an intractable unilateral seizure disorder, particularly one that manifests with epilepsia partialis continua, points to the diagnosis. The progressive nature of the condition and the progressive changes on neuroimaging confirm the diagnosis.

Therapy with anticonvulsant drugs is usually unsuccessful, but hemispherectomy has proved beneficial in the majority of patients (1460,1461). Selected cases have responded to chronic corticosteroid therapy (1462), intravenous gamma globulin (1463), intraventricular alpha-interferon (1458), or plasmapheresis (1464). Ganciclovir therapy also has been reported to be of benefit (1465). In the majority of children hemispherectomy is required. The response to the procedure is generally satisfactory. The use of hemispherectomy in the treatment of intractable focal seizures is covered more extensively in Chapter 14.

Thrombotic Thrombocytopenic Purpura and Hemolytic-Uremic Syndrome

Thrombotic thrombocytopenic purpura (TTP) and hemolytic-uremic syndrome (HUS) are two closely related conditions that may in fact represent differing clusters of manifestations of a single disease process. TTP is marked by the combination of fever, hemolytic anemia, renal failure, and neurologic dysfunction in association with widespread hyaline thrombosis of small blood vessels. HUS may have any or all of these same findings. In fact, no objective criteria except age distinguish these two illnesses. When the patient is younger (e.g., younger than 5 years of age) and renal abnormalities are predominant, HUS is usually diagnosed. TTP is rare in children, but when the patient is older and neurologic findings are predominant, TTP is usually diagnosed (1466).

TTP and HUS appear to have common mechanisms, and it is not known why there is age-related variation in organ involvement. Patients with recurrent illness may have manifestations suggesting HUS on one exacerbation and TTP on another (1467).

Both illnesses appear to be mediated by inflammatory or toxic vascular endothelial injury. Antiendothelial antibodies may play a role in TTP (1468), whereas circulating bacterial toxins may mediate injury in HUS (1469,1470). The epidemic form of HUS has been associated with a verocytotoxin-producing *E. coli,* notably *E. coli* O157:H7, or *Shigella dysenteriae* type 1 infection (1471). This toxin kills mammalian cells by inhibiting protein synthesis and is thought to initiate HUS by damaging vascular endothelial cells (1472). Verocytotoxin is composed of five B subunits and one A subunit. The B subunits bind to Gb_3 ganglioside in the cell membrane. After endocytosis the A unit enzymatically inactivates the 60S ribosomal subunit, thus blocking protein synthesis (1472). The mechanism by which verocytotoxins produce disease are not fully understood (1471). An overwhelming amount of unusually large multimeric forms of von Willebrand factor is produced (1473). TNF and IL-1 induce expression of the verocytotoxin receptor globotriaosylceramide in human endothelial cells (1474). Thrombin generation (probably due to accelerated thrombogenesis) and inhibition of fibrinolysis precede renal injury and may be the cause of such injury (1475). Shiga lipopolysaccharide (endotoxin) and TNF, but not IL-1, augment the cytotoxicity of Shiga toxin (1476). Other factors also may be involved because female gender, use of antimotility drugs, and increased hemoglobin level are associated with an increased risk for developing a neurologic manifestation, whereas prior administration of a blood product is associated with a decreased risk (1477). In addition, it is possible that patients are rendered more vulnerable to either HUS or TTP because they are deficient in a plasma factor that regulates endothelial prostacyclin synthetase. Circulating factors related to platelet adhesion that also may be of importance include a calcium-activated cysteine protease and unusually large von Willebrand factor multimers. The von Willebrand multimers, produced by megakaryocytes or endothelial cells, may react with circulating adenosine diphosphate, calcium, or abnormalities of fluid shear forces and result in platelet aggregation. Some patients may lack a component of plasma that is involved in the reduction of large circulating multimers of von Willebrand factor. Persistence of these multimers in circulation may be of particular importance in recurrence of TTP or HUS (1478,1479).

Although TTP is often idiopathic, it can develop in association with a variety of inflammatory diseases (e.g., rheumatoid arthritis, polyarteritis nodosa, systemic lupus erythematosus, Sjögren syndrome), lymphoma, endocarditis, puerperium, and drugs and poisons (i.e., sulfa, cyclosporine, iodine, birth control pills) (1480,1481). TTP is slightly more common in girls than in boys (ratio 3:2). Congenital TTP should be considered in the differential diagnosis for newborns presenting with severe hyperbilirubinemia, anemia, and thrombocytopenia (1482,1483).

HUS develops in approximately 1% of patients treated with cyclosporine. On rare occasions the condition is associated with *Salmonella typhi* infection, pneumococcal sepsis caused by neuraminidase-producing organisms, and *Campylobacter* enteritis (1484). It also is seen as a complication of pneumococcal meningitis or pneumococcal pneumonia (1485).

Although the peak incidence of TTP is in the third decade, it can occur in neonates and young children

(1486). The illness may be monophasic or may recur. The tendency to recur is not predictable on either a clinical or a laboratory basis. Some studies have suggested an autosomal recessive trait that predisposes patients to TTP, conceivably genetic deficiency of one of the factors noted previously, such as prostacyclin synthetase (1487).

By contrast, HUS develops in infants and young children. It is manifested by a prodromal period of vomiting, bloody diarrhea, and abdominal pain lasting an average of 1 week. Occasionally, an antecedent urinary tract infection occurs (1488). Severe pneumococcal disease may also trigger HUS (1489). Then, after a silent period of several days, children have acute renal insufficiency, hemolytic anemia, and thrombocytopenia. A subgroup of pediatric patients with atypical and nonpostdiarrheal HUS have von Willebrand factor–cleaving protease deficiency much like what is seen in congenital TTP (1466,1490). There is a close relation between systemic lupus erythematosus and TTP in childhood (1491).

Neurologic symptoms, which can be the presenting feature, appear during the third phase in as many as 20% to 50% of patients (1473,1492,1493). They are believed in part to be caused by azotemia, hyponatremia, and hypocalcemia. In addition, a thrombotic microangiopathy occurs, with areas of reduced cerebral perfusion seen on SPECT (1494). Some 3% to 5% of patients develop focal areas of infarction surrounded by edema and necrosis. Thrombi are usually located in arterioles and capillary–postcapillary venular complexes. Two patterns can be distinguished. One is a loose fibrin meshwork with entrapped leukocytes and erythrocytes and the other is a course granular aggregation of eosinophilic material that is often acellular (1495). Large thrombotic strokes also have been reported (1496).

Neurologic manifestations include changes in consciousness and generalized or partial seizures (1484, 1493,1494). Seizures can occur in the absence of uremia or hypertension (1495). Less common are transient or permanent hemipareses, decerebrate or dystonic posturing, cortical blindness, and transient hallucinations (1494,1497). CNS symptoms can be aggravated by complications of systemic involvement such as hyponatremia, uremia, and severe hypertension (1498).

The EEG can show a unique pattern with epochs of diffuse slowing alternating with epochs of classic burst suppression. Infusion of fresh-frozen plasma improves this tracing before any clinical improvement (1499). Neuroimaging studies disclose large vessel infarctions or multiple small infarcts, often in conjunction with diffuse cerebral edema or multiple hemorrhages (1493). Basal ganglia involvement is common and often associated with other cerebral pathologies (1500).

Treatment of the neurologic symptoms requires correction of any electrolyte imbalance and cerebral edema and control of seizures. Hemolysis can cause significant anemia and hyperkalemia. Seizures, which may be caused by cerebral structural damage, electrolyte imbalance, hypertension, or severe azotemia, require specific therapy but generally respond to diazepam and phenytoin (1484). Plasmapheresis, the standard therapy for TTP, is effective in achieving remission in most patients, and the addition of vincristine and cyclosporine may be effective in refractory patients (1501).

In the majority of children, neurologic symptoms recede, and the prognosis is that of renal insufficiency, which is usually self-limiting. Factors associated with a poor prognosis are elevated polymorphonuclear leukocyte count, short duration of prodrome, bloody diarrhea, hypocalcemia, and oliguria detected within 48 hours of hospital admission (1473). Children with neurologic involvement are more likely to develop residual hypertension or chronic renal failure or to die, suggesting that neurologic involvement is associated with increased severity of the syndrome (1502). Coma and increased CSF protein are more common in patients with a poor outcome (1462). However, even prolonged coma can be compatible with good outcome (1503).

ACKNOWLEDGEMENT

The authors thank G. Ellis Ziel, Virginia Williams and Erin Forsbey for their technical assistance.

REFERENCES

1. Saez-Llorens X, McCracken GH Jr. Bacterial meningitis in children. *Lancet* 2003;361:2139–2148.
2. Stephens DS, Farley MM. Pathogenic events during infection of the human nasopharynx with *Neisseria meningitidis* and *Haemophilus influenzae*. *Rev Infect Dis* 1991;13:22–33.
3. Quagliarello V, Scheld WM. Bacterial meningitis: pathogenesis, pathophysiology, and progress. *N Engl J Med* 1992;327:864–872.
4. Tunkel AR, Scheld WM. Alterations in the blood–brain barrier in bacterial meningitis: *in vivo* and *in vitro* models. *Pediatr Infect Dis J* 1989;8:911–912.
5. Ring A, Weiser JN, Tuomanen EI. Pneumococcal trafficking across the blood–brain barrier: molecular analysis of a novel bidirectional pathway. *J Clin Invest* 1998;102:347–360.
6. Wispelwey B, Hansen EJ, Scheld WM. *Haemophilus influenzae* outer membrane vesicle-induced blood–brain barrier permeability during experimental meningitis. *Infect Immun* 1989;57:2559–2562.
7. Paul R, Lorenzl S, Koedel U, et al. Matrix metalloproteinases contribute to the blood-brain barrier disruption during bacterial meningitis. *Ann Neurol* 1998;44:592–600.
8. Schiffer MS, Oliveira E, Glode MP, et al. A review: relation between invasiveness and the K-1 capsular polysaccharide of *Escherichia coli*. *Pediatr Res* 1976;10:82–87.
9. Schuchat A, Robinson K, Wenger JD, et al., for the Active Surveillance Team. Bacterial meningitis in the United States in 1995. *N Engl J Med* 1997;337:970–976.
10. Saez-Llorens X, Ramilo O, Mustafa MN, et al. Molecular pathophysiology of bacterial meningitis: current concepts and therapeutic implications. *J Pediatr* 1990;116:671–684.
11. Smith AL. Bacterial meningitis. *Pediatr Rev* 1993;14:11–18.
12. Tunkel AR, Scheld WM. Pathogenesis and pathophysiology of bacterial meningitis. *Annu Rev Med* 1993;44:103–120.

13. Tunkel AR, Scheld WM. Acute bacterial meningitis. *Lancet* 1995;346:1675–1680.
14. Sze G, Zimmerman RD. The magnetic resonance imaging of infections and inflammatory diseases. *Radiol Clin North Am* 1988;26:839–859.
15. Smith JF, Landing BH. Mechanism of brain damage in *Haemophilus influenzae* meningitis. *J Neuropathol Exp Neurol* 1960;19:248–265.
16. Gallin GI, Goldstein IM, Snyderman R. *Inflammation. Basic principles and clinical correlates*, 2nd ed. New York: Raven Press, 1992.
17. Syrogiannopoulos GA, Hansen EJ, Erwin AL. *Haemophilus influenzae* type B lipooligosaccharide induces meningeal inflammation. *J Infect Dis* 1988;157:237–244.
18. Perry VH, Gordon S. Microglia and macrophages. In: Keane RW, Hickey WF, eds. *Immunology of the nervous system*. Oxford: Oxford University Press, 1997: 155–172.
19. Mustafa MM, Ramilo O, Saez-Llorens X, et al. Prostaglandins E2 and I2, interleukin 1-b and tumor necrosis factor in cerebrospinal fluid in infants and children with bacterial meningitis. *Pediatr Infect Dis J* 1989;8:921–922.
20. Liles WC, Van Voorhis WC. Review: Nomenclature and biologic significance of cytokines involved in inflammation and the host immune response. *J Infect Dis* 1995;172:1573–1580.
21. Saukkonen K, Sande S, Cioffe C, et al. The role of cytokines in the generation of inflammation and tissue damage in experimental gram-positive meningitis. *J Exp Med* 1990;171:439–448.
22. Mustafa MM, et al. Cerebrospinal fluid prostaglandins, interleukin 1 beta, and tumor necrosis factor in bacterial meningitis. Clinical and laboratory correlations in placebo-treated and dexamethasone-treated patients. *Am J Dis Child* 1990;144:883–887.
23. Van Furth AM, Roord JJ, van Furth R. Roles of proinflammatory and anti-inflammatory cytokines in pathophysiology of bacterial meningitis and effect of adjunctive therapy. *Infect Immun* 1996;64:4883–4890.
24. Lopez-Cortes LF, Ramilo O, Saez-Llorens X, et al. Measurement of levels of tumor necrosis factor-alpha and interleukin-1 beta in the CSF of patients with meningitis of different etiologies: utility in the differential diagnosis. *Clin Infect Dis* 1993;16:534–539.
25. Ramilo O, et al. Tumor necrosis factor-alpha, cachectin, and interleukin 1-beta initiate meningeal inflammation. *J Exp Med* 1990;172:497–507.
26. Rusconi F, et al. Interleukin 6 activity in infants and children with bacterial meningitis. The Collaborative Study on Meningitis. *Pediatr Infect Dis* 1991;10:117–121.
27. Kanoh Y, Ohtani H. Levels of interleukin-6, CRP, and alpha 2 macroglobulin in cerebrospinal fluid (CSF) and serum as indicator of blood–SCF barrier damage. *Biochem Mol Biol Int* 1997;43:269–278.
28. Hashim IA, et al. Cerebrospinal fluid interleukin-6 and its diagnostic value in the investigation of meningitis. *Ann Clin Biochem* 1995;32:289–296.
29. Gallo P, et al. Intrathecal synthesis of interleukin-10 (IL-10) in viral and inflammatory diseases of the central nervous system. *J Neurol Sci* 1994;126:48–53.
30. Arditi M, Manogue KR, Caplan M, et al. Cerebrospinal fluid cachectin/tumor necrosis factor-alpha and platelet-activating factor concentrations and severity of bacterial meningitis. *Microb Pathog* 1995;19:245–255.
31. Glimaker M, et al. Tumor necrosis factor-alpha (TNF alpha) in cerebrospinal fluid from patients with meningitis of different etiologies: high levels of TNF alpha indicate bacterial meningitis. *J Infect Dis* 1993;167:882–889.
32. Moller B, et al. Bioactive and inactive forms of tumor necrosis factor-alpha in spinal fluid from patients with meningitis. *J Infect Dis* 1991;163:886–889.
33. Ossege LM, Voss B, Wiethege T, et al. Detection of transforming growth factor beta 1 mRNA in cerebrospinal fluid cells of patients with meningitis by non-radioactive in situ hybridization. *J Neurol* 1994;242:14–19.
34. Quagliarello VJ, et al. Recombinant human interleukin-1 induces meningitis and blood–brain barrier injury in the rat. Characterization and comparison with tumor necrosis factor. *J Clin Invest* 1991;87:1360–1366.
35. Selmaj KW, Raine CS. Tumor necrosis factor mediates myelin and oligodendrocyte damage in vitro. *Ann Neurol* 1988;23:339–346.
36. Glimaker M, et al. Tumor necrosis factor (TNF)-a in cerebrospinal fluid from patients with meningitis of different etiologies. High levels of TNF-a indicate bacterial meningitis. *J Infect Dis* 1993;167:882–889.
37. Dulkerian S, Kilpatrick L, Costarino AT Jr., et al. Cytokine elevations in infants with bacterial and aseptic meningitis. *J Pediatr* 1995;126:872–876.
38. Sapolsky R, Rivier C, Yamamoto G, et al. Interleukin-1 stimulates the secretion of hypothalamic corticotropin-releasing factor. *Science* 1987;238:522–524.
39. McCracken GH, Mustafa MM, Ramilo O, et al. Cerebrospinal fluid interleukin 1-b and tumor necrosis factor concentrations and outcome from neonatal gram-negative enteric bacillary meningitis. *Pediatr Infect Dis J* 1989;8:155–159.
40. Moser R, Schlieffenbaum B, Groscurth P, et al. Interleukin-1 and tumor necrosis factor stimulate human vascular endothelial cells to promote transendothelial neutrophil passage. *J Clin Invest* 1989;83:444–455.
41. Torre D, Zeroli C, Ferraro G, et al. Cerebrospinal fluid levels of IL-6 in patients with acute infections of the central nervous system. *Scand J Infect Dis* 1992;24:787–791.
42. Ostergaard C, Benfield TL, Sellebjerg F, et al. Interleukin-8 in cerebrospinal fluid from patients with septic and aseptic meningitis. *Eur J Clin Microbiol Infect Dis* 1996;15:166–169.
43. Anthony D, Fearn S, Dempster R, et al. CXC chemokines generate age-related increases in neutrophil-mediated brain inflammation and blood–brain barrier breakdown. *Curr Biol* 1998;923–926.
44. Tani M, Fuentes ME, Peterson JW, et al. Neutrophil infiltration, glial reaction, and neurological disease in transgenic mice expressing the chemokine N51/KC in oligodendrocytes. *J Clin Invest* 1996;98:529–539.
45. Tang T, Frenetle PS, Hynes RO, et al. Cytokine-induced meningitis is dramatically attenuated in mice deficient in endothelial selectins. *J Clin Invest* 1996;97:2485–2490.
46. Lipton SA, Cho YB, Pan ZH, et al. A redox based mechanism for the neuroprotective and neurodestructive effects of nitric oxide and related nitroso-compounds. *Nature* 1993;364:626–632.
47. Moncada S, Higgs A. The L-arginine-nitric oxide pathway. *N Engl J Med* 1993;329:2002–2012.
48. Buster BL, Mattes KA, Scheld WM. Potential role of nitric oxide in the pathophysiology of experimental bacterial meningitis in rats. *Infect Immun* 1995;63:3835–3839.
49. Stahel PF, Nadai D, Pfister HW, et al. Complement C3 and factor B cerebrospinal fluid concentrations in bacterial and aseptic meningitis. *Lancet* 1997;349:1886–1887.
50. Goitein KJ, Tamir I. Cerebral perfusion pressure in central nervous system infections of infancy and childhood. *J Pediatr* 1983;103:40–43.
51. Fishman RA, Sligar K, Hake RB. Effects of leukocytes on brain metabolism in granulocytic brain edema. *Ann Neurol* 1977;2:89–94.
52. Chan PH, Fishman RA, Caronna J, et al. Induction of brain edema following intracerebral injection of arachidonic acid. *Ann Neurol* 1983;13:625–632.
53. Ducker TB, Simmons RL. The pathogenesis of meningitis: systemic effects of meningococcal endotoxin within the cerebrospinal fluid. *Arch Neurol* 1968;18:123–128.
54. McCracken GH Jr. Endotoxin concentrations in cerebrospinal fluid correlate with clinical severity and neurologic outcome of *Haemophilus influenzae* type B meningitis. *Am J Dis Child* 1991;145:1099–1103.
55. Goh D, Minns RA. Cerebral blood flow velocity monitoring in pyogenic meningitis. *Arch Dis Child* 1993;68:111–119.
56. Paulson OB, Hansen EL, Kristensen HS, et al. Cerebral blood flow, cerebral metabolic rate of oxygen and CSF acid-base parameters in patients with acute pyogenic meningitis and with acute encephalitis. *Acta Neurol Scand Suppl* 1972;51:407–408.

57. Ashwal S, Peabody JL, Schneider S, et al. Cerebral blood flow and carbon dioxide reactivity in children with bacterial meningitis. *J Pediatr* 1990;117:523–530.
58. Goitein KJ, Amit Y, Mussaffi H. Intracranial pressure in central nervous system infections and cerebral ischaemia of infancy. *Arch Dis Child* 1983;58:184–186.
59. Swartz MH, Dodge PR. Bacterial meningitis: a review of selected aspects. I. General clinical features, special problems and unusual meningeal reactions mimicking bacterial meningitis. *N Engl J Med* 1965;272:725–731, 779–787, 842–848, 898–902.
60. Durand ML, Calderwood SB, Webber DJ, et al. Acute bacterial meningitis in adults. A review of 493 episodes. *N Engl J Med* 1993;328:21–28.
61. Vincent J, Thomas K, Mathew O. An improved clinical method for detecting meningeal irritation. *Arch Dis Child* 1993;68:215–218.
62. Dodge PR, Swartz MN. Bacterial meningitis: a review of selected aspects. II. Special neurologic problems, post-meningitic complications and clinicopathological correlations. *N Engl J Med* 1965;272:954–960, 1003–1010.
63. Samson JH, Apthorp J, Finley A. Febrile seizures and purulent meningitis. *JAMA* 1969;10:1918–1919.
64. Rutter N, Smales OR. Lumbar puncture in children with convulsions. *Lancet* 1977;2:190–191.
65. Green SM, Rotnrock SG, Clern KJ, et al. Can seizures be the sole manifestation of meningitis in febrile children? *Pediatrics* 1993;92:527–534.
66. Rivner MH, Jay WM, Green JB, et al. Opsoclonus in *Haemophilus influenzae* meningitis. *Neurology* 1982;32:661–663.
67. Eavey RD, Gao YZ, Schuknecht HF, et al. Otologic features of bacterial meningitis of childhood. *J Pediatr* 1985;106:402–407.
68. Comis SD, Osborne MP, Stephen J, et al. Cytotoxic effects on hair cells of guinea pig cochlea produced by pneumolysin, the thiolactivated toxin of *Streptococcus pneumoniae*. *Acta Otolaryngol Stockh* 1993;113:152–159.
69. Jeffery H, Scott J, Chandler D, et al. Deafness after bacterial meningitis. *Arch Dis Child* 1977;52:555–559.
70. Fortnum H, Davis A. Hearing impairment in children after bacterial meningitis: incidence and resource implications. *Br J Audiol* 1993;27:43–52.
71. Jiang ZD, Liu XY, Wu YY, et al. Long-term impairments of brain and auditory functions of children recovered from purulent meningitis. *Dev Med Child Neurol* 1990;32:473–480.
72. Richard MP, et al. Otoacoustic emissions as a screening test for hearing impairment in children recovering from acute bacterial meningitis. *Pediatrics* 1998;102:1364–1368.
73. Green JP, Newman NJ, Winterkorn JS. Paralysis of downward gaze in two patients with clinical-radiologic correlation. *Arch Ophthalmol* 1993;111:219–222.
74. Yabek SM. Meningococcal meningitis presenting as acute cerebellar ataxia. *Pediatrics* 1973;52:718–720.
75. Thun-Hohenstein L, Schmitt B, Steinlin H, et al. Cortical visual impairment following bacterial meningitis: magnetic resonance imaging and visual evoked potentials findings in two cases. *Eur J Pediatr* 1992;15:779–782.
76. Holmes RD, Kuhns LR, Oliver WJ. Widened sutures in childhood meningitis, unrecognized sign of an acute illness. *Am J Roentgenol* 1977;128:977–979.
77. Snyder RD. Ventriculomegaly in childhood bacterial meningitis. *Neuropediatrics* 1984;15:136–138.
78. Mace JW, Peters ER, Mathies AW Jr. Cranial bruits in purulent meningitis in childhood. *N Engl J Med* 1968;278:1420–1422.
79. Berman PH, Banker BQ. Neonatal meningitis: a clinical and pathological study of 29 cases. *Pediatrics* 1966;38:6–24.
80. Salmon JH. Ventriculitis complicating meningitis. *Am J Dis Child* 1972;124:35–40.
81. Snedeker JD, Kaplan SL, Dodge PR, et al. Subdural effusion and its relationship with neurologic sequelae of bacterial meningitis in infancy: a prospective study. *Pediatrics* 1990;86:163–170.
82. Bok AP, Peter JC. Subdural empyema: burr hole or craniotomy?—a retrospective computerized tomography-era analysis of treatment in 90 cases. *J Neurosurg* 1993;78:574–578.
83. Matson DD. *Neurosurgery of infancy and childhood*, 2nd ed. Springfield, IL: Charles C Thomas, 1969.
84. Chen CY, Huang CC, Chang YC, et al. Subdural empyema in 10 infants: US characteristics and clinical correlates. *Radiology* 1998;207:609–617.
85. Rabe EF, Flynn RE, Dodge PR. Subdural collections of fluids in infants and children: a study of 62 patients with special reference to factors influencing prognosis and efficacy of various forms of therapy. *Neurology* 1968;18:559–570.
86. Kaplan SL, Feigin RD. The syndrome of inappropriate secretion of antidiuretic hormone in children with bacterial meningitis. *J Pediatr* 1978;92:758–761.
87. Fajardo JE, Stafford EM, Bass JW, et al. Inappropriate antidiuretic hormone in children with viral meningitis. *Pediatr Neurol* 1989;5:37–40.
88. Decaux G, Waterlot Y, Genette F, et al. Treatment of the syndrome of inappropriate secretion of antidiuretic hormone with furosemide. *N Engl J Med* 1981;304:329–330.
89. Lieb G, Krauss J, Collmann H, et al. Recurrent bacterial meningitis. *Eur J Pediatr* 1996;155:26–30.
90. Cherry JD, Sheenan CP. Bacteriologic relapse in *Haemophilus influenzae* meningitis: inadequate ampicillin therapy. *N Engl J Med* 1968;278:1001–1003.
91. Klein JO, Feigin RD, McCracken GH Jr. Report of the task force on diagnosis and management of meningitis. *Pediatrics* 1986;78:959–982.
92. Feigin RD, McCracken GH Jr, Klein JO. Diagnosis and management of meningitis. *Pediatr Infect Dis J* 1992;11:785–814.
93. Archer BD. Computed tomography before lumbar puncture in acute meningitis: a review of the risks and benefits. *Can Med Assoc J* 1993;148:961–965.
94. Quagliarello VJ, Scheld WM. Treatment of bacterial meningitis. *N Engl J Med* 1997;336:708–716.
95. Ni H, Knight AI, Cartwright K, et al. Polymerase chain reaction for diagnosis of meningococcal meningitis. *Lancet* 1992;340:1432–1434.
96. Narita M, Matsuzono Y, Shibata M, et al. Nested amplification protocol for the detection of *Mycobacterium tuberculosis*. *Acta Paediatr* 1992;81:997–1001.
97. Hansen K. Lyme neuroborreliosis. Improvements of the laboratory diagnosis and a survey of epidemiological and clinical features in Denmark 1985–1990. *Acta Neurol Scand* 1994; 899Suppl 151):6–44.
98. Troendle-Atkins J, Demmler GJ, Buffone GJ. Rapid diagnosis of herpes simplex virus encephalitis by using the polymerase chain reaction. *J Pediatr* 1993;123:376–380.
99. Jeffery KJM, et al. Diagnosis of viral infections of the central nervous system: clinical interpretation of PCR results. *Lancet* 1997;349:313–317.
100. Mandal BK. The dilemma of partially treated bacterial meningitis. *Scand J Infect Dis* 1976;8:185–188.
101. Talan DA, Hoffman JR, Yoshikawa TT, et al. Role of empiric parenteral antibiotics prior to lumbar puncture in suspected bacterial meningitis: state of the art. *Rev Infect Dis* 1988;10:365–376.
102. Rosenthal J, Golan A, Dagan R. Bacterial meningitis with initial normal cerebrospinal fluid findings. *Isr J Med Sci* 1989;25:186–188.
103. Milne A, Hamilton W. Developing or normocellular meningitis. *N Z Med J* 1976;84:6–8.
104. Ismail Y, Arsura EL. Eosinophilic meningitis associated with coccidioidomycosis. *West J Med* 1993;158:300–301.
105. Donald PR, Malan C, van der Walt A. Simultaneous determination of cerebrospinal fluid glucose and blood glucose concentrations in the diagnosis of bacterial meningitis. *J Pediatr* 1983;103:413–415.
106. Lichtheim L. Bei Gehirnkrankheiten durch die Punktion der Subarachnoidalräume auf der Höhe des dritten Lendenwirbels und Entziehung von Liquor cerebrospinalis therapeutisch einzugreifen [Abstract]. *Dtsch Med Wochenschr* 1893;19:12–34.
107. Menkes JH. The causes for low spinal fluid sugar in bacterial meningitis—another look. *Pediatrics* 1969;44:1–3.
108. Prockop LD, Fishman RA. Experimental pneumococcal meningitis. Permeability changes influencing the concentration of sugars and macromolecules in the cerebrospinal fluid. *Arch Neurol* 1968;19:449–463.

109. Wolf SM. Decreased cerebrospinal fluid glucose level in herpes zoster meningitis. Report of a case. *Arch Neurol* 1974;30:109.
110. Shaaban SY, Girgis NI, Mansour MM, et al. Prognostic value of cerebrospinal fluid protein content and leukocyte count in infants and childhood bacterial meningitis. *J Egypt Public Health Assoc* 1991;66:345–355.
111. Contronі G, et al. Cerebrospinal fluid lactic acid levels in meningitis. *J Pediatr* 1977;91:379–384.
112. Gould IM, Irwin WJ, Wadhwani RR. The use of cerebrospinal fluid lactate determination in the diagnosis of meningitis. *Scand J Infect Dis* 1980;12:185–188.
113. Bland RD, Lister RC, Ries JP. Cerebrospinal fluid lactic acid levels and pH in meningitis. AIDS in differential diagnosis. *Am J Dis Child* 1974;128:151–156.
114. Converse GM, Gwaltney JM Jr., Strassburg DA, et al. Alteration of cerebrospinal fluid findings by partial treatment of bacterial meningitis. *J Pediatr* 1973;83:220–225.
115. Riordan FAI, et al. Does computed tomography have a role in the evaluation of complicated acute bacterial meningitis in childhood? *Dev Med Child Neurol* 1993;35:275–276.
116. Rennick G, Shann F, de Campo J. Cerebral herniation during bacterial meningitis in children. *BMJ* 1993;306:953–955.
117. Benjamin CM, Newton RW, Clark MA. Risk factors for death from meningitis. *BMJ (Clin Res Ed)* 1988;296:20.
118. Feske SK, Carrazana EJ, Kupsky WJ, et al. Uncal herniation secondary to bacterial meningitis in a newborn. *Pediatr Neurol* 1992;8:142–144.
119. Feigin RD, Pearlman E. Bacterial meningitis beyond the neonatal period. In: Feigin RD, Cherry JD, eds. *Textbook of pediatric infectious diseases,* 4th ed. Philadelphia: Saunders, 1998: 400–429.
120. Wubbel L, McCracken GH Jr. Management of bacterial meningitis. *Pediatr Rev* 1998;19:78–84.
121. American Academy of Pediatrics. Pickering LK, ed. *2003 Red book: report of the Committee on Infectious Diseases*, 26th ed. Elk Grove Village, IL: Author, 2003.
122. Friedland IR, McCracken GH Jr. Management of infections caused by antibiotic-resistant *Streptococcus pneumoniae*. *N Engl J Med* 1994;331:377–382.
123. Kaplan SL, Fishman MA. Supportive therapy for bacterial meningitis. *Pediatr Infec Dis J* 1987;6:670–677.
124. Roos KL, Tunkel AR, Scheld WM. Acute bacterial meningitis in children and adults. In: Scheld WM, Whitley RJ, Durack DT, eds. *Infections of the central nervous system*. New York: Raven Press, 1991: 335–409.
125. Lebel MH, Freij BJ, Syrogiannopoulos GA, et al. Dexamethasone therapy for bacterial meningitis. Result of two double-blind, placebo-controlled trials. *N Engl J Med* 1988;319:964–971.
126. Schaad UB, Lips U, Gnehm HE, et al. Dexamethasone therapy for bacterial meningitis in children. Swiss Meningitis Study Group. *Lancet* 1993;342:457–461.
127. Syrogiannopoulos GA, Lourida AN, Theodoridov MC, et al. Dexamethasone therapy for bacterial meningitis in children: 2- versus 4-day regimen. *J Infect Dis* 1994;169:8553–8858.
128. Schaad UB, Kaplan SL, McKracken GH Jr. Steroid therapy for bacterial meningitis. *Clin Infect Dis* 1995;20:685–690.
129. Dodge PR. Sequelae of bacterial meningitis. *Pediatr Infect Dis J* 1986;5:618–620.
130. Radetsky M. Duration of symptoms and outcome in bacterial meningitis: an analysis of causation and the implications of a delay in diagnosis. *Pediatr Infect Dis J* 1992;11:694–698.
131. Kresky B, Buchbinder S, Greenberg IM. The incidence of neurologic residua in children after recovery from bacterial meningitis. *Arch Pediatr* 1962;79:63–71.
132. Thomas DG. Outcome of paediatric bacterial meningitis 1979–1989. *Med J Aust* 1992;157:519–520.
133. Grimwood K, Anderson VA, Bond L, et al. Adverse outcomes of bacterial meningitis in school-age survivors. *Pediatrics* 1995;95: 646–656.
134. Anderson V, Bond L, Catroppa C, et al. Childhood bacterial meningitis: impact of age at illness and acute medical complications on long term outcome. *J Int Neuropsychol Soc* 1997;3:147–158.
135. MacDonald JT, Feinstein S. Hearing loss following *Haemophilus influenzae* meningitis in infancy. Diagnosis by evoked response audiometry. *Arch Neurol* 1984;41:1058–1059.
136. Bao X, Wong V. Brainstem auditory-evoked potential evaluation in children with meningitis. *Pediatr Neurol* 1998;19:109–112.
137. Dodge PR, Davis H, Feigin RD, et al. Prospective evaluation of hearing impairment as a sequela of acute bacterial meningitis. *N Engl J Med* 1984;311:869–874.
138. Annegers JF, Hauser WA, Beghi E, et al. The risk of unprovoked seizures after encephalitis and meningitis. *Neurology* 1988;38:1407–1410.
139. Marks DA, Kim J, Spencer DD, et al. Characteristics of intractable seizures following meningitis and encephalitis. *Neurology* 1992;42:1513–1518.
140. Baraff LJ, Lee SI, Schriger DL. Outcomes of bacterial meningitis in children: a meta-analysis. *Pediatr Infect Dis J* 1993;12:389–394.
141. Wehrle PF, Leedom JM, Mathies AW. Treatment of meningococcal meningitis. *Mod Treatment* 1967;4:929–938.
142. Westendorp RGJ, Langermans JA, Huizinga TW, et al. Genetic influences on cytokine production and fatal meningococcal disease. *Lancet* 1997;349:170–173.
143. Fijen CA, Kuijper EJ, Tjia HG, et al. Complement deficiency predisposes to meningitis due to nongroupable meningococci and *Neisseria*-related organisms. *Clin Infect Dis* 1994;18:780–784.
144. Feigin RD, San Joaquin VS, Middlekamp JN. *Purpura fulminans* associated with *Neisseria catarrhalis* septicemia and meningitis. *Pediatrics* 1969;44:120–123.
145. Demmler GJ, Couch RS, Taber LH. *Neisseria subflava* bacteremia and meningitis in a child: report of a case and review of the literature. *Pediatr Infect Dis* 1985;4:286–288.
146. Swierczewski JA, Mason EJ, Cabrera PB, et al. Fulminating meningitis with Waterhouse-Friderichsen syndrome due to *Neisseria gonorrhoeae*. *Am J Clin Pathol* 1970;54:202–203.
147. Dalldorf FG, Jennette JC. Fatal meningococcal septicemia. *Arch Pathol Lab Med* 1977;101:6–9.
148. Astiz ME, Rackow EC. Septic shock. *Lancet* 1998;351:1501–1505.
149. Parrillo JE. Pathogenetic mechanisms of septic shock. *N Engl J Med* 1993;328:1471–1477.
150. Bass JL, Nuss R, Mehta KA, et al. Recurrent meningococcemia associated with IgG2-subclass deficiency [Letter]. *N Engl J Med* 1983;309:430.
151. Davis CA, Shurin SB, Pate K, et al. Neutrophil function in a patient with meningococcal meningitis and C7 deficiency. *Am J Dis Child* 1983;137:404–406.
152. Williams DN, Geddes AM. Meningococcal meningitis complicated by pericarditis, panophthalmitis, and arthritis. *Br Med J* 1970;2:93.
153. Hardman JM, Earle KM. Myocarditis in 200 fatal meningococcal infections. *Arch Pathol* 1969;87:318–325.
154. Mayatepek E, Grauer M, Sonntag HG. Deafness after meningococcal meningitis. *Lancet* 1991;338:13–31.
155. Cuevas L, Hart CA. Chemoprophylaxis of bacterial meningitis. *J Antimicrob Chemother* 1993;3([Suppl B):79–91.
156. Adams WG, Deaver KA, Cochi SL, et al. Decline of childhood *Haemophilus influenzae* type B (Hib) disease in the Hib vaccine era. *JAMA* 1993;269:221–226.
157. Schoendorf KC, Adams WG, Kiely JL, et al. National trends in *Haemophilus influenzae* meningitis mortality and hospitalization among children 1980 through 1991. *Pediatrics* 1994;93:663–668.
158. Nizet V, Colina KF, Aimquist JR, et al. A virulent nonencapsulated *Haemophilus influenzae*. *J Infect Dis* 1996;173:180–186.
159. A survey of invasive *Haemophilus influenzae* infections—England and Wales. *Can Comm Dis Rep* 1992;18:42–47.
160. Falla TJ, Dobson SR, Crook DW, et al. Population-based study of non-typable *Haemophilus influenzae* invasive disease in children and neonates. *Lancet* 1993;341:851–854.
161. Smith ER. An adult with *Haemophilus meningitis*: case report. *N Z Med J* 1976;83:367–368.
162. Granoff DM, Squires JE. *Haemophilus meningitis*: new developments in epidemiology, treatment and prophylaxis. *Semin Neurol* 1982;2:151–165.
163. Taylor HG, Michaels RH, Mazur PM, et al. Intellectual, neuropsychological, and achievement outcomes in children six to eight

years after recovery from *Haemophilus influenzae* meningitis. *Pediatrics* 1984;74:198–205.
164. Tepperberg J, Nussbaum E, Feldman F. Cortical blindness following meningitis due to *Haemophilus influenzae* type B. *J Pediatr* 1977;91:434–435.
165. Dunn DW, Daum RS, Weisberg L, et al. Ischemic cerebrovascular complications of *Haemophilus influenzae* meningitis. The value of computed tomography. *Arch Neurol* 1982;39:650–652.
166. Headings DL, Glasgow LA. Occlusion of the internal carotid artery complicating *Haemophilus influenzae* meningitis. *Am J Dis Child* 1977;131:854–856.
167. Morriss JH, Gillette PC, Barrett FF. Atrioventricular block complicating meningitis: treatment with emergency cardiac pacing. *Pediatrics* 1976;58:866–868.
168. Granoff DM, Nankervis GA. Cellulitis due to *Haemophilus influenzae* type B. Antigenemia and antibody responses. *Am J Dis Child* 1976;130:1211–1214.
169. Scheld WM. Bacterial meningitis in the patient at risk: intrinsic risk factors and host defense mechanisms. *Am J Med* 1984;76:193–207.
170. Brandtzaeg P, Mollnes TE, Kierulf P. Complement activation and endotoxin levels in systemic meningococcal disease. *J Infect Dis* 1989;160:58–65.
171. Griesemer DA, Winkelstein JA, Luddy R. Pneumococcal meningitis in patients with a major sickle hemoglobinopathy. *J Pediatr* 1978;92:82–84.
172. Tuomanen E, Masure R. The molecular and cell biology of pneumococcal infection. *Microb Drug Resist* 1997;3:297–308.
173. Tuomanen E, Liu H, Hengstler B, et al. The induction of meningeal inflammation by components of the pneumococcal cell wall. *J Infect Dis* 1985;151:859–868.
174. Winter A, Cornis SD, Osborne MP, et al. A role for pneumolysin but not neuraminidase in the hearing loss and cochlear damage induced by experimental pneumococcal meningitis in guinea pigs. *Infect Immun* 1997;65:4411–4418.
175. Kornelisse RF, Westerbeek CM, Spoor AB, et al. Pneumococcal meningitis in children: prognostic indicators and outcome. *Clin Infect Dis* 1995;21:1390–1397.
176. Arditi M, Mason EO Jr., Bradley JS, et al. Three-year multicenter surveillance of pneumococcal meningitis in children: clinical characteristics, and outcome related to penicillin susceptibility and dexamethasone use. *Pediatrics* 1998;102:1087–1097.
177. Kim JH, Vander Horst C, Mulrow CD, et al. *Staphylococcus aureus* meningitis: review of 28 cases. *Rev Infect Dis* 1989;11:698–706.
178. Givner LB, Kaplan SL. Meningitis due to *Staphylococcus aureus* in children. *Clin Infect Dis* 1993;16:766–771.
179. Ziment I. Nervous system complications in bacterial endocarditis. *Am J Med* 1969;47:593–607.
180. Jensen AG, Espersen F, Skinhoj P, et al. *Staphylococcus aureus* meningitis. A review of 104 nation-wide, consecutive cases. *Arch Int Med* 1993;153:1902–1908.
181. Diaz-Mitoma F, Harding GK, Hoban DJ, et al. Clinical significance of a test for slime production in ventriculoperitoneal shunt infections caused by coagulase-negative staphylococci. *J Infect Dis* 1987;156:555–560.
182. Holt R. The classification of staphylococci from colonized ventriculo-atrial shunts. *J Clin Pathol* 1969;22:475–482.
183. Shurtleff DB, Christie D, Faltz EL. Ventriculoauriculostomy-associated infection. A 12-year study. *J Neurosurg* 1971;35:686–694.
184. deLouvois J. Acute bacterial meningitis in the newborn. *J Antimicrob Chemother* 1994;34(Suppl A):61–73.
185. Dyggve H. Prognosis in meningitis neonatorum. *Acta Pediatr Scand* 1962;51:303–312.
186. McCrory JH, Au-Yeung B, Sugg VM, et al. Recurrent group B streptococcal infection in an infant: ventriculitis complicating type Ib meningitis. *J Pediatr* 1978;92:231–238.
187. Bates HA, Controni G, Elliot N, et al. Septicemia and meningitis in a newborn due to *Pasteurella multocida*. *Clin Pediatr* 1965;4:668–670.
188. Mann JM, Shandler L, Cushing AH. Pediatric plague. *Pediatrics* 1982;69:762–767.
189. Kostiala AA, Westerstrahle M, Muttilainen M. Neonatal salmonella Panama infection with meningitis. *Acta Paediatr* 1992;81:856–858.
190. Jones RN, Slepack J, Eades A. Fatal neonatal meningococcal meningitis. Association with maternal cervicalvaginal colonization. *JAMA* 1976;236:2852–2853.
191. Unhanand M, Mustafa MM, McCracken GH Jr, et al. Gram-negative enteric bacillary meningitis: a twenty-one-year experience. *J Pediatr* 1993;122:15–21.
192. Siitonen A, Takala A, Ratiner YA, et al. Invasive *Escherichia coli* infections in children: bacterial characteristics in different age groups and clinical entities. *Pediatr Inf Dis J* 1993;12:606–612.
193. Overall JC Jr. Neonatal bacterial meningitis. Analysis of predisposing factors and outcome compared with matched control subjects. *J Pediatr* 1970;76:499–511.
194. St.Geme JW Jr, Murray DL, Carter J, et al. Perinatal bacterial infection after prolonged rupture of membranes. Analysis of risk and management. *J Pediatr* 1984;104:608–613.
195. Visser VE, Hall RT. Lumbar puncture in the evaluation of neonatal sepsis. *J Pediatr* 1980;96:1063–1067.
196. Groover RV, Sutherland JM, Landing BH. Purulent meningitis of newborn infants: eleven year experience in the antibiotic era. *N Engl J Med* 1961;264:1115–1121.
197. Weiss MG, Ionides SP, Anderson CL. Meningitis in premature infants with respiratory distress: role of admission lumbar puncture. *J Pediatr* 1991;119:973–975.
198. Sarff LD, Platt LH, McCracken GH Jr. Cerebrospinal fluid evaluation in neonates: Comparison of high-risk infants with and without meningitis. *J Pediatr* 1976;88:473–477.
199. Hristeva L, Bowler I, Booy R, et al. Value of cerebrospinal fluid examination in the diagnosis of meningitis in the newborn. *Arch Dis Child* 1993;69:514–517.
200. Baker CJ, Barrett FF, Gordon RC, et al. Suppurative meningitis due to streptococci of Lancefield group B. A study of 33 infants. *J Pediatr* 1973;82:724–729.
201. Haslam RH, Allen JR, Dorsen MM, et al. The sequelae of group B b hemolytic meningitis in early infancy. *Am J Dis Child* 1977;131:845–849.
202. Baker CJ, Kasper DL. Immunological investigation of infants with septicemia or meningitis due to group B streptococcus. *J Infect Dis* 1977;136:(Suppl):S98–S104.
203. Booy R, Kroll S. Bacterial meningitis in children. *Curr Opin Pediatr* 1994;6:29–35.
204. Hristeva L, Booy R, Bowler I, et al. Prospective surveillance of neonatal meningitis. *Arch Dis Child* 1993;69(1 Spec No):14–18.
205. Medical Research Council Tuberculosis and Chest Diseases Unit. Tuberculosis in children: a national survey of notifications in England and Wales in 1983. *Arch Dis Child* 1988;63:266–276.
206. Kopanoff DE. A continuing survey of tuberculosis primary drug resistance in the United States: March 1975 to November 1977. A United States Public Health Service cooperative study. *Am Rev Respir Dis* 1978;118:835–842.
207. Yaramis A, Gurkan F, Elevli M, et al. Central nervous system tuberculosis in children: a review of 214 cases. *Pediatrics* 1998;102:E49.
208. Dastur DK, Lalitha VS, Udani PM, et al. The brain and meninges in tuberculous meningitis: gross pathology in 100 cases and pathogenesis. *Neurology* (India) 1970;18:86–100.
209. Critchley M. Brain tumors in children: their general symptomatology. *Br J Child Dis* 1925;22:251–264.
210. Lincoln EM. Tuberculous meningitis in children. I. Tuberculous meningitis. *Am Rev Tuberc Pulm Dis* 1946: 56:75–94.
211. Idriss ZH, Sinno AA, Kronfol NM. Tuberculous meningitis in childhood. Forty-three cases. *Am J Dis Child* 1976;130:364–367.
212. Narotam PK, Kemp M, Buck R, et al. Hyponatremic natriuretic syndrome in tuberculous meningitis: the probable role of atrial natriuretic peptide. *Neurosurgery* 1994;34:982–998.
213. Whitener DR. Tuberculous brain abscess. Report of case and review of the literature. *Arch Neurol* 1978;35:148–155.
214. Lees AJ, McLeod AF, Marshall J. Cerebral tuberculomas developing during treatment of tuberculous meningitis. *Lancet* 1980;1:1208–1211.
215. Teoh R, Humphries MJ, O'Mahoney G. Symptomatic intracranial tuberculoma developing during treatment of tuberculosis:

a report of 10 patients and a review of the literature. *QJM* 1987;63:449–460.
216. Chambers ST, Hendrickse WA, Record C, et al. Paradoxical expansion of intracranial tuberculomas during chemotherapy. *Lancet* 1984;2:181–184.
217. Gourie-Devi M, Satishchandra P. Hyaluronidase as an adjuvant in the management of tuberculous spinal arachnoiditis. *J Neurol Sci* 1991;102:105–111.
218. Davis LE, Rastogi KR, Lambert LC, et al. Tuberculous meningitis in the southwest United States: a community-based study. *Neurology* 1993;43:1775–1778.
219. Lincoln EH, Sewell EM. *Tuberculosis in children*. New York: McGraw-Hill, 1963.
220. Kent SJ, Crowe SM, Yung A, et al. Tuberculous meningitis: a 30-year review. *Clin Infect Dis* 1993;17:987–994.
221. Seth V, Kabra SK, Beotra A, et al. Tuberculous meningitis in children: manifestation of an immune compromised state. *Indian Pediatr* 1993;30:1181–1186.
222. Zarabi M, Sane S, Girdany BR. The chest roentgenogram in the early diagnosis of tuberculous meningitis in children. *Am J Dis Child* 1971;121:389–392.
223. Narita M, Matsuzono Y, Shibata M, et al. Nested amplification protocol for the detection of *Mycobacterium* tuberculosis. *Acta Paediatr* 1992;81:997–1001.
224. Hernandez R, Muñoz O, Guiscafre H. Sensitive enzyme immunoassay for early diagnosis of tuberculous meningitis. *J Clin Microbiol* 1984;20:533–535.
225. Larsson L, Mardh P, Odham G, et al. Use of selected ion monitoring for detection of tuberculostearic and C32 mycocerosic acid in mycobacteria and in five-day-old cultures of sputum specimens from patients with pulmonary tuberculosis. *Acta Pathol Microbiol Scand B* 1981;89:245–251.
226. Hinman AR. Tuberculous meningitis at Cleveland Metropolitan General Hospital 1959–1963. *Am Rev Respir Dis* 1975;670–673.
227. Weiss IK, Krogstad PA, Botero C, et al. Fatal *Mycobacterium avium* meningitis after mis-identification of *M. tuberculosis. Lancet* 1995;305:991–992.
228. Chandra B. Some aspects of tuberculous meningitis in Surabaya. *Proc Aust Assoc Neurol* 1976;13:73–81.
229. Shanley DJ. Computed tomography and magnetic resonance imaging of tuberculous meningitis. *J Am Osteopathic Assoc* 1993;93:497–501.
230. Bhargava S, Gupta AK, Tandon PN. Tuberculous meningitis—a CT study. *Br J Radiol* 1982;55:189–196.
231. Gupta RK, Pandey R, Kahn EM, et al. Intracranial tuberculomas: MRI signal intensity correlation with histopathology and localised proton spectroscopy. *Magn Reson Imaging* 1993;11:443–449.
232. Durfee NL, et al. The treatment of tuberculosis in children. *Am Rev Respir Dis* 1969;99:304–307.
233. American Academy of Pediatrics. Tuberculosis. In: Peter G, ed. *1997 Red book: report of the Committee onInfectious Diseases*, 24th ed. Elk Grove Village, IL: Author, 1997: 541–562.
234. Kaojarern S, Supmonchai K, Phuapradit P, et al. Effect of steroids on cerebrospinal fluid of antituberculous drugs in tuberculous meningitis. *Clin Pharmacol Ther* 1991;49:6–12.
235. Rozwarski DA, Grant GA, Barton DH, et al. Modification of the NADH of the isoniazid target (InhA) from *Mycobacterium tuberculosis*. *Science* 1998;279:99–102.
236. Iseman MD. Treatment of multidrug-resistant tuberculosis. *N Engl J Med* 1993: 329:784–791.
237. Schoeman JF, Van Zyl LE, Laubscher JA, et al. Effect of corticosteroids on intracranial pressure, computed tomographic findings, and clinical outcome in young children with tuberculous meningitis. *Pediatrics* 1997;99:226–231.
238. Alzeer AH, Fitzgerald JM. Corticosteroids and tuberculosis: risks and use as adjunct therapy. *Tuberc Lung Dis* 1993;74:6–11.
239. O'Toole RD, Thornton GF, Mukherjee MK, et al. Dexamethasone in tuberculous meningitis. Relationship of cerebrospinal fluid effects to therapeutic efficacy. *Ann Intern Med* 1969;70:39–48.
240. Watson JD, Schnier RC, Seale JP. Central nervous system tuberculosis in Australia: a report of 22 cases. *Med J Aust* 1993;158:408–413.
241. Damany BJ. Surgery in tuberculous meningitis. *Prog Pediatr Surg* 1982;15:181–185.
242. Bullock MR, Van Dellen Jr. The role of cerebrospinal fluid shunting in tuberculous meningitis. *Surg Neurol* 1982;18:274–277.
243. Peacock WJ, Deenny JE. Improving the outcome of tuberculous meningitis in childhood. *S Afr Med J* 1984;66:597–598.
244. Bhagwati SN, Parulekar GD. Management of intracranial tuberculomas in children. *Childs Nerv Syst* 1986;2:232–234.
245. Todd RM, Neville JG. Sequelae of tuberculous meningitis. *Arch Dis Child* 1964;39:213–225.
246. Deeny JE, Walker MJ, Kibel MA, et al. Tuberculous meningitis in children in the Western Cape. Epidemiology and outcome. *S Afr Med J* 1985;68:75–78.
247. Lorber J. Long-term follow up of 100 children who recovered from tuberculous meningitis. *Pediatrics* 1961;28:778–791.
248. Drury MI, O'Lochlainn S, Sweeney E. Complications of tuberculous meningitis. *BMJ* 1968;1:842.
249. Lam KS, Sham MM, Tam SC, et al. Hypopituitarism after tuberculosis in childhood. *Ann Intern Med* 1993;118:701–706.
250. Lorber J. The results of treatment of 549 cases of tuberculous meningitis. *Am Rev Tuberc Pulm Dis* 1954;69:13–25.
251. Mann JM, Shandler L, Cushing AH. Pediatric plague. *Pediatrics* 1982;69:762–767.
252. Lavetter A, Leedom JM, Mathies AW Jr., et al. Meningitis due to *Listeria monocytogenes*. A review of 25 cases. *N Engl J Med* 1971;285:598–603.
253. Brook I. *Listeria monocytogenes* meningitis. *N Y State J Med* 1980;80:1845–1846.
254. Armstrong RW, Fung PC. Brainstem encephalitis (rhombencephalitis) due to *Listeria monocytogenes:* case report and review. *Clin Infect Dis* 1993;16:689–702.
255. Levey HL, Ingall D. Meningitis in neonates due to *Proteus mirabilis*. *Am J Dis Child* 1967;14:320–324.
256. Graber CD, Higgins LS, Davis JS. Seldom-encountered agents of bacterial meningitis. *JAMA* 1965;192:956–960.
257. Tahernia AC, Hashemi G. Survival in anthrax meningitis. *Pediatrics* 1972;50:329–333.
258. Kolyvas E, Sorger S, Marks MI, et al. *Pasteurella ureae* meningoencephalitis. *J Pediatr* 1978;92:81–82.
259. Foreman SD, Smith EE, Ryan NJ, et al. Neonatal *Citrobacter* meningitis: pathogenesis of cerebral abscess formation. *Ann Neurol* 1984;16:655–659.
260. Omar FZ, Zuberi S, Minns RA. Neurobrucellosis in childhood: six new cases and a review of the literature. *Dev Med Child Neurol* 1997;39:762–765.
261. Lubani MM, Dudin KI, Araj GF, et al. Neurobrucellosis in children. *Pediatr Infect Dis* 1989;8:79–82.
262. McLean DR, Russel N, Khan MY. Neurobrucellosis: clinical and therapeutic features. *Clin Infect Dis* 1992;15:582–590.
263. Cover TL, Aber RC. *Yersinia enterocolitica*. *N Engl J Med* 1989;321:16–24.
264. Saez-Llorens X. Brain abscess in children. *Semin Pediatr Infect Dis* 2003;14(2):108–114.
265. Ersahin Y, Mutluer S, Guzelbag E. Brain abscess in infants and children. *Childs Nerv Syst* 1994;10:185–189.
266. Goodkin HP, Harper MB, Pomeroy SL. Intracerebral abscess in children: historical trends at Children's Hospital Boston. *Pediatrics* 2004;113:1765–1770.
267. Fischer EG, Schwachman H, Wepsic JG. Brain abscess and cystic fibrosis. *J Pediatr* 1979;95:385–388.
268. Jadavji T, Humphreys RB, Prober CG. Brain abscesses in infants and children. *Pediatr Infect Dis* 1985;4:394–398.
269. Tekkok IH, Erbengi A. Management of brain abscess in children: review of 130 cases over a period of 21 years. *Childs Nerv Syst* 1992;8:411–416.
270. Byrne E, Brophy BP, Perrett LV. Nocardial cerebral abscess: new concepts in diagnosis, management, and prognosis. *J Neurol Neurosurg Psychiatry* 1979;11:1038–1045.
271. McLeod R, Berry PF, Marshall WH Jr., et al. Toxoplasmosis presenting as brain abscesses. Diagnosis by computerized tomography and cytology of aspirated purulent material. *Am J Med* 1979;67:711–714.

272. Brook I. Aerobic and anaerobic bacteriology of intracranial abscesses. *Pediatr Neurol* 1992;8:210–214.
273. Rau CS, Chang WN, Lin YC, et al. Brain abscess caused by aerobic Gram-negative bacilli: clinical features and therapeutic outcomes. *Clin Neurol Neurosurg* 2002;105:60–65.
274. Raimondi AJ, Matsumoto S, Miller RA. Brain abscess in children with congenital heart disease. I. *J Neurosurg* 1965;23:588–595.
275. Fischer EG, McLennan JE, Suzuki Y. Cerebral abscess in children. *Am J Dis Child* 1981;135:746–749.
276. Domingue JN, Wilson CB. Pituitary abscesses. Report of seven cases and review of literature. *J Neurosurg* 1977;46:601–608.
277. Candon E, Frerebeau P. Abcès bactériens de la moelle épinière. Revue de la littérature (73 cas). *Rev Neurol* (Paris) 1994;150:370–376.
278. Mampalam TJ, Rosenblum ML. Trends in the management of bacterial brain abscess: a review of 102 cases over 17 years. *Neurosurgery* 1988;23:451–458.
279. Smith RR. Neuroradiology of intracranial infection. *Pediatr Neurosurg* 1992;18:92–104.
280. Segall HD, Rumbaugh CL, Bergeron RT, et al. Neuroradiology in infections of the brain and meninges. *Surg Neurol* 1973;1:178–186.
281. Heinz ER, Cooper RD. Several early angiographic findings in brain abscess including the "ripple sign." *Radiology* 1968;90:735–739.
282. Mishra AM, Gupta RK, Jaggi RS, et al. Role of diffusion-weighted imaging and *in vivo* proton magnetic resonance spectroscopy in the differential diagnosis of ring-enhancing intracranial cystic mass lesions. *J Comput Assist Tomogr* 2004;28:540–547.
283. Teixeira J, Zimmerman RA, Haselgrove JC, et al. Diffusion imaging in pediatric central nervous system infections. *Neuroradiology* 2001;43:1031–1039.
284. Desbarats LN, Herlidou S, de Marco G, et al. Differential MRI diagnosis between brain abscesses and necrotic or cystic brain tumors using the apparent diffusion coefficient and normalized diffusion-weighted images. *Magn Reson Imaging* 2003;21:645–650.
285. Cartes-Zumelzu FW, Stavrou I, Castillo M, et al. Diffusion-weighted imaging in the assessment of brain abscesses therapy. *Am J Neuroradiol* 2004;25:1310–1317.
286. Tyler HR, Clark DB. Cerebrovascular accidents in patients with congenital heart disease. *Arch Neurol Psychiatr* 1957;77:483–489.
287. Clark DB. Brain abscess and congenital heart disease. *Clin Neurosurg* 1966;14:274–287.
288. Rosenblum ML, Hoff JT, Norman D, et al. Nonoperative treatment of brain abscesses in selected high-risk patients. *J Neurosurg* 1980;52:217–225.
289. Hirsch JF, Roux FX, Sainte-Rose C, et al. Brain abscess in childhood. A study of 34 cases treated by puncture and antibiotics. *Childs Brain* 1983;10:251–265.
290. Psiachou-Leonard E, Sidi V, Tsivitanidou M, et al. Brain abscesses resulting from *Bacillus cereus* and *Aspergillus*-like mold. *J Pediatr Hematol/Oncol* 2002;24:569–571.
291. Ciurea AV, Stoica F, Vasilescu G, et al. Neurosurgical management of brain abscesses in children. *Childs Nerv Syst* 1999;15:309–317.
292. Agrawal D, Suri A, Mahapatra AK. Primary excision of pediatric posterior fossa abscesses—towards zero mortality? A series of nine cases and review. *Pediatr Neurosurg* 2003;38:63–67.
293. Fuentes S, Bouillot P, Regis J, et al. Management of brain stem abscess. *Br J Neurosurg* 2001;15:57–62.
294. Moylett EH, Pacheco SE, Brown-Elliot BA, et al. Clinical experience with linezolid for the treatment of *Nocardia* infection. *Clin Infect Dis* 2003;36:313–318.
295. Editorial. Treatment of brain abscess. *Lancet* 1988;1:219–220.
296. Wright RL, Ballantine HT Jr. Management of brain abscesses in children and adolescents. *Am J Dis Child* 1967;114:113–122.
297. Berlit P, Fedel C, Tornow K, et al. Bacterial brain abscess: a review of 67 patients in Germany. *Fortschr Neurol Psychiatr* 1996;64:297–306.
298. Jennett WB, Barker J, Fitch W, et al. Effect of anaesthesia on intracranial pressure in patients with space-occupying lesions. *Lancet* 1969;1:61–64.
299. Berg B, Franklin G, Cuneo R, et al. Non-surgical cure of brain abscess. Early diagnosis and follow-up with computerized tomography. *Ann Neurol* 1978;3:474–478.
300. Boom WH, Tauazon CU. Successful treatment of multiple brain abscess with antibiotic alone. *Rev Infect Dis* 1985;7:189–199.
301. Bambakidis NC, Cohen AR. Intracranial complications of frontal sinusitis in children: Pott's puffy tumor revisited. *Pediatr Neurosurg* 2001;35:82–89.
302. Legg NJ, Gupta PC, Scott DF. Epilepsy following cerebral abscess. *Brain* 1973;96:259–268.
303. Tekkok IH, Erbengi A. Management of brain abscess in children: review of 130 cases over a period of 21 years. *Childs Nerv Syst* 1992;8:411–416.
304. Galbraith JG, Barr VW. Epidural abscess and subdural empyema. *Adv Neurol* 1974;6:257–267.
305. Farmer TW, Wise GR. Subdural empyema in infants, children and adults. *Neurology* 1973;23:254–261.
306. Skelton R, Maixner W, Isaacs D. Sinusitis induced subdural hematoma. *Arch Dis Child* 1992;67:1478–1480.
307. Ogilvy CS, Chapman PH, McGrail K. Subdural empyema complicating bacterial meningitis in a child: enhancement of membranes with gadolinium on magnetic resonance imaging in a patient without enhancement on computed tomography. *Surg Neurol* 1992;37:138–141.
308. Wong AM, Zimmerman RA, Simon EM, et al. Diffusion-weighted MR imaging of subdural empyemas in children. *Am J Neuroradiol* 2004;25:1016–1021.
309. Tewari MK, Sharma RR, Shiv VK, et al. Spectrum of intracranial subdural empyemas in a series of 45 patients: current surgical options and outcome. *Neurol India* 2004;52:346–349.
310. Nathoo N, Nadvi SS, Gouws E, et al. Craniotomy improves outcomes for cranial subdural empyemas: computed tomography-era experience with 699 patients. *Neurosurgery* 2001;49:872–878.
311. Nielsen H, Gyldensted C, Harmsen A. Cerebral abscess. Aetiology and pathogenesis, symptoms, diagnosis and treatment. A review of 200 cases from 1935–1976. *Acta Neurol Scand* 1982;65:609–622.
312. Smith HP, Hendrick EB. Subdural empyema and epidural abscess in children. *J Neurosurg* 1983;58:392–397.
313. Baker AS, Ojemann RG, Swartz MN, et al. Spinal epidural abscess. *N Engl J Med* 1975;293:463–468.
314. Heran NS, Steinbok P, Cochrane DD. Conservative neurosurgical management of intracranial epidural abscesses in children. *Neurosurgery* 2003;53:893–898.
315. Reynolds DJ, Kodsi SR, Rubin SE, et al. Intracranial infection associated with preseptal and orbital cellulitis in the pediatric patient. *J AAPOS* 2003;7:413–417.
316. Tsai YD, Chang WN, Shen CC, et al. Intracranial suppuration: a clinical comparison of subdural empyemas and epidural abscesses. *Surg Neurol* 2003;59:191–196.
317. Auletta JJ, John CC. Spinal epidural abscesses in children: a 15-year experience and review of the literature. *Clin Infect Dis* 2001;32:9–16.
318. Kost-Byerly S, Tobin JR, Greenberg RS, et al. Bacterial colonization and infection rate of continuous epidural catheters in children. *Anesth Analg* 1998;86:712–716.
319. DiTullio MV Jr. Intramedullary spinal abscess: a case report with a review of 53 previously described cases. *Surg Neurol* 1977;7:351–354.
320. Leahy AL, Fogarty EE, Fitzgerald RJ, et al. Discitis as a cause of abdominal pain in children. *Surgery* 1984;95:412–414.
321. Garcia FF, et al. Diagnostic imaging of childhood spinal infection. *Orthop Rev* 1993;22:321–327.
322. Boston HC Jr, Bianco AJ Jr, Rhodes KH. Disc space infections in children. *Orthop Clin North Am* 1975;6:953–964.
323. Spiegel PG, Kengla KW, Isaacson AS, et al. Intervertebral disc-space inflammation in children. *J Bone Joint Surg* 1972;54A:284–296.
324. Jansen BR, Hart W, Schreuder O. Discitis in childhood. 12–35-year follow-up of 35 patients. *Acta Orthop Scand* 1993;64:33–36.
325. Ryoppy S, Jaaskelainen J, Rapola J, et al. Nonspecific diskitis in children, a nonmicrobial disease? *Clin Orthop* 1993;297:95–99.
326. Nahmias AJ. The TORCH complex. *Hosp Pract* 1974(May): 65–72.

327. Bale JF J, ed. Congenital infections of the central nervous system. *Sem Pediatr Neurol* 1994: 1:1–70.
328. Ueda K, Nishida Y, Oshmia K, et al. Congenital rubella syndrome: correlation of gestational age at time of maternal rubella with type of defect. *J Pediatr* 1979;94:763–765.
329. Alkalay AL, Pomerance JJ, Rimoin DL. Fetal varicella syndrome. *J Pediatr* 1987;111:320–323.
330. Swisher C, Boyer K, McLoed R. Congenital toxoplasmosis. *Sem Pediatr Neurol* 1994;1:4–25.
331. Demmler GJ. Summary of a workshop on surveillance of congenital cytomegalovirus disease. *Rev Infect Dis* 1991;13:315–329.
332. Ho M. *Cytomegalovirus: biology and infection*. New York: Plenum Press, 1982.
333. Hayward JC, Titelbaum DS, Clancy RR, et al. Lissencephaly-pachygyria associated with congenital cytomegalovirus infection. *J Child Neurol* 1991;6:109–114.
334. Iasnnetti P, Nigro G, Spalice, et al. Cytomegalovirus infection and schizencephaly: case reports. *Ann Neurol* 1998;43:123–127.
335. Pass RF, August AM, Dworsky M, et al. Cytomegalovirus infection in a day care center. *N Engl J Med* 1982;307:477–479.
336. Murph JR, Baron JC, Brown CK, et al. The occupational risk of cytomegalovirus among day care providers. *JAMA* 1991;265:603–608.
337. Stagno S, Pass RF, Cloud G, et al. Primary cytomegalovirus infection in pregnancy: incidence, transmission to fetus, and clinical outcome. *JAMA* 1986;256:1904–1908.
338. Boppana SB, Rivera LB, Fowler KB, et al. Intrauterine transmission of cytomegalovirus to infants of mothers with preconceptional immunity. *N Engl J Med* 2001;344:1366–1371.
339. Istas AS, Demmler GJ, Dobbins JG, et al. Surveillance for congenital cytomegalovirus disease: a report from the National Congenital Cytomegalovirus Disease Registry. *Clin Infect Dis* 1995;20:665–670.
340. Boppana SB, Pass RF, Britt WJ, et al. Symptomatic congenital cytomegalovirus infection: neonatal morbidity and mortality. *Pediatr Infect Dis J* 1992;11:93–99.
341. Koskiniemi M, Lappalainen M, Hedman K. Toxoplasmosis needs evaluation: An overview and proposals. *Am J Dis Child* 1989;143:724–728.
342. Couvreur J, Desmonts G. Congenital and maternal toxoplasmosis. *Dev Med Child Neurol* 1962;4:519–530.
343. McAuley J, Boyer K, Patel D, et al. Early and longitudinal evaluations of treated infants and children and untreated historical patients with congenital toxoplasmosis. The Chicago Collaborative Treatment Trial. *Clin Infect Dis* 1994;18:38–72.
344. Noyola DE, Demmler GJ, Nelson CT, et al. Early predictors of neurodevelopmental outcome in symptomatic congenital cytomegalovirus infection. *J Pediatr* 2001;138:325–331.
345. Boppana SB, Fowler KB, Vaid Y, et al. Neuroradiographic findings in the newborn period and long term outcome in children with symptomatic congenital cytomegalovirus infection. *Pediatrics* 1997;99:409–414.
346. Adler SP, Finney JW, Manganello AM, et al. Prevention of child-to-mother transmission of cytomegalovirus by changing behaviors: a randomized controlled trial. *Pediatr Infect Dis J* 1996;15:240–246.
347. Baril L, Ancelle T, Goulet V, et al. Risk factors for *Toxoplasma* infection in pregnancy: a case control study in France. *Scand J Infect Dis* 1999;31:305–308.
348. Kimberlin DW, Lin CY, Sanchez PJ, et al. Effect of ganciclovir therapy on hearing in symptomatic congenital cytomegalovirus infection involving the central nervous system: a randomized, controlled trial. *J Pediatr* 2003: 143:16–25.
349. Dahle AJ, Fowler KB, Wright JD, et al. Longitudinal investigation of hearing disorders in children with congenital cytomegalovirus. *J Am Acad Audiol* 2000;11:283–290.
350. Pass RF, Stagno S, Meyers GJ, et al. Outcome of symptomatic congenital cytomegalovirus infection: results of long-term, longitudinal follow-up. *Pediatrics* 1980;66:758–762.
351. Jones JL, Kruszon-Moran D, Wilson D, et al. *Toxoplasma gondii* infection in the United States: seroprevalence and risk factors. *Am J Epidemiol* 2001;154:352–365.
352. Mara M, Hsu HW, Eaton RB, et al. Epidemiology of congenital toxoplasmosis identified by population-based newborn screening in Massachusetts. *Pediatr Infect Dis J* 2001;20:1132–1135.
353. Couvreur J. Problems of congenital toxoplasmosis: evolution over four decades. *Presse Med* 1999;28:753–757.
354. Naessens A, Jenum PA, Pollak A, et al. Diagnosis of congenital toxoplasmosis in the neonatal period: a multicenter evaluation. *J Pediatr* 1999;135:714–719.
355. Boyer KM. Diagnostic testing for congenital toxoplasmosis. *Pediatr Infect Dis J* 2001;20:59–60.
356. Johnson J, Butcher P, Savva D, et al. Application of the polymerase chain reaction to the diagnosis of human toxoplasmosis. *J Infect* 1993;26:147–158.
357. Lopez A, Dietz VJ, Wilson M, et al. Preventing congenital toxoplasmosis. *MMWR Recomm Rep* 2000;49 (RR-2):59–68.
358. Wallon M, Liou C, Garner P, et al. Congenital toxoplasmosis: systematic review of evidence of efficacy of treatment in pregnancy. *BMJ* 1999;318:1511–1514.
359. Gilbert R, Gras L, Wallon M, et al. Effect of prenatal treatment on mother to child transmission of *Toxoplasma gondii*: retrospective cohort study of 554 mother–child pairs in Lyon, France. *Int J Epidemiol* 2001;30:1303–1308.
360. Guerina N, Hsu H, Mcissner H, et al. Neonatal serologic screening and early treatment for congenital *Toxoplasma gondii* infection. *N Engl J Med* 1994;330:1858–1863.
361. Armstrong GL, Schillinger J, Markowitz L, et al. Incidence of herpes simplex virus type 2 infection in the Unites States. *Am J Epidemiol* 2001;153:912–920.
362. Buchacz K, McFarland W, Hernandez M, et al. Prevalence and correlates of herpes simplex virus type 2 infection in a population-based survey of young women in low-income neighborhoods of Northern California. The Young Women's Survey Team. *Sex Transm Dis* 2000;27:393–400.
363. Brown ZA, Selke S, Zeh J, et al. The acquisition of herpes simplex virus during pregnancy. *N Engl J Med* 1997;337:509–515.
364. Grose C. Congenital infections caused by varicella-zoster virus and herpes simplex virus. *Semin Pediatr Neurol* 1994;1:43–49.
365. Baldwin S, Whitley RJ. Intrauterine herpes simplex virus infections. *Teratology* 1989;39:1–10.
366. Hutto C, Arvin A, Jacobs R, et al. Intrauterine herpes simplex virus infections. *J Pediatr* 1987;110:97–101.
367. Hoppen T, Eis-Hubinger AM, Schild RL, et al. Intrauterine herpes simplex virus infection. *Klin Padiatr* 2001;213:63–68.
368. Jacobs RF. Neonatal herpes simplex virus infections. *Semin Perinatol* 1998;22:64–71.
369. Kimberlin DW, Lin CY, Jacobs RF, et al. Safety and efficacy of high-dose intravenous acyclovir in the management of neonatal herpes simplex virus infections. *Pediatrics* 2000;108:230–238.
370. American Academy of Pediatrics. Rubella. In: Pickering LK, ed. *2003 Red book: report of the Committee on Infectious Diseases*, 26th ed. Elk Grove Village, IL: Author, 2003:538.
371. Brunell P. Varicella in pregnancy, the fetus, and the newborn: problems in management. *J Infect Dis* 1992;166:42–47.
372. Pastuszak A, Levy M, Schick B, et al. Outcome after maternal varicella infection in the first 20 weeks of pregnancy. *N Engl J Med* 1994;330:901–905.
373. Jones KL, Johnson KA, Chambers CA. Offspring of women infected with varicella during pregnancy: a prospective study. *Teratology* 1994;49:29–32.
374. Paryani SG, Arvin AM. Intrauterine infection with varicella-zoster virus after maternal varicella. *N Engl J Med* 1986;14:1542–1546.
375. Cuthbertson G, Weiner C, Giller R, et al. Clinical and laboratory observations: Prenatal diagnosis of second-trimester congenital varicella syndrome by virus-specific immunoglobulin M. *J Pediatr* 1987;111:592–595.
376. Isada NB, Paar DP, Johnson MP, et al. *In utero* diagnosis of congenital varicella-zoster virus infection by chorionic villus sampling and polymerase chain reaction. *Am J Obstet Gynecol* 1991;165:1727–1730.
377. Bale JF, Murph JR. Infections of the central nervous system of the newborn. *Clin Perinatol* 1997;24:787–806.
378. American Academy of Pediatrics. Varicella-zoster virus. In: Pickering LK, ed. *2003 Red book: report of the Committee on Infectious Diseases*, 26th ed. Elk Grove Village, IL: Author, 2003: 678–680.

379. Barton LL, Mets MB. Congenital lymphocytic choriomeningitis virus infection: decade of rediscovery. *Clin Infect Dis* 2001;33:370–374.
380. Childs JE, Glass GE, Korch GW, et al. Lymphocytic choriomeningitis virus and house mouse (*Mus musculus*) distribution in urban Baltimore. *Am J Trop Med Hyg* 1992;47:27–34.
381. Park JY, Peters CJ, Rollin PE, et al. Age distribution of lymphocytic choriomeningitis virus serum antibody in Birmingham, Alabama: evidence of a decreased risk of infection. *Am J Trop Med Hyg* 1997;57:37–41.
382. Marie TJ, Saron MF. Seroprevalence of lymphocytic choriomeningitis virus in Nova Scotia. *Am J Trop Med Hyg* 1998;58:47–49.
383. Ambrosio AM, Feuillade MR, Gamboa GS, et al. Prevalence of lymphocytic choriomeningitis virus infection in a human population in Argentina. *Am J Trop Med Hyg* 1994;50:381–386.
384. Childs JE, Glass GE, Ksiazek TG, et al. Human–rodent contact and infection with lymphocytic choriomeningitis and Seoul viruses in an inner-city population. *Am J Trop Med Hyg* 1991;44:117–121.
385. Wright R, Johnson D, Neumann M, et al. Congenital lymphocytic choriomeningitis virus syndrome: a disease that mimics congenital toxoplasmosis or cytomegalovirus infection. *Pediatrics* 1997;100:9.
386. Cochi SI, Edmonds LE, Dyer K, et al. Congenital rubella syndrome in the United States, 1970–1985. *Am J Epidemiol* 1989;129:349–361.
387. Schluter WW, Reer SE, Redd SC, et al. Changing epidemiology of congenital rubella syndrome in the United States. *J Infect Dis* 1998;178:636–641.
388. Reef SE, Plotkin S, Cordero JF, et al. Preparing for elimination of congenital rubella syndrome (CRS). summary of a workshop on CRS elimination in the United States. *Clin Infect Dis* 2000;31:85–95.
389. Gregg NM. Congenital cataract following German measles in the mother. *Trans Ophthal Soc Aust* 1941;3:35–41.
390. Dudgeon J. Congenital rubella. *J Pediatr* 1975;87:1078–1086.
391. Givens KT, Lee DA, Jones T, et al. Congenital rubella syndrome: ophthalmic manifestations and associated systemic disorders. *Br J Ophthalmol* 1993;77:358–363.
392. Souza I, Bale JF Jr. The diagnosis of congenital infections: contemporary strategies. *J Child Neurol* 1995;10:271–282.
393. Desmond MM, Fisher ES, Vorderman AL, et al. The longitudinal course of congenital rubella syndrome in nonretarded children. *J Pediatr* 1979;93:584–391.
394. Desmond MM, Wilson CW, Vorderman AL. The health and educational status of adolescents with the congenital rubella syndrome. *Dev Med Child Neurol* 1985;27:721–729.
395. Forrest JM, Turnbull FM, Sholler GF, et al. Gregg's congenital rubella patients 60 years later. *Med J Aust* 2002;177:664–671.
396. Nakashima AK, Rolfs RT, Flock ML, et al. Epidemiology of syphilis in the United States, 1941–1993. *Sex Transm Dis* 1996;23:16–23.
397. Centers for Disease Control and Prevention. Congenital syphilis-United States, 1998. *MMWR Morb Mortal Wkly Rep* 1999;48:757–761.
398. Sison CG, Ostrea EM, Reyes MP, et al. The resurgence of congenital syphilis: a cocaine-related problem. *J Pediatr* 1997;130:289–292.
399. Hollier LM, Cox SM. Syphilis. *Semin Perinatol* 1998;22:323–331.
400. Murph JR. Rubella and syphilis: continuing causes of congenital infection in the 1990s. *Sem Pediatr Neurol* 1994;1:26–35.
401. Ikeda MK, Jenson HB. Evaluation and treatment of congenital syphilis. *J Pediatr* 1990;117:843–852.
402. American Academy of Pediatrics. Syphilis. In: Pickering LK, ed. *2003 Red book: report of the Committee on Infectious Diseases*, 26th ed. Elk Grove Village, IL: Author, 2003: 596–603.
403. Bittencourt AL. Congenital Chagas disease. *Am J Dis Child* 1975;130:97–103.
404. Howard J, Rubio M. Congenital Chagas' disease. *Bol Chil Parasitol* 1968;23:107–112.
405. Schenone J, Gaggero M, Sapunar J, et al. Congenital Chagas disease of second generation in Santiago, Chile: report of two cases. *Rev Inst Med Trop Sao Paulo* 2001;43:231–232.
406. Koskiniemi M, Rautonen J, Laipio ML, et al. Epidemiology of encephalitis in children: a 20-year survey. *Ann Neurol* 1991;29:492–497.
407. Johnson RT. The pathogenesis of acute viral encephalitis and postinfectious encephalomyelitis. *J Infect Dis* 1987;155:359–364.
408. Gonzalez-Scarano F, Tyler KL. Molecular pathogenesis of neurotropic viral infections. *Ann Neurol* 1987;22:565–574.
409. Leist TP, Frei K, Kam-Hansen S, et al. Tumor necrosis factor in the cerebrospinal fluid during bacterial, but not viral meningitis. Evaluation in murine model infections and in patients. *J Exp Med* 1988;167:1743–1748.
410. Ramilo O, Mustafa MM, Porter J, et al. Detection of interleukin-1-β but not tumor necrosis factor-α in the cerebrospinal fluid of children with aseptic meningitis. *Am J Dis Child* 1990;144:349–352.
411. Matsuo M, Hamasaki Y, Masuyama T, et al. Leukotriene B4 and C4 in cerebrospinal fluid from children with meningitis and febrile seizures. *Pediatr Neurol* 1996;14:121–124.
412. Hoke CH Jr, Vaughn DW, Nisalak A, et al. Effect of high-dose dexamethasone on the outcome of acute encephalitis due to Japanese encephalitis virus. *J Infect Dis* 1992;165:631–637.
413. Reiser H, Stadecker MJ. Costimulatory B7 molecules in the pathogenesis of infectious and autoimmune diseases. *N Engl J Med* 1996;335:1369–1377.
414. Razvi ES, Welsh RM. Apoptosis in viral infections. *Adv Virus Res* 1995;45:1–60.
415. Rantala H, Uhari M, Uhari M, et al. Outcome after childhood encephalitis. *Dev Med Child Neurol* 1991;33:858–867.
416. Rotenone J, Koskiniemi M, Vaheri A. Prognostic factors in childhood acute encephalitis. *Pediatr Infect Dis J* 1991;10:461–466.
417. Mustonen K, Mustakangas P, Uotila L, et al. Viral infections in neonates with seizures. *J Perinat Med* 2003;31:75–80.
418. Berlin LE, Rorabaugh ML, Heldrich F, et al. Aseptic meningitis in infants <2 years of age: diagnosis and etiology. *J Infect Dis* 1993;169:888–892.
419. Fukushima K, Ishiguro A, Shimbo T. Transient elevation of granulocyte-stimulating factor levels in cerebrospinal fluid at the initial stage of aseptic meningitis in children. *Pediatr Res* 1995;37:160–164.
420. Whitley RJ, Gnann JW. Viral encephalitis: familiar infections and emerging pathogens. *Lancet* 2002;359:507–514.
421. Klein SK, Hom DL, Anderson MR, et al. Predictive factors of short-term neurologic outcome in children with encephalitis. *Pediatr Neurol* 1994;11:308–312.
422. Launes J, Siren J, Valanne L, et al. Unilateral hyperperfusion in brain-perfusion SPECT predicts poor prognosis in acute encephalitis. *Neurology* 1997;48:1347–1351.
423. Koelfen W, Freund M, Guckel F, et al. MRI of encephalitis in children: comparison of CT and MRI in the acute stage with long-term follow-up. *Neuroradiology* 1996;38:73–79.
424. Koskiniemi M, Vaheri A. Effect of measles, mumps, rubella vaccination on pattern of encephalitis in children. *Lancet* 1989;1:31–34.
425. Cassady KA, Whitley RJ. Pathogenesis and pathophysiology of viral infections of the central nervous system. In: Scheld WM, Whitley RJ, Durack DT, eds. *Infections of the central nervous system*. Philadelphia: Lippincott–Raven, 1997: 7–22.
426. Johnson RT. Acute encephalitis. *Clin Infect Dis* 1996;23:219–226.
427. Modlin JF. Update on enterovirus infections in infants and children. In: Aronoff SC, Hughes WT, Kohl S, et al., eds. *Advances in pediatric infectious diseases*. St Louis, MO: Mosby, 1996;12:155–180.
428. Cherry JD. Enteroviruses: coxackieviruses, echoviruses, and polioviruses. In: Feigin RD, Cherry JD, eds. *Textbook of pediatric infectious diseases*, 4th ed. Philadelphia: Saunders, 1998: 1787–1839.
429. Thoelen I, Lemey P, Van Der Donck I, et al. Molecular typing and epidemiology of enteroviruses identified from an outbreak of aseptic meningitis in Belgium during the summer of 2000. *J Med Virol* 2003;70:420–429.

430. Dagan R, Jenista JA, Menegus MA. Association of clinical presentation, laboratory findings, and virus serotypes with the presence of meningitis in hospitalized infants with enterovirus infections. *J Pediatr* 1988;113:975–978.
431. Berlin LE, Rorabaugh ML, Heldrich F, et al. Aseptic meningitis in infants <2 years of age: diagnosis and etiology. *J Infect Dis* 1993;169:888–892.
432. Rorabaugh ML, Berlin LE, Heldrich F, et al. Aseptic meningitis in infants younger than 2 years of age: acute illness and neurologic complications. *Pediatrics* 1993;92:206–211.
433. Komatsu I, et al. Outbreak of severe neurologic involvement associated with enterovirus 71 infection. *Pediatr Neurol* 1999;20:17–23.
434. Huang CC, Liu CC, Chang YC, et al. Neurological complications in children with enterovirus 71 infection. *N Engl J Med* 1999;341:936–942.
435. Lin TY, Hsia SH, Huang YC, et al. Proinflammatory cytokine reactions in enterovirus 71 infections of the central nervous system. *Clin InfectDis* 2003;36:269–274.
436. Chang LY, Tsao KC, Hsia SH, et al. Transmission and clinical features of enterovirus 71 infections in household contacts in Taiwan. *JAMA* 2004;291:222–227.
437. Lu HK, Lin TY, Hsia SH, et al. Prognostic implications of myoclonic jerk in children with enterovirus infection. *J Microbiol Immunol Infect* 2004;37:82–87.
438. Prager P, Nolan M, Andrews IP, et al. Neurologic pulmonary edema in enterovirus 71 encephalitis is not uniformly fatal by causes severe morbidity in survivors. *Pediatr Crit Care Med* 2003; 4:377–381.
439. Lum LCS, Chua KB, McMinn PC. Echovirus 7 associated encephalomyelitis. *J Clin Virol* 2002;23:153–160.
440. Wang SM, Lei HY, Huang KJ, et al. Pathogenesis of enterovirus 71 brainstem encephalitis in pediatric patients: roles of cytokines and cellular immune activation in patients with pulmonary edema. *J Infect Dis* 2003;188:564–570.
441. Modlin JD, et al. Focal encephalitis with enterovirus infections. *Pediatrics* 1991;88:841–845.
442. Romero JR. Pleconaril: a novel antipicornaviral drug. *Expert Opin Investig Drugs* 2001;10:369–379.
443. Wadia NH, Wadia PN, Katrak SM, et al. A study of the neurological disorder associated with acute hemorrhagic conjunctivitis due to enterovirus 70. *J Neurol Neurosurg Psychiatry* 1983;46:599–610.
444. Katiyar BC, Misra S, Singh RB, et al. Neurological syndromes after acute epidemic conjunctivitis. *Lancet* 1981;2:866–867.
445. Wadia NH, Irani PF, Katrak SM. Lumbosacral radiculomyelitis associated with pandemic acute hemorrhagic conjunctivitis. *Lancet* 1973;1:350–352.
446. Bowles NE, Dubowitz V, Sewry CA, et al. Dermatomyositis, polymyositis, and coxsackie-B-virus infection. *Lancet* 1987;1: 1004–1007.
447. Jadoul C, Van Goethem J, Martin JJ. Myelitis due to coxsackievirus B infection. *Neurology* 1995;45:1626–1627.
448. Chang LY, Huang YC, Lin TY. Fulminant neurogenic pulmonary oedema with hand, foot, and mouth disease. *Lancet* 1998;352:367–368.
449. Lum LCS, Wong KT, Lam SK, et al. Neurogenic pulmonary oedema and enterovirus 71 encephalomyelitis [Letter]. *Lancet* 1998;352:13–91.
450. Modlin JD. Neonatal enterovirus infections. In: Feigin RD, ed. *Seminars in pediatric infectious diseases, Vol. 5, No. 1.* Philadelphia: Saunders, 1994: 70–77.
451. Lake AM, Lauer BA, Clark JC, et al. Enterovirus infections in neonates. *J Pediatr* 1976;89:787–791.
452. Hosoya M, Sato M, Honzumi K, et al. Association of nonpolio enteroviral infection in the central nervous system of children with febrile seizures. *Pediatrics* 2001;107:e12.
453. Shattuck KE, Chonmaitree T. The changing spectrum of neonatal meningitis over a fifteen-year period. *Clin Pediatr Phila* 1992;31:130–136.
454. Aintablian N, Pratt RD, Sawyer MH. Rapidly recurrent enteroviral meningitis in non-immunocompromised infants caused by different viral strains. *J Med Virol* 1995;47:126–129.
455. Sells CJ, Carpenter RL, Ray CG. Sequelae of central-nervous-system enterovirus infections. *N Engl J Med* 1975;293:1–4.
456. Wilfert CM, Thompson RJ Jr., Sunder TR, et al. Longitudinal assessment of children with enteroviral meningitis during the first three months of life. *Pediatrics* 1981;67:811–815.
457. Bergman I, Painter MJ, Wald ER, et al. Outcome in children with enteroviral meningitis during the first year of life. *J Pediatr* 1987;110:705–709.
458. Baker RC, Kummer AW, Schultz JR, et al. Neurodevelopmental outcome of infants with viral meningitis in the first three months of life. *Clin Pediatr Phila* 1996;35:295–301.
459. Wilfert CM, Buckley RH, Mohanakumar T, et al. Persistent and fatal central-nervous-system echovirus infections in patents with agammaglobulinemia. *N Engl J Med* 1977;296:1485–1489.
460. Sawyer MH. Enterovirus infections: diagnosis and treatment. *Semin Pediatr Infect Dis* 2002;13:40–47.
461. Foray S, Pailloud F, Thouvenot D, et al. Evaluation of combining upper respiratory tract swab samples with cerebrospinal fluid examination of the diagnosis of enteroviral meningitis in children. *J Med Virol* 1999;57:193–197.
462. Rotbart HA, Ahmed A, Hickey S, et al. Diagnosis of enterovirus infection by polymerase chain reaction of multiple specimen samples. *Pediatr Infect Dis J* 1997;16:409–411.
463. Guney C, Ozkaya E, Yapar M, et al. Laboratory diagnosis of enteroviral infections of the central nervous system by using a nested RT-polymerase chain reaction (PCR) assay. *Diagn Microbiol Infect Dis* 2003;47:557–562.
464. Heine J. *Beobachtungen über Lähmungszustände der unteren Extremitäten und deren Behandlung*. Stuttgart, Germany: Kohler, 1840.
465. Kew OM, Wright PF, Agol VI, et al. Circulating vaccine-derived polioviruses: current state of knowledge. *Bull WHO* 2004;82:16–23.
466. John TJ. A developing country perspective on vaccine-associated paralytic poliomyelitis. *Bull WHO* 2004;82:53–58.
467. Center for Disease Control. Poliomyelitis prevention in the United States: introduction of a sequential vaccination schedule of inactivated poliovirus vaccine followed by oral polio vaccine. Recommendations of the Advisory Committee on Immunization Practices (ACIP). *MMWR Morb Mortal Wkly Rep* 1997;46 (Suppl RR-3):1–25.
468. Baker AB, Cornwell S, Tichy F. Poliomyelitis IX. The cerebral hemispheres. *Arch Neurol Psychiatr* 1954;71:435–454.
469. Heyes MP, Saito K, Major EO, et al. A mechanism of quinolinic acid formation by brain in inflammatory neurological disease. Attenuation of synthesis from l-tryptophan by 6-chlorotryptophan and 4-chloro-3 hydroxyanthranilate. *Brain* 1993;116:1425–1450.
470. Baker AB, Cornwell S, Tichy F. Poliomyelitis X. The cerebellum. *Arch Neurol Psychiatr* 1954;71:455–465.
471. Horstmann DM, Paul JR. The incubation period in human poliomyelitis and its implications. *JAMA* 1947;135:11–14.
472. Horstmann DM. Poliomyelitis: severity and type of disease in different age groups. *Ann N Y Acad Sci* 1955;61:956–967.
473. Abramson H, Greenberg M. Acute poliomyelitis in infants under one year of age: epidemiological and clinical features. *Pediatrics* 1955;16:478–487.
474. Wernstedt W. Epidemiologische Studien über die zweite grosse Poliomyelitisepidemie in Schweden 1911–1913. *Ergebn Inn Med Kinderheilkd* 1924;26:248–350.
475. Strebel PM, Ion-Nedelcu N, Baughman AL, et al. Intramuscular injections within 30 days of immunization with oral poliovirus vaccine—risk factor for vaccine-associated paralyatic poliomyelitis. *N Engl J Med* 1995;332:500–506.
476. Hill AB, Knowelden J. Inoculation and poliomyelitis: statistical investigation in England and Wales in 1946. *BMJ* 1950;2:16.
477. Leon-Monzon ME, Illa I, Dulakas MC. Expression of poliovirus receptor in human spinal cord and muscle. *Ann N Y Acad Sci* 1995;753:48–57.
478. Lawson RB, Garvey FK. Paralysis of the bladder in poliomyelitis. *JAMA* 1947;135:93–94.
479. Minnesota Poliomyelitis Research Commission. The bulbar form of poliomyelitis. Diagnosis and the correlation with physiologic and pathologic manifestations. *JAMA* 1947;134:757–762.

480. Baker AB, Matzke HA, Brown JR. Poliomyelitis III. Bulbar poliomyelitis: a study of medullary function. *Arch Neurol Psychiatr* 1950;63:257–281.
481. Baker AB. Poliomyelitis: a study of pulmonary edema. *Neurology* 1957;7:743–751.
482. Baker AB, Cornwell S, Brown IA. Poliomyelitis VI. The hypothalamus. *Arch Neurol Psychiatr* 1952;68:16–36.
483. Merritt HH, Fremont-Smith F. *The cerebrospinal fluid*. Philadelphia: Saunders, 1937.
484. Rotbart HA. Enteroviral infections of the central nervous system. *Clin Infect Dis* 1995;20:971–981.
485. Sharland M, Hodgson J, Davies EG, et al. Enteroviral pharyngitis diagnosed by reverse transcriptase-polymerase chain reaction. *Arch Dis Child* 1996;74:462–463.
486. Chezzi C. Rapid diagnosis of poliovirus infection by PCR amplification. *J Clin Microbiol* 1996;34:1722–1725.
487. Centers for Disease Control and Prevention. Recommendation of the international task force for disease eradication. *MMWR Morb Mortal Wkly Rep* 1993;42:10.
488. Nkowane RM, et al. Vaccine-associated paralytic poliomyelitis. United States: 1973–1984. *JAMA* 1987;257:1335–1340.
489. Gaebler JW, Kleiman MB, French ML, et al. Neurologic complications in oral polio vaccine recipients. *J Pediatr* 1986;108:878–881.
490. Groom SN, Clewley J, Litton PA, et al. Vaccine-associated poliomyelitis. *Lancet* 1994;343:609–610.
491. Otelea D, Guillot S, Furione M, et al. Genomic modifications in naturally occurring neurovirulent revertants of Sabin 1 polioviruses. *Dev Biol Stand* 1993;78:33–38.
492. Yohannan MD, Ramia S, al-Frayh AR. Acute paralytic poliomyelitis presenting as Guillain-Barré syndrome. *J Infect* 1991;22:129–133.
493. Hahn AF. Guillain-Barré syndrome. *Lancet* 1998;352:635–641.
494. Wong M, Connolly AM, Noetzel MJ. Poliomyelitis-like syndrome associated with Epstein-Barr infection. *Pediatr Neurol* 1999;20:235–237.
495. Likar M, Dane DS. An illness resembling acute poliomyelitis caused by a virus of the Russian spring-summer encephalitis louping ill group in Northern Ireland. *Lancet* 1958;1:456–458.
496. Hopkins IJ. A new syndrome: poliomyelitis-like illness associated with acute asthma in childhood. *Aust Paediatr* 1974;10:273–276.
497. Kyllerman MG, Herner S, Bergstrom TB, et al. PCR diagnosis of primary herpesvirus type I in poliomyelitis-like paralysis and respiratory tract disease. *Pediatr Neurol* 1993;9:227–229.
498. Sabin AB. My last will and testament on rapid elimination and ultimate eradication of poliomyelitis and measles. *Pediatrics* 1992;90(Suppl):162–169.
499. McKhann GM, Cornblath DR, Ho T, et al. Clinical and electrophysiological aspects of acute paralytic disease of children and young adults in northern China. *Lancet* 1991;338:593–597.
500. Gear JH. Nonpolio causes of polio-like paralytic syndromes. *Rev Infect Dis* 1984;6(Suppl 2):S379–S384.
501. Bodian D, Howe HA. Experimental non-paralytic poliomyelitis. Frequency and range of pathological involvement. *Bull Johns Hopkins Hosp* 1945;76:1–17.
502. Bukh N. Muscle recovery of poliomyelitis. *Acta Orthop Scand* 1968;39:579–592.
503. Sharief MK, Hentges R, Ciardi M. Intrathecal immune response in patients with the post-polio syndrome. *N Engl J Med* 1991;325:749–755.
504. Dalakas MC, Bartfeld H, Kurland LT, eds. *The post-polio syndrome. Advances in the pathogenesis and treatment*. New York: New York Academy of Sciences, 1995.
505. Waring WP, Davidoff G, Werner R. Serum creatine kinase in the post-polio population. *Am J Phys Med Rehabil* 1989;68:86–90.
506. Windebank AJ, Litchy WJ, Daube JR, et al. Late effects of paralytic poliomyelitis in Olmsted County, Minnesota. *Neurology* 1991;41:501–507.
507. Dean AC, Graham BA, Dalakas M, et al. Sleep apnea in patients with postpolio syndrome. *Ann Neurol* 1998;43:661–664.
508. Dalakas MC. Why drugs fail in postpolio syndrome. Lessons from another clinical trial. *Neurology* 1999;53:1166–1167.
509. American Academy of Pediatrics. Poliovirus infections. In: Peter G, ed. *1997 Red book: report of the Committee on Infectious Diseases*, 24th ed. Elk Grove Village, IL: Author, 1997:424–433.
510. Salk J, Salk D. Control of influenza and poliomyelitis with killed virus vaccines. *Science* 1977;195:834–847.
511. Kuban KC, Ephros MA, Freeman RL, et al. Syndrome of opsoclonus-myoclonus caused by coxsackie B3 infection. *Ann Neurol* 1983;13:69–71.
512. Chalhub EG, Devivo DC, Siegel BA, et al. Coxsackie A9 focal encephalitis associated with acute infantile hemiplegia and porencephaly. *Neurology* 1977;27:574–579.
513. Moossy J, Geer JC. Encephalomyelitis, myocarditis and adrenal cortical necrosis in coxsackie B3 virus infection. Distribution of the central nervous system lesions. *Arch Pathol* 1960;70:614–622.
514. Walker SH, Togo Y. Encephalitis due to group B, type 5 coxsackievirus. *Am J Dis Child* 1963;105:209–212.
515. Walters JH. Post-encephalitic Parkinson syndrome after meningoencephalitis due to coxsackievirus group B, type 2. *N Engl J Med* 1960;263:744–747.
516. Casals J, Clarke DH. Arboviruses: group A. In: Horsfall FL, Tamm I, eds. *Viral and rickettsial infections of man*, 4th ed. Philadelphia: Lippincott, 1965: 583–605.
517. Modlin JF. Coxsackieviruses, echoviruses, and newer enteroviruses. In: Mandell G, Bennett J, Dolin R, eds. *Principles and practice of infectious* diseases, 4th ed. New York: Churchill Livingstone, 1995: 1620–1636.
518. Casteels-van Daele M, et al. Basilar migraine and viral meningitis [Letter]. *Lancet* 1981;1:13–66.
519. Karzon DT, Hayner NS, Winkelstein W Jr., et al. An epidemic of aseptic meningitis syndrome due to ECHO virus type 6. II. A clinical study of ECHO 6 infection. *Pediatrics* 1962;29:418–431.
520. Marzetti G, Midulla M. Acute cerebellar ataxia associated with Echo 6 infection in two children. *Acta Paediatr Scand* 1967;56:547–551.
521. Forbes SJ, Brumlik J, Harding HB. Acute ascending polyradiculomyelitis associated with ECHO 9 virus. *Dis Nerv Syst* 1967; 28:537–540.
522. Freund A, Zass R, Kurlemann G, et al. Bilateral oedema of the basal ganglia in echovirus type 21 infection: complete clinical and radiological normalization. *Dev Med Child Neurol* 1998;40:421–423.
523. Haddad J, Messer J, Gut JP, et al. Neonatal echovirus encephalitis with white matter necrosis. *Neuropediatrics* 1990;21:215–217.
524. Roberton DM, Jack I, Joshi W, et al. Failure of intraventricular gamma globulin and a-interferon for persistent encephalitis in congenital hypogammaglobulineamia. *Arch Dis Child* 1988;63: 948–952.
525. Kondoh H, Kobayashi K, Sugio Y, et al. Successful treatment of echovirus meningoencephalitis in sex-linked agammaglobulinaemia by intrathecal and intravenous injection of high titer gamma globulin. *Eur J Pediatr* 1987;146:610–612.
526. Ogra PL. Distribution of echovirus antibody in serum, nasopharynx, rectum, and spinal fluid after natural infection with echovirus type 6. *Infect Immun* 1970;2:150–155.
527. Lum LCS, Wong KT, Lam SK, et al. Fatal enterovirus 71 encephalomyelitis. *J Pediatr* 1998;133:795–798.
528. Johansson PJ, Sveger T, Ahlfors K, et al. Reovirus type 1 associated with meningitis. *Scand J Infect Dis* 1996;28:117–120.
529. Davis D, Henslee PJ, Markesbery WR. Fatal adenovirus meningoencephalitis in a bone marrow transplant patient. *Ann Neurol* 1988;23:385–389.
530. Kim KS, Gohd RS. Acute encephalopathy in twins due to adenovirus type 7 infection. *Arch Neurol* 1983;40:58–59.
531. Straussberg R, Harel L, Levy Y, et al. A syndrome of transient encephalopathy associated with adenovirus infection. *Pediatrics* 2001;107:e69.
532. Osamura T, Mizuta R, Yoshioka H, et al. Isolation of adenovirus type 11 from the brain of a neonate with pneumonia and encephalitis. *Eur J Pediatr* 1993;152:496–499.
533. Suga S, Yoshikawa T, Asano Y, et al. Clinical and virological analyses of 21 infants with exanthem subitum (roseola infantum) and central nervous system complications. *Ann Neurol* 1993;33:597–603.

534. Caserta MT, Hall CB, Schanbel K, et al. Primary human herpesvirus 7 infection: a comparison of human herpesvirus 7 and human herpesvirus 6 infections in children. *J Pediatr* 1998;133: 386–389.
535. Cherry JD. Contemporary infectious exanthems. *Clin Infect Dis* 1993;16:199–207.
536. Huang LM, Lee CY, Lee PI, et al. Meningitis caused by human herpesvirus-6. *Arch Dis Child* 1991;66:1443–1444.
537. Kamei A, Ichinohe S, Onuma R, et al. Acute disseminated demyelination due to primary herpesvirus-6 infection. *Eur J Pediatr* 1997;156:709–712.
538. Huang LM, Lee CY, Lee PI, et al. Meningitis caused by human herpesvirus-6. *Arch Dis Child* 1991;66:1443–1444.
539. Asano Y, Yoshikawa T, Suga S, et al. Clinical features of infants with primary human herpesvirus 6 infection (exanthum subitum, roseola infantum). *Pediatrics* 1994;93:104–108.
540. Hall CB, Long CE, Schnabel KC, et al. Human herpesvirus-6 infection in children—a prospective study of complications and reactivation. *N Engl J Med* 1994;331:432–438.
541. Kondo K, et al. Association of human herpesvirus 6 infection of the central nervous system with recurrence of febrile convulsions. *J Infect Dis* 1993;167:1197–1200.
542. Caserta MT, Mock DJ, Dewhurst S. Human herpesvirus 6. *Clin Infect Dis* 2001;33:829–833.
543. Yoshikawa T, Nakashima T, Suga S, et al. Human herpesvirus-6 DNA in cerebrospinal fluid of a child with exanthem subitum and meningoencephalitis. *Pediatrics* 1992;89:888–890.
544. Osman H. Human herpesvirus 6 and febrile convulsions. *Herpes* 2000;7:33–37.
545. van den Berg JSP, van Zeijl JH, Rotteveel JJ, et al. Neuroinvasion by human herpesvirus type 7 in a case of exanthem subitum with severe neurologic manifestations. *Neurology* 1999;52:1077–1079.
546. Torigoe S, Koide W, Yamada M, et al. Human herpesvirus 7 infection associated with central nervous system manifestations. *J Pediatr* 1996;129:301–305.
547. Pohl-Koppe A, Blay M, Jager G, et al. Human herpes virus type 7 DNA in the cerebrospinal fluid of children with central nervous system diseases. *Eur J Pediatr* 2001;160:351–358.
548. Agut H, Collandre H, Aubin JT, et al. *In vitro* sensitivity of human herpesvirus-6 to antiviral drugs. *Res Virol* 1989;140:219–228.
549. Rehle TM. Classification, distribution, and importance of arboviruses. *Trop Med Parisitol* 1989;40:391–395.
550. American Academy of Pediatrics. Arboviruses. In: Peter G, ed. *1997 Red book: report of the Committee on Infectious Diseases*, 24th ed. Elk Grove Village, IL: Author, 1997;137–141.
551. *MMWR Morb Mortal Wkly Rep* 1999;47:1119.
552. Jones TF, Erwin PC, Craig AS, et al. Serological survey and active surveillance for La Crosse virus infections among children in Tennessee. *Clin Infect Dis* 2000;31:1284–1287.
553. Chun RW, Thompson WH, Grabow JD, et al. California arbovirus encephalitis in children. *Neurology* 1968;18:369–375.
554. Sokol DK, Kleiman MB, Garg BP. LaCrosse viral encephalitis mimics herpes simplex viral encephalitis. *Pediatr Neurol* 2001;25:413–415.
555. Hardin SG, Erwin PC, Patterson L, et al. Clinical comparisons of La Crosse encephalitis and enteroviral central nervous system infections in a pediatric population: 2001 surveillance in East Tennessee. *Am J Infect Control* 2003;31:508–510.
556. Monath TP, Nuckolls JG, Berall et al. Studies on California encephalitis in Minnesota. *Am J Epidemiol* 1970;92:40–50.
557. Johnson KP, Lepow ML, Johnson RT. California encephalitis. I. Clinical and epidemiological studies. *Neurology* 1968;18:250–254.
558. Tsai TF. Arboviral infections in the United States. *Infect Dis Clin North Am* 1991;5:73–102.
559. Balfour HH Jr, Siem RA, Bauer H, et al. California arbovirus (La Crosse) infections. I. Clinical and laboratory findings in 66 children with meningoencephalitis. *Pediatrics* 1973;52:680–691.
560. McJunkin JE, de los Reyes EC, Irazuzta JE, et al. La Crosse encephalitis in children. *N Engl J Med* 2001;344:801–807.
561. Grabow JD, Matthews CG, Chun RW, et al. The electroencephalogram and clinical sequelae of California arbovirus encephalitis. *Neurology* 1969;19:394–404.
562. Chun RW. Clinical aspects of La Crosse encephalitis: neurological and psychological sequelae. *Prog Clin Biol Res* 1983;123:193–200.
563. Matthews CG, Chun RW, Grabow JD, et al. Psychological sequelae in children following California arbovirus encephalitis. *Neurology* 1968;18:1023–1030.
564. Rie HE, Hilty MD, Cramblett HG. Intelligence and coordination following California encephalitis. *Am J Dis Child* 1973;125:824–827.
565. McJunkin JE, Kahn R, de los Reyes EC, et al. Treatment of severe La Crosse encephalitis with intravenous Ribavirin following diagnosis by brain biopsy. *Pediatrics* 1997;99:261–267.
566. Cassidy LF, Patterson JL. Mechanism of La Crosse virus inhibition by ribavirin. *Antimicrob Agents Chemother* 1989;33:2009–2011.
567. Bailey CL, Eldridge BF, Hayes DE, et al. Isolation of St. Louis encephalitis virus from overwintering *Culex pipiens* mosquitoes. *Science* 1978;199:1346–1349.
568. McCordock HA, Collier W, Gray SH. The pathologic changes of the St. Louis type of acute encephalitis. *JAMA* 1934;103:822–825.
569. Barrett FF, Yow MD, Phillips CA. St. Louis encephalitis in children during the 1964 epidemic. *JAMA* 1965;193:381–385.
570. Powell KE, Blakey DL. St. Louis encephalitis. The 1975 epidemic in Mississippi. *JAMA* 1977;237:2294–2298.
571. Estrin WJ. The serologic diagnosis of St. Louis encephalitis in a patient with the syndrome of opsoclonia, body tremulousness, and benign encephalitis. *Ann Neurol* 1977;1:596–598.
572. Pranzatelli MR, Mott SH, Pavlakis SG, et al. Clinical spectrum of secondary parkinsonism in childhood: a reversible disorder. *Pediatr Neurol* 1994;10:131–140.
573. Kaplan AM, Koveleski JT. St. Louis encephalitis with particular involvement of the brain stem. *Arch Neurol* 1978;35:45–46.
574. Zentay PJ, Basman J. Epidemic encephalitis type B in children. *J Pediatr* 1939;14:323–332.
575. Azar GJ, et al. Follow-up studies of St. Louis encephalitis in Florida. Sensorimotor findings. *Am J Public Health* 1966;56:1074–1081.
576. Smadel JE, Bailey P, Baker AB. Sequelae of the arthropod-borne encephalitides. *Neurology* 1958;8:873–896.
577. Rozdilsky B, Robertson HE, Chorney J. Western encephalitis: a report of eight fatal cases. *Can Med Assoc J* 1965;98:79–86.
578. Herzon H, Shelton JT, Bruyn HG. Sequelae of western equine and other arthropod-borne encephalitides. *Neurology* 1957;7:535–548.
579. Schultz DR, Barthal JS, Garrett C. Western equine encephalitis with rapid onset of Parkinsonism. *Neurology* 1977;27:1095–1096.
580. Finley KH, Fitzgerald LH, Richter RW, et al. Western encephalitis and cerebral ontogenesis. *Arch Neurol* 1967;16:140–164.
581. Noran HH, Baker AB. Western equine encephalitis: the pathogenesis of the pathological lesions. *J Neuropathol Exp Neurol* 1945;4:269–276.
582. Reeves WC, Hammon WM. Epidemiology of the arthropod-borne viral encephalitides in Kern County, California 1943–1952. *Univ Calif Public Health Rep* 1962;4:1–257.
583. Kokernot RH, Shinefield HR, Longshore WA Jr. The 1952 outbreak of encephalitis in California: differential diagnosis. *Calif Med* 1953;79:73–77.
584. Feemster RF. Equine encephalitis in Massachusetts. *N Engl J Med* 1957;257:701–704.
585. Johnson RT. Eastern encephalitis virus. In: Johnson RT, ed. *Viral infections of the nervous system*. New York: Raven Press, 1982: 109.
586. Deresiewicz RL, Thaler SJ, Hsu L, et al. Clinical and neuroradiographic manifestations of eastern equine encephalitis. *N Engl J Med* 1997;336:1867–1874.
587. Weaver SC, Salas R, Rico-Hesse R, et al. Re-emergence of epidemic Venezuelan equine encephalomyelitis in South America. *Lancet* 1996;348:436–440.
588. Bowen GS, Calisher CH. Virological and serological studies of Venezuelan equine encephalomyelitis in humans. *J Clin Microbiol* 1976;4:22–27.
589. Chaudhuri N, Shaw BP, Mondal KC, et al. Epidemiology of Japanese encephalitis. *Indian Pediatr* 1992;29:861–865.

590. Poneprasert B. Japanese encephalitis in children in northern Thailand. *Southeast Asian J Trop Med Public Health* 1989;20:599–603.
591. Arya SC. Japanese encephalitis virus and poliomyelitis-like illness. *Lancet* 1998;351:1964.
592. McCallum JD. Japanese encephalitis in southeastern Nepal: clinical aspects in the 1986 epidemic. *J R Army Med Corps* 1991;137: 8–13.
593. Kumar R, Mathur A, Singh KB, et al. Clinical sequelae of Japanese encephalitis in children. *Indian J Med Res* 1993;97:9–13.
594. Kalita J, Misra UK, Pandey S, et al. A comparison of clinical and radiological findings in adults and children with Japanese encephalitis. *Arch Neurol* 2003;60:1760–1764.
595. Ravi V, Parida S, Desai A, et al. Correlation of tumor necrosis factor levels in the serum and cerebrospinal fluid with clinical outcome in Japanese encephalitis patients. *J Med Virol* 1997;51:132–136.
596. Winter PM, Dung NM, Loan HT, et al. Proinflammatory cytokines and chemokines in humans with Japanese encephalitis. *J Infect Dis* 2004;190:1618–1626.
597. Abe T, Kojima K, Shoji H, et al. Japanese encephalitis. *J Magn Reson Imaging* 1998;8:755–761.
598. Kumar S, Misra UK, Kalita J, et al. MRI in Japanese encephalitis. *Neuroradiology* 1997;39:180–184.
599. Prakash M, Kumar S, Gupta RK. Diffusion-weighted MR imaging in Japanese encephalitis. *J Comput Assist Tomogr* 2004;28:756–761.
600. Tiroumourougane SV, Raghava P, Srinivasana S. Management parameters affecting the outcome of Japanese encephalitis. *J Trop Pediatr* 2003;49:153–156.
601. Kumar P, Sulochana P, Nirmala G, et al. Impaired T helper 1 function of nonstructural protein 3-specific T cells in Japanese patients with encephalitis with neurological sequelae. *J Infect Dis* 2004;189:880–891.
602. Kalita J, Misra UK. Neurophysiological changes in Japanese encephalitis. *Neurol India* 2002;50:262–266.
602a. Yim, R, Posfay-Babe KM, Nolt, De et al. Spectrum of clinical manifestations of West Nile Virus Infection in Children. *Pediatrics* 2004;114:1673–1675.
602b. Sejvar JJ. West Nile virus and "poliomyelitis." *Neurology* 2004;63:206–207.
602c. Fratkin JD, Leis AA, Stokic DS, et al. Spinal cord neuropathology in human West Nile virus infection. *Arch Pathol Lab Med.* 2004;128:533–537.
602d. Kraushaar G, Patel R, Stoneham GW. West Nile Virus: a case report with flaccid paralysis and cervical spinal cord: MR imaging findings. *AJNR Am J Neuroradiol* 2005;26:26–29.
603. Lessell S, Collins TE. Ophthalmoplegia in Powassan encephalitis. *Neurology* 2003;60:1726–1727.
604. White, NJ. Variation in virulence of dengue virus. *Lancet* 1999;354:1401–1402.
605. Cam BV, Fonsmark L, Hue NB, et al. Prospective case–control study of encephalopathy in children with dengue hemorrhagic fever. *Am J Trop Med Hyg* 2001;65:848–851.
606. Monath TP. Early indicators in acute dengue infection. *Lancet* 1997;350:1719–1720.
607. Richter RW, Shimojyo S. Neurologic sequelae of Japanese B encephalitis. *Neurology* 1961;11:553–559.
608. Ishii T, Matsushita M, Hamada S. Characteristic residual neuropathological features of Japanese B encephalitis. *Acta Neuropathol (Berl)* 1977;38:181–186.
609. Braito A, Corbisiero R, Corradini S, et al. *Toscana* virus infections of the central nervous system in children: a report of 14 cases. *J Pediatr* 1998;132:144–148.
609a. Mackenzie JS, et al. Australian encephalitis in Western Australia. *Med J Aust* 1993;158:591–595.
609b. Burrow JN, Whelan PI, Kilburn CJ, et al. Australian encephalitis in the Northern Territory: clinical and epidemiological features, 1987–1996. *Aust N Z J Med* 1998;28:590–596.
609c. Robertson EG. Murray Valley encephalitis: pathological aspects. *M J Aust* 1952:1:107–110.
610. Hloucal L. Tick-borne encephalitis as observed in Czechoslovakia. *J Trop Med Hyg* 1960;63:293–296.
611. Gesikova M, Kaluzova M. Biology of tick-borne encephalitis virus. *Acta Virol* 1997;41:115–124.
612. Pavri K. Clinical, clinicopathologic, and hematologic features of Kyasanur Forest disease. *Rev Infect Dis* 1989;11(Suppl 4):S854–S859.
613. Kolski H, Ford-Jones EL, Richardson S, et al. Etiology of acute childhood encephalitis at The Hospital for Sick Children, Toronto, 1994–1995. *Clin Infect Dis* 1998;26:398–409.
613a. Silver HK, Meiklejohn G, Kempe CH. Colorado tick fever. *Am J Dis Child* 1961;101:30–36.
614. Johnson AJ, Karabatsos N, Lanciotti RS. Detection of Colorado tick fever virus by using reverse transcriptase PCR and application of the technique in laboratory diagnosis. *J Clin Microbiol* 1997;35:1203–1208.
615. Wahlberg P, Saikku P, Brummer-Korvenkontio M. Tick-borne viral encephalitis in Finland. The clinical features of Kumlinge disease during 1959–1987. *J Intern Med* 1989;225:173–177.
616. Davidson MM, Williams H, Macleod JA. Louping ill in man: a forgotten disease. *J Infect* 1991;23:241–242.
617. Meegan JM, Shope RE. Emerging concepts on Rift Valley fever. In: *Perspectives in neurology, Vol. II.* New York: Alan R. Liss, 1981: 267.
618. Sonmez FM, Odemis E, Ahmetoglu A, et al. Brainstem encephalitis and acute disseminated encephalomyelitis following mumps. *Pediatr Neurol* 2004;30:132–134.
619. Russell RR, Donald JC. The neurological complications of mumps. *BMJ* 1958;2:27–30.
620. Levitt LP, Rich TA, Kinde SW, et al. Central nervous system mumps. A review of 64 cases. *Neurology* 1970;20:829–834.
621. Azimi PH, Cramblett HG, Haynes RE. Mumps meningoencephalitis in children. *JAMA* 1969;207:509–512.
622. Wilfert CM. Mumps meningoencephalitis with low cerebrospinal fluid glucose, prolonged pleocytosis and elevation of protein. *N Engl J Med* 1969;280:855–859.
623. Koskiniemi M, Donner M, Pettay O. Clinical appearance and outcome in mumps encephalitis in children. *Acta Paediatr Scand* 1983;72:603–609.
624. Oldfelt V. Sequelae of mumps meningoencephalitis. *Acta Med Scand* 1949;134:405–415.
625. Leheup BP, Feillet F, Roland J, et al. Lésions des noyeaux gris centraux au cours des oreillons. Evolution clinique et neuroradiologique d'un cas. *Rev Neurol* 1987;143:301–303.
626. Haginoya K, Ike K, Iinuma K, et al. Chronic progressive mumps virus encephalitis in a child. *Lancet* 1995;346:50.
627. Murray H, Fuld CM, McLeod W. Mumps meningoencephalitis. *BMJ* 1960;1:1850–1853.
628. Vandvik B, Norrby E, Steen-Johnsen J, et al. Mumps meningitis: prolonged pleocytosis and occurrence of mumps virus-specific oligoclonal IgG in the cerebrospinal fluid. *Eur Neurol* 1978;17:13–22.
629. Chomel JJ, Robin Y, Durdilly R, et al. Rapid direct diagnosis of mumps meningitis by ELISA capture technique. *J Virol Meth*1997;68:97–104.
630. Tarr RW, Edwards KM, Kessler RM, et al. MRI of mumps encephalitis: comparison with CT evaluation. *Pediatr Radiol* 1987;17:59–62.
631. Nahmias AJ, Roizman B. Infections with herpes simplex viruses 1 and 2. *N Engl J Med* 1973;289:667–674, 719–725, 781–789.
632. Plummer G, Waner JL, Phuangsab A, et al. Type 1 and type 2 herpes simplex viruses: serological and biological differences. *J Virol* 1970;5:51–59.
633. Dowdle WR, Nahmias AJ, Harwell RW, et al. Association of antigenic type of herpes-virus hominis with site of viral recovery. *J Immunol* 1967;99:974–980.
634. Johnson RT, Mims CA. Pathogenesis of viral infections of the nervous system. *N Engl J Med* 1968;278:23–30, 84–92.
635. DeBiasi RL, Kleinschmidt-DeMasters BK, Richardson-Burns S, et al. Central nervous system apoptosis in human herpes simplex virus and cytomegalovirus encephalitis. *J Infect Dis* 2002;186:1547–1557.
636. Tan JCH, Byles D, Stanford MR, et al. Acute retinal necrosis in children caused by herpes simplex virus. *Retina* 2001;21:344–347.

637. Enquist LW, Husak PJ, Banfield BW, et al. Infection and spread of alpha-herpesviruses in the nervous system. *Adv Virus Res* 1999;51:237–347.
638. Drachman DA, Adams RD. Herpes-simplex and acute inclusion-body encephalitis. *Arch Neurol* 1962;7:45–63.
639. Baringer JR, Swoveland P. Recovery of herpes-simplex virus from human trigeminal ganglions. *N Engl J Med* 1973;228:648–650.
640. Baringer JR. Recovery of herpes-simplex virus from sacral ganglions. *N Engl J Med* 1974;291:828–830.
641. Liedtke W, Opalka B, Zimmermann CW, et al. Age distribution of latent herpes simplex virus 1 and varicella-zoster virus genome in human nervous tissue. *J Neurol Sci* 1993;116:6–11.
642. Leider W, et al. Herpes-simplex-virus encephalitis: its possible association with reactivated latent infection. *N Engl J Med* 1965;273:341–347.
643. Crompton MR, Teare RD. Encephalitis after reduction of steroid maintenance therapy. *Lancet* 1965;2:1318–1320.
644. Prober CG, Hensleigh PA, Boucher FD, et al. Use of routine viral cultures at delivery to identify neonates exposed to herpes simplex virus. *N Engl J Med* 1988;318:887–891.
645. Craig CP, Nahmias AJ. Different patterns of neurologic involvement with herpes simplex virus types 1 and 2: isolation of herpes simplex virus 2 from the buffy coat of two adults with meningitis. *J Infect Dis* 1973;127:365–372.
646. Whitley RJ, Soong SJ, Linneman C Jr., et al. Herpes simplex encephalitis. Clinical assessment. *JAMA* 1982;247:317–320.
647. Olson LC, Buescher EL, Artenstein MS, et al. Herpesvirus infections of the human central nervous system. *N Engl J Med* 1967;277:1271–1277.
648. Illis LS, Gostling JV. *Herpes simplex encephalitis*. Bristol, PA: Scientechnica, 1972.
649. van der Poel JC, Haenggeli CA, Overweg-Plandsoen WCB. Operculum syndrome: unusual feature of herpes simplex encephalitis. *Pediatr Neurol* 1995;12:246–249.
650. Shanks DE, Blasco PA, Chason DP. Movement disorder following herpes simplex encephalitis. *Dev Med Child Neurol* 1991;33:348–352.
651. Mikati M, Krishnamoorthy KS. Hypoglycorrhachia in neonatal herpes simplex meningoencephalitis. *J Pediatr* 1985;107:746–748.
652. Upton A, Gumpert J. Electroencephalography in diagnosis of herpes-simplex encephalitis. *Lancet* 1970;1:650–652.
653. Smith JB, Westmoreland BF, Reagan TJ, et al. A distinctive clinical EEG profile in herpes simplex encephalitis. *Mayo Clin Proc* 1975;50:469–474.
654. Kowal-Vern A, Patel J, Kneger P, et al. Magnetic resonance imaging in an unusual presentation of herpes encephalitis. *Neuropediatrics* 1988;19:49–51.
655. Schroth G, Gawehn J, Thron A, et al. Early diagnosis of herpes simplex encephalitis by MRI. *Neurology* 1987;37:179–183.
656. Troendle-Atkins J, Demmler GJ, Buffone GJ. Rapid diagnosis of herpes simplex virus encephalitis by using the polymerase chain reaction. *J Pediatr* 1993;123:376–380.
657. Sauerbrei A, Wutzler P. Laboratory diagnosis of central nervous system infections caused by herpesviruses. *J Clin Virol* 2002;25:S45–S51.
658. Lakeman FD, Whitley RJ. The National Institute of Allergy and Infectious Diseases Collaborative Antiviral Study Group. Diagnosis of herpes simplex encephalitis: application of polymerase chain reaction to cerebrospinal fluid from brain-biopsied patients and correlation with disease. *J Infect Dis* 1995;171:857–863.
659. Wildemann B, Ehrhart K, Storch-Hagenlocher B, et al. Quantitation of herpes simplex virus type 1 DNA in cells of cerebrospinal fluid of patients with herpes simplex virus encephalitis. *Neurology* 1997;48:1341–1346.
660. Kimura H, Futamura M, Kito H, et al. Detection of viral DNA in neonatal herpes simplex virus infections: frequent and prolonged presence in serum and cerebrospinal fluid. *J Infect Dis* 1991;164:289–293.
661. Levine DP, Lauter CB, Lerner AM. Simultaneous serum and cerebrospinal fluid antibodies in herpes simplex virus encephalitis. *JAMA* 1978;240:356–360.
662. Koskiniemi M, Vaheri A, Taskinen E. Cerebrospinal fluid alterations in herpes simplex virus encephalitis. *Rev Infect Dis* 1984;6:608–618.
663. Hanada N, Kido S, Terashima M, et al. Non-invasive method for early diagnosis of herpes simplex encephalitis. *Arch Dis Child* 1988;63:1470–1473.
664. Arvin AM, Johnson RT, Whitley RT, et al. Consensus: management of the patient with herpes simplex encephalitis. *Pediatr Infect Dis* 1987;6:2–5.
665. Anderson NE, et al. Brain biopsy in the management of focal encephalitis. *J Neurol Neurosurg Psychiatry* 1991;54:1001–1003.
666. Nahmias AJ, Whitley RJ, Visintine AN, Takei Y, et al. Herpes simplex virus encephalitis: laboratory evaluations and their diagnostic significance. *J Infect Dis* 1982;145:829–836.
667. Whitley RJ, Soong SJ, Hirsch MS, et al. Herpes virus encephalitis. Vidarabine therapy and diagnostic problems. *N Engl J Med* 1981;304:313–318.
668. Soo MS, Tien RD, Gray L, et al. Mesenrhomboencephalitis: MR findings in nine patients. *Am J Roentgenol* 1993;160:1089–1093.
669. Johns DR, Stein AG, Wityk R. MELAS syndrome masquerading as herpes simplex encephalitis. *Neurology* 1993;43:2471–2473.
670. Whitley RJ, Gnann JW Jr. Acyclovir: a decade later. *N Engl J Med* 1992;327:782–789.
671. Wade JC, Meyers JD. Neurologic symptoms associated with parenteral acyclovir treatment after marrow transplantation. *Ann Int Med* 1983;98:921–925.
672. Erlich KS, Mills J, Chatis P, et al. Acyclovir-resistant herpes simplex infections in patients with the acquired immunodeficiency syndrome. *N Engl J Med* 1989;320:293–296.
673. Burns WH, Saral R, Santos GW, et al. Isolation and characterisation of resistant herpes simplex virus after acyclovir therapy. *Lancet* 1982;1:421–423.
674. Wutzler P. Antiviral therapy of herpes simplex and varicella-zoster virus infections. *Intervirology* 1997;40:343–356.
675. Tyler KL. Herpes simplex virus infections of the central nervous system: encephalitis and meningitis, including Mollaret's. *Herpes* 2004;11(Suppl 2):57A–64A.
676. Najioullah F, Bosshard S, Thouvenot D, et al. Diagnosis and surveillance of herpes simplex virus infection of the central nervous system. *J Med Virol* 2000;61:468–473.
677. Togashi T, Matsuzono Y, Narita M, et al. Influenza-associated acute encephalopathy in Japanese children in 1994–2002. *Virus Res* 2004;103:75–78.
678. Kohl S. Effectiveness of adenine arabinoside therapy for herpes simplex infections. *J Infect Dis* 1984;150:777–778.
679. Pike MG, Kennedy CR, Neville BG, et al. Herpes simplex encephalitis with relapse. *Arch Dis Child* 1991;66:1242–1244.
680. Hargrave DR, Webb DW. Movement disorders in association with herpes simplex virus encephalitis in children: a review. *Dev Med Child Neurol* 1998;40:640–642.
681. Prober CG, Sullender WM, Yasukawa LL, et al. Low risk of herpes simplex virus infections in neonates exposed to the virus at the time of vaginal delivery to mothers with recurrent genital herpes simplex virus infections. *N Engl J Med* 1987;316:240–244.
682. Corey L, Whitley RJ, Stone EF, et al. Difference between herpes simplex virus type 1 and type 2 neonatal encephalitis in neurologic outcome. *Lancet* 1988;1:1–4.
683. Whitley RJ. Neonatal herpes simplex virus infections: pathogenesis and therapy. *Pathol Biol* (Paris) 1992;40:729–734.
684. Malm G, Forsgren M, el Azazi M, et al. A follow-up study of children with neonatal herpes simplex virus infections with particular regard to late nervous disturbances. *Acta Paediatr Scand* 1991;80:226–234.
685. Studahl M. Influenza virus and CNS manifestations. *J Clin Virol* 2003;28:225–232.
686. Stevens D, Burman D, Clarke SK, et al. Temporary paralysis in childhood after influenza B. *Lancet* 1974;2:1354–1355.
687. Paisley JW, Bruhn FW, Lauer BA, et al. Type A2 influenza viral infections in children. *Am J Dis Child* 1978;132:34–36.
688. Fujii Y, Kuriyama M, Konishi Y, et al. MRI and SPECT in influenzal encephalitis. *Pediatr Neurol* 1992;8:133–136.
689. Protheroe SM, Mellor DH. Imaging of influenza A encephalitis. *Arch Dis Child* 1991;66:702–705.

690. Kawashima H, Morishima T, Togashi T, et al. Extraordinary changes in excitatory amino acid levels in cerebrospinal fluid of influenza-associated encephalopathy of children. *Neurochem Res* 2004;29:1537–1540.
691. Nakai Y, Itoh M, Mizuguchi M, et al. Apoptosis and microglial activation in influenza encephalopathy. *Acta Neuropathol* 2003; 105:233–239.
692. McCarthy VP, Zimmerman AW, Miller CA. Central nervous system manifestations of parainfluenza virus type 3 infections in childhood. *Pediatr Neurol* 1990;6:197–201.
693. Craver RD, Gohd RS, Sundin DR, et al. Isolation of parainfluenza virus type 3 from cerebrospinal fluid associated with aseptic meningitis. *Am J Clin Pathol* 1993;99:705–707.
694. Lindquist SW, Darnule A, Istas A, et al. Parainfluenza virus type-4 infections in pediatric patients. *Pediatr Infect Dis J* 1997;16:34–38.
695. Tsolia M, Skardoutsou A, Tsolas G, et al. Pre-eruptive neurologic manifestations associated with multiple cerebral infarcts in varicella. *Pediatr Neurol* 1995;12:165–168.
696. Yilmaz K, Caliskan M, Askdeniz C, et al. Acute childhood hemiplegia associated with chickenpox. *Pediatr Neurol* 1998;18:256–261.
697. Tsolia, M, et al. Pre-eruptive neurologic manifestations associated with multiple cerebral infarcts in varicella. *Pediatr Neurol* 1995;12:165–168.
698. Amlie-Lefond C, Kleinschimdt-Demasters BK, Mahalingam R, et al. The vasculopathy of varicella-zoster virus encephalitis. *Ann Neurol* 1995;37:784–790.
699. Downie AW. Chickenpox and zoster. *Br Med Bull* 1959;15:197–200.
700. Croen KD, Straus SE. Varicella-zoster virus latency. *Ann Rev Microbiol* 1991;45:265–282.
701. Arvin AM, Koropchak CM, Wittek AE. Immunologic evidence of reinfection with varicella-zoster virus. *J Infect Dis* 1983;148:200–205.
702. Gilden D. Varicella-zoster virus and central nervous system syndromes. *Herpes* 2004;11(Suppl 2):89A–94A.
703. Hardy I, Gershon AA, Steinberg SP, et al. Varicella Vaccine Collaborative Study Group. The incidence of zoster after immunization with live attenuated varicella vaccine. A study of children with leukemia. *N Engl J Med* 1991;325:1545–1550.
704. Denny-Brown D, Adams RD, Fitzgerald PJ. Pathologic features of herpes zoster. A note on "geniculate herpes." *Arch Neurol Psychiatry* 1944;51:216–231.
705. McCormick WF, Rodnitzky RL, Schochet SS Jr., et al. Varicella-zoster encephalomyelitis—a morphologic and virologic study. *Arch Neurol* 1969;21:559–570.
706. Schmidbauer M, Budka H, Pilz P, et al. Presence, distribution and spread of productive varicella-zoster virus infection in nervous tissues. *Brain* 1992;115:383–398.
707. Hope-Simpson RE. The nature of herpes zoster. A long-term study and a new hypothesis. *Proc R Soc Med* 1965;58:9–20.
708. DeMorgas JM, Kierland RR. The outcome of patients with herpes zoster. *Arch Dermatol* 1957;75:193–196.
709. Kost RG, Straus SE. Drug therapy: postherpetic neuralgia—pathogenesis, treatment, and prevention. *N Engl J Med* 1996;335: 32–42.
710. Oaklander AL, Romans K, Horasek S, et al. Unilateral postherpetic neuralgia is associated with bilateral sensory neural damage. *Ann Neurol* 1998;44:789–795.
711. Baron R, Saguer M. Postherpetic neuralgia. *Brain* 1993;116:1477–1496.
712. Kleinschmidt-DeMasters BK, Gilden DH. Varicella-zoster virus infections of the nervous system: clinical and pathologic correlates. *Arch Pathol Lab Med* 2001;125:770–780.
713. Rose FC, Brett EM, Burston J. Zoster encephalomyelitis. *Arch Neurol* 1964;11:155–172.
714. Rosenfeld J, Taylor CL, Atlas SW. Myelitis following chickenpox: a case report. *Neurology* 1993;43:1834–1836.
715. Eidelberg D, Sotrel A, Horoupian DS, et al. Thrombotic cerebral vasculopathy associated with herpes zoster. *Ann Neurol* 1986;19:7–14.
716. Reshef E, Greenberg SB, Jankovic J. Herpes zoster ophthalmicus followed by contralateral hemiparesis: report of two cases and review of the literature. *J Neurol Neurosurg Psychiatry* 1985;48:122–127.
717. Bodensteiner JB, Hille MR, Riggs JE. Clinical features of vascular thrombosis following varicella. *Am J Dis Child* 1992;146:100–102.
718. Merselis JG Jr, Kaye D, Hooke EW. Disseminated herpes zoster: a report of 17 cases. *Arch Intern Med* 1964;113:679–686.
719. Feldman S, et al. A viremic phase for herpes zoster in children with cancer. *J Pediatr* 1977;91:557–560.
720. Hung PY, Lee WT, Shen YZ. Acute hemiplegia associated with herpes zoster infection in children: report of one case. *Pediatr Neurol* 2000;23:345–348.
721. Horten B, Price RW, Jiminez D. Multifocal varicella-zoster virus leukoencephalitis temporally remote from herpes zoster. *Ann Neurol* 1981;9:251–266.
722. Gnann JW, Whitley RJ. Neurologic manifestations of varicella and herpes zoster. In: Scheld WM, Whitley RJ, Durack DT, eds. *Infections of the central nervous system*, 2nd ed. Philadelphia: Lippincott–Raven, 1997: 91–105.
723. Echevarria JM, Martinez-Martin P, Tellez A, et al. Aseptic meningitis due to varicella-zoster virus: serum antibody levels and local synthesis of specific IgG, IgM, and IgA. *J Infect Dis* 1987;155:959–967.
724. Peterslund NA. Herpes zoster associated encephalitis: clinical findings and acyclovir treatment. *Scand J Infect Dis* 1988;20:583–592.
725. Mayo DR, Booss J. Varicella-zoster-associated neurologic disease without skin lesions. *Arch Neurol* 1989;46:313–315.
726. Silliman CC, Tedder D, Ogle JW, et al. Unsuspected varicella-zoster virus encephalitis in a child with acquired immunodeficiency syndrome. *J Pediatr* 1993;123:418–422.
727. Persaud D, Chandwani S, Rigaud M, et al. Delayed recognition of human immunodeficiency virus infection in preadolescent children. *Pediatrics* 1992;90:688–691.
728. Keidan SE, Mainwaring D. Association of herpes zoster with leukemia and lymphoma in children. *Clin Pediatr* 1965;4:13–17.
729. Hunt JR. On herpetic inflammations of the geniculate ganglion: a new syndrome and its complications. *J Nerv Ment Dis* 1907;34:73–96.
730. Terada K, Niizumu T, Kawano S, et al. Detection of varicella-zoster virus DNA in peripheral mononuclear cells from patients with Ramsay Hunt syndrome or zoster sine herpete. *J Med Virol* 1998;56:359–363.
731. Berrettini S, Bianchi MC, Segnini G, et al. Herpes zoster oticus: correlations between clinical and MRI findings. *Eur Neurol* 1998;39:26–31.
732. Murakami S, Hato N, Horiuchi J, et al. Treatment of Ramsay Hunt syndrome with acyclovir-prednisone: significance of early diagnosis and treatment. *Ann Neurol* 1997;41:353–357.
733. Gershon A, Steinberg S, Greenberg S, et al. Varicella-zoster-associated encephalitis: detection of specific antibody in cerebrospinal fluid. *J Clin Microbiol* 1980;12:764–769.
734. Casas I, Pozo F, Trallero G, et al. Viral diagnosis of neurological infection by RT multiplex PCR: a search for entero- and herpesviruses in a prospective study. *J Med Virol* 1999;57:145–151.
735. Echevarria JM, Casas I, Martinez-Martin P, et al. Infections of the nervous system caused by varicella-zoster virus: a review. *Intervirology* 1997;40:72–84.
736. Koskiniemi M, Piiparinen H, Rantalaiho T, et al. Acute central nervous system complications in varicella-zoster virus infections. *J Clin Virol* 2002;25:293–301.
737. Wood MJ, Johnson RW, McKendrick MW, et al. A randomized trial of acyclovir for 7 or 21 days with and without prednisolone for treatment of acute herpes zoster. *N Engl J Med* 1994;330:896–900.
738. Hay J, Arvin AM. Varicella-zoster virus infection: new insights into pathogenesis and post-herpetic neuralgia. *Ann Neurol* 1994;35(Suppl):S1–S72.
739. de Silva SM, Mark AS, Gilden DH, et al. Zoster myelitis: improvement with antiviral therapy in two cases. *Neurology* 1996;47:929–931.
740. Whitley RJ, Gnann JW Jr., Hinthorn D, et al. Disseminated herpes zoster in the immunocompromised host: a comparative trial of acyclovir and vidarabine. *J Infect Dis* 1992;165:450–455.

741. Otero J, et al. Response to acyclovir in two cases of herpes zoster leukoencephalitis and review of the literature. *Eur J Clin Microbiol Infect Dis* 1998;17:286–289.
742. Segal AZ, Rordorf G. Gabapentin as a novel treatment for post herpetic neuralgia. *Neurology* 1996;46:1175–1176.
743. Pasteur L. Méthode pour prevenir la rage après morsure. *C R Acad Sci Paris* 1885;101:765–774.
744. Fishbein DB, Robinson LE. Rabies. *N Engl J Med* 1993;329:1632–1638.
745. Plotkin SA, Clark HF. Rabies. In: Feigin RD, Cherry JD, eds. *Textbook of pediatric infectious diseases*, 4th ed. Philadelphia: Saunders, 1998: 2111–2125.
746. American Academy of Pediatrics. Rabies. In: Peter G, ed. *1997 Red book: report of the Committee on Infectious Diseases*, 24th ed. Elk Grove Village, IL: Author, 1997: 435–442.
747. Dupont JR, Earle K. Human rabies encephalitis. A study of forty-nine fatal cases and a review of the literature. *Neurology* 1965; 15:1023–1034.
748. McKendrick AG. A ninth analytical review of reports from Pasteur Institutes on the results of anti-rabies treatment. *Bull Health Org League Nations* 1940;9:31–78.
749. Lentz TL, Burrage TG, Smith AL, et al. The acetylcholine receptor as a cellular receptor for rabies virus. *Yale J Biol Med* 1983;56:315–322.
750. Schindler R. Studies on the pathogenesis of rabies. *Bull WHO* 1961;25:119–126.
751. Gonzalez-Angulo A, Marquez-Monter H, Feria-Velasco A, et al. The ultrastructure of Negri-bodies in Purkinje neurons in human rabies. *Neurology* 1970;20:323–328.
752. Jackson AC, Ye H, Ridaura-Sanz C, et al. Quantitative study of the infection in brain neurons in human rabies. *J Med Virol* 2001;65:614–618.
753. Mrak RE, Young L. Rabies encephalitis in humans: pathology, pathogenesis and pathophysiology. *J Neuropathol Exp Neurol* 1994;53:1–10.
754. Anonymous. Human rabies: strain identification reveals lengthy incubation period [Editorial]. *Lancet* 1991;337:822–823.
755. Anderson LJ, Nicholson KG, Tauxe RV, et al. Human rabies in the United States, 1960–1979: epidemiology, diagnosis and prevention. *Ann Intern Med* 1984;100:728–735.
756. Bhatt DR, Hattwick MA, Gerdsen R, et al. Human rabies. *Am J Dis Child* 1974;127:862–869.
757. Blatt ML, Hoffman SJ, Schneider M. Rabies: report of twelve cases, with a discussion of prophylaxis. *JAMA* 1938;111:688–691.
758. Desai RV, Jain V, Singh P, et al. Radiculomyelitic rabies: Can MR imaging help? *Am J Neuroradiol* 2002;23:632–634.
759. Blattner RJ. Bats and rabies. *J Pediatr* 1955;46:612–614.
760. Cheetham HD, Hart J, Coghill NF, et al. Rabies with myocarditis. Two cases in England. *Lancet* 1970;1:921–922.
761. Perl DP, Good PF. The pathology of rabies in the central nervous system. In: Baer GM, ed. *The natural history of rabies*, 2nd ed. Boca Raton, FL: CRC Press, 1991: 164–190.
762. Cereghino JJ, Osterud HT, Pinnas JL, et al. Rabies: a rare disease but a serious pediatric problem. *Pediatrics* 1970;45:839–844.
763. Johnson HN. Rabies virus. In: Lennette EH, Schmidt NJ, eds. *Diagnostic procedures for viral, rickettsial and chlamydial infections*, 5th ed. Washington, DC: American Public Health Association 1979: 843–877.
764. Whitley RJ. Rabies. In: Scheld WM, Whitley RJ, Durack DT, eds. *Infections of the central nervous system*. New York: Lippincott-Raven, 1997: 181–198.
765. Hattwick MA, Weiss TT, Stechschulte CJ, et al. Recovery from rabies. A case report. *Ann Intern Med* 1972;76:931–942.
766. Vodopija I, Soreau P, Smerdel S. Current issues in human rabies immunization. *Rev Infect Dis* 1988;10(Suppl 4):S758–S763.
767. Fishbein DB, Sawyer LA, Reid-Senden FL, et al. Administration of human diploid-cell rabies vaccine in the gluteal area [Letter]. *N Engl J Med* 1988;318:124–125.
768. Mortiere MD, Falcone AL. An acute neurological syndrome temporally associated with postexposure treatment of rabies. *Pediatrics* 1997;100:720–721.
769. Park JY, Saron MF. Age distribution of lymphocytic choriomeningitis virus serum antibody in Birmingham, Alabama: evidence of a decreased risk of infection. *Am J Trop Hyg* 1997;57:37–41.
770. Marrie TJ, Saron MF. Seroprevalence of lymphocytic choriomeningitis virus in Nova Scotia. *Am J Trop Hyg* 1998;58:47–49.
771. Howard ME. Infection with the virus of choriomeningitis in man. *Yale J Biol Med* 1940;13:161–180.
772. Baker AB. Chronic lymphocytic choriomeningitis. *J Neuropathol Exp Neurol* 1947;6:253–264.
773. Brezin AP, Thulliez P, Cisneros B, et al. Lymphocytic choriomeningitis virus chorioretinitis mimicking ocular toxoplasmosis in two otherwise normal children. *Am J Ophthalmol* 2000;130:245–247.
774. Baum SG, Lewis AM Jr., Rowe WP, et al. Epidemic nonmeningitic lymphocytic-choriomeningitis-virus infection. An outbreak in a population of laboratory personnel. *N Engl J Med* 1966;274:934–936.
775. Lewis JM, Utz JP. Orchitis, parotitis and meningoencephalitis due to lymphocytic-choriomeningitis virus. *N Engl J Med* 1961;265:776–780.
776. Green WR, Sweet LK, Prichard RW. Acute lymphocytic choriomeningitis: a study of 21 cases. *J Pediatr* 1949;35:688–701.
777. Adair CV, Gauld RL, Smadel JE. Aseptic meningitis, a disease of diverse etiology: clinical and etiologic studies on 854 cases. *Ann Intern Med* 1953;39:675–704.
778. Wright R, Johnson D, Neumann M, et al. Congenital lymphocytic meningitis virus syndrome: a disease that mimics congenital toxoplasmosis or cytomegalovirus infection. *Pediatrics* 1997;100:E9.
779. Park JY, Peters CJ, Rollin PE, et al. Development of a reverse transcription-polymerase chain reaction assay for the diagnosis of lymphocytic choriomeningitis virus infection and its use in a prospective surveillance study. *J Med Virol* 1997;51:107–114.
780. Yamamoto M, Ohga S, Ohnishi Y, et al. Optic disk vasculitis associated with chronic active Epstein-Barr virus infection. *Ophthalmologica* 2002;216:221–225.
781. Gautier-Smith PC. Neurological complications of glandular fever (infectious mononucleosis). *Brain* 1965;88:323–334.
782. Silverstein A, Steinberg G, Nathanson M. Nervous system involvement in infectious mononucleosis. The heralding and/or major manifestation. *Arch Neurol* 1972;26:353–358.
783. Wong M, Connolly AM, Noetzel MJ. Poliomyelitis-like syndrome associated with Epstein-Barr virus infection. *Pediatr Neurol* 1999;20:235–237.
784. Pedneault L, Katz BZ, Miller G, et al. Detection of Epstein-Barr virus in the brain by polymerase chain reaction. *Ann Neurol* 1992;32:184–192.
785. Halsted CC, Chang RS, et al. Infectious mononucleosis and encephalitis: recovery of EB virus from spinal fluid. *Pediatrics* 1979;64:257–258.
786. Domachowske JB, Cunningham CK, Cummings DL, et al. Acute manifestations and neurologic sequelae of Epstein-Barr virus encephalitis in children. *Pediatr Infect Dis J* 1996;15:871–875.
787. Majid A, Galetta SL, Sweeney CJ, et al. Epstein-Barr virus myeloradiculitis and encephalomyeloradiculitis. *Brain* 2002;125(Pt 1): 159–165.
788. Grose C, Henle W, Horwitz MS, et al. Primary Epstein-Barr infections in acute neurologic diseases. *N Engl J Med* 1975;292:392–395.
789. Erzurum S, Kalavsky SM, Watanakunakorn C. Acute cerebellar ataxia and hearing loss as initial symptoms of infectious mononucleosis. *Arch Neurol* 1983;40:760–762.
790. North K, de Silva L, Procopis P. Brain-stem encephalitis caused by Epstein-Barr virus. *J Child Neurol* 1993;8:40–42.
791. Connelly PD, DeWitt LD. Neurologic complications of infectious mononucleosis. *Pediatr Neurol* 1994;10:181–184.
792. Schellinger PD, Sommer C, Leithauser F, et al. Epstein-Barr virus meningoencephalitis with a lymphoma-like response in an immunocompetent host. *Ann Neurol* 1999;45:659–662.
793. Shechter FR, Lipsius EI, Rasansky HN. Retrobulbar neuritis. A complication of infectious mononucleosis. *Am J Dis Child* 1955;89:58–61.
794. Gross C, et al. Bell's palsy and infectious mononucleosis. *Lancet* 1973;2:231–232.

795. Parano E, Giuffrida S, Restivo D, et al. Reversible palsy of the hypoglossal nerve complicating infectious mononucleosis in a young child. *Neuropediatrics* 1998;29:46–47.
796. Erwin W, Weber RW, Manning RT. Complications of infectious mononucleosis. *Am J Med Sci* 1959;238:699–712.
797. Walsh FC, Poser CM, Carter S. Infectious mononucleosis encephalitis. *Pediatrics* 1954;13:536–543.
798. Pejme J. Infectious mononucleosis. A clinical and hematological study of patients and contacts, and a comparison with healthy subjects. *Acta Med Scand* 1964;413(Suppl):183.
799. Tselis A, Duman R, Storch GA, et al. Epstein-Barr virus encephalomyelitis diagnosed by polymerase chain reaction: detection of the genome in the CSF. *Neurology* 1997;48:1351–1355.
800. Weinberg A, Li S, Palmer M, Tyler KL. Quantitative CSF PCR in Epstein-Barr virus infections of the central nervous system. *Ann Neurol* 2002;52:543–548.
801. Gerber MA, Shapiro ED, Ryan RW, et al. Evaluations of enzyme-linked immunosorbent assay procedure for determining specific Epstein-Barr virus serology and of rapid test kits for diagnosis for infectious mononucleosis. *J Clin Microbiol* 1996;34:3240–3241.
802. Hausler M, Ramaekers VT, Doenges M, et al. Neurological complications of acute and persistent Epstein-Barr virus infection in paediatric patients. *J Med Virol* 2002;68:253–263.
803. Hongou K, Konishi T, Yagi S, et al. Rotavirus encephalitis mimicking afebrile benign convulsions in infants. *Pediatr Neurol* 1998;18:354–357.
804. Morrison C, Gilson T, Nuovo GJ. Histologic distribution of fatal rotaviral infection: an immunohistochemical and reverse transcriptase *in situ* polymerase chain reaction analysis. *Hum Pathol* 2001;32:216–221.
805. Lajo A, Borque C, Del Castillo F, et al. Mononucleosis caused by Epstein-Barr virus and cytomegalovirus in children: a comparative study of 124 cases. *Pediatr Infect Dis J* 1994;13:56–60.
806. Studahl M, Ricksten A, Sandberg T, et al. Cytomegalovirus encephalitis in four immunocompetent patients. *Lancet* 1992;340:1045–1046.
807. Kabins S, Keller R, Peitchel R, et al. Acute idiopathic polyneuritis caused by cytomegalovirus. *Arch Intern Med* 1976;136:100–101.
808. Takahashi M, Yamada T, Nakajima S, et al. The substantia nigra is a major target for neurovirulent influenza A virus. *J Exp Med* 1995;181:2161–2169.
809. Schmitz H, Enders G, et al. Cytomegalovirus as a frequent cause of Guillain-Barré syndrome. *J Med Virol* 1977;1:21–27.
810. Power C, Poland SD, Blume WT, et al. Cytomegalovirus and Rasmussen's encephalitis. *Lancet* 1990;336:1282–1284.
811. Middleton PJ, Alexander RM, Szymanski MT. Severe myositis during recovery from influenza. *Lancet* 1970;2:533–535.
812. Cinque P, Marenzi R, Ceresa D, et al. Cytomegalovirus infection of the central nervous system in patients with AIDS: diagnosis by PCR amplification from cerebrospinal fluid. *J Infect Dis* 1992;166:1408–1411.
813. Vancikova Z, Dvorak P. Cytomegalovirus infection in immunocompetent and immunocompromised individuals—a review. *Curr Drug Targets Immune Endocr Metabol Disord* 2001;1:179–187.
814. Debré R, et al. La maladie des griffes de chat. *Sem Hop Paris* 1950;26:1895–1904.
815. Parrot JH, Dure L, Sullender W. Central nervous system infection with *Bartonella quintana*: a report of two cases.1997;100:403–408.
816. Zangwill KM, Hamilton DH, Perkins BA, et al. Cat scratch disease in Connecticut. Epidemiology, risk factors and evaluation of a new diagnostic test. *N Engl J Med* 1993;329:8–13.
817. Adal KA, Cockerell CJ, Petri WA Jr. Cat scratch disease, bacillary angiomatosis, and other infections due to rochalimaea. *N Engl J Med* 1994;330:1509–1515.
818. Wear DJ, Margileth AM, Hadfield TL, et al. Cat scratch disease: a bacterial infection. *Science* 1983;221:1403–1405.
819. Regnery RI, Andersen BE, Clarridge JE III. Characterization of a novel *Rochalimaea* species, *R. Henselae* sp. nov., isolated from blood of a febrile, human immunodeficiency virus-positive patient. *J Clin Microbiol* 1992;30:265–274.
820. Carithers HA, Margileth AM. Cat-scratch disease: acute encephalopathy and other neurologic manifestations. *Am J Dis Child* 1991;145:98–101.
821. Margileth AM. Cat scratch disease. *Adv Pediatr Infect Dis* 1993; 8:1–21.
822. Lewis DW, Tucker SH. Central nervous system involvement in cat scratch disease. *Pediatrics* 1986;77:714–721.
823. Carithers H. A. Cat-scratch disease: an overview based on a study of 1,200 patients. *Am J Dis Child* 1985;139:1124–1133.
824. Tsao CY. Generalized tonic-clonic status epilepticus in a child with cat-scratch disease and encephalopathy. *Clin Electroencephalogr* 1992;23:65–67.
825. Drancour M, Birtles R, Chaumentin G, et al. New serotype of *Bartonella henselae* in endocarditis and cat-scratch disease. *Lancet* 1996;347:441–443.
826. Patnaik M, Schwartzman WA, Barka NE, et al. Possible role of *Rochalimaea henselae* in pathogenesis of AIDS encephalopathy. *Lancet* 1992;340:971.
827. Regnery RL, Olson JG, Perkins BA, et al. Serological response to "*Rochalimaea henselae*" antigen in suspected cat-scratch disease. *Lancet* 1992;339:1443–1445.
828. Weston KD, Tran T, Kimmel KN, et al. Possible role of high-dose steroids in the treatment of cat-scratch disease encephalopathy. *J Child Neurol* 2001;16:762–763.
829. Sigurdsson B. Rida, a chronic encephalitis of sheep. With general remarks on infections which develop slowly and some of their special characteristics. *Br Vet J* 1954;110:341–358.
830. Prusiner SB. Prions. *Proc Natl Acad Sci USA* 1998;95:13363–13383.
831. Prusiner SB. The prion diseases. *Brain Pathol* 1998;8:499–513.
832. Klein MA, Frigg R, Flechsig E, et al. A crucial role for B cells in neuroinvasive scrapie. *Nature* 1997;390:687–690.
833. Prusiner SB, DeArmond SJ. Prion diseases and neurodegeneration. *Annu Rev Neurosci* 1994;17:311–339.
834. Prusiner SB. Prion diseases and the BSE crisis. *Science* 1997; 278:245–251.
835. Hill AF, Desbruslais M, Joiner S, et al. The same prion strain causes vCJD and BSE. *Nature* 1997;389:448–450.
836. Haywood AM. Transmissible spongiform encephalopathies. *N Engl J Med* 1997;337:1821–1828.
837. Mestel R. Putting prions to the test. *Science* 1996;273:184–189.
838. DeArmond SJ, Mobley WC, DeMott DL, et al. Changes in the localization of brain prion proteins during scrapie infection. *Neurology* 1987;37:1271–1280.
839. Kristensson K, Feuerstein B, Taraboules A, et al. Scrapie prions alter receptor-mediated calcium responses in cultured cells. *Neurology* 1993;43:2335–2341.
840. Collinge J, Whittington MA, Sidle KC, et al. Prion protein is necessary for synaptic function. *Nature* 1994;370:295–297.
841. Kovacs GG, Kalev O, Budka H. Contribution of neuropathology to the understanding of human prion disease. *Folia Neuropathol* 2004;42(Suppl A):69–76.
842. Weissmann C. The state of the prion. *Nat Rev Microbiol* 2004;2: 861–871.
843. Ito M, Okuno T, Mikawa H, et al. Chronic mumps virus encephalitis. *Pediatr Neurol* 1991;7:467–470.
844. Ogawa M, Okubo H, Tsuji Y, et al. Chronic progressive encephalitis occurring 13 years after Russian spring-summer encephalitis. *J Neurol Sci* 1973;19:363–373.
845. Sharma S, Mathur A, Prakash V, et al. Japanese encephalitis virus latency in peripheral blood lymphocytes and recurrence of infection in children. *Clin Exp Immunol* 1991;85:85–89.
846. Pantaleo G, Graziosi C, Fauci AS. The immunopathogenesis of human immunodeficiency virus infection. *N Engl J Med* 1993;328:327–335.
847. Greene WC. The molecular biology of human immunodeficiency virus type 1 infection. *N Engl J Med* 1991;324:308–317.
848. Levy JA. Infection by human immunodeficiency virus—CD4 is not enough. *N Engl J Med* 1996;335:1528–1530.
849. Human immunodeficiency virus. In: Johnson RT. *Viral infections of the nervous system*, 2nd ed. Philadelphia: Lippincott–Raven, 1998: 287–313.
850. Merril JE, Jonakait M. Interactions of the nervous and immune

systems in development, normal brain homeostasis, and disease. *FASEB J* 1995;9:611–618.
851. Pulliam L, Gascon R, Stubblebine M, et al. Unique monocyte subset in patients with AIDS dementia. *Lancet* 1997;349:692–695.
852. Tyor WR, Glass JD, Baumrind N, et al. Cytokine expression of macrophages in HIV-1-associated vacuolar myelopathy. *Neurology* 1993;43:1002–1009.
853. Kolson DL, Lavi E, Gonzàlez-Scarano F. The effects of human immunodeficiency virus in the central nervous system. *Adv Virus Res* 1998;50:1–47.
854. Lipton SA, Gendelman HE. Dementia associated with the acquired imunodeficiency syndrome. *N Engl J Med* 1995;332:934–944.
855. Davis LE, Hjelle BL, Miller VE, et al. Early viral brain invasion in iatrogenic human immunodeficiency virus infection. *Neurology* 1992;42:1736–1739.
856. Chamberlain MC, Nichols SL, Chase CH. Pediatric AIDS: comparative cranial MRI and CT scans. *Pediatr Neurol* 1991;7:357–362.
857. Epstein LG, Sharer LR, Oleske JM, et al. Neurologic manifestations of human immunodeficiency virus infection in children. *Pediatrics* 1986;78:678–687.
858. Brown MM. Retroviruses and diseases of the nervous system. *J R Soc Med* 1989;82:306–309.
859. Childs EA, Lyles RH, Selnes OA, et al. Plasma viral load and CD4 lymphocytes predict HIV-associated dementia and sensory neuropathy. *Neurology* 1999;52:607–613.
860. Dickson DW, Llena JF, Nelson SJ, et al. Central nervous system pathology in pediatric AIDS: an autopsy study. *APMIS* 1989;8(Suppl):40–57.
861. Donaldson YK, Bell JE, Ironside JW. Redistribution of HIV outside the lymphoid system with onset of AIDS. *Lancet* 1994;343:382–385.
862. Falloon J, Eddy J, Wiener L, et al. Human immunodeficiency virus infection in children. *J Pediatr* 1989;114:1–30.
863. Spencer DC, Price RW. Human immunodeficiency virus and the central nervous system. *Annu Rev Microbiol* 1992;46:655–693.
864. Petito CK. What causes brain atrophy in human immunodeficiency virus infection? *Ann Neurol* 1993;34:128–129.
865. Kure K, Weidenheim KM, Lyman WD, et al. Morphology and distribution of HIV-1 gp41-positive microglia in subacute AIDS encephalitis. Pattern of involvement resembling a multisystem degeneration. *Acta Neuropathol* 1990;80:393–400.
866. Giangaspero F, Scanabissi E, Balduci MC, et al. Massive neuronal destruction in human immunodeficiency virus (HIV) encephalitis. A clinico-pathological study of a pediatric case. *Acta Neuropathol* 1989;78:662–665.
867. Evans BK, Donley DK, Whitaker JN. Neurological manifestations of infection with the human immunodeficiency viruses. In: Scheld WM, Whitley RJ, Durack DT, eds. *Infections of the central nervous system*. New York: Raven Press, 1991:201–232.
868. Gray F, et al. Neuropathology of early HIV-1 infection. *Brain Pathol* 1996;6:1–15.
869. Adamson DC, Wildemann B, Sasaki M, et al. Immunologic NO synthase: elevation in severe AIDS dementia and induction by HIV-1 gp41. *Science* 1996;274:1917–1921.
870. Markham RB, Coberly J, Ruff AJ, et al. Maternal IgG1 and IgA antibody to the V3 loop consensus sequence and maternal-infant HIV-1 transmission. *Lancet* 1994;343:390–391.
871. Blanche S, Mayaux MJ, Rouzioux C, et al. Relation of the course of HIV infection in children to the severity of the disease in their mothers at delivery. *N Engl J Med* 1994;330:308–312.
872. Sperling RS, Shapiro DE, Coombs RW, et al. Maternal viral load, zidovudine treatment, and the risk of transmission of human immunodeficiency virus type 1 from mother to infant. *N Engl J Med* 1996;335:1621–1629.
873. Landesman SH, Kalish LA, Burns DN, et al. Obstetrical factors and the transmission of human immunodeficiency virus type 1 from mother to child. *N Engl J Med* 1996;334:1617–1623.
874. Newell ML. Mechanisms and timing of mother-to-child transmission of HIV-1. *AIDS* 1998;12:831–837.
875. Pantaleo G, Graziosi C, Demarest JF. HIV infection is active and progressive in lymphoid tissue during the clinically latent stage of disease. *Nature* 1993;362:355–358.
876. Fauci AS. Multifactorial nature of human immunodeficiency virus disease: implications for therapy. *Science* 1993;262:1011–1018.
877. Civitello LA. Neurologic complications of HIV infection of children. *Pediatr Neurosurg* 1991;17:104–112.
878. Belman AL, Diamond G, Dickson D, et al. Pediatric acquired immunodeficiency syndrome: neurologic syndromes. *Am J Dis Child* 1988;142:29–35.
879. Belman AL, Muenz LR, Marcus JC, et al. Neurologic status of human immunodeficiency virus 1-infected infants and their controls: a prospective study from birth to 2 years. Mothers and Infants Cohort Study. *Pediatrics.* 1996: 98:1109–1118.
880. Roy S, Geoffroy G, LaPointe N, et al. Neurological findings in HIV-infected children: a review of 49 cases. *Can J Neurol Sci* 1992;19:453–457.
881. Cooper ER, Hanson C, Diaz C, et al. Encephalopathy and progression of human immunodeficiency virus disease in a cohort of children with perinatally acquired human immunodeficiency virus infection. Women and Infants Transmission Study Group. *J Pediatr* 1998;132:808–812.
882. Kahn JO, Walker BD. Acute human immunodeficiency virus type 1 infection. *N Engl J Med* 1998;339:33–39.
883. Morriss MC, et al. Progressive multifocal leukoencephalopathy in an HIV-infected child. *Neuroradiology* 1997;39:142–144.
884. Epstein LG, Gelbard HA. HIV-1-induced neuronal injury in the developing brain. *J Leukoc Biol* 1999;65:453–457.
885. Bale JF Jr., Contant CF, Garg B, et al. Neurologic history and examination results and their relationship to human immunodeficiency virus type 1 serostatus in hemophilia subjects: results from the Hemophilia Growth and Development Sudy. *Pediatrics* 1993;91:736–741.
886. Mitchell WG, Lynn H, Bale JF Jr., et al. Longitudinal follow-up of a group of HIV-seropositive and HIV-seronegative hemophiliacs: results from the Hemophilia Growth and Development Study. *Pediatrics* 1997;100:817–824.
887. Misdrahi D, Vila G, Funk-Brentano I. DSM-IV mental disorders and neurological complications in children and adolescents with human immunodeficiency virus type 1 infection (HIV-1). *Eur Psychiatry* 2004;19:182–184.
888. Mitchell W. Neurological and developmental effects on HIV and AIDS in children and adolescents. *MRDD Res Rev* 2001;7:211–216.
889. DeCarli C, Civitello LA, Brouwers P, et al. The prevalence of computerized tomographic abnormalities of the cerebrum in 100 consecutive children symptomatic with the human immunodeficiency virus. *Ann Neurol* 1993;34:198–205.
890. Post MJ, Tate LG, Quencer RM, et al. CT, MR, and pathology in HIV encephalitis and meningitis. *Am J Roentgenol* 1988;151:373–380.
891. Scarmato V, Frank Y, Rozenstein A, et al. Central brain atrophy in childhood AIDS encephalopathy. *AIDS* 1996;10:1227–1231.
892. Angelini L, Zibordi F, Triulzi F, et al. Age-dependent neurologic manifestations of HIV infection in childhood. *Neurol Sci* 2000;21:135–142.
893. States LJ, Zimmerman RA, Rutstein RM. Imaging of pediatric central nervous system HIV infection. *Neuroimaging Clin North Am* 1997;7:321–339.
894. Pavlakis SG, Lu D, Frank Y, et al. Brain lactate and N-acetylaspartate in pediatric AIDS encephalopathy. *Am J Neuroradiol* 1998;19:383–385.
895. Salvan AM, Lamoureax S, Michael G, et al. Localized proton magnetic resonance spectroscopy of the brain in children infected with human immunodeficiency virus with and without encephalopathy. *Pediatr Res* 1998;44:755–762.
896. Miles SA, Balden E, Magpantay L, et al. Rapid serologic testing with immune-complex-dissociated HIV p24 antigen for early detection of HIV infection in neonates. *N Engl J Med* 1993;328:297–302.
897. Dunn DT, Brandt CD, Krivine A, et al. The sensitivity of HIV-1 DNA polymerase chain reaction in the neonatal period and the relative contributions of intra-uterine and intra-partum transmission. *AIDS* 1995;9:7–11.

898. McIntosh K, Pitt J, Brambilla D, et al. Blood culture in the first 6 months of life for diagnosis of vertically transmitted human immunodeficiency virus infection. The Woman and Infant Study Group. *J Infect Dis* 1994;170:996–1000.
899. Public Health Service Task Recommendations. Guidelines for the use of antiretroviral agents in pediatric HIV infection. *MMWR Morb Mortal Wkly Rep* 1998;47(RR-4):1–34.
900. Burgard M, Mayaux MJ, Blarche S, et al. The use of viral culture and p24 antigen testing to diagnose human immunodeficiency virus infection in neonates. *N Engl J Med* 1992;327:1192–1197.
901. Sei S, Sandelli SL, Theafan G, et al. Evaluation of human immunodeficiency virus (HIV) type 1 RNA levels in cerebrospinal fluid and viral resistance to zidovudine in children with HIV encephalopathy. *J Infect Dis* 1996;174:1200–1206.
902. McCoig C, Castrejon MM, Saavedra-Lozano J, et al. Cerebrospinal fluid and plasma concentrations of proinflammatory mediators in human immunodeficiency virus-infected children. *Pediatr Infect Dis J* 2004;23:114–118.
903. Sanchez-Ramon S, Bellon JM, Resino S, et al. Low blood CD8+ T-lymphocytes and high circulating monocytes are predictors of HIV-1-associated progressive encephalopathy in children. *Pediatrics* 2003;111:E168–E175.
904. Sanchez-Ramon S, Canto-Nogues C, Munoz-Fernandez MA. Reconstructing the course of HIV-1-associated progressive encephalopathy in children. *Med Sci Monit* 2002;8:RA249–RA252.
905. McFarlin DE. Neurological disorders related to HTLV-I and HTLV-II. *J Acquir Immune Defic Syndr* 1993;6:640–644.
906. Gessain A, Gout O. Chronic myelopathy associated with human T-lymphotropic virus type I (HTLV-I). *Ann Intern Med* 1992;117:933–946.
907. Harrington WJ Jr, Sheremata W, Hjelle B, et al. Spastic ataxia associated with human T-cell lymphotropic virus type II infection. *Ann Neurol* 1993;33:411–414.
908. Sheremata, WA, Harrington WJ Jr., Bradshaw PA, et al. Association of '(tropical) ataxic neuropathy' with HTLV-II. *Virus Res* 1993;29:71–77.
909. Levin MC, et al. Immunologic analysis of a spinal cord biopsy specimen from a patient with human T-cell lymphotropic virus type I-associated neurologic disease. *N Engl J Med* 1997;336:839–845.
910. Moritoyo T, Reinhart TA, Moritoyo H, et al. Human T-lymphotrophic virus type I myelopathy and *tax* gene expression in CD4+ T lymphocytes. *Ann Neurol* 1996;40:84–86.
911. Leon-Monzon M, Illa I, Dalakas MC. Polymyositis in patients infected with human T-cell leukemia virus type I: the role of virus in the cause of the disease. *Ann Neurol* 1994;36:643–649.
912. Izumo S, Goto I, Itoyama Y, et al. Interferon-alpha is effective in HTLV-I-associated myelopathy: a multicenter, randomized, double-blind, controlled trial. *Neurology* 1996;46:1016–1021.
913. Gibbs CJ Jr, Joy A, Heffner R, et al. Clinical and pathological features and laboratory confirmation of a Creutzfeldt-Jakob disease in a recipient of pituitary-derived human growth hormone. *N Engl J Med* 1985;313:734–738.
914. Rappaport EB, Graham DJ. Pituitary growth hormone from human cadavers: neurologic disease in ten recipients. *Neurology* 1987;37:1211–1213.
915. Brown P, Gibbs CJ Jr., Rodgers-Johnson P, et al. Human spongiform encephalopathy: the National Institutes of Health series of 300 cases of experimentally transmitted disease. *Ann Neurol* 1994;35:513–529.
916. Swerdlow AJ, Higgins CD, Adlard P, et al. Creutzfeldt-Jakob disease in United Kingdom patients treated with human pituitary growth hormone. *Neurology* 2003;61:783–791.
917. Monreal J, Collins GH, Masters CL, et al. Creutzfeldt-Jakob disease in an adolescent. *J Neurol Sci* 1981;52:341–350.
918. Brown P, Preece M, Brandel JP, et al. Iatrogenic Creutzfeldt-Jakob disease: an example of the interplay between ancient genes and modern medicine. *Neurology* 1994;44:291–293.
919. Chretien F, Le Pavec G, Vallat-Decouvelaere AV, et al. Expression of excitatory amino acid transporter-1 (EAAT-1) in brain macrophages and microglia of patients with prion diseases. *J Neuropathol Exp Neurol* 2004;63:1058–1071.
920. Deslys JP, Lasmizas C, Dormont D. Selection of specific strains in iatrogenic Creutzfeldt-Jakob disease. *Lancet* 1994;343:848–849.
921. Hayashi R, Hanyu N, Kuwabara T, et al. Serial computed tomographic and electroencephalographic studies in Creutzfeldt-Jakob disease. *Acta Neurol Scand* 1992;85:161–165.
922. Zerr I, Bodemer M, Otto M, et al. Diagnosis of Creutzfeldt-Jakob disease by two-dimensional gel electrophoresis of cerebrospinal fluid. *Lancet* 1996;348:846–849.
923. Hsich G, Kenney K, Gibbs CJ, et al. The 14-3-3 protein in cerebrospinal fluid as a marker for transmissible spongiform encephalopathies. *N Engl J Med* 1996;335:924–930.
924. Berndt RM. Reaction to contact in the eastern highlands of New Guinea. *Oceania* 1954;24:206.
925. Gajdusek DC. Unconventional viruses and the origin and disappearance of Kuru. *Science* 1977;197:943–960.
926. Gajdusek DC, Zigas V. Kuru. *Am J Med* 1959;26:442–469.
927. Gajdusek DC, Gibbs CJ Jr. Transmission of Kuru from man to Rhesus monkey (*Macaca mulatta*) eight and one-half years after inoculation. *Nature* 1972;240:351.
928. Grabow JD, Campbell RJ, Okazaki H, et al. A transmissible subacute spongiform encephalopathy in a visitor to the eastern highlands of New Guinea. *Brain* 1976;99:637–658.
929. Kompoliti K, Goetz CG, Gajdusek DC, Cubo E. Movement disorders in Kuru. *Mov Disord* 1999;14:800–804.
930. Gajdusek DC, Zigas V. Degenerative disease of the central nervous system in New Guinea: the endemic occurrence of "Kuru" in the native population. *N Engl J Med* 1957;257:974–978.
931. Hilton DA, Fathers E, Edwards P, et al. Prion immunoreactivity in appendix before clinical onset of variant Creutzfeldt-Jakob disease. *Lancet* 1998;352:703–704.
932. Aguzzi A. Neuro-immune connection in spread of prions in the body? *Lancet* 1997;349:742–743.
933. Zeidler M, Ironside JW, et al. New variant Creutzfeldt-Jakob disease: neurological features and diagnostic tests. *Lancet* 1997;350:903–907.
934. Zeidler M, Johnstone EC, Bamber RW, et al. New variant Creutzfeldt-Jakob disease: psychiatric features. *Lancet* 1997;350: 908–910.
935. Collee JG, Bradley R. BSE: a decade on—part 1 and 2. *Lancet* 1997;349:636–641, 715–721.
936. Medori R, Montagna P, Tritschuer HJ, et al. Fatal familial insomnia, a prion disease with a mutation at codon 178 of the prion protein gene. *N Engl J Med* 1992;326:444–449.
937. Dawson JR Jr. Cellular inclusions in cerebral lesions of epidemic encephalitis. *Arch Neurol Psychiatr* 1934;31:685–700.
938. Bergamini F, Defanti CA, Ferrante P. *Subacute sclerosing panencephalitis: a reappraisal.* New York: Elsevier, 1986: 440.
939. Case 15-1998. Case records of the Massachusetts General Hospital. *N Engl J Med* 1998;338:1448–1456.
940. Herndon RM, Rubinstein LJ. Light and electron microscopy observation on the development of viral particles in the inclusions of Dawson's encephalitis (subacute sclerosing panencephalitis). *Neurology* 1968;18:8–20.
941. Ohya T, et al. Subacute sclerosing panencephalitis: correlation of clinical, neurophysiologic and neuropathologic findings. *Neurology* 1974;24:211–218.
942. Shapshak P, Tourtellotte WW, Nakamura S, et al. Subacute sclerosing panencephalitis: measles virus matrix protein nucleic acid sequences detected by *in situ* hybridization. *Neurology* 1985;35:1605–1609.
943. Hirano A, Wang AH, Gombart AF, et al. The matrix proteins of neurovirulent subacute sclerosing panencephalitis virus and its acute measles progenitor are functionally different. *Proc Natl Acad Sci U S A* 1992;89:8745–8749.
944. Schmid A, et al. Subacute sclerosing panencephalitis is typically characterized by alterations in the fusion protein cytoplasmic domain of the persisting measles virus. *Virology* 1992;188:910–915.
945. Hirano A, Ayata M, Wang AH, et al. Functional analysis of matrix proteins expressed from cloned genes of measles virus variants that cause subacute sclerosing panencephalitis reveals a common defect in nucleocapside binding. *J Virol* 1993;67:1848–1853.
946. Mehta PD, Thormar H, Wisniewski HM. Oligoclonal IgG bands with and without measles antibody activity in sera of patients

with subacute sclerosing panencephalitis (SSPE). *J Immunol* 1982;129:1983–1985.
947. Mehta PD, Kulczycki J, Mehta SP, et al. Increased levels of b_2-microglobulin, soluble interleukin-2 receptor, and soluble CD8 in patients with subacute sclerosing panencephalitis. *Clin Immunol Immunopathol* 1992;65:53–59.
948. Miller C, Farrington CP, Harbert K. The epidemiology of subacute sclerosing panencephalitis in England and Wales 1970–1989. *Int J Epidemiol* 1992;21:998–1006.
949. Kornberg AJ, Harvey AS, Shield LK. Subacute sclerosing panencephalitis presenting as simple partial seizures. *J Child Neurol* 1991;6:146–149.
950. Robb RM, Watters GV. Ophthalmic manifestations of sub-acute sclerosing panencephalitis. *Arch Ophthalmol* 1970;83:426–435.
951. Jabbour JT, Garcia JH, Lemmi H, et al. Subacute sclerosing panencephalitis: a multidisciplinary study of eight cases. *JAMA* 1969;207:2248–2254.
952. Cochereau-Massin I, Gaudric A, Reinert P, et al. Changes in the fundus in subacute sclerosing panencephalitis. Apropos of 23 cases. *J Fr Ophthalmol* 1992;15:255–261.
953. Freeman JM. The clinical spectrum and early diagnosis of Dawson's encephalitis. *J Pediatr* 1969;75:590–603.
954. Grünewald T, Lampe J, Weissbrich B, et al. A 35-year-old bricklayer with hemi-myoclonic jerks. *Lancet* 1998;351:1926.
955. PeBenito R, Naqvi SH, Arca MM, et al. Fulminating subacute sclerosing panencephalitis: case report and literature review. *Clin Pediatr* 1997;36:149–154.
956. Huber M, Pawlik G, Bamborsch Ke S, et al. Changing patterns of glucose metabolism during the course of subacute sclerosing panencephalitis as measured with ^{18}FDG-positron-emission tomography. *J Neurol* 1992;293:157–161.
957. Pedersen H, Wulff CH. Computed tomographic findings in early subacute sclerosing panencephalitis. *Neuroradiology* 1982;23:31–32.
958. Winer JB, Pires M, Kermode A, et al. Resolving MRI abnormalities with progression of subacute sclerosing panencephalitis. *Neuroradiology* 1991;33:178–180.
959. Anlar B, Saatci I, Kose G, et al. MRI findings in subacute sclerosing panencephalitis. *Neurology* 1996;47:1278–1283.
960. Brismar J, Gascon GG, von Steyem KV, et al. Subacute sclerosing panencephalitis: evaluation with CT and MR. *AJNR Am J Neuroradiol* 1996;17:761–772.
961. Wulff CH. Subacute sclerosing panencephalitis: serial electroencephalographic studies. *J Neurol Neurosurg Psychiatry* 1982;45:418–421.
962. Yagi S, Miuru Y, Kataoka N, et al. The origin of myoclonus and periodic synchronous discharges in subacute sclerosing panencephalitis. *Acta Paediatr Jpn* 1992;34:310–315.
963. Giminez-Roldan S, Martin M, Mateo D, et al. Preclinical EEG abnormalities in subacute sclerosing panencephalitis. *Neurology* 1981;31:763–767.
964. Johnson RT. Subacute measles encephalitis with immunosuppression. In: Johnson RT, ed. *Viral infections of the nervous system*. New York: Raven Press, 1982: 247.
965. Kim TM, Brown HR, Lee SH, et al. Delayed acute measles body encephalitis in a 9-year-old girl: ultrastructural, immunohistochemical, and in situ hybridization studies. *Mod Pathol* 1992;5:348–352.
966. Baczko K, Liebert UG, CaHaneo R, et al. Restriction of measles virus gene expression in measles inclusion body encephalitis. *J Infect Dis* 1988;158:144–150.
967. DuRant RH, Dyken PR. The effect of inosiplex on the survival of subacute sclerosing panencephalitis. *Neurology* 1983;33:1053–1055.
968. Anlar B, Yalaz K, Oktem F, et al. Long-term follow-up of patients with subacute sclerosing panencephalitis treated with intraventricular gamma-interferon. *Neurology* 1997;48:526–528.
969. Yoshioka H, Nishimura O, Nakagawa M, et al. Administration of human leukocyte interferon to patients with subacute sclerosing panencephalitis. *Brain Dev* 1989;11:302–307.
970. Hayashi T, Ichiyama T, Nishikawa M, et al. Carbamazepine and myoclonus in SSPE subacute sclerosing panencephalitis. *Pediatr Neurol* 1996;346:346.
971. Weil ML, Itabashi H, Cremer NE, et al. Chronic progressive panencephalitis due to rubella virus simulating subacute sclerosing panencephalitis. *N Engl J Med* 1975;292:994–998.
972. Wolinsky J. Subacute sclerosing panencephalitis, progressive rubella panencephalitis, and multifocal leukoencephalopathy. *Res Publ Assoc Res Nerv Ment Dis* 1990;68:259–268.
973. Townsend JJ, Stroop WG, Baringer JR, et al. Neuropathology of progressive rubella panencephalitis after childhood rubella. *Neurology* 1982;32:185–190.
974. Vandvik B, Weil ML, Grandien M, et al. Progressive rubella panencephalitis: synthesis of oligoclonal virus-specific antibodies and free light chains in the central nervous system. *Acta Neurol Scand* 1978;57:53–64.
975. Wolinsky JS, Berg BO, Maitland CJ. Progressive rubella panencephalitis. *Arch Neurol* 1976;33:722–723.
976. Weil ML, Itabashi H, Cremer NE, et al. Chronic progressive panencephalitis due to rubella virus. *Arch Neurol* 1975;32:501.
977. Wolinsky JS, Dau PC, Buimovlci-Klein E, et al. Progressive rubella panencephalitis: immunovirological studies and results of isoprinosine therapy. *Clin Exp Immunol* 1979;35:397–404.
978. Noorden SK, Lopez-Bravo L, Sundaresan TK. Estimated number of leprosy cases in the world. *Bull WHO* 1992;70:7–10.
979. Britton WJ, Lockwood DNJ. Leprosy. *Lancet* 2004;363:1209–1219.
980. Smith WCS. The epidemiology of disability in leprosy including risk factors. *Lepr Rev* 1992;63(Suppl):23–30.
981. Centers for Disease Control. Public Health Service. Mosquitoes carry Hansen's disease. *US Dep Health Education Welfare Vet PublicHealth Notes* 1975;90:183.
982. Jacobson RR, Krahenbuhl JL. Leprosy. *Lancet* 1969;353:655–660.
983. Pfaltzgraff RE, Bryceson A. Clinical leprosy. In: Hastings RC, ed. *Leprosy*. Edinburgh: Churchill Livingstone, 1985: 134–176.
984. Yamamura M, Uyemura K, Deans RJ. Defining protective responses to pathogens: cytokine profiles in leprosy lesions. *Science* 1991;254:277–279.
985. van Voorhis WC, et al. The cutaneous infiltrates of leprosy. Cellular characteristics and the predominant T-cell phenotypes. *N Engl J Med* 1982;307:1593–1597.
986. Wallach D, Cottenot F, Bach M. Imbalance in T cell subpopulations in lepromatous leprosy. *Int J Lepr* 1982;50:282–290.
987. Job CK, Desikan KV. Pathological changes and their distribution in peripheral nerves in lepromatous leprosy. *Int J Lepr* 1968;36:257–270.
988. Miko TL, Maitre CL, Kinfu Y. Damages and regeneration of peripheral nerves in advanced treated leprosy. *Lancet* 1993; 3442:521–525.
989. Bullock WE. *Mycobacterium leprae*. In: Mandel CL, Douglas RG, Bennett JE, eds. *Principles and practice of infectious diseases*, 3rd ed. New York: Churchill Livingstone, 1990: 1906–1914.
990. Wall JR, Wright DM. Antibodies against testicular germinal cells in lepromatous leprosy. *Clin Exp Immunol* 1974;17:51–54.
991. Bullock WE. Studies of immune mechanisms in leprosy. Depression of delayed allergic responses to skin test antigens. *N Engl J Med* 1968;278:298–301.
992. Flaguel B, Wallach D, Vignon-Pennamer M. Late onset reversal reaction in borderline leprosy. *J Am Acad Dermatol* 1989;20:857–860.
993. Pearson JMH, Ross WX. Nerve involvement in leprosy: pathology, differential diagnosis and principles of management. *Lepr Rev* 1975;46:199–207.
994. Crawford CL. Neurological lesions in leprosy. *Lepr Rev* 1968;39: 9–13.
995. Monrad-Krohn GH. *The neurological aspect of leprosy*. Chicago: Chicago Medical Book, 1923.
996. Browne SG. Some less common neurological findings in leprosy. *J Neurol Sci* 1965;2:253–261.
997. Dash MS. A study of the mechanisms of cutaneous sensory loss in leprosy. *Brain* 1968;91:379–392.
998. Job CK, Karat AB, Karat S, et al. Leprous myositis—a histopathological and electron microscopic study. *Lepr Rev* 1969;40:9–16.
999. Editorial. Ocular complications of leprosy. *Lancet* 1992;340:642–643.

1000. Richardus JH, Nicholls PG, Croft RP, et al. Incidence of acute nerve function impairment and reactions in leprosy: a prospective cohort analysis after 5 years of follow-up. *Int J Epidemiol* 2004;33:337–343.
1001. Daniel E, Koshy S, Rao GS, et al. Ocular complications in newly diagnosed borderline lepromatous and lepromatous leprosy patients: baseline profile of the Indian cohort. *Br J Ophthalmol* 2002;86:1336–1340.
1002. Martinoli C, Derchi LE, Bertolotto M, et al. US and MR imaging of peripheral nerves in leprosy. *Skeletal Radiol* 2000;29:142–150.
1003. Singh N, Malik A, Arora VK, et al. Fine needle aspiration cytology of leprous neuritis. *Acta Cytol* 2003;47:368–372.
1004. Nations SP, Katz JS, Lyde CB, et al. Leprous neuropathy: an American perspective. *Semin Neurol* 1998;18:113–124.
1005. Willcox ML. The impact of multiple drug therapy on leprosy disabilities. *Lepr Rev* 1997;68:350–366.
1006. Manandhar R, Shrestha N, Butlin CR, et al. High levels of inflammatory cytokines are associated with poor clinical response to steroid treatment and recurrent episodes of type 1 reaction in leprosy. *Clin Exp Immunol* 2002;128:333–338.
1007. Katz AR, Ansdell VE, Effler PV, et al. Assessment of the clinical presentation and treatment of 353 cases of laboratory-confirmed leptospirosis in Hawaii, 1974–1998. *Clin Infect Dis* 2001;33:1834–1841.
1008. Meites E, Jay MT, Deresinski S, et al. Reemerging leptospirosis, California. *Emerg Infect Dis* 2004;10:406–412.
1009. Lopes AA, Costa E, Costa YA, et al. Comparative study of the in-hospital case-fatality rate of leptospirosis between pediatric and adult patients of different age groups. *Rev Inst Med Trop Sao Paulo* 2004;46:19–24.
1010. Hubbert WT, Humphrey GL. Epidemiology of leptospirosis in California: a cause of aseptic meningitis. *Calif Med* 1968;108:113–117.
1011. Lecour H, et al. Human leptospirosis: a review of 50 cases. *Infection* 1989;17:10–14.
1012. Edwards GA, Domm BM. Human leptospirosis. *Medicine* 1960;39:117–156.
1013. Watt G, Manaloto C, Hayes CG. Central nervous system leptospirosis in the Philippines. *Southeast Asian J Trop Med Public Health* 1989;20:265–269.
1014. Verma B, Daga SR, Sawant D. Leptospirosis in children. *Indian Pediatr* 2003;40:1081–1083.
1015. American Academy of Pediatrics. Leptospirosis. In: Peter G, ed. *1997 Red book: report of the Committee on Infectious Diseases*, 24th ed. Elk Grove Village, IL: Author, 1997: 326–327.
1016. Sehgal SC, Sugunan AP, Murhekar MV, et al. Randomized controlled trial of doxycycline prophylaxis against leptospirosis in an endemic area. *Int J Antimicrob Agents* 2000;13:249–255.
1017. Christian CW, Lavelle J, Bell LM. Preschoolers with syphilis. *Pediatrics* 1999;103:E4.
1018. Han JH, Lee CC, Crupi RS. Meningovascular syphilis and improvement with tissue-plasminogen activator (t-PA). *Am J Emerg Med* 2004;22:426–427.
1019. Merritt HH, Adams RD, Solomon HC. *Neurosyphilis*. New York: Oxford University Press, 1946.
1020. Marcus JC. Congenital neurosyphilis: a re-appraisal. *Neuropediatrics* 1982;13:195–199.
1021. Hallgren B, Hollström E. Congenital syphilis: a follow-up study with reference to mental abnormalities. *Acta Psychiatr Neurol Scand* 1954;93(Suppl):1–81.
1022. Sanchez PJ, Wendel GD Jr, Grimprel E, et al. Evaluation of molecular methodologies and rabbit infectivity testing for the diagnosis of congenital syphilis and neonatal central nervous system invasion by *Treponema pallidum*. *J Infect Dis* 1993;167:148–157.
1023. Jordan KG. Modern neurosyphilis—a critical analysis. *West J Med* 1988;149:47–157.
1024. Davis LE, Sperry S. The CSF-FTA test and the significance of blood contamination. *Ann Neurol* 1979;6:68–69.
1025. Davis LE, Schmitt JW. Clinical significance of cerebrospinal fluid tests for neurosyphilis. *Ann Neurol* 1989;25:50–55.
1026. Michelow IC, Wendel GD, Norgard MV, et al. Central nervous system infection in congenital syphilis. *N Engl J Med* 2002;346:1792–1798.
1027. Burstain JM, Grimprel E, Lukehart SA, et al. Sensitive detection of *Treponema pallidum* by using the polymerase chain reaction. *J Clin Microbiol* 1991;29:62–69.
1028. Rosen EU, Richardson NJ. A reappraisal of the value of the IgM fluorescent treponemal antibody absorption test in the diagnosis of congenital syphilis. *J Pediatr* 1975;87:38–42.
1029. American Academy of Pediatrics. Syphilis. In: Peter G, ed. *1997 Red book: report of the Committee on Infectious Diseases*, 24th ed. Elk Grove Village, IL: Author, 1997: 504–514.
1030. Parish JL. Treponemal infections in the pediatric population. *Clin Dermatol* 2000;18:687–700.
1031. Pfister HW, Wilske B, Weber K. Lyme borreliosis: basic science and clinical aspects. *Lancet* 1994;343:1013–1016.
1032. Hengge UR, Tannapfel A, Tyring SK, et al. Lyme borreliosis. *Lancet Infect Dis* 2003;3:489–500.
1033. Pachner AR, Dail D, Bai Y, et al. Genotype determines phenotype in experimental lyme borreliosis. *Ann Neurol* 2004;56:361–370.
1034. Steere AC, Grodzicki RL, Kornblatt AN, et al. The spirochetal etiology of Lyme disease. *N Engl J Med* 1983;308:733–740.
1035. Spach DH, Liles WC, Campbell GL, et al. Tick-borne diseases in the United States. *N Engl J Med* 1993;329:936–947.
1036. Reik L, Burgdorfer W, Donaldson JO. Neurological abnormalities in Lyme disease without erythema chronicum migrans. *Am J Med* 1986;81:73–78.
1037. Christen HJ, Hanefeld F, Eiffert H, et al. Epidemiology and clinical manifestations of Lyme borreliosis in childhood. A prospective multicentre study with special regard to neuroborreliosis. *Acta Paediatr* 1993;386(Suppl):176.
1038. Oksi J, Kalimo H, Marttila RJ, et al. Inflammatory brain changes in Lyme borreliosis: a report of three patients and review of literature. *Brain* 1996;119:2143–2154.
1039. Sigal LH, Tatum AH. Lyme disease patients' serum contains IgM antibodies to *Borrelia burgdorferi* that cross-react with neuronal antigens. *Neurology* 1988;38:1439–1442.
1040. Szer IS, Taylor E, Steere AC. The long-term course of Lyme arthritis in children. *N Engl J Med* 1991;325:159–163.
1041. Glasscock ME III, et al. Lyme disease. A cause of bilateral facial paralysis. *Arch Otolaryngol* 1985;111:47–49.
1042. Darras BT, Annunziato D, Leggiadro RJ. Lyme disease with neurologic abnormalities. *Pediatr Infect Dis* 1983;2:47–49.
1043. Krejcova H, Bojar M, Jerabek J, et al. Otoneurological symptomatology in Lyme disease. *Adv Otorhinolaryngol* 1988;42:210–212.
1044. Belman AL, Iyer M, Coyle PK, et al. Neurologic manifestations in children with North American Lyme disease. *Neurology* 1993;43:2609–2614.
1045. Jörbeck HJ, Gustafsson PM, Lind HC, et al. Tick-borne *Borrelia*-meningitis in children. An outbreak in the Kolmar area during the summer of 1984. *Acta Paediatr Scand* 1987;76:228–233.
1046. Hansen K, Lebech AM. The clinical and epidemiological profile of Lyme neuroborreliosis in Denmark 1985–90. A prospective study of 187 patients with *Borrelia burgdorferi* specific intrathecal antibody production. *Brain* 1992;115:399–423.
1047. Sterman AB, Nelson S, Barclay P. Demyelinating neuropathy accompanying Lyme disease. *Neurology* 1982;32:1302–1305.
1048. Kan L, Sood SK, Maytal J. Pseudotumor cerebri in Lyme disease: a case report and review of the literature. *Pediatr Neurol* 1998;18:439–441.
1049. Moses JM, Riseberg RS, Mansbach JM. Lyme disease presenting with persistent headache. *Pediatrics* 2003;112:e477–e479.
1050. Ryberg B, Nilsson B, Burgdorfer W, et al. Antibodies to Lyme-disease spirochaete in European lymphocytic meningoencephalitis (Bannwarth's syndrome) [Letter]. *Lancet* 1983;2:519.
1051. Feder HM, Zalneraitis EL, Reik L Jr. Lyme disease: acute focal meningoencephalitis in a child. *Pediatrics* 1988;82:931–934.
1052. Pfister HW, Preac-Mursic V, Wilske B, et al. Catatonic syndrome in acute severe encephalitis due to *Borrelia burgdorferi* infection. *Neurology* 1993;43:433–435.
1053. Eppes SC, Nelson DK, Lewis LL, et al. Characterization of Lyme meningitis and comparison with viral meningitis in children. *Pediatrics* 1999;103:957–960.

1054. Ackermann R, Rehse-Kupper B, Gollmer E, et al. Chronic neurologic manifestations of erythema migrans borreliosis. *Ann N Y Acad Sci* 1988;539:16–23.
1055. Bensch J, Olcen P, Hagberg L. Destructive chronic *Borrelia* meningoencephalitis in a child untreated for 15 years. *Scand J Infect Dis* 1987;19:697–700.
1056. Halperin JJ, Volkman DJ, Wu P. Central nervous system abnormalities in Lyme neuroborreliosis. *Neurology* 1991;41:1571–1582.
1057. Martin R, Martins U, Stricht-Groh V, et al. Persistent intrathecal secretion of oligoclonal, *Borrelia burgdorferi*–specific IgG in chronic meningoradiculomyelitis. *J Neurol* 1988;235:229–233.
1058. Halperin JJ, Luft BJ, Anand AK, et al. Lyme neuroborreliosis: central nervous system manifestations. *Neurology* 1989;39:753–759.
1059. Hirai K, Takemori N, Yanagawa N, et al. *Borrelia burgdorferi* and Shulman syndrome [Letter]. *Lancet* 1992;340:1472.
1060. Hansen K, Lebech AM. The clinical and epidemiological profile of Lyme neuroborreliosis in Denmark 1985–1990. A prospective study of 187 patients with *Borrelia burgdorferi* specific intrathecal antibody. *Brain* 1992;115:399–423.
1061. Albisetti M, Schaer GH, Good M, et al. Diagnostic value of cerebrospinal fluid examination in children with peripheral facial palsy and suspected Lyme borreliosis. *Neurology* 1997;49:817–824.
1062. Belman AL, Coyle PK, Roque C, et al. MRI findings in children infected by *Borrelia burgdorferi*. *Pediatr Neurol* 1992;8:428–431.
1063. Ustymowicz A, Tarasow E, Zajkowska J, et al. Proton MR spectroscopy in neuroborreliosis: a preliminary study. *Neuroradiology* 2004;46:26–30.
1064. Hattingen E, Weidauer S, Kieslich M, et al. MR imaging in neuroborreliosis of the cervical spinal cord. *Eur Radiol* 2004;14:2072–2075.
1065. Dattwyler RJ, Volkman DJ, Luft BJ, et al. Seronegative Lyme disease. Dissociation of specific T- and B-lymphocyte responses to *Borrelia burgdorferi*. *N Engl J Med* 1988;319:1441–1446.
1066. Tumani H, Nölker G, Reiber H. Relevance of cerebrospinal fluid variables for early diagnosis of neuroborreliosis. *Neurology* 1995;45:1663–1670.
1067. Rose CD, Fawceh PT, Singsen BH, et al. Use of Western blot and enzyme-linked immunosorbent assay in the diagnosis of Lyme disease. *Pediatrics* 1991;88:465–470.
1068. Halperin JJ, Heyes MP. Neuroactive kynurenines in Lyme borreliosis. *Neurology* 1992;42:43–45.
1069. Karlssen M, Hammers-Berggen S, Lindquist L, et al. Comparison of intravenous penicillin G and oral doxycycline for treatment of Lyme neuroborreliosis. *Neurology* 1994;44:1203–1207.
1070. American Academy of Pediatrics. Lyme disease. In: Peter G, ed. *1997 Red book: report of the Committee on Infectious Diseases*, 24th ed. Elk Grove Village, IL: Author, 1997: 329–333.
1071. Weber K, Pfister HW. Clinical management of Lyme borreliosis. *Lancet* 1994;343:1016–1017.
1072. Salazar JC, Gerber MA, Goff CW. Long-term outcome of Lyme disease in children given early treatment. *J Pediatr* 1993;122:591–593.
1073. Crisp D, Ashby P. Lyme radiculoneuritis treated with intravenous immunoglobulin. *Neurology* 1996;46:1174–1175.
1074. Benke T, Gasse T, Hittmair-Delazer M, et al. Lyme encephalopathy: long-term neuropsychological deficits years after neuroborreliosis. *Acta Neurol Scand* 1995;91:353–357.
1075. Tager FA, Fallon BA, Keilp J, et al. A controlled study of cognitive deficits in children with chronic Lyme disease. *J Neuropsychiatry Clin Neurosci* 2001;13:500–507.
1076. Vazquez M, Sparrow SS, Shapiro ED. Long-term neuropsychologic and health outcomes of children with facial nerve palsy attributable to Lyme disease. *Pediatrics* 2003;112:e93–e97.
1077. Kisinza WN, McCall PJ, Mitani H, et al. A newly identified tick-borne *Borrelia* species and relapsing fever in Tanzania. *Lancet* 2003;362:1283–1284.
1078. Dworkin MS, Shoemaker PC, Fritz CL, et al. The epidemiology of tick-borne relapsing fever in the United States. *Am J Trop Med Hyg* 2002;66:753–758.
1079. Fritz CL, Bronson LR, Smith CR, et al. Isolation and characterization of *Borrelia hermsii* associated with two foci of tick-borne relapsing fever in California. *J Clin Microbiol* 2004;42:1123–1128.
1080. Southern PM Jr, Sanford JP. Relapsing fever: a clinical and microbiological review. *Medicine* 1969;48:129–149.
1081. Lehtokoski-Lehtiniemi E, Koskiniemi ML. *Mycoplasma pneumoniae* encephalitis: a severe entity in children. *Pediatr Inf Dis J* 1989;8:651–653.
1082. Pellegrini M, O'brien TJ, Hoy J, et al. *Mycoplasma pneumoniae* infection associated with an acute brainstem syndrome. *Acta Neurol Scand* 1996;93:203–206.
1083. Candler PM, Dale RC. Three cases of central nervous system complication associated with *Mycoplasma pneumoniae*. *Pediatr Neurol* 2004;31:133–138.
1084. Socan M, Ravnik I, Bencina D, et al. Neurological symptoms in patients whose cerebrospinal fluid is culture- and/or polymerase chain reaction-positive for *Mycoplasma pneumoniae*. *Clin Infect Dis* 2001;32:e31–e35.
1085. Cherry JD, Hurwitz ES, Welliver RC. *Mycoplasma pneumoniae* infections and exanthems. *J Pediatr* 1975;87:369–373.
1086. Lerer RJ, Kalavsky SM. Central nervous system disease associated with *Mycoplasma pneumoniae* infection: report of five cases and review of literature. *Pediatrics* 1973;52:658–668.
1087. Bruch LA, Jefferson RJ, Pike MG, et al. *Mycoplasma pneumoniae* infection, meningoencephalitis, and hemophagocytosis. *Pediatr Neurol* 2001;25:67–70.
1088. Narita M, Yamada S. Two distinct patterns of central nervous system complications due to *Mycoplasma pneumoniae* infection. *Clin Infect Dis* 2001;33:916.
1089. Bencina D, Dove P, Mueller-Premru M, et al. Intrathecal synthesis of specific antibodies in patients with invasion of the central nervous system by *Mycoplasma pneumoniae*. *Eur J Clin Microbiol Infect Dis* 2000;19:521–530.
1090. Al-Mateen M, Gibbs M, Dietrich R, et al. Encephalitis lethargica-like illness in a girl with mycoplasma infection. *Neurology* 1988;38:1155–1158.
1091. Pongsakdi V, Chiemchanya S, Sirinavin S. Internal carotid artery occlusion associated with *Mycoplasma pneumoniae* infection. *Pediat Neurol* 1992;8:237–239.
1092. Siber GR, Alpert S, Smith AL, et al. Neonatal central nervous system infection due to *Mycoplasma hominis*. *J Pediatr* 1977;90:625–627.
1093. McDonald JC, Moore DL. *Mycoplasma hominis* meningitis in a premature infant. *Pediatr Infect Dis J* 1988;7:795–798.
1094. Gilbert GL, Law F, Macinnes SJ, et al. Chronic *Mycoplasma hominis* infection complicating severe intraventricular hemorrhage, in a premature neonate. *Pediatr Infect Dis J* 1988;7:817–818.
1095. Hulihan JF, Bebin EM, Westmoreland BF. Bilateral periodic lateralized epileptiform discharges in *Mycoplasma* encephalitis. *Pediatr Neurol* 1992;8:292–294.
1096. MacFarlane PI, Miller V. Transverse myelitis associated with *Mycoplasma pneumoniae*. *Arch Dis Child* 1984;59:80–82.
1097. Francis DA, Brown A, Miller DH, et al. MRI appearances of the CNS manifestations of *Mycoplasma pneumoniae*: a report of two cases. *J Neurol* 1988;235:441–443.
1098. Maida E, Kristoferitsch W. Cerebrospinal fluid findings in *Mycoplasma pneumoniae* infections with neurological complications. *Acta Neurol Scand* 1982;65:524–538.
1099. Murray HW, Masur H, Senterflt LB, et al. The protean manifestations of *Mycoplasma pneumoniae* infection in adults. *Am J Med* 1975;58:229–242.
1100. Vikerfors T, Brodin G, Grandien M, et al. Detection of specific IgM antibodies for the diagnosis of *Mycoplasma pneumoniae* infections: a clinical evaluation. *Scand J Infect Dis* 1988;20:601–610.
1101. Narita M, Matsuzono Y, Togashi T, et al. DNA diagnosis of central nervous system infection by *Mycoplasma pneumoniae*. *Pediatrics* 1992;90:250–253.
1102. Fetter BF, Klintworth GK, Hendry WS. *Mycoses of the central nervous system*. Baltimore: Williams & Wilkins, 1967.
1103. Kozinn PJ, Taschdjian CL, Pishvazadeh P, et al. *Candida* meningitis successfully treated with amphotericin B. *N Engl J Med* 1963;268:881–884.

1104. Chesney PJ, Teets KC, Mulvihill JJ, et al. Successful treatment of *Candida* meningitis with amphotericin B and 5-fluorocytosine in combination. *J Pediatr* 1976;89:1017–1019.
1105. Kourtopoulos H, Holm SE. Treatment of *Candida* ventriculitis and septicemia with 5-fluoro-cytosine. Combined peroral and intraventricular administration. *Neuropaediatrie* 1976;7:356–361.
1106. Lunel FMV, Voss A, Kuijper EJ, et al. Detection of the *Candida* antigen mannan in cerebrospinal fluid specimens from patients suspected of having *Candida* meningitis. *J Clin Microbiol* 2004;42:867–870.
1107. Roessmann U, Friede RL. Candidal infection of the brain. *Arch Pathol* 1967;84:495–498.
1108. Zaoutis TE, Greves HM, Lautenbach E, et al. Risk factors for disseminated candidiasis in children with candidemia. *Pediatr Infect Dis J* 2004;23:635–641.
1109. Chesney PJ, Justman RA, Bogdanowicz WM. *Candida* meningitis in newborn infants: a review and report of combined amphotericin B-flucytosine therapy. *Johns Hopkins Med J* 1978;142:155–160.
1110. Como JA, Dismukes WE. Oral azole drugs as systemic antifungal therapy. *N Engl J Med* 1993;330:263–272.
1111. Kovacicova G, Hanzen J, Pisarcikova M, et al. Nosocomial fungemia due to amphotericin B-resistant *Candida* spp. in three pediatric patients after previous neurosurgery for brain tumors. *J Infect Chemother* 2001;7:45–48.
1112. Conant NF. Medical mycology. In: Dubos RJ, Hirsch JG, eds. *Bacterial and mycotic infections of man*. Philadelphia: Lippincott, 1965: 825–885.
1113. Caudill RG, Smith CE, Reinarz JA. Coccidioidal meningitis. A diagnostic challenge. *Am J Med* 1970;49:360–365.
1114. McCullough DC, Harbert JC. Isotope demonstration of CSF pathways. Guide to antifungal therapy in coccidioidal meningitis. *JAMA* 1969;209:558–560.
1115. Wrobel CJ, Meyer S, Johnson RH, et al. MR findings in acute and chronic coccidioidomycosis meningitis. *Am J Neuroradiol* 1992;13:1241–1245.
1116. Wrobel CJ, Chappell ET, Taylor W. Clinical presentation, radiological findings, and treatment results of coccidioidomycosis involving the spine: report on 23 cases. *J Neurosurg Spine* 2001;95:33–39.
1117. Reeves DL. Chronic coccidioidal meningitis. Report of two cases. *J Neurosurg* 1968;28:383–386.
1118. American Academy of Pediatrics. Systemic treatment with amphotericin B. In: Peter G, ed. *1997 Red book: report of the Committee on Infectious Diseases*, 24th ed. Elk Grove Village, IL: Author, 1997: 630–631.
1119. Galgiani JN, Catanzaro A, Cloud GA, et al. Fluconazole therapy for coccidioidal meningitis. The NIAID-Mycosis Study Group. *Ann Int Med* 1993;119:28–35.
1120. Kauffman CA. Role of azoles in antifungal therapy. *Clin Infect Dis* 1996;22(Suppl 2):S148–S153.
1121. Patel R. Antifungal agents. Part I. Amphotericin B preparations and flucytosine. *Mayo Clin Proc* 1998;73:1205–1225.
1122. Galgiani JN, Catanzaro A, Cloud GA, et al. Comparison of oral fluconazole and itraconazole for progressive, nonmeningeal coccidioidomycosis: a randomized, double-blind trial. *Ann Intern Med* 2000;133:676–686.
1123. Tucker RM, Denning DW, Dupont B, et al. Itraconazole therapy for chronic coccidiodal meningitis. *Ann Intern Med* 1990; 112:108–112.
1124. Crum NF, Lederman ER, Stafford CM, et al. Coccidioidomycosis: a descriptive survey of a reemerging disease. Clinical characteristics and current controversies. *Medicine* (Baltimore) 2004;83:149–175.
1125. Connelly MB, Zerella JT. Surgical management of coccidioidomycosis in children. *J Pediatr Surg* 2000;35:1633–1634.
1126. Knapp S, Turnherr M, Dekan G, et al. A case of HIV-associated cerebral histoplasmosis successfully treated with fluconazole. *Eur J Clin Microbiol Infect Dis* 1999;18:658–661.
1127. Cooper RA Jr, Goldstein E. Histoplasmosis of the central nervous system. Report of two cases and review of the literature. *Am J Med* 1963;35:45–57.
1128. Saccente M, McDonnell RW, Baddour LM, et al. Cerebral histoplasmosis in the azole era: report of four cases and review. *South Med J* 2003;96:410–416.
1129. Couch JR, Abdou NI, Sagawa A. *Histoplasma* meningitis with hyperactive suppressor T cells in cerebrospinal fluid. *Neurology* 1978;28:119–123.
1130. Wheat LJ, Batteiger BE, Sathapatayavongs B. *Histoplasma capsulatum* infections of the central nervous system. A clinical review. *Medicine* 1990;69:244–260.
1131. Klein CJ, Dinapoli RP, Temesgen Z, et al. Central nervous system histoplasmosis mimicking a brain tumor: difficulties in diagnosis and treatment. *Mayo Clin Proc* 1999;74:803–807.
1132. Rivera IV, Curless RG, Indacochea FJ, et al. Chronic progressive CNS histoplasmosis presenting in childhood: response to fluconazole therapy. *Pediatr Neurol* 1992;8:151–153.
1133. Haynes RR, Connolly PA, Durkin MM, et al. Antifungal therapy for central nervous system histoplasmosis, using a newly developed intracranial model of infection. *J Infec t Dis* 2002;185:1830–1832.
1134. LeMonte AM, Washum KE, Smedema ML, et al. Amphotericin B combined with itraconazole or fluconazole for treatment of histoplasmosis. *J Infect Dis* 2000;182:545–550.
1135. Gonzalez-Amaro R, Salazar-Gonzalez JF, Baranda L, et al. Natural killer cell-mediated cytotoxicity in cryptococcal meningitis. *Rev Invest Clin* 1991;43:133–138.
1136. Mirza SA, Phelan M, Rimland D, et al. The changing epidemiology of cryptococcosis: an update from population-based active surveillance in 2 large metropolitan areas, 1992–2000. *Clin Infect Dis* 2003;36:789–794.
1137. Husain S, Wagener MM, Singh N. *Cryptococcus neoformans* infection in organ transplant recipients: variables influencing clinical characteristics and outcome. *Emerg Infect Dis* 2001;7:375–381.
1138. Goldman DL, Khine H, Abadi J, et al. Serologic evidence for *Cryptococcus neoformans* infection in early childhood. *Pediatrics* 2001;107:e66.
1139. Shih CC, Chen YC, Chang SC, et al. Cryptococcal meningitis in non-HIV-infected patients. *Q J Med* 2000;93:245–251.
1140. Gumbo T, Kadzirange G, Mielke J, et al. *Cryptococcus neoformans* meningoencephalitis in African children with acquired immunodeficiency syndrome. *Pediatr Infect Dis J* 2002;21:54–56.
1141. Woodall WC III, Bertorini TE, Bakhtian BJ, et al. Spinal arachnoiditis with *Cryptococcus neoformans* in a nonimmunocompromised child. *Pediatr Neurol* 1990;6:206–208.
1142. Gordon MA, Vedder DK. Serologic tests in diagnosis and prognosis of cryptococcosis. *JAMA* 1966;197:961–967.
1143. McIntyre HB. Cryptococcal meningitis. A case successfully treated by cisternal administration of amphotericin B with a review of the recent literature. *Bull Los Angeles Neurol Soc* 1967;32:213–219.
1144. Sarosi GA, Parker JD, Doto IL. Amphotericin B in cryptococcal meningitis: long-term results of treatment. *Ann Intern Med* 1969;71:1079–1087.
1145. Goodman JS, Kaufman L, Koenig MG. Diagnosis of cryptococcal meningitis. Value of immunologic detection of cryptococcal antigen. *N Engl J Med* 1971;285:434–436.
1146. Correa MPSC, Severo LC, Oliveira FM, et al. The spectrum of computerized tomography (CT) findings in central nervous system (CNS) infection due to *Cryptococcus neoformans* var. *gatti* in immunocompetent children. *Rev Inst Med Trop S Paulo* 2002;44:283–287.
1147. Dismukes WE, Cloud G, Gallis HA, et al. Treatment of cryptococcal meningitis with combination amphotericin B and flucytosine for four as compared with six weeks. *N Engl J Med* 1987;317:334–341.
1148. American Academy of Pediatrics. In Peter G, ed. *1997 Red book: report of the Committee on Infectious Diseases*, 24th ed. Elk Grove Village, IL: Author, 1997: 184–185.
1149. Leake HA, Appleyard MN, Hartley JP. Successful treatment of resistant cryptococcal meningitis with amphotericin B lipid emulsion after neurotoxicity with conventional intravenous amphotericin B. *J Infect* 1994;28:319–322.
1150. Laing RB, Milne LJ, Leen CL, et al. Anaphylactic reactions to liposomal amphotericin [Letter]. *Lancet* 1994;344:682.

1151. Saag MS, Powderly WG, Cloud GA, et al. Comparison of amphotericin B with fluconazole in the treatment of acute AIDS-associated cryptococcal meningitis. *N Engl J Med* 1992;326:83–89.
1152. Pappas PG, Perfect JR, Cloud GA, et al. Cryptococcosis in human immunodeficiency virus-negative patients in the era of effective azole therapy. *Clin Infect Dis* 2001;33:690–699.
1153. Barter AP, Falconer MA. Actinomycosis of the brain. *Guy Hosp Rep* 1955;104:135–145.
1154. Iyer S, Dodge PR, Adams RD. Two cases of *Aspergillus* infection of the central nervous system. *J Neurol Neurosurg Psychiatry* 1952;15:152–163.
1155. Mukoyama M, Gimple AB, Poser CM. Aspergillosis of the central nervous system. Report of a brain abscess due to *A. fumigatus* and a review of the literature. *Neurology* 1969;19:967–974.
1156. Koh S, Ross LA, Gilles FH, et al. Myelopathy resulting from invasive aspergillosis. *Pediatr Neurol* 1998;19:135–138.
1157. Gonyea EF. The spectrum of primary blastomycotic meningitis: a review of central nervous system blastomycosis. *Ann Neurol* 1978;3:26–39.
1158. Papadatos C, Pavlatou M, Alexiou D. *Cephalosporium* meningitis. *Pediatrics* 1969;44:749–751.
1159. Landau JW, Newcomer VD. Acute cerebral phycomycosis (mucormycosis). Report of a pediatric patient successfully treated with amphotericin B and cycloheximide and review of the pertinent literature. *J Pediatr* 1962;61:363–385.
1160. Blodi FC, Hannah FT, Wadsworth JA. Lethal orbitocerebral phycomycosis in otherwise healthy children. *Am J Ophthalmol* 1969;67:698–705.
1161. Smego RA Jr, Moeller MB, Gallis HA. Trimethoprimsulfamethoxazole therapy for *Nocardia infections*. *Arch Intern Med* 1983;143:711–718.
1162. Ballenger CN Jr, Goldring D. Nocardiosis in childhood. *J Pediatr* 1957;50:145–169.
1163. Lope ES, Gutierrez DC. *Nocardia asteroides* primary cerebral abscess and secondary meningitis. *Acta Neurochir* 1977;37:139–145.
1164. Silpapojakul K, Varachit B, Silpapojakul K. Paediatric scrub typhus in Thailand: a study of 73 confirmed cases. *Trans R Soc Trop Med Hyg* 2004;98:354–359.
1165. Watt G, Parola P. Scrub typhus and tropical rickettsioses. *Curr Opin Infect Dis* 2003;16:429–436.
1166. Zavala-Velazquez JE, Ruiz-Sosa JA, Sanchez-Elias RA, et al. *Rickettsia felis* rickettsiosis in Yucatan. *Lancet* 2000;356:1079–1080.
1167. Abrahamian FM. Consequences of delayed diagnosis of Rocky Mountain spotted fever in children—West Virginia, Michigan, Tennessee, and Oklahoma, May-July 2000. *Ann Emerg Med* 2001;37:537–540.
1168. Treadwell TA, Holman RC, Clarke MJ, et al. Rocky Mountain spotted fever in the United States, 1993–1996. *Am J Trop Med Hyg* 2000;63:21–26.
1169. Spach DH, Liles WC, Campbell GL, et al. Tick-borne diseases in the United States. *N Engl J Med* 1993;329:936–947.
1170. Miller JQ, Price TR. The nervous system in Rocky Mountain fever. *Neurology* 1972;22:561–566.
1171. Horney LF, Walker DH. Meningoencephalitis as a major manifestation of Rocky Mountain spotted fever. *South Med J* 1988;81:915–918.
1172. Bell WE, Lascari AD. Rocky Mountain spotted fever. Neurological symptoms in the acute phase. *Neurology* 1970;20:841–847.
1173. Hornaday CA, Kernodle DS, Curry WA. Neurogenic bladder in Rocky Mountain spotted fever. *Arch Intern Med* 1983;143:365.
1174. Miller JQ, Price TR. Involvement of the brain in Rocky Mountain spotted fever. *South Med J* 1972;65:437–439.
1175. Raab EL, Leopold IH, Hodes HL. Retinopathy in Rocky Mountain spotted fever. *Am J Ophthalmol* 1969;68:42–46.
1176. Rosenblum MJ, Masland RL, Harrell GT. Residual effects of rickettsial disease on the central nervous system. Results of neurologic examinations and electroencephalograms following Rocky Mountain spotted fever. *Arch Intern Med* 1952;90:444–455.
1177. O'Reilly M, Paddock C, Elchos B, et al. Physician knowledge of the diagnosis amd management of Rocky Mountain spotted fever: Mississippi, 2002. *Ann N Y Acad Sci* 2003;990:295–301.
1178. Wright L. Intellectual sequelae of Rocky Mountain spotted fever. *J Abnorm Psychol* 1972;80:315–316.
1179. Centers for Disease Control and Prevention (CDC). Fatal cases of Rocky Mountain spotted fever in family clusters—three states, 2003. *MMWR Morb Mortal Wkly Rep* 2004;53(19):407–410.
1180. Haynes RE, Sanders DY, Cramblett HG. Rocky Mountain spotted fever in children. *J Pediatr* 1970;76:685–693.
1181. Marshall GS, Stout GG, Jacobs RF, et al. Antibodies reactive to *Rickettsia rickettsii* among children living in the southeast and south central regions of the United States. *Arch Pediatr Adolesc Med* 2003;157:443–448.
1182. American Academy of Pediatrics. Rocky mountain spotted fever. In: Peter G, ed. *1997 Red book: report of the Committee on Infectious Diseases*, 24th ed. Elk Grove Village, IL: Author, 1997: 452–454.
1183. Noad KB, Haymaker W. Neurological features of tsutsugamushi fever with special reference to deafness. *Brain* 1953;76:113–131.
1184. Herman E. Neurological syndromes in typhus fever. *J Nerv Ment Dis* 1949;109:25–36.
1185. Watt G, Chouriyagune C, Ruangweerayud R, et al. Scrub typhus infections poorly responsive to antibiotics in northern Thailand. *Lancet* 1996;348:86–89.
1186. Maltezou HC, Raoult D. Q fever in children. *Lancet Infect Dis* 2002;2:686–691.
1187. Case records of the Massachusetts General Hospital. Case 38-1996. *N Engl J Med* 1996;335:1829–1834.
1188. Most H. Treatment of common parasitic infections of man encountered in the United States. *N Engl J Med* 1972;287:495–498, 698–702.
1189. Brown WJ. Cysticercosis. In: Brown WJ, Voge M, eds. *Neuropathology of parasitic infections*. New York: Oxford University Press, 1982: 108.
1190. Kramer LD, Locke GE, Byrd SE, et al. Cerebral cysticercosis: documentation of natural history with CT. *Radiology* 1989;171:459–462.
1191. Rosenfeld E. Neurocysticercosis update. *Pediatr Infect Dis J* 2003;22:181–182.
1192. Singhi P, Singhi S. Neurocysticercosis in children. *J Child Neurol* 2004;19:482–492.
1193. Virmani V, Roy S, Kamala G. Periodic lateralised epileptiform discharges in a case of diffuse cerebral cysticercosis. *Neuropaediatrie* 1977;8:196–203.
1194. Kalra V, Sethi A. Childhood neurocysticercosis—epidemiology, diagnosis and course. *Acta Paediatr Jpn* 1992;34:365–370.
1195. Lopez-Hernandez A, Garaizar C. Childhood cerebral cysticercosis: clinical features and computed tomographic findings in 89 Mexican children. *Can J Neurol Sci* 1982;9:401–407.
1196. Thompson AJG. Neurocysticercosis: experience at the teaching hospitals of the University of Cape Town. *S Afr Med J* 1993;83:332–334.
1197. Zhu L, Weng X, Shi Y, et al. CSF-VP shunt placement and albendazole therapy for cerebral cysticercosis. *Chin Med J* 2002;115(6):936–938.
1198. Garg RS. Neurocysticercosis. *Postgrad Med J* 1998;74:321–326.
1199. Liu LX, Weller PF. Antiparasitic drugs. *N Engl J Med* 1996; 334:1178–1184.
1200. Bale Jr JF. Cysticercosis. *Curr Treat Options Neurol* 2000;2:355–360.
1201. Mitchell WG, Crawford TO. Intraparenchymal cerebral cysticercosis in children: diagnosis and treatment. *Pediatrics* 1988;82:76–82.
1202. Rajshekhar V. Albendazole therapy for persistent, solitary cysticercosis granulomas in patients with seizures. *Neurology* 1993;43:1238–1240.
1203. Dalessio DJ, Wolff HG. *Trichinella spiralis* infection of the central nervous system. Report of a case and review of the literature. *Arch Neurol* 1961;4:407–417.
1204. Tatatuto AL, Venturiello SM. Trichinosis. *Brain Pathol* 1997;7:663–672.
1205. Kramer MD, Aita JF. Trichinosis with central nervous system involvement. A case report and review of the literature. *Neurology* 1972;22:485–491.
1206. Lopez-Lozano JJ, Garcia-Merino JA, Liano H. Bilateral facial

paralysis secondary to trichinosis. *Acta Neurol Scand* 1988; 78:194–197.
1207. Evans RW, Pattern BM. Trichinosis associated with superior sagittal sinus thrombosis. *Ann Neurol* 1982;11:216–217.
1208. Gay T, Pankey GA, Beckman EN, et al. Fatal CNS trichinosis. *JAMA* 1982;127:1024–1025.
1209. American Academy of Pediatrics. Trichinosis (*Trichinella spiralis*). In: Peter G, ed. *1997 red Book: report of the Committee on Infectious Diseases*, 24th ed. Elk Grove Village, IL: Author, 1997: 535–536.
1210. Zucker JR, Campbell CC. Malaria: principles of prevention and treatment. *Infect Dis Clin North Am* 1993;7:547–567.
1211. Phillips RE, Solomon T. Cerebral malaria in children. *Lancet* 1990;336:1355–1360.
1212. Warrell DA. Cerebral malaria. *Q J Med* 1989;71:369–371.
1213. Brewster DR, Kwiatkowski D, White NJ. Neurological sequelae of cerebral malaria in children. *Lancet* 1990;336:1039–1043.
1214. van Hensbroek MB, Palmer A, Jaffar S, et al. Residual neurologic sequelae after childhood cerebral malaria. *J Pediatr* 1997;131:125–129.
1215. Turner G. Cerebral malaria. *Brain Pathol* 1997;7:569–582.
1216. MacPherson GG, Warrell MJ, White NJ, et al. Human cerebral malaria. A quantitative ultrastructural analysis of parasitized erythrocyte sequestration. *Am J Pathol* 1985;119:385–401.
1217. Aikawa M, Iseki M, Barnwell JW, et al. The pathology of human cerebral malaria. *Am J Trop Hyg* 1990;43:30–37.
1218. Nakamura K, Hasler T, Morehead K, et al. *Plasmodium falciparum*-infected erythrocyte receptor(s) for CD36 and thrombospondin are restricted to knobs on the erythrocyte surface. *J Histochem Cytochem* 1992;40:1419–1422.
1219. Newbold C, Warn P, Black G, et al. Receptor-specific adhesion and clinical disease in *Plasmodium falciparum*. *Am J Trop Med Hyg* 1997;57:389–398.
1220. Fernandez-Reyes D, Craig AG, Kyes SA, et al. A high frequency African coding polymorphism, in the N-terminal domain of ICAM-1 predisposing to cerebral malaria in Kenya. *Hum Mol Genet* 1997;6:1357–1360.
1221. Urban BC, et al. *Plasmodium falciparum*–infected erythrocytes modulate the maturation of dendritic cells. *Nature* 1999;400:73–77.
1222. Johnson JK, Swerlick RA, Grady KK, et al. Cytoadherence of *Plasmodium falciparum*–infected erythrocytes to microvascular endothelium is regulatable by cytokines and phorbol ester. *J Infect Dis* 1993;167:698–703.
1223. Clark IA, Chaudhri G, Cowden WB. Roles of tumor necrosis factor in the illness and pathology of malaria. *Trans R Soc Trop Med Hyg* 1989;83:436–440.
1224. Clark IA, Rockett KA, Cowden WB. Possible central role of nitric oxide in conditions clinically similar to cerebral malaria. *Lancet* 1992;340:894–896.
1225. Kwiatkowski D, Hill AV, Sambou I, et al. TNF concentration in fatal malaria, non-fatal cerebral, and uncomplicated *Plasmodium falciparum* malaria. *Lancet* 1990;336:1201–1204.
1226. Grau GE, Taylor TE, Molyneux ME, et al. Tumor necrosis factor and disease severity in children with falciparum malaria. *N Engl J Med* 1989;320:1586–1591.
1227. Grau GE, Piguet PF, Vassalli P, et al. Tumor necrosis factor and other cytokines in cerebral malaria. Experimental and clinical data. *Immunol Rev* 1989;112:49–70.
1228. Kwiatkowski D, Molyneux ME, Stephens S, et al. Anti-TNF therapy inhibits fever in cerebral malaria. *Q J Med* 1993;86:91–98.
1229. Molyneux ME, Taylor TE, Wirima JJ, et al. Clinical features and prognostic indicators in paediatric cerebral malaria: a study of 131 comatose Malawian children. *Q J Med* 1989:71:441–459.
1230. Jaffar S, van Hensbroek MB, Palmer A, et al. Predictors of a fatal outcome following childhood cerebral malaria. *Am J Trop Med Hyg* 1997;57:20–24.
1231. Maitland K, Marsh K. Pathophysiology of severe malaria in children. *Acta Tropica* 2004;90:131–140.
1232. Taylor TE, Borgstein A, Molyneux ME. Acid-base status in paediatric *Plasmodium falciparum* malaria. *Q J Med* 1993;86:99–109.
1233. Burgner D, Xu W, Rockett K, et al. Inducible nitric oxide synthase polymorphism and fatal cerebral malaria. *Lancet* 1998; 232:1193–1194.
1234. Looareesuwan S, Wilairatana P, Krishna S, et al. Magnetic resonance imaging of the brain in patients with cerebral malaria. *Clin Infect Dis* 1995;21:300–309.
1235. Miller LH, Good MF, Milon G. Malaria pathogenesis. *Science* 1994;264:1878–1883.
1236. Wright PW, Avery WG, Ardill WD, et al. Initial clinical assessment of the comatose patient: cerebral malaria vs. meningitis. *Pediatr Infect Dis J* 1993;12:37–41.
1237. White NJ, Krishna S, Looareesuwan S. Encephalitis, not cerebral malaria, is likely cause of coma with negative blood smears. *J Infect Dis* 1992;166:1195–1196.
1238. Newton CRJC, Warrell DA. Neurological manifestations of falciparum malaria. *Ann Neurol* 1998;43:695–702.
1239. Lewallen S, Taylor TE, Molyneux ME, et al. Ocular fundus findings in Malawian children with cerebral malaria. *Ophthalmology* 1993;100:857–861.
1240. Stauffer W, Fischer PR. Diagnosis and treatment of malaria in children. *Clin Infect Dis* 2003;37:1340–1348.
1241. White NJ, Warrell DA, Chanthavanich P, et al. Severe hypoglycemia and hyperinsulinemia in falciparum malaria. *N Engl J Med* 1983;309:61–66.
1242. White NJ, Looareesuwan S, Warrell DA, et al. Quinine loading dose in cerebral malaria. *Am J Trop Med Hyg* 1983;332:1–5.
1243. Phillips RE, Warrell DA, White NJ, et al. Intravenous quinidine for the treatment of severe falciparum malaria. Clinical and pharmacokinetic studies. *N Engl J Med* 1985;312:1273–1278.
1244. Shwe T, Myint PT, Myint W, et al. Clinical studies on treatment of cerebral malaria with artemether and mefloquine. *Trans R Soc Trop Med Hyg* 1989;83:489.
1245. Taylor TE, Wills BA, Kazembe P, et al. Rapid coma resolution with artemether in Malawian children with cerebral malaria. *Lancet* 1993;341:661–662.
1246. Van Hensbroek MB, Onyiorah E, Jaffar S. A trial of artemether or quinine in children with cerebral malaria. *N Engl J Med* 1996;335:69–75.
1247. White NJ, Nosten F, Looareesuwan S, et al. Averting a malaria disaster. *Lancet* 1999;353:1965–1967.
1248. White NJ. The treatment of malaria. *N Engl J Med* 1996;335:800–806.
1249. Moyou-Somo R, Tietche F, Ondoa M, et al. Clinical trial of beta-arteether versus quinine for the treatment of cerebral malaria in children in Yaounde, Cameroon. *Am J Trop Med Hyg* 2001;64:229–232.
1250. Goka BQ, Adabayeri V, Ofori-Adjei E, et al. Comparison of chloroquine with artesunate in the treatment of cerebral malaria in Ghanaian children. *J Trop Pediatr* 2001;47:165–169.
1251. Thuma PE, Bhat GJ, Mabeza GF, et al. A randomized controlled trial of artemotil (beta-arteether) in Zambian children with cerebral malaria. *Am J Trop Med Hyg* 2000;62:524–529.
1252. Satti GM, Elhassan SH, Ibrahim SA. The efficacy of artemether versus quinine in the treatment of cerebral malaria. *J Egypt Soc Parasitol* 2002;32:611–623.
1253. Huda SN, Shahab T, Ali SM, et al. A comparative clinical trial of artemether and quinine in children with severe malaria. *Indian Pediatr* 2003;40:939–945.
1254. Medana IM, Day NP, Hien TT, et al. Axonal injury in cerebral malaria. *Am J Pathol* 2002;160:655–666.
1255. Gordeuk V, Thuma P, Brittenham G, et al. Effect of iron chelation therapy on recovery from deep coma in children with cerebral malaria. *N Engl J Med* 1992;327:1473–1477.
1256. Brandts CH, Ndjave M, Grahinger W, et al. Effect of paracetamol on parasite clearance time in *Plasmodium falciparum* malaria. *Lancet* 1997;350:704–709.
1257. Lyke KE, Diallo DA, Dicko A, et al. Association of intraleukocytic *Plasmodium falciparum* malaria pigment with disease severity, clinical manifestations, and prognosis in severe malaria. *Am J Trop Med Hyg* 2003;69:253–259.
1258. Ala-Odera VM, Snow RW, Newton CRJC. The burden of the neurocognitive impairment associated with *Plasmodium falciparum* malaria in sub-Saharan Africa. *Am J Trop Med Hyg* 2004;71: 64–70.

1259. Carter JA, Neville BG, White S, et al. Increased prevalence of epilepsy associated with severe falciparum malaria in children. *Epilepsia* 2004;45:978–981.
1260. Mai NTH, et al. Post-malaria neurological syndrome. *Lancet* 1996;348:917–921.
1261. Lell B, Luckner D, Ndjave M, et al. Randomised placebo-controlled study of atovaquone plus proguanil for malaria prophylaxis in children. *Lancet* 1998;351:709–713.
1262. Power J. Sleeping sickness research and control. *TDR News* 1989: 28:3.
1263. Kuzoe FA. Current knowledge on epidemiology and control of sleeping sickness. *Ann Soc Belg Med Trop* 1989;69:217–220.
1264. Hajduk SL, Englund PT, Smith DH. African trypanosomiasis. In: Warren KS, Mahmoud AAF, eds. *African trypanosomiasis*. New York: McGraw-Hill, 1990: 268–281.
1265. Mhlanga JD, Bentivoglio M, Kristensson K. Neurobiology of cerebral malaria and African sleeping sickness. *Brain Res Bull* 1997;44:579–589.
1266. Bentivoglio M, Grassi-Zucconi G, Kristensson K, et al. *Trypanosoma brucei* and the nervous system. *Trends Neurosci* 1994;17:325–329.
1267. Poltera AA, Owor R, Cox JN. Pathological aspects of human African trypanosomiasis in Uganda. A postmortem survey of 14 cases. *Virchows Arch* 1976;373:249–265.
1268. Adams JH, Hallen L, Boa FY. African trypanosomiasis: a study of 16 fatal cases with some observations on acute reactive arsenical encephalopathy. *Neuropathol Appl Neurobiol* 1986;12:81–94.
1269. Asongonyi T, Lando G, Ngu JL. Serum antibodies against human brain myelin proteins in Gambian trypanosomiasis. *Ann Soc Beg Med Trop* 1989;69:213–221.
1270. Poltera AA. Immunopathological and chemotherapeutic studies in experimental trypanosomiasis with special reference to the heart and brain. *Trans R Trop Med Hyg* 1980;74:706–715.
1271. Wellde BT, Chumo DA, Hockmeyer WT. Sleeping sickness in the Lambwe Valley in 1978. *Ann Trop Med Parasitol* 1989;83: 21–27.
1272. Lambo TA. Neuropsychiatric syndromes associated with human trypanosomiasis in tropical Africa. *Acta Psychiatrica Scand* 1966;42:474–484.
1273. Calwell HG. The pathology of the brain in Rhodesian trypanosomiasis. *Trans R Soc Trop Med Hyg* 1937;30:611–624.
1274. Van Meirvenne N, Le Ray D. Diagnosis of African and American trypanosomiasis. *Br Med Bull* 1985;41:156–161.
1275. Lejon V, Reiber H, Legros D, et al. Intrathecal immune response pattern for improved diagnosis of central nervous system involvement in trypanosomiasis. *J Infect Dis* 2003;187:1475–1483.
1276. Gutteridge WE. Trypanosomiasis: existing chemotherapy and limitations. *Br Med Bull* 1985;41:162–168.
1277. Arroz JO. Melarsoprol and reactive encephalopathy in *Trypanosoma brucei* rhodesiense infection. *Trans R Soc Trop Med Hyg* 1987;81:192.
1278. McCann PP, Bitoniti AJ, Bacchi CJ. Use of difluoromethylornithine (DFMO, eflornithine) for late stage trypanosomiasis. *Trans R Soc Trop Med Hyg* 1987;81:701–702.
1279. Pitella JEH. Brain involvement in the chronic cardiac form of Chagas disease. *J Trop Med Hyg* 1985;88:313–317.
1280. Cegielski JP, Durack DT. Protozoal infections of the central nervous system. In: Scheld WM, Whitley RJ, Durack DT, eds. *Infections of the central nervous system*. New York: Raven Press, 1991: 767–800.
1281. Leiguarda R, Roncoroni A, Taratuto AI. Acute CNS infection by *trypanosoma cruzi* in immunosuppressed patients. *Neurology* 1990;40:850–851.
1282. Carrea R, Dowling E Jr, Guevara JA. Surgical treatment of hydatid cysts of the central nervous system in the pediatric age (Dowling's technique). *Childs Brain* 1975;1:4–21.
1283. Boles DM. Cerebral echinococciasis. *Surg Neurol* 1981;16:280–282.
1284. Radford AJ. Hydatid disease. In: Weatherall DJ, Ledingham JGG, Warrell DA, eds. *Oxford textbook of medicine*, 2nd ed. Oxford: Oxford University Press, 1988: 561–565.
1285. Banerjee AK, Bhatnagar RK, Bhusnurmath SR. Secondary cerebral amoebiasis. *Trop Geogr Med* 1993;35:333–336.
1286. Cegielski JP, Durack DT. Protozoal infections of the central nervous system. In: Scheld WM, Whitley RJ, Durack DT, eds. *Infections of the central nervous system*. New York: Raven Press, 1991: 767–800.
1287. Turgut M. Hydatidosis of central nervous system and its coverings in the pediatric and adolescent age groups in Turkey during the last century: a critical review of 137 cases. *Childs Nerv Syst* 2002;18:670–683.
1288. Tuzun M, Altinors N, Arda IS, et al. Cerebral hydatid disease: CT and MR findings. *J Clin Imaging* 2002;26:353–357.
1289. Becker GL, Knep S, Lance KP. Amoebic abscess of the brain. *Neurosurgery* 1980;6:192–194.
1290. Barnett ND, Kaplan AM, Hopkin RJ, et al. Primary amoebic meningoencephalitis with *Naegleria fowleri*: clinical review. *Pediatr Neurol* 1996;15:230–234.
1291. Visuesuara GS, Callaway CS. Light and electron microscopic observation on the pathogenesis of *Naeglaria fowleri* in mouse brain and tissue culture. *J Protozool* 1990;21:239–250.
1292. Thong YH, Ferrante A. Migration patterns of pathogenic and nonpathogenic *Naegleria* spp. *Infect Immun* 1986;51:177–180.
1293. Rutherford GS. Amoebic meningo-encephalitis due to free living amoeba. *S Afr Med J* 1986;69:52–55.
1294. Kilvington S, Beeching J. Identification and epidemiological typing of *Naegleria fowleri* with DNA probes. *Appl Environ Microbiol* 1995;61:2071–2078.
1295. Brown RL. Successful treatment of primary amoebic meningoencephalitis. *Arch Intern Med* 1991;151:1201–1202.
1296. Slater CA, Sickel JZ, Visvesvara GS, et al. Brief report: successful treatment of disseminated acanthamoeba infection in an immunocompromised patient. *N Engl J Med* 1994;331:85–87.
1297. Koo J, Dien F, Kliks MM. Angiostrongylus eosinophilic meningitis. *Rev Infect Dis* 1988;10:1155–1162.
1298. Chye SM, Lin SR, Chen YL, et al. Immuno-PCR for detection of antigen to *Angiostrongylus cantonensis* circulating fifth-stage worms. *Clin Chem* 2004;50:51–57.
1299. Kliks MM, Kroenke K, Handman JM. Eosinophilic radiculomyelo-encephalitis. *J Trop Med Hyg* 1982;31:1114–1122.
1300. Lowichik A, Ruff AJ. Parasitic infections of the central nervous system in children. Part II: disseminated infections. *J Child Neurol* 1995;10:77–87.
1301. Diaz Camacho SP, Zazueta Ramos M, Ponce Torrecillas E, et al. Clinical manifestations and immunodiagnosis of gnathostomiasis in Culiacan, Mexico. *Am J Trop Med Hyg* 1998;59:908–915.
1302. Chitanondh H, Rosen L. Fatal eosinophilic encephalomyelitis caused by the nematode *Gnathostoma spinigerum*. *Am J Trop Med Hyg* 1967;16:638–645.
1303. Schmutzhand E, Boorgind P, Veijjava A. Eosinophilic meningitis in Thailand caused by CNS invasion of *Gnathostoma spinigerum* and *Angiostrongylus cantonensis*. *J Neurol Neurosurg Psychiatry* 1988;51:80–87.
1304. Sawanyawisuth K, Tiamkao S, Kanpittaya J, et al. MR imaging findings in cerebrospinal gnathostomiasis. *Am J Neuroradiol* 2004;25:446–449.
1305. Hill IR, Denham DA, Scholtz CL. *Toxocara canis* larvae in the brain of a British child. *Trans R Soc Trop Med Hyg* 1985;79:351–354.
1306. Mikhael NZ, Montpetit UJA, Orizaga M. *Toxocara canis* infestation with encephalitis. *Can J Neurol Sci* 1974;1:114–120.
1307. Moreira-Silva SF, Rodrigues MG, Pimenta JL, et al. Toxocariasis of the central nervous system: with report of two cases. *Rev Soc Bras Med Trop* 2004;37:169–174.
1308. Vidal JE, Sztajnbok J, Seguro AC. Eosinophilic meningoencephalitis due to *Toxocara canis*: case report and review of the literature. *Am J Trop Med Hyg* 2003;69:341–343.
1309. Glickman L, Cypress RH, Crumrine PK, et al. *Toxocara* infection and epilepsy in children. *J Pediatr* 1979;94:75–78.
1310. Bachli H, Minet JC, Gratzl O. Cerebral toxocariasis: a possible cause of epileptic seizure in children. *Childs Nerv Syst* 2004;20:468–472.
1311. Pitella JE. Neuroschistosomiasis. *Brain Pathol* 1997;7:649–662.
1312. Scrimgeour EM, Gajdusek DC. Involvement of the central nervous system in *Schistosoma mansoni* and *S. haematobium* infection. *Brain* 1985;108:1023–1038.

1313. Anonymous. Acute schistosomiasis with transverse myelitis in American students returning from Kenya. *MMWR Morb Mortal Wkly Rep* 1984;33:445–447.
1314. Boyce TG. Acute transverse myelitis in a 6-year-old girl with schistosomiasis. *Pediatr Infect Dis J* 1990;9:279–284.
1315. Pitella JE, Lana-Peixoto MA. Brain involvement in hepatosplenic *Schistosomiasis mansoni*. *Brain* 1981;104:621–632.
1316. Bennett G, Provenzale JM. Schistosomal myelitis: finding at MR imaging. *Eur J Radiol* 1998;27:268–270.
1317. Ferrari TC, Moreira PR, Oliveira RC, et al. The value of an enzyme-linked immunosorbent assay for the diagnosis of *Schistosomiasis mansoni* myeloradiculopathy. *Trans R Soc Trop Med Hyg* 1995;89:496–500.
1318. Watt E, et al. Praziquantel in the treatment of cerebral schistosomiasis. *Lancet* 1986;2:529–532.
1319. Jankovic D, Wynn TA, Kullberg MC, et al. Optimal vaccination against *Schistosoma mansoni* requires the induction of both B cell- and IFN-gamma-dependent effector mechanisms. *J Immunol* 1999;162:345–351.
1320. La Flamme AC, Ruddenklau K, Backstrom BT. Schistosomiasis decreases central nervous system inflammation and alters the progression of experimental autoimmune encephalomyelitis. *Infect Immun* 2003;71:4996–5004.
1321. La Flamme AC, Canagasabey K, Harvie M, et al. Schistosomiasis protects against multiple sclerosis. Mem Inst Oswaldo Cruz. (Rio de Janeiro) 2004;99:33–36.
1322. Higashi K, Aoki H, Tatebayashi K, et al. Cerebral paragonimiasis. *J Neurosurg* 1971;34:515–527.
1323. Oh SJ. Spinal paragonimiasis. *J Neurol Sci* 1968;6:125–140.
1324. Oh SJ. Ophthalmological signs in cerebral paragonimiasis. *Trop Geogr Med* 1968;20:13–20.
1325. Chang KH, Han MH. MRI of CNS parasitic diseases. *J Magn Reson Imaging* 1998;8:297–307.
1326. Newman LS, Rose CS, Maier LA. Sarcoidosis. *N Engl J Med* 1997;336:1224–1234.
1327. Baumann RJ, Robertson Jr WC. Neurosarcoid presents differently in children than in adults. *Pediatrics* 2003;112:e480–e486.
1328. Johns CJ, Scott PP, Schonfeld SA. Sarcoidosis. *Annu Rev Med* 1989;40:353–371.
1329. Jefferson M. Sarcoidosis of the nervous system. *Brain* 1957;80:540–556.
1330. Symonds C. Recurrent multiple cranial nerve palsies. *J Neurol Neurosurg Psychiatry* 1958;21:95–100.
1331. Heerfordt CF. Über eine, "Febris uveoparotidea sub chronica" an der Glandula parotis und der Uvea des Auges lokalisiert und häufig mit Paresen cerebrospinaler Nerven kompliziert. *Arch Ophthalmol* (Leipzig) 1889;70:254–273.
1332. McGovern JP, Merritt DH. Sarcoidosis in childhood. *Adv Pediatr* 1956;8:97–135.
1333. Rubinstein I, Hiss J, Baum GL. Intramedullary spinal cord sarcoidosis. *Surg Neurol* 1984;21:272–274.
1334. Kinnman J, Link H. Intrathecal production of oligoclonal IgM and IgG in CNS sarcoidosis. *Acta Neurol Scand* 1984;69:97–106.
1335. Borucki SJ, Nguyen BV, Ladoulis CT, et al. Cerebrospinal fluid immunoglobulin abnormalities in neurosarcoidosis. *Arch Neurol* 1989;46:270–273.
1336. Koné-Paut I, Portas M, Wechsler B, et al. The pitfall of silent neurosarcoidosis. *Pediatr Neurol* 1999;20:215–218.
1337. Miller DH, Kendall BE, Barter S, et al. Magnetic resonance imaging in central nervous system sarcoidosis. *Neurology* 1988;38:378–383.
1338. Scott TF. Neurosarcoidosis: progress and clinical aspects. *Neurology* 1993;43:8–12.
1339. Reye RD, Morgan G, Baral J. Encephalopathy and fatty degeneration of the viscera. A disease entity in childhood. *Lancet* 1963;2:749–752.
1340. Pollack JD, ed. *Reye's syndrome*. New York: Grune and Stratton, 1975.
1341. Hardie RM, Newton LH, Bruce JC, et al. The changing clinical pattern of Reye's syndrome 1982–1990. *Arch Dis Child* 1996;74:400–405.
1342. Jenkins R, Dvorak A, Patrick J. Encephalopathy and fatty degeneration of the viscera associated with chickenpox. *Pediatrics* 1967;39:769–771.
1343. Casteels-Van Daele M, Van Geet C, Wouters C, et al. Reye syndrome revisited: a descriptive term covering a group of heterogenous disorders. *Eur J Pediatr* 2000;159:641–648.
1344. Kurup RK, Kurup PA. The isoprenoid pathway and the pathogenesis of Reye's syndrome. *Pediatr Pathol Mol Med* 2003;22:423–434.
1345. Powell HC, Rosenberg RN, McKellar B. Reye's syndrome: isolation of parainfluenza virus. Report of three cases. *Arch Neurol* 1973;29:135–139.
1346. Olson LC, Bourgeois CH Jr., Cotton RB, et al. Encephalopathy and fatty degeneration of the viscera in northeastern Thailand. Clinical syndrome and epidemiology. *Pediatrics* 1971;47:707–716.
1347. Editorial. Reye's syndrome and aspirin. Epidemiological associations and inborn errors of metabolism. *Lancet* 1987;2:429–431.
1348. Partin JC, Schubert WK, Partin JS. Mitochondrial ultrastructure in Reye's syndrome. *N Engl J Med* 1971;285:1339–1343.
1349. Lovejoy FH Jr., Smith AL, Bresnan MJ, et al. Clinical staging in Reye's syndrome. *Am J Dis Child* 1974;128:36–41.
1350. Aoki Y, Lombroso CT. Prognostic value of electroencephalography in Reye's syndrome. *Neurology* 1973;23:333–343.
1351. Ey JL, Smith SM, Fulginiti VA. Varicella hepatitis without neurologic symptoms or findings. *Pediatrics* 1981;67:285–287.
1352. Venes JL, Shaywitz BA, Spencer DD. Management of severe cerebral edema in the metabolic encephalopathy of Reye-Johnson syndrome. *J Neurosurg* 1978;48:903–915.
1353. Brunner RL, O'Grady DJ, Partin JC, et al. Neuropsychologic consequences of Reye's syndrome. *J Pediatr* 1979;95:706–711.
1354. Benjamin PY, Levinsohn M, Drotar D, et al. Intellectual and emotional sequelae of Reye's syndrome. *Crit Care Med* 1982;10:583–587.
1355. Reitman MA, Casper J, Coplan J, et al. Motor disorders of voice and speech in Reye's syndrome survivors. *Am J Dis Child* 1984;138:1129–1131.
1356. Glasgow JFT, Middleton B. Reye syndrome—insights on causation and prognosis. *Arch Dis Child* 2001;85:351–353.
1357. Levin M, Hjelm M, Kay JD, et al. Haemorrhagic shock and encephalopathy: a new syndrome with a high mortality in young children. *Lancet* 1983;2:64–67.
1358. Whittington LK, Roscelli JD, Parry WH. Hemorrhagic shock and encephalopathy: further description of a new syndrome. *J Pediatr* 1985;106:599–602.
1359. Jardine DS, Winters WD, Shaw DW. CT scan abnormalities in a series of patients with hemorrhagic shock and encephalopathy syndrome. *Pediatr Radiol* 1997;27:540–544.
1360. Thebaud B, Husson B, Navelet Y, et al. Haemorrhagic shock and encephalopathy syndrome: neurological course and predictors of outcome. *Intensive Care Med* 1999;25:293–299.
1361. Ince E, Kuloglu Z, Akinci Z. Hemorrhagic shock and encephalopathy syndrome: neurologic features. *Pediatr Emerg Care* 2000;16:260–264.
1362. Sofer S, Yerushalmi B, Shahak E, et al. Possible aetiology of haemorrhagic shock and encephalopathy syndrome in the Negev area of Israel. *Arch Dis Child* 1996;75:332–334.
1363. Bacon CJ, Bell SA, Gaventa JM, et al. Case control study of thermal environment preceding haemorrhagic shock encephalopathy syndrome. *Arch Dis Child* 1999;81:155–158.
1364. Behçet H. Über rezidivierende Aphthöse durch ein Virus verursachte Geschwüre am Mund, am Auge, und an den Genitalien. *Dermatol Monatsschr* 1937;105:1152–1157.
1365. Devlin T, Gray L, Allen NB, et al. Neuro-Behçet's disease: factors hampering proper diagnosis. *Neurology* 1995;45:1754–1757.
1366. Lewis MA, Priestley BL. Transient neonatal Behcet'sdisease. *Arch Dis Child* 1986;61:805–806.
1367. Sakane T, Takeno M, Suzuki N, et al. Behcet's disease. *N Engl J Med* 1999;341:1284–1291.
1368. Arbesfeld SJ, Kurban AK. Behçet's disease. New perspectives on an enigmatic syndrome. *J Am Acad Dermatol* 1988;19:767–779.
1369. Allen NB. Miscellaneous vasculitic syndromes including Behcet's disease and central nervous system vasculitis. *Curr Opin Rheumatol* 1993;5:51–56.

1370. Martinez JM, Barraquer-Bordas L, Ferrer I, et al. Anatomoclinical study of Behcet's syndrome with involvement of the central nervous system. *Rev Neurol* (Paris) 1988;144:130–135.

1371. Karakucuk S, Baskol G, Oner AO, et al. Serum paraoxonase activity is decreased in the active stage of Behcet's disease. *Br J Ophthalmol* 2004;88:1256–1258.

1372. Wolf SM, Schotland DL, Phillips LL. Involvement of nervous system in Behçet syndrome. *Arch Neurol* 1965;12:315–325.

1373. Gokcay F, Celebisoy N, Kisabay A, et al. P300 and neuropsychological evaluation in Behcet's disease with and without neurological manifestations. *J Neurol* 2004;251:676–679.

1374. Iseki E, Iwabuchi K, Yagishita S, et al. Two necropsy cases of chronic encephalomyelitis: variants of neuro-Behcet's syndrome? *J Neurol Neurosurg Psychiatry* 1988;51:1084–1087.

1375. Wechsler B, et al. Cerebral venous thrombosis in Behçet's syndrome. A clinical study and long term follow-up of 25 cases. *Neurology* 1992;42:614–618.

1376. Vignola S, Nobili F, Picco P, et al. Brain perfusion SPECT in juvenile neuro-Behcet's disease. *J Nucl Med* 2001;42:1151–1157.

1377. Al-Kawi MZ, Bohlega S, Banna M. MRI findings in neuro-Behçet's disease. *Neurology* 1991;41:405–408.

1378. Yurdakul S, Gunaydin I, Tuzun Y, et al. The prevalence of Behçet's syndrome in a rural area in northern Turkey. *J Rheumatol* 1988;15:820–822.

1379. Rakover Y, Adar H, Tal I, et al. Behçet disease: long-term follow-up of three children and review of the literature. *Pediatrics* 1989;83:986–992.

1380. Hatzinikolaou P, Vaiopoulos G, Mavropoulos S, et al. Adamantiadis–Behçet's syndrome: central nervous system involvement. *Acta Neurol Scand* 1993;87:290–293.

1381. Feron EJ, Rothova A, van Hagen PM, et al. Interferon-a-2b for refractory ocular Behçet's disease [Letter]. *Lancet* 1994;343:14–28.

1382. Riehl JL, Andrews JM. The uveomeningoencephalitic syndrome. *Neurology* 1966;16:603–609.

1383. Goldberg AC, Yamamoto JH, Chiarella JM, et al. HLA-DRB1*0405 is the predominant allele in Brazilian patients with Vogt-Koyanagi-Harada disease. *Hum Immunol* 1998;59:183–188.

1384. Moorthy RS, Inomata H, Rao NA. Vogt-Koyanagi-Harada syndrome. *Surv Ophthalmol* 1995;39:265–292.

1385. Pezzi PP, Paroli MP, Priori R, et al. Vogt-Koyanagi-Harada syndrome and keratoconjunctivitis sicca. *Am J Ophthalmol* 2004;137:769–770.

1386. Kimura R, Kasai M, Shaji K, et al. Swollen ciliary processes as an initial symptom in Vogt-Koyanagi-Harada disease. *Am J Ophthalmol* 1983;95:402–403.

1387. Takeshita T, Nakazawa M, Murakami K, et al. A patient with long standing melanin laden macrophages in cerebrospinal fluid in Vogt-Koyanagi-Harada syndrome. *Br J Ophthalmol* 1997;81:11–14.

1388. Gocho K, Kondo I, Yamaki K. Identification of autoreactive T cells in Vogt-Koyanagi-Harada disease. *Invest Ophthalmol Vis Sci* 2001;42:2004–2009.

1389. Brazis PW, Stewart M, Lee AG. The uveomeningeal syndromes. *Neurologist* 2004;10:171–184.

1390. Ohno C, Char DH, Kimura SJ, et al. Vogt-Koyanagi-Harada syndrome. *Am J Ophthalmol* 1977;83:735–740.

1391. Beniz J, Forster DJ, Lean JS, et al. Variations in clinical features of the Vogt-Koyanagi-Harada syndrome. *Retina* 1991;11:275–280.

1392. Belfort R Jr, et al. Vogt-Koyanagi-Harada's disease in Brazil. *Jpn J Ophthalmol* 1988;32:344–347.

1393. Gruich MJ, Evans OB, Storey JM, et al. Vogt-Koyanagi-Harada syndrome in a 4-year-old child. *Pediatr Neurol* 1995;13:50–51.

1394. Brouzas D, Chatzoulis D, Galina E, et al. Corneal anesthesia in a case with Vogt-Koyanagi-Harada syndrome. *Acta Ophthalmol Scand* 1997;75:464–465.

1395. Maruyama Y& Kishi S. Tomographic features of serous retinal detachment in Vogt-Koyanagi-Harada syndrome. *Ophthalmic Surg Lasers Imaging* 2004;35:239–242.

1396. Ikeda M, Tsukagoshi H. Vogt-Koyanagi-Harada disease presenting meningoencephalitis. Report of a case with magnetic resonance imaging. *Eur Neurol* 1992;32:83–85.

1397. Helveston WR, Gilmore R. Treatment of Vogt-Koyanagi-Harada syndrome with intravenous immunoglobulin. *Neurology* 1996;46:584–585.

1398. Andrade RE, Muccioli C, Farah ME, et al. Intravitreal triamcinolone in the treatment of serous retinal detachment in Vogt-Koyanagi-Harada syndrome. *Am J Ophthalmol* 2004;137:572–574.

1399. Tabbara KF, Chavis PS, Freeman WR. Vogt-Koyanagi-Harada syndrome in children compared to adults. *Acta Ophthalmol Scand* 1998;76:723–726.

1400. Sheu SJ, Kou HK, Chen JF. Significant prognostic factors for Vogt-Koyanagi-Harada disease in the early stage. *Kaohsiung J Med Sci* 2004;20:97–105.

1401. Keino H, Goto H, Usui M. Sunset glow fundus in Vogt-Koyanagi-Harada disease with or without chronic ocular inflammation. *Graefes Arch Clin Exp Ophthalmol* 2002;240:878–882.

1402. Read RW, Rechodouni A, Butani N, et al. Complications and prognostic factors in Vogt-Koyanagi-Harada disease. *Am J Ophthalmol* 2001;131:599–606.

1403. Picard FJ, Dekaban GA, Silva J, et al. Mollaret's meningitis associated with herpes simplex type 2 infection. *Neurology* 1993;43:1722–1727.

1404. Achard JM, Lallement PY, Veyssier P. Recurrent aseptic meningitis secondary to intracranial epidermoid cyst and Mollaret's meningitis: two distinct entities or a single disease? A case report and a nosologic discussion. *Am J Med* 1990;89:807–810.

1405. Mollaret P. La meningite endothelioleucocytaire multiricurrente binigne. Syndrome nouveau ou maladie nouvelle? Documents humoraux et microbiologiques. *Ann Inst Pasteur* 1945;71:1–17.

1406. Cohen BA, Rowley AH, Long CM. Herpes simplex type 2 in a patient with Mollaret's meningitis: demonstration by polymerase chain reaction. *Ann Neurol* 1994;35:112–116.

1407. Mirakhur B, McKenna M. Recurrent herpes simplex type 2 virus (Mollaret) meningitis. *J Am Board Fam Pract* 2004;17:303–305.

1408. Hermans PE, Goldstein NP, Wellman WE. Mollaret's meningitis and differential diagnosis of recurrent meningitis. Report of case, with review of literature. *Am J Med* 1972;52:128–150.

1409. Haynes BF, Wright R, McCracken JP. Mollaret meningitis—a report of three cases. *JAMA* 1976;236:1967–1969.

1410. Iivanainen M. Benign recurrent aseptic meningitis of unknown aetiology (Mollaret's meningitis). *Acta Neurol Scand* 1973;49:133–138.

1411. Blumenfeld H, Cha JH, Cudkowicz ME. Trimethoprim and sulfonamide-associated meningoencephalitis with MRI correlates. *Neurology* 1996;46:556–558.

1412. Yamamoto LJ, Tedder DG, Ashley R, et al. Herpes simplex virus type 1 DNA in the cerebrospinal fluid of a patient with Mollaret's meningitis. *N Engl J Med* 1991;325:1082–1085.

1413. Choung YH, Park K, Moon SK, et al. Various causes and clinical characteristics in vertigo in children with normal eardrums. *Int J Pediatr Otorhinolaryngol* 2003;67:889–894.

1414. Drigo P, Carli G, Laverda AM. Benign paroxysmal vertigo of childhood. *Brain Dev* 2001;23:38–41.

1415. Uneri A, Turkdogan D. Evaluation of vestibular functions in children with vertigo attacks. *Arch Dis Child* 2003;88:510–511.

1416. Pederson E. Epidemic vertigo. Clinical picture, epidemiology and relation to encephalitis. *Brain* 1959;82:566–580.

1417. Basser LS. Benign paroxysmal vertigo of childhood. (A variety of vestibular neuronitis.) *Brain* 1964;87:141–152.

1418. Koenigsberger MR, et al. Benign paroxysmal vertigo of childhood. *Neurology* 1968;18:301–302.

1419. Eviatar L, Eviatar A. Vertigo in children: differential diagnosis and treatment. *Pediatrics* 1977;59:833–838.

1420. Morgon A. Vertigo in children. *Ann Pediatr* (Paris) 1992;39:519–522.

1421. Ravid S, Bienkowski R, Eviatar L. A simplified diagnostic approach to dizziness in children. *Pediatr Neurol* 2003;29:317–320.

1422. von Economo C. *Encephalitis lethargica: its sequelae and treatment*. London: Oxford University Press, 1931.

1423. Rail D, Scholtz C, Swash M. Post-encephalitic parkinsonism: current experience. *J Neurol Neurosurg Psychiatry* 1981;44:670–676.

1424. Association for Research in Nervous and Mental Disease. *Acute epidemic encephalitis*. New York: Paul B. Hoeber, 1921.

1425. Hohman LB. Post-encephalitic behavior disorders in children. *Bull Johns Hopkins Hosp* 1922;33:372–375.
1426. Sissons JGP. Superantigens and infectious disease. *Lancet* 1993;341:1627–1629.
1427. Leung DYM, Meissner HC, Fulton DR, et al. Toxic shock syndrome toxin-secreting *Staphylococcus aureus* in Kawasaki disease. *Lancet* 1993;342:1385–1388.
1428. Nigro G, Zerbini M, Krzysztofiak A. Active or recent parvovirus B19 infection in children with Kawasaki disease. *Lancet* 1994;343:1260–1261.
1429. Kuijpers TW, Tija KL, de Jager F, et al. A boy with chickenpox whose fingers peeled. *Lancet* 1998;351:1782.
1430. Yokota S, Tsubaki K, Kuriyama T, et al. Presence in Kawasaki disease of antibodies to mycobacterial heat-shock protein HSP65 and autoantibodies to epitopes of human HSP65 cognate antigen. *Clin Immunol Immunopathol* 1993;67:163–170.
1431. Okada Y, Shinohara M, Kobayashi T, et al. Effect of corticosteroids in addition to intravenous gamma globulin therapy on serum cytokine levels in the acute phase of Kawasaki disease in children. *J Pediatr* 2003;143:363–367.
1432. Quasney MW, Bronstein DE, Cantor RM, et al. Increased frequency of alleles associated with elevated tumor necrosis factor-alpha levels in children with Kawasaki disease. *Pediatr Res* 2001;49:686–690.
1433. Gupta M, Noel GJ, Schaefer M, et al. Cytokine modulation with immune gamma globulin in peripheral blood of normal children and its implications in Kawasaki disease treatment. *J Clin Immunol* 2001;21:193–199.
1434. Uehara R, Yashiro M, Nakamura Y, et al. Kawasaki disease in parents and children. *Acta Paediatr* 2003;92:694–697.
1435. Chang RKR. Hospitalizations for Kawasaki disease among children in the United States, 1988–1997. *Pediatrics* 2002;109:e87–e93.
1436. Stockheim JA, Innocentini N, Shulman ST. Kawasaki disease in older children and adolescents. *J Pediatr* 2000;137:250–252.
1437. Gama C, Breeden K, Miller R. Myositis in Kawasaki disease. *Pediatr Neurol* 1990;6:135–136.
1438. Bushara K, Wilson A, Rust RS. Facial palsy in Kawasaki syndrome. *Pediatr Neurol* 1997;17:362–364.
1439. Melish ME. Kawasaki syndrome (the mucocutaneous lymph node syndrome). *Annu Rev Med* 1982;33:569–585.
1440. Dengler LD, Capparelli EV, Bastian JF, et al. Cerebrospinal fluid profile in patients with acute Kawasaki disease. *Pediatr Infect Dis J* 1998;17:478–481.
1441. American Academy of Pediatrics. Kawasaki disease. In: Peter G, ed. *1997 Red book: report of the Committee on Infectious Diseases*, 24th ed. Elk Grove Village, IL: Author, 1997: 316–319.
1442. Takei S, Arora YK, Walker SM. Intravenous immunoglobulin contains specific antibodies inhibitory to activation of T cells by staphylococcal toxin superantigens. *J Clin Invest* 1993;91:603–607.
1443. Newburger JW. Treatment of Kawasaki disease. *Lancet* 1996;347: 11–28.
1444. Takagi N, Kihara M, Yamaguchi S, et al. Plasma exchange in Kawasaki disease. *Lancet* 1995;346:1307.
1445. Rasmussen T, Olszewski J, Lloyd-Smith D. Focal seizures due to chronic localized encephalitis. *Neurology* 1958;8:435–445.
1446. Antel JP, Rasmussen T. Rasmussen's encephalitis and the new hat. *Neurology* 1996;46:9–11.
1447. Power C, Poland SD, Blume WT, et al. Cytomegalovirus and Rasmussen's encephalitis. *Lancet* 1990;336:1282–1284.
1448. Andrews JM, Thompson JA, Pysher TJ, et al. Chronic encephalitis, epilepsy and cerebrovascular immune complex deposits. *Ann Neurol* 1990;28:88–90.
1449. Jay V, Becker LE, Otsubo H, et al. Chronic encephalitis and epilepsy (Rasmussen's encephalitis): Detection of cytomegalovirus and herpes simplex virus 1 by the polymerase chain reaction and *in situ* hybridization. *Neurology* 1995;45:108–117.
1450. Rogers SW, Andrews PI, Gahring LC, et al. Autoantibodies to glutamate receptor GluR3 in Rasmussen's encephalitis. *Science* 1994;265:648–651.
1450a. Watson R, Jiang Y, Bermudez I, et al. Absence of antibodies to glutamate receptor type 3 (GlueR3) in Rasmussen encephalitis. *Neurology* 2004;63:43–50.
1451. Whitney KD, Andrews PL, McNamara JO. Immunoglobulin G and complement immunoreactivity in the cerebral cortex of patients with Rasmussen's encephalitis *Neurology* 1999;53:699–708.
1452. Aguilar MJ, Rasmussen T. Role of encephalitis in pathogenesis of epilepsy. *Arch Neurol* 1960;2:663–676.
1453. Piatt JH Jr, Hwang PA, Armstrong DC, et al. Chronic focal encephalitis (Rasmussen's syndrome): six cases. *Epilepsia* 1988;29:268–279.
1454. Hart YM, Andremann F, Robitaille Y, et al. Chronic encephalitis and epilepsy in adults and adolescents: a variant of Rasmussen's syndrome? *Neurology* 1997;48:418–424.
1455. Tien RD, Ashdown BC, Lewis DV Jr., et al. Rasmussen's encephalitis: neuroimaging findings in four patients. *Am J Roentgenol* 1992;158:1329–1332.
1456. Kim SJ, Park YD, Pillai JJ, et al. A longitudinal MRI study in children with Rasmussen syndrome. *Pediatr Neurol* 2002;27:282–288.
1457. Fiorella DJ, Provenzale JM, Coleman RE, et al. 18F-Fluorodeoxyglucose positron emission tomography and MR imaging findings in Rasmussen encephalitis. *Am J Neuroradiol* 2001;22:1291–1299.
1458. Maria BL, Ringdahl DM, Mickle JP, et al. Intraventricular alpha interferon therapy for Rasmussen's syndrome. *Can J Neurol Sci* 1993;20:333–336.
1459. Cendes F, Andremann F, Silver K, et al. Imaging of axonal damage *in vivo* in Rasmussen's syndrome. *Brain* 1995;118:753–758.
1460. Vining EP, Freeman JM, Pillas DJ, et al. Why would you remove half a brain? The outcome of 58 children after hemispherectomy—the Johns Hopkins experience. *Pediatrics* 1997;100:163–171.
1461. Vining EP, Freeman JM, Brandt J, et al. Progressive unilateral encephalopathy of childhood (Rasmussen's syndrome): a reappraisal. *Epilepsia* 1993;34:639–650.
1462. Krauss GL, Campbell ML, Roche KW, et al. Chronic steroid-responsive encephalitis without antibodies to glutamate receptor GluR3. *Neurology* 1996;46:247–249.
1463. Wise MS, Rutledge SL, Kuzniecky RI. Rasmussen syndrome and long-term response to gamma globulin. *Pediatr Neurol* 1996;14:149–152.
1464. Andrews PI, Dichter MA, Berkovic SF, et al. Plasmapheresis in Rasmussen's encephalitis. *Neurology* 1996;46:242–246.
1465. McLachlan RS, Levin S, Blume WT. Treatment of Rasmussen's syndrome with ganciclovir. *Neurology* 1996;47:925–928.
1466. Veyradier A, Obert B, Haddad E, et al. Severe deficiency of the specific von Willebrand factor–cleaving protease (ADAMTS-13) activity in a subgroup of children with atypical hemolytic uremic syndrome. *J Pediatr* 2003;142:310–317.
1467. Ruggenenti P, Remuzzi G. Thrombotic microangiopathies. *Crit Rev Oncol Hematol* 1991;11:243–265.
1468. Wall RT, Harker LA. The endothelium and thrombosis. *Annu Rev Med* 1980;31:361–371.
1469. Karmali MA, Steele BT, Petric M, et al. Sporadic cases of haemolytic-uraemic syndrome associated with faecal cytotoxin and cytotoxin-producing *Escherichia coli* in stools. *Lancet* 1983;1:619–620.
1470. Akashi, S, Joh K, Tsuji A, et al. A severe outbreak of haemorrhagic colitis and haemolytic uraemic syndrome associated with *Escherichia coli* O157:H7 in Japan. *Eur J Pediatr* 1994;153:650–655.
1471. Rondeau E, Peraldi M-N. *Escherichia coli* and the hemolytic-uremic syndrome. *N Engl J Med* 1996;335:660–662.
1472. Mead PS, Griffin PM. *Escherichia coli* O157:H7. *Lancet* 1998;352:1207–1212.
1473. Moake JL. Haemolytic-uremic syndrome: basic science. *Lancet* 1994;343:393–397.
1474. van de Kar NC, Monnens LA, Karmail MA, et al. Tumor necrosis factor and interleukin-1 induce expression of the verocytotoxin receptor globotriaosylceramide on human endothelial cells: implications for the pathogenesis of the hemolytic uremic syndrome. *Blood* 1992;80:2755–2764.
1475. Chandler WL, Jelacic S, Boster DR, et al. Prothrombotic

coagulation abnormalities preceding the hemolytic-uremic syndrome. *N Engl J Med* 2002;346:23–32.
1476. Louise CB, Obrig TG. Shiga toxin-associated hemolytic uremic syndrome: combined cytotoxic effects of shiga toxin and lipopolysaccharide (endotoxin) on human vascular endothelial cells in vitro. *Infect Immun* 1992;60:1536–1543.
1477. Cimolai N, Morrison BJ, Carter JE. Risk factors for the central nervous system manifestations of gastroenteritis-associated hemolytic-uremic syndrome. *Pediatrics* 1992;90:616–621.
1478. Moake JL. The role of von Willebrand factor (vWF) in thrombotic thrombocytopenic purpura (TTP) and the hemolytic-uremic syndrome (HUS). *Prog Clin Biol Res* 1990;337:135–140.
1479. Moake JL. Recent observations on the pathophysiology of thrombotic thrombocytopenic purpura and the hemolytic-uremic syndrome. *Hematol Pathol* 1990;4:197–201.
1480. Remuzzi G. HUS and TTP; variable expression of a single entity. *Kidney Int* 1987;32:292–308.
1481. Teshima T, Miyoshi T, Ono M. Cyclosporine-related encephalopathy following allogeneic bone marrow transplantation. *Int J Hematol* 1996;63:161–164.
1482. Schiff DE, Roberts WD, Willert J, et al. Thrombocytopenia and severe hyperbilirubinemia in the neonatal period secondary to congenital thrombotic thrombocytopenic purpura and ADAMTS13 deficiency. *J Pediatr Hematol Oncol* 2004;26:535–538.
1483. Schneppenheim R, Budde U, Hassenpflug W, et al. Severe ADAMTS-13 deficiency in childhood. *Semin Hematol* 2004;41:83–89.
1484. Siegler RL. Management of hemolytic-uremic syndrome. *J Pediatr* 1988;112:1014–1020.
1485. Cabrera GR, Fortenberry JD, Warshaw BL, et al. Hemolytic uremic syndrome associated with invasive *Streptococcus pneumoniae* infection. *Pediatrics* 1998;101:699–703.
1486. Kennedy SS, Zacharski LR, Beck JR. Thrombotic thrombocytopenic purpura: analysis of 48 unselected cases. *Semin Thromb Hemost* 1980;6:341–349.
1487. Fuchs WE, George JN, Dotin LN, et al. Thrombotic thrombocytopenic purpura. Occurrence two years apart during late pregnancy in two sisters. *J Am Med Assoc* 1976;235:2126–2127.
1488. Tarr PI, Fouser LS, Stapleton AE, et al. Hemolytic-uremic syndrome in a six-year old girl after a urinary tract infection with shiga-toxin-producing *Escherichia coli* 0103:H2. *N Engl J Med* 1996;335:635–638.
1489. Brandt J, Wong C, Mihm S, et al. Invasive pneumococcal disease and hemolytic uremic syndrome. *Pediatrics* 2002;110:371–376.
1490. Moake JL. Thrombotic thrombocytopenic purpura and the hemolytic uremic syndrome. *Arch Pathol Lab Med* 2002;126:1430–1433.
1491. Brunner HI, Freedman M, Silverman ED. Close relationship between systemic lupus erythematosus and thrombotic thrombocytopenic purpura in childhood. *Arthritis Rheum* 1999;42:2346–2355.
1492. Bale JF Jr, Brasher C, Siegler RL. CNS manifestations of the hemolytic-uremic syndrome: relationship to metabolic alterations and prognosis. *Am J Dis Child* 1980;134:869–872.
1493. Hahn JS, Havens PL, Higgins JJ, et al. Neurological complications of hemolytic-uremic syndrome. *J Child Neurol* 1989;4:108–113.
1494. Siegler RL. Spectrum of extrarenal involvement in postdiarrheal hemolytic-uremic syndrome. *J Pediatr* 1994;125:511–518.
1495. Upadhyaya K, Barwick K, Fishaut M, et al. The importance of nonrenal involvement in the hemolytic-uremic syndrome. *Pediatrics* 1980;65:115–120.
1496. Travathan E, Dooling EC. Large thrombotic strokes in hemolytic-uremic syndrome. *J Pediatr* 1987;111:863–866.
1497. Gianantonio C, Vitacco M, Mendilaharzu F. et al. The hemolytic-uremic syndrome. *J Pediatr* 1964;64:478–491.
1498. Neild GH. Haemolytic-uraemic syndrome in practice. *Lancet* 1994;343:398–401.
1499. Pascual-Leone A, Dhuna AK, Janousek ST, et al. EEG correlation of improvement in hemolytic-uremic syndrome after plasma infusion. *Pediatr Neurol* 1990;6:269–271.
1500. Theobald I, Kuwertz-Broking E, Schiborr M, et al. Central nervous system involvement in hemolytic uremic syndrome (HUS)—a retrospective analysis of cerebral CT and MRI studies. *Clin Nephrol* 2001;56:S3–S8.
1501. Jayabose S, Levendoglu-Tugal O, Ozkayanak MF, et al. Use of vincristine and cyclosporine in childhood thrombotic thrombocytopenic purpura. *J Pediatr Hematol Oncol* 2003;25:421–425.
1502. Martin DL, MacDonald KL, White KE, et al. The epidemiology and clinical aspects of the hemolytic-uremic syndrome in Minnesota. *N Engl J Med* 1990;323:1161–1167.
1503. Steele BT, Murphy N, Chuang SH, et al. Recovery from prolonged coma in hemolytic-uremic syndrome. *J Pediatr* 1983;102:402–404.

Autoimmune and Postinfectious Diseases

Agustín Legido, Silvia N. Tenembaum, Christos D. Katsetos, and John H. Menkes

This chapter considers several groups of neurologic diseases believed to result from a failure of the normal mechanisms of self-tolerance. One group consists of the primary demyelinating diseases of the central nervous system (CNS), the second the immunologically mediated diseases affecting CNS gray matter, the third the immunologically mediated demyelinating diseases of the peripheral nervous system, and the last the primary and secondary systemic vasculitides with nervous system manifestations. Myasthenia gravis, another autoimmune condition, is discussed in Chapter 16. The paraneoplastic processes are so uncommon in the pediatric age group that they do not warrant discussion here.

EXPERIMENTAL MODELS FOR INFLAMMATORY DEMYELINATING DISEASE

Experimental allergic encephalomyelitis (EAE) and Theiler murine encephalomyelitis virus (TMEV) disease have been used as experimental animal models to study viral and autoimmune pathogenetic mechanisms in multiple sclerosis (MS) (1). The neuropathologic features and immunopathologic mechanisms responsible for inflammatory demyelination in EAE and TMEV are in many respects different. However, the models share certain similarities at the cellular and clinical levels insofar as they recall changes seen in human MS and acute disseminated encephalomyelitis (ADEM), for which they may serve as the two best experimental models (1–3).

Experimental Allergic Encephalomyelitis

Experimental allergic encephalomyelitis, also referred to as experimental autoimmune encephalomyelitis (4), has served for many decades as a useful animal model for the development and evolution of autoimmune diseases that affect the CNS. The EAE model was identified through efforts to elucidate the nature of a disseminated encephalomyelitis developing after human inoculation with Pasteur rabies vaccine (5). Because the vaccine was produced from virally infected neural tissue, animals were inoculated either with the vaccine or, for controls, uninfected neural tissue (5). However, during this exercise it was determined that some of the animals receiving uninfected neural tissue also developed encephalomyelitis (1,6).

Rivers and Schwentker were first to note that repeated injection of brain tissue into monkeys induced an inflammatory demyelinating encephalomyelitis (7).

Similar lesions have been produced consistently in other mammalian species; their appearance is enhanced by the addition of Freund's adjuvant, which is a commonly used emulsion of water, oil, and killed acid-fast organisms added to the antigenic material. Its mode of action is unknown, but is believed to be a slow release of antigen inducing an inflammatory reaction that attracts mononuclear cells. In the original studies by Wolf and coworkers (8), 90% of monkeys developed EAE in 2 to 8 weeks after the first of an average of three weekly subcutaneous inoculations. The characteristic clinical features of this monophasic disease included paresis of the extremities, ataxia, nystagmus, and blindness. The disease was usually fatal, but some animals had mild symptoms that often subsided. A chronic and a relapsing disease marked by exacerbations and remissions reminiscent of the clinical picture of MS was produced subsequently in several animal species, including nonhuman primates (9,10).

Since then, the EAE model has been studied extensively owing to its clinical and histopathologic similarities to the human demyelinating diseases, especially ADEM (3) and multiple sclerosis (MS) (4,11,12).

Pathology

Postmortem neuropathologic examination of animals with EAE reveals multiple, multifocal areas of demyelination distributed throughout the neuraxis. Histologically, the demyelinating lesions exhibit a distinctive angiocentric predilection and are accompanied by perivascular accumulations of mononuclear inflammatory cells (lymphocytes and monocytes) and perivascular microhemorrhages (13).

In addition, recent studies have demonstrated a range of axonal changes in EAE including axonal remodeling at multiple levels consistent with a highly plastic response of the motor system to inflammatory demyelinating insults (14). A comparative evaluation of acute axonal injury based on immunohistochemical reactivity for β-amyloid-precursor protein as a marker for dystrophic axons demonstrated similarities between patterns of axonal pathology in rats with myelin-oligodendrocyte glycoprotein (MOG)–induced chronic active EAE and human MS (15). The highest incidence of acute axonal injury was found during active demyelination, which was associated with axonal damage around demyelinating lesions and in the normal-appearing white matter of actively demyelinating cases. In addition, low but significant axonal injury was also observed in inactive demyelinated plaques. In contrast, no significant axonal damage was found in remyelinated shadow plaques (15).

Pathogenesis

EAE in the laboratory rat gives rise to an acute paralytic disease from which most animals recover spontaneously. The disease can be induced in genetically susceptible inbred Lewis and DA rats by direct immunization with myelin basic protein (MBP), encephalitogenic MBP peptides, or several other encephalitogenic proteins derived from myelin components, administered in complete Freund's adjuvant (4). In addition, the disease can be adoptively transferred to syngeneic recipients with primed T cells [adoptive transfer of antimyelin-specific CD4+ T cells (16,17)] that have been reactivated *in vitro* with antigen (4).

Considerable variations in the susceptibility of various animals have been described, which are largely attributed to genotypic attributes, especially to the major histocompatibility complex (MHC) gene repertoire of the animal strain (18). That said, it should be noted that EAE is not a naturally occurring autoimmune disease except in genetically modified animal models such as in antimyelin-specific TCR/RAG−/− transgenic mice (19).

Studies of EAE in susceptible rats have provided many important insights into the interactions of T cells and accessory cells that culminate in the induction of the autoimmune response leading to inflammatory demyelination (4).

EAE immunopathogenesis revolves around predominantly cell-mediated autoimmune mechanisms. T cells are thought to play a pivotal role in initiating and perpetuating the myelinoclastic inflammatory process associated with EAE (5). The disease of the CNS is regarded as Th1 MHC class II restricted and CD4+ T cell mediated (5). EAE is mediated by CD4+ T cells that secrete cytokines (1,4,5). After stimulation and activation, T cells upregulate key adhesion molecules, facilitating their entry into the CNS (1). Moreover, Th1 proinflammatory cytokines secreted by CD4+ T lymphocytes augment the recruitment of mononuclear inflammatory cells in the CNS (4). In turn, cytotoxic T cells, activated monocytes/macrophages, and/or glial cells secrete cytotoxic factors leading to demyelination in conjunction with humoral responses in which B cells secrete antibodies against myelin antigens (1,4,5). Spontaneous remission is associated with CD4+ T cells that secrete transforming growth factor-beta (TGF-β) (4).

T cells recognizing antigenic determinants of myelin such as myelin basic protein (MBP), proteolipid protein (PLP), or myelin oligodendrocyte glycoprotein (MOG) are activated in the periphery and are subsequently recruited to the CNS through the action of chemokines to cause inflammation leading to neurologic signs including paralysis (20).

Normal individuals may harbor autoreactive CD4+ T cells, which, however, exist, as a rule, in a steady state of clonal deletion, T-cell anergy, and immunologic ignorance (5). Moreover, the peripheral immune system is endowed with a series of regulatory mechanisms that afford protection against both the generation of self-directed active immune responses and the initiation of autoimmune diseases (5). For example, CD4+ CD25+ regulatory T (Treg) cells can suppress such autoreactive T cells in EAE (21–24). Interestingly, alterations of such regulatory T cells were recently found in MS patients (25). In addition, the CNS is regarded as an "immunologically privileged" system, which is protected against peripheral immune responses by the tight endothelial junctions of the blood–brain barrier (BBB), the absence of dendritic cells in CNS parenchyma, and the presence of an immunosuppressive microenvironment (5). The latter is characterized by the secretion of anti-inflammatory cytokines and the expression of Fas ligand (CD154), which promotes T-cell apoptosis (5). However, this immunologic CNS homeostasis is perturbed and ultimately overcome when the CNS is exposed to inflammation, which causes opening of the BBB. The processes underlying T-cell priming and/or autoreactive T-cell dysregulation are unknown. T cell–mediated immune responses lead to the alteration of the BBB, facilitating the recruitment of other inflammatory cells, such as monocytes, as well as components of the humoral response (B cells and complement factors) in the CNS (26,27). In addition, cytokines produced by activated T cells in the lesions induce the activation of macrophages and local microglia effector cells, leading to the increase of their destructive activity, which is responsible for demyelination and tissue damage in MS (28).

Recent studies using genetically modified animals have elucidated two distinct clinical phenotypes of EAE in BALB interferon (IFN)-γ knockout mice immunized with different residues of encephalitogenic peptides of MBP: (a) conventional disease, characterized by ascending weakness and paralysis, marked histologically by spinal cord inflammatory demyelination; and (b) a distinctive disease phenotype, characterized by uncontrolled axial rotation, involving demyelination of lateral medullary areas of brain (29). The type of disease is determined entirely by the inducing T cells, attesting to several divergent T cell–initiated effector pathways potentially involved in the pathogenesis of inflammatory demyelination (29).

Although our current understanding of autoimmune inflammatory demyelinating disease of the CNS points to a role of regulatory T cells in EAE (21–23,30) and in MS patients (31), other regulatory mechanisms may also be involved in the immunopathogenesis of these disorders. These include the role of natural killer (NK) cells, natural killer T (NKT) cells, mast cells, B cells, and antibody responses in EAE and MS (5). The presumptive role played by B cells in the immunopathogenesis of MS is supported to some extent by the oligoclonal pattern of immunoglobulin production in the CSF in MS (32) and increased intrathecal immunoglobulin synthesis (33). As mentioned prevously, the disruption of the BBB that occurs in EAE and MS may facilitate the entry of B cells, antibodies, and complement into the CNS (5). B cells may then be activated or reactivated following T-cell interactions and become antibody-secreting cells (5). It is speculated that the demyelination observed during MS and EAE may represent an immunopathogenic synergy between autoimmune T and B cells through CD40–CD40L interactions, which underlie the development of humoral immunity (5,34,35). However, the significance of the presence of B cells and antibodies in the CNS is controversial and seems to be dependent on the experimental model used.

In summary, current understanding of the pathogenetic model of EAE and MS conforms to the following scheme of autoimmunity: Autoantigens are presented to T cells in a MHC context by antigen-presenting cells (APCs) such as dendritic cells in lymph nodes. Cooperation between T helper cells and B cells results in the recruitment of B-cell repertoires specific to autoantigens. Activated T cells are recruited to the CNS via chemoattraction and are reactivated by local or infiltrating APCs, resulting in the release of proinflammatory and cytotoxic mediators, leading to cellular injury. Vascular inflammation causes disruption of the BBB, which further facilitates the migration of T and B lymphocytes and monocytes and perpetuates recurrent immune-mediated injury to the CNS. The myelin sheath is damaged by several compounding mechanisms mediated by cytokines, complement, digestion of surface myelin antigens by activated macrophages, and direct damage by CD4+ and CD8+ T cells (5). Collectively, these pathways lead to cell death, including apoptosis, of oligodendrocytes and microglia (5) and axonal injury (15).

The usefulness of EAE as an experimental model for MS is likely to continue in the years to come. In particular, the reproduction of EAE in a nonhuman-primate model in the common marmoset (*Callithrix jacchus*), bridging the phylogenetic gap between rodents and humans, may further facilitate the elucidation of novel immunopathogenetic mechanisms and the development of more effective therapeutic strategies in MS and allied disorders (36).

Theiler Murine Encephalomyelitis Virus (TMEV) Infection

TMEV, DA strain, induces a biphasic disease in susceptible strains of mice (such as SJL), consisting of an early acute meningo-polioencephalomyelitis involving predominantly cerebral and spinal cord gray matter followed by a late chronic demyelinating disease with spinal cord white matter involvement akin to MS (2).

Pathology

In the early phase of infection, the disease is characterized by variously dense and multifocal inflammatory infiltrates involving cerebral and spinal cord gray matter (37). The inflammatory infiltrates are mononuclear and consist of lymphocytes (predominantly T cells) and monocytes/macrophages. Although there is lymphocytic infiltration of the leptomeninges and the cerebral cortex, most of the inflammation is present in the deep gray nuclei and mesotemporal region, especially in the thalamus, basal ganglia, and hippocampus (2). In the spinal cord, the inflammation is predominantly seen in the anterior horns, although infiltration of the leptomeninges is also present (2,38). During the acute early phase, there is sparing of the white matter throughout the neuraxis. The inflammatory infiltrates consist predominantly of perivascular CD3+ T cells and to lesser degree monocytes/macrophages. There is also evidence of incipient vasculitis in some small to medium-sized blood vessels (2).

Approximately 3 weeks after initial infection, there is infiltration of the spinal white matter by lymphocytes and monocytes/macrophages, which coincides with the onset of the chronic demyelinating phase of the disease marked by vacuolar change of the white matter, myelin loss, and aggregates of myelin-laden macrophages (2). Axonal swellings (spheroids) are detected in demyelinating lesions during the advanced stages of chronic disease. The demyelinating process is multifocal and involves all funiculi of the spinal cord (37). Demyelinating lesions are associated with perivascular and parenchymal inflammatory infiltrates comprised of CD4+ and CD8+ T cells, macrophages, and a few B cells, which are present predominantly in the spinal cord (37). There is widespread inflammatory infiltration of the spinal leptomeninges.

In the advanced chronic phase of the demyelinating disease (100 to 200 days postinfection) there is marked spinal cord atrophy without a concomitant increase in spinal cord demyelination (39). McGavern and colleagues (39) demonstrated a statistically significant loss of medium-sized and large myelinated axons only after the demyelinating phase of the disease is established. They speculate that following myelin denudation the naked axons are vulnerable to further inflammation and undergo dystrophic changes as a consequence of secondary damage (39). However, it is unclear whether the axonal damage in TMEV is the result of direct (inflammatory) injury or delayed wallerian or "dying-back" type of degeneration (39). On the other hand, Tsunoda and Fujinami (40) hypothesized that in TMEV, axonal injury is accompanied by oligodendrocyte apoptosis, which precedes demyelination, suggesting that an inciting axonal injury may be responsible for triggering demyelination.

The comparative neuropathology of TMEV-induced demyelinating disease in mice and MS in humans was discussed in the review article by Oleszak and colleagues (2).

Pathogenesis

Early acute disease is characterized by replication of the virus in gray matter (41,42). This phase of disease is associated with neuronophagia and inflammatory infiltrates in the cerebral cortical and deep gray matter as well as anterior horn cells of spinal cord (43). Infection with live TMEV is an essential component of TMEV demyelinating disease. TMEV-specific cellular and humoral immunity and apoptosis of infected cells eliminate virus from the gray matter of the CNS during the acute phase of TMEV disease (1,44). In particular, the virus is partially cleared from the CNS by CD3+ T cells, which undergo activation-induced apoptotic cell death, leading to resolution of the inflammatory response (44). Within 2 to 3 weeks the virus is partially cleared, and approximately 35 days postinfection susceptible mice develop late chronic demyelinating disease. In contrast to the acute phase, during the chronic phase, TMEV persistently infects glial cells and/or macrophages in the white matter (1,2,37,42,43,45,46). At the same time, recruitment of macrophages and T cells and generation of antibodies lead to inflammation and demyelination (1,2,44). Unlike the acute phase of TMEV infection, only very few mononuclear inflammatory cells (lymphocytes and macrophages) undergo apoptosis in the late phase of the disease, leading to the accumulation of these cells in the CNS, particularly in the spinal cord. It is believed that clonal expansions of T cells resistant to apoptotic clearance may play a pivotal role in the pathogenesis of demyelinating disease (2,44).

The fact that resistant strains of mice (such as C57BL/6) develop only early acute disease, are capable of clearing the virus completely, and do not develop delayed demyelination underscores the importance of genetic susceptibility, in the context of MHC genes, underlying the pathogenesis of TMEV-induced demyelinating disease (2,38,44). These strain-dependent, genetically determined immune responses to TMEV infection are also illustrated in the differential expression of proinflammatory cytokines in demyelinating disease–prone (SJL) versus disease-resistant (B6) mouse strains.

During early acute disease, there is a robust proinflammatory (Th1) cytokine response in the CNS of both TMEV-infected SJL and B6 mice, evidenced by the increased expression of polymerase chain reaction (PCR) transcripts for IFN-γ, interleukin (IL)-1, IL-6, IL-12p40, and tumor necrosis factor (TNF)-α (47). In the subacute phase of TMEV infection (8 days postinfection) TGF-β1 and TNF-α transcripts were present at significantly higher levels in the CNS of SJL susceptible mice as compared to resistant B6 mice (48). Concomitantly, TGF-β protein expression was demonstrated by immunohistochemical staining in leptomeningeal inflammatory cell infiltrates in brain sections of SJL mice but not in B6 mice. Chang and coworkers speculated that TGF-β may be responsible for the failure of SJL mice to mount an effective anti-TMEV circulating T-lymphocyte response (48). During late chronic demyelinating disease, there is an increase of proinflammatory Th1 cytokines in the CNS of disease-sensitive SJL mice as compared to disease-resistant B6 mice (48). Interestingly, increased expression of anti-inflammatory cytokine transcripts [IL-4, IL-5, and IL-10 (Th2 cytokines) and TGF-β] has been detected in the spinal cord of TMEV-infected SJL mice with chronic demyelinating disease as compared to the spinal cord of B6 mice. These anti-inflammatory cytokines may represent a compensatory mechanism of the host (disease prone SJL mice) in an attempt to downregulate proinflammatory cytokine responses in the CNS (48).

Thus, although oligodendrocytes and/or myelin may be damaged by a direct attack of cytotoxic T cells, other cells, including CD4+ T cells, activated macrophages, and microglia, may contribute to myelin destruction by the production of cytokines as well as reactive oxygen and reactive nitrogen species.

The role of inducible nitric oxide synthase (iNOS) has been investigated during early acute and late chronic TMEV-induced demyelinating disease. Both iNOS transcripts and protein have been detected in brains and spinal cords of TMEV-infected SJL mice during early acute disease, with significant decline during the chronic demyelinating phase of the disease (2,38,49). Immunohistochemically, iNOS has been detected in reactive astrocytes and in some monocytes during the acute phase of the disease but is distinctly absent in myelin-laden foamy macrophages in chronic demyelinating lesions (38). A similar trend has been observed in acute versus chronic human MS cases (50). It has been suggested that blockade of nitric oxide by treatment of TMEV-infected SJL mice with amino guanidine (AG), a specific nitric oxide inhibitor, results in delay of late chronic demyelinating disease (51). However, this protective effect may depend on the temporal phase of the disease (early versus late), the type of cells expressing iNOS, and the time of administration of the nitric oxide inhibitor (49). It is speculated that nitric oxide production during early acute disease may be beneficial to the host through induction of apoptosis of infiltrating T cells and resolution of encephalitis, but its role in the pathogenesis of myelin or oligodendrocyte injury during late chronic demyelinating disease is unclear and may depend on other contributory factors (2,49).

TMEV-induced late chronic demyelinating disease is an excellent animal model for human MS (52), which, together with EAE, is likely to provide further critical insights into the pathogenesis and therapy of autoimmune demyelinating CNS disease in humans.

PRIMARY DEMYELINATING DISEASES OF THE CENTRAL NERVOUS SYSTEM

In Western countries with temperate climates, acute disseminating encephalomyelitis (ADEM), multiple sclerosis (MS), and optic neuritis are the three most frequently encountered primary demyelinating illnesses of the CNS (53). The concept of primary demyelination implies the destruction of the myelin sheets, oligodendrocytes, and Schwann cells with relative preservation of other components of the CNS (54). However, axonal injury is a common finding in demyelinating lesions, which correlates well with permanent functional deficits (55–58).

The demyelinating diseases of the CNS can be the consequence of (a) an immune-mediated inflammatory process resulting in destruction of the normally developed myelin (demyelinating or myelinoclastic diseases), (b) metabolic and genetic disorders of myelin metabolism, which embody abnormally formed myelin (dysmyelinating diseases) (3,59–62), or (c) a primary demyelinating process that occurs as a result of cerebral hypoxic-ischemic insults and certain forms of poisoning (54). Table 8.1 displays the classification of CNS myelin disorders.

TABLE 8.1 Classification of Central Nervous System Myelin Disorders

Noninfectious Inflammatory, Probably Autoimmune
Acute demyelinating encephalomyelitis
Acute hemorrhagic encephalomyelitis
Multiple sclerosis
Marburg disease
Optic neuromyelitis or Devic disease
Concentric sclerosis or Baló disease
Diffuse cerebral sclerosis or Schilder disease
Optic neuritis
Transverse myelitis
Postinfectious cerebellitis
Postinfectious brainstem encephalitis
Inflammatory or Infectious Demyelinating Disorders
Progressive multifocal leukoencephalitis
Subacute sclerosing panencephalitis
Progressive rubella panencephalitis
Human immunodeficiency virus subacute encephalitis
Cytomegalovirus subacute encephalitis
Toxic and Metabolic Disorders
CO poisoning
Vitamin B_{12} deficiency
Folate deficiency
Mercury poisoning
Post–hypoxic-ischemic newborn leukoencephalopathy
Central pontine and extrapontine myelinolisis
Marchiafava-Bignami disease
Radiation-induced leukoencephalopathy
Hereditary Disorders of Myelin Metabolism (Dysmyelinating Diseases)
Adrenoleukodystrophy
Metachromatic leukodystrophy
Multiple sulfatase deficiency
Krabbe disease
Alexander disease
Canavan disease
Pelizaeus-Merzbacher disease
Phenylketonuria
Tay-Sachs disease
Niemann-Pick disease
Gangliosidosis G_{M1} and G_{M2}
Fabry disease
Peroxisomal Disorders
Mitochondrial leukoencephalopathies
Vascular
Vasculitis

ADEM is more common in children under the age of 12 years; MS is more common in adolescents and adults. Difficulty in distinguishing ADEM from the first bout of MS is among the most important reasons for the requirement of a second distinct episode occurring at least 1 month after the first for diagnosis of MS. It remains controversial as to whether "relapsing ADEM" should be distinguished from MS, but it appears likely that this distinction is ill defined in prepubertal children. Optic neuritis and the combination of optic neuritis and transverse myelitis (Devic disease) usually occur as manifestations of ADEM or MS, but pure transverse myelitis seems to be a distinctive nosologic entity, which may result from other type of illnesses (53).

An area of semiologic overlap exists between ADEM and Guillain-Barré syndrome (GBS). This area of overlap includes some or possibly all patients who manifest the clinical findings of Miller Fisher syndrome. It also includes the minority of ADEM cases that manifest diminished or absent muscle stretch reflexes in combination with weakness and sensory changes referable to peripheral nerve dysfunction. The designation of encephalomyelo-radiculoneuropathy (EMRN) may be applied to cases exhibiting this overlap of central and peripheral demyelinating manifestations. Other considerably less common primary demyelinating conditions that may occur in children and are often difficult to accurately classify include acute (Marburg type) MS, myelinoclastic diffuse sclerosis (Schilder disease), and concentric sclerosis (Baló disease). The disease encountered in infants younger than 2 years of age, who may experience a single bout of severe demyelination with edema, should be termed either acute MS or, perhaps more appropriately, severe ADEM (53).

The etiology and pathogenesis of these various primary demyelinating illnesses are incompletely understood. Moreover, the degree of pathogenetic overlap among MS, ADEM, and other demyelinating diseases such as Devic disease and transverse myelitis is unknown. Both MS and ADEM are regarded as autoimmune diseases that involve cellular and humoral responses that are directed, at least in part, against myelin antigens. The onset of MS does not have a clear etiologic relationship to a preceding infection, and clinically discernible bouts of the disease are typically associated with detectable oligoclonal immunoglobulin production in the cerebrospinal fluid (CSF). ADEM appears in many cases to be provoked by an antecedent infectious illness and is accompanied by elevated CSF concentrations of immunoglobulins or immunoglobulin oligoclonality only in a minority of cases. Normal CSF immunoglobulin profiles are characteristic of recurrences of ADEM, as compared with a greater than 94% likelihood of abnormality in association with an MS recurrence (53).

A small minority of individuals who have experienced typical cases of ADEM in early childhood ultimately satisfy the clinical criteria for diagnosis of MS during adolescence, whereas others satisfy criteria for the diagnosis of MS with either relapsing-remitting or steadily progressive manifestations of primary central demyelination. There are no specific diagnostic tests or disease biomarkers to differentiate between ADEM and MS in the pediatric setting, and a number of other conditions must be excluded before entertaining either of these diagnoses. It may be particularly difficult to distinguish ADEM and related forms of inflammation from encephalitis. Indeed, some forms of encephalitis (such as those caused by herpes or measles viruses) may share overlapping clinicopathologic abnormalities with ADEM (53).

Multiple Sclerosis

Historical Aspects

MS is the principal immune-mediated demyelinating illness of humans (63,64). The pathologic lesions of MS were described by Cruveilhier and Carswell early in the nineteenth century. Frerichs was the first to make a clinical diagnosis of MS, in 1840. Charcot's extensive studies of the clinical manifestations and natural history of MS resulted in diagnostic criteria for a coherent clinical entity designated disseminated sclerosis or *sclérose en plaques disseminées*, or Charcot disease (60). This condition was recognized at the outset exclusively among young adults. The occurrence of MS in children has been a topic for discussion for more than 50 years (53,60)

In 1922, Wechsler rejected most of the cases reported in pediatric populations but stated that "authentic cases of MS in children, in spite of their rarity, can occur (64a)." After that some isolated pediatric cases or small groups of affected children were reported (65). However, in that pre–computed tomography era, there was little evidence to identify the distinguishing characteristics of the condition in children. In 1948, Kabat and colleagues (66). reported increases in oligoclonal immunoglobulins in the cerebrospinal fluid of patients with MS, providing tangible evidence for an immunologically mediated inflammatory nature of the disease. In 1965, the diagnostic criteria of Schumacher and coworkers (67) established the age of debut of MS as being between 10 and 59 years, acknowledging that the condition does indeed occur below the age of 16 years.

A better understanding of the natural history of MS during the last 40 years has been made possible by important advances in neuroimmunology, molecular genetics, and biochemistry as well as the development of magnetic resonance imaging (MRI) techniques, which have allowed for an excellent and accurate anatomic visualization of the white matter *in vivo*. As a consequence, metabolic and infectious-inflammatory causes of demyelination have been delineated and the diagnosis of MS in children corroborated. Several retrospective studies were published in the 1980s and early 1990s, including those of adult patients with MS whose symptoms had been initiated during adolescence; the description of prepubertal patients was exceptional (68–74).

Today, it is generally accepted that MS can occur in children and even infants (75,76), although the distinctive characteristics of the disease at this age are not well established. It has been estimated that between 2.7% and 5.6% of patients with MS show symptoms attributable to the disease before 16 years of age (71,77–83). The frequency of MS beginning in early childhood has been calculated as 0.2% to 0.7% (71,84). According to these percentages, the corresponding prevalence of pediatric MS would be 1.35 to 2.5 per 100,000 people and that of the early infantile form would be 0.4 to 1.4 per 100,000 (85), although wider ranges. From 0.8 to 248 per 100,000 people, have been reported in Japan and Canada, respectively (77). Girls and women are at 1.5-fold to 2-fold greater risk than boys or men. Light-skinned individuals are at greater risk than more heavily pigmented individuals (64). However, MS can occur in black children, where it seems to have a rapidly progressive course (86). Residence in a northern climate before the age of 15 years confers an increased risk of developing the disease, although immigration to a southern climate at an early age substantially lowers the risk (87).

Pathogenesis

MS is clinicopathologically defined as a primary inflammatory demyelinating disease of the CNS. Although its etiology is unknown MS is widely regarded as an autoimmune disease involving predominantly abnormal cellular immune responses to putative (but not fully elucidated) autoantigens of central myelin (88). Over the years, two experimental animal models of MS have helped to better understand the pathogenetic mechanisms of this condition (see prior discussion of EAE and TMEV).

Epidemiologic data support the association of MS with hitherto unknown environmental factor(s) encountered during early childhood that after years of latency trigger the disease or contribute to its development. Three main groups of factors have been postulated in the immunopathogenesis of MS: (a) environmental factors, particularly the persistence of a viral infection, (b) immunologic factors involving autoimmune mechanisms with loss of tolerance to myelin antigens or molecular mimicry of viral antigens and myelin (or other host) proteins (2,88,89), and (c) genetic factors inducing a genetic predisposition to immunologic dysfunction.

Environmental Factors

Many investigators consider a viral infection to be the most likely environmental factor explaining the pathogenesis of MS. Indirect evidence supporting this theory comes from the particular distribution of the disease, with areas of high and low risk; serologic studies; isolation of viral proteins and genomic material from the brain of patients with MS; and different viral experimental models causing CNS lesions similar to MS pathology. Viruses probably related to MS include herpesvirus (in particular herpes human type 6), Epstein-Barr virus, paramyxovirus, and retrovirus. The recently discovered human endogenous retrovirus (HERV)-W family has an extracellular particle, named HSRV, that is associated to MS. Recent studies have shown that CSF levels of MSRV are related to the degree of CNS inflammation, and, even if this were an epiphenomenon, it could be used as a clinical prognostic marker of early MS (88).

Immunologic Factors

It is generally accepted that in addition to an early viral infection, there must be an autoimmune reaction that attacks some of the components of the myelin (2,88,90). Most patients exhibit T-cell reactivity to a number of myelin antigens, suggesting that by the time a patient develops clinical MS there has been epitope spreading with reactivity to multiple myelin epitopes (90). T cells that can react against myelin antigens are normally present in the immune system. These cells escaped thymic mechanisms of control such as clonal deletion.

A nontolerant, peripherally activated CD4+ T cell recognizes its autoantigen within the CNS parenchyma in the context of class II MHC molecules expressed by both local glial antigen-presenting cells (88) and dendritic cells (91), which commit T cells toward a Th1 phenotype. Activated Th1 cells cause myelin disruption and the release of new potential CNS autoantigens.

Secreted proinflammatory cytokines, such as IFN-γ and TNF-α, and chemokines recruit additional nonspecific inflammatory cells and specific antimyelin antibody–forming B cells, which exacerbate tissue injury (88,92,93). Finally, the apoptotic clearance of T cells and their conversion toward a Th2 phenotype modulates the outcome of the lesion (94). Additional cells are necessary for the development of typical MS lesions, such as the cytotoxic CD8+ cells, which show a more prominent clonal expansion within MS plaques and correlate better than CD4+ cells with the extent of acute axonal injury (95,96).

The cascade of inflammatory events that culminates in demyelination of axons depends on the peripheral activation of T lymphocytes (97). Interactions of lymphocytes with the vascular endothelium are required for lymphocyte trafficking into the CNS (2). Adhesion molecules play a critical role in this process and are pivotal in lymphocytes infiltrating the CNS through the BBB (98). One such molecule is the intercellular adhesion molecule-1 (ICAM-1), a glycoprotein that interacts with many α_2-integrins such as lymphocyte function–associated antigen-1 (LFA-1) on T cells and CD11b/CD18 on monocytes (99,100). Other adhesion molecules mediating the interactions between lymphocytes and endothelial cells are very late antigen 4/vascular cell adhesion molecule-1 (VCAM-1), L-selectin (on lymphocytes) and E-selectin (on endothelial cells) (101,102).

Genetic Factors

Genetic factors have also been postulated to be contributors to the pathogenesis of MS, based on different studies. Prevalence rates for MS among first-degree relatives of individuals with MS are approximately 20-fold greater than those of other individuals from the same region (53). The risk of developing MS in the general population of 1 in 1,000 increases to 20 to 40 in 1,000 for first-degree relatives (87). In a pediatric series of 44 children with MS, 10 (23%) had a positive family history of MS in a first-degree relative (1 child), a second-degree relative (5 children), or their extended family (4 children). This is very similar to the 15% to 20% rate of a positive family history reported in an adult MS series (77). Identical twins have a 25% to 35% concordance rate for MS, as compared to 0.5% for offspring (possibly much higher for daughters of mothers with MS), 0.6% for parents, 1.2% for siblings, and 2% to 4% for dizygotic twins (87,103,104).

Guided by the considerations related to the presumptive immunopathogenesis of the disease, candidate gene searches have been focused on genes of the T cell–mediated immune response and of myelin proteins. Negative results have been found for the genes for T-cell receptor-α, complement, chemokine receptors, interferons, other cytokine receptors, and the cytotoxic T-lymphocyte antigen 4 (CTL4), a gene located in the HLA class I region (88,103). There is a highly significant association of MS with HLA-DR2 and a weaker association with HLA-A3 and B7 in whites. Other candidates such as HLA class II have yielded positive results, especially when subtyped into HLA DRB1*1501, DQA*0102, and DQB1*0602 extended haplotype, although the estimated relative risk is only 2 to 4 (77,103,105). HLA-DR15 has been specifically associated with an earlier onset of MS in a large study of more than 900 patients (106).

Recent analysis of markers of microsatellite polymorphisms in populations of different sizes and ethnicities identified chromosome regions of interest in MS susceptibility: chromosome 6 within the MHC and chromosomes 3q21–q24, 18p11, and 17q22–q24; a later meta-analysis, however, indicated the highest consensus evidence for linkage at 17p11 (107). All studies are concordant with the conclusion that HLA contributes, although modestly, to overall susceptibility and that a relatively large number of other MHC and non-HMC genes with individually small epistatic effects may be responsible for predisposition to MS. This implies a number of genes with interacting effects and suggests a polygenic inheritance of the disease. For example, the ApoE4 haplotype is also a genetic factor determining MS severity; these patients have a twofold higher likelihood of developing "black holes" on MRI and have an approximately fivefold greater rate of brain atrophy (108,109). It is probable that the expression of the implicated genes depends on environmental factors (88,103).

In summary, there is credence in the long-standing tenet of MS pathogenesis that the disease is produced by an environmental agent acting on a genetically susceptible individual in whom there are impaired immune responses.

Pathology

MS is defined as an inflammatory demyelinating disease of the CNS characterized by inflammation, demyelination, and axonal damage (58,95,110). The histologic hallmark of the disease, the MS plaque, is thought to be an end-point lesion. MS plaques reflect a continuum of immunologic activity encompassing inflammatory and secondary cellular changes in the affected brain. Morphologically, plaques are classified as acute (active), chronic active, chronic inactive, and "shadow" type (58,111). The histologic variability and the age of the plaques may be part of a temporospatial gradient of morphologic changes reflecting different immunologic mechanisms of cellular injury (95,111).

Plaque morphogenesis and evolution embody the interaction of immunologic and metabolic factors including the effects of cytotoxic T cells, antibodies, toxic metabolites derived from activated monocytes/macrophages, and metabolic derangements of oligodendrocytes (95,110,112–115). Our understanding of the pathogenesis of myelin destruction in MS is in keeping with the notion that plaques may represent a common morphologic end point of divergent immunologic pathways of myelin and axonal damage (114,116,117).

Gross Topography

The external appearance of the brain in patients with MS may be unremarkable. In the chronic cases, signs of atrophy with widening of sulci and slight enlargement of the ventricular system can be observed. When sectioning the brain, it is possible to identify firm, gray lesions on the surface of the brainstem, spinal cord, and optic nerves and multiple plaques of variable diameter in the white matter (118). Inflammatory demyelinating lesions are typically disseminated throughout the neuraxis, but are more frequently encountered in certain anatomic sites relating to recognizable patterns of neurologic semiology. Although the distribution of the plaques varies among patients, the preferential locations are: periventricular white matter, floor of the aqueduct and fourth ventricle (brain stem), cerebellar peduncles, cervical spinal cord, and optic nerves (Fig. 8.1).

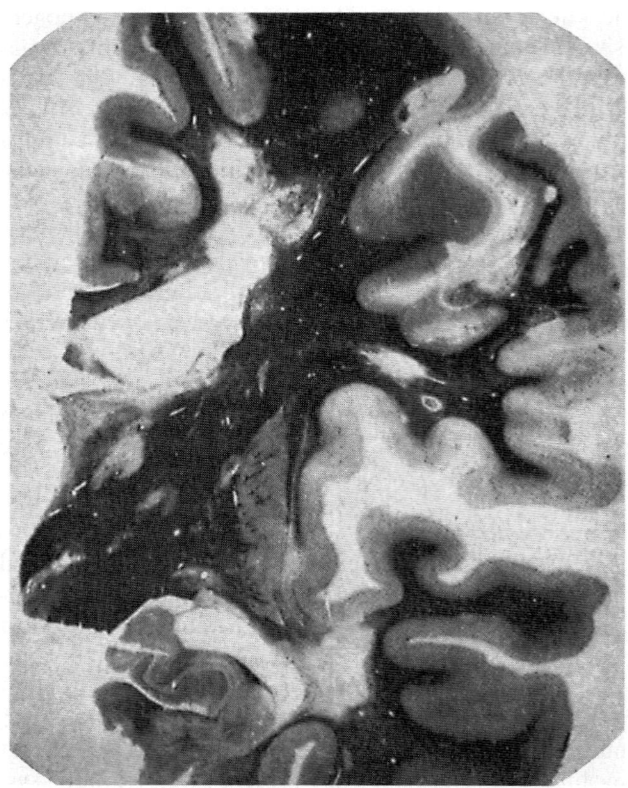

FIGURE 8.1. Multiple sclerosis. Disseminiated area of demyelination in white and gray matter of cerebral hemispheres. Myelin stain. (From Merritt HJ. *Textbook of neurology*, 5th ed. Philadelphia, Lea and Febiger, 1973. With permission.)

Distinctive anatomic correlates are encountered in certain variants, such as the neuromyelitis optica or Devic type. Even though in the cerebral hemispheres the lesions have a periventricular predilection, an important proportion of lesions can be observed in other locations of central white matter and the gray–white matter junction (119–121). Lesions involving convolutional white matter typically spare the U fibers. There are instances in which white matter lesions extend into the contiguous cortex gray matter or deep gray nuclei (basal ganglia and thalami) (119,120). Subpial and intracortical plaque formation has been described and may represent an important correlate of neurologic disability (56). Exceptionally, large, spherical, tumor-like lesions are encountered (122), but such lesions are most commonly seen in conjunction with myelinoclastic diffuse sclerosis (Schilder disease) (see later discussion).

Histopathology

The MS plaques can be classified into four categories encompassing cellular changes that reflect disease activity or quiescence:

1. Acute (fresh) lesions: These are the early plaques characterized by perivascular inflammation (comprising predominantly lymphocytes and monocytes/macrophages), edema, myelin swelling, and activation of endothelial cells (58,95,110,111,119,120). Variable, often pronounced depletion of oligodendrocytes is present (58,123–125). Plasma cells are infrequent. There is apparent preservation of axons; however, incipient axonal injury may be present (57,58).
2. Chronic active lesions: These are full-blown plaques marked by active inflammation and demyelination, typically at their margins (i.e., interfaces with normal-appearing white matter). The following morphologic changes are present: perivascular lymphocytic infiltrates, ongoing myelin breakdown, myelin-laden macrophages, oligodendrocyte depletion, and reactive astrocytosis. The lymphocytic infiltrates may extend beyond the plaque margins (58,111,119–121). Ostensibly, there is sparing of axons, but variable degrees of axonal damage may be present (57,58,126).
3. Chronic inactive lesions: These are old, "burnt-out" plaques or quiescent lesions tantamount to glial scars (hence the classical use of the term sclerosis). They are sharply delimited from the adjacent, normally myelinated white matter. There is prominent astrocytic gliosis, loss of oligodendrocytes, and variable axonal damage ranging from dystrophic neurites to overt transection of axons and dendrites (58,111,119–121,126). Scant perivascular lymphocytic cuffs, monocytes, and/or plasma cells may be focally present. The walls of the blood vessels are sclerotic and hyalinized, pointing to antecedent inflammatory vascular injury. A thin rim of perivascular collagenous fibrosis may be present in long-standing lesions. The blood–brain barrier is disrupted (127).
4. Shadow plaques: These represent a variously sized and ill-defined zone of partially demyelinated or incompletely remyelinated tissue surrounding, and occasionally "overshadowing," the principal plaque (128). Their occurrence in chronic MS is unpredictable, ranging from absent to frequent. There are no known clinical correlates, but "shadow plaques" may underlie a distinctive pathogenetic pathway (111).

Occasionally, the lesions are so severe that they evolve into cysts. It is classic to observe in the same patient lesions in different stages of progression.

Immunopathology

There are two integral components of MS lesions, perivascular inflammation and demyelination. It has long been hypothesized that inflammatory demyelination is the result of immune-mediated responses to myelin antigens in the myelin sheaths of axons and/or at the level of myelin-forming oligodendrocytes (95,110,119). Destruction of myelin and oligodendrocytes is not uniform in MS plaques (111,119). The morphogenesis of plaques is not fully understood, although circumstantial evidence points to early inflammatory damage of the BBB and infiltration by monocytes and lymphocytes, predominantly T cells (58,95,110,119). BBB disruption signals the onset of clinical symptoms, but a correlation between symptoms and inflammatory demyelination is not clear-cut.

Four distinct pathogenetic patterns of demyelination (I through IV) have been proposed (113). The first two focus on the concept that inflammation causes demyelination by direct and/or indirect mechanisms. Lymphocytes contribute to the pathologic process through cellular- and humoral-mediated immunologic responses (presumptive direct mechanisms) or by production of lymphokines and cytokines (indirect mechanisms). It follows then that patterns I and II exhibit remarkable similarities to either T cell–mediated or T cell plus antibody–mediated autoimmune encephalomyelitis (113). Monocytes/macrophages contribute to the demyelinating process in a twofold manner. First, through their traditional phagocytic role, cells of the monocyte/macrophage lineage, including hematogenously derived and activated resident microglia of the CNS, are potent effectors of axonal myelin and oligodendrocyte damage (58). Monocytes contribute to demyelination by way of production of cytokines, nitric oxide, and proteases and/or by directly targeting oligodendrocytes at the border of MS lesions (58,101,119). Activated CNS resident microglia play a role in the early stages of demyelination through cell-to-cell contact interactions with myelin internodes of the axons at the edges of active and chronic active MS lesions (58,119).

The other two patterns (III and IV) are consistent with a primary oligodendrocyte pathology (dystrophy) reminiscent of direct viral- or toxin-induced demyelination as opposed to bona fide autoimmune mechanisms (113). Over the years, various theories have been brought forward concerning the nature of oligodendrocyte damage in MS lesions. It is believed that this damage is incurred through a variety of immunologic mechanisms, including anti-MOG antibodies, cytokines produced by monocytes/macrophages and lymphocytes, T cell–mediated injury, immunoglobulins and components of activated complement, apoptosis, and a variety of other cytotoxic factors (58,114,115,129,130). In pattern III there is loss of myelin proteins in the distalmost (periaxonal) cell processes of oligodendrocytes, which is associated with apoptotic cell death (114,130,131). This mechanism has been previously defined as "distal" or "dying-back" oligodendrogliopathy (132) and is akin to oligodendroglial injury incurred during early hypoxic-ischemic demyelination of the white matter (130). In pattern IV there is cell death of oligodendrocytes in the white matter near active lesions (113). In this regard, it has been shown that activated monocytes/microglia expressing VCAM-1 selectively target oligodendrocytes at the border of MS lesions (101).

Axonal damage in the form of axonal swellings (dystrophic neurites) and transections has emerged as a major component of the disease (55,57,58,133,134). Axonal injury correlates with certain parameters of functional MR imaging (reduction of *N*-acetylaspartate) and certain patterns of neurologic disability in MS (15,114,126,135). Axonal pathology, evidenced by immunohistochemical staining for amyloid precursor protein (APP) in postmortem specimens, is more prominent in active MS lesions than in chronic inactive plaques (15).

Hypoxic-ischemic damage is an important but somewhat underrated aspect of MS neuropathology. Inflammatory damage of the vessel wall, endothelium, and BBB by T cells and monocyes (111,136–138) resembles the injury caused by angiocentric T-cell infiltrates in human immunodeficiency virus-1 (HIV-1)–associated CNS disease in children (139). The latter, compounded by edema and disturbance of the cerebral microcirculation, may impart damage to myelin, axons, and oligodendrocytes.

Disturbances in oxidative metabolism in MS reminiscent of hypoxia-ischemia may result from vascular factors (i.e., vascular inflammation) and/or the release of toxic metabolites associated with hypoxia-ischemia (130,140). Interestingly, overt ischemic damage has been demonstrated in severe cases of acute MS of the Marburg type, Baló concentric sclerosis, and neuromyelitis optica (141–143). It is hypothesized that certain active MS lesions may represent a form of "sublethal" hypoxic injury reminiscent of an ischemic white matter penumbra. Evidence of hypoxia-like metabolic tissue injury in MS due to the liberation of excitotoxins, reactive oxygen species, and nitric oxide lends further credence to this postulate (50,130,144–146).

In summary, current understanding of neuropathogenetic mechanisms in MS supports the hypothesis that white matter demyelination, axonal damage, dendritic transection, and apoptotic loss of neurons in the cerebral cortex contribute to neurologic dysfunction in MS patients (56).

Clinical Manifestations

Bauer and Hanefeld (147) classified MS according to the age at presentation: early infantile MS (EIMS), beginning between 1 and 5 years of age; delayed infantile or infantile MS (DIMS), beginning between 5.1 and 10 years; and juvenile MS (JMS), beginning between 10.1 and 16 years.

The clinical characteristics of 51 pediatric patients seen by one of us (S.N.T) (82,83) who fulfilled the MS diagnostic criteria of Poser and coworkers (148) are shown in Table 8.2. In 13 children disease was initiated before 5 years of age, and in another 13 it was initiated between 5 and 10 years. The youngest patient was an 18-month-old girl who has been followed for 16 years. So far, the youngest patient described in the literature is an 11-month-old infant (76).

The higher prevalence of infantile MS in girls was established in the series from Göttingen (147,149), which

TABLE 8.2 Clinical Data and Symptoms at the Time of the Initial Presentation of Multiple Sclerosis in 51 Children

	EIMS n = 13	DIMS n = 13	JMS n = 25	Total %
Clinical Data				
Age (years, mean)	3.4	7.1	13.5	
Gender (ratio female:male)	3:10	6:7	16:9	
Monosymptomatic	2	2	19	45
Polysymptomatic	11	11	6	55
Symptoms				
Pyramidal syndrome	12	9	16	73
Paresthesias	1	2	16	37
Myelopathy	4	5	6	29
Brainstem dysfunction	6	5	3	29
Impairment of consciousness	5	6	3	27
Ataxia	6	5	2	25
Loss of vision[a]	3	3	4	20
Meningeal signs	5	3	2	20
Seizures[b]	3	—	—	6
Aphasia	1	1	—	4
Extrapyramidal signs	—	1	1	4

Pediatric patients from Children's Hospital "Dr. J. P. Garrahan," Buenos Aires, Argentina (82,83). EIMS, early infantile multiple sclerosis; DIMS, delayed infantile or infantile multiple sclerosis; JMS, juvenile multiple sclerosis.

[a] Optic neuritis, bilateral in 8, unilateral in 2.

[b] Partial secondary generalized status.

included 20 children, with a ratio of 2.3:1. In our experience, this ratio was 1:3.3 in EIMS, 1:1.2 in DIMS, and 1.8:1 in JMS, the latter within the 1.5:1 to 1.9:1 ratio observed in adults (150). This finding suggests that hormonal changes related to puberty can interact with the immune and neuroendocrine systems and influence the course of some autoimmune diseases by modifying the humoral and cellular immune responses (151).

The most frequent clinical presentation in children with EIMS and DIMS is an acute encephalopathy with multifocal deficits, more frequently acute hemiparesis with unilateral or bilateral pyramidal signs (81%). Other neurologic signs and symptoms present in 30% to 40% of patients include altered mental status, headache, vomiting, brainstem dysfunction, cerebellar ataxia, and meningeal signs. Most of the children recover from this dramatic picture after treatment with corticosteroids or may be left with mild residual deficits.

The patients with JMS, however, present isolated demyelinating syndromes, the most frequent one being the sensory hemisyndrome (64%), with or without associated motor findings, frequently without signs of acute diffuse encephalopathy. Acute loss of vision due to optical neuritis is observed more frequently as an initial symptom in children younger than 10 years of age (23%) than in those with JMS (16%). Seizures are infrequent (6% in our experience), and they present only in children less than 5 years of age, as part of the acute encephalopathy. Nevertheless, seizure frequency as high as 22% has been reported in early infantile forms of MS (80). Sensory findings, as indicated, are a frequent finding in these patients, and should suggest the diagnosis of MS. Paraparesis is often associated with abnormalities of posterior column function, which is often overlooked in adolescents because of an inadequate examination (53,64). Sometimes patients feel transient paroxysmal sensory phenomena such as sensation of a constricting truncal band or unexplained momentary exacerbation of sensory disturbance, associated or not with weakness, l'Hermitte sign (electric shock–like painful sensations spreading from the spine down into the extremities), and the Uhthoff phenomenon [transient appearance or worsening of neurologic dysfunction in association with exercise or exposure to hot ambient temperatures (atmospheric or while showering or bathing)] (53,64).

Children with MS more frequently present with a polysymptomatic form of the disease (43%) than a monosymptomatic one (36%), whereas the opposite is true for adults (35% and 65%, respectively) (77). Both children and adults commonly develop pyramidal signs, paresthesias, or myelopathy, but adults have a high incidence of brainstem and cerebellar signs and rarely manifest an acute encephalopathy (82,152,153).

Other symptoms that pediatric patients may experience as a consequence of MS include fatigue, spasticity, school difficulties, and emotional liability. Fatigue is described as "a subjective lack of physical or mental energy of sufficient severity as to interfere with the child's ability to complete requisite school work, engage in extracurricular activities, or interact socially with peers" (77). Spasticity is one of the most common symptoms of MS; it hinders functional mobility, and is related to the course of the disease. Therefore it is more prominent in adults than children (154). Cognitive impairment has been demonstrated in pediatric MS patients (155,156). Adolescents with MS report difficulty with higher-order concepts and with organization of multiple tasks (77). The psychological impact of MS on the child or adolescent may be profound, although most children cope well with their diagnosis (77). More serious neuropsychiatric manifestations are seen in adults (157). Bowel and bladder dysfunction can also be an issue, although it is much less frequent in children than in adult patients (77). Epilepsy usually appears late in the course of the disease and, therefore, it is usually not seen in children with MS. Sometimes seizures may herald the onset of the condition or a relapse; they have a good prognosis (158–160).

Diagnosis

The diagnosis of MS in children is essentially clinical. It is supported by the neurologic examination, which reveals signs of white matter involvement with a defined temporal and spatial course, following the diagnostic criteria of Poser and colleagues (148). Additional studies, including MRI, CSF, and brain evoked potentials, complete the diagnostic process according to the new guidelines from the International Panel on the Diagnosis of MS (161) (Table 8.3)

Immunologic Studies

Immunologic abnormalities can be found both in the serum and the CSF. Dysfunction of cellular immunity is represented by an increase in the circulating CD4+ T-helper/inducer to CD8+ T-suppressor/cytotoxic cell ratio during MS relapses (53,162,163). Molecular markers of apoptosis (i.e., regulator CD95, caspases 8 and 10), and cytokine IL-10 and TNF-α in peripheral blood mononuclear cells correlate inversely with new MRI inflammatory activity, indicating that the CD95-dependent pathway plays a complex role in the regulation of survival of activated immune cells in MS (164).

CSF abnormalities in MS patients are characteristic, although neither specific nor pathognomonic. During the acute phase of demyelination there is lymphocytic pleocytosis of variable degree (30% to 70%), not generally exceeding 50 cells/mm^3 (65,71,165,166). Dysfunction of the humoral immunity is a consistent finding in patients with MS and is represented by the almost universal presence in the CSF of (a) detectable oligoclonal immunoglobulins by electrophoresis, (b) elevated rates of synthesis and concentrations

TABLE 8.3 Diagnostic Criteria of Multiple Sclerosis

Clinical Presentation	*Additional Data Needed for MS Diagnosis*
Two or more attacks; objective clinical evidence of two or more lesions	None[a]
Two or more attacks; objective clinical evidence of one lesion	Dissemination in space demonstrated by MRI[b] or Two or more MRI lesions consistent with MS plus positive CSF[c] *or* Await further clinical attack at a different site
One attack; objective clinical evidence of two or more lesions	Dissemination in time, demonstrated by MRI[d] *or* Second clinical attack
One attack; objective clinical evidence of one lesion (monosymptomatic presentation; clinically isolated syndrome)	Dissemination in space demonstrated by MRI[b] *or* two or more MRI lesions consistent with MS plus positive CSF[c] *and* Dissemination in time, demonstrated by MRI[d] *or* Second clinical attack
Insidious neurologic progression suggestive of MS	Positive CSF[c] *and* Dissemination in space, demonstrated by (a) nine or more T2 lesions in brain *or* (b) two or more lesions in spinal cord, or (c) four to eight brain plus one spinal cord lesion *or* Abnormal VEP[e] associated with four to eight brain lesions, with fewer than four brain lesions plus one spinal cord lesion on MRI *and* Dissemination in time, demonstrated by MRI[d] *or* Continued progression for 1 year

MS, multiple sclerosis; MRI, magnetic resonance imaging; CSF, cerebrospinal fluid; VEP, visual-evoked potential.
[a]No additional tests are required, but if MRI and CSF studies are done and are negative, alternative diagnoses must be considered.
[b]MRI must fulfill criteria of space dissemination (see text).
[c]Presence of oligoclonal bands different from any such bands in serum, or by a raised immunoglobulin index.
[d]Presence of a new gadolinium-enhancing lesion at least 3 months later.
[e]Abnormal visual-evoked potential: delay with a well-preserved waveform.
From McDonald WI, Compston A, Edan G, et al. Recommended diagnostic criteria for multiple sclerosis: guidelines from the International Panel on the Diagnosis of Multiple Sclerosis. *Ann Neurol* 2001;50:121–127. With permission.

in the CSF of intrathecally generated immunoglobulin G (IgG) and IgM with varied or unknown epitopic specificity, and (c) increased levels of immunoglobulin components such as kappa chains (53,65,71,165–169). The finding of oligoclonal bands (OCB) of IgG present in the CSF and absent in blood has been described in 65% to 95% of adult patients with MS (33,166,170,171). The reported frequency of OCB in children with MS is variable, which is probably a reflection of the different methodologies used (172). With the isoelectric approach followed by inmunofixation, Tenembaum and colleagues (82,83) detected positive CSF OCB in 27 of 51 (53%) children with MS. The detection rates for the three clinical forms, EIMS, DIMS, and JMS, were, respectively, 46%, 38%, and 64%. Recently, the serum analysis of antimyelin antibodies, notably anti-MOG and anti-MBP, has been shown to be relatively effective in predicting the progression of isolated demyelinating syndromes to full blown MS (173). Rejdak and collaborators (174) reported increased CSF levels of nitric oxide metabolites (nitrite and nitrate levels) in adult MS patients, which correlated with clinical and MRI progression of the disease over a 3-year follow-up. Sueoka and colleagues (175) found selective CSF synthesis of antibodies against ribonucleoprotein B1 in adults with relapsing-remitting MS, suggesting that they could be a disease marker for MS.

Neurophysiology

Neurophysiologic studies are not specific. The electroencephalogram (EEG) can show changes corresponding to the epilepsy diagnosed in some patients (148,158, 160). Aphasic status epilepticus, epilepsia partialis continua, and periodic lateralized epileptiform discharges have been reported (176–178). Prolonged treatment with corticosteroids induces changes of the sleep EEG in MS patients similar to the changes observed in patients with an acute depressive episode (179). Evoked potentials (EPs) provide information about dissemination of demyelinating disease within the CNS (77). Visual and somatosensory EPs can demonstrate a second lesion (180). Although their usefulness in pediatric MS has yet to be formally evaluated, abnormalities in visual and somatosensory EPs have been demonstrated (68) and are likely to be of similar diagnostic significance as in adult MS patients (181–183).

Anatomic Neuroimaging

Brain and spinal cord MRI are the neuroimaging modalities of choice for evaluating children with demyelinating disorders in general and MS in particular. The typical MRI lesions described in adult patients with relapsing-remitting MS are round or oval plaques, bright or hyperintense on T2-weighted, proton density, and fluid-attenuated inversion recovery (FLAIR) images. They are variable in number and distributed in the white matter of the centrum semiovale, adjacent to the ventricles, and in the corpus callosum, brainstem, cerebellum, optic nerves, and spinal cord (118,181). These lesions are perpendicular to the lateral ventricles, are usually small (less than 5 mm), and show an incomplete, nonuniform enhancement with gadolinium. In the experience of one of us (S.N.T.) the cerebral images of patients with juvenile MS are not different from this classic description at the time of the initial presentation or during relapses (82,83) (Fig. 8.2A).

In contrast, brain MRIs performed during the initial demyelinating episode in children younger than 10 years of age show large multifocal demyelinating plaques with a tendency to coalesce (Fig. 8.2B) in 80% of cases (83), a finding that is somewhat underrated (72). These lesions can have a tumefactive (tumor-like) appearance with variable mass effect. Usually these can be differentiated from tumors by the lesser amount of edema around the lesions frequently (but not invariably) in association with other typical, smaller lesions (184) (Fig. 8.2C). That said, there are reported cases of infantile MS with a solitary plaque associated with perilesional edema (185). The enhancement with gadolinium can be helpful for establishing this difference because the demyelinating plaque usually shows an enhancement pattern of incomplete "hoop" or "open ring" (186). Up to 15% of patients with juvenile MS may have tumefactive lesions on the MRI at the time of the initial attack. The presence of "black holes" on unenhanced T1-weighted images and signs of brain atrophy, like widened subarachnoid spaces, ventriculomegaly, and thinning of the corpus callosum, have not been frequently described in the pediatric literature, but these findings are clearly seen in children with secondarily progressive clinical forms of MS (82).

The MRI images observed in children with an initial attack of EIMS or DIMS recall the images of patients with ADEM (187,188). Characteristic lesions are large and disseminated in the subcortical white matter, but also in the cortex and deep gray nuclei, without the distribution and morphology observed in juvenile and adult MS. As a rule, only if subsequent studies at the time of clinical follow-up or relapses show new lesions that enhance with gadolinium can the diagnosis of MS can confirmed (161,189,190). With this in mind, it should be recognized that ADEM can be accompanied usually by one or several episodes of relapse (biphasic or multiphasic ADEM) (161,189,190), but successive MRIs will reveal active lesions only in the context of a concomitant clinical attack; in other words, "subclinical" or "silent" lesions exhibiting active MRI changes (that are typical of MS) are not seen in ADEM (188,191).

According to the new guidelines from the International Panel on the Diagnosis of MS, (161,192), in certain clinical situations, MRI lesions must fulfill the diagnostic criteria of space dissemination, which include three of the following four: (a) one gadolinium-enhancing lesion or nine T2 hyperintense lesions if there is no gadolinium enhancement, (b) at least one infratentorial lesion, (c) at least one juxtacortical lesion, and (d) at least three periventricular lesions. One spinal cord lesion can be substituted for one brain lesion (161). However, these criteria may not apply as well to the pediatric MS population. Children with MS appear to have fewer white matter lesions at the time of their MS diagnosis than do newly diagnosed adults. Moreover, because myelinogenesis is incomplete in childhood, this may influence lesion appearance, size, and distribution within the CNS. Further studies are necessary to develop MRI diagnostic criteria that are validated in the pediatric MS population (193).

MRI and MR spectroscopy (MRS) in patients with MS for less than 5 years shows brain atrophy and loss of axonal integrity. Although the exact mechanisms underlying CNS atrophy in MS patients are largely unknown, evidence exists that atrophy may be secondary to the repeated effects of inflammatory demyelination, axonal injury, including dystrophic changes and frank axonal transection, wallerian degeneration, and neuronal loss (56,194, 195).

Functional Neuroimaging

Although routine MRI is the mainstay of diagnosis of MS, there is increasing interest in using quantitative MRI methods to better understand pathology in gray matter and normal-appearing white matter. Magnetization-transfer MRI and diffusion-weighted MRI are techniques that provide additional useful information about the process of demyelination and remyelination in MS (196). In addition, functional neuroimaging studies like MRS, functional MRI (fMRI), single photon emission computed tomography (SPECT), and positron emission tomography (PET) allow a better study of the CNS dysfunction secondary to the pathologic changes of the disease (194,196).

MRS of the cerebral demyelinating plaques in children shows a spectrum of alterations with reduction of *N*-acetylaspartate (NAA) and creatine and increase of choline and myo-inositol compared with age-specific controls (71,197). MRS in adults with MS may also show elevation of lactate in the acute demyelinating plaque, but this finding has not been reported in children (74). The white matter adjacent to the plaques that has a normal appearance on MRI has a normal metabolic pattern on MRS, but the adjacent gray matter usually shows a decrease in NAA (197). These data are similar to the findings in adult patients, and are the consequence of neuronal, including axonal, injury in addition to myelin damage that occurs early as a result of repeated inflammatory demyelinating insults (194,196).

fMRI is being used in clinical research to study the neuronal mechanisms that underlie CNS function and to define abnormal patterns of brain activation that arise from

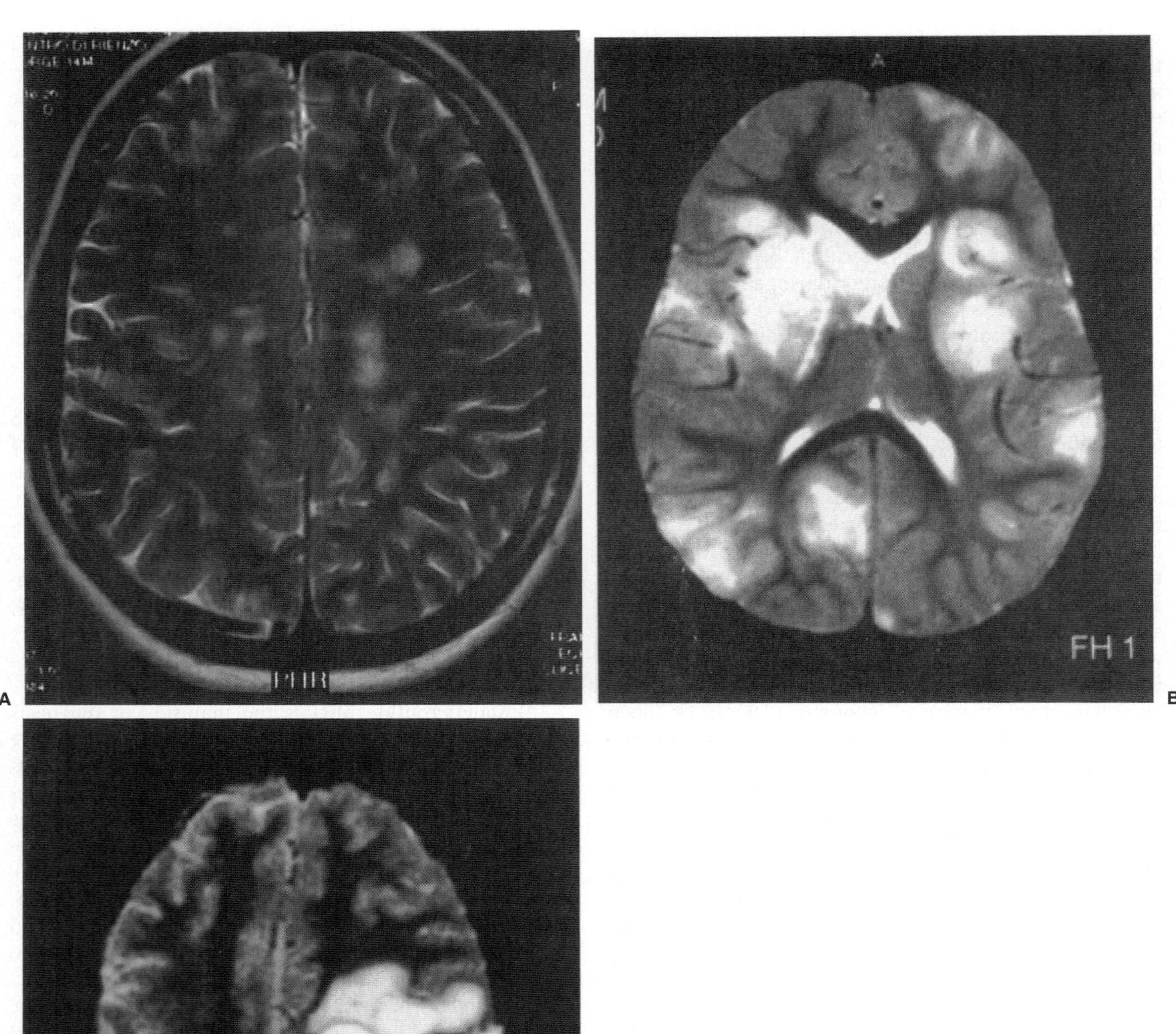

FIGURE 8.2. **A:** Juvenile MS. Axial T2-weighted magnetic resonance imaging (MRI) showing small, hyperintense lesions in the periventricular white matter. **B:** Early infantile multiple sclerosis (MS). Axial T2-weighted MRI with numerous bilateral, predominantly subcortical demyelinating lesions. Right thalamic lesion shows expansive effect with partial ventricular collapse. **C:** Juvenile MS. Axial T2-weighted MRI, with extensive tumefactive lesion in the left frontoparietal white matter. A "satellite" small lesion can be observed in the contralateral white matter.

disease (196,198). A changed pattern of cortical activation, mainly characterized by increased activation of the contralateral primary sensorimotor cortex, has been found in MS patients with clinically isolated syndromes when they do a simple motor task (199). A strong correlation has also been found between the extent of activation of the contralateral primary sensory motor cortex and the reduction of the whole-brain NAA concentration, which suggests that functional cortical reorganization might contribute to the maintenance of normal cortical function in the early stages of MS. Increased activation of several sensorimotor areas, mainly in the cerebral hemisphere ipsilateral to the extremity used to do the task, has also been reported in patients with early MS and preceded by an episode of hemiparesis (200). In patients with similar characteristics but with optic neuritis as their first clinical manifestation, sensorimotor areas mainly located in the contralateral cerebral hemisphere were recruited (201). Abnormal brain activation of the prefrontal/frontal lobe has been demonstrated in MS patients with fMRI during specific tasks; the dysfunction normalizes with rivastigmine, a central cholinesterase inhibitor (202).

New functional MRI techniques are being developed to study *in vivo* CNS diseases at a molecular level (194). Experimental studies with Theiler murine encephalomyelitis virus have investigated MRI techniques using antibodies linked to superparamagnetic particles directed against immune-specific immune determinants. This allows selective imaging of CD4+ T cells, CD8+ T cells, and Mac1+ cells in the CNS (203). Being able to monitor dynamically the activity of specific classes of inflammatory cells in MS will provide an important way of understanding the evolution of pathology and the effects of interventions (194).

In a study of 17 MS patients, ^{99m}Tc-D,L-hexamethylpropylene amine oxime (99m Tc-HmPAO) SPECT showed reduced ratios of regional to whole-brain activity in the frontal lobes and left temporal lobe (204). A relationship was found between left temporal lobe abnormality and deficit in verbal fluency and verbal memory. SPECT is also useful in evaluating MS patients with depressive disorders (205) and in establishing the differential diagnosis of tumor-like lesions (206).

PET studies have demonstrated that global and regional cortical glucose metabolism is significantly reduced in MS patients compared with normal controls. Such a decrease correlates with number of relapses, total lesion area on MRI, and cognitive dysfunction, indicating that MRI white lesion burden causes deterioration of cortical cerebral neural function (207–209). Hypometabolism is widespread, including the cerebral cortex (frontal, parietal, occipital), supratentorial white matter (parietal), and infratentorial structures (pons) (208,210). Using a radioligand for the peripheral benzodiazepine receptor, PET has allowed the visualization of microglia and its involvement in the inflammatory processes causing MS (211).

Neuroimaging techniques will continue to develop in the future to provide not only more accurate diagnosis of MS, but also important prognostic information (194,196).

Differential Diagnosis

The differential diagnosis of MS is broad. Although the clinical signs and symptoms, the MRI changes, and the CSF findings are characteristic of MS, they are not specific and can be found in other inflammatory or infectious conditions, as given in Table 8.4.

TABLE 8.4 Differential Diagnoses of Multiple Sclerosis

Acute CNS Infection
Acute viral encephalitis (i.e., HSV, enterovirus)*
HTLV-1 infection (tropical spastic paraparesis)
CNS tuberculosis
Progressive multifocal leukoencephalopathy
Neuro-AIDS
Neuroborreliosis (Lyme disease)
Subacute sclerosing panencephalitis
Postinfectious Conditions
Acute disseminated encephalomyelitis*
Bi- or multiphasic encephalomyelitis*
Transverse myelitis
Postinfectious cerebellitis
Postinfectious brainstem encephalitis
Vasculitis
Systemic lupus erythematosus*
Behçet disease
Sjögren syndrome
Isolated CNS vasculitis*
Prothrombotic States
Antiphospholipid syndrome
Ischemic vascular disease
Moyamoya disease
Intracranial Tumors
Gliomatosis cerebri*
Hereditary Metabolic Disorders
Leukodystrophies (i.e., adreno-, metachromatic-)
Mitochondrial encephalomyopathy*
Beta-oxidation disorders
Acute, Subacute, or Chronic Spinal Cord Disorders
Tumor
Syringomyelia
Anchored marrow
Arteriovenous malformation
Subacute combined degeneration (B_{12} deficiency)
Arnold-Chiari malformation
Vascular Headache (i.e., Migraine)
Chronic Inflammatory Demyelinating Polyneuropathy
Leber Optic Atrophy

The asterisk denotes more common differential diagnoses.
HSV, herpes simplex virus; HTLV-1, human T-cell lymphotropic virus-1; CNS, central nervous system; AIDS, acquired immune deficiency syndrome.

Treatment

The treatment of MS in children, as in adults, must include the suppression of the inflammatory immune responses during relapses and the amelioration of the associated inter-relapse symptoms (i.e., fatigue, spasticity, urinary tract infections) (77).

Initial treatment consists of the administration of corticosteroids, either orally or intravenously (212). The use of an intravenous (IV) pulse of methylprednisolone is indicated in severe attacks, characterized by marked involvement of mental status, optic nerves, or spinal cord, or in cases with tumefactive lesions on MRI (213). The recommended dose is 30 mg/kg per day to 1 g/day, administered as a 1-hour infusion on 3 to 5 consecutive days, followed by oral administration of methylprednisone, 1 mg/kg per day in the morning during the next 10 days, followed by tapering over a 3-week period. Administration of IV methylprednisolone hastens recovery from acute exacerbations of the disease (77). Recent studies have shown that methylprednisolone suppresses the expression of genes associated with T-cell differentiation and activation, which may contribute to its beneficial effect in relapses of MS (214). Treatment with corticosteroids requires careful monitoring of blood pressure, urine glucose, and serum potassium and administration of gastric protection.

Relapses that are not as severe can be treated with oral methylprednisone at a dose of 1 to 2 mg/kg per day for 10 to 15 days. By and large, very mild exacerbations manifested only by sensory symptoms like paresthesias do not require treatment. Chronic administration of corticosteroids is not indicated because it has been shown that they do not modify the natural history of the disease in adult patients and can cause serious side effects in children (213).

Some children who do not respond to IV corticosteroids may benefit from IV immunoglobulin (IVIG) (77). The recommended dose is 2 mg/kg in divided doses over 2 to 5 days. There are no studies of IVIG efficacy in pediatric MS. Its efficacy in adults was recently reviewed in a meta-analysis, which suggested a potential role for IVIG in patients with high relapse frequency (215). Similarly, IVIG treatment for the first year from onset of the first neurologic event suggestive of MS significantly lowers the incidence of a second attack and reduces disease activity as measured by MRI (216). In a single-blind study of adolescents and adults, IVIG showed a similar efficacy to INF-β1a in decreasing the relapse rate in relapsing-remitting MS (217). In contrast, IVIG did not show any clinical benefit in a group of adult patients with secondary progressive MS (218).

The efficacy and long-term benefits of other immunosuppressive agents in MS are unclear. In this regard, there are only a few trials in adults and none in children. Azathioprine has been used alone and in combination with IVIG (217) or IFN-β1b (219). Although this immunosuppressive agent appears to reduce the relapse rate in MS patients, its effect on disease progression and neurologic disability has not been established (220). Methotrexate may alter the course of disease favorably in patients with progressive MS, but the evidence is tenuous (215).

Cyclophosphamide has been used in adults with variable success. It appears to be more efficient in the early stage of progressive MS independent of age, relapses, or neurologic disability scale (221). The preliminary analysis of a randomized, single-blind, parallel-group, multicenter trial in MS patients of pulse cyclophosphamide demonstrated it to be a therapeutic option as rescue therapy for patients who are IFN nonresponders (222). In addition to having a general immunosuppressant effect, cyclophosphamide has selective immunosuppressant effects in MS by suppressing IL-12 Th1-type responses and enhancing Th2/Th3 responses (IL-4, IL-10) (223). Cyclophosphamide has been used in a few children with very aggressive MS after failed IVIG and IFN therapies. Potential risks of immunosuppression, malignancy, and infertility should be carefully weighted against potential benefits and be thoroughly discussed with the patient and family (77).

Mitoxantrone is another potent immunosuppressive agent used to treat MS in adults. In a study of 94 patients followed for 3 years, it was effective in improving or stabilizing the course of the disease, particularly in patients with a low rate of relapses (224).

Plasmapheresis has shown efficacy in some studies of adult MS patients (225–227). However, its efficacy in the treatment of MS is controversial (228).

The usefulness of immunomodulatory treatments, which have been demonstrated to improve the natural history of MS in adults, such as IFNs (229–232) and glatiramer acetate (copolymer 1, or Copaxone) (233), has not been investigated with controlled studies in children, although there is evidence of success in isolated cases (77). IFN-β1b (Betaseron, Betaferon) is tolerated well and has been shown to produce clinical benefit in children with MS (234–236). Tenembaum and colleagues (213,237) reported their experience treating 31 children with IFN-β1a (Avonex) 30 μg once a week, IFN-β1a (Rebif) 22 μg three times a week, IFN-β1b (Betaseron), 250 μg every other day, and glatiramer acetate (Copaxone) 20 mg daily. The tolerance to the four treatments was similar to that reported in adult patients. Children showed flulike symptoms in 61% of cases, reactions at the site of injection in 39%, migraines in 29%, and systemic transient reaction in 6%; these symptoms gradually decreased until their disappearance in a few months. The doses were titrated according to age, weight, and clinical response. Analysis of the efficacy showed a significant reduction of the rates of relapse in 94% of patients with relapsing-remitting MS and in 33% of patients with secondary progressive MS.

Preliminary clinical trials suggest that combination therapy in MS does not increase the side effects of approved monotherapy; its efficacy over monotherapy should therefore be tested (238).

Natalizumab (Tysabri) is an anti-α4-integrin monoclonal antibody that blocks $\alpha 4\beta 1$-integrin–mediated leukocyte migration. The latter binds to vascular cell adhesion molecule-1, which is expressed at high levels in the blood vessels in the CNS during MS exacerbations (239). An open-label studied of 38 patients with relapsing-remitting MS stable on treatment with IFN-β1a demonstrated the safety of this combination (240), and a large multicenter study provided efficacy results sufficient for the U.S. Food and Drug Administration to approve Tysabri in 2004 as an IV formulation for the treatment of multiple sclerosis (and Crohn disease) in adults.

Other therapeutic approaches that are being investigated and may provide new therapeutic alternatives for MS in the future are (a) selective immunosuppression against T-cell homing (241); (b) immunomodulation using new drugs like statins (242) or targeting new mechanisms like chemokine receptors or dendritic cells that inhibit T cells (243,244), neuroprotective agents like erythropoietin (245), or T-cell migration per se with antimetalloproteinases (246) or antioxidants (247); (c) interventions aimed at iron and iron-mediated production of free radicals (248); (d) T-cell vaccination (249); (e) stem cell transplantation (250); and (f) gene therapy (251)

Symptomatic treatment is paramount to improving the quality of life of patients with MS (252). Modafinil and amantadine are effective in treating fatigue (253). Exercise and yoga (52) have also demonstrated a beneficial effect. Depression responds well to pharmacotherapy (253a). Spasticity (154) and epilepsy (158–160) should be treated with the appropriate specific medications.

A multidisciplinary approach to the care of these children and their families through assessment, support, education, advocacy, referral, and coordination of care is ideal for the best control of the disease and the best quality of life (254).

Prognosis

In adult patients, the clinical course of the disease is highly variable. Relapsing-remitting MS is the most frequent form of progression (80%), followed by secondary progressive MS after an initial period of frequent bouts (26%) and primary progressive MS (6% to14%).

There is a scarcity of information about the clinical course and prognosis of MS in children. In a study of 296 children having a first episode of acute CNS inflammatory demyelination, the rate of a second attack was higher in patients with age at onset older than 10 years, MS-suggestive initial MRI, or optic nerve lesion and lower in patients with myelitis or mental status change (255). In the series of one of us (S.N.T.) (83) the clinical course of a group of children with an established diagnosis of MS was relapsing-remitting (73%) or secondary progressive (25%). No patient developed primary progressive MS. Other authors have published similar findings (78,256)

The natural history of MS in adults shows that in the long term the frequency of disease exacerbations decreases spontaneously (257). In the experience of Tenembaum and colleagues (83) the mean number of bouts per year was 2, 2.3, and 2.2 for EIMS, DIMS, and JMS, respectively, during the first year of disease. These figures decreased to 0.9, 1.4, and 1.5, respectively, at the time of 4 to 8 years follow-up. These findings indicate that children with MS have a tendency to undergo more relapses of demyelination than adults, although they also show a spontaneous reduction of the frequency of relapses with time.

Relapses can be provoked by acute febrile viral illnesses. Bacterial infections, typically those involving the urinary tract of girls or women with MS, may provoke a relapse, but it is more likely that they worsen the degree of already existing disease activity. There is no proof that live-virus vaccine or influenza vaccine provokes relapses. Other factors that may be associated with a relapse include stress, physical trauma, surgery, and spinal anesthesia (53).

As the frequency of relapses increases, recovery is hampered and deficits may become cumulative. As a rule, the longer the bout, the greater is the likelihood that recovery will be incomplete (53). The evaluation of neurologic disability is usually performed utilizing the Expanded Disability Status Scale (EDSS) of Kurztke (258,259). However, this method, which is widely used in adults, shows clear limitations in children. In the series of Tenembaum and colleagues (83), after a mean follow up of 6.6 years, 70% of children with MS had an EDSS score of 3.5, that is, they were ambulatory without assistance; 9% had scores between 4 and 4.5, indicating moderate disability with limitations, but still ambulatory; 15% had scores ranging from 6 to 9.5, meaning that they ambulated with assistance or were wheelchair bound. These data demonstrate that MS in children, both the infantile and juvenile variants, cannot be considered a benign disease because its clinical course can be aggressive and cause significant physical handicap.

Children in the series of Mikaeloff and coworkers (255) were followed up for a mean of 3 years. Ninety percent had no or minor disability. Occurrence of severe disability was associated with a polysymptomatic onset, sequelae after the first attack, further relapses, and progressive MS.

The mortality rate in pediatric MS has been reported to range from 10% to 40% during the first 5 years of disease (147,260). In the experience of one of us (S.N.T.), 3 of 51 children (6%) with progressive secondary MS died after a period of 3 to 12 years of disease (83).

Variants of Multiple Sclerosis

Three variants of MS that have attracted considerable attention among neurologists are Schilder disease (myelinoclastic diffuse cerebral sclerosis), Devic disease (neuromyelitis optica), and Baló disease (encephalitis periaxialis concentrica).

Schilder Disease (Myelinoclastic Diffuse Cerebral Sclerosis, Encephalitis Periaxialis Diffusa)

Myelinoclastic diffuse sclerosis (MDS) is a rare demyelinating disorder of the CNS that affects mainly children but also adults (3,261,262). The disease was originally described by Paul Schilder in 1912 under the name encephalitis periaxialis diffusa (263). Schilder subsequently used the same designation to describe two additional cases in 1913 (264) and 1924 (265). However, in the intervening years, the term Schilder disease was applied to a variety of fundamentally disparate CNS diseases affecting myelin. These include MDS (the type in Schilder's original 1912 case), which exemplifies the nosologic position of this disease entity as a variant of MS; leukodystrophies (Schilder's 1913 case); instances of postmeasles subacute sclerosing panencephalitis (SSPE) (Schilder's 1924 case); and atypical cases of ADEM (3,266). This nosologic confusion was eventually clarified in 1956 by Poser and von Bogaert (267), who after analyzing the cases compiled by Bouman in his extensive monograph of the disease (268), found that more than one-half of cases described as Schilder disease or MDS were in fact leukodystrophies, ischemic demyelinations attributed to hypoxic-ischemic encephalopathies, or SSPE. Subsequently, Poser (261) showed that in many cases of MDS, typically scattered lesions of MS also existed in addition to the larger areas of demyelination, attesting to the fact that Schilder's 1912 case was indeed another form of MS, more commonly seen in the young (3). In recent years, additional confusion has been introduced by indiscriminately applying the diagnosis of Schilder disease to cases characterized by large areas of increased signal intensity on T2-weighted MRIs that actually represent instances of ADEM (269).

Currently, Schilder disease (or MDS) is considered to be an inflammatory demyelinating disease of unknown etiology, which constitutes a distinctive clinicopathologic variant of MS affecting the white matter of the cerebrum and the entire neuraxis (119,262,270). The disease is distinguished by two features: First, there is a propensity to produce one or more fairly symmetric, large, often spherical and tumefactive demyelinating lesions in the centrum ovale and central white matter with sparing of the subcortical U fibers (271). Second, there is an exquisite sensitivity to treatment with corticosteroids (272).

Pathology

On anatomic examination of the sectioned brain, the most striking alteration is the grossly discernible demyelination of the central hemispheric white matter. Typically, the plaques are fewer and larger than in classical MS and their deep location with sparing of the U fibers at the gray–white junction serves as a topographic distinguishing feature from ADEM. Remarkably, even in the most severely affected white matter with near total loss of myelin, a narrow band of subcortical, convolutional white matter is usually spared (Fig. 8.3). The lesions are most common in the frontal and posterior parietal/occipital lobes, but can involve any part of the cerebral hemispheres, brain stem, cerebellum, and spinal cord (119).

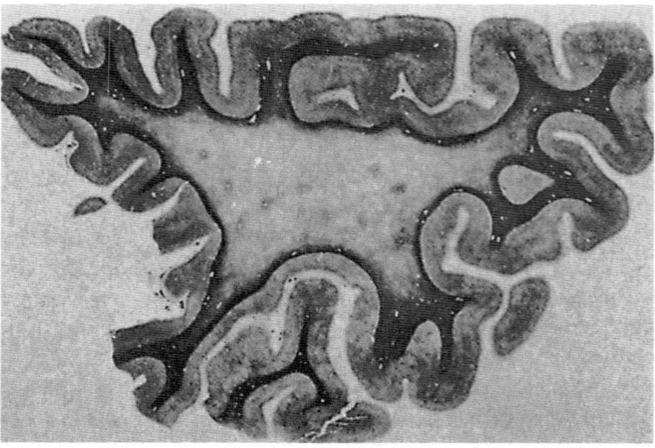

FIGURE 8.3. Diffuse cerebral sclerosis (Schilder disease). Myelin preparation of the frontal lobe demonstrating demyelination. The arcuate fibers are characteristically spared. (Courtesy of the late Dr. D. B. Clark, University of Kentucky, Lexington. KY.)

Histopathologically, the lesions are indistinguishable from active inflammatory demyelinating lesions of MS (262) or ADEM, although there is a distinctive tendency for central necrosis and cavitation especially within larger lesions (119). Histologic sections of the gross specimen confirm the presence of an inflammatory demyelinating process. As a rule in autopsy cases, lesions are of the same age. When they are extensive, multifocal, and confluent they are typically characterized by massive accumulations of foamy or myelin-laden macrophages imperceptibly merging with hypertrophic reactive astrocytes. The former are highlighted by immunohistochemistry using macrophage markers such HAM-56 and CD68, whereas the latter are delineated by robust staining for glial fibrillary acidic protein (GFAP) (50). Focal perivascular mononuclear, lymphocytic-monocytic infiltrates are present.

The pathogenesis of MDS is unknown, but it likely involves similar immunopathogenetic mechanisms to those of MS. As indicated in the discussion of MS pathogenesis, an inflammatory-type oxidative stress injury marked by increased expression of iNOS and nitrotyrosine has also been reported in cases of MDS (50).

Clinical Manifestations

The illness tends to present in children between the ages of 4 and 13 years, although it can be seen in adolescents and adults (53). Onset is often subacute and presents with some combination of headache, lethargy, behavioral and cognitive disturbances, personality changes, progressive clumsiness, and ataxia. Most cases exhibit hemiparesis or asymmetric double hemiparesis, variously combined with aphasia, visual disturbances, dysarthria, oropharyngeal dysfunction, bilateral pyramidal signs, ataxia, or pseudobulbar manifestations (271,273–276). Elevated intracranial pressure with papilledema is occasionally encountered. Unlike ADEM, there is usually no history of prodromal illness or fever (53).

Recently, optic neuritis has been reported as a novel mode of presentation in Schilder disease (277)

Diagnosis

The subacute onset of focal neurologic signs and increased intracranial pressure often suggests a space-occupying lesion, namely a brain tumor or an abscess (278,279). The CSF protein levels are usually within normal range, as is the CD4/CD8 ratio. Oligoclonal bands are detected in some cases (262,276).

Extensive hypodense areas are typically seen on computed tomography (CT). MRI shows massive involvement by either single, albeit large, or multiple areas of cerebral white matter disease consistent with demyelination. Multiple lesions in Schilder disease are characteristically bilateral, but exceptionally multiple unilateral lesions may occur (278). The typical large lesions are usually clearly visible as areas of hyperintense bright signal on T2-weighted images. Some lesions have a tumefactive (tumor-like) cystic appearance, with a peripheral rim enhancing with gadolinium (122,271,276,278,279).

The absence of significant perilesional edema, the irregular and incomplete ring enhancement, and the discrepancy between size of the lesions and the associated mass effect may help differentiate Schilder disease from a neoplastic or pyogenic process (278). As a rule, neuroimaging studies exclude the diagnosis of a tumor or abscess and point to a demyelinating process. The diagnosis of diffuse sclerosis can be made with a high degree of certainty because no other demyelinating condition can progress relatively rapidly to produce edema.

It is important to emphasize that the diagnosis of Schilder disease cannot be made unless adrenoleukodystrophy (ADL) has been ruled out by analysis of the long-chain fatty acids of plasma cholesterol esters (262,280) (see Chapter 3). ADL, which occasionally can progress relatively rapidly, can be distinguished by the presence of very long chain fatty acids in the serum. In addition, ring enhancement distinguishes the lesions of Schilder disease from the myelin abnormalities observed in ADL, which is usually found in the parieto-occipital white matter (281).

MDS must be included in the differential diagnosis in young patients with a brain tumor with atypical neuroimaging features (279,282). Many of these lesions are subjected to open craniotomy and resection because of the suspicion of tumor (278,279,282,283). Biopsy and frozen sections of these are often misinterpreted as astrocytoma. However, the inflammatory nature of the lesion dominated by macrophages, perivascular mononuclear cuffs, and reactive astrocytes is more easily recognized in paraffin-embedded material, especially with the aid of immunohistochemical markers (50,278).

Treatment

Immunosuppression with corticosteroids (methylprednisolone) or with a combination of cyclophosphamide and adrenocorticotrophic hormone (ACTH) has been reported to induce rapid, often dramatic and unequivocal improvement in the majority of cases, with complete or near-complete resolution of the MRI lesions (275,276). In the series by Barth and coworkers, all 5 patients did well after corticosteroid therapy (273).

The rapid early improvement of the clinical manifestations and neuroimaging changes after administration of corticosteroids is a characteristic feature of Schilder disease. Maximal recovery may require weeks or months of treatment and can often be incomplete. The time for discontinuing steroids is not clear-cut and may be dictated by the clinical picture. It may vary from 4 to 6 months (279). The benefit of adding intravenous immunoglobulin to the regimen in patients who attained only partial response to corticosteroid therapy is uncertain (279), and more studies are needed in this regard. The precise effect of corticosteroids in achieving maximal recovery or preventing progression to MS is unclear. Although some uncertainty exists about the optimal dose, it is generally agreed that high doses should be administered intravenously for 3 to 5 days followed by an oral taper. Although the MRI appearances usually improve, abnormalities may persist for years, especially if there is necrosis or cavitation in large tumor-like lesions. In some cases surgical decompressive aspiration of large lesions may improve the recovery (284).

The majority of patients appear to experience prolonged remissions after treatment; however, occasionally there are recurrences (275). As in MS, it is important to distinguish exacerbation caused by tapering of steroids from true recurrences.

Garell and coworkers suggested that there may be two clinical subsets of the disease: (a) a self-limiting, monophasic type, in which patients do well after the first brief episode, and (b) a progressive type, which is less responsive to treatment and may result in severe neurologic deficits or death (279). It is unclear whether these apparently divergent courses in the natural history of the disease represent inherent variations in the nosologic spectrum of MDS or are the result of early or efficacious treatment. Interestingly, in Garell's small series, consisting of only 3 patients, the patient who underwent gross full resection did considerably better than the 2 patients who were treated only medically (279).

Fatal cases of Schilder disease present as a rapidly progressive, unremitting white matter disease resembling acute MS (Marburg type), with diffuse cerebral and spinal cord involvement (50,119).

Neuromyelitis Optica (Devic Disease)

In 1894, Eugene Devic described the case of a 45-year-old woman suffering from bilateral optic neuritis associated with acute transverse myelitis (285). Later, his student F. Gault reviewed 16 patients described in the literature with the same symptoms (285a). Since then, the association of optic neuritis and acute transverse myelitis is known as the syndrome of neuromyelitis optica (NMO) or Devic disease, where both clinical manifestations appear simultaneously or within several weeks or months of one another (53,64,286,287).

NMO is a rare condition in the Western world, although it is not uncommon in Asia (50). It is more frequent in adults (median age of onset is in the fourth decade) and more prevalent in women (288), but it can present in children as well (289–292). Whether NMO is a subtype of MS or a distinct entity is controversial (292). For some authors, NMO is a form of MS, probably modified by histocompatibility antigens or by external factors (53). But it can also be associated with ADEM, systemic lupus erythematosus (SLE), and Sjögren syndrome, infectious diseases, and immunizations (286,288,289). Although familial cases have been reported, NMO is generally a sporadic disease (288).

Pathogenesis

The immunopathogenesis of NMO is unclear. Inflammation plays a major role in NMO, where BBB damage and inflammatory cells prevail, although these changes can fluctuate. The lesions are mostly inflammatory at onset and may undergo necrotizing changes over time (293). Stansbury proposed in 1949 that perivascular inflammation is the initial stage in the pathogenesis of NMO lesions (294). Autopsy studies of patients with NMO have shown abnormal vasculature in the spinal cord (295). The latter may be a target for autoimmune inflammation, with participation of immunoglobulins, activated complement (C9 neoantigen), and macrophages immunoreactive for myelin proteins, including MOG; in addition, T cells and monocytes/macrophages may contribute to the myelin damage (142,286,288). Moreover, eosinophils may play a significant role in the destructive inflammatory process of NMO (142).

Pathology

The most typical neuropathologic features of the lesions are demyelination associated with inflammatory necrosis, a topographic distribution restricted to the anterior part of the optic tract (optic nerve and usually the chiasm) and the spinal cord without any signs of other lesions elsewhere. The spinal lesions are located in one or several segments. They sometimes extend to the whole spinal cord, but usually are not multicentric (296). The lesions progress through a series of stages (294):

1. Acute inflammation with prominent perivascular exudates. Subsequently, inflammatory infiltrates consist mainly of macrophages and microglia, with B lymphocytes also prominent, but few CD3+ or CD8+ T lymphocytes. Early lesions are also characterized by the combined presence of eosinophilic and granulocyte perivascular infiltration (142).
2. Tissue destruction and demyelination.
3. Coalescence of small lesions into larger ones, involving gray and white matter, and necrosis.
4. Reactive microglial changes.
5. Astrocytosis and formation of glial scars. Glial scarring is less frequent and usually only partial, in contrast to typical MS plaques.

The presence of hyalinized medium-sized spinal cord arteries is very characteristic (288,291). The selective localization of NMO lesions may be explained by the vulnerability of the spinal cord and optic nerve to antibody-mediated injury due to inherent susceptibility of the BBB at these sites or less likely by the fact that the latter regions of the neuraxis may harbor anatomically restricted neural or vascular antigen(s) (142).

Clinical Manifestations

Clinically, ON attacks are generally severe and exhibit poor recovery; a minority of patients experience simultaneous bilateral ON. Myelitis attacks are often fulminant, bilateral, complete acute transverse myelitis (ATM) and accompanied by pain and a great degree of residual neurologic impairment (287,288,296). The clinical course is monophasic in about 35% of patients, where there is a single episode of ON and ATM and several years of follow-up that reveals no further exacerbations. Most patients experience a relapsing course, where ON and ATM may be many weeks or even years apart but attacks recur over the next months or years (288,297); 55% of relapses occur within the first year after the initial clinical event, 78% at 3 years, and 90% at 5 years (298).

Diagnosis

The diagnosis is based on the typical association of ON and ATM (see Table 8.5)

The differential diagnosis with connective tissue diseases and MS may be difficult in some cases at the time of the first clinical attack. Early diagnosis and treatment are very important to reduce morbidity of NMO (288,299). Recently, Lennon and collaborators (299) described NMO-IgG, a serum autoantibody against a putative target autoantigen of NMO, associated with both the subarachnoid glia limitans and Virchow-Robin spaces and the

TABLE 8.5 Diagnostic Criteria of Neuromyelitis Optica (Devic Disease)

Absolute criteria	Optic neuritis Acute myelitis No evidence of clinical disease outside the optic nerve or spinal cord
Major supportive criteria	Negative MRI at onset Spinal cord MRI with signal Abnormality extending three or more vertebral segments CSF pleocytosis of >50 WBC/mm^3 or >5 neutrophils/mm^3
Minor supportive criteria	Bilateral optic neuritis Severe optic neuritis with fixed visual acuity <20/200 in at least one eye Severe, fixed, attack-related weakness in one or more limb

MRI, magnetic resonance imaging; CSF, cerebrospinal fluid; WBC, white blood cells.
From Wingerchuk DM, Hogancamp WF, O'Brien PC, et al. The clinical course of neuromyelitis optica (Devic's disease). *Neurology* 1999;53:1107–1114. With permission.

extracellular matrix or parenchymal-penetrating microvessels in the CNS. This antibody was detected in almost three-fourth of patients with NMO, in nearly half of those at high risk of developing NMO, and in about one-tenth of those showing ON or ATM as the initial manifestation of MS. However, it was negative in all patients with classic MS. The authors concluded that NMO-IgG is a specific marker autoantibody of NMO, which is useful for establishing a differential diagnosis with MS and for monitoring the progression of ONM and its response to treatment (299). Patients with ONM also have a high seropositivity for multiple markers of autoimmunity such as antinuclear antibody (ANA), extractable antinuclear antigen (ENA), and thyroid antibodies (288,289).

The CSF is often abnormal with mild elevation of protein and pleocytosis, including neutrophils, up to 3,000 cells/mm^3. Pleocytosis can vary depending on the phase of the disease, being relevant during the acute symptomatic event(s) and normalizing during the stationary phase. Oligoclonal bands may be present, but less often than in typical MS, and, if they are present, they usually disappear in the course of the disease, contrary to what happens in MS (286,289,290,293). In patients with relapsing NMO total IgG concentration is elevated, as in MS patients, but the percentage of IgG1 and IgG1 index are increased only in patients with MS; these findings suggest less Th1 immunity in relapsing NMO and may also explain the rarity of oligoclonal bands in patients with this disease (300).

Brain MRI in NMO patients shows no focal white matter lesion suggestive of MS, whereas spinal cord MRI displays extensive cervical or thoracic confluent, longitudinally extensive lesions, usually longer than two vertebral segments. They are T1 hypointense, which distinguishes them from those described in MS, which are hyperintense in T2-weighted sequences and enhance with gadolinium (288–290,293).

In selected cases, leptomeningeal biopsy shows increased vascularization and thickened hyalinized vessel walls (291).

Treatment

The treatment of choice for acute attacks in NMO is intravenous methylprednisolone for 5 days followed by prednisone taper. In patients refractory to corticosteroids, intravenous IVIG has been used with some success (286,288,291). Plasmapheresis, in a randomized, double-blind, crossover trial in patients with idiopathic inflammatory demyelinating disease, showed moderate or marked improvement in 6 of 10 patients with severe, corticosteroid-refractory NMO (301).

Case series of NMO patients suggest that azathioprine and prednisone may reduce relapse frequency and protect optic nerve and spinal cord function more effectively (302). The use of other immunosuppressive drugs like cyclophosphamide and mycophenolate mofetil has been limited (286,288). The role of immunotherapy with interferons or glatiramer acetate is unclear, but anecdotal evidence has been discouraging (288). Based on knowledge about the immunopathogenesis of NMO, B-cell modulators should be investigated as possible therapeutic agents (288).

Prognosis

The prognosis of patients with NMO has been well studied in adults, and is related to the severity and clinical course of the disease (288–290). In the experience of the Mayo Clinic, patients with monophasic NMO have more severe acute ON and ATM, but the long-term neurologic impairment and disability is significantly less than in patients with a relapsing course. Although 22% of them may remain legally blind at least in one eye, more than 50% recover to 20/30 visual acuity or better. Neurologic impairment is mainly related to sequelae of ATM; most patients experience at least a moderate degree of both limb weakness and sphincter dysfunction. Five-year survival in this group is 90%, and the cause of death is unrelated to NMO or its complications (288). A relapsing course of NMO is more likely to occur if patients are of female gender, are older at disease onset, and have less severe motor impairment with the first ATM attack and there is a longer interval between the first and the second attacks. The prognosis is worse in these patients: at 5 years of follow-up more than 50% will be legally blind in at least one eye. In addition, with each relapse the motor disability increases. Life expectancy is seriously affected: Almost one-third of patients die secondary to recurrent myelitis with respiratory failure and attendant medical complications. The presence of autoimmune disease, the degree of motor recovery after the initial myelitis event, and a higher attack frequency in the first 2 years of disease all predict a shorter survival (288,292,297). Other series of patients with NMO reported similar prognostic data (289,290).

Encephalitis Periaxialis Concentrica (Baló Disease)

Encephalitis periaxialis concentrica was first described in 1927 by Josef Baló in Hungary and was published in the English-language literature in 1928 (303). The characteristic pathologic findings are alternating rings of myelin preservation or remyelination and myelin loss, consistent with demyelination, involving the cerebral hemispheres, cerebellum, brainstem, spinal cord, and optic chiasm (303,304). Lesions show sharp edges, and in almost all cases there are separate small plaques of demyelination (3). Both findings are typically seen in MS, and, therefore, Baló disease is now considered a variant of MS (53).

The exact mechanism for the peculiar configuration of the plaques is unclear, but it has been suggested that it represents a local phenomenon (3). Although the initial triggering event is unknown, a centrifugally spreading band of lymphocytes emanates from the initial site. The polarity of the demyelinating bands suggests that the demyelinating activity is periodically reactivated and then fades in strength as it migrates from the center (304). Candidate modulators of immune activity include the cytokines, some of which undergo periodic level fluctuations (304,305).

The disease appears to be more common in persons of Asian descent, suggesting a genetic predisposition (3,304). It usually has an acute or subacute onset and follows a monophasic course over a period of weeks or months, suggesting a space-occupying lesion (3,304). Frequently, the clinical picture is indistinguishable from that of ADEM (see later discussion) (53).

MRI plays a central role in antemortem diagnosis of this rare disease. The typical findings consist of concentric rings or a whorled appearance on T2-weighted and contrast-enhanced T1-weighted images, which corresponds to pathologic findings (304,306,307). Serial MRI studies demonstrated that concentric lesions do not occur simultaneously, but develop in a stepwise and distinctive centrifugal fashion (308). Brain MRS performed in some patients shows increased choline peak and decreased *N*-acetylaspartate peak, findings similar to the ones described in MS patients (71,197). In some unclear cases, a brain biopsy may be necesary to exclude tumefactive processes such as neoplasm or abscess (304).

High doses of intravenous corticosteroids produce significant improvement of the neurologic symptoms and signs (304,307). Recent reports show a benign course of the disease, without relapses after responding to treatment (304,309,310). This is in contrast with the classic description of patients with a progressive and fatal course diagnosed at autopsy. Therefore, it is likely that benign cases were missed or misdiagnosed before the availability of MRI (304).

Acute Disseminated Encephalomyelitis

Acute disseminated encephalomyelitis (ADEM) is an immune-mediated inflammatory disorder of the CNS, which is commonly preceded by an infection and predominantly affects the white matter of the brain and spinal cord (64,188,311–314).

Although the literature indicates that ADEM is not frequent, it is difficult to establish its real incidence because only isolated cases or small series of patients are usually reported. Leake and colleagues reported an overall incidence of 0.4 in 100,000 per year (315). The incidence of ADEM quadrupled during 1998 through 2000 as compared with earlier years, but this may be attributed to the widespread use of MRI, which has facilitated a more accurate identification of this condition, otherwise frequently diagnosed as "acute nonspecific meningoencephalitis" (188). It has been estimated that ADEM represents approximately one-third of all the patients diagnosed as having encephalitis in the United States (316,317).

ADEM can occur at any age, but it is much more frequent in children probably because of a higher exposure to infections and immunizations. In our experience, the mean age of patients is 5 years, with a male preponderance (188). The presentation may be acute or subacute, and it is typically monophasic, although recurrent or relapsing forms have been reported (190).

Historical Aspects

Illnesses recognizable as ADEM were first described in the late nineteenth century by Osler and others, who were particularly struck by the occasional child who showed remarkable recovery from severe, acute, multifocal encephalitic illnesses. Many cases occurred in association with epidemics of viral illnesses that spread through Europe in the wake of World War I. The characteristic pathology was described almost simultaneously in the late 1920s and early 1930s in children who had died of ADEM after measles, chickenpox, influenza, smallpox, and/or vaccinations (53,313,318).

Over the years, this disorder has received different names, reflecting different salient aspects of the disease:

1. Triggering events: postinfectious or postvaccinial encephalomyelitis (319).
2. Histopathologic features and distribution of lesions: acute perivascular myelinoclasia (320), perivenous encephalitis (321), disseminated vasculomyelinopathy (322).

3. Probable immunopathogenetic mechanisms: acute demyelinating encephalomyelitis (323), hyperergic encephalomyelitis (324), postvaccinial perivenous encephalitis (325).

Based on our clinicopathologic understanding of the disease, ADEM is probably the most appropriate nosologic designation because the precipitating infective event may be absent and the various underlying disease mechanisms are unclear.

Pathogenesis

The pathogenesis of ADEM is thought to be due to disseminated multifocal inflammation and patchy demyelination associated with autoimmune mechanisms in the CNS (53,64,326). Attempts to recover viruses or to demonstrate the presence of viral particles or antigens in the lesions have been unsuccessful. The absence of the typical pathologic findings seen in viral infections indicates that a direct viral invasion of the CNS is not the cause of the disease. The presence of a "silent" (clinically asymptomatic) interval between an antecedent of infection or immunization and the beginning of the encephalopathy, along with the presence of pathologic changes similar to the ones observed in EAE, supports an autoimmune mechanism (2) (see later discussion).

The occurrence of ADEM in humans exposed to rabies vaccine contaminated with brain tissue lends credence to the usefulness of EAE as an experimental model for ADEM and MS (2,312,313,327). The autoimmune hypothesis indicates that T cells directed against viral or bacterial antigens recognize sequences of amino acids shared with myelin proteins (2,328). Activated T cells cross the BBB, facilitating the recruitment and migration of other inflammatory cells, which would contribute to the demyelinating process. Target antigens include basic myelin protein (MBP), proteolipid protein (PLP), myelin oligodendrocyte protein (MOP), myelin associated glycoprotein (MAG), oligodendrocyte basic protein, and others (2,64,311,312,329). Humoral immunity may also play a role. Dale and colleagues (330) demonstrated autoantibodies reactive against putative basal ganglionic antigens in poststreptococcal ADEM associated with dystonia and lesions in the basal ganglia. Autoimmunity can be triggered by several mechanisms, including molecular mimicry, bystander activation, epitope spreading, and "mistaken self" (331). The degree to which these different autoimmune mechanisms are operative in ADEM is not known (313).

The exact molecular mechanisms that cause death of oligodendrocytes in ADEM and its variants are not known; however cytokines, chemokines, and adhesion molecules may collectively contribute to the pathogenesis of inflammatory encephalomyelitis (311,312). TNF-α is considered an important factor in the pathogenesis of EAE (332). It has been suggested that upregulation of Fas ligand (FasL) on autoreactive infiltrating T cells together with upregulation of Fas in resident oligodendroglial cells may account for neural tissue damage via an apoptotic pathway (333).

Genetic susceptibility explains why encephalomyelitic complications develop only in a small percentage of patients who have infections or receive immunizations Among candidate polymorphic MHC and non-MHC genes that contribute to disease susceptibility, including those that encode for effector (cytokines and chemokines) or receptor molecules within the immune system, human leukocyte antigen class II genes have the most significant influence (312,334). Active nitrogen species are overproduced in EAE and nitric oxide has been shown to mediate the death of oligodendrocytes (335). Other suggested mechanisms include oxidative stress–induced cell death of premature oligodendrocytes (336) and excitotoxicity (337).

Pathology

Macroscopic examination of the brain can be essentially unremarkable, although frequently there is edema, with signs of cerebral congestion. The distinguishing histopathologic feature of ADEM is demyelination with perivascular, particularly perivenous inflammation, involving predominantly white matter areas of the cerebral hemispheres, brainstem, cerebellum, spinal cord, and optic nerves (312). The inflammatory process is characterized by a perivascular infiltration of inflammatory mononuclear cells (lymphocytes and monocytes), typically around veins and venules and reactive microglial proliferation. Not infrequently, instances of frank vasculitis, with or without segmental necrotizing changes, marked by transmural inflammatory involvement are encountered. There is associated vasogenic edema, which causes variable degrees of brain and spinal cord swelling. It is significant that the inflammatory process involves both white and gray matter, although the former exhibits more prominent involvement and more severe changes. Within the lesions there is myelin fragmentation with relative preservation of axons, but there may be substantial axonal damage (338). The lesions can be confluent, forming large demyelinating areas. The leptomeninges and the Virchow-Robin spaces show cellular infiltrates of lymphocytes, plasma cells, and, occasionally, neutrophils during the initial stages of the disease. In the late stages, the inflammatory response is replaced by fibrillary gliosis (339).

Clinical Manifestations

Neurologic manifestations begin 3 days to 4 weeks (mean 12 days) following a precipitating event, which can be identified in as many as three-fourths of patients in the experience of one of us (S.N.T.) (Table 8.2) (183).

According to the literature, the viral agents most frequently related to ADEM are influenza A and B, parainfluenza, mumps, rubella, varicella, herpes simplex type 1 (HSV), human herpesvirus-6, Epstein-Barr virus, cytomegalovirus (CMV), hepatitis A and B, and coxsackie virus (311–313,315,328,340–343). Measles infection poses the highest risk for development of ADEM: 1 in 400 to 1 in 1,000 cases, as compared with 1 in 10,000 cases for varicella and 1 in 20,000 cases for rubella (342,344). Less frequently, bacterial infections are implicated in the development of ADEM, including *Mycoplasma pneumoniae*, *Borrelia bugdorferi*, *Chlamydia*, *Campylobacter*, *Rickettsia rickettsii*, *Streptococcus pyogenes*, *Streptococcus* β-hemolytic group A, and *Bartonella henselae* (342,345–347). Immunizations linked to the development of ADEM are those against measles, mumps, rubella, diphtheria-pertussis-tetanus (DPT), varicella, mumps parotitis, rubeola, influenza, Japanese encephalitis type B, and poliomyelitis (311–313,346,348–352). However, the only pathologically proven causal association has been with the old antirabies vaccine, which it is not currently used (327).

Initially the patient may complain of nonspecific symptoms such as headache, low-grade fever, myalgia, and malaise. These are followed by a rapid onset of overt neurologic manifestations including acute encephalopathy coupled with a triad of focal neurologic deficits (hemiparesis, quadriparesis), ataxia, and change in mental status (sleepiness, stupor, or coma). Other symptoms and signs include cranial nerve involvement, meningismus, convulsions, migraine, myelopathy, optic neuritis, aphasia, involuntary movements, and paresthesias (64,188,311–313, 353,354).

Acute severe combined demyelination is characterized by combined findings of central and peripheral demyelination. These patients fulfill the clinical and electrophysiologic diagnostic criteria of Guillain-Barré syndrome, they develop acute change in mental status and multiple cranial nerve palsies, and their neuroimaging studies show white matter abnormalites characteristic of ADEM (355,356).

Diagnosis

The diagnosis of ADEM is based on MRI evidence of multifocal white matter demyelination of a patient in whom there is acute onset of neurologic dysfunction after a latent period preceded by a systemic infection, usually viral, or an immunization (64,188,311,312,314,315,326,357,358).

Immunologic Studies

The peripheral blood counts may be within normal range, although they can also show leukocytosis with lymphocytosis. The CSF is essentially unremarkable in one-half of the patients, whereas in the other half it may show a mild to moderate pleocytosis, rarely, though, above 100 cells/mm^3. Glucose is usually within normal range and protein is moderately elevated (64,188,311,312,314,315, 326,357,358).

The presence of IgG oligoclonal bands or increased IgG index in the CSF, indicating intrathecal synthesis of immunoglobulins, is a rare occurrence (311–313,357). In a series of 84 patients previously reported by one of us (S.N.T.), only 2 patients showed presence of oligoclonal bands; both patients had developed ADEM following HSV encephalitis (188). The finding of increased CSF MBP is an indicator of the destruction of myelin and depends on the timing of performing the spinal tap and on the extent of the demyelinating lesions and has no clinical diagnostic value. High levels of IL-6 (311) and low levels of IL-10 and TNF-α (315) have recently been reported in the CSF of ADEM patients.

A recent study by Yoshikawa and colleagues (359) found low levels of hypocretin in the CSF of ADEM patients that correlated with excessive daytime sleepiness during the course of the disease. The authors suggested that a dysfunction of hypothalamic hypocretin-peptide neurotransmission is involved in the altered state of alertness in these patients.

Neurophysiology

Neurophysiologic studies show nonspecific abnormalities. The EEG performed during the acute phase of the disease shows generalized or focal slowing, with high-amplitude theta and delta waves (188,311,312,326). The observed prolonged latencies in the evoked potentials are nondiagnostic because they can be seen in other acute encephalopathies. However, they correlate well with the clinical and neuroimaging data and can be useful in evaluating the course of the disease. It is important to emphasize that the evoked potentials do not reveal subclinical involvement of functional systems in ADEM, in contrast to MS (311,312).

Anatomic Neuroimaging

MRI examination of the CNS is the investigation of choice for establishing the diagnosis of ADEM (64,315, 360,361), which should be suspected on the basis of the clinical history and neurologic evaluation. Demyelinating lesions are hypointense on T1 and inversion-recovery sequences and hyperintense on T2, proton density, and FLAIR images. Lesions are usually asymmetric and variable in number and size (187,213,311–313,326, 357,362,363). The absence of periventricular changes is one of the key features that help to distinguish ADEM from a first clinical presentation of MS (313,353). The lesions involve the deep white matter with variable compromise of the subcortical white matter of the cerebral hemispheres, cerebellum, brainstem, and spinal cord. However, cortical and deep gray matter involvement is a commonly reported finding (189,313,364). The corpus callosum is usually not

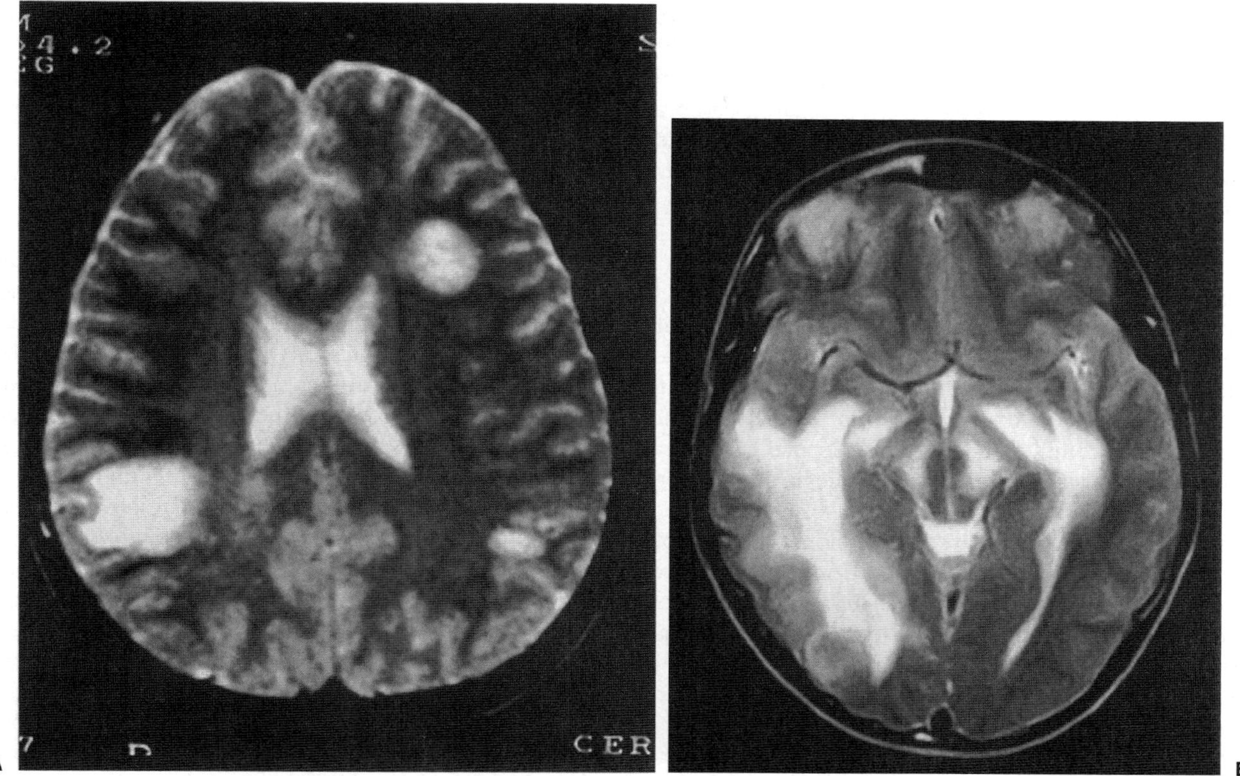

FIGURE 8.4. **A:** Acute disseminated encephalomyelitis (ADEM). Axial T2-weighted magnetic resonance imaging (MRI) showing small, bilateral, hyperintense lesions in the periventricular white matter. **B:** ADEM. Axial T2-weighted MRI with extensive bihemispheric demyelinating lesions involving the white matter and basal ganglia, extending into the mesencephalon.

involved in ADEM; infrequently, its involvement has been reported, suggesting extensive lesion load (312,353). Lesions may not enhance after the administration of gadolinium, or, more often, may enhance in a homogeneous fashion, which indicates that they are in the same phase of progression (365,366). Different patterns of enhancement can be observed, including ring shaped, nodular, incomplete ringlike, and complete-ring shaped (367). Although multifocal or disseminated lesions are characteristic of ADEM, there have been instances with solitary CNS lesions (122,368,369).

Tenembaum and colleagues (188) developed a classification of MRI lesions in ADEM, which include the following groups: A (62%), with small demyelinating lesions (less than 5 mm) (Fig. 8.4A); B (24%) with larger demyelinating plaques (greater than 5 mm or confluent), an asymmetric distribution, and variable tumefactive effect ("pseudotumoral ADEM") (Fig. 8.4B); C (12%), with additional, symmetric, bilateral thalamic involvement; and D (2%): acute hemorrhagic encephalomyelitis (HAEM) or Hurst disease, with large plaques showing some evidence of hemorrhage.

The diffusion-weighted imaging (DWI)-MRI technique adds to the diagnostic power of MRI in patients with ADEM, and may help to elucidate different overlapping phases in CNS inflammation (362,370–372). Diffusion tensor MRI (DT-MRI) measures diffusibility or microscopic random translational motion of molecules and water, which provides information about the orientation, size, shape, and geometry of brain structures. DT-MRI of the basal ganglia has demonstrated that patients with ADEM have a high mean diffusibility (microscopic random translational motion of molecules and water), in contrast to MS patients, suggesting that deep gray matter tissue damage occurs in ADEM patients. DT-MRI may be useful for establishing a differential diagnosis between ADEM and MS (373).

Functional Neuroimaging

Studies with quantitative proton MR spectroscopy reveal low levels of *N*-acetylaspartate (NAA), without increase in choline, and elevated lactate within the regions of prolonged T2 MRI signal, which recover with normalization of clinical and MRI findings (369,371,374).

99m Tc-HmPAO SPECT studies have shown areas of hypoperfusion that are more extensive than the MRI lesions (375–378). SPECT also reflects better the clinical course than the time course of MRI abnormalities; in spite of

MRI becoming normal, SPECT detects persistent cerebral circulatory impairment probably contributing to cognitive and language deficits observed in these patients (376). Similarly, PET scan demonstrated global decreased cerebral metabolism in both hemispheric white and gray matter in a case where MRI showed a focal right frontoparietal demyelinating lesion (378).

Differential Diagnosis

The differential diagnosis of ADEM is broad. In patients presenting with acute changes in mental status, motor focal findings, fever, and partial seizures one is required to rule out acute viral meningoencephalitis, in particular due to HSV. It is recommended to initiate specific antiviral treatment (acyclovir) until MRI and virologic studies confirm or rule out HSV infection (53).

The cases of ADEM with large MRI lesions with variable mass effect need to be differentiated from primary cerebral tumors or Schilder disease (262,368). MRI resolution with corticosteroid treatment in patients with a monophasic disease will support the diagnosis of ADEM but this is not entirely clear-cut given the responsiveness of cases of Schilder disease to steroid treatment.

The use of MR spectroscopy can be of value in supporting the diagnosis of gliomatosis cerebri because it shows high choline/creatine and choline/NAA ratios (379). Clinical and radiologic recovery after a pulse of corticosteroids is diagnostic of demyelinating disease (ADEM or Schilder disease) as opposed to tumor.

The metabolic leukoencephalopathies, such as metachromatic leukodystrophy, Krabbe disease, and adrenoleukodystrophy, as well as mitochondrial disorders should be included in the differential diagnosis (313). However, the clinical course in these disorders is different than in ADEM.

Isolated angiitis of the CNS and macrophage activation syndromes (i.e., familial hemophagocytic lymphohistiocytosis) should also be considered in the differential diagnosis (380).

In patients with bithalamic MRI involvement one has to rule out acute necrotizing encephalopathy of childhood, which presents with a severe, acute neurologic dysfunction and bilateral thalamic necrosis with cavitation (381,382). Patients with ADEM show complete resolution of the bithalamic lesions without cerebral atrophy or gliosis (188,383–385). A similar neuroradiologic pattern can be observed in patients with deep cerebral venous thrombosis (386), but a careful observation of T1 and T2 MRI images in sagittal views makes it possible to rule out this condition when not showing signal changes in the deep cerebral veins and straight sinus. Infantile striatal necrosis and other forms of encephalitis involving the basal ganglia should also be considered in the differential diagnosis of patients with bilateral bright MRI signal in the caudate and lenticular nucleus (387).

Finally, the biphasic or multiphasic clinical forms of ADEM raise the issue of risk of developing MS (188,311, 312,387) (see later discussion).

Treatment

There are no controlled clinical trials investigating therapies for ADEM. Several studies have reported spontaneous and rapid improvement in untreated patients with ADEM (342,357,364,374). Low-dose corticosteroids have no beneficial effect and may be contraindicated (313). However, the use of high doses of corticosteroids during the acute period of the disease is considered the specific treatment directed against the inflammatory immune process. The efficacy of this regimen has been shown in several reports in that it shortens the duration and severity of the encephalopathy (64,188,311,326,357,388,389). The use of intravenous pulses of methylprednisolone is particularly indicated in the clinical forms with severe impairment of consciousness or involvement of the optic nerves or spinal cord and in the neuroradiologic forms with pseudotumor-like or expansive effect (93). The recommended dose of methylprednisolone is 30 mg/kg per day for children less than 30 kg and 1 g/day for those above this weight, for 3 to 5 consecutive days. In patients with a less severe clinical picture one can use oral corticosteroids such as methylprednisone at 2 mg/kg per day or deflazacort at 3 mg/kg per day, for 10 to 15 consecutive days. In every case the discontinuation of the corticosteroids should be gradual over a period of 4 to 6 weeks.

The use of intravenous IgG has been reported in a few case studies and in a small series of children with satisfactory results, particularly in severe cases who did not respond to corticosteroids (326,358,390–392). The experience using plasmapheresis in the treatment of ADEM is limited (226,326,393–395). In our hands, plasmapheresis has been demonstrated to be a good treatment option for patients with a fulminant form of the disease who do not improve on steroids and immunoglobulin (326).

Other alternative therapies deserve to be mentioned. One patient with a fulminant form of ADEM responded to treatment with hypothermia (396). Experimental studies suggest that cyclosporine and NOX-100, a novel nitric oxide scavenger, may have a potential therapeutic application (397,398).

Medical support is an important aspect of the treatment of patients with ADEM. It should include mechanical ventilation in the cases with severe brainstem dysfunction, correction of electrolyte derangements, treatment of the fever, use of antiepileptic drugs in the cases that present seizures, treatment of neurogenic bladder if present, use of antibiotics to treat secondary respiratory, and urinary tract infections and administration of intravenous acyclovir at 30 mg/kg per day when viral herpes encephalitis has not been ruled out (311).

Prognosis

In spite of the dramatic clinical and neuroradiologic presentation, ADEM is considered a relatively benign condition; a full recovery is attained by up to 90% of patients (64,188,314,326,357,358,361,399). However, high mortality rates (10% to 30%) have been reported during the first week of the disease, particularly in cases of ADEM following measles (64,313,400) and in the hemorrhagic form (188,401). The early and aggressive use of corticosteroids and improvement in the care of neurologically critically ill patients have improved the prognosis in ADEM. Patients with poor response to the treatment probably have sustained irreversible structural damage prior to the initiation of therapy.

ADEM is, by definition, a monophasic disease in approximately 90% of patients, who will never have a similar neurologic episode. However, there have been instances of patients diagnosed with ADEM who developed clinical relapses (188,311,313,326,344,380,385,399,402–404). A relapse is characterized by a neurologic dysfunction, usually different than the one present during the previous episode, following an interval of at least 1 month, in a patient with partial or complete recovery. The MRI shows demyelinating lesions in a different location than the one observed during the initial episode (161,313,405). However, cases of recurrence at the previously affected brain site have been reported (406). The frequency of the biphasic (a single relapse during the follow-up) or multiphasic (more than one relapse) ADEM variants ranges between 10% and 20%; recurrences usually occur within 6 months following the initial episode (188,189,399). Biphasic or multiphasic forms of ADEM need to be differentiated from steroid dependency, which is present in patients whose lesions reactivate and whose clinical symptoms recur when stopping the treatment with corticosteroids (188,402).

The clinical variants of ADEM with one or multiple relapses raises a diagnostic problem because a demyelinating disease characterized by a clinical course of relapses and remissions is, by definition, MS. It is useful to consider the following characteristics of ADEM relapses when establishing a differential diagnosis with MS (118,188–190): (a) The clinical relapses are polysymptomatic, (b) the clinical follow-up confirms the absence of multiple new relapses, (c) repeated MRIs do not show new demyelinating lesions and the previous plaques resolve partially or totally, and (d) the CSF does not demonstrate the presence of oligoclonal bands (326).

The possibility of long-term progression of ADEM to MS in children seems low, although there are no series with prolonged follow-up. Tenembaum and colleagues (188) followed 8 children with biphasic ADEM for 3 to 16 years and none of them had further recurrences. The series of Anlar and collaborators (399) consisted of 46 patients followed for 3 months to 10 years; 9 of them had one relapse and 4 had multiple relapses, but no patient was diagnosed with MS. In the series of Hynson and coworkers (357), 4 of 31 children had relapses and 3 showed involvement of the corpus callosum, a feature suggestive of MS, but none of them were diagnosed as having MS. Leake and colleagues (315) followed 42 children diagnosed with ADEM over a 10-year period and found that 4 of them (9.5%) were subsequently diagnosed with MS after multiple episodes of demyelination. This is in contrast to what has been reported in adults. Schwarz and collaborators (407) followed 40 patients aged 15 to 68 years (mean 35.5 years) with ADEM, of whom 14 (35%) developed clinically definite MS. In all of the patients diagnosed with MS, the second episode occurred within the first year of initial presentation. In the longest follow-up (8 years) of 11 patients with final diagnosis of ADEM, none experienced a new clinical attack, and new white matter MRI lesions were seen in only 1 patient.

Although the neurologic recovery in ADEM is good in the majority of patients and the risk of MS is low, neurocognitive deficits are common long-term sequelae. Hahn and coworkers (408) studied 6 children followed for a mean of 4 years after the diagnosis of ADEM and found impairment of tests of attention and executive functions and lower performance than verbal IQ. Similarly, Jacobs and colleagues (409) reported that children with ADEM, particularly those who sustain the illness before 5 years of age, are vulnerable to impairments in both cognitive and social domains and present a high incidence of severe behavioral and emotional problems (409).

Acute Hemorrhagic Leukoencephalitis (Hurst Disease)

This condition is a fulminant variant of ADEM. It is rapidly progressive, causing death usually in the first week of disease due to severe brain edema. However, some patients may survive with an early and aggressive treatment with corticosteroids, cyclophosphamide, and plasmapheresis (188,410–412)

The gross brain may be variably swollen. Histologically, there are numerous, multifocal small hemorrhages in the white matter, with sparing of the cerebral cortex and basal ganglia. However, these microhemorrhages may also become confluent and form lobar-like hemorrhages, which are not usually massive. The microscopic examination demonstrates abnormalites predominantly in the small veins and small arteries. There is necrosis of the walls of the vessels, with fibrinous exudates, perivascular edema, hemorrhage, and scanty neutrophil infiltration (119). The demyelination is perivascular and can even be observed surrounding ostensibly normal vessels. There is substantial axonal damage (338). Genetic susceptibility is a possible determining factor (312,354).

Optic Neuritis

Optic neuritis (ON) is an acute inflammatory condition affecting the optic nerve (413). In the majority of cases it probably has an autoimmune pathogenesis (313). The disease may occur in isolation or in association with other inflammatory demyelinating disorders such as MS with a predilection for spinal cord involvement akin to transverse myelitis (Devic type), classical MS, ADEM, and collagen vascular diseases (53,313). Such an association is more frequently seen in older children and adolescents (414). ON has an incidence of 1 to 5 in 100,000 per year; the incidence is highest in whites, in countries at high altitude, and in spring. Individuals aged 20 to 49 years are most at risk (415). Overall, ON is rare in children, although childhood cases have been described since the late nineteenth century. In the pediatric age group the mean age of onset is 9 to 10 years, and most patients are older than 5 years, but cases as young as 21 months have been reported (416). No gender predilection is seen in prepubertal children, but there is a 2:1 female predominance after the onset of puberty (413,416–418).

Clinical Manifestations

About two-thirds of patients, particularly those younger than 14 years, have a history of an infectious illness within 2 weeks prior to the onset of symptoms (417,419,420). Infections linked to ON include those related to adenovirus, measles, mumps, chickenpox, EBV (53,413), human herpes virus 7 (421), human parvovirus B19 (422), *Mycoplasma* (423), pertussis, and Lyme disease (413). ON may also occur following immunizations, especially for measles, mumps, rubella, hepatitis B, tetanus, rabies, diphtheria, and smallpox (413).

Prodromal symptoms and signs at onset may include fever, frontal or retro-orbital headache accompanied by scintillating scotomata, and painful eye movements (53,64,419,420). In 10% of patients no pain is reported, and in the rest its severity varies, although it does not interfere with sleep (416). A sudden impairment of visual acuity typically follows (413,416–418,420). Initially, the disturbance may be limited to mere visual blurring with progression over several days to partial or complete visual loss (53,64,418). In some instances, the disease becomes biocular a few days or weeks after involvement of one eye. Bilateral ocular involvement is commonly encountered in younger children, as compared to monocular disease, which is seen in adolescents and adults (53,413,414,416,420). In part this tendency may reflect the ability of small children to ignore unilateral visual loss (53). Light flashes (phosphenes or photopsias) might be seen by the patient on eye movement (416). Some patients have subclinical symptoms only manifested as Unthoff phenomenon (visual deterioration on getting warm or during exercise) (416).

Children with ON may also have neurologic deficits, including seizures or signs of cerebellar dysfunction (413,424).

The initial visual acuity ranges from 20/15 all the way to no light perception; however, profound visual loss at onset is more common in children than in adults (413,417). A vision of 20/200 or worse, including counting fingers, has been reported in 84% to 100% of cases in several series (416,417,420,425).

Children with ON usually also have severe visual field defects, including central and cecocentral scotomata, contraction, and other types of defects (arcuate, altitudinal, or vertical) (413,415,417,420).

Color vision abnormalities are common, although color vision testing is limited in very young children (415,420). There is loss of red vision (red desaturation) and loss of duration or variety of the flight of colors that occurs when the eye is closed after a period of bright illumination of the retina (53,64,415,420).

In cases with greater visual impairment, patients present an afferent pupillary defect (loss of the reflexive constriction of the contralateral pupil when the retina of the affected eye is illuminated) (53,64,415). Funduscopic examination is abnormal in 64% to 87% of cases and more commonly shows swelling (anterior neuritis or papillitis), which is usually seen in prepubertal children. Other, more striking abnormalities like optic atrophy, hemorrhages at the optic nerve margin, vascular tortuosity, or sheathing of veins can also be seen (53,64,413,417–420,424). A normal fundus can be observed when the optic nerve is involved proximal to the optic disc (retrobulbar neuritis). This finding is more common in children over 14 years of age (53,64,413,416,417).

Diagnosis

The diagnosis of ON in children is made on the basis of a combination of clinical and laboratory findings. The differential diagnosis in children includes optic neuropathy secondary to sinusitis, orbital cellulitis, optic nerve/optic nerve sheath tumors, neuroblastoma, leukemia, orbital pseudotumor, other demyelinating conditions, and malingering (53,413,416).

CSF examination is frequently unremarkable. However, it can show mild pleocytosis and elevated protein content (416,417,419,420,424). Immune-function studies (IgG index, IgG synthesis rate, oligoclonal bands) may be positive, but are of limited value in differentiating isolated ON from other demyelinating conditions (64,420,424). A major reason to examine the CSF in these patients is to rule out other neurologic disorders that may cause visual disturbances and optic disc changes simulating idiopathic ON (420).

Visual-evoked potentials (VEPs) are helpful in establishing the diagnosis in equivocal cases and in determining the degree of visual dysfunction (53,415,416). During the acute phase of the illness, VEPs are abnormal in almost all of the cases (absent, attenuated, or delayed P100). The abnormality may be present even in patients without evident clinical signs (418,426). After a few days, when the visual acuity improves, VEPs return to normal amplitudes in parallel with the recovering of vision, although decreased amplitude or prolonged latencies may remain in some patients for months or years, even with a good clinical recovery (53,415,426). VEP is superior to MRI for determining chronic optic nerve involvement (427). The combination of VEPs with pattern electroretinogram (PERG) can be useful in differentiating macular from optic nerve disorder: In retinal disorders, both the P50 (early) and N95 (late) components of the PERG are abnormal, whereas in optic nerve disorders, only the N95 component is abnormal (416).

Contrast-enhanced high-resolution CT with fine cuts through the orbits will show up most compressive lesions (416). However, MRI is preferable because it also shows any intrinsic optic nerve lesions, as arise in ON (416). Patients should receive triple-dose gadolinium-enhanced MRI of the brain and orbits. T2-weighted, FLAIR sequence, or fat suppression are also useful techniques (428–430). MRI shows signal abnormalities in 84% of the symptomatic and 20% of the asymptomatic optic nerves with ON (431). Disseminated abnormal MRI signals may be detected in the cerebral white matter of as many as 72% of patients (432). They may resolve, but in a subset of patients with monosymptomatic ON, MRI signal abnormalities may accumulate without causing any clinical manifestations of MS even when the patient is followed up for more than a decade (433). The use of serial MRIs following the mean cross-sectional area of the intraorbital portion of the optic nerve demonstrates a decline over time. This observation indicates that optic nerve atrophy occurs following ON and may continue to develop over the years (430).

Treatment

In adults, the Optic Neuritis Treatment Trial (ONTT) has provided the most comprehensive information regarding the treatment of acute ON (428). Based on data from the ONTT (434–436) and similar trials (437), there is no treatment for acute demyelinating ON that affects long-term visual outcome or visual prognosis compared to placebo. It has been suggested that such a lack of long-term beneficial effect might be because the corticosteroids were given too late to provide neuroprotection; treatment trials in the hyperacute phase are required to address this issue (416).

The most commonly used treatment, IV methylprednisolone (1 g/day for 3 days) followed by oral prednisone, may hasten visual recovery by 2 to 3 weeks when started within 1 to 2 weeks of symptom onset. In monosymptomatic, high-risk patients (two or more white matter lesions), IV methylprednisolone may also delay the onset of MS within the first 2 years. Oral prednisone alone may increase the risk of recurrent ON and should be avoided in patients with typical acute demyelinating ON (423). A Practice Parameter published by the American Academy of Neurology Quality Standards Subcommittee offers similar recommendations (438).

The treatment of pediatric ON with corticosteroids is controversial (416), considering the visual prognosis is good even without treatment regardless of laterality or localization (papillitis vs. retrobulbar) (413). As in adults, intravenous methylprednisolone is recommended (30 mg/kg per day for 3 to 5 days) to hasten recovery of debilitating bilateral visual loss (439), but it does not seem to have an impact on the final visual outcome (416,417). Relapse is frequent in children if the steroids are tapered too quickly, and therefore this should be done over a longer period of time than in adults (at least 4 weeks) (413).

In adult patients who have a severe form of ON unresponsive to corticosteroids, IVIG and plasmapheresis have been used. In a recent study, plasmapheresis was associated with an improvement in visual acuity in 7 of 10 patients with ON largely unresponsive to previous treatments (440).

Among patients with ON at high risk for developing MS (two or more white matter lesions 3 mm or larger in diameter, at least one lesion periventricular or ovoid), treatment with IFN-β1a (Avonex) following acute ON significantly reduced the 3-year cumulative probability of MS (441, 442).

Gene therapy techniques have been applied to experimental models of ON, like EAE. In this model reactive oxygen species contribute to optic nerve demyelination and free-radical scavengers such catalase prevent this process. Catalase gene delivery by using viral vectors could be a potential therapeutic strategy in the futures for patients with severe progressive ON (443).

Prognosis

The prognosis of childhood ON is excellent, particularly when it is bilateral, and the overwhelming majority of children recover their vision completely within weeks or months. The most common sequelae include optic nerve atrophy and impairments of color and stereoscopic vision (53,417,429,443,444). Permanent, severe visual loss is quite exceptional (53). Factors that are associated with a better prognosis in adults are (a) having a short acute lesion on triple-dose gadolinium-enhanced imaging, (b) having higher VEP amplitudes during recovery, and (c) having a steep gradient of the initial improvement in visual acuity (429). In children, younger age, bilateral disease, and a normal MRI portend a better outcome (416).

The risk of recurrent ON after 5 years of follow-up in the ONTT was 19% for the affected eye, 17% for the unaffected eye, and 30% for either eye. The risk was twice as great in patients who had developed MS and was also higher in those who were initially treated with oral prednisone (416,429).

A frequently asked question of concern with prognostic implications for patients with ON and their families pertains to the risk of developing MS at a later time. In adults the rate of progression varies among series, gender, geographic region, and duration of follow-up, ranging from 34% to 74% in New England (445) to 11% in Brazil (446). In children the figures vary from 4% to 26% (420,447–449). Most patients who develop MS following an initial episode of ON will have a relatively benign course for at least10 years (433). Factors that increase the risk of developing MS are bilateral sequential or recurrent ON, Uhthoff symptom, presence of oligoclonal bands in the CSF, and abnormal brain MRI (53,449,450). Conversely, presence of infection within 2 weeks before the onset of ON decreases the risk. Gender, age, funduscopic findings, visual acuity, and family history do not predict subsequent development of MS (420,449). Genetic predisposition may be an important factor in the progression of ON to MS. A recent study conducted in an Iranian cohort of ON patients showed that the HLA class II alleles DR2, A23, and B21 are strongly associated with developing MS (451).

Acute Transverse Myelitis

Acute transverse myelitis (ATM) is a condition characterized by the sudden onset of rapidly progressive weakness of the lower extremities, accompanied by loss of sensation and sphincter control, and often preceded by a respiratory infection (53). ATM has been recognized for more than 100 years. An excellent description of the clinical picture was given by Gowers in 1886 (452). Before then many diseases of the spinal cord were termed myelitis. Only subsequent to the description of MS by Cruveilhier, tabes by Duchenne, Todd, and Romberg, and syringomyelia by Gull and Hallopeau did this entity gain recognition. Its first description in this century is that by Foix and Alajouanine (453). In 1928, it was first postulated that many cases of acute myelitis were postinfectious (rather than infectious) because for many patients the "fever had fallen and the rash had begun to fade" when the myelitis symptoms began (454). It was in 1948 that the term "acute transverse myelitis" was used in reporting a case of fulminant inflammatory myelopathy complicating pneumonia (455).

Pathology and Pathogenesis

Pathologic abnormalities during the acute phase invariably include focal infiltration by monocytes and lymphocytes (CD4+/CD8+ T cells) into segments of the spinal cord and perivascular spaces accompanied by astroglial and microglial activation. During the subacute phase prominent monocyte/macrophage infiltration is observed. The presence of white matter changes, demyelination, and axonal injury is prominent in postinfectious myelitis. It is noteworthy that involvement of the gray matter is also marked in some cases (456,457). In patients with autoimmune disorders such as SLE, there are typical vasculitic lesions that produce focal areas of spinal cord ischemia without overt inflammation (457,458).

The pathogenesis of ATM is believed to be immune mediated. In 30% to 60% of idiopathic ATM cases, there is an antecedent respiratory, gastrointestinal, or systemic illness (456,457). In the majority of infections, mechanisms of autoimmunity, such as molecular mimicry and superantigen-mediated disease, account for the pathologic damage characteristic of ATM (456).

Molecular mimicry may occur in ATM. A variety of infectious agents possess antigenic determinants (i.e., proteins, glycolipids, proteoglycans) that resemble self-antigens in the spinal cord. Generation of cellular and humoral immune responses results in cross-reactive immune activation against cellular targets of the spinal cord itself (89,457,458). It is also possible that autoantibodies may initiate a direct injury to neurons. A particular pentapeptide sequence found on microbial agents is also present in the extracellular region of the glutamate receptor subunits NR2a and NR2b, present on neurons in the CNS, and can induce neuronal death (456,459). In addition, high levels of even normal circulating antibodies may cause damage in ATM (451). A patient with high levels of antibodies against hepatitis B surface antigen developed recurrent ATM; circulating immune complexes containing hepatitis B surface antigen were detected in the serum and CSF, and their disappearance after treatment correlated with functional recovery (460).

Another autoimmune mechanism may be mediated by the fulminant activation of lymphocytes by microbial superantigens. These are microbial peptides that can stimulate large numbers of lymphocytes, which trigger autoimmune disease by activating autoreactive T-cell clones (461)

Additionally, immune derangements involving ILs may participate in the inflammatory mechanism of ATM. Marked upregulation of IL-6 with increased NO production has been mechanistically linked to tissue injury in ATM (457).

Humoral derangements may also be involved in some cases of ATM (456). A group of patients with allergy to house mites and who developed ATM had high total and specific serum IgE levels, antibody deposition within the spinal cord, perivascular lymphocyte cuffing, and infiltration of eosinophils (462). It was postulated that eosinophils recruited to the spinal cord degranulated and induced neuronal injury (457).

The inflammatory process induced by the immunopathogenic mechanisms may cause vasculitis and secondary ischemic damage of the spinal cord (53,463).

Clinical Manifestations

ATM has an incidence of 1 to 4 new cases per million people per year, affecting individuals of all ages, with bimodal peaks between the ages of 10 and 19 years and 30 and 39 years (464–466) ATM is rare in childhood; in the first 10 years of life there are substantially fewer children affected than in the second decade. Most affected children are older than 5 years (465,467), although the condition can occur even in young infants (467,468). The male-to-female ratio in pediatric series varies form 0.5:1 to 0.9:1 (463,467,469); there is no familial predisposition (457).

Approximately two-thirds of diagnosed children have a history of a recent or a concurrent infection, which is more frequently observed around the summer months (53,467). Viruses etiologically linked to ATM include herpes simplex, herpes zoster, cytomegalovirus, Epstein-Barr, echo, coxsackie, hepatitis B, hepatitis A, influenza, measles, mumps, rubella, varicella, human T-cell lymphotropic virus-1 (HTLV-1), and HIV. Bacteria that may cause ATM are *Borrelia burgdorferi*, *Mycoplasma pneumoniae*, *Yersenia enterocolitica*, *Chlamydia psittaci*, *Rochalimaea henselae*, mycobacteria, and *Listeria monocytogenes*. Parasites can also cause ATM, including schistosoma, cysticercus, toxocara, and toxoplasma (470–474). ATM has also been associated with immunizations for rabies, tetanus toxoid, flu, measles, smallpox, and hepatitis B (53,456,467) and with SLE and antiphospholipid syndrome (458,472,475).

The time from infection to neurologic symptoms is usually 5 to 10 days (467,469). As a general rule, the rate of onset is proportional to the intensity of the initial discomfort (53). Before the onset of acute loss of spinal cord function, there are often nonspecific symptoms such as nausea, muscle aches, and fever. The latter may be present in up to 60% of patients (463,469,474). Occasionally, cases are preceded by relatively trivial blunt trauma to the spine (53). The neurologic picture is most frequently characterized by the presence of back pain and pain in the lower extremities, gait disturbance due to weakness, paraplegia, and paresthesias. Sphincter dysfunction is frequent, and it may be present in up to 90% of children, at times manifested as urinary retention. Other symptoms are neck stiffness in one-half of patients and respiratory insufficiency, particularly if there is cervical compromise, which can cause cardiopulmonary arrest (53). In a few cases a urinary tract infection may herald the diagnosis of ATM (467). The full-blown disease is reached 4 weeks after disease onset at the latest, and in more than 80% of cases the peak is seen within the first 3 or 10 days in hyperacute and acute cases, respectively (463,466,469,474); in subacute ATM, it may take several days or weeks for the maximal deficits to occur (53,467).

The neurologic examination demonstrates the dysfunction of the motor and sensory spinal cord pathways. Motor exam shows paresis usually involving the legs, although in some instances it may involve the legs and arms sequentially. The weakness is initially flaccid (hypotonia, hypo- or areflexia), but later it evolves into a spastic paresis with upper motor neuron signs (hypertonia, hyperreflexia, clonus, and Babinski sign). Superficial reflexes (abdominal, cremasteric, bulbocavernosus) are absent (53). Sensory examination is characterized by involvement of pain and temperature, whereas posterior column function (vibration and proprioception) is generally spared. A sensory level can be found in almost all the children, particularly if examining cold sensation (53). In 70 children from three pediatric series of ATM, the sensory level was located in the upper thoracic region in 37% of cases, in the lower thoracic in 37%, in the cervical in 14%, and in the lumbar in 10% (463,467,469). Abnormal rectal tone is a frequent finding (467).

Diagnosis

The diagnosis of ATM is mostly clinical. Recently, the Transverse Myelitis Consortium Working Group proposed specific criteria for the diagnosis of ATM (Table 8.6). A diagnosis of idiopathic ATM should require that all of the inclusion criteria and none of the exclusion criteria be fulfilled. A diagnosis of disease-associated ATM should require that all the inclusion criteria are met and that the patient is identified as having an underlying condition listed in the disease-specific exclusions (464).

Serology

Serologic evaluation for specific antibodies may be helpful in identifying a specific infectious agent (467). CSF findings vary depending on the time of lumbar puncture in the course of the disease (474). Abnormalities are found in more than half of patients and include moderate lymphocytic pleocytosis and high protein level (53,467,474). Myelin basic protein is elevated in cases of postinfectious ATM (53,463,476). IgG index may be increased (457). CSF viral studies or molecular investigations (e.g., PCR for Lyme disease) will confirm an etiologic diagnosis in some patients.

TABLE 8.6 Diagnostic Criteria of Idiopathic Acute Transverse Myelitis

Inclusion Criteria	*Exclusion Criteria*
Development of sensory, motor, or autonomic dysfunction attributable to the spinal cord	History of previous radiation to the spine within the last 10 years
Bilateral signs and/or symptoms (though not necessarily symmetric)	Clear arterial distribution clinical deficit consistent with thrombosis of the anterior spinal artery
Clear defined sensory level	
Exclusion of extra-axial compressive etiology by neuroimaging (MRI or myelography; CT of spine not adequate)	Abnormal flow voids on the surface of the spinal cord consistent with AVM
Inflammation within the spinal cord demonstrated by CSF pleocytosis or elevated IgG index or gadolinium enhancement; if none of the inflammatory criteria are met at symptom onset, repeat MRI and lumbar puncture evaluation between 2 and 7 days following symptom onset	Serologic or clinical evidence of connective tissue disease (sarcoidosis, Behçet's disease, Sjögren's syndrome, SLE, mixed connective tissue disorder, etc.)[a]
	CNS manifestations of syphilis, Lyme disease, HIV, HTLV-1, *Mycoplasma,* other viral infection (i.e., HSV-1, HSV-2, VZV, EBV, CMV, HHV-6, enteroviruses)[a]
Progression to nadir between 4 hours and 21 days following the onset of symptoms (if patient awakens with symptoms, symptoms must become more pronounced from point of awakening)	Brain MRI abnormalities suggestive of MS[a]
	History of clinically apparent optic neuritis[a]

MRI, magnetic resonance imaging; CT, computed tomography; CSF, cerebrospinal fluid; IgG, immunoglobulin G; AVM, arteriovenous malformation; SLE, systemic lupus erythematosus; HIV, human immunodeficiency virus; HTLV-1, human T-cell lymphotropic virus-1; HSV, herpes simplex virus; VZV, varicella-zoster virus; EBV, Epstein-Barr virus; CMV, cytomegalovirus; HHV, human herpes virus; MS, multiple sclerosis

[a]Do not exclude disease-associated acute transverse myelitis.

From Transverse Myelitis Consortium Working Group. Proposed diagnostic criteria and nosology of acute transverse myelitis. *Neurology* 2002;59:499–505. With permission.

Neurophysiology

Clinical neurophysiologic studies are important in distinguishing central versus peripheral nervous system dysfunction (474). Although peripheral nerve conduction velocity is normal, compound muscle action potential amplitudes may be affected if segmental anterior-horn cells are affected. Missing F waves or prolonged F latencies, indicating root involvement, occur in Guillain-Barré syndrome and in anterior spinal artery infarction. Prolonged or absent somatosensory-evoked potentials (SEPs) in conjunction with normal sensory nerve action potentials indicate a CNS lesion, for example, in the spinal cord as in ATM (474). Magnetic motor-evoked potentials (MEPs) are not very useful in children because their absence is physiologic before 12 years (477), but they may be helpful in adolescent patients (478).

In a study of 39 adult patients with ATM, abnormal central motor conduction time to tibialis anterior was the most frequent abnormality (90%), followed by abnormal tibial SEP (77%). Central motor time to abductor digiti minimi was abnormal in 30% and median SEP in 15% of patients. Evidence of denervation on electromyography (EMG) was present in 51% of patients. MEPs and SEPs had a good correlation with motor or sensory findings, respectively (479). Unrecordable, prolonged, or normal EPs reflect the decreasing severity of spinal cord involvement. Unrecordable motor and sensory EPs may be due to necrosis, edema, and severe demyelination resulting in conduction block. The prolongation of central conduction time may be due to dispersion and/or demyelination. The normal EPs may be due to milder involvement or sparing of fast-conducting motor or sensory pathways (479). In cases of mild ATM with normal SEPs and spinal cord MRI, the diagnostic segmental EPs need to be performed to confirm the diagnosis (A.L., personal experience). Visual evoked potentials (VEPs) are useful for ruling out or ruling in MS (53).

Neuroimaging

MRI results are relatively variable and nonspecific in ATM. The value of MRI is to exclude other conditions that cause paraparesis, particularly space-occupying lesions that require emergency surgical treatment (467,474). In post–infectious/immunization ATM the most frequent findings are spinal cord swelling, longitudinal fusiform-like diffuse hyperintensities on T2-weighted images, and presence of gadolinium enhancement in a nodular, diffuse, or peripheral pattern. The lesions are solitary in more than 80% of cases and frequently extend over several vertebral segments (467,474,480–482). When ATM is associated with SLE, the MRI findings are similar to those found in MS, sometimes with overlap features called "lupoid sclerosis" (482). After clinical remission of ATM with residual symptoms, atrophy of the spinal cord can be found on T1-weighted images and with low intensity on T2-weighted images. Brain MRI may show clinically silent T2 bright lesions (483), the significance of which is unclear, and, as in ON, should not necessarily suggest a diagnosis of MS (53).

The first step in the algorithm of differential diagnosis of ATM is to consider whether it is idiopathic or disease associated (Table 8.6). Specific tests will confirm the diagnosis (464). Then ATM should be differentiated from other acute myelopathies such as spinal cord compression by a tumor or abscess, arteriovenous malformation, hemorrhage, stroke (myelomalacia), or radiation injury (53,472); MRI is the test of choice for clarifying the diagnosis (481,482). Tropical spastic paraparesis is a progressive myelopathy caused by HTLV-1 infection, which may produce MRI changes similar to ATM, although its neurologic progression is much slower than that of ATM (53). Sometimes MS can present with a clinical picture similar to ATM. In MS, spinal MRI is abnormal in only 5% to 12% of cases if the brain MRI is normal. In MS, spinal cord lesions rarely extend more than two vertebrae; they may be multifocal; spinal cord enlargement is rare; and MRI may show typical diagnostic high-signal T2 lesions (474). Devic disease requires the diagnosis of associated ON. The differential diagnosis of an acutely presenting Guillain-Barré syndrome (GBS) and the initial phase of ATM may be difficult in some cases. The presence of CSF albumino-cytologic dissociation and abnormal peripheral nerve conduction velocity are the keys supporting the diagnosis of GBS (484).

Treatment

There is no treatment that has clearly demonstrated the ability to modulate the outcome in patients with ATM. Considering the diverse pathogenetic mechanisms, it may be that distinct treatment options should be used for different subsets of patients with ATM (456).

The usefulness of corticosteroids in the treatment of ATM in children is controversial (156,485,486). Lahat and coworkers (486) performed a pilot study in 10 children with ATM and demonstrated that treatment with high-dose intravenous methylprednisolone significantly shortened motor recovery (5.5 days) compared with a historical control group receiving either no treatment or low-dose steroids (23 days). Defresne and collaborators (485), in a multicenter, controlled study, evaluated 12 children with severe ATM treated with methylprednisolone (1 g/1.73 m2 per day for 3 to 5 days followed by 2 to 3 weeks of prednisone taper) and found that this protocol increased the percentage of patients who walked independently after 1 month (66% vs. 18% in a historical control group) and the percentage of patients making a full recovery (55% vs. 12%) and decreased the median time to independent walking (25 vs. 120 days). On the other hand, Kalita and Misra (156) did not find a beneficial role of intravenous methylprednisolone, 500 mg for 5 days, on the 3-month outcome of 9 patients with ATM evaluated clinically and with neurophysiologic studies. SEPs and MPs may be useful for monitoring the effect of steroids on ATM (479).

Other possibly useful immunosuppressant treatments are cyclophosphamide, which has been used together with steroids in lupus-associated ATM (487), and IVIG, which has been successful in preventing ATM attacks in Devic disease (488). Azathioprine, methotrexate, and mycophenolate are also used by some authors (457). Plasmapheresis is recommended in those patients who fail to improve after high-dose corticosteroid treatment; the use of seven courses has been recommended after other causes for the white matter disease are excluded (489,490). A randomized trial of plasma exchange in acute CNS inflammatory demyelinating disease showed important neurologic recovery in a subgroup of patients with ATM (490). Future therapeutic alternatives are CSF fluid filtration, which has been effective in GBS (491), and immunization (456). The latter is supported by experimental studies in which active or passive immunization of animals against CNS antigens resulted in improved functional status and diminished neuronal death after spinal cord contusion (492,493), maybe because the removal of damaged tissue facilitates enhanced recovery (456).

Long-term management of ATM patients requires attention to a number of issues. They require rehabilitative care to prevent secondary complications of immobility and to improve their functional skills. Spasticity is often a very difficult problem to manage and requires antispasticity drugs (baclofen, diazepam, dantrolene), botulinum toxin injections, and baclofen pump or surgery in selected cases. Another major area of concern is effective management of bowel and bladder function (360,457,494).

Prognosis

ATM is usually a monophasic disease, but in some cases it is associated with recurrent bouts. Many patients have underlying diseases such as MS, SLE, vascular malformations in the spinal cord, or antiphospholipid syndrome (495), but cases of idiopathic recurrent ATM have been described, raising the question of whether this is a genetically, immunologically, and clinicopathologically different disease (496).

The outcome of ATM is variable (313). Based on several series, the prognosis can be summarized as follows: Good outcome occurs in 44% of cases. Such patients who have no residual symptoms or mildly disturbed micturation only, minimal sensory loss, or pyramidal tract signs. Fair outcome occurs in 33% of patients. These have spastic paresis, sensory loss, and transient sphincter disturbances, but are able to walk without aid. Approximately 23% have a poor outcome, meaning that they show severe neurologic symptoms and signs, are unable to walk, and have no bladder or rectal control (463,466,467,469,474,497). The neurologic improvement starts within 1 month and usually continues up to 6 months, although there are patients who can regain function as late as 2 years after the onset of symptoms (467,469,474). The incidence of MS in several series of pediatric ATM patients is low (463,467,469); in a retrospective study of MS patients whose symptoms started before 16 years of age, only 3% had presented with ATM (71). Mortality is a rare outcome (313,467).

Factors associated with an unfavorable outcome are younger age, acute onset of symptoms with maximal deficit reached within 24 hours, backache as the first symptom, complete paraplegia, absence of pyramidal signs, and sensory disturbances up to the level of cervical dermatomes (53,467,474,497). Favorable outcome is related to a plateau shorter than 8 days, presence of supraspinal symptoms, time to independent walking shorter than 1 month, and maybe treatment with high-dose intravenous methylprednisolone (360,467,485,486,494).

Acute Cerebellar Ataxia

Acute cerebellar ataxia (ACA) is a clinical syndrome characterized by the sudden onset of ataxia following an infectious illness, usually viral, which manifests primarily as gait disturbance and incoordination It is a relatively common condition, representing 0.4% of all children evaluated for neurologic problems at a children's hospital (498). ACA was first described by Batten in 1905 (499), who described the usual clinical course as follows:

> A child perfectly healthy and of good intellectual development is taken ill with some acute febrile disease. The child is kept in bed and seems to be making a normal convalescence. When, however, the child is sat up in bed it is found that he is unable to maintain his balance.

Etiology

The cause of the condition is probably heterogeneous, with a number of infectious agents being directly or indirectly responsible. ACA occurs after exanthematous diseases, most commonly varicella, less often rubella. It is also associated with other viral infections, including poliovirus type I, influenza A, influenza B, mumps, EBV, parvovirus B19, and hepatitis A. In other patients, echovirus type 9 and coxsackievirus type B have been isolated from CSF (53). Other infectious etiologies that can cause ACA are typhoid fever, *Mycoplasma*, malaria, *Legionella*, and meningococcal meningitis. ACA may also occur after vaccination (500,501). It is noteworthy that acute and transient cerebellar ataxia can also be the presenting symptom of childhood MS (53) (Table 8.2). The association of acute cerebellar ataxia with occult neuroblastoma has been observed on many occasions (502,503).

In 136 patients with ACA combined from the series of Connolly and collaborators (498), Iff and coworkers (504), and Nussinovitch and colleagues (500), the percentage distribution of etiologies was as follows: varicella (34%), viral (32%), idiopathic (23%), mumps (6%), EBV (2%), mycoplasma (1.5%), and vaccine (1.5%).

Pathogenesis

It is probable that in some instances acute cerebellar ataxia is caused by direct viral invasion of the cerebellum, whereas in others it is the result of an autoimmune response to a variety of agents. It is uncertain whether the principal site of CNS injury is the neuronal cell body (perikaryon) or the axodendritic compartments (53). Because ACA is not a fatal condition, its descriptive pathologic anatomy is unknown (53).

Antineuronal antibodies were reported by Ito and coworkers in 1994 (505) in a case of postinfectious cerebellar ataxia following EBV infection. In another study, two children with ataxia and other CNS manifestations following *Mycoplasma pneumoniae* infection were found to have antibodies directed to centrioles (506). The finding of oligoclonal bands in the CSF and development of ACA in patients with varicella infections suggests that autoantibodies may be responsible for at least part of the clinical picture (507). Adams and coworkers (508) demonstrated the presence of serum autoantibodies against cerebrum and cerebellum in 3 of 8 patients with postvaricella and 1 with post-EBV ACA. Viral antigen staining was colocalized with cytoplasmic immunoreactivity using antibodies to the centrosome protein pericentrin. Similarly, Fritzler and collaborators (509) found antibodies to pericentrin in the serum of patients with ACA, 5 of 12 postvaricella and 1 post-EBV. Cells stained by antibodies to pericentrin were distributed throughout the cerebellum, including those in the nuclear and granular layers. Therefore, in addition to being a component of centrosomes, pericentrin exists as particles in the cytoplasm. Certain Purkinje cells contain numerous particles and more than one centrosome ("supernumerary centrosomes"), indicating that these neurons may have ploidy abnormalities (509).

The observation that children with ataxia produce antibodies to centrosome proteins, including pericentrin, and that Purkinje cells may exhibit genomic instability raises the question of the vulnerability of these cells to autoimmune attacks (509). Of interest in this regard is the paper by Ploubidou and coworkers (510) indicating that newly assembled viruses disrupt microtubule organization as well as centrosome duplication and function (511). Of possible relevance is the recent finding that the centrosome may be an important locus for MHC class I antigen processing and that targeting of antigens on the centrosome may enhance the immune response (512).

The origin of centrosome autoantibodies as sequelae of varicella (or other viral) infections and the potential pathogenetic role of antibodies to pericentrin await further elucidation (509).

Clinical Manifestations

By definition, the onset of ataxia is always acute, although approximately one-half of the children experience a nonspecific infectious illness within 3 weeks before the onset of neurologic symptoms (53,500,503,504). ACA is seen in children of all ages, but in the experience of Weiss and Carter (513), it occurred most commonly between 1 and 2 years of age. In 112 patients combined from the series of Connolly and collaborators (498) and Nussinovitch and colleagues (500), the mean age at presentation was 7.5 years, but 50% of the cases occurred before 4 years of age. The latency between prior infection or immunization and initiation of ataxia ranged from 1 to 21 days.

The clinical picture is marked by truncal ataxia and dysmetria. The ataxia is usually emphasized during walking as compared to sitting, thus representing a manifestation of gait ataxia (498). Nystagmus is encountered in 8% to 50% of patients (498,501), whereas a number of children have other ocular disturbances, including sudden random motions of the eyes during voluntary movements (504). Speech is often affected. Hypotonia, tremor of the extremities, head, and trunk, and depressed level of consciousness are seen less often (53,504). Other neurologic signs that may be present are dizziness, headache, photophobia, and myoclonic movements of the head and arms. Brainstem signs are present occasionally (53). Vomiting frequently accompanies the neurologic picture, and fever is documented in 3% to 25% of patients (498,504).

Diagnosis

Acute cerebellar ataxia is diagnosed by the clinical history and physical and neurologic examination. Complementary tests may be helpful.

The CSF is usually unremarkable, although a mild pleocytosis is found in up to 50% of cases (498). The CSF protein content can be normal on initial taps but may become elevated late in the course of the illness (498,500,504). Oligoclonal bands may be positive, particularly in patients with postvaricella ACA (498).

Neuroimaging studies have shown parenchymal swelling of the cerebellum coupled with a transiently increased signal in the cerebellar cortex or the brainstem (511,514,515). When MRI abnormalities are confined to the brainstem, the condition resembles brainstem encephalitis, except that in the latter disease cerebellar symptoms are accompanied by clinical evidence of widespread CNS involvement.

SPECT scan has shown decreased (516,517) or increased (518–520) blood flow to the cerebellum.

Electrical cerebellar stimulation may be abnormal in cases with normal CT, MRI, and SPECT neuroimaging studies (521).

Differential Diagnosis

Although ACA is a descriptive clinical diagnosis, the differential diagnosis is broad, and in many cases the diagnosis is confirmed mainly by exclusion (53,498,501).

Ataxia can develop in the course of acute viral diseases of the CNS, notably varicella, mumps, poliomyelitis, and West Nile virus (522). The nosologic distinction between these cases and the usual cases of acute cerebellar ataxia may be especially difficult and to some degree a question of semantics. In general, if a causative agent can be proven, the condition is termed cerebellar encephalitis; otherwise the term cerebellar ataxia of unknown cause is used.

ACA needs to be differentiated from acute cerebellitis (AC), defined by Horowitz and colleagues (523) as a neurologic condition consisting of nausea, headache, and altered mental status, including loss of consciousness and convulsions, in addition to the acute onset of cerebellar symptoms. According to these authors fever and signs of meningeal irritation were excluded from the diagnostic criteria for AC because in such instances either infective meningoencephalitis or ADEM needs to be ruled out. With this in mind, fever and signs of meningeal irritation can be observed in patients with AC (524).

Sudden onset of ataxia may also be caused by posterior fossa tumors, occult neuroblastoma (autoimmune basis), acute labyrynthitis, and drug intoxications (53).

Although the onset of ataxia in a posterior fossa tumor is rarely sudden, imaging studies to exclude a mass lesion are indicated. The presence of papilledema and a history of headache or vomiting point to a posterior fossa tumor or, more rarely, to a tumefactive demyelinating lesion.

Neuroblastoma should be investigated using specific diagnostic techniques (see the later discussion of the opsoclonus-myoclonus syndrome).

Acute labyrynthitis (vestibular neuronitis or epidemic vertigo) is not easily distinguishable from ataxia, particularly in an uncooperative youngster. It is usually associated with nausea, intense vertigo, and abnormal tests of labyrinthine function, particularly an absence of caloric responses (525,526).

ACA can also be seen after the ingestion of a variety of toxins, particularly alcohol, medications, thallium, and organic mercurials (see Chapter 10). It can also happen as a consequence of heat stroke, as a result of hyperthermia-induced cerebellar degeneration (527).

Acute cerebellar ataxia, often precipitated by a respiratory infection, accompanies a number of metabolic disorders, including various mitochondrial disorders, Hartnup disease, and the intermittent forms of maple syrup urine disease (see Chapter 1). Recurrent attacks of ataxia can be transmitted as an autosomal dominant trait (episodic ataxia). Two forms of this condition have been delineated: type 1, caused by missense mutations in the potassium-channel gene *KCNA1*, and type 2, caused by missense and nonsense mutation in the calcium-channel gene *CACNA1A*. These ion channels are crucial for both central and peripheral neurotransmission. These entities have been recently reviewed by Baloh and Jen (528), and are covered more extensively in Chapter 3.

Some children with minor motor seizures suddenly develop ataxia that probably results from frequent transitory impairment of consciousness. EEG signs of a seizure disorder should readily distinguish this entity (53).

In a significant percentage of children who develop MS, ataxia is the first sign of the disease. Diagnostic studies to exclude this entity are therefore indicated in the appropriate clinical context (53).

Ataxia associated with the various cerebellar degenerations develops gradually and should cause little diagnostic confusion. Apparent ataxia can be the consequence of generalized weakness (i.e., in acute infectious polyneuritis). In acute cerebellar ataxia, hypotonia is associated with normal or increased deep tendon reflexes, whereas in polyneuritis, the reflexes are either reduced or absent (53).

Treatment

In the majority of cases, the disease is self-limiting and therefore it does not require any treatment. Thus, the major focus of care should be on the identification and treatment of alternate diagnoses that carry the potential for greater morbidity and mortality (501).

However, because an autoimmune pathogenesis has been implicated in ACA, immunosuppression therapies have been tried in selected cases, with promising results, although generally based on small series or anecdote (501). A good symptomatic response has been seen with the use of steroids (520,529,530). High-dose steroids are particularly of marked benefit in cases of ACA associated with cerebellar swelling resulting in brainstem compression as well as upward or downward cerebellar herniation (531). Case reports (516,518) have presented patients who quickly improved with IVIG, suggesting that this treatment is worth considering when there is no response to corticosteroids.

Due to the association with varicella, antiviral therapy with acyclovir is often used in immunocompromised patients (501).

Prognosis

In approximately two-thirds of children, the ataxia resolves completely, with an average duration of cerebellar signs of approximately 2 months. Some mildly affected children recover completely within 1 week. Nearly 90% of children improve completely over weeks to months. More than 2 months is required for recovery of 18% to 33% of children with viral prodromata and 50% of those without prodromata. In the series of Nussinovitch and coworkers (500), improvement was more rapid, and full gait recovery was seen on the average in less than 2 weeks.

Persistence of major neurologic deficits is noted in approximately one-third of children. These deficits include ataxia of trunk and extremities, speech impairment, mental retardation, and behavioral abnormalities (53,498,500). A poorer prognosis is associated with older age and an EBV infection (498,501). In addition, the presence of lesions on MRI seems to be associated with an increased chance of residual deficits (501).

In rare cases, acute cerebellar ataxia can have a relapsing course, which requires ruling out an underlying metabolic disorder (530). According to Connolly and collaborators (498), the risk of recurrence is associated with a longer latency between the prodrome and development of the initial attack of ataxia. One patient with recurrent ataxia in Connolly's series (498) developed residual attention-deficit hyperactivity disorder and cognitive impairment. One of us (J.H.M.) also encountered at least two children whose cerebellar ataxia recurred over several years, with exacerbations often preceded by a mild respiratory illness. These bouts could be distinguished from the aggravation of the ataxia expected in any uncoordinated patient experiencing an acute febrile episode. Both patients were left with mental retardation.

Soussan and colleagues (532) reported their experience with the prognostic value of MRI in a series of 8 children with ACA. Neuroimaging was abnormal in 4 of them (high T2 cerebellar signal) during the acute phase and in 7 after at least 1 month of evolution (cerebellar atrophy). After 1 to 6 years of follow-up, 4 children had clinical sequelae, including 3 of the 4 patients with initially abnormal MRI. Conversely, the 2 patients with initially normal MRI had a good clinical recovery. The authors concluded that MRI is a useful prognostic tool in ACA.

SPECT may also be useful in monitoring ACA clinical course (518). Cerebellar electrical stimulation may be informative in the follow-up evaluation of cerebellar function in patients who had ACA (521).

Opsoclonus-Myoclonus Syndrome (Myoclonic Encephalopathy)

In 1962, Kinsbourne described a syndrome of myoclonic encephalopathy in infants and young children characterized by multidirectional, chaotic eye movements (opsoclonus), myoclonus, and ataxia (OMS) (533).

Pathogenesis

The underlying disease mechanism of OMS is likely to be immune mediated, either as a postinfectious process or as a neuroimmunologic complication of neuronal/

neuroblastic tumors, most commonly, neuroblastoma (534).

Several immunologic abnormalities have been found in patients with OMS. In peripheral blood, they have T-cell abnormalities of mononuclear cells, the most robust of which is the reduction of the CD4+ T-cell subset and the CD4/CD8 ratio (535).

In the CSF, they have a lower percentage of CD4+ T cells and CD4/CD8 ratio and higher levels of B cells, including CD5+ and CD5− B-bell subsets, which correlate with neurologic severity, suggesting that CSF B-cell expansion is a biomarker of disease activity (536,537). A transient intrathecal increase of IgM and a persistent elevation of IgG have been found (538). In addition, an increasing number of oligoclonal IgG bands, indicative of expanding local autoantibody production in the intrathecal compartment, has been reported (538).

IgM and IgG autoantibodies from sera derived from patients with myoclonic encephalopathy, regardless of its underlying cause, bind to cerebellar Purkinje cell perikaryal cytoplasm and axons. A high-molecular-weight subunit of neurofilaments appears to be one of the major targets (507). Interestingly, Prassanan and colleagues (539) recently identified β-tubulin isoforms as tumor antigens in neuroblastoma, β-tubulin being an integral component of microtubules (540).

In a study of 64 children with neuroblastoma, 16 with OMS and 48 age-matched controls, antineuronal antibodies were found in 81% of patients with OMS and in 25% of those only with neuroblastoma (541). However, the frequency and specificity of those autoantibodies and their relationship to relapses are unclear. Fisher and coworkers (542) demonstrated the presence of anti-Hu antibodies in a patient with neuroblastoma-OMS. In the study by Antunes and collaborators (541) anti-Hu antibodies were detected in 10 serum samples (4 with OMS), but no other specific immunoreactivity profiles were identified. In contrast, Pranzatelli and colleagues (543) studied 18 children with symptomatic low-grade neuroblastoma-OMS and found that all of them were seronegative for anti-Hu, anti-Ri, and anti-Yo. Recently, Bataller and coworkers (544) emphasized the possible role of the proteins of the postsynaptic density (PSD) as a frequent source of autoantigens in OMS. PSD is a complex of protein associated with the glutamate *N*-methyl-D-aspartate receptor and includes membrane proteins (such as receptors, ion channels, and adhesion molecules) that are attached to a network of intracellular scaffold, signaling, and cytoskeletal proteins. However, these authors believed that the occasional identification of antibodies to Hu and other proteins most likely represents cancer-induced immunity unrelated to the neurologic symptoms of OMS (544).

A frequent histologic feature of neuroblastic tumors with OM is the presence of diffuse and variously extensive lymphocytic infiltration with lymphoid follicles. This observation also supports an immune-mediated mechanism for this paraneoplastic syndrome (545,546)

It is postulated that the pathophysiologic-anatomic correlate of this syndrome may be the cerebellum or the brainstem (547,548). Studies with functional MRI support a crucial role of the fastigial nucleus in opsoclonus (547). Recently, the Nova onconeural antigens have been implicated in the pathogenesis of OMS (549-551). Nova is a neuron-specific RNA-binding protein, which is characterized by failure of inhibition of brainstem and spinal motor systems (549). In mice, Nova-1–null animals die postnatally from a motor deficiency associated with apoptotic death of spinal and brainstem neurons. They show specific splicing defects in two inhibitory receptor pre-mRNAs, glycine alpha2 exon3A (GlyRalpha2E3A) and GABA (A) exon gamma 2L. The defect in splicing in Nova-1–null mice provides a model for understanding the motor dysfunction in OMS (550).

Clinical Manifestations

Children, commonly below 3 years of age, present with acute or subacute manifestations of the typical triad: (a) opsoclonus, a chaotic irregularity of eye movements in which the globes are in a state of constant agitation with rapid and unequal movements that usually take place in the horizontal plane; (b) polymyoclonus and shocklike myoclonic contractions, which persist when the affected part is at rest, producing total disorganization of willed movements; and (c) cerebellar ataxia (53,543).

Frequently, the symptoms follow an infectious process. However, in approximately 50% of cases OMS presents as a paraneoplastic syndrome, which is more frequently associated with an underlying peripheral sympathoadrenal neuroblastoma (548).

The clinical course is variable and unpredictable. There may be spontaneous remissions, which may be partial or complete. In some cases the syndrome progresses with recurrences characterized by worsening of symptoms, which are usually precipitated by intercurrent respiratory infections or tapering of the treatment (552).

Diagnosis

Neuroblastoma is found in approximately one-half of the cases. However, because of the high incidence of spontaneous regression or maturation in neuroblastomas, the actual percentage of OMS cases linked to extracranial neuronal tumors may be somewhat underestimated (553).

In a retrospective questionnaire survey of 105 patients, the mean delay in diagnosis was 11 weeks, and 17 weeks in initiation of treatment (553). The tumor is often not apparent at the onset of the illness and is uncovered only after persistent diagnostic investigation (548,553). Palpation of the abdomen, rectal examination, and computed tomography and/or ultrasonography of the chest and abdomen are the most useful procedures. In the experience of Boltshauser and colleagues, bone marrow examination, skeletal surveys, and urinary vanillylmandelic acid (VMA) assays were only rarely helpful (554). This is unlike the experience of Tuchman and coworkers (555), who analyzed random urine specimens in a large series of patients with no false-positive and some 7% false-negative results. Metaiodobenzylguanidine (MIBG) total-body scintigraphy may be ultimately required for revealing occult neuroblastoma in OMS (556). Because OMS may precede the appearance of an underlying tumor by several months, the diagnostic work-up may need to be repeated (548).

Aside from neuroblastoma, myoclonic encephalopathy has been linked to many other etiologies, including infectious causes. Conditions that have been related to OMS include EBV, enterovirus (polio, coxsackie), mumps, St. Louis encephalitis virus, salmonellosis, *Mycobacterium* tuberculosis, rickettsia, and malaria (53,548). Intracranial tumors, various intoxicants, and hydrocephalus are other, albeit considerably rarer, causes (53).

Treatment

The treatment consists of ACTH, corticosteroids, or high doses of IVIG. Immunosuppressants (azathioprine) and chemotherapeutic agents (cyclophosphamide) have also been used (543,548,557–559). Plasmapheresis is an effective therapeutic alternative in those patients who fail to respond to steroids and IVIG (560,561). Pranzatelli and collaborators (562), based on their finding of CSF B-cell expansion (536,537), suggested the use of monoclonal anti–B cell antibodies (rituximab) to treat patients with OMS. In some cases, symptomatic treatment of myoclonus is necessary (563,564).

Prognosis

The condition is self-limiting, and in a substantial proportion of children, aggressive treatment induces a dramatic improvement (53). Nevertheless, the long-term outcome is not always favorable or totally innocuous, insofar as more than one-half of the children are left with neurologic deficits, cognitive impairment, abnormalities in motor performance, and language, psychosocial, and behavioral problems (559,565–568) According to Mitchell and coworkers (559), the increased deficits in older children raise the concern that OMS is a progressive encephalopathy rather than a time-limited single insult.

The clinical course, response to corticosteroid therapy, and long-term prognosis of myoclonic encephalopathy–associated neuroblastoma are the same as in children with myoclonic encephalopathy who do not harbor a tumor. Interestingly, for reasons as yet unknown, the survival rate of children with myoclonic encephalopathy and neuroblastoma is far better than that of the general population of children with neuroblastoma (568).

Spasmus Nutans

Spasmus nutans is an unusual but generally benign condition described in 1897 by Raudnitz (569). It presents in late infancy (1 to 15 months), often in late winter or early spring, and is characterized by anomalous head positions, head nodding, and small-amplitude, dissociated, pendular nystagmus, which can be conjugate, dysconjugate, or uniocular (53,570). When visual targets such as a picture book are presented, children start to nod or the amplitude of the nystagmus becomes larger. Straightening the tilted head or fixing the head also increases the amplitude of the nystagmus (53). For these reasons, some authors believe the head nodding is compensatory to the nystagmus (571,572).

In the majority of cases the cause is unknown. Raudnitz (569) described an association of spasmus nutans with inadequate exposure to light and rickets, which was also supported by several studies in the early 1900s. In these studies onset of nystagmus was more frequent in darker months of the year, and social and hygienic conditions were poor (573). A recent controlled study found that low socioeconomic status is a risk factor for the development of spasmus nutans (574). For unknown reasons, the condition appears to be far more common in the eastern United States than in the southwest of the country (53). It has also been postulated that spasmus nutans could be the sequel to a viral illness (575,576).

The diagnosis is established by the constancy of the characteristic triad and the elimination of other causes of nystagmus (571). Congenital nystagmus usually starts before 6 months of age and is associated with abnormal visual acuity or optic nerve anomalies in approximately 90% of children. In these cases, an evaluation with VEPs and electroretinogram is important to confirm the diagnosis of spasmus nutans (577–580). The differential diagnosis should also be established with bobble-head syndrome (571).

An increasing number of reports have linked spasmus nutans to gliomas of the optic nerve and chiasm (577,581) or thalamus (582), even though their estimated prevalence is less than 1.4% (573). In particular, when spasmus nutans–like symptoms begin after late infancy a brain tumor should be suspected (583). In other cases, spasmus nutans has been associated with other conditions such as Leigh disease (584), Bardet-Biedl syndrome (585), opsoclonus-myoclonus (586), arachnoid or porencephalic cysts (587), and ocular motor apraxia with cerebellar vermian hypoplasia (588). Therefore, MRI studies of the optic nerves and of the CNS are indicated. In spasmus nutans MRI is invariably normal.

The condition is self-limiting, resolves after a period of 4 months to 6 years and is not associated with any visual deficits. In most children a subclinical nystagmus persists for many years (571,589). There is also a high incidence of strabismus and amblyopia (590).

IMMUNOLOGICALLY MEDIATED DISEASES AFFECTING CENTRAL NERVOUS SYSTEM GRAY MATTER

Rheumatic Fever (Sydenham Chorea)

Sydenham chorea, also historically known as "St. Vitus dance," is one of the major clinical manifestations of acute rheumatic fever and its principal neurologic manifestation. It is the most common form of acquired chorea in childhood (chorea minor; for many years the term chorea magna was used to designate chorea of hysterical nature) (591). The incidence is 0.2 to 0.8 in 100,000 per year in developed countries; this represents between 10% and 40% of those who develop rheumatic fever (591).

This condition was first defined by Sydenham in 1684 (592):

> Chorea Sancti Viti is a sort of Convulsion, which chiefly invades Boys and Girls, from ten Years of Age to Puberty: First it shews its self by a certain Lameness, or rather Instability of one of the Legs, which the Patient drags after him like a Fool; afterward it appears in the hand of the same side; which he that is affected with this Disease, can by no means keep in the same Posture for one moment, if it be brought to the Breast, or any other Part, but it will be distorted to another Position or Place by a certain Convulsion, let the Patient do what he can. If a Cup of Drink be put into his Hand he represents a thousand Gestures, like Juglers, before he brings it to his Mouth in a right line, his Hand being drawn hither and thither by the Convulsion, he turns it often about for some time, till at length happily raching his Lips, he flings it suddenly into his Mouth, and drinks it greedily, as if the poor Wretch designed only to make sport. For as much as this Disease seems to me to proceed from some Humour rushing in upon the Nerves, which provoke such Preternatural Motions, I think the curative Indications are first to be directed to the lessening of those Humours by bleeding and purging, and then to the strengthening the Genus Nervosum, in order to which I use this method: I take seven Ounces of Blood from the Arm, more or less, according the Age of the Patient; the next Day I prescribe half, or somewhat more, (according to the Age, or the more or less disposition of the Body to bear purging) of the common purging Potion above-described, of Tamarinds, Sena etc. In the Evening I give the following Draught:
>
> Take of Black-cherry-water one Ounce, of Langius's Epileptick-water three Drachms, of old Venice-Treacle one Scruple, of Liquid Laudanum eight Drops; make a Draught.

Etiology and Pathology

The relationship of Sydenham chorea to rheumatic fever was first suggested by Stoll in 1780 (593) and gained general acceptance by the medical profession in the nineteenth century. Most cases of chorea are preceded by a streptococcal infection or rheumatic fever; however, the interval between the bacterial infection and the onset of neurologic symptoms is between 2 and 7 months, so that in one study, serologic evidence of the streptococcal infection was no longer demonstrable in 27% of the children who had chorea as the only clinical manifestation of rheumatic disease (594). In approximately one-third of choreic patients, rheumatic heart disease or other major manifestations of rheumatic fever develop after the onset of chorea (595). Conversely, Sydenham chorea has been seen in approximately one-third of rheumatic fever cases (596). In a series of rheumatic fever patients from Brazil reported in 1997, chorea was seen in 26% (597).

Sydenham chorea is hypothesized to occur when antibodies against group A β-hemolytic *Streptococcus* cross-react with epitopes on neurons via a mechanism of molecular mimicry. The M protein on the surface of group A streptococci has been suggested to be the antigen that triggers the autoimmune response (591). Using immunofluorescent staining techniques, Husby and coworkers (598) demonstrated that sera from 46% of children with Sydenham chorea contain IgG antibodies that react with neuronal cytoplasmic antigens located preferentially in the region of the caudate and subthalamic nuclei. Staining of neurons probably represents a cross-reaction between neuronal cytoplasm and antigens present in the membrane of group A streptococci. These antibodies bind to the caudate nucleus and are less prevalent and are of lower titer in children with active rheumatic fever without chorea and in controls (598,599). Kirvan and associates (600) linked these antibodies to neuronal cell surface antigens and found that they appeared to activate CaM kinase II (calcium/calmodulin protein–dependent kinase II), an enzyme involved in intracellular signaling. This observation increases the likelihood that antibodies documented in Sydenham chorea lead to the release of dopamine, as has been shown in brain slices, and to an imbalance of neurotransmitters (601).

Genetic factors also operate in inducing rheumatic fever. A family history of rheumatic fever can be elicited in 26% of choreic patients, and Sydenham chorea is found in 3.5% of parents and 2.1% of siblings of choreic patients (595). Emotional trauma also can be important in the development of chorea, for the onset of neurologic symptoms is sometimes closely correlated with experiences that cause obvious psychic trauma (602,603).

The pathology in Sydenham chorea primarily affects the basal ganglia (591). Neuropathologic studies have been singularly uninformative. The few persons who have died during the illness, often because of other rheumatic manifestations, have shown an arteritis with a mild perivascular cellular infiltration and a diffuse loss of nerve cells not only from the basal ganglia, but also from the cortex and cerebellum. No typical Aschoff bodies have been found in the brain (604).

Neurochemically, Sydenham chorea has been postulated to be a dopaminergic dysfunction, based on the findings of elevation of homovanillic acid in the CSF as well as on the clinical response to dopamine antagonists and agents that deplete presynaptic dopamine (591). The ultimate underlying neurochemistry has not been well studied (591).

Clinical Manifestations

Up to the last 25 years, Sydenham chorea had become a rare condition in the Western world (605), but in the 1980s and 1990s the number of cases of acute rheumatic fever increased greatly. This increase occurred against a backdrop of no particular increase in the rate of group A streptococcal pharyngitis. The microbiologic and host reasons for this resurgence are not completely understood; they are reviewed by Kaplan (606). In part, the resurgence is believed to result from the appearance of certain serologic types of group A streptococci that produce pyrogenic exotoxin, particularly toxin A, which had been uncommon for many years. In a 1987 report from Ohio, some 17% of children with acute rheumatic fever presented with choreic manifestations. Many of these patients came from middle- or upper-middle-class homes, making invalid the previously noted predisposition for occurrence in low-income groups and crowded housing (607).

The condition begins between ages 3 and 13 years and is somewhat more common in girls. In the Brazilian series the mean age of onset was 9.2 years and the female-to-male ratio was 1.16:1 (597). An adage cited by Wilson (608) is that

> the child with Sydenham chorea is punished three times before the diagnosis is made: once for general fidgetiness, once for breaking crockery, and once for making faces at his grandmother. In part, this adage illustrates the three major clinical features of Sydenham chorea: spontaneous movements, incoordination of voluntary movements, and muscular weakness.

Chorea usually occurs between 1 and 6 months after acute streptococcal infection (591). The involuntary movements affect mainly the face, hands, and arms. At first inconspicuous and usually best observed when the patient is under stress, they are abrupt and short, but gradually they become more frequent and extensive, ultimately becoming almost continuous, disappearing only during sleep and sedation. Chorea interrupts the voluntary movements and is particularly prominent during skilled motor acts and speech. Muscular weakness can be profound and is sometimes the most prominent aspect of the disorder.

The child with pronounced Sydenham chorea is not difficult to recognize. He or she is restless and emotional. Involuntary movements are continuous, quick, and random. They involve mainly the face and the distal portion of the extremities. Speech is jerky, indistinct, and at times completely absent. Willed acts also are performed abruptly; as quickly as the tongue is protruded, it returns into the mouth ("chameleon tongue"). Muscular hypotonia and weakness result in the characteristic pronator sign: When the patient holds the arms above the head, the palms turn outward. Hypotonia also can be demonstrated when the arms are extended in front of the body. The wrist is flexed, and the metacarpophalangeal joints are overextended ("choreic hand"). The child is unable to maintain muscular contraction, and the grip waxes and wanes abruptly ("milkmaid's grip"). The deep tendon reflexes are usually normal, but the patellar reflex is often "hung up." With the legs hanging down, the contraction of the quadriceps elicited by the tap is maintained, causing the leg to be briefly held outstretched before it falls back down (53).

Occasional variants of chorea provide a diagnostic problem. The most common is hemichorea, in which the movements are confined to or are more marked on one side of the body. Hemichorea was seen in 18% of choreic patients reviewed by Aron and associates (595). In a more recent series reported from Chile, hemichorea was seen in 54% of patients (609). In paralytic chorea, the hypotonia and muscular weakness are sufficiently pronounced to obscure the presence of choreiform movements (53).

MRI studies often show increased signal on T2-weighted images in the head of the caudate and in other portions of the basal ganglia, notably the putamen (610). Quantitative MRI demonstrates an increase in the size of the caudate, putamen, and globus pallidus, consistent with the presence of an antibody-mediated inflammation of this region (611). These abnormalities resolve with clinical improvement, but they may be permanent in patients who tend to suffer prolonged attacks and a greater number of recurrences (612). SPECT has shown a marked increase in perfusion of the thalamus and striatum during the stage of active chorea (613,614), which may evolve to baseline (613) or to a hypoperfusion state around the second to third week after the appearance of the initial symptoms (614).

Chorea lasts from 1 month to 2 years. Approximately one-third of patients have a single attack; the remainder have up to five or even more recurrences, despite adequate penicillin prophylaxis. In the series of Diaz-Grez and coworkers (609), 18% of patients had between 2 and 10 recurrences. In a series reported from Israel, 42% of patients developed recurrences any time up to 10 years after the initial episode (615). It is not clear whether these recurrences represent exacerbations of chronic low-grade choreiform activity, the response to transient, mild streptococcal infections, or the response to other, nonstreptococcal stimuli (616). It might represent a primary underlying abnormality that renders patients susceptible to developing chorea or the outcome of permanent subclinical damage to the basal ganglia following the initial episode (615). According to Harrison and coworkers (617), the absence of anti–basal ganglia antibodies in some of the patients with recurrent Sydenham chorea suggests a dopamine hypersensitivity of chronically damaged basal ganglia neurons. If the patient has been free of symptoms for 1 to 2 years, there is little likelihood of relapse.

Complications of Sydenham chorea are rare. Occlusion of the central retinal artery and pseudotumor cerebri are unusual associated conditions (618). Although complete recovery without gross neurologic residua is the rule in Sydenham chorea, minor neurologic signs, notably tics or other adventitious movements, tremor, and impaired coordination, can persist (603). Some of the signs, such as an unusual abruptness of voluntary movements, can be apparent long after the chorea has disappeared. Furthermore, convalescents can develop choreic reactions to a variety of drugs, notably methylphenidate, phenylethylamines, and dextroamphetamine (619).

Behavioral disturbances, including personality changes, irritability, distractibility, age-regressed behaviors, and, notably, obsessive-compulsive disorder (OCD) are common; in many instances, these had been noted weeks to months before the onset of chorea (53,591). Recurrence of Sydenham chorea episodes may result in a cumulative effect, thus increasing the risk of appearance and intensification of OCD (620).

Diagnosis

The major causes for chorea are presented in Table 8.7 (621,622). The diagnosis of Sydenham chorea is based on clinical observation and lack of evidence for other conditions (53,591). Chorea must be differentiated from tics and from a variety of other movement disorders (see Introduction chapter). Additionally, Sydenham chorea should be distinguished from chorea that results from a variety of other causes, notably perinatal asphyxia, Huntington disease, SLE, and chorea that is an expression of the motor impersistence of sensorimotor and cognitive immaturity (minimal brain dysfunction).

Tics, unlike true chorea, are abrupt, repetitive, and patterned, involving the same muscle groups repeatedly. They do not interfere with coordination and are not

TABLE 8.7 Major Causes of Chorea

	Reference
Onset Before 3 Years of Age	
Physiologic chorea of infancy	Freud (621)
Perinatal asphyxia	Chapter 6
Kernicterus	Chapter 10
Postcardiopulmonary bypass	Chapter 17
Onset in Childhood	
"Minimal brain dysfunction"	Prechtl and Stremmer (622)
Genetic	
Disorders of intermediary metabolism	
Glutaric acidemia type 1	Chapter 1
δ-Glyceric acidemia	
Sulfite oxidase deficiency	
G_{M1} gangliosidosis	
G_{M2} gangliosidosis	
Lesch-Nyhan syndrome	
Leigh syndrome	
Heredodegenerative disorders	
Ataxia-telangiectasia	Chapter 12
Familial nonprogressive choreoathetosis	Chapter 3
Paroxysmal dyskinesia	Chapter 3
Toxic	
Neuroleptics (tardive dyskinesia)	Chapter 3
Anticonvulsants (phenytoin, carbamazepine)	Chapter 14
Metals (thallium, manganese)	Chapter 10
Isoniazid, reserpine	
Metabolic	
Hepatic encephalopathy	Chapter 17
Renal encephalopathy	Chapter 17
Hypoparathyroidism	Chapter 17
Pseudohypoparathyroidism	Chapter 17
Hyponatremia and hypernatremia	Chapter 17
Post–protein-calorie malnutrition	Chapter 10
Infectious	
Viral encephalitis	Chapter 7
Behçet disease	
Immunologic	
Systemic lupus erythematosus	Chapter 8
Sydenham chorea	
Trauma	Chapter 9
Onset in Adolescence	
Heredodegenerative diseases	
Wilson disease	Chapter 1
Huntington disease	Chapter 3
Hallervorden-Spatz disease	Chapter 3
Pellzaeus-Merzbacher disease	Chapter 3
Toxic	
Metabolic	
Infectious	
Immunologic	
Trauma	

associated with muscular hypotonia. To complicate the differentiation between chorea and tics, preexisting motor tics can merge into Sydenham chorea after a streptococcal infection (623). Sydenham chorea also should be distinguished from the various pediatric autoimmune neuropsychiatric diseases associated with streptococcal infection (PANDAS; discussed later in this chapter). The differentiation of chorea that develops as a symptom of SLE and Sydenham chorea rests on the presence of antinuclear and anti-DNA antibodies in the former entity. Antibodies against streptococcal DNAase are particularly useful for the diagnosis of Sydenham chorea because they tend to remain elevated for some 6 months after a streptococcal infection. Additionally, increased expression of the D8/17 B-cell alloantigen is seen in patients with Sydenham chorea and rheumatic fever, but not in SLE (624).

Choreic movements resulting from perinatal asphyxia generally become apparent between the first and the third years of life (see Chapter 6), an earlier age than in Sydenham chorea. The movements are usually slower and tend to be more evident in the larger proximal musculature. Like the involuntary movements of Sydenham chorea, they are exaggerated by fatigue and emotion. In most cases, choreiform movements are accompanied by other involuntary movements, principally athetosis.

The differential diagnosis between children with mild choreiform movements owing to Sydenham chorea and those whose choreiform movements are based on minimal brain dysfunction (see Chapter 18) is difficult because children with Sydenham chorea also have a high incidence of preexisting learning and personality problems. Resolution of the chorea in a matter of months suggests Sydenham chorea, as does the absence of clear-cut cognitive immaturities.

Huntington disease is rarely seen in children (see Chapter 3). The involuntary movements predominantly involve the proximal musculature, and, although abrupt, they are more extensive than those of Sydenham chorea. In particular, twisting movements of the shoulders and trunk are characteristic of Huntington disease. Mental deterioration or seizures, commonly found in Huntington disease and not observed in Sydenham chorea, and a history of autosomal dominant transmission are further clinical diagnostic aids.

Numerous drugs, notably haloperidol, isoniazid, reserpine, phenytoin, and phenothiazines such as prochlorperazine, also can induce choreiform movements. The various forms of paroxysmal choreoathetosis, a subgroup of the paroxysmal dyskinesias, can be distinguished by the sudden onset of choreiform movements in a child who has few, if any, involuntary movements between attacks (see Chapter 3). Familial benign choreoathetosis is a rare condition that begins in the first two decades of life. It is characterized by choreiform movements of the hands, shoulders, arms, and legs and by a combined resting and intention tremor (see Chapter 3). The disorder is transmitted in an autosomal dominant manner.

Treatment

Since Sydenham's 1684 recommendation of bleeding, purges, and laudanum (alcoholic tincture of opium) for the treatment of chorea, a large number of therapeutic regimens have been suggested. The variability in the duration of untreated chorea makes evaluation difficult, and the effectiveness of salicylates, cortisone, or ACTH in shortening the length of the illness has not been proven (53).

Currently, the optimal form of treatment is bed rest in a darkened, quiet room. For children whose movements are severe, drug therapy is necessary. In the past, phenobarbital, chlorpromazine, or haloperidol was used (53,591). Sodium valproate (15 to 25 mg/kg per day) appears to be equally efficacious and controls the involuntary movements in 5 to 10 days (625,626). The mechanism by which it works remains a matter of speculation. The drug is gradually withdrawn after 2 to 6 months. Should symptoms recur, it is restarted. Carbamazepine may be equally effective in the treatment of chorea (627,628). Cardoso and coworkers (629) suggested that intravenous methylprednisolone followed by oral prednisone be given to patients whose chorea remains refractory to the more conventional medication. Other immunomodulatory therapies, including IVIG and plasmapheresis, have been used successfully (591).

Even when streptococci cannot be isolated from throat cultures, a course of penicillin is indicated as soon as the diagnosis of Sydenham chorea is made. The patient is given a single intramuscular dose of 1.2 million U of benzathine penicillin, or an oral penicillin dose of 200 to 250 mg is given four times daily for 10 days (53).

The subsequent occurrence of rheumatic complications in many patients with Sydenham chorea dictates the prophylactic use of antimicrobial agents: the oral administration of penicillin (200,000 U two or three times daily) or clindamycin (75 mg two or three times daily) (630). The antibiotic is given for several years, or at least until the patient has completed high school.

Sydenham chorea remains an important public health problem, and there is no consensus regarding appropriate treatment other than penicillin prophylaxis. Therefore, a decision to treat should be based on patient disability and an awareness of the risk–benefit and side-effect profiles of the various treatment options (591).

Pediatric Autoimmune Neuropsychiatric Diseases Associated with Streptococcal Infection

The term PANDAS has been used to designate a group of neuropsychiatric disorders, notably tic disorders, Tourette syndrome, and OCD, that are believed to be related to an antecedent streptococcal infection and for which an autoimmune pathogenesis has been postulated (631,632). The condition began to be recognized in the early 1990s. Whether it had been present before then and not recognized or is of new onset is unknown. In fact, there is considerable controversy as to the actual existence of this entity (633).

The current understanding of its pathogenesis indicates that the process begins with a group A β-hemolytic streptococcal (GAS) infection in a susceptible host who produces antibodies to GAS that cross-react with the cellular components of the basal ganglia, particularly in the caudate nucleus and putamen (632). No unique strain of *Streptococcus* has been identified as trigger (634). Serum antineuronal antibodies that cross-react with caudate nucleus and other brain tissue have been found in Tourette syndrome and OCD (635), but their levels do not appear to differ from controls (636). However, patients with OCD or Tourette syndrome are frequently positive for B lymphocytes that express an epitope reactive with a D8/17 monoclonal antibody, the same antibody whose expression is increased in rheumatic fever and Sydenham chorea (637). Infantile bilateral striatal necrosis can occur following a streptococcal infection, and such patients harbor antibodies directed against neurons of the basal ganglia. By immunohistochemistry these antibodies exhibit specificity for large-size striatal neurons (638). Recently, Pavone and colleagues (639) suggested that anti–basal ganglia antibodies are present in children with PANDAS that cannot be explained merely by a history of GAS infection. As in chorea, expanded expression of D8/17 B-cell monoclonal antibody is found in PANDAS; thus, it is found in 85% of cases compared to 17% of normal individuals (634).

The clinical characteristics for the diagnosis of PANDAS have been listed by Swedo and colleagues (640,641). They are (a) presence of OCD, a tic disorder, or both; (b) onset between 3 years of age and puberty; (c) episodic course with abrupt onset or dramatic exacerbation of symptoms; (d) symptom exacerbations temporally related to group A β-hemolytic streptococcal infections, as demonstrated by a positive throat culture result, elevated antistreptococcal antibody titers, or both; and (e) association with neurologic abnormalities, notably choreiform movements during periods of symptom exacerbation. PANDAS is not a rare disorder, and the characteristic patient demonstrates a combination of choreiform movements and a tic disorder that has had an abrupt onset or a marked worsening in the wake of a streptococcal infection. Characteristically, there is no evidence for rheumatic carditis (642).

The diagnosis is suggested by a positive throat culture result or by positive antistreptococcal antibodies (Snider, Singer). Many questions about this disorder remain, notably how to treat it, and, most important, well-controlled studies are required to verify the relationship between streptococcal infection and the movement disorder (643,644). Dale and coworkers (645) reviewed the various movement disorders and psychiatric manifestations that follow streptococcal infections.

Various clinical recommendations have been proposed. These include laboratory testing of children for streptococcal infections and use of antibiotics directed against the putative inciting streptococcal organisms. These are coupled with the management of the various neuropsychiatric symptoms by means of serotonin-reuptake blockers and behavioral therapies (646). A randomized, placebo-controlled trial of IVIG (1 g/kg for 2 consecutive days) and plasmapheresis (five to six procedures performed on alternate days) resulted in significant and persistent improvement. When children are given IVIG, improvement is seen 3 weeks after treatment or even later and persists for 1 or more years (647). With plasma exchange, symptom improvement is noted toward the end of the first week of treatment and persists for 1 year or longer (647). In the experience of Perlmutter and colleagues, tic symptoms are more effectively treated with plasma exchange, whereas IVIG and plasma exchange appear almost equally effective for symptoms of OCD (647). Tonsillectomy may also represent an effective treatment option in children severely affected by PANDAS (634,648).

Rasmussen Syndrome

Rasmussen syndrome or encephalitis is a rare, progressive gray matter disease of children. It is marked by an onset in the first decade of life with intractable focal epilepsy, progressive hemiparesis, atrophy of the involved cerebral hemisphere, and dementia (649,650). Serum G1uR3 antibodies (651,652) and cytotoxic T cells (653,654) have been found in a small proportion of patients with Rasmussen syndrome, and both humoral and cellular immunologic mechanisms have been implicated in its pathogenesis. A good, albeit transient, response to immunomodulatory therapy, including IVIG and plasmapheresis, has been reported (649–651,655,656). All these findings support the notion that this condition represents an immune-mediated disease. Rasmussen syndrome is more fully described in Chapter 7.

Other Types of Epilepsy

A relationship between the immune system and epilepsy is also suggested by immunologic data available in other types of epilepsy (657). GluR3 antibodies are not specific for Rasmussen's encephalitis, and they have also been demonstrated in patients with partial or generalized epilepsy, particularly with severe early-onset disease and intractable seizures (658–660). Other autoantibodies that have been found in different types of epilepsy, which may be pathogenetically related to it, include antibodies against G_{M1} gangliosides in cryptogenic partial epilepsies (661), glutamic acid decarboxylase in refractory epilepsy (662,663), antiphospholipid in multiple, frequent seizures (664), and temporal cortex in Landau-Kleffner syndrome (665). Immunomodulatory therapy, including corticosteroids and immunoglobulins, has been used successfully in specific epileptic syndromes and in refractory epilepsies (666,667).

Experimental studies have also demonstrated the immunopathogenesis of different animal models of epilepsy and have suggested that the immune system can be used to target epilepsy (668,669).

IMMUNOLOGICALLY MEDIATED DEMYELINATING DISEASES OF THE PERIPHERAL NERVOUS SYSTEM

Guillain-Barré Syndrome

Guillain-Barré syndrome is an acquired, immune-mediated polyradiculoneuropathy causing dysfunction, segmental demyelination, and/or axonal degeneration in peripheral nerves, spinal sensory and motor nerve roots, and, occasionally, cranial nerves. Although GBS has been traditionally viewed as a unitary disorder with variations, recent research indicates that the syndrome includes several distinctive subtypes (484,670–672). These are classified as follows: (a) Sporadic GBS, which is most common, accounting for some 85% to 90% of cases, has been termed acute inflammatory demyelinating polyneuropathy (AIDP); (b) acute motor-sensory axonal neuropathy (AMSAN); (c) acute motor-axonal neuropathy (AMAN); (d) Miller Fisher syndrome: and (e) chronic inflammatory demyelinating polyneuropathy (CIDP). AIDP or GBS, terms that are still used interchangeably, is by far the most common cause of immune-mediated peripheral nerve disease in children, and with the near disappearance of poliomyelitis, is responsible for the great majority of cases of acute flaccid, areflexic paralysis. The condition is characterized by progressive weakness, which usually appears a few days to weeks after a nonspecific infection and is accompanied by mild sensory disturbances and a so-called "albumino-cytologic dissociation" (high protein but normal cell count) in the CSF (53,484,670–672).

The first cases were recorded in 1859 by Landry (673), who noted that the disorder can produce both motor and sensory symptoms (especially motor) that involve the distal parts of the limbs and that in some instances can become generalized by a sequential ascent of the neuraxis. Guillain et al. stressed the presence of "albumino-cytologic dissociation" (674).

GBS occurs year-round at a rate of 1 or 2 cases per 100,000 population per year in North America and South America, whereas the incidence is lower in Northern Europe (0.4 per 100,000 per year). For the United States and Canada this amounts to 3,500 cases per year. Male and female individuals are similarly at risk, and children are less frequently affected than adults (670,675,676). GBS occurs evenly throughout the Western hemisphere, without geographic clustering and with only minor seasonal variations. GBS has become the leading cause of acute flaccid paralysis in countries where widespread public health immunization programs have virtually eliminated epidemic polyneuritis (675).

Pathology

The pathology varies according to the clinical subtype (670,677). In the classic form of GBS, AIDP, both motor and sensory fibers are affected, although the anatomic structures mainly involved are the roots, motor in particular, and the adjacent proximal plexuses (484,670). The pathologic features are characterized by a marked segmental inflammatory demyelination, with focal and diffuse mononuclear, predominantly T-lymphocytic and monocytic/macrophage infiltration of all levels of the peripheral nervous system, from the anterior and posterior roots to the terminal twigs, and involving at times also the sympathetic chain and ganglia and the cranial nerves (670,677–679). Inflammatory cells are usually clustered around the endoneurial and epineurial vessels, particularly the small veins. T-lymphocyte infiltration appears to be preceded by a complement-mediated antibody binding to epitopes on the surface membrane of Schwann cells, resulting in their damage and vesicular demyelination (680). Segmental demyelination occurs in the areas infiltrated by inflammatory cells, whereas interruption of the axonal cylinders with subsequent wallerian degeneration is generally less extensive and is related to the intensity of the inflammatory response (670,678). The number of Schwann cells is increased, representing a reactive, possibly a reparative response. Ultrastructural studies reveal that macrophages are the major effectors of demyelination, and that neither Schwann cells nor myelin sheaths show significant primary damage, except where they are in direct contact with or are encroached on by activated monocytes/macrophages (681). In a minority of cases, a predominantly macrophage-associated demyelination occurs characterized by a paucity of lymphocytes (682).

In Miller Fisher syndrome, the reported pathologic changes appear to be similar to those reported in AIDP (670).

In the axonal variants of GBS, AMAN and AMSAN, in contrast to the demyelinating forms of GBS, there are no inflammatory features, and the primary effect on nerve fibers is axonal degeneration (670). In AMAN, the primary immune attack appears to be on the motor nodes of Ranvier. Motor fiber damage can be seen in ventral roots, peripheral nerves, and preterminal intramuscular motor nerve twigs (670). In AMAN, the primary attack is more widely distributed at both the motor and sensory nerve nodes of Ranvier, but the sequence of complement activation, macrophage attachment at nodes, opening of periaxonal spaces, and concurrent axonal shrinkage and axonal degeneration is the same in AMAN and AMSAN (670,683,684).

In the CNS, the alterations are essentially secondary to axonal degeneration. Most common is central chromatolysis involving the anterior horn cells in the spinal gray matter and neurons of the motor cranial nerve nuclei in the brainstem. Long-standing cases may show some features of degeneration of the posterior columns (678).

Pathogenesis

The morphologic alterations in the AIDP and CIDP forms of GBS resemble those found in experimental autoimmune neuritis (EAN), which is induced in animals by immunization with peripheral nerve homogenates (685) or, more specifically, by peptides P2 (686) and P0 (687), which are derived from peripheral nerve myelin protein. Immunization of rabbits with brain gangliosides G_{M1} also produces a motor axonal neuropathy with flaccid paralysis of the hind limbs (688). The role of T cells in the pathogenesis of EAN has been clearly shown in adoptive transfer EAN by the transfer of a T-cell line specific for P2 protein (677,689,690). Recent studies in mice have suggested that apolipoprotein E (apoE) acts as an inhibitor of the inflammatory and demyelinating process seen in EAN (691).

The current understanding of GBS is that it is an acquired immune-mediated neuropathy resulting from an aberrant immune response to an antecedent event, whether infection, immunization, or another immune-activating event (672,677,689), that eventually leads to autoimmune-mediated tissue injury through molecular mimicry, superantigen mechanisms, or cytokine stimulation, individually or in concert (672,692). In the AMAN form of GBS, the infecting organisms probably share homologous epitopes to a component of the peripheral myelin, myelin-producing Schwann cells, or axons (molecular mimicry). In AIDP, the antigen on the Schwann cell membrane that is involved in GBS is believed to be a glycoconjugate. In AMAN, the target molecules are likely to be gangliosides G_{M1}, G_{M1b}, G_{D1a}, and GalNAc-G_{D1a} expressed on the motor axolemma (672,676,677,689,693).

Antecedents

An antecedent acute infectious illness has been documented in approximately two-thirds of children who develop GBS (484,670–672,677). Most commonly, it is a respiratory tract infection or gastroenteritis. Several agents have been implicated in these infections (694–702). Of these, *Campylobacter jejuni* infection has become recognized as the most common bacterial antecedent of GBS (484,670,672,696,698,701). In various series it accounted for 23% to 41% of sporadic cases (698,701). Other responsible agents include cytomegalovirus, which has been implicated in 8% to 22% of GBS cases (696,701), and the Epstein-Barr virus, which is responsible for up to 2% to 10% of cases (696,697). Primary infection with herpes zoster has been noted in nearly 5% of childhood cases of GBS in some series (702). Other viruses implicated in the evolution of GBS are listed in Table 8.8. The chief feature shared by most of these is that they have a viral envelope. GBS has also been associated with *Mycoplasma pneumoniae* (703) and *Haemophilus influenzae* (704) infections.

Several vaccines have been related to the evolution of GBS. Of these, the best substantiated is the rabies vaccine as prepared from brain tissue and probably contaminated with myelin antigens (705,706). The swine-flu influenza vaccine, as administered in 1976 and 1977, was also responsible for numerous cases of GBS (646). Furthermore, it has been suggested that GBS is associated with other immunizations, including those for tetanus (707), polio (oral vaccine) (708), influenza (709), mumps, measles, and rubella (MMR) (710), hepatitis A (711), hepatitis B (712), and *H. influenza* type b (713). The most reasonable conclusion we can draw today from all available data is that a causal relationship between immunization and GBS has not convincingly been established, but cannot be excluded (672).

The association of GBS with trauma or surgical procedures purportedly precipitating stressful immunologic events is probably anecdotal (53).

Humoral Immunity

There is ongoing debate as to whether the primary effector mechanism of autoimmune injury is antibody mediated, T cell driven, or both (672).

The first step in GBS immunopathogenesis is the presentation of antigen to "naive" T cells resulting in their activation. The activated T cells circulate in the bloodstream and attach to the venular endothelium of peripheral nerves. T cells need to traverse the blood–nerve barrier. They migrate through the endothelial lining to a perivascular location into the endoneurium with the participation of a pathway of adhesion molecules, including selectins and leukocyte integrins and their counter-receptors on endoneurial vascular endothelial cell walls (672,689). The role of integrins (a family of cell adhesion molecules) in the development of inflammation in experimental allergic neuritis and GBS and subsequent remyelination is critically reviewed by Archelos and colleagues (714).

The last step of the pathogenetic events occurs when activated T cells and autoantibody enter the endoneurium along with macrophages, where both antibody and T cell–targeting mechanisms identify autoantigens on axonal or Schwann cell constituents, resulting in tissue injury accompanied by active phagocytosis by cells of the monocyte/macrophage lineage (670,672,677,689,715). A series of serum antibodies have been extensively studied, both in the clinical and experimental settings; however, their role in the pathogenesis of GBS is unclear.

TABLE 8.8 Infectious Organisms Associated with Guillain-Barré Syndrome or Acute Disseminated Encephalomyelitis

	Envelope	*Guillain-Barré Syndrome*	*Acute Disseminated Encephalomyelitis*	*Encephalitis*
DNA Viruses				
Adenoviridae				
Adenovirus		x	x	x
Herpesviridae				
Cytomegalovirus	x	x	x	x
Epstein-Barr virus	x	x	x	x
Herpes simplex viruses I, II	x	x	x	x
Human herpesvirus 6	x	x	?	x
Varicella-zoster virus	x	x	x	
Poxviridae				
Vaccinia	x	x		
Variola	x	x		
RNA Viruses				
Flaviviridae				
Japanese encephalitis virus		x		x
Orthomyoxoviridae				
Influenza viruses A and B	x	x		x
Paramyxoviridae				
Measles virus		x	x	x
Mumps virus		x	x	x
Picornaviridae (enteroviruses)				
Coxsackievirus		x		x
Echovirus		x		x
Retroviridae				
Human immunodeficiency viruses	x	x		x
Coronavirus				
Hepatitis viruses A, B, C				
Parainfluenza viruses I, II, III			x	
Parvovirus B19			x	
Respiratory syncytial virus				

C. jejuni is the reported causal agent in one-third of patients with GBS, and molecular mimicry between the gangliosides and the lipopolysaccharide (LPS) of the bacterium is considered to contribute to the generation of antiganglioside antibodies (670,672,677,716–718). G_{M1}, G_{M1b}, G_{D1a}, G_{Q1b}, and GalNAc-G_{D1a} epitopes are expressed in the LPSs of *C. jejuni* isolated from patients with GBS, and a single strain of *C. jejuni* has several ganglioside-like LPSs (676,689,693,718–720). Antiganglioside antibodies are detected in high titers in serum samples of approximately 40% of patients with GBS, and they are of the three major subclasses, IgM, IgG, and IgA (721). These antibodies are believed to react with epitopes located mainly in the axoplasmic compartment of axons, but also, to a lesser degree, in the myelin sheaths. Immunization of mice with *C. jejuni* LPS generates a monoclonal antibody that reacts with G_{M1} and binds to the peripheral nerves (720).

It has become increasingly apparent that the antigenic structure of the antecedent infectious agent determines the clinical manifestations of GBS. Patients whose sera have anti-G_{M1} antibodies (IgG) tend to develop the acute motor axonal neuropathy form of GBS (718,721,722), whereas those who specifically develop antibodies to G_{M1b} (723) or to anti–GalNAc-G_{D1a} (724,725) tend to have a more rapidly progressive, more severe form of disease with predominantly distal weakness. *C. jejuni* also has been implicated in the demyelinating form of GBS (726). More than of 90% of patients with Miller Fisher syndrome have elevated serum antibodies against the G_{Q1b} ganglioside (677,693,721,727). However, different phenotypes of the anti G_{Q1b} IgG antibody syndrome can occur at different times in the same patient, showing that this syndrome may be a distinct entity with a wide clinical spectrum on a unique immunologic background. Patients with anti G_{T1a} IgG, which cross-reacts with G_{Q1b} in 75% of cases, often have cranial nerve palsy (728). CMV infection is related to ganglioside G_{M2} (729), which is preferentially expressed in sensory nerves and causes a motor and sensory neuropathy (721); *M. pneumoniae* ganglioside GalC triggers antibodies that cause a poorly known neuropathy (721).

The pathogenicity of ganglioside-specific antibody (IgG) has been suggested lie in its capacity to reduce nerve conduction velocity (730) and activate phagocytes via IgG receptors (FcγR) (731). It has also been suggested that the participation of complement in the ganglioside-antibody reaction could lead to events that damage ion channels because there is experimental evidence that anti-G_{M1} antibodies can cause ion channel dysfunction (670). Taguchi and collaborators (732) showed that GalNAc-G_{D1a} antibodies may block neuromuscular transmission by affecting the ion channels in the presynaptic motor axon. Similarly, in the study of Yuki and coworkers previously cited (720), the monoclonal antibody induced by *C. jejuni* LPS and anti-G_{M1} IgG from patients with GBS does not induce paralysis, but blocks muscle action potentials in a muscle–spinal cord coculture (720).

Alternatively, other microbial structures rather than gangliosides per se may influence antigen presentation, thereby facilitating the proliferation of ganglioside-specific B- and T-cell clones. These are the so-called "superantigens," which are molecules capable of activating lymphocytes, bypassing the classic interaction of T-cell receptors with MHC-antigen complexes and B-cell receptors with antigens (721,733).

Another postulated immunopathogenetic mechanism in GBS is the "heterotypic cross-linking of specific and innate leukocyte receptors" (721,733). Interaction of mucosal lymphocytes with GBS-associated pathogens may trigger an engagement of leukocyte pattern recognition receptors (PRR) in addition to ganglioside-specific B- and T-cell receptors. PRR are potent immune modulatory molecules recognizing prototypical bacterial or viral structures. Cross-linking of both PRR and B-cell receptors has been shown to induce B-cell activation (734).

Cellular Immunity

T cell–mediated pathways are clearly also involved in the pathogenesis of the autoimmune injury of peripheral nerves in GBS (672,677,689). This assertion is supported by several lines of evidence derived from immunopathologic findings in GBS patients: (a) Cellular infiltrates, mainly macrophages, but also CD4− and CD8+ T lymphocytes, are seen in nerve biopsies (735), (b) there is systemic T-cell activation: T cells reactive to nerve antigens are found in peripheral blood (736), (c) *C. jejuni* DNA has been detected in myelomonocytic cells, suggesting that neuritogenic antigens may be presented by MHC class II to T cells (737), (d) a T-cell subset that expresses Vγ8/δ1 T-cell receptor phenotype has recently been isolated from sural nerve, lending credence to the hypothesis that *C. jejuni* could stimulate such receptors in the gut, hence becoming neuritogenic (738), and (e) there is evidence of a T cell-dependent serum antibody response to gangliosides (739). This body of evidence points to selective recruitment of macrophages and T lymphocytes causing damage to the peripheral nervous system. To this end, cytokines and chemokines are active participants in this inflammatory process (677,689).

Cytokines and Chemokines

Cytokines regulate the amplitude and the duration of the immune-inflammatory responses (677,689). Once the immune cells are drawn into the peripheral nerves in GBS patients, cytokines are released by them and also by the Schwann cells. Recent studies have confirmed the immune capabilities of Schwann cells, which can initiate, regulate, and terminate the immune response. They are able to participate in the processes of antigen presentation and secretion of pro- and anti-inflammatory cytokines, chemokines, and neurotrophic factors. The discovery of the purinergic receptor $P2X_7$ in Schwann cells may help to explain how their secretion of cytokines is regulated (740). Some of the cytokines implicated in the pathogenesis of GBS include IL-18, IL-12, IL-10, leukemia inhibitory factor (LIF), and TNF-α (677,741,742). Cytokines induce the production of proinflammatory mediators such as granulocyte-macrophage colony-stimulating factor (GM-CSF), chemokines (MIP-1), prostaglandins, and nitric oxide (NO) (677,743). The importance of NO in the pathogenesis of axon damage in GBS has recently been emphasized (744). Cytokines also regulate the generation of effector T and B lymphocytes (677). The serum levels of some cytokines, for examples, TNF-α (745), correlate with neurophysiologic evidence of demyelination.

Chemokines are low-molecular-weight cytokines involved in chemotaxis and activation of phagocytes and lymphocytes (677). In GBS patients, high levels of chemokines have been demonstrated, like monocyte chemoattractant protein (MCP-1) in serum (746) and IFN-inducible protein (IP-10) in CSF (747). In addition, the expression of chemokines is increased in nerve biopsies of animals with EAN (748) and in GBS patients (747). Further evidence of the role of chemokines in GBS pathogenesis is provided by the work of Zou and coworkers (749), who demonstrated that the injection of anti–CCL-3 (MIP-1α) antibody ameliorates the clinical course of EAN induced in the Lewis rat.

Genetics

Unlike autoimmune disorders where a genetic predisposition to develop the disease has been proved, the role of genetic factors in GBS is unclear. Disease heterogeneity and varying associations of preceding infections, antibody responses, and neurologic damage may be secondary to immunogenetic factors that direct the host immune response (689). Attempts to identify an immunogenetic susceptibility factor have largely focused on the HLA system. A study of HLA antigens in GBS by Adams and colleagues in 1977 (750) showed that the appearance of the disease is not influenced by genes associated with the

HLA-A or HLA-B locus. Other studies, however, reported an association between HLA-54, HLA-CW1, and HLA-DQB*3 antigens and GBS or Miller Fisher syndrome (751,752). In a British study, HLA-DQB1*03 was highly associated with a preceding infection with *C. jejuni* (751), whereas one Japanese study reported a high frequency of HLA-Bw54 in a clinically similar patient group (752). Recently, Magira and colleagues (753) demonstrated a positive association of AIDP with the DQB1*0401 allele with the unique DQβED$^{70-71}$ epitope and a negative association with the alleles AQB1*0503, DQB1*0601, DQB1*0602, and DQB1*0603, characterized by the epitope RDP$^{55-57}$. Moreover, the study revealed a differential distribution of HLA-DQB epitopes between AMAN and AIDP, providing immunogenetic evidence for differentiating these two GBS entities. Geleijns and coworkers (754) found that HLA-DRB1*01 is increased in patients who need mechanical ventilation. In this study, there was also a tendency toward an association between certain HLA alleles and several antiganglioside antibodies. Overall, these findings suggest that HLA class may be determinant in distinct groups of GBS, but that there is a need for further exploration in large-scale studies. In addition, information about the genetics of GBS has been provided by a recent study of GBS within 12 Dutch families, which concluded that GBS is a complex genetic disorder and its outcome is determined by both environmental and genetic factors. The genealogy and molecular genetics of a large number of families with GBS may give more insight into host factors determining an individual's susceptibility to the condition (755).

Clinical Manifestations

Acute Inflammatory Demyelinating Polyneuropathy (AIDP)

This is the traditionally recognized hallmark phenotype of GBS, and it is the most common clinical presentation among affected children in developed countries (670,672). Clinical symptoms result from disturbed saltatory conduction through myelinated axons (conduction block). GBS can occur at any time during childhood, but is most frequent between the ages of 4 and 9 years (756). A prodromal respiratory illness or gastroenteritis occurs in approximately two-thirds of the patients, approximately within 2 weeks before the onset of weakness (Table 8.9) (756,757).

Neurologic symptoms usually appear fairly suddenly (53). In a large proportion of cases, 89% of adult patients in the series of Moulin and colleagues (758), paralysis was accompanied by pain or paresthesias. In 47%, pain was severe and was described as a deep, aching pain in back and legs. Visceral pain was noted in 20%. In children, pain is also a prominent feature at presentation in 50% to 80% of cases and paresthesias in 18%(672).

The paralysis usually begins in the lower extremities, then ascends. Characteristically, it is symmetric, although minor differences between the sides are not rare. In approximately 50% of patients, the weakness is mostly distal, whereas in approximately 15%, the proximal musculature is more extensively involved (see Table 8.9). Ataxia is also common in children, and was present in 44% of patients in the series of Sladky (672). Cranial nerve palsies can appear at any time during the illness with variable frequency, from 15% to 43%. The facial nerve is most commonly affected; it was involved in more than one-half of patients in the series of Winer and colleagues (700). Papilledema is relatively rare. Although its appearance correlates well with increased intracranial pressure (759), papilledema is not always accompanied by elevation in CSF protein, and its pathogenesis is unexplained (760).

TABLE 8.9 Clinical Characteristics of 56 Children with Acute Infectious Polyneuritis

Characteristic	Percentage
Antecedent infection	70
Distal weakness predominantly	44
Proximal weakness predominantly	14
Cranial nerve weakness	43
Facial nerve	32
Spinal accessory nerve	21
Papilledema	5
Paresthesia and pain	43
Loss of vibratory or position sense or both	34
Meningeal irritation	17
Cerebrospinal fluid protein more than 45 mg/dL	88
Mortality	4
Full recovery or mild impairment	77
Relapses	7
Asymmetry of involvement	9

Data from Low NL, Schneider J, Carter S. Polyneuritis in children. *Pediatrics* 1958;22:972; and Peterman AF, Daly D, Dion FR, et al. Infectious neuronitis (Guillain-Barré syndrome) in children. *Neurology* 1959;9:533.

Paralysis of the respiratory muscles is a common complication in severely affected patients, but even in the absence of respiratory symptoms, vital capacity can be impaired with consequent carbon dioxide retention. Involvement of the sympathetic nervous system can produce a variety of dysautonomic abnormalities, including profuse sweating, hypertension, and postural hypotension, which often are predictors of a fatal cardiac arrhythmia (672,761). Sphincter disturbances are noted in up to one-third of patients (672,700).

Position sense is the sensory function most frequently impaired, followed by vibration, pain, and touch, in descending order of frequency. The deep tendon reflexes are generally absent, although increased reflexes and extensor plantar responses are occasionally recorded during the initial days of the illness (53). Recently, several adult patients with GBS exhibiting marked, persistent hyperreflexia were reported (762,763).

An elevation in the CSF protein content is characteristic. This exceeds 45 mg/dL in 88% of affected children (see Table 8.9) and peaks by 4 to 5 weeks, thereafter gradually returning to normal. However, in the first 2 to 3 days the CSF protein level is not elevated in most cases, and the appearance of the electrodiagnostic features of demyelination–remyelination tend to lag behind clinical evolution (670). The CSF cell count is usually normal, although significant pleocytosis (100+ cells/mL) occurs in approximately 5% of patients (53).

Electromyography reveals a picture compatible with involvement of the lower motor neurons or peripheral nerves. Abnormalities in nerve conduction are the most specific electrophysiologic findings. The most characteristic is the presence of conduction block. These features include prolongation of distal latencies or F-wave latencies, conduction velocity greater than 5 m/sec among comparable nerve segments, and dispersion of proximally evoked compound motor action potentials (672).There is a reduction in amplitude of the muscle action potential after stimulation of the distal, as compared to proximal, portion of the nerve. Approximately 80% of patients have nerve conduction block or slowing at some time during the illness. Not infrequently, the conduction velocity does not become abnormal until several weeks into the illness (764,765). When axonal degeneration is the primary feature of GBS, the severity of axonal loss correlates well with the prognosis. Profound reduction in compound motor action potential amplitudes usually is associated with a prolonged, incomplete recovery (672).

This neurologic picture evolves rapidly, and paralysis can be maximal within a few hours of the initial symptoms. More commonly, however, the paralysis becomes more extensive over 1 to 2 weeks, often, as in the classic Landry type of paralysis, progressively affecting the trunk, upper extremities, and cranial nerves. After the paralysis reaches a plateau, clinical improvement is usually first noted by the second to fourth weeks of the illness, and the majority of children experience complete recovery. Recovery is usually achieved within 2 months, although it can take as long as 18 months (53).

Some patients, approximately 10% of the Dublin series of Briscoe and coworkers (766) and 5% in the series of Das and collaborators (767), experience one or more relapses over the subsequent 2 months to several years. Such patients are considered to have CIDP. This condition is covered in a subsequent section.

Acute Motor-Sensory Axonal Neuropathy (AMSAN)

Feasby and coworkers (768,769) first described a subgroup of patients who developed a fulminant, extensive, and severe weakness with delayed and incomplete recovery. Electrophysiologic studies in these patients suggested a primary axonal degeneration, which was confirmed by nerve biopsy performed on patients who died shortly after the onset of their illness. This demonstrated severe axonal degeneration with little demyelination and scanty lymphocytic infiltration, an indication that in this condition the primary insult is to motor and sensory nerve axons (683). In these patients the earliest identifiable changes are in the nodes of Ranvier of motor fibers (770). Patients with this form of neuropathy are much more likely to have experienced an antecedent *C. jejuni* infection than control populations and are more likely to have high titers of serum anti-$G_D$la antibodies (722,771). This subtype is thought to be a more severe and widespread (both sensory and motor) version of acute motor-axonal neuropathy (670). The clinical presentation is indistinguishable from that of AIDP, but the prognosis is worse; therefore, elucidation of this diagnosis is clinically important (672). Electrophysiologic testing will confirm the presence of markedly decreased compound motor action potential and sensory-evoked potential amplitude and widespread denervation on EMG (672).

Acute Motor-Axonal Neuropathy

A pure motor axonal neuropathy has been reported from Mexico, China, and India, and is increasingly recognized in the Western world. In the Chinese cases, the disease appeared in annual summer epidemics and manifested as a severe motor neuropathy, with involvement of the proximal portion of the motor neurons or cell bodies and good recovery. Electrophysiologic studies show decreased motor action potential amplitude, preservation of motor nerve conduction velocities, denervation on EMG, and normal sensory nerve conduction velocities (672,772,773). In the Indian paralytic disease, fever and hemorrhagic conjunctivitis occur at the onset of the illness, the weakness is asymmetric, and the CSF demonstrates a pleocytosis. This form of neuropathy also is closely associated with *C. jejuni* infection (698,721).

Miller Fisher Syndrome (MFS)

Another variant of GBS, MFS, was first described by Fisher in 1956 (774). It is characterized by the evolution, within approximately 1 week, of external ophthalmoplegia, ataxia, and areflexia (670,672). The first symptom is usually diplopia, with bilateral facial paresis being present in approximately one-half of the affected children (775). Internal ophthalmoplegia is present in approximately two-thirds.

The CSF shows a mild elevation in protein content and, occasionally, pleocytosis, but typical albumino-cytologic dissociation, as seen in AIDP, can be present (672). Electrophysiologic testing shows abnormalites confined to sensory axonal populations. Some patients may exhibit slowing of motor and sensory nerve conduction (672). In a recent study of 6 patients with MFS, 5 had electrophysiologic evidence of an axonal, predominantly sensory polyneuropathy characterized by reduced amplitude or absent sensory responses, accentuated in their arms, and mild F-wave abnormalities. However, 3 patients had the patterns of low median, normal sural responses, raising the possibility of demyelinating neuropathy. Needle EMG found patchy fibrillation in 2 patients (776). The EEG can show excessive slow-wave activity or can be normal (777). Neuroimaging studies exclude a mass lesion (778,779).

Symptoms remain severe for 1 to 2 weeks before recovery commences. Recovery proceeds at a variable rate, but generally is complete.

The Miller Fisher syndrome is associated with strains of *C. jejuni* that have the ability to induce antibodies against ganglioside G_{Q1b} (677,693,721,780,781). Such antibodies can be demonstrated in 95% of patients with MFS, and their titers parallel the course of the disease. These antibodies have the ability to block the release of acetylcholine from motor nerve terminals, with oculomotor fibers having the highest concentration of G_{Q1b}-reactive antigens (693,773,782,783). The effect resembles that induced by α-latrotoxin (784) (see Table 10.6).

It is a matter of dispute whether Miller Fisher syndrome should be distinguished from brainstem encephalitis, as delineated by Bickerstaff and others (785,786). According to some, ataxia in Miller Fisher syndrome is caused entirely by peripheral nerve involvement, and pathologic changes are restricted to the peripheral nervous system (787). Others believe that the CNS also is involved and that in some cases a combined central and peripheral demyelination exists. MRI studies do not appear to help in the differential diagnosis. Whereas the MRI is normal in some cases of MFS, in others T2-weighted images demonstrate areas of increased signal in the brainstem. Conversely, there are several instances of clinically diagnosed brainstem encephalitis in which electrophysiologic evidence exists for involvement of the peripheral nerves (788). MFS also must be distinguished from posterior fossa tumors. Before neuroimaging studies this differentiation was difficult. However, the constellation of a severe and sometimes complete external ophthalmoplegia, ataxia, and loss of deep tendon reflexes in a fairly alert child is unique (53).

Chronic Inflammatory Demyelinating Polyradiculoneuropathy (CIDP)

CIDP has a childhood incidence of 0.5 in 100,000 per year. It can occur as early as in infancy, frequently with motor delay. Usually children present with a subacute onset of symmetric proximal weakness that progresses over at least 2 months (789). CIDP has some of the clinical features of GBS, but the evolution of the neurologic symptoms is slower, a matter of weeks or months rather than days. The motor component of the picture is usually predominant (716,790), and weakness is greatest in the distal muscles. Fatigue and sensory symptoms, including dysesthesias and sensory loss, are common (789). Some children progress to maximal weakness over the course of 3 months or less and tend to have a monophasic course. Recovery with long-term remission is common in this group. Some other children have a chronic fluctuating course without complete recovery between exacerbations (789,791,792). The initiating factor responsible for CIDP is unknown in most children, although evidence suggests an immune-mediated mechanism. There is presence of T cells, predominantly CD8+, in the endoneurium, which correlates with the activity of demyelination, suggesting that a T cell-mediated process is of pathogenetic significance in CIDP (689,793). Antibodies directed at G_{M1}, G_D1b, and asialo-G_{M1} glycolipids have been identified in some cases, suggesting that the galactosyl (α1-3) *N*-acetogalactosaminyl moiety of myelin may be an important target antigen in some cases (794). Connolly and Pestronk (795) reported selective polyclonal β-tubulin (epitope 301–314) autoantibodies in about one-half of patients with CIDP; the pathogenic significance of these antibodies is unclear. The 301-314 tubulin epitope has sequence homology to several human viruses, including herpes simplex and CMV, but no homologies to sequences have been indentified in any myelin surface component. Unlike GBS, in which no association with histocompatibility antigens has been established, CIDP has been shown to be associated with haplotypes B8, Cw7, DR3, and Dw3 (796,797).

The diagnostic clinical research criteria include (a) progressive or relapsing motor and sensory dysfunction of more than one limb and (b) hyporeflexia or areflexia, which usually involves all four limbs (798) The CSF shows albumino-cytologic dissociation, and in some cases oligoclonal bands and IgG synthesis may be identified (789,799). Electrophysiologic studies must fulfill three of the following four criteria for research diagnosis (798): (a) a slowing of motor conduction velocity, (b) partial conduction block, abnormal temporal dispersion in one or two motor nerves, (c) prolonged distal latencies in two or more nerves, and (d) absent or prolonged minimal F-wave latencies. In a series of 18 patients from Brazil, electrophysiologic studies revealed demyelination in all of them and axonal damage in 94% (800). On biopsy, the peripheral nerves show mononuclear infiltrates, a segmental demyelination, and increased numbers of Schwann cells, with subsequent remyelination of various proportions. Their processes are arranged in whorls around the demyelinated axons. Termed onion bulbs, they are characteristic of not only the hereditary peripheral neuropathies (see Chapter 3), but also of most chronic recurrent neuropathies, and their presence correlates with the duration of symptoms (801). Table 8.10 shows the differential diagnosis of CIDP of childhood, together with some salient diagnostic features of each of the major entities.

TABLE 8.10 Differential Diagnosis of Chronic Polyneuritis of Childhood

Condition	Diagnostic Features
Lead poisoning	Blood lead levels; basophilic stippling of erythrocytes
Arsenic poisoning	Elevated arsenic in hair, nails
Thiamine deficiency	Transketolase deficiency
Polyarteritis nodosa	Muscle biopsy
Systemic lupus erythematosus	Antinuclear antibodies Antiphospholipid antibodies Familial history
Hereditary motor and sensory neuropathies	Sural nerve biopsy; motor and sensory conduction times on patient and on parents
Refsum disease (ataxia polyneuritiformis)	Elevated blood phytanic acid
Metachromatic leukodystrophy	Intellectual deterioration; absent urinary and tissue arylsulfatase
Globold cell leukodystrophy (Krabbe)	Early onset, intellect deteriorates, nerve biopsy, galactocerebroside galactosidase assays in serum
Chronic polyneuritis of unknown cause	Exclusion of above

Modified from Byers RK, Taft LT. Chronic multiple neuropathy in childhood. *Pediatrics* 1957;20:517.

Unusual Clinical Variants

Ropper in 1986 (802) and 1994 (803) described a series of patients who did not strictly fulfill the diagnostic criteria of GBS but had clinical and neurophysiologic characteristics compatible with GBS. The latter included acute monophasic polyneuropathy followed by improvement or remission, CSF with albumino-cytologic dissociation, and electrophysiologic findings of demyelinating or axonal pattern of nerve damage. The diagnoses established by Ropper included: (a) pharyngeal-cervical-brachial weakness (PCBW), (b) paraparesis, (c) severe ptosis without ophthalmoplegia, (d) facial diplegia and paresthesias, and (e) combination of MFS and PCBW. Recently, the pediatric neurology group from the Garrahan Hospital in Buenos Aires, Argentina, described (804), for the first time in children, a series of patients with similar diagnoses to the ones described by Ropper (802,803). In addition, the authors described a new variant, the so-called "saltatoria" ("jumping") form, in a patient who presented as a classic AIDP but progressed to lower cranial nerve paresis without compromising the upper limbs. Recently, MacLeann and colleagues described one case of PCBW variant in a 12-year-old, emphasizing that this diagnosis should be considered in a child presenting with bulbar palsy and/or respiratory failure (805). Whether the concept of variant polyneuritis can be extended to explain pure multiple cranial nerve palsies as an "oligosymptomatic" form of GBS or these should be classified separately is unclear (803). Osaki and coworkers (806) reported a case of asymmetric PCBW with anti-G_{T1a} IgG antibody. Further studies with antiganglioside antibodies should help to better define these unusual GBS variants and clarify their pathogenesis (804).

Diagnosis

The criteria for the clinical diagnosis of classical GBS were established in 1978 by the National Institute of Neurological and Communicative Disorders and Stroke (NINDS) (807) and were updated in 1990 by Asbury and Cornblath (764). They are presented in Table 8.11. In essence they rest on the gradual development of symmetric muscular weakness, which is often worse over the distal portion of the lower extremities, the presence of areflexia, and the aforementioned CSF and electrodiagnostic abnormalities (484,670–672). Selective contrast enhancement of anterior

TABLE 8.11 Guillain-Barré Syndrome Study Group Diagnostic Criteria

Required for Diagnosis
Progressive motor weakness involving more than one extremity
Areflexia or marked hyporeflexia
No more than 50 monocytes or two granulocytes per μL cerebrospinal fluid
Strongly Supportive of Diagnosis
Initial absence of fever
Progression over days to a few weeks
Onset of recovery 2 to 4 weeks after cessation of progression
Relatively symmetric weakness
Mild sensory signs and symptoms
Cranial nerve signs
Elevation of cerebrospinal fluid protein after 1 week of symptoms
Slowed nerve conduction velocity or prolonged F waves
Autonomic dysfunction

From National Institute of Neurologic and Communicative Disorders and Stroke. Ad hoc Committee. Criteria for diagnosis of Guillain-Barré syndrome. *Ann Neurol* 1978;3:565, With permission.

spinal nerve roots on MRI has been reported as a neuroimaging feature suggestive of GBS (808–810).

In the presence of sensory changes, usually little doubt exists about the diagnosis. On the other hand, when sensory changes are absent, a number of other entities must be considered in the context of differential diagnosis (671,672). In poliomyelitis, the onset of paralysis is accompanied by fever and evidence of a systemic illness. Although poliomyelitis due to poliovirus has been practically eliminated through effective immunization programs, West nile virus, and enteroviruses, particularly enterovirus 71, can cause infection of anterior horn neurons, resulting in acute paralysis (811). Yet, muscle involvement is rarely symmetric in poliomyelitis, and CSF pleocytosis is common during the initial stages of the illness (see Chapter 7). Polymyositis, seen mainly in adults, can be confused with GBS. The distribution of muscular weakness in polymyositis tends to be proximal, and the CSF protein content remains normal. The presence of hypokalemia in the occasional patient with GBS calls for consideration of hypokalemic paralysis in the differential diagnosis. This condition usually carries a family history, and the ECG is abnormal during a paralytic attack (114,812). The differential diagnosis of ATM and GBS has been noted already. Other less common conditions that induce progressive muscular weakness of rapid onset are described in Chapter 16.

Treatment

Taking into account the autoimmune-mediated pathogenesis of GBS, the approach to treatment includes immunosuppressants and immunomodulators (484,670–672,689,772,813–815).

Corticosteroids

Steroids have been shown to be not beneficial in the treatment of GBS and possibly are contraindicated (772,813,814,816). A Cochrane systematic review published in 1999 and including all trials in which any form of corticosteroid or ACTH treatment was used for the management of patients with GBS evaluated the results of six randomized studies. The authors concluded that there was no difference in the Improvement in Disability Scale, which was the primary outcome. There was also no significant difference between the groups for secondary outcome measures of recovery, time to recovery of unaided walking, time to discontinue ventilation in the subgroup who needed it, mortality, and combined mortality and disability after 1 year.

A comparison of a series of corticosteroid-treated patients with historical controls pointed to a beneficial effect from corticosteroids when given in combination with IVIG (817). However, a double-blind, placebo-controlled, multicenter, randomized study of 233 GBS patients showed no significant difference in disability score between patients treated with IVIG alone and those treated with combination of IVIG and methylprednisolone (818). In conclusion, corticosteroids are not recommended for the treatment of patients with GBS (816).

In contrast, many patients who experience CIDP show a clear-cut response to corticosteroids (772,814,819). Thus, Dyck and colleagues (820) reported that prednisone treatment beginning at a daily dose of 120 mg and slowly tapered over 13 weeks led to a small but statistically significant improvement in adult patients compared to those receiving no drug treatment. Patients began to improve after 2 weeks and had a maximum response after 6 months.

Immunoglobulin

Treatment with IVIG has shown in case reports, case series, and retrospective reviews to accelerate recovery from GBS. Although no placebo-controlled trials have been performed, IVIG has been compared with plasmapheresis or plasma exchange (PE) in controlled clinical trials. The predominant mechanisms by which IVIG therapy exerts its action appears to be a combined effect of complement inactivation, neutralization of idiotypic antibodies, cytokine inhibition, and saturation of Fc receptors on macrophages (676). The most likely mechanism is that it modulates the immune response in GBS by selective suppression of the proinflammatory cytokines (821).

The results of the first large, randomized trial comparing IVIG and PE in treating GBS in adults were published in 1992 (822). In this Dutch study, 150 GBS patients who were unable to walk independently were randomized to treatment with IVIG, 0.4 mg/kg per day for 5 days, or PE, 200 to 250 mL/kg, within 2 weeks of symptom onset. Patients treated with IVIG showed a greater and faster improvement than those subjected to PE. Moreover, there was significantly less need for assisted ventilation and fewer complications in the IVIG group. A recent Cochrane Database System Review by Hughes and collaborators (823) evaluated through a meta-analysis 536 GBS patients, mostly adults, from six randomized trials comparing IVIG and PE. Patients were unable to walk unaided and had been ill for less than 2 weeks. The authors concluded that IVIG hastens recovery from GBS as much as PE. Giving IVIG after PE is not significantly better than PE alone. However, in the study of Hadden and coworkers (696) in adult GBS patients, those with pure motor GBS had a better outcome if treated with both IVIG and PE compared with PE alone. Other reports have suggested that IVIG is superior to PE in GBS patients with a preceding *C. jejuni* infection and a predominantly motor syndrome and G_{M1} and G_{M1b} antibodies. However, none of these correlations is absolute, and testing for ganglioside antibodies and preceding infections is not warranted for guiding therapeutic decisions (689).

Because of inconsistencies in reporting, it is not clear whether adverse events are more common with IVIG or PE (816). The possible side effects of IVIG include fever, myalgia, headache, hypotension, meningismus, urticaria, eczema, and, rarely, renal tubular necrosis, thromboembolic events, pancytopenia, alopecia, and anaphylaxis. IVIG probably has a higher risk of infection transmission than PE (824). There have been reports of patients whose symptoms may worsen during and after the infusion or who may suffer relapses (825,826).

Randomized trials are needed to decide the effect of IVIG in children, in adults with mild disease, and in adults who start treatment after more than 2 weeks (827).

High-dose IVIG has also been effective in the treatment of CIDP (689,772,789,791,813,814).

Plasma Exchange

PE has been extensively used in the treatment of GBS; however, since the introduction of IVIG to treat this condition, the indication for PE has decreased (828). Controlled studies have confirmed that in pediatric patients PE shortens the interval to independent ambulation (829) and the duration of mechanical ventilation (830). One study, involving patients older than 16 years, indicated that for mild cases of GBS two exchanges are better than none. For moderate or severe cases, four exchanges, conducted in the course of 1 week, are better than two. The use of more than four exchanges does not confer additional benefits (831).

PE is also useful in the treatment of CIDP (689,772,789,791,813,814). A recent Cochrane Database Systematic Review by Mehndiratta and colleagues (832) concluded that evidence from two small trials show significant short-term benefit of PE in about two-thirds of patients with CIDP, but rapid deterioration may occur afterward. More research is needed to identify agents that may prolong the beneficial effect of PE.

The report on immunotherapy for GBS of the Quality Standards Subcommittee of the American Academy of Neurology concluded the following (816):

1. PE is recommended for nonambulatory adult patients who seek treatment within 4 weeks of the onset of neuropathic symptoms. PE should also be considered for patients who were ambulatory and were examined within 2 weeks of the onset of neuropathic sympotoms.
2. IVIG is recommeneded for nonambulatory adult patients within 2 weeks, and possibly 4 weeks, of the onset of neuropathic symptoms. The effects of PE and IVIG are equivalent.
3. Corticosteroids are not recommended for treatment.
4. Sequential treatment with PE followed by IVIG or immunoabsorption followed by IVIG is not recommended.
5. PE and IVIG are treatment options for children with severe symptoms.

Other Therapies

Filtration of CSF has been investigated in a small prospective study of 37 GBS patients (491). The repeated removal of small volumes of CSF through a lumbar catheter followed by filtration through a Millipore filter and reinfusion through the same catheter is well tolerated and equally effective to conventional PE. The rationale for this therapeutic approach rests on the notion that the nerve roots are prominently affected in GBS cases and, therefore, filtration of CSF rather than whole PE might be more efficient (689).

Immunosuppressive drugs have been used successfully in the treatment of CIDP, including azathioprine, cyclophosphamide, and cyclosporine. Other immunomodulatory therapies that may be useful in CIDP are mycophenolate and interferon-β (772,789,813,814). In refractory patients, Rosenberg and colleagues (833) reported good response in 3 of 4 patients subjected to total lymphoid irradiation (200 rads). Vermeulen and Van Oers (834) described the remarkable improvement of a patient with CIDP after undergoing autologous stem-cell transplantation.

In the future, a better understanding of the immunopathogenesis of GBS and its clinical variants will improve our therapeutic intervention (672). Possible strategies may include using monoclonal antibodies against B cells, modifying agents of the macrophage Fcγ.

Management

Optimal proactive management and treatment of GBS is critically important. The neuropathy can progress rapidly, so that the potential for paralysis of the respiratory muscles should be considered in each patient, and facilities for tracheostomy and mechanical ventilation should be readily available. Generally, these measures should be instituted when impaired vital capacity first becomes apparent rather than after the patient has obvious respiratory compromise. A reduction of vital capacity to approximately one-half the norm for the patient's age calls for immediate consideration of tracheostomy. Signs of autonomic dysfunction should be carefully monitored because fluctuations in blood pressure and hemodynamic instability are common. Oropharyngeal weakness may increase salivation and compromise oral intake. Careful attention should be paid to nutritional requirements, both during the acute treatment in the intensive care unit and after discharge to the floor. Diligent nursing care is mandatory. Early introduction of physical and occupational therapy to prevent musculoskeletal and skin complications is paramount. Both active and passive exercises should be graduated as recovery progresses (53,670–672).

Prognosis

In general, the outlook, including prospects for recovery, is better in children than in adults. During the course of the acute illness, about 40% of children become either bed or wheelchair bound and approximately 15% of them require mechanical ventilatory support. However, 90% to 95% of patients make a complete recovery within 6 to 12 months; the remainder are expected to be ambulatory with only minor residual neurologic deficits (672).

The greatest life-threatening dangers during the acute phase of GBS are respiratory paralysis and cardiac arrhythmias. Cardiac arrhythmias can be brought on by manipulation of the patient, such as from changing a tracheotomy tube (839). Mortality was reported to be 4% in the combined series of Low and colleagues (756) and Peterman and coworkers (757) (Table 8.9). However, with improvement in supportive care, fatalities are rare nowadays. In the pediatric age group, there is generally no correlation between the severity of the illness and the long-term outcome (839).

Some studies suggest that an antecedent *C. jejuni* infection correlates with a disease in which there is axonal degeneration and a poor outcome (670,696,698). In adults, other disease factors associated with a worse prognosis are the fulminance and severity of the attack, diarrhea, marked reduction of compound action motor potentials, raised soluble interleukin-2 receptor (sIL-2R), and absence of IgM antibodies to gangliosides G_{M1} (670,696). Studies in adults have shown the patients may have residual fatigue, which persists for a long time and reduce the quality of life, but responds well to physical training (840). Electrophysiologic studies carried out in adult patients demonstrate persistent abnormalities indicating axonal loss and compensatory reinnervation, more frequent than in patients who were severely affected at nadir (841). These findings underscore the disabling nature of the disease in some patients and further point to the need for developing treatments aimed at neuroprotection and the promotion of regeneration (841).

Bell's Palsy

An acute paralysis of the face, often after a mild infection, was first described by Bell in 1829 (842):

> Cases of this partial paralysis must be familiar to every medical observer. It is very frequent for young people to have what is vulgarly called a blight, by which is meant a slight palsy of the muscles on one side of the face, and which the physician knows is not formidable.
> Inflammations of glands seated behind the angle of the jaw will sometimes produce this.... The patient has a command over the muscles of the face; he can close the lips, and the features are duly balanced; but the slightest smile is immediately attended with distortion, and in laughing and crying the paralysis becomes quite distinct.

Because the process is often partly or wholly reversible, little is known about the acute pathology or pathophysiology, which is assumed to be inflammatory. The essential anatomic changes of the seventh nerve in Bell's palsy are under considerable dispute. Most authors agree that during the acute phase of the illness, patients have considerable edema of the nerve and venous congestion in the facial canal. A few microscopic hemorrhages occur, but little inflammatory reaction.

In 73% of patients, there is an antecedent upper respiratory infection or exposure to cold drafts; these causes were the most frequently implicated during the nineteenth century (843). More recently, a variety of infectious agents have been suggested. On the basis of antibody levels, the list includes Epstein-Barr virus (in some 20% of patients) (844), mumps, and possibly herpes simplex and herpes zoster (845). Facial palsy caused by Lyme disease is particularly frequent in Scandinavia and other endemic areas. In one series, 60% of children with Bell's palsy had specific IgM antibodies for the spirochete in CSF (846). Lymphocytes from patients with Bell's palsy have been found to respond specifically to a basic protein (P1) isolated from human peripheral myelin. No response could be elicited to the P2 protein implicated in GBS (847). Additionally, T lymphocytes, mainly T-helper cells, are depressed during the first 2 weeks of the disease (848). Facial palsy has also been associated with elevation of antiglycolipid IgM antibodies against G_{M2} and LM1 (849). Kanoh and colleagues (850) emphasized ischemia as an important pathogenetic factor. A genetic predisposition also appears to be relevant (851).

Clinical Manifestations

Any aspects of facial nerve function may be involved. This includes facial motor movement, notably facial expression and lid closure; the tensor tympani, resulting in impaired dampening of eardrum reaction to loud noises; taste sensation of the anterior two-thirds of the tongue; and autonomic regulation of lachrymal and salivary glands. The site of dysfunction determines which modalities are involved. Although potential sites include any point from the pontine nucleus to distal portions of nerve within canaliculi of the skull, the most common site is within the facial canal of the temporal bone (53).

Bell's palsy occurs in 2.7 in 100,000 children younger than 10 years of age and 10.1 in 100,000 children older than 10 years of age. As is the case for GBS and ADEM, Bell's palsy commonly follows an upper respiratory illness. Whereas most childhood cases are unilateral, asymmetric bilateral Bell's palsy occasionally is encountered; usually this is a manifestation of GBS (53).

In many cases, pain localized in the ear or surrounding area is the initial symptom. This is followed by a rapid evolution of the paralysis, which reaches its full extent in a few hours. Characteristically, paralysis involves the musculature of the forehead, cheek, and perioral region. Approximately one-half of patients lose taste sensation. Lacrimation is retained in the great majority of children (852). The pain, which can reflect trigeminal nerve involvement, usually disappears quickly.

Auditory-evoked potentials and trigeminal nerve-evoked potentials indicate that in a considerable proportion of patients, Bell's palsy is not a mononeuropathy, but is accompanied by subclinical involvement of the trigeminal and auditory pathways (853,854). Rarely, there is a familial predisposition to facial nerve palsy; in these cases, facial nerve weakness can be accompanied by oculomotor paralyses (855).

The CSF is usually normal or shows a slight pleocytosis. In cases that evolve as a complication of Lyme disease, pleocytosis is often striking (846,856). MRI demonstrates enhancement of the intrameatal segment of the facial nerve on T1-weighted images. On T2-weighted images enlargement of the intrameatal segment can be seen with three-dimensional imaging (857).

In most children, recovery begins within a few weeks and reaches its maximum in 1 to 9 weeks (852). The patient can be expected to recover completely when the palsy is partial, as is the case in 80% of children (858,859), or when evoked EMG shows an incomplete denervation of the facial nerve. When denervation is complete, the onset of recovery is delayed for approximately 6 weeks and its maximal extent is not achieved until 6 months (860). In such instances, return of muscle function is usually incomplete. In 7% of children, facial paralysis recurs (861,862). In some, it is part of Melkersson syndrome. This condition is characterized by recurrent facial palsy that is often associated with swelling of the lips, tongue, cheeks, or eyelids and, less commonly, furrowing of the tongue (863). With each attack of Melkersson syndrome, facial nerve function becomes progressively more impaired, and paralysis ultimately can be nearly complete (864). Treatment with methylprednisolone and lymecycline has been suggested (865,866).

Diagnosis

The diagnosis of Bell's palsy rests on the exclusion of other causes of isolated facial paralysis (Table 8.12).

Facial nerve palsy caused by otitis media, with or without mastoiditis, is relatively common (860). A number of intracranial neoplasms, particularly those involving the brainstem, can result in the sudden onset of facial weakness (see Chapter 11). In some instances, transient improvement can be observed before other neurologic signs appear. Isolated facial nerve palsy can be seen with a variety of viral encephalitides, notably those due to mumps, varicella, and the enteroviruses (see Chapter 7). It also is a concomitant to osteomyelitis of the skull, pseudotumor cerebri, and systemic hypertension (867,868). The cause of the facial palsy in systemic hypertension is not clear but is believed to be induced by hemorrhages within the facial canal. The facial palsy can be the presenting feature of hypertension, and it is often intermittent and unrelated to the level of hypertension. In children, facial palsy is rarely caused by herpes zoster of the geniculate ganglion (Ramsay Hunt syndrome) (860). Another unusual cause for facial nerve palsy is the presence of an intra-aural tick. The salivary gland of the tick secretes a toxin that interferes with the synthesis or liberation of acetylcholine at the motor end plates of facial muscle fibers (869).

TABLE 8.12 Causes of Isolated Facial Paralysis, 1957 Through 1972

	Number of Cases	
Cause	***Paine (852)***	***Manning and Adour (860)***
Congenital		
Congenital anomaly	15	2
Birth trauma	18	5
Postnatal		
Idiopathic (Bell's)	19	37
With upper respiratory infection	9	
Without upper respiratory infection	10	
Otitis media	16	6
Surgical trauma	2	
Other trauma	3	2
Intracranial tumor	2	
Extracranial tumor	1	
Hypertension	2	
Polymyelitis	2	
Histiocytosis X		2
Varicella		1
Herpes zoster (Ramsay Hunt)		1
Mumps		1
Postimmunization (diphtheria-pertussis-tetanus and polio)		1

Treatment and Prognosis

A number of therapeutic approaches have been suggested (53), and their selection varies among physicians (870).

Administration of corticosteroids to reduce the edema within the facial canal has been used for several years. In view of the high recovery rate of untreated children, its evaluation is difficult. An analysis of all available studies led Huizing and coworkers (871), Holland and Weiner (872), and Ünüvar and coworkers (873) to conclude that therapy was no better than placebo. In many instances, however, one has the clinical impression that treatment with corticosteroids within several days of the onset of symptoms is beneficial. Nevertheless, Salman and MacGregor, who performed a systematic review of pediatric cases, concluded that the use of steroids is not recommended (874). At this time, however, a randomized, multicenter trial of the early administration of steroids has not been concluded (875). There is also no evidence for the effectiveness of antiviral agents. In any case late treatment is certainly of no value.

Decompression of the facial nerve from the stylomastoid foramen through its pyramidal portion has been advised for patients who show complete denervation on evoked EMG, although no evidence indicates that this procedure is effective in either children or adults, and the procedure is not offered routinely (872,876).

In children whose facial function recovers only partially, contractures can be expected. Misdirection of growth results in facial mass action in which attempted activity of one muscle group produces movements in several different muscle groups (synkinesis). Misdirection of growth also can result in tics or in the syndrome of crocodile tears. In this syndrome, food in the mouth or the smell of food is followed by lacrimation rather than salivation (877).

Varieties of cosmetic surgical procedures have been described, but these should be deferred until facial growth is complete. Facial retraining with biofeedback has also been recommended (878). Artificial tears and eye patches should be supplied to all children whose Bell's palsy results in incomplete eye closure, particularly during sleep.

Generally, the younger the patient, the more likely it is there will be a good recovery. Other favorable factors include the absence of hyperacusis and relatively normal minimal excitability values for the affected facial nerve. These values are obtained by electrical stimulation of the branches of the nerve just anterior to the ear and measurement of the minimal current required to effect a visible contraction of the muscle. The excitability study must be done within the first few days of the onset of paralysis; if corticosteroid therapy has been chosen, the dose of corticosteroids can be modified according to the values obtained (879).

Postinfectious Abducens Palsy

A painless palsy of the abducens nerve that clears without residua can develop in children of any age 7 to 21 days after a nonspecific febrile illness or upper respiratory infection. The paralysis is often complete but unassociated with any other cranial nerve palsy or neurologic signs. Improvement becomes evident in 3 to 6 weeks, and the palsy clears completely in 2 to 3 months. Except for the CSF, which can occasionally show a mild lymphocytosis, all laboratory and radiologic study results are normal (880). The various infectious agents that have been implicated include Epstein-Barr virus, cytomegalovirus, and *Mycoplasma pneumoniae* (881). Postinfectious abducens palsy is diagnosed by exclusion of abducens palsy secondary to increased intracranial pressure, tumors of the brainstem, brainstem encephalitis, and Gradenigo syndrome (882). The last, caused by an osteomyelitis of the apex of the petrous bone, is characterized by abducens palsy after otitis media; it is accompanied by pain in the distribution of the homolateral trigeminal nerve.

Rarely, abducens palsy may recur, with the episodes occurring on the same side. A variety of events can precede the palsy. These include a febrile illness, trauma, and diphtheria-pertussis-tetanus (DPT) immunization (883).

Other Postinfectious Cranial Neuropathies

An isolated temporary paralysis of the glossopharyngeal nerve has been reported. The presenting symptoms in children were dysphagia and nasal speech. CSF examination was normal, and the condition cleared completely within 1 to 2 months (884).

Other postinfectious cranial neuropathies include an isolated hypoglossal nerve palsy, asymmetric palatal paresis, and involvement of the trigeminal sensory nerve (885–888).

Cranial polyneuropathy is generally idiopathic. It is probably related to the Miller Fisher syndrome, and *C. jejuni* has been isolated from the stool in several patients who had elevated serum anti-G_{Q1b} antibodies (889,890). Trigeminal sensory neuropathy has also been associated with antiglycolipid IgM antibodies against G_{M2} and LM1 (849).

NERVOUS SYSTEM VASCULITIS

Introduction

Vasculitis of the nervous system refers to a spectrum of pathogenetically and nosologically heterogeneous disorders characterized by inflammation of the blood vessels, including arteries and veins of all calibers, which result in a variety of clinical neurologic manifestations related to ischemic and/or hemorrhagic parenchymal damage (891) (Table 8.13). If unrecognized and, consequently, untreated, vasculitis of the CNS leads to permanent neurologic injury and disability, thus the utmost importance of the accurate diagnosis and management of each one of the different entities comprising this variant group of disorders (891). CNS vasculitis (plural, vasculitides) may be primary (also known as "isolated," meaning that it is manifest exclusively in the CNS without an identifiable etiology or pathogenesis) or secondary (occurring as a result of an underlying systemic infectious, noninfectious immunologic, neoplastic, or other etiology).

There is considerable overlap among the various types of vasculitis involving either primarily and/or exclusively the nervous system. In addition, there are instances

TABLE 8.13 Clinicopathologic Classification of Nervous System Vasculitides in Childhood Based on Putative Etiology and Immunopathogenesis

Primary Angiitis of the Central Nervous System (PACNS) (Unknown Immunopathogenesis)
Granulomatous angiitis of the CNS (GACNS)
Benign angiopathy of the CNS (BACNS)
Secondary CNS Vasculitis in Children
Infective (owing to direct infection; may be accompanied by autoimmune mechanisms involving both cellular and humoral arms of immunity)
Bacterial (e.g., *Neisseria meningitidis*)
Mycobacterial (e.g., *Mycobacterium tuberculosis*)
Spirochetal (e.g., Lyme disease, syphilis)
Rickettsial (e.g., Rocky Mountain spotted fever)
Fungal (e.g., aspergillosis, mucormycosis)
Viral (e.g., HZV/VZV, HIV, hepatitis C)
Parasitic (e.g., *Toxoplasma gondii*)
Primarily immunologic
Systemic vasculitis
Anti–neutrophil cytoplasmic autoantibody (ANCA) mediated
Wegener granulomatosis
Microscopic polyangiitis (microscopic polyarteritis)
Churg-Strauss syndrome
Direct antibody attack mediated
Kawasaki disease (antiendothelial antibodies)
Immune complex mediated
Henoch-Schönlein purpura
SLE and rheumatoid arthritis (see below, collagen vascular diseases)
Drug induced
Cryoglobulinemia
Serum sickness
Unknown immunopathogenesis
Giant cell (temporal) arteritis
Takayasu arteritis
Polyarteritis nodosa (classic polyarteritis nodosa)
Collagen vascular diseases
Systemic lupus erythematosus (immune complex mediated)
Juvenile rheumatoid arthritis (immune complex mediated)
Adamantiades-Behçet syndrome
Dermatomyositis
Sjögren syndrome
Primarily cell mediated
Graft-versus-host disease
Inflammatory bowel disease
Vascular injury
Dissection
Irradiation
Drugs
Amphetamines
Contraceptives
Paraneoplastic vasculitis

HZV/VZV, herpes zoster virus/varicella-zoster virus; HIV, human immunodeficiency virus; SLE, systemic lupus erythematosus. Modified after Benseler S, Schneider R. Central nervous system vasculitis in children. *Curr Opin Rheumatol* 2004;16:43–50; and Jeannette JC, Fulk RJ. Update on the pathobiology of vasculitis. In: Schoen FJ, Gimbone MA, (eds.) *Cardiovascular pathology: clinicopathologic correlations and pathogenetic Mechanisms.* Philadelphia: Williams & Wilkins, 1995:156.

in which a systemic vasculitis may initially present predominantly with neurologic manifestations, which may antecede systemic manifestations, prompting clinical and laboratory evaluation of systemic organs and tissues.

Both inflammatory and noninflammatory diseases of CNS blood vessels (vasculopathies) share clinical and neuroimaging (including angiographic) features, which may potentially give rise to diagnostic difficulties. In such instances the diagnosis ultimately rests on further clinical and laboratory correlations as well as on the pathologic examination of biopsy specimens obtained from systemic tissues (skin, skeletal muscle, kidney) or directly from the CNS lesions by brain and/or meningeal biopsy.

General Pathogenetic Mechanisms of CNS Vasculitis

CNS vasculitis is characterized by transmural inflammation of cerebral blood vessels of all types and sizes that involves the endothelial lining and/or the cellular components of the vascular wall. Vascular inflammation is generated as a result of immune-mediated mechanisms involving both the cellular and humoral arms of immunity. The mounting of angiocentric inflammatory responses may be triggered by antigenic determinants of microbial pathogens or by altered host proteins mimicking pathogenic antigens (molecular mimicry) (139).

The subsequent inflammatory damage of cerebral blood vessels and disruption of the BBB may either be due to direct targeting of infected vascular elements (endothelium or smooth muscle cells of the vascular wall) or occur in a secondary "bystander" fashion (139). The latter refers to vascular injury in which inflammatory cells, such as cytotoxic lymphocytes, exert secondary vascular damage after having been initially recruited by, and directed against, antigens presented by infected monocytes/macrophages infiltrating either the subarachnoid or the perivascular (Virchow-Robin) spaces of intraparenchymal CNS vessels (139).

The resultant inflammation is accompanied by increased expression of proinflammatory cytokines, monocyte-produced proteases, and nitric oxide–mediated cellular injury signaling the production of oxygen free radicals and oxidative stress. In addition, prothrombotic phenomena, through alterations of the vascular adhesion molecules and upregulation of vascular endothelial growth factors and endothelins in the affected endothelium, compromise the vascular lumens and produce BBB damage and local hemodynamic derangements. These factors collectively culminate in perfusion deficits and hypoxic-ischemic injury to the surrounding nervous tissue (892).

Immunopathogenesis

Three immunopathogenetic mechanisms are usually involved: (a) antibody mediated, (b) immune complex mediated, and (c) cell mediated. It should be noted that some vasculopathies traditionally classified as "noninflammatory" may be preceded by an inflammatory phase in which elements of the endothelium and vascular wall may be damaged giving rise to reactive changes or impaired cellular responses.

Neuropathogenesis

The main pathologic correlate of vasculitis-related neurologic dysfunction is hypoxic-ischemic injury of the CNS parenchyma. Vascular inflammation causes local hemodynamic derangements leading to luminal compromise, vasospasm, distal embolization arising from necrotic vascular endothelium, and perifocal tissue injury attributed to proinflammatory soluble factors, such as nitric oxide, cytokines, and proteases produced by the infiltrating inflammatory cells and/or by the injured brain vascular endothelial cells. Secondary posthypoxic and/or postictal (excitotoxic) mechanisms, such as nitric oxide–mediated elevations of intracellular calcium in neurons and initiation of pronecrotic or proapoptotic cascades of cell death, may also contribute to the neuropathogenesis of vasculitis.

At the histopathologic level, ischemic necrosis in the context of infarction, apoptosis of neurons and glia in the surrounding penumbra zone, and white matter rarefaction or postischemic myelin loss may be encountered. In addition, a number of cases may present with perivascular hemorrhages, which may, on occasion, become confluent and culminate in spontaneous lobar hemorrhages (see the discussion of acute hemorrhagic leukoencephalitis, Hurst disease).

It should be noted that occasionally patients with systemic vasculitides might experience neurologic dysfunction as a result of impaired function of systemic organs such as the heart, lungs, liver, and/or kidneys.

In the peripheral nervous system (PNS), vasculitides may give rise to distinctive patterns such as mononeuritis multiplex, polyneuropathy, radiculopathy, or even plexopathy. Motor, sensory, and autonomic systems may be variously affected, often in overlapping or protean patterns.

Epidemiology

The incidence of CNS vasculitis in children is unknown. This is attributable, in large part, to the fact that the disease is rare, but also because there is no general agreement regarding the criteria of diagnosis (893). The youngest child reported in the series by Benseler and colleagues (893) was 7 months, whereas the youngest patient in our experience is 3 months of age.

Primary Systemic Vasculitides

Of the various primary systemic vasculitides, Vogt-Koyanagi-Harada syndrome is covered in Chapter 7. Giant cell arteritis, Churg-Strauss vasculitis, Takayashu disease, and Cogan syndrome are rarely seen in the pediatric population. These conditions are summarized in Table 8.14.

Primary Angiitis of the Central Nervous System

Since its original description as "granulomatous angiitis" by Cravioto and Feigin in 1959 (894), primary CNS vasculitis has been described by various designations, used interchangeably, such as isolated CNS angiitis, intracranial vasculitis, idiopathic or noninfectious granulomatous angiitis of the CNS, and primary angiitis of the CNS

TABLE 8.14 Vasculitides Affecting the Nervous System

Disease	*Systemic Manifestations*	*Characteristic Laboratory Features*	*Neurologic Symptoms*
Churg-Strauss syndrome	Lungs primarily	Peripheral hypereosinophilia	Peripheral neuropathy
Cogan syndrome	Interstitial keratitis, aortic valvulitis	Cerebrospinal fluid pleocytosis	Progressive deafness, vestibular abnormalities, encephalopathy
Takayasu disease	Aortic arch affected predominantly, female individuals affected mainly	Elevated erythrocyte sedimentation rate	Vascular accidents, vision loss
Temporal arteritis	In pediatric population affects temporal arteries and external carotids	Elevated serum levels of elastin peptide	Headaches, painful nodule of superficial temporal artery, vision loss
Wegener granulomatosis	Small vessels of respiratory tract and kidneys	Elevated erythrocyte sedimentation rate, thrombocytosis	Peripheral neuropathy
Mixed connective tissue disease	Skin lesions of dermatomyositis, scleroderma	Antibodies directed at the ribonuclease-sensitive component of extractable nuclear antigen	Headache, seizures, aseptic meningitis

(PACNS). The term PACNS was first introduced by Calabrese and colleagues (895) as an operational diagnosis encompassing cases of CNS vasculitis without an identifiable etiology and/or pathogenesis (893). PACNS constitutes a heterogeneous group of vasculitides, of which two distinct nosologic categories warrant distinction, namely granulomatous angiitis of the CNS (GACNS) and benign angiopathy of the CNS (BACNS) (896). However, it is unclear whether the adult and childhood forms of PACNS are part of the same disease spectrum or are in fact biologically and/or nosologically different (893).

The literature considers PACNS a rare disease in children, although one should keep in mind the paucity of data in this regard (893). The problem of nosologic definition of PACNS in children is further complicated by the method by which diagnosis is made. Although earlier case reports were mainly based on histopathologic data derived from autopsy and biopsy specimens, the recent clinical literature relies heavily on angiographic criteria for diagnosis (897,898). The use of elective surgical biopsy to rule out PACNS has only rarely been undertaken (898).

Current clinical practice uses the same diagnostic criteria in children as in adults. Accordingly, the diagnosis of PACNS must satisfy the following three criteria proposed by Calabrese and colleagues (895): (a) an acquired neurologic deficit that remains unexplained after a thorough initial work-up, (b) either angiographic or histopathologic evidence of angiitis in the CNS, and (c) no evidence of systemic vasculitis or any other condition to which the angiographic or pathologic features may be construed as secondary (893).

Clinical Features

The clinical presentation of CNS vasculitis is heterogeneous and may be in the form of a diffuse encephalopathy with headache, stroke, and/or seizures. The clinical presentation of childhood PACNS is highly variable and often nonspecific, some children presenting with a rapidly progressive neurologic deficit and others exhibiting slowly evolving diffuse or focal lesions (893). It is believed that the type of neurologic manifestation may correlate with the size of blood vessel involvement as well as with the distribution and degree of luminal compromise of the affected vessels. Two groups of patients are identified on clinicopathologic grounds: those with predominant involvement of small vessels and those with predominant involvement of large to medium-sized arteries (897,898).

As a rule, in PACNS affecting the small vessels, the clinical picture is more "encephalopathic," and the disease course tends to be variable but on the whole less fulminant. Such patients typically present with headaches, behavioral changes, multifocal neurologic deficits, and/or seizures. Occasionally, multifocal infarcts and "tumor-like" lesions may be detected on MRI (898). In contrast, in PACNS affecting large and/or medium-sized arteries, children present with either transient ischemic attacks or strokes (predominantly of an ischemic and to a lesser extent hemorrhagic nature) (898).

The most common presentations, in descending order of frequency, are acute severe headache (80% of cases), focal neurologic deficit (78%), gross motor deficit or hemiparesis (62%), cranial nerve involvement (59%), and cognitive dysfunction, including mood and behavioral changes (54%). Conversely, new onset of seizures (18%), movement abnormalities, and constitutional symptoms such as fever, fatigue, and weight loss (18%) are less common in children than adults (893,899). Mental status may range from normal with irritability to various degrees of confusion and obtundation. In some cases ischemic strokes, single or multiple cranial nerve palsies, or spinal cord syndromes are either the preponderant or the sole manifestations of PACNS (900). In other instances, children with PACNS can present with acute loss of consciousness or with symptoms and signs of increased intracranial pressure owing to edema or spontaneous parenchymal and/or subarachnoid hemorrhage (893,901). The latter are similar to those described in adult patients with PACNS (902,903).

Diagnosis

PACNS is a diagnosis of exclusion, and a thorough search of a host of mimicking conditions, especially infections, is mandatory in every case in which suspicion for CNS vasculitis exists on clinical and/or angiographic grounds (896). Some cases may present with what is described as "vanishing" saccular- or mycotic-like aneurysms (904,905). Despite certain apparent similarities, pediatric cases frequently have different or atypical clinical, anatomic, and angiographic features than those in adults. To this end, PACNS in children may exhibit a proclivity for large-vessel involvement and unilateral disease based on angiography (897). Mention should be made of a number of diseases that can mimic childhood PACNS (893). These include secondary vasculitides involving the CNS (see later discussion), cases of migraine or vasospasm, hemoglobinopathies (sickle cell anemia and thalassemia), thromboembolism (906), antiphospholipid antibody syndrome (907), metabolic diseases (908), moyamoya disease (909), and fibromuscular dysplasia (910). In cases with seizures, PACNS may also be mimicked by Rasmussen encephalitis (911).

Laboratory Investigations. Clinical pathology evaluations are essentially nonspecific and of limited diagnostic value other than in excluding identifiable disease states, such as infections or systemic vasculitides associated with immunologic abnormalities in the context of recognizable clinical syndromes. With this in mind, the overall lack of positive proinflammatory biomarkers in pediatric PACNS should not rule against the diagnosis of active CNS vasculitis.

Patients may have mildly elevated erythrocyte sedimentation rate (ESR), C-reactive protein (CRP) levels, white blood cell (WBC) counts, and C3 complement and IgG levels (893,897,898). Low anticardiolipin antibodies have been reported in about half of children with PACNS, but their detection is neither consistent nor specific (893). Some patients may exhibit positive antinuclear antibodies (ANAs) (897), but antineutrophil cytoplasmic antibodies (ANCAs) are usually not detectable nor is there a disease-specific or disease-suggestive autoantibody profile trend associated with childhood PACNS (893).

Although CSF examination is not in itself sensitive or specific for establishing the diagnosis of PACNS, its value is important to the extent that it yields WBC counts, cell morphology, and protein levels. This important information is useful for confirming or ruling out an active inflammatory process or CNS infection. Moreover, CSF analysis lends itself to traditional and molecular microbiologic approaches, which may contribute to diagnosis and/or potentially shed light on the infectious or immunologic pathogenesis of PACNS.

According to Calabrese (896), approximately 90% of adults with biopsy-proven PACNS exhibited CSF abnormalities in the form of elevated protein levels or pleocytosis. Stone and colleagues (912) concluded that in the context of PACNS, the sensitivity of abnormal CSF findings is significantly lower if diagnosed by angiography as compared to biopsy-based histopathologic evidence of vasculitis. CSF analysis in children with PACNS is highly variable and may be normal (904,913) or show protein elevation (911), pleocytosis, or both (893). The detection of significantly higher concentrations of cytoskeletal proteins of the intermediate filament type associated with neurons (neurofilament protein) and glia (glial fibrillary acidic protein) in the CSF of patients with CNS vasculitis holds promise as a potential diagnostic biomarker system (914).

In contrast to adults, the CSF findings in the pediatric literature with respect to angiographically confirmed CNS vasculitis are scanty and highly variable, ranging from essentially normal (most cases) to markedly abnormal (evidence of significant CSF pleocytosis) (897,898). In a recent small series of 4 children with angiography-negative, biopsy-positive childhood PACNS reported by Benseler and colleagues (915), all patients exhibited lymphocytic pleocytosis and/or increased protein levels. CSF opening pressure may be increased and should be determined and recorded with all lumbar puncture procedures (893).

It should be emphasized that although initial CSF analysis may be normal, CSF abnormalities may still be present in follow-up analyses and reflect disease progression (893).

Neuroimaging and Angiography. MRI is superior to CT for both initial diagnosis and monitoring of the disease (916). In fact, CT may be unremarkable in more than half of adult patients with PACNS (912). That said, neither the specificity nor the sensitivity of MRI has been established in pediatric patients with PACNS (917). CT of the brain is much less sensitive as compared to MRI.

The main body of neuroradiologic literature on PACNS is derived from adult cases, where characteristic MRI patterns have been described (918,919) and are thought to correlate with the distribution of angiographic findings (920). A near absolute MRI sensitivity has been reported in biopsy-proven PACNS cases (918). With this in mind, there are instances of PACNS in which MRI was essentially negative in the face of abnormal angiographic findings (921,922). Collectively taken, the combination of unremarkable CSF and brain MRI studies confers a high negative predictive value for PACNS (893).

With respect to the topographic distribution of MRI lesions in children with PACNS, these may be solitary (less common) or multifocal (more common) and may involve one or both hemispheres (897). The most characteristic finding is the presence of multifocal lesions involving both gray and white matter. They typically exhibit the following characteristics: (a) a distinctive hyperintensity in T2-weighted images, (b) fluid-attenuated inversion recovery, and (c) gadolinium enhancement in T1-weighted images (893). The distinct quality of hyperintensity in T2-weighted images includes widespread small, irregular tufts of T2 bright signal that suggests vasculitis rather than ADEM; moreover, the discrete ("plaquelike") lesions at the gray–white matter junction that are so characteristic of ADEM are usually not present in CNS vasculitis. However, the predictive value of MRI patterns, including the roles of fluid-attenuated inversion recovery, diffusion-weighted images, and gadolinium enhancement, is not fully established (923).

Current clinical practice indicates that conventional angiography is the mainstay for the diagnosis of PACNS in both adults and children (893,897). The procedure appears to be a safe in children (893). A "high-probability angiogram" in the context of PACNS reveals alternating areas of stenosis and ectasia in more than one vascular bed (924). Even though angiography is widely regarded as the gold standard of diagnosis, the fact remains that it alone is neither sufficiently sensitive nor entirely specific for the diagnosis of CNS vasculitis (896). This is particularly true in adults, where there is a lack of sensitivity, let alone specificity, in this regard (924,925). These limitations underscore the importance of biopsy and histopathologic confirmation in establishing a firm diagnosis (896).

Because several adult diseases mimicking CNS vasculitis, such as atherosclerosis/arteriosclerosis and vasospasm (896), are comparatively uncommon in children and because of the inherent risks of brain biopsy, the diagnosis of CNS vasculitis rests to a large extent on conventional angiography. Yet neither the sensitivity nor the specificity of the latter modality has been determined in the setting of childhood PACNS (893).

In most reported cases of CNS vasculitis, arterial stenosis involves predominantly the middle cerebral artery and its branches and less commonly the branches of the anterior and posterior cerebral arteries. Most pediatric patients exhibit involvement of more than one vascular beds in a manner analogous to that seen in adult PACNS patients (924).

In recent years, magnetic resonance angiography (MRA) has emerged as a promising noninvasive diagnostic tool both in the initial evaluation and the subsequent monitoring of CNS vasculitis. Notwithstanding the fact that MRA is frequently used in this clinical setting, its sensitivity and specificity for the diagnosis of PACNS are unknown (893). A 75% correlation between MRA and conventional angiography has been reported in a series of adult PACNS cases (926).

Considering the pathologic sequels of postinflammatory vasculopathy, including obliterative changes or poststenotic dilatation, it becomes apparent that angiographic abnormalities may persist after resolution of the clinical findings or parenchymal lesions as determined by MRI (893). Likewise, disease progression may be characterized by worsening of luminal compromise and/or new obliterative changes in previously unaffected parenchymal blood vessels (893).

Diffusion-weighted imaging (DWI) may be useful in the diagnosis of PACNS and other systemic vasculitides affecting the CNS and has emerged as an important diagnostic neuroimaging modality that may also be informative in patient follow-up, including assessment of treatment efficacy and disease outcome (927).

Transcranial Doppler ultrasonography may be valuable in monitoring disease-related changes involving large intracranial vessels (928) but has limited usefulness in small-vessel cerebrovascular disease (929).

Brain Biopsy. Biopsy of the brain and leptomeninges is considered the ultimate approach for the diagnosis of PACNS (925,930,931). Brain biopsies are primarily undertaken in the clinical and radiologic setting of atypical, and therefore problematic, cases to rule out infectious or neoplastic processes mimicking CNS vasculitis, which would require a diametrically different approach to therapy. As a rule, where there is a high index of suspicion for small-vessel involvement, brain and/or leptomeningeal biopsies may be required because neither MRA nor conventional angiography is sufficiently sensitive or specific for the accurate detection of vasculitic changes in small-caliber parenchymal vessels (898). Conversely, in cases in which there is large and/or medium-sized vascular involvement, the diagnostic fidelity of angiographic and MRA studies is significantly higher (897).

That said, brain biopsies are not free of pitfalls, and the threshold for the performance of brain biopsies in children is generally high (893). Vasculitic changes may be segmental, multifocal, and/or discontinuous, and, as such, brain biopsies may not always be diagnostic. The frequency of false-negative brain biopsies in adults with CNS vasculitis is significant and ranges from 17% to 53% (925) with the average realistic figure being closer to 25% (896).

The possibility of a false-negative brain biopsy coupled with procedure-related morbidity risks has dampened enthusiasm for the use of brain biopsy in children (893,896,897). With this in mind, the morbidity related to brain biopsies performed in adults is slightly over 3%, which may even be lower in children due to the absence of comorbidity factors in the latter population (893). It has been shown that the morbidity associated with aggressive immunosuppression is in fact significantly greater than that associated with cerebral angiography or brain biopsy (925). Brain biopsy should therefore be strongly considered in a child with typical clinical features and suggestive MRI lesions but normal angiography; in addition, biopsy of surgically accessible brain parenchymal or leptomeningeal lesions is recommended (893).

Most of the clinicopathologic studies on the subject have been conducted in adult cases and unfortunately there are no comparable studies in children. In a clinicopathologic study of 30 adult PACNS cases, the predictive value of brain biopsy was found to be significantly higher than those of angiography or MRI (925). In a subsequent large clinicopathologic study conducted in 61 consecutive brain biopsies from adult patients suspected of having PACNS, the latter diagnosis was confirmed by biopsy-based histopathology only in 36% of cases. The remainder of the cases were found to be of infectious, neoplastic, or demyelinating/degenerative nature, and one-fourth of the biopsies were not diagnostic (930). The latter finding underscores the difficulties of biopsy sampling. This is due in large part to the patchy distribution of the lesions (893) and also because certain larger focal lesions may be situated in eloquent regions of the brain and may therefore not be surgically accessible. Another potential caveat is that large-vessel inflammation demonstrated by angiography may not necessarily be associated with small-vessel involvement in a biopsy sample (893).

Surgical pathology experience with childhood PACNS is severely limited owing to the fact that elective brain biopsies have only rarely been performed in children with PACNS (898). Histologically, most adult cases of PACNS (80%) exhibit a segmental necrotizing and/or frequently overt granulomatous angiitis with giant cells (925,931,932). A predominantly lymphocytic vasculitis involving small vessels has been described in children with unremarkable angiography (898,913). Evidence of large-vessel necrotizing granulomatous angiitis has been established in neuropathologic studies from fatal childhood cases examined at autopsy (901,904,905,933,934).

From a clinicopathologic perspective, a predominantly lymphocytic vasculitis is more likely to be associated with early or innocuous disease, whereas a florid granulomatous inflammation (comprising predominantly activated monocytes-macrophages) with fibrinoid necrosis of the vessel wall is consistent with a more aggressive or advanced disease (898).

Treatment

Untreated PACNS is a potentially fulminant disease that can be fatal. Currently, therapeutic recommendations for childhood PACNS are made from earlier experience in adults (935), and on the basis of case reports or small series of pediatric cases (893,936). In view of the rarity of the disease and because of inherent difficulties and pitfalls in diagnosis, no controlled clinical trials have been conducted (893,896). In a small series of 5 pediatric patients with PACNS affecting large and medium-sized arteries and in which none of the children received immunosuppressive treatment, 4 patients succumbed within 10 days from the onset of neurologic manifestations, whereas 1 child died 7 years after initial presentation (898). Notwithstanding the likelihood of biologic heterogeneity within the spectrum of pediatric PACNS, patients treated with corticosteroids and cyclophosphamide exhibited improvement both with respect to clinical outcome and resolution of neuroimaging findings (897). Taken collectively, these observations speak in favor of use of immunosuppressive therapy.

Therapy is twofold and is aimed at suppressing or abrogating immune-mediated inflammation of brain blood vessels and preventing thrombotic phenomena. Therapeutic recommendations are as follows.

Immunosuppression Therapy. Remission or even cure may be attained in patients who are treated with the combination of oral prednisone and cyclophosphamide, as outlined by Woolfenden and colleagues (937). The combination therapy should be continued for at least 1 year. At that time, if angiographic evaluation of patients who previously displayed angiographic abnormalities shows resolution, cyclophosphamide can be discontinued and the prednisone can be tapered over 3 to 6 months. PACNS should be suspected in children who are thought to have steroid-responsive forms of ADEM that relapse as long-term corticosteroid monotherapy is weaned to low doses.

The usual threshold for relapse is at prednisone equivalents of approximately 12 to 16 mg administered on alternate days (932). Along the lines of combined immunosuppressive therapy, a modified protocol was recently proposed that entails combination of high-dose steroids and monthly intravenous cyclophosphamide (893).

Alternative approaches to the management of childhood PACNS consist of intravenous monthly cyclophosphamide (500 to 1,000 mg/m2) or bimonthly high-dose intravenous cyclophosphamide (10 m/kg per dose) (897). Oral cyclophosphamide (2 mg/kg per day) has also been used in children either with refractory disease or relapses, whereas some children have attained remission after treatment with corticosteroids only (898). Azathioprine and low-dose weekly methotrexate have also been used to maintain remission but their efficacy is unknown (893).

Antithrombotic Therapy. The role of antithrombotic therapy and prophylaxis in the management of CNS vasculitis is controversial. PACNS is accompanied by a proclivity for generalized thrombosis, thromboembolism, and/or perfusion defects attributed to widespread stenosis of blood vessels of all calibers, which may warrant anticoagulation prophylaxis.

The administration of coumadin or low-molecular-weight heparin should be tailored taking into consideration potential risks and benefits for each individual patient. Prophylactic administration of low-dose acetylsalicylic acid (3 to 5 mg/kg per day) should be considered in patients who have not developed any of the aforementioned conditions or complications (893).

Disease Monitoring

A thorough follow-up is mandatory particularly during the first year and should include determination of biomarkers of inflammation (especially if these were elevated from the outset) and sequential neuroimaging. In addition, CSF examination should be repeated, especially if abnormalities were detected in the initial analysis, because they may be serve as indices of relapse (893).

Prognosis

The prognosis of children with CNS vasculitis is unknown and largely unpredictable. Early reports in the literature pointed to an overall poor prognosis in both adults and children (901,904,905,913,934,938). Predictably, large ischemic strokes result in variably severe and permanent neurologic deficits; however, it should be noted that a number of patients also have made remarkable recoveries (893).

The long-term cognitive or behavioral outcomes are unknown, and no longitudinal studies have been conducted in pediatric populations (893). In a relatively large cohort of 41 adult PACNS patients with a mean follow-up of 4 years, the rate of relapse was 29%, whereas 80% of patients had an overall favorable outcome; the mortality rate was 10% (939).

Benign Angiopathy of the CNS

Benign angiopathy of the CNS (BACNS), also known as transient angiopathy and/or benign CNS angiitis, refers to an ill-defined subgroup of adult patients with PACNS presenting at a younger age with a monophasic (predominantly nonrelapsing) disease devoid of inflammatory CSF changes (940). The term transient cerebral arteriopathy was used to describe 9 children in a cohort of 34 patients with ischemic stroke (941). It should be emphasized that the spectrum of the disease is variable and ranges from self-limiting CNS events to either slowly or rapidly progressive CNS vasculitis with fatal outcomes. Consequently, the designations "benign" and "transient"are somewhat misleading because they do not necessarily imply prognostically favorable outcomes (940).

Experience with the management of childhood BACNS is limited, but adult patients either do not receive immunosuppressive treatment (942) or are given a short course of corticosteroids (902). Hajj-Ali and colleagues reported favorable neurologic outcomes in 8 of 16 adult patients with BACNS, with only 1 patient having relapsed, and no deaths (902).

Secondary Systematic Vasculitides

CNS vasculitis in children may be secondary to infections or a number of immunologically-defined systemic conditions classified under the clinical rubric of systemic vasculitides.

CNS Vasculitis Secondary to Infections

Microbial pathogens capable of causing secondary CNS vasculitis in children include viruses, mycobacteria, spirochetes, bacteria, fungi, and rickettsia. Direct inflammation of the cerebral blood vessels caused by infectious agents constitutes a distinct nosologic group within the spectrum of vasculitides and accounts of one of the major mechanisms of stroke in children (943). For the most part, infective vasculitis is more likely to result in ischemic stroke (cerebral infarction) than hemorrhagic stroke in children. A number of infectious agents causing meningoencephalitis are associated with a proclivity for angiocentric inflammation and vasculitis often complicated by cerebral infarction. These include mycobacteria such as *Mycobacterium tuberculosis* (944,945), spirochetes such as *Treponema pallidum* (syphilis) (946), *Borrelia burgdorferi* (Lyme disease) (400,947), atypical bacteria such *Mycoplasma pneumoniae* (948), fungi such as *Cryptococcus neoformans* (945), zygomycetes, and *Aspergillus fumigatus*, as well as viruses. Among viral agents, herpes-zoster virus (HZV), also known as varicella-zoster virus (VZV) (949–952), Japanese encephalitis virus (953), and human immunodeficiency virus (HIV) (139,954,955) are nosologically significant in the context of CNS vasculitis and stroke in children (943). Finally, inflammation of the leptomeningeal and intracerebral vessels contributes to the pathogenesis of ischemic stroke associated with pyogenic bacterial meningitis (956) (see Chapter 7).

Although hemorrhagic stroke is significantly less frequent than ischemic stroke in children, intracranial aneurysms complicating infection of cerebral vessels (mycotic aneurysms), such as those arising in the setting of vasoinvasive fungal infections (957,958) or viral infections, can lead to potentially catastrophic hemorrhagic stroke with devastating neurologic deficits (943). In addition, aneurysms arising in the background of HZV vasculopathy (959), HIV vasculopathy (960,961), or PACNS (901) are liable of undergoing spontaneous rupture causing massive subarachnoid hemorrhage and attendant complications.

Among CNS vasculitides associated with viral infections, two postviral syndromes warrant special attention in the neuropediatric setting: HZV CNS vasculitis and HIV CNS vasculitis.

Post–Herpes-Zoster Virus CNS Vasculitis-Vasculopathy

The clinical, microbiologic, and pathologic aspects of varicella and HZV infection of the nervous system were reviewed extensively by Kleinschmidt-DeMasters and Gilden (962). HZV infection can give rise to a wide range of neurologic manifestations and complications. The latter include aseptic meningitis/meningoencephalitis (including cerebellitis), ventriculitis, multifocal leukoencephalopathy, transverse myelitis, postherpetic neuralgia, neuritis/peripheral neuropathy, and, rarely, Reye encephalopathy (943,962).

The neurologic features of HZV CNS vasculopathy are protean, and the onset of neurologic manifestations often occurs months after clinically apparent disease and in fact occasionally without any history of cutaneous rash (963). In immunocompromised patients, reactivation of HZV from dorsal ganglia roots can lead to serious neurologic complications including disseminated leukoencephalopathy and ventriculitis (964). CNS vasculitis can be the result of primary varicella infection and/or HZV reactivation either spontaneously or in the setting of immunocompromise.

Varicella (chickenpox) has been implicated in the pathogenesis of ischemic stroke in children and is regarded as a major risk factor for cerebral infarction in the pediatric population (949,965). The absolute risk of HZV-associated stroke in children is 1 in 15,000 (949). As varicella is becoming increasingly recognized as a significant cause of stroke in children, the frequency of this causal relationship in the pediatric population is considered to be relatively high and therefore, to have been underestimated in the past (943).

CNS vasculitis following HZV infection typically presents with occlusive stroke as a result of large-vessel involvement (952). However, it should be emphasized that HZV CNS vasculopathy may, in addition to its preponderant large-vessel involvement, affect small cerebral blood vessels (963). As a rule, large-vessel disease is most common in immunocompetent individuals and small-vessel disease is more likely to be encountered in immunocompromised patients, although a subset of patients may have dual large- and small-vessel involvement (963) (see later discussion).

The approach to diagnosis is threefold and comprises MRI, cerebral angiography, and examination of CSF with molecular virologic testing (966). The diagnosis of post-HZV CNS vasculitis/vasculopathy is contingent on three criteria: (a) HZV infection within the preceding 12 months, (b) evidence of unilateral, proximal large-vessel stenosis, and (c) detection of HZV DNA by polymerase chain reaction (PCR) and/or HZV IgG in the CSF (952,962,965,967). However, it should be pointed out that not all patients with HZV vasculopathy exhibit PCR amplification of HVZ DNA sequences in the CSF, in which case the diagnosis can be confirmed by the detection of anti-HZV antibody in CSF along with reduced serum-to-CSF ratios of HZV IgG as compared to albumin or total IgG (963,968).

The pathogenesis of the post-HZV CNS vasculitis appears to be different in immunocompetent versus immunocompromised patients. In immunocompetent individuals, the disease mechanism is due to transaxonal spread of reactivated HZV originating from the trigeminal ganglion, a known site of viral latency, and subsequent invasion of the virus in cerebral blood vessels resulting in infection of smooth muscle cells (969). The spread of the virus occurs predominantly along the ophthalmic branch of the trigeminal nerve as compared to maxillary or mandibular branches (943). Post-HZV large-vessel giant cell vasculitis accompanied by secondary thromboses and attendant local hemodynamic derangements leading to stroke is also known to involve the main branches of the internal carotid arteries, especially the middle cerebral artery (950). Granulomatous CNS vasculitis has also been reported in adults as a complication of herpes-zoster ophthalmicus, a well-known syndrome of stroke associated with HZV (970). Herpes-zoster ophthalmicus is uncommon in children and its outcome is reportedly poor (952).

In the immunocompromised group of patients, notably in children with HIV/AIDS, the presumptive mode of spread is direct infection of the blood vessel walls by HZV. Again, in the setting of coinfection with HIV, there may be dual large- and small-vessel involvement, which may also contribute to the pathogenesis of cerebral infarcts and/or multifocal leukoencephalopathy (971,972).

Morphologically, viral infection of arterial smooth muscle cells is accompanied by granulomatous inflammation (950) in the context of a delayed hypersensitivity reaction. The classic histologic feature of post-HZV CNS vasculitis from autopsy-based neuropathologic studies performed on fatal childhood cases is granulomatous angiitis characterized by mononuclear inflammatory cell infiltrates, numerous giant cells, fragmentation of the internal elastic lamina, and intimal fibrosis affecting predominantly large intracranial blood (950). The localization of HZV antigen has been detected by immunohistochemistry in the smooth muscle cells of the arterial walls (950).

The outcome of post-HZV CNS vasculitis is variable and unpredictable, ranging from rapid resolution and an overall good prognosis (941) to instances of fatal outcome (950,973,974). The extent of neurologic morbidity is illustrated in a large controlled study by Askalan and colleagues (949) demonstrating a substantial recurrence rate of stroke (estimated at 45%) and residual neurologic deficits present in as many as 68% of patients (949). That said, the HZV vasculitis-vasculopathy sequence may not be necessarily irreversible or invariably progressive. Significant resolution of stenosis in the middle cerebral artery, determined by serial contrast-enhanced MRI and MRA, has been documented over a period of several months in a child with HZV-associated cerebral infarction in the territorial distribution of this artery (975). The latter suggests that the post-HZV large cell vasculopathy may be partially reversible, possibly as part of the natural history of the disease process.

Against this background, the therapeutic approach to post-HZV CNS vasculitis in children is controversial (893). In adult patients, treatment is anticoagulation with low-dose aspirin with or without low-molecular-weight heparin, acyclovir for 7 to 10 days, and a short course (3 to 5 days) of oral corticosteroids (964). However, neither anticoagulation nor steroid treatment was found to have a clear therapeutic benefit in a cohort of 28 children with HZV-related stroke (952). The fact that patients may have detectable HZV DNA sequences in their CSF (as determined by PCR) several months after the onset of clinical neurologic manifestations raises the conjecture that the persistence of HZV infection in the cerebral vessels could be a possible mechanism of continuous or recurrent vascular injury. It follows then that treatment with acyclovir or other antiviral agents may provide therapeutic benefit by preventing the progression of the vasculitic changes that have been reported in some fatal cases (943). Yet, based on a review of the literature, the outcome was found to be variable, and many patients were found to have residual motor deficits following HZV-associated stroke (952). However, the neurologic morbidity in this regard may be complicated by collateral factors, and the therapeutic benefit of antiviral drugs in the management of the HZV vasculitis-vasculopathy sequence remains open to further investigation. It is generally held that when HZV vasculopathy develops months after zoster, antiviral treatment is often effective (963).

Recently, the International Herpes Management Forum (IHMF) proposed the following guidelines regarding diagnosis and management of CNS syndromes associated with HZV by placing special emphasis on VZV vasculopathy (966). Early diagnosis of HZV vasculopathy and potentially associated serious complications is paramount because aggressive antiviral treatment has been shown to be effective in this clinical setting (966). Children with focal vasculopathy due to HZV should undergo treatment with intravenous acyclovir (500 mg/m^2 body surface area) for 7 days (966). It should be noted that patients who are immunocompromised may require longer treatment, but antiviral therapy should be discontinued should both CSF HZV DNA and anti-HZV antibody be negative (966). In addition, corticosteroids (prednisone 60 to 80 mg/day for 3 to 5 days) should be considered because they may contribute to the amelioration of HZV-associated CNS vasculitis (966).

HIV-Associated CNS Vasculitis-Vasculopathy

CNS vasculitis may be encountered in the clinical setting of HIV/AIDS, often in association with stroke (139,955) or aneurysmal arteriopathy (960). CNS vasculitis in children with HIV/AIDS may be primary, that is, HIV associated (139), or secondary owing to coinfection with other viruses such as HZV.

Angiocentric mononuclear inflammatory cell infiltrates with transmural vascular involvement have been described in both adults (891) and children (139,954) with HIV infection in whom there is no evidence of opportunistic infection (139,891).

An increased incidence of cerebrovascular disease is present in children infected with HIV. Most index cases appear to acquire HIV through vertical transmission or during perinatal infection. Among 426 HIV-infected pediatric patients with comparative neuroimaging studies who were evaluated at the National Cancer Institute from 1986 to June 2001 for participation in approved therapeutic research trials, 11 (2.6%) were found to have cerebrovascular lesions (976). Most patients had advanced HIV disease and had received antiretroviral treatment (976). Earlier studies reported incidence rates ranging from 4% to 29% in adult patients with HIV/AIDS (977,978), but the true incidence of HIV-associated cerebrovascular complications in children is unclear. This may be attributed in part to underrecognition in cases that do not present with neurologic manifestations, especially focal signs, but also to the shifting clinicopathologic patterns of the disease following efficacious treatment of antiretroviral agents, particularly highly active antiretroviral therapy, in Western countries.

HIV-associated CNS vasculitis, together with other coinfections exhibiting a tropism for blood vessels such as HZV, as well as cardiogenic thromboemboli and autoimmune thombocytopenia may contribute to an increased incidence of cerebrovascular complications in pediatric patients with neuro-AIDS. These include aneurysmal vasculopathy (960,961,971,979–981), cerebral infarction (139,977,982–986), and hemorrhage. In addition, small-vessel CNS vasculitis may be responsible for the calcific vasculopathy underlying CNS perfusion deficits and the mineralizations of the basal ganglia and thalami that are commonly encountered by neuroimaging in children with HIV/AIDS (139).

A significant proportion of brain samples from fatal childhood cases of HIV/AIDS in the 1990s that were evaluated histologically at autopsy showed evidence of angiocentric inflammation in the form of perivascular and/or transmural mononuclear-cell infiltrates (139). Perivascular infiltrates consist of CD3+ T cells and equal or greater proportions of CD68+ monocytes/macrophages. Transmural (including endothelial) infiltrates comprise predominantly CD3+ T cells and small or, in certain vessels, approximately equal proportions of CD68+ monocytes/macrophages. In some cases there is a clear preponderance of CD3+ CD8+ T cells on the endothelial side of the transmural infiltrates. The majority of CD3+ cells have been found to be also CD8+ and CD45RO+, consistent with activated cytotoxic T lymphocytes (139). In some cases, scattered perivascular monocytes/macrophages in areas of florid vasculitis have been shown to express the p24 core protein of HIV (139) (Fig. 8.5). In a small autopsy series of fatal childhood cases not previously treated with protease inhibitors, we demonstrated that 5 of 6 patients with angiocentric infiltrates had evidence of calcific vasculopathy, but only 2 exhibited concomitant histologic hallmarks of HIV encephalitis. One patient had multiple subacute cerebral and brainstem infarcts associated with a widespread and fulminant mononuclear-cell vasculitis. A second patient had an old brain infarct associated with fibrointimal thickening of large leptomeningeal vessels (139). Sharer and collaborators (987) reported vascular or perivascular inflammation involving small or medium-sized arteries or veins in the brains of 5 of 11 HIV-1–infected children (ages 4 months to 11 years). CNS vasculitis in the context of HIV-associated CNS disease in both children and adults may also exhibit features of overt granulomatous angiitis (akin to GACNS described in the context of PACNS) comprised principally of cells of the monocyte-macrophage lineage (891,988). A difference in neuropathologic findings between adult patients and children infected with HIV-1 is that in the latter group of patients a predominantly lymphocytic vasculitis of the CNS is more prevalent than bona fide granulomatous angiitis (139,983,987,989–991).

It should be noted that in children with HIV/AIDS, cerebral vascular inflammation has been demonstrated without any evidence of an infectious cause other than HIV-1 infection (971,992,993). However, it should be equally emphasized that HIV-associated CNS vasculitis per se is clinicopathologically distinct from the more common HIV encephalitis. Morphologically the latter is characterized by microglial nodules, perivascular multinucleated syncytial giant cells, and immunohistochemical localization of HIV core antigens in monocytes, which taken together are indicative of productive HIV infection (139). Moreover, these angiocentric mononuclear inflammatory cell infiltrates may be transient, and therefore their

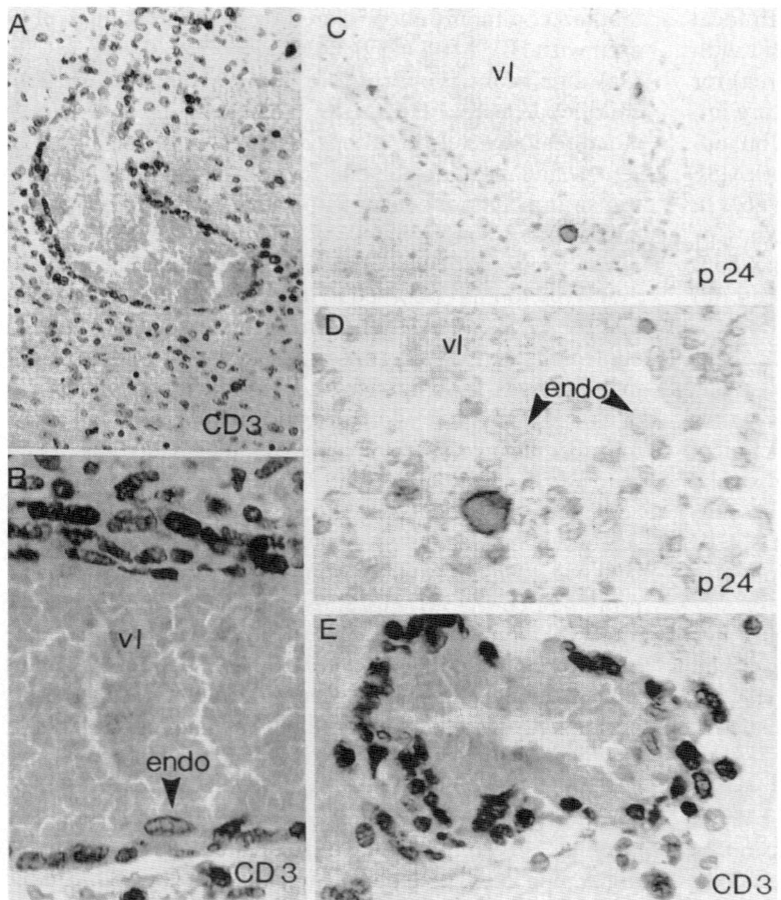

FIGURE 8.5. Immunohistochemical localization of CD3 antigen (T-cell marker) and HIV-1 p24 core antigen in foci of central nervous system vasculitis affecting medium-sized and cerebral vessels in a 2-year-old HIV-1–infected child who succumbed after suffering multiple cerebral infarcts. T-lymphocytic (CD3+) infiltrates traverse the walls and endothelial lining (endo) of parenchymal veins. The contiguous perivascular rim is comprised of CD3+ T cells intermingled with monocytes/macrophages. Panels A, B, and E show transmural vascular inflammation (vasculitis-endotheliitis), which consists predominantly of CD3+ T lymphocytes, whereas the surrounding neuropil is dominated by cells of the monocyte/macrophage lineage and contains only scarce CD3+ T cells. Panels C and D depict the localization of HIV-1 p24 core protein in scattered perivascular monocytes/macrophages bordering a blood vessel affected by florid inflammatory changes. The angiocentric inflammatory infiltrate consists predominantly of lymphocytes. Note the close, abutting relationship of p24-positive monocytes, p24-negative lymphocytes, and p24-negative endothelial cells (*arrowheads*). Avidin–biotin complex peroxidase method with hematoxylin (A, B, E) or methyl green (C, D) counterstains. vl, vascular lumen. (From Katsetos CD, Fincke JE, Legido A, et al. Angiocentric CD3(+) T-cell infiltrates in human immunodeficiency virus type 1-associated central nervous system disease in children. *Clin Diagn Lab Immunol* 1999;6:105–114. With permission.)

presence does not necessarily mirror productive HIV infection in the CNS. That said, there are instances in which CNS vasculitis and HIV encephalitis may in fact overlap (139). From a clinicopathologic perspective, the role of this vasculitis-vasculopathy sequence may be important in the morphogenesis of the various types of HIV-associated vasculopathy including the calcific vasculopathy that contributes to the mineralization of the basal ganglia. It is possible that the hypoxia-ischemia ensuing from HIV vasculopathy is an additional mechanism of neuronal injury in HIV encephalopathy by stimulating glutamate receptors and intracellular penetration of calcium (139,540).

Calcific Vasculopathy as a Histologic Correlate of Mineralization of the Basal Ganglia. The presence of mineralization (calcification) of the basal ganglia and of the frontal white matter, which is seen in greater than 85% of cases examined at autopsy, is one of the most characteristic neuropathologic features of progressive HIV-associated CNS disease in children (987,994). In a large proportion of HIV-infected children, perivascular and, in certain cases, transmural mononuclear-cell infiltrates (vasculitis) consisting primarily of lymphocytes are encountered concomitantly with mineralization of blood vessels of all calibers (calcific vasculopathy) (983,987,991,992). It is postulated that calcific vasculopathy is a sequel of the vasculitis-vasculopathy pathogenetic sequence in which vascular inflammation triggered by an immune response precedes dystrophic mineralization of the damaged walls of the blood vessels (139,955,983,987,991,992). In addition, intimal fibroplasia of large and medium-sized leptomeningeal arteries is also found in HIV-1–infected children, albeit less frequently (983,987,989,991,992). Calcific vasculopathy in the context of pediatric neuro-AIDS is frequently associated with HIV encephalitis.

In summary, HIV-associated CNS vasculitis may be triggered either by HIV or other coinfections in the context of HIV/AIDS or through autoimmune mechanisms (139). Although the incidence of CNS vasculitis in the context of childhood HIV/AIDS is thought to be relatively low, its frequency may be underestimated because the pathologic process may go unrecognized (139). We previously suggested that CNS vasculitis may be an antecedent of calcific vasculopathy, fibrointimal fibroplasia, and aneurysmal arteriopathy contributing to the disruption of BBB, endothelial cell injury, prothrombotic phenomena, and vascular stenosis, collectively, accounting for perfusion deficits and stroke in children (139,955). Interestingly, instances of recurrent stroke in the setting of adult HIV infection may carry the diagnosis of PACNS based on autopsy neuropathologic studies in which other coinfections known to produce CNS vasculitis have been ruled out (995).

Treatment. Because the majority of HIV-infected children asymptomatic during the early stages of the disease, screening of high-risk children, preferably by MRI, is advisable for the early detection of cerebrovascular abnormalities (976). However, the role of prophylaxis with antiretroviral agents in diminishing the incidence and possibly the severity of cerebral vasculopathy remains to be determined (976).

HIV-Associated Vasculitic Peripheral Neuropathy

Even though immune-mediated disorders (principally demyelinating processes) account for nearly half of peripheral neuropathies in childhood, peripheral neuropathy appears to be rare in association with HIV infection in children (996,997).

On the other hand, peripheral nerve vasculitis is more common in adults with HIV/AIDS, where it is often the first manifestation of HIV disease, but also occurs after AIDS has developed, and may be manifest as a symmetric sensorimotor neuropathy or as an overlapping mononeuritis multiplex syndrome. Interestingly, the inflammatory infiltrates usually consist of CD8 T cells and macrophages (998,999) similar to the angiocentric T-cell infiltrates in the CNS (139). It is also of interest that HIV antigens have also been detected in perivascular macrophages in peripheral nerve biopsies (1000) similar to the localization of the p24 core antigen in perivascular macrophages of the CNS (139). Pathologic findings in HIV-associated peripheral neuropathy are diverse and include necrotizing arteritis of the epineurial vessels that is reminiscent, but not identical, to polyarteritis nodosa. It should be noted that necrotizing vasculitis can be seen also in muscle biopsies of patients with peripheral nerve vasculitis, calling for a combined muscle–nerve biopsy examination in all clinically suspected cases (891). Muscle biopsy is also important to rule out myopathic or neuropathic changes secondary to antiretroviral therapy. There are reported cases of cryoglobulinemia in adult patients with HIV infection and mononeuritis multiplex (891), but not in children. Mononeuritis multiplex refers to involvement of several or many individual nerves either simultaneously or metachronously at different times in the course of the disease (1001).

Less Common Secondary Systemic Vasculitides

CNS vasculitis may occur in the setting of less common systemic vasculitides encountered in the pediatric age group (1002,1003), including bona fide "collagen vascular diseases."

Polyarteritis Nodosa

The polyarteritis nodosa (PAN) group of systemic necrotizing vasculitides comprises a series of clinicopathologic entities typified by a necrotizing arteritis involving small and medium-sized muscular arteries (1002). Members of the group include the classic PAN, microscopic polyangiitis, Churg-Strauss syndrome (allergic granulomatosis), overlap syndrome, and the mucocutaneous lymph node syndrome (MLNS, Kawasaki disease) (1002). As a nosologic entity PAN accounts for approximately 15% of all cases of systemic vasculitis (1004). The incidence is approximately 0.7 to 1.8 per 100,000 per year, the prevalence is approximately 5 in 100,000, and boys are twice as likely to have PAN as girls. Most cases occur in adults, and most childhood cases occur in older children and adolescents. However, the disease has been described in children as young as 6 years of age.

Pathogenesis

PAN has diverse etiologic correlates and underlying immunologic disease mechanisms. The most important underlying pathogenetic correlates are viral infection, hepatitis B, hepatitis C (often in association with essential mixed cryoglobulinemia), HIV infection (rare, see prior discussion), and occult cancer (1002). Before the widespread implementation of hepatitis B vaccination programs, up to 40% of adult patients with PAN were chronic carriers of hepatitis B, and circulating immune complexes involving the hepatitis B antigen could be involved in the immunopathogenesis of PAN in some patients (1005). An immune complex–mediated vasculitis appears to be involved in at least one-half of the cases with detectable circulating immune complexes, deposition of viral antigen–antibody complexes in the vessel walls, and reductions of serum complement (1002).

Familial Mediterranean fever, an autosomal-recessive illness characterized by recurrent but self-limited fever and polyserositis, is yet another disease entity that has been associated with the development of PAN. In such instances the Mediterranean fever tends to manifest before 12 years of age and PAN shortly thereafter (1006,1007). During the last decade, there has been evidence of antibodies against endothelial antigens and the role of T-cell infiltrates, implicating cell-mediated cytotoxic mechanisms in the immunopathogenesis of vasculitic neuropathy in PAN (1002,1008).

Neuropathology

The early PAN lesions consist predominantly of polymorphonuclear leukocytes (PMNs) involving all three arterial layers accompanied by fibrinoid necrosis and thrombosis. The inflammatory infiltrates of subacute/chronic PAN lesions are comprised predominantly of lymphocytes and monocytes accompanied by fibrosis and endothelial proliferation with compromise of the vascular lumens (obliterative endarteritis). Necrotizing arteritis may lead to the formation of microaneurysms and attendant neuropathologic complications such as stroke (1009).

In the CNS, there is consistent involvement of the small meningeal arteries with a lesser involvement of the parenchymal arteries. In a fatal pediatric case of polyarteritis nodosa, the autopsy revealed characteristic focal segmental necrotizing CNS vasculitis (1010).

Segmental necrotizing inflammation of small epineurial arteries typically characterizes the ischemic lesions affecting cranial and peripheral nerves (vasculitic neuropathy).

Clinical Manifestations

PAN may give rise to diverse neurologic manifestations in up to 80% of patients (1001,1011) reflecting the frequent involvement of both the PNS and CNS in this disease. In adults, PNS involvement in the form of multiple mononeuropathies (mononeuritis multiplex) and/or symmetric polyneuropathies is more common than CNS manifestations. The latter have been reported in 3% to 41% of PAN patients, where in most patients the disease process is limited to peripheral nerve and skeletal muscle (1002). Subclinical muscle involvement may be as high as in 80% of PAN patients (1002). CNS involvement in PAN has been described in 10% of adult patients and is generally considered to be a poor prognostic factor (1012).

PAN is uncommon in the pediatric population. Although many of the clinical features of the disease appear to cross age groups, children are more likely to present with skin rashes, calf pain, arthritis, and/or arthralgias, myalgias, abdominal pain, hypertension, and Raynaud's phenomenon. It is important to note that seizures are considerably more common in children, whereas peripheral neuropathy is less common in the pediatric population than in adults (1002). Two distinct syndromes are recognized: an infantile form and a late juvenile form. The former is associated with seizures and aseptic meningitis (1013). Children with this form of PAN often present with viral exanthems and are at risk of sudden death during convalescence owing to necrotizing vasculitis of the coronary arteries (1002). This clinicopathologic variant of pediatric PAN has a predilection for the coronary arteries and is probably the same as the mucocutaneous lymph node syndrome (MLNS) or Kawasaki disease (Kawasaki disease is more fully discussed in Chapter 7).

In older children, the disease resembles that seen in adults. In the series by Ozen and colleagues (1003), severe myalgia refractory to analgesia was seen as the presenting complaint in three-fourths of cases. Peripheral nerve involvement marked by numbness and paresthesias was noted in 13%. Encephalitic symptoms including seizures, cranial nerve palsies, and hemiplegia are also encountered (1010). Multiple mononeuropathies in the context of mononeuritis multiplex are considered to be characteristic of this condition. The peripheral nerves most frequently affected are the branches of the popliteal nerve (1014). Mononeuritis multiplex is an early manifestation and a clue for diagnosis of PAN, and usually manifests by rapid onset of focal neuritic pain associated with sensorimotor deficits (1002). Remissions and relapses are common. Coalescence of multiple peripheral nerve lesions is usually seen at a late stage of the disease and may even result in a symmetric or asymmetric polyneuropathy. Practically every cranial nerve has been reported to be involved, but there is a predilection for cranial nerves III and VIII.

Ocular manifestations of PAN in children may be due to ischemic lesions of cranial nerve nuclei and visual cortex (1015,1016) or the retina. Patients may present with cranial nerve palsies, nystagmus, and visual field defects in association with additional focal or diffuse neurologic deficits (893). Asymmetric shrinkage of visual fields, scotomata, decreased visual acuity, and total blindness may occur as a consequence of proliferative retinitis and retinal hemorrhage. Appropriate funduscopic changes should be sought. Papilledema may develop in PAN patients with raised intracranial pressure and especially those with concomitant systemic hypertension, who are at great risk for retinal hemorrhage (1017).

Diagnosis

The diagnosis of PAN should be considered in those patients whose obscure febrile illness is linked with CNS or PNS manifestations and in whom antinuclear and anti-DNA antibodies are negative. In the series of Ozen (1003), hepatitis B antigen was only present in 10% of cases. Neuroimaging studies may be unremarkable or may demonstrate bland or hemorrhagic infarction, focal or generalized encephalomalacia, or intraparenchymal or subarachnoid hemorrhage. Cerebral angiography may be normal early in the course of the illness, but segmental narrowing of small and medium-sized vessels is often found after weeks or months of illness. Microaneurysms involving superficial or deep small or medium-sized cerebral arteries are less common (1003).

Diagnosis usually requires angiography of the liver, kidney, and gut in combination with biopsy of symptomatic organs. Renal, skin, muscle, and peripheral nerve biopsies may be especially useful in confirming the diagnosis. The pathognomonic findings on renal angiography are segmental narrowing and/or microaneurysmal dilatation of medium-sized renal arteries associated with focal hypoperfusion. Renal biopsy demonstrates necrotizing arteritis or diffuse glomerulonephritis. Because renal vasculitis may be patchy, a negative result by no means excludes the diagnosis.

Laboratory features may include elevated erythrocyte sedimentation rate, leukocytosis, and CSF pleocytosis. MRI and traditional angiography may show ischemic CNS lesions and intracranial hemorrhage secondary to stenosis of medium-sized and large blood vessels and to intracranial aneurysms (1018).

Treatment

Evaluation of the effectiveness of therapy is complicated by the natural fluctuations of the disease. Use of corticosteroids combined with immunosuppressive agents is the preferred treatment (1005). A combination of high-dose corticosteroids and cyclophosphamide (1012) may result in improvement of the clinical and MRI findings, but the therapeutic response may not be lasting (1015). Cyclophosphamide may lead to sterility, and caution should be used when administering this immunosuppressive agent to children or adolescents (1002).

Prognosis

The prognosis of childhood cases is poor, and the disease tends to take a steady downhill course (1013). In the series of Ozen (1003), complete remission was achieved in only 13% of children.

Two relatively common systemic vasculitides of childhood, notably Henoch-Schönlein purpura and Kawasaki disease, have been shown to have CNS involvement (1019–1021). Although angiography or brain biopsy confirming vasculitis has only seldom been reported, focal neurologic findings and MRI lesions in both diseases are likely to be related to CNS vasculitis (893).

Kawasaki Disease

This is a predominantly childhood disease, which has also been reported in adults. The annual incidence of the disorder is 5.3 to 8.5 in 100,000 in children younger than 4 years of age in the United States and 46 to 195 in 100,000 in Japan (1002).

The initial illness lasts for 1 to 2 weeks and is characterized by conjuctivitis, marked dryness, redness, and fissuring of the lips ("strawberry tongue"), marked edema of the hands and feet, erythema and excoriation of volar and plantar surfaces, variegated exanthema of the torso (without vesicles or crusts), and cervical lymphadenopathy. Up to one-third of patients develop myocarditis, coronary artery aneurysms, and, less often, pericarditis or cardiac valve disease. Coronary artery involvement is the hallmark feature of vascular disease, a consistent pathologic finding that is present in all autopsy cases. There may be variable, albeit lesser, involvement of other systemic blood vessels.

Kawasaki disease has been shown to have CNS involvement (1021). The most common manifestations are aseptic meningitis (5%) and encephalopathy. Stroke, seizures, retinal vasculitis, cranial nerve palsies, polyneuropathy, and myositis have been reported but are less frequent (1002). Although angiography or brain biopsy confirming vasculitis has only seldom been reported, focal neurologic findings and MRI lesions are likely to be related to CNS vasculitis (893).

High-dose aspirin (80 to 100 mg/kg per day) for 14 days in conjunction with IVIG administration in a single dose of 2 g/kg appears to be highly effective in ameliorating the arteritis and myocardial complications (1022–1024). The condition is covered more extensively in Chapter 7.

Wegener's Granulomatosis and ANCA Vasculitides

CNS vasculitis in children may also occur in the setting of antineutrophil cytoplasmic antibody (ANCA)–positive vasculitides (1025–1027). In Wegener granulomatosis, inflammatory lesions of the upper respiratory tract and lungs are accompanied by vasculitis of the small and medium-sized arteries and veins. CNS involvement is seen in approximately 5% of adults (1026), and childhood cases are rare (1027). In the series of Rottem and colleagues (1028), neurologic symptoms including a peripheral neuropathy, multiple cranial nerve palsies, and seizures were seen in 17%. The presence of ANCA indicates the diagnosis.

Collagen Vascular Diseases

The central and peripheral nervous systems are frequently involved in systemic collagen vascular (autoimmune) diseases affecting children and adolescents. Among them, systemic lupus erythematosus (SLE), dermatomyositis, and Adamantiades-Behçet disease appear to be the most frequently encountered autoimmune disorders in the pediatric neurology setting nowadays (1029). Neurologic complications of childhood dermatomyositis are discussed in Chapter 16. Briefly, there are rare instances of previously healthy children with dermatomyositis who died after a fulminant CNS vasculitis characterized by endothelial necrosis (1030). Juvenile rheumatoid arthritis, though it only rarely affects the nervous system in children, may occasionally have devastating neurologic sequelae. Conventional and newer biologically targeted therapies are of pivotal importance in disease amelioration and prevention of long-term neurologic disability and psychiatric sequelae (1029).

Acute Rheumatic Fever

Patients with acute rheumatic fever exhibit disseminated, unstable, and transient neuropsychiatric manifestations (1031). The characteristic histopathologic lesion of acute rheumatic fever is a rheumatic proliferative endarteritis. Although there is a paucity of neuropathologic descriptions in patients with acute rheumatic fever, long-term involvement of the CNS results from disseminated, recurrent obliterative endarteritis and/or microemboli in the terminal blood vessels of the cerebral cortex and the leptomeninges causing focal ischemic damage (1031).

Infantile Multisystem Inflammatory Disease

Neonatal/infantile-onset multisystem inflammatory disease, or chronic, infantile onset multisystem inflammatory disease (CINCA), is a rare, multisystem inflammatory disease characterized by neonatal onset of urticarial symptoms, persistent rash, ocular inflammatory lesions, characteristic deforming arthropathy, and neurologic involvement (1032–1034). The latter includes chronic meningitis, a persistently open fontanel, papilledema, and seizures. Psychomotor development may be slow, and cerebral atrophy may be apparent on brain imaging (53,1034). The condition must be differentiated from juvenile rheumatoid arthritis and from Behçet syndrome (53,1033). Recently, mutations in the *NALP3/CIAS1/PYPAF1* gene have been associated with CINCA (808,1032,1035). It has been sugested that IL-1β may be involved in the pathogenesis of inflammation seen in CINCA and similar conditions, like Muckle-Wells syndrome (MWS) and familial cold autoinflammatory syndrome (FCAS), because of the response of MWS to anakinra (1035) a nonglycosylated form of the human interleukin-1 receptor antagonist (IL-1Ra).

Juvenile Rheumatoid Arthritis (JRA)

Rheumatoid vasculitis affecting the CNS is rare and may present clinically with seizures, dementia, hemiparesis, cranial nerve palsy, blindness, hemispheric dysfunction, cerebellar ataxia, or dysphasia (1036–1038). Except for fatigue, irritability, myalgia, or disuse atrophy, neurologic dysfunction is uncommon in JRA. Focal neurologic disturbances that may occur are produced most commonly as a consequence of articular or soft tissue inflammation or treatment regimens (1039). A small percentage of patients with JRA develop encephalopathy (1040), which can take the form of meningismus and seizures. In a milder form, patients have irritability and drowsiness and display diffuse EEG abnormalities. Progression to decorticate posturing and coma have been reported.

A symmetric, ascending, sensorimotor polyneuropathy has been reported in some cases of JRA or scleroderma (1041). This is probably a vasculitic neuropathy owing to inflammation of the vasa nervorum and generally carries a poor prognosis. The CSF may show protein elevation and, less commonly, mild pleocytosis. Rarely, JRA patients develop immune-mediated diseases of the neuromuscular system, notably myositis, myasthenia gravis, or inflammatory neuropathy (1042).

Most neurologic complications of JRA improve once the underlying systemic JRA is brought under control. Many cases respond to aspirin and nonsteroidal anti-inflammatory agents. There are instances in which corticosteroids, IVIG, parenteral gold salts, penicillamine, or immunosuppressive agents are required (1043). Cyclophosphamide is being used increasingly in the management of extraarticular manifestations in RA (1044); however, TNF inhibitors such as infliximab infusions hold promise in RA-associated vasculitis refractory to conventional treatment (1045).

Appropriate physical and occupational therapy can alleviate pain and assist in the management of spinal cord muscular dysfunction or peripheral nerve entrapment (1046).

Scleroderma

Two forms of scleroderma occur in childhood: focal scleroderma and childhood progressive systemic sclerosis. Both are chronic systemic diseases that involve integument and connective tissues as well as joints and viscera organs. Typical dermal histologic features include increased thickness and density of subepidermal collagen associated with scattered foci of perivascular mononuclear infiltrate (53,1047).

The chief manifestations of focal scleroderma, peculiarly a disease of childhood and adolescence, are morphea and linear scleroderma. Both of these lesions initially present with edema and induration with subsequent sclerotic atrophy and the development of associated hyperpigmentation. Focal scleroderma is associated with abnormalities of esophageal peristalsis, chronic recurrent sinusitis, and hemiatrophy. Renal and cardiac abnormalities often remain subclinical (53,1047).

CNS involvement of scleroderma is rare in children (1047). Neurologic complications include headache, seizures, and a variety of ophthalmologic disturbances that range from diplopia to indistinct or diminished vision. Some of these cases have developed vasculitic changes in the small or medium-sized cerebral or meningeal vessels underlying linear scleroderma or morphea of the face or scalp. Localized scleroderma en coup de sabre is associated with focal brain lesions, which may be epileptogenic and/or progressive (1048), the latter culminating in cerebral atrophy (1049). Contralateral hemiatrophy, hemiparesis, and focal seizures may develop in such cases. This condition should be differentiated from facial hemiatrophy (see Chapter 3). The possible pathogenetic relationship of localized scleroderma en coup de sabre to brain calcifications is conjectural (1050). The neuroimaging and clinical features of this form of scleroderma have been recently reappraised by Appenzeller and colleagues (1048). SPECT is a sensitive modality in revealing brain functional deficits in approximately half of patients with systemic sclerosis who may be otherwise free of neurologic manifestations (1051). Peripheral neuropathy, possibly the result of involvement of endoneurial blood vessels, and inflammatory myopathy resembling polymyositis may also develop (1052).

Sjögren Syndrome

Sjögren syndrome, characterized by xerostomia, recurrent lymphocytic inflammation of the salivary glands, and keratoconjunctivitis sicca, rarely affects children (1053). No neurologic complications have been noted in the few childhood cases that have occurred, primarily adolescent girls (53).

Mixed Connective Tissue Disease

This collagen vascular disease combines the features of progressive systemic sclerosis with those of polymyositis and SLE. It is uncommon in children. The most common complication of neurologic interest in this condition is inflammatory muscle disease (myositis). Other complications of mixed connective tissue disease include headache, seizures, elevation of CSF protein, and aseptic meningitis (1054).

Adamantiades-Behçet Disease (Neuro-Behçet Disease)

Adamantiades-Behçet disease is a systemic vascular inflammatory disease of unknown etiology characterized by ocular inflammation (uveitis), oral and genital ulcers, skin lesions (erythema nodosum), vasculitis, and articular, gastrointestinal, and nervous system involvement (1037,1055,1056). An association with HLA-B51 has been reported, particularly in severe cases (1057). The CNS may be affected in 10% to 49% of patients (1058,1059). The syndrome is rare, and patients are generally young adults (1056).

Neurologic manifestations in Adamantiades-Behçet disease (a presentation also referred to as "neuro-Behçet" disease) are relatively rare in children (1055,1060), but when present they can present diagnostic challenges. The syndrome is part of the differential diagnosis of MS, ADEM, stroke, or even tumor, especially in a child or a young adult (1056). Proper diagnosis may be hampered by inadequate history and physical examination and lack of awareness of the condition in children coupled with failure to recognize the underlying systemic syndrome and its relationship to the neurologic manifestations (1061). The diagnosis may also be confounded by the fact that CSF studies may be intermittently unremarkable and also by incomplete neuroimaging studies (1061).

The initial symptoms and signs in children are oral ulcers plus cutaneous lesions, genital ulcers, and headache (1055). However, the clinical expression of the disease may be incomplete and highly variable (1055). Some pediatric patients may present from the outset with arthritis, abdominal pain, eye inflammation, and neurologic manifestations. Others may have a complete form of the disease encompassing ocular, neurologic, and/or vascular abnormalities, whereas others may exhibit an incomplete form of the syndrome with mucocutaneous, gastrointestinal, or articular involvement occurring either singly or in combination (1055). Family history of Adamantiades-Behçet disease may be positive in some cases (1055).

Neuropathology. Histologically, there is vascular and perivascular inflammation (vasculitis) involving arteries (panarteritis) and veins of all sizes (panphlebitis). Different stages of vascular inflammation may be encountered. In the acute phase there is a predominantly neutrophil-mediated vasculitis devoid of fibrinoid necrosis or microthrombi (1062), whereas in the later phase of the disease lymphocytic infiltrations may predominate. Parenchymal changes result either from primary inflammation (including inflammatory demyelination) or vasculitis of predominantly venous and to a lesser extent arterial elements, culminating in ischemic stroke (1037,1059,1063). Intracerebral hemorrhage is rare (1064).

Clinical Manifestations. Two major neurologic forms of the disease are recognized, which do not usually occur in the same individual and probably involve different pathogenetic mechanisms (1056). One comprises focal or multifocal CNS lesions owing to vasculitis and inflammatory changes in the parenchyma. The other form, which may be caused by isolated cerebral venous sinus thrombosis and elevated intracranial pressure, is characterized by few symptoms and a more favorable neurologic prognosis (1056).

Headaches are the most frequent, albeit nonspecific neurologic symptom of the disease. They may be primary, exhibiting a nonstructural recurrent, bifrontal, vascular quality, or secondary to ocular inflammation, meningoencephalitis, or dural sinus thrombosis (1056). The most common presentation of parenchymal CNS involvement in all ages is an acute or, more often, a subacute brainstem syndrome accompanied by cranial neuropathies, dysarthria, and cerebellar/peduncular and/or descending tract signs (1037,1056,1065). Less frequently, patients may present with features of stroke, seizures (indicating cortical inflammatory or ischemic involvement), and neuropsychiatric manifestations (1037,1065).

An uncommon but highly suggestive presentation *de novo* that may unveil the systemic disease is cerebral venous sinus thrombosis (1066). The latter usually develops slowly, giving rise to symptoms and signs of elevated intracranial pressure such as headache, nausea and vomiting, and bilateral papilledema (1059).

From the neuropediatric perspective, there are reports of patients exhibiting a picture of ADEM associated with (or in some cases actually unmasking) ophthalmic and/or mucocutaneous lesions that typify Adamantiades-Behçet disease (1065,1067). Other neurologic presentations include meningoencephalitis and language deficits (1065). Chorea has been described in adult patients but not in children (1068). Rarely, cerebral hemorrhage has been reported in adults, and its causation may either be related to or compounded by underlying cyclosporine treatment (1064). Often neuro-Behçet syndrome may mimic

MS both in terms of MRI findings and clinical course (i.e., primary progressive, relapsing-remitting, or secondary progressive), prompting a thorough systemic work-up (1037,1056,1069,1070). To this end, patients with Behçet disease display a serum and CSF cytokine and chemokine profile akin to nonspecific inflammation that differs from that seen in MS and other autoimmune disorders (1071).

Behavioral manifestations (such as psychosis), pure spinal cord (myelopathy), or peripheral nervous system involvement are relatively uncommon (1056,1063). Skeletal muscle involvement in the form of necrotizing myositis with vasculitis and vascular deposition of immune complexes is rare but recognized (1072). The possibility of myositis should be entertained in patients presenting with myalgia and swelling of the lower limbs (1072).

Neuroimaging. Neuroimaging findings are highly variable and may imitate other vasculitic and demyelinating processes. Venous thrombosis is a classic complication of Adamantiades-Behçet disease that can occasionally unmask the underlying systemic disease. Cerebral venous thrombosis is a finding associated with neuro-Behcet disease (1073). Sagittal sinus thrombosis may occasionally, albeit rarely, present as the first manifestation of the disease in children (1066) MRI, if performed during the acute illness, may exhibit an abnormally high signal on the T2-weighted sequences in the occluded sinus and may also show minor flow abnormalities suggestive of partial recanalization of the sinus at a later clinical stage (1073). To this end, MRI can be an alternative, noninvasive, neurodiagnostic modality to intravenous cerebral angiography (1073).

MRI may show focal (solitary, often tumefactive) or multifocal, disseminated lesions. Anatomically, diffuse lesions in the brainstem, basal ganglia, and diencephalon (predominantly thalamic nuclei) are the most common (1058,1073,1074). MRI performed during the acute illness may show multiple scattered hyperintense lesions on T2-weighted sequences, which are usually multifocal and/or confluent and measure less than 5 mm in greatest diameter. These lesions are most commonly distributed in the cerebral hemispheric white matter and the brainstem (1073,1074). Lesions are also seen in the cerebral cortex, cerebellum, optic nerves, and spinal cord (1073,1074). Less common lesions have been described, including a hyperintense MRI lesion of the corpus callosum (1067) and multiple cortical calcifications on CT (1065).

Typically, brain MRI is abnormal in most patients with CNS involvement and is only rarely so in patients with features of the systemic disease but without CNS manifestations (1074). MRI abnormalities are usually associated with corresponding clinical deficits, but are often larger and more disseminated than the clinical semiology indicates (1073). As a rule, the cerebral white matter lesions are asymptomatic and usually small, whereas the brainstem lesions are frequently expansive and symptomatic (1074). Isolated, tumor-like (tumefactive) lesions are not uncommon in this disease setting (1075–1078). In a follow-up study of 2 patients in the series by Morrissey and colleagues (1074) who presented with brainstem syndromes and were treated with immunosuppressive regimens, 1 showed resolution of a large lesion concomitant with clinical remission, whereas the other developed marked brainstem atrophy and became severely disabled. Brain perfusion abnormalities (hypoperfusion) have been reported involving cerebral cortex, basal ganglia, and thalamus (927,1051,1079).

Neurophysiology. Abnormal brainstem auditory-, visual-, and somatosensory-evoked potentials were described in a series of 44 patients with Adamantiades-Behçet disease, including children (1080).

Treatment. Primary headaches may be treated symptomatically, including with tricyclic antidepressants or valproic acid, whereas triptans should be reserved for intractable headaches refractory to conventional treatment (1081). Topiramate has been effective in a case of intracranial hypertension associated with Behçet disease purportedly by virtue of reducing CSF production (1082). Treatment of CNS parenchymal lesions entails high-dose corticosteroid pulse therapy followed by long-term immunosuppression.

Potent cytotoxic agents such as cyclophosphamide are reserved for more severe cases refractory to steroid treatment (1037,1057). A frequent side effect in patients with active disease who are on high-dose steroids is impairment of long-term verbal and nonverbal memory and visuospatial skills (1037,1083).

This condition is covered further in Chapter 7.

Systemic Lupus Erythematosus

SLE is a systemic inflammatory disease affecting multiple organs and tissues including blood vessels. The annual incidence of SLE in North America is approximately 5 in 100,000 and the prevalence is 45 to 50 in 100,000 (1084). Neurologic complications, occurring either as presenting symptoms or some time during the course of the illness, occur in 10% to 45% of children affected by SLE (1085,1086). There is a female predilection.

Neuropathology and Pathogenesis. In the CNS, SLE lesions are focal, diffuse, or both and are produced by several mechanisms (1087). Neuropathologic studies reveal a wide range of brain abnormalities including multifocal microinfarcts, cortical atrophy, gross infarcts, hemorrhages, ischemic demyelination, and patchy multiple sclerosis–like demyelination (1088).

A bona fide, histopathologically defined CNS vasculitis is relatively rare and has been documented in only

7% to16% of fatal cases of CNS SLE evaluated at autopsy (1089,1090). The most common morphologic finding is a vasculopathy devoid of inflammatory infiltrates and characterized by mural hyalinization, intimal proliferation, and luminal compromise of small cerebral and meningeal arteries often resulting in multiple ischemic lesions (infarcts) (1091,1092). Gliosis of the neuropil around arterioles or capillaries, microinfarcts, and microhemorrhages are also commonly seen.

The paucity of inflammatory infiltrates does not necessarily preclude an inciting inflammatory process, because the vasculopathy may represent the chronic or end stage of an obliterative endarteritic damage conceivably preceded by an inflammatory (vasculitic) phase. In addition to CNS SLE-associated vasculitis/vasculopathy, embolic brain infarcts of cardiac origin (demonstrated in 20% of cases in a major autopsy series) (1093) as well as thrombotic thrombocytopenic purpura (1093) and a variety of infective (bacterial and fungal) microorganisms are capable of causing CNS pathology in SLE. Gross intracranial hemorrhages arising from microaneurysmal dilatations secondary to arteritis are reported in as many as 10% of cases with CNS SLE.

Immunopathogenesis. The underlying neuropathogenesis of CNS SLE centers on two distinctive but not necessarily mutually exclusive mechanisms: (a) hypoxic-ischemic parenchymal injury secondary to immunologically mediated CNS microvascular damage with attendant disruption of the BBB and (b) direct immune-mediated neuronal injury by antineuronal autoantibodies. However, the precise immunopathogenesis of CNS SLE is uncertain; it is complex and multifactorial. It may involve a range of immunologic abnormalities, including, but not limited to, autoantibody production targeting specific cell types in the CNS, immune complex depositions, microangiopathy, and intrathecal production of proinflammatory cytokines (1094). Recently, it has been shown that CNS SLE is associated with apolipoprotein E polymorphism (1095).

Antiphospholipid Antibodies. The most clinically important autoantibodies in CNS SLE are the prothrombotic antiphospholipid antibodies. Potential targets of antiphospholipid antibodies are endothelial cell antigens, prostacyclin, protein C, the protein C-S complex, and platelets (1094). However, the pathogenetic mechanism underlying the association between thromboembolic disease and antiphospholipid antibodies is uncertain (1094).

Cerebrovascular disease is one of the most common clinical presentations in SLE, only second to deep vein thrombosis (1096). Antiphospholipid antibodies have been causally linked to ischemic and hemorrhagic strokes, transient ischemic attacks, venous sinus thrombosis, amaurosis fugax, and acute subdural hematomas (1094). Elevated serum levels of intercellular adhesion molecule-1, vascular cell adhesion molecule-1, and E-selectin have been shown to correlate with antiphospholipid antibody titers (1097). Furthermore, the upregulation of adhesion molecule expression by antiphospholipid antibodies has both prothrombotic and proinflammatory effects (1094).

Anti–Ribosomal P Antibodies. A strong relationship exists between anti–ribosomal P antibodies and CNS SLE (1098–1104). Increases of ribosomal P antibodies are associated with neuropsychiatric manifestations, especially psychosis (1098), and mark disease activity in SLE (1101,1103). P protein is present in neurons and may be one of the antigenic determinants preferentially targeted in the context of immune-mediated responses in SLE (1105).

Antineuronal Antibodies. The occurrence of antineuronal antibodies relates to a clinical subset of CNS SLE characterized by encephalopathy and seizures (1094). It has been shown that a subset of anti-DNA antibodies cross-reacts with *N*-methyl-D-aspartate receptors and can signal neuronal death through an excitotoxic mechanism (459).

A recent study showed that serum autoantibodies to a neuronal protein, microtubule-associated protein-2, appear to be a robust and especially promising biomarker for CNS SLE (1106).

Cytokines. There is evidence of increased production of proinflammatory cytokines in the CSF of patients with CNS SLE. These include increased levels of CSF IL-1 (1107), IL-6 (1108), IL-1β, IL-6, IL-10, and TNF-α (1109), IL-10 and IFN-γ (1110), IL-6 and IL-8 (1111,1112), and TGF-β (1094). IL-8 is a chemokine that alters the permeability of the BBB and attracts B and T cells to the site of inflammation. IL-6 is an important growth factor for activated B cells (1112).

Elevated levels of prostaglandin E2 have been found in the CSF of CNS SLE patients (1113). In addition, significantly increased CSF and serum concentrations of kinins (high-molecular-weight kininogen, low-molecular-weight kininogen, prekallikrein, tissue kallikrein, and kininase II) have been reported in CNS-SLE patients (1109).

Brain-reactive antibodies (antineuronal antibodies, antiglial antibodies, anti-G_{M1} ganglioside, and anti–ribosomal P protein) have been implicated in immunopathogenesis of CNS lupus and may serve as disease biomarkers for CNS SLE (1098,1114,1115). There are elevated titers of antineuronal antibodies in the CSF of patients with CNS SLE but not in those who have SLE without neuropsychiatric manifestations. Anti–ribosomal P antibody titers are more likely to be elevated in pediatric SLE patients with psychosis than in SLE patients without psychosis (1116).

The presence of circulating antiphospholipid antibodies is associated with arterial or venous thromboses, giving rise to transient ischemic attacks (TIAs) or stroke (1117).

TABLE 8.15 Neuropsychiatric Symptoms Encountered in Systemic Lupus Erythematosus

Central Nervous System
Aseptic meningitis
Cerebrovascular disease
Demyelinating syndrome
Headache (including migraine and benign intracranial hypertension)
Movement disorder (chorea)
Myelopathy
Seizure disorder
Acute confusional state
Anxiety attacks
Cognitive dysfunction
Mood disorder
Psychosis
Peripheral Nervous System
Guillain-Barré syndrome
Autonomic disorder
Motor neuropathy, single/multiplex
Myasthenia gravis
Neuropathy, cranial
Plexopathy
Polyneuropathy

From Ad Hoc Committee on Neuropsychiatric Lupus Nomenclature. The American College of Rheumatology nomenclature and case definition for neuropsychiatric lupus syndromes. *Arthritis Rheum* 1999;42:599–608. With permission.

Antiphospholipid antibodies interfere with the protein C activation pathway, resulting in prolonged and sustained procoagulant activation after small blood vessel damage and thrombosis. In addition, antiphospholipid antibodies contribute to the immunopathogenesis of endocardiac and valvular heart disease as well as thrombocytopenia (1118). The diverse pathogenetic effects of antiphospholipid antibodies were critically reviewed by Mackworth-Young (1119).

Clinical Manifestations. There is a wide range of neuropsychiatric manifestations of SLE and the symptoms and signs are typically protean and progressive (1094) (Table 8.15). The majority of patients present with mental changes, namely, psychosis, mood disturbance, particularly depression, confusion, and/or hallucinations, though a significant percentage of patients may also exhibit concomitant neurologic manifestations (1120,1121). The latter include generalized seizures, encephalopathy (acute confusional state or cognitive decline), headaches, including migraine, movement disorders particularly chorea/hemichorea, and ischemic and/or hemorrhagic stroke (ischemic and hemorrhagic). Many patients exhibit abnormal EEGs (1120–1122).

In addition, myelopathy, cranial neuropathies, peripheral neuropathies, and myasthenia have been described in association with SLE (1094). Peripheral neuropathy may not be clinically manifest, but a significant number of patients may have neurophysiologic evidence of a neuropathy. In rare instances, neurologic symptoms may be the first manifestation of the disease. Intracranial hemorrhage is a rare but potentially fatal complication. A subset of children may display residual neuropsychiatric sequelae despite treatment (1120).

Neuroimaging. The course of CNS SLE is largely unknown. New imaging techniques are available to assist in monitoring the disease course (1123). Neuroimaging modalities include CT, MRI, MRS, magnetization transfer imaging (MTI), DWI, and SPECT (927,1121,1123).

Cerebral atrophy is found by CT scans in a number of children. MRI reveals new lesions or abatement of previous lesions. MRS reveals evidence of inflammation and metabolically compromised tissue denoting neuronal damage or loss whereas MTI reflects changes in whole-brain lesion load (1123). DWI is capable of detecting small and active ischemic changes not visible on conventional MRI, and it distinguishes cytotoxic from vasogenic edema. Recent studies indicate that DWI may be particularly useful in the diagnosis and monitoring of CNS vasculitis or vasculopathy in the setting of SLE, Behçet disease, Churg-Strauss disease, and PACNS (927).

Diagnosis. Cases of pediatric CNS SLE must fulfill the 1997 revised diagnostic criteria spelled out by the American College of Rheumatology. Standard laboratory studies are warranted in all suspected cases. These include routine laboratory and immunologic tests and antinuclear antibodies, anti–double-stranded DNA, anti-Smith, antiphospholipid antibodies, antineuronal antibodies, and complement components C3 and C4 (1121,1124). In addition to serum and CSF immunologic studies, neurodiagnostic studies should include EEG, MRI, CT, and SPECT (1124).

SPECT, in conjunction with antineuronal antibodies, helps to confirm CNS involvement in children with SLE and neuropsychiatric manifestations. There is persuasive data to support that serum antineuronal antibodies are positive with onset of symptoms and decline with clinical improvement (1121).

In many instances, recurrent and progressive neurologic manifestations such as seizures may occur even after years after initial presentation and despite adequate treatment. In addition, MS-like lesions have been described in the pediatric setting of CNS SLE (1123), underscoring the potential for overlapping patterns of inflammatory and demyelinating CNS injury, which may be traceable, at least in part, to vascular hypoxic-ischemic insults.

Treatment. Early aggressive treatment with combined intravenous methylprednisolone (1 to 2 mg/kg) and cyclophosphamide followed by monthly intravenous cyclophosphamide for at least 3 months, and then every 2 and/or 3 months according to the clinical response, may be an effective therapy for severe childhood neuropsychiatric SLE/CNS SLE (1124).

Recently, a study intended to evaluate the short-term effect of therapeutic plasma exchange in children with active SLE revealed a benefit for patients with CNS manifestations (1125).

NEUROLOGIC COMPLICATIONS OF IMMUNIZATIONS

Active immunization of children has proven highly effective in that it has practically eliminated poliomyelitis, measles, rubella, tetanus, *Haemophilus influenzae* type b, and other infectious or communicable diseases in the United States and other developed countries (1127). Individual vaccines, however, have the potential of giving rise to adverse systemic reactions that range from relatively minor to severe. In rare instances such adverse reactions involve the nervous system.

Major neurologic complications related to immunizations are manifested by seizures, shock, and encephalopathy and, in exceptional instances, are terminated by a fatal outcome (1127). A number of reporting systems have been put in place aimed at monitoring adverse events that may follow immunization (1128).

In recent years, immunization programs have also generated considerable controversy, as evidenced by recent concerns of the public regarding claims of a possible relationship between vaccines or their constituents and neurologic diseases such as autism or MS (1127,1129). Vaccine constituents with potential neurotoxic and myotoxic properties include thimerosal and aluminum, macrophagic myofasciitis, the latter being associated with (1128).

Postvaccinal Encephalomyelitis

Although no longer encountered, the neurologic complications after smallpox vaccination can be considered as a prototype for complications encountered after various other immunizations in which a live organism is introduced into the human host. Neurologic complications were seen after either primary or repeat vaccination. Their average incidence was 2.9 in 1,000,000 vaccinations, with the highest frequency in younger vaccinated individuals (53).

Two clinical pictures were observed. Postvaccinal encephalomyelitis was an acute illness that began during the second week after the successful vaccination of a nonimmune individual (1130,1131). Its pathologic picture was highlighted by perivascular demyelination and is identical to the postexanthematous encephalitides.

The other postvaccinial complication was termed postvaccinial encephalopathy. It commonly affected infants younger than 2 years old and followed a variable incubation period of 1 to 24 days. The condition was heralded by a prolonged generalized convulsion. The CSF was normal, and aside from cerebral edema, no striking pathologic alterations were encountered (53).

Post–Rabies Vaccination Encephalopathy

Because rabies immunization by the use of either a duck embryo vaccine or vaccines grown in human diploid cell culture (preparations with a low content of nervous tissue antigen) has become common practice in Western countries, the incidence of postvaccinial complications has fallen markedly. The current estimated rate is less than 1 in 100,000 individuals, contrasted with 1 in 300 to 1 in 7,000 at a time when the neural vaccines were being used (1132). In developing countries, vaccines grown in brain or spinal cord are still in vogue, and the most recently reported incidence of encephalomyelitis was 1 in 220, with a 17% mortality (1133).

Neurologic symptoms appear 8 to 21 days after the first injection of the vaccine. Their onset is marked by chills, fever, headache, myalgia, vomiting, and changes in mental status. The most common neurologic complications are encephalitis and meningitis. Each of these was encountered in one-third of patients in a series from Thailand published in 1987 (1134). Less frequently, patients develop transverse myelitis, usually involving the thoracic or lumbar segments of the spinal cord, or neuritis of the peripheral and, less often, of the cranial nerves (1133,1134). A postvaccination GBS also has been encountered (705). High titers of IgG and IgM antibodies to G_{M1} and G_{D11} ganglioside have been detected in patients with neuroparalytic complications, suggesting that these antibodies play a pathogenetic role in postvaccine demyelination (1135). Genetic susceptibility also may play a role in the pathogenesis of the encephalopathy (1136).

The CSF usually shows lymphocytic pleocytosis and increased protein content. CSF MBP is elevated within 1 day after the onset of the neurologic symptoms, and lymphocytes demonstrate a positive response to purified myelin in approximately one-half of patients (1134). The MRI demonstrates multiple white matter lesions in the cerebrum, cerebellar peduncles, and brainstem, which resolve in parallel with clinical improvement (1137). Although relapses occur occasionally, the disease is usually monophasic. Treatment with dexamethasone has been recommended. Patients usually recover in 1 to 2 weeks. In the Thailand series, recovery was complete in 83% of patients.

Post–Influenza Vaccination Complications

Before 1976, when a federal program of immunization against swine flu was initiated, complications of influenza immunization were rare. The incidence of post–influenza vaccination encephalitis is uncertain. In the cases reported to the surveillance group, almost all patients developed systemic and neurologic symptoms in 5 hours to 4 days after the immunization. The neurologic picture was characterized by a change in consciousness and occasionally by brainstem dysfunction. The CSF showed significant pleocytosis in approximately one-half the instances. In the majority of cases, recovery was reported to be complete.

A GBS-like polyneuropathy was observed more often, occurring in 1 in 100,000 immunizations. It began between 5 and 10 weeks after the immunization (1138). The clinical course of this complication was similar to that seen after viral infections.

Other reported complications included brachial plexus neuropathy, transverse myelitis, optic neuritis, and other cranial neuropathies (1138).

Encephalopathy after Pertussis Vaccination

Hardly any other subject in pediatric neurology has evoked more controversy in both professional and lay groups than the neurologic complications after immunization with whole-cell pertussis vaccine (1138–1140).

Although the earliest reports date back to 1933, Byers and Moll (1141) were the first to document a severe encephalopathy after prophylactic pertussis vaccination in infants. Between that time and up to the introduction of acellular vaccine numerous reports were made of children who experienced seizures and encephalopathy soon after their pertussis immunization. A variety of neurologic complications has been recorded.

The use of whole-cell pertussis vaccine has been associated with febrile and afebrile seizures, which are generalized and typically occur within 72 hours after immunization (1139,1140). Febrile seizures and a hypotonic hyporesponsive state are temporary neurologic complications. In the prospective study of Cody and coworkers, both were encountered with a frequency of 1 in 1,750 immunizations, or approximately in 1 in 650 infants immunized (1142). Although some of the infants who experienced a febrile seizure within 48 hours of their vaccination were younger than 5 to 6 months of age and below the age range during which simple febrile seizures are generally encountered (see Chapter 14), the failure to document seizure recurrence or any permanent adverse effects in the majority of these infants suggests that a pyrogen in the whole-cell vaccine preparation evoked the seizure response. There has been a reduction in postvaccination febrile seizures since the introduction of acellular pertussis vaccine (1143). Approximately 10% of children who experience seizures within 48 hours of diphtheria- pertussis-tetanus (DPT) vaccination have afebrile convulsions (1144).

Hypotonic hyporesponsive episodes occur within 24 hours, with a mean interval of 12 hours from immunization. Approximately one-half of infants are febrile, and the episode subsides in minutes to at most 4 hours, leaving no apparent residua (1144). Additionally, persistent or high-pitched crying was seen in 3.2% of DPT-immunized infants and drowsiness was seen in approximately 32%. These complications were far less common following the use of a diphtheria-tetanus (DT) vaccine (1130). A smaller study, conducted in the United Kingdom using aluminum hydroxide–adsorbed DPT, failed to demonstrate any difference between DPT and DT vaccines with respect to the incidence of convulsions and other neurologic complications (1145). Follow-up studies on the infants initially reported by Cody and associates did not uncover any apparent evidence of major neurologic damage (1146). A transient increase in intracranial pressure, manifested by a bulging fontanel, has been encountered after both whole-cell DPT and DT immunizations. Its mechanism is unknown (1147). No long-term follow-up studies of infants with "minor" neurologic complications after whole-cell DPT administration have been carried out, but they would be important to determine whether such complications are precursors to hyperactivity, learning disorders, or perceptual handicaps.

Permanent neurologic disability directly attributable to the pertussis vaccine is rare and the risk–benefit ratio for all three immunizations is favorable when compared to the risks from serious complications related to the natural history of these infections (1139,1140). Several seemingly permanent neurologic syndromes develop soon after whole-cell pertussis immunization. An encephalopathy characterized by generalized febrile or nonfebrile convulsions, altered consciousness, and serious neurologic or neuropsychologic residua can occur within 72 hours of immunization. The encephalopathy's incidence has been estimated at 1 in 165,000 immunizations (1148). The prognosis for survival is good, but most children, 77% in the series of Miller and colleagues, are left with major neurologic residua, retardation, or recurrent seizures (1149,1150). A similar high incidence of these complications was found in the older series of Byers and Moll (1141) and Kulenkampff and coworkers (1151). More commonly, the first seizure, febrile or afebrile, occurs within 24 hours of immunization, and the infants, usually without fully recovering to their preimmunization levels of functioning, develop a chronic mixed major and minor motor seizure disorder clinically related to Brett epileptogenic encephalopathy, severe myoclonic epilepsy, or the Lennox-Gastaut syndrome (see Chapter 14). In the experience of Miller and associates, 85% of children who developed afebrile seizures and 44% of children who developed prolonged febrile convulsions within 7 days of their vaccination died or were left with neurologic dysfunction. A serious seizure disorder commencing within 24 hours of immunization was recorded in 1 in 106,000 patients in a retrospective study conducted by Walker and coworkers (1152).

Pathologic examination of the brain in infants who died shortly after their pertussis immunization has not been contributory. Some have a diffuse neuronal necrosis with nonspecific gliosis; in others, the changes were minimal beyond cerebral edema. Neither an acute encephalitis with perivascular infiltration nor demyelination were detected (1153). The histologic picture thus differs from that seen in the encephalopathy following smallpox vaccination, although the neuropathologic data are relatively too scarce to enable a clear-cut or compelling distinction between the two postvaccination syndromes on morphologic grounds. Experimental data indicate that pertussis toxin can attach itself to neuronal membrane receptors and, by ADP-ribosylation, modify the adenylate cyclase system so that the action of inhibitory neurotransmitters is impaired and the action of excitatory neurotransmitters is enhanced (325,1154–1156). Whereas in the vast majority of cases the blood–brain barrier prevents entry of the toxin into the brain, its temporary disruption with a concurrent viral disease or fever or as a response to the endotoxin present in the vaccine could well facilitate access of pertussis toxin to the nerve cells. Such a disruption has been seen in pertussis encephalopathy, in which high CSF antibody titers to pertussis toxin have been demonstrated (1157).

None of the numerous epidemiologic studies has exonerated or implicated pertussis vaccine in these more serious adverse responses (1158). All are confounded by the relatively low incidence of these complications and by the differences in whole-cell pertussis vaccines as used at different times and in different countries. Whole-cell vaccines were not only not standardized between manufacturers, but also, one suspects, varied with the same manufacturer from one lot to the next. This is reflected in the marked differences in antibody response to pertussis vaccination (1159).

From the wealth of case reports and studies attempting to understand the relationship, if any, between whole-cell pertussis immunization and permanent brain damage, the Institute of Medicine has offered three conclusions: (a) DPT administration causes a serious acute neurologic illness and subsequent permanent neurologic dysfunction in children who otherwise would not have experienced either acute or chronic neurologic illness; (b) DPT vaccination triggers an acute and subsequently a chronic neurologic illness in children with an underlying brain abnormality; and (c) DPT vaccination causes an acute neurologic illness in children with underlying brain abnormalities that would eventually have led to chronic neurologic disease even in the absence of the acute, DPT-initiated neurologic illness (1159a).

Choosing among these three alternatives depends a great deal on whether one sets out from the proposition that whole-cell pertussis vaccine can or cannot cause permanent neurologic damage in previously healthy children. There is of course no reason why the same alternative should be operative for all children with suspected vaccine reactions.

Although child neurologists should recommend the use of pertussis vaccine for brain-damaged infants with known static or chronic (progressive) brain syndromes, immunization should be delayed or be omitted in those cases in which the nature of the neurologic illness is equivocal (1139,1140).

Major neurologic reactions to acellular pertussis vaccine have been reported significantly less frequently than those following whole-cell vaccine (1160,1161).

Other Immunizations

Neurologic adverse reactions to the other immunizations are less controversial. The most common reaction to measles, mumps, and rubella (MMR) immunization is mumps meningoencephalitis. Depending on the strain of vaccine used, its incidence ranges from 1 in 11,000 to 1 in 100,000 doses, with symptoms beginning between 15 and 35 days after immunization (1162). Like meningitis induced by the wild mumps virus, the outcome is generally excellent (1163).

Acute encephalopathy can follow immunization with live attenuated monovalent measles vaccine or measles vaccine in combination with mumps vaccine, rubella vaccines, or both (1164,1165). The condition develops between 2 and 15 days after immunization, with the peak onset of encephalopathy on days 8 and 9. It is marked by seizures, altered behavior or consciousness, and ataxia. Death or mental regression is common. No cases of encephalopathy have been identified after administration of monovalent mumps or rubella vaccines (1165).

The association of MMR vaccination and autism or pervasive developmental disorders and Crohn disease (1166) has not been confirmed; in fact, there was no sudden increase of autism in the United Kingdom after the introduction of MMR vaccine (1167). In addition, several epidemiologic studies suggest that there is no association between MMR immunization and encephalitis or aseptic meningitis (1127,1164,1168–1170). Still, public fears for neurologic complications have led to a significant decrease in the uptake of MMR immunization in the United Kingdom, from a peak of 92% in the mid-1990s to a national level of 82% in 2003, to less than 75% in London (1129). This trend may potentially give rise to significant risk of measles outbreaks (1129). In a similar vein, the proportion of parents opting out of regulations requiring immunization as a condition of school entry has recently increased significantly in some areas of the United States (1129).

The administration of tetanus toxoid has been reported to be followed after some 10 to 14 days by polyneuritis, transverse myelitis, optic neuritis, or an encephalopathy (1128,1138,1171).

The anterior horn disease that follows immunization with attenuated oral poliovirus is covered in Chapter 7. In some children recovering from an acute episode of asthma, a flaccid paralysis resembling poliomyelitis has been encountered. This condition, first reported from Australia in 1974 (1172), has been termed Hopkins syndrome (see Chapters 16 and 17). No consistent virus has been cultured from such patients, who generally have been successfully vaccinated against poliomyelitis. The disorder primarily involves the anterior horn cells. A rapid progression of paralysis usually affects one limb, leaving the child with a severe and permanent weakness. No sensory involvement occurs. The CSF usually shows moderate mononuclear pleocytosis, and the protein content can be slightly elevated (1173). Some of the children have evidence for an underlying immune deficiency (1174).

It should be noted that paralytic disease or other neurologic complications have not been reported with the use of inactivated poliovirus vaccine (1127).

Neurologic complications may also be encountered, albeit rarely, with other commonly administered immunizations. These include demyelinating lesions resembling ADEM or MS (hepatitis B vaccine), meningoencephalitis (Japanese encephalitis vaccine), GBS and giant cell arteritis (influenza vaccine), and untoward reactions after exposure to animal rabies vaccine (1127,1128). Neurologic complications associated with varicella vaccination are exceptionally rare, including a single case report of acute cerebellar ataxia ascribed to varicella vaccination (1127,1128).

REFERENCES

1. Tsunoda I, Fujinami RS. Two models for multiple sclerosis: experimental allergic encephalomyelitis and Theiler's murine encephalomyelitis virus. *J Neuropathol Exp Neurol* 1996;55:673–686.
2. Oleszak EL, Chang JR, Friedman H, et al. Theiler's virus infection: a model for multiple sclerosis. *Clin Microbiol Rev* 2004;17:174–207.
3. Poser CM, Brinar VV. The nature of multiple sclerosis. *Clin Neurol Neurosurg* 2004;106:159–171.
4. Swanborg RH. Experimental autoimmune encephalomyelitis in the rat: lessons in T-cell immunology and autoreactivity. *Immunol Rev* 2001;184:129–135.
5. Behi ME, Dubucquoi S, Lefranc D, et al. New insights into cell responses involved in experimental autoimmune encephalomyelitis and multiple sclerosis. *Immunol Lett* 2005;96:11–26.
6. Fressinaud C, Sarlieve LL, Vincendon G. Multiple sclerosis: review of main experimental data and pathogenic hypotheses [in French]. *Rev Med Interne* 1990;11:201–208.
7. Rivers TM, Schwentker FF. Encephalomyelitis accompanied by myelin destruction experimentally produced in monkeys. *J Exp Med* 1935;61:689–702.
8. Wolf A, Kabat EA, Bezer AE. The pathology of acute disseminated encephalomyelitis produced experimentally in Rhezus monkey and its resemblance to human demyelinating disease. *J Neuropathol Exp Neurol* 1947;6:333–357.
9. Ferraro ACC. Chronic experimental allergic encephalomyelitis in monkeys. *J Neuropathol Exp Neurol* 1948;7:235–260.
10. Shaw CM, Alvord EC Jr, Hruby S. Chronic remitting-relapsing experimental allergic encephalomyelitis induced in monkeys with homologous myelin basic protein. *Ann Neurol* 1988;24:738–748.
11. Alvord EC. *Experimental allergic encephalomyelitis: a useful model for multiple sclerosis*. New York: Liss, 1984.
12. Swanborg RH. Experimental autoimmune encephalomyelitis in rodents as a model for human demyelinating disease. *Clin Immunol Immunopathol* 1995;77:4–13.
13. Brown A, McFarlin DE, Raine CS. Chronologic neuropathology of relapsing experimental allergic encephalomyelitis in the mouse. *Lab Invest* 1982;46:171–185.
14. Kerschensteiner M, Bareyre FM, Buddeberg BS, et al. Remodeling of axonal connections contributes to recovery in an animal model of multiple sclerosis. *J Exp Med* 2004;200:1027–1038.
15. Kornek B, Storch MK, Weissert R, et al. Multiple sclerosis and chronic autoimmune encephalomyelitis: a comparative quantitative study of axonal injury in active, inactive, and remyelinated lesions. *Am J Pathol* 2000;157:267–276.
16. Ben-Nun A, Wekerle H, Cohen IR. The rapid isolation of clonable antigen-specific T lymphocyte lines capable of mediating autoimmune encephalomyelitis. *Eur J Immunol* 1981;11:195–199.
17. Pettinelli CB, McFarlin DE. Adoptive transfer of experimental allergic encephalomyelitis in SJL/J mice after *in vitro* activation of lymph node cells by myelin basic protein: requirement for Lyt 1+ 2-T lymphocytes. *J Immunol* 1981;127:1420–1423.
18. Petry KG, Boullerne AI, Pousset F, et al. Experimental allergic encephalomyelitis animal models for analyzing features of multiple sclerosis. *Pathol Biol (Paris)* 2000;48:47–53.
19. Goverman J, Woods A, Larson L, et al. Transgenic mice that express a myelin basic protein-specific T cell receptor develop spontaneous autoimmunity. *Cell* 1993;72:551–560.
20. Mor F, Kantorowitz M, Cohen IR. The dominant and the cryptic T cell repertoire to myelin basic protein in the Lewis rat. *J Neurosci Res* 1996;45:670–679.
21. Furtado GC, Olivares-Villagomez D, Curotto de Lafaille MA, et al. Regulatory T cells in spontaneous autoimmune encephalomyelitis. *Immunol Rev* 2001;182:122–134.
22. Hori S, Haury M, Coutinho A, et al. Specificity requirements for selection and effector functions of CD25+ 4+ regulatory T cells in anti-myelin basic protein T cell receptor transgenic mice. *Proc Natl Acad Sci USA* 2002;99:8213–8218.
23. Kohm AP, Carpentier PA, Anger HA, et al. Cutting edge: CD4+ CD25+ regulatory T cells suppress antigen-specific autoreactive immune responses and central nervous system inflammation during active experimental autoimmune encephalomyelitis. *J Immunol* 2002;169:4712–4716.
24. Zhang X, Koldzic DN, Izikson L, et al. IL-10 is involved in the suppression of experimental autoimmune encephalomyelitis by CD25+ CD4+ regulatory T cells. *Int Immunol* 2004;16:249–256.
25. Viglietta V, Baecher-Allan C, Weiner HL, et al. Loss of functional suppression by CD4+ CD25+ regulatory T cells in patients with multiple sclerosis. *J Exp Med* 2004;199:971–979.
26. Kubes P, Ward PA. Leukocyte recruitment and the acute inflammatory response. *Brain Pathol* 2000;10:127–135.
27. Zhang L, Looney D, Taub D, et al. Cocaine opens the blood-brain barrier to HIV-1 invasion. *J Neurovirol* 1998;4:619–626.
28. Compston A, Coles A. Multiple sclerosis. *Lancet* 2002;359:1221–1231.
29. Abromson-Leeman S, Bronson R, Luo Y, et al. T-cell properties determine disease site, clinical presentation, and cellular pathology of experimental autoimmune encephalomyelitis. *Am J Pathol* 2004;165:1519–1533.
30. Zang YC, Li S, Rivera VM, et al. Increased CD8+ cytotoxic T cell responses to myelin basic protein in multiple sclerosis. *J Immunol* 2004;172:5120–5127.
31. Kohm AP, Williams JS, Miller SD. Cutting edge: ligation of the glucocorticoid-induced TNF receptor enhances autoreactive CD4+ T cell activation and experimental autoimmune encephalomyelitis. *J Immunol* 2004;172:4686–4690.
32. Walsh MJ, Tourtellotte WW. Temporal invariance and clonal uniformity of brain and cerebrospinal IgG, IgA, and IgM in multiple sclerosis. *J Exp Med* 1986;163:41–53.
33. McLean BN, Luxton RW, Thompson EJ. A study of immunoglobulin G in the cerebrospinal fluid of 1007 patients with suspected

neurologicalneurologic disease using isoelectric focusing and the Log IgG-Index. A comparison and diagnostic applications. *Brain* 1990;113 (Pt 5):1269–1289.

34. Gerritse K, Laman JD, Noelle RJ, et al. CD40-CD40 ligand interactions in experimental allergic encephalomyelitis and multiple sclerosis. *Proc Natl Acad Sci USA* 1996;93:2499–2504.
35. Girvin AM, Dal Canto MC, Miller SD. CD40/CD40L interaction is essential for the induction of EAE in the absence of CD28-mediated co-stimulation. *J Autoimmun* 2002;18:83–94.
36. t Hart BA, Laman JD, Bauer J, et al. Modelling of multiple sclerosis: lessons learned in a non-human primate. *Lancet Neurol* 2004;3:588–597.
37. Rodriguez M, Oleszak E, Leibowitz J. Theiler's murine encephalomyelitis: a model of demyelination and persistence of virus. *Crit Rev Immunol* 1987;7:325–365.
38. Oleszak EL, Katsetos CD, Kuzmak J, et al. Inducible nitric oxide synthase in Theiler's murine encephalomyelitis virus infection. *J Virol* 1997;71:3228–3235.
39. McGavern DB, Murray PD, Rivera-Quinones C, et al. Axonal loss results in spinal cord atrophy, electrophysiological abnormalities and neurological deficits following demyelination in a chronic inflammatory model of multiple sclerosis. *Brain* 2000;123(Pt 3):519–531.
40. Tsunoda I, Fujinami RS. Inside-out versus outside-in models for virus induced demyelination: axonal damage triggering demyelination. *Springer Semin Immunopathol* 2002;24:105–125.
41. Dal Canto MC, Lipton HL. Multiple sclerosis. Animal model: Theiler's virus infection in mice. *Am J Pathol* 1977;88:497–500.
42. Oleszak EL, Kuzmak J, Good RA, et al. Immunology of Theiler's murine encephalomyelitis virus infection. *Immunol Res* 1995;14:13–33.
43. Lipton HL. Theiler's virus infection in mice: an unusual biphasic disease process leading to demyelination. *Infect Immun* 1975;11:1147–1155.
44. Oleszak EL, Hoffman BE, Chang JR, et al. Apoptosis of infiltrating T cells in the central nervous system of mice infected with Theiler's murine encephalomyelitis virus. *Virology* 2003;315:110–123.
45. Brahic M, Stroop WG, Baringer JR. Theiler's virus persists in glial cells during demyelinating disease. *Cell* 1981;26:123–128.
46. Lindsley MD, Rodriguez M. Characterization of the inflammatory response in the central nervous system of mice susceptible or resistant to demyelination by Theiler's virus. *J Immunol* 1989;142:2677–2682.
47. Chang JR, Zaczynska E, Katsetos CD, et al. Differential expression of TGF-beta, IL-2, and other cytokines in the CNS of Theiler's murine encephalomyelitis virus-infected susceptible and resistant strains of mice. *Virology* 2000;278:346–360.
48. Chang A, Nishiyama A, Peterson J, et al. NG2-positive oligodendrocyte progenitor cells in adult human brain and multiple sclerosis lesions. *J Neurosci* 2000;20:6404–6412.
49. Oleszak EL, et al. iNOS in TMVE infection. In: C.C. Lavi E Constantinesau CS, ed. *Experimental models of multiple sclerosis*. Norwell, MA: Kluwer, 2005: (In Press).
50. Oleszak EL, Zaczynska E, Bhattacharjee M, et al. Inducible nitric oxide synthase and nitrotyrosine are found in monocytes/macrophages and/or astrocytes in acute, but not in chronic, multiple sclerosis. *Clin Diagn Lab Immunol* 1998;5:438–445.
51. Rose JW, Hill KE, Wada Y, et al. Nitric oxide synthase inhibitor, aminoguanidine, reduces inflammation and demyelination produced by Theiler's virus infection. *J Neuroimmunol* 1998;81:82–89.
52. Oken BS, Kishiyama S, Zajdel D, et al. Randomized controlled trial of yoga and exercise in multiple sclerosis. *Neurology* 2004;62:2058–2064.
53. Rust R, Menkes JH. Autoimmune and postinfectious diseases. In: Menkes JH, Sarnat HB, eds. *Child neurology*. Philadelphia: Lippincott Williams & Wilkins, 2000: 627–691.
54. Lassmann H. Classification of demyelinating diseases at the interface between etiology and pathogenesis. *Curr Opin Neurol* 2001;14:253–258.
55. Kornek B, Lassmann H. Axonal pathology in multiple sclerosis. A historical note. *Brain Pathol* 1999;9:651–656.
56. Peterson JW, Bo L, Mork S, et al. Transected neurites, apoptotic neurons, and reduced inflammation in cortical multiple sclerosis lesions. *Ann Neurol* 2001;50:389–400.
57. Trapp BD, Peterson J, Ransohoff RM, et al. Axonal transection in the lesions of multiple sclerosis. *N Engl J Med* 1998;338:278–285.
58. Trapp BD, Bo L, Mork S, Chang A. Pathogenesis of tissue injury in MS lesions. *J Neuroimmunol* 1999;98:49–56.
59. Adams RD, Richardson EPJ. The demyelinative diseases of the human nervous system: a classification; a review of salient neuropathologic findings; comments on recent biochemical studies. In: J. Folchi-Pi , ed. *Chemical pathology of the nervous system*. New York: Pergamon Press, 1961:162–196.
60. DeJong RN. Multiple sclerosis: history, definition and general considerations. In: Vinken PJ, Bruyn GW, eds. *Handbook of clinical neurology*. Amsterdam: North-Holland, 1970;9:45–62.
61. Poser C. Diseases of the myelin sheath. In: J. Minckler, ed. *Pathology of the nervous system*. New York: McGraw-Hill, 1968:767–778.
62. Poser CM. Leukodystrophy and the concept of dysmyelination. *Arch Neurol* 1961;4:323–332.
63. Matthews WB. *McAlpine's Multiple sclerosis*. Edinburgh: Churchill Livingstone, 1991.
64. Rust RS. Multiple sclerosis, acute disseminated encephalomyelitis, and related conditions. *Semin Pediatr Neurol* 2000;7:66–90.
64a. Wechsler IS. Statistics of multiple sclerosis including a study of the infantile, congenital, familial hereditary froms and the mental and psychic symptoms. *Arch Neurol Psychiatry* 1922;8:59–75.
65. Gall JC Jr, Hayles AB, Siekert RG, et al. Multiple sclerosis in children; a clinical study of 40 cases with onset in childhood. *Pediatrics* 1958;21:703–709.
66. Kabat EA, Glusman M, Knaub V. Quantitative estimation of the albumin and gamma globulin in normal and pathologic cerebrospinal fluid of one hundred cases of multiple sclerosis and other diseases. *Am J Med Sci* 1948;219:55–64.
67. Schumacker GA, Beebe G, Kibler RF, et al. Problems of experimental trials of therapy in multiple sclerosis: report by the Panel on the Evaluation of Experimental Trials of Therapy in Multiple Sclerosis. *Ann N Y Acad Sci* 1965;122:552–568.
68. Boutin B, Esquivel E, Mayer M, et al. Multiple sclerosis in children: report of clinical and paraclinical features of 19 cases. *Neuropediatrics* 1988;19:118–123.
69. Bye AM, Kendall B, Wilson J. Multiple sclerosis in childhood: a new look. *Dev Med Child Neurol* 1985;27:215–222.
70. Cole GF, Stuart CA. A long perspective on childhood multiple sclerosis. *Dev Med Child Neurol* 1995;37:661–666.
71. Duquette P, Murray TJ, Pleines J, et al. Multiple sclerosis in childhood: clinical profile in 125 patients. *J Pediatr* 1987;111:359–363.
72. Hanefeld FA. Characteristics of childhood multiple sclerosis. *Int MS J* 1995;1:91–97.
73. Mattyus A, Veres E. Multiple sclerosis in childhood: long term katamnestic investigations. *Acta Paediatr Hung* 1985;26:193–204.
74. Hanefeld F, Bauer HJ, Christen HJ, et al. Multiple sclerosis in childhood: report of 15 cases. *Brain Dev* 1991;13:410–416.
75. Hanefeld FA, Christen HJ, Kruse B, Bauer HJ. Childhood and juvenile multiple sclerosis. In: Bauer HJ, Hanefeld FA, eds. *Multiple sclerosis. Its impact from childhood to old age*. Philadelphia: Saunders, 1993:14–52.
76. Shaw CM, Alvord EC Jr. Multiple sclerosis beginning in infancy. *J Child Neurol* 1987;2:252–256.
77. Banwell BL. Pediatric multiple sclerosis. *Curr Neurol Neurosci Rep* 2004;4:245–252.
78. Ghezzi A, Deplano V, Faroni J, et al. Multiple sclerosis in childhood: clinical features of 149 cases. *Mult Scler* 1997;3:43–46.
79. Lowis GW. The social epidemiology of multiple sclerosis. *Sci Total Environ* 1990;90:163–190.
80. Ruggieri M, Polizzi A, Pavone L, Grimaldi LM. Multiple sclerosis in children under 6 years of age. *Neurology* 1999;53:478–484.
81. Sindern E, Haas J, Stark E, et al. Early onset MS under the age of 16: clinical and paraclinical features. *Acta Neurol Scand* 1992;86:280–284.
82. Tenembaum S, Chamoles N, Segura M. Clinical and neuroimaging features of 18 patients with childhood and juvenile multiple sclerosis. *Mult Scler* 1998;4:316. (Abstract)
83. Tenembaum S, Segura M, Miranda M. Clinical and paraclinical

differences between childhood and juvenile multiple sclerosis. *Neurology* 1999;52(Suppl 2):500. (Abstract)
84. Compston A, Ebers GC, Lassmann H, et al. *McAlpine's Multiple sclerosis*. London: Churchill Livingstone, 1998.
85. Gadoth N. Multiple sclerosis in children. *Brain Dev* 2003;25:229–232.
86. Zelnik N, Gale AD, Shelburne SA Jr. Multiple sclerosis in black children. *J Child Neurol* 1991;6:53–57.
87. Hawker K, Frohman E. Multiple sclerosis. *Prim Care* 2004;31: 201–226.
88. Sotgiu S, Pugliatti M, Fois ML, et al. Genes, environment, and susceptibility to multiple sclerosis. *Neurobiol Dis* 2004;17:131–143.
89. Levin MC, Lee SM, Kalume F, et al. Autoimmunity due to molecular mimicry as a cause of neurological disease. *Nat Med* 2002;8:509–513.
90. Hafler DA. Multiple sclerosis. *J Clin Invest* 2004;113:788–794.
91. Pashenkov M, Teleshova N, Link H. Inflammation in the central nervous system: the role for dendritic cells. *Brain Pathol* 2003;13:23–33.
92. Kouwenhoven M, Ozenci V, Tjernlund A, et al. Monocyte-derived dendritic cells express and secrete matrix-degrading metalloproteinases and their inhibitors and are imbalanced in multiple sclerosis. *J Neuroimmunol* 2002;126:161–171.
93. Teleshova N, Pashenkov M, Huang YM, et al. Multiple sclerosis and optic neuritis: CCR5 and CXCR3 expressing T cells are augmented in blood and cerebrospinal fluid. *J Neurol* 2002;249:723–729.
94. Link H. The cytokine storm in multiple sclerosis. *Mult Scler* 1998;4:12–15.
95. Lassmann H. Neuropathology in multiple sclerosis: new concepts. *Mult Scler* 1998;4:93–98.
96. Neumann H. Molecular mechanisms of axonal damage in inflammatory central nervous system diseases. *Curr Opin Neurol* 2003;16:267–273.
97. Compston A. The pathogenesis and basis for treatment in multiple sclerosis. *Clin Neurol Neurosurg* 2004;106:246–248.
98. Dietrich JB. The adhesion molecule ICAM-1 and its regulation in relation with the blood-brain barrier. *J Neuroimmunol* 2002;128:58–68.
99. Diamond MS, Staunton DE, Marlin SD, et al. Binding of the integrin Mac-1 (CD11b/CD18) to the third immunoglobulin-like domain of ICAM-1 (CD54) and its regulation by glycosylation. *Cell* 1991;65:961–971.
100. Marlin SD, Springer TA. Purified intercellular adhesion molecule-1 (ICAM-1) is a ligand for lymphocyte function-associated antigen 1 (LFA-1). *Cell* 1987;51:813–819.
101. Peterson JW, Bo L, Mork S, et al. VCAM-1-positive microglia target oligodendrocytes at the border of multiple sclerosis lesions. *J Neuropathol Exp Neurol* 2002;61:539–546.
102. Tedder TF, Steeber DA, Chen A, et al. The selectins: vascular adhesion molecules. *FASEB J* 1995;9:866–873.
103. Dyment DA, Ebers GC, Sadovnick AD. Genetics of multiple sclerosis. *Lancet Neurol* 2004;3:104–110.
104. Ebers GC. Genetics and multiple sclerosis: an overview. *Ann Neurol* 1994;36:S12–S14.
105. Barcellos LF, Oksenberg JR, Green AJ, et al. Genetic basis for clinical expression in multiple sclerosis. *Brain* 2002;125:150–158.
106. Masterman T, Ligers A, Olsson T, et al. HLA-DR15 is associated with lower age at onset in multiple sclerosis. *Ann Neurol* 2000;48:211–219.
107. GAMES and the Transatlantic Multiple Sclerosis Genetics Cooperative. A meta-analysis of whole genome linkage screens in multiple sclerosis. *J Neuroimmunol* 2003;143:39–46.
108. Enzinger C, Ropele S, Smith S, et al. Accelerated evolution of brain atrophy and "black holes" in MS patients with APOE-epsilon 4. *Ann Neurol* 2004;55:563–569.
109. Evangelou N, Jackson M, Beeson D, et al. Association of the APOE epsilon4 allele with disease activity in multiple sclerosis. *J Neurol Neurosurg Psychiatry* 1999;67:203–205.
110. Lassmann H. Pathology of multiple sclerosis. In: Compston A, Ebers GC, Lassmann H, eds. *McAlpine's Multiple sclerosis*. London: Churchill Livingstone, 1998: 323–358.
111. Hickey WF. The pathology of multiple sclerosis: a historical perspective. *J Neuroimmunol* 1999;98:37–44.
112. Archelos JJ, Storch MK, Hartung HP. The role of B cells and autoantibodies in multiple sclerosis. *Ann Neurol* 2000;47:694–706.
113. Lucchinetti C, Bruck W, Parisi J, et al. Heterogeneity of multiple sclerosis lesions: implications for the pathogenesis of demyelination. *Ann Neurol* 2000;47:707–717.
114. Lucchinetti C, Bruck W, Noseworthy J. Multiple sclerosis: recent developments in neuropathology, pathogenesis, magnetic resonance imaging studies and treatment. *Curr Opin Neurol* 2001;14:259–269.
115. Neumann H, Medana IM, Bauer J, et al. Cytotoxic T lymphocytes in autoimmune and degenerative CNS diseases. *Trends Neurosci* 2002;25:313–319.
116. Lucchinetti CF, Bruck W, Rodriguez M, et al. Distinct patterns of multiple sclerosis pathology indicates heterogeneity on pathogenesis. *Brain Pathol* 1996;6:259–274.
117. Paz Soldan MM, Rodriguez M. Heterogeneity of pathogenesis in multiple sclerosis: implications for promotion of remyelination. *J Infect Dis* 2002;186(Suppl 2):S248–S253.
118. van der Knaap MS, Vallk J. Multiple sclerosis. In: van der Knaap MS, Valk J, eds. *Magnetic resonance of myelin, myelination and myelin disorders*. Berlin: Springer-Verlag, 1995:297–313.
119. Prineas JW, McDonald WI. Demyelinating diseases. In: Graham DI, Lantos PL, eds. *Greenfield's Neuropathology*. London: Arnold, 1997:813–896.
120. Raine CS. The neuropathology of multiple sclerosis. In: Raine CS, McFarland HF, Tourtellotte WW, eds. *Multiple sclerosis clinical and pathogenetic basis*. London: Chapman and Hall, 1997:149–172.
121. Raine CS. Demyelinating diseases. In: Davis RL, Robertson DM, eds. *Textbook of neuropathology*, 3rd ed. Baltimore: Williams & Wilkins, 1997:627–714.
122. Kepes JJ. Large focal tumor-like demyelinating lesions of the brain: intermediate entity between multiple sclerosis and acute disseminated encephalomyelitis? A study of 31 patients. *Ann Neurol* 1993;33:18–27.
123. Ozawa K, Suchanek G, Breitschopf H, et al. Patterns of oligodendroglia pathology in multiple sclerosis. *Brain* 1994;117 (Pt 6):1311–1322.
124. Prineas JW, Barnard RO, Kwon EE, et al. Multiple sclerosis: remyelination of nascent lesions. *Ann Neurol* 1993;33:137–151.
125. Prineas JW, Barnard RO, Revesz T, et al. Multiple sclerosis. Pathology of recurrent lesions. *Brain* 1993;116 (Pt 3):681–693.
126. Bjartmar C, Kidd G, Mork S, et al. Neurological disability correlates with spinal cord axonal loss and reduced *N*-acetyl aspartate in chronic multiple sclerosis patients. *Ann Neurol* 2000;48:893–901.
127. Kwon EE, Prineas JW. Blood-brain barrier abnormalities in longstanding multiple sclerosis lesions. An immunohistochemical study. *J Neuropathol Exp Neurol* 1994;53:625–636.
128. Raine CS. Multiple sclerosing and chronic relapsing EAE: comparative ultrastructural neuropathology. In: Hallpike JF, Adams CWM, Tourtellotte WW, eds. *Multiple sclerosis, pathology, diagnosis and management*. Baltimore: Williams & Wilkins, 1983:413–460.
129. Genain CP, Cannella B, Hauser SL, et al. Identification of autoantibodies associated with myelin damage in multiple sclerosis. *Nat Med* 1999;5:170–175.
130. Lassmann H. Hypoxia-like tissue injury as a component of multiple sclerosis lesions. *J Neurol Sci* 2003;206:187–191.
131. Itoyama Y, Sternberger NH, Webster HD, et al. Immunocytochemical observations on the distribution of myelin-associated glycoprotein and myelin basic protein in multiple sclerosis lesions. *Ann Neurol* 1980;7:167–177.
132. Ludwin SK, Johnson ES. Evidence for a "dying-back" gliopathy in demyelinating disease. *Ann Neurol* 1981;9:301–305.
133. Ferguson B, Matyszak MK, Esiri MM, et al. Axonal damage in acute multiple sclerosis lesions. *Brain* 1997;120 (Pt 3):393–399.
134. Grigoriadis N, Ben-Hur T, Karussis D, et al. Axonal damage in multiple sclerosis: a complex issue in a complex disease. *Clin Neurol Neurosurg* 2004;106:211–217.

135. Lovas G, Szilagyi N, Majtenyi K, et al. Axonal changes in chronic demyelinated cervical spinal cord plaques. *Brain* 2000;123 (Pt 2): 308–317.
136. Allen I, Brankin B. Pathogenesis of multiple sclerosis—the immune diathesis and the role of viruses. *J Neuropathol Exp Neurol* 1993;52:95–105.
137. Guseo A, Jellinger K. The significance of perivascular infiltrations in multiple sclerosis. *J Neurol* 1975;211:51–60.
138. Lumsden CE. The neuropathology of multiple sclerosis. In: Vinken PJ, Bruyn GW, eds. *Handbook of clinical neurology*. Amsterdam: North-Holland, 1970:217–319.
139. Katsetos CD, Fincke JE, Legido A, et al. Angiocentric CD3(+) T-cell infiltrates in human immunodeficiency virus type 1-associated central nervous system disease in children. *Clin Diagn Lab Immunol* 1999;6:105–114.
140. Putnam TJ. The pathogenesis of multiple sclerosis: a possible vascular factor. *N Engl J Med* 1933;209:786–790.
141. Courville CB. Acute lesions of multiple sclerosis—possible significance of vascular changes. *J Neuropathol Exp Neurol* 1968;27:159.
142. Lucchinetti CF, Mandler RN, McGavern D, et al. A role for humoral mechanisms in the pathogenesis of Devic's neuromyelitis optica. *Brain* 2002;125:1450–1461.
143. Wakefield AJ, More LJ, Difford J, et al. Immunohistochemical study of vascular injury in acute multiple sclerosis. *J Clin Pathol* 1994;47:129–133.
144. Bo L, Dawson TM, Wesselingh S, et al. Induction of nitric oxide synthase in demyelinating regions of multiple sclerosis brains. *Ann Neurol* 1994;36:778–786.
145. De Groot CJ, Ruuls SR, Theeuwes JW, et al. Immunocytochemical characterization of the expression of inducible and constitutive isoforms of nitric oxide synthase in demyelinating multiple sclerosis lesions. *J Neuropathol Exp Neurol* 1997;56:10–20.
146. Liu JS, Zhao ML, Brosnan CF, Lee SC. Expression of inducible nitric oxide synthase and nitrotyrosine in multiple sclerosis lesions. *Am J Pathol* 2001;158:2057–2066.
147. Bauer HJ, Hanefeld FA. Multiple Sklerose im Kindesalter. In: Hanefeld FA, Rating D, Christen HJ, eds. *Aktuelle Neuropädiatrie*. Berlin: Springer-Verlag, 1989:285–298.
148. Poser CM, Paty DW, Scheinberg L, et al. New diagnostic criteria for multiple sclerosis: guidelines for research protocols. *Ann Neurol* 1983;13:227–231.
149. Bauer HJ. Multiple sclerosis in Europe. *J Neurol* 1987;234:195–206.
150. Weinshenker BG, Bass B, Rice GP, et al. The natural history of multiple sclerosis: a geographically based study. I. Clinical course and disability. *Brain* 1989;112 (Pt 1):133–146.
151. Duquette P, Girard M. Hormonal factors in susceptibility to multiple sclerosis. *Curr Opin Neurol Neurosurg* 1993;6:195–201.
152. Kurtzke JF, Beebe GW, Norman JE, Jr. Epidemiology of multiple sclerosis in U.S. veterans: 1. Race, sex, and geographic distribution. *Neurology* 1979;29:1228–1235.
153. Kurtzke JF, Page WF, Murphy FM, Norman JE, Jr. Epidemiology of multiple sclerosis in US veterans. 4. Age at onset. *Neuroepidemiology* 1992;11:226–235.
154. Rizzo MA, Hadjimichael OC, Preiningerova J, et al. Prevalence and treatment of spasticity reported by multiple sclerosis patients. *Mult Scler* 2004;10:589–595.
155. Banwell BL, Anderson PE. Neuropsychological features of pediatric multiple sclerosis. *Neurology* 2002;58:A173.
156. Kalita J, Misra UK. Is methyl prednisolone useful in acute transverse myelitis? *Spinal Cord* 2001;39:471–476.
157. Feinstein A. The neuropsychiatry of multiple sclerosis. *Can J Psychiatry* 2004;49:157–163.
158. Nyquist PA, Cascino GD, Rodriguez M. Seizures in patients with multiple sclerosis seen at Mayo Clinic, Rochester, Minn, 1990–1998. *Mayo Clin Proc* 2001;76:983–986.
159. Poser CM, Brinar VV. Epilepsy and multiple sclerosis. *Epilepsy Behav* 2003;4:6–12.
160. Striano P, Orefice G, Brescia Morra V, et al. Epileptic seizures in multiple sclerosis: clinical and EEG correlations. *Neurol Sci* 2003;24:322–328.
161. McDonald WI, Compston A, Edan G, et al. Recommended diagnostic criteria for multiple sclerosis: guidelines from the International Panel on the Diagnosis of Multiple Sclerosis. *Ann Neurol* 2001;50:121–127.
162. Gran B, Hemmer B, Vergelli M, et al. Molecular mimicry and multiple sclerosis: degenerate T-cell recognition and the induction of autoimmunity. *Ann Neurol* 1999;45:559–567.
163. Weiner HL, Hafler DA, Fallis RJ, et al. T cell subsets in patients with multiple sclerosis. An overview. *Ann N Y Acad Sci* 1984;436:281–293.
164. Gomes AC, Morris M, Stawiarz L, et al. Decreased levels of CD95 and caspase-8 mRNA in multiple sclerosis patients with gadolinium-enhancing lesions on MRI. *Neurosci Lett* 2003;352:101–104.
165. Hauser SL, Bresnan MJ, Reinherz EL, et al. Childhood multiple sclerosis: clinical features and demonstration of changes in T cell subsets with disease activity. *Ann Neurol* 1982;11:463–468.
166. Johnson KP, Nelson BJ. Multiple sclerosis: diagnostic usefulness of cerebrospinal fluid. *Ann Neurol* 1977;2:425–431.
167. Mehta PD. Diagnostic usefulness of cerebrospinal fluid in multiple sclerosis. *Crit Rev Clin Lab Sci* 1991;28:233–251.
168. Olsson T. Immunology of multiple sclerosis. *Curr Opin Neurol Neurosurg* 1992;5:195–202.
169. Rudick RA, Medendorp SV, Namey M, et al. Multiple sclerosis progression in a natural history study: predictive value of cerebrospinal fluid free kappa light chains. *Mult Scler* 1995;1:150–155.
170. Link H. Contribution of CSF studies to diagnosis of multiple sclerosis. *Ital J Neurol Sci* 1987;6:57–69.
171. Taylor-Robinson SD. Grand rounds–Hammersmith Hospitals: distinguishing acute disseminated encephalomyelitis from multiple sclerosis. *BMJ* 1996;313:802–804.
172. Verbeek MM, de Reus HP, Weykamp CW. Comparison of methods for the detection of oligoclonal IgG bands in cerebrospinal fluid and serum: results of the Dutch Quality Control survey. *Clin Chem* 2002;48:1578–1580.
173. Berger T, Rubner P, Schautzer F, et al. Antimyelin antibodies as a predictor of clinically definite multiple sclerosis after a first demyelinating event. *N Engl J Med* 2003;349:139–145.
174. Rejdak K, Eikelenboom MJ, Petzold A, et al. CSF nitric oxide metabolites are associated with activity and progression of multiple sclerosis. *Neurology* 2004;63:1439–1445.
175. Sueoka E, Yukitake M, Iwanaga K, et al. Autoantibodies against heterogeneous nuclear ribonucleoprotein B1 in CSF of MS patients. *Ann Neurol* 2004;56:778–786.
176. Gandelman-Marton R, Rabey JM, Flechter S. Periodic lateralized epileptiform discharges in multiple sclerosis: a case report. *J Clin Neurophysiol* 2003;20:117–121.
177. Striano P, Striano S, Carrieri PB, et al. Epilepsia partialis continua as a first symptom of multiple sclerosis: electrophysiological study of one case. *Mult Scler* 2003;9:199–203.
178. Trinka E, Unterberger I, Spiegel M, et al. *De novo* aphasic status epilepticus as presenting symptom of multiple sclerosis. *J Neurol* 2002;249:782–783.
179. Antonijevic IA, Steiger A. Depression-like changes of the sleep-EEG during high dose corticosteroid treatment in patients with multiple sclerosis. *Psychoneuroendocrinology* 2003;28:780–795.
180. Gronseth GS, Ashman EJ. Practice parameter: the usefulness of evoked potentials in identifying clinically silent lesions in patients with suspected multiple sclerosis (an evidence-based review): report of the Quality Standards Subcommittee of the American Academy of Neurology. *Neurology* 2000;54:1720–1725.
181. Anlar O, Kisli M, Tombul T, Ozbek H. Visual evoked potentials in multiple sclerosis before and after two years of interferon therapy. *Int J Neurosci* 2003;113:483–489.
182. Leocani L, Martinelli V, Natali-Sora MG, et al. Somatosensory evoked potentials and sensory involvement in multiple sclerosis: comparison with clinical findings and quantitative sensory tests. *Mult Scler* 2003;9:275–279.
183. Spiegel J, Hansen C, Baumgartner U, et al. Sensitivity of laser-evoked potentials versus somatosensory evoked potentials in patients with multiple sclerosis. *Clin Neurophysiol* 2003;114:992–1002.
184. Rusin JA, Vezina LG, Chadduck WM, et al. Tumoral multiple sclerosis of the cerebellum in a child. *AJNR Am J Neuroradiol* 1995;16:1164–1166.

185. Brunot E, Marcus JC. Multiple sclerosis presenting as a single mass lesion. *Pediatr Neurol* 1999;20:383–386.
186. Masdeu JC, Moreira J, Trasi S, et al. The open ring. A new imaging sign in demyelinating disease. *J Neuroimaging* 1996;6:104–107.
187. Kesselring J, Miller DH, Robb SA, et al. Acute disseminated encephalomyelitis. MRI findings and the distinction from multiple sclerosis. *Brain* 1990;113(Pt 2):291–302.
188. Tenembaum S, Chamoles N, Fejerman N. Acute disseminated encephalomyelitis: a long-term follow-up study of 84 pediatric patients. *Neurology* 2002;59:1224–1231.
189. Dale RC, de Sousa C, Chong WK. Acute disseminated encephalomyelitis, multiphasic disseminated encephalomyelitis and multiple sclerosis in children. *Brain* 2000;123:2407–2422.
190. Tenembaum S, Galicchio S, Granana N. Multiphasic disseminated encephalomyelitis and multiple sclerosis in children: diagnostic clues. *J Neurol Sci* 1997;150(Suppl):S230. (Abstract)
191. Ebner F, Millner MM, Justich E. Multiple sclerosis in children: value of serial MR studies to monitor patients. *AJNR Am J Neuroradiol* 1990;11:1023–1027.
192. Miller DH, Filippi M, Fazekas F, et al. Role of magnetic resonance imaging within diagnostic criteria for multiple sclerosis. *Ann Neurol* 2004;56:273–278.
193. Hahn CD, Shroff MM, Blaser SI, et al. MRI criteria for multiple sclerosis: Evaluation in a pediatric cohort. *Neurology* 2004;62:806–808.
194. Matthews PM. An update on neuroimaging of multiple sclerosis. *Curr Opin Neurol* 2004;17:453–458.
195. Minagar A, Toledo EG, Alexander JS, Kelley RE. Pathogenesis of brain and spinal cord atrophy in multiple sclerosis. *J Neuroimaging* 2004;14:5S–10S.
196. Filippi M, Rocca MA, Comi G. The use of quantitative magnetic-resonance–based techniques to monitor the evolution of multiple sclerosis. *Lancet Neurol* 2003;2:337–346.
197. Bruhn H, Frahm J, Merboldt KD, et al. Multiple sclerosis in children: cerebral metabolic alterations monitored by localized proton magnetic resonance spectroscopy *in vivo*. *Ann Neurol* 1992;32:140–150.
198. Filippi M, Rocca MA. Disturbed function and plasticity in multiple sclerosis as gleaned from functional magnetic resonance imaging. *Curr Opin Neurol* 2003;16:275–282.
199. Rocca MA, Mezzapesa DM, Falini A, et al. Evidence for axonal pathology and adaptive cortical reorganization in patients at presentation with clinically isolated syndromes suggestive of multiple sclerosis. *Neuroimage* 2003;18:847–855.
200. Pantano P, Iannetti GD, Caramia F, et al. Cortical motor reorganization after a single clinical attack of multiple sclerosis. *Brain* 2002;125:1607–1615.
201. Pantano P, Mainero C, Iannetti GD, et al. Contribution of corticospinal tract damage to cortical motor reorganization after a single clinical attack of multiple sclerosis. *Neuroimage* 2002;17:1837–1843.
202. Parry AM, Scott RB, Palace J, et al. Potentially adaptive functional changes in cognitive processing for patients with multiple sclerosis and their acute modulation by rivastigmine. *Brain* 2003;126:2750–2760.
203. Rausch M, Hiestand P, Baumann D, et al. MRI–based monitoring of inflammation and tissue damage in acute and chronic relapsing EAE. *Magn Reson Med* 2003;50:309–314.
204. Pozzilli C, Passafiume D, Bernardi S, et al. SPECT, MRI and cognitive functions in multiple sclerosis. *J Neurol Neurosurg Psychiatry* 1991;54:110–115.
205. Sabatini U, Pozzilli C, Pantano P, et al. Involvement of the limbic system in multiple sclerosis patients with depressive disorders. *Biol Psychiatry* 1996;39:970–975.
206. Terada H, Kamata N. Contribution of the combination of (201)Tl SPECT and (99m)T(c)O(4)(−) SPECT to the differential diagnosis of brain tumors and tumor-like lesions. A preliminary report. *J Neuroradiol* 2003;30:91–94.
207. Blinkenberg M, Jensen CV, Holm S, et al. A longitudinal study of cerebral glucose metabolism, MRI, and disability in patients with MS. *Neurology* 1999;53:149–153.
208. Blinkenberg M, Rune K, Jensen CV, et al. Cortical cerebral metabolism correlates with MRI lesion load and cognitive dysfunction in MS. *Neurology* 2000;54:558–564.
209. Sun X, Tanaka M, Kondo S, et al. Clinical significance of reduced cerebral metabolism in multiple sclerosis: a combined PET and MRI study. *Ann Nucl Med* 1998;12:89–94.
210. Bakshi R, Miletich RS, Kinkel PR, et al. High-resolution fluorodeoxyglucose positron emission tomography shows both global and regional cerebral hypometabolism in multiple sclerosis. *J Neuroimaging* 1998;8:228–234.
211. Debruyne JC, Versijpt J, Van Laere KJ, et al. PET visualization of microglia in multiple sclerosis patients using [11C]PK11195. *Eur J Neurol* 2003;10:257–264.
212. Iannetti P, Marciani MG, Spalice A, et al. Primary CNS demyelinating diseases in childhood: multiple sclerosis. *Childs Nerv Syst* 1996;12:149–154.
213. Tenembaum S, Segura M, Fejerman N. Disease-modifying therapies in childhood and juvenile multiple sclerosis. *Mult Scler* 2001;7:S57.
214. Airla N, Luomala M, Elovaara I, et al. Suppression of immune system genes by methylprednisolone in exacerbations of multiple sclerosis. Preliminary results. *J Neurol* 2004;251:1215–1219.
215. Sorensen PS. The role of intravenous immunoglobulin in the treatment of multiple sclerosis. *J Neurol Sci* 2003;206:123–130.
216. Achiron A, Kishner I, Sarova-Pinhas I, et al. Intravenous immunoglobulin treatment following the first demyelinating event suggestive of multiple sclerosis: a randomized, double–blind, placebo–controlled trial. *Arch Neurol* 2004;61:1515–1520.
217. Kalanie H, Gharagozli K, Hemmatie A, et al. Interferon beta-1a and intravenous immunoglobulin treatment for multiple sclerosis in Iran. *Eur Neurol* 2004;52:202–206.
218. Hommes OR, Sorensen PS, Fazekas F, et al. Intravenous immunoglobulin in secondary progressive multiple sclerosis: randomised placebo–controlled trial. *Lancet* 2004;364:1149–1156.
219. Fernandez O, Guerrero M, Mayorga C, et al. Combination therapy with interferon beta-1b and azathioprine in secondary progressive multiple sclerosis. A two-year pilot study. *J Neurol* 2002;249:1058–1062.
220. Fernandez O, Fernandez V, De Ramon E. Azathioprine and methotrexate in multiple sclerosis. *J Neurol Sci* 2004;223:29–34.
221. Delmont E, Chanalet S, Bourg V, et al. Treatment of progressive multiple sclerosis with monthly pulsed cyclophosphamide–methylprednisolone: predictive factors of treatment response [in French]. *Rev Neurol (Paris)* 2004;160:659–665.
222. Smith D. Preliminary analysis of a trial of pulse cyclophosphamide in IFN-beta–resistant active MS. *J Neurol Sci* 2004; 223:73–79.
223. Weiner HL. Immunosuppressive treatment in multiple sclerosis. *J Neurol Sci* 2004;15:1–11.
224. Debouverie M, Vandenberghe N, Morrissey SP, et al. Predictive parameters of mitoxantrone effectiveness in the treatment of multiple sclerosis. *Mult Scler* 2004;10:407–412.
225. Khatri BO, McQuillen MP, Harrington GJ, et al. Chronic progressive multiple sclerosis: double–blind controlled study of plasmapheresis in patients taking immunosuppressive drugs. *Neurology* 1985;35:312–319.
226. Meca–Lallana JE, Rodriguez–Hilario H, Martinez–Vidal S, et al. Plasmapheresis: its use in multiple sclerosis and other demyelinating processes of the central nervous system. An observation study [in Spanish]. *Rev Neurol* 2003;37:917–926.
227. Medenica RD, Mukerjee S, Alonso K, et al. Plasmapheresis combined with interferon: an effective therapy for multiple sclerosis. *J Clin Apheresis* 1994;9:222–227.
228. McLeod BC. Plasmapheresis in multiple sclerosis. *J Clin Apheresis* 2003;18:72–74.
229. Confavreux C, Vukusic S. Non-specific immunosuppressants in the treatment of multiple sclerosis. *Clin Neurol Neurosurg* 2004;106:263–269.
230. Kappos L, Weinshenker B, Pozzilli C, et al. Interferon beta-1b in secondary progressive MS: a combined analysis of the two trials. *Neurology* 2004;63:1779–1787.
231. Rudick RA, Lee JC, Simon J, et al. Defining interferon beta response status in multiple sclerosis patients. *Ann Neurol* 2004;56:548–555.

232. Russo P, Paolillo A, Caprino L, et al. Effectiveness of interferon beta treatment in relapsing-remitting multiple sclerosis: an Italian cohort study. *J Eval Clin Pract* 2004;10:511–518.
233. Arnon R, Aharoni R. Mechanism of action of glatiramer acetate in multiple sclerosis and its potential for the development of new applications. *Proc Natl Acad Sci USA* 2004;101(Suppl 2):14593–14598.
234. Adams AB, Tyor WR, Holden KR. Interferon beta-1b and childhood multiple sclerosis. *Pediatr Neurol* 1999;21:481–483.
235. Mikaeloff Y, Moreau T, Debouverie M, et al. Interferon-beta treatment in patients with childhood-onset multiple sclerosis. *J Pediatr* 2001;139:443–446.
236. Schilling S, Haertel C, Sperner J. Follow-up of Interferon beta-1b treatment in a 15-year-old patient with secondary progressive multiple sclerosis. *Neuropediatrics* 2002;33:A1–A36.
237. Tenembaum S. Clinical effects of disease-modifying therapies in early-onset multiple sclerosis. *Neurology* 2004;62:A488.
238. Gonsette RE. Combination therapy for multiple sclerosis. *Int MS J* 2004;11:10–21.
239. Adis International Limited. Natalizumab: AN 100226, anti-4alpha integrin monoclonal antibody. *Drugs R D* 2004;5:102–107.
240. Vollmer TL, Phillips JT, Goodman AD, et al. An open-label safety and drug interaction study of natalizumab (Antegren) in combination with interferon-beta (Avonex) in patients with multiple sclerosis. *Mult Scler* 2004;10:511–520.
241. Gonsette RE. New immunosuppressants with potential implication in multiple sclerosis. *J Neurol Sci* 2004;223:87–93.
242. Neuhaus O, Stuve O, Zamvil SS, et al. Are statins a treatment option for multiple sclerosis? *Lancet Neurol* 2004;3:369–371.
243. Rose JW, Watt HE, White AT, et al. Treatment of multiple sclerosis with an anti–interleukin-2 receptor monoclonal antibody. *Ann Neurol* 2004;56:864–867.
244. Adorini L. Immunotherapeutic approaches in multiple sclerosis. *J Neurol Sci* 2004;223:13–24.
245. Li W, Maeda Y, Yuan RR, et al. Beneficial effect of erythropoietin on experimental allergic encephalomyelitis. *Ann Neurol* 2004;56:767–777.
246. Nygardas PT, Gronberg SA, Heikkila J, et al. Treatment of experimental autoimmune encephalomyelitis with a neurotropic alphavirus vector expressing tissue inhibitor of metalloproteinase-2. *Scand J Immunol* 2004;60:372–381.
247. Marracci GH, McKeon GP, Marquardt WE, et al. Alpha lipoic acid inhibits human T-cell migration: implications for multiple sclerosis. *J Neurosci Res* 2004;78:362–370.
248. Levine SM, Chakrabarty A. The role of iron in the pathogenesis of experimental allergic encephalomyelitis and multiple sclerosis. *Ann N Y Acad Sci* 2004;1012:252–266.
249. Achiron A, Lavie G, Kishner I, et al. T cell vaccination in multiple sclerosis relapsing-remitting nonresponders patients. *Clin Immunol* 2004;113:155–160.
250. Fassas A, Nash R. Stem cell transplantation for autoimmune disorders. Multiple sclerosis. *Best Pract Res Clin Haematol* 2004;17:247–262.
251. Chernajovsky Y, Gould DJ, Podhajcer OL. Gene therapy for autoimmune diseases: quo vadis? *Nat Rev Immunol* 2004;4:800–811.
252. Lobentanz IS, Asenbaum S, Vass K, et al. Factors influencing quality of life in multiple sclerosis patients: disability, depressive mood, fatigue and sleep quality. *Acta Neurol Scand* 2004;110: 6–13.
253. Zifko UA. Management of fatigue in patients with multiple sclerosis. *Drugs* 2004;64:1295–1304.
253a. Benedetti F, Campori E, Colombo C, Smeraldi E. Fluvoxamine treatment of major depression associated with multiple sclerosis. *J Neuropsychiatry Clin Neurosc* 2004;16:364–366.
254. Boyd JR, MacMillan LJ. Multiple sclerosis in childhood: understanding and caring for children with an "adult" disease. *Axone* 2000;22:15–21.
255. Mikaeloff Y, Suissa S, Vallee L, et al. First episode of acute CNS inflammatory demyelination in childhood: prognostic factors for multiple sclerosis and disability. *J Pediatr* 2004;144:246–252.
256. Sevon M, Sumelahti ML, Tienari P. Multiple sclerosis in childhood and its prognosis. *Int MS J* 2001;8:29–33.
257. Kremenchutzky M. The natural history of multiple sclerosis. *Rev Neurol* 2000;30:967–972.
258. Kurtzke JF. Further notes on disability evaluation in multiple sclerosis, with scale modifications. *Neurology* 1965;15:654–661.
259. Kurtzke JF. Rating neurologic impairment in multiple sclerosis: an expanded disability status scale (EDSS). *Neurology* 1983;33:1444–1452.
260. Sheremata W, Brown SB, Curless RR. Childhood multiple sclerosis: a report of 12 cases. *Ann Neurol* 1981;10:304.
261. Poser CM. Diffuse-disseminated sclerosis in the adult. *J Neuropathol Exp Neurol* 1957;16:61–78.
262. Poser CM, Goutieres F, Carpentier MA, Aicardi J. Schilder's myelinoclastic diffuse sclerosis. *Pediatrics* 1986;77:107–112.
263. Schilder P. Zur Kenntnis der sogenannten diffusen sklerose (Über encephalitis periaxialis diffusa). *Z Ges Neurol Psychiatr* 1912;10:1–60.
264. Schilder P. Zur Frage der Encephalitis periaxialis diffusa (sogenannte diffuse sklerose). *Z Ges Neurol Psychiatr* 1913;15:359–376.
265. Schilder P. Die Encephalitis periaxialis diffusa. *Arch Psychiat* 1924;71:327–356.
266. Devries E. *Postvaccinal perivenous encephalitis. A pathological anatomical study on the place of postvaccinal perivenous encephalitis in the group encephalitides*. Amsterdam: Elsevier, 1960.
267. Poser CM, Van Bogaert L. Natural history and evolution of the concept of Schilder's diffuse sclerosis. *Acta Psychiatr Neurol Scand* 1956;31:285–331.
268. Bouman L. *Diffuse sclerosis,* Bristol, UK: John Wright, 1934.
269. Fitzgerald MJ, Coleman LT. Recurrent myelinoclastic diffuse sclerosis: a case report of a child with Schilder's variant of multiple sclerosis. *Pediatr Radiol* 2000;30:861–865.
270. Leuzzi V, Lyon G, Cilio MR, et al. Childhood demyelinating diseases with a prolonged remitting course and their relation to Schilder's disease: report of two cases. *J Neurol Neurosurg Psychiatry* 1999;66:407–408.
271. Mehler MF, Rabinowich L. Inflammatory myelinoclastic diffuse sclerosis. *Ann Neurol* 1988;23:413–415.
272. Pretorius ML, Loock DB, Ravenscroft A, et al. Demyelinating disease of Schilder type in three young South African children: dramatic response to corticosteroids. *J Child Neurol* 1998;13:197–201.
273. Barth PG, Derix MM, de Krom MC, et al. Schilder's diffuse sclerosis: case study with three years' follow-up and neuro-imaging. *Neuropediatrics* 1989;20:230–233.
274. Fernandez-Jaen A, Martinez-Bermejo A, Gutierrez-Molina M, et al. Schilder's diffuse myelinoclastic sclerosis [in Spanish]. *Rev Neurol* 2001;33:16–21.
275. Konkol RJ, Bousounis D, Kuban KC. Schilder's disease: additional aspects and a therapeutic option. *Neuropediatrics* 1987;18:149–152.
276. Kurul S, Cakmakci H, Dirik E, et al. Schilder's disease: case study with serial neuroimaging. *J Child Neurol* 2003;18:58–61.
277. Afifi AK, Follett KA, Greenlee J, et al. Optic neuritis: a novel presentation of Schilder's disease. *J Child Neurol* 2001;16:693–696.
278. Afifi AK, Bell WE, Menezes AH, et al. Myelinoclastic diffuse sclerosis (Schilder's disease): report of a case and review of the literature. *J Child Neurol* 1994;9:398–403.
279. Garell PC, Menezes AH, Baumbach G, et al. Presentation, management and follow-up of Schilder's disease. *Pediatr Neurosurg* 1998;29:86–91.
280. Martin JJ, Guazzi GC. Schilder's diffuse sclerosis. *Dev Neurosci* 1991;13:267–273.
281. Aicardi J. *Diseases of the nervous system in childhood*. London: MacKeith Press, 1992.
282. Obara S, Takeshima H, Awa R, et al. Tumefactive myelinoclastic diffuse sclerosis—case report. *Neurol Med Chir* (Tokyo) 2003;43:563–566.
283. Kotil K, Kalayci M, Koseoglu T, et al. Myelinoclastic diffuse sclerosis (Schilder's disease): report of a case and review of the literature. *Br J Neurosurg* 2002;16:516–519.
284. Nejat F, Eftekhar B. Decompressive aspiration in myelinoclastic diffuse sclerosis or Schilder disease. Case report. *J Neurosurg* 2002;97:1447–1449.

285. Devic E. Myelite aubaigue compliquée de neurite optique. *Bull Med* 1894;8:1033–1034.
285a. Gault F. De la neuromyelite optique aigue. Lyon: Thesis, 1894.
286. Cree BA, Goodin DS, Hauser SL. Neuromyelitis optica. *Semin Neurol* 2002;22:105–122.
287. Fardet L, Genereau T, Mikaeloff Y, et al. Devic's neuromyelitis optica: study of nine cases. *Acta Neurol Scand* 2003;108:193–200.
288. Wingerchuk DM. Neuromyelitis optica: current concepts. *Front Biosci* 2004;9:834–840.
289. de Seze J, Stojkovic T, Ferriby D, et al. Devic's neuromyelitis optica: clinical, laboratory, MRI and outcome profile. *J Neurol Sci* 2002;197:57–61.
290. Ghezzi A, Bergamaschi R, Martinelli V, et al. Clinical characteristics, course and prognosis of relapsing Devic's neuromyelitis optica. *J Neurol* 2004;251:47–52.
291. Milani N, Zibordi F, Erbetta A, et al. Neuromyelitis optica in a child with atypical onset and severe outcome. *Neuropediatrics* 2004;35:198–201.
292. Wingerchuk DM, Hogancamp WF, O'Brien PC, et al. The clinical course of neuromyelitis optica (Devic's syndrome). *Neurology* 1999;53:1107–1114.
293. Bergamaschi R. Importance of cerebrospinal fluid examination in differential diagnosis of Devic's neuromyelitis optica by multiple sclerosis. *Neurol Sci* 2003;24:95–96.
294. Stansbury F. Neuromyelitis optica (Devic's disease): presentation of five cases with pathology study and review of the literature. *Arch Ophthalmol* 1949;43:292–235.
295. Lefkowitz D, Angelo JN. Neuromyelitis optica with unusual vascular changes. *Arch Neurol* 1984;41:1103–1105.
296. Baudoin D, Gambarelli D, Gayraud D, et al. Devic's neuromyelitis optica: a clinicopathological review of the literature in connection with a case showing fatal dysautonomia. *Clin Neuropathol* 1998;17:175–183.
297. Wingerchuk DM, Weinshenker BG. Neuromyelitis optica: clinical predictors of a relapsing course and survival. *Neurology* 2003;60:848–853.
298. Kalita J, Misra UK, Mandal SK. Prognostic predictors of acute transverse myelitis. *Acta Neurol Scand* 1998;98:60–63.
299. Lennon VA, Wingerchuk DM, Kryzer TJ, et al. A serum autoantibody marker of neuromyelitis optica: distinction from multiple sclerosis. *Lancet* 2004;364:2106–2112.
300. Nakashima I, Fujihara K, Fujimori J, et al. Absence of IgG1 response in the cerebrospinal fluid of relapsing neuromyelitis optica. *Neurology* 2004;62:144–146.
301. Keegan M, Pineda AA, McClelland RL, et al. Plasma exchange for severe attacks of CNS demyelination: predictors of response. *Neurology* 2002;58:143–146.
302. Mandler RN, Ahmed W, Dencoff JE. Devic's neuromyelitis optica: a prospective study of seven patients treated with prednisone and azathioprine. *Neurology* 1998;51:1219–1220.
303. Balo JA. Encephalitis periaxialis concentrica. *Arch Neurol* 1928;19:242–264.
304. Karaarslan E, Altintas A, Senol U, et al. Balo's concentric sclerosis: clinical and radiologic features of five cases. *AJNR Am J Neuroradiol* 2001;22:1362–1367.
305. Moore GR, Neumann PE, Suzuki K, et al. Balo's concentric sclerosis: new observations on lesion development. *Ann Neurol* 1985;17:604–611.
306. Gharagozloo AM, Poe LB, Collins GH. Antemortem diagnosis of Balo concentric sclerosis: correlative MR imaging and pathologic features. *Radiology* 1994;191:817–819.
307. Murakami Y, Matsuishi T, Shimizu T, et al. Balo's concentric sclerosis in a 4-year-old Japanese infant. *Brain Dev* 1998;20:250–252.
308. Chen CJ, Chu NS, Lu CS, et al. Serial magnetic resonance imaging in patients with Balo's concentric sclerosis: natural history of lesion development. *Ann Neurol* 1999;46:651–656.
309. Bolay H, Karabudak R, Tacal T, et al. Balo's concentric sclerosis. Report of two patients with magnetic resonance imaging follow-up. *J Neuroimaging* 1996;6:98–103.
310. Yao DL, Webster HD, Hudson LD, et al. Concentric sclerosis (Balo): morphometric and *in situ* hybridization study of lesions in six patients. *Ann Neurol* 1994;35:18–30.
311. Dale RC. Acute disseminated encephalomyelitis. *Semin Pediatr Infect Dis* 2003;14:90–95.
312. Garg RK. Acute disseminated encephalomyelitis. *Postgrad Med J* 2003;79:11–17.
313. Jones CT. Childhood autoimmune neurologic diseases of the central nervous system. *Neurol Clin* 2003;21:745–764.
314. Murthy SN, Faden HS, Cohen ME, Bakshi R. Acute disseminated encephalomyelitis in children. *Pediatrics* 2002;110:e21.
315. Leake JA, Albani S, Kao AS, et al. Acute disseminated encephalomyelitis in childhood: epidemiologic, clinical and laboratory features. *Pediatr Infect Dis J* 2004;23:756–764.
316. Behan P, Currie S. Acute disseminated encephalomyelitis. In: *Clinical neuroimmunology*. London: Saunders, 1978: 49–61.
317. Vinken PJ, Bruyn GW, Klawans HL. Demyelinating diseases. In: Vinken PJ, Bruyn GW, eds. *Handbook of clinical neurology*. New York: Elsevier, 1985: 474–494.
318. Greenfield JG. Acute disseminated encephalomyelitis and sequela to influenza. *J Pathol Bacteriol* 1930;33:453–462.
319. Van Bogaert L. Post-infectious encephalomyelitis and multiple sclerosis; the significance of perivenous encephalomyelitis. *J Neuropathol Exp Neurol* 1950;9:219–249.
320. Marsden JP, Hurst EW. Acute perivascular myelinoclasis (acute disseminated encephalomyelitis) in small pox. *Brain* 1932;55:181–193.
321. Carpenter S, Lampert PW. Postinfectious perivenous encephalitis and acute hemorrhagic leukoencephalitis. In: Minckler J, ed. *Pathology of the nervous system*. New York: McGraw-Hill, 1968: 2260–2269.
322. Poser CM. Disseminad vasculomyelinopathy. A review of the clinical and pathologic reactions of the nervous system in hyperergic diseases. *Acta Neurol Scand* 1969;(Suppl 37):33–44.
323. Davison C, Brock S. Acute demyelinating encephalomyelitis following respiratory disease. *Bull Neurolog Inst New York* 1937;6:504–514.
324. Ferraro A, Roizin L. Hyperergic encephalomyelitides following exanthematic diseases, infectious diseases and vaccination. *J Neuropathol Exp Neurol* 1957;16:423–445.
325. De Vries. *Postvaccinal perivenous encephalitis*. Amsterdam: Elsevier, 1960.
326. Khurana DS, et al. Acute disseminated encephalomyelitis in children: discordance of MRI and therapeutic role of plasmapheresis. *Pediatrics* 2005:in press.
327. Scott TF. Postinfectious and vaccinal encephalitis. *Med Clin North Am* 1967;51:701–717.
328. Oleszak EL, Lin WL, Legido A, et al. Presence of oligoclonal T cells in cerebrospinal fluid of a child with multiphasic disseminated encephalomyelitis following hepatitis A virus infection. *Clin Diagn Lab Immunol* 2001;8:984–992.
329. Ter Meulen V. Virus-induced cell-mediated autoimmunity. In: Notkins A, Oldstone M, eds. *Concepts in viral pathogenesis*. New York: Springer-Verlag, 1989: 297–303.
330. Dale RC, Church AJ, Cardoso F, et al. Poststreptococcal acute disseminated encephalomyelitis with basal ganglia involvement and auto-reactive antibasal ganglia antibodies. *Ann Neurol* 2001;50:588–595.
331. Stocks M. Genetics of childhood disorders: XXIX. Autoimmune disorders, part 2: molecular mimicry. *J Am Acad Child Adolesc Psychiatry* 2001;40:977–980.
332. Liu J, Marino MW, Wong G, et al. TNF is a potent anti-inflammatory cytokine in autoimmune-mediated demyelination. *Nat Med* 1998;4:78–83.
333. Sabelko-Downes KA, Russell JH, Cross AH. Role of Fas–FasL interactions in the pathogenesis and regulation of autoimmune demyelinating disease. *J Neuroimmunol* 1999;100:42–52.
334. Hart BA, Brok HP, Amor S, et al. The major histocompatibility complex influences the ethiopathogenesis of MS-like disease in primates at multiple levels. *Hum Immunol* 2001;62:1371–1381.
335. Boullerne AI, Nedelkoska L, Benjamins JA. Role of calcium in nitric oxide–induced cytotoxicity: EGTA protects mouse oligodendrocytes. *J Neurosci Res* 2001;63:124–135.
336. van der Goes A, Brouwer J, Hoekstra K, et al. Reactive oxygen species are required for the phagocytosis of myelin by macrophages. *J Neuroimmunol* 1998;92:67–75.

337. Matute C, Alberdi E, Domercq M, et al. The link between excitotoxic oligodendroglial death and demyelinating diseases. *Trends Neurosci* 2001;24:224–230.
338. Ghosh N, DeLuca GC, Esiri MM. Evidence of axonal damage in human acute demyelinating diseases. *J Neurol Sci* 2004;222:29–34.
339. Herndon RM, Rudick R. Multiple sclerosis and related conditions. In: Herndon RM, Rudick R, eds. *Clinical neurology on CD-ROM*. Philadelphia: Lippincott Raven, 1996.
340. Abramson JS, Roach ES, Levy HB. Postinfectious encephalopathy after treatment of herpes simplex encephalitis with acyclovir. *Pediatr Infect Dis* 1984;3:146–147.
341. Ichiyama T, Hayashi T, Yamaguchi E, et al. Involvement of the white matter in the initial stage of herpes simplex encephalitis. *Pediatr Radiol* 1992;22:145.
342. Johnson RT, Griffin DE, Gendelman HE. Postinfectious encephalomyelitis. *Semin Neurol* 1985;5:180–190.
343. Okuno T, Takao T, Ito M, et al. Contrast enhanced hypodense areas in a case of acute disseminated encephalitis following influenza A virus. *Comput Radiol* 1982;6:215–217.
344. Shoji H, Kusuhara T, Honda Y, et al. Relapsing acute disseminated encephalomyelitis associated with chronic Epstein-Barr virus infection: MRI findings. *Neuroradiology* 1992;34:340–342.
345. Fernandez CV, Bortolussi R, Gordon K, et al. *Mycoplasma pneumoniae* infection associated with central nervous system complications. *J Child Neurol* 1993;8:27–31.
346. Hall MC, Barton LL, Johnson MI. Acute disseminated encephalomyelitis-like syndrome following group A beta-hemolytic streptococcal infection. *J Child Neurol* 1998;13:354–356.
347. Munn R, F, Barrell K, Cimolai N. Acute encephalomyelitis: extending the neurological manifestations of acute rheumatic fever? *Neuropediatrics* 1992;23:196–198.
348. Miller JR, Freddo L. Corticosteroid-sensitive encephalomyelopathy following influenza vaccination. *Ann Neurol* 1989;26:176.
349. Ohtaki E, Murakami Y, Komori H, et al. Acute disseminated encephalomyelitis after Japanese B encephalitis vaccination. *Pediatr Neurol* 1992;8:137–139.
350. Ohtaki E, Matsuishi T, Hirano Y, et al. Acute disseminated encephalomyelitis after treatment with Japanese B encephalitis vaccine (Nakayama-Yoken and Beijing strains). *J Neurol Neurosurg Psychiatry* 1995;59:316–317.
351. Ozawa H, Noma S, Yoshida Y, et al. Acute disseminated encephalomyelitis associated with poliomyelitis vaccine. *Pediatr Neurol* 2000;23:177–179.
352. Saito H, Endo M, Takase S, Itahara K. Acute disseminated encephalomyelitis after influenza vaccination. *Arch Neurol* 1980;37:564–566.
353. Brass SD, Caramanos Z, Santos C, et al. Multiple sclerosis vs acute disseminated encephalomyelitis in childhood. *Pediatr Neurol* 2003;29:227–231.
354. Scully RE, Mark EJ, McNeely WF. Case records of the Massachussetts General Hospital, case 1-1999. *N Engl J Med* 1999;340:127–135.
355. Amit R, Glick B, Itzchak Y, et al. Acute severe combined demyelination. *Childs Nerv Syst* 1992;8:354–356.
356. Nadkarni N, Lisak RP. Guillain-Barré syndrome (GBS) with bilateral optic neuritis and central white matter disease. *Neurology* 1993;43:842–843.
357. Hynson JL, Kornberg AJ, Coleman LT, et al. Clinical and neuroradiologic features of acute disseminated encephalomyelitis in children. *Neurology* 2001;56:1308–1312.
358. McGovern RA, DiMario FJ. Acute disseminated encephalomyelitis: A retrospective pediatric series. *Ann Neurol* 2003;54:S129.
359. Yoshikawa S, Suzuki S, Kanbayashi T, et al. Hypersomnia and low cerebrospinal fluid hypocretin levels in acute disseminated encephalomyelitis. *Pediatr Neurol* 2004;31:367–370.
360. Ganesan V, Borzyskowski M. Characteristics and course of urinary tract dysfunction after acute transverse myelitis in childhood. *Dev Med Child Neurol* 2001;43:473–475.
361. Gupte G, Stonehouse M, Wassmer E, et al. Acute disseminated encephalomyelitis: a review of 18 cases in childhood. *J Paediatr Child Health* 2003;39:336–342.
362. Mader I, Wolff M, Niemann G, Kuker W. Acute haemorrhagic encephalomyelitis (AHEM): MRI findings. *Neuropediatrics* 2004;35:143–146.
363. Miller DH, Robb SA, Ormerod IE, et al. Magnetic resonance imaging of inflammatory and demyelinating white-matter diseases of childhood. *Dev Med Child Neurol* 1990;32:97–107.
364. Kimura S, Nezu A, Ohtsuki N, et al. Serial magnetic resonance imaging in children with postinfectious encephalitis. *Brain Dev* 1996;18:461–465.
365. Caldemeyer KS, Harris TM, Smith RR, et al. Gadolinium enhancement in acute disseminated encephalomyelitis. *J Comput Assist Tomogr* 1991;15:673–675.
366. van der Meyden CH, de Villiers JF, Middlecote BD, et al. Gadolinium ring enhancement and mass effect in acute disseminated encephalomyelitis. *Neuroradiology* 1994;36:221–223.
367. Lim KE, Hsu YY, Hsu WC, et al. Multiple complete ring-shaped enhanced MRI lesions in acute disseminated encephalomyelitis. *Clin Imaging* 2003;27:281–284.
368. Miller DH, Scaravilli F, Thomas DC, et al. Acute disseminated encephalomyelitis presenting as a solitary brainstem mass. *J Neurol Neurosurg Psychiatry* 1993;56:920–922.
369. Tan HM, Chan LL, Chuah KL, et al. Monophasic, solitary tumefactive demyelinating lesion: neuroimaging features and neuropathological diagnosis. *Br J Radiol* 2004;77:153–156.
370. Bernarding J, Braun J, Koennecke HC. Diffusion- and perfusion-weighted MR imaging in a patient with acute demyelinating encephalomyelitis (ADEM). *J Magn Reson Imaging* 2002;15:96–100.
371. Harada M, Hisaoka S, Mori K, et al. Differences in water diffusion and lactate production in two different types of postinfectious encephalopathy. *J Magn Reson Imaging* 2000;11:559–563.
372. Kuker W, Ruff J, Gaertner S, et al. Modern MRI tools for the characterization of acute demyelinating lesions: value of chemical shift and diffusion-weighted imaging. *Neuroradiology* 2004;46:421–426.
373. Holtmannspotter M, Inglese M, Rovaris M, et al. A diffusion tensor MRI study of basal ganglia from patients with ADEM. *J Neurol Sci* 2003;206:27–30.
374. Bizzi A, Ulug AM, Crawford TO, et al. Quantitative proton MR spectroscopic imaging in acute disseminated encephalomyelitis. *AJNR Am J Neuroradiol* 2001;22:1125–1130.
375. Broich K, Horwich D, Alavi A. HMPAO-SPECT and MRI in acute disseminated encephalomyelitis. *J Nucl Med* 1991;32:1897–1900.
376. Okamoto M, Ashida KI, Imaizumi M. Hypoperfusion following encephalitis: SPECT with acetazolamide. *Eur J Neurol* 2001;8:471–474.
377. San Pedro EC, Mountz JM, Liu HG, et al. Postinfectious cerebellitis: clinical significance of Tc-99m HMPAO brain SPECT compared with MRI. *Clin Nucl Med* 1998;23:212–216.
378. Tabata K, Shishido F, Uemura K, et al. Positron emission tomography in acute disseminated encephalomyelitis: a case report [in Japanese]. *Kaku Igaku* 1990;27:261–265.
379. Bendszus M, Warmuth-Metz M, Klein R, et al. MR spectroscopy in gliomatosis cerebri. *AJNR Am J Neuroradiol* 2000;21:375–380.
380. Tardieu M, Mikaeloff Y. What is acute disseminated encephalomyelitis (ADEM)? *Eur J Paediatr Neurol* 2004;8:239–242.
381. Mizuguchi M, Abe J, Mikkaichi K, et al. Acute necrotising encephalopathy of childhood: a new syndrome presenting with multifocal, symmetric brain lesions. *J Neurol Neurosurg Psychiatry* 1995;58:555–561.
382. Mizuguchi M. Acute necrotizing encephalopathy of childhood: a novel form of acute encephalopathy prevalent in Japan and Taiwan. *Brain Dev* 1997;19:81–92.
383. Cusmai R, Bertini E, Di Capua M, et al. Bilateral, reversible, selective thalamic involvement demonstrated by brain MR and acute severe neurological dysfunction with favorable outcome. *Neuropediatrics* 1994;25:44–47.
384. Marcu H, Hacker H, Vonofakos D. Bilateral reversible thalamic lesions on computed tomography. *Neuroradiology* 1979;18:201–204.
385. Suwa K, Yamagata T, Momoi MY, et al. Acute relapsing encephalopathy mimicking acute necrotizing encephalopathy in a 4-year-old boy. *Brain Dev* 1999;21:554–558.

386. Ruggieri M, Polizzi A, Pavone L, et al. Thalamic syndrome in children with measles infection and selective, reversible thalamic involvement. *Pediatrics* 1998;101:112–119.
387. Roig M, Macaya A, Munell F, et al. Acute neurologic dysfunction associated with destructive lesions of the basal ganglia: a benign form of infantile bilateral striatal necrosis. *J Pediatr* 1990;117:578–581.
388. Pasternak JF, De Vivo DC, Prensky AL. Steroid-responsive encephalomyelitis in childhood. *Neurology* 1980;30:481–486.
389. Straub J, Chofflon M, Delavelle J. Early high-dose intravenous methylprednisolone in acute disseminated encephalomyelitis: a successful recovery. *Neurology* 1997;49:1145–1147.
390. Nishikawa M, Ichiyama T, Hayashi T, et al. Intravenous immunoglobulin therapy in acute disseminated encephalomyelitis. *Pediatr Neurol* 1999;21:583–586.
391. Pradhan S, Gupta RP, Shashank S, et al. Intravenous immunoglobulin therapy in acute disseminated encephalomyelitis. *J Neurol Sci* 1999;165:56–61.
392. Straussberg R, Schonfeld T, Weitz R, et al. Improvement of atypical acute disseminated encephalomyelitis with steroids and intravenous immunoglobulins. *Pediatr Neurol* 2001;24:139–143.
393. Balestri P, Grosso S, Acquaviva A, et al. Plasmapheresis in a child affected by acute disseminated encephalomyelitis. *Brain Dev* 2000;22:123–126.
394. Kanter DS, Horensky D, Sperling RA, et al. Plasmapheresis in fulminant acute disseminated encephalomyelitis. *Neurology* 1995;45:824–827.
395. Miyazawa R, Hikima A, Takano Y, et al. Plasmapheresis in fulminant acute disseminated encephalomyelitis. *Brain Dev* 2001;23:424–426.
396. Takata T, Hirakawa M, Sakurai M, et al. Fulminant form of acute disseminated encephalomyelitis: successful treatment with hypothermia. *J Neurol Sci* 1999;165:94–97.
397. Jolivalt CG, Howard RB, Chen LS, et al. A novel nitric oxide scavenger in combination with cyclosporine A ameliorates experimental autoimmune encephalomyelitis progression in mice. *J Neuroimmunol* 2003;138:56–64.
398. McCombe PA, Harness J, Pender MP. Effects of cyclosporin A treatment on clinical course and inflammatory cell apoptosis in experimental autoimmune encephalomyelitis induced in Lewis rats by inoculation with myelin basic protein. *J Neuroimmunol* 1999;97:60–69.
399. Anlar B, Basaran C, Kose G, et al. Acute disseminated encephalomyelitis in children: outcome and prognosis. *Neuropediatrics* 2003;34:194–199.
400. Johnson RT, Griffin DE, Hirsch RL, et al. Measles encephalomyelitis—clinical and immunologic studies. *N Engl J Med* 1984;310:137–141.
401. Hurst EW. Acute hemorrhagic leukoencephalitis: a previously undefined entity. *Med J Aust* 1941;1:1–6.
402. Khan S, Yaqub BA, Poser CM, et al. Multiphasic disseminated encephalomyelitis presenting as alternating hemiplegia. *J Neurol Neurosurg Psychiatry* 1995;58:467–470.
403. Revel-Vilk S, Hurvitz H, Klar A, et al. Recurrent acute disseminated encephalomyelitis associated with acute cytomegalovirus and Epstein-Barr virus infection. *J Child Neurol* 2000;15:421–424.
404. Tsai ML, Hung KL. Multiphasic disseminated encephalomyelitis mimicking multiple sclerosis. *Brain Dev* 1996;18:412–414.
405. Poser CM. The epidemiology of multiple sclerosis: a general overview. *Ann Neurol* 1994;36(Suppl 2):S180–S193.
406. Cohen O, Steiner-Birmanns B, Biran I, et al. Recurrence of acute disseminated encephalomyelitis at the previously affected brain site. *Arch Neurol* 2001;58:797–801.
407. Schwarz S, Mohr A, Knauth M, et al. Acute disseminated encephalomyelitis: a follow-up study of 40 adult patients. *Neurology* 2001;56:1313–1318.
408. Hahn CD, Miles BS, MacGregor DL, et al. Neurocognitive outcome after acute disseminated encephalomyelitis. *Pediatr Neurol* 2003;29:117–123.
409. Jacobs RK, Anderson VA, Neale JL, et al. Neuropsychological outcome after acute disseminated encephalomyelitis: impact of age at illness onset. *Pediatr Neurol* 2004;31:191–197.
410. Klein CJ, Wijdicks EF, Earnest Ft. Full recovery after acute hemorrhagic leukoencephalitis (Hurst's disease). *J Neurol* 2000;247:977–979.
411. Rosman NP, Gottlieb SM, Bernstein CA. Acute hemorrhagic leukoencephalitis: recovery and reversal of magnetic resonance imaging findings in a child. *J Child Neurol* 1997;12:448–454.
412. Seales D, Greer M. Acute hemorrhagic leukoencephalitis. A successful recovery. *Arch Neurol* 1991;48:1086–1088.
413. Boomer JA, Siatkowski RM. Optic neuritis in adults and children. *Semin Ophthalmol* 2003;18:174–180.
414. Adler IN, James CA, Glasier CM. Ophthalmologic disease in children. *Magn Reson Imaging Clin N Am* 2001;9:191–206.
415. Hickman SJ, Dalton CM, Miller DH, et al. Management of acute optic neuritis. *Lancet* 2002;360:1953–1962.
416. Brady KM, Brar AS, Lee AG, et al. Optic neuritis in children: clinical features and visual outcome. *J AAPOS* 1999;3:98–103.
417. Morales DS, Siatkowski RM, Howard CW, et al. Optic neuritis in children. *J Pediatr Ophthalmol Strabismus* 2000;37:254–259.
418. Tekavcic-Pompe M, Stirn-Kranjc B, Brecelj J. Optic neuritis in children—clinical and electrophysiological follow-up. *Doc Ophthalmol* 2003;107:261–270.
419. Franco AF, Cabrera D, Carrizosa J, et al. Clinical characteristics of optical neuritis in children [in Spanish]. *Rev Neurol* 2003;36:208–211.
420. Lana-Peixoto MA, Andrade GC. The clinical profile of childhood optic neuritis. *Arq Neuropsiquiatr* 2001;59:311–317.
421. Yoshikawa T, Yoshida J, Hamaguchi M, et al. Human herpesvirus 7–associated meningitis and optic neuritis in a patient after allogeneic stem cell transplantation. *J Med Virol* 2003;70:440–443.
422. Barash J, Dushnitzky D, Sthoeger D, et al. Human parvovirus B19 infection in children: uncommon clinical presentations. *Isr Med Assoc J* 2002;4:763–765.
423. Candler PM, Dale RC. Three cases of central nervous system complications associated with *Mycoplasma pneumoniae*. *Pediatr Neurol* 2004;31:133–138.
424. Riikonen R, Donner M, Erkkila H. Optic neuritis in children and its relationship to multiple sclerosis: a clinical study of 21 children. *Dev Med Child Neurol* 1988;30:349–359.
425. Kennedy C, Carroll FD. Optic neuritis in children. *Arch Ophthalmol* 1960;63:747–755.
426. Frederiksen JL, Petrera J. Serial visual evoked potentials in 90 untreated patients with acute optic neuritis. *Surv Ophthalmol* 1999;44 (Suppl 1):S54S–62.
427. Acar G, Ozakbas S, Cakmakci H, et al. Visual evoked potential is superior to triple dose magnetic resonance imaging in the diagnosis of optic nerve involvement. *Int J Neurosci* 2004;114:1025–1033.
428. Balcer LJ, Galetta SL. Treatment of acute demyyelinating optic neuritis. *Semin Ophthalmol* 2002;17:4–10.
429. Hickman SJ, Toosy AT, Miszkiel KA, et al. Visual recovery following acute optic neuritis—a clinical, electrophysiological and magnetic resonance imaging study. *J Neurol* 2004;251:996–1005.
430. Hickman SJ, Toosy AT, Jones SJ, et al. A serial MRI study following optic nerve mean area in acute optic neuritis. *Brain* 2004;127:2498–2505.
431. Miller DH, Newton MR, van der Poel JC, et al. Magnetic resonance imaging of the optic nerve in optic neuritis. *Neurology* 1988;38:175–179.
432. Scholl GB, Song HS, Wray SH. Uhthoff's symptom in optic neuritis: relationship to magnetic resonance imaging and development of multiple sclerosis. *Ann Neurol* 1991;30:180–184.
433. Beck RW, Smith CH, Gal RL, et al. Neurologic impairment 10 years after optic neuritis. *Arch Neurol* 2004;61:1386–1389.
434. Beck RW, Cleary PA, Anderson MM Jr, et al. A randomized, controlled trial of corticosteroids in the treatment of acute optic neuritis. The Optic Neuritis Study Group. *N Engl J Med* 1992;326:581–588.
435. Cole SR, Beck RW, Moke PS, et al. The National Eye Institute Visual Function Questionnaire: experience of the ONTT. Optic Neuritis Treatment Trial. *Invest Ophthalmol Vis Sci* 2000;41:1017–1021.
436. Trobe JD, Sieving PC, Guire KE, et al. The impact of the optic neuritis treatment trial on the practices of ophthalmologists and neurologists. *Ophthalmology* 1999;106:2047–2053.

437. Wakakura M, Mashimo K, Oono S, et al. Multicenter clinical trial for evaluating methylprednisolone pulse treatment of idiopathic optic neuritis in Japan. Optic Neuritis Treatment Trial Multicenter Cooperative Research Group (ONMRG). *Jpn J Ophthalmol* 1999;43:133–138.
438. Kaufman DI, Trobe JD, Eggenberger ER, et al. Practice parameter: the role of corticosteroids in the management of acute monosymptomatic optic neuritis. Report of the Quality Standards Subcommittee of the American Academy of Neurology. *Neurology* 2000;54:2039–2044.
439. Farris BK, Pickard DJ. Bilateral postinfectious optic neuritis and intravenous steroid therapy in children. *Ophthalmology* 1990;97:339–345.
440. Ruprecht K, Klinker E, Dintelmann T, et al. Plasma exchange for severe optic neuritis: treatment of 10 patients. *Neurology* 2004;63:1081–1083.
441. CHAMPS Study Group. Interferon beta-1a for optic neuritis patients at high risk for multiple sclerosis. *Am J Ophthalmol* 2001;132:463–471.
442. Foroozan R, Buono LM, Savino PJ, et al. Acute demyelinating optic neuritis. *Curr Opin Ophthalmol* 2002;13:375–380.
443. Martin KR, Quigley HA. Gene therapy for optic nerve disease. *Eye* 2004;18:1049–1055.
444. Parkin PJ, Hierons R, McDonald WI. Bilateral optic neuritis. A long-term follow-up. *Brain* 1984;107 (Pt 3):951–964.
445. Rizzo JF 3rd, Lessell S. Risk of developing multiple sclerosis after uncomplicated optic neuritis: a long-term prospective study. *Neurology* 1988;38:185–190.
446. Lana-Peixoto MA, Lana-Peixoto MI. The risk of multiple sclerosis developing in patients with isolated idiopathic optic neuritis in Brazil. *Arq Neuropsiquiatr* 1991;49:377–383.
447. Kennedy C, Carter S. Relation of optic neuritis to multiple sclerosis in children. *Pediatrics* 1961;28:377–387.
448. Kriss A, Francis DA, Cuendet F, et al. Recovery after optic neuritis in childhood. *J Neurol Neurosurg Psychiatry* 1988;51:1253–1258.
449. Lucchinetti CF, Kiers L, O'Duffy A, et al. Risk factors for developing multiple sclerosis after childhood optic neuritis. *Neurology* 1997;49:1413–1418.
450. Tumani H, Tourtellotte WW, Peter JB, et al. Acute optic neuritis: combined immunological markers and magnetic resonance imaging predict subsequent development of multiple sclerosis. The Optic Neuritis Study Group. *J Neurol Sci* 1998;155:44–49.
451. Kheradvar A, Tabassi AR, Nikbin B, et al. Influence of HLA on progression of optic neuritis to multiple sclerosis: results of a four-year follow-up study. *Mult Scler* 2004;10:526–531.
452. Gowers WR. *A manual of disease of the nervous system*. London: J. A. Churchill, 1886.
453. Foix C, Alajouanine T. La myelite necrotique subaguë. *Rev Neurol* 1926;33:1–42.
454. Ford FR. The nervous complications of measles: with a summary of literature and publications of 12 additional case reports. *Bull Johns Hopkins Hosp* 1928;43:140–184.
455. Suchett-Kaye AI. Acute transverse myelitis complicating pneumonia. *Lancet* 1948;255:417.
456. Kerr DA, Ayetey H. Immunopathogenesis of acute transverse myelitis. *Curr Opin Neurol* 2002;15:339–347.
457. Kroshnan C, Kaplin AI, Dehpande DM. Transverse myelitis: pathogenesis, diagnosis and treatment. *Front Biosci* 2004;9:1483–1499.
458. D'Cruz DP, Mellor-Pita S, Joven B, et al. Transverse myelitis as the first manifestation of systemic lupus erythematosus or lupus-like disease: good functional outcome and relevance of antiphospholipid antibodies. *J Rheumatol* 2004;31:280–285.
459. DeGiorgio LA, Konstantinov KN, Lee SC, et al. A subset of lupus anti-DNA antibodies cross-reacts with the NR2 glutamate receptor in systemic lupus erythematosus. *Nat Med* 2001;7:1189–1193.
460. Matsui M, Kakigi R, Watanabe S, et al. Recurrent demyelinating transverse myelitis in a high titer HBs-antigen carrier. *J Neurol Sci* 1996;139:235–237.
461. Vanderlugt CL, Begolka WS, Neville KL, et al. The functional significance of epitope spreading and its regulation by co-stimulatory molecules. *Immunol Rev* 1998;164:63–72.
462. Kikuchi H, Osoegawa M, Ochi H, et al. Spinal cord lesions of myelitis with hyperIgEemia and mite antigen specific IgE (atopic myelitis) manifest eosinophilic inflammation. *J Neurol Sci* 2001;183:73–78.
463. Paine RS, Byers RK. Transverse myelopathy in childhood. *AMA Am J Dis Child* 1953;85:151–163.
464. Roman GC. Proposed diagnostic criteria and nosology of acute transverse myelitis. *Neurology* 2002;59:499–505.
465. Berman M, Feldman S, Alter M, et al. Acute transverse myelitis: incidence and etiologic considerations. *Neurology* 1981;31:966–971.
466. Jeffery DR, Mandler RN, Davis LE. Transverse myelitis. Retrospective analysis of 33 cases, with differentiation of cases associated with multiple sclerosis and parainfectious events. *Arch Neurol* 1993;50:532–535.
467. Defresne P, Hollenberg H, Husson B, et al. Acute transverse myelitis in children: clinical course and prognostic factors. *J Child Neurol* 2003;18:401–406.
468. Garcia-Zozaya IA. Acute transverse myelitis in a 7-month-old boy. *J Spinal Cord Med* 2001;24:114–118.
469. Dunne K, Hopkins IJ, Shield LK. Acute transverse myelopathy in childhood. *Dev Med Child Neurol* 1986;28:198–204.
470. Andersen O. Myelitis. *Curr Opin Neurol* 2000;13:311–316.
471. Antal EA, Loberg EM, Bracht P, et al. Evidence for intraaxonal spread of *Listeria monocytogenes* from the periphery to the central nervous system. *Brain Pathol* 2001;11:432–438.
472. Correia de Farias Brito J, Virgolino da Nóbrega P. Myelopathy: clinical considerations and etiological aspects. *Arq Neuropsiquiatr* 2003;61:1–11.
473. Galanakis E, Bikouvarakis S, Mamoulakis D, et al. Transverse myelitis associated with herpes simplex virus infection. *J Child Neurol* 2001;16:866–867.
474. Knebusch M, Strassburg HM, Reiners K. Acute transverse myelitis in childhood: nine cases and review of the literature. *Dev Med Child Neurol* 1998;40:631–639.
475. Sherer Y, Hassin S, Shoenfeld Y, et al. Transverse myelitis in patients with antiphospholipid antibodies—the importance of early diagnosis and treatment. *Clin Rheumatol* 2002;21:207–210.
476. Linssen WH, Gabreels FJ, Wevers RA. Infective acute transverse myelopathy. Report of two cases. *Neuropediatrics* 1991;22:107–109.
477. Linden D, Berlit P. Magnetic motor evoked potentials (MEP) in diseases of the spinal cord. *Acta Neurol Scand* 1994;90:348–353.
478. Noguchi Y, Okubo O, Fuchigami T, et al. Motor-evoked potentials in a child recovering from transverse myelitis. *Pediatr Neurol* 2000;23:436–438.
479. Kalita J, Misra UK. Neurophysiological studies in acute transverse myelitis. *J Neurol* 2000;247:943–948.
480. Andronikou S, Albuquerque, JG, Wilmshurst J, et al. MRI findings in acute idiopathic transverse myelopathy in children. *Pediatr Radiol* 2003;33:624–629.
481. Isoda H, Ramsey RG. MR imaging of acute transverse myelitis (myelopathy). *Radiat Med* 1998;16:179–186.
482. Scotti G, Gerevini S. Diagnosis and differential diagnosis of acute transverse myelopathy. The role of neuroradiological investigations and review of the literature. *Neurol Sci* 2001;22(Suppl 2):S69–S73.
483. Miller DH, McDonald WI, Blumhardt LD, et al. Magnetic resonance imaging in isolated noncompressive spinal cord syndromes. *Ann Neurol* 1987;22:714–723.
484. Newswanger DL, Warren CR. Guillain-Barré syndrome. *Am Fam Physician* 2004;69:2405–2410.
485. Defresne P, Meyer L, Tardieu M, et al. Efficacy of high dose steroid therapy in children with severe acute transverse myelitis. *J Neurol Neurosurg Psychiatry* 2001;71:272–274.
486. Lahat E, Pillar G, Ravid S, et al. Rapid recovery from transverse myelopathy in children treated with methylprednisolone. *Pediatr Neurol* 1998;19:279–282.
487. Mok CC, Lau CS, Chan EY, et al. Acute transverse myelopathy in systemic lupus erythematosus: clinical presentation, treatment, and outcome. *J Rheumatol* 1998;25:467–473.
488. Bakker J, Metz L. Devic's neuromyelitis optica treated with intravenous gamma globulin (IVIG). *Can J Neurol Sci* 2004;31:265–267.

489. Celik Y, Tabak F, Mert A, et al. Transverse myelitis caused by varicella. *Clin Neurol Neurosurg* 2001;103:260–261.
490. Weinshenker BG, O'Brien PC, Petterson TM, et al. A randomized trial of plasma exchange in acute central nervous system inflammatory demyelinating disease. *Ann Neurol* 1999;46:878–886.
491. Wollinsky KH, Hulser PJ, Brinkmeier H, et al. CSF filtration is an effective treatment of Guillain-Barré syndrome: a randomized clinical trial. *Neurology* 2001;57:774–780.
492. Hauben E, Butovsky O, Nevo U, et al. Passive or active immunization with myelin basic protein promotes recovery from spinal cord contusion. *J Neurosci* 2000;20:6421–6430.
493. Hauben E, Agranov E, Gothilf A, et al. Posttraumatic therapeutic vaccination with modified myelin self-antigen prevents complete paralysis while avoiding autoimmune disease. *J Clin Invest* 2001;108:591–599.
494. Cheng W, Chiu R, Tam P. Residual bladder dysfunction 2 to 10 years after acute transverse myelitis. *J Paediatr Child Health* 1999;35:476–478.
495. Kim JH, Lee SI, Park SI, et al. Recurrent transverse myelitis in primary antiphospholipid syndrome—case report and literature review. *Rheumatol Int* 2004;24:244–246.
496. Kim KK. Idiopathic recurrent transverse myelitis. *Arch Neurol* 2003;60:1290–1294.
497. Miyazawa R, Ikeuchi Y, Tomomasa T, et al. Determinants of prognosis of acute transverse myelitis in children. *Pediatr Int* 2003;45:512–516.
498. Connolly AM, Dodson WE, Prensky AL, et al. Course and outcome of acute cerebellar ataxia. *Ann Neurol* 1994;35:673–679.
499. Batten FE. Ataxia in childhood. *Brain* 1905;28:487–505.
500. Nussinovitch M, Prais D, Volovitz B, et al. Post-infectious acute cerebellar ataxia in children. *Clin Pediatr* (Phila) 2003;42:581–584.
501. Davis DP, Marino A. Acute cerebellar ataxia in a toddler: case report and literature review. *J Emerg Med* 2003;24:281–284.
502. Wolff M, Schoning M, Niemann G, et al . Late detection of neuroblastoma in a patient with prolonged cerebellar ataxia without opsoclonus. *Neuropediatrics* 2001;32:101–103.
503. Yeung WL, Li CK, Nelson EA, et al. Unusual neurological presentation of neuroblastoma. *Hong Kong Med J* 2003;9:142–144.
504. Iff T, Donati F, Vassella F, et al. Acute encephalitis in Swiss children: aetiology and outcome. *Eur J Paediatr Neurol* 1998;2:233–237.
505. Ito H, Sayama S, Irie S, et al. Antineuronal antibodies in acute cerebellar ataxia following Epstein-Barr virus infection. *Neurology* 1994;44:1506–1507.
506. Cimolai N, Mah D, Roland E. Anticentriolar autoantibodies in children with central nervous system manifestations of *Mycoplasma pneumoniae* infection. *J Neurol Neurosurg Psychiatry* 1994;57:638–639.
507. Connolly AM, Pestronk A, Mehta S, et al. Serum autoantibodies in childhood opsoclonus-myoclonus syndrome: an analysis of antigenic targets in neural tissues. *J Pediatr* 1997;130:878–884.
508. Adams C, Diadori P, Schoenroth L, et al. Autoantibodies in childhood post-varicella acute cerebellar ataxia. *Can J Neurol Sci* 2000;27:316–320.
509. Fritzler MJ, Zhang M, Stinton LM, et al. Spectrum of centrosome autoantibodies in childhood varicella and post-varicella acute cerebellar ataxia. *BMC Pediatr* 2003;3:11.
510. Ploubidou A, Moreau V, Ashman K, et al. Vaccinia virus infection disrupts microtubule organization and centrosome function. *EMBO J* 2000;19:3932–3944.
511. Bakshi R, Bates VE, Kinkel PR, et al. Magnetic resonance imaging findings in acute cerebellitis. *Clin Imaging* 1998;22:79–85.
512. Hung CF, Cheng WF, He L, et al. Enhancing major histocompatibility complex class I antigen presentation by targeting antigen to centrosomes. *Cancer Res* 2003;63:2393–2398.
513. Weiss S, Carter S. Course and prognosis of acute cerebellar ataxia in children. *Neurology* 1959;9:711–721.
514. Groen RJ, Begeer JH, Wilmink JT, et al. Acute cerebellar ataxia in a child with transient pontine lesions demonstrated by MRI. *Neuropediatrics* 1991;22:225–227.
515. Maggi G, Varone A, Aliberti F. Acute cerebellar ataxia in children. *Childs Nerv Syst* 1997;13:542–545.
516. Go T. Intravenous immunoglobulin therapy for acute cerebellar ataxia. *Acta Paediatr* 2003;92:504–506.
517. Nagamitsu S, Matsuishi T, Ishibashi M, et al. Decreased cerebellar blood flow in postinfectious acute cerebellar ataxia. *J Neurol Neurosurg Psychiatry* 1999;67:109–112.
518. Daaboul Y, Vern BA, Blend MJ. Brain SPECT imaging and treatment with IVIg in acute post-infectious cerebellar ataxia: case report. *Neurol Res* 1998;20:85–88.
519. Park JW, Choi YB, Lee KS. Detection of acute Epstein Barr virus cerebellitis using sequential brain HMPAO-SPECT imaging. *Clin Neurol Neurosurg* 2004;106:118–121.
520. Yazawa S, Ohi T, Sugimoto S, et al. A case of acute cerebellar ataxia with abnormal single photon emission computed tomography [in Japanese]. *Rinsho Shinkeigaku* 1995;35:424–427.
521. Matsunaga K, Uozumi T, Hashimoto T, et al. Cerebellar stimulation in acute cerebellar ataxia. *Clin Neurophysiol* 2001;112:619–622.
522. Kanagarajan K, Ganesh S, Alakhras M, et al. West Nile virus infection presenting as cerebellar ataxia and fever: case report. *South Med J* 2003;96:600–601.
523. Horowitz MB, Pang D, Hirsch W. Acute cerebellitis: case report and review. *Pediatr Neurosurg* 1991;17:142–145.
524. Sawaishi Y, Takada G. Acute cerebellitis. *Cerebellum* 2002;1:223–228.
525. Basser LS. Benign paroxysmal vertigo of childhood (a variety of vestibular neuronitis). *Brain* 1964;87:141–152.
526. Pedersen E. Epidemic vertigo, Clinical picture, epidemiology and relation to encephalitis. *Brain* 1959;82:566–580.
527. Freedman DA, Schenthal JE. A parenchymatous cerebellar syndrome following protracted high body temperature. *Neurology* 1953;3:513–516.
528. Baloh RW, Jen JC. Genetics of familial episodic vertigo and ataxia. *Ann N Y Acad Sci* 2002;956:338–345.
529. Kato Z, Shimozawa N, Kokuzawa J, et al. Magnetic resonance imaging of acute cerebellar ataxia: report of a case with gadolinium enhancement and review of the literature. *Acta Paediatr Jpn* 1998;40:138–142.
530. Visudtibhan A, Visudhiphan P, Chiemchanya S. Recurrent acute cerebellar ataxia of childhood following nonspecific respiratory tract infection. *J Med Assoc Thai* 1998;81:1015–1018.
531. Gohlich-Ratmann G, Wallot M, Baethmann M, et al. Acute cerebellitis with near-fatal cerebellar swelling and benign outcome under conservative treatment with high dose steroids. *Eur J Paediatr Neurol* 1998;2:157–162.
532. Soussan V, Husson B, Tardieu M. Description and prognostic value of cerebellar MRI lesions in children with severe acute ataxia [in French]. *Arch Pediatr* 2003;10:604–607.
533. Kinsbourne M. Myoclonic encephalopathy of infants. *J Neurol Neurosurg Psychiatry* 1962;25:271–276.
534. Dale RC. Childhood opsoclonus myoclonus. *Lancet Neurol* 2003;2:270.
535. Pranzatelli MR, Travelstead AL, Tate ED, et al. Immunophenotype of blood lymphocytes in neuroblastoma-associated opsoclonus-myoclonus. *J Pediatr Hematol Oncol* 2004;26:718–723.
536. Pranzatelli MR, Travelstead AL, Tate ED, et al. CSF B-cell expansion in opsoclonus-myoclonus syndrome: a biomarker of disease activity. *Mov Disord* 2004;19:770–777.
537. Pranzatelli MR, Travelstead AL, Tate ED, et al. B- and T-cell markers in opsoclonus-myoclonus syndrome: immunophenotyping of CSF lymphocytes. *Neurology* 2004;62:1526–1532.
538. Bartos A, Pitha J. Opsoclonus-myoclonus-dysequilibrium syndrome: cytological and immunological dynamics in the serial cerebrospinal fluid in two patients. *J Neurol* 2003;250:1420–1425.
539. Prasannan L, Misek DE, Hinderer R, et al. Identification of beta-tubulin isoforms as tumor antigens in neuroblastoma. *Clin Cancer Res* 2000;6:3949–3956.
540. Katsetos CD, Legido A, Perentes E, et al. Class III beta-tubulin isotype: a key cytoskeletal protein at the crossroads of developmental neurobiology and tumor neuropathology. *J Child Neurol* 2003;18:851–866; discussion 867.
541. Antunes NL, Khakoo Y, Matthay KK, et al. Antineuronal antibodies in patients with neuroblastoma and paraneoplastic

opsoclonus-myoclonus. *J Pediatr Hematol Oncol* 2000;22:315–320.

542. Fisher PG, Wechsler DS, Singer HS. Anti-Hu antibody in a neuroblastoma-associated paraneoplastic syndrome. *Pediatr Neurol* 1994;10:309–312.
543. Pranzatelli MR, Tate ED, Wheeler A, et al. Screening for autoantibodies in children with opsoclonus-myoclonus-ataxia. *Pediatr Neurol* 2002;27:384–387.
544. Bataller L, Rosenfeld MR, Graus F, et al. Autoantigen diversity in the opsoclonus-myoclonus syndrome. *Ann Neurol* 2003;53:347–353.
545. Cooper R, Khakoo Y, Matthay KK, et al. Opsoclonus-myoclonus-ataxia syndrome in neuroblastoma: histopathologic features—a report from the Children's Cancer Group. *Med Pediatr Oncol* 2001;36:623–629.
546. Gambini C, Conte M, Bernini G, et al. Neuroblastic tumors associated with opsoclonus-myoclonus syndrome: histological, immunohistochemical and molecular features of 15 Italian cases. *Virchows Arch* 2003;442:555–562.
547. Helmchen C, Rambold H, Sprenger A, et al. Cerebellar activation in opsoclonus: an fMRI study. *Neurology* 2003;61:412–415.
548. Ramos S, Temudo T. Opsoclonus myoclonus syndrome: how long are we going to go on researching? [in Spanish]. *Rev Neurol* 2002;35:322–325.
549. Dredge BK, Darnell RB. Nova regulates GABA(A) receptor gamma2 alternative splicing via a distal downstream UCAU-rich intronic splicing enhancer. *Mol Cell Biol* 2003;23:4687–4700.
550. Jensen KB, Dredge BK, Stefani G, et al. Nova-1 regulates neuron-specific alternative splicing and is essential for neuronal viability. *Neuron* 2000;25:359–371.
551. Musunuru K, Darnell RB. Determination and augmentation of RNA sequence specificity of the Nova K-homology domains. *Nucleic Acids Res* 2004;32:4852–4861.
552. Pranzatelli MR, Tate ED, Kinsbourne M, et al. Forty-one year follow-up of childhood-onset opsoclonus-myoclonus-ataxia: cerebellar atrophy, multiphasic relapses, and response to IVIG. *Mov Disord* 2002;17:1387–1390.
553. Tate ED, Allison TJ, Pranzatelli MR, et al. Neuroepidemiologic trends in 105 US cases of pediatric opsoclonus-myoclonus syndrome. *J Pediatr Oncol Nurs* 2005;22:8–19.
554. Boltshauser E, Deonna T, Hirt HR. Myoclonic encephalopathy of infants or "dancing eyes syndrome". Report of 7 cases with long-term follow-up and review of the literature (cases with and without neuroblastoma). *Helv Paediatr Acta* 1979;34:119–133.
555. Tuchman M, Ramnaraine ML, Woods WG, et al. Three years of experience with random urinary homovanillic and vanillylmandelic acid levels in the diagnosis of neuroblastoma. *Pediatrics* 1987;79:203–205.
556. Swart JF, de Kraker J, van der Lely N. Metaiodobenzylguanidine total-body scintigraphy required for revealing occult neuroblastoma in opsoclonus-myoclonus syndrome. *Eur J Pediatr* 2002;161:255–258.
557. Blaes F. Immunotherapeutic approaches to paraneoplastic neurological disorders. *Expert Opin Biol Ther* 2002;2:419–430.
558. Glatz K, Meinck HM, Wildemann B. Parainfectious opsoclonus-myoclonus syndrome: high dose intravenous immunoglobulins are effective. *J Neurol Neurosurg Psychiatry* 2003;74:279–280.
559. Mitchell WG, Davalos-Gonzalez Y, Brumm VL, et al. Opsoclonus-ataxia caused by childhood neuroblastoma: developmental and neurologic sequelae. *Pediatrics* 2002;109:86–98.
560. Sheela SR, Mani PJ. Opsoclonus myoclonus syndrome: response to plasmapheresis. *Indian Pediatr* 2004;41:499–502.
561. Yiu VW, Kovithavongs T, McGonigle LF, et al. Plasmapheresis as an effective treatment for opsoclonus-myoclonus syndrome. *Pediatr Neurol* 2001;24:72–74.
562. Pranzatelli MR, Tate ED, Travelstead AL, et al. Immunologic and clinical responses to rituximab in a child with opsoclonus-myoclonus syndrome. *Pediatrics* 2005;115:e115–e119.
563. Caviness JN, Brown P. Myoclonus: current concepts and recent advances. *Lancet Neurol* 2004;3:598–607.
564. Moretti R, Torre P, Antonello RM, et al. Opsoclonus-myoclonus syndrome: gabapentin as a new therapeutic proposal. *Eur J Neurol* 2000;7:455–456.
565. Hayward K, Jeremy RJ, Jenkins S, et al. Long-term neurobehavioral outcomes in children with neuroblastoma and opsoclonus-myoclonus-ataxia syndrome: relationship to MRI findings and anti-neuronal antibodies. *J Pediatr* 2001;139:552–559.
566. Papero PH, Pranzatelli MR, Margolis LJ, et al. Neurobehavioral and psychosocial functioning of children with opsoclonus-myoclonus syndrome. *Dev Med Child Neurol* 1995;37:915–932.
567. Plantaz D, Michon J, Valteau-Couanet D, et al. Opsoclonus-myoclonus syndrome associated with non-metastatic neuroblastoma. Long-term survival. Study of the French Society of Pediatric Oncologists [in French]. *Arch Pediatr* 2000;7:621–628.
568. Rudnick E, Khakoo Y, Antunes NL, et al. Opsoclonus-myoclonus-ataxia syndrome in neuroblastoma: clinical outcome and antineuronal antibodies—a report from the Children's Cancer Group Study. *Med Pediatr Oncol* 2001;36:612–622.
569. Raudnitz RW. Zur Lehre vom Spasmus nutans. *Jahrb Kinderheilkd* 1897:145–176.
570. Weissman BM, Dell'Osso LF, Abel LA, et al. Spasmus nutans. A quantitative prospective study. *Arch Ophthalmol* 1987;105:525–528.
571. Doummar D, Roussat B, Beauvais P, et al. arch. Pediatr. Spasmus nutans: a propos of 16 cases. 1998;5:264–268.
572. Gottlob I, Zubcov AA, Wizov SS, et al. Head nodding is compensatory in spasmus nutans. *Ophthalmology* 1992;99:1024–1031.
573. Herman C. Head shaking with nystagmus in infants. A study of sixty four cases. *Trans Am Pediatr Soc* (Chicago) 1918;30:180–184.
574. Wizov SS, Reinecke RD, Bocarnea M, Gottlob I. A comparative demographic and socioeconomic study of spasmus nutans and infantile nystagmus. *Am J Ophthalmol* 2002;133:256–262.
575. Hoefnagel D. Spasmus nutans. *Dev Med Child Neurol* 1968;10:32–35.
576. Norton WD. Spasms nutants: clinical study of 120 cases followed two years or more since onset. *AMA Arch Ophthalmol* 1954;52:442–446.
577. Farmer J, Hoyt CS. Monocular nystagmus in infancy and early childhood. *Am J Ophthalmol* 1984;98:504–509.
578. Lambert SR, Newman NJ. Retinal disease masquerading as spasmus nutans. *Neurology* 1993;43:1607–1609.
579. Shaw FS, Kriss A, Russell-Eggitt I, et al. Diagnosing children presenting with asymmetric pendular nystagmus. *Dev Med Child Neurol* 2001;43:622–627.
580. Smith DE, Fitzgerald K, Stass-Isern M, et al. Electroretinography is necessary for spasmus nutans diagnosis. *Pediatr Neurol* 2000;23:33–36.
581. Arnoldi KA, Tychsen L. Prevalence of intracranial lesions in children initially diagnosed with disconjugate nystagmus (spasmus nutans). *J Pediatr Ophthalmol Strabismus* 1995;32:296–301.
582. Baram TZ, Tang R. Atypical spasmus nutans as an initial sign of thalamic neoplasm. *Pediatr Neurol* 1986;2:375–376.
583. Newman SA, Hedges TR, Wall M, et al. Spasmus nutans—or is it? *Surv Ophthalmol* 1990;34:453–456.
584. Sedwick LA, Burde RM, Hodges FJ 3rd. Leigh's subacute necrotizing encephalomyelopathy manifesting as spasmus nutans. *Arch Ophthalmol* 1984;102:1046–1048.
585. Gottlob I, Helbling A. Nystagmus mimicking spasmus nutans as the presenting sign of Bardet-Biedl syndrome. *Am J Ophthalmol* 1999;128:770–772.
586. Allarakhia IN, Trobe JD. Opsoclonus-myoclonus presenting with features of spasmus nutans. *J Child Neurol* 1995;10:67–68.
587. King RA, Nelson LB, Wagner RS. Spasmus nutans. A benign clinical entity? *Arch Ophthalmol* 1986;104:1501–1504.
588. Kim JS, Park SH, Lee KW. Spasmus nutans and congenital ocular motor apraxia with cerebellar vermian hypoplasia. *Arch Neurol* 2003;60:1621–1624.
589. Gottlob I, Wizov SS, Reinecke RD. Spasmus nutans. A long-term follow-up. *Invest Ophthalmol Vis Sci* 1995;36:2768–2771.
590. Young TL, Weis JR, Summers CG, et al. The association of strabismus, amblyopia, and refractive errors in spasmus nutans. *Ophthalmology* 1997;104:112–117.
591. Jordan LC, Singer HS. Sydenham chorea in children. *Curr Treat Options Neurol* 2003;5:283–290.

592. Sydenham T. *The whole works of that excellent practical physician Dr. Thomas Sydenham*. London: R. Wellington, 1705: 422–423.
593. Stoll M. *Rationis medendi in Nosocomio Practico Vindobonensis, parst tertia*. Vienna: Sumptibus A. Bernardi, 1780.
594. Taranta A, Stollerman GH. The relationship of Sydenham's chorea to infection with group A streptococci. *Am J Med* 1956;20:170–175.
595. Aron AM, Freeman JM, Carter S. The natural history of Sydenham's chorea. Review of the literature and long-term evaluation with emphasis on cardiac sequelae. *Am J Med* 1965;38:83–95.
596. Westlake RM, Graham TP, Edwards KM. An outbreak of acute rheumatic fever in Tennessee. *Pediatr Infect Dis J* 1990;9:97–100.
597. Cardoso F, Eduardo C, Silva AP, et al. Chorea in fifty consecutive patients with rheumatic fever. *Mov Disord* 1997;12:701–703.
598. Husby G, van de Rijn I, Zabriskie JB, et al. Antibodies reacting with cytoplasm of subthalamic and caudate nuclei neurons in chorea and acute rheumatic fever. *J Exp Med* 1976;144:1094–1110.
599. Singer HS, Loiselle CR, Lee O, et al. Anti–basal ganglia antibody abnormalities in Sydenham chorea. *J Neuroimmunol* 2003;136:154–161.
600. Kirvan CA, Swedo SE, Heuser JS, et al. Mimicry and autoantibody-mediated neuronal cell signaling in Sydenham chorea. *Nat Med* 2003;9:914–920.
601. Page G, Barc-Pain S, Pontcharraud R, et al. The up-regulation of the striatal dopamine transporter's activity by cAMP is PKA-, CaMK II- and phosphatase-dependent. *Neurochem Int* 2004;45:627–632.
602. Bird MT, Palkes H, Prensky AL, et al. A follow-up study of Sydenham's chorea. *Neurology* 1976;26:601–606.
603. Freeman JM, Aron AM, Collard JE, et al. The emotional correlates of Sydenham's chorea. *Pediatrics* 1965;35:42–49.
604. Buchanan DN. Pathologic changes in chorea. *Am J Dis Child* 1941;62:443–445.
605. Nausieda PA, Grossman BJ, Koller WC, et al. Sydenham chorea: an update. *Neurology* 1980;30:331–334.
606. Kaplan EL. Recent epidemiology of group A streptococcal infections in North America and abroad: an overview. *Pediatrics* 1996;97:945–948.
607. Hosier DM, Craenen JM, Teske DW, et al. Resurgence of acute rheumatic fever. *Am J Dis Child* 1987;141:730–733.
608. Wilson SK. *Neurology,* 2nd ed. New York: Hafner Press, 1969.
609. Diaz-Grez F, Lay-Son L, del Barrio-Guerrero E, et al. Sydenham's chorea. A clinical analysis of 55 patients with a prolonged follow-up [in Spanish]. *Rev Neurol* 2004;39:810–815.
610. Heye N, Jergas M, Hotzinger H, et al. Sydenham chorea: clinical, EEG, MRI and SPECT findings in the early stage of the disease. *J Neurol* 1993;240:121–123.
611. Giedd JN, Rapoport JL, Kruesi MJ, et al. Sydenham's chorea: magnetic resonance imaging of the basal ganglia. *Neurology* 1995;45:2199–2202.
612. Faustino PC, Terreri MT, da Rocha AJ, et al. Clinical, laboratory, psychiatric and magnetic resonance findings in patients with Sydenham chorea. *Neuroradiology* 2003;45:456–462.
613. Lee PH, Nam HS, Lee KY, et al. Serial brain SPECT images in a case of Sydenham chorea. *Arch Neurol* 1999;56:237–240.
614. Citak EC, Gucuyener K, Karabacak NI, et al. Functional brain imaging in Sydenham's chorea and streptococcal tic disorders. *J Child Neurol* 2004;19:387–390.
615. Korn–Lubetzki I, Brand A, Steiner I. Recurrence of Sydenham chorea: implications for pathogenesis. *Arch Neurol* 2004;61:1261–1264.
616. Berrios X, Quesney F, Morales A, et al. Are all recurrences of "pure" Sydenham chorea true recurrences of acute rheumatic fever?. *J Pediatr* 1985;107:867–872.
617. Harrison NA, Church A, Nisbet A, et al. Late recurrences of Sydenham's chorea are not associated with anti–basal ganglia antibodies. *J Neurol Neurosurg Psychiatry* 2004;75:1478–1479.
618. Chun RW, Smith NJ, Forster FM. Papilledema in Sydenham's chorea. *Am J Dis Child* 1961;101:641–644.
619. Nausieda PA, Bieliauskas LA, Bacon LD, et al. Chronic dopaminergic sensitivity after Sydenham's chorea. *Neurology* 1983;33:750–754.
620. Asbahr FR, Ramos RT, Negrao AB, et al. Case series: increased vulnerability to obsessive-compulsive symptoms with repeated episodes of Sydenham chorea. *J Am Acad Child Adolesc Psychiatry* 1999;38:1522–1525.
621. Freud S. Die infantile Cerebrallähmung. In: Nothnagel H, ed. *Spezielle Pathologie und Therapie,* Vol. 9, Part 3. Vienna: Alfred Holder, 1897:853–254.
622. Prechtl HF, Stemmer J. The choreiform syndrome in children. *Dev Med Child Neurol* 1962;4:119–127.
623. Kerbeshian J, Burd L, Pettit R. A possible post-streptococcal movement disorder with chorea and tics. *Dev Med Child Neurol* 1990;32:642–644.
624. Feldman BM, Zabriskie JB, Silverman ED, et al. Diagnostic use of B-cell alloantigen D8/17 in rheumatic chorea. *J Pediatr* 1993;123:84–86.
625. Dhanaraj M, Radhakrishnan AR, Srinivas K, et al. Sodium valproate in Sydenham's chorea. *Neurology* 1985;35:114–115.
626. Alvarez LA, Novak G. Valproic acid in the treatment of Sydenham chorea. *Pediatr Neurol* 1985;1:317–319.
627. Genel F, Arslanoglu S, Uran N, et al. Sydenham's chorea: clinical findings and comparison of the efficacies of sodium valproate and carbamazepine regimens. *Brain Dev* 2002;24:73–76.
628. Pena J, Mora E, Cardozo J, et al. Comparison of the efficacy of carbamazepine, haloperidol and valproic acid in the treatment of children with Sydenham's chorea: clinical follow-up of 18 patients. *Arq Neuropsiquiatr* 2002;60:374–377.
629. Cardoso F, Maia D, Cunningham MC, et al. Treatment of Sydenham chorea with corticosteroids. *Mov Disord* 2003;18:1374–1377.
630. Massell BF. Prophylaxis of streptococcal infections and rheumatic fever: a comparison of orally administered clindamycin and penicillin. *JAMA* 1979;241:1589–1594.
631. Singer HS, Loiselle C. PANDAS: a commentary. *J Psychosom Res* 2003;55:31–39.
632. Snider LA, Swedo SE. PANDAS: current status and directions for research. *Mol Psychiatry* 2004;9:900–907.
633. Kurlan R, Kaplan EL. The pediatric autoimmune neuropsychiatric disorders associated with streptococcal infection (PANDAS) etiology for tics and obsessive-compulsive symptoms: hypothesis or entity? Practical considerations for the clinician. *Pediatrics* 2004;113:883–886.
634. van Toorn R, Weyers HH, Schoeman JF. Distinguishing PANDAS from Sydenham's chorea: case report and review of the literature. *Eur J Paediatr Neurol* 2004;8:211–216.
635. Kiessling LS, Marcotte AC, Culpepper L. Antineuronal antibodies in movement disorders. *Pediatrics* 1993;92:39–43.
636. Singer HS, Loiselle CR, Lee O, et al. Anti–basal ganglia antibodies in PANDAS. *Mov Disord* 2004;19:406–415.
637. Swedo SE, Leonard HL, Mittleman BB, et al. Identification of children with pediatric autoimmune neuropsychiatric disorders associated with streptococcal infections by a marker associated with rheumatic fever. *Am J Psychiatry* 1997;154:110–112.
638. Dale RC, Church AJ, Benton S, et al. Post-streptococcal autoimmune dystonia with isolated bilateral striatal necrosis. *Dev Med Child Neurol* 2002;44:485–489.
639. Pavone P, Bianchini R, Parano E, et al. Anti-brain antibodies in PANDAS versus uncomplicated streptococcal infection. *Pediatr Neurol* 2004;30:107–110.
640. Swedo SE, Leonard HL, Garvey M, et al. Pediatric autoimmune neuropsychiatric disorders associated with streptococcal infections: clinical description of the first 50 cases. *Am J Psychiatry* 1998;155:264–271.
641. Swedo SE, Leonard HL, Rapoport JL. The pediatric autoimmune neuropsychiatric disorders associated with streptococcal infection (PANDAS) subgroup: separating fact from fiction. *Pediatrics* 2004;113:907–911.
642. Snider LA, Sachdev V, MacKaronis JE, et al. Echocardiographic findings in the PANDAS subgroup. *Pediatrics* 2004;116:e748–751.
643. Kurlan R. Tourette's syndrome and 'PANDAS': will the relation bear out? Pediatric autoimmune neuropsychiatric disorders associated with streptococcal infection. *Neurology* 1998;50:1530–1534.
644. Shulman ST. Pediatric autoimmune neuropsychiatric disorders

associated with streptococci (PANDAS). *Pediatr Infect Dis J* 1999;18:281–282.

645. Dale RC, Heyman I, Surtees RA, et al. Dyskinesias and associated psychiatric disorders following streptococcal infections. *Arch Dis Child* 2004;89:604–610.
646. Safranek TJ, Lawrence DN, Kurland LT, et al. Reassessment of the association between Guillain-Barré syndrome and receipt of swine influenza vaccine in 1976–1977: results of a two-state study. Expert Neurology Group. *Am J Epidemiol* 1991;133:940–951.
647. Perlmutter SJ, Leitman SF, Garvey MA, et al. Therapeutic plasma exchange and intravenous immunoglobulin for obsessive-compulsive disorder and tic disorders in childhood. *Lancet* 1999;354:1153–1158.
648. Heubi C, Shott SR. PANDAS: pediatric autoimmune neuropsychiatric disorders associated with streptococcal infections—an uncommon, but important indication for tonsillectomy. *Int J Pediatr Otorhinolaryngol* 2003;67:837–840.
649. Granata T. Rasmussen's syndrome. *Neurol Sci* 2003;24(Suppl 4):S239–S243.
650. Hart Y. Rasmussen's encephalitis. *Epileptic Disord* 2004;6:133–144.
651. Andrews PI, Dichter MA, Berkovic SF, et al. Plasmapheresis in Rasmussen's encephalitis. 1996. *Neurology* 2001;57:S37–S41 .
652. Rogers SW, Andrews PI, Gahring LC, et al. Autoantibodies to glutamate receptor GluR3 in Rasmussen's encephalitis. *Science* 1994;265:648–651.
653. Bauer J, Bien CG, Lassmann H. Rasmussen's encephalitis: a role for autoimmune cytotoxic T lymphocytes. *Curr Opin Neurol* 2002;15:197–200.
654. Bien CG, Bauer J, Deckwerth TL, et al. Destruction of neurons by cytotoxic T cells: a new pathogenic mechanism in Rasmussen's encephalitis. *Ann Neurol* 2002;51:311–318.
655. Geller E, Faerber EN, Legido A, et al. Rasmussen encephalitis: complementary role of multitechnique neuroimaging. *AJNR Am J Neuroradiol* 1998;19:445–449.
656. Granata T, Fusco L, Gobbi G, et al. Experience with immunomodulatory treatments in Rasmussen's encephalitis. *Neurology* 2003;61:1807–1810.
657. Aarli JA. Epilepsy and the immune system. *Arch Neurol* 2000;57:1689–1692.
658. Ganor Y, Goldberg-Stern H, Amromd D, et al. Autoimmune epilepsy: some epilepsy patients harbor autoantibodies to glutamate receptors and dsDNA on both sides of the blood–brain barrier, which may kill neurons and decrease in brain fluids after hemispherotomy. *Clin Dev Immunol* 2004;11:241–252.
659. Mantegazza R, Bernasconi P, Baggi F, et al. Antibodies against GluR3 peptides are not specific for Rasmussen's encephalitis but are also present in epilepsy patients with severe, early onset disease and intractable seizures. *J Neuroimmunol* 2002;131:179–185.
660. Wiendl H, Bien CG, Bernasconi P, et al. GluR3 antibodies: prevalence in focal epilepsy but no specificity for Rasmussen's encephalitis. *Neurology* 2001;57:1511–1514.
661. Bartolomei F, Boucraut J, Barrie M, et al. Cryptogenic partial epilepsies with anti-GM1 antibodies: a new form of immune-mediated epilepsy? *Epilepsia* 1996;37:922–926.
662. Kwan P, Sills GJ, Kelly K, et al. Glutamic acid decarboxylase autoantibodies in controlled and uncontrolled epilepsy: a pilot study. *Epilepsy Res* 2000;42:191–195.
663. Peltola J, Kulmala P, Isojarvi J, et al. Autoantibodies to glutamic acid decarboxylase in patients with therapy-resistant epilepsy. *Neurology* 2000;55:46–50.
664. Eriksson K, Peltola J, Keranen T, et al. High prevalence of antiphospholipid antibodies in children with epilepsy: a controlled study of 50 cases. *Epilepsy Res* 2001;46:129–137.
665. Connolly AM, Chez MG, Pestronk A, et al. Serum autoantibodies to brain in Landau-Kleffner variant, autism, and other neurologic disorders. *J Pediatr* 1999;134:607–613.
666. Prasad AN, Stafstrom CF, Holmes GL. Alternative epilepsy therapies: the ketogenic diet, immunoglobulins, and steroids. *Epilepsia* 1996;37(Suppl 1):S81–S95.
667. Villani F, Avanzini G. The use of immunoglobulins in the treatment of human epilepsy. *Neurol Sci* 2002;23(Suppl 1):S33–S37.
668. During MJ, Symes CW, Lawlor PA, et al. An oral vaccine against NMDAR1 with efficacy in experimental stroke and epilepsy. *Science* 2000;287:1453–1460.
669. Young D, During MJ. Using the immune system to target epilepsy. *Adv Exp Med Biol* 2004;548:134–144.
670. Asbury AK. New concepts of Guillain-Barré syndrome. *J Child Neurol* 2000;15:183–191.
671. Jones HR Jr. Guillain-Barré syndrome: perspectives with infants and children. *Semin Pediatr Neurol* 2000;7:91–102.
672. Sladky JT. Guillain-Barré syndrome in children. *J Child Neurol* 2004;19:191–200.
673. Landry O. Note sur la paralyse ascendante aigué. *Gaz Hebd Med Chir* 1859;6:472–474.
674. Guillain G, Barré JA, Strohl A. Sur un syndrome de radiculonévrite avec hyperalbuminose du liquide céphalorachidien sans réaction cellulaire: remarques sur les caracteres cliniques et graphiques des réflexes tendineux. *Bull Soc Med Hop Paris* 1916;40:1462–1470.
675. Molinero MR, Varon D, Holden KR, et al. Epidemiology of childhood Guillain-Barré syndrome as a cause of acute flaccid paralysis in Honduras: 1989—1999. *J Child Neurol* 2003;18:741–747.
676. Kuwabara S. Guillain-Barré syndrome: epidemiology, pathophysiology and management. *Drugs* 2004;64:597–610.
677. Tsang RS, Valdivieso-Garcia A. Pathogenesis of Guillain-Barré syndrome. *Expert Rev Anti Infect Ther* 2003;1:597–608.
678. Asbury AK, Arnason BG, Adams RD. The inflammatory lesion in idiopathic polyneuritis. Its role in pathogenesis. *Medicine* (Baltimore) 1969;48:173–215.
679. Haymaker W, Kernohan JW. The Landry-Guillain Barré syndrome: a clinical pathologic report of 50 fatal cases and a review of the literature. *Medicine* 1949;28:59–141.
680. Hafer-Macko CE, Sheikh KA, Li CY, et al. Immune attack on the Schwann cell surface in acute inflammatory demyelinating polyneuropathy. *Ann Neurol* 1996;39:625–635.
681. Prineas JW. Immune attack on the Schwann cell surface in acute inflammatory demyelinating polyneuropahy. *Ann Neurol* 1981;9:S6–19.
682. Honavar M, Tharakan JK, Hughes RA, et al. A clinicopathological study of the Guillain-Barré syndrome. Nine cases and literature review. *Brain* 1991;114 (Pt 3):1245–1269.
683. Griffin JW, Li CY, Ho TW, et al. Pathology of the motor-sensory axonal Guillain-Barré syndrome. *Ann Neurol* 1996;39:17–28.
684. McKhann GM, Cornblath DR, Griffin JW, et al. Acute motor axonal neuropathy: a frequent cause of acute flaccid paralysis in China. *Ann Neurol* 1993;33:333–342.
685. Waksman BH, Adams RD. Allergic neuritis: an experimental disease of rabbits induced by the injection of peripheral nervous tissue and adjuvants. *J Exp Med* 1955;102:213–236.
686. Rostami A, Brown MJ, Lisak RP, et al. The role of myelin P2 protein in the production of experimental allergic neuritis. *Ann Neurol* 1984;16:680–685.
687. Zhu J, Pelidou SH, Deretzi G, et al. P0 glycoprotein peptides 56–71 and 180–199 dose-dependently induce acute and chronic experimental autoimmune neuritis in Lewis rats associated with epitope spreading. *J Neuroimmunol* 2001;114:99–106.
688. Yuki N, Yamada M, Koga M, et al. Animal model of axonal Guillain-Barré syndrome induced by sensitization with GM1 ganglioside. *Ann Neurol* 2001;49:712–720.
689. Kieseier BC, Kiefer R, Gold R, et al. Advances in understanding and treatment of immune-mediated disorders of the peripheral nervous system. *Muscle Nerve* 2004;30:131–156.
690. Linington C, Izumo S, Suzuki M, et al. A permanent rat T cell line that mediates experimental allergic neuritis in the Lewis rat *in vivo*. *J Immunol* 1984;133:1946–1950.
691. Yu S, Duan RS, Chen Z, et al. Increased susceptibility to experimental autoimmune neuritis after upregulation of the autoreactive T cell response to peripheral myelin antigen in apolipoprotein E-deficient mice. *J Neuropathol Exp Neurol* 2004;63:120–128.
692. Dalakas MC. Basic aspects of neuroimmunology as they relate to immunotherapeutic targets: present and future prospects. *Ann Neurol* 1995;37(Suppl 1):S2–S13.
693. Willison HJ, Yuki N. Peripheral neuropathies and anti-glycolipid antibodies. *Brain* 2002;125:2591–2625.

694. Abbott NJ, Mendonca LL, Dolman DE. The blood-brain barrier in systemic lupus erythematosus. *Lupus* 2003;12:908–915.
695. Church Potter R, Kaneene JB. A descriptive study of Guillain-Barré syndrome in high and low *Campylobacter jejuni* incidence regions of Michigan: 1992–1999. *Neuroepidemiology* 2003;22:245–248.
696. Hadden RD, Karch H, Hartung HP, et al. Preceding infections, immune factors, and outcome in Guillain-Barré syndrome. *Neurology* 2001;56:758–765.
697. Jacobs BC, Rothbarth PH, van der Meche FG, et al. The spectrum of antecedent infections in Guillain-Barré syndrome: a case–control study. *Neurology* 1998;51:1110–1115.
698. Rees JH, Soudain SE, Gregson NA, et al. *Campylobacter jejuni* infection and Guillain-Barré syndrome. *N Engl J Med* 1995; 333:1374–1379.
699. Visser LH, van der Meche FG, Meulstee J, et al. Cytomegalovirus infection and Guillain-Barré syndrome: the clinical, electrophysiologic, and prognostic features. Dutch Guillain-Barré Study Group. *Neurology* 1996;47:668–673.
700. Winer JB, Hughes RA, Osmond C. A prospective study of acute idiopathic neuropathy. I. Clinical features and their prognostic value. *J Neurol Neurosurg Psychiatry* 1988;51:605–612.
701. Hahn AF. Guillain-Barré syndrome. *Lancet* 1998;352:635–641.
702. Rantala H, Uhari M, Niemela M. Occurrence, clinical manifestations, and prognosis of Guillain-Barré syndrome. *Arch Dis Child* 1991;66:706–708; discussion 708–709.
703. Kusunoki S, Shiina M, Kanazawa I. Anti–Gal-C antibodies in GBS subsequent to mycoplasma infection: evidence of molecular mimicry. *Neurology* 2001;57:736–738.
704. Mori M, Kuwabara S, Miyake M, et al. *Haemophilus influenzae* has a GM1 ganglioside–like structure and elicits Guillain-Barré syndrome. *Neurology* 1999;52:1282–1284.
705. Hemachudha T, Griffin DE, Chen WW, et al. Immunologic studies of rabies vaccination–induced Guillain-Barré syndrome. *Neurology* 1988;38:375–378.
706. Udawat H, Chaudhary HR, Goyal RK, et al. Guillain-Barré syndrome following antirabies semple vaccine—a report of six cases. *J Assoc Physicians India* 2001;49:384–385.
707. Tuttle J, Chen RT, Rantala H, et al. The risk of Guillain-Barré syndrome after tetanus-toxoid–containing vaccines in adults and children in the United States. *Am J Public Health* 1997;87:2045–2048.
708. Anlar O, Tombul T, Arslan S, et al. Report of five children with Guillain-Barré syndrome following a nationwide oral polio vaccine campaign in Turkey. *Neurol India* 2003;51:544–545.
709. Haber P, DeStefano F, Angulo FJ, et al. Guillain-Barré syndrome following influenza vaccination. *JAMA* 2004;292:2478–2481.
710. Bino S, Kakarriqi E, Xibinaku M, et al. Measles–rubella mass immunization campaign in Albania, November 2000. *J Infect Dis* 2003;187(Suppl 1):S223–S229.
711. Blumenthal D, Prais D, Bron-Harlev E, et al. Possible association of Guillain-Barré syndrome and hepatitis A vaccination. *Pediatr Infect Dis J* 2004;23:586–588.
712. Seti NK, Reddi R, Anand I, et al. Guillain-Barré syndrome following vaccination with hepatitis B vaccine. *J Assoc Physicians India* 2002;50:989.
713. Nejmi SE, Tajri M, Laraki M, et al. Guillain-Barré syndrome following immunization against *Haemophilus influenzae* type b [in French]. *Arch Pediatr* 2001;8:894–895.
714. Archelos JJ, Previtali SC, Hartung HP. The role of integrins in immune-mediated diseases of the nervous system. *Trends Neurosci* 1999;22:30–38.
715. Hughes RA, Hadden RD, Gregson NA, et al. Pathogenesis of Guillain-Barré syndrome. *J Neuroimmunol* 1999;100:74–97.
716. Odaka M, Yuki N, Hirata K. Patients with chronic inflammatory demyelinating polyneuropathy initially diagnosed as Guillain-Barré syndrome. *J Neurol* 2003;250:913–916.
717. Ogawara K, Kuwabara S, Koga M, et al. Anti–GM1b IgG antibody is associated with acute motor axonal neuropathy and *Campylobacter jejuni* infection. *J Neurol Sci* 2003;210:41–45.
718. Yuki N. Molecular mimicry between gangliosides and lipopolysaccharides of *Campylobacter jejuni* isolated from patients with Guillain-Barré syndrome and Miller Fisher syndrome. *J Infect Dis* 1997;176(Suppl 2):S150–S153.
719. Odaka M, Koga M, Yuki N, et al. Longitudinal changes of anti-ganglioside antibodies before and after Guillain-Barré syndrome onset subsequent *to Campylobacter jejuni* enteritis. *J Neurol Sci* 2003;210:99–103.
720. Yuki N, Susuki K, Koga M, et al. Carbohydrate mimicry between human ganglioside GM1 and *Campylobacter jejuni* lipooligosaccharide causes Guillain-Barré syndrome. *Proc Natl Acad Sci USA* 2004;101:11404–11409.
721. van Sorge NM, van der Pol WL, Jansen MD, et al. Pathogenicity of anti-ganglioside antibodies in the Guillain-Barré syndrome. *Autoimmun Rev* 2004;3:61–68.
722. Ho TW, Willison HJ, Nachamkin I, et al. Anti-GD1a antibody is associated with axonal but not demyelinating forms of Guillain-Barré syndrome. *Ann Neurol* 1999;45:168–173.
723. Yuki N, Ang CW, Koga M, et al. Clinical features and response to treatment in Guillain-Barré syndrome associated with antibodies to GM1b ganglioside. *Ann Neurol* 2000;47:314–321.
724. Ang CW, Yuki N, Jacobs BC, et al. Rapidly progressive, predominantly motor Guillain-Barré syndrome with anti-GalNAc-GD1a antibodies. *Neurology* 1999;53:2122–2127.
725. Hao Q, Saida T, Yoshino H, et al. Anti-GalNAc-GD1a antibody-associated Guillain-Barré syndrome with a predominantly distal weakness without cranial nerve impairment and sensory disturbance. *Ann Neurol* 1999;45:758–768.
726. Vriesendorp FJ, Mishu B, Blaser MJ, et al. Serum antibodies to GM1, GD1b, peripheral nerve myelin, and *Campylobacter jejuni* in patients with Guillain-Barré syndrome and controls: correlation and prognosis. *Ann Neurol* 1993;34:130–135.
727. Willison HJ, Veitch J, Paterson G, et al. Miller Fisher syndrome is associated with serum antibodies to GQ1b ganglioside. *J Neurol Neurosurg Psychiatry* 1993;56:204–206.
728. Koga M, Yoshino H, Morimatsu M, et al. Anti–GT1a IgG in Guillain-Barré syndrome. *J Neurol Neurosurg Psychiatry* 2002;72:767–771.
729. Ang CW, Jacobs BC, Brandenburg AH, et al. Cross-reactive antibodies against GM2 and CMV-infected fibroblasts in Guillain-Barré syndrome. *Neurology* 2000;54:1453–1458.
730. Weber F, Rudel R, Aulkemeyer P, et al. Anti-GM1 antibodies can block neuronal voltage-gated sodium channels. *Muscle Nerve* 2000;23:1414–1420.
731. van Sorge NM, van den Berg LH, Geleijns K, et al. Anti-GM1 IgG antibodies induce leukocyte effector functions via Fcgamma receptors. *Ann Neurol* 2003;53:570–579.
732. Taguchi K, Ren J, Utsunomiya I, et al. Neurophysiological and immunohistochemical studies on Guillain-Barré syndrome with IgG anti-GalNAc-GD1a antibodies—effects on neuromuscular transmission. *J Neurol Sci* 2004;225:91–98.
733. Silverman GJ. B-cell superantigens. *Immunol Today* 1997;18:379–386.
734. Leadbetter EA, Rifkin IR, Hohlbaum AM, et al. Chromatin–IgG complexes activate B cells by dual engagement of IgM and Toll-like receptors. *Nature* 2002;416:603–607.
735. Schmidt B, Toyka KV, Kiefer R, et al. Inflammatory infiltrates in sural nerve biopsies in Guillain-Barré syndrome and chronic inflammatory demyelinating neuropathy. *Muscle Nerve* 1996;19:474–487.
736. Khalili-Shirazi A, Hughes RA, Brostoff SW, et al. T cell responses to myelin proteins in Guillain-Barré syndrome. *J Neurol Sci* 1992;111:200–203.
737. Van Rhijn I, Bleumink-Pluym NM, Van Putten JP, et al. *Campylobacter* DNA is present in circulating myelomonocytic cells of healthy persons and in persons with Guillain-Barré syndrome. *J Infect Dis* 2002;185:262–265.
738. Cooper JC, Ben-Smith A, Savage CO, et al. Unusual T cell receptor phenotype V gene usage of gamma delta T cells in a line derived from the peripheral nerve of a patient with Guillain-Barré syndrome. *J Neurol Neurosurg Psychiatry* 2000;69:522–524.
739. Ilyas AA, Chen ZW, Cook SD, et al. Immunoglobulin G subclass distribution of autoantibodies to gangliosides in patients with Guillain-Barré syndrome. *Res Commun Mol Pathol Pharmacol* 2001;109:115–123.

740. Colomar A, Marty V, Combe C, et al. The immune status of Schwann cells: what is the role of the P2X7 receptor? [in French]. *J Soc Biol* 2003;197:113–122.
741. Yu S, Chen Z, Mix E, et al. Neutralizing antibodies to IL-18 ameliorate experimental autoimmune neuritis by counter-regulation of autoreactive Th1 responses to peripheral myelin antigen. *J Neuropathol Exp Neurol* 2002;61:614–622.
742. Zhu J, Bai XF, Mix E, et al. Cytokine dichotomy in peripheral nervous system influences the outcome of experimental allergic neuritis: dynamics of mRNA expression for IL-1 beta, IL-6, IL-10, IL-12, TNF-alpha, TNF-eta, and cytolysin. *Clin Immunol Immunopathol* 1997;84:85–94.
743. Hu W, Mathey E, Hartung HP, et al. Cyclo-oxygenases and prostaglandins in acute inflammatory demyelination of the peripheral nerve. *Neurology* 2003;61:1774–1779.
744. Kapoor R, Davies M, Blaker PA, et al. Blockers of sodium and calcium entry protect axons from nitric oxide–mediated degeneration. *Ann Neurol* 2003;53:174–180.
745. Sharief MK, Ingram DA, Swash M. Circulating tumor necrosis factor-alpha correlates with electrodiagnostic abnormalities in Guillain-Barré syndrome. *Ann Neurol* 1997;42:68–73.
746. Orlikowski D, Chazaud B, Plonquet A, et al. Monocyte chemoattractant protein 1 and chemokine receptor CCR2 productions in Guillain-Barré syndrome and experimental autoimmune neuritis. *J Neuroimmunol* 2003;134:118–127.
747. Kieseier BC, Tani M, Mahad D, et al. Chemokines and chemokine receptors in inflammatory demyelinating neuropathies: a central role for IP-10. *Brain* 2002;125:823–834.
748. Kieseier BC, Krivacic K, Jung S, et al. Sequential expression of chemokines in experimental autoimmune neuritis. *J Neuroimmunol* 2000;110:121–129.
749. Zou LP, Pelidou SH, Abbas N, et al. Dynamics of production of MIP-1alpha, MCP-1 and MIP-2 and potential role of neutralization of these chemokines in the regulation of immune responses during experimental autoimmune neuritis in Lewis rats. *J Neuroimmunol* 1999;98:168–175.
750. Adams D, Gibson JD, Thomas PK, et al. HLA antigens in Guillain-Barré syndrome. *Lancet* 1977;2:504–505.
751. Koga M, Yuki N, Kashiwase K, et al. Guillain-Barré and Fisher's syndromes subsequent to *Campylobacter jejuni* enteritis are associated with HLA-54 and Cw1 independent of anti-ganglioside antibodies. *J Neuroimmunol* 1998;88:62–66.
752. Rees JH, Vaughan RW, Kondeatis E, et al. HLA-class II alleles in Guillain-Barré syndrome and Miller Fisher syndrome and their association with preceding *Campylobacter jejuni* infection. *J Neuroimmunol* 1995;62:53–57.
753. Magira EE, Papaioakim M, Nachamkin I, et al. Differential distribution of HLA-DQ beta/DR beta epitopes in the two forms of Guillain-Barré syndrome, acute motor axonal neuropathy and acute inflammatory demyelinating polyneuropathy (AIDP): identification of DQ beta epitopes associated with susceptibility to and protection from AIDP. *J Immunol* 2003;170:3074–3080.
754. Geleijns K, Schreuder GM, Jacobs BC, et al. HLA class II alleles are not a general susceptibility factor in Guillain-Barré syndrome. *Neurology* 2005;64:44–49.
755. Geleijns K, Brouwer BA, Jacobs BC, et al. The occurrence of Guillain-Barré syndrome within families. *Neurology* 2004;63:1747–1750.
756. Low NL, Schneider J, Carter S. Polyneuritis in children. *Pediatrics* 1958;22:972–990.
757. Peterman AF, Daly D, Dion FR, et al. Infectious neuronitis (Guillain-Barré syndrome) in children. *Neurology* 1959;9:533–539.
758. Moulin DE, Hagen N, Feasby TE, et al. Pain in Guillain-Barré syndrome. *Neurology* 1997;48:328–331.
759. Morley JB, Reynolds EH. Papilloedema and the Landry-Guillain-Barré syndrome. Case reports and a review. *Brain* 1966;89:205–222.
760. Sullivan RL Jr, Reeves AG. Normal cerebrospinal fluid protein, increased intracranial pressure, and the Guillain-Barré syndrome. *Ann Neurol* 1977;1:108–109.
761. Winer JB, Hughes RA. Identification of patients at risk of arrhythmia in the Guillain-Barré syndrome. *Q J Med* 1988;68:735–739.
762. Kuwabara S, Nakata M, Sung JY, et al. Hyperreflexia in axonal Guillain-Barré syndrome subsequent to *Campylobacter jejuni* enteritis. *J Neurol Sci* 2002;199:89–92.
763. Susuki K, Atsumi M, Koga M, et al. Acute facial diplegia and hyperreflexia: a Guillain-Barré syndrome variant. *Neurology* 2004;62:825–827.
764. Asbury AK, Cornblath DR. Assessment of current diagnostic criteria for Guillain-Barré syndrome. *Ann Neurol* 1990;27:S21–S24.
765. Ropper AH. The Guillain-Barré syndrome. *N Engl J Med* 1992; 326:1130–1136.
766. Briscoe DM, McMenamin JB, O'Donohoe NV. Prognosis in Guillain-Barré syndrome. *Arch Dis Child* 1987;62:733–735.
767. Das A, Kalita J, Misra UK. Recurrent Guillain-Barré syndrome. *Electromyogr Clin Neurophysiol* 2004;44:95–102.
768. Feasby TE, Gilbert JJ, Brown WF, et al. An acute axonal form of Guillain-Barré polyneuropathy. *Brain* 1986;109 (Pt 6):1115–1126.
769. Feasby TE, Hahn AF, Brown WF, et al. Severe axonal degeneration in acute Guillain-Barré syndrome: evidence of two different mechanisms? *J Neurol Sci* 1993;116:185–192.
770. Griffin JW, Li CY, Macko C, et al. Early nodal changes in the acute motor axonal neuropathy pattern of the Guillain-Barré syndrome. *J Neurocytol* 1996;25:33–51.
771. Hughes RA, Rees JH. Clinical and epidemiologic features of Guillain-Barré syndrome. *J Infect Dis* 1997;1769 Suppl 20:S92–S98.
772. Bertorini T, Narayanaswami P. Autoimmune neuropathies. *Compr Ther* 2003;29:194–209.
773. Ho TW, McKhann GM, Griffin JW. Human autoimmune neuropathies. *Annu Rev Neurosci* 1998;21:187–226.
774. Fisher M. An unusual variant of acute idiopathic polyneuritis (syndrome of ophthalmoplegia, ataxia and areflexia). *N Engl J Med* 1956;255:57–65.
775. Becker WJ, Watters GV, Humphreys P. Fisher syndrome in childhood. *Neurology* 1981;31:555–560.
776. Scelsa SN, Herskovitz S. Miller Fisher syndrome: axonal, demyelinating or both? *Electromyogr Clin Neurophysiol* 2000;40: 497–502.
777. Bell W, Van Allen M, Blackman J. Fisher syndrome in childhood. *Dev Med Child Neurol* 1970;12:758–766.
778. Landau WM, Glenn C, Dust G. MRI in Miller Fisher variant of Guillain-Barré syndrome. *Neurology* 1987;37:1431.
779. Shuaib A, Becker WJ. Variants of Guillain-Barré syndrome: Miller Fisher syndrome, facial diplegia and multiple cranial nerve palsies. *Can J Neurol Sci* 1987;14:611–616.
780. Jacobs BC, Endtz H, van der Meche FC, et al. Serum anti-GQ1b antibodies recognize surface epitopes on *Campylobacter jejuni* from patients with Miller Fisher syndrome. *Ann Neurol* 1995;37:260–264.
781. Nagashima T, Koga M, Odaka M, et al. Clinical correlates of serum anti-GT1a IgG antibodies. *J Neurol Sci* 2004;219:139–145.
782. Chiba A, Kusunoki S, Obata H, et al. Ganglioside composition of the human cranial nerves, with special reference to pathophysiology of Miller Fisher syndrome. *Brain Res* 1997;745: 32–36.
783. Roberts M, Willison H, Vincent A, et al. Serum factor in a variant of Guillain-Barré syndrome and neurotransmitter release. *Lancet* 1994;343:454–455.
784. Plomp JJ, Molenaar PC, O'Hanlon GM, et al. Miller Fisher anti-GQ1b antibodies: alpha-latrotoxin–like effects on motor end plates. *Ann Neurol* 1999;45:189–199.
785. Bickerstaff ER. Brain-stem encephalitis; further observations on a grave syndrome with benign prognosis. *Br Med J* 1957;1384–1387.
786. Odaka M, Yuki N, Yamada M, et al. Bickerstaff's brainstem encephalitis: clinical features of 62 cases and a subgroup associated with Guillain-Barré syndrome. *Brain* 2003;126:2279–2290.
787. Jamal GA, Ballantyne JP. The localization of the lesion in patients with acute ophthalmoplegia, ataxia and areflexia (Miller Fisher syndrome). A serial multimodal neurophysiological study. *Brain* 1988;111(Pt 1):95–114.
788. Petty RK, Duncan R, Jamal GA, et al. Brainstem encephalitis and the Miller Fisher syndrome. *J Neurol Neurosurg Psychiatry* 1993;56:201–203.

789. Connolly AM. Chronic inflammatory demyelinating polyneuropathy in childhood. *Pediatr Neurol* 2001;24:177–182.
790. Byers RK, Taft LT. Chronic multiple peripheral neuropathy in childhood. *Pediatrics* 1957;20:517–537.
791. McCombe PA, Pollard JD, McLeod JG. Chronic inflammatory demyelinating polyradiculoneuropathy. A clinical and electrophysiological study of 92 cases. *Brain* 1987;110(Pt 6):1617–1630.
792. Tasker W, Chutorian AM. Chronic polyneuritis of childhood. *J Pediatr* 1969;74:699–708.
793. Matsumuro K, Izumo S, Umehara F, et al. Chronic inflammatory demyelinating polyneuropathy: histological and immunopathological studies on biopsied sural nerves. *J Neurol Sci* 1994;127:170–178.
794. Yoshino H, Inuzuka T, Miyatake T. IgG antibody against GM1, GD1b and asialo-GM1 in chronic polyneuropathy following *Mycoplasma pneumoniae* infection. *Eur Neurol* 1992;32: 28–31.
795. Connolly AM, Pestronk A. Anti-tubulin autoantibodies in acquired demyelinating polyneuropathies. *J Infect Dis* 1997;176 (Suppl 2):S157–S159.
796. Tiwari JL, Terasaki PI. *HLA and disease associations*. New York: Springer-Verlag, 1985.
797. Vaughan RW, Adam AM, Gray IA, et al. Major histocompatibility complex class I and class II polymorphism in chronic idiopathic demyelinating polyradiculoneuropathy. *J Neuroimmunol* 1990;27:149–153.
798. Subcommittee of the American Academy of Neurology AIDS Task Force. Research criteria for diagnosis of chronic inflammatory demyelinating polyneuropathy (CIDP). *Neurology* 1991;41:617–618.
799. Burns TM. Chronic demyelinating polyradiculoneuropathy. *Arch Neurol* 2004;973–975.
800. Calia LC, Oliveira AS, Gabbai AA. Chronic inflammatory demyelinating polyradiculoneuropathy. Study of 18 cases [in Portuguese]. *Arq Neuropsiquiatr* 1997;55:712–721.
801. Pleasure DE, Towfighi J. Onion bulb neuropathies. *Arch Neurol* 1972;26:289–301.
802. Ropper AH. Unusual clinical variants and signs in Guillain-Barré syndrome. *Arch Neurol* 1986;43:1150–1152.
803. Ropper AH. Further regional variants of acute immune polyneuropathy. Bifacial weakness or sixth nerve paresis with paresthesias, lumbar polyradiculopathy, and ataxia with pharyngeal-cervical-brachial weakness. *Arch Neurol* 1994;51:671–675.
804. Buompadre MC, Ganez LA, Miranda M, et al. Unusual variants of Guillain-Barré syndrome in children. *Rev Neurol* 2005:in press.
805. MacLennan SC, Fahey MC, Lawson JA. Pharyngeal-cervical-brachial variant Guillain-Barré syndrome in a child. *J Child Neurol* 2004;19:626–627.
806. Osaki Y, Koga M, Matsubayashi K, et al. Asymmetric pharyngeal-cervical-brachial weakness associated with anti-GT1a IgG antibody. *Acta Neurol Scand* 2002;106:234–235.
807. National Institute of Neurological and Communications Disorders and Stroke. Criteria for diagnosis of Guillain-Barré syndrome. *Ann Neurol* 1978;3:565–566.
808. Landry O. Note sur la paralysie ascendante aiguë. *Gaz Hebd Med Chir* 1859;6:472–474.
809. Berciano J, Pascual J. Selective contrast enhancement of anterior spinal nerve roots on magnetic resonance imaging: a suggestive sign of Guillain-Barré syndrome and neurobrucellosis. *J Peripher Nerv Syst* 2003;8:135.
810. Coskun A, Kumandas S, Pac A, et al. Childhood Guillain-Barré syndrome. MR imaging in diagnosis and follow-up. *Acta Radiol* 2003;44:230–235.
811. Alexander JP Jr, Baden L, Pallansch MA, et al. Enterovirus 71 infections and neurologic disease—United States, 1977–1991. *J Infect Dis* 1994;169:905–908.
812. Haddad S, Arabi Y, Shimemeri AA. Hypokalemic paralysis mimicking Guillain-Barré syndrome and causing acute respiratory failure. *Middle East J Anesthesiol* 2004;17:891–897.
813. Czaplinski A, Steck AJ. Immune mediated neuropathies—an update on therapeutic strategies. *J Neurol* 2004;251:127–137.
814. Donofrio PD. Immunotherapy of idiopathic inflammatory neuropathies. *Muscle Nerve* 2003;28:273–292.
815. Kieseier BC, Hartung HP. Therapeutic strategies in the Guillain-Barré syndrome. *Semin Neurol* 2003;23:159–168.
816. Hughes RA, Wijdicks EF, Barohn R, et al. Practice parameter: immunotherapy for Guillain-Barré syndrome: report of the Quality Standards Subcommittee of the American Academy of Neurology. *Neurology* 2003;61:736–740.
817. The Dutch Guillain-Barré Study Group. Treatment of Guillain-Barré syndrome with high-dose immune globulins combined with methylprednisolone: a pilot study. *Ann Neurol* 1994;35:749–752.
818. van Koningsveld R, Schmitz PI, Meche FG, et al. Effect of methylprednisolone when added to standard treatment with intravenous immunoglobulin for Guillain-Barré syndrome: randomised trial. *Lancet* 2004;363:192–196.
819. Austin JH. Recurrent polyneuropathies and their corticosteroid treatment; with five-year observations of a placebo-controlled case treated with corticotrophin, cortisone, and prednisone. *Brain* 1958;81:157–192.
820. Dyck PJ, O'Brien PC, Oviatt KF, et al. Prednisone improves chronic inflammatory demyelinating polyradiculoneuropathy more than no treatment. *Ann Neurol* 1982;11:136–141.
821. Sharief MK, Ingram DA, Swash M, et al. I. v. immunoglobulin reduces circulating proinflammatory cytokines in Guillain-Barré syndrome. *Neurology* 1999;52:1833–1838.
822. van der Meché FGA, Schmitz PIM, and the Dutch Guillain-Barré Study Group. A randomized trial comparing intravenous immune globulin and plasma exchange in Guillain-Barré syndrome. *N Engl J Med* 1992;326:1123–1129.
823. Hughes RAC, Raphaël JC, Swan AV, et al. Intravenous immunoglobulin for Guillain-Barré syndrome. *Cochrane Database Syst Rev* 2004;4:CD002063.
824. Dalakas MC. Intravenous immunoglobulin in the treatment of autoimmune neuromuscular diseases: present status and practical therapeutic guidelines. *Muscle Nerve* 1999;22:1479–1497.
825. Bleck TP. IVIg for GBS: potential problems in the alphabet soup. *Neurology* 1993;43:857–858.
826. Castro LH, Ropper AH. Human immune globulin infusion in Guillain-Barré syndrome: worsening during and after treatment. *Neurology* 1993;43:1034–1036.
827. Hughes RAC, Raphael JC, van Doorn PA. Intravenous immunoglobulin for Guillain-Barré syndrome. *Cochrane Database Syst Rev* 2004;1:CD002063.
828. Korach JM, Petitpas D, Paris B, et al. Plasma exchange in France: epidemiology 2001. *Transfus Apheresis Sci* 2003;29:153–157.
829. Epstein MA, Sladky JT. The role of plasmapheresis in childhood Guillain-Barré syndrome. *Ann Neurol* 1990;28:65–69.
830. Jansen PW, Perkin RM, Ashwal S. Guillain-Barré syndrome in childhood: natural course and efficacy of plasmapheresis. *Pediatr Neurol* 1993;9:16–20.
831. The French Cooperative Group on Plasma Exchanges in Guillain-Barré syndrome. Appropriate number of plasma exchanges in Guillain-Barré syndrome. *Ann Neurol* 1997;41:298–306.
832. Mehndiratta MM, Hughes RA, Agarwal P. Plasma exchange for chronic inflammatory demyelinating polyradiculoneuropathy. *Cochrane Database Syst Rev* 2004;CD003906.
833. Rosenberg NL, Lacy JR, Kennaugh RC, et al. Treatment of refractory chronic demyelinating polyneuropathy with lymphoid irradiation. *Muscle Nerve* 1985;8:223–232.
834. Vermeulen M, Van Oers MH. Successful autologous stem cell transplantation in a patient with chronic inflammatory demyelinating polyneuropathy. *J Neurol Neurosurg Psychiatry* 2002;72:127–128.
835. Clynes R. Immune complexes as therapy for autoimmunity. *J Clin Invest* 2005;115:25–27.
836. Creange A, Chazaud B, Plonquet A, et al. IFN-beta decreases adhesion and transmigration capacities of lymphocytes in Guillain-Barré syndrome. *Neurology* 2001;57:1704–1706.
837. Creange A, Chazaud B, Sharshar T, et al. Inhibition of the adhesion step of leukodiapedesis: a critical event in the recovery of Guillain-Barré syndrome associated with accumulation of proteolytically active lymphocytes in blood. *J Neuroimmunol* 2001;114:188–196.

838. Kieseier BC, Seifert T, Giovannoni G, et al. Matrix metalloproteinases in inflammatory demyelination: targets for treatment. *Neurology* 1999;53:20–25.
839. Cole GF, Matthew DJ. Prognosis in severe Guillain-Barré syndrome. *Arch Dis Child* 1987;62:288–291.
840. Garssen MP, Bussmann JB, Schmitz PI, et al. Physical training and fatigue, fitness, and quality of life in Guillain-Barré syndrome and CIDP. *Neurology* 2004;63:2393–2395.
841. Dornonville de la Cour C, Andersen H, Stalberg E, et al. Electrophysiological signs of permanent axonal loss in a follow-up study of patients with Guillain-Barré syndrome. *Muscle Nerve* 2005;31:70–77.
842. Bell C. On the nerves of the face, being a second paper on that subject. *Phil Trans* 1829;111:317–339.
843. Zülch KJ. Idiopathic facial paresis. In: Vinken PJ, Bruyn GW, eds. *Handbook of clinical neurology*, Vol. 8: *Diseases of nerves*, Part 2. Amsterdam: Elsevier Science, 1968: 241–302.
844. Grose C, Henle W, Henle G, et al. Primary Epstein-Barr-virus infections in acute neurologic diseases. *N Engl J Med* 1975;292:392–395.
845. Berry C, MacKie RM. A case of facial diplegia associated with herpes simplex reactivation. *Eur J Neurol* 1998;5:305–307.
846. Christen HJ, Bartlau N, Hanefeld F, et al. Peripheral facial palsy in childhood—Lyme borreliosis to be suspected unless proven otherwise. *Acta Paediatr Scand* 1990;79:1219–1224.
847. Abramsky O, Webb C, Teitelbaum D, Arnon R. Cellular immune response to peripheral nerve basic protein in idiopathic facial paralysis (Bell's palsy). *J Neurol Sci* 1975;26:13–20.
848. Jonsson L, Sjoberg O, Thomander L. Activated T cells and Leu-7+ cells in Bell's palsy. *Acta Otolaryngol* 1988;105:108–113.
849. Kunishige M, Mitsui T, Yoshino H, et al. Isolated cranial neuropathy associated with anti-glycolipid antibodies. *J Neurol Sci* 2004;225:51–55.
850. Kanoh N, Nomura J, Satomi F. Nocturnal onset and development of Bell's palsy. *Laryngoscope* 2005;115:99–100.
851. Alter M. Familial aggregation of Bell's palsy. *Arch Neurol* 1963;8:557–564.
852. Paine RS. Facial paralysis in children; review of the differential diagnosis and report of ten cases treated with cortisone. *Pediatrics* 1957;19:303–316.
853. Benatar M, Edlow J. The spectrum of cranial neuropathy in patients with Bell's palsy. *Arch Intern Med* 2004;164:2383–2385.
854. Hanner P, Badr G, Rosenhall U, et al. Trigeminal dysfunction in patients with Bell's palsy. *Acta Otolaryngol* 1986;101:224–230.
855. Rousseau JJ, Godfroi ME, Husquinet H. Recurrent familial idiopathic facial paralysis [in French]. *Acta Neurol Belg* 1983;83: 23–28.
856. Roberg M, Ernerudh J, Forsberg P, et al. Acute peripheral facial palsy: CSF findings and etiology. *Acta Neurol Scand* 1991;83:55–60.
857. Sartoretti-Schefer S, Kollias S, Wichmann W, et al. T2-weighted three-dimensional fast spin-echo MR in inflammatory peripheral facial nerve palsy. *AJNR Am J Neuroradiol* 1998;19:491–495.
858. Salam EA, Elyahky WS. Evaluation of prognosis and treatment in Bell's palsy in children. *Acta Paediatr Scand* 1968;57:468–472.
859. Skogman BH, Croner S, Odkvist L. Acute facial palsy in children—a 2-year follow-up study with focus on Lyme neuroborreliosis. *Int J Pediatr Otorhinolaryngol* 2003;67:597–602.
860. Manning JJ, Adour KK. Facial paralysis in children. *Pediatrics* 1972;49:102–109.
861. Eidlitz-Markus T, Gilai A, Mimouni M, et al. Recurrent facial nerve palsy in paediatric patients. *Eur J Pediatr* 2001;160:659–663.
862. Park HW, Watkins AL. Facial paralysis; analysis of 500 cases. *Arch Phys Med Rehabil* 1949;30:749–762.
863. Wadlington WB, Riley HD Jr, Lowbeer L. The Melkersson-Rosenthal syndrome. *Pediatrics* 1984;73:502–506.
864. Stevens H. Melkersson's syndrome. *Neurology* 1965;15:263–266.
865. Kesler A, Vainstein G, Gadoth N. Melkersson-Rosenthal syndrome treated by methylprednisolone. *Neurology* 1998;51:1440–1441.
866. Pigozzi B, Fortina AB, Peserico A. Successful treatment of Melkersson-Rosenthal syndrome with lymecycline. *Eur J Dermatol* 2004;14:166–167.
867. Chutorian AM, Gold AP, Braun CW. Benign intracranial hypertension and Bell's palsy. *N Engl J Med* 1977;296:1214–1215.
868. Siegler RL, Brewer ED, Corneli HM, et al. Hypertension first seen as facial paralysis: case reports and review of the literature. *Pediatrics* 1991;87:387–389.
869. Indudharan R, Dharap AS, Ho TM. Intra-aural tick causing facial palsy. *Lancet* 1996;348:613.
870. Shaw M, Nazir F, Bone I. Bell's palsy: a study of the treatment advice given by neurologists. *J Neurol Neurosurg Psychiatry* 2005;76:293–294.
871. Huizing EH, Mechelse K, Staal A. Treatment of Bell's palsy. An analysis of the available studies. *Acta Otolaryngol* 1981;92:115–121.
872. Holland NJ, Weiner GM. Recent developments in Bell's palsy. *BMJ* 2004;329:553–557.
873. Ünüvar E, Oguz F, Sidal M, et al. Corticosteroid treatment of childhood Bell's palsy. *Pediatr Neurol* 1999;21:814–816.
874. Salman MS, MacGregor DL. Should children with Bell's palsy be treated with corticosteroids? A systematic review. *J Child Neurol* 2001;16:565–568.
875. Sullivan F, Daly F, Swan I. Recent developments in Bell's palsy: trial for Bell's palsy is in progress in Scotland. *BMJ* 2004;329:1103–1104.
876. May M, Klein SR, Taylor FH. Idiopathic (Bell's) facial palsy: natural history defies steroid or surgical treatment. *Laryngoscope* 1985;95:406–409.
877. Ford FR. Paroxysmal lacrimation during eating as a sequel of facial palsy (syndrome of crocodile tears): report of 4 cases with possible interpretation and comparison with auriculotemporal syndrome. *Arch Neurol Psychiatr* 1933;1279–1288.
878. Beurskens CH, Heymans PG. Positive effects of mime therapy on sequelae of facial paralysis: stiffness, lip mobility, and social and physical aspects of facial disability. *Otol Neurotol* 2003;24:677–681.
879. Devi S, Challenor Y, Duarte N, et al. Prognostic value of minimal excitability of facial nerve in Bell's palsy. *J Neurol Neurosurg Psychiatry* 1978;41:649–652.
880. Knox DL, Clark DB, Schuster FF. Benign VI nerve palsies in children. *Pediatrics* 1967;40:560–564.
881. Wang CH, Choud ML, Huang CH. Benign isolated abducens nerve palsy in *Mycoplasma pneumoniae* infection. *Pediatr Neurol* 1998;18:71–72.
882. Gradenigo G. Uber circumscripte leptomeningitis mit spinalen symptomen und uber paralyse des n. abducens ototischen ursprungs. *Arch Ohrenh* 1904;51:255–270.
883. Afifi AK, Bell WE, Bale JF, et al. Recurrent lateral rectus palsy in childhood. *Pediatr Neurol* 1990;6:315–318.
884. Edin M, Sveger T, Tegner H, et al. Isolated temporary pharyngeal paralysis in childhood. *Lancet* 1976;1:1047–1049.
885. Auberge C, Ponsot G, Gayraud P, et al. Acquired isolated velopalatine hemiparalysis in children [in French]. *Arch Fr Pediatr* 1979;36:283–286.
886. Blau JN, Harris M, Kennett S. Trigeminal sensory neuropathy. *N Engl J Med* 1969;281:873–876.
887. Roberton DM, Mellor DH. Asymmetrical palatal paresis in childhood: a transient cranial mononeuropathy? *Dev Med Child Neurol* 1982;24:842–846.
888. Wright GD, Lee KD. An isolated right hypoglossal nerve palsy in association with infectious mononucleosis. *Postgrad Med J* 1980;56:185–186.
889. Kuroki S, Saida T, Nukina M, et al. Three patients with ophthalmoplegia associated with *Campylobacter jejuni*. *Pediatr Neurol* 2001;25:71–74.
890. Lyu RK, Chen ST. Acute multiple cranial neuropathy: a variant of Guillain-Barré syndrome? *Muscle Nerve* 2004;30:433–436.
891. Younger DS. Vasculitis of the nervous system. *Curr Opin Neurol* 2004;17:317–336.
892. Schoen FJ, Cotran RS. Blood vessels. In: Cotran RS, Kumar V, Collins T, eds. *Robbin's Pathologic basis of disease*. Philadelphia: Saunders, 1999: 515–524.
893. Benseler S, Schneider R. Central nervous system vasculitis in children. *Curr Opin Rheumatol* 2004;16:43–50.

894. Cravioto H, Feigin I. Noninfectious granulomatous angiitis with a predilection for the nervous system. *Neurology* 1959;9:599–609.
895. Calabrese LH, Furlan AJ, Gragg LA, et al. Primary angiitis of the central nervous system: diagnostic criteria and clinical approach. *Cleve Clin J Med* 1992;59:293–306.
896. Calabrese L. Primary angiitis of the central nervous system: the penumbra of vasculitis. *J Rheumatol* 2001;28:465–466.
897. Gallagher KT, Shaham B, Reiff A, et al. Primary angiitis of the central nervous system in children: 5 cases. *J Rheumatol* 2001;28:616–623.
898. Lanthier S, Lortie A, Michaud J, et al. Isolated angiitis of the CNS in children. *Neurology* 2001;56:837–842.
899. Ilhan A, Budak F. Primary angiitis of the central nervous system: unusual clinical presentation. *Int J Angiol* 2000;9:23–26.
900. Caccamo DV, Garcia JH, Ho KL. Isolated granulomatous angiitis of the spinal cord. *Ann Neurol* 1992;32:580–582.
901. Kumar R, Wijdicks EF, Brown RD Jr, et al. Isolated angiitis of the CNS presenting as subarachnoid haemorrhage. *J Neurol Neurosurg Psychiatry* 1997;62:649–651.
902. Hajj-Ali RA, Furlan A, Abou-Chebel A, et al. Benign angiopathy of the central nervous system: cohort of 16 patients with clinical course and long-term followup. *Arthritis Rheum* 2002;47:662–669.
903. Moore PM. Diagnosis and management of isolated angiitis of the central nervous system. *Neurology* 1989;39:167–173.
904. Nishikawa M, Sakamoto H, Katsuyama J, et al. Multiple appearing and vanishing aneurysms: primary angiitis of the central nervous system. Case report. *J Neurosurg* 1998;88:133–137.
905. Shuangshoti S. Localized granulomatous (giant cell) angiitis of brain with eosinophil infiltration and saccular aneurysm. *J Med Assoc Thai* 1979;62:281–289.
906. Cognard C, Weill A, Lindgren S, et al. Basilar artery occlusion in a child: "clot angioplasty" followed by thrombolysis. *Childs Nerv Syst* 2000;16:496–500.
907. Kwon SU, Koh JY, Kim JS. Vertebrobasilar artery territory infarction as an initial manifestation of systemic lupus erythematosus. *Clin Neurol Neurosurg* 1999;101:62–67.
908. Roach ES. Cerebrovascular disorders and trauma in children. *Curr Opin Pediatr* 1993;5:660–668.
909. Aydin K, Okuyaz C, Gucuyener K, et al. Moyamoya disease presented with migrainelike headache in a 4-year-old girl. *J Child Neurol* 2003;18:361–363.
910. Mettinger KL, Ericson K. Fibromuscular dysplasia and the brain. I. Observations on angiographic, clinical and genetic characteristics. *Stroke* 1982;13:46–52.
911. Derry C, Dale RC, Thom M, et al. Unihemispheric cerebral vasculitis mimicking Rasmussen's encephalitis. *Neurology* 2002;58:327–328.
912. Stone JH, Pomper MG, Roubenoff R, et al. Sensitivities of noninvasive tests for central nervous system vasculitis: a comparison of lumbar puncture, computed tomography, and magnetic resonance imaging. *J Rheumatol* 1994;21:1277–1282.
913. Matsell DG, Keene DL, Jimenez C, et al. Isolated angiitis of the central nervous system in childhood. *Can J Neurol Sci* 1990;17:151–154.
914. Nylen K, Karlsson JE, Blomstrand C, et al. Cerebrospinal fluid neurofilament and glial fibrillary acidic protein in patients with cerebral vasculitis. *J Neurosci Res* 2002;67:844–851.
915. Benseler S, Tsang LM, Tyrell PN, et al. Primary CNS vasculitis in children. *Arthritis Rheum* 2002;46:S311.
916. Yuh WT, Ueda T, Maley JE. Perfusion and diffusion imaging: a potential tool for improved diagnosis of CNS vasculitis. *AJNR Am J Neuroradiol* 1999;20:87–89.
917. Wasserman BA, Stone JH, Hellmann DB, et al. Reliability of normal findings on MR imaging for excluding the diagnosis of vasculitis of the central nervous system. *AJR Am J Roentgenol* 2001;177:455–459.
918. Calabrese LH, Duna GF. Evaluation and treatment of central nervous system vasculitis. *Curr Opin Rheumatol* 1995;7:37–44.
919. Greenan TJ, Grossman RI, Goldberg HI. Cerebral vasculitis: MR imaging and angiographic correlation. *Radiology* 1992;182:65–72.
920. Pomper MG, Miller TJ, Stone JH, et al. CNS vasculitis in autoimmune disease: MR imaging findings and correlation with angiography. *AJNR Am J Neuroradiol* 1999;20:75–85.
921. Alhalabi M, Moore PM. Serial angiography in isolated angiitis of the central nervous system. *Neurology* 1994;44:1221–1226.
922. Imbesi SG. Diffuse cerebral vasculitis with normal results on brain MR imaging. *AJR Am J Roentgenol* 1999;173:1494–1496.
923. Sener RN. Diffusion MRI findings in isolated intracranial angiitis. *Comput Med Imaging Graph* 2002;26:265–269.
924. Duna GF, Calabrese LH. Limitations of invasive modalities in the diagnosis of primary angiitis of the central nervous system. *J Rheumatol* 1995;22:662–667.
925. Chu CT, Gray L, Goldstein LB, et al. Diagnosis of intracranial vasculitis: a multi-disciplinary approach. *J Neuropathol Exp Neurol* 1998;57:30–38.
926. Schluter A, Hirsch W, Jassoy A, et al. MR angiography in diagnosis of vasculitis and benign angiopathies of the central nervous system [in German]. *Rofo Fortschr Geb Rontgenstr Neuen Bildgeb Verfahr* 2001;173:522–527.
927. Moritani T, Hiwatashi A, Shrier DA, et al. CNS vasculitis and vasculopathy: efficacy and usefulness of diffusion-weighted echoplanar MR imaging. *Clin Imaging* 2004;28:261–270.
928. Hirsch W, Hiebsch W, Teichler H, et al. Transcranial Doppler sonography in children: review of a seven-year experience. *Clin Radiol* 2002;57:492–497.
929. Ritter MA, Dziewas R, Papke K, et al. Follow-up examinations by transcranial Doppler ultrasound in primary angiitis of the central nervous system. *Cerebrovasc Dis* 2002;14:139–142.
930. Alrawi A, Trobe JD, Blaivas M, et al. Brain biopsy in primary angiitis of the central nervous system. *Neurology* 1999;53:858–860.
931. Lie JT. Primary (granulomatous) angiitis of the central nervous system: a clinicopathologic analysis of 15 new cases and a review of the literature. *Hum Pathol* 1992;23:164–171.
932. Vollmer TL, Guarnaccia J, Harrington W, et al. Idiopathic granulomatous angiitis of the central nervous system. Diagnostic challenges. *Arch Neurol* 1993;50:925–930.
933. Lasner TM, Sutton LN, Rorke LB. Multifocal noninfectious granulomatous encephalitis in a child. Case report. *J Neurosurg* 1997;86:1042–1045.
934. Panda KM, Santosh V, Yasha TC, et al. Primary angiitis of CNS: neuropathological study of three autopsied cases with brief review of literature. *Neurol India* 2000;48:149–154.
935. Cupps TR, Moore PM, Fauci AS. Isolated angiitis of the central nervous system. Prospective diagnostic and therapeutic experience. *Am J Med* 1983;74:97–105.
936. Barron TF. Isolated angiitis of CNS: treatment with pulse cyclophosphamide. *Pediatr Neurol* 1993;9:73–75.
937. Woolfenden AR, Tong DC, Marks MP, et al. Angiographically defined primary angiitis of the CNS: is it really benign? *Neurology* 1998;51:183–188.
938. Shukla G, Deol PS, Arora R, et al. Isolated angiitis of the central nervous system: report of a patient with an unusually prolonged course. *Eur Neurol* 2001;46:162–163.
939. Hajj-Ali RA, Villa-Forte AL, Abou-Chebel A. Long term outcome of patients with primary angiitis of the central nervous system (PACNS). *Arthritis Rheum* 2000;43:S162.
940. Calabrese LH, Gragg LA, Furlan AJ. Benign angiopathy: a distinct subset of angiographically defined primary angiitis of the central nervous system. *J Rheumatol* 1993;20:2046–2050.
941. Chabrier S, Rodesch G, Lasjaunias P, et al. Transient cerebral arteriopathy: a disorder recognized by serial angiograms in children with stroke. *J Child Neurol* 1998;13:27–32.
942. Berger JR, Romano J, Menkin M, et al. Benign focal cerebral vasculitis: case report. *Neurology* 1995;45:1731–1734.
943. Takeoka M, Takahashi T. Infectious and inflammatory disorders of the circulatory system and stroke in childhood. *Curr Opin Neurol* 2002;15:159–164.
944. Dastur DK, Manghani DK, Udani PM. Pathology and pathogenetic mechanisms in neurotuberculosis. *Radiol Clin North Am* 1995;33:733–752.
945. Lan SH, Chang WN, Lu CH, et al. Cerebral infarction in chronic meningitis: a comparison of tuberculous meningitis and cryptococcal meningitis. *QJM* 2001;94:247–253.

946. Johns DR, Tierney M, Parker SW. Pure motor hemiplegia due to meningovascular neurosyphilis. *Arch Neurol* 1987;44:1062–1065.
947. Wilke M, Eiffert H, Christen HJ, et al. Primarily chronic and cerebrovascular course of Lyme neuroborreliosis: case reports and literature review. *Arch Dis Child* 2000;83:67–71.
948. Socan M, Ravnik I, Bencina D, et al. Neurological symptoms in patients whose cerebrospinal fluid is culture- and/or polymerase chain reaction–positive for *Mycoplasma pneumoniae*. *Clin Infect Dis* 2001;32:E31–35.
949. Askalan R, Laughlin S, Mayank S, et al. Chickenpox and stroke in childhood: a study of frequency and causation. *Stroke* 2001;32:1257–1262.
950. Berger TM, Caduff JH, Gebbers JO. Fatal varicella-zoster virus antigen–positive giant cell arteritis of the central nervous system. *Pediatr Infect Dis J* 2000;19:653–656.
951. Hattori H, Higuchi Y, Tsuji M. Recurrent strokes after varicella. *Ann Neurol* 2000;47:136.
952. Moriuchi H, Rodriguez W. Role of varicella-zoster virus in stroke syndromes. *Pediatr Infect Dis J* 2000;19:648–653.
953. Rohatgi A, Monga R, Goyal D. Japanese encephalitis with movement disorder and atypical magnetic resonance imaging. *J Assoc Physicians India* 2000;48:834–835.
954. Hoffmann M, Berger JR, Nath A, et al. Cerebrovascular disease in young, HIV-infected, black Africans in the KwaZulu Natal province of South Africa. *J Neurovirol* 2000;6:229–236.
955. Legido A, Lischner HW, De Chadarevian JP, et al. Stroke in pediatric HIV infection. *Pediatr Neurol* 1999;21:588.
956. Kaplan SL, Fishman MA. Update on bacterial meningitis. *J Child Neurol* 1988;3:82–93.
957. Allison JW, Davis PC, Sato Y, et al. Intracranial aneurysms in infants and children. *Pediatr Radiol* 1998;28:223–229.
958. Amacher LA, Drake CG. Cerebral artery aneurysms in infancy, childhood and adolescence. *Childs Brain* 1975;1:72–80.
959. O'Donohue JM, Enzmann DR. Mycotic aneurysm in angiitis associated with herpes zoster ophthalmicus. *AJNR Am J Neuroradiol* 1987;8:615–619.
960. Dubrovsky T, Curless R, Scott G, et al. Cerebral aneurysmal arteriopathy in childhood AIDS. *Neurology* 1998;51:560–565.
961. Fulmer BB, Dillard SC, Musulman EM, et al. Two cases of cerebral aneurysms in HIV+ children. *Pediatr Neurosurg* 1998;28:31–34.
962. Kleinschmidt-DeMasters BK, Gilden DH. Varicella-zoster virus infections of the nervous system: clinical and pathologic correlates. *Arch Pathol Lab Med* 2001;125:770–780.
963. Gilden DH, Mahalingam R, Cohrs RJ, et al. The protean manifestations of varicella-zoster virus vasculopathy. *J Neurovirol* 2002;8(Suppl 2):75–79.
964. Gilden DH, Kleinschmidt-DeMasters BK, LaGuardia JJ, et al. Neurologic complications of the reactivation of varicella-zoster virus. *N Engl J Med* 2000;342:635–645.
965. Sebire G, Meyer L, Chabrier S. Varicella as a risk factor for cerebral infarction in childhood: a case–control study. *Ann Neurol* 1999;45:679–680.
966. Gilden D. Varicella zoster virus and central nervous system syndromes. *Herpes* 2004;11(Suppl 2):89A–94A.
967. deVeber G. Stroke and the child's brain: an overview of epidemiology, syndromes and risk factors. *Curr Opin Neurol* 2002;15:133–138.
968. Gilden DH, Bennett JL, Kleinschmidt–DeMasters BK, et al. The value of cerebrospinal fluid antiviral antibody in the diagnosis of neurologic disease produced by varicella zoster virus. *J Neurol Sci* 1998;159:140–144.
969. Melanson M, Chalk C, Georgevich L, et al. Varicella-zoster virus DNA in CSF and arteries in delayed contralateral hemiplegia: evidence for viral invasion of cerebral arteries. *Neurology* 1996;47:569–570.
970. Doyle PW, Gibson G, Dolman CL. Herpes zoster ophthalmicus with contralateral hemiplegia: identification of cause. *Ann Neurol* 1983;14:84–85.
971. Frank Y, Lim W, Kahn E, et al. Multiple ischemic infarcts in a child with AIDS, varicella zoster infection, and cerebral vasculitis. *Pediatr Neurol* 1989;5:64–67.
972. Frank Y, Lu D, Pavlakis S, et al. Childhood AIDS, varicella zoster, and cerebral vasculopathy. *J Child Neurol* 1997;12:464–466.
973. Alehan FK, Boyvat F, Baskin E, et al. Focal cerebral vasculitis and stroke after chickenpox. *Eur J Paediatr Neurol* 2002;6:331–333.
974. McKelvie PA, Collins S, Thyagarajan D, et al. Meningoencephalomyelitis with vasculitis due to varicella zoster virus: a case report and review of the literature. *Pathology* 2002;34:88–93.
975. Singhal AB, Singhal BS, Ursekar MA, et al. Serial MR angiography and contrast-enhanced MRI in chickenpox-associated stroke. *Neurology* 2001;56:815–817.
976. Patsalides AD, Wood LV, Atac GK, et al. Cerebrovascular disease in HIV–infected pediatric patients: neuroimaging findings. *AJR Am J Roentgenol* 2002;179:999–1003.
977. Connor MD, Lammie GA, Bell JE, et al. Cerebral infarction in adult AIDS patients: observations from the Edinburgh HIV Autopsy Cohort. *Stroke* 2000;31:2117–2126.
978. Gillams AR, Allen E, Hrieb K, et al. Cerebral infarction in patients with AIDS. *AJNR Am J Neuroradiol* 1997;18:1581–1585.
979. Husson RN, Saini R, Lewis LL, et al. Cerebral artery aneurysms in children infected with human immunodeficiency virus. *J Pediatr* 1992;121:927–930.
980. Kure K, Park YD, Kim TS, et al. Immunohistochemical localization of an HIV epitope in cerebral aneurysmal arteriopathy in pediatric acquired immunodeficiency syndrome (AIDS). *Pediatr Pathol* 1989;9:655–667.
981. Mazzoni P, Chiriboga CA, Millar WS, et al. Intracerebral aneurysms in human immunodeficiency virus infection: case report and literature review. *Pediatr Neurol* 2000;23:252–255.
982. Moriarty DM, Haller JO, Loh JP, et al. Cerebral infarction in pediatric acquired immunodeficiency syndrome. *Pediatr Radiol* 1994;24:611–612.
983. Park YD, Belman AL, Kim TS, et al. Stroke in pediatric acquired immunodeficiency syndrome. *Ann Neurol* 1990;28:303–311.
984. Picard O, Brunereau L, Pelosse B, et al. Cerebral infarction associated with vasculitis due to varicella zoster virus in patients infected with the human immunodeficiency virus. *Biomed Pharmacother* 1997;51:449–454.
985. Shah SS, Zimmerman RA, Rorke LB, et al. Cerebrovascular complications of HIV in children. *AJNR Am J Neuroradiol* 1996;17:1913–1917.
986. Visudtibhan A, Visudhiphan P, Chiemchanya S. Stroke and seizures as the presenting signs of pediatric HIV infection. *Pediatr Neurol* 1999;20:53–56.
987. Sharer LR, Epstein LG, Cho ES, et al. Pathologic features of AIDS encephalopathy in children: evidence for LAV/HTLV–III infection of brain. *Hum Pathol* 1986;17:271–284.
988. Younger DS, Calabrese LH, Hays AP. Granulomatous angiitis of the nervous system. *Neurol Clin* 1997;15:821–834.
989. Dickson DW, Belman AL, Park YD, et al. Central nervous system pathology in pediatric AIDS: an autopsy study. *APMIS Suppl* 1989;8:40–57.
990. Sharer LR, Cho ES. Neuropathology of HIV infection: adults versus children. *Prog AIDS Pathol* 1989;1:131–141.
991. Sharer LR, Saito Y, Blumberg BM. Neuropathology of human immunodeficiency virus-1 infection of the brain. In: Berger JR, Levy RM, eds. *AIDS and the nervous system*. Philadelphia: Lippincott–Raven, 1997: 461–471.
992. Price RW. Neurological complications of HIV infection. *Lancet* 1996;348:445–452.
993. Yankner BA, Skolnik PR, Shoukimas GM, et al. Cerebral granulomatous angiitis associated with isolation of human T-lymphotropic virus type III from the central nervous system. *Ann Neurol* 1986;20:362–364.
994. Calabrese LH, Estes M, Yen-Lieberman B, et al. Systemic vasculitis in association with human immunodeficiency virus infection. *Arthritis Rheum* 1989;32:569–576.
995. Nogueras C, Sala M, Sasal M, et al. Recurrent stroke as a manifestation of primary angiitis of the central nervous system in a patient infected with human immunodeficiency virus. *Arch Neurol* 2002;59:468–473.
996. Raphael SA, Price ML, Lischner HW, et al. Inflammatory demyelinating polyneuropathy in a child with symptomatic human immunodeficiency virus infection. *J Pediatr* 1991;118:242–245.
997. Sladky JT. Immune neuropathies in childhood. *Baillieres Clin Neurol* 1996;5:233–244.

998. Gherardi RK, Chretien F, Delfau-Larue MH, et al. Neuropathy in diffuse infiltrative lymphocytosis syndrome: an HIV neuropathy, not a lymphoma. *Neurology* 1998;50:1041–1044.
999. Younger DS, Rosoklija G, Neinstedt LJ, et al. HIV-1 associated sensory neuropathy: a patient with peripheral nerve vasculitis. *Muscle Nerve* 1996;19:1364–1366.
1000. Younger DS, Rposoklija G, Hays AP. Sensory neuropathy in AIDS: demonstration of vasculitis and HIV antigens in peripheral nerve. *J Neurol* 1994;241:S17.
1001. Ford RG, Siekert RG. Central nervous system manifestations of periarteritis nodosa. *Neurology* 1965;15:114–122.
1002. Nadeau SE. Neurologic manifestations of systemic vasculitis. *Neurol Clin* 2002;20:123–150.
1003. Ozen S. The spectrum of vasculitis in children. *Best Pract Res Clin Rheumatol* 2002;16:411–425.
1004. Hunder GG, Arend WP, Bloch DA, et al. The American College of Rheumatology 1990 criteria for the classification of vasculitis. Introduction. *Arthritis Rheum* 1990;33:1065–1067.
1005. Ronco P, Verroust P, Mignon F, et al. Immunopathological studies of polyarteritis nodosa and Wegener's granulomatosis: a report of 43 patients with 51 renal biopsies. *Q J Med* 1983;52:212–223.
1006. Ozdogan H, Arisoy N, Kasapcapur O, et al. Vasculitis in familial Mediterranean fever. *J Rheumatol* 1997;24:323–327.
1007. Said R, Hamzeh Y, Said S, et al. Spectrum of renal involvement in familial Mediterranean fever. *Kidney Int* 1992;41:414–419.
1008. Kissel JT, Riethman JL, Omerza J, et al. Peripheral nerve vasculitis: immune characterization of the vascular lesions. *Ann Neurol* 1989;25:291–297.
1009. Malamud NA. A case of periarteritis nodosa with decerebrate rigidity and extensive encephalomalacia in a five-year-old child. *J Neuropathol Exp Neurol* 1945;4:88–92.
1010. Engel DG, Gospe SM Jr, Tracy KA, et al. Fatal infantile polyarteritis nodosa with predominant central nervous system involvement. *Stroke* 1995;26:699–701.
1011. Moore PM, Fauci AS. Neurologic manifestations of systemic vasculitis. A retrospective and prospective study of the clinicopathologic features and responses to therapy in 25 patients. *Am J Med* 1981;71:517–524.
1012. Guillevin L, Cohen P, Mahr A, et al. Treatment of polyarteritis nodosa and microscopic polyangiitis with poor prognosis factors: a prospective trial comparing glucocorticoids and six or twelve cyclophosphamide pulses in sixty-five patients. *Arthritis Rheum* 2003;49:93–100.
1013. Ettlinger RE, Nelson AM, Burke EC, et al. Polyarteritis nodosa in childhood a clinical pathologic study. *Arthritis Rheum* 1979;22:820–825.
1014. Bleehen SS, Lovelace RE, Cotton RE. Mononeuritis multiplex in polyarteritis nodosa. *Q J Med* 1963;32:193–209.
1015. Morfin-Maciel B, Medina A, Espinosa Rosales F, et al. Central nervous system involvement in a child with polyarteritis nodosa and severe atopic dermatitis. *Rev Alerg Mex* 2002;49:189–195.
1016. Ragge NK, Harris CM, Dillon MJ, et al. Ocular tilt reaction due to a mesencephalic lesion in juvenile polyarteritis nodosa. *Am J Ophthalmol* 2003;135:249–251.
1017. Magilavy DB, Petty RE, Cassidy JT, et al. A syndrome of childhood polyarteritis. *J Pediatr* 1977;91:25–30.
1018. Oran I, Memis A, Parildar M, et al. Multiple intracranial aneurysms in polyarteritis nodosa: MRI and angiography. *Neuroradiology* 1999;41:436–439.
1019. Bulun A, Topaloglu R, Duzova A, et al. Ataxia and peripheral neuropathy: rare manifestations in Henoch-Schonlein purpura. *Pediatr Nephrol* 2001;16:1139–1141.
1020. Suda K, Matsumura M, Ohta S. Kawasaki disease complicated by cerebral infarction. *Cardiol Young* 2003;13:103–105.
1021. Tabarki B, Mahdhaoui A, Selmi H, et al. Kawasaki disease with predominant central nervous system involvement. *Pediatr Neurol* 2001;25:239–241.
1022. Calabro JJ, Londino A Jr, Weber CA. Preventing coronary involvement in Kawasaki disease. *JAMA* 1986;255–200.
1023. Koren G, Rose V, Lavi S, et al. Probable efficacy of high-dose salicylates in reducing coronary involvement in Kawasaki disease. *JAMA* 1985;254:767–769.
1024. Newburger JW, Takahashi M, Beiser AS, et al. A single intravenous infusion of gamma globulin as compared with four infusions in the treatment of acute Kawasaki syndrome. *N Engl J Med* 1991;324:1633–1639.
1025. Deshpande PV, Gilbert R, Alton H, et al. Microscopic polyarteritis with renal and cerebral involvement. *Pediatr Nephrol* 2000;15:134–135.
1026. Nishino H, Rubino FA, Parisi JE. The spectrum of neurologic involvement in Wegener's granulomatosis. *Neurology* 1993;43:1334–1337.
1027. von Scheven E, Lee C, Berg BO. Pediatric Wegener's granulomatosis complicated by central nervous system vasculitis. *Pediatr Neurol* 1998;19:317–319.
1028. Rottem M, Fauci AS, Hallahan CW, et al. Wegener granulomatosis in children and adolescents: clinical presentation and outcome. *J Pediatr* 1993;122:26–31.
1029. Schor NF. Neurology of systemic autoimmune disorders: a pediatric perspective. *Semin Pediatr Neurol* 2000;7:108–117.
1030. Jimenez C, Rowe PC, Keene D. Cardiac and central nervous system vasculitis in a child with dermatomyositis. *J Child Neurol* 1994;9:297–300.
1031. Halbreich U, Assael M, Kauly N, et al. Rheumatic brain disease: a disease in its own right. *J Nerv Ment Dis* 1976;163:24–28.
1032. Aksentijevich I, Nowak M, Mallah M, et al. *De novo* CIAS1 mutations, cytokine activation, and evidence for genetic heterogeneity in patients with neonatal-onset multisystem inflammatory disease (NOMID): a new member of the expanding family of pyrin-associated autoinflammatory diseases. *Arthritis Rheum* 2002;46:3340–3348.
1033. de Boeck H, Scheerlinck T, Otten J. The CINCA syndrome: a rare cause of chronic arthritis and multisystem inflammatory disorders. *Acta Orthop Belg* 2000;66:433–437.
1034. Leone V, Presani G, Perticarari S, et al. Chronic infantile neurological cutaneous articular syndrome: CD10 over-expression in neutrophils is a possible key to the pathogenesis of the disease. *Eur J Pediatr* 2003;162:669–673.
1035. Hawkins PN, Lachmann HJ, Aganna E, et al. Spectrum of clinical features in Muckle-Wells syndrome and response to anakinra. *Arthritis Rheum* 2004;50:607–612.
1036. Ando Y, Kai S, Uyama E, et al. Involvement of the central nervous system in rheumatoid arthritis: its clinical manifestations and analysis by magnetic resonance imaging. *Intern Med* 1995;34:188–191.
1037. Chin RL, Latov N. Central nervous system manifestations of rheumatologic diseases. *Curr Opin Rheumatol* 2005;17:91–99.
1038. Vollertsen RS, Conn DL. Vasculitis associated with rheumatoid arthritis. *Rheum Dis Clin North Am* 1990;16:445–461.
1039. Yamashita Y, Takahashi M, Sakamoto Y, et al. Atlantoaxial subluxation. Radiography and magnetic resonance imaging correlated to myelopathy. *Acta Radiol* 1989;30:135–140.
1040. Jan JE, Hill RH, Low MD. Cerebral complications in juvenile rheumatoid arthritis. *Can Med Assoc J* 1972;107:623–625.
1041. Sundelin F. Investigations of the cerebrospinal fluid in cases of rheumathoid arthritis. *Am J Med* 1947;2:579–587.
1042. Carbajal-Rodriguez L, Perea-Martinez A, Loredo-Abdala A, et al. Neurologic involvement in juvenile rheumatoid arthritis [in Spanish]. *Bol Med Hosp Infant Mex* 1991;48:502–508.
1043. Fink CW. Medical treatment of juvenile arthritis. *Clin Orthop* 1990;60–69.
1044. Turesson C, Matteson EL. Management of extra-articular disease manifestations in rheumatoid arthritis. *Curr Opin Rheumatol* 2004;16:206–211.
1045. Unger L, Kayser M, Nusslein HG. Successful treatment of severe rheumatoid vasculitis by infliximab. *Ann Rheum Dis* 2003;62:587–588.
1046. Rhodes VJ. Physical therapy management of patients with juvenile rheumatoid arthritis. *Phys Ther* 1991;71:910–919.
1047. Foeldvari I. Scleroderma in children. *Curr Opin Rheumatol* 2002;14:699–703.
1048. Appenzeller S, Montenegro MA, Dertkigil SS, et al. Neuroimaging findings in scleroderma en coup de sabre. *Neurology* 2004;62:1585–1589.
1049. Grosso S, Fioravanti A, Biasi G, et al. Linear scleroderma associated with progressive brain atrophy. *Brain Dev* 2003;25:57–61.

1050. Kasapcopur O, Ozkan HC, Tuysuz B. Linear scleroderma en coup de sabre and brain calcification: is there a pathogenic relationship? *J Rheumatol* 2003;30:2724–2725.
1051. Nobili F, Cutolo M, Sulli A, et al. Brain functional involvement by perfusion SPECT in systemic sclerosis and Behcet's disease. *Ann N Y Acad Sci* 2002;966:409–414.
1052. Poncelet AN, Connolly MK. Peripheral neuropathy in scleroderma. *Muscle Nerve* 2003;28:330–335.
1053. Cimaz R, Casadei A, Rose C, et al. Primary Sjogren syndrome in the paediatric age: a multicentre survey. *Eur J Pediatr* 2003;162:661–665.
1054. Oetgen WJ, Boice JA, Lawless OJ. Mixed connective tissue disease in children and adolescents. *Pediatrics* 1981;67:333–337.
1055. Kone-Paut I, Bernard JL. Behcet disease in children in France [in French]. *Arch Fr Pediatr* 1993;50:561–565.
1056. Siva A, Altintas A, Saip S. Behcet's syndrome and the nervous system. *Curr Opin Neurol* 2004;17:347–357.
1057. Gold R, Fontana A, Zierz S. Therapy of neurological disorders in systemic vasculitis. *Semin Neurol* 2003;23:207–214.
1058. Akman-Demir G, Bahar S, Coban O, et al. Cranial MRI in Behcet's disease: 134 examinations of 98 patients. *Neuroradiology* 2003;45:851–859.
1059. Al-Araji A, Sharquie K, Al-Rawi Z. Prevalence and patterns of neurological involvement in Behcet's disease: a prospective study from Iraq. *J Neurol Neurosurg Psychiatry* 2003;74:608–613.
1060. Lampert F, Belohradsky BH, Forster C, et al. Letter: Infantile chronic relapsing inflammation of the brain, skin, and joints. *Lancet* 1975;1:1250–1251.
1061. Devlin T, Gray L, Allen NB, et al. Neuro-Behcet's disease: factors hampering proper diagnosis. *Neurology* 1995;45:1754–1757.
1062. Hadfield MG, Aydin F, Lippman HR, et al. Neuro-Behcet's disease. *Clin Neuropathol* 1997;16:55–60.
1063. Akman–Demir G, Serdaroglu P, Tasci B. Clinical patterns of neurological involvement in Behcet's disease: evaluation of 200 patients. The Neuro-Behcet Study Group. *Brain* 1999;122(Pt 11):2171–2182.
1064. Kikuchi S, Niino M, Shinpo K, et al. Intracranial hemorrhage in neuro-Behcet's syndrome. *Intern Med* 2002;41:692–695.
1065. Grippo J, Zocchi G, Fleiderman S, et al. Behcet's disease in children: cortical calcifications [in Spanish]. *Rev Neurol* 2002;35:209–211.
1066. Humberclaude V, Vallee L, Sukno S, et al. Cerebral venous thrombosis disclosing Behcet disease. *Arch Fr Pediatr* 1993;50:603–605.
1067. Lackmann GM, Lyding S, Scherer A, et al. Acute disseminated encephalomyelitis and mucocutaneous ulcerations. *Neuropediatrics* 2004;35:253–254.
1068. Kuriwaka R, Kunishige M, Nakahira H, et al. Neuro-Behcet's disease with chorea after remission of intestinal Behcet's disease. *Clin Rheumatol* 2004;23:364–367.
1069. Ashjazadeh N, Borhani Haghighi A, Samangooie S, et al. Neuro-Behcet's disease: a masquerader of multiple sclerosis. A prospective study of neurologic manifestations of Behcet's disease in 96 Iranian patients. *Exp Mol Pathol* 2003;74:17–22.
1070. Motomura S, Tabira T, Kuroiwa Y. A clinical comparative study of multiple sclerosis and neuro-Behcet's syndrome. *J Neurol Neurosurg Psychiatry* 1980;43:210–213.
1071. Saruhan-Direskeneli G, Yentur SP, Akman-Demir G, et al. Cytokines and chemokines in neuro-Behcet's disease compared to multiple sclerosis and other neurological diseases. *J Neuroimmunol* 2003;145:127–134.
1072. Worthmann F, Bruns J, Turker T, et al. Muscular involvement in Behcet's disease: case report and review of the literature. *Neuromuscul Disord* 1996;6:247–253.
1073. Wechsler B, Dell'lsola B, Vidailhet M, et al. MRI in 31 patients with Behcet's disease and neurological involvement: prospective study with clinical correlation. *J Neurol Neurosurg Psychiatry* 1993;56:793–798.
1074. Morrissey SP, Miller DH, Hermaszewski R, et al. Magnetic resonance imaging of the central nervous system in Behcet's disease. *Eur Neurol* 1993;33:287–293.
1075. Imoto H, Nishizaki T, Nogami K, et al. Neuro-Behcet's disease manifesting as a neoplasm-like lesion—-case report. *Neurol Med Chir* (Tokyo) 2002;42:406–409.
1076. Kermode AG, Plant GT, MacManus DG, et al. Behcet's disease with slowly enlarging midbrain mass on MRI: resolution following steroid therapy. *Neurology* 1989;39:1251–1252.
1077. Park JH, Jung MK, Bang CO, et al. Neuro-Behcet's disease mimicking a cerebral tumor: a case report. *J Korean Med Sci* 2002;17:718–722.
1078. Tuzgen S, Kaya AH, Erdincler D, et al. Two cases of neuro-Behcet's disease mimicking cerebral tumor. *Neurol India* 2003;51:376–378.
1079. Vignola S, Nobili F, Picco P, et al. Brain perfusion spect in juvenile neuro-Behcet's disease. *J Nucl Med* 2001;42:1151–1157.
1080. Stigsby B, Bohlega S, al-Kawi MZ, et al. Evoked potential findings in Behcet's disease. Brain-stem auditory, visual, and somatosensory evoked potentials in 44 patients. *Electroencephalogr Clin Neurophysiol* 1994;92:273–281.
1081. Evans RW, Akman-Demir G. Behcet syndrome and headache. *Headache* 2004;44:102–104.
1082. Palacio E, Rodero L, Pascual J. Topiramate-responsive headache due to idiopathic intracranial hypertension in Behcet syndrome. *Headache* 2004;44:436–437.
1083. Monastero R, Camarda C, Pipia C, et al. Cognitive impairment in Behcet's disease patients without overt neurological involvement. *J Neurol Sci* 2004;220:99–104.
1084. Brown MM, Swash M. Systemic lupus erythematosus. In: Vinken PJ, Bruyn GW, Klawans HL, eds. *Handbook of clinical neurology, revised series, vascular diseases,* Part III, Vol. 55. Amsterdam: Elsevier, 1989: 369–385.
1085. King KK, Kornreich HK, Bernstein BH, et al. The clinical spectrum of systemic lupus erythematosus in childhood. *Arthritis Rheum* 1977;20:287–294.
1086. Yancey CL, Doughty RA, Athreya BH. Central nervous system involvement in childhood systemic lupus erythematosus. *Arthritis Rheum* 1981;24:1389–1395.
1087. Moore PM, Lisak RP. Systemic lupus erythematosus: immunopathogenesis of neurologic dysfunction. *Springer Semin Immunopathol* 1995;17:43–60.
1088. Hanly JG, Walsh NM, Sangalang V. Brain pathology in systemic lupus erythematosus. *J Rheumatol* 1992;19:732–741.
1089. Belmont HM, Abramson SB, Lie JT. Pathology and pathogenesis of vascular injury in systemic lupus erythematosus. Interactions of inflammatory cells and activated endothelium. *Arthritis Rheum* 1996;39:9–22.
1090. Wallace DJ, Metzger AL. Systemic lupus and the nervous system. In: Wallace DJ, Han BH, eds. *Dubois' Lupus erythematosus,* 4th ed. Philadelphia: Lea & Febiger, 1993: 370–385.
1091. Ellis SG, Verity MA. Central nervous system involvement in systemic lupus erythematosus: a review of neuropathologic findings in 57 cases, 1955–1977. *Semin Arthritis Rheum* 1979;8:212–221.
1092. Malamud N, Saver G. Neuropathologic findings in disseminated lupus erythematosus. *AMA Arch Neurol Psychiatry* 1954;71:723–731.
1093. Devinsky O, Petito CK, Alonso DR. Clinical and neuropathological findings in systemic lupus erythematosus: the role of vasculitis, heart emboli, and thrombotic thrombocytopenic purpura. *Ann Neurol* 1988;23:380–384.
1094. Trysberg E, Tarkowski A. Cerebral inflammation and degeneration in systemic lupus erythematosus. *Curr Opin Rheumatol* 2004;16:527–533.
1095. Pullmann R Jr, Skerenova M, Hybenova J, et al. Apolipoprotein E polymorphism in patients with neuropsychiatric SLE. *Clin Rheumatol* 2004;23:97–101.
1096. Cervera R, Piette JC, Font J, et al. Antiphospholipid syndrome: clinical and immunologic manifestations and patterns of disease expression in a cohort of 1,000 patients. *Arthritis Rheum* 2002;46:1019–1027.
1097. Zaccagni H, Fried J, Cornell J, et al. Soluble adhesion molecule levels, neuropsychiatric lupus and lupus-related damage. *Front Biosci* 2004;9:1654–1659.
1098. Bonfa E, Golombek SJ, Kaufman LD, et al. Association between lupus psychosis and anti-ribosomal P protein antibodies. *N Engl J Med* 1987;317:265–271.
1099. Isshi K, Hirohata S. Differential roles of the anti-ribosomal P antibody and antineuronal antibody in the pathogenesis of central

nervous system involvement in systemic lupus erythematosus. *Arthritis Rheum* 1998;41:1819–1827.
1100. Nojima Y, Minota S, Yamada A, et al. Correlation of antibodies to ribosomal P protein with psychosis in patients with systemic lupus erythematosus. *Ann Rheum Dis* 1992;51:1053–1055.
1101. Sato T, Uchiumi T, Ozawa T, et al. Autoantibodies against ribosomal proteins found with high frequency in patients with systemic lupus erythematosus with active disease. *J Rheumatol* 1991;18:1681–1684.
1102. Schneebaum AB, Singleton JD, West SG, et al. Association of psychiatric manifestations with antibodies to ribosomal P proteins in systemic lupus erythematosus. *Am J Med* 1991;90:54–62.
1103. Tzioufas AG, Tzortzakis NG, Panou-Pomonis E, et al. The clinical relevance of antibodies to ribosomal-P common epitope in two targeted systemic lupus erythematosus populations: a large cohort of consecutive patients and patients with active central nervous system disease. *Ann Rheum Dis* 2000;59:99–104.
1104. Yoshio T, Masuyama J, Ikeda M, et al. Quantification of antiribosomal P0 protein antibodies by ELISA with recombinant P0 fusion protein and their association with central nervous system disease in systemic lupus erythematosus. *J Rheumatol* 1995;22:1681–1687.
1105. Koren E, Reichlin MW, Koscec M, et al. Autoantibodies to the ribosomal P proteins react with a plasma membrane–related target on human cells. *J Clin Invest* 1992;89:1236–1241.
1106. Williams RC Jr, Sugiura K, Tan EM. Antibodies to microtubule-associated protein 2 in patients with neuropsychiatric systemic lupus erythematosus. *Arthritis Rheum* 2004;50:1239–1247.
1107. Alcocer-Varela J, Aleman-Hoey D, Alarcon-Segovia D. Interleukin-1 and interleukin-6 activities are increased in the cerebrospinal fluid of patients with CNS lupus erythematosus and correlate with local late T-cell activation markers. *Lupus* 1992;1:111–117.
1108. Hirohata S, Tanimoto K, Ito K. Elevation of cerebrospinal fluid interleukin-6 activity in patients with vasculitides and central nervous system involvement. *Clin Immunol Immunopathol* 1993;66:225–229.
1109. Dellalibera-Joviliano R, Dos Reis ML, Cunha Fde Q, et al. Kinins and cytokines in plasma and cerebrospinal fluid of patients with neuropsychiatric lupus. *J Rheumatol* 2003;30:485–492.
1110. Svenungsson E, Andersson M, Brundin L, et al. Increased levels of proinflammatory cytokines and nitric oxide metabolites in neuropsychiatric lupus erythematosus. *Ann Rheum Dis* 2001;60:372–379.
1111. Trysberg E, Carlsten H, Tarkowski A. Intrathecal cytokines in systemic lupus erythematosus with central nervous system involvement. *Lupus* 2000;9:498–503.
1112. Trysberg E, Nylen K, Rosengren LE, et al. Neuronal and astrocytic damage in systemic lupus erythematosus patients with central nervous system involvement. *Arthritis Rheum* 2003;48:2881–2887.
1113. Tsai CY, Wu TH, Tsai ST, et al. Cerebrospinal fluid interleukin-6, prostaglandin E2 and autoantibodies in patients with neuropsychiatric systemic lupus erythematosus and central nervous system infections. *Scand J Rheumatol* 1994;23:57–63.
1114. Kelly MC, Denburg JA. Cerebrospinal fluid immunoglobulins and neuronal antibodies in neuropsychiatric systemic lupus erythematosus and related conditions. *J Rheumatol* 1987;14:740–744.
1115. Zvaifler NJ, Bluestein HG. The pathogenesis of central nervous system manifestations of systemic lupus erythematosus. *Arthritis Rheum* 1982;25:862–866.
1116. Press J, Palayew K, Laxer RM, et al. Antiribosomal P antibodies in pediatric patients with systemic lupus erythematosus and psychosis. *Arthritis Rheum* 1996;39:671–676.
1117. Levine SR, Kieran S, Puzio K, et al. Cerebral venous thrombosis with lupus anticoagulants. Report of two cases. *Stroke* 1987;18:801–804.
1118. van Dam AP. Diagnosis and pathogenesis of CNS lupus. *Rheumatol Int* 1991;11:1–11.
1119. Mackworth-Young C. Antiphospholipid antibodies: more than just a disease marker? *Immunol Today* 1990;11:60–65.
1120. Loh WF, Hussain IM, Soffiah A, et al. Neurological manifestations of children with systemic lupus erythematosus. *Med J Malaysia* 2000;55:459–463.
1121. Turkel SB, Miller JH, Reiff A. Case series: neuropsychiatric symptoms with pediatric systemic lupus erythematosus. *J Am Acad Child Adolesc Psychiatry* 2001;40:482–485.
1122. Trysberg E, Hoglund K, Svenungsson E, et al. Decreased levels of soluble amyloid beta-protein precursor and beta-amyloid protein in cerebrospinal fluid of patients with systemic lupus erythematosus. *Arthritis Res Ther* 2004;6:R129–R136.
1123. Steens SC, Bosma GP, ten Cate R, et al. A neuroimaging follow up study of a patient with juvenile central nervous system systemic lupus erythematosus. *Ann Rheum Dis* 2003;62:583–586.
1124. Baca V, Lavalle C, Garcia R, et al. Favorable response to intravenous methylprednisolone and cyclophosphamide in children with severe neuropsychiatric lupus. *J Rheumatol* 1999;26:432–439.
1125. Wright EC, Tullus K, Dillon MJ. Retrospective study of plasma exchange in children with systemic lupus erythematosus. *Pediatr Nephrol* 2004;19:1108–1114.
1126. Karassa FB, Ioannidis JP, Boki KA, et al. Predictors of clinical outcome and radiologic progression in patients with neuropsychiatric manifestations of systemic lupus erythematosus. *Am J Med* 2000;109:628–634.
1127. Bale JF Jr. Neurologic complications of immunization. *J Child Neurol* 2004;19:405–412.
1128. Piyasirisilp S, Hemachudha T. Neurological adverse events associated with vaccination. *Curr Opin Neurol* 2002;15:333–338.
1129. Fitzpatrick M. MMR: risk, choice, chance. *Br Med Bull* 2004;69:143–153.
1130. Adams RD, Kubik CS. The morbid anatomy of the demyelinative disease. *Am J Med* 1952;12:510–546.
1131. Spillane JD, Wells CE. The neurology of Jennerian vaccination. A clinical account of the neurological complications which occurred during the smallpox epidemic in South Wales in 1962. *Brain* 1964;87:1–44.
1132. Cereghino JJ, Osterud HT, Pinnas JL, et al. Rabies: a rare disease but a serious pediatric problem. *Pediatrics* 1970;45:839–844.
1133. Mozar HN, Finnigan FB, Petzold H, et al. Myelopathy after duck embryo rabies vaccine. *JAMA* 1973;224:1605–1607.
1134. Hemachudha T, Phanuphak P, Johnson RT, et al. Neurologic complications of Semple-type rabies vaccine: clinical and immunologic studies. *Neurology* 1987;37:550–556.
1135. Laouini D, Kennou MF, Khoufi S, et al. Antibodies to human myelin proteins and gangliosides in patients with acute neuroparalytic accidents induced by brain-derived rabies vaccine. *J Neuroimmunol* 1998;91:63–72.
1136. Piyasirisilp S, Schmeckpeper BJ, Chandanayingyong D, et al. Association of HLA and T-cell receptor gene polymorphisms with Semple rabies vaccine–induced autoimmune encephalomyelitis. *Ann Neurol* 1999;45:595–600.
1137. Murthy JM. MRI in acute disseminated encephalomyelitis following Semple antirabies vaccine. *Neuroradiology* 1998;40:420–423.
1138. Fenichel GM. Neurological complications of immunization. *Ann Neurol* 1982;12:119–128.
1139. Fenichel GM. Pertussis: the disease and the vaccine. *Pediatr Neurol* 1988;4:201–206.
1140. Fenichel GM, Lane DA, Livengood JR, et al. Adverse events following immunization: assessing probability of causation. *Pediatr Neurol* 1989;5:287–290.
1141. Byers RK, Moll FC. Encephalopathies following prophylactic pertussis vaccine. *Pediatrics* 1948;1:437–457.
1142. Cody CL, Baraff LJ, Cherry JD, et al. Nature and rates of adverse reactions associated with DTP and DT immunizations in infants and children. *Pediatrics* 1981;68:650–660.
1143. Morris SA, Bernstein HH. Immunizations, neonatal jaundice, and animal-induced injuries. *Curr Opin Pediatr* 2004;16:450–460.
1144. Blumberg DA, Lewis K, Mink CM, et al. Severe reactions associated with diphtheria-tetanus-pertussis vaccine: detailed study of children with seizures, hypotonic-hyporesponsive episodes, high fevers, and persistent crying. *Pediatrics* 1993;91:1158–1165.
1145. Pollock TM, Miller E, Mortimer JY, et al. Symptoms after primary immunisation with DTP and with DT vaccine. *Lancet* 1984;2:146–149.

1146. Baraff LJ, Shields WD, Beckwith L, et al. Infants and children with convulsions and hypotonic-hyporesponsive episodes following diphtheria-tetanus-pertussis immunization: follow-up evaluation. *Pediatrics* 1988;81:789–794.
1147. Gross TP, Milstien JB, Kuritsky JN. Bulging fontanelle after immunization with diphtheria–tetanus–pertussis vaccine and diphtheria–tetanus vaccine. *J Pediatr* 1989;114:423–425.
1148. Stewart GT. Vaccination against whooping-cough. Efficacy versus risks. *Lancet* 1977;1:234–237.
1149. Miller D, Madge N, Diamond J, et al. Pertussis immunisation and serious acute neurological illnesses in children. *BMJ* 1993;307:1171–1176.
1150. Murphy JV, Sarff LD, Marquardt KM. Recurrent seizures after diphtheria, tetanus, and pertussis vaccine immunization. Onset less than 24 hours after vaccination. *Am J Dis Child* 1984;138:908–911.
1151. Kulenkampff M, Schwartzman JS, Wilson J. Neurological complications of pertussis inoculation. *Arch Dis Child* 1974;49:46–49.
1152. Walker AM, Jick H, Perera DR, et al. Neurologic events following diphtheria-tetanus-pertussis immunization. *Pediatrics* 1988;81:345–349.
1153. Corsellis JA, Janota I, Marshall AK. Immunization against whooping cough: a neuropathological review. *Neuropathol Appl Neurobiol* 1983;9:261–270.
1154. Black WJ, Munoz JJ, Peacock MG, et al. ADP-ribosyltransferase activity of pertussis toxin and immunomodulation by *Bordetella pertussis*. *Science* 1988;240:656–659.
1155. Dolphin AC, Scott RH. Modulation of Ca2+ channel currents in sensory neurons by pertussis toxin-sensitive G-proteins. *Ann N Y Acad Sci* 1989;560:387–390.
1156. Koulen P, Liu J, Nixon E, Madry C. Interaction between mGluR8 and calcium channels in photoreceptors is sensitive to pertussis toxin and occurs via G protein {beta}{gamma} subunit signaling. *Invest Ophthalmol Vis Sci* 2005;46:287–291.
1157. Grant CC, McKay EJ, Simpson A, et al. Pertussis encephalopathy with high cerebrospinal fluid antibody titers to pertussis toxin and filamentous hemagglutinin. *Pediatrics* 1998;102:986–990.
1158. Howson CP, Howe CJ, Fineberg HV. *Adverse effects of pertussis and rubella vaccines*. Washington, DC: National Academic Press, 1991.
1159. Edwards KM, Decker MD, Halsey NA, et al. Differences in antibody response to whole-cell pertussis vaccines. *Pediatrics* 1991;88:1019–1023.
1159a. Institute of Medicine. DPT vaccine and chronic nervous system dysfunction: a new analysis. Washington, DC: 1994, National Academy Press.
1160. Geier DA, Geier MR. An evaluation of serious neurological disorders following immunization: a comparison of whole-cell pertussis and acellular pertussis vaccines. *Brain Dev* 2004;26:296–300.
1161. Kuno-Sakai H, Kimura M. Safety and efficacy of acellular pertussis vaccine in Japan, evaluated by 23 years of its use for routine immunization. *Pediatr Int* 2004;46:650–655.
1162. Miller D, Madge N, Diamond J, et al. Pertussis immunisation and serious acute neurological illnesses in children. *BMJ* 1993;307:1171–1176.
1163. Gray JA, Burns SM. Mumps meningitis following measles, mumps, and rubella immunisation. *Lancet* 1989;2:98.
1164. Kennedy RC, Byers VS, Marchalonis JJ. Measles virus infection and vaccination: potential role in chronic illness and associated adverse events. *Crit Rev Immunol* 2004;24:129–156.
1165. Weibel RE, Caserta V, Benor DE, et al. Acute encephalopathy followed by permanent brain injury or death associated with further attenuated measles vaccines: a review of claims submitted to the National Vaccine Injury Compensation Program. *Pediatrics* 1998;101:383–387.
1166. Wakefield AJ, Much SH, Anthony A, et al. Ileal-lymphoid-nodular hyperplasia, non-specific colitis, and pervasive developmental disorder in children. *Lancet* 1998;351:637–641.
1167. Taylor B, Miller E, Farrington CP, et al. Autism and measles, mumps, and rubella vaccine: no epidemiological evidence for a causal association. *Lancet* 1999;353:2026–2029.
1168. Chez MG, Chin K, Hung PC. Immunizations, immunology, and autism. *Semin Pediatr Neurol* 2004;11:214–217.
1169. Madsen KM, Hviid A, Vestergaard M, et al. A population-based study of measles, mumps, and rubella vaccination and autism. *N Engl J Med* 2002;347:1477–1482.
1170. Makela A, Nuorti JP, Peltola H. Neurologic disorders after measles-mumps-rubella vaccination. *Pediatrics* 2002;110:957–963.
1171. Read SJ, Schapel GJ, Pender MP. Acute transverse myelitis after tetanus toxoid vaccination. *Lancet* 1992;339:1111–1112.
1172. Hopkins IJ. A new syndrome: poliomyelitis-like illness associated with acute asthma in childhood. *Aust Paediatr J* 1974;10:273–276.
1173. Beede HE, Newcomb RW. Lower motor neuron paralysis in association with asthma. *Johns Hopkins Med J* 1980;147:186–187.
1174. Manson JI, Thong YH. Immunological abnormalities in the syndrome of poliomyelitis-like illness associated with acute bronchial asthma (Hopkin's syndrome). *Arch Dis Child* 1980;55:26–32.

Chapter 9

Postnatal Trauma and Injuries by Physical Agents

John H. Menkes and Richard G. Ellenbogen

CRANIOCEREBRAL TRAUMA

In the Western world, accidents constitute the major cause of death of children between the ages of 5 and 19 years (Table 9.1) (1). From 1951 to 1971, the number of children with head injuries admitted to hospitals in Newcastle-upon-Tyne, United Kingdom, increased sixfold, reaching 13.9% of all admissions to pediatric wards (2). This increase probably was partially caused by a change in policy such that more apparently minor injuries were admitted for observation. In the United States, the situation is similar; cranial and major facial injuries are responsible for 3.6% of hospital admissions and 3.3% of days spent in the hospital, and they are the most common neurologic conditions requiring hospital admission for patients younger than 19 years of age (3). Head injury is now the most common cause of death and disability of children in the United States, causing death in approximately 7,000 children each year (4). It is also the cause of significant cognitive and motor-sensory dysfunction in the pediatric population, with an estimated economic burden approximating $10 billion a year in the United States alone (5).

A high proportion of head injuries cause death at the site of the accident or on the way to the hospital, so admission figures reflect only part of the incidence. In the San Diego Prospective Survey, as many as 85% of fatalities occurred at these times (6). Since the 1980s, child abuse has been recognized increasingly. The incidence of reported cases rose from 10.1 in 1,000 children in 1976 to 39 in 1,000 children in 1990 (7), with one of the more recent estimates of the incidence of fatal abuse in children younger than 4 years of age being at least 10 in 100,000 (8). As the reported frequency of maltreatment has risen, it has become an important cause of head injury. In one series, in infants younger than age 1 year, 36% of all head injuries and 95% of injuries resulting in intracranial hemorrhage or other major cerebral complications were caused by child abuse (9). In older children, the proportion of injury from abuse is lower, but still significant. In addition, children who were hospitalized as a consequence of child abuse remained in the hospital more than twice as long as other hospitalized children (10).

Although no accurate data exist, cranial trauma commonly occurs in childhood sports. Brain concussion occurs in an estimated 19 in 100 American football players per year. Bicycling is probably the second-most-common sport leading to head injury. In an Australian series published in 1987, bicycling was responsible for more than 20% of all head injuries in children (11). The remarkable effectiveness of bicycle helmets in preventing head injuries in children has been attested to in several studies (12,13).

This chapter presents only postnatal injuries; perinatal injuries are described in Chapter 6. This chapter discusses the diagnosis and nonsurgical management of head injuries and considers their pathophysiology and pathology based on the severity of the craniocerebral trauma and the complications and sequelae of head injuries.

Dynamics and Pathophysiology

The adverse effects of head injury are primary and secondary. The primary effects are the result of physical forces, mainly acceleration and deceleration, that act on the brain through shear-strain deformation (a change in shape without a change in volume) and through compression-rarefaction strain (a change in volume without a change in shape). The brain is injured through these two mechanisms acting alone, in combination, or in succession (14–16). Secondary effects result from the various processes that complicate the injury.

Shear-Strain Deformation

Shear strain occurs when two layers slide on each other, moving in parallel in opposite directions (16). The injury from shearing or tearing is responsible for most lesions, especially in an infant or a young child, whose skull is more easily deformed than an adult's. Deformation

TABLE 9.1 Causes of Death in Children in 1986

Cause of Death	Age <5 years	5–9 years	10–14 years	15–19 years
All causes	46,371	4,082	4,706	16,224
Accidents	5.5%	20.6%	18.3%	10.8%
Motor vehicle accidents	2.6%	26.2%	27.2%	43.1%
Influenza and pneumonia	0.9%	1.2%	0.9%	0.5%
Congenital anomalies	19.7%	6.3%	0.1%	1.6%
Malignant neoplasms	2.3%	21.3%	15.8%	7.1%

From U.S. Department of Health, Education and Welfare, Public Health Service, *Vital statistics of the United States*. Washington, DC: Author, 1986.

absorbs much of the energy of impact, reducing the adverse effects of acceleration and deceleration but adding to the risk of tearing of blood vessels. Because of its elasticity and ability to undergo a greater degree of deformation, the skull of an infant absorbs the energy of the physical impact and protects the brain better than the skull of an older person.

The relationship between stress waves and deformity depends mainly on the momentum of the head and of the object at the instant of impact. In a child with intact reflexes, a free fall probably causes more injury to the brain than an aimed object striking the head with even greater speed. Approximately 70% of shear-strain deformation skull fractures are linear and single; the rest are depressed fractures. The faster moving the object delivering the blow, the more likely it is that a depressed fracture will result; a lower-velocity impact with the same momentum tends to produce deformity and linear fracture, sometimes distant from the point of impact but at a weak part of the cranial vault where distortion can occur. In addition, the size of the object that strikes the skull is important. Objects smaller than 5 cm^2 tend to produce a depressed fracture; larger objects tend to produce a linear fracture (16). A linear fracture is usually not important in management of the child because outcome of the injury and its complications are determined by damage to the intracranial contents at the moment of impact; an injury can be fatal in the absence of a fracture.

Compression-Rarefaction Strains

In an acceleration injury, in which the momentary compression is greatest, the effects of compression-rarefaction strains are usually maximal at the point of impact; at the same time, an area of low pressure or rarefaction occurs contralaterally, the site of the familiar contrecoup injury (13,14), Thus, a blow to the occiput can result in the major damage in the frontal and temporal regions. Contrecoup injuries generally occur on the undersurface and poles of the frontal and temporal lobes (16). They are relatively rare in infants and young children, presumably because skull distortion rather than pressure waves predominate (19). Contrecoup injuries are most likely to occur when the impact is to the occiput or to the side of the head (16). Distortion of the brainstem is particularly likely in deceleration injuries such as those that occur in falls; any resulting loss of function in this area is liable to have serious or fatal consequences.

Magnetic resonance imaging (MRI) has allowed a better understanding of the lesions that can result from head injury. These were grouped into primary and secondary lesions by Gentry and coworkers (20) (Table 9.2). The injuries expected from various accident mechanisms are depicted in Table 9.3.

TABLE 9.2 Classification of Traumatic Intracranial Lesions

Primary Lesions
- Intraaxial
  - Diffuse axonal injury
  - Cortical contusion
  - Subcortical matter injury
  - Primary brainstem injury
- Extraaxial hematomas
  - Extradural
  - Subdural
- Diffuse hemorrhage
  - Subarachnoid
  - Intraventricular
- Primary vascular injuries

Secondary Lesions
- Pressure necrosis (secondary to brain displacement and herniations)
- Tentorial arterial infarction
- Diffuse hypoxic injury
- Diffuse brain swelling
- Boundary and terminal zone infarction
- Others
  - Fatty embolism
  - Secondary hemorrhage
  - Infection

From Gentry LR, Godersky JC, Thompson B. MR imaging of head trauma: review of the distribution and radiopathologic features of traumatic lesions. *AJR Am J Roentgenol* 1988;15:663. With permission.

TABLE 9.3 Expected Injury Types Associated with Accident Mechanisms in Young Children

Mechanism	*Injury Types*
Fall <4 ft	Concussion/soft tissue injury Linear fracture Epidural hematoma Ping-pong fracture ? Depressed fracture[a]
Fall >4 ft	Injuries listed for fall <4 ft plus the following: Depressed fracture Basilar fracture Multiple fractures Subarachnoid hemorrhage Contusion ? Subdural hematoma[a] ? Stellate fracture[a]
Motor vehicle accident	Injuries listed for falls plus the following: Subdural hematoma Diffuse axonal injury

[a]Injury types are uncommonly associated with the given mechanism.
From Dumaine AC. Head injury in very young children. *Pediatrics* 1992;90:184. With permission.

Diffuse Axonal Injury

The term *diffuse axonal injury* (DAI) refers to a clinical-pathologic-radiologic entity that clinically manifests itself by loss or impairment of consciousness.

The lesion usually is not the result of a fall, except when the fall occurs from a considerable height. Instead, it results from severe angular acceleration-deceleration forces (21) and is believed to induce coma through disconnection of the cortex from the lower centers. It is responsible for severe, irreversible, and potentially fatal brain damage occurring at the moment of injury. DAI is frequently unaccompanied by skull fracture, increased intracranial pressure, or cerebral contusion (21).

As viewed microscopically, the hallmark of DAI is the presence of axonal retraction balls identified by silver stains or, as in more recent studies, immunohistochemical staining for beta-amyloid precursor protein (16,22). Postmortem examinations have demonstrated axonal lesions in the inferior portion of the corpus callosum and the dorsolateral quadrant of the rostral brainstem, notably in the region of the superior cerebellar peduncles, and throughout the cerebral hemisphere and cerebellum (23–25). Damage to the superior cerebellar peduncles, which are particularly vulnerable to rotational injuries, is responsible for the ataxia commonly observed after major head injuries (26).

The microscopic picture of axonal lesions was first described by Strich (27), who proposed that the shearing forces sustained during injury cause stretching of axons, which might be sufficient to prevent them from functioning. The more subtle changes that precede this final state have been studied in animals by electron microscopy and through the use of immunocytochemical labeling techniques. Although the exact time course for humans has not been determined, in animals an alteration in the structure of the nodes of Ranvier occurs within 15 minutes of the injury (28). This is followed some 12 to 24 hours later by an interruption of antegrade and retrograde axonal transport, the loss of microtubules, and the gradual development of axonal swelling. When axonal swelling exceeds a certain critical level, effective transection of the axon occurs, although without evident tearing or damage to adjacent blood vessels. DAI is frequently accompanied by evidence of neuronal injury (29).

It is unclear how mechanical forces induce the instantaneous perturbation of the cell membrane that in turn initiates these axonal changes. Wolf and coworkers proposed that traumatic deformation of axons induces abnormal sodium influx through mechanically sensitive Na^+ channels. This influx subsequently triggers an increase in intraaxonal calcium through the opening of the voltage-gated calcium channel (30). This can result in activation of calmodulin and an increase of extracellular potassium at the damaged node (31). Intracellular calcium, in turn, increases the activity of proteolytic enzymes that disrupt axonal cytoarchitecture. Over time, the swollen axons either degenerate or undergo regenerative changes, as shown by sprouting and growth cones (32).

On MRI, axonal damage is best visualized by diffusion tensor imaging (DTI) or high-spatial-resolution susceptibility-weighted imaging techniques (33,34). By these techniques diffuse axonal injury appears as small, oval, focal abnormalities in white matter tracts, usually adjacent to cortical gray matter, but sometimes in the splenium of the corpus callosum (20). Proton magnetic resonance spectroscopy can provide further information on the extent of axonal injury. A lowered ratio of *N*-acetylaspartate (NAA) to creatine is believed to be indicative of axonal injury, but there does not appear to be any elevation of tissue lactate (35).

Cortical Contusion

The second-most-common type of brain injury visualized by MRI of patients with severe head trauma is cortical contusions, which tend to be multiple and represent bruises on the surface of the brain. As verified by both imaging and pathologic studies, points of predilection for contusions are the crests of gyri on the orbital surfaces of the frontal lobes and the inferolateral aspect of the temporal lobes. Contusions consist mainly of petechial hemorrhages in the superficial cortical layers occurring at the site of impact (coup injuries) or at contrecoup areas (Fig. 9.1). Impact on the forehead or vertex can send the initial pressure wave caudally, leading to downward displacement of the brain toward and into the tentorial opening. This

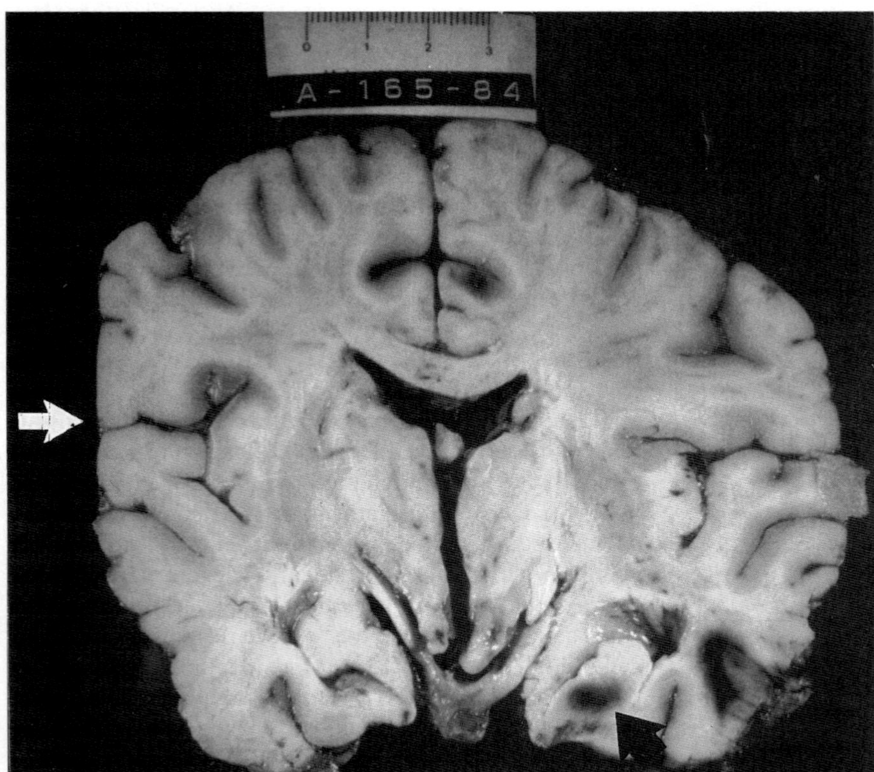

FIGURE 9.1. Contrecoup injury. A left-sided epidural hematoma not seen in the picture caused severe compression of the left cerebral hemisphere (*white arrow*). Hemorrhage in the right inferior temporal lobe (*black arrow*) probably represents a contrecoup injury. (Courtesy of Dr. Harry V. Vinters, Division of Neuropathology, UCLA Center for the Health Sciences, Los Angeles, CA.)

displacement can result in contusions of the hippocampal gyrus, particularly the uncus, the basal ganglia, and the upper part of the brainstem (36). The severity of brain damage caused by contusion depends on the extent of vascular injury. Damage tends to be less common in infants and small children than in older children or adults subjected to comparable trauma. Instead, contusions in infants consist of slitlike tears in the cerebral white matter of the frontal and temporal lobes (16,37). One of the major clinical issues in the management of contusions is their tendency to increase in size, coalesce, or cause a mass effect, especially after the first day following injury. Therefore, a follow-up imaging study is often useful.

Cerebral Laceration

Cerebral lacerations are usually the result of damage from penetrating wounds or depressed skull fractures, but they can occur without fracture in small children, whose skulls tend to become more grossly distorted at the moment of injury. Lacerations frequently involve the frontal and temporal poles and are associated primarily with tears of the dura and tears or other injuries of the major vessels and secondarily with thromboses, hemorrhages, or focal cerebral ischemia. Tears in the white matter are seen commonly in infants after blunt trauma even without fracture (38) (Fig. 9.2). They result from the soft consistency of the poorly myelinated cerebrum and from the pliancy of the immature skull.

MRI has demonstrated that macroscopic traumatic injuries to subcortical structures such as the thalamus and to the brainstem are rare. Instead, the pathologic change that results in the clinical picture generally attributed to primary brainstem damage is diffuse axonal injury.

Concussion

The physical processes within the skull caused by trauma induce numerous changes within the brain. The most common is concussion. Although there is some disagreement with respect to the definition of concussion, the American Academy of Neurology defines it as a trauma-induced alteration in mental status with or without loss of consciousness (39). In addition, there also can be post-traumatic amnesia for the moment of injury and for a variable period before it (retrograde amnesia).

The pathogenesis of concussion is under debate. From a structural viewpoint, concussion is believed to result from minor degrees of diffuse axonal injury. With more severe concussive injuries, there is a massive release of excitatory neurotransmitters, notably glutamate (40). As a result, there is a synchronized depolarization of neuronal membranes with subsequent increase of extracellular potassium (41), resulting in a functional deafferentation of the cortex (42). Compounding the disruption of ionic homeostasis is an imbalance between energy demands and supply, a loss of cerebral autoregulation in a significant proportion of patients with minor head injuries

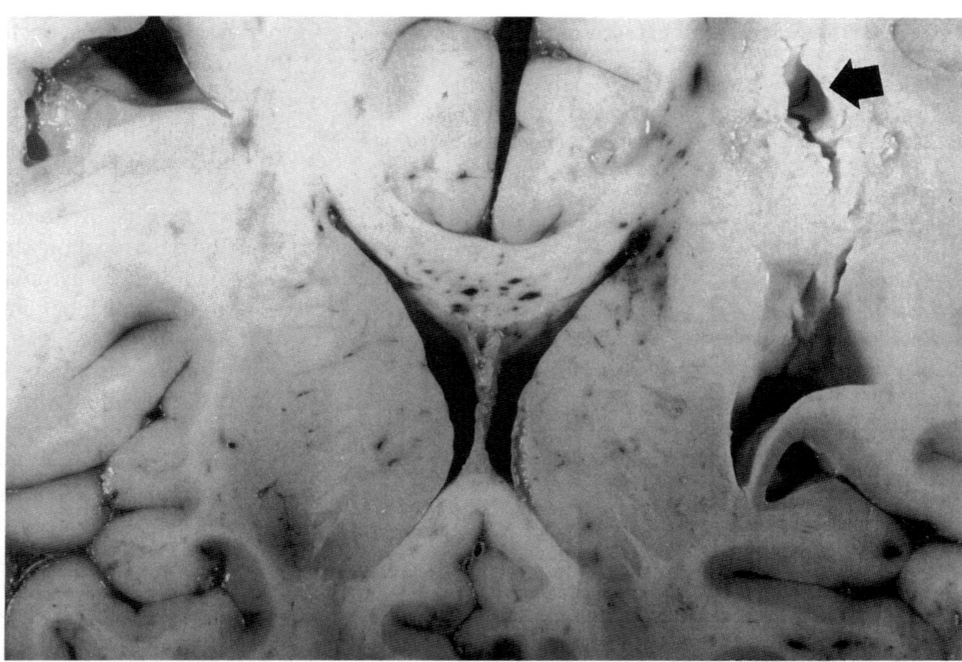

FIGURE 9.2. Closed head injury. Note the petechial hemorrhages in the corpus callosum and a tear in the white matter of the right centrum semiovale (*arrow*). (Courtesy of Dr. Harry V. Vinters, Division of Neuropathology, UCLA Center for the Health Sciences, Los Angeles, CA.)

(43), the presence of vasospasm, and a global increase in intracranial pressure, which reduce the supply of substrates to the tissue.

From a clinical point of view, concussion is marked by the immediate loss of consciousness, a suppression of reflexes, a transient arrest in respiration, accompanied by bradycardia and a fall in blood pressure. Vital signs quickly stabilize, and there is a gradual return of consciousness. However, neuropsychologic testing will show deficits for as long as 15 minutes after the injury. With increasing injury, the loss of consciousness is prolonged and there is an increasing duration of post-traumatic amnesia (44). The clinical features of postconcussion syndrome are covered in another part of this chapter.

Secondary Effects of Brain Trauma

Secondary effects of trauma develop as a consequence of at least five factors: cerebrovascular dysregulation, excitotoxicity, free radical formation leading to oxidative stress, energy failure, and inflammation (Fig. 9.3; Table 9.4) (45). Cerebrovascular dysregulation, excitotoxicity, and energy failure are of primary importance in the evolution of cerebral swelling. This condition has been defined as an

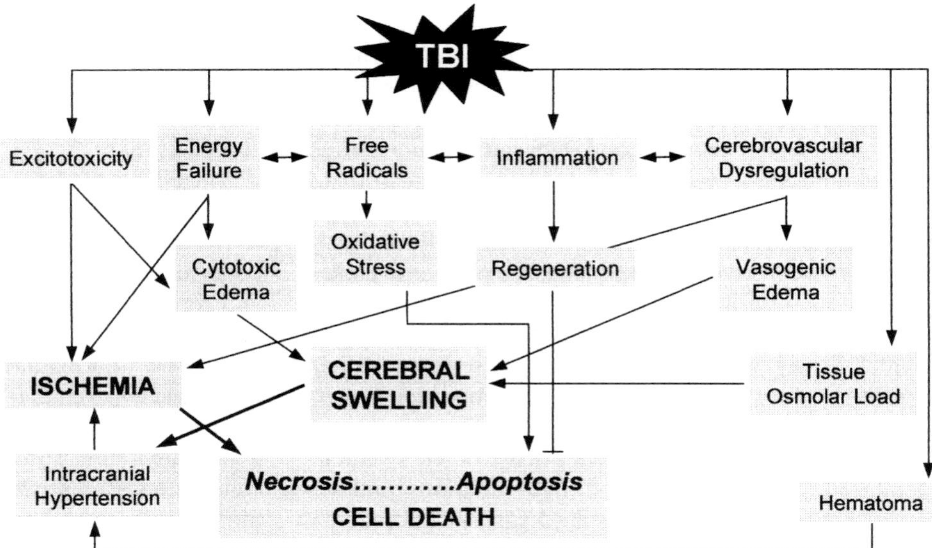

FIGURE 9.3. Proposed mechanisms for secondary damage after traumatic brain injury (TBI). (From Bayir H, Kochanek PM, Clark RS. Traumatic brain injury in infants and children: mechanisms of secondary damage and treatment in the intensive care unit. *Crit Care Clin* 2003;19:529–549. With permission.)

TABLE 9.4 Secondary Effects of Brain Trauma

Cerebral Blood Flow Dysregulation
Hypoperfusion in the first 24 hours following trauma
Reduced response to endogenous vasodilators (adenosine, nitric oxide, cyclic AMP)
Reduced NO production
Increased production of endogenous vasoconstrictors (endothelin-1)
Excitotoxicity
Increased glutamate after head injury
Causes sodium-dependent neuronal swelling
Followed by calcium-dependent activation of intracellular proteases, lipases
Production of reactive oxygen nitrogen species (free radicals)
Results in mitochondrial and DNA damage
Oxidative Stress
Free radical production important in early neuronal and vascular damage
Inflammation
Increase in cytokines, soluble adhesion molecules
Apoptosis
Activated by mitochondrial or DNA damage
Cerebral Swelling
Due to cellular swelling, injury to blood–brain barrier, osmolar swelling
Results in intracranial hypertension, secondary ischemia

increase in volume caused by an increase in brain water and sodium content. Brain swelling results from increased cerebral blood volume, cerebral edema, or a combination of the two (45).

Fishman distinguished three major categories of cerebral edema: vasogenic edema, cytotoxic or cellular edema, and interstitial edema (46). Vasogenic edema is characterized by increased permeability of brain capillary endothelial cells. This results from defects in the tight endothelial cell junctions and an increased number of pinocytic vesicles, which are responsible for the transport of macromolecules across the blood–brain barrier. Vasogenic edema fluid is extracellular and accumulates primarily in white matter because resistance to fluid flow is less in white matter than in gray matter. It occurs around brain tumors, notably glioblastomas and metastatic tumors, after cerebral infarction, and in lead encephalopathy. Cytotoxic edema is marked by swelling of all cellular elements of the brain with reduction in the volume of extracellular fluid. This last form of edema is characteristic of energy depletion such as occurs during the initial stages of cerebral hypoxia. Fishman postulated a third form of brain edema in which there is an increase in water and sodium content of periventricular white matter (46). This condition is seen in obstructive hydrocephalus.

In brain trauma, the prominence of astrocytic swelling, the integrity of the interepithelial tight junctions, and the relative paucity of protein-rich fluid suggest that edema is mainly cytotoxic (47), although massive swelling of perivascular astrocytic foot processes can compress the microvasculature and reduce tissue perfusion, inducing secondary vasogenic edema.

The importance of cytotoxic edema has been confirmed by diffusion-weighted MRI performed on experimental animals. These studies demonstrate that immediately after injury, there is predominantly vasogenic edema, which, over the next few hours to days, becomes superseded and overshadowed by cytotoxic edema (48).

A number of biochemical changes follow severe traumatic head injury (Fig. 9.3, Table 9.4). In both clinical and experimental settings, good correlation exists between the severity of traumatic brain injury and the amount of neuroexcitatory amino acids, such as glutamate and aspartate, that are released (40,49). As a result, neuronal membranes depolarize with subsequent increase of extracellular potassium (42). This is accompanied by the entry of calcium into nerve terminals and is followed by further glutamate release and potassium flux. At the same time, arachidonic acid is released, which in turn induces a cascade of reactions with the ultimate formation of free radicals (50). These changes are accompanied by increased energy demands as brain cells attempt to reinstate normal ionic membrane balance (51). With an increase in energy consumption there is a rapid decrease in adenosine triphosphate (ATP) and an increase in lactic acid (52). These biochemical alterations, which suggest impaired mitochondrial function, are confirmed by the electron microscopic observations of swollen neuronal mitochondria and an increased permeability of the organelles' outer membranes (53). These factors all contribute to astrocytic swelling, as does an energy shortage–induced failure of the sodium pump (54). In addition, there is a local inflammatory response with complement and microglial activation and an increased release into cerebrospinal fluid (CSF) of a variety of cytokines (interleukin-1, interleukin-6, and interleukin-10) (56). These substances also contribute to the evolution of diffuse cerebral edema. The role of a trauma-induced upregulation of aquaporins, a family of transmembrane proteins that selectively allow the passage of water through the plasma membrane, in the formation of brain edema has not been fully clarified (56a).

The effects of traumatic brain injury on cerebral blood flow are critical to the development of cerebral edema. Early after severe traumatic brain injury, marked hypoperfusion develops with reduction in oxygen delivery and cerebral ischemia (57). Some 24 hours later cerebral blood flow increases, and there is uncoupling of cerebral blood flow and oxidative cerebral metabolism (1). Posttraumatic hyperemia is more common in infants and children than in adults and is probably the consequence of a loss of cerebral autoregulation (45). Hyperemia in turn contributes to massive brain swelling, which is not uncommon in infants and young children and has been termed *malignant brain edema* (58).

Anatomically, cerebral edema involves principally the subcortical white matter and the centrum semiovale. Less often, cerebral edema surrounds an area of contusion or an intracerebral hematoma. Brain swelling also can occur in response to the evacuation of a large extracerebral clot or after other major intracranial surgery (59).

When the additive effects of injury and brain swelling are severe, a self-perpetuating sequence develops, which can lead to further increases of intracranial pressure, with collapse of cerebral venules. This collapse in turn reduces cerebral perfusion and causes tissue hypoxia. This leads to further cerebral edema (60). A loss of selective permeability of cell membranes results, with increased loss of fluid from the vascular compartment into the parenchyma, thereby increasing cerebral swelling. Recovery has not been seen when intracranial pressure equals or exceeds mean systemic arterial pressure, at which point cerebral perfusion ceases.

Numerous changes occur secondary to cerebral edema. Herniation of the uncus over the tentorial edge compresses the midbrain and often occludes the posterior cerebral arteries. Edema and infarction of the occipital poles can occur, contributing further to supratentorial pressure and thus to herniation. Petechial hemorrhages develop in the midbrain and pons, with infarctions in the areas of the basal ganglia supplied by the anterior choroidal artery. A decrease in blood pressure, commonly seen with a severe injury, potentiates the vicious circle.

Clinical Conditions

Closed Head Injury

More than 90% of major pediatric head injuries are nonpenetrating and closed (i.e., no scalp wound exists). The clinical picture is highlighted by alterations in consciousness (14). As is the case for head injuries at all ages, boys are involved three times more often than girls.

Clinical Manifestations

When the injury is mild, initial unconsciousness is brief and is followed by confusion, somnolence, and listlessness. Vomiting, pallor, and irritability are common, and particularly in infants can occur in the apparent absence of an initial loss of consciousness. By definition, except for transient nystagmus or extensor plantar responses, neurologic signs are not observed in concussion. As a rule, a computed tomography (CT) scan clarifies the differential diagnosis of contusion, cerebral laceration, or other complications of closed head injury, and a lumbar puncture is not warranted without specific indications.

From 7% to 40% of children with mild head injuries have associated linear fractures of the skull (61). These fractures are most common in the parietal region. According to most authorities, such fractures do not, by themselves, affect the clinical course or prolong the period of morbidity; children with and without simple fractures have the same incidence of serious sequelae (14,61,62).

Electroencephalography (EEG), when performed soon after injury, can reveal striking abnormalities, such as generalized and focal slowing, prolonged reaction to hyperventilation, and even hypsarrhythmia. In milder head injuries, these changes tend to be transient. Taking into account the time elapsed between injury and recording, Mizrahi and Kellaway found that the degree of EEG abnormality correlated with the severity of the injury (63). Nevertheless, the EEG does not predict the development of post-traumatic epilepsy, and there is no correlation between the appearance of the EEG immediately after the head injury and development of early post-traumatic epilepsy (64). Proton resonance spectroscopy appears to be more valuable in predicting outcome. In the experience of Ashwal and coworkers, the presence of lactate had a poor prognosis in that 91% of head-injured infants and 80% of head-injured children with poor outcomes had a lactate peak; conversely, none of the infants and children with good outcome showed the presence of lactate (65).

In major closed head injuries, consciousness is interrupted more profoundly and for longer periods than in minor head injuries, and focal neurologic signs point to localized brain contusion. The clinical picture in such cases is outlined in Table 9.5 (66). Generally, the greatest neurologic deficit is found at the time of injury. New neurologic

TABLE 9.5 Clinical Findings in 4,465 Children with Major Closed Head Injuries

Finding	*Percentage*
Initial level of consciousness	
Normal	56.0
Drowsy, confused	30.2
Major impairment	13.8
Vomiting	30.3
Skull fractures	26.6
Linear	72.8
Depressed	27.2
Compound	19.7
Seizures	7.4
Paralyses	3.8
Retinal hemorrhages	2.3
Pupillary abnormalities	3.6
Papilledema	1.5
Extradural hematoma	0.9
Subdural hematoma	5.2
Mortality	5.4
Major neurologic residua	5.9

This series includes 243 infants with major birth injuries. This group had 50% mortality and a higher incidence of paralyses, retinal hemorrhages, and major residua.

From Hendrick EB, Harwood-Nash DC, Hudson AR. Head injuries in children: a survey of 4,465 consecutive cases at the Hospital for Sick Children, Toronto, Canada. *Clin Neurosurg* 1963;11:46. With permission.

signs appearing subsequently indicate progressive brain swelling or, if localized, indicate secondary intracranial hemorrhage, vasospasm, or thrombosis. The duration of coma depends on the site and severity of injury.

The clinical picture follows one of several courses (67). Many children die without recovering consciousness. In a smaller group of patients, coma persists. Prognosis for survival is relatively good in children alive 48 hours after injury. In one-half of the surviving children, consciousness is regained in less than 24 hours. Recovery is often complete or nearly complete, although transient sequelae are not unusual. These include CSF leakage often complicated by secondary meningitis, post-traumatic epilepsy, and the development of a carotid artery–cavernous sinus fistula. Communicating hydrocephalus resulting from subarachnoid bleeding more commonly follows perinatal trauma and is discussed in Chapters 5 and 6.

Nonaccidental trauma

Child abuse is the most common cause of head injury in infants younger than 2 years of age. In the experience of Duhaime and coworkers, in 24% of infants admitted to hospital with head injuries the injuries were presumed to have been inflicted, and in another 32% the injuries were suspicious for child abuse (68). Although the term "shaken baby" has been used in the past, pathologic data collected on a larger Scottish series has made it clear that a whiplash shaking injury could be documented in only 6% of cases (69). The hyperextension and hyperflexion whiplashing forces injure the brainstem or upper cervical spinal cord with consequent acute respiratory failure, hypoxia, and brain swelling. Subdural bleeding was generally trivial. These pathologic findings are commensurate with the clinical presentation of collapse or respiratory arrest (70). Shannon and Becker also stressed the frequency of brainstem and spinal cord injuries in infantile child abuse (71).

The more commonly encountered clinical picture is characterized by depressed consciousness, increased intracranial pressure, seizures, and subdural and retinal hemorrhages. These symptoms are frequently accompanied by other nonaccidental injuries and an inconsistent or unreliable medical history. This constellation of symptoms has been termed the shaken impact syndrome. The encephalopathy developed acutely in 53% of the Scottish cases, subacutely in 19%, and chronically in 22% (69). The less acute the presentation, the better is the outcome with respect to long-term morbidity. In the series of Bechtel and coworkers, the clinical picture of nonaccidental head injury could be distinguished from that seen in accidental head injury by more frequent bilateral retinal hemorrhages, a greater likelihood of presenting with an altered mental state and seizures, and a lesser incidence of scalp hematomas (71a).

Pathologic examination of the brain of infants subjected to nonaccidental head injury disclosed skull fractures in 36%, acute subdural bleeding in 72%, and retinal hemorrhages in 71% (70). Severe hypoxic brain damage was present in 77%, and the usual cause of death, seen in 82%, was increased intracranial pressure. Eighty-five percent of the children had signs of impact to the head at autopsy, and 51% had significant extracranial injuries (70). The clinical presentation of infants who showed no signs of impact was of collapse or respiratory arrest; the pathologic picture did not differ from the majority of infants who showed evidence of impact (72).

There is considerable uncertainty as to the mechanism of brain damage in shaken impact syndrome, and according to Donohoe there is inadequate scientific evidence to come to a firm conclusion on most aspects of causation (73). Geddes and Plunkett (74) shared this skepticism and stressed that although most infants do indeed show signs of inflicted violence, serious injury or death from a low-level fall is possible, and contrary to Harding and coworkers, who believed that retinal hemorrhages result from rotational acceleration and deceleration forces (75), they doubted that shaking can induce the characteristic retinal hemorrhages.

The combination of a subdural hematoma and retinal hemorrhages can also result from a variety of bleeding disorders. It is also encountered in Menkes disease and in type 1 glutaric aciduria (see Chapter 1) (76).

Nonsurgical Treatment

Major Head Injury

A recommended sequence consists of the following four steps: a rapid initial evaluation, resuscitation, a more extensive secondary evaluation including radiologic assessment, and definitive treatment (1,45,76a). In many instances of major closed head injury, diagnosis of the injury is performed in parallel with emergency treatment.

Because in children the clinical condition can change rapidly and frequently, a high degree of alertness and preparedness is required of both medical and nursing attendants.

Neurologic Examination

Careful, but not elaborate, neurologic examination must be made and recorded, with particular emphasis on the state of consciousness; pupillary size, equality, and response to light; the extent and symmetry of spontaneous movements; and the reflex responses. Recording of blood pressure, pulse, and respiration is likewise essential. Caloric and optokinetic responses are useful for evaluating brainstem function. Some or all of these observations, especially the level of consciousness and motor activity, are principally of value when made serially at intervals that

TABLE 9.6 Pediatric Coma Scale

Eyes Open	
Spontaneously	4
To speech	3
To pain	2
Not at all	1
Best Verbal Response	
Oriented	5
Words	4
Vocal sounds	3
Cries	2
None	1
Best Motor Response	
Obeys commands	5
Localizes pain	4
Flexion to pain	3
Extension to pain	2
None	1
Normal Aggregate Score	
Birth to 6 months	9
6–12 months	11
1–2 years	12
2–5 years	13
Older than 5 years	14

Modified from Simpson D, Reilly P. Pediatric coma scale. *Lancet* 1982;2:450.

can be as often as every 5 minutes. Such examinations allow trends away from or toward normal functioning to be detected, thus providing warning of any need to intervene surgically.

Several pediatric modifications of the Glasgow Coma Scale (77), which is widely used for the assessment of head-injured adults, have been proposed. One example is presented in Table 9.6 (78).

The Glasgow Coma Scale measures three neurologic responses: eye opening, verbal response, and limb movement. Each response is given a score; the higher the score, the better is the condition of the patient.

Additionally, the extent of retrograde and post-traumatic amnesia should be recorded when possible. Spontaneous or provoked episodes of decerebrate activity or hypotonia are associated with a poor outcome (79); the length of pre- and post-traumatic amnesia is a useful indicator of the severity of the head injury (80).

Maintenance of Airway and Circulation

After the immediate evaluation of the child's general condition, an adequate airway should be established and maintained. Airway obstruction is the most frequent cause of respiratory failure. Maintenance of patency requires suction of mouth or pharyngeal contents or endotracheal intubation followed, when necessary, by artificial respiration. Tracheostomy may be indicated to bypass mechanical obstruction of the airway caused by facial or mandibular injuries. Because an injury to the cervical spine must be presumed until proven absent, the neck must be stabilized while an airway is established. Arterial pressure is monitored by cannulation of a peripheral artery and maintained by administration of crystalloid, colloid, or blood products. Gas exchange also must be monitored.

Shock in closed head injuries is usually caused by blood loss elsewhere in the body. Rarely, it indicates damage to the medullary cardiovascular centers. Infants and young children have a higher incidence of shock than those in older age groups (1). In infants, in particular, subgaleal, subperiosteal, subdural, or extradural hemorrhages can be sufficiently extensive to induce shock. The injured brain is highly susceptible to episodes of systemic hypotension, in part because cerebral edema in conjunction with systemic hypotension lowers cerebral blood flow, and perhaps because an impairment of autoregulation of cerebral blood flow also occurs. Whatever the physiologic mechanism, when head injury is accompanied by systemic hypotension, the outcome is significantly worse (81).

After the initial emergency measures have been completed, the child's neurologic status should be reevaluated. The importance of repeated observations of vital signs and neurologic status cannot be overemphasized. Slowing of the pulse rate and widening of pulse pressure often accompany an increase of intracranial pressure (Cushing effect) (see Chapter 11). An irregular respiratory pattern is also common after severe head injuries (82).

Neuroimaging Studies

CT of the head has revolutionized the clinical assessment of head injuries, and it is the most appropriate study for the assessment of intracranial complications, taking precedence over skull radiography and MRI. The need for and timing of such imaging studies depend mainly on the clinical findings. A suggested strategy is outlined in Table 9.7 (83). Some centers suggest that in children who show signs of brainstem compression and a Glasgow coma score of 3, precious time can be saved by foregoing CT and proceeding directly with exploratory surgery to remove a hematoma. Although emergency trephination may benefit the occasional patient, scanning is still the most important diagnostic study for the majority of children (84).

CT can delineate the presence and the extent of fractures and can demonstrate the presence of diffuse cerebral swelling and hyperemia of the brain (85), hemorrhages in the epidural and subdural space, and intracerebral hemorrhages (Fig. 9.4) (86).

In some injuries, the condition of the sinuses should be noted for evidence of a fracture, which makes the injury compound, or the presence of blood. Ethmoid and maxillary sinuses are pneumatized at birth, the sphenoid sinuses become pneumatized at approximately 5 years of age, and the frontal sinuses, the last to develop, are not visualized until 4 to 6 years of age (87).

TABLE 9.7 Management Strategy for Radiographic Imaging in Pediatric Patients with Head Trauma

Low-Risk Group	*Moderate-Risk Group*	*High-Risk Group*
Possible findings	**Possible findings**	**Possible findings**
Asymptomatic	Change of consciousness at time of injury or subsequently	Depressed or decreasing level of consciousness
Headache	Unreliable history	Focal neurologic signs
Dizziness	Younger than 2 years of age	Penetrating skull injury
Scalp laceration	Post-traumatic seizure	Depressed fracture
Scalp hematoma	Vomiting	
	Signs of basilar skull fracture	
	Fracture into an air sinus	
	Possible depressed fracture	
	Suspected child abuse	
Recommendations	**Recommendations**	**Recommendations**
Observation	Hospitalization	Emergency CT scan
Discharge with head injury information sheet, and have family observe child	Close observation	Neurosurgical consultation
	CT scan and neurosurgical consultation	

CT, computed tomography.
Adapted from Masters SJ, McLean PM, Arcarese JS, et al. Skull x-ray examinations after head trauma. Recommendations by a multi-disciplinary panel and validation study. *N Engl J Med* 1987;316:84–91.

MRI usually contributes little to the initial management of major closed head injury. It is, however, more sensitive than CT in detecting an extraaxial hematoma, particularly a chronic subdural hematoma (88). Additionally, MRI provides better visualization of subacute and chronic contusions and of shearing lesions of the white matter such as result from child abuse (89). MR angiography (MRA), performed at a subsequent time, can be of use in delineating such vascular abnormalities as arteriovenous fistulae, venous sinus occlusion, and arterial occlusions.

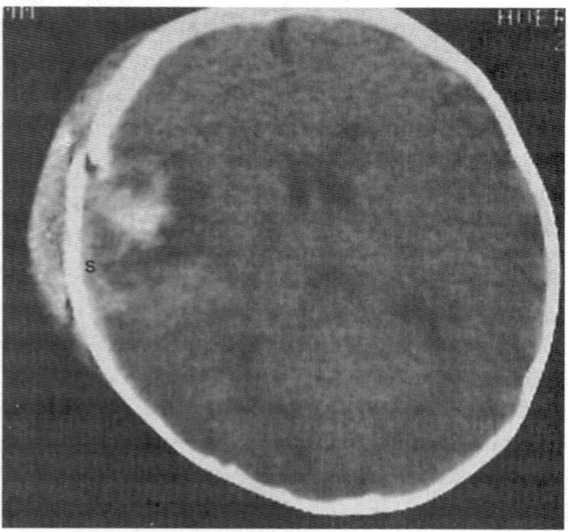

FIGURE 9.4. Computed tomographic scan after head trauma. Head injury shown by computed tomographic scan without contrast. The soft tissue swelling and the left parietal skull fracture are readily evident. An intracerebral hematoma is seen with surrounding cerebral edema resulting in ventricular compression and shift. A small subdural hematoma (*s*) is also evident.

One must guard against excessive complacency on the basis of a single normal CT obtained in the early hours after an injury because hemorrhagic complications can evolve subacutely after an interval of several hours or days. A repeat CT is indicated under the following circumstances: (a) when doubt exists about the presence of a mass lesion, (b) when intracranial pressure monitoring demonstrates an increase in pressure, (c) when a patient is unconscious despite an initial benign-appearing CT, and (d) when a contusion is accompanied by a neurologic deficit. A normal CT result also does not exclude the presence of cerebral edema. In the series of O'Sullivan and coworkers, 88% of head-injured patients with a Glasgow coma score of 8 or less and no evidence of cerebral edema by CT had increased intracranial pressure when recorded directly (90).

Fluid and Electrolytes

The appropriate fluid management of the hypovolemic head-injured patient remains controversial, although both clinical and experimental studies indicate that the most important goals are to correct any hypovolemia and prevent reduction of osmolality. A period of hyponatremia with natriuresis is a common response to brain injury (91). Hyponatremia can result from either a cerebral salt-wasting syndrome characterized by hypovolemia or from an inappropriate excess of antidiuretic hormone that causes water retention (syndrome of inappropriate antidiuretic hormone secretion [SIADH]). Whereas the cerebral salt-wasting syndrome is treated by fluid and salt supplementation, SIADH requires fluid restriction. In the majority of patients, hyponatremia during the first week after a head injury is caused by excessive antidiuretic hormone, whereas hyponatremia that develops later probably results from chronic salt-wasting (92). Berkenbosch and colleagues advocated the measurement of urine output to distinguish between the two conditions. In SIADH, urine output is reduced, and at times there is a frank oliguria, whereas cerebral salt-wasting syndrome is marked by polyuria (93).

The relationship between fluid load, sodium balance, and intracranial pressure is unclear. The traditional view is that during the early post-traumatic period, there is a danger of overloading the patient with fluids, which can increase intracranial pressure and thus diminish the level of consciousness. Therefore, fluid intake for the first 2 to 4 days should be between 35% and 50% of the average normal daily fluid requirements, as long as urine volume remains adequate (94). This view has been challenged, and more recent work indicates that rapid, continuous infusion of hypertonic (3%) saline with a view of maintaining intracranial pressure below 20 mm Hg is safely tolerated and possibly improves the outcome of severely brain injured children without incurring a significant risk for renal failure or extrapontine myelinolysis (95). Most neurosurgeons currently recommend that hypertonic crystalloid solutions be given intravenously to maintain a normal intravascular volume and adequate cerebral perfusion pressure (96). Both clinical and experimental studies suggest that glucose-containing solutions should be avoided because these tend to increase cerebral lactic acidosis (97).

Despite the evidence of sodium retention in the early post-traumatic period, salt should be administered to avoid hypotonicity of extracellular fluids. A total of 30 mEq of sodium chloride per liter of calculated fluid requirements meets the usual electrolyte requirements. As a result of a catecholamine-induced intracellular potassium shift, hypokalemia can accompany severe head injuries (98). Although hypokalemia was documented in 7% of traumatic brain injuries admitted to the Boston Children's Hospital, it corrected spontaneously, and in almost all instances did not require potassium supplementation (99).

Less commonly, hypernatremia and dehydration follow closed head injury. These are occasionally seen in a subfrontal injury that has caused hypothalamic damage and diabetes insipidus, or they are the result of a failure in the thirst response or inadequate hydration of an unconscious patient.

Coagulation Defects

A significant proportion of patients with head injuries severe enough to result in destruction of brain tissue show clinical and laboratory evidence of impaired coagulation (100). This results from structural damage, hypoxia, or elevated catecholamine and steroid levels. These patients have low fibrinogen levels, diminished amounts of factors V and VIII, and thrombocytopenia. Treatment can require emergency replacement of hemostatic factors with fresh-frozen plasma or recombinant activated factor VII (101). Disseminated intravascular coagulation was seen in approximately one-third of children evaluated within 2 hours of major head injury (102).

Seizures

Seizures can occur shortly after the injury or can appear after an interval of days to years. Seizures appearing during the acute stage can increase intracranial pressure by Valsalva effects. They can increase cerebral blood flow, cause the release of neuroexcitatory transmitters, and aggravate any preexisting hypoxia. They generally are managed with intravenous phenytoin (5 mg/kg loading dose). Intramuscular phenytoin, which can crystallize within muscles, is unreliable. Diazepam (0.1 to 0.3 mg/kg) and lorazepam (0.05 to 0.25 mg/kg) are suitable alternatives. Some authorities are loath to administer phenytoin to infants and toddlers, preferring carbamazepine. In adults, phenytoin appears to reduce the likelihood of early post-traumatic seizures but does not decrease the risk of late post-traumatic epilepsy (103,104). EEG monitoring is desirable to detect electrical seizures even when paralysis of the patient prevents overt seizures. The role of anticonvulsants in the treatment of post-traumatic seizures is discussed in Chapter 14. In view of the relative rarity of post-traumatic seizures, we do not advocate preventive anticonvulsant therapy, except in the presence of a major brain laceration. Chadwick is of the same opinion (103). For this purpose we prefer carbamazepine or valproate to phenytoin.

Increased Intracranial Pressure

Children tend to have a lower incidence of surgically treatable mass lesions than adults (less than 10% in a CT-verified series) but a higher incidence of increased intracranial pressure (105). Therefore, in the infant or child who has sustained a severe head injury, control of increased intracranial pressure becomes the most important problem of medical management. For this purpose, continuous pressure monitoring is necessary for the more seriously injured patients and for infants who are more likely to experience increased intracranial pressure (1,45,94). A variety of monitoring techniques are in use, each with its advantages and disadvantages. These include an indwelling ventriculostomy with direct monitoring from the ventricular system; monitoring from the subarachnoid, subdural, and epidural spaces (106); and fiberoptic monitoring by placement of a device into the frontal parenchyma (107). Of these methods, subdural monitoring using the Camino or Codman fiber-optic pressure transducer is preferred at the University of California, Los Angeles, and the University of Washington. This allows an indirect, continuous measurement of intracranial pressure, which, when combined with the value of mean arterial blood pressure, permits calculation of cerebral perfusion pressure (cerebral perfusion pressure equals mean systemic arterial blood pressure minus intracranial pressure). When possible, estimation or measurement of cerebral blood flow allows detection of global cerebral ischemia, which generally worsens the clinical course and outcome (108). Focal cerebral ischemia is more difficult to assess. After major head injuries, some regions of the brain may require higher levels of cerebral perfusion pressure to maintain adequate cerebral blood flow.

In some head-injured children CSF drainage via a ventriculostomy is a useful adjunct for controlling elevated intracranial pressure in those patients whose ventricles can safely be cannulated. Ventriculostomy remains the most effective way to monitor intracranial pressure and treat elevated pressure via continuous or intermittent CSF drainage. In selected patients who do not have mass lesions but have elevated intracranial pressures that are refractory to all other therapies, treatment with controlled lumbar CSF drainage has been encouraging (109).

Continuous monitoring of jugular venous oxygen saturation using an indwelling fiber-optic catheter also has been suggested, but the usefulness of this technique in the pediatric population has yet to be assessed (1). Venous oxygen saturation in the adult should lie between 55% and 85%, and values below 45% indicate global cerebral ischemia (110).

Intracranial pressure is usually maintained below 15 mm Hg, although temporary increases to 20 mm Hg are often unavoidable and can occur in the course of nursing procedures. The initial step in lowering intracranial pressure is to induce hypocarbia by hyperventilation and reduce the carbon dioxide partial pressure (pCO_2) to between 25 and 30 mm Hg. With profound hyperventilation and pCO_2 values below 25 mm Hg, cerebral ischemia can develop (111).

Historically, hyperventilation has been part of the treatment algorithm for trauma patients with elevated intracranial pressures. This maneuver causes cerebral vasoconstriction, thereby decreasing cerebral blood flow and volume. The response to hyperventilation is rapid but short lived, and hyperventilation must be continued or increased to remain effective. Studies show that the prolonged and routine use of hyperventilation may be deleterious in some patients by exacerbating ischemic brain injuries. Therefore, in the absence of elevated intracranial pressure, we no longer recommend the routine use of hyperventilation. Substantial beneficial effects can be realized when refractory elevated intracranial pressure is treated by moderate hyperventilation, accomplished by maintaining the arterial carbon dioxide pressure between 28 and 35 mm Hg. This therapy can be administered safely, with careful monitoring to avoid the complications associated with prolonged, profound hyperventilation, notably cerebral ischemia (112,113). Should hyperventilation be ineffective in reducing increased intracranial pressure, other measures must be undertaken.

Raising the head between 0 and 30 degrees in the neutral, midline position is commonly performed after severe head injury. This maneuver facilitates cerebral venous drainage and thus theoretically decreased intracranial pressure. Feldman and coworkers showed in their randomized study of head position of the trauma patient that by elevating the head from 0 to 30 degrees, the intracranial pressure was decreased without a decrease in cerebral perfusion pressure of cerebral blood flow (114). When the head is raised approximately 60 degrees, there appears to be a deleterious effect on cerebral blood flow. However, these studies have not been confirmed for children. Thus, the most advantageous head position in a child with an intracranial pressure monitor (i.e., the best way to maximize cerebral perfusion pressure) can be determined by raising the head and observing the concomitant change in intracranial pressure and cerebral perfusion pressure.

Diuretics are used in a number of centers. Mannitol and urea are the most commonly used osmotic diuretics. Mannitol, given in amounts of 1.5 to 2.0 g/kg body weight in the form of a 20% solution, has a slower effect than urea, but maintains the lowered intracranial pressure at its minimum level for 2 to 4 hours. It has the disadvantage of leaking into the brain through areas where injury has damaged the blood–brain barrier and thus inducing local edema. In addition, by slowly diffusing into the intercellular space, mannitol carries water with it, thereby inducing a rebound effect. For these reasons diuretics are used mainly as a temporary measure to gain time while the patient and the operating room are being readied for surgery, while diagnostic studies are being performed, or for acute control of elevated intracranial pressure. Mannitol, furosemide, or both are favored in most institutions; however, there are few well-controlled studies to show their effectiveness in the pediatric population (45). One appropriate dosing regimen for furosemide is 0.5 to 1.0 mg/kg administered every 4 to 6 hours.

Several well-controlled clinical studies have failed, however, to demonstrate any significant effectiveness of corticosteroids in counteracting brain swelling in head-injured children. The agents did not improve outcome or lower intracranial pressure and in some cases may have been deleterious. For these reasons, corticosteroids are not routinely employed in the treatment of pediatric head injuries. A multicenter, randomized, placebo-controlled trial of corticosteroids after significant head injury in adults with a Glasgow Coma Score of 14 or less within 8 hours of injury actually demonstrated an increase in mortality with methylprednisolone (114a,114b).

The clinical effectiveness of various oxygen-derived free radical scavengers, when given to patients with severe head injuries within 8 to 12 hours of the injury, has not been established in terms of improving neurologic outcome (115). Agents that inhibit lipid peroxidation, block excitotoxicity, and block apoptosis or promote brain cell regeneration have been employed in various experimental situations, but as yet have no clinical application.

High doses of barbiturates, generally pentobarbital, have been advocated whenever intracranial pressure does not respond to other forms of therapy. However, there is no convincing evidence that barbiturate coma improves outcome, and the initial enthusiasm for this form of treatment has waned because barbiturates can cause myocardial depression (1,116). For this reason barbiturates require cautious use in children, especially those with hemodynamic instability. Currently, barbiturates are used as a last resort to help control intractable elevations of intracranial pressure and to help place patients who are in status epilepticus into EEG burst suppression. Under these circumstances, bedside EEG monitoring is mandatory.

Sedation with pharmacologically induced paralysis is often used in the treatment of the severely head-injured child. This reduces the increase in intracranial pressure associated with agitation, suctioning, and ventilation. In our institutions, sedation and paralysis is titrated with intracranial pressure. Intravenous narcotics in small doses by continuous or bolus infusion, short-acting benzodiazepines, and nondepolarizing muscle relaxants are used effectively for this purpose. Titration of short-acting drugs permits intermittent examinations and rapid reversal, when necessary. In nonventilated, awake, but intermittently confused patients, medication is used sparingly because the neurologic examination is the most important parameter for the management of the head-injured patient. Small boluses of narcotics and short-acting benzodiazepines are used in some institutions to sedate the agitated pediatric patient without a mass lesion, but this issue remains controversial among neurosurgeons and critical care physicians.

Induced mild hypothermia (cooling to 32°C to 33°C) in conjunction with hyperventilation (pCO_2 between 25 and 30 mm Hg) and barbiturates (4 to 6 mg/kg intravenous thiopental, followed by 6 to 8 mg/kg per hour of continuous thiopental) has reemerged as another measure to lower increased intracranial pressure and increase cerebral perfusion by lowering metabolic demands (45). Hypothermia attenuates the increases of excitatory amino acids, decreases endogenous antioxidant consumption, and has antiinflammatory effects. The effectiveness of this measure in the pediatric population has not been clearly demonstrated (45). Preliminary results suggest that this method can improve neurologic outcome in younger patients, particularly those who were already hypthermic on admission. From these studies it is not clear whether this represents a beneficial effect of early hypothermia or a detrimental effect of passively warming a previously hypothermic patient (117).

Neurogenic pulmonary edema is a rare and potentially fatal complication of head injury. Its pathogenesis is unknown, but focal brainstem lesions, particularly in the region of the nucleus solitarius, can increase pulmonary arterial pressure and capillary permeability. Symptoms appear within the first day after injury and are managed with diuretics and positive end-expiratory pressure (118).

More detailed treatment schedules for the child with a major closed head injury are given by Jennett and Teasdale (119) and Bayir and colleagues (45). All infants with head injuries and all older children with severe head injuries, as defined by a Glasgow coma score of 8 or less, or who have sustained a major skull fracture should be seen by a neurosurgeon.

Minor Head Injury

The American Academy of Pediatrics issued guides for the management of minor head treauma in children older than age 2 years (120) and younger than age 2 years (121). These are summarized in Table 9.8. Considerable judgment is

TABLE 9.8 Guidelines for Management of Children with Minor Head Injuries

Children Older Than 2 Years of Age
Minor closed head injury—no loss of consciousness
History
Physical and neurologic examinations
Observation
Minor closed head injury—loss of consciousness less than 1 minute
History
Physical and neurologic examinations
Computed tomography scan
Children Younger Than 2 Years of Age
Low-risk group: falls less than 3 feet, no signs or symptoms 2+ hours after injury
Observation
Intermediate-risk group: loss of consciousness less than 1 minute, episodes of vomiting, lethargy resolved by time of exam, behavior not at baseline
Prolonged observation (4 to 6 hours) OR computed tomography scan
High-risk group: depressed mental status, focal neurologic signs, irritability, full fontanel
Computed tomography scan
Neurosurgical consultation

Adapted from Committee on Quality Improvement, American Academy of Pediatrics. The management of minor closed head injury in children. *Pediatrics* 1999;104:1407–1415; and Shutzman SA, Barnes P, Duhaime AC, et al. Evaluation and management of children younger than two years old with apparently minor head trauma: Proposed guidelines. *Pediatrics* 2001;107:983–993.

required to avoid unnecessary hospitalization and expensive diagnostic studies, at the same time keeping in mind the possibility of post-traumatic complications that require emergency surgery. In general, children who have experienced only a momentary loss of consciousness are better managed at home. Parents are instructed to note at regular intervals the child's state of alertness and ability to move his or her extremities. The parents should be told to contact the physician if diminished consciousness or limb weakness occurs.

The role of routine CT in the management of the child with minor head injuries continues to be controversial. As indicated in Tables 9.7 and 9.8, the infant younger than 2 years of age or the child who sustains loss of consciousness should undergo CT. The younger the child, the lower the threshold should be for imaging studies. In the small infant the incidence of significant intracranial injuries is greater, and there is a higher likelihood of asymptomatic intracranial injuries (121). The cost-effectiveness of CT as a screening for safe discharge as compared with hospitalization for observation has been affirmed in a number of centers both in the United States and Europe (122–124). These studies have not addressed the costs of follow-up visits for false-positive imaging studies or the costs of return visits and subsequent hospitalization for a youngster who is handled with observation only (120). The use of skull radiography as a screening device for children with minor head injuries has serious limitations and should no longer be used inasmuch as a CT with bone windows to show the presence of fractures is superior diagnostically (122). According to some authorities, the presence of a linear skull fracture should not influence the decision about whether to send the child home; others suggest that a child found to have a skull fracture is at increased risk for an extradural hematoma and therefore should be observed in the hospital (125). We believe that whenever the fracture line crosses the groove of the middle meningeal artery or crosses the path of the sagittal or other major venous sinus, the possibility of an extradural hemorrhage is increased, so that the child should be hospitalized for the initial 24 hours. If the fracture involves an air sinus, checking for the next 10 days for signs of intracranial infection is recommended even if the child is not hospitalized.

The rehabilitation of a child with a major head injury is summarized in Table 9.9. A more detailed discussion is presented in a book edited by Ylvisaker (126).

Prognosis

There has been continuing improvement in terms of mortality and ultimate neurologic status in the outcome of severely brain-injured infants and children as defined by a postresuscitation Glasgow coma score of 8 or less (127). The outlook for full intellectual function in children experiencing minor head injuries (i.e., head injuries without associated neurologic manifestations) is generally excellent (128). The prognosis for major head injuries, although less certain, is far better in children than in infants or adults. As a rule, prediction of outcome with respect to the severity of ultimate disability is accurate in only 70% by the end of the first week after the injury (129). In the experience of the Traumatic Coma Data Bank, children younger than age 4 years who have sustained a severe head injury have a cumulative mortality of 62% during the first year after their injury. This compares with a mortality during the same period of 22% in children aged 5 to 10 years and 48% in adults (130). In this series, only 1 in 5 infants had a favorable outcome. These figures, published in 1992, should be contrasted with a mortality of 10% in a cohort gathered in the years 1994 to 1996 (127). A low postresuscitation Glasgow coma score and the presence of cerebral swelling, particularly when it is accompanied by a shift of midline structures, are indices for a poor outcome. These indices have not changed in the last few decades. The poor outcome in infants in all series probably reflects the higher incidence of child abuse and multiple injuries during the first year of life. Keenan and colleagues, working in North Carolina, found that 53% of serious or fatal head injuries incurred by infants younger than 2 years of age were caused by child abuse (131).

In a series of children treated for major head injuries at the Johns Hopkins Hospital and reported in 1983, 29% were normal on follow-up and 53% had returned to school with mild behavioral or cognitive problems. In the latter group, however, 61% had shown evidence of significant language delay, minimal cerebral dysfunction, and learning problems before the accident (132). The outcome tended to be worse in children who sustained prolonged coma. When outcome is stratified according to age, all studies show that morbidity as well as mortality are greater when the injury is experienced in infancy or in early childhood.

Generally, children with only behavioral abnormalities during the early post-traumatic period later achieve normal functioning. No significant improvement in cognitive function can be expected after the first 6 to 12 months after injury. Improvement in speech and motor function, however, can continue for several years (133,134). Decerebrate rigidity during the early postinjury phase, although associated with an early mortality in 25% to 50% of patients, by itself does not preclude functional survival; approximately one-half of survivors have a fairly good quality of life (134). Excessive daytime sleepiness is fairly common after head trauma, especially in adolescents. In some of these, notably when there has been an associated whiplash injury, sleep apnea is responsible; in others, the condition resembles narcolepsy (see Chapter 15) (135). In the experience of Guilleminault and coworkers, daytime sleepiness

TABLE 9.9 Rehabilitation of Head Injuries at Each Level of Consciousness

Level[a]	*Neurologic Characteristic*	*Therapeutic Intervention*
V	No response to stimuli Glasgow coma score 3	Keep patient in intensive care unit
IV	Responds to pain by flexor withdrawal or increased extensor tone; no visual response to light or threat Glasgow coma score 4–6	Maintain clear airway and prevent pulmonary complications Control hypertension and tachycardia Institute seizure prophylaxis Institute nasogastric tube feeding Prevent contractures (range of motion, casting, splinting, medication to reduce spasticity) Get child out of bed; provide sensory stimulation Continue crisis intervention counseling with family
III	Responds to visual stimuli by blinking to light or threat or tracking Shows nonpurposeful movements of extremities Glasgow coma score 8–10	Decrease agitation (do not use drugs) Stimulate visual and auditory responses Facilitate purposeful movements Improve head and trunk control Begin feeding program (delay gastronomy, try nasogastric tube feeding) Continue family support
II	Coma ends Demonstrates purposeful movements Follows commands, imitates gestures, responds verbally Glasgow coma score 12–14	Reinforce appropriate behavior and decrease agitation Improve gross and fine motor skills Begin transfers and ambulation training Start self-care and self-feeding program Evaluate for developmental and perceptual deficits Improve child's speech, language, and cognitive performance: auditory processing, orientation, attention span Continue family support Plan discharge
I	Is oriented to person, time, and place; may still have cognitive and perceptual deficits Glasgow coma score 15	Refine motor skills, community ambulation Increase independence in self-care and community-living skills Improve orientation, verbal expression, and cognitive and perceptual skills Assess vision and hearing Perform neuropsychologic assessment Complete discharge planning Continue family preparation and training, adaptive equipment, outpatient medical and therapy follow-up, school placement, involvement with community agencies

[a]Depending on the severity of the injury, progress can stop at any of these levels.
Adapted from Brink J. *Case management of head injuries.* With permission of the author.

can persist for months to years, and its duration correlates with the severity of the initial head trauma (135). Methylphenidate or amphetamine appear to be the most effective medications. A significant postural and intention tremor affecting primarily the upper extremities has been observed in a substantial number of children recovering from a serious head injury. In the series of Johnson and Hall, the tremor appeared within 2 months of the injury in 49% of their patients and between 2 and 12 months of the injury in 40%. It subsided spontaneously in 54% (136). Hyperekplexia and myoclonic twitches have also been seen (137). The cause of this complication is not clear, but based on radiouptake studies, it probably reflects striatal dopaminergic denervation (138).

A substantial proportion of survivors from major head injuries experience subsequent emotional and psychiatric disorders. These are covered in another section of this chapter.

Skull Fractures

Linear Fractures

The immature and more flexible skull of the child can sustain a greater degree of deformation than that of an adult. Most skull fractures are linear and asymptomatic and, in the older child, are readily diagnosed by CT using bone windows. In infants, fractures tend to be irregular, so that on plain skull films they are sometimes confused with a suture or wormian bone (Fig. 9.5). In early childhood the fracture can be diastatic and usually involves the lambdoid suture. The separation of the bones indicates that the intracranial pressure increased at the moment of impact.

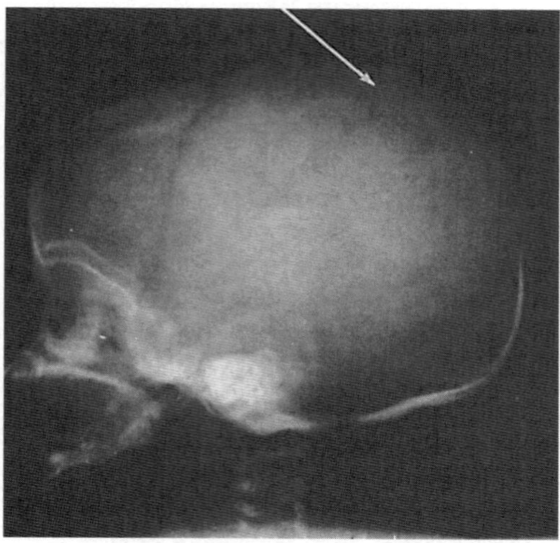

FIGURE 9.5. Depressed frontal fracture and linear parietal fracture (*arrow*) on plain skull films of a newborn infant who had undergone a difficult forceps delivery. Associated left-sided epidural hematoma was demonstrated at angiography.

Often a subperiosteal or subgaleal hematoma, termed *cephalhematoma*, in the newborn infant accompanies a linear skull fracture. Palpation of the hematoma may falsely lead the examiner to think a depressed skull fracture exists. Imaging studies disclose the underlying linear fracture. A small number of these hematomas calcify (see Fig. 6.1). There rarely is an indication for aspiration of a traumatic hematoma, and insertion of a needle or drain only increases the risk of introducing an infection into the hematoma cavity (see Chapter 6 for further discussion of this complication).

Closed linear fractures generally heal in 3 to 4 months and, except for breaks crossing the path of major vessels or entering the paranasal sinuses, do not require special therapy or observations.

An infrequent complication of a closed head injury with a linear fracture in an infant is the diastatic or *growing* fracture (139). It occurs in less than 1% of all fractures and usually represents a complication of a serious head injury (140). It occurs when the fracture tears the dura causing the arachnoid to be trapped in the fracture (16). Rare after age 3 years, it is thought to be more common in victims of child abuse, but its appearance is not confined to victims of nonaccidental trauma (140). Dural tears responsible for a growing fracture occur mostly in the parietal area; their presence, unrecognized because the scalp is intact, leads to the development of a CSF-filled cyst between the cortex and the overlying bone. At the same time, the bone edges along the fracture do not unite, apparently prevented by their direct contact with fluid. The bone is resorbed, so that plain skull radiography or CT scans taken after an interval of several months show an irregular bone defect with scalloped edges that is an elliptical erosive cranial defect (139).

In many instances, an associated cortical injury occurs and beneath the area of the cyst there is usually a porencephalic diverticulum of the lateral ventricle, producing a palpable and sometimes visible bone defect and occasionally leading to seizures and progressive hemiparesis. Leptomeningeal cysts should be differentiated from an encephalocele, which is congenital, usually located in the occipital midline, and associated with a regular bone defect. A growing fracture does not resolve spontaneously and must be treated surgically. Treatment, which should be begun as early as possible, involves the surgical separation of the bone from underlying arachnoid, dural repair or replacement, and closure of the bone defect with autologous bone, bone source, or cranioplasty. In rare cases, normal-pressure hydrocephalus develops, which requires a ventriculoperitoneal shunt.

Basal Skull Fractures

Basal skull fractures involve the floor of the anterior, middle, or posterior fossae; they are uncommon in children. Their presence can be suspected when the child has signs of bleeding from the nasopharynx or the middle ear or has postauricular ecchymoses (Battle's sign) (141). Epistaxis is frequent in childhood head injury, however, because of the high incidence of nasal fractures.

Fractures of the base of the anterior fossa can lead to hemorrhage into the orbit. Under these circumstances a subconjunctival hemorrhage represents a forward extension of blood behind the optic globe, in contrast to an anterior hemorrhage, which arises from a direct blow to the eye. Exophthalmos and subconjunctival hemorrhage occur in conjunction with "raccoon eyes." Fractures of the mastoid portion of the temporal bone result in postauricular ecchymoses.

Distinctive unilateral fresh purpuric hemorrhages in the antitragus, triangular fossa, and helix of the ear have been termed the "tin ear syndrome" (142). The condition can be associated with retinal hemorrhages and an ipsilateral subdural hematoma, a syndrome considered to be pathognomonic of child abuse. Rotational acceleration of the head produced by blunt trauma to the ear is believed to produce this syndrome (142).

CSF rhinorrhea can accompany a fracture of the floor of the anterior fossa that has involved the cribriform plate. It represents a rare complication of head trauma in children, but the high risk of intracranial infections (20% to 37% as reported by Wilson and coworkers) makes its recognition imperative (143).

CSF rhinorrhea usually appears within the first 2 days after the injury, but it may not become apparent for up to several years. In 70% of cases, it ceases within 1 week, and in a large proportion of the remainder, it ends within 6 months. It is accompanied by anosmia in approximately 75% of cases (144). Because the glucose content of nasal discharge (40 mg/dL) differs little from that of CSF, glucose determinations are of no value in distinguishing CSF rhinorrhea from ordinary nasal discharge (145).

Several imaging modalities have been evaluated for their ability to pinpoint the site of CSF leakage. High-resolution CT and MR cisternography using a water-soluble nonionic contrast medium appear to be equally accurate in localizing the site and the extent of the CSF fistula (146,147) and are superior to CT cisternography (148). In our institutions, high-resolution CT and CT cisternography have proven to be adequate for pinpointing the site of CSF leakage.

When rhinorrhea has not ceased within 1 week to 10 days, surgical repair of the dural and bony defect is usually indicated, inasmuch as any CSF leak, particularly one that results in CSF rhinorrhea, predisposes to meningitis (143). The infecting agents are a variety of gram-positive cocci and gram-negative bacilli (149). Conservative management of CSF fistulas is successful in most instances. Bedrest with the head of the bed elevated is usually sufficient. Continuous lumbar or ventricular drainage often works in persistent CSF fistulas. If conservative treatment fails, surgical repair (intradural, extradural, or both) is required.

Whether chemoprophylaxis should be used on all patients with basal skull fractures has been the subject of considerable debate. Prospective studies have shown that prophylactic ampicillin does not reduce the risk of meningitis but can change the flora so that gram-negative organisms become the infecting agents (150). We therefore prefer to withhold antibiotics until careful observation has revealed evidence of infection. Lumbar puncture to obtain CSF and ascertain the presence of an infection is unwise because it can facilitate the entry of organisms into the anterior fossa by lowering intracranial pressure. The patient should be observed carefully, with therapy undertaken only when indicated by symptoms and subsequently by the CSF examination.

Injury to the cranial nerves, particularly the olfactory, facial, and acoustic nerves, can accompany basal fractures. Complete loss of the sense of smell is usually permanent; 90% of facial nerve injuries recover spontaneously (151). Deafness can be a temporary or permanent sequela to temporal bone fractures.

Labyrinthine disorders, notably vertigo and spontaneous or positional nystagmus, are common. In the experience of Eviatar and coworkers, more than 50% of children who had experienced a head injury complained of dizziness, headache, or both (152). The condition is usually transient. In approximately one-half of the cases, electronystagmography provides objective evidence of the presence of an injury to the labyrinth (152). Less commonly, one may encounter episodic vertigo that resembles Ménierè disease. It can result either from fistulization of the bony labyrinth with disturbed perilymph-endolymph pressure relationship or from direct injury to the membranous labyrinth or to the endolymphatic draining system (153).

CSF otorrhea is seen in approximately 0.5% of childhood head injuries, but in approximately 95% of cases it stops spontaneously within 7 to 10 days. Unlike CSF rhinorrhea, recurrence of leakage is rare (151). Rarely, transient total blindness can follow an apparently mild blunt head injury. The onset can be immediate or can be delayed for days or weeks (154). The child may not complain of vision loss, but can appear restless and disoriented and have an unsteady gait. The cause for blindness is uncertain, and outlook for recovery is poor. In some children the event may recur (155,156).

The diagnosis of basal fractures often depends on the clinical findings because in many instances, the fracture is not readily demonstrated by imaging studies. As a rule, the child with a basal fracture associated with hematotympanum or Battle's sign is hospitalized and observed. However, when the neurologic examination is normal and imaging studies do not show an intracranial injury, hospitalization might not be required (157). Because the incidence of meningitis in children with basilar skull fractures is only 1%, antibiotics should be withheld.

When meningitis is associated with a CSF leak, antibiotic treatment should be continued well after the leak stops.

Air within the cranial cavity (pneumocele) or air within the brain (pneumocephalus) rarely complicates head injury (158). When it does occur, it most commonly follows a fracture into the frontal sinuses and is usually an incidental finding on radiography. Pneumocephalus can denote either extradural or intradural air. Intradural air is of concern because it signifies a dural tear that can require surgical repair. Extradural air often denotes an air sinus disruption that may well resolve spontaneously. However, follow-up imaging is essential in all cases of pneumocephalus. Because meningitis develops occasionally, some centers suggest prophylactic antibiotic therapy until the air has resolved. Tension pneumocephalus is even more rare; it presents a neurosurgical emergency because of the rapid increase in intracranial pressure (159).

Depressed Fractures

Depressed fracture is a common consequence of perinatal injury, often the result of a difficult forceps delivery (ping-pong fracture; see Chapter 6). It also can occur with any localized skull trauma in later childhood in which there is an impact with a small surface with sufficient force to depress fragments of the inner table by at least the thickness of the skull (16). It is often associated with a break in the skin (compound fracture) and localized cerebral injury. The extent of the bony injury is best diagnosed by CT. In the past, elevation and examination of the underlying dura was recommended if the depression was greater than approximately 3 mm and the fracture did not reduce spontaneously. Steinbok and coworkers adopt a more conservative approach, reserving surgery for infants with compound depressed fractures or those with focal neurologic signs. The outcome appears to be the same with or without surgery (160). Ersahin and colleagues concur and suggest that conservative treatment is indicated whenever there is no underlying hematoma and the depression is less than 1 cm (161). We believe that a case can be made for elevating on cosmetic grounds a deep or unsightly depression, particularly when it is located in the frontal region.

Compound Fractures

Compound fractures of the skull are seen in approximately 20% of children with major head trauma (66). In this kind of injury, medical treatment is limited to an initial cleansing of the scalp, institution of antibiotics, and tetanus prophylaxis. Anticonvulsant therapy is used routinely when the bony fragments have penetrated beyond the dura. Traditionally, phenytoin has been the preferred drug. Its use requires an intravenous loading dose of 10 mg/kg and subsequent oral doses to maintain a blood level between 12 and 20 μg/mL. In children, maintaining this level is usually difficult and requires careful, repeated determinations of blood levels and adjustments of dose (162). Because of the unreliability of phenytoin in infants and small children and its relatively high incidence of side reactions, we prefer to use carbamazepine as a maintenance anticonvulsant.

Scalp Lacerations

Scalp lacerations can cause considerable blood loss. If any doubt exists about the presence of a scalp injury, the child's hair should be clipped and the area around the wound widely shaved. If examination and radiography do not show an underlying fracture, the wound should be closed in anatomic layers after careful débridement with strict adherence to aseptic techniques. Closure of the galeal layer to stem hemorrhage and protect from infection is optimal. Tetanus immunization should be administered.

Complications

Extradural Hematoma

An extradural or epidural hematoma is a localized accumulation of blood between the skull and the dura. It occurs in approximately 1.0% to 3.4% of children hospitalized for head trauma (66,163). According to Matson, nearly one-half of childhood cases occur during the first 2 years of life (164). In this age group, the injury is usually the result of a fall of less than 4 to 5 feet, and no other significant injuries are seen (68,165). In the experience of Shugerman and coworkers, 47% of children who developed an epidural hematoma had falls of 6 feet or less and skull fractures were seen in only 18%. Nonaccidental trauma was diagnosed in only 6% (165).

Pathogenesis

An extradural hematoma develops at or near the point of traumatic impact, usually in the temporoparietal region, less commonly in the frontal region. It is nearly always unilateral. In adults, the hematoma is almost invariably caused by a laceration of the middle meningeal artery or one of its branches. In children, extradural bleeding can be the consequence of even mild injury that has produced a tear in the dural veins, a scenario seen in 15% of patients in Matson's series (164), in the meningeal artery or its branches, in the accompanying middle meningeal veins (60% of cases), or in the smaller emissary veins of the dural sinuses (15%). The stripping of the dura from the skull successively tears more vessels, contributing to the enlargement of the hematoma. This successive tearing of dural vessels is probably why Mazza and coworkers were unable to identify a source in some 20% of their cases (166). Arterial bleeding results in a rapid deterioration of the clinical condition as the hematoma enlarges and produces acute cerebral compression (Fig. 9.6A and B). The severity of symptoms depends on the size of the hematoma, the speed of its evolution, and the development of transtentorial herniation. Transtentorial herniation is more likely when cerebral edema accompanies the hematoma. When bleeding arises from veins, neurologic symptoms progress gradually, a feature more common to the extradural hematomas of childhood than to those of adult life (167). Rarely, the hematoma can stop growing; it can then resolve or ultimately calcify.

The effects of transtentorial herniation accompanying an epidural hematoma are similar to those seen with other space-occupying lesions and are considered in Chapter 11.

Clinical Manifestations

In adults, an extradural hematoma characteristically is preceded by a temporary loss of consciousness followed by partial or full recovery, with subsequent deterioration of sensorium and appearance of focal neurologic signs. This sequence is rare in children; it did not appear in any of Mealey's 20 children with extradural hematoma (14). It appeared in only one-third of 125 cases reported by McKissock and colleagues (168) and in 40% of Mazza's 62 cases (166). More commonly, the child appears to be little affected by the initial injury or, at worst, has a brief period of unconsciousness. After an interval of minutes to

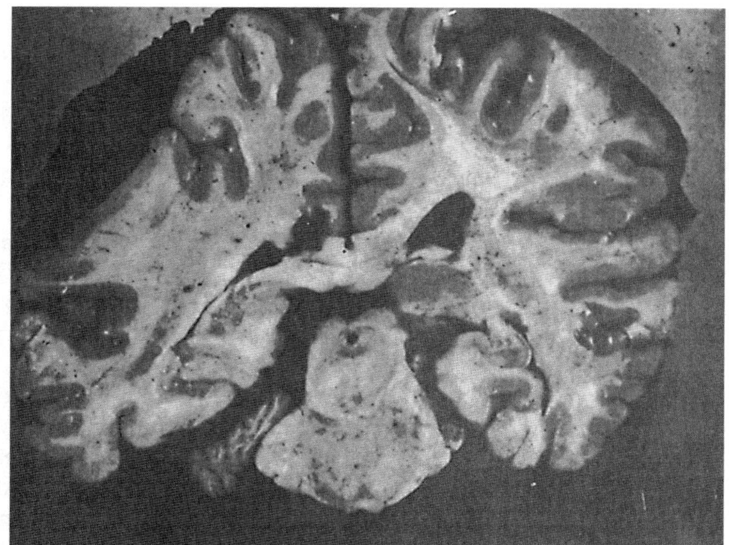

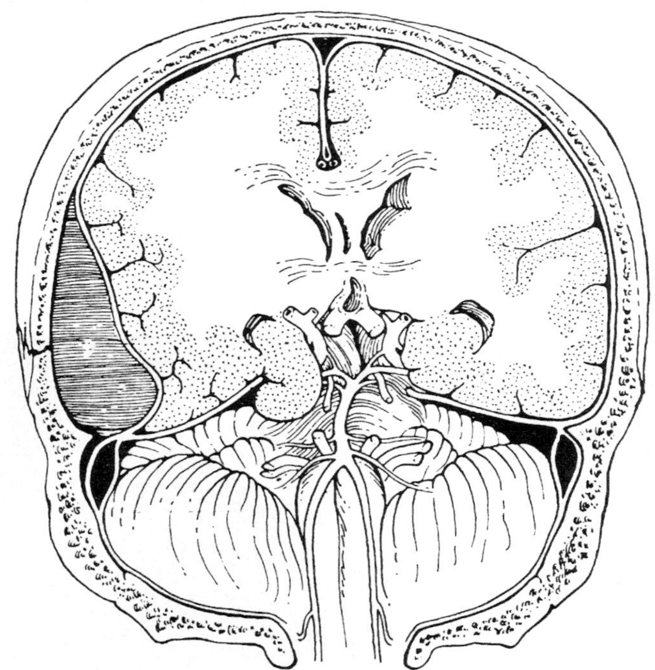

FIGURE 9.6. Cerebral compression and tentorial pressure cone owing to extradural hematoma. **A:** Coronal section of the brain. **B:** Diagram illustrating the swelling and displacement of the involved cerebral hemisphere with distortion of brainstem structures. (From Mealey J. *Pediatric head injuries*. Springfield, IL: Charles C. Thomas, 1968. With permission.)

several days, a progressive impairment of consciousness develops and neurologic signs appear. Of the children reported by McKissock and colleagues, the condition took this course in 67% (167). In general, the younger the child, the longer is the latency. In Mealey's series, 50% of children younger than 6 years of age remained asymptomatic for 12 hours or longer (14). The clinical picture of extradural hematoma is summarized in Table 9.10.

Aside from the delayed progressive impairment of consciousness, the most significant neurologic signs are pupillary inequality, hemiparesis, papilledema, and changes in vital signs. As the hematoma enlarges, signs of transtentorial herniation appear. The earliest of these signs is a dilated pupil that soon becomes unreactive to light and, in approximately 90% of instances, is on the side of the lesion (167). This dilation is followed by hemiparesis, usually contralateral to the hematoma, and finally by decerebrate rigidity and cardiovascular signs of decompensated increased intracranial pressure. Ipsilateral hemiparesis can develop caused by compression of the cerebral peduncle against the tentorial edge by a contralateral mass, and, in the days before neuroimaging, resulted in a false localizing sign (Kernohan sign) (168). Blood loss in infants can be sufficient to produce shock. When the latency period in infants is as long as days or weeks, progressive anemia can provide a clue to the diagnosis. Seizures resulting from an

TABLE 9.10 Common Clinical Features of Extradural Hematoma

Symptom[a]	*Percentage of Patients*
Vomiting	62.5
Unequal pupils	55.0
Delayed loss of consciousness	48.7
Skull fracture, all types	40.0
Hemiparesis	25.0
Papilledema	22.5
Depressed skull fracture	20.0
Third-nerve paresis, other than pupillary dilation	17.5
Retinal hemorrhages	12.5

[a]Symptoms listed occur with a significantly greater frequency in children with extradural hematomas than in the general head trauma series.
Modified from Hendrick EB, Harwood-Nash DC, Hudson AR. Head injuries in children: a survey of 4,465 consecutive cases at the Hospital for Sick Children. Toronto, Canada. *Clin Neurosurg* 1963;11:46.

epidural hematoma are rare and were present in only 7.5% of children seen by Hendrick and colleagues (66).

Occasionally, an extradural hematoma develops in the posterior fossa (169,170). Bleeding usually arises from the lateral dural sinuses, and fracture lines crossing the lateral sinus are seen nearly always. In almost all instances the history includes a severe fall on the occiput, followed by persistent impairment of consciousness, headache, vomiting, and neck stiffness. Only approximately one-half of the children have such posterior fossa signs as nystagmus, cerebellar ataxia, and cranial nerve palsies. Evacuation of a posterior fossa hematoma generally constitutes an emergency procedure.

Diagnosis

The diagnosis of an extradural hematoma rests principally on the clinical picture, and in some cases surgical treatment is so urgent that there is no time for imaging studies (84). Extradural hematoma must be differentiated from an acute subdural hematoma, an intracerebral hematoma, and severe brain swelling with or without contusion. Because both an acute extradural hematoma and an acute subdural hematoma require immediate surgical evacuation, the distinction between these two entities is academic. CT almost always detects the extradural hematoma, except when the collection of blood is very thin (Fig. 9.7). The usual appearance on CT scanning is a lenticular hyperdense lesion that crosses the suture lines (Fig. 9.8A). This is in contrast to a subdural hematoma, which tends to be crescent shaped and interdigitates with the cortical gyri (Fig. 9.8B). MRI is equal or superior to CT but is rarely indicated because of the time constraints associated with treating an acute injury. In 20% to 40% of children with extradural hematoma, a skull fracture is not

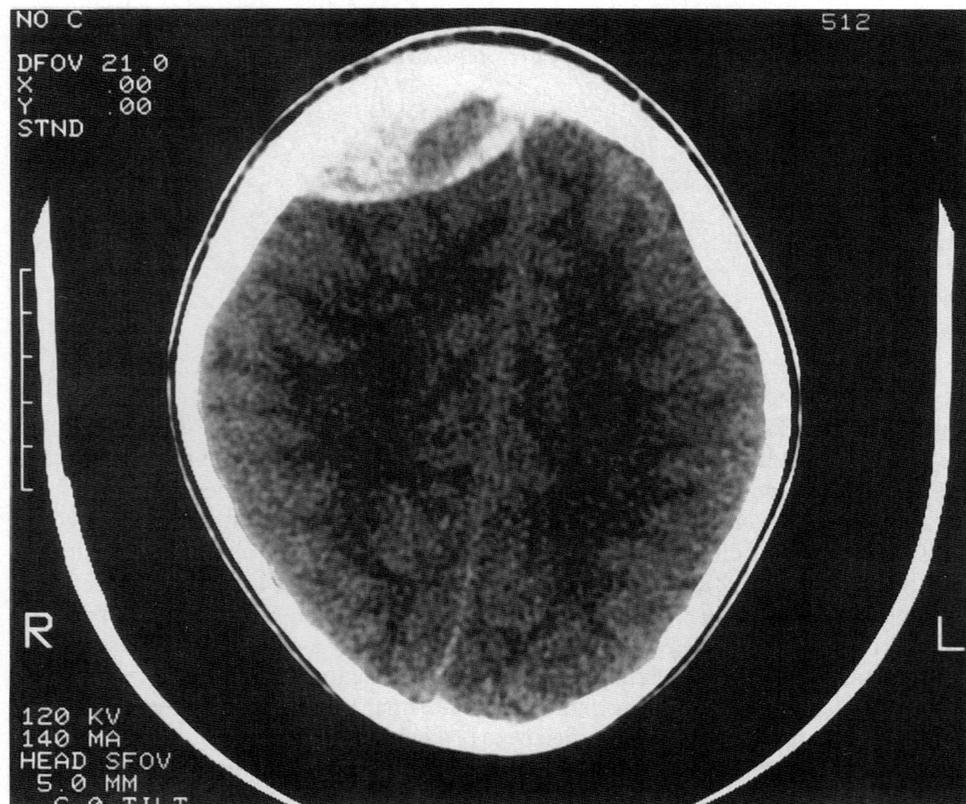

FIGURE 9.7. Extradural hematoma in a victim of child abuse. The lentiform shape of the hematoma and the fact that the collection of blood crosses to the opposite side are consistent with the presence of an extradural hematoma. Bone films (not shown) disclosed an underlying skull fracture. (Courtesy of Dr. Franklin G. Moser, Division of Neuroradiology, Cedars-Sinai Medical Center, Los Angeles, CA.)

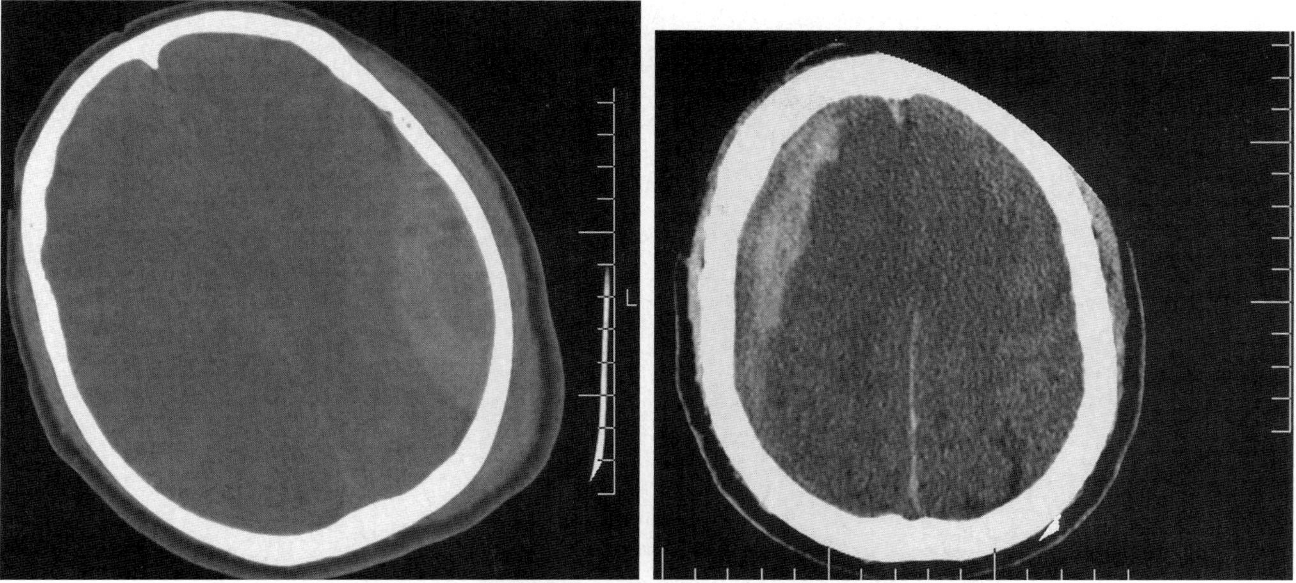

FIGURE 9.8. **A:** Left extradural hematoma in a teenager after a skateboard accident. Note the lentiform shape of the lesion. Epidural blood dissects the dura from the skull and causes this lenticular appearance, which spans the dural attachments between suture lines. **B:** Right subdural hematoma. Note that the bleeding interdigitates with the cortical sulci along the periphery of the hemisphere. The blood has extravasated into the subdural space between the arachnoid and the pia mater.

detectable by radiographic examination or even at operation (14), so that time should not be spent on searching for the fracture. EEG and MRI, which are also time-consuming procedures, should not be used to further delineate the hematoma.

Posterior fossa extradural hematomas are more difficult to recognize. The biconvex and more focal configuration of the extradural hematoma frequently permits the CT to distinguish between extradural and subdural accumulations.

Treatment

Operative removal of the clot can be performed occasionally through burr holes, but usually requires a craniotomy for complete removal and arrest of the bleeding. If the child's condition does not allow time for imaging studies, a low temporal burr hole is made for confirmation of the diagnosis and rapid removal of the clot. Further burr holes or craniectomy might then be needed. For details of the neurosurgical procedure, see Marshall (171) and Jennett and Teasdale (119). Repeat CTs are useful in assessing a patient after surgical evacuation of a hematoma.

Prognosis

Although the majority of patients show dramatic improvement, the general prognosis of extradural hematoma is grave if the condition is not treated in a timely fashion. Surgery for a large acute extradural hematoma is a life-saving procedure when performed within the first few hours of injury. In Matson's series, published in 1969, the mortality was nearly 10%, with another 20% of patients being left with major neurologic residua (164). Generally, infants fare worse than older children. In a 1986 series of children younger than 2 years of age reported by Choux and coworkers, 68% were left without apparent sequelae, some 10% died, and 12% had major residua (172). As a rule, the likelihood for sequelae increases if the child deteriorates acutely or had a depressed level of consciousness or neurologic abnormalities by the time of surgery. Posterior fossa extradural hematomas also have a grave prognosis, partly because they tend to progress rapidly (173). Despite the ready availability of imaging, the mortality in one series was 35%, and 20% of patients were left with a moderate disability (169). In more recently compiled cases the outlook was better, and in the series of Berker and coworkers from Turkey, 87% of children had a favorable outcome (170). It is clear that the prognosis for survival and the extent of the neurologic deficit are related to the early diagnosis of this complication and the presence of any associated brain damage.

Subdural Hematoma

A subdural hematoma is a collection of bloody fluid between the dura and the arachnoid over the cerebral mantle. It is a relatively common complication of recognized and unrecognized head trauma of childhood and represents one of the two major neurosurgical problems of

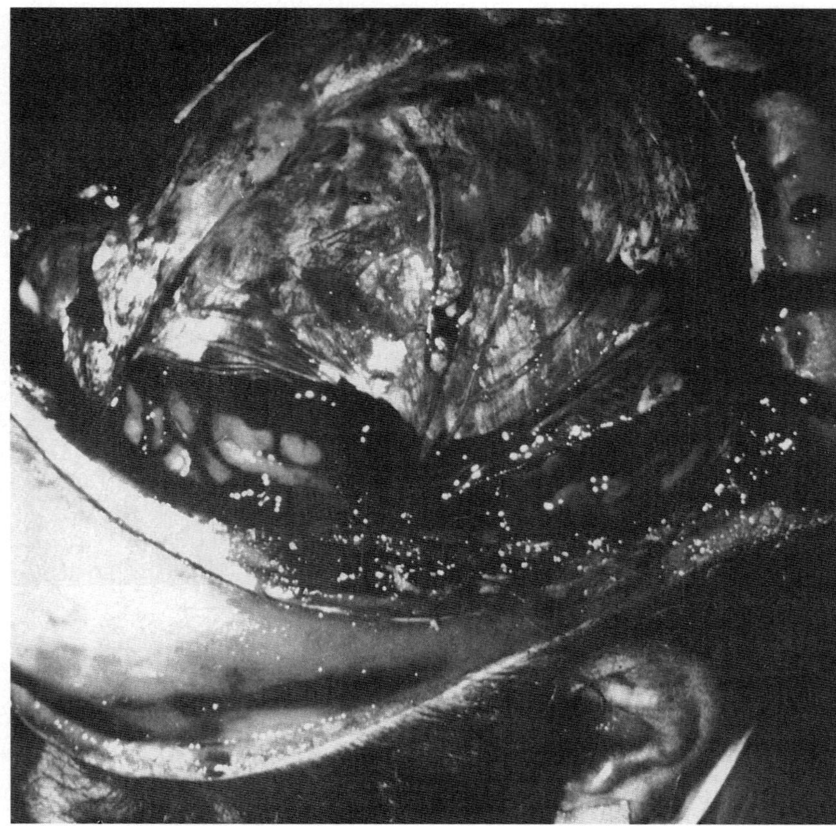

FIGURE 9.9. Subacute subdural hematoma. Gross appearance of the brain. Note blood oozing from the subdural compartment. (Courtesy of Dr. Harry V. Vinters, Division of Neuropathology, UCLA Center for the Health Sciences, Los Angeles, CA.)

infancy. In the series of Choux and coworkers, this complication was seen in 4.3% of children with head trauma; 73% of cases occurred in children younger than 2 years of age (172). A subdural hematoma should be distinguished from a postmeningitic subdural effusion containing clear or xanthochromic fluid with a high protein concentration. The etiology and the course of treatment of a postmeningitic subdural effusion differ from those of a subdural hematoma and are discussed in Chapter 7.

Pathogenesis

Subdural bleeding usually arises from the veins that pass from the cerebral cortex to the dural sinuses, bridging the potential subdural space. Skull distortion at the moment of injury, particularly in infants, and possibly the relative movement of the brain within the skull can so stretch these veins that they rupture and bleed beneath the dura, separating the dura from the underlying arachnoid membrane. It is also likely that a tear of the arachnoid allows CSF to leak into the subdural space. Venous bleeding also can arise from a laceration of the dura or from a direct injury to a dural sinus, as can happen with depressed fractures. Less often, the bleeding originates from cortical arteries and is associated with cerebral contusion (16). In 80% to 85% of infants, the hematoma is bilateral and located in the frontoparietal region. In a large percentage of infants whose hematomas result from postnatal trauma, parental abuse can be suspected from evidence of soft tissue bruising and radiographic evidence of multiple episodes of skeletal trauma (174,175).

The appearance of the hematoma varies with the age of the lesion (Fig. 9.9). In the acute stage (less than 48 hours), the fluid is composed of blood and clot. Subsequently, in the subacute stage (2 to 14 days), the formed elements break down, producing a fluid that is a mixture of clot and fluid and changes in color from chocolate to straw. It contains few red cells but large amounts of methemoglobin and bilirubin. Within approximately 1 week, a membrane forms from the inner surface of the dura and ultimately envelops the clot or fluid collection. After about 14 days the hematoma is chronic and consists solely of fluid blood (16). Eventually, the lesion can enlarge, probably from the leakage of albumin from the thin-walled and abnormally permeable vessels of the outer subdural membrane (176). The accumulation of albumin in the subdural pocket increases the osmotic pressure and causes an influx of water. The evolution of a subdural hematoma can be documented by CT; it is depicted in Fig. 9.10. Acute lesions tend to be hyperdense, and lesions that have produced symptoms for more than 3 weeks are usually hypodense; when symptoms have been present for 1 to 3 weeks, the fluid collection tends to be isodense. Under these circumstances the

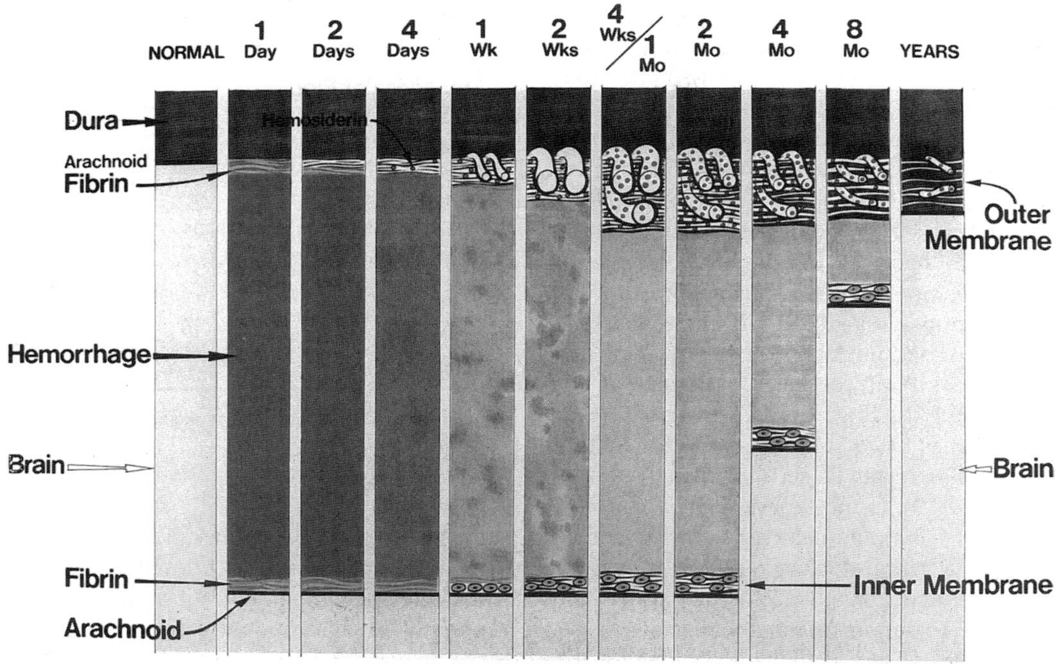

FIGURE 9.10. Temporal evolution of a subdural hematoma. (Courtesy of Dr. E.C.Alvord, Jr., Department of Pathology, University of Washington, Seattle, WA).

hematoma is recognized by ventricular compression and distortion.

Although the enlarging subdural hematoma can produce symptoms of increased intracranial pressure, no evidence exists that the presence of either a hematoma or the membranes interferes with brain development. Instead, any permanent neurologic deficit results from the original trauma that caused the hematoma. Additionally, often a diffuse damage occurs secondary to increased intracranial pressure and diminished cerebral perfusion. Single photon emission CT (SPECT) scanning has been of assistance in demonstrating both regional and diffuse abnormalities in cerebral perfusion (177). In experimental animals, focal ischemic damage in the hemisphere underlying the subdural hematoma is believed to result from the release of vasogenic substances from the hematoma that enhance vasoconstriction and attenuate vasodilatation (178). The focal ischemia, in turn, induces localized cytotoxic edema and the release of free radicals (179). The biochemical changes of the underlying parietal white matter show an accumulation of lactate and a loss of *N*-acetylaspartate. The severity of these alterations is believed to be prognostic of the outcome (180).

Unlike subdural hematomas in older children and in adults, the post-traumatic subdural hematoma of infants tends to recollect repeatedly, even after total evacuation. Mealey attributed the reaccumulation of fluid to the disproportion between the enlarged skull and the previously compressed brain (14). Most investigators now believe that rebleeding is the principal cause for recurrence and persistence of the subdural hematoma (181). Although it is unlikely that a subdural hematoma inhibits brain growth, it produces an enlargement of the skull and creates a pocket that tends to refill with blood. A similar disproportion between the volume of the brain and the skull increases the incidence of subdural hematomas in infants with congenital or acquired cerebral atrophy (14).

Clinical Manifestations

To a great extent, clinical manifestations depend on the patient's age. In older children, as in adults, the disorder can be acute or chronic. In both groups, symptoms of increased intracranial pressure predominate.

When a subdural hematoma after a serious head injury takes an acute course, symptoms develop within the first day or two. Venous bleeding usually does not produce symptoms unless it is accompanied by a major cerebral contusion or laceration. In these conditions, the hematoma is only one of several components of the injury, and its evacuation is not usually followed by rapid recovery (182). In part, the poor outlook reflects the aforementioned reduction of cerebral blood flow and metabolic rate throughout the hemisphere underlying the hematoma. Brain injury, usually in the form of an acute subdural hematoma, is seen in a significant proportion of battered babies, and an acute subdural hematoma is the most common cause of death or physical disability in infants; it must, therefore, be sought in all victims of child abuse.

Chronic subdural hematomas are the consequence of one of three scenarios: trauma, a complication of ventricular shunt placement, and the consequence of an infectious or parainfectious process (181).

A post-traumatic chronic subdural hematoma is most commonly seen in infants. It is usually encountered between ages 2 and 6 months, the average age at admission being 4 months. In this age group, the lesions are bilateral in approximately 80% of cases. In some 60% of infants, the environmental history or other evidence of recent unreported physical trauma suggests child abuse (68,183). The more serious the head injury, the greater is the likelihood of abuse. Of 45 infants younger than 1 year of age who sustained a skull fracture, only 11% were victims of child abuse, whereas of 19 infants who had a subdural hematoma or other forms of serious intracranial injury, 95% were abused (9). In the experience of Bruce and Zimmerman, 80% of traumatic deaths occurring in children younger than 2 years of age were nonaccidental; in fact, infants rarely sustain an accidental injury that is sufficiently severe to render them unconscious (184). Harcourt and Hopkins observed that intraocular hemorrhages in the absence of subdural effusions and external evidence of ocular trauma are commonly encountered in battered children. They postulated that these hemorrhages result from the gravitational effects of swinging the infant around by its feet (185). Additionally, compression of the thorax inducing an abrupt increase in intracranial pressure can play a role. Whether the abused infant is injured by these means or by violent to and fro shaking has since been disputed: Much greater gravitational forces can be generated by striking the infant's head against a mattress (183).

A chronic subdural hematoma can also develop in older children, especially during adolescence. In the latter age group, the clinical picture is one of a gradual change in personality and alertness, headaches, and, ultimately, seizures or rapid deterioration of consciousness. Often, there is no history of antecedent head trauma. The hematoma is unilateral in 80% of instances, and its differentiation from a tumor of the cerebral hemispheres is difficult clinically. The diagnosis is usually made by imaging studies. MRI permits better delineation of small subdural hematomas, hematomas that are adjacent to the falx or the tentorium, and isodense accumulations. MRI also delineates any associated cerebral injuries and assists in timing the lesion (89).

Occasionally, an arachnoid cyst in the middle fossa can predispose to a chronic subdural hematoma. The management of this condition is discussed by Swift and McBride (181) and Parsch and coworkers (186).

CT and MRI can be of considerable assistance in confirming that a child has been battered (86,187,188). An interhemispheric subdural hematoma in the subtemporal or the parieto-occipital region accompanied by a skull fracture can be documented in more than 50% of abused children, whereas in trauma unrelated to abuse, bleeding in this region accompanied by a skull fracture is seen in only 13% (187,189). Additionally, the presence of both acute and chronic hematomas supports the diagnosis of child abuse.

TABLE 9.11 Clinical Features of 116 Cases of Infantile Subdural Hematoma

Symptom of Finding	*Percentage of Infants*
Tense anterior fontanelle	73
Vomiting	70
Seizures	60
Retinal or subhyaloid hemorrhages	54
Abnormal skull circumference	40
Impaired consciousness	22
Papilledema	12
Skull fracture	13
Other fractures	17

Modified from Till K. Subdural haematoma and effusion in infancy. *BMJ* 1968;2:400.

An interhemispheric subdural hematoma should be distinguished from an interhemispheric subarachnoid hemorrhage (falx sign), which can be seen after perinatal trauma. In interhemispheric subarachnoid hemorrhage, the hemorrhage tends to extend along the entire interhemispheric fissure (190).

Although in infancy a chronic subdural hematoma lacks a characteristic clinical picture, certain features should suggest the condition. Lethargy and seizures are the most common presenting features. Seizures occur in approximately one-half of the patients; they are focal or, more commonly, generalized. Vomiting, fever, and hyperirritability or lethargy are other common clinical features (Table 9.11) (191,192). Most often, the infant's history includes failure to gain weight; refusal of feedings followed by frequent episodes of vomiting, some of which might be projectile; irritability; progressive enlargement of the head; and, ultimately, a seizure. Often, symptoms are present for several months before a diagnosis is made.

On examination, the infant can be febrile as a result of dehydration or blood within the cranial cavity. The head is enlarged, with a prominent parietal or biparietal bulge. The fontanelle is full, and a setting-sun sign of the eyes might be noted. Funduscopy can reveal retinal hemorrhages, subhyaloid hemorrhages, or, less commonly, papilledema. Retinal hemorrhages have been found in more than 50% of infants with a subdural hematoma, and almost invariably indicate a nonaccidental injury (164,174). Focal neurologic signs, including hemiparesis or facial palsy, are present in 15% to 25% of patients.

Laboratory studies are usually of little help in establishing the diagnosis, although approximately 50% of the infants are anemic. It is important to exclude a bleeding disorder, and various inborn errors of metabolism, notably kinky hair disease (Menkes disease), a sex-linked disorder of copper transport, and glutaric aciduria type 1, which can present with a subdural hematoma and subperiosteal bleeding (76,193). Lumbar puncture can reveal grossly bloody or xanthochromic fluid, evidence of an associated cerebral injury. The protein level can be elevated, and a pleocytosis can be present if the hematoma has been long-standing. The EEG is of little assistance in either the diagnosis or localization of a subdural hematoma and frequently fails to show any focal abnormality.

Diagnosis

A chronic subdural hematoma should be suspected in an irritable infant who has failed to gain weight and has developed an enlarged head and a tense fontanelle. Characteristically, the head assumes a biparietal bulge that differs from the frontal bulge of early hydrocephalus. Confirmation of the diagnosis and determination of the size of the hematoma and of any associated brain damage rest on CT and, if necessary, MRI.

Treatment

Several regimens have been proposed for the treatment of post-traumatic infantile subdural hematoma. These are based on the classic work of Sherwood (194) and Ingraham and Heyl (195), and are summarized by Swift and McBride (181) and in greater detail in a symposium edited by El-Kadi and Kaufman (196).

We have found that with serial subdural taps the collection of fluid dries up completely in selected patients, thus eliminating the need for a surgical procedure. When fluid re-forms between tapping or when imaging studies reveal the presence of a subdural clot, surgical intervention must be considered. This occurs in approximately 50% of cases. In the remainder of instances, fluid formation gradually decreases and the membranes disappear. However, this does not happen when the brain and skull are disproportionate, as is the case in cerebral atrophy. The operative removal of subdural membranes can never be complete. It is no longer practiced except when craniotomy is being performed for the removal of a large blood clot, which seldom is present in the chronic stage of infantile subdural hematoma. Instead, a subdural-peritoneal shunt (119,197) using simple tubes without valves allows the drainage of fluid and reduces the volume of dead space, allowing it to be obliterated by the growing brain. A unilateral shunt is sufficient in many cases (181,192). Subdural membranes completely disappear and the vascularity becomes reduced with time as long as the subdural space is adequately drained. Improvement can be confirmed by repeated imaging studies. Continuous external subdural drainage is also useful in selected patients before subdural-peritoneal shunting because in approximately one-half of the children the procedure makes it possible to avoid shunt placement (198).

Chronic subdural hematomas occurring in older children and adolescents are drained through burr holes (199). At this age, too, the fluid collection is frequently bilateral.

Prognosis

The prognosis for an infant with a subdural hematoma correlates with the extent of damage sustained by the brain rather than with the volume of subdural fluid itself. If brain injury has been extensive, the brain does not expand and the hematoma can calcify or ossify. Removal of a calcified subdural hematoma is of no advantage (200).

The prognosis for children whose subdural hematoma resulted from nonaccidental trauma has been shown to be relatively poor (201,202). Even when no gross neurologic deficits are present, abused children have a higher incidence of neurologic residua, significantly lower IQ scores, growth failure, and a significantly higher incidence of emotional handicaps compared to children with accidental subdural hematoma (203). These differences may result in part from the repetitive rotational forces experienced by the brain during shaking and in part from the socioeconomic environment of children who have experienced abuse (201,203).

Post-Traumatic Epilepsy

Seizures associated with trauma have been classified according to their time of onset into immediate, early, and late types (64,204). A few patients experience seizures 1 or 2 seconds after their head trauma. Such immediate seizures are most probably the result of direct mechanical stimulation of cerebral tissue having a low seizure threshold.

Seizures can appear during the first week after major cerebral trauma (early post-traumatic seizures). These arise from cerebral edema or from intracranial hemorrhage, contusion, laceration, or necrosis. The convulsions are usually generalized, but unilateral seizures and focal twitching (epilepsia partialis continua) can be seen. Generally, early post-traumatic epilepsy is more common in children than in adults, and in the experience of Jennett it was encountered in approximately 10% of head-injured children aged 5 years or younger (204). A history of prior seizures or developmental abnormalities is seen in approximately one-half of cases (205). Status epilepticus occurs in approximately one-fifth of children and is most likely to occur during the first hour after trauma (64). In the experience of Hendrick and his group, 7.4% of children with head trauma requiring hospitalization had seizures during the early post-traumatic period (66). The incidence was highest in infants younger than 1 year of age; those subjected to perinatal injury were particularly susceptible (see Chapter 6).

In the experience of Hendrick and colleagues, 24% of patients with early post-traumatic seizures had an associated skull fracture (66). Closed and compound depressed fractures are particularly common, together accounting for approximately one-half the fractures seen in patients with early post-traumatic epilepsy. Seizures, and even status epilepticus, are far more likely to occur in children who sustained relatively minor head trauma than in adults with similar trauma.

Late post-traumatic seizures tend to develop within the first 2 years after the injury. The mechanisms that cause post-traumatic epilepsy are poorly understood. In some instances seizures are believed to originate from a cerebromeningeal scar, with the epileptic focus localized to grossly normal tissue (206). Experimental studies show that head trauma induces long-term alterations in both the excitatory and inhibitory circuits in the hippocampus, resulting in a persistent decrease of the seizure threshold (207). Approximately 75% of children with late post-traumatic seizures had no significant deficits at the time of the injury (208). In approximately 50% of cases, seizures appear during the first 12 months after trauma (64). The overall incidence of late post-traumatic epilepsy is difficult to estimate because the figure is lowered by the inclusion of mild head injuries in any prospective series. In the series of Annegers and colleagues, which included both children and adults, the 5-year and 30-year cumulative incidence after severe head injury was 10% and 16.7%, respectively. It is of note that after severe injury the incidence of new-onset seizures remained elevated throughout the follow-up period, an indication that the interval between serious head injury and the onset of post-traumatic seizures can be many years (209).

According to Jennett, the likelihood of late post-traumatic epilepsy is increased by the presence of any of three factors: an acute hematoma, a depressed skull fracture, and early epilepsy (64). Temkin arrived at similar risk factors (210). These conclusions, derived from his experience with a mixed adult and pediatric population, need some amplification. Annegers and colleagues found that in children the presence of early post-traumatic epilepsy did not predict late post-traumatic epilepsy (205), and Jennett noted that when early focal seizures occured in children, the incidence of late post-traumatic seizures did not increase significantly (64). It is not clear whether the location of brain injury, as judged from the fracture site, affects the likelihood of late epilepsy. Most authorities agree, however, that injuries to the parietal lobe and to the anterior and medial parts of the temporal lobe are most likely to be followed by late post-traumatic epilepsy (210).

In Jennett's data, only 2% of children who retained consciousness after head trauma developed post-traumatic epilepsy (64). The percentage rose to 5% to 10% when consciousness was lost for 1 hour or longer. By comparison, children who sustained brain laceration had a 30% incidence of post-traumatic epilepsy. In general, if the dura is penetrated, the incidence of post-traumatic epilepsy increases at least twofold. Temkin confirmed these data (210). Another factor that influences the incidence of late epilepsy is the duration of post-traumatic amnesia; late epilepsy is twice as common in children with more than 24 hours of post-traumatic amnesia.

Seizures can take several clinical forms. They can be generalized or focal with secondary generalization. Focal seizures can be preceded by an aura consisting of motor phenomena such as clonic movements of an extremity or by somatosensory phenomena. The seizures also can be focal without secondary generalization, but petit mal (absence) attacks do not occur as a result of trauma (64,211). The EEG has proved to be uniformly unsuccessful in predicting post-traumatic epilepsy in children (64,212).

The diagnosis of post-traumatic epilepsy depends on the antecedent history of head trauma and the absence of any pretraumatic seizure history. The possibility of an intracranial hematoma should always be excluded using imaging studies.

Treatment of post-traumatic epilepsy is similar to that used for focal or generalized seizures of unknown cause (see Chapter 14). Although prophylactic phenytoin and other anticonvulsants reduce seizures during the first week after injury, they do not prevent late post-traumatic seizures (213).

Generally, the prognosis of post-traumatic seizures is good. The clinical impression that seizures that begin within 2 years of trauma have a better likelihood of subsiding than those with a later onset has not been proven by more recent studies. Jennett and Teasdale concluded that once a patient has developed late post-traumatic epilepsy, the patient will always remain prone to a seizure disorder, even though he or she can experience remissions of 2 years or longer (119). In approximately 20% to 50% of all patients, seizures gradually become less frequent after the third year and finally cease completely (64,214). In all instances, medical therapy should be used first, but surgery for excision of the meningocerebral scar and any underlying cysts or gliosis should be considered in patients whose seizures persist for 2 or more years despite adequate anticonvulsant therapy.

Some children are subject to profound but temporary alterations of consciousness after relatively mild head trauma. The attacks, similar to complicated migraine, are marked by a scotoma or other visual symptoms, including cortical blindness, hemianopsia, brainstem signs, confusion or depression of consciousness, headache, nausea, and vomiting (215,216). Convulsions can develop after the onset of the migraine-like symptoms, as can a hemiparesis. Attacks do not develop immediately after head trauma, but rather after a symptom-free interval of several minutes to an hour. The great majority of attacks resolve completely within 24 hours. During an attack, EEG tracings show symmetric or asymmetric slowing, whereas cerebral angiography and neuroimaging are generally normal. The mechanism for the attacks is unknown (216).

Major Vascular Injuries

Blunt or penetrating injuries to the major vessels of the head or neck are relatively uncommon in children who have experienced trauma to that area. Blunt carotid injuries can result in a contusion or tear of the wall of the internal carotid artery, with a subsequent dissecting aneurysm, or in a carotid-cavernous fistula (217,218,219). A traumatic carotid-cavernous fistula can also be caused by a sphenoid bone fracture that lacerates the internal carotid artery as it passes through the cavernous sinus. Symptoms include unilateral pulsating exophthalmos, an intracranial bruit, and paralysis of the cranial nerves, most commonly the sixth (220). Traumatic thrombosis of the internal carotid artery has been reported in children as a result of relatively minor injuries to the head or neck, such as following puncture of the soft palate by a lollipop stick (221). Internal carotid artery dissection can appear immediately after what often is relatively minor trauma or can develop after a few hours or days (222,223). Spontaneous internal carotid artery dissection is an important cause of cerebrovascular accidents in children (see Chapter 13). Symptoms include focal ischemia or a headache accompanied by an objective and subjective bruit and by Horner syndrome. Internal carotid artery dissection is treated by anticoagulation and early thrombectomy if the site of obstruction is accessible (223).

Trauma to the cervical spine can produce stretching of the vertebral arteries, with disruption of the endothelium and subsequent arterial dissection. Symptoms of intermittent brainstem and cerebellar dysfunction can develop and last for months or years. When, as often occurs, the patient has no history of antecedent trauma, cervical spinal trauma is difficult to differentiate from complicated migraine (224–226). MRI of the upper cervical spine and foramen magnum region and MR angiography can assist in the diagnosis (227). Basilar artery migraine is covered in Chapter 15.

Delayed Deterioration after Mild Head Injury

A relatively common, potentially fatal complication of head injury in the pediatric age group is one of rapid secondary deterioration occurring within minutes or hours after relatively minor trauma and after a lucid interval or a period of improved consciousness (228). A significant proportion of children with this symptom complex have early post-traumatic seizures, sometimes with focal or generalized status epilepticus. The syndrome also has been encountered in youngsters who have experienced repeated concussive injuries in sports ("second-impact syndrome") (229).

The mechanism underlying this phenomenon is not fully understood. Kors and coworkers noted that in at least some patients with delayed post-traumatic cerebral edema have a mutation in the gene that encodes the α_{1A} subunit of a neuronal calcium channel that is primarily involved in the release of neurotransmitters (*CACNA1A*) (230). Mutations of this gene are responsible for familial hemiplegic migraine and episodic ataxia.

In the series of Bruce and colleagues, diffuse cerebral swelling after minor head injury was encountered in 15% of children and adolescents whose Glasgow coma scores on admission were 8 or better (231). Most likely, the swelling results from vasodilatation and hyperemia, which is probably the indirect consequence of a channelopathy. This in turn, disrupts neurotransmitter release and causes the loss of cerebral vascular autoregulation, with a subsequent increase in brain bulk. Treatment is directed at constricting brain vascular volume. This is best accomplished by prolonged (24 to 48 hours) hyperventilation of the intubated youngster coupled with the treatment scheme for cerebral edema described elsewhere in this chapter. Kors and coworkers also proposed the use of acetazolamide (230).

Post-Traumatic Mental Disturbances

Whereas it has been argued that because of its greater plasticity the brain of a child recovers more fully after injury than that of an adult, this is true only in terms of gross neurologic function. It is now becoming apparent that early brain damage limits intellectual capacity and, in so doing, constrains the formation of new cognitive products over the remaining years of brain growth and maturation (231a). Furthermore, numerous studies now indicate that the younger the child subjected to head injury, the more likely it is that cognitive and academic development will be compromised, and the more significant will be the long-term consequences of the head injury (232).

In the experience of Koskiniemi and colleagues, who studied the long-term outcome of severe head injury incurred by preschool children, 30% had a below-normal IQ when tested in adulthood (233). Only 21% of those with normal IQ were able to work full time outside the home. None of the children who experienced the head injury before 4 years of age were able to work independently. A secondary attention-deficit hyperactivity disorder is commonly seen in children who suffered head injuries. In the recent series of Max and collaborators, it was encountered in 38% of children with severe head injuries and in 8% of children with mild to moderate head injuries. In some of the latter group the attention-deficit hyperactivity disorder was preexisting (233a).

As a rule, the capacity for new learning is more affected than retention of previously learned information. Perceptual-motor and spatial skills appear to be particularly susceptible to early insult. These deficits are most marked in children who sustained their injury at a young age and are proportional to the duration of impaired consciousness (233). Attention and verbal and written language abilities are also compromised (234). Deficits in verbal and visual recognition memory are particularly evident in younger children and are proportional to the duration of impaired consciousness. Although severity of injury is an important predictor of outcome, age at insult and psychosocial variables must all be acting both independently and interactively to determine prognosis (235). From these data one must conclude that a child is better able to compensate for focal brain injury than an adult, but tolerates less well a diffuse injury that interferes with learning capacities (231a). Skills that are not yet well developed at the time of the head injury are more susceptible to disruption than those that are already well established (234). The effects of brain trauma on an established skill are illustrated in Fig. 9.11A. Improvements in performance with age occur at a growth rate *b*. At some point of time t_2 recovery reaches a plateau, leaving a residual deficit *c*. When the brain injury affects a developing skill, as illustrated in Fig. 9.11B, the deficit may not be apparent at time t_1. This is because the skill has not yet emerged. Sequelae, however, become more marked over time as the child fails to acquire skills at an expected rate. With further time, the disparity between a normal child and a child who has acquired brain trauma may become even more striking as a skill becomes more complex or as new learning is required (232).

Neuroimaging studies, notably positron emission tomography scans and SPECT scans, can corroborate the various cognitive deficiencies by showing areas of hypoperfusion, but these tests do not assist with prognosis (237).

One of the most obvious cognitive deficits is post-traumatic amnesia, an inability to recall events as a result of injury. In most cases, the length of post-traumatic amnesia is proportional to the severity of brain damage (80,236). One of the common features of concussion injuries is a failure to recall events that occurred just before the injury (retrograde amnesia). Here, too, a relationship exists between the length of time before the accident for which memory is impaired and the severity of the brain injury. Post-traumatic amnesia is usually more extensive than retrograde amnesia (238). When a patient has unusually extensive retrograde amnesia, trauma to the limbic system, particularly the hippocampal formation and the mamillary bodies, should be suspected. We and others have encountered the occasional child in whom a mild head injury triggers a profound global and retrograde amnesia. Whether this represents a form of traumatic migraine is unresolved (239). Generally, the rate of recovery from amnesia is faster in children than in adults; however, in the experience of Harris, major post-traumatic psychological difficulties persisted in one-half of the 13% of children who manifested prolonged retrograde amnesia (240).

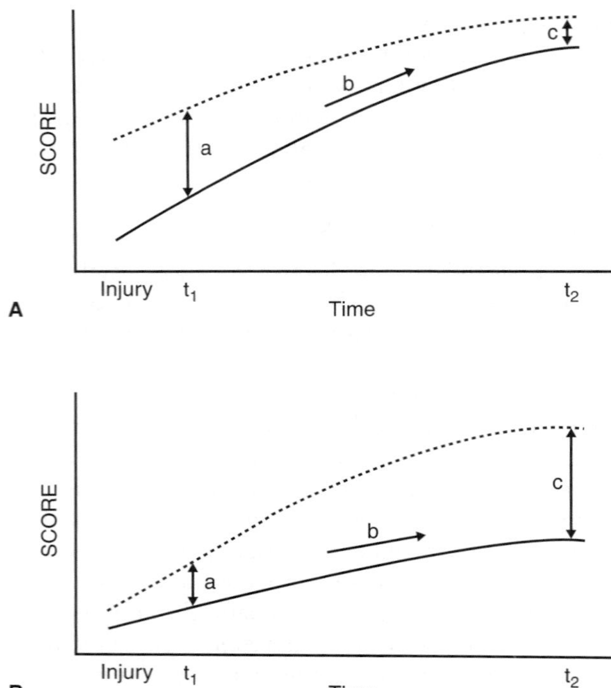

FIGURE 9.11. **A:** Hypothetical developmental changes in established skills in children with brain insults (*solid line*) and in unaffected children (*dotted line*). **B:** Hypothetical developmental changes in to-be-acquired skills in children with brain insults (*solid line*) and in unaffected children (*dotted line*). (From Taylor HG, Alden J. Age-related differences in outcomes following childhood brain insults: An introduction and overview. *J Internat Neuropsychol Soc* 1997;3:555–557. Courtesy Dr. H.Gerry Taylor, Department of Pediatrics, Rainbow Babies & Childrens Hospital, Cleveland. OH.)

The effects of a mild head injury, that is, an injury that is sufficiently severe for the child to be seen in the emergency room but not severe enough to require hospitalization, have been studied extensively. It is the current consensus that if the injury occurs at an important developmental age, children may fail to develop certain skills such as reading abilities as quickly as controls (241,242).

In many instances, however, the appearance of major psychiatric disorders after head injury, including lability of mood, outbursts of anger, increased aggressiveness, sleep disturbances, nightmares, and enuresis, is unrelated to the injury itself, but reflects the child's family and social environment. In this respect, it is undoubtedly significant that a large proportion of children showing these posttraumatic behavior disturbances had a history of previous accidents requiring medical treatment, and that approximately 25% were either mentally retarded or had required psychiatric therapy before their head injury. In the experience of Mahoney and colleagues (132), and Hjern and Nylander (247), the overwhelming majority of children with persistent psychiatric symptoms had similar problems before their accident, which only served to aggravate symptoms. Other studies however, have not found any significantly higher than normal rates of preinjury problems in children who suffered mild head injuries (242a). It does appear however, that head injury increases a child's vulnerability to subsequent environmental stresses (243). It is also significant that when head injuries are incurred during sports, the clinical picture of the postconcussion syndrome, although similar to that seen after potentially litigious injuries, is strikingly brief (244). This observation lends support to the view that the postconcussion syndrome results from environmental, psychological, and physiologic factors. These are reviewed by Nylander and Rydelius (245), and by McClelland and colleagues (246).

Psychiatric symptoms of head injury can frequently be avoided by giving parents, particularly mothers, reassurance or extensive supportive therapy at an early stage, preferably as soon as the child is admitted to the hospital (247). We have most of our patients return to school as soon as feasible but recommend limiting academic demands, increasing them gradually as warranted by the child's adjustment and school performance. Based on the considerable evidence that the effects of repeated concussion are additive, children who have had two or more episodes of head injury associated with loss of consciousness or amnesia should not be allowed to participate in contact sports (228). This is consistent with the practice parameters issued by the American Academy of Neurology (248).

In summary, the long-term outcome of severe head injuries is poor when incurred in infancy or during the preschool years in terms of both gross neurologic deficits and developmental delays. In infants, the results of the ocular examination, part of the pediatric Glasgow coma score assessed on admission, appear to be most predictive of the outcome. Additionally, when an initial CT scan demonstrates cerebral swelling and a midline shift, a poor outcome can be expected. The outcome for older children is better; it is a function of the condition of the child on admission to the hospital, the severity of increased intracranial pressure, and the duration of coma. Even prolonged coma is consistent with recovery without major neurologic deficits. For instance, in one study, 26% of children who were in coma longer than 24 hours died and 61% had a good outcome from a gross neurologic standpoint (132).

PERSISTENT VEGETATIVE STATE

Persistent vegetative state (PVS) is a relatively rare sequela to major head trauma in the pediatric population. As defined by Jennett and Plum (249), in this state the patient exhibits periods of apparent wakefulness during which the eyes open and move and responsiveness is limited to primitive postural and reflex movements of the limbs.

In the majority of instances, patients blink in response to painful stimuli, exhibit spontaneous eye movements, and show a sleep–wake periodicity. Less often, yawning, chewing, and eye-following movements occur. Meaningless laughter and weeping are not unusual. Decerebrate rigidity is seen in approximately one-half of cases and reflects damage to the midbrain and pons. This is confirmed by MRI studies that show diffuse axonal injury localized in the majority of instances to the corpus callosum and the dorsolateral aspect of the rostral brainstem (250). PVS should be distinguished from the minimally conscious state in which there is minimal behavioral evidence of self or environmental awareness (251).

Higashi and coworkers proposed three levels of PVS (252). Level I is marked by the presence of a sleep–wake cycle and emotional expression, level II is marked by a sleep–wake cycle without emotional expression, and level III is marked by the absence of the sleep–wake cycle. The EEG does not correspond to the severity of damage or to changes in the clinical status; in fact, 25% of patients demonstrate a significant amount of activity.

The prognosis of PVS in the pediatric patient when it follows head trauma is significantly better than when it follows hypoxic brain injury (253). In the experience of Heindl and Laub, 84% of children who had been in post-traumatic PVS for at least 30 days had left PVS 19 months after the injury. Of all children in post-traumatic PVS, 16% were able to become independent. However, after 9 months in PVS less than 5% were able to leave this state (253). Survival in PVS is conditional on the age of the youngster, with infants younger than 1 year of age having a mean survival of 2.6 years, as contrasted with 5.2 years in children aged 2 to 6 years and 7.0 years in children aged 7 to 18 years (254). The same group found that life expectancy doubled between the 1980s and 1993 to 1996, so that in 1993 life expectancy for a 15-year-old in PVS was 10.5 to 12.2 years. For a 1-year-old it was 7.2 years (255). See Chapter 17 for a discussion of the diagnosis of brain death in infants and children.

SPINAL CORD INJURIES

Because of the spinal cord's protected location, a considerable amount of direct trauma is required to injure it. In children, therefore, injuries to the spinal cord are relatively uncommon. Most frequently, they are the result of indirect trauma. This is seen in accidents marked by sudden hyperflexion or hyperextension of the neck or by vertical compression of the spine resulting from falls on the head or buttocks, as can occur from surfing, diving into shallow water, falling from a horse, or various other athletic accidents (256). In physically abused infants, spinal cord injuries can be induced by violent shaking of the head. Obstetric spinal cord injuries are covered in Chapter 6.

Pathology and Pathophysiology

Based on gross pathologic findings, Norenberg and coworkers divided spinal cord injuries into four groups (257). Most common is contusion of the cord with cavity formation. In this type of injury there is no disruption of the surface anatomy, but there are areas of hemorrhage and necrosis that ultimately evolve into cysts. Laceration of the cord induces a clear disruption of the surface anatomy. This injury is usually caused by sharp fragments of bone. In massive compression of the cord the injury is caused by direct compression from without by bone and intervertebral disc or from within by a hematoma. Solid cord injury refers to a cord that grossly appears normal but on histologic examination shows gross disruption of the normal architecture.

The importance of vascular changes in the induction of spinal cord injury has only recently become evident. In particular, post-traumatic ischemia is of major importance in the evolution of spinal cord lesions (258). The anterior spinal artery and its sulcal branches seem particularly vulnerable; the vascular shed in the upper thoracic cord and the ventral radicular artery (artery of Adamkiewicz), which usually feeds the cord at approximately the tenth thoracic vertebra, are other favorite sites for interruption of the blood supply (259). Relatively minor trauma to this area or to the cervical spine can, on occasion, result in an infarction of the spinal cord, with ensuing paraparesis or quadriparesis, respectively (260). Such injuries constituted 8% of spinal cord injuries at the Toronto Hospital for Sick Children (261). Symptoms do not appear immediately, but after a latent period of some 2 hours to 4 days. Paraplegia or tetraplegia is usually profound and recovery is unlikely. Imaging study results are generally normal, although spinal angiography occasionally visualizes an occlusion of the anterior spinal artery (261).

When the patient survives major spinal cord injury for a long time, the damaged area is found to be softened, gray and white matter are poorly delineated, the myelin sheaths are destroyed, and all cellular elements are lost extensively. Replacement by cavities or fibrous gliosis occurs ultimately. In less than 5% of paraplegics, this leads to post-traumatic syringomyelia with worsening of symptoms starting one to several years after the initial injury. There is dispute as to the mechanism of the syringomyelic cavity (262). It can arise from a hematoma at the site of the original injury or from softening of the cord and liquefaction, or it may result from the cord being pulled open by meningeal fibrosis or arachnoiditis. If the injury is symptomatic and of significant diameter, most authorities advise syringo-subarachnoid or syringo-pleural drainage, although others prefer a wide opening of the subarachnoid spaces to allow free CSF movement past the area of cord damage (263).

In many patients in whom an accident produced early paraplegia, the spinal cord does not show any gross pathologic abnormality. Termed *spinal concussion*, this condition is characterized by transient loss of spinal cord function (264). The mechanism inducing spinal concussion is not clear, but is believed to involve changes in the microvasculature and in neurotransmitters.

Common sites for childhood spinal cord injuries are the second cervical vertebra (27%), followed by the tenth thoracic vertebra (13%), the seventh thoracic vertebra (6%), and the first lumbar segment (6%) (265). Fractures of the twelfth thoracic and first lumbar vertebrae are relatively common and can produce a conus medullaris and cauda equina syndrome.

In the experience of Hamilton and Myles, fracture of the vertebral body or posterior elements without subluxation was the most common pediatric spinal injury. It was seen in 56% of patients (256). Fracture with subluxation was seen in 29% and subluxation without fracture in only 2%. Major spinal cord injury without any radiologic abnormalities was seen in 13% of children. It was the most common form of spinal injury in children younger than 9 years of age, being encountered in 42% of spinal cord injuries.

With the increased use of lap belts in cars, children can incur a horizontal splitting of the spine, also known as a Chance fracture, in the course of a motor vehicle accident. The typical fracture involves L1 with a transverse fracture through the vertebra, with compression of the anterior portion of the body, and vertical distraction posteriorly. Intraabdominal injuries are common, but the spinal canal can be compromised with resultant spinal cord injury and paraplegia (266). The radiographic findings are often subtle and are best visualized on lateral lumbar spine views (267).

Because of the mobility of the neck, the lower cervical region is particularly prone to fracture and dislocation injuries. Direct violence along the axis of the vertebral column can produce fractures of the vertebral bodies, and the spinal cord can be injured by fragments of bone that enter the vertebral canal.

Discussion of the acute and secondary pathophysiologic responses of the spinal cord to injury, in particular, the contributions of calpain activation, inflammation, oxygen radical formation, and lipid peroxidation to cell damage and death, are beyond the scope of this text. This topic is reviewed by Carlson and Gorden (268) and Dumont and coworkers (269).

Clinical Manifestations

The clinical picture depends on the severity of the injury and its location. Concussion can result from apparently minor falls on the back and is characterized by a temporary and completely reversible loss of function below the injured segment. With more extensive injuries, recovery is only partial and permanent residua can be expected.

Evaluation of the patient who has sustained injury to the spinal cord has been facilitated by a grading system devised by Frankel and coworkers (270) and more recently modified by the American Spinal Injury Association (271). The Frankel scheme describes four levels: (a) no sensory or motor function; (b) incomplete sensory function, no motor function; (c) incomplete sensory function, no useful motor function; and (d) normal function with some spasticity.

When the cord is seriously compromised, the clinical picture is highlighted by spinal shock. Spinal shock is described in the classic experimental studies of Sherrington (272) and their clinical application by Riddock (273). The condition is marked by the loss of all reflex function distal to the injury, with the segments closest to the injury being the most severely affected. Spinal shock represents a transient decrease of synaptic excitability of neurons distal to the injury. It is caused by loss of supraspinal impulses, which normally produce a background of partial depolarization of the spinal neurons. Clinically, spinal shock can persist for days or weeks and can be prolonged by sepsis, particularly urinary tract infection. The evolution of spinal shock to the return of reflexes and progression to spasticity is reviewed by Ditunno and coworkers (274). This process probably reflects a reorganization of receptors (275,276).

Immediately after the injury, the patient experiences complete loss of motor and sensory function in the segments caudal to the injury (277). There is complete areflexia of variable duration, usually for at least 2 to 6 weeks. A delayed plantar response, a slow flexion, and relaxation of the toes in response to a very strong stroking from the heel toward the toes along the lateral side of the foot can often be elicited (274). Should reflex activity not return, probably the distal spinal cord has been destroyed as the result of vascular insufficiency.

During the first stage of spinal shock, the stage of flaccidity, complete bladder paralysis, and urinary retention occur (273, 278). Gradually, a muscular response of the lower extremities can be elicited in response to stimulation of the skin or the deeper structures. The earliest movements occur in the legs and are flexor. The deep tendon reflexes reappear and soon become hyperactive. Abdominal reflexes also can return. A typical extensor plantar response can be induced and is often accompanied by flexor withdrawal movements of the foot, ankle, and, subsequently, the knee and hips. Contraction of the extensor muscles of the crossed limb frequently accompanies the mass flexion reflex (273,279). During this stage, the bladder empties automatically, although never completely.

In the majority of patients, extensor reflexes involving the quadriceps and other extensor muscles ultimately appear, becoming the dominant reflex activity. Stimuli eliciting the extensor reflex are more complicated than those inducing the flexion response. They include extension of the thigh, as is seen when the patient shifts from a sitting to a supine position, and squeezing of the thigh.

Depending on the severity of the spinal cord injury, the ultimate result can be purely reflex activity of the isolated cord. With less extensive injuries, muscular function or subjective sensation can return over the course of the next few months up to 1 year.

The neurologic picture of the most common spinal cord injuries is summarized in Table 9.12.

An unusual clinical picture that occurs exclusively in children is a transient apparent subluxation of the atlantoaxial joint, which often follows an upper respiratory infection or trauma, especially sports-related trauma (279,280). It is called *rotary atlantoaxial luxation*. Children present with a head tilt to the affected side, the "cock robin sign," after its similarity to the appearance of the bird. The neck is tender laterally and posteriorly over C1 and C2. The bulge of the anterior dislocation can be felt by the examiner through the posterior pharyngeal wall, but is best diagnosed by cine-CT scan. This study demonstrates that the subluxed axis and atlas move as a unit during neck rotation (280). The condition is associated only rarely with root or cord signs and usually resolves with traction and immobilization. When the subluxation is persistent or recurrent, as happens in the occasional patient, surgical immobilization is required.

Dislocation of the atlantoaxial joint and an increased atlantoaxial interval are seen with particular frequency in Down syndrome (see Chapter 4). It is also encountered in neurofibromatosis (NF-1) (281), Marfan syndrome, and Arnold-Chiari malformation type I.

Diagnosis

The history of trauma is usually readily elicitable, and the most common diagnostic problem is to establish the site and extent of the injury. In small children, the physician can best perform a sensory examination by demonstrating impairment of autonomic response. Shortly after the injury, the dermatomes below the lesion are dry and often have a defective vasomotor response. Evaluation of reflexes and motor function should not be particularly difficult because reflex withdrawal is not seen during the acute phase of spinal shock.

TABLE 9.12 Clinical Features of Spinal Cord Injuries

Injury	*Neurologic Features*
Transverse Injuries	
T12–1.1	Flaccid paralysis of lower extremities
	Loss of sphincter control
	Loss of sensation below inguinal ligament
C5–6	Flaccid quadriparesis
	Sparing of diaphragmatic movements
	Sensory level at second rib, with preservation of sensation over upper lateral aspect of arm
	Bilateral Horner syndrome
	Loss of sphincter control
C1–4	Respiratory paralysis, complete quadriplegia
	Rapid death
Conus Medullaris	
Cauda equina syndrome	Urinary retention
	Disturbance of renal sphincter
	Loss of sensation over lumbosacral dermatomes
	Flaccid paralysis of lower extremities
Brown-Séquard Syndrome	Unilateral muscular paresis
	Contralateral disturbances of superficial sensitivity, especially pain and temperature
	Incomplete forms far more common than classic syndrome
Central Cord Lesion	Disproportionately more motor impairment of upper extremities (caused by involvement of the more medial segments of the lateral corticospinal tracts)
	Lower motor neuron lesion of upper extremities; upper motor neuron lesion of lower extremities
	Bladder dysfunction (usually urinary retention)
	Varying degrees of sensory loss, usually pain and temperature below level of lesion
	Relatively good prognosis
	Motor power returns first to lower extremities

The patient with a suspected cervical spinal cord injury must be moved to the radiography unit with utmost care. After plain films of the spine, including lateral films of the cervical spine, are evaluated, it is usually necessary to establish the presence or absence of a subarachnoid block, which can be caused by bone fragments, disc material, hematoma, or swelling of neural tissues (Fig. 9.12). CT or MRI of the involved and adjacent spinal levels provides the most complete information on the status of the spinal column and on the extent to which the spinal cord and canal have been compromised by the injury (282).

Generally, MRI centers are not equipped to image patients with multisystem injuries and needing complex life support systems, so that this procedure is usually deferred until the patient is stabilized. Each imaging study has its advantages. CT provides a better picture of fractures and of trauma to the osseous elements, whereas MRI is better suited to view disc protrusions and the spinal cord itself and any associated bleeding or edema (Fig. 9.13). MRA can be used to screen the status of the vasculature, in particular, the vertebral arteries, although angiography is the definitive diagnostic procedure.

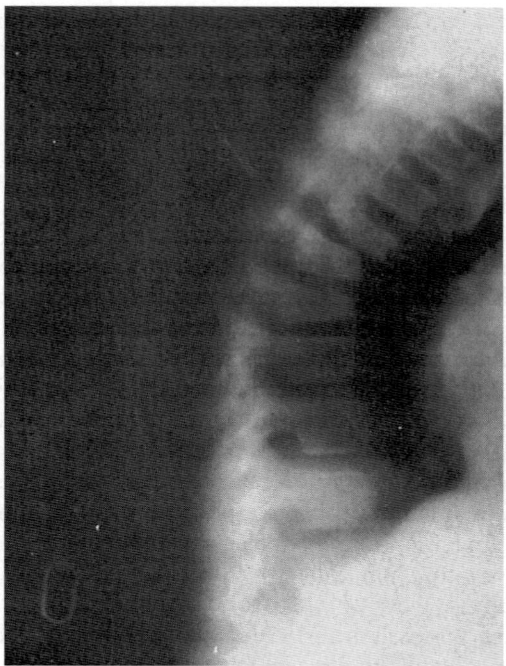

FIGURE 9.12. Compression fracture of thoracic spine (T6, T7, and T8) with anterior displacement of T6 on T7. This patient was a 9-year-old girl who fell from a tree and had an immediate total motor and sensory paralysis below the level of the injury.

Analogous to the changes seen in craniocerebral trauma, three types of abnormalities of the cord can be distinguished. The most common is hyperintensity on T2-weighted images, represented by edema of the cord. Less often, one sees a central hypointensity on T1-weighted images, which evolves to a hypointensity on T2-weighted images surrounded by a ring of hyperintensity. This finding is consistent with an intramedullary hemorrhage and is a poor prognostic sign. In some 16% to 21% of children, all imaging study results are completely normal (256,259,283).

The radiologic diagnosis of a dislocated cervical spine has many pitfalls (284). A marked anterior displacement of C2 on C3 can be seen in 20% of all children younger than 7 years of age. This variant is particularly common during the first 3 years of life. Displacement of C3 on C4 is also common, as is an apparent hypermobility of the atlas on the axis.

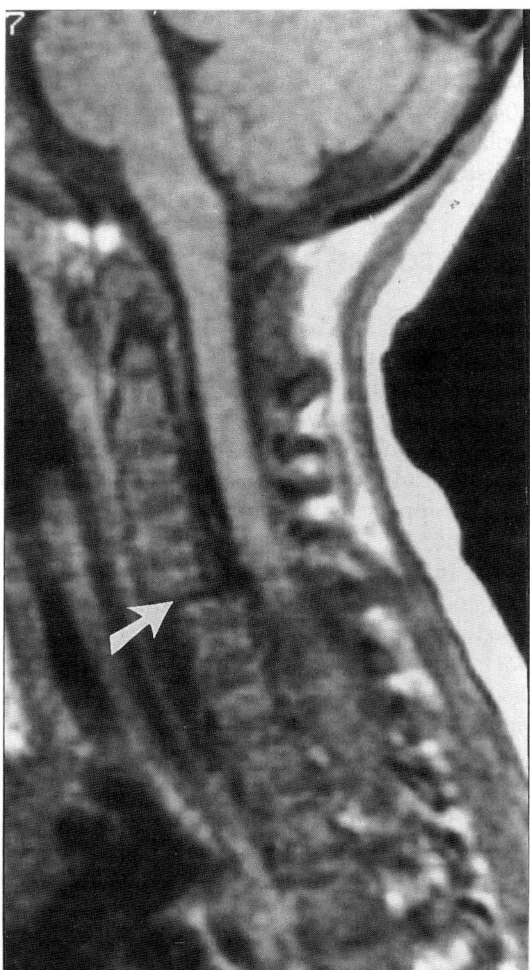

FIGURE 9.13. Spinal cord trauma. A sagittal T1-weighted magnetic resonance image (600/15/2) demonstrates vertebral subluxation at the C4 to C5 level (*arrow*). The cord at and below the bony injury is expanded and hypointense. This 2-year-old boy was wrenched from his mother's lap and thrown around the vehicle in a motor vehicle accident. He was rendered quadriparetic. (Courtesy of Dr. John G. Curran, Department of Neuroradiology, Childrens Memorial Hospital, Chicago, IL.)

The severity of the injury often cannot be determined immediately. An early return of reflex activity, particularly of extensor movements, is encouraging. In general, sensory changes give a clearer indication of the level of the lesions than do motor changes. In cervical cord injuries, bilateral meiosis is a bad prognostic sign because it indicates extensive cord damage (285). Prognosis is better when the cord lesion is incomplete. For instance, in the experience of Hamilton and Myles, 74% of children with a physiologically incomplete spinal cord deficit improved by one or two Frankel levels, with 59% experiencing complete recovery (256). When the spinal cord injury was physiologically complete, only 10% improved by one or two Frankel levels. In this study, the absence of radiologic abnormalities did not influence the outcome.

Treatment

Treatment of the child with a spinal cord injury is essentially surgical, but not always operative, and involves a multidisciplinary approach. Intravenous fluids, colloids, and vasopressors are administered to maintain arterial blood pressure. Guttman advanced the conservative, postural treatment of the patient with spinal cord injury and believed that operative procedures for decompression and stabilization should be used only in selected cases (286). Because excessive movement is likely to aggravate spinal cord injury, special care is required in the handling of the patient, and only the absolutely essential diagnostic studies should be done. In injuries of the cervical spine, the head should be maintained in neutral position (287,288). Skeletal traction, usually by means of tongs inserted into the skull, is required for hyperflexion injuries of the cervical spine, whereas mild traction using a canvas sling is used in hyperextension injuries. The management of cervical spine injuries is reviewed by Sypert (289). Injuries of the lumbar spine and thoracolumbar junction are best stabilized in slight hyperextension.

All patients with open wounds of the spine, with injuries in which imaging studies reveal bony fragments within the spinal canal, and with an apparent total block in the presence of an incomplete transection of the cord should undergo surgery, including débridement, removal of bone fragments, laminectomy, and dural repair, if necessary. Any patient whose neurologic deficit increases after initial assessment, either by extending cephalad or by becoming more complete, also should have the benefit of an exploratory laminectomy. Surgical intervention is needed for dislocations of the spine that cannot be reduced adequately by traction and immobilization and for injuries of the spine known by past experience to be unstable; the surgical intervention often need not be immediate. Reduction of dislocations and internal stabilization are then carried out as indicated.

A number of treatments have been proposed to reverse secondary pathophysiologic processes such as ischemia, excitotoxicity, and lipid peroxidation (290). A high dose of methylprednisolone, a synthetic glucocorticoid drug, given within 8 hours of the injury as a 30-mg/kg bolus, followed by 5.4 mg/kg per hour for 23 hours, induces greater improvement in motor and sensory functions than does placebo in patients with complete and incomplete spinal cord deficits (291). At these doses, methylprednisolone may act as an antioxidant or as a free radical scavenger. The monosialoganglioside G_{M1}, which experimentally has been observed to increase neurite outgrowth and to prevent cell death by inhibiting glutamate-induced neuronal excitotoxicity, has been found to improve lower limb function after spinal cord injury. The drug is started within 19 to 72 hours after the injury and is administered at 100 mg/day for 18 to 32 days (292). Optimal doses of these drugs, their optimal initiation time, and duration of therapy are not known, and neither treatment has been approved by the U.S. Food and Drug Administration. Many other drugs, notably estrogens, calpain, other free radical inhibitors, and tirilazad mesylate, a 21-amino corticosteroid that acts as a potent antioxidant with no glucocorticoid receptor activity, await preclinical and clinical investigations (293).

There has been considerable interest in the prospects of functional spinal cord regeneration. Although axons of injured spinal neurons cannot regrow within the spinal cord, they can grow long distances in peripheral nerves outside the cord. The reason for this discrepancy is the presence within spinal cord of myelin-associated neurite growth inhibitors (294,295). The various interventional strategies and the problems that prevent their current clinical applications are reviewed by Bregman and coworkers (296).

The long-term care of the paraplegic child is beyond the scope of this book. It is reviewed by Guttman (286), Short and colleagues (297), and Piepmeier (298). The management of the quadriplegic patient is considered by Whiteneck (299). Generally, the patient requires care of the skin overlying the paralyzed part and prevention of decubitus lesions. Also needed is care of the urinary system (300). During the acute phase, urinary retention is treated by intermittent catheterization or insertion of an indwelling catheter, preferably one with a separate irrigating arm (three-way Foley). Additionally, the child needs regular enemas to treat fecal retention; automatic sphincter function can develop. Ileus, when present, can be relieved with neostigmine or with an indwelling rectal tube.

The ultimate outlook for spinal cord function after injury depends on the extent of the injury. The immediate loss of function is caused by both anatomic alteration and impaired physiologic function of the cord. In general, much of the improvement occurs during the first 6 months after the injury and at a much slower pace from 6 months to 2 years after the injury. As a rule, muscles with no initial motor power have a longer period of recovery than those in which there was some initial motor power. The mechanisms underlying the improvement are not clear; certainly, resolution of edema cannot account for the slow recovery. In rare instances, a progressive myelopathy can be caused by a nonunited or malunited dens fracture (301).

Herniated Intervertebral Disc

Although common in the adult, this entity is rare in children, with most cases occurring during adolescence, usually after trauma (302).

Injuries at L4 to L5 and L5 to S1 occur with approximately equal frequency. Many affected children have an underlying malformation of the vertebral column, most often spondylolisthesis or spina bifida. Herniation of intervertebral discs also has been noted in achondroplasia (303,304). Because the presenting symptoms of extradural neoplasms can be similar, MRI is indicated for all suspected disc lesions.

INJURIES TO THE CRANIAL NERVES

Injury to the cranial nerves is a relatively common complication of head injuries. The mechanisms of cranial nerve paralysis are multiple. As listed by Friedman and Merritt (305), they include injury to the nerve by bony fragments, laceration of the nerve when a fracture involves the canal by which the cranial nerve leaves the cranial cavity, tears or stretching, compression by hemorrhage, edema or arachnoiditis, contusion, and injury to the motor cells in the brainstem. Injuries to the olfactory nerves are the most common and are generally bilateral. They are believed to be caused by trauma to the frontal poles or by tearing of the olfactory filaments. Facial and abducens nerve injuries are also encountered, as are palsies of the trochlear nerve. They are generally accompanied by evidence of fracture of middle fossa. Seventh- and eighth-nerve palsies result from a fracture of the petrous ridge. In children, trauma is the most common cause of isolated, acquired, unilateral, or bilateral trochlear nerve palsy (306). In the experience of Friedman and Merritt, the onset of cranial nerve palsy was immediate in 68% of case and was delayed for several days in the remainder (305). In the majority of instances, dysfunction is permanent when the palsy is immediate. The likelihood for recovery is significantly greater when the palsy is delayed (307).

INJURIES TO THE PERIPHERAL NERVES

Peripheral nerve injuries are relatively uncommon in childhood. The most common postnatal injuries are of the brachial plexus and are caused by severe trauma to the shoulder or sudden traction to the arm. Other injuries include division of the ulnar and median nerves at the wrist, the result of pushing the hand through a pane of glass; division of the radial nerve in the upper arm, associated with fracture of the humerus; division of the ulnar nerve with fracture or dislocation of the medial epicondyle; injury of one or both branches of the sciatic nerve as a consequence of injections into the buttocks; and division of the common peroneal nerve in fractures at the neck of the fibula. Peripheral neuropathies are relatively common in Ehlers-Danlos syndrome, with both brachial plexus palsy and lumbosacral plexus palsies developing because of increased ligament laxity (308).

Pathology

The pathologic changes in an injured peripheral nerve depend on whether the axon remains intact. When the axon is destroyed at the site of injury, wallerian degeneration is induced in the peripheral segment of the nerve. The pathologic, neurophysiologic, and biochemical alterations accompanying wallerian degeneration are reviewed by Stoll and coworkers (309).

Stretch injuries of the peripheral nerves result from damage to the perineurium and the blood vessels (vasa nervorum). Ischemic peripheral nerve injuries also are produced by impairment of the blood supply to the nerves via these vessels. Regeneration of the injured nerve starts from the proximal end of the axon and begins shortly after injury, proceeding in children at approximately 2.5 to 3.0 mm/day. The speed and extent of recovery depend on whether the sheaths of the nerve remain intact; these provide a continuous channel for the young neurites sprouting from the proximal axonal end. When the gap between nerve ends is wide, and particularly when the ends are separated by fibrous tissue, a neuroma can form proximally and spontaneous anastomosis can be delayed or prevented.

Clinical Manifestations

The salient clinical features of the most frequent peripheral nerve lesions of childhood are presented in Table 9.13. In general, symptoms consist of weakness and sensory disturbances in the area supplied by the individual nerve. Muscular weakness and wasting are characteristic for peripheral nerve injuries. Contractures develop through overaction of unopposed muscle groups.

TABLE 9.13 Clinical Features of Common Peripheral Nerve Injuries

Nerve Injury	*Predisposing Factors*	*Clinical Features*
Brachial plexus upper root (Erb-Duchenne)	Sudden traction to arm	Arm internally rotated at shoulder, pronated at forearm Paralysis of spinati, deltoid, biceps, brachialis, brachio-radialis, extensor carpi radialis Sensory disturbance minimal or absent Biceps and supinator jerks lost, triceps preserved
Lower root (Klumpke paralysis)	Violent upward pull of shoulder	Arm flexed at elbow, forearm supinated, fingers extended, edema and cyanosis of hand Paralysis of small muscles of hand, finger flexors Sensory loss of ulnar aspects of fingers, hand, and forearm Horner syndrome if root avulsed
Long thoracic nerve	Carrying heavy weights on shoulder Postimmunization	Paralysis of serratus magnus with or without trapezius No sensory symptoms
Circumflex nerve	Fracture of humerus (crutch palsy)	Paralysis of deltoid Sensory loss of upper and outer part of arm
Radial nerve	Fracture of humerus (Saturday night palsy)	Paralysis of triceps uncommon, only if nerve damaged in axilla Paralysis of brachioradialis, extensors of wrist and fingers Sensory loss inconstant
Median nerve (310)	Cuts at wrist, mucolipidosis III	Atrophy of thenar eminence Paralysis of pronation beyond midposition Paralysis of flexor of index finger, impaired flexion, and opposition of thumb Sensory loss of radial aspect of palm
Ulnar nerve	Fractures at lower end of humerus Pressure palsy at elbow	Flattened hypothenar eminence, claw hand Paralysis of ulnar flexors at wrist and fingers, interossei, adductor of thumb Sensory loss of ulnar side of arm, hand
Sciatic nerve [common peroneal and posterior tibial nerve (311)]	Intramuscular injuries (common peroneal component injured more frequently)	Foot drop, paralysis of peronei, anterior tibialis, extensors of toe Sensory loss of anterior aspect of lower leg and foot Absent ankle jerk
Femoral nerve (312)	Hemorrhagic disease (hemophilia)	Paralysis and atrophy of quadriceps Defective sensation, anterior and anterior medial aspect of thigh
Common peroneal nerve	Fracture at neck of fibula	Stepping gait Loss of dorsiflexion (anterior tibialis) eversion at ankle (peronei), extensors of toe
	Incorrectly fitted leg cast	Sensory deficit, dorsum of foot and outer side of leg Achilles tendon reflex lost or reduced

When a nerve regenerates, manual pressure on the nerve at the level to which axons have regrown can induce a tingling pain referred distally to an area that is still anesthetic (Tinel's sign). Pain and paresthesia can be generalized or can be referred to one site along the course of the nerve. These symptoms are aggravated by touch or muscular contractions.

Deep tendon reflexes are diminished or abolished in the affected area. A number of vasomotor symptoms, including mottling and thinning of the skin, edema, cyanosis, and impaired sweating, also are observed.

Diagnosis

Examination of the child with a peripheral nerve injury is directed toward determining the cause and the anatomic site of the injury. Several manuals detail the neurologic examination of such a patient (313). Generally, evaluation of motor function and sensory deficits is more important in the diagnosis of peripheral nerve injuries than is the status of reflexes because the presence or absence of reflexes does not depend on the integrity of a single nerve.

Tinel's sign, which originally was believed to be evidence of regeneration, does not have much prognostic significance during the first month of injury, unless the most distal point at which it can be elicited moves further down the nerve trunk on progressive examinations.

Electrical studies can delineate the extent of the nerve injury. Somatosensory-evoked potentials can delineate the extent of the injury and distinguish between peripheral nerve and spinal cord injuries (314). Electromyography indicates fibrillation potentials of denervated muscles. Nerve conduction times are either impossible to elicit or reduced. The ability of the nerve below the lesion to respond to direct electrical stimulation despite motor paralysis indicates absence of wallerian degeneration and is a favorable prognostic sign. In the course of regeneration, the conduction times, which initially are impossible to determine, are slow at first and subsequently regain as much as 60% of the original velocity (315). CT myelography and MRI have been used for the diagnosis of cervical root evulsion in brachial plexus injury (316). MR neurography has shown great promise in the diagnosis and management of patients with peripheral nerve pathology (317).

Treatment

Surgical treatment may not be required during the early phase of peripheral nerve injuries. Clean lacerations of a nerve are suitable for early repair. In other types of nerve injury, nothing is gained by immediate exploration of the site. If the nerve presents readily in the wound, a single stainless-steel marking suture can facilitate subsequent repair. Secondary disability, such as contractures or injury of the paralyzed muscles by excess stretching, should be prevented by splinting the affected limb. Electrostimulation of the paralyzed muscles is of no advantage. A severed nerve should be explored and reapproximated 3 weeks after injury, provided the wound is healed. At this time, the extent of nerve injury can be defined more clearly and suturing is technically more satisfactory. A nerve that is known to have been traumatized but not severed should be explored if recovery of motor and sensory functions does not take place or is less complete than anticipated. External and internal neurolysis of such a nerve trunk can allow further recovery of function. A neuroma in continuity can require resection and reanastomosis if nerve function is absent or poor.

Prognosis

The prognosis depends on the extent and nature of the nerve injury. Pressure palsies almost invariably recover. If electrical studies indicate wallerian degeneration of the distal segment, recovery is delayed until the regenerating fibers reach the muscles they innervate. If no recovery can be documented after 3 months by either clinical or electrical examinations, the ultimate prognosis is poor, and few patients benefit from surgical exploration. Different nerves have different capacities for regeneration. Generally, radial nerve injuries fare best and sciatic nerve injuries worst. Spontaneous recovery from sciatic nerve injuries can be extremely slow, but can continue for 1 to 2 years.

COMPLEX REGIONAL PAIN SYNDROME (REFLEX SYMPATHETIC DYSTROPHY)

Complex regional pain syndrome (CRPS) type I is the new designation for what was formerly termed reflex sympathetic dystrophy. It is an an occasional sequela to trauma affecting the limbs without obvious peripheral nerve injury. Whereas in CRPS I, the more commonly encountered syndrome, the pain is not limited to the distribution of a single peripheral nerve, CRPS II, formerly termed causalgia, is a condition that develops following nerve injury. Causalgia was first defined in adults by Mitchell (318) and has been encountered in children, predominantly in girls (319,320). The condition is characterized by constant burning pain and hyperesthesia in an extremity. Most often, the lower extremities, notably the ankle and foot, are affected. Pain is accompanied by swelling, sweating, vasomotor instability, and sometimes trophic changes. There may not be a history of antecedent trauma, or the injury may have been considered minor. Psychological disturbances are common and can become the most important part of the clinical picture. An important early sign of reflex sympathetic dystrophy is piloerection over the hairy aspect of the affected limb (321). Often, associated muscle spasms, myoclonus, or focal dystonia occurs (322,323). When dystonia is part of the condition, it can appear at the same time as the causalgia or up to many months later.

Many theories exist as to etiology, none of them well supported by clinical evidence. A disorder of the sympathetic system, release of a pain substance, or supersensitivity to neurotransmitters are the most likely (320); however, in many instances surgical or chemical sympathectomy does not relieve the pain, an indication that pain is independent of sympathetic function (324). Pathologic examination of nerve and muscle taken from the affected limb suggest a microangiopathy (325). Symptoms of causalgia can last a few days to as long as a year. A number of therapies have been suggested; none is infallible. The response to intensive physical therapy is often excellent in children (321). Analgesics, nonsteroidal inflammatory drugs, antidepressants, narcotics, and corticosteroids all have their advocates. Blockage of the sympathetic chain with paravertebral or epidural anesthetics has been tried, as has surgical sympathectomy (326). No treatment for the movement disorder has been effective; an occasional patient recovers spontaneously after a few years (322).

INJURIES BY PHYSICAL AGENTS

Injuries of the Nervous System by X-Ray Irradiation

Radiation damage to the central nervous system can occur before birth and can result in a variety of gross and microscopic malformations of the brain. These are discussed in Chapter 5.

The neurologic complications of therapeutic irradiation for intracranial tumors are discussed in Chapter 11.

Heatstroke (Sunstroke)

Heatstroke results from prolonged exposure to direct sunlight and heat, with subsequent failure of the body's heat-regulating mechanism. Cells respond to excessive heat by producing heat-shock proteins. These function as molecular chaperones and bind to partially folded or misfolded proteins and prevent their irreversible denaturation (327). Presence of hyperpyrexia distinguishes heat stroke from symptoms resulting from sodium loss caused by excessive sweating.

The clinical and pathologic picture of heatstroke results from a combination of hyperpyrexia and shock. Sunlight contributes to the heat load, but probably does not affect the brain directly. In fatal cases, examination of the brain reveals generalized edema and degeneration of cerebellar neurons, particularly the Purkinje cells and the cells of the dentate nucleus, with lesser degrees of neuronal loss in other areas of the neuraxis (328,329).

Clinically, brain dysfunction can range from subtle to severe. The patient has sudden onset of coma, cyanosis, impaired sweating, and hyperpyrexia (330). Generalized or focal seizures may occur, especially during cooling (327). Rhabdomyolysis, hyperkalemia, and metabolic acidosis can complicate the picture. Clinical heatstroke can be associated with an underlying abnormality of skeletal muscle similar to that of malignant hyperthermia (330). Cerebellar symptoms can be evident with recovery. They usually improve considerably in time.

Treatment of the acute condition involves removing the child from the sun, reducing body temperature, and providing intravenous fluids. Seizure control is best achieved with benzodiazepines (327).

Electrical Injuries of the Nervous System

Electrical injuries to children can be caused by household current or lightning. Lightning is responsible for approximately one-fourth of all fatal electrical accidents. Cherington described four clinical pictures. Most often, the patient either dies at once as a result of cardiac arrest or recovers fully. Neurologic symptoms may be immediate and permanent, or they may be delayed or progressive (332). The progressive neurologic signs include hemiparesis, cerebellar deficits, paraplegia, cranial nerve palsies, and other focal neurologic signs. Increased intracranial pressure also has been observed (333,334). Long-term behavioral changes, including disturbances in affect, memory, and mood, are not unusual and can last for months, out of proportion to the duration of any cardiorespiratory arrest (332,334a). Kotagal and colleagues suggested they are the consequence of a direct injury to the limbic system (335).

Neurologic Complications of Burns

Approximately 5% of children develop encephalitic symptoms within the first few weeks after they sustain severe burns. As a rule, these represent complications from the burn. These symptoms include changes in level of consciousness, seizures, aphasia, extrapyramidal disorders, and impaired intellectual function, which result from infections, metabolic encephalopathies, and cerebrovascular accidents. Neurologic symptoms during the first 3 days after the burn are generally caused by shock and derangements of electrolytes. Infections are responsible for neurologic symptoms after the first week after the burn in what is essentially an immunocompromised host. They are most common during the second to third weeks after the injury. Three organisms are usually responsible: *Candida*, *Pseudomonas aeruginosa*, and *Staphylococcus aureus*. Almost invariably they enter the nervous system from a systemic source. Microabscesses of the brain are most likely to be caused by candidiasis, with *S. aureus* a less common culprit. Meningitis or septic infarcts are caused by *P. aeruginosa*. Intracranial hemorrhages are less common than infarcts and generally result from disseminated intravascular coagulation or serum hyperosmolarity. Central pontine myelinolysis and cerebral edema also can develop, the latter generally caused by anoxia (336,337).

Despite the number of potentially irreversible neurologic complications, the majority of children experience full neurologic recovery (338).

Neurologic Injury from Undersea Diving

Underwater diving places the teenager or young adult at risk for two major types of neurologic injuries. The most common is decompression sickness that results from a too rapid decompression on ascent. It mainly affects the spinal cord and results in a unique multilevel spinal cord disease, with deficits consisting of pain, sensory loss, and motor weakness (339). The condition usually resolves with administration of oxygen and recompression, although there may be a residual patchy sensory loss. Arterial gas embolism, a much rarer condition, is the most serious complication of self-contained underwater breathing apparatus (scuba) diving. It results from pulmonary overpressure on ascent with extravasation of air into the arterial system and occlusion of a major cerebral artery. The first sign of the condition is usually a seizure. This can be quickly followed by an acute, strokelike picture marked by hemiparesis, aphasia, and cortical blindness. It is the major cause of death in diving accidents. MRI studies of the head show ischemic changes in a vascular distribution (340). By contrast, imaging study of brain and spinal cord are usually normal in decompression sickness, although on rare occasions studies demonstrate a swollen spinal cord with increased signal posteriorly on T2-weighted images (341).

REFERENCES

1. Adelson PD, Kochanek PM. Head injuries in children. *J Child Neurol* 1998;13:2–15.
2. Craft AW, Shaw DA, Cartlidge NE. Head injuries in children. *Br Med J* 1972;4:200–203.
3. North AF. When should a child be in the hospital? *Pediatrics* 1976;57:540–543.
4. Kraus JF, Rock A, Hemyari P. Brain injuries among infants, children, adolescents and young adults. *Am J Dis Child* 1990;144:684–691.
5. Frankowski RF, Annegers JF, Whitman S. Epidemiological and descriptive studies. Part 1. The descriptive epidemiology of head trauma in the U.S. In: Becker DP, Povlishok JT, eds. *Central nervous system trauma, status report 1985*. Bethesda, MD: NIH, NINCDS., 1985:33–43.
6. Klauber MR, Marshall LF, Barrett-Connor E, et al. The epidemiology of head injury: a prospective study of an entire community—San Diego County, CA, 1978. *Am J Epidemiol* 1981;113:500–509.
7. Leventhal JM, Horwitz SM, Rude C, et al. Maltreatment of children born to teenage mothers: a comparison between the 1960s and 1980s. *J Pediatr* 1993;122:314–319.
8. McClain PW, Sacks JJ, Froehlke RG, et al. Estimates of fatal child abuse and neglect, United States, 1979 through 1988. *Pediatrics* 1993;91:338–343.
9. Billmire ME, Myers PA. Serious head injury in infants: accident or abuse. *Pediatrics* 1985;75:340–342.
10. Rovi S, Chen PH, Johnson MS. The economic burden of hospitalizations associated with child abuse and neglect. *Am J Public Health* 2004;94:586–590.
11. O'Rourke NA, Costello F, Yelland JD, et al. Head injuries to children riding on bicycles. *Med J Aust* 1987;146:619–621.
12. Attewell RG, Glase K, McFadden M. Bicycle helmet efficacy: a meta-analysis. *Accid Anal Prev* 2001;33:345–352.
13. Kopjar B, Wickizer TM. Age gradient in the cost-effectiveness of bicycle helmets. *Prev Med* 2000;30:401–406.
14. Mealey J. *Pediatric head injuries*. Springfield, IL: Charles C. Thomas, 1968.
15. Graham DI. Neuropathology of head injury. In Narayan RK, Wilberger JE, Povlishock JT, eds. *Neurotrauma*. McGraw-Hill, New York, 1996:43–59.
16. Pearl GS. Traumatic neuropathology. *Clin Lab Med* 1998;18:39–64.
17. Stålhammar D. Experimental models of head injury. *Acta Neurochirurg* 1986;36(Suppl):33–46.
18. Ommaya AK, Goldsmith W, Thibault L. Biomechanics and neuropathology of adult and paediatric head injury. *Br J Neurosurg* 2002;16:220–242.
19. Berney J, Froidevaux AC, Favier J. Paediatric head trauma: influence of age and sex. II. Biomechanical and anatomo-clinical correlations. *Childs Nerv Syst* 1994;10:517–523.
20. Gentry LR, Godersky JC, Thompson B. MR imaging of head trauma: review of the distribution and radiopathologic features of traumatic lesions. *Am J Roentgenol* 1988;15:663–672.
21. Adams JH, Graham DI, Gennarelli TA, et al. Diffuse axonal injury in nonmissile head injuries. *J Neurol Neurosurg Psychiatr* 1991;54:481–483.
22. Reichard RR, White CL, Hladik CL, et al. Beta-amyloid precursor protein staining of nonaccidental central nervous system injury in pediatric autopsies. *J Neurotrauma* 2003;20:347–355.
23. Adams JH, Mitchell DE, Graham DI, et al. Diffuse brain damage of immediate impact type: Its relationship to "primary brain-stem damage" in head injury. *Brain* 1977;100:489–502.
24. Adams JH, Graham DI, Murray LS, et al. Diffuse axonal injury due to nonmissile head injury in humans. An analysis of 45 cases. *Ann Neurol* 1982;12:557–563.
25. Yamaki T, Murakami N, Iwamotor Y, et al. Pathological study of diffuse axonal injury patients who died shortly after impact. *Acta Neurochir* 1992;119:153–158.
26. Chester CS, Reznick BR. Ataxia after severe head injury: the pathological substrate. *Ann Neurol* 1987;22:77–79.
27. Strich SJ. Diffuse degeneration of the cerebral white matter in severe dementia following head injury. *J Neurol Neurosurg Psychiat* 1956;19:163–185.
28. Graham DI, McIntosh TK, Maxwell WL, et al. Recent advances in neurotrauma. *J Neuropathol Exp Neurol* 2000;59:641–651.
29. Singleton RH, Povlishock JT. Identification and characterization of heterogenous neuronal injury and death in regions of diffuse brain injury: evidence for multiple independent injury phenotypes. *J Neurosci* 2004;24:3543–3553.
30. Wolf JA, Stys PK, Lusardi T, et al. Traumatic axonal injury induces calcium influx modulated by tetrodotoxin-sensitive sodium channels. *J Neurosci* 2001;21:1923–1930.
31. Maxwell WL, Povlishock JT, Graham DL. A mechanistic analysis of nondisruptive axonal injury: a review. *J Neurotrauma* 1997;14:419–440.
32. Povlishock JT, Becker DP. Fate of reactive axonal swellings induced by head injury. *Lab Invest* 1985;52:540–552.
33. Huisman TA, Schwamm, LH, Schaefer PW, et al. Diffusion tensor imaging as potential biomarker of white matter injury in diffuse axonal injury. *Am J Neuroradiol* 2004;25:370–376.
34. Tong KA, Ashwal S, Holshouser BA., et al. Hemorrhagic shearing lesions in children and adolescents with posttraumatic diffuse axonal injury: improved detection and initial results. *Radiology* 2003;227:332–339.
35. Cecil KM, Hills EC, Sandel ME, et al. Proton magnetic resonance spectroscopy for detection of axonal injury in the splenium of the corpus callosum of brain-injured patients. *J Neurosurg* 1998;88:795–801.
36. Lindenberg R. Significance of the tentorium in head injuries from blunt forces. *Clin Neurosurg* 1964;12:129–142.

37. Freytag E. Autopsy findings in head injuries from blunt forces. *Arch Pathol* 1963;75:402–413.
38. Calder IM, Hill I, Scholtz CL. Primary brain trauma in nonaccidental injury. *J Clin Pathol* 1984;37:1095–1100.
39. American Academy of Neurology: Practice parameter: the management of concussion in sports (summary statement). Report of the Quality Standards Subcommittee of the American Academy of Neurology. *Neurology* 1997;48:581–585.
40. Bullock R, Zauner A, Woodward JJ, et al. Factors affecting excitatory amino acid release following severe human head injury. *J Neurosurg* 1998;89:507–518.
41. Shaw NA. The neurophysiology of concussion. *Prog Neurobiol* 2002;67:281–344.
42. Katayama Y, Becker DP, Tamura T, Hovda DA. Massive increases in extracellular potassium and the indiscriminate release of glutamate following concussive brain injury. *J Neurosurg* 1990;73:889–900.
43. Junger EC, Newell DW, Grant GA, et al. Cerebral autoregulation following minor head injury. *J Neurosurg* 1997;86:425–432.
44. McCrea M, Kelly JP, Randolph C, et al. Immediate neurocognitive effects of concussion. *Neurosurgery* 2002;50:1032–1042.
45. Bayir H, Kochanek PM, Clark RS. Traumatic brain injury in infants and children: mechanisms of secondary damage and treatment in the intenisve care unit. *Crit Care Clin* 1003;19:529–549.
46. Fishman RA. *Cerebrospinal fluid in diseases of the nervous system*, 2nd ed. Philadelphia: WB Saunders, 1992:116–138.
47. Bullock R, Maxwell WL, Graham DI, et al. Glial swelling following human cerebral contusion: an ultrastructural study. *J Neurol Neurosurg Psychiatry* 1991;54:427–434.
48. Barzo P, Marmarou A, Fatouros P, et al. Contribution of vasogenic and cellular edema to traumatic brain swelling measured by diffusion-weighted imaging. *J Neurosurg* 1997;87:900–907.
49. Ruppel RA, Kochanek PM, Adelson PD, et al. Excitatory amino acid concentrations in ventricular cerebrospinal fluid after severe traumatic brain injury in infants and children. The role of child abuse. *J Pediatr* 2001;138:18–25.
50. Becker DP, Verity MA, Povlishock J, et al. Brain cellular injury and recovery—horizons for improving medical therapies in stroke and trauma. *West J Med* 1988;148:670–684.
51. Kawamata T, Katayama Y, Hovda DA, et al. Administration of excitatory aminoacid antagonists via microdialysis attenuates the increase in glucose utilization seen following concussive brain injury. *J Cereb Blood Flow Metab* 1992;12:12–24.
52. Hovda DA, Becker DP, Katayama Y. Secondary injury and acidosis. *J Neurotrauma* 1992;9(Suppl 1):S47–S60.
53. Bakay L, Lee JC, Lee GR, et al. Experimental cerebral concussion. Part I: An electron microscopic study. *J Neurosurg* 1977;47:525–531.
54. Kempsky O. Cerebral edema. *Semin Nephrol* 2001;21:303–307.
55. Bell MJ, Kochanek PM, Doughty LA, et al. Comparison of the interleukin-6 and interleukin-10 response in children after severe traumatic brain injury or septic shock. *Acta Neurochir Suppl (Vienna)* 1997;70:96–97.
56. Papadopoulos MC, Krishna S, Verkman AS. Aquaporin water channels and brain edema. *Mt Sinai J Med* 2002;69:242–248.
56a. Griesdale DE, Honey CR. Aquaporins and brain edema. *Surg Neurol* 2004;61:418–421.
57. Adelson PD, Clyde B, Kochanek PM, et al. Cerebrovascular response in infants and young children following severe traumatic brain injury: a preliminary report. *Pediatr Neurosurg* 1997;26:200–207.
58. Bruce DA, Alavi A, Bilaniuk L, et al. Diffuse cerebral swelling following head injuries in children. The syndrome of "malignant brain edema." *J Neurosurg* 1981;54:170–178.
59. Langfitt TW, Gennarelli TA, Obrist WD, et al. Prospects for the future in the diagnosis and management of head injury: pathophysiology, brain imaging, and population based studies. *Clin Neurosurg* 1982;29:353–376.
60. Cruz J, Gennarelli TA, Alves WM. Continuous monitoring of cerebral hemodynamic reserve in acute brain injury: relationship to changes in brain swelling. *J Trauma* 1992;32:629–635.
61. Choux M. Incidence, diagnosis and management of skull fractures. In: Raimondi AS, Choux M, DiRocco C, eds. *Head injuries in the newborn and infant*. New York: Springer-Verlag, 1986:163–182.
62. Lloyd DA, Carty H, Patterson M, et al. Predictive value of skull radiography for intracranial injury in children with blunt head injury. *Lancet* 1997;349:821–824.
63. Mizrahi EM, Kellaway P. Cerebral concussion in children: assessment of injury by electroencephalography. *Pediatrics* 1984;73:419–425.
64. Jennett B. *Epilepsy after nonmissile head injuries*, 2nd ed. Chicago: Year Book, 1975.
65. Ashwal S, Holshouser BA, Shu SK, et al. Predictive value of proton magnetic resonance spectroscopy in pediatric head injury. *Pediatr Neurol* 2000;23:114–125.
66. Hendrick EB, Harwood-Nash DC, Hudson AR. Head injuries in children: a survey of 4465 consecutive cases at the Hospital for Sick Children, Toronto, Canada. *Clin Neurosurg* 1963;11:46–65.
67. Raimondi AJ, Hirschauer J. Head injury in the infant and toddler—coma scoring and outcome scale. *Childs Brain* 1984;11:12–35.
68. Duhaime AC, Alario AJ, Lewander WJ, et al. Head injury in very young children: mechanisms, injury types, and ophthalmologic findings in 100 hospitalized patients younger than 2 years of age. *Pediatrics* 1992;90:179–185.
69. Minns RA, Busuttil A. Patterns of presentation of the shaken baby syndrome. *BMJ* 2004;328:766.
70. Geddes JF, Hackshaw AK, Vowles GH, et al. Neuropathology of inflicted head injury in children. I. Patterns of brain damage. *Brain* 2001;124:1290–1298.
71. Shannon P, Becker L. Mechanisms of brain injury in infantile child abuse. *Lancet* 2001;358:686–687.
71a. Bechtel K, Stoessel K, Leventhal JM, et al. Characteristics that distinguish accidental from abusive injury in hospitalized young children with head trauma. *Pediatrics* 2004;114:165–168.
72. Geddes JF, Vowles GH, Hackshaw AK, et al. Neuropathology of inflicted head injury in children. II. Microscopic brain injury in infants. *Brain* 2001;124:1299–1306.
73. Donohoe M. Evidence-based medicine and shaken baby syndrome. Part I. Literature review, 1966-1998. *Am J Forensic Med Pathol* 2003;24:239–242.
74. Geddes JF, Plunkett J. The evidence base for shaken baby syndrome. *BMJ* 2004;328:719–720.
75. Harding B, Risdon RA, Krous HF. Shaken baby syndrome. *BMJ* 2004;328:720–721.
76. Menkes JH. Subdural haematoma, non-accidental head injury. *Eur J Paediatr Neurol* 2001;5:175–176.
76a. Jaffe D, Wesson D. Current concepts: emergency management of blunt trauma in children. *N Engl J Med* 1991;324:1477–1482.
77. Teasdale G, Jennett B. Assessment of coma and impaired consciousness. A practical scale. *Lancet* 1974;2:81–84.
78. Simpson D, Reilly P. Pediatric coma scale. *Lancet* 1982;2:450.
79. Overgaard J, Hvid-Hansen O, Land AM, et al. Prognosis after head injury based on early clinical examination. *Lancet* 1973;2:631–635.
80. Russell WR. *The traumatic amnesias*. London: Oxford University Press, 1971.
81. Chesnut RM. Management of brain and spine injuries. *Crit Care-Clin* 2004;20:25–55.
82. Plum FB, Posner JB. *Diagnosis of stupor and coma*, 3rd ed. Philadelphia: Davis, 1980.
83. Masters SJ, McClean PM, Arcarese JS, et al. Skull x-ray examinations after head trauma. Recommendations by a multidisciplinary panel and validation study. *N Engl J Med* 1987;316:84–91.
84. Johnson DL, Duma C, Sivit C. The role of immediate operative intervention in severely head-injured children with a Glasgow Coma Scale score of 3. *Neurosurgery* 1992;30:320–324.
85. Zimmerman RA, Bilaniuk LT, Bruce D, et al. Computed tomography of pediatric head trauma: acute general cerebral swelling. *Radiology* 1978;126:403–408.
86. Johnson MH, Lee SH. Computed tomography of acute cerebral trauma. *Radiol Clin North Am* 1992;30:325–352.
87. Ginsburg CM. Frontal sinus fractures. *Pediatr Rev* 1997;18:120–121.
88. Sklar EML, Quencer RM, Bowen BC, et al. Magnetic resonance applications in cerebral injury. *Radiol Clin North Am* 1992;30:353–356.

89. Kelly AB, Zimmerman RD, Snow RB, et al. Head trauma: comparison of MR and CT—experience in 100 patients. *Am J Neuroradiol* 1988;9:699–708.
90. O'Sullivan MG, Statham PF, Jones PA, et al. Role of intracranial pressure monitoring in severely head-injured patients without signs of intracranial hypertension on initial computerized tomography. *J Neurosurg* 1994;80:46–50.
91. Sivakumar V, Rajshekhar V, Chandy MJ. Management of neurosurgical patients with hyponatremia and natriuresis. *Neurosurgery* 1994;34:269–274.
92. Vingerhoets F, de Tribolet N. Hyponatremia hypo-osmolarity in neurosurgical patients. "Appropriate secretion of ADH" and "cerebral salt-wasting syndrome." *Acta Neurochir* 1988;91:50–54.
93. Berkenbosch JW, Lentz CW, Jimenez DF, et al. Cerebral salt wasting syndrome following brain injury in three pediatric patients: suggestions for rapid diagnosis and therapy. *Pediatr Neurosurg* 2002;36:75–79.
94. Pascucci RC. Head trauma in the child. *Intensive Care Med* 1988;14:185–195.
95. Khanna S, Davis D, Peterson B, et al. Use of hypertonic saline in the treatment of severe refractory postraumatic intracranial hypertension in pediatric traumatic brain injury. *Crit Care Med* 2000;28:1144–1151.
96. Adelson PD, Bratton SL, Carney NA, et al. Guidelines for the acute medical management of severe traumatic brain injury in infants, children, and adolescents. Chapter 11. Use of hyperosmolar therapy in the management of severe pediatric traumatic brain injury. *Pediatr Crit Care Med* 2003;4(3 Suppl):S40–S44.
97. Feldman Z, Zachari S, Reichenthal E, et al. Brain edema and neurological status with rapid infusion of lactated Ringer's or 5% dextrose solution following head trauma. *J Neurosurg* 1995;83:1060–1066.
98. Schaefer M, Link J, Hannemann L, et al. Excessive hypokalemia and hyperkalemia following head injury. *Intensive Care Med* 1995;21:235–237.
99. MacDonald JS, Atkinson CC, Mooney DP. Hypokalemia in acutely ill children: a benign laboratory abnormality. *J Trauma* 2003;54:197–198.
100. Brohi K, Singh J, Heron M, et al. Acute traumatic coagulopathy. *J Trauma* 2003;54:1127–1130.
101. Morenski JD, Tobias JD, Jimenez DF. Recombinant activated factor VII for cerebral injury–induced coagulopathy in pediatric patients. Report of three cases and review of the literature. *J Neurosurg* 2003;98:611–616.
102. Miner ME, Kaufman HH, Graham SH, et al. Disseminated intravascular coagulation fibrinolytic syndrome following head injury in children: frequency and prognostic implications. *J Pediatr* 1982;100:687–691.
103. Chadwick D. Seizures and epilepsy after traumatic brain injury. *Lancet* 2000;355:334–335.
104. Chang BS, Lowenstein DH. Practice parameter: antiepileptic drug prophylaxis in severe traumatic brain injury. *Neurology* 2003;60:10–16.
105. Zimmerman RA, Bilaniuk LT. Computed tomography in pediatric head trauma. *J Neuroradiol* 1981;8:257–271.
106. Kanter MJ, Narayan RK. Intracranial pressure monitoring. *Neurosurg Clin North Am* 1991;2:257–265.
107. Jensen RL, Hahn YS, Ciro E. Risk factors of intracranial pressure monitoring in children with fiberoptic devices: a critical review. *Surg Neurol* 1997;47:16–22.
108. Bouma GJ, Muizelaar JP, Choi SC, et al. Cerebral circulation and metabolism after severe traumatic brain injury: the elusive role of ischemia. *J Neurosurg* 1991;75:685–693.
109. Levy DI, Recate HL, Cherny WB, et al. Controlled lumbar drainage in pediatric head injury. *J Neurosurg* 1995;83:453–460.
110. Miller JD. Head injury. *J Neurol Neurosurg Psychiatr* 1993;56:440–447.
111. Muizelaar JP, Marmarou A, Ward JD, et al. Adverse effects of prolonged hyperventilation in patients with severe head injury: a randomized clinical trial. *J Neurosurg* 1991;75:731–739.
112. Marion DW, Firlik A, McLaughlin MR. Hyperventilation therapy for severe traumatic brain injury. *New Horizons* 1995;3:439–447.
113. Cruz J, Raps EC, Hoffstad OJ, et al. Cerebral oxygen monitoring. *Crit Care Med* 1993;21:1242–1246.
114. Feldman Z, Kanter MJ, Robertson CS, et al. Effect of head elevation on intracranial pressure, cerebral perfusion pressure, and cerebral blood flow in head-injured patients. *J Neurosurg* 1992;76:207–211.
114a. Roberts I, Yates D, Sandercock P, et al. Effect of intravenous corticosteroids on death within 14 days in 10008 adults with clinically significant head injury (MRC CRASH trial): randomised placebo-controlled trial. *Lancet* 2004;364:1321–1328.
114b. Alderson P, Roberts I. Corticosteroids for acute traumatic brain injury. *Cochrane Database Syst Rev* 2005;25:CD 000196.
115. Young B, Runge JW, Waxman KS, et al. Effects of pegorgotein on neurologic outcome of patients with severe head injury. A multicenter, randomized controlled trial. *J Am Med Assoc* 1996;276:538–543.
116. Ward JD, Becker DP, Miller, JD, et al. Failure of prophylactic barbiturate coma in the treatment of severe head injury. *J Neurosurg* 1985;62:383–388.
117. Clifton GL, Miller ER, Choi SC, et al. Hypothermia on admission in patients with severe brain injury. *J Neurotrauma* 2002;19:293–301.
118. Rubin DM, McMillan CO, Helfaer MA, et al. Pulmonary edema associated with child abuse: case reports and review of the literature. *Pediatrics* 2001;108:769–775.
119. Jennett B, Teasdale G. *Management of head injuries*. Philadelphia: Davis, 1981.
120. Committee on Quality Improvement, American Academy of Pediatrics. The management of minor closed head injury in children. *Pediatrics* 1999;104:1407–1415.
121. Shutzman SA, Barnes P, Duhaime AC, et al. Evaluation and management of children younger than two years old with apparently minor head trauma: Proposed guidelines. *Pediatrics* 2001;107:983–993.
122. Stein SC, O'Malley KF, Ross SE. Is routine computed tomography scanning too expensive for mild head injury? *Ann Emerg Med* 1991;20:1286–1289.
123. Davis RL, Hughes M, Gubler KD, et al. The use of cranial CT scans in the triage of pediatric patients with mild head injury. *Pediatrics* 1995;95:345–349.
124. Ingebrigtsen T, Romner B. Routine early CT-scan is cost saving after minor head injury. *Acta Neurol Scand* 1996;93:207–210.
125. Rosenthal BW, Bergman I. Intracranial injury after moderate head trauma in children. *J Pediatr* 1989;115:346–350.
126. Ylvisaker M, ed. *Traumatic brain injury rehabilitation: children and adolescents,* 2nd ed. Boston: Butterworth–Heinemann, 1997.
127. Levi L, Guilburd JN, Bar-Josef G, et al. Severe head injury in children—analyzing the better outcome over a decade and the role of major improvements in intensive care. *Childs Nerv Syst* 1998; 14:195–202.
128. Bijur PE, Haslum M, Golding J. Cognitive and behavioral sequelae of mild head injury in children. *Pediatrics* 1990;86:337–344.
129. Hall DMB, Johnson SL, Middleton J. Rehabilitation of head injured children. *Arch Dis Child* 1990;65:553–556.
130. Levin HS, Aldrich EF, Saydjari C., et al. Severe head injury in children: experience of the Traumatic Coma Data Bank. *Neurosurgery* 1992;31:435–443.
131. Keenan HT, Runyan DK, Marshall SW, et al. A population-based study of inflicted traumatic brain injury in young children. *JAMA* 2003;290:621–626.
132. Mahoney WJ, D'Souza BJ, Haller JA, et al. Long-term outcome of children with severe head trauma and prolonged coma. *Pediatrics* 1983;71:756–762.
133. Hjern B, Nylander I. Late prognosis of severe head injuries in childhood. *Arch Dis Child* 1962;37:113–116.
134. Costeff H, Groswasser Z, Goldstein R. Long-term follow-up review of 31 children with severe closed head trauma. *J Neurosurg* 1990;73:684–687.
135. Guilleminault C, Faull KF, Miles, L, et al. Posttraumatic excessive daytime sleepiness: a review of 20 patients. *Neurology* 1983;33:1584–1589.
136. Johnson SL, Hall DM. Posttraumatic tremor in head-injured children. *Arch Dis Child* 1992;67:227–228.

137. Kruass JK, Trankle R, Kopp KH. Posttraumatic movement disorders after moderate or mild head injury. *Mov Disord* 1997;12:428–431.
138. Zijlmans J, Booij J, Valk J, et al. Posttraumatic tremor without parkinsonism in a patient with complete contralateral loss of the nigrostriatal pathway. *Mov Disord* 2002;17:1086–1088.
139. Kingsley D, Till K, Hoare RD. Growing fractures of the skull. *J Neurol Neurosurg Psychiatr* 1978;41:312–318.
140. Muhonen MG, Piper JG, Menezes AH. Pathogenesis and treatment of growing skull fractures. *Surg Neurol* 1995;43:367–373.
141. Battle WH. *Hunterian lectures*. London: Royal College of Surgeons of England, 1890.
142. Hanigan WC, Peerson RA, Njus G. Tin ear syndrome: rotational acceleration in pediatric head injuries. *Pediatrics* 1987;80:618–622.
143. Wilson NW, Copeland B, Bastian JF. Posttraumatic meningitis in adolescents and children. *Pediatr Neurosurg* 1990–1991;16:17–20.
144. Ommaya AK. Spinal fluid fistulae. *Clin Neurosurg* 1976;23:363–392.
145. Hull HF, Morrow G. Glucorrhea revisited: prolonged promulgation of another plastic pearl. *JAMA* 1975;234:1052–1053.
146. El Gammal T, Sobol W, Wadlington VR, et al. Cerebrospinal fluid fistula: detection with MR cisternography. *Am J Neuroradiol* 1998;19:627–631.
147. Shetty PG, Shroff MM, Sahani DV, et al. Evaluation of high-resolution CT and MR cisternography in the diagnosis of cerebrospinal fluid fistula. *Am J Neuroradiol* 1998;19:633–639.
148. Eberhardt KE, Hollenbach HP, Deimling, M, et al. MR cisternography: a new method for the diagnosis of CSF fistulae. *Eur Radiol* 1997;7:1485–1491.
149. Baltas I, Tsoulfa S, Sakellariiou P, et al. Posttraumatic meningitis: bacteriology, hydrocephalus, and outcome. *Neurosurgery* 1994;35:422–426.
150. Rathore MH. Do prophylactic antibiotics prevent meningitis after basilar skull fracture? *Pediatr Infect Dis J* 1991;10:87–88.
151. Davis RE, Telischi FF. Traumatic facial nerve injuries: review of diagnosis and treatment. *J Craniomaxillofac Trauma* 1995;1:30–41.
152. Eviatar L, Bergtraum M, Randel RM. Posttraumatic vertigo in children: a diagnostic approach. *Pediatr Neurol* 1986;2:61–66.
153. Shea JJ, Ge X, Orchik DJ. Traumatic endolympathic hydrops. *Am J Otol* 1995;16:235–240.
154. Erdilitz-Markus T, Shuper A, Schwartz M, et al. Delayed posttraumatic visual loss: a clinical dilemma. *Pediatr Neurol* 2000;22:133–135.
155. Griffith JF, Dodge PR. Transient blindness following head injury in children. *N Engl J Med* 1968;278:648–651.
156. Eldridge PR, Punt JAG. Transient traumatic cortical blindness in children. *Lancet* 1988;1:815–816.
157. Kadish HA, Schunk JE. Pediatric basilar skull fracture: do children with normal neurologic findings and no intracranial injury require hospitalization? *Ann Emerg Med* 1995;26:37–41.
158. Dandy WE. Pneumocephalus (intracranial pneumatocele or aerocele). *Arch Surg* 1926;12:949–982.
159. Keskil S, Baykamer K, Ceviker N, et al. Clinical significance of acute traumatic intracranial pneumocephalus. *Neurosurg Rev* 1998;21:10–13.
160. Steinbok P, Flodmark O, Martens D, et al. Management of simple depressed skull fractures in children. *J Neurosurg* 1987;66:506–510.
161. Ersahin Y, Mutluer S, Mizai H, et al. Pediatric depressed skull fractures: analysis of 530 cases. *Childs Nerv Syst* 1996;12:523–531.
162. Foy PM, Chadwick DW, Rajgopalan N, et al. Do prophylactic anticonvulsants alter the pattern of seizures after craniotomy? *J Neurol Neurosurg Psychiatry* 1992;55:753–757.
163. Dhellemmes P, Lejeune JP, Christiaens JL, et al. Traumatic extradural hematoma in infancy and childhood. *J Neurosurg* 1985;62:861–864.
164. Matson DD. Extradural hematoma. In: Matson DD. *Neurosurgery of infancy and childhood,* 2nd ed. Springfield, IL: Charles C. Thomas, 1969:316–327.
165. Shugerman RP, Paez A, Grossman DC, et al. Epidural hemorrhage: is it abuse? *Pediatrics* 1996;97:664–668.
166. Mazza, C, Pasqualin A, Feriotti G, et al. Traumatic extradural haematoma in children: experience with 62 cases. *Acta Neurochir* 1982;65:67–80.
167. McKissock W, Taylor JC, Bloom WH, Till K. Extradural haematoma: observations on 125 cases. *Lancet* 1960;2:167–172.
168. Kernohan JW, Woltman HW. Incisura of the crus due to contralateral brain tumor. *Arch Neurol Psychiatr* 1929;21:274–278.
169. Holtzschuh M, Schuknecht B. Traumatic epidural haematomas of the posterior fossa: 20 new cases and a review of the literature since 1961. *Br J Neurosurg* 1989;3:171–180.
170. Berker M, Cataltepe O, Ozcan OE. Traumatic epidural haematoma of the posterior fossa in childhood: 16 new cases and a review of the literature. *Br J Neurosurg* 2003;17:226–229.
171. Marshall LF. Surgical treatment of extracerebral lesions in head injury. In: Pitts LH, Wagner FC, eds. *Craniospinal trauma*. New York: Thieme, 1990:37–48.
172. Choux M, Lena G, Genitori L. Intracranial hematomas. In: Raimondi AJ, Choux M, DiRocco C, eds. *Head injuries in the newborn and infant*. New York: Springer-Verlag, 1986:203–216.
173. Neubauer UJ. Extradural hematoma of the posterior fossa. Twelve years experience with CT-scan. *Acta Neurochir* 1987;87:105–111.
174. Duhaime AC, Gennarelli TA, Thibault LE, et al. The shaken baby syndrome. A clinical, pathological, and biomechanical study. *J Neurosurg* 1987;66:409–415.
175. Wilkins B. Head injury—abuse or accident? *Arch Dis Child* 1997;76:393–396.
176. Rabe EF, Flynn RC, Dodge PR. A study of subdural effusions in an infant with particular reference to the mechanisms of their persistence. *Neurology* 1962;12:79–92.
177. Provencale J. The current role of SPECT in imaging subdural hematoma. *J Nucl Med* 1992;33:248–250.
178. Yakubu MA, Leffler CW. 5-Hydroxytryptamine–induced vasoconstriction after cerebral hematoma in piglets. *Pediatr Res* 1997;41:317–320.
179. Duhaime AC, Gennarelli LM, Yachnis A. Acute subdural hematoma: is the blood itself toxic? *J Neurotrauma* 1994;11:669–678.
180. Haseler LJ, Arcinue E, Danielsen ER, et al. Evidence from proton magnetic resonance spectroscopy for a metabolic cascade of neuronal damage in shaken baby syndrome. *Pediatrics* 1997;99:4–14.
181. Swift DM, McBride L. Chronic subdural hematoma in children. *Neurosurg Clin North Am* 2000;11:439–446.
182. McLaurin RL, Tutor FT. Acute subdural hematoma: review of ninety cases. *J Neurosurg* 1961;18:61–67.
183. Litovsky NS, Raffel C, McComb JG. Management of symptomatic chronic extra-axial fluid collections in pediatric patients. *Neurosurgery* 1992;31:445–450.
184. Bruce DA, Zimmerman RA. Shaken impact syndrome. *Pediatr Ann* 1989;18:482–494.
185. Harcourt B, Hopkins D. Ophthalmic manifestations of the battered-baby syndrome. *Br Med J* 1971;3:398–401.
186. Parsch CS, Krass J, Hoffmann E., et al. Arachnoid cysts associated with subdural hematomas and hygromas: Analysis of 16 cases, long-term follow-up, and review of literature. *Neurosurgery* 1997;40:482–490.
187. Barlow KM, Gibson RJ, McPhillips M, et al. Magnetic resonance imaging in acute non-accidental head injury. *Acta Paediatr* 1999;88:734–740.
188. Harwood-Nash DC. Abuse to the pediatric central nervous system. *Am J Neuroradiol* 1992;13:569–575.
189. Zimmerman RA, Bilaniuk LT, Bruce D, et al. Computed tomography of craniocerebral injury in the abused child. *Radiology* 1979;130:687–690.
190. Dolinskas CA, Zimmerman RA, Bilaniuk LT. A sign of subarachnoid bleeding on computed tomograms of pediatric head trauma patients. *Radiology* 1978;126:409–411.
191. Parent AD. Pediatric chronic subdural hematoma: a retrospective comparative analysis. *Pediatr Neurosurg* 1992;18:266–271.
192. Till K. Subdural haematoma and effusion in infancy. *Br Med J* 1968;2:400–402.
193. Hoffmann GF, Naughten ER. Abuse or metabolic disorder? *Arch Dis Child* 1998;78:199.
194. Sherwood D. Chronic subdural hematoma in infants. *Am J Dis Child* 1930;39:980–1021.

195. Ingraham FD, Heyl HL. Subdural hematoma in infancy and childhood. *JAMA* 1939;112:198–204.
196. El-Kadi H, Kaufman HH, eds. Chronic subdural hematoma. *Neurosurg Clin North Am* 2000;11.
197. Sauter KL. Percutaneous subdural tapping and subdural peritoneal drainage for the treatment of subdural hematoma. *Neurosurg Clin North Am* 2000;11:519–524.
198. Ersahin Y, Mutluer S, Koraman S. Continuous external subdural drainage in the management of infantile subdural collections: a prospective study. *Childs Nerv Syst* 1997;13:526–529.
199. Tabaddor K, Shulman K. Definitive treatment of chronic subdural hematoma by twist-drill craniostomy and closed-system drainage. *J Neurosurg* 1977;46:220–226.
200. McLaurin RL, McLaurin KS. Calcified subdural hematomas in childhood. *J Neurosurg* 1966;24:648–655.
201. Haviland J, Russell RI. Outcome after severe non-accidental head injury. *Arch Dis Child* 1997;77:504–507.
202. Martin HP, Beezley P, Conway EF, et al. The development of abused children. *Adv Pediatr* 1974;21:25–73.
203. Elmer E. A follow-up study of traumatized children. *Pediatrics* 1977;59:273–279.
204. Jennett WB. Trauma as a cause of epilepsy in childhood. *Dev Med Child Neurol* 1973;15:56–62.
205. Annegers JF, Grabow JD, Groover RV, et al. Seizures after head trauma: a population study. *Neurology* 1980;30:683–689.
206. Hendrick E, Harris L. Posttraumatic epilepsy in children. *J Trauma* 1968;8:547–556.
207. Santhakumar V, Ratzliff ADH, Jeng J, et al. Long-term hyperexcitability in the hippocampus after experimental head trauma. *Ann Neurol* 2001;50:708–717.
208. Hendrick E, Harris L. Posttraumatic epilepsy in children. *J Trauma* 1968;8:547–556.
209. Annegers J, Hauser WA, Coan SP, et al. A population-based study of seizures after traumatic brain injuries. *N Engl J Med* 1998;338: 20–24.
210. Temkin NR. Risk factors for posttraumatic seizures in adults. *Epilepsia* 2003;44(Suppl 10):18–20.
211. Caveness WF, Meirowski AM, Rish BL, et al. The nature of posttraumatic epilepsy. *J Neurosurg* 1979;50:545–553.
212. Walton JW, Barwick DD, Longley BP. The electroencephalogram in brain injury. In: Rowbotham GF, ed. *Acute injuries of the head: their diagnosis, treatment, complications and sequels*. Baltimore: Williams & Wilkins, 1964.
213. Temkin NR. Antiepileptogenesis and seizure prevention trials with antiepileptic drugs: meta-analysis of controlled trials. *Epilepsia* 2001;42:515–524.
214. Walker AE. Posttraumatic epilepsy: an inquiry into the evolution and dissolution of convulsions following head injury. *Clin Neurosurg* 1958;6:69–103.
215. Jan MS, Camfield PR, Gordon K, et al. Vomiting after mild head injury is related to migraine. *J Pediatr* 1997;130:134–137.
216. Haas DC, Lourie H. Trauma-triggered migraine: an explanation for common neurological attacks after mild head injury. *J Neurosurg* 1988;68:181–188.
217. Dandy WE, Follis RH Jr. On the pathology of carotidcavernous aneurysms (pulsating exophthalmos). *Am J Ophthalmol* 1941;24:365–385.
218. Fattahi TT, Brandt MT, Jenkins WS, et al. Traumatic carotid-cavernous fistula: pathophysiology and treatment. *J Craniofac Surg* 2003;14:240–246.
219. Desal H, Leaute F, Auffray-Calvier E, et al. Fistule carotido-caverneuse directe, études clinique, radiologique et thérapeutique. Ápropos de 49 cas. *J Neuroradiol* 1997;24:141–154.
220. Berger G, Bonilha L, Santos SF, et al. Thrombosis of the internal carotid artery secondary to soft palate injury in children and childhood. Report of two cases. *Pediatr Neurosurg* 2000;32:150–153.
221. Mokri B, Piepgras DG, Houser OW. Traumatic dissections of the extracranial internal carotid artery. *J Neurosurg* 1988;68:189–197.
222. Payton TF, Siddiqui KM, Sole DP, et al. Traumatic dissection of the internal carotid artery. *Pediatr Emerg Care* 2004;20:27–29.
223. Chabrier S, Lasjaunias P, Husson B, et al. Ischaemic stroke from dissection of the craniocervical arteries in childhood: report of 12 patients. *Eur J Paediatr Neurol* 2003;7:39–42.
224. Ganesan V, Chong WK, Cox TC, et al. Posterior circulation stroke in childhood: risk factors and recurrence. *Neurology* 2002;59:1552–1556.
225. Khurana DS, Bonnemann CG, Dooley EC, et al. Vertebral artery dissection: issues in diagnosis and management. *Pediatr Neurol* 1996;14:255–258.
226. Hasan I, Wapnick, S, Tenner MS, et al. Vertebral artery dissection in children: a comprehensive review. *Pediatr Neurosurg* 2002;37:168–177.
227. Auer A, Felber S, Schmidauer C, et al. Magnetic resonance angiographic and clinical features of extracranial vertebral artery dissection. *J Neurol Neurosurg Psychiatry* 1998;64:474–481.
228. Snoek JW, Minderhoud JM, Wilmink JT. Delayed deterioration following mild head injury in children. *Brain* 1984;107:15–36.
229. McCrory PR, Berkovic SF. Second impact syndrome. *Neurology* 1998;50:677–683.
230. Kors EE, Terwind GM, Vermeulen FLMG, et al. Delayed cerebral edema and fatal coma after minor head trauma: Role of the *CACNA1A* calcium channel subunit gene and relationship with familial hemiplegic migraine. *Ann Neurol* 2001;49:753–760.
231. Bruce DA, Alavi A, Bilaniuk L, et al. Diffuse cerebral swelling following head injuries in children: the syndrome of malignant brain edema. *J Neurosurg* 1981;54:170–178.
231a. Levin HS. Neuroplasticity following non-penetating traumatic brain injury. *Brain Injury* 2003;17:665–674.
232. Taylor HG, Alden J. Age-related differences in outcomes following childhood brain insults: An introduction and overview. *J Int Neuropsychol Soc* 1997;3:555–567.
233. Koskiniemi M, Kyykka T, Nybo T, Jarho L. Long-term outcome after severe head injury in preschoolers is worse than expected. *Arch Pediatr Adolesc Med* 1995;149:249–254.
233a. Max JE, Lansing AE, Koele SL, et al. Attention deficit hyperactivity disorder in children and adolescents following traumatic brain injury. *Dev Neuropsychol* 2004;25:159–177.
234. Hawley CA, Ward AB, Magnay AR, et al. Outcomes following childhood head injury: A population study. *J Neurol Neurosurg Psychiatry* 2004;75:737–742.
235. Ewing-Cobbs L, Barnes M, Fletcher JM. Modeling of longitudinal academic achievement scores after pediatric traumatic brain injury. *Dev Neuropsychol* 2004;25:107–133.
236. Anderson VA, Morse SA, Klug, G, et al. Predicting recovery from head injury in young children: A prospective study. *J Int Neuropsychol Soc* 1997;3:568–580.
237. Mitchener A, Wyper DJ, Patterson J, et al. SPECT, CT, and MRI in head injury: acute abnormalities followed up at six months. *J Neurol Neurosurg Psychiatry* 1997;62:633–636.
238. Symonds C. Disorders of memory. *Brain* 1966;89:625–644.
239. Haas DC, Ross GS. Transient global amnesia triggered by mild head trauma. *Brain* 1986;109:251–257.
240. Harris P. Head injuries in childhood. *Arch Dis Child* 1957;32:488–491.
241. Gronwall D, Wrightson P, McGinn V. Effect of mild head injury during the preschool years. *J Int Neuropsychol Soc* 1997;3:592–597.
242. Wrightson P, McGinn V, Gronwall D. Mild head injury in preschool children: Evidence that it can be associated with a persistent cognitive deficit. *J Neurol Neurosurg Psychiatr* 1995;59:375–380.
242a. Pelco L, Sawyer M, Duffield G, et al. Premorbid emotional and behavioral adjustment in children with mild head injuries. *Brain Inj* 1992;6:26–37.
243. McKinlay A, Dalrymple-Alford JC, Horwood LJ, et al. Long term psychosocial outcomes after mild head injury in early childhood. *J Neurol Neurosurg Psychiatry* 2002;73:281–288.
244. Chadwick O. Psychological sequelae of head injury in children. *Dev Med Child Neurol* 1985;27:72–75.
244a. Cook JB. The effects of minor head injuries sustained in sport and the postconcussion syndrome. In: Walker AE, Caveness WF, Critchley M, eds. *The late effects of head injury*. Springfield, IL: Charles C. Thomas, 1969;408–413.
245. Nylander I, Rydelius PA. Post-concussion syndrome. Brain damage, consitutional characterics and environmental reactions. *Acta Paediatr Scand* 1988;77:475–477.

246. McClelland RJ, Fenton GW, Rutherford W. The postconcussional syndrome revisited. *J R Soc Med* 1994;87:508–510.
247. Hjern B, Nylander I. Acute head injuries in children: traumatology, therapy and prognosis. *Acta Paediatr* 1964(Suppl):152.
248. American Academy of Neurology. Practice parameter: the management of concussion in sports. *Neurology* 1997;48:581–585.
249. Jennett B, Plum F. Persistent vegetative state after brain damage. A syndrome in search of a name. *Lancet* 1972;1:734–737.
250. Kampfl A, Franz G, Aichner F, et al. The persistent vegetative state after closed head injury: clinical and magnetic resonance imaging findings in 42 patients. *J Neurosurg* 1998;88:809–816.
251. Ashwal S. Medical aspects of the minimally conscious state in children. *Brain Dev* 2003;25:535–545.
252. Higashi K, Sakata Y, Hatano M, et al. Epidemiological studies on patients with a persistent vegetative state. *J Neurol Neurosurg Psychiatry* 1977;40:876–885.
253. Heindl UT, Laub MC. Outcome of persistent vegetative state following hypoxic or traumatic brain injury in children and adolescents. *Neuropediatrics* 1996;27:94–100.
254. Ashwal S, Eyman RK, Call TL. Life expectancy in a persistent vegetative state. *Pediatr Neurol* 1994;10:27–33.
255. Strauss DJ, Shavelle RM, Ashwal S. Life expectancy and median survival time in the permanent vegetative state. *Pediatr Neurol* 1999;21:626–631.
256. Hamilton MG, Myles ST. Pediatric spinal injury: review of 174 hospital admissions. *J Neurosurg* 1992;77:700–704.
257. Norenberg MD, Smith J, Marcillo A. The pathology of human spinal cord injury: Defining the problems. *J Neurotrauma* 2004;21:429–440.
258. Tator CH, Fehlings MG. Review of the secondary injury theory of acute spinal cord trauma with emphasis on vascular mechanisms. *J Neurosurg* 1991;75:15–26.
259. Bischof W, Nittner K. Zur Klinik und Pathogenese der vaskular bedingten Myelomalazien. *Neurochirurgie* 1965;8:215–231.
260. Ahmann PA, Smith SA, Schwartz JF, et al. Spinal cord infarction due to minor trauma in children. *Neurology* 1975;25:301–307.
261. Choi JU, Hoffman HJ, Hendrick EB, et al. Traumatic infarction of the spinal cord in children. *J Neurosurg* 1986;65:608–610.
262. Williams B. Pathogenesis of posttraumatic syringomyelia. *Br J Neurosurg* 1992;6:517–520.
263. La Haye PA, Batzdorf U. Posttraumatic syringomyelia. *West J Med* 1988;148:657–663.
264. Zwimpfer TJ, Bernstein M. Spinal cord concussion. *J Neurosurg* 1990;72:894–900.
265. Ruge JR, Sinson GP, McLone DG, Cerullo IJ. Pediatric spinal injury: the very young. *J Neurosurg* 1988;68:25–30.
266. Greenwald TA, Mann DC. Pediatric seatbelt injuries: diagnosis and treatment of lumbar flexion-distraction injuries. *Paraplegia* 1994;32:743–751.
267. Taylor GA, Eggli KD. Lap-belt injuries of the lumbar spine in children: a pitfall in CT diagnosis. *Am J Roentgenol* 1988;150:1355–1358.
268. Carlson GD, Gorden C. Current developments in spinal cord injury research. *Spine J* 2002;2:116–128.
269. Dumont RJ, Okonkwo DO, Verma S, et al. Acute spinal cord injury, part I: pathophysiologic mechanisms. *Clin Neuropharmacol* 2001;24:254–264.
270. Frankel HL, Hancock DO, Hyslop G, et al. The value of postural reduction in the initial management of closed injuries of the spine with paraplegia and tetraplegia. *Paraplegia* 1969;7:179–192.
271. Ditunno JF, Young W. Donovan WH, et al. The international standards booklet for neurological and functional classification of spinal cord injury. American Spinal Injury Association. *Paraplegia* 1994;32:70–80.
272. Sherrington CS. *The integrative action of the nervous system*. New York: Scribner, 1906.
273. Riddock G. The reflex functions of the completely divided spinal cord in man, compared with those associated with less severe lesions. *Brain* 1917;40:264–402.
274. Ditunno JF, Little JW, Tessler A, et al. Spinal shock revisited: a four-phase model. *Spinal cord* 2004;42:383–395.
275. Atkinson PP, Atkinson JLD. Spinal shock. *Mayo Clin Proc* 1996;71:384–389.
276. Hiersemenzel, LP, Curt A, Dietz V. From spinal shock to spasticity. Neuronal adaptations to a spinal cord injury. *Neurology* 2000;54:1574–1582.
277. Chiles BW, Cooper PR. Acute spinal injury. *N Engl J Med* 1996;514–520.
278. Kuhn RA. Functional capacity of the isolated human spinal cord. *Brain* 1950;73:1–51.
279. Sullivan AW. Subluxation of atlanto-axial joint. *J Pediatr* 1949;35:451–464.
280. Menezes AH, Mohonen M. Management of occipito-cervical instability. In: Cooper PR, ed. *Neurosurgical topics,* Vol. 1. Baltimore: Williams & Wilkins, 1990:65–76.
281. Veras LM, Castellanos J, Ramirez G, et al. Atlanto axial instability due to neurofibromatosis: case report. *Acta Orthop Belg* 2000;66:392–396.
282. Controversies in imaging acute cervical spine trauma. *Am J Neuroradiol* 1997;18:1866–1868.
283. Hadley MN, Zabramski JM, Browner CM, et al. Pediatric spinal trauma. Review of 122 cases of spinal cord and vertebral column injuries. *J Neurosurg* 1988;68:18–24.
284. Cattell HS, Filtzer DL. Pseudosubluxation and other normal variations in the cervical spine in children. *J Bone Joint Surg* 1965;47A:1295–1309.
285. Jefferson G. Concerning injuries of the spinal cord. *Br Med J* 1936;2:1125–1130.
286. Guttman L. *Spinal cord injuries,* 2nd ed. Oxford: Blackwell, 1976.
287. Sonntag VKH, Hadley MN. Nonoperative management of cervical spine injuries. *Clin Neurosurg* 1988;34:630–649.
288. Vale FL, Burns J, Jackson AB, et al. Combined medical and surgical treatment after acute spinal cord injury: results of a prospective pilot study to assess the merits of aggressive medical resuscitation and blood pressure management. *J Neurosurg* 1997;87:239–246.
289. Sypert GW. Stabilization and management of cervical injuries. In: Pitts LH, Wagner FC, eds. *Craniospinal trauma*. New York: Thieme, 1990:171–185.
290. Becker D, Sadowsky CL, McDonald JW. Restoring function after spinal cord injury. *Neurologist* 2003;9:1–15.
291. Bracken MB. Methylprednisolone and acute spinal cord injury: an update of the randomized evidence. *Spine* 2001;26(24 Suppl):S47–S54.
292. Geisler FH, Dorsey FC, Coleman WP. Recovery of motor function after spinal cord injury—a randomized, placebo-controlled trial with GM1 ganglioside. *N Engl J Med* 1991;324:1829–1838.
293. Geisler FH. Clinical trials of pharmacotherapy for spinal cord injury. *Ann N Y Acad Sci* 1998;845:374–381.
294. Kapfhammer JP. Axon sprouting in the spinal cord: growth promoting and growth inhibitory mechanisms. *Anat Embryol* 1997;196:417–426.
295. Okada S, Nakamura M, Mikami Y, et al. Blockade of interleukin-6 receptor suppresses reactive astrogliosis and ameliorates functional recovery in experimental spinal cord injury. *Neurosci Res* 2004;76:265–276.
296. Bregman BS, Coumans JV, Dai HN., et al. Transplants and neurotrophic factors increase regeneration and recovery of function after spinal cord injury. *Prog Brain Res* 2002;137:257–273.
297. Short DJ, Frankel HL, Bergstrwöm EMK. Injuries of the spinal cord in children. In: Vinken GW, Bruyn GW, Klawans HL, et al, eds. *Spinal cord trauma. Handbook of clinical neurology,* Rev. Ser. 17, Vol. 61. Amsterdam: Elsevier, 1992:233–252.
298. Piepmeier JM. Late sequelae of spinal cord injury. In: Narayan RK, Wilberger JE Jr, Povlikshock JT, eds. *Neurotrauma*. New York: McGraw-Hill, 1996:1237–1244.
299. Whiteneck G, Lammertse DP, Manley S, et al., eds. *The management of high quadriplegia*. New York: Demos, 1989.
300. Lightner DJ. Contemporary urologic management of patients with spinal cord injury. *Mayo Clin Proc* 1998;73:434–438.
301. Crockard HA, Heilman AE, Stevens JM. Progressive myelopathy secondary to odontoid fractures: clinical, radiological and surgical features. *J Neurosurg* 1993;78:579–586.
302. Martinez-Lage JF, Fernandez Cornejo V, Lopez F, et al. Lumbar disc herniation in early childhood: case report and literature review. *Child Nerv Syst* 2003;19:258–260.

303. Epstein JA, Lavine LS. Herniated lumbar intervertebral disks in teenage children. *J Neurosurg* 1964;21:1070–1075.
304. Kahanovitz N, Rimoin DL, Sillence DO. The clinical spectrum of lumbar spine disease in achondroplasia. *Spine* 1982;7:137–140.
305. Friedman AP, Merritt HH. Damage to cranial nerves resulting from head injury. *Bull Los Angeles Neurol Soc* 1944;9:135–139.
306. Brazis PW. Palsies of the trochlear nerve: diagnosis and localization—recent concepts. *Mayo Clin Proc* 1993;68:501–509.
307. McKennan KX, Chole RA. Facial paralysis in temporal bone trauma. *Am J Otol* 1992;13:167–172.
308. Galan E, Kousseff BG. Peripheral neuropathy in Ehlers-Danlos syndrome. *Pediatr Neurol* 1995;12:242–245.
309. Stoll G, Jander S, Myers RR. Degeneration and regeneration of the peripheral nervous system: from Augustus Waller's observations to neuroinflammation. *J Peripher Nerv Syst* 2002;7:13–27.
310. Manabe Y, Sakai K, Kashihara K, et al. Presumed venous infarction in spinal decompression sickness. *Am J Neuroradiol* 1998;19:1578–1580.
311. Van Meir N, De Smet L. Carpal tunnel syndrome in children. *Acta Orthop Belg* 2003;69:387–395.
312. Villarejo FJ, Pascual AM. Injection injury of the sciatic nerve (370 cases). *Childs Nerv Syst* 1993;9:229–232.
313. Medical Research Council. *Aids to the examination of peripheral nerve injuries*. London: Balliere Tindall, 1986.
314. Papazian O, Alfonso I, Yaylali I, et al. Neurophysiological evaluation of children with traumatic radiculopathy, plexopathy, and peripheral neuropathy. *Semin Pediatr Neurol* 2000;7:26–35.
315. Hodes R, Larrabee MG, German W. The human electromyogram in response to nerve stimulation and the conduction velocity of motor axons: studies on normal and on injured peripheral nerves. *Arch Neurol Psychiatry* 1948;60:340–365.
316. Carvalho GA, Nikkhah G, Matthies C, et al. Diagnosis of root avulsions in traumatic brachial plexus injuries: value of computerized tomography myelography and magnetic resonance imaging. *J Neurosurg* 1997;86:69–76.
317. Aagaard BD, Maravilla KR, Kliot M. Magnetic resonance neurography: magnetic resonance imaging of peripheral nerves. *Neuroimaging Clin North Am* 2001;11:131–146.
318. Mitchell SW. *Injuries of nerves and their consequences*. Philadelphia: Lippincott, 1972.
319. Matsui M, Ito M, Tomoda A, et al. Complex regional pain syndrome in childhood: report of three cases. *Brain Dev* 2000;22:445–448.
320. Gordon N. Reflex sympathetic dystrophy. *Brain Dev* 1996;18:257–262.
321. Hannington-Kiff JG. Reflex sympathetic dystrophy. *J R Soc Med* 1987;80:605.
322. Bhatia KP, Bhatt MH, Marsden CD. The causalgia-dystonia syndrome. *Brain* 1993;116:843–851.
323. Birklein F, Riedl B, Sieweke N., et al. Neurological findings in complex regional pain syndromes–analysis of 145 cases. *Acta Neurol Scan* 2000;101:262–269.
324. Goldstein DS, Tack C, Li, ST. Sympathetic innervation and function in reflex sympathetic dystrophy. *Ann Neurol* 2000;48:49–59.
325. van der Laan L, ter Laak HJ, Gabreels-Festen A, et al. Complex regional pain syndrome type I (RSD). Pathology of skeletal muscle and peripheral nerve. *Neurology* 1998;51:20–25.
326. Honjyo K, Hamasaki Y, Kita M, et al. An 11-year-old girl with reflex sympathetic dystrophy successfully treated by thoracoscopic sympathectomy. *Acta Paediatr* 1997;86:903–905.
327. Bouchama A, Knochel JP. Heat stroke. *N Engl J Med* 1002;346:1978–1988.
328. Malamud N, Haymaker W, Custer RP. Heat stroke: a clinicopathologic study of 125 fatal cases. *Milit Surg* 1946;99:397–449.
329. Freedman D, Schenthal J. A parenchymatous cerebellar syndrome following protracted high body temperature. *Neurology* 1953;3:513–516.
330. Chavez-Carballo E, Bouchama A. Fever, heatstroke, and hemorrhage shock and encephalopathy. *J Child Neurol* 1998;13:286–287.
331. Hopkins PM, Ellis FR, Halsall PJ. Evidence for related myopathies in exertional heat stroke and malignant hyperthermia. *Lancet* 1991;338:1491–1492.
332. Cherington M. Neurologic manifestations of lightning strike. *Neurology* 2003;60:182–185.
333. Critchley M. Neurological effects of lightning and of electricity. *Lancet* 1934;1:68–72.
334. Silversides J. The neurological sequelae of electrical injury. *Can Med Assoc J* 1964;91:195–204.
334a. Duff K, MacCaffrey RJ. Electrical injury and lightning injury: a review of their mechanisms and neuropsychological, psychiatric and neurological sequelae. *Neuropsychol Rev* 2001;11:101–116.
335. Kotagal S, Rawlings CA, Chen SC, et al. Neurologic, psychiatric and cardiovascular complications in children struck by lightning. *Pediatrics* 1982;70:190–192.
336. Winkelman MD, Galloway PG. Central nervous system complications of thermal burns. A postmortem study of 139 patients. *Medicine* 1992;71:271–283.
337. Mohnot D, Snead OC, Benton JW. Burn encephalopathy in children. *Ann Neurol* 1982;12:42–47.
338. Antoon AY, Volpe JJ, Crawford JD. Burn encephalopathy in children. *Pediatrics* 1972;50:609–616.
339. Greer HD. Neurologic consequences. In: Bove AA, ed. *Diving medicine,* 3rd ed. Philadephia: Saunders, 1997:258–269.
340. Reuter M, Tetzlaff K, Hutzelmann A, et al. MR imaging of the central nervous system in diving-related decompression illness. *Acta Radiol* 1997;38:940–944.
341. Deymeer F, Jones HR. Pediatric median mononeuropathies: a clinical and electromyelographic study. *Muscle Nerve* 1994;17:755–762.

Chapter 10

Toxic and Nutritional Disorders

John H. Menkes

TOXIC DISORDERS

Neurotoxins are endogenous or environmental. Various sections of this text consider the endogenous neurotoxins, notably the excitatory neurotransmitters. These substances are implicated in cell death from asphyxia and hypoglycemia, following uncontrolled seizures, and possibly in some of the heredodegenerative disorders. This chapter discusses environmental toxins. Almost all environmental toxins induce neurologic symptoms if ingested in sufficient quantity. This chapter considers only those that are encountered in clinical practice commonly and for which the nervous system is a primary site of action. They are discussed in ascending order of their chemical complexity.

Drug intoxications that are encountered less commonly by the practitioner are not considered in detail. The reader is referred to Table 10.1 (1–24) for a summary of their neurologic complications and treatment.

In addition, the reader is directed to the comprehensive text on medical toxicology edited by Ellenhorn and colleagues (25), and a book on neurotoxicology edited by Spencer and coworkers (26).

The incidence of the various drug intoxications in an Australian pediatric population during the years 1977 through 1981 is depicted in Table 10.2 (27). A series compiled from the Children's Hospital of the University of Antwerp for the years 1980 through 1988 shows a similar distribution (28).

Metallic Toxins

Lead

Although some of the toxic actions of lead have been known since antiquity, the understanding of the clinical picture of lead poisoning is based on the classic studies of Tanquerel des Planches (29), Blackfan (30), and Holt (31). As a result of the considerable advances in the prevention of lead exposure, cases of acute lead encephalopathy have all but disappeared from the United States. Nevertheless, children with increased blood lead levels are still being encountered with considerable frequency, and the effect of elevated blood lead levels on neurocognitive and neurobehavioral function has been the subject of considerable recent controversy.

Pharmacology

One of the major sources of lead continues to be exterior and, to a lesser extent, interior lead-based paint, which remains as an environmental hazard in some 3.8 million homes in the United States housing children 7 years of age or younger (32). Lead can be absorbed by water with a low mineral content as it passes through lead pipes or lead-soldered copper pipes. It also can be ingested when water is boiled in soldered electric kettles. Until the 1990s, organic lead also was ingested from roadside dust contaminated with automobile emissions, or by habitual sniffing of leaded gasoline. Less common sources of lead include lead arsenate insecticides; lead solder, which in the United States has been virtually eliminated from the seams of food and beverage cans; ancient pewter; imperfectly glazed ceramics; painted jewelry; and eye shadow, which in some developing countries is applied to infant boys and girls. One form of lead poisoning, once relatively common in nursing infants, was caused by prolonged use of lead nipple shields.

The gastrointestinal tract of infants and children absorbs approximately 40% of ingested lead, with the remainder being excreted. Approximately 90% of inhaled lead is absorbed. Iron deficiency and constipation encourage absorption; diarrhea has the reverse effect. Lead and calcium compete for a common transport mechanism; reduced calcium intake and low serum levels of 25-hydroxy vitamin D_1 increase lead absorption. The vitamin D receptor gene is involved in calcium absorption and, if lead is present, will also absorb lead, and genotype variants of the vitamin D receptor gene may influence the degree of lead absorption (33). After absorption, lead is distributed into three compartments: Some enters a rapidly exchangeable pool in the liver and kidney and from there binds to a low-molecular-weight protein of erythrocytes (34); some enters a rapidly exchangeable pool in soft tissue and is loosely bound to bone; and the major portion (60% to 90%) is

TABLE 10.1 Neurotoxic Complications of Some Drugs

Drug	Neurologic Symptoms	Reference
Antihistamine	Tonic-clonic seizures	Hestand and Tesky (1), Goetz, et al. (2)
Atropine (jimson weed, thornapple, deadly nightshade)	Dilated pupils, slurred speech, ataxia, seizures	Priest (Down syndrome) (3), Amitai et al. (4)
Boric acid	Seizures	Valdez-Dapena and Arey (5), Cheng (6)
Codeine	Respiratory depression	von Muhlendahl et al. (7)
Dextromethorphan (Coricidin)	Dystonia	Warden et al. (8), Kirages et al. (9)
Diphenoxylate (Lomotil)	Excitement, hypotonia, rigidity, cortical blindness, cerebral edema	McCarron et al. (10)
Ferrous sulfate	Vomiting, diarrhea, seizures, lethargy	Robotham and Leitman (11), Mann et al. (12)
Hexachlorophene	Seizures, blindness, spastic paraparesis	Martínez et al. (13), Martin-Bouyer et al. (14)
Hydroxyquinolines (clioquinol)	Optic neuritis, myelitis, peripheral neuropathy	Oakley (15), Selby (16), Shigematsu and Yanagawa (17)
Imipramine and other tricyclic antidepressants	Clonic movements, seizures, coma	McFee et al. (18), Saraf et al. (19)
Phenylpropanolamine	Cerebral vasculitis, intracranial hemorrhage	Forman et al. (20)
Piperazine	Impaired coordination, chorea, encephalopathy	Parsons (21)
Propoxyphene (Darvon)	Lethargy, seizures	Lovejoy et al. (22)
Sympathomimetics (dextroamphetamine)	Agitation, seizures	Espelin and Done (23), Alldredge et al. (24)

tightly bound as the insoluble and nontoxic lead triphosphate in the skeleton, notably in the epiphyseal portion of growing bone. Lead also is deposited in hair and nails and crosses the placenta. Only a small amount of lead enters the brain; the major portion is found in gray matter and the basal ganglia (35,36). High phosphate and high vitamin D intakes favor skeletal storage of lead, whereas parathormone, low phosphate intake, and acidosis promote its release into the bloodstream. Almost all the absorbed lead is excreted in urine; fecal lead represents the unabsorbed fraction. The half-life of lead in blood is 1 to 2 months; it is 20 to 30 years in bone (36). Excretion is so slow that even a slight increase in the average daily intake above 0.3 mg/day, the maximum permissible level for adults, can ultimately induce poisoning.

TABLE 10.2 Agents Accidentally Ingested by Children (0 Through 12 Years) Resulting in Hospital Admission

Agent	Number of Patients	Percent of Accidental Ingestions
Petroleum distillates	255	13
Antihistaminics	186	9
Benzodiazepines	182	9
Bleach, detergents	142	7
Aspirin, acetaminophen	117	6
Camphor, mothballs	117	6
Barbiturates	97	5
Caustic soda	69	3
Painting chemicals	61	3
Noxious plants	49	2
Tricyclics	45	2
Phenytoin	40	2
Iron tablets	36	2
Sympathomimetics	36	2

Data from Brisbane, Australia, 1977–1981. From Pearn J. et al. Accidental poisoning in childhood. Five year urban population study with 15 year analysis of fatality. *BMJ* 1984;288:45. With permission.

The levels of lead in blood and urine are an index of the degree of exposure to the toxin. Although blood lead levels below 10 μg/dL are currently considered acceptable, δ-aminolevulinic acid dehydratase (ALAD) activity is significantly inhibited at blood lead levels of 5 to 10 μg/dL (37), and abnormalities in auditory and visual-evoked potentials have been demonstrated at levels below 10 μg/dl. (38). Measurement of hair lead is an unreliable indicator of the severity of lead exposure, whereas the reliability of tooth lead content is still under debate (39). As yet, the threshold level for neurotoxicity is unknown. The American Academy of Pediatrics has stated that concentrations of 25 μg/dL or higher are certain to be toxic, and the average blood lead level in American children is 2.6 μg/dL (40).

Pathology

Almost all organs are affected by lead poisoning, with damage caused by heavy metal inhibition of numerous sulfhydryl enzymes and its ability to substitute for calcium, and perhaps zinc (38). One of the earliest manifestations of lead intoxication is anemia, induced by a disturbance in heme synthesis and by shortening of red cell life span. Lead impairs heme synthesis at several points, with globin synthesis also being disrupted at higher lead levels (36,41).

Within the central nervous system (CNS), lead acts primarily on capillary endothelium. It causes extravasation of plasma, followed by endothelial, microglial, and astrocytic proliferation and widespread interstitial edema (42). Neuronal degeneration is also widespread, with the neocortex and cerebellum being affected most prominently; neocortical degeneration also can reflect agonal anoxia, rather than a direct effect of lead. Experimental work suggests that the immature cerebral vasculature is particularly sensitive to lead, and that neurotoxicity is the result of multifactorial events. Lead interrupts the cellular calcium pump in mitochondria with a resultant calcium-mediated cell death in the cerebrovascular endothelium (43). Chronic exposure to lead interferes with calmodulin-dependent processes resulting in abnormal post-translational modifications of cytoskeletal proteins. In addition, lead inhibits acetylcholine release and enhances the release of dopamine and norepinephrine (44). These multiple neurotoxic effects of lead are reviewed by Lidsky and Schneider (38).

In peripheral nerves, axonal degeneration occurs with loss of large myelinated fibers, but with no demyelination (45). Occasionally, the anterior horn cells also are degenerated. Chronic, low-level exposure, as is seen in industrial workers, can produce paranodal demyelination and internodal remyelination (46). No explanation exists for the preferential involvement of nerves in the upper extremity.

Pathologic changes within other organs, notably the liver and kidney, have been described in a classic publication by Blackman (47).

Clinical Manifestations

Neurologic symptoms of lead poisoning form a continuum from the most minor to the most severe (48). In the classic form of severe lead encephalopathy, symptoms progress insidiously, first becoming apparent in late summer in some 80% of cases. Before then, there is usually a prodromal period of several weeks or months during which the child is pale, irritable, listless, and without appetite. Epigastric pain, vomiting, and constipation are common. These nonspecific symptoms are often interrupted by the sudden onset of a series of generalized convulsions or by depression of consciousness (Table 10.3) (49,50).

Seizures are common and resist anticonvulsant therapy. They can be followed by hemiplegia or other neurologic sequelae.

The child with lead encephalopathy demonstrates increased intracranial pressure. Less frequent is cerebellar ataxia and palsies of the sixth and seventh cranial nerves. Nuchal rigidity is fairly common and can be related to tonsillar herniation. Patients in some parts of the world have a high incidence of optic neuritis with profound vision loss, acute communicating hydrocephalus, and tremors (51).

In children, peripheral neuritis caused by lead poisoning is rare. When seen, it almost invariably occurs in subjects with sickle cell anemia (52).

Anemia and deranged renal tubular function usually accompany the neurologic symptoms. Red cells in peripheral blood and bone marrow can show basophilic stippling, and the presence of a large number of such cells is almost invariable in chronic poisoning caused by inorganic lead, although not in poisoning with organic (tetraethyl) lead. Basophilic stippling, however, is not specific for lead intoxication.

Radiologic findings in acute lead encephalopathy are characteristic (53). Most prominent is the presence of a dense, radiopaque band at the metaphyses of numerous long bones. Less commonly, radiopaque particles are

TABLE 10.3 Signs and Symptoms of Overt Lead Poisoning in Children (Chicago, 1955–1957)

Prodromal Symptoms	*Number of Cases*	*Overt Symptom*	*Number of Cases*
Irritability	20	Convulsions	11
Pallor	16	Lethargy	7
Vomiting	16	Sixth nerve palsy	7
Constipation	11	Ataxia	2
Weight loss	7		
	2-Year follow-up of 14 patients		
	13/46	Fatal	
	3/14	Retarded motor development	
	7/14	Retarded language development	

Adapted from Mellins RB, Jenkins CD. Epidemiologic and psychological study of lead poisoning in children. *JAMA* 1955;158:15; and Jenkins CD, Mellins RB. Lead poisoning in children. *Arch Neurol Psychiatry* 1957;77:70.

found within the gastrointestinal tract as evidence of recent plaster ingestion.

Although lead encephalopathy and peripheral neuritis represent the classic and severe form of lead intoxication, neurobehavioral symptoms as a consequence of lesser degrees of exposure are now far more common, and have, in the last few years, become a contentious issue for health care workers.

A large number of epidemiologic studies designed to examine the effects of low-level lead exposure on the nervous system differ with respect to the measures selected to reflect the amount of lead to which the developing brain has been exposed. They also differ in the areas of cognitive and neurologic performance chosen to measure the effects of lead intoxication. In almost every study, the results have been confounded by the association between increased lead intake and disadvantaged family and home environment. Smith (54) and Pocock and colleagues (39) have extensively and dispassionately reviewed these issues.

I concur with their conclusions that from the current state of knowledge one is unable to say whether low-level lead exposure affects performance or behavior of children, or whether a reverse causality exists (i.e., children with lower IQs or aberrant behavior patterns have increased lead uptake). In either case, in cases in which effects of environmental lead are found, they are likely to be small and are overshadowed by the effects that result from the child's socioeconomic status, quality of home environment, and parental intelligence (39,54,55). In addition, the effects of genetic and dietary factors on lead absorption and neurocognition have not been clarified. Most significantly, a blood lead level below which lead exposure has absolutely no effect on neurocognitive function has not yet been established (56). Finally, we also do not know what role, if any, intrauterine exposure to lead plays in inducing cognitive deficits (39,55). Thus, in the Australian study of Baghurst and coworkers, no significant relation existed between IQ at 57 months of age and antenatal or perinatal blood lead concentrations (55).

A further discussion on the interrelation between lead exposure and cognitive function can be found in Chapter 18.

Diagnosis

Even though lead encephalopathy has become extremely rare, the appearance of seizures and increased intracranial pressure in a young child should always suggest this condition. Posterior fossa tumors rarely produce seizures, and tumors of the cerebral hemispheres are rare in toddlers. Lead lines on radiographic examination and basophilic stippling in a blood smear offer a presumptive diagnosis even in the absence of a history of pica.

The differential diagnosis between a sickle cell crisis that produces neurologic symptoms and lead poisoning can be difficult because both can produce cramping abdominal pains and seizures. Generally, neurologic signs in sickle cell crisis are caused by cerebrovascular occlusion and thus result in lateralizing findings, which are generally absent in lead encephalopathy.

Currently, the most widely used test to detect chronic low-grade exposure to lead is the whole blood lead level, with the analysis being performed by atomic absorption spectrophotometry. Capillary blood can be used for diagnosis and surveillance (57), and for screening purposes, a filter paper blood test has been found to be reliable (58). An increased hair lead level has been suggested as an indicator for the timing of increased exposure to lead. This measurement, however, is unreliable in that hair lead concentrations can vary in different hairs from the same individual. It also is difficult to remove surface contaminants without removing lead from within the hair. The lead contact of teeth has been used as an indicator of cumulative lead exposure, but this test is obviously impractical for the routine diagnosis of lead poisoning (59).

Because peripheral nerve conduction times are slowed in many youngsters with even inapparent neuropathy, peripheral nerve conduction studies can provide an ancillary indication of subclinical lead intoxication (52).

Treatment and Prognosis

Because recurrent exposure is common, and because neurologic damage caused by lead poisoning is probably progressive rather than all or none, the source of the ingested lead must be ascertained and eliminated before the child returns home from the hospital. The recommended practice is to forego treatment for children whose blood lead level is less than 25 μg/dL. Children with blood lead levels between 25 and 45 μg/dL require their immediate removal from lead exposure, but neither chelation therapy nor dietary calcium supplementation is indicated (60,61). Chelation therapy is indicated for patients with blood lead levels over 45 μg/dL. Two parenteral and two oral chelation agents are currently available. The former are dimercaprol (BAL) and calcium disodium ethylenediaminetetraacetic acid (EDTA). Oral chelation agents are succimer, a water-soluble analogue of BAL, and D-penicillamine. A full discussion of dosages, duration of therapy, and adverse reactions is beyond the scope of this text. They are detailed in the treatment guidelines prepared by the American Academy of Pediatrics, Committee on Drugs (62), in a publication by Piomelli (63), and in a review by Henretig (64). Case management and pitfalls in the treatment of children with severe lead poisoning are discussed by Friedman and Weinberger (65).

Even with the best therapy, the prognosis for complete recovery in children with lead encephalopathy is not good, and by the time symptoms become overt, lasting CNS damage has already been incurred.

Thallium

Children can accidentally ingest thallium-containing pesticides. How the metal damages the nervous system is still unknown (66). One likely possibility is that thallium replaces potassium in the activation of potassium-dependent enzymes, notably pyruvate kinase and succinate dehydrogenase. In fatal cases, one sees white matter edema and degenerative changes in the nerve cells of the cerebral and cerebellar cortex, hypothalamus, olivary nuclei, and the corpus striatum. In peripheral nerves, there is a loss of myelinated fibers and degeneration of the central axons of sensory ganglion cells (67).

Depending on the dose ingested, intoxication can be fatal during the acute phase by causing renal and cardiac failure. In less severe intoxications, neurologic symptoms appear 2 to 6 days after ingestion, including a motor neuropathy that principally affects the lower extremities. Hair fibers in the growing stage, which constitute between 80% and 90% of scalp hair, and large-diameter fibers are most vulnerable to thallium intoxication (68). Subsequently, cerebellar ataxia can develop, accompanied by somnolence or seizures. A characteristic depilation resembling that seen after vincristine therapy begins within 2 weeks. Less commonly, there are retrobulbar neuritis and cranial nerve palsies (69).

Approximately one-half of the survivors have persistent neurologic deficits, most commonly mental retardation and ataxia. The diagnosis suggested by neurologic symptoms in the presence of depilation can be confirmed by the detection of thallium in urine using atomic absorption spectroscopy and emission spectrography (70).

Chelating agents such as diethyl dithiocarbamate or dimercaptosuccinic acid are ineffective in the treatment of thallium poisoning. Although they increase thallium excretion, the chelate formed is lipophilic and crosses the blood–brain barrier. As a consequence, neurologic symptoms worsen (71). Prussian blue, however, does have some value, having induced clinical improvement in a number of patients (72).

Arsenic

In the Western world, arsenic poisoning in the pediatric population most commonly results from the accidental ingestion of pesticides, notably ant poison (73). Since 1980, arsenic toxicity has become a major health problem in some developing countries with arsenic contaminating drinking water obtained from wells. The metal can arise from natural geological sources such as iron-pyrite as a result of overexploitation of ground water as well as from contamination induced by mining and other industrial processes. Arsenic poisoning is particularly common in Bangladesh and West Bengal, where up to 6% of children demonstrate symptoms of arsenic poisoning (74,75). The pathologic changes in the brain have been reviewed in a classic paper by Russell (76). They include generalized edema and pericapillary hemorrhages within white matter, with foci of demyelination. Nerve biopsies show axonal degeneration (77). The toxicity of arsenic probably lies in its ability to inactivate up to 200 sulfhydryl enzymes, notably those involved in the cellular energy pathways and DNA synthesis and repair (74,78).

Symptoms of arsenic poisoning in the pediatric population are more likely to be gastrointestinal than dermatological (pigmentation and keratosis) or neurologic (75,79). After acute arsenic ingestion, they can take the form of a violent attack of vomiting and bloody diarrhea. Chronic arsenic intake induces intermittent gastrointestinal upsets. In children, anemia is not unusual. Neurologic symptoms are mainly those of a peripheral sensory neuritis; numbness and severe paresthesias of the distal portion of the extremities predominate. Distal weakness of the lower extremities follows and can extend to involve the upper extremities.

For the treatment of acute arsenic toxicity, BAL is the drug of choice. For patients with subacute or chronic toxicity, succimer or 2,3-dimercapto-1-propanesulfonate (DMPS) are preferred (80). Their mode of administration to children is described by Ford (81).

Mercury

Mercury poisoning can result from exposure to elemental mercury in the form of its vapor, inorganic mercury salts, and organic mercury, most commonly as methylmercury. Because of their ability to affect neuronal cell division and migration, organic mercury compounds are highly toxic to the fetus and the early developing postnatal brain.

Mercury vapor poisoning has been reported to induce seizures. Pink disease (acrodynia), once relatively common owing to ingestion of calomel (mercuric chloride) teething powders (82), is now much rarer but has been observed after exposure to latex paint, which up to 1990 contained phenylmercuric acetate. Mercury is released from surfaces coated with this paint after it has dried (83). Only a small proportion of exposed infants and young children become symptomatic. Clinical manifestations are marked by erythema, most intense over the fingertips and toes; profound weakness of all extremities; hyperesthesia; extreme irritability; and changes in consciousness.

Intoxication with organic mercury compounds derived from the fungicides or methylmercury was responsible for outbreaks of poisoning in Iraq (84), whereas ingestion of methylmercury-contaminated fish resulted in Minamata disease, an encephalopathy encountered along Minamata Bay in Japan. The neurologic picture of organic mercury poisoning in children is complex. Tingling and other sensory disturbances and progressive visual impairment, taking the form of constriction of visual fields, tunnel vision, or complete blindness, are almost invariable. Ataxia, tremor, impaired hearing, and mental deterioration also are encountered. A variety of involuntary movements are less common (85). Magnetic resonance imaging (MRI) shows atrophy of the ventral portion of the calcarine sulcus (86). Although neurological degeneration was progressive in the Japanese epidemic, the more recently affected Iraqi children have had considerable functional recovery (84,87).

Methylmercury compounds also have been held responsible for congenital mercury poisoning. Affected infants show tremors, hypotonia, myoclonic jerks, and microcephaly (88,89). Researchers have studied the role of prenatal and early postnatal exposure to methylmercury derived from fish and other seafood—where it is found coordinated with an aliphatic thiol, most likely cysteine—on early development and neurocognitive functions.Whereas studies from the Faeroe Islands and New Zealand (90) have shown subtle but significant adverse effects in school-age children accompanied by abnormalities of the brainstem auditory-evoked potentials (91), the more recently conducted studies from the Seychelles Islands found no developmental effect of prenatal mercury exposure (92). The different outcomes could in part reflect the different concentrations of methylmercury consumed in these areas, since in the Seychelles, seafood has lower concentrations of methylmercury than in the other two regions (92). In addition, the Faroese population was exposed to polychlorinated biphenyls (PCP) and other organic pollutants that can act synergistically with mercury (92a).

Thimerosal, a mercury-containing compound that is degraded to ethylmercury and until the early 1990s was used as a preservative in various vaccines, has been implicated in neurodevelopmental disorders, particularly regressive autism (see Chapter 18). At present, the body of existing data is not consistent with an association between thimerosal-containing vaccines and autism or neurodevelopmental disorders (93,93a,94,94a).

The neuropathology of organic mercury poisoning in children has been described by Takeuchi and coworkers (95). It consists of focal cerebral and cerebellar atrophy with the axonal retraction bulbs (torpedoes) on Purkinje cells resembling those seen in Menkes disease (see Chapter 1).

The diagnosis of mercury poisoning depends on the measurement of urinary mercury concentrations. Treatment is by oral administration of 2,3-dimercaptosuccinic acid (succimer) (96). It is ineffective if not started promptly after exposure to mercury (97).

Manganese

Whereas in the adult population manganese intoxication is mainly incurred as a consequence of chronic inhalation of the metal dust by welders or miners, in the pediatric age group, this condition is seen in patients who have been receiving long-term parenteral nutrition, particularly in the presence of chronic hepatic disease. Manganese exposure leads to a selective dopaminergic dysfunction, neuronal loss, and gliosis in the basal ganglia. Astrocytes appear to be particularly vulnerable in that they have a specific transport system for manganese facilitating its uptake and sequestration in mitochondria (98). The condition results in a variety of movement disorders, notably a parkinsonian picture, seizures, or myoclonus (99). The MRI studies are characteristic. They demonstrate hyperintensities in the globus pallidus on T1-weighted images (100). Chelation treatment is said to be beneficial and results in improvement of symptoms and the neuroradiologic abnormalities.

Aluminum

Aluminum intoxication, usually caused by the ingestion of aluminum hydroxide, has been implicated in the pathogenesis of progressive dementia and seizures in children with chronic renal failure, whether or not they are undergoing maintenance dialysis. Aluminum intoxication is discussed more fully in Chapter 17.

Organic Toxins

Carbon Monoxide

Carbon monoxide poisoning is one of the major causes of death caused by toxins. In infants and small children, the majority of cases results from faulty home heaters or, as in the Orient, the use of anthracite coal briquettes. The brain and the myocardium are most vulnerable to carbon monoxide. The principal effect of carbon monoxide is to interfere with tissue oxygenation by reducing the capacity of blood to transport oxygen and by shifting the blood oxyhemoglobin saturation curve, thus requiring blood oxygen tension to decrease to lower than normal values before a given amount of oxygen is released from hemoglobin. Carbon monoxide also reduces oxygen delivery to tissue by reducing cardiac output. In addition, carbon monoxide binds directly to iron-rich brain regions, notably the globus pallidus and the pars reticulata of the substantia nigra (101).

Neurological symptoms of carbon monoxide toxicity include irritability, lethargy, and coma. In the Korean series of Kim and Coe, 14% of children presented with convulsions, in 13% there was neck stiffness, and 3% had blindness on admission. Computed tomographic scans showed diffuse cerebral edema and low-density areas in the basal ganglia, notably, the globus pallidus (102). On T2-weighted MRI, increased signal is seen in the basal ganglia and white matter (102a). Chronic carbon monoxide poisoning can result from poorly ventilated heating systems and inadequately ventilated housing. Symptoms include hyperactivity, sleepiness, and headaches (103).

After apparent recovery, some 10% to 30% of patients, most of them of advanced age, who have had moderate to severe carbon monoxide poisoning develop delayed neurologic sequelae some 3 to 240 days after intoxication (104,105,106). The sequelae include a variety of extrapyramidal symptoms, notably tremor, rigidity, and choreoathetosis. Additionally, Kim and Coe encountered mental retardation, seizures, mutism, hemiparesis, and paraplegia (102). MRI in such patients shows a progressive demyelinating process (107). The underlying mechanism for the delayed neurologic symptoms is currently believed to involve carbon monoxide–mediated brain lipid peroxidation (106,108).

The pros and cons for the treatment of children suffering from carbon monoxide poisoning with hyperbaric oxygen are beyond the scope of this book and are reviewed by Liebelt (109). The biological effects of carbon monoxide on pregnant mothers, fetuses, and newborn infants are reviewed by Ginsberg and Myers (110) and Longo (111).

Alcohol

Fetal Alcohol Syndrome

Alcohol is believed to affect the immature nervous system through chronic *in utero* exposure or through acute maternal intoxication.

In 1851, over 2000 years after Plutarch noted "one drunkard begets another" and Aristotle observed that "drunken women bring forth children like to themselves," Carpenter reviewed the then current data on alcohol use during pregnancy and concluded that offspring can experience mental and behavioral disabilities (112). More than 100 years later, French (113,114) and American (115) clinicians described a craniofacial and neurologic disorder with growth and psychomotor retardation called the *fetal alcohol syndrome* (FAS). Its frequency, as estimated by Clarren and Smith in 1978, is between 1 and 2 in 1,000 live births, with partial expression of the syndrome, the fetal alcohol effects syndrome (FES), occurring in 3 to 5 in 1,000 live births (115). A survey published in 1997 indicated that the combined rate of FAS and FES was at least 9.1 in 1,000 live births (116).

Data obtained from a variety of experimental models suggest that alcohol, or a metabolic product thereof, such as acetaldehyde, can adversely affect the developing brain through multiple mechanisms. These include direct effects such as a transient impairment in uterine blood flow, vasoconstriction of uterine vessels, and reduced fetal cerebral metabolic rate. In addition, alcohol, which acts as an *N*-methyl-D-aspartate (NMDA) antagonist and has GABA-mimetic properties, is capable of triggering apoptotic neurodegeneration (117). The various potential mechanisms by which alcohol can damage the developing nervous system have been reviewed by West and colleagues (118), Shibley and Pennington (119), and Davies (120).

Despite the wealth of experimental data, considerable debate surrounds the pathogenesis of FAS and FES. On the one hand, some researchers question whether there is a threshold amount of alcohol intake, beyond which fetal abnormalities can develop, and suggest that even the smallest amount of alcohol can be dangerous to the fetus. On the other hand, it is not known what role several other variables play in the production of FAS and FES. These variables include the type and quality of the alcoholic beverage consumed (particularly the presence of contaminants in illicitly procured alcohol), associated food and vitamin deficiencies, binge drinking, smoking during pregnancy, drug intake, low plasma zinc levels, and the stage of pregnancy when exposure occurred (121–123). Furthermore, we do not know whether there are certain alleles of alcohol dehydrogenase that are protective or, conversely, place the fetus at increased risk for FAS (124). Also not established is whether the same dysmorphology can occur in the absence of maternal alcohol intake. Lacking such data, it is unclear whether alcohol per se causes FAS and FES, or whether high maternal alcohol intake is but a reflection of other environmental or genetic causes of mental retardation.

Neuropathologic features of FAS include neuroglial and leptomeningeal heterotopias with aberrant neural and glial tissue incorporated within arachnoid and meninges (125). Lissencephaly, cerebellar dysplasia, and agenesis of the corpus callosum also have been described, and migration anomalies can involve the cerebellum and brainstem as well as the cerebrum (126). MRI studies have delineated the variety of anomalies that can be encountered in FAS (127,128). Using material obtained for the most part during voluntary medical abortions, Konovalov and colleagues have shown that the proportion of fetuses showing these abnormalities in brain development increases with an increase in maternal ethanol intake (129), being lowest in women who were binge drinking during the first 3 months of pregnancy. They suggest that the teratogenic period for induction of the brain defects involves the initial 3 to 6 weeks of brain morphogenesis. These observations are at variance with those of Autti-Rämö and colleagues, who found that the number of physical anomalies was significantly increased in infants exposed to alcohol throughout gestation, but not when heavy alcohol consumption, defined as in excess of 140 g per week, was limited to the first or to the first and second trimesters (130).

The diagnosis of FAS is based entirely on history and the physical appearance of the child. In addition to confirmation of maternal alcohol abuse, the diagnostic criteria recommended by the Research Society on Alcoholism Fetal Alcohol Study Group require the following three: (a) the presence of prenatal or postnatal growth retardation; (b) CNS dysfunction such as developmental delay or

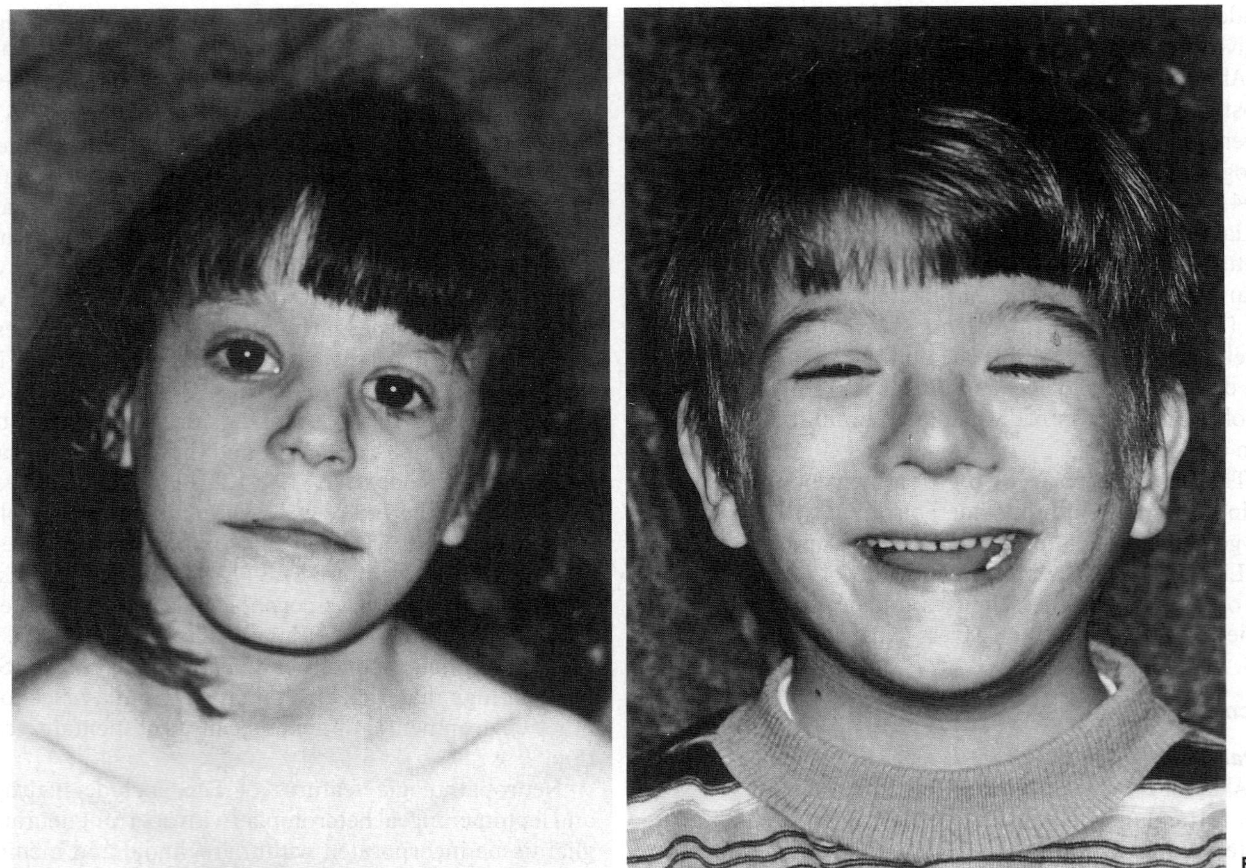

FIGURE 10.1. **A:** Fetal alcohol effects. This eight-year-old girl is mildly retarded and growth-deficient, with facial features typical of fetal alcohol syndrome: short palpebral fissures, short nose with flat nasal bridge, and thin lips with a smooth philtrum. **B:** This eight-year-old boy shows similar facial features. He is mildly retarded and growth-deficient. He weighed 2 kg at birth after a term gestation in a gravida 5, para 4, abortus 1, 28-year-old woman who drank one-fifth of hard liquor every one to two days during the first four months of pregnancy. (Courtesy of Dr. John Graham, Cedars-Sinai Medical Center.)

intellectual impairment; and (c) at least two of the following: microcephaly, microphthalmia, short palpebral fissures, or all three, and hypoplastic philtrum with thin upper lip and flattening of the maxillary area (131) (Fig. 10.1 A,B). When a child demonstrates two of the three criteria, the condition is diagnosed with *fetal alcohol effect* (FAE). The use of this term has been challenged by Aase and colleagues on the basis of its imprecision, and that by labeling a child as having FAE, health workers presuppose that maternal alcohol abuse is the major or only cause of the child's problems (132).

Optic nerve hypoplasia is seen in up to one-half of children born to alcoholic mothers (133). Other ocular anomalies include microphthalmia, glaucoma, and cataracts (134). Less often, a sensorineural hearing loss and a variety of other minor physical anomalies occur (130). Outside the nervous system, abnormalities of the heart (notably ventricular septal defects), joints (e.g., congenital dislocation of the hips and flexion-extension deformities), genitalia, or skeleton occur (135,136).

A considerable amount of work has been done to ascertain the long-term cognitive development of children diagnosed in infancy as having FAS or FAE. Two such studies can be cited as examples of the problems encountered in this endeavor. In the Finnish study of Autti-Rämö and colleagues, children who were subjected to heavy alcohol exposure throughout gestation had significantly lower scores on the Bayley Mental Scale and the Reynell Verbal Comprehension Test at 27 months of age. This study, however, failed to find any significant effect on intellectual development when heavy prenatal alcohol exposure was restricted to the first trimester. In this study, as in many others, social class and maternal education could have been confounding variables (137). In the German study of Spohr and coworkers, children were reexamined more than 10 years after their initial diagnosis (138). Many of the features of FAS and some of the minor physical anomalies had disappeared in the interval, so it became difficult to diagnose FAS in a substantial proportion of children who initially had a mild expression of FAS. In severely affected children with FAS, the features of the condition tended to persist. In this series (138), 88% of FAS children were microcephalic at the first assessment at 3 years of age and 65% at the second assessment at approximately 11 years of age. There was little improvement in IQ scores, and 69% of children had an IQ of 85 or less. It was noteworthy that not all children with mild morphologic damage had normal intelligence, and not all children with severe morphologic changes were mentally retarded. These findings are at variance with the observations of Mattsen and colleagues (139), who found that alcohol-exposed children displayed significant deficits in overall IQ measures even in the absence of any dysmorphic features.

Several other studies purport to demonstrate that even children whose IQs fall within the normal range have deficits in cognitive function, particularly in language development, and that school performance tends to deteriorate with time (138,140,141). It is quite likely that an adverse social environment contributes substantially to these features.

Acute Alcohol Poisoning

Acute alcohol intake by infants and young children initially induces a depression of the CNS, and if untreated, it causes marked hypoglycemia and convulsions several hours after ingestion (142–144). The mechanism for hypoglycemia is not completely understood. Wilson and coworkers suggest that ethanol inhibits hepatic gluconeogenesis because of an increase in the ratio of nicotinamide-adenine dinucleotide (reduced form) (NADH) to nicotinamide-adenine dinucleotide (NAD), and possibly also because it inhibits the carboxylation of pyruvate to oxaloacetate (144).

Theophylline (Aminophylline)

Theophylline, like other alkylxanthines, lowers the seizure threshold by antagonizing the anticonvulsant effect of endogenous adenosine (145). Neurological symptoms can result from administration of a toxic dose of the drug, or from a therapeutic dose in children who have a lowered seizure threshold as a result of a preexisting seizure disorder or other previous brain injury or disease (146). Seizures are usually the most serious complication. These are often accompanied by cerebral vasoconstriction and ischemia. Ataxia, visual hallucinations, dyskinesias, and infantile spasms also have been reported as complications of theophylline toxicity (147–149). In premature infants, toxic effects include tachycardia, jitteriness, clonic posturing, and generalized seizures (150). Treatment of seizures involves the various anticonvulsants used for status epilepticus (see Chapter 14). Exchange transfusions also have been used in neonates given toxic dosages of theophylline.

Barbiturates

With the increased availability of other sedatives, the incidence of barbiturate intoxication in infants and children has diminished substantially since the 1980s.

Pharmacology

Barbiturates are general depressants. The mechanism of their action has been reviewed by Olsen and coworkers (151). In essence, toxic effects on the central nervous system (CNS) result from the particular sensitivity of the reticular activating system to barbiturates. On a subcellular basis, barbiturates act on the γ-aminobutyric acid ($GABA_A$) receptor sites of postsynaptic neurons to increase the GABA-induced chloride current, thus potentiating the inhibitory effects of GABA. In addition, they inhibit excitatory α-amino-3-hydroxy-5-methyl-4-isoxazole propionate (AMPA) receptors.

The severity of intoxication induced by a given dose of barbiturate varies considerably. At comparable blood levels, slow-acting barbiturates are less toxic than rapid-acting thiobarbiturates. Other factors affecting the severity of clinical symptoms are the development of tolerance, as occurs in children treated with barbiturates for a convulsive disorder, and the rapidity with which the drug is metabolized by the liver.

Clinical Manifestations

Clinical symptoms of barbiturate intoxication are mainly those of CNS depression. A modified Glasgow Coma Scale, which scores both the level of consciousness and vital signs (respiratory rate, blood pressure, and hypothermia), has been suggested as a means of grading the severity of barbiturate intoxication (152). In severe intoxication, the child is comatose, although the deep tendon reflexes can persist and the plantar reflex is often positive. Barbiturates are respiratory depressants; they impair respiratory drive and the mechanisms responsible for rhythmic respiratory movements. Respiratory centers become insensitive to increased CO_2, and respiratory control becomes dependent on hypoxic drive, which, in turn, fails with progressively increasing barbiturate levels. As a consequence, respiration is affected early, and breathing becomes slow and shallow. Blood pressure decreases as a direct action of the drug on the myocardium and the depression of the medullary centers. A central antidiuretic action depresses urine formation. Hypoxia and pulmonary complications are common with severe barbiturate poisoning. Neuropathologic findings closely resemble those of fatal anoxia.

Diagnosis

The diagnosis of barbiturate intoxication in a child with severe CNS depression or coma rests on the history of drug ingestion or, in the absence of such a history, on the exclusion of other causes for coma and on the positive identification of the toxin.

The physical examination, which must be performed expeditiously, should be directed toward the exclusion of infectious, traumatic, metabolic, and vascular causes for the child's condition. Nuchal rigidity and focal neurologic signs make drug ingestion unlikely. Mitchell and colleagues (153) have stressed the frequency of miosis in children who are comatose owing to barbiturate intoxication and noted that miosis is usually absent in children admitted in coma as a consequence of head trauma or infection. The physician must always consider the possibility of nonaccidental barbiturate ingestion, which is an increasing form of child abuse (154).

A number of rapid urinary screening tests are available that produce characteristic color reactions in the presence of barbiturates or other toxins.

Treatment

Because barbiturate levels in brain correlate poorly with those in serum, serum barbiturate levels can only serve as a guide to assess the severity of intoxication. If the drug was ingested shortly before the child is examined, gastric lavage is done. When respirations are depressed, an airway is instituted, and artificial respiration is used whenever necessary to maintain normal blood CO_2 and pH levels. Circulatory collapse, the chief cause of death in barbiturate intoxication, is prevented with plasma expanders or whole blood. Vasopressors are of relatively little value except in the initial management of severe hypotension (155). Forced diuresis with fluid loading and alkalinization by the intravenous administration of sodium bicarbonate facilitate urinary excretion of phenobarbital and other long-lasting barbiturates. Renal failure and hypothermia are other potentially serious complications of barbiturate intoxication (156).

In severe intoxication, or in children who because of renal or hepatic disease have impaired drug elimination, hemodialysis or peritoneal dialysis is the most effective means of removing the drug from the bloodstream (157). The effectiveness of peritoneal dialysis depends on the blood barbiturate level, which is usually high when long-acting barbiturates are ingested. Multiple doses of charcoal appear to be of little benefit.

Detoxification with hemoperfusion through charcoal coated with acrylic hydrocarbons and exchange transfusion also has been suggested (158). The use of analeptics such as picrotoxin has been abandoned because they were found to induce cardiac arrhythmias and convulsions.

The presentation of benzodiazepine overdose is similar to that of barbiturate intoxication, and treatment is analogous, except that diuresis and forced alkalinization are unnecessary, because diazepines are metabolized by the liver. As a class, benzodiazepines are safer than barbiturates, and the mortality for intoxications is far smaller (156).

Phenothiazines

The neurotoxic actions of phenothiazines result from either an overdose or idiosyncratic adverse reactions to therapeutic dosages. The toxic responses include depression of consciousness, seizures, hypotension, loss of temperature control, and movement disorders. In the series of James and coworkers, 90% of children who accidentally ingested phenothiazines or other psychotropic medications presented with depressed consciousness, while 51% developed dystonia (159). Movement disorders constitute the major adverse effects of therapeutic doses of phenothiazines. Although all phenothiazines can produce movement disorders, the extrapyramidal signs in children occur most commonly with prochlorperazine, haloperidol, thioridazine, chlorpromazine, and clozapine (160). They are less likely to occur with olanzapine and risperidone.

Several kinds of movement disorders have been encountered. Younger children tend to have generalized manifestations, whereas adolescents tend to have signs localized to the face and trunk (160). The most common are sudden episodes of opisthotonus accompanied by marked deviation of the eyes and torticollis without loss of consciousness. Dystonic movements of the tongue, face, and neck muscles, drooling, trismus, ataxia, tremor, episodic rigidity, and oculogyric crises also are seen. Seizures are rare but can be mimicked by violent dystonic movements.

Tardive dyskinesia is a late appearing neurological syndrome seen with the use of phenothiazines and other neuroleptic drugs, and is believed to be the consequence of hypersensitivity of dopamine receptors in the basal ganglia secondary to prolonged blockade of the receptors by the medication. The condition is relatively uncommon in children, and there is less risk with olanzepine and the other atypical antipsychotic agents. Tardive dyskinesia is characterized by stereotypic choreiform movements of the face, eyelids, mouth, and tongue and less so of the trunk and extremities. Dystonic movements also can be seen, as can a tardive akathisia, an unpleasant sensation of internal restlessness that is relieved by volutional movements.

The condition persists even following withdrawal of the offending medication. In the Queen Square series of Kiriakakis, remission occurred after a mean of 5.2 years following onset (161). A large number of agents have been used to treat this condition, notably tocopherol, propanolol, lithium, and clonidine, but none of these appears to have a convincing benefit. Most recently, branched-chain amino acids have been suggested for the treatment of tardive dyskinesia in children and adolescents (162). Tardive dyskinesia is also discussed in Chapter 3.

A neuroleptic malignant syndrome has occasionally been encountered. The most common inciting drugs are haloperidol, phenothiazines, butyrophenones, and thioxanthines. The condition generally develops 3 to 9 days after initiation of neuroleptic treatment. It manifests by hyperthermia, muscular rigidity, extrapyramidal signs, opisthotonus, altered consciousness, and autonomic disturbances. Hyperthermia does not always have to be present (163). Serum creatine phosphokinase is elevated, and myoglobinuria is common. The condition lasts approximately 7 to 10 days (164). In contrast to its frequency in patients who have ingested toxic doses of phenothiazines, drowsiness is rare when symptoms are caused by an idiosyncratic reaction to the drug. Persistence of the dyskinesias after withdrawal of the drug is relatively common in young adults, but rare in children (165).

Extrapyramidal movements have been reported in newborns whose mothers received phenothiazines during pregnancy. The movement disorder is accompanied by hypertonia, tremor, and a poor suck reflex. It can persist for up to 12 months (166).

Diagnosis of phenothiazine intoxication depends on the history of drug ingestion. The most common appearance of the extrapyramidal disorder, namely as episodes of opisthotonus, trismus, and dystonic posturing, is distinctive. Paroxysmal choreoathetosis can present a similar picture, but its onset is gradual with a prolonged history of recurrent attacks.

Diphenylhydramine in a dose of 2 mg/kg, given intravenously over the course of 5 minutes, is an effective antidote for the extrapyramidal disorder appearing at therapeutic doses, and it often produces a dramatic response. Benztropine mesylate (0.5 mg/kg), given intravenously, or diazepam also is effective (160).

Neuroleptic malignant syndrome is treated by discontinuation of the neuroleptic, reduction of hyperthermia by means of cooling blankets, and support of respiratory and cardiovascular status. The administration of dantrolene (0.5 mg/kg every 12 hours) or bromocriptine has been suggested, but controlled studies do not appear to show that either drug administered singly or in combination shortens the illness (167).

Antibacterial Agents

The increasing number of antibacterial agents used by clinicians for the treatment of various infectious diseases also has increased the incidence of neurologic complications associated with antibacterial therapy. The various clinical syndromes of neurotoxicity are shown in Table 10.4.

TABLE 10.4 Neurotoxicity of Antibacterial Therapy

Syndrome	*Drugs*
Seizures, encephalopathy, organic brain syndrome	Cephalosporins
	Erythromycin
	Metronidazole
	Penicillins
	Rifampin
Cerebellar ataxia	Metronidazole
Pseudotumor cerebri	Nalidixic acid
	Nitrofurantoin
	Tetracyclines
	Trimethoprim-sulfamethoxazole
Aseptic meningitis	Trimethoprim-sulfamethoxazole
Myasthenic syndrome	Aminoglycosides
	Ampicillin
	Clindamycin
	Erythromycin
	Lincomycin
	Polymyxins
	Tetracycline
Optic neuritis	Chloramphenicol
	Ethambutol
	Isoniazid
Cochlear toxicity	Aminoglycosides
Vestibular toxicity	Aminoglycosides
	Erythromycin
	Tetracyclines
Peripheral neuropathy	Chloramphenicol
	Colistin
	Dapsone
	Ethionamide
	Isoniazid
	Metronidazole
	Nitrofurantoin

Adapted from Thomas RJ. Neurotoxicity of antibacterial therapy. *South Med J* 1994;9:869.

They also have been reviewed by Thomas (168) and Wallace (169).

Encephalopathy/Seizures

The β-lactam antibiotics, notably penicillins, cephalosporins, and carbapenems, can manifest significant neurotoxicity. Studies on animal models have shown the toxic effect of penicillins to be caused by a dose-dependent inhibition of the GABA-gated chloride ion influx (168,170).

The principal manifestations of β-lactam toxicity are seizures. The major risk factors for development of seizures are high-dose intravenous use of the antibiotic, impaired renal function, a preexisting or concurrent CNS disorder such as meningitis, and the concomitant use of drugs such as theophylline, which can lower the seizure threshold (169). In addition to seizures, the β-lactams can cause hallucinations, and in the case of ceftazidime, absence status epilepticus (169).

Cochlear and Vestibular Damage

Several aminoglycoside antibiotics can induce damage to the eighth nerve. Gentamicin and tobramycin can damage both cochlear and vestibular components, whereas neomycin, kanamycin, and amikacin affect the auditory component predominantly. These complications are less common in children than in adults. Routine studies of brainstem auditory-evoked potentials during aminoglycoside therapy can detect high-frequency hearing loss as an early sign of ototoxicity (171). The development of ototoxicity is related to the dosage and duration of aminoglycoside therapy, the presence of impaired renal function, and a genetic predisposition to aminoglycoside susceptibility, notably a mitochondrial ribosomal RNA mutation (172). Symptomatic hearing loss is seen initially as reduced high-frequency acuity, followed by impairment of lower-frequency hearing, damage to the hair cells, and complete destruction of the organ of Corti with ultimate eighth nerve damage.

Neuromuscular Blockage

A myasthenic syndrome has been encountered in children treated with neomycin, ampicillin, gentamicin, and other aminoglycoside antibiotics. These drugs should therefore be used cautiously in children with neuromuscular disease, notably myasthenia gravis (173).

Pesticides

Organophosphates

Organophosphate insecticides are widely used on food crops throughout the world. These chemicals inhibit acetylcholinesterase and result in an accumulation of acetylcholine and overstimulation of the muscarinic postganglionic fibers of the parasympathetic nervous system. When ingested or inhaled, manifestations are of three types: acute, intermediate, and delayed. The acute syndrome represents a cholinergic crisis with headache, abdominal pain, irritability, sweating, miosis, and muscular twitching (174). After recovery, which generally occurs within 24 to 96 hours of the poisoning, an intermediate syndrome develops in many patients. This is characterized by profound muscular weakness, affecting predominantly the proximal and respiratory muscles, and often accompanied by cranial nerve palsies. Dystonia was seen in approximately 20% of Sri Lanka patients (175). Symptoms resolve within 1 to 5 weeks. A delayed polyneuropathy appears 2 to 3 weeks after the poisoning and often blends into the intermediate phase (176). It primarily affects the distal musculature, with recovery in 6 to 12 months. Controversy exists as to whether neurobehavioral effects persist after recovery (177).

Atropine has been recommended for treatment during the acute phase. For children younger than 12 years of age, the dose is 0.05 mg/kg, given intravenously. This is followed by a maintenance dosage of 0.02 to 0.05 mg/kg every 10 to 30 minutes until the cholinergic signs are no longer present or until pupils become dilated. Pralidoxime, given intravenously over the course of 15 to 30 minutes in a dose of 25 to 50 mg/kg, also has been recommended (178).

Organochlorines

Endrin is the most toxic of the organochlorine pesticides and has been responsible for several epidemics throughout the world. Symptoms are caused by CNS excitation. This results from suppression of the GABA-induced chloride current, and with it, suppression of the GABA-mediated synaptic inhibition (179). Symptoms occur within 12 hours of the poisoning. Convulsions are frequently the presenting symptom. Older children report headache, nausea, and muscle spasms just before the seizures (180). Phenobarbital or benzodiazepines are generally effective in controlling seizures, although recurrent convulsions are not unusual (181).

Lindane, another chlorinated hydrocarbon, has been used extensively in the form of Kwell for the treatment of scabies, and its accidental ingestion by toddlers is not unusual. If ingested in sufficient amounts, the substance can induce depression of consciousness, coma, and major motor seizures (182). The clinical picture of exposure to the various types of pesticides is reviewed by O'Malley (177).

Psychedelic Drugs

Fashions occur in psychedelic drugs, as they do in clothes. Currently, the use of 3,4-methylenedioxymethamphetamine, also known as *ecstasy*, among college students and adolescents continues to exceed that of lysergic acid diethylamine and cocaine (183). A recently published American survey indicated that 5% of tenth graders had used ecstasy within the last year, and 2% reporting using it within the last month (184). Data obtained from New Zealand show a comparable incidence. Accidental poisoning with psychedelic drugs is uncommon in small children and is generally not life threatening, although subarachnoid hemorrhage following use of the drug has been reported (185).

Intoxication with phencyclidine often is produced by passive inhalation (186,187). The psychosis seen in older subjects is less common in small children than a depressed sensorium, hypotonia, dystonia or opisthotonus, and ataxia. Seizures as well as opisthotonus and a variety of ocular signs, notably horizontal or vertical nystagmus and miosis, can be encountered after phencyclidine or ecstasy ingestion (186,188). Treatment is symptomatic, and observation of the intoxicated youngster usually suffices. A variety of barbiturates or phenothiazines can be used for sedation.

Hexachlorophene

Hexachlorophene—a chlorinated phenolic compound widely used as an antiseptic until 1972, when it became a prescription drug—has been shown to induce seizures when absorbed through burned or extensively excoriated skin. Significant amounts also are absorbed through the intact skin of premature neonates (189).

Accidental ingestion of hexachlorophene by older children results in vomiting, hypotension, and a neurologic picture characterized by total blindness caused by deterioration of the optic nerves (190). Additionally, behavioral changes, convulsions, increased intracranial pressure, paralysis, and spastic paraparesis or paraplegia can occur (191).

Mepivacaine

In the past, the use of mepivacaine hydrochloride to induce paracervical or pudendal block in the course of labor resulted in accidental poisoning of the newborn by direct injection of the anesthetic. The clinical picture was reduced responsiveness, bradycardia, apnea, hypotonia, and seizures that commenced within 6 hours, usually between 1 and 3 hours of age. Mepivacaine intoxication is differentiated from perinatal asphyxia by the earlier onset of seizures and the abnormality of oculomotor reflexes, which in asphyxia tend to be preserved for the first few hours of life. The condition is self-limiting, and if asphyxia is prevented, infants return to normal by 18 hours of age (192).

Salicylate

A less widespread use of salicylates in this country has resulted in a significant reduction in the incidence of salicylate intoxication. Currently, most acute intoxications are the outcome of attempted suicide with aspirin or methylsalicylate (193). Both acute and chronic salicylate intoxication are associated with mental status depression whose severity is usually proportionate to the serum salicylate level (194). Additionally, a delayed encephalopathy owing to cerebral edema can develop. In some instances, this encephalopathy is associated with a rapid decrease in serum sodium concentrations, the consequence of inappropriate antidiuretic hormone secretion resulting from the action of salicylates on the brain (195). The administration of salicylates in a patient with an influenza virus or varicella infection can initiate Reye syndrome (see Chapter 7).

Eosinophilia-Myalgia Syndrome

Eosinophilia-myalgia syndrome is characterized by eosinophilia, myalgia, and a progressive neuropathy. Muscle biopsy demonstrates a perivascular eosinophilic infiltrate; sural nerve biopsy documents a demyelinating neuropathy with axonal degeneration (196). Involvement of the CNS includes seizures, dementia, and vascular infarctions (197). The condition is induced by consumption of tryptophan contaminated with 3-(phenylamino) alanine. This substance is chemically similar to 3-phenylamino-1,2-propanediol, an aniline derivative believed to be responsible for the contamination of rapeseed oil, which caused the toxic oil syndrome seen during 1981 in the central region of Spain (198). Cooking oil contaminated with polychlorinated biphenyls has been responsible for mass poisoning in Japan and central Taiwan. Neurologic symptoms include polyneuropathy. Children who were *in utero* when their mothers consumed contaminated oil were prone to severe developmental deficits (199).

Neonatal Drug Addiction

The increasing prevalence of drug abuse among women of childbearing age has made relatively common the problem of neonates born to mothers addicted to cocaine, methamphetamine, heroin, or other opiates, or who receive methadone as part of a drug treatment program.

Cocaine

Four aspects of the effect of cocaine on the developing nervous system are considered: teratogenic effects, acute effects evident during the neonatal period, long-term effects on cognition, and accidental intoxication.

The most common teratogenic effect of cocaine is a reduction in head circumference. When cocaine-exposed infants are compared with control infants, head circumferences of the former group are significantly smaller. This observation in drug-exposed infants is probably significant because it persists when birth weight and other confounding variables are controlled and shows a dose-response effect (200,201,202). Reports of other malformations are more anecdotal. These include disorders of midline prosencephalic development, septo-optic dysplasia, agenesis of the corpus callosum, and neuronal heterotopias (203). The mechanism for the teratogenic effects of cocaine is not clear.

The clinical picture of the drug-exposed neonate results from the effects of these drugs on intrauterine development and postnatal withdrawal.

Cocaine is passed to the fetus through the maternal circulation during pregnancy and in breast milk. It acts as a sympathomimetic agent and impairs the reuptake of norepinephrine and epinephrine by presynaptic nerve endings, activating the adrenergic system and inducing vasoconstriction. Cocaine also impairs dopamine and serotonin reuptake. The vasoconstriction and reduced cerebral blood flow induced by cocaine probably are direct effects of the alkaloid and are not caused by an increase in catecholamines.

A neonate exposed *in utero* to cocaine can be born prematurely or be small for gestational age. As a rule, when newborns have been exposed to lows levels of cocaine *in utero*, growth retardation is symmetric, as contrasted to the asymmetric growth retardation seen with maternal malnutrition. By contrast, newborns exposed to a high level of cocaine exhibit asymmetric growth retardation with the head circumference disproportionately smaller than would be predicted from the birth weight (202). A number of physical and behavioral disturbances are common during the first few days of life. These include excessive jitteriness, tachycardia, tremors, irritability, poor feeding, an increased startle response, and abnormal sleep patterns, with excessive drowsiness after the hyperirritable stage (201,204,205). Seizures were observed in 81% of the neonates of Kramer and coworkers. They developed within 36 hours of birth (206). A transient dystonic reaction also has been reported (207). Cerebrospinal fluid (CSF) examination and neuroimaging study results are generally normal, although cerebral infarction has been encountered. The electroencephalogram (EEG) tends to be abnormal during the first few weeks of life, with multifocal bursts of spikes and sharp waves. Neurologic and electrical abnormalities are transient and usually do not continue beyond 3 weeks, although in the series of Kramer and colleagues, collected from Watts, California, one-half of the infants went on to develop epilepsy (206). The reason for persistence of seizures is unclear.

In utero exposure to cocaine has been implicated in several instances of cerebral infarction, usually in the distribution of the middle cerebral artery. Cerebral blood flow velocity is increased in the anterior cerebral artery for the first 2 days of life, an observation consistent with the presence of vasoconstriction (201). Although Dixon and Bejar have reported an abnormal cranial ultrasound in 41% of term cocaine-exposed newborns (208), the controlled study by King and coworkers found no difference in the incidence of neurosonographic abnormalities between cocaine-exposed infants and controls (201).

The effects of maternal drug addiction on the ultimate physical and cognitive development of offspring have not been completely clarified. The catch-up in weight and length is analogous to that seen in small-for-date infants due to other causes. The effect of intrauterine cocaine exposure on head circumference becomes progressively less significant during the first and second years of postnatal life (200). When adequately controlled for socioeconomic status, most studies do not find a significant impairment of intelligence or language function by the time children reach school years (209–211). In their review of the cognitive development of offspring of mothers with drug and alcohol abuse, Zuckerman and Bresnahan concluded that such infants are clearly at risk for developmental and behavioral problems but that it is difficult to separate the biological vulnerability caused by prenatal drug exposure from the environmental vulnerability caused by an environment formed by drug use (122).

The clinical manifestations of accidental cocaine ingestion are a function of the age of the child when ingestion occurs. In the experience of Mott and colleagues, children younger than 7 years of age present with seizures, whereas in older children, obtundation or delirium are the characteristic presenting symptoms (212).

Opiates

The effect of opiates on the fetus and on the newborn has been well studied. As a rule, symptoms are more severe than those resulting from exposure to cocaine. Approximately one-half of infants born to addicted mothers weigh less than 2,500 g, and many of these are small for their gestational age. Additionally, 40% have a head circumference below the tenth percentile (213). Approximately two-thirds of infants born to heroin-addicted mothers develop symptoms (214). These symptoms generally become apparent during the first 48 hours of life. In order of frequency of occurrence, they are fist sucking, irritability, tremors, vomiting, high-pitched cry, sneezing, hypertonia, and abnormal sleep patterns (215,216). Seizures are relatively uncommon (214). The severity of the clinical course is related to the length of maternal addiction, the length of time from the last dose to delivery, the magnitude of the drug doses taken, and the gestational age of the infant, with withdrawal symptoms being more severe in term infants (216). For reasons as yet undetermined, the incidence of intraventricular hemorrhage is less in neonates of opiate-dependent mothers than in infants of comparable weight born to nonaddicted mothers (217). To my knowledge this observation has not been confirmed.

Untreated, opiate withdrawal syndrome has a significant mortality. Administration of benzodiazepines is of considerable benefit. Clonidine, phenothiazines, barbiturates, methadone, and paregoric also have been recommended. Dosages and modes of administration of these drugs are reviewed by Yaster and coworkers (218).

Follow-up studies on infants of opiate- and methadone-addicted mothers indicate that the effects on growth parameters resolve by 1 to 2 years of age (219) and that antenatal exposure to illicit drugs does not increase infant mortality (220). Developmental scores and overall IQ are normal, but children have a higher incidence of behavioral abnormalities, notably temper tantrums and impulsivity, than children matched for socioeconomic status (221–223). As is the case for children of cocaine- and alcohol-addicted mothers, the developmental outcome is influenced more by the home environment than by exposure of the developing brain to toxin (223).

Kernicterus

The term *kernicterus*, originally coined by Schmorl in 1903 (224), has been used both pathologically and clinically. Pathologically, it indicates a canary yellow staining of circumscribed areas of the basal ganglia, brainstem, and cerebellum; clinically, it describes a syndrome consisting of athetosis, impaired vertical gaze, and auditory loss or imperception.

Up to 1990, kernicterus had nearly disappeared; its reemergence is probably the result of a shortened hospital stay for term neonates and a decreased concern about jaundice when it develops in breast-fed infants.

Pathology and Pathogenesis

On gross inspection, deposition of deep yellow pigment is noted in the meninges, choroid plexus, and numerous areas of the brain itself (225). The unique topography of neuronal damage in kernicterus is essentially the same in full-term and premature infants. As visualized on neuropathological examination, the regions most commonly affected are the basal ganglia (particularly the globus pallidus), the subthalamic nucleus, the dentate nuclei, the cerebellar vermis, sectors H2 and H3 of the hippocampus, and the cranial nerve nuclei (notably the oculomotor, vestibular, and cochlear nuclei). The cerebral cortex is spared.

The microscopic alterations point to the cell membrane as the primary site of damage, with mitochondrial changes being secondary to disorganization of the cytoplasmic membranes.

Two distinct pathologic entities can be distinguished. In brains that are grossly stained yellow, the most frequently observed abnormality is a spongy degeneration and gliosis. In others, there is neuronal degeneration and deposition of the pigment within neurons, their processes, and the surrounding glial cells (226). Neurons can be in various stages of degeneration, the severity of degeneration being proportional to the age of the patient. A marked neuronal loss with demyelination and astrocytic replacement is observed in patients who die after the first month of kernicterus. Studies on cultures of newborn rodent neurons indicate that low and moderate unconjugated bilirubin concentrations induce early necrosis followed by late apoptosis, whereas higher bilirubin concentrations induce a rapid necrotic neuronal death (226a)

Although the exact pathogenesis of kernicterus in the term infant is far from clear, several factors acting in concert are involved. They include hyperbilirubinemia, serum albumin levels, reduced albumin bilirubin-binding capacity, the presence of acidosis and/or hypoxia, opening of the blood–brain barrier, clearance of bilirubin from brain, and duration of contact between free or bound bilirubin and brain endothelium. These are reviewed by Hascoet (227).

The role of hyperbilirubinemia in the production of kernicterus has been known since the classic studies of Hsia and coworkers at Boston Children's Hospital (228). High bilirubin levels can be caused not only by Rh incompatibility but by several other conditions as well. These include prematurity, sepsis, and the presence of significant hemorrhage such as occurs in a large cephalhematoma or in subgaleal bleeding. The causes of neonatal hyperbilirubinemia and guidelines for treatment have been reviewed by Newman and Maisels (229) and Johnson and colleagues (230).

Considerable evidence suggests that hyperbilirubinemia alone, even when extreme, is not sufficient for the production of kernicterus. Hyperbilirubinemia unaccompanied by isoimmunization or other adverse factors usually has no detrimental effect on motor and cognitive development or on hearing when these parameters are tested after the first year of life (231). At bilirubin levels of 30 mg/dL or higher, the likelihood of developing kernicterus is no greater than 50%. Thus, in a series of 105 full-term and 24 premature babies whose peak indirect bilirubin levels were between 20 and 30.8 mg/dL, only seven, two of them preterm, were found to have abnormal results on neurologic and psychological examination some 5 years later. Of these, one infant's jaundice was the result of Rh incompatibility. ABO incompatibility, sepsis, and unknown factors were responsible for jaundice in the remainder (232).

These observations, published in 1967, have since been amply verified from a number of centers (233). However, they must be qualified by the observation that kernicterus can develop in breast-fed infants in the absence of isoimmune or hemolytic disease (234). Kernicterus is extremely rare in adults, even when massive elevation of indirect serum bilirubin occurs. Patients with a congenital deficiency of glucuronyl transferase (the Crigler-Najjar I syndrome), whose indirect bilirubin levels typically range from 10 to 44 mg/dL, have been known to be free of neurologic symptoms for many years before developing a rapidly progressive extrapyramidal disorder, often after an infection (235). The clinical manifestations of Crigler-Najjar syndromes are reviewed by Kadakol and colleagues (236) and Shevell and colleagues (237). Fox and coworkers have suggested this condition be treated by infusion of hepatocytes (238).

Currently, the most plausible theory is that the clinical and pathologic picture of kernicterus results from antecedent or concomitant damage to the CNS with breakdown of the blood–brain barrier accompanied by a level of unconjugated bilirubin that exceeds the binding capacity of serum albumin and permits bilirubin to cross the blood–brain barrier and injure neurons. A number of factors, present singly or in concert, can act as noxious agents on the blood–brain barrier and nerve cells. Some of these, notably Rh hemolytic disease, ABO incompatibility, and hyperosmolarity, can do so by damaging the vascular endothelium of the brain, whereas prenatal and perinatal anoxia, sepsis, and acidosis can damage the nerve cell directly (239,240). Sepsis appears to be a particularly important factor. In the series of Pearlman and associates, two-thirds of infants who died of sepsis had kernicterus, as evidenced by yellow discoloration of the susceptible nuclei and neuronal degeneration and necrosis in the stained lesions. In these infants, none of whom had any characteristic clinical abnormalities for kernicterus, neither acidosis nor the use of antibiotics known to displace bilirubin from albumin appeared to be responsible for the evolution of kernicterus (239).

The role of bilirubin-albumin binding in facilitating the entry of bilirubin into the brain is stressed by the observation that analbuminemic individuals do not develop kernicterus (241). In experimental animals, bilirubin deposited in the brain is derived not only from the free fraction, but to a significant extent (30% to 60%) from the albumin-bound fraction. Whatever the source of the bilirubin, on theoretical grounds, free bilirubin is cytotoxic and induces an immediate and marked disturbance of brain energy metabolism. The exact mechanism by which bilirubin induces mitochondrial dysfunction is unknown. Experimental data show that membranes are the primary target for unconjugated bilirubin, which disrupts the mitochondrial membrane lipid and protein structure with consequent release of apoptotic factors (242).

In premature infants, relatively low serum bilirubin levels are associated with the subsequent development of kernicterus, and there is a direct correlation between peak bilirubin values and abnormal neurological outcome (243,244). However, other studies have failed to demonstrate an association between low-level hyperbilirubinemia (5.8 to 14.6 mg/dl) and neurodevelopmental outcome of extremely low birth weight infants (245). It therefore appears likely that other factors in addition to an elevated serum bilirubin level are important in causing kernicterus in premature infants. In the course of the 1980s and 1990s, the incidence of kernicterus in premature infants coming to autopsy, which up to then had been approximately 25%, decreased significantly to approximately 4% for the period of 1983 to 1993 (246,247). The reasons for this decline are unclear. Jardine and Rogers have suggested that it is related to the discontinuation of benzyl alcohol, a bacteriostatic agent added to intravenous fluids and medications that competes with bilirubin for albumin binding (248).

Clinical Manifestations

The jaundiced term infant developing kernicterus becomes drowsy by the second to fifth day of life and begins to nurse poorly. The infant develops fever, has a monotonous cry, and loses the Moro reflex (249). Approximately 10% of infants who go on to develop kernicterus have no clinical manifestations during the neonatal period.

TABLE 10.5 Clinical Picture of Patients with Kernicterus

Number of children with severe neonatal jaundice due to Rh factor	248
Athetosis	93%
Gaze palsy	91%
Dental enamal dysplasia	83%
Auditory imperception	43%
Extrapyramidal rigidity	5%

From Peristein MA. The clinical syndrome of kernicterus. In: American Academy for Cerebral Palsy. *Kernicterus and its importance in cerebral palsy.* Springfield, IL: Charles C Thomas, 1961;268. With permission.

By 2 weeks of age, the infant usually has developed hypertonia, with opisthotonus, extensor spasms, and in approximately 10% of cases, clonic convulsions. Over the ensuing months, the infant becomes hypotonic, and by 4 years of age the syndrome characteristic of kernicterus has evolved. The striking constancy of neurologic symptoms in the older child with kernicterus is evident from Table 10.5 (250).

Athetosis is present almost invariably, often with dystonia, rigidity, and tremors. Gaze palsy can involve movements in all directions, but vertical gaze is by far the most commonly involved. Auditory imperception can take the form of a hearing loss, a receptive aphasia, or a combination of both. In a number of patients, the vestibular portion of the eighth nerve also is involved (232). Severe mental retardation is relatively uncommon in youngsters with kernicterus, although impaired hearing and gaze paralysis make psychometric testing extremely difficult. Of surviving children with kernicterus who could be tested, Byers and colleagues found 47% to have IQs between 90 and 110, and 27% between 70 and 90. The remainder (27%) had an IQ below 70 (251).

The auditory system is highly sensitive to bilirubin toxicity. Bilirubin can damage the brainstem auditory nuclei, the auditory nerve, and the spiral ganglion containing cell bodies of the primary auditory neurons (252). As a consequence, auditory dysfunction can occur in the presence or absence of kernicterus. When brainstem auditory-evoked potentials are used to screen high-risk infants, some studies have noted a correlation between maximum unbound bilirubin levels and abnormal central conduction times (253), whereas others have failed to do so (254). It is becoming evident that any hearing loss in high-risk infants reflects both the severity and duration of hyperbilirubinemia and, more importantly, any associated hypoxia and respiratory acidosis (255).

MRI in children with kernicterus caused by Rh isoimmunization shows a symmetric increased signal in the globus pallidus on T2-weighted images (Fig. 10.2) (256).

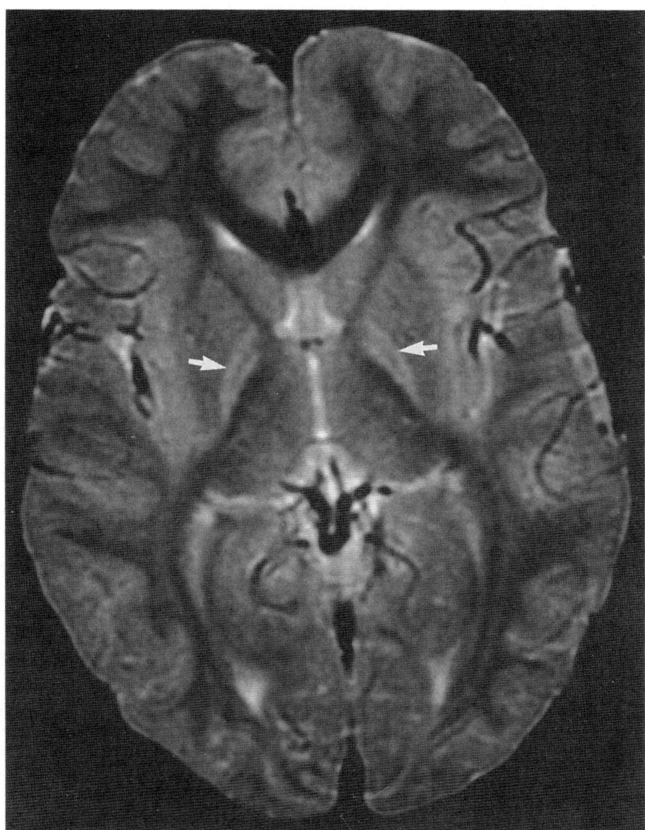

FIGURE 10.2. Magnetic resonance imaging in kernicterus. T2-weighted images, 1.5T. The globus pallidus (*arrows*) is bilaterally demonstrated by both posteromedial and lateral outlines of high signal density. (Courtesy of Dr. Kenji Yokochi, Ohzora Hospital, Shizuoka, Japan.)

Some cases also show increased signal in the globus pallidus on T1-weighted images (257).

Diagnosis

The diagnosis of kernicterus in a term infant during the neonatal period rests on changes in body tone, abnormalities in eye movements, loss of the Moro reflex, and an abnormal cry, all in the presence of hyperbilirubinemia. The combination of extrapyramidal signs, ocular disturbances, and impaired hearing, although characteristic for kernicterus caused by isoimmunization, also can be seen in children who are only mildly jaundiced and also have a history of prematurity and perinatal anoxia.

Treatment and Prognosis

The treatment of kernicterus rests on the prevention of severe hyperbilirubinemia. As pointed out by Maisels, it is known how, but not when, to treat hyperbilirubinemia. The role of exchange transfusions, multiple intrauterine transfusions, and phototherapy in the current treatment of isoimmunization and hyperbilirubinemia is discussed by Newman and Maisels (229) and Gourley (257). The use of metalloporphyrins for the prevention of neonatal jaundice has been reviewed by Gourley (257).

Bacterial Toxins

The most potent nerve poisons known are produced by two anaerobic, spore-forming bacteria, *Clostridium botulinum* and *Clostridium tetani*.

Botulism

Botulism is induced by the ingestion of preserves and other canned goods in which *C. botulinum* has grown and produced toxin. The organism produces seven antigenically distinct protein toxins, of which A, B, and E are most commonly responsible for human disease.

The toxins produced by *C. botulinum* are lethal at the lowest dose per kilogram of body weight of any of the known poisons. Calculated from data obtained in mice, the lethal dose for an adult is approximately 0.12 mg. Chemically, botulism toxin A, the most studied substance, is a simple polypeptide of known sequence with 33% homology to tetanus toxin. Its toxicity is lost with heat denaturation. Both botulinus and tetanus neurotoxins block the release of neurotransmitters. Whereas tetanus neurotoxin acts mainly on CNS synapses, the botulinum neurotoxins act peripherally on the terminal unmyelinated motor nerve fibrils blocking the release of acetylcholine. Three steps are involved: (a) irreversible binding of the toxin to the presynaptic nerve surface, (b) crossing of the toxin into the nerve terminal, probably by receptor-mediated endocytosis, and (c) disabling the release of acetylcholine by zinc-dependent proteolysis of three synaptic proteins—the SNARE proteins (SNAP-25, VAMP, and syntaxin)—involved in the exocytosis of neurotransmitters. A second, nonproteolytic inhibitory mechanism of action is believed to involve the activation of neuronal transglutaminases (258). The result is an interruption of transmission of the nerve impulse, producing a myasthenia-like syndrome. The actions of botulinum and tetanus toxins are reviewed by Lalli and coworkers (259).

Symptoms appear between 12 and 48 hours after ingestion of contaminated food. A prodromal period of nonspecific gastrointestinal symptoms is followed by the evolution of neurologic dysfunction (260). Initial symptoms include blurring of vision, impaired pupillary reaction to light, diplopia, and progressive weakness of the bulbar musculature. Paralysis of the major skeletal muscles follows, with death caused by respiratory arrest. In patients who do not die, convalescence is slow, and complete recovery of a totally paralyzed muscle can take as long as 1 year.

The clinical picture of botulism can be distinguished from various viral encephalitides by the early appearance in botulism of internal and external ophthalmoplegia, ptosis, and paralysis of the pupillary accommodation reflex. Electromyography (EMG) shows the motor unit action potentials to be brief and of small amplitude. Fibrillation potentials, consistent with functional denervation, are observed in approximately one-half of patients (261). Although the response to repetitive nerve stimulation is diagnostic for botulism, it may be normal in mild cases, and incremental responses do not occur at slower rates of stimulation (5 Hz). In severe intoxication, transmitter release is blocked to such an extent that no increment occurs, even at rapid rates of stimulation (50 Hz) (262).

Infantile Botulism

This condition has its onset between ages 3 and 18 weeks and is characterized by hypotonia, hyporeflexia, and weakness of the cranial musculature. Infants often have an antecedent history of constipation and poor feeding, and a significantly large proportion (44%) has been fed honey (263).

Symptoms range from a mild disorder to one that resembles sudden infant death syndrome (SIDS). Bulbar signs predominate. These include a poor cry, poor sucking, an impaired pupillary light response, and external ophthalmoplegia. As the illness progresses, a flaccid paralysis develops. Autonomic dysfunction can be present; cardiovascular symptoms are absent, however, and the ECG remains normal (264). Almost all infants recover completely, with the illness lasting between 3 and 20 weeks. In 5% of infants, relapses occur 1 to 2 weeks after hospital discharge. The second bout of infantile botulism is just as severe or even more severe than the first attack (265).

The EMG results are similar to those seen in older individuals with botulism. It typically shows a pattern of brief duration, small-amplitude potentials with decremental response at low-frequency (3 to 10 Hz) repetitive stimulation, and an incremental (*staircase*) response at high-frequency (20 to 50 Hz) repetitive stimulation (266). The incremental response may not be seen in all muscles and is not as apparent at slower frequencies of nerve stimulation. Anticholinesterase medications should be withdrawn at least 8 hours before the study (266). When present, the finding of an incremental response to nerve stimulation is diagnostic because the only other condition in which it is observed is Lambert-Eaton syndrome, an entity not seen in infants (267). The diagnosis can be confirmed by demonstrating the organism or toxin in stool (268).

Whereas botulism in older children and adults is generally, but not invariably, caused by the ingestion of preformed toxin, infant botulism results from the colonization of the gut with type A or type B spores of *C. botulinum* and from the subsequent release of the toxin, which has been demonstrated in feces (269). Because spores of *C. botulinum* are ubiquitous and most individuals ingest *C. botulinum* without adverse effects, the cause for the illness is still obscure. A number of host factors, possibly constipation, immune deficiency, or unusual gut flora, also must be present to permit germination of the spores and production of the toxin within the gastrointestinal tract (270).

The diagnosis of infantile botulism is difficult to establish because the condition mimics septicemia, viral encephalitis, neonatal myasthenia gravis, and infectious polyneuritis. The predominance of bulbar symptoms in an infant who appears fairly aware of the surroundings should alert the clinician to the diagnosis and prompt the performance of an EMG.

In most cases, including all those of infant botulism, antitoxin administration is ineffective by the time botulism is diagnosed, and symptomatic therapy, including respiratory support and nasogastric feeding, must suffice. Recovery is slow. In the series of Schreiner and coworkers, the average duration of hospitalization in patients who required mechanical ventilation was 23 days (271). When treating with antibiotics, aminoglycosides that potentiate the paralysis must be avoided.

Tetanus

Tetanus is the result of an infection of wounded or damaged tissue by the spores of *Clostridium tetani*. It is still widely encountered and is believed to cause between 800,000 and 1 million deaths each year (272). Under anaerobic conditions, the spores germinate, and the vegetative forms multiply to produce two toxins: a hemolysin and a neurotoxin.

The crystalline neurotoxin, tetanospasmin, is a 150,000-dalton protein, ranking second in potency only to botulism toxin. When tetanospasmin is treated with formalin, two molecules of protein polymerize to form toxoid, a nontoxic dimer with intact antigenicity that is used for immunizations.

Tetanus toxin enters the nervous system by binding to peripheral sensory, motor, and autonomic nerve terminals that are unprotected by the blood–brain barrier and traveling centrally by intra-axonal transport. The toxin binds to a highly specific protein receptor, with lesser affinity to disialogangliosides and trisialogangliosides localized on the cell membrane (273). The toxin is then taken up by endocytosis and is transported retrograde via an intra-axonal transport system to the corresponding cell bodies—in the case of a peripheral injury, the α-motoneurons. When the toxin reaches the perikarya of motor neurons, it is passed trans-synaptically to the surrounding presynaptic terminals, including the afferent fibers of the glycinergic inhibitors (274). The exact subcellular mechanism of action is similar to that of botulinum toxin in that it blocks exocytosis by proteolysis of synaptobrevin, a membrane component of synaptic vessicles and one of the proteins involved in vesicle exocytosis (272,275).

The manifestations of tetanus result from the action of the toxin within the spinal cord and brainstem. The toxin blocks the release of GABA and glycine from the presynaptic terminals of the inhibitory polysynaptic circuits surrounding the motor neurons. Abolition of the inhibitory influence of afferent fibers on the motor neurons produces uncontrolled firing, which results in paroxysmal muscle spasms (276). At high toxin concentrations, excitatory transmission also is reduced, and the toxin prevents release of acetylcholine from the neuromuscular junction, thereby producing flaccid paralysis. Additionally, elevation of serum creatine phosphokinase and fluorescent binding techniques provide evidence that tetanospasmin produces direct injury to skeletal muscles.

Clinical Manifestations

Most commonly, symptoms appear approximately 1 week after injury. A number of authors have noted that the shorter the incubation period, the graver the infection. The incubation period reflects the amount of toxin released and the distance between the site of injury and the CNS. Trismus or stiffness of the neck and back is generally the earliest symptom. A characteristic retraction of the angles of the mouth has been termed *risus sardonicus* (Fig. 10.3). Rigidity becomes generalized, and tetanic spasms develop. These can be induced by various sensory stimuli or passive movements of the limbs, or they can occur spontaneously. Sudden respiratory failure, obstruction of the airway, and bronchopneumonia account for most deaths.

In some patients, muscular rigidity is initially localized to the area of the wound and only slowly extends to other muscles.

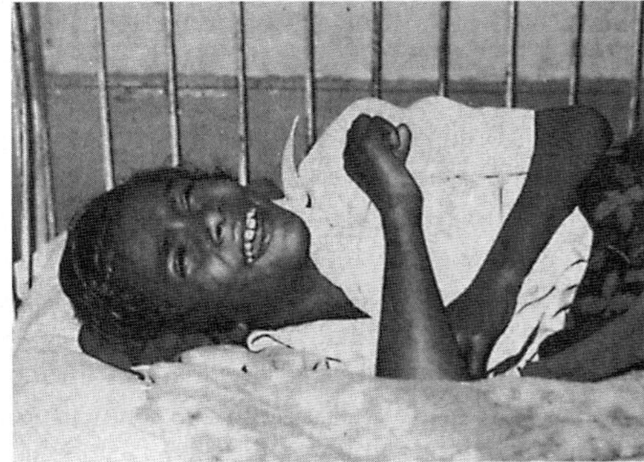

FIGURE 10.3. Risus sardonicus in tetanus, causing an increased tone of all facial muscles, interfering with speech. Patient is a 6-year-old Pakistani boy after 7 days of therapy. (Courtesy of Dr. Muhammed Ibrahim Memon, Professor of Paediatric Medicine, Liaquat Medical College, Jamshoro, Sindh, Pakistan.)

Tetanus owing to clostridial otitis media is distinctive in that trismus and risus sardonicus predominate over generalized spasms and rigidity.

Treatment of tetanus requires maintenance of an airway and adequate ventilation, administration of antitoxin as quickly as possible, debridement of the site of infection, treatment with an antibiotic such as penicillin to eradicate both vegetative and spore forms from the site of infection, and use of a sedative such as diazepam or phenobarbital. The effectiveness of any of these measures has not been subjected to rigid, controlled studies. Patients who do not respond to any of these measures require neuromuscular blockade with curarelike agents. Despite these measures, the mortality of tetanus in children who demonstrate the full clinical picture is still high. In a 1987 series from Bombay, the overall mortality was 12%, and mortality in severe cases was 23%, with death being caused by unexpected cardiac arrest caused by arrhythmias and to sudden hyperthermia and circulatory collapse (277).

Recovery from tetanus is slow. Approximately one-fourth of patients have major sleep disturbances for approximately 1 to 3 years. In approximately one-half, seizures, often accompanied by myoclonus, occur 1 to 2 months after apparent recovery and persist for 6 months to 1 year, with an average frequency of one major attack every 2 months (278).

Tetanus Neonatorum

Tetanus neonatorum is responsible for at least 500,000 deaths a year, most of them in developing countries, where umbilical cord sepsis and lack of maternal immunity contribute to its high incidence. It is the most under-reported fatal infectious disease. In the United States, cases have been encountered in infants born to immigrant families (279).

The condition develops between the fourth and eighth day of life, with the more severe cases having a shorter incubation period. Irritability and trismus, with consequent inability to suck, are usually the earliest signs. As the disease progresses, infants develop opisthotonus and generalized tetanic spasms. These can be induced by stimulation or, in the more severe cases, appear spontaneously. In the most severe cases, the spasms become continuous and are accompanied by apneic episodes (280–282).

Treatment of neonatal tetanus is difficult even in technically more advanced countries. In their series of five patients, Adams and associates used nasotracheal intubation, mechanical ventilation, and neuromuscular blockade with pancuronium bromide to permit ventilatory control (283). Andersson has been successful with a relatively simple method of treatment. This consists of an initial intramuscular injection of diazepam (10 mg), followed by 5 to 10 mg of diazepam given by nasogastric tube four times daily, with additional diazepam administered rectally or intramuscularly as needed to maintain the infant free of spasms. Early nasogastric feedings are started to maintain the nutritional status of the infant. Diazepam is tapered when spasms and rigidity start to subside. This usually occurs after 10 to 21 days (284). Metronidazole is preferred to penicillin or ampicillin, which like tetanus toxin are known antagonists of GABA (285). Einterz and Bates have reported on a similar regimen that they used in Nigeria in a series of 237 cases of neonatal tetanus. They also have used phenobarbital (15 mg three times daily) via nasogastric tube (286). Other sedatives, including propanolol and paraldehyde, also have been recommended. Tetanus antiserum (30,000 to 40,000 U) is administered subcutaneously around the umbilicus, and 1,500 U are given intravenously, although Daud and colleagues believe that the mode of administering the antitoxin does not affect the outcome (287). Large amounts of intramuscular pyridoxine (100 mg/day) are said to lower mortality significantly (288). Even so, a series of some 200 cases of neonatal tetanus reported from developing countries indicates a mortality of at least 25%, and as recently as 1991, neonatal tetanus accounted for 30% to 70% of neonatal deaths in Africa (286). As is the case for older children and adults, the shorter the incubation period the more severe the disease, and the likelihood for survival increases when the incubation period is greater than 6 days.

Symptoms gradually abate after 25 to 45 days. The effect of the disease on cognitive function is uncertain. In the experience of Anlar and colleagues, who studied Turkish children, mental and physical retardation were relatively common in survivors (289).

Diphtheria

Although diphtheria is exceedingly rare in western countries as a result of widespread immunization programs, it still occurs with sufficient frequency in some of the developing countries to warrant mentioning its neurologic features (290). The clinical and pathologic features of diphtheria from the viewpoint of neurologists are reviewed in the classic publication by Fisher and Adams (291).

Diphtheria results from an infection with *Corynebacterium diphtheriae*, which establishes itself on the mucous membranes of the throat or nasopharynx and can synthesize a potent, heat-labile toxin. This substance, a low-molecular-weight protein, interrupts the incorporation of amino acids into proteins (292). Once absorbed, the toxin is bound to membrane receptors and is transported intracellularly by endocytosis. The toxin does not cross the blood–brain barrier; its major effect is on the peripheral nervous system.

Neurologic symptoms are seen in 3% to 5% of children, with the incidence depending on the severity of the disease (290). The two types of symptoms are local paralyses and a polyneuropathy. Paralyses develop between the fifth and twelfth days of the illness and are marked by paralysis of the palate with a nasal voice, nasal regurgitation, dysphagia, and weakness of the neck extensors. Hoarseness, numbness of the face, and ciliary paralysis with loss of accommodation ensue (291). Less often, the extraocular muscles are involved. Symptoms involving the other cranial nerves, such as deafness or loss of taste, have been noted on rare occasions. These deficits last 1 to 2 weeks, then gradually resolve.

A gradual evolution of a combined sensory and motor demyelinating, noninflammatory polyneuropathy, which affects mainly the lower extremities, can appear 5 to 8 weeks after the initial infection (291,293). The polyneuropathy progresses for 2 weeks, then resolves completely. The segmental demyelination responsible has a unique topography in that it is most marked in the anterior and posterior roots near the sensory ganglion. No inflammatory cells are evident (291).

Cardiac symptoms have been attributed to a toxin-induced myocarditis or to an involvement of the vagus nerve.

All these complications are preventable by early antitoxin therapy. Once symptoms have developed, treatment is nonspecific. Even so, most patients experience complete or functionally complete remission of symptoms.

Tick Paralysis

A progressive symmetric paralysis, associated with the bite of a wood or dog tick, is endemic in the Rocky Mountain and Appalachian regions of the United States. A similar condition also has been encountered in the Australian states of Victoria, Tasmania, and New South Wales; in Israel; and in South Africa (294,295). It is usually seen in children under five years of age. The disease also has been seen in one-humped Sudanese camels, llamas, and the red wolf (296). Symptoms are produced by a neurotoxin, secreted by the insect, that probably blocks depolarization in the terminal portions of the motor nerves and, in a manner as yet undelineated, also affects the large myelinated motor and sensory axons (297).

After a prodrome of a viral-like illness, the condition manifests by an unsteady gait, an ascending flaccid paralysis, and commonly internal and external ophthalmoplegia (295). The paralysis can extend to involve the bulbar musculature. It is accompanied by areflexia and numbness or tingling of face and extremities.

Neurophysiologic studies disclose low-amplitude compound muscle action potentials with normal motor and sensory conduction velocities (295).

Neither clinical nor electrodiagnostic findings differentiate this condition from acute infectious polyneuritis (298). Infant botulism usually is seen in younger children and is not associated with ophthalmoplegia. Because scalp hair is one of the favorite sites for a tick, a thorough search

TABLE 10.6 Neurologic Symptoms of Animal Venoms

Animals	*Symptoms*	*Action of Venom*	*Reference*
Coelentarata, jellyfish	Muscular weakness, respiratory paralysis	Unknown	306,307a
Mollusca, bivalve (infected by flagellate plankton, paralytic shellfish poisoning)	Ataxia, ascending paralysis, paresthesia	Binding to voltage-activated Na channel; blockade of nerve and muscle action potentials	307
Mussels (contaminated)	Confusion, memory loss, seizures, distal atrophy, alternating hemiparesis, ophthalmoplegia	Domoic acid, neuroexcitatory transmitter at glutamate receptor	308,309a
Reptiles			
Crotalidae (rattlesnakes, water moccasins, copperheads)	Progressive paralysis	Mosaic of antigens, direct action on central nervous system; inhibits neuromuscular transmission at motor end-plate, damages muscle	309,310
Elapidae (coral snakes, cobras)	Progressive paralysis, rapid onset	Competitive block of muscle nicotinic acetylcholine receptors	311,311a, 312,313
Viperidae (vipers)	Cerebral infarction	Thrombinlike enzyme, causes vasculitis	315,315a
Arthropods			
Spiders, *Latrodectus* (black widow)	Local pain, abdominal rigidity, muscle spasms, convulsions	Massive exocytotic transmitter release followed by depletion and irreversible block	314,315,316, 317,317a
Centruroides (scorpions)	Muscle spasms, convulsions	Several toxins depending on species; some act on Na channels, others on Ca-activated K channels	318,319, 320a,321
Chordata			
Chondrichthyes (stingray)	Muscle spasms, convulsions	Unknown	320
Osteichthyes (stonefish)	Local pain, paralysis, convulsions, slow recovery	Stonustoxin acts as cytolytic toxin liberates nitric oxide–synthase	322,322a, 322b,323a
Puffer (ingestion of ovaries, liver)	Ataxia, paresthesias, muscular twitching, paralysis	Neuromuscular block, binds to voltage sensitive Na channel, blocks Na flux	323,325a
Ciguatera (reef fish)	Gastrointestinal symptoms, tingling of mouth, dizziness, ataxia, hallucinations, transient blurred vision or blindness, peripheral muscular weakness	Ciguatoxin from blue-green algae is nutritional source for ciguatera Excitatory agent acts on Na channels	324,325,343

for the insect should be conducted in children who have had a recent onset of a progressive weakness resembling infectious polyneuritis (298,299). After removal of the tick, recovery has been prompt in the North American cases, but in the Australian cases, there can be worsening of the paralysis over the subsequent 24 to 48 hours (295). Full recovery can be expected but often requires weeks to months.

Animal Venoms

Neurologic symptoms induced through the bite or sting of venomous animals usually are caused by impaired neuromuscular transmission and take the form of weakness or painful muscle spasms. In recent years, considerable interest has focused on the molecular mechanisms of the various animal venoms and their specific interactions with the various ion channels within the CNS and the neuromuscular junction. The chemistry and molecular biology of the various toxins are summarized by Adams and Swanson (300); the clinical picture by Russell (301), Southcott (302), and Campbell (303); and treatment by Auerbach (304) and Gold and coworkers (305). A review of the more toxic animals and pertinent references are presented in Table 10.6.

Plant Toxins

The neurologic symptoms of some of the more frequently encountered plant toxins are presented in Table 10.7. A complete and up-to-date review of the clinical presentation and management of plant toxins is given by Furbee and Wermuth (340).

Neurolathyrism

Neurolathyrism is probably the most common plant toxin–induced neurological disorder. It is an upper motor neuron disease that affects the anterior horn cells of the

TABLE 10.7 Neurologic Symptoms Resulting from Ingestion of Plant Toxins

Plant	*Symptoms*	*Toxin and Action*
Mushroom		
Amanita phalloides	Gastrointestinal symptoms, hepatic and renal dysfunction, hemorrhagic encephalopathy	Amatoxins inhibit RNA polymerase, phalloidin disrupts membranes (327a,328,331a,332a)
Amanita muscaria	Dizziness, ataxia, convulsions	Mucimol activates γ-aminobutyric acid receptors ibotenic acid acts as glutamate receptor agonist (327,327a,331a)
Inocybes	Perspiration, salivation, lacrimation, blurring of vision	Muscarine, a parasympathomimetic (326,327)
Psilocybes	Psychotropic effects	Psilocybin (326,327)
Gyromitra (brain fungus)	Gastrointestinal symptoms, renal and hepatic failure	Monomethyl hydrazine (326)
Buckthorn	Flaccid quadriparesis, bulbar weakness	Segmental demyelination caused by at least four neurotoxins (329)
Nutmeg	Flushing, gastrointestinal symptoms, drowsiness or hyperactivity, hallucinations	Amino-derivatives of elemicin and myristicin (330)
Ricin (castor bean)	Hemorrhagic gastroenteritis, stupor, seizures	Ricin: ? proteolytic enzyme (331,332)
Jimsonweed (locoweed, thornapple)	Flushed face, dilated pupils, bizarre behavior, visual hallucinations, urinary retention	Atropine and scopolamine, anticholinergic action (333,334)
Pokeweed	Abdominal cramps, vomiting, diaphoresis, dizziness, lethargy, seizures	Phytolaccine (335)
Unripe akee nut	Jamaican vomiting sickness; symptoms similar to Reye syndrome (see Chapter 7)	Hypoglycin A, a cyclopropyl propionic acid (336,337,341a)
Sugarcane (mildewed)	Impaired consciousness, seizures, delayed dystonia after recovery; computed tomography: bilateral hypodensities in putamen, globus pallidus	3-Nitropropionic acid (338)
Ginkgo seed	Vomiting, diarrhea, repetitive convulsions	4-methoxypyridoxine (339)

lumbar spinal cord. It is induced by overconsumption of a grass pea (*Lathyrus sativus*) that contains the neurotoxin β-oxalylaminoalanine. The toxin causes neuronal damage in part through excitation of the α-amino-3-hydroxy-5-methyl-4-isoxazole propionic acid (AMPA) subtype of the ionotropic glutamate receptor (341). The prevalence of this condition is as high as 12 of 1000 persons in Pakistan, 6 of 1000 persons in Ethiopia, and 5.3 of 1000 persons in India.

Males are twice as commonly affected than females, and in the Ethiopian epidemic of 1995 to 1999, boys aged 10 to 14 years were most affected. Symptoms appear suddenly, or subacutely, and are highlighted by a progressive upper motor neuron paralysis affecting the lower extremities. There are no sensory deficits, and bladder function remains intact (342). The deficits are irreversible, and apart from muscle relaxants, there is no effective treatment. Clinically, this condition is indistinguishable from konzo (see later discussion).

NUTRITIONAL DISORDERS

Malnourished children constitute approximately 75% of the preschool population in developing countries. Grossly insufficient quantities of food, dietary imbalances, poor protein intake, lack of essential fatty acids and vitamins, climate, intercurrent bacterial or parasitic infections, and emotional deprivation all combine to predispose a child to nutritional diseases. Additionally, inadequate prenatal and perinatal care also can contribute to the final clinical picture.

Protein-Energy Malnutrition

Protein-energy malnutrition (also called protein-calorie malnutrition) refers to the severe clinical syndromes of marasmus and kwashiorkor, and to milder, often unappreciated cases of nutritional deficiencies. These entities are common in Third World countries, and a recent Nigerian survey indicated that some 41% of children were affected. Kwashiorkor was first described in 1935 by Williams working in the Gold Coast, now Ghana (344). The word *kwashiorkor* means "sickness the older child gets when the next baby is born" in the Ga tribe dialect of Ghana. Kwashiorkor and marasmus are interrelated syndromes of malnutrition that in their most severe stages are distinct, with different causes and different metabolic pictures. Marasmus, primarily caused by caloric insufficiency, is of early onset and develops when infants are weaned before the end of their first year or when the available breast milk is reduced markedly. It is characterized by emaciation and growth failure (345,346). Kwashiorkor, an edematous form of malnutrion, is most common in children between 1 and 4 years of age, and frequently it is triggered by measles or various bacterial or parasitic infections. The condition results from a diet containing adequate calories but insufficient protein. Golden (347) and others have stressed the important role of antioxidant deficiency in producing kwashiorkor, in that affected children lack albumin, one of the most important plasma antioxidants. In addition, the children are deficient in glutathione, vitamin E, selenium, and polyunsaturated fatty acids (348). Conversely nitrogen monoxide (NO) concentrations are increased, aiding in the depletion of glutathione and other antioxidants (348), and inflammatory markers such as prostaglandin E2 are elevated (349). Thus, kwashiorkor is the result of multiple factors (350). These not only include dietary deficiencies and imbalances, but also multiple infections, parasitic infestations, dietary toxins such as aflatoxins (351), and maternal deprivation (352). Finally, it should be stressed that in many areas of the world, symptoms of kwashiorkor develop in a child who already has demonstrated retarded growth and mental development.

Clinical Manifestations

In mild to moderate forms of protein-energy malnutrition, a clinical distinction between marasmus and kwashiorkor is impossible. In certain areas of the world, diets giving rise to kwashiorkor also can be deficient in one or more vitamins, and signs of vitamin deficiency can accompany the more advanced stages. In West Africa, for instance, riboflavin deficiency is common; in Southeast Asia, thiamine deficiency can induce a mixed picture of protein-energy malnutrition and beriberi.

Certain changes in protein metabolism, notably a reduced serum albumin concentration, a reduced serum concentration of all essential amino acids except phenylalanine and histidine, reduced glutathione levels, and a normal or even higher than normal concentration of nonessential amino acids, are characteristic for kwashiorkor and can be used in making a biochemical diagnosis.

The clinical picture of kwashiorkor varies from one region of the world to another. The four basic symptoms and signs are edema, growth failure, behavioral changes, and muscle wasting. Other relatively common features include dyspigmentation of hair and skin, dermatitis, anemia, and hepatomegaly. In particular, a flaky paint type of dermatosis is said to be diagnostic of kwashiorkor (350).

Neurologic Features

The effects of undernutrition on the immature nervous system have been the subject of intensive investigation. Neuropathologic studies reveal the brain of a malnourished infant to be small for the infant's chronologic age, and its number of neurons, degree of myelination, and total cerebral lipid content to be reduced (353,354). In interpreting these findings, one must note that in almost all instances, these autopsies have been performed on children who died as a result of an infection in addition to protein and calorie deprivation.

Physiologic studies on children with severe protein-energy malnutrition conducted by Mehta and colleagues, including myself, indicated that the proportion of glucose undergoing aerobic oxidation by the brain is reduced, and that a significant proportion is converted to long-chain fatty acids (355).

Although these findings provide a biochemical basis for both the loss in myelination and the ultimate cognitive deficits of malnourished infants, the time during which the human brain is vulnerable to nutritional insults is still uncertain. Animal experiments indicate that a severe nutritional insult early in brain development can have a permanent adverse effect on cerebral structure and function. Periods of CNS growth spurt (in humans between 15 and 20 weeks' gestation, when neuronal multiplication is maximal, and between 30 weeks' gestation and the end of the first year of extrauterine life, when glial division occurs) are times when the brain is particularly vulnerable to experimental nutritional deficiency (356). As yet, these experimental data cannot be correlated with clinical experience.

Apathy is the most constant and earliest neurologic feature and is usual in children who weigh less than 40% of the expected amount (357). In the Indian series of Sachdeva and colleagues, 87% of children admitted for treatment of protein-energy malnutrition showed mental changes, 77% had muscle wasting, 70% weakness, and 40% hyporeflexia (358). More recent data from the Indian clinic of Chopra and his group are comparable (359). Most studies show that head circumference varies directly with nutritional status and is often below the third percentile for American children. It is less affected than height and weight. Hypotonia and reduced deep tendon reflexes are common; they are more marked in the lower extremities, particularly in the proximal musculature (360). "Soft" neurologic signs, notably impaired fine motor coordination and the presence of choreoathetoid movements, are seen far more commonly in malnourished children than in control children with normal nutritional status.

The EEG has been studied by several groups. Generally, it demonstrates nonspecific abnormalities such as diffuse slowing. These are more commonly seen in malnourished than in control children (361). Nerve conduction times are significantly delayed in both the marasmic and the kwashiorkor forms of protein-energy malnutrition, even in the absence of overt associated vitamin deficiencies. As a rule, the degree of delay correlates with the duration and the severity of the protein-energy malnutrition, and thus is more marked in marasmus (360). Approximately one-half of patients with the more severe forms of protein-energy malnutrition have segmental demyelination; when malnutrition is severe and long-standing, an arrest in myelination of peripheral nerves occurs, with a persistence of the small myelinated fibers and a relative lack of the large myelinated fibers (359).

Neuroimaging studies demonstrate widened cortical sulci, widened cerebellar folia, and enlarged ventricles. These abnormalities resolve quickly with nutritional rehabilitation, suggesting that they do not represent cerebral atrophy, but rather ventricular dilatation and enlargement of sulci as a consequence of a decrease in plasma proteins and reduced colloid osmotic pressure (362). It is of note that in the South African series of Gunston and coworkers, myelination was age appropriate even in children with severe kwashiorkor (362).

Treatment

The medical and social aspects of treatment of protein-energy malnutrition are reviewed by Torun (346). It is of note that with nutritional rehabilitation, there is a rapid and striking increase in head circumference. This may become sufficiently marked to result in splitting of sutures and papilledema, suggesting the presence of pseudotumor cerebri.

Approximately one-fifth of children with kwashiorkor become drowsy 3 to 4 days after being started on a normal diet. Although the condition is most often self-limited, it is occasionally accompanied by asterixis and can progress to coma with fatal outcome (363). The nature of this complication is unknown, but it is believed to reflect hepatic failure resulting from the ingestion of relatively large amounts of protein. Even more rarely, a transient syndrome marked by coarse tremors, parkinsonian rigidity, bradykinesia, and myoclonus has been observed in children with kwashiorkor 6 days to several weeks after starting a corrective high-protein diet (364). This condition is distinct from the infantile tremor syndrome (see later discussion).

Prognosis

Follow-up studies on children who experienced protein-energy malnutrition indicate that the younger the child at the time of the hospitalization for malnutrition, the more likely the child is to have a variety of cognitive deficits (365–367). Growth-retarded children who received supplementary feedings had higher verbal intelligence than their undernourished sibling controls, a difference that could not be accounted for by socioeconomic factors (368). These benefits are not sustained however, and the greatest postnatal influence on cognitive performance comes not from nutrition but from social stimulation, in particular from the combination of psychosocial stimulation and nutritional supplementation (369). When children are subjected to either nutritional or social stimulation, the effect becomes evident within 18 months; it is almost immediate when both interventions are made available to them (Fig. 10.4) (370).

Summarizing sometimes contradictory data, one can conclude that when intellectual inadequacy follows malnutrition in early life, it occurs not only as the result of protein-energy malnutrition, but because the infant's nervous system and its social environment are inadequate and interfere with normal neurodevelopment.

Vitamin Deficiencies

The action of a vitamin in intermediary metabolism can be disturbed by its deficiency, by abnormally high vitamin requirements such as are seen in a variety of bacterial and parasitic infections, and by the inhibitory action of various antivitamin substances. Dietary factors antagonistic

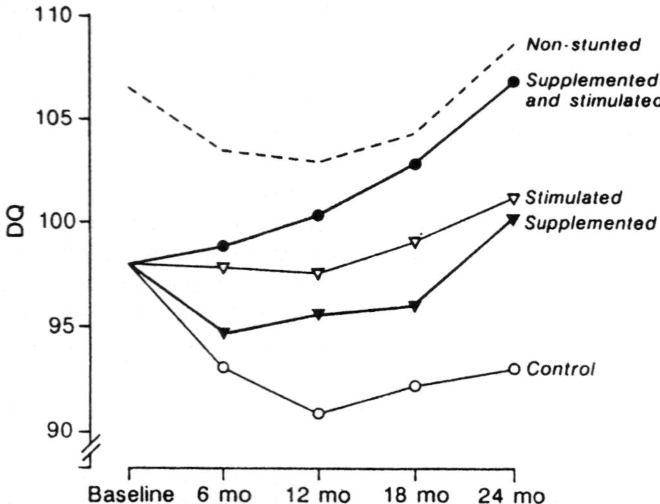

FIGURE 10.4. Recovery from malnutrition in 129 Jamaican infants, aged 9 to 24 months, with stunted growth (length less than 2 standard deviations below the mean). The effect of nutritional supplementation is compared with that of psychosocial stimulation, combined nutritional and psychosocial interventions, and controls. A group of 32 nonstunted Jamaican infants served as reference. (DQ, developmental quotient.) (From Grantham-McGregor SM, Powell CA, Walker SP, et al. Nutritional supplementation, psychosocial stimulation, and mental development of stunted children: the Jamaican Study. *Lancet* 1991;338:15. With permission.)

to the action of a vitamin include avidin (found in raw egg white), which is an antagonist to biotin, and the enzyme thiaminase (present in raw fish), which destroys dietary thiamine.

Although a deficiency in almost any of the vitamins can directly or indirectly affect the CNS, only components of the B complex group are known to be involved directly in brain function.

Deficiency of vitamin A can produce increased intracranial pressure, which can be reversed by dietary treatment (371). Chronic vitamin A intoxication induces increased intracranial pressure as well, which is accompanied by craniotabes and cortical hyperostosis (372).

Vitamin E (tocopherol) deficiency is encountered in severe cases of cystic fibrosis and in other malabsorptive conditions. The syndrome of spinocerebellar degeneration and peripheral neuropathy occurring as a complication of tocopherol deficiency is described in the section on gastrointestinal diseases in Chapter 17.

The role of vitamin supplementation in preventing neural tube defects is covered in Chapter 5.

Thiamine Deficiency

The discovery of how thiamine participates in cerebral metabolism was an important part of the early history of neurochemistry and is reviewed by Peters (373) and Haas (374).

Thiamine functions in the form of pyrophosphate, which acts as a coenzyme for many enzyme systems. Generally speaking, thiamine pyrophosphate is involved in oxidative decarboxylation, nonoxidative decarboxylation, and various ketolases, notably the conversion of 5-carbon to 6-carbon sugars by means of the enzyme transketolase.

Pyruvate and α-ketoglutarate, whose decarboxylations are two integral steps of the Krebs cycle, exemplify enzymes responsible for oxidative decarboxylation. In thiamine deficiency, oxidation of pyruvate and α-ketoglutarate by the brain is reduced. As a consequence, cerebral oxygen and glucose consumption are lowered, and the concentrations of the two ketoacids (pyruvate and α-ketoglutarate) are increased in various tissues, including blood (375). When a thiamine-deficient individual is presented with a glucose load, the concentration of serum ketoacids increases to abnormal levels and remains elevated for several hours. At the same time, there is an increase in serum and CSF lactic and pyruvic acids.

Transketolase has been found to be more susceptible to thiamine deprivation than are the ketoacid decarboxylases, and the decrease in transketolase activity during induced thiamine deficiency is greater than the decrease of pyruvate decarboxylase activity (376). Dreyfus and Hauser postulated that failure in transketolase represents the basic biochemical lesion of thiamine deficiency, although the increase in transketolase activity with administration of thiamine was insufficient to account for the clinical improvement (377). In experimental studies, thiamine-deficient rats had a low glucose metabolic rate and limited glial proliferation in the vestibular nuclei. Both abnormalities were reversed by thiamine supplementation (378).

Thiamine deficiency is seen in breast-fed infants, whose mothers, themselves, could have been thiamine deficient during pregnancy, and whose breast milk consequently contains inadequate amounts of thiamine. It is also seen in critically ill infants on prolonged enteric feeding, in children with malignancies, in children receiving intensive chemotherapy, and in anorexia nervosa (379–381). Thiamine deficiency due to inadequate diets occurs principally in Asia, where the milling of rice grain or the use of soda in the baking of bread excludes the vitamin from the diet. Extensive outbreaks of beriberi are still being reported from Africa (382).

Two symptom complexes are seen: infantile beriberi and Wernicke-Korsakoff syndrome. Infantile beriberi appears suddenly, often after a bout of gastroenteritis, and is marked by weakness owing to acute peripheral neuritis, neck stiffness, and aphonia (voiceless cry) (383). Cardiac symptoms are not common in infants. The diagnosis can be established by the depressed thiamine concentrations in whole blood and CSF and by the low red cell ketolase activity (384). The experiences of Haridas in Malaya (383) and DeSilva in Sri Lanka (345) illustrate the differential diagnosis and treatment of childhood thiamine deficiency in developing countries.

A neurologic picture resembling that seen in adults with Wernicke-Korsakoff syndrome is rare in children. More often, one sees a relatively nonspecific picture of lethargy, apneic spells, hypothermia, and deteriorating cardiovascular function (385,386). Generally, Wernicke-Korsakoff syndrome is clinically unsuspected and can develop rapidly in the absence of parenteral vitamin supplementation (387). MRI studies are diagnostic in that they demonstrate increased signal on T2-weighted images in the medial aspects of the thalamus, the diencephalon and mesencephalon, the mammillary bodies, and the floor of the hypothalamus (388). These lesions are reversed by thiamine therapy. In many instances, however, the diagnosis is made only on postmortem examination by noting the characteristic spongy changes in the mamillary bodies, hypothalamus, midbrain, and pons.

Infantile subacute necrotizing encephalopathy (Leigh syndrome), a familial neurologic degenerative condition with pathologic changes reminiscent of Wernicke disease, has been termed *pseudo-Wernicke syndrome*. This disease is the result of mitochondrial dysfunction and is more fully discussed in Chapter 2.

Pyridoxine Deficiency

Pyridoxine (vitamin B_6) in the form of its aldehyde derivative, pyridoxal-5-phosphate, is a coenzyme for numerous essential metabolic reactions within the nervous system. Both decarboxylation of glutamic acid to GABA, a neurotransmitter, and transamination of glutamic acid to α-ketoglutaric acid are impaired in animals receiving a pyridoxine-deficient diet. Several other amino acid decarboxylases, several transaminases, and serine hydroxymethyltransferase also are pyridoxine dependent. Pyridoxine also is involved in synaptogenesis, dendritic arborization, and the maintenance of the normal neurotransmitter balance within the CNS.

In at least three conditions, a relative deficiency of pyridoxine is related to the appearance of seizures and potentially permanent neurologic deficits.

Dietary Pyridoxine Deficiency

Pyridoxine deficiency appears at 1 to 12 months of age in a significant proportion of infants whose intake of the vitamin is below 0.1 mg/day. Aside from seizures and hyperirritability, other symptoms of vitamin deficiency, notably anemia, can sometimes also be documented (389). Pyridoxine deficiency unaccompanied by other nutritional deficits is rarely encountered, even in the developing countries. A series of cases was seen, however, in the United States between 1952 and 1953 in a small percentage of infants fed a pyridoxine-deficient proprietary formula (390). More recently, prolonged seizures that were unresponsive to treatment with the usual anticonvulsant medications but responded to pyridoxine (100 mg) were seen in an infant fed powdered goat's milk, a preparation devoid of pyridoxine and folic acid (391). Seizures owing to pyridoxine deficiency also are seen in infants who have been breastfed exclusively for longer than 6 months and in those who have had a jejunoileal bypass (392).

Pyridoxine Dependency

A familial pyridoxine dependency syndrome is marked by the evolution of seizures *in utero*, at birth, or at any time up to the end of the second year of life (393,394). The condition was first described by Hunt and colleagues (395) and is transmitted as an autosomal recessive trait, with the gene having been mapped to chromosome 5q31.2–31.3 (396). It is a relatively uncommon entity but one of the important causes for intractable seizures. Seizures can be generalized or focal with secondary generalization or can take the form of infantile spasms. They are almost immediately arrested by the administration of intramuscular or intravenous pyridoxine (50 to 200 mg). Subsequently, infants are often hypotonic and unresponsive (397). Microcephaly, if present, is corrected with pyridoxine treatment. Thus, pyridoxine dependency, like protein-energy malnutrition, is a rare cause of reversible microcephaly. The EEG usually shows a variety of paroxysmal discharges, including hypsarrhythmia and also normalizes promptly with pyridoxine administration. The dose of pyridoxine required to control seizures, and dramatically reverse the EEG abnormalities, ranges from 0.2 to 50 mg/day. This dosage is many times the minimum daily requirement for the vitamin. MRI shows diffuse cortical atrophy, most marked in the frontal regions, and positron emission tomographic scan reveals a widespread cerebral hypometabolism (398).

CSF GABA levels are markedly reduced, and CSF glutamate levels are markedly elevated (397). Both levels return to normal with treatment. On autopsy, the GABA content of cerebral cortex has been found to be low, whereas the content of glutamic acid is elevated (399). The locus for the defect does not correspond to that of either of the genes for glutamic acid decarboxylase (GAD) or that for GABA transaminase (400,401), and the gene defect remains unknown.

The diagnosis of pyridoxine dependency rests on the presence of seizures that are intractable to the usual anticonvulsant medications, the prompt cessation of seizures with parenteral or oral pyridoxine administration, and, optimally, the recurrence of seizures after pyridoxine withdrawal.

Life-long continuous treatment with pyridoxine is necessary to prevent seizures and severe mental retardation. The dosage required for seizure control ranges between 0.2 and 30 mg/kg per day (402). Larger amounts of pyridoxine have been given in some instances, but the vitamin can induce a reversible sensory neuropathy (403). The optimal dose of pyridoxine appears to vary between families, and regulation of pyridoxine dosage by aiming at normalization of the EEG is probably indicated.

Hydrazine Toxicity

Treatment with isoniazide (INH), penicillamine, or other hydrazides capable of reacting with the aldehyde group of pyridoxal can induce symptoms of B_6 deficiency (404). With the increased prevalence of tuberculosis, and with INH being one of the first-line antituberculous drugs, the incidence of INH poisoning has increased to the point where INH together with diphenhydramine and theophylline has become one of the three major causes for drug-induced seizures in the pediatric population (405,406). Dosages of INH greater than 30 mg/kg can produce seizures. In addition, the characteristic clinical picture is that of a metabolic acidosis and coma (406). Seizures are often refractory to commonly used anticonvulsants, including intravenous benzodiazepines, and parenteral pyridoxine is necessary to control them (406).

Pellagra

Although pellagra is considered a multiple-deficiency disease, the main clinical manifestations—dermatitis, diarrhea, and diffuse cerebral disease—respond to therapy with nicotinic acid (niacin) or tryptophan. Pellagra is endemic to areas where corn, a poor source of nicotinic acid, is the staple food, and where intake of meat, which provides tryptophan needed for the biosynthesis of nicotinic acid, also is low (407). Approximately one-half of the human minimum daily requirement of nicotinic acid is synthesized from tryptophan by micro-organisms, either in tissues or in the intestinal tract. Nicotinic acid is an integral component of two coenzymes involved in electron transfer, nicotinamide adenine dinucleotide and nicotinamide adenine dinucleotide phosphate. Both are essential for a variety of enzymatic reactions in carbohydrate and fatty acid metabolism. Since isoniazide inhibits the conversion of tryptophan to niacin, pellagra has been encountered in poorly nourished tuberculous patients who had been on isoniazide therapy (408).

Children who are mildly deficient in nicotinic acid are irritable or apathetic. With severe involvement, they become delirious or mentally obtunded, and they can show spasticity, coarse tremors of the face and hands, polyneuritis, and optic atrophy. In the experience of Malfait and colleagues, working in Malawi, dermatitis of the areas exposed to sunlight, particularly of the chest, arms, and neck (Casal's necklace), was seen in 80% of nicotinic acid–deficient subjects (409). Stomatitis was present in 60%, diarrhea in 20%, and mental disorders in 10%. Histologic examination of the brain shows degeneration of Betz cells of the motor cortex and, to a lesser extent, of the cerebellar Purkinje cells. In the spinal cord, degeneration of the posterior columns and the pyramidal and spinocerebellar tracts is seen. Demyelination of the peripheral nerves is common (410).

The experience of Spies and colleagues (411) in Alabama during the 1930s and the review by Lanska (412) provide the reader with an idea of the problems inherent in the differential diagnosis of pellagra and its therapy. Despite the availability of chemical assays for nicotinic acids and its metabolites, the diagnosis of the condition of pellagra rests on the clinical pictures and the prompt response to administration of nicotinic acid. A pellagralike skin rash also is seen in Hartnup disease and in some other genetic defects of tryptophan and kynurenine metabolism (see Chapter 1).

Subacute Combined Degeneration

Degeneration of the posterior and lateral columns of the spinal cord owing to deficiency of vitamin B_{12} (cobalamin) is rare in childhood. When seen, it can accompany one of the several forms of congenital pernicious anemia. The most likely form of subacute combined degeneration to be encountered in childhood is caused by a congenital defect of transcobalamin II, a plasma globulin that promotes the cellular uptake of the vitamin by receptor-mediated endocytosis. The condition is an autosomal recessive disorder that generally presents with megaloblastic anemia, which if inadequately treated can progress to impaired mental development (413). Congenital intrinsic factor deficiency is less common. It presents during the first two to three years of life with a similar neurologic picture (414,415). The condition can be associated with intestinal disease, regional ileitis, or celiac syndrome. The various congenital disorders of cobalamin metabolism are covered in Chapter 1.

Many reports have described vitamin B_{12} deficiency in infants of mothers with undiagnosed pernicious anemia and in exclusively breast-fed infants whose mothers are vegans, who exclude from the diet not only meat, but also eggs and dairy products, or vegans, who exclude all three (416,417). Megaloblastic anemia, always present with subacute combined degeneration in children, is accompanied by apathy, developmental regression, athetoid movements, and tremor (418). Alterations in sensorium can progress to coma (419). In older children, the presenting signs and symptoms of the condition are ataxia, spasticity, weakness of the lower extremities, loss of vibratory sensation, and mental retardation. Plasma homocysteine is increased, and plasma methionine is reduced. Excretion of methylmalonic acid and homocysteine is increased (420).

Somatosensory-evoked potentials reveal the presence of CNS involvement even when overt clinical signs are absent (421). MRI studies show a loss of volume and delayed myelination, while proton resonance spectroscopy displays an accumulation of lactate in gray and white matter and a depletion of choline-containing compounds, suggesting a disturbance in oxidative energy metabolism (422). Vitamin B_{12} administration quickly corrects the hematologic abnormalities. EEG and neuroimaging abnormalities also are reversible with treatment. However, cognitive and language development frequently remains delayed, particularly when neurologic symptoms appear during the first year of life (416,423). A combination tremor and myoclonus affecting the face, tongue, and pharynx can appear after the initiation of treatment with cobalamin (418,424). It is said to respond to the administration of clonazepam (424). A similar neurologic picture has been encountered in children with ifosfamide (425). In the experience of Pearson and colleagues, folic acid therapy often aggravates neurologic symptoms (426).

The pathogenesis of neurologic deficits is still not understood. Hall has reviewed the role of vitamin B_{12} in normal nervous system function (427).

Infantile Tremor Syndrome

Infantile tremor syndrome is fairly common in India. It is seen in children between ages 6 months and 2 years with a history of developmental delay and severe malnutrition. Symptoms, which commence between May and July, include a tremor that can be generalized or confined to one or more extremities. The tremor is rapid, rhythmic, and coarse, and it disappears during sleep. It can be accompanied by myoclonic jerks, epilepsia partialis continua, or choreic movements. Affected children are pale and apathetic and have sparse, light-colored hair and prominent pigmentation over the knuckles. Despite treatment, the outcome is poor, and the majority is left with subnormal intelligence (428,429).

A number of deficiencies have been documented. These include a magnesium deficiency, and, more recently, a deficiency of vitamin B_{12} and zinc (429). In a series by Garewal and coworkers, concomitant malnutrition was documented in 82%, and an antecedent viral illness in 91% (430). The condition also was noted in infants of mothers who were strict vegetarians. Low serum B_{12} levels and a megaloblastic erythropoiesis could be demonstrated in 87%. In other series, magnesium deficiency with low CSF and urine magnesium levels was apparently well documented. The cause of this distinctive condition is still not clear, but tremors respond to supplementation with vitamin B_{12} or magnesium (428,430).

Tropical Myeloneuropathies

Several forms of progressive myeloneuropathies have been described in Third World countries, notably India and Africa. They fall into two clinical types with overlapping features: tropical spastic paraparesis and tropical ataxic neuropathy. Tropical spastic paraparesis is a slowly progressive spastic paraplegia that affects the pyramidal tracts and, to a lesser degree, the sensory systems and is often accompanied by optic atrophy and a peripheral neuropathy. The condition is caused by the human T-cell lymphotropic virus 1 and is considered more extensively in Chapter 7.

Outbreaks of another form of acute spastic paraparesis, termed *konzo,* have been reported from a variety of areas in Africa, notably Tanzania, Mozambique, and Zaire, where cassava is the main staple crop. The condition affects boys predominantly, with its onset generally between 5 and 15 years of age. The onset is abrupt with difficulty in walking. This progresses over the course of 1 to 3 days to a complete and symmetric paraparesis with hyper-reflexia and extensor plantar responses. In the majority of cases, some degree of slow functional improvement occurs (431). Clinically, this entity is indistinguishable from neurolathyrism, considered at another point in this chapter.

The cause for konzo is uncertain. High cyanide intake from the consumption of inadequately processed cassava has been proposed as one etiology. No antibodies to human T-cell lymphotropic virus 1 have been found.

Tropical ataxic neuropathy (nonspastic paraparesis), seen in the western parts of Nigeria, differs from the various forms of tropical spastic paraparesis. Its diagnosis is based on the presence of two of the following symptoms: bilateral optic atrophy, neurosensory deafness, the loss of proprioception and vibratory sensation, and a distal symmetric sensory polyneuropathy (432,433). It is rarely encountered in the first two decades of life (433). Several exogenous factors have been proposed as causes for the condition. Ingestion of cassava beans and a consequent chronic cyanide toxicity plays an important role in some epidemics (434) but not in others (435). The role of the human T-cell lymphotropic virus 2 in the etiology of the condition has not been clarified.

A discussion of the amyotrophic lateral sclerosis–Parkinson disease–dementia complex seen in Guam and the other Mariana Islands and of the role of a plant excitant neurotoxin in causing this neurologic picture and those of the other toxic upper motor neuron diseases is outside the scope of this text. The reader is referred to reviews by Spencer and colleagues (436) and Cox and Sax (437).

REFERENCES

1. Hestand HE, Teske DW. Diphenhydramine hydrochloride intoxication. *J Pediatr* 1977;90:1017–1018.
2. Goetz CM, Lopez G, Dean BS, et al. Accidental childhood death from diphenhydramine overdosage. *Am J Emerg Med* 1990;8:321–322.
3. Priest JH. Atropine response of eyes in mongolism. *Am J Dis Child* 1960;100:869–972.
4. Amitai Y, Almog S, Singer R, et al. Atropine poisoning in children during the Persian Gulf crisis. A national survey in Israel. *J Am Med Assoc* 1992;268:630–632.
5. Valdes-Dapena MA, Arey JB. Boric acid poisoning: three fatal cases with pancreatic inclusion and review of literature. *J Pediatr* 1962;61:531–546.
6. Cheng CT. Perak, Malaysia, mass poisoning. Tale of the nine emperor gods and rat tail noodles. *Am J Forensic Med Pathol* 1992;13:261–263.
7. von Muhlendahl KE, Scherf-Rahne B, Krienke EG, et al. Codeine intoxication in childhood. *Lancet* 1976;2:303–305.
8. Warden CR, Diekema DS, Robertson WO. Dystonic reaction associated with dextromethorphan ingestion in a toddler. *Pediatr Emerg Care* 1997;13:214–215.
9. Kirages TJ, Sule HP, Mycyk MB. Severe manifestations of coricidin intoxication. *Am J Emerg Med* 2003;21:473–475.
10. McCarron MM, Challoner KR, Thomson GA. Diphenoxylate-atropine (Lomotil) overdose in children: an update. *Pediatrics* 1991;87:694–700.
11. Robotham JL, Leitman PS. Acute iron poisoning. A review. *Am J Dis Child* 1980;134:875–879.
12. Mann KV, Piciotti MA, Spevack TA, et al. Management of acute iron overdose. *Clin Pharm* 1989;8:428–440.
13. Martinez AJ, Boehm R, Hadfield MG. Acute hexachlorophene encephalopathy: cliniconeuropathological correlation. *Acta Neuropathol* 1974;28:93–103.
14. Martin-Bouyer G, Lebreton R, Toga M, et al. Outbreak of accidental hexachlorophene poisoning in France. *Lancet* 1982;1:91–95.
15. Oakley CP Jr. The neurotoxicity of the halogenated hydroxyquinolines. *JAMA* 1983;225:395–397.
16. Selby G. Subacute myelo-optic neuropathy in Australia. *Lancet* 1972;1:123–125.
17. Shigematsu I, Yanagawa H. Data on clinoquinol and S.M.O.N. *Lancet* 1978;2:945.
18. McFee RB, Caraccio TR, Mofenson HC. Selected tricyclic antidepressant ingestions involving children 6 years old or less. *Acad Emerg Med* 2001;8:139–144.
19. Saraf KR, Klein DF, Gittelman-Klein R, et al. Imipramine side effects in children. *Psychopharmacologia* 1974;37:265–274.
20. Forman HP, Levin S, Steward B, et al. Cerebral vasculitis and hemorrhage in an adolescent taking diet pills containing

phenylpropanolamine: case report and review of the literature. *Pediatrics* 1989;83:737–741.
21. Parsons AC. Piperazine neurotoxicity: worm wobble. *BMJ* 1971;4:792.
22. Lovejoy FH Jr, Mitchell AA, Goldman P. The management of propoxyphene poisoning. *J Pediatr* 1974;85:98–100.
23. Espelin D, Done A. Amphetamine poisoning. Effectiveness of chlorpromazine. *N Engl J Med* 1968;278:1361–1365.
24. Alldredge BK, Lowenstein DH, Simon RP. Seizures associated with recreational drug abuse. *Neurology* 1989;39:1037–1039.
25. Ellenhorn MJ, Schonwalf S, Ordog G, et al., eds. *Medical toxicology: diagnosis and treatment of human poisoning*. Baltimore: Williams & Wilkins, 1997.
26. Spencer PS, Schaumburg HH, Ludolph AC. *Experimental and clinical neurotoxicology*, 2nd ed. New York: Oxford University Press, 2000.
27. Pearn J, Nixon J, Ansford A, et al. Accidental poisoning in childhood. Five year urban population study with 15 year analysis of fatality. *BMJ* 1984;288:44–46.
28. Melis K, Bochener A. Acute poisoning in a children's hospital: an 8 year experience. *Acta Clin Belgica* 1990;13[Suppl.]:98 100.
29. Dana SL. *Lead diseases, a treatise from the French of L. Tanquerel des Planches*. Lowell, MA: D. Bixby Co, 1848.
30. Blackfan KD. Lead poisoning in children with especial reference to lead as a cause of convulsions. *Am J Med Sci* 1917;153:877–887.
31. Holt LE. Lead poisoning in infancy. *Am J Dis Child* 1923;25:229–233.
32. Mahaffey KR. Exposure to lead in childhood—the importance of prevention. *N Engl J Med* 1992;327:1308–1309.
33. Haynes EN, Kalwarf HJ, Hornung R, et al. Vitamin D receptor Fok1 polymorphism and blood lead concentration in children. *Environ Health Perspect* 2003;111:1665–1169.
34. Raghavan SRV, Gonick HC. Isolation of a low-molecular-weight lead-binding protein from human erythrocytes. *Proc Soc Exp Biol Med* 1977;155:164–167.
35. Rabinovitz MB, Wetherill GW, Kopple JD. Lead metabolism in the normal human. Stable isotope studies. *Science* 1973;182:725–727.
36. Klaassen CD. Heavy metals and heavy-metal antagonists. In: Hardman JG, Limbird LE, Gilman AG, eds. *Goodman and Gilman's the pharmacologic basis of therapeutics*, 10th ed. New York: McGraw-Hill, 2001:1851–1857.
37. Landrigan PJ, Graef JW. Pediatric lead poisoning in 1987: the silent epidemic continues. *Pediatrics* 1987;79:582–583.
38. Lidsky TI, Schneider JS. Lead neurotoxicity in children: basic mechanisms and clinical correlates. *Brain* 2003;126:5–19.
39. Pocock SJ, Smith M, Baghurst P. Environmental lead and children's intelligence: a systematic review of the epidemiological evidence. *BMJ* 1994;309:1189–1197.
40. American Academy of Pediatrics, Committee on Environmental Hazards. Statement on childhood lead poisoning. *Pediatrics* 1987;79:457–465.
41. Warren MJ, Cooper JB, Wood SP, et al. Lead poisoning, haem synthesis and 5-aminolaevulinic acid dehydratase. *Trends Biochem Sci* 1998:23:217–221.
42. Pentschew A. Morphology and morphogenesis of lead encephalopathy. *Acta Neuropathol* 1965;5:133–160.
43. Verity MA. Comparative observations on inorganic and organic lead neurotoxicity. *Environ Health Persp* 1990;89:43–48.
44. Winder C, Garten LL, Lewis PD. The morphological effects of lead on the developing central nervous system. *Neuropath Appl Neurobiol* 1983;9:87–108.
45. Behse F, Carlsen F. Histology and ultrastructure of alterations in neuropathy. *Muscle Nerve* 1978;1:368–374.
46. Thomas PK, Landon DN, King R. Diseases of the peripheral nerves. In: Graham DI, Lantos PL, eds. *Greenfield's neuropathology*, 6 th ed. London: Edward Arnold, Ltd., 1997:417–419.
47. Blackman SS. Intranuclear inclusion bodies in the kidney and liver caused by lead poisoning. *Bull Johns Hopkins Hosp* 1936;58:384–403.
48. Freeman R. Chronic lead poisoning in children: a review of 90 children diagnosed in Sydney 1948–1967. 2. Clinical features and investigations. *Med J Aust* 1970;1:648–651.
49. Mellins RB, Jenkins CD. Epidemiologic and psychological study of lead poisoning in children. *JAMA* 1955;158:15–20.
50. Jenkins CD, Mellins RB. Lead poisoning in children. *Arch Neurol Psychiatry* 1957;77:70–78.
51. Mirando EH, Ranasinghe L. Lead encephalopathy in children: uncommon clinical aspects. *Med J Aust* 1970;2:966–968.
52. Imbus CE, Warner J, Smith E, et al. Peripheral neuropathy in lead-intoxicated sickle cell patients. *Muscle Nerve* 1978;1:168–171.
53. Park EA, Jackson D, Kajdi L. Shadows produced by lead in x-ray pictures of growing skeleton. *Am J Dis Child* 1931;41:485–499.
54. Smith M. The effects of low-level lead exposure on children. In: Smith MA, Grant LD, Sors AI, eds. *Lead exposure and child development: an international assessment*. London: Kluwer Academic Publishers, 1989:347.
55. Baghurst PA, McMichael AJ, Wigg NR, et al. Environmental exposure to lead and children's intelligence at the age of seven years. The Port Pirie Cohort Study. *N Engl J Med* 1992;327:1279–1284.
56. Canfield RL, Henderson CR, Cory-Slechta DA, et al. Intellectual impairment in children with blood lead concentrations below 10 microg per deciliter. *N Engl J Med* 2003;348:1517–1526.
57. Graziano JH. Validity of lead-exposure markers in diagnosis and surveillance. *Clin Chem* 1994;40:1387–1390.
58. Stanton NV, Jones R. Evaluation of filter paper blood lead methods: results of a pilot proficiency testing program. *Clin Chem* 1999;45:2229–2235.
59. de la Burde B, Choat MS. Early asymptomatic lead exposure and development at school age. *J Pediatr* 1975;87:638–642.
60. Markowitz ME, Sinnett M, Rosen JF. A randomized trial of calcium supplementation for childhood lead poisoning. *Pediatrics* 2004;113(1Pt 1):e34–39.
61. Rogan WE, Dietrich KN, Ware JH, et al. The effect of chelation therapy with succimer on neuropsychological development in children exposed to lead. *N Engl J Med* 2001;344:1421–1426.
62. Committee on Drugs, American Academy of Pediatrics. Treatment guidelines for lead exposure in children. *Pediatrics* 1995;96:155–260.
63. Piomelli S. Childhood lead poisoning. *Pediatr Clin North Am* 2002;49:1285–1304.
64. Henretig FN. Lead. In: Goldfrank LR, Flomenbaum NE, Lewin NA, et al., eds. *Goldfrank's Toxicologic Emergencies*, 7th ed. New York: McGraw-Hill, 2002:1200–1227.
65. Friedman JA, Weinberger HL. Six children with lead poisoning. *J Pediatr* 1988;112:799–804.
66. Cavanagh JB. What have we learned from Graham Fredrick Young? Reflections on the mechanism of thallium neurotoxicity. *Neuropath Appl Neurobiol* 1991;17:3–9.
67. Bank WJ, Pleasure DE, Suzuki K, et al. Thallium poisoning. *Arch Neurol* 1972;26:456–464.
68. Yokoyama K, Araki S, Abe H. Distribution of nerve conduction velocities in acute thallium poisoning. *Muscle Nerve* 1990;13:117–120.
69. Cavanagh JB, Fuller NH, Johnson HR, et al. The effects of thallium salts, with particular reference to the nervous system changes. *Quart J Med* 1974;43:293–319.
70. Meggs WJ, Hoffman RS, Shi RD, et al. Thallium poisoning from maliciously contaminated food. *J Toxicol Clin Toxicol* 1994;32:723–730.
71. Wainwright AP, Kox WJ, House IM, et al. Clinical features and therapy of acute thallium poisoning. *Quart J Med* 1988;69:939–944.
72. Pai V. Acute thallium poisoning. Prussian blue therapy in 9 cases. *West Indian Med J* 1987;36:256–258.
73. Kersjes MP, Maurer JR, Trestrail JH, et al. An analysis of arsenic exposures referred to the Blodget Regional Poison Center. *Vet Hum Toxicol* 1987;29:75–78.
74. Ratnaike RN. Acute and chronic arsenic toxicity. *Postgrad Med J* 2003;79:391–396.
75. Rahman MM, Chowdhury UK, Mukherjee SC, et al. Chronic arsenic toxicity in Bangladesh and West Bengal, India—a review and commentary. *J Toxicol Clin Toxicol* 2001;39:683–700.
76. Russell DS. Changes in the central nervous system following arsphenamine medication. *J Pathol* 1937;45:357–366.
77. Ohta M. Ultrastructure of sural nerve in a case of arsenic neuropathy. *Acta Neuropathol* 1970;16:233–242.

78. Gorby MS. Arsenic poisoning. *West J Med* 1988;49:308–315.
79. Cullen NM, Wolf LR, St Clair D. Pediatric arsenic ingestion. *Am J Emerg Med* 1995;13:432–435.
80. Mazumder G, De BK, Santra A, et al. Randomized placebo-controlled trial of 2,3-dimercapto-1-propanesulfonate (DMPS) in therapy of chronic arsenicosis due to drinking arsenic-contaminated water. *J Toxicol Clin Toxicol* 2001;39:665–674.
81. Ford MD. Arsenic. In: Goldfrank LR, Flomenbaum NE, Lewin NA, et al., eds. *Goldfrank's Toxicologic Emergencies*, 7th ed. New York: McGraw-Hill, 2002:1183–1195.
82. Cheek DB. Pink disease (infantile acrodynia). *J Pediatr* 1953;42: 239–260.
83. Agocs MM, Etzel RA, Parrish RG, et al. Mercury exposure from interior latex paint. *N Engl J Med* 1990;323:1096–1101.
84. Amin-Zaki L, Majeed MA, Clarkson TW, et al. Methylmercury poisoning in Iraqi children: clinical observation over 2 years. *BMJ* 1978;1:613–616.
85. Elhassani SB. The many faces of methylmercury poisoning. *J Toxicol Clin Toxicol* 1983;19:875–906.
86. Korogi Y, Takahashi M, Hirai T, et al. Representation of the visual field in the striate cortex: comparison of MR findings with visual field deficits in organic mercury poisoning. *Am J Neuroradiol* 1997;18:1127–1130.
87. Kurland LT, Faro SN, Siedler H. Minimata disease. *World Neurol* 1960;1:370–395.
88. Snyder RD. Congenital mercury poisoning. *N Engl J Med* 1971;284:1014–1016.
89. Marsh DO, Turner MD, Smith JC, et al. Fetal methylmercury poisoning: clinical and toxicological data on 29 cases. *Ann Neurol* 1980;7:348–353.
90. Steuerwald U, Weihe R, Jurgensen PJ, et al. Maternal seafood diet, methylmercury exposure, and neonatal neurologic function. *J Pediatr* 2000:136:599–605.
91. Murata K, Weihe P, Budtz-Jorgensen E, et al. Delayed brainstem auditory evoked potential latencies in 14-year-old children exposed to methylmercury. *J Pediatr* 2004;144:177–183.
92. Myers G, Davidson PW, Cox C, et al. Prenatal methylmercury exposure from ocean fish consumption in the Seychelles child development study. *Lancet* 2003;361:1686–1692.
92a. Risher JF, Murray E, Prince GR. Organic mercury compounds: human exposure and its relevance to public health. *Toxicology Industr Health* 2002;18:109–160.
93. Ball LK, Ball R, Pratt RD. An assessment of thimerosal use in childhood vaccines. *Pediatrics* 2001;107:1147–1154.
93a. Andrews N, Miller E, Grant A, et al. Thiomerosal exposure in infants and developmental disorders: a retrospective cohort study in the United Kingdom does not support a causal association. *Pediatrics* 2004;114:584–591.
94. Nelson KB, Bauman ML. Thimerosal and autism. *Pediatrics* 2003;111:674–679.
94a. Parker SK, Schwartz B, Todd J, et al. Thimerosal-containing vaccines and autistic spectrum disorder: a critical review of published original data. *Pediatrics* 2004;114:793–804.
95. Takeuchi T, Eto N, Eto K. Neuropathology of childhood cases of methylmercury poisoning (Minimata disease) with prolonged symptoms, with particular reference to the decortication syndrome. *Neurotoxicology* 1979;1:120.
96. Aposhian HV. DMSA and DMPS—water soluble antidotes for heavy metal poisoning. *Annu Rev Pharmacol Toxicol* 1983;23:193–215.
97. Nierenberg DW, Nordgren RE, Chang MB, et al. Delayed cerebellar disease and death after accidental exposure to dimethylmercury. *N Engl J Med* 1998;338:1672–1676.
98. Normandin L, Hazell AS. Manganese neurotoxicity: an update of pathophysiologic mechanisms. *Metab Brain Dis* 2002;17:375–387.
99. Fell JM, Reynolds AP, Meadows N, et al. Manganese toxicity in children receiving long-term parenteral nutrition. *Lancet* 1996;374:1218–1221.
100. Lucchini R, Albini E, Placidi D, et al. Brain magnetic resonance imaging and manganese exposure. *Neurotoxicology* 2000;21:769–775.
101. Auer RN, Benveniste H. Hypoxia and related conditions. In: Graham DI, Lantos PL, eds. *Greenfield's neuropathology*, 6 th ed. London: Edward Arnold, Ltd., 1997:275–276.
102. Kim JK, Coe CJ. Clinical study on carbon monoxide intoxication in children. *Yonsie Med J* 1987;28:266–273.
102a. Prockop LD. Carbon monoxide brain toxicity: clinical, magnetic resonance imaging, magnetic resonance spectroscopy, and neuropsychological effects in 9 people. *J Neuroimaging* 2005;15:144–149.
103. Khan K, Sharief N. Chronic carbon monoxide poisoning in children. *Acta Paediatr* 1995;84:742.
104. Zimmerman SS, Truxal B. Carbon monoxide poisoning. *Pediatrics* 1981;68:215–224.
105. Choi IS. Delayed neurologic sequelae in carbon monoxide intoxication. *Arch Neurol* 1983;40:433–435.
106. Ernst A, Zibrak JD. Carbon monoxide poisoning. *N Engl J Med* 1998;339:1603–1608.
107. Kim JH, Chang KH, Song IC, et al. Delayed encephalopathy of acute carbon monoxide intoxication: diffusivity of cerebral white matter lesions. *Am J Neuroradiol* 2003;24:1592–1597.
108. Thom SR. Carbon monoxide–mediated brain lipid peroxidation in the rat. *J Appl Physiol* 1990;68:997–1003.
109. Liebelt EL. Hyperbaric oxygen thrapy in childhood carbon monoxide poisoning. *Curr Opin Pediatr* 1999;11:259–264.
110. Ginsberg MD, Myers RE. Fetal brain injury after maternal carbon monoxide intoxication. Clinical and neuropathologic aspects. *Neurology* 1976;26:15–23.
111. Longo LD. The biological effects of carbon monoxide on the pregnant woman, fetus and newborn infant. *Am J Obstet Gynecol* 1977;129:69–103.
112. Carpenter WV. *Use and abuse of alcoholic liquors*. Boston: Crosby & Nichols, 1851.
113. Heuyer G, Mises R, Dereux JF, et al. La descendance des alcooliques. *La Presse Med* 1957;29:657–658.
114. Lemoine P, Harousseau H, Borteyru J. Les enfants de parents alcooliques: anomalies observées. *Ouest Médicale* 1968;25:476–482.
115. Clarren SK, Smith DW. The fetal alcohol syndrome. *N Engl J Med* 1978;298:1063–1067.
116. Sampson PD, Streissguth AP, Bookstein FL, et al. Incidence of fetal alcohol syndrome and prevalence of alcohol-related neurodevelopmental disorder. *Teratology* 1997;56:317–326.
117. Olney JW, Wozniak DF, Jevtovic-Todorovic V, et al. Drug-induced apoptotic neurodegeneration in the developing brain. *Brain Pathol* 2002;12:488–498.
118. West JR, Chen WJ, Pantazis NJ. Fetal alcohol syndrome: the vulnerability of the developing brain and possible mechanisms of damage. *Metab Brain Dis* 1995;9:291–322.
119. Shibley IA, Pennington SN. Metabolic and mitotic changes associated with the fetal alcohol syndrome. *Alcohol Alcohol* 1997;32:423–434.
120. Davies M. The role of $GABA_A$ receptors in mediating the effects of alcohol in the central nervous system. *J Psychiatry Neurosci* 2003;28:263–274.
121. Forrest F, Florey C. The relation between maternal alcohol consumption and child development: the epidemiological evidence. *J Publ Health Med* 1991;13:247–255.
122. Zuckerman B, Bresnahan K. Developmental and behavioral consequences of prenatal drug and alcohol exposure. *Pediatr Clin North Am* 1991;38:1387–1406.
123. Day NL, Richardson GA. Prenatal alcohol exposure: a continuum of effects. *Semin Perinatol* 1991;15:271–279.
124. Chambers CD, Jones KL. Is genotype important in predicting the fetal alcohol syndrome? *J Pediatr* 2002;141:751–752.
125. Wisniewski K, Dambska M, Sher JH, et al. A clinical neuropathological study of the fetal alcohol syndrome. *Neuropediatrics* 1983;14:197–201.
126. Ferrer I, Galofre E. Dendritic spine anomalies in fetal alcohol syndrome. *Neuropediatrics* 1987;18:161–163.
127. Archibald SL, Fennema-Notestine C, Gamst A, et al. Brain dysmorphology in individuals with severe prenatal alcohol exposure. *Dev Med Child Neurol* 2001;43:148–154.
128. Autti-Rämö I, Autti T, Korkman M, et al. MRI findings in children with school problems who had been exposed prenatally to alcohol. *Dev Med Child Neurol* 2002;44:98–106.

129. Konovalov HV, Kovetsky NS, Bobryshev YK, et al. Disorders of brain development in the progeny of mothers who used alcohol during pregnancy. *Early Human Development* 1997;48:153–166.
130. Autti-Rämö I, Gaily E, Granström M-L. Dysmorphic features in offspring of alcoholic mothers. *Arch Dis Child* 1992;67:712–716.
131. Sokol RJ, Clarren SK. Guidelines for use of terminology describing the impact of prenatal alcohol on the offspring. *Alcoholism* 1989;13:597–598.
132. Aase JM, Jones KL, Clarren SK. Do we need the term "FAE"? *Pediatrics* 1995;95:428–430.
133. Pinazo-Duran MD, Renau-Piqueras J, Guerri C, et al. Optic nerve hypoplasia in fetal alcohol syndrome: an update. *Eur J Ophthalmol* 1997;7:262–270.
134. Strömland K, Hellström A. Fetal alcohol syndrome—an opthalmological and socioeducational prospective study. *Pediatrics* 1996;97:845–850.
135. Peiffer J, Majewski F, Fischbach H, et al. Alcohol embryo- and fetopathy. *J Neurol Sci* 1979;41:125–137.
136. Nitowsky HM. Fetal alcohol syndrome and alcohol-related birth defects. *NY State J Med* 1982;82:1214–1217.
137. Autti-Rämö I, Korkman M, Hilakivi-Clarke L, et al. Mental development of 2-year-old children exposed to alcohol *in utero*. *J Pediatr* 1992;120:740–746.
138. Spohr H-L, Willms J, Steinhausen H-C. Prenatal alcohol exposure and long-term developmental consequences. *Lancet* 1993;341:907–910.
139. Mattsen SN, Riley EP, Gramling L, et al. Heavy prenatal alcohol exposure with or without physical features of fetal alcohol syndrome leads to IQ deficits. *J Pediatr* 1997;131:718–721.
140. Shaywitz SE, Caparulo B, Hodgson ES. Developmental language disability as a result of prenatal exposure to ethanol. *Pediatrics* 1981;68:850–855.
141. Larsson G, Bohlin A-B, Tunell R. Prospective study of children exposed to variable amounts of alcohol in utero. *Arch Dis Child* 1985;60:316–321.
142. Vogel C, Caraccio T, Mofenson H, et al. Alcohol intoxication in young children. *J Toxicol Clin Toxicol* 1995;33:25–33.
143. Cummins LH. Hypoglycemia and convulsions in children following alcohol ingestion. *J Pediatr* 1961;58:23–26.
144. Wilson NM, Brown PM, Juul SM, et al. Glucose turnover and metabolic and hormonal changes in ethanol-induced hypoglycaemia. *BMJ* 1981;282:849.
145. Young D, Dragunow M. Status epilepticus may be caused by loss of adenosine anticonvulsant mechanisms. *Neuroscience* 1994;58:245–261.
146. Bahls FH, Ma KK, Bird TD. Theophylline-associated seizures with "therapeutic" or low toxic serum concentrations: risk factors for serious outcome in adults. *Neurology* 1991;41:1309–1312.
147. Baker MD. Theophylline toxicity in children. *J Pediatr* 1986;109: 538–542.
148. Pranzatelli MR, Albin RL, Cohen BH. Acute dyskinesias in young asthmatics treated with theophylline. *Pediatr Neurol* 1991;7:216–219.
149. Shields MD, Hicks EM, Macgregor DF, et al. Infantile spasms associated with theophylline toxicity. *Acta Paediatr* 1995;84:215–217.
150. Skopnik H, Bergt U, Heimann G. Neonatal theophylline intoxication: pharmacokinetics and clinical evaluation. *Eur J Pediatr* 1992;151:221–224.
151. Olsen RW, Sapp DM, Bureau MH, et al. Allosteric actions of central nervous system depressants including anesthetics on subtypes of the inhibitory g-aminobutyric acid A receptor-chloride channel complex. *Ann NY Acad Sci* 1991;625:145–154.
152. McCarron MM, Schulze BW, Walberg CB, et al. Short-acting barbiturate overdosage. Correlation of intoxication score with serum barbiturate concentration. *JAMA* 1982;248:55–61.
153. Mitchell AA, Lovejoy FH, Goldman P. Drug ingestions associated with miosis in comatose children. *J Pediatr* 1976;89:303–305.
154. Lorber J, Reckless JPD, Watson JBG. Nonaccidental poisoning: the elusive diagnosis. *Arch Dis Child* 1980;55:643–647.
155. Mann JB, Sandberg DH. Therapy of sedative overdosage. *Pediatr Clin North Am* 1970;17:617–628.
156. Bertino JS Jr, Reed MD. Barbiturate and nonbarbiturate sedative hypnotic intoxication in children. *Pediatr Clin North Am* 1986;33:703–722.
157. Palmer BF. Effectiveness of hemodialysis in the extracorporeal therapy of phenobarbital overdose. *Am J Kidney Dis* 2000;36:640–643.
158. Sancak R, Kucukoduk S, Tasdemir HA, et al. Exchange transfusion treatment in a newborn with phenobarbital intoxication. *Pediatr Emerg Care* 1999;15:268–270.
159. James LP, Abel K, Wilkinson J, et al. Phenothiazine, butyrophenone, and other psychotropic medication poisonings in children and adolescents. *J Toxicol Clin Toxicol* 2000:38:615–623.
160. Knight ME, Roberts RJ. Phenothiazine and butyrophenone intoxication in children. *Pediatr Clin North Am* 1986;33:299–309.
161. Kiriakakis V, Bhatia KP, Quinn NP, et al. The natural history of tardive dystonia. A long-term follow-up study of 107 cases. *Brain* 1998;121:2053–2066.
162. Richardson MA, Small AM, Read LL, et al. Branched chain amino acid treatment of tardive dyskinesia in children and adolescents. *J Clin Psychiatry* 2004;65:92–96.
163. Lev R, Clark RF. Neuroleptic malignant syndrome presenting without fever: case report and review of the literature. *J Emerg Med* 1994;12:49–55.
164. Heiman-Patterson TD. Neuroleptic malignant syndrome and malignant hyperthermia. Important issues for the medical consultant. *Med Clin North Am* 1993;77:477–492.
165. Shields WD, Bray PF. A danger of haloperidol therapy in children. *J Pediatr* 1976;88:301–303.
166. Guze BH, Guze PA. Psychotropic medication use during pregnancy. *West J Med* 1989;151:296–298.
167. Rosebush PI, Stewart T, Mazurek MF. The treatment of neuroleptic malignant syndrome. Are dantrolene and bromocriptine useful adjuncts to supportive care? *Br J Psychiatry* 1991;159:709–712.
168. Thomas RJ. Neurotoxicity of antibacterial therapy. *Southern Med J* 1994;87:869–874.
169. Wallace KL. Antibiotic-induced convulsions. *Crit Care Clin* 1997;13:741–762.
170. Tsuda A, Ito M, Kishi K, et al. Effect of penicillin on GABA-gated chloride ion influx. *Neurochem Res* 1994;19:1–4.
171. Fausti SA, Larson VD, Noffsinger D, et al. High frequency audiometric monitoring for early detection of aminoglycoside ototoxicity. *J Infect Dis* 1992;165:1026–1032.
172. Guan MX, Fischel-Ghodsian N, Attardi G. A biochemical basis for the inherited susceptibility to aminoglycoside ototoxicity. *Hum Mol Genet* 2000;22:1787–1793.
173. Kaeser HE. Drug-induced myasthenic syndromes. *Acta Neurol Scand Suppl* 1984;100:39–47.
174. Zwiener RJ, Ginsberg CM. Organophosphate and carbamate poisoning in infants and children. *Pediatrics* 1988;81:121–126.
175. Senanayake N, Karalliede L. Neurotoxic effects of organophosphorus insecticides. An intermediate syndrome. *N Engl J Med* 1987;316:761–763.
176. Moretto A, Lotti M. Poisoning by organophosphorus insecticides and sensory neuropathy. *J Neurol Neurosurg Psychiatry* 1998;64:463–468.
177. O'Malley M. Clinical evaluation of pesticide exposure and poisonings. *Lancet* 1997;349:1161–1166.
178. Mortenson ML. Management of acute childhood poisoning caused by selected insecticides and herbicides. *Pediatr Clin North Am* 1986;33:421–445.
179. Narahashi T, Frey JM, Ginsburg KS, et al. Sodium and GABA-activated channels as the targets of pyrethroids and cyclodienes. *Toxicol Lett* 1992;64–65:429 436.
180. Waller K, Predergast TJ, Slagle A, et al. Seizures after eating a snack food contaminated with the pesticide endrin. The tale of toxic taquitos. *West J Med* 1992;157:648–651.
181. Rowley DL, Rab MA, Hardjotanojo W, et al. Convulsions caused by endrin poisoning in Pakistan. *Pediatrics* 1987;79:928–934.
182. Aks SE, Krantz A, Hryhrczuk DO, et al. Acute accidental lindane ingestion in toddlers. *Ann Emerg Med* 1995;26:647–651.
183. Schwartz RH, Miller NS. MDMA (ecstasy) and the rave: a review. *Pediatrics* 1997;100:705–708.
184. Yacoubian GS. Correlates of ecstasy use among tenth graders

surveyed though Monitoring the Future. *J Psychoactive Drugs* 2002;34:225–230.

185. Auer J, Berent R, Weber T, et al. Subarachnoid haemorrhage with "Ecstasy" abuse in a young adult. *Neurol Sci*. 2002;23:199–201.
186. Kulberg A. Substance abuse: clinical identification and management. *Pediatr Clin North Am* 1986;33:325–361.
187. Schwartz RH, Einhorn A. PCP intoxication in seven young children. *Pediatr Emerg Care* 1986;2:238–241.
188. Cooper AJ, Egleston CV. Accidental ingestion of ecstasy by a toddler: unusual cause for convulsion in a febrile child. *J Acid Emerg Med* 1997;14:183–184.
189. Kimbrough RD. Review of recent evidence of toxic effects of hexachlorophene. *Pediatrics* 1973;51:391–394.
190. Martinez AJ, Boehm R, Hadfield MG. Acute hexachlorophene encephalopathy: cliniconeuropathological correlation. *Acta Neuropathol* 1974;28:92–103.
191. Martin-Bouyer G, Lebreton R, Toga M, et al. Outbreak of accidental hexachlorophene poisoning in France. *Lancet* 1982;28:93–103.
192. Hillman LS, Hillman RE, Dodson WE. Diagnosis, treatment and follow-up of neonatal mepivacaine intoxication secondary to paracervical and pudendal blocks during labor. *J Pediatr* 1979;95:472–477.
193. Chan TY. The risk of severe salicylate poisoning following the ingestion of topical medicaments or aspirin. *Postgrad Med J* 1996;72:109–112.
194. Done AK. Aspirin overdosage: incidence, diagnosis, and management. *Pediatrics* 1978;62[5 Pt 2 Suppl.]:890 897.
195. Dove DJ, Jones T. Delayed coma associated with salicylate intoxication. *J Pediatr* 1982;100:493–496.
196. Heiman-Patterson TD, Bird SJ, Parry GJ, et al. Peripheral neuropathy associated with eosinophilia-myalgia syndrome. *Ann Neurol* 1990;28:522–528.
197. Tolander LM, Bamford CR, Yoshino MT, et al. Neurologic complications of the tryptophan-associated eosinophilia-myalgia syndrome. *Arch Neurol* 1991;48:436–438.
198. de la Paz P, Philen RM, Borda AI. Toxic oil syndrome: the perspective after 20 years. *Epidemiol Rev* 2001;23:231–247.
199. Tilson HA, Jacobson JL, Rogan WJ. Polychlorinated biphenyls and the developing nervous system: cross-species comparisons. *Neurotoxicol Teratol* 1990;12:239–248.
200. Chasnoff IJ, Griffith DR, Freier C, et al. Cocaine/polydrug use in pregnancy: two-year follow-up. *Pediatrics* 1992;89:284–289.
201. King TA, Perlman JM, Laptook AR, et al. Neurologic manifestations of *in utero* cocaine exposure in near-term and term infants. *Pediatrics* 1995;96:259–264.
202. Bateman DA, Chiriboga CA. Dose-response effect of cocaine on newborn head circumference. *Pediatrics* 2000;106:E33.
203. Dominguez R, Vila-Coro A, Slopis JM, et al. Brain and ocular abnormalities in infants with in utero exposure to cocaine and other street drugs. *Am J Dis Child* 1991;145:688–695.
204. Oro AS, Dixon SD. Perinatal cocaine and methamphetamine exposure: maternal and neonatal correlates. *J Pediatr* 1987;111:571–578.
205. Doberczak TM, Shanzer S, Senie RT, et al. Neonatal neurologic and electroencephalographic effects of intrauterine cocaine exposure. *J Pediatr* 1988;113:354–358.
206. Kramer LD, Locke GE, Ogunyemi A, et al. Neonatal cocaine-related seizures. *J Child Neurol* 1990;5:60–64.
207. Beltran RS, Coker SR. Transient dystonia of infancy, a result of intrauterine cocaine exposure? *Pediatr Neurol* 1995;12:354–356.
208. Dixon SD, Bejar R. Echoencephalographic findings in neonates associated with maternal cocaine and methamphetamine use: incidence and clinical correlates. *J Pediatr* 1989;115:770–778.
209. Wasserman GA, Kline JK, Baeman DA, et al. Prenatal cocaine exposure and school-age intelligence. *Drug Alchol Depend* 1998;50:203–210.
210. Frank DA, Augustyn M, Knight WG, et al. Growth, development, and behavior in early childhood following prenatal cocaine exposure: a systematic review. *J Am Med Assoc* 2001;285:1613–1625.
211. Hurt H, Malmud E, Betancourt I, et al. Children with *in utero* cocaine exposure do not differ from control subjects on intelligence testing. *Arch Pediatr Adolesc Med* 1997;151:1237–1241.
212. Mott SH, Packer RJ, Soldin SJ. Neurologic manifestations of cocaine exposure in children. *Pediatrics* 1994;93:557–560.
213. Vargas GC, Pildes RS, Vidyasagar D, et al. Effect of maternal heroin addiction on 67 liveborn neonates. *Clin Pediatr* 1975;14:751–753.
214. Zelson C, Rubio E, Wasserman E. Neonatal narcotic addiction: 10-year observation. *Pediatrics* 1971;48:178–189.
215. Schulman CA. Alterations of the sleep cycle in heroin addicted and "suspect" newborns. *Neuropädiatrie* 1969;1:89–100.
216. Ostrea EM, Chavez CJ, Strauss ME. A study of factors that influence the severity of neonatal narcotic withdrawal. *J Pediatr* 1976;88:642–645.
217. Cepeda EE, Lee MI, Mehdizadeh B. Decreased incidence of intraventricular hemorrhage in infants of opiate dependent mothers. *Scand Acta Paediatr* 1987;76:16–18.
218. Yaster M, Kost-Byerly S, Berde C, et al. The management of opioid and benzodiazepine dependence in infants, children and adolescents. *Pediatrics* 1996;98:135–140.
219. Vance JC, Chant DC, Tudehope DI, et al. Infants born to narcotic dependent mothers: physical growth patterns in the first 12 months of life. *J Paediatr Child Health* 1997;33:504–508.
220. Ostrea EM, Ostrea AR, Simpson PM. Mortality within the first 2 years in infants exposed to cocaine, opiate, or cannabinoid during gestation. *Pediatrics* 1997;100:79–83.
221. Kaltenbach K, Finnegan LP. Perinatal and developmental outcome of infants exposed to methadone *in utero*. *Neurotoxicol Teratol* 1987;9:311–313.
222. Wilson GS, McCreary R, Kean J, et al. The development of preschool children of heroin-addicted mothers: a controlled study. *Pediatrics* 1979;63:135–141.
223. Ornoy A, Michailevskaya V, Lukashov I, et al. The developmental outcome of children born to heroin-dependent mothers, raised at home or adopted. *Child Abuse Negl* 1996;20:385–396.
224. Schmorl G. Zur Kenntnis des Ikterus neonatorum insbesondere der dabei auftretenden Gehirnveränderungen. *Verh Dtsch Ges Pathol* 1903;6:109–115.
225. Haymaker W, et al. Pathology of kernicterus and posticteric encephalopathy. In: American Academy for Cerebral Palsy. *Kernicterus and its importance in cerebral palsy*. Springfield, IL: Charles C Thomas, 1961:210–228.
226. Turkel SB, Miller CA, Guttenberg ME, et al. A clinical pathologic reappraisal of kernicterus. *Pediatrics* 1982;69:267–272.

226a. Hanko E, Hansen WR, Almaas R, et al. Bilirubin indices apoptosis and necrosis in human NT2-N neurons. *Pediatr Res* 2005;57:179–184.

227. Hascoet JM. Control of brain intracellular bilirubin levels. *Pediatr Res* 2003;54:439–440.
228. Hsia DYY, Allen FH Jr, Gellis SS, et al. Erythroblastosis fetalis. VIII. Studies of serum bilirubin in relation to kernicterus. *N Engl J Med* 1952;247:668–671.
229. Newman TB, Maisels MJ. Evaluation and treatment of jaundice in the term newborn: a kinder, gentler approach. *Pediatrics* 1992;89:809–818.
230. Johnson LH, Bhutani VK, Brown AK. System-based approach to management of neonatal jaundice and prevention of kernicterus. *J Pediatr* 2002;140:396–403.
231. Rubin RA, Balow B, Fisch RO. Neonatal serum bilirubin levels related to cognitive development at ages 4 through 7 years. *J Pediatr* 1979;94:601–604.
232. Johnston WH, Angara V, Baumal R, et al. Erythroblastosis fetalis and hyperbilirubinemia: a five-year follow-up with neurological, psychological and audiological evaluation. *Pediatrics* 1967;39:88–92.
233. Scheidt PC, Graubard BI, Nelson KB, et al. Intelligence at six years in relation to neonatal bilirubin level: follow-up of the National Institute of Child Health and Human Development clinical trial of phototherapy. *Pediatrics* 1991;87:797–805.
234. Maisels MJ, Newman TB. Kernicterus in otherwise healthy, breast-fed term newborns. *Pediatrics* 1995;96:730–733.
235. Blumenschein SD, Kallen RJ, Storey B, et al. Familial nonhemolytic jaundice with late onset of neurological damage. *Pediatrics* 1968;42:786–792.
236. Kadakol A, Ghoss SS, Sappal BS, et al. Genetic lesions of bilirubin uridine-diphosphoglucuronate glucuronosyltransferase

(UGT1A1) causing Crigler-Najjar and Gilbert syndromes: correlation of genotype to phenotype. *Hum Mutat* 2000;16:297–306.
237. Shevell MI, Majnemer A, Schiff D. Neurologic perspectives of Crigler-Najjar syndrome type I. *J Child Neurol* 1998;13:265–269.
238. Fox IJ, Chowdhury JR, Kaufman SS, et al. Treatment of the Crigler-Najjar syndrome Type I with hepatocyte transplantation. *N Engl J Med* 1998;338:1422–1426.
239. Pearlman MA, Gartner LM, Lee K, et al. The association of kernicterus with bacterial infection in the newborn. *Pediatrics* 1980;65:26–29.
240. Bratlid D, Cashore WJ, Oh W. Effect of serum hyperosmolality on opening of blood–brain barrier for bilirubin in rat brain. *Pediatrics* 1983;71:909–912.
241. Levine RL, Fredericks WR, Rapoport SI. Entry of bilirubin into the brain due to opening of the blood–brain barrier. *Pediatrics* 1982;69:255–259.
242. Rodrigues CM, Sola S, Brites D. Bilirubin induces apoptosis via the mitochondrial pathway in developing rat brain neurons. *Hepatology* 2002;35:1186–1195.
243. Oh W, Tyson JE, Fanaroff AA, et al. Association between peak serum bilirubin and neurodevelopmental outcomes in extremely low birth weight infants. *Pediatrics* 2003;112:773–779.
244. Van der Bor M, Ens-Dokkum M, Schreuder AM, et al. Hyperbilirubinema in low birth weight infants and outcome at 5 years of age. *Pediatrics* 1992;89:359–364.
245. O'Shea TM, Dillard RG, Klinepeter KL, et al. Serum bilirubin levels, intracranial hemorrhage, and the risk of developmental problems in very low birth weight neonates. *Pediatrics* 1992;90:888–892.
246. Ahdab-Barmada M, Moossy J. The neuropathology of kernicterus in the premature neonate: diagnostic problems. *J Neuropath Exp Neurol* 1984;43:45–56.
247. Watchko JF, Classen D. Kernicterus in premature infants: current prevalence and relationship to NICHD Phototherapy Study Exchange Criteria. *Pediatrics* 1994;93:996–999.
248. Jardine DS, Rogers K. Relationship of benzyl alcohol to kernicterus, intraventricular hemorrhage, and mortality in preterm infants. *Pediatrics* 1989;83:153–160.
249. Boreau T, Mensch-Dechene J, Roux-Doutheret F. Etude clinique de 34 cas d'ictere nucléaire par maladie hémolytique néonatale et de leur évolution. *Arch Fr Pediatr* 1964;21:43–85.
250. Perlstein MA. The clinical syndrome of kernicterus. In: American Academy for Cerebral Palsy. *Kernicterus and its importance in cerebral palsy*. Springfield, IL: Charles C Thomas, 1961:268–279.
251. Byers RK, Paine RS, Crothers B. Extrapyramidal cerebral palsy with hearing loss following erythroblastosis. *Pediatrics* 1955;15:248–254.
252. Shapiro SM, Nakamura H. Bilirubin and the auditory system. *J Perinatol* 2001;21[Suppl. 1]:52 55.
253. Nakamura H, Takada S, Shimabuko R, et al. Auditory nerve and brainstem responses in newborn infants with hyperbilirubinemia. *Pediatrics* 1985;75:703–708.
254. Ogun B, Serbetcioglu B, Duman N, et al. Long-term outcome of neonatal hyperbilirubinaemia: subjective and objective audiological measures. *Clin Otolaryngol* 2003;28:507–513.
255. deVries LS, Laray S, Dubowitz LMS. Relationship of serum bilirubin to ototoxicity and deafness in high-risk low-birth-weight infants. *Pediatrics* 1985;76:351–354.
256. Yokochi K. Magnetic resonance imaging in children with kernicterus. *Acta Paediatr* 1995;84:937–939.
257. Gourley GR. Bilirubin metabolism and kernicterus. *Adv Pediatr* 1997;44:173–229.
258. Tonello F, Morante S, Rosetto O, et al. Tetanus and botulism neurotoxins: a novel group of zinc-endopeptidases. *Adv Exp Med Biol* 1996;389:251–260.
259. Lalli G, Bohnert S, Deinhart K, et al. The journey of tetus and botulinum neurotoxin in neurons. *Trends Microbiol* 2003:11:431–437.
260. Goldfrank LR, Flomenbaum NE. Botulism. In: Goldfrank LR, Flomenbaum NE, Lewin NA, et al., eds. *Goldfrank's Toxicologic Emergencies*, 7th ed. New York: McGraw-Hill, 2002:1100–1111.
261. Oh SJ. Botulism: electrophysiological studies. *Ann Neurol* 1977;1:481–485.
262. Keesey JC. Electrodiagnostic approach to defects in neuromuscular transmission. *Muscle Nerve* 1989;12:613–626.
263. Arnon SS. Infant botulism. *Annu Rev Med* 1980;31:541–560.
264. Clay SA, Ramseyer JC, Fishman LS, et al. Acute infantile motor unit disorder. Infantile botulism? *Arch Neurol* 1977;34:236–243.
265. Ravid S, Maytal J, Eviatar L. Biphasic course of infant botulism. *Pediatr Neurol* 2000;23:338–340.
266. Graf WD, Hays RM, Astley SJ, et al. Electrodiagnosis reliability in the diagnosis of infant botulism. *J Pediatr* 1992;120:745–749.
267. Cornblath DR, Sladky JT, Sumner A. Clinical electrophysiology of infantile botulism. *Muscle Nerve* 1983;6:448–452.
268. Cox N, Hinkle R. Infant botulism. *Am Fam Physician* 2002;65:1388–1392.
269. Arnon SS. Infant botulism: anticipating the second decade. *J Infect Dis* 1986;154:201–206.
270. Tardo C, Steele RW. Infant botulism. *Clin Pediatr* 1997;36:592–594.
271. Schreiner MS, Field E, Ruddy R. Infant botulism: a review of 12 years' experience at the Children's Hospital of Philadelphia. *Pediatrics* 1991;87:159–165.
272. Farrar JJ, Yen LM, Cook T, et al. Tetanus. *J Neurol Neurosurg Psychiatry* 2000:69:292–301.
273. Pierce EJ, Davison MD, Parton RG, et al. Characterization of tetanus toxin binding to rat brain membranes. Evidence for a high-affinity proteinase-sensitive receptor. *Biochem J* 1986;236:845–852.
274. Schwab ME, Suda K, Thoenen N. Selective retrograde transsynaptic transfer of a protein, tetanus toxin, subsequent to retrograde axonal transport. *J Cell Biol* 1979;82:798–810.
275. Ahnert-Hilger G, Bigalke H. Molecular aspects of tetanus and botulinum neurotoxin poisoning. *Prog Neurobiol* 1995;46:83–96.
276. Bergey GK, Bigalke H, Nelson PG. Differential effects of tetanus toxin on inhibitory and excitatory synaptic transmission in mammalian spinal cord neurons in culture: a presynaptic locus of action for tetanus toxin. *J Neurophysiol* 1987;57:121–131.
277. Udwadia FE, Lall A, Udwadia ZF, et al. Tetanus and its complications: intensive care and management experience in 150 Indian patients. *Epidemiol Infect* 1987;99:675–684.
278. Illis LS, Taylor FM. Neurological and electroencephalographic sequelae of tetanus. *Lancet* 1971;1:826–830.
279. Craig AS, Reed GW, Mohon RT, et al. Neonatal tetanus in the United States: a sentinel event in the foreign-born. *Pediatr Infect Dis J* 1997;16:955–959.
280. Salimpour R. Cause of death in tetanus neonatorum. Study of 233 cases with 54 necropsies. *Arch Dis Child* 1977;52:587–594.
281. Tompkins AB. Tetanus in African children. *Arch Dis Child* 1959;34:398–405.
282. Pinheiro D. Tetanus of the newborn infant. *Pediatrics* 1964;34:32–37.
283. Adams JM, Kenny JD, Rudolph AJ. Modern management of tetanus neonatorum. *Pediatrics* 1979;64:472–477.
284. Andersson R. High dose oral diazepam and early full alimentation in neonatal tetanus. *Tropical Doct* 1991;21:172–173.
285. Sanford JP. Tetanus—forgotten but not gone. *N Engl J Med* 1995;332:812–813.
286. Einterz EM, Bates ME. Caring for neonatal tetanus patients in a rural primary care setting in Nigeria: a review of 237 cases. *J Trop Pediatr* 1991;37:179–181.
287. Daud S, Mohammad T, Ahmad A. Tetanus neonatorum. *J Trop Pediatr* 1981;27:308–311.
288. Godel JC. Trial of pyridoxine therapy for tetanus neonatorum. *J Infect Dis* 982;145:547 549.
289. Anlar B, Yalaz K, Dizmen R. Long-term prognosis after neonatal tetanus. *Dev Med Child Neurol* 1989:31:76–80.
290. Singh M, Saidali A, Bakhtiar A, et al. Diphtheria in Afghanistan—review of 155 cases. *J Trop Med Hyg* 1985;88:373–376.
291. Fisher CM, Adams RD. Diphtheritic polyneuritis—a pathological study. *J Neuropath Exp Neurol* 1956;15:243–268.
292. London E. Diphtheria toxin: membrane interaction and membrane translocation. *Biochim Biophys Acta* 1992;1113:25–51.
293. Solders G, Nennesmo I, Persson A. Diphtheritic neuropathy, an analysis based on muscle and nerve biopsy and repeated neurophysiological and autonomic function tests. *J Neurol Neurosurg Psychiatry* 1989;52:876–880.
294. Tibballs J, Cooper SJ. Paralysis with Ixodes cornuatus envenomation. *Med J Aust* 1986;145:37–38.

295. Grattan-Smith PJ, Morris JG, Johnston HM, et al. Clinical and neurophysiological features of tick paralysis. *Brain* 1997;120:1975–1987.
296. Beyer AB, Grossman M. Tick paralysis in a red wolf. *J Wildl Dis* 1997;33:900–902.
297. Kincaid JC. Tick bite paralysis. *Semin Neurol* 1990;10:32–34.
298. Vedanarayanan VV. Evans OB, Subramony SH. Tick paralysis in children: electrophysiology and possibility of misdiagnosis. *Neurology* 2002;39:1088–1090.
299. Mushatt DM, Hyslop NE Jr. Neurologic aspects of North American zoonoses. *Infect Dis Clin North Am* 1991;5:703–731.
300. Adams ME, Swanson G. *Neurotoxins*, 2 nd ed. *Trends Neurosci* 1996;17[Suppl.]:S1–37.
301. Russell FE. *Snake venom poisoning*. Great Neck, NY: Scholium International, 1983.
302. Southcott RV. The neurologic effects of noxious marine creatures. In: Hornabrook RW, ed. *Topics on tropical neurology*. Philadelphia: FA Davis, 1975:165–258.
303. Campbell CH. The effects of snake venoms and their neurotoxins on the nervous system of man and animals. In: Hornabrook RW, ed. *Topics on tropical neurology*. Philadelphia: FA Davis, 1975:259–294.
304. Auerbach PS, ed. *Wilderness medicine: management of wilderness and environmental emergencies*, 4th ed. St. Louis: Mosby, 2001.
305. Gold BS, Dart RC, Barish RA. Bites of venomous snakes. *N Engl J Med* 2002:347:347–356.
306. Burnett JW, Bloom DA, Imafuku S, et al. Coelenterate venom research 1991–1995: clinical, chemical and immunological aspects. *Toxicon* 1996;34:1377–1383.
307. Gessner BD, Middaugh JP, Doucette GJ. Paralytic shellfish poisoning in Kodiak, Alaska. *West J Med* 1997;167:351–353.
307a. Nimorakiotakis B, Winkel KD. Marine envenomations. Part I—Jellyfish. *Aust Fam Physician* 2003;32:969–974.
308. Teitelbaum JS, Zatorre RJ, Carpenter S, et al. Neurologic sequelae of domoic acid intoxication due to the ingestion of contaminated mussels. *N Engl J Med* 1990;322:1781–1787.
309. Holstege CP, Miller MB, Wermuth M, et al. Crotalid snake envenomation. *Crit Care Clin* 1997;13:888–921.
309a. Stommel EW, Watters MR. Marine neurotoxins: ingestible toxins. *Curr Treat Options Neurol* 2004;6:105–114.
310. Weber RA, White RR. Crotalidae envenomation in children. *Ann Plast Surg* 1993;31:141–145.
311. Watt G, Theakston RD, Hayes CG, et al. Positive response to edrophonium in patients with neurotoxic envenoming by cobras (*Naja naja philippinensis*). A placebo-controlled study. *N Engl J Med* 1986;315:1444–1448.
311a. Roberts JR, Otten EJ. Snakes and other reptiles. In: Goldfrank LR, Flomenbaum NE, Lewin NA, et al., eds. *Goldfrank's Toxicologic Emergencies,*, 7th ed. New York: McGraw-Hill, 2002:1552–1557.
312. Vijayaraghavan S, Pugh PC, Zhang ZW, et al. Nicotinic receptors that bind α-bungarotoxin on neurons raise intracellular free $Ca2^+$. *Neuron* 1992;8:353–362.
313. Britt A, Burkhart K. Naja naja cobra bite. *Am J Emerg Med* 1997;15:529–531.
314. Moss HS, Binder LS. A retrospective review of black widow spider envenomation. *Ann Emerg Med* 1987;16:188–192.
315. Ushkaryov YA, Petrenko AG, Geppert M, et al. Neurexins: synaptic cell-surface proteins related to the α-latrotoxin receptor and laminin. *Science* 1992;257:50–56.
315a. Lee BC, Hwang SH, Bae JC, et al. Brainstem infarction following Korean viper bite. *Neurology* 2001;56:1244–1245.
316. Davletov BA, Krasnoperov V, Hata Y, et al. High affinity binding of alpha-latrotoxin to recombinant neurexin I alpha. *J Biol Chem* 1995;270:23903–23905.
317. Woestman R, Perkin R, Van Stralen D. The black widow: is she deadly to children? *Pediatr Emerg Care* 1996;12:360–364.
317a. Sudhof TC. Alpha-latrotoxin and its receptors: neurexins and CIRL/latrophilins. *Annu Rev Neurosci* 2001;24:933–962.
318. Berg RA, Tarantino MD. Envenomation by the scorpion centuroides exilicauda (*C. sculpturatus*): severe and unusual manifestations. *Pediatrics* 1991;87:930–933.
319. Mazzei de Davila CA, Parra M, Feunmayor A, et al. Scorpion envenomation in Merida, Venezuela. *Toxicon* 1997;35:1459–1462.
320. Russell FE. Stingray juices: a review and discussion of their treatment. *Am J Med Sci* 1953;226:611.
320a. Bentur Y, Taitelman U, Aloufy A. Evaluation of scorpion stings: the poison center perspective. *Vet Hum Toxicol* 2003;45:108–111.
321. Kizer KW, McKinney HE, Auerbach PS. Scorpaenidae envenomation. A five year poison center experience. *JAMA* 1985;253:807–810.
321a. Isbister GK. Venomous fish stings in tropical northern Australia *Am J Emerg Med* 2001;19:561–565.
322. Ghadessy FJ, Chen DS, Kini RM, et al. Stonustoxin is a novel lethal factor from stonefish (*Synanceja horrida*) venom. CDNA cloning and characterization. *J Biol Chem* 1996;271:25575–25581.
322a. Khoo HE, Chen D, Yuen R. Role of free thiol groups in the biological activities of stonustoxin, a lethal factor from stonefish (*Synanceja horrida*) venom. *Toxicon* 1998;36:469–476.
322b. Weisman RS. Marine Envenomations. In: Goldfrank LR, Flomenbaum NE, Lewin NA, et al., eds. *Goldfrank's Toxicologic Emergencies*, 7th ed. New York: McGraw-Hill, 2002:1592–1597.
323. Mills AR, Pasmore R. Pelagic paralysis. *Lancet* 1988;1:161–164.
323a. Breton P, Delamanche I, Buee J, et al. Evidence for a neurotoxic activity in crude venom of the stonefish (*Synanceia verrucosa*). *J Nat Toxins* 2002;11:305–313.
324. Cameron J, Flowers AE, Capra MF. Electrophysiological studies on ciguatera poisoning in man (Part II). *J Neurol Sci* 1991;101:93–97.
325. Williams RK, Palafox NA. Treatment of pediatric ciguatera fish poisoning. *Am J Dis Child* 1990;144:747–748.
325a. Isbister GK, Son J, Wang F, et al. Puffer fish poisoning: a potentially life-threatening condition. *Med J Aust* 2002;177:650–653.
326. DeWolfe FA. Neurologic aspects of mushroom intoxications. In: Vinken PJ, Bruyn GW, eds. *Intoxications of the nervous system, part I. Handbook of clinical neurology*. Vol. 36. Amsterdam: North-Holland, 1979:529–546.
327. McPartland JM, Vilgalys RJ, Cubeta MA. Mushroom poisoning. *Am Fam Phys* 1997;55:1797–1800.
327a. Tunik MG, Goldfrank LR. Food Poisoning. In: Goldfrank LR, Flomenbaum NE, Lewin NA, et al., eds. *Goldfrank's Toxicologic Emergencies,* 7th ed. New York: McGraw-Hill, 2002:1085–1099.
328. Pond SM, Olson KR, Woo OF, et al. Amatoxin poisoning in Northern California, 1982–1983. *West J Med* 1986;145:204–209.
329. Villalobos R, Santos MA. Karwinskia palsy in childhood. *Acta Neuropediatr* 1996;2:154–159.
330. Mack RB. Toxic encounters of the dangerous kind. The nutmeg connection. *North Car Med J* 1982;43:439.
331. Mack RB. Toxic encounters of the dangerous kind. The baddest seed-ricin poisoning. *North Car Med J* 1982;43:584–589.
331a. Goldfrank LR. Mushrooms. In: Goldfrank LR, Flomenbaum NE, Lewin NA, et al., eds. *Goldfrank's Toxicologic Emergencies,* 7th ed. New York: McGraw-Hill, 2002:1115–1128.
332. Lond JM, Roberts LM, Robertus JD. Ricin: structure, mode of action, and some current applications. *FASEB J* 1994;8:201–208.
332a. Benjamin DR. Mushroom poisoning in infants and childen: the *Amanita Pantheria/Muscaria group*. *J Toxicol Clinc Toxicol* 1992;30:13–22.
333. Mack RB. Toxic encounters of the dangerous kind. "Loco" weed and the anticholinergic syndrome. *North Car Med J* 1982;43:650.
334. Savitt DL, Roberts JR, Seigel EG. Anisocoria from jimson weed. *JAMA* 1986;255:1439–1440.
334a. Martinez HR, Bermudez MV, Rangel-Guerra RA, et al. Clinical diagnosis in Karwinskia humboldtiana polyneuropathy. *J Neurol Sci* 1998;154:49–54.
335. Mack RB. Toxic encounters of the dangerous kind. Poke-weed. *North Car Med J* 1982;43:365.
336. Tanaka K. Jamaican vomiting sickness. In: Vinken PJ, Bruyn GW, eds. *Intoxications of the nervous system, part II. Handbook of clinical neurology*, Vol. 37. Amsterdam: North-Holland, 1979:511–539.
337. Trost LC, Lemasters JJ. The mitochondrial permeability transition: a new pathophysiological mechanism for Reye's syndrome and toxic liver injury. *J Pharmacol Exp Therap* 1996;278:1000–1005.
338. He F, Zhang GS, Qian F, Zhang C. Delayed dystonia with striatal CT lucencies induced by a mycotoxin (3-nitropropionic acid). *Neurology* 1995;45:2178–2183.
339. Kajiyama Y, Fujii K, Takeuchi H, et al. Ginkgo seed poisoning. *Pediatrics* 2002;109:325–327.

340. Furbee B, Wermuth M. Life-threatening plant poisoning. *Crit Care Clin* 1997;13:849–888.
341. Spencer PS. Food toxins, AMPA receptors and motor neuron diseases. *Drug Metabolism Reviews* 1999;31:561–587.
341a. Meda HA, Diallo B, Buchet JP, et al. Epidemic of fat encephalopathy in preschool children in Burkina and consumption of unripe ackee (*Blighia sapida*) fruit. *Lancet* 1999;353:536–540.
342. Getahun H, Lambein F, Vanhoorne M, et al. Pattern and associated factors of the neurolathyrism epidemic in Ethiopia. *Trop Med Internat Health* 2002;7:118–124.
343. Williams RK, Palafox NA. Treatment of pediatric ciguatera fish poisoning. *Am J Dis Child* 1990;144:747–748.
344. Williams CD. Kwashiorkor—a nutritional disease of children associated with a maize diet. *Lancet* 1935;2:1151–1152.
345. DeSilva CC. Common nutritional disorders of childhood in the tropics. *Adv Pediatr* 1964;13:213–264.
346. Torun B. Protein-energy malnutrition. In: Strickland GT, ed. *Hunter's tropical medicine and emerging infectious diseases*, 8th ed. Philadelphia: WB Saunders, 2000:927–940.
347. Golden MH. Oedematous malnutrition. *Br Med Bull* 1998;54:433–444.
348. Fechner A, Böhme CC, Grohmer S, et al. Antioxidant status and nitric oxide in the malnutrition syndrome kwashiorkor. *Pediatr Res* 2001;49:237–243.
349. Iputo JE, Sammon AM, Tindimwebwa G. Prostaglandin E2 is raised in kwashiorkor. *S Afr Med J* 2002;92:310–312.
350. Krawinkel M. Kwashiorkor is still not fully understood. *Bull World Health Organ* 2003;81:910–911.
351. Hendrickse RG. Kwashiorkor: the hypothesis that incriminates aflatoxins. *Pediatrics* 1991;88:376–379.
352. Jelliffe DB, Jelliffe EFP. Causation of kwashiorkor: toward a multifactorial consensus. *Pediatrics* 1992;90:110–113.
353. Harper C, Butterworth R. Nutritional and metabolic disorders. In: Graham DI, Lantos PL, eds. *Greenfields's neuropathology*, 6th ed. London: Edward Arnold, Ltd., 1997:601–655.
354. Udani PM. Protein energy malnutrition (PEM), brain and various facets of child development. *Indian J Pediatr* 1992;59:165–186.
355. Mehta S, Kalsi HK, Nain CK, et al. Energy metabolism of brain in human protein-calorie malnutrition. *Pediatr Res* 1977;11:290–293.
356. Dobbing J. Undernutrition and developing brain. *Am J Dis Child* 1970;120:411–415.
357. Udani PM. Neurological manifestations in kwashiorkor. *Indian J Child Health* 1960;9:103–112.
358. Sachdeva KK, Taori GM, Pereira SM. Neuromuscular status in protein-calorie malnutrition. Clinical, nerve conduction and electromyographic studies. *Neurology* 1971;21:801–805.
359. Chopra JS, Dhand UK, Mehta S, et al. Effect of protein calorie malnutrition on peripheral nerves. A clinical, electrophysiological and histopathological study. *Brain* 1986;109:307–323.
360. Chopra JS, Sharma A. Protein energy malnutrition and the nervous system. *J Neurol Sci* 1992;110:8–20.
361. Agarwal KN, Das D, Agarwal DK, et al. Soft neurological signs and EEG pattern in rural malnourished children. *Acta Paediatr Scan* 1989;78:873–878.
362. Gunston GD, Burkimsher D, Malan H, et al. Reversible cerebral shrinkage in kwashiorkor: an MRI study. *Arch Dis Child* 1992;67:1030–1032.
363. Balmer S, Howells G, Wharton B. The acute encephalopathy of kwashiorkor. *Dev Med Child Neurol* 1968;10:766–771.
364. Kahn E, Falcke HC. A syndrome simulating encephalitis affecting children recovering from malnutrition (kwashiorkor). *J Pediatr* 1956;49:37–45.
365. Birch HG, Pineiro C, Alcalde E, et al. Relation of kwashiorkor in early childhood and intelligence at school age. *Pediatr Res* 1971;5:579–585.
366. Eichenwald HF, Fry PC. Nutrition and learning. *Science* 1969;163:644–648.
367. Beckman DSD, Lescano AG, Gilman RH, et al. Effects of stunting, diarrhoeal disease, and parasitic infection during infancy on cognition in late childhood: a follow-up study. *Lancet* 2002;359:564–571.
368. Evans D, Hansen JD, Moodie AD, et al. Intellectual development and nutrition. *J Pediatr* 1980;97:358–363.
369. Walker SP, Grantham-McGregor SM, Powell CA, et al. Effects of growth restriction in early childhood on growth, IQ, and cognition at age 11–12 years and the benefits of nutritional supplementation and psychosocial stimulation. *J Pediatr* 2000;137:36–41.
370. Grantham-McGregor SM, Powell CA, Walker SP, et al. Nutritional supplementation, psychosocial stimulation, and mental development of stunted children: the Jamaican study. *Lancet* 1991;338:15.
371. Keating JP, Feigin RD. Increased intracranial pressure associated with probable vitamin A deficiency in cystic fibrosis. *Pediatrics* 1970;46:41–46.
372. Snodgrass SR. Vitamin neurotoxicity. *Mol Neurobiol* 1992;6:41–73.
373. Peters RA. Significance of thiamine in the metabolism and function of the brain. In: Elliott KA, Page IH, Quastel JH, eds. *Neurochemistry*. Springfield, IL: Charles C Thomas, 1962:267
374. Haas RH. Thiamine and the brain. *Ann Rev Nutr* 1988;8:483–515.
375. Shimojyo S, Scheinberg P, Reinmuth O. Cerebral blood flow and metabolism in the Wernicke-Korsakoff syndrome. *J Clin Invest* 1967;46:849–854.
376. McCandless DW, Schenker S. Encephalopathy of thiamine deficiency: studies of intracerebral mechanisms. *J Clin Invest* 1968;47:2268–2280.
377. Dreyfus PM, Hauser G. The effect of thiamine deficiency on the pyruvate decarboxylase system of the central nervous system. *Biochem Biophys Acta* 1965;104:78–84.
378. Sharp FR, Bolger E, Evans K. Thiamine deficiency limits glucose utilization and glial proliferation in brain lesions of symptomatic rats. *J Cereb Blood Flow Metab* 1982;2:203–207.
379. Vasconcelos MM, Silva KP, Vidal G, et al. Early diagnosis of pediatric Wernicke's encephalopathy. *Pediatr Neurol* 1999;20:289–294.
380. Hahn JS, Berquist W, Alcorn DM, et al. Wernicke encephalopathy and beriberi during total parenteral nutrition attributable to multivitamin infusion shortage. *Pediatrics* 1998;101:E10.
381. Seear M, Lockitch G, Jacobson B, et al. Thiamine, riboflavin, and pyridoxine deficiencies in a population of critically ill children. *J Pediatr* 1992;121:533–538.
382. Tang CM, Rolfe M, Wells JC, et al. Outbreak of beri-beri in The Gambia. *Lancet* 1989;2:206–207.
383. Haridas L. Infantile beriberi in Singapore. *Arch Dis Child* 1947;22:23–33.
384. Wyatt DT, Noetzel MJ, Hillman RE. Infantile beriberi presenting as subacute necrotizing encephalomyelopathy. *J Pediatr* 1987;110:888–892.
385. Pihko M, Saarinen V, Paetau A. Wernicke encephalopathy: a preventable cause of death—report of two children with malignant disease. *Pediatr Neurol* 1989;5:237–242.
386. Seear MD, Norman MG. Two cases of Wernicke's encephalopathy in children: an underdiagnosed complication of poor nutrition. *Ann Neurol* 1988;24:85–87.
387. Barrett TG, Forsyth JM, Nathavitharana KA, et al. Potentially lethal thiamine deficiency complicating parenteral nutrition in children. *Lancet* 1993;341:901.
388. Sparacia G, Banco A, Lagalla R. Reversible MRI abnormalities in an unusual paediatric presentation of Wernicke's encephalopathy. *Pediatr Radiol* 1999;29:381–384.
389. Bessey OA, Adam DJ, Hansen AE. Intake of vitamin B_6 and infantile convulsions. A first approximation of requirements of pyridoxine in infants. *Pediatrics* 1957;20:33–44.
390. Molony CJ, Parmelee AH. Convulsions in young infants as a result of pyridoxine (vitamin B_6) deficiency. *JAMA* 1954;154:405–406.
391. Johnson GM. Powdered goat's milk. *Clin Pediatr* 1982;21:494–495.
392. Heiskanen K, Siimes MA, Perheentupa J, et al. Risk of low vitamin B_6 status in infants breast-fed exclusively beyond six months. *J Pediatr Gastroenterol Nutr* 1996;23:38–44.
393. Coker SB. Postneonatal vitamin B_6-dependent epilepsy. *Pediatrics* 1992;90:221–223.
394. Baxter P. Pyridoxine-dependent and pyridoxine-responsive seizures. *Dev Med Child Neurol* 2001;43:416–420.
395. Hunt AD, Stokes J, McCrory WW, et al. Pyridoxine dependency: report of a case of intractable convulsions in an infant controlled by pyridoxine. *Pediatrics* 1954;13:140–145.
396. Cormier-Daire V, Dagoneau N, Nabbout R, et al. A gene for pyridoxine-dependent epilepsy maps to chromosome 5p31. *Am J Hum Genet* 2000;67:991–993.

397. Baumeister FAM, Gsell W, Shin YS, et al. Glutamate in pyridoxine-dependent epilepsy: neurotoxic glutamate concentration in the cerebrospinal fluid and its normalization by pyridoxine. *Pediatrics* 1994;94:318–321.
398. Shih JJ, Kornblum H, Shewmon DA. Global brain dysfunction in an infant with pyridoxine dependency: evaluation with EEG, evoked potentials, MRI and PET. *Neurology* 1996;47:824–826.
399. Kurlemann G, Menges EM, Palm DG. Low levels of GABA in CSF in vitamin B_6-dependent seizures. *Dev Med Child Neurol* 1991:33:749–750.
400. Lott IT, Coulombe T, Di Paolo RV, et al. Vitamin B_6-dependent seizures. Pathology and chemical findings in brain. *Neurology* 1978;28:47–54.
401. Battaglioli G, Rosen DR, Gospe SM, et al. Glutamate decarboxylase is not genetically linked to pyridoxine-dependent seizures. *Neurology* 2000;55:309–311.
402. Grillo E, da Silva RJ, Barbato JH Jr. Pyridoxine-dependent seizures responding to extremely low-dose pyridoxine. *Dev Med Child Neurol* 2001:43:413–415.
403. McLachlan RS, Brown WF. Pyridoxine dependent epilepsy with iatrogenic sensory neuronopathy. *Can J Neurol Sci* 1995;22:50–51.
404. Jaffe KA, Altman K, Merryman P. The antipyridoxine effect of penicillamine in man. *J Clin Invest* 1964;43:1869–1873.
405. Olson KR, Kearney TE, Dyer JE, et al. Seizures associated with poisoning and drug overdose. *Am J Emerg Med* 1994;12:392–395.
406. Shah BR, Santucci K, Sinert R, et al. Acute isoniazide neurotoxicity in an urban hospital. *Pediatrics* 1995;95:700–704.
407. Spillane JD. *Nutritional disorders of the nervous system*. Edinburgh: E & S Livingstone, 1947.
408. Ishii N, Nishihara V. Pellagra encephalopathy among tuberculous patients: its relation to isoniazid therapy. *J Neurol Neurosurg Psychiatry* 1985;48:628–634.
409. Malfait P, Moren A, Dillon JC, et al. An outbreak of pellagra related to changes in dietary niacin among Mozambican refugees in Malawi. *Int J Epidemiol* 1993;22:504–511.
410. Meyer A. On parenchymatous systemic degeneration mainly in the central nervous system. *Brain* 1901;24:47–115.
411. Spies TD, Walker AA, Wood AW. Pellagra in infancy and childhood. *JAMA* 1939;113:1481–1483.
412. Lanska DJ. Stages in the recognition of epidemic pellagra in the United States: 1865–1960. *Neurology* 1996;47:829–834.
413. Hall CA. The neurologic aspects of transcobalamin II deficiency. *Br J Haematol* 1992;80:80;117–120.
414. Kapadia CR. Vitamin B_{12} in health and disease: part I—inherited disorders of function, absorption, and transport. *Gastroenterologist* 1995;3:329–344.
415. Gordon MM, Brada N, Remacha A, et al. A genetic polymorphism in the coding region of the gastric intrinsic factor gene (GIF) is associated with congenital intrinsic facor deficiency. *Hum Mutat* 2004;23:85–91.
416. Graham SM, Arvela OM, Wise GA. Long-term neurologic consequences of nutritional vitamin B_{12} deficiency in infants. *J Pediatr* 1992;121:710–714.
417. Kuhne T, Bubl R, Baumgartner R. Maternal vegan diet causing a serious infantile neurological disorder due to vitamin B_{12} deficiency. *Eur J Pediatr* 1991;150:205–208.
418. Grattan-Smith PJ, Wilcken B, Procopis PG, et al. The neurological syndrome of infantile cobalamin deficiency: developmental regression and involuntary movements. *Mov Disord* 1997;12:39–46.
419. Davis JR, Goldenring J, Lubin BH. Nutritional vitamin B_{12} deficiency in infants. *Am J Dis Child* 1981;135:566–567.
420. McNicholl B, Egan B. Congenital pernicious anemia: effects of growth, brain, and absorption of B_{12}. *Pediatrics* 1968;42:149–156.
421. Zegers de Beyl D, Delecluse F, Verbanck P, et al. Somatosensory conduction in vitamin B_{12} deficiency. *Electroencephal Clin Neurophysiol* 1988;69:313–318.
422. Horstmann M, Neumaeier-Probst E, Lukacs Z, et al. Infantile cobalamin deficiency with cerebral lactate accumulation and sustained choline depletion. *Neuropediatrics* 2003:34:261–264.
423. von Schenck U, Bender-Gotze C, Koletzko B. Persistence of neurological damage induced by dietary vitamin B_{12} deficiency in infancy. *Arch Dis Child* 1997;77:137–139.
424. Ozer EA, Turker M, Bakiler AR, et al. Involuntary movements in infantile cobalamin deficiency appearing after treatment. *Pediatr Neurol* 2001:25:81–83.
425. Shuper A, Stein J, Goshen J, et al. Subacute central nervous system degeneration in a child: an unusual manifestation of ifosfamide intoxication. *J Child Neurol* 2000:15:481–483.
426. Pearson HA, Vinson R, Smith RT. Pernicious anemia with neurologic involvement in childhood. *J Pediatr* 1964;65:334–339.
427. Hall CA. Function of vitamin B_{12} in the central nervous system as revealed by congenital defects. *Am J Hematol* 1990;34:121–127.
428. Sharda B, Bhandari B. Infantile tremor syndrome. *Indian Pediatr* 1987;24:415–421.
429. Vora RM, Tullu MS, Bartakke SP, et al. Infantile tremor syndrome and zinc deficiency. *Indian J Med Sci* 2002;56:69–72.
430. Garewal G, Narang A, Das KC. Infantile tremor syndrome: a vitamin B_{12} deficiency syndrome in infants. *J Trop Pediatr* 1988;34:174–178.
431. Howlett WP, Brubaker GR, Mlingi N, et al. Konzo, an epidemic upper motor neuron disease studied in Tanzania. *Brain* 1990;113:223–235.
432. Kazadi K, Garin B, Goussard B, et al. Nonspastic paraparesis associated with HTLV-I. *Lancet* 1990;336:260.
433. Oluwole OS, Onabolu AO, Link H, et al. Persistence of tropical ataxic neuropathy in a Nigerian community. *J Neurol Neurosurg Psychiatry* 2000;69:96–101.
434. Roman GC, Spencer PS, Schoenberg BS. Tropical myeloneuropathies. The hidden endemias. *Neurology* 1985;35:1158–1170.
435. Carton H, Kayembe K, Kabeya O, et al. Epidemic spastic paraparesis in Bandundu (Zaire). *J Neurol Neurosurg Psychiatr* 1986;49: 620–627.
436. Spencer PS, Nunn PB, Hugon J, et al. Guam amyotrophic lateral sclerosis-Parkinson-dementia linked to a plant excitant neurotoxin. *Science* 1987;237:517–522.
437. Cox PA, Sacks OW. Cycad neurotoxins, consumption of flying foxes, and ALS-PDC disease in Guam. *Neurology* 2002;58:956–959.

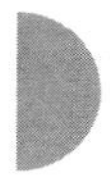

Chapter 11

Tumors of the Nervous System

Bernard L. Maria and John H. Menkes

BRAIN TUMORS

Incidence

Tumors of the central nervous system (CNS) occur relatively frequently during the early years of life. They are the most common solid tumors of childhood and afflict approximately 1,500 patients every year in the United States (1,2). Reported incidence rates have varied from 20 to 50 per 1,000,000 children (3). Representing 20% of all malignancies, they are second only to leukemia in overall cancer incidence and account for a high proportion of deaths (4). CNS tumors in infants less than one year old account for about 10% of all intracranial tumors occurring in the pediatric population (5). Males and white, non-Hispanics have a higher incidence of CNS tumors compared with females and other ethnic groups, respectively (6). The nadir in incidence of CNS neoplasms between the ages 0 and 44 years occurs in the 15- to 29-year age group, at a rate of 22.3 per million (5).

Although the incidence of leukemia has remained relatively stable, the incidence of brain tumors has increased approximately 2% per year in the past 20 years (7). A review of earlier studies on the incidence of intracranial space-occupying lesions indicates that the relative frequencies of pathologic varieties have changed. Critchley, writing in 1925, found tuberculoma to be the most common intracranial tumor of childhood (8). Subsequent surveys by Bailey and associates (9) and Cuneo and Rand (10) stressed the preponderance of gliomas. Meningiomas and neurinomas were virtually absent, except in association with neurofibromatosis (11). Tuberculomas are now rare in the developed countries, but a series of 107 cases was reported from India as recently as 1965 (12). Data from the National Cancer Institute Surveillance, Epidemiology, and End-Results (SEER) from 1975 to 1998 showed that the incidence of CNS tumors in people age 0 to 44 years increased over time, mainly due to an increased incidence of "other glioma" (5). From 1981 through 1993, the incidence of primitive neuroectodermal tumor/medulloblastoma (PNET/MB), the most common malignant posterior fossa tumor, rose more than 4% per year (Table 11.1). This trend has not been fully explained, but improved detection through sensitive and specific neuroimaging technology, such as magnetic resonance imaging (MRI), may account for much of the increase (13). Inherited conditions such as neurofibromatosis, tuberous sclerosis, basal cell nevus syndrome, Von Hippel–Lindau disease, Li-Fraumeni syndrome (p53 mutation), Gorlin syndrome (PATCHED mutation), and Turcot syndrome (APC mutation) account for a small percent of CNS tumors (14–21). In addition to inherited conditions, ionizing radiation delivered in the past for tinea capitis or for leukemia and brain tumors is a known risk factor for CNS tumors (22–24). Various risk factors including nitrosamine/micronutrient intake, pesticide/fertilizer exposure, and parental occupation in chemical industries have been inconsistently associated with childhood brain tumors (25). Thus, the etiology for the vast majority of CNS tumors is unknown and there is no conclusive data to show that toxic waste, air and water pollutants, and electromagnetic fields and irradiation in local environments are tumorigenic (26). Furthermore, environmental influences ordinarily are expected to be gender blind, and thus could not account for the 4% increase in PNET/MB, which elicits a male-to-female gender ratio of approximately 2.5:1. Epidemiological investigations and population-based case-control studies are needed to determine how genes, environment, and lifestyle influence risk and may combine to cause CNS tumors in children (27).

Pediatric brain tumors include a spectrum of both glial and nonglial tumors that differ significantly in location and biologic behavior from that of adults (Table 11.2) (28,29). Subtentorial tumors constitute more than 50% of all intracranial space-occupying lesions in children; in adults, only 25% to 30% of tumors originate below the tentorium. In children younger than age 1 year, as in adults, supratentorial tumors are most frequent; in infancy these often arise from hamartomas or other congenital malformations (1).

TABLE 11.1 Florida Childhood Cancer Incidence 1981–1993, 0–14 Years

Tumor	Number of Cancers	Annual % Change
All	4,174	0.91
Leukemias	1,257	−0.31
Brain tumors	769	1.92
Glioma WM	214	3.36
Glioma WF	188	1.10
PNET	163	4.19
Neuroblastoma	293	3.25

PNET, primitive neuroectodermal tumor; WF, white female; WM, white male.
Table adapted from Roush SW, et al. The incidence of pediatric cancer in Florida, 1981 ot 1986. *Cancer* 1992;69:2212–2219.

Pathogenesis

A discussion of the molecular origins of neoplasia within the nervous system is far beyond the scope of this text. However, in recent years, real progress has been made in our understanding of the molecular genetic abnormalities that govern the initiation and/or progression of these tumors (30). Suffice it to say that the uncontrolled proliferation of a population of somatic cells is basically a genetic disorder, with multiple genetic abnormalities preceding the neoplastic transformation of normal tissue. Most tumors of childhood are derived from the neuroectoderm, and there is evidence that transcription factors expressed by neural crest cells correlate with phenotype in neurorectodermal tumors (31). Two distinct fundamental mechanisms appear to be operative. One is associated with the activation or overexpression of growth-promoting factors such as proto-oncogenes, and the other is the result of loss or inactivation of genes that normally regulate or suppress cell growth, the tumor-suppressor genes. The mutation of the proto-oncogene to an oncogene has a dominant effect; only one of the cell's two gene copies needs to undergo the mutation. The inactivation of a tumor-suppressor gene is recessive, which means that both gene copies must be inactivated. Inactivation of tumor-suppressor genes is believed to be responsible for the development of tumors in neurofibromatosis and tuberous sclerosis (see Chapter 12).

TABLE 11.2 Incidence of Brain Tumors in the Pediatric Population Younger Than 15 Years of Age Versus All Ages[a]

Tumors	All Ages (%)	Children (%)
Glioma	45	70
Astrocytoma	15	30
Glioblastoma	15	5
Oligodendroglioma	8	1
Medulloblastoma	4	20
Ependymoma	4	10
Meningioma	15	1
Neurinoma	6	<0.5
Pituitary adenoma	6	1
Metastases	5–20	<0.5
Craniopharyngioma	3	10

[a]Figures are estimates and are based on reports collected from the literature.
Table adapted from Tobias J, Hayward RD. Brain and spinal cord tumours in children. In: Thomas DGT, ed. *Neuro-oncology: primary malignant brain tumours.* Baltimore: The Johns Hopkins University Press, 1990:164–192.

The role of tumor viruses in CNS neoplasia of childhood is less clear. However, one-half of choroid plexus tumors and most ependymomas contain and express a segment of a gene related to the monkey polyoma virus (SV40). This virus, which is highly tumorigenic in rodents, could have an etiologic role in the development of some childhood neoplasms. The JC virus a human neurotropic polyomavirus, which causes progressive multifocal leukoencephalopathy and is closely related to SV40, has been detected in ependymomas and choroid plexus papilloma, but not medulloblastoma or pilocytic astrocytoma (32). It is also possible that certain human neoplasms provide a favorable microenvironment for viral replication in tissue that is latently infected with SV40 (33). From the data currently available, it is clear that the combination of accumulating events is distinct for each tumor type; what is still unknown is which molecular abnormality is the rate-limiting step that leads to neoplastic transformation.

Cytogenetic analysis of glial tumors has identified a variety of gross chromosomal abnormalities (Table 11.3) (34,35–43). Gains of chromosome 7 and losses of 9 and 10 have been reported in adult high-grade astrocytomas, but pediatric astrocytomas may also be associated with gains in chromosomes 1q and 2 (44). Other genomic imbalances include extra copies of chromosome 8q, loss of 6, 8, 10q, 11, 13, 17p, or 22, and structural abnormalities of chromosome 9p and 19q. Deletions of the short arm of chromosome 17 (17p13.3) is seen in approximately 40% to 50% of primary PNET/MB (30,45). Such deletions of 17p may occur in the absence of other gross abnormalities of 17, as a component of an isochromosome of 17q [i(17q)]. The molecular consequences of chromosomal loss in medulloblastoma are still being elucidated, but loss of 17p13.3, high-frequency MYC amplification, and Survivin expression are associated with a poor prognosis (45–47). Dysregulation of the hedgehop, PTCH, neurotrophin, ErbB receptor, adenomatous polyposis coli gene, and the Wnt signalling pathways that are important in CNS development has been shown in embryonal tumors, and current evidence favors site-specific origin of such tumors (48–50). ErbB2 is undectable in developing cerebellum but is expressed in 40% of medulloblastomas and is associated with a poor clinical outcome (51). The epigenetic silencing of tumor-suppressor gene expression by aberrant methylation (e.g., promoter hypermethylation) has emerged

TABLE 11.3 Chromosomal and Genetic Alterations Characteristic of Specific Types of Brain Tumors

Tumor Type	*Chromosomal or LOH Abnormality*	*Genetic Alteration*	*Reference*
Astrocytoma/glioblastoma	+7p	*EGFR* gene amplification and rearrangement	35–37
	−9p	CDKN2A, CDKN2B, *p14*^{ARF} gene deletion	
	−1p	?Expression of neuron-related genes	
	−17p	*p53* gene mutation	
	+8	Unknown	
	−10	PTEN mutation, DMBT1 deletion	
Oligodendroglioma	−1p	?Expression of neuron-related genes	38,39
	−19q	Unknown	
	−10q	DMBT1 deletion	
Ependymoma	−22	?*NF2* gene mutation	40
Medulloblastoma	−8p	Unknown	41
	−17p	Unknown	
	Dmins	c-*myc*, N-*myc* gene amplification	
Meningioma	−22q	*NF2* gene mutation	42,43
	−1p	Unknown	
	−9p	CDKN2A	
	−7p	Unknown	
Schwannoma	−22q	*NF2* gene mutation	

recently as a major mechanism of tumorigenesis (52,53). *P53* pathway dysfunction may also be abrogated in pediatric CNS tumors (54,54a). Moroever, polymorphisms among the genes involved in the folate pathway may significantly affect the risk for developing a childhood brain tumor (25). The molecular biology of tumors has been reviewed by Bigner and colleagues (34), Santarius and colleagues (55), and Ng and Lam (56). Complete and detailed reviews of newer developments in tumor cell culture, the effect of animal models on brain tumor research, and basic discoveries in neuro-oncology are also available elsewhere (57,58).

From a clinical point of view, the importance of genetic factors in the development of brain tumors is significant. Surveys of the incidence of tumors in relatives of brain tumor patients have demonstrated a higher incidence of CNS neoplasms and of leukemia, but no greater incidence of other malignancies (59). Craniopharyngiomas and some of the PNET/MBs are congenital and arise from an area of maldevelopment. Craniopharyngiomas arise from persistent remnants of the craniopharyngeal (Rathke's) pouch and PNET/MBs usually from primitive cell rests in the posterior medullary velum.

Postnatal factors, trauma in particular, have not proven significant in the development of brain tumors in children. In a few instances, irradiation has been implicated in the appearance of malignant mesodermal tumors at the radiation site. In one study, radiation for ringworm of the scalp was associated with an increased incidence of brain tumors occurring after an interval that ranged from 7 to 21 years (60).

Symptoms and Signs

Neurologic symptoms produced by brain tumors are general or local. General symptoms result from increased intracranial pressure, which results directly from progressive enlargement of the tumor within the limited volume of the cranial vault; local symptoms are due to the effects of the tumor on contiguous areas of the brain.

Pathophysiology

An intracranial mass produces cerebral compression by its intrinsic volume; by its encroachment on the ventricular system, obstructing the flow of cerebrospinal fluid (CSF) and producing ventricular dilatation; and particularly when malignant, by its ability to produce edema in white matter adjacent to the expanding mass.

As the tumor enlarges, the intracranial contents, primarily the ventricular spaces, are initially compressed. The duration of the initial asymptomatic period depends on the rate of tumor expansion and on whether the tumor's location causes it to compromise the circulation of CSF.

When the intracranial pressure approaches or equals the systemic arterial pressure, it causes the systemic arterial pressure to increase. Cushing noted that systemic hypertension was accompanied by bradycardia and slow irregular respirations (Cushing triad) (61,62). Compression of the venous channels, especially the large, draining venous sinuses, reduces cerebral blood flow. The resulting cerebral anoxia in turn produces vascular dilatation and a further increase in intracerebral volume and pressure (63).

A number of experiments have proven Cushing's contention that the pressure threshold for the induction of the vasopressor response is reached when intracranial pressure is at the level of systemic arterial pressure. Clinical experience, however, suggests that arterial hypertension first appears at lower pressures, particularly when a pressure differential exists above and below the tentorium. Under these instances, the pressure response can be triggered by local ischemia of the cerebral hemispheres or by distortion of the brainstem and subsequent medullary ischemia. With a further increase in intracranial pressure, the vasopressor mechanism fails, arterial pressure decreases, and cerebral blood flow is substantially reduced (64,65).

Pulmonary edema can accompany increased intracranial pressure (neurogenic pulmonary edema). Its pathogenesis is poorly understood; most likely, the edema is the direct result of an elevated pulmonary capillary pressure. Whether this elevation results from an increase in left atrial pressure (the consequence of left ventricular failure), as has been postulated for some years, or from a disturbance in hypothalamic function (with a consequent massive α-adrenergic discharge) has not been clarified (66). The rapid evolution of pulmonary edema after severe head trauma makes the latter alternative more attractive.

Increased intracranial pressure decreases cerebral blood flow when perfusion pressure (the difference between arterial pressure and intracranial pressure) decreases to approximately 40 mm Hg. At perfusion pressures below 40 mm Hg, cerebral blood flow decreases abruptly, and it eventually ceases completely (67). Additionally, asphyxia or shifts in the brainstem or in the cerebral hemispheres that arise from the mass effects of a tumor can affect cerebrovascular autoregulation and induce a decrease in cerebral blood flow at perfusion pressures higher than 40 mm Hg.

Aside from these circulatory disturbances, an expanding tumor produces a variety of mechanical deformations of the brain, especially in adults or in older children whose sutures cannot widen and whose cranium cannot enlarge in response to a prolonged increase in intracranial pressure.

Clinically, the most significant of these mechanical deformations are the various herniations, notably herniation of the cerebellar tonsils through the foramen magnum, a feature of infratentorial tumors, and herniation of the hippocampal gyrus, particularly the uncus, down through the tentorial opening (Fig. 11.1). This herniation is observed with supratentorial masses, especially ipsilateral temporal lobe tumors.

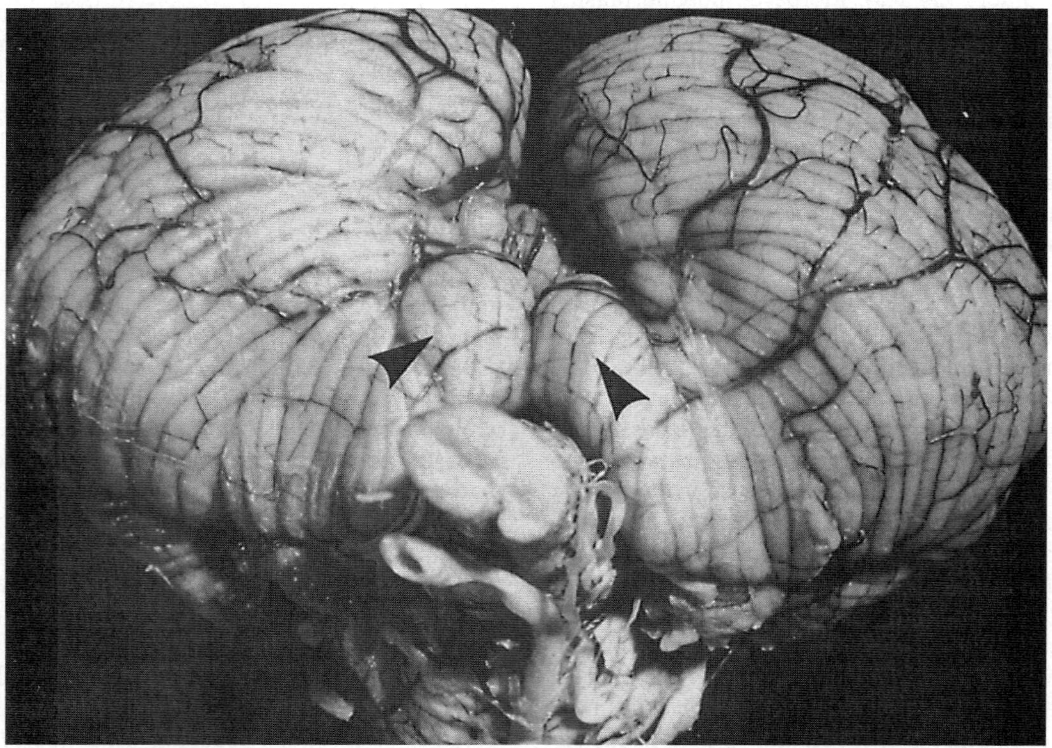

FIGURE 11.1. Herniation of cerebellar tonsils. The view from the posterior aspect of the cerebellum demonstrates caudal displacement of the cerebellar tonsils resulting from increased intracranial pressure. The cone of herniated tonsillar tissue (*arrows*) impinges on the dorsal surface of the cervical spinal cord. (From Bell WE, McCormick WF. *Increased intracranial pressure in children,* 2nd ed. Philadelphia: Saunders, 1978. With permission.)

Both types of herniations can produce secondary brainstem dysfunction, most probably by circulatory impairment and edema.

Clinical signs of occipital lobe infarction from increased intracranial pressure are less frequent. This condition results from kinking of the posterior cerebral arteries as they become wedged against the rigid tentorial edge (68). Because arterial pressure usually exceeds intracranial pressure, even in the presence of a mass lesion, local or systemic circulatory disturbances contribute to the development of arterial insufficiency.

Impaired cranial nerve function commonly accompanies increased intracranial pressure (69). The abducens nerve can become compressed between the anteroinferior cerebellar artery and the pons, producing weakness or paralysis of the lateral rectus muscle. This cause of sixth nerve paralysis was originally suggested by Cushing (70) and Collier (71) as a "false localizing sign." The nerve also may be stretched as a result of transtentorial herniation, or it may be compressed directly against the clivus. Although its vulnerability to increased intracranial pressure has commonly been attributed to its length, anatomic studies have shown that the abducens nerve is approximately one-third the length of the trochlear nerve (71a). Involvement of the oculomotor nerve can accompany uncal herniations. The oculomotor nerve, particularly its pupillomotor fibers, can be compressed by the posterior cerebral artery. Pressure on the nerve can produce transitory circulatory disturbances or actual grooving of the nerve with distal petechial hemorrhages from the vasa nervorum.

Clinical Manifestations

Increased intracranial pressure produces headaches, vomiting, impaired vision, and changes in consciousness, and, when sutures have not fused, an enlarging head.

Headache

Headache, a constant feature of increased intracranial pressure in adults, is less common in children, being noted in 70% of the series of Bailey and coworkers (9), and in approximately 50% of children younger than age 13 years (72). However, headache is the most frequent presenting symptom in pediatric CNS tumors (73). Headaches from brain tumors result from traction on the dura and blood vessels at the base of the brain. Pain may be generalized or localized and worsen with exertion. In children, the site of the pain, most commonly bifrontal, rarely assists in localizing the site of the tumor. Posterior fossa tumors, however, can produce irritation of the posterior roots of the upper cervical cord, resulting in pain in the back of the head and neck. Stiffness of the neck and a persistent head tilt, which can be adopted to avoid diplopia, also indicate a mass in the posterior fossa. Most commonly, the headache is transitory, occurring in the morning or awakening the child during the night. In children younger than age 12 years, it can disappear temporarily with widening of the sutures, only to recur with further growth of the mass lesion. The majority of children who develop headache as a consequence of a brain tumor have it as their first symptom, though few have it as their only symptom. It has been reported that children with brain tumors have had headache for less than 4 months (95%) or 2 months (85%) (74,75). In a recent retrospective study of 200 children with brain tumors in the United Kingdom, 36% had headache for more than 4 months (73), and a dirunal pattern of headache was present in two-thirds. The longer the headache is present, the greater the likelihood of associated vomiting (77%), visual difficulties (57%), unsteadiness (45%), behavioral change (32%), and disturbed sleep (26%) (73). Thus, if headache has been present for 4 months or longer and the neurologic and ophthalmologic examinations are normal, it is unlikely the child has a brain tumor.

Vomiting

Vomiting is one of the most constant signs of increased intracranial pressure in children. It occurred in 84% of patients in the series of Bailey and associates (9), in 61% of children younger than 13 years of age in the 1975 series of Till (72), and in 51% in the series of Ferris (73). The reduced incidence of vomiting in the more recent series probably reflects an earlier referral. Vomiting can result from both increased intracranial pressure and from irritation of the brainstem by tumors of the posterior fossa. Contrary to general belief, vomiting in these patients is often not projectile, and it can be accompanied by nausea. Parents often note that vomiting relieves the headache. Like headaches, vomiting is most prominent in the morning and is unrelated to eating. Widening of the sutures can afford transitory relief.

Impaired Vision

Diplopia is usually the result of paralysis of one or both lateral recti muscles. Strabismus can be most striking at the end of a day and occasionally can fluctuate in parallel with the degree of increased intracranial pressure (Fig. 11.2). Visual problems were noted in 39% of children with brain tumors in Ferris's series; the median duration of visual symptoms was 3 weeks. Cranial nerve abnormalities were the most common finding (49%) on neurological examination (73).

Papilledema

Bailey and coworkers noted papilledema in 80% of children with brain tumors (9), whereas in the later series of Till compiled in 1975, it was absent in 45% of children younger than 13 years of age (72). In the latest series of Ferris and coworkers, published in 2004 (73), it was

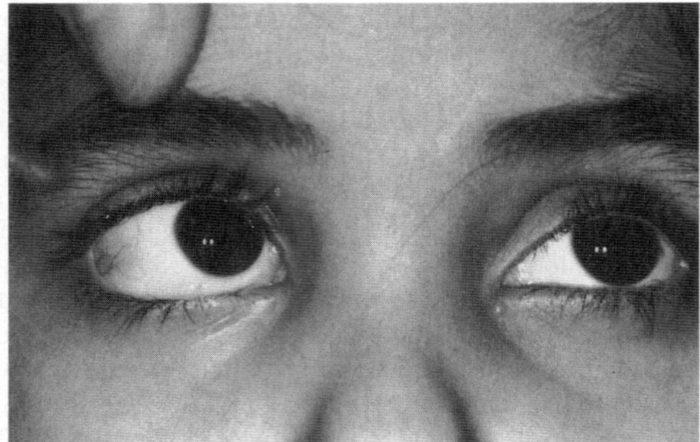
A

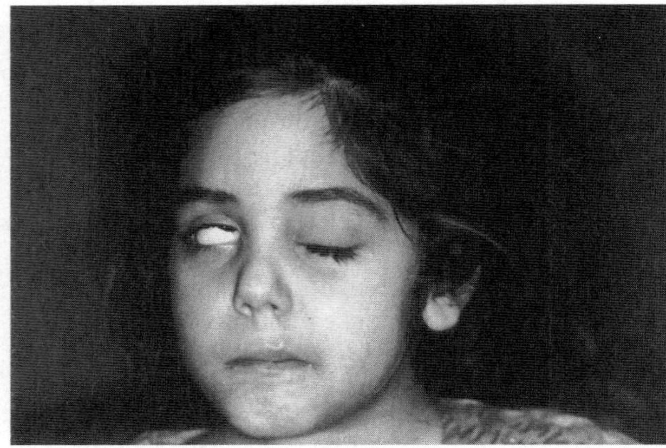
B

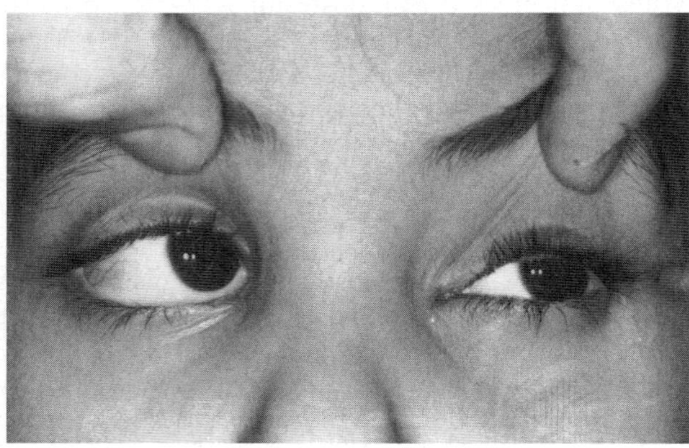
C

FIGURE 11.2. Right-gaze palsy **(A)** caused by involvement of paramedian pontine reticular formation and of the abducens nucleus itself is present in this child with brainstem glioma. As compared with intact left gaze **(C),** there is complete inability to move either eye to the right past the midline. Profound right peripheral facial paresis **(B)** is noted, with associated facial asymmetry and right orbicularis oculi weakness.

absent in 62% of children. This trend of decreasing prevalence of papilledema at the time of diagnosis may reflect more readily available neuroimaging modalities to evaluate headache. Papilledema represents an abnormal elevation of the nerve head. Obliteration of the disk margins and absent pulsations of the central veins are the earliest and most important ophthalmoscopic findings. When increased intracranial pressure has developed acutely, vascular congestion with hemorrhages and exudates also are conspicuous (Fig. 11.3).

Papilledema should be distinguished from pseudopapilledema. Pseudopapilledema is a congenital anomaly associated with small anomalous disks, less commonly with drusen (hyaline bodies) buried below the surface of the disks and resulting in excessive glial proliferation at the disk margins. The nerve fibers appear raised, creating a blurred disk with or without vascular tortuosity. This anomaly can be transmitted as a dominant trait, and frequently it accompanies hyperopia or congenital malformations of the skull, such as brachycephaly. The clinical diagnosis of pseudopapilledema is often difficult and rests on the absence of physiologic cups, and the normal central emergence of vessels, and most important, the absence of other signs of increased intracranial pressure (76,77). Although examination of the visual fields demonstrates a normal blind spot, in contrast to the increased blind spot

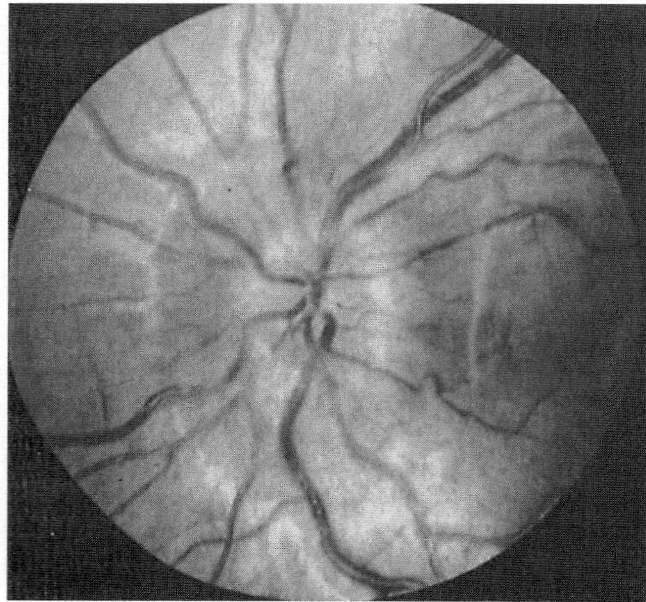

FIGURE 11.3. Papilledema in 10-year-old girl with pseudotumor cerebri. The disc margins are elevated, and the retinal veins are tortuous and distended. (Courtesy of Dr. Robert Hepler, Department of Ophthalmology, University of California, Los Angeles, UCLA School of Medicine.)

seen in true papilledema, this test is difficult to perform in young children.

Fluorescein fundus angiography has been advocated for distinguishing papilledema from pseudopapilledema. After the injection of fluorescein, the papilledematous optic disk discloses an increased capillary network, the presence of microaneurysms, and most significantly, persistence of fluorescence at the disk margins or over the edematous disk area. Generally, these changes are not observed in pseudopapilledema (78).

In papilledema, visual symptoms usually are insignificant or limited to transient attacks of blurred vision. The concentric enlargement of the blind spot, detected when charting of visual fields is possible, is always asymptomatic.

Increased intracranial pressure is an important factor in the production of papilledema, but other causes can contribute. Papilledema can occur with normal intracranial pressure, as in infectious polyneuritis. Conversely, it sometimes fails to appear despite a prolonged increase in intracranial pressure.

The most favored hypothesis to explain the mechanism for papilledema is that the subarachnoid spaces surrounding the optic nerves, which are continuous with those inside the skull, allow a free transmission of intracranial pressure. When pressure is elevated, optic nerve tissue pressure increases. If communication between the ventricular and the perioptic spaces is blocked, as occurs in some patients with hydrocephalus, then papilledema does not develop, even after a long-standing elevation of intracranial pressure. The increased pressure within the optic nerve in turn interferes with axoplasmic flow and causes stasis at the optic nerve head. This produces axonal swelling and the clinical appearance of papilledema. Compression of vessels over the surface of the disk results in their dilatation and in the formation of microaneurysms and hemorrhages. Obstruction of venous and lymphatic drainage is probably secondary to the increase in optic nerve pressure, rather than being its cause (77,79).

Although the presence of papillédema makes an intracranial mass highly probable, a number of other conditions must be excluded. In particular, choked optic disks also are encountered in pseudotumor cerebri, a condition characterized by increased intracranial pressure in the absence of a mass lesion.

Papilledema also can be found in the presence of subdural hematoma and in such systemic diseases as infectious polyneuritis, poliomyelitis, hypoparathyroidism, carbon dioxide retention, hypervitaminosis A, severe anemia, and lead poisoning.

Enlargement of the Head

Enlargement of the head is characteristic of a longstanding increase in intracranial pressure in infants and young children. In a series of brain tumors appearing during the first 2 years of life, an enlarging head was the most frequent presenting sign and was noted in 76% of infants (80). Enlargement of the head is not solely caused by brain tumors, but can occur in any child who has increased intracranial pressure and open sutures. Percussion of the head gives a high-pitched sound, termed *cracked pot* or *Macewen's sign*.

TABLE 11.4 Location of Tumors Producing Seizures in Children

Location	*Number of Cases*
Temporal lobe	10
Frontal lobe	2
Parietal lobe	8
Entire hemisphere (diffuse or multiple tumors)	3
Other sites	5

Adapted from Low NL, Correll JW, Hammill JF. Tumors of the cerebral hemispheres in children. *Arch Neurol* 1965;13:547.

Seizures

Seizures are rarely an early indication of mass lesion; in one series, they represented the initial symptom in approximately 15% of children with supratentorial lesions (81). Conversely, less than 1% of children with new onset seizures have a brain tumor as the etiology (82). Seizures become more frequent as the tumor grows and can be a late sign even in tumors of the posterior fossa. When seizures are caused by a brain tumor, patients rarely have other associated symptoms or signs of increased intracranial pressure. A complex partial seizure is the most common seizure type seen with intracranial masses, and the temporal lobe is the most common site for tumors producing seizures early in the course of illness (Table 11.4) (81).

Disturbances of Affect and Consciousness

Although mental disturbances or psychiatric disorders are fairly common with brain tumors in adults and indicate lesions of the frontal or temporal lobe, they are rarely observed in children. Children occasionally develop drowsiness, changes in personality, and irrational behavior, suggesting hypothalamic or thalamic involvement; changes in sleep patterns or in appetite are relatively common in frontal tumors. A progressive depression of consciousness resulting in drowsiness, stupor, and coma reflects increased intracranial pressure and compression of the reticular activating system. This compression can involve the reticular activating system in the upper brainstem when there is downward uncal or transtentorial herniation, or when, as a consequence of unilateral mass lesions, compression of the lower thalamus with horizontal displacement of the midbrain is seen (83).

Diagnosis

The diagnostic evaluation of the child suspected of harboring a brain tumor has undergone drastic changes since the 1970s. Classic texts, such as those by Bailey, Buchanan, and Bucy (9), published in 1939, bear witness to the early diagnostic difficulties presented by intracranial mass lesions. Formerly, initial evaluation involved the use of plain skull films and electroencephalography (EEG), followed by invasive procedures such as pneumoencephalography, ventriculography, and arteriography. This regimen has been superseded by various neuroimaging studies.

Diagnostic Neuroimaging

Advances in computer technology have helped to establish more effective methods of identifying and characterizing pediatric brain tumors (12,84). The primary objective for any diagnostic MRI or computed tomographic (CT) study is to distinguish between normality and abnormality, and to determine the relevance of the findings on neuroimaging to the clinical situation. Establishing normality is typically more difficult than recognizing obvious pathology. Once a lesion is observed, the role of imaging shifts toward more specialized tasks, including interpreting the nature of the lesion, establishing the spatial relationship between the mass and eloquent areas of the brain, and staging the extent of disease.

In the initial evaluation of a child with a brain tumor, careful staging is particularly essential to appropriate treatment decisions. This process is critical, as the initial surgical resection may be the only time some tumors can be cured. Therefore, it is imperative that the full extent of the lesion is appreciated. Additionally, cytoreductive surgical intervention may not be warranted if evidence exists of distant spread. Several factors contribute to assisting the radiologist with the differential diagnosis of a particular tumor: the age of the patient (Table 11.5), the location of the tumor (Table 11.6), and the inherent imaging features (Tables 11.7 and 11.8).

Unlike in adults, many masses in children are not actually tumors, and a variety of pathologic lesions can mimic the picture of a brain tumor on neuroimaging (Table 11.9). Some tumors are indolent, exhibiting virtually static biologic growth characteristics (85), whereas other mass lesions can display a mixture of both true tumor and cortical dysplastic features in the same region (86).

CT is used effectively for imaging the skull base, where the natural contrast of bone, air (paranasal sinuses), fat (nasopharyngeal/retrobulbar orbit), or CSF provides inherent contrast resolution. CT also is used whenever an imaging study is performed on an urgent basis. However, some tumors, especially those in the posterior fossa or temporal fossa, are best visualized with MRI and are occasionally missed by CT imaging (Fig. 11.4). This is particularly the case when the tumor is isodense and thus requires contrast infusion for its delineation (Fig. 11.5). In a brainstem glioma, for instance, sagittal scans demonstrate the rostrocaudal extent of the tumor (Fig. 11.6). Tumors involving the sella or the chiasmatic cistern are also more readily delineated by MRI than by CT because interference

TABLE 11.5 Pediatric Brain Tumors and Age at Presentation

Age	*Benign Masses*	*Malignant Tumors*
0–3 yr	Optic nerve and chiasm glioma, CPP, DIG, low-grade astrocytoma	Ependymoma, PNET/MB, CPC, teratoma, intermediate- and high-grade gliomas
4–12 yr	Migrational abnormalities, JPA, DNT, craniopharyngioma, cerebellar astrocytoma	High-grade gliomas, PNET/MB, ependymoma, BSG, ATT/RhT, germinoma
13–21 yr	Ganglioglioma, PXA, schwannoma, pituitary adenoma	High-grade gliomas, PNET/MB

ATT/RhT, atypical teratoid/rhabdoid tumor; BSG, brainstem glioma; CPC, choroid plexus carcinoma; CPP, choroid plexus papilloma; DIG, desmoplastic infantile ganglioglioma; DNT, dysembryoplastic neuroepithelial tumor; JPA, juvenile pilocytic astrocytoma; PNET/MB, primitive neuroectodermal tumor/medulloblastoma; PXA, pleomorphic xanthoastrocytoma.
Adapted from Quisling RG. Imaging for pediatric brain tumors. *Semin Pediatr Neurol* 1997;4:254–272.

TABLE 11.6 Pediatric Brain Tumors and Central Nervous System Location

Intra-axial cerebrum	Low- and high-grade gliomas, CPP, CPC, DIG, DNT, PXA, PNETs (such as cerebral PNET or pineoplastoma)
Intra-axial cerebellum	JPA, PNET/MB, ependymoma, ATT/RhT
Intra-axial brainstem	Pilocytic or diffuse BSG, ganglioglioma, dorsally exophytic glioma, invasion by ependymomas, PNET/MB
Suprasellar region	Craniopharyngioma, optic pathway glioma, ectopic germ cell tumors, histiocytosis, lipodermoid, arachnoid cyst, adenoma dermoid/epidermoid, tuber cinereum hamartoma
Pineal region	Germ cell tumors, exophytic tectal glioma, exophytic vermic glioma, trilateral retinoblastoma, PNET, teratoma

ATT/RhT, atypical teratoid/rhabdoid tumor; BSG, brainstem glioma; CPC, choroid plexus carcinoma; CPP, choroid plexus papilloma; DIG, desmoplastic infantile ganglioglioma; DNT, dysembryoplastic neuroepithelial tumor; JPA, juvenile pilocytic astrocytoma; PNET/MB, primitive neuroectodermal tumor/medulloblastoma; PXA, pleomorphic xanthoastrocytoma.
Adapted from Quisling RG. Imaging for pediatric brain tumors. *Semin Pediatr Neurol* 1997;4:254–272.

TABLE 11.7 Magnetic Resonance Imaging Features of Benign Tumors

Little to no growth on serial imaging.
Epicenter in gray matter.
Unenhanced signal (in the solid portion) is similar in intensity to gray matter.
Cysts may be present, but necrosis is absent.
Calcification (except in pineal region).
No contrast enhancement in DNTs.
Contrast enhancement in a mural nodule.
Tumor margins on T1 and T2 images correspond anatomically (T1/T2 concordance).

DNT, dysembryoplastic neuroepithelial tumor.

from surrounding bone limits the accuracy of CT. In the experience of Sartor and coworkers, who compared the accuracy of CT scanning with MRI in delineating mass lesions in the sellar region, MRI was equivalent to CT scanning in 54% of cases, superior in 41%, and inferior in only 5% (87).

Because CT imaging concepts are similar to standard radiologic acquisitions, and CT is less often required for neuroaxis tumor imaging, most of the following discussion focuses on MRI.

An understanding of the nature of a brain tumor and its location requires knowledge of T1, T2, and gadolinium-enhanced T1-weighted information (88). Unenhanced

TABLE 11.8 Magnetic Resonance Imaging Features of Malignant Tumors

Growth on serial imaging.
Evidence of tumor necrosis.
T1 and T2 spatial discordance.
Calcification in a pineal region tumor.
Malignant pattern of gadolinium enhancement:
Subpial or subependymal enhancement suggesting tumor infiltration.
Extension of a white matter centered mass through the gray matter cortical mantle.
Multicentricity or satellite lesions in the primary site or in more distant locations remote from the epicenter.
Distant spread in neuraxis. Such lesions can be shown by using a body coil and obtaining post contrast, sagittal, spin echo T1-weighted sequences followed by sagittal gradient using parameters that provide "white" CSF (a myelogram effect). Axial, postcontrast, T1-weighted images are then obtained in the regions often involved by drop metastases, the cervical plexus and cauda equina regions. If any abnormality is observed on the sagittal images, then axial or coronal images would be obtained in these regions as well.

CNS, central nervous sysem; CSF, cerebrospinal fluid.
Note: Clinical history is important to the radiologist evaluating a CNS lesion and the probability that it is malignant. Patients with associated immune system dysfunction are at risk of having malignant tumors such as lymphoma. In addition, prior radiotherapy and chemotherapy increase the probability that a CNS lesion is malignant.

TABLE 11.9 Pediatric Brain Tumor Mimics

Inflammatory	Tumefactive multiple sclerosis, myelin basic protein hypersensitivity, adrenoleukodystrophy
Infectious	Progressive multifocal leukoencephalopathy (papovavirus), tuberculoma, cryptococcoma, neurocystercercosis, chronic empyema
Postsurgical	Reaction to shunt material, seroma, chronic hematoma
Postradiation	Radiation effect, radiation necrosis
Postchemotherapy	Progressive necrotizing leukoencephalopathy
Developmental	Cortical, subcortical, and periventricular heteropias, tuberous sclerosis
Dishistiogenesis	Neurofibromatosis, neurocutaneous melanosis
Vascular	Giant arterial or venous aneurysms (e.g., vein of Galen aneurysms), thrombosed vascular malformations, cavernous angioma, sequestered stroke

Adapted from Quisling RG. Imaging for pediatric brain tumors. *Semin Pediatr Neurol* 1997;4:254–272.

T1-weighted images can reveal areas of pathology that differ from normal brain by being either hyperintense or hypointense when compared with contiguous normal brain. Hyperintensity on T1-weighted images implies the presence of substances that naturally increase proton relaxation, such as methemoglobin (subacute residua of hemorrhage), melanin, dilute amounts of interstitial or intracellular calcification (postradiotherapy), and hyperconcentrated proteins (as might occur in a colloid-containing mass or hypercellular tumors). T1 hypointensity suggests changes related to either anisotropic effects (by structures containing either very large or rigidly bound molecules, as seen in intratumoral desmoplasia or matrix calcification) or, alternatively, tissue containing unbound water (as seen in peritumoral edema, necrosis, or cyst formation) (89,90). T1 hypointensity reflects both extremes of hydrogen states: too tightly bound or too loosely bound compared with protons in adjacent brain parenchyma.

Information from T2-weighted sequences differs from T1-weighted data. In physical terms, T2 rate reflects the time required for the signal to degrade or to disappear from the image. It is a measure of loss of coherence of the magnetic vectors that had been refocused by the second radiofrequency pulse in spin echo sequences or by gradient applications in gradient echo imaging. Tissue with faster T2 rates disperses its signal faster than tissue with slower T2 rates, and hence exhibits less signal intensity on the image. Tissue in which the water molecules are bound within large complex molecules or within rigid tissue has faster T2 rates, and therefore destroys its signal more quickly (T2 hypointensity). Abnormal T2 hypointensity implies a more restricted bulk water pool. The latter occurs in fibrosis, ossification, and dehydrated tissues. Tissues that

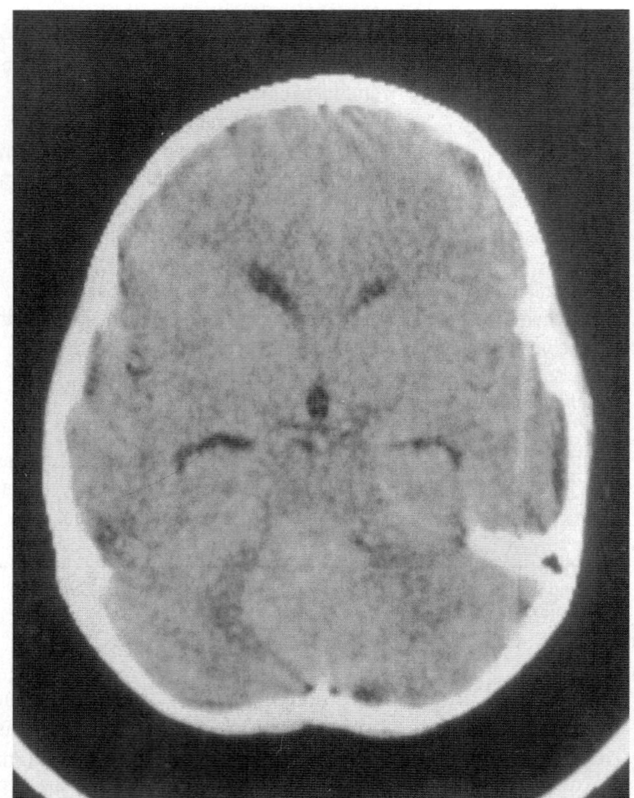

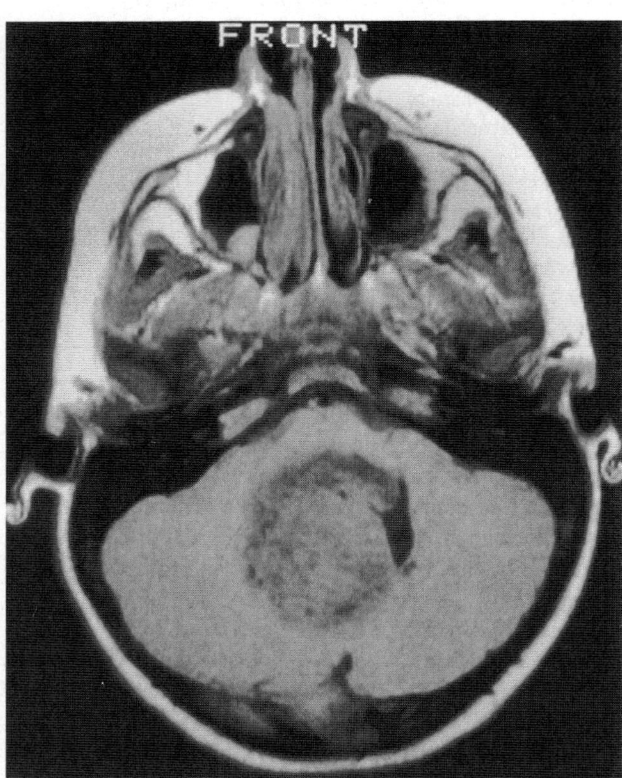

A B

FIGURE 11.4. **A:** Computed tomographic scan of head shows ill-defined posterior fossa density that obliterates the fourth ventricle. **B:** Magnetic resonance imaging shows a well-defined midline posterior fossa tumor in the same patient. Magnetic resonance imaging is clearly superior to computed tomographic scanning in visualizing the tumor.

possess more unbound water molecules (such as CSF or vasogenic edema) have slower T2 rates and therefore exhibit a brighter signal. Abnormal T2 hyperintensity implies an increase in bulk tissue water.

For most intra-axial brain or spinal cord tumors, the T2-weighted sequences more accurately predict the extent of tumor infiltration. Although peritumoral tissue edema may not always contain tumor cells, the correlation is high. The zone of abnormality on standard spin echo T2-weighted images is a good measure of tumor infiltration.

Use of intravenously injected gadolinium (gadopentetate dimeglumine at 0.1 mmol/kg) or other paramagnetic compounds significantly improves the resolution of many brain tumors (86). T1-weighted, gadolinium-enhanced imaging is generally acquired in two orthogonal planes to ensure full appreciation of a tumor's margins. The optimal planes of section, however, depend on the location of the tumor. Gadolinium enhancement arises whenever the capillary bed is expanded or vessels leak contrast through their walls. It assists in defining areas of edema and necrosis, cyst formation, spinal cord metastases, and extension of tumor to the leptomeninges or ependyma. High-grade tumors such as glioblastomas, ependymoblastomas, and PNET/MBs tend to enhance, whereas surrounding edema does not. Lack of enhancement increases the likelihood that the tumor is benign. MRI with gadolinium enhancement also is of considerable value in postoperative follow-up studies in distinguishing residual or recurrent tumor from edema, granulation tissue, and necrosis. As a rule, any structure that enhances with iodine on CT enhances on MRI with gadolinium; the reverse is not always the case. In a recent series of 225 patients by Laughton and colleagues (91), MRI linear enhancement following surgery almost always resolved or improved within 12 weeks. Increasing enhancing tissue at the surgical site correlated with local recurrence. The persistence of enhancing tissue beyond 12 weeks was usually due to residual tumor. The development of enhancing foci in the previously nonenhancing tumor was due to radionecrosis or histological change in the grade of the original tumor. Finally, nodular postsurgical enhancement was nonspecific and secondary to postsurgical changes, residual tumor, or occasionally, choroid plexus.

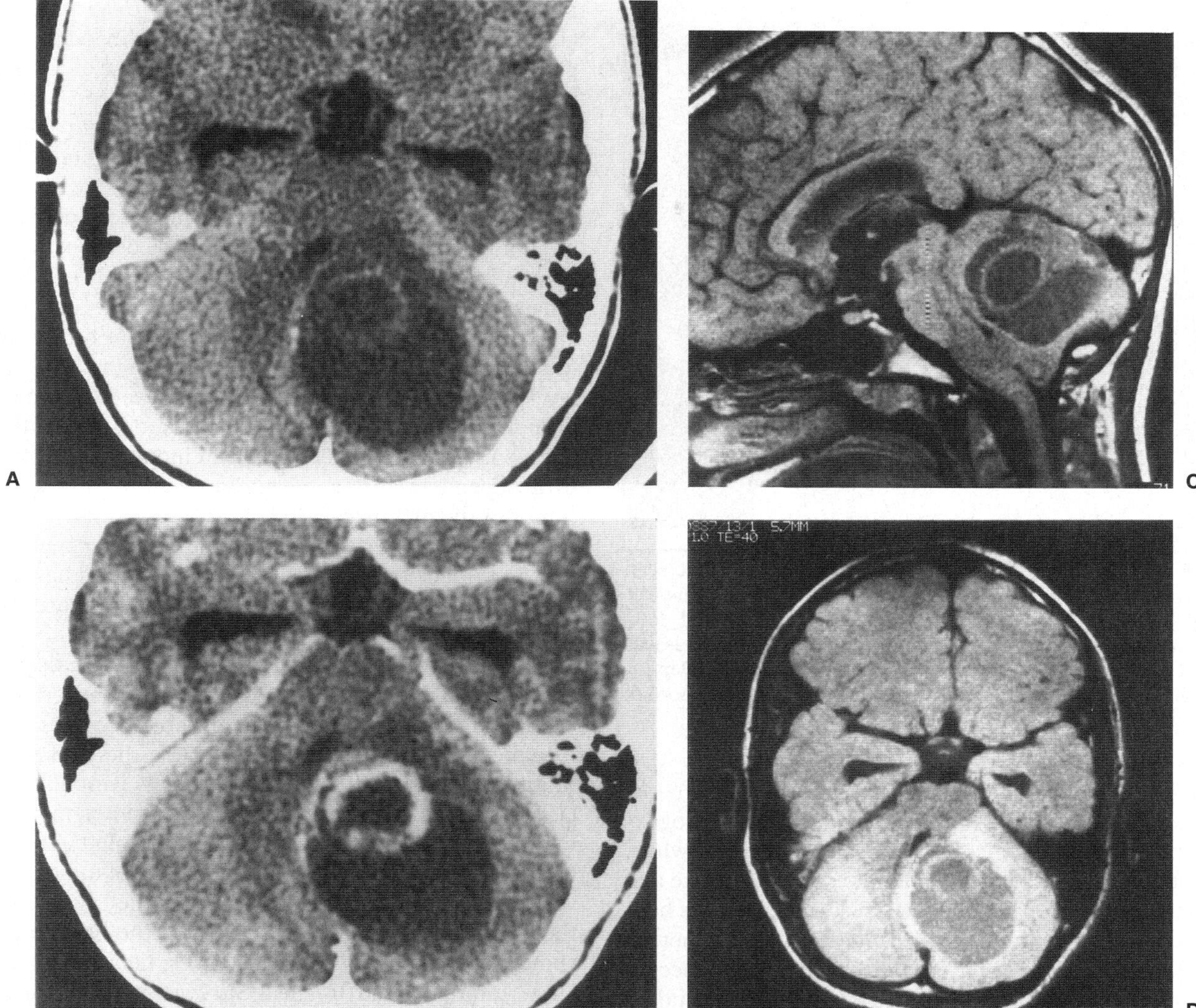

FIGURE 11.5. Computed tomographic scans revealing cerebellar cystic astrocytoma in a 13-year-old boy. Computed tomographic scans before **(A)** and after **(B)** injection of iodinated contrast material show a large lesion predominantly involving the left cerebellar hemisphere but extending to the vermis. The large, well-demarcated macrocyst contains proteinaceous fluid, which accounts for the high density of the cyst fluid compared with CSF in the suprasellar cistern, temporal horns, and third ventricle. **A:** A small fleck of calcium is noted medially within the wall of the macrocyst on the noncontrast computed tomography. An enhancing tumor nodule projects into the anterior portion of the macrocyst; some areas of the macrocyst wall are enhanced as well. T1-weighted magnetic resonance images in the sagittal **(C)** and axial **(D)** planes also are shown. These noncontrast magnetic resonance studies were done before gadolinium-diethylenetriaminepenta-acetic acid was approved for use in children. The magnetic resonance findings are concordant with the computed tomographic scan changes. If gadolinium-diethylenetriaminepenta-acetic acid could have been used, it probably would have enhanced abnormalities comparable with iodinated contrast on the computed tomographic scan. At surgery, a middle-grade astrocytoma was found. The macrocyst contained yellow fluid; small cysts and necrotic areas were found within the mural nodule. (Courtesy of Drs. Hervey D. Segall, Marvin D. Nelson, Jr., and Corey Raffel, Children's Hospital, Los Angeles.)

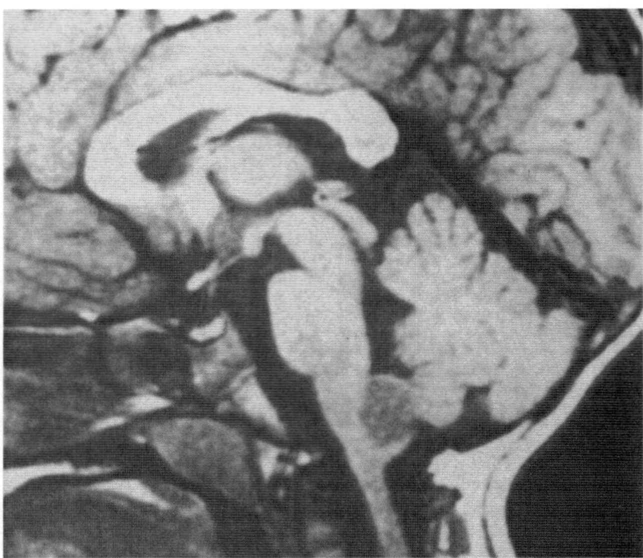

FIGURE 11.6. Sagittal T1-weighted magnetic resonance scan showing a posterior exophytic brainstem glioma in a 6-year-old girl. The scan shows a rounded, sharply marginated, low-intensity tumor projecting posteriorly from the medulla. This was a grade II astrocytoma. (Courtesy of Dr. Hervey D. Segall, Department of Radiology, University of Southern California School of Medicine.)

Fluid-attenuated inversion recovery (FLAIR) sequences, which are now preferred by many radiologists to distinguish pathologic tissue edema in locations where CSF abuts brain, especially along the cortical surface and within the depths of sulci. Since fast scan techniques have been applied in conjunction with the FLAIR parameters, they have become the preferred imaging sequence in neuro-oncology. Other imaging techniques, including diffusion imaging, perfusion imaging, and functional imaging (such as MR spectroscopy) are increasingly used in neuro-oncology (92–96). Newer technologic developments are constantly unfolding to characterize tumor burden and the effects of tumor and therapies on brain structure and function (97,98). There is evidence that combining positron-emission tomography (PET) to image-guided surgical tumor resection provides contour to achieve total resection of ill-defined tumors and better resolution of residual disease following surgery (99–101). Methionine-PET is useful in distinguishing between benign and malignant CNS lesions (102). MRI diffusion, perfusion, and spectroscopy imaging tools are increasingly incorporated into clinical trials in pediatric neuro-oncology (103).

Other Studies

Ancillary studies are often used to further delineate the nature and the extent of the tumor. MR arteriography, or conventional arteriography using digital subtraction techniques, helps delineate the blood supply to the mass lesion (104). Additionally, these procedures can indicate the degree of malignancy and exclude the presence of a vascular malformation (105).

The dangers attending lumbar puncture in the presence of increased intracranial pressure preclude its use as part of the initial evaluation of a child with a suspected brain neoplasm. Because the presence and location of an intracranial abscess can readily be demonstrated by gadolinium-enhanced MRI, examination of the CSF is no longer used for this purpose. The appearance and composition of CSF in brain tumor patients were presented by Merritt in his classic study (106). Although CSF glucose level is almost always normal, it is reduced in some children with leukemic or lymphosarcomatous infiltration of the meninges and in meningeal carcinomatosis secondary to an ependymoma, a melanosarcoma, or a malignant tumor of the meninges (107).

Cytology can be performed on the CSF after centrifugation and can help determine whether the tumor has spread to the meninges or to the spinal subarachnoid space, as can occur in a PNET/MB (108).

The presence of malignant cells in the CSF indicates extensive seeding of the leptomeninges. In the experience of Glass and associates, such results were encountered only in patients with lymphomas and were the consequence of mistakenly identifying lymphocytes as lymphoma cells (108). False-negative results are fairly common in all types of tumors, with the exception of acute lymphatic leukemia (108). They are the result of the adherance of tumor cells to various structures of the CNS, such as the cauda equina, the cranial nerves, and the surface of the brain and the spinal cord (108a). In some instances, neuroimaging can show tumor spread to the CSF even when cytology is normal.

A less beneficial adjunct to the localization of an intracranial mass lesion is the EEG. Its greatest value lies in suggesting the presence of temporal lobe tumors in children with complex partial seizures. In such patients, the persistence of local slow-wave activity, overshadowing the spike and sharp-wave activity usually associated with seizures, points to a space-occupying lesion and calls for more definitive imaging studies.

Plain skull films can suggest an intracranial mass lesion if they show separation of sutures, erosion or enlargement of the sella turcica, or osteoporosis, especially thinning of the sphenoid ridge. Because the bones of the vault become more firmly joined, separation of sutures is rare in children older than 10 years of age and is practically nonexistent beyond age 20 years. In young children, sutures can spread after increased intracranial pressure lasting 10 days or even less, though suture separation takes longer to develop in older children (109). Radiographic evidence of calcification can be seen in 15% to 20% of intracranial tumors of childhood, mostly in the form of clusters of multiple specks. Approximately 50% of oligodendrogliomas, a rare tumor in childhood, develop radiologic signs of calcification (110). The most common tumor to produce suprasellar calcification is the craniopharyngioma, and it does so in approximately 70% to 80% of cases, usually along the superior aspect of the mass. In tuberous sclerosis, multiple calcifications varying in size from specks to up to 1 cm are usually located along the ventricular walls, less often within the cerebrum and the posterior fossa.

The use of ultrasound in the detection of intracranial tumors is limited to neonates and infants with an open fontanelle (111).

Positron-emission tomography has considerable potential in delineating brain tumors. Primary brain tumors show good correlation between the uptake of labeled fluorodeoxyglucose (FDG) and the malignancy of the tumor as verified by its histology. Differences in uptake of FDG or labeled methionine also can assist in defining the site for a stereotactic biopsy (99–101). Additionally, the rate of FDG uptake after tumor irradiation generally allows one to differentiate between tumor recurrence, in which uptake is increased, and radiation necrosis, in which it is reduced (112). Corticosteroid therapy does not alter the PET scan. Thus, in the experience of Glantz and coworkers, 95% of patients with hypermetabolic abnormalities on the postoperative PET scan had recurrence of their tumor. Abscesses were, however, indistinguishable from recurrent tumors (113). The role of metabolic brain imaging as an adjunct to structural imaging is further discussed in the subsequent section dealing with radiotherapy.

MR spectroscopy has been used to determine the response of tumors to radiation or chemotherapy. As experience has grown with spectroscopy, it has increasingly been used in characterizing brain tumors at diagnosis and in follow-up (92–96).

Differential Diagnosis

Increased intracranial pressure is encountered not only in brain tumors, but also in various other mass lesions within the cranium. In infants, brain tumors cause increased intracranial pressure less commonly than do hydrocephalus, intracranial hemorrhage, and infections. Beyond 2 years of age, brain tumors become a progressively more frequent cause of increased intracranial pressure. Infections are encountered less often.

A brain abscess can act as a space-occupying lesion. It can arise from the direct spread of bacteria from an infected ear, mastoid, or paranasal sinus, or by hematogenous dissemination from a distant source. Brain abscesses are liable to occur in patients with congenital heart disease, particularly in those who have a significant right-to-left shunt. The presence of increased intracranial pressure in patients with congenital heart disease should arouse immediate suspicion of a brain abscess. Only approximately 30% of these children have fever, so its absence does not distinguish an abscess from a tumor. In most instances, MRI or CT scanning with contrast infusion is diagnostic of abscesses.

In pseudotumor cerebri, intracranial pressure is elevated in the absence of a mass lesion. No localizing signs are present, the spinal fluid is normal, and imaging studies show the ventricular system to be normal or smaller than normal, but not displaced or distorted.

In the past, one of the differential diagnoses was lead encephalopathy. This was particularly the case when generalized convulsions coincided with a clinical picture of a posterior fossa tumor (see Chapter 10).

The clinical differentiation of hydrocephalus of nonneoplastic origin from midline brain tumors usually requires MRI. Like hydrocephalus, mass lesions can produce striking cranial enlargement during the early months of life, and a gradually expanding periaqueductal tumor, such as a fibrillary astrocytoma of the quadrigeminal plate, can produce aqueductal stenosis and ultimately complete obstruction. MRI demonstrates not only the distortion of the ventricular system that can accompany a brain tumor, but also any small mass that might have produced aqueductal obstruction (114). Normally, CSF flow through the aqueduct produces a signal void on T2-weighted images (i.e., an area of blackness); absence of the void indicates cessation of flow and partial or complete obstruction.

Severe herpes simplex encephalitis can simulate a rapidly expanding temporal lobe lesion because of the massive edema that accompanies the infection and because of its predilection for the temporal lobe. Additionally, a small proportion of children with cerebral degenerative diseases, notably acute disseminated encephalomyelitis (ADEM) and subacute sclerosing panencephalitis, can develop increased intracranial pressure and papilledema. When these signs are accompanied by predominantly unilateral signs, as they frequently are, the clinical diagnosis of brain tumor is unavoidable and is refuted only by neuroimaging studies that demonstrate white matter edema (115).

Treatment

Surgical extirpation remains the mainstay of treatment for pediatric brain tumors. The advent of the operating microscope, laser beam, and ultrasonographic methods have made it possible to increase the number of children having safe and complete tumor resections.

Most patients harboring a brain tumor rapidly improve with the administration of dexamethasone at a 0.1 to 0.5 mg/kg starting dose. This reduces increased intracranial pressure and allows the surgeon a much less explosive environment in which to radically resect the tumor. Then, if necessary, the child should be immediately transported to a brain tumor center. Other medications, such as phenytoin or fosphenytoin, can be used prophylactically in the perioperative period. The pediatric neurosurgeon is more than a technician in brain tumor surgery because the surgeon can provide vital information about extent of infiltration of the nervous system by direct observation of the brain tumor. Experience is the key to radical resection with low morbidity. The adaptation of the operating microscope to microneurosurgery, ultrasonic aspiration, and stereotaxis have made it possible to operate on brain tumors with minimal morbidity. The role of CT- and MRI-guided stereotactic biopsies in childhood brain tumors is appropriate and preferable to open biopsy in tumors involving the basal ganglia, thalamus, and midbrain. This simple, precise diagnostic test can provide an accurate diagnosis in approximately 95% of cases, with morbidity in the 2% to 5% range (116).

The main goal of brain tumor surgery has remained constant: to maximize resection while preserving function. Patients with benign tumors such as pilocytic astrocytomas of the posterior fossa are often cured by complete resections. However, one of most common errors made during surgery is the discontinuation of a procedure when a tumor such as an astrocytoma, ependymoma, or PNET/MB is perceived to be emanating from the floor of the fourth ventricle (117). Commonly, these tumors involve the middle cerebellar peduncle adjacent to the fourth ventricle and should be totally resectable. For PNET/MB, it is widely accepted that the degree of tumor resection is important prognostically. Ependymoma can insinuate itself into an enlarged foramen of Luschka, but the surgical attempt will be discontinued inappropriately when the surgeon perceives the lesion to be invading the brainstem. Although the posterior fossa poses a considerable challenge to the neurosurgeon, new techniques such as intraoperative imaging with MRI are having a favorable impact on the safety of tumor resection (118). Whether such techniques will decrease the incidence of cerebellar mutism postoperatively remains to be seen.

Establishing the correct neuropathologic diagnosis of a pediatric brain tumor is critical in directing subsequent therapeutic efforts. Neuroimaging studies and perioperative frozen sections and touch preparations may be highly suggestive of a particular histologic type of tumor. However, a final diagnosis of surgically resected material often requires immunohistochemistry, flow cytometry, and electron microscopy. Therefore, it is best to wait 48 to 72 hours postoperatively for a final neuropathologic interpretation before discussing prognosis and any adjuvant treatment plans with the family.

Postsurgical Neuroimaging

The most important role of neuroimaging after surgery is to determine whether a mass has been completely resected and to assess the extent of any residual tumor. This information is most readily provided by serial imaging studies. Consequently, an immediate (24 to 48 hours) postoperative baseline study should be obtained. A variety of abnormalities can be observed. Postoperative edema can be present for days. Blood products can be seen for months. Tumor bed granulation tissue may be seen for years and can mimic residual tumor. MRI shows encephalomalacia, non-nodular contrast enhancement conforming to the encephalomalacia (granulation tissue), and hypodense susceptibility artifact in the same region as the enhancement on T2-weighted images. The reduced T2 signal is believed to be the result of microhemorrhages and hemosiderin deposition. Presence of nodular hyperintense abnormalities on T2-weighted sequences should raise the suspicion of residual neoplasia. Special attention to the depths of the middle fossa and to the cribriform plate is important because subarachnoid space extends to these regions and may harbor metastatic tumor.

Another surgically related abnormality is dural thickening and enhancement associated with the presence of an indwelling ventricular-peritoneal shunt catheter. The dural changes may occur near the entrance of the shunt or in a more diffuse fashion overlying the surface of the brain. Benign dural thickening is not nodular and generally ranges from 1 to 3 mm. The ventricular-peritoneal shunt typically reduces the volume of the ipsilateral lateral ventricle more so than the contralateral side. The value of surveillance brain imaging varies by tumor type. The purpose of serial imaging is to document the response to treatment and make a diagnosis of recurrence or complications as soon as possible (119).

Radiotherapy

Radiotherapy can be used either as an adjuvant to surgery or for definitive therapy when complete resection is not feasible. Standard techniques of pediatric CNS radiotherapy, such as limited-field radiotherapy and craniospinal radiotherapy, have offered curative therapy for low-grade gliomas, PNET/MB, germinoma, and other tumor types. Advanced radiotherapy techniques, including conformal therapy, fractionated stereotactic radiotherapy, and stereotactic radiosurgery, are improving survival and reducing neurotoxicity. Many factors must be considered in deciding precisely how to safely use radiotherapy.

Within cells, the most abundant molecule is water. In addition, lipids, proteins, carbohydrates, and nucleotides are present. When ionizing radiation interacts with a cell, reactive species are created that damage cellular DNA (120). Tumor cells are particularly vulnerable to such damage because of aberrant cell cycle control mechanisms and because radiotherapy technique (multiple beams of radiation) delivers more radiation to the tumor site than to normal brain.

For each histologically defined pediatric brain tumor, there are critical radiation treatment parameters, such as total dose, time, and volume of tissue treated. Slow-growing focal tumors such as pilocytic and low-grade fibrillary astrocytomas may require limited-field radiation, whereas infiltrative tumors such as PNET/MB, germinoma, and atypical teratoid/ rhabdoid tumor require craniospinal radiation.

Another important factor in determining a treatment approach for pediatric brain tumors is whether radiation is used as a single modality or in its more common role as a component of multimodal therapy. Timing of treatment and the dose delivered are affected by adjuvant chemotherapy, surgery, or both. Furthermore, patient age and tumor location in relationship to dose-limiting critical neural structures significantly influence the anticipated sequelae of treatment.

Modern brain imaging machines have made the use of stereotactic radiotherapy techniques possible and have allowed for the delivery of large single doses of radiation to well-defined intracranial targets (121). In addition, radiation scatter is limited and thus, theoretically, should reduce late cognitive or endocrine effects from limited-field radiation of brain tumors. Advances in stereotactic treatment methods may soon supplant standard external-beam radiation, which has been used for decades (121).

In models of external-beam radiotherapy, treatment planning begins with construction of a face mask for reproducible position. Using this system along with standard relocation technologies such as laser beams, a patient can be repositioned daily with an accuracy of 3 to 9 mm (122). Stereotactic radiosurgery requires placement of a stereotactic head ring, which is attached to the patient's skull. Imaging in reference to the ring can then identify mathematical coordinates for each pixel in the CT or MRI images that directly corresponds to points in the patient positioned in the ring. Treatment planning identifies a coordinate at the center of a treatment plan, and data can be transferred to a treatment delivery machine with high accuracy (123). The technique uses the equivalent of hundreds of radiation beams delivered with circular fields via multiple arcs of treatment. This allows the radiation dose to be delivered accurately and to fall off optimally outside the treatment volume. Although a large single-dose treatment has radiobiologic disadvantages for more malignant tumors, the advantage of accurate avoidance of normal tissue with steep dose gradients has made this a proven therapy for several entities, including arteriovenous malformations ependymomas, acoustic schwannomas, metastases, and meningiomas (124,125).

Use of stereotactic radiosurgery in benign and malignant tumors in children has been less well defined than in adults, although experience in pediatrics is increasing. Stereotactic radiosurgery has been a valuable adjunctive strategy in the management of recurrent or unresectable pediatric astrocytomas (126). Further details of this procedure are provided by Bova and coworkers (127), Flickinger and coworkers (128), and Murthy and colleagues for posterior fossa tumors (129). Proton radiation therapy enables the radiation oncologist to conform the radiation dose around even highly irregular tumor volumes with homogeneous dose distribution throughout. Hug and colleagues have reported use of conformal proton radiation therapy for pediatric low-grade astrocytomas (130). Proton radiation therapy may also allow reduction of the cochlear dose of radiation associated with sensorineural hearing loss that is a significant late effect from treatment of brain tumors (131).

Immediate and Long-Term Effects of Radiation Therapy

As improved surgical and radiation techniques have lengthened survival of children with brain tumors, concern has grown about the quality of life in survivors and about the nature and extent of radiation-induced deficits.

Pathologic and experimental studies indicate that the major pathophysiology of radiation-induced brain damage results from damage to the vascular endothelium, tissue that is more radiosensitive than neurons. This results in obstruction of small and medium-sized blood vessels with ensuing thrombosis and infarction of deep white matter, but relative sparing of cortex and subcortical white matter. Large vessel injury is far less common (132). Additional or alternative mechanisms of brain injury have been proposed. These involve direct injury to glia and axons, and, less likely, an autoimmune vasculitis (133). Vasogenic edema is probably responsible for acute reactions that develop within a few weeks of radiation.

Neurologic symptoms can develop during radiation, or shortly thereafter, or have their onset after an interval of many months or years.

Acutely, craniospinal radiation may produce nausea and vomiting within 2 to 6 hours of treatment because the radiation beam exits through the stomach and bowel. In contrast, some children exhibit anticipatory nausea and vomiting that occurs before or within 2 hours of treatment. Symptoms are typically well controlled with antiemetics such as prochlorperazine, but occasionally require newer, more potent agents such as ondansetron.

Several weeks after the start of radiotherapy, patients lose hair and complain of skin soreness, erythema, and sore throat. These side effects begin to abate 1 to 2 weeks after therapy. Use of topical cream should be avoided unless the radiation oncologist is consulted because many are oil-based and contain metal, which increases the surface radiation dose during therapy. After therapy is complete, aloe-based creams are recommended, and occasionally corticosteroid-based creams or newer matrix gels are used. Craniospinal radiation can cause thrombocytopenia, leukopenia, and anemia; thrombocytopenia delays completion of radiation treatment. Thus, complete blood counts should be obtained weekly during radiotherapy. If a delay is necessary, any limited-field external beam boost or fractionated stereotactic approaches may be used in the interim. These regionally limited treatments allow bone marrow recovery without placing the patient at risk for future tumor progression.

Acute radiation encephalopathy occurs in the course of treatment whenever large daily fraction doses are administered. The underlying pathology is that of cerebral edema caused by vascular damage and an ensuing increase in vessel wall permeability, which in turn produces perivascular edema, and in the most severe cases, microhemorrhage and thrombi. Cortical neurons disappear, and fibrillary gliosis extends from the cortical surface into the deeper layers of gray matter. Radiation injury to brain parenchyma results in intravascular and perivascular microcalcifications. These are most common at the junction of cortical gray and white matter and the basal ganglia (134).

The clinical picture varies. In general, it consists of lethargy, nausea and vomiting, seizures, and an exacerbation of pre-existing neurologic deficits. MRI shows focal, multifocal, or diffusely increased signal in white matter on T2-weighted images (135). Lesions tend to start as small foci that progress with time. They are irreversible and do not correlate well with neurologic or developmental deficits (136). Acute radiation encephalopathy can be treated with corticosteroids, but it is preferable to prevent complications by administering low daily dosages, particularly in the rare instance in which radiotherapy is considered essential in infants and young children.

During therapy, some children are fatigued and do not make optimal effort in cognitive testing. Thus, it is best to complete radiation treatment before assessing cognition. Fatigue usually diminishes weeks to months after therapy, although many patients experience an early delayed response termed the *somnolence syndrome* in the 6 weeks to 3 months after radiotherapy.

The late effects of radiotherapy include impaired cognition, defective endocrine function, and the development of a second neoplasia.

A reduction of cognitive function is encountered in children irradiated for supratentorial and infratentorial tumors (120). Retrospective studies indicate that between 10% and 80% of surviving children who have undergone either local or whole-brain radiation therapy demonstrate a significant loss in full-scale IQ (134). Craniospinal radiation can be expected to lower IQ by 10 to 20 points (137). In a study by Spiegler and colleagues, results showed a 2- to 4-point decline per year in intelligence scores, with more rapid declines over the first few years (138). In addition, almost all children who have retained a normal IQ can be found to have some degree of attention and memory deficit (137). Visual perceptual skills, learning abilities, memory, and adaptive behavior also are adversely affected (138–140). These cognitive deficits are most evident in children younger than 7 years of age and appear to progress over the course of several years after completion of radiotherapy (141,142). Infants younger than 3 years of age have the worst prognosis in terms of intellectual development (143,144). Adjuvant chemotherapy, particularly intraventricular or intrathecal methotrexate, is believed to increase the risk for the development of dementia, as does a tumor localized to the cerebral hemispheres or the hypothalamus (137,145). Thus, the commonly used regimen of cranial irradiation and methotrexate can induce a necrotizing encephalopathy several months to years after completion of treatment. The incidence of necrotizing encephalopathy is dose related with respect to methotrexate and irradiation. However, children under age 10 years with brain tumors treated without radiation have a stable IQ (146). It is too early to know if hyperfractionated and reduced boost radiotherapy will decrease cognitive effects in children with PNET/MB without increasing the risk of tumor recurrence. Children with ependymoma who receive local radiotherapy are at much lower risk for worsening cognition, but postoperative neurological deficits are strongly correlated with poor intellectual outcome (147).

Neuroimaging studies in children with reduced cognition demonstrate white matter damage. On MRI, increased signal is seen in the periventricular white matter on FLAIR or T2-weighted images. The involved area has a scalloped appearance; often it extends to the gray-white matter junction (148). Zimmerman and colleagues have graded the white matter changes observed on MRI (149). There appears to be a direct relationship between the volume of brain irradiated and the development of white matter changes (150); the correlation between the severity of white matter involvement and the neurologic and cognitive deficits is not as good. This is particularly true for young children whose abnormalities on MRI tend to be less pronounced than those of older children (151). A longitudinal MRI study showed a decline in corpus callosum volumes in posterior subregions that receive the highest total dose of irradiation in treatment of PNET/MB (152).

Because of these sequelae, hyperfractionated approaches to treatment have been designed for treatment of the youngest children who must receive radiotherapy for tumor control. Careful attention to obtaining baseline studies before beginning radiotherapy is essential, as is recognition that the tumor itself plus surgery, chemotherapy, and psychosocial factors all contribute to function and coping.

A second important late effect of irradiation of the craniospinal axis is a disturbance in various growth and endocrine functions. This is seen in some 70% to 90% of patients (144,153). Although acutely not problematic, pituitary function can decline with time in 50% to 70% of patients, depending on the radiation dose and fractionation used. As a rule, the hypothalamus is more sensitive to radiation than the pituitary, and growth hormone secretion is affected first (134). An irreversible growth hormone deficiency becomes apparent 1 or more years after completion of irradiation and produces a gradual diminution of growth rate (154,155). In the series of Constine and coworkers, only 36% of children who received cranial irradiation, and 25% of children who received craniospinal irradiation, attained a height greater than the third percentile (153). Irradiation of the spine significantly affects the overall crown-rump height of a young patient. Furthermore, the musculature and size of the vertebral bodies and sternum may be affected by treatment. These growth anomalies yield a characteristic body habitus (120). In addition, cranial treatment in young children can affect skull growth. These growth anomalies are important to recognize because musculoskeletal function and appearance are important determinants of self-esteem, coping, and social function in children and adolescents. Gonadotropin deficiency with delayed or precocious puberty also is encountered. Seventy percent of irradiated postpubertal girls had oligomenorrhea, and 30% of postpubertal boys had low testosterone levels. Symptoms of hypothyroidism were seen in 28%, and 62% had low total or free serum thyroxine levels (153). Interestingly, a recent report from Massimino and colleagues showed that thyroid stimulating hormone (TSH) suppression through I-thyroxin medication had protective activity on thyroid function at three years following radiotherapy for PNET/MB (156). Diabetes insipidus owing to irradiation has not been reported (154). In a recently reported series of survivors of pediatric brain tumors (a mix of patients having had surgery, radiotherapy, and chemotherapy), 85.3% had hypothyroidism, 73.5% had proven/probable growth hormone deficiency, 44.1% had adrenal insufficiency, 38.2% had hypogonadism, 34% had diabetes insipidus, and 8.8% had precocious puberty; 32.4% of patients with neuroendocrine sequelae had panhypopituitarism (157). However, in a study by Spoudeas and colleagues of children with posterior fossa tumors, there was a low incidence of anterior pituitary hormone deficiencies (158). Regrettably, radiation to the hypothalamic-pituitary axis and/or whole brain radiation seems to have little effect on the high prevalence of body mass indexes above the 95th percentile in children with brain tumors (31.5%) (159).

Replacement of growth, thyroid, adrenal, and sex hormones should be overseen by an endocrinologist (160,161). No conclusive data show an increased risk of tumor recurrence with growth hormone replacement. As an extra precaution, however, it is common practice for endocrinologists to ensure that there has been no residual tumor or evidence of tumor progression for at least 2 years before starting growth hormone therapy. In addition, many recommend more frequent brain imaging in the first year of growth hormone therapy.

An uncommon but devastating late effect is a second unrelated malignancy within or outside the CNS (162–164). It is estimated that one in six children who have had a brain tumor develop this complication years after radiation (165,166). A different type of cancer found within a radiation field at a significant interval after completion of treatment is considered a radiation-induced malignancy (164). In the series of Meadows and colleagues (153), 68% of tumors developed in radiation-exposed tissue. Tumors result not only from prior radiation, but also reflect a genetic predisposition to malignancies. These second cancers can be highly malignant and respond poorly to available therapies (162,167).

Children treated with high-dose radiation also are at a ninefold increase in risk for developing second, unrelated CNS tumors. These appear at intervals of years to decades after irradiation and are often highly malignant (134). In a study at St. Jude Children's Research Hospital (168), the 15-year cumulative incidence of second neoplasm and second malignant neoplasm was 5.3% and 4%, respectively (168). Young patients and patients with choroid plexus tumors appear to have an increased risk of second neoplasms that is associated with genetic factors (169).

Late radiation encephalopathy is a much less common complication. It develops several months to years after completion of treatment and is caused by brain necrosis or atrophy. The clinical picture is highlighted by headaches, seizures, and focal neurologic signs, notably hemiparesis. The course is slowly progressive. Imaging studies demonstrate low-density lesions within the brain. Symptomatic intraparenchymal hemorrhages outside the primary brain tumor site also have been recorded as a late complication (170). The exact cause of late radiation encephalopathy is unknown, but it is believed to result from a large total radiation dosage or large daily fractions (171).

Rarely, one observes a transitory episode of demyelination that appears some 2 to 3 months after completion of radiation and slowly resolves over the course of 6 to 8 weeks.

A late-onset myelopathy is another rare complication. Symptoms can be acute or chronically progressive. They range in severity from mild sensory signs, or lower motor neuron disease, to an acute paraplegia or quadriplegia (172). Cerebrovascular disease, manifested by strokes or transient ischemic attacks, can develop years to decades after completion of radiotherapy, particularly when radiotherapy is combined with chemotherapy. Damage to medium or large vessels—-in particular, the carotid artery and its major branches—-often can be documented (173). Recurrent attacks of migraine-like headaches lasting 2 to 24 hours and associated with focal symptoms such as aphasia or hemiparesis can represent a late complication of irradiation and chemotherapy (174). Children respond to propanolol or other antimigraine medications. Cerebral arteriography can trigger such an attack in these children.

In view of the high incidence of serious complications, there has been a trend toward delaying radiotherapy in

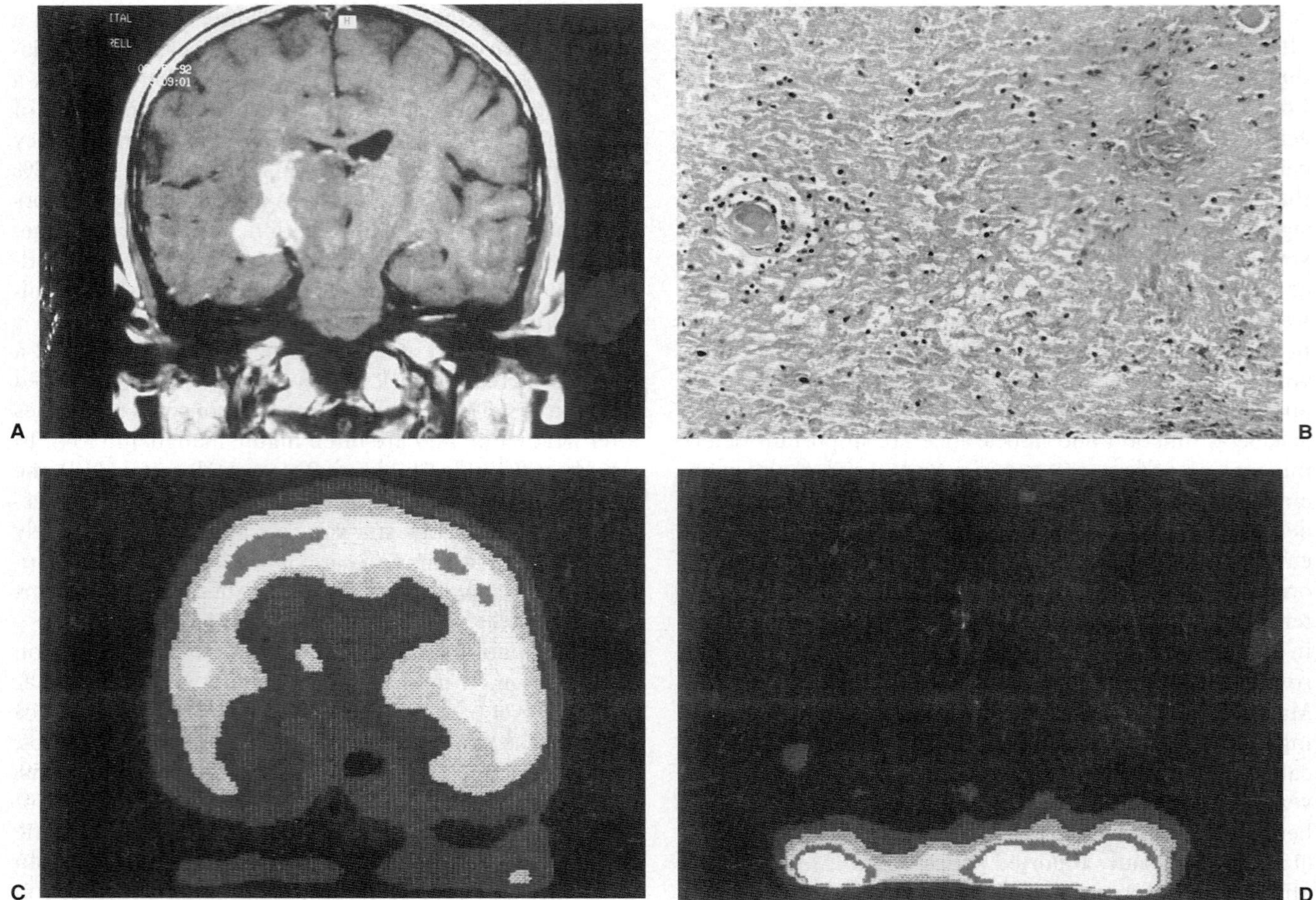

FIGURE 11.7. T1-weighted coronal magnetic resonance imaging with gadolinium demonstrates deep white matter enhancing lesion in right hemisphere **(A).** ^{99m}Tc HMPAO uptake **(B)** was decreased and ^{201}Tl uptake was absent **(D).** Histologic preparation **(C)** reveals coagulative necrosis, consistent with radiation effect, and no evidence of tumor (hematoxylin and eosin, original magnification x66). The patient was originally thought to have had a low-grade glioma and thus received radiotherapy. The patient is free of tumor more than 8 years from diagnosis.

patients younger than 3 years of age; prolonged postoperative chemotherapy is the preferred treatment. Such a regimen appears to be well tolerated, and its results compare favorably with those obtained in children treated with postoperative radiation and adjuvant chemotherapy. It appears, therefore, that postponement of radiation therapy is a feasible alternative for small children and infants (175).

Neuroimaging After Radiotherapy

Neuroimaging can disclose a variety of changes consequent to radiotherapy. Most commonly, one sees mucositis within the paranasal sinuses and mastoid air cells and replacement of fat in marrow space. T2 hyperintensity may persist for months after stereotactic radiotherapy or radiosurgery. Standard-dose craniospinal radiotherapy produces few acute or subacute changes. Patients receiving whole-brain or craniospinal radiation may, after a period of several months, develop mild diffuse brain or spinal cord atrophy and chronic ischemic demyelination.

Radiation dosages that exceed neural tolerance produce radiation necrosis or progressive necrotizing leukoencephalopathy. The latter is usually seen when radiation therapy is used in conjunction with chemotherapy. The appearance of radiation necrosis on MRI and CT studies mimics residual or recurrent tumor (Fig. 11.7). Metabolic imaging tools such as 2-fluoro-2-deoxy-D-glucose (FDG) positron emission tomography, or thallium 201 single-photon emission CT (SPECT) can characterize metabolic activity within lesions (176–179). Neoplastic lesions have increased uptake of FDG and thallium, whereas radiation necrosis has decreased FDG metabolism as compared with normal surrounding brain; no thallium uptake occurs on SPECT imaging (179). Evidence exists that thallium is a more sensitive marker of viable tumor, whereas FDG provides information about metabolic activity in brain surrounding tumor (179). Despite these advances in metabolic characterization of lesions that arise after radiotherapy, biopsy is still the diagnostic gold standard.

Chemotherapy

One of the concerns about using chemotherapy in treating brain tumors has been the fact that chemotherapy drugs cannot penetrate the blood–brain barrier with ease. However, blood vessels within tumors, particularly malignant lesions, are much more permeable than normal vessels, thus allowing entry of drugs. The heterogeneity of tumors and their vasculature probably accounts for incomplete entry of drugs in different regions of a mass lesion; invading tumor cells at a distance from the primary mass are less likely to encounter cytotoxic chemotherapy because surrounding vessels retain their blood–brain barrier. Despite these limitations, clinical trials have shown safety and efficacy of chemotherapy in pediatric brain tumors, such as PNET/MB, germinoma, and pilocytic astrocytoma, and in infants with various malignant lesions. To overcome the blood–brain barrier, strategies have been designed to concentrate chemotherapy agents within brain tumors. One of the proposed strategies is to implant a pump that administers chemotherapy. The pump is a self-contained delivery system connected to the brain or spinal cord. Although pumps have the capacity to deliver drugs more uniformly than pills or injections and to bypass the blood–brain barrier, their overall effectiveness for managing brain tumors remains inconclusive (180).

Another approach is the use of polymer matrixes (plastic) to improve local therapy of malignant brain tumors. The new plastics enable the drugs to diffuse into the tumor bed in a continuous, uniform fashion. The plastic casings also protect unstable drugs from the body's own enzymes that may prematurely break them down. The pliability of plastics enables them to be molded into a variety of shapes and sizes that can be surgically implanted or injected into precise locations in the body (180). Langer and colleagues demonstrated that polymer systems can be used to treat malignant adult brain tumors (180). Carmustine (BCNU)–containing polymer disks have been implanted to deliver tumor-killing doses of BCNU even after 4 weeks. Preliminary evidence suggests that implanting a BCNU polymer disk into the area where a tumor has been resected reduces the recurrence rate of such tumors (180,181). No studies have as yet tested pumps or polymer systems in malignant pediatric brain tumors.

Another option has been the use of chemotherapy in conjunction with drugs such as mannitol to disrupt the blood–brain barrier and thus permit better access of systemic chemotherapy to tumor cells. Preliminary experiments have shown that this approach results in a high incidence of seizures and other complications without demonstrating evidence of better tumor control. The approach has not been tested for safety or efficacy in children with malignant brain tumors.

It has become clear that chemotherapy increases disease-free survival in some children (78). As a consequence, by using chemotherapy, radiation can be delayed and neurotoxicity ameliorated in many infants (182). Chemotherapy can reduce the size of low-grade glioma, optic glioma, and oligodendroglioma (183). High-grade glioma and ependymoma, however, are relatively chemoresistant (184). It is important to recognize that the chemosensitivity of brain tumors varies greatly among tumor types and among patients with a particular histologic type. High-dose chemotherapy with autologous stem cell rescue has increasingly been used in clinical trials to improve the dismal prognosis of young patients with malignant supra and infratentorial tumors (185–200). A discussion of the safety, toxicity, and efficacy of high-dose chemotherapy in brain tumors is far beyond the scope of this text. This area has been reviewed by Wolff and Finlay (200a).

Chemotherapeutic agents are toxic not only to malignant cells, but also to normal ones (201). Because they are carried out by the blood circulation, they can affect any tissue in the body. Most drugs have preferential activity for rapidly proliferating cells such as hair follicles (alopecia), bone marrow (anemia, thrombocytopenia, granulocytopenia), intestinal mucosa, and gonads. In many cases, the effects are temporary when used in conventional doses. The spectrum of systemic side effects from chemotherapy is dependent on agent and dosage (202).

Almost all agents cause transient alopecia, which begins within a month of starting treatment and resolves when treatment is discontinued. Chemotherapy can affect all three hematologic cell lines. Anemia and thrombocytopenia may require transfusions. Weekly blood counts are indicated in most cases. Nausea and vomiting are common within 4 to 5 hours of administration and may persist for a few days. These symptoms are best controlled with the serotonin antagonist ondansetron. Stomatitis, glossitis, and proctitis occur with the beginning of neutropenia and disappear once the blood count recovers.

Vincristine frequently causes transient constipation and jaw pain (203). Virtually all patients develop hyporeflexia or areflexia. Less common side effects include foot drop, wrist drop, cranial nerve palsies, and vocal cord paralysis. Seizures with hyponatremia and inappropriate secretion of antidiuretic hormone can occur. Cisplatin can produce irreversible hearing loss in the high-frequency range. It also can cause severe hearing loss in the normal speech frequency range, especially if combined with radiotherapy. The dose-limiting toxicity of cisplatin is nephrotoxicity, and most patients ultimately have a permanent reduction of the glomerular filtration rate. More complete and detailed accounts of the systemic and neurotoxic complications of chemotherapy alone or in combination with radiotherapy are discussed in several excellent texts and reviews (204,205).

Neuroimaging After Chemotherapy

Chemotherapy can produce a variety of changes in the brain, ranging from mild atrophy to a destructive encephalopathy. The most severe complication of chemotherapy, usually seen in tandem with radiotherapy, is progressive necrotizing leukoencephalopathy (PNL) (206). PNL is characterized on MRI and CT as multicentric areas of contrast enhancement scattered randomly throughout cerebral white matter. The sites of the lesions do not necessarily correspond anatomically with the site of the primary tumor or the epicenter of radiotherapy. The findings may be more intense along the tract of an Ommaya reservoir catheter, presumably because of a higher concentration of chemotherapy from intraventricular injections. In time, the lesions calcify, and their widespread presence is associated with diminished IQ, neurobehavioral disturbances, and neuroendocrine sequelae (Fig. 11.8).

Brain changes have been associated with the use of specific chemotherapeutic agents (e.g., cyclosporine) that have been given intravenously rather than intrathecally. These agents can infrequently produce a zone of infarction in deep capillary beds. For the most part, these have occurred in the parieto-occipital regions and produced vision loss. The mechanism is presumed to be related to a regional vasculopathy, platelet activation, and capillary zone infarction.

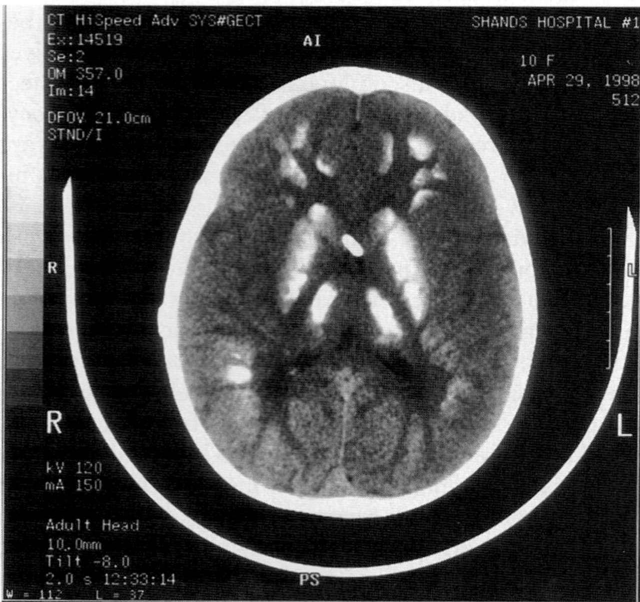

FIGURE 11.8. Computed tomographic scan in axial plane shows widespread calcifications in both cerebral hemispheres resulting from radiotherapy and chemotherapy treatment.

Cutting-Edge Therapies

Advanced therapies for brain tumors are being designed to block tumor cell-surface receptors, inhibit signal transduction, inhibit tumor infiltration and metastasis, or inhibit the angiogenesis that is so essential to tumor survival. For example, therapeutic agents that inhibit the activation of tyrosine kinase receptors that mediate tumor growth (EGFR, HER2) and survival (TrkA, IGF1) are being developed. The primary challenges to developing effective targeted molecular therapies include the heterogeneity of tumors and their variability of receptor expression, limited specificity of agents for targeted receptors, and multiple pathways to signal transduction.

One of the more compelling approaches is that of targeting microvessels in evolving tumors. As tumors progress, they have redundant growth factor capacity; such growth factors such as bFGF and aFGF are more dominant in pediatric tumors during progression (207). Thus, agents that would modulate relevant growth factors and genes that contribute to angiogenesis in pediatric brain tumors could be highly effective. Over 30 antiangiogenesis agents are in clinical trials in the United States (approximately 70 worldwide) for treatment of a variety of malignancies. So far, there are no studies reporting results from use of antiangionesis agents in pediatric brain tumors. Gene therapy has been one of the most intellectually satisfying approaches. This modality offers hope for ultimately treating the root cause of the problem by replacing defective genes, amplifying the immune response to neoplasia, and sensitizing tumor cells to systemic therapies (suicide gene therapy).

Gene therapy involves the transfer of one or more genes and the sequences controlling their expression into target cell populations. Theoretically, gene therapy replaces defective genes, alters the immune response, and inserts drug-sensitizing genes. Currently, the most efficient delivery systems to transfer genes intracellularly are viral vectors such as adenovirus, adeno-associated virus, and retrovirus.

Insertion of the thymidine kinase gene from herpesvirus into tumor cells can sensitize them to intravenous ganciclovir (208,209). A replication-incompetent retrovirus (murine leukemia virus) contained within vector-producer cells (fibroblast vector-producer cells) is used to deliver thymidine kinase gene from herpesvirus. This gene therapy strategy is the most mature innovative approach and has been tested *in vitro*, in animals, and in a series of adult and pediatric clinical trials (209). Pivotal to the thymidine kinase gene from herpesvirus strategy is the *bystander effect*, which results in a larger number of tumor cells being killed than those that have been genetically altered.

Immunocompetence and the presence of gap junctions between tumor cells are required experimentally to obtain the bystander effect. The various hurdles inherent to the strategy of gene therapy are reviewed by Maria and colleagues (208–210). Limited clinical studies conducted in children with recurrent brain tumors have not shown an improved outcome with the various newer treatment modalities.

For the time being, however, surgery, radiotherapy, and chemotherapy continue to be the mainstays of pediatric brain tumor management, and despite the many promising approaches, the problem with treating deep or inaccessible tumors still remains.

SPECIFIC TUMOR TYPES

There have been many attempts to classify CNS tumors based not only on traditional morphology, but also on their biologic, immunopathologic, and genetic features. The most recently updated classification was published by the World Health Organization in 1993 and was based, whenever possible, on the histiogenesis of tumors and their biologic behavior (211–214). Because the same type of tumor can produce totally different clinical pictures depending on its site, this chapter, for the greater part, adheres to a location-based classification. A standardized method for grading adult neuroglial tumors is based on the presence or absence of four histologic features: endothelial proliferation, necrosis, mitosis, and nuclear atypia. This scheme has been determined to be inappropriate for assesssing childhood supra- and infratentorial neuroglial tumors and adds little in terms of prognostic information (214a,214b).

Pediatric brain tumors include a spectrum of both glial and nonglial tumors that differ significantly in location and biologic behavior from those found in adults. Brain tumors in infants and children most often arise from central neuroepithelial tissue, whereas a significant number of adult tumors arise from CNS coverings (e.g., meningioma) or adjacent tissue (e.g., pituitary adenoma) or are metastases.

Tumors of the Posterior Fossa

Cerebellar Tumors

The cerebellum can be the site of various neoplastic processes, three of which are particularly common in children. These are the cerebellar pilocytic astrocytoma, a generally benign tumor arising from the cerebellar hemispheres or vermis, the PNET/MB, a malignant invasive tumor arising from the fetal cerebellar granular layer of the anterior and posterior medullary vela, and the ependymoma, which arises from the ependymal layer of the fourth ventricle (215). The incidence of the various neoplasms in the infratentorial compartment is shown in Table 11.10 (216).

TABLE 11.10 Frequencies of Common Pediatric Brain Tumors in the Infratentorial Compartment

Tumor	%
Medulloblastoma	32.4
(desmoplastic medulloblastoma)	5.4
Pilocytic astrocytoma	28.3
Ependymoma	12.0
Fibrillary astrocytoma	3.8
Astrocytoma, NOS	3.7
Protoplasmic astrocytoma	2.5
Anaplastic astrocytoma	2.4

NOS, not otherwise specified.
Adapted from Gilles FH. Pediatric brain tumors: classification. In: Morantz RA, Walsh JW, eds. *Brain tumors. A comprehensive text.* New York: Marcel Dekker Inc, 1994:109–134.

Pathology

Astrocytomas. These tumors are derived from the astrocytic neuroglial cells and can arise from either the vermis or the lateral lobes of the cerebellum. They are almost always well circumscribed and tend to be cystic, with the neoplasm confined to a small intramural nodule (see Fig. 11.9). Occasionally, astrocytomas form a solid tumor mass involving the cerebellum, vermis, and their brainstem connections.

The microscopic appearance of cerebellar astrocytomas varies considerably even within the same tumor. On the basis of histologic characteristics, Gilles and his group distinguished two tumor types whose resectability and long-term survival can be predicted (216,217). The *pilocytic astrocytoma* represents a distinct subtype of glioma that is most common in children and is genetically and biologically distinct from the diffuse, infiltrating gliomas that affect both adults and children. It constitutes approximately two-thirds of all cerebellar astrocytomas and 28% of posterior fossa tumors (216). On gross inspection, the tumor arises most commonly from the cerebellum, where it frequently projects as a mural nodule into a macroscopically well-circumscribed fluid-filled cyst (Fig. 11.9). Solid (noncystic) variants also are encountered. Microscopically, the tumor is characterized by a "biphasic" pattern that consists of areas containing tightly packed, piloid ("hairlike") tumor cell processes alternating with areas having numerous microscopic cysts. The latter often coalesce to form larger cysts. Nonspecific changes of astrocytic cell processes such as eosinophilic granular bodies and Rosenthal fibers also are characteristic. The latter are intracytoplasmic, opaque, homogeneous, strongly eosinophilic beaded masses that stain deep purple with Mallory's phosphotungstic acid–hematoxylin. Their presence indicates a degenerative change, and they can be found in other tumors, notably in craniopharyngiomas. In an otherwise typical pilocytic astrocytoma, the presence of vascular proliferation

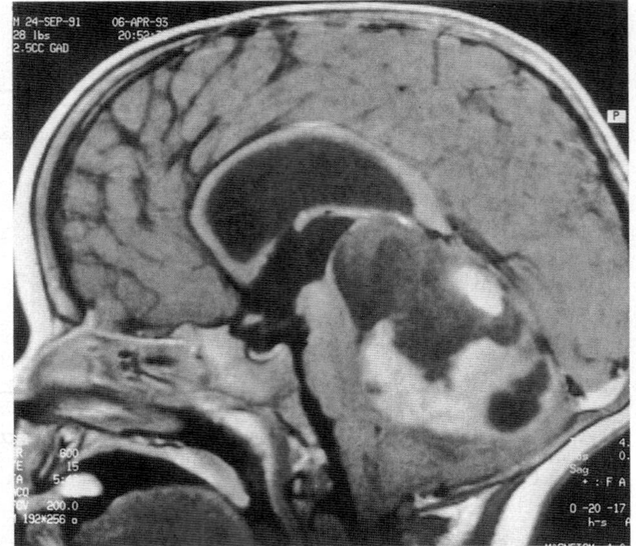

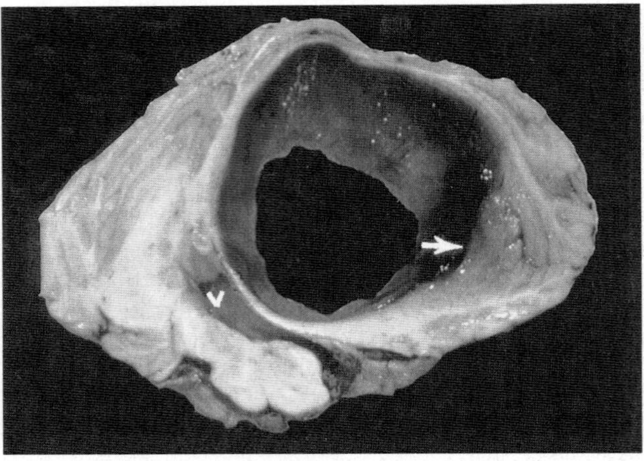

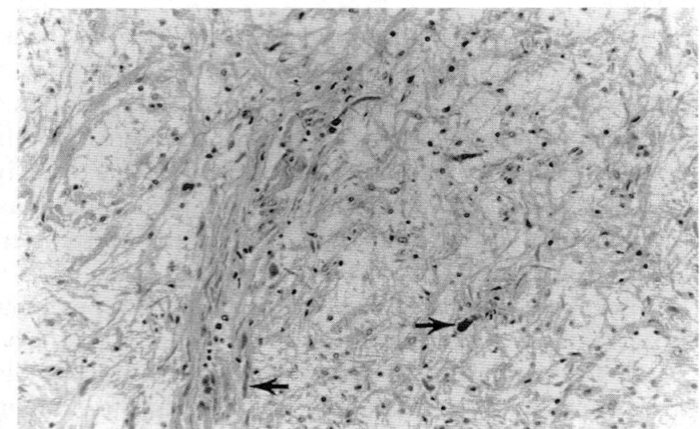

FIGURE 11.9. Cerebellar pilocytic astrocytoma consisting of a large, well-circumscribed tumor that compresses the fourth ventricle (v) **(A** and **B)**. Arrow **(B)** indicates a mural nodule of solid tumor. **C:** The histologic section from the mural nodule of a pilocytic astrocytoma. The tumor contains abundant piloid (hair-like) processes and microscopic cysts. Arrows indicate Rosenthal fibers (hematoxylin and eosin, original magnification ×200).

or nuclear atypia does not correlate with aggressive behavior as it does in diffuse astrocytomas. Mitoses are rare. Although grossly circumscribed, these tumors may locally infiltrate adjacent tissues and may extend into the adjacent subarachnoid space. Neither of these features suggests a tendency for aggressive behavior. Anaplastic (malignant) pilocytic astrocytomas are rare (218). Although most pilocytic astrocytomas have normal karyotypes (219), deletions on the long arm of chromosome 17 have been reported (220). A *p53* mutation (exon 9, codon 324) was identified in one of seven pilocytic astrocytomas, but this was a silent mutation, and its significance is uncertain (221).

Diffuse astrocytomas can occur anywhere in the CNS and are as common in the posterior fossa as in the supratentorial space (222). Diffuse astrocytomas constitute a spectrum of infiltrating astroglial tumors that display increasing grades of anaplasia and include the low-grade diffuse (fibrillary) astrocytoma, anaplastic (intermediate grade) astrocytoma, and glioblastoma multiforme (high grade). Collectively, these tumors account for 12.4% of pediatric infratentorial tumors (216). These intra-axial tumors are similar in histology and biological behavior to those affecting adults (215,222,223). Common pathologic features of this group are extensive infiltration of CNS tissue and a tendency of lower grade lesions to progress to higher grade lesions. Diffuse (fibrillary) astrocytomas tend to arise in white matter and often extensively invade adjacent gray matter structures. In contrast to the pilocytic astrocytoma, these tumors are difficult to eradicate by surgery alone because of poor demarcation between tumor and surrounding normal tissues, and a higher biologic propensity for regrowth.

Histologically malignant astrocytomas (anaplastic astrocytoma and glioblastoma multiforme) of childhood are infiltrative, biologically aggressive neoplasms (Figs. 11.10 and 11.11) (224). Microscopically, they are characterized by perivascular pseudorosette formation, necrosis, high cell density or mitotic figures, and calcifications, which usually are minute. In this type of glioma, microcyst formation is less common (occurring in 23% of cases).

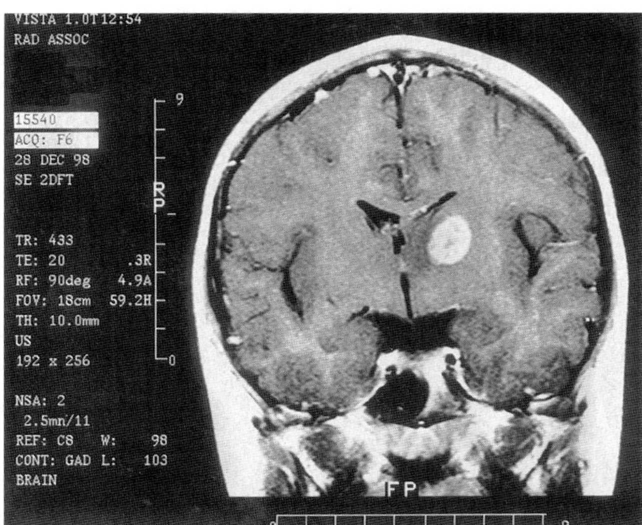

FIGURE 11.10. Coronal magnetic resonance imaging with contrast shows inhomogenously enhancing left thalamic anaplastic astrocytoma in a 9-year-old child with a 3-month history of right hand tremor.

Cytogenetic characteristics of pediatric malignant astrocytomas differ from those most commonly encountered in adults. Structural abnormalities in chromosomes 9, 13, 17, and double minutes were observed in malignant astrocytomas (anaplastic astrocytoma and glioblastoma) of childhood, whereas the most common chromosomal abnormalities in adult glioblastomas are losses of chromosomes 10 and 19q or gains in chromosome 7 (219). Furthermore, to date, the chromosomal abnormalities found in malignant astrocytomas of childhood are similar to those reported in a genetically distinct subset of glioblastomas that was found to arise in young adults (225).

Distinguishing between these various tumor types is difficult in many cases, and changes from one type of tumor to another have been noted with tumor recurrence (226). Additionally, spinal seeding with astrocytomas that appear benign on histologic examination has been observed (227).

Calcification of cerebellar tumors is usually minute but was seen in 26% of patients in Russell and Rubinstein's series (215).

Primitive Neuroectodermal Tumor/Medulloblastoma. The PNET/MB is the prototype of embryonal brain tumors and is among the most common malignant solid tumors of childhood. It accounts for 38% of pediatric infratentorial tumors (216). Unlike astrocytomas, MBs are derived from primitive neurons, the neuroblasts. Most of the laterally placed tumors arise from the fetal granular layer, a superficial layer of the cerebellar cortex present at birth, which disappears during the first year of life. The more numerous midline tumors are believed to arise from embryonal cell rests in the posterior medullary velum, the site of a germinal bud from which the external granular layer is derived (228). In some instances, the origin of the tumor has been traced back to the thirteenth week of gestation, a period of active cerebellar histiogenesis (229).

Macroscopically, these tumors are soft, friable, and moderately well demarcated from the remainder of the cerebellum. In general, they infiltrate the floor or lateral wall of the fourth ventricle and extend into its cavity (Fig. 11.12). The tumor grows backward, occluding the foramen magnum and infiltrating the meninges. It can metastasize by way of the CSF into the subarachnoid space of the spinal canal, with spinal ("drop") metastasis characteristic. Less commonly, the tumor spreads over the cerebral convexity (Fig. 11.13). In the spinal canal, the cord

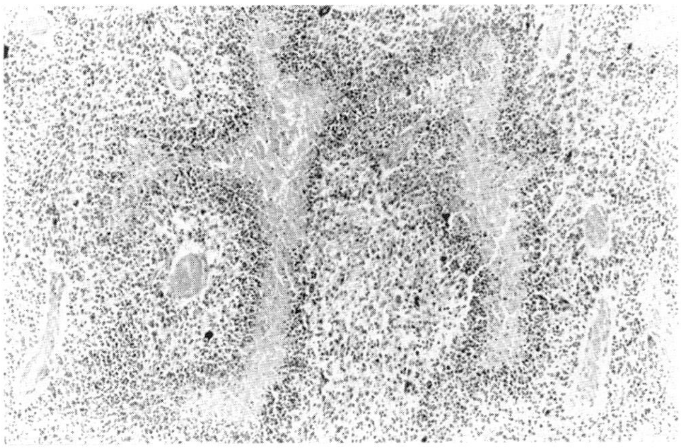

FIGURE 11.11. Histologic section demonstrates increased cellularity and classic pseudopalisading necrosis of glioblastoma multiforme.

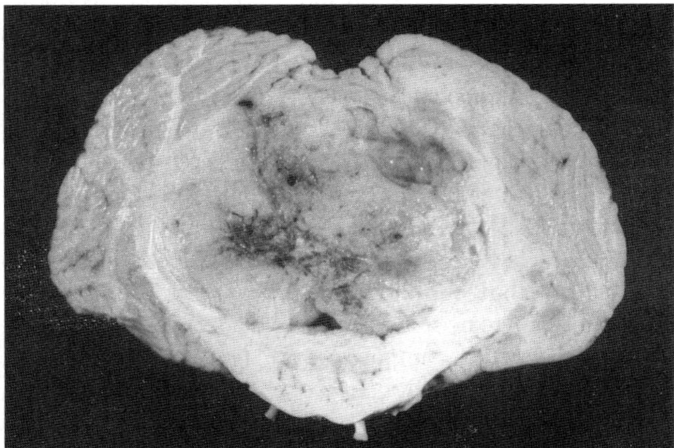

FIGURE 11.12. Primitive neuroectodermal tumor/medulloblastoma invading the fourth ventricle and the midline cerebellum.

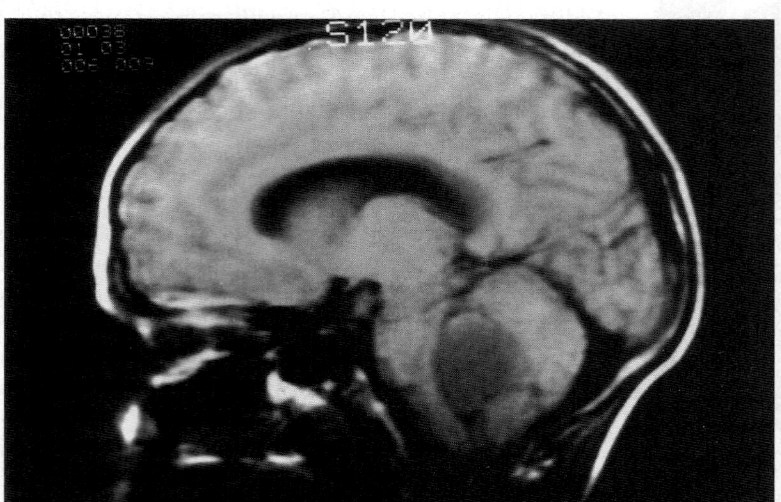

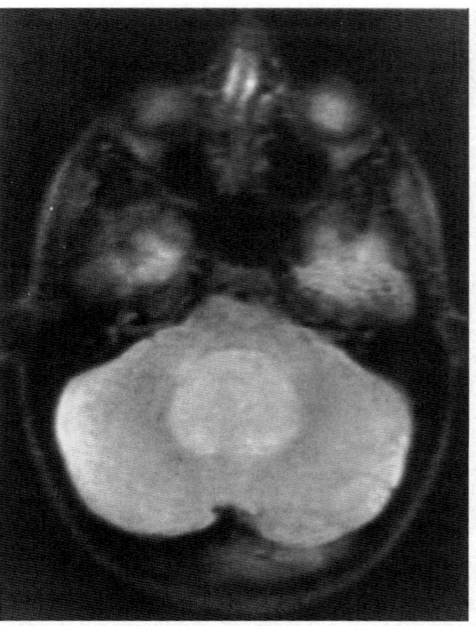

FIGURE 11.13. Primitive neuroectodermal tumor/medulloblastoma containing astrocytic elements. Sagittal **(A)** and axial **(B)** magnetic resonance images in this boy show a tumor within the fourth ventricle. It is of low signal intensity (darker than brain, but less dark than CSF) on the T1-weighted imaging **(A)**. The lesion appeared to arise from the roof of the fourth ventricle. Although the neoplasm compressed the posterior aspect of the pons and medulla, it seemed separable from the brainstem. This was confirmed at surgery. (Courtesy of Drs. Hervey D. Segall and J. Gordon McComb, Departments of Radiology and Neurosurgery, Children's Hospital, Los Angeles.)

and cauda equina become coated with metastatic tumor deposits. The site most frequently involved is the lower end of the spinal cord.

Histologically, PNET/MBs are highly cellular and are composed of small- to medium-sized cells with round to oval, often molded (carrot-shaped) hyperchromatic nuclei and poorly defined cell borders. Homer Wright rosettes (ring-like accumulations of tumor cell nuclei around a neurophil-containing or fibrillary core) are occasionally observed (Fig. 11.14). These tumors express a variety of neuronal/neuroendocrine markers, including synaptophysin (a 38-kd synaptic vesicle protein) and neurofilament proteins (230,231). Photoreceptor differentiation (retinal S-antigen and rhodopsin) is identified in 27% to 50% of these tumors (223,232). Glial fibrillary acidic protein (GFAP) has been reported in some 13% to 62% of PNET/MBs (233). One study found that patients with PNET/MBs that contained sheets or clumps of GFAP-immunoreactive neoplastic cells had a threefold increased risk of recurrence compared with those tumors without GFAP immunoreactivity. However, the prognostic value of immunohistochemical data has been controversial. Approximately 15% to 20% of children with PNET/MB have an anaplastic phenotype with a worse prognosis (234). In contrast, PNET/MBs with extreme nodularity have a more favorable prognosis (226,235). It also is important to know that posterior fossa PNET/MB and supratentorial PNET are molecularly distinct entities, although their histopathological analysis overlaps (236).

The most common molecular genetic abnormality identified to date in PNET/MB is loss of heterozygosity for the short arm of chromosome 17 [i(17q)], which occurs

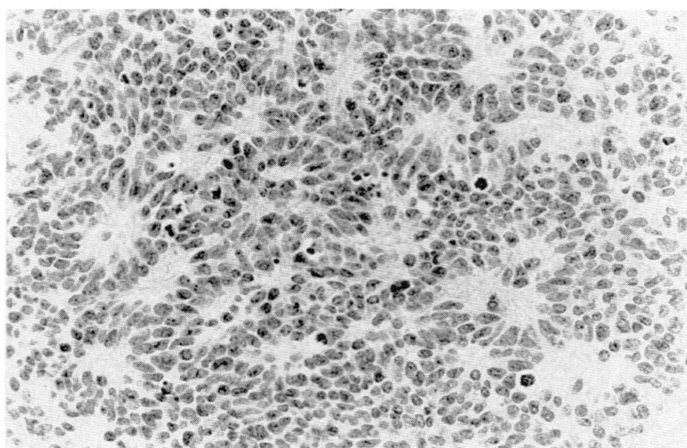

FIGURE 11.14. Histology of primitive neuroectodermal tumor of the cerebellum (primitive neuroectodermal tumor/medulloblastoma) with several Homer Wright rosettes (hematoxylin and eosin, original magnification ×1,000).

in 30% to 50% of cases; more recent studies indicate that i(17q) is not an independent prognostic factor, but may be a marker for uncontrolled cell proliferation (237). Other common losses of heterozygosity involve 8p and 11p, 10p, 11q, 16q, 20q, and 20p. Gains have been found at 7q, 17q, 18q, 7p, 13q, 18p, and the like (238). Flow cytometric analyses have indicated a worse prognosis for DNA diploid tumors, whereas aneuploid tumors have a better prognosis (239,240). Several biological factors have been studied as candidate progonostic factors in PNET/MB: GFAP expression, calbindin-positivity, HER2/HER4 coexpression, MIB-1 proliferation index, mitotic index, TrkC mRNA expression and MYC mRNA expression (241,242). Of these, TrkC mRNA and MYC mRNA expression seem to be the most potent prognostic factors (243).

The desmoplastic variant of PNET/MB is found in approximately 10% of PNET/MBs and tends to affect an older age group. In contrast to the classic midline form, it often arises laterally in a cerebellar hemisphere. The presence of reticulin-free "pale islands" is a characteristic histopathologic feature (244). Zacharoulis and colleagues have shown that desmoplastic pathology is more common in younger patients (median age 4.5 years for desmoplastic vs. 8.0 years for nondesmoplastic) and in the absence of other risk factors may be associated with a better prognosis, even for patients younger than three years of age (245).

Ependymomas. Ependymomas are the third most common brain tumor after cerebellar astrocytoma and PNET/MB. They account for 6% to 15% of brain tumors in children (246). Although these tumors can arise from any part of the ventricular system, the roof and the floor of the fourth ventricle are the most common sites of origin in childhood (Fig. 11.15A). Grossly, fourth ventricular ependymomas are exophytic growths that arise from the ventricular floor and fill the ventricle. Tumor may extend into the basal subarachnoid space through the foramina of Lushka or protrude into the cisterna magna. Ependymomas invade adjacent parenchymal structures but are less overtly infiltrative than high-grade astrocytomas. In appearance, ependymomas are gray-tan, granular, and may contain cysts and areas of hemorrhage. Microscopically, the tumor is composed of a uniform population of cells with round to oval nuclei and fibrillary processes; the latter directed toward abundant intratumoral blood vessels forming a distinct perivascular pseudorosette pattern (Fig. 11.15B). Better differentiated examples may contain tubular structures and canals. Although ependymal tumors with increased cellularity, pleomorphism, mitoses, and necrosis have been termed *anaplastic* or *malignant*, such histological features have been less predictive of aggressive behavior than they are in diffuse astrocytomas (247). The association of a high number of mitoses and high cell density with incomplete pseudorosettes allows one to make the diagnosis of the anaplastic variant in

A

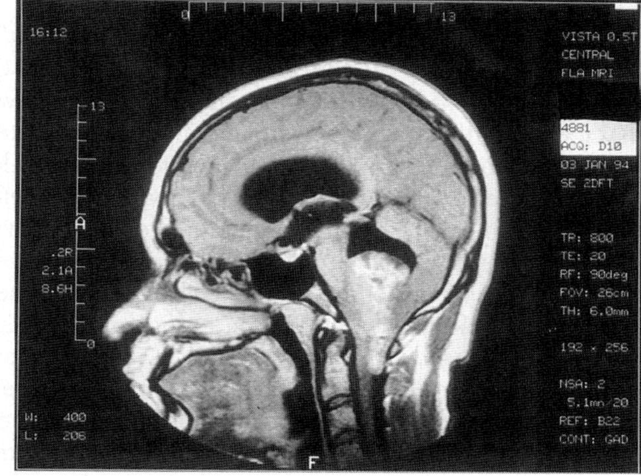

B

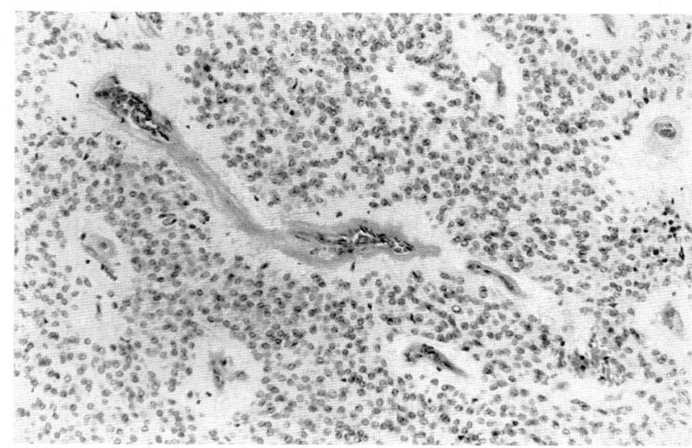

FIGURE 11.15. **A:** Sagittal magnetic resonance imaging shows large contrast-enhancing ependymoma filling most of fourth ventricle. **B:** Histologic section of ependymoma shows a uniform population of cells with round to slightly oval nuclei and indistinct cell borders. Perivascular clear areas (*pseudorosettes*) represent tumor cell processes oriented perpendicular to intratumoral vessels (hematoxylin and eosin, original magnification ×500).

supratentorial ependymomas (248). It is important to note that histologically benign ependymomas can hemorrhage and invade the brainstem (85). Paradoxically, the presence of calcifications in the tumor has a poor prognosis. Conversely, high cell density and nuclear polymorphism suggest a good prognosis (249). There is a paucity of histological markers in ependymoma that have strong predictive validity.

Chromosomal abnormalities identified in ependymomas include monosomy and deletions of chromosome 22, trisomy of chromosome 7, loss of sex chromosomes, and structural rearrangements of chromosome 2 (223). In addition, chromosomes 9 and 11 may harbor genes involved in the pathogenesis of ependymoma. Integrative profiling of chromosome copy number abnormalities and gene expression is being developed to discriminate genetically between supratentorial and infratentorial ependymomas, and between classical and anaplastic variants (250). A germ-line mutation of the tumor-suppressor gene *p53* has been implicated in the pathogenesis of anaplastic ependymoma (251). Gaspar and colleagues have shown that the *p53* pathway in ependymoma might be abrogated without *p53* mutation, mdm2 overexpression, $p14^{ARF}$ deletion, or increased pax5 protein expression (54). A deletion of chromosome 1 has been identified in the myxopapillary ependymoma, a distinct subtype that arises in the filum terminale. Korshunov and colleagues examined gene expression patterns in relation to biologic behavior (252). Interestingly, spinal, supratentorial, and infratentorial ependymomas had different patterns of gene expression that could implicate a multistep transformation process leading to aggressive biologic behavior in some patients. It seems that the heterogeneity that applies at the chromosomal level also applies at the molecular level in ependymomas.

Other Tumors. Other tumor types involving the cerebellum and its contiguous structures include undifferentiated sarcomas, some of which are of leptomeningeal origin, glioblastomas, and cerebellar hemangioblastoma, which is discussed in Chapter 12 under von Hippel–Lindau disease. Some of the uncommon CNS tumors are reviewed in Table 11.11 (253–278).

Acoustic nerve tumors, which are common in adults, are rare in children; when seen, they are usually bilateral and a manifestation of neurofibromatosis 2 (see Chapter 12).

Clinical Manifestations

The three tumors described previously are frequently indistinguishable clinically. Intracranial pressure is increased, and the cerebellum and its contiguous structures are involved.

In cerebellar tumors, the growing mass soon obstructs the ventricular system, making increased intracranial pressure a common presenting sign (Table 11.12). Early on, headaches are generally unlocalized or frontal; subsequently, they are suboccipital. When the tumor is unilateral, the child often holds the head tilted, with the head bent toward the more involved hemisphere while the chin points to the other side.

Vomiting is the most common presenting sign of cerebellar tumors. Usually, it results from increased intracranial pressure, but at times it can be caused by direct pressure on the medullary vagal nuclei or the vomiting center.

The progressive evolution of cerebellar signs was described by Cushing in 1931 (279):

> A child apparently healthy in all respects begins toward the end of the first decade, possibly after a fall

TABLE 11.11 Some Less Common Central Nervous System Tumors of Childhood

Tumor	Most Common Site	Characteristics	Reference
Pleomorphic xanthoastrocytoma	Temporal lobe	Slow growing, may exhibit anaplastic features, can undergo malignant transformation	253–258
Ganglioglioma	Temporal lobe (38%), parietal lobe (30%), frontal lobe (18%), cerebellum, brainstem, spinal cord	Slow growing, benign, often cystic; associated with cortical dysplasia, neoplastic astroglial elements and ganglion cells	259–262
Desmoplastic infantile ganglioglioma	Supratentorial with frontoparietal predilection, often involves leptomeninges	Benign, partially cystic, extensive deposition of stromal collagen	263–265
Dysembryoplastic neuroepithelial tumor	Temporal lobe, caudate nucleus	Slow growing and benign, bundles of axons attached to oligodendroglial-like cells, cystic areas, adjacent cortical dysplasia	266–269
Medulloepithelioma	Supratentorial and infratentorial	Responds poorly to treatment; tumor cells and vesicular structures resembling embryonic neural tube	270
Atypical teratold/malignant rhabdoid tumors	Posterior fossa (65%), other areas of neuraxis	Highly malignant; histologically mixed with primitive neuroectodermal tumor and rhabdoid elements; prognosis worse than primitive neuroectodermal tumor/medulloblastoma	271–275
Dermoids and epidermoids	Extradural: scalp, skull; intradural: temporal lobe, posterior fossa, suprasellar region	Arise from trapped pouches of ectoderm; epidermoids have squamous epithelium, dermoids contain squamous epithelium, hair, sebaceous and sweat glands	276, 277
Central neurocytoma	Supratentorial ventricular system	Generally benign, uniform round cells, with evidence of neuronal differentiation	278

TABLE 11.12 Presenting Manifestations in Patients 18 Years of Age or Less with Cerebellar Tumors

Initial Signs or Symptoms	*Medulloblastoma*	*Astrocytoma*
Vomiting	29	34
Headaches	10	38
Unsteadiness	22	15
Visual impairment	1	1
Strabismus	5	7
Enlarging head	0	1
Pain or stiffness of neck	1	3
Others (head tilt, malaise, dizziness, lumbar pain, hemiparesis)	8	4

From Cushing H. Experiences with the cerebellar astrocytomas. *Surg Gynecol Obstet* 1931;52:129. With permission.

or an attack of whooping cough, to have early morning headaches and vomiting. Nothing much is made of this by the family doctor, should he be called in, for the child subsequently feels perfectly well, has had breakfast, and wants to go out and play. This daily performance may continue for a considerable time, the child even going to school meanwhile. There may then be a remission of weeks or perhaps months and the episode be forgotten. On their reoccurrence, the symptoms are likely to be more pronounced and are apt to be ascribed to some gastrointestinal disturbance. This appears the more probable since the child finds that straining at stool brings on a headache and there is a tendency to become constipated. What is more, a mild daily laxative usually serves completely to mask the symptoms.

This sort of thing continues off and on until it becomes evident that the child is a little clumsy at play and gets knocked over easily. Very possibly, before this, the periodic headache and vomiting will have ceased completely or at least have occurred at much longer intervals; and if parents are observant they may notice that the child's head in the interim has increased in size more rapidly than it should. This, however, is usually discounted for the child meanwhile has become free from complaints and in all respects appears alert and well.

Matters may run on in this way for an indefinite time, possibly with some increase in clumsiness of movement or in some instances with no noticeable change whatever until it suddenly becomes apparent, perhaps at school, that the child's sight is poor. To counteract this, glasses are usually prescribed; but even should an ophthalmoscope be resorted to, a child's retina is less easily examined than that of an adult and, because of the decompressive effects of the enlarging head, the optic papillae often show no measurable swelling and the fact of their being pale and with margins blurred may easily pass unrecognized.

The length of time that a child with a cerebellar neoplasm is symptomatic before being hospitalized is a function of the malignancy of tumor and the readiness of the primary physician to request a consultation or perform imaging studies. In the experience of Park and coworkers, who in 1983 reported on a series of children with PNET/MB compiled between 1950 and 1980, the clinical history lasted less than 6 weeks in 51% of cases and less than 12 weeks in 76% of cases (280). By contrast, in the 1987 experience of Diebler and Dulac, the mean interval between the first signs of a cerebellar astrocytoma and diagnosis was approximately 4 months, and approximately 3 months for children with an ependymoma (281).

The most common cerebellar symptom is unsteadiness of gait, owing to involvement of the vermis. The child stands with the feet widely separated and quickly loses balance if the center of gravity is displaced. On attempting to walk, the child sways and staggers. Often, the impairment in gait is at its worst on awakening and lessens with prolonged activity. Disturbances of speech indicate more advanced involvement of the vermis. Speech is slow and monotonous, and syllables are uttered in a jerky, explosive manner.

Disorders of limb movement (dysmetria, adiadochokinesia or slowing and dissociation of rapid alternating movements, and intention tremor) and disorders of posture (hypotonia), both of which indicate involvement of the cerebellar hemispheres, are seen less commonly during the early stages of the process. Some tumors located exclusively along the midline, notably PNET/MBs arising from the vermis, can elicit no localizing symptoms. Hypotonia is more marked on the ipsilateral side. As a consequence, the child tends to stagger to the side of the lesion. The rebound phenomenon, the pendular deep tendon reflexes, and other evidence of postural instability are also more marked on the side of the lesion.

Nystagmus, although in general a classic sign of cerebellar disease, usually occurs late in children with posterior fossa tumors. When present, it is almost always bilateral and more noticeable with lateral than with vertical gaze. Although nystagmus is usually conjugate, the rapid phase is occasionally more evident in the direction of the predominantly involved hemisphere, with a slow drift back to the midline. The oscillations are slow (2 to 3 per second) and coarse.

Seizures are rare in cerebellar tumors, although Hughlings Jackson (281a), Stewart, Gordon, Holmes (282), and numerous other, older authors have described tonic cerebellar seizures with retraction of the head, arching of the back, flexion of the elbows, and rigid extension of the legs. These episodes are accompanied by disorders of respiration and can terminate fatally. They do not represent true seizures, but result from compression of the vermis or lower brainstem.

Diagnosis

The only distinguishing feature in the clinical course of the three major cerebellar tumors is the duration of symptoms before hospitalization. If symptoms have lasted more than 12 months, a benign cerebellar astrocytoma is most likely. With symptoms of more recent onset, clinical differentiation might not be possible. Although the CT scan was once considered a nearly flawless means of localizing a cerebellar tumor and was a guide to tumor type, MRI, particularly with gadolinium-diethylenethriaminepenta-acetic acid (DTPA) enhancement, provides an excellent and generally preferable diagnostic means.

An PNET/MB presents as a centrally located, generally uniformly homogeneous, dense tumor on precontrast scans, but after administration of contrast, material shows homogeneous enhancement with sharp borders. The pilocytic astrocytoma presents as a uniform zone of low density with sharp borders; an enhanced tumor nodule is observed in the majority of instances. The diffuse astrocytoma has a low density on precontrast scans but tends to become enhanced. Calcification within a mass located near the fourth ventricle should suggest the diagnosis of an ependymoma or, in children from Third World countries, a tuberculoma (283).

The MRI characteristics of the various posterior fossa tumors are shown in Table 11.13. Little difference is seen in unenhanced T1-weighted signal intensity between benign and malignant tumors (284,285). Most posterior fossa tumors enhance after the administration of gadolinium contrast, so the presence or absence of enhancement provides no clue as to tumor type in posterior fossa neoplasms. On T2-weighted images, the PNET/MB is isointense to gray matter, whereas all types of astrocytomas are hyperintense (286) (see Fig. 11.13). Generally, there is no clear demarcation between the tumor itself and any surrounding edema. The increased protein content of a cyst results in a high-intensity signal on T2-weighted images. This increased signal is usually readily differentiated from the tumor itself.

Some children with posterior fossa PNET/MBs show evidence of metastases. In the series of Park and associates (280), these were localized to the supratentorial region in 15% of patients with, most commonly, the frontal lobes being invaded. Clinically silent spinal cord metastases were detected in 19% of patients in a more recent series (287). When symptomatic, the child complains of pain, spinal tenderness, urinary symptoms, and, in the most advanced stage, spinal cord compression and paraplegia. Systemic metastases, mainly to the skeleton, were seen in 10% of PNET/MBs.

Occasionally, tumors outside the posterior fossa induce signs simulating cerebellar involvement. A long-standing increase in intracranial pressure can result in ataxia and unsteadiness of gait. Frontal lobe tumors, rare in childhood, also can produce ataxia. In contrast to cerebellar ataxia, dysmetria and adiadochokinesia are absent in approximately 40% of patients with frontal lobe ataxia, and nystagmus is absent in approximately 65%. The ataxia is generally thought to arise from interruption of frontopontocerebellar fibers or interruption of afferent cerebellar fibers in the dentatorubrothalamocortical system (288). Craniopharyngiomas rarely can show predominantly cerebellar signs. Involuntary movements, consisting of rhythmic myoclonus of the face and arms, have been seen in an occasional child with a posterior fossa neoplasm (288). Although the diagnosis of posterior fossa masses with such unusual clinical features was difficult at one time, neuroimaging studies now readily localize the responsible lesion.

An unusual tumor of the cerebellum that produces prolonged and slowly progressive cerebellar signs was first described by Lhermitte and Duclos (289). The most striking feature of this condition is the replacement of the granular cell layer by a hamartomatous mass of pleiomorphic ganglion cells. Although the condition usually presents in adult life, it probably represents an abnormality in cell migration or a phakomatosis (290). Examination of tissue by

TABLE 11.13 Magnetic Resonance Characteristics of Specific Histologic Types of Posterior Fossa Tumors

	Hypointense on T1	*Hyperintense on T2*	*Enhanced on T1*	*Cystic Component*
Medulloblastoma	42/42	0/42	20/22	0/42
Pilocytic astrocytoma	23/23	23/23	23/23	18/23
Malignant glioma	17/17	17/17	6/17	1/17
Fibrillary astrocytoma	8/8	8/8	4/8	0/8
Astrocytoma	7/7	7/7	5/7	1/7
Ganglioglioma	1/1	1/1	1/1	1/1
Ependymoma	8/10	6/10	9/10	0/10

Note: The signal intensity change is relative to that of normal gray matter. The numbers indicate the proportion of cases showing such change.

Adapted from Zimmerman RD, Bilaniuk LT, Rebsamen S. Magnetic resonance imaging of pediatric posterior tossa tumors. *Pediatr Neurosurg* 1992;18:58.

immunohistochemistry shows that most of the abnormal neurons in the lesion are derived from granule cells, with a small subpopulation of cells demonstrating Purkinje cell–specific monoclonal and polyclonal antibodies (291). MRI discloses nonenhancing gyriform patterns with enlargement of the cerebellar folia (290). Lhermitte-Duclos disease is occasionally associated with Cowden syndrome, a rare autosomal dominant condition manifested by multiple hamartomas and other neoplasms (290a,292). A mutation of the PTEN/MMAC 1 gene, a tumor-suppressor gene, has been found in some patients with Lhermitte-Duclos disease (293,293a).

Treatment and Prognosis of Posterior Fossa Tumors

Astrocytomas. The treatment for pilocytic astrocytomas is gross total resection, whenever possible. Some surgeons prefer to place a shunt before performing surgery to diminish the volume of the excessively dilated ventricle. Evacuation of an associated cyst can relieve symptoms for long periods, but does not prevent ultimate refilling. After resection, patients should have an MRI and neurologic examination every 6 months for the first 2 years. With total tumor resection, the outcome for the cystic variety of type A glioma is extremely good; in fact, in a series reported by Matson as early as 1956, the cure rate was 94% (294). With better surveillance, disease-free survival rates are equally good (295). If the resection is partial, as is often the case for midline supratentorial lesions, radiotherapy is recommended, and more frequent MRIs and neurologic examinations are indicated. In children younger than 3 years of age with partially resected or progressive supratentorial pilocytic astrocytomas, chemotherapy is recommended. As a rule, fibrillary astrocytomas are less responsive to chemotherapy than pilocytic astrocytomas.

Gross surgical excision of the diffuse astrocytoma is far more difficult. These tumors tend to arise in white matter and often extensively invade adjacent gray matter structures. In contrast to the pilocytic astrocytoma, there is a poor demarcation between tumor and surrounding normal tissues, and the tumor has a higher biologic propensity for regrowth. In the series of Schneider and colleagues, total resection was achieved in only 37.5% (296). In children who underwent partial tumor resection followed by postoperative radiotherapy, the 5-year and 10-year survival rates were 70% and 63%, respectively (297). A study by Desai and colleagues of prognostic factors for cerebellar astrocytomas in children showed that the location of the tumor, its histological grade, and the extent of tumor resection had a significant and definitive relationship to the length of survival (298).

It is as yet an unresolved question whether postoperative radiotherapy decreases the recurrence rate and improves survival of children with subtotally removed cerebellar astrocytomas. The difficulty of assessing the benefits of radiotherapy are because of the long survival of children in whom subtotal resection was the only therapy and the lack of uniformity in radiation dosages and techniques. However, the adverse effects of radiation to the developing brain are clearly known, particularly when radiation is administered to children younger than age 3 years. It is, therefore, our recommendation that radiation therapy is best deferred in small children, even if tumor resection is incomplete, and that children be followed closely with imaging studies and not be irradiated unless tumor progression is documented (299). In all instances, MRI studies and neurologic examinations are required every 2 to 4 months in the first 2 years from diagnosis. Generally, a child can be considered cured of his or her neoplasm if the child remains free of any evident recurrence for a period equivalent to his or her age at diagnosis plus 9 months (Collins' law) (300). The effectiveness of chemotherapy on this tumor is still uncertain, and more studies are needed before specific agents and dosages can be routinely recommended for treatment of diffuse astrocytomas in children.

Management of Primitive Neuroectodermal Tumor/Medulloblastoma. Management of PNET/MB is a far more difficult task, but in the course of the past two decades, survival for children with this type of tumor has gradually improved (301). Advances in surgical technique, radiotherapy, and chemotherapy have culminated in 5-year progression-free survival rates as high as 85% (302). A number of studies have concluded that survival is improved with gross total resection, especially in patients with localized disease at the time of diagnosis (301,303,304). However, although 5-year survival rates have climbed to more than 50%, late recurrences have been reported, and late effects of therapy are common (305).

The decision of what treatment to recommend after surgery of PNET/MB is difficult because of conflicting results from clinical trials around the world. The value of chemotherapy, given before or after radiotherapy, is under investigation, with several ongoing study groups using different regimens. The results of studies conducted in the last few years show that adjuvant chemotherapy used with 36Gy of craniospinal radiation (54 Gy posterior fossa boost) is beneficial in high-risk disease, namely those with ≥ 1.5 cm^3 residual disease), those younger than 3 years of age, and those with presence of metastatic disease (306,307). Results of a randomized study of preradiation chemotherapy versus radiotherapy alone showed an advantage for chemotherapy compared with radiotherapy alone (308). Some studies have tested myeloablative chemotherapy in combination with radiotherapy in high-risk disease to improve survival (195). Others are examining reduced-dose radiotherapy (18 Gy craniospinal radiotherapy) followed by high-dose chemotherapy to decrease late effects of radiotherapy (309).

Conversely, low-risk patients are those in whom more than 75% of the tumor is resected surgically, as confirmed by imaging studies, who have a negative spinal cord MRI study result and CSF cytology, have no evidence of CNS or extraneural metastases, and who are older than 2 years of age (310). Because of the high prevalence of late effects in survivors, a current trend favors decreasing doses of craniospinal radiotherapy (23.4 Gy vs. 36 Gy) but maintaining a posterior fossa boost to 54 Gy, in combination with chemotherapy in children with low-risk disease.

In the experience of Packer and colleagues, reported in 1991, chemotherapy did not improve 5-year disease-free survival of children with standard risk for disease. However, there was a significant 5-year survival advantage from using chemotherapy in high-risk groups, as based on tumor size, degree of brainstem involvement, and evidence of CSF dissemination (302). Other studies also have reported a significantly better event-free survival in high-risk patients receiving chemotherapy (311). A randomized postoperative trial in which adjuvant postradiation chemotherapy (nitrogen mustard, vincristine, procarbazine, and prednisone) was tested against radiotherapy (312) showed that both groups had almost identical overall and event-free survival at 10 years postdiagnosis (312).

Based on available information on surgery, radiotherapy, and chemotherapy, the following recommendations can be made. The goal should be to achieve a gross total resection of the PNET/MB, but the risks of surgical mortality and morbidity from removing brainstem components of the tumor probably outweigh the benefits of a complete excision. There is a survival advantage to total resection, but 15% to 20% of patients will develop posterior fossa mutism, with 50% experiencing permanent sequelae (313,314). PNET/MB is often large in the area of the roof of the fourth ventricle and requires extensive suboccipital craniectomy and incision through the vermis for total microsurgical resection. Probably fewer benefits accrue from achieving a gross total surgical resection in patients with CSF dissemination of tumor. A critical aspect to defining the risk of tumor recurrence is determining the extent of invasion of the floor of the fourth ventricle by microscopic inspection of the ependymal lining. Postoperative craniospinal imaging and CSF cytology are required to determine if CSF and neuroaxis spread have occurred (315).

After near total resection, current therapy includes reduced-dose (craniospinal 23.4 Gy, posterior fossa boost to 54 Gy) radiotherapy followed by chemotherapy (316). It is well established that the entire neuroaxis must be treated with radiotherapy (317,318). If the resection is partial or the patient has other, aforementioned risk factors for tumor recurrence, 36 Gy craniospinal radiotherapy is recommended, followed by chemotherapy. It is premature to consider using low-dose craniospinal radiotherapy (e.g., 23.4 Gy or 18 Gy) in high-risk disease until more information is available from ongoing clinical trials using high-dose chemotherapy. Taken together, the results from the studies on chemotherapy in PNET/MB suggest that cisplatin, etoposide, vincristine, and cyclophosphamide produce the greatest survival benefit to patients with high-risk disease. Optimal combinations of existing agents and doses, relation to radiotherapy, and new agents must be studied before they can be routinely recommended for high-risk patients. All children should have MRIs and neurologic examinations every 3 to 4 months in the first 2 years after diagnosis. Careful attention to growth, development, endocrine function, behavior, and cognition are pivotal in long-term follow-up. The overall event-free 5-year survival rate in PNET/MB is 60% to 70% in most clinical trials. However, after recurrence, less than 25% of children will be alive without progression of disease at 5 years.

Management of Ependymomas. The management of ependymoma is controversial, and tumor histology is not as predicitive of outcome as it is for posterior fossa astrocytoma. However, total surgical resection of ependymomas arising from the floor of the fourth ventricle is recognized as a favorable prognostic factor, though it is difficult and dangerous. In fact, improvement in survival statistics since 1980 is probably because of improved surgical technique and lower perioperative deaths (319). Evidence exists that patients undergoing a radical resection have twice the survival rate as those receiving a partial resection (320). Complete resection of posterior fossa ependymoma should be followed by limited-field radiotherapy (321). For nondisseminated low-grade infratentorial ependymoma, the radiotherapy volume does not need to include the entire posterior fossa, and conformal radiotherapy should be used to treat a local field (322). For incomplete resections, a recent study showed that preirradiation chemotherapy (cisplatin, vincristine, cyclophosphamide, and etoposide) in combination with focal radiation had the same event-free survival than patients with complete resections (323). Second-look surgeries are being incorporated into new clinical trials in incompletely resected posterior fossa ependymoma.

For supratentorial ependymomas, limited-field radiotherapy and chemotherapy are recommended (324,325). For posterior fossa anaplastic ependymomas, craniospinal radiotherapy and chemotherapy are recommended, although symptomatic spinal seeding is rare (326–329).

One prospective randomized trial, conducted in the 1980s, to evaluate the value of chemotherapy in ependymomas showed no improvement in outcome (330). Interestingly, infants with ependymomas showed a significant response to chemotherapy (175,331), and a more recent trial (323) showed that chemotherapy was of benefit in patients with incomplete tumor resections. In view of the observation that infants who received 2 years of chemotherapy have a lower 5-year survival than those who only receive 1 year of chemotherapy, Duffner and coworkers recommend that after maximal surgical resection, radiation therapy should not be delayed more than 1 year (332).

MRIs and neurologic examinations are required every 2 to 4 months in the first 2 years from diagnosis. As the 5-year survival for infants and children harboring an ependymoma is only 35% to 50%, it will be necessary to test the safety and efficacy of new radiotherapy strategies and chemotherapy agents (246,333,334). When possible, a complete surgical excision is desirable.

As already mentioned, cerebellar mutism has been encountered following the resection of a posterior fossa tumor. It occurs within a few hours to up to 9 days after surgery and can last as long as 20 weeks (335). The nature of the condition is poorly understood. It may be related to the degree of disruption of cerebellar function or neuronal circuits and appears to be associated with a transient oral apraxia or a loss of ability to initiate oral movements (336). Persistent neurocognitive deficits and, rarely, transient visual impairment are seen in a substantial minority of children with cerebellar mutism (337). In a study reported by Misakyan and colleagues, mutism was evident in 38% of patients assessed at a median of 3.9 weeks after posterior fossa tumor surgery (338). These patients continued to demonstrate impairments following speech recovery, including deficits in oral motor control (100%), reduced rates of conversational speech and production of alternating speech sounds (78% and 68%, respectively), and reduced intelligibility of speech (56%). However, children who did not experience mutism also demonstrated significant impairments in oral motor control and speech. The pathogenesis of these deficits needs to be defined and remedies proposed because they are associated with significant long-term impairments in communication.

Brainstem Tumors

Diffuse infiltrative tumors of the brainstem produce a clinical picture with a variable initial presentation but a uniformly fatal progression. It is appropriate to think of diffuse infiltrating brain stem gliomas much like one thinks of highly malignant gliomas without the marginal benefit of surgical resection. They account for 10% of pediatric CNS neoplasms (339,340). Although nearly all brainstem gliomas are malignant by virtue of their location, morphologic studies show them to be a nonhomogeneous group, with a variety of appearances ranging from the benign, well-differentiated astrocytoma to the highly malignant glioblastoma.

Pathology

Most commonly, tumor of the brainstem arises from the pons and appears as a symmetric enlargement of the brainstem, bulging into the floor of the fourth ventricle, a pathologic feature termed *pontile hypertrophy* (Fig. 11.16). Approximately 80% of pediatric brainstem gliomas are diffusely infiltrating astrocytomas and, of these, approximately 50% are histologically malignant at presentation (340). Extensive infiltration of tumor along white matter tracts is typical. Characteristically, cells grow by insinuating themselves between pre-existing structures, separating but not destroying them; hence, the relative paucity of signs in the earlier stages of tumor growth.

Microscopic examination shows the glioma to be composed of elongated bipolar cells that resemble a fibrillary astrocytoma (339). Like astrocytomas of the cerebral hemispheres, but in contrast to cerebellar astrocytomas, brainstem tumors tend to show anaplasia, and certain areas, primarily those deep in the tumor, ultimately resemble glioblastoma multiforme. In their series of 21 tumors, Berger and coworkers found that all but one had the microscopic appearance of an anaplastic astrocytoma or a glioblastoma multiforme and that frequently what appeared to be a benign tumor harbored highly malignant cells (341). Metastasis and invasion of the meninges are rare, but dissemination into the subarachnoid space of the spinal cord is well documented. Based on combined CT and morphologic studies, the Toronto group proposed the following classification (342):

- Group I tumors arise from the floor of the fourth ventricle with exophytic growth into the fourth ventricle, with only limited brainstem infiltration. This type of a

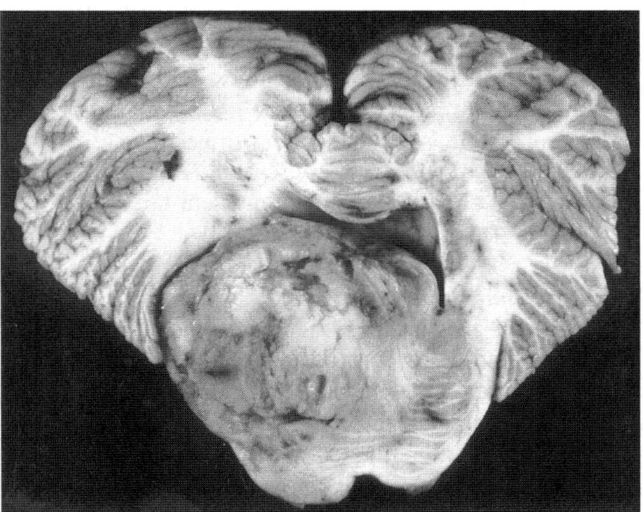

FIGURE 11.16. Brainstem glioma diffusely expanding the pons and effacing normal structures.

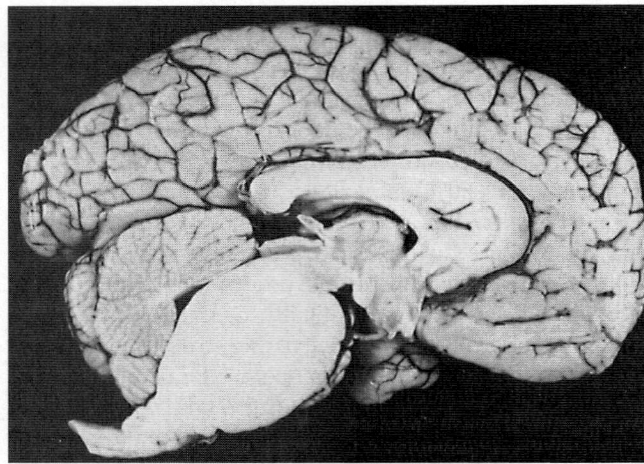

FIGURE 11.17. Glioma of the brainstem. The tumor has diffusely infiltrated the brainstem, producing *hypertrophy*. Note the relative lack of dilatation of lateral ventricles. (Courtesy of Dr. P. Cancilla, Department of Pathology, University of California, Los Angeles, UCLA School of Medicine.)

tumor constituted 22% of pediatric brainstem gliomas. Histologically, it generally is a grade I to II astrocytoma.

- Group II tumors, which constituted 51% of brainstem gliomas in the Toronto series, are intrinsic and diffusely infiltrative. Histologically, they are grade III astrocytomas or glioblastomas.
- Group III tumors, which constituted 8% of brainstem gliomas, have a cystic component.
- Group IV tumors, constituting 18% of the series, are focal tumors intrinsic to the brainstem, commonly located in the cervicomedullary area. They tend to be low-grade astrocytomas.

Von Deimling and colleagues and Louis and colleagues reported losses of portions of chromosome 17p, mutations of *p53*, and allelic losses of chromosome 10q in brainstem gliomas, a pattern similar to a subset of supratentorial glioblastomas that occurs in young adults (225,343). Because the expression or *erbB1* and *TP53* is increased in brain stem glioma, they may represent targets for new therapies.

Clinical Manifestations

Brainstem gliomas present with an insidious onset of symptoms and signs that have remained unchanged in the many series published since the 1930s (9,344) (Table 11.14). In contrast to the comparatively uniform evolution of the clinical picture in cerebellar tumors, the initial symptoms of a brainstem neoplasm are variable. The most commonly encountered brainstem tumor (group II, using the Toronto terminology) is characterized by the presence of four major features: cranial nerve palsies, pyramidal tract signs, cerebellar signs, and progression to advanced stages, usually without increase in intracranial pressure (342,344). In most patients, the period from onset of symptoms to diagnosis is less than 6 months, and it is usually under 2 months (345,346). Manifestations appear at 2 to 12 years of age, with peak incidence at 6 years. Vomiting and disturbances of gait are the most common presenting complaints. Less frequent is the gradual or rapid onset of a hemiparesis or evidence of cranial nerve involvement, especially facial weakness, strabismus, or difficulties in swallowing. The presence of a head tilt and changes in personality are other relatively common early signs (see Table 11.14).

TABLE 11.14 Incidence of Neurologic Signs and Symptoms in Children with Brainstem Tumors

Sign/Symptom	*Incidence/Number of Patients*
Gait disturbance	47/48
Squinting	25/48
Vomiting	22/48
Headache	21/48
Dysarthria	19/48
Facial weakness	15/48
Personality change	11/48
Dysphagia	10/48
Drowsiness	10/48
Head tilt	5/48
Hearing loss	4/48
Pyramidal tract signs	41/48
Cranial nerve involvement	
VII	64/78
IX and X	54/78
VI	48/78
V (sensory)	38/78
V (motor)	13/48
XII	13/48
VIII	12/78
Cerebellar signs	62/78
Nystagmus	
Horizontal	26/48
Vertical	14/14
Papilledema	24/78
Gaze paralysis	
Horizontal	22/48
Vertical	5/48
Hemisensory deficit	5/48

Adapted from Bray PF, Carter S, Taveras JM. Brainstem tumors in children. *Neurology* 1958;8:17; and Matson DD. *Neurosurgery of infancy and childhood.* Springfield, IL: Charles C Thomas, 1969.

Vomiting, unaccompanied by headache, is caused not by increased intracranial pressure, but by direct infiltration of the medullary vomiting center. Impairment of gait is caused in part by involvement of the cerebellum or its peduncles, and in part by hemiparesis. Various neurologic signs found in affected children result from involvement of the major structures within the brainstem: the pyramidal tracts, nuclei of the various cranial nerves, and corticopontocerebellar fibers. Corticospinal tracts are usually involved early. Patients develop a spastic hemiparesis, increased deep tendon reflexes, and an extensor plantar response.

The cranial nerves most commonly affected by the neoplasm are the seventh and the sixth. Because the nucleus of the facial nerve is involved, facial weakness is almost invariably of lower motor neuron type. Dysfunction of the ninth and tenth nerves leads to drooling, difficulty in swallowing, and often insidious loss of weight. Sixth nerve weakness often is associated with horizontal conjugate gaze palsy. It is, therefore, caused by involvement of the brainstem, rather than being a false localizing sign resulting from increased intracranial pressure.

Functions of some of the other structures within the brainstem, notably the sensory pathways within the medial lemniscus, appear to be more resistant to tumor encroachment, and hemisensory deficits are rare. Infiltration of the reticular substances occasionally produces alterations in personality and changes in eating and sleeping patterns. In contrast to cerebellar tumors, impairment of consciousness is less common.

The progression of symptoms is relentless. As one cranial nerve after another becomes involved, patients become unable to swallow or speak, the extremities become completely paralyzed, and finally, the patient has impairment of consciousness with deepening coma and respiratory or cardiac irregularities ending in death. The average survival time for the untreated patient is approximately 15 months from the date of the patient's first hospitalization (347).

Symptoms and signs of group I tumors differ from those of group II tumors in that hydrocephalus is seen in 75% of the patients, as compared with 16% of children with group II tumors. Hydrocephalus results from the tumor's extension into the fourth ventricle and its obstruction of CSF circulation. Cerebellar deficits are also more common than in group II tumors; long tract signs are rare (Table 11.15) (348).

TABLE 11.15 Incidence of Neurologic Signs and Symptoms in 16 Patients with Dorsally Exophytic Brainstem Gliomas (Group I)

Sign/Symptom	Number of Patients
Hydrocephalus	12
Ataxia	11
Cranial nerve signs	8
Headache	6
Failure to thrive	5
Nystagmus	4
Long tract signs	1

Modified from Stroink AR, Hoffman HJ, Hendrick EB, et al. Transependymal benign dorsally exophytic brainstem gliomas in childhood: diagnosis and treatment recommendations. *Neurosurgery* 1987;20:439–444.

Diagnosis

The diagnosis suggested by the clinical features of a brainstem neoplasm can be confirmed by imaging studies. MRI, which has the capability of imaging in any plane and provides sagittal views of the posterior fossa, is the preferred procedure for characterization of the neoplasm. Imaging typically shows a diffuse, infiltrative, variable-enhancing tumor that enlarges and distorts the brainstem (Fig. 11.18). The technique provides excellent visualization of exophytic tumors and delineation of intrinsic brainstem tumors, with sagittal views often clearly showing the rostrocaudal extent of the mass (349). The neoplasm is almost always hypointense on T1-weighted images and, in the experience of Barkovich and colleagues, was always hyperintense on T2-weighted images (350). MRI indicates the presence and extent of tumor spread and allows visualization of areas of necrotic degeneration. Necrotic degeneration indicates a particularly poor prognosis, even if it appears after radiotherapy (351).

Several clinical entities should be considered in the differential diagnosis. These include a brain abscess, cysticercosis, tuberculoma, vascular malformation, and dermoid and epidermoid cysts (352). The appearance of these lesions on MRI is often difficult to distinguish from a neoplasm, and serial studies or a biopsy of the lesion is

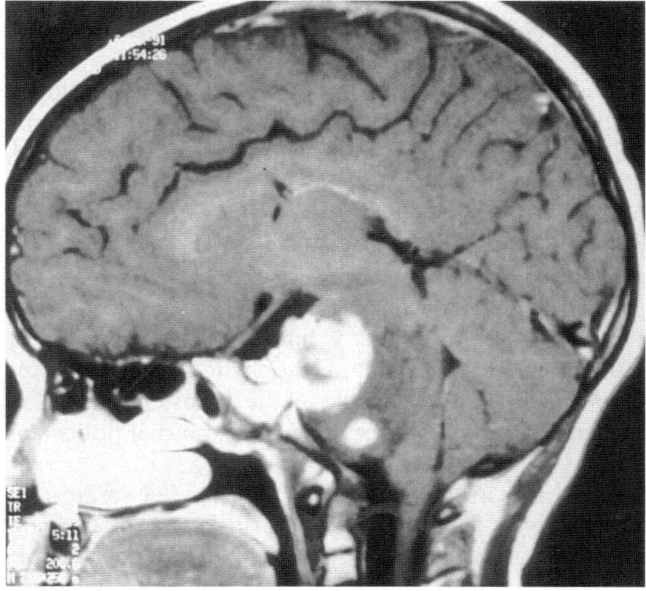

FIGURE 11.18. Sagittal magnetic resonance imaging shows enlarged pons and contrast-enhancing malignant glioma with associated edema.

sometimes necessary. In some instances, symptoms and signs of a brainstem glioma have receded spontaneously, leading to complete recovery. This condition has been termed *brainstem encephalitis*. It is probably identical to the Miller Fisher syndrome, a variant of infectious polyneuritis (353). Another important condition in the differential diagnosis of brainstem glioma is the diffuse cerebellar astrocytoma that displaces and sometimes invades the brainstem. Such tumors may radiologically mimic intrinsic diffuse brainstem gliomas, but, in contrast, are amenable to near complete resections and may not require further therapy.

Treatment of Brainstem Gliomas

Treatment of brainstem gliomas depends on the tumor group. For group I tumors, Stroink and coworkers advocate subtotal resection, with radiotherapy being used only when tumor recurs (348). Generally, the morphologic appearance of the tumor correlates with survival time (354), and in the case of the diffuse brainstem gliomas, there is no evidence that microscopic examination of tissue obtained by stereotactic biopsy is a better predictor of clinical progression than neuroimaging (355). The use of combined PET and MRI improves radiological interpretation of a mass lesion in the brainstem (356). Magnetic resonance spectroscopy may offer additional information about prognosis, but such technologies have not been validated as prognostic tools in large clinical studies (357). The presence of lower brainstem dysfunction is an important absolute contraindication to biopsy because patients will likely require tracheostomy postoperatively. Astrocytic tumors involving the midbrain have a much better prognosis than those involving the pons; medullary lesions have a somewhat better prognosis than pontine lesions.

Less common forms of brainstem glioma include focal, cystic, cervicomedullary, and tectal types (Toronto groups III and IV). In contrast to the diffuse type, these tumors tend to be well circumscribed and exophytic, and display histologic and biologic characteristics of pilocytic astrocytomas. Such tumors may have a much more favorable prognosis than diffuse brainstem gliomas and can be approached surgically with the intent to safely resect the lesions. However, morbidity is high, with the exception of lesions that are predominantly exophytic, and rare focal tumors that extend to the surface of the brainstem and can be shelled out without surgically incising normal brainstem tissue.

The principles of surgical excision of brainstem gliomas, whether exophytic or intrinsic, entail adequate exposure and visualization with an operating microscope. The concept is to excise the offending, noninfiltrating component of this lesion, which is best done with bipolar coagulation and suction. Use of ultrasonic aspirators and laser probes can aid in the early excision of these lesions, but once the tumor–brainstem interface is reached, careful tactile monitoring is required. The glial tumor in the cerebellum proper should be excised totally, and this entails staying in a plane of normal brain tissue surrounding the tumor. Again, this resection is best done with tactile feedback to the surgeon because visualization becomes confusing when tissue becomes charred and discolored using the laser. Focal pilocytic brainstem gliomas that have been excised can be followed conservatively with MRI every 3 to 4 months in the first 2 years. In the absence of clinical or radiographic recurrence, radiotherapy and chemotherapy should be deferred. Nonpilocytic focal brainstem gliomas or partially resected pilocytic brainstem gliomas should be treated with conformal or stereotactic radiotherapy. Progressive pilocytic lesions in infants should be treated with chemotherapy rather than radiotherapy. There have been no controlled clinical trials examining the benefits and risks of radiotherapy or chemotherapy in focal brainstem gliomas.

For group II tumors, a surgical approach is impossible, leaving radiotherapy and chemotherapy as principal treatments. The prognosis for these children is, to say the least, discouraging, regardless of the histology at the time of biopsy.

Radiation therapy produces transient clinical remissions in approximately 60% of this group, with initial improvement being noted some 3 to 6 weeks after the onset of treatment, most commonly as partial clearing of cranial nerve signs. Mean survival is between 6 and 12 months. Tumors that arise from the mesencephalon or those that extend into the cerebellopontine and prepontine cisterns fare a little better (342). The response to a second course of irradiation is usually poor (358,359).

Hyperfractionated radiotherapy, which entails the use of a large number of smaller fractions given in the same overall treatment time and allows a higher total dose to be directed at the tumor, has been tested and found ineffective in prolonging event-free survival or overall survival in brain stem glioma (360). Rather, the radiation necrosis encountered at high doses caused neurologic morbidity and high-dose steroid dependence (361,362).

Few studies have evaluated the efficacy of chemotherapy in brainstem gliomas backed by objective neuroimaging (363). A number of chemotherapeutic agents have been tried, notably BCNU, lomustine (CCNU), vincristine, cisplatin, carboplatin, and various alkylators. To date, when responses to chemotherapy do occur, they are of short duration, although exceptions have been encountered (339,364,365). For example, one study reported 80% partial response (four of five) to high-dose cyclophosphamide (366). This has not been corroborated by other investigators. One of us (B.M.) has treated six newly diagnosed children having diffuse brainstem gliomas with high-dose cyclophosphamide and thiotepa followed by bone marrow reinfusion. One patient had a partial response, and one had minor response to chemotherapy (339,367). On recovery, they were given hyperfractionated radiotherapy.

The patient with a partial response to chemotherapy has then achieved a complete response and is free of disease or late effects 11 years from diagnosis (367). Kretschmar and colleagues evaluated high-dose cyclophosphamide and cisplatin and radiotherapy before radiation in 32 pediatric patients (368). Of 32 patients, 3 had a partial response, 23 had stable disease, and 6 had progressive disease. Median survival was 9 months. Two arms of preradiation chemotherapy did not improve outcome in the Children's Cancer Group group-wide phase II trial in brain stem glioma (369). Overall, there is little evidence that chemotherapy is effective in the treatment of diffuse infiltrative brain stem gliomas (370).

Neither brachytherapy, the implant of ^{125}I into the tumor, or immunotherapy, in the form of intraventricular interleukin-2 or interferon-β, have improved survival significantly (371). The direct transfer by means of a retroviral vector of specific tumor-suppressor genes, of genes that encode a product toxic to tumors, or of genes whose products induce apoptosis in tumors, are new therapeutic approaches that are still experimental (372,373). It is clear that new treatment strategies are required to reduce the high mortality of diffuse brainstem gliomas. Once hydrocephalus is diagnosed in the progressive clinical course of brain stem glioma, CSF diversion should be performed promptly (374).

Midline Tumors

A number of pathologically diverse tumors arising from the midline of the supratentorial region are grouped together because their initial clinical pictures share several features. These include the insidious development of increased intracranial pressure often caused by hydrocephalus, as well as by the bulk of the tumor, visual impairment, abnormalities of endocrine or metabolic function, and alterations of consciousness or personality.

Most common of these midline tumors are the craniopharyngioma (55% of midline lesions, and 5% to 6% of all pediatric intracranial tumors) and the glioma of the optic nerve (19% of midline lesions) (375). Other tumors, such as pinealomas, and various intraventricular neoplasms, such as colloid cysts of the third ventricle, papillomas of the choroid plexus, and ependymomas of the lateral or third ventricle, are much rarer (Table 11.16).

TABLE 11.16 Frequencies of Common Pediatric Brain Tumors in the Suptratentorial Compartment

Tumor	*Percent*
Craniopharyngioma	14.9
Anaplastic astrocytoma	12.5
Pilocytic astrocytoma	12.2
Fibrillary astrocytoma	8.9
Unclassifiable or unknown	8.5
Germ cell tumors (including teratomas)	5.3
Ependymoma	5.0
Choroid plexus papilloma (including anaplastic varieties)	4.4

Adapted from Gilles FH. Pediatric brain tumors: classification. In: Morantz RA, Walsh JW, eds. *Brain tumors. A comprehensive text.* New York: Marcel Dekker; 1994:109.

Craniopharyngioma

Pathology

The craniopharyngioma is located in the suprasellar region in 43% of patients, and in both intrasellar and suprasellar regions in 53%. Purely intrasellar craniopharyngiomas are rare in childhood. The tumor is believed to arise from small rests of squamous cells, normally encountered where the stalk joins with the pars distalis of the pituitary gland and is considered to represent remnants of the embryonal Rathke's pouch. If so, the tumor would be present at birth, but because of its slow growth, symptoms can be delayed for years to several decades. An adamantinomatous type usually is seen in children. Grossly, this neoplasm is characterized by the presence of cysts containing viscous material, and calcifications. A *papillary* variant, lacking calcifications, occurs almost exclusively in adults (376). β-Catenin gene mutations have been found in adamantinomatous but in none of the papillary craniopharyngiomas (377). However, chromosomal imbalances are a rare event in both adamantinomatous and papillary craniopharyngiomas (378).

As the craniopharyngioma expands forward, it begins to compress the optic chiasm. With downward expansion, the pituitary gland is compressed; with upward expansion, the third ventricle becomes distorted (Fig. 11.19A). Posterior expansion occurs into the posterior fossa but rarely causes posterior fossa signs. Large tumors are partly or completely cystic and contain a cloudy brown fluid with a high concentration of cholesterol often seen as floating crystals. Growth pattern is closely correlated to the origin of the tumor, whether it is above or below the diaphragm sellae. In craniopharyngiomas with prechiasmatic growth, the major portion of the tumor can be resected by traction. These tumors are candidates for the transphenoidal approach if the sphenoid sinus is pneumatized (379). Tumors with retrochiasmatic growth, which are not covered by diaphragm sellae and contact brain tissue directly, are easily torn by traction, and the tumor-glial interface should be carefully dissected under direct vision (380).

Microscopically, the tumor's appearance can vary greatly. In some areas, the cysts are lined with stratified squamous epithelium with peripheral accumulation of tumor cells and more internally situated loose, degenerative-appearing epithelium called *stellate reticulum*. Plump deposits of so-called wet keratin that may undergo dystrophic

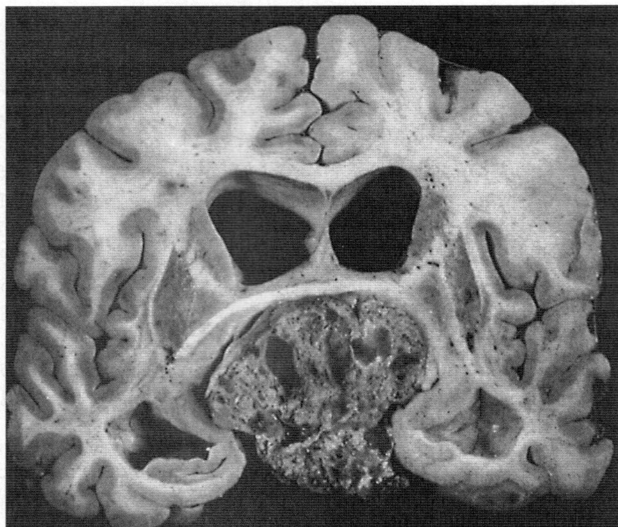

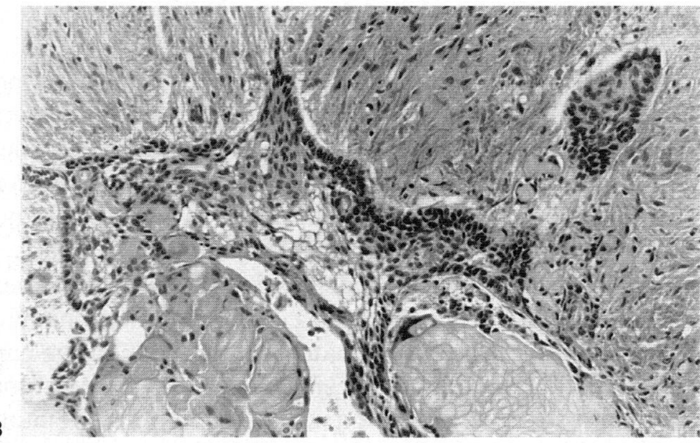

FIGURE 11.19. **A:** Craniopharyngioma. Large tumor obstructing the third ventricle and causing hydrocephalus. (From Merritt HH. *A textbook of neurology*, 7th ed. Philadelphia: Lea & Febiger, 1984. With permission.) **B:** Note intraepithelial vacuolated areas (*stellate reticulum*) and islands of wet keratin (hematoxylin and eosin, original magnification ×500).

calcification are typical (Fig. 11.19B). Deposition of lamellar bone also can occur. In other areas, the tumor consists of epithelial masses with poorly cellular connective tissue, resembling the enamel pulp of developing teeth and termed *adamantinoma* because of its resemblance to a similar tumor arising from the jaw. Craniopharyngiomas are locally invasive and the adjacent brain tissue usually shows an exuberant reactive gliosis. The latter may contain large numbers of Rosenthal fibers that also can be seen in juvenile pilocytic astrocytomas (222).

On the basis of morphologic appearance and growth characteristics in tissue culture, Liszczak and colleagues distinguished two tumor types (381). In the majority of specimens, cells have the typical appearance and growth characteristics of epithelioid cells, with a smooth cell surface demonstrable by electron microscopy. Cells from atypical tumors contain cholesterol crystals and demonstrate some features characteristic of neoplastic transformation, with surface microvilli being evident on electron microscopy. Clinically, patients with atypical tumors tend to be younger and are more likely to experience early tumor recurrence.

Clinical Manifestations

In craniopharyngioma, as in many other midline neoplasms, the availability of imaging studies has facilitated diagnosis and, hence, significantly reduced the duration of symptoms before diagnosis. Whereas Northfield, compiling a series of patients in 1957 (382), recorded an interval of between 2 and 5 years between onset of symptoms and diagnosis, time before diagnosis is now shorter. As a consequence, treatment occurs sooner and increased intracranial pressure is seen less frequently, and when present, it is less marked.

In approximately one-half of the younger patients, presenting symptoms are those of increased intracranial pressure, whereas in older children, visual complaints and endocrine abnormalities are common (Table 11.17) (383,384).

A variety of visual disturbances can be encountered, depending on the location of the tumor and the direction of its expansion. They include unilateral and bilateral optic atrophy and various field deficits. Unilateral or bilateral temporal field cuts are the most common disturbance, often commencing as field cuts in both upper bitemporal quadrants. Homonymous hemianopia (Fig. 11.20) and unilateral blindness also are noted (383). The hemianopia is the result of direct encroachment of the tumor on the optic chiasm or optic tracts. It should be noted that the craniopharyngioma is the intracranial tumor that causes the greatest loss of vision and the most extensive field

TABLE 11.17 Presenting Signs and Symptoms in Children with Craniopharyngiomas

	Percent of Children	
Sign/Symptom	***1968***	***1980***
Increased intracranial pressure	65	24
Impaired vision or field defects	62	57
Endocrine abnormalities	41	53
Papilledema	41	9
Ataxia	9	0
Intracranial calcification	79	86
Erosion of sella	50	Large majority
Psychologic symptoms	24	—

Adapted from Richmond IL, Wilson CB. Parasellar tumors in children. I. Clinical presentation, preoperative assessment, and differential diagnosis. *Childs Brain* 1980;7:73; and Bingas B, Wolter M. Das Kraniopharyngiom. *Fortschr Neurol Psychiatr* 1968;36:117.

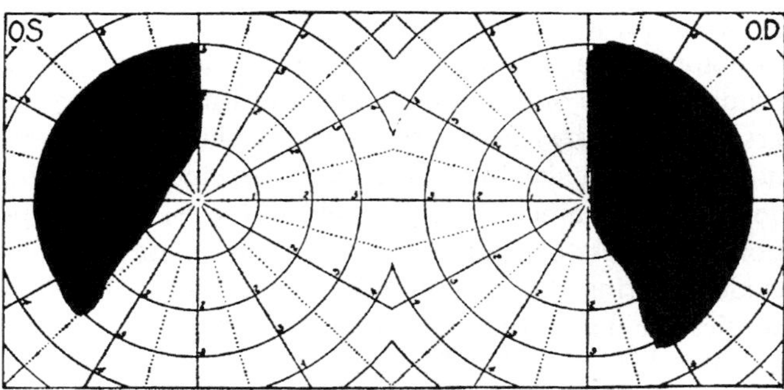

FIGURE 11.20. Craniopharyngioma. Bitemporal hemianopia is almost complete. (OS, left eye; OD, right eye.) (Courtesy of Dr. Robert Hepler, Department of Ophthalmology, UCLA Center for the Health Sciences, Los Angeles.)

cut even though the optic disks remain normal for a long time.

Disturbances in endocrine function result from either compression of the pituitary itself by a tumor both above and within the sella or hypothalamic involvement by a suprasellar tumor.

In the experience of Imura and coworkers, hypopituitarism was seen in 91% of patients with craniopharyngioma (385). Most had multiple hormone deficiencies. Delayed growth is the most common result of the endocrine disturbance, and growth hormone deficiency can be documented in more than one-half of affected children (383,386). A low gonadotropin level is found in approximately one-half of the pubertal patients. The failure of gonadotropic activity results in a reduced output of 17-ketosteroids and delayed or absent secondary sexual development. Abnormalities in follicle-stimulating hormone and luteinizing hormone output are seen in approximately one-third of patients, as are an elevation of prolactin and a reduction in thyroid-stimulating hormone (383,385).

Diabetes insipidus is a less common preoperative finding and is seen in 10% to 20% of children. Hypotension is seen occasionally and is sometimes related to hyponatremia owing to chronic adrenal insufficiency. A rare patient has oliguria with an inappropriate output of antidiuretic hormone. Precocious puberty was not seen in the series of Imura and coworkers. Nevertheless, the question of CNS lesions is frequently raised in patients with true precocious puberty. In boys, congenital or acquired disorders of the CNS can be implicated in 80% to 90% of these cases, whereas in girls, CNS lesions, most frequently a hypothalamic hamartoma, are responsible for 20% to 30% (387).

Disturbances of personality or dementia are not unusual and include periods of visual and olfactory hallucinations, abnormalities of sleep cycle, and dementia. These symptoms are believed to arise from hypothalamic involvement, although in some instances, they can reflect a chronic increase of intracranial pressure. Seizures caused by impingement of the tumor on the medial aspect of the temporal lobe are seen on occasion. Attacks of shivering or of falling without apparent loss of consciousness are somewhat rarer but still characteristic.

A confusing finding is the occasional presence of cerebellar signs resulting from involvement of the red nucleus and its connections (388). Should cerebellar signs be accompanied by increased intracranial pressure, the erroneous clinical diagnosis of a posterior fossa tumor is almost inevitable, unless one keeps in mind that cerebellar signs occur late in the clinical course of a craniopharyngioma, but relatively early in posterior fossa tumors.

Diagnosis

The craniopharyngioma is characterized by a gradual development of increased intracranial pressure, visual disturbances, and endocrine dysfunction. Plain radiographs of the skull, at one time used as the initial diagnostic procedure, usually revealed eroded clinoid processes. Approximately 80% of children had curvilinear areas of suprasellar calcification. The tumor is readily demonstrable by imaging studies. CT scan reveals the cyst, with the increased density of its capsule, accompanied by calcifications (Fig. 11.21). Even though MRI does not reveal calcifications, sagittal views provide better information about the location, extent, and vascular relationships of the

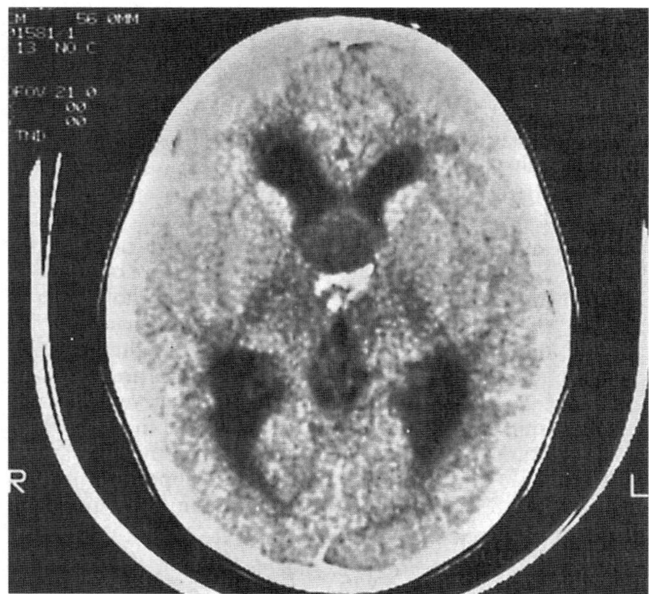

FIGURE 11.21. Craniopharyngioma. Computed tomographic scan without contrast. The tumor consists of a cyst anteriorly and a calcified area posteriorly. The ventricular system—in particular, the third ventricle—is somewhat enlarged. This 10-year-old boy had a 1-year history of growth failure and several months of intermittent headaches and vomiting. Papilledema and a field cut were seen on initial examination. The tumor could be only partially resected.

tumor. The size of the cyst and its proportions of keratin and cholesterol also can be determined. Cysts of Rathke's pouch are more likely to be hyperintense on T1-weighted images owing to the high cholesterol content of the cyst and the presence of methemoglobin (389). The signal on T2-weighted images is variable. When the optic tracts show increased signal on T2-weighted images, as is occasionally the case, and astrocytic gliosis is adjacent to the tumor as a result of an inflammatory response to the leaking contents of the cyst, the neoplasm can be misinterpreted as a glioma (390).

Other diagnostic studies are not helpful. The EEG either is normal or shows diffuse slowing. Of Russell and Pennybacker's patients, 75% had elevated spinal or ventricular fluid protein content (391).

Differential Diagnosis

Imaging studies readily differentiate between a craniopharyngioma and the various other commonly encountered space-occupying lesions in the sellar and suprasellar areas, notably optic glioma, chordoma, suprasellar arachnoid cyst, and the rare suprasellar meningioma. Even without their assistance, the clinical picture can provide important clues about the nature of the underlying neoplasm.

In an optic glioma, vision is lost early, and there is a high incidence of neurofibromatosis 1 (von Recklinghausen disease).

Chordomas are rare tumors in this region. They are believed to arise from notochord rest cells and in the majority of cases are located along the clivus (392). Those arising from the superior portion of the clivus can involve the chiasm and thus their clinical picture can mimic a craniopharyngioma. Chordomas that arise from the inferior portion of the clivus have a clinical picture suggesting a brainstem glioma with cranial nerve involvement and cerebellar deficits. In childhood, the course of these tumors is usually acute, and they tend to metastasize to the lungs (393,394).

Pinealomas, particularly those with extensions or implantations into the anterior portion of the third ventricle, can be mistaken clinically for suprasellar cysts. These tumors tend to compress the upper part of the mesencephalon and produce paralysis of upward gaze, impaired pupillary light reaction, and precocious puberty. At other times, the presenting symptom is increased intracranial pressure owing to meningeal invasion.

The most common presenting symptoms of chromophobe and eosinophilic adenomas include pituitary hypersecretion and failure of sexual maturation.

Suprasellar arachnoid cysts also present with midline tumor symptoms (395). In order of frequency, symptoms of these cysts include hydrocephalus (87% of affected children), increased head size (57%), vision loss (30%), and ataxia (28%). Additionally, some children with this condition develop the *bobble-head* syndrome (396).

When tumors of the anterior third ventricle become symptomatic in infancy, they produce the diencephalic syndrome. The outstanding features of this condition, as first described by Russell (397), are emaciation in spite of normal food intake, hypoglycemia, hyperkinetic behavior, vomiting, a characteristic pale, elflike facies, and exceptional alertness or euphoria. Visual impairment becomes evident during the later months of the illness. Imaging studies are diagnostic and reveal the tumor encroaching into the third ventricle. Tumors producing this syndrome are usually astrocytomas of the third ventricle or optic gliomas.

Treatment and Prognosis

With earlier diagnosis now possible, with a better understanding of preoperative, intraoperative, and postoperative hormonal and fluid requirements, and with the availability of microsurgical techniques, total resection of the tumor as verified by postoperative neuroimaging can be achieved with minimal neurologic and endocrine damage in 70% to 90% of patients (398,399). Nevertheless, the respective roles of radical surgery and limited surgery with radiotherapy continue to be debated. In some series, the results of the two approaches are equivalent or show long-term results of combined surgery and radiation to be better than results with total resection alone (400–402). At the Medical University of South Carolina and at the UCLA Center for Health Sciences, we favor radical surgery. As a rule, total removal is easier in children than in adults because in adults chronic leakage of cyst fluid often results in the formation of dense adhesions (398,403).

There is no clear consensus on the best therapeutic approach to craniopharyngioma. Therapeutic alternatives include total resection, subtotal resection with observation, subtotal resection with postoperative radiotherapy, cyst aspiration, and instillation of intracavitary radiation or bleomycin (404). The neurosurgical approach differs for each case and depends on the location of the tumor. If total removal is impossible, as is the case when the tumor is large or when neighboring brain is invaded, surgery is limited to partial removal to avoid high morbidity and mortality. Under these circumstances, tumor recurrence is likely. As a rule, complete tumor removal also is less likely the more marked the ventricular dilatation at the time of surgery (405). Because regrowth of the tumor is often delayed for many years, and because of the deleterious effects of radiotherapy on the developing brain, we believe that the status of the tumor should be followed with imaging studiesand that radiotherapy be delayed until necessary, even when tumor removal has been shown to be subtotal (406,407). Recurrences can be treated by another attempt at surgery or a combination of radiotherapy and surgery. In the experience of Jose and coworkers, 72% of patients with recurrent tumor treated with combined radiotherapy and surgery experienced a 10-year progression-free survival (400). Brachytherapy with stereotactic instillation of ^{32}P or bleomycin into the cyst also have been advocated (408–410). It appears to be effective when more than 50% of the tumor bulk is cystic (411).

Vision does not improve, and endocrine disturbances are generally exacerbated after surgical treatment (405). All children in the series of Lyen and Grant had hormonal deficiencies, most commonly (100% in Lyen and Grant's series) impaired growth hormone secretion (412). A defect in the output of gonadotropins is seen in 93%, and reduced adrenocorticotropic hormone (ACTH) and thyroid-stimulating hormone output also is observed in most affected children. Up to three-fourths of the children develop diabetes insipidus, which is usually permanent and can be accompanied by an absent or impaired sense of thirst (405,413). Poor postoperative control of this condition can lead to cerebral vein thrombosis. Morbid postoperative obesity is common and interferes with social adaptation (414,415). In obese patients, there is MRI evidence of preoperative hypothalamic damage (414). As a rule, absence of calcification on neuroimaging is associated with a significantly better progression-free survival (406). Postoperative endocrine therapy and its results are reviewed by Lyen and Grant (412) and de Vile and associates (405). It is of note that no significant difference in morbidity was seen after complete tumor excision without radiotherapy or subtotal excision with adjuvant irradiation (405). In the series of Fahlbusch and colleagues, which comprised both children and adults, the 10-year recurrence-free survival rate was 83% after what was deemed total removal and 50.5% after subtotal removal. Tumor recurrences occurred mostly within the first 5 years after surgery (416). Without adequate hormone replacement, minor infections can lead to rapid deterioration or sudden death.

A variety of psychological deficits can be seen in subjects who have undergone surgical treatment of craniopharyngioma. These include visual perceptual dysfunction and frontal lobe deficits, notably a lack of inhibitory control and perseveration. The frontal lobe deficits can be caused by hypothalamic injury rather than direct trauma to the frontal lobes by surgery (417). Patients with craniopharyngioma rated their health-related quality of life as considerably lower than healthy controls; the domains of social and emotional functioning can be particularly affected (418,419).

TUMORS OF THE OPTIC PATHWAY

Pathology

This heterogenous group of tumors represent 3% to 6% of pediatric brain tumors. Approximately one-third affect the optic nerve and the remainder involve the optic chiasm, hypothalamus, third ventricle, and optic tracts, singly or in combination. Tumors that arise from the optic nerve are histologically similar to the cerebellar pilocytic astrocytoma. They occur within or outside the orbit as a fusiform dilatation of the nerve. Neoplasms arising within the orbit tend to spread through the optic foramina and expand into the cranium in a dumbbell fashion. Tumors arising from the optic chiasm or hypothalamus can invade the third ventricle or grow inferiorly to compress the pituitary gland (420). On histologic examination, the neoplasm consists of oligodendroglia or astrocytes similar to the glial tumors arising from the cerebral hemispheres. Many optic nerve tumors are associated with neurofibromatosis. In this condition, the neoplasm is usually a glioma, less often a meningioma of the optic sheath (7).

Clinical Manifestations

A strong association exists between gliomas of the optic nerve and neurofibromatosis type 1; between 33% and 70% of patients with chiasmal gliomas have the clinical features of neurofibromatosis type 1 (421,422). Conversely, optic gliomas are the most common intracranial tumors in neurofibromatosis type 1.

The various signs and symptoms seen in patients with gliomas of the optic nerve are depicted in Table 11.18 (423). A more recent clinical series compiled in 1981 by Iraci and coworkers (424) indicates little difference in the initial clinical presentation as a consequence to the ready availability of the newer imaging techniques. In approximately one-half of patients, poor vision is the presenting symptom. In infancy, it can become evident as searching nystagmus or failure to fix on and follow objects. Deterioration of eyesight can progress so insidiously that children can have an apparent sudden loss of vision. Exophthalmos

TABLE 11.18 Symptoms and Signs in 56 Children with Optic Glioma

Symptom/Sign	*Determined by Patient History*	*Determined by Physical Examination*
Diminished visual acuity	28	53
Exophthalmos	25	29
Nystagmus	8	14
Strabismus	6	17
Field cut	1	12
Disc change		
Pallor		36
Pallor and blurring		11
Blurring		8
Increased intracranial pressure	3	15
Enlarged head	1	4
Multiple café au lait spots		12
Hemiparesis		4

From Chutorian AM, Schwartz JF, Evans RA, et al. Optic gliomas in children. *Neurology* 1964;14:83–95. With permission.

develops when the tumor grows anteriorly. Because exophthalmos is easily recognized, affected patients have a relatively shorter illness before hospitalization than those whose tumor expands posteriorly into the third ventricle.

Other ocular symptoms, such as strabismus, are less frequent presenting symptoms and are usually secondary to impaired vision. Increased intracranial pressure and endocrine abnormalities such as precocious puberty, diabetes insipidus, and growth retardation are uncommon early symptoms of optic gliomas. They indicate that the tumor has extended into the area surrounding the third ventricle and, therefore, are associated with a poor prognosis.

Almost all children with gliomas have abnormalities of the optic disks. These consist of primary optic atrophy, papilledema, or a mixture of the two abnormalities. These findings accompany a variety of visual field defects.

Diagnosis

Neuroimaging imaging studies readily detect gliomas of the optic nerve and delineate their extent (Fig. 11.22). An optic nerve sheath meningioma is distinguished by an increased signal on T1-weighted, gadolinium-enhanced images, with the hyperintensity sharply delineated from the optic nerve, which does not appear enlarged (425). They can be solitary or a component of NF-1. If bilateral, they are considered to be pathognomonic of NF-1 (426). The clinical course of optic pathway tumors detected in the context of NF-1 is often benign (427) (see Chapter 12).

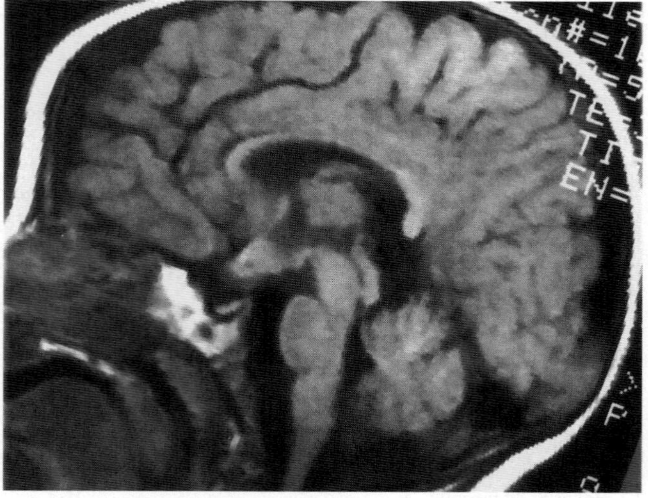

FIGURE 11.22. Glioma of optic nerve and chiasm. Sagittal view on a T1-weighted magnetic resonance scan in a 6-month-old boy. A mass compresses and obliterates the optic and infundibular recesses of the anterior portion of the third ventricle. From there, the tumor extends anteroinferiorly. (Courtesy of Drs. Hervey D. Segall, William Kneeland, and William Bank, Children's Hospital, Los Angeles.)

Treatment and Prognosis

Because the natural progression of this tumor is so variable, there is considerable controversy as to its best management (428). Some tumors remain static for years, and others progress rapidly. Consequently, no uniform management exists, and observation, chemotherapy, radiotherapy, and surgeries have been suggested by various authorities (429). We believe that the unilateral tumor confined to the optic nerve and producing a severely proptotic blind eye should be removed with the globe left in place. This allows the physician to monitor for tumor growth by either funduscopy or neuroimaging. The prognosis for patients with this type of tumor presentation is excellent, and the likelihood of posterior extension was only 5% in the series of Alvord and Lofton (430,431). In a multivariate analysis of optic gliomas conducted by Khafaga and colleagues, only age over 3 years emerged has a significant determinant for progression-free survival (432).

Treatment of bilateral tumor or a tumor that involves the optic chiasm and structures posterior to the chiasm is more uncertain (421). Tao and coworkers have demonstrated that radiotherapy can shrink the tumor and stabilize vision in 88% of patients, and provide a 10-year freedom from disease progression in 100% of 29 children (433). Even so, many clinicians, including ourselves, believe that the benefits of radiotherapy are difficult to prove (433). Using a regimen of 5,000 to 5,500 cGy given over the course of 6 to 8 weeks, Tenny and associates recorded a 50% survival over a mean follow-up period of 13 years (434). This figure, however, should be compared with a 64% survival of untreated patients with chiasmal gliomas followed by Imes and Hoyt for a median of 20 years (421), and a 10-year survival rate of 83% in untreated patients reported by Jenkin and colleagues (435). If treatment is decided on, children younger than age 5 years should receive chemotherapy in preference to radiotherapy (434) because the former preserves intellectual function (436). Stereotactic radiosurgery and proton radiation therapy decrease doses of radiation to brain adjacent to tumor. These technologies increase the feasibility of safely considering radiotherapy in selected cases (437,438).

The benefits of chemotherapy, however, are equally uncertain. Packer and coworkers using a combination of actinomycin-D and vincristine for patients with chiasmatic pilocytic astrocytomas induced significant tumor shrinkage (439). Petronio and colleagues used a five-drug regimen that included 6-thioguanine, procarbazine, dibromodulcitol, BCNU, and vincristine (440). Ten of 19 patients had a partial response and five had disease stabilization. Packer and colleagues treated 23 children with recurrent and 37 with newly diagnosed low-grade glioma using a 10-week induction cycle of carboplatin and vincristine, followed by maintenance treatment with the same drugs (441). Of newly diagnosed patients 62% had an objective response, and of children with recurrent disease, 52% of had an objective response. DNA topoisomerase IIα correlates with tumor cell proliferation, but its expression does not correlate with patient survival (442). A similar partial response was seen by Chamberlain and colleaguestreated recurrent chiasmatic-hypothalamic gliomas with 21-day courses of oral etoposide (443), a DNA topoisomerase II–inhibiting drug.

From these data we can conclude that chemotherapy can result in low-grade glioma shrinkage in more than one-half of patients treated (441) and should be used for tumors that are not surgically resectable and in young children (younger than age 3 years) for whom radiotherapy is contraindicated. In all cases, glioma of the optic chiasm or posterior structures should be treated only when its growth has been documented by neuroimaging studies or by progression of clinical symptoms, particularly deterioration of vision. In patients with neurofibromatosis, there is a higher risk of vasculopathy complicating radiotherapy; thus, chemotherapy should be strongly considered in such patients (444).

Optic gliomas associated with neurofibromatosis type 1 are no more aggressive than those unaccompanied by neurofibromatosis type 1, and from the wealth of conflicting follow-up studies, one gathers that the outlook for patients with optic gliomas and neurofibromatosis type 1 is no worse than for those without neurofibromatosis type 1 with respect to morbidity or mortality from the optic glioma. Patients with neurofibromatosis type 1, however, have an increased likelihood of succumbing to tumors arising from other sites in the body.

PINEAL TUMORS

Tumors of the pineal region account for 3% to 10% of all pediatric intracranial tumors (445,446). On histologic examination, at least four types of pineal tumors can be distinguished: (a) germ cell tumors, including germinomas, benign and malignant teratomas, and choriocarcinomas, which arise from the pineal body or structures immediately surrounding it; (b) pinealomas, which arise from the pineal parenchyma cells; (c) epidermoid cysts; and (d) gliomas. Russell and Sachs, Jooma and Kendall, and the Toronto Neurosurgical Group have observed the germinoma to be the most common, accounting for approximately one-half of pineal neoplasms (447–449). Germinomas are biphasic tumors consisting of a neoplastic component of large, glycogen-rich, germ cells with large nuclei and prominent nucleoli, and a nonneoplastic component of small mature lymphocytes. The germ cell component is immunoreactive for placental alkaline phophatase. Approximately 5% to 50% of germinomas contain syncytiotrophoblastic tumor giant cells that elaborate β-human choriogonadotropic hormone. The presence of such cells in an otherwise typical germinoma does not indicate the presence of a choriocarcinoma element.

Other germ cell tumors, including the embryonal carcinoma, endodermal sinus tumor (yolk sac tumor), choriocarcinoma, and teratoma (mature and immature), are much less common than germinomas and tend to occur as mixed tumors rather than one particular type.

Primary tumors of the pineal parenchyma are rare and include the pineocytoma, pineoblastoma (PNET), intermediate, and mixed types. Details of the pathology and patient outcomes have been reported recently by Schild and colleagues (450). Pineal tumors should be distinguished from a benign pineal cyst. This lesion shows a rim of calcification and enhances with contrast. It is a relatively common, nonneoplastic entity that is usually asymptomatic and is often discovered serendipitously on MRI (451,452).

Clinical Manifestations

Germ cell tumors occur predominantly in male subjects. In the series of Hiraga and colleagues, 74% of patients presenting before 15 years of age were male; when presentation was after 15 years of age, 92% were male (453). Both the incidence of CNS germ cell tumors and the male predominance increase about the time of puberty (454). The peak incidence in the SEER database (3.8 per million population) occurs in the 15 to 19 year old age group, and the greatest male to female ratio (19.5:1) is seen in the 20 to 24 year old age group. Initial symptoms depend to some extent on the nature of the tumor. In the series of Kageyama and coworkers, the predominant symptoms of patients with a pineal germinoma include Parinaud's sign (paralysis of conjugate upward gaze) (76%), increased intracranial pressure (67%), Argyll Robertson pupil (46%), diplopia (32%), diabetes insipidus (32%), and hypopituitarism (24%) (455). Increased intracranial pressure often arises acutely as a result of aqueductal obstruction or meningeal infiltration. The other neurologic signs, notably the limitation of conjugate upward gaze, impaired pupillary light reaction in the presence of an intact accommodative response (Argyll Robertson pupil), and central deafness, are caused by pressure on the corpora quadrigemina (Table 11.19) (456).

Cerebellar signs, resulting from transmitted pressure, were seen in 14% of the Japanese series of Kageyama (455). An abnormally calcified pineal body is seen in approximately 20% of patients with pinealoma, but precocious puberty is relatively uncommon; it was seen in only 3% and 14%, respectively, of the two Japanese series of Kageyama and colleagues and Hiraga and colleagues (453,455). It is far more common in boys harboring a malignant teratoma or in choriocarcinoma (448,453). Calcifications are common in more malignant tumors. Some 70% of patients with

TABLE 11.19 Eye Signs in Pineal Tumors

Sign	Percent
Dilated pupils	31
Impaired light reaction	50
Diplopia	25
Nystagmus	38
Limitation of upward gaze	31
Papilledema	56
Abducens palsy	25

From Posner M, Horrax G. Eye signs in pineal tumors. *J Neurosurg* 1946;3:15. With permission.

malignant teratomas have other signs of hypothalamic disturbance, including obesity, somnolence, polyphagia, and diabetes insipidus. The mechanism whereby pineal tumors produce precocious puberty is still unclear and probably is not uniform.

A greater than chance association between bilateral retinoblastoma and a midline intracranial malignancy, most commonly a malignant pinealoma, has been reported (trilateral syndrome). In the series of Pesin and Shields, the retinoblastoma was diagnosed between 4 years before and 5 months after the diagnosis of the intracranial tumor (457).

Diagnosis

Increased intracranial pressure in the presence of pupillary abnormalities and impaired upward gaze in a male subject should always suggest a pineal tumor. Imaging studies are highly accurate in detecting and characterizing these tumors (458). The sagittal cut on MRI is optimal for visualizing the extent of the tumor, whereas CT scanning is generally superior to MRI for characterizing its histology, in that CT scanning is able to demonstrate the presence of calcifications, an indication of a benign or malignant teratoma (459). Normally, a calcified pineal body is rarely seen in a child younger than age 10 years. In the experience of Zimmerman, the youngest normal child with a calcified pineal body was 6 years old (458).

Increased secretion of β-human chorionic gonadotropins and α-fetoprotein has been noted in patients with pinealoma. Generally, their presence indicates a malignant teratoma rather than a germinoma (460).

Treatment and Prognosis

Despite the availability of human choriogonadotropic and α-fetoprotein markers and imaging studies, it is not always possible to differentiate preoperatively between germinomas, which are not amenable to total excision, and teratomas, which are amenable if benign (460). Therefore, tissue diagnosis is important, and the preferred treatment is definitive surgery for benign tumors (461).

No consensus exists on optimal therapy for germinomas (461,462). Craniospinal radiotherapy has been perceived as the gold standard treatment for localized intracranial germinoma, but because of the high prevalence of late effects from craniospinal radiotherapy, there is a trend to reduce the irradiation volume (463). It is appropriate to offer a CT- or MRI-guided biopsy and carboplatin-base chemotherapy and ventricular/tumor bed irradiation at 24 Gy. This approach has a low operative risk and a high cure rate while maintaining pituitary function (464). The alternative surgical approach is to perform a craniotomy and resect the tumor, but unlike PNET/MBs, there is no evidence that gross tumor resection produces a more favorable outcome in germinomas. The outcome is relatively good for germinomas, and 70% to 100% 5-year survival rates are commonly reported for localized tumors (452,461,465).

Other tumors, particularly the nongerminomatous germ cell tumors in the pineal region in which α-fetoprotein or human choriogonadotropic can be detected in serum or CSF, have a much lower 5-year survival rate than germinomas. Treatment for the more malignant germ cell tumors consists of debulking, followed by multidrug chemotherapy; the attainment of a complete response to chemotherapy prior to radiotherapy may improve progression-free survival (466). Most patients harboring a pineal tumor do not require ventricular-peritoneal shunting after surgery and craniospinal radiotherapy. Occasionally, endoscopic third ventriculostomy is required (467). Edwards and associates have suggested prophylactic spinal irradiation for nongerminomatous germ cell tumors (461). Marker response [α-fetoprotein (AFP) and human choriogonadotropic (HCG)] may be seen in the absence of radiologic response, and the risk of systemic dissemination of tumor is small (466).

TUMORS OF LATERAL AND THIRD VENTRICLES

Intraventricular tumors are rare in children. The most common histologic types encountered are papillomas of the choroid plexus of the lateral ventricles, colloid cysts arising from the third ventricle, and ependymomas.

Choroid Plexus Papillomas

Choroid plexus papillomas are intraventricular tumors that arise as cauliflowerlike masses that histologically can resemble normal choroid plexus. They are seen most frequently in the lateral ventricles, followed by the fourth ventricle and third ventricle, in order of decreasing frequency (468). These papillary neoplasms show increased cell density and low mitotic activity. Increased mitotic activity, lack of the papillary architecture, and evidence of invasion suggest a potential for local recurrence and aggressive behavior. Like ependymomas, choroid plexus carcinomas are most common in young children, usually the age of 3 years (469,470). The clinical picture is generally a progressive increase in intracranial pressure and hydrocephalus caused by increased CSF production and blockage of CSF flow. This is accompanied by ataxia and an organic mental syndrome.

Choroid plexus tumors can occur in various familial syndromes, including von Hippel–Lindau, Li-Fraumeni, and Aicardi's syndromes, but consistent abnormal genetic loci have not yet been identified (471,472). Although abnormal polyoma virus sequences have been associated with these tumors, a definitive role in pathogenesis remains uncertain.

Choroid plexus papillomas that are surgically resected may not require further therapy. The most common surgical approach is to first interrupt the vascular supply and then remove the tumor by a transventricular approach. More recently, endoscopic contact coagulation of the hyperplastic choroid plexus has been proposed to reduce the risk of transventricular surgery (473). Several chromosomal imbalances are common in choroid plexus papillomas (474) and recurrent papillomas or more malignant carcinomas may have gains of chromosomes 7 and 12 (475); they should be treated with chemotherapy followed by reoperation and limited-field radiotherapy (476). The most effective chemotherapy seems to be platinum-based regimens (e.g., cisplatin, bleomycin, vinblastine), as first suggested by Maria and colleagues (477).

Colloid Cysts of the Third Ventricle

Colloid cysts of the third ventricle constitute between 0.5% to 1.0% of brain tumors (478). Unlike choroid plexus papillomas, they do not show any predilection for early childhood; in the series of Mathiesen and coworkers, only 8% of patients were younger than 15 years (478). On microscopic examination, the cyst is lined by cuboidal, pseudostratified, or columnar ciliated and mucous-secreting epithelial cells (479). Headache was the principal symptom in all children. In some instances, particularly when the cyst is located in the vicinity of the foramen of Monro, symptoms appear acutely or intermittently with paroxysmal attacks of headache and vomiting, terminated by a brief period of unconsciousness, with complete but transient recovery (480–482).

The diagnosis is readily made by CT or MRI. On CT scans, most are slightly hyperdense with respect to the brain, but may occasionally be hypodense or isodense. On MRI, colloid cysts have a variable appearance. About 50% of colloid cysts are hyperintense on T1-weighted images, and the rest are either isointense or hypointense. On T2-weighted images, most colloid cysts are hypointense to the brain. Isointense cysts may be difficult to identify on MRI and may be more easily seen on CT scans (483). Microsurgical removal of these tumors is currently preferred though their deep midline location is challenging (484,485). Damage to the left fornix in the course of surgery can impair verbal memory, whereas bilateral fornix damage can induce amnesia (486).

Tumors of the Pituitary

Pituitary adenomas are uncommon in children; in the large pediatric series of Rorke and colleagues, they accounted for only 1.1% of all intracranial tumors with the majority occurring around or after puberty (85). They arise from the adenohypophysis and are histologically monomorphous and benign appearing (487). The most frequently encountered neoplasm is a prolactin-secreting adenoma (488). This tumor is more common in girls and manifests by amenorrhea, usually accompanied by galactorrhea (489). Headaches and visual disturbances are occasionally present. Some of the prolactin-secreting adenomas are invasive and extend into the suprasellar cisterns. ACTH-secreting tumors are next most common, producing the clinical picture of Cushing disease (488). ACTH-secreting microadenomas might not be detected by imaging studies, even if MRI with gadolinium enhancement is used.

Microadenomas can be removed by transsphenoidal microsurgery (490). The procedure is preferable to irradiation, which induces pituitary-hypothalamic dysfunction. Macroadenomas cannot be cured surgically (491). Endocrinologic follow-up is critical to successful management of such patients.

TUMORS OF THE CEREBRAL HEMISPHERES

Tumors of the cerebral hemispheres are less frequent in children than in adults and account for approximately 40% of brain tumors (492). In children, it is often difficult to arrive at an early diagnosis because increased intracranial pressure appears late, focal signs are difficult to elicit, and the relatively high incidence of idiopathic epilepsy in childhood makes the appearance of seizures less alarming than when their onset is at a later age. Before the advent of imaging studies, tumors of the cerebral hemispheres commonly grew to enormous sizes before diagnoses were made, and, not surprisingly, surgical therapy was often unsuccessful.

Pathology

Histologically, the most common types of tumors, accounting for 30% of neoplasms in the series of Gjerris (492), are the astrocytomas, in pure form or in conjunction with other cell types, such as oligodendrogliomas, and the malignant glioblastomas. The microscopic classification of childhood astrocytomas, used at University of California, Los Angeles, takes into account the cellularity of the neoplasm, its vascularity, nuclear detail, and the presence and amount of necrosis.

Four grades of *astrocytomas* are distinguished: Grade I, the most benign, has hypercellularity as its major feature. Grade I astrocytomas must be differentiated from astrocytosis. Grade II is marked by the presence of vascular proliferation and pleomorphism. Grade III demonstrates hyperchromatic nuclei and malignant cytologic features such as mitosis. As in adults, the histologically malignant astrocytomas (anaplastic astrocytoma and glioblastoma multiforme, grade IV gliomas) of childhood are infiltrative, biologically aggressive neoplasms characterized by a marked variation in cell size and areas of necrosis. Cytogenetic characteristics of pediatric malignant astrocytomas differ from those most commonly encountered in adults. Structural abnormalities in chromosomes 9, 13, 17, and double minutes were observed in malignant astrocytomas (anaplastic astrocytoma and glioblastoma) of childhood, whereas the most common chromosomal abnormalities in adult glioblastomas are losses of chromosomes 10 and 19q or gains in chromosome 7 (219). Furthermore, to date, the chromosomal abnormalities found in malignant astrocytomas of childhood are similar to those reported in a genetically distinct subset of glioblastomas that was found to arise in young adults (225).

Oligodendrogliomas are infiltrative glial neoplasms composed primarily of oligodendrocytes. They account for only approximately 2% of pediatric intracranial tumors (85). They arise most commonly in the frontal lobe but may occur anywhere in the neuroaxis (493). These frequently calcified tumors are composed of a uniform population of round cells with clear perinuclear cytoplasm (494,495).

Tumors are usually permeated by a delicate meshwork of angulated capillaries. Allelic deletions of chromosomes 1p and 19q appear to occur preferentially in oligodendrogliomas (496,497), and they are statistically significant predictors of both chemosensitivity and longer overall survival (498).

Less commonly encountered tumors of the cerebral hemispheres include epidermoid cysts, sarcomas, and ganglion cell tumors. The ganglion cell tumors include a spectrum of brain tumors that have in common a population of neoplastic or hamartomatous mature neurons, termed *ganglion cells*.

The *ganglioglioma* is the prototype of this group (499). Approximately 75% of gangliogliomas are in the temporal lobe. Less common locations include the brainstem, spinal cord, optic nerve and chiasm, pineal gland, and cerebellum. These slowly growing neoplasms are usually well circumscribed, often cystic, and may be associated with adjacent areas of cortical dysplasia (500,501). Gangliogliomas are composed of two histologic components: a neoplastic astroglial element that tends to be well differentiated (low grade) and a population of ganglion cells. The latter have features of mature neurons including large vesicular nuclei, prominent nucleoli, cytoplasmic Nissl substance, immunoreactivity for neuronal antigens such as neurofilament protein and synaptophysin, and little proliferative activity (500). Abnormal ganglion cells of a ganglioglioma tend to occur in clusters, have abnormally oriented cell processes, and may occasionally be binucleated (Fig. 11.23A) (502). Varying degrees of calcification, desmoplasia, lymphocytic infiltration, and pilocytic differentiation also may be observed. Although rare malignant degeneration has been described, surgical resection is the treatment of choice and is curative in many cases (502). No consistent genetic abnormalities have been reported, but the reelin and tuberin/insulin growth receptor

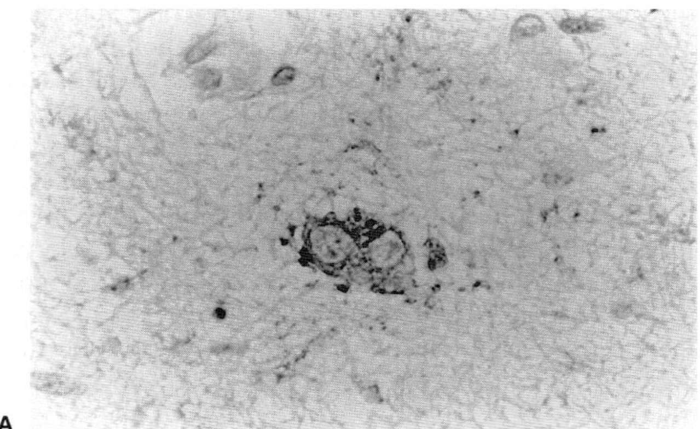

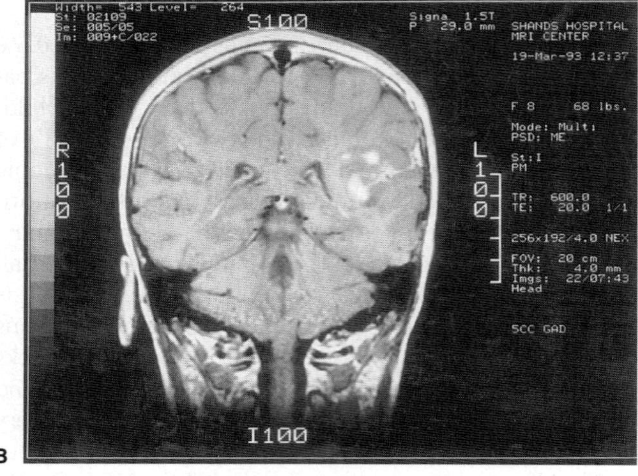

FIGURE 11.23. **A:** Histology shows ganglioglioma with binucleate ganglion cells immunostained for synaptophysin. Unstained cells at upper right-hand corner are of astrocytic lineage (original magnification ×1,200). **B:** Coronal magnetic resonance imaging with contrast shows ganglioglioma surrounding the left sylvian fissure.

pathways have been implicated in ganglioglioma development (503).

In the temporal lobe, these tumors can be missed with CT scanning because they are often isodense with brain. MRI clearly shows gangliogliomas (Fig. 11.23B). In the brainstem, these tumors can be focal. In the area of the medulla, they can be found in the area postrema. Rarely, posterior fossa ganglioglioma can seed into the CSF and spread through the neuroaxis. Radiotherapy is often recommended postoperatively in posterior fossa gangliogliomas, although no clinical trials have been conducted.

Meningiomas are rare during childhood, and meningeal tumors are often highly malignant meningeal sarcomas (504,505). A number of children with a meningioma have clinical or pathologic evidence of neurofibromatosis or tuberous sclerosis. Metastatic tumors are rare in childhood. The only form that seeds into the CNS with any frequency is the neuroblastoma.

Clinical Manifestations

The clinical picture depends on the location of the tumor rather than on its histologic characteristics (81). Signs of increased intracranial pressure, headaches, and vomiting occur in approximately 50% of patients and are the initial complaints in approximately 25% of affected children. Seizures occur in approximately 50% of patients, most commonly in children with temporal lobe tumors. Many patients exhibit a combination of different seizure patterns; nearly 50% of seizure patients experience complex partial seizures, either alone or in combination with generalized seizures or have generalized seizures with a focal component. Absence attacks are rarely seen (Table 11.20).

Patients experiencing uncinate seizures (i.e., complex partial seizures with olfactory or gustatory hallucinations) are no more likely to harbor a temporal lobe glioma than those with other forms of complex partial epilepsy (506). A prolonged history of often intractable seizures can precede demonstration of a tumor (see Chapter 14) (507,508). Children who experience seizures owing to an underlying tumor tend to be normal on neurologic examination and are of normal intelligence. Additionally, neurologic evaluation uncovers no other plausible cause for their seizures; however, the EEG demonstrates persistent focal slowing (508).

Other symptoms are related to the presence of hemiparesis. Hemisensory signs and aphasia are rare. Approximately 15% of patients show ataxia, usually as the outcome of involvement of the frontopontocerebellar pathways but often clinically misinterpreted as being caused by a posterior fossa mass.

Supratentorial malignant tumors are relatively rare in early childhood; they occur predominantly in older children and adolescents. Most commonly, they represent a malignant degeneration of previously diagnosed low-grade astrocytomas appearing at the irradiated site, or occurring in patients who received prophylactic whole-brain radiation for acute lymphoblastic leukemia (162,167). Malignant gliomas are also more likely to develop in children with neurofibromatosis. Leptomeningeal spread is seen in approximately 30% of these tumors, usually in conjunction with tumor recurrence. An intratumoral hemorrhage occurred in 18% of children followed by Dropcho and coworkers at the Sloan-Kettering Cancer Center (509).

TABLE 11.20 Characteristics of Seizures in 49 Patients with Tumors of the Cerebral Hemispheres

	Percent
Seizure type	
Generalized	49
Generalized with focal components	25
Psychomotor	39
Focal	39
Petit mal	0
Other seizure forms	6
Duration of seizures before diagnosis of tumor	
<6 mo	39
6–12 mo	6
1–3 yr	18
3–5 yr	12
5–10 yr	20
>10 yr	2
Location of tumor producing seizures	
Temporal lobe	36
Frontal lobe	7
Parietal lobe	29
Other sites or diffuse	29

Adapted from Low NL, Correll JW, Hammill JF. Tumors of the cerebral hemispheres in children. *Arch Neurol* 1965;13:547.

Diagnosis

Imaging studies, in particular MRI, confirm the clinical diagnosis of a cerebral hemisphere tumor. Calcifications within the tumor, which were found in 23% of children reported by Low and associates (81), are best demonstrated by CT scan. When CT scanning is performed with contrast material, it usually is definitive, although, on occasion, it fails to disclose a tumor that is subsequently discovered with MRI or on surgical resection of an epileptic focus. For this reason, MRI with gadolinium enhancement is the preferred study for youngsters with seizure disorders who are suspected as harboring a neoplasm.

For the initial diagnostic evaluation, EEG can help localize a structural lesion to some extent, particularly with tumors of the temporal lobe. The CSF can be under increased pressure with increased protein content.

Treatment and Prognosis

Low-grade gliomas have a relatively good prognosis, with 5-year survival ranging from 75% to 85% (510–512). Patients typically present with hemiparesis and seizures that can be managed with anticonvulsants after gross total resection. If seizures are a major component of the clinical course, then intraoperative corticography helps reduce the incidence of postoperative seizures (513). Image-guided surgery and intraoperative monitoring of evoked potentials is useful in reducing morbidity in these cortical and white matter resections (514). After a partial resection, limited-field radiotherapy is currently the standard of care. It is important that every effort be made to distinguish pilocytic astrocytoma from low-grade fibrillary astrocytoma because pilocytic tumors are often curable by surgery alone.

Diffuse astrocytomas of the cerebral hemispheres, even when localized to the periphery of the cerebrum and appearing well circumscribed, infiltrate adjacent tissues so readily that complete surgical removal is often impossible. In the large series by Gjerris, collected in 1978 before MRI, 45% of tumors were believed to have been totally removed, yet less than one-half of these children were alive 15 years later (492). Frontal lobe tumors can be treated by lobectomy and, therefore, have a better prognosis. Intermediate- or high-grade astrocytic tumors are best treated with radical resection followed by limited-field radiotherapy and chemotherapy. In all series, the most important prognostic factor for a given patient was the extent of tumor resection (515). In a large multi-institutional study by Weisfeld-Adams and colleagues, the extent of surgical resection and tumor location significantly and independently influenced long-term outcome in children with consensus panel diagnoses of high-grade glioma (516); the effect of resection was greatest in children with glioblastoma multiforme (overall survival: $29 \pm 4\%$ vs. $3 \pm 1.5\%$, $p = 0.0091$).

Chemotherapy should be used first in children younger than 3 years of age so as to minimize the late effects of radiotherapy. Clinical trials show that radiotherapy can be averted altogether in some cases, although the event-free survival and overall survival rates in children under 3 years of age and from 3 to 6 years of age are well below 50% (517–518).

On the whole, chemotherapy has produced but modest improvement in survival of patients with anaplastic astrocytoma and has failed to make a significant difference in the outcome of children with glioblastoma multiforme. The best results are obtained when children are treated with a combination of radiotherapy followed by chemotherapy (519–520). The nitrosoureas and temozolamide are among the most commonly used agents for patients with high-grade gliomas (521). The best overall survival at 1-year is 60% to 65%; over one-third of patients develop metastatic disease and two-thirds develop progressive thalamic disease.

MRIs and neurologic examinations are required every 2 to 4 months in the first 2 years from diagnosis. More studies are needed before specific agents and doses can be routinely recommended for treatment of diffuse astrocytomas in children.

Low-grade oligodendrogliomas that have been totally resected may be followed conservatively without further therapy. If the resection is partial, then limited-field radiotherapy should be given. For anaplastic oligodendrogliomas, surgery should be followed by limited-field radiotherapy and chemotherapy. Because oligodendrogliomas are relatively rare in children, most of the information available on chemotherapy safety and efficacy comes from adult clinical trials. These have shown malignant oligodendrogliomas to be chemosensitive and responsive to nitrosourea-based therapy (522). MRIs and neurologic examinations are required every 2 to 4 months in the first 2 years from diagnosis. For patients who relapse, melphalan may be tried with strong consideration of consolidating responders with high-dose chemotherapy and stem cell rescue (523,524).

Brachytherapy is one of the newer therapeutic approaches designed to improve the poor prognosis of the more malignant hemisphere tumors. It involves the stereotactic implantation into the tumor of a source of high radioactivity, such as ^{125}I or yttrium 90 (371,408,524). This therapeutic regimen can offer significantly prolonged survival times for children with highly anaplastic lesions, in particular those that have a significant cystic component. Stereotactic radiosurgery (gamma knife) is the precise delivery of a single fraction of radiation to an imaging-defined target. The technique has found little application for nonmetastatic malignant tumors, and lesions greater than 35 mm are poor candidates because with larger lesions there is an increase in radiation-related complications (525,526). Clinical trials with cytokines and other angiogenesis inhibitors are in their preliminary stages (527). Most other new agents are disappointing, as is neutron therapy, and the disruption of the blood–tumor barrier by the administration of hyperosmolar mannitol. Locally directed immunotherapy, in the form of lymphokine-activated killer cells and interleukin-2 instilled into the glioma, results in cerebral edema and neurologic side effects (527).

BRAIN TUMORS IN CHILDREN YOUNGER THAN 3 YEARS OF AGE

The most common histologic types of tumors occurring in children younger than 3 years of age are ependymomas, PNET/MBs, choroid plexus papillocarcinomas, astrocytomas, and teratomas (134,143,528). Thus, most tumors are malignant and require multimodal therapy. The 5-year survival rate for young children with brain tumors is poor, ranging from 20% to 40% (529,530). Late effects are common, with endocrinopathies in 70%, neurologic sequelae in 65%, and cognitive decline in 85% of infants (144). Radiotherapy has been implicated as a primary factor in the high incidence of mental retardation because of its effects on axonal growth, dendritic arborization, and synaptogenesis. Studies, therefore, have been initiated to determine the efficacy of postoperative chemotherapy in halting tumor progression in children younger than 3 years of age (531).

Clinical trials of postoperative chemotherapy in children younger than 3 years of age with malignant brain tumors at the MD Anderson Cancer Center, St. Jude Children's Hospital, and the Children's Hospital of Philadelphia provided preliminary data suggesting that chemotherapy could effectively defer radiotherapy (311,532,533). Subsequent studies have confirmed that chemotherapy can be an effective substitute to radiotherapy in preventing progression of malignant brain tumors in a minority of children under age 3 years with malignant brain tumors. In the Children's Cancer Group "eight-drugs-in-1-day" treatment series, the 3-year progression-free survival was 22% for PNET/MBs, 0% for pineal PNETs, 55% for supratentorial nonpineal PNETs, and 26% for ependymomas (534). In the French Society of Pediatric Oncology (BBSFOP) study (535), half of the children with completely resected PNET/MB were cured with conventional chemotherapy; radiotherapy was not administered. For children with metastatic disease or partial resection, chemotherapy alone was not sufficient. However, in the Head Start study (187), overall survival was 55% at 3 years in patients with disseminated PNET/MB receiving an intensified chemotherapy regimen. Approximately one-third of children with relapses of localized or disseminated PNET/MB can be salvaged by high-dose chemotherapy and/or focal or craniospinal radiotherapy; regrettably, the prognosis in recurrent ependymoma is worse than in PNET/MB (200,536,536). New therapeutic strategies that are being planned incorporate intrathecal therapy plus the early introduction of limited-field radiation therapy in an attempt to control leptomeningeal disease without the toxicities associated with neuraxis radiation. Whereas young children with standard-risk PNET/MB who receive chemotherapy alone have a good cognitive outcome (median IQ $\approx$ 90), there is significantly more dysfunction in those having received cranial radiotherapy (median IQ $\approx$ 60–70).

These studies show that chemotherapy can be an effective substitute to radiotherapy in preventing progression of malignant brain tumors in the minority of children younger than 3 years of age with malignant brain tumors and that omission of radiotherapy clearly contributes to a better quality of life in young children cured from the disease (537). More time, however, is needed to assess the late effects of such therapy in long-term survivors and to see whether radiotherapy is ultimately required to maintain tumor control. Because radiotherapy has such detrimental effects on cognition in young children, more effective treatment strategies are required that limit the use of radiotherapy.

High-Dose Chemotherapy

High-dose chemotherapy followed by reinfusion of autologous stem cells (harvested from the bone marrow or the peripheral blood) holds promise to further improve survival in children with malignant brain tumors and may produce sustained remissions in patients with selected tumor types who are at high risk for tumor progression (538,539). Effective use of autologous peripheral blood stem cells rather than bone marrow has enhanced hematologic recovery from high-dose therapy and has decreased the risk of life-threatening complications (540). Several high-dose chemotherapy protocols have shown efficacy in treating poor-prognosis malignant pediatric brain tumors (189,191–193,195,541). A discussion of chemotherapy agents and specific protocol design is far beyond the scope of this text. However, much more information about safety and efficacy is required before high-dose chemotherapy can be routinely recommended in the treatment of malignant pediatric brain tumors.

SPINAL CORD TUMORS

In childhood, spinal cord neoplasms are less common than brain tumors. Although the exact prevalence of spinal tumors is uncertain owing to varying criteria used in published accounts, they represent approximately 10% to 20% of CNS tumors. An estimated 1 in 400 new patients referred to a child neurology center has a spinal cord tumor (542). Most series report an equal distribution across sexes (543,544), and in the series of Pascual-Castroviejo, most patients were younger than 7 years old (542–546). A comprehensive review of spinal cord tumors has been edited by Pascual-Castroviejo (547) and Jallo (548).

Pathology

Spinal cord tumors can arise anywhere along the neuraxis. They have been categorized as extradural extramedullary, intradural extramedullary, or intramedullary (Table 11.21). Extradural tumors were the most common (43%) among the 1,234 spinal tumors in a series reported by DiLorenzo and colleagues (543). In the extradural space, the most common tumors are neuroblastomas,

TABLE 11.21 Tumors of the Spinal Cord

Intramedullary Tumors	*Intradural Extramedullary Tumors*	*Extradural Tumors*
Astrocytoma	Spinal teratoma	Peripheral nerve tumors
Ependymoma	Dermoid and epidermoid cyst	Neurofibroma
Medulloblastoma	Spinal neurenteric cyst	Lymphoma
Others	Intraspinal cyst	Osseous tumors
	Meningioma	
	Schwannoma (neurinoma)	
	Neurofibroma	
	Spinal hemangioma	
	Extraneural (lymphoma)	

Adapted from Escalona-Zapata J. Epidemiology of spinal cord tumors in children. In: Pascual-Castroviejo I, ed. *International review of child neurology series: spinal tumors in children and adolescents.* New York; Raven, 1990:11.

sarcomas, and other primary tumors of bone (546). Benign tumors, such as neurofibromas, dermoid cysts, and teratomas, are usually extradural or intradural extramedullary (549,550). The two most common intramedullary tumors are low-grade astrocytomas followed by ependymomas and other gliomas (Fig. 11.24) (551,552). Rarely, primitive neuroectodermal tumors or malignant gliomas can arise from a child's spinal cord and seed the neuroaxis (553–555). Intramedullary tumors occasionally are associated with a cystic cavity that does not communicate with the spinal subarachnoid space.

During the first 3 years of life, a variety of tumors are encountered. These include teratomas, lipomas, neuroblastomas, dermoids, and epidermoids (552). The most frequent benign histologic types, in decreasing order, are histiocytosis X, osteoid osteoma, and aneurysmal cyst (514).

Pathologic features have been reviewed by Escalona-Zapata (553) and cytogenetic studies reported by Chadduck and colleagues (556).

Clinical Manifestations

Clinical presentation of spinal cord tumors depends on the location of the lesion. Most tumors are slow growing, and it is not unusual for symptoms to exist for several months before diagnosis. Whereas intramedullary lesions usually produce symmetric weakness and atrophy of the affected segments, extramedullary tumors tend to affect nerve roots before the spinal cord and, therefore, begin with unilateral pain in a segmental distribution. This pain is often described as sharp "electric-like," radiating down

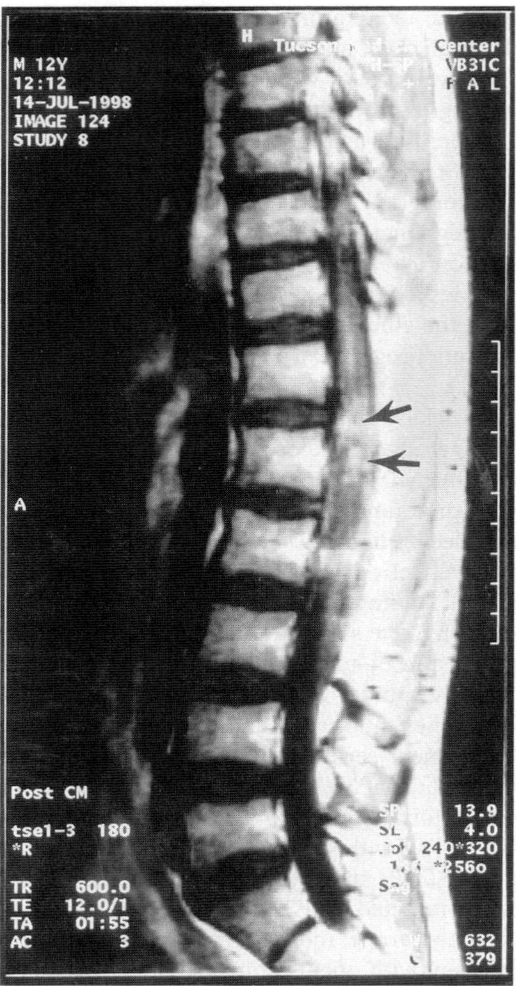

FIGURE 11.24. Sagittal magnetic resonance imaging of spinal cord shows intramedullary ependymoma (*arrows*).

a limb. It is accompanied by paresthesias and numbness (557). Valsalva maneuvers (coughing, sneezing, straining) frequently cause or exacerbate back pain in patients with extramedullary lesions. Extramedullary lesions must be large before they produce upper motor neuron weakness or a sensory level. When weakness does occur, it is typically unilateral. In both extramedullary and intramedullary tumors, impaired gait and stiffness as well as pain in the back or the legs is a common early complaint and can precede the onset of neurologic signs by a long time (558).

Intramedullary lesions produce bilateral weakness, spasticity, atrophy, a sensory level, sphincter disturbance, and hyper-reflexia. In a study by Constantini and colleagues, the most common reasons for radiologic investigation in infants with intramedullary lesions were pain (42%), motor regression (36%), gait abnormalities (27%), torticollis (27%), and progressive kyphoscoliosis (24%) (559).

On examination, two types of neurologic findings can be elicited: those that result from segmental spinal cord involvement, and those that result from interruption of ascending and descending tracts within the cord. Segmental weakness, atrophy, hyporeflexia, and sensory changes are caused by involvement of central gray matter or nerve roots. Spasticity, sensory deficits to a definable spinal cord level, and sphincteric involvement are caused by interruption of long tracts. Extramedullary tumors can cause Brown-Séquard syndrome [6% of patients in the series of Levy and coworkers (557)]. Classically, this syndrome follows hemisection of the spinal cord after trauma and includes homolateral weakness, spasticity, ataxia, and contralateral loss of pain and temperature sensation. Incomplete forms of this syndrome, however, are more common in patients with spinal cord tumors.

In infants and small children, an absolute loss of response to pinprick below a specific spinal level usually cannot be established. Diminished or absent sweating below the appropriate level, however, is frequently demonstrable on examination or by the iodine starch sweat test, particularly with intramedullary lesions (560). Somatosensory-evoked potentials can further delineate the sensory level of spinal cord tumors. Deep tendon reflexes below the level of the lesion are exceptionally brisk in tumors compressing the spinal cord, and an extensor plantar response occurs. Impaired bladder function is a late finding that dictates emergency surgery. Initial bladder symptoms are increased urgency followed by incontinence or retention of urine (561,562).

Nystagmus or papilledema can accompany spinal cord tumors. In some instances, the papilledema is caused by impaired CSF absorption, a consequence of the mucinous protein material that is formed by the degenerative changes within the tumor. Other factors also can operate in the production of papilledema; these include infiltration of the meninges by tumor, subarachnoid hemorrhage, and hydrocephalus, the last caused by Arnold-Chiari malformations (563,564). The unusual combination of papilledema and hydrocephalus should alert the clinician to an associated spinal cord tumor, particularly a teratoma.

Diagnosis

Spinal cord tumors are rare in childhood, so early recognition hinges on careful neurologic examination and localization of the offending lesion. Neurologic condition on admission, regardless of specific tumor type, is an important prognostic factor for functional recovery after therapy (565,566). Local spinal pain is a rare complaint in childhood; if present, a neurologic examination must be performed to evaluate neural function in tissue underlying the painful bony segment (567). The sudden onset of back pain is more likely caused by trauma or infection (e.g., empyema). The spine should be examined for point tenderness by gently percussing vertebral tips with a large soft rubber reflex hammer. Any scoliosis or limitation in flexion and extension of the pediatric spine is suspect for the presence of a spinal mass. Eeg-Olofsson and coworkers have noted that recurrent abdominal pain can be the first symptom of a thoracic intramedullary spinal cord tumor (568). Another finding that points to a spinal cord neoplasm is the presence of a painful scoliosis, with pain elicited or aggravated by physical effort, coughing, sneezing, or flexion of neck or back (569). The neurologic examination of motor and sensory function is intended to identify the likely diseased segment so that spinal imaging is directed to the epicenter of the neoplasm. Examination of the anus for gaping is important in evaluating medullary function.

MRI has replaced plain films, myelography, and CT as the preferred imaging study when spinal tumor is suspected (570). Faster imaging technologies have made motion artifacts uncommon, especially when a particular spinal segment is suspect. MRI is useful in separating neoplasms from edema or syrinx. Once the site and extent of the lesion are localized and defined by MRI with gadolinium enhancement, it is important to also image the cranium. Malignant pediatric brain tumors (e.g., PNET/MB, ependymoma) can present with gross spinal subarachnoid metastasis before the appearance of symptoms pointing to a lesion above the foramen magnum. In addition, intramedullary spinal tumors may be associated with rostral extension of hydromyelia into the brainstem that can produce lower cranial nerve dysfunction. Rarely, as occurs in neurofibromatosis, a patient has spinal and intracranial tumors (e.g., schwannomas, meningiomas). Detailed aspects of imaging parameters (plane, slice thickness, weighting) best suited to viewing CNS tumors are reviewed by Quisling (571). As a rule, sagittal images are the most important plane for screening the spine.

Treatment and Prognosis

The treatment of spinal neoplasms depends on the involved segment (cervical, thoracic, lumbar, sacral), the location of the tumor (intradural vs. extradural), tumor type (benign vs. malignant), and tumor extent (localized vs. infiltrative). Extramedullary tumors that can be totally removed surgically have an excellent prognosis. Even partial removal of a tumor is compatible with long periods of partial or complete symptomatic relief, particularly when surgery is followed by radiotherapy. Intramedullary tumors can sometimes be removed by microsurgical techniques (572). Because there is a higher incidence of incomplete excision of benign intramedullary tumors, treatment for this type of tumor is more controversial. The goal of therapy is to remove as much of the tumor as possible to improve neurologic function, and to reduce the

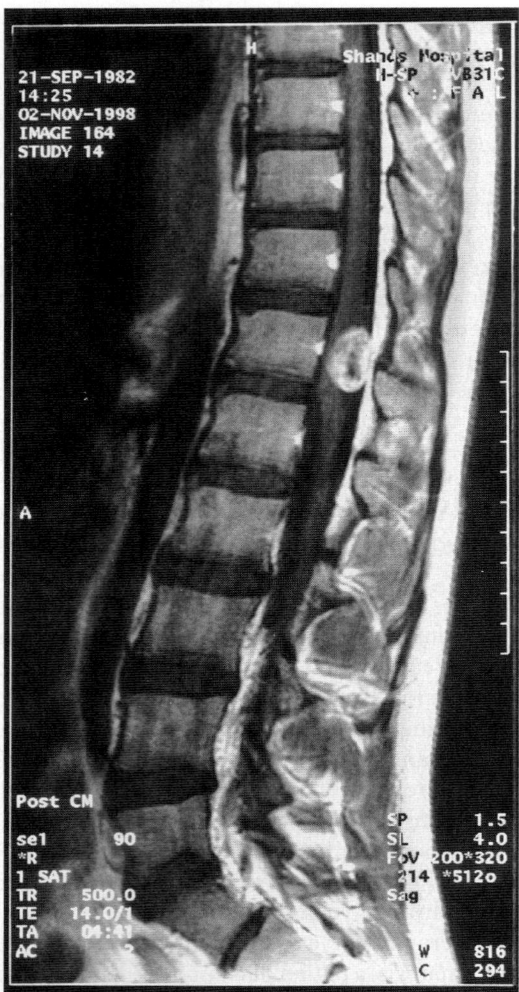

FIGURE 11.25. Sagittal magnetic resonance imaging shows well-circumscribed spinal cord schwannoma.

risk of local recurrence and metastasis. For histologically benign extradural tumors (osteoid osteoma, aneurysmal bone cyst), intradural extramedullary tumors (dermoids, epidermoids, meningiomas, schwannomas), or intramedullary tumors (low-grade astrocytomas, lipomas), the prognosis is excellent after tumor removal by microsurgical techniques (Fig. 11.25). For intramedullary surgery, intraoperative spinal cord monitoring has a favorable effect on neurologic outcome (573). Surgical technique is reviewed in detail by Epstein (574) and Mottl and Koutecky (575).

Spinal column deformity after laminectomy can be a serious long-term problem for children in whom a curative tumor operation has been performed. Radiotherapy has been associated with an excellent outcome in patients with intramedullary tumors (astrocytomas, ependymomas), but there have been no controlled studies testing the safety and efficacy of radiotherapy in children with intramedullary spinal cord tumors. Thus, most neuro-oncology centers favor surgery alone (574–576). In addition, radiotherapy increases the risk of spinal column deformity in the growing child (559). Other complications of irradiation of the spinal cord include an acute reaction, a transient postirradiation myelopathy, or an irreversible myelomalacia (577).

Postirradiation myelopathy appears several months after irradiation and is characterized by transient paresthesias and by sensations similar to electric shock in the extremities, precipitated by flexion of the cervical spine (Lhermitte's sign). Symptoms tend to resolve in the course of several months. Myelomalacia can result in a rapidly evolving paraplegia, the consequence of pathology in capillaries and small arteries (578). The time-dose relationship producing these complications has not been fully established, but, as in postirradiation encephalopathy, the complications have been encountered even after conservative doses, notably in infants and small children (579). Unusual complications of cord irradiation include amyotrophy, acute transverse myelitis, and slowly progressive myelopathy that advances to complete or incomplete transverse myelitis (577).

Radiotherapy and chemotherapy are targeted at malignant spinal tumors after surgery, but the prognosis is poor for malignant gliomas, neuroblastomas, and sarcomas (566). There is no evidence that the extent of surgical resection affects outcome in children with histologically malignant lesions. Even low-grade spinal neoplasms can be associated with extensive subarachnoid dissemination (580). Every effort must be made to preserve neurologic function and to tailor radiotherapy and chemotherapy to the patient's age, pathology, tumor extent, and functional status.

PSEUDOTUMOR CEREBRI (IDIOPATHIC INTRACRANIAL HYPERTENSION, BENIGN INTRACRANIAL HYPERTENSION)

Pseudotumor cerebri (idiopathic intracranial hypertension, benign intracranial hypertension), in which increased intracranial pressure occurs in the absence of a space-occupying lesion, was first recognized by Quincke in 1893 (581).

Pathology and Pathophysiology

Pseudotumor cerebri is a result of various causes. Johnston and Paterson, who in 1974 compiled one of the largest reported series, found middle ear infection to be responsible for 24.3% of cases, nonspecific infections responsible for 13.9%, minor head injuries responsible for 4.4%, and withdrawal from corticosteroid therapy responsible for 1.2% (582). Pseudotumor cerebri also has been seen secondary to hypo- and hypervitaminosis A, and after the administration of isoretinoin for acne, nitrofurantoin for urinary tract infection, chlortetracycline, minocycline, and tetracycline (584,585). It may follow varicella as a consequence of transient protein S deficiency caused by the presence of an anti–protein S antibody (586). Other, more unusual causes include profound iron deficiency anemia, hypoparathyroidism, Addison disease, disseminated lupus erythematosus, and carbon dioxide retention secondary to chronic lung disease (587). Some of these associations, however, may exist coincidentally. In children younger than 10 years of age, thrombosis of one or more of the dural sinuses, particularly the lateral sinus, as a sequel to otitis or mastoiditis, is probably still one of the most common abnormalities (588,589). The term *otitic hydrocephalus*, which has been used to designate this condition, is inappropriate because the ventricular system is always normal or even small. In older subjects, the cause of increased intracranial pressure is usually obscure. Endocrine disturbances also have been implicated in view of the relationship of pseudotumor cerebri to menarche, disorders of the menstrual cycle, obesity, and rapid discontinuation of prolonged corticosteroid therapy (590).

The pathophysiology for increased intracranial pressure is still unclear, and it is likely that more than one mechanism is at fault. Three major factors are an increased resistance to CSF absorption, increased CSF production, and increased venous sinus pressure (583,583a). Johnston and Paterson postulated that an increase in the volume of CSF is responsible (582). Because CSF formation in pseudotumor cerebri is diminished, there probably is increased resistance to its absorption, possibly at the level of the arachnoid villi. McComb points out that if this were indeed the case, there should be a progressive accumulation of CSF, with a new equilibrium established at a larger volume and at a higher pressure of CSF, which is not the case in pseudotumor cerebri (591). Anatomic examinations have revealed increased brain water content in some instances. MRI studies performed on obese young women with pseudotumor cerebri have confirmed the presence of increased white matter water. Additionally, the most severely affected patients show areas of increased signal intensity on T2-weighted images, an indication of focal areas of edema (592). Increased brain water content may decrease brain compliance, resulting in normal-size ventricles, despite elevated CSF pressure.

Corbett and Digre have stressed the importance of elevated venous sinus pressure and suggest that there is evidence that all cases of pseudotumor cerebri have increased venous sinus pressure (583). Using gadolinium-enhanced MR venography, Farb and coworkers have found transverse dural sinus stenosis in over 90% of patients with pseudotumor cerebri (592a). This phenomenon however is probably not a primary event but most likely is secondary to the elevated intracranial pressure (592b).

Clinical Manifestations

Patients develop nonspecific signs of increased intracranial pressure, such as intermittent headaches, vomiting, blurred vision, and diplopia. In otitic hydrocephalus, these symptoms are often preceded by a partially treated otitis (593–594). Headaches tend to worsen at night, and in the child with migraine pseudotumor cerebri aggravates a typical migrainous attack.

Papilledema is evident in the majority of cases; it was present in 82% in the series of Soler and colleagues (585). Visual impairment is usually slight, particularly in patients whose intracranial pressure has been elevated for only a short time. In contrast to patients with increased intracranial pressure secondary to mass lesions, the level of consciousness and intellectual functioning remains normal (594). A variety of cranial nerve palsies have been encountered (595). Most common is sixth nerve palsy, which is seen in up to one-half of children (596). An occasional patient has third, fourth, or hypoglossal nerve palsy (597).

Diagnosis

The diagnosis of pseudotumor cerebri is made after exclusion of other causes for increased intracranial pressure, particularly mass lesions localized to the midline or to the silent areas of the brain such as the frontal lobes. Friedman and Jacobson stress that the diagnosis should not be made in the absence of papilledema, unless there is an associated condition such as optic atrophy that precludes the formation of papilledema (597a). Generally, imaging studies reveal a ventricular system that is midline and normal or somewhat reduced in size (592,598).

The CSF is generally normal, although mild pleocytosis is not unusual. In a few instances, obstruction of the lateral sinus has been documented by carotid angiography or retrograde jugular venography.

Treatment and Prognosis

Although there are no randomized controlled studies and the natural course of the condition is unknown, treatment is directed toward maintaining the intracranial pressure within near normal limits to reduce the danger of permanent visual damage (599).

Twice daily serial lumbar punctures have been used; in the experience of Soler and colleagues, the increased CSF pressure resolved in 18% of children after one lumbar puncture. Acetazolamide was effective in 55% of the children who did not respond to the lumbar puncture (585). Some of the unresponsive children obtained symptomatic relief with 1 to 2 weeks of corticosteroid therapy. The remainder, some 23% in the series of Soler and colleagues, required surgery. Optic nerve sheath fenestration or lumboperitoneal shunts are the most commonly used procedures. Because of the significant incidence of shunt failures and other complications, optic nerve sheath fenestration is probably the procedure of choice (600). Corbett and Thompson believe that an asymptomatic patient with no visual field loss and normal visual acuity should not be treated, rather the patient should be followed by a neurologist and an ophthalmologist (601). We personally would prefer more frequent follow-up examinations than at intervals of 6 to 12 months as suggested by Corbett and Thompson. Indications for surgery are a loss of visual field or visual acuity or a severe headache that does not respond to medication or lumbar puncture. The various treatment methods have been reviewed by Baker and coworkers (602). Recurrences are rare: They were recorded in some 10% of subjects in Johnston and Paterson's series (582) and in only one patient in Grant's series of 79 patients (603). Some 10% of patients are left with visual defects that are permanent or require more than a year to resolve (583,604). These appear to be most common in women with systemic hypertension (605). Surgery is indicated for patients at risk for severe visual loss. Thus, indications for surgery include:

- Progressive visual loss despite maximal tolerated medical treatment
- Severe visual loss at presentation
- Severe papilledema or chronic atrophic papilledema, especially in children who are too young to perform reliable visual field testing

Surgical options include optic nerve sheath fenestration (ONSF) and lumbar peritoneal (LP) shunt (606,607). These procedures rapidly reduce papilledema, although complete resolution may take several weeks. ONSF involves making multiple slits in the perioptic meninges behind the globe. This allows the egress of CSF through the perioptic nerve sheath and reduces pressure at the optic nerve head. ONSF effectively treats papilledema, stabilizing or improving visual function in children with visual loss from pseudotumor cerebri. Unilateral ONSF will eliminate papilledema of both discs in approximately 50% of cases and reduce headache symptoms in some patients. Complications, including ischemic optic neuropathy, transient blindness, pupillary dilation, and retrobulbar hemorrhage, are infrequent. However, there is a high rate of failure with long-term follow-up.

LP shunting reduces intracranial pressure (ICP) and therefore treats the headaches and relieves the pressure on both optic nerves (607). This procedure effectively resolves papilledema and stabilizes vision in children with visual loss from pseudotumor cerebri. However, low-pressure headaches associated with an acquired Arnold-Chiari malformation type I tonsillar herniation may occur. Shunt failures are frequent, and the procedure may need to be repeated many times over several years. Other complications include shunt infections, abdominal pain, CSF leak, and migration of the peritoneal catheter.

ONSF should be considered for patients with progressive visual loss after apparently successful LP shunting. Similarly, an LP shunt should be considered for patients with progressive visual loss after an ONSF.

Bariatric surgery effectively reduces ICP in severely obese patients with pseudotumor cerebri and has the added advantage of reducing comorbidity associated with excessive weight (608). Although bariatric surgery is most commonly performed on adults, it has been used to treat severely obese adolescents. The weight loss and reduction of ICP occurs gradually over several months. Therefore, this is not the treatment of choice for patients with acute visual deterioration.

REFERENCES

1. Cohen ME, Duffner PK, eds. *Brain tumors in children. Principles of diagnosis and treatment*. New York: Raven Press, 1994.
2. Maria BL, ed. Teamwork in pediatric neuro-oncology. In: Bodensteiner JB, ed. *Seminars in pediatric neurology*. Philadelphia: WB Saunders Co, 1997:251–253.
3. Miltenburg D, Louw DF, Sutherland GR. Epidemiology of childhood brain tumors. *Can J Neurol Sci* 1996;23:118–122.
4. Pollack IF. Brain tumors in children. *N Engl J Med* 1994;331:1500–1507.
5. Di Rocco C, Massimi L. Caldarelli M, et al. Cerebral tumors in children less than one year old. *Neuro-Oncology* 2004;6:419.
6. Bendel A, Ries L, Beaty O, et al. CNS tumor epidemiology and outcome in adolescents and young adults in the United States, 1975–1998. *Neuro-Oncology* 2004;6:416.
7. Roush SW, Krisher JB, Cox MW, et al. Progress in childhood cancer care in Florida. 1970–1992. *J Fla Med Assoc* 1993;80:747–751.
8. Critchley M. Brain tumours in children: their general symptomatology. *Br J Child Dis* 1925;22:251–264.
9. Bailey P, Buchanan DN, Bucy PC. Intracranial tumors of infancy and childhood. Chicago: University of Chicago Press, 1939.
10. Cuneo HM, Rand CW. *Brain tumors of childhood*. Springfield, IL: Charles C Thomas, 1952.
11. Crouse SK, Berg BO. Intracranial meningiomas in childhood and adolescence. *Neurology* 1972;22:135–141.
12. Dastur HM, Desai AD. Comparative study of brain tuberculomas and gliomas based on 107 case records of each. *Brain* 1965;88:375–396.
13. Roush SW, Krisher JP, Pollock NC, et al. The incidence of pediatric cancer in Florida, 1981 to 1986. *Cancer* 1992;69:2212–2219.
14. Mapstone TB. Neurofibromatosis and central nervous system tumors in childhood. *Neurosurg Clin N Am* 1992;3:771–779.
15. Cooper JR. Brain tumors in hereditary multiple system hamartomatosis (tuberous sclerosis). *J Neurosurg* 1971;34(2 Pt 1):194–202.
16. Hemminki K, Li X. Association of brain tumours with other neoplasms in families. *Eur J Cancer* 2004;40:253–259.
17. Birch JM, Alston RD, McNally RJ, et al. Relative frequency and morphology of cancers in carriers of germline TP53 mutations. *Oncogene* 2001;20:4621–4628.
18. Evans DG, Farndon PA, Burnell LD, et al. The incidence of Gorlin syndrome in 173 consecutive cases of medulloblastoma. *Br J Cancer* 1991;64:959–961.
19. Miyaki M, Nishio J, Konishi M, et. al. Drastic genetic instability of tumors and normal tissues in Turcot syndrome. *Oncogene* 1997;15:2877–2881.
20. Aliani S, Brunner J, Graf N, et al. Medulloblastoma with extensive nodularity in nevoid basal cell carcinoma syndrome. *Med Pediatr Oncol* 2003;40:266–267.
21. Amlashi SF, Riffaud L, Brassier G, et al. Nevoid basal cell carcinoma syndrome: relation with desmoplastic medulloblastoma

in infancy. A population-based study and review of the literature. *Cancer* 2003;98:618–24.
22. Prasad KN, Cole WC, Hasse GM. Health risks of low dose ionizing radiation in humans: a review. *Exp Biol Med* 2004;229:378–382.
23. Snyder AR. Review of radiation-induced bystander effects. *Hum Exp Toxicol* 2004;23:87–89.
24. Little MP. Risks associated with ionizing radiation. *Br Med Bull* 2003;68:259–275.
25. Van Tornout JM, Tu W, Gilinsky S, et al. Genetic polymorphisms in folate metabolizing genes as risk factor for childhood primitive neuroectodermal and astrocytic tumors. *Neuro-Oncology* 2004;6:415.
26. Packer RJ. Brain tumors in children. *Arch Neurol* 1999;56:421–425.
27. Fisher PG, Preston-Martin S, Wrensch MR, et al. Biologic and environmental risk factors for childhood brain tumors: the California Childhood Brain Tumor study. *Neuro-Oncology* 2004;6:426.
27a. Nobel M, Dietrich J. The complex identity of brain tumors: emerging concerns regarding origin, diversity and plasticity. *Trends Neurosci* 2004;27:148–154.
28. Bleyer WA. The U.S. pediatric cancer clinical trials programmes: international implications and the way forward. *Eur J Cancer* 1997;33:1439–1447.
29. Tobias J, Hayward RD. Brain and spinal cord tumours in children. In: Thomas DGT, ed. *Neuro-oncology: primary malignant brain tumours*. Baltimore: The Johns Hopkins University Press, 1990:164–192.
30. Gilbertson R. Paediatric embryonic brain tumours: biological and clinical relevance of molecular genetic abnormalities. *Eur J Cancer* 2002;38:675–685.
31. Gershon TR, Chin SS. Transcription factors expressed by neural crest cells correlate with phenotype in development and in neuroectodermal tumors. *Neuro-Oncology* 2004;6:407.
32. Mineta T, Okamoto H, Ueda S, et al. Detection of JC virus DNA sequences in pediatric brain tumors. *Neuro-Oncology* 2004;6:411.
33. Huang H, Reis R, Yonekawa Y, et al. Identification in human brain tumors of DNA sequences specific for SV40 large T antigen. *Brain Pathol* 1999;9:33–44.
34. Bigner SH, et al. Brain tumors. In: Vogelstein B, Kintzler KW, eds. *The genetic basis of human cancer*. New York: McGraw-Hill, 1998:661–670.
35. Pang JC, Dong Z, Zhang R, et al. Mutation analysis of DMBT1 in glioblastoma, medulloblastoma and oligodendroglial tumors. *Int J Cancer* 2003;105:76–81.
36. Krupp W, Geiger K, Schober R, et al. Cytogenetic and molecular cytogenetic analyses in diffuse astrocytomas. *Cancer Genet Cytogenet* 2004;153:32–38.
37. Collins VP. Cellular mechanisms targeted during astrocytoma progression. *Cancer Letters* 2002;188:1–7.
38. Mukasa A, Ueki K, Ge X, et al. Selective expression of a subset of neuronal genes in oligodendroglioma with chromosome 1p loss. *Brain Pathol* 2004;14:34–42.
39. Sanson M, Leuraud P, Aguirre-Cruz L, et al. Analysis of loss of chromosome 10q, DMBT1 homozygous deletions, and PTEN mutations in oligodendrogliomas. *J Neurosurg* 2002;97:1397–1401.
40. Kraus JA, de Millas W, Sorensen N, et al. Indications for a tumor suppressor gene at 22q11 involved in the pathogenesis of ependymal tumors and distinct from hSNF5/INI1. *Acta Neuropathol* 2001;102:69–74.
41. Yin XL, Pang JC, Ng HK. Identification of a region of homozygous deletion on 8p22–23.1 in medulloblastoma. *Oncogene* 2002;21:1461–1468.
42. Zang KD. Meningioma: a cytogenetic model of a complex benign human tumor, including data on 394 karyotyped cases. *Cytogenet Cell Genet* 2001;93:207–220.
43. Henn W, Neidermayer I, Ketter R, et al. Monosomy 7p in meningiomas: a rare constituent of tumor progression. *Cancer Genet Cytogenet* 2003;144:65–68.
44. Dyer S, Prebble E, Brundler M, et al. Genomic imbalances in high- and low-grade paediatric astrocytomas. *Neuro-Oncology* 2004;6:405.
45. Ellison DW, Lamont JM, McManamy CS, et al. Combined histopathological and molecular cytogenetic stratification defines a high-risk subset of patients with medulloblastoma—a United Kingdom Children's Cancer Group study. *Neuro-Oncology* 2004;6:405.
46. Fangusaro J, Jiang Y, Singh V, et al. Survivin and survivin isoforms in medulloblastoma show unique patterns of expression and prognostic value. *Neuro-Oncology* 2004;6:405.
47. Nakahara Y, Shiraisi T, Mineta T, et al. Analysis of genome-wide copy number profiles of medulloblastomas using array-based comparative genomic hybridization. *Neuro-Oncology* 2004;6:411.
48. Lawman MJ, Braccili SC, Tebbi CK, et al. Post-transcriptional silencing of genes involved in the development of medulloblastoma. *Neuro-Oncology* 2004;6:410.
49. Pietsch T, Raso A, Capra V, et al. Clinical and genetic studies of medulloblastoma with extensive nodularity (NMB) in patients with and without Gorlin's syndrome. *Neuro-Oncology* 2004;6:412.
50. Tamburrini G, Chiaretti A, Piastra M, et al. Neurotrophic factors expression in childhood low-grade astrocytomas and ependymomas. *Neuro-Oncology* 2004;6:415.
51. Calabrese C, Hernan R, Sherr C, et al. Transgenic mouse model of ERBB2 overexpression in cerebellar granule neuron precursor cells. *Neuro-Oncology* 2004;6:403.
52. Clifford SC, Lindsey JC, Lusher ME, et al. Identification of tumour suppressor genes in childhood medulloblastoma by promoter hypermethylation profiling. *Neuro-Oncology* 2004;6:404.
53. Frühwald MC, Muhlisch J, Sorensen N, et al. Gene specific aberrant methylation in medulloblastomas (MB), anaplastic ependymomas (AE), and stPNET of childhood. *Neuro-Oncology* 2004;6:406.
54. Gaspar N, Geoerger B, Grill J, et al. Pathway dysfunction in primary childhood ependymomas and xenografts. *Neuro-Oncology* 2004;6:406.
54a. Pollack IF, Finkelstein SD, Woods J, et al. Expression of *p53* and prognosis in children with malignant glioma. *N Engl J Med* 2002;346:420–427.
55. Santarius T, Kirsch M, Rossi ML, et al. Molecular aspects of neuro-oncology. *Clin Neurol Neurosurg* 1997;99:184–195.
56. Ng HK, Lam PY. The molecular genetics of central nervous system tumors. *Pathology* 1998;30:196–202.
57. Muir DF. Translational research models in neuro-oncology. In: Bodensteiner JB, Maria BL, eds. *Seminars in pediatric neurology*. Philadelphia: WB Saunders, 1997:292–303.
58. Kornblith PL, Walker MD, eds. *Advances in neuro-oncology II*. Armack: Futura Publishing Co Inc, 1997.
59. Farwell J, Flannery JT. Cancer in relatives of children with central-nervous-system neoplasms. *N Engl J Med* 1984;311:749–753.
60. Modan B, Baidatz D, Mart H, et al. Radiation-induced head and neck tumours. *Lancet* 1974;1:277–279.
61. Cushing H. Concerning a definite regulatory mechanism of the vasomotor center which controls blood pressure during cerebral compression. *Bull Johns Hopkins Hosp* 1901;12:290–292.
62. Cushing H. Some experimental and clinical observations concerning states of increased intracranial tension. *Am J Med Sci* 1902;124:375–400.
63. Marmarou A, Tabaddo RK. Intracranial pressure: physiology and pathophysiology. In: Cooper PR, ed. *Head injury*, 3rd ed. Baltimore: Williams & Wilkins, 1993:203–224.
64. Kety SS, Shenkin HA, Schmidt CF. The effects of increased intracranial pressure on cerebral circulatory function in man. *J Clin Invest* 1948;27:493–510.
65. Langfitt TW, Weinstein JD, Kassell NF. Cerebral vasomotor paralysis produced by intracranial hypertension. *Neurology* 1965;15:622–641.
66. Theodore J, Robin ED. Speculations on neurogenic pulmonary edema (NPE). *Annu Rev Resp Dis* 1976;113:405–411.
67. Miller JD. Disorders of cerebral blood flow and intracranial pressure after head injury. *Clin Neurosurg* 1982;29:162–173.
68. Lindenberg R. Compression of brain arteries as pathogenetic factor for tissue necroses and their areas of predilection. *J Neuropathol Exp Neurol* 1955;14:223–243.
69. McNealy DE, Plum F. Brain stem dysfunction with supratentorial mass lesion. *Arch Neurol* 1962;7:10–32.
70. Cushing H. Strangulation of the nervi abducentes by lateral branches of the basilar artery in cases of brain tumour. With an

explanation of some obscure palsies on the basis of arterial constriction. *Brain* 1910;33:204–235.

71. Collier J. The false localizing signs of intracranial tumour. *Brain* 1904;27:490–508.

71a. Hanson RA, Ghosh S, Gonzalez-Gomez I, et al. Abducens length and vulnerability? *Neurology* 2004;62:33–36.

72. Till K. *Paediatric neurosurgery*. Oxford: Blackwell Scientific Publications, 1975.

73. Ferris R, Kennedy C, Nathwani A. Presenting features of brain tumors. *Neuro-Oncology* 2004;6:420.

74. Honig PJ, Charney EB. Children with brain tumor headaches. Distinguishing features. *Am J Dis Child* 1982;136:121–124.

75. The epidemiology of headache among children with brain tumor. Headache in children with brain tumors. The Childhood Brain Tumor Consortium. *J Neurooncol* 1991;10:31–46.

76. Savino PJ, Glaser JS. Pseudopapilledema versus papilledema. *Int Ophthalmol Clin* 1977;17:115–137.

77. Sanders MD. Papilloedema: "the pendulum of progress." *Eye* 1997;11:267–294.

78. Anmarkrud N. The value of fluorescein fundus angiography in evaluating optic disc oedema. *Acta Ophthalmol* 1977;55:605–615.

79. Hayreh SS. Optic disc edema in raised intracranial pressure. V. Pathogenesis. *Arch Ophthalmol* 1977;95:1553–1565.

80. Gordon GS, Wallace SJ, Neal JW. Intracranial tumours during the first two years of life: presenting features. *Arch Dis Child* 1995;73:345–347.

81. Low NL, Correll JW, Hammill JF. Tumors of the cerebral hemispheres in children. *Arch Neurol* 1965;13:547–554.

82. Burton LJ, Quinn B, Pratt-Cheney JL, et al. Headache etiology in a pediatric emergency department. *Pediatr Emerg Care* 1997;13:1–4.

83. Ropper AH. Lateral displacement of the brain and level of consciousness in patients with an acute hemispheral mass. *N Engl J Med* 1986;314:953–958.

84. Kuttesch JF. Advances and controversies in the management of childhood brain tumors. *Curr Opin Oncol* 1997;9:235–240.

85. Rorke LB. Pathology of brain tumors in infants and children. In: Tindall GT, Cooper PR, Barrow DL, eds. *The practice of neurosurgery*. Baltimore: Williams & Wilkins, 1996:733–754.

86. Tovi M, Lilja A, Bergstrom M, et al. Delineation of gliomas with magnetic resonance imaging using Gd-DTPA in comparison with computed tomography and positron emission tomography. *Acta Radiol* 1990;31:417–429.

87. Sartor K, Karnaze MG, Winthrop JD, et al. MR imaging in infra-, para-, and retrosellar mass lesions. *Neuroradiology* 1987;29:19–29.

88. Knopp MV, Essig M, Hawighorst H, et al. Functional neuroimaging in the assessment of CNS neoplasms. *Eur Radiol* 1997;7[Suppl 5]:209–215.

89. Brant-Zawadzki M, Berry I, Osaki L, et al. Gd-DTPA in clinical MR of the brain: 1. Intraaxial lesions. *AJR Am J Roentgenol* 1986;147:1223–1230.

90. Dean BL, Drayer BP, Bird CK, et al. Gliomas: classification with MR imaging. *Radiology* 1990;174:411–415.

91. Laughton SJ, Pereira JK, Bland EA, et al. MRI enhancement patterns in follow up imaging of childhood brain tumours. *Neuro-Oncology* 20046:432.

92. Jurkiewicz E, Pakula-Kosciescza J, Malczyk K, et al. Usefulness of proton magnetic resonance spectroscopy (MRS) in differentiation of pathologic lesions in neurofibromatosis type 1 (NF1) in children. *Neuro-Oncology* 2004;6:432.

93. Krieger MD, Panigrahy A, McComb JG, et al. PNET histology can be non-invasively predicted by elevated taurine levels detected by proton magnetic resonance spectroscopy. *Neuro-Oncology* 2004;6:432.

94. Peet A, Garala P, MacPherson L, et al. Mobile lipids detected by short echo time H magnetic resonance spectrosocopy correlate with malignancy in childhood brain tumors. *Neuro-Oncology* 2004;6:432.

95. Shimoda KC, Wolters P, Warren K. A pilot study of proton magnetic resonance spectroscopic imaging in the evaluation of neurotoxicity in cancer patients: neuropsychological functioning. *Neuro-Oncology* 2004;6:434.

96. Warren K, Hill R, Black J, et al. Evaluating neurotoxicity in cancer patients. *Neuro-Onocology* 2004;6:435.

97. Kramer ED, Vezina LG, Packer RJ, et al. Staging and surveillance of children with central nervous system neoplasms: recommendations of the neurology and tumor imaging committees of the Children's Cancer Group. *Pediatr Neurosurg* 1994;20:254–263.

98. Rydberg JN, Hammond CA, Grimm RC, et al. Initial clinical experience in MR imaging of the brain with a fast fluid-attenuated inversion-recovery pulse sequence. *Radiology* 1994;193:173–180.

99. Pirotte B, Goldman S, Wikler D, et al. Combined stereotactic positron emission tomography and magnetic resonance imaging for image-guided surgical resection of brain tumors in children. *Neuro-Oncology* 2004;6:433.

100. Pirotte B, Lubansu A, Goldman S, et al. Impact on the surgical strategy of integrating positron emission tomography in the diagnostic imaging of pediatric brain lesions. *Neuro-Oncology* 2004;6:433.

101. Pirotte B, Lubansu A, Levivier M, et al. Postoperative positron emission tomography imaging for the evaluation of surgical resection in pediatric brain tumors. *Neuro-Oncology* 2004;6:433.

102. Tsuyuguchi N, Sunada I, Hara M. Methionine positron emission tomography for brain tumor in children. *Neuro-Oncology* 2004;6:434.

103. Young-Poussaint T, Ramamurthy U, Boyett J, et al. Analysis of correlative MRI perfusion and diffusion in a phase I trial of the anti-angiogenesis agent SU5416 in children with refractory or progressive brain tumors: a report from the pediatric brain tumor consortium (PBTC). *Neuro-Oncology* 2004;6:435.

104. Mistretta CA, Crummy AB, Strother CM. Digital angiography: a perspective. *Radiology* 1981;139:273–276.

105. Brody AS. New perspectives in CT and MR imaging. *Neurol Clin* 1991;9:273–286.

106. Merritt HH. The cerebrospinal fluid in cases of tumors of the brain. *Arch Neurol Psychiatry* 1935;34:1175–1187.

107. Berg L. Hypoglycorrhachia of noninfectious origin. Diffuse meningeal neoplasia. *Neurology* 1953;3:811–824.

108. Glass JP, Melamed M, Chernik NL, et al. Malignant cells in cerebrospinal fluid (CSF): the meaning of a positive CSF cytology. *Neurology* 1979;29:1369–1375.

108a. DeAngelis LM, Cairncross JG. A better way to find tumor in CNS. *Neurology* 2002;58:339–340.

109. Taveras JM, Wood EH. *Diagnostic neuroradiology*, 2nd ed. Baltimore: Williams & Wilkins, 1976:131.

110. Weir B, Elvidge AR. Oligodendrogliomas. An analysis of 63 cases. *J Neurosurg* 1968;29:500–505.

111. Babcock DS, Han BK. The accuracy of high resolution, real-time ultrasonography of the head in infancy. *Radiology* 1981;139:665–676.

112. Janus TJ, Kim EE, Tilbury R, et al. Use of [18_F] fluorodeoxyglucose positron emission tomography in patients with primary malignant brain tumors. *Ann Neurol* 1993;33:540–548.

113. Glantz MJ, Hoffman JM, Coleman RE, et al. Identification of early recurrence of primary central nervous system tumors by [18_F] fluorodeoxyglucose positron emission tomography. *Ann Neurol* 1991;29:347–355.

114. Kemp SS, Zimmerman RA, Bilaniuk LT, et al. Magnetic resonance imaging of the cerebral aqueduct. *Neuroradiology* 1987;29:430–436.

115. Kazner E, Lanksch W, Steinhoff H. Cranial computerized tomography in the diagnosis of brain disorders in infants and children. *Neuropaediatrie* 1976;7:136–174.

116. Mickle JP. Neurosurgery for pediatric brain tumors. *Semin Pediatr Neurol* 1997;4:273–281.

117. D'Angio GJ, Rorke LB, Packer R, et al. Key problems in the management of children with brain tumors. *Int J Radiat Oncol Biol Phys* 1990;18:805–810.

118. Shulder M, Carmel PW. Intraoperative magnetic resonance imaging: impact on brain tumor surgery. *Cancer Control* 2003;10:115–124.

119. Steinbok P, Hentschel S, Cochrane DD, et al. Value of postoperative surveillance imaging in the management of children with some common brain tumors. *J Neurosurg* 1996;84:726–732.

120. Buatti JM, Meeks SL, Marcus RB Jr, et al. Radiotherapy for pediatric brain tumors. *Semin Pediatr Neurol* 1997;4:304–319.

121. Friedman WA, Bova FJ. Stereotactic radiosurgery. *Contemp Neurosurg* 1989;11:1–7.

122. Rabinowitz I, Broomberg J, Goitein M, et al. Accuracy of radiation

field alignment in clinical practice. *Int J Radiat Oncol Biol Phys* 1985;11:1857–1867.
123. Friedman WA, Bova FJ, Spiegelmann R. Linear accelerator radiosurgery at the University of Florida. *Neurosurg Clin N Am* 1992;3:141–166.
124. Auchter RM, Lamond JP, Alexander E, et al. A multiinstitutional outcome and prognostic factor analysis of radiosurgery for resectable single brain metastasis. *Int J Radiat Oncol Biol Phys* 1996;35:27–35.
125. Lunsford LD. Contemporary management of meningiomas: radiation therapy as an adjuvant and radiosurgery as an alternative to surgical removal. *J Neurosurg* 1994;80:187–190.
126. Hadjipanayis CG, Kondziolka D, Gardner P, et al. Stereotactic radiosurgery for pilocytic astrocytoma when multimodal therapy is necessary. *J Neurosurg* 2002;97:56–64.
127. Bova FJ, Buatti JM, Friedman WA, et al. The University of Florida frameless high-precision stereotactic radiotherapy system. *Int J Radiat Oncol Biol Phys* 1997;38:875–882.
128. Flickinger JC, Kondziolka D, Lunsford LD. Clinical applications of stereotactic radiosurgery. *Cancer Treat Res* 1998;93:283–297.
129. Murthy V, Jalali R, Sarin R, et al. Stereotactic conformal radiotherapy for posterior fossa tumours: a modelling study for potential improvement in therapeutic ratio. *Radiother Oncol* 2003;67:191–198.
130. Hug EB, Muenter MW, Archambeau JO, et al. Conformal proton radiation therapy for pediatric low-grade astrocytomas. *Strahlenterapie und Onkologie* 2002;178:10–17.
131. Chen Y-L, Yock T, Butler W, et al. Reduction of cochlear dose using proton boost for pediatric medulloblastoma. *Neuro-Oncology* 2004;6:450.
132. Benson PJ, Sung JH. Cerebral aneurysms following radiotherapy for medulloblastoma. *J Neurosurg* 1989;70:545–550.
133. Ball WS, Prenger EC, Ballard ET. Neurotoxicity of radio/chemotherapy in children: pathologic and MR correlation. *Am J Neuroradiol* 1992;13:761–776.
134. Duffner PK, Cohen ME. The long-term effects of central nervous system therapy on children with brain tumors. *Neurol Clin* 1991;9:479–495.
135. Curran WJ, Hecht-Leavitt C, Schut L, et. al. Magnetic resonance imaging of cranial radiation lesions. *Int J Radiat Oncol Biol Phys* 1987;13:1093–1098.
136. Kramer JH, Norman D, Brant-Zawadski M, et al. Absence of white matter changes on magnetic resonance imaging in children treated with CNS prophylactic therapy for leukemia. *Cancer* 1988;61:928–930.
137. Ellenberg L, McComb JG, Siegel SE, et al. Factors affecting intellectual outcome in pediatric brain tumor patients. *Neurosurgery* 1987;21:638–644.
138. Spiegler BJ, Bouffet E, Greenberg ML, et al. Change in neurocognitive functioning after treatment with cranial radiation in childhood. *J Clin Oncol* 2004;22:706–713.
139. Glauser TA, Packer RJ. Cognitive deficits in long-term survivors of childhood brain tumors. *Childs Nerv Syst* 1991;7:2–12.
140. Armstrong C, Ruffer J, Corn B, et al. Biphasic patterns of memory deficits following moderate-dose partial-brain irradiation: neuropsychologic outcome and proposed mechanisms. *J Clin Oncol* 1995;13:2263–2271.
141. Duffner PK, Cohen ME, Parker MS. Prospective intellectual testing in children with brain tumors. *Ann Neurol* 1988;23:575–579.
142. Radcliffe J, Packer RJ, Atkins TE, et al. Three- and four-year cognitive outcome in children with noncortical brain tumors treated with whole-brain-radiotherapy. *Ann Neurol* 1992;32:551–554.
143. Cohen BH, Packer RJ, Siegel KR, et al. Brain tumors in children under 2 years: treatment, survival and long-term prognosis. *Pediatr Neurosurg* 1993;19:171–179.
144. Suc E, Kalifa C, Brauner R, et al. Brain tumours under the age of three. The price of survival. A retrospective study of 20 long-term survivors. *Acta Neurochir* 1990;106:93–98.
145. Jannoun L, Bloom HJG. Long-term psychological effects in children treated for intracranial tumors. *Int J Radiat Oncol Biol Phys* 1990;18:747–753.
146. Ater J, Copeland D, Moore B III. Longitudinal neuropsychological study of children with medulloblastoma. *Neuro-Oncology* 2004;6:436.
147. Ittner K, Renaux VK, Levy-Piebois C, et al. Neuropsychological outcome after local posterior fossa radiation for ependymoma. *Neuro-Oncology* 2004;6:439.
148. Curnes JT, Laster DW, Ball MR, et al. MRI of radiation injury to the brain. *AJR Am J Roentgenol* 1986;147:119–124.
149. Zimmerman RD, Fleming CA, Lee BC, et al. Periventricular hyperintensity as seen by magnetic resonance: prevalence and significance. *AJR Am J Neuroradiol* 1986;7:13–20.
150. Constine LS, Konski A, Ekholm S, et al. Adverse effects of brain irradiation correlated with MR and CT imaging. *Int J Radiat Oncol Biol Phys* 1988;15:319–330.
151. Tsuruda JS, Kortman KE, Bradley WG. Radiation effects on cerebral white matter: MR evaluations. *AJR Am J Neuroradiol* 1987;8:431–437.
152. Palmer SL, Reddick WE, Glass JO, et al . Decline in corpus callosum volume among pediatric patients with medulloblastoma: longitudinal MR imaging study. *Am J Neuroradiol* 2002;23:1088–1094.
153. Constine LS, Woolf PD, Cann D, et al. Hypothalamic-pituitary dysfunction after radiation for brain tumors. *N Engl J Med* 1993; 328:87–94.
154. Rappaport R, Brauner R. Growth and endocrine disorders secondary to cranial irradiation. *Pediatr Res* 1989;25:561–567.
155. Cassady JR. Developmental toxicity: unique radiation toxicity in children which deserves study. *Radiat Oncol Invest* 1993;1:77–80.
156. Massimino M, Gandola L, Serra A, et al. Protection by hypothyroidism due to craniospinal irradiation in medulloblastoma patients. *Neuro-Oncology* 2004;6:440.
157. Ali K, Jones A, Riddell B, et al. Neuroendocrine sequelae in survivors of pediatric brain tumors in Saskatchewan, Canada: 1984–2000. *Neuro-Oncology* 2004;6:436.
158. Spoudeas HA, Charmandari E, Brook CGD. Hypothalamo-pituitary-adrenal axis integrity after cranial irradiation for childhood posterior fossa tumours. *Med Pediatr Oncol* 2003;40:224–229.
159. Howell DL, Janss AJ, Meacham LR. Incidence and trends of overweight and at risk for overweight among pediatric central nervous system (CNS) tumor patients. *Neuro-Oncology* 2004;6:438.
160. Samaan NA, Vieto R, Schultz PN, et al. Hypothalamic, pituitary and thyroid dysfunction after radiotherapy to the head and neck. *Int J Radiat Oncol Biol Phys* 1982;8:1857–1867.
161. Awwad S, Gregor A. Hormonal abnormalities in survivors of primary brain tumors. *Radiother Oncol* 1993;27:171–172.
162. Meadows AT, Baum E, Fossati-Bellani F, et al. Second malignant neoplasms in children: an update from the Late Effects Study Group. *J Clin Oncol* 1985;3:532–538.
163. Malone M, Lumley H, Erdohazi M. Astrocytoma as a second malignancy in patients with acute lymphoblastic leukemia. *Cancer* 1986;57:1979–1985.
164. Harrison MJ, Wolfe DE, Lau TS, et al. Radiation-induced meningiomas: experience at the Mount Sinai Hospital and review of the literature. *J Neurosurg* 1991;75:564–574.
165. Ater JL, van Eys J, Woo SY, et al. MOPP chemotherapy without irradiation as primary postsurgical therapy for brain tumors in infants and young children. *J Neurooncol* 1997;32:243–252.
166. Stavrou T, Bromley CM, Nicholson HS, et al. Prognostic factors and secondary malignancies in childhood medulloblastomas. *J Pediatr Hematol Oncol* 2001;23:431–436.
167. Walter AW, Hancock ML, Pui CH, et al. Secondary brain tumors in children treated for acute lymphoblastic leukemia at St. Jude Children's Research Hospital. *J Clin Oncol* 1998;16:3761–3767.
168. Broniscer A, Ke W, Fuller CE, et al. Second neoplasms (SN) in pediatric patients with primary central nervous system (CNS) tumors: the St. Jude Children's Research Hospital experience. *Neuro-Oncology* 2004;6:436.
169. Broniscer A, Ke W, Fuller CE, et al. Second neoplasms in pediatric patients with primary central nervous system tumors. *Cancer* 2004;100:2246–2252.
170. Allen JC, Miller DC, Budzilovich GN, et al. Brain and spinal cord hemorrhage in long-term survivors of malignant pediatric brain tumors: a possible late effect of therapy. *Neurology* 1991;41:148–150.
171. Sheline GE. Irradiation injury of the human brain: a review of clinical experience. In: Gilbert HA, Kagan AR, eds. *Radiation damage to the nervous system*. New York: Raven Press, 1980:39.

172. Duffner PK, Cohen ME. Long-term consequences of CNS treatment for childhood cancer. Part II. Clinical consequences. *Pediatr Neurol* 1991;7:237–242.
173. Mitchell WG, Fishman LS, Miller JH, et al. Stroke as a late sequela of cranial irradiation for childhood brain tumors. *J Child Neurol* 1991;6:128–133.
174. Shuper A, Packer RJ, Vezina LG, et al. "Complicated migraine-like episodes" in children following cranial irradiation and chemotherapy. *Neurology* 1995;45:1837–1840.
175. Duffner PK, Kun LE, Burger PC, et al. Postoperative chemotherapy and delayed radiation in children less than three years of age with malignant brain tumors. *N Engl J Med* 1993;328:1725–1731.
176. Maria BL, Drane WE, Quisling RG. Metabolic imaging in children with brain tumors. *Int Pediatr* 1993;8:233–238.
177. Maria BL, Drane WE, Quisling RG, et al. Value of ^{201}Thallium SPECT imaging in childhood brain tumors. *Pediatr Neurosurg* 1994;20:11–18.
178. Maria BL, Drane WB, Quisling RJ, et al. Correlation between gadolinium-DTPA contrast enhancement and thallium-201 chloride uptake in pediatric brainstem gliomas. *J Child Neurol* 1997;12:341–348.
179. Maria BL, Drane WE, Mastin ST, et al. Comparative value of thallium and glucose SPECT imaging in childhood brain tumors. *Pediatr Neurol* 1998;19:351–357.
180. Langer LF, Brem H, Langer R. New technologies for fighting brain disease. *Technol Rev* 1991;94:62.
181. Mitchell MS. Combining chemotherapy with biological response modifiers in treatment of cancer. *J Natl Cancer Inst* 1988;80:1445–1450.
182. Kuhl J, Gnekow H, Havers W, et al. Primary chemotherapy after surgery and delayed irradiation in children under three years of age with medulloblastoma-pilot trial of the German pediatric brain tumor study group. *Med Pediatr Oncol* 1992;20:387.
183. Levin VA, ed. *Cancer in the nervous system*. New York: Churchill Livingstone Inc, 1996.
184. Evans AE, Anderson JR, Lefkowitz-Boudreaux-IB, et. al. Adjuvant chemotherapy of childhood posterior fossa ependymoma: craniospinal irradiation with or without adjuvant CCNU, vincristine, and prednisone: a Children's Cancer Group study. *Med Pediatr Oncol* 1996;27:8–14.
185. Vassal G, Tranchand D, Valteau-Couanet D, et al. Pharmacodynamics of tandem high-dose melphalan with peripheral blood stem cell transplantation in children with neuroblastoma and medulloblastoma. *Bone Marrow Transplantation* 2001;27:471–477.
186. Perez-Martinez A, Quintero V, Vincent MG, et al. High-dose chemotherapy with autologous stem cell rescue as first line of treatment in young children with medulloblastoma and supratentorial primitive neuroectodermal tumors. *J Neurooncol* 2004;67:101–106.
187. Chi SN, et al. Newly diagnosed high-risk malignant brain tumors with leptomeningeal dissemination in young children: response to "Head Start" induction chemotherapy intensified with high-dose methotrexate. *Neuro-Oncology* 2004;6:451.
188. Chintagumpala M, Morriss M, Chiu J, et al. Intensity modulated radiation therapy (IMRT) induces changes that mimic new leptomeningeal disease in patients with medulloblastoma. *Neuro-Oncology* 2004;6:451.
189. Dunkel I, Gardner S, Garvin J, et al. High-dose carboplatin, thiotepa, and etoposide with autologous stem cell rescue (ASCR) for recurrent medulloblastoma. *Neuro-Oncology* 2004;6:453.
190. Foreman N, Le T, Orsini E, et al. Peripheral hematopoietic progenitor cell harvests in pediatric brain tumor patients undergoing high dose chemotherapy: experience with patients weighing less than 15 kg. *Neuro-Oncology* 2004;6:453.
191. Foreman N, Handler M, Schissel D, et al. A study of sequential high dose cyclophosphamide and high dose carboplatin with peripheral stem cell rescue in resistant or recurrent pediatric brain tumors. *Neuro-Oncology* 2004;6:454.
192. Gajjar A, Chintagumpala M, Kellie S, et al. Excellent event free survival (EFS) in newly diagnosed high risk (HR) medulloblastoma (MB) treated with craniospinal radiation (CSI) therapy followed by 4 cycles of high-dose chemotherapy and stem cell rescue: results of a prospective multicenter trial (SJMB 96). *Neuro-Oncology* 2004;6:455.
193. Gardner S, Baker D, Belasco J, et al. Phase I dose escalation of temozolomide with thiotepa and carboplatin with autologous stem cell rescue (ASCR) in patients with recurrent/refractory central nervous system (CNS) tumors. *Neuro-Oncology* 2004;6:455.
194. Gardner S, Diez B, Green A, et al. Intensive induction chemotherapy followed by high dose chemotherapy with autologous stem cell rescue (ASCR) in young children newly diagnosed with central nervous system (CNS) atypical teratoid rhabdoid tumors (ATT/RT)—the "Head Start" regimens. *Neuro-Oncology* 2004;6:455.
195. Garrè ML, Dallorso S, Milanaccio C, et al. Myeloablative chemotherapy with peripheral blood stem cells rescue before craniospinal radiotherapy in patients with medulloblastoma with post-operative residual or metastatic disease. Results of a mono-institutional study in Italy. *Neuro-Oncology* 2004;6:455.
196. Kato K, Inao S, Ikeda H, et al. High-Dose chemotherapy with peripheral blood stem cell transplantation in patients with pediatric malignant brain tumors. *Neuro-Oncology* 2004;6:460.
197. Massimino M, Ganlola L, Spreafico F, et al. High-dose chemotherapy is not enough to cure supratentorial PNET(S-PNET). *Neuro-Oncology* 2004;6:462.
198. Ridola V, Doz F, Frappaz D, et al. High dose chemotherapy and posterior fossa radiotherapy for children less than 3–5 years with localized high risk medulloblastoma at diagnosis or at relapse the SFOP experience. *Neuro-Oncology* 2004;6:465.
199. Terasaki M, Eguchi H, Nakagawa S, et al. High-dose chemotherapy with peripheral blood stem cell transplantation for medulloblastoma in children. *Neuro-Oncology* 2004;6:467.
200. Ziegler DS, Cohn RJ, McCowage G, et al. Efficacy of high dose cyclophosphamide with etoposide and vincristine ("vetopec") in very high risk paediatric brain tumors. *Neuro-Oncology* 2004;6:469.
200a. Wolff JE, Finlay JL. High-dose chemotherapy in childhood brain tumors. *Onkolie* 2004;27:239–245.
201. Kolker JD, Weichselbaum RR. Radiobiology update. In: Kornblith PL, Walker MD, eds. *Advances in neuro-oncology II*. Armack: Futura Publishing Co Inc, 1997.
202. Maria BL. *Brain tumors: current management in child neurology*. Maria BL, ed. Hamilton, Ontario, Canada: BC Decker Inc, 1999:336–341.
203. Rowinski EK, Donehower RC. Vinca alkaloids and epipodophyllotoxins. In: Perry MC, ed. *The chemotherapy source book*. Baltimore: Williams & Wilkins: 1992:359–383.
204. Green DM, D'Angio GJ, eds. *Late effects of treatment for childhood cancer*. New York: Wiley-Liss Inc, 1992.
205. Perry MC, ed. *The chemotherapy source book*. Baltimore: Williams & Wilkins, 1996.
206. Maria BL, Dennis M, Obonsawin M. Severe permanent encephalopathy in acute lymphoblastic leukemia. *Can J Neurol Sci* 1993;20:199–205.
207. Aonuma M, Iwahana M, Nakayama Y, et al. Tumorigenicity depends on angiogenic potential of tumor cells: dominant role of vascular endothelial growth factor and/or fibroblast growth factors produced by tumor cells. *Angiogenesis* 1998;2:57–66.
208. Maria BL, Medina CD, Hoang KB, et al. Gene therapy for neurologic disease: benchtop discoveries to bedside applications. 1. The bench. *J Child Neurol* 1997;12:1–12.
209. Maria BL, Medina CD, Hoang KB, et al. Gene therapy for neurologic disease: benchtop discoveries to bedside applications. 2. The bedside. *J Child Neurol* 1997;12:77–84.
210. Maria BL, Friedman T. Gene therapy in neuro-oncology: lessons learned from pioneering studies. In: Bodensteiner JB, Maria BL, eds. *Seminars in pediatric neurology*. Philadelphia: WB Saunders, 1997:333–339.
211. Kleihues P, Louis DN, Scheithauer BW, et al. The WHO classification of tumors of the nervous system. *J Neuropathol Exp Neurol* 2002;61:215–225.
212. Burger PC, Fuller GN. Pathology—trends and pitfalls in histologic diagnosis, immunopathology, and applications of oncogene research. *Neurol Clin* 1991;9:249–271.
213. Vagner-Capodano AM, Gentet JC, Gambarelli D, et al. Cytogenic studies in 45 pediatric brain tumors. *Pediatr Hematol Oncol* 1992;9:223–235.

214. Bigner SH, McLendon RE, Fuchs H, et al. Chromosomal characteristics of childhood brain tumors. *Cancer Genet Cytogenet* 1997;97:125–134.

214a. Brown WD, Gilles FH, Tavare CJ, et al. Prognostic limitations of the Daumas-Duport grading scheme in childhood supratentorial astroglial tumors. *J Neuropathol Exp Neurol* 1998;57:1035–1040.

214b. Gilles FH, Tavaré CJ, Leviton A, et al. Prognostic limitations of the Daumas-Duport grading scheme in infratentorial neuroglial tumors in children. *Pediat Devel Pathol* 2004;7:138–147.

215. Russell DS, Rubinstein LJ, eds. *Pathology of tumours of the nervous system*, 5th ed. London: E. Arnold, 1989.

216. Gilles FH. Pediatric brain tumors: classification. In: Morantz RA, Walsh JW, eds. *Brain tumors. A comprehensive text*. New York: Marcel Dekker Inc, 1994:109–134.

217. Gilles FH, Winston K, Fulchiero A, et al. Histologic features and observational variation in cerebellar gliomas in children. *Natl Cancer Inst Monogr* 1977;58:175–181.

218. Tomlinson FH, Scheithauer BW, Hayostek CJ, et al. The significance of atypia and histologic malignancy in pilocytic astrocytoma of the cerebellum: a clinicopathologic and flow cytometric study. *J Child Neurol* 1994;9:301–310.

219. Agamanolis DP, Malone JM. Chromosomal abnormalities in 47 pediatric brain tumors. *Cancer Genet Cytogenet* 1995;81:125–134.

220. von Deimling A, Louis DN, Menon AG, et al. Deletions on the long arm of chromosome 17 in pilocytic astrocytoma. *Acta Neuropathol (Berl)* 1993;86:81–85.

221. Patt S, Gries H, Giraldo M, et al. *p53* gene mutations in human astrocytic brain tumors including pilocytic astrocytomas. *Hum Pathol* 1996;27:586–589.

222. Burger PC, Scheithauer BW. Tumors of the nervous system. In: *Atlas of tumor pathology*, third series, fascicle 10. Washington, DC: Armed Forces Institute of Pathology, 1994.

223. Lantos PL, Vandenberg SR, Kleihues P. Tumors of the nervous system. In: Graham DI, Lantos PL, eds. *Greenfield's neuropathology*, 6th ed. London: Arnold, 1997:583–879.

224. Maria BL,Cafferty LL, Singer HS, et al. Diffuse leptomeningeal seeding from a malignant spinal cord astrocytoma in a child with neurofibromatosis. *J Neurooncol* 1986;4:159–163.

225. von Deimling A, von Ammon K, Schoenfeld D, et al. Subsets of glioblastoma multiforme defined by molecular genetic analysis. *Brain Pathol* 1992;3:19–26.

226. Shapiro K, Katz M. The recurrent cerebellar astrocytoma. *Childs Brain* 1983;10:168–176.

227. Civitello LA, Packer REJ, Rorke LB, et al. Leptomeningeal dissemination of low-grade gliomas in childhood. *Neurology* 1988;38:562–566.

228. Rubinstein LJ. Cytogenesis and differentiation of primitive central neuroepithelial tumors. *J Neuropathol Exp Neurol* 1972;31:7–26.

229. Rorke LB. Origin and histogenesis of medulloblastoma. In: Zeltxer PM, Pochedly C, eds. *Medulloblastomas in children*. New York: Praeger, 1986:14–21.

230. Schwechheimer K, Wiedenmann B, Franke WW. Synaptophysin: a reliable marker for medulloblastomas. *Virchows Arch A Pathol Anat Histopathol* 1987;411:53–59.

231. Molenaar WM, Trojanowski JO. Biological markers of glial and primitive tumors. In: Salcman M, ed. *Neurobiology of brain tumors: concepts in neurosurgery*. Vol. 4. Baltimore: Williams & Wilkins, 1991:185–210.

232. Maraziotis J, Perentes E, Karamitopoulou E, et al. Neuron-associated class III beta-tubulin isotype, retinal S-antigen, synaptophysin and glial fibrillary acidic protein in human medulloblastomas: a clinicopathological analysis of 36 cases. *Acta Neuropathol* 1992;84:355–363.

233. Janss AJ, Yachnis AT, Silbert JH, et al. Glial differentiation predicts poor clinical outcome in primitive neuroectodermal brain tumors. *Ann Neurol* 1996;39:481–489.

234. McManamy CS, Lamont JM, Taylor RE, et al. Morphophenotypic variation predicts clinical behavior in childhood non-desmoplastic medulloblastomas. *J Neuropathol Exp Neurol* 2003;62:627–632.

235. Giangaspero F, Perilongo G, Fondelli MP, et al. Medulloblastoma with extensive nodularity: a variant with favorable prognosis. *J Neurosurg* 1999;91:971–977.

236. Pomeroy SL, Tamayo P, Gaasenbeek M, et al. Prediction of central nervous system embryonal tumour outcome based on gene expression. *Nature* 2002;415:436–442.

237. Dechiara C, Borghese A, Fiorillo A, et al. Cytogenetic evaluation of isochromosome 17q in posterior fossa tumors of children and correlation with clinical outcome in medulloblastoma. *Childs Nerv Syst* 2002;18:380–384.

238. Michiels EM, Weiss MM, Hoovers JM, et al. Genetic alterations in childhood medulloblastoma analyzed by comparative genomic hybridization. *J Pediatr Hematol Oncol* 2002;24:205–210.

239. Gajjar AJ, Heideman RL, Douglass EC, et al. Relation of tumor-cell ploidy to survival in children with medulloblastoma. *J Clin Oncol* 1993;11:2211–2217.

240. del Charco JO, Bolek TW, McCollough WM, et al. Medulloblastoma: time-dose relationship based on a 30-year review. *Int J Radiat Oncol Biol Phys* 1998;42:147–154.

241. Grotzer MA, Hogarty MD, Janss AJ, et al. MYC messenger RNA expression predicts survival outcome in childhood primitive neuroectodermal tumor/medulloblastoma. *Clin Cancer Res* 2001;7:2425–2433.

242. Pelc K, Vincent S, Ruchoux MM, et al. Calbindin-D_{28k} a marker of recurrence for medulloblastomas. *Cancer* 2002;95:410–419.

243. Herms J, Neidt I, Luscher B, et al. C-MYC expression in medulloblastoma and its prognostic value. *Int J Cancer (Ped Oncol)* 2000;89:395–402.

244. Katsetos CD, Herman MM, Frankfurter A, et al. Cerebellar desmoplastic medulloblastomas. A further immunohistochemical characterization of the reticulin-free pale islands. *Arch Pathol Lab Med* 1989;113:1019–1029.

245. Zacharoulis S, et al. Desmoplastic Versus Non-desmoplastic medulloblastoma: differences in clinical outcome? *Neuro-Oncology* 2004;6(4).

246. Undjian S, Marinov M. Intracranial ependymomas in children. *Childs Nerv Syst* 1990;6:131–134.

247. Reyes-Mugica M, Chou PM, Myint MM, et al. Ependymomas in children: histologic and DNA-flow cytometric study. *Pediatr Pathol* 1994;14:453–466.

248. Schiffer D, Chio A, Giordana MT, et al. Histologic prognostic factors in ependymoma. *Childs Nerv Syst* 1991;7:177–182.

249. Rorke LB. Relationship of morphology of ependymoma in children to prognosis. *Prog Exp Tumor Res* 1987;30:170–174.

250. Sheldon M, Johnson RH, Lu Y, et al. Integrative profiling of chromosomal copy number abnormalities and gene expression in pediatric ependymomas. *Neuro-Oncology* 2004;6:414.

251. Tominaga T, Kayama T, Kumabe T, et al. Anaplastic ependymomas: clinical features and tumour suppressor gene *p53* analysis. *Acta Neurochir (Wien)* 1995;135:163–70.

252. Korshunov A, Neben K, Wrobel G, et al. Gene expression patterns in ependymomas correlate with tumor location, grade, and patient age. *Am J Pathol* 2003;163:1721–1727.

253. Kepes JJ, Rubenstein LJ, Eng LF. Pleomorphic xanthoastrocytoma: a distinctive meningocerebral glioma of young subjects with relatively favorable prognosis: a study of 12 cases. *Cancer* 1979;44:1839–1852.

254. Kepes J. Pleomorphic xanthoastrocytoma: the birth of a diagnosis and a concept. *Brain Pathol* 1993;3:269–274.

255. Kordek R, Biernat W, Sapieja W, et al. Pleomorphic xanthoastrocytoma with a gangliomatous component: an immunohistochemical and ultrastructural study. *Acta Neuropathol (Berl)* 1995;89:194–197.

256. Powell SZ, Yachnis AT, Rorke LB, et al. Divergent differentiation in pleomorphic xanthoastrocytoma. Evidence for a neuronal element and possible relationship to ganglion cell tumors. *Am J Surg Pathol* 1996;20:80–85.

257. Paulus W, Lisle DK, Tonn JC, et al. Molecular genetic alterations in pleomorphic xanthoastrocytoma. *Acta Neuropathol (Berl)* 1996;91:293–297.

258. Tonn JC, Paulus W, Warmuth-Metz M, et al. Pleomorphic xanthoastrocytoma: report of six cases with special consideration of diagnostic and therapeutic pitfalls. *Surg Neurol* 1997;47:162–169.

259. Wolf HK, Muller MB, Spanle M, et al. Ganglioglioma: a detailed histopathological and immunohistochemical analysis of 61 cases. *Acta Neuropathol (Berl)* 1994;88:166–173.

260. Miller DC, Lang FF, Epstein FJ. Central nervous system gangliogliomas. Part 1 :pathology. *J Neurosurg* 1993;79:859–866.
261. Jay V, Squire J, Becker LE, et al. Malignant transformation in a ganglioglioma with anaplastic neuronal and astrocytic components. Report of a case with flow cytometric and cytogenetic analysis. *Cancer* 1994;73:2862–2868.
262. Johnson JH Jr, Hariharan S, Berman J, et al. Clinical outcome of pediatric gangliogliomas: ninety-nine cases over 20 years. *Pediatr Neurosurg* 1997;27:203–207.
263. Vandenberg SR. Desmoplastic infantile ganglioglioma and desmoplastic cerebral astrocytoma of infancy. *Brain Pathol* 1993;3:275–281.
264. Taratuto AL, Monges J, Lylyk P, et al. Superficial cerebral astrocytoma attached to dura. Report of six cases in infants. *Cancer* 1984;54:2505–2512.
265. Sperner J, Gottschalk J, Neumann K, et al. Clinical, radiological and histological findings in desmoplastic infantile ganglioglioma. *Child Nerv Syst* 1994;10:458–462.
266. Daumas-Duport C, Scheithauer BW, Chodkiewicz JP, et al. Dysembryoplastic neuroepithelial tumor: a surgically curable tumor of young patients with intractable partial seizures. Report of thirty-nine cases. *Neurosurgery* 1988;23:545–556.
267. Daumas-Duport C. Dysembryoplastic neuroepithelial tumors. *Brain Pathol* 1993;3:283–295.
268. Hirose T, Scheithauer BW, Lopes MB, et al. Dysembryoplastic neuroepithelial tumor (DNT): an immunohistochemical and ultrastructural study. *J Neuropathol Exp Neurol* 1994;53:184–195.
269. Cervera-Pierot P, Varlet P, Chodkiewicz JP, et al. Dysembryoplastic neuroepithelial tumors located in the caudate nucleus area: report of four cases. *Neurosurgery* 1997;40:1065–1069.
270. Molloy PT, Yachnis AT, Rorke LB, et al. Central nervous system medulloepithelioma: a series of eight cases including two arising in the pons. *J Neurosurg* 1996;84:430–436.
271. Rorke LB, Packer RJ, Biegel JA. Central nervous system atypical teratoid/rhabdoid tumors of infancy and childhood: definition of an entity. *J Neurosurg* 1996;85:56–65.
272. Rorke LB, Packer RJ, Biegel JA. Central nervous system atypical teratoid/rhabdoid tumors of infancy and childhood. *J Neurooncol* 1995;24:21–28.
273. Haas JE, Palmer NF, Weinberg AG, et al. Ultrastructure of malignancy rhabdoid tumor of the kidney. A distinctive renal tumor of children. *Hum Pathol* 1981;12:646–657.
274. Biegel JA, Burk CD, Parmiter AH, et al. Molecular analysis of a partial deletion of 22q in a central nervous system rhabdoid tumor. *Genes Chromosomes Cancer* 1992;5:104–108.
275. Yachnis AT, Neubauer D, Muir D, et al. Characterization of a primary central nervous system atypical teratoid/rhabdoid tumor and derivative cell line: immunophenotype and neoplastic properties. *J Neuropathol Exp Neurol* 1998;57:961–971.
276. Smirniotopoulos JG, Chiechi MV. Teratomas, dermoids, and epidermoids of the head and neck. *Radiographics* 1995;15:1437–1455.
277. Gormley WB, Tomecek FJ, Qureshi N, Malik GM. Craniocerebral epidermoid and dermoid tumours: a review of 32 cases. *Acta Neurochir* 1994;128:115–121.
278. Mackenzie IR. Central neurocytoma: histologic atypia, proliferation potential, and clinical outcome. *Cancer* 1999;85:1606–1610.
279. Cushing H. Experiences with the cerebellar astrocytomas. *Surg Gynecol Obstet* 1931;52:129–204.
280. Park TS, Hoffman HJ, Hendrick EB, et al. Medulloblastoma: clinical presentation and management. Experience at the Hospital for Sick Children, Toronto, 1950–1980. *J Neurosurg* 1983;58:543–552.
281. Diebler C, Dulac O. *Pediatric neurology and neuroradiology*. Berlin: Springer-Verlag, 1987:296.
281a. Hughlings Jackson J. On Tumours of the Cerebellum. In: Selected Writings, Hodderaud Stoughton, Ltd, London, 1932, Volume 2, 328–333.
282. Stewart TG, Holmes G. Symptomatology of cerebellar tumours: a study of forty cases. *Brain* 1904;27:522–591.
283. Welchman JM. Computerized tomography of intracranial tuberculomata. *Clin Radiol* 1979;30:567–573.
284. Komiyama M, Yagura H, Baba M, et al. MR imaging: possibility of tissue characterization of brain tumors using T1 and T2 values. *Am J Neuroradiol* 1987;8:65–70.
285. Stack JP, Antoun NM, Jenkins JP, et al. Gadolinium-DTPA as a contrast agent in magnetic resonance imaging of the brain. *Neuroradiology* 1988;30:145–154.
286. Zimmerman RD, Bilaniuk LT, Rebsamen S. Magnetic resonance imaging of pediatric posterior fossa tumors. *Pediatr Neurosurg* 1992;18:58–64.
287. O'Reilly G, Hayward RD, Harkness WF. Myelography in the assessment of children with medulloblastoma. *Br J Neurosurg* 1993;7:183–188.
288. Grant FC. Cerebellar symptoms produced by supratentorial tumors: further report. *Arch Neurol Psychiatry* 1928;20:292–308.
289. Lhermitte J, Duclos P. Sur un ganglioneurome diffus du cortex du cervelet. *Bull Assoc Franc Cancer* 1920;9:99–107.
290. Nowak DA, Trost HA. Lhermitte-Duclos disease (dysplastic cerebellar gangliocytoma): a malformation, hamartoma or neoplasm? *Acta Neurol Scand* 2002;105:137–145.
290a. Perez-Nunez A, Lagares A, Benitez J, et al. Lhermitte-Duclos disease and Cowden disease: clinical and genetic study in five patients with Lhermitte-Duclose disease and lieterature review. *Acta Neurochir* 2004;146:679–690.
291. Hair LS, Symmans F, Powers JM, Carmel P. Immunohistochemistry and proliferative activity in Lhermitte-Duclos disease. *Acta Neuropathol (Berl)* 1992;84:570–573.
292. Koch R, Scholz M, Nelen MR, et al. Lhermitte-Duclos disease as a component of Cowden's syndrome. Case report and review of the literature. *J Neurosurg* 1999;90:776–779.
293. Sutphen R, Diamond TM, Minton SE, et al. Severe Lhermitte-Duclos disease with unique germline mutation of PTEN. *Am J Med Genet* 1999;82:290–293.
293a. Waite KA, Eng C. Protean PTEN: form and function. *Am J Hum Genet* 2002:70:829–844.
294. Matson DD. Cerebellar astrocytomas in childhood. *Pediatrics* 1956;18:150–158.
295. Warnick RE, Edwards MS. Pediatric brain tumors. *Curr Probl Pediatr* 1991;21:129–173.
296. Schneider JH, Raffel C, McComb JG. Benign cerebellar astrocytomas of childhood. *Neurosurgery* 1992;30:58–63.
297. Bloom HJ, Glees J, Bell J. The treatment and long-term prognosis of children with intracranial tumors: a study of 610 cases, 1950 to 1981. *Int J Radiat Oncol Biol Phys* 1990;18:723–745.
298. Desai KI, Nadkarni TD, Muzumdar DP, Goel A. Prognostic factors for cerebellar astrocytomas in children: a study of 102 cases. *Pediatr Neurosurg* 2001;35:311–317.
299. Wallner KE, Gonzales MF, Edwards MS, et al. Treatment results of juvenile pilocytic astrocytoma. *J Neurosurg* 1988;69:171–176.
300. Collins VP, Loeffler RK, Tivey H. Observations on growth rates of human tumors. *AJR Am J Roentgenol* 1956;76:988–1000.
301. Packer RJ. Chemotherapy for medulloblastoma/primitive neuroectodermal tumors of the posterior fossa. *Ann Neurol* 1990;28:823–828.
302. Packer RJ, Sutton LN, Goldwein JW, et al. Improved survival with the use of adjuvant chemotherapy in the treatment of medulloblastoma. *J Neurosurg* 1991;74:433–440.
303. Evans AE, Jenkin RD, Sposto R, et al. The treatment of medulloblastoma. Results of a prospective randomized trial of radiation therapy with and without CCNU, vincristine, and prednisone. *J Neurosurg* 1990;72:572–582.
304. Johnson DL, McCabe MA, Nicholson HS, et al. Quality of long-term survival in young children with medulloblastoma. *J Neurosurg* 1994;80:1004–1010.
305. Duffner PK, Krischer JP, Horowitz ME, et al. Second malignancies in young children with primary brain tumors following treatment with prolonged postoperative chemotherapy and delayed irradiation: a Pediatric Oncology Group study. *Ann Neurol* 1998;44:313–316.
306. Chintagumpala M, Berg S, Blaney SM. Treatment controversies in medulloblastoma. *Curr Opin Oncol* 2001;13:154–159.
307. Freeman CR, Taylor RE, Kortmann RD, Carrie C. Radiotherapy for medulloblastoma in children: a perspective on current international clinical research efforts. *Med Pediatr Oncol* 2002;39:99–108.
308. Taylor RE, Bailey CC, Robinson K, et al. Results of a randomized

study of preradiation chemotherapy versus radiotherapy alone for nonmetastatic medulloblastoma: the International Society of Paediatric Oncology/United Kingdom Children's Cancer Study Group PNET-3 study. *J Clin Oncol* 2003;21:1581–1591.
309. Hara J. Pilot study of reduced-dose craniospinal radiotherapy followed by high-dose chemotherapy consisting of thiotepa and melphalan in children with M1/2/3 medulloblastoma. *Neuro-Oncology* 2004;6:458.
310. Levin VA, Rodriguez LA, Edwards MS, et al. Treatment of medulloblastoma with procarbazine, hydroxyurea, and reduced radiation doses to whole brain and spine. *J Neurosurg* 1988;68:383–387.
311. Tait DM, Thornton-Jones H, Bloom HJ, et al. Adjuvant chemotherapy for medulloblastoma: the first multicentre control trial of the International Society of Pediatric Oncology (SIOP 1). *Eur J Cancer* 1990;26:464–469.
312. Krischer JP, Ragab AH, Kun L, et al. Nitrogen mustard, vincristine, procarbazine, and prednisone as adjuvant chemotherapy in the treatment of medulloblastoma. *J Neurosurg* 1991:74:905–909.
313. Steinbok P, Cochrane DD, Perrin R, Price A. Mutism after posterior fossa tumour resection in children: incomplete recovery on long-term follow-up. *Pediatr Neurosurg* 2003;39:179–183.
314. Steinlin M, Imfeld S, Zulauf P, et al. Neuropsychological long-term sequelae after posterior fossa tumour resection during childhood. *Brain* 2003;126:1998–2008.
315. Prayson RA, Fischler DF. Cerebrospinal fluid cytology. An 11-year experience with 5951 specimens. *Arch Pathol Lab Med* 1998;122: 47–51.
316. Douglas JG, Barker JL, Ellenbogen RG, Geyer JR. Concurrent chemotherapy and reduced-dose cranial spinal irradiation followed by conformal posterior fossa tumor bed boost for average-risk medulloblastoma: efficacy and patterns of failure. *Int J Radiat Oncol Biol Phys* 2004;58:1161–1164.
317. Salazar OM. Primary malignant cerebellar astrocytomas in children: a signal for postoperative craniospinal irradiation. *Int J Radiat Oncol Biol Phys* 1981;7:1661–1665.
318. Keene DL, Hsu E, Ventureyra E. Brain tumors in childhood and adolescence. *Pediatr Neurol* 1999;20:198–203.
319. Jayawickreme DP, Hayward RD, Harkness WF. Intracranial ependymomas in childhood: a report of 24 cases followed for 5 years. *Childs Nerv Syst* 1995;11:409–413.
320. Undjian S, Marinov M. Intracranial ependymomas in children. *Childs Nerv Syst* 1990;6:131–134.
321. Furie DM, Provenzale JM. Supratentorial ependymomas and subependymomas: CT and MR appearance. *J Comput Assist Tomogr* 1995;19:518–526.
322. Paulino AC. The local field in infratentorial ependymoma: does the entire posterior fossa need to be treated? *Int J Radiat Oncol Biol Phys* 2001;49(3):757–761.
323. Garvin J, et al. Childhood ependymoma: improved survival for patients with incompletely resected tumors with the use of pre-irradiation chemotherapy. *Neuro-Oncology* 2004;6:456.
324. Palma L, Celli P, Cantore G. Supratentorial ependymomas of the first two decades of life. Long-term follow-up of 20 cases (including two subependymomas). *Neurosurgery* 1993;32:169–175.
325. Ernestus RI, Schroder R, Stutzer H, Klug N. Prognostic relevance of localization and grading in intracranial ependymomas of childhood. *Childs Nerv Syst* 1996;12:522–526.
326. Lyons MK, Kelly PJ. Posterior fossa ependymomas: report of 30 cases and review of the literature. *Neurosurgery* 1991;28:659–664.
327. Rousseau P, Habrand JL, Sarrazin D, et al. Treatment of intracranial ependymomas of children: review of a 15-year experience. *Int J Radiat Oncol Biol Phys* 1994;28:381–386.
328. McLaughlin MP, Marcus RB Jr, Buatti JM, et al. Ependymoma: results, prognostic factors, and treatment recommendations. *Int J Rad Oncol Biol Phys* 1998;40:845–850.
329. Spagnoli D, Tomei G, Ceccarelli G, et al. Combined treatment of fourth ventricle ependymomas: report of 26 cases. *Surg Neurol* 2000;54:19–26.
330. Evans AE, Anderson JR, Lefkowitz-Boudreaux IB, Finlay JL. Adjuvant chemotherapy of childhood posterior fossa ependymoma: cranio-spinal irradiation with or without adjuvant CCNU, vincristine, and prednisone: a Children's Cancer Group study. *Med Pediatr Oncol* 1996;27:8–14.
331. Geyer JR, Zeltzer PM, Boyett JM, et al. Survival of infants with primitive neuroectodermal tumors or malignant ependymomas of the CNS treated with eight drugs in 1 day: a report from the children's cancer group. *J Clin Oncol* 1994;12:1607–1615.
332. Duffner PK, Krischer JP, Sanford RA, et al. Prognostic factors in infants and very young children with intracranial ependymomas. *Pediatr Neurosurg* 1998;28:215–222.
333. Chiu JK, Woo SY, Ater J, et al. Intracranial ependymoma in children: analysis of prognostic factors. *J Neurooncol* 1992;13:283–290.
334. Zorlu AF, Atahan IL, Akyol FH, et al. Intracranial ependymomas: treatment results and prognostic factors. *Radiat Med* 1994;12:269–272.
335. van Mourik M, Catsman-Berrevoets CE, van Dongen HR, Neville BG. Complex orofacial movements and the disappearance of cerebellar mutism: report of five cases. *Dev Med Child Neurol* 1997;39:686–690.
336. Dailey AT, McKhann GM, Berger MS. The pathophysiology of oral pharyngeal apraxia and mutism following posterior fossa tumor resection in children. *J Neurosurg* 1995;83:467–475.
337. Liu GT, Phillips PC, Molloy PT, et al. Visual impairment associated with mutism after posterior fossa surgery in children. *Neurosurgery* 1998;42:253–256.
338. Misakyan T, et al. Speech and language functioning following surgery for posterior fossa tumors. *Neuro-Oncology* 2004;6:440.
339. Maria BL, Rehder K, Eskin TA, et al. Brainstem glioma: I. Pathology, clinical features, and therapy. *J Child Neurol* 1993;8:112–128.
340. Mantravadi RV, Phatak R, Bellur S, et al. Brainstem glioma: an autopsy study of 25 cases. *Cancer* 1982;49:1294–1296.
341. Berger MS, Edwards MS, LaMasters D, et al. Pediatric brain stem tumors: radiographic, pathological and clinical correlations. *Neurosurgery* 1983;12:298–302.
342. Stroink AR, Hoffman HJ, Hendrick EB, Humphreys RP. Diagnosis and management of pediatric brain-stem gliomas. *J Neurosurg* 1986;65:745–750.
343. Louis DN, Rubio MP, Correa KM, et al. Molecular genetics of pediatric brain stem gliomas. Application of PCR techniques to small and archival brain tumor specimens. *J Neuropathol Exp Neurol* 1993;52:507–515.
344. Bray PF, Carter S, Taveras JM. Brainstem tumors in children. *Neurology* 1958;8:1–7.
345. Flores LE, Williams DL, Bell BA, et al. Delay in the diagnosis of pediatric brain tumors. *Am J Dis Child* 1986;140:684–686.
346. Cohen ME, Duffner PK, Heffner RR, et al. Prognostic factors in brainstem gliomas. *Neurology* 1986;36:602–605.
347. Panitch HS, Berg BO. Brain stem tumors of childhood and adolescence. *Am J Dis Child* 1970;119:465–472.
348. Stroink AR, Hoffman HJ, Hendrick EB, et al. Transependymal benign dorsally exophytic brain stem gliomas in childhood: diagnosis and treatment recommendations. *Neurosurgery* 1987;20:439–444.
349. Packer RJL. Brainstem gliomas of childhood: magnetic resonance imaging. *Neurology* 1985;35:397–401.
350. Barkovich AJ, Krischer J, Kun LE, et al. Brainstem gliomas: a classification based on magnetic resonance imaging. *Pediatr Neurosurg* 1990;16:73–83.
351. Nelson MD Jr, Soni D, Baram TZ. Necrosis in pontine gliomas: radiation induced or natural history? *Radiology* 1994;191:279–282.
352. Caldarelli M, Colosimo C, Di Rocco C. Intra-axial dermoid/epidermoid tumors of the brainstem in children. *Pediatr Neurosurg* 2001;56:97–105.
353. Schain RJ, Wilson G. Brain stem encephalitis with radiographic evidence of medullary enlargement. *Neurology* 1971;21:537–539.
354. Albright AL, Guthkelch AN, Packer RJ, et al. Prognostic factors in pediatric brain-stem gliomas. *J Neurosurg* 1986;65:751–755.
355. Albright AL, Packer RJ, Zimmerman R, et al. Magnetic resonance scans should replace biopsies for the diagnosis of diffuse brain stem gliomas: a report from the Children's Cancer Group. *Neurosurgery* 1993;33:1026–1029.
356. Massager N, David P, Goldman S, et al. Combined magnetic resonance imaging and positron emission tomography–guided stereotactic biopsy in brainstem mass lesions: diagnostic yield in a series of 30 patients. *J Neurosurg* 2000;93:951–957.

357. Curless RG, Bowen BC, Pattany PM, et al. Magnetic resonance spectroscopy in childhood brainstem tumors. *Pediatric Neurology* 2002;26:374–378.
358. Edwards MS, Levin VA, Wilson CB. Chemotherapy of pediatric posterior fossa tumors. *Childs Brain* 1980;7:252–260.
359. Wilson CB. Diagnosis and treatment of childhood brain tumors. *Cancer* 1975;35:950.
360. Mandell LR, Kadota R, Freeman C, et al. There is no role for hyperfractionated radiotherapy in the management of children with newly diagnosed diffuse intrinsic brainstem tumors: results of a pediatric oncology group phase III trial comparing conventional vs. hyperfractionated radiotherapy. *Int J Radiat Oncol Biol Phys* 1999;43:959–964.
361. Edwards MS, Wara WM, Urtasun RC, et al. Hyperfractionated radiation therapy for brain-stem gliomas: a phase I–II trial. *J Neurosurg* 1989;70:691–700.
362. Freeman CR, Krischer J, Sanford RA, et al. Hyperfractionated radiation therapy in brain stem tumors. *Cancer* 1991;68:474–481.
363. Finlay JL, Boyett JM, Yates AJ, et al. Randomized phase III trial in childhood high-grade astrocytoma comparing vincristine, lomustine, and prednisone with the eight-drugs-in-1-day regimen. *J Clin Oncol* 1995;13:112–123.
364. Zeltzer PM, Epport K, Nelson MD Jr, et al. Prolonged response to carboplatin in an infant with brainstem glioma. *Cancer* 1991;67: 43–47.
365. Gaynon PS, Ettinger LJ, Baum ES, et al. Carboplatin in childhood brain tumors. A Children's Cancer Study Group phase II trial. *Cancer* 1990;66:2465–2469.
366. Allen JC, Helson L. High-dose cyclophosphamide chemotherapy for recurrent CNS tumors in children. *Am J Pediatr Hematol Oncol* 1990;112:297–300.
367. Kedar A, Maria BL, Graham-Pole J, et al. High-dose chemotherapy with marrow reinfusion and hyperfractionated irradiation for children with brainstem glioma. *Proc Am Soc Clin Oncol* 1994;177:428–436.
368. Kretschmar CS, Tarbell NJ, Barnes PD, et al. Pre-irradiation chemotherapy and hyperfractionated radiation therapy 66 Gy for children with brain stem tumors: a phase II study of the Pediatric Oncology Group Protocol 8833. *Cancer* 1993;72:1404–1413.
369. Jennings MT, Sposto R, Boyett JM, et al. Preradiation chemotherapy in primary high-risk brainstem tumors: phase II study CCG-9941 of the Children's Cancer Group. *J Clin Oncol* 2002;20:3431–3437.
370. Freeman CR, Perilongo G. Chemotherapy for brain stem gliomas. *Childs Nerv Syst* 1999;15:545–553.
371. Chuba PJ, Zamarano L, Hamre M, et al. Permanent I-125 brain stem implants in children. *Childs Nerv Syst* 1998;14:570–577.
372. Culver KW, Ram Z, Wallbridge S, et al. In vivo gene transfer with retroviral vector-producer cells for treatment of experimental brain tumors. *Science* 1992;256:1550–1552.
373. Fueyo J, Gomez-Manzano C, Yung WK, Kyritsis AP. Targeting in gene therapy for gliomas. *Arch Neurol* 1999;56:445–448.
374. Amano T, Inamura T, Nakamizo A, et al. Case management of hydrocephalus associated with the progression of childhood brain stem gliomas. *Childs Nerv Syst* 2002;18:599–604.
375. Richmond IL, Wilson CB. Parasellar tumors in children. I. Clinical presentation, preoperative assessment, and differential diagnosis. *Childs Brain* 1980;7:73–84.
376. Crotty TB, Scheithauer BW, Young WF, et al. Papillary craniopharyngioma: a clinicopathological study of 48 cases. *J Neurosurg* 1995;83:206–214.
377. Sekine S, Shibata T, Kokubu A, et al. Craniopharyngiomas of adamantinomatous type harbor beta-catenin gene mutations. *Am J Pathol* 2002;161:1997–2001.
378. Rickert CH, Paulus W. Lack of chromosomal imbalances in adamantinomatous and papillary craniopharyngiomas. *J Neurol Neurosurg Psychiatry* 2003;74:260–261.
379. Maira G, Anile C, Albanese A, et al. The role of transsphenoidal surgery in the treatment of craniopharyngiomas. *J Neurosurg* 2004;100:445–451.
380. Wang KC, Kim SK, Choe G, et al. Growth patterns of craniopharyngioma in children: role of the diaphragm sellae and its surgical implication. *Surg Neurol* 2002;57:25–33.
381. Liszczak T, Richardson EP Jr, Phillips JP, et al. Morphological, biochemical, ultrastructural, tissue culture and clinical observations of typical and aggressive craniopharyngiomas. *Acta Neuropathol* 1978;43:191–203.
382. Northfield DWC. Rathke-pouch tumours. *Brain* 1957;80:293–312.
383. Epstein F, McCleary EL. Intrinsic brain-stem tumors of childhood. Surgical indications. *J Neurosurg* 1986;64:11–15.
384. Bingas B, Wolter M. Das Kraniopharyngiom. *Fortschr Neurol Psychiatr* 1968;36:117–195.
385. Imura H, Kato Y, Nakai Y. Endocrine aspects of tumors arising from suprasellar, third ventricular regions. *Prog Exp Tumor Res* 1987;30:313–324.
386. Newman CB, Levine LS, New MI. Endocrine function in children with intrasellar and suprasellar neoplasms. *Am J Dis Child* 1981;135:259–262.
387. Cacciari E, Frejaville E, Cicognani A, et al. How many cases of true precocious puberty are idiopathic? *J Pediatr* 1983;102:357–360.
388. Bailey P. Concerning the cerebellar symptoms produced by suprasellar tumors. *Arch Neurol Psychiatry* 1924;11:137–150.
389. Ito H, Shoin K, Hwang WZ, et al. Preoperative diagnosis of Rathke's cleft cyst. *Childs Nerv Syst* 1987;3:225–227.
390. Brummitt ML, Kline LB, Wilson ER. Craniopharyngioma: pitfalls in diagnosis. *J Clin Neuroophthalmol* 1992;12:77–81.
391. Russell RWR, Pennybacker JB. Craniopharyngioma in the elderly. *J Neurol Neurosurg Psychiatry* 1961;24:1–13.
392. Watkins L, Khudados ES, Kaleoglu M, et al. Skull base chordomas: a review of 38 patients, 1958–1988. *Br J Neurosurg* 1993;7:241–248.
393. Kaneko Y, Sato Y, Iwaki T, et al. Chordoma in early childhood: a clinicopathological study. *Neurosurgery* 1991;29:442–446.
394. Matsumoto J, Towbin RB, Ball WS. Cranial chordomas in infancy and childhood: a report of two cases and review of the literature. *Pediatr Radiol* 1989;20:28–32.
395. Hoffman HJ, Hendrick EB, Humphreys RP, et al. Investigation and management of suprasellar arachnoid cysts. *J Neurosurg* 1982;57:597–602.
396. Nellhaus G. The bobble-head doll syndrome. A "tic" with a neuropathologic basis. *Pediatrics* 1967;40:250–253.
397. Russell A. A diencephalic syndrome of emaciation in infancy and childhood [Abstract]. *Arch Dis Child* 1951;26:74.
398. Shillito J. Treatment of craniopharyngioma. *Clin Neurosurg* 1986;33:533–546.
399. Yasargil MG, Curcic M, Kis M, et al. Total removal of craniopharyngiomas. Approaches and long-term results in 144 patients. *J Neurosurg* 1990;73:3–11.
400. Jose CC, Rajan B, Ashley S, et al. Radiotherapy for the treatment of recurrent craniopharyngioma. *Clin Oncol (R Coll Radiol)* 1992;5:287–289.
401. Rajan B, Ashley S, Gorman C, et al. Craniopharyngioma—long-term results following limited surgery and radiotherapy. *Radiother Oncol* 1993;26:1–10.
402. Regine WF, Kramer S. Pediatric craniopharyngiomas: long-term results of combined treatment with surgery and radiation. *Int J Radiat Oncol Biol Phys* 1992;24:611–617.
403. Hoffman HJ. Craniopharyngiomas. *Can J Neurol Sci* 1985;12:348–352.
404. Stripp DCH, Maity A, Janss AJ, et al. Surgery with or without radiation therapy in the management of craniopharyngiomas in children and young adults. *Int J Radiat Oncol Biol Phys* 2004;58:714–720.
405. de Vile CJ, Grant DB, Kendall BE, et al. Management of childhood craniopharyngioma: can the morbidity of radical surgery be predicted? *J Neurosurg* 1996;85:73–81.
406. Fisher PG, Jenab J, Gopldthwaite PT, et al. Outcomes and failure patterns in childhood craniopharyngiomas. *Childs Nerv Syst* 1998;14:558–563.
407. Richmond IL, Wilson CB. Parasellar tumors in children. II. Surgical management, radiation therapy and follow-up. *Childs Brain* 1980;7:85–94.
408. Bernstein M, Laperriere NJ. A critical appraisal of brachytherapy for pediatric brain tumors. *Pediatr Neurosurg* 1990–91;16:213–218.
409. Van den Berge JH, Blaauw G, Breeman WA, et al. Intracavitary brachytherapy of cystic craniopharyngiomas. *J Neurosurg* 1992;77:545–550.

410. Mottolese C, Stan H, Hermier M, et al. Intracystic chemotherapy with bleomycin in the treatment of cranipharyngiomas. *Childs Nerv Syst* 2001;17:724–730.
411. Backlund EO. Colloidal radioisotopes as part of a multi-modality treatment of craniopharyngiomas. *J Neurol Sci* 1989;33:95–97.
412. Lyen KR, Grant DB. Endocrine function, morbidity and mortality after surgery for craniopharyngioma. *Arch Dis Child* 1982;57:837–841.
413. Honegger J, Buchfelder M, Fahlbusch R. Surgical treatment of craniopharyngiomas: endocrinological results. *J Neurosurg* 1999;90:251–257.
414. de Vile CJ, Grant DB, Hayward RD, et al. Obesity in childhood craniopharyngioma: relation to post-operative hypothalamic damage shown by magnetic resonance imaging. *J Clin Endocrin Metab* 1996;81:2734–2737.
415. Srinivasan S, Ogle GD, Garnett SP, et al. Features of the metabolic syndrome after childhood craniopharyngioma. *J Clin Endocrinol Metab* 2004;89:81–86.
416. Fahlbusch R, Honegger J, Paulus W, et al. Surgical treatment of craniopharyngiomas: experience with 168 patients. *J Neurosurg* 1999;90:237–250.
417. Anderson CA, Wilkening GN, Filley CM, et al. Neurobehavioral outcome in pediatric craniopharyngioma. *Pediatr Neurosurg* 1997;26:255–260.
418. Poretti A, Grotzer MA, Ribi K, et al. Outcome of craniopharyngioma in children: long-term complications and quality of life. *Dev Med Child Neurol* 2004;46:220–229.
419. Kalapurakal JA, Goldman S, Hsieh YC, et al. Clinical outcome in children with craniopharyngioma treated with primary surgery and radiotherapy deferred until relapse. *Med Pediatr Oncol* 2003;40:214–218.
420. Martin P, Cushing H. Primary gliomas of chiasm and optic nerves in their intracranial portion. *Arch Ophthalmol* 1923;52:209–241.
421. Imes RK, Hoyt WF. Childhood chiasmal gliomas. Update on the fate of patients in the 1969 San Francisco study. *Prog Exp Tumor Res* 1987;30:108–112.
422. Listernick R, Charrow J. Neurofibromatosis type 1 in childhood. *J Pediatr* 1990;116:845–853.
423. Chutorian AM, Schwartz JF, Evans RA, et al. Optic gliomas in children. *Neurology* 1964;14:83–95.
424. Iraci G, Gerosa M, Tomazzoli L, et al. Gliomas of the optic nerve and chiasm: a clinical review. *Childs Brain* 1981;8:326–349.
425. Lindblom B, Truwit CL, Hoyt WF. Optic nerve sheath meningioma. Definition of intraorbital, intracanalicular, and intracranial components with magnetic resonance imaging. *Ophthalmology* 1992;99:560–566.
426. Hollander MD, FitzPatrick M, O'Connor SG, et al. Imaging in ophthalmology II optic gliomas. *Radiol Clin North Am* 1999;37:60–72.
427. Chateil JF, Soussotte C, Pedespan JM, et al. MRI and clinical differences between optic pathway tumours in children with and without neurofibromatosis. *Brit J Radiol* 2001;74:24–31.
428. Dunn DW, Purvin V. Optic pathway gliomas in neurofibromatosis. *Dev Med Child Neurol* 1990;32:820–824.
429. Hoffman HJ, Humphreys RP, Drake JM, et al. Optic pathway/hypothalamic gliomas: a dilemma in management. *Pediatr Neurosurg* 1993;19:186–195.
430. Alvord EC, Lofton S. Gliomas of the optic nerve or chiasm. *J Neurosurg* 1988;68:85–98.
431. Tow SL, Chandela S, Miller NR, et al. Long-term outcome in children with gliomas of the anterior visual pathway. *Pediatric Neurology* 2003;28:262–270.
432. Khafaga Y, Hassounah M, Kandil A, et al. Optic gliomas: a retrospective analysis of 50 cases. *Int J Radiat Oncol Biol Phys* 2003;56:807–812.
433. Tao ML, Barnes PD, Billett AL, et al. Childhood optic chasm gliomas: radiographic response following radiotherapy and long-term clinical outcome. *Int J Radiat Oncol Biol Phys* 1997;39:579–587.
434. Tenny RT, Laws ER Jr, Younge BR, et al. The neurosurgical management of optic glioma. Results in 104 patients. *J Neurosurg* 1982;57:452–458.
435. Jenkin D, et al. Optic glioma in childhood. Resection, irradiation or surveillance? The University of Toronto experience [Abstract]. *Pediatric Neurosurg* 1990–91;16:1–27.
436. Lacaze E, Kieffer V, Streri A, et al. Neuropsychological outcome in children with optic pathway tumours when first-line treatment is chemotherapy. *Brit J Cancer* 2003;89:2038–2044.
437. Stafford SL, Pollock BE, Leavitt JA, et al. A study on the radiation tolerance of the optic nerves and chiasm after stereotactic radiosurgery. *Int J Radiat Oncol Biol Phys* 2003;55:1177–1181.
438. Fuss M, Hug EB, Schaefer RA, et al. Proton radiation therapy (PRT) for pediatric optic pathway gliomas: comparison with 3D planned conventional photons and a standard photon technique. *Int J Radiat Oncol Biol Phys* 1999;45:1117–1126.
439. Packer RJ, Sutton LN, Bilaniuk LT, et al. Treatment of chiasmatic/hypothalamic gliomas of childhood with chemotherapy: an update. *Ann Neurol* 1988;23:79–85.
440. Petronio J, Edwards MS, Prados M, et al. Management of chiasmal and hypothalamic gliomas of infancy and childhood with chemotherapy. *J Neurosurg* 1991;74:701–708.
441. Packer RJ, Lange B, Ater J, et al. Carboplatin and vincristine for recurrent and newly diagnosed low-grade gliomas of childhood. *J Clin Oncol* 1993;11:850–856.
442. Bredel M, Slavc I, Birner P, et al. DNA topoisomerase IIα expression in optic pathway gliomas of childhood. *Eur J Cancer* 2002;38:393–400.
443. Chamberlain MC, Grafe MR. Recurrent chiasmatic-hypothalamic glioma treated with oral etoposide. *J Clin Oncol* 1995;13:2072–2076.
444. Osztie E, Varallyay P, Doolittle ND, et al. Combined intraarterial carboplatin, intraarterial etoposide phosphate, and IV cytoxan chemotherapy for progressive optic-hypothalamic gliomas in young children. *AJNR Am J Neuroradiol* 2001;22:818–823.
445. Vaquero J, Ramiro J, Martínez R. Clinicopathological experience with pineocytomas: report of five surgically treated cases. *Neurosurgery* 1990;27:618–619.
446. Edwards MSB, Hudgins RJ, Wilson CB. Pineal region tumors in children. *J Neurosurg* 1988;68:689–696.
447. Russell WO, Sachs E. Pinealoma: a clinicopathologic study of seven cases with a review of the literature. *Arch Pathol* 1943; 35:869–888.
448. Jooma R, Kendall BE. Diagnosis and management of pineal tumors. *J Neurosurg* 1983;58:654–665.
449. Hoffman HJ, Yoshida M, Becker LE, et al. Experience with pineal region tumors in childhood. *Neurol Res* 1984;6:107–112.
450. Schild SE, Scheithauer BW, Schomberg PJ, et al. Pineal parenchymal tumors: clinical, pathologic, and therapeutic aspects. *Cancer* 1994;72:870–880.
451. Bodensteiner JB, Schaefer GB, Keller GM, et al. Incidental pineal cysts in a prospectively ascertain normal cohort. *Clin Pediatr* 1996;35:277–279.
452. Stein BM, Bruce JN. Surgical management of pineal region tumors. *Clin Neurosurg* 1992;39:509–532.
453. Hiraga S, Arita N, Ohnishi T, et al. A study of 31 juvenile patients with primary intracranial germ cell tumor [Abstract]. *Pediatr Neurosurg* 1990–91;16:118.
454. Chuba PJ, Severson RK, Bhambani K, et al. Male predominance in CNS germ cell tumors: analysis of SEER data. *Neuro-Oncology* 2004;6:418.
455. Kageyama N, Kobayashi T, Kida Y, et al. Intracranial germinal tumors. *Prog Exp Tumor Res* 1987;30:255–267.
456. Posner M, Horrax G. Eye signs in pineal tumors. *J Neurosurg* 1946;3:15–24.
457. Pesin SR, Shields JA. Seven cases of trilateral retinoblastoma. *Am J Ophthalmol* 1989;107:121–126.
458. Zimmerman RA. Computed tomography on pineal, parapineal and histologically related tumors. *Radiology* 1980;137:669–677.
459. Ganti SR, Hilal SK, Stein BM, et al. CT of pineal region tumors. *Am J Neuroradiol* 1986;7:97–104.
460. Hoffman HJ. Pineal region tumors. *Prog Exp Tumor Res* 1987;30:281–288.
461. Edwards MSB, Hudgins RJ, Wilson CB. Pineal region tumors in children. *J Neurosurg* 1988;68:689–696.
462. Matsutani M. Multi-institutional cooperative clinical study for intracranial germ cell tumors in Japan. *Neuro-Oncology* 2004;6:462.

463. Saran FH, Rogers SJ. Pattern of relapse after irradiation alone in localised intracranial germinoma. *Neuro-Oncology* 2004;6:423.
464. Alapetite C, Ricardi U, Saran F, et al. Combined approach with ventricular irradiation for CNS germinoma: the SIOP European Consensus. *Neuro-Oncology* 2004;6:449.
465. Vaquero J, Ramiro J, Martínez R. Clinicopathological experience with pineocytomas: report of five surgically treated cases. *Neurosurgery* 1990;27:618–619.
466. Robertson P, Siffert J, Jakacki R, et al. Multimodality therapy for CNS non-germinoma germ cell tumors (NGGCT): results of a phase II consortium. *Neuro-Oncology* 2004;6:465.
467. Husain M, Jha D, Thaman D, et al. Ventriculostomy in a tumor involving the third ventricular floor. *Neurosurg Rev* 2004;27:70–72.
468. Shin JH, Lee HK, Jeong AK, et al. Choroid plexus papilloma in the posterior cranial fossa MR, CT, and angiographic findings. *Clin Imaging* 2001:25:154–162.
469. Packer RJ, Perilongo G, Johnson D, et al. Choroid plexus carcinoma of childhood. *Cancer* 1992;69:580–585.
470. Pierga JY, Kalifa C, Terrier-Lacombe MJ, et al. Carcinoma of the choroid plexus: a pediatric experience. *Med Pediatr Oncol* 1993;21:480–487.
471. Zwetsloot CP, Kros JM, Pay y, Gueze HD. Familial occurrence of tumors of the choroid plexus. *J Med Genet* 1991;28:492–494.
472. Trifiletti RR, Incorpora G, Polizzi A, et al. Aicardi syndrome with multiple tumors: a case report with literature review. *Brain Dev* 1995;17:283–285.
473. Erman T, Gocer AI, Erdogan S, et al. Choroid plexus papilloma of bilateral lateral ventricle. *Acta Neurochir* 2003;145:139–143.
474. Rickert CH, Wiestler OD, Paulus W. Chromosomal imbalances in choroid plexus tumors. *Am J Pathol* 2002;160:1105–1113.
475. Grill J, Avet-Loiseau H, Lellouch-Tubiana A, et al. Comparative genomic hybridization detects specific cytogenetic abnormalities in pediatric ependymomas and choroid plexus papillomas. *Cancer Genet Cytogenet* 2002;136:121–125.
476. Johnson DL. Management of choroid plexus tumors in children. *Pediatr Neurosci* 1989;15:195–206.
477. Maria BL, Graham ML, Strauss LC, et al. Response of a recurrent choroid plexus tumor to combination chemotherapy. *J Neurooncol* 1985;3:259–262.
478. Mathiesen T, Grane P, Lindgren L, et al. Third ventricle colloid cysts: a consecutive 12-year series. *J Neurosurg* 1997;86:5–12.
479. Macaulay RJ, Felix I, Jay V, et al. Histological and ultrastructural analysis of six colloid cysts in children. *Acta Neuropathol* 1997;93:271–276.
480. Teng P, Papatheodorou C. Tumors of cerebral ventricles in children. *J Nerv Ment Dis* 1966;142:87–93.
481. Antunes JL, Louis KM, Ganti SR. Colloid cysts of the third ventricle. *Neurosurgery* 1980;7:450–455.
482. Kava MP, Tullu MS, Deshmukh CT, et al. Colloid cyst of the third ventricle: a cause of sudden death in a child. *In J Cancer* 2003;40:31 33.
483. Armao D, Castillo M, Chen H, et al. Colloid cyst of the third ventricle: imaging-pathologic correlation. *Am J Neuroradiol* 2000;21:1470–1477.
484. Solaroglu I, Beskonakli E, Kaptanoglu E, et al. Transcortical-transventricular approach in colloid custs of the third ventricle: surgical experience with 26 cases. *Neurosurg Rev* 2004;27:89–92.
485. Desai KI, Nadkarni TD, Muzumdar DP, et al. Surgical management of colloid cyst of the third ventricle—a study of 105 cases. *Surg Neurol* 2002;57:295–304.
486. McMackin D, Cockburn J, Anslow P, et al. Correlation of fornix damage with memory impairment in six cases of colloid cyst removal. *Acta Neurochir* 1995;13:12–18.
487. Arafah BM, Nasrallah MP. Pituitary tumors: pathophysiology, clinical manifestations, and management. *Endocr Relat Cancer* 2001;8:287–305.
488. Styne DM, Grumbach MM, Kaplan SL, et al. Treatment of Cushing's disease in childhood and adolescence by transsphenoidal microadenomectomy. *N Engl J Med* 1984;310:889–893.
489. Cannavo S, Venturino M, Curto L, et al. Clinical presentation and outcome of pituitary adenomas in teenagers. *Clin Endocrinol* 2003;58:519–527.
490. Hagiwara A, Inoue Y, Wakasa K, et al. Comparison of growth hormone-producing and non-growth hormone-producing pituitary adenomas: imaging characteristics and pathologic correlation. *Radiology* 2003;228:533–538.
491. Kanter SL, Mickle JP, Hunter SB, et al. Pituitary adenomas in pediatric patients: are they more invasive? *Pediatr Neurosci* 1985;12:202–204.
492. Gjerris F. Clinical aspects and long-term prognosis in supratentorial tumors in infancy and childhood. *Acta Neurol Scand* 1978;57:445–470.
493. Fountas KN, Karampelas I, Nikolakakos LG, et al. Primary spinal cord oligodendroglioma: case report and review of the literature. *Childs Nerv Syst* 2004;[Epub ahead of print].
494. Jacob R, Jyothirmayi R, Dalal Y, et al. Oligodendroglioma: clinical profile and treatment results. *Neurol India* 2002;50:462–466.
495. Leonardi MA, Lumenta CB. Oligodendrogliomas in the CT/MR era. *Acta Neurochir* 2001;143:1195–1203.
496. Reifenberger J, Reifenberger G, Liu L, et al. Molecular genetic analysis of oligodendroglial tumors shows preferential allelic deletions on 19p and 1p. *Am J Pathol* 1994;145:1175–1190.
497. Kraus JA, Koopmann J, Kaskel P, et al. Shared allelic losses on chromosomes 1p and 19q suggest a common origin of oligodendroglioma and oligoastrocytoma. *J Neuropathol Exp Neurol* 1995;54:91–95.
498. Hashimoto N, Murakami M, Takahashi Y, et al. Correlation between genetic alteration and long-term clinical outcome of patients with oligodendroglial tumors, with identification of a consistent region of deletion on chromosome arm 1p. *Cancer* 2003;97:2254–2261.
499. Sutton LN, Packer RJ, Zimmerman RA, et al. Cerebral gangliogliomas of childhood. *Prog Exp Tumor Res* 1987;30:239–246.
500. Wolf HK, Muller MB, Spanle M, et al. Ganglioglioma: a detailed histopathological and immunohistochemical analysis of 61 cases. *Acta Neuropathol (Berl)* 1994;88:166–173.
501. Miller DC, Lang FF, Epstein FJ. Central nervous system gangliogliomas. Part 1. Pathology. *J Neurosurg* 1993;79:859–866.
502. Jay V, Squire J, Becker LE, et al. Malignant transformation in a ganglioglioma with anaplastic neuronal and astrocytic components. Report of a case with flow cytometric and cytogenetic analysis. *Cancer* 1994;73:2862–2868.
503. Blümcke I, Wiestler OD. Gangliogliomas: an intriguing tumor entity associated with focal epilepsies. *J Neuropathol Exp Neurol* 2002;61:575–584.
504. Cooper M, Dohn DF. Intracranial meningiomas in childhood. *Clev Clin Quart* 1974;41:197–204.
505. Merten DF, Gooding CA, Newton TH, et al. Meningiomas of childhood and adolescence. *J Pediatr* 1974;84:696–700.
506. Howe JG, Gibson JD. Uncinate seizures and tumors, a myth reexamined. *Ann Neurol* 1982;12:2–27.
507. Page LK, Lombroso CT, Matson DD. Childhood epilepsy with late detection of cerebral glioma. *J Neurosurg* 1969;31:253–261.
508. Blume WT, Girvin JP, Kaufmann JCE. Childhood brain tumors presenting as chronic uncontrolled focal seizure disorders. *Ann Neurol* 1982;12:538–541.
509. Dropcho EJ, Wisoff JH, Walker RW, et al. Supratentorial malignant gliomas in childhood: a review of fifty cases. *Ann Neurol* 1987;22:355–364.
510. Laws ER Jr, Taylor WF, Bergstralh EJ, et al. Neurosurgical management of low-grade astrocytoma of the cerebral hemispheres. *J Neurosurg* 1984;61:665–673.
511. Gajjar A, Heideman RL, Kovnar EH, et al. Response of pediatric low grade gliomas to chemotherapy. *Pediatr Neurosurg* 1993;19:113–120.
512. North CA, North RB, Epstein JA, et al. Low-grade cerebral astrocytomas. Survival and quality of life after radiation therapy. *Cancer* 1990;66:6–14.
513. Berger MS, Ojemann GA, Lettich E. Neurophysiological monitoring during astrocytoma surgery. *Neurosurg Clin N Am* 1990;1:65–80.
514. Black PM. The present and future of cerebral tumor surgery in children. *Childs Nerv Syst* 2000;16:821–828.
515. Sposto R, Ertel IJ, Jenkin RD, et al. The effectiveness of chemotherapy for treatment of high grade astrocytoma in children: results of a randomized trial. *J Neurooncol* 1989;7:165–177.
516. Weisfeld-Adams J, Murphy DM, Wisoff JH, et al. The impact of

extent of surgical resection of consensus-reviewed pediatric intracranial high-grade glioma on outcome: a report of the Children's Cancer Group trial no. CCG-945. *Neuro-Oncology* 2004;6:468.
517. Batra V, Sposto R, Geyer JR, et al. Long-term outcome for children less than six years of age with diagnosis of consensus reviewed high-grade gliomas: a report of the CCG-945 study. *Neuro-Oncology* 2004;6:450.
518. Dufour C, Grill J, Lellouch-Tubiana A, et al. High-grade gliomas (HGG) in children below 5 years of age: results of a chemotherapy only approach with the BBSFOP protocol. A multicenter trial of the French Society of Pediatric Oncology. *Neuro-Oncology* 2004;6:453.
519. Mahaley MS Jr, Mettlin C, Natarajan N, et al. National survey of patterns of care for brain-tumor patients. *J Neurosurg* 1989;71:826–836.
520. Phuphanich S, Edwards MS, Levin VA, et al. Supratentorial malignant gliomas of childhood. Results of treatment with radiation therapy and chemotherapy. *J Neurosurg* 1984;60:495–499.
521. Jakacki R, Prados M, Yates A, et al. A phase I trial of temozolomide and CCNU in pediatric patients with newly diagnosed incompletely resected non-brainstem high-grade gliomas (HGG): a Children's Oncology Group study. *Neuro-Oncology* 2004;6:459.
522. Cairncross JG, Macdonald DR. Successful chemotherapy for recurrent malignant oligodendroglioma. *Ann Neurol* 1988;23:260–364.
523. Mahoney DH Jr, Strother D, Camitta B, et al. High-dose melphalan and cyclophosphamide with autologous bone marrow rescue for recurrent/progressive malignant brain tumor in children: a pilot pediatric oncology group study. *J Clin Oncol* 1996;14:382–388.
524. Sneed PK, Russo C, Scharfen CO, et al. Long-term follow-up after high-activity ^{125}I brachytherapy for pediatric brain tumors. *Pediatr Neurosurg* 1996;24:314–322.
525. Coffey RJ, Lunsford LD, Flickinger JC. The role of radiosurgery in the treatment of malignant brain tumors. *Neurosurg Clin N Am* 1992;3:231–244.
526. Pollock BE, Gorman DA, Schomberg PJ, et al. The Mayo Clinic gamma knife experience: indications and initial results. *Mayo Clin Proc* 1999;74:5–13.
527. Fathallah-Shaykh H. New molecular strategies to cure brain tumors. *Arch Neurol* 1999;56:449–453.
528. Tomita T, McLone DG. Brain tumors during the first twenty-four months of life. *Neurosurgery* 1985;17:913–919.
529. Deutsch M. Radiotherapy for primary brain tumors in very young children. *Cancer* 1982;50:2785–2789.
530. Jooma R, Kendall BE, Hayward RD. Intracranial tumors in neonates: a report of seventeen cases. *Surg Neurol* 1984;21:165–170.
531. Strauss LC, Killmond TM, Carson BS, et al. Efficacy of postoperative chemotherapy using cisplatin plus etoposide in young children with brain tumors. *Med Pediatr Oncol* 1991;19:16–21.
532. Krischer JP, Regab AH, Kun L, et al. Nitrogen mustard, vincristine, procarbazine, and prednisone as adjuvant chemotherapy in the treatment of medulloblastoma. *J Neurosurg* 1991;74:905–909.
533. Kovnar EH, Kellie SJ, Horowitz ME, et al. Preirradiation cisplatin and etoposide in the treatment of high-risk medulloblastoma and other malignant embryonal tumors of the central nervous system: a phase II study. *J Clin Oncol* 1990;8:330–336.
534. Finlay J, Boyett JM, Yates AJ, et al. Randomized phase III trial in childhood high-grade astrocytomas comparing vincristine, lomustine and prednisone with eight-drug-in-one-day regimen. *J Clin Oncol* 1995;13:112–123.
535. Grill J, Sainte-Rose C, Jouvet A, et al. Localized medulloblastomas can be cured without recourse to craniospinal irradiation provided complete surgery can be carried out: final results of the first french prospective study in children below five years of age (BBSFOP). *Neuro-Oncology* 2004;6:457.
536. Ridola V, Doz F, Frappaz D, et al. High dose chemotherapy and posterior fossa radiotherapy for children less than 3–5 years with localized high risk medulloblastoma at diagnosis or at relapse. The SFOP experience. *Neuro-Oncology* 2004;6:465.
537. Rutkowski S, Bode U, Deinlein F, et al. Cure of children less than three years of age with medulloblastoma (M0/M1-stage) by postoperative chemotherapy only: final results of the HIT-SKK'92 study. *Neuro-Oncology* 2004;6:469.
538. Maria BL. High dose chemotherapy in the treatment of children with infiltrative brain tumors. *Int Pediatr* 1993;8:244–249.
539. Kedar A, Maria BL, Graham-Pole J, et al. High-dose chemotherapy with marrow reinfusion and hyperfractionated irradiation for children with high-risk brain tumors. *Med Pediatr Oncol* 1994;23:428–436.
540. Shen V, Woodbury C, Killen R, et al. Collection and use of peripheral blood stem cells in young children with refractory solid tumors. *Bone Marrow Transplant* 1997;19:197–204.
541. Picton S, Robinson K, Weston C, et al. A UKCCSG study of the treatment of relapsed CNS primitive neuroectodermal tumours using high dose chemotherapy. *Neuro-Oncology* 2004;6:464.
542. Pascual-Castroviejo I. Epidemiology of spinal cord tumors in children. In: Pascual-Castroviejo I, ed. *International review of child neurology series: spinal tumors in children and adolescents*. New York: Raven Press, 1990:1–10.
543. Di Lorenzo N, Giuffre R, Fortuna A. Primary spinal neoplasms in childhood: analysis of 1234 published cases (including 56 personal cases) by pathology, sex, age and site. Differences from the situation in adults. *Neurochirurgia (Stuttg)* 1982;25:153–164.
544. Arseni C, Horvath L, Iliescu D. Intraspinal tumours in children. *Psychiatr Neurol Neurochir* 1967;70:123–133.
545. Stella G, De Sanctis N, Boero S, et al. Benign tumors of the pediatric spine: statistical notes. *Chir Organi Mov* 1998;83:15–21.
546. Murovic J, Sundaresan N. Pediatric spinal axis tumors. *Neurosurg Clin N Am* 1992;3:947–958.
547. Pascual-Castroviejo I, ed. *Spinal tumors in children and adolescents*. New York: Raven Press, 1990.
548. Jallo GI, Freed D, Epstein F. Intramedullary spinal cord tumors in children. *Childs Nerv Syst* 2003;19:641–649.
549. Sharma MC, Aggarwal M, Ralte AM, et al. Clinicopathological study of spinal teratomas. A series of 10 cases. *J Neurosurg Sci* 2003;47:95–100.
550. Kluwe L, Mautner V, Heinrich B, et al. NF1 mutations and clinical spectrum in patients with spinal neurofibromatosis. *J Med Genet* 2003;40:368–371.
551. Steinbok P, Cochrane DD, Poskitt K. Intramedullary spinal cord tumors in children. *Neurosurg Clin N Am* 1992;3:931–945.
552. O'Sullivan C, Jenkin RD, Doherty MA, et al. Spinal cord tumors in children: long-term results of combined surgical and radiation treatment. *J Neurosurg* 1994;81:507–512.
553. Escalona-Zapata J. Epidemiology of spinal cord tumors in children. In: Pascual-Castroviejo I, ed. *International review of child neurology series: spinal tumors in children and adolescents*. New York: Raven Press, 1990:11–34.
554. Kwon OK, Wang KC, Kim CJ, et al. Primary intramedullary spinal cord primitive neuroectodermal tumor with intracranial seeding in an infant. *Childs Nerv Syst* 1996;12:633–636.
555. Nam DH, Cho BK, Kim YM, et al. Intramedullary anaplastic oligodendroglioma in a child. *Childs Nerv Syst* 1998;14:127–130.
556. Chadduck WM, Frederick AB, Sawyer JR. Cytogenetic studies of pediatric brain and spinal cord tumors. *Pediatr Neurosurg* 1991–92;17:57–65.
557. Levy WJ, Bay J, Dohn D. Spinal cord meningioma. *J Neurosurg* 1982;57:804–812.
558. Richardson FL. A report of 16 tumors of the spinal cord: the importance of spinal rigidity as an early sign of disease. *J Pediatr* 1960;57:42–54.
559. Constantini S, Houten J, Miller DC, et al. Intramedullary spinal cord tumors in children under the age of 3 years. *J Neurosurg* 1996;85:1036–1043.
560. Buchanan DN. Tumors of the spinal cord in infancy [Abstract]. *Arch Neurol Psychiatry* 1950;63:835.
561. Haft H, Ransohoff J, Carter S. Spinal cord tumors in children. *Pediatrics* 1959;23:1152–1159.
562. Ross AT, Bailey OT. Tumors arising within the spinal canal in children. *Neurology* 1953;3:922–930.
563. Oi S, Raimondi AJ. Hydrocephalus associated with intraspinal neoplasms in childhood. *Am J Dis Child* 1981;135:1122–1124.
564. Rifkinson-Mann S, Wisoff JH, Epstein F. The association of hydrocephalus with intramedullary spinal cord tumors: a series of 25 patients. *Neurosurgery* 1990;27:749–754.
565. Innocenzi G, Raco A, Cantore G, et al. Intramedullary astrocytomas and ependymomas in the pediatric age group: a retrospective study. *Childs Nerv Syst* 1996;12:776–780.

566. Bouffet E, Pierre-Kahn A, Marchal JC, et al. Prognostic factors in pediatric spinal cord astrocytoma. *Cancer* 1998;83:2391–2399.
567. Robertson PL. Atypical presentations of spinal cord tumors in children. *J Child Neurol* 1992;7:360–363.
568. Eeg-Olofsson O, Carlsson E, Jeppson S. Recurrent abdominal pains as the first symptom of spinal cord tumor. *Acta Paediatr Scand* 1981;70:595–597.
569. Taylor LJ. Painful scoliosis: a need for further investigation. *BMJ* 1985;292:120–122.
570. Blaser S, Harwood-Nash D. Pediatric spinal neoplasms. *Top Magn Reson Imaging* 1993;5:190–202.
571. Quisling RG. Imaging for pediatric brain tumors. *Semin Pediatr Neurol* 1997;4:254–272.
572. Epstein FJ, Farmer JP, Schneider SJ. Intraoperative ultrasonography: an important surgical adjunct for intramedullary tumors. *J Neurosurg* 1991;74:729–733.
573. Kothbauer K, Deletis V, Epstein FJ. Intraoperative spinal cord monitoring for intramedullary surgery: an essential adjunct. *Pediatr Neurosurg* 1997;26:247–254.
574. Epstein FJ. Surgical treatment of intramedullary spinal cord tumors of childhood. In: Pascual-Castroviejo I, ed. *International review of child neurology series: spinal tumors in children and adolescents*. New York: Raven Press, 1990:51–70.
575. Mottl H, Koutecky J. Treatment of spinal cord tumors in children. *Med Pediatr Oncol* 1997;29:293–295.
576. Goh KY, Velasquez L, Epstein FJ. Pediatric intramedullary spinal cord tumors: is surgery alone enough? *Pediatr Neurosurg* 1997;27:34–39.
577. Godwin-Austin RB, Howell DA, Worthington B. Observations in radiation myelopathy. *Brain* 1975;98:557–568.
578. DiChiro G, Herdt JR. Angiographic demonstration of spinal cord arterial occlusion in post-radiation myelomalacia. *Radiology* 1973;106:317–319.
579. Wara WM, Phillips TL, Sheline GE, et al. Radiation tolerance of the spinal cord. *Cancer* 1975;35:1558–1562.
580. Perilongo G, Gardiman M, Bisaglia L, et al. Spinal low-grade neoplasms with extensive leptomeningeal dissemination in children. *Childs Nerv Syst* 2002;18:505–512.
581. Quincke H. Ueber Meningitis serosa. *Volkmann's Sammlung klinischer Vorträge*. N F 1893, Nr. 67. Cited In: Quincke H. Ueber Meningitis serosa und verwandte Zustände. *Deutsch Z Nervenheilk* 1897;9:149–168.
582. Johnston I, Paterson A. Benign intracranial hypertension. I. Diagnosis and prognosis. *Brain* 1974;97:289–300.
583. Corbett JJ, Digre K. Idiopathic intracranial hypertension. An answer to "the chicken or the egg?" *Neurology* 2002;58:5–6.
583a. Binder DK, et al. Idiopathic intracranial hypertension. *Neurosurgery* 2004;54:538–551.
584. Feldman MH, Schlezinger NS. Benign intracranial hypertension associated with hypervitaminosis A. *Arch Neurol* 1970;22:1–7.
585. Soler D, Cox T, Bullock P, et al. Diagnosis and management of benign intracranial hypertension. *Arch Dis Child* 1998;78:89–94.
585a. Tabassi A, Salmasi AH, Jalali M. Serum and CSF vitamin A concentrations in idiopathic intracranial hypertension. *Neurology* 2005;64:1893–1896.
586. Konrad D, Kuster H, Hunziker UA. Pseudotumour cerebri after varicella. *Eur J Pediatr* 1998;157:904–906.
587. Walker AE, Adamkiewicz JJ. Pseudotumor cerebri associated with prolonged corticosteroid therapy: reports of four cases. *JAMA* 1964;188:779–784.
588. Gills JP, Kapp JP, Odom GL. Benign intracranial hypertension: pseudotumor cerebri from obstruction of dural sinuses. *Arch Ophthalmol* 1967;78:592–595.
589. Rush JA. Pseudotumor cerebri: clinical profile and visual outcome in 63 patients. *Mayo Clin Proc* 1980;55:541–546.
590. Greer M. Benign intracranial hypertension. IV. Menarche. *Neurology* 1964;14:569–573.
591. McComb JG. Recent research into the nature of cerebrospinal fluid formation and absorption. *J Neurosurg* 1983;59:369–383.
592. Moser FG, Hilal SK, Abrams G, et al. MR imaging of pseudotumor cerebri. *Am J Radiol* 1988;4:903–909.
592a. Farb RI, Vanek I, Scott JN, et al. Idiopathic intracranial hypertension. The prevalence and morphology of sinovenous stenosis. *Neurology* 2003;60:1418–1424.
592b. King JO, Mitchell PJ, Thompson KR, et al. Manometry combined with cervical puncture in idiopathic intracranial hypertension. *Neurology* 2002;58:26–30.
593. Foley J. Benign forms of intracranial hypertension—"toxic" and "otitic" hydrocephalus. *Brain* 1955;78:1–41.
594. Greer M. Benign intracranial hypertension. I. Mastoiditis and lateral sinus obstruction. *Neurology* 1962;12:472–476.
595. Phillips, Paul H. Pseudotumor cerebri: Idiopathic intracranial hypertension. In: *Current management in child neurology*, 2nd ed. Bernard L. Maria, ed. London: BC Decker Inc, 2002:503–508.
596. Babikian P, Corbett J, Bell W. Idiopathic intracranial hypertension in children: the Iowa experience. *J Child Neurol* 1994;9:144–149.
597. Speer C, Pearlman J, Phillips PH, et al. Fourth cranial nerve palsy in pediatric patients with pseudotumor cerebri. *Am J Ophthalmol* 1999;127:236–237.
597a. Friedman DI, Jacobson DM. Diagnostic criteria for idiopathic intracranial hypertension. *Neurology* 2002;59:1492–1495.
598. Jacobson DM, Karanjia PN, Olson KA, et al. Computed tomography ventricular size has no predictive value in diagnosing pseudotumor cerebri. *Neurology* 1990;40:1454–1455.
599. Cinciripini GS, Donahue S, Borchert MS. Idiopathic intracranial hypertension in prepubertal pediatric patients: characteristics, treatment, and outcome. *Am J Ophthalmol* 1999;127:178–82.
600. Rosenberg ML, Corbett JJ, Smith C, et al. Cerebrospinal fluid diversion procedures in pseudotumor cerebri. *Neurology* 1993;43:1071–1072.
601. Corbett JJ, Thompson HS. The rational management of idiopathic intracranial hypertension. *Arch Neurol* 1989;46:1049–1051.
602. Baker RS, Baumann RJ, Buncic JR. Idiopathic intracranial hypertension (pseudotumor cerebri) in pediatric patients. *Pediatr Neurol* 1989;5:5–11.
603. Grant DN. Benign intracranial hypertension. A review of 79 cases in infancy and childhood. *Arch Dis Child* 1971;46:651–655.
604. Guidetti B, Giuffre R, Gambacorta D. Follow-up study of 100 cases of pseudotumor cerebri. *Acta Neurochir* 1968;18:259–267.
605. Corbett JJ, Savino PJ, Thomson HS, et al. Visual loss in pseudotumor cerebri. Follow up of 57 patients from 5 to 41 years and a profile of 14 patients with permanent severe visual loss. *Arch Neurol* 1982;39:461–474.
606. Brazis PW, Lee AG. Elevated intracranial pressure and pseudotumor cerebri. *Curr Opin Ophthalmol* 1998;9(6):27 32.
607. Rekate HL, Wallace D. Lumboperitoneal shunts in children. *Pediatr Neurosurg* 2003;38:41–46.
608. Sugerman HJ, Sugerman EL, DeMaria EJ, et al. Bariatric surgery for severely obese adolescents. *J Gastrointest Surg* 2003;7:102–107.

Chapter 12

Neurocutaneous Syndromes

Bernard L. Maria and John H. Menkes

The neurocutaneous syndromes are marked by the conjoined abnormalities of skin and nervous system. The term *phakomatoses* (*phakomatosis* from fakos, Greek for *lentil*) is reserved for a group of diseases in which the subject is predisposed to tumors of the skin, nervous system, and other organs. The major entities included among the phakomatoses are the neurofibromatoses, tuberous sclerosis (TS), Sturge-Weber syndrome (SWS), von Hippel–Lindau disease, ataxia-telangiectasia (AT), and hypomelanosis of Ito (HI).

Additionally, numerous other conditions exist, many of uncertain heredity and some extremely rare, in which abnormalities of skin are linked with those of the nervous system. These are detailed in a book edited by Gomez (1).

Though a common pathogenesis of all neurocutaneous syndromes has eluded investigators for a century because the various diseases in this category have very different clinical presentations, genetic transmissions, and pathological findings, a unifying etiology has recently been proposed. This suggests that all neurocutaneous syndromes are disorders of neural crest (i.e., neurocristopathies) that can affect all three primitive germ layers. The known genes that regulate neural crest formation, migration or terminal differentiation also serve as tumor-suppressor genes (e.g., NF1, TSC1,2), hence the high incidence of neoplasms, both benign and malignant, in these diseases (1a).

NEUROFIBROMATOSIS (VON RECKLINGHAUSEN DISEASE)

No longer considered to be a single disorder, neurofibromatosis has been divided into at least two genetically distinct forms. The common form, once known as *peripheral neurofibromatosis*, is called *neurofibromatosis 1* (NF1). The other, rarer form, once termed *central neurofibromatosis*, is now called *neurofibromatosis 2* (NF2). Additionally, several authorities distinguish segmental neurofibromatosis, in which the features of NF1 are confined to one part of the body; spinal neurofibromatosis, characterized by the late appearance of spinal cord tumors; and a condition marked by autosomal dominant café au lait spots. Oh and colleagues have recently reported that a subset of patients may meet diagnostic criteria for both NF1 and NF2 (2).

Neurofibromatosis 1

NF1 is characterized by multiple tumors within the central and peripheral nervous systems, cutaneous pigmentation, and lesions of the vascular system and viscera. Additionally, a tendency exists for a variety of tissues to undergo malignant transformation. Although it was described initially in the eighteenth century, and more succinctly in 1849 by Smith (3), von Recklinghausen in 1882 first combined the various features of the condition and termed it *neurofibromatosis* (4). The disease occurs in approximately 2 to 3 per 10,000 live births and is transmitted as a dominant trait with variable expression but virtually complete penetrance by the age of 5 years (5). It is the most common single-gene defect to affect the nervous system. Approximately one-half of the cases appear to be sporadic, and the mutation rate has been estimated at 1 in 10,000 gametes per generation, one of the highest mutation rates in humans (6). Stephens and coworkers found that 93% of new mutations were in the paternally derived chromosome (7). For as yet unknown reasons, no parental age effect occurs. As determined by linkage analysis and translocation breakpoints, the gene for NF1 is located on the long arm of chromosome 17, near the centromere (q11.2). It has been cloned and consists of 60 exons that are spread out over 350 kb of genomic DNA and gives rise to three alternative-spliced messenger RNA transcripts (8,9). NF1 is heterogeneous at the mutation level, with more than 300 independent mutations having been reported (10). The gene encodes a cytoplasmic protein, named *neurofibromin*, which contains a 2818 amino acid segment whose only demonstrated function is down-regulation of the Ras signal transduction. The peptide domain encoded by exons 21 to 27 activates the intrinsic guanosine triphosphatase of Ras proteins (N-, K-, and H-ras), which leads to hydrolysis of bound guanosine triphosphate and inactivation of downstream signaling. Neurofibromin inactivates the tumor gene *p21ras* by stimulating its GTPase activity and converting the active form of *p21ras* into its inactive form. Inasmuch as the active form of *p21ras* is a specific growth regulator for astrocytes, the NF1 gene functions as a tumor-suppressor gene (11–13). This is confirmed by the observation that loss of NF1 gene expression occurs in at least some neurofibroma, in neurosarcoma, and in leukemic cells derived from NF1 subjects (11,14,15). Neurofibromin also has been shown to be associated with cytoplasmic microtubules in the brain and is believed to be involved in signaling within the central nervous system (CNS).

The NF1 gene is large and is intrinsically hypermutable; more than 300 mutations have been described, and only rarely has the same mutation been identified in unrelated patients. Mutations include large deletions seen in 7.5% to 17% of patients (16,17), frame shifts, stop mutations, and point mutations. The majority (60% to 70%) of mutations result in the formation of truncated and nonfunctioning neurofibromin. Somatic mosaicism is fairly common; its exact frequency has not been ascertained (16). NF1 gene expression is complex and is modulated post-transcriptionally by numerous alternative splicings and RNA editing (18). Some of the alternative transcripts lack tumor suppressor activity and are developmentally regulated. Their role in producing the clinical phenotype of NF1 is not understood (9,18,19).

It, therefore, comes as no surprise that there is much variability in the expression of NF1, even within the same family. Since the NF1 gene was cloned in 1990, two major pathogenetic mechanisms have been considered: (a) loss of NF1 function as a tumor suppressor gene, and (b) heterozygous mutation of the gene leads to haploinsufficiency of the gene product (20). A detailed review of the pathogenesis is beyond the scope of this text. The interested reader is referred to a chapter by Huson and Korf (5).

Correlation between the genetic mutation and the clinical expression is still poor. However, a significant proportion of subjects with severe manifestations, including dysmorphic features, have large deletions in the NF1 gene (21).

Pathology

The most striking neuropathologic feature of neurofibromatosis 1 is the presence of tumors along the major peripheral nerves, with the ulnar and radial nerves being involved most frequently. Neurofibromas are the most common tumor type, but schwannomas also can be seen. Tumors that are prone to develop within the CNS include primarily optic gliomas; pilocytic astrocytomas of the third ventricle, cerebellum, and spinal cord; and high-grade astrocytomas (22,23). Additionally, neurofibromatosis has been associated with a number of other neoplastic processes with a greater than random frequency (24). These include leukemia, Wilms tumor, neuroblastoma, and pheochromocytoma (25). A syndrome of multiple endocrine neoplasia characterized by bilateral pheochromocytomas, medullary thyroid carcinoma, and multiple neuromas and café au lait lesions has been delineated (26). Although generally benign, both central and peripheral neurofibromas can undergo malignant degeneration. This is particularly likely to occur with the plexiform neurofibroma, for which the risk for malignant transformation to neurofibrosarcoma has been estimated at 5% (27).

Clinical Manifestations

NF1 is a progressive disease process that can affect almost every organ. When many peripheral lesions are present, few lesions tend to be within the CNS. The reverse also is true (28).

The most common skin lesions are the café au lait spots. These are numerous light brown areas, usually located over the trunk, with smooth, well-defined borders and uniform pigmentation. They are seen in virtually every patient with NF1, and they result from an aggregation of neural crest-derived pigmented melanoblasts in the basal layer of the epidermis (5). They are present at birth, and their number and size increase until puberty. According to Crowe and associates, at least six such lesions are necessary for a diagnosis of NF1 (29). There is no correlation between the number of spots and the severity of the NF1. Less frequent are diffuse freckling, freckling in the armpits and groin that tends to begin between 3 and 5 years of age, and large areas of faintly increased pigmentation (melanoderma). Although usually present before the onset of neurologic symptoms, these pigmentary abnormalities are not striking during infancy but intensify with age, particularly after puberty.

Various types of cutaneous tumors can be found (Fig. 12.1). The most characteristic for NF1 is the pedunculated molluscum fibrosum and the subcutaneous neurofibromas. The latter consist of an overgrowth of Schwann cells admixed with tortuous nerve fibers and perineural fibroblasts. The number of neurofibromas is highly variable, and they are located singly or in groups along nerve trunks. Generally, cutaneous tumors tend to enlarge slowly throughout life, and they occur at an unpredictable rate (20). Plexiform neurofibromas can occur in all affected tissues and lead to exophthalmos, or defects of the skull and orbit, or hypertrophy of one or more extremity, sometimes with overlying hyperpigmentation. Plexiform neurofibromas can be quite extensive and infiltrative and can be associated with soft tissue overgrowth. There is a risk that a neurofibroma will transform into a malignant peripheral nerve sheath tumor, which is associated with anaplastic changes and multiple mitoses. The lifetime risk for malignant peripheral nerve sheath tumor is estimated to be 5 to 10% (30).

Multiple nodules within the iris (iris hamartomas) (Fig. 12.2) were first described by Lisch (31). Lisch nodules are seen in almost all affected individuals aged 21 or more

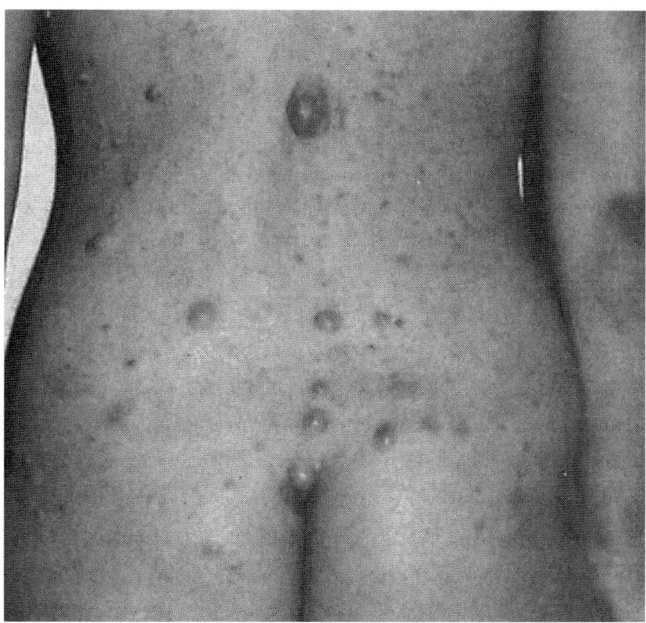

FIGURE 12.2. Neurofibromatosis. Posterior view demonstrating various types of cutaneous tumors. These include the pedunculated molluscum fibrosum and subcutaneous neurofibromas. Note the area of hyperpigmentation of the right elbow and a typical café au lait lesion. (Courtesy of Dr. V. M. Riccardi, Neurofibromatosis Institute, La Crescenta, CA.)

years, but only in one-half of children aged 5 to 6 years (32). Initially light colored, these melanocytic hamartomas become darker with time. They do not affect vision, but they are helpful diagnostic markers (32).

Short stature is common. It was seen in 31.5% of patients in the series of Huson and Korf (5). In some children, a number of risk factors, including suprasellar lesions and skeletal deformities are responsible. In addition, growth hormone deficiency can be common; Vassilopoulou-Sellin and coworkers found defective growth hormone levels in 79% of children who had no obvious medical or radiologic lesions to account for their short stature (33).

Macrocephaly is common, and 16% of children in Riccardi's series (27), 45% of children in the series of Huson and Korf (5), and 38% of children in Young and coworkers (35) series had a head circumference at or above the 98th percentile (34). Only rarely is there associated hydrocephalus, typically owing to aqueductal stenosis. Various skeletal abnormalities not associated with tumors have been described. The most common location for dysplasia of a long bone is the tibia, although other long bones can be affected (36). Low cervical or thoracic kyphoscoliosis can result in a narrow angulation of the spine that may require surgery in 5% of patients (35,37). Scoliosis was noted in 32% of children in the series of Holt, and its incidence increases with age (38). Less commonly, one observes scalloping of the posterior portion of the vertebral bodies. This scalloping is caused by a dural ectasia, the

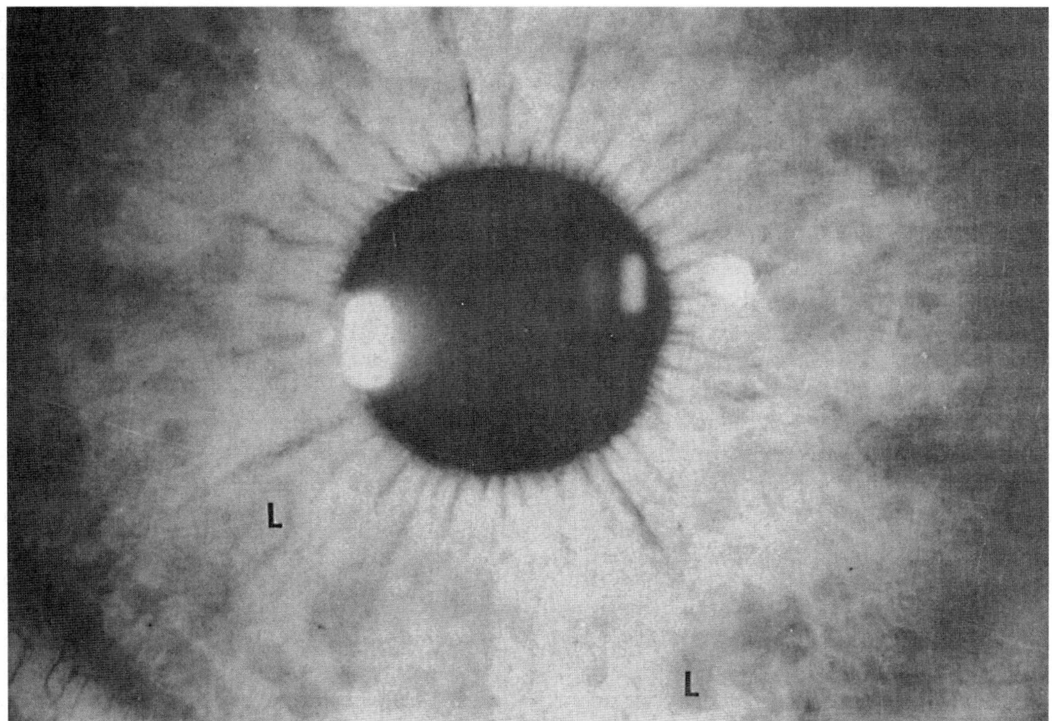

FIGURE 12.1. Lisch nodules of iris (L). (Courtesy of Dr. Bronwyn Bateman, Department of Ophthalmology, University of Colorado School of Medicine, Denver.)

consequence of congenital weakness of the dura and the resulting pressure on the vertebral bodies. Anterior and lateral meningoceles, which are more common in adults, also result from the dural weakness. Bony rarefactions, the consequence of subperiosteal neurofibromas, can arise within the spine, the pelvis, particularly the iliac wings, or the skull. These rarefactions can induce pathologic fractures. Bony overgrowth, often with contiguous elephantiasis, is seen in approximately 10% of patients. Radiographic findings are reviewed by Holt (38), Klatte and coworkers (39) and Ippolito and coworkers (40).

Headache is common in children with NF1 and usually occurs in the absence of structural lesions (41). Severe migrainelike headache occurs in 20% to 25% of children with NF1, but because of the risk of CNS tumors, prompt neuroimaging with MRI is warranted. Hypertension can develop owing to the presence of a pheochromocytoma, which is seen in 1% to 4% of subjects. It also can be the result of renal artery stenosis, the most common of a variety of arterial abnormalities seen in neurofibromatosis (42,43). The microscopic picture of these arterial abnormalities is one of an intense subintimal proliferation of the spindle cells, which are believed to be of Schwann cell origin. Congenital heart disease has been reported in NF1 as well.

Neurologic manifestations can be grouped into five major categories (44,45).

Cognitive Disabilities

Although as many as 30% to 60% of children with neurofibromatosis have learning disabilities, only a small proportion are severely retarded (27,34,46). Thus, in the series of Ferner and colleagues, only 8% of patients with NF1 had an IQ below 70 (47). All studies designed to investigate the cognitive deficits of NF1 subjects have shown a significant lowering in full-scale IQ when compared with unaffected siblings. As a rule, children tend to do better on verbal tasks rather than performance tasks and show deficits in visuospatial areas, attention, short-term memory, and reading (47,48). Both nonverbal and verbal learning problems occur, and the children may be easily distractible and poorly organized (49). Mental retardation is only slightly more common in patients with NF1 than in the general population (4% to 8%) (46). These deficits are believed to result from cortical heterotopias and other malformations of cerebral architecture such as glial nodules and other hamartomatous lesions (50) as well as from the presence of abnormal myelin. Studies conducted by Costa and Silva suggest that learning disabilities associated with NF1 are associated with excessive Ras activity that leads to increased γ-aminobutyric acid (GABA) inhibition and to decreased long-term potentiation (51).

Malformations have been demonstrated by magnetic resonance imaging (MRI) as small focal areas of increased signal (*unidentified bright objects*—UBOs) on T2-weighted scans in 60% to 70% of patients with neurofibromatosis (35,52). Areas of increased signal (isointense on T1-weighted images) are located with particular frequency in the globus pallidus, brainstem, optic tracts, thalamus, and cerebellum (53,53a). They exert no mass effect, do not enhance with contrast, and are not visible on CT scan; they are asymptomatic and unrelated to the presence of macrocephaly. UBOs tend to diminish or disappear over the years and are rare in subjects older than 30 years of age. In the experience of DiMario and Ramsby, lesions in the basal ganglia and cerebellum decrease in size and number over time, whereas lesions in the brainstem tended to increase in both number and size (54). Pathologic studies suggest that these hyper-intense areas on MRI may represent dysmyelination or increased water content in the brain. Jurkiewicz and colleagues have shown that proton magnetic resonance spectroscopy may distinguish UBOs from astrocytomas in NF1 (55). Studies present conflicting data as to whether the number of abnormalities seen on MRI correlate with the severity of cognitive deficits (49,56). The most recent series, published in 2003 by Feldmann and colleagues, suggest that as a rule, patients with focal areas of increased signal on T2-weighted MRI studies do worse on cognitive and fine motor performance than NF-1 patients who do not show these lesions (56a). When lesions are seen in the brainstem, they should not be confused with a neoplasm (50).

Intracranial Tumors

Children with NF1 are at risk for optic pathway gliomas and brainstem gliomas. In addition, there appears to be an increased risk for the occurrence of benign and malignant neoplasms in other locations (the cerebrum or cerebellum), ependymomas, meningiomas, PNET/MBs, and malignant schwannomas arising from the cranial nerves (57).

Optic Pathway Gliomas. Intracranial tumors can arise at any time of life, the optic pathway being the most common and the earliest site of involvement (58). In the series of Holt, optic pathway gliomas were found in 23% of children with neurofibromatosis (38). This compares with an incidence of 15% in the series of Huson and Korf (5) 20% in the series of Poyhonen (58a), and 19% in the series of Listernick and colleagues (59). The tumor is benign and histologically corresponds to a pilocytic astrocytoma. It is more common in girls, with a female to male ratio of 2:1 (59). Approximately one-half of patients who harbor optic pathway tumors develop signs or symptoms, and the tumor can involve any portion of the optic pathway (60). Bilateral optic nerve gliomas are seen almost exclusively in NF1 (61). Although optic pathway gliomas are an incidental finding in the majority of children with NF1, these neoplasms occasionally enlarge to distort and compress local structures, causing decreased visual acuity, visual field cuts, afferent papillary defect, decreased color vision, proptosis, strabismus, papilledema, optic nerve atrophy, and optic disk pallor. Precocious puberty is seen in approximately 40% of subjects and results from compression of the hypothalamus and interference with the tonic central nervous system inhibition of the hypothalamic-pituitary-gonadal axis. The presence of precocious puberty in a child with NF1, therefore, should always arouse the suspicion of an enlarging chiasmatic glioma. The diencephalic syndrome also may be seen but is much more common in hypothalamic tumors in patients without NF1 (62).

Decreased visual acuity is rarely a presenting complaint in children, even though it can be demonstrated by examination. The natural history of these optic pathway tumors in subjects with NF1 is not known, and their growth rate differs considerably from one patient to the next. In the series of Listernick and colleagues (59), no tumor growth was seen as determined by MRI over a mean interval of 2.4 years. Only a small proportion of intraorbital tumors progress, whereas tumors that involve the optic chiasm are more likely to progress. The consensus statement from the NF1 Optic Pathway Glioma Task Force has concluded that MRI screening of children with NF1 for optic pathway gliomas has only limited value, and even though asymptomatic tumors are often found, these only rarely progress. Riccardi believes that if an MRI study does not demonstrate an optic glioma by one year of age, these studies will remain negative (62a). Optic pathway gliomas also have been noted to spontaneously regress in patients with and without NF1, providing further evidence of their benign nature. Serial visual acuity examinations in asymptomatic children with NF1 under age 6 years and in symptomatic children are preferable and less costly than repeated MRIs. Accelerated linear growth or the appearance of premature secondary sexual characteristics should prompt an immediate work-up. Listernick and colleagues recommend that even for stable lesions, an MRI should be performed at 3, 9, 15, 24, and 36 months after diagnosis. Ophthalmologic exams should be performed at 3, 6, 12, 18, 24, and 36 months (63).

It is unusual for optic pathway gliomas to become aggressive, and tumors may even regress though they are symptomatic. One must carefully weigh the risks and benefits of any intervention in these children, attempting to preserve visual function while causing the least amount of harm. Treatment options include surgery, radiation, and chemotherapy, alone or in combination (23). The benefits of radical versus conservative surgery in these tumors have been debated in the literature (64). Radiotherapy has been shown to halt tumor progression, but there has been concern that it could transform the tumor to a higher-grade glioma and cause a vasculopathy (63). Reservations regarding the dangers of surgical resection and the potential toxicities of radiation therapy have led to the use of chemotherapy in progressive chiasmatic/hypothalamic gliomas, as reviewed by Rosser and Packer (23).

Focal or generalized seizures can appear early in childhood and were seen in 7% of patients in the series of Huson and Korf (5). Some of these patients had an electroencephalographic picture consistent with hypsarrhythmia. Because a significant proportion of patients with seizures and neurofibromatosis are ultimately found to have intracranial tumors, a child with cutaneous neurofibromatosis and seizures should be suspected of harboring a tumor and should receive imaging studies.

Brainstem Gliomas. The true incidence of brainstem gliomas in NF1 is difficult to estimate because they are often mistaken for brainstem and cerebellar UBOs (65). Brainstem gliomas in NF1 cause neurologic symptoms such as headaches, hydrocephalus, and cranial neuropathies in 88% of patients. The medulla represents the primary tumor site in 80% of patients. Patients may require cerebrospinal fluid diversion, but unlike brainstem glioma in non-NF1 patients, radiotherapy or chemotherapy is rarely required. In fact, such tumors behave much like optic pathway gliomas in NF1 in that they have a relatively benign course and can regress spontaneously after becoming symptomatic. Pollack and colleagues reviewed the course of 21 children (mean age 9.5 years) with NF1 and brainstem gliomas (66). Twelve patients (57%) had clinically symptomatic lesions, with cranial neuropathies and hydrocephalus as most common symptoms. Only 4 children required specific intervention such as biopsy, resection, or adjuvant radiation. All children were alive at the time of the report, and radiographic progression was seen in only 9 children (3 clinically deteriorated).

Tumors of the Peripheral Nerves

Tumors of the peripheral nerves can arise at any age and can involve any of the major nerves. Even though these tumors are occasionally painful, surgical removal must be weighed carefully against the possibility of the procedure producing considerable neurologic deficit. Malignant degeneration of neurofibromas occurs in less than 3% of children, but appears more frequently in adults (27). Tumors also can arise within the autonomic nerve supply of various viscera. According to Kissel and Schmitt, the stomach, tongue, mediastinum, large intestines, and adrenal medulla are the most common sites (67). Treatment options for patients with progressive plexiform neurofibromas have been limited, with surgery as the only proven modality. Trials that have evaluated antihistamines, maturation agents, and antiangiogenic agents have had mixed results that are difficult to interpret, and therapy is moving toward a more biologically based approach (68).

Intraspinal Tumors

Intraspinal tumors are generally slower to develop than intracranial tumors, and asymptomatic spinal cord tumors are commonly detected on routine neuroimaging studies. The youngest patient with a symptomatic intraspinal tumor in Canale's series was 20 years of age (44). Approximately one-half of intraspinal tumors are multiple, and occasionally, they are accompanied by malformations

TABLE 12.1 Neurological Complications in Patients with NF-1

Complication	Incidence (%)
Educational difficulties	62
Cutaneous neurofibroma	59
High signals on T2 MRI	54
Macrocephaly (≥2 SD)	29
Optic gliomas (ascertained by neuroimaging)	20
Plexiform neurofibroma	15
Epilepsy	5.6
Spinal neurofibroma	5.0
Visceral neurofibroma	3.0
Astrocytomas	1.5
Other CNS tumors	4.0
Aqueductal stenosis	1.2
Vestibular schwannoma	0

SD = standard deviation.
After Pyhonen (58a), and McGaughran et al. (72a).

such as syringomyelia. Familial spinal neurofibromatosis is a variant of NF1. The condition is marked by the development of multiple spinal cord tumors during adult life (67,69,70).

Cerebral Infarction

Cerebral infarctions are common and can be responsible for the abrupt evolution of neurologic signs. They result from cerebrovascular occlusive disease and most commonly affect the supraclinoid portion of the internal carotid artery or one of its major branches (71,72). More than one-half of the patients with occlusive disease of the internal carotid have the arteriographic picture of moyamoya disease (71,72).

The incidence of some of the neurologic complications encountered in NF1 and NF2 is presented in Table 12.1 (58a,72a).

Several conditions are related to NF1. Watson syndrome—characterized by dominantly transmitted pulmonary valve stenosis, café au lait spots, and low to normal intelligence—is believed to be allelic with NF1 (73). The concurrence of Noonan syndrome with NF1 may represent either a contiguous gene syndrome or the coincidental segregation of two autosomal dominant conditions (see Chapter 4 (73a)).

Diagnosis

Despite the advances in understanding the molecular biology for NF1 and NF2, the diagnosis for both conditions is still largely based on clinical criteria. The diagnosis of NF1 cannot be made with certainty before 1 year of age in almost half of affected children with a negative family history (74). The appearance of most signs of NF1 is age dependent, and reliability of diagnostic criteria improves as the child grows older (75). At this time, expert consensus does not support the use of UBOs as a diagnostic criterion because adding it the the National Institutes of Health (NIH) Diagnostic Criteria does not improve their sensitivity significantly (74a). The NIH diagnostic criteria for NF1 are two or more of the following:

- Six or more café au lait macules whose greatest diameter is more than 5 mm in prepubertal patients and more than 15 mm in postpubertal patients
- Two or more neurofibromas of any type, or one or more plexiform neurofibroma
- Freckling in the axillary or inguinal region (Crowe's sign)
- An optic pathway tumor
- Two or more Lisch nodules (iris hamartomas)
- A distinctive osseous lesion such as sphenoid wing dysplasia or thinning of the cortex of the long bones (with or without pseudoarthrosis)
- A first-degree relative (parent, sibling, or offspring) with NF1 according to the previously mentioned criteria (76–79).

At the moment, DNA-based testing is unnecessary to make a diagnosis if the NIH criteria are met. DNA testing for the diagnosis of NF1 is limited because present techniques detect only approximately 70% of mutations (5), and detection of a specific mutation does not predict the severity of the disease. Although a solitary café au lait spot can occur in the normal population, the incidence of more than four such lesions in nonaffected persons is low, and in the absence of other symptoms of neurofibromatosis, the lesions can indicate a partial penetrance of the disease (80). Conversely, some 75% of individuals with proven NF1 have six or more café au lait spots 1 cm or more at the largest diameter (29).

Both parents should be examined with particular attention to the presence of café au lait spots, subcutaneous neurofibromas, and Lisch nodules. Detection of Lisch nodules often requires slit-lamp examination by an ophthalmologist. If one parent has the stigmata of NF1, the condition in the offspring is not a new mutation, and a 50% chance exists for it to occur in each subsequent sibling. The risk for the patient's own potential offspring is the same. If neither parent has any abnormalities, a new mutation is presumed, and the recurrence risk for NF1 is no greater than in the general population. Prenatal diagnosis of the condition can be made by linkage analysis, if two or more family members are affected (79).

Treatment and Prognosis

Therapy is symptomatic. Most pediatric patients with NF1 should be seen in a multispecialist clinic at intervals of at least 6 months to 1 year to detect and manage the various potential complications. The necessity or value of routine cranial MRI scans is a matter of debate because it is becoming apparent that the detection of asymptomatic lesions may not alter clinical management (79). However, the detection of asymptomatic optic pathway gliomas may alter the intensity of ophthalmologic monitoring. When tumors are confined to peripheral nerves, the long-term prognosis is generally good. The prognosis for intracranial tumors depends on their location and whether they are single or multiple. In a follow-up study of patients with NF1 first reported in 1951, Sorensen and coworkers found that survival was limited by an incidence of neoplasms that was four times greater than seen in the normal population. Thus, 84% of patients developed a glioma, and second tumors were seen five to eight times more frequently than expected. Malignancies were encountered in one-third of the cohort, with female subjects having a higher incidence than male subjects. Second neoplasms were seen in 83% of patients with optic gliomas and in 43% of patients with other types of gliomas (81). NF1 is a progressive disease, and more manifestations are usually present in older patients. The clinical variability and natural history of the burden of disease in NF1 has been reviewed by Friedman (75) and Young, Hyman, and North (35).

Neurofibromatosis 2

NF2 is genetically and clinically distinct from NF1. It is far less common, with an estimated incidence of 1 in 33,000 to 40,000, and it is characterized by the development of CNS tumors, notably bilateral vestibular schwannomas (77). The gene for NF2 has been mapped to the long arm of chromosome 22 (22q11) and has been cloned. Its gene product, merlin (schwannomin), shares significant homology with several actin-associated proteins (78). Merlin is localized to the cell membrane and is believed to act as a membrane-cytoskeletal linker. It serves as a tumor suppressor by playing a role in the regulation of cell-cell adhesion and in the reorganization of the actin cytoskeleton in response to growth factors, confluency, and changes in the shape of the cell (82,83). Merlin is widely expressed in human brain; it is absent from almost all schwannomas and from many meningiomas and ependymomas isolated from subjects with NF2 (83a). A large number of gene mutations have been documented. Some 90% of patients have gross truncations of merlin as a result of nonsense or frame-shift mutations (84). These patients tend to be younger at onset of symptoms and at diagnosis and tend to harbor a large number of tumors (85).

Clinical Manifestations

In contrast to NF1, clinical manifestations and age of onset are similar within a given family, but differ considerably between families (86). The clinical manifestations of NF2 are highlighted by the presence of bilateral vestibular schwannomas (acoustic neuromas), which become manifest in more than 95% of genetically affected subjects (87). Generally, these tumors become symptomatic at puberty or thereafter. In addition, schwannomas occur in the other cranial nerves and the spinal and cutaneous nerves. Other tumors of the CNS seen in this condition include cranial and spinal meningiomas and multiple tumors of glial and meningeal origin. These tumors are readily detectable by imaging studies, with the acoustic neuromas appearing as a mass in the cerebellopontine angles or enlargement of the gasserian ganglia (52,88). As a rule, the mean age of onset of symptoms is in the second decade of life. In the series of Mautner and colleagues it was 17 years, with the age ranging from 2 to 36 years (88). In the same series, 44% of patients presented with deafness. Café au lait lesions were present in only 43% and in this series as in others they rarely number more than six (89,90). Cataracts (posterior subcapsular or cortical) were seen in 81%, and seizures were presenting complaints in 8%. Peripheral nerve tumors were seen in 68%. These are predominantly schwannomas, but also can be neurofibromas (89). These appear as discrete, well-circumscribed slightly raised lesions with a roughened, slightly pigmented surface. Other skin lesions such as nodular tumors or neurofibromas also are less common than in NF1. According to Riccardi, acoustic neuromas and optic glioma never coexist in a patient (27). The various neurological complications are summarized in Table 12.2 (90a).

TABLE 12.2 Neurological Complications in Patients with NF-2

	Incidence (%)
Presentation at 15 years or less	18
Presentation at 10 years or less	9
Complications in Children 15 years or less	
Vestibular schwannoma (Hearing loss, tinnitus, facial palsy)	43
Meningioma (Headaches, seizures)	31
Spinal tumor	11
Unilateral facial palsy	10

From Evans et al. (90a).

Diagnosis

As is the case for NF1, the diagnosis of NF2 rests on clinical grounds. The criteria for NF2 are one or more of the following conditions:

- Bilateral eighth nerve masses (vestibular schwannomas) seen with imaging techniques
- A parent, sibling, or child with NF2 and either unilateral eighth nerve mass or any two of the following conditions: neurofibroma, meningioma, glioma, schwannoma, or juvenile posterior subcapsular lenticular opacity (76,89,91)
- Patients with unilateral vestibular schwannomas and cataracts, or meningioma, glioma, or schwannoma are suspect for NF2, as are patients with multiple meningiomas plus unilateral vestibular schwannoma, cataracts, or glioma (89).

- In 10% of cases of NF2, there is an identifiable mutation in merlin; for the remainder of patients, prenatal diagnosis requires a linkage study using DNA derived from at least two affected family members, if these are available.

Tuberous Sclerosis

Although the earliest report of a patient with TS is said to have been made by von Recklinghausen in 1863 (92), its first complete, albeit mainly pathologic, description is attributed to Bourneville, who, in 1880, was the first to call it TS (93). This is a protean disorder, chiefly manifested by mental deficiency, epilepsy, and skin lesions. It occurs with a frequency of 1 in 6,000 to 9000 and is transmitted as an autosomal dominant gene (94–97). Approximately one-third of cases have inherited a mutated TS gene from one of the parents; the rest are new mutations.

TS is genetically heterogeneous, with loci on chromosome 9q34.3 (*TSC1*), and 16p13.3 (*TSC2*) near the mapped location of the adult polycystic kidney disease gene (*APKD1*). Each locus accounts for approximately 50% of familial cases (96). The phenotypic expression of the two genetic defects appears to be similar, aside from the observation that TSC2 patients appear more prone to neurologic problems. *TSC1* codes for hamartin, a 130-kd protein with no significant homology to any other known vertebrate protein (98). *TSC2* codes for tuberin, a 200-kd protein, which functions as a tumor-suppressor gene (99). It acts as a GTPase activator for *rap1*, which is an effective proliferation signal, expressed in several tissues, notably astrocytes. *Rap1* also is involved in morphogenesis and cell migration (100). Tuberin is most abundant in cerebral gray matter and increases during prenatal and postnatal development (101). The protein also may be involved in neuronal differentiation (102). The similarity in phenotypes produced by mutations in the *TSC1* and *TSC2* genes suggests that the genes somehow function together, and direct interaction between the two proteins has been shown (103). Hamartin and tuberin associate physically *in vivo*, and inactivation of either is believed to prevent the formation of a functional protein complex that regulates cell growth and proliferation (104,105). Nearly 1,000 mutations have been discovered to date, and genotype/phenotype correlation studies could provide guidance for optimal medical care in affected individuals. Relevant animal models, including conventional and conditional knockout mice, are valuable tools for studying the normal functions of tuberin and hamartin and how disruption of their expression gives rise to the variety of clinical features that characterize TS.

Mutations in the *TSC2* genes are more readily detected in sporadic than in familial cases (106). Penetrance is variable. No family with two or more affected offspring has been encountered in which one parent did not have adenoma sebaceum or some other skin lesion characteristic for TS (107). Conversely, the risk of having more than one affected child is low when both parents are clinically unaffected because under such circumstances, the condition is probably a new mutation.

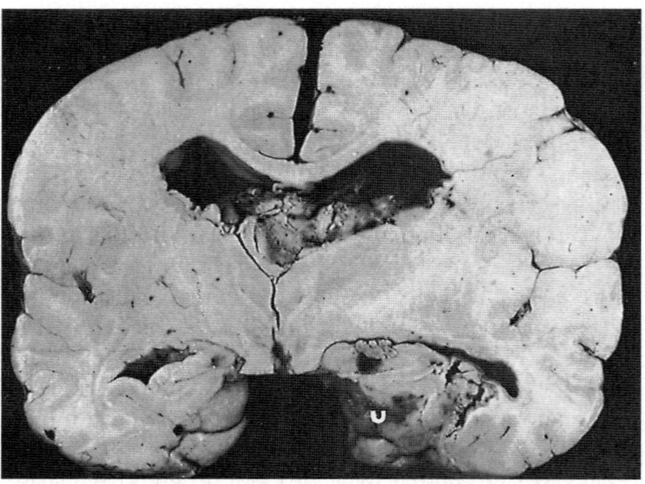

FIGURE 12.3. Tuberous sclerosis. A large intraventricular tuber produces increased intracranial pressure, flattening of the gyri, and herniation of the right temporal uncus (U). (Courtesy of Dr. P. Cancilla, Department of Pathology, University of California, Los Angeles, UCLA School of Medicine.)

Pathology

Abnormalities can be found in the brain, eyes, skin, kidneys, bones, heart, and lungs. In the brain, three types of abnormalities occur: cortical tubers, subependymal nodules, and disorders of myelination. The most characteristic gross abnormality is the presence of tubers. These are numerous hard areas of gliotic tissue of varying size, after which this condition is named. Tubers can be located in the convolutions of any part of the cerebral hemispheres (Fig. 12.3). Less commonly, they are in the cerebellum, brainstem, or spinal cord. The highest frequency of tubers is in the frontal lobes, but the highest density is in the parietal regions (108). On histologic examination, tubers are sclerotic areas that consist of an overgrowth of atypical giant cells that exhibit cytomegaly (109) and express both gial and neuronal markers. Adjacent to these giant cells are dysplastic neurons that are characterized by aberrant dendritic arborizations and a dysmorphic cell body. Tubers may be dynamic lesions characterized by populations of cells undergoing proliferation, migration, and death. Crino recently showed that there is cell-specific activation of the mTOR/p70-S6 kinase/ribosomal S6 cascade in tubers and that giant cells express activated (phosphorylated) p70-S6-kinase and ribosomal S6 protein (110). The tuberin/hamartin complex regulates mTOR, and Rheb (Ras homologue enriched in brain), a Raslike GTPase, has been identified as a target of tuberin GAP activity (111–116). These findings support impaired hamartin/tuberin–mediated mTOR pathway and Rheb regulation.

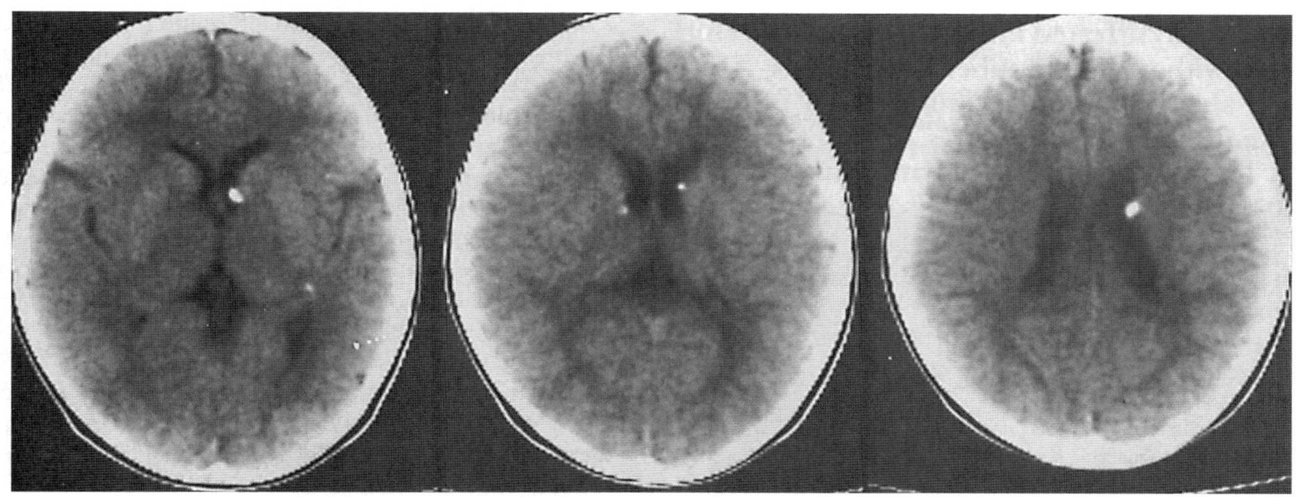

FIGURE 12.4. Noncontrast computed tomographic scan of tuberous sclerosis, taken at several levels, shows typical calcified subependymal tubers at the margins of the lateral ventricles and projecting slightly into the ventricles. (Courtesy of Dr. Hervey D. Segall, Children's Hospital of Los Angeles.)

Tubers likely form a constitutive activation of mTOR cascade during brain development as a consequence of impaired hamartin (*TSC1*) or tuberin (*TSC2*) function.

Rapamycin, a specific inhibitor of mTOR, is currently in clinical trials and may prove useful in some TS-related tumors, including those that affect the brain. Similarly, farnesyltransferase inhibitors may prove useful in disrupting Rheb activation (117). Blood vessels in sclerotic regions show hyaline degeneration of their walls. In approximately one-half of subjects, calcium is deposited within the gliotic areas to an extent as to be visible on plain radiography of the skull or on computed tomographic (CT) scanning (Fig. 12.4). Subependymal nodules are found in the caudate nucleus and the ventricular walls, particularly in the region of the foramen of Monro. Tuber and nodule volumes are significantly positively correlated. Subependymal nodules are multiple small, tumorlike nodules that project into the ventricles and that because of their appearance on pneumoencephalography were described as "candle drippings." Calcification of these nodules is common and increases with age. Subependymal giant cell astrocytomas arise from subependymal nodules, particularly in the area surrounding the foramen of Monro, and transitions between gliosis and astrocytomas are common. Their incidence in TS is approximately 10% to 15% (118). Although only rarely malignant, they often obstruct the foramen of Monro. It is of note that approximately one-half of high-grade and low-grade sporadic adult astrocytomas show reduced or absent expression of tuberin (119). In the remainder, the majority have an increased expression of *rap1*.

Myelination usually is diminished in the gliotic areas within and surrounding the cortical tubers. In addition, islets occur consisting of heterotopic cells within white matter. These are distributed in a linear pattern that follows the normal migratory path of primitive neurons between the germinal layer of the ventricles and the cortical surface.

Tumors also can arise from various viscera. In the heart, the characteristic lesion is the rhabdomyoma. The incidence of these tumors in children with TS can be as high as 50%. Characteristically, they are multiple and well circumscribed. Rhabdomyomas cause as many as one-fourth of infants to die from circulatory failure during the first few days of life, well before developing other stigmata of TS. Between 50% and 80% of patients develop multiple renal tumors, which are usually benign and of mixed embryonal type. Lungs are rarely involved, but when lesions are present in the lungs, they are usually cystic or fibrous. Other organs can be the seat of fibrocellular hamartomas (1). The pathologic features of the disease are extensively reviewed by Bender and Yunis (120).

Clinical Manifestations

Manifestations of TS vary considerably with respect to age of onset, severity, and rate of progression, and natural history studies have yet to be conducted to investigate cell lineage and identify the point at which cortical development of TS is initiated as well as determine whether these lesions continue to evolve after birth. The four main types of manifestations are mental retardation, seizures, cutaneous lesions, and tumors in various organs including the brain. The frequency of the major signs and symptoms is given in Table 12.3 (121).

The degree of mental retardation varies widely, and for unknown reasons, a significant proportion of youngsters develops autistic features. Approximately one-third of patients diagnosed as having TS on the basis of other clinical manifestations maintain a normal intelligence. In the most

TABLE 12.3 Clinical Picture in 71 Patients with Tuberous Sclerosis

Manifestation	43 Patients with Mental Retardation	26 Patients with Average Intelligence
Seizures	43	26
Major motor seizures	19	6
Minor seizures	6	5
Major and minor seizures	7	3
Seizure onset before 1 year of age	28	4
Seizure onset before 5 years of age	38	8
Adenoma sebaceum (facial angiofibroma)	37	22
Appearance of skin lesion before 2 years of age	17	9
Appearance of skin lesion after 9 years of age	2	3
Retinal tumors	21	13
Intracranial calcifications	20	15

From Lagos JC, Gomez MR. Tuberose sclerosis: reappraisal of a clinical entity. *Mayo Clin Proc* 1967;42:26. With permission.

recent population-based study, 55% of those with TS had an IQ >70, while 30.5% had an estimated IQ <21 (122). Individuals with TS in the normal range of intellectual abilities showed a normal distribution of IQ, but with a mean IQ 12 points lower than their unaffected siblings. Even normal-intelligent individuals with TS without a lifetime history of seizures had mean IQs below that of their non-TS siblings. In others, language and perceptual development is slowed. Of retarded patients studied by Borberg, 15% developed normally for the first few years of life, showing the first signs of intellectual deterioration between 8 and 14 years of age (123). This deterioration can be the consequence of either frequent, uncontrolled seizures or the development of increased intracranial pressure caused by an obstruction at the foramen of Monro. In some series, the number of tubers is greater in subjects with mental retardation than in those with normal intelligence, whereas in others, there is no consistent relationship between intelligence and the number of tubers, and mental retardation reflects the early onset of seizures (118,124). In addition to the concerns of global inellectual problems, there is a higher prevalence of behavioral problems, psychiatric diagnoses, learning disorders, and specific neuropsychologic deficits. The behavioral and cognitive aspects of TS have been recently reviewed by Prather and Petrus (125). Because of the potential for behavioral and cognitive regression in TS, most experts in the field recommend that children with TS have a neuropsychologic evaluation when entering school, in the fourth grade, and again in the ninth grade.

Seizures, the most common presenting complaint in all patients with TS, occur at some time in all patients who are retarded. Almost all seizure types are seen in TS though typical absence seizures are not observed. Infantile spasms are the most common seizures during infancy (126). Between one-fourth and one-half of children presenting with this type of seizure ultimately develop TS (127). Later, generalized convulsions or focal seizures can occur. Seizures can appear as early as the first week of life. The earlier the onset of seizures, the more likely the infant is to be mentally retarded (Table 12.3). Of 90 children whose seizures began before 1 year of age, only 8% were deemed to have average intelligence (128). Gomez and colleagues have postulated the presence of an epileptogenic factor, independent of cerebral TS, that facilitates the early onset of seizures and, in turn, impairs normal CNS development (129). Abnormalities in glutamatergic and γ-aminobutyric acid (GABA) receptor subunits have been identified in cortical tuber samples, and abnormal glutamatergic transport in astrocytes had been observed in mouse models of TS (130,131). Several studies have characterized the neurophysiologic activity of cortical tubers at the time of epilepsy surgery, with some studies finding cortical tubers electrically silent, but others finding frequent epileptiform activity associated with the tuber or the region around the tuber (132,133). The severity of the seizures is unpredictable (134). Interestingly, up to 10% of individuals with TS and intractable epilepsy have normal brain MRI scans, with no evidence of cortical tubers or other dysgenetic features (125). As is discussed in Chapter 14, vigabatrin (150 mg/kg per day) is extremely effective in the management of infantile spasms caused by TS and is now considered to be the treatment of choice (135).

Autism or pervasive developmental disorder is a prominent feature of TS (136). In a series of TS patients from the University of California, Los Angeles, 28.5% satisfied the clinical features for autism, and a further 14.2% met the criteria for pervasive developmental disorder (137). In other series of patients with TS, the incidence of autistic disorders was even higher (138). Bolton and Griffiths have commented on the association of autism with tubers within the temporal lobes (139). In a later report of a larger series, Bolton and coworkers stated that risk factors for autism spectrum disorders were temporal lobe tubers associated with temporal lobe epileptiform activity and infantile spasms having an early onset and persistence (140).

Adenoma sebaceum (angiofibroma) is the characteristic cutaneous lesion of TS (Fig. 12.5). These lesions consist of a red, papular rash over the nose, chin, cheeks, and malar region, appearing between ages 1 and 5 years. In the experience of Pampiglione and Moynahan, 12% of affected children developed this skin lesion by 1 year of age, and 40% by 3 years of age (141). Depigmented nevi, resembling vitiligo, in the form of oval areas with irregular margins (*ash leaf*) over the trunk and extremities are equally

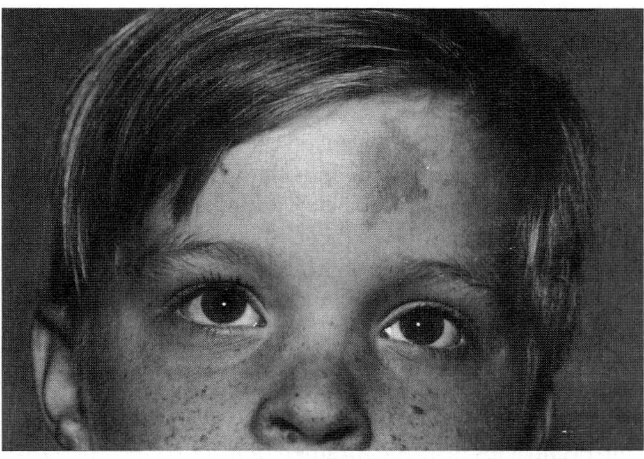

FIGURE 12.5. Tuberous sclerosis. Characteristic fibrous plaque of the forehead and facial angiofibroma in a boy with an early stage of the condition. (From Gomez MR, ed. *Neurocutaneous diseases. A practical approach*. Boston: Butterworths, 1987. With permission.)

common. Generally, they appear earlier than the adenoma sebaceum. They can be noted at birth and are seen before 2 years of age in more than one-half of the subjects (141,142). They are more readily visualized when the skin is illuminated with ultraviolet light (Wood lamp). Depigmented nevi differ from vitiligo in that in vitiligo, the melanocytes are absent, whereas in depigmented macules, the melanocytes are normal but the melanosomes are reduced and contain less melanin. Hypopigmented macules are seen in 0.8% of apparently healthy newborns (143).

Of the other cutaneous abnormalities, flattened fibromas are the most common. They appear in a variety of areas, including the trunk, gingivae, and periungual regions. In some infants, fibromas are found along the hairline or eyebrows. Another striking, but less common, lesion is the shagreen patch. This is an uneven thickening of skin, grayish green or light brown, raised above the surrounding surface, usually in the posterior lumbosacral region. Café au lait spots are seen in 7% to 16% of subjects. Their incidence is not much greater than in the general population, and their presence in isolation should not prompt the diagnosis of neurofibromatosis. A significant percentage of subjects have patches of gray or white hair. Their presence can precede that of the depigmented nevi and thus can be the earliest clinical manifestation of TS (144). The abnormality is seen in 0.3% of apparently healthy newborns (143).

Intracranial tumors are less frequent in TS than in neurofibromatosis, but occurred in 15% of the series of Kapp and coworkers (145). Although the numerous intraventricular nodules are technically tumors, they usually do not grow to the extent of producing increased intracranial pressure. Tumors are found in the neighborhood of the foramen of Monro, arising from either the walls of the lateral ventricles or the anterior portion of the third ventricle. On the basis of their histology, they have been classified as giant cell astrocytomas.

The usual symptoms indicating the presence of an expanding mass in a patient with TS are headache, vomiting, and diminished vision. Papilledema is common, and occasionally lateralizing signs such as hemiparesis can develop. In as many as 50% of patients, tumors are detected in the retina, where they usually arise from the nerve head (146). Other common retinal anomalies are hyaline or cystic nodules (147). Further sites for neoplasms include the skin, lung, kidneys, bone, liver, and spleen (148,149). Patients require lifelong follow-up for early detection of potentially life-threatening conditions. The major causes of death include status epilepticus, renal disease, brain tumors, and lymphangiomyomatosis of the lung (150).

The non-neurologic manifestations of TS often present in adulthood. After neurologic manifestations, renal lesions are the most common cause of morbidity and mortality in TS. Two types of renal involvement are seen. Polycystic kidney disease occurs in 3% to 5% of individuals and reflects a contiguous gene syndrome with involvement of the *APKD1* gene adjacent to the *TSC2* gene on chromosome 16. Such patients develop progressive renal failure and require transplantation. More commonly, patients with TS and renal disease have single or multiple renal cysts that may be associated with angiomyolipomas and do not cause renal failure (151). Pulmonary disease in TS includes lymphangiomyomatosis of the lung, a progressive and often fatal disease seen almost exclusively in women; approximately 40% of women with TS develop the condition, and screening high-resolution chest CTs are recommended in adult women with TS. TS patients also may have pulmonary disease with multifocal micronodular pneumocyte hyperplasia and clear cell tumors of the lung, both of which are benign conditions detected radiographically. Cardiac lesions occur in 50% of all individuals with TS, but in contrast to lymphangiomyomatosis and angiomyolipomas, such lesions are of maximal size and clinically symptomatic during intrauterine life or in early infancy; they are rich in glycogen and usually regress spontaneously within 2 to 3 years (151,97). Patients with TS develop gingival fibromas and dental pits and craters.

Diagnosis

As a rule, the diagnosis of TS is based on the characteristic skin lesions, seizures, and intellectual impairment or deterioration. In infants, the combination of depigmented areas of skin, infantile spasms, and delayed development is diagnostic. Griffiths and Martland suggest that the role of neuroimaging is to confirm the clinical suspicion of TS, evaluate the extent of the abnormality, look for associated but clinically unsuspected abnormalities, and follow the progression of the disease (152). Definite TS, as defined

TABLE 12.4 Diagnostic Features of Tuberous Sclerosis

Major features
Skin Manifestions
Facial angiofibromas
Ungual fibroma
More than three hypomelanotic macules
Shagreen patch
Brain Lesions
Cortical tuber
Subependymal nodules
Subependymal giant cell astrocytoma
Eye Lesions
Multiple retinal nodual hamartomas
Tumors of Other Organs
Cardiac rhabdomyoma
Lymphangioleiomyomatosis
Renal angiomyolipoma
Minor features
Multiple randomly distributed pits in dental enamel
Rectal polyps
Bone cysts
Cerebral white matter migration abnormalties on brain imaging
Gingival fibromas
Non-renal hamartomas
Retinal achromic patches
Confetti skin lesions
Multiple renal cyts

From Roach ES, Sparagana SP. Diagnosis of tuberous sclerosis complex. *J Child Neurol* 2004;19:643–649.

by the 1998 consensus conference sponsored by the TS Alliance and the National Institutes of Health, is diagnosed when at least two major, or one major and two minor, features are present. Probable TS includes one major and one minor feature. Possible TS includes one major or two or more minor features Table 12.4) (153). The 1998 criteria do not include symptoms such as seizures or mental retardation, to avoid "double counting" (i.e., central nervous system lesions cause seizures, and including both in the criteria leads to counting the same symptom twice) (153). Associated neurologic features include seizures, autism or pervasive developmental disorders, mental retardation, and various learning and behavioral disorders (97).

The clinical criteria outlined above are useful, despite the availability of a genetic test for TS, because they are quick, accurate, and inexpensive. Phenotypic variability may be related to the following factors: (1) the stronger phenotypic presentation in patients with *TSC2* gene mutations, (2) somatic mosaicism, and (3) the specific type of genetic mutation. Genetic testing for *TSC1* and *TSC2* mutations has been available since 2002. Confirmatory testing for TS is helpful in individuals who fail to meet the criteria for definite TS as well as to improve genetic counseling. Prenatal genetic testing for TS also is possible when there is a defined TS mutation in a specific family. Preimplantation genetic diagnosis testing also is feasible (154–156). Genetic testing for TS has a false negative rate of 15% to 20%.

MRI is the simplest way to confirm the diagnosis of TS. Ninety percent of people with TS exhibit at least one supratentorial brain lesion, including cortical tubers, subependymal nodules, subependymal giant cell astrocytoma, white matter linear migration lines, corpus callosum agenesis or dysplasia, and transmantle cortical dysplasia (157). Infratentorial brain lesions are seen in less than 2% of patients. CT scanning demonstrates multiple scattered calcium deposits varying in size up to several centimeters and located close to the wall of the lateral and third ventricles near the foramen of Monro (see Fig. 12.4). In the series of Kingsley and coworkers, only 5% of patients with clinical features of TS had a normal CT scan result (118). Calcified masses within the cortex and white matter also are seen, as is cerebral cortical atrophy and ventricular dilatation, but the CT does not show cortical tubers unless they have become calcified (118). Whereas MRI is inferior to CT scanning for the detection of calcified lesions, it is preferable for the visualization of cortical tubers, the various white matter lesions, areas of heterotopias, and hamartomas. MRI also demonstrates islets of abnormal heterotopic giant cells that extend radially from the ependyma to the cortex. These are particularly common in the frontal lobes and the cerebellum (53,158). Cortical tubers can be found in 95% to 100% of patients with TS. They appear as thickened cortical gray matter that is hyperintense on T2-weighted images with indistinct gray-white differentiation. Fluid attenuated inversion recovery (FLAIR) sequences, which suppress the signal from cerebrospinal fluid (CSF), can be used to demonstrate smaller tubers (159). Subependymal nodules are hypointense on T1-weighted images. They are seen in approximately 95% of TS subjects, with the amount of calcification increasing with age. Gadolinium-enhanced MRI can be helpful in distinguishing a subependymal giant cell astrocytoma from a benign subependymal nodule (53,160) (Fig. 12.6). Hence, both CT and MRI studies are necessary for the complete evaluation of the child with TS, particularly for the detection of the heterotopias, which in our experience have proven to be troublesome seizure foci. There is evidence that the number of subependymal nodules and tubers is associated with increased frequency of seizures, cognitive impairment, and adaptive functioning (157).

Equally diagnostic for TS are the cystlike foci in the phalanges in approximately two-thirds of subjects. These are not seen at birth, but appear around puberty. A periungual or subungual fibroma (Koenen tumor), also characteristically appearing after puberty, is virtually diagnostic of TS, as are retinal hamartomas, which can be visualized in approximately one-half of patients (128).

Electroencephalography and the CSF are of relatively little diagnostic importance. Approximately one-third of

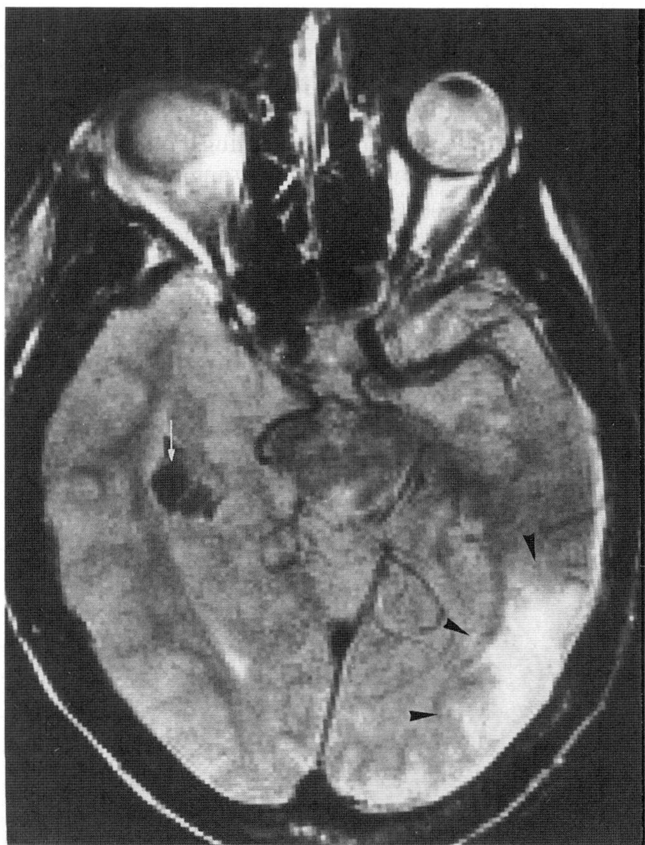

FIGURE 12.6. Magnetic resonance imaging of tuberous sclerosis. A large cortical tuber is seen as a signal void corresponding to the calcification seen on computed tomographic scan. This area is surrounded by a fine hyperintense rim (*white arrow*). An area of high signal intensity with blurred margins corresponds to another large cortical tuber (*arrowheads*). (Courtesy of Dr. Nadine Martin, Départment de Neuroradiologie, Capital Beaujon, Clichy, France.)

children have hypsarrhythmia, which can persist in a modified form in patients up to 8 years of age (141). Focal and multifocal paroxysmal discharges and diffuse slowing also are seen. Slow-wave abnormalities are often indicative of large intracerebral calcifications or masses.

The CSF protein content can be elevated, particularly in patients in whom intraventricular nodules have expanded, interfering with CSF circulation.

In numerous patients, incomplete forms of TS have been recognized by means of genetic surveys. These include isolated adenoma sebaceum, isolated retinal hamartomas, adenoma sebaceum with intracranial tumors but no seizures or intellectual deterioration, and visceral tumors without cerebral involvement (107,121,134). In the experience of Roach, who used MRI to screen apparently normal parents of children with TS, only 0.8% of the parents had typical MRI findings but a normal physical examination (161). Thus, a careful physical examination of parents is nearly as sensitive and much more cost effective than imaging studies. Incompletely affected individuals can have children with complete TS, a fact that should be kept in mind when offering genetic counseling. When both parents appear to be unaffected, the recurrence risk for a second child with TS has been calculated to be 1 in 22 after one affected offspring and 1 in 3 after two affected offspring (5).

The genetic diagnosis of TS has limited application. Two-thirds of the cases are sporadic, and a substantial fraction of even the most severe cases could be caused by mosaicism and missed by screening of leukocytes (162). Genetic testing has not been used routinely for the prenatal diagnosis of TS.

Treatment and Prognosis

No specific treatment for TS is available. As stated elsewhere in this section, seizures are managed with anticonvulsant medications. Although vigabatrin's availability is limited in the United States because of its retinal toxicity and nonapproval by the Food and Drug Administration, it is the most effective antiepileptic drug in children with infantile spams and TS. In selected patients, resection of a single cortical epileptogenic tuber by stereotactic techniques or open craniotomy can result in a marked reduction of seizure frequency (163). Studies are currently under way to examine the impact of neurosurgery on the quality of life in TS. Whether pertussis immunizations provoke the onset of infantile spasms in subjects with TS predisposed to such seizures is a matter of considerable controversy (164). In view of studies that suggest as much and the observations of Gomez and associates that pertussis immunization can precede the onset of infantile spasms by less than 24 hours in infants with TS, pertussis immunization with whole cell vaccine is best withheld (129).

Resection of intraventricular tumors is reserved for children who develop ventricular obstruction. In view of the long survival of patients who do not receive radiation therapy for their mass lesions, we cannot draw any conclusions about its usefulness as an adjunct to surgery.

Whether patients should undergo periodic neuroimaging to detect the development of subependymal giant cell astrocytomas is a matter of debate (165). Whatever position a clinician wishes to take on this issue, regular neurologic examinations of the patient with TS are indicated. The management of cardiac rhabdomyomas and the various renal tumors that can develop in TS is outside the scope of this text.

Sturge-Weber Syndrome

Sturge-Weber Syndrome (SWS), as described by Sturge in 1879 (166) and Kalischer in 1897 (167), is a sporadic condition characterized by a port-wine vascular nevus on the upper part of the face, saltatory neurologic deterioration, and eventual neurodevelopmental delay. No convincing evidence for hereditary transmission has been found. The hallmark intracranial vascular anomaly is a leptomeningeal angiomatosis that involves one or more lobes in one or both hemispheres (166). Although a port-wine stain on the face is a relatively common malformation, occurring in approximately 3 in 1,000 births (frequency of 1/50,000), only 5% of infants affected with this type of a cutaneous lesion have SWS (168). Conversely, 13% of patients with cerebral manifestations of SWS do not have a facial nevus (169).

Pathogenesis and Pathology

In SWS, abnormalities of the skin, leptomeninges, choroid, and cortex can be traced to malformation of an embryonic vascular plexus, arising within the cephalic mesenchyme between the epidermis (neuroectoderm) and the telencephalic vesicle. Interference with the development of vascular drainage of these areas at approximately 5 to 8 weeks of gestation subsequently affects the face, eye, leptomeninges, and brain. Imaging findings in SWS can best be explained by the model of low-flow angiomatosis involving the leptomeninges (170). The angiomatosis is accompanied by poor superficial cortical venous drainage, with enlarged regional transmedullary veins developing as alternate pathways (Fig. 12.7). The ipsilateral choroid plexus may become engorged. Vascular stasis promotes chronic hypoxia of both cortex and underlying white matter. Ultimately, tissue loss and dystrophic calcification occur. Key radiologic features, therefore, are leptomeningeal enhancement of the angiomatosis, enlarged transmedullary

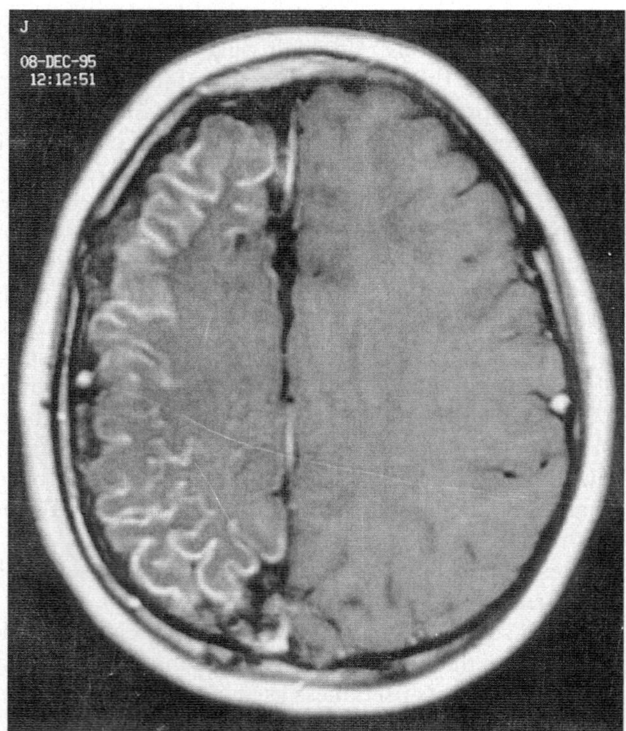

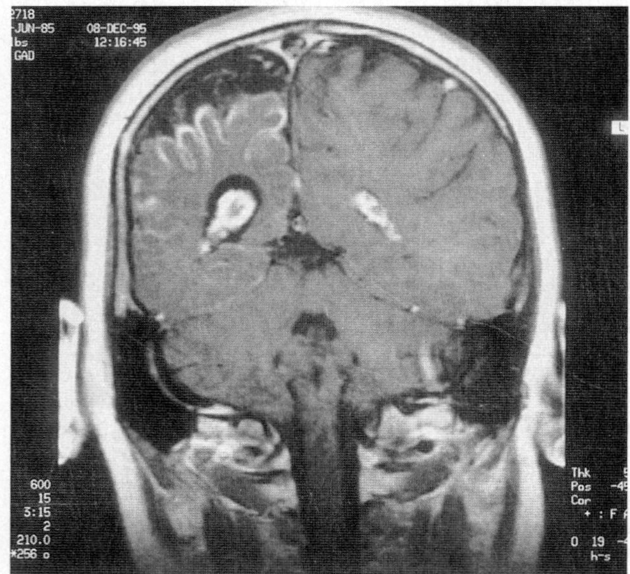

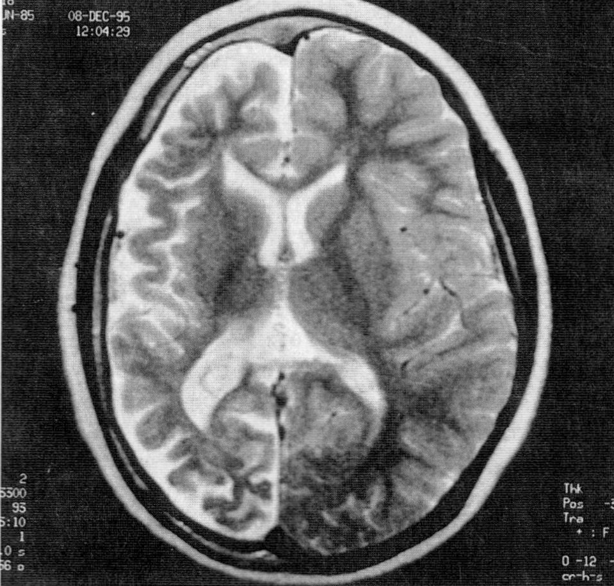

FIGURE 12.7. Magnetic resonance imaging **(A)** in axial plane shows contrast-enhancing angiomatosis overlying the right cerebral hemisphere. Note hypertrophy of the choroid plexus in the coronal section **(B)**. Axial T2-weighted magnetic resonance imaging **(C)** shows widespread atrophy of the right hemisphere.

veins, enlarged choroid plexus, white matter abnormalities, atrophy, and cortical calcifications.

Two structural aspects of SWS compromise cerebral blood flow. First, obstruction in the angiomatosis creates stasis, decreased venous return, and hypoxia. Under such conditions, neuronal metabolism suffers. Second, the lack of normal leptomeningeal vessels hinders neuroglial oxygenation, particularly at times of increased demand, such as when seizures occur. The resulting hypoxia is associated with several physiologic changes: abnormal drainage into the deep plexus and hypertrophy of the choroid plexus, increased capillary permeability, alterations in pH, calcium deposition, cerebral atrophy, and disruption of the blood–brain barrier (171–173). Poor venous drainage in one or both hemispheres is indicated by the presence of enlarged cortical vessels that extend beyond the borders of the leptomeningeal angiomatosis (174). The vascular compromise accounts for neurologic deterioration and eventual neurodevelopmental delay. The phenomenon of saltatory neurologic deterioration has been explained by the development of repeated thromboses, which are caused by microcirculatory stasis in the leptomeningeal angiomatosis. The stasis results in progressive, recurrent infarction that underlies loss of neurologic function.

On pathologic examination of the brain, the essential feature is a leptomeningeal angiomatosis with a predilection for the occipital or occipitoparietal region of one cerebral hemisphere (175). On microscopic examination, the walls of these vessels are encrusted with iron and calcium deposits. Cortical calcifications usually are found in the degenerated cortex underneath the vascular malformations; in the less affected areas, calcifications are localized to the cortical tissue surrounding the walls of the smaller blood vessels. Calcification of microglia and neurons is a less common finding.

Clinical Manifestations

SWS is a progressive disease. The cutaneous port-wine nevus is present at birth and involves at least one eyelid or the supraorbital region of the face (172). It is initially pale red and gradually assumes the deep port-wine color. The angiomas also commonly affect the mucous membranes of the pharynx and other viscera. An angioma of the choroid membrane of the eye is often associated with unilateral congenital glaucoma and buphthalmos. Bilateral facial nevi are not uncommon and were seen in 33% of patients in the series of Pascual-Castroviejo and colleagues (176). Approximately one-fourth of these patients had bilateral cerebral lesions on imaging studies. It is important to note that most children with a facial cutaneous vascular malformation do not have SWS. When the cutaneous malformation is unilateral or bilateral and includes the ophthalmic division of the trigeminal nerve, the likelihood of SWS increases. The overall risk of SWS associated with any kind of facial cutaneous vascular malformation is approximately 8%. Children with involvement of the eyelids are at elevated risk for eye and brain disease (177). Rarely, some children with SWS lack a facial cutaneous vascular malformation but have the neurologic and/or ophthalmic components. The intracranial leptomeningeal angiomatosis is a key diagnostic feature in SWS.

Some 75% to 90% of affected patients develop focal or generalized seizures (178,179). These are usually the initial neurologic manifestation and frequently begin in the first year of life. Seizures can progressively become more refractory to medication and can be followed by transient or permanent hemiparesis. Hemiparesis, often with homonymous hemianopia, ultimately develops. In the Mayo Clinic series, some 67% of patients with a unilateral lesion and seizures were mentally handicapped (169). This is comparable with the data of Sujansky and Conradi, who found that 71% of SWS subjects with seizures required special education (178), and that of Pascual-Castroviejo and colleagues, who found that the IQ of 70% of SWS subjects was less than 90 (176). By contrast, all patients without seizures were mentally normal (169,178). Of the longitudinal studies published, none shows that early onset of seizures indicates poor prognosis. In fact, retrospective studies do not support the widely held belief that seizure frequency early in life in patients who have SWS is a prognostic indicator. However, some patients do develop intractable epilepsy, permanent weakness, hemiatrophy, and visual field cuts, glaucoma, and mental retardation (180,181). The hemiparesis and hemiatrophy are thought to arise from chronic cerebral hypoxia. Other findings common to patients with SWS are vascular headache (40% to 60%), developmental delay and mental retardation (50% to 75%), glaucoma (30% to 70%), hemianopsia (40% to 45%), and hemiparesis (25% to 60%) (182).

Diagnosis

Diagnosis of SWS is made on the basis of the presence or absence of ophthalmologic or neurologic disease. The disease course, however, is variable, and the patient must be continually monitored for complications. Glaucoma can be present at birth or develop over the years in up to 60% of patients (178). Less commonly, symptoms owing to hemangiomas involve the viscera. These include hematuria and gastrointestinal hemorrhages. Intracranial hemorrhages are rare.

Most port-wine stains occur as an isolated anomaly. However, the coincidence of a facial vascular nevus and seizures should suggest SWS. Neuroimaging studies document the gradual but inexorable progression of the disease. This is particularly true for those children who develop seizures. MRI is presently the diagnostic modality of choice. In infants, the unenhanced MRI can be normal, and the most reliable diagnostic features are leptomeningeal enhancement on MRI after gadolinium administration, enlarged transmedullary veins, and unilateral hypertrophy of

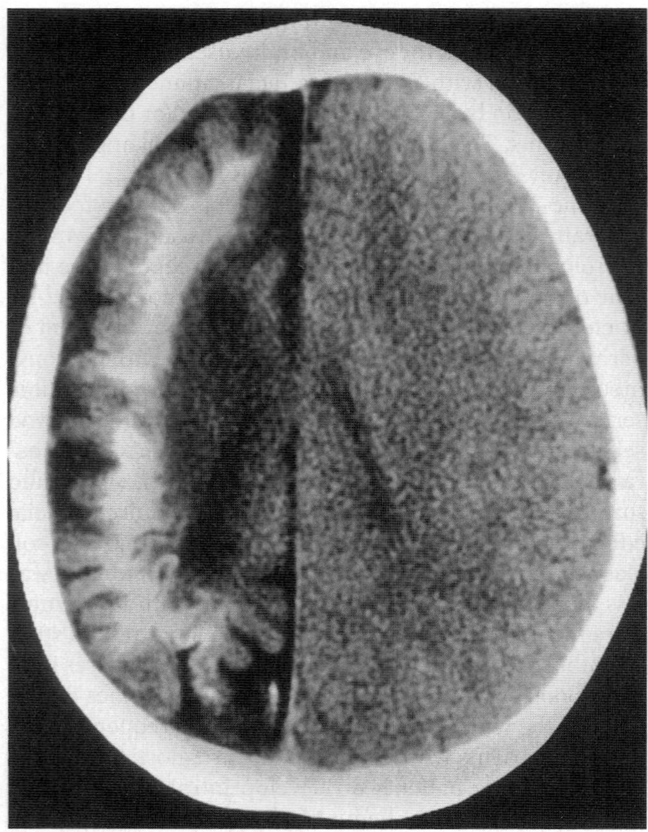

FIGURE 12.8. Computed tomographic scan in axial plane shows widespread calcification in right hemisphere of the same patient in Figure 12.7.

the choroid plexus (see Fig. 12.7) (179,183,184). CT scan can reveal the localization and extent of intracranial calcifications (Fig. 12.8). Rarely present at birth, these become evident in nearly 90% of patients by the end of the second decade of life (169). Characteristically, calcifications are arranged in parallel lines ("railroad tracks") or serpentine convolutions that are most striking in the occipital and parieto-occipital areas (see Fig. 12.8). In older subjects, MRI not only shows the pial angiomatosis, but also adjacent cerebral atrophy and enlargement of the lateral ventricles ipsilateral to the vascular nevus. Depending on the age when the study is performed, arteriography or MR arteriography can demonstrate abnormalities in approximately 50% of subjects. These include venous angiomas, thrombotic lesions, and other vascular anomalies (185,186). Functional cerebral imaging by means of a positron emission tomography (PET) or a single photon emission CT (SPECT) scan shows hypometabolism and hypoperfusion (Fig. 12.9) (187). The affected area is more extensive than the area of CT or MRI abnormalities (184). In infants who have not yet experienced a seizure, generally accelerated myelination and hyperperfusion of the affected region is seen (174,184,188).

The characteristic intracranial calcifications and seizures unaccompanied by a facial nevus also are seen in some patients with celiac disease (189). This condition is covered in Chapter 17.

Klippel-Trenaunay syndrome is a nonhereditary condition that shares a number of clinical features with SWS. In essence, it consists of cutaneous vascular nevi, which can appear at any site of the body and vary in size, venous varicosities, and hypertrophy of the bone and soft tissues (190,191). In some instances, the syndrome is associated with seizures, facial hemihypertrophy, and intracerebral calcifications (192) (see Chapter 13).

An association of large facial hemangiomas and abnormalities of the posterior fossa, notably the Dandy-Walker syndrome, posterior fossa arachnoid cyst, or cerebellar hypoplasia, has been recorded (193). There also is an autosomal dominant condition characterized by cerebral or cerebellar arteriovenous malformations, cutaneous vascular malformations, and seizures (194).

Treatment

Patients with SWS require consistent and thorough monitoring for development of glaucoma, seizures, headache, and strokelike episodes. Medical and surgical management of glaucoma associated with SWS continues to be challenging. Lifelong medical treatment coupled with frequent surgeries is standard. The goal is to control intraocular pressure in order to prevent optic nerve damage. Medications should be given to decrease the production of aqueous fluid or promote the outflow of aqueous fluid. Beta-antagonist eye drops, adrenergic eye drops, and carbonic anhydrase inhibitors are the treatments of choice. Trabeculectomy and goniotomy are typical surgical options.

Laser therapy for facial cutaneous vascular malformation should be started soon after diagnosis for the best prospect of success. A vascular-specific pulsed dye laser can improve the appearance of the facial cutaneous vascular malformation, typically within 10 treatments. The location of the facial cutaneous vascular malformation predicts the response to laser therapy. Central forehead lesions respond best, whereas central facial lesions do not respond as well (195–199). Many patients benefit psychologically from removal of the facial cutaneous vascular malformation (200). Without laser therapy, the lesion grows and typically darkens, developing vascular ectasias that promote nodularity and superficial blebbing. This may lead to overgrowth of the soft tissue and bone beneath the lesion. Hypertrophy and nodularity within the lesion develop in 65% of patients by the fifth decade (200).

Prevention of recurrent seizures may diminish effects of hypometabolism and hypoxia; therefore, the goal is complete seizure control. Management principles for recurrent seizures associated with other conditions also apply to seizure prophylaxis in SWS (see Chapter 14). Children who

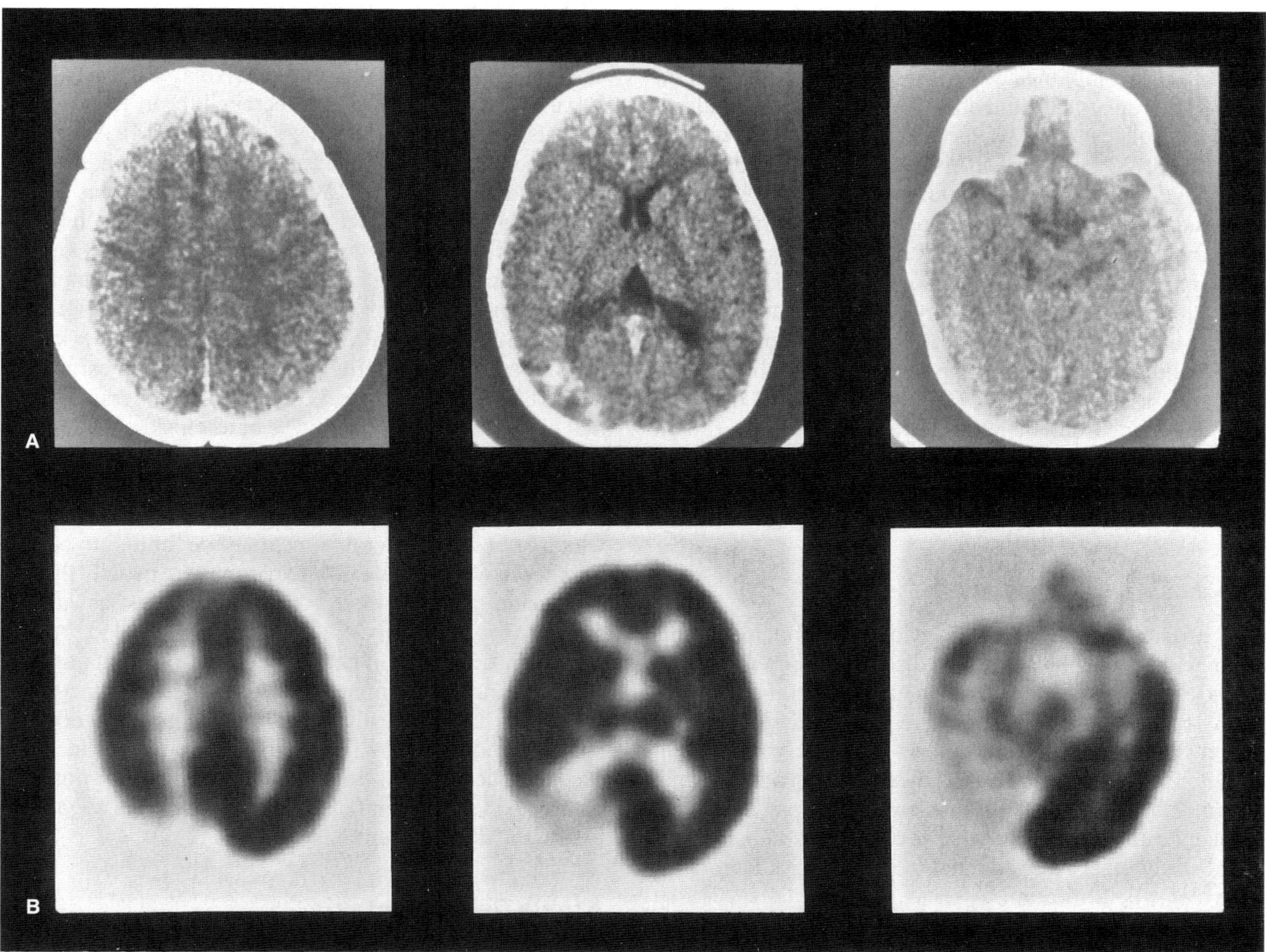

FIGURE 12.9. Sturge-Weber disease. Computed tomographic scan and fluorodeoxyglucose positron emission tomography scans of a 13-month-old girl with bilateral capillary hemangiomas affecting all three divisions of the fifth cranial nerve. The hemangioma was more intense on the left, and there was left-sided glaucoma. Seizures began at 1 year of age, developmental milestones were normal, and no hemiparesis was seen. **A:** Computed tomographic scan showing early left occipital calcifications. **B:** Positron emission tomography scan indicating marked hypometabolism of occipital, temporal, and posterior parietal regions of the left hemisphere. (Courtesy of Dr. Harry Chugani, Division of Pediatric Neurology, Wayne State University, Detroit, MI.)

receive no relief from frequent, debilitating seizures are candidates for epilepsy surgery. Although there is no conclusive evidence that surgical management in infancy provides a better prognosis, delay of surgical treatment may result in further cognitive deterioration (201). A retrospective clinicopathologic review of infants requiring epilepsy surgery indicated that in 7 of 8 patients, epilepsy was absent or significantly diminished postoperatively, supporting the benefits of early surgery (202). Arzimanoglou and colleagues had similar good results with surgery. They found that almost all patients benefited. All children with a pre-existing hemiparesis became seizure-free following hemispherectomy (202a). However, most candidates for the procedure have significant developmental delay, and there is a significant operative risk (203). Few data are available, but anecdotal experience suggests that surgical relief of catastrophic epilepsy may result in resumption of developmental progression. For each patient, the timing of surgery must be carefully considered after fully assessing the procedure's relative risks and benefits (204). The retrospective study of Kossoff and colleagues showed that the age when hemispherectomy was performed or the type of surgical procedure did not affect the outcome (205).

Transient focal deficits presenting with hemiparesis or visual field defects not directly linked to epileptic incidences should be monitored diligently. Prophylactic aspirin is recommended for the prevention of these episodes. Aspirin may delay the neurologic deterioration that often accompanies SWS. Anecdotal data suggest that aspirin therapy is safe and effective. However, no randomized, controlled clinical trials have tested its use in children with SWS. We recommend the antiplatelet dose of 3 to 5 mg/kg/d for children with recurrent strokelike episodes.

Headaches can be debilitating in patients with SWS. The frequency and severity of headaches is higher in SWS than in the general population. Many children report a temporal relationship between their headaches and seizure activity. The leptomeningeal angioma may predispose children to neuronal hyperexcitability, which could account for the migraines. Children with SWS often respond to standard abortive and preventive migraine management in order to cope with headaches. To the best of knowledge, there are no reported serious adverse events from the use of triptans in SWS.

Prognosis

The prognosis in SWS varies widely. Although patients with widespread hemispheric disease or bihemispheric disease are at greatest risk for neurologic complications, many function virtually normally. Clearly, a subgroup of patients with limited central nervous system involvement as defined by neuroimaging studies has a particularly malignant clinical course, with intractable epilepsy, headache, strokelike episodes, and cognitive deterioration. A longitudinal study must be conducted to identify risk factors for neurologic deterioration.

Von Hippel–Lindau Disease

The association of cerebellar hemangioblastomas with angiomas of the spinal cord, multiple congenital cysts of the pancreas, and kidney and renal carcinoma was first recorded by Lindau in 1926 (206), although retinal hemangiomas had already been described by Collins (207) and more definitively by von Hippel in 1904 (208). The condition is transmitted as a dominant trait with variable penetrance. Its prevalence is 1 in 40,000 to 50,000 (209). The von Hippel–Lindau (*VHL*) gene has been localized to the tip of the short arm of chromosome 3 (3p25–p26). It codes for two different tumor-suppressor proteins (210,210a,211).

As a rule, VHL disease does not present during the pediatric years, although cerebellar hemangioblastomas can be seen as early as 9 years of age (211a). More often symptoms are delayed until the second or third decade. They can be referred to the eye with sudden intraocular hemorrhage or to the posterior fossa with increased intracranial pressure or cerebellar signs (212). Of the gene carriers, 51% have retinal hemangiomatosis, and 46% have CNS hemangioblastoma. Most commonly (52% of cases), the neoplasm is located in the cerebellum. It can be found in the spinal cord in 44% and in the brainstem in 18% of patients with CNS hemangioblastoma (213). Vortmeyer and colleagues found angiomesenchymal tumorlets in the nerve roots, spinal cord, and cerebellum in postmortem CNS tissue from four patients with VHL (214). Antiangiogenic treatments with interferons and thalidomide are being tested in progressive CNS hemangioblastomas (215).

Associated with the retinal and cerebral lesions are a number of systemic lesions that tend to progress and become apparent during adult life. These include pancreatic cysts, found in 72% of autopsied patients with VHL, and various other pancreatic endocrine lesions (216); kidney cysts, seen in 59% of autopsies; juvenile renal carcinoma (217); liver cysts, seen in 17% of autopsies; and epididymal cystoadenomas, seen in 7% of autopsies. VHL also is associated with the adult form of renal carcinoma, seen in 45% of autopsies, and pheochromocytomas, seen in 17% of autopsies. The high incidence of pheochromocytomas, which are often bilateral, appears to be limited to certain families in whom pheochromocytomas are usually the first expression of the disease, becoming manifest as early as 5 years of age (218).

A high CSF protein content is seen in the majority of subjects, and approximately 50% of patients with cerebellar tumors have polycythemia, the consequence of erythropoietin production by the tumor. MRI appears to be an excellent means for screening and follow-up examinations of affected family members in that it can detect neoplasms before the development of symptoms (219).

Ataxia-Telangiectasia

Ataxia-telengiectasia (AT) is characterized by slowly progressive cerebellar ataxia, ocularmotor apraxia, choreoathetosis, telangiectasis of the skin and conjunctivae, susceptibility to sinobronchopulmonary infections, lymphoreticular neoplasia, other malignancies, and sensitivity to ionizing radiation (220). It was described by Syllaba and Henner in 1926 (221), by Louis-Bar in 1941 (222), and more definitively in 1958 by Boder and Sedgwick (223), who presented the first clinical and neuropathologic delineation of the disease and named it AT. AT has a frequency of approximately 1 in 40,000 births in the United States.

Pathology and Pathogenesis

The gene for AT (*ATM*, *AT*, mutated) has been mapped to the long arm of chromosome 11 (11q23.3). It has been cloned, and it codes for a nuclear serine/threonine protein kinase ATM, which activates the cellular response to double-stranded breaks in the DNA (224,225). These proteins are involved in the cellular responses to DNA damage, cell-cycle control, and maintaining telomere length (226,227). The ATM protein is localized in both the nucleus and cytoplasm. Screening for the gene has disclosed a large variety of mutations, most of which are unique for a given family, with nonconsanguinous patients being compound heterozygotes (226,228). The majority of mutations give rise to a truncated and nonfunctioning protein (228). As a result, a number of biochemical and cellular abnormalities occur.

One basic lesion results in a marked increase in cellular sensitivity to ionizing radiation. This sensitivity is accompanied by a normal response to ultraviolet irradiation. Radiosensitivity of AT cells appears to result from an inability to recognize and respond to the presence of DNA damage by inhibition of DNA synthesis. In normal cells, reduced DNA synthesis provides time for DNA repair before DNA synthesis is resumed at its preinjury rate. Although there is no defect in the ability to repair or remove strand breaks, fibroblasts derived from patients with AT contain increased amounts of topoisomerase II, an enzyme involved in inducing the transient breaks in double-stranded DNA (229).

Another feature of AT that arises from cellular sensitivity to ionizing radiation is the increased incidence of chromosomal breaks and rearrangements. Spontaneous intrachromosomal recombination rates are 30 to 200 times higher in fibroblasts derived from patients with AT than in normal cells (230). Translocations between chromosomes 7 and 14 are particularly frequent and can occur in the vicinity of the genes that code for the T-cell receptor and IgG genes (226).

Another basic characteristic of AT is a variety of immunologic abnormalities involving both the cellular and the humoral arms of the immune system (226). Low levels of serum and secretory IgA are found in 70% to 80% of patients (231). Additionally, low or borderline values for IgG_2 and IgG_4 are almost invariable (232). IgE is decreased or absent in 80% to 90% of patients, whereas IgM, IgG_1, and IgG_3 levels tend to be high (232). In most subjects, the deficiency of IgA and IgE results from impaired synthesis, although a high catabolic rate, the consequence of circulating anti-IgA antibodies, also has been noted (233). As a consequence of these humoral deficits, antibody response to various bacterial and viral antigens is deficient. Impaired cellular immunity is common in older children and is reflected in hypoplastic, embryonic-appearing tonsils, adenoids, and lymphoid tissue. In spite of the high prevalence of laboratory immunologic abnormalities, systemic bacterial, severe viral, and opportunistic infections are uncommon in AT, and the immune defect is rarely progressive (234).

ATM protein is believed to also be involved in a complex system that prevents apoptosis after DNA damage (235). A defect in this system could be responsible for cell death within the nervous system as well as within the thymus and the vascular endothelium (226,236).

Such a cell loss is the most striking finding on neuropathologic examination. This is most clearly seen in the cerebellar cortex where extensive loss of both Purkinje cells and internal granular cells occurs. Surviving Purkinje cells contain eosinophilic cytoplasmic inclusion bodies. Older patients show demyelination of the posterior columns and the dorsal spinocerebellar tracts (237,238). In some instances, loss of anterior horn cells also occurs. Examination of peripheral nerves can reveal lipid inclusions in Schwann cells and a slight degree of axonal degeneration (238). Vascular malformations have been found inconsistently within the nervous system and the meninges (239).

Clinical Manifestations

AT is not a rare condition. Next to tumors of the posterior fossa, it is the most common cause for progressive ataxia in children younger than 10 years of age.

Cerebellar signs appear in infancy or early childhood. The telangiectases, which are characteristically located over the exposed areas, bulbar conjunctivae, bridge of the nose, ears, neck, and antecubital fossae, are first seen at between 3 and 10 years of age (Fig. 12.10) and become more marked with exposure to sunlight (240,241). Thinning and premature graying of the hair and loss of skin elasticity and subcutaneous fat also are prominent.

Approximately 85% of patients develop choreoathetosis, apraxia of eye movements, and nystagmus. Hypotonia, diminished reflexes, and generalized muscular weakness also have been observed and occur later. Imaging studies show cerebellar atrophy. Although normal initially, intelligence usually becomes impaired as the illness progresses, perhaps owing to diminished stimulation. Most patients experience recurrent sinopulmonary infections. Neoplastic disease is common. In particular, children

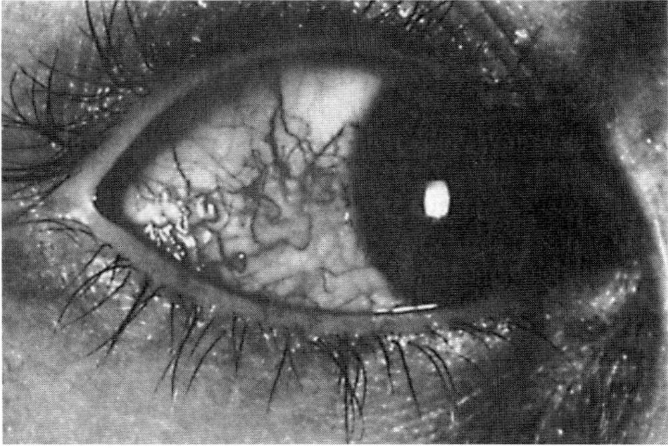

FIGURE 12.10. Telangiectasia of the bulbar conjunctiva in a 12-year-old child with ataxia-telangiectasia. (From Boder E, Sedgwick RP. Ataxia-telangiectasia. In: Goldensohn ES, Appel S, eds. *Scientific approaches to clinical neurology*. Philadelphia: Lea & Febiger, 1977. With permission.)

with AT are 40 to 100 times more likely to develop lymphoma, leukemia, lymphosarcoma, and Hodgkin's disease than their peers (242). Other associated neoplasms include basal cell carcinoma, adenocarcinoma of the stomach, ovarian dysgerminoma, and a variety of brain tumors. In obligatory heterozygotes, the incidence of malignancies is increased threefold, with breast cancer being the most likely malignancy to be encountered in an AT heterozygote (243,244). Approximately one-half of patients develop an unusual form of diabetes in adolescence, characterized by hyperglycemia with only rare glycosuria, absence of ketosis, hypersecretion of insulin, and peripheral resistance to the action of insulin (245).

As expected from their *in vitro* fibroblast radiation sensitivity, children with AT are unusually sensitive to radiotherapy (246). It is unknown whether this radiosensitivity extends to the malignant cell lines derived from AT subjects.

Generally, the clinical course is downhill, although neurologic deterioration decelerates after adolescence. Death results from bronchopulmonary infection or malignancies.

Diagnosis

The diagnosis of AT is not difficult when the oculocutaneous lesions and the neurologic picture, particularly the oculomotor apraxia, are fully developed. In their absence, a young child often presents with progressive cerebellar ataxia. Friedreich ataxia, the late infantile or juvenile neuronal ceroid lipofuscinoses, Refsum disease, and abetalipoproteinemia must all be considered.

Several laboratory tests assist in the diagnosis. A clinical diagnosis can now be confirmed by radiosensitivity testing (colony survival assay), immunoblotting, and mutation detection (247). Elevated α-fetoprotein levels are found in up to 95% of patients and precede by several years the appearance of telangiectases (248,249). An elevated carcinoembryonic antigen also was present in nearly all patients with AT. The characteristic defect in serum immunoglobulins, the demonstration of impaired delayed hypersensitivity responses, and the demonstration of spontaneous chromosome breaks also can assist in the diagnosis. MRI of the brain shows cerebellar atrophy. Prenatal diagnosis of the disease is available by showing mutations in the AT gene (250).

Milder forms of AT have been recognized (251). These patients have a later onset of neurologic symptoms, absence of telangiectatic lesions, less severe ataxia, and a longer life span (228). In these patients, the ATM protein is present but in reduced amounts.

The Nijmegen breakage syndrome (NBS) is an autosomal recessive disorder characterized by microcephaly, a birdlike facies, growth retardation, immune deficiency, an increased incidence of lymphoid cancers, and cellular sensitivity to ionizing radiation. The gene (*NBS1*) for this disorder differs from the AT gene; it has been localized to chromosome 8q21 (252). It encodes a protein called *nibrin*, which is involved in the repair of DNA double-stranded breaks. The pathologic characteristic of this disorder is an oligyric microcephaly, an indication that the *NBS1* gene is involved in corticogenesis (252a). While ATM and NBS regulate several genes in common, both of these proteins have distinct patterns of gene regulation—findings consistent with the functional overlap and distinctiveness of these two conditions (235).

Treatment

No specific treatment prevents the neurologic progress of AT. Intercurrent sinopulmonary infections can be prevented by γ-globulin therapy or treated with antibiotics and postural drainage using a regimen similar to that used for cystic fibrosis.

Incontinentia Pigmenti and Hypomelanosis of Ito

Incontinentia pigmenti and hypomelanosis of Ito (HI) have considerable clinical similarity. Incontinentia pigmenti (Bloch-Sulzberger syndrome) is an X-linked disorder with lethality in male subjects. It is characterized by incontinence of melanin from the melanocytes in the basal layer of the epidermis into the superficial dermis. The skin lesions are erythematous and bullous at birth, crusting with residual pigmentation. They tend to follow a dermatome distribution. Neurologic symptoms are seen in up to 30% of patients (253). These include seizures, spasticity, microcephaly, and mental retardation (254). MRI discloses a variety of abnormalities. These include hypoplasia of the corpus callosum, neuronal heterotopias, and small or large vessel occlusion (255).

HI is characterized by hypopigmented lesions occurring in whorls and located on the trunk, head, or extremities, following a dermatome distribution, the lines of Blaschko. In the series of Pascual-Castroviejo and colleagues, mental retardation and seizures were found in 76% of subjects, macrocephaly in 23%, and hemihypertrophy in 20% (256). Some 10% of patients showed infantile spasms during the first year of life, and another 10% had autistic behavior. In addition, a variety of ophthalmologic abnormalities occur, notably microphthalmos and choroidal atrophy. Gray matter heterotopias, cerebellar atrophy, and intracranial arteriovenous malformations are occasionally seen on imaging studies (257). The disorder is probably heterogeneous, and in some instances, the phenotype may result from the loss of pigmentation genes (258).

Recent evidence convincingly indicates that HI is not a discrete disorder as originally believed but instead is a nonspecific pigmentary disorder caused by chromosomal mosaicism. It almost always occurs sporadically, and it

TABLE 12.5 Some Neurocutaneous Syndromes

Condition	Signs and Symptoms	Reference
Angiomatoses		
Wyburn-Mason syndrome	Facial nevus flammeus, telangiectases intracranial cirsoid aneurysm, racemose angioma of retina, seizure disorder, and variable degree of mental retardation	259,260
Cutaneomeningospinal angiomatosis (Cobb syndrome)	Vascular skin nevus at birth, angioma of spinal cord, neurologic symptoms appearing in childhood (see Chapter 12)	261
Riley-Smith syndrome	Macrocephaly, pseudopapilledema, multiple hemangiomas	262,263
Osler-Weber-Rendu disease	Telangiectases on tongue, face, mucous membranes, liver, and brain, epistaxes, intracranial hemorrhage, autosomal dominant hereditary pattern	Chapter 13
Gass syndrome	Cavernous hemangiomas of retina, intracranial cavernous hemangiomas, angiomatous hamartomas of skin	264
Linear nevus sebaceus	Yellow papules in linear patches (may be evident at birth), mental retardation, seizures, various developmental and vascular anomalies of CNS	265,266
Leopard syndrome	Lentigenes, electrocardiographic abnormalities, ocular hypertelorism, pulmonic stenosis, abnormal genitalia, retardation, sensorineural deafness, autosomal dominant gene	269,271 270
Xeroderma pigmentosum (De Sanctis–Cacchione syndrome)	Neurologic abnormalities (20%; 90% in Japan), microcephaly, mental deterioration, ataxia, choreoathetosis sensorineural hearing loss, peripheral neuropathy	Chapter 4
Klippel-Trenaunay syndrome	Capillary hemangioma, lymphedema, angioma of gut and bladder, hypertrophy of long bones, macrocephaly, intracranial and intraspinal angiomas	Chapter 13
Neurocutaneous melanosis	Multiple pigmented skin nevi present at birth, meningeal melanosis tending to become malignant, hydrocephalus, seizures	267,268

seems to be caused by a *de novo* mutation in early embryogenesis. Although HI is often considered the fourth most common neurocutaneous syndrome, it is an uncommon condition, with only 1 affected individual in every 600 to 1,000 new patients in a pediatric neurology service.

Treatment for HI is symptomatic. The skin lesions require no special treatment, and individuals do not have to take extra precautions with exposure to ultraviolet light. For children without additional neurologic manifestations, an annual follow-up appointment is recommended. The hypopigmented lesions tend to darken with time. Children with HI and neurologic complications will benefit from special education services. Dentists can frequently treat abnormalities of the teeth. Surgery, corrective glasses, vision therapy, and medication may help some of the ophthalmologic conditions seen in HI. Patients suffering from seizures may benefit from antiepileptic drugs, but almost 30% of patients with HI have refractory epilepsy.

Some of the other less common neurocutaneous syndromes are presented in Table 12.5 (259–271).

REFERENCES

1. Gomez MR, ed. *Neurocutaneous diseases. A practical approach*. Boston: Butterworths, 1987.

1a. Sarnat H, Flores-Sarnat L. *J Child Neurol* 2005; (In press).

2. Oh BC, Krieger MD, Sandberg DI, et al. Neurofibromatosis 3: a report of patients meeting diagnostic criteria for both neurofibromatosis 1 and 2. *Neuro-Oncology* 2004;6:412.
3. Smith RW. *A treatise on the pathology diagnosis and treatment of neuroma*. Dublin: Hodgis and Smith, 1849.
4. von Recklinghausen FD. *Ueber die multiplen Fibrome der Haut und ihre Beziehung zu den multiplen Neuromen*. Berlin: A. Hirschwald, 1882.
5. Huson SM, Korf BR. The phakomatoses. In: Rimoin DL, Connor JM, Pyeritz RE, et al., eds. *Principles and practice of medical genetics*, 4th ed. New York: Churchill Livingstone, 2002:3162–3202.
6. Huson SM, Compston DA, Harper PS. A genetic study of von Recklinghausen neurofibromatosis in Southeast Wales. I. Prevalence, fitness, mutation rate, and effect of parental transmission on severity. *J Med Genet* 1989;26:704–711.
7. Stephens K, Kayes L, Ricardi VM, et al. Preferential mutation of the neurofibromatosis type 1 gene in paternally derived chromosomes. *Hum Genet* 1992;88:279–282.
8. Li Y, O'Connell P, Breidenbach HH, et al. Genomic organization of the neurofibromatosis 1 gene (NF1). *Genomics* 1995;25:9–18.
9. Viskochil D. Genetics of neurofibromatosis 1 and the NF1 gene. *J Child Neurol* 2002;17:562–570.
10. Thomson SAM, Fishbein L, Wallace MR. NF1 mutations and molecular testing. *J Child Neurol* 2002;17:555–561.
11. Legius E, Marchuk DA, Collins FS, et al. Somatic deletion of the neurofibromatosis type 1 gene in a neurofibrosarcoma supports a tumour suppressor gene hypothesis. *Nat Genet* 1993;3:122–126.
12. Brodeur GM. The NF1 gene in myelopoiesis and childhood myelodysplastic syndromes. *N Engl J Med* 1994;330:637–639.
13. Gutmann DH. Recent insights into neurofibromatosis type 1: clear genetic progress. *Arch Neurol* 1998;55:778–780.
14. Sawada S, Florell S, Purandare SM, et al. Identification of NF1 mutations in both alleles of a dermal neurofibroma. *Nat Genet* 1996;14:110–112.
15. Side L, Taylor B, Cayouette M, et al. Homozygous inactivation of the NF1 gene in bone marrow cells from children with neurofibromatosis type 1 and malignant myeloid disorders. *N Engl J Med* 1997;336:1713–1720.
16. Rasmussen SA, Colman SD, Ho VT, et al. Constitutional and mosaic large NF1 gene deletions in neurofibromatosis type 1. *J Med Genet* 1998;35:468–471.
17. Tonsgard JH, Yelavarthi KK, Cushner S, et al. Do NF1 deletions result in a characteristic phenotype? *Am J Med Genet* 1998;73:80–86.
18. Skuse GR, Cappione AJ. RNA processing and clinical variability

in neurofibromatosis type I (NF1). *Hum Mol Genet* 1997;6: 1707–1712.
19. Gutmann DH. Recent insights into neurofibromatosis type 1. *Arch Neurol* 1998;55:778–780.
20. Korf BR. Clinical features and pathobiology of neurofibromatosis 1. *J Child Neurol* 2002;17:573–577.
21. Wu BL, Schneider GH, Korf BR. Deletion of the entire NF1 gene causing distinct manifestations in a family. *Am J Med Genet* 1997;69:98–101.
22. Pearce J. The central nervous system pathology in multiple neurofibromatosis. *Neurology* 1967;17:691–697.
23. Rosser T, Packer RJ. Intracranial neoplasms in children with neurofibromatosis 1. *J Child Neurol* 2002;17:630–637.
24. Hope DG, Mulvihill JJ. Malignancy in neurofibromatosis. In: Riccardi VM, Mulvihill JJ, eds. *Advances in neurology. Neurofibromatosis (von Recklinghausen disease)*. New York: Raven Press, 1981: 33–55.
25. Poyhonen M, Niemela S, Herva R. Risk of malignancy and death in neurofibromatosis. *Arch Pathol Lab Med* 1997;121:139–143.
26. Schimke RN, Hartmann WH, Prout TE, et al. Syndrome of bilateral pheochromocytoma, medullary thyroid carcinoma and multiple neuromas. A possible regulatory defect in the differentiation of chromaffin tissue. *N Engl J Med* 1968;279:1–7.
27. Riccardi VM. *Neurofibromatosis: phenotype, natural history, and pathogenesis*, 2nd ed. Baltimore: Johns Hopkins University Press, 1992.
28. Huson SM, Hughes RAC, eds. *The neurofibromatoses: pathogenetic and clinical overview*. London: Chapman-Hall, 1994.
29. Crowe F, Scholl W, Neel J. *Clinical, pathological and genetic study of multiple neurofibromatosis*. Springfield, IL: Charles C Thomas, 1956.
30. Baser ME, Friedman JM, Aeschliman D, et al. Predictors of the risk of mortality in neurofibromatosis 2. *Am J Hum Genet* 2002;71: 715–723.
31. Lisch K. Über Beteilung der Augen, insbesondere das Vorkommen von Irisknötchen bei der Neurofibromatose (Recklinghausen). *Z Augenheilk* 1937;93:137–143.
32. Lubs ME, Bauer MS, Formas ME, et al. Lisch nodules in neurofibromatosis type 1. *N Engl J Med* 1991;324:1264–1266.
33. Vassilopoulou-Sellin R, Klein MJ, Slopis JK. Growth hormone deficiency in children with neurofibromatosis type 1 without suprasellar lesions. *Pediatr Neurol* 2000;22:355–358.
34. Huson SM, Harper PS, Compston DAS. Von Recklinghausen neurofibromatosis: a clinical and population study in southeast Wales. *Brain* 1988;111:1355–1381.
35. Young H, Hyman S, North K. Neurofibromatosis 1: clinical review and exceptions to the rules. *J Child Neurol* 2002;17:613–621.
36. Hefti F, Bollini G, Dungl P, et al. Congenital pseudoarthrosis of the tibia: history, etiology, classification and epidemiologic data. *J Pediatr Orthop B* 2000;9:11–15.
37. Durrani AA, Crawford AH, Chouhdry SN, et al. Modulation of spinal deformities in patients with neurofibromatosis type 1. *Spine* 2000;25:69–75.
38. Holt JF. Neurofibromatosis in children. *Am J Radiol* 1978;130: 615–639.
39. Klatte EC, Franken EA, Smith JA. The radiographic spectrum in neurofibromatosis. *Semin Roentgenol* 1976;11:17–33.
40. Ippolito E, Corsi A, Grill F, et al. Pathology of bone lesions associated with congenital pseudoarthrosis of the leg. *J Pediatr Orthop B* 2000;9:3–10.
41. North KN. Clinical aspects of neurofibromatosis 1. *Eur J Paediatr Neurol* 1998;2:223–231.
42. Pellock JM, Kleinman PK, McDonald BM, et al. Childhood hypertensive stroke with neurofibromatosis. *Neurology* 1980;30: 656–659.
43. Zachos M, Parkin PC, Babyn PS, et al. Neurofibromatosis type 1 vasculopathy associated with lower limb hypoplasia. *Pediatrics* 1997;100:395–398.
44. Canale D, Bebin Y, Knighton RS. Neurologic manifestations of von Recklinghausen's disease of the nervous system. *Confin Neurol* 1964;24:359–403.
45. Michaux L, Feld M, eds. *Les phakomatoses cérébrales*. Paris: Droust, 1963.
46. North KN, Riccardi V, Samango-Sprouse, et al. Cognitive function and academic performance in neurofibromatosis 1: consensus statement from the NF1 Cognitive Disorders Task Force. *Neurology* 1997;48:1121–1127.
47. Ferner RE, Hughes RA, Weinman J. Intellectual impairment in neurofibromatosis 1. *J Neurol Sci* 1996;138:125–133.
48. Hofman KJ, Harris EL, Bryan RN, et al. Neurofibromatosis type 1: the cognitive phenotype. *J Pediatr* 1994;124:S1–S8.
49. North K, Joy P, Juille D, et al. Specific learning disability in children with neurofibromatosis type 1: significance of MRI abnormalities. *Neurology* 1994;44:878–883.
50. Duffner PK, Cohen ME, Seidel FG, et al. The significance of MRI abnormalities in children with neurofibromatosis. *Neurology* 1989;39:373–378.
51. Costa RM, Silva AJ. Molecular and cellular mechanisms underlying the cognitive deficits associated with neurofibromatosis 1. *J Child Neurol* 2002;17:622–626.
52. Bognanno JR, Edwards MK, Lee TA, et al. Cranial MR imaging in neurofibromatosis. *Am J Neuroradiol* 1988;9:461–468.
53. Truhan AP, Filipek PA. Magnetic resonance imaging. Its role in the neuroradiologic evaluation of neurofibromatosis, tuberous sclerosis, and Sturge–Weber syndrome. *Arch Dermatol* 1993;129: 219–226.
53a. Wang PY, Kaufmann WE, Koth CW, et al. Thalamic involvement in neurofibromatosis type 1: evaluation with protein magnetic resonance spectroscopic imaging. *Ann Neurol* 2000;47:477–484.
54. DiMario FJ, Ramsby G. Magnetic resonance imaging lesion analysis in neurofibromatosis type 1. *Arch Neurol* 1998;55:500–505.
55. Jurkiewicz E, Pakula-Kosciesza I, Malczyk K, et al. Usefulness of proton magnetic resonance spectroscopy (MRS) in differentiation of pathologic lesions in neurofibromatosis type 1 (NF1) in children. *Neuro-Oncology* 2004;6:432.
56. Legius E, Descheemaeker MJ, Steyaert J, et al. Neurofibromatosis type 1 in childhood: correlation of MRI findings with intelligence. *J Neurol Neurosurg Psychiatry* 1995;59:638–640.
56a. Feldmann R, Denecke J, Grenzebach M, et al. Neurofibromatosis type 1: motor and cognitive function and T2-weighted MRI hyperintensities. *Neurology* 2003;61:1725–1728.
57. Korf BR. Malignancy in neurofibromatosis type 1. *Oncologist* 2000;5:477–485.
58. Rodriguez HA, Berthrong M. Multiple primary intracranial tumors in von Recklinghausen's neurofibromatosis. *Arch Neurol* 1966;14:467–475.
58a. Poyhonen M. A clinical assessment of neurofibromatosis type 1 (NF1) and segmental NF in northern Finland. *J Med Genet* 2000; 37:e43 (December).
59. Listernick R, Charrow J, Greenwald M, et al. Natural history of optic pathway tumors in children with neurofibromatosis type 1: a longitudinal study. *J Pediatr* 1994;125:63–66.
60. Riccardi VM. Type 1 neurofibromatosis and the pediatric patient. *Curr Probl Pediatr* 1992;22:66–106.
61. Listernick R, Darling C, Greenwald M, et al. Optic pathway tumors in children: the effect of neurofibromatosis type 1 on clinical manifestations and natural history. *J Pediatr* 1995;127:718–722.
62. Johnston MV. Developmental disorders of activity dependent neuronal plasticity. *Indian J Pediatr* 2001;68:423–426.
62a. Riccardi VM. Personal communication, 2004.
63. Listernick R, Louis DN, Packer RJ, et al. Optic pathway gliomas in children with neurofibromatosis 1: consensus statement from the NF1 Optic Pathway Glioma Task Force. *Ann Neurol* 1997;41: 143–149.
64. Janss AJ, Grundy R, Cnaan, et al. Optic pathway and hypothalamic/chiasmatic gliomas in children younger than age 5 years with a 6-year follow-up. *Cancer* 1995;75:1051–1059.
65. Molloy PT, Bilaniuk LT, Vaughan SN, et al. Brainstem tumors in patients with neurofibromatosis type 1: a distinct clinical entity. *Neurology* 1995;45:1897–1902.
66. Pollack IF, Shultz B, Mulvihill JJ. The management of brainstem gliomas in patients with neurofibromatosis 1. *Neurology* 1996; 46:1652–1660.
67. Kissel P, Schmitt J. Les formes viscerales des phakomatoses. In: Michaux L, Feld M, eds. *Les phakomatoses cérébrales*. Paris: Droust, 1963.

68. Packer RJ, Rosser T. Therapy for plexiform neurofibromas in children with neurofibromatosis type 1: an overview. *J Child Neurol* 2002;17:638–641.
69. Ars E, Kruyer H, Gaona A, et al. A clinical variant of neurofibromatosis type 1: familial spinal neurofibromatosis with a frameshift mutation in the NF1 gene. *Am J Hum Genet* 1998;62:834–841.
70. Poyhonen M, Leisti EL, Kytola S, et al. Hereditary spinal neurofibromatosis: a rare form of NF1? *J Med Genet* 1997;34:184–187.
71. Taboada D, Alonso A, Moreno J, et al. Occlusion of the cerebral arteries in Recklinghausen's disease. *Neuroradiology* 1979;18: 281–284.
72. Hilal SK, Solomon GE, Gold AP, et al. Primary cerebral arterial occlusive disease in children. II. Neurocutaneous syndromes. *Radiology* 1971;99:87–93.
72a. McGaughran JM, Harris DI, Donnai D, et al. A clinical study of type 1 neurofibromatosis in north west England. *J Med Genet* 1999;36: 197–203.
73. Riccardi VM. Genotype, malleotype, phenotype, and randomness: lessons from neurofibromatosis-1 (NF-1). *Am J Hum Genet* 1993;53:301–304.
73a. Bertola DR, Pereira AC, Passetti F, et al. Neurofibromatosis-Noonan syndrome: Molecular evidence of the concurrence of both disorders in a patient. *Am J Med Genet A.* 2005;136:242–245.
74. DeBella K, Szudek J, Friedman JM. Use of the National Institutes of Health criteria for diagnosis of neurofibromatosis 1 in children. *Pediatrics* 2000;105:608–614.
74a. DeBella K, Poskitt K, Szudek J, et al. Use of "unidentified bright objects" on MRI for diagnosis of neurofibromatosis 1 in children. *Neurology* 2000;54:1646–1651.
75. Friedman JM. Neurofibromatosis 1: clinical manifestations and diagnostic criteria. *J Child Neurol* 2002;17:548–554.
76. Listernick R, Charrow J. Neurofibromatosis type 1 in childhood. *J Pediatr* 1990;116:845–853.
77. Evans DGR, Huson SM, Donnai D, et al. A genetic study of type 2 neurofibromatosis in the United Kingdom. I. Prevalence, mutation rate, fitness, and confirmation of maternal transmission effect on severity. *J Med Genet* 1992;29:841–846.
78. Gutmann DH, Sherman L, Seftor L, et al. Increased expression of the NF2 tumor suppressor gene product, merlin, impairs cell motility, adhesion and spreading. *Hum Mol Genet* 1999;8:267–275.
79. Gutmann DH, Aylsworth A, Carey JC, et al. The diagnostic evaluation and multidisciplinary management of neurofibromatosis 1 and neurofibromatosis 2. *JAMA* 1997;278:51–57.
80. Whitehouse D. Diagnostic value of the café-au-lait spot in children. *Arch Dis Child* 1966;41:316–319.
81. Sorensen SA, Mulvihill JJ, Nielsen A. Long-term follow-up of von Recklinghausen neurofibromatosis: survival and malignant neoplasms. *N Engl J Med* 1986;314:1010–1015.
82. Shaw RJ, McCatchey AI, Jacks T. Regulation of the neurofibromatosis type 2 tumor suppressor protein, merlin, by adhesion and growth arrest stimuli. *J Biol Chem* 1998;273:7757–7764.
83. Scoles DR, Huynh DP, Morcos PA, et al. Neurofibromatosis 2 tumour suppressor schwannomin interacts with beta II-spectrin. *Nat Genet* 1998;18:354–359.
83a. Gronholm M, Teesalu T, Tyynela J, et al. Characterization of the NF2 protein merlin and the ERM protein ezrin in human, rat, and mouse central nervous system. *Mol Cell Neurosci* 2005;28:683–693.
84. MacCollin M, Braverman BN, Viskochil D, et al. A point mutation associated with a severe phenotype of neurofibromatosis 2. *Ann Neurol* 1996;40:440–445.
85. Parry DM, MacCollin MM, Kaiser-Kupfer MI, et al. Germ-line mutations in the neurofibromatosis 2 gene: correlations with disease severity and retinal abnormalities. *Am J Hum Genet* 1996;59: 529–539.
86. Parry DM, Eldridge R, Kaiser-Kupfer MI, et al. Neurofibromatosis 2 (NF2): clinical characteristics of 63 affected individuals and clinical evidence for heterogeneity. *Am J Med Genet* 1994;52:450–461.
87. Wertelecki W, Rouleau GA, Superneau DW, et al. Neurofibromatosis 2: clinical and DNA linkage studies of a large kindred. *N Engl J Med* 1988;319:278–283.
88. Mautner VF, Lindenau M, Baser ME, et al. The neuroimaging and clinical spectrum of neurofibromatosis 2. *Neurosurgery* 1996;38:880–885.
89. Mautner VF, Lindenau M, Baser ME, et al. Skin abnormalities in neurofibromatosis 2. *Arch Dermatol* 1997;133:1539–1543.
90. Evans DG, Huson SM, Donnai D, et al. A clinical study of type 2 neurofibromatosis. *QJM* 1992;84:603–618.
90a. Evans DGR, Birch JM, Ramsden RT. Paediatric presentation of type 2 neurofibromatosis. *Arch Dis Child* 1999;81:496–499.
91. Martuza RL, Eldridge R. Neurofibromatosis 2 (bilateral acoustic neurofibromatosis). *N Engl J Med* 1988;318:684–688.
92. von Recklinghausen FD. Ein Herz von einen Neugeborenen welches mehrere theils nach aussen, theils nach den Höhlen prominierende Tumoren (Myomen) trug. *Verh Berl Ges Geburtsh* 1863;15:73.
93. Bourneville DM. Contributions a l'étude de l'idiotie. III. Sclerose tubereuse des circonvolutions cérébrales. *Arch Internat Neurol (Paris)* 1880;1:81–91.
94. Hunt A, Lindenbaum RH. Tuberous sclerosis: a new estimate of prevalence within the Oxford region. *J Med Genet* 1984;21: 272–277.
95. Editorial. Progress in tuberous sclerosis. *Lancet* 1990;336:598–599.
96. Kwiatkowski DJ, Dib C, Slaugenhaupt SA, et al. An index marker map of chromosome 9 provides strong evidence for positive interference. *Am J Hum Genet* 1993;53:1279–1288.
97. Maria BL, Deidrick KM, Roach ES, et al. Tuberous sclerosis complex: pathogenesis, diagnosis, strategies, therapies, and future research directions. *J Child Neurol* 2004;19:632–642.
98. Van Slegtenhorst M, de Hoogt R, Hermans C, et al. Identification of the tuberous sclerosis gene TSC1 on chromosome 9q34. *Science* 1997;277:805–808.
99. Jin F, Wienecke R, Xiao GH, et al. Suppression of tumorigenicity by the wild-type tuberous sclerosis 2 (Tsc2) gene and its C-terminal region. *Proc Natl Acad Sci USA* 1996;93:9154–9159.
100. Asha H, de Ruiter ND, Wang MG, et al. The Rap1 GTPase functions as a regulator of morphogenesis in vivo. *EMBO J* 1999;18:605–615.
101. Mizuguchi M, Kato M, Yamanouchi H, et al. Loss of tuberin from cerebral tissues with tuberous sclerosis and astrocytoma. *Ann Neurol* 1996;40:941–944.
102. Soucek T, Holzl G, Bernaschek G, et al. A role of the tuberous sclerosis gene-2 product during neuronal differentiation. *Oncogene* 1998;16:2197–2204.
103. Au KS, Williams AT, Gambello MJ, et al. Molecular genetic basis of TSC: from bench to bedside. *J Child Neurol* 2004;19:699–709.
104. Van Slegtenhorst M, Nellist M, Nagelkerken B, et al. Interaction between hamartin and tuberin, the TSC1 and TSC2 gene products. *Hum Mol Genet* 1998;7:1053–1057.
105. Scheidenhelm DK, Gutmann DH. Mouse models of tuberous sclerosis complex. *J Child Neurol* 2004;19:725–733.
106. Au KS, Rodriguez JA, Finch JL, et al. Germ-line mutational analysis of the TSC2 gene in 90 tuberous sclerosis patients. *Am J Hum Genet* 1998;62:286–294.
107. Bundy S, Evans K. Tuberous sclerosis: a genetic study. *J Neurol Neurosurg Psychiatry* 1969;32:591–603.
108. Ridler K, Suckling J, Higgins N, et al. Standardized whole brain mapping of tubers and subependymal nodules in tuberous sclerosis complex. *J Child Neurol* 2004;19:658–665.
109. Richardson EP. Pathology of tuberous sclerosis. *Ann NY Acad Sci* 1991;615:128–139.
110. Crino PB. The molecular pathogenesis of tuber formation in the tuberous sclerosis complex. *J Child Neurol* 2004;19:716–725.
111. Garami A, Zwartkruis FJT, Nobukuni T, et al. Insulin activation of Rheb, a mediator of mTOR/S6K/4E-BP signaling, is inhibited by TSC1 and 2. *Mol Cell* 2003;11:1457–1466.
112. Castro AR, Rebhun JF, Clark GJ, et al. Rheb binds TSC2 and promotes S6 kinase activation in a rapamycin and farnestylation-dependent manner. *J Biol Chem* 2003;278:32493–32496.
113. Inoki K, Li Y, Xu T, et al. Rheb GTPase is a direct target of TSC2 GAP activity and regulates mTOR signaling. *Genes Dev* 2003;17: 1829–1835.
114. Tabancay AP, Gau CL, Machado IMP, et al. Identification of dominant negative mutants of Rheb GTPase and their use to implicate the involvement of human Rheb in the activation of p70S6K. *J Biol Chem* 2003;278:39921–39930.
115. Tee AR, Manning BD, Roux PP, et al. Tuberous sclerosis complex gene products, tuberin and hamartin control mTOR signaling by

acting as a GTPase-activating protein complex toward Rheb. *Curr Biol* 2003;13:1259–1268.
116. Zhang Y, Gao X, Saucedo LJ, et al. Rheb is a direct target of the tuberous sclerosis tumor suppressor proteins. *Nat Cell Biol* 2003;5:578–581.
117. Haluska P, Dy GK, Adjei AA. Farnesyl transferase inhibitors as anticancer agents. *Eur J Cancer* 2002;38:1685–1700.
118. Kingsley DPE, Kendall BE, Fitz CR. Tuberous sclerosis: a clinicoradiological evaluation of 110 cases with particular reference to atypical presentation. *Neuroradiology* 1986;28:38–46.
119. Wienecke R, Guha A, Maize JC Jr, et al. Reduced TSC2 RNA and protein in sporadic astrocytomas and ependymomas. *Ann Neurol* 1997;42:230–235.
120. Bender BL, Yunis EJ. The pathology of tuberous sclerosis. *Pathol Annu* 1982;17:339–382.
121. Lagos JC, Gomez MR. Tuberose sclerosis: reappraisal of a clinical entity. *Mayo Clin Proc* 1967;42:26–49.
122. Joinson C, O'Callaghan FJ, Osborne JP, et al. Learning disability and epilepsy in an epidemiological sample of individuals with tuberous sclerosis. *Psychol Med* 2003;32:335–344.
123. Borberg A. Clinical and genetic investigation into tuberous sclerosis and Recklinghausen's neurofibromatosis: contribution to elucidation of interrelationship and eugenics of the syndromes. *Acta Psychiatr Neurol Scand* 1951;71[Suppl]:11–239.
124. Shepherd CW, Houser OW, Gomez MR. MR findings in tuberous sclerosis complex and correlation with seizure development and mental impairment. *Am J Neuroradiol* 1995;16: 149–155.
125. Prather P, Petrus JV. Behavioral and cognitive aspects of tuberous sclerosis (TSC). *J Child Neurol* 2004;19:666–674.
126. Roth JC, Epstein CJ. Infantile spasms and hypopigmented macules: early manifestations of tuberous sclerosis. *Arch Neurol* 1971;25:547–551.
127. Della Rovere M, Hoare RD, Pampiglione G. Tuberose sclerosis in children: an EEG study. *Dev Med Child Neurol* 1964;6:149–157.
128. Gomez MR, ed. *Tuberous sclerosis*, 2nd ed. New York: Raven Press, 1988.
129. Gomez MR, Kuntz NL, Westmoreland BF. Tuberous sclerosis, early onset of seizures, and mental subnormality: study of discordant monozygous twins. *Neurology* 1982;32:604–611.
130. White R, Hua Y, Scheithauer B, et al. Selective alterations in glutamate and GABA receptor subunit mRNA expression in dysplastic neurons and giant cells of cortical tubers. *Ann Neurol* 2001;49: 67–78.
131. Wong M, Ess KC, Uhlmann EJ, et al. Impaired glial glutamate transport in a mouse tuberous sclerosis epilepsy model. *Ann Neurol* 2003;54:251–256.
132. Asano E, Chugani DC, Juhasz C, et al. Epileptogenic zones in tuberous sclerosis complex: subdural EEG versus MRI and FDG PET. *Epilepsia* 2000;41(Suppl 17):128.
133. Koh S, Jayakar P, Dunoyer C, et al. Epilepsy surgery in children with tuberous sclerosis complex: presurgical evaluation and outcome. *Epilepsia* 2000;41:1206–1213.
134. Critchley M, Earl CJ. Tuberose sclerosis and allied conditions. *Brain* 1932;55:311–346.
135. Chiron C, Dumas C, Jambaque I, et al. Randomized trial comparing vigabatrin and hydrocortisone in infantile spasms due to tuberous sclerosis. *Epilepsy Res* 1997;26:389–395.
136. Wiznitzer M. Autism and tuberous sclerosis. *J Child Neurol* 2004;19:675–679.
137. Gutierrez GC, Smalley SL, Tanguey PE. Autism in tuberous sclerosis complex. *J Autism Dev Disord* 1998;28:97–103.
138. Gillberg IC, Gillberg C, Ahlsén G. Autistic behaviour and attention deficits in tuberous sclerosis: a population-based study. *Dev Med Child Neurol* 1994;36:50–56.
139. Bolton PF, Griffiths PD. Association of tuberous sclerosis of temporal lobes with autism and atypical autism. *Lancet* 1997;349: 392–395.
140. Bolton PF, Park RJ, Higgins JNP, et al. Neuro-epileptic determinants of autism spectrum disorders in tuberous sclerosis complex. *Brain* 2002;125:1247–1255.
141. Pampiglione G, Moynahan EJ. The tuberous sclerosis syndrome: clinical and EEG studies in 100 children. *J Neurol Neurosurg Psychiatry* 1976;39:666–673.
142. Gold AP, Freeman JM. Depigmented nevi: the earliest sign of tuberose sclerosis. *Pediatrics* 1965;35:1003–1005.
143. Alper JC, Holmes LB. The incidence and significance of birthmarks in a cohort of 4641 newborns. *Pediatr Dermatol* 1983;1:58–68.
144. McWilliam RC, Stephenson JBP. Depigmented hair. The earliest sign of tuberous sclerosis. *Arch Dis Child* 1978;53:961–963.
145. Kapp JP, Paulson GW, Odom GL. Brain tumors with tuberose sclerosis. *J Neurosurg* 1967;26:191–202.
146. McLean JM. Glial tumors of the retina. In relation to tuberous sclerosis. *Am J Ophthalmol* 1956;41:428–432.
147. Grover WD, Harley RD. Early recognition of tuberous sclerosis by funduscopic examination. *J Pediatr* 1969;75:991–995.
148. Dawson J. Pulmonary tuberose sclerosis and its relationship to other forms of the disease. *QJM* 1954;47:113–145.
149. Reed WB, Nickel WR, Campion G. Internal manifestations of tuberous sclerosis. *Arch Dermatol* 1963;87:715–728.
150. Shepherd CW, Gomez MR, Lie JT, et al. Causes of death in patients with tuberous sclerosis. *Mayo Clin Proc* 1991;66:792–796.
151. Franz, DN. Non-neurologic manifestations of tuberous sclerosis complex. *J Child Neurol* 2004;19:690–698.
152. Griffiths PD, Martland TR. Tuberous sclerosis complex: the role of neuroradiology. *Neuropediatrics* 1997;28:244–252.
153. Roach ES, Sparagana SP. Diagnosis of tuberous sclerosis complex. *J Child Neurol* 2004;19:643–649.
154. Harper JC, Wells P, Piyamongkol W, et al. Preimplantation genetic diagnosis for single gene disorders: experience with five single gene disorders. *Prenat Diagn* 2002;22:525–533.
155. ESRHE PGD Consortium Committee: ESHRE preimplantation genetic diagnosis consortium: data collection III. *Hum Reprod* 2002;17:233–246.
156. Tachataki M, Winston RML, Taylor DM. Evaluation of RT-PCT as a clinical tool for diagnosis in PGD: a model study on the expression of the tuberous sclerosis genes throughout human preimplantation embryo development. *Hum Reprod* 2001;16:12.
157. DiMario, FJ. Brain abnormalities in tuberous sclerosis complex. *J Child Neurol* 2004;19:650–657.
158. Inoue Y, Nemoto Y, Murata R, et al. CT and MR imaging of cerebral tuberous sclerosis. *Brain Dev* 1998;20:209–221.
159. Takanashi J, Sugita K, Fujii K, et al. MR evaluation of tuberous sclerosis: increased sensitivity with fluid-attenuated inversion recovery and relation to severity of seizures and mental retardation. *Am J Neuroradiol* 1995;16:1923–1928.
160. Martin N, Debussche C, De Broucker T, et al. Gadolinium-DTPA enhanced MR imaging in tuberous sclerosis. *Neuroradiology* 1990;31:492–497.
161. Roach ES. Diagnosis and management of neurocutaneous syndromes. *Semin Neurol* 1988;8:83–96.
162. Kwiatkowska J, Wigowska-Sowinska J, Napierala D, et al. Mosaicism in tuberous sclerosis as a potential cause of the failure of molecular diagnosis. *N Engl J Med* 1999;340:703–707.
163. Bebin EM, Kelly PJ, Gomez MR. Surgical treatment for epilepsy in cerebral tuberous sclerosis. *Epilepsia* 1993;651–657.
164. Goodman M, Lamm SH, Bellman MH. Temporal relationship modeling: DTP or DT immunizations and infantile spasms. *Vaccine* 1998;16:225–231.
165. Webb DW, Fryer AE, Osborne JP. Morbidity associated with tuberous sclerosis: a population study. *Dev Med Child Neurol* 1996;38:146–155.
166. Sturge WA. A case of partial epilepsy apparently due to a lesion of one of the vasomotor centres of the brain. *Trans Clin Soc Lond* 1879;12:162–167.
167. Kalischer S. Demonstration des Gehirns eines Kindes mit Teleangiectasie der linksseitgen Gesichts-Kopfhaut und Hirnoberfläche. *Berl Klin Wchnschr* 1897;34:10–59.
168. Tan OT, Sherwood K, Gilchrist BA. Treatment of children with port-wine stains using the flashlamp-pulsed tunable dye laser. *N Engl J Med* 1989;320:416–421.
169. Gomez MR, Bebin EM. Sturge-Weber syndrome. In: Gomez MR, ed. *Neurocutaneous disease. A practical approach*. Boston: Butterworths, 1987:356–367.
170. Maria BL, Hoang KBN, Robertson RL, et al. Imaging CNS pathology in Sturge-Weber syndrome. In: Bodensteiner JB, Roach SE. *Sturge-Weber syndrome*. Mt. Freedom, NJ: The Sturge-Weber Foundation, 1999.

171. Norman MG, Schoene WC. The ultrastructure of Sturge-Weber disease. *Acta Neuropathol (Berl)* 1977;37:199–205.
172. Alexander GL, Norman RM. *The Sturge-Weber syndrome*. Bristol: John Wright and Sons Ltd, 1960.
173. Sperner J, Schmauser I, Bittner R, et al. MR-imaging findings in children with Sturge-Weber syndrome. *Neuropediatrics* 1990;21: 146–152.
174. Segall HD, Ahmadi J, McComb JG, et al. Computed tomographic observations pertinent to intracranial venous thrombotic and occlusive disease in childhood. State of the art, some new data, and hypothesis. *Radiology* 1982;143:441–449.
175. Wohlwill FJ, Yakovlev PI. Histopathology of meningo-facial angiomatosis (Sturge-Weber disease). *J Neuropathol Exp Neurol* 1957;16:341–364.
176. Pascual-Castroviejo I, Diaz-Gonzalez C, Garcia-Melian RM, et al. Sturge-Weber syndrome: study of 40 patients. *Pediatr Neurol* 1993;9:283–288.
177. Tallman B, Tan OT, Morelli JG, et al. Location of port-wine stains and the likelihood of ophthalmic and/or central nervous system complications. *Pediatrics* 1991;87:323–327.
178. Sujansky E, Conradi S. Outcome of Sturge-Weber syndrome in 52 adults. *Am J Med Genet* 1995;57:35–45.
179. Pinton F, Chiron C, Enjolras O, et al. Early single photon emission computed tomography in Sturge-Weber syndrome. *J Neurol Neurosurg Psychiatry* 1997;63:616–621.
180. Boltshauser E, Wilson J, Hoare RD. Sturge-Weber syndrome with bilateral intracranial calcification. *J Neurol Neurosurg Psychiatry* 1976;39:429–435.
181. Bebin EM, Gomez MR. Prognosis in Sturge-Weber disease: comparison of unihemispheric and bihemispheric involvement. *J Child Neurol* 1988;3:181–184.
182. Rivello JJ. Sturge-Weber syndrome. *Emedicine* [serial online] 2001 Oct [cited 2004 Aug 15]:1(1):[47 screens]. Available from URL: http://www.emedicine.com/neuro/topic356.htm
183. Griffiths P, Blaser S, Boodram MB, et al. Choroid plexus size in young children with Sturge-Weber syndrome. *Am J Neuroradiol* 1996;17:175–180.
184. Benedikt RA, Brown DC, Walker R, et al. Sturge-Weber syndrome: cranial MR imaging with Gd-DTPA. *Am J Neuroradiol* 1993;14: 409–415.
185. Bentson JR, Wilson GH, Newton TH. Cerebral venous drainage pattern of the Sturge-Weber syndrome. *Radiology* 1971;101: 111–118.
186. Vogl TJ, Stemmler J, Bergman C, et al. MR and MR angiography of Sturge-Weber syndrome. *Am J Neuroradiol* 1993;14:417–425.
187. Chugani HT, Mazziotta JC, Phelps ME. Sturge-Weber syndrome: a study of cerebral glucose utilization with positron emission tomography. *J Pediatr* 1989;114:244–253.
188. Adamsbaum C, Stemmler J, Bergman C, et al. Accelerated myelination in early Sturge-Weber syndrome: MRI-SPECT correlations. *Pediatr Radiol* 1996;26:759–762.
189. Tiacci C, D'Alessandro P, Cantisani TA, et al. Epilepsy with bilateral occipital calcifications: Sturge-Weber variant or a different encephalopathy? *Epilepsia* 1993;34:528–539.
190. Kramer W. Klippel-Trenaunay syndrome. In: Vinken PS, Bruyn GW, eds. *Handbook of clinical neurology*, Vol. 14. Amsterdam: North-Holland Publishing, 1968:390–404.
191. Barek L, Ledor S, Ledor K. The Klippel-Trenaunay syndrome: a case report and review of the literature. *Mt Sinai J Med (NY)* 1982;49:66–70.
192. Heuser M. De l'entité nosologique des angiomatoses neurocutanées (Sturge-Weber et Klippel-Trénaunay). *Rev Neurol* 1971;124:213–228.
193. Reese V, Frieden IJ, Paller AS, et al. Association of facial hemangiomas with Dandy-Walker and other posterior fossa malformations. *J Pediatr* 1993;122:379–384.
194. Leblanc R, Melanson D, Wilkinson RD. Hereditary neurocutaneous angiomatosis. Report of four cases. *J Neurosurg* 1996;85:1135–1142.
195. Fitzpatrick RE, Lowe NJ, Goldman MP, et al. Flashlamp-pumped pulsed dye laser treatment of port-wine stains. *J Dermatol Surg Oncol* 1994;20:743–748.
196. Morelli JG, Weston WL, Huff JC, et al. Initial lesion size as a predictive factor in determining the response of port-wine stains in children treated with the pulsed dye laser. *Arch Pediatr Adolesc Med* 1995;149:1142–1144.
197. Nguyen CM, Yohn JJ, Huff C, et al. Facial port-wine stains in childhood: prediction of the rate of improvement as a function of the age of the patient, size and location of the port-wine stain and the number of treatments with the pulsed dye (585 nm) laser. *Br J Dermatol* 1998;138:821–825.
198. Renfro L, Geronemus RG. Anatomical differences of port-wine stains in response to treatment with the pulsed dye laser. *Arch Dermatol* 1993;129:182–188.
199. Batta K. Management of large birthmarks. *Semin Neonatol* 2000;5:325–532.
200. Geronemus RG, Ashinoff R. The medical necessity of evaluation and treatment of port-wine stains. *J Dermatol Surg Oncol* 1991;17:76–79.
201. Kramer U, Kahana E, Shorer Z, et al. Outcome of infants with unilateral Sturge-Weber syndrome and early onset seizures. *Dev Med Child Neurol* 2000;42:756–759.
202. Prayson RA. Clinicopathological findings in patients who have undergone epilepsy surgery in the first year of life. *Pathol Int* 2000;50:620–625.
202a. Arzimanoglou AA, Andermann F, Aicardi J, et al. Sturge-Weber syndrome: indications and results of surgery in 20 patients. *Neurology* 2000;55:1472–1479.
203. Maria BL, Olson LL, Comi AM. Sturge-Weber Syndrome. *Current management in child neurology*. 3rd Ed., Hamilton, London: BC Decker, 2005:470–475.
204. Saneto RP, Wyllie E. Epilepsy surgery in infancy. *Semin Pediatr Neurol* 2000;7:187–193.
205. Kossoff EH, Buck C, Freeman JM. Outcomes of 32 hemispherectomies for Sturge-Weber syndrome worldwide. *Neurology* 2002;59:1735–1738.
206. Lindau A. Studien über Kleinhirncysten: Bau, Pathogenese und Beziehungen zur Angiomatosis retinae. *Acta Pathol Microbiol Scand* 1926;[Suppl 1]:1–128.
207. Collins ET. Intra-ocular growths. I. Two cases, brother and sister, with peculiar vascular new growth, probably primarily retinal, affecting both eyes. *Trans Ophthalmol Soc UK* 1894;14:141–149.
208. von Hippel, E. Ueber eine sehr seltene Erkrankung der Netzhaut. *Acta Ophthalmol* 1904;59:83–103.
209. Neumann HPH, Eggert HR, Scheremet R, et al. Central nervous system lesions in von Hippel–Lindau syndrome. *J Neurol Neurosurg Psychiatry* 1992;55:898–901.
210. Pause A, Lee S, Lonergan KM, et al. The von Hippel–Lindau tumor suppressor gene is required for cell cycle exit upon serum withdrawal. *Proc Natl Acad Sci USA* 1998;95:993–998.
210a. Joerger M, Koeberle D, Neumann HP, Gillessen S. Von Hippel-Lindau disease—a rare disease important to recognize. *Onkologie* 2005;28:159–163.
211. Schoenfeld A, Davidowitz EJ, Burk RD. A second major native von Hippel–Lindau gene product initiated from an internal translation start site, functioning as a tumor suppressor. *Proc Natl Acad Sci USA* 1998;95:8817–8822.
211a. Lonser RR, Glenn GM, Walther M, et al. von Hippel-Lindau disease. *Lancet* 2003;361:2059–2067.
212. Maher ER, Yates JR, Harries R, et al. Clinical features and natural history of von Hippel–Lindau disease. *QJM* 1990;77:1151–1163.
213. Filling-Katz MR, Choyke PL, Oldfield E, et al. Central nervous system involvement in von Hippel–Lindau disease. *Neurology* 1991;41:41–46.
214. Vortmeyer AO, Yuan Q, Lee YS, et al. Developmental effects of von Hippel–Lindau gene deficiency. *Ann Neurol* 2004;55(5):721–728.
215. Piribauer M, Czech T, Dieckmann K, et al. Stabilization of progressive hemangioblastoma under treatment with thalidomide. *J Neurooncol* 2004;66:295–299.
216. Chetty R, Kennedy M, Ezzat S, et al. Pancreatic endocrine pathology in von Hippel–Lindau disease: an expanding spectrum of lesions. *Endocr Pathol* 2004;15(2):141–148.
217. Granata A, Sessa A, Righetti M, et al. Juvenile renal cell carcinoma as first manifestation of von Hippel–Lindau disease. *J Nephrol* 2004;17:306–310.
218. Atuk NO, McDonald T, Wood T, et al. Familial pheochromocytoma, hypercalcemia, and von Hippel–Lindau disease. *Medicine (Baltimore)* 1979;58:209–218.

219. Sato Y, Waziri M, Smith W, et al. Hippel–Lindau disease: MR imaging. *Radiology* 1988;166:241–246.
220. Chun HH, Gatti RA. Ataxia-telangiectasia, an evolving phenotype. *DNA Repair* 2004;3:1187–1196.
221. Syllaba L, Henner K. Contribution à l'indépendance de l'athétose double idiopathique et congénitale. *Rev Neurol (Paris)* 1926;45:541–562.
222. Louis-Bar D. Sur un syndrome progressif comprenant des télangiectasies capillaires cutanées et conjonctivale symétriques à disposition naevoïde et des troubles cérébelleux. *Confin Neurol* 1941;4:32–42.
223. Boder E, Sedgwick RP. Ataxia-telangiectasia. A familial syndrome of progressive cerebellar ataxia, oculocutaneous telangiectasia and frequent pulmonary infection. *Pediatrics* 1958;21:526–554.
224. Shiloh Y, Andegeko Y, Tsarfaty I. In search of drug treatment for genetic defects in the DNA damage response: the example of ataxia-telangiectasia. *Semin Cancer Biol* 2004;14:295–305.
225. Goodarzi AA, Lees-Miller SP. Biochemical characterization of the ataxia-telangiectasia mutated (ATM) protein from human cells. *DNA Repair* 2004;3:753–767.
226. Lavin MF, Shiloh Y. The genetic defect in ataxia-telangiectasia. *Annu Rev Immunol* 1997;15:177–202.
227. Kastan M. Ataxia-telangiectasia—broad implications for a rare disorder. *N Engl J Med* 1995;333:662–663.
228. Gilad S, Chessa L, Khosravi R, et al. Genotype-phenotype relationships in ataxia-telangiectasia and variants. *Am J Hum Genet* 1998;62:551–561.
229. Epstein RJ. Topoisomerases in human disease. *Lancet* 1988;1:521–524.
230. Meyn MS. High spontaneous intrachromosomal recombination rates in ataxia-telangiectasia. *Science* 1993;260:1327–1330.
231. McFarlin DE, Strober W, Waldmann TA. Ataxia-telangiectasia. *Medicine (Baltimore)* 1972;51:281–314.
232. Oxelius VA, Berkel AI, Hanson LA. IgG2 deficiency in ataxia-telangiectasia. *N Engl J Med* 1982;306:515–517.
233. Strober W, Wochner RD, Barlow MH, et al. Immunoglobulin metabolism in ataxia-telangiectasia. *J Clin Invest* 1968;47:1905–1915.
234. Nowak-Wegrzyn, Crawford TO, Winkelstein JA, et al. Immunodeficiency and infections in ataxia-telangiectasia. *J Pediatr* 2004;144:505–511.
235. Jang ER, Lee JH, Lim DS, et al. Analysis of ataxia-telangiectasia mutated (ATM) and Nijmegen breakage syndrome (NBS)—regulated gene expression patterns. *J Cancer Res Clin Oncol* 2004;130:225–234.
236. Meyn MS. Ataxia-telangiectasia and cellular responses to DNA damage. *Cancer Res* 1995;55:5991–6001.
237. Solitare GB, Lopez VF. Louis-Bar's syndrome (ataxia-telangiectasia): neuropathologic observations. *Neurology* 1967;17:23–31.
238. De Leon GA, Grover WD, Huff DS. Neuropathologic changes in ataxia-telangiectasia. *Neurology* 1976;26:947–951.
239. Agamanolis DP, Greenstein JL. Ataxia-telangiectasia. Report of a case with Lewy bodies and vascular abnormalities within cerebral tissue. *J Neuropathol Exp Neurol* 1979;38:475–488.
240. Reed WB, Epstein WL, Boder E, et al. Cutaneous manifestations of ataxia-telangiectasia. *JAMA* 1966;195:746–753.
241. Sedgwick RP, Boder E. Ataxia-telangiectasia. In: Vinken PJ, Bruyn GW, eds. *Handbook of clinical neurology*, Vol. 14. Amsterdam: North-Holland Publishing Co, 1972:267–339.
242. Toledano SR, Lange BJ. Ataxia-telangiectasia and acute lymphoblastic leukemia. *Cancer* 1980;45:1675–1678.
243. Swift M, Reitnauer PJ, Morrell D, et al. Breast and other cancers in families with ataxia-telangiectasia. *N Engl J Med* 1987;316:1289–1294.
244. Swift M, Morrell D, Massey RB, et al. Incidence of cancer in 161 families affected by ataxia-telangiectasia. *N Engl J Med* 1991;325:1831–1836.
245. Schalch DS, McFarlin DE, Barlow MH. An unusual form of diabetes mellitus in ataxia-telangiectasia. *N Engl J Med* 1970;282:1396–1402.
246. Pritchard J, Sandland MR, Breatnach FB, et al. The effects of radiation therapy for Hodgkin's disease in a child with ataxia-telangiectasia. A clinical, biological and pathological study. *Cancer* 1982;50:877–886.
247. Perlman S, Becker-Catania S, Gatti RA. Ataxia-telangiectasia: diagnosis and treatment. *Semin Pediatr Neurol* 2003;10:173–182.
248. Boder E. Ataxia-telangiectasia. In: Gomez MR, ed. *Neurocutaneous diseases. A practical approach*. Boston: Butterworths, 1987:95–117.
249. Cabana MD, Crawford TO, Winkelstein JA, et al. Consequences of the delayed diagnosis of ataxia-telangiectasia. *Pediatrics* 1998;102:98–100.
250. Gatti RA, Peterson KL, Novak J, et al. Prenatal genotyping of ataxia-telangiectasia. *Lancet* 1993;342:376.
251. Taylor AM, Groom A, Byrd PJ. Ataxia-telangiectasia–like disorder (ATLD)—its clinical presentation and molecular basis. *DNA Repair* 2004;3:1219–1225.
252. Cerosaletti KM, Lange E, Stringham HM, et al. Fine localization of the Nijmegen breakage syndrome gene to 8q21: evidence for a common founder haplotype. *Am J Hum Genet* 1998;63:125–134.
252a. Lammens M, Hiel JAP, Gabreëls FJM, et al. Nijmegen breakage syndrome: a neuropathological study. *Neuropediatrics* 2003;34:189–193.
253. Landy SJ, Donnai D. Incontinentia pigmenti (Bloch-Sulzberger syndrome). *J Med Genet* 1993;30:53–59.
254. O'Doherty NJ, Norman RM. Incontinentia pigmenti (Bloch-Sulzberger syndrome) with cerebral malformation. *Dev Med Child Neurol* 1968;10:168–174.
255. Lee AG, Goldberg MF, Gillard JH, et al. Intracranial assessment of incontinentia pigmenti using magnetic resonance imaging, angiography, and spectroscopic imaging. *Arch Pediatr Adolesc Med* 1995;149:573–580.
256. Pascual-Castroviejo I, Roche C, Martinez-Bermejo A, et al. Hypomelanosis of Ito. A study of 76 infantile cases. *Brain Dev* 1998;20:36–43.
257. Pini G, Faulkner LB. Cerebellar involvement in hypomelanosis of Ito. *Neuropediatrics* 1995;26:208–210.
258. Pellegrino JE, Schnur RE, Kline R, et al. Mosaic loss of 15q11q13 in a patient with hypomelanosis of Ito: is there a role for the P gene? *Hum Genet* 1995;96:485–489.
259. Wyburn-Mason R. Arteriovenous aneurysm of mid-brain and retina, facial naevi, and mental changes. *Brain* 1943;66:163–209.
260. Patel U, Gupta SC. Wyburn-Mason syndrome: a case report and review of the literature. *Neuroradiology* 1990;31:544–546.
261. Kissel P, Dureux JB. Cobb syndrome. Cutaneomeningospinal angiomatosis. In: Vinken PJ, Bruyn GW, eds. *Handbook of clinical neurology*, Vol. 14. Amsterdam: North-Holland Publishing Co, 1972:429–445.
262. Riley HD, Smith WR. Macrocephaly, pseudopapilledema and multiple hemangiomata. A previously undescribed heredofamilial syndrome. *Pediatrics* 1960;26:293–300.
263. Arch EM, Goodman BK, Van Wesep RA, et al. Deletion of PTEN in a patient with Bannayan-Riley-Ruvalcaba syndrome suggests allelism with Cowden disease. *Am J Med Genet* 1997;71:489–493.
264. Gass JDM. Cavernous hemangioma of the retina. A neuro-oculocutaneous syndrome. *Am J Ophthalmol* 1971;71:799–814.
265. Pavone L, Curatolo P, Rizzo R, et al. Epidermal nevus syndrome: a neurologic variant with hemimegalencephaly, gyral malformations, mental retardation, seizures, and facial hemihypertrophy. *Neurology* 1991;41:266–271.
266. Prensky AL. Linear sebaceous nevus. In: Gomez MR, ed. *Neurocutaneous diseases*. Boston: Butterworths, 1987:335–344.
267. Di Rocco F, Sabatino G, Koutzoglou M, et al. Neurocutaneous melanosis. *Childs Nerv Syst* 2004;20:23–28.
268. Demirci A, Kawamura Y, Sze G, et al. MR of parenchymal neurocutaneous melanosis. *Am J Neuroradiol* 1995;16:603–606.
269. Coppin BD, Temple IK. Multiple lentigines syndrome (LEOPARD syndrome or progressive cardiomyopathic lentiginosis). *J Med Genet* 1997;34:582–586.
270. Robbins JH, Brumback RA, Mendiones M, et al. Neurological disease in xeroderma pigmentosum. Documentation of a late onset type of the juvenile onset form. *Brain* 1991;114:1335–1361.
271. Sarkozy A, Conti E, Digilio MC, et al. Clinical and molecular analysis of 30 patients with multiple lentigines LEOPARD syndrome. *J Med Genet* 2004;41:e68.

Chapter 13

Cerebrovascular Disorders

Cesar C. Santos, Harvey B. Sarnat and E. Steve Roach

Cerebrovascular disorders are now frequently recognized in children, probably because of increased awareness of these conditions by clinicians; the widespread application of noninvasive diagnostic studies such as magnetic resonance imaging (MRI), magnetic resonance angiography (MRA), computed tomography (CT); and, in the neonate, cranial ultrasound studies (1). These studies allow confirmation of a diagnosis that in previous years would have been missed or at least not recognized as a vascular lesion. Additionally, the number of children who develop cerebrovascular lesions from certain risk factors may have increased, as more effective treatments for some causes of stroke have allowed patients to survive long enough to develop vascular complications.

The most important distinction between cerebrovascular diseases in children and those of adults is the variety of conditions that cause stroke in children versus adults (Table 13.1) (1,2). Congenital heart disease and sickle cell disease, for example, are common causes of ischemic stroke in children, while atherosclerosis is rare in children. Treatment of the risk factors is essential if subsequent strokes are to be prevented, and it is sometimes the underlying condition that determines the patient's outcome.

Recent advances in diagnosis notwithstanding, cerebrovascular lesions are often more difficult to diagnose in children, particularly in very young children who are unable to adequately describe their symptoms and who are sometimes less cooperative during an examination. Once the diagnosis is considered, however, these difficulties can usually be solved with careful observation and diagnostic studies.

STROKE

Incidence

Schoenberg and colleagues studied the incidence of cerebrovascular disease in the children of Rochester, Minnesota, from 1965 through 1974 (3,4). Excluding strokes related to birth, intracranial infection, and trauma, they identified three hemorrhagic strokes and one ischemic stroke in a risk population of 15,834, for an estimated annual incidence of 1.89/100,000/year and 0.63/100,000/year for hemorrhagic and ischemic strokes, respectively. The overall average annual incidence for children through 14 years of age in this study was 2.52/100,000/year. In this well-defined population, hemorrhagic strokes were seen more commonly than ischemic strokes, while in the Mayo Clinic referral population, ischemic strokes were more common. Several years later, Broderick and coworkers found a similar 2.7 pediatric stroke cases/100,000/year (5).

These earlier estimates may be low. One report on the incidence of vascular disease in Dijon, France, between the years 1985 and 1993 found childhood stroke in 13.0/100,000 children/year (6). Stroke is among the top ten causes of death in children in the United States (7), and the 1998 estimated mortality rate from stroke in children below one year of age was 7.8/100,000 children (7). The risk of stroke seems to be particularly high among neonates, patients who were not included in the earlier surveys. Cerebral ischemic infarction is recognized in 12% to 14% of neonates with seizures (8), and neonates comprise one-fourth of all childhood strokes (9). Data from the National Hospital Discharge Survey conducted from 1980 through 1998 indicate a stroke rate during the first month of life of 26.4/100,000; hemorrhagic stroke occurred in 6.7/100,000 and ischemic stroke occurred in 17.8/100,000. Based on these numbers, stroke in neonates occur in approximately 1 per 4,000 live births per year (10).

Clinical Manifestations

The clinical presentation depends on the child's age, the presence of underlying risk factors, the location of the lesion, and the type of stroke. The diagnosis of stroke is often missed or delayed in children. In one retrospective study of children with stroke, the average time from the onset of symptoms until diagnosis was 35.7 hours (11). Some neonates initially appear normal but neurological impairment is recognized months later after they develop premature handedness or delayed milestones (12). In general,

TABLE 13.1 Risk Factors for Pediatric Stroke[1]

Congenital heart disease	**Vasospastic disorders**
Ventricular septal defect	Migraine
Atrial septal defect	Ergot poisoning
Patent ductus arteriosus	Vasospasm & subarachnoid bleed
Aortic stenosis	**Hematologic disorders/coagulopathies**
Mitral stenosis	Hemoglobinopathies (sickle cell anemia, sickle cell–hemoglobin C)
Coarctation	Immune thrombocytopenic purpura
Cardiac rhabdomyoma	Thrombotic thrombocytopenic purpura
Complex congenital heart defects	Thrombocytosis
Acquired heart disease	Polycythemia
Rheumatic heart disease	Disseminated intravascular coagulation
Prosthetic heart valve	Leukemia or other neoplasm
Libman-Sacks endocarditis	Congenital coagulation defects
Bacterial endocarditis	Oral contraceptive use
Cardiomyopathy	Pregnancy/postpartum period
Myocarditis	Antithrombin III deficiency
Atrial myxoma	Factor V Leiden
Arrhythmia	Protein S deficiency
Systemic vascular disease	Protein C deficiency
Systemic hypertension	Congenital serum C2 deficiency
Systemic hypotension	Liver dysfunction–coagulopathy
Hypernatremia	Vitamin K deficiency
Superior vena cava syndrome	Lupus anticoagulant
Diabetes	Anticardiolipin antibodies
Vasculitis	**Structural anomalies**
Meningitis	Arterial fibromuscular dysplasia
Systemic infection	Agenesis or hypoplasia of the internal carotid or vertebral artery
Systemic lupus erythematosus	Arteriovenous malformation
Polyarteritis nodosa	Hereditary hemorrhagic telangiectasia
Granulomatous angiitis	Sturge-Weber syndrome
Takayasu's arteritis	Intracranial aneurysm
Rheumatoid arthritis	**Trauma**
Dermatomyositis	Child abuse
Inflammatory bowel disease	Fat or air embolism
Drug abuse (cocaine, amphetamines)	Foreign body embolism
Hemolytic-uremic syndrome	Carotid ligation (eg, ECMO)
Vasculopathies	Vertebral occlusion after abrupt cervical rotation
Ehlers-Danlos syndrome	Post-traumatic arterial dissection
Homocystinuria	Blunt cervical arterial trauma
Moyamoya syndrome	Arteriography
Fabry disease	Carotid cavernous fistula
Malignant atrophic papulosis	Coagulation defect with minor trauma
Pseudoxanthoma elasticum	Amniotic fluid/placental embolism
NADH-CoQ reductase deficiency	Penetrating intracranial trauma
Williams syndrome	

[1]Modified from Roach and Riela. *Pediatric cerebrovascular disorders.* New York: Futura Publishing Co., 1995. With permission.

stroke occurs more often in boys and in African American children, even after adjusting for trauma and for sickle cell disease (12,13).

Ischemic Infarction

It is often impossible to determine whether an ischemic infarction has resulted from an embolism or a thrombosis on purely clinical grounds. Sudden-onset symptoms suggest an embolism, but the precise onset of the symptoms is often unknown, especially in very young children. Specific risk factors sometimes suggest whether the stroke has resulted from an embolus or a thrombus. Cardiac disease, for example, results in embolism more often than thrombosis, while the presence of cerebral arteritis would favor thrombosis.

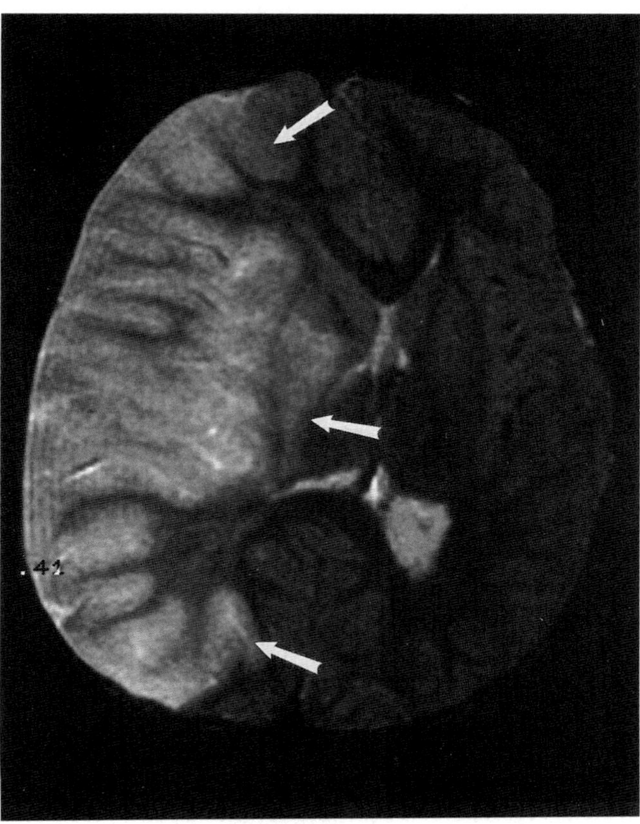

FIGURE 13.1. An MRI showing an acute embolic infarction (*arrows*) of most of the right cerebral hemisphere with mass effect.

The specific signs and symptoms of an ischemic infarction depend on the size and location of the lesion. The anterior circulation is affected more often than the vertebrobasilar system. The basal ganglia and thalamus are together the most frequent location for ischemic infarction in children (Fig. 13.1) (14). An infarction in this region results directly from occlusion of the small penetrating arteries that supply this area, but in many cases, an ipsilateral carotid or middle cerebral artery is occluded. Infarction in these individuals is limited to the basal ganglia because this area lacks the collateral blood flow that rescues the nearby cortex. Because the vessels most often occluded are the supraclinoid internal carotid arteries and the branches of the middle cerebral arteries, typical signs include hemiparesis, hemianesthesia, and aphasia. However, a wide array of signs and symptoms are possible depending on the area of the brain affected. Hemichorea also has been described in children with basal ganglia infarction (15). Epileptic seizures are common. In one report of 43 children from 1 to 16 years of age, the most common presenting symptom was weakness followed by seizures (16). Acute ataxia and other cerebellar and brain stem findings occur in patients with a posterior circulation infarction.

Neonatal Infarction

Although not nearly as common as the germinal matrix hemorrhage in premature patients, ischemic infarction in term neonates may occur more often than previously suspected (see Chapter 6). The infarction typically occurs in a term baby after an uneventful pregnancy and a routine delivery. The infarction is often identified after the onset of focal seizures, and most of the time, the physical findings are nonspecific with only mild lethargy, irritability, hypotonia, or subtle hemiparesis. Focal motor seizures more often involve the right body because about three-fourths of single infarcts occur in the left cerebral hemisphere. The initial radiographic appearance of the lesion sometimes suggests that the infarction occurred even before birth. Some babies with cerebral infarction are probably missed because the findings are often subtle, and not all babies develop seizures. Similar lesions of long-standing duration are sometimes discovered in older children who are being evaluated for epileptic seizures or developmental delay.

Most neonatal infarctions probably result from emboli. Systemic emboli can occasionally be demonstrated in these neonates, and the left hemisphere predominance is more easily explainable by embolic than by thrombotic infarction. Interruption of aortic laminar flow by blood from the still patent ductus arteriosus might explain emboli being preferentially directed to the left hemisphere. The source of the emboli is not known with certainty, but they may arise from degenerating placental vessels or the just-activated pulmonary vascular bed.

Watershed infarcts are frequent in the neonate. Two patterns are found. The first is similar to watershed infarcts in the adult, in areas between the territories of the anterior and middle cerebral arteries and between the middle and posterior cerebral arteries. The difference from adults is that in term neonates, about one-third of such supratentorial watershed infarcts are hemorrhagic, whereas in the adult nearly all are ischemic infarcts without hemorrhage. In preterm infants of less than 35 weeks gestation, two-thirds of cerebral cortical watershed infarcts are hemorrhagic, so that there is a shift in watershed infarcts toward coagulation necrosis as the brain matures. The second pattern is that of symmetrical tegmental infarcts in the brainstem. They involve the superior and inferior colliculi and tegmentum of the midbrain, pons, and medulla oblongata near the floor of the fourth ventricle. This tegmental watershed zone is between the territories of the paramedian penetrating arteries and the long circumferential arteries, both arising on each side from the basilar artery as a series of 25 to 30 sets, hence the infarction as a longitudinal column. Because tegmental structures in this zone include the fasciculus and nucleus solitarius (central "pneumotaxic" center of respiratory drive) and the nucleus ambiguous (somatic vagal component of muscles of deglutition), clinical manifestations include lack of central respiratory drive and dysphagia, in addition to multiple cranial neuropathies, Möbius syndrome, and sometimes micrognathia and ankylosis of the jaw because of infarction including the motor trigeminal nucleus (16a) (see Chapter 5).

Venous Occlusion

Cortical vein and dural sinus thrombosis can be difficult to recognize because the clinical findings are sometimes less dramatic than those of arterial occlusion. Focal or generalized seizures are common with cortical vein thrombosis, and dural sinus thrombosis often leads to increased intracranial pressure. In the face of seizures, focal neurological dysfunction due to sinovenous occlusion is easily mistaken for postictal deficit. Venous occlusion is frequently associated with a nearby infection such as chronic otitis, sinusitis, or orbital cellulitis; it also is seen in children with hemoglobinopathy, congestive heart failure, polycythemia, and dehydration.

Etiology

The risk factors for stroke in children (Table 13.1) are different from those of adults, although there is some overlap (1,2). Even after a thorough diagnostic evaluation, about one-fourth of children with ischemic infarction have no obvious cause for stroke, and others have suspected risk factors that may or may not explain the infarction. On the other hand, a likely cause for intracranial hemorrhage is usually found after a complete evaluation, including a cerebral angiogram.

Cardiac Disorders

The most common cause of ischemic infarction in children is congenital or acquired heart disease (17), although the likelihood of stroke due to heart disease seems to have decreased in recent years as newer and more effective treatments have become available. In the Canadian Pediatric Ischemic Stroke Registry, cardiac disease occurred in 24% of children with arterial stroke, and stroke in 20% and 17% of cases following cardiac surgery and catheterization, respectively. Complex cardiac anomalies are by far the biggest problem, but any cardiac lesion can lead to stroke. Particularly concerning are the cyanotic cardiac lesions associated with polycythemia, which increase the risk of both thrombosis and embolism. If a right-to-left cardiac shunt is present, a venous (paradoxical) embolus can bypass the pulmonary circulation and reach the brain. Many patients are already known to have heart disease prior to stroke, but in other instances, a less obvious cardiac lesion is discovered only after stroke. Surgical correction of congenital heart disease decreases the risk of stroke, although risk of embolism in these children remains higher than normal. Rheumatic valvular heart disease and other acquired cardiac conditions are known to cause stroke in children. Some children with congenital heart disease seem to have an increased risk for intracranial aneurysms and arterial dissection (18). Cerebral embolism has been reported in patients with cardiac rhabdomyomas, atrial myxomas, and primary cardiac lymphomas (19–21).

Hematological Disorders

Although stroke is occasionally linked to other hemoglobinopathies and to sickle cell trait, homozygous sickle cell disease (SCD) accounts for most of the individuals with stroke. The cumulative risk of having stroke increases with age: 11% by age 20, 15% by age 30, and 24% by age 45 (22). Moreover, after the first sickle cell–related stroke, that individual's risk of having a second stroke soars to over 50%. Stroke accounts for 12% of deaths in individuals with sickle cell disease (23). Most sickle cell–related strokes are ischemic, but both intraparenchymal and subarachnoid hemorrhages occur. Stroke is somewhat more likely during a thrombotic crisis, but most of the time, an infarction occurs in an otherwise asymptomatic individual. Silent infarction, evident with MRI in an individual without an obvious neurologic deficit, occurs in 22% of children with homozygous SCD (24). See Chapter 17.

Although both large and small cerebral arteries are affected by SCD, the distal internal carotid arteries and their immediate branches are usually involved (25,26). Elevated cerebral blood flow velocity measured by transcranial Doppler (TCD) predicts a much higher stroke risk due to SCD. A randomized multicenter controlled study (the STOP trial) compared prophylactic blood transfusion with standard medical care in individuals at high risk for stroke based on TCD measurements (27). This study showed conclusively that the time-averaged mean blood flow velocity measured by TCD indicates a higher stroke risk due to SCD and demonstrated that prophylactic blood transfusion reduces the occurrence of first stroke by over 90% (28,29). The neurologic complications of sickle cell disease and the other hemoglobinopathies are further discussed in Chapter 17.

Coagulation Defects

As many as one-half of children with ischemic cerebral infarction have a prothrombotic disorder (30), although many of these patients also have other risk factors (31). Protein C, protein S, and antithrombin III (AT-III) are naturally occurring anticoagulants, and deficiency states may be either inherited or acquired as a result of kidney or liver disease and pregnancy (Table 13.2) (32,33). Additionally, protein C deficiency has been described in children using valproic acid and L-asparaginase (34,35). Low levels of protein C impair the inactivation of activated factors V and VIII and promote excessive fibrin formation, increasing the likelihood of thrombosis. Heterozygous protein C deficiency has variable expressivity (36), but newborns with homozygous deficiency present with severe and typically fatal thrombotic disease (37). Protein C can be transiently

TABLE 13.2 Acquired and Inherited Prothrombotic Disorders

Common gene mutations
Factor V Leiden mutation (APC resistance)
MTHFR C677T (Homocystinuria)
Prothrombin G20210A mutation
Rare genetic deficiency
Protein C
Protein S
Antithrombin III
Plasminogen
Acquired risk factor
Antiphospholipid antibodies
Genetic thrombophilia
Homocysteine
Lipoprotein(a)
Other risk factors
Increased fibrinogen
Increased factor IX
Increased factor VIIIC
Decreased factor XII

diminished following a stroke, but if the deficiency persists after several months and there is no evidence of an acquired deficiency, then hereditary protein C deficiency is likely.

Antithrombin (AT) III is a serine proteinase inhibitor that acts as a heparin cofactor to inactivate thrombin (38). Its importance is well illustrated in the finding that mutant mice null for ATIII die *in utero* (39). Two subtypes of ATIII deficiency exist. Type I is more strongly correlated with venous thrombosis (38). Patients with type I deficiency have heterozygous mutation resulting in a 50% reduction of ATIII. Type II deficiency, on the other hand, is usually due to single amino acid substitution, which results in a normal AT level but an AT that is physiologically ineffective (40). To date, there are several dozen reported mutations affecting the ATIII gene causing venous thrombosis (41). ATIII deficiency also can be associated with multiple congenital anomalies due to interstitial 1q deletion (42). Heterozygous ATIII deficiency is more commonly seen in young adults (43). In children, this is rare, and it usually occurs in association with other risk factors (44). The estimated prevalence of heterozygous ATIII deficiency in the general population is 1:550 (45). Homozygous ATIII deficiency, on the other hand, is extremely rare. Kuhle and coworkers reported five patients from three families with homozygous ATIII deficiency type II with both venous and arterial thromboembolism (46).

A mutation of the factor V gene results in resistance to activated protein C (47). Known as factor V Leiden, it occurs in 5% to 8% of Caucasian individuals but is less common in other races (48,49). The risk of an individual with the mutation having a thrombotic complication is not precisely known, but it is generally agreed that the risk for venous thrombosis is higher than the risk for arterial occlusion (49). As well, the role of factor V Leiden has not been fully established in children and adolescents (50). In one series, no individuals with factor V Leiden mutation were identified among 22 children with arterial or cerebral venous thrombosis (51). Other studies documented the mutation in 20% to 38% of children (52,53). Factor V Leiden mutation may be associated with an adverse maternal or fetal outcome (10).

Prothrombin G20210A gene mutation is the second most common hereditary cause of venous thrombosis. Whether *de novo* or hereditary, it is a known risk factor for extracerebral venous thrombosis as well as venous sinus thrombosis both in adults and children including neonates (54–56). Its exact role in ischemic stroke is unknown, and arguments showing both a strong association and the lack of one exist (50). One study of 50 children with stroke did not show an increased odds ratio (57).

Antiphospholipid antibodies, which include lupus anticoagulant and anticardiolipin antibodies, are antibodies against anionic phospholipids or protein-phospholipid complexes (58). These antibodies are commonly seen in patients with antiphospholipid syndrome, which in addition is characterized by thrombosis and recurrent fetal death (59). Both arterial and venous thromboses have been reported. The most common sites of venous thrombosis are the deep veins of the lower extremities (60). Arterial involvement, on the other hand, is commonly manifested by ischemic stroke or transient ischemic attacks (61). Children with antiphospholipid antibodies have an increased risk for both venous and arterial thrombosis, and up to 50% of these can occur in the central nervous system (62). Lupus anticoagulant is a double misnomer; first because most patients with lupus anticoagulant do not have lupus, and second, it is a procoagulant rather than an anticoagulant (58). The presence of lupus anticoagulant is associated with a 30% lifetime risk of thrombotic event (63). Anticardiolipin antibodies are either of the IgG or IgM variety. However, only the IgG class, especially IgG_2, has been linked to stroke (64). Both antibodies can be seen in (a) primary antiphospholipid antibody syndrome (PAPS), where thromboses occur in the absence of a collagen vascular disease; (b) secondary antiphospholipid antibody syndrome associated with lupus and other collagen vascular disease; (c) the elderly with atherosclerosis, where it is considered to be an epiphenomenon; and (d) infectious diseases such as syphilis, malaria, and parasitic and viral infections as well as medication exposure (50,65,66). In young adults, antiphospholipid antibodies could be seen in up to 40% of patients with a first stroke (67). Compare this with the study by Angelini and colleagues, which documented the presence of antiphospholipid antibodies in 75% of children with idiopathic cerebral ischemia (68). Neonates with antiphospholipid antibodies appear to be at risk for developing neonatal stroke. Antibody titers greater than 1:100 are more common in children with cerebral palsy as compared with controls (69).

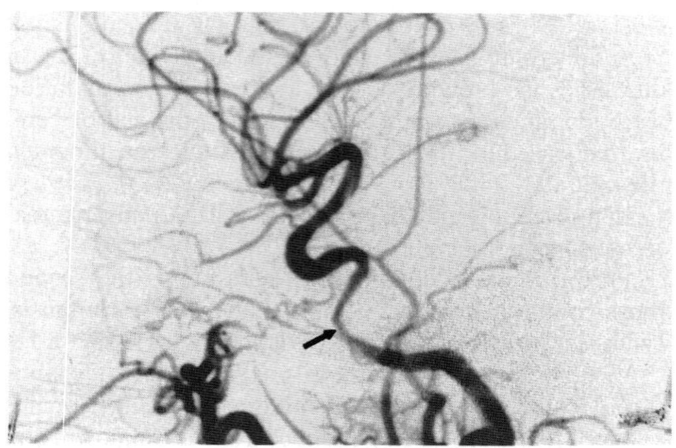

FIGURE 13.2. Cerebral arteriography demonstrates narrowing of the internal carotid artery from a traumatic dissection (*arrow*).

Other causes for symptomatic venous and arterial thromboses in children include elevated D-dimer levels (D-dimer is a fibrin fragment in plasma that is a marker of fibrin formation and reactive fibrinolysis; its levels are elevated during acute thromboembolic episodes). Elevations in plasma factor VIII also are associated with thrombotic events, and persistent elevation of these two factors after anticoagulant therapy predicts a poor outcome, notably recurrent thromboses and lack of thrombus resolution (70).

Arterial Dissection

Arterial dissection is increasingly recognized as a cause of stroke in children. Although trauma is the usual etiology, the preceding injury can be trivial or occur spontaneously, suggesting an underlying defect of the involved artery (71). The initial injury, whether traumatic or spontaneous, is an intimal tear that permits blood to penetrate between the layers of the arterial wall, resulting in stenosis or occlusion of the lumen (Fig. 13.2). Neurologic deficits can either begin immediately if the artery is occluded or occur later from an embolism arising at the dissection site (72). In one pediatric study of 59 children with cerebral arterial infarction, the incidence of arterial dissection was reported to be 20% (73).

Carotid dissection after peritonsillar trauma is well documented in children; the injury typically results from a fall onto an ice cream stick, toothbrush, pen, or similar object inside the mouth (74). Intimal damage from blunt trauma initiates the dissection, usually without penetrating the artery.

In a review of 118 patients less than 18 years of age with arterial dissection, Fullerton and colleagues found that 74% had an anterior circulation dissection and that all patients had evidence of cerebral ischemia at the time of presentation. None of the individuals with posterior circulation dissection had a recurrent dissection (versus 10% when the anterior circulation was involved), and 87% of the patients with posterior circulation dissection were male. The most common level of vertebral artery dissection is at the level of C1-C2 vertebral bodies, similar to what occurs in adults (75). In contrast to children who suffered strokes affecting the anterior circulation, over 90% of children in the series of Ganesan and coworkers who experienced posterior circulation strokes were previously normal. It is of note that MRA has poor sensitivity and specificity for the posterior circulation, and if MRI and MRA do not exclude vertebral artery dissection, cerebral angiography is necessary (76).

Vasculitis

Intracranial vasculitis in children can cause arterial thrombosis, venous thrombosis, or intraparenchymal or subarachnoid hemorrhage. Bacterial meningitis is the most common cause of intracranial arteritis in children. In a recent study, 10% of children with culture-proven meningitis had cerebral infarction (77). In infants with meningitis, the risk is even greater: Up to 92% have diffusion-weighted imaging evidence of multiple cerebral infarctions, typically involving the frontal lobes (78). The intracranial vessels evidently become inflamed due to their close proximity to the inflamed meninges (79). Factors that predict cerebral infarction in children with bacterial meningitis include an age of less than 1 year, the occurrence of seizures, hydrocephalus, altered consciousness at the time of presentation, and a high CSF lactate concentration. The frequency of stroke due to meningitis has waned in concert with the decline of *Haemophilus influenzae* meningitis, which has been dramatically reduced by widespread vaccination. In one recent series, the most commonly isolated organisms were *Salmonella* and *Streptococcus pneumoniae*, which together accounted for 57% of cases (77). Tuberculous meningitis is uncommon in the United States, but large series of children with tuberculous meningitis document the frequent occurrence of secondary vascular occlusion. In children less than 14 years of age with tuberculosis, stroke was documented in 25 of 65 individuals (38%) (80). Cerebral infarction from tuberculous meningitis occurs more frequently in children than adults. Inflammation of the intracranial arteries and veins can be demonstrated in the majority of autopsied cases and is sometimes associated with thrombosis and infarction.

Other infectious causes of cerebral vasculitis include meningovascular syphilis, fungal meningoencephalitides, and varicella-zoster virus encephalitis (33). Varicella-zoster virus infects multiple different types of cells in the neuraxis, which could explain the multitude of clinical neurologic dysfunction associated with the virus. One well-defined although rare complication of varicella-zoster infection is cerebral arteritis, which is usually a large-vessel disease, with stroke (81).

Human immunodeficiency virus (HIV) can cause cerebral vasculitis and subsequent stroke, probably as a result of direct invasion of HIV (32). In addition, aneurysms can result from HIV-induced vasculopathy, and intracerebral hemorrhage can develop as a result of HIV-induced immune thrombocytopenia (82). Between 10% and 30% of pediatric HIV patients have evidence of cerebral infarction at autopsy (82–84). The vascular complications of the various bacterial and viral meningitides are more extensively covered in Chapter 7.

Cerebral vasculitis and stroke occur with many systemic inflammatory diseases, including polyarteritis nodosa, Churg-Strauss angiitis, Wegener's granulomatosis, Henoch-Schonlein purpura, cryglobulinemia, systemic lupus erythematosus, rheumatoid arthritis, Beçet's disease, sarcoidosis, and Kawasaki disease (33,35). As mentioned previously, some patients with systemic lupus erythematosus also have a hypercoagulable state due to antiphospholipid antibodies.

Isolated angiitis of the central nervous system presents in children with either small or large vessel involvement (85). The diagnosis of isolated angiitis should be confirmed by leptomeningeal biopsy prior to initiation of immunosuppressive treatment (85a). Homocystinuria is an autosomal recessive disorder of methionine metabolism that has long been recognized as a cause of stroke in children. This condition is covered in Chapter 1.

Metabolic Stroke

"Metabolic" stroke or "strokelike" episodes occur in association with several different metabolic disorders, including mitochondrial myopathy, encephalopathy, lactic acidosis, and strokelike episodes (MELAS); Leigh syndrome; organic and aminoacidurias; carbohydrate-deficiency glycoprotein syndrome; and carnitine deficiency (35), usually with the onset of symptoms during childhood or early adulthood. These conditions are presented more completely in Chapter 2.

BRAIN HEMORRHAGE

Structural vascular anomalies collectively constitute the largest cause of nontraumatic intraparenchymal and subarachnoid hemorrhage in children (Table 13.3). In the Wake Forest series of 68 children with nontraumatic hemorrhage, 26 children (41.2%) had some type of congenital vascular anomaly, with arteriovenous malformation and arteriovenous fistula together accounting for about one-third of the children (Fig. 13.3). Arterial aneurysm was documented in four (5.9%) children; three of these four children had a saccular aneurysm, and one had a mycotic aneurysm (18).

Nine of the 68 children (13.2%) presented with clinical and radiographic signs of intraparenchymal hemorrhage but were eventually found to harbor a brain tumor. However, none of the patients in this series had long-

TABLE 13.3 Risk Factors for Intraparenchymal Hemorrhage

Risk factor	N (%)
Vascular malformation/fistula	22 (32.4%)
Cavernous malformation	2 (2.9%)
Aneurysm	4 (5.9%)*
Brain tumor	9 (13.2%)
Hematologic	12 (17.6%)
Sickle cell disease	3 (4.4%)
Thrombocytopenia	8 (11.8%)
Bone marrow transplant	1 (1.5%)
Coagulopathy	10 (14.7%)
Factor VII deficiency	3 (4.4%)
Factor XIII deficiency	1 (1.5%)
Liver failure	2 (2.9%)
Warfarin therapy	1 (1.5%)
Protein C deficiency	1 (1.5%)
Protein S deficiency	1 (1.5%)
Vitamin K deficiency	1 (1.5%)
Hemorrhagic infarct	6 (8.8%)
Spontaneous dissection	2 (2.9%)
Miscellaneous	4 (5.9%)
ACTH	1 (1.5%)
HIV infection	1 (1.5%)
Systemic lupus erythematosus	1 (1.5%)
Herpes encephalitis	1 (1.5%)
Systemic hypertension	0 (0%)
No risk factors found	7 (10.3%)

N = 68; some patients had more than 1 risk factor.
*One patient had a mycotic aneurysm; the others had saccular aneurysms.
From Al-Jarallah, Al-Rifai T, Riela AR, et al. Spontaneous intraparenchymal hemorrhage in children: a study of 68 patients. *J Child Neurol* 2000;15:284–289. With permission.

standing systemic hypertension or markedly elevated blood pressure readings at the time of the hemorrhage (86).

Clinical Manifestations

Intraparenchymal Brain Hemorrhage

Not surprisingly, most children with intraparenchymal brain hemorrhage present with pain or symptoms of increased intracranial pressure (87). In the Wake Forest series of 68 children with spontaneous brain hemorrhage, for example, 40 children (58.8%) presented with dominant symptoms of headache or vomiting, and six others (8.8%) presented with irritability (86). Coma occurred in only two of these 68 children, and there were various focal neurological deficits. Twenty-five of the 68 children (36.8%) developed focal or generalized epileptic seizures acutely after the hemorrhage (86). Neonates can present only with tense and bulging fontanelle (88).

Subarachnoid Hemorrhage

Subarachnoid hemorrhage classically produces sudden severe headache, vomiting, meningismus, and alteration of consciousness. The clinical picture may be less distinct in

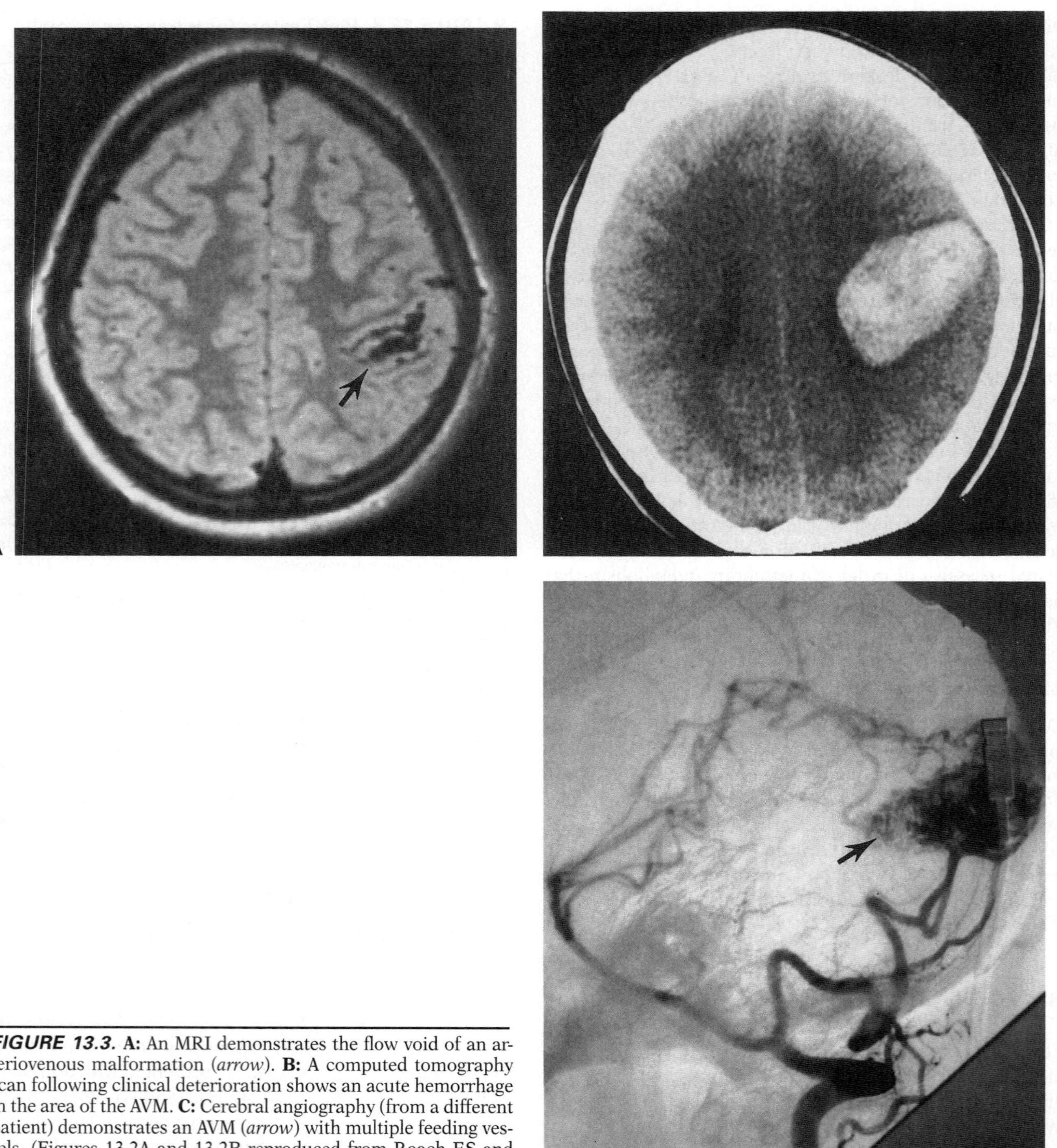

FIGURE 13.3. **A:** An MRI demonstrates the flow void of an arteriovenous malformation (*arrow*). **B:** A computed tomography scan following clinical deterioration shows an acute hemorrhage in the area of the AVM. **C:** Cerebral angiography (from a different patient) demonstrates an AVM (*arrow*) with multiple feeding vessels. (Figures 13.2A and 13.2B reproduced from Roach ES and Riela AR. *Pediatric cerebrovascular disorders*. New York: Futura Publishers, 1995. With permission.)

younger children, who can present with unexplained irritability, vomiting, photophobia or seizures. The site of the headache does not predict the site of bleeding, but more severe hemorrhage tends to produce more impairment of consciousness. Focal or generalized seizures occur in about one-fifth of patients, and signs of increased intracranial pressure are typical.

Subarachnoid hemorrhage is the most common presentation of an intracranial aneurysm. Headache also can result from expansion of an aneurysm, a small subarachnoid hemorrhage ("sentinel headache"), or, if the aneurysm is large, increased intracranial pressure from mass effect or obstruction of the cerebrospinal fluid (89).

Etiology

Thrombocytopenia

Thrombocytopenia most often results from either immune thrombocytopenic purpura (ITP) or the combined effects of leukemia or its treatment. Regardless of the cause, intracranial hemorrhage is the most feared complication of thrombocytopenia (90). Nontraumatic brain hemorrhage due to reduced platelets does not usually occur with counts above 20,000 to 30,000, and even with lower counts, spontaneous hemorrhage is uncommon. In the Wake Forest series of 68 patients involving children and adolescents with nontraumatic intraparenchymal brain hemorrhage, thrombocytopenia was the most common hematologic risk factor for brain hemorrhage, occurring in 11.8% of cases (86). Brain hemorrhage later in the course of ITP frequently coincides with a systemic viral infection, probably because the infection stimulates the production of antiplatelet antibodies and produces a further drop in the number of platelets. Patients with thrombocytopenia should avoid aspirin or other antiplatelet drugs, especially during viral infections (for ITP patients) as well as situations that are likely to produce head trauma, although most hemorrhages occur without trauma.

Bleeding Disorders

Hemophilia A (factor VIII deficiency) and B (factor IX deficiency) are the two most common hereditary bleeding disorders that cause intracranial hemorrhage, although intracranial bleeding has been less often attributed to various other disorders (e.g., factor XIII deficiency, factor V deficiency, and congenital afibrinogenemia). Among patients with a given disorder, it is generally the severity of the bleeding tendency rather than the specific defect that determines the risk of intracranial hemorrhage. In the Wake Forest series of 68 children with nontraumatic hemorrhage, 10 children (14.7%) had some type of congenital or acquired coagulation defect. Three of these 10 children had factor VII deficiency, two had coagulopathy from hepatic failure, and one took warfarin (86).

Acquired coagulation defects also can cause intracranial hemorrhage. Vitamin K deficiency results in decreased factors II, VII, IX, and X. The routine use of vitamin K injections in newborns has virtually eliminated vitamin K deficiency as a cause of hemorrhage in neonates in the United States. Infants born to mothers taking anticonvulsants sometimes bleed excessively, apparently due to reduction of vitamin K–dependent coagulation factors. These neonates may require a higher dose of vitamin K after birth in order to prevent bleeding, and vitamins during the last trimester of pregnancy may be of value. Rarely, children taking antiepileptic medications develop a vitamin K–responsive coagulopathy. Hepatic disease, malabsorption, and various other disorders promote vitamin K deficiency and need to be considered in patients with abnormal coagulation (1).

INTRACRANIAL ANEURYSM

Approximately 7% of the population develops an aneurysm 2 mm or larger by the time of death (91). Inasmuch as the vast majority of aneurysms are not congenital but are acquired during life, the condition is rare in children (92). Although aneurysms are approximately one-tenth as frequent as arteriovenous malformations (AVM), they have a greater tendency to rupture. Of patients younger than 20 years of age who have experienced a spontaneous subarachnoid hemorrhage, 40% have an aneurysm, and 27% have an AVM. In the remaining 33% of patients, the bleeding is of unknown origin (93). In the series of Sedzimir and Robinson, only 10% of patients developed symptoms before 10 years of age (93).

From these data, it is obvious that when a preadolescent patient develops a spontaneous intracranial hemorrhage, it is far more likely to be caused by an AVM rather than an aneurysm.

Aneurysms in childhood have no gender or racial predilection, and their rupture bears little relationship to systemic hypertension or physical activity. Whereas aneurysms in adults are usually located on or adjacent to the circle of Willis, in children, 50% of aneurysms originate from the carotid bifurcation, 25% from the anterior cerebral artery, and 12.5% from the posterior cerebral artery (94). The majority of childhood aneurysms are of the giant type, and only 25% of them have the small, saccular shape that is typical in adults. Fusiform aneurysm of the basilar artery, which is not an uncommon form in adults with arteriosclerosis, is extremely unusual in children (95). Multiple aneurysms were only seen in 3% of children (96). The pathology of these malformations is reviewed by Rorke (97).

Pathogenesis

In aneurysms appearing during childhood, the most common cause is a congenital weakness of the vascular media. Familial occurrence has been reported, and in 6% to 20%, two or more cases of intracranial aneurysms are confirmed (98). In some families, the transmission of the disorder is compatible with an autosomal dominant trait (99) and autosomal recessive in others (100). Among first-degree relatives of patients with an aneurysmal subarachnoid hemorrhage, the risk of a ruptured intracranial aneurysm is four times higher than in the general population (101). In a cooperative screening study using MRA published in 1999, unruptured aneurysms were found in 4% of first-degree relatives. In 48%, aneurysms were less than 5 mm in diameter. In view of the substantial risks of prophylactic therapy, the risk of rupture must be weighed against the adverse psychological and functional risks of a diagnostic study and subsequent surgery (102).

In the 1973 series of Thompson and coworkers (103), only 9% of childhood aneurysms were mycotic. These usually were more peripheral and were most commonly encountered in children with congenital heart disease. A traumatic origin could be documented in 14%. In 12% of instances, intracranial aneurysms, usually of the saccular type, were associated with coarctation of the aorta and in 4% with bilateral polycystic kidneys (104,105).

The larger the aneurysm, the more likely it is to rupture. This is particularly true for aneurysms larger than 1 cm in diameter, the size at which they tend to become symptomatic during childhood.

Clinical Manifestations

There is a biphasic presentation of saccular aneurysms during the first two decades, with the lesions most often becoming symptomatic before age 2 or after age 10 (106). Sudden massive intracranial hemorrhage is by far the most common clinical manifestation in children. The ruptured aneurysm spills blood into the subarachnoid space, providing sudden severe headache, vomiting, meningeal irritation, and increased intracranial pressure. With progressive bleeding, focal neurologic deficits, seizures, impaired consciousness, and retinal hemorrhages can occur. Retinal hemorrhages can be flame shaped and localized near blood vessels or ovoid and near or on the optic disc (101). They can dissect between retinal layers (subhyaloid hemorrhage). An intracerebral hematoma occurs in one-fourth to one-half of children and can produce a sudden increase in intracranial pressure. Other clinical manifestations, such as cranial nerve palsies and focal neurologic deficits consequent to embolization, are almost always confined to adults. In the experience of Patel and Richardson (104), 11 out of 58 youngsters with ruptured intracranial aneurysms had a prior history of headaches; in only one did these headaches take the form of the classic migraine. A more recently conducted prospective study of patients presenting with acute serious headache and proven to have a subarachnoid hemorrhage did not uncover any minor, premonitory hemorrhages (107).

Diagnosis

Bruits are seldom heard in the unruptured aneurysm. Whenever the sudden onset of a severe headache associated with vomiting and photophobia implies a ruptured aneurysm, a CT scan is the first diagnostic procedure. If both the CT scan, performed within 12 hours of the onset of symptoms, and a subsequent cerebrospinal (CSF) examination are normal, angiography will probably not uncover an aneurysm (108). Aneurysms larger than 5 mm can be seen by MRI or MRA (96). MRI is superior to CT scanning for demonstrating the aneurysm and for delineating the various complications of an aneurysmal bleed, such as an intraventricular hemorrhage, a subdural hemorrhage (which is a relatively common complication in infants), an intracerebral hematoma, or acute hydrocephalus (109). When none of these study results is positive, digital subtraction cerebral angiography remains as the most definitive diagnostic procedure (110).

Treatment

A ruptured cerebral aneurysm has traditionally been treated by a neurosurgeon. Considerable controversy surrounds the clinical management of vasospasm resulting from the extravasated blood and the timing of the operation. The results of elective surgery are excellent in terms of morbidity and mortality, but mortality is high among patients awaiting elective aneurysm clipping. Because the mortality of early surgery is no longer as prohibitive as it was a decade or two ago, and because early surgery seems to prevent the delayed cerebral vasospasm, many authorities now opt for early surgery (101). Clipping of the aneurysm, endovascular therapy by insertion of a soft metallic coil, or a combination of the two procedures are the most commonly used approaches.

When an aneurysm is detected during an evaluation for headache or when it is encountered adventitiously, surgery is indicated if the aneurysm is greater than 1 cm in diameter. Such an aneurysm is likely to rupture—a generally fatal event (111). Aneurysms at the juncture of the internal carotid and posterior communicating arteries and aneurysms within the vertebrobasilar system have a higher rate of rupture than other aneurysms (112). Conversely, aneurysms smaller than 1 cm are not likely to subsequently rupture or to be responsible for neurologic symptoms.

Children appear to tolerate surgery better than adults, particularly when it is performed with the patient in a satisfactory state of alertness (94). Although operative mortality is low, many of the survivors are left with significant cognitive deficits, primarily because of a high incidence of cerebral infarction resulting from the delayed vasospasm. For patients who survive the initial hemorrhage, every effort must be made to avoid rebleeding until the diagnosis can be confirmed and the aneurysm treated (113,114).

The technology of endovascular treatment of intracranial aneurysms is changing rapidly and has been reviewed by McDougall and colleagues (115). For further discussion of the problem of intracranial aneurysms, which is primarily one of adult neurology and neurosurgery, the reader should consult various current neurosurgical texts.

Mycotic aneurysms have become less common with the decrease in rheumatic heart disease, the earlier treatment of congenital heart disease, and the use of antibiotics for bacterial suspected endocarditis. Nevertheless, the occurrence of subarachnoid or intracerebral hemorrhage in an individual with a structural heart lesion, chronic pulmonary infection, or a history of intravenous drug abuse should suggest a mycotic aneurysm. Multiple septic emboli can produce multiple mycotic aneurysms. Less virulent organisms tend to produce mycotic aneurysms, while more virulent strains are more likely to produce abscess or meningitis. Because mycotic aneurysms are often located in the peripheral branches of the vasculature, hemorrhage into the brain parenchyma occurs more often than with saccular aneurysms (116). Some mycotic aneurysms resolve with antibiotics and do not rupture. Persistence of an aneurysm after two months of an antibiotic regimen or the development of symptoms are indications for surgery (117).

Disorders Associated with Aneurysms

The association of aneurysms with neuroepithelial cysts, agenesis of the corpus callosum, and other cerebral malformations suggests that congenital factors operate in the formation of some aneurysms (118). The best established of these conditions are coarctation of the aorta, adult polycystic renal disease, and fibromuscular dysplasia. Tyler and Clark found only three patients with definite and two patients with probable cerebral aneurysm among 200 individuals with aortic coarctation (119), but the true aneurysm frequency is probably higher because some of their patients were young, and others might have had an asymptomatic aneurysm. Cerebral aneurysms in patients with coarctation of the aorta do not usually become symptomatic until adolescence or adulthood; the average age for rupture of the aneurysm is 25 years. The incidence of aneurysm in individuals with autosomal dominant polycystic renal disease is lower, and again, it is unusual to develop symptoms until after the second decade. The estimated frequency of intracranial aneurysms in adults with arterial fibromuscular dysplasia is 30% to 50%, but aneurysms in affected children are much less common.

A deficiency of type III collagen has been demonstrated to be responsible for the various vascular defects observed in the severe, autosomal recessive form of Ehlers-Danlos disease type IV (120,121) and for at least a significant proportion of patients diagnosed as having a congenital cerebral aneurysm (122). Hyperelastic skin and hyperextensible joints are not prominent features of type IV Ehlers-Danlos syndrome, and diagnosis is sometimes delayed in these individuals until after major vascular complications occur. The intracranial portion of the internal carotid artery is the most common site for an aneurysm to develop (Fig. 13.4). Individuals with pseudoxanthoma elasticum have an increased risk of intracranial aneurysm. As with Ehlers-Danlos syndrome, most of the aneurysms involve the distal internal carotid artery, and it is unusual to develop symptoms from the aneurysm before adulthood (120,123). Aneurysms also have been reported in Pompe disease (glycogenosis type 2) (124) and in various disorders of connective tissue, including the more benign autosomal dominant form of Marfan syndrome and in pseudoxanthoma elasticum. In our opinion, this last association is so rare that it might be no more than coincidental.

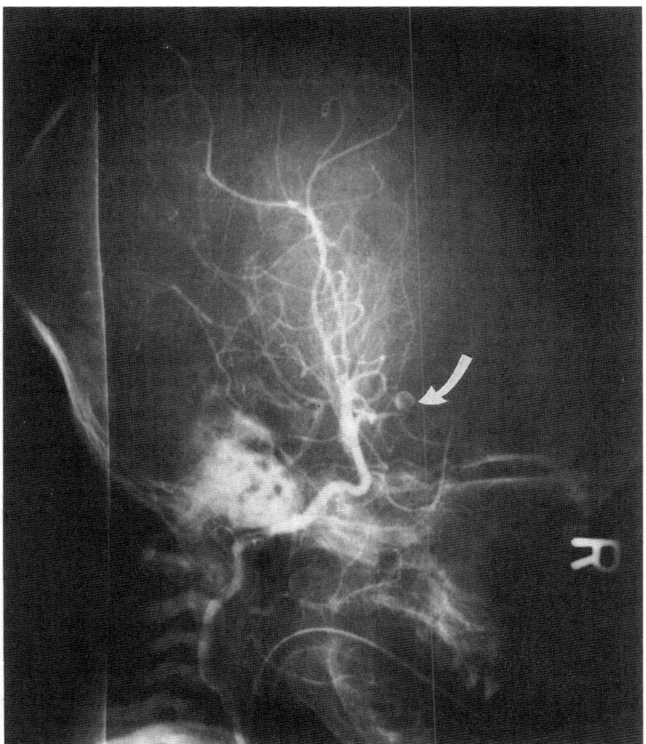

FIGURE 13.4. Cerebral angiography shows a saccular aneurysm (curved arrow) of the anterior communicating artery in an infant. (Reproduced from Roach ES and Riela AR. *Pediatric cerebrovascular disorders*. New York: Futura Publishers, 1995. With permission.)

ARTERIOVENOUS MALFORMATIONS

Pathogenesis

AVMs result from the embryonic failure of capillary development between artery and vein. This malformation in turn produces an enlargement of the vessels and abnormal shunting of blood. On gross examination of the brain, the lesion has a "bag of worms" appearance, which is caused by the tangled mass of dilated veins, the frequently enlarged and tortuous arteries feeding these venous channels, and the interposed thickened, dilated, and hyalinized vessels. The malformation can extend from the cortical meningeal surface through the parenchyma to the ventricular cavity, and its size can vary from 1 mm to more than 10 cm. Calcifications within the walls of the vessel and the

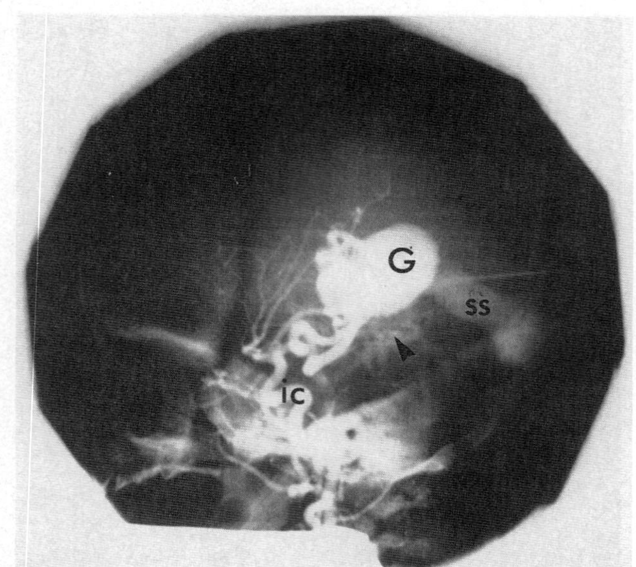

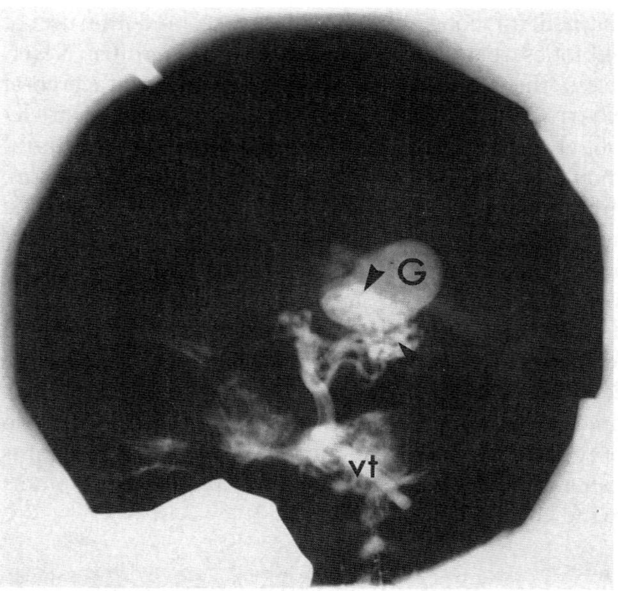

FIGURE 13.5. Term neonate with vein of Galen malformation, presenting with high-output congestive heart failure and hydrocephalus. Left lateral views of arteriograms by selective catheterization and injection of the **(A)** left internal carotid (ic) and **(B)** left vertebral (vt) arteries. From both anterior (carotid) and posterior (vertebrobasilar) circulatory sources, while contrast material is still seen in these major vessels during the infusion, a large aneurysmal sac, representing the dilated vein of Galen (G), is seen filling with contrast and blood. Even the straight sinus (ss) is visualized at the same time, indicating a large component of arteriovenous fistulous shunt. In addition, aggregates of numerous smaller pathologic vessels (*arrowheads*) are seen, another component of this complex vascular malformation. The right carotid injection in this child (not shown) yielded similar results to the left carotid injection. The blood supply to this congenital vascular malformation was therefore from all three major vessels, both carotids and the basilar artery, making surgical treatment extremely difficult.

surrounding parenchyma are common, and some ossification can be present. Hemosiderin can be found in the gliotic parenchyma as a consequence of extravasated blood. The pathology of these lesions has been reviewed by Rorke (97). In the pediatric series of Kondziolka and colleagues, 67% of malformations were in the cerebral hemispheres, 13% in the cerebellum, 11% in the brainstem, and 5% in the thalamus or basal ganglia (125). The distribution of lesions is similar for other series.

AVMs must be differentiated from the rarely encountered carotid-cavernous fistula, which almost always is traumatic in origin (see Chapter 9). Spontaneous carotid-cavernous fistulas have been reported, however, in patients with type IV Ehlers-Danlos syndrome (126,127).

Clinical Manifestations

Only one-half of AVMs are symptomatic, and the presentation of an AVM can vary with age. Symptomatic neonates often present with unexplained high-output cardiac failure or, occasionally, with intraparenchymal hemorrhage or hydrocephalus. Neonates with congestive heart failure tend to have larger vascular lesions than those who present in some other fashion. Infants especially can develop hydrocephalus, particularly when they have a posterior fossa AVM with secondary aneurysmal dilatation of the vein of Galen (Fig. 13.5). In our experience, small lesions are often deep and silent and bleed massively. Large lesions are characterized by seizures and focal neurologic signs and bleed less extensively. In most large studies of symptomatic AVMs, 10% become clinically manifest during the first decade, and up to 45% are evident by the second or third decade (128). These lesions are seen twice as frequently in male subjects. In the overwhelming majority, 79% in the series of Kondziolka and colleagues (125), intracranial hemorrhage is the initial presentation. In 23% of patients, the hemorrhage recurs from a few days to many years after the first event (129). A chronic seizure disorder, recurrent headache, and progressive neurologic deficits are less common presentations. Progressive neurologic deficits can result from the AVM acting as a space-occupying lesion or, more commonly, are caused by arterial steal away from normal surrounding brain into a high-flow AVM or venous hypertension transmitted from the malformation into the surrounding brain (130). Rarely, the condition is familial, being transmitted as an autosomal dominant disorder accompanied by polycystic kidneys (131).

When a hemorrhage develops, it is generally parenchymal, but depending on the location of the AVM, blood can dissect into the subarachnoid space and the ventricular system. The most frequent clinical picture is that of a child who either has been completely asymptomatic or has experienced periodic migrainelike headaches, and who suddenly has a severe headache, vomiting, nuchal rigidity, and seizures (128,132,133). As a consequence of massive bleeding, the patient can develop signs and symptoms of increased intracranial pressure with transtentorial or foramen magnum pressure cones. The mortality from a hemorrhage depends on the location of the AVM. In the series of Kondziolka and colleagues, it was 4.5% for cerebral AVMs, but 57% when the hemorrhage arose from a cerebellar malformation (125).

Less commonly (12% to 22% of children), an AVM presents with a focal or generalized seizure (125,133). The seizure focus is typically near the malformation, and the seizure type is most often focal motor or complex partial. Generalized tonic-clonic seizures are seen in some 20% of subjects (134). Control of seizures is relatively easy, and in the experience of Murphy, some 50% of patients were free of seizures for a minimum of 2 years (134). Other symptoms include progressive hemiparesis, behavioral abnormalities, and dementia. Intracranial bruits were found in only 25% of patients with AVMs reported by Kelly and coworkers (133). Rarely, an AVM can thrombose and produce ischemic focal neurologic deficits.

Relatively more common in the adult, AVMs in the posterior fossa become manifest before 20 years of age in less than 10% to 25% of cases (125,135). Symptoms are those of a cerebellar or brainstem lesion. Because most AVMs in this region are small, usually less than 2 cm in diameter, intracranial bruits are rarely heard. A pontine angioma can mimic a similarly placed neoplasm by presenting with insidious and progressive brainstem deficits (135). Hydrocephalus can complicate this type of AVM (136).

A spinal cord syndrome owing to an AVM is rare in childhood. Symptomatic spinal cord AVMs are more frequent in the cervical region, whereas in adults, they are more likely to be located in the thoracolumbar region (137). In the pediatric series of Aminoff and Edwards (138), 55% of children presented with a subarachnoid hemorrhage. Symptoms are marked by sudden severe pain at the site of the hemorrhage, which spreads to involve the entire back. Older children and adults often experience impairment of motor function, usually coming on after physical effort, and recurrent pain and paresthesias of girdle or root distribution. Sensory symptoms can present as fluctuating lower abdominal pain or sciatica and can last from several minutes to hours. Symptoms are produced by small hemorrhages, and stepwise progression of long tract signs below the lesion follows each attack. In 34%, a spinal cord AVM coexists with a cutaneous angioma in the same or an adjacent dermatome (139,140). The skin lesions include port-wine–stained angiomas (Cobb syndrome) (141) or telangiectasia (Osler-Weber-Rendu syndrome). An important clinical decision must be made in managing children with facial angiomas with respect to which patients to investigate for intracranial vascular lesions. Port-wine stains involving the cutaneous distribution of the ophthalmic branch of the trigeminal nerve are most likely to be associated with intracranial vascular malformations, especially if they are extensive; those involving two or more trigeminal branches nearly always have intracranial components (142).

Osler-Weber-Rendu syndrome (OWRS) (hereditary hemorrhagic telangiectasia) consists of a group of autosomal dominant disorders, the gene for the most common of which is located on the long arm of chromosome 9 (9q33-q34). The gene encodes endoglin, a component of the transforming growth factor-b_1 receptor (TGF) complex (143,144). TGF inhibits growth of many cell types, including hematopoietic cells and lymphocytes. Less often the defective gene codes for an activin receptor-like kinase, a member of the serine-threonine kinase receptor family, expressed in endothelium (144a). The clinical manifestations of OWRS involve vascular abnormalities of the nose, skin, gastrointestinal tract, lung, and brain. In the nose, telangiectases result in epistaxis, whereas in the lungs, there are AVMs (145). In the experience of Putman and colleagues, who systematically screened subjects with OWRS with MRI, 23% had abnormalities suggesting a vascular malformation. Follow-up angiography showed that all subjects had at least one AVM, and 39% had three or more AVMs (146). These lesions can result in subarachnoid hemorrhage, seizures, and, if the AVM involves the spinal cord, paraparesis (139,146,147). Brain abscess can develop in the presence of pulmonary AVM and right-to-left shunt (148).

In Klippel-Trenaunay syndrome, which occurs sporadically, a spinal cord AVM is associated with hypertrophy of one or more limbs or of the face as well as with generally unilateral hemangiomas of the skin (see Chapter 12). Less often, a spinal cord AVM coexists with an AVM of the brain (140,149). Vertebral angiomas behave as extradural mass lesions, producing spinal cord and nerve root compression syndromes and deficits (150).

Should an AVM become symptomatic in infancy, its initial manifestations can be increased intracranial pressure and hydrocephalus. These result from the mass effect of the lesion itself, from an intracerebral hematoma, intraventricular hemorrhage, or dissection of a superficial cortical hemorrhage into the subdural space.

Diagnosis

When confronted with clinical evidence of a sudden intracranial hemorrhage—namely, severe headache, vomiting, and nuchal rigidity—the physician must consider the presence of an AVM or, less likely, an aneurysm. An intracranial bruit, which should always be listened for, is heard in a significant percentage of patients with AVMs. The incidence varies markedly from one series to the next and probably reflects the care with which the skull is auscultated. Unlike a benign bruit, it is accompanied by a thrill and has a much louder and harsher quality. Intracranial bruits are heard in a significant percentage of normal children (see Introductory chapter) and in a variety of conditions characterized by increased cerebral blood flow. These include anemia, thyrotoxicosis, and meningitis. Bruits also accompany hydrocephalus and some, not necessarily vascular, intracranial tumors.

Although plain skull radiography has revealed intracranial calcifications in up to 10% of children with AVMs (133), currently, the initial diagnostic procedure of choice in the child who presents emergently with an acute intracranial hemorrhage is a CT scan. Contrast enhancement identifies virtually all vascular lesions larger than 1.5 mm in diameter (151) and can even detect angiographically occult vascular malformations. The CT scan also can determine the presence and extent of hydrocephalus and a secondary intracerebral hematoma and, hence, is immediately helpful in the surgical management of a pressure cone (152). Both MRI and MRA are invaluable for the more definitive evaluation of AVMs. MRI can show the presence and extent of any associated hematomas and the relationship of the angioma to the ventricular system but does not obviate the need for angiography (153). Angiography remains the definitive diagnostic procedure and is invariably required before a nonemergency surgical procedure. When angiography is performed, bilateral carotid and vertebral studies are indicated, inasmuch as other vascular malformations can coexist with the malformation responsible for neurologic symptoms. Additionally, saccular aneurysms can coexist with AVMs in some 4% to 10% of patients (128,129,133). In planning the angiographic procedure, one must remember that a small fraction of AVMs is supplied exclusively by the external carotid artery (154). But even angiography may not show a small malformation, particularly in the acute stage when obscured by hemorrhage and edema, and it may need to be repeated after resolution of the acute hemorrhage.

CSF examination is of little value. In the patient who is deteriorating acutely as a consequence of an expanding hematoma or intraventricular dissection of blood and who has signs of tentorial or foramen magnum herniation, it is contraindicated.

Spinal cord AVMs are difficult to document. CT has been of little help. When the malformation has a significant intramedullary component, MRI or MRA can identify the presence and the location of the malformation. When the AVM is localized to the dura of the spinal cord, the lesion cannot usually be demonstrated by these procedures. In such cases, a dilated epidural venous plexus can sometimes be demonstrated by an MRI of the spinal cord (137).

Treatment

Children with AVMs should be treated aggressively because of the risk of future catastrophic hemorrhage (125). Surgical removal of an AVM is indicated if the operative risk is less than the risk determined by the natural history of the AVM. Spetzler and his group have proposed a grading system for AVMs that takes into account the size of the malformation, whether venous drainage occurs through the cortical venous system or through deep veins such as the internal cerebral veins, and the location of the lesion with reference to areas whose injury results in a disabling neurologic deficit (155,156). In their experience, grade I and II AVMs, which constitute 26% of all AVMs, were removed without difficulty, with neither mortality nor major neurologic deficit. Grade IV and V AVMs, which constitute 38% of all AVMs, often require preoperative and intraoperative embolization and a multistaged surgical removal. Preoperative embolization changes a vascular lesion into an avascular tangle of thrombosed vessels and thereby facilitates their surgical removal. Embolization alone has been tried, but the cure rate with this procedure has been between 8% and 16% (130). Complications from embolization include transient neurologic deficits, stroke, and hemorrhage.

Stereotactic radiosurgical treatment (Gamma knife) is a minimally invasive and effective alternative to surgical removal of an AVM. The effectiveness of this procedure partially depends on the size of the AVM; the smaller the lesion, the higher the rate of obliteration (157). The risk of hemorrhage following this procedure is significantly reduced, in part because radiosurgery induces a progressive thickening of the intimal wall that develops three months or so after surgery (157a). In addition, thrombosis of the irradiated vessels decreases the number of patent vessels in the malformation. In children, most neurosurgeons opt for a definitive procedure designed to completely remove or obliterate the malformation (158,159).

The outcome depends on the size and location of the malformation. After surgery, 10% of patients with grade I and II AVMs were left with major neurologic deficits and 20% with minor ones. Complete surgical removal almost certainly prevents recurrence, whereas incomplete removal and ligation of feeding vessels does not. Incomplete obliteration by embolization also fails to provide protection from recurrent hemorrhage, even if follow-up angiography appears to show complete obliteration of the lesion (160).

Contrasted with this surgical experience are the data indicating that the mortality for the initial hemorrhage is greater in children than in adults, ranging between 7.1% and 13.3%. In children, a ruptured AVM has approximately a 2% to 4% risk of recurrence per year, whereas an unruptured AVM has a 32% risk of bleeding by 10 years of age and an 85% risk by 25 years of age (161). The latter values are significantly higher than those for adults (162). In particular, even trivial head trauma incurred during sports participation can result in rupture of an AVM (163). One must, therefore, conclude that surgery is indicated whenever an AVM is detected in children, even when there has been no antecedent hemorrhage (164).

The results of surgical resection when performed for seizure control are under dispute. In the experience of Murphy, the results were not good, and seizure control was not improved after resection of the AVM. In some cases, seizures began following surgery (134). By contrast, Kondziolka and coworkers found that excision of an AVM responsible for a chronic seizure disorder produced complete seizure control without use of anticonvulsants in 73% of children (125).

The current consensus is that the younger the child, the greater the indication for attempted resection of an accessible lesion because of the longer period the child is vulnerable to either rupture or gliosis and atrophy of the surrounding parenchyma. In inoperable lesions, stereotactic radiosurgery offers another therapeutic approach (157,158,165). This subject has been reviewed extensively by Fleetwood and Steinberg (166).

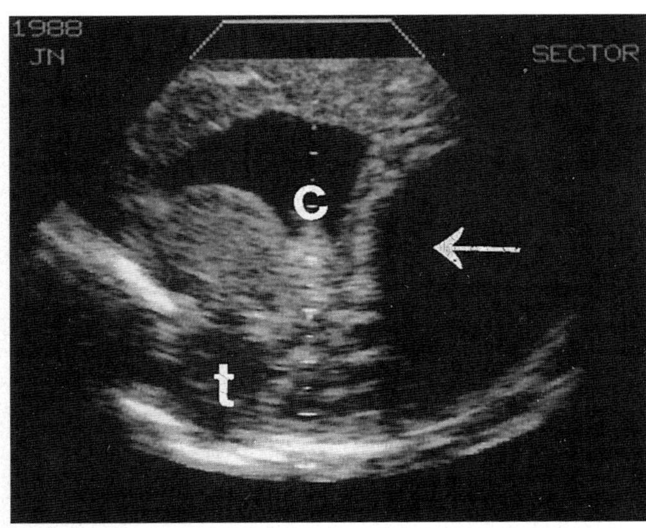

FIGURE 13.6. Vascular malformation of the vein of Galen in a 3-day-old child. This full-term infant presented with a sudden change in level of consciousness, tachycardia, tachypnea, and cyanosis. There was a loud bruit over the cranium. Ultrasonography, sagittal view, demonstrates a massive malformation (*arrow*) that has pushed the choroid plexus (c) anteriorly. The right lateral ventricle and the temporal horn (t) are enlarged.

VEIN OF GALEN MALFORMATIONS

The great vein of Galen is a single midline vein lying in the subarachnoid space dorsal to the midbrain. It is formed by the union of the paired internal cerebral veins that course in the medial wall of the thalamus, the basal veins of Rosenthal, and the superior cerebellar vein. Joining the inferior sagittal sinus soon after its origin, the vein of Galen empties into the straight sinus. It drains the medial deep nuclei of the forebrain, the medial surfaces of the occipital and temporal lobes, and the superior surface of the cerebellum.

Malformations of the vein of Galen are complex and are sometimes called *aneurysms of the vein of Galen* because of the great dilatation caused by the arteriovenous fistula component, but this term is not entirely accurate because the angiomatous portion is equally important and creates an AVM (167). Some malformations represent direct fistulas between the arteries and veins; others have an intervening vascular cluster or represent a venous malformation without arteriovenous shunting (see Fig. 13.5; Fig. 13.6) (168,169). Neuropathologic studies of the vein of Galen malformation show intimal thickening of the abnormal vascular channels, which could produce higher vascular resistance (170).

Three distinct age-dependent presentations occur (171). Generally, the larger the arteriovenous shunt, the earlier the lesion becomes manifest clinically. Signs appearing during the neonatal period are primarily those of congestive heart failure (169,171,172). Shunting of a large volume of blood results in increased peripheral resistance and increased cardiac output. This produces high-output heart failure with cardiomegaly, a wide arterial pulse pressure, and a narrow arteriovenous oxygen difference (171). A loud, harsh, systolic or systolic-diastolic intracranial bruit, which is often heard without auscultation, is noted in a large proportion of neonates and in nearly every symptomatic infant.

When signs of a vein of Galen malformation appear during early infancy, initial manifestations take the form of hydrocephalus (42%), seizures (26%), or distention and tortuosity of scalp veins (26%) (169). Hydrocephalus is caused by aqueductal obstruction by the vein of Galen or by subarachnoid adhesions associated with intracranial hemorrhage. The older child with a malformation of the vein of Galen presents with an acute subarachnoid hemorrhage, focal seizures, or headaches. Because in this age group the arteriovenous flow is relatively small, intracranial bruits are rare (169). Cerebral atrophy and periventricular leukomalacia are not unusual and can be the result of a "steal phenomenon" (172).

Both MRI and MRA demonstrate the malformation. MRA is able to distinguish the high flow arterial feeding vessels from the low flow venous lesions. Conventional arteriography is performed as the initial component of the interventional procedure. In the neonate, the presence of a malformation of the vein of Galen can often be demonstrated by ultrasonography (see Fig. 13.6).

Surgical treatment of the malformation has had poor results, with only 10% of infants surviving ligation of the feeding vessels. One-half of these infants were neurologically impaired (173). The poor outcome is in part

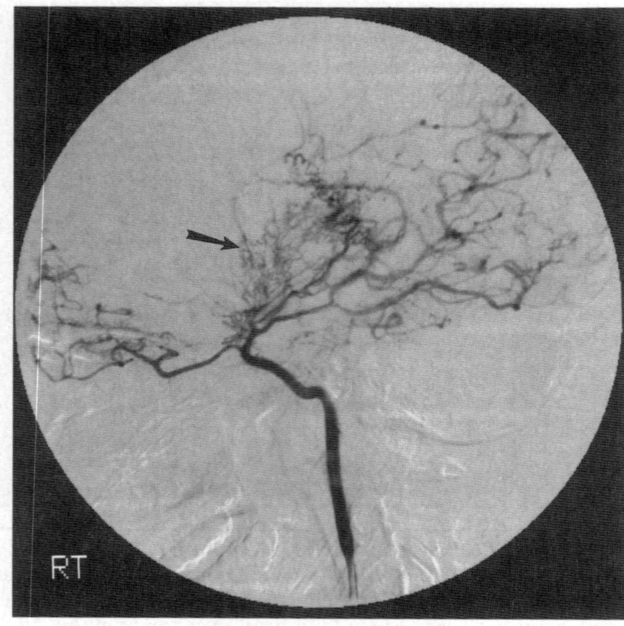

A

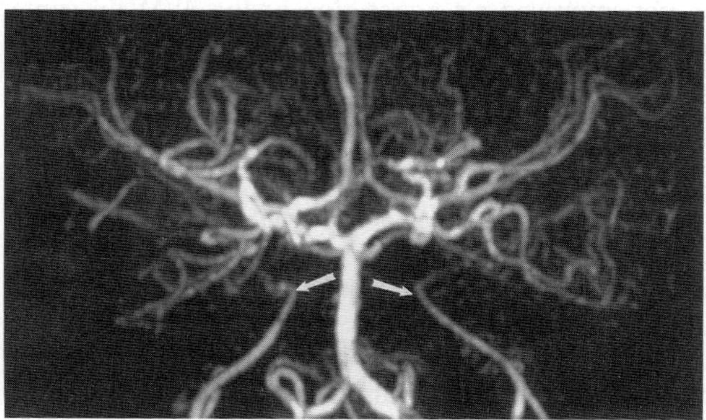

B

FIGURE 13.7. **A:** Internal carotid angiogram demonstrating moyamoya syndrome (following irradiation) with complete carotid artery occlusion and distal collateral vessels (*arrow*). **B:** Anterior view MRA (from a different patient) shows occlusion of both internal carotid arteries (*arrows*) with filling of both middle cerebral arteries via the basilar artery. (Figure 13.7A reproduced from Roach ES and Riela AR. *Pediatric cerebrovascular disorders*, New York: Futura Publishers, 1995. With permission.)

because the vascular lesion is fed by all major cerebral vessels, both carotids and the vertebrobasilar circulation (see Fig. 13.5). With the development of precise invasive radiologic procedures for controlled transarterial embolization of synthetic cyanoacrylate compounds, the vascular malformation may be reduced significantly in size in some children (174). A minority of patients experience spontaneous thrombosis of the malformation in childhood without treatment (174,175), and rarely, adults have thrombosis of the straight sinus as late as 64 years of age (170).

At present, endovascular techniques with transarterial embolization of the malformation represent the primary treatment (177,178). Infants who present during the neonatal period fare less well than those who present later in infancy or in childhood (179), and this procedure is more successful in older infants (180). Even though in many instances embolization does not produce a cure, it still allows the neonate to develop to an age when more definitive surgical treatment can be attempted (181). When hydrocephalus develops, as it does not infrequently, the complication is treated by placement of a ventriculoperitoneal shunt (178).

MOYAMOYA SYNDROME

Moyamoya syndrome is a vasculopathy of the cranial arteries, typically the carotids, leading to progressive intracranial arterial occlusion with distal telangiectatic collateral vessels. These collateral vessels are visible as an angiographic blush distal to the occluded large artery (Fig. 13.7). This condition was first described by Takeuchi in 1963 and more fully delineated by Suzuki (182). [*Moya-moya* is a Japanese term, first used by Kudo. It refers to something hazy, "just like a puff of cigarette smoke drifting in the air" (183).]

Moyamoya disease is not a single entity but is best considered to be a syndrome. Takeuchi and associates (184) and Gadoth and Hirsch (185) distinguished two forms, primary and secondary (moyamoya syndrome). Since then, moyamoya has been more accurately classified as a radiographic syndrome rather than a specific disease entity; often the term *moyamoya disease* is applied to children with no defined cause of their vasculopathy, and moyamoya syndrome is reserved for individuals with a known risk factor for the condition. Primary moyamoya disease with a strong hereditary predisposition is fairly common among Japanese patients (0.1 in 100,000 per year), and 10% of Japanese cases are familial, with transmission being autosomal dominant inheritance with low penetrance has been reported (186,187). Linkage in these families to 3p24.2-26 (*MYMY1*), 17q25 (*MYMY2*), and 8q24 (*MYMY3*) has been described (187–189,189a).

Although moyamoya is more common in Asians, it has now been recognized in most populations. The nationwide Japanese survey conducted in 1995 suggested that there were around 4,000 individuals with moyamoya disease in Japan. The syndrome has occurred with several

TABLE 13.4 Moyamoya Syndrome Risk Factors

Trauma
Basilar meningitis
Tuberculous meningitis
Leptospirosis
Cranial radiation therapy for optic pathway glioma
Neurofibromatosis
Tuberous sclerosis
Brain tumors
Fibromuscular dysplasia
Polyarteritis nodosa
Marfan syndrome
Pseudoxanthoma elasticum
Hypomelanosis of Ito
Williams syndrome
Cerebral dissecting and saccular aneurysms
Sickle cell anemia
β-thalassemia
Fanconi anemia
Apert syndrome
Factor XII deficiency
Type I glycogenosis
NADH-coenzyme Q reductase deficiency
Renal artery stenosis
Down syndrome
Coarctation of the aorta

From Broderick J, Talbot T, Prenger E, et al. Stroke in children within a major metropolitan area: the surprising importance of intracerebral hemorrhage. *J Child Neurol* 1993;8:250–255. With permission.

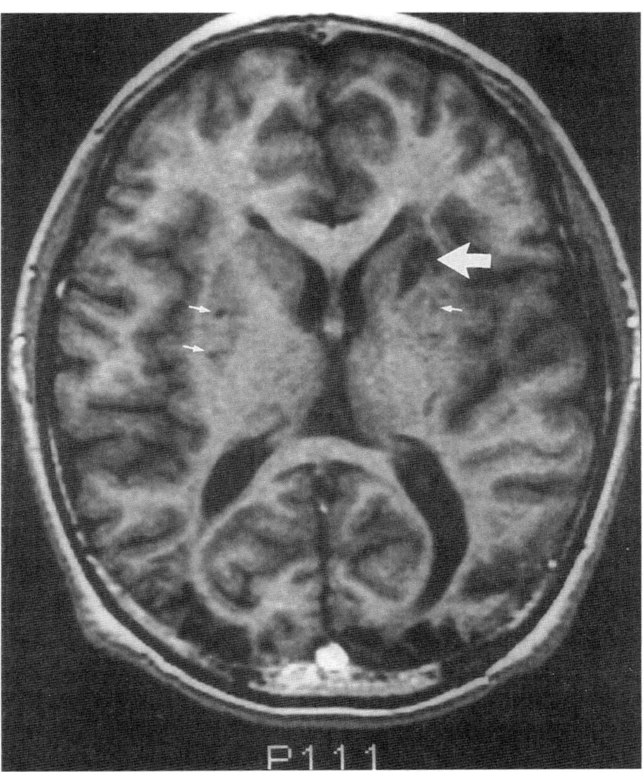

FIGURE 13.8. Moyamoya disease. Axial T1-weighted magnetic resonance imaging in a 13-year-old with moyamoya. An infarct is visible on the left, at the border between the caudate nucleus and the internal capsule (*arrow*). Prominent signal voids are seen in the basal ganglia (*small arrows*). (Courtesy of Dr. John Curran, Dept. Neuroradiology, Children's Memorial Hospital, Chicago.)

other conditions, some of which may prove coincidental (Table 13.4).

The pathophysiology of moyamoya is unknown and may be multifactorial. The clinical features of moyamoya are both variable and nonspecific, depending in part on the rapidity of vascular occlusion, the availability of collateral flow, and the anatomic site of the infarction. Various focal neurological deficits are described, and the findings may be exacerbated by hyperventilation (190). Mental retardation is present in more than one-half of the cases, and patients with onset of cerebral ischemia before 4 years of age usually develop progressive mental retardation (191). Adults with moyamoya, on the other hand, more often develop an intracranial hemorrhage (190). About 20% to 30% of cases present with seizures (190).

Initial diagnosis and periodic screening of moyamoya can be accomplished by MRI and MRA (Fig. 13.8). Standard angiography is useful especially when revascularization procedures are being contemplated.

Untreated, transient ischemic attacks tend to lessen over the years, but intellectual deterioration and persistent motor deficits become progressively worse. Intellectual deterioration was noted in 65% of children who had moyamoya disease for longer than 5 years (192). Early onset of symptoms and hypertension were related to a poor prognosis, whereas the presence of seizures was not. Conversely, children with the transient ischemic attack form of moyamoya disease tend to do somewhat better in terms of mental status and activities of daily living (193).

A variety of extracranial-intracranial bypass procedures have been proposed as treatment for moyamoya disease. These procedures produce direct, indirect, or combined anastomotic revascularization. Direct revascularization includes anastomosis of the superficial temporal artery or the occipital artery to the middle cerebral artery. Indirect bypasses, which are more or less effective, are encephalo-duro-arterio-synangiosis (EDAS), in which a piece of galea with a still-attached branch of the superficial temporal artery is fixed to the dura to provide another conduit for collateral blood flow, and encephalo-arteriosynangiosis, in which branches of the scalp arteries are used as donor arteries. Currently, most younger children who require surgery undergo EDAS. Older patients with larger arteries often undergo a direct bypass attaching the superficial temporal artery–middle cerebral artery (STA-MCA) bypass (194,195). Other indirect bypasses include encephalo-myo-synangiosis (EMS), in which a pedunculated temporalis muscle flap is placed over the temporoparietal lobe and omental transplantation. These procedures are often combined with direct or other indirect revascularization procedures. Indirect revascularization, technically less difficult, is used first in most Japanese centers, with direct anastomosis reserved for patients whose symptoms persist (196).

Fukui presented data from 821 patients in the Japanese moyamoya registry. Just over two-thirds of these patients were treated with various surgical procedures, while the remaining 23% were treated medically, and there was no difference in the outcome of the two groups (197). Thus, without controlled studies, it is hard to determine if any of the operations improve the outcome. Given that some patients do well without surgery, one sensible approach is to follow the cerebral blood flow reserve with single photon emission tomography (SPECT) or positron emission tomography (PET) and perform surgery on those who become symptomatic or whose blood flow reserve dips beneath a certain level (195,198).

CAVERNOUS ANGIOMA

Cavernous angioma is frequently clinically silent, detected only incidentally by CT scan or MRI. Unlike other vascular malformations, cavernous angiomas have a significant familial incidence, compatible with transmission as a dominant trait (199,200). Three genes are associated with the familial cavernous angioma. *CCM1* is responsible for some 40% to 50% of cases (201). It has been mapped to the long arm of chromosome 7q11.2-21 (202). It encodes a protein (Krit1) that appears to function as a tumor supressor and regulates angiogenesis (201,203). Other loci have been mapped to chromosome 7 p15-13 (*CCM2*), and 3q25.2-q27 (*CCM3*). When families carrying the *CCM1* mutation are investigated with MRI, both clinical and radiological penetrance are generally found to be incomplete (204,205).

Most cavernous angiomas in children occur in the cerebral hemispheres, and the long-term results of surgical resection are generally good (205). Surgery should be considered once the diagnosis is established in order to prevent catastrophic subsequent intracerebral hemorrhages. In the brainstem, once they become symptomatic, cavernous angiomas also may cause progressive morbidity from repeated hemorrhages and can even be fatal (206). After surgical resection, the vascular malformation may regrow and again become symptomatic, but complete excision is feasible, safe, and potentially curative in lesions located superficially and away from the floor of the fourth ventricle (206).

Cavernous angiomas usually do not become clinically apparent until adult life. They were first described by Virchow in 1863 (206a). They are endothelial-lined vascular channels, variable in size and devoid of mature vessel wall elements, such as internal elastic, muscular, or adventitial layers; the thin-walled channels are separated by collagenous stroma and are filled with blood at various stages of thombosis and organization (206b,c). Patients generally present with seizures, less commonly as vascular accidents or severe headache. The lesion is responsible for 12% of intracranial hemorrhages owing to vascular anomalies (207). Most cavernous angiomas are located in the cerebral hemispheres. Typically, they involve the rolandic area (Fig. 13.9) and can accompany similar lesions in the retina, liver, kidneys, or skin (199,208).

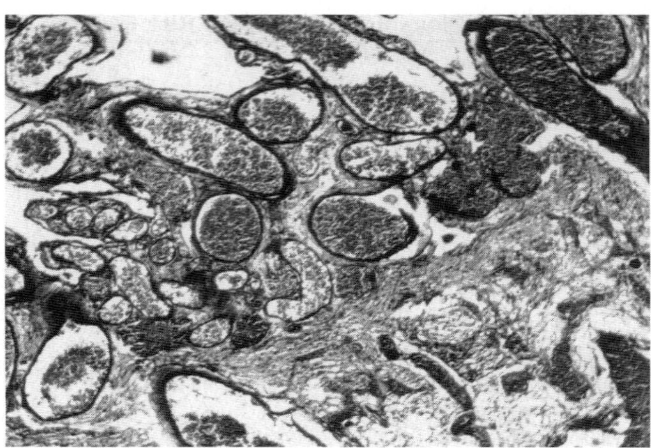

FIGURE 13.9. Histopathologic section of a cavernous hemangioma within the brain parenchyma in the parietal lobe of a 7-year-old girl. Multiple closely clustered thin-walled vascular channels are seen that vary greatly in size but lack the muscular walls of arterioles, arteries, or veins. The lumina are filled with blood. Because of the large diameter and thin walls of these pathologic vessels, they are subject to rupture, causing intracerebral and subarachnoid hemorrhage (Verhoeff–van Gieson stain, ×250 original magnification).

CAPILLARY ANGIOMAS AND TELANGIECTASIA

Though the terms *capillary angioma* and *telangiectasis* (plural, *telangiectasia*) are used interchangeably by some authors, there is an important distinction both pathologically and in biological behavior (209). The neural tissue between the pathologic vessels in capillary angiomas is usually gliotic and contains no neurons; the cerebral parenchyma between vessels in telangiectasia is normal and includes normal neurons, a normal concentration of glial cells, and normal fibers, the ratios depending on the involved region of the brain. The vessels themselves are more constant in size and are morphologically consistent with capillaries in telangiectasia, whereas in angiomas, the vessels are more variable in diameter and many are thin-walled, resembling the smaller vessels of cavernous angiomas (see Fig. 13.9). Unlike capillary angiomas, telangiectasia always remain asymptomatic and never cause intraparenchymal hemorrhage, result in neurologic deficits, or behave as neuronal irritants to cause seizures. The most common site of telangiectasia is in the basis pontis, where they are usually discovered in children or adults as an unsuspected, incidental finding at autopsy.

Much smaller than either AVMs or venous angiomas, capillary angiomas are usually found in the posterior fossa, particularly in the pons or medulla, occasionally in the cerebellum (67). This lesion, admixed with a venous angioma, constitutes the basic abnormality in Sturge-Weber syndrome (see Chapter 12). Capillary angiomas also can be found in the subependymal deep cortical region, where they tend to be solitary and often are discovered incidentally postmortem. Because of their location in the brainstem or subependymal region, they can be responsible for massive and catastrophic hemorrhage in these regions.

VASCULAR MALFORMATIONS CAUSED BY PERSISTENT OR ANOMALOUS

The pattern of cerebrovascular circulation in the embryo and early fetus differs from the mature pattern because of the sequence of development of major cerebral arteries, which also results in changes in direction of blood flow in the basilar artery in particular. The changes in ontogenesis are illustrated in Fig. 13.10 and are explained in the legend.

In addition to the maturational changes of major cerebral arteries, the microcirculation of the brain also undergoes an important developmental evolution (210,211). This evolution affects the vulnerability of the fetus and preterm infant to lesions seen rarely after 36 weeks' gestation, such as extensive white matter infarcts, periventricular leukomalacia, and germinal matrix hemorrhages. The penetrating vessels supplying the white matter of the cerebral mantle are mostly end-arterioles with few anastomoses, hence little collateral circulation, in the fetus and premature. The vascular channels of the germinal matrix are immature, thin-walled vessels rather than mature capillaries. Their thin endothelial cells are easily damaged by hypoxia and acidosis and often rupture during reperfusion after an episode of transient systemic hypotension. These factors are discussed more extensively in Chapter 5.

Striatal arteries develop a muscularis wall at approximately 24 weeks' gestation, but most other cerebral vessels do not form a smooth muscular wall until the last few weeks of fetal life, and the muscularization of intracerebral arteries occurs in a centripetal direction (210).

An uncommon and usually clinically silent anomaly sometimes discovered in the course of cerebral angiography and at times by MRA is a persistence of one of the three major transitory embryonic arteries that communicates between the internal carotid arteries and the basilar artery before the vertebral arteries are established (see Fig. 13.10A,B). The most rostral of this group of paired vessels, the trigeminal artery, is the most common (212–214) (Fig. 13.11), but persistence of the otic and hypoglossal arteries also occurs, either individually or conjointly (215–218). Persistence of paired embryonic vessels may be unilateral or bilateral. Many variants are seen: The trigeminal artery may form mainly an anastomosis between the internal carotid and the superior or inferior cerebellar arteries (219–223). Although usually occurring as anomalies in patients with otherwise normal brains, a persistent

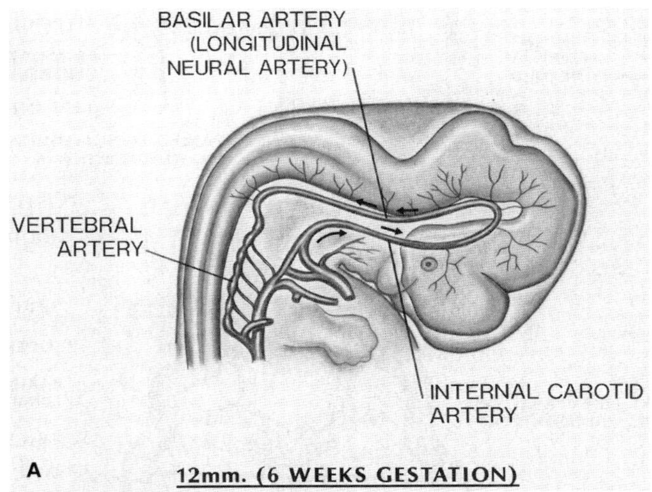

FIGURE 13.10. **A and B.** Diagrams showing the changes in the posterior circulation of the developing human embryonic (6 weeks' gestation), fetal circulation. The carotid arterial system develops sooner than does the vertebrobasilar system, and the anterior part of the circle of Willis also develops late. The basilar artery forms by the fusion of a pair of parallel adjacent vessels at the base of the embryonic brain, the paired longitudinal neural arteries, to create the single, midline vessel at the base of the brainstem, by approximately 6 weeks' gestation. Blood flow in the paired longitudinal neural arteries, and initially in the basilar artery, is rostrocaudal from the internal carotid arteries through a series of paired, transitory embryonic arteries that connect the carotid and basilar arteries; these vessels are called the trigeminal, otic, and hypoglossal arteries, named for the nerves with which they are associated anatomically. The posterior communicating arteries of the circle of Willis are not yet formed. Because of the embryonic pontine and cervical flexures, the carotid and basilar arteries are oriented nearly parallel and in close proximity, unlike the adult, facilitating the development of the embryonic communicating (i.e., trigeminal, otic, and hypoglossal) arteries; this relationship is best appreciated in the lateral view. The vertebral arteries form from a coalescence of paired plexuses of small, immature vessels, associated temporally with the formation of the vertebral neural arches, but they are not ready to provide complete blood flow into the basilar artery until approximately 8 weeks' gestation. At that time, a reversal of blood flow occurs in the basilar artery from rostrocaudal to caudorostral, the mature state. As this new direction of flow becomes established, the transient trigeminal, otic, and hypoglossal arteries progressively atrophy and disappear by approximately 9 weeks' gestation.

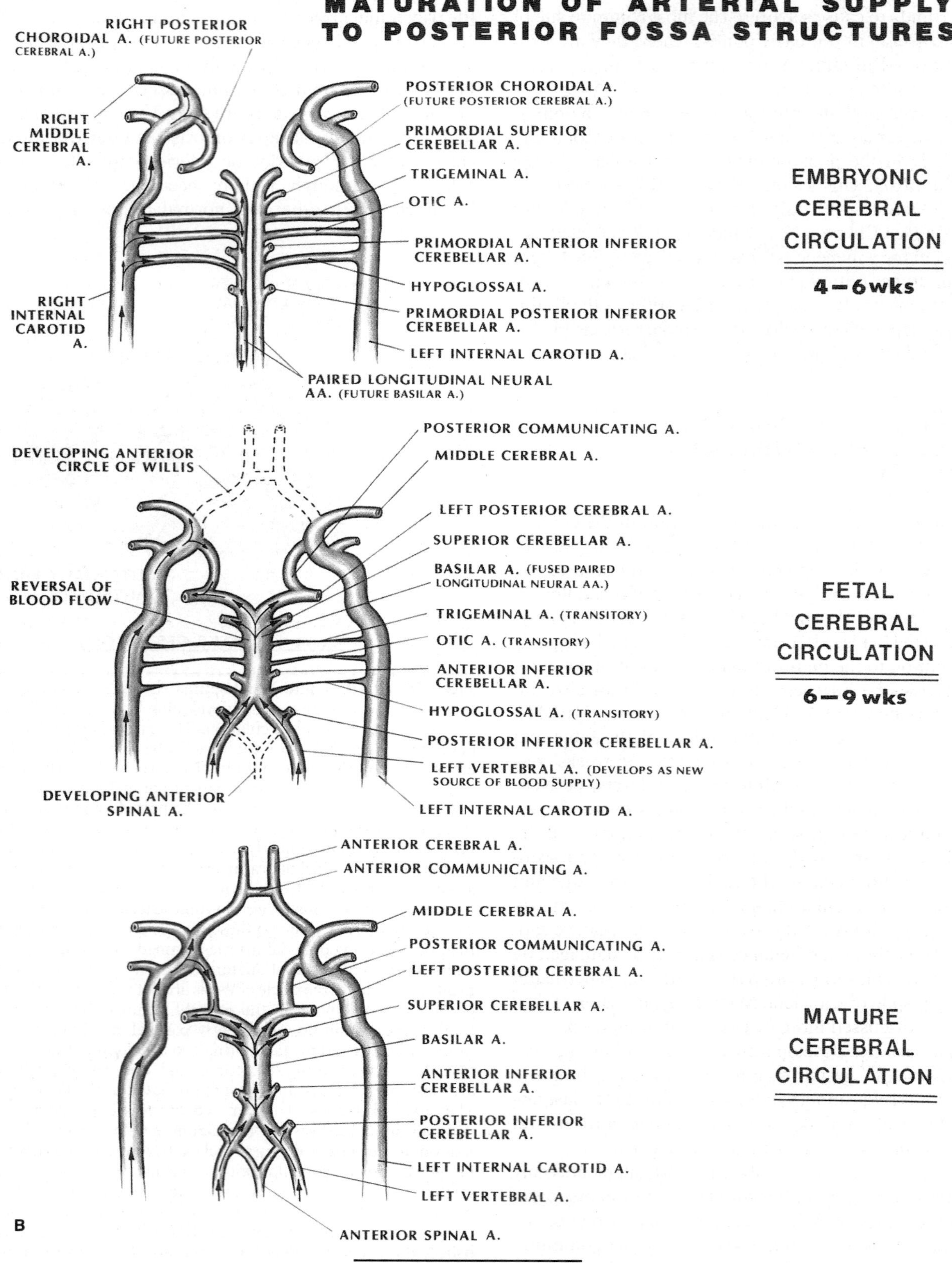

FIGURE 13.10. (Continued)

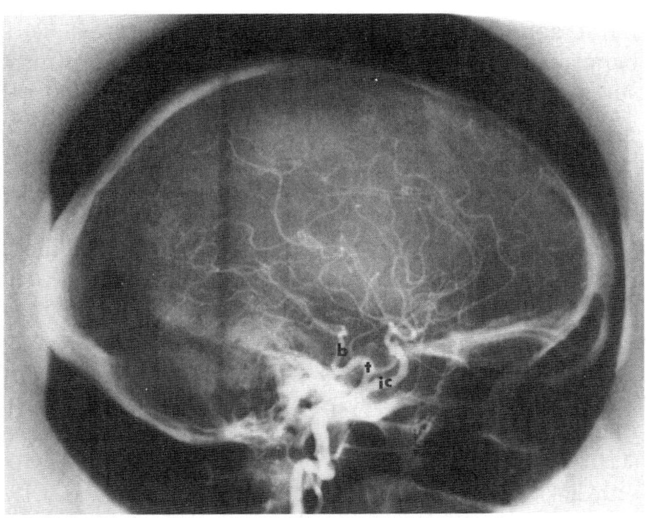

FIGURE 13.11. Persistent embryonic trigeminal artery in a 46-year-old woman. Left lateral views of left internal carotid injection of cerebral angiogram by selective catheterization. A large trigeminal artery (t) appears as an aberrant communication between the internal carotid (ic) and basilar (b) arteries. Distal arterial blood flow is seen in both the anterior (middle and anterior cerebral) and posterior (posterior cerebral) circulations after carotid injection. After vertebral injection, only a small amount of flow was seen in the basilar artery and posterior cerebral circulation, and the right internal carotid injection showed a pattern similar to that shown by the left carotid injection, demonstrating that the carotid arteries supply nearly all of the blood to the brain in this anomalous condition, as in the embryo. This circulatory pattern was entirely asymptomatic, and the woman was neurologically normal; this arteriogram was performed because of an unrelated small anterior communicating aneurysm (not shown) causing a mild subarachnoid hemorrhage for the first time in her life.

trigeminal artery occurs with greater frequency in holoprosencephaly (224). In other cases, it is reported in association with cerebellar malformations or hypoplasias (225).

Although not a cause of neurologic deficit or symptoms in themselves, these anomalies of persistent fetal cerebral arteries render such patients vulnerable to more extensive and often life-threatening infarction in the event of carotid artery thrombosis because the carotid artery provides the main blood supply to posterior fossa structures and to the posterior cerebral artery territory as well as to its normal distribution to the middle and anterior cerebral territories. Carotid occlusion is most commonly caused by trauma or infection in childhood and to atherosclerosis in older adults. In some patients, a persistent trigeminal artery coexists with a saccular aneurysm or with an angioma to produce deficits of cranial nerves III, IV, V, or VI, and the associated vascular lesions may cause spontaneous subarachnoid hemorrhage (226,227). In rare cases, multifocal AVMs of the brain have been described with persistent fetal carotid-basilar anastomoses (228).

Agenesis of the carotid arteries is another developmental malformation that leads to either an aberrant blood supply of the internal carotid territories or to neurologic deficits resulting from poor development of supratentorial structures (227–230). It is important to recognize that the anterior and middle cerebral arteries develop embryologically as isolated vessels and only later acquire their connection with the internal carotid artery. The anterior cerebral artery develops in pharyngeal pouch 1 (somitomeres 3–4) and the middle cerebral artery in pharyngeal pouch 2 (somitomeres 5–6) (231). Stenoses, congenital aneurysms, and other defects at the branch points or connections but not involving the rest of the vessel more distally thus may have an ontogenetic basis in the sequence of development and the different genes that regulate their formation.

Bilateral dissecting aneurysms of the internal carotid arteries might be a result of hypoplasia of these vessels or at least of stenosis of the supraclinoid segment (232). Various anomalous loops, kinks, or tortuosities in the internal carotid artery may occur during development and may cause neurologic symptoms secondary to ischemic atrophy of the involved hemisphere (233). Developmental dysplasias of the cerebrum are reported rarely in association with carotid agenesis, accompanied by facial hemangioma (234). True developmental agenesis of the carotid arteries, in contrast to acquired occlusions later in fetal or postnatal life, is generally associated with absence of the carotid canals at the base of the skull, which may be demonstrated radiographically or by CT scan (235).

Anomalies of the circle of Willis are extremely common, being encountered in nearly 50% of autopsy cases; however, these are probably of no clinical significance in children.

EVALUATION OF THE INFANT OR CHILD WITH A CEREBROVASCULAR DISORDER

The diagnostic evaluation should confirm the presence of a cerebrovascular lesion and perhaps identify the cause of the stroke. A child at increased risk for stroke faces decades of increased susceptibility, making the identification and treatment of risk factors relatively more important in children than adults. There are many known or suspected risk factors for cerebrovascular disease in children (Table 13.1), and it is not possible to discuss each in detail. Even a thorough diagnostic evaluation fails to identify a known risk factor in about one-third of the children with an ischemic infarction. A complete evaluation for hemorrhagic lesions, in contrast, is usually successful. Sometimes, a likely cause of the stroke is apparent from the start, as in a youngster already known to have sickle cell disease or congenital heart disease. In some individuals, multiple risk factors are present.

The evaluation should begin with simple noninvasive tests with low cost and high yield. A complete blood count, for example, provides clues to a wide array of conditions such as polycythemia, hemoglobinopathy, infections, or isoimmune thrombocytopenic purpura. Hemoglobin electrophoresis should be done on patients at risk for hemoglobinopathy who have not had the test already.

Computed tomography is quickly done and readily available after hours. It will distinguish hemorrhagic from ischemic lesions but may fail to identify smaller ischemic lesions, especially soon after they occur. MRI is superior to CT for infarctions, and MRA is able to show abnormalities of the larger cerebral vessels. Doing both studies at times provides complementary information, but generally a CT is not necessary if MRI is available.

Given the frequency of cardiac lesions in children with ischemic stroke, we usually consult a pediatric cardiologist and arrange for an electrocardiogram and chest x-ray. Ambulatory cardiac rhythm monitoring and echocardiography are sometimes useful, but their yield is low if the cardiac examination and earlier cardiac studies are normal.

Lumbar puncture should be considered in children with acute focal deficit who do not have significant mass effect and when the earlier evaluation has failed to establish a cause. A lumbar puncture is key to the diagnosis of nonvascular disorders such as herpes simplex encephalitis that can mimic a vascular lesion. CSF analysis is particularly important in a stroke patient with unexplained fever or signs of central nervous system infection. Chronic meningitis or early tuberculous meningitis can present with stroke; bacterial meningitis often causes stroke, but not typically as the presenting sign. Syphilis serology is appropriate in adolescents with infarction; recent reports also link HIV to cerebrovascular dysfunction.

MRA is ideal for patients at additional risk from standard angiography or for those whose diagnosis is already suspected. In children with sickle cell disease, for example, standard angiography could induce sickling of red blood cells, and an MRA may be adequate. A youngster with an unexplained intracerebral or subarachnoid hemorrhage, on the other hand, should almost always undergo standard angiography because the risk of rebleeding from a missed AVM or aneurysm is far higher than that of an angiogram.

TREATMENT OF THE INFANT OR CHILD WITH A CEREBROVASCULAR DISORDER

In some children, the underlying cause of stroke may be a greater initial management concern than the stroke itself, and with few exceptions, evidence-based treatment strategies are not yet possible. Supportive treatment should begin even before the diagnosis of cerebrovascular disease is established, since large lesions can generate increased intracranial pressure and brainstem lesions, or extensive hemispheric lesions can lead to herniation. Special measures to control increased intracranial pressure are not usually indicated unless the patient is deteriorating from extensive edema. As with increased intracranial pressure from other causes, rapid reduction of the $PaCO_2$ by hyperventilation is the quickest way to lower intracranial pressure. Patients with a large cerebral hemorrhage and those with a cerebellar infarction or hemorrhage may benefit from surgical evacuation of the lesion. Steroids are not effective for cytotoxic edema and are not ordinarily used in stroke patients.

The risk of seizures following an ischemic stroke is low. In a recent study of 581 adult ischemic stroke patients, a seizure occurred during the first week after the stroke in only 2.4% of patients. The risk of later seizures was 3.1% at one year and 5.5% within three years (236). Risks factors predictive of late seizures from this study included early acute seizures, presence of cortical signs, and large (more than one-half of the hemisphere). When these factors are considered, the risk of seizure at one year could range from 0% in those with no risk factors to as high as 33.3% when all three are present. Based in part on these data, we do not begin antiepileptic medication after an ischemic stroke. When seizures occur, a nonsedating antiepileptic medication is preferable. Children with subarachnoid hemorrhage due to an aneurysm or an AVM, on the other hand, should receive a prophylactic anticonvulsant because a seizure could increase the risk of rebleeding.

Anticoagulation

The usefulness of anticoagulation in children with cerebral infarction depends on the likelihood a second infarction that might be prevented by treatment and on the risk of inducing a hemorrhage due to anticoagulation. Unfortunately, there currently are no published controlled treatment trials in children, but limited experience with anticoagulants and antithrombotic agents has shown that these agents can be safely used in children (237–240). Most of the time, either heparin is used initially followed by warfarin or the patient is maintained on low-molecular weight-heparin (LMWH) injections. How long to continue anticoagulation is usually arbitrarily decided, based on whether complications have occurred and on estimation of the degree of ongoing risk.

Based partly on the approach used in adults, anticoagulation is often used in children with arterial dissection, dural sinus thrombosis, hypercoagulable disorders, or a high risk of embolism. Although intraparenchymal hemorrhage is common distal to a thrombosed sinus, there is little indication that anticoagulation worsens the bleeding, and there is increasing evidence for improved outcome. The strategy for using warfarin in children with cerebrovascular disorders also resembles that used in adults.

Low-molecular-weight heparin (Lovenox, Rhone-Poulenc) can be given to children subcutaneously in two divided doses of 1 mg/kg/dose (or in neonates, 1.5 mg/kg every 12 hours) (240,241). Monitoring antifactor Xa activity and platelet counts are recommended (242). The loading dose of heparin is 75 units/kg intravenously followed by 20 units/kg/hour for children over 1 year of age (or 28 units/kg/hour below 1 year of age). The target activated partial thromboplastin time (APTT) is 60 to 85 seconds. Platelet count should be monitored because of the associated risk of heparin-induced thrombocytopenia (243). An international normalized ration (INR) of 2.0 to 3.0 is appropriate for most children on warfarin; for children with mechanical heart valves, the INR should be 2.5 to 3.5 (244).

Transfusion

The risk of a second stroke due to sickle cell disease exceeds 50%, and individuals with very abnormal blood flow velocities on transcranial Doppler exhibit a 10% per year stroke risk (123–125). This increased stroke risk can be dramatically reduced by repeated transfusions to suppress the production of sickle hemoglobin below 30%, but eventual iron overload is a major concern that is only partially addressed by iron chelation. A less intense transfusion program designed to maintain a slightly higher percent of hemoglobin S (50% instead of 30%) may reduce the stroke rate yet delay the iron overload, but if transfusions are completely halted, the stroke risk evidently returns to a higher level. Hydroxyurea has shown some promise but is still under investigation.

Thrombolytic Agents

There is little information about the effectiveness or risks of thrombolytic agents such as recombinant tissue plasminogen activator (rTPA) in children, and there are reports of both dramatic successes and serious hemorrhagic complications from thrombolytic agents. If these agents are to be considered for use in children, they should as a minimum be subject to the same exclusions that apply to adults. Individuals with hemorrhagic infarction or those whose stroke began more than 3 hours earlier are typically excluded. Unfortunately, most children with ischemic infarction are not evaluated quickly enough to qualify for treatment even if there were good evidence of efficacy.

Antiplatelet Agents

Aspirin is the commonly used antiplatelet agent in children, although none of these agents has been thoroughly studied in children (245). Nevertheless, aspirin is being used more and more in the routine clinical care of children with cerebral ischemic disorders, and daily low-dose aspirin seems to be fairly safe. Long-term aspirin has been recommended in older infants and children with ischemic infarction, whose stroke recurrence risk could be as high as 20% (10). On the other hand, just how well aspirin works in children and how much aspirin to use remain unanswered questions. Aspirin's effect on platelets does not begin for several days, so aspirin should not substitute for heparin when there is a high risk of a second embolus. A daily aspirin dose of 3 to 5 mg/kg/day administered acutely in children with stroke may reduce early recurrence. This dose can be reduced to 1 to 3 mg/kg for long-term prophylaxis.

REFERENCES

1. Roach ES, Riela AR. *Pediatric cerebrovascular disorders*, 2nd ed. New York: Futura Publishing, 1995.
2. Riela AR, Roach ES. The etiology of stroke in children. *J Child Neurol* 1993;8:201–220.
3. Schoenberg BS, Mellinger JF, Schoenberg DG. Cerebrovascular disease in infants and children: a study of incidence, clinical features, and survival. *Neurology* 1978;28:763–768.
4. Schoenberg BS. Risk factors for stroke in infants and children. *Adv Neurol* 1979;25:313–324.
5. Broderick J, Talbot T, Prenger E, et al. Stroke in children within a major metropolitan area: the surprising importance of intracerebral hemorrhage. *J Child Neurol* 1993;8:250–255.
6. Giroud M, Lemesle M, Gouyon JB, et al. Cerebrovascular disease in children under 16 years of age in the city of Dijon, France: a study of incidence and clinical features from 1985 to 1993. *J Clin Epidemiol* 1995;48:1343–1348.
7. Murphy S. Deaths: final data for 1998. National Vital Statistics Reports. Hyattsville, MD: National Center for Health Statistics, 2000.
8. Levy SR, Abroms IF, Marshall PC, et al. Seizures and cerebral infarction in the full-term newborn. *Ann Neurol* 1985;17:366–370.
9. DeVeber G. Arterial ischemic strokes in infants and children: an overview of current approaches. *Semin Thromb Hemost* 2003;29:567–573.
10. Estan J, Hope P. Unilateral neonatal cerebral infarction in full term infants. *Arch Dis Child Fetal Neonatal Ed* 1997;76:F88–F93.
11. Gabis LV, Yangala R, Lenn NJ. Time lag to diagnosis of stroke in children. *Pediatrics* 2002;110:924–928.
12. Lynch JK, Hirtz DG, DeVeber G, et al. Report of the National Institutes of Neurological Disorders and Stroke workshop on perinatal and childhood stroke. *Pediatrics* 2002;109:116–123.
13. Fullerton HJ, Wu YW, Zhao S, et al. Risk of stroke in children: ethnic and gender disparities. *Neurology* 2003;61:189–194.
14. Brower MC, Rollins N, Roach ES. Basal ganglia and thalamic infarction in children: cause and clinical features. *Arch Neurol* 1996;53:1252–1256.
15. Riela A, Roach ES. Choreoathetosis in an infant with tuberculous meningitis. *Arch Neurol* 1982;39:596.
16. Nagaraja D, Verma A, Taly AB, et al. Cerebrovascular disease in children. *Acta Neurol Scand* 1994;90:251–255.

16a. Sarnat HB. Watershed infarcts in the fetal and neonatal brainstem. An aetiology of central hypoventilation, dysphagia, Möbius syndrome and micrognathia. *Eur J Paediatr Neurol* 2004;8:71–87.

17. deVeber G, Roach ES, Riela AR, et al. Stroke in children: recognition, treatment, and future directions. *Semin Pediatr Neurol* 2000;7:309–317.
18. Schievink WI, Mokri B, Piepgras DG, et al. Intracranial aneurysms and cervicocephalic arterial dissections associated with congenital heart disease. *Neurosurgery* 1996;39:685–689.
19. Poole GV Jr, Breyer RH, Holliday RH, et al. Tumors of the heart: surgical considerations. *J Cardiovasc Surg* 1984;25:5–11.
20. Al-Mateen M, Hood M, Trippel D, et al. Cerebral embolism from arterial myxoma in pediatric patients. *Pediatrics* 2003;112:162–167.
21. Quigley MM, Schwartzman E, Boswell PD, et al. A unique atrial primary cardiac lymphoma mimicking myxoma presenting with embolic stroke: a case report. *Blood* 2003;101:4708–4710.

22. Ohene-Frempong K, Weiner SJ, Sleeper LA, et al. Cerebrovascular accidents in sickle cell disease: rates and risk factors. *Blood* 1998;91:288–294.
23. Leikin SL, Gallagher D, Kinney TR, et al. Cooperative study of sickle cell disease. Mortality in children and adolescents with sickle cell disease. *Pediatrics* 1989;84:500–508.
24. Pegelow CH, Macklin EA, Moser FG, et al. Longitudinal changes in brain magnetic resonance imaging findings in children with sickle cell disease. *Blood* 2002;99:3014–3018.
25. Rothman SM, Fulling KH, Nelson JS. Sickle cell anemia and central nervous system infarction: a neuropathological study. *Ann Neurol* 1986;20:684–690.
26. Hillery CA, Panepinto JA. Pathophysiology of stroke in sickle cell disease. *Microcirculation* 2004;11:195–208.
27. Adams RJ, McKie VC, Hsu L, et al. Prevention of first stroke by transfusion in children with sickle cell anemia and abnormal results on transcranial Doppler utrasonography. *N Engl J Med* 1998;339:5–11.
28. Adams RJ, Pavlakis S, Roach ES. Sickle cell disease and stroke: primary prevention and transcranial Doppler. *Ann Neurol* 2003;54:559–563.
29. Adams RJ, Brambilla DJ, Granger S, et al. Stroke and conversion to high risk in children screened with transcranial Doppler ultrasound during the STOP trial. *Blood* 2004;103:3689–3694.
30. Ganesan V, Prengler M, McShane MA, et al. Investigation of risk factors in children with arterial ischemic stroke. *Ann Neurol* 2003;53:167–173.
31. Chan AK, deVeber G. Prothrombotic disorders and ischemic stroke in children. *Semin Pediatr Neurol* 2000;7:301–308.
32. Carlin TM, Chanmugam MD. Stroke in children. *Emerg Med Clin N Am* 2002;20:671–685.
33. Kasner SE. Stroke treatment—specific considerations. *Stroke* 2000;19:399–417.
34. Gruppo R, DeGrauw A, Fogelson H. Protein C deficiency related to valproic acid therapy: a possible association with childhood stroke. *J Pedaitr* 2000;137:714–718.
35. Carvalho KS, Garg BP. Arterial strokes in children. *Neurol Clin N Am* 2002;20:1079–1100.
36. Broekmans AW, Veltkamp JJ, Bertina RM. Congenital protein C deficiency and venous thromboembolism. *N Engl J Med* 1983;309:340–344.
37. Tarras S, Gadia C, Meister L, et al. Homozygous protein C deficiency in a newborn: clinicopathologic correlation. *Arch Neurol* 1988;45:214–216.
38. Quinsey NS, Greedy AL, Bottomley SP, et al. Antithrombin: in control of coagulation. *Int J Biochem Cell Biol* 2004;36:386–389.
39. Isiguro K, Kojima T, Kadomatsu K, et al. Complete antithrombin deficiency in mice results in embryonic lethality. *J Clin Invest* 2000;106:873–878.
40. Stein PE, Carrell RW. What do dysfunctional serpins tell us about molecular mobility and disease? *Nat Struc Biol* 1995;2:96–113.
41. Nagaizumi K, Inaba H, Amano K, et al. Five novel and four recurrent point mutations in the antithrombin gene causing venous thrombosis. *Int J Hematol* 2003;78:79–83.
42. Pallota R, Dalpra L, Miozzo M, et al. A patient defines the interstitial 1q deletion syndrome characterized by antithrombin III deficiency. *Am J Med Genet* 2001;104:282–286.
43. Thaaler E, Lechner K. Antithrombin III deficiency and thromboembolism. *Clin Haematol* 1981;10:369–390.
44. Andrew M, Monagle PT, Brooker LA. Congenital prothrombotic disorders. In: *Thromboembolic complications during infancy and childhood*. Hamilton: BC Decker 2000:47–110.
45. Tait RC, Walker ID, Perry DJ, et al. Prevalence of antithrombin deficiency in the healthy population. *Br Med J Haematol* 1994;87: 106–112.
46. Kuhle S, Lane DA, Jochmanns K, et al. Homozygous antithrombin deficiency type II (99 Leu to Phe mutation) and childhood thromboembolism. *Thromb Haemost* 2001;86:1007–1011.
47. Simioni P, Prandoni P, Lensing AWA, et al. The risk of venous thromboembolism in patients with an Arg506 -> Gln mutation in the gene for factor V (factor V Leiden). *N Engl J Med* 1997;336: 399–403.
48. Rees DC, Coz M, Clegg JB. Worldwide distribution of factor V Leiden. *Lancet* 1995;348:1133–1134.
49. Ridker PM, Hennekens CH, Lindpaintner K, et al. Mutation in the gene coding for coagulation factor V and the risk of myocardial infarction, stroke, and venous thrombosis in apparently healthy men. *N Engl J Med* 1995;332:912–917.
50. Moster ML. Coagulopathies and arterial stroke. *J Neuro-Ophthalmol* 2003;23:63–67.
51. deVeber GA, Monagle P, Chan A, Fischer M. Prothrombotic disorders in infants and children with cerebral thromboembolism. *Arch Neurol* 1998;55:1539–1543.
52. Halbmayer WM, Haushofer A, Schon R, et al. The prevalence of poor anticoagulant response to activated protein C (APC resistance) among patients suffering from stroke or venous thrombosis and among healthy subjects. *Blood Coag Fibrinolysis* 1994;5:51–57.
53. Nowak-Gottl U, Koch HG, Aschka I, et al. Resistance to activated protein C (APCR) in children with venous or arterial thromboembolism. *Br J Haematol* 1996;92:992–998.
54. Swarte R, Appel I, Lequin M, et al. Factor II gene (prothrombin G20210A) mutation and neonatal cerebrovenous thrombosis. *Thromb Haemost* 2004;92:719–721.
55. Junker R, Koch HG, Auberger K, et al. Prothrombin G20210A gene mutation and further prothrombotic risk factors in childhood thrombophilia. *Arterioscler Thromb Vasc Biol* 1999;19:2568–2572.
56. Klein L, Bhardwaj V, Gebara B. Cerebral venous sinus thrombosis in a neonate with homozygous prothrombin G20210A genotype. *J Perinatol* 2004;24:797–799.
57. McColl MD, Chalmers EA, Thomas A, et al. Factor V Leiden, prothrombin 20210G-A and the MTHFR C677T mutations in childhood stroke. *Thromb Haemost* 1999;81:690–694.
58. Keswani SC, Chauhan N. Antiphospholipid syndrome. *J R Soc Med* 2002;95:336–342.
59. Harris EN. Syndrome of the black swan. *Br J Rheumatol* 1987;26:324–326.
60. Black RL, Jakway J, Baker WF. Deep vein thrombosis: prevalence of etiologic factors and results of management in 100 consecutive patients. *Semin Thromb Hemost* 1992;18:267–274.
61. Levine SR. Antiphospholipid syndromes and the nervous system: clinical features, mechanism and treatment. *Semin Neurol* 1994;14:168–176.
62. deVeber G, Monagle P, Chan A, et al. Prothrombotic disorders in infants and children with cerebral thromboembolism. *Arch Neurol* 1998;55:1539–1543.
63. Lechner K, Pabinger-Fashing IP. Lupus anticoagulant and thrombosis. A study of 25 cases and review of the literature. *Haemostasis* 1985;15:252–262.
64. Sammaritano LR, Ng S, Sobel R, et al. Anticardiolipin IgG subclasses; association of IgG2 with arterial and/or venous thrombosis. *Arthritis Rheum* 1997;40:1998–2006.
65. Triplett DA, Brandt JT. The relationship between lupus anticoagulants and antibodies to phospholipids. *JAMA* 1988;259:550–554.
66. Vita P, Hernandez MC, Lopez-Fernandez MF. Prevalence, follow-up and clinical significance of the anticardiolipin antibodies in normal subjects. *Thromb Haemost* 1994;72:209–213.
67. Brey RL, Hart RG, Sherman DJ, et al. Antiphospholipid antibodies and cerebral ischemia in young people. *Neurology* 1990;40: 1190–1196.
68. Angelini L, Ravelli A, Caporali R, et al. High prevalence of antiphospholipid antibodies in children with idiopathic cerebral ischemia. *Pediatrics* 1994;94:500–503.
69. Nelson KB, Dambrosia JM, Grether JK, et al. Neonatal cytokines and coagulation factors in children with cerebral palsy. *Ann Neurol* 1998;44:665–675.
70. Goldenberg NA, Knapp-Clevenger R, Manco-Johnson MJ, et al. Elevated plasma factor VIII and D-dimer levels as predictors of poor outcomes of thrombosis in children. *N Engl J Med* 2004;351: 1081–1088.
71. Adelman LS, Doe FD, Sarnat HB. Bilateral dissecting aneurysms of the internal carotid arteries. *Acta Neuropathol(Berl)* 1974;29: 93–97.
72. Lucas C, Moulin T, Deplanque D, et al. Stroke patterns of internal carotid artery dissection in 40 patients. *Stroke* 1998;29:2646–2648.
73. Chabrier S, Husson B, Lasjaunias P, et al. Stroke in childhood: outcome and recurrence risk by mechanism in 59 patients. *J Child Neurol* 2000;15:290–294.
74. Schievink WI, Morki B, Piepgras DG. Spontaneous dissections of

the cervicocephalic arteries in childhood and adolescence. *Neurology* 1994;44:1607–1612.

75. Fullerton HJ, Johnston SC, Smith WS. Arterial dissection and stroke in children. *Neurology* 2001;57:1155–1160.
76. Ganesan V, Chong WK, Cox TC, et al. Posterior circulation stroke in childhood: risk factors and recurrence. *Neurology* 2002;59: 1552–1556.
77. Chang CJ, Chang WN, Huang LT, et al. Cerebral infarction in perinatal and childhood bacterial meningitis. *Quart J Med* 2003;96:755–762.
78. Jan W, Zimmerman RA, Bilaniuk LT, et al. Diffusion-weighted imaging in acute bacterial meningitis in infancy. *Neuroradiology* 2003;45:634–639.
79. Takeoka M, Takahashi T. Infectious and inflammatory disorders of the circulatory system and stroke in childhood. *Curr Opin Neurol* 2002;15:159–164.
80. Leiguarda R, Berthier M, Starkstein S, et al. Ischemic infarction in 25 children with tuberculous meningitis. *Stroke* 1988;19:200–204.
81. Kleinschmidt-DeMasters BK, Gilden DH. Varicella-zoster virus infections of the nervous system: clinical and pathologic correlates. *Arch Pathol Lab Med* 2001;125:770–780.
82. Park YD, Belman AL, Kim TS, et al. Stroke in pediatric acquired immunodeficiency syndrome. *Ann Neurol* 1990;28:303–311.
83. Ferrera PC, Curran CB, Swanson H. Etiology of pediatric ischemic stroke. *Am J Emerg Med* 1997;15:671–679.
84. Moriarty DM, Haller JO, Loh JP, et al. Cerebral infarctions in pediatric acquired immunodeficiency syndrome. *Pediatr Radiol* 1994;24:611–612.
85. Lanthier S, Lortie A, Michaud J, et al. Isolated angiitis of the CNS in children. *Neurology* 2001;56:837–842.

85a. Volcy M, Toro ME, Uribe CS, Toro G. Primary angiitis of the central nervous system: report of five biopsy-confirmed cases from Colombia. *J Neurol Sci* 2004;227:85–89.

86. Al-Jarallah M, Al-Rifai T, Riela AR, et al. Spontaneous intraparenchymal hemorrhage in children: a study of 68 patients. *J Child Neurol* 2000;15:284–289.
87. Eeg-Olofsson O, Ringheim Y. Stroke in children. *Acta Pediatr Scand Care* 1983;72:391–395.
88. Calder K, Kokorowski P, Tran T, et al. Emergency department presentation of pediatric stroke. *Pediatr Emerg Care* 2003;19:320–328.
89. Verweij RD, Wijdicks EFM, van Gijn J. Warning headache in aneurysmal subarachnoid hemorrhage. A case-control study. *Arch Neurol* 1994;45:1019–1020.
90. Krivit W, Tate D, White JG, et al. Idiopathic thrombocytopenic purpura and intracranial hemorrhage. *Pediatrics*67:570–571.
91. McCormick WF. Vascular disorders of nervous tissue: anomalies, malformations and aneurysms. In: Bourne GH, ed. *The structure and function of nervous tissue*. New York: Academic Press, 1969.
92. Storrs BB, Humphreys RP, Hendrick EB, et al. Intracranial aneurysms in the pediatric age-group. *Childs Brain* 1982;9: 358–361.
93. Sedzimir CB, Robinson J. Intracranial hemorrhage in children and adolescents. *J Neurosurg* 1973;38:269–281.
94. Heiskanen O, Vilkki J. Intracranial arterial aneurysms in children and adolescents. *Acta Neurochir* 1981;59:55–63.
95. Read D, Esiri MM. Fusiform basilar artery aneurysm in a child. *Neurology* 1979;29:1045–1049.
96. Zimmerman RA, Atlas S, Bilaniuk LT, et al. Magnetic resonance imaging of cerebral aneurysm. *Acta Radiol* 1987;369:108–109.
97. Rorke LB. Pathology of cerebral vascular disease in children. In: Edwards MSB, Hoffman HJ, eds. *Cerebral vascular disease in children and adolescents*. Baltimore: Williams & Wilkins, 1989:95–138.
98. Ronkainen A, Hernesniemi J, Puranen M, et al. Familial intracranial aneurysm. *Lancet* 1997;349:380–384.
99. ter Berg HWM, Bijlsma JB, Willemse J. Familial occurrence of intracranial aneurysms in childhood: a case report and review of the literature. *Neuropediatrics* 1987;18:227–230.
100. Bromberg JEC, Rinkel GJ, Algra A, et al. Familial subarachnoid hemorrhage, distinctive features and patterns of inheritance. *Ann Neurol* 1995;38:929–934.
101. Schievink WI. Intracranial aneurysms. *N Engl J Med* 1997;336: 28–40.
102. The Magnetic Resonance Angiography in Relatives of Patients with Subarachnoid Hemorrhage Study Group. Risks and benefits of screening for intracranial aneurysms in first-degree relatives of patients with sporadic subarachnoid hemorrhage. *N Engl J Med* 1999;341:1344–1350.
103. Thompson JR, Harwood-Nash DC, Fitz CR. Cerebral aneurysms in children. *Am J Roentgenol* 1973;118:163–175.
104. Patel AN, Richardson AE. Ruptured intracranial aneurysm in the first two decades of life. A study of 58 patients. *J Neurosurg* 1971;35:571–576.
105. Chapman AB, Rubinstein D, Hughes R, et al. Intracranial aneurysms in autosomal dominant polycystic kidney disease. *N Engl J Med* 1992;327:916–920.
106. Orozco M, Trigueros F, Quintana F, et al. Intracranial aneurysms in early childhood. *Surg Neurol* 1978;9:247–252.
107. Linn FH, Wijdicks EF, van der Graaf Y, et al. Prospective study of sentinel headache in aneurysmal subarachnoid haemorrhage. *Lancet* 1994;344:590–593.
108. Editorial. Headaches and subarachnoid haemorrhage. *Lancet* 1988;1:80.
109. Jenkins A, Hadley DM, Teasdale GM, et al. Magnetic resonance imaging of acute subarachnoid hemorrhage. *J Neurosurg* 1988;68:731–763.
110. Weisberg LA. Computed tomography in aneurysmal subarachnoid hemorrhage. *Neurology* 1979;29:802–808.
111. Wiebers DO, Whisnant JP, Sundt TM Jr, et al. The significance of unruptured intracranial saccular aneurysms. *J Neurosurg* 1987;66:23–29.
112. Caplan LR. Should intracranial aneurysms be treated before they rupture? *N Engl J Med* 1998;339:1774–1775.
113. Vermeulen M, Lindsay KW, van Gijn J. *Subarachnoid hemorrhage*. London: W. B. Saunders Company, 1992.
114. Kassell NF, Torner JC, Haley EC Jr., et al. The international cooperative study on the timing of aneurysm surgery. Part 1: overall management results. *J Neurosurg* 1990;73:18–36.
115. McDougall CG, Halbach VV, Dowd CF, et al. Endovascular treatment of basilar tip aneurysms using electrolytically detached coils. *J Neurosurg* 1996;84:393–399.
116. Barrow DL, Prats AR. Infectious intracranial aneurysms: comparison of groups with and without endocarditis. *Neurosurgery* 1990;27:562–573.
117. Ahmadi J, Tung H, Giannotta SL, et al. Monitoring of infectious intracranial aneurysms by sequential computed tomographic/magnetic resonance imaging studies. *Neurosurgery* 1993;32:45–50.
118. Shuanghoti S, Netsky MG, Switter DJ. Combined congenital vascular anomalies and neuroepithelial (colloid) cysts. *Neurology* 1978;28:552–555.
119. Tyler HR, Clark DB. Neurologic complications in patients with coarctation of aorta. *Neurology* 1958;8:712–718.
120. Roach ES, Zimmerman CF. Ehlers-Danlos syndrome. In: Roach ES, Miller VS, eds. *Neurocutaneous disorders*. London: Cambridge University Press, 2004:144–149.
121. North KN, Whiteman DA, Pepin MG, et al. Cerebrovascular complications in Ehlers-Danlos syndrome type IV. *Ann Neurol* 1995;38:960–964.
122. Hegedüs K. Some observations on reticular fibers in the media of the major cerebral arteries. A comparative study of patients without vascular diseases and those with ruptured berry aneurysms. *Surg Neurol* 1984;22:301–307.
123. Kato T, Hattori H, Yorifuji T, et al. Intracranial aneurysms in Ehlers-Danlos syndrome type IV in early childhood. *Pediatr Neurol* 1001;25:336–339.
124. Braunsdorf WE. Fusiform aneurysm of basilar artery and ectatic internal carotid arteries associated with glycogenosis type 2 (Pompe's disease). *Neurosurgery* 1987;21:748–749.
125. Kondziolka D, Humphreys RP, Hoffmann HJ, et al. Arteriovenous malformations of the brain in children: a forty year experience. *Can J Neurol Sci* 1992;19:40–45.
126. Schoolman A, Kepes JJ. Bilateral spontaneous carotid-cavernous fistulae in Ehlers-Danlos syndrome. *J Neurosurg* 1967;26:82–86.
127. Lach B, Nair SG, Russell NA, et al. Spontaneous carotid-cavernous fistula and multiple arterial dissections in type IV Ehlers-Danlos syndrome. Case report. *J Neurosurg* 1987;66:462–467.

128. Paterson JH, McKissock WA. A clinical survey of intracranial angiomas with special reference to their mode of progression and surgical treatment. A report of 110 cases. *Brain* 1956;79:233–266.
129. Michelson WJ. Natural history and pathophysiology of arteriovenous malformations. *Clin Neurosurg* 1979;26:307–313.
130. Halbach VV, Higashida RT, Hieshima GB. Interventional neuroradiology. *Am J Radiol* 1989;153:467–476.
131. Proesmans W, Van Damme B, Casaer P, et al. Autosomal dominant polycystic kidney disease in the neonatal period: association with a cerebral arteriovenous malformation. *Pediatrics* 1982;70:971–975.
132. Henderson WR, Gomez RD. Natural history of cerebral angiomas. *BMJ* 1967;4:571–574.
133. Kelly JJ, Mellinger JF, Sundt TM. Intracranial arteriovenous malformations in childhood. *Ann Neurol* 1978;3:338–343.
134. Murphy MJ. Long-term follow-up of seizures associated with cerebral arteriovenous malformations. *Arch Neurol* 1985;42:477–479.
135. Zeller RS, Chutorian AM. Vascular malformations of the pons in children. *Neurology* 1975;25:776–780.
136. McCormick WF, Hardman JF, Boulter TR. Vascular malformations ("angiomas") of the brain with special reference to those occurring in the posterior fossa. *J Neurosurg* 1968;28:241–251.
137. Detwiler PW, Porter RW, Spetzler RF. Spinal arteriovenous malformations. *Neurosurg Clin N Am* 1999;10:89–100.
138. Aminoff MS, Edwards MSB. Spinal arteriovenous malformations. In: Edwards MSB, Hoffman HJ, eds. *Cerebral vascular disease in children and adolescents*. Baltimore: Williams & Wilkins, 1989: 321–335.
139. Riché MC, Modenesi-Freitas J, Djindjian M, et al. Arteriovenous malformations (AVM) of the spinal cord in children. Review of 38 cases. *Neuroradiology* 1982;22:171–180.
140. Wyburn-Mason R. *The vascular abnormalities and tumours of the spinal cord and its membranes*. London: Kimpton, 1943.
141. Kissel P, Dureux JB. Cobb syndrome: cutaneomeningospinal angiomatosis. In: Vinken PJ, Bruyn GW, eds. *Handbook of clinical neurology*, Vol. 14. New York: Elsevier, 1972:429–445.
142. Pascual-Castroviejo I. The association of extracranial and intracranial vascular malformations in children. *Can J Neurol Sci* 1985;12:139–148.
143. Pece N, Vera S, Cymerman U, et al. Mutant endoglin in hereditary hemorrhagic telangiectasia type 1 is transiently expressed intracellularly and is not a dominant negative. *J Clin Invest* 1997;100: 2568–2579.
144. Letteboer TG, Zewald RA, Kamping EJ, et al. Hereditary hemorrhagic telangiectasia: ENG and ALK-1 mutations in Dutch patients. *Hum Genet* 2005;116:8–16.
144a. Abdalla SA, Cymerman U, Rushlow D, et al. Novel mutations and polymorphisms in genes causing hereditary hemorrhagic telangiectasis. *Hum Mutat* 2005;25:320–321.
145. Guttmacher AE, Marchuk DA, White RI. Hereditary hemorrhagic telangiectasia. *N Engl J Med* 1995;333:918–924.
146. Putman CM, Chaloupka JC, Fulbright RK, et al. Exceptional multiplicity of cerebral arteriovenous malformations associated with hereditary hemorrhagic telangiectasia (Osler-Weber-Rendu syndrome). *Am J Neuroradiol* 1996;17:1733–1742.
147. Sobel D, Norman D. CNS manifestations of hereditary hemorrhagic telangiectasia. *Am J Neuroradiol* 1984;5:569–573.
148. Roman G, Fisher M, Perl DP, et al. Neurological manifestations of hereditary hemorrhagic telangiectasia (Rendu-Osler-Weber disease): report of 2 cases and review of the literature. *Ann Neurol* 1978;4:130–144.
149. Hoffman HJ, Mohr G, Kusunoki T. Multiple arteriovenous malformations of the spinal cord and brain in a child. Case report. *Childs Brain* 1976;2:317–324.
150. McAllister VL, Kendall BE, Bull JWD. Symptomatic vertebral haemangiomas. *Brain* 1975;98:71–80.
151. Bergström M, Riding M, Greitz T. The limitations of definition of blood vessels with computer intravenous angiography. *Neuroradiology* 1976;11:35–40.
152. Leblanc R, Ethier R, Little JR. Computerized tomography in arteriovenous malformations of the brain. *J Neurosurg* 1979;51:765–772.
153. Young IR, Bydder GM, Hall AS, et al. NMR imaging in the diagnosis and management of intracranial angiomas. *Am J Neuroradiol* 1983;4:837–838.
154. Holla PS, et al. Radiographic features of vascular malformations. In: Smith RR, Haerer A, Russell WF, eds. *Vascular malformations and fistulas of the brain*. New York: Raven Press, 1982.
155. Spetzler RF, Martin NA. A proposed grading system for arteriovenous malformations. *J Neurosurg* 1986;65:476–483.
156. Hamilton MG, Spetzler RF. The prospective application of a grading system for arteriovenous malformations. *Neurosurgery* 1994;34:2–7.
157. Shin M, Maruyama K, Kurita H, et al. Analysis of nidus obliteration rates after gamma knife surgery for arteriovenous malformations based on long-term follow-up data: the University of Tokyo experience. *J Neurosurg* 2004;101:18–24.
157a. Maruyama K, Kawahara N, Shin M, et al. The risk of hemorrhage after radiosurgery for cerebral arteriovenous malformations. *N Engl J Med*. 2005;352:146–153.
158. Lunsford LD. Stereotactic radiosurgical procedures for arteriovenous malformations of the brain. *Mayo Clin Proc* 1995;70: 305–307.
159. Kiris T, Sencer A, Sahinbas M, et al. Surgical results in pediatric Spetzler-Martin grades I-III intracranial arteriovenous malformations. *Childs Nerv Syst* 2005;21:69–74.
160. Fournier D, TerBrugge KG, Willinsky R, et al. Endovascular treatment of intracerebral arteriovenous malformations: experience in 49 cases. *J Neurosurg* 1991;75:228–233.
161. Celli P, Ferrante L, Palma L, et al. Cerebral arteriovenous malformations in children: clinical features and outcome of treatment in children and in adults. *Surg Neurol* 1984;22:43–49.
162. Wilkins RH. Natural history of intracranial vascular malformations: a review. *Neurosurgery* 1985;16:421–430.
163. Nishi T, Matsukado Y, Marubayashi T, et al. Ruptures of arteriovenous malformations in children associated with trivial head trauma. *Surg Neurol* 1987;28:451–457.
164. Brown RD, Wiebers DO, Forbes G, et al. The natural history of unruptured intracranial arteriovenous malformations. *J Neurosurg* 1988;68:352–357.
165. Loeffler JS, Rossitch E Jr, Siddon R, et al. Role of stereotactic radiosurgery with a linear accelerator in treatment of intracranial arteriovenous malformations and tumors in children. *Pediatrics* 1990;85:774–782.
166. Fleetwood IG, Steinberg GK. Arteriovenous malformations. *Lancet* 2002;359:863–873.
167. Challa VR, Moody DM, Brown WR. Vascular malformations of the central nervous system. *J Neuropathol Exp Neurol* 1995;54: 609–621.
168. Litvak J, Yahr MD, Ransohoff J. Aneurysms of the great vein of Galen and midline cerebral arteriovenous anomalies. *J Neurosurg* 1960;17:945–954.
169. Gold AP, Ransohoff J, Carter S. Vein of Galen malformation. *Acta Neurol Scand* 1964;40[Suppl 11]:131.
170. Yamashita Y, Nakamura Y, Okudera T, et al. Neuroradiological and pathological studies on neonatal aneurysmal dilation of the vein of Galen. *J Child Neurol* 1990;5:45–48.
171. Holden AM, Fyler DC, Shillito J Jr, et al. Congestive heart failure from intracranial arteriovenous fistula in infancy. Clinical and physiological considerations in eight patients. *Pediatrics* 1972;49:30–39.
172. Pasqualin A, Mazza C, Da Pian R, et al. Midline giant arteriovenous malformations in infants. *Acta Neurochir* 1982;64:259–271.
173. Johnston IH, Whittle IR, Besser M, et al. Vein of Galen malformation: diagnosis and management. *Neurosurgery* 1987;20:747–758.
174. Lasjaunias P, Garcia-Monaco R, Rodesch G, et al. Vein of Galen malformation. *Childs Nerv Syst* 1991;7:360–367.
175. Gangemi M, Maiuri F, Donati PA, et al. Spontaneous thrombosis of aneurysm of the vein of Galen. *Acta Neurol (Napoli)* 1988;10: 113–118.
176. Mayberg MR, Zimmerman C. Vein of Galen aneurysm associated with dural AVM and straight sinus thrombosis. *J Neurosurg* 1988;68:288–291.
177. Chisholm CA, Kuller JA, Katz VL, et al. Aneurysm of the vein of Galen: prenatal diagnosis of perinatal management. *Am J Perinatol* 1996;13:503–506.
178. Jones BV, Ball WS, Tomsick TA, et al. Vein of Galen aneurysmal malformation: diagnosis and treatment of 13 children with

extended clinical follow-up. *AJNR Am J Neuroradiol* 2002;23: 1717–1724.
179. Fullterton HJ, Aminoff AR, Ferriero DM, et al. Neurodevelopmental outcome after endovascular treatment of vein of Galen malformation. *Neurology* 2003;61:1386–1390.
180. Borthne A, Carteret M, Baraton J, et al. Vein of Galen vascular malformations in infants: clinical, radiological and therapeutic aspect. *Eur Radiol* 1997;7:1252–1258.
181. Moriarty JL, Steinberg GK. Surgical obliteration for vein of Galen malformation: a case report. *Surg Neurol* 1995;44:365–369.
182. Suzuki J. *Moyamoya disease*. Berlin: Springer-Verlag, 1986.
183. Kudo T. Spontaneous occlusion of the circle of Willis. A disease apparently confined to Japanese. *Neurology* 1968;18:485–496.
184. Takeuchi K, Hara M, Yokota H, et al. Factors influencing the development of moyamoya phenomenon. *Acta Neurochir* 1981;59: 79–86.
185. Gadoth N, Hirsch M. Primary and acquired forms of moyamoya syndrome: a review and three case reports. *Isr J Med Sci* 1980;16:370–377.
186. Wakai K, Tamakoshi A, Ikesaki K, et al. Epidemiological features of moyamoya disease in Japan: findings from a nationwide survey. *Clin Neurol Neurosurg* 1997;99(Suppl 2):S1–5.
187. Yamauchi T, Mitsuhiro T, Kiyohiro H, et al. Linkage of familial moyamoya disease (spontaneous occlusion of the circle of Willis) to chromosome 17q25. *Stroke* 2000;31:930–935.
188. Ikeda H, Sasaki T, Yoshimoto T, et al. Mapping of a familial Moyamoya disease gene to chromosome 3p24.2-p26. *Am J Hum Gen* 1999;64:533–537.
189. Inoue TK, Ikezaki K, Sasazuki T, et al. Linkage analysis of moyamoya disease on chromosome 6. *J Child Neurol* 2000;15:179–182.
189a. Sakurai K, Horiuchi Y, Ikeda H, et al. A novel susceptibility locus for moyamoya disease on chromosome 8q23. *J Hum Genet* 2004;49:278–281.
190. Yonekawa Y, Kahn N. Moyamoya disease. *Adv Neurol* 2003;92: 113–118.
191. Moritake K, Handa H, Yonekawa Y, et al. Follow-up study on the relationship between age at onset of illness and outcome in patients with moyamoya disease. *No Shinnkei Geka* 1986;14:957–963.
192. Kurokawa T, Tomita S, Ueda K, et al. Prognosis of occlusive disease of the Circle of Willis (Moyamoya disease) in children. *Pediatr Neurol* 1985;1:274–277.
193. Imaizumi T, Hayashi K, Saito K, et al. Long-term outcomes of pediatric moyamoya disease monitored to adulthood. *Pediatr Neurol* 1998;18:321–325.
194. Matsushima T, Inoue TK, Suzuki SO, et al. Surgical techniques and the results of a fronto-temporo-parietal combined indirect bypass procedure for children with Moyamoya disease: a comparison with the results of encephalo-duro-arteriosynangiosis alone. *Clin Neurol Neurosurg* 1997;99(Suppl 2):S123–S127.
195. Ikezaki K, Loftus CM, eds. *Moyamoya disease*. Rolling Meadows, IL: American Association of Neurological Surgeons, 2001.
196. Miyamoto S, Kikuchi H, Karasawa J, et al. Pitfalls in the surgical treatment of moyamoya disease. Operative techniques for refractory cases. *J Neurosurg* 1988;68:537–543.
197. Fukui M. Current state of study on moyamoya disease in Japan. *Surg Neurol* 1997;47:138–143.
198. Roach ES. Immediate surgery for moyamoya syndrome: not necessarily. *Arch Neurol* 2001;58:130–131.
199. Dobyns WB, Michels VV, Groover RV, et al. Familial cavernous malformations of the central nervous system and retina. *Ann Neurol* 1987;21:578–583.
200. Labauge P, Laberge S, Brunereau L, et al. Hereditary cerebral cavernous angiomas: clinical and genetic features in 57 French families. *Lancet* 1998;352:1892–1897.
201. Verlaan DJ, Davenport WJ, Stefan H, et al. Cerebral cavernous malformations. Mutations in Krit 1. *Neurology* 2002;58:853–857.
202. Gil-Nagel A, Dubovsky J, Wilcox KJ, et al. Familial cerebral cavernous angioma: a gene localized to a 15-cM interval on chromosome 7q. *Ann Neurol* 1996;39:807–810.
203. Laberge-le Couteulx S, Jung HH, Labauge P, et al. Truncating mutations in CCM1, encoding KRIT1, cause hereditary cavernous angiomas. *Nat Genet* 1999;23:189–193.
204. Rigamonti D, Hadley MN, Drayer BP, et al. Cerebral cavernous malformations: incidence and familial occurrence. *N Engl J Med* 1988;319:343–347.
205. Scott RM, Barnes P, Kupsky W, et al. Cavernous angiomas of the central nervous system in children. *J Neurosurg* 1992;76:38–46.
206. Zimmerman RS, Spetzler RF, Lee S, et al. Cavernous malformations of the brain stem. *J Neurosurg* 1991;75:32–39.
206a. Virchow R. Die krankhhaften Geschwülste. *Berlin*. August Slirschwald, 1863;Bd 1:325.
206b. Maraire JN, Awad IA. Intracranial cavernous malformations: lesion behavior and management strategies. *Neurosurgery* 1995;37: 591–605.
206c. Pascual-Castroviejo I, Pascual-Pascual SI. Congenital vascular malformations in childhood. *Semin Pediatr Neurol* 2002;9: 254–273.
207. Ochiai C, Saito I, Sano K. Intracranial hemorrhage with cerebral vascular malformation. In: Smith RR, Haerer A, Russell WF, eds. *Vascular malformations and fistulas of the brain*. New York: Raven Press, 1982.
208. Russell DS, Rubinstein LJ. *The pathology of tumours of the nervous system*, 4th ed. London: E Arnold, 1977.
209. Challa VR, Moody DM, Brown WR. Vascular malformations of the central nervous system. *J Neuropathol Exp Neurol* 1995;54: 609–621.
210. Kuban KC, Gilles FH. Human telencephalic angiogenesis. *Ann Neurol* 1985;17:539–548.
211. Norman MG, O'Kusky JR. The growth and development of microvasculature in human cerebral cortex. *J Neuropathol Exp Neurol* 1986;45:222–232.
212. Morris ED, Moffat DB. Abnormal origin of the basilar artery from the cervical part of the internal carotid and its embryological significance. *Anat Rec* 1956;125:701–711.
213. Tibbs PA, Walsh JW, Minix WB. Persistent primitive trigeminal artery and ipsilateral acquired blepharoptosis. *Arch Neurol* 1981;38:323–324.
214. Saltzman G. Patent primitive trigeminal artery studied by cerebral angiography. *Acta Radiol* 1959;51:329–336.
215. Bruetman ME, Fields WS. Persistent hypoglossal artery. *Arch Neurol* 1963;8:369–372.
216. Anderson RA, Sondheimer FK. Rare carotid-vertebrobasilar anastomoses with notes on the differentiation between proatlantal and hypoglossal arteries. *Neuroradiology* 1976;11:113–118.
217. Khodadad G. Persistent hypoglossal artery in the fetus. *Acta Anat* 1977;99:477–481.
218. Garza-Mercado R, Cavazos E, Urrutia G. Persistent hypoglossal artery in combination with multifocal arteriovenous malformations of the brain: case report. *Neurosurgery* 1990;26:871–876.
219. Teal JS, Rumbaugh CL, Bergeron RT, et al. Persistent carotid-superior cerebellar artery anastomosis: a variant of persistent trigeminal artery. *Neuroradiology* 1972;103:335–341.
220. Chambers AA, Lukin R. Trigeminal artery connection to the posterior inferior cerebellar arteries. *Neuroradiology* 1975;9:121–123.
221. Haughton VM, Rosenbaum AE, Pearce J. Internal carotid artery origins of the inferior cerebellar arteries. *AJR Am J Roentgenol* 1978;130:1191–1192.
222. Siqueira M, Piske R, Ono M, et al. Cerebellar arteries originating from the internal carotid artery. *Am J Neuroradiol* 1993;14: 1229–1235.
223. Zingesser LH, Schechter MM, Medina A. Angiographic and pneumoencephalographic features of holoprosencephaly. *AJR Am J Roentgenol* 1966;97:5651–574.
224. Pascual-Castroviejo I, Tendero A, Martinez-Bermejo JM, et al. Persistence of the hypoglossal artery and partial agenesis of the cerebellum. *Neuropediatrics* 1975;6:184–189.
225. Wise BL, Palubinskas AJ. Persistent trigeminal artery (carotid-basilar anastomosis). *J Neurosurg* 1964;21:199–206.
226. Turnbull I. Agenesis of the internal carotid artery. *Neurology* 1962;12:588–590.
227. Hussain SA, Araj JS, Forman JF, et al. Congenital absence of the internal carotid artery. *Arch Pathol* 1968;90:265–270.
228. Cali RL, Berg R, Rama K. Bilateral internal carotid artery agenesis: a case study and review of the literature. *Surgery* 1993;113: 227–233.
229. Yokochi K, Iwase K. Bilateral internal carotid artery agenesis in

a child with psychomotor developmental delay. *Pediatr Neurol* 1996;15:76–78.

230. Carstens MH. Neural tube programming and craniofacial cleft formation. I. The neuromeric organization of the head and neck. *Eur J Paediatr Neurol* 2004;8:181–210.
231. Adelman LS, Doe FD, Sarnat HB. Bilateral dissecting aneurysms of the internal carotid arteries. *Acta Neuropathol* 1974;29:93–97.
232. Sarkari NBS, Holmes JM, Bickerstaff ER. Neurological manifestations associated with internal carotid loops and kinks in children. *J Neurol Neurosurg Psychiatry* 1970;33:194–200.
233. Pascual-Castroviejo, Viaño J, Pascual-Pascual SI, et al. Facial haemangioma, agenenesis of the internal carotid artery and dysplasia of cerebral cortex: case report. *Neuroradiology* 1995;37:692–695.
234. Quint DJ, Silbergleit R, Young WC. Absence of the carotid canals at skull base CT. *Radiology* 1992;182:477–481.
235. Lamy C, Domingo V, Semah F, et al. Early and late seizures after cryptogenic ischemic stroke in young adults. *Neurology* 2003;60:400–404.
236. Michelson AD, Bovill E, Monagle P, et al. Antithrombotic therapy in children. *Chest* 1998;114(Suppl 5):748S–769S.
237. deVeber G, Chan A, Monagle P, et al. Anticoagulation therapy in pediatric patients with sinovenous thrombosis: a cohort study. *Arch Neurol* 1998;55:1533–1537.
238. Massicotte P, Adams M, Marzinotto V, et al. Low-molecular-weight heparin in pediatric patients with thrombotic disease: a dose finding study. *J Pediatr* 1996;128:313–318.
239. Dix D, Andrew M, Marzinotto V, et al. The use of low-molecular-weight heparin in pediatric patients. A prospective cohort study. *J Pediatr* 2000;136:439–445.
240. Hofman S, Knoefler R, Lorenz N, et al. Clinical experience with low-molecular-weight heparins in pediatric patients. *Thromb Res* 2001;103:345–353.
241. Nowak-Gottl U, Gunther G, Kurnik K, et al. Arterial ischemic stroke in neonates, infants, and children: an overview of underlying conditions, imaging methods, and treatment modalities. *Semin Thromb Hemost* 2003;29:405–414.
242. Schmugge M, Risch L, Huber AR, et al. Heparin-induced thrombocytopenia-associated thrombosis in pediatric intensive care patients. *Pediatrics* 2002;109:U69–U72.
243. Massicotte P, Marzinotto V, Vegh P, et al. Home monitoring of warfarin therapy in children with a whole blood prothrombin time monitor. *J Pediatr* 1995;127:389–394.
244. Strater R, Kurnik K, Heller C, et al. Aspirin versus low-molecular-weight heparin: antithrombotic therapy in pediatric patients. A prospective follow-up study. *Stroke* 2001;32:2554–2558.

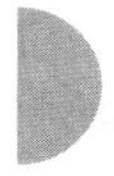

Paroxysmal Disorders

Raman Sankar, Susan Koh, Joyce Wu, and John H. Menkes

This chapter discusses conditions manifested by sudden, recurrent, and potentially reversible epileptic alterations of brain function.

EPILEPSY

Epilepsy was known to the ancient Babylonians and was described by Hippocrates, who considered it a disease of the brain. Its history, related by Tempkin, spans that of medicine itself (1). Hughlings Jackson concisely defined epilepsy as "an occasional excessive and disordered discharge of nerve tissue" (2). More recently, epilepsy has been defined as recurrent convulsive or nonconvulsive seizures caused by partial or generalized epileptogenic discharges in the cerebrum.

The epilepsies represent a group of diseases for which recurrent seizures represent their principal manifestation.

Estimates of the incidence of epilepsy depend on whether a single convulsive or nonconvulsive episode and febrile seizures are included in the definition. According to Millichap, febrile seizures account for 2% of all childhood illnesses (3). More recent estimates of the prevalence of single and recurrent nonfebrile seizures in children younger than 10 years of age range from 5.2 to 8.1 per 1,000 (4,5). By age 40 years, the cumulative incidence is 1.7% to 1.9% (4,5).

Classification

The epilepsies have been designated as primary (idiopathic), secondary (symptomatic), or reactive (Table 14.1). The term *primary* implies that, with the present knowledge, no structural or biochemical cause for the recurrent seizures can be found. In general, the primary epilepsies are genetically transmitted, and they tend to have a better prognosis for seizure control. The term *secondary* (symptomatic) epilepsy indicates that the cause of the seizure can be discovered. Such seizures are the principal manifestation of many diseases. They occur in the course of many congenital or acquired conditions of the nervous system, or they can complicate systemic disease. The designation of an epileptic condition as cryptogenic implies that the underlying etiology is symptomatic, but not readily demonstrable by available diagnostic techniques (6). In the reactive epilepsies, seizures are the consequence of an abnormal reaction of an otherwise normal brain to physiologic stress or transient insult. A notable example is febrile seizures. Not all epilepsies can be categorized conveniently. Some are atypical, others are rare, and for a significant proportion data necessary for classification are inadequate or incomplete.

The characteristics for all epilepsies are recurrent convulsive or nonconvulsive seizures. The 1989 classification scheme of the International League Against Epilepsy (ILAE) elected a hierarchy of dichotomies in which the initial categorization is based on whether the epilepsy is localization-related or generalized (6). This distinction was, in fact, made by Hughlings Jackson more than 100 years ago (7) (Table 14.2). Localization-related epilepsies (partial or focal) seizures are classified into simple, complex, and secondarily generalized. Simple partial seizures involve preserved consciousness, whereas complex partial seizures are those with impaired consciousness. The prevalence of the various seizure types is presented in Table 14.3.

The descriptive classification of epileptic syndromes is extremely useful clinically. The so-called epileptic syndromes are distinctive in that they demonstrate characteristic age of onset, seizure types, electroencephalographic (EEG) features, and prognosis. This is particularly valuable in pediatric epileptology because the immature brain often produces stereotypic epileptic behaviors that are a function of its stage of development, rather than etiology. Childhood syndromes can be considered as benign or catastrophic based on their responsiveness to treatment, the possibility of remission of seizures, and the long-term prognosis for normal cognitive development.

Etiology

Recurrent seizures are thought to result from a genetic predisposition, underlying neuropathologic changes, and chemicophysiologic alterations in the nerve cell and its

TABLE 14.1 Scheme for Organizing Epileptic Conditions

	With Generalized Seizures	*With Partial (Focal) Seizures*
Primary (idiopathic) epilepsies		
Without structural lesions; benign; genetic	Absence (petit mal) epilepsy Juvenile absence epilepsy Many generalized tonic-clonic seizures Juvenile myoclonic epilepsy Benign neonatal seizures	Benign epilepsy with centrotemporal spikes (rolandic epilepsy) Childhood epilepsy with occipital spikes
Secondary (symptomatic) epilepsies		
With anatomic or known biochemical lesions	Infantile spasms Lennox-Gastaut syndrome	Temporal lobe (psychomotor) epilepsy Epilepsies caused by gray matter heterotopias, polymicrogyria Epilepsies caused by focal postasphyxial gliosis
Conditions with reactive seizures		
Abnormal reaction of an otherwise normal brain to physiologic stress or transient epileptogenic insult	Febrile seizures Most toxic- and metabolic-induced seizures Many isolated tonic-clonic seizures Early post-traumatic seizures	Partial seizures occur when conditions with reactive seizures are superimposed on transient or preexisting nonepileptogenic brain injury, as often seen with head trauma, hypernatremia, hypoglycemia

Adapted from Engel J. *Seizures, epilepsies and the epileptic patient.* Philadelphia: FA Davis, 1989.

TABLE 14.2 Classification of Epileptic Seizures

- **I. Partial (focal or local) seizures**
  - Simple partial seizures
    - Seizures with motor signs
    - Seizures with somatosensory or special sensory symptoms
    - Seizures with autonomic symptoms or signs
    - Seizures with psychic symptoms
  - Complex partial (psychomotor) seizures
    - Simple partial onset followed by impairment of consciousness
    - Seizures with impairment of consciousness at outset
  - Partial (focal) seizures evolving to secondarily generalized (tonic-clonic, grand mal) seizures
    - Simple partial (focal) seizures evolving to generalized (grand mal) seizures
    - Complex partial (psychomotor) seizures evolving to generalized (grand mal) seizures
    - Simple partial (focal) seizures evolving to complex partial psychomotor seizures evolving to generalized seizures
- **II. Generalized seizures (convulsive and nonconvulsive)**
  - Absence seizures
    - Typical absences (petit mal attacks)
    - Atypical absences (atypical petit mal attacks)
  - Myoclonic seizures
  - Clonic seizures
  - Tonic seizures
  - Tonic-clonic seizures (grand mal seizures)
  - Atonic seizures (akinetic or astatic seizures)
- **III. Unclassified epileptic seizures**

From Commission on Classification and Terminology of the International League Against Epilepsy. Proposal for revised clinical and electroencephalographic classification of epileptic seizures. *Epilepsia* 1981;22:489. With permission.

connections. Each of these factors is considered in turn. Attributed causes for epilepsy in children and adolescents are presented in Table 14.4 (8).

Genetic Factors

Numerous studies suggest that the genetic susceptibility to seizures is normally distributed in the general population, and that there is a threshold above which the condition becomes clinically evident.

An interaction between one or more genes and various nongenetic events operates in several conditions accompanied by seizures. These include head trauma, brain tumors, and congenital hemiplegia (9,10). Genetic factors appear to be most significant in patients with the various primary epilepsies (11). The various nonprogressive hereditary epilepsies are summarized in Table 14.5 (12–30). In one study, Lennox and Lennox found a 70% concordance for monozygotic twins and 5.6% concordance for dizygotic twins for epilepsies without organic brain lesions (31). Metrakos and Metrakos found a 12% incidence of seizures among parents and siblings of children with absence seizures; 45% of siblings had an abnormal EEG. They proposed that this EEG abnormality is an expression of an autosomal dominant gene with nearly complete penetrance during childhood and low penetrance in infancy and adult life (32). Gerken and Doose, interpreting data derived from their clinic, concluded that it was unlikely that a single autosomal dominant gene was responsible for the 3-Hz spike and wave trait and suggested a polygenic inheritance with neurophysiologic and genetic heterogeneity (33). Indeed, at least three genes for absence epilepsy have been mapped at this point in time (see Table 14.5) (34,35).

TABLE 14.3 Prevalence Rates Per 1,000 of Specific Seizure Types in Children Aged Newborn to 9 Years

Seizure Type	*Ohtahara et al. (1981)[a]*	*Cowen et al. (1989)*	*Kurland (1959)*
All types	8.21 (n = 2,378)	5.24 (n = 626)	5.79 (n = 29)
Generalized	2.57	2.22	—
Primary generalized	1.99	1.29	—
Grand mal	1.82	1.18	3.20
Petit mal	0.11	0.06	1.20
Myoclonus	0.07	0.05	—
Secondary generalized	0.58	0.94	—
Lennox-Gastaut syndrome	0.29	0.13	—
Infantile spasms (West syndrome)	0.14	0.19	—
Others	0.14	0.61	—
Partial	3.60	1.17	—
With elementary symptomatology	0.71	0.43	0.60
With complex symptomatology	0.21	0.30	0.40
Secondarily generalized	2.68	0.43	—
Mixed	0.12	0.02	—
Unclassified	1.92	1.82	0.40

[a]n, total number of prevalent cases in children aged 0 to 9 years. Includes single and recurrent afebrile seizures.
From Cowen LD, Bodensteiner JB, Leviton A, et al. Prevalence of the epilepsies in children and adolescents. *Epilepsia* 1989;30:94. With permission.

In families with centrotemporal spikes or sharp-wave discharges and rolandic seizures, EEG abnormalities are transmitted in a dominant manner with age-dependent penetrance (11). Only 12% of relatives with EEG abnormalities, however, develop clinically apparent seizures. This type of seizure has been mapped to chromosome 10q22-q24, with the defective gene being LGI1 (36). A significant genetic predisposition also occurs in juvenile myoclonic epilepsy, in photosensitive seizures, and in the various other primary generalized epilepsies. In seizures

TABLE 14.4 Attributed Causes for Epilepsy in Children and Adolescents by Sex: Prevalent Cases, 1983

	Male		*Female*		*Total*	
Cause	*Number*	*Percent*	*Number*	*Percent*	*Number*	*Percent*
Idiopathic	428	68	375	70	803	69
Congenital	17	3	19	4	36	3
CNS malformation	9	1	11	2	20	2
MH, DD	5	<1	6	1	11	1
Phacomatoses	3	<1	1	<1	4	<1
Other	—	—	1	<1	1	<1
CNS infection	19	3	14	3	33	3
Toxic/metabolic	15	2	11	2	26	2
CNS neoplasm	2	<1	1	<1	3	<1
Perinatal	45	7	36	7	81	7
Birth trauma	9	1	1	<1	10	1
Asphyxia/hypoxia	17	3	21	4	38	3
Other perinatal	9	1	2	<1	11	1
Multiple perinatal	10	2	12	2	22	2
Traumatic	23	4	20	4	43	4
Other and multiple	77	12	57	11	134	12
Total	626	100	533	100	1,159	100

CNS, central nervous system; DD, developmental delay (includes the diagnoses of mental retardation, psychomotor retardation, failure to thrive, and developmental delay); MH, motor handicap (includes the diagnoses of cerebral palsy, monoplegia, diplegia, hemiplegia, and quadriplegia).
From Cowen LD, Bodensteiner JB, Leviton A, et al. Prevalence of the epilepsies in children and adolescents. *Epilepsia* 1989;30:94. With permission.

TABLE 14.5 Genetically Transmitted Nonprogressive Epilepsies

Syndrome	*Locus*	*Gene*	*Clinical Manifestations*	*Ref*
Benign familial neonatal seizure (EBN1)	20q13.3	KCNQ2	AD, neonatal seizures, clear spontaneously, normal development	36,38
Benign familial neonatal seizures (EBN2)	8q24	KCNQ3	AD, similar clinically to EBN1	12,13,40
Benign familial neonatal seizures (EBN3)	Pericentric inversion 5		AD, similar to EBN1	14
Benign familial neonatal-infantile seizures	2q23–q24.3	SCN2A1	AD, afebrile seizures during first year of life, remission by 1 year	15
Generalized epilepsy with febrile seizure + type 1	19q13	SCN1B	AD, highly variable, febrile seizures, variety of afebrile seizures	16
Generalized epilepsy with febrile seizure + type 2	2q24	SCN1A	AD, variable, febrile seizure, seizures triggered by fever, partial seizures, also severe myoclonic epilepsy of infancy	17,18,23
Generalized epilepsy with febrile seizure + type 3	2q23–q24.3	SCN2A	AD, intractable epilepsy, mental deterioration	22
Generalized epilepsy with febrile seizure + type 3	5q31.1–q33.1	GABRG2	AD, some have febrile seizures, others afebrile, allelic with ECA2	19
Benign familial infantile convulsions (BFIS1)	19q		Onset of seizures at 6 months, resolve at 1 year, normal development	20
Benign familial infantile convulsions (BFIS2)	16p		AD, a variety of seizure types	21
Nocturnal frontal lobe epilepsy — type 1	20q13.2–q13.3	CHRNA4	AD, onset in second month, occur during sleep, persist into adult life	24
Nocturnal frontal lobe epilepsy — type 2	15q24			
Nocturnal frontal lobe epilepsy — type 3	1q21	CHRNB2	AD, onset in first decade	26b
Familial temporal lobe seizures with aphasia	10q22–q24	LGI1	AD, partial seizures, auditory symptoms, aphasia with attacks	25
Myoclonic epilepsy and spasticity	Xp22.13	ARX	Myoclonic epilepsy, mental retardation, spasticity, allelic with X-linked infantile spasms	26
Absence epilepsy (ECA1)	8q24			
Absence epilepsy (ECA2)	5q31.1	GABRG2	Absence seizure, allelic with generalized epilepsy with febrile seizures + type 3	26a
Absence epilepsy (ECA3)	3q26	CLCN2		34
Infantile spasms, X-linked		STK9		34
Familial hemiplegic migraine and benign infantile convulsions	1q23	ATP1A	Family members have familial hemiplegic migraine, infantile convulsions, or both.	35
Juvenile absence epilepsy	5q34–q35 3q26–qter 2q22–q23	GABRA1 CLCN2 CACNB4	Sudden myoclonic jerks after awakening and grand mal attacks. Transmission is still uncertain.	See text
Juvenile myoclonic epilepsy (JME)	6p12–p11 15q14 6 p21	EFHC1 ? ?		See text
Febrile seizure (FEB 1)	8q13–21	?	AD, high penetrance	27
Febrile seizure (FEB 2)	19p3	?	AD	28
Febrile seizure (FEB 3)	2q23–24	?	Identical with generalized epilepsy with febrile seizure + type 3	29
Febrile seizure (FEB 4)	5q14–q15	?	AD	30
Febrile seizure susceptibility locus	18p11.2	? IMPA2		30a

Abbreviations: AD, autosomal dominant; ARX, aristaless homeobox gene; CACNB, calcium channel voltage-dependent, beta subunit; CHRNA, cholinergic receptor nicotinic, alpha polypeptide; CLCN, chloride channel gene; GABRG, gamma-aminobutyric acid receptor, gamma subunit; GABRA, gamma-aminobutyric acid receptor, alpha subunit; KCN, potassium channel; IMPA2-gene encodes myo-inositol monophosphatase, LGI, leucine-rich gene, glioma inactivated; SCN, sodium channel (A and B refer to alpha and beta subunit genes); STK, serine-threonine kinase.

with secondary generalization, the genetic factors, although demonstrable through controlled twin studies, are not as striking as in the primary generalized epilepsies. However, even in absence epilepsy, in which the genetic factor is most prominent, the overall risk of developing seizures is only 8% for siblings of affected subjects and 2% in as yet unaffected siblings older than 6 years of age (37). For offspring of subjects with absence seizures, the risk for EEG abnormalities is 64% and for seizures is 6.7% (38). When promazine is used to activate the EEG, 73.5% of 7- to 14-year-old siblings of subjects with idiopathic absence seizures develop an abnormal EEG (39).

Several other genes responsible for epilepsy have been mapped and cloned. The first epilepsy gene to be cloned was one of three genes responsible for autosomal dominant nocturnal frontal lobe epilepsy (24,40). It has been mapped to chromosome 20q13.2-13.3 and encodes the nicotinic acetylcholine receptor alpha-4 subunit (CHRNA 4). The same authors later reported a different mutation in the same gene for a different pedigree with this syndrome (41). Two other genes for this condition have been mapped to chromosome 15q24 and chromosome 1 (24). The discovery of mutations in this gene was perplexing to many because this receptor has not been considered to be involved in the modulation of neuronal excitability relevant to seizure disorders.

The finding that benign familial neonatal convulsions are attributable to mutations of voltage-gated potassium channels, KCNQ2 (12,13,42,43) and KCNQ3 (44), is more in tune with our understanding of the mechanisms of excitability. Altered K^+-channel function could impair neuronal repolarization and thus contribute toward increased excitability. The extremely transient nature of this disorder suggests that compensatory changes probably take place in other genes controlling excitatory or inhibitory ion channels.

The relationship between the genotype and the phenotypic expression of the gene disorder is complex and is complicated by phenotypic convergence—that is, two different genetic mutations can induce the same clinical picture. Thus, afebrile seizures during the first year of life can result not only from mutations in the sodium channel gene, SCN2A1, but also from mutations in the GABA receptor gene, GABRG2. Conversely, there is phenotypic divergence, and different mutations of the same calcium channel gene CACNA1A are associated with familial hemiplegic migraine, episodic ataxia, and epilepsy (45). Mutations in LGI1 can be associated with a variety of phenotypes: partial epilepsy with auditory features, mesial temporal lobe epilepsy, temporal lobe epilepsy with febrile seizures, and temporal lobe epilepsy with developmental delay (36). Mutations in SCN1A are associated with a clinical continuum, including severe myoclonic epilepsy of infancy, generalized epilepsy with febrile seizures plus, and intractable childhood epilepsy with tonic-clonic seizures as well milder forms such as classical "febrile seizures"(46). Likewise, mutations in the chloride channel gene CLCN2 can be found in childhood absence epilepsy, juvenile myoclonic epilepsy, or epilepsy with grand mal upon awakening (46a). The reasons that underlie this clinical diversity are unclear. It is likely that additional genes contribute and modify the phenotypic expression. Indeed, Durner and colleagues found statistical support for a major susceptibility gene for idiopathic generalized epilepsy and different modifying genes (47).

Neuropathologic Factors

Seizures can occur in patients with almost any pathologic process that affects the brain. Two types of abnormalities are seen: those that are responsible for recurrent seizures, and those that are the consequence of recurrent seizures.

Gowers stated more than 100 years ago that seizures beget seizures (48). The question whether lesions produce seizures or seizures produce lesions has been extensively investigated.

Lesions Responsible for Recurrent Seizures

A variety of morphologic changes can cause recurrent seizures. They range from the most obvious, such as some of the major developmental anomalies (see Chapter 5) or postasphyxial changes (see Chapter 6), to minor dysgenetic lesions such as the gray matter heterotopias (see Chapter 5). Although morphologic alterations would not be expected to be found in the primary epilepsies, sometimes they are (49). Mutations in the gene *filamin A*, that codes for a protein with a role in actin cross-linking and membrane stabilization have been reported to be responsible for the aberrance in migration that results in periventricular heterotopia (50,51). A number of authors have called attention to minor developmental anomalies in the molecular layer of the cerebral cortex and in the cerebellar cortex, some of which are clearly the result of disturbed cell migration (52). Malformations, notably gray matter heterotopias, *cryptic tubers*, or angiomas arising within the temporal lobe, can cause recurrent seizures. Such lesions also can be found in other areas of the brain (53,54). The genetic basis of some of the dramatic cerebral malformations associated with severe epilepsies of early childhood, such as the double cortex syndrome or band heterotopia, are also beginning to be understood (55,56) (see Chapter 5).

Altered neuronal migration that results in granule cell disorganization in the dentate gyrus has been seen in tissue resected from patients with temporal lobe epilepsy (57). Although initially this was thought to be a congenital lesion, provocative data from Parent demonstrates that, even in mature animals, status epilepticus can result in neurogenesis in the dentate gyrus, and that the nascent granule cells may migrate aberrantly. The data suggest that aberrant synapse formation by these cells could contribute to abnormal excitability (58–60).

The role of infectious processes in the pathogenesis of epilepsy has received relatively little attention since Aguilar and Rasmussen established that some epileptic patients with focal seizures, slowly progressive intellectual deterioration, and cerebral atrophy demonstrate a pathologic picture consistent with a viral encephalitis (61). Attempts at viral isolation have been unsuccessful in these cases. Nevertheless, it is likely that not only focal epilepsy, but also other forms of seizure disorders, particularly disorders beginning in early childhood in previously healthy children (such as epileptogenic encephalopathy or progressive facial hemiatrophy), are caused by a smoldering viral disease within the brain (see Chapter 7).

Lesions Secondary to Recurrent Seizures

Among the lesions considered to be secondary to recurrent seizures are those that result from the physical trauma that often attends seizures, and those that result from hypoxia, vascular alterations, or the action of the excitatory neurotransmitters.

Meldrum and colleagues (62) explored the possibility that the seizure itself, rather than systemic changes, was responsible for brain damage. They showed that brain damage occurred in the absence of systemic abnormalities in paralyzed, ventilated, adolescent baboons that were subjected to prolonged, bicuculline-induced seizures. Although the neurochemical changes attending cell death owing to prolonged seizures are similar to those seen in ischemia and hypoglycemia, significant differences in the time course and anatomic distribution of brain damage occur (see Table 17.1).

Under clinical conditions, damage results from a combination of the increased metabolic demands that accompany excessive neuronal activity and the reduced circulation and substrate supply induced by the combination of hyperthermia, hypoglycemia, hypotension, and hypoxia. Cell death under these conditions occurs through a process that resembles cell death in asphyxia, namely through the release of excitotoxins that increase intracellular calcium in the course of prolonged seizures. A more extensive discussion of this process can be found in Chapter 6.

Several areas of the brain, especially the hippocampus, appear to be particularly vulnerable to recurrent and prolonged seizures. Anatomic manifestations of cell damage to the hippocampus include loss of interneurons in the hilus, pyramidal cell loss within the Sommer's sector (prosubiculum and subfield CA1 of Ammon's horn), and subfield CA3, with consequential glial scarring and atrophy (63,64). Using Golgi techniques to study the hippocampus and dentate nucleus, Scheibel and associates have observed loss of dendritic spines and deformation of the dendritic shaft (65). This selective hippocampal vulnerability has been postulated to result from a high density of excitatory receptors on nerve cells in Sommer's sector (66). Other factors also could be operative. Using *in situ* hybridization techniques, Sommer and coworkers showed unique developmental patterns in the mRNA expression of the Glu R-1, -2, and -3 glutamate receptor subunits in CA1, CA3, and the dentate gyrus. Differences in receptor structure could result in differences in receptor function and differences with maturation in resistance of the hippocampus to epileptic damage (67). The protective role of calbindin, a calcium-binding protein, from glutamate-induced neurotoxicity also could account for the selective nerve cell loss (68).

Within the gray matter of the cerebral hemispheres, neuronal cell loss is most likely to occur in laminae 3 and 4, where the thalamocortical afferents terminate. Damage also occurs in the pars reticularis of the substantia nigra, globus pallidus, and thalamus. In animal models, the substantia nigra has been demonstrated to play an

TABLE 14.6 Possible Etiologic Factors for Complex Partial Seizures

Factor	Mesial Temporal Sclerosis, 47[a] Cases	Small Tumors, 21 (24) Cases	Miscellaneous Lesions, 10 (13) Cases	Equivocal Lesions, 22 Cases	Totals, 100 Cases
Positive family history	6	0	2 (4)	0	8
Difficult or precipitate birth	7	4	3	7	21
Infantile convulsions	13	1	1	1	16
Difficult/precipitate birth and infantile convulsions	6	1	0	0	7
Head injury	5	6	3 (5)	5	19
Other factors[b]	11	1 (2)	4	4	20
None of above factors	5	10	2	7	—

[a]The figures without parentheses refer to pure cases of each subgroup, and those with parentheses refer to cases with a dual pathology, including mesial temporal sclerosis.
[b]For example, meningitis, mastoid disease, febrile illnesses in infancy without convulsions.
Modified from Falconer MA, Serafetinides EA, Corsellis JAN. Etiology and pathogenesis of temporal lobe epilepsy. *Arch Neurol* 1964;10:233.

important role in the propagation of seizures, and damage to this structure could conceivably contribute to increased propensity for seizures (69). The caudate nucleus appears to be spared (70).

There is controversy as to the effect of seizures on the immature brain and whether brief but repetitive seizures can induce brain damage. One of us (R.S.) has reviewed the arguments for both sides in this controversial issue (71,72). Some types of experimental seizures fail to produce histologic lesions (71). This observation gave rise to the argument that the immature brain is not vulnerable to seizure-induced damage. This argument runs contrary to the observations on surgically resected tissue from epileptic children that show structural alterations that can be attributed to seizures (73,74). More recent work has shown that the effect of seizures on the developing brain is age- and model-specific, and also that both prolonged and brief and repetitive seizures are associated with the induction of neuronal apoptosis in specific cell populations in human and experimental animals (75–78).

Brief but recurrent seizures induced by pentylenetetrazol have been shown to contribute to morphologic and functional alterations in neonatal rat pups (79–81). The question whether brief but recurrent seizures also have a similar potential to induce brain damage cannot be answered with assurance in humans. In terms of clinical practice, patients with recurrent seizures are invariably treated with antiepileptic drugs, which on their own can affect development (82); the natural history of the condition without treatment is, therefore, impossible to study. Autopsy material does not permit an easy distinction of the pathology that caused the frequent seizures from the effect of the seizures themselves.

The studies of Shewmon and Erwin are more directly applicable to the clinical problem. These workers have demonstrated that interictal spikes, when followed by prominent inhibitory after potentials, can transiently disrupt cortical function. Thus, frequent interictal spikes could interfere with modality-specific learning (83). Presumably, recurrent electrical discharges could influence activity-dependent plasticity of the developing brain.

Mesial Temporal Sclerosis (Ammon's Horn Sclerosis, Hippocampal Sclerosis)

The damage seen in the hippocampus obtained by surgical resection in chronic temporal lobe epilepsy differs from that seen in postmortem specimens after status epilepticus (84,85). In contrast to the selective damage seen after status epilepticus, the hippocampus of subjects with chronic temporal lobe epilepsy shows more widespread damage throughout the CA1, CA2, and CA3 subfields as well as the dentate granule cells (84). Hippocampal cell loss ranges from mild and random to almost complete. Although initially the changes have a bilateral distribution, with time, one hemisphere becomes more affected (86). This pathologic abnormality has been designated as mesial temporal sclerosis (MTS) or hippocampal sclerosis. It was seen in 47% of resected temporal lobes in the series of Falconer and associates (Table 14.6) (87), and in 64% of a more recent series compiled by Engel and associates (88). Cell loss and gliosis in the amygdala also has been observed and can occur in the absence of significant hippocampal changes (89). In more severe cases, nerve cell loss and gliosis involves not only the entire hippocampus, but also the uncus, amygdala, and adjacent cortex (Fig. 14.1). Atrophic changes in the cerebellum or the thalamus are not uncommon.

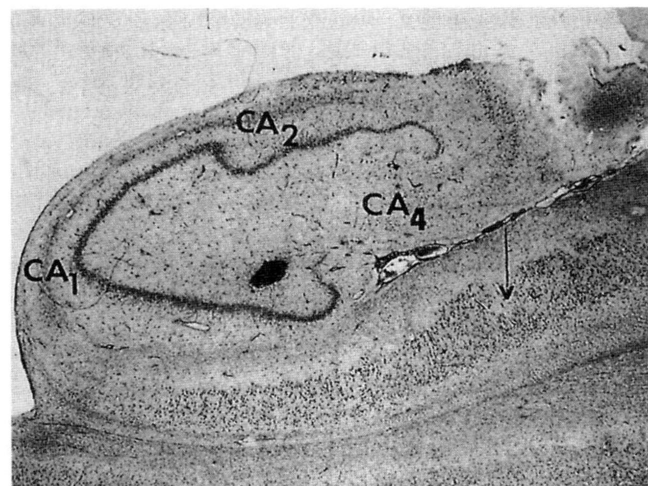

FIGURE 14.1. Mesial temporal sclerosis in 23-year-old man. Onset of complex partial seizures began at age 6 years, with a frequency of up to seven per day. A few major motor seizures occurred each year. Cross-section of the cornu Ammonis shows the extent of injury of the pyramidal cell layer. Neurons of areas CA_4, CA_2, and CA_1 are markedly reduced in number. There are also focal areas of cell loss in the subiculum (*arrow*) (Gridley stain, ×10). (Courtesy of the late Dr. W. Jann Brown, Department of Pathology, University of California, Los Angeles, UCLA School of Medicine.)

The cause or causes of MTS are still unresolved. MTS has been seen as early as 1 year of age, and combined morphologic and electrophysiologic studies suggest that the seizure focus is generated in part when abnormal, recurrent, monosynaptic excitatory synapses are formed after damage to normal intrahippocampal synapses (90). A detailed analysis of the epileptogenic potential of the lesions produced by intrahippocampal or systemic kainic acid or by ischemia led Franck to conclude that hippocampal sclerosis and seizures are both symptoms of an underlying pathology, and that although MTS may be produced by seizures, the development of epilepsy as a syndrome does not depend on cell loss or plasticity in the hippocampus (91). Neuroimaging studies performed within 48 hours of a prolonged febrile convulsion indicate the presence of hippocampal edema that resolves within a few days, and that in some instances is replaced by hippocampal atrophy (92,92a). These studies do not resolve the questions of whether a pre-existing hippocampal abnormality predisposed to the prolonged febrile convulsion and whether the anatomic features of MTS may become incorporated into, and sustain, an epileptic focus. In this regard, the identification of an interleukin gene polymorphism identified with both prolonged febrile convulsions and temporal lobe epilepsy with hippocampal sclerosis is quite interesting (92b).

Vascular, metabolic, genetic, and immunologic factors, acting singly or in concert, can be responsible for MTS (93,94). Epidemiologic studies have been used to ascertain risk factors for this condition. Febrile convulsions were seen in 20% of subjects, as compared with 2% of controls. The majority experienced at least one complicated febrile seizure. An increased incidence of head trauma and neonatal convulsions also could be documented. Additionally, there was a significant association with maternal seizures (95). In a significant population of patients, the brain, after a lifetime of recurrent epileptic attacks, shows neither gross nor microscopic abnormalities. This observation reflects the current limitation of morphologic studies in furthering our understanding of the epilepsies.

Basic Mechanisms of Epileptogenesis

> We must notice what the normal function of nerve tissue is. Its function is to store up and expend force.
> —*H. Jackson, 1873 (96)*

It should be stated at the outset that modulation of transmitter effects, of voltage-gated channels, and of cell electrical properties involves processes that occur continually during normal brain function. This plasticity is the basis of the cortex to learn from experience. It seems that the same plastic mechanisms are involved in epileptogenicity. One extreme result of such plasticity is the hyperexcitability and hypersynchrony that characterize epileptiform activities. The risk of epileptiform activity is the price that has to be paid for a nervous system that is so adaptive (97).

Each clinical form of epilepsy is generated by a different set of mechanisms. In general, there is greater understanding presently of generators of focal epileptiform activity than generalized epileptiform activities. Cellular aspects of epileptogenesis are reviewed by DeLorenzo (98) and Velísek and Moshé (99).

Neurophysiology and Neurochemistry

From a neurophysiologic point of view, an epileptic seizure has been defined as an alteration of central nervous system (CNS) function resulting from spontaneous electrical discharge in a diseased neuronal population of cortical gray matter or the brainstem.

Epileptogenesis requires a set of epileptogenic neurons, the presence of disinhibition, and circuitry to permit synchronization.

Partial Epilepsies

An epileptic neuron has, among other characteristics, an increased electric excitability and the ability to sustain an autonomous paroxysmal discharge that can be influenced from the outside by synaptic activity. Intracellular recordings within an epileptic focus reveal that during the time when an interictal discharge is recorded on the scalp EEG, a compact population of neurons displays a stereotyped abnormality called paroxysmal depolarization shift (PDS) in intracellular recordings. A PDS is characterized by a sudden, large, and sustained (approximately 30 mV for 70 to 150 msec) depolarization that is synchronized in many neurons. Multiple, high-frequency action potentials are superimposed on the PDS. The PDS and the interictal spike on scalp EEG, which represents that synchronized PDS of a local population of neurons can occur spontaneously or can be triggered by afferent stimuli. The PDS is followed by a hyperpolarization of 10 to 20 mV below the resting potential that lasts 700 msec or longer. During this period, the focus is refractory to afferent stimulation.

The large and lasting depolarization that characterizes a PDS is attributed to the triggering of voltage-gated calcium channels by the incoming action potential. This depolarizing calcium conductance is mediated by a subtype of excitatory amino acid receptor, which is characterized by its high affinity to *N*-methyl-D-aspartate (NMDA). The calcium channel is regulated by magnesium through a voltage-dependent block that can be removed by the initial sodium influx triggered by the action potential. The rise in intracellular calcium in turn triggers the opening of a specific type of potassium channel that initiates the hyperpolarization phase.

Ictogenesis is the spread of localized epileptic discharges to induce a clinical seizure during which thousands of neurons fire synchronously for prolonged periods. Several experimental systems have been used to study how localized discharges are able to spread. In a nonepileptic brain, an area of neuronal hyperpolarization, the inhibitory surround, surrounds the region of synchronous paroxysmal discharges. This inhibitory surround limits the duration of the interictal discharge, determines its frequency, and prevents its progression into a full-blown seizure. Neurons can become hyperpolarized by several processes that can differ from one set of neurons to another.

The mechanisms responsible for this transition from interictal to ictal period probably involve nonsynaptic processes such as electrical field effects (ephaptic interactions) and electrotonic coupling via gap junctions (100). Changes in the extracellular environment, such as K^+ and Ca^{2+} concentrations, also can affect the excitability of neuronal populations (101,102), suggesting that astrocytes also may play important roles in this process.

The observation that the normal limbic system can become epileptogenic by repeated stimulation, a process termed *kindling*, has provided a model for the study of the development of complex partial epilepsy (103,104). Kindling refers to a process by which brief trains of subconvulsive electrical stimuli are repeatedly delivered at appropriate intervals to a susceptible area of the brain. Initially, these stimuli produce after-discharges, which become progressively more prolonged until they give rise to limbic and clonic motor seizures. When stimulations are continued for even longer periods, spontaneous seizures appear. Once established, the effects of kindling are permanent. Kindling also can be achieved by chemical stimulation of the cortex.

During kindling, the mossy fiber pathway (efferent from the granule cells of the dentate gyrus) undergoes reorganization of its synaptic connections (105). The resulting recurrent excitatory connections have been implicated in the progressive development of hypersynchronous discharge. Such synaptic reorganization associated with loss of pyramidal cells in the CA3 subfield has been demonstrated in human epileptic tissue (106–108). Sloviter has suggested that the recurrent mossy fiber terminals include synapses on inhibitory interneurons (109).

Using his perforant path stimulation model of status epilepticus, Sloviter has studied the development of mossy fiber sprouting, chronic epilepsy, and time-dependent alterations in dentate inhibition. He suggested that the recurrent mossy fiber terminals include synapses on inhibitory interneurons (109,110). In his conceptualization, the hilar basket cells [inhibitory, g-aminobutyric acid (GABA)-ergic] are deafferented by the loss of another group of cells, the mossy cells (excitatory, glutamatergic), which normally receive mossy fiber input, and drive the inhibitory basket cells (Fig. 14.2); hence the term *dormant basket cell hypothesis* for this concept. Mossy fiber sprouting compensates for the loss of drive to the basket cells. GABAergic cells, indeed, appear to be preserved in human epileptic tissue (111) and also in animal models (110), thus supporting this concept.

Studies have compared the expression of excitatory amino acid receptor subunits and glutamic acid dehydrogenase (GAD) (presynaptic marker for GABA terminals) to the extent of mossy fiber sprouting in tissue from patients who underwent surgery. Patients' granule cell KA2 and GluR5 mRNA levels were increased in association with aberrant fascia dentata mossy fiber sprouting; however, increased glutamic acid dehydrogenase immunoreactivity also was present in such tissue (112,113).

The preceding discussions pertain to the structural (network) plasticity that may be associated with focal epileptogenesis. There also is evidence for functional plasticity of synapses. Excitatory synapses show robust enhancement when they undergo repetitive high-frequency activation (114). This includes facilitation during the course of sustained stimulation and long-term potentiation that lasts hours to days after such a burst of activity in excitatory synapses. In contrast, similar repetitive high-frequency driving diminishes the efficacy of inhibitory (GABAergic) synapses (115,116).

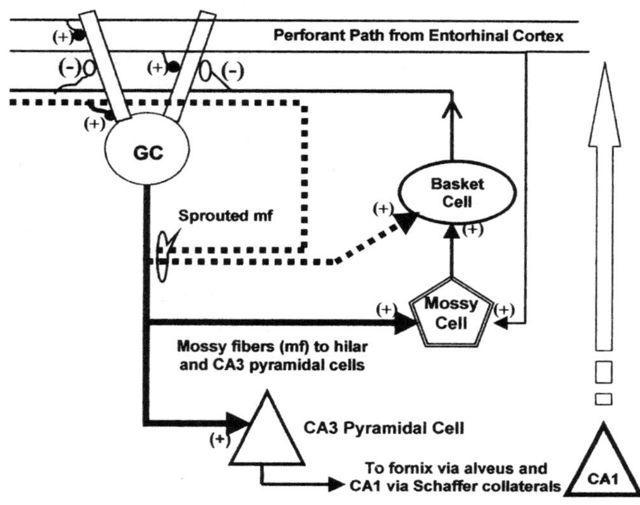

FIGURE 14.2. Hippocampal circuitry and seizure-induced circuit reorganization. Granule cells (GC) receive their major input via the perforant path. The perforant path also stimulates hilar interneurons (such as mossy cells and basket cells) to provide feed-forward inhibition of the granule cells. Granule cell axons, the mossy fibers, make synaptic contact with CA3 pyramidal cells. Mossy fiber collaterals innervate the hilar interneurons, such as the mossy cell shown in the diagram. Mossy cells are excitatory to GABAergic basket cells, which provide feedback inhibition to the granule cell. Sprouting of mossy fibers (in response to seizure-induced loss of CA3 pyramidal cells and hilar mossy cells) can result in enhanced excitation by forming autapses (an axon sprout synapsing with the dendrites of the same cell) and can augment synchronization by stimulating neighboring granule cells (not shown), thus contributing to epileptogenicity. It also has been suggested that the sprouted mossy fibers may restore inhibition lost after seizure-induced death of hilar mossy cells by direct stimulation of deafferented (dormant) basket cells.

Evidence has emerged to suggest that the epileptogenic process also may involve cellular plasticity in addition to synaptic and network plasticity. Lasting changes in the subunit composition of hyperpolarization-induced, cyclic nucleotide-activated cation channels (HCN), which regulate cellular excitability, have been noted after hyperthermic convulsions in rodents (117). HCN channel plasticity also has been demonstrated in resected hippocampal tissue from humans (118). Alterations in channels that mediate low-threshold calcium currents (T-calcium channels) also has been demonstrated in both experimental and resected human hippocampi (119).

Three factors determine whether a focal seizure will become generalized. The first is the excitability of the epileptic neurons, the second is the ease with which an electric discharge can be propagated from the focus, and the third is the threshold of the brainstem centers for disseminating an electric discharge. The last is believed to reflect in part a genetic predisposition, and in part the frequency with which the brainstem centers are activated by the primary epileptic focus.

Current concepts propose that a secondarily generalized tonic-clonic seizure results from the axonal propagation of the cortical ictal discharge to the contralateral cortex, and to subcortical structures via intrahemispheric and interhemispheric association pathways. The substantia nigra, in particular, appears to be involved, at least in the control of experimental seizures (120).

Once neuronal excitation derived from the epileptic cortical focus spreads to involve the brainstem, particularly the midbrain and the pontine reticular formation, a generalized seizure develops almost instantly. These areas are responsible for the dissemination of epileptic potentials (121,122). With the subcortical neurons involved by the epileptic discharge, a positive excitatory feedback circuit is established between the cortex and the subcortical neurons, inducing discharges at a rate of 10 to 40 Hz. This circuit is responsible for the tonic phase of the focal motor seizure. As inhibitory neurons are recruited, a negative inhibitory feedback circuit develops, which periodically interrupts the excitatory activity and produces the clonic phase of the seizure. When the negative feedback wins ascendancy, the seizure subsides, leaving the neuronal membrane in a far greater hyperpolarized state than before the onset of the seizure.

Considerable evidence suggests that postictal (Todd's) paralysis, a common sequel to a focal seizure, is caused by persistence of the active inhibitory state, rather than by metabolic exhaustion of epileptic neurons (123).

The various areas of the cortex differ in their potential for secondary generalization. A number of areas including the temporal, frontal, and prefrontal cortex have particularly strong corticofugal projections to the centrencephalic system, and focal lesions within them readily induce a generalized seizure discharge (124,125). By contrast, the potential for secondary generalization is low in the motor strip. Additionally, small cortical lesions are more likely to induce a focally restricted seizure, whereas multiple or diffuse cortical lesions are more likely to result in a generalized seizure.

Primary Generalized Epilepsies

The pathophysiology of the primary generalized epilepsies is less well understood, and much of the experimental data is based on animal models that might not be applicable to the human epilepsies. In the 1940s, Penfield introduced the concept of centrencephalic epilepsy. This idea was that a generalized spike and wave discharge, such as occurs in absence epilepsy, originates in the rostral brainstem structures and the diencephalon, with the thalamus being responsible for the sudden generalized cortical discharge (126).

Gloor and Fariello postulate that in the primary generalized epilepsies, the cortex is in a diffusely hyperexcitable state, perhaps as a result of the discharge of a group of excitatory neurons. As a result, an epileptic discharge can be triggered by excitation of the brainstem and the midline thalamic reticular system induced by thalamocortical input (127). Engel suggests that the firing of a small group of excitatory neurons stimulates a set of inhibitory neurons that have connections throughout the cortex. A second burst of properly timed excitatory impulses then produces a synchronized discharge over a wide area of the cortex (128). Thus, the spike-wave discharges arise from the rhythmic, reverberatory interactions between interconnected thalamic and cortical neurons.

The oscillations in the thalamocortical circuits rely in part on the intrinsic membrane properties of the involved thalamic neurons. These neurons undergo slow, calcium-dependent depolarizations, attributed to the so-called T-channel (129). These low-threshold calcium currents provide the pacemaker quality to these cells that forms the basis of the thalamocortical reverberations. These spike-wave paroxysms are abolished by substances such as trimethadione or ethosuximide, which have a specific effect of abolishing calcium currents associated with the T-channel (129).

Clinically, such a discharge produces grand mal or absence epilepsy. In the latter condition, quick excitation of a neuronal inhibitory system prevents a prolonged clinical seizure and the development of the tonic-clonic components. These seizures can occur without known cerebral injury or disease, and, as indicated previously, they have a high rate of genetic transmission.

Views on the propagation of cortical electrical discharges have been considerably modified in the last few years, and the importance of the cortex in the production of both primary and secondarily generalized seizures has become increasingly evident from implanted or surface electrodes and from ictal and interictal PET scanning. These techniques also have shown the marked discrepancies between the scalp EEG and the actual seizure focus in approximately one-third of patients with refractory seizures (130,131).

Excitatory and Inhibitory Neurotransmitters

Excitatory neurotransmitters can play a role in the development of seizure discharges. Glutamate and aspartate are the major excitatory neurotransmitters found in the mammalian brain (132). Focal application of glutamate to hippocampal slices induces a calcium ion current and depolarizes the neuron. Another excitatory neurotransmitter system, the cholinergic system, has been successfully manipulated to produce experimental limbic seizures (133). Although the development of antiepileptic drugs based on their action at excitatory amino acid receptors is an active area of current research, presently available antimuscarinic agents are not likely to be useful as anticonvulsants because of their widespread central and peripheral sites of action.

Nicotinic receptors have not been thought to be important in the mechanisms underlying seizures. The recent finding of an association between autosomal dominant nocturnal frontal lobe epilepsy and mutations in the gene for a nicotinic cholinergic receptor subunit (CHRNA4) was thus surprising to investigators (24).

GABA has been shown to have inhibitory postsynaptic activity and is one of the principal inhibitory neurotransmitters in the mammalian brain. The role of inhibitory GABA-releasing neurons in producing hyperpolarization has been well established, and temporary disinhibition might predispose a normal neuronal population to epileptiform activity. The GABA receptor has been found in all areas of the brain (134). This receptor is coupled to the chloride channel (chloride ionophore), so that GABA binding to its receptor results in a rapid opening of the chloride channel, with an ensuing increase in the postsynaptic membrane conductance to chloride. Increased chloride ion permeability stabilizes the cell near its resting membrane potential and reduces its response to excitatory inputs. Modulation of the GABA receptor-chloride ionophore complex mediates the actions of benzodiazepines and barbiturates as well as the convulsant effect of picrotoxin and its analogues (135). Interactions at the GABA receptor-chloride ionophore complex also underlie some of the mechanisms of action of felbamate and topiramate. These substances all have receptor sites on the GABA receptor complex. The receptor protein has been isolated and purified, and the genes coding for its five subunits have been cloned (136,137). The physiology and pharmacology of the receptor assembly depend on the subunit composition (137–139). No genetic diseases resulting from a defect in these genes have been demonstrated as yet.

Convulsions can be induced by substances that block the biosynthesis of GABA. Allylglycine, an inhibitor of glutamic acid decarboxylase, the enzyme promoting conversion of glutamic acid to GABA, is a potent epileptogenic compound (94). Inhibition of GABA binding to its receptor by bicuculline and inhibition of the postsynaptic GABA-chloride conductance responses by picrotoxin also induces convulsions. When GABAergic inhibition is progressively blocked with picrotoxin, stimulation of one neuron excites more and more neurons until neuronal behavior begins to resemble a seizure. Conversely, a number of compounds that elevate nerve-terminal GABA concentrations are potential anticonvulsants (140). These include such inhibitors of GABA transaminase as γ-vinyl-GABA (vigabatrin) and valproate. It is unclear, however, whether the anticonvulsant effects of valproate are indeed related to its elevation of brain GABA because this effect is seen only at supratherapeutic levels.

Magnetic resonance (MR) spectroscopy has provided evidence that gabapentin and topiramate also measurably increase brain concentrations of GABA even though they do not inhibit GABA transaminase (141,142). Extracellular (presumably also synaptic) concentration of GABA is increased by tiagabine, a nipecotic acid derivative (143).

Pyridoxine functions as a coenzyme for glutamic acid decarboxylase. Consequently, an increased glutamic acid to GABA ratio is expected in pyridoxine deficiency, a state marked by prolonged seizures. In pyridoxine dependency, an autosomal recessive disorder also characterized by seizures, the GABA content of brain is reduced, and brain glutamic acid concentration is elevated (144). Even though skin fibroblasts show reduced activity of pyridoxal-dependent glutamic acid decarboxylase, no abnormality in the two genes coding for glutamic acid decarboxylase, the biosynthetic enzyme for GABA, has been documented (145).

This relatively simple model for the epileptogenicity of insufficient inhibition and excessive excitation may, however, not hold true. Strong inhibition can predispose to hypersynchronization, and in petit mal seizures, hyperfunction of GABAergic inhibitory pathways is evident (146). Brainstem and diencephalic influences, which normally induce slow-wave sleep, also increase cortical neuronal synchronization and raise the potential for epileptogenicity. In some of the experimental epilepsies, notably the reflex epilepsy of Mongolian gerbils, the number of GABAergic neurons is increased (147).

A role for other inhibitory neurotransmitters, notably the opioid peptides, in the production of interictal inhibition, and a role for postictal depression have been suggested from various animal models (148). At low dosages, morphine and other opioids have anticonvulsant activity that is reversed by naloxone, whereas at higher dosages, they act as convulsants, producing a petit mal–like seizure disorder. The relevance of these observations to human petit mal is uncertain, although positron emission tomography (PET) has revealed increased opiate receptor binding in the temporal cortex in patients with complex partial seizures (149).

Adenosine is another potent inhibitor of cortical neurons, acting primarily by depressing spontaneous neuronal firing or synaptic transmission through its inhibition of the presynaptic release of excitatory neurotransmitters. In a rat model of limbic status epilepticus, an adenosine A1 receptor agonist antagonized the development of status (150). Evidence from *in vivo* microdialysis experiences, performed intraoperatively on humans, suggests that adenosine may be a potential mediator of seizure arrest and postictal refractoriness (151). The clinical use of adenosine and of adenosine analogues has not been investigated extensively (152), and there is evidence that systemically administered adenosine analogues do not cross the blood–brain barrier (153). Moreover, the widespread effects of adenosine in the brain may not permit the development of a highly specific anticonvulsant with minimal CNS side effects.

Catecholamines and Indolamines

Adrenergic neurotransmitters are believed to play a significant role in the regulation of cortical excitability; consequently, a number of laboratories have searched for abnormalities in this system. Brain norepinephrine levels are low in several species of epileptic animals, and a decrease in brain norepinephrine concentration increases their seizure susceptibility. Conversely, an increase in brain norepinephrine levels decreases seizure severity (154). The lesioning of noradrenergic projections from the locus ceruleus lowers the threshold for forebrain and brainstem seizures (155). The importance of the role of brain stem catecholaminergic projections also is suggested by experiments in cats invoving the vagus nerve stimulator (VNS). The efficacy of VNS was lost when the locus coeruleus was lesioned by 6-hydroxydopamine (156).

The serotonergic system also influences the expression of seizures. In view of the recent popularity of highly selective serotonin-uptake antagonists as antidepressants, it is of interest that fluoxetine (Prozac) appears to have anticonvulsant effects (157–159). Experiments have suggested that the antiepileptic action of fluoxetine on CA1 neurons is caused by an enhancement of endogenous serotonin that in turn seems mediated by 5-hydroxytryptamine-1A ($5\text{-HT}1_A$) receptor (160,161). Interestingly, in a genetic rat model of absence epilepsy, a $5\text{-HT}1_A$ agonist increased spike waves in a dose-dependent manner (162). Genetically altered mice lacking the gene for $5\text{-HT}2_C$ receptor seem to exhibit spontaneous seizures, while the wild type background could be made to mimic such behavior by the administration of a specific $5\text{-HT}2_C$ antagonist (163).

Biochemical Alterations Induced by Seizures

During a brief seizure, the brain undergoes several biochemical alterations. Cerebral oxygen and glucose consumption increase strikingly, but with maintenance of adequate ventilation, the increase in cerebral blood flow is sufficient to meet the increased metabolic requirements of the brain.

These studies, derived from experimental animals, have been confirmed in the epileptic human by PET. Autoradiography using labeled 2-deoxyglucose as a substrate provides excellent information on the local cerebral glucose metabolism. Using this technique, cerebral metabolism is generally found to be increased in the area of the epileptic focus during a seizure. In some instances, the area of increased metabolic activity extends to adjacent tissue and into areas of neuronal projection (164). In absence seizures, a marked and diffuse increase in cerebral metabolic rate occurs (165). The hypermetabolism probably reflects the enhanced excitatory and inhibitory neuronal activity during a seizure.

By contrast, the interictal metabolic picture reveals areas of hypometabolism (128,166). These observations, important to the localization of epileptic foci, are discussed in a subsequent section of this chapter.

When a generalized seizure lasts 30 minutes or longer, it is usually accompanied by apnea. Apnea induces hypoxia and carbon dioxide retention. As a result of the energy demands of the convulsing muscles, the subject becomes hypoxic and hyperpyrexic (167). Oxygen tension within the brain decreases, a shift toward anaerobic metabolism occurs, and lactic acid accumulates (168). MR spectroscopy performed on rabbits subjected to status epilepticus corroborates these data. Phosphocreatine levels decrease, inorganic phosphorus levels increase, lactate increases, and intracellular pH decreases within 30 minutes of the onset of seizures (169). The increase in cerebral lactate after prolonged seizures results from activation of phosphofructokinase, which is a primary regulatory enzyme for cerebral glycolysis (169).

Clinical Manifestations

To facilitate presentation of the clinical manifestations of seizures, which vary even in a given patient, each of the common epilepsies is discussed. A miscellaneous group of less common epilepsies is then covered, with literature references for more extensive reading. Finally, the discussion turns to febrile seizures and the problem of seizures during the neonatal period.

Epilepsies Characterized by Generalized Tonic-Clonic (Grand Mal) Seizures

A generalized tonic-clonic seizure, occurring as a manifestation of primary generalized epilepsy, occurring as a secondary generalization of a partial epilepsy, or alternating with other seizure forms is the most common epileptic manifestation of childhood (see Table 14.3) (170). These conditions do not represent a homogeneous group but are seen in a variety of clinical settings.

The seizure can be primary generalized or secondarily generalized. A primary generalized seizure can occur without warning, whereas a secondarily generalized seizure can be preceded by an aura. Occasionally, the child might be irritable or might manifest unusual behavior for several hours before the seizure. In localizing the epileptic focus, the aura offers the most important clinical clue, more reliable at times than the EEG. The examining physician should always try to elicit its history. The most common epileptic aura is a sensation of dizziness or an unusual feeling of ascending abdominal discomfort. These sensations have been attributed to a discharge in the area of visceral sensory representation but offer less evidence for the site of the epileptic focus than do focal sensory symptoms (171).

In the classic form of an attack, the aura, if present, can be followed by rolling up of the eyes and loss of consciousness. A generalized tonic contraction of the entire body musculature occurs, and the child can utter a piercing, peculiar cry, after which he or she becomes apneic and cyanotic. With the onset of the clonic phase of the convulsion, the trunk and extremities undergo rhythmic contraction and relaxation. As the attack ends, the rate of clonic movements slows, and finally, the movements cease abruptly. The duration of a seizure varies from a few seconds to half an hour or more. In the series of Shinnar and coworkers, new-onset seizures lasted longer than 5 minutes in 50% of children. In 29% of children, they lasted longer than 10 minutes; in 16%, they lasted longer than 20 minutes; and in 12%, they lasted longer than 30 minutes. The authors pointed out that the longer a seizure lasts, the less likely it will stop spontaneously (172). This is commensurate with our experience.

A series of attacks at intervals too brief to allow the child to regain consciousness between attacks is known as status epilepticus. Because status epilepticus is one of the few neurologic conditions requiring emergency treatment, it will be referred to again in the section on treatment.

After the seizure, the child can remain semiconscious and then confused for several hours. When examined soon after an attack, he or she is poorly coordinated, with mild impairment of fine movements. Truncal ataxia, increased deep tendon reflexes, clonus, and extensor plantar responses can be present. Occasionally, the child appears blind and speechless. Postictally, he or she may vomit or complain of severe headache.

The major motor attack has numerous variations. Occasionally, particularly when drug therapy has been partly effective in controlling a secondarily generalized seizure, a typical aura occurs but is not followed by a seizure. In other patients, either the tonic or the clonic phase is too brief to be noted. Attacks can occur at any time of the day or night, although their frequency is somewhat greater shortly before or after the child falls asleep or awakens. Approximately one-fourth of patients experience nocturnal seizures; the remainder experience diurnal or mixed seizures. Generally, patients who for 1 year or more have experienced seizures only during sleep are unlikely to have attacks at other times of the day. In the experience of D'Allessandro and colleagues, who studied both pediatric and adult patients, the risk of a daytime seizure during a six-year follow-up was 13% (173). In some girls, seizures occur a few days before or shortly after their menstrual period.

A generalized tonic-clonic seizure or other epileptic manifestations can be precipitated by infection and fever, fatigue, emotional disturbances, hyperventilation and alkalosis, and drugs.

Fever can induce a seizure not only in children experiencing febrile seizures, but also in patients who previously had recurrent epileptic attacks unassociated with fever. In some children, dehydration and ketosis accompanying an acute infectious illness decrease seizure frequency.

In a few children, excessive fatigue or lack of sleep appears to precede a seizure but probably does not represent an important precipitating factor. Considerable clinical evidence indicates that epileptic children have fewer seizures when engaged in regular strenuous physical activity. Although fatigue seems to have little effect on the EEG, sleep deprivation can activate the EEG of epileptic patients and can precipitate seizures (174).

Parents often believe that emotional disturbances precipitate seizures in epileptic children. No evidence supports this idea, however, and there is no justification for parents' failing to set limits to the behavior of their epileptic child.

Hyperventilation and alkalosis induce absence attacks in approximately 90% of patients subject to them but are less effective in precipitating other seizure forms.

A variety of drugs can induce single seizures or status epilepticus. In the experience of Messing and coworkers, isoniazid and psychotropic medications accounted for approximately one-half of cases (175). Other drugs implicated in bringing on seizures include cocaine (176), theophylline, and penicillin. Isoniazid (INH) antagonizes glutamic acid decarboxylase by binding with its cofactor, pyridoxal phosphate, thus interfering with the biosynthesis of GABA. Demonstrable decreases in brain GABA levels result from INH administration. An increasing number of patients has presented with status epilepticus and encephalopathy attributable to INH overdoses (176–177). In these cases, immediate administration of pyridoxal (vitamin B_6) is crucial. Theophylline acts as an adenosine antagonist, whereas penicillin acts as a GABA antagonist and interferes with benzodiazepine binding in the brain (152). For INH and theophylline, the convulsive effects tend to be dose related (175). Various anticonvulsants, notably phenytoin, when given in toxic amounts, increase seizure frequency. Trimethadione, which was formerly used in the treatment of absence epilepsy, occasionally precipitated a grand mal seizure within 1 to 2 days of first being administered. The sudden withdrawal of anticonvulsant medication, particularly barbiturates and benzodiazepines, is the most common cause for status epilepticus. Finally, adolescent patients should be warned against excessive alcohol consumption.

Spontaneous variations in the frequency of attacks are common and must be taken into account when judging the effectiveness of anticonvulsant medication. In the experience of van Donselaar and colleagues, who studied untreated tonic-clonic seizures in children younger than 16 years of age, 42% showed a decelerating pattern, and ultimately became seizure free even in the absence of anticonvulsant treatment. An accelerating pattern of seizure frequency was seen in only 20% of children with four or more untreated seizures (178). Some children have seizures during early childhood, then remain asymptomatic until puberty, when their attacks recur for 4 to 7 years.

Epilepsies with Typical Absence (Petit Mal) Seizures

Typical absence seizures are most commonly identified with absence (petit mal) epilepsy. In its pure form, an absence (petit mal) attack was defined by Gowers as a "transient loss of consciousness without conspicuous convulsions" (48). Absence seizures are relatively uncommon; they comprise between 2 and 11 percent of seizure types in all ages (179).

The onset of seizures is usually abrupt, and the child suddenly develops an estimated 20 or more attacks each day. The characteristic attack is a brief arrest of consciousness, usually lasting 5 to 10 seconds, appearing without warning or aura. There can be a slight loss of body tone, causing the child to drop objects from his or her hand, but this loss is rarely profound enough to induce a fall. Minor movements occur in approximately 70% of patients; these are usually lip-smacking or twitching of the eyelids or face, often at the three-per-second frequency of the EEG abnormality (Fig. 14.3). Urinary incontinence is rare (180). The seizure terminates abruptly, and the patient is often unaware of the lapse of consciousness. The occurrence and duration of a lapse can be determined by reciting to the child a series of numbers during the attack and asking the child to repeat them when consciousness appears to have returned. Attacks first appear during childhood; in 64% of instances, they begin between 5 and 9 years of age. They are more common in girls; Dalby's series had 99 female and 62 male subjects (181).

When attacks are frequent, the child's intellectual processes are slowed and, often, the first indication of the presence of absence seizures is a deterioration in schoolwork and behavior (182). Responsiveness to auditory stimuli is impaired in the majority of patients in 0.1 to 0.4 seconds after the onset of a generalized spike-wave

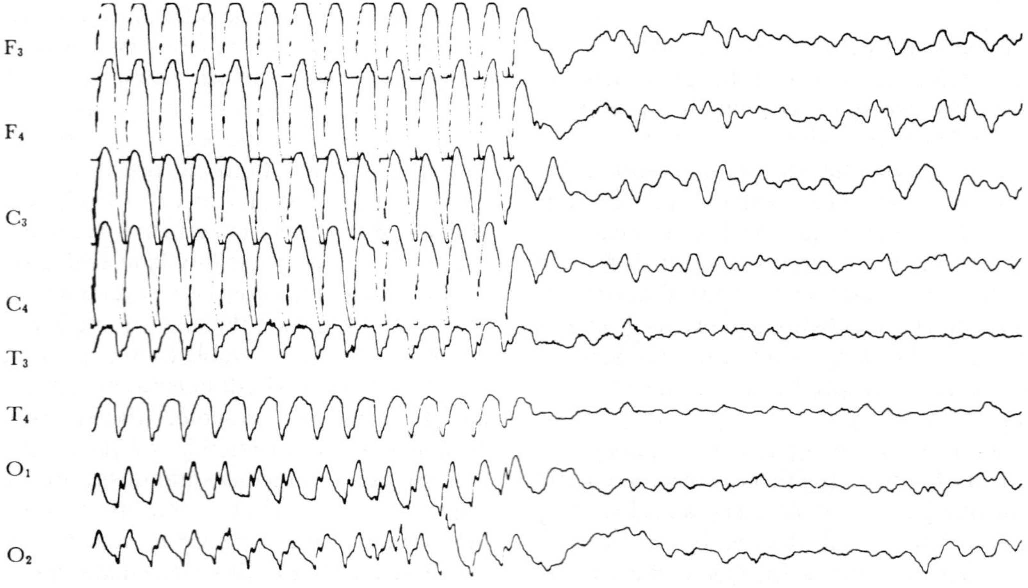

FIGURE 14.3. Three-hertz (three per second) spike-wave discharges in an 11-year-old girl with frequent absence (petit mal) attacks. In this instance, a clinically evident seizure lasting 19 seconds was induced by hyperventilation. (F_3, left frontal; F_4, right frontal; C_3, left central; C_4, right central; T_3, left temporal; T_4, right temporal; O_1, left occipital; O_2, right occipital.)

paroxysm, but it recovers in 2 to 3 seconds after the cessation of the attack. Extrapolations from spike-wave discharges associated with focal epilepsies have implicated the slow-wave component of the spike-wave complex in the interrupted cognitive function (83). Even brief and clinically undetectable attacks can impair intellectual performance.

Some absence attacks are more complex, and their appearance can be difficult to differentiate from complex partial seizures. They involve brief behavioral automatisms or, less commonly, prolonged symmetric myoclonic movements of the head or extremities (myoclonic petit mal). In the series of Sato and coworkers, some 40% of patients with typical absence seizures also experienced a grand mal attack, either before or after the onset of their absence attack (183). This figure is probably high and perhaps reflects the patterns of referral to a university center.

On a clinical basis, absence attacks must be distinguished from brief complex partial seizures and daydreaming. Complex partial seizures are often preceded by an aura and followed by postictal depression. Additionally, brief complex partial seizures tend to be less frequent and clustered and rarely will occur more than twice a day. Routine EEG studies in most instances clarify the situation. In a child with typical absence attacks, the EEG demonstrates a 3-Hz spike-wave discharge, which occasionally slows as the seizure progresses. The interictal EEG is normal in approximately one-half of patients, and the background EEG frequency is generally age appropriate (184). Approximately 10% of children with clinical and EEG features of typical absence attacks have a focal onset to their EEG seizures and demonstrate focal cortical lesions (185). Attacks of daydreaming also can occur several times a day and can last for several seconds to minutes. Automatisms are absent, there is no postictal depression, and attacks are not induced by hyperventilation or photic stimulation. The EEG is normal.

Typical absence seizures also should be differentiated from atypical absence attacks, which are associated with the Lennox-Gastaut syndrome (atypical petit mal, petit mal variant). This relatively common seizure type is associated with a variety of CNS insults, and the majority of affected children have a significant developmental delay. Unlike typical absence attacks, the frequency of atypical attacks is cyclic, in that seizure-free periods alternate with days or weeks of a high seizure frequency. The EEG shows complexes occurring at 1.5 to 2.5 Hz or multiple spike and wave discharges. Diffuse slowing of background activity was seen in 85% of children in the series of Holmes and coworkers (184).

Absence attacks are a common prelude to juvenile absence epilepsy and start about one to nine years earlier. Its characteristic features consist of typical absence attacks, seen in approximately one-third of patients and commencing later than those of typical childhood absence epilepsy. Brief myoclonic jerks that generally occur on awakening usually develop around 15 years of age (i.e., several years after the appearance of absence attacks), and tonic-clonic seizures follow some months thereafter. Attacks tend to occur much less frequently than they do in absence seizures, usually once a day or less (185). Intelligence is preserved. The interictal EEG in juvenile absence epilepsy demonstrates discharges not only at 3 Hz, but also at 4 to 6 Hz (186–189). The background activity is usually normal. In the series of Appleton and coworkers, photosensitivity was seen in 90% of patients (190).

Experimental studies designed to clarify the mechanism for absence seizures have already been reviewed (127,128,191).

Epilepsies with Complex Partial Seizures (Psychomotor Seizures, Temporal Lobe Seizures)

Complex partial seizures have been defined as seizures that arise from a limited area of one cerebral hemisphere and produce a period of impaired consciousness that varies from mild to profound. Although these seizures are most characteristically associated with lesions of the temporal lobe and have been called temporal lobe seizures, they also can be associated with lesions of the frontal (192) or occipital lobes (193). As the terminology indicates, they are focal seizures.

The epilepsies characterized by this seizure type are heterogeneous. Pathologic alterations seen within the surgically resected temporal lobe have been summarized in Table 14.6 (194).

The most common abnormality is MTS (Ammon's horn sclerosis or hippocampal sclerosis). In the series of Harvey and colleagues, it was seen in 21% of children aged 15 years or younger with new-onset temporal lobe epilepsy (195). The association of this characteristic lesion with both epileptogenicity and seizure-related damage has been discussed in the Neuropathologic Factors section of this chapter. Less commonly, 13% of cases in the series of Harvey and colleagues (195), a variety of tumors in the epileptogenic cortex can occur. These include hamartomas, which occasionally undergo malignant transformation, small gliomatous nodules, hemangiomas, and lesions suggestive of tuberous sclerosis (196,197). In early childhood, however, tumors are the most common etiology for complex partial seizures. Thus, in the series of Wyllie and colleagues, comprising children younger than 12 years of age who underwent temporal lobectomy, tumors were seen in 64%, as compared with MTS, seen in 29%. It is of note that 75% of children with MTS in the series of Wyllie and coworkers had a history of previous febrile convulsions (198). When bilateral MTS develops early in life, usually after prolonged seizures or status epilepticus, the clinical picture is marked by loss of language, or failure of language development, and impaired social and adaptive learning (199).

In a significant proportion of patients with complex partial seizures, focal abnormalities are found outside the hippocampus, in the limbic portion of the frontal lobes, in the lateral temporal lobe, and in nonlimbic areas outside the temporal lobe (200). In these instances, the ictal discharge probably spreads from the focus to involve the temporal lobe.

Even though seizures start before 10 years of age in approximately 75% of children (95), typical complex partial seizures are rarely seen until 10 years of age. Rather, children who later develop complex partial attacks can have an antecedent history of convulsive seizures associated with chewing, lip-smacking, or other oral automatisms (201). Additionally, they can experience a variety of behavior disorders, enuresis, nightmares, and sleepwalking (202).

Seizure manifestations in older children are presented in Table 14.7. The aura can consist of a variety of subjective phenomena. In children, Glaser and Dixon have found intense anxiety usually associated with visceral sensations to be the most common antecedent to complex partial seizures (203). Wyllie and colleagues have noted that a large proportion of children complain of a "funny" or bad taste (198). An epigastric "rising" sensation also is common. Olfactory hallucinations (uncinate fits) are usually described as unpleasant but unidentifiable odors. Their association with temporal lobe tumors is a matter of some dispute. In Daly's series, almost 40% of 55 patients who experienced this aura were found to have neoplasms (204). Similarly, in the series of Acharya and colleagues, 73% of patients with such an aura harbored a tumor (205). By contrast, Howe and Gibson found a tumor incidence of only 8.1% in their series of 37 patients, which is comparable with the 9.1% overall incidence of gliomas in patients with temporal lobe seizures (206).

TABLE 14.7 Clinical Manifestation of Complex Partial Seizures in Childhood

Seizure Manifestation	Number of Patients With Manifestations (Total 25)		
	Age 1–6	Age 7–16	Total
Aura	6	10	16
Altered consciousness	12	13	25
Change in position of body or limbs	10	11	21
Integrated but confused activity	8	11	19
Staring or dazed expression	10	8	18
Epigastric sensation, nausea, vomiting	9	5	14
Oral movements, drooling	8	5	13
Muttering, mumbling, hissing	5	5	10
Walking, wandering	4	6	10
Pallor or flushing	5	4	9
Rubbing or fumbling	4	5	9
Speech (usually irrelevant or incoherent)	3	5	8
Affective disturbance (fear, anger)	5	3	8
Stiffening of body or limbs	5	3	8
Falling	4	3	7
Aggressive activity	4	3	7
Dreamy state	2	3	5
Forced thinking or ideational blocking	1	4	5
Searching or orienting movements	1	3	4
Abdominal pain	3	1	4
Incontinence (urinary)	2	1	3
Perceptual disturbance (visual, auditory)	0	3	3

Modified from Glaser GH, Dixon MS. Psychomotor seizures in chilhood: a clinical study. *Neurology* 1956;6:646.

Hallucinatory experiences, most commonly a feeling of déjà vu, an adventitious sense of familiarity, and visual hallucinations, have been reported by children with complex partial seizures (207). According to Mullan and Penfield, they occur more frequently when the focus is in the nondominant temporal lobe (208).

Paroxysmal emotional states, particularly fear, are not rare in children and are commonly reported by parents. Rage reactions or temper tantrums are unusual auras of a complex partial seizure, and purposeful aggressive acts are uncommon in the course of seizure. A detailed history of the aura can assist in localizing the seizure focus, but does not help in lateralizing it. Whereas experiential auras, such as fear and déjà vu, almost invariably originate from the temporal lobes, notably the neocortex (200), cephalic auras, such as a sensation of dizziness or lightheadedness are of less localizing value and can emanate from either frontal or temporal areas. Viscerosensory auras were found to accompany a temporal lobe focus in 76% of subjects, and somatosensory auras accompanied a parieto-occipital focus in 62% (209).

On the basis of the initial seizure manifestations, Escueta and associates have divided complex partial seizures into two types (210). In the more common form, type I, the seizure originates from the temporal lobe. Patients briefly stop all activity after their aura. They stand still, stare, or turn pale. Shortly thereafter, minor motor acts are initiated. Prolonged postictal confusion is common in these patients. In type II, seizures originate from outside the temporal lobe, most commonly from the frontal lobe. In this type, automatisms initiate the attack. Commonly, these involve chewing and smacking movements, purposeless fumbling or patting of the hands, and picking at clothes. Postictal confusion is brief in this group of patients. Drop attacks as part of temporal lobe seizures are unusual in childhood (211).

The final part of the seizure generally involves more complex motor acts. The child might move about the room, begin to undress, and occasionally utter stereotyped or nonsensical phrases. In the majority of cases, these automatisms usually do not last longer than 5 minutes, although reliable observers have recorded prolonged complex partial seizures. Complex partial status epilepticus (psychomotor status) is extremely rare, and to our knowledge, it has never initiated complex partial epilepsy (212,213). In children, the condition manifests by impaired consciousness with intermittent staring and wandering eye movements and intermittent automatisms, such as picking at clothes. At other times, it can result in a prolonged period of amnesia. The condition should be differentiated from absence status or hysterical amnesia. Depth electrode studies suggest that the seizure focus is more commonly within the frontal lobes (214). A variety of electrocardiographic abnormalities can accompany complex partial seizures. These can be responsible for some of the sudden deaths seen in inadequately treated epileptic patients (215).

Following the seizure, the patient experiences postictal confusion, drowsiness, or clouding of consciousness. When fully recovered, the child has complete amnesia for the entire attack.

As with major motor seizures, the frequency of complex partial seizures varies, but in contrast to typical absence attacks, more than one to two attacks a day is uncommon (203).

The possibility of complex partial seizures is often raised in a child with behavior problems who has an abnormal EEG result. Aird and Yamamoto examined this question and found that approximately one-half of children with behavior problems have an abnormal EEG result. Of all patients studied, 27% had EEG foci primarily involving the temporal lobe (216). Although some authors vigorously dispute this predilection to behavior disturbances (217), others support it and have found behavior disturbances to be three times as common in this as in the other types of epilepsy (218). Additionally, symptoms suggesting complex partial seizures are highly prevalent among violent juveniles (219). Several further studies have confirmed these observations. In a series published in 1980, the incidence of abnormal behavior was 36% (220). Schoenfeld and coworkers, however, found that children with complex partial seizures are not aggressive or delinquent. Rather they suffer from social withdrawal, various somatic complaints, anxiety, and depression (221). The cause of the seizures, their duration, and the presence of associated grand mal attacks do not seem to affect the likelihood of psychiatric disturbances; however, the frequency of seizures and early seizure onset do (221). Boys whose seizure focus is located in the dominant hemisphere and whose seizures commence between 5 and 10 years of age appear to be particularly vulnerable (218). In most instances, the psychiatric illness commences during adolescence; its manifestation before 12 years of age is unusual.

The basis for these psychiatric phenomena has undergone considerable speculation. The most attractive hypothesis states that recurrent complex partial seizures kindle a limbic dopamine system, whose paroxysmal activity does not produce seizures but does produce serious behavior disturbances (222). The role of limbic kindling in the genesis of psychiatric illness is outside the scope of this text. Adamec and Stark-Adamec and Weiss and Post review this subject (223,224).

Epilepsies Characterized by Simple Partial Seizures (Focal Seizures, Partial Seizures with Elementary Symptoms)

Focal seizures are characterized by the development of localized motor or sensory symptoms without impairment of consciousness. In a large proportion of children, these seizures spread to other parts of the body, ultimately becoming generalized with loss of consciousness. On rare occasions, progression follows an orderly sequence, a phenomenon known as the *jacksonian march*. This type of a seizure is generally considered to be symptomatic of a structural cortical lesion.

Perhaps the most common focal attack observed in children is the versive seizure (225). These seizures begin in or spread to area 8, the frontal eye field, and the supplementary motor area or the mesial part of the premotor area. They are manifested most often by a turning of the eyes, or the eyes and head, away from the side of the focus. In some patients, the upper extremity on the side toward which the head turns is abducted and extended, and the fingers are clenched. Thus, the child appears to look at his closed fist.

The patient may be aware of this movement or may simultaneously lose consciousness. By means of combined telemetry and EEG monitoring, the cortical areas of discharge responsible for this form of seizure have been found to be either the contralateral temporal lobe or the contralateral frontal lobe, anterior to the rolandic gyrus. Patients whose seizure starts with versive movements and who retain awareness of them tend to have a frontal lobe seizure focus. Patients whose seizure starts with staring and automatisms tend to have a temporal lobe focus (210, 226,227). EEG changes, as recorded on scalp electrodes, are seen in only approximately one-third of patients during telemetry-verified attacks of a variety of simple partial seizures. Therefore, the presence of an unaltered EEG does not speak against the diagnosis (228).

Focal motor seizures are particularly common in hemiplegic children. The epileptic movements are usually clonic and begin in the hemiplegic hand, often heralded by localized sensory symptoms. The clonic movements spread over the entire affected side, ultimately becoming generalized in many cases. Postictal weakness (Todd's paralysis) commonly follows this kind of seizure and can last for several hours or for a day or more. In the experience of Kellinghaus and Kotagal, Todd's paralysis was contralateral to the epileptiform focus in 93% of subjects (229).

Whereas adults have a high positive correlation between Todd's paralysis and a structural cortical lesion, children do not, and often attacks of alternating left- and right-sided focal seizures with postictal paralyses are the initial events in a child with apparently idiopathic epilepsy. This observation probably reflects a smaller and less readily detectable focus in the pediatric population.

A heterogeneous group of conditions are characterized by focal (simple partial) seizures. In approximately one-half of patients, one can document an underlying structural lesion. These lesions include developmental malformations, notably gray matter heterotopias and localized pachygyria, gliosis resulting from asphyxial damage or perinatal and postnatal physical trauma, and a variety of space-occupying lesions. In the remainder of patients with simple partial seizures, no obvious etiology can be demonstrated. Several clinically distinct types of these idiopathic focal epilepsies have been recognized. They are characterized by the absence of anatomic or functional focal lesions and by a benign course with normal intellectual development and spontaneous cure. Aside from febrile seizures and a family history of seizures for approximately one-third of children, no obvious antecedents exist. The frequency of these conditions is difficult to ascertain. Roger and Bureau believe they constitute some 60% of partial epilepsies seen in school-aged children (230).

Rolandic Epilepsy

The most common and most clearly delineated of the idiopathic focal epilepsies is midtemporal epilepsy (sylvian epilepsy, rolandic epilepsy, benign childhood epilepsy with centrotemporal spikes). In the experience of Loiseau and coworkers, it represented 10.7% of children seen in a specialized private practice (231). A high incidence of similar seizures occurs in first-degree relatives, and an autosomal dominant form of rolandic epilepsy has been reported (see Table 14.5) (25,232). In approximately 75% of children, this type of a seizure commences between ages 5 and 10 years. Seizures are infrequent, in the majority of cases occurring less than three or four times a year, and are generally brief. Most characteristically, attacks commence with a somatosensory aura, usually referred to the tongue, cheek, or gums and less often to the abdomen. As a result of motor interference, speech is arrested, the child salivates, and tonic or tonic-clonic movements involve the face. Consciousness is preserved in some 60% of children. Because approximately three-fourths of the attacks occur during sleep, a good patient history is difficult to obtain. The interictal EEG shows midtemporal spikes, probably a reflection of discharges arising from the rolandic cortex (233,234). In about 30% of cases, spikes are only seen during sleep (235). The spikes in this syndrome display a horizontal dipole with maximum negativity in the centrotemporal regions and positivity over the superior frontal area (236). In contrast to other seizures having a temporal spike focus, the prognosis in this condition is excellent (237); most children respond well to anticonvulsant therapy. In the experience of Lombroso, almost 50% were seizure free within 3 years of their first attack, and in more than 30%, the EEG reverted to normal as well (233). Beaussart and Faou share this optimism. In their series of 334 cases, no patient had seizures after age 13 years, even when anticonvulsants had been withdrawn (238).

Benign Epilepsy of Childhood with Occipital Focus (Panayiotopoulos Syndrome)

Benign epilepsy with an occipital focus (239) is somewhat less common, accounting for 6% of all children with seizures (240). The age of onset is variable; ranging between 15 months and 17 years, with the peak age being 5 years (239,240). Seizures are infrequent and tend to mainly occur at night. Attacks during the day are initiated by hemianopia, phosphenes (white or colored luminous spots), or visual hallucinations. Amaurosis or nonvisual symptoms follow. The latter include unilateral convulsions, automatisms, or generalized tonic-clonic seizures. Aphasia is not unusual. Ictal deviation and vomiting may be seen, and in about one-half of children, there is postictal migraine (241). The interictal EEG most commonly demonstrates nearly continuous unilateral or bilateral high-voltage spike-wave discharges from the occipital or posterior temporal regions. This is generally suppressed by opening of the eye. The prognosis is excellent with or without anticonvulsant therapy, and all children in Beaumanoir's series were seizure free with a normal EEG by 9 to 13 years of age (239). The experience of Panayiotopoulos is similar, with 89% of children gaining remission (242).

Focal Epilepsy with Midtemporal Spikes and Affective Symptoms

European epileptologists also distinguish a focal epilepsy with midtemporal spikes and affective symptoms. Seizures commence with a sensation of fear or terror and proceed with chewing and swallowing movements and speech arrest. Consciousness is depressed. Unlike complex partial seizures, seizures cease with therapy, and no evidence for a focal lesion can be found on clinical examination or by imaging studies (228).

Lennox-Gastaut Syndrome (Myoclonic-Astatic Petit Mal)

The epileptic syndromes considered in this section share an early onset, an EEG picture characterized by slow spike-wave forms at a frequency lower than the regular 3 Hz, and poor prognosis, in terms of both seizure control and ultimate intellectual development. Livingston and associates have used the term *minor motor seizures* to designate the epilepsies described in this section (243). This term has been abandoned in recent years; not only is there nothing minor about these seizures, but the term is overly broad and encompasses a variety of seizures with limited expression, regardless of their etiology and EEG features.

The causes for Lennox-Gastaut syndrome (LGS) are multiple. In the experience of Lennox and Davis, compiled in 1950, 50% of patients had a history of perinatal cerebral injury, another 20% might have had an attack of encephalitis or meningitis, and 13% had major complications of gestation (244). Currently, complications of gestation appear to be the most significant cause, with perinatal asphyxia, infections, and genetic factors following in order of importance.

Types of Seizures

Based on the different clinical manifestations of the epileptic attacks, at least four seizure types can be distinguished: atonic (astatic or akinetic) seizures, brief tonic seizures, atypical petit mal seizures, and myoclonic seizures (245).

Atonic (Akinetic) Seizures. Atonic seizures are characterized by a sudden, momentary loss of posture or muscle tone. In the infant who is able to sit but cannot yet stand, atonic spells consist of a sudden dropping forward of the head and neck, the *salaam seizure*, such as is seen as part of infantile spasms. In older children, the loss of postural tone precipitates the child violently to the ground. Consciousness is lost only momentarily, but the force of the fall commonly produces injuries to the face and head. Atonic spells recur frequently during the course of a day and are particularly common during the morning hours and shortly after the child awakens.

Tonic Seizures. Tonic seizures are characterized by a brief generalized increase in muscle tone. These seizures are frequent during non–rapid eye movement (NREM) sleep and generally are the most common form of seizure in LGS as well as the type most resistant to anticonvulsant therapy (246).

Atypical Petit Mal Seizures. Atypical petit mal seizures are characterized by absence seizures that, unlike true petit mal, tend to occur in cycles and can disappear for periods of several days (247). These seizures can occur by themselves or can be accompanied by grand mal or complex partial seizures.

Myoclonic Seizures. The term *myoclonic seizure* includes a variety of seizures characterized by myoclonus, that is, single or repetitive contractures of a muscle or a group of muscles. For therapeutic and prognostic purposes, myoclonus has been classified into two forms: epileptic and nonepileptic (248). Myoclonic seizures account for approximately 7% of the epilepsies that have an onset during the first 3 years of life (249). In primary generalized epileptic myoclonus, the myoclonic jerks consist of small, random, recurring twitches, most evident in the fingers and hands. They synchronously involve muscles on both sides of the body. An EEG abnormality, originating most commonly from the frontal leads, precedes the myoclonus, suggesting that a hyperexcitable cortex responds to a subcortical input with the paroxysm. This form of myoclonus usually is seen with chronic epileptic disorders. In the series of Wilkins and associates, it was part of LGS in more than one-half of the subjects (250).

Onset of LGS seizures ranges from age 6 months to approximately age 16 years. In some two-thirds of instances, the onset is between 2 and 14 years of age (251). In some patients, 6% of Kruse's series, LGS follows infantile spasms (251). In approximately one-half of the children, one or more major motor attacks, with or without fever, precede the illness. Brett delineated a group of children who experience a sudden onset of major seizures that, after a seizure-free interval of approximately 1 week, are followed by LGS and progressive intellectual deterioration (252). This entity, termed *epileptogenic encephalopathy* by Brett, is not rare. Its cause is unknown, but in view of the occasional cerebrospinal fluid (CSF) pleocytosis, it might be infectious. The association of Ohtahara syndrome or early infantile epileptic encephalopathy (EIEE) to West syndrome and LGS has been documented (253). Atonic, myoclonic, or atypical absence seizures can continue throughout the patient's lifetime. In three-fourths of patients, generalized tonic-clonic or focal seizures also can appear.

LGS syndrome correlates with an EEG result that Lennox and Davis termed the *petit mal variant* (Fig. 14.4) (244). It is an asymmetric, sometimes lateralized, slow (2.0 to 2.5 Hz) polyspike-wave discharge (atypical spike-wave discharge), which, in contrast to the 3-Hz synchronous discharge of petit mal, is less likely to be provoked by hyperventilation.

Mental development of the child with LGS is usually slow. In part, this reflects the underlying brain disease, and in part, it is the result of the frequency of seizures. Characteristically, the earlier motor milestones are attained at the expected age, but subsequent evaluations reveal subnormal intelligence in a large proportion of affected children. In the series of Blume and associates, 35% of patients attained an IQ of 75 or above, and only 10% scored above 100 on psychometric testing (254). In the experience of Chevrie and Aicardi, the incidence of retardation was even higher (224).

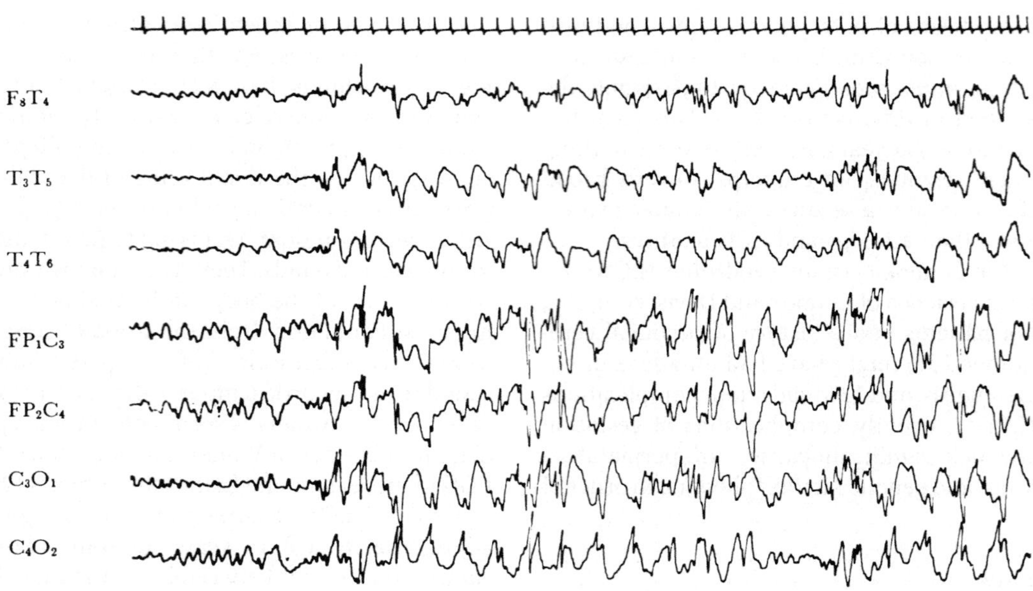

FIGURE 14.4. Atypical polyspike-wave discharge. Photically (5 Hz) induced myoclonic seizure in a 14-year-old girl. The electroencephalogram shows 3-Hz multiple spike-wave discharges. (F_8T_4, right frontotemporal; T_3T_5, left frontotemporal; T_4T_6, right temporal; FP_1C_3, left frontopolar-central; FP_2C_4, right frontopolar-central; C_3O_1, left central-occipital; C_4O_2, right central-occipital. Top lead is photostimulator.)

Differential Diagnosis of Myoclonic Seizures

Pseudo-Lennox syndrome is a condition that was first described by Aicardi and Chevrie under the term *atypical benign partial epilepsy of childhood*. It is marked by generalized minor seizures, such as atonic seizures, atypical absences, and myoclonic seizures, and focal sharp slow waves and spikes with generalization during sleep. Seizure onset peaked at about three years of age (255). In contrast to LGS, prognosis in terms of seizure remission is good. In the series of Hahn and coworkers, 84% of children with this condition ultimately went into remission (256). However, over 50% of children were attending schools for the mentally handicapped.

Myoclonic seizures also are seen as a nonspecific symptom in several forms of viral encephalitis, metabolic disturbances such as uremia, and progressive cerebral degenerative diseases such as the various lysosomal storage diseases, some of the leukodystrophies, Menkes disease, and Unverricht-Lundberg disease (see Chapter 3).

Several types of nonepileptic myoclonus have been recognized. Cortical reflex myoclonus is believed to result from hyperexcitability of a small region of the sensory portion of the sensorimotor cortex. The muscular contractions are irregular and are precipitated or aggravated by sensory stimuli, most commonly by light, noise, or tapping on the face or chest. Postural changes intensify the contractions. The movements disappear in sleep. The EEG is clearly abnormal, and a paroxysm precedes both the spontaneous and the reflex-induced myoclonic jerks. Giant somatosensory-evoked potentials are characteristic for this type of myoclonus (257).

In reticular reflex myoclonus, the myoclonic jerks affect the entire body, with the flexor muscles being more involved than the extensors. The seizures are believed to be the result of hyperexcitability of the caudal brainstem reticular formation, possibly the nucleus reticularis gigantocellularis (248). An EEG spike usually follows the first electromyographic evidence of myoclonus. Another nonepileptic form of myoclonus is considered to be of spinal cord or brainstem origin. The muscular contractions are rhythmic and are unaffected by sensory stimuli. They persist during sleep. The EEG can be normal or abnormal, and response to anticonvulsant medication is poor.

Nonepileptic myoclonus also is encountered in the context of involuntary movements in some of the disorders of the extrapyramidal system. It is seen in normal individuals while falling asleep. Rarely, frequent but nonprogressive myoclonic movements occur unaccompanied by other types of epileptic attacks or intellectual subnormality. This condition is termed *paramyoclonus multiplex* or *essential myoclonus*. It is probably identical to myoclonic dystonia (DYT 11) and is considered with the various dystonias covered in Chapter 3 (258). Closely related to this condition is the exaggerated startle response (hyperekplexia), conditions also considered in Chapter 3. In hyperekplexia, patients exhibit momentary muscular stiffness and loss of voluntary postural control without loss of consciousness.

Other features of this condition include transient hypertonia during infancy, nocturnal jerking of the legs, and insecure gait. No other epileptic phenomena occur, although the EEG can have paroxysmal features. Minor, quantitatively less severe forms of this condition also have been observed. The condition should be distinguished from startle epilepsy, a type of reflex epilepsy (259).

Infantile Spasms (West Syndrome)

Infantile spasms most commonly develop between 3 and 8 months of age, with only 8% of cases first being encountered in infants older than 2 years of age. It occurs somewhat more frequently in male infants. Attacks are characterized by a series of sudden muscular contractions by which the head is flexed, the arms are extended, and the legs are drawn up. A cry or giggling can precede or follow the seizure, and the infant can flush or can turn pale or cyanotic.

Other clinical presentations of infantile spasms occur less commonly. They include head nodding and extensor spasms characterized by extension rather than flexion of arms, legs, and trunk. Rarely, the attacks are concluded by a brief clonic seizure.

Lightning attacks (Blitzkrämpfe) (260) are a variant involving a single, momentary, shocklike contraction of the entire body (261).

Clusters of seizures recur frequently, particularly on waking, and some children have 50 to 100 each day. In Jeavons and Bower's series of 112 children, mental development was normal up to the onset of seizures in 52% and was definitely or probably delayed in the remainder (262). More recent series have had a higher incidence of delayed mental development before the onset of seizures. In 66% of patients, the EEG has the characteristics of hypsarrhythmia, namely diffuse dysrhythmia with high-voltage slow waves and multiple spike-wave discharges (Fig. 14.5) (262). This unique electrical pattern is seen in the early stages of the disorder, becoming apparent after 3 to 4 months of age. In some infants, it is most evident in non-REM sleep. During REM sleep and immediately after arousal from REM or non-REM sleep, the EEG can be normal for up to several minutes (263). The discharges tend to favor the posterior areas of the brain. This contrasts with the paroxysmal discharges in LGS, which are most evident anteriorly. The significance of this finding is not clear, particularly because many children with infantile spasms progress to LGS. To our knowledge, there has not been a systematic study of EEG maturation in infantile spasms. Variations in this pattern are common (modified hypsarrhythmia). They include hypsarrhythmia with a focus of abnormal discharge, hypsarrhythmia with increased interhemispheric synchronization, hypsarrhythmia with little spike or sharp-wave activity, and hypsarrhythmia with episodes of voltage attenuation, a variant termed *suppression burst variant* by Hrachovy and coworkers (263).

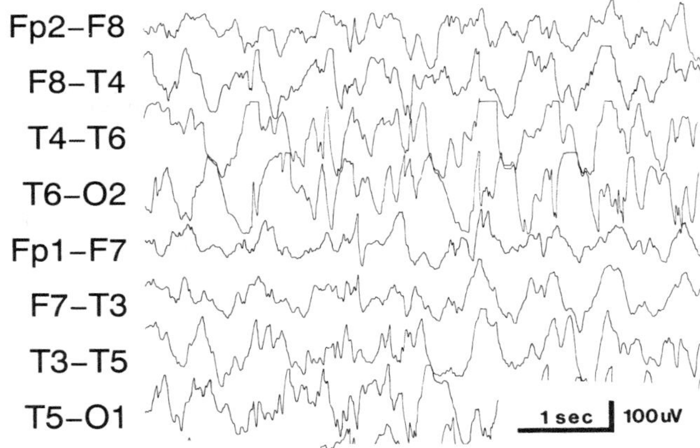

FIGURE 14.5. Hypsarrhythmia in a 6-month-old girl with infantile spasms. The record is characterized by mountainous slow waves, multifocal spikes, and sharp waves. (Fp2–F8, right frontopolar-frontal; F8–T4, right frontotemporal; T4–T6, right temporal; T6–O2, right temporal-occipital; Fp1–F7, left frontopolar-frontal; F7–T3, left frontotemporal; T3–T5, left temporal; T5–O1, left temporal-occipital.)

Hypsarrhythmia persists for some years, then is superseded by a variety of other paroxysmal abnormalities. These include focal discharges, most commonly arising from the temporal areas, multifocal spike discharges, and an atypical spike-wave pattern. The evolution of infantile spasms to LGS was commented upon earlier in the discussion of the latter syndrome.

Attacks of spasms are often associated with a discharge of multiple spike-wave or polyspikes. Sudden suppression of electric activity begins with an attack and persists briefly after its completion.

Although infantile spasms are considered as a generalized epilepsy, the neuroanatomic substrates responsible for them are poorly understood (264). A marked decrease in REM sleep has led to the proposal that the basic abnormality is at the pontile level in proximity to centers regulating sleep cycles (265). This hypothesis is supported by the finding on interictal PET scan of hypermetabolism of the brainstem. Additionally, hypermetabolism of the lenticular nucleus occurs, which suggested to Chugani and coworkers a neuronal circuitry involving cortex, lenticular nucleus, and brainstem in the generation of infantile spasms (266).

Infantile spasms are classified as cryptogenic or symptomatic. Cryptogenic spasms, a minority of the cases of infantile spasms [less than 15% in the series of Riikonen (267)], occur in infants with normal birth and development until the onset of seizures, in whom no obvious cause for the convulsions can be demonstrated. A variety of prenatal and perinatal insults are responsible for the majority of cases in the symptomatic group. Abnormalities of gestation, manifested by a history of maternal infection and prematurity, are particularly common. Perinatal asphyxia or traumatic birth injuries are seen less often. Neonatal seizures are a common precursor, and symptomatic neonatal hypoglycemia is encountered in some 18% of infants (267). In the remainder of the infants, tuberous sclerosis is the major etiologic factor, with intracerebral calcifications detectable by CT scanning in up to 25%. Infantile spasms also are seen in neurofibromatosis, agenesis of the corpus callosum, and metabolic diseases such as phenylketonuria, maple syrup urine disease, and pyridoxine dependency (268). In a small group of infants, spasms begin shortly after pertussis immunization with the whole cell vaccine. Whether this association is fortuitous, as suggested by Bellman and coworkers (269), or whether pertussis vaccine indeed represents a rare cause for infantile spasms will probably never be resolved, and with the switch to acellular pertussis vaccine, this question has become moot (270).

As might be expected, a variety of neuropathologic findings have been reported. These include structural malformations of cortical gray matter. The most commonly observed abnormality observed in surgically resected specimens is a focal cortical dysplasia (271). Other alterations include hamartomatous proliferation of multipotential neuroectodermal cells (272), ulegyria, lissencephaly, unilateral megalencephaly, and pachygyria (273). Focal areas of cortical microdysgenesis are not readily detectable by magnetic resonance imaging (MRI) during the first few months of life but can be visualized indirectly in subsequent studies by a focal delay in maturation of subcortical white matter. This can only be visualized by repeated imaging studies (274). Tumors, cytomegalovirus infection (275) and spongy degeneration of gray and white matter are less common (271,276).

In most children, the outlook for normal intellectual development is poor, even though in approximately 50%, infantile spasms have ceased by 3 years of age or are replaced by the LGS or by major motor attacks (277). According to Jeavons and Bower, none of the patients whose development was already retarded when infantile spasms began had a subsequent normal intellectual development, whereas 29% of infants believed to have developed normally up to the onset of seizures (cryptogenic infantile spasms) were found to be neurologically intact and intellectually in the normal or low-normal range when their infantile spasms disappeared (262). More recent series, such as those of Riikonen (267) and Gaily and coworkers (278), present comparable results. The latter workers observed 67% of infants with cryptogenic infantile spasms to have normal intelligence when tested between the ages of 4 and 6 years. Specific cognitive deficits were found in 42% of children in this group. In the series of Kivity and coworkers, the outcome of children with cryptogenic infantile spasms treated with high doses of adrenocorticotropic hormone prior to mental deterioration was uniformly excellent (279). Riikonen found that in children whose infantile spasms are attributed to tuberose sclerosis, the long-term prognosis is worse than in other symptomatic or cryptogenic cases of infantile spasms (280). By contrast, the prognosis is relatively good when infantile spasms accompany neurofibromatosis (281).

Differential Diagnosis

A condition that has a similar ominous prognosis as infantile spasms, and also is marked by frequent minor generalized seizures is Ohtahara syndrome (282) Onset of seizures is earlier than in infantile spasms and is usually prior to three months. The main seizure type is tonic spasms with or without clustering. The EEG is characteristic. It consists of high voltage bursts interspersed with a nearly flat pattern. The condition results from a variety of brain malformations, notably focal cortical dysplasias. It is more resistant to treatment than infantile spasms, and the prognosis for mental function is poor. In many instances, the tonic spasms evolve into infantile spasms, and like infantile spasms into LGS (283).

Treatment

The relationship between treatment regimens and outcome is controversial, and the recommendations prepared by the American Academy of Pediatrics and the Child Neurology Society are too conservative to clarify the situation. These bodies concluded that adrenocorticotropic hormone (ACTH) is "probably an effective agent" for the short-time treatment of infantile spasms. They also concluded that there was insufficient evidence to state that successful treatment of infantile spasms improves the long-term prognosis (284). The Israeli group under Lerman and Kivity, however, found that optimal results are obtained when treatment is initiated within a month after the onset of seizures and when high doses are given for a prolonged period (259,285), and as already noted, their results with early treatment of infants with cryptogenic infantile spasms were uniformly excellent in terms of mental development and seizure control. The series of Glaze and coworkers did not have a sufficient number of cryptogenic cases to determine the benefit of early therapy (286). The more recent series of Askalan and coworkers also is too small and included infants who already had shown developmental regression before treatment (286a). Certainly, early ACTH therapy does not alter the uniformly poor outcome of symptomatic infantile spasms (286). In this respect, it is of interest that the relapse after ACTH treatment is much higher in patients with tuberose sclerosis than in other forms of symptomatic infantile spasms

(280). Even when treatment does not improve mental functioning, it can have a beneficial effect on seizure control and on the EEG in over one-half of the cases.

Many regimens for ACTH treatment have been proposed. As a rule, at higher ACTH doses, there is a greater proportion of remissions but also a higher incidence of major adverse reactions. One convenient treatment schedule follows: ACTH is given intramuscularly in a daily dose of 80 to 120 U. This dose is maintained until spasms and hypsarrhythmia disappear. If a response is noted, the dose is changed to 40 to 80 U every other day and then gradually reduced to half that dose. This is maintained for approximately 3 more months. Thereafter, the dosage is reduced further by 10 U at 2-month intervals until the drug is completely withdrawn or the minimal dosage for seizure control is reached. One of us (JHM) has recommended a starting dose of 40 U, which is increased at weekly increments to 60 U and 80 U if there has not been any response. A prospective study has indicated that there is no difference in the effectiveness of high-dose and low-dose regimens with respect to seizure control and normalization of the EEG (287). Ito and coworkers have suggested a starting dose of 20 U of synthetic ACTH for infants over 1 year of age and 10 U for infants under 1 year of age (288). On this dosage, excellent seizure control was seen in 76% of patients, and normalization of EEG was seen in 38%. Outcome in terms of mental function was poor, however, with only 6% of subjects being normal.

Side reactions to ACTH include hypertension, which can become apparent at a dosage of 80 U per day, gastroenteritis, sepsis, osteoporosis, and unexplained CNS hemorrhage. The incidence of these complications varies considerably and probably reflects the different treatment schedules. In some series, it can be as high as 37% (289), whereas others have not shown any serious morbidity (290). One interesting concomitant to ACTH therapy is an enlargement of the cerebral ventricular system, which is disclosed by serial neuroimaging studies. This enlargement, which is occasionally permanent (perhaps as a result of abnormalities predating the onset of infantile spasms), is believed to reflect loss of water, owing to altered CSF absorption (291).

The mechanism by which ACTH controls infantile spasms is a matter of some debate, and Snead has reviewed the various hypotheses (292). Baram and colleagues have shown that in infantile spasms, CSF levels of ACTH and cortisol are reduced and have postulated that there is an increased synthesis of corticotropin-releasing hormone (CRH), which in infant rats has been shown to induce seizures originating from the amygdala. They suggest that ACTH desensitizes the CRH receptors and thus induces a negative feedback on CRH release (293). ACTH also could modulate second messenger systems or increase the expression of several genes and thus accelerate myelination, in this manner shortening a vulnerable, hyperexcitable period (294). In that respect, it is significant that several studies, as well as our own experience, indicate that ACTH is a potent anticonvulsant for Lennox-Gastaut syndrome (290,295).

Of the other medications recommended for the treatment of infantile spasms, vigabatrin appears to be the most effective. In an uncontrolled study, Mitchell and Shah started patients on 125 to 250 mg per day, with gradual increments to a target dose of 100 mg/kg per day or any lower effective dose (296). In this unselected series, 60% responded with cessation of spasms and resolution of hypsarrhythmia. Appleton recommends starting at 25 to 50 mg/kg per day and increasing the dosage to a maximum of 80 to 120 mg/kg per day. In their group of children, making up 81% of symptomatic infantile spasms, 81% experienced total cessation of spasms. On follow-up 2 years later, 67% had remained seizure free (297). Chiron and coworkers have used vigabatrin with considerable success in the treatment of infantile spasms associated with tuberose sclerosis (298). In a retrospective study by Cossette and colleagues, vigabatrin was found to be as effective as ACTH in terms of controlling seizures and offering a good developmental outcome. Side effects were less frequent in vigabatrin-treated children than in those who received ACTH (299). Their results are at variance with those of Lux and colleagues, who found that synthetic adrenocorticotropic hormone and prednisolone were more likely to induce cessation of spasms than vigabatrin given in minimal doses of 100 mg/kg per day (299a). The high incidence of visual field defects seen on even low doses of vigabatrin has raised concerns with respect to the safety of the medication. On that account, Riikonen believes that the benefits of vigabatrin do not outweigh the risks of irreversible visual changes (300). In spite of these drawbacks, vigabatrin has become the first-line drug in other clinics for the treatment of infantile spasms, particularly when these occur in a setting of tuberose sclerosis (301,302).

Oral steroids are probably not as effective for infantile spasms as ACTH. In a prospective, randomized study, high-dose ACTH (150 U/m^2 per day) was more effective than prednisone by both clinical and EEG criteria (303). Prats and coworkers have suggested treating infantile spasms with extremely high doses of sodium valproate (100 to 300 mg/kg per day). According to their protocol, the anticonvulsant is given for 21 days or until the EEG resolves. Then, the medication is reduced to 25 to 50 mg/kg per day (304). Although their results require confirmation, the outcome of children treated with valproate appears to be as good or better than those treated with ACTH both in terms of seizure control and normal intellectual development.

Kossoff and coworkers have used the ketogenic diet to treat infantile spasms and found the response rate to be significant, with 46% being more than 90% improved and

100% of subjects being more than 50% improved in terms of EEGs and parent reports (305).

Many other treatment regimens have been suggested. In Japan, large doses of pyridoxine are preferred by the majority of institutions, followed by the combination of pyridoxine and valproate, and valproate monotherapy (306). Combined treatment with vigabatrin and topiramate has been used in Italy (307). Zonisamide has been found to be effective in one-fourth to one-third of patients with infantile spasms (308–310).

As ominous as are infantile spasms in terms of ultimate mental development, Lombroso and Fejerman were able to distinguish a benign form (311). In this condition, myoclonic attacks are accompanied by normal intellectual development and a normal EEG, in contrast to infantile spasms in which the EEG is abnormal at the onset of seizures or becomes abnormal within a few months, as is the case in young infants. In the benign form of the condition, myoclonus ceases before 2 years of age, and no other seizures supervene.

Attacks characterized by shuddering and resembling myoclonic seizures can occur in monosodium glutamate poisoning and also can be noted as a prelude to familial (essential) tremor (see Chapter 3).

A syndrome of infantile spasms, mental retardation, chorioretinitis, colobomas of the retina, and agenesis of the corpus callosum limited to female subjects was first described by Aicardi and coworkers (Aicardi syndrome) (see Chapter 4) (312–314).

Juvenile Absence Epilepsy; Juvenile Myoclonic Epilepsy

Juvenile absence epilepsy and Juvenile myoclonic epilepsy (JME) are two clinically related conditions that are genetically heterogeneous, probably transmitted as a dominant trait. Several genes have been implicated in this condition. One of them encodes the GABA receptor (*GABABR1*) and has been mapped to chromosome 6p21.3 (Table 14.5) (315,316). Another gene (*EFHC1*) has been mapped to chromosome 6p12–p11 and encodes a protein with an EF-hand motif. EF hands are Ca(2+) binding motifs that are widely distributed throughout the entire animal kingdom (317).

Juvenile myoclonic epilepsy has a prevalence of 0.5 to 1.0 per 1,000 and represents some 4% of the primary generalized epilepsies (189).

Symptoms usually become apparent in adolescence, with age of onset between 12 and 18 years (189). Seizures are characterized by sudden myoclonic jerks of shoulders and arms that usually appear shortly after awakening. A majority of patients also experience grand mal attacks. As a rule, myoclonic jerks precede grand mal seizures. Up to one-third of patients also experience absence attacks, which tend to precede the onset of myoclonic jerks (189). Intelligence remains normal. The interictal EEG is characteristic, in that it demonstrates 4- to 6-Hz polyspike and wave complexes, with photosensitivity in approximately 30% (318). Valproic acid is effective in up to 90% of subjects but has to be continued for the remainder of the patient's life because withdrawal of anticonvulsants results in seizure recurrence in some 90% of patients, even after many years of complete control (319). Alternatives to valproate therapy with newer anticonvulsant medications are being explored and are reviewed by one of us (R.S.) (320).

Miscellaneous Seizure Forms

A number of epileptic conditions are manifested by unusual seizure forms. These are seen too rarely to warrant more than a brief description. The following types deserve mention.

Abdominal Seizures

Paroxysmal attacks of abdominal pain can occur as an aura for a major motor attack or can be the only manifestation of a seizure. The abdominal pain is usually periumbilical, radiating to the epigastrium. In the majority of cases, it lasts 5 to 10 minutes, but it can persist for 24 to 36 hours. It is usually associated with disturbed awareness (321).

The pediatrician often sees a child who has recurrent bouts of paroxysmal abdominal pain accompanied by vomiting and in whom the usual gastrointestinal evaluation result has been normal. Only a small proportion of these children has abdominal epilepsy. A more common cause of this complaint is childhood migraine. A history of pain and vomiting is common in small children who subsequently develop the usual clinical picture of migraine. The diagnosis of abdominal epilepsy rests on the presence of other epileptic manifestations, usually complex partial seizures, an abnormal EEG pattern during or between attacks, and, less convincingly, a favorable response to anticonvulsants, usually carbamazepine, valproate, or phenytoin (322).

Epilepsia Partialis Continua

Epilepsia partialis continua, a variant of a simple partial (focal) seizure, is characterized by clonic movements, usually localized to the face or upper extremities, that persist over long periods either continuously or with only brief interruptions. Consciousness is not impaired, but postictal weakness is usually evident. We have seen several children with this condition who had an underlying chronic encephalitis of the kind described by Aguilar and Rasmussen (61) and Rasmussen and McCann (323). Rasmussen syndrome was the most common cause for epilepsia partialis continua in the series of Thomas and coworkers (324). This condition, and its relationship to immune disorders and a

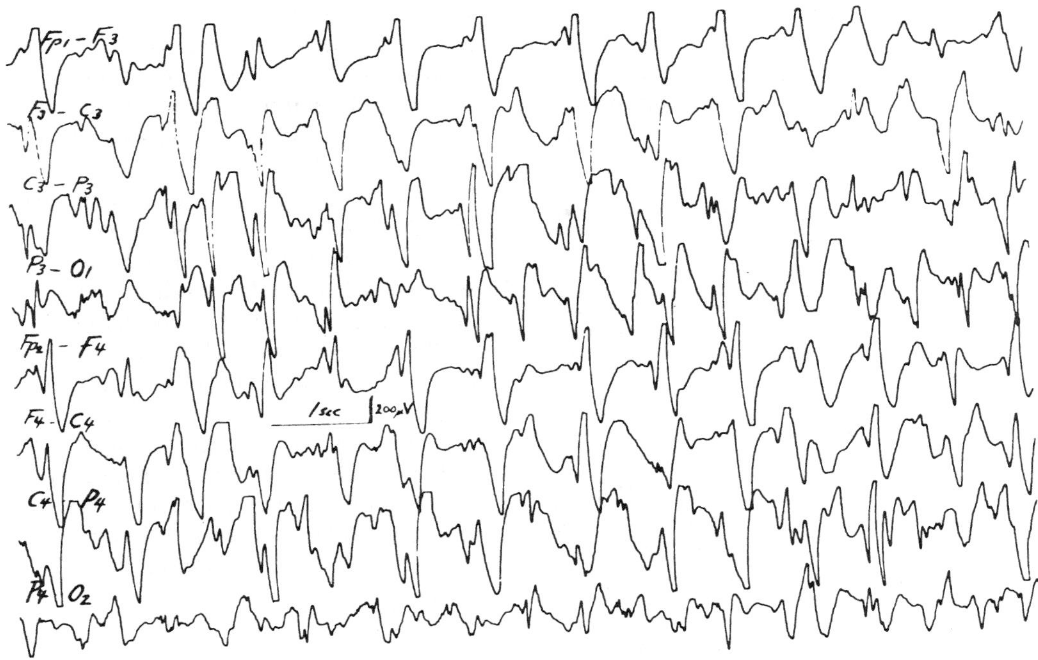

FIGURE 14.6. Absence status (generalized nonconvulsive status) in a 26-month-old girl with mild retardation and 14-day history of drowsiness. Note the enormously high voltage of the spike and sharp waves. (C, central; F, frontal; O, occipital; P, parietal.) (Marker indicates 200 μV.) (Courtesy of Dr. E. Niedermeyer, Johns Hopkins Hospital, Baltimore, MD.)

variety of infectious agents, and its treatment is considered in Chapter 8.

Various space-occupying lesions, including tumor, abscess, and cerebral cysticercosis, are less frequent causes for epilepsia partialis continua. Epilepsia partialis continua also has been encountered in various metabolic disorders, notably nonketotic hyperglycinemia (see Chapter 1).

Nonconvulsive Status Epilepticus, Absence Status (Generalized Nonconvulsive Status Epilepticus, Petit Mal Status)

Several types of nonconvulsive status epilepticus (NCSE) have been recognized: a generalized form, also termed *absence status* or *petit mal status*, and a partial type, termed *complex partial status epilepticus*; NCSE in patients with learning difficulties—including status epilepticus during sleep, atypical absence status epilepticus, and tonic status epilepticus—and NCSE in coma (325,326). NCSE is frequently seen in patients who are critically ill, such as in end-stage renal disease, or who have other major medical problems and can arise from treatment with cephalosporins, cefepine, isfosfamide, or tiagabine or upon acute withdrawal of diazepines, such as lorazepam.

Absence status is the most common form of nonconvulsive status epilepticus. It is characterized by a prolonged state of clouded mental activity usually accompanied by an EEG picture of atypical, slow spike-wave complexes and polyspike discharges. Untreated, the condition can last from several hours to as long as 2 years (327). Absence status almost always occurs in children with pre-existing organic cerebral lesions, a history of intellectual retardation, and a variety of other seizure forms (Fig. 14.6) (328). Approximately one-fourth of children with Lennox-Gastaut syndrome enter absence status one or more times during their lifetime (251).

Farran and coworkers have suggested that absence status is seen in patients with cerebellar anomalies and a consequent defect in the inhibitory system mediated by the Purkinje cells (329). The PET scan obtained during an attack fails to confirm this supposition in that it demonstrates only diffuse hypometabolism of fluorodeoxyglucose (330).

Complex partial status epilepticus is characterized by altered mentation, with impaired or absent language function, and a variable degree of responsiveness. The EEG during an attack shows various abnormalities, ranging from focal temporal spike and wave discharges to rhythmic slowing.

Benzodiazepines (lorazepam or diazepam) or valproate are the best drugs for treatment of both forms of nonconvulsive status, followed by institution or resumption of long-term anticonvulsant therapy (331). There is no conclusive evidence that prolonged NCSE can induce brain damage, and Kaplan cautions against overtreatment of the condition (332).

Landau-Kleffner Syndrome

Landau-Kleffner syndrome, which has attracted considerable attention in recent years, is marked by an acquired aphasia in children who have had normal language and motor development (333). Symptoms develop between 4 and 7 years of age. A variety of seizures accompany this condition in approximately 80% of cases. They can be rare and can disappear completely before adolescence. The EEG abnormalities are diagnostic. They include bilateral independent temporal or temporoparietal spikes, or spike and wave discharges, and in a large proportion of children, a continuous spike and wave discharge during as much as 90% of the sleeping state (334). Neuroimaging study results are normal. The aphasia frequently fluctuates in severity, but as a rule, the younger the age when symptoms start, the worse the prognosis in terms of language function (335). Other aspects of higher cortical function are preserved. Although in the initial report the condition was seen in two brothers, the etiology remains totally unknown.

Valproate, ethosuximide, and the benzodiazepines can improve the condition; phenobarbital and carbamazepine are generally ineffective. ACTH or corticosteroids also can be partially effective (336). Other therapeutic approaches include the use of intravenous immunoglobulins, which can be effective in some patients (337), and multiple subpial transections (338). As a rule, the EEG abnormalities regress with time, leaving the child with a severe receptive and expressive aphasia.

Landau-Kleffner syndrome has much in common with a condition in which subclinical electrical status epilepticus occurs during slow-wave sleep; continuous spike-wave discharges during slow-wave sleep (ESES) (339,340). This is a relatively rare seizure disorder. It is marked by partial or generalized seizures that are usually nocturnal, associated with reduction in language function, reduced attention span, and a variety of behavior disorders (341,342). The characteristic EEG pattern appears with onset of sleep and consists of spike-wave discharges, usually at 1.5 to 2 Hz, that persist throughout slow-wave sleep. During REM sleep, the frequency of spike and wave discharges is the same as during the waking state.

Treatment of the EEG abnormalities is not successful, although a number of anticonvulsants and corticosteroids have been used (341). In distinction from Landau-Kleffner syndrome, where there is an isolated disturbance of language function, other cognitive functions also are affected in ESES. The clinical course and response to anticonvulsants is similar for the two conditions, and many workers consider ESES to be a variant of the Landau-Kleffner syndrome or to represent a clinical continuum (334,340).

Other Seizures

Rarer seizure forms are summarized in Table 14.8 (343–351). The most likely of these to be encountered are the *reflex seizures*. This term denotes seizures that are repeatedly initiated by clearly defined stimuli. Reflex epilepsies account for some 5% of all epilepsies, with visually induced reflex (photogenic) epilepsy being the most common form, constituting 53% of Forster's series (352). Visual reflex epilepsy includes television epilepsy and video game epilepsy as well as most cases of epilepsy in which the child induces his or her own seizures by looking at a light source and rapidly moving the hand back and forth in front of the eyes ("fanning") (353,354). Other patients, not included in the group of reflex epileptic patients, can have both photogenic and nonphotogenic seizures or, even more

TABLE 14.8 Unusual Seizure Forms

Seizure Type	*Characteristics*	*Ref*
Gelastic	Paroxysmal laughter associated with transitory loss of consciousness	Gascon and Lombroso (343)
Reflex	Seizures evoked by a number of specific sensory stimuli:	
	Light	Jeavons and Harding (344)
	Language	Geschwind and Sherwin (345)
	Sound	Forster (346)
	Music	Critchley (347)
	Somatosensory stimulus (e.g., tapping, brushing teeth)	Forster (346), Calderon-Gonzalez, et al (348)
	Decision making (e.g., chess)	Ingvar and Nyman (349)
	Reading	Critchley, et al. (350)
Running	Episodic alteration of awareness associated with running; running may occur in an ictal twilight state, postictally, as a preconvulsive phenomenon, and possibly as an attack of paroxysmal compulsive behavior	Strauss (357)

commonly, can show only a photoconvulsive response on the EEG (355).

The mechanism for reflex seizures is unclear. The most attractive theory is that the attacks are caused by hyperexcitability of the sensory cortex, perhaps combined with a lack of cortical inhibition for a certain type of afferent input.

Treatment consists of avoiding the specific stimulus that induces seizures and administering anticonvulsants, preferably valproate or clonazepam. It is of note that the frequency of the TV or video game screen is important in provoking a seizure, with a 100-Hz screen being significantly safer than a 50-Hz screen. In addition, the distance of the child from the screen also is important, in that 1 m is safer than 50 cm (354).

Diagnosis

The diagnostic process in a child with epileptic seizures has two phases: the ascertainment of the type of seizure and its focus, if any, and an attempt to understand the cause for the attacks. Evaluation of the child with the first nonfebrile seizure has been reviewed by Hirtz and coworkers (356). They recommend the following steps: (a) determine whether a seizure has occurred, and (b) determine the cause of the seizure.

A thorough history, taken not only from the parent but also from the child, is crucial for arriving at a diagnosis. Usually, the physician is not able to witness an attack, and hospitalizing the child in the hopes of recording a seizure is financially prohibitive, although in some instances, it ultimately may be necessary.

Differential Diagnosis

The diagnosis of a generalized tonic-clonic seizure is usually made without much difficulty, although psychogenic seizures (hysteric seizures) also should be kept in mind despite their current relative rarity (357). The best discussion of the differential diagnosis between the two conditions is by Gowers, who emphasized the following points (48):

1. In the hysteric convulsion, the aura is absent or consists of palpitation, malaise, or a choking sensation.
2. During a hysteric attack, consciousness is impaired rather than lost.
3. The movements accompanying a hysteric seizure are somewhat coordinated but lack the definite sequence of a true tonic-clonic seizure. Tonic spasms are long and severe, often associated with opisthotonus or brief and irregular clonic movements.
4. Micturition and tongue biting are rarely seen in a hysteric attack.
5. The hysteric attack terminates suddenly, and the patient often resumes his or her former activities.

To these criteria, distinguishing hysteric seizures, proposed more than 100 years ago, can now be added the absence of abnormalities on EEG or video-telemetry EEG recordings during a hysteric attack (357,358).

Childhood hysteria can be encountered as early as 6 years of age. Although it is still more common in girls, in children younger than 10 years of age, the sexes are affected equally (359).

Lazare has listed several psychological criteria for the diagnosis of a conversion symptom, such as a hysterical seizure (360):

1. A disorder of somatization (i.e., long-standing psychosomatic symptoms affecting several organ systems)
2. An associated psychopathology (e.g., depression, personality disorder, schizophrenia)
3. A model for the symptom, based on the patient's own previous illness or on that of an important figure in the patient's life

Less important criteria for the diagnosis of a conversion reaction are emotional stress before the onset of symptoms, a disturbed sexuality (i.e., a history of seduction or incest), and the patient's being the youngest child. These considerations do not always allow a definite diagnosis, and it is important to remember that casual evaluation can lead to an erroneous diagnosis.

Grand mal attacks also should be differentiated from syncope. Syncope is rare in childhood, being more common in adolescence, particularly in girls. The attacks usually occur in the upright position and are preceded by fatigue or emotional stress. Syncopal attacks are occasionally terminated by a brief generalized tonic or tonic-clonic convulsion, probably the result of cerebral anoxia. An EEG recording during a syncopal attack, if available, shows diffuse electric slowing rather than seizure activity (361).

Another condition requiring differentiation from grand mal attacks is breath-holding. Breath-holding spells are limited to children younger than age 6 years. They are precipitated by crying in response to emotional upsets. The attack is usually brief and accompanied by intense cyanosis or pallor. The child can be limp or opisthotonic. A short clonic convulsion induced by cerebral anoxia can terminate the spell.

Tharp has listed a variety of other disorders that mimic seizures (Table 14.9) (362).

A few comments with respect to some of the more commonly encountered diagnostic problems follow.

The differentiation between a prolonged absence seizure with motor accompaniments and a brief complex partial seizure should take the following items into account: that a complex partial seizure lasts longer and includes a greater variety of movements; that absence attacks do not have an aura, occur far more frequently than psychomotor seizure, and can often be elicited by

TABLE 14.9 Episodic Disorders that Mimic Seizures

Benign neonatal sleep myoclonus
Normal but excessive motor activity during active (rapid eye movement) sleep in infants
Jitteriness of newborns (including drug withdrawal in maternal addiction)
Breath-holding spells
Gastroesophageal reflux (Sandifer syndrome)
Sleep disorders, including pavor nocturnus, sleep mycoclonus, and narcolepsy
Familial essential myoclonus
Familial paroxysmal hypnogenic dystonia
Familial paroxysmal dyskinesias
Abnormal startle reaction (hyperekplexia)
Infantile shuddering attacks (see Chapter 3)
Nocturnal paroxysmal dystonia
Transient paroxysmal dystonia of infancy
Migraine and syncope
Habit spasms, tics, Gilles de la Tourette syndrome
Pseudoseizures
Benign paroxysmal vertigo of childhood (see Chapter 7)

From Tharp BR. An overview of pediatric seizure disorders and epileptic syndromes. *Epilepsia* 1987;28[Suppl 1]:S36. With permission.

hyperventilation; that the patient with a complex partial seizure has partial clouding of consciousness for a brief period after the seizure has ended; and that the interictal EEG abnormalities in absence epilepsy are generally diagnostic.

Pavor nocturnus (night terror) should be distinguished from nocturnal complex partial seizures or major motor seizures. Pavor nocturnus is a paroxysmal sleep disturbance occurring during arousal from slow-wave sleep. The child appears agitated or leaves bed crying and in apparent terror. Heart rate and respiratory rate are increased. The episode is brief, often lasting less than a minute, and the child returns to sleep. Generally, efforts to rouse the child fail, and the child has no recollection of the attack. The EEG during pavor nocturnus is normal (363), and children generally outgrow this condition (see Chapter 15).

Myoclonic seizures of the body or extremities commonly occur when a child drops off to sleep and in a few families can be unusually violent. The syndrome of severe nocturnal myoclonus, although benign and not amenable to drug therapy, must be differentiated from a true nocturnal epileptic seizure (364).

Tics are usually distinguished from myoclonic seizures because the patient is able to control tics voluntarily, they consist of the same movement each time, and they occur in patients who manifest other evidence of psychological disturbance and are aggravated by emotional strain.

Spasmus nutans (see Chapter 8) is often confused with epileptic seizures, particularly salaam seizures. Unlike in salaam seizures, children with spasmus nutans do not lose consciousness during an attack, and intellectual development remains normal. Vertical or horizontal nystagmus affecting one or both eyes is a common feature of spasmus nutans. Head thrusts and blinking observed in congenital ocular motor apraxia have been mistaken for the seizure manifestations of Lennox-Gastaut syndrome (365).

Patient History

Because the diagnosis of a seizure disorder relies to a great extent on the history furnished to the physician, an intentionally falsified history leads to the erroneous diagnosis of epilepsy. Over the last decades, we have seen an increasing number of children with Munchausen disease by proxy who have been brought in with a history of a seizure disorder or recurrent apnea (366). *Fictitious epilepsy*, the term used by Meadow, is a not at all rare form of child abuse and can lead to years of unwarranted invalidism (367). Its diagnosis is difficult but should be considered when, in addition to epilepsy, the youngster suffers from other disorders equally difficult to document. These include diarrhea and food allergies, hematuria and hematemesis, and apneic episodes. Additionally, the patient often has an inexplicable mixture of overdosing and undertreatment, as verified by blood anticonvulsant levels. When fictitious epilepsy is suspected, verification of the history from individuals outside the family (e.g., teachers) and observation in the hospital are indicated.

Physical Examination

The physical examination in a patient with a seizure disorder can be abnormal when the patient has underlying cerebral pathology (Fig. 14.7). A small fraction of children with long-standing seizure disorders unaccompanied by neurologic abnormalities harbor a cerebral tumor. Although

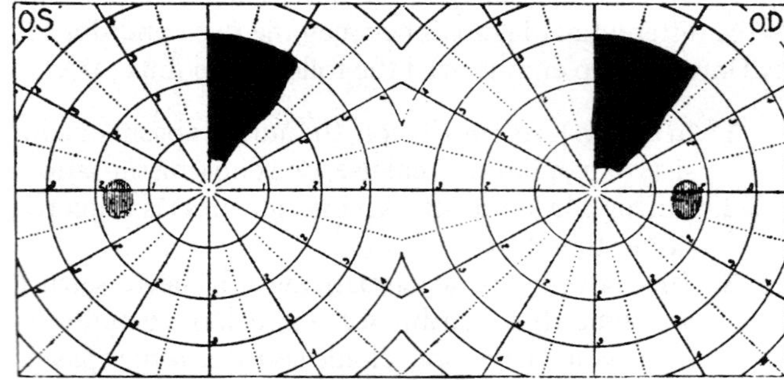

FIGURE 14.7. Visual field defect in child with complex partial seizures and temporal lobe tumor. The child has a superior quadrantal hemianopia with sparing of the macula. (OD, right eye; OS, left eye.) (Courtesy of Dr. R. Hepler, Department of Ophthalmology, University of California, Los Angeles, UCLA School of Medicine.)

TABLE 14.10 Warning Signs of Cerebral Neoplasms in 23 Children with Long-Standing Seizure Disorder and Brain Tumor

Parameter	Time Before Diagnosis of Tumor 6–24 mo	Time Before Diagnosis of Tumor Less Than 6 mo
Deterioration of behavior and school performance	9	3
Slow wave focus on electroencephalography	8	11
Seizure pattern changed or increased in frequency	8	5
Abnormalities on plain skull film	3	9
Specific neurologic signs	1	13
Signs reflecting increased intracranial pressure	0	12

Modified from Page LK, Lombroso CT, Matson DD. Childhood epilepsy with late detection of cerebral glioma. *J Neurosurg* 1969;31:253.

imaging studies, especially MRI, disclose the neoplasm, it is impractical and far too costly to subject every child who has experienced a seizure to imaging studies. What makes the diagnosis even more difficult is the fact that in most of the children with an underlying tumor, neither the type of seizure nor the initial EEG suggests a focal disorder; even a CT scan performed as part of an initial evaluation can be normal. Page and associates compiled the clinical features that they consider indicative of a cerebral tumor in children with a seizure disorder (Table 14.10) (368). The physician must keep in mind that the physical examination also can be abnormal when the patient is examined shortly after a seizure, and when cerebral dysfunction results from recurrent seizures or is the consequence of anticonvulsant medication.

The patient may be confused following a severe seizure, and transient neurologic signs, including intention tremor, incoordination, weakness of one or more extremities, and pathologic exaggeration of reflexes, are common. When convulsions recur at brief intervals, these signs can persist for prolonged periods.

Cerebral damage can result from recurrent seizures. Usually, this damage takes the form of intellectual deterioration and emotional disturbance. The incidence of these complications is treated in the section on Prognosis.

A number of anticonvulsants can induce neurologic abnormalities (Table 14.11).

Laboratory Tests

Laboratory studies are directed toward uncovering the cause of the seizures. Various diagnostic procedures are customarily performed on patients with seizures who lack a history or neurologic findings that point to a diagnosis.

Blood Chemistries

Serum glucose and calcium levels are obtained for all infants with seizures and for older children whose histories raise the possibility of a metabolic disturbance (see Chapter 17). In neonates, an evaluation of renal function also is indicated. Serum electrolyte disturbances are rare in patients with recurrent seizures, but hyponatremia (sodium of less than 125 meq/l) was associated with seizures in 70% of infants under 6 months of age (356). In children with seizures owing to hypernatremia, the history

TABLE 14.11 Neurologic Complications of Commonly Used Antiepileptic Drugs

Drug	Most Common Neurologic Complications
Phenobarbital	Hyperkinetic behavior, drowsiness
Methylphenobarbital	Hyperkinetic behavior, drowsiness
Primidone	Drowsiness, ataxia, dizziness, dysarthria, diplopia, nystagmus, personality changes
Phenytoin	Nystagmus on vertical and horizontal gaze, truncal ataxia, intention tremor, dysarthria, aggravation of seizures, permanent cerebellar degeneration, personality disturbances
Ethosuximide	Headache, dizziness, hiccups, personality disturbances
Diazepam	Drowsiness, ataxia, hallucinations, blurred vision, diplopia, headaches, slurred speech, tremors, extrapyramidal movements
Clonazepam	Ataxia, drowsiness, dysarthria, irritability, belligerence, and other behavior disturbances
Carbamazepine	Diplopia, disturbed coordination, drowsiness, headaches, visual hallucinations, peripheral neuritis or paresthesias, extrapyramidal movements
Valproic acid	Ataxia, tremor (dose-related), asterixis, drowsiness, or stupor (when given in conjunction with phenobarbital)
Vigabatrin	Dyskineslas, visual field defects
Topiramate	Dizziness, ataxia, somnolence, psychomotor slowing, impaired memory
Lamotrigine	Dizziness, ataxia, somnolence, diplopia, blurred vision
Gabapentin	Somnolence, dizziness, ataxia
Felbamate	Insomnia, somnolence, mononeuritis, choreoathetosis

usually suggests a fluid imbalance. A toxicology study also is indicated.

Electroencephalography

The EEG can be useful in determining the type of seizure the patient experiences. It differentiates between absence and complex partial seizures, and between absence attacks and atypical petit mal. Occasionally, it can assist in establishing a diagnosis when the history is inadequate or not diagnostic. It also is the best predictor of the likelihood of recurrence. The EEG must be interpreted in conjunction with the patient's history. A normal EEG, seen in approximately one-half of epileptic patients, does not exclude the diagnosis of epilepsy, nor does an abnormal EEG necessarily establish it. King and colleagues have found that it is easier to differentiate between a primary generalized and a secondarily generalized seizure disorder if the initial EEG is performed within 24 hours of the seizure. They also recommend that should the initial EEG be normal, a second, sleep-deprived EEG should be performed (369). Hirtz and colleagues also state that an EEG obtained within 24 hours of a seizure is more likely to show epileptiform abnormalities and can guide the physician as to whether neuroimaging is necessary (356).

Electric abnormalities can be seen during an overt attack as well as between seizures. Generalized tonic-clonic seizures arising from subcortical excitation can be recorded on the EEG, but the abnormalities are usually obscured by movement artifacts. One exception is the major seizure with a focal cortical origin. In this condition, random focal spiking or spike-wave discharges that had already been seen during the interseizure period increase in frequency and amplitude and spread both contiguously and via subcortical centers. Generalization can occur within a fraction of a second after the onset of the focal seizure; less commonly, it develops slowly over as long as 20 seconds. Following the seizure, electric activity is depressed. Recovery starts with slow waves, normal cortical activity first appearing contralateral to the epileptic focus, then ipsilateral, and finally over the focus itself.

Less commonly, the ictal tracing is marked by suppression of electrical activity, or low-voltage fast activity, an indication of disinhibition.

The EEG during an absence attack shows bilateral high-voltage synchronous alternating spike-wave complexes, most commonly 3 to 4 Hz (see Fig. 14.3). The discharge frequency can be increased by hyperventilation. As the discharge continues, the frequency of the spike-wave complexes tends to slow down.

In most patients with complex partial seizures, the EEG patterns accompanying the seizure are slow, rhythmic, and usually bilaterally synchronous, 4- to 6-Hz discharges, most prominent in the frontal and temporal areas but becoming generalized as the seizure progresses. At the conclusion of the attack, the EEG is featureless, and recovery of normal activity is delayed for many minutes.

The interseizure record in patients with major motor attacks can be normal or can demonstrate a number of nonspecific abnormalities, including disorganization, spike discharges, loss of a-rhythm or loss of the highest expected frequency activity for the child's age, and, occasionally, continuous or intermittent focal slowing. This last finding, particularly when it is continuous, should always raise the possibility of an underlying tumor or other structural lesion and indicates the need for imaging studies.

In complex partial seizures, the interseizure tracing is normal or shows nonspecific abnormalities or spike foci, which usually arise from the anterior portions of the temporal lobes (Fig. 14.8). Often, the seizure focus is apparent only during the transition between wakefulness and sleep, and a combined wake and sleep tracing should always be obtained from children suspected of having complex partial seizures. In approximately 80% of children with this condition, three serial wake and sleep recordings uncover an abnormality. In a number of patients, secondary spike foci can be recorded from the opposite temporal lobe. It is rare to find focal temporal spike discharges in children younger than 8 years of age, even in those with a classic clinical picture of complex partial seizures.

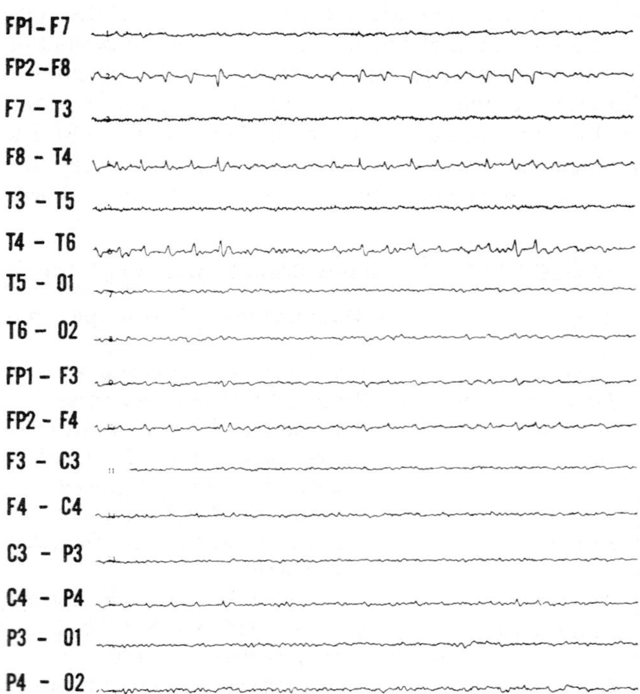

FIGURE 14.8. Right anterior temporal spike discharge in patient with complex partial seizures. (C, central; F, frontal; FP, frontopolar; O, occipital; P, parietal; T, temporal.) (Courtesy of Dr. Gregory Walsh, Department of Neurology, University of California, Los Angeles, UCLA School of Medicine.)

Atypical spike-wave discharges (i.e., spike-wave discharges at a frequency less than 2.5 Hz) and polyspike-wave discharges are common in children with Lennox-Gastaut syndrome. They indicate a poor prognosi in terms of seizure control and normal intellectual function. The high positive correlation between hypsarrhythmia and infantile spasms has already been discussed.

With EEG maturation, the EEG in patients with seizure disorders can undergo significant changes. Focal spike activity tends to migrate from the occipital to the midtemporal and ultimately to the anterior temporal leads (370). In patients with 3-Hz generalized spike-wave discharges, an improvement in clinical status can be associated with the disappearance of the abnormal EEG pattern, which is often replaced by a wandering spike focus (371). In patients with focal seizure discharges, mirror spike activity can appear. In some, this second focus is suppressed by anticonvulsants; in others, it becomes the only active focus (371).

For further information on the clinical aspects of EEG, the reader is referred to one of the several standard EEG texts.

Lumbar Puncture

Lumbar puncture is not performed routinely in patients with seizure disorders. Because a significant proportion of infants with bacterial or tuberculous meningitis have a febrile seizure as their initial symptom (see Chapter 7), we believe a lumbar puncture is indicated in patients who have experienced their first febrile seizure and in all infants having their first seizure.

Although the CSF is by definition normal in the majority of patients with idiopathic epilepsy, minor abnormalities were found in the classic study of Lennox and Merritt (372). In 4% of their patients, pleocytosis was slight (5 to 10 cells/μL), and in 10%, protein content was increased (45 to 85 mg/dL). Both abnormalities were believed to be related to the presence of small areas of cerebral contusion that resulted from a fall attending the seizure. They had disappeared when the spinal tap was repeated several weeks later. More recent studies are consistent with these observations (373,374). Wong and coworkers, who examined the CSF of children within 24 hours of a seizure, found a normal range of 0 to 12 cells in infants under 4 months of age, and a range of 0 to 8 cells in infants over 4 months. The normal postictal protein was less than 100 mg/dl in infants less than 2 months, less than 60 mg/dl between 2 and 4 months, and less than 35 mg/dl in infants over 4 months of age (375). We suspect that abnormalities in cell count and protein level, when present, reflect the cerebral edema, disturbed autoregulation, and the breakdown of the blood–brain barrier that attend a prolonged seizure and that have been documented by MRI (376). In contrast to adults, seizure-induced neuronal injury is not marked by an increase in neuron-specific enolase; rather, increases reflect the presence of metabolic or genetic abnormalities (377).

Imaging Studies

MRI and CT scans are the procedures currently used in the initial evaluation of a child with a seizure disorder. The question as to whether an emergent imaging study should be performed as part of the evaluation of the child that presents with an afebrile seizure has been considered by several authors. In the experience of Maytal and coworkers, only 6% of children who presented with cryptogenic seizures had an abnormal CT. By contrast, the CT was abnormal in 60% of children whose seizures were considered to be symptomatic (378). Similar results were obtained by Sharma and coworkers (379). From studies such as these, it is evident that neuroimaging of children with the first afebrile seizure should be reserved for those who have conditions that place him or her at an increased risk for neuroimaging abnormalities. These include an abnormal neurologic examination, a history of malignancy, sickle cell disease, bleeding disorder, a closed head injury, or travel to an area endemic for cysticercosis (379). Infants under 33 months with focal seizures should undergo imaging as well. In this group, in the experience of Sharma and coworkers, CT abnormalities were seen in 29% (379). By contrast, only 2% of CTs were abnormal in children with nonfocal seizures and no predisposing conditions (379). Hirtz and colleagues found that the yield of abnormalities on CT scan is low in the presence of a normal EEG and a normal neurological examination, and that abnormalities when present do not influence treatment (356).

An imaging study is indicated for the child with recurrent seizures under several circumstances: in the presence of an abnormal neurologic examination, including dysmorphic features, or skin lesions suggestive of a phakomatosis (64%); in the presence of focal EEG abnormalities, particularly focal slowing (63%); with a history of neonatal seizures (100%); and with a history compatible with simple partial or complex partial seizures (52% and 30%, respectively). The numbers in parentheses represent percentage of positive CT scan results seen by Yang and coworkers in their series of seizure patients (380); the percentages of positive combined CT and MRI studies would undoubtedly have been higher.

Whether imaging studies also are indicated for children who by history and examination do not fulfill these criteria is a matter of individual judgment. Children whose neurologic examination and EEG are normal have a low yield of positive scan results (356), as do children with primary generalized seizures [5% and 8%, respectively, in the series of Yang and coworkers (380)]. In confirmation of this experience, King and coworkers found no MRI abnormalities in any of their patients with EEG-confirmed primary generalized seizures (369).

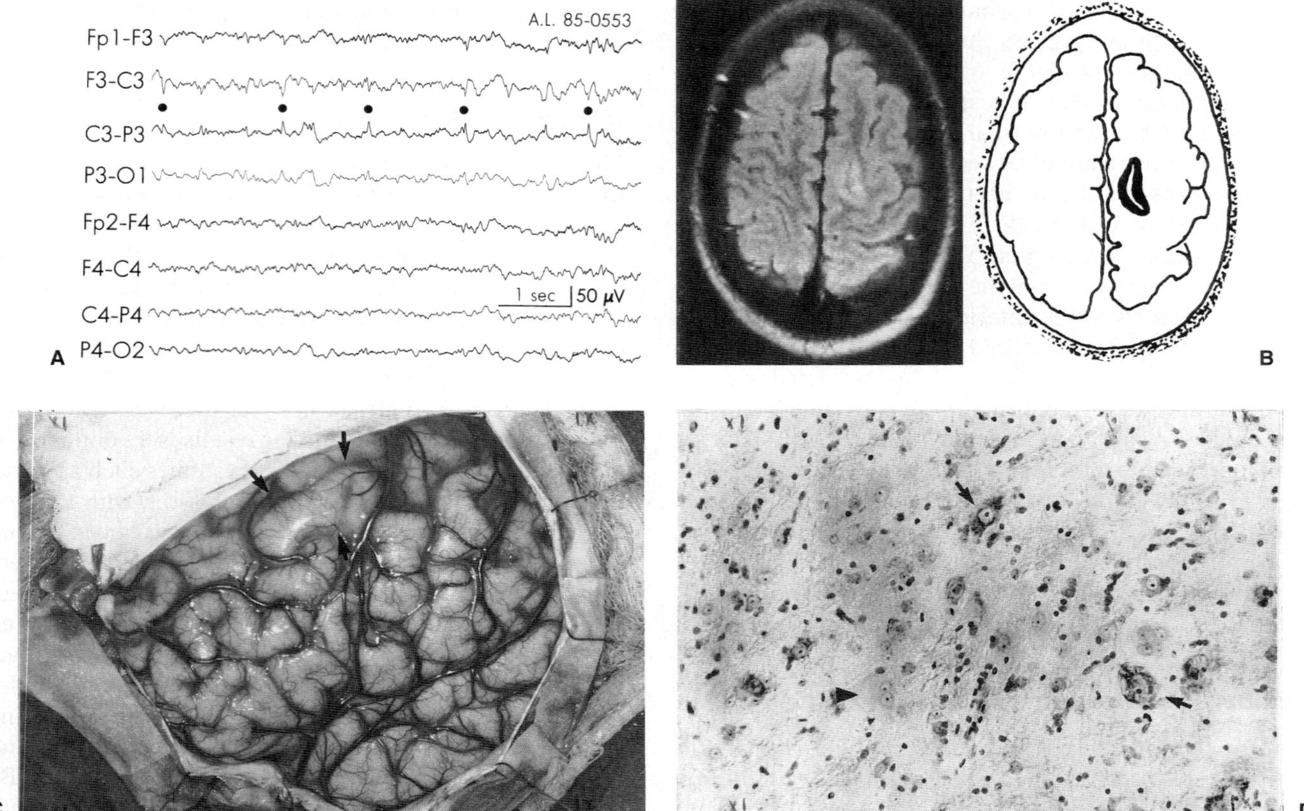

FIGURE 14.9. An 18-year-old girl with onset at 6 years of age of focal myoclonus involving right arm and shoulder and right hemiparesis. **A:** Representative section of electroencephalogram showing frequent sharp waves with phase reversals over the left central region (C3). (C, central; F, frontal; O, occipital; P, parietal.) **B:** Magnetic resonance imaging showing left hemiatrophy and an area of slightly increased signal corresponding to the abnormal gyrus (see adjacent diagram). **C:** Left cerebral hemisphere at operation. Note enlarged gyrus (*black arrows*). **D:** Microscopic section at junction of cortex and white matter showing disruption of cortical lamination with abnormally large dysplastic neurons (*arrows*) and large astrocytes (*arrowhead*) (Luxol fast blue, ×130). (Courtesy of Drs. R. Kuzniecky and F. Andermann, Department of Neurology, McGill University, Montreal, Canada.)

Several studies have compared CT scans and MRI for their respective advantages and disadvantages in evaluating a seizure patient. Although the two procedures occasionally provide complementary information, MRI is the preferred initial screening procedure. Unlike CT scanning, MRI detects congenital malformations of the cortex, gray matter heterotopias, and a large proportion of arteriovenous malformations, some of which can be angiographically occult. MRI also is an excellent screening test for detecting neoplasms, particularly when it is used with gadolinium enhancement. On the other hand, CT scans are more sensitive for small foci of calcification.

The joint use of EEG and imaging studies has been applied most successfully in the evaluation of patients with focal seizure disorders. MRI is effective in detecting underlying abnormalities in the cortical architecture of children with simple partial epilepsies (369,381) (Fig. 14.9). In young children with intractable partial epilepsies, malformations of the cortex are detectable on MRI. These abnormalities are most common in the central cortical area, particularly in the region of the operculum. The complexity of cortical gyration makes difficult the detection of subtle abnormalities, and when MRI is correlated with pathologic examination of brain tissue resected from epileptic seizure foci, only approximately one-half of the malformations were detected before surgery by MRI (382). MRI results are abnormal in most patients with severe mesial temporal sclerosis as well as in a large proportion of subjects with pathologically proven mild to moderate sclerosis (383,384). These abnormalities are best demonstrated with T2-weighted or fluid-attenuated inversion recovery (FLAIR) images. Additionally, MRI can detect small epileptogenic lesions in the temporal lobe, notably hamartomas and low-grade gliomas (385,386). When children with newly diagnosed epilepsy were subjected to both MRI

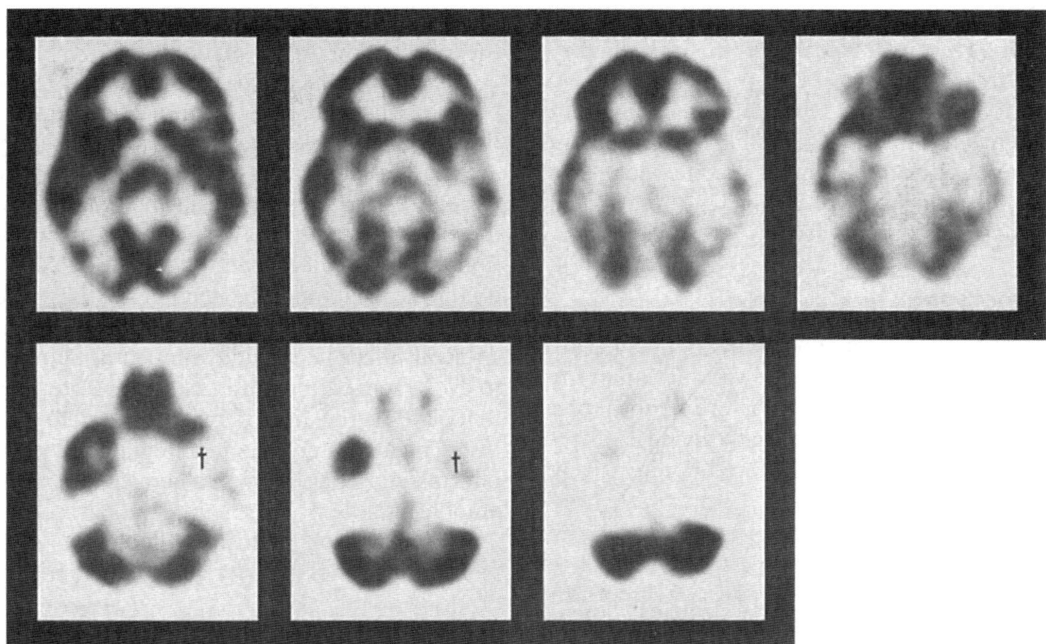

FIGURE 14.10. Positron emission tomography using labeled fluorodeoxyglucose. Interictal scan in a patient with complex partial seizures since age 5 years. There is a zone of relative hypometabolism in the left temporal lobe (t). The electroencephalogram on this patient showed a left mesial temporal spike focus. Computed tomographic scans showed possible enlargement of the left temporal horn, but angiographic and pneumoencephalographic studies were normal. Pathologic examination following left temporal lobectomy revealed a mesial temporal lobe sclerosis. (From Engel J, Crandall PH, Rausch R. The partial epilepsies. In: Rosenberg RN, et al., eds. *The clinical neurosciences*, Vol. 2. *Neurology/neurosurgery*. New York: Churchill Livingstone, 1983. With permission.)

and CT, both studies were abnormal in 83%, and in the remainder, the CT was normal but the MRI was abnormal. The MRI also found a number of incidental abnormalities, such as Chiari 1 malformations, pineal cysts, and arachnoid cysts (387).

Transient abnormalities at the site of an actively discharging epileptic focus can be visualized by MRI, particularly on T2-weighted images (388). These abnormalities can reflect hyperemia or can be caused by a shift of water from the extracellular compartment into dendrites or glia (389). Similar changes also can be visualized on CT scans. The abnormalities take from 1 to 48 hours to develop and can resolve within 1 week or as late as 12 weeks (390). Additionally, some drugs, notably digoxin and heparin, can increase the signal intensity on MRI (391).

PET scanning provides three-dimensional functional images of the brain. Although in most centers PET scanning is still a research study, this procedure has become part of the diagnostic evaluation of a youngster with focal seizures or with intractable generalized seizures and assists in the surgical treatment of intractable epilepsies (392). Fluorodeoxyglucose, which measures glucose metabolism, is the most commonly used tracer. The interictal PET scan demonstrates focal areas of hypometabolism corresponding to the site of the epileptic focus as determined by EEG, and to focal changes on MRI (393) (Fig. 14.10). Juhasz and coworkers have noted, however, that the hypomtabolic area itself is not involved in epileptic activity, but rather arises from the surrounding cortex (394). During a seizure, this area of hypometabolism becomes hypermetabolic. When the seizure is generalized, such as in children with absence attacks, hypermetabolism is generalized (395). Focal areas of hypometabolism have been found in children with infantile spasms and in the Lennox-Gastaut syndrome (304). The relative value of localizing a seizure focus by means of EEG, MRI, and PET has been a matter of some debate. Most centers, including ours, consider PET to be more likely to detect a focal temporal abnormality than structural imaging studies, and we have seen a number of patients with PET abnormalities in whom MRI had been normal (396). The experiences of Won and colleagues with respect to the comparative ability of MRI, interictal PET, and ictal single photon emission CT (SPECT) show that PET was the best study to correctly localize the epileptic focus. SPECT and MRI were equally useful (397). In our experience, and that of Theodore and colleagues, the anatomic distribution of neuronal cell loss correlates poorly with the degree and the spatial extent of PET hypometabolism (398).

The advantages and drawbacks of SPECT in the localization of epileptic foci are considered in the Introductory chapter.

In the majority of instances, abnormal imaging studies do not influence treatment of the child with a seizure disorder. For the physician who must practice defensive medicine under the legal sword of Damocles, these logical guidelines are, however, of little help.

Cerebral Angiography

Cerebral angiography, requiring hospitalization, is hardly ever indicated, except to determine the vascular anatomy as part of the preoperative evaluation before removal of a seizure focus. In many cases, exceptionally vivid visualization of vascular structures can be achieved noninvasively with spiral (helical) CT (399).

Magnetoencephalography

In contrast to EEG, which records the electrical potentials, magnetoencephalography (MEG) records the magnetic fields generated by the brain. Although these fields are extremely small, the magnetic fields generated by epileptiform discharges can be localized three-dimensionally, particularly when the focus is in the more superficial areas of the cortex. At this time, the procedure is primarily a research tool, and because of its high cost and complexity of equipment, the procedure does not yet offer any significant advantages over other routine diagnostic studies (400,401). However, it has been the experience of most centers involved in the surgical treatment of epilepsy that the combination of EEG and MEG is superior to each in isolation in terms of localizing the site of a seizure discharge.

Telemetry and Other Tests to Determine Focal or Generalized Cerebral Dysfunction

A number of tests can be used to localize an epileptogenic focus in patients whose seizures have remained intractable with standard medical therapy or in whom the epileptic nature of recurrent episodes has not been clarified. Several techniques have been used for long-term EEG monitoring. The most commonly employed is a combined EEG telemetry and video monitoring (402). For this procedure, the child is admitted to the hospital and is continuously monitored until enough ictal events have been recorded to determine the epileptic nature of the attacks, the epileptic seizure type, and the site of onset. Because the monitoring system is portable, the child is free to move around the ward and can engage in usual ward activities (403). Prolonged (8- to 10-hour) EEG recordings in the laboratory are somewhat simpler but require considerable cooperation by the patient. An ambulatory cassette recorder allows the child to remain at home or attend school, while the parent or teacher keeps a log of the activities. We have found the ambulatory technique useful to determine whether or not recurrent episodes are epileptic but of lesser value in the localization of the seizure focus.

Sphenoidal electrodes have been used to localize epileptic discharges generated by mesial temporal sclerosis in patients with complex partial seizures. Although electrodes are fairly easily placed in the cooperative adult, their use in children requires analgesia and sedation. Once in place, the electrodes are generally well tolerated. For most situations, anterior cheek electrodes provide adequate sensitivity for mesial temporal discharges. Other procedures used to localize an epileptic discharge and select patients for surgical ablation include thiopental activation intended to evoke focal attenuation of barbiturate-induced fast activity (404), the use of methohexital to distinguish between primary and secondary epileptic foci (405), and the pharmacologic ablation of a hemisphere with intracarotid amobarbital.

The activation of focal epileptiform discharges with pentylenetetrazol is no longer done in most institutions.

Metabolic Screening Studies and Cytogenetics

Metabolic screening studies and cytogenetics are performed when seizures are coupled with mental retardation of indiscernible cause or are associated with periods of prolonged impairment of consciousness. Generally, screening of plasma amino acids and other metabolites is combined with determination of urine organic acids, blood ammonia levels, and blood and CSF lactate and pyruvate levels. Several cytogenetic abnormalities are coupled with a seizure disorder. These are reviewed in Chapter 4.

Treatment

Clinical Aspects of Treatment

The objective in the treatment of the epileptic patient is complete control of seizures, or at least a reduction in their frequency to the point at which they no longer interfere with physical and social well-being. Two aspects of therapy are discussed: who to treat and how to treat.

Candidates

Although all authorities agree that all patients with recurrent seizures should be treated as soon as the diagnosis is established, considerable controversy surrounds the optimal method of dealing with certain groups of patients.

Febrile Seizures

The treatment of febrile seizures is discussed in the section on Specific Seizure Types.

Isolated Tonic-Clonic (Grand Mal) Seizure

We believe that treatment of this type of seizure is optional and depends on the risk for recurrence and a variety of social factors, notably patient and family anxiety, and compliance.

Several studies have attempted to assess the recurrence risk after a first seizure. Generally, the risk is a function of the type of seizure and the time interval between the first seizure and the patient's visit to the doctor. Recurrence rates for a generalized tonic-clonic seizure have ranged from 24% to 71%. Hauser and associates reported a recurrence risk of 24% for idiopathic, mainly generalized tonic-clonic seizures. Patients who had experienced two or more seizures by the time they were first diagnosed were excluded from the study (406). When patients are seen within 1 day of their first tonic-clonic seizure, the recurrence risk is much greater. In the experience of Elwes and coworkers, the cumulative probability of recurrence in untreated children and adults was 20% by 1 month, 32% by 3 months, 46% by 6 months, 62% by 1 year, and 71% by 3 to 4 years (407). These statistics are consistent with a recurrence risk of 84% obtained in a demographic survey in Kent, England (5). In the experience of Shinnar and coworkers, who followed children for a mean of 9.6 years, the risk for a second seizure was 29%, 37%, 43%, and 46% at one, two, five, and ten years, respectively (408). Of those children who experienced a second seizure, 72% experienced a third seizure, 58% had four or more seizures, and 29% had ten or more seizures. Recurrence is most likely in children with neurologic or developmental abnormalities, complex partial seizures, recurrence of the second seizure within six months of the first seizure, and a paroxysmal EEG (408,409). In the experience of Hauser and coworkers (406), recurrence also was likely for children whose seizures were idiopathic, and for those who had a parent or sibling with nonfebrile seizures (406,410). A history of an antecedent febrile seizure or the age when the initial seizure was experienced does not affect the likelihood of recurrence (409,410).

In children, one-half of the observed recurrences were encountered during the first 6 months of follow-up (410). An overall incidence of 48.3% for recurrences of childhood generalized motor seizures was obtained in a prospective study of both treated and untreated subjects (410).

In view of these relatively optimistic experiences, and a 30% incidence of significant side reactions to anticonvulsant therapy, we are reluctant to treat the youngster who has suffered a first isolated idiopathic grand mal seizure and whose neurologic examination and EEG are normal, except on insistence of the family. Other authorities are of a similar opinion, but consensus suggests that if two or more tonic-clonic seizures occur in a period of less than 1 year, treatment is indicated.

Breath-Holding Spells

We have found antiepileptic drugs to be of no value in preventing recurrence of attacks. Our experience is shared by Stephenson, who recommends a trial of atropine for breath-holding spells, and for resistant reflex anoxic seizures (411). For a further discussion of breath-holding spells, see Chapter 15.

Syncopal Attacks

Anticonvulsant therapy is of little use in preventing either the attack or the clonic seizure that can terminate it. For a further discussion of syncopal attacks, see Chapter 15.

One or More Episodes the Epileptic Nature of Which Cannot Be Established with Certainty

Three options are open for the management of one or more episodes the epileptic nature of which cannot be established with certainty. One can defer therapy until the clinical picture becomes clear. If the patient probably experienced a seizure equivalent, one can institute a clinical trial with carbamazepine, which is relatively more effective in seizure equivalents than most other anticonvulsants. If the episodes are sufficiently frequent, inpatient telemetry or outpatient ambulatory cassette EEG monitoring are invaluable (403,412).

Drugs

Principles

Once treatment has been decided on, several therapeutic principles should be kept in mind.

1. The selection of the preferred drug is based on the type of seizure and on the potential toxicity of the drug.
2. Treatment should begin with one drug, its dosage being increased until seizures are controlled or the child develops toxicity (caveat: see below). If the drug does not control seizures, it is discontinued gradually, while a second drug is instituted and its dosage is increased.

   This concept of monotherapy (i.e., the preferential use of a single anticonvulsant in the treatment of seizures) has gained considerable support from a number of clinical studies. These have documented various disadvantages of polytherapy (413,414). First, chronic toxicity is directly related to the number of drugs consumed by the child. Even though none of them may be present in toxic level, their effect, particularly on sensorium and intellectual performance, is cumulative. Second, drug interactions might not only enhance toxicity, but might lead to loss of seizure control. Third, polytherapy can aggravate seizures in a significant proportion of patients. Finally, polytherapy makes it difficult to identify the cause of an adverse reaction.

   In the experience of Reynolds and Shorvon (413), the conversion of polytherapy to monotherapy is associated with improved seizure control and intellectual performance. One of us (J.H.M.) had made comparable observations many years before (415). In approximately one-fourth of patients, a single anticonvulsant, however, does not control seizures, and two drugs are required.

Having stated the traditional teachings regarding monotherapy until toxicity to the first agent, one of us (R.S.) has been making the observation that the conventional wisdom against polypharmacy was attained during an era of anticonvulsants that had low therapeutic indices (phenytoin, carbamazepine), high protein binding (phenytoin, valproic acid), and the ability to induce hepatic microsomal enzymes (barbiturates, hydantoins), thus creating a setting for adverse drug-drug interactions without frank synergy (phenytoin and carbamazepine). Most new generation medications, developed more recently than the 1990s, lack protein binding, ability to induce hepatic microsomal enzymes, and display a richness in mechanistic diversity that tempts one to explore synergy. Some of these medications also display a wide therapeutic index, such that the greatest efficacy is achieved at a relatively modest dose, and increasing the dose to toxicity may not be very useful.

3. Alterations in drug dosage should be made gradually, usually not more frequently than once every 5 to 7 days.
4. The chance of controlling epilepsy with a lesser known drug when first-line medications have failed is small. Conversely, the chances of inducing perplexing side reactions with a new or rarely used drug are great.
5. Once seizures are controlled, the medication should be continued for a time that can be determined by the syndromic diagnosis (some idiopathic epilepsies of childhood remit in a predictable duration) and resolution of certain types of EEG abnormalities. It is customary to plan on two years of seizure freedom and a normal EEG as the trigger to initiate a discussion about discontinuation of medication.
6. The value of anticonvulsant blood levels is considerable for patients receiving phenobarbital, phenytoin, carbamazepine, and ethosuximide (Table 14.12). Plasma levels of these drugs should be monitored regularly for the following reasons: (a) to establish the baseline effective blood level, (b) to evaluate potential causes for lack of efficacy (e.g., fast metabolizer, noncompliance), (c) to evaluate potential causes for toxicity (e.g., altered drug utilization, slow metabolizer, pathologic conditions such as uremia or hepatic disease), (d) to evaluate causes for loss of efficacy, and (e) for judging whether there is "room to move" or "time to change" (416). The relationship between drug dosage and blood levels is variable, particularly in the case of valproate, clonazepam, and phenytoin, and there is no correlation between valproate toxicity and serum levels (417). With respect to the newer anticonvulsants (felbamate, gabapentin, lamotrigine, levetiracetam, tiagabine, topiramate, vigabatrin, and zonisamide), there are at present few studies that correlate serum concentrations and effectiveness. The one exception to this is oxcarbazepine, for which there

TABLE 14.12 Which Anticonvulsants Should Be Monitored?

Drug	*Therapeutic levels*[a] *μmol/L (μg/mL)*	*Value Rating*[b]	*Comments*
Phenytoin	40–80 (10–20)	*****	Monitoring essential for good therapy. Accurate dosing difficult without serum levels because of saturable metabolism. Low therapeutic ratio, disguised toxicity, and frequency of drug interactions add weight to the case of routine monitoring.
Carbamazepine	20–40 (5–10)	***	Monitoring useful. Clinical symptoms (especially eye symptoms) are often helpful in determining dose limit, but water intoxication and increase in fit frequency may be caused by high serum level. Standardization of sampling time advisable.
Ethosuximide	350–750 (50–100)	***	Monitoring in children is less acceptable but can be helpful as a guide to correct dose.
Phenobarbital	70–180 (15–40)	**	Tolerance develops and, therefore, therapeutic range difficult to define.
Primidone (unchanged)		*	Phenobarbitone is major metabolite; therefore, this should be monitored if indicated. Occasional measurement of primidone useful in slow metabolizers.
Valproic acid	350–700 (50–100)	*	Timed specimens essential. Little evidence that management is improved by monitoring. Possibility of *hit and run* effect.
Clonazepam		*	Sedation is usually dose limiting; serum levels unhelpful because of development of receptor tolerance.

[a]Evidence for these ranges is, in some cases, inadequate.
[b]The greater the number of asterisks, the greater the value of monitoring.
From Richens A. *Textbook of epilepsy,* 4th ed. Edinburgh: Churchill, 1993. With permission.

appears to be a dose-response relationship at the doses used. With respect to gabapentin, the correlation between dose and blood levels is highly variable because of a saturable transporter needed for absorption that results in decreased bioavailability with increasing dosage. Therapeutic blood levels for the more commonly monitored anticonvulsants are listed in Table 14.12 (418–422). In clinical interpretation of blood anticonvulsant levels, the physician should remember Kutt's statement that there are "as many therapeutic plasma levels as there are patients," a statement that has been unalloyed by time (423). Whether drug levels should be determined routinely in seizure-free patients is a matter of some debate (424,425). Despite evidence that epileptic drug monitoring does not improve the overall degree of seizure control, we believe that the metabolic changes in a growing youngster who is receiving one of the readily monitored anticonvulsants dictate obtaining levels at regular intervals.

7. Routine hematologic and hepatic evaluations have been suggested on the assumption that the serious hematologic and hepatic abnormalities, which occasionally develop in patients receiving anticonvulsants, are preceded by an asymptomatic phase that can be detected by laboratory examinations. This is not the case, and we believe that there is little value in routine blood counts and liver function tests. Wyllie and Wyllie have pointed out that if every patient receiving anticonvulsants were to be monitored as suggested by the *Physicians' Desk Reference*, the annual costs of epileptic therapy would be astronomic (426).
8. Anticonvulsant medication should be withdrawn gradually. Sudden withdrawal of medication, particularly barbiturates, is one of the most common causes of status epilepticus.
9. The initial choice of an anticonvulsant should be based on the best available data on the efficacy for the specific epilepsy syndrome that is being treated, a consideration of the toxicities associated with the medications (idiosyncratic organ toxicities, treatment-emergent toxicities), with an appreciation of the comorbidities that may exist in the child with epilepsy and paying careful attention to the effect of the drug on cognition and behavior. One of us (R.S.) has completed a detailed review of this approach (427).

Mechanism of Action of Anticonvulsant Drugs: Cellular and Animal Models

The history of modern pharmacologic treatment of the epilepsies can be said to have started in the middle of the nineteenth century, when bromides were tried with some success for the control of convulsions. This approach predates the treatises on epilepsy by John Hughlings Jackson (2,96) and William Gowers (48). Bromides were first used in 1857 by Sir Charles Locock, Queen Victoria's physician accoucheur, in treating eclamptic seizures and catamenial seizures (427a).

Phenobarbital was adopted in 1912 after Hauptmann observed its ability to suppress seizures when he used it to sedate a ward of noisy psychiatric and epileptic patients during the night (427b). Introduction of more specific anticonvulsants for clinical application followed the availability of the first animal seizure model, the maximal electroshock (MES) model (428). The history and principles of the development of anticonvulsants has been reviewed by one of us (R.S.) (429).

As newer antiepileptic drugs with a variety of different mechanisms of action become available, it becomes important to categorize these agents in a manner consistent with preclinical and clinical pharmacology. Preclinical pharmacology involves an understanding of the cellular mechanisms of action, usually at the level of membrane ion channels. This information is correlated with the expression of seizures in animal models. Finally, the action of antiepileptic drugs at cellular and experimental levels must be correlated with their action in the epileptic patient. The principal molecular actions of the major anticonvulsants are presented in Table 14.13.

It is beyond the scope of this text to detail the large number of animal models that have been developed to study the various types of epilepsy; these have been reviewed by Fisher (430). Two models important in the development of antiepileptic drugs are the MES model, which is highly predictive of antiepileptic drug activity against tonic-clonic seizures, and the pentylenetetrazol or metrazol (MET) model, which is useful in the development of compounds with activity against absence seizures. The prototypical compounds active in the MES model are phenytoin and carbamazepine. The compound in current use that typifies activity in the MET model is ethosuximide. In our discussion, we categorize antiepileptic drugs according to their activity in the MES and MET animal models.

On a cellular level, the activity of antiepileptic drugs results from their action on cellular (neuronal) excitability, in particular, their effects on various ion channels, either directly or through a neurotransmitter system. These aspects are covered by Rho and Sankar in a current and comprehensive review (431).

Several antiepileptic drugs, classically phenytoin and carbamazepine, reduce sustained, high-frequency, repetitive firing (SRF) of cortical neurons in a use-dependent manner. This effect is attributable to the antagonism of Na^+ conductance in voltage-gated channels. Both phenytoin and carbamazepine are active in the MES model and are inactive in the MET animal model. They protect humans against tonic-clonic seizures but can exacerbate absence seizures. Use-dependent blockade of voltage-dependent sodium channels is demonstrated also by valproic acid, felbamate, lamotrigine, and topiramate.

TABLE 14.13 Principal Molecular Actions Of Clinically Important Anticonvulsants

	PHT CBZ	*BZD*	*PB*	*ESM*	*VPA*	*AZM*	*FBM*	*GBP*	*LTG*	*TPM*
Inhibits voltage-gated sodium channels	+				+		+		+	
Inhibits sodium currents through non-NMDA receptors										
Inhibits calcium currents through NMDA receptors							+			
Inhibits low-threshold T-type voltage-gated calcium channels				+	+?					
Enhances $GABA_A$-receptor mediated chloride currents		+	+				+			+
Inhibits presynaptic GABA reuptake										
Increases brain GABA by inhibiting GABA transaminase					+					
Increases brain GABA through unknown mechanisms								+		
Inhibits brain carbonic anhydrase activity						+				
Novel actions not yet clearly defined					+			+		
Decreases dendritic excitability									+	
Inhibits ligand-gated Na^+ channels to AMPA glutamate receptor										+

AZM, acetazolamide; BZD, benzodiazepines; CBZ, carbamazepine; ESM, ethosuximide; FBM, felbamate; GABA, γ-aminobutyric acid; GBP, gabapentin; NMDA, *N*-methyl-D-aspartate; PB, phenobarbital; PHT, phenytoin; LTG, lamotrigine; TPM, topiromate; VPA, valproic acid.

Trimethadione and ethosuximide possess the specific ability to block low-threshold T-type calcium currents exhibited by rhythmically firing thalamic neurons. This action of trimethadione and ethosuximide is attributed to their activity against MET-induced spike and wave epilepsy in animal models and may explain their activity against absence epilepsy. The newer anticonvulsant zonisamide has activity against both voltage-gated sodium channels and T-calcium channels.

Barbiturates and benzodiazepines function by enhancing GABA-mediated chloride currents and thus hyperpolarize the neuronal membrane. They bind to different sites on the GABA-receptor, chloride ionophore complex, and enhance the action of GABA. Benzodiazepines increase the frequency of channel openings, whereas barbiturates enhance the duration of an individual channel opening. Both felbamate and topiramate have the ability to enhance GABA-mediated Cl^- currents. The kinetics of felbamate action resemble that of barbiturates (432), whereas the kinetics of topiramate-induced Cl^- channel openings resemble that of benzodiazepines (433). The activity of topiramate at this site is not antagonized by the benzodiazepine antagonist flumazenil, suggesting that this is a novel site on this receptor-ionophore complex. However, the ability of topiramate to enhance GABA-mediated Cl^- currents is highly subunit-specific, and thus topiramate cannot be considered to have an effect resembling barbiturates or benzodiazepines in the forebrain. All such compounds tend to have some activity in both MES and MET models and tend to be active against a wide variety of human epilepsies.

Other ways exist to influence GABAergic activity than by direct binding to the GABA receptor. Tiagabine functions by antagonizing the reuptake of GABA, whereas vigabatrin, an investigational agent in the United States, functions by inhibiting GABA transaminase, the enzyme that inactivates GABA by converting it to succinic semialdehyde. The anticonvulsant effect of valproic acid is still unexplained, and at therapeutic dosages, its action on GABAergic systems is probably not significant.

It is appropriate at this juncture to distinguish between two distinct types of inhibition mediated by GABA receptors, based on their subunit composition and their anatomic localization to synaptic versus extrasynaptic sites. Recent studies suggest that α_4-containing $GABA_A$ receptors are predominantly extrasynaptic and may have their principal role in mediating tonic inhibition, rather than the better understood phasic inhibition resulting from presynaptically released GABA acting on postsynaptic receptors containing the α1-subunit (434). Further, these extrasynaptic receptors, which tend to contain the δ-subunit (rather than γ) along with α4 or α6, exhibit much higher affinity for GABA than those that mediate synaptic inhibition, and they do not inactivate rapidly like the latter. Thus, drugs that increase brain GABA may disproportionately increase tonic inhibition, promote synchronization, and may contribute to increased spike-wave incidence and duration. This might explain in part the clinical observation that vigabatrin and tiagabine exacerbate spike-wave epilepsies.

Several new anticonvulsants that act on the excitatory amino acid receptors and their associated ion channels are being developed, but to date, few have made it into clinical practice. Two antiepileptic drugs in current use have activity against excitatory amino acid sites. At least one mechanism of action of felbamate has been shown to involve a dose-dependent antagonism of ligand-gated calcium currents mediated by glutamate at the NMDA receptor (432,435). Topiramate, on the other hand, shows activity against Na^+ currents triggered by the binding of glutamate to non-NMDA receptors, such as the kainate- or AMPA-sensitive sites, in addition to its antagonism of voltage-gated Na^+ channels.

Several new targets for anticonvulsant action have been identified in recent years, many of which are discussed in greater detail by one of us (R.S.) recently (436,437). These include the discovery of the action of lamotrigine on HCN channels to increase dendritic $I_h$currents (438) and the novel targets for levetiracetam (439).

Levetiracetam has been shown to block synchronization in brain slice experiments in which conventional antiepileptic drugs (AED) such as valproic acid, benzodiazepines, and carbamazepine were inactive (440,441). Klitgaard and coworkers also have confirmed this finding by *in vivo* recordings in the rat pilocarpine model of temporal lobe epilepsy (441). This is quite exciting because conventional AEDs impact mainly neuronal hyperexcitability, even though the two *sine qua non* conditions of the epileptic state are hypersynchrony and hyperexcitability. How does levetiracetam accomplish this? Could it be antagonizing currents mediated by gap-junctions that are responsible for "local" synchrony? We do not know for certain.

Mossy fiber synapses release zinc, and zinc antagonizes GABA-mediated inhibition. Coulter and colleagues have shown that the GABA receptors in the granule cells of the epileptic hippocampus have undergone subunit changes that render them even more sensitive to the antagonism of GABAergic inhibition by zinc (442). Levetiracetam can reverse the inhibitory effect of zinc on GABA-mediated currents (443). This observation is one possible explanation for how levetiracetam may be ineffective in acute seizure models and yet antagonize seizure activity in chronic models.

A synaptic vesicle protein has been identified as a neuronal binding site for levetiracetam (444), and the affinity to this site seems to correlate with the ability to block audiogenic seizures.

Selection of Anticonvulsant

Since 1993, eight new anticonvulsant drugs have become available in the United States. As a consequence, deciding which drug to use to treat a patient with a seizure disorder has become more difficult. In part, the choice is dictated by the type of seizure or epilepsy syndrome. Preferred drugs are presented in Table 14.14.

At the time of the first visit of a patient with recurrent seizures, we have made it a practice to outline in the chart the proposed course of therapy and the drugs we intend to use in order of preference.

Phenobarbital. Phenobarbital is an effective anticonvulsant in the treatment of generalized tonic-clonic (grand mal) and simple partial (focal) seizures. The therapeutic dosage of phenobarbital varies from patient to patient. Therefore, we prefer to start at approximately 4 to 5 mg/kg per day, given in two divided doses. Svensmark and Buchthal have shown that in most patients with major motor seizures controlled by phenobarbital, the drug was effective at serum levels of 10 to 15 μg/mL. These levels were achieved by an oral dose of 2 to 3 mg/kg in children weighing 10 to 20 kg and approximately 2 mg/kg in larger children (445).

Toxic levels of phenobarbital vary between individuals, but generally, no permanent sedation is seen with levels below 35 μg/mL. There is considerable variability in the extent of tolerance that develops with prolonged use of the drug. In some instances, the administration of phenobarbital induces an elevation of transaminase activity. As confirmed by electron microscopy on liver biopsies, this elevation is the consequence of enzyme induction, rather than cellular damage (446).

The major side reactions encountered with phenobarbital are drowsiness and hyperactivity; however, the long-term effect of phenobarbital and the other anticonvulsants on intellectual performance is a matter of much debate. As documented by PET scanning, performed before and after withdrawal of therapeutic doses, phenobarbital produces a significant (37%) reduction in local glucose cerebral metabolism (447). Some authors have found that the drug induces a major depressive disorder (448), disturbances in sleep, fussiness, and impaired concentration, whereas others, confirming an initial impairment in cognitive functions, show that these side effects disappear after the first year of therapy (449,450). Mitchell and coworkers found that when phenobarbital levels were in the middle of the therapeutic range, there was little dose-dependent effect on reaction time, attention, and impulsivity (451). Farwell and colleagues, in a double-blind, counter-balanced, crossover study of children receiving

TABLE 14.14 Summary of Pediatric Epilepsy Syndromes and Treatments

Syndrome	*Treatment*
Neonatal seizures	Phenobarbital and phenytoin commonly used, but more than 50% of cases do not respond to either drug used alone, and potential adverse effects on the immature brain are a concern. There are only anecdotal reports of nasogastric or oral use of topiramate or levetiracetam in neonates.
Febrile convulsions	Long-term prophylactic therapy after simple febrile seizures is not recommended. Families can be advised to have rectal diazepam available for use as needed.
Infantile spasms	See text.
Lennox-Gastaut syndrome	Lamotrigine and topiramate are broad-spectrum AEDs with demonstrated efficacy in Lennox-Gastaut syndrome in clinical trials. Lamotrigine may exacerbate myoclonic seizures in some patients. Therapy can begin with topiramate, and low to moderate doses of lamotrigine may then be considered for synergistic action.
BECTS (rolandic epilepsy)	Carbamazepine is commonly used. Gabapentin was shown to be efficacious in one controlled trial and may be first choice because of lack of toxicity compared with carbamazepine. Sulthiame also efficacious in a controlled trial but not available in United States.
Childhood and juvenile absence epilepsy	Ethosuximide, valproic acid, and lamotrigine are commonly used; insufficient evidence is available to guide choice in clinical practice. Initial choice may be based on perception of tolerability, potential cognitive effects and systemic toxicity, and urgency of need for rapid control.
Juvenile myoclonic epilepsy	Valproic acid is currently the drug of choice. Among newer agents, there is evidence of effectiveness of lamotrigine as monotherapy and of topiramate as adjunctive therapy (with insufficient data to evaluate topiramate monotherapy).
Partial seizures	Phenytoin rarely used as first-line agent in children because of toxicity. Carbamazepine considered an acceptable first drug by many, followed by oxacarbazepine, lamotrigine, or topiramate, with choice based on tolerability and comorbidities.
Generalized tonic-clonic (GTC) seizures	Strongest evidence favors topiramate among the newer AEDs. Two studies have shown efficacy of the older AEDs in pediatric patients, and one trial showed equivalent efficacy of oxcarbazepine and phenytoin. Lamotrigine was shown to be efficacious for GTC seizures in Lennox-Gastaut syndrome. One trial showing equivalent efficacy of topiramate, valproic acid, and carbamazepine included children with GTC seizures. Selection may be shaped by tolerability and comorbidities in the individual patient.

AAN, American Academy of Neurology; CNS, Child Neurology Society; ACTH, adrenocorticotropic hormone; BECTS, benign epilepsy of childhood with centrotemporal spikes; AED, antiepileptic drug.
From Sankar R. Initial treatment of epilepsy with antiepileptic drugs. *Neurology* 2004;63[Suppl 4]:S30–S39. With permission.

phenobarbital for prevention of febrile convulsions, found that children receiving phenobarbital performed significantly poorer than patients receiving placebo in measurements of cognitive function and behavior (452). These observations are supported by a study of de Silva and colleagues, who found that 60% of children receiving phenobarbital for the treatment of generalized tonic-clonic or partial seizures developed side effects leading to drug withdrawal. This was in contrast to 4% to 9% of unacceptable side effects for phenytoin, carbamazepine, or sodium valproate (453).

Methylphenobarbital. Methylphenobarbital has been used in the place of phenobarbital because it was believed to have fewer side effects. Because methylphenobarbital is demethylated to phenobarbital in the liver, we would not expect it to have any advantages over phenobarbital in terms of seizure control.

Primidone. In the past, primidone was used as an effective anticonvulsant for generalized tonic-clonic, simple partial seizures and complex partial seizures. Unlike phenobarbitol, primidone, by itself, has no effect on postsynaptic GABA responses on Cl^- currents. It behaves much like phenytoin in abolishing sustained, repetitive firing in cultured neurons, presumably antagonizing Na^+ currents. Because of the marked sedation that often occurs when the drug is started, primidone has fallen into disfavor, and currently, it is not considered a first-line choice for any particular pediatric epilepsy syndrome and is mainly used for the treatment of familial tremor (see Chapter 3).

Phenytoin. Phenytoin is as effective as phenobarbital and carbamazepine in controlling tonic-clonic seizures. It has, however, lost considerable favor as a long-term anticonvulsant for use in pediatric practice because of the wide variability in its absorption, the effect of other anticonvulsants and even mild intercurrent illnesses on its rate of metabolism, and the relatively high incidence of adverse reactions (454).

Depending on the size of the child, the average effective dose of phenytoin is 5 to 10 mg/kg per day, with clinically effective phenytoin levels ranging from 10 to 20 μg/mL. The drug is slowly absorbed from the gastrointestinal tract, and at a dose of 4 to 6 mg/kg per day, equilibrium levels in the blood are established between 7 and 10 days after initiation of therapy (455). The daily fluctuations in serum concentrations in children who weigh less than 30 kg are sufficiently large to require the drug to be administered at approximately 8-hour intervals (456). Phenytoin is metabolized in the liver, mainly by the P450 mixed function oxidase system, which hydroxylates the drug at the para-position (457). Phenytoin produces a number of untoward reactions; in many instances, these are related to overdosage and can be relieved by reducing the drug intake.

Nystagmus at lateral gaze appears with blood levels of 15 to 30 μg/mL, ataxia appears at above 30 μg/mL, and lethargy or aggravation of seizures appears at levels of 40 μg/mL or higher (458). Irreversible degeneration of the cerebellar Purkinje cells can occur after chronic intoxication or severe acute intoxication (459), and cerebellar atrophy has been demonstrable by imaging studies.

The rate of phenytoin metabolism varies considerably and appears to be under polygenetic control. Small infants eliminate only 1% to 20% of the drug in a 24-hour period and often develop toxic side effects (456).

One of the major drawbacks of phenytoin therapy is a long and worrisome list of common side reactions.

Approximately 2% to 5% of patients receiving phenytoin develop fever, a morbilliform rash, and lymphadenopathy within 2 weeks of the start of therapy. The drug is known to induce a variety of severe hypersensitivity reactions, including antinuclear antibodies, a lupuslike disease, and Stevens-Johnson syndrome (460). Antinuclear antibodies have been detected not only in patients receiving phenytoin, but also in those receiving phenobarbital or ethosuximide exclusively. According to Kapur and associates, 93% of patients with phenytoin levels between 10 and 20 μg/mL develop gum hyperplasia, and 75% of patients develop hirsutism (461). Gum hyperplasia can be reduced by strict oral hygiene, daily gum massage, and repeated excision of hyperplastic tissue. Coarsening of facial features and increased skin pigmentation are other, relatively common, adverse effects of phenytoin therapy. Patients on prolonged phenytoin therapy can develop megaloblastic anemia and lowered serum folate concentrations, which respond to folic acid therapy (462,463). Although prolonged folate deficiency can induce an organic brain syndrome in the absence of subacute combined degeneration of the cord, folate therapy has no effect on the behavior or mental function of chronic epileptic patients (464).

A disturbed vitamin D metabolism resulting in hypocalcemic rickets, decreased serum calcium and phosphorus, and increased alkaline phosphatase is seen in some ambulatory, noninstitutionalized patients after long-term therapy with phenytoin, primidone, or phenobarbital (465,466). Peripheral neuropathy also can result from prolonged anticonvulsant therapy. Deep tendon reflexes are lost in approximately one-half of patients receiving phenytoin for longer than 15 years (467).

The teratogenic effect of phenytoin and other anticonvulsants has attracted considerable attention. As delineated by Hanson and Smith (468), the fetal hydantoin syndrome is characterized by intrauterine and postnatal growth deficiency, mental retardation, hypoplasia of the distal phalanges with small nails, ocular hypertelorism, a low and broad nasal bridge, and a bowed upper lip. Studies on offspring of mothers who were receiving mainly phenytoin monotherapy and whose blood levels were carefully monitored and maintained in the low therapeutic range found a 1% to 2% risk of serious developmental anomalies, a value slightly greater than the risk in the general population (469). The suggestion that mutations in the gene for microsomal epoxide hydrolase are responsible for anticonvulsant teratogenicity or hypersensitivity reactions has not been confirmed. It is nevertheless the present consensus that not only phenytoin, but other hydantoins, as well as phenobarbital, valproate, and carbamazepine, increase the incidence of fetal malformations, particularly when combinations of anticonvulsants are being used (470,471).

Mephenytoin. Mephenytoin, which is chemically related to phenytoin, was once used in the treatment of generalized tonic-clonic and complex partial seizures. Unlike phenytoin, it did not appear to cause hirsutism, gingival hyperplasia, or many of the cerebellar deficits associated with the use of phenytoin (472).

Carbamazepine. Carbamazepine is an iminostilbene, chemically unrelated to any of the other major anticonvulsants. It appears to function by antagonizing sodium currents in a manner similar to phenytoin (473).

Children with complex partial and tonic-clonic seizures are most likely to benefit from the drug (474). The starting dosage in children aged 6 to 12 years is 10 to 25 mg/kg per day, and maximum dosage for effective seizure control in that age range is approximately 600 to 800 mg per day. The suggested starting dosage for children younger than 6 years of age is 10 mg/kg per day. Although optimal therapeutic levels are generally stated to be between 4 and 12 μg/mL (475), carbamazepine-plasma protein binding and the conversion of carbamazepine to a pharmacologically active 10,11-epoxide, which cannot readily be assayed, complicate the interpretation of serum concentrations in children (476). Ratios of carbamazepine to its epoxide range from 4 to 1 in children receiving carbamazepine monotherapy to 3 to 1 in those receiving other anticonvulsants as well (474). The ratio between the epoxide and carbamazepine tends to decrease with increasing age (477). The ratio between the dosage of carbamazepine and the blood concentration is linear for any given child, but the ratio varies considerably among children. On the average, dosage increments of 2 mg/kg increase carbamazepine concentration by 1 μg/mL (474). The drug is given two to four times daily. Two sustained-release preparations, Tegretol-XR and Carbatrol, are available in the United States. The latter is a sprinkle preparation. Oxcarbazepine, a keto-substituted analogue, has a pharmacologic spectrum and potency similar to that of carbamazepine but a lower incidence of side reactions (478).

Clearance of carbamazepine increases for the first month after initiation of therapy as a consequence of induction of the metabolic enzymes. When carbamazepine is used in conjunction with another drug, notably valproic acid, protein binding is decreased, with an ensuing increase in unbound carbamazepine and toxicity at lower blood levels (474). Since valproic acid is an inhibitor of epoxide hydrolase and of UDP-glucuronyl transferase, the concentration of the carbamazepine-10,11-epoxide tends to increase, further contributing to neurotoxicity.

Diplopia is the most common side reaction encountered in patients receiving carbamazepine. It can disappear spontaneously or after reduction of drug dosage. Lesser and coworkers, however, found no clear relationship between such toxic side effects and either free or total plasma carbamazepine levels (414). Transient drowsiness, incoordination, and vertigo can be seen with initiation of therapy or when the dosage is increased too rapidly (479).

Other side reactions include a variety of rashes, hyponatremia, hepatic dysfunction, and leukopenia (480). Rashes are undoubtedly the most common and were encountered in 5% of children in the series of Pellock (479). Hyponatremia is believed to result from an antidiuretic effect of carbamazepine or an excessive release of antidiuretic hormone. It is usually mild and reversible with fluid restriction (481). A stable, nonprogressive leukopenia is not rare. In the series of Pellock, a leukopenia of less than 4,000 per μL was seen in 12.7% of children; only 2.3% had counts below 3,000 (479). These cases of leukopenia were not progressive and therefore did not require discontinuation of the drug; blood counts reversed spontaneously in 75% of children. In some of these patients, a minor viral illness can induce the decrease in the number of white cells. The experiences of Camfield and coworkers have been similar. In their series, 9% of children on carbamazepine also had an elevated aspartate aminotransferase level (482). Isolated cases of rash followed by acute hepatic failure during the first few weeks of carbamazepine therapy have been reported, as have a few instances of systemic lupus erythematosus (483).

Administration of therapeutic doses of carbamazepine to children with atypical absence and other minor motor seizures can aggravate the seizure disorder or induce absence status; less often a continuous, nonepileptic myoclonus is seen (484,485). Less commonly encountered side reactions include dystonic movements. The concurrent administration of other drugs can induce carbamazepine neurotoxicity by inhibiting its metabolism. These drugs include calcium channel blockers such as diltiazem and verapamil, propoxyphene hydrochloride, isoniazid, and erythromycin (486).

Despite the various potential side reactions, carbamazepine has the advantage over phenobarbital or phenytoin in that it improves cognitive functions and makes patients feel brighter and more alert (451,487). Additionally, behavior was thought to be improved in 15% of children in Pellock's series (479). The experience of Forsythe and his group differs from these studies, in that patients receiving carbamazepine monotherapy demonstrated impairment in recent recall and slowed information processing at therapeutic drug levels (488). The most recent studies performed on well-controlled epileptic patients show that carbamazepine induces small long-term neurocognitive impairment (489).

We therefore conclude that carbamazepine does result in slight cognitive impairment, which is often counterbalanced by the improvement induced by seizure control.

Generic substitution for carbamazepine raises problems in patients in whom the therapeutic to toxic window is narrow because of the reduced shelf-life of some products and a relatively large range in bioavailability of the various generic preparations. These concerns have been reviewed by Nuwer and colleagues (490). Grapefruit juice, which inhibits carbamazepine metabolism by P-450 isozyme, can induce significant increases in drug levels and effects (491).

Oxcarbazepine. Oxcarbazepine, a keto-substituted, saturated analogue of carbamazepine that is devoid of the ability to be transformed to the 10,11-epxide, has a pharmacologic spectrum and potency similar to that of carbamazepine, but a lower incidence of side reactions (478). In a series of well-controlled studies, its effectiveness in controlling partial seizures and primary generalized tonic clonic seizures was found to be equivalent to phenytoin, valproic acid, and carbamazepine. French and the members of the Therapeutics and Technology Subcommittee of the American Academy of Neurology and the American Epilepsy Society have concluded that oxcarbazepine was equivalent to phenytoin and carbamazepine in terms of efficacy, but superior in dose-related tolerance, and equivalent in both efficacy and tolerability to valproate (492). Like carbamazepine, it can induce hyponatremia by a mechanism that is as yet unexplained (493).

Ethosuximide. Ethosuximide has a long history as a specifically antiabsence drug. In experimental models, the drug blocks pentylenetetrazol-induced seizures. Starting dosages for children are 250 mg twice daily or 20 mg/kg per day. Optimal therapeutic plasma levels are between 40 and 100 μg/mL (420). We use ethosuximide by itself in the treatment of absence attacks unless the patient has had a history of other seizure types, in which case valproate or lamotrigine monotherapy can be used.

Phenytoin, which increases the frequency of absence attacks, should not be used in the patient with combined major and absence seizures. Side effects of ethosuximide are generally minor. They include gastrointestinal upsets, usually during the first few days of drug therapy, skin rashes, headaches, and, occasionally, hematologic abnormalities, principally a reversible leukopenia (420).

Trimethadione. Until the introduction of ethosuximide in 1958, trimethadione had been the drug of choice in the treatment of absence attacks. Like ethosuximide, it blocks pentylenetetrazol seizures. Its tendency to predispose patients to major motor seizures and the induction of bone marrow depression in approximately 5% of patients made it inferior to ethosuximide.

Valproic Acid. Since its introduction into clinical practice in the 1970s, valproic acid (VPA), either as its sodium or magnesium salt or as a free acid, has proven highly effective for all seizure types (494).

The exact mechanism of drug action is unknown, and the drug probably acts through a combination of several mechanisms (495). VPA increases GABA synthesis and release and reduces the release of the epileptogenic amino acid γ-hydroxybutyric acid. It also is believed to potentiate the postsynaptic GABA inhibitory effect, block spike generation, and inhibit the excitatory neuronal pathways (496,497). It also may inhibit GABA-transaminase and succinic semialdehyde dehydrogenase activities and thus elevate GABA concentrations in CSF and within the brain. There is, however, considerable doubt whether increased GABA concentrations are important for anticonvulsant action because VPA demonstrates an antiepileptic effect before brain GABA levels increase. Modulation of the low-threshold calcium current could be one way that VPA disrupts generalized spike and wave discharges (498).

Starting dosages for children are 15 to 20 mg/kg per day given two to three times a day, with the dose increased at weekly intervals to an amount that provides seizure control, usually in the range of 20 to 70 mg/kg per day. Serum VPA levels and anticonvulsant action are poorly correlated, and there is considerable fluctuation in VPA levels because of the short half-life. Even though several authorities consider 50 to 100 μg/mL to represent optimal drug levels, we have found that fasting VPA levels are not reproducible and only monitor VPA concentrations to verify compliance. Bourgeois (499) and a *Lancet* editorial (500) have taken the same position.

The dose-serum concentration relationship is complex, in part because of the short half-life of VPA, and in part because of its high degree of plasma protein binding. At low plasma VPA levels, protein binding is 90% to 95%, but with increasing dosages, the proportion of VPA bound to protein decreases progressively, and as a consequence, the total serum concentration of VPA does not increase in proportion to the dose (419). The concentration of valproate in brain tissue resected from patients with chronic epilepsy is extremely low. In part, the low concentrations reflect the fact that valproate is not bound to lipids; in part, they can be accounted for by gliosis in the surgical specimens (501).

Although the plasma half-life is short (i.e., 6 to 15 hours when VPA is administered alone, and even less when VPA is given in combination with other anticonvulsants), the practice of administering the drug in two to four daily doses might not be required; twice-daily administration of enteric-coated VPA or once-daily divalproex sodium extended-release tablets appears to provide equally good seizure control (502). Absorption of VPA sprinkles is slower but is as complete as the syrup. Because there is less fluctuation in the serum levels, this preparation of VPA can be given every 12 hours (503).

With the widespread use of VPA, numerous adverse effects have been encountered. The majority of these are listed in Table 14.15. The most common of these are a variety of gastrointestinal upsets (494). In part, these can be

TABLE 14.15 Adverse Effects of Valproic Acid Therapy

Neurologic
Tremor
Asterixis
Drowsiness, lethargy, confusion
Reversible dementia
Nonconvulsive status epilepticus
Gastrointestinal
Nausea, vomiting, anorexia
Weight gain
Abdominal pain
Hepatotoxicity
Pancreatitis
Elevated serum amylase
Parotid gland swelling
Hematologic
Thrombocytopenia
Decreased platelet aggregation
Reduced factor VIII/von Willebrand factor complex
Metabolic/endocrinologic
Hyperammonemia
Hypocarnitinemia
Hyperglycinemia
Polycystic ovaries
Menstrual irregularities
Fanconi syndrome
Miscellaneous
Hair loss and changes in hair texture
Edema of face and limbs
Teratogenicity
Hypoplasia of midface
Neural tube defects
Mental retardation

reduced by taking the medication after meals, by a gradual increase in dosage, or by the use of an enteric-coated preparation. Increased appetite is another common side reaction, seen in 11% of patients receiving enteric-coated VPA in the Collaborative Study Group (504). Wirrell has noted mild to moderate weight gain in 58% of children placed on VPA, with the only predictor of significant weight gain being children who are already overweight or who have the potential for weight gain at initiation of therapy (505). We have noted that significant weight gain is encountered in the patients who respond best to the drug. Thinning of hair is encountered less often (1% of patients in the Collaborative Study Group).

The effects of VPA on liver function have generated serious concern (499,506). Dose-related elevations of liver enzymes are seen in up to 44% of patients receiving VPA as the sole anticonvulsant. Usually, these abnormalities are transient or resolve with dosage reduction. Far more serious is a Reye syndrome–like hepatic failure usually encountered during the first 3 months of therapy. This complication is unrelated to VPA dosage, and its incidence is highest (1 in 543) in children younger than 2 years of age receiving polytherapy (506). Infants with mental retardation and those with medical conditions other than epilepsy are particularly prone to fatal hepatic failure. Children younger than 2 years of age who were on monotherapy had an incidence of 1 in 8,213, whereas those older than 2 years of age on monotherapy had an incidence of 1 in 45,000 (507). In the United Kingdom's surveillance of fatal suspected adverse drug reactions for the years 1964 to 2000, there were 64 fatalities due to anticonvulsant therapy. Of these, 30 were caused by hepatic failure. VPA monotherapy was implicated in 21 of these cases and VPA polytherapy in another 2 cases (508).

The cause for VPA-induced acute hepatic failure is still unclear, although an unsaturated metabolite of VPA, 2-n-propyl-4-pentenoic acid, is believed to be indirectly responsible. This substance inhibits hepatic cytochrome P450, inhibits fatty acid b-oxidation, and induces hepatic microvesicular steatosis, the characteristic cellular abnormality in VPA-induced liver injury. Liver microsomes from phenobarbital-treated rats catalyzed the desaturation of VPA to 2-n-propyl-4-pentenoic acid, implying that patients who concurrently receive VPA and phenobarbital are at particular risk for hepatic failure (509). Inasmuch as 2-n-propyl-4-pentenoic acid is seen in approximately 10% of children on VPA, its presence cannot be used to predict fatal hepatotoxicity (510). In any case, there is no continuum between those patients who show an elevation in serum liver enzymes and those who develop hepatic failure. Thus, routine monitoring of liver function does not prevent hepatic failure (511). Treatment with L-carnitine, preferably given intravenously, appears to provide the best chance for survival in VPA-induced hepatotoxicity (512). There is no evdience that carnitine supplementation prevents hepatic dysfunction or failure (513,514). Many pediatric neurologists will, however, give carnitine to infants and young children on VPA therapy.

We should point out that valproate hepatotoxicity should be distinguished from the syndrome of progressive cerebral degeneration, which is associated with liver disease (see Chapter 3) (515). Adverse effects of VPA are not limited to the liver, and microvesicular lipid droplets also are seen between myofibrils near mitochondria (516).

Hyperammonemia is a common accompaniment of VPA therapy. Laub encountered fasting ammonia levels between 33 and 143 μg/mL in otherwise asymptomatic patients receiving therapeutic dosages of VPA. Following protein load, ammonia levels rose even further (58 to 426 μg/mL). There is no correlation between elevated ammonia levels and hepatic failure, and finding high blood ammonia should not prompt discontinuation of VPA therapy (517).

Sedation owing to VPA is seen in some 10% of patients (504). When it occurs, it is self-limiting and is often attributable to other, concurrently administered anticonvulsants. Episodes of stupor also have been encountered. These are almost invariably seen in children being treated for complex partial seizures with VPA, either exclusively or in combination with other anticonvulsants (518). Whether hyperammonemia has a role in the development of stupor is unclear (519). What has been amply demonstrated, however, is that VPA elevates serum levels of a variety of other anticonvulsants, notably phenobarbital (520), ethosuximide (521), primidone, and carbamazepine, and markedly increases the half-life of lamotrigine. VPA lowers total phenytoin concentrations, but by displacing phenytoin from its plasma binding sites, it increases the proportion of free phenytoin; thus, toxicity is encountered at lower phenytoin levels (522). The combination of VPA and clonazepam has strong hypnotic effects, and in some instances, it induces absence status.

Tremor and asterixis have been encountered in patients receiving VPA (494). We, and others, have seen that in most instances, tremor develops only at doses greater than 40 to 50 mg/kg per day and is reduced or cleared by lowering the dosage (523). Some of these children have a family history of essential tremor. Asterixis is rare and is associated with polytherapy (524). A decrease in platelet count, which is often transient, also is dose related. It appears to have an autoimmune basis and, in general, is not sufficiently severe to require reduction or withdrawal of VPA. The thrombocytopenia can be aggravated with infections and at such times can result in bruising or minor bleeding phenomena (525). In a large proportion of children receiving VPA, one observes a reduction in factor VIII/von Willebrand factor complex. This results in a prolonged bleeding time, but aside from nosebleeds, or mild bleeding from the gums or skin, this defect is generally asymptomatic. It is unrelated to VPA dosage or whether the child is on monotherapy or polytherapy (526). Many epilepsy centers discontinue VPA before surgical procedures. Ward and coworkers, however, have shown that surgical blood loss in the course of temporal lobectomy was no greater in patients receiving VPA than in those who were not (527).

Much rarer side reactions to VPA therapy include hyperglycinemia (528) and pancreatitis (529,530). Hyperglycinemia is believed to be caused by inhibition of the glycine cleavage system by valproic acid, valproyl-CoA, or both (528). Pancreatitis manifests by epigastric pain, nausea, and vomiting. It is unrelated to dosage but is more commonly encountered in patients who are on polytherapy. In most instances, this complication develops during the first few months of therapy. In the series of Asconape, an asymptomatic elevation of serum amylase levels was seen in 11% of patients receiving valproate (531). Edema of face and limbs has been encountered in children receiving valproate for more than a year. The reason for this complication is not clear (532). One of us (J.H.M.) has seen asymptomatic but persistent bilateral parotid gland swelling with elevation of serum amylase.

A variety of endocrine disorders has been described. These include centripetal obesity and menstrual disorders. In women who have been on long-term VPA therapy, obesity, polycystic ovaries, and hyperandrogenism are a frequent occurrence (533).

VPA therapy lowers serum free carnitine levels, although the exact mechanism is still unclear. Valproic acid, a C8 fatty acid, forms carnitine esters that are readily excreted in urine. Additionally, VPA reduces hepatic β-oxidation of fatty acids, which are then excreted as acylated carnitine. There is no correlation between VPA dosage and carnitine levels or between carnitine and ammonia levels. Because children with low carnitine levels are asymptomatic, dietary carnitine supplementation is not required (514), and in a double-blind, placebo-controlled study, the administration of carnitine in children receiving VPA monotherapy or polytherapy was no more effective than placebo in relieving nonspecific symptoms such as hypotonia and lethargy (534).

Maternal intake of VPA increases significantly the likelihood of congenital malformations in offspring (535). Affected infants have a characteristic facial appearance with trigonocephaly, a small and broad nose, small ears, medial deficits of eyebrows, anteverted nares, and a shallow philtrum. Gross abnormalities of the brain and neural tube defects are less common (536,537).

Despite these side reactions, VPA is an excellent anticonvulsant, not only because it provides better seizure control, but because it does so without sedating the child. Nevertheless, patients on this drug should be seen by a physician at regular intervals, and routine blood studies, particularly platelet counts, should be obtained at every visit. Whether liver function tests are needed is more problematic.

Benzodiazepine Anticonvulsants. Several benzodiazepine agents are used in the treatment of epilepsy. In experimental models, all of them have been shown to enhance the GABA-mediated chloride currents.

Clonazepam. In our experience, clonazepam is an effective anticonvulsant for most types of minor motor seizures. It is instituted in gradually increasing dosages beginning at 0.05 mg/kg per day in three or four divided doses and increased by 0.05 mg/kg every fifth to seventh day until seizures are controlled or until a dose of 0.25 mg/kg is reached. Thereafter, the dose is increased more slowly to 0.5 mg/kg if needed or until side effects are encountered. Side effects include ataxia, drowsiness, dysarthria, irritability or belligerence, and excessive weight gain (538,539). Emotional disturbances that occur commonly with this drug are often aggravated when it is combined with barbiturates or other benzodiazepines (540). Although seizure control is exceedingly good when clonazepam is first initiated, the drug's effectiveness is lost within a few weeks or months in approximately one-third to one-half of subjects. Olsen suggested that the receptor-chloride channel complex is directly involved in the development of tolerance, or that an endogenous benzodiazepine antagonist is produced (135). Clonazepam is most effective in akinetic seizures and atypical petit mal. It is ineffective for infantile spasms.

Nitrazepam. Nitrazepam, a benzodiazepine, which differs from clonazepam by its lack of a chlorine atom, is an effective anticonvulsant for the Lennox-Gastaut syndrome, generalized tonic-clonic, myoclonic, atypical absence, and partial seizures (541,542). It also is as effective as ACTH for acute treatment of infantile spasms (543). Because elevated hepatic enzymes are seen in approximately one-half of patients, its use has been restricted in the United States to compassionate grounds. The drug is readily available in Europe and Latin America, however. Nitrazepam induces cricopharyngeal incoordination with impaired swallowing and aspiration. Its use has been coupled with sudden death probably caused by aspiration in infants who were on dosages higher than 0.8 mg/kg per day and who had intractable epilepsy (544,545).

Clorazepate. Clorazepate appears to be another potentially useful benzodiazepine for the treatment of various seizure disorders. Clorazepate is a prodrug. It is converted to *N*-desmethyldiazepam, a long-acting metabolite, whose half-life has been estimated to be between 30 and 150 hours (546). Its usefulness as an adjunctive agent in a variety of seizure types has been reported, and the data has been summarized by Ko and colleagues (547). In our service at UCLA, we have used it as a well-tolerated adjunct in refractory patients and as monotherapy in treating transient seizure problems in organ transplant recipients to avoid pharmacokinetic interactions of antiepileptic drugs with drugs used to prevent rejection of transplanted organs. The latter use is being replaced with gabapentin.

Midazolam. The use of midazolam for the treatment of acute seizures and status epilepticus is increasing (548–550). The recommended dose is 0.15 to 0.2 mg/kg per minute initially, followed by 1 to 7 μg/kg per minute. Compared with barbiturates, which are mitochondrial toxins at high doses, the use of midazolam in the induction of coma is likely to result in much less cardiac toxicity that necessitates the use of pressors and inotropes to support the patient. O'Regan and colleagues have described the intranasal use of midazolam to treat acute seizures successfully in the emergency department (551). Chamberlain and associates found that intramuscular use of midazolam achieved a more rapid cessation of seizures in an emergency room setting than diazepam administered after placement of intravenous access (552).

Diazepam and Lorazepam. Diazepam and lorazepam are used mainly for the treatment of status epilepticus and febrile convulsions. They are discussed under these sections. We have had no experience with other benzodiazepines, notably clobazam, which is being used extensively in Europe and Canada. In the experience of the Canadian Study Group, clobazam is as effective as carbamazepine or phenytoin for the treatment of partial and some generalized childhood epilepsies, with no greater adverse cognitive effects than are encountered with carbamazepine (553,554).

Acetazolamide. Acetazolamide has been viewed favorably as an anticonvulsant in the treatment of refractory childhood seizures, including absence seizures, menstruation-related generalized seizures, and complex partial seizures, by a group of epileptologists, notably Millichap (555). Because of tolerance, it usually becomes ineffective with prolonged use. In menstruation-related generalized seizures, we start the drug approximately 5 to 10 days before the expected menses and continue it until its end.

Felbamate. Felbamate is effective in both the MET and MES animal models. It also inhibits NMDA currents and facilitates GABA currents. Up to 1994, the drug had been used widely as an add-on anticonvulsant or as monotherapy for both refractory partial-onset seizures and the Lennox-Gastaut syndrome (556,557). The drug is started at 15 mg/kg per day in three to four divided doses, with the dose increased by 15 mg/kg per day at weekly intervals to 45 mg/kg per day or higher (up to 200 mg/kg per day) should there be no clinical response and no adverse reactions. Valproate, phenytoin, and carbamazepine epoxide steady-state plasma concentrations increase with the addition of felbamate; therefore, when felbamate is used as adjunctive therapy, the present antiepileptic drug dosage is reduced by approximately 20%, and plasma levels of the other anticonvulsant should be verified during the initial stages of felbamate treatment.

Several cases of a sometimes irreversible aplastic anemia, some in patients on felbamate monotherapy, have been reported. The incidence of this complication in approximately 1 in 10,000 patients is far higher than background incidence of aplastic anemia. Thompson and colleagues have suggested that some patients may have an increased propensity to form a reactive metabolite, 3-carbamoyl-2-phenylpropionaldehyde, which is readily transformed to atropaldehyde, a compound proposed to play a role in the development of toxicity during felbamate therapy (558). In addition, several cases of severe and sometimes fatal hepatotoxicity have been encountered, with the overall risk being about the same as that associated with valproate (559). As a consequence of these adverse reactions, the use of felbamate has been restricted to patients who absolutely require this drug for seizure control. Other, less severe reactions seen in children include rash, insomnia, and loss of appetite. The American Academy of Neurology has recommended the use of felbamate for patients with the Lennox-Gastaut syndrome who are older than 4 years of age, and who have been unresponsive to primary antiepileptic drugs. The drug is recommended also for intractable partial seizures in patients older than age 18 years who have failed standard antiepileptic drug therapy. The drug may be continued in those patients who have been receiving it for more than 18 months. The use of felbamate is optional in children with intractable partial epilepsy, primary generalized epilepsy unresponsive to primary anticonvulsants, children younger than 4 years of age with Lennox-Gastaut syndrome, and in those patients who experience unacceptable sedative or cognitive side effects with traditional antiepileptic drugs (560).

Gabapentin. Although designed as a GABA agonist, the mode of action of this anticonvulsant, a structural analogue of GABA, is still uncertain. Significant elevations in brain GABA levels as measured by MR spectroscopy have been demonstrated in epileptic patients treated with gabapentin (561). Binding to the $\alpha 2/\delta$ subunit of the voltage-activated calcium channel also has been demonstrated. The drug is effective for monotherapy in newly diagnosed epilepsy at dosages of 900 mg and 1800 mg per day (562). It also is effective in reducing seizure frequency as adjunctive therapy in patients with refractory partial seizures but is no more active than placebo in monotherapy for refractory partial seizures (563,564). Gabapentin is usually given to adults in dosages of 2,400 to 3,600 mg per day, but much higher dosages appear to be well tolerated. To date, reported side effects include somnolence, fatigue, dizziness, and weight gain (492,564,565). The advantages of gabapentin are that it is not bound by plasma albumin, does not undergo hepatic metabolism, and does not induce cytochrome P450 isoenzymes. Therefore, it can be added to other regimens without concern regarding pharmacokinetic interactions. It also is devoid of problems with hypersensitivity reactions and bone marrow toxicity.

Based on experience with animal models (566), gabapentin should not be used in primary generalized spike-wave epilepsies. This is confirmed by its lack of efficacy in absence seizures (567) and its exacerbation of symptomatic generalized epilepsy of the Lennox-Gastaut type (568).

Lamotrigine. Lamotrigine resembles phenytoin and carbamazepine in animal models, being most effective in the MES model (569). The drug reduces sustained repetitive firing in cultured neurons (570) and blocks the use- and voltage-dependent sodium channels with the rapidly and repetitively firing neurons being most susceptible. Its ability to decrease dendritic excitability by increasing I_h currents distinguishes it from phenytoin and carbamazepine (571). Since this current is important in oscillatory circuits, this action might contribute to lamotrigine's antiabsence activity (572,573). Lamotrigine appears to have activity against partial and generalized tonic-clonic seizures (492,574). Its efficacy against refractory partial seizures has been demonstrated in a monotherapy trial in which this antiepileptic drug appeared to be well tolerated (575).

Lamotrigine also has been shown to be useful in the Lennox-Gastaut syndrome (576,577), juvenile myoclonic epilepsy (578), and typical and atypical absence seizures (579,580).

When lamotrigine is used as monotherapy, optimal doses range between 3 and 6 mg/kg per day, with the starting dose approximately one-fourth of that amount. When lamotrigine is given to a child who is already receiving valproate, a starting dose of 0.1 to 0.2 mg/kg per day is recommended, with the dosage being built up slowly to a maximum of 5 mg/kg. Because valproate inhibits lamotrigine metabolism, higher doses produce severe toxicity (581,582). This is particularly evident in children receiving both lamotrigine and valproate. When lamotrigine is added to carbamazepine, phenytoin, or phenobarbital, drugs that induce hepatic enzymes, the half-life of lamotrigine is decreased, and higher lamotrigine dosages are required 5 to 15 mg/kg per day (573,583).

The most commonly encountered side effects of lamotrigine are dizziness, somnolence, nausea, vomiting, and headache (573). In about 3% to 14% of patients receiving lamotrigine as add-on therapy, a variety of rashes developed, including severe reactions such as Stevens-Johnson syndrome or toxic epidermal necrolysis and disseminated intravascular coagulation (492,584). The risk for rash is increased with a high starting dose as well as when VPA is used concomitantly (585). Schlienger and colleagues also found that 74% of the patients who had a severe skin reaction to lamotrigine (Stevens-Johnson syndrome or toxic epidermal necrolysis) were comedicated with valproic acid (584). In adults, the incidence of such reactions appears to be in the same order of magnitude as with phenytoin and carbamazepine. The estimated incidence of these severe reactions in children has resulted in the manufacturer and the U.S. Food and Drug Administration suggesting that lamotrigine not be used as first-line therapy of seizures in children.

A slow titration rate, beginning at 25 mg every other day, has been proposed as a means to minimize the chance of developing a rash. Buchanan suggests that patients on lamotrigine monotherapy be started on 12.5 mg per day, with the dosage increased by 12.5 mg every 2 weeks. Patients who are on a combination of valproate and lamotrigine should be started on a dosage of 12.5 mg every 3 days for 2 weeks, then increased to 12.5 mg every 2 days for 2 weeks, then 12.5 mg per day, with further dosage increases every 2 weeks (586). Less commonly encountered side reactions include a syndrome of multiorgan dysfunction and disseminated intravascular coagulation after a flulike illness in children who received a combination of lamotrigine and valproate (587). No controlled studies on the cognitive side effects of the drugs are as yet available, but the drug does not appear to have any long-term effects in healthy adults (588,589).

Topiramate. Topiramate, a sulfamate-substituted fructose derivative, has demonstrated potent anticonvulsant activity in several animal models, with the exception of those involving seizures induced by chemoconvulsants (590). Its mechanisms of action include activity against ligand-gated Na^+channels linked to AMPA-Kainate subtypes of glutamate receptors and, to a limited extent, blockade of voltage-dependent Na^+ channels as well as enhancement of GABA-mediated Cl^- currents (431). In addition, topiramate also seems to elevate brain GABA levels (591,592) and acts as a weak carbonic anhydrase inhibitor.

Topiramate has been demonstrated to be effective against partial seizures and generalized seizures as well as the drop attacks and major motor seizures in the Lennox-Gastaut syndrome (593–595). The American Academy of Neurology–American Epilepsy Society task force headed by French and coworkers found topiramate to be the only new generation AED with convincing evidence for efficacy against generalized tonic-clonic seizures (492,564). The possibility of synergy with lamotrigine and the potential for this specific combination has been reviewed (320).

Topiramate is associated with weight loss and paresthesias. The major side effect of the drug is its adverse action on cognitive function. A number of studies have shown that topiramate was associated with declines in verbal fluency and other language skills, attention, and concentration, with subjects performing worse on tests of verbal memory and psychomotor speed (596). These deficits and assoicated behavioral problems result in over 50% of children ceasing the medication (589,597). Some studies have suggested that pre-existing conditions could determine the incidence and severity of cognitive deficits. Thus, Mula and coworkers found that patients with complex partial seizures and hippocampal sclerosis were more prone to develop adverse cognitive events than patients with cryptogenic temporal lobe epilepsy (598). In addition, the titration rate appears to have an important effect on the incidence of cognitive deficits. These studies are consistent with clinical observations from many centers including our own.

Recent studies investigating monotherapy have found that even a 50 mg per day dose to be highly efficaceous in providing freedom from seizures for 6 or 12 months in new-onset epilepsy (599). Wheless and colleagues recommend a daily dose of 100 mg or 2 mg/kg per day in children based on a comparative monotherapy study with carbamazepine and valproate, taking into account comparative efficacy and tolerability (600). In that study, 100 mg per day of topiramate provided the same efficacy rates as either 200 mg per day of topiramate or 600 mg per day of carbamazepine or 1250 mg per day of valproic acid. Studies reporting high discontinuation rates typically employed higher doses and titration rates, since topiramate was initially prescribed at a dose of 6 mg/kg per day in adults and 10 mg/kg per day in children. Recognition of lowered target dose for topiramate is paramount to implementing successful therapy with this highly potent agent devoid of hepatotoxicity, hematopoietic toxicity, or risk for rash.

Topiramate therapy has been associated with nephrolithiasis and hypohidrosis (600a,b). Acute closed angle glaucoma has been encountered very rarely and typically occurs during the first few weeks of therapy. A well-documented side effect is weight loss, typically about 10%, and is generally greater in those with a higher body mass index (601). The weight loss is not associated with long-term adverse effects on growth and development (602). This side effect may be seen as a benefit for some children in an era of increasing obesity and incidence of type 2 diabetes in children.

Topiramate, like valproic acid, can be useful in managing patients with epilepsy who also experience migraines. Migraines are a common comorbidity in epilepsy, and there is an even stronger association between some benign childhood epilepsies and migraine (see Chapter 15).

Vigabatrin. Vigabatrin (γ-vinyl GABA), an irreversible inhibitor of GABA transaminase, was first licensed as an antiepileptic agent in Britain and the Republic of Ireland in 1989 (603). It binds irreversibly to GABA transaminase (GABA-T), the enzyme that breaks down GABA. This action increases the brain levels of GABA, increasing inhibition in the brain and thereby decreasing the likelihood of seizures.

Vigabatrin has been approved for treatment in nearly 50 countries worldwide, but its approval in the United States has stalled because of concerns regarding toxicity to the visual system (604). These concerns include reports of severe, persistent visual field defects noted in association with use of vigabatrin. In the pediatric series of Gross-Tsur and colleagues, visual field constriction was seen in 65% of children who were able to undergo perimetric studies (605). In most instances, the defect was bilateral symmetrical constriction with relative temporal sparing. In addition, visual-evoked potentials were abnormal in 33%, and electroretinography (ERG) was abnormal in 36% of children (606,607). These studies indicate that vigabatrin not only impairs the peripheral, cone-derived function, but also affects the rod-derived visual fields. Anatomic studies suggest that there is a loss in the ganglion cells of the retina. In patients who were continued on vigabatrin, there was no further worsening of visual acuity or visual field constriction (608). Discontinuation of vigabatrin does not improve the visual field defect, but does result in improved ERG. Other reported adverse effects include weight gain, behavioral disturbances, and depression (585).

The clinical efficacy of vigabatrin in partial seizures has been documented in several studies, summarized by one of us (R.S.) (603). The most promising effect of the drug is in infantile spasms, especially its unique and extraordinary efficacy in the subset whose spasms are caused by tuberous sclerosis (609,610). Its dramatic efficacy in this subpopulation, when compared with the poor responses of these patients to ACTH (280), mandates a separate risk to benefit analysis of this medication in pediatric patients (611). Vigabatrin is not effective in children with Lennox-Gastaut syndrome (612).

The recommended starting dose is 40 mg/kg per day, which is increased to 80 to 100 mg/kg per day, as required. In infantile spasms, dosages of more than 100 mg/kg per day have been used with some effect (298). Side effects include drowsiness, agitation and confusion, and a variety of dyskinesias such as akathisia, hyperkinesia, and forced laughter (613).

Tiagabine. Tiagabine is a designer drug that blocks GABA uptake by presynaptic neurons and glial cells. The drug appears to be effective for add-on therapy for intractable partial seizures (564). Doses used for these studies ranged from 16 to 56 mg per day (0.37 to 1.25 mg/kg per day). The most common side effects are dizziness, somnolence, and weakness. The drug does not affect visual fields or the ERG (614). Several reports have implicated tiagabine therapy with nonconvulsive status epilepticus (615).

Levetiracetam. Levetiracetam is novel in its drug-development heritage as well as in its mode of action. Its heritage is unique because it survived the anticonvulsant screening process in spite of its lack of activity in the electroshock convulsive model and the threshold pentylenetetrazol model (616).

The drug is effective as an add-on agent in refractory partial epilepsy (564,617). In these trials, dosages of

1000 to 3000 mg per day were used. There were no major side effects, but irritability and behavior changes were noted. Reports of class I evidence in support of the pediatric use of levetiracetam are pending, but observational studies are supportive of its use (618,619). One of us (R.S.) has summarized the pediatric experience with this novel anticonvulsant (620).

Levetiracetam appears to have broad spectrum potential. Reports exist in the literature of efficacy in generalized spike-wave epilepsy (621), myoclonic epilepsies (622,623), and childhood syndromes such as rolandic epilepsy (624).

Advantages of levetiracetam include high water solubility, linear pharmacokinetics with renal clearance, and lack of protein-binding and hepatic enzyme induction as well as being devoid of hepatic or hematopoietic toxicity. Sedation can be dose-limiting during titration, and there have been reports of psychiatric adverse effects such as irritability and psychosis in some patients (625). The overall tolerability of levetiracetam is generally considered to be high.

Zonisamide. Zonisamide is a sulfonamide derivative with a structural similarity to serotonin. It blocks voltage-dependent sodium channels, low threshold Ca^{++} channels, and binds to a chloride channel associated with the GABA receptor as well as a weak carbonic anhydrase inhibitor (626). It has been in use in Japan for nearly a decade, and in that country, it is one of the first-line agents for the treatment of epilepsy in adults and children. Treatment is started at 100 mg per day, or 1.5 mg/kg per day, and gradually increased to a maximum of 400 mg to 600 mg per day. In controlled studies, the drug was effective as add-on therapy for patients with refractory partial epilepsy (564,627,628). Side reactions include somnolence, renal calculi, hyperhidrosis, irritability, and photosensitivity. Language impairment similar to that observed with topiramate also has been recorded (492,629). Zonisamide also has been used with some benefit in the progressive myoclonus epilepsies (630).

Advantages of zonisamide include long half-life, linear pharmacokinetics, low protein binding, and lack of hepatic enzyme induction. It is generally easy to add to an existing anticonvulsant and is generally well tolerated.

Other Anticonvulsants. Older anticonvulsants, notably stiripentol, have been used as add-on to VPA or clobazam for the treatment of severe myoclonic epilepsy in infancy (631). Other drugs, such as phenacemide, paramethadione, and methsuximide, are rarely used in the treatment of seizures.

Ketogenic Diet

Although the value of fasting in the treatment of seizures has been recognized since biblical times, the ketogenic diet, which attempts to reproduce the ketosis and acidosis of starvation, was introduced only in 1921 (632). Despite the development of a variety of new and effective anticonvulsants in this country and abroad, it remains an attractive alternate means for the treatment of Lennox-Gastaut syndrome and other intractable seizures (633). The diet involves restricting protein and carbohydrate intake and supplying 80% to 90% of caloric intake through fats. The mechanism by which this regimen controls convulsions is still unknown. It is independent of respiratory or metabolic acidosis and of the accumulation of ketone bodies, and the anticonvulsant effects do not result from the direct effect of ketone bodies on voltage- and ligand-gated ion channels (634). Caloric restriction as well as the ketogenic diet reduce neuronal excitability, perhaps by inducing the activity of D-3-hydroxybutyrate dehydrogenase and allowing the brain to metabolize ketone bodies (635). It is still unclear if the benefits of the diet in seizure disorders stem primarily from the switch in cerebral metabolism involving the use of β-hydroxybutyrate instead of glucose as an energy substrate. In that respect, it is of interest that the Atkins diet also can reduce seizure frequency in focal and multifocal epilepsy (636). As well, there is accumulating experience suggesting that a low-glycemic diet may provide seizure control without a high degree of ketosis (637). A novel hypothesis has been advanced that lowering the rate of glycolysis decreases the production of cytosolic ATP, which inhibits current mediated by K^+ channels that are sensitive to that nucleotide trophosphate. Increased outward K^+ currents through these channels provides a hyperpolarizing mechanism. Research is under way to clarify this concept. The metabolic and endocrine aspects of this diet have been reviewed in detail by one of us (R.S.) (638).

The diet is most effective in children with minor motor seizures between 2 and 5 years of age. Older children do not respond as well because they fail to maintain an adequate degree of ketosis. We reserve the ketogenic diet for children who have been unable to tolerate anticonvulsant drugs because of multiple allergies. Details of the induction and maintenance of the diet are presented by Nordli and De Vivo (639). Medium-chain triglycerides as a substitute for a ketogenic diet have been advocated by Huttenlocher and associates (640). We have had relatively little experience with this regimen, but it appears to be as effective as the ketogenic diet and is better tolerated by some children. The need for initial fasting and fluid restriction has been questioned by Kim and coworkers, who find that the percentage of patients who become seizure-free for at least three months after institution of a non-fasting diet (34.1%) is no less than that obtained by using a fasting protocol (34.9%) (640a).

The increasing popularity of the diet in the 1990s prompted a multicenter study to evaluate its effectiveness (641). This study found that 10% of the patients became free of seizures on the diet. One-half the patients received considerable benefit from the diet, whereas the other one-half had dropped out of the diet by the end of the year, either because of lack of efficacy or adverse effects. There have been concerns among clinicians as how to best screen patients for safety with this diet. To state that physicians should avoid placing a child with seizures on the diet if the child also demonstrates hypotonia and developmental delay, with metabolic acidosis and abnormalities of organic or amino acids, is too general to provide adequate guidance. A child with such a presentation could have pyruvate dehydrogenase deficiency, and hence may stand to benefit significantly from the ketogenic diet. On the other hand, a child with a primary or acquired carnitine deficiency or a defect in the β-oxidation of fatty acids sustains significant morbidity if fasted or placed on the diet. If a patient has undergone a muscle biopsy earlier in the workup for hypotonia and weakness, a biopsy showing a few ragged-red fibers may not be a contraindication to the diet, but the appearance of a lipid myopathy is. Increased serum pyruvate and lactate along with alaninuria may not be a problem, but increased dicarboxylic acid excretion points to a potential for trouble. We, therefore, suggest that in the presence of an abnormal pattern of urinary organic acids, the type of dicarboxylic aciduria should be determined before the child is started on a ketogenic diet. We should point out that dicarboxylic aciduria and carnitine deficiency can occur in a patient who is on both valproic acid and the ketogenic diet. In addition, children who present with a history of seizures and intermittent encephalopathy in the course of minor infections should be carefully evaluated for the nature of the metabolic abnormality before considering the ketogenic diet.

We agree with Demeritte and colleagues (642) that organic acid screening be done before and after the initiation of the ketogenic diet. However, we do not recommend that patients on the diet be supplemented routinely with carnitine. Rather, we agree with recommendations from a roundtable discussion on the role of L-carnitine supplementation in children with epilepsy that suggests that carnitine supplementation be reserved for children with demonstrable carnitine deficiency (643). Even though most centers offering the ketogenic diet have patients who also are on valproate, one study has hinted at the added risk for complications in such patients (644). Other complications include the development of renal calculi, osteoporosis, hypoglycemia, and, in about one-third of children, increased bruising with a prolonged bleeding time (645).

Anticonvulsants in Children Suffering from Systemic Disease

Phenobarbital can be administered in the presence of severe hepatic disease. Even though hepatic hydroxylation of the drug is impaired, with consequent doubling of its half-life, increased renal elimination of unchanged phenobarbital reduces the importance of hepatic metabolism.

Carbamazepine levels are altered in hepatic disease. Metabolism of the drug is reduced significantly, reducing its clearance. This effect is counteracted by reduced plasma binding and increased free carbamazepine. Generally, however, levels tend to increase and must be monitored carefully, keeping in mind that the free carbamazepine fraction is higher than normal.

No modification of clearance or bioavailability of carbamazepine has been observed in renal failure. In cardiac failure, carbamazepine absorption, which is normally erratic, is reduced. However, the drug is metabolized more slowly than usual, thus reducing its clearance. Carbamazepine can cause increased sodium and water retention, which may aggravate cardiac symptoms.

In cirrhosis and renal disease, the free fraction of valproic acid increases two- to threefold. The intrinsic metabolism of the drug is reduced, however, so that the actual clearance remains essentially normal.

Among the newer agents, gabapentin, topiramate, levetiracetam, zonisamide, oxcarbazepine, and lamotrigine offer the benefits of not having significant systemic toxicity, protein binding, or hepatic induction. Of those, oxcarbazepine and higher doses of topiramate have the potential to induce to some measure cytochrome P-450 C3A4 isoenzyme, while there is some chance of a rash with zonisamide, and even more so with lamotrigine. Thus, we prefer the use of levetiracetam, topiramate, or gabapentin in children who are transplant recipients maintained on immunosuppressants with brittle pharmacokinetic properties. In renal disease, it is important to recognize that the clearance of these three agents is increased with a concommitant decrease in their half-life, necessitating dose and dosage interval adjustments.

Summary

In summarizing medical therapy for seizure disorders, we would like to point out several common errors.

1. The physician fails to diagnose correctly the type of seizure experienced by the child. This failure is almost always because an inadequate history was obtained. Misinterpretation of EEGs also contributes to the failure to diagnose the seizure syndrome.
2. Traditional anticonvulsants are not given in sufficiently high dosage. No drug should be abandoned unless the physician is certain that it has no beneficial effects and unless toxic symptoms are verified.
3. Some of the newer anticonvulsants (topiramate, levetiracetam) may produce most of their beneficial effects at doses lower than initially recommended by the manufacturer, and increasing the dose often produces a disproportionate increase in adverse effects, while rational polypharmacy may exploit synergies (646) and reduced adverse events. The

protective effect of lamotrigine on lowering psychiatric adverse events due to topiramate (647) and levetiracetam (648) has already been addressed.

4. Frequent changes in medication and alterations of the dosage of more than one drug at the same time should be avoided.
5. Finally, the tendency for polytherapy by *serial addition of numerous agents* to increase seizure frequency has been insufficiently appreciated. Such an approach does not constitute rational polypharmacy. Many years ago, one of us (J.H.M.) found that complete discontinuation of anticonvulsant medication can produce significant, and sometimes permanent, improvement in approximately one-third of patients with Lennox-Gastaut syndrome, and we believe that periodic withdrawal or reduction of anticonvulsants is indicated in such patients whose seizures remain under poor control (415). This interdiction of polytherapy does not apply to the newer anticonvulsants, and there have numerous well-documented instances where polytherapy is more effective than monotherapy and where tolerability of anticonvulsants can be improved by polypharmacy at lower doses.

Surgical Procedures

When epilepsy is intractable to medical treatment, surgical resection of the tissue responsible for the epilepsy should be considered. Epilepsy is considered medically intractable when a child continues to experience seizures despite adequate trials of three or more anticonvulsant medications, used either alone or in combination therapy (649). Ko and Holmes found symptomatic etiology, early age of onset, the presence of tonic seizures and/or simple partial seizures to be predictive of evolution to intractability (649). Diffuse slowing in the EEG and focal spike and wave activity were electrographic predictors. Kwan and Brodie (650) estimated that slightly greater than one-third of all the patients with new-onset epilepsy became medically intractable. Camfield and coworkers found the response of children to the first medication to be useful in predicting intractability (651). The fraction of their overall population that became intractable was only 8.4%, but the study defined seizure control without incorporating tolerability to the treatment. The number reflects the fact that many children present with seizure syndromes that may remit with time. However, when children present with complex partial seizures, they are much more likely to become intractable. Dlugos and colleagues found 37.5% of their pediatric patients with temporal lobe epilepsy to be refractory at 2 years after initiation of treatment (652). Only about one-third of medically refractory patients may be amenable to surgical therapy.

It is thought that at least 60% of all seizures are partial seizures arising from a single location in the cortex and that 30% of these partial seizures are intractable (653). Of these intractable partial seizure patients, many are not referred to epilepsy surgery centers. It is estimated that approximately 5,000 new patients annually in the United States may benefit from epilepsy surgery, but only one-third receive treatment (654). Much of this is related to a lack of education among primary physicians in referring patients for epilepsy surgery. This is especially true for pediatric epilepsy patients, as many pediatric neurologists are concerned about surgical risk in children and are reluctant to send patients to epilepsy surgery centers.

There are many benefits associated with epilepsy surgery, such as less morbidity and mortality due to intractable epilepsy and status epilepticus, less anticonvulsants used, improved quality of life, and improved cognition and development. It is common knowledge that the earlier surgery is performed, the better chance for developmental gains to occur (653). However, some studies recently have shown that the cognitive improvement after surgery may only be modest and is dependent on the etiology of the epilepsy (655). The complications for surgery include bleeding, risk for infection, cranial nerve dysfunction, increased intracranial pressure, and stroke. These complications are more prevalent for children due to the smaller body volume as well as extensive types of surgeries that are performed, such as hemispherectomy (656). However, iatrogenic residual deficits such as a hemianopsia or hemiplegia resulting from hemispherectomy may be indicated in cases where there is a catastrophic childhood illness in which the natural course of the disease would be worse than the resultant deficit. For example, a disease such as Rasmussen syndrome can eventually lead to the same deficit such as hemiparesis, but early surgery will prevent cognitive delay that occurs with the disease. Unlike in adults, some concerns regarding language lateralization do not apply to very young children due to plasticity in language development. Children younger than 10 years of age can transfer their language to the side contralateral to the resected side, if the resection involves the language dominant side.

For some patients, especially in temporal lobectomies, surgery is felt to be curative if the epileptogenic focus is localized to an area that is easily accessible and not involved in critical function (657). In fact, seizure freedom after surgery depends on whether or not the entire focus can be resected (658). If any area is left, there is a greater chance of seizure recurrence. However, there are many cases where the patient has diffuse areas of involvement that cannot be fully resected. This is especially true for mentally retarded children, considering that dysfunction involves both hemispheres. With these children, palliative surgery aids with decreased seizure frequency but provides no seizure freedom. For example, patients who have drop attacks may benefit from corpus callosotomy, where the risk for head injury is lessened, although the other seizures will not stop.

Surgical Candidacy

Whether a surgery is for palliative reasons or curative reasons, medical intractability of seizures is important to establish (654). Many children are thought to be intractable, but on further surgical evaluation such as long-term videotelemetry, it is found that these children have nonepileptic events. Children who are surgical candidates must have partial-onset seizures. Medical intractability for partial seizures should include a substantial trial of anticonvulsant therapy. Some feel that this includes a trial of at least three anticonvulsants, one of which is a newer anticonvulsant such as felbamate, lamotrigine, topiramate, zonisamide, or levetiracetam. The seizures should be frequent, occurring at least monthly. Many feel that recurrent status epilepticus or regression in cognitive skills with less frequent seizures also should be a criterion, since the frequent seizures or frequent epileptiform discharges interfere with the functions of the healthy brain and therefore will cause cognitive decline to progress. Finally, if a patient has a catastrophic illness where the prognosis for cognition and seizure control is poor, then this would be strong criterion for surgery, regardless of whether the patient has failed three anticonvulsants. These catastrophic diseases include Rasmussen syndrome, Sturge-Weber syndrome, and hemimegalencephaly.

Contraindications to surgery include benign childhood epilepsy syndromes, presence of neurodegenerative disease, and lack of adequate demonstration of medical intractability. There are some controversial contraindications as well. One is intercurrent psychiatric illness. There have been reports that surgery worsens a psychiatric illness such as psychosis, depression, or mania. Yet, there also have been reports in the literature stating that surgery may improve these conditions. Others believe that mental retardation may be a contraindication for surgery, since diffuse involvement of both hemispheres is implied. However, in many children with mental retardation, surgery is used as a palliative treatment for their disabling seizures. Shewmon engaged the question as to whether bilateral interictal discharges were a contraindication to surgery (659). It was felt that this does not represent widespread disease in younger children and therefore, if a focal region can be proved, the patient may still benefit from surgery. Finally, some feel that a lack of social support may be a contraindication if the child will not be able to participate in the intensive rehabilitation that is required for some surgeries, such as a hemispherectomy.

Neuroimaging aspects of presurgical evaluation of candidates have been reviewed (660,661), and the special considerations for presurgical noninvasive and semi-invasive neurophysiologic tests are outlined by Duchowny and colleagues (662). In neuroimaging infants with cortical microdysplasias, the timing of the MRI is of crucial importance because of the progression of myelination affecting the MR signal characteristics. One of us (R.S.) has demonstrated that even microscopic cortical abnormalities may become discernible by changes in the maturation of the adjacent white matter (274). Thus, an infant with West syndrome and a normal MRI at the age of 4 to 6 months may have to be reimaged several months later if the clinical course warrants considering surgical treatment.

Scalp EEG

Long-term video-EEG evaluation is preferred to routine scalp EEG in order to establish whether an event is actually a seizure and to interpret the semiology that determines the origin of the seizure. The interictal background as well as the ictal onset of at least two typical seizures should be captured. If mesial temporal lobe sclerosis is considered, then sphenoidal electrodes or cheek electrodes should be placed. In addition, the timing of the seizure electrographically as well as the semiology can aid in determining whether the seizure starts in a deep focus (where there are EEG changes prior to the semiology change). Ictal epileptiform abnormalities are sometimes not clearly lateralized in children; for example, in infantile spasms, the ictal EEG tends to be generalized even when a lateralized zone of cortical abnormality exists. However, the nonepileptiform abnormalities, such as focal bursts of slowing or asymmetry in the generation of beta rhythms in response to barbiturates, or asymmetry of sleep spindles can suggest the presence of an underlying lateralized zone of cortical abnormality (659). In addition, the ictal onset is often subtle and vague in children when compared with adults. For these reasons, interpretation of the video-EEG recordings should be performed by a pediatric electroencephalographer, if possible.

Neuroimaging

With recent advances in MRI, using stronger magnet strengths and novel and varied pulse sequences, more abnormalities are evident than were seen in the past. A high resolution MRI is the preferred neuroimaging for epilepsy surgery evaluation, as it provides details of neuroanatomy that are not discernible on a CT scan. However, CT is still used occasionally, especially in etiologies where there are calcifications such as in tuberous sclerosis or cystircercosis, which is difficult to pick up on MRI. The MRI should involve FLAIR sequences and T2 coronal sequences with thin cuts (1mm) through the temporal lobe in order to clearly visualize mesial temporal lobe sclerosis. Many children evaluated for epilepsy surgery may harbor cortical dysplasia where gyral thickening and/or gray white matter blurring may be discerned. Sometimes, the dysplasia is not noticeable if the MRI is performed early, such as at 4 to 6 months of age. A child may need to be reimaged several months later in order to determine whether there is a subtle dysplasia (274).

Positron Emission Tomography

The utility of ^{18}F-fluorodeoxyglucose positron emission tomography (^{18}FDG-PET) to map regional cerebral glucose metabolism in presurgical evaluation for temporal lobe epilepsy was established in the early 1980s at UCLA (663). Use of newer ligands such as the benzodiazepine receptor ligand ^{11}C-flumazenil have not significantly improved the utility of PET scanning compared with traditional interictal metabolic mapping with PET using ^{18}F-fluorodeoxyglucose (664). However, tracers such as α-methyl-L-tryptophan (AMT) have been found to be more reliable for specific illnesses such as tuberous sclerosis (665), although the AMT tracer is less available than FDG.

Single Photon Emission Computerized Tomography

Single photon emission computerized tomography (SPECT) also is a nuclear medicine study where hexylmethylprophylene amineoxine (HMPAO) is injected. Unlike PET, SPECT is based on cerebral blood flow to determine where the seizures originate. Seizure origin utilizes increased blood flow compared with other areas of the brain. Also unlike PET, SPECT is more reliable when it is an ictal study (666,667) Therefore, the injection must be given within 30 seconds of the onset of the seizure in order to be valid.

The regional blood flow data determined by interictal SPECT can be combined with either ictal or postictal studies to generate a subtraction SPECT. The coregistration of subtraction data with the MRI significantly enhances the sensitivity and specificity of localization (668,669).

Other modes of evaluation include proton magnetic resonance spectroscopy (MRS) and functional MRI. MRS is not commonly used in children because it is mainly helpful for temporal lobe epilepsy patients. This utilizes *N*-acetyl aspartate (NAA) and creatinine, which are increased in cortical damage that is seen especially in hippocampal sclerosis (670–673).

Functional MRI uses rapid scanning techniques to find areas with low deoxyhemoglobin concentration that correlate with increased cerebral blood flow. Ictal onset can be determined because blood flow increases in areas where the seizure starts. It also can be used for localization of frequent interictal spiking if performed with concurrent EEG. Finally, functional MRI demonstrates areas of critical function such as motor or language (674) and may surpass the intracarotid amytal testing for the determination of language dominance. A subject is monitored while performing a task as well as at rest, which is subtracted from each other; this leaves an image of where the blood flow is located for areas of critical function. The main problem with functional MRI in children is that it is difficult for them to cooperate during a task and remain motionless in the gantry since they cannot be sedated. Also, the paradigms that are used for language tasks may cause different areas of the brain to interact and, therefore, produce different results.

There are newer techniques, such as diffusion tensor imaging (DTI) and diffusion-weighted magnetic resonance imaging (DWI), that are currently being studied. DTI suppresses gray matter on the image and allows for easier observation of the white matter tracts (675). Thus, cortical dysplasia close to the gray-white margin is easily enhanced. DWI uses a similar technique and may offer help in determining seizure origin in a multifocal disease such as tuberous sclerosis (676).

Magnetoencephalography

Over the last decade, magnetoencephalography (MEG) is increasingly utilized for presurgical localization of epileptiform discharges, presurgical localization of the sensorimotor or visual cortex for epilepsy and tumor surgery, and for preoperative planning to guide the placement of a grid for epilepsy surgery. Similar to EEG, MEG is another tool to assess functional and dynamic cortical activity. In fact, EEG and MEG are the only neurophysiologic techniques that provide information specifically for epilepsy, namely the measurement of epileptiform discharges. They are also the only methods that have a temporal resolution in the order of milliseconds, which is essential for evaluating the dynamic processes underlying human epilepsy. While EEG is a measure of the electrical currents, the MEG detects and amplifies the magnetic field generated by the same electrical currents. The two essential problems of detecting such weak magnetic fields in the midst of such strong competing magnetic noise (such as the earth's own magnetic field) were solved by first, a magnetically shielded room, and second, the development of extremely sensitive measurement devices. These superconducting quantum inference devices (SQUIDs) are based on the physical principle of superconductivity and were a major breakthrough in the investigation of the brain's magnetic field. To maintain superconductivity, SQUIDs require an operating temperature of 4° Kelvin by immersion in a helium-containing cryogenic vessel. Detection of extracranial magnetic field, generated by intracranial electrical current, occurs when the patient's head rests in a helmet-shaped device.

Compared with other modalities of epilepsy mapping, MEG provides one of the best temporal and spatial resolutions, without the invasiveness. The signal can be superimposed on MEG and is not distorted by intervening layers of skull and scalp, as it occurs with electrical signals. Another advantage is that the localization is achieved with interictal recordings, which are logistically easier. It is much more sensitive to superficial activity and is thus best suited for neocortical epilepsy (rather than limbic epilepsy with deep sources).

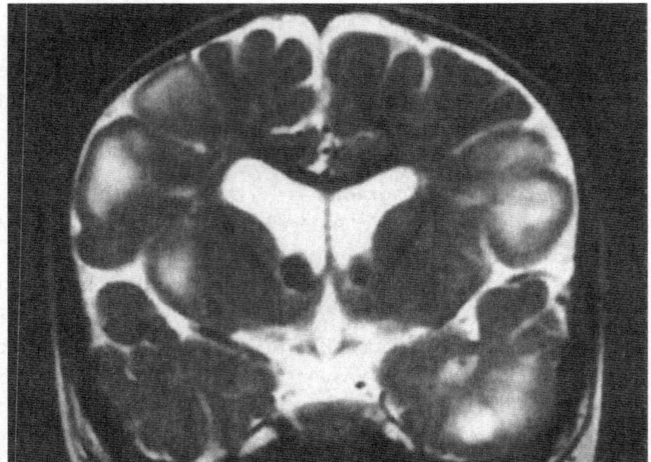
A

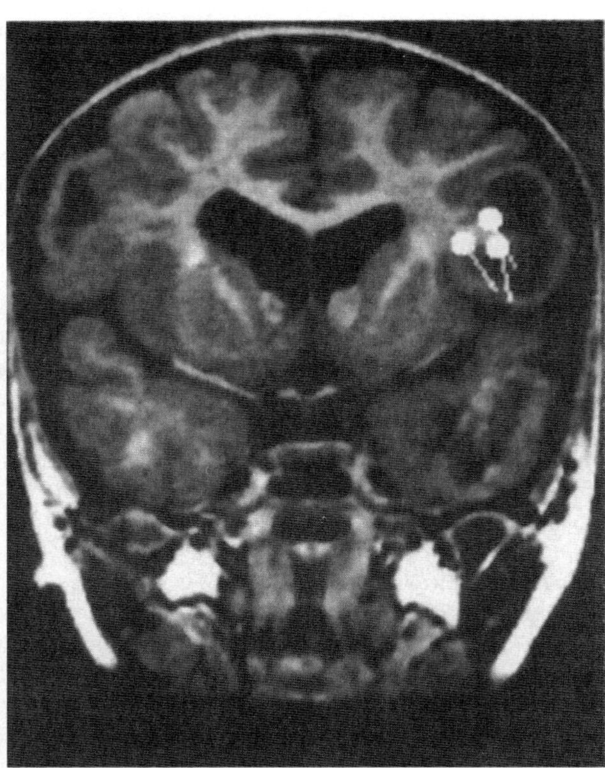
B

FIGURE 14.11. Magnetoencephalography in surgical evaluation of seizures. **A:** T2 image showing multiple tubers. **B:** MEG identifies one tuber as epileptogenic and is concordant with surface EEG ictal onset and was confirmed by intraoperative recordings. This youngster had the tubers resected and has been seizure free for the past three years.

In one study, MEG correctly localized the epileptogenic zone with an excellent surgical outcome in 44% of patients with extratemporal epilepsy (677). As well, MEG performed best in epileptogenic zone localization among the noninvasive studies, outperforming interictal scalp EEG (33%), ictal scalp EEG (20%), and MRI (31%); MEG was second only to the invasive interictal (75%) and ictal (81%) intracranial recording. Mamelak and coworkers (678) have found magnetic source imaging to provide unique localizing data that is not available by other noninvasive means. We have found this technology to be especially useful in assisting in the localization of epileptogenic tubers in children with multiple tubers of tuberous sclerosis (Fig. 14.11).

Knowlton and Shih have provided a recent review of the scope of this modality (679).

Invasive Procedures

After localizing the epileptogenic zone through surgical evaluations, other invasive studies are performed in order to confirm the location or to tailor the resection further. In addition, if there is a concern that the epileptogenic focus is involved in critical function such as motor or language, functional mapping also is executed.

Electrocorticography

In electrocorticography (ECoG), the skull and dura are removed, and subdural electrodes are placed on the area thought to be the origin of the seizure. An interictal background is recorded, which means that seizure onsets are sometimes not captured. Anesthesia is usually weaned off to increase the yield for interictal abnormalities and provoke seizures (680). Interictal spike discharges are not as revealing as the slowing and attenuation in the background. Somatosensory-evoked potentials are performed prior to ECoG in order to determine where the motor strip is located. For a temporal lobe focus in adults or older children or when there are multiple foci involved, chronic recordings from stereotactically implanted depth electrodes are helpful (681). However, depth electrodes are rarely used in children because most children do not have mesial temporal lobe sclerosis but instead have neocortical epilepsy, which is easily accessed by grid.

Subdural Grid Monitoring

Chronic subdural grid recordings in children are another option where the patient is implanted with subdural grid electrodes in areas where the seizure is thought to originate. The patient is monitored in the pediatric intensive care unit (PICU) for seizure onset and mapping of the critical cortex. Subdural grids provide accurate information for children, especially in cases where other evaluations such as scalp EEG is nonlocalizing or vague and/or if the neuroimaging is nonlesional. Also, if the surgical evaluations provide noncongruent results, then subdural grid monitoring can provide more accurate information. A grid is used when there are multiple foci seen, such as in tuberous sclerosis. Finally, grid monitoring provides confirmation as to where the language and motor cortex are located in comparison to the seizure origin through functional mapping. Here, the subdural electrodes are directly stimulated while the patient is talking or reading or is observed for movements (682). Problems with subdural grid electrodes in children include the need for sedation and steroids while in the PICU because young children may pull their subdural electrodes out, or swelling and infection may occur with the implantation of hardware. In addition, there are times when the grid is placed incorrectly away from the origin, causing an "edge of the grid" phenomena where the grid looks diffusely involved.

Types of Surgery

Temporal Lobectomy

Temporal lobe seizures are not common in children as compared with adults. If they occur, they tend to be neocortical rather than mesial temporal and are more widespread than the typical mesial temporal sclerosis. Therefore, temporal lobectomies may involve larger areas than just the standard temporal lobectomies found in adults. A standard anterior temporal lobectomy usually involves 4 to 5 cm of the dominant lobe or 6 to 7 cm of the nondominant lobe in order to avoid language areas. A total temporal lobe resection includes the amygdala and 1 to 2 cm of hippocampus (683). Usually, a selective amygdalohippocampectomy (684) or selective lateral neocortical resections sparing the amygdala and the hippocampus (685) are not performed because children do not have discrete lesions involving these locations and therefore have poor seizure control if these techniques are utilized. Other than surgical complications, main problems with extensive temporal lobectomies include superior quadrantanopsia due to resection of Meyer's loop in the temporal white matter, transient anomies due to swelling, and memory difficulties.

The outcome of anterior temporal lobectomy is excellent for seizure control when epileptiform discharges originate within the hippocampus or amygdala (686). Conversely, when the epileptic focus is outside the hippocampus or amygdala, response to this type of surgery is not as good (687). These results have been challenged by other workers and need to be confirmed. A consensus, however, suggests that the longer seizure control remains complete, the less likely is a recurrence. Improvement in the behavior disorder that often accompanies complex partial seizures usually parallels seizure control but can take considerable time to become apparent. Results with children suggest that performing a temporal lobectomy at an early age leads to a better outcome than when the procedure is done during the adult years (688) Postoperatively, there appears to be a decrease in immediate and delayed verbal memory scores in preadolescent children. This is particularly evident in those who performed above the median preoperatively. Immediate verbal memory was more affected in those children who had a left temporal lobectomy (689).

Extratemporal Lobectomy

Extratemporal seizures such as frontal, parietal, and occipital seizures are more common in children than adults, with frontal seizures being the most prevalent. Extratemporal lobectomies occur predominantly in older children rather than younger children who often suffer from multilobar epilepsy. Unlike in temporal lobectomies, language and motor function are more at risk. There may be more of a need for invasive monitoring with subdural grids to define a focus and stimulation studies to define and map eloquent areas (690). There can be temporal mutism or motor apraxia with removal of the supplementary motor area, abulia in frontal resections, neglect in parietal resections, or visual loss in occipital resections.

Results from the Montreal Neurological Institute suggest that the outcome of frontal resections is not nearly as good as that of central, parietal, or occipital resections, probably because the epileptogenic area cannot be resected completely without sacrificing eloquent cortex (691). The percentage of patients who became completely free of seizures subsequent to surgery was 26% in frontal resections, as compared with 34% in central, parietal, and occipital resections. These figures contrast with a 70% seizure-free rate after temporal lobectomies (691,692).

Multilobar/Hemispherectomy

Multiple lobe involvement is the most common epilepsy surgery for young children with catastrophic illnesses that tend to involve diffuse areas. Multilobar resections often carry more surgical complications due to bleeding and the potential for neurologic deficits. Temporal-occipital-parietal (TOP) resections are performed but are less effective than hemispherectomy, with poor long-term seizure control. However, a TOP resection can save motor function.

Hemispherectomies involves the removal of the entire hemisphere, and there are two predominant types. With an anatomical removal, the entire hemisphere is removed with sparing of the basal ganglia. Functional removal involves removal of the temporal and/or parietal lobes with disconnection of the white matter tracts between the frontal and occipital lobes (693,694). Anatomical removal is less common than functional removal because with the former, there are significant side effects involved such as increased risk of bleeding, subdural hematomas, increased intracranial pressure requiring VP shunt, and more long-term side effects such as hemosiderosis, which was seen in as many as one-third of patients after many seizure-free years. It was believed to result from a lack of adequate support for the remaining hemispheres and from consequent bouts of small bleeds into the intracranial cavity (695). After hemispherectomy, dense hemiparesis and visual field loss occurs. However, in children who receive intense rehabilitation, the hemiparesis involves mainly fine motor movement of the fingers, and truncal control remains intact. The patient can still run with a hemiparetic gait while using the arm as a helper hand (696). There is potential for incomplete disconnection of white matter tracts due to the difficulties involved with the surgery, especially in very young patients who have undergone functional hemispherectomy. Therefore, patients may start having seizures again, which requires a subsequent operation.

In terms of seizure control, there are many outcome studies that have shown improvement with hemispherectomy in terms of seizure control and developmental quotients. The Montreal Neurological Institute found that seizures remained totally controlled over an average follow-up period of 7 years in 78% of patients, and IQ improved significantly without worsening of the hemiparesis (695). At UCLA, seizure freedom and antiepileptic drug usage after resective surgery for symptomatic cortical dysplasia and noncortical dysplasia etiologies was comparable with complex partial temporal lobe epilepsy cases up to 2 years postsurgery (697). Furthermore, at 5 years postsurgery, patients with cortical dysplasia had outcomes better than presurgery but worse than temporal lobe epilepsy cases. Similar results have been reported from the Cleveland Clinic (698). A recent study also found that developmental quotient increased depending on the pathology, with hemimegalencephaly performing the worst (699). Chugani and coworkers believe that the degree of functional recovery is greater if the procedure is performed early in life rather than if it is delayed (700).

Corpus Callosotomy

Corpus callosotomy is performed as a palliative procedure because it is only helpful for drop attacks and not for other types of seizures (701–703). The theory is to interrupt the spread of epileptic discharges from one hemisphere to the other (704). Transection of the anterior two-thirds of the corpus callosum as well as complete transection have been used, with the latter procedure generally being more effective (705). Complete transection of the corpus callosum and the anterior and hippocampal commissures produces a disconnection syndrome. Patients experience difficulties performing tasks in which the sensory inflow is restricted to one hemisphere, and in which the response involves the hand for which the cortical representation is in the opposite hemisphere. Transient mutism also is encountered after surgery (706,707). At UCLA, the number of callosotomy procedures has decreased in recent years because of the reemergence of the ketogenic diet and the availability of vagus nerve stimulation.

Multiple Subpial Transactions

Multiple subpial transactions use a probe that is swept along the pial surface perpendicular to the long axis of the gyrus and disconnects the horizontal fibers while leaving the vertical fibers intact. Theoretically, this will prevent seizures from spreading but will leave the function of the area intact. Therefore, it is often used where there is involvement of eloquent cortex. In practice, this type of procedure is not effective in eliminating seizures in many patients, especially with those who have cortical dysplasia. In addition, there have been complications described such as temporal mutism due to edema postoperatively or stroke due to excessive bleeding.

Other Surgical Options

There are other options considered for epilepsy surgery. One option is gamma knife, which is a stereotactic radiation treatment usually reserved for deep lesions that are surgically difficult to approach, such as hypothalamic harmatomas (708). The side effects of chronic radiation exposure and efficacy rates have not yet been elucidated. There also is some discussion regarding the use of deep brain stimulation of the caudate, thalamus, or cerebellum as a potential treatment for seizures. Although there are some case reports of implantation in adults, none has been documented in children (709).

Vagal Nerve Stimulation

Intermittent stimulation of the vagus nerve using a neurocybernetic prosthesis is an approach to achieving seizure control that has been approved in the United States, Canada, and several European Union countries. The mechanism of action of vagal nerve stimulation is poorly understood. The vagus nerve consists of approximately 80% afferent fibers, and these fibers terminate in the nucleus of the solitary tract. Axons from this nucleus project to a number of cortical and subcortical structures, including the amygdala, hippocampus, hypothalamus, thalamus, and the insular cortex.

Even though acute changes in neurotransmitter metabolites have been demonstrated in the CSF (710), the gradual increase in efficacy of chronic stimulation suggests some plastic changes in circuitry. Indeed, Henry and associates have shown that the increases in acute blood flow in the thalamus correlate with chronic efficacy of vagal nerve stimulation in reducing seizure frequency (711).

The programmable pulse generator (neurocybernetic prosthesis) is implanted in the patient's chest on the upper left side. The signals are conveyed to the vagus nerve by leads that terminate in helical, bipolar stimulating electrodes. Stimulation parameters are adjusted noninvasively via a radio frequency programming wand from a PC-compatible computer. The adjustable stimulation parameters include signal frequency (typically set at 30 Hz), signal pulse width (typically 500 μs), signal on time (typically 30 s), signal off time (typically 5 minutes), and the output current that is gradually increased over several visits in increments of 0.25 mA in the range of 0.25 to 4.0 mA. In our practice, most children who receive benefit with the device do so between 1.5 and 3.0 mA. Those who have an aura can activate the device by a handheld magnet, if they perceive the aura between stimulations in the duty cycle to attempt aborting the seizure.

Clinical efficacy has been demonstrated in adults (712–714) and in children (715). Experience thus far suggests that partial as well as idiopathic and symptomatic generalized epilepsies are responsive. Efficacy is seen within 6 months after implantation and seems to improve up to 18 months. This method is especially valuable for children who remain refractory to available medical therapy or who exhibit severe adverse reactions to antiepileptic drugs and whose epilepsies are not amenable to resective surgical therapy.

Treatment of Status Epilepticus (Convulsive Status Epilepticus)

A patient is said to be in status epilepticus when seizures occur so frequently that over the course of 30 or more minutes, he or she has not recovered from the coma produced by one attack before the next attack supervenes. Status epilepticus is one of the few true emergencies in the practice of pediatric neurology. Consensus states that the more prolonged the status, the worse the outcome.

As has been reviewed elsewhere in this chapter, experimental studies indicate that convulsions lasting longer than 20 to 30 minutes can induce brain damage. Several systemic factors, acting singly or in concert, are believed to be responsible. During the initial stages of status (i.e., for the first 30 minutes or so), cardiac output increases. Tachycardia and systemic hypertension lead to a two- to threefold increase in cerebral blood flow, with a marked increase in cerebral oxygen consumption. During this period, plasma glucose and glucose uptake by the brain is increased. In due time, the brain requirements for oxygen outstrip its supply, and when status lasts longer than 30 to 60 minutes, decompensation sets in (716–718). From that time on, cerebral autoregulation breaks down, cardiac output decreases, and there is arterial hypotension and reduced cerebral perfusion. With increased oxygen demands and inadequate oxygen delivery to the brain, cellular metabolism energy fails, and with mitochondrial damage, the organ reverts to anaerobic metabolism with consequent cellular acidosis, increased CSF lactate, and cerebral edema. Ultimately, there is respiratory failure and hyperthermia (716).

Additionally, prolonged and abnormal electrical discharges, by themselves, can cause neuronal damage. The mechanism by which this occurs has not been fully substantiated but involves enhanced glutaminergic excitatory transmission that leads to excessive depolarization of neurons and increased intracellular calcium and sodium. These ion changes initiate a cascade of events that lead to cell death (719). This subject also is reviewed in Chapters 6 and 17.

Status epilepticus is not part of the natural history of the epilepsies, but rather is a complication induced by changes in medication or intercurrent infections. Its incidence has increased with the advent of the newer anticonvulsant drugs, and in a study published in 1989, 3.7% of epileptic patients experienced one or more bouts of status epilepticus (720). In children, 85% of status epilepticus develops during the first 5 years of life and 25% during the first year of life (717).

Status epilepticus also can occur as an isolated phenomenon, particularly in children experiencing viral encephalitis or brain abscess or can occur after an open head injury, especially of the frontal lobes. It can be the initial epileptic attack in patients with secondary (symptomatic) epilepsy or can appear in the course of chronic primary (idiopathic) epilepsy. Maytal and coworkers (720) analyzed the causes of status epilepticus in children. In their series, approximately one-fourth of cases occurred without an obvious precipitating cause in patients who had a prior CNS insult. One-fourth were precipitated by fever and thus represented febrile convulsions, and one-fourth were caused by an acute neurologic insult, such as meningitis, trauma, and anoxia or were due to withdrawal of anticonvulsants. In approximately one-fourth, the precipitant for status was unknown.

Four sequential aspects to the management of the patient in status should be followed. They are (a) maintenance of vital functions, (b) institution of drug therapy to control convulsions, (c) diagnosis of the cause for the condition, and (d) prevention of further convulsions (721).

The physician who treats a child in status should act promptly to maintain an adequate airway, prevent aspiration of mucus, and secure the child from injury induced by the violence of the convulsions. Hyperthermia and hypotension should be corrected.

Several modes of therapy have been used, each with its advantages and disadvantages. We currently favor the use of lorazepam as the first-line anticonvulsant. The drug is highly lipid soluble and penetrates rapidly into the brain. In our experience and that at other centers, lorazepam is superior to diazepam in that fewer seizure recurrences follow lorazepam, and fewer repeat dosages are required (722). Whether the use of lorazepam is accompanied by a lower incidence of respiratory depression has not been clarified (723).

Lorazepam is administered as an intravenous bolus at a dosage of 0.1 mg/kg, up to a maximum of 4 mg, or 0.06 mg/kg for children older than 13 years of age (724). The drug is administered over the course of 3 or more minutes. Should seizures continue for more than 10 minutes, the initial dose is repeated (725). In most children with generalized or focal status epilepticus, seizures stop within 5 minutes of the administration of lorazepam. The principal side effect is respiratory depression, which can require assisted ventilation. Unlike with diazepam, the likelihood of this complication is not increased by concurrent or antecedent administration of barbiturates. The serum half-life of lorazepam is approximately 15.7 hours (724), and sequential doses of lorazepam are often necessary; in the Los Angeles Children's Hospital series, sequential doses were used in 30% of cases (724). Stewart and coworkers believe that the incidence of respiratory depression is increased by the use of multiple doses of benzodiazepines (723). The effectiveness of lorazepam diminishes with successive doses.

Diazepam is another effective agent in the treatment of status epilepticus. Like lorazepam it is highly lipid soluble and as judged from concurrent EEGs the drug enters the brain in 1.0 to 9.5 minutes (726). It is highly protein bound, and its redistribution within the body limits its duration of action within the brain to less than 30 minutes. This contrasts with an 8- to 12-hour duration of CNS action of lorazepam (727). Diazepam is administered intravenously at a dosage of 0.3 to 0.5 mg/kg, up to a maximum of 20 mg, and at a rate of 1 to 2 mg per minute (725). In one-third of patients, seizures stop within 3 minutes after diazepam is injected, and in the majority within 5 minutes (728). From the range of suggested dosages and from clinical experience, it is apparent that the amount of medication required for seizure control varies considerably among individuals. The principal advantages of diazepam are its rapid effectiveness, its margin of safety, and its ability to control seizures of cortical as well as of centrencephalic origin (729). The principal side effects of diazepam are respiratory depression and hypotension. They are most likely to occur in patients receiving a combination of drugs, particularly diazepam and phenobarbital, and multiple doses, often at the low end or less than the recommended dose (723,730).

Rectal diazepam (0.5 mg/kg for children aged 2 to 5 years, 0.3 mg/kg for children aged 6 years or older) is administered by means of a rubber tube inserted 4 to 5 cm beyond the anus. It appears to be a simple and safe means of controlling prolonged major motor seizures (731,732).

The use of intravenous phenytoin in the treatment of status epilepticus has been advocated by several groups (718,733). Phenytoin enters the brain more rapidly than phenobarbital, but not as rapidly as diazepam. Once phenytoin has controlled the seizures, immediate recurrence is unlikely. The major drawbacks to phenytoin are its delivery into the circulation and the side effects caused by its high pH level as well as the propylene glycol content needed to increase its solubility (734). Phenytoin is given as an initial intravenous bolus of 10 mg/kg. To prevent cardiovascular toxicity, the drug is given at a rate of less than 1 mg/kg per minute (725,733). A second bolus of 5 mg/kg is given an hour later. This is followed by an intravenous maintenance dose of 10 mg/kg per 24 hours. Shorvon and Richard and coworkers recommend a somewhat higher loading dose (15 mg/kg), with subsequent intravenous doses adjusted according to blood levels obtained at 2 and 8 hours (718,735). The former group recommends changing to oral maintenance phenytoin at 28 hours. We prefer the use of carbamazepine or valproate for maintenance after status, particularly in infants and small children.

The main advantages of phenytoin are a half-life of 24 or more hours and lack of significant CNS depression. For this reason, the drug is usually preferred for patients with status following a head injury, in whom preservation of consciousness is desirable. The anticonvulsant should not be administered intramuscularly because it is absorbed too slowly to result in effective anticonvulsant serum and tissue levels (736).

Fosphenytoin, a disodium phosphate ester of phenytoin, has found wide acceptance for the treatment of status and in many centers has replaced phenytoin. The drug is completely water soluble and is rapidly and completely converted to phenytoin. It can be administered both intravenously at a dosage of 10 to 20 mg/kg or intramuscularly (733,737). Holmes and Riviello recommend its use in children whose status has lasted longer than 10 minutes (738). Evrard and colleagues recommend prompt combined treatment with a benzodiazepine such as lorazepam, which has GABAergic action and counteracts the excitatory effect of released glutamate, with fosphenytoin, which antagonizes the release of excitatory amino acids, and believe that these two drugs have a synergistic effect (739).

Another means of controlling status epilepticus is by the use of sodium phenobarbital. The initial dose of 15 mg/kg is administered intravenously at a rate of 2 mg/kg per minute, intramuscularly, or even subcutaneously. Because the drug requires 15 minutes to penetrate the blood–brain barrier regardless of its mode of administration, the rate at which seizures are controlled is slower than with lorazepam or diazepam, and it is now reserved for those children whose seizures have failed to respond to a benzodiazepine within 15 to 40 minutes after its administration (738).

If phenobarbital is to be used as a backup to a benzodiazepine, the child must be intubated. Aside from its slow rate of action, the disadvantages of phenobarbital are the depression of consciousness and respiration when the drug is used in dosages required for the control of status epilepticus (740).

Refractory seizures are seizures that have continued for 60 minutes or longer despite adequate anticonvulsant therapy. They frequently develop in the presence of acute CNS injury or a neurodegenerative disease. When brain edema is suspected, as is the case when status follows a head injury, corticosteroids or other antiedematous agents should be given. In addition, one may have to resort to midazolam or pentobarbital. Midazolam, an injectable benzodiazepine, is given in a bolus dose of 0.2 mg/kg, followed by an infusion of 1 to 5 μg/kg per minute (741,742). Pentobarbital is given in a loading dose of 5 to 15 mg/kg, followed by a maintenance infusion of 1 to 5 mg/kg per hour (738), with the dosages of pentobarbital being adjusted to maintain an EEG burst suppression pattern (743). Although monitoring the electrical activity of the brain whenever a patient is in status is always desirable, this measure becomes mandatory in the patient with refractory status (725,738).

Other drugs that have been used for the treatment of status epilepticus include intravenous valproate (10 to 20 mg/kg) and lidocaine (744,745). Intravenous valproic acid is given at a dosage of 25 mg/kg for patients who have not been on previous anticonvulsants and 10 mg/kg for patients with a breakthrough seizure. The average infusion rate is 2.5 to 3.0 mg/kg per minute (746). In the United States, clinical experience with long-term use of lidocaine has been limited. According to a survey, 76% of U.S. neurologists use intravenous lorazepam for the treatment of status epilepticus. If this fails, 95% use phenytoin or fosphenytoin. Thereafter, 43% would give phenobarbital, 16% would give intravenous valproic acid, and 19% would give continuous infusion of either pentobarbital, midazolam, or propofol (747).

Whatever the means for treating status, the physician must keep in mind that the intravenous route is the preferred way to administer anticonvulsants; that the most common mistake is to give repeated, yet insufficient, doses of anticonvulsants; and that he or she should avoid using more than one anticonvulsant drug. Transient abnormalities on neuroimaging studies, particularly on MRI, have been seen by us and have been reported in the literature (748). They may raise the suspicion of a neoplastic lesion, but in most instances, they resolve completely.

Following termination of status, the patient is maintained on parenteral anticonvulsant therapy until the patient has regained consciousness. Oral medication is then resumed. With successive doses, the effectiveness of lorazepam and diazepam is progressively reduced, and these agents cannot be used for long-term seizure control.

With prompt and appropriate therapy, mortality owing to status has fallen to essentially nil. However, a significant percentage of patients can die as a consequence of the condition that precipitated status. In the 1989 series of Maytal and coworkers, no deaths occurred in 137 children with unprovoked or febrile status (720). In the series of Phillips and Shanahan, also published in 1989, only 1% of patients died (749). With current therapy, the incidence of residua is low and is essentially nil when status results from a febrile seizure. Although some 9% of children are left with new motor or cognitive deficits, these usually are the consequence of the underlying neurologic condition that caused status. In terms of outcome, the duration of status is less important than its etiology (720). The clinician who cares for children who have experienced an episode of status should keep in mind that such children have a 4% to 6% likelihood of experiencing one or more additional episodes of status, and that children who have had more than one episode of status have approximately a one in three risk of further episodes (750).

Prognosis

Up to 30% of children with epilepsy do not have remission of their seizures despite apparently adequate treatment. One important, recently uncovered factor in the development of refractory epilepsy is the overexpression of a variety of drug resistance proteins or their genes in brain tissue. This overexpression has been observed in brain tissue taken from areas of cortical dysplasia, hippocampal sclerosis, and tubers from patients with refractory epilepsy. Several proteins have been implicated to date, and all belong to the ATP-binding cassette superfamily that also has been associated with resistance of cancer cells to antineoplastic agents. They are the multidrug resistance gene-1 P-glycoprotein (MDR1), multidrug resistance-associated proteins (MRP1 and MRP2), and the major vault protein (MVP). By contrast, control tissue have no or low expression of these four types of proteins (751–753). Because these multidrug transporters restrict the entry of lipophilic molecules such as many of the antiepileptic drugs into brain, their overexpression reduces effective drug concentration at target sites. Genetic factors may well be implicated in whether there is overexpression of one or more of these proteins, and Siddiqui and coworkers have identified a polymorphism in the gene encoding MDR1 in subjects who did not respond to anticonvulsant medications (754). It is not clear, however, whether overexpression of these proteins is the cause or the result of intractable seizures. In experimental animals, recurrent seizures have been shown to induce multidrug resistance genes, and antiepileptic drugs can up-regulate MDR1 and some of the other multidrug transporters. From these data, we suspect that there also could be a genetic contribution to drug-resistant epilepsy.

In addition to these newly uncovered genetic factors, the success of medical therapy in epilepsy depends on the type of seizure and its natural course (755). Several studies have demonstrated that the response to the first drug trial predicts the success of anticonvulsant therapy. Thus, Dlugos and coworkers found that in children with temporal lobe epilepsy, failure to respond to the first anticonvulsant drug was highly predictable for refractory epilepsy (652). MacDonald and colleagues found that the number of seizures experienced by a child during the first six months after presentation predicts the likelihood of remission. Thus, the patient who has experienced two seizures during the first 6 months of observation has a 47% chance of five years' remission, whereas a patient who experienced 10 or more seizures during this period only has a 24% chance of five years' remission (756).

As mentioned previously, the series of Kwan and Brodie working in Glasgow confirm these observations. In their experience, 47% of patients became seizure-free during treatment with their first antiepileptic drug, and only a further 14% became seizure-free during treatment with a second or third drug. In 3%, treatment with two drugs succeeded in controlling seizures (650). Among patients who failed to respond to the first anticonvulsant, only 11% became seizure free when treatment failure was due to lack of efficacy rather than due to intolerable side effects of an idiosyncratic reaction.

Generally, spontaneous remission or control of seizures by anticonvulsants is greatest in children with idiopathic seizures and age of onset between 2 and 12 years (757). Clinically, such children have normal intellect, no abnormalities on neurologic examination, and no focal lesions on imaging studies. In the experience of Camfield and coworkers, who studied children with generalized tonic-clonic, partial, and partial with secondarily generalized seizures, 83% were successfully treated with a single anticonvulsant. Treatment was more likely to be successful in children with generalized tonic-clonic seizures, and treatment failures were more likely in children with complex partial seizures. Of the 17% of children who did not respond to the first anticonvulsant, only 42% ultimately became free of seizures and were in remission at the end of four or more years (651). As in most other studies, the success of anticonvulsant treatment for children with neurologic deficits was significantly less than in the remainder of the study group.

Between 25% and 83% of children younger than 16 years of age who have had a single nonfebrile seizure experience a recurrence, with the median time to recurrence being 5.7 months. In the series of Shinnar and colleagues, 88% of recurrences occurred within 2 years, and only 3% recurred after 5 years (758). The lower recurrence figures are derived from prospective studies (759), whereas the higher figures are derived from retrospective studies (760). As many as 70% of the group with recurrent seizures had only a small number of further attacks before going into remission, which in approximately 90% was permanent (761). In 30% of subjects, seizures continued. These chronic cases constitute the mainstay of a pediatric neurologist's practice. With successful treatment of children in this group, some 30% enter a long remission, whereas 70% continue to experience occasional seizures despite adequate therapy and compliance.

Generally, the longer the period between the onset of seizures and their control, the less likely the chance for significant remissions. The remission rate is 60% if seizures do not come under control within a year of their onset. This contrasts with a remission rate of 10% if seizures remain uncontrolled for more than 4 years and 5% for those who continue to experience seizures for 10 or more years after their diagnosis (762). However, even in medically intractable seizures, the frequency of attacks tends to diminish over the years, especially in those who maintain a normal IQ (763).

Some clinical features can be singled out for prognostic significance.

Remissions occurred in 13% of neurologically intact children with grand mal epilepsy who had experienced fewer than 20 such seizures (764) and in 75% to 80% of children with childhood absence (petit mal) epilepsy (765). In our experience, it is the rare child with normal intelligence whose seizures are not completely or nearly completely controlled with adequate medical supervision and good compliance. Despite good seizure control, the social outcome is not as favorable. In part, this is because of associated learning disorders and, in part, the consequence of a chronic illness (766).

Adverse prognostic factors include partial or mixed seizures, an abnormal neurologic examination, mental retardation, and inadequate seizure control during the early years of the disorder (767). Complete remission is least likely in children with minor motor attacks.

A particularly favorable prognosis is seen in the following seizures:

- Sylvian seizures (i.e., attacks in which the EEG demonstrates a centrotemporal spike discharge) and the other benign partial epilepsies of childhood (768). Otsubo and coworkers have, however, described what they term a *malignant* sylvian epilepsy, with a similar EEG picture to Sylvian seizures but unresponsiveness to anticonvulsants, cognitive deficits, and requiring cortical excision and multiple subpial transections. The underlying cause was a neuronal migration disorder or gliosis in that region (769).
- Partial seizures on falling asleep or waking, absences, or brief atonic and myoclonic seizures in which the EEG demonstrates continuous, generalized spike-wave paroxysmal activity during sleep
- Benign myoclonic seizures
- Nocturnal myoclonus

Absence seizures also have a favorable prognosis. In a follow-up performed 15 years after seizure onset, 65% of patients were in remission, and 18% were taking anticonvulsants. Of the latter group, 38% were seizure free. Seventeen percent were not taking anticonvulsants and continued to experience seizures. Of the total cohort, 15% had progressed to juvenile myoclonic epilepsy. The factors that predicted treatment failure included the presence of cognitive problems, development of nonconvulsive status, the appearance of tonic-clonic seizures after the onset of anticonvulsant therapy, an abnormal EEG background, and a history of generalized seizures in first-degree relatives (770).

Of patients with complex partial seizures, 84% experienced complete seizure control at the end of the first year (651); 61% were in remission at the end of 4 or more years; 35% experienced sporadic seizures, and 4% had intractable epilepsy. Favorable predictive factors in complex partial seizures are good intelligence, a family history of seizures, and a right temporal seizure focus. According to Lindsay and colleagues, unfavorable factors include early onset of seizures, frequent grand mal seizures, an associated hyperkinetic syndrome, and attacks of rage during childhood (771).

Approximately one-eighth of patients with nocturnal tonic-clonic seizures ultimately can be expected to experience daytime attacks as well (772). Although there are no controlled studies that determine whether early and effective anticonvulsant therapy influences the chances for a spontaneous remission, Reynolds and other members of his group, including Shorvon, believe that epilepsy must be treated early and effectively to preclude the evolution of a chronic epileptic condition (761,773). We agree with their position.

Aside from dying from unrelated disorders, epileptic patients can die in status epilepticus as a consequence of their underlying brain disease (e.g., tumor or a CNS degenerative disorder), accidentally as a result of a seizure, and, most perplexing, without any apparent cause (774). The majority of children in the last group had a severe handicap, and death in children with absence epilepsy or partial and primary generalized epilepsy was between 1% and 2% (775). In the series of Donner and coworkers, 52% of children with sudden unexplained death had symptomatic epilepsy that appeared to have been relatively well controlled. In pediatric patients, 60% had therapeutic anticonvulsant blood levels at the time of death (774). Low serum anticonvulsant levels and polytherapy, which are considered to be risk factors in adults, are not significant in the pediatric population. The most likely explanation for their demise is that it is a seizure-related event, such as aspiration, or possibly neurogenic pulmonary edema (775–777).

The question whether recurrent seizures can cause neuronal injury and intellectual deterioration has yielded conflicting results. This is not surprising when one considers the various confounding factors: the heterogeneity of the conditions that induce epilepsy, the effect of subclinical seizures and interictal epileptiform activity, the various comorbidities, the effect of many different treatment regimens, and the genetically determined susceptibilities (778). Neuropathologic examinations of the human brain suggest that recurrent seizures are associated with neuronal injury and reactive changes in the hippocampus. This evidence must be qualified by the lack of data on the effect of chronic epilepsy on the neocortex and cerebellum.

There are longitudinal studies indicating that recurrent seizures are accompanied by a decline in cognitive function, notably an impairment of memory, and more importantly, for the pediatric age group by disruptive behavior. Thus, in a longitudinal study conducted by Austin and Dunn, children with recurrent seizures had worse behavior scores than those children whose seizures were controlled. This study was confounded by the effects of the underlying neurologic dysfunction that resulted in treatment-resistant seizures (779). Neuroimaging studies used to identify structural changes in the brain that might objectify brain damage leading to intellectual deterioration have yielded conflicting results. Most studies have examined the effect of recurrent temporal lobe epilepsy on the hippocampal volume. Studies with contrasting results have been published. In a cross-sectional study, Cendes and coworkers could not find an effect of the duration of epilepsy and seizure frequency with the volume of the hippocampus or amygdala (780). A similar result was obtained by Liu and coworkers, who were unable to correlate changes that developed in the hippocampus, the cerebellum, or the neocortex over the course of several years with the frequency or severity of overt seizures (781). Van Paesschen and colleagues obtained conflicting data. These workers found that the severity of hippocampal damage correlated with the duration of epilepsy and the number of secondarily generalized seizures (782). In a longitudinal study, Briellmann and coworkers found that the hippocampal volume loss over the course of 3 to 4 years correlated with the number of secondarily generalized seizures between scans (783). In other studies, significant atrophy of hippocampus, neocortex, or cerebellum developed in the course of $3^1/_2$ years in 16% of chronic epilepsy patients as compared with 3% of controls. However, the number of overt seizures had no effect on brain volume (778). Other cross-sectional studies have shown that childhood onset temporal lobe epilepsy was associated with a reduced volume of the corpus callosum, particularly its posterior portion (784). The reliability of functional imaging techniques such as MRS, PET, and SPECT for ascertaining cerebral damage following seizures has not been confirmed.

Several cross-sectional and longitudinal studies have found a progressive decline in cognitive function, particularly in memory in both adult and pediatric patients with poorly controlled temporal lobe epilepsy (785,786). In children with rolandic or occipital lobe epilepsy, mild and transient cognitive difficulties were documented, which

Deonna and coworkers felt had a direct relationship to the presence of paroxysmal EEG activity (787).

There is considerable evidence that implicates various drug regimens in causing intellectual deterioration of epileptic patients (788). In the experience of Trimble, some 15% of patients with recurrent seizures deteriorate intellectually over time (789). Examination of patients in Trimble's group revealed that patients with intellectual deterioration had significantly higher serum levels of phenytoin and primidone and lower folic acid levels than the group who did not experience deterioration. When seizure frequency was factored out, these findings still persisted with respect to phenytoin and folic acid (789). Other studies also have implicated polytherapy in intellectual deterioration. Addy concluded that an association between poor cognitive function and phenobarbital or phenytoin intake has been reported too often to continue considering them as first-line anticonvulsants for the pediatric population (790). Trimble and his group have demonstrated that phenobarbital and phenytoin, given singly or jointly, impair immediate and delayed memory and interfere with performance on visual and auditory scanning tasks (789). Eliminating polytherapy or changing the anticonvulsant to carbamazepine tended to improve cognitive function within 3 months. Even with therapeutic anticonvulsant levels of drugs such as phenobarbital, children experience subtle cognitive effects (791). Lamotrigine, carbamazepine, and valproic acid produce less striking cognitive impairment than phenobarbital.

Behavior disturbances are common in epileptic children. In part, they stem from the deleterious effects of a chronic illness, but frequently they, too, are induced by drug therapy and disappear spontaneously once the offending anticonvulsant is withdrawn (792). Additionally, it is likely that children with complex partial seizures are particularly prone to disordered behavior. Abnormal behavior or psychoses also can be part of the ictal phenomenon, as in some patients with absence status, or they can follow a seizure (793).

In view of the adverse effects of long-term anticonvulsant therapy, medication should be withdrawn as soon as feasible. There has been considerable controversy about when drugs should be discontinued after prolonged seizure control. Several studies have attempted to answer this question and have found that recurrence risks are similar after seizure-free intervals of 2, 3, or 4 years (757,794,795).

Holowach-Thurston and coworkers discontinued anticonvulsants after 4 years of seizure control and encountered a relapse rate of 28%, which increased by another 4% when the follow-up was extended to 15 years (796). More than one-half of recurrences were seen during the first year after anticonvulsant withdrawal, and 85% had occurred within 5 years of withdrawal. Other studies have come up with similar recurrence rates, even though in some studies, drug withdrawal was started after a 2-year seizure-free interval (764,797). Neither the sex of the patient nor the age when drugs are withdrawn affect the relapse rate. Children with neurologic dysfunction or an abnormal neurologic examination have a higher incidence of recurrence. The relapse rate is highest in children with juvenile myoclonic epilepsy and complex partial seizures and lowest in benign rolandic epilepsy and absence seizures (797). These results probably reflect the relatively high proportion of patients with idiopathic epilepsy in the last two groups. In the experience of some workers, the age of seizure onset also influences the likelihood of relapse. The prognosis is poorest for those with onset younger than 2 years of age, less so for those with seizure onset at age 12 years or older, and best for those with onset between 2 and 12 years of age (757). Children with seizure onset after 12 years of age have a higher risk for recurrence (795). By contrast, Gherpelli and colleagues noted that the age of seizure onset did not influence the likelihood for recurrence after anticonvulsant withdrawal but found that in their series, the greater the number of seizures experienced by the patient before control, the greater the likelihood for relapse (798).

Whether the EEG can predict a relapse is still unresolved. Whereas Holowach-Thurston and coworkers (796) did not consider EEG findings to be an important predictor of seizure recurrence, Peters and colleagues, Shinnar and coworkers, and Tennison and coworkers did (795,797,799). In the experience of Shinnar and coworkers, EEG slowing, but not epileptiform features, signaled an increased risk for relapse (979). Peters and colleagues and Tennison and coworkers found that the presence of paroxysmal EEG discharges was predictive for recurrence (795,799). As a rule, the EEG is more predictive for relapse in children with idiopathic epilepsy than in those with epilepsy secondary to a known CNS abnormality (794). In all studies, risk of recurrence has been highest during the first few months after withdrawal, with 50% or more of recurrences taking place within 6 months after initiation of withdrawal (794,978). Callaghan and coworkers found that the factors predictive for relapse are the same as in an adult population (800). The rate of anticonvulsant withdrawal does not appear to influence the frequency of relapse, although withdrawal over the course of less than a month is inadvisable, and abrupt withdrawal is known to initiate status epilepticus (799).

Based on these studies, we consider withdrawal of anticonvulsants after approximately 2 years of seizure control. Generally, we withdraw medication over 2 to 3 months. When the child has been on polytherapy, one drug is completely stopped before the other is tapered.

Drug withdrawal after successful epilepsy surgery has been proposed after the patient has been seizure- and aura-free for more than one year. The recurrence rate appears to be unrelated to the duration of seizure-free postoperative anticonvulsant therapy, and in the series compiled by Schiller and coworkers was 14% at two years and 36% at five years following complete anticonvulsant withdrawal. Even after 5 to 6 years of being seizure free on anticonvulsants, patients ran a 33% risk of seizure recurrence (801).

The social problems incurred by an epileptic child in terms of his or her relationship to family and peers are so considerable that they are beyond the scope of this book. The reader is referred to books by O'Donohoe (170) and the chapter by Craig and Oxley in the volume by Laidlaw and colleagues (802) for a more extensive discussion.

In our opinion, epileptic children should participate in all normal activities, including sports. The hyperventilation incurred in the more strenuous athletics is accompanied by a buildup of carbon dioxide and, therefore, should not induce seizures. However, the more hazardous contact sports, such as high school football, are best avoided and should be reserved for nonepileptic youngsters. As well, epileptic children should be permitted to swim with a friend under competent adult supervision (802,803). Kemp and Sibert, who reviewed drowning accidents in epileptic children, found that no child who participated in supervised swimming drowned (804). Most states and countries restrict an epileptic patient from driving a car. Considering the likelihood that a youngster who has been seizure free for 2 or more years will continue to be seizure free, we have no hesitation in recommending such a patient for a driver's license. When it comes to withdrawing medication in such a youngster, we are reluctant to do so, for fear that seizure recurrence will result in loss of the license. The dilemma between maintaining anticonvulsants for longer than necessary and inducing a serious social inconvenience requires an individualized decision.

Specific Seizure Types

Febrile Seizures

The term *febrile seizure* is used to designate seizures associated with fever, usually occuring between three months and five years of age, and excluding those caused by infections of the CNS or other defined causes. Although not part of the definitions used by the National Institutes of Health or the International League Against Epilepsy, in most instances, a minimum body temperature of 37.8° to 38.5°C or 100.1° to 101.4°F is required for a seizure to be considered febrile.

Febrile seizures represent one of the most common neurologic disorders of childhood. In 1924, Patrick and Levy found an incidence of 4.2% of febrile seizures in an unselected group of children attending well baby clinics (805). Subsequent studies have shown an incidence between 2% and 4% (806–808). In Japanese children, the incidence is about 7%, and in Guam, it is as high as 14%. The condition is somewhat more common in male subjects.

Etiology and Clinical Manifestations

The cause for febrile seizures is still unknown. To date, at least three autosomal dominant genes for febrile seizures have been mapped by genetic linkage studies (Table 14.5). In the series of Berg and colleagues (808), 24% of children with febrile seizures had a first-degree relative with febrile seizures; only 20% had no family history of febrile seizures. The reported incidence of frequency of febrile seizures in siblings of children with febrile seizures ranges from 9% to 22% (809). In the families for whom the gene has been mapped, an autosomal dominant mode of inheritance has been established.

From clinical and genetic studies, it has become evident that the genes for febrile seizures differ from those causing afebrile seizures. In the prospective study of Berg and colleagues, only 4% of children with febrile seizures had a first-degree relative with afebrile seizures (808). Berg also pointed out that if febrile seizures were a manifestation of epilepsy, the risk for a second febrile seizure would equal the risk for a second afebrile seizure. In actuality, the risk for the former was 34% as compared with a risk of 2% to 3% for afebrile seizures. Additionally, the factors that predict recurrent febrile seizures, namely young age and a family history of febrile seizures, do not predict occurrence of subsequent afebrile seizures (810).

In most patients, the height of body temperature appears to be an important factor in triggering the seizures, and Millichap has postulated a convulsive threshold beyond which the seizure is precipitated (3,811). Although the rate at which body temperature increases has been frequently cited as a contributing factor in the development of seizures, EEG data obtained on children with artificially induced fever indicate that this is not the case (812). What appears clear, however, is that in a significant proportion of infants, a febrile seizure occurs at the same time or shortly after fever is recognized. In the series of Berg and colleagues, 44% of infants had experienced less than 1 hour of fever at the time of their febrile convulsion; only 13% had fever of more than 24 hours' duration (808). Other authors concur with this observation. In the experience of Autret and colleagues, a febrile seizure was the first manifestation of an illness in 42% of infants treated for febrile seizures (813). Infants who develop a febrile seizure at a relatively low temperature tend to present with a focal febrile seizure and are at risk for a second febrile seizure during the same illness (814).

Aside from human herpesvirus 6 infections and roseola (exanthema subitum), which are responsible for some one-third of first-time febrile seizures (807,815), epidemic diseases are a relatively infrequent cause of febrile seizures. More commonly, a convulsion accompanies an upper respiratory infection or severe gastroenteritis, particularly when caused by *Shigella* (816,817). In none of the infectious illnesses has there been evidence for direct involvement of the brain by the organisms. From these data, the best conclusion is that febrile seizures occur when, as a result of genetic predisposition, the immature neuronal membrane is particularly susceptible to temperature elevations and responds by breaking down. The role of the cytokine network, particularly interferon-alpha, in the pathogenesis of febrile seizures has not been clarified (818).

The first febrile seizure occurs between 6 months and 3 years of age in 93% of affected children (3). Generally, patients with febrile seizures are considered to consist of two distinct groups: the majority (96.9%) has an entity designated by Livingston as a simple febrile seizure (819). The remainder (3.1%) had complex (complicated) febrile seizures. These are defined as seizures of greater than 30 minutes' duration, seizures repeated within the same day, or having focal features either at the onset of the seizure or during the seizure and recurring within 24 hours or within the same febrile illness.

Diagnosis

In the child who has just experienced a first febrile seizure, the clinician is frequently called on to make a decision with respect to obtaining a lumbar puncture, neuroimaging studies, and a subsequent EEG.

Whether the infant who has just experienced his or her first febrile seizure should undergo a lumbar puncture has been a matter of some debate. Despite Lorber and Sunderland's advocacy for a selective lumbar puncture (820), we believe that the diagnostic skills required to ascertain whether an infant is more ill than his or her physical signs suggest are so considerable that it is best to err on the side of safety and perform the tap. This is particularly so for infants younger than 2 months of age, and the study of Green and coworkers documenting the low incidence of occult meningitis in children between the ages of 2 months and 15 years does little to alter our stance (821). Waruiru and Appleton suggest that in children under two years of age, there should be a low threshold for considering meningitis or encephalitis, and a lumbar puncture should be performed, particularly when there is a prior history of irritability, decreased feeding, or lethargy; when a seizure has been complicated; when there has been a prolonged postictal alteration of consciousness or neurologic deficits; when the child has been pretreated with antibiotics; and, of course, when there are physical findings pointing to meningitis or encephalitis (809).

We do not believe that the neurologically healthy child who has experienced his or her first febrile seizure should undergo neuroimaging studies. Freeman and Vining concur with our position (822). However, in the presence of a recurrent febrile seizures, or if the neurologic examination is abnormal, neuroimaging is indicated.

The EEG is of little value in predicting recurrence of febrile seizures or the evolution of afebrile seizures (823). In the Bulgarian series of Sofijanov and colleagues, the EEG, taken 7 to 20 days after a febrile seizure, was normal or nonspecifically abnormal in 78% of children (824). A paroxysmal abnormality was found in 20%, with a generalized or focal fast spike and wave discharge being the most commonly observed paroxysmal abnormality. Stores found a far lower incidence of paroxysmal discharges (1.4% to 3.0%). Their presence was of no predictive value, and he believes that the procedure made more trouble than it was worth (825). Freeman and Vining also consider an EEG to be unnecessary after a first febrile seizure (822). Freeman further states that in his experience, the results of an EEG rarely affect the decision whether or not to treat and that, consequently, an EEG can be deferred for a few weeks (826). We, too, believe that the EEG only rarely contributes to the management of infants with febrile seizures, but find that, in general, the medically sophisticated population in southern California expects or even demands this procedure.

Treatment

Treatment of the febrile seizure consists of controlling the convulsion with anticonvulsants in dosages analogous to those recommended for the treatment of status epilepticus, reduction of body temperature by conductive or evaporative cooling of the patient, and treatment of the acute infection responsible for the fever.

Over the last few years, there has been a fair degree of concensus as to the management of a child who has experienced his or her first febrile seizure. One-third of children will experience one or more further febrile convulsions. More than one-half of recurrences are experienced during the first year following the initial febrile seizure, and over 90% develop within two years. The risk for recurrence is greatest in the first 6 to 12 months after the initial seizure, and the likelihood for recurrence is enhanced in infants who convulse at temperatures below 40°C. A family history for either febrile or afebrile seizures makes a recurrence more likely, as do multiple seizures during the same febrile episode, and an initial febrile seizure at an early age, the last factor simply by increasing the length of time during which the child is susceptible to further febrile convulsions (827,828). The duration of the initial seizure does not influence the likelihood of a recurrent febrile seizure (827). The evidence is overwhelming that neither antipyretics, phenobarbital, nor oral diazepam (0.2 mg/kg) given singly or in combination at the time of another febrile episode can prevent a recurrence (829–831). Administration of rectal diazepam (0.33 to 0.5 mg/kg) at the onset of a febrile illness reduces significantly the risk for a subsequent febrile seizure but does not prolong the time between the first febrile seizure and the next breakthrough (832). Many physicians are, however, concerned that the drowsiness and ataxia induced by diazepam might interfere with their ability to distinguish a benign febrile illness from a potentially more serious condition (809).

Administration of rectal phenobarbital at the onset of a febrile illness is ineffective (833).

It is important to realize that most febrile seizures are self-limited, but should a seizure not stop within five minutes, prompt administration of rectal diazepam is indicated.

Continuous prophylactic anticonvulsant therapy has been considered for children without risk factors. However, with only a 30% likelihood of a recurrence of the first febrile seizure, and no evidence that treatment of febrile seizures prevents subsequent afebrile (i.e., epileptic) seizures or that recurrent febrile seizures have an adverse effect on intellect, the only rationale for treating febrile seizures in such children is to allay family anxiety. Current consensus as formulated by Baumann and Duffner for the American Academy of Pediatrics proposes that even though continuous prophylactic treatment with phenobarbital or valproic acid does reduce the risk for recurrence, the side effects of phenobarbital and the potential toxicity of valproate outweigh the relatively minor risks of recurrent febrile convulsions (834). When treatment has been elected for children who are developmentally delayed or who have an abnormal neurologic examination, phenobarbital is given for approximately 1 to 2 years, during which time blood levels should be monitored. If side effects are encountered, we change to oral or rectal diazepam (0.5 mg/kg per day) to be given at the onset of subsequent fevers.

Prognosis

In addition to the likelihood of further febrile convulsions, two other aspects of prognosis are usually of concern to the family and to the physician: the likelihood of subsequent afebrile seizures, and the likelihood that a prolonged febrile seizure will induce permanent neurologic or intellectual damage.

Five risk factors predispose the child with febrile seizures to subsequent epilepsy (817,835–838). In order of importance, they are antecedent neurologic or developmental abnormalities, epilepsy in a first-degree relative, complex febrile seizures, onset of febrile seizures before 1 year of age, and multiple recurrences of febrile seizures (839). The importance of prior neurologic deficits in increasing the likelihood for subsequent afebrile seizures has been stressed by Maytal and Shinnar, who noted that a complex febrile seizure does not increase the risk for subsequent afebrile seizures in an infant who is neurologically normal (840). Other studies, including the British cohort study of Verity and colleagues, have come to similar conclusions (841).

In the collaborative study conducted under the auspices of the National Institutes of Health, the incidence of epilepsy by 7 years of age was 1.1% in children with febrile seizures who did not have any of the previously mentioned risk factors. This compared with an incidence of 0.5% in the general population. In the Mayo Clinic study by Annegers and coworkers, the cumulative risk for subsequent epilepsy in children with febrile seizures was 2.4% (838). In children whose neurologic status before their first febrile seizure was not normal, and whose first febrile seizure was severe, the incidence of epilepsy rose to 9.2% (835). A similar greater risk for afebrile seizures is seen in children with focal, prolonged, or repeated febrile seizures, being 50% when all these factors were combined (838). Probably a pre-existing brain abnormality predisposes to both complex febrile seizures and subsequent afebrile seizures.

TABLE 14.16 Time of Appearance of Spontaneous Nonfebrile Seizures in Relation to Onset of Febrile Seizures in 313 Patients with Both Types of Seizures

Time of Appearance of Nonfebrile Seizures	*Patients with Febrile Seizures*	
	Number	***Percent***
Before febrile seizures	20	6.4
Close to febrile seizures	21	6.7
Years after febrile seizures	147	46.9
1 mo to 1 yr		
1–4	54	17.3
5–9	47	15.1
10–14	14	4.5
15–35	10	3.1

Modified from Lennox WG. Significance of febrile convulsions. *Pediatrics* 1953;11:341.

Afebrile seizures after febrile seizures are usually major motor and tend to appear within 1 year after the first febrile seizures (Table 14.16) (835,838,842). The relationship between febrile seizures and subsequent temporal lobe epilepsy remains controversial. As many as 40% of adults with intractable temporal lobe epilepsy have a history of prolonged febrile convulsions during childhood (843,844). On the other hand, prospective and controlled population-based studies—perhaps not conducted over a sufficiently long period—have failed to find this association (845). Relevant to this discussion is the recent discovery of polymorphisms in the interleukin gene that links prolonged febrile convulsions with temporal lobe epilepsy with hippocampal sclerosis (846).

Autopsy studies performed on the rare infant who died after a prolonged febrile seizure reveal anoxic changes affecting the hippocampus, neocortex, thalamus, and cerebellum. It is not clear whether these alterations represent precursors to mesial temporal sclerosis, which is a common pathologic finding in patients with complex partial seizures (194). MRI studies are commensurate with pathologic examination. In adults with temporal lobe epilepsy who provided a history of prolonged febrile seizures, neuroimaging uncovered a higher incidence of atrophy of the amygdala and mesial temporal sclerosis than in patients with temporal lobe seizures who had not experienced prolonged febrile convulsions (843). Fernández and coworkers suggest that in familial febrile convulsions, a subtle pre-existing malformation of the hippocampus, possibly a migrational disturbance, is a prerequisite for the development of hippocampal sclerosis after febrile convulsions (847). Based on work performed on animal models, Bender and colleagues suggest that synaptic reorganization of granule cells and alteration in the expression of various genes resulting from prolonged febrile convulsions could lead to epileptogenesis (848).

Although intuitively one would expect that prolonged febrile seizures are detrimental to ultimate intellectual function, the IQs of children who were developmentally normal before their first seizure and who did not have any subsequent afebrile seizures were no lower than the IQs of their asymptomatic siblings, regardless of the duration of the first febrile seizure (849,850). These observations are confirmed by more recent studies published in 1998 (851).

Complications of febrile seizures are extremely rare: Death occurs in 0.08%, and persistent hemiplegia is unusual (817,835,852). Subsequent mental retardation was noted in only 1% of 400 children with febrile seizures; in none did the febrile seizure last longer than 5 minutes, and one-half of the mentally retarded children already had a history of delayed milestones before their first febrile seizure (833,853).

Neonatal Seizures

Because seizures occur with relatively high frequency during the neonatal period and present special problems for diagnosis and treatment, they are considered separately.

Etiology

The incidence rate of seizures during the neonatal period ranges between 2.0 and 2.8 in 1,000 live births for term neonates. It is 13.5 in 1,000 live births for infants weighing less than 2,500 g and 57.5 in 1,000 for infants weighing less than 1,500 g (854,855). The various causes for seizures during the newborn period and their relative frequency as determined by autopsy are presented in Table 14.17 (856). Currently, the most common identifiable causes are hypoxic-ischemic encephalopathy and infections, especially sepsis and bacterial meningitis (see Chapter 7). In the study of Ronen and coworkers, prenatal, perinatal, and postnatal hypoxic ischemic encephalopathy accounted for 40% of neonatal seizures, and infections for 20% of neonatal seizures (855). Subdural hemorrhage and intracerebral and intraventricular hemorrhages are less common. Developmental anomalies of the brain are probably more common than would appear from the data of Mizrahi (856) and the autopsy series of Volpe (857) because a large proportion of infants with these anomalies do not die from them, and others who have a poor Apgar score are frequently included in the group with hypoxic-ischemic encephalopathy.

TABLE 14.17 Etiology of Neonatal Seizures (1971 and 1986)

Etiology	*Percent (1986)*	*Percent (1971)*
Hypoxic-ischemic encephalopathy	46	36
Infection	17	4
Intracerebral hemorrhage	7	
Intraventricular hemorrhage	6	
Infarction	6	
Hypoglycemia	5	5
Congenital anomaly of CNS	4	6
Inborn errors of metabolism	4	
Subarachnoid hemorrhage	2	
Unknown	2	23
Hypocalcemia	0	31

Modified from Mizrahi EM. Neonatal seizures: problems in diagnosis and classification. *Epilepsia* 1987;28[Suppl]:S46.

Characteristically, seizures owing to perinatal asphyxia and its complications start within the first 24 hours of life. According to Volpe, 60% of asphyxiated infants who experience a seizure have their first seizure within 12 hours of birth (857). Neonatal seizures induced by developmental defects also start in the first 3 days of life; the age when seizures start, therefore, will not assist in diagnosing their etiology or, in the case of a perinatal asphyxial insult, its timing (858).

Hypoglycemic seizures are relatively common during the neonatal period, but as shown in Table 14.17, hypocalcemic seizures have become extremely rare over the last three decades. In the series of Ronen and colleagues, collected in Newfoundland and published in 1999, seizures caused by hypocalcemia or hypomagnesemia accounted for 5.6% of neonatal seizures (855). Hypoglycemic seizures are more common in infants who are small for gestational age and offspring of diabetic mothers, and generally, they appear during the second day of life. In the majority of these children, hypoglycemia is preceded by perinatal asphyxia or other causes for perinatal stress (855). A more extensive discussion of these seizures can be found in Chapter 17.

The narcotic withdrawal syndrome in newborn infants of mothers who are narcotic addicts has been recognized with increased frequency in recent years. Although seizures are uncommon among these infants, they have been observed in the most severely affected. Seizures are most likely to be encountered in infants born to mothers taking barbiturates, particularly the short-acting type; in neonates passively addicted to alcohol; and in infants born to methadone-addicted mothers (859). Signs of neonatal withdrawal usually appear during the first or second day of life but can be delayed for up to several days.

In rare instances, various genetic disorders can induce seizures during the neonatal period. These are listed in Table 14.5. In exceptional instances, inborn errors of metabolism are responsible for neonatal seizures (see Chapter 1).

Clinical Manifestations

Only a small fraction of neonates experience classic tonic-clonic convulsions (860). Rather, neonatal seizures are difficult to recognize, and their appearance reflects the immature nervous system of the newborn infant and its inability to propagate epileptic discharges. Volpe delineated these various seizure types in order of decreasing frequency: subtle, tonic, multifocal clonic, focal clonic, and generalized focal or multifocal myoclonic seizures (857,861). In the EEG-monitored series of Scher and colleagues, subtle seizures also were the most common and accounted for 71% of seizures seen in term infants and 68% of seizures seen in preterm infants (858). Other workers have encountered a much lower incidence of subtle seizures (855,862). It is possible that because of their unimpressive clinical appearance, subtle seizures are frequently overlooked. Subtle seizures (or motor automatisms) are characterized by rhythmic eye movement, chewing, or unusual rowing; swimming; or pedaling movements of arms and legs. These movements can frequently be provoked by stimulation and are suppressed by restraint or repositioning (860).

Tonic seizures can be generalized or focal. Generalized tonic seizures are more common and are marked by sustained hyperextension of the upper and lower extremities or of the trunk and neck. Focal or multifocal clonic movements of the extremities are usually at one to three jerks per second. They can be distinguished from tremor or jitteriness, which is observed in approximately one-half of healthy neonates, by the fact that in the latter condition, the rate of rhythmic movements is faster, usually five to six per second. The movements and jitteriness are of equal amplitude around a fixed axis and can be stopped by restraining or repositioning the limb (863).

Other seizure forms include symmetric posturing of limbs or trunk and atonic attacks characterized by arrest of movement, with the infant becoming limp and unresponsive. In the experience of Mizrahi and Kellaway, apnea was never seen as the sole seizure manifestation (860). In the series of Ronen and colleagues, apneic seizures were more frequently seen in infants of less than 38 weeks' gestation (855).

When seizures are correlated with simultaneously recorded EEG, it becomes evident that not all seizure types are accompanied by cortical seizure activity and that not all electrocortical seizures are clinically manifest (electroclinical disassociation) (860,864). In particular, motor automatisms and generalized tonic seizures can occur without associated EEG seizure activity, implying that these movements originate from subcortical gray matter or that they represent brainstem-release phenomena. Mizrahi and Kellaway favor the latter alternative and argue against treatment of these phenomena with anticonvulsants for fear of further depression of the higher centers (860).

Although these various seizure forms cannot yet be related to gestational age or to etiology, seizures without corresponding EEG abnormalities are more likely to be seen after hypoxic-ischemic encephalopathy and are a poor prognostic sign. In a significant proportion of nonparalyzed term infants, EEG seizures occur in the absence of obvious clinical findings. In the series of Connell and coworkers, clinical seizures accompanied EEG seizures in only 47% of term infants; in approximately two-thirds of these, the clinical evidence for seizures was not at all obvious (862). As many as 70% of preterm infants do not show any clinical evidence for seizures despite a concurrent paroxysmal EEG (862).

Evaluation

The evaluation of the neonate with seizures requires obtaining the basic clinical and laboratory data, including blood chemistries, a septic workup, and imaging for structural brain abnormalities. The value of each of the various available imaging techniques is covered in Chapter 6. Electroencephalography plays a central role in evaluation and management of the infant, and EEG video monitoring has become an important diagnostic tool (865). It can be used to determine the severity and, hence, the prognosis of cerebral dysfunction, and with an amplitude-integrated EEG using the cerebral function monitor, it is a valuable monitoring device (866). A survey of the various EEG patterns in the neonate is far beyond the scope of this text. The interested reader is referred to a text by Mizrahi and coworkers (867).

Treatment

The primary concern of the physician treating the neonate with seizures is the immediate identification of those causes that are amenable to specific treatment. Therefore, appropriate studies must be performed to exclude sepsis, meningitis, hypoglycemia, hyponatremia, hypocalcemia, and hypomagnesemia. Intramuscular pyridoxine (25 to 50 mg) also should be given as a therapeutic trial to exclude pyridoxine dependency (868).

When the underlying cause for seizures cannot be treated specifically, the physician must be content with symptomatic therapy. Phenobarbital is the anticonvulsant most commonly used during the neonatal period. The drug is administered in an intramuscular or intravenous loading dose of 20 mg/kg, with the intravenous dose being given over the course of 15 minutes. This is followed by additional increments of 10 mg/kg as required to achieve serum barbiturate levels between 20 and 40 μg/ml. Donn and coworkers have found that loading doses of up to 30 mg/kg are well tolerated (869). Peak barbiturate concentrations are reached within 1 to 6 hours, and maintenance dosages of 3 to 4 mg/kg per day are initiated once the blood barbiturate level falls below 15 to 20 μg/mL. Because the drug has a half-life of more than 6 days in the neonate, this usually does not occur until 5 to 7 days of age (869–871). These drug schedules apply irrespective of the gestational age of the infant at the time of birth. Nevertheless, for optimal seizure control, daily or twice daily barbiturate levels must be secured, with optimal levels being between 16 and 40 μg/mL (861,864).

We have not had much success controlling neonatal seizures using oral or parenteral phenytoin. However, Painter and coworkers have found intravenous phenytoin to be equally effective as phenobarbital in controlling seizures (872). In our experience, the relation between drug dosage and serum levels is unpredictable, and toxic reactions are common, probably because of the immaturity of the hepatic hydroxylating system responsible for phenytoin detoxification. Bourgeois and Dodson recommend administering the drug orally or parenterally in dosages of 5 to 15 mg/kg per day (873). Mizrahi and Kellaway recommend a loading dose of 20 mg/kg to achieve serum levels between 15 and 20 μg/ml (874). The experience with fosphenytoin has been similar in that therapeutic serum phenytoin levels are difficult to maintain (875).

Diazepam given intravenously (0.5 mg/kg) also has been suggested as an anticonvulsant in the newborn infant, although it is no better than phenobarbital for the treatment of neonatal seizures (857). Also, its short half-life (18 hours in term infants) makes it a poor drug for maintenance (875).

In summary, as one of us (R.S.) has recently pointed out, fewer than one-half of infants treated with either phenobarbital or phenytoin responded with electrographic cessation of seizures (876). What is even more worrisome is that experimental studies suggest that the traditional anticonvulsants such as phenytoin, which block voltage-dependent sodium channels, or phenobarbital, which enhances chloride flux through the GABA A receptor, can produce widespread apoptosis of neurons (877). Midazolam, another GABA agonist, has been suggested as alternative anticonvulsant in infants who fail to respond to phenobarbital or phenytoin and has been widely used in the United Kingdom (878). There is good likelihood that AMPA-antagonist anticonvulsants such as topiramate will be more effective in controlling neonatal seizures without potential long-term side-effects.

Infants with electrocortical paroxysmal discharges but no apparent clinical seizures present a therapeutic dilemma. Although considerable experimental evidence suggests that uncontrolled seizures have a deleterious effect on the developing brain, so does chronic administration of phenobarbital (79). Not wishing to treat an EEG abnormality, we prefer to delay the use of anticonvulsants under such circumstances until clinical evidence for seizures exists. Volpe is of the same opinion (857,861). On the other hand, PET and nuclear MR (NMR) studies suggest that seizures documented by EEG exacerbate the brain damage produced by the underlying insult (879).

Prognosis

As a rule, the prognosis for neonatal seizures depends on the underlying cause. Follow-up studies on infants with neonatal seizures are summarized in Table 14.18. In a series from Pittsburgh, compiled by Bergman and coworkers, 47% of infants were normal at 1 to 5 years of age, and 24.7% died (880). Infants with seizures caused by perinatal asphyxia or malformations of the CNS have a fair prognosis for survival, but not for normal intellectual development and freedom from subsequent seizures (881). In a series of neonates with EEG-confirmed seizures, 70% of infants who survived perinatal asphyxia experienced epilepsy, developmental delay, or cerebral palsy (879). In the relatively current experience of Volpe (857), 50% of infants with neonatal seizures had normal development, whereas only 10% of infants whose seizures were the result of intraventricular hemorrhage, and none of those with congenital anomalies of the brain, escaped intellectual deficits (857). It should be noted that every patient who experienced a chronic seizure disorder secondary to hypoxic-ischemic encephalopathy also had cerebral palsy or mental retardation (879). The incidence of permanent neurologic sequelae is similar in other studies, although results from the Collaborative Project are somewhat more optimistic in that 70% of 7-year-old children who had experienced seizures during the neonatal period were neurologically and intellectually intact (882). The differences in outcomes could reflect the inclusion of hypocalcemic seizures in the Collaborative Project. When neonatal seizures recur in later life, they usually do so before the third year, and preventive therapy with phenobarbital appears to be ineffectual. Infantile spasms or minor motor seizures are particularly common and were seen in approximately one-half of children who experienced a recurrence of their neonatal seizures (883).

The clinical appearance of the child can provide important prognostic clues. Prolonged and repetitive seizures are associated with a bad outcome, either in terms of mortality or significant neurologic residua. A persistently abnormal neurologic examination—in particular, abnormalities of eye movements—suggests a poor prognosis, as does the presence of subtle seizures. The interictal EEG also is of considerable prognostic help. The presence of burst-suppression patterns, low voltage background, or multifocal sharp waves are particularly ominous findings; only 12% of infants showing multifocal sharp waves achieved normal development (884).

TABLE 14.18 Outcome of 131 Infants with Neonatal Seizures

Cause	Number of Patients	Death or Severe or Moderate Impairment	Normal or Mild Impairment
Hypoxia-ischemia, intracranial hemorrhage, or both[a]	77	41	34
≤31 wk[b]	28	16	11
32–36 wk	14	10	4
≥37 wk[b]	35	15	19
16			
Infection, bacterial or viral[c]	16	7	9
Metabolic			
Hypoglycemia	7	2	5
Hypocalcemia	2	0	2
Hyperbilirubinemia	1	1	0
Transient hyperammonemia	1	1	0
Brain malformations/genetic syndromes	5	5	0
Trauma	4	0	4
Narcotic withdrawal	2	0	3
Unknown	16	4	12
Total	**131**	**61**	**68**

[a]Outcome unknown for two patients with hypoxic-ischemic seizures.
[b]Gestational age.
[c]Twelve meningitis and four sepsis.
From Bergman L, Painter MJ, Hirsch RP, et al. Outcome in neonates with convulsions treated in an intensive care unit. *Ann Neurol* 1983;14:642–647. With permission.

The outlook is better for the infant who is seizure free at discharge. In the experience of Painter and coworkers (885), only 6% of neonates who had experienced a seizure but were free of seizures at the time of hospital discharge had a recurrence. Bad prognostic factors are a 5-minute Apgar score of less than 7, seizures lasting more than 30 minutes, and the need for prolonged resuscitation (886).

Considerable controversy exists, but little data, regarding how long anticonvulsants should be given to an infant who has experienced neonatal seizures. Although experimental data derived from rats suggest an adverse effect of phenobarbital on the developing nervous system, the applicability of these results to the human, whose brain is more mature at birth, has not been demonstrated unequivocally.

We maintain adequate phenobarbital blood levels for the first 3 months of life. Thereafter, in the presence of normal development, continued freedom from seizures, and a normal EEG, we allow the infant to outgrow the phenobarbital dosage so that when blood levels drop below 15 μg/mL, the drug can be discontinued.

Differential Diagnosis of Neonatal Seizures

A syndrome of infantile epileptic encephalopathy was first described by Ohtahara and colleagues (887). The condition is marked by severe and recurrent seizures, mainly tonic spasms or partial motor seizures and a striking and persistent burst-suppression EEG. It is discussed in another part of this chapter.

A syndrome, termed *benign idiopathic neonatal seizures*, is characterized by the onset of seizures during the latter part of the first week of life. In the experience of Volpe (857), 5% of term infants fell into this group. The seizures are generally multifocal clonic and last less than 24 hours (888). Their cause is as yet unexplained, and almost all infants become seizure free with normal intellectual development.

The rare and genetically heterogeneous conditions, termed *benign familial neonatal convulsions*, are characterized by the occurrence of focal or generalized clonic seizures during the second or third day of life (889,890). The interictal EEG is normal, and seizures usually stop by 6 months of age. These conditions were summarized in Table 14.5.

REFERENCES

1. Tempkin O. *The falling sickness*, 2nd ed. Baltimore: The Johns Hopkins University Press, 1971.
2. Jackson HJ. On convulsive seizures. *BMJ* 1890;1:703–707,765–771,821–827.
3. Millichap JG. *Febrile convulsions*. New York: Macmillan, 1968.
4. Baumann RJ. Classification and population studies of epilepsy. In: Anderson VA, et al., eds. *Genetic basis of the epilepsies*. New York: Raven Press, 1982:11–20.
5. Goodridge DMG, Shorvon SD. Epileptic seizures in a population of 6000. I. Demography, diagnosis and classification, and role of the hospital services. *BMJ* 1983;287:641–645.
6. Commission on Classification and Terminology of the International League Against Epilepsy. Proposal for revised classification

of epilepsies and epileptic syndromes. *Epilepsia* 1989;30:389–399.

7. Hughlings-Jackson J. On right- or left-sided spasm at the onset of epileptic paroxysms, and on crude sensation warnings, and elaborate mental states. *Brain* 1880;3:192–206.
8. Cowan LD, Bodensteiner JB, Leviton A, et al. Prevalence of the epilepsies in children and adolescents. *Epilepsia* 1989;30:94–106.
9. AndermannE. Multifactorial inheritance of generalized and focal epilepsy. In: Anderson VE, et al., eds. *Genetic basis of the epilepsies*. New York: Raven Press, 1982:355–374.
10. Hauser WA, Hesdorffer DC. *Epilepsy: frequency, causes and consequences*. New York: Demos Publications, 1990.
11. Blandfort M, Tsuboi T, Vogel F. Genetic counseling in the epilepsies. I. Genetic risks. *Hum Genet* 1987;76:303–331.
12. Jouvenceau A, Eunson LH, Spauschus A, et al. Human epilepsy associated with dysfunction of the brain P/Q-type calcium channel. *Lancet* 2001;358:801–807.
13. Heron SE, Crossland KM, Andermann E, et al. Sodium-channel defects in benign familial neonatal-infantile seizures. *Lancet* 2002; 360:851–852.
14. Concolino D, Iembo MA, Rossi E, et al. Familial pericentric inversion of chromosome 5 in a family with benign neonatal convulsions. *J Med Genet* 2002;39:214–216.
15. Berkovic SF, Heron SE, Giordano L, et al. Benign familial neonatal-infantile seizures: characterization of a new sodium channelopathy. *Ann Neurol* 2004;55:550–557.
16. Audenaert D, Claes L, Ceulemans B, et al. A deletion in SCN1B is associated with febrile seizures and early-onset absence epilepsy. *Neurology* 2003;61:854–856.
17. Escayg A, MacDonald BT, Meisler MH, et al. Mutations of SCN1A, encoding a neuronal sodium channel, in two families with GEFS+2. *Nat Genet* 2000;24:343–345.
18. Baulac S, Gourfinkel-An I, Picard F, et al. A second locus for familial generalized epilepsy with febrile seizures plus maps to chromosome 2q21–q33. *Am J Hum Genet* 1999;65:1078–1085.
19. Baulac S, Huberfeld F, Gourfinkel-An I, et al. First genetic evidence of GABA(A) receptor dysfunction in epilepsy: a mutation in the gamma2-subunit gene. *Nat Genet* 2001;28:46–48.
20. Echenne R, Humbertclaude V, Rivier F, et al. Benign infantile epilepsy with autosomal dominant inheritance. *Brain Dev* 1994;16:108–111.
21. Weber YG, Berger A, Bebek N, et al. Benign familial infantile convulsions: linkage to chromosome 16p12–q12 in 14 families. *Epilepsia* 2004;45:601–609.
22. Kamiya K, Kaneda M, Sugawara T, et al. A nonsense mutation of the sodium channel gene SCN2A in a patient with intractible epilepsy and mental decline. *J Neurosci* 2004;24:2690–2698.
23. Nabbout R, Gennaro E, Della Bernardina B, et al. Spectrum of SCN1A mutations in severe myoclonic epilepsy of infancy. *Neurology* 2003;60:1961–1967.
24. Gambardella A, Annesi G, De Fusco M, et al. A new locus for autosomal dominant nocturnal frontal lobe epilepsy maps to chromosome 1. *Neurology* 2000;55:1467–1471.
25. Go W, Brodtkorb E, Steinlein OK. LGI1 is mutated in familial temporal lobe epilepsy characterized by aphasic seizures. *Ann Neurol* 2002;52:364–367.
26. Scheffer IE, Wallace RH, Phillips FL, et al. X-linked myoclonic epilepsy with spasticity and intellectual disability: mutation in the homeobox gene ARX. *Neurology* 2002;59:348–356.

26a. Wallace RH, Marini C, Petrou S, et al. Mutant GABA(A) receptor gamma2-subunit in childhood absence epilepsy and febrile seizures. *Nat Genet* 200l;28:49–52.

26b. Fusco MD, Becchetti A, Patrignani A, et al. The nicotinic receptor beta 2 subunit is mutant in nocturnal frontal lobe epilepsy. *Nat Genet* 2000;26:275–276.

27. Wallace RH, Berkovic SF, Howell RA, et al. Suggestion of a major gene for familial febrile convulsions mapping to 8q13–21. *J Med Genet* 1996;33:308–312.
28. Johnson EW, Dubowsky J, Rich SS, et al. Evidence for a novel gene for familial febrile convulsions, FEB2, linked to chromosome 19p in an extended family from the Midwest. *Hum Mol Genet* 1998;7:63–67.
29. Peiffer A, Thompson J, Charlier C, et al. A locus for febrile seizures (FEB3) maps to chromosome 2q23–24. *Ann Neurol* 46:671–678.
30. Nakayama J, Hamano K, Iwasaki N, et al. Significant evidence for linkage of febrile seizures to chromosome 5q14–q15. *Hum Mol Genet* 2000;9:87–91.

30a. Nakayama J, Yamamoto N, Hamano K, et al. Linkage and association of febrile seizures to the IMPA2 gene on human chromosome 18. *Neurology* 2004;63:1803–1807.

31. Lennox WG, Lennox MA. *Epilepsy and related disorders*. Boston: Little, Brown and Company, 1960.
32. Metrakos K, Metrakos JD. Genetics of convulsive disorders. II. Genetic and electroencephalographic studies in centrencephalic epilepsy. *Neurology* 1961;11:474–483.
33. Gerken H, Doose H. On the genetics of EEG-anomalies in childhood. III. Spike and waves. *Neuropädiatrie* 1973;4:88–97.
34. Guitierrez-Delicado E, Serratosa JM. Genetics of the epilepsies. *Curr Opin Neurol* 2004;17:147–153.
35. Vanmolkot KR, Kors EE, Hottenga JJ, et al. Novel mutations in the Na^+, K^+-ATPase pump gene ATP1A2 associated with familial hemiplegic migraine and benign familial infantile convulsions. *Ann Neurol* 2003;54:360–366.
36. Berkovic SF, Izzillo P, McMahon JM, et al. LGI1 mutations in temporal lobe epilepsies. *Neurology* 2004;62:1115–1119.
37. Metrakos JD, Metrakos K. Childhood epilepsy of subcortical ("centrencephalic") origin. *Clin Pediatr* 1966;5:537–542.
38. Tsuboi T. Seizures of childhood. A population-based and clinic-based study. *Acta Neurol Scand* 1986;74[Suppl 110]:12–37.
39. Degen R, Degen H-E, Roth C. Some genetic aspects of idiopathic and symptomatic absence seizures: waking and sleep EEG in siblings. *Epilepsia* 1990;31:784–794.
40. Steinlein OK, Mulley JC, Propping P, et al. A missense mutation in the neuronal nicotinic acetylcholine receptor alpha 4 subunit is associated with autosomal dominant nocturnal frontal lobe epilepsy. *Nat Genet* 1995;11:201–203.
41. Steinlein OK, Magnusson A, Stoodt J, et al. An insertion mutation of the CHRNA4 gene in a family with autosomal dominant nocturnal frontal lobe epilepsy. *Hum Mol Genet* 1997;6:943–947.
42. Biervert C, Schroeder BC, Kubisch C, et al. A potassium channel mutation in neonatal human epilepsy. *Science* 1998;279:403–406.
43. Singh NA, Charlier C, Stauffer D, et al. A novel potassium channel gene, KCNQ2, is mutated in an inherited epilepsy of newborns. *Nat Genet* 1998;18:25–29.
44. Charlier C, Singh NA, Ryan SG, et al. A pore mutation in a novel KQT-like potassium channel gene in an idiopathic epilepsy family. *Nat Genet* 1998;18:53–55.
45. Kullmann DM. The neuronal channelopathies. *Brain* 2002;125: 1177–1195.
46. Scheffer IE. Severe infantile epilepsies: molecular genetics challenge clinical classification. *Brain* 2003;126:513–514.

46a. Haug K, Warnstedt M, Alekov AK, et al. Mutations in CLCN2 encoding a voltage-gated chloride channel are associated with idiopathic generalized epilepsies. *Nat Genet* 2003;33:527–532.

47. Durner M, Keddache MA, Tomasini L, et al. Genome scan of idiopathic generalized epilepsy: evidence for major susceptibility gene and modifying genes influencing the seizure type. *Ann Neurol* 2001;49:328–335.
48. Gowers WR. *Epilepsy and other chronic convulsive diseases: their causes, symptoms, and treatment*. London: William Wood and Co, 1885.
49. Giza CC, Kuratani JD, Cokely H, et al. Periventricular nodular heterotopia and childhood absence epilepsy. *Pediatr Neurol* 1999;20:315–318.
50. Fox JW, Lamperti ED, Eksioglu YZ, et al. Mutations in filamin 1 prevent migration of cerebral cortical neurons in human periventricular heterotopia. *Neuron* 1998;21:1315–1325.
51. Sampson LJ, Leyland ML, Dart C. Direct interaction between the actin-binding protein filamin-A and the inwardly rectifying potassium channel, Kir2.1. *J Biol Chem* 2003;278:41988–41997.
52. Meencke HJ, Janz D. Neuropathological findings in primary generalized epilepsy: a study of eight cases. *Epilepsia* 1984;25:8–21.
53. Corsellis JA, Falconer MA. "Cryptic tubers" as a cause of focal epilepsy [Abstract]. *J Neurol Neurosurg Psychiatry* 1971;34:104–105.

54. Pollen DA, Trachtenberg MC. Neuroglia: gliosis and focal epilepsy. *Science* 1970;167:1252–1253.
55. Gleeson JG, Allen KM, Fox JW, et al. Doublecortin, a brain-specific gene mutated in human X-linked lissencephaly and double cortex syndrome, encodes a putative signaling protein. *Cell* 1998;92:63–72.
56. Gleeson JG, Minnerath SR, Fox JW, et al. Characterization of mutations in the gene doublecortin in patients with double cortex syndrome. *Ann Neurol* 1999;45:146–153.
57. Houser CR. Granule cell dispersion in the dentate gyrus of humans with temporal lobe epilepsy. *Brain Res* 1990;535:195–204.
58. Parent JM. The role of seizure-induced neurogenesis in epileptogenesis and brain repair. *Epilepsy Res* 2002;50:179–189.
59. Sankar R, Shin D, Liu H, et al. Granule cell neurogenesis after status epilepticus in the immature rat brain. *Epilepsia* 2000;41[Suppl 6]:S53–S56.
60. Scharfman HE. Functional implications of seizure-induced neurogenesis. *Adv Exp Med Biol* 2004;548:192–212.
61. Aguilar NJ, Rasmussen T. Role of encephalitis in pathogenesis of epilepsy. *Arch Neurol* 1960;2:663–676.
62. Meldrum BS, Vigouroux RA, Brierley JB. Systemic factors and epileptic brain damage: prolonged seizures in paralyzed, artificially ventilated baboons. *Arch Neurol* 1973;29:82–87.
63. Corsellis JAN, Bruton CJ. Neuropathology of status epilepticus in humans. *Adv Neurol* 1983;34:129–139.
64. Wasterlain CG, Fujikawa DG, Penix L, et al. Pathophysiological mechanisms of brain damage from status epilepticus. *Epilepsia* 1993;34[Suppl 1]:S37–53.
65. Scheibel ME, Crandall PH, Scheibel AB. The hippocampus-dentate complex in temporal lobe epilepsy. A Golgi study. *Epilepsia* 1974; 15:55–80.
66. Greenamyre JT, Olson JM, Penney JB Jr, et al. Autoradiographic characterization of *n*-methyl-D-aspartate, quisqualate- and kainate-sensitive glutamate binding sites. *J Pharmacol Exp Ther* 1985;233:254–263.
67. Sommer B, Keinanen K, Verdoorn TA, et al. Flip and flop: a cell-specific functional switch in glutamate-operated channels of the CNS. *Science* 1990;249:1580–1584.
68. Goodman JH, Wasterlain CG, Massarweh WF, et al. Calbindin-D28k immunoreactivity and selective vulnerability to ischemia in the dentate gyrus of the developing rat. *Brain Res* 1993;606:309–314.
69. Iadarola MJ, Gale K. Substantia nigra: site of anticonvulsant activity mediated by gamma-aminobutyric acid. *Science* 1982; 218:1237–1240.
70. Auer RN, Siesjö BK. Biological differences between ischemia, hypoglycemia, and epilepsy. *Ann Neurol* 1988;24:699–707.
71. Sankar R, Wasterlain, CG, Sperber EF. Seizure-induced changes in the immature brain. In: Schwartzkroin PA, Moshe SL, Noebels JL, et al., eds. *Brain development and epilepsy*. Oxford: Oxford University Press, 1995:268–288.
72. Wasterlain CG, Niquet J, Thompson KW, et al. Seizure-induced neuronal death in the immature brain. *Prog Brain Res* 2002; 135:335–353.
73. Represa A, Robain O, Tremblay E, et al. Hippocampal plasticity in childhood epilepsy. *Neurosci Lett* 1989;99:351–355.
74. Mathern GW, Leite JP, Pretorius JK, et al. Children with severe epilepsy: evidence of hippocampal neuron losses and aberrant mossy fiber sprouting during postnatal granule cell migration and differentiation. *Dev Brain Res* 1994;78:70–80.
75. Sankar R, Shin DH, Liu H, et al. Patterns of status epilepticus-induced neuronal injury during development and long-term consequences. *J Neurosci* 1998;18:8382–8393.
76. Sankar R, Shin DH, Wasterlain CG. Serum neuron-specific enolase is a marker for neuronal damage following status epilepticus in the rat. *Epilepsy Res* 1997;28:129–136.
77. Holmes GL. Seizure-induced neuronal injury: animal data. *Neurology* 2002;59[9 Suppl 5]:S3–S6.
78. Shinoda S, Schindler CK, Meller R, et al. Bim regulation may determine hippocampal vulnerability after injurious seizures and in temporal lobe epilepsy. *J Clin Invest* 2004;113:1059–1068.
79. Holmes GL, Ben-Ari Y. Seizures in the developing brain: perhaps not so benign after all. *Neuron* 1998;21:1231–1234.
80. Holmes GL, Gairsa JL, Chevassus-Au-Louis N, et al. Consequences of neonatal seizures in the rat: morphological and behavioral effects. *Ann Neurol* 1998;44:845–857.
81. Holmes GL, Sarkisian M, Ben-Ari Y, et al. Mossy fiber sprouting after recurrent seizures during early development in rats. *J Comp Neurol* 1999;404:537–553.
82. Holmes GL. The long-term effect of seizures on the developing brain: clinical and laboratory issues. *Brain Dev* 1991;13:393–409.
83. Shewmon DA, Erwin RJ. Focal spike-induced cerebral dysfunction is related to the after-coming slow wave. *Ann Neurol* 1988;23: 131–137.
84. Meldrum BS. Excitotoxicity and epileptic brain damage. *Epilepsy Res* 1991;10:55–61.
85. DeGiorgio CM, Tomiyasu U, Gott PS, et al. Hippocampal pyramidal cell loss in human status epilepticus. *Epilepsia* 1992;33: 23–27.
86. Bruton C. *The neuropathology of temporal lobe epilepsy*. New York: Oxford University Press, 1988.
87. Falconer MA, Serafetinides EA, Corsellis JAN. Etiology and pathogenesis of temporal lobe epilepsy. *Arch Neurol* 1964;10:233–248.
88. Engel J, Brown WJ, Kuhl DE, et al. Pathological findings underlying focal temporal lobe hypometabolism in partial epilepsy. *Ann Neurol* 1982;12:518–528.
89. Hudson LP, Munoz DG, Miller L, et al. Amygdaloid sclerosis in temporal lobe epilepsy. *Ann Neurol* 1993;33:622–631.
90. Babb TL, Pretorius JK, Kupfer WR, et al. Glutamate decarboxylase-immunoreactive neurons are preserved in human epileptic hippocampus. *J Neurosci* 1989;9:2562–2574.
91. Franck JE. Cell death, plasticity, and epilepsy. In: Schwartzkroin PA, ed. *Epilepsy: models, mechanisms, and concepts*. Cambridge: Cambridge University Press, 1993:281–303.
92. Scott RC, King MD, Gadian DG, et al. Hippocampal abnormalities after prolonged febrile convulsion: a longitudonal MRI study. *Brain* 2003;126:2551–2557.
92a. VanLandingham KE, Heinz ER, Cavazos JE, et al. Magnetic resonance imaging evidence of hippocampal injury after prolonged focal febrile convulsions. *Ann Neurol* 1998;43:413–426.
92b. Kanemoto K, Kawasaki J, Yuasa S, et al. Increased frequency of interleukin-1beta-511T allele in patients with temporal lobe epilepsy, hippocampal sclerosis, and prolonged febrile convulsion. *Epilepsia* 2003;44:796–799.
93. Engel J. Epileptic brain damage: how much excitement can a limbic neuron take? *Trends Neurosci* 1983;6:356–357.
94. Meldrum BS, Horton RW, Brierley JB. Epileptic brain damage in adolescent baboons following seizures induced by allylglycine. *Brain* 1974;97:407–418.
95. Rocca WA, Sharbrough FW, Hauser WA, et al. Risk factors for complex partial seizures: a population-based case-control study. *Ann Neurol* 1987;21:22–31.
96. Taylor J. *Selected writings of John Hughlings Jackson*. Vol. 1. London: Hodder & Stoughton, 1931.
97. Schwartzkroin PA. "Normal" brain mechanisms that support epileptiform activities. In: Schwartzkroin PA, ed. *Epilepsy: models, mechanisms, and concepts*. Cambridge: Cambridge University Press, 1993:358–370.
98. DeLorenzo RJ. Ion channels, membranes, and molecules in epilepsy and neuronal excitability. In: Pellock JM, Dodson WE, Bourgeois BFD, eds. *Pediatric epilepsy*, 2nd ed. New York: Demos, 2001:25–36.
99. Velísek L, Moshé S. Pathophysiology of seizures and epilepsy in the immature brain: cells, synapses, and circuits. In: Pellock JM, Dodson WE, Bourgeois BFD, eds. *Pediatric epilepsy*, 2nd ed. New York: Demos, 2001:1–24.
100. Dudek FE, Snow RW, Taylor CP. Role of electrical interactions in synchronization of epileptiform bursts. *Adv Neurol* 1986;44:593–617.
101. Heinemann U. Changes in the neuronal micro-environment and epileptiform activity. In: Wieser HG, Speckman EJ, Engel J, eds. *Current problems in epilepsy 3: the epileptic focus*. London: John Libbey & Co Ltd, 1987:27–44.
102. Prince DA, Schwartzkroin PA. Non-synaptic mechanisms in epileptogenesis. In: Chalozonitis N, Boiusson M, eds. *Abnormal neuronal discharges*. New York: Raven Press, 1978:1–12.

103. Goddard GV, McIntyre DC, Leech CK. A permanent change in brain function resulting from daily electrical stimulation. *Exp Neurol* 1969;25:295–330.
104. McNamara J. Kindling: an animal model of complex partial epilepsy. *Ann Neurol* 1984;16[Suppl]:S72–S76.
105. Sutula T, He XX, Cavazos J, et al. Synaptic reorganization in the hippocampus induced by abnormal functional activity. *Science* 1988;239:1147–1150.
106. Sutula T, Cascino G, Cavazos J, et al. Mossy fiber synaptic reorganization in the epileptic human temporal lobe. *Ann Neurol* 1989;26:321–330.
107. Houser CR, Miyashiro JE, Swartz BE, et al. Altered patterns of dynorphin immunoreactivity suggest mossy fiber reorganization in human temporal lobe epilepsy. *J Neurosci* 1990;276–282.
108. Babb TL, Kupfer WR, Pretorius JK, et al. Synaptic reorganization by mossy fibers in human epileptic fascia dentata. *Neuroscience* 1991;42:351–363.
109. Sloviter RS. Possible functional consequence of synaptic reorganization in the dentate gyrus of kainic acid–treated rats. *Neurosci Lett* 1992;137:91–96.
110. Sloviter RS. Permanently altered hippocampal structure, excitability, and inhibition after experimental status epilepticus in the rat: the "dormant basket cell" hypothesis and its possible relevance to temporal lobe epilepsy. *Hippocampus* 1991;1:46–66.
111. Babb TL, Pretorius JK, Kupfer WR, et al. Glutamate decarboxylase–immunoreactive neurons are preserved in human epileptic hippocampus. *J Neurosci* 1989;9:2562–2574.
112. Mathern GW, Pretorius JK, Kornblum HI, et al. Altered hippocampal kainate-receptor mRNA levels in temporal lobe epilepsy patients. *Neurobiol Dis* 1998;5:151–176.
113. Mathern GW, Mendoza D, Lozada A, et al. Hippocampal GABA and glutamate transporter immunoreactivity in patients with temporal lobe epilepsy. *Neurology* 1999;52:453–472.
114. Zucker RS. Frequency dependent changes in excitory synaptic efficacy. In: Dichter MA, ed. *Mechanisms of epileptogenesis—the transition to seizure*. New York: Plenum Publishing, 1988:163–168.
115. Dichter MA. Modulation of inhibition and the transition to seizures. In: Dichter MA, ed. *Mechanisms of epileptogenesis—the transition to seizure*. New York: Plenum Publishing, 1988:169–182.
116. Kapur J, Stringer JL, Lothman LW. Evidence that repetitive seizures in the hippocampus cause a lasting reduction of GABAergic inhibition. *J Neurophysiol* 1989;61:417–426.
117. Brewster A, Bender RA, Chen Y, et al. Developmental febrile seizures modulate hippocampal gene expression of hyperpolarization-activated channels in an isoform- and cell-specific manner. *J Neurosci* 2002;22:4591–4599.
118. Bender RA, Soleymani SV, Brewster AL, et al. Enhanced expression of a specific hyperpolarization-activated cyclic nucleotide-gated cation channel (HCN) in surviving dentate gyrus granule cells of human and experimental epileptic hippocampus. *J Neurosci* 2003;23:6826–6836.
119. Su H, Sochivko D, Becker A, Chen J, et al. Upregulation of a T-type $Ca2^{+}$ channel causes a long-lasting modification of neuronal firing mode after status epilepticus. *J Neurosci* 2002;22:3645–3655.
120. Gale K. Progression and generalization of seizure discharge: anatomical and neurochemical substrates. *Epilepsia* 1988;29 [Suppl 2]:S15–S34.
121. Burnham WM. Core mechanisms in generalized convulsions. *Fed Proc* 1985;44:2442–2445.
122. Browning RA. Role of the brain-stem reticular formation in tonic-clonic seizures: lesion and pharmacological studies. *Fed Proc* 1985;44:2425–2431.
123. Efron R. Post-epileptic paralysis: theoretical critique and report of a case. *Brain* 1961;84:381–394.
124. Niedermeyer E, Laws ER Jr, Walker AE. Depth EEG findings in epileptics with generalized spike-wave complexes. *Arch Neurol* 1969;21:51–58.
125. Goldring S. The role of prefrontal cortex in grand mal convulsion. *Arch Neurol* 1972;26:109–119.
126. Penfield W. Epileptic automatism and the centrencephalic integrating system. *Assoc Res Nerv Ment Dis* 1952;30:513–528.
127. Gloor P, Fariello RG. Generalized epilepsy: some of its cellular mechanisms differ from those of focal epilepsy. *Trends Neurosci* 1988;11:63–68.
128. Engel J. *Seizures, epilepsy and the epileptic patient*. Philadelphia: FA Davis Co, 1989.
129. Coulter DA, Haguenard JR, Prince DA. Characterization of ethosuximide reduction of low-threshold calcium currents in thalamic neurons. *Ann Neurol* 1989;25:582–593.
130. Engel J, Kuhl DE, Phelps ME, et al. Interictal cerebral glucose metabolism in partial epilepsy and its relation to EEG changes. *Ann Neurol* 1982;12:510–517.
131. Spencer SS, Spencer DD, Williamson PD, et al. The localizing value of depth electroencephalography in 32 patients with refractory epilepsy. *Ann Neurol* 1982;12:248–253.
132. Cotman CW, Iverson LL. Excitatory amino acids in the brain-focus on NMDA receptors. *Trends Neurosci* 1987;10:263–265.
133. Turski WA, Cavalheiro EA, Schwarz M, et al. Limbic seizures produced by pilocarpine in rats: a behavioral, electroencephalographic, and neuropathological study. *Behav Brain Res* 1983;9:315–335.
134. Olsen RW, Wamsley JK, Lee RJ, et al. Benzodiazepine/barbiturate/GABA receptor-chloride ionophore complex in a genetic model for generalized epilepsy. *Adv Neurol* 1986;44:365–378.
135. Olsen RW. GABA-drug interactions. *Prog Drug Res* 1987;31:223–341.
136. Schofield PR, Darlison MG, Fujita N, et al. Sequence and functional expression of the GABA A receptor shows a ligand-gated receptor super-family. *Nature* 1987;328:221–227.
137. Pritchett DB, Sontheimer H, Shivers BD, et al. Importance of a novel GABA A receptor subunit for benzodiazepine pharmacology. *Nature* 1989;338:582–584.
138. Sigel E, Baur R, Trube G, et al. The effect of subunit composition of rat brain GABA A receptors on channel function. *Neuron* 1990;5:703–711.
139. Macdonald RL, Twyman RE, Ryan-Jastrow T, et al. Regulation of GABA A receptor channels by anticonvulsant and convulsant drugs and by phosphorylation. *Epilepsy Res Suppl* 1992;265–277.
140. Gale K, Iadarola MJ. Seizure protection and increased nerve-terminal GABA: delayed effects of GABA transaminase inhibition. *Science* 1980;208:288–291.
141. Petroff OA, et al. Human brain GABA and homocarnosine increased after starting topiramate. *Neurology* 1998;50[Suppl 4]:A312.
142. Petroff OAC, Hyder F, Mattson RH, et al. Topiramate increases brain GABA, homocarnosine, and pyrrolidinone in patients with epilepsy. *Neurology* 1999;52:473–478.
143. During M, Mattson R, Scheyer C, et al. The effect of tiagabine hydrochloride on extracellular GABA levels in the human hippocampus. *Epilepsia* 1992;33[Suppl 3]:83.
144. Lott IT, Coulombe T, Di Paolo RV, et al. Vitamin B6–dependent seizures: pathology and chemical findings in brain. *Neurology* 1978;28:47–54.
145. Gospe SM, Olin KL, Keen CL. Reduced GABA synthesis in pyridoxine-dependent seizures. *Lancet* 1994;343:1133–1134.
146. Fromm GH. Role of inhibitory mechanisms in staring spells. *J Clin Neurophysiol* 1986;3:297–311.
147. Peterson GM, Ribak CE, Oertel WH. A regional increase in the number of hippocampal GABAergic neurons and terminals in the seizure-sensitive gerbil. *Brain Res* 1985;340:384–389.
148. Engel J Jr, Ackermann RF, Caledcott-Hazard S, et al. Do altered opioid mechanisms play a role in human epilepsy? In: Fariello RF, Morselli PL, Lloyd KG, et al. *Neurotransmitters, seizures and epilepsy*. New York: Raven Press, 1984:263–274.
149. Frost JJ, Mayberg HS, Fisher RS, et al. μ-Opiate receptors measured by positron emission tomography are increased in temporal lobe epilepsy. *Ann Neurol* 1988;23:231–237.
150. Handforth A, Treiman DM. Effect of an adenosine antagonist and an adenosine agonist on status entry and severity in a model of limbic status epilepticus. *Epilepsy Res* 1994;18:29–42.
151. During MJ, Spencer DD. Adenosine: a potential mediator of seizure arrest and postictal refractoriness. *Ann Neurol* 1992;32:618–624.
152. Dragunow M. Purinergic mechanisms in epilepsy. *Progr Neurobiol* 1988;31:85–108.

153. Chin JH. Adenosine receptors in brain: neuromodulation and role in epilepsy. *Ann Neurol* 1989;26:695–698.
154. Jobe PC, Laird HE. Neurotransmitter abnormalities as determinants of seizure susceptibility and intensity in the genetic models of epilepsy. *Biochem Pharmacol* 1981;30:3137–3144.
155. Mishra PK, Burger RL, Bettendorf AF, et al. Role of norepinephrine in forebrain and brainstem seizures. Chemical lesioning of locus ceruleus with DSP4. *Exp Neurol* 1994;125:58–64.
156. Krahl SE, Clark KB, Smith DC, et al. Locus coeruleus lesions suppress the seizure-attenuating effects of vagus nerve stimulation. *Epilepsia* 1998;39:709–714.
157. Prendiville S, Gale K. Anticonvulsant effect of fluoxetine on focally evoked limbic motor seizures in rats. *Epilepsia* 1993;34:381–384.
158. Leander JD. Fluoxetine, a selective serotonin-uptake inhibitor, enhances the anticonvulsant effects of phenytoin, carbamazepine, and ameltolide (LY201116). *Epilepsia* 1992;33:573–576.
159. Favale E, Rubino V, Mainardi P, et al. Anticonvulsant effect of fluoxetine in humans. *Neurology* 1995;45:1926–1927.
160. Salgado-Commissariat D, Alkadhi KA. Serotonin inhibits epileptiform discharge by activation of 5-HT1A receptors in CA1 pyramidal neurons. *Neuropharmacology* 1997;36:1705–1712.
161. Lu KT, Gean PW. Endogenous serotonin inhibits epileptiform activity in rat hippocampal CA1 neurons via 5-hydroxytryptamine 1A receptor activation. *Neuroscience* 1998;86:729–737.
162. Gerber K, Filakovszky J, Halasz P, et al. The 5-HT_{1A} agonist 8-OH-DPAT increases the number of spike-wave discharges in a genetic rat model of absence epilepsy. *Brain Res* 1998;807:243–245.
163. Applegate CD, Tecott LH. Global increases in seizure susceptibility in mice lacking 5-HT2C receptors: a behavioral analysis. *Exp Neurol* 1998;154:522–530.
164. Engel J, Kuhl DE, Phelps ME, et al. Local cerebral metabolism during partial seizures. *Neurology* 1983;33:400–413.
165. Engel J, Kuhl DE, Phelps ME. Patterns of human local cerebral glucose metabolism during epileptic seizures. *Science* 1982;218:64–66.
166. Engel J, Kuhl DE, Phelps ME, et al. Comparative localization of epileptic foci in partial epilepsy by PCT and EEG. *Ann Neurol* 1982;12:529–537.
167. Meldrum BS, Horton RW. Physiology of status epilepticus in primates. *Arch Neurol* 1973;28:19.
168. Beresford HR, Posner JB, Plum F. Changes in brain lactate during induced cerebral seizures. *Arch Neurol* 1969;20:243–248.
169. Petroff OAC, Prichard JW, Ogino T, et al. Combined ^{1}H and ^{31}P nuclear magnetic resonance spectroscopic studies of bicuculline-induced seizures in vivo. *Ann Neurol* 1986;20:185–193.
170. O'Donohoe NV. *Epilepsies of childhood*, 3rd ed. Oxford: Butterworth–Heinemann, 1994.
171. Van Buren JM. The abdominal aura. A study of abdominal sensations occurring in epilepsy and produced by depth stimulation. *Electroencephalogr Clin Neurophysiol* 1963;15:119.
172. Shinnar S, Berg AT, Moshe SL, et al. How long do new-onset seizures in children last? *Ann Neurol* 2001;49:659–664.
173. D'Allessandro R, Guarino M, Greco G, et al. Risk of seizures while awake in pure sleep epilepsies: a prospective study. *Neurology* 2004;62:254–257.
174. Mattson RH, Pratt KL, Calverley JR. Electroencephalograms of epileptics following sleep deprivation. *Arch Neurol* 1965;13:310–315.
175. Messing RO, Closson RG, Simon RP. Drug-induced seizures: a 10-year experience. *Neurology* 1984;34:1582–1586.
176. Olson KR, Kearney TE, Dyer JE, et al. Seizures associated with poisoning and drug overdose. *Am J Emerg Med* 1994;12:392–395.
177. Blanchard PD, Yao JD, McAlpine DE, et al. Isoniazid overdose in the Cambodian population of Olmstead County, Minnesota. *JAMA* 1986;256:3131–3133.
178. Van Donselaar CA, Brouwer OF, Geerts AT, et al. Clinical course of untreated tonic-clonic seizures in childhood: prospective hospital based study. *Brit Med J* 1997;314:401–404.
179. Pearl PL, Holmes GL. Absence seizures. In: Pellock JM, Dodson WE, Bourgeois BFD, eds. *Pediatric epilepsy*, 2nd ed. New York: Demos, 2001:219–231.
180. Gastaut H, Roger J, Favel F. La miction au cours des absences petit mal. Le petit mal enuretique. *Rev Neurol* 1960;103:53–58.
181. Dalby MA. Epilepsy and 3 per second spike and wave rhythms. *Acta Neurol Scand* 1969;40[Suppl]:3.
182. Lennox WG. The petit mal epilepsies: their treatment with Tridione. *JAMA* 1945;129:1069–1074.
183. Sato S, Dreifuss FE, Penry JK. Prognostic factors in absence seizures. *Neurology* 1976;26:788–796.
184. Holmes GL, McKeever M, Adamson M. Absence seizures in children: clinical and electroencephalographic features. *Ann Neurol* 1987;21:268–273.
185. Berkovic SF, Andermann F, Andermann E, et al. Concepts of absence epilepsies: discrete syndromes or biological continuum? *Neurology* 1987;37:993–1000.
186. Panayiotopoulos CP, Obeid T, Waheed G. Differentiation of typical absence seizures in epileptic syndromes. *Brain* 1989;112:1039–1053.
187. Taylor I, Marini C, Johnson MR, et al. Juvenile myoclonic epilepsy and idiopathic photosensitive occipital lobe epilepsy: is there overlap? *Brain* 2004;127:1878–1876.
188. Janz D. Epilepsy with impulsive petit mal (juvenile myoclonic epilepsy). *Acta Neurol Scand* 1985;72:449–459.
189. Delgado-Escueta AV, Serratosa JM, Medina MT. Juvenile myoclonic epilepsy. In: Wyllie E, ed. *The treatment of epilepsy: principles and practice*, 2nd ed. Baltimore: Williams & Wilkins, 1996:484–501.
190. Appleton R, Beirne M, Acomb B. Photosensitivity in juvenile myoclonic epilepsy. *Seizure* 2000;9:108–111.
191. Prevett MC, Duncan JS, Jones T, et al. Demonstration of thalamic activation during typical absence seizures using $H_2{}^{15}O$ and PET. *Neurology* 1995;45:1396–1402.
192. Williamson PD, Spencer DD, Spencer SS, et al. Complex partial seizures of frontal lobe origin. *Ann Neurol* 1985;18:497–504.
193. Williamson PD, Thadani VM, Darcey TM, et al. Occipital lobe epilepsy: clinical characteristics, seizure spread patterns and results of surgery. *Ann Neurol* 1992;31:3–13.
194. Falconer MA, Serafitinides EA, Corsellis JAN. Etiology and pathogenesis of temporal lobe epilepsy. *Arch Neurol* 1964;10:233–248.
195. Harvey AS, Berkovic SF, Wrennall JA, et al. Temporal lobe epilepsy in childhood. Clinical, EEG, and neuroimaging findings and syndrome classification in a cohort with new-onset seizures. *Neurology* 1997;49:960–968.
196. Cavanagh JB. On certain small tumours encountered in the temporal lobe. *Brain* 1958;81:389–405.
197. Malamud N. The epileptogenic focus in temporal lobe epilepsy from a pathological standpoint. *Arch Neurol* 1966;14:190–195.
198. Wyllie E, Chee M, Granstrom ML, et al. Temporal lobe epilepsy in early childhood. *Epilepsia* 1993;34:859–868.
199. DeLong GR, Heinz ER. The clinical syndrome of early-life bilateral hippocampal sclerosis. *Ann Neurol* 1997;42:11–17.
200. Pacia SV, Devinsky O, Perrine K, et al. Clinical features of neocortical temporal lobe epilepsy. *Ann Neurol* 1996;40:724–730.
201. Yamamoto N, Watanabe K, Negoro T, et al. Complex partial seizures in children: ictal manifestations and their relation to clinical course. *Neurology* 1987;37:1379–1382.
202. Aird RB, Venturini AM, Spielman PM. Antecedents of temporal lobe epilepsy. *Arch Neurol* 1967;16:67–73.
203. Glaser GH, Dixon MS. Psychomotor seizures in childhood: a clinical study. *Neurology* 1956;6:646–655.
204. Daly DD. Uncinate fits. *Neurology* 1958;8:250–260.
205. Acharya V, Acharya J, Lüders H. Olfactory epileptic auras. *Neurology* 1998;51:56–61.
206. Howe JG, Gibson JD. Uncinate seizures and tumors, a myth reexamined. *Ann Neurol* 1982;12:227.
207. Penfield W, Perot P. The brain's record of auditory and visual experience. A final summary and discussion. *Brain* 1963;86:595–616.
208. Mullan S, Penfield W. Illusions of comparative interpretation and emotion; production by epileptic discharge and by electrical stimulation in the temporal cortex. *Arch Neurol Psychiatry* 1959;81:269–284.
209. Palmini A, Gloor P. The localizing values of auras in partial seizures: a prospective and retrospective study. *Neurology* 1992;42:801–809.

210. Escueta AVD, Enrile BF, Treiman DM. Complex partial seizures on closed-circuit television and EEG: a study of 691 attacks in 79 patients. *Ann Neurol* 1982;11:292–300.
211. Gambardella A, Reutens DC, Andermann F, et al. Late-onset drop attacks in temporal lobe epilepsy: a reevaluation of the concept of temporal lobe syncope. *Neurology* 1994;44:1074–1078.
212. Markand ON, Wheeler GL, Pollack SL. Complex partial status epilepticus (psychomotor status). *Neurology* 1978;28:189–196.
213. McBride MC, Dooling EC, Oppenheimer EY. Complex partial status epilepticus in young children. *Ann Neurol* 1981;9:526–530.
214. Williamson PD, Spencer DD, Spencer SS, et al. Complex partial status epilepticus: a depth-electrode study. *Ann Neurol* 1985;18:647–654.
215. Blumhardt LD, Smith PE, Owen L. Electrocardiographic accompaniments of temporal lobe epileptic seizures. *Lancet* 1986;1:1051–1056.
216. Aird RB, Yamamoto T. Behavior disorders of childhood. *Electroenceph Clin Neurophysiol* 1966;21:148–156.
217. Stevens JR, Hermann BP. Temporal lobe epilepsy, psychopathology, and violence: the state of the evidence. *Neurology* 1981;31:1127–1132.
218. Rutter M, Graham P, Yule W. A neuro-psychiatric study in childhood. In: Rutter M, Graham P, Yule W. *Clinics in developmental medicine*. London: Butterworth–Heinemann, 1970:35–36.
219. Pincus JH. Can violence be a manifestation of epilepsy? *Neurology* 1980;30:304–307.
220. Pritchard PB, Lombroso CT, McIntyre M. Psychological complications of temporal lobe epilepsy. *Neurology* 1980;30:227–232.
221. Schoenfeld J, Seidenberg M, Woodard A, et al. Neuropsychological and behavioral status of children with complex partial seizures. *Dev Med Child Neurol* 1999;41:724–731.
222. Stevens JR, Livermore A. Kindling in the mesolimbic dopamine system: animal model of psychosis. *Neurology* 1978;28:36–46.
223. Adamec RE, Stark-Adamec C. Limbic kindling and animal behavior—implications for human psychopathology associated with complex partial seizures. *Biol Psychiatry* 1983;18:269–293.
224. Weiss SR, Post RM. Kindling: separate vs. shared mechanisms in affective disorders and epilepsy. *Neuropsychobiology* 1998;38:167–180.
225. Ochs R, Gloor P, Quesney F, et al. Does head-turning during a seizure have lateralizing or localizing significance? *Neurology* 1984;34:884–890.
226. Wyllie E, Luders H, Morris HH, et al. The lateralizing significance of versive head and eye movements during epileptic seizures. *Neurology* 1986;36:606–611.
227. McLachlan RS. The significance of head and eye turning in seizures. *Neurology* 1987;37:1617–1619.
228. Devinsky O, Kelley K, Porter RJ, et al. Clinical and electroencephalographic features of simple partial seizures. *Neurology* 1988;38:1347–1352.
229. Kellinghaus C, Kotagal P. Lateralizing value of Todd's palsy in patients with epilepsy. *Neurology* 2004;62:289–291.
230. Roger J, Bureau M. Les épilepsies partielles idiopathiques de l'enfant (épilepsies partielles bénignes or primaries). *Rev Neurol* 1987;143:381–391.
231. Loiseau P, Duché B, Loiseau J. Classification of epilepsies and epileptic syndromes in two different samples of patients. *Epilepsia* 1991;32:303–309.
232. Scheffer IE, Jones L, Pozzebon M, et al. Autosomal dominant rolandic epilepsy and speech dyspraxia: a new syndrome with anticipation. *Ann Neurol* 1995;38:633–642.
233. Lombroso CT. Sylvian seizures and midtemporal spike foci in children. *Arch Neurol* 1967;17:52–59.
234. Loiseau P, Beaussart M. The seizures of benign childhood epilepsy with Rolandic paroxysmal discharges. *Epilepsia* 1973;14:381–389.
235. Blom S, Heijbel J. Benign epilepsy of children with centro-temporal EEG foci. Discharge rate during sleep. *Epilepsia* 1975;16:133–140.
236. Gregory DL, Wong PK. Topographical analysis of the centrotemporal discharges in benign rolandic epilepsy of childhood. *Epilepsia* 1984;25:705–711.
237. Loiseau P, Pestre M, Dartigues JF, et al. Long-term prognosis in two forms of childhood epilepsy: typical absence seizures and epilepsy with rolandic (centrotemporal) EEG foci. *Ann Neurol* 1983;13:642–648.
238. Beaussart M, Faou R. Evolution of epilepsy with rolandic paroxysmal foci: a study of 324 cases. *Epilepsia* 1978;19:337–342.
239. Beaumanoir A. Infantile epilepsy with occipital focus and good prognosis. *Eur Neurol* 1983;22:43–52.
240. Ferrie CD, Grünewald RA. Panayiotopoulos syndrome: a common and benign childhood epilepsy. *Lancet* 2001;357:821–823.
241. Caraballo R, Cersosimo R, Medina C, et al. Panayiotopoulos-type benign childhood occipital epilepsy: a prospective study. *Neurology* 2000;55:1096–1100.
242. Panayiotopoulos CP. Benign childhood epilepsy with occipital paroxysms: a 15-year prospective study. *Ann Neurol* 1989;26:51–56.
243. Livingston S, Eisner V, Pauli L. Minor motor epilepsy: diagnosis, treatment and prognosis. *Pediatrics* 1958;21:916–928.
244. Lennox WG, Davis JP. Clinical correlates of fast and slow spike-wave electroencephalogram. *Pediatrics* 1950;5:626–644.
245. Menkes JH. Diagnosis and treatment of minor motor seizures. *Pediatr Clin North Am* 1976;23:435–442.
246. Chevrie JJ, Aicardi J. Childhood epileptic encephalopathy with slow spike-wave. A statistical study of 80 cases. *Epilepsia* 1972;13:259–271.
247. Janz D. *Die epilepsien*. Stuttgart: Georg Thieme Verlag, 1969.
248. Hallett M. The pathophysiology of myoclonus. *Trends Neurosci* 1987;10:69–73.
249. Hurst DL. Epidemiology of myoclonic epilepsy of infancy. *Epilepsia* 1990;31:397–400.
250. Wilkins D, Hallett M, Erba G. Primary generalised epileptic myoclonus: a frequent manifestation of minipolymyoclonus of central origin. *J Neurol Neurosurg Psychiatry* 1985;48:506–516.
251. Kruse R. *Das myoklonisch-astatische Petit Mal*. Berlin: Springer-Verlag, 1968.
252. Brett EM. On a peculiar mode of onset of epilepsy in childhood: epileptogenic encephalopathy. *J Neurol Sci* 1967;4:315–338.
253. Kurokawa T, Goya N, Fukuyama Y, et al. West syndrome and Lennox-Gastaut syndrome: a survey of natural history. *Pediatrics* 1980;65:81–88.
254. Blume WT, David RB, Gomez MR. Generalized sharp and slow wave complexes—associated clinical features and long-term follow-up. *Brain* 1973;96:289–306.
255. Aicardi J, Chevrie JJ. Atypical benign partial epilepsy of childhood. *Dev Med Child Neurol* 1982;24:281–292.
256. Hahn A, Pistohl J, Neubauer BA, et al. Atypical "benign" partial epilepsy or pseudo-Lennox syndrome. Part I. Symptomatology and long-term prognosis. *Neuropediatrics* 2001;32:1–8.
257. Rothwell JC, Obeso JA, Marsden CD. On the significance of giant somatosensory evoked potentials in cortical myoclonus. *J Neurol Neurosurg Psychiatry* 1984;47:33–42.
258. Muller U, Steinberger D, Nemeth AH. Clinical and molecular genetics of primary dystonias. *Neurogenetics* 1998;1:165–177.
259. Aguglia U, Tinuper P, Gastaut H. Startle-induced epileptic seizures. *Epilepsia* 1984;25:712–720.
260. Asal B, Moro E. Über bösartige Nickkrämpfe in frühen Kindesalter. *Jahrb Kinderheilk* 1924;107:1–17.
261. Druckman RD, Chao D. Massive spasms in infancy and childhood. *Epilepsia* 1955;4:61–72.
262. Jeavons PM, Bower BD. *Infantile spasms*. London: The Spastics Society Medical Education and Information Unit in association with Butterworth–Heinemann, 1964:12.
263. Hrachovy RA, Frost JD, Kellaway P. Hypsarrhythmia: variations on the theme. *Epilepsia* 1984;25:317–325.
264. Hrachovy RA, Frost JD. Infantile epileptic encephalopathy with hypsarrhythmia (infantile spasms/West syndrome). *J Clin Neurophysiol* 2003;20:408–425.
265. Hrachovy RA, Frost JD Jr, Kellaway P. Sleep characteristics in infantile spasms. *Neurology* 1981;31:688–694.
266. Chugani HT, Shewmon DA, Sankar R, et al. Infantile spasms: II. Lenticular nuclei and brain stem activation on positron emission tomography. *Ann Neurol* 1992;31:212–219.
267. Riikonen R. A long-term follow-up study of 214 children with the syndrome of infantile spasms. *Neuropediatrics* 1982;13:14–23.

268. Baxter P. Epidemiology of pyridoxine dependent and pyridoxine response seizures in the U.K. *Arch Dis Child* 1999;81:431–433.
269. Bellman MH, Ross EM, Miller DL. Infantile spasms and pertussis immunization. *Lancet* 1983;1:1031–1034.
270. Geier DA, Geier MR. An evaluation of serious neurological disorders following immunization: a comparison of whole-cell pertussis and acellular pertussis vaccines. *Brain Dev* 2004;26:296–300.
271. Vinters HV. Histopathology of brain tissue from patients with infantile spasms. *Int Rev Neurobiol* 2002;49:63–76.
272. Vinters HV, Fisher RS, Cornford ME, et al. Morphologic substrates of infantile spasms: studies based on surgically resected cerebral tissue. *Childs Nerv Syst* 1992;8:8–17.
273. Jellinger K. Neuropathologic aspects of hypsarrhythmia. *Neuropädiatrie* 1970;1:277–294.
274. Sankar R, Curran JG, Kevill JW, et al. Microscopic cortical dysplasia in infantile spasms: evolution of white matter abnormalities. *Am J Neuroradiol* 1995;16:1265–1272.
275. Midulla M, Balducci L, Iannetti P, et al. Infantile spasms and cytomegalovirus infection. *Lancet* 1976;2:377.
276. Poser C, Low NL. Autopsy findings in three cases of hypsarrhythmia (infantile spasms with mental retardation). *Acta Paediatr Scand* 1960;49:695–706.
277. Jeavons PM, Harper JR, Bower BD. Long-term prognosis in infantile spasms: a follow-up report on 112 cases. *Dev Med Child Neurol* 1970;12:413–421.
278. Gaily E, Appelqvist K, Kantola-Sorsa E, et al. Cognitive deficits after cryptogenic infantile spasms with benign seizure evolution. *Dev Med Child Neurol* 1999;41:660–664.
279. Kivity S, Lerman P, Ariel R, et al. Long-term cognitive outcomes of a cohort of children with cryptogenic infantile spasms treated with high-dose adrenocorticotropic hormone. *Epilepsia* 2004;45:255–262.
280. Riikonen R, Simell O. Tuberous sclerosis and infantile spasms. *Dev Med Child Neurol* 1990;32:203–209.
281. Workshop on infantile spasms. *Epilepsia* 1992;33:195.
282. Ohtahara S, Yamatogi Y. Severe encephalopathic epilepsy in early infancy. In: Pellock JM, Dodson WE, Bourgeois BFD, eds. *Pediatric epilepsy*, 2nd ed. New York: Demos, 2001:193–199.
283. Ohtahara S, Ohtsuka Y, Yamatogi Y, et al. The early-infantile epileptic encephalopathy with suppression-bursts: developmental aspects. *Brain Dev* 1987;9:371–376.
284. Mackay MT, Weiss SK, Adams-Webber T, et al. Practice parameter: medical treatment of infantile spasms: report of the American Academy of Neurology and the Child Neurology Society. *Neurology* 2004;62:1668–1681.
285. Lerman P, Kivity S. The efficacy of corticotropin in primary infantile spasms. *J Pediatr* 1982;101:294–296.
286. Glaze DG, Hrachovy RA, Frost JD, et al. Prospective study of outcome of infants with infantile spasms treated during controlled studies of ACTH and prednisone. *J Pediatr* 1988;112:389–396.
286a. Askalan R, Mackay M, Brian J, et al. Prospective preliminary analysis of the development of autism and epilepsy in children with infantile spasms. *J Child Neurol* 2003;18:165–170.
287. Hrachovy RA, Frost JD, Glaze DG. High-dose, long-duration versus low-dose, short-duration corticotropin therapy for infantile spasms. *J Pediatr* 1994;124:803–806.
288. Ito M, Aika H, Hashimoto K, et al. Low-dose ACTH therapy for West syndrome: initial effects and long-term outcome. *Neurology* 2002;58:110–114.
289. Riikonen R, Donner MA. ACTH therapy in infantile spasms: side effects. *Arch Dis Child* 1980;55:664–672.
290. Snead OC, Benton JW, Myers GJ. ACTH and prednisone in childhood seizure disorders. *Neurology* 1983;33:966–970.
291. Carollo C, Marin G, Scanarini M, et al. CT and ACTH treatment in infantile spasms. *Childs Brain* 1982;9:347–353.
292. Snead OC. How does ACTH work against infantile spasms? From bedside to bench. *Ann Neurol* 2001;49:288–289.
293. Baram T, Mitchell WG, Hanson RA, et al. Cerebrospinal fluid corticotropin and cortisol are reduced in infantile spasms. *Pediatr Neurol* 1995;13:108–113.
294. Baram TZ. Pathophysiology of massive infantile spasms: perspective on the putative role of the brain adrenal axis. *Ann Neurol* 1993;33:231–236.
295. Charuvanij A, Ouvrier RA, Procopis PG, et al. ACTH treatment in intractable seizures of childhood. *Brain Dev* 1992;14:102–106.
296. Mitchell WG, Shah NS. Vigabatrin for infantile spasms. *Pediatr Neurol* 2002;27:161–164.
297. Appleton RF. A simple, effective and well-tolerated treatment regime for West syndrome. *Dev Med Child Neurol* 1995;37:185–187.
298. Chiron C, Dulac O, Beaumont D, et al. Therapeutic trial of vigabatrin in refractory infantile spasms. *J Child Neurol* 1991; 2[Suppl]:S52–S59.
299. Cossette P, Riviello JJ, Carmant L. ACTH versus vigabatrin in infantile spasms: a retrospective study. *Neurology* 1999;52:1691–1694.
299a. Lux AL, Edwards SW, Hancock E, et al. The United Kingdom Infantile Spasms Study comparing vigabatrin with prednisolone or tetracosactide at 14 days: a multicentre, randomised controlled trial. *Lancet* 2004;364:1773–1778.
300. Riikonen RS. Steroids or vigabatrin in the treatment of infantile spasms? *Pediatr Neurol* 2000;23:403–408.
301. Wohlrab G, Boltshauser E, Schmitt B. Vigabatrin as a first-line drug in West syndrome: clinical and electroencephalographic outcome. *Neuropediatrics* 1998;29:133–136.
302. Vigevano F, Cilio MR. Vigabatrin versus ACTH as first-line treatment for infantile spasms: a randomized, prospective study. *Epilepsia* 1997;38:1270–1274.
303. Baram TZ, Mitchell WG, Tournay A, et al. High-dose corticotropin (ACTH) versus prednisone for infantile spasms: a prospective, randomized, blinded study. *Pediatrics* 1996;97:375–379.
304. Prats JM, Garaizar C, Rua MJ, et al. Infantile spasms treated with high doses of sodium valproate: initial response and follow-up. *Dev Med Child Neurol* 1991;33:617–625.
305. Kossoff EH, Pyzik PL, McGrogan JR, et al. Efficacy of the ketogenic diet for infantile spasms. *Pediatrics* 2002;109:780–783.
306. Ito M, Seki T, Takuma Y. Current therapy for West syndrome in Japan. *J Child Neurol* 2000;15:424–428.
307. Buoni S, Zannolli R, Strambi M, et al. Combined treatment with vigabatrin and topiramate in West syndrome. *J Child Neurol* 2004;19:385–386.
308. Yanai S, Hanai T, Narazaki O. Treatment of infantile spasms with zonisamide. *Brain Dev* 1999;21:157–61.
309. Suzuki Y. Zonisamide in West syndrome. *Brain Dev* 2001;23:658–661.
310. Lotze TE, Wilfong AA. Zonisamide treatment for symptomatic infantile spasms. *Neurology* 2004;62:296–298.
311. Lombroso CT, Fejerman N. Benign myoclonus of early infancy. *Ann Neurol* 1977;1:138–143.
312. Aicardi J, Lefebvre J, Lerique-Koechlin A. A new syndrome: spasm in flexion, callosal agenesis, ocular abnormalities. *Electroencephalogr Clin Neurophysiol* 1965;19:609–610. [Abstract].
313. Dennis J, Bower BD. The Aicardi syndrome. *Dev Med Child Neurol* 1972;14:392–390.
314. Goutieres F, Aicardi J, Barth PG, et al. Aicardi-Goutieres syndrome: an update and results of interferon-alpha studies. *Ann Neurol* 1998;44:900–907.
315. Sander T, Bockenkamp B, Hildmann T, et al. Refined mapping of the epilepsy susceptibility locus EJM1 on chromosome 6. *Neurology* 1997;19:842–847.
316. Cossette P, Liu L, Brisebois K, et al. Mutation of GABRA1 in an autosomal dominant form of juvenile myoclonic epilepsy. *Nat Genet* 2002;31:184–189.
317. Suzuki T, Delgado-Escueta AV, Aguan K, et al. Mutations in EFHC1 cause juvenile myoclonic epilepsy. *Nat Genet* 2004;36:842–849.
318. Wolf P, Goosses R. Relation of photosensitivity to epileptic syndromes. *J Neurol Neurosurg Psychiatry* 1986;49:1386–1391.
319. Grünewald RA, Chroni E, Panayiotopoulos CP. Delayed diagnosis of juvenile myoclonic epilepsy. *J Neurol Neurosurg Psychiatry* 1992;55:497–499.
320. Sankar R. Initial treatment of epilepsy with antiepileptic drugs: pediatric issues. *Neurology* 2004;63(10 Suppl 4):S30–39.
321. Douglas EF, White PT. Abdominal epilepsy—a reappraisal. *J Pediatr* 1971;78:59–67.
322. Schäffler L, Karbowski K. Rezidivierende paroxysmale abdominale Schmerzen zerebraler Genese. *Schweiz Med Wschr* 1981;111:1352–1360.

323. Rasmussen T, McCann W. Clinical studies of patients with focal epilepsy due to "chronic encephalitis." *Trans Am Neurol Assoc* 1968;93:89–94.
324. Thomas JE, Reagan TJ, Klass DW. Epilepsia partialis continua. A review of 32 cases. *Arch Neurol* 1977;34:266–275.
325. Cascino GD. Nonconvulsive status epilepticus in adults and children. *Epilepsia* 1993;34[Suppl 1]:S21–S28.
326. Walker MC. Diagnosis and treatment of nonconvulsive status epilepticus. *CNS Drugs* 2001;15:931–939.
327. Brett EM. Minor epileptic status. *J Neurol Sci* 1966;3:52–75.
328. Niedermeyer E, Khalifeh R. Petit mal status ("spike-wave stupor"). An electro-clinical appraisal. *Epilepsia* 1965;6:250–262.
329. Farran RD, McIntyre HB, Itabashi HH. Pathogenesis of spike-wave status: a clinical-pathological study implicating cerebellar disturbance. *Bull Los Angeles Neurol Soc* 1975;40:153–159.
330. Chugani HT, Mazziotta JC, Engel J Jr, et al. The Lennox-Gastaut syndrome: metabolic subtypes determined by 2-deoxy-2[^{18}F]fluoro-D-glucose positron emission tomography. *Ann Neurol* 1987;21:413.
331. Kaplan PW. Intravenous valproate treatment of generalized nonconvulsive status epilepticus. *Clin Electroencephalogr* 1999;30:1–4.
332. Kaplan PW. No, some types of nonconvulsive status epilepticus cause little permanent neurologic sequelae (or: "the cure may be worse than the disease"). *Neurophysiol Clin* 2000;30:377–382.
333. Landau WM, Kleffner FR. Syndrome of acquired aphasia with convulsive disorder in children. *Neurology* 1957;7:523–530.
334. Hirsch E, Marescaux C, Maquet P, et al. Landau-Kleffner syndrome: a clinical and EEG study of five cases. *Epilepsia* 1990;31: 756–767.
335. Paquier PF, Van Dongen HR, Loonen MCB. The Landau-Kleffner syndrome or "acquired aphasia with convulsive disorder." Long-term follow-up of six children and a review of the recent literature. *Arch Neurol* 1992;49:354–359.
336. Marescaux C, Marescaux C, Maquet P, et al. Landau-Kleffner syndrome: a pharmacologic study of five cases. *Epilepsia* 1990;31:768–777.
337. Lagae LG, Silberstein J, Gillis PL, et al. Successful use of intravenous immunoglobulin in Landau-Kleffner syndrome. *Pediatr Neurol* 1998;18:165–168.
338. Grote CL, Van Slyke P, Hoeppner JA. Language outcome following multiple subpial transection for Landau-Kleffner syndrome. *Brain* 1999;122:561–566.
339. Jayakar PB, Seshia SS. Electrical status epilepticus during slow-wave sleep: a review. *J Clin Neurophysiol* 1991;7:299–311.
340. Rossi PG, Parmeggiani A, Posar A, et al. Landau-Kleffner syndrome (LKS): long-term follow-up and links with electrical status epilepticus during sleep (ESPS). *Brain Dev* 1999;21:90–98.
341. Galanopoulou AS, Bojko A, Lado F, et al. The spectrum of neuropsychiatric abnormalities associated with electrical status epilepticus in sleep. *Brain Dev* 2000;22:279–295.
342. Smith MC, Hoeppner TJ. Epileptic encephalopathy of late childhood: Landau-Kleffner syndrome and the syndrome of continuous spike and waves during slow-wave sleep. *J Clin Neurophysiol* 2003;20:462–472.
343. Gascon GG, Lombroso CT. Epileptic (gelastic) laughter. *Epilepsia* 1971;12:63–76.
344. Jeavons PM, Harding GF. *Photosensitive epilepsy*. Spastics Int Med Publ. London: William Heinemann Medical Books Ltd, 1975.
345. Geschwind N, Sherwin I. Language-induced epilepsy. *Arch Neurol* 1967;16:25–31.
346. Forster FM. *Reflex epilepsy, behavioral therapy and conditioned reflexes*. Springfield, IL: Charles C Thomas Publisher, 1977.
347. Critchley MacD. Musicogenic epilepsy. *Brain* 1937;60:13–27.
348. Calderon-Gonzalez R, Hopkins I, McLean WT. Tap seizures. A form of sensory precipitation epilepsy. *JAMA* 1966;198:521–523.
349. Ingvar DH, Nyman GE. Epilepsia arithmetices. A new psychological mechanism in a case of epilepsy. *Neurology* 1962;12:282–287.
350. Critchley MacD, Cobb W, Sears TA. On reading epilepsy. *Epilepsia* 1959;1:403–417.
351. Strauss H. Paroxysmal compulsive running and the concept of epilepsia cursiva. *Neurology* 1960;10:341–344.
352. Forster FM. *Reflex epilepsy, behavioral therapy and conditioned reflexes*. Springfield, IL: Charles C Thomas Publisher, 1977.
353. Darby CE, de Korte RA, Binnie CD, et al. The self-induction of epileptic seizures by eye closure. *Epilepsia* 1980;21:31–42.
354. Badinand-Hubert N, Bureau M, Hirsch E, et al. Epilepsies and video games: results of a multicentric study. *Electroencephalogr Clin Neurophysiol* 1998;107:422–427.
355. Newmark ME, Penry JK. *Photosensitivity and epilepsy: a review*. New York: Raven Press, 1979.
356. Hirtz D, Ashwal S, Berg A, et al. Practice parameters: Evaluating a first nonfebrile seizure in children. Report of the Quality Standards Subcommittee of the American Academy of Neurology, the Child Neurology Society, and the American Epilepsy Society. *Neurology* 2000;55:616–623.
357. Wyllie E, Friedman D, Rothner AD, et al. Psychogenic seizures in children and adolescents: outcome after diagnosis by ictal video and electroencephalographic recording. *Pediatrics* 1990;85:480–484.
358. Williams DT, Spiegel H, Mostofsky DI. Neurogenic and hysterical seizures in children and adolescents: differential diagnostic and therapeutic considerations. *Am J Psychiatry* 1978;135:82–86.
359. Schneider S, Rice DR. Neurologic manifestations of childhood hysteria. *J Pediatr* 1979;94:153–156.
360. Lazare A. Conversion symptoms. *N Engl J Med* 1981;305:745–748.
361. Gastaut H, Fischer-Williams M. Electroencephalographic study of syncope: its differentiation from epilepsy. *Lancet* 1957;2:1018–1025.
362. Tharp BR. An overview of pediatric seizure disorders and epileptic syndromes. *Epilepsia* 1987;28[Suppl. 1]:S36–S45.
363. Tassinari CA, Mancia D, Bernardina BD, et al. Pavor nocturnus of non-epileptic nature in epileptic children. *Electroencephalogr Clin Neurophysiol* 1972;33:603–607.
364. Symonds CP. Nocturnal myoclonus. *J Neurol Neurosurg Psychiatry* 1953;16:166–171.
365. Altrocchi PH, Menkes JH. Congenital ocular motor apraxia. *Brain* 1960;83:579–588.
366. Mitchell I, Brummitt J, DeForest J, et al. Apnea and factitious illness (Münchausen syndrome) by proxy. *Pediatrics* 1993;92:810–814.
367. Meadow R. Fictitious epilepsy. *Lancet* 1984;2:25–28.
368. Page LK, Lombroso CT, Matson DD. Childhood epilepsy with late detection of cerebral glioma. *J Neurosurg* 1969;31:253–261.
369. King MA, Newton MR, Jackson GD, et al. Epileptology of the first-seizure presentation: a clinical, electroencephalographic, and magnetic resonance imaging study of 300 consecutive patients. *Lancet* 1998;352:1007–1011.
370. Gibbs EL, Gillen HW, Gibbs FA. Disappearance and migration of epileptic foci in children. *Am J Dis Child* 1954;88:596–603.
371. Strobos RJ, Kavallinis GP. Changes in repeat electroencephalograms in epileptics. *Neurology* 1968;18:622–633.
372. Lennox WG, Merritt HH. Cerebrospinal fluid in "essential" epilepsy. *J Neurol Psychopathol* 1936;17:97–106.
373. Edwards R, Schmidley JW, Simon RP. How often does a CSF pleocytosis follow generalized convulsions? *Ann Neurol* 1983;13:460–462.
374. Barry E, Hauser WA. Pleocytosis after status epilepticus. *Arch Neurol* 1994;51:190–193.
375. Wong M, Schlaggar BL, Landt M. Postictal cerebrospinal fluid abnormalities in children. *J Pediatr* 2001;138:373–377.
376. Yaffe K, Ferriero D, Barkovich AJ, et al. Reversible MRI abnormalities following seizures. *Neurology* 1995;45:104–108.
377. Wong M, Ess K, Landt M. Cerebrospinal fluid neuron-specific enolase following seizures in children: role of etiology. *J Child Neurol* 2002;17:261–264.
378. Maytal J, Krauss JM, Novak G, et al. The role of brain computed tomography in evaluating children with new onset of seizures in the emergency department. *Epilepsia* 2000;41:950–954.
379. Sharma S, Riviello JJ, Harper MB, et al. The role of emergent neuroimaging in children with new-onset afebrile seizures. *Pediatrics* 2003;111:1–5.
380. Yang PJ, Berger PE, Cohen ME, et al. Computed tomography and childhood seizure disorders. *Neurology* 1979;29:1084–1088.
381. Kuzniecky R, Berkovic S, Andermann F, et al. Focal cortical myoclonus and rolandic cortical dysplasia: clarification by magnetic resonance imaging. *Ann Neurol* 1988;23:317–325.

382. Kuzniecky R, Murro A, King D, et al. Magnetic resonance imaging in childhood intractable partial epilepsies: pathologic correlations. *Neurology* 1993;43:681–687.
383. Kuzniecky R, de la Sayette V, Ethier R, et al. Magnetic resonance imaging in temporal lobe epilepsy: pathological correlations. *Ann Neurol* 1987;22:341–347.
384. Williamson PD, French JA, Thadani VM, et al. Characteristics of medial temporal lobe epilepsy: I. Interictal and ictal scalp electroencephalography, neuropsychological testing, neuroimaging, surgical results, and pathology. *Ann Neurol* 1993;34:781–787.
385. Theodore WH, Katz D, Kufta C, et al. Pathology of temporal lobe foci: correlation with CT, MRI and PET. *Neurology* 1990;40:797–803.
386. Kuzniecky R, Garcia JH, Faught E, et al. Cortical dysplasia in temporal lobe epilepsy: magnetic resonance imaging correlations. *Ann Neurol* 1991;29:293–298.
387. Berg AT, Testa FM, Levy SR, Shinnar S. Neuroimaging in children with newly diagnosed epilepsy: a community-based study. *Pediatrics* 2000;106:527–532.
388. Kramer RE, Luders H, Lesser RP, et al. Transient focal abnormalities of neuroimaging studies during focal status epilepticus. *Epilepsia* 1987;28:528–532.
389. McLachlan RS, Karlik SJ, Myles V. Nuclear magnetic resonance relaxometry in a penicillin model of focal epilepsy. *Epilepsia* 1988;29:396–400.
390. Sammaritano M, Andermann F, Melanson D, et al. Prolonged focal cerebral edema associated with partial status epilepticus. *Epilepsia* 1985;26:334–339.
391. Karlik SJ. Common pharmaceuticals alter tissue proton NMR relaxation properties. *Magn Reson Imaging Med* 1986;3:181–193.
392. Juhasz C, Chugani HT. Imaging the epileptic brain with positron emission tomography. *Neuroimaging Clin N Am* 2003;13:705–716.
393. Abou-Khalil BW, Siegel GJ, Sackellares JC, et al. Positron emission tomography studies of cerebral glucose metabolism in chronic partial epilepsy. *Ann Neurol* 1987;22:480–486.
394. Juhasz C, Chugani DC, Muzik O, et al. Is epileptogenic cortex truly hypometabolic on interictal positron emission tomography? *Ann Neurol* 2000;48:88–96.
395. Engel J, Lubens P, Kuhl DE, et al. Local cerebral metabolic rate for glucose during petit mal absences. *Ann Neurol* 1985;17:121–128.
396. Olson DM, Chugani HT, Shewmon DA, et al. Electrocorticographic confirmation of focal positron emission tomographic abnormalities in children with intractable epilepsy. *Epilepsia* 1990;31:731–739.
397. Won HJ, Chang KH, Cheon JE, et al. Comparison of MR imaging with PET and ictal SPECT in 118 patients with intractable epilepsy. *Am J Neuroradiol* 1999;20:593–599.
398. Theodore WH, Sato S, Kufta C, et al. Temporal lobectomy for uncontrolled seizures: the role of positron emission tomography. *Ann Neurol* 1992;32:789–794.
399. Hoh BL, Cheung AC, Rabinov JD, et al. Results of a prospective protocol of computed tomographic angiography in place of catheter angiography as the only diagnostic and pretreatment planning study for cerebral aneurysms by a combined neurovascular team. *Neurosurgery* 2004;54:1329–40.
400. Sutherling WW, Crandall PH, Cahan LD, et al. The magnetic field of epileptic spikes agrees with intracranial localizations in complex partial epilepsy. *Neurology* 1988;38:778–786.
401. Wheless JW, Willmore LJ, Breier JI, et al. A comparison of magnetoencephalography, MRI and V-EEG in patients evaluated for epilepsy surgery. *Epilepsia* 1999;40:931–941.
402. Scott CA, Fish DR, Smith SJ, et al. Presurgical evaluation of patients with epilepsy and normal MRI: role of scalp video-EEG telemetry. *J Neurol Neurosurg Psychiatry* 1999;66:69–71.
403. Gotman J, Ives JR, Gloor P, eds. Long-term monitoring in epilepsy. *Electroenceph Clin Neurophysiol* 1985;[Suppl 37].
404. Engel J, Driver MV, Falconer MA. Electrophysiological correlates of pathology and surgical results in temporal lobe epilepsy. *Brain* 1975;98:129–156.
405. Morrell F, Ford E, Bergen D, et al. Diagnostic value of the methohexital suppression test for differentiating independent secondary foci. *Neurology* 1984;34[Suppl 1]:124.
406. Hauser WA, Rich SS, Lee JR, et al. Risk of recurrent seizures after two unprovoked seizures. *N Engl J Med* 1998;338:429–434.
407. Elwes RDC, Chesterman P, Reynolds EH. Prognosis after a first untreated tonic-clonic seizure. *Lancet* 1985;2:752–753.
408. Shinnar S, Berg AT, O'Dell C, et al. Predictors of multiple seizures in a cohort of children prospectively followed from the time of their first unprovoked seizure. *Ann Neurol* 2000;48:140–147.
409. Camfield PR, Camfield CS, Dooley JM, et al. Epilepsy after a first unprovoked seizure in childhood. *Neurology* 1985;35:1657–1660.
410. Hirtz DG, Ellenberg JH, Nelson KB. The risk of recurrence of nonfebrile seizures in children. *Neurology* 1984;34:637–641.
411. Stephenson JBP. *Fits and faints. Clinics in developmental medicine*. Oxford: MacKeith Press, 1990:109.
412. Ebersole JS, Leroy RF. Evaluation of ambulatory cassette EEG monitoring. III. Diagnostic accuracy compared to intensive inpatient EEG monitoring. *Neurology* 1983;33:853–860.
413. Reynolds EH, Shorvon SD. Monotherapy or polytherapy for epilepsy? *Epilepsia* 1981;22:110.
414. Lesser RP, Pippenger CE, Luders H, et al. High-dose monotherapy in treatment of intractable seizures. *Neurology* 1984;34:707–711.
415. Hanson RA, Menkes JH. Iatrogenic perpetuation of epilepsy. *Trans Am Neurol Assoc* 1972;97:290–291.
416. Glauser TA, Pippinger CE. Controversies in blood-level monitoring: reexamining its role in the treatment of epilepsy. *Epilepsia* 2000;41[Suppl 8]:S6–S15.
417. Choonara IA, Rane A. Therapeutic drug monitoring of anticonvulsants: state of the art. *Clin Pharmacokinet* 1990;18:318–328.
418. Curless RG, Walson PD, Carter DE. Phenytoin kinetics in children. *Neurology* 1976;26:715–720.
419. Laidlaw J, Richens A, Chadwick D. *A textbook of epilepsy*, 4th ed. Edinburgh: Churchill Livingstone, 1993.
420. Browne TR, Dreifuss FE, Dyken PR, et al. Ethosuximide in the treatment of absence (petit mal) seizures. *Neurology* 1975;25:515–524.
421. Bourgeois BFD. Phenobarbital and primidone. In: Wyllie E, ed. *The treatment of epilepsy: principles and practice*, 2nd ed. Baltimore: Williams & Wilkins, 1996:845–855.
422. Johannessen SI, Battino D, Berry DJ, et al. Therapeutic drug monitoring of the newer antiepileptic drugs. *Ther Drug Monit* 2003;25:347–363.
423. Kutt H. Relation of plasma concentration to seizure control. In: Woodbury DM, Penry JK, Pippenger CE, eds. *Antiepileptic drugs*, 2nd ed. New York: Raven Press, 1982:241–246.
424. Chadwick DW. Overuse of monitoring of blood concentrations of antiepileptic drugs. *BMJ* 1987;294:723–724.
425. Pellock JM, Willmore LJ. A rational guide to routine blood monitoring in patients receiving antiepileptic drugs. *Neurology* 1991;41:961–964.
426. Wyllie E, Wyllie R. Routine laboratory monitoring for serious adverse effects of antiepileptic medications: the controversy. *Epilepsia* 1991;32[Suppl 5]:S74–S79.
427. Sankar R. Initial treatment of epilepsy with antiepileptic drugs: pediatric issues. *Neurology* 2004;63[10 Suppl 4]:S30–S39.
427a. Pearce, JMS. Bromide, the first effective antiepileptic agent. *J Neurol Neurosurg Psychiatry* 2002;72:412.
427b. Hauptmann A. Luminal bei Epilepsie. *Munchn Medizin Wochenschrift* 1912;59:1907–9.
428. Merritt HH, Putnam TJ. A new series of anticonvulsant drugs tested by experiments on animals. *Arch Neurol Psychiatry* 1938;38:1003–1015.
429. Sankar R, Weaver DF. Basic principles of medicinal chemistry. In: Engel J Jr, Pedley TA, eds. *Epilepsy: a comprehensive textbook*. Philadelphia: Lippincott-Raven Publishers, 1998:1393–1403.
430. Fisher RS. Animal models of the epilepsies. *Brain Res Rev* 1989;14:245–278.
431. Rho JM, Sankar R. The pharmacologic basis of antiepileptic drug action. *Epilepsia* 1999;40:1471–1483.
432. Rho JM, Donevan SD, Rogawski MA. Mechanism of action of the anticonvulsant felbamate: opposing effects on *N*-methyl-D-aspartate and γ-aminobutyric acid A receptors. *Ann Neurol* 1994;35:229–234.
433. White HS, Brown SD, Woodhead JH, et al. Topiramate enhances GABA-mediated chloride flux and GABA-evoked chloride currents

in murine brain neurons and increases seizure threshold. *Epilepsy Res* 1997;28:167–179.

434. Nusser Z, Mody I. Selective modulation of tonic and phasic inhibitions in dentate gyrus granule cells. *J Neurophysiol* 2002;87:2624–2628.
435. Rho JM, Donevan SD, Rogawski MA. Barbiturate-like actions of the propanediol dicarbamates felbamate and meprobamate. *J Pharmacol Exp Ther* 1997;280:1383–1391.
436. Sankar R, Rho JM. Ontogeny of molecular targets of antiepileptic drugs: impact on drug choice. InRho JM, Sankar R, Cavazos JE, eds. *Epilepsy: scientific foundations of clinical practice.* New York: Marcel Dekker, 2004.
437. Sankar R, Holmes GL. Mechanisms of action for the commonly used antiepileptic drugs: relevance to antiepileptic drug-associated neurobehavioral adverse effects. *J Child Neurol* 2004; 19[Suppl 1]:S6–S14.
438. Poolos NP, Migliore M, Johnston D. Pharmacological upregulation of h-channels reduces the excitability of pyramidal neuron dendrites. *Nat Neurosci* 2002;5:767–774.
439. Sankar R, Shields WD. Levetiracetam. In: Dodson WE, Bourgeois BF, Pellock JM, eds. *Pediatric epilepsy: diagnosis and therapy*, 2nd ed. New York: Demos Medical Publishing, 2000;2003.
440. Margineanu D, Klitgaard H. Inhibition of neuronal hypersynchrony in vitro differentiates levetiracetam from classical antiepileptic drugs. *Pharmacol Res* 2000;42:281–285.
441. Klitgaard H, Matagne A, Grimee R, et al. Electrophysiological, neurochemical and regional effects of levetiracetam in the rat pilocarpine model of temporal lobe epilepsy. *Seizure* 2003;12:92–100.
442. Coulter DA. Mossy fiber zinc and temporal lobe epilepsy: pathological association with altered "epileptic" gamma-aminobutyric acid A receptors in dentate granule cells. *Epilepsia* 2000;41[Suppl 6]:S96–S99.
443. Rigo JM, Hans G, Nguyen L, et al. The anti-epileptic drug levetiracetam reverses the inhibition by negative allosteric modulators of neuronal GABA- and glycine-gated currents. *Br J Pharmacol* 2002;136:659–672.
444. Lynch BA, Lambeng N, Nocka K, et al. The synaptic vesicle protein SV2A is the binding site for the antiepileptic drug levetiracetam. *Proc Natl Acad Sci USA* 2004;101:9861–9866.
445. Svensmark O, Buchthal F. Diphenylhydantoin and phenobarbital. Serum levels in children. *Am J Dis Child* 1964;108:82–87.
446. Aiges HW, Daum F, Olson M, et al. The effects of phenobarbital and diphenylhydantoin on liver function and morphology. *J Pediatr* 1980;97:22–26.
447. Theodore WH, DiChiro G, Margolin R, et al. Barbiturates reduce human cerebral glucose metabolism. *Neurology* 1986;36:60–64.
448. Brent DA, Crumrine PK, Varma RR, et al. Phenobarbital treatment and major depressive disorder in children with epilepsy: a naturalistic follow-up. *Pediatrics* 1990;85:1086–1091.
449. Camfield CS, Chaplin S, Doyle AB, et al. Side effects of phenobarbitone in toddlers: behavioral and cognitive aspects. *J Pediatr* 1979;95:361–365.
450. Hellstrom B, Barlach-Christoffersen M. Influence of phenobarbital on the psychomotor development and behaviour in preschool children with convulsions. *Neuropädiatrie* 1980;11:151–160.
451. Mitchell WG, Zhou Y, Chavez JM, et al. Effects of antiepileptic drugs on reaction time, attention and impulsivity in children. *Pediatrics* 1993;91:101–105.
452. Farwell JR, et al. Phenobarbital for febrile seizures—effects on intelligence and on seizure recurrence. *N Engl J Med* 1990;322:364–369.
453. de Silva M, MacArdle B, McGowan M, et al. Randomized comparative monotherapy trial of phenobarbitone, phenytoin, carbamazepine or sodium valproate for newly diagnosed childhood epilepsy. *Lancet* 1996;347:709–713.
454. Dodson WE. Nonlinear kinetics of phenytoin in children. *Neurology* 1982;32:42–48.
455. Buchthal F, Svensmark O. Aspects of the pharmacology of phenytoin (Dilantin) and phenobarbital relevant to their dosage in the treatment of epilepsy. *Epilepsia* 1960;1:373–384.
456. Buchthal F, Svensmark O. Serum concentrations of diphenylhydantoin (phenytoin) and phenobarbital and their relation to therapeutic and toxic effects. *Psychiatr Neurol Neurochir* 1971;74:117–136.
457. Browne TR, Change T. Phenytoin: biotransformation. In: Levy R, Mattson RH, Meldrum BS, eds. *Antiepileptic drugs*, 3rd ed. New York: Raven Press, 1989:197–214.
458. Kutt H, McDowell F. Management of epilepsy with diphenylhydantoin sodium. Dosage regulation for problem patients. *JAMA* 1968;203:969–972.
459. Kokenge R, Kutt H, McDowell F. Neurological sequelae following Dilantin overdose in a patient and in experimental animals. *Neurology* 1965;15:823–829.
460. Beernink DH, Miller JJ. Anticonvulsant-induced antinuclear antibodies and lupus-like disease in children. *J Pediatr* 1973;82:113–117.
461. Kapur RN, Girgis S, Little TM, et al. Diphenylhydantoin-induced gingival hyperplasia: its relationship to dose and serum level. *Dev Med Child Neurol* 1973;15:483–487.
462. Reynolds EH. Folate metabolism and anticonvulsant therapy. *Proc R Soc Med* 1974;67:68.
463. Weber TH, Knuutila S, Tammisto P, et al.Long term use of phenytoin: effects on whole blood and red cell folate and haematological parameters.*Scand J Haematol* 1977;18:81–85.
464. Reynolds EH. Anticonvulsants, folic acid, and epilepsy. *Lancet* 1973;1:1376–1378.
465. Crosley CJ, Chee C, Berman PH. Rickets associated with long-term anticonvulsant therapy in a pediatric outpatient population. *Pediatrics* 1975;56:52–57.
466. Morijiri Y, Sato T. Factors causing rickets in institutionalized handicapped children on anticonvulsant therapy. *Arch Dis Child* 1981;56:446–449.
467. Lovelace RE, Horwitz SJ. Peripheral neuropathy in long-term diphenylhydantoin therapy. *Arch Neurol* 1968;18:69–77.
468. Hanson JW, Smith DW. The fetal hydantoin syndrome. *J Pediatr* 1975;87:285–290.
469. Gaily E, Granstrom ML, Hiilesmaa V, et al. Minor anomalies in offspring of epileptic mothers. *J Pediatr* 1988;112:520–529.
470. Meadow SR. Anticonvulsant drugs in pregnancy. *Arch Dis Child* 1991;66:62–65.
471. Moore SJ, Turnpenny P, Quinn A, et al. A clinical study of 57 children with fetal anticonvulsant syndromes. *J Med Genet* 2000;37:489–497.
472. Troupin AS, Friel P, Lovely MP, et al. Clinical pharmacology of mephenytoin and ethotoin. *Ann Neurol* 1979;6:410–414.
473. Reckziegel G, Beck H, Schramm J, et al. Carbamazepine effects on Na^+ currents in human dentate granule cells from epileptogenic tissue. *Epilepsia* 1999;40:401–407.
474. Dodson WE. Carbamazepine efficacy and utilization in children. *Epilepsia* 1987;28[Suppl 3]:S17–S24.
475. Troupin A, Ojemann LM, Halpern L, et al. Carbamazepine—a double-blind comparison with phenytoin. *Neurology* 1977;27:511–519.
476. Westenberg HG, van der Kleijn E, Oei TT, et al. Kinetics of carbamazepine and carbamazepine epoxide, determined by use of plasma and saliva. *Clin Pharmacol Ther* 1978;23:320–328.
477. Bertilsson L, Tomson T. Clinical pharmacokinetics and pharmacological effects of carbamazepine and carbamazepine-10, 11-epoxide. An update. *Clin Pharmacokinet* 1986;11:177–198.
478. Dam M, Ekberg R, Loyning Y, et al. A double-blind study comparing oxcarbazepine and carbamazepine in patients with newly diagnosed previously untreated epilepsy. *Epilepsy Res* 1989;3: 70–76.
479. Pellock JM. Carbamazepine side effects in children and adults. *Epilepsia* 1987;28[Suppl 3]:S64–S70.
480. Perucca E, Garratt A, Hebdige S, et al. Water intoxication in epileptic patients receiving carbamazepine. *J Neurol Neurosurg Psychiatry* 1978;41:713–718.
481. Van Amelsvoort T, Bakshi R, Devaux CB, et al. Hyponatremia associated with carbamazepine and oxcarbazepine therapy: a review. *Epilepsia* 1994;35:181–188.
482. Camfield C, Camfield P, Smith E, et al. Asymptomatic children with epilepsy: little benefit from screening for anticonvulsant-induced liver, blood, or renal damage. *Neurology* 1986;36:838–841.

483. Hadzic N, Portmann B, Davies ET, et al. Acute liver failure induced by carbamazepine. *Arch Dis Child* 1990;65:315–317.
484. Snead OC, Hosey LC. Exacerbation of seizures in children by carbamazepine. *N Engl J Med* 1985;313:916–921.
485. Aguglia U, Zappia M, Quattrone A. Carbamazepine-induced nonepileptic myoclonus in a child with benign epilepsy. *Epilepsia* 1987;28:515–518.
486. Macphee GJ, McInnes GT, Thompson GG, et al. Verapamil potentiates carbamazepine neurotoxicity: a clinically important inhibitory interaction. *Lancet* 1986;1:700–703.
487. Dodrill CB, Troupin AS. Psychotropic effects of carbamazepine in epilepsy: a double blind comparison with phenytoin. *Neurology* 1977;27:1023–1028.
488. Forsythe I, Butler R, Berg I, et al. Cognitive impairment in new cases of epilepsy randomly assigned to carbamazepine, phenytoin and sodium valproate. *Dev Med Child Neurol* 1991;33:524–534.
489. Pieters MS, van Steveninck AF, Schoemaker RC, et al. The psychomotor effect of carbamazepine in epileptic patients and healthy volunteers. *J Psychopharmacol* 2003;17:269–272.
490. Nuwer MR, Browne TR, Dodson WE, et al. Generic substitutions for antiepileptic drugs. *Neurology* 1990;40:1647–1651.
491. Fuhr U. Drug interaction with grapefruit juice. Extent, probable mechanism and clinical relevance. *Drug Safety* 1998;18:251–272.
492. French JA, Kanner AM, Bautista J, et al. Efficacy and tolerability of the new antiepileptic drugs I: treatment of new onset epilepsy. *Neurology* 2004;62:1252–1260.
493. Sachdeo RC, Wasserstein A, Mesenbrink PJ, et al. Effects of oxcarbazepine on sodium concentration and water handling. *Ann Neurol* 2002;51:613–620.
494. Dean JC. Valproate. In: Wyllie E, ed. *The treatment of epilepsy: principles and practice*, 2nd ed. Baltimore: Williams & Wilkins, 1996:824–832.
495. Loscher W. Valproate: a reappraisal of its pharmacodynamic properties and mechanisms of action. *Prog Neurobiol* 1999;58:31–59.
496. Buchhalter JR, Dichter MA. Effects of valproic acid in cultured mammalian neurons. *Neurology* 1986;36:259–262.
497. Johnston D. Valproic acid: update on its mechanisms of action. *Epilepsia* 1984;25[Suppl 1]:S1–S4.
498. Sankar R, Holmes GL. Mechanisms of action for the commonly used antiepileptic drugs (AEDs): relevance to AED-associated neurobehavioral adverse dvents. *J Child Neurol* 2004;19[Suppl 1]:S6–S14.
499. Bourgeois BFD. Valproate. In: Pellock JM, Dodson WE, Bourgeois BFD, eds. *Pediatric epilepsy*, 2nd ed. New York: Demos, 2001:433–446.
500. Editorial. Sodium valproate. *Lancet* 1988;2:1229–1232.
501. Shen DD, Ojemann GA, Rapport RL, et al. Low and variable presence of valproic acid in human brain. *Neurology* 1992;42:582–585.
502. Dutta S, Zhang Y, Conway JM, et al. Divalproex-ER pharmacokinetics in older children and adolescents. *Pediatr Neurol* 2004;30:330–337.
503. Cloyd JC, Kriel RL, Jones-Saete CM, et al. Comparison of sprinkle versus syrup formulations of valproate for bioavailability, tolerance, and preference. *J Pediatr* 1992;120:634–638.
504. Collaborative Study Group, Bourgeois B, et al. Monotherapy with valproate in primary generalized epilepsies. *Epilepsia* 1987;28[Suppl 2]:S8–S11.
505. Wirrell EC. Valproic acid–associated weight gain in older children and teens with epilepsy. *Pediatr Neurol* 2003;28:126–129.
506. Bryant AE, Dreifuss FE. Valproic acid hepatic fatalities. III. U.S. experience since 1986. *Neurology* 1996;48:465–469.
507. Dreifuss FE, Langer DH, Moline KA, et al. Valproic acid hepatic fatalities. II. U.S. experience since 1984. *Neurology* 1989;39:201–207.
508. Clarkson A, Choonara I. Surveillance for fatal suspected adverse drug reactions in the UK. *Arch Dis Child* 2002;87:462–466.
509. Rettie AE, Rettenmeier AW, Howald WN, et al. Cytochrome P-450-catalyzed formation of delta-4-VPA, a toxic metabolite of valproic acid. *Science* 1987;235:890–893.
510. Tennison MB, Miles MV, Pollack GM, et al. Valproate metabolites and hepatotoxicity in an epileptic population. *Epilepsia* 1988;29:543–547.
511. Jeavons PM. Sodium valproate and acute hepatic failure. *Dev Med Child Neurol* 1980;22:547–548.
512. Bohan TP, Helton E, McDonald I, et al. Effect of L-carnitine treatment for valproate-induced hepatotoxicity. *Neurology* 2001; 56:1405–1409.
513. Murphy JV, Groover RV, Hodge C. Hepatotoxic effects in a child receiving valproate and carnitine. *J Pediatr* 1993;123:318–320.
514. Laub MC, Paetzke-Brunner I, Jaeger G. Serum carnitine during valproic acid therapy. *Epilepsia* 1986;27:559–562.
515. Lenn NJ, Ellis WG, Washburn ER, et al. Fatal hepatocerebral syndrome in siblings discordant for exposure to valproate. *Epilepsia* 1990;31:578–583.
516. Melegh B, Trombitás K. Valproate treatment induces lipid globule accumulation with ultrastructural abnormalities of mitochondria in skeletal muscle. *Neuropediatrics* 1997;28:257–261.
517. Laub MC. Nutritional influence on serum ammonia in young patients receiving sodium valproate. *Epilepsia* 1986;27:55–59.
518. Marescaux C, Warter JM, Micheletti G, et al. Stuporous episodes during treatment with sodium valproate: report of seven cases. *Epilepsia* 1982;23:297–305.
519. Coulter DL, Allen RJ. Secondary hyperammonaemia: a possible mechanism for valproate encephalopathy. *Lancet* 1980;1:1310–1311.
520. Bruni J, Wilder BJ, Perchalski RJ, et al. Valproic acid and plasma levels of phenobarbital. *Neurology* 1980;30:94–97.
521. Mattson RH, Cramer JA. Valproic acid and ethosuximide interaction. *Ann Neurol* 1980;7:583–584.
522. Patsalos PN, Lascelles PT. Effect of sodium valproate on plasma protein binding of diphenylhydantoin. *J Neurol Neurosurg Psychiatry* 1977;40:570–574.
523. Hyman NM, Dennis PD, Sinclair KG. Tremor due to sodium valproate. *Neurology* 1979;29:1177–1180.
524. Bodensteiner JB, Morris HH, Golden GS. Asterixis associated with sodium valproate. *Neurology* 1981;31:194–195.
525. Barr RD, Copeland SA, Stockwell ML, et al. Valproic acid and immune thrombocytopenia. *Arch Dis Child* 1982;57:681–684.
526. Kreuz W, Linde R, Funk M, et al. Valproate therapy induces von Willebrand disease type I. *Epilepsia* 1992;33:178–184.
527. Ward M, Barbaro NM, Laxer KD, et al. Preoperative valproate administration does not increase blood loss during temporal lobectomy. *Epilepsia* 1996;37:98–101.
528. Mortensen PB, Kolvraa S, Christensen E. Inhibition of the glycine cleavage system: hyperglycinemia and hyperglycinuria caused by valproic acid. *Epilepsia* 1980;21:563–569.
529. Parker PH, Helinek GL, Ghishan FK, et al. Recurrent pancreatitis induced by valproic acid. A case report and review of the literature. *Gastroenterology* 1981;80:826–828.
530. Grauso-Eby NL, Goldfarb O, Feldman-Winter LB, et al. Acute pancreatitis in children from valproic acid: case series and review. *Pediatr Neurol* 2003;28:145–148.
531. Asconape JJ, Penry JK, Dreifuss FE, et al. Valproate-associated pancreatitis. *Epilepsia* 1993;34:177–183.
532. Ettinger A, Moshe S, Shinnar S. Edema associated with long-term valproate therapy. *Epilepsia* 1990;31:211–213.
533. Isojärvi JIT, Laatikainen TJ, Knip M, et al. Obesity and endocrine disorders in women taking valproate for epilepsy. *Ann Neurol* 1996;39:579–584.
534. Freeman JM, Vining EP, Cost S, et al. Does carnitine administration improve the symptoms attributed to anticonvulsant medications? A double-blinded, crossover study. *Pediatrics* 1994;93:893–895.
535. Wide K, Winblath B, Kallen B. Major malformations in infants exposed to antiepileptic drugs in utero, with emphasis on carbamazepine and valproic acid: a nation-wide, population-based register study. *Acta Paediatr* 2004;93:174–176.
536. Kozma C. Valproic acid embryopathy: report of two siblings with further expansion of the phenotypic abnormalities and review of the literature. *Am J Med Genet* 2001;98:168–175.
537. Malm H, Kajantie E, Kivirikko S, et al. Valproate embryopathy in three sets of siblings: further proof of hereditary susceptibility. *Neurology* 2002;59:630–633.
538. Hansen RA, Menkes JH. A new anticonvulsant in the management of minor motor seizures. *Dev Med Child Neurol* 1972;14:3–14.
539. Farrell K. Benzodiazepines in the treatment of children with epilepsy. *Epilepsia* 1986;27[Suppl 1]:S45–S51.

540. Martin D, Hirt HR. Clinical experience with clonazepam (Rivotril) in the treatment of epilepsies in infancy and childhood. *Neuropädiatrie* 1973;4:245–266.
541. Markham CH. The treatment of myoclonic seizures of infancy and childhood with LA-1. *Pediatrics* 1964;34:511–518.
542. Hosain SA, Green NS, Solomon GE, et al. Nitrazepam for the treatment of Lennox-Gastaut syndrome. *Pediatr Neurol* 2003;28:16–19.
543. Mikati MA, Lepejian GA, Holmes GL. Medical treatment of patients with infantile spasms. *Clin Neuropharmacol* 2002;25:61–70.
544. Murphy JV, Sawasky F, Marquardt KM, et al. Deaths in young children receiving nitrazepam. *J Pediatr* 1987;111:145–147.
545. Rintahaka PJ, Nakagawa JA, Shewmon DA, et al. Incidence of death in patients with intractable epilepsy during nitrazepam treatment. *Epilepsia* 1999;40:492–496.
546. Wretlind M, Pilbrant A, Sundwall A, et al. Disposition of three benzodiazepines after single oral administration in man. *Acta Pharmacol Toxicol* 1977;40:28–39.
547. Ko DY, Rho JM, De Giorgio CM, et al. Benzodiazepines. In: Engel J Jr, Pedley TA, eds. *Epilepsy: a comprehensive textbook*. Philadelphia: Lippincott-Raven, 1998:1475–1489.
548. Kumar A, Bleck TP. Intravenous midazolam for the treatment of refractory status epilepticus. *Crit Care Med* 1992;20:483–488.
549. Parent JM, Lowenstein DH. Treatment of refractory generalized status epilepticus with continuous infusion of midazolam. *Neurology* 1994;44:1837–1840.
550. Koul R, Chacko A, Javed H, et al. Eight-year study of childhood status epilepticus:midazolam infusion in management and outcome. *J Child Neurol* 2002;17:908–910.
551. O'Regan ME, Brown JK, Clarke M. Nasal rather than rectal benzodiazepines in the management of acute childhood seizures? *Dev Med Child Neurol* 1996;38:1037–1045.
552. Chamberlain JM, Altieri MA, Futterman C, et al. A prospective, randomized study comparing intramuscular midazolam with intravenous diazepam for the treatment of seizures in children. *Pediatr Emerg Care* 1997;13:92–94.
553. Clobazam has equivalent efficacy to carbamazepine and phenytoin as monotherapy for childhood epilepsy. Canadian Study Group for Childhood Epilepsy. *Epilepsia* 1998;39:952–959.
554. Bawden HN, Camfield CS, Camfield PR, et al. The cognitive and behavioural effects of clobazam and standard monotherapy are comparable. Canadian Study Group for Childhood Epilepsy. *Epilepsy Res* 1999;33:133–143.
555. Millichap JG. Acetazolamide in treatment of epilepsy [Letter]. *Neurology* 1991;41:764.
556. The Felbamate Study Group in Lennox-Gastaut Syndrome. Efficacy of felbamate in childhood epileptic encephalopathy (Lennox-Gastaut syndrome). *N Engl J Med* 1993;328:29–33.
557. Faught E, Sachdeo RC, Remler MP, et al. Felbamate monotherapy for partial-onset seizures: an active-control trial. *Neurology* 1993;43:688–692.
558. Thompson CD, Barthen MT, Hopper DW, et al. Quantification in patient urine samples of felbamate and three metabolites: acid carbamate and two mercapturic acids. *Epilepsia* 1999;40:769–776.
559. Pellock JM. Felbamate. *Epilepsia* 1999;40[Suppl 5]:S57–S62.
560. French J, Smith M, Faught E, et al. Practice advisory: the use of felbamate in the treatment of patients with intractable epilepsy. *Neurology* 1999;52:1540–1545.
561. Petroff OA, Rothman DL, Behar KL, et al. The effect of gabapentin on brain gamma-aminobutyric acid in patients with epilepsy. *Ann Neurol* 1996;39:95–99.
562. Chadwick DW, Anhut H, Greiner MJ, et al. A double-blind trial of gabapentin monotherapy for newly diagnosed partial seizures. International Gabapentin Monotherapy Study Group. *Neurology* 1998;51:1282–1288.
563. Leach JP, Girvan J, Paul A, et al. Gabapentin and cognition: a double-blind, dose-ranging, placebo controlled study in refractory epilepsy. *J Neurol Neurosurg Psychiatry* 1997;62:372–376.
564. French JA, Kanner AM, Bautista J, et al. Efficacy and tolerability of the new antiepileptic drugs II. Treatment of refractory epilepsy. *Neurology* 2004;62:1261–1273.
565. UK Gabapentin Study Group. Gabapentin in partial epilepsy. *Lancet* 1990;335:1114–1117.
566. Hosford DA, Wang Y. Utility of the lethargic (lh/lh) mouse model of absence seizures in predicting the effects of lamotrigine, vigabatrin, tiagabine, gabapentin, and topiramate against human absence seizures. *Epilepsia* 1997;38:408–414.
567. Trudeau V, Myers S, LaMoreaux L, et al. Gabapentin in naive childhood absence epilepsy: results from two double-blind, placebo-controlled, multicenter studies. *J Child Neurol* 1996;11:470–475.
568. Vossler DG. Exacerbation of seizures in Lennox-Gastaut syndrome by gabapentin. *Neurology* 1996;46:852–853.
569. Miller AA, Wheatley P, Sawyer DA, et al. Pharmacological studies on lamotrigine, a novel potential antiepileptic drug: I. Anticonvulsant profile in mice and rats. *Epilepsia* 1986;27:483–489.
570. Cheung H, Kamp D, Harris E. An in vitro investigation of the action of lamotrigine on neuronal-activated sodium channels. *Epilepsy Res* 1992;13:107–112.
571. Poolos NP, Migliore M, Johnston D. Pharmacological upregulation of h-channels reduces the excitability of pyramidal neuron dendrites. *Nat Neurosci* 2002;5:767–774.
572. Lang DG, Wang CM, Cooper BR. Lamotrigine, phenytoin and carbamazepine interactions on the sodium current in N4TG1 Neuroblastoma cells. *J Pharmacol Exp Ther* 1993;266:820–835.
573. Duchowny M, Gilman J, Messenheimer J, et al. Long-term tolerability and efficacy of lamotrigine in pediatric patients with epilepsy. *J Child Neurol* 2002;17:278–285.
574. Beran RG, Berkovic SF, Dunagan FM, et al. Double-blind, placebo-controlled, crossover study of lamotrigine in treatment-resistant generalised epilepsy. *Epilepsia* 1998;39:1329–1333.
575. Gilliam F, Vazquez B, Sackellares JC, et al. An active-control trial of lamotrigine monotherapy for partial seizures. *Neurology* 1998;51:1018–1025.
576. Dulac O, Kaminska A. Use of lamotrigine in Lennox-Gastaut and related epilepsy syndromes. *J Child Neurol* 1997;12[Suppl 1]:S23–S28.
577. Motte J, Trevathan E, Arvidsson JF, et al. Lamotrigine for generalized seizures associated with the Lennox-Gastaut syndrome. Lamictal Lennox-Gastaut Study Group. *New Engl J Med* 1997; 337:1807–1812.
578. Buchanan N. The use of lamotrigine in juvenile myoclonic epilepsy. *Seizure* 1996;5:149–151.
579. Besag FMC, Wallace SJ, Dulac O, et al. Lamotrigine for the treatment of epilepsy in childhood. *J Pediatr* 1995;127:991–997.
580. Frank LM, Enlow T, Holmes GL, et al. Lamictal (lamotrigine) monotherapy for typical absence seizures in children. *Epilepsia* 1999;40:973–979.
581. Battino D, Buti D, Croci D, et al. Lamotrigine in resistant childhood epilepsy. *Neuropediatrics* 1993;24:332–336.
582. Yuen AWC, Land G, Weatherley BC, et al. Sodium valproate acutely inhibits lamotrigine metabolism. *Br J Clin Pharmacol* 1992;33:511–513.
583. Gram L. Potential antiepileptic drugs. Lamotrigine. In: Levy R, Mattson RH, Meldrum BS, eds. *Antiepileptic drugs*. New York: Raven Press, 1989:947–953.
584. Schlienger RG, Shapiro LE, Shear NH. Lamotrigine-induced severe cutaneous adverse reactions. *Epilepsia* 1998;39[Suppl 7]:S22–S26.
585. Brodie MJ, French JA. Management of epilepsy in adolescents and adults. *Lancet* 2000;356:323–329.
586. Buchanan N. Lamotrigine: clinical experience in 200 patients with epilepsy with follow-up to four years. *Seizure* 1996;5:209–214.
587. Chattergoon DS, McGuigan MA, Koren G, et al. Multiorgan dysfunction and disseminated intravascular coagulation in children receiving lamotrigine and valproic acid. *Neurology* 1997;49:1442–1444.
588. Martin R, Kuzniecky R, Ho S, et al. Cognitive effects of topiramate, gabapentin, and lamotrigine in healthy young adults. *Neurology* 1999;52:321–327.
589. Aldencamp AP, De Krom M, Reijs R. Newer antiepileptic drugs and cognitive issues. *Epilepsia* 2003;44[Suppl 4]:S21–S29.
590. Kramer LD, Reife RA. Topiramate. In: Engel J Jr, Pedley TA, eds. *Epilepsy: a comprehensive textbook*. Philadelphia: Lippincott-Raven Publishers, 1998:1593–1598.
591. Kuzniecky R, Hetherington H, Ho S, et al. Topiramate increases cerebral GABA in healthy humans. *Neurology* 1998;51:627–629.
592. Petroff OAC, Hyder F, Mattson RH, et al. Topiramate increases brain GABA, homocarnosine, and pyrrolidinone in patients with epilepsy. *Neurology* 1999;52:473–478.

593. Gilliam FG, Veloso F, Bomhof MAM, et al. A dose-comparison trial of topiramate as monotherapy in recently diagnosed partial epilepsy. *Neurology* 2003;60:196–201.
594. Sachdeo RC, Glauser TA, Ritter F, et al. A double-blind, randomized trial of topiramate in Lennox-Gastaut syndrome. Topiramate YL Study Group. *Neurology* 1999;52:1882–1887.
595. Glauser TA, Levisohn PM, Ritter F, et al. Topiramate in Lennox-Gastaut syndrome: open-label treatment of patients completing a randomized controlled trial. Topiramate YL Study Group. *Epilepsia*. 2000;41[Suppl 1]:S86–S90.
596. Lee S, Sziklas V, Andermann F, et al. The effects of adjunctive topiramate on cognitive function in patients with epilepsy. *Epilepsia* 2003;44:339–347.
597. Reith D, Burke C, Appleton DB, et al. Tolerability of topiramate in children and adolescents. *J Paediatr Child Health* 2003;39:416–419.
598. Mula M, Trimble MR, Sander JW. The role of hippocampal sclerosis in topiramate-related depression and cognitive deficits in people with epilepsy. *Epilepsia* 2003;44:1573–1577.
599. Arroyo S, Squires L, Wang S, et al. Topiramate (TPM): effective as monotherapy in dose-response study in newly diagnosed epilepsy. *Epilepsia* 2002;43[Suppl 7]:241.
600. Wheless JW, Neto W, Wang S; EPMN-105 Study Group. Topiramate, carbamazepine, and valproate monotherapy: double-blind comparison in children with newly diagnosed epilepsy. *J Child Neurol* 2004;19:135–141.
600a. Lamb EJ, Stevens PJ, Nashef L. Topiramate increases biochemical risk of nephrolithiasis. *Ann Clin Biochem* 2004;41:166–169.
600b. Galicia CS, Lewis SL, Metman LV. Severe Topiramate-induced hyperthermia resulting in persistent neurological dysfunction. *Clin Neuropharmacol* 2005;28:94–95.
601. Reiter E, Feucht M, Hauser E, et al. Changes in body mass index during long-term topiramate therapy in paediatric epilepsy patients—a retrospective analysis. *Seizure* 2004;13:491–493.
602. Levisohn PM. Safety and tolerability of topiramate in children. *J Child Neurol* 2000;15 [Suppl 1]:S22–S26.
603. Sankar R, Derdiarian AT. Vigabatrin. *CNS Drug Rev* 1998;4:260–274.
604. Spence SJ, Sankar R. Visual field defects with vigabatrin. *Drug Saf* 2001;24:385–404.
605. Gross-Tsur V, Banin E, Shahar E, et al. Visual impairment in children with epilepsy treated with vigabatrin. *Ann Neurol* 2000;48:60–64.
606. Krauss GL, Johnson MA, Miller NR. Vigabatrin-associated retinal cone system dysfunction: electroretinogram and ophthalmologic findings. *Neurology* 1998;50:614–618.
607. Kälviäinen R, Nousiainen I, Mantyjarvi M, et al. GABAergic antiepileptic drug vigabatrin causes concentric visual field defects. *Neurology* 1999;53:922–926.
608. Paul SR, Krauss GL, Miller NR, et al. Visual function is stable in patients who continue long-term vigabatrin therapy: implications for clinical decision making. *Epilepsia* 2001;42:525–530.
609. Chiron C, Dumas C, Jambaque I, et al. Randomized trial comparing vigabatrin and hydrocortisone in infantile spasms due to tuberous sclerosis. *Epilepsy Res* 1997;26:389–395.
610. Hancock E, Osborne JP. Vigabatrin in the treatment of infantile spasms in tuberous sclerosis: literature review. *J Child Neurol* 1999;14:71–74.
611. Sankar R, Wasterlain CG. Is the devil we know the lesser of two evils? Vigabatrin and visual fields. [Editorial]. *Neurology* 1999;52:1537–1538.
612. Gibbs JM, Appleton RE, Rosenbloom L. Vigabatrin in intractable childhood epilepsy: a retrospective study. *Pediatr Neurol* 1992;8:338–340.
613. Jongsma MJ, Laan LA, van Emde Boas W, et al. Reversible motor disturbances induced by vigabatrin. *Lancet* 1991;338:893.
614. Krauss GL, Johnson MA, Sheth S, et al. A controlled study comparing visual function in patients treated with vigabatrin and tiagabine. *J Neurol Neurosurg Psychiatry* 2003;74:339–343.
615. Mangano S, Cusumano L, Fontana A. Non-convulsive status epilepticus associated with tiagabine in a pediatric patient. *Brain Dev* 2003;25:518–521.
616. Klitgaard H, Matagne A, Gobert J, et al. Evidence for a unique profile of levetiracetam in rodent models of seizures and epilepsy. *Eur J Pharmacol* 1998;353:191–206.
617. Cereghino JJ, Biton V, Abou-Khalil B, et al. Levetiracetam for partial seizures: results of a double-blind, randomized clinical trial. *Neurology* 2000;55:236–242.
618. Glauser TA, Dulac O. Preliminary efficacy of levetiracetam in children. *Epileptic Disord* 2003;5[Suppl 1]:S45–S50.
619. Tan MJ, Appleton RE. Efficacy and tolerability of levetiracetam in children aged 10 years and younger: a clinical experience. *Seizure* 2004;13:142–145.
620. Sankar R, Shields WD. Levetiracetam. In: Dodson WE, Bourgeois BF, Pellock JM, eds. *Pediatric epilepsy: diagnosis and therapy*, 2nd ed. New York: Demos Medical Publishing, 2003.
621. Gallagher MJ, Eisenman LN, Brown KM, et al. Levetiracetam reduces spike-wave density and duration during continuous EEG monitoring in patients with idiopathic generalized epilepsy. *Epilepsia* 2004;45:90–91.
622. Genton P, Gelisse P. Suppression of post-hypoxic and post-encephalitic myoclonus with levetiracetam. *Neurology* 2001;57: 1144–1145.
623. Magaudda A, Gelisse P, Genton P. Antimyoclonic effect of levetiracetam in 13 patients with Unverricht-Lundborg disease: clinical observations. *Epilepsia* 2004;45:678–681.
624. Bello-Espinosa LE, Roberts SL. Levetiracetam for benign epilepsy of childhood with centrotemporal spikes-three cases. *Seizure* 2003;12:157–159.
625. Kossoff EH, Bergey GK, Freeman JM, et al. Levetiracetam psychosis in children with epilepsy. *Epilepsia* 2001;42:1611–1613.
626. Fisher RS, Kerrigan JF, Pellock JM. Zonisamide. In: Pellock JM, Dodson WE, Bourgeois BFD, eds. *Pediatric epilepsy*, 2nd ed. New York: Demos, 2001:509–512.
627. Sackellares JC, Ramsay RE, Wilder BJ, et al. Randomized, controlled clinical trial of zonisamide as adjunctive treatment for refractory partial seizures. *Epilepsia* 2004;45:610–617.
628. Faught E, Ayala R, Mountouris GG, et al. Randomized controlled trial of zonisamide for the treatment of refractory partial-onset seizures. *Neurology* 2001;57:1774–1779.
629. Ojemann LM, Ojemann GA, Dodrill CB, et al. Language disturbances as side effects of topiramate and zonisamide therapy. *Epilepsy Behav* 2001;2:579–584.
630. Kyllerman M, Ben-Menachem E. Zonisamide for progressive myoclonus epilepsy: long-term observations in seven patients. *Epilepsy Res* 1998;29:109–114.
631. Chiron C, Marchand MC, Tran A, et al. Stiripentol in severe myoclonic epilepsy in infancy: a randomized placebo-controlled syndrome-dedicated trial. STICLO study group. *Lancet* 2000; 356:1638–1642.
632. Wilder RM. The effects of ketonuria on the course of epilepsy. *Mayo Clin Proc* 1921;2:307–308.
633. Kinsman SL, Vining EP, Quaskey SA, et al. Efficacy of the ketogenic diet for intractable seizure disorders: review of 58 cases. *Epilepsia* 1992;33:1132–1136.
634. Thio LL, Wong M, Yamada KA, et al. Ketone bodies do not directly alter excitatory or inhibitory hippocampal synaptic transmission. *Neurology* 2000;54:325–331.
635. Bough KJ, Schwartzkroin PA, Rho JM. Calorie restriction and ketogenic diet diminish neuronal excitability in rat dentate gyuris in vivo. *Epilepsia* 2003;44:752–760.
636. Kossoff EH, Krauss GL, McGrogan JR, et al. Efficacy of the Atkins diet as therapy for intractable epilepsy. *Neurology* 2003;61:1789–1791.
637. Dr. Elizabeth Thiele, personal communications (2005).
638. Sankar R, Sotero de Menezes M. Metabolic and endocrine aspects of the ketogenic diet. *Epilepsy Res* 1999;37:191–201.
639. Nordli DB, De Vivo DC. The ketogenic diet. In: Pellock JM, Dodson WE, Bourgeois BFD, eds. *Pediatric epilepsy*, 2nd ed. New York: Demos, 2001:549–554.
640. Huttenlocher PR, Wilbourn AJ, Signore JM. Medium-chain triglycerides as a therapy for intractable childhood epilepsy. *Neurology* 1971;21:1097–1103.
640a. Kim DW, Kang HC, Park JC, Kim HD. Benefits of the nonfasting ketogenic diet compared wtih the initial fasting ketogenic diet. *Pediatrics* 2004;114:1627–1630.
641. Vining EP, Freeman JM, Ballaban-Gil K, et al. A multicenter study of the efficacy of the ketogenic diet. *Arch Neurol* 1998;55:1433–1437.

642. Demeritte EL, Ventimiglia J, Coyne M, Nigro MA. Organic acid disorders and the ketogenic diet. *Ann Neurol* 1996;40:305.
643. De Vivo DC, Bohan TP, Coulter DL, et al. L-carnitine supplementation in childhood epilepsy: current perspectives. *Epilepsia* 1998;39:1216–1225.
644. Ballaban-Gil K, Callahan C, O'Dell C, et al. Complications of the ketogenic diet. *Epilepsia* 1998;39:744–748.
645. Berry-Kravis E, Booth G, Taylor A, et al. Bruising and the ketogenic diet: evidence for diet-induced changes in platelet function. *Ann Neurol* 2001;49:98–103.
646. Stephen LJ, Sills GJ, Brodie MJ. Lamotrigeine and topiramate may be a useful combination. *Lancet* 1998;351:958–959.
647. Mula M, Trimble MR, Lhatoo SD, et al. Topiramate and psychiatric adverse events in patients with epilepsy. *Epilepsia* 2003;44:659–663.
648. Mula M, Trimble MR, Yuen A, et al. Psychiatric adverse events during levetiracetam therapy. *Neurology* 2003;61:704–706.
649. Ko T-S, Holmes GL. EEG and clincial predictors of medically intractable childhood epilepsy. *Clin Neurophysiol* 1999;110:1245–1251.
650. Kwan P, Brodie MJ. Early identification of refractory epilepsy. *N Engl J Med* 2000;342:314–319.
651. Camfield PR, Camfield CS, Gordon K, et al. If a first antiepileptic drug fails to control a child's epilepsy, what are the chances of success with the next drug? *J Pediatr* 1997;131:821–824.
652. Dlugos DJ, Sammel MD, Strom BL, et al. Response to first drug trial predicts outcome in childhood temporal lobe epilepsy. *Neurology* 2001;57:2259–2264.
653. Fusco L, Vigevano F. Indications for surgical treatment of epilepsy in childhood: a clinical and neurophysiological approach. *Acta Pediatr Supp* 2004;93(445):28–31.
654. Duchowny MS, et al. Indications and criteria for surgical intervention. In: Engle J Jr, Pedley TA, eds. *Epilepsy: a comprehensive textbook*. Philadelphia: Lippincott-Raven Publishers, 1998:1677–1685.
655. Pusifer MB, Brandt J, Salorio CF, et al. The cognitive outcome of hemispherectomy in 71 children. *Epilepsia* 2004;45:243–254.
656. Piastra M, Pietrini D, Caresta E, et al. Hemispherectomy procedures in children: hematological issues. *Childs Nerv Syst* 2004;20:453–458.
657. Andermann F. Identification of candidates for surgical treatment of epilepsy. In: Engel J Jr, ed. *Surgical treatment of the epilepsies*. New York: Raven Press, 1987:51–70.
658. Paolicchi JM, Jayakar P, Dean P, et al. Predictors of outcome in pediatric epilepsy surgery. *Neurology* 2000;54:642–647.
659. Shewmon DA, Shields WD, Chugani HT, et al. Contrasts between pediatric and adult epilepsy surgery: rationale and strategy for focal resection. *J Epilepsy* 1990;3[Suppl]:141–155.
660. Sankar R, Chugani HT. Strategies for diagnosis and treatment of childhood epilepsy. *Curr Opin Neurol Neurosurg* 1993;6:398–402.
661. Chugani HT, Shewmon DA, Shields WD, et al. Surgery for intractable infantile spasms: neuroimaging perspectives. *Epilepsia* 1993;34:764–771.
662. Duchowny MS, Shewmon DA, Wyllie E, et al. Special considerations for preoperative evaluation in childhood. In: Engel J Jr, ed. *Surgical treatment of the epilepsies*, 2nd ed. New York: Raven Press, 1993:415–428.
663. Mazziotta JC, Engel J Jr. The use and impact of positron computed tomography scanning in epilepsy. *Epilepsia* 1984;25[Suppl 2]:S86–S104.
664. Debets RM, Sadzot B, van Isselt JW, et al. Is ^{11}C-flumazenil PET superior to 18_FDG PET and 123_I-iomazenil SPECT in presurgical evaluation of temporal lobe epilepsy? *J Neurol Neurosurg Psychiatry* 1997;62:141–150.
665. Chugani DC, Chugani HT, Muzik O, et al. Imaging epileptogenic tubers in children with tuberous sclerosis complex using alpha-[11C]methyl-L-tryptophan positron emission tomography. *Ann Neurol* 1998;44:858–866.
666. Markand ON, Salanova V, Worth R, et al. Comparative study of interictal PET and ictal SPECT in complex partial seizures. *Acta Neurol Scand* 1997;95:129–136.
667. Ho SS, Berkovic SF, Berlangieri SU, et al. Comparison of ictal SPECT and interictal PET in the presurgical evaluation of temporal lobe epilepsy. *Ann Neurol* 1995;37:738–745.
668. O'Brien TJ, So EL, Mullan BP, et al. Subtraction SPECT coregistered to MRI improves postictal SPECT localization of seizure foci. *Neurology* 1999;52:137–146.
669. O' Brien TJ, So EL, Cascino GD, et al. Subtraction SPECT coregistered to MRI in focal malformation cortical development: localization of the epileptogenic zone in epilepsy surgery candidates. *Epilepsia* 2004;45:367–376.
670. Jack CR, Sharbrough FW, Twomey CK. Temporal lobe seizures: lateralization with MR volume measurements of hippocampal formation. *Radiology* 1990;175:423–429.
671. Lencz T, McCarthy G, Bronen RA, et al. Quantitative magnetic resonance in temporal lobe epilepsy: relationship to neuropathology and neuropsychological function. *Ann Neurol* 1992;31:629–637.
672. Bernasconi N, Bernasconi A, Andermann F, et al. Entorhinal cortex in temporal lobe epilepsy. *Neurology* 1999;52:1870–1876.
673. Lawson JA, Nguyen W, Bleasel AF, et al. ILAE-defined epilepsy syndromes in children: correlation with quantitative MRI. *Epilepsia* 1998;39:1345–1349.
674. Brey R, Laxer KD. Type I/II complex partial seizures: no correlation with surgical outcome. *Epilepsia* 1985;26:657–660.
675. Nimsky C, Ganslandt O, Hastreiter P, et al. Intraoperative diffusion-tensor MR imaging: shifting of white matter tracts during neurosurgical procedures—initial experience. *Radiology* 2004;234:218–225.
676. Jansen FE, Braun KP, van Nieuwenhuizen O, et al. Diffusion-weighted magnetic resonance imaging and identification of the epileptogenic tuber in patients with tuberous sclerosis. *Arch Neurol* 2003;60:1580–1584.
677. Wheless JW, Willmore LJ, Breier JI, et al. A comparison of magnetoencephalography, MRI, and V-EEG in patients evaluated for epilepsy surgery. *Epilepsia* 1999;40:931–941.
678. Mamelak AN, Lopez N, Akhtari M, et al. Magnetoencephalography-directed surgery in patients with neocortical epilepsy. *J Neurosurg* 2002;97:865–873.
679. Knowlton RC, Shih J. Magnetoencephalography in epilepsy. *Epilepsia* 2004;45[Suppl 4]:61–71.
680. Asano E, Benedek K, Shah A, et al. Is intraoperative electrocorticography reliable in children with intractable neocortical epilepsy? *Epilepsia* 2004;45:1091–1099.
681. So N, Gloor P, Quesney LF, et al. Depth electrode investigations in patients with bitemporal epileptiform abnormalities. *Ann Neurol* 1989;25:423–431.
682. Jayakar P. Invasive EEG monitoring in children: when, where and what? *J Clin Neurophysiol* 1999;16:408–418.
683. Brey R, Laxer KD. Type I/II complex partial seizures: no correlation with surgical outcome. *Epilepsia* 1985;26:657–660.
684. Wieser HG, Siegel AM, Yasargil GM. The Zurich amygdalohippocampectomy series: a short up-date. *Acta Neurochir Suppl (Wien)*. 1990;50:122–127.
685. Keogan M, McMackin D, Peng S, et al. Temporal neocorticectomy in the management of intractable epilepsy: long-term outcome and predictive factors. *Epilepsia* 1992;33:852–861.
686. Delgado-Escueta AV, Walsh GO. Type I complex partial seizures of hippocampal origin. Excellent results of anterior temporal lobectomy. *Neurology* 1985;35:143–154.
687. Walsh GO, Delgado-Escueta AV. Type II complex partial seizures: poor results of anterior temporal lobectomy. *Neurology* 1984; 34:113.
688. Shields WD, Duchowny MS, Holmes GL. Surgically remediable syndromes of infancy and early childhood. In: Engel J Jr, ed. *Surgical treatment of the epilepsies*, 2nd ed. New York: Raven Press, 1993:35–48.
689. Szabo CA, Wyllie E, Stanford LD, et al. Neuropsychological effect of temporal lobe resection in preadolescent children with epilepsy. *Epilepsia* 1998;39:814–819.
690. Peacock WJ, Comair Y, Hoffman HJ, et al. Special consideration for epilepsy surgery in childhood. In: Engel J Jr, ed. *Surgical treatment of the epilepsies*, 2nd ed. New York: Raven Press, 1993: 541–548.
691. Rasmussen T. Surgery for epilepsy arising in regions other than

the temporal and frontal lobes. In: Purpura DP, et al., eds. *Neurosurgical management of epilepsies. Adv Neurol* 1975;8:207–226.
692. Olivier A. Surgery of extratemporal epilepsy. In: Wyllie E, ed. *The treatment of epilepsy: principles and practice*, 2nd ed. Baltimore: Williams & Wilkins, 1997:1060–1073.
693. Rasmussen T. Hemispherectomy for seizures revisited. *Can J Neurosci* 1983;10:71–78.
694. Ville mure JG, Mascott C. Hemispherotomy: the peri-insular approach. Technical aspects. *Epilepsia* 1993;34[Suppl 6]:48.
695. Tinuper P, Andermann F, Villemure JG, et al. Functional hemispherectomy for treatment of epilepsy associated with hemiplegia: rationale, indications, results, and comparison with callosotomy. *Ann Neurol* 1988;24:27–34.
696. van Empelen R, Jennekens-Schinkel A, Buskens E, et al. Functional consequences of hemispherectomy. *Brain* 2004;127:2071–2079.
697. Mathern GW, Giza CC, Yudovin S, et al. Postoperative seizure control and antiepileptic drug use in pediatric epilepsy surgery patients: the UCLA experience, 1986–1997. *Epilepsia* 1999;40:1740–1749.
698. Wyllie E, Comair YG, Kotagal P, et al. Seizure outcome after epilepsy surgery in children and adolescents. *Ann Neurol* 1998;44:740–748.
699. Jonas, R, Nguyen S, Hu B, et al. Cerebral hemispherectomy: hospital course, seizure, developmental, language and motor outcomes. *Neurology* 2004;62:1712–17221.
700. Chugani HT, Shewmon DA, Peacock WJ, et al. Surgical treatment of intractable neonatal-onset seizures: the role of positron emission tomography. *Neurology* 1988;38:1178–1188.
701. Wyllie E. Corpus callosotomy for intractable generalized epilepsy. *J Pediatr* 1988;113:255–261.
702. Spencer SS. Corpus callosum section and other disconnection procedures for medically intractable epilepsy. *Epilepsia* 1988; 29[Suppl 2]:S85–S99.
703. Gates JR. Surgery in Lennox-Gastaut syndrome. Corpus callosum division for children. *Adv Exp Med Biol*. 2002;497:87–98.
704. Blume WT. Corpus callosum section for seizure control: rationale and review of experimental and clinical data. *Cleve Clin Q* 1984;51:319–332.
705. Black MP, Holmes G, Lombroso C. Corpus callosum section for intractable epilepsy in children. *Pediatr Neurosurg* 1992;18:298–304.
706. Brey R, Laxer KD. Type I/II complex partial seizures: no correlation with surgical outcome. *Epilepsia* 1985;26:657–660.
707. Gazzaniga MS, Bogen JE, Sperry RW. Observations on visual perception after disconnexion of the cerebral hemisphere in man. *Brain* 1965;88:221–236.
708. Dunoyer C, Ragheb J, Resnick T, et al. The use of stereotactic radiosurgery to treat intractable childhood partial epilepsy. *Epilepsia* 2002;43:292–300.
709. Chabardes S, Kahane P, Minotti L, et al. Deep brain stimulation in epilepsy with particular references to the subthalamic nucleus. *Epileptic Disord* 2002;4[Suppl 3]:S83–93.
710. Hammond EJ, Uthman BM, Wilder BJ, et al. Neurochemical effects of vagus nerve stimulation in humans. *Brain Res* 1992;583: 300–303.
711. Henry TR, Votaw JR, Pennell PB, et al. Acute blood flow changes and efficacy of vagus nerve stimulation in partial epilepsy. *Neurology* 1999;52:1166–1173.
712. Uthman B, Wilder BJ, Penry JK, et al. Treatment of epilepsy by stimulation of the vagus nerve. *Neurology* 1993;43:1338–1345.
713. Ben-Menachem E, Manon-Espaillat R, Ristanovic R, et al. Vagus nerve stimulation for treatment of partial seizures: 1. A controlled study of effect on seizures. *Epilepsia* 1994;35:616–626.
714. Handforth A, DeGiorgio CM, Schachter SC, et al. Vagus nerve stimulation therapy for partial-onset seizures. A randomized active control trial. *Neurology* 1998;51:48–55.
715. Murphy JV. Left vagal nerve stimulation in children with medically refractory epilepsy. The Pediatric VNS Study Group. *J Pediatr* 1999;134:563–566.
716. Lothman E. The biochemical basis and pathophysiology of status epilepticus. *Neurology* 1990;40[Suppl 2]:13–23.
717. Brown JK, Hussain IHM. Staus epilepticus: I. Pathogenesis. *Dev Med Child Neurol* 1991;33:317.
718. Shorvon S. Tonic clonic status epilepticus. *J Neurol Neurosurg Psychiatry* 1993;56:125–134.
719. Holmes GL. Epilepsy in the developing brain: lessons from the laboratory and clinic. *Epilepsia* 1997;38:12–30.
720. Maytal J, Shinnar S, Moshe SL, et al. Low morbidity and mortality of status epilepticus in children. *Pediatrics* 1989;83:323–331.
721. Payne TA, Black TP. Status epilepticus. *Crit Care Clin* 1997;13:17–38.
722. Cock HR, Schapia AH. A comparison of lorazepam and diazepam as initial therapy in convulsive status epilepticus. *Quart J Med* 2002;95:225–231.
723. Stewart WA, Harrison R, Dooley JM. Respiratory depression in the acute management of seizures. *Arch Dis Child* 2002;57:225–226.
724. Crawford TO, Mitchell WG, Snodgrass SR. Lorazepam in childhood status epilepticus and serial seizures: effectiveness and tachyphylaxis. *Neurology* 1987;37:190–195.
725. Brown JK, Hussain IHM. Status epilepticus: II. Treatment. *Dev Med Child Neurol* 1991;33:97–109.
726. Franzoni E, Carboni C, Lambertini A. Rectal diazepam: a clinical and EEG study after a single dose in children. *Epilepsia* 1981;24:35–41.
727. Leppik IE. Status epilepticus. In: Wyllie E, ed. *The treatment of epilepsy: principles and practice*. Philadelphia: Lea & Febiger, 1993:678–685.
728. Delgado-Escueta AV, Wasterlain C, Treiman DM, et al. Current concepts in neurology. Management of status epilepticus. *N Engl J Med* 1982;306:1337–1340.
729. Lombroso CT. Treatment of status epilepticus with diazepam. *Neurology* 1966;16:629–634.
730. Bell DS. Dangers of treatment of status epilepticus with diazepam. *BMJ* 1969;1:159–161.
731. Kriel RL. Home use of rectal diazepam for cluster and prolonged seizures. Efficacy, adverse reactions, quality of life, and cost analysis. *Pediatr Neurol* 1991;7:13–17.
732. Dreifuss FE, Rosman NP, Cloyd JC, et al. A comparison of rectal diazepam gel and placebo for acute repetitive seizures. *N Engl J Med* 1998;338:1869–1875.
733. Runge JW, Allen FH. Emergency treatment of status epilepticus. *Neurology* 1996;46[Suppl 1]:S20–S23.
734. Wheeles JW. Pediatric use of intravenous and intramuscular phenytoin: lessons learned. *J Child Neurol* 1998;13[Suppl 1]:S11–S14.
735. Richard MO, Chiron C, d'Athis P, et al. Phenytoin monitoring in status epilepticus in infant and children. *Epilepsia* 1993;34:144–150.
736. Wilensky AJ, Lowden JA. Inadequate serum levels after intramuscular administration of diphenylhydantoin. *Neurology* 1973;23: 318–324.
737. Pellock JM. Fosphenytoin use in children. *Neurology* 1996; 46[Suppl 1]:S14–S16.
738. Holmes GL, Riviello JJ. Midazolam and pentobarbital for refractory status epilepticus. *Pediatr Neurol* 1999;20:259–264.
739. Evrard P, Arzimanoglou A, Husson H, et al. Management of status epilepticus in the pediatric age group. In: Treiman DM, Wasterlain CG, eds. *Status epilepticus: mechanisms and management*. MIT Press Cambridge, MA 2006; (in press).
740. Shaner DM, McCurdy SA, Herring MO, et al. Treatment of status epilepticus: a prospective comparison of diazepam and phenytoin versus phenobarbital and optional phenytoin. *Neurology* 1988;38:202–207.
741. Koul RL, Raj Aithala G, Chacko A, et al. Continuous midazolam infusion as treatment of status epilepticus. *Arch Dis Child* 1997;76:445–448.
742. Singhi S, Murthy A, Singhi P, et al. Continuous midazolam versus diazepam infusion for refractory convulsive status epilepticus. *J Child Neurol* 2002;17:106–110.
743. Van Ness PC. Pentobarbital and EEG burst suppression in treatment of status epilepticus refractory to benzodiazepines and phenytoin. *Epilepsia* 1990;31:61–67.
744. Mitchell WG. Status epilepticus and acute repetitive seizures in

children, adolescents, and young adults: etiology, outcome, and treatment. *Epilepsia* 1996;37[Suppl 1]:S74–S80.
745. Kobayashi K, Ito M, Miyajima T, et al. Successful management of intractable epilepsy with intravenous lidocaine and lidocaine tapes. *Pediatr Neurol* 1999;21:476–480.
746. Yu KT, Mills S, Thompson M, Cunanan C. Safety and efficacy of intravenous valproate in pediatric status epilepticus and acute repetitive seizures. *Epilepsia* 2003;44:724–726.
747. Classen J, Hirsch LJ, Mayer SA. Treatment of status epilepticus: a survey of neurologists. *J Neurol Sci* 2003;211:37–41.
748. Cohen-Gadol AA, Britton JW, Worrell GA, Meyer FB. Transient cortical abnormalities on magnetic resonance imaging after status epilepticus: case report. *Surg Neurol* 2004;61:479–482.
749. Phillips SA, Shanahan RJ. Etiology and mortality of status epilepticus in children. A recent update. *Arch Neurol* 1989;46:74–76.
750. Berg AT, Shinnar S, Levy SR, et al. Status epilepticus in children with newly diagnosed epilepsy. *Ann Neurol* 1999;45:618–623.
751. Sisodiya SM, Lin WR, Harding BN, et al. Drug resistance in epilepsy: expression of drug resistance proteins in common causes of refractory epilepsy. *Brain* 2002;125:22–31.
752. Pedley TA, Hirano M. Is refractory epilepsy due to genetically determined resistance to antiepileptic drugs? *N Engl J Med* 2003;348:1480–1482.
753. Lazarowski A, Lubieniecki F, Camarero S, et al. Multidrug resistance proteins in tuberous sclerosis and refractory epilepsy. *Pediatr Neurol* 2004;30:102–106.
754. Siddiqui A, Kerb R, Weale ME, et al. Association of multidrug resistance in epilepsy with a polymorphism in the drug-transporter gene ABCB1. *N Engl J Med* 2003;348:1442–1448.
755. Rodin EA. *The prognosis of patients with epilepsy*. Springfield, IL: Charles C Thomas Publisher, 1968.
756. MacDonald BK, Johnson AL, Goodridge DM, et al. Factors predicting prognosis of epilepsy after presentation with seizures. *Ann Neurol* 2000;48:833–841.
757. Shinnar S, et al. Discontinuing antiepileptic drugs in children with epilepsy after a seizure free period: effect of age on outcome. *Epilepsia* 1991;32[Suppl. 3]:69–70.
758. Shinnar S, Berg AT, Moshe SL, et al. The risk of seizure recurrence after a first unprovoked afebrile seizure in childhood: an extended follow-up. *Pediatrics* 1996;98:216–225.
759. Hauser WA, Anderson VE, Loewenson RB, et al. Seizure recurrence after a first unprovoked seizure: an extended follow-up. *Neurology* 1990;40:1163–1170.
760. Sander JW, Hart YM, Johnson AL, et al. National General Practice Study of Epilepsy: newly diagnosed epileptic seizures in a general population. *Lancet* 1990;336:1267–1271.
761. Shorvon SD. The temporal aspects of prognosis in epilepsy. *J Neurol Neurosurg Psychiatry* 1984;47:1157–1165.
762. Annegers JF, Hauser WA, Elveback LR. Remission of seizures and relapse in patients with epilepsy. *Epilepsia* 1979;20:729–737.
763. Huttenlocher PR, Hapke RJ. A follow-up study of intractible seizures in childhood. *Ann Neurol* 1990;28:699–705.
764. Emerson R, D'Souza BJ, Vining EP, et al. Stopping medication in children with epilepsy. *N Engl J Med* 1981;304:1125–1129.
765. Sato S, Dreifuss FE, Penry JK, et al. Long-term follow-up of absence seizures. *Neurology* 1983;33:1590–1595.
766. Camfield C, Camfield P, Smith B, et al. Biologic facts as predictors of social outcome of epilepsy in intellectually normal children: a population-based study. *J Pediatr* 1993;122:869–873.
767. Reynolds EH, Elwes RD, Shorvon SD. Why does epilepsy become intractable? Prevention of chronic epilepsy. *Lancet* 1983;2:952–954.
768. Aicardi J. *Epilepsy in children*, 2nd ed. New York: Raven Press, 1994.
769. Otsubo H, Chitoku S, Ochi A, et al. Malignant rolandic-sylvian epilepsy in children: diagnosis, treatment, and outcome. *Neurology* 2001;57:590–596.
770. Wirrell EC, Camfield CS, Camfield PR, et al. Long-term prognosis of typical childhood absence epilepsy. Remission or progression to juvenile myoclonic epilepsy. *Neurology* 1996;47:912–918.
771. Lindsay J, Ounsted C, Richards P. Long-term outcome in children with temporal lobe seizures. I. Social outcome and childhood factors. *Dev Med Child Neurol* 1979;21:285–298.
772. D'Allessandro R, Guarino M, Greco G, et al. Risk of seizures while awake in pure sleep epilepsies: a prospective study. *Neurology* 2004;62:254–257.
773. Reynolds EH. Early treatment and prognosis of epilepsy. *Epilepsia* 1987;28:97–106.
774. Donner EJ, Smith CR, Snead OC. Sudden unexplained death in children with epilepsy. *Neurology* 2001;57:430–434.
775. Camfield CS, Camfield PR, Veugelers PJ. Death in children with epilepsy: a population-based study. *Lancet* 2002;359:1891–1895.
776. Terrence CF, Rao GR, Perper JA. Neurogenic pulmonary edema in unexpected, unexplained death of epileptic patients. *Ann Neurol* 1981;9:458–464.
777. Nilsson L, Farahmand BY, Persson PG, et al. Risk factors for sudden unexplained death in epilepsy: a case-controlled study. *Lancet* 1999;353:888–893.
778. Duncan JS. Seizure-induced neuronal injury: human data. *Neurology* 2002;59[9 Suppl 5]:S15–S20.
779. Austin JK, Dunn DW. Progressive behavioral changes in children with epilepsy. *Prog Brain Res* 2002;135:419–428.
780. Cendes K, Andermann F, Gloor P, et al. Atrophy of mesial structures in patients with temporal lobe epilepsy: cause or consequence of repeated seizures? *Ann Neurol* 1993;34:795–801.
781. Liu RS, Lemieux L, Bell GS, et al. The structural consequences of newly diagnosed seizures. *Ann Neurol* 2002;52:573–580.
782. Van Paesschen W, Connelly A, King MD, et al. The spectrum of hippocampal sclerosis: a quantitative magnetic resonance imaging study. *Ann Neurol* 1997;41:41–51.
783. Briellmann RS, Berkovic SF, Syngeniotis A, et al. Seizure-associated hippocampal volume loss: a longitudinal magnetic resonance study of temporal lobe epilepsy. *Ann Neurol* 2002;51:641–644.
784. Hermann B, Hansen R, Seidenberg M, et al. Neurodevelopmental vulnerability of the corpus callosum in childhood onset localization-related epilepsy. *Neuroimage* 2003;18:284–292.
785. Helmstaedter C, Kurthen M, Lux S, et al. Chronic epilepsy and cognition: a longitudinal study in temporal lobe epilepsy. *Ann Neurol* 2003;54:425–432.
786. Hermann BP, Seidenberg M, Bell B. The neurodevelopmental impact of childhood onset temporal lobe epilepsy on brain structure and function and the risk of progressive cognitive effects. *Prog Brain Res* 2002;135:429–438.
787. Deonna T, Zesiger P, Davidoff V, et al. Benign partial epilepsy of childhood: a longitudinal neuropsychological and EEF study of cognitive function. *Dev Med Child Neurol* 2000;42:595–603.
788. Meador KJ. Cognitive outcomes and predictive factors in epilepsy. *Neurology* 2002;58[8 Suppl 5]:S21–S26.
789. Trimble MR. Cognitive hazards of seizure disorders. *Epilepsia* 1988;29[Suppl 1]:S19–S24.
790. Addy DP. Cognitive function in children with epilepsy. *Dev Med Child Neurol* 1987;29:394–397.
791. Vining EPG, Mellitis ED, Dorsen MM, et al. Psychological and behavioral effects of antiepileptic drugs in children: a double-blind comparison between phenobarbital and valproic acid. *Pediatrics* 1987;80:165–174.
792. Trimble MR, Reynolds EH. Anticonvulsant drugs and mental symptoms: a review. *Psychol Med* 1976;6:169–178.
793. Goldensohn ES, Gold AP. Prolonged behavioral disturbances as ictal phenomena. *Neurology* 1960;10:19.
794. Gross-Tsur V, Shinnar S. Discontinuing antiepileptic drug treatment. In: Wyllie E, ed. *The treatment of epilepsy: principles and practice*, 2nd ed. Baltimore: Williams & Wilkins, 1997:799–807.
795. Peters ACB, Brouwer OF, Geerts AT, et al. Randomized prospective study of early discontinuation of antiepileptic drugs in children with epilepsy. *Neurology* 1998;50:724–730.
796. Holowach-Thurston JH, Thurston DL, Hixon BB, et al. Prognosis in childhood epilepsy: additional follow-up of 148 children 15 to 23 years after withdrawal of anticonvulsant therapy. *N Engl J Med* 1982;306:831–836.
797. Shinnar S, Berg AT, Moshe SL, et al. Discontinuing antiepileptic drugs in children with epilepsy: a prospective study. *Ann Neurol* 1994;35:534–535.
798. Gherpelli JLD, Kok F, dal Forno S, et al. Discontinuing medication

in epileptic children: a study of risk factors related to recurrence. *Epilepsia* 1992;33:681–686.
799. Tennison M, Greenwood R, Lewis D, et al. Discontinuing antiepileptic drugs in children. A comparison of a six-week and a nine-month taper period. *N Engl J Med* 1994;330:1407–1410.
800. Callaghan N, Garret A, Goggin T. Withdrawal of anticonvulsant drugs in patients free of seizures for two years: a prospective study. *N Engl J Med* 1988;318:942–946.
801. Schiller Y, Cascino GD, So EL, et al. Discontinuation of antiepileptic drugs after successful epilepsy surgery. *Neurology* 2000;54:346–349.
802. Craig A, Oxley J. Emotional and psychiatric aspects of epilepsy. In: Laidlaw J, Richens A, Chadwick D, eds. *A textbook of epilepsy*, 3rd ed. Oxford: Butterworth–Heinemann, 1994:186–200.
803. O'Donohoe NV. What should the child with epilepsy be allowed to do? *Arch Dis Child* 1983;58:934–937.
804. Kemp AM, Sibert JR. Epilepsy in children and the risk of drowning. *Arch Dis Child* 1993;68:684–685.
805. Patrick HT, Levy DM. Early convulsions in epileptics and in others. *JAMA* 1924;82:375–381.
806. Wallace SJ. *The child with febrile seizures*. London: John Wright, 1988.
807. Vanden-Berg BJ, Yerushalmy J. Studies on convulsive disorders in young children. I. Incidence of febrile and nonfebrile convulsions by age and other factors. *Pediatr Res* 1969;3:298–304.
808. Berg AT, Shinnar S, Hauser WA, et al. A prospective study of recurrent febrile seizures. *N Engl J Med* 1992;327:1122–1127.
809. Waruiru C, Appleton R. Febrile seizures: an update. *Arch Dis Child* 2004;89:751–756.
810. Berg AT. Febrile seizures and epilepsy: the contribution of epidemiology. *Paediatr Perinat Epidemiol* 1992;6:145–152.
811. Berg AT, Shinnar S, Shapiro ED, et al. Risk factors for a first febrile seizure: a matched case-control study. *Epilepsia* 1995;36:334–341.
812. Baird HW III, Garfunkel JM. Electroencephalographic changes in children with artificially induced hyperthermia. *J Pediatr* 1956;48:28–33.
813. Autret E, Billard C, Bertrand P, et al. Double-blind, randomized trial of diazepam versus placebo for prevention of recurrence of febrile seizures. *J Pediatr* 1990;117:490–494.
814. Berg AT, Shinnar S. Complex febrile seizures. *Epilepsia* 1996;37: 126–133.
815. Hall CB, Long CE, Schnabel KC, et al. Human herpesvirus-6 infections in children. A prospective study of complications and reactivation. *N Engl J Med* 1994;331:432–438.
816. Fischler E. Convulsions as a complication of shigellosis in children. *Helv Paediatr Acta* 1962;17:389–394.
817. Lennox-Buchthal MA. Febrile convulsions. A reappraisal. *Electroencephalogr Clin Neurophysiol* 1973;[Suppl 32].
818. Masuyama T, Matsuo M, Ichimaru T, et al. Possible contribution of interferon-alpha to febrile seizures in influenza. *Pediatr Neurol* 2002;27:289–292.
819. Livingston S. *Comprehensive management of epilepsy in infancy, childhood, and adolescence.* Springfield IL: Charles C Thomas Publisher, 1972.
820. Lorber J, Sunderland R. Lumbar puncture in children with convulsions associated with fever. *Lancet* 1980;1:785–786.
821. Green SM, Rothrock SG, Clem KJ, et al. Can seizures be the sole manifestation of meningitis in febrile children? *Pediatrics* 1993;92:527–534.
822. Freeman JM, Vining EPG. Decision making and the child with febrile seizures. *Pediatr Rev* 1992;13:298–310.
823. Maytal J, Steele R, Eviatar L, et al. The value of early postictal EEG in children with complex febrile seizures. *Epilepsia* 2000;41:219–221.
824. Sofijanov N, Emoto S, Kuturec M, et al. Febrile seizures: clinical characteristics and initial EEG. *Epilepsia* 1992;33:52–57.
825. Stores G. When does the EEG contribute to the management of febrile seizures? *Arch Dis Child* 1991;66:554–557.
826. Freeman JM. Less testing is needed in the emergency room after a first febrile seizure. *Pediatrics* 2003;111:194–196.
827. Offringa M, Bossuyt PM, Lubsen J, et al. Risk factors for seizure recurrence in children with febrile seizures: a pooled analysis of individual patient data from five studies. *J Pediatr* 1994;124:574–584.
828. Al-Eissa YA. Febrile seizures: rate and risk factors of recurrence. *J Child Neurol* 1995;10:315–319.
829. Camfield PR, Camfield CS, Gordon K, et al. Prevention of recurrent febrile seizures. *J Pediatr* 1995;126:929–930.
830. Wolf SM, Carr A, Davis DC, et al. The value of phenobarbital in the child who has had a single febrile seizure: a controlled prospective study. *Pediatrics* 1977;59:378–385.
831. Uhari M, Rantala H, Vainionpaa L, et al. Effect of acetaminophen and low intermittent doses of diazepam on prevention of recurrences of febrile seizures. *J Pediatr* 1995;126:991–995.
832. Rosman NP, Colton T, Labazzo J, et al. A controlled trial of diazepam administered during febrile illnesses to prevent recurrence of febrile seizures. *N Engl J Med* 1993;329:79–84.
833. Wolf SM, Forsythe A. Epilepsy and mental retardation following febrile seizures in childhood. *Acta Paediatr Scand* 1989;78:291–295.
834. Baumann RJ, Duffner PK. Treatment of children with simple febrile seizures: the AAP practice parameter. *Pediatr Neurol* 2000;23:11–17.
835. Nelson KB, Ellenberg JH. Predictors of epilepsy in children who have experienced febrile seizures. *N Engl J Med* 1976;295:1029–1033.
836. Tsuboi T, Endo S. Febrile convulsions followed by nonfebrile convulsions. A clinical, electroencephalographic and follow-up study. *Neuropädiatrie* 1977;8:209–223.
837. Nelson KB, Ellenberg JH. Prognosis in children with febrile seizures. *Pediatrics* 1978;61:720–727.
838. Annegers JF, Hauser WA, Shirts SB, et al. Factors prognostic of unprovoked seizures after febrile convulsions. *N Engl J Med* 1987;316:493–498.
839. Berg AT, Shinnar S. Unprovoked seizures in children with febrile seizures: short-term outcome. *Neurology* 1996;47:562–568.
840. Maytal J, Shinnar S. Febrile status epilepticus. *Pediatrics* 1990;86: 611–617.
841. Verity CM, Ross EM, Golding J. Outcome of childhood status epilepticus and lengthy febrile convulsions: findings of national cohort study. *Brit Med J* 1993;307:225–228.
842. Lennox WG. Significance of febrile convulsions. *Pediatrics* 1953; 11:341–357.
843. Cendes F, Andermann F, Dubeau F, et al. Early childhood prolonged febrile convulsions, atrophy and sclerosis of mesial structures, and temporal lobe epilepsy; an MRI volumetric study. *Neurology* 1993;43:1083–1087.
844. Trinka E, Unterrainer J, Haberlandt UE, et al. Childhood febrile convulsion—which factors determine the subsequent epilepsy syndrome? A retrospective study. *Epilepsy Res* 2002;50:283–292.
845. Tarkka R, Paakko E, Phytinen J, et al. Febrile seizures and mesial temporal lobe sclerosis: no association in a long-term follow-up study. *Neurology* 2003;60:215–218.
846. Kanemoto K, Kawasaki J, Yuasa S, et al. Increased frequency of interleukin-1 beta-511T allele in patients with temporal lobe epilepsy, hippocampal sclerosis, and prolonged febrile convulsion. *Epilepsia* 2003;44:796–799.
847. Fernández G, Effenberger O, Vinz B, et al. Hippocampal malformation as a cause of familial febrile convulsions and subsequent hippocampal sclerosis. 1998. *Neurology* 2001;57[11 Suppl 4]:S13–S21.
848. Bender RA, Dube C, Baram TZ. Febrile seizures and mechanisms of epileptogenesis: insights from an animal model. *Adv Exp Med Biol* 2004;548:213–225.
849. Ellenberg JH, Nelson KB. Febrile seizures and later intellectual performance. *Arch Neurol* 1978;35:17–21.
850. Verity CM, Butler NR, Golding J. Febrile convulsions in a national cohort followed up from birth. II. Medical history and intellectual ability at 5 years of age. *BMJ* 1985;290:1311–1315.
851. Verity CM, Greenwood R, Golding J. Long-term intellectual and behavioral outcomes of children with febrile convulsions. *N Engl J Med* 1998;338:1723–1728.
852. Wolf SM. Controversies in the treatment of febrile convulsions. *Neurology* 1979;29:287–290.
853. Baram TZ, Shinnar S. Do febrile seizures improve memory? *Neurology* 2001;57:7–8.

854. Lanska MJ, Lanska DJ, Baumann RJ, et al. A population-based study of neonatal seizures in Fayette County, Kentucky. *Neurology* 1995;45:724–732.
855. Ronen GM, Penney S, Andrews W. The epidemiology of clinical neonatal seizures in Newfoundland: a population-based study. *J Pediatr* 1999;143:71–75.
856. Mizrahi EM. Neonatal seizures: problems in diagnosis and classification. *Epilepsia* 1987;28[Suppl 1]:S46–S55.
857. Volpe JJ. *Neurology of the newborn*, 4th ed. Philadelphia: WB Saunders, 2001:178–214.
858. Scher MS, Aso K, Beggarly M, et al. Electrographic seizures in preterm and full-term neonates: clinical correlates, associated brain lesions, and risk for neurologic sequelae. *Pediatrics* 1993;91:128–134.
859. Herzlinger RA, Kandall SR, Vaughan HG. Neonatal seizures associated with narcotic withdrawal. *J Pediatr* 1977;91:638–641.
860. Mizrahi EM, Kellaway P. Characterization and classification of neonatal seizures. *Neurology* 1987;37:1837–1844.
861. Volpe JJ. Neonatal seizures: current concepts and revised classification. *Pediatrics* 1989;84:422–428.
862. Connell J, Oozeer R, de Vries L, et al. Continuous EEG monitoring of neonatal seizures: diagnostic and prognostic considerations. *Arch Dis Child* 1989;64:452–458.
863. Parker S, Zuckerman B, Bauchner H, et al. Jitteriness in full-term neonates: prevalence and correlates. *Pediatrics* 1990;85:17–23.
864. Scher MS. Neonatal seizures. In: Wyllie E, ed. *The treatment of epilepsy: principles and practice*, 2nd ed. Baltimore: Williams & Wilkins, 1996:600–621.
865. Mizrahi EM. Pediatric electroencephalographic video monitoring. *J Clin Neurophysiol* 1999;16:100–110.
866. Toet MC, van der Meij W, de Vries LS, et al. Comparison between simultaneously recorded amplitude integrated electroencephalogram (cerebral function monitor) and standard electroencephalogram in neonates. *Pediatrics* 2002;109:772–779.
867. Mizrahi EM, Hrachovy RA, Kellaway P. *Atlas of neonatal electroencephalography*, 3rd ed. Lippincott, Williams and Wilkins, Philadelphia, 2003.
868. Waldinger C, Berg RB. Signs of pyridoxine dependency manifest at birth in siblings. *Pediatrics* 1963;32:161–168.
869. Donn SM, Grasela TH, Goldstein CW. Safety of a higher loading dose of phenobarbital in the term newborn. *Pediatrics* 1985; 75:1061–1064.
870. Painter MJ, Pippenger C, MacDonald H, Pitlick W. Phenobarbital and diphenylhydantoin levels in neonates with seizures. *J Pediatr* 1978;92:315–319.
871. Lockman LA, Kriel R, Zaske D, et al. Phenobarbital dosage for control of neonatal seizures. *Neurology* 1979;29:1445–1449.
872. Painter MJ, Scher MS, Stein AD, et al. Phenobarbital compared with phenytoin for the treatment of neonatal seizures. *N Engl J Med* 1999;341:485–489.
873. Bourgeois BFD, Dodson WE. Phenytoin elimination in newborns. *Neurology* 1983;33:173–178.
874. Mizrahi EM, Kellaway P. Neonatal seizures. In: Pellock JM, Dodson WE, Bourgeois BFD, ed. *Pediatric epilepsy*, 2nd ed. New York: Demos, 2001:145–161.
875. Takeoka M, Krishnamoorthy KS, et al. Fosphenytoin in infants. *J Child Neurol* 1998;13:537–540.
876. Sankar R, Painter MJ. Neonatal seizures: after all these years we still love what doesn't work. *Neurology* 2005;64:776–777.
877. Bittigau P, Sifringer M, Genz K. et al. Antiepileptic drugs and apoptotic neurodegeneration in the developing brain. *Proc Natl Acad Sci USA* 2002;99:15089–15094.
878. Castro Coinde JR, Hernández Borges AA, Doménech Martínez E, et al. Midazolam in neonatal seizures with no response to phenobarbital. *Neurology* 2005;64:876–879.
879. Legido A, Clancy RR, Berman PH. Neurologic outcome after electroencephalographically proven neonatal seizures. *Pediatrics* 1991;88:583–596.
880. Bergman I, Painter MJ, Hirsch RP, et al. Outcome in neonates with convulsions treated in an intensive care unit. *Ann Neurol* 1983;14:642–647.
881. Dennis J. Neonatal convulsions: aetiology, late neonatal status and long-term outcome. *Dev Med Child Neurol* 1978;20:143–158.
882. Holden KR, Mellits ED, Freeman JM. Neonatal seizures. I. Correlation of prenatal and perinatal events with outcomes. *Pediatrics* 1982;70:165–176.
883. Clancy RR, Legido A. Postnatal epilepsy after EEG-confirmed neonatal seizures. *Epilepsia* 1991;32:69–76.
884. Rose AL, Lombroso CT. Neonatal seizure states: a study of clinical, pathological and electroencephalographic features in 137 full-term babies with long-term follow-up. *Pediatrics* 1970;45:404–425.
885. Painter MJ, Bergman I, Crumrine P. Neonatal seizures. *Pediatr Clin North Am* 1986;33:91–109.
886. Mellits ED, Holden KR, Freeman JM. Neonatal seizures. II. A multivariate analysis of factors associated with outcome. *Pediatrics* 1982;70:177–185.
887. Ohtahara S, Yamatogi Y. Severe encephalopathic epilepsy in early infancy. In: Pellock JM, Dodson WE, Bourgeois BFD, eds. *Pediatric epilepsy: diagnosis and treatment*, 2nd ed. New York: Demos, 2001:103–199.
888. Pryor DS, Don N, Macourt DC. Fifth day fits: a syndrome of neonatal convulsions. *Arch Dis Child* 1981;56:753–758.
889. Quattlebaum TG. Benign familial convulsions in the neonatal period and early infancy. *J Pediatr* 1979;95:257–259.
890. Alfonso I, Hahn JS, Papazian O, et al. Bilateral tonic-clonic epileptic seizures in non-benign familial neonatal convulsions. *Pediatr Neurol* 1997;16:249–251.

Chapter 15

Headaches and Nonepileptic Episodic Disorders

A. David Rothner and John H. Menkes

HEADACHES IN CHILDREN AND ADOLESCENTS

Headache is common problem affecting a significant number of children and adolescents. In one recent report, 59% of boys and 84% of girls between the ages of 13 and 18 reported having experienced a headache within the past month (1). Headaches may be a primary disorder, such as migraine, tension type, or cluster, or they may be secondary to a systemic illness or primary central nervous system disorder. The vast majority of headaches in children and adolescents are not due to serious underlying problems. When evaluating a youngster with headaches, both physical factors and emotional factors must be considered in order to arrive at the correct diagnosis and to initiate appropriate treatment.

The historical aspects of headache have been reviewed by several authors (2). Hippocrates described *migraine* more than 25 centuries ago, and Galen coined the term *hemicrania*. The modern era of headaches in children was initiated by Bille in 1962 (3). He reported on the incidence and nature of headaches in over 9,000 children. Shortly thereafter, three textbooks dealing with headaches in children appeared (4–6). The past five years have shown not only an increase in articles dealing with the epidemiology, diagnosis, evaluation, and treatment of various headache types, but also four additional textbooks and two significant practice parameters (7–10). The first practice parameter, published in 2002, dealt with the evaluation of children and adolescents with recurrent headaches (11). The second, published in 2004, dealt with the pharmacologic treatment of migraine headache in children and adolescents (12). Discussions of headache as a symptom of general pediatric disorders and specific neurologic disorders are presented elsewhere in this text.

Epidemiology

The modern era of the study of headaches in children and adolescents was initiated by Bille in 1962 (3). He reported data gathered from a population of 9,000 Scandinavian school children. He stated that by age 7, 1.4% of children had experienced episodic migraine, and 2.5% had frequent nonmigrainous headaches. An additional 35% had experienced infrequent headaches of other varieties. By age 15 years, 5.3% of children and adolescents had experienced migraine, 15.7% had experienced frequent nonmigrainous headaches, and 54% had infrequent nonmigrainous headaches. Further communications from Bille suggested that the frequent nonmigrainous headaches are tension-type headaches (13,14). In a study conducted in a prepaid health plan, 80% of all enrolled children were examined for headache during a six-year period. The incidence of new cases of migraine with aura was 6.6/1,000 in males, and the incidence of migraine without aura was 10/1,000 in males. In females, the incidence was 14/1,000 of migraine with aura and 18/1,000 of migraine without aura. The overall prevalence of headaches increases quite strikingly from preschool children through high school. Prevalence of headaches by age 7 ranges from 37% to 51%. From ages 7 to 15, the range increases from 57% to 82%. Recent studies have suggested that the prevalence of headaches in general and migraine in particular may be increasing compared with studies done 10 to 20 years ago. The epidemiology of headaches in children has been reviewed in detail by Lipton (15,16).

Classification

Various methods of classifying headaches both in adults and children have been published. Prior to 1988, the classification of headache was not uniform, and diagnostic criteria were not based on operational rules. In 1988, the International Headache Society (IHS) instituted a classification system for headache that has become the standard for headache diagnosis and clinical research (17). The second edition of this classification was published in 2004 (18). Numerous pediatric authors have reviewed the initial IHS classification and have suggested that it is not appropriate for use in children and adolescents. They have

TABLE 15.1 Proposed Revision to the Internal Headache Society Diagnostic Criteria for Pediatric Migraine Without Aura

A. At least five attacks fulfilling B through D.
B. Headache attack lasts 1 to 48 hours.
C. Headache has at least two of the following:
   a. Either bilateral or unilateral (frontal/temporal) location
   b. Pulsating quality
   c. Moderate to severe intensity
   d. Aggravation by routine physical activity
D. During headache, at least one of the following:
   a. Nausea and/or vomiting
   b. Photophobia and/or phonophobia

From Lewis DW, Diamond S, Scott D, et al. Prophylactic treatment of pediatric migraine. *Headache* 2004;44:230–237.

proposed several modifications (19,20). No papers have been published evaluating the second edition of the IHS criteria, as it is too recent. Unfortunately, that edition contains little regarding modifications of the criteria as they apply to children and adolescents.

Prior to and along with these IHS classifications, other clinical methods of classifying pediatric and adolescent headache have been proposed, the most prominent of these by Vahlquist (21) and Prensky and Sommer (22). Winner and Rothner proposed a clinical classification utilizing both the temporal pattern of a child's headache plotted against its severity over time (7). Five patterns were identified, including acute, acute recurrent, chronic progressive, chronic nonprogressive, and "mixed" or comorbid headaches. A proposed revision of the classification of pediatric headaches is shown in Table 15.1 (23).

An *acute headache* is a single event with no history of a previous similar event. It may be generalized or localized. It may be associated with neurologic symptoms and signs or seen in the absence of neurologic symptoms or signs. If an acute headache is noted in a critically ill child, a diagnosis needs to be made quickly, and intervention may be lifesaving. The differential diagnosis of acute headaches involves a wide variety of general medical as well as central nervous system etiologies (Table 15.2).

Acute recurrent headaches are periodic headaches that are separated by pain-free intervals. When an acute recurrent headache is associated with nausea, vomiting, photophobia, and phonophobia, the headaches are usually migrainous in nature.

Chronic progressive headaches are headaches that worsen in frequency and severity over time. The progression may occur rapidly or slowly. These headaches may be accompanied by symptoms and signs of increased intracranial pressure or progressive neurologic disease. The neurologic examination is frequently abnormal. An organic process is usually present, and further testing is usually indicated.

TABLE 15.2 Differential Diagnosis of Headaches

Acute generalized headaches
- Fever
- Systemic infection
- CNS infection
- Toxins (CO, amphetamines)
- Postictal
- Hypertension
- Shunt malfunction
- Hypoxia
- Hypoglycemia
- Post-lumbar puncture
- Trauma
- CNS hemorrhage
- Embolus
- Exertion
- Electrolyte imbalance

Focal acute headaches
- Trauma
- Sinusitis
- Otitis
- Pharyngitis
- Chiari malformation
- Glaucoma
- Other ocular disorders
- Temporomandibular joint disorder
- Dental disorders
- Occipital neuralgia

Acute recurrent headaches
- Migraine
- Hypertension
- Vasculitis
- Substance abuse
- Shunt malfunction
- Arteriovenous malformation
- MELAS
- Postictal
- Hypoglycemia
- Exertion
- Colloid cyst of third ventricle
- Dialysis

Chronic progressive headaches
- Hydrocephalus
- Subdural hematoma
- Neoplasm
- Abscess
- Dandy-Walker complex
- Chiari malformation
- Subdural empyema
- Pseudotumor cerebri

Chronic nonprogressive headaches have been referred to under a variety of names, including tension-type headaches, muscle contraction headaches, chronic daily headaches, and chronic nonprogressive headaches. Silberstein and Lipton have recently subdivided chronic daily headaches into chronic tension-type headaches,

TABLE 15.3 Silberstein and Lipton's Classification of Chronic Daily Headache

Chronic daily migraine (transformed migraine)
Chronic tension-type headache
New persistent daily headache
Hemicrania continua

From Silberstein SD, Lipton RB. Chronic daily headache. *Curr Opin Neurol* 2000;13:277–283.

hemicrania continua, transformed migraine, and new daily persistent headaches (Table 15.3) (24). Chronic tension-type headaches may occur several times a week, more than 15 days per month, or may be constant. They are usually not associated with symptoms of increased intracranial pressure or progressive neurologic disease. The neurologic examination is normal. Factors relating to school, stress, family dysfunction, and medication overuse are frequently noted. Excessive school absences are common.

Much dispute surrounds the entity of "the *mixed* headache syndrome" also known as *comorbid headaches*. Some feel that these are the transformed migraine or chronic migraine as described by other authors. In the latter two entities, the patients begin having episodic migraine, and a number of years later, depending on medication overuse as well as headache frequency, the headaches evolve into a daily vascular headache (24a). Chronic daily headaches are one of the most frequent types of headaches seen in the adolescent population as well as in adults seen at tertiary headaches centers. In our opinion, the condition consists of a combination of acute recurrent headaches, which are migrainous and superimposed on a pattern of chronic nonprogressive daily headaches. At times, it is difficult to differentiate between chronic daily headaches, comorbid headaches, transformed migraine, and chronic migraine. In all of these, however, symptoms of increased intracranial pressure and progressive neurologic disease are absent. The neurologic examination is normal. Laboratory testing is not diagnostic.

Over the years, clinicians have found that the added dimensions of severity and duration as well as the periodicity of the headache are useful in evaluating patients seen in a pediatric or pediatric neurology setting.

Pathophysiology of Headache

If indeed there are various distinct classes of headache, the pathophysiology of each type of headache must be discussed separately. Both extracranial and intracranial structures are sensitive to pain. The sensitive extracranial structures include the skin, subcutaneous tissues, muscles, mucous membranes, teeth, and some of the larger vessels. Pain-sensitive intracranial tissues include the vascular sinuses, larger veins, and dura surrounding these structures and arteries at the base of the brain. Pain from extracranial and intracranial structures in and about the face and from the front half of the skull is mediated via the fifth cranial nerve. Smaller areas are innervated by branches of seventh, ninth, and tenth cranial nerves. Pain from the posterior aspect of skull and upper neck are mediated via the upper cervical nerves. The brain itself and most of the dura, ependyma, and choroid plexus are insensitive to pain. Any process causing inflammation, displacement, irritation, traction, dilation, or physical invasion of any of these pain-sensitive structures will cause pain referred to either the face, top of the head, back of the head, or neck. The pain, at times, may have localizing value. The perception of this pain is certainly modified by the patient's age, previous experience with pain, and psychologic state, among other factors. The severity of the pain may not be an indication of the severity of the disease.

Pathophysiology of Migraine

There have been numerous advances in the understanding of the pathophysiology of migraine. The initial concept was that migraine was secondary to dysfunction of the central nervous system. In 1938, Graham and Wolff proposed the vascular theory of migraine (25). This theory of migraine pathophysiology held that an attack has two phases. The prodromal phase, marked by an aura, was believed to be characterized by vasospasm that induces cerebral ischemia and the various transient focal symptoms that initiate the attack. The second phase, characterized by extracranial vasodilatation, was thought to be responsible for the pulsating headache, which is generally felt in the distribution of the trigeminal nerve and the upper cervical roots (26). It now has been shown that the aura is rarely accompanied by ischemia and that the onset of headache occurs at a time when cortical blood flow is reduced and therefore not caused by vasodilatation (27). The vascular theory has been supplemented by a theory that combines the vascular theory and the neuronal theory and is generally referred to as the *trigemino-vascular theory*. The elements required to understand this concept include the anatomy of head pain, the physiology and pharmacology of the peripheral branches of the trigeminal nerve and the trigeminal cervical complex, the modification of these systems by brain stem and diencephalic structures, the further connections of these structures to thalamic and cortical areas, and the secondary vascular responses producing plasma protein extravasation.

The trigemino-vascular theory proposes that classical migraine (i.e., migraine preceded by an aura or other focal symptoms) is related to a paroxysmal depolarization of cortical neurons. During the initial phase of the attack, a cortical spreading depression is elicited at the occipital pole of the brain. The term *cortical spreading depression* is used to describe a depression of spontaneous EEG and other cortical electrical activities spreading across the cerebral cortical surface in the wake of a variety of noxious stimuli (28). The cortical spreading depression moves anteriorly in the course of the attack at a rate of approximately 2 mm per minute. At the wave front, transient ionic changes cause neurons and glia to depolarize with ensuing neuronal silence. Associated with these changes are dramatic alterations in the ion distribution between intracellular and extracellular departments. These changes are believed to trigger the migraine aura and to induce a 20% to 35% reduction in posterior cerebral cortical blood flow (29). The factors that induce the onset of cortical spreading depression are multiple and also are not well clarified. No doubt, they are both exogenous and endogenous. In part, they include any disturbance of K^+ homeostasis, genetic predisposition, stress, and dietary factors as well as the antidromic release of vasoactive peptides from the trigeminovascular system (30,31).

Cerebral ischemia is probably the result of arteriolar vasoconstriction and, in most instances, is not of primary importance in the induction of the migraine aura or of focal neurologic symptoms. Generally, oligemia in the posterior part of the brain is the most characteristic alteration of regional cerebral blood flow in attacks of classical migraine (32). Cerebral blood flow in the areas of the brain not affected by cortical spreading depression remains normal. Regional blood flow in the brainstem is increased, however, with maximal increase in the region corresponding to the dorsal raphe nucleus and the locus caeruleus (33). The course followed by the spreading oligemia is independent of vascular patterns and appears to be related to neuronal cytoarchitecture (30). As a rule, the cortical spreading depression stops at the central sulcus. Ventral propagation of the cortical spreading depression to the pain-sensitive meningeal trigeminal fibers that innervate the intracranial and dural blood vessels is believed to induce the headache. Stimulation of the trigeminal sensory neurons results in the release of a number of vasoactive substances. These include vasoactive intestinal peptide, substance P, and calcitonin gene-related peptides. These substances interact with blood vessel walls and induce vascular dilatation, plasma protein extravasation, and platelet activation and induce neurogenic inflammation (34). Neurogenic inflammation sensitizes nerve fibers to the point that they respond to previously innocuous stimuli such as blood vessel pulsations (35). Trigeminal sensitization is probably responsible for the cutaneous allodynia that patients frequently develop in the course of an attack of migraine and whose presence inhibits the effectiveness of triptans (36).

In migraine without an antecedent aura (common migraine), there are no consistent changes in cerebral blood flow (37), and the mechanisms other than cortical spreading depression that are responsible for this form of migraine are poorly understood. They could involve extracranial and intracranial arterial dilatation (38).

In addition to the vascular changes seen in classical migraine, there are a variety of abnormalities in the metabolism and concentrations of neurotransmitters, notably serotonin and its metabolites. At the onset of an attack, serotonin is released from platelets, and during an attack, there is a transient reduction in serotonin turnover (38,39). Between attacks, there appears to be an enhancement in serotonin turnover (40). This observation corresponds to the finding obtained by PET of an increased serotonin synthesis capacity in all brain regions in patients having migraine without aura (40). Of the various serotonin receptors, 5-HT1, 5-HT2, and 5-HT_3 are involved in the pathophysiology of migraine. The 5-HT1 receptors are inhibitory. The postsynaptic 5-HT1_B receptor is located on intracranial blood vessels, whereas the presynaptic receptor, 5-HT1_D, is located on the trigeminal nerve ending. Most of the drugs used for the acute treatment of migraine are 5-HT1_B/5-HT1_D agonists, whereas medications such as propanolol and methysergide are antagonists to the excitatory 5-HT2 receptors (41).

A number of substances can initiate an attack of migraine. These include prostaglandin E_1, tyramine, and phenylethylamine. Tyramine and phenylethylamine can be found in a variety of foods, notably cheese and chocolate, and are responsible for consistently initiating migraine attacks in a significant proportion of adults. In children, however, these amines are of lesser import (42). Considerable evidence suggests that the brain is not the only organ affected during an attack of migraine; alterations in renal functions, particularly polyuria and increased histidine excretion, have been demonstrated (34).

Pathophysiology of Tension–Type Headache

The term *tension-type headache* implies that the basis of the pain seen in this disorder is related to muscle. This is not really the case. Chronic tension-type headaches have many of the same features of migraine but lack the severe problem with nausea, sensitivity to light and sound, as well as movement. They also lack the usual triggering association such as menses, missing meals, or altering sleep patterns. Possible mechanisms include genetic aspects, muscle mechanisms, and central and/or peripheral sensitization (43,44). A few studies have suggested that there are genetic factors that play a role in chronic tension-type headaches (45). Stress also is identified as a trigger, but neither of these two triggers helps us to understand the basic pathophysiology better. Various experiments of injecting substances into muscle have reproduced pain, as has direct electrical stimulation of muscles. However, these types of pain do not seem to produce the same dull bifrontal headache that is seen in chronic tension-type headaches. Muscles that seem to be more sensitive to touch than normal controls have not been found to be different when studied neurophysiologically. Whether "anoxia" or nitric oxide generation plays a role in causing muscle pain remains to be proven. EMG data is controversial. Initial perceptions were that muscle contraction generates the pain seen in tension-type headaches. Although EMG activity tends to be higher in patients than in controls, there is no increased EMG activity during a headache, compared with EMG activity in the absence of a headache (46,47). Until the clinical definition is better clarified, the pathophysiology of chronic tension-type headaches will not be elucidated.

Neurophysiology of Cluster Headache

Cluster headaches are a clinically well-defined disorder. The clinical condition closely resembles other disorders, such as paroxysmal hemicrania or SUNCT (short-lasting unilateral neuralgiform headache with conjunctival injection and tearing). There are three major aspects to the pathophysiology of this disorder—the trigeminal distribution of the pain, the autonomic features associated with the pain, and the episodic pattern of the attacks (48). The majority of patients affected are males, and the neuroendocrine abnormalities of testosterone levels altered during cluster headaches have been known for over 30 years (49). Other interesting observations relating to cortisol, growth hormone, and prolactin also have been published (49). The hypothalamus as well has been implicated, since these headaches characteristically awaken patients at the same time each night. Imaging studies indicate increased activation of the anterior cingula and the contralateral frontal cortex, insula, and thalamus (50). The ipsilateral hypothalamic gray matter becomes activated during cluster headaches. Vascular changes seem to be secondary to the above. Additionally, there is some initial data suggesting that in a small percentage of cluster patients, genetics are implicated (48).

Genetics

The familial transmission of migraine has been known for centuries. Although in the past the condition was considered to be transmitted as an autosomal dominant disorder, current genetic data do not support this pattern. Almost all genetic studies have been confounded by the high prevalence of migraine in the general population, which facilitates a chance familial occurrence. In addition, inclusion of a family history of migraine as a diagnostic criterion, differences in migraine case definition, and variation in case ascertainment (referral to a clinic vs. a population survey) all have hindered valid genetic studies. However, over the last few years, several studies have shed light on the genetics of the disorder. Twin studies have supported a strong genetic component in the etiology of migraine, with a significantly higher concordance rate among monozygotic twins as compared with dizygotic twins (51–53). Subjects with classical migraine are more likely to have first-degree relatives with classical migraine than with common migraine, and vice versa. From data such as these, it has become evident that migraine with aura (classical migraine) and migraine without aura (common migraine) are genetically distinct entities (54). Although some authors have postulated an autosomal recessive model with reduced penetrance, it is more likely that both migraine entities have a multifactorial inheritance and that there is no evidence for any specific Mendelian transmission (55–57). In any case, the frequency of migraine indicates that in the future, multiple genes will almost certainly be implicated. Familial hemiplegic migraine has offered the most fruitful lines of genetic research. This condition is covered in another section of this chapter.

Clinical Manifestations

An excellent review of the clinical presentations can be found in the monograph by Winner and Rothner (7).

PATIENT EVALUATION

The key to a correct diagnosis is a properly obtained history and a thoroughly performed general physical and neurological examination. Because of the role of stress-related and psychologic factors, a private interview with the adolescent patient is helpful. General pediatric questions relating to pregnancy, labor, delivery, growth and development, past medical history, review of systems, and school and behavior are directed toward the parents with the patient making some contribution. However, when it comes to a good understanding of the headache itself, the questions should be directed at the patient with the parent not participating until the entire history has been obtained from the patient. Patients as young as 4 or 5 years of age may contribute significantly to a better understanding of their headache disorder.

Specific questions, as contained in the Headache Data Base, help clinicians to arrive at a specific headache diagnosis (Table 15.4) (7). Other questions that are related to the presence or absence of increased intracranial pressure, progressive neurologic disease, quality of life, and impact upon daily activities follow.

Important clues regarding potentially ominous headaches include the severity of the headache, a headache that occurs in the absence of previous headaches, changes in a chronic headache pattern, consistently localized pain, pain that awakens the patient at night, pain associated with straining, pain associated with neurologic symptoms or signs, and the patient declaring that "this is the worst pain I have ever had." The family history is quite important from both a genetic and environmental perspective. Migraine is recognized as a familial disorder. Both migraine and chronic nonprogressive headaches

TABLE 15.4 Headache Data Base

1. Do you have one or more types of headache?
2. When did your headache(s) start?
3. How did your headaches begin?
4. How often do your headaches occur?
5. Are your headaches occurring more often?
6. Are your headaches becoming more severe?
7. Does anything special bring them on?
8. Can you tell 15 to 30 minutes before that a headache is coming? How?
9. Where is your pain?
10. What does the pain feel like?
11. Do you have other symptoms when you get a headache?
12. What do you do when you get a headache?
13. What makes your headache worse? Better?
14. Do you take anything for your headache?
15. How long does your headache last?
16. Does anyone else in the family have headaches?
17. Do you have any other medical problems?
18. Are you taking any medications regularly?
19. Do you have any neurologic symptoms in between your headaches?
20. How many days of school have you missed because of your headache?
21. How often do you take medication to relieve your headache?
22. What do you think is causing your headaches?

From Rothner AD. Evaluation of headache. In Winner P, Rothner AD. *Headache in children and adolescents.* Hamilton, London: BC Decker, 2001;7:21–23.

often have a stress-related component, and the latter occurs more frequently in dysfunctional families.

The general physical examination may disclose abnormalities that are related to or causing the headache. The patient with primary headaches such as migraine or tension-type headaches has a normal examination. Specific areas of concern on the general examination include elevated temperature or blood pressure, the presence of café-au-lait spots or other diagnostic skin abnormalities, short stature, and tenderness over a specific localized area of the scalp or skull.

The neurologic examination should seek out signs of trauma, nuchal rigidity, head circumference, the presence of bruits, and abnormalities of eye movements and/or the fundus. The patient's strength, muscle bulk, tone, and reflexes should be carefully examined, and any asymmetry should be noted. If the neurologic examination is abnormal, an underlying primary or secondary neurologic disorder should be suspected. The patient's affect should be monitored throughout the examination and may be suggestive of a stress- or psychologically related problem. Once again, in the majority of patients with migraine or stress-related headaches, both the general physical and the neurologic examinations are normal.

A more in-depth discussion of the neurologic history and examination as it relates to children and adolescents with headaches can be found in the Introduction of this text.

After the initial history, physical examination, and neurologic examination are completed, a differential diagnosis should be considered. Combining the above with the clinical classification as outlined previously, the tentative diagnosis is made. If a patient has intermittent headaches with nausea and vomiting and no neurologic symptoms or signs, if these headaches are indeed intermittent and separated by pain-free intervals, and if there is a positive family history of migraine, the diagnosis of migraine should be suspected, and no further laboratory interventions are needed. On the other hand, if the patient has a relatively short history of a headache that is worsening quickly over time and is associated with neurologic symptoms and/or abnormalities on the neurologic examination, an organic disorder should be suspected. Further laboratory tests are generally indicated. When a patient tells you that the headache is severe and at the same time appears to be in no distress, has no symptoms of increased intracranial pressure or progressive neurologic disease, and has a normal neurologic examination, then stress-related chronic daily nonprogressive headaches should be suspected.

Laboratory tests should be ordered based upon the history, character and temporal pattern of the headache, physical and neurologic examinations, and differential diagnosis. The choice of which of the many laboratory tests should be ordered rests upon this differential diagnosis. Routine testing such as complete blood count, metabolic survey or SMA-17, sedimentation rate, thyroid function, and ANA profile are rarely of value. Routine urine analysis is not indicated. Guidelines regarding the ordering of specific imaging tests have been discussed in detail elsewhere (11).

On the other hand, if a patient is clinically ill, in the emergency room, or the history suggests the presence of an underlying systemic disease or a neurologic disease, further laboratory studies may be indicated. These may include the tests mentioned above or serum lead level, toxicology screen, neurologic testing for autoimmune disease, testing for metabolic disorders, coagulation studies, and titers for infectious diseases. Imaging studies also may be useful in such a situation.

The EEG is of limited value in the routine evaluation of headaches in children (58). Nonspecific abnormalities are frequently found in normal children as well as in children who are ill (59). Benign rolandic epileptiform discharges may be seen in as many as 9% of patients, even in the absence of seizures, and are most likely an epiphenomenon and not related to the patient's underlying disorder (60). EEG abnormalities do not constitute an indication for the use of antiepileptic drugs in such headache patients. If there are abnormal movements or alteration of consciousness, an EEG may be of value.

CT scanning is a useful diagnostic procedure, especially under emergent circumstances, and should be used to identify subarachnoid hemorrhage, ventricular enlargement, abscess, mass lesion, and hemorrhage secondary to trauma (61). If, however, the diagnosis of a central nervous system lesion is suspected and the situation is not urgent, magnetic resonance imaging (MRI) at times coupled with magnetic resonance angiography (MRA) and/or magnetic resonance venography (MRV) should be considered. It should be noted that as many as 40% of individuals imaged for headache may have nonspecific abnormalities, including abnormalities of the sinuses, nonspecific white matter abnormalities, arachnoid cysts, pineal cysts, venous angiomas, and Chiari malformations (62). Although these abnormalities are of interest, most often they are unrelated and not the cause of the patient's headache. Indications for, results of, and usefulness of such imaging studies in children and adolescents with headache have been studied extensively and reviewed elsewhere (11,63).

Lumbar puncture is useful when one suspects an infectious disorder or the diagnosis of pseudotumor cerebri. If possible, an imaging procedure should precede a lumbar puncture to make sure a mass lesion has been excluded.

Both psychologic evaluation and psychologic testing are useful in individuals with headache (64). If the patient has an associated learning disability, which is proving stressful to the patient and his or her family, a complete evaluation for learning disabilities may be indicated. If the patient has a chronic nonprogressive headache, comes from a dysfunctional home, and a psychologic or psychiatric disorder is suspected, a psychologic interview along with personality testing, anxiety testing, and evaluation for depression may be quite useful.

At the conclusion of the history and physical examination, a specific headache type and its presumptive etiology should be suspected.

Only after a diagnosis has been established can treatment be considered. This may include patient education, simple observation and maintenance of a headache diary, judicious avoidance of specific foods or triggers, and the occasional utilization of over-the-counter medication. A return visit 6 to 8 weeks after the initial visit is useful, since educated observation may clarify the etiology of the patient's headache.

SPECIFIC HEADACHE SYNDROMES

The general pediatrician sees both a combination of headache secondary to other conditions as well as primary headache syndromes. The most common forms of secondary headache seen in the primary care physician's office in children and adolescents include headache related to infectious disorders such as viral infections with fever, sinusitis, otitis, pharyngitis, and infectious mononucleosis. In addition, headaches due to mild head trauma and exertion are also often seen. The most common primary headaches seen in the general physician's office are migraine and stress-related headaches.

The pediatric neurologist sees headaches in the setting of primary neurologic disorders, primary headache disorders, and headaches secondary to underlying medical disorders such as collagen vascular disease, congenital heart disease, and hypertension.

Acute generalized headache is most often seen by the general pediatrician unless neurological symptoms and signs are present. The patient with acute generalized headache who has abnormal neurologic symptoms or signs is often referred to the emergency room or a pediatric neurologist. An isolated acute generalized headache in an otherwise well child is frequently associated with fever or infectious disease. If the headache is associated with an infection, simple analgesics at times combined with an antibiotic are usually sufficient to remediate the headache. In a viral illness, analgesics and antipyretics as well as time frequently results in resolution of the headache. Exertional headaches are common and are discussed later.

An acute localized headache should arouse concern about a localized pathologic process, such as sinusitis, otitis, ocular disorder, dental problems, or temporal mandibulor joint (TMJ) dysfunction, or minor head trauma. It should be noted that many patients have abnormal sinus imaging and that such imaging abnormalities may or may not be related to the patient's headache. Their relationship to one another is often not clear. The lay public feels that ocular abnormalities are frequently the cause of children's headaches. Although definitive studies are lacking, ophthalmologic examination is usually normal, and astigmatism and refractive errors are rarely the cause of headaches. Glaucoma, optic neuritis, and orbital cellulitis are rare.

Headache may be associated with mild head trauma, which can be one of the many triggers of migraine, and well-documented trauma can trigger the first attack of migraine in a susceptible individual (65,66). This disorder is discussed in Chapter 9. If a patient is seen with chronic daily headache and reports a history of mild or serious head trauma in the past, a re-evaluation is indicated. If the history is negative for symptoms of increased intracranial pressure or progressive neurologic disease, and the general physical and neurologic examinations are normal, the patient most often has chronic nonprogressive headaches. Frequently, in view of our litigious society, reimaging is indicated. Once no abnormality is demonstrated, overuse of over-the-counter medication, excessive school absenteeism, and psychologic issues should be addressed and remediated. Patients should be treated as if they have chronic nonprogressive headaches. The pain usually resolves over time.

Approximately 2% to 6% of all emergency room visits by children and adolescents are because of headache. Four studies of headaches seen in emergency rooms have been carried out (67,68). These indicate that the majority of pediatric and adolescent patients who come to the emergency room with headaches do not have serious underlying disorders. Disorders can be divided into those associated with infectious illnesses such as viral respiratory illnesses, otitis, or sinusitis. Another large group has primary headaches that have exacerbated and/or that have not been properly remediated until that evening and are either migraine or tension-type headaches. Only 2% to 16% of pediatric and adolescent patients who come to the emergency room have headaches secondary to primary or secondary neurologic disorders. These include aseptic meningitis/meningitis/encephalitis, shunt malfunction, hydrocephalus, brain tumors, and the like. Once again, the overwhelming majority of headaches in this situation are related to minor generalized illness or primary headaches. If the patient has elevated temperature or blood pressure, nuchal rigidity, papilledema, retinal hemorrhage, focal neurologic signs, altered affect or consciousness, rapid intervention, and evaluation is needed (68).

From their temporal patterns, one of us (A.D.R.) has distinguished four categories of headaches in older children: acute, paroxysmal and recurrent, chronic and progressive, and chronic and nonprogressive (7). He separates acute headaches into those in which the pain is generalized and those in which it is localized. Although the causes for acute generalized headache are multiple, ranging from the first attack of migraine to a subarachnoid hemorrhage, thorough physical and neurologic examinations and some basic laboratory studies provide a diagnosis in almost every instance. Acute localized headaches can be caused by head trauma; 12% of children seen by Chu and Shinnar had post-traumatic headaches (69). In the Winnipeg series, post-traumatic headaches accounted for only 3% of patients (19). Other causes include sinusitis, glaucoma, optic neuritis, and a variety of atypical facial pains, some of which are caused by temporomandibular joint dysfunction (70).

Acute Recurrent Headaches

The migraine syndrome is the classic example of an acute recurrent headache. Episodic migraine is characterized by episodic, periodic, paroxysmal attacks of throbbing headache, which may be unilateral or bilateral. The attacks are separated by pain-free intervals. They are often preceded by pallor and behavioral change and are often associated with decreased appetite, nausea, vomiting, phonophobia, and photophobia. They are frequently relieved by sleep.

Migraine is relatively common in children. A survey published in 1997 of 3- to 11-year-old children in a British general practice using a questionnaire and a structured interview disclosed that depending on the diagnostic criteria, 3.7% to 4.9% of children experienced migraine. Of these, 1.5% had migraine with aura (71).

Migraine begins surprisingly early in life. Initial complaints are paroxysmal and recurrent abdominal pain, restlessness, head banging, or sudden alterations in personality. A history of motion sickness or carsickness can be elicited in approximately two-thirds of patients (72). Because these symptoms are nonspecific, the diagnosis of migraine is generally not made until the child is old enough to relate the symptoms. Approximately one out of five patients has the first attack before age 5 years (73). Prior to puberty, boys are affected almost twice as often as girls (74).

As already noted, headaches are characteristically paroxysmal and are separated by symptom-free intervals. Commonly, particularly in teenagers, an attack begins in the early morning hours, often awakening the child. In younger children, the attacks tend to start in the afternoon. In the classic form of migraine, many attacks of headache are preceded by an aura. The most common symptoms in children involve nausea, vomiting, abdominal pain, and disturbances of vision. Some of the older children describe scintillating scotomata moving across one or both visual fields, and in adults, visual symptoms are the most common manifestation of the aura (75). Vision is blurred, and the child can have a transient hemianopsia or even complete blindness in one eye (amaurosis fugax). Both can terminate with the onset of contralateral headache or can last for several days unaccompanied by head pain (76). A family history of the disorder can be elicited in over one-half of the patients and was found in 72% in the data compiled by Prensky (74).

Other symptoms preceding the headache include numbness and tingling in one arm or over the entire side, hemiplegia, aphasia, or apraxia (77). In most instances, symptoms appearing during the preheadache phase are completely reversible, but in some children, function returns slowly, and an occasional case of persistent hemianopsia or hemiparesis has been reported (78,79). Some of the latter cases undoubtedly were subjects with familial hemiplegic migraine.

In younger children, migraine headache is bifrontal or poorly localized and is almost invariably accompanied by pallor, nausea, and vomiting (5). Occasionally, vomiting can be sufficiently intense and prolonged to induce acidosis and mimic cyclic vomiting. The relationship between migraine and cyclic vomiting is not clear. Some patients with cyclic vomiting have a strong family history of migraine, and a significant proportion develop migraine in adult life (80,81). An attack of migraine lasts anywhere from half an hour to several days.

In a small proportion of children, focal neurologic symptoms that are present during an attack persist beyond the headache phase. The term *complicated migraine* has been applied to forms of migraine that include those of the hemiplegic and basilar artery migraine. Ophthalmoplegic migraine is no longer considered a complicated form of migraine. The authors feel that any attack of migraine associated with even transient neurologic disturbances requires further thought and investigation. The neurologic syndromes associated with migraine are defined by their vascular territories. In the majority of patients, complete recovery is the rule. Certainly, any patient left with neurologic deficits requires further investigation if the initial investigation has not been carried out. Structural abnormalities may on occasion mimic migraine. It is best to think of a patient with migraine and neurologic features as having an underlying neurologic disorder until proven otherwise. A noninvasive evaluation that includes MRI should be utilized prior to the diagnosis of complicated migraine. Invasive angiographic studies are only uncommonly needed.

Basilar Artery Migraine

Basilar artery migraine was originally described by Bickerstaff (82). It is a recurrent dysfunction referable to the brain stem, cerebellum, and parieto-occipital and inferotemporal cortices. The condition manifests itself by vertigo, tinnitus, ataxia, dysarthria, and diplopia that can precede the onset of headache. The symptoms are quite variable and also may include blurred vision or tunnel vision, variable visual field cuts, paresthesias, dizziness, hemiparesis, obtundation, quadriparesis, loss of consciousness, and aphasia. The usual attacks, however, are not this severe. They may be associated with occipital headaches, nausea, and vomiting and may overlap with the symptoms seen in occipital epilepsy. The neurologic symptoms are usually of short duration. Although symptoms clear after an hour to several hours, residua after multiple attacks have been reported (83). The condition is most common in adolescent females, with the first attack occurring at any time from infancy to adolescence. In our experience, attacks tend to recur as frequently as once a month but are ultimately replaced by typical migraine.

The differential diagnosis is quite large and includes a variety of disorders such as seizures, demyelinating disease, vertebral artery dissection, or abnormalities of the bony structures of the occipital cervical junction. Individuals with this disorder should be studied further if the diagnosis is not clear.

Ophthalmoplegic Migraine

Ophthalmoplegic migraine has been reclassified in the 2004 IHS classification as a cranial neuralgia (84). The condition manifests itself by the association of orbital or frontal pain with a complete or incomplete third nerve palsy. The headache may precede, accompany, or follow the ophthalmoplegia. The third nerve dysfunction and, at times, fourth and sixth nerve dysfunction frequently outlast the headache. In the initial attacks, the paralysis lasts for only a few hours. With repeated bouts, it can persist for weeks or months or can even become permanent. The cause for the ophthalmoplegia is unknown (85).

Patients with this disorder require further evaluation, as the differential diagnosis includes aneurysm at the junction of the internal carotid and posterior communicating arteries, the Tolosa-Hunt syndrome, and a complication of diabetes mellitus (86). Preventive treatment has not been well studied, but acute treatment with steroids reduces both the pain and the duration of the ophthalmoplegia (87).

In the past, a disorder called *confusional migraine* has been included in the classification of complicated migraine (79,88). It is not a specific syndrome, but confusion can occur in migraine often in the setting of basilar artery migraine, hemiplegic migraine, and migraine with aura. In some instances, a period of confusion is triggered by a relatively minor head injury. This leads to an obvious but false diagnosis of an epidural or subdural hematoma (90). If a patient arrives at the emergency room with a past history of migraine and a current history of severe headache as well as confusion, agitation, or altered sensation, an evaluation for drug abuse and other causes of encephalopathy should be carried out. If it is migraine with confusion, the neurologic deficits usually clear within 4 to 6 hours. During the acute episode, the patient with confusion-related migraine has focal slowing on the electroencephalogram (EEG) and does not have MRI abnormalities. Confusional attacks tend to recur, but are eventually replaced by typical migraine (88).

Migraine Variants

Migraine variants imply episodic recurrent or transient neurologic dysfunction in patients who are known to have migraine, who have a family history of migraine, or who are destined to have migraine. In these syndromes, headache may not be prominent. The most common forms of migraine variants include benign paroxysmal vertigo of childhood, benign paroxysmal torticollis, abdominal migraine, and cyclic vomiting. The Alice In Wonderland syndrome is now considered an aura and not a migraine variant.

Benign paroxysmal vertigo is common, although incidence figures are not available. Typically, a child between the ages of 1 and 2 will develop a sudden, unsteady gait, and they will be confused and grab on to a nearby object or person for stability and/or fall to the ground. Consciousness is not lost. Nystagmus may be noticed. The patient may or may not have a headache and may or may not have vomiting. The spells are short, lasting only a few minutes, and the children will often sleep afterwards (91,92). Often, they return to their normal activities without an interval period of sleep. The spells seem to come in clusters and occur several times per day or per week, then disappear for weeks to months at a time (93).

Benign paroxysmal vertigo may occur in a milder form in older school-age children. The spells probably represent a form of basilar artery migraine. During follow-up studies, it has been demonstrated that benign paroxysmal vertigo often evolves into typical migraine. Evaluation should include an MRI scan to rule out posterior fossa abnormality if the spells are severe or persistent and recurrent. Vestibular dysfunction can be documented in a significant proportion of subjects (94). Since the spells are variable in frequency and severity, many patients will do fine without any sort of treatment. Other patients may respond to as-needed dosages of diphenhydramine.

Benign paroxysmal torticollis is a rare paroxysmal disorder characterized by attacks of head tilt in infants or head tilt accompanied by vomiting (95). The spells may last longer than those in benign paroxysmal vertigo from hours to days. The frequency is quite variable. Other dystonic features may coexist. The etiology of this disorder is felt to be similar to migraine (96). However, in some families, the condition has been linked to a CACNA1A mutation causing familial hemiplegic migraine (97). The differential diagnosis includes gastroesophageal reflux and torsion dystonia. Evaluation of the intracranial contents to rule out a posterior fossa or craniocervical junction abnormality should be considered. Once again, the frequency of this disorder is variable, and very little data are available regarding its treatment.

Abdominal migraine is a poorly understood and even more poorly characterized condition. It presents in childhood with repeated stereotyped bouts of unexplained abdominal pain, nausea and vomiting. The diagnosis can only be entertained after exhaustive gastrointestinal and metabolic evaluations have been unrevealing. The condition could be a variant of the cyclic vomiting syndrome (97a). *Cyclic vomiting* is considered at another point of this chapter.

Epilepsy and migraine have been discussed in relationship to one another extensively. They have many features in common, including the fact that both are familial and that there is an increased frequency of migraine in epilepsy patients and an increased incidence of epilepsy in migraine patients. Both are chronic disorders that are paroxysmal and episodic in nature. The clinical scenarios may be similar, including an aura, loss of consciousness, motor dysfunction, and an associated headache.

Both have been discussed as having both a neuronal and vascular pathogenesis and are secondary to neuronal hyperexcitability. Both have EEG abnormalities of different natures, and the etiology has been related to neurotransmitters and channel pathologies in both disorders. Both disorders respond to hormones, and both disorders may respond to antiepileptic drugs. Their pathophysiology and genetics have many things in common as well.

Andermann and Andermann have described eight migraine epilepsy syndromes, including epileptic seizures induced by classical migraine aura; epilepsy with seizures no longer triggered by migrainous aura; epilepsy due to gross cerebral lesions caused by migraine; benign occipital epilepsy of childhood as well as the spectrum of occipital epilepsies; benign rolandic epilepsy; malignant migraine related to mitochondrial myopathy, encephalopathy, lactic acidosis, and strokelike episodes (known better as MELAS); migraine attacks following complex partial seizures; and alternating hemiplegia of childhood (98).

Pediatric neurologists should be familiar with these connections, and when patients with epilepsy have frequent and severe postictal headaches, they should be treated appropriately.

Other types of headache syndromes, some not at all uncommon, are summarized in Table 15.5 (70,99–103).

Children with migraine often show a characteristic personality. They are meticulous, compulsive, and unusually mature for their age, striving to excel at school and to please the family at home. Additionally, they have considerable difficulty in expressing anger or rage (104).

Diagnosis

The differential diagnosis of headache in a child is a common task for the clinician. In the series of children younger than age 7 years evaluated for headaches, Chu and Shinnar found that 75% were experiencing migraine. Common

TABLE 15.5 Less Common Headache Syndromes in Children and Adolescents

Syndrome	*Symptoms*	*References*
Occipital neuralgia	Unilateral or bilateral pain in posterior part of head, infrequent to continuous.	Rothner (99)
Temporal manibular joint	Dull, aching unilateral pain below ear, frequently aggravated by chewing.	Belfer ML, Kaban LB. (70)
Exertional headaches	Headaches precipitated by coughing, sneezing, laughing, or sports. Pain is generalized and lasts from 15 minutes to 12 hours.	Symonds C. (100)
Hemicrania continua	Steady, severe headache over frontal area, unaccompanied by nausea. Good response to indomethacin.	Rothner (99)
Ice cream headache	Cold-indudced, severe but of short duration.	Raskin NH, Knittle SC. (101)
Ice pick headache	Single or repeated episodes of brief, sharp, jabbing pain over orbit, temple or parietal area.	Fuh et al. (102) Raskin NH, Schwartz RK. (103)

TABLE 15.6 Headache Classification

Primary migraine
With aura
Without aura
Periodic syndromes
Tension-type
Episodic
Chronic
Cluster
Secondary migraine
Trauma
Vascular
Intracranial disorders
Substance abuse
Infection
Homeostasis
Cranial structure
Neuralgia

Modified from IHS criteria, 2004 (18).

migraine was the most frequent form, and only 17% of children could relate the presence of an aura (69). In 72 patients from the Winnipeg pediatric neurologic outpatient service, which handled referrals up to 18 years of age, common migraine (migraine without aura) also was the most frequently seen form of headache and accounted for 61% of patients (19). Migraine with aura accounted for 15% of children, tension-type headaches for 3% of children, and mixed migraine and tension-type headaches were seen in 15%. There was only one patient with sinus headaches. In pediatric neurology headache clinics, tension-type headaches and mixed headaches are seen frequently.

The diagnosis of migraine rests on the periodicity of the paroxysmal headaches and, at times, their initiation by stress. The diagnostic criteria for migraine that have been established for adults by the International Headache Society have been modified for children. In a simplified form, they are summarized in Table 15.6. In the experience of Maytal and coworkers, the IHS criteria are satisfactory for the diagnosis of pediatric migraine with aura (classical migraine), but when applied to children suffering from migraine without aura (common migraine), these criteria have a high specificity but a poor sensitivity when the clinical diagnosis is used as a gold standard (19). A number of clinical diagnostic criteria have been delineated (105): An aura, generally visual, is seen in 10% to 50% of children (73); gastrointestinal symptoms, mainly nausea and vomiting but also anorexia and abdominal pain in 70% to 100%; a positive family history in 44% to 87%; unilateral headaches (less common in children than in adults) in 25% to 66%; and a history of motion sickness in 45% to 65%.

As mentioned previously, EEG abnormalities are not unusual in the child with migraine headaches. They were found in 27% of Holguin and Fenichel's series (73), in 20% of patients in the series of Chu and Shinnar (69), and in 23% of the series of Friedman and Pampiglione (106). In the experience of Kramer and colleagues, epileptiform EEG abnormalities were encountered in 11% in both migraine and tension-type headaches (107). In such instances, one must consider the possibility that the headache represents a true epileptic equivalent, an aura of a major motor seizure, or a postictal state of a clinically inapparent seizure (108). We have treated a few of these patients with anticonvulsants, notably carbamazepine or phenytoin, and, contrary to the observations of Friedman and Pampiglione, have occasionally found them to be beneficial (106). We should point out that the practice parameters of the American Academy of Neurology do not recommend an EEG in the routine evaluation of a child with recurrent headaches (11).

Even though the history of migraine headache might be convincing, the possibility of an underlying space-occupying lesion should not be forgotten. We have seen several children in whom the appearance of a malignant posterior fossa tumor aggravated long-standing migraine. Paroxysmal headaches also can be caused by intraventricular tumors, such as a colloid cyst of the third ventricle (see Chapter 11) (109).

The question as to whether neuroimaging should be part of the workup for a child presenting with recurrent headache has already been considered. In the series of Chu and Shinnar (69), some 30% of 104 children younger than the age of 7 years who presented with headache underwent imaging. In only one instance, a child with Chiari I malformation, did these studies uncover a previously unknown finding. In the series of Maytal and coworkers, neuroimaging studies disclosed cerebral abnormalities in 3% of pediatric headache patients. All abnormalities were deemed to be unrelated to the presenting complaint (110). In older children and adolescents, the incidence of abnormal findings in the face of a normal neurologic examination is even lower. It is, therefore, our policy to defer neuroimaging, unless there is excessive parental concern. McAbee and coworkers, who have studied the value of MRI in children with migraine, concur (111). The question of how to go about finding the rare youngster in whom headache is the first and only sign of an intracerebral tumor has been addressed by several groups, most recently by Straussberg and Amir, who recommend performing imaging studies on youngsters younger than 4 years of age in whom headache is accompanied by vomiting, even when the neurologic examination is normal (112). Battistella and colleagues found that headache was the first symptom in 27% of children with brain tumors and the only presenting symptom in 10%. The authors noted that headache associated with brain tumors had a high incidence of projectile vomiting, nocturnal or morning onset, and a lack of triggering factors. Also of note was that rest or sleep failed to relieve the pain and that nausea, photophobia, and phonophobia infrequently accompanied headaches associated with brain tumors (113). The practice parameters of the American Academy of Neurology do not recommend neuroimaging in children with recurrent headaches and a normal neurologic examination. They do recommend that such studies be considered in the child with the recent onset of severe headaches or when there is a change in the type or quality of the headache (11).

On rare occasion, attacks of migraine that are accompanied by temporary unilateral sensory symptoms, aphasia, or motor deficits are associated with a cerebrospinal fluid lymphocytic pleocytosis and an aseptic inflammation of the leptomeningeal vasculature (114).

Treatment

The treatment of migraine is symptomatic or prophylactic. It is based on the patient's age as well as the frequency of attacks and the severity and disability caused by the migraine. The presence of an aura, the location of the patient at the time of the attack, his or her age and reliability, and the family's attitude toward the use of medication also are important. Often, when the patient and his or her family are reassured that this is a migraine and there is no serious underlying disorder, the attacks seem to become fewer and less distressing. Patients are most interested in having a better understanding of what causes their attacks—being reassured that their attacks are not serious and will not result in prominent neurologic dysfunction—and, very importantly, finding relief from their symptoms (11).

Both nonpharmacologic methods and pharmacologic methods are useful in dealing with migraine. General nonpharmacologic methods include patient and parent education, the maintenance of a diary, and the elimination of trigger factors. A regular diet, sufficient sleep, and exercise also may be helpful. Stress reduction is important, if present. Additional nonpharmacologic methods may include counseling and biofeedback. Food allergies are commonly believed to trigger attacks. A double-blind study suggests that some foods, notably cow's milk, eggs, chocolate, oranges, wheat, benzoic acid, cheese, tomatoes, and rye, can provoke attacks and that their exclusion results in improvement in the majority of children (115).

A number of other activities and measures have been proposed to relieve migraine. These include yoga, karate, and biofeedback. Despite many examples of dramatic effectiveness, none of these techniques can be shown to work consistently. The effectiveness of any form of intervention in a disease that exhibits as much periodicity as does migraine can be evaluated only through long-term studies.

Pharmacologic Treatment

Rare patients require no pharmacologic intervention if the attacks are short, not severe, and quickly relieved by vomiting or sleep. However, if nausea, vomiting and pain are severe and/or prolonged, symptomatic medications such as analgesics, antiemetics, and sedatives play an important role. Acetaminophen and the nonsteroidal anti-inflammatory drugs (NSAID) have been well studied in children and adolescents. In most studies, NSAIDs seem to be more successful than acetaminophen in relieving pain. In the experience of Hämäläinen and coworkers, acetaminophen (15 mg/kg) is effective for moderate to severe attacks (116). Other medications used for severe attacks include naproxen (Aleve) and ibuprofen (Motrin, Advil). Butalbital (Fiorinal), phenacetin, or caffeine singly or in combination are less often recommended (5,117).

A suggestion has been made that liquid medication is absorbed quicker since there is gastroparesis during a migraine attack. This phenomenon has not been well studied. Some patients respond to one versus the other in a better fashion, and it is not known why. These medications have different pharmacologic bases of activity and can be used simultaneously or successively.

When pain is severe, these medications can be combined with abortive medications such as triptans. The authors, in milder cases, begin with rest, followed by an antiemetic; 5 to 10 minutes later, a sedative such as diphenhydramine and an analgesic such as an NSAID is given. Two hours later, if the patient is not better, the sedative is repeated, and a different analgesic such as acetaminophen is used. If this fails on two successful attacks, triptans are introduced.

Nausea and vomiting are a frequent part of an attack of migraine and are more common in the younger patient. Both nausea and vomiting often impede the ability of the youngsters to accept oral medications; therefore, many individuals are treated with antiemetics initially followed 15 to 30 minutes later by analgesics. The most commonly used antiemetics include suppositories, such as Tigan, and oral antiemetics. More recently, the use of oral medications seen in chemotherapy such as ondansteron, which melts under the tongue, have been useful, although these have not been specifically studied in the treatment of pediatric or adolescent migraine.

It has long been noted by parents that once a patient sleeps, the headache is often relieved. We find the addition of a sedative to be quite useful in the treatment of an acute attack. The sedative may range from a simple antihistamine such as diphenhydramine to a medicine used in the prophylaxis of migraine, cyproheptadine, to a benzodiazepine. After several attacks, the patient and his or her parents may determine which of the above modalities—an analgesic, an antiemetic, and/or sedative—is most useful.

In some patients, all three are used; in others, one or two are utilized (118).

In the past, patients with infrequent episodes were treated with ergotamines. Currently, this is not commonly utilized in pediatric and adolescent practice. There is a form of dihydroxyergotamine that can be given nasally in the form of Migranal. This medication has been utilized in adolescents with success, especially if they are unresponsive to triptans (119). If patients require acute treatment and the usual symptomatic and/or abortive medications including triptans are not useful, Migranal should be considered and is generally well tolerated, although not approved by the Food and Drug Administration (FDA) for the pediatric population. The previous use of a combination medication, Midrin, which contains isometheptane mucate, dichloralphenazone, and acetaminophen, is no longer used frequently and has in many patients been replaced by the use of triptans. However, it seems to be useful for some patients.

The introduction of triptans for the treatment of migraine represented a significant step in their remediation. Unfortunately, these medications have not been approved as of yet for use in youngsters 17 years or younger in the United States even though they are approved in other countries. Despite their nonapproval, numerous trials have demonstrated both their effectiveness and their safety, and they are often used by experienced clinicians. The recently published practice parameter, however, has concluded that for acute treatment of migraine in children and adolescents, ibuprofen is effective, and acetaminophen is probably effective. For adolescents, sumatriptan nasal spray is effective and should be considered. There were conflicting or insufficient data to warrant recommending any other medication for the acute treatment of migraine (11). For preventive treatment, flunarizine was found to be probably effective. This corroborates the results from studies conducted in Europe (120,121). Data for the other prophylactic medications listed in Table 15.7 were either insufficient, conflicting, or did not show efficacy.

Nevertheless, there is now extensive data available regarding the safety of the various triptans. There are five short-acting triptans and two longer-acting triptans. Head-to-head trials have not been carried out, so it is impossible to recommend one over the other. The lowest dose of triptan that can be used in young children is the 5 mg sumatriptan nasal spray. In addition, the 2.5 mg zolmitriptan tablet can be split. Utilizing the short-acting triptans in addition to the symptomatic medications mentioned above is often useful. If the patient is no better in two hours and there have been no adverse effects, these triptans can be repeated (122). Utilization of the longer-acting triptans Amerge and Frova has not been extensively studied in the pediatric and adolescent population. Administration of triptans must be timely; once the migraine attack has proceeded to the point where cutaneous allodynia has developed, the effectiveness of triptans drops dramatically (123). In the series of Burstein and coworkers, triptans were effective in only 15% of migraine attacks that were accompanied by cutaneous allodynia, in contrast to 93% of subjects who had not developed allodynia when the triptan was taken (123). The effectiveness of the various triptans in pediatric migraine has been reviewed by Major and coworkers (124).

TABLE 15.7 Medications Used for Preventive Therapy of Migraine

Agent Class	Dosage Range
Antihistamine	
Cyproheptadine (Periactin)	2 mg bid or 4 mg hs
Beta-blockers	
Propanolol (Inderal)	1 mg/kg, up to 10 mg bid
Atenonol	0.8–2.0 mg/kg per day
Tricyclic antidepressants	
Amitriptyline (Elavil)	0.25–0.5 mg/kg, up to 10 mg hs
Nortriptyline (Pamelor)	0.25–0.5 mg/kg, up to 10 mg hs
Anticonvulsants	
Divalproex sodium (Depakote)	10 mg/kg, up to 125 mg per day
Topiramate (Topamax)	50 mg to 100 mg per day
Levitiracetam (Keppra)	1000 mg per day
Calcium-channel blockers	
Verapamil	4.0–7.0 mg/kg per day
Nifedipine	0.5–1.0 mg/kg per day
Flunarizine	5 mg per day

Please review dosages, indications, contraindications, and side effects carefully before using. Many of these medications are not FDA approved for these indications and/or in these age groups.

Prophylactic medication should be considered when children or adolescents have either frequent migraine that is unresponsive to acute measures or migraine that is occurring so frequently that it results in days lost from school and other activities. In addition, it should be considered if the patient has a comorbid headache disorder and is utilizing over-the-counter medication in an inappropriate fashion. Prophylactic medications that have been utilized include NSAIDs, antihistamines, beta-blockers, calcium-channel blockers, and antiepileptic medications. Once again, these medications have not yet been approved by the FDA. The most commonly used prophylactic medications are listed in Table 15.7.

Propranolol has been advocated as a preventive for childhood migraine. In children who weigh less than 35 kg, the maximum dosage is 20 mg three times daily; in those weighing more than 35 kg, it is 40 mg three times daily. Although this drug is a fairly good prophylactic, many children complain of difficulty in falling asleep (125). This drug should be used with considerable caution in asthmatic children and in childhood diabetes.

Divalproex (Depakote) also has been used as a migraine preventive in children and adults (126,127). It is given in dosages of 10 to 20 mg/kg per day. In a single-blind, placebo-controlled study performed on adults, it was as effective as propranolol in the prophylaxis of migraine without aura (128). A second medication that we find useful, especially in adolescents who may be overweight, is topiramate. The dosages used in the treatment of migraine seem to be lower than those used in the treatment of epilepsy (129). At these low dosages, side effects are less than those reported in epilepsy (130,131). An associated beneficial side effect is that of weight loss, which is useful in adult patients. This medication also is not FDA approved for use in the treatment of pediatric migraine.

Methysergide (Sansert), a 5-HT2 antagonist, is rarely used in children or adults because of its propensity to induce thrombophlebitis and pleuroperitoneual fibrosis (132). The use of tricyclics or monoamine oxidase inhibitors such as phenelzine (Nardil) has not been fully explored in a pediatric population. One of us (A.D.R) finds amitriptyline, a tricyclic antidepressant agent, to be the drug of choice for the prophylactic treatment of migraine. It is utilized only at night. Many physicians, because of its potential effect on the heart rhythm, prefer to do an EKG prior to initiating medication. A.D.R begins the medication at a low dose (5 mg) and at two weekly intervals slowly increases the medication to 20 to 30 mg nightly. The most common bothersome side effects include sedation and increased appetite.

Flunarizine, a calcium-channel blocker, available in Europe and Canada but not in the United States, given in doses of 5 mg per day, also has been used with some effect as a preventive in children with common and classical migraine (133,134). No data on the effectiveness of other calcium-channel blockers in children are available, and the rationale for their effectiveness is still speculative (135).

One of us (A.D.R) prefers to use antihistamines exclusively at night in younger children, especially if they are thin. Cyproheptadine should not be used in younger patients who are overweight.

The use of calcitonin gene-related peptide (CGRP) receptor antagonists in the treatment of migraine is still in its experimental stages (136), as is the use of angiotensin II receptor blocker (137). The use of Botox as a preventive for adult migraine has had increasing application. As yet, there are no good controlled studies to determine its effectiveness in children. The various migraine preventives have been reviewed by Lewis and coworkers (11).

Prognosis

The outlook for the patient with migraine headaches is excellent, and in most instances, the condition does not interfere with schoolwork. In approximately two-thirds of children, attacks persist throughout life, although many patients are intermittently free from them for long periods or their headaches are at least partly relieved by medication or a less stressful family and school environment (42,138).

Status Migrainosus

Status migrainosus is a migraine attack lasting longer than 72 hours. We begin to think about this diagnosis if a migraine attack has disabled the patient for longer than 24 hours. It most commonly occurs in patients with preexisting migraine and only rarely is the first manifestation of migraine (139). Careful attention must be paid to differentiating between a true attack of status migrainosis from patients with chronic daily headache and severe prolonged exacerbation of that chronic daily headache. In true status migrainosus, the patients have failed to respond to their usual acute medication and/or prophylactic medication. Most require parenteral medications as well as intravenous fluids. In our practice, an infusion suite is available on a daily basis for such patients. Patients are sedated, given intravenous fluids and antiemetics. They are then given a variety of medication, administered intravenously, in an attempt to abort their attacks. These include magnesium, valproic acid, sedatives, and dihydroxyergotamine. Management of this disorder in adolescents and children is different from that in adults, and very little data is available.

Chronic Progressive Headache

The presence of a chronic and progressive headache implies a disorder that is worsening over time. Frequently, there are abnormal neurologic symptoms or symptoms of increased intracranial pressure. In addition, the patient frequently has abnormalities of the neurologic examination. Prominent in this group of disorders are hydrocephalus, brain tumors, pseudotumor cerebri, brain abscess, and chronic subdural hematoma. These conditions are considered in various other chapters of this text.

Chronic Nonprogressive Headache

The term *chronic nonprogressive headache* denotes a headache that has been present for longer than six weeks to three months. It occurs almost daily or daily and usually presents in the absence of an overt etiology. Symptoms of increased intracranial pressure and progressive neurologic disease are absent. Silberstein and Lipton have divided this disorder into chronic tensiontype headaches, hemicrania continua, new-onset daily persistent headaches, and transformed or chronic migraine (24) (Table 15.3). These disorders seem to be less common in children under the ages of 10 and become more frequent in adolescents. In all of these disorders, females are more frequently affected. The frequent nonmigrainous headaches originally described by Bille are muscle contraction headaches and are probably related to stress (13,14).

Chronic tension-type headaches or chronic muscle contraction headaches have been studied in adolescents. Symptoms are similar to those seen in adults. There is no aura. The pain seems to be less severe than with migraine. It is bitemporal or bifrontal and is rarely associated with nausea or vomiting (140). Headaches occur greater than 15 times per month. Many of these patients will have excessive school absences or have overused over-the-counter medications and/or prescription analgesics (24a). Many have stress-related problems or come from dysfunctional families. The patients describe the headache in a nonspecific manner and may have mild associated symptoms such as blurred vision, fatigue, and dizziness. Previous behavioral difficulties are not uncommon. Laboratory tests, if done, are noncontributory. MRI shows no abnormality. An interview with a psychologist is frequently helpful. Both the parents and the patient should be interviewed separately as well as together. Additional testing for anxiety, learning disabilities, and the like is sometimes indicated.

Moderate depression may be a concomitant of chronic nonprogressive headaches. Manifestations of depression in adolescents include withdrawal, poor school performance, sleep disturbance, a change in behavior, somatic complaints, lack of energy, mood changes, weight loss, and school phobia.

If a patient has had minor head trauma and presents with headaches of this nature that have been present for several months, a repeat MRI should be done, then the patient should be evaluated and treated as if he or she has a chronic tension-type headache.

If the headache has been present for more than 8 to 12 weeks in the absence of neurologic symptoms and signs and the physical and neurologic examinations are normal, the headache is usually not found to be secondary to a structural abnormality. This is especially true if coupled with over-the-counter medication and excessive school absences. This diagnosis should then be discussed openly with the patient and parents. Investigations should be minimal, and evaluation by a counselor should be scheduled. Treatments include discontinuation of over-the-counter medications, return to school, counseling, and one of us (A.D.R.) has found low-dose amitriptyline to be useful. Little definitive data is available regarding the outcome of these children. In the experience of Moore and Shevell, about one-half of children experienced complete resolution of their headaches within two to 48 months (24a).

Hemicrania continua is a headache disorder that is indeed rare in adolescents. It is a strictly unilateral continuous headache with multiple daily painful exacerbations accompanied by autonomic features lasting approximately 30 minutes. The exacerbations occur anywhere from 2 to 3 times per day to 2 to 3 times per week, and on rare occasion, they can occur up to 30 times per day. This type of headache is associated with unilateral autonomic features, including tearing, nasal stuffiness, ptosis, conjunctival injection, and rhinorrhea as well as migrainous symptoms such as nausea, photophobia, phonophobia, or stabs and jabs (141). The autonomic and migrainous features are absent during the continuous baseline headache. Nocturnal exacerbations are common. The mean age of onset in adults is 28 years, but several cases have been reported in adolescents. Indomethacin is the drug treatment of choice, and it has been proven to provide complete relief of symptoms in most cases of hemicrania continua within 72 hours. The usual dosage is in the vicinity of 100 to 225 mg given in two to three divided doses. Patients using indomethacin must be monitored on a regular basis, as side effects may occur. Hemicrania continua must be differentiated from other unilateral headache disorders such as cluster and SUNCT (short-lasting unilateral neuralgiform headache with conjunctival injection and tearing) (142). The prognosis of this disorder is not well known.

Chronic migraine/transformed migraine indicates a disorder in which the headache syndrome begins as episodic migraine. Over time, and often complicated by excessive over-the-counter medications and frequent intake of caffeine-containing beverages, the patient's headaches become less severe but more frequent until they merge into a daily headache syndrome. This disorder can at times be difficult to differentiate from chronic tension-type headaches, but many adult headache authorities feel that most chronic headaches seen in their practices have evolved from intermittent migraine into transformed or chronic migraine (24a,143). This is a primary headache disorder in which no underlying etiology can be found. Treatment is difficult but requires discontinuation of excessive over-the-counter and prescription medications as well as and withdrawal of caffeine-containing beverages (144,145). This type of headache disorder is one of the most frequent headache disorders seen in most large referral headache clinics. It is significant that many of these patients have comorbidities such as low back pain, stomachaches, and frequent sore throats and that they are experiencing a high level of psychosocial difficulties (146).

Miscellaneous Headache Syndromes

There are several headache syndromes that do not fit into the usual classifications and are less commonly encountered in the pediatric population than the syndromes already mentioned. The majority of these conditions are not associated with structural brain disease. Proper identification may lead to specific treatment, resulting in dramatic relief of symptoms.

Cluster Headaches

Two forms of cluster headaches can occur: episodic and chronic. The episodic form is defined by frequent headaches lasting for periods from one to three months, followed by periods of remission lasting from months to years. Episodic cluster affects 80% of cluster headache patients. In 20%, however, chronic cluster headache occurs. Chronic cluster headaches are defined as headaches that occur for more than 1 year without remission or with remissions that last less than 2 weeks. These types of headaches are difficult to treat, and generally do not respond to preventive medications.

Cluster headaches primarily affect males, although it is increasingly being recognized in females. The mean onset is in the third decade of life, although adolescents have been described by Maytal (147). In Sweden, 1% of 18-year-old men are diagnosed with cluster headaches. The typical attack occurs 2 to 10 times daily and lasts 10 minutes to 3 hours. The average length is 45 minutes. Many occur at the same time during sleep, waking the patient during the first phase of rapid eye movement sleep. The intensity is severe. The pain is unilateral and rarely, if ever, changes sides. It is localized in or about the eye and is associated with ipsilateral lacrimation, rhinorrhea, and nasal stuffiness. Ptosis and miosis also may occur. Patients frequently get up and walk around, as they are unable to lie down and rest. The attacks can be provoked by alcohol. The genetic implications are less important than in migraine. The acute treatment includes oxygen, triptans, and/or cafergot. Prophylactic medications have included methysergide, verapamil, lithium, and prednisone.

Indomethacin-Sensitive Headache

There are four types of headache syndromes that are infrequently seen in pediatric practice and are specifically responsive to indomethacin. They are usually severe and unilateral. On close questioning, they are different from migraine and muscle contraction headaches.

Chronic paroxysmal hemicrania is characterized by multiple daily attacks that last from 5 to 30 minutes. They are persistently unilateral. The pain is described as severe, and other symptoms are usually lacking. It is usually localized to an eye or forehead above the eye and may be precipitated by head movement. It is more common in females. It is less frequent in children and adolescents. The neurologic examination between attacks is normal. During the attacks, the children are uncomfortable, and the pathogenesis of this disorder is unknown (148). Response to indomethacin usually occurs within 72 hours.

Exertional headaches are not uncommon in adolescents and are precipitated by exertion, including coughing, running, swimming, and sexual activity (149). In athletes, these headaches may interfere with training and performance. They can occur during the initiation of an activity, during the middle of an activity, or after an activity is completed. The headaches may be migrainous in nature, associated with nausea and vomiting, and may be so severe as to suggest a life-threatening disorder. The headache may be brief and generalized or localized or may last hours. Although the majority of these headaches are benign, patients must be evaluated to rule out a structural abnormality, especially the Chiari malformations (150). Exertional headaches also may be seen in patients residing in high altitudes as well as in migraine patients.

Once a structural abnormality has been ruled out treatment should be conservative. In many patients, the headache disappears spontaneously. Beta-blockers cannot be used in athletes, as they decrease athletic performance. NSAIDs prior to an activity or indomethacin should be attempted if the patient's headache does not respond to simpler means.

Cyclic migraine is a form of migraine that comes in cycles (151). It has not been well reported in the pediatric and adolescent population and is rare even in adults. It also has been called *cluster migraine*, but it is not a form of cluster headache. The headache cycle averages anywhere from 2 to 10 to 12 weeks, with an average of 6 weeks. During the cycle, the migraine headache occurs daily or several times per week. At times when the migraine is not present, there may be a low-intensity, constant headache. The majority of cycles are followed by headache-free intervals lasting for months. The majority of patients are female. The headache may begin in the first or second decade, and there may be a strong family history of migraine. Once again, a structural abnormality is not usually present. The treatment of cyclic migraine has included both indomethacin and lithium carbonate. The pathogenesis of this disorder is unknown.

Hemicrania continua is marked by a steady, nonparoxysmal, severe hemicrania localized to the frontal part of the head and not associated with nausea or autonomic symptoms (152). The majority of affected subjects are female, and the condition can commence during adolescence (153).

Familial Hemiplegic Migraine

In some families, transient attacks of hemiplegia followed by contralateral headache are transmitted as an autosomal dominant trait (154,155). Attacks generally start with numbness of the hand, accompanied by a homonymous hemianopsia, and spreading to involve the face, tongue, and the remainder of the body. Aphasia and weakness are common. Migrainelike headache can precede or follow the neurologic symptoms. Full neurologic recovery can take 24 hours or longer. In a large proportion of patients, attacks are triggered by relatively minor head injuries (155). In approximately 20% of patients, familial hemiplegic migraine is accompanied by progressive cerebellar ataxia (156).

The elucidation of the molecular genetics of this condition represents one of the major recent advances in the understanding of the pathophysiology of migraine. Familial hemiplegic migraine is a heterogenic condition, and to date, two genes have been implicated (157,158,158a). In approximately one-half of the families with familial hemiplegic migraine, the condition has been mapped to chromosome 19p13 and codes for a brain-specific P/Q type calcium-channel alpha$_1$-subunit gene (CACNL1A4)

(FHM1) (158,159). This condition is allelic with episodic ataxia type 2, and all cases of familial hemiplegic migraine with progressive ataxia map to this site (see Chapter 3). A number of mutations in the gene have been documented; a considerable proportion of mutation carriers are asymptomatic (160). A second locus has been mapped to the long arm of chromosome 1q23 (FHM2), and the affected gene encodes a P-type Na^+, K^+-ATPase. This ATPase exchanges three intracellular sodium ions for two extracellular potassium ions and may be essential for maintaining sodium ion gradients that facilitate the export of intracellular calcium (161). In some families, both loci have been excluded, an observation that underlines the heterogeneity of the condition (162).

Cyclic Vomiting

Although in most instances cyclic vomiting is not a paroxysmal disorder, it is considered here because of its relationship to migraine. Gee characterized the condition as producing fits of vomiting that recur after intervals of uncertain lengths and continue for a few hours or several days (163). Cyclic vomiting is neither uncommon nor benign. Its incidence can be as high as 10% of unselected schoolchildren, with peak occurrence between ages 6 and 11 years (80).

As delineated in a 1999 consensus conference, attacks are stereotypic (164). They start as early as 1 year of age; in 82%, the first attack occurs before age 6 years (165). Aside from vomiting, symptoms include headache (seen in 36% of children in the series of Hoyt and Stickler) (165), fever (43%), and abdominal pain (18%). Hypertension also can be present. Curiously, there appears to be a high incidence of prematurely gray hair in affected children and their mothers (81). The EEG is more likely to be abnormal than in the general population, but there is no evidence that the condition represents a seizure equivalent or that it responds to anticonvulsants (166). Recent work suggests that there is a significant mitochondrial component in the pathogenesis of this condition and that sequence variation in the mitochondrial control region could constitute a risk for the development of the disease (167).

In 64% of children, attacks last 4 days or less; in 11%, they last longer than 1 week (165). A variety of medications have been suggested, but none is convincingly effective. Thus, treatment is directed toward maintaining fluid and electrolyte balance. Because a variety of emotional stresses are believed to trigger attacks, psychotherapy is considered an important therapeutic adjunct (168).

Important in understanding the nature of the condition is the widespread observation that children with cyclic vomiting become adults with migraine and have a positive family history of migraine (80,81,169). In the series of Hammond, 75% of adults who experienced cyclic vomiting during childhood suffered from migraine. Approximately two-thirds still have recurrent bouts of vomiting (80). A high percentage of children in this group respond favorably to antimigraine therapy, notably sumatriptan (170). Anticonvulsants, inderal, and carnitine also have been suggested.

Cyclic vomiting must be distinguished from several other entities. Most commonly, recurrent vomiting occurs in severely retarded youngsters. In many instances, this vomiting is the consequence of gastroesophageal reflux (171). Symptoms can respond to small feedings and antacid therapy. The effectiveness of postprandial upright positioning is a matter of dispute. In some instances, even fundal plication is ineffective. Other neurologic conditions inducing recurrent vomiting include dysautonomia, the various disorders of urea cycle, and organic acid metabolism, notably dicarboxylic aciduria (see Chapter 1), mitochondrial DNA mutations, and abdominal epilepsy (172,173). Additionally, functional disorders are common in children older than 5 years of age. Less often, one encounters the irritable bowel syndrome, lactose intolerance, inflammatory bowel disease, and *Giardia* infections. In infants, intussusception, constipation, and urinary tract infections must be excluded.

SYNCOPE

Syncope or fainting is characterized by transient loss of consciousness resulting from inadequate cerebral perfusion and from anoxia. Four major causes can be distinguished: (a) vasovagal, (b) reflex, (c) decreased venous return, and (d) cardiac.

In the first three entities, syncope results from a sudden decrease in systolic and diastolic blood pressure in a child who is upright. In vasovagal syncope, which accounts for approximately 75% of instances, the attack is triggered by pain or some obvious emotional upset. In reflex syncope, the event is precipitated by hyperventilation, violent coughing, hot baths, defecation, or micturition (174). Syncope resulting from Valsalva maneuver is probably the consequence of reduced venous return. Adolescents subject to postural hypotension can faint when maintaining an upright posture for long periods.

Loss of consciousness during vasovagal syncope is probably caused by cerebral hypoperfusion, which is due to an impairment of cerebral vascular autoregulation . This results in a failure to maintain adequate cerebral blood flow and occurs when a drop in systemic blood pressure is induced by a transient decompensation of the autonomic nervous system. Transcranial Doppler studies show a sudden increase in cerebrovascular resistance, probably due to arteriolar constriction concomitant with the loss of consciousness (175–177). During presyncope, systolic and diastolic blood pressure decline, accompanied by a fall in total peripheral resistance, whereas heart rate may slow or remain constant. These phenomena are accompanied by dizziness, nausea, diaphoresis, and diplopia or blurred vision. The cause for the impaired cerebral autoregulation remains unclear. Follow-up studies have shown that patients with vasovagal syncope have no increased risk of cardiovascular morbidity or mortality (178).

Cardiac syncope is seen in children with cardiac asystole (Stokes-Adams syndrome), paroxysmal changes in cardiac rhythm, obstruction to left ventricular outflow, or anemia. Syncopal attacks caused by a prolonged QT interval have a familial incidence and occasionally present with a seizure. Attacks are frequently induced by exercise or excitement (179).

Two clinical entities marked by a prolonged QT interval have been described. The Romano-Ward syndrome is an autosomal dominant condition caused by a mutation in the KCNQ1 gene mapped to chromosome 11p15.5. In the Jervell-Lange-Nielsen syndrome, an autosomal recessive condition caused by a homozygous mutation of a cardiac potassium channel gene (KVLQT1) or by a mutation in the KCNE1 gene, prolongation of the QT interval is accompanied by congenital deafness (180,181). Heterozygotes for this entity have a prolonged QT interval.

Syncope preceded by dyspnea also can be seen in systemic mastocytosis. Because skin involvement is not invariable, this condition must be kept in mind under such circumstances (182).

Syncope is rare in childhood and more common during adolescence, particularly in girls, and it is seen in about 15% of individuals under the age of 18 years. Fainting spells consist of an initial period during which the patient experiences a number of premonitory symptoms, including restlessness, pallor, sweating, and reduction in vision. These are followed by loss of consciousness. In two-thirds of the patients followed by Livingston for recurrent syncope, unconsciousness lasted less than 5 minutes; in the remainder, it persisted for 5 to 30 minutes (183). Approximately 40% of syncopal attacks are accompanied by a convulsion. Usually this is a tonic spasm followed by confusion lasting several minutes. Less often, there are clonic movements or a tonic-clonic convulsion. Subjects who experience convulsive syncope have a normal EEG and a negative family history for seizure disorders. Their blood pressure and heart rate during an attack do not differ significantly from subjects who experience uncomplicated syncope, and the cause of the seizure is unknown (184).

The differentiation between syncope and epilepsy is difficult and has already been discussed. The differential diagnosis is reviewed in a highly readable manner by Stephenson (185).

The most important investigation in a child with recurrent syncope is electrocardiographic monitoring and echocardiography to exclude a long QT interval. As a rule, these studies are more valuable than EEG, which will generally be normal. McLeod considers neuroimaging to be an expensive waste of time (186). A tilt-table test is probably of limited value in the usual clinical setting (187). McLeod provides a protocol for this procedure that is tolerated by most children over the age of 6 years (186). The child rests supine for 15 minutes and is then tilted to 60° head-up for a maximum of 45 minutes. During this time, blood pressure is continuously but noninvasively monitored, and an ECG is continuously recorded. The most common positive response is a combination of hypotension with or without bradycardia. In the vasoconstrictive form of syncope, symptoms arise from cerebral vasoconstriction without bradycardia or hypotension. In such subjects, the EEG will be abnormal during the tilt test ###(187). In the experience of McLeod, approximately 50% of children with a good history of vasovagal syncope will have a positive test (186).

In some instances, differentiation between a syncopal and an epileptic attack is not simple. In general, the longer the period of unconsciousness, the greater the likelihood of an epileptic equivalent. In such patients, anticonvulsant therapy is often beneficial in reducing the frequency of attacks. Finally, syncope can precipitate a convulsion in an epileptic individual (188).

Reassurance is the best treatment for syncope. The likelihood of recurrent attacks is proportional to the number of attacks the child has experienced prior to evaluation. Many pharmacologic agents have been suggested, but to date, none has been adequately evaluated, and probably all have a significant placebo effect. Volume expansion with salt tablets or electrolyte-containing beverages and educating the youngster on how to perform isometric arm contractions and/or leg crossing in order to abort impending syncope also are important. Tilt-training has demonstrated benefit in several clinical studies. When symptoms remain despite the above-noted interventions, pharmacologic therapy with fludrocortisone (100 μg per day), vasoconstrictors such as midodrine, or a nonselective β-blocker can be considered (189).

Psychogenic pseudosyncopal attacks are not unusual in adolescents. Admission to the hospital with cardiac and EEG monitoring will frequently assist in making this diagnosis.

BREATH-HOLDING SPELLS

It is common for a small child to hold his or her breath when crying. These episodes, termed *breath-holding spells*, are seen in about one-third of healthy children. Like syncope, the underlying cause is believed to be a dysfunctional autonomic nervous system. In the opinion of Shore and Painter (190) and McLeod (186), pallid breath-holding spells represent a form of vasovagal syncope. The finding of increased QT dispersion also points to an abnormality in central autonomic regulation (191,192).

Attacks follow a distinct clinical pattern. In a typical attack, the infant who has been frightened or frustrated begins to cry and ceases breathing. Usually the breath is held in expiration, and after a few seconds, the infant becomes cyanotic to varying degrees. Consciousness is lost; the infant becomes limp and can experience a few clonic convulsions of the extremities. Lombroso and Lerman found breath-holding spells in 4.6% of infants, with the majority of spells (76%) beginning in infants between 6 and 18 months of age (193). In a large number, the first attack was observed during the neonatal period. The frequency of attacks varies considerably. Approximately 10% of patients experience two or more attacks a day, and another 20% experience an average of one spell a day. A family history of breath-holding spells can be elicited in a significant number of first-degree relatives. In the series of DiMario and Sarfarazi, 27% of parents and 21% of siblings had current or prior breath-holding spells. These authors suggest that the condition is transmitted as an autosomal dominant with reduced penetrance (194,195).

With increasing age, spells become less common; in almost all instances, they finally disappear by age 5 to 6 years. Lombroso and Lerman believe that infants with breath-holding spells can be divided into two well-defined groups of approximately equal size: one group in which spells are conspicuously cyanotic and another in which they are characterized by pallor (193). The latter group is particularly sensitive to vagal stimulation as elicited by ocular compression, which induces a prolonged asystole and an occasional seizure. McLeod considers that the distinction between the two groups is more blurred than is often realized (186).

A breath-holding spell accompanied by a seizure can be differentiated from an epileptic convulsion (apneic seizure) in that an obvious precipitating factor that has induced the child to cry can almost always be elicited in the former. Cyanosis generally follows the onset of convulsions in an epileptic attack, but it precedes breath-holding spells (196). Finally, the interictal EEG is invariably normal in patients with breath-holding spells. Apneic seizures, which represent true epileptic attacks probably arising from the limbic system, can occur during both the waking and sleeping state. They are generally seen in neurologically damaged infants and are accompanied by EEG abnormalities. Treatment with anticonvulsants can be effective in apneic seizures.

In the experience of Daoud and colleagues, iron therapy significantly reduced the frequency of breath-holding spells, even though not all children who responded were iron deficient and not all iron-deficient children responded (197). Their results have since been confirmed by Mocan and colleagues (198). Drug therapy for breath-holding spells is neither indicated nor effective, although atropine is said to be helpful in the pallid type of breath-holding spell. Donma, however, has found piracetam, a cyclic derivative of GABA, to be extremely effective in the control of breath-holding spells (199). These observations have still not been confirmed.

Basically, breath-holding spells are triggered by a disciplinary conflict between parent and child, with the child using the attacks or the threat of an attack to assert him- or herself and to express anger. Proper family counseling and assurance to parents that the attacks do not represent any danger to the child are often effective in stopping them (196).

Although breath-holding spells disappear spontaneously in every case, many patients become prone to syncope and develop behavior disturbances, particularly temper tantrums. The incidence of true epilepsy in children with breath-holding spells, however, is no greater than is found in the general population.

One of the most difficult problems confronting the clinician is the patient with paroxysmal episodes of aggressive and explosive behavior, a condition commonly termed *episodic dyscontrol* or *intermittent explosive disorder*. In a significant proportion of cases, the first attack follows a head injury; in other instances, there is an antecedent history of temper tantrums, learning disabilities, and isolated seizures. The neurologic aspects of this entity are reviewed more extensively by Rickler (200).

NARCOLEPSY

Narcolepsy is characterized by paroxysmal attacks of irrepressible sleep. The somnolence is occasionally associated with transient loss of muscular tone or cataplexy. There is strong familial clustering, and the major histocompatibility complex (MHC) class II molecule DQ0602 confers strong susceptiblity to the condition.

Pathogenesis

Narcolepsy was first described by Westphal in 1877 (201); its neurophysiologic basis has been found to represent abnormal recurrent episodes of REM sleep. Healthy subjects always go into non-REM sleep first, changing to REM sleep after a variable period, that averages 140 minutes in children 19 to 45 months of age (202). By contrast, the sleep attack of most typical narcoleptic subjects shows an appearance of REM sleep within 5 minutes. The cataplectic attack often associated with narcolepsy has been explained as resulting from the intrusion into wakefulness of the motor inhibitory process that is an essential part of normal REM periods; whenever cataplexy is not interrupted, it goes on into REM sleep.

There is a strong genetic predisposition to narcolepsy, and almost 100% of patients with narcolepsy and cataplexy have first-degree relatives similarly affected (203). Because monozygotic twins have a significant rate of discordance, the condition is believed to be multifactorial.

The pathogenesis of narcolepsy is still not clear (204). Saper and coworkers have reviewed the pathways involved in normal wakefulness, non-REM sleep, and REM sleep (205). Considerable evidence suggests that most of the REM-on cells are cholinergic or cholinoceptive neurons in the laterodorsal and pedunculopontine tegmental nuclei of the dorsal pons that activate the thalamus during REM sleep. REM-off cells (cells that fire most rapidly during the waking state, slower in non-REM sleep, and become silent in REM sleep) include noradrenergic neurons of the locus coeruleus, serotonergic neurons of the dorsal raphe, and histaminergic neurons of the tuberomammillary nucleus (205,206). Dopaminergic neurons also may promote wakefulness, and lesions of dopaminergic cells in the ventral midbrain can reduce wakefulness in experimental animals (206).

Orexin (Hypocretin), a recently discovered neuropeptide, is believed to play a key role in regulating the various systems that interact to produce the waking state, REM sleep, and non-REM sleep (207). Orexin-containing neurons are found in the posterior and lateral hypothalamus; they ennervate and excite the aminergic and cholinergic neurons of the locus coeruleus, raphe, and tuberomammillary nucleus that promoke wakefulness. These neurons are active during the waking state and suppress REM sleep by inhibiting the REM-inducing neurons of the laterodorsal and pedunculopontine tegmental nuclei (208,208a). The release of orexins is under the control of the suprachiasmatic nucleus, and lesions in that region suppress the daily rhythm of orexin release (209).

About 84% of narcoleptic subjects with cataplexy have extremely low or absent orexin A (hypocretin-1) levels in CSF (210). Orexin A and orexin B are two neuropeptides derived from the same precursor gene. By contrast, nearly all narcoleptic subjects without cataplexy have normal orexin A levels in CSF (211).

Neuropathologic studies have shown that the marked decrease in CSF orexin in subjects who had suffered from narcolepsy with cataplexy is caused by a striking and highly selective loss of orexin-producing neurons. By contrast, subjects who during their lifetime had suffered from narcolepsy without cataplexy had the greatest number of remaining orexin neurons. The loss of orexin-containing neurons is accompanied by an increased amount of hypothalamic gliosis, a finding that points to an initiating cytotoxic or immunologically mediated attack that is focused on one of the orexin receptors (212). Interestingly, the DQB1*0602 allele provides strong protection against type 1 diabetes (213).

Although narcolepsy in dogs and mice can be caused by mutations of genes for the orexin precursor or orexin receptors, only one case of human narcolepsy caused by a mutation in the gene for the orexin precursor has been documented (214,215). Whether narcolepsy with cataplexy and narcolepsy without cataplexy represent the same or different diseases has not been resolved.

Clinical Manifestations

Narcolepsy is common, with a prevalence of just under 0.1% (216). It first appears during the late second or third decade of life, although spells can develop as early as 2 to 3 years of age (217,218). As a rule, there is a stronger family history in subjects with an early onset, and the condition tends to be more severe (219). In preschool children, unexpected, abrupt falls are the most common initial complaint; in older children, these are accompanied by chronic sleepiness, repetitive falling asleep in class, difficulty waking in the morning, and abnormal behavior in school, notably hyperactivity and an attention deficit disorder (220). Attacks of sleep usually occur while the child is at rest. Although the patient can resist them, he or she can do so only briefly. If not disturbed, sleep lasts from a few minutes to half an hour, after which the patient awakens and is completely alert. Narcoleptic sleep is usually shallow, and the patient can easily be aroused.

Cataplexy is associated with narcolepsy in approximately 75% of children. In general, the history indicates that during an emotional reaction, particularly laughter, anger, or surprise, the child loses all muscular tone and falls to the ground but retains consciousness. The attack may begin with clonic inhibitory movement leading to the fall, followed by a period of atonia and areflexia that rarely lasts more than a minute.

Some children experience both narcolepsy and cataplexy on separate occasions; others experience somnolence as a result of excitement, and if sleep occurs, they undergo a cataplectic attack. The condition persists throughout adult life, the frequency of attacks varying over the years without showing a definite trend toward improvement or worsening.

A narcoleptic attack is distinguished from a true seizure in that the patient is easily aroused and once awake does not show postictal confusion, which is a common sequel to an epileptic attack.

Diagnosis

The diagnosis of narcolepsy is based on the clinical history and is confirmed by an overnight polysomnogram, followed by a multiple sleep latency test in which the subject is given four or five opportunities to nap every two hours. Normal subjects fall asleep in 10 to 15 minutes, whereas narcoleptic patients generally fall asleep in less than five minutes, and their naps often include REM sleep. Sleep-onset REM periods also are seen in sleep deprivation or sleep apnea (203,206,218,220).

Additionally, HLA typing demonstrates the presence of DQB1*0602, a DQ1 subtype allele, in 88% to 98% of narcoleptic subjects, as compared with an incidence of 12% of white American and 38% of African American controls (221). However, more than 99% of DQB1*0602-positive subjects do not have narcolepsy (206).

It has been shown that some children who present with hyperactivity and attention deficit disorders or with various learning disabilities experience underlying narcolepsy or other sleep disorders, but how commonly this occurs has not been determined (222).

Narcolepsy should be differentiated from idiopathic hypersomnia, a condition that can make its onset as early as 6 years of age. It is marked by deep, excessively long periods of sleep and difficulty in waking. In distinction from narcolepsy, naps are not refreshing, and the multiple sleep latency test is normal. The condition is frequently preceded by viral illnesses or head trauma. CSF orexin levels in these subjects tend to be lower than normal (211,223).

Narcolepsy also should be distinguished from the excessive somnolence of the patient with obesity and carbon dioxide retention due to a low level of ventilation (Pickwickian syndrome) (224,225).

Treatment

Narcolepsy requires long-term treatment. Methylphenidate or dextroamphetamine are the drugs that have been used traditionally to combat sleep attacks. Modafinil (100 mg to 400 mg q am), a psychostimulant, is believed to be equally effective (227). Pemoline is generally used in younger children. Monoamine inhibitors suppress REM sleep for extended periods. Their adverse effects, including insomnia, hypotension, and alterations in personality, limit their usefulness (228). A child with narcolepsy tolerates large doses of these drugs (40 to 60 mg methylphenidate per day), but the drugs rarely give complete relief, although 50% of patients report a reduction in frequency and severity of attacks.

Cataplexy frequently does not respond to these psychostimulant drugs. Imipramine, clomipramine, and fluoxetine inhibit REM sleep and are effective in treating cataplexy (203,204,228). More recently, γ-hydroxybutyrate (1.5 gm to 4.5 gm given at bedtime) also has been found to be of considerable help (206). Frequent brief daytime naps should be encouraged, as they reduce the dose of stimulants required to keep the child awake. Teachers and family should be made to understand that narcolepsy is a chronic physical illness and that sleep attacks cannot be controlled by the child.

KLEINE-LEVIN SYNDROME

The Kleine-Levin syndrome of recurrent hypersomnia, morbid hunger, and behavioral changes, which is occasionally encountered in adolescence, is unrelated to narcolepsy (229,230). The condition is sporadic and is seen more commonly in boys. The mean onset is at 15 years of age, and on the average, subjects experience four episodes a year, with a duration of 12 ± 8 days (231). Pathologic examination of the brain shows infiltrates of inflammatory microglia in thalamus, diencephalon, and midbrain. The locus coeruleus is reduced in size, and there is diminished pigmentation of the substantia nigra. CSF orexin concentration is normal between attacks, but one patient, also affected with Prader-Willi syndrome experienced a twofold decrease during a symptomatic episode (232). Like narcolepsy, Kleine-Levin syndrome is now believed to represent an autoimmune disorder.

PARASOMNIAS

The term *parasomnia* refers to a variety of motor and autonomic disturbances in sleep that do not represent abnormalities of the processes responsible for the sleep and waking states, but that still repesent undesirable physical phenomena that occur predominantly during sleep. They are relatively common in childhood. They include somniloquy, infantile myoclonic jerks, bruxism, head banging, leg restlessness, sleepwalking, enuresis, and night terrors (pavornocturnus) (203,233).

Somniloquy is the most common of the parasomnias. It was seen in 55.5% of boys and girls in data collected by Laberge and coworkers (234). Restless legs were seen in 31.7% of children and night terrors in 17.3%.

Infantile myoclonic jerks are seen during stage 1 and 2 of non-REM sleep. They consist of rhythmic jerks of the limbs that usually subside in one to three minutes but can last up to 30 minutes and be severe enough to interfere with sleep. The condition tends to be familial and subsides within the first 2 years, although in some families, it persists throughout life. Attacks are not stimulus sensitive and because the EEG during an attack is normal, telemetry readily distinguishes infantile myoclonic jerks from a nocturnal myoclonic seizure (235). The condition also should be distinguished from benign myoclonic epilepsy of infancy, which is seen also in healthy infants. Attacks of benign myoclonic epilepsy have their onset between 6 months and 3 years; they are brief and involve the upper extremities and the head (236). Unlike sleep myoclonus, this condition can appear throughout the day; the EEG taken during an attack always shows bursts of generalized spike-wave and polyspike-wave discharges. Photic or unexpected tactile or auditory stimuli can provoke these seizures (237).

Bruxism and head banging also occur before sleep or during stages 1 and 2 of non-REM sleep. These phenomena are relatively common in infants and young children, with the incidence of bruxism being 28.1% and head banging as high as 15% (238,239). Both entities are more common in blind, mentally retarded, or autistic infants. Onset of head banging is generally in the latter half of the first year of life, and the condition is transient in most healthy infants, disappearing in a few months or, at the latest, before 4 years of age. The most plausible cause for head banging is that the condition is stress related, and that infants experience a need for motor release. Treatment for head banging is usually unnecessary, and head injury does not often occur; when it does, child abuse should be suspected. If excessive, both head banging and bruxism can require the bedtime use of chloral hydrate or benzodiazepines. High anxiety scores have been found in many of the children who suffer from parasomnias (238), and when the condition persists, psychiatric evaluation should be considered.

Some 15% of healthy children sleepwalk (234). This phenomenon generally occurs during stages 3 and 4 of non-REM sleep. In some, sleepwalking alternates with episodes during which the child sits up in bed and performs semipurposive movements. If awakened, the child is transiently confused. Attacks last from a few seconds to a few minutes, rarely up to an hour (240,241). An EEG taken during the episode shows it to commence with paroxysmal bursts of slow-wave activity and to continue with a mixture of wake and sleep activity. Sleepwalking tends to be familial, occurs more frequently during periods of stress, and often is found in conjunction with night terrors, somniloquy, and sleep-disordered breathing (242,243). Guilleminault and coworkers have stressed that polysomnography should be used for the diagnosis of sleep-disordered breathing, and if present, the condition should be treated. In their experience, treatment results in clear and prompt improvement (218).

A discussion of night terrors and the various other sleep disorders is outside the scope of this text. The interested reader is referred to reviews by Vgontzas and Kales (203), Dahl (244), Rosen (245), and Woody (246) and to a book by Sheldon and coworkers (240).

REFERENCES

1. Zwart JA, Dyb G, Holmen TL, et al. The prevalence of migraine and tension-type headaches among adolescents in Norway. The Nord-Trondelag Health Study (Head-HUN Study), a large population-based study. *Cephalalgia* 2004;24:373–379.
2. Isler H. Retrospect: the history of thought about migraine from Aretaeus to 1920. In: Blau JN, ed. *Migraine*. London: Chapman and Hall, 1987:659–674.
3. Bille BS. Migraine in school children. A study of the incidence and short-term prognosis, and a clinical, psychological and electroencephalographic comparison between children with migraine and matched controls. *Acta Paediatr* 1962;51[Suppl 136]:1–151.
4. Friedman AP.Harms E. *Headaches in children*. Springfield, IL: CC Thomas, 1967.
5. Barlow CF. *Headaches and migraine in childhood*. Philadelphia and Oxford: Blackwell, 1984.
6. Hockaday JM, ed. *Migraine in childhood*. London: Butterworth, 1988.
7. Winner P, Rothner AD, eds. *Headache in children and adolescents*. Hamilton and London: B.C. Decker, 2001.
8. McGrath PA, Hillier LM, ed. *The child with headache: diagnosis and treatment*. Seattle: IASP Press, 2001.
9. Abu-Arafeh I. *Childhood headache*. London: Mac Keith Press, 2002.
10. Guidetti V, Sillanpaa M, Russell G, et al. *Headache and migraine in childhood and adolescence*. London: Martin Dunitz, Ltd., 2002.
11. Lewis DW, Ashwal S, Dahl G, et al. Practice parameter: evaluation of children and adolescents with recurrent headaches: report of the Quality Standards Subcommittee of the American Academy of Neurology and the Practice Committee of the Child Neurology Society. *Neurology* 2002;59:490–498.
12. Lewis D, Ashwal S, Hershey A, et al. Practice parameter: pharmacological treatment of migraine headache in children and adolescents: report of the American Academy of Neurology Quality Standards Subcommittee and the Practice Committee of the Child Neurology Society. *Neurology* 2004;63:2215–2224.
13. Bille BS. Migraine and tension-type headache in children and adolescents. *Cephalalgia* 1996;16:78.
14. Bille BS. Migraine in childhood and its prognosis. *Cephalalgia* 1981;1:71–75.
15. Lipton RB, Stewart WF. Migraine headaches: epidemiology and comorbidity. *Clin Neurosci* 1998;5:2–9.
16. Lipton RB, Stewart WF, Diamond S, et al. Prevalence and burden of migraine in the United States: data from the American Migraine Study II. *Headache* 2001;41:646–657.
17. Headache Classification Committee of the International Headache Society. Classification and diagnostic crieteria for headache disorders, cranial neuralgia, and facial pain. *Cephalalgia* 1988;8:1–96.
18. Headache Classification Committee. The international classification of headache disorders, 2nd ed. *Cephalalgia* 2004;24:1–160.
19. Maytal J, Young M, Schechter A, et al. Pediatric migraine and the International Headache Society (IHS) criteria. *Neurology* 1997; 48:602–607.
20. Seshia S, Wolstein J, Adams C, et al. The International Headache Society criteria and childhood migraine. *Dev Med Child Neurol* 1994;36:419–428.
21. Vahlquist B. Migraine in children. *Int Arch Allergy* 1955;7:348–352.
22. Prensky AL, Sommer D. Diagnosis and treatment of migraine in children. *Neurology* 1979;29:506–510.
23. Lewis DW, Diamond S, Scott D. Prophylactic treatment of pediatric migraine. *Headache* 2004;44:230–237.
24. Silberstein SD, Lipton RB. Chronic daily headache. *Curr Opin Neurol* 2000;13:277–283.

24a. Moore AJ, Shevell M. Chronic daily headaches in pediatric neurology practice. *J Child Neurol* 2004;19:925–929.

25. Graham JR, Wolff HG. Mechanism of migraine headache and action of ergotamine tartrate. *Arch Neurol Psychiatry* 1938;39:737–763.
26. Silberstein SB, Lipton RB, Dalessio DJ. *Wolff's headache and other head pain*. New York: Oxford University Press, 2001.
27. Pietrobon D, Striessnig J. Neurobiology of migraine. *Nat Rev Neurosci* 2003;4:386–398.
28. Bures J, Buresova O, Krivanek J. *The mechanism and applications of Leao's spreading depression of electroencephalographic activity*. New York: Academic Press, 1974.
29. Oleson J. Cerebral and extracranial circulatory disturbances in migraine: pathophysiological implications. *Cerebrovasc Brain Metab Rev* 1991;3:1–28.
30. Lauritzen M. Pathophysiology of the migraine aura. The spreading depression therapy. *Brain* 1994;117:199–210.
31. Lance JW. Current concepts of migraine pathogenesis. *Neurology* 1993;43[Suppl 3]:S11–S15.
32. Oleson J, Edvinsson L. Migraine: a research field matured for the basic neurosciences. *Trends Neurosci* 1991;14:3–5.
33. Weiller C, May A, Limmroth V, et al. Brain stem activation in spontaneous human migraine attacks. *Nature Med* 1995;1:658–660.
34. Silberstein SD. Migraine. *Lancet* 2004;363:381–391.
35. Strassman AM, Raymond SA, Burstein R. Sensitization of meningeal sensory neurons and the origin of headaches. *Nature* 1996;384:560–564.
36. Burstein R, Collins B, Bajwa Z, et al. Triptan therapy can abort migraine attacks if given before the establishment or in the absence of cutaneous allodynia and central sensitization: clinical and preclinical evidence. *Headache* 2002;42:390.
37. Ferrari MD, Haan J, Blokland JA, et al. Cerebral blood flow during migraine attacks without aura and effect of sumatriptan. *Arch Neurol* 1995;52:135–139.
38. Woods RP, Iacoboni M, Mazziotta JC. Bilateral spreading cerebral hypoperfusion during spontaneous migraine headache. *N Engl J Med* 1994;331:1689–1692.
39. Ferrari MD, Odink J, Tapparelli C, et al. Serotonin metabolism in migraine. *Neurology* 1989;39:1239–1242.

40. Chugani DC, Niimura K, Chaturvedi S, et al. Increased brain serotonin synthesis in migraine. *Neurology* 1999;53:1473–1479.
41. Peroutka SJ. Antimigraine drug interactions with serotonin receptor subtypes in human brain. *Ann Neurol* 1988;23:500–504.
42. Congden PJ, Forsythe WI. Migraine in childhood: a study of 300 children. *Dev Med Child Neurol* 1979;21:209–216.
43. Antilla P. Tension-type headache in children and adolescents. *Curr Pain Headache Rep* 2004;8:500–504.
44. Bendtsen L. Central and peripheral sensitization in tension-type headache. *Curr Pain Headache Rep* 2003;7:760–765.
45. Jensen R. Pathophysiological mechanisms of tension-type headache: a review of epidemiological and experimental studies. *Cephalalgia* 1999;19:602–621.
46. Ulrich V, Gervil M, Olesen J. The relative influene of environment and genes in episodic tension-type headache. *Neurology* 2004;62:2065–2069.
47. Ong JC, Nicholson RA, Gramling SE. EMG reactivity and oral habits among young adult headache sufferers and painfree controls in a scheduled-waiting task. *Appl Psychophysiol Biofeedback* 2003;28:255–265.
48. Russell MB. Epidemiology and genetics of cluster headaches. *Lancet Neurol* 2004;3:279–283.
49. Leone M, Bussone G. A review of hormonal findings in cluster headache. Evidence for hypothalamic involvement. *Cephalalgia* 1993;13:309–317.
50. May A, Bahra A, Buchel C, et al. PET and MRA findings in cluster headache and MRA in experimental pain. *Neurology* 2000;55:1328–1335.
51. Larsson B, Bille B, Pederson N. Genetic influence in headaches: a Swedish twin study. *Headache* 1995;35:513–519.
52. Ulrich V, Gervil M, Kyvik KO, et al. The inheritance of migraine with aura estimated by means of structural equation modelling. *J Med Genet* 1999;36:225–227.
53. Gervil M, Gervil M, Kyvik KO, et al. Migraine without aura: a population-based twin study. *Ann Neurol* 1999;46:606–611.
54. Russell MB, Olesen J. Migrainous disorder and its relation to migraine without aura and migraine with aura. A genetic epidemiological study. *Cephalalgia* 1996;16:431–435.
55. Russell MB, Iselius L, Olesen J. Inheritance of migraine investigated by complex segregation analysis. *Hum Genet* 1995;96:726–730.
56. Ulrich V, Russell MB, Ostergaard S, Olesen J. Analysis of 31 families with an apparently autosomal-dominant transmission of migraine with aura in the nuclear family. *Am J Med Genet* 1997; 74:395–397.
57. Sandor PS, Ambrosini A, Agosti RM, Schoenen J. Genetics of migraine: possible links to neurophysiological abnormalities. *Headache* 2002;42:365–377.
58. DeRomanis F, Buzzi MG, Assensa S, et al. Basilar migraine with electroecenphalographic findings of occipital spike-wave complexes: a long-term study in seven children. *Cephalalgia* 1993; 13:192–196.
59. Eeg-Olofsson O. The development of the electroencephalogram in normal children and adolescents from the age of 1 through 21 years. *Acta Paediatr Scand Suppl* 1970;[Suppl 208]:1.
60. Kinast M, Lueders H, Rothner AD, et al. Benign focal epileptiform discharges in childhood migraine (BFEDC). *Neurology* 1982; 32:1309–1311.
61. Dooley JM, Camfield PR, O'Neill M, et al. The value of CT scans for children with headaches. *Can J Neurol Sci* 1990;17:309–310.
62. Osborn RE, Alder DC, Mitchell CS. MR imaging of the brain in patients with migraine headaches. *AJNR Am J Neuroradiol* 1991;12:521–524.
63. Practice parameter: the utility of neuroimaging in the evaluation of headache in patients with normal neurologic examinations (summary statement). Report of the Quality Standards Subcommittee of the American Academy of Neurology. *Neurology* 1994;44:1353–1354.
64. Harrison RH. Psychological testing in headache: a review. *Headache* 1975;14:177–185.
65. Weiss HD, Stern BJ, Goldberg J. Post-traumatic migraine: chronic migraine precipitated by minor head or neck trauma. *Headache* 1991;31:157–158.
66. Solomon S. Posttraumatic migraine. *Headache* 1998;38:772–778.
67. Burton LJ, Quinn B, Pratt-Chenye IL, et al. Headache etiology in a pediatric emergency room. *Pediatr Emerg Care* 1997;13:1–4.
68. Lewis DW, Qureshi FA. Acute headache in the pediatric emergency department. *Headache* 2000;40:200–203.
69. Chu ML, Shinnar S. Headaches in children younger than 7 years of age. *Arch Neurol* 1992;49:79–82.
70. Belfer ML, Kaban LB. Temporomandibular joint dysfunction with facial pain in children. *Pediatrics* 1982;69:564–567.
71. Mortimer MJ, Kay J, Jaron A. Epidemiology of headache and childhood migraine in an urban general practice using ad hoc, Vahlquist and IHS criteria. *Dev Med Child Neurol* 1992;34:1095–1101.
72. Baloh RW. Neurotology of migraine. *Headache* 1997;37:615–621.
73. Holguin J, Fenichel G. Migraine. *J Pediatr* 1967;70:290–297.
74. Prensky AL. Migraine and migrainous variants in pediatric patients. *Pediatr Clin North Am* 1976;23:461–471.
75. Russell MB, Olesen J. A nosographic analysis of the migraine aura in a general population. *Brain* 1996;119:355–361.
76. Hachinski VC, Porchawka J, Steele JC. Visual symptoms in the migraine syndrome. *Neurology* 1973;23:570–579.
77. Rossi LN, Mumenthaler M, Vassella F. Complicated migraine (migraine accompagnée) in children. *Neuropädiatrie* 1980;11:27–35.
78. Kupersmith MJ, Warren FA, Hass WK. The non-benign aspects of migraine. *Neuro-ophthalmology* 1987;7:1–10.
79. Editorial. Migraine-related stroke in childhood. *Lancet* 1991;337: 825–826.
80. Hammond J. The late sequelae of recurrent vomiting of childhood. *Dev Med Child Neurol* 1974;16:15–22.
81. Smith CH. Recurrent vomiting in children. Its etiology and treatment. *J Pediatr* 1937;10:719–742.
82. Bickerstaff ER. Basilar artery migraine. *Lancet* 1961;1:15–17.
83. Golden GS, French JH. Basilar artery migraine in young children. *Pediatrics* 1975;56:722–726.
84. Kuzemko JA, Young W. Ophthalmoplegic migraine. A case report. *Dev Med Child Neurol* 1967;9:427–429.
85. Weiss AH, Phillips JO. Ophthalmoplegic migraine. *Pediatr Neurol* 2004;30:64–66.
86. Gladstone JP, Dodick DW. Painful ophthalmoplegia: overview with a focus on Tolosa-Hunt syndrome. *Curr Pain Headache Rep* 2004;8:321–329.
87. Levin M, Ward TM. Ophthalmoplegic migraine. *Curr Pain Headache Rep* 2004;8:306–309.
88. Ehyai A, Fenichel GM. The natural history of acute confusional migraine. *Arch Neurol* 1978;35:368–369.
89. Gascon G, Barlow CE. Juvenile migraine, presenting as acute confusional states. *Pediatrics* 1970;45:628–635.
90. Haas DC, Pineda GS, Lourie H. Juvenile head trauma syndromes and their relationship to migraine. *Arch Neurol* 1975;32:727–730.
91. Fenichel GM. Migraine as a cause of benign paroxymal vertigo of childhood. *J Pediatr* 1967;71:114–115.
92. Basser LS. Benign paroxysmal vertigo of childhood. *Brain* 1964;87: 141–152.
93. Lanzi G, Ballottin U, Fazzi E, et al. Benign paroxysmal vertigo of childhood: a long-term follow-up. *Cephalalgia* 1994;14:458–460.
94. Uneri A, Turkdogan D. Evaluation of vestibular functions in children with vertigo attacks. *Arch Dis Child* 2003;88:510–511.
95. Chutorian AM. Benign paroxysmal toticollis, tortipelvis and retrocollis of infancy. *Neurology* 1974;24:366–367.
96. Chavez-Carballo E. Paroxysmal torticollis. *Semin Pediatr Neurol* 1996;3:255–256.
97. Giffin NJ, Benton S, Goadsby PJ. Benign paroxysmal torticollis of infancy: four new cases and linkage to CACNA1A mutation. *Dev Med Child Neurol* 2002;44:490–493.
97a. Plunkett A, Beattie RM. Recurrent abdominal pain in childhood. *J Roy Soc Med* 2005;98:101–106.
98. Andermann F, Andermann E. Migraine and epilepsy, with special reference to the benign epilepsies of childhood. *Epilepsy Res Suppl.* 1992;6:207–214.
99. Rothner AD. Miscellaneous headache syndromes in children and adolescents. *Semin Pediatr Neurol* 1995;2:159–164.
100. Symonds C. Cough headaches. *Brain* 1956;79:557–568.
101. Raskin NH, Knittle SC. Ice cream headaches and orthostatic symptoms in patients with migraine. *Headache* 1976;16:222–225.

102. Fuh JL, Wang SJ, Lu SR, Juang KD. Ice-cream headache—a large survey of 8359 adolescent. *Cephalalgia* 2003;977–981.
103. Raskin NH, Schwartz RK. Icepick-like pain. *Neurology* 1980;30: 203–205.
104. Menkes MM. Personality characteristics and family roles of children with migraine. *Pediatrics* 1974;53:560–564.
105. Barabas G, Matthews WS, Ferrari M. Childhood migraine and motion sickness. *Pediatrics* 1983;72:188–190.
106. Friedman E, Pampiglione G. Recurrent headache in children (a clinical and electroencephalographic study). *Arch de Neurobiol* 1974;37[Suppl]:115–176.
107. Kramer U, Nevo Y, Neufeld MY, Harel S. The value of EEG in children with chronic headache. *Brain Dev* 1994;16:304–306.
108. Schon F, Blau JN. Postepileptic headache and migraine. *J Neurol Neurosurg Psychiatry* 1987;50:1148–1152.
109. Young WB, Silberstein SD. Paroxysmal headache caused by colloid cyst of the third ventricle: case report and review of the literature. *Headache* 1997;37:15–20.
110. Maytal J, Bienkowski RS, Patel M, et al. The value of brain imaging in children with headaches. *Pediatrics* 1995;96:413–416.
111. McAbee GN, Siegel SE, Kadakia S, et al. Value of MRI in pediatric migraine. *Headache* 1993;33:143–144.
112. Straussberg R, Amir J. Headaches in children younger than 7 years: are they really benign? *Arch Neurol* 1993;50:130–131.
113. Battistella PA, Naccarella C, Soriani S, and Perilongo G. Headache and brain tumors: different features versus primary forms in juvenile patients. *Headache Q* 1998;9:245–248.
114. Gomez-Aranda F, Canadillas F, Marti-Masso JF, et al. Pseudomigraine with temporary neurological symptoms and lymphocytic pleocytosis. A report of 50 cases. *Brain* 1997;120:1105–1113.
115. Egger J, Carter CM, Wilson J, et al. Is migraine a food allergy? *Lancet* 1983;2:865–869.
116. Hämäläinen ML, Hoppu K, Valkeila E, et al. Ibuprofen or acetaminophen for the acute treatment of migraine in children. A double-blind, randomized, placebo-controlled, crossover study. *Neurology* 1997;48:103–107.
117. Capobianco DJ, Cheshire WP, Campbell JK. An overview of the diagnosis and pharmacologic treatment of migraine. *Mayo Clin Proc* 1996;71:1055–1066.
118. Linder SL. Treatment of childhood headache with dihydroergotamine mesylate. *Headache* 1994;34:995–997.
119. Von Seggern RL, Adelman JU. Cost considerations in headache treatment. Part 2: Acute migraine treatment. *Headache* 1996;36: 493–502.
120. Akova-Ozturk E, Evers S. Flunarizine in the prophylactic treatment of childhood migraine. *MMW Fortschr Med* 2004;146:48.
121. Diener HC, Matias-Guiu J, Hartung E, et al. Efficacy and tolerability in migraine prophylaxis of flunarizine in reduced doses: a comparison with propranolol 160 mg daily. *Cephalalgia* 2002;22:209–221.
122. Ferrari MD, Roon KI, Lipton RB, et al. Oral triptans (serotonin 5-$HT_{1B/1D}$agonists) in acute migraine treatment: a meta-analysis of 53 trials. *Lancet* 2001;358:1668–1675.
123. Burstein R, Collins B, Jakubowski M. Defeating migraine pain with triptans: a race against the development of cutaneous allodynia. *Ann Neurol* 2004;55:19–26.
124. Major PW, Grubisa HS, Thie NM. Triptans for treatment of acute pediatric migraine: a systematic literature review. *Pediatr Neurol* 2003;29:425–429.
125. Ludvigsson J. Propranolol used in prophylaxis of migraine in children. *Acta Neurol Scand* 1974;50:109–115.
126. Mathew NT, Saper JR, Silberstein SD, et al. Migraine prophylaxis with divalproex. *Arch Neurol* 1995;52:281–286.
127. Chronicle E, Mulleners W. Anticonvulsant drugs for migraine prophylaxis. *Cochrane Data Base System Rev*. 2004;(3):CD003226.
128. Kaniecki RG. A comparison of divalproex with propanolol and placebo for the prophylaxis of migraine without aura. *Arch Neurol* 1997;54:1141–1145.
129. Silberstein SD. Topiramate in migraine prevention: evidence-based medicine from clinical trials. *Neurol Sci* 2004;25[Suppl 2]:S244–S245.
130. Mei D, Capuano A, Vollono C, et al. Topiramate in migraine prophylaxis: a randomized double-blind versus placebo study. *Neurol Sci* 2004;25:245–250.
131. Brandes JL, Saper JR, Diamond M, et al. Topiramate for migraine prevention. A randomized controlled trial. *JAMA* 2004;291:965–973.
132. Fenichel GM, Battiata S. Thrombophlebitis secondary to methysergide maleate therapy. *J Pediatr* 1966;68:632–634.
133. Andersson KE, Vinge E. β-Adrenoreceptor blockers and calcium antagonists in the prophylaxis and treatment of migraine. *Drugs* 1990;39:355–373.
134. Sorge F, De Simone R, Marano E, et al. Flunarizine in prophylaxis of childhood migraine: a double-blind, placebo-controlled study. *Cephalalgia* 1987;7[Suppl 6]:385–386.
135. Igarashi M, May WN, Golden GS. Pharmacologic treatment of childhood migraine. *J Pediatr* 1992;120:652–657.
136. Arulmani U, Maassenvandenbrink A, Villalon CM, et al. Calcitonin gene-related peptide and its role in migraine pathophysiology. *Eur J Pharmacol* 2004;500:315–330.
137. Tronvik E, Stovner LJ, Helde G, et al. Prophylactic treatment of migraine with an angiotensin II receptor blocker: a randomized controlled trial. *JAMA* 2003;289:65–69.
138. Hinrichs WL, Keith HM. Migraine in childhood: a follow-up report. *Mayo Clin Proc* 1965;40:593–596.
139. Akhtar ND, Murray MA, Rothner AD. Status migrainosus in children and adolescents. *Semin Pediatr Neurol* 2001;8:27–33.
140. Esposito SB, Gherpelli JL. Chronic daily headaches in children and adolescents: a study of clinical characteristics. *Cephalalgia* 2004;24:476–482.
141. Moorjani BI, Rothner AD. Indomethacin-responsive headaches in children and adolescents. *Semin Pediatr Neurol* 2001;8:40–45.
142. May A, Bahra A, Buchel C, et al. Functional magnetic resonance imaging in spontaneous attacks of SUNCT; short-lasting neuralgiform headache with conjunctival injection and tearing. *Ann Neurol* 1999;46:791–763.
143. Esposito SP, Gherpelli JL. Chronic daily headaches in children and adolescents: a study of clinical characteristics. *Cephalalgia* 2004;24:476–482.
144. Hering-Hanit R, Gadoth N. Caffeine-induced headaches in children and adolescents. *Cephalalgia* 2003;23:332–335.
145. Hering-Hanit R, Gadoth N, Cohen A, et al. Successful withdrawal from analgesic abuse in a group of youngsters with chronic daily headache. *J Child Neurol* 2001;16:448–449.
146. Jones GT, Watson KDF, Silman AJ, et al. Predictors of low back pain in British school children: a population-based prospective cohort study. *Pediatrics* 2003;111:822–828.
147. Maytal J. Childhood onset of cluster headaches. *Headache* 1992;275–279.
148. Sjaastad O, Dale I. Evidence for a new (?), treatable headache entity. *Headache* 1976;14:105–108.
149. Rooke DE. Benign exertional headaches. *Med Clin North Am* 1968;52:801–808.
150. Buzzi MG, Formisano R, Colonnese C, et al. Chiari-associated exertional, cough, and sneeze headache responsive to medical therapy. *Headache* 2003;43:404–406.
151. Medina JL, Diamond S. Cyclical migraine. *Arch Neurol* 1981;38: 343–344.
152. Sjaasstad O, Spierings ELH. "Hemicrania continua": another headache absolutely responsive to indomethacin. *Cephalalgia* 1984;4:65–70.
153. Zuckerman E, Hannuch SN, Carvalho D, et al. "Hemicrania continua": a case report. *Cephalalgia* 1987;7:171–173.
154. Glista GG, Mellinger JF, Rooke ED. Familial hemiplegic migraine. *Mayo Clin Proc* 1975;50:307–311.
155. O'Hare JA, Feely MJ, Callaghan N. Clinical aspects of familial hemiplegic migraine in two families. *Irish Med J* 1981;74:291–295.
156. Ophoff RA, Terwindt GM, Vergouwe MN, et al. Familial hemiplegic migraine and episodic ataxia type 2 are caused by mutations in the Ca (2^+) channel gene CACNL1A4. *Cell* 1996;87:543–552.
157. Gardner K, Barmada MM, Ptacek LJ, et al. A new locus for hemiplegic migraine maps to chromosome 1q31. *Neurology* 1997; 49:1231–1238.
158. Wessman M, Kaunisto MA, Kallela M, et al. The molecular genetics of migraine. *Ann Med* 2004;36:462–473.
158a. Haan J, Kors EE, Vanmolkot KR, et al. Migraine genetics: an update. *Curr Pain Headache Rep* 2005;9:213–220.
159. Kors EE, Haan J, Giffin J, et al. Expanding the phenotypic

spectrum of the CACNA1A gene T666M mutation. A description of 5 families with familial hemiplegic migraine. *Arch Neurol* 2003;60:684–688.
160. Denier C, Ducros A, Vahedi K, et al. High prevalence of CACNA1A truncations and broader clinical spectrum in episodic ataxia type 2. *Neurology* 1999;52:1816–1821.
161. Estevez M, Gardner KL. Update on the genetics of migraine. *Hum Genet* 2004;114:225–235.
162. Ducros A, Joutel A, Vahedi K, et al. Mapping of a second locus for familial hemiplegic migraine to 1q21–q23 and evidence of further heterogeneity. *Ann Neurol* 1997;42:885–890.
163. Gee S. On fitful or recurrent vomiting. *St. Bartholomew's Hospital Reports* 1882;18:1–6.
164. Li BU, Issenman RM, Sarna SK. Consensus statement—2nd International Scientific Symposium on CVS. Faculty of the 2nd International Scientific Symposium on cyclic vomiting syndrome. *Dig Dis Sci* 1999;44:9S–11S.
165. Hoyt CS, Stickler GB. A study of 44 children with the syndrome of recurrent (cyclic) vomiting. *Pediatrics* 1960;25:775–780.
166. MacKeith RCM, Pampiglione G. The recurrent syndrome in children. Clinical and EEG observations in 52 cases [Abstract]. *Electroenceph Clin Neurophys* 1956;8:161.
167. Wang Q, Ito M, Adams K, et al. Mitochondrial DNA control region sequence variation in migraine headache and cyclic vomiting syndrome. *Am J Med Genet* 2004;131A:50–58.
168. Reinhart JB, Evans SL, McFadden DL. Cyclic vomiting in children: seen through the psychiatrist's eye. *Pediatrics* 1977;59:371–377.
169. Li BU, Misiewicz L. Cyclic vomiting syndrome: a brain-gut disorder. *Gastroenterol Clin North Am* 2003;32:997–1019.
170. Li UK, Murray RD, Heitlinger LA, et al. Is cyclic vomiting syndrome related to migraine? *J Pediatr* 1999;134:567–572.
171. Sondheimer JM, Morris BA. Gastroesophageal reflux among severely retarded children. *J Pediatr* 1979;94:710–714.
172. Li UK, Murray RD, Heitlinger LA, et al. Heterogeneity of diagnoses presenting as cyclic vomiting. *Pediatrics* 1998;102:583–587.
173. Boles RG, Chun N, Senadheera D, et al. Cyclic vomiting and mitochondrial DNA mutations. *Lancet* 1997;350:1299–1300.
174. Katz RM. Cough syncope in children with asthma. *J Pediatr* 1970;77:48–51.
175. Carey BJ, Manktelow BN, Panerai RB, et al. Cerebral autoregulatory responses to head-up tilt in normal subjects and patients with recurrent vasovagal syncope. *Circulation* 2001;104:898–902.
176. Sung RYT, Du ZD, Yu CW, et al. Cerebral blood flow during vasovagal syncope induced by active standing or head up tilt. *Arch Dis Child* 2000;82:154–158.
177. Grubb BP. Cerebral syncope: new insights into an emerging entity. *J Pediatr* 2000;136:431–432.
178. Soteriades ES, Evans JC, Larson MG, et al. Incidence and prognosis of syncope. *N Engl J Med* 2002;347:878–885.
179. Garson A. Medicolegal problems in the management of cardiac arrhythmias in children. *Pediatrics* 1987;79:84–88.
180. Gospe SM, Choy M. Hereditary long Q-T syndrome presenting as epilepsy: electroencephalography laboratory diagnosis. *Ann Neurol* 1989;25:514–516.
181. Splawski I, Timothy KW, Vincent GM, et al. Molecular basis of the long-QT syndrome associated with deafness. *N Engl J Med* 1997;336:1562–1567.
182. Travis WD, Li CY, Bergstralh EJ, et al. Systemic mast cell disease. Analysis of 58 cases and literature review. *Medicine* 1988;67:345–368.
183. Livingston S. *Comprehensive management of epilepsy in infancy, childhood and adolescence*. Springfield, IL: Charles C Thomas, 1972.
184. Lin JTY, Ziegler DK, Lai CW, et al. Convulsive syncope in blood donors. *Ann Neurol* 1982;11:525–528.
185. Stephenson JBP. *Fits and faints*. London: MacKeith Press, 1990.
186. McLeod KA. Syncope in childhood. *Arch Dis Child* 2003;88:350–353.
187. Lerman-Sagie T, Rechavia E, Strasberg B, et al. Head-up tilt for the evaluation of syncope of unknown origin in children. *J Pediatr* 1991;118:676–679.
188. Stephenson J, Breningstall G, Steer C, et al. Anoxic-epileptic seizures: home video recordings of epileptic seizures induced by syncopes. *Epileptic Disord* 2004;6:15–19.
189. Melby DP, Cytron JA, Benditt DG. New approaches to the treatment and prevention of neurally mediated reflex (neurocardiogenic) syncope. *Curr Cardiol Rep*. 2004;6:385–90.
190. Shore PM, Painter M. Adolescent asystolic syncope. *J Child Neurol* 2002;17:395–397.
191. Di Mario FJ. Increased QT dispersion in breath-holding spells. *Acta Paediatr* 2004;93:728–730.
192. Akalin F, Turan S, Guran T, et al. Increased QT dispersion in breath-holding spells. *Acta Paediatr* 2004;93:770–774.
193. Lombroso CT, Lerman P. Breathholding spells (cyanotic and pallid infantile syncope). *Pediatrics* 1967;39:565–581.
194. DiMario FJ, Sarfarazi M. Family pedigree analysis of children with severe breath-holding spells. *J Pediatr* 1997;130:647–651.
195. DiMario FJ. Prospective study of children with cyanotic and pallid breath-holding spells. *Pediatrics* 2001;107:265–269.
196. Livingston S. Breath-holding spells in children: differentiation from epileptic attacks. *J Am Med Assoc* 1970;212:2231–2235.
197. Daoud AS, Batieha A, al-Sheyyab M, et al. Effectiveness of iron therapy on breath-holding spells. *J Pediatr* 1997;130:547–550.
198. Mocan H, Yildiran A, Orhan F, et al. Breath holding spells in 91 children and response to treatment with iron. *Arch Dis Child* 1999;261–262.
199. Donma MM. Clinical efficacy of piracetam in treatment of breath-holding spells. *Pediatr Neurol* 1998;18:41–45.
200. Rickler KB. Episodic dyscontrol. In: Benson DF, Blumer D, eds. *Psychiatric aspects of neurologic disease*. New York: Grune & Stratton, 1982:49–73.
201. Westphal C. Zwei Krankheitsfälle. II. Eigenthümliche mit Einschlafen verbundene Anfälle. *Arch Psychiat Nervenkr* 1877;7:631–635.
202. Ornitz EM, Ritvo ER, Brown MB, et al. The EEG and rapid eye movements during REM sleep in normal and autistic children. *Electroencephalogr Clin Neurophysiol* 1969;26:167–175.
203. Vgontzas AN, Kales A. Sleep and its disorders. *Ann Rev Med* 1999;50:387–400.
204. Guilleminault C, Heinzer R, Mignot E, et al. Investigations into the neurologic basis of narcolepsy. *Neurology* 1998;50[2 Suppl 1]: S8–S15.
205. Saper CB, Chou TC, Scammell TE. The sleep switch: hypothalamic control of sleep and wakefulness. *Trends Neurosci* 2001;24:726–731.
206. Scammel TE. The neurobiology, diagnosis, and treatment of narcolepsy. *Ann Neurol* 2003;53:154–166.
207. Willie JT, Chemelli RM, Sinton CM, et al. To eat or to sleep? Orexin in the regulation of feeding and wakefulness. *Annu Rev Neurosci* 2001;24:429–458.
208. Taheri S, Zeitzer JM, Mignot E. The role of hypocretins (orexins) in sleep regulation and narcolepsy. *Annu Rev Neurosci* 2002;25: 283–313.
208a. Lee MG, Hassani OK, Jones BE. Discharge of identified orexin/hypocretin neurons across the sleep-waking cycle. *J Neurosci* 2005;25:6716–6720.
209. Zhang S, Zeitzer JM, Yoshida Y, et al. Lesions of the suprachiasmatic nucleus eliminate the daily rhythm of hypocretin-1 release. *Sleep* 2004;27:619–627.
210. Nishino S, Ripley B, Overeem S, et al. Low cerebrospinal fluid hypocretin (Orexin) and altered energy homeostasis in human narcolepsy. *Ann Neurol* 2001;50:381–388.
211. Mignot E, Lammers GJ, Ripley B, et al. The role of cerebrospinal fluid hypocretin measurement in the diagnosis of narcolepsy and other hypersomnias. *Arch Neurol* 2002;59:1553–1562.
212. Thannickal TC, Siegel JM, Nienhuis R, et al. Pattern of hypocretin (orexin) soma and axon loss, and gliosis, in human narcolepsy. *Brain Pathol* 2003;13:340–351.
213. Siebold C, Hansen BE, Wyer JR, et al. Crystal structure of HLA-DQ0602 that protects against type 1 diabetes and confers strong susceptibility to narcolepsy. *Proc Nat Acad Sci USA* 2004;101:1999–2004.
214. Peyron C, Faraco J, Rogers W, et al. A mutation in a case of early onset narcolepsy and a generalized absence of hypocretin peptides in human narcoleptic brains. *Nature Med* 2000;6:991–997.
215. Mignot E. Sleep, sleep disorders and hypocretin (orexin). *Sleep Med* 2004;5[Suppl 1]:S2–S8.
216. Broughton RJ. Polysomnography: principles and applications in

sleep and arousal disorders. In: Niedermeyer E, Lopes da Silva F, eds. *Electroencephalography*, 3rd ed. Baltimore: Williams & Wilkins, 1993:765–802.
217. Yoss RE, Daly DD. Narcolepsy in children. *Pediatrics* 1960;25: 1025–1033.
218. Guilleminault C, Pelayo R. Narcolepsy in prepubertal children. *Ann Neurol* 1997;43:135–142.
219. Dauvilliers Y, Montplaisir J, Molinari N, et al. Age at onset of narcolepsy in two large populations of patients in France and Quebec. *Neurology* 2001;57:2029–2033.
220. Kotagal S, Hartse KM, Walsh JK. Characteristics of narcolepsy in children. *Pediatrics* 1990;85:205–209.
221. Mignot E, Lin L, Rogers W, et al. Complex HLA-DR and –DQ interactions confer risk of narcolepsy-cataplexy in three ethnic groups. *Am J Hum Genet* 2001;68:686–699.
222. Chervin RD, Dillon JE, Bassetti C, et al. Symptoms of sleep disorders, inattention, and hyperactivity in children. *Sleep* 1997;20: 1185–1192.
223. Bassetti C, Aldrich MS. Idiopathic hypersomnia. A series of 42 patients. *Brain* 1997;120:1423–1435.
224. Ward WA Jr, Kelsey WM. The Pickwickian syndrome: a review of the literature and report of a case. *J Pediatr* 1962;61:745–750.
225. Erler T, Paditz E. Obstructive sleep apnea syndrome in children: a state-of-the-art review. *Treat Respirat Med* 2004;3:107–122.
226. Beusterien KM, Rogers AE, Walsleben JA, et al. Health-related quality of life effects of modafinil for treatment of narcolepsy. *Sleep* 1999;22:757–765.
227. Littner M, Johnson SF, McCall WV, et al. Practice parameters for the treatment of narcolepsy: an update for 2000. *Sleep* 2001;24: 451–466.
228. Shapiro WR. Treatment of cataplexy with clomipramine. *Arch Neurol* 1975;32:653–656.
229. Critchley M. Periodic hypersomnia and megaphagia in adolescent males. *Brain* 1962;85:627–656.
230. Orlosky MJ. The Kleine-Levin syndrome: a review. *Psychosomatics* 1982;23:609–621.
231. Dauvilliers Y, Mayer G, Lecendreux M, et al. Kleine-Levin syndrome: an autoimmune hypothesis based on clinical and genetic analyses. *Neurology* 2002;59:1739–1745.
232. Dauvilliers Y, Baumann CR, Carlander B, et al. CSF hypocretin-1 levels in narcolepsy, Kleine-Levin syndrome, and other hypersomnias and neurological conditions. *J Neurol Neurosurg Psychiatry* 2003;74:1667–1673.
233. D'Cruz OF, Vaughn BV. Parasomnias—an update. *Semin Pediatr Neurol* 2001;8:251–257.
234. Laberge L, Tremblay RE, Vitaro F, et al. Development of parasomnias from childhood to early adolescence. *Pediatrics* 2000;106:67–74.
235. Resnick TJ, Moshe SL, Perotta L, Chambers HJ. Benign neonatal sleep myoclonus: relationship to sleep states. *Arch Neurol* 1986;43:266–268.
236. Ricci S, Cusmai R, Fusco L, et al. Reflex myoclonic epilepsy in infancy: a new age-dependent idiopathic epileptic syndrome related to startle reaction. *Epilepsia* 1995;36:342–348.
237. Zafeiriou D, Vargiami E, Kontopoulos E. Reflex myoclonic epilepsy in infancy: a benign age-dependent idiopathic startle epilepsy. *Epileptic Disord* 2003;5:121–122.
238. Vinson RP, Gelinas-Sorell DF. Head banging in young children. *Am Fam Physician* 1991;43:1625–1628.
239. Dyken ME, Lynn-Dyken DC, Yamada T. Diagnosing rhythmic motor movement disorders with video-polysomnography. *Pediatr Neurol* 1997;16:37–41.
240. Sheldon SH, Spire J-P, Levy HB. *Pediatric sleep medicine*. Philadelphia: WB Saunders, 1992.
241. Masand P, Popli AP, Weilburg JB. Sleepwalking. *Am Fam Physician* 1995;51:649–654.
242. Kales A, Soldatos CR, Bixler EO, et al. Hereditary factors in sleepwalking and night terrors. *Br J Psychiatry* 1980;137:111–118.
243. Guilleminault C, Palombini L, Pelayo R, Chervin RD. Sleep walking and sleep terrors in prepubertal children: what triggers them? *Pediatrics* 2003;111:e17–25.
244. Dahl RE. The development and disorders of sleep. *Adv Pediatr* 1998;45:73–90.
245. Rosen CL. Sleep disorders in infancy, childhood, and adolescence. *Curr Opin Pulm Med* 1997;3:449–455.
246. Woody RC. Sleep disorders in children. *Semin Neurol* 1988;8: 71–77.

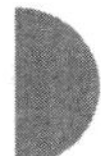

Chapter 16

Diseases of the Motor Unit

Harvey B. Sarnat and John H. Menkes

> But this form of myopathy, this pseudo-hypertrophic paralysis which was described by Duchenne (of Boulogne), that great worker in neuro-nosography, is so different in its clinical characters from the progressive spinal amyotrophies that they have rarely been confused clinically. Pseudo-hypertrophic paralysis is a disease of early youth. It is scarcely ever met with after twenty years of age. It is noticed that the child becomes clumsy in his walk, that he is more easily fatigued than the other children of his age; for it is always, quoting from Duchenne's description, in the lower extremities where it commences. Then the upper extremities may be attacked in their turn; but, whatever be the degree of the affection, the hands are generally absolved. Finally the muscles attacked, or at least a great number of them, present an augmentation of volume, an enormous increase in size, giving to the limb, or a segment of the limb, Herculean proportions. Anatomically this hypertrophy is characterized by lesions of the interstitial tissue, such as does not exist in the same degree in spinal amyotrophies. Moreover, and this is a peculiarity which is not found in Duchenne-Aran disease, heredity plays a great part in the development of pseudo-hypertrophic paralysis of the muscles. It often happens that several children are attacked in one family, and that some of their relatives may present the same affection.
>
> *J. M. Charcot, Clinical Lectures on Diseases of the Nervous System, 1889.*

The *motor unit* consists of the motor neuron, its axon, the neuromuscular junction, and muscle fibers that this single motor neuron innervates. The size of the motor unit varies greatly: Finely tuned small muscles, such as the extraocular muscles or the stapedius, have a 1:1 ratio, whereas large muscles not requiring such refined control, such as the glutei or quadriceps femoris, have a ratio of 1:200 or more. This chapter discusses disorders of the motor unit, or neuromuscular disorders, and excludes suprasegmental disorders of cerebral origin, such as spasticity, ataxia, and dyskinesias, that are not primary disturbances of the motor unit even though they may profoundly affect muscular function.

Neuromuscular disorders have a limited clinical expression with considerable overlap of symptoms and signs; hence, their definitive diagnosis depends in part on the proper application of laboratory techniques. The procedures used most are serum myogenic enzymes, imaging of muscle, electromyography (EMG), electrophysiologic measurement of motor and sensory nerve conduction velocities, and muscle biopsy. The latter procedure involves histochemistry, immunocytochemistry, biochemistry, and electron microscopy. Advances in genetics now provide molecular genetic markers for many specific diseases that may be diagnosed from a blood sample. Examples include many muscular dystrophies, spinal muscular atrophy (SMA), and several metabolic myopathies. The clinician must decide which of these procedures provides the needed information in the least invasive manner. At times, two procedures are complementary rather than competitive: Nerve conduction velocity and nerve biopsy provide different information. At other times, one procedure confirms another: A blood polymerase chain reaction for Duchenne dystrophy is nondiagnostic in approximately one-third of cases, but the more precise dystrophin immunoreactivity of the muscle biopsy is diagnostic in all cases. Several excellent texts and review chapters deal with disorders of muscle: Engel and Franzini-Armstrong (1), Brooke (2), Dubowitz (3), Swash (4), and Sarnat (5). The best current monograph on pediatric disorders of peripheral nerve is by Ouvrier and colleagues (6).

LABORATORY INVESTIGATION OF NEUROMUSCULAR DISEASE

Muscle Enzymes

Degenerating or necrotic myofibers release several enzymes into the serum because of loss of integrity of the sarcolemmal membrane. These provide useful markers in blood for a few neuromuscular diseases, but not for those in which no degenerative changes occur or the process is so mild that renal clearance can compensate.

The gold standard of muscle enzymes is creatine kinase (CK), previously known as creatine phosphokinase. This enzyme of striated muscle is shared by only two other organs—the cardiac muscle and central nervous system (CNS)—and not by the liver, pancreas, or other viscera. If elevated, isoenzymes may be measured in blood to separate the source: The MM band is striated muscle, MB band is heart, and BB is brain or spinal cord. The upper range of normal serum CK in childhood is approximately 180 IU/L, and the CK usually must be approximately three times normal to be considered significant. Strenuous physical activity always results in a transient increase in serum CK, as shown in studies of athletes, so the enzyme should be measured after a period of relative rest. It also is elevated after traumatic injury of muscle; hence, it should not be measured for at least a week after muscle biopsy or EMG. It is transiently elevated in neonates because of minor contusions of muscle during labor and delivery, but is not elevated in infants delivered by cesarean section unless they have suffered prolonged labor and arrested descent within the maternal pelvis.

The serum CK may be mildly elevated (in the hundreds) in some neuromuscular disorders (e.g., SMA, limb-girdle muscular dystrophy), greatly elevated (in the thousands) in others (e.g., Duchenne and Becker muscular dystrophy, rhabdomyolysis), and remains normal in most (e.g., the congenital myopathies, mitochondrial cytopathies). In some myopathies, it is variable from normal to high (e.g., polymyositis, dermatomyositis), depending on the activity of the inflammation and necrosis. The serum CK is, therefore, not a screening test for neuromuscular diseases, but a normal CK level always excludes Duchenne muscular dystrophy, even in the presymptomatic neonate.

Other *muscle enzymes* are not as specific as CK and may be misleading. The first such serum enzyme discovered was aldolase, but this enzyme is expressed in many tissues, including in red blood cells where it is present in high concentrations. An elevated aldolase out of proportion to CK in the same sample is usually an artifact caused by hemolysis. The transaminases (e.g., aspartate aminotransferase, alanine aminotransferase), often regarded as *liver enzymes*, also are present in muscle, and some children with myopathy have undergone unnecessary liver biopsy for unexplained high liver enzymes because CK was not also measured. Enzymes other than CK rarely contribute to the diagnosis if CK is available.

Imaging of Muscle

In recent years, ultrasonography, computed tomography, and magnetic resonance imaging (MRI) have been applied to muscle in various neuromuscular diseases and indeed may be helpful at times in diagnosing fatty or fibrous connective tissue replacement of muscle and distinguishing edematous or mostly dystrophic myofibers from normal muscle. The most useful of these methods is ultrasound. It is probably the simplest, least invasive, and least expensive (7,8). Plain roentgenography of the extremities may provide useful information about the ratio of the *muscle cylinder* and subcutaneous fat pad and about intramuscular calcifications, but ultrasonography should be reserved for soft tissues, not for bone as in the usual radiographs of the extremities.

Cardiac Evaluation

In some myopathies, cardiomyopathy may be present as well as involvement of striated muscle (e.g., Duchenne muscular dystrophy, Emery-Dreifuss muscular dystrophy, some cases of nemaline rod myopathy), or there may be a disturbance in the Purkinje conduction system (e.g., myotonic muscular dystrophy). Electrocardiography, roentgenography of the chest, and echocardiography may be indicated in selected cases. In muscular dystrophies in which cardiac involvement to some degree is almost universal at some stage in the disease, early consultation with a pediatric cardiologist should be requested, even if the patient is asymptomatic, as a baseline for anticipated future problems.

Molecular Genetic Markers

Several molecular genetic DNA markers in blood now provide definitive diagnoses in specific diseases such as SMA and some cases of Duchenne dystrophy, and may obviate the need for more invasive diagnostic tests such as muscle biopsy. Muscle dystrophin is characterized and quantitated by means of the Western blot test or quantitated by immunohistochemistry or enzyme-linked immunosorbent assay (ELISA) (9). The polymerase chain reaction (PCR) blood test for Duchenne dystrophy is falsely normal, however, in approximately one-third of cases, but the more specific immunocytochemistry of antibodies against various portions of the dystrophin molecule is diagnostic in all cases and must be performed on frozen sections of muscle biopsy tissue. The ratio of myofibers expressing or not expressing dystrophin shown by specific antibodies to the rod domain, N-terminus, and C-terminus of the dystrophin molecule distinguishes Duchenne from Becker dystrophies and also detects the female carrier state and mildly affected girls. Immunocytochemical markers in the muscle biopsy for merosin (congenital muscular dystrophy), the family of sarcoglycans (limb-girdle muscular dystrophy), dystroglycans, collagen VI, dysferlin, caveolin-3 and others are now available as well. Genetic markers for many other diseases undoubtedly will become commercially available in the next few years. These markers have an additional importance in prenatal diagnosis and for the detection of carrier states.

Electrophysiologic Studies

Motor and sensory nerve conduction velocities (NCV) are valuable diagnostic studies of children with neuropathies. They also help to distinguish motor neuron disease from peripheral neuropathy and axonal degeneration from primary demyelination. NCV can be measured in the facial nerve and the phrenic nerve as well as those of the extremities. NCV usually can be performed with surface electrodes on the skin, without the use of needles, and hence are less frightening to the child and are not painful.

EMG requires needle insertion into muscle and is less useful in pediatric conditions than in those of adults. EMG may provide useful information in distinguishing myopathy from neuropathy, but does not generally distinguish the exact type of myopathy; therefore, it is not an alternative to the more specific muscle biopsy in most cases. EMG has the advantage of being able to sample several muscles at one examination, to compare distal and proximal muscles, upper and lower extremities and axial muscles, and any presence of left and right asymmetries. In myopathies, the EMG characteristically shows a shortened mean duration and lower amplitude of the motor unit action potentials. A unique pattern is found in myotonic conditions. In contrast to myopathies, neuropathic patterns are characterized by spontaneous activity at rest and motor unit action potentials of increased duration and amplitude.

EMG with repetitive nerve stimulation (i.e., evoked potential EMG) is a highly specific diagnostic test for myasthenia and is an example of one condition in which EMG is more definitive than the muscle biopsy. Other specialized EMG studies such as macro-EMG and single-fiber EMG recording are available in some centers but are not generally used for clinical diagnosis.

Muscle Biopsy

A muscle biopsy has become the most essential diagnostic procedure in evaluating a child with neuromuscular disease. It is a simple procedure generally performed in day-surgery under local anesthesia with a regional nerve block and does not require a general anesthetic. Needle biopsy has become popular in some centers. It can be performed percutaneously and has the advantage that repeated biopsies may be performed, if necessary (10). However, an open biopsy usually provides a better quality specimen for pathology and any biochemical studies.

The first decision is to choose the muscle to undergo biopsy. The selected muscle should be affected clinically, but not to such an advanced degree that all muscle tissue has degenerated beyond recognition. Additionally, the muscle should not have been subjected to EMG study in the previous 4 to 6 weeks. Because all muscles do not normally have the same ratio of fiber types, this is an additional consideration. The deltoid, for example, normally expresses a 60% to 80% predominance of type I fibers, which at times can complicate interpretation of neurogenic changes. The muscle most studied and generally suitable for the diagnosis of most generalized neuromuscular diseases is the vastus lateralis (i.e., quadriceps femoris), a large proximal muscle not in the region of large blood vessels or major nerves.

The muscle sample is divided, and portions are used for routine examination, histochemistry, electron microscopy, and biochemical or enzymatic studies. For routine histologic examination, a portion of the specimen can be fixed in 10% buffered formalin and embedded in paraffin. For histochemical and most histologic studies, the tissue is frozen in liquid nitrogen and then stored at −70°C. A separate piece of the biopsy should be frozen directly and preserved for possible biochemical studies.

The histochemical reactions generally used, together with their indications, are shown in Table 16.1. Histochemical studies have shown that muscle fibers in human skeletal muscle can be differentiated into two types: type I fibers, which are rich in oxidative enzymes but poorer in glycogen and phosphorylase, and type 2 fibers, weaker in oxidative enzymatic activities but rich in glycogen and phosphorylase. Calcium-mediated myofibrillar adenosine triphosphatase (ATPase) is equally strong in both fiber types, but epitopes are selectively inhibited by changing the pH of preincubation, so that at alkaline pH (10.4 or 9.8) type 2 fibers appear darker than type 1, and at acid pH (4.7 and 4.3) type 1 fibers are darker, with subtypes of 2 appearing as intermediate intensity of staining and thus providing a

TABLE 16.1 Histochemical Reactions for Muscle Biopsies

Stain	*Indication*
Hematoxylin and eosin	General survey
Modified Gomori trichrome	Intermyofibrillar network; Z-bands and nemaline rods
Nicotinamide-adenine dinucleotide (reduced form) dehydrogenase	Mitochondrial respiratory complex I
Succinate dehydrogenase	Mitochondrial respiratory complex II
Cytochrome-c oxidase	Mitochondrial respiratory complex IV
Myofibrillar (calcium-mediated) ATPase; preincubation at pH 4.3, 4.7, and 10.2 (or 9.8)	Fiber types and subtypes
Heavy-chain myosin	Fiber types (applicable to paraffin sections)
Acid phosphatase	Lysosomal enzyme
Alkaline phosphatase	Lysosomal enzyme
Periodic acid–Schiff	Glycogen and polysaccharides
Oil red O	Neutral lipids
Acridine orange fluorochrome	Nucleic acids, regenerating and denervated myofibers
Acetylcholinesterase	Nerve terminals

convenient marker of these subtypes. Type 2C fibers are the least mature type and represent about 5% of fibers in term neonates, more in preterm infants and are infrequent in adult muscle. Normal muscle of children and adults presents a mosaic of both types 1 and 2 fibers. A fuller discussion of histochemical techniques, the histochemistry of developing muscles, and the histologic changes in neurogenic muscular atrophies is presented by Dubowitz (3), Sarnat (5), and Engel and Franzini-Armstrong (1).

Immunocytochemistry has become important in muscle biopsy diagnosis only in the past few years. Frozen sections are required for sarcolemmal region proteins, such as dystrophin, spectrin, merosin, and the sarcoglycans (11). Intermediate filament proteins such as vimentin and desmin are important in some congenital myopathies and can be demonstrated both in frozen and paraffin sections. Heavy-chain myosin immunocytochemistry is the first technique to reliably distinguish fiber types in paraffin sections. Other special purpose immunocytochemical methods include antibodies against actin, tropomyosin, and for marking T and B lymphocytes and macrophages to help distinguish different types of inflammatory myopathies.

Electron microscopy is needed only in selected cases, particularly when there is a question of a mitochondrial myopathy (see Chapter 2). However, tissue submitted for electron microscopy can be used to prepare 1-μ epoxy resin-embedded sections that are suitable for examination in the light microscope after staining with toluidine blue. These thin sections are valuable to confirm the presence of inclusions, such as those seen in a variety of storage diseases, and other details. Thinner sections for electron microscopy usually are stained with uranyl acetate and lead citrate.

Biochemical Studies

In metabolic myopathies, particularly in the glycogenoses and lipid storage myopathies, quantitative assays may be performed on frozen muscle biopsy tissue for specific enzymatic activities, such as acid maltase, myophosphorylase, brancher and debrancher enzymes, phosphofructokinase, and carnitine palmitoyl-transferase. Total muscle glycogen and fat and muscle carnitine content also may be measured. These tests are expensive and not routine; they are requested only if the clinical suspicion is strong and especially if the muscle biopsy histochemistry and ultrastructure support the diagnosis.

The increased awareness of mitochondrial diseases and the large number of different deletions and point mutations involving mtDNA have resulted in a much larger number of muscle biopsies now being performed with the specific question of ruling out a mitochondrial cytopathy. Quantitative analysis of each of the mitochondrial respiratory chain enzymes and of mtDNA can be performed on freshly frozen muscle biopsy tissue if there is sufficiently strong clinical or histochemical and ultrastructural evidence. A few mitochondrial cytopathies fail to exhibit morphologic or histochemical changes, so normal routine biopsy results do not definitively exclude mitochondrial disease, but these cases are only a minority of the mitochondrial cytopathies. Frozen tissue remaining on the block after cutting frozen sections is not suitable for the quantitative analysis of mitochondrial respiratory complexes because the isopentane used to preserve the histologic detail and prevent ice crystal artifacts during the freezing process in liquid nitrogen interferes with the determination of complexes I through III and gives falsely low values. A portion of the muscle biopsy should be freshly frozen directly for possible later biochemical study (see Chapter 2).

DISEASES OF THE MOTOR NEURON

In children, the most common entity affecting the motor neuron in the brainstem and spinal cord is the SMAs. Poliomyelitis, once seen in epidemic proportions, is a rarity in Western countries. Other neurotropic agents including West Nile virus (12) and other enteroviruses that, like poliomyelitis, produce transient or permanent paralysis are considered in Chapter 7. A flaccid paralysis resembling poliomyelitis has been seen in some children who are recovering from an acute episode of asthma (Hopkins syndrome) (see Chapter 17). A familial degenerative disease resembling the adult form of amyotrophic lateral sclerosis (ALS) is encountered rarely in pediatric practice. It is characterized by degeneration of the pyramidal tracts and the motor cells of the spinal cord and brainstem (see Chapter 3). Involvement of the motor neurons as part of generalized storage diseases is observed in some hereditary metabolic diseases such as GM_1 gangliosidosis, Hurler syndrome, infantile Gaucher disease, glycogenosis type II (Pompe), and neuronal ceroid-lipofuscinosis. These entities are considered under their appropriate sections in Chapter 1.

Spinal Muscular Atrophies

The SMAs are a group of relatively common diseases occurring in infancy or early childhood, transmitted by an autosomal recessive gene and manifested by widespread muscular denervation and atrophy (13). Carrier frequency has been estimated to fall between 1 in 50 to 80, and the disease has an overall incidence of 1 in 10,000 to 25,000, making it the second most common hereditary neuromuscular disease after Duchenne dystrophy. Three forms of SMA have been recognized. These are the infantile, acute form (SMA type 1 or Werdnig-Hoffmann disease), the intermediate form (SMA type 2), and the juvenile form (SMA type 3 or Kugelberg-Welander disease). Some workers also have delineated an adult form of SMA (SMA type 4), in which symptoms start after 30 years of age. A severe fetal form of SMA is described as type 0. The muscle biopsy in this entity may present a picture of centronuclear myopathy, thus confusing the diagnosis (13a,b). Approximately one-fourth of cases of SMA fall into the type 1 variety, approximately one-half into type 2, and the remainder into type 3 (2). All three forms are caused by mutations in a gene, the telomeric survival motor neuron gene (*SMN1*) (14). Two copies of the gene are normally present, a telomeric copy, *SMN1*, and a centromeric copy, *SMN2*. The two genes have greater than 99% homology, and their exons differ in but two nucleotides (15). *SMN1* produces a majority of full-length SMN transcript, whereas *SMN2* generates mostly a nonfunctional isoform lacking the carboxy-terminal amino acids encoded by exon 7.

Pathologic Anatomy and Pathogenesis

Both Guido Werdnig, an Austrian neurologist from the University of Graz (16), and Johan Hoffmann, a German neurologist (17), in their original descriptions of the infantile form of SMA, pointed to the conspicuous loss of ventral horn cells along the entire length of the spinal cord. Some of the residual motor neurons are in the process of degenerating or are being phagocytized by microglial cells. Motor neurons in the brainstem, notably in the hypoglossal and motor trigeminal nuclei also are affected. Those cranial nerves innervating extraocular muscles and sacral motor nerves innervating the striated muscle of the urethral and rectal sphincters are selectively spared. Some authors describe suprasegmental lesions, including loss of large pyramidal cells from layers 5 and 6 of the motor cortex. These findings must be interpreted in light of the severe agonal anoxia that is commonly encountered. In general, the absence of upper motor neuron involvement is an important clinical feature that distinguishes SMAs from degenerative motor neuron diseases such as ALS.

More than 95% of patients experiencing the various forms of SMA have a homozygous deletion or absence of exons 7 and 8 for both copies of the *SMN1* gene (13). Subjects who do not have detectable deletions have microdeletions or point mutations in the gene, or have their *SMN1* gene converted to *SMN2* (18,19). In some patients with SMA types 2 and 3, *SMN1* is not deleted; rather, it is replaced by *SMN2*, the reverse form of "gene conversion" (19,20). Two other genes have been mapped to the SMA critical region. Homozygous deletions of neuronal apoptosis inhibitory protein gene (*NAIP*) are seen in up to 69% of patients with SMA type 1. By contrast, only some 12% to 18% of patients with SMA types 2 and 3 are deleted for this gene (21). A third gene in this region, shown to encode a subunit of the basal transcription factor (*TFIIH*) is deleted in approximately 15% of all types of SMA (21). *NAIP* and *TFIIH* as well as a multicopy microsatellite marker in close proximity to *SMN1* have been proposed as SMA-modifying genes (22,23).

The genetic basis for the phenotypic variability of SMA is not completely clear. About one-half of severely affected *SMA1* children also miss both homologues of a neighboring gene, the gene for neuronal apoptosis inhibitory protein (*NAIP*). Milder forms of SMA appear to have more than two copies of *SMN2*, and in asymptomatic or late-onset subjects with homozygous deletion of the *SMN1* gene, there were four copies of the *SMN2* gene (24,25).

The SMN protein is widely expressed in the cytoplasm and nucleus of brain, the motor neurons, and in a variety of non-CNS tissues (26). In the nucleoplasm the SMN protein is localized to discrete bodies called "gems" where it forms a stable complex with a group of proteins called the gamins (27). This complex is intimately involved in the assembly of spliceosomal small nuclear ribonucleoproteins, which function in the splicing of RNA. The reason for the effect of gene mutation on the spinal motor neurons is still unclear, and it is not known whether symptoms result from deficiencies in SMA functions that are specific to the motor neuron, or common to all cells but at a higher demand in the motor neuron. One attractive hypothesis is that SMN protein has an antiapoptotic effect (28), suggesting that that SMA is a primary disorder of apoptosis, with the condition representing a physiologic process that becomes pathologic because of continued degeneration of motor neurons in late fetal life as well as postnatally (29,30).

Prominent glial proliferation often occurs in the proximal portion of the anterior spinal roots, an abnormality initiated in fetal life, and which was thought to induce secondary neuronal degeneration (31). In some instances, the glial bundles also are demonstrated in the posterior roots, accompanied by shrinkage of the dorsal root ganglion cells (32). An inconstant finding in SMA is loss of myelin from the posterior columns of thoracic and lumbar segments and in the corticospinal tracts (33). These phenomena are now believed to be secondary reactive changes. Removal of the peripheral target of the anterior horn cells accentuates the normal process of motor neuron apoptosis (34–36), but there is no evidence that the primary disorder in this disease is in the muscle target or that there is a distal-to-proximal *dying-back* axonal degeneration in the nerve.

There is selective loss of the large motor neurons, but a striking preservation of several types of motor neurons, notably some of the cervical cord (37) and those innervating extraocular muscles. This histologic contrast is expressed clinically as preservation of normal eye movements, even in late stages of the disease. Some genes that program the differentiation and maintenance of motor neurons are expressed in all motor neurons, whereas others are expressed only in certain motor neurons and may provide a protective effect on oculomotor neurons by the principle of genetic redundancy (see Chapter 5 on neuroembryology).

Clinical Manifestations

The clinical picture of SMA is marked by reduction of muscle power and spontaneous movement (38). Muscle

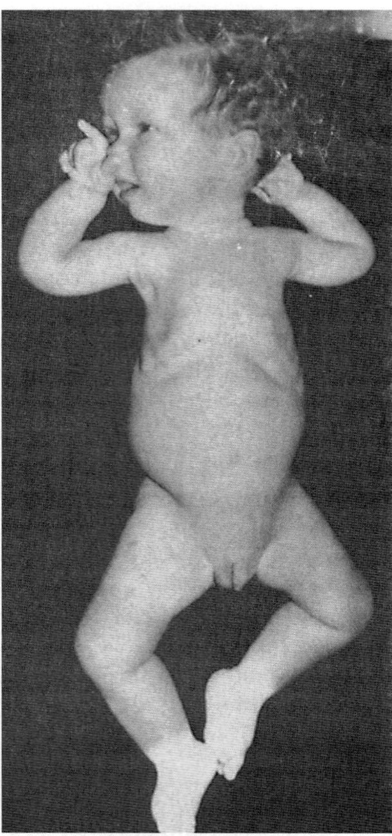

FIGURE 16.1. A 1-year-old infant with severe spinal muscular atrophy showing intercostal recession and diaphragmatic breathing. Note frog-leg posture, ability to flex elbows and move hands, and normal facial expression. (Courtesy of Professor Victor Dubowitz, Royal Postgraduate Medical School, London.)

weakness is symmetric and is more extensive in the proximal part of the limbs, and what little movement is left to the child is found in the small muscles of the hands and feet. At the same time, the affected muscles undergo atrophy, although this is concealed by the subcutaneous fat normally seen at this age. Muscles of the trunk, neck, and thorax are affected equally, but the diaphragm generally is spared until the late stages of the disease (39) (Fig. 16.1). Cardiac and smooth muscles are usually spared as well. With progression of the disease, involvement of bulbar musculature becomes more prominent, and atrophy and fasciculation of the tongue are noted. Deep tendon reflexes are nearly always markedly reduced or absent. There is no intellectual retardation or sphincter disturbance. Sensory nerve involvement has been demonstrated by nerve conduction studies and confirmed by demonstration of axonal loss on sural nerve biopsy and autopsy. Hypertrophy of unmyelinated axons of the sural nerve also is frequent (29). These sensory nerve changes have not been observed in SMA types 2 and 3 (40,41).

TABLE 16.2 Age of First Clinical Manifestations in Infantile Spinal Muscular Atrophy

Age	*Percent of Cases*
Newborn	37
0–1 month	10
1–3 months	12
3–6 months	6
6–9 months	12
9–12 months	9
More than 1 year	8

Modified from Brandt S. *Werdnig-Hoffmann's infantile progressive muscular atrophy.* Copenhagen: Ejnar Munksgaard, 1950.

The age at which the first clinical manifestations become apparent is presented in Table 16.2. It is evident from this table that there are at least two populations, one with onset of symptoms before 6 months of age, SMA type 1, and another with its onset after 6 months of age, SMA types 2 and 3. About 10% of infants with SMA type 1 are born with arthrogryposis, and this may indicate the severe fetal form recently designated type 0 (13a,b).

In SMA type 1 (infantile SMA, Werdnig-Hoffmann disease), the onset is acute, and the disease progresses rapidly. Infants who were already severely hypotonic at birth rarely survive the first year of life, whereas those whose weakness appears postnatally tend to deteriorate more slowly (42,43). Some infants can even experience transient improvement. This improvement is partly caused by a true stationary period in the disease, such as was already noted by Hoffmann in one of his earliest patients (17). Maturation of partially paralyzed muscles also can give the impression of improvement. In most instances, however, the disease is fatal by 3 years of age, with death generally resulting from a respiratory infection.

Children who experience SMA type 2 [29% in Brandt's series (38), 47% in the more recent series (2)] develop normally for the first 6 months of life, but by 18 months of age experience an arrest of their motor milestones. These children generally lack bulbar symptoms, and their disease has a less malignant course (43). One unusual feature of this form of SMA is the presence of a tremor that affects the upper extremities (44) and can even be recorded on the electrocardiogram as a tremor of the baseline (45). Serum CK activity is elevated to approximately five times normal in approximately one-half of these patients but is never in the thousands of units as in muscular dystrophy; hypertrophy of the gastrocnemius is not unusual (46).

SMA type 3, a milder form of SMA consistent with survival into adult life, was first described by Wohlfart and coworkers (47) and by Kugelberg and Welander (48). Muscular weakness develops after 18 months of age, and in some patients does not manifest until adult life. Adult onset SMA is referred to as SMA type 4. It is characterized by involvement of the predominantly proximal muscles and thus bears close clinical resemblance to the muscular dystrophies. Unlike SMA types 1 and 2, impaired joint mobility is relatively common. The condition is differentiated from Duchenne muscular dystrophy by a less striking elevation in muscle enzymes, and from the other types of muscular dystrophies by the alterations seen on muscle biopsy (see Muscle Biopsy, later in this chapter). In some families, SMA types 1 and 2, or types 2 and 3, coexist. This observation represents a genetic puzzle because haplotype analysis has shown that this variability cannot be accounted for by different alleles at the SMA locus (49).

In some families, a condition that clinically resembles Kugelberg-Welander disease is transmitted in an autosomal dominant manner (50). X-linked pedigrees also have been reported. Hexosaminidase A deficiency can resemble Kugelberg-Welander disease, but patients demonstrate mental deterioration (51) (see Chapter 1).

A condition in which spinal muscular atrophy presents with early respiratory distress, and in which there also is intrauterine growth retardation, foot deformities, early involvement of the diaphragm, and a predominance of distal muscular weakness can be distinguished from SMA type 1. The gene for this condition has been mapped to chromosome 11 q13–q21. It encodes the immunoglobulin binding protein 2 (52).

Diagnosis

Genetic Studies

The definitive diagnosis may now be made by the marker in blood of the *SMN* gene that usually shows deletions of exons 7 and 8 (18). Thus, in the series of van der Steege and colleagues, the *SMN1* gene, as determined by PCR, was homozygously absent or interrupted in 98.6% of SMA patients (53). An additional gene mapped to 11q13–q21 in SMA may help explain early respiratory failure in some patients (53a). Muscle biopsy, which until only recently had been the diagnostic standard, can therefore be avoided in most patients, with exception of the small fraction whose molecular genetic test results are negative or uninformative.

Biochemical Studies

The study of serum enzymes is important in the differential diagnosis of motor neuron disease. Serum CK is often normal in SMA type 1 but may be elevated in the hundreds, although never in the thousands. It usually is normal or only slightly elevated in the other types. The excretion of amino acids and creatine is generally normal during the early stages of the illness. None of these features is definitively diagnostic of SMA.

Neurophysiologic Studies

EMG findings help to confirm the clinical diagnosis of motor neuron disease. Characteristically, the denervated muscles contract spontaneously, involving single muscle fibers (fibrillation) or entire motor units (fasciculation) (54). The finding most specific for the disease and not observed in any other condition marked by muscular denervation is the presence of spontaneous, rhythmic muscle activity at a frequency of 5 to 15 per second, which can be activated by voluntary effort. This abnormality can be recorded in approximately 75% of patients, irrespective of age or severity of disease (55). In addition, the residual motor unit potentials are polyphasic and increased in amplitude and duration. With increased muscular effort, little increase occurs in the frequency of discharge and recruitment is impaired. Conduction velocity in the motor nerves is decreased in the more severely affected children (56). This is because of the preferential involvement of the largest motor neurons, which also have the most myelinated and fastest-conducting axons.

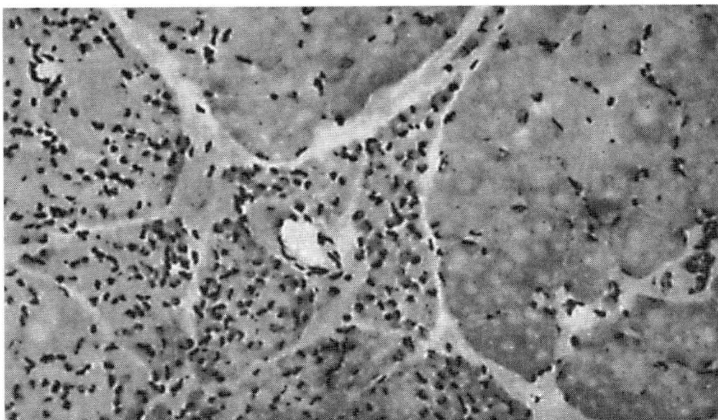

FIGURE 16.2. Transverse section of muscle from a patient with Werdnig-Hoffmann disease. Note the relative preservation of muscle fibers in the right side of the field and atrophy of fibers on the left (hematoxylin and eosin, × 20). (Courtesy of Dr. P. Cancilla, Department of Pathology, University of California, Los Angeles, UCLA School of Medicine.)

Muscle Biopsy

Chemical analyses for glycogen, lipids, glycolytic enzymes, and mitochondrial enzymes are performed, with the selection of assays dictated by the clinical presentation.

In SMAs, a biopsy shows the classic features of denervation atrophy (Fig. 16.2), but perinatal denervation shows unique features not seen in neurogenic atrophy of mature muscle. Large patches of small, atrophic fibers of both histochemical types are present, and both scattered and grouped muscle fibers of exclusively type I also are present. The normal mosaic or *chessboard* pattern is lost. This uniformity of fiber type reflects an ongoing compensatory reinnervation (3). Electron microscopy adds little additional diagnostic information except to demonstrate scattered immature myofibers including myotubes (29, 54a). The myofilaments are loosened, and mitochondria are diminished in number and show atrophic cristae. Muscle biopsies showing the perinatal pattern of denervation-reinnervation nearly always signify SMA but are not definitively diagnostic because rare perinatal polyneuropathies may yield a similar picture.

TABLE 16.3 Diagnosis of 107 Cases of Floppy Infant[a]

Diagnosis	Number of Cases
Infantile muscular atrophy	67
Congenital muscular dystrophy	3
Polymyositis	1
Myasthenia gravis	1
Scurvy	2
Cerebral disease (atonic cerebral palsy)	14
"Benign congenital hypotonia"	17

[a]Complete recovery in eight patients.
Modified from Walton JH. The limp child. *J Neurol Neurosurg Psychiatry* 1957;20:144.

Differential Diagnosis

The presenting signs of the infant with SMA type 1 (Werdnig-Hoffmann disease) are poor muscle tone and a marked delay in motor development. Because a variety of well-defined diseases present the picture of the floppy infant (Table 16.3), differential diagnosis on purely clinical grounds can be difficult. Unlike Walton writing in 1957 (57), we have found the most common cause for diminished muscle tone in a small infant to be *atonic cerebral palsy*, often secondary to cerebellar hypoplasia. Hypotonia also may result from major abnormalities of the cerebrum, both developmental malformations and disorders acquired in the perinatal period. Invariably, affected infants have considerable intellectual retardation. Spontaneous movements are present, and the tendon reflexes are easily elicited. Often when the infant is lifted by the trunk, the legs promptly become rigid, and a striking accentuation of the extensor thrust reflex is seen. Although some of these children remain hypotonic, others develop dyskinesias or a clear-cut hypertonia within 1 to 3 years. A more extensive discussion of this condition is found in Chapter 6.

Amyotonia congenita, now an obsolete term, was a clinical syndrome reported briefly in a single case by Oppenheim in 1900 (58). It represents a number of unrelated disease processes. It is important to differentiate these entities, now collectively termed *congenital myopathies* (benign congenital hypotonias), from the usually fatal SMA type 1. The term *congenital myopathy* is used to describe floppy infants with a marked delay in motor development. Some of these children recover completely, whereas others can be considered to have a stationary or, at worst, a slowly progressive muscular disorder. In these infants, the muscles are soft and flabby, and a remarkable range of passive movement is possible. Deep tendon reflexes are elicitable, and spontaneous movements are more prominent than in SMA type 1. Respiratory muscles are involved only slightly, and intellectual development is usually normal. Histochemical and electron microscopic studies of muscle biopsies have delineated numerous distinct entities, many of which demonstrate specific genetic mutations (see Congenital Myopathies, later in this chapter).

A relatively common clinical problem is that of a floppy infant with delayed gross motor milestones, notably delayed walking, but with normal or nearly normal fine motor development and speech and no demonstrable muscular disorder. This heterogeneous entity, termed *congenital laxity of ligaments* by the late Dr. Frank Ford (59), has more recently been designated as *dissociated motor development* (60) or *benign maturation delay* (61).

In a series of such infants reported by Lundberg, 52% achieved normal development between 17 months and 6 years of age (60). A further 24% continued to have delayed motor milestones without any apparent cause. Ultimately, 15% were found to have mild mental retardation. The remaining infants experienced various neuromuscular disorders, notably congenital deafness with hypoactive labyrinths and macrocephaly (61,62). Muscle biopsy revealed fiber size disproportion and showed a predominance of type 1 fibers, which persisted despite clinical improvement (61). Dissociated motor development should be distinguished from the less common Ehlers-Danlos syndromes, which are characterized by marked hyperelasticity of skin.

The syndrome of congenital fiber type disproportion (Table 16.4) (63–84) is part of a broader spectrum of muscle dysmaturation. Type 1 fibers are uniformly small and also more numerous than type 2 fibers that often exhibit compensatory hypertrophy. Many infants who demonstrate dysmaturation of muscle, particularly when type 2 fibers are affected, also have significant developmental retardation (85).

Rarer causes for infantile hypotonia include various forms of congenital or neonatal myasthenia gravis, some of which can be diagnosed by the striking improvement in muscle strength after administration of an anticholinesterase drug. For diagnostic purposes, a slowly metabolized drug, such as neostigmine administered subcutaneously or intramusculary, but never intravenously, is more suitable for infants than edrophonium chloride, whose effectiveness is often too fleeting to allow correct sequential assessment of muscle strength. Muscular dystrophy is only rarely seen in a small infant, but in no other condition is a significant elevation in serum enzymes, particularly in CK, common. In the absence of a family history of a dystrophic process, the diagnosis depends mainly on a muscle biopsy.

Finally, infantile botulism (see Chapter 10), Down syndrome, transection of the spinal cord, congenital polyneuritis, muscular hypotonia owing to Marfan syndrome or Prader-Willi syndrome, various chronic illnesses, malnutrition, or metabolic disorders (e.g., organic acidurias and mitochondrial disorders) also must be considered in the differential diagnosis of the hypotonic child.

TABLE 16.4 Some Congenital Myopathies

Myopathy	*Characteristic Clinical Features*	*Muscle Biopsy Abnormalities*	*Reference*
Nemaline	Dominant or recessive sporadic transmission; associated skeletal dysmorphism; respiratory problems	Rodlike expansions of Z-band	Shy et al. (63)
Central core disease	Dominant or sporadic transmission; associated congenital dislocation of hips	Central area of fiber devoid of mitochondria; myofibril disruption variable; defect in muscle ryanodine receptor	Shuaib et al. (64), Lynch et al. (65)
Myotubular (centronuclear)	Ptosis; weak external ocular muscles; usually sex-linked	Most fibers with one or more central nuclei	Spiro et al. (66), Kioschis et al. (67)
Multicore (minicore) disease	Nonprogressive proximal weakness; neck muscle weakness	Multiple small areas of severe filament disruption devoid of mitochondrial enzymes	Heffner et al. (68)
Congenital fiber type disproportion	Variable clinical picture; muscle contractures; congenital dislocation of hips; facial weakness; high palate; hypotonia more marked than weakness; may be autosomal recessive, autosomal dominant, or sporadic	Type 1 fibers uniformly smaller than type 2; increased variability in fiber diameter; also seen in Krabbe leukodystrophy, fetal alcohol syndrome, Pompe disease, myotonic dystrophy, result of abnormal suprasegmental influence on fetal motor unit (e.g., cerebellar hypoplasia)	Dubowitz (45), Cavanagh et al. (69), Dehkharganl et al. (70), Sarnat (71)
Fingerprint	Tremors; mental retardation	Subsarcolemmal inclusions resembling fingerprints; also found in myotonic dystrophy; dermatomyositis	Engel et al. (72)
Sarcotubular	None	Dilated and fragmented sarcotubules in type 2 fibers	Jerusalem et al. (73)
Zebra body	None	Unique bodies on electron microscopy	Lake and Wilson (74)
Reducing body	None	Inclusions rich in sulfhydryl groups and RNA	Brooke and Neville (75)
Trilaminar	Rigidity of muscle tone gradually disappearing with age; increased serum creatine kinase	Distinctive three-zone fibers by histochemistry and electron microscopy	Ringel et al. (76)
Tubular aggregate	Cramps; muscle pain; proximal limb weakness; autosomal dominant	Tubular aggregates in subsarcolemmal region	Rohkamm et al. (77)
Cytoplasmic body	Progressive proximal muscle weakness; autosomal dominant or recessive	Inclusions in subsarcolemmal region	Goebel et al. (78), Mitrani-Rosenbaum et al. (79)
Cylindrical spiral	Cramps; percussion myotonia; autosomal dominant	Cylindric spirals	Bove et al. (80)
Myopathy with excessive autophagy	Early onset; affects proximal muscles; slow progresion, marked creatine kinase elevation; sex-linked	Increased number of autophagic vacuoles	Kalimo et al. (81)
Polysaccharide storage myopathy	Proximal myopathy; no demonstrable abnormality of glycogen pathway	Branched-chain polysaccharides and mucoprotein storage	Thompson et al. (82)
Desmin storage myopathy	Congenital proximal myopathy; cardiomyopathy starting at any age; autosomal dominant distal myopathy	Intrasarcoplasmic accumulation of electron-dense granulofilamentous material, staining for desmin, an intermediate filament protein	Horowitz and Schmalbruch (83), Goldfarb et al. (84)

Several rare conditions are transmitted as autosomal recessive traits in which amyotrophy of the limbs and of the bulbar musculature are combined with progressive pyramidal tract symptoms (juvenile ALS). These conditions are reviewed in Chapter 3.

Treatment

Treatment for SMA is purely symptomatic and is of no value in altering the course of infantile SMA type 1. In the forms with slower progression, treatment should be directed at maintaining joint mobility and avoiding contractures. The child should be fitted with a lightweight support for the spine to prevent kyphoscoliosis. If at all possible, the youngster should be encouraged to walk with braces. Active exercise can help strengthen still functioning muscles (2,45). Dysphagia may be a late complication in some patients, and aspiration is a risk.

Several workers have suggested that *SMN2* gene expression can be increased by administration of 4-phenylbutyrate, an inhibitor of histone deacetylase, an enzyme that promotes transcriptional repression (86). This compound has been proposed for the treatment of SMA 1.

Arthrogryposis

Arthrogryposis refers to a syndrome of multiple congenital and nonprogressive contractures of the joints that are fixed in flexion or, less commonly, in extension, accompanied by diminution and wasting of skeletal muscle. The term is derived from the Greek "hooked joint." The condition can be seen in isolation or can be accompanied by a variety of other congenital malformations, particularly clubfoot and cerebral maldevelopment (87,88).

Arthrogryposis appears to have several causes, all involving impaired fetal mobility (89). These can be categorized as myopathic, neuropathic, connective tissue disorders, and exogenous effects. Hall has classified arthrogryposis into conditions where there is primarily limb involvement, those in which there is limb involvement plus other body areas, and those in which there is limb and CNS involvement (88). In one group of infants (25% of an English series) (90), the neuromuscular apparatus was normal, and arthrogryposis was caused by external mechanical factors. Such factors include a malformed uterus (e.g., bicornuate uterus), the treatment of maternal tetanus with muscle relaxants, or oligohydramnios (e.g., Potter syndrome). In the majority of infants, arthrogryposis results from a neuromuscular or a combined cerebral and neuromuscular disorder (89,90). The most common of these disorders is one in which the large anterior horn cells are markedly reduced, the muscle fibers are small and often hyalinized, and the EMG abnormalities are consistent with denervation (91). In contrast to the SMAs, no gliosis occurs, and the small neurons in the ventral horn of the spinal cord are preserved or even increased in number (92). In the experience of Quinn and colleagues, neurogenic arthrogryposis constituted 30% of cases (93). A neurogenic arthrogryposis with velopharyngeal incompetence is associated with a deletion at 22q11.2 (93a).

In other cases of arthrogryposis, the changes are compatible with congenital muscular dystrophy (94), congenital myotonic dystrophy (95), congenital myasthenic syndrome (96), fibrosis of the anterior spinal roots, or evidence of embryonic denervation and maturation arrest of muscle (95). Such cases constituted 60% of subjects with arthrogryposis who came to autopsy (93).

The prevalence of the condition varies considerably, ranging from 1:3000 in Canada to 1:12,000 in Western Australia to 1:56,000 in Edinburgh (87,97). Even though autosomal dominant, autosomal recessive, and X-linked transmission have been well documented, a viral or toxic etiology is likely in the majority of cases. In at least one instance, maternal antibodies against the fetal form of the acetylcholine receptor (AChR) were demonstrated, and plasma from anti-AChR antibody–positive mothers who had borne offspring with severe arthrogryposis induced fixed joints in neonatal mice when injected into pregnant dams (98).

Arthrogryposis is marked by multiple and severe flexion and extension contractures of all extremities, notably the hips, elbows, and fingers. Skin creases are absent, an indication of early intrauterine onset (87), and approximately one-fourth of affected infants have contractures of the temporomandibular joint. These contractures produce the typical round face and micrognathia (99). In one variant, amyoplasia, the shoulders are internally rotated, the elbows are extended, the wrists are flexed, and the hands are clenched. In the lower extremities, the knees are generally flexed, and the feet are maintained in an equinovarus position. Some 10% to 30% of patients have various superimposed developmental malformations of the CNS (89).

In Pena-Shokeir syndrome I, a heterogeneous condition, arthrogryposis is accompanied by facial anomalies, pulmonary hypoplasia, intrauterine growth retardation, and a variety of cerebral malformations. There is a paucity of motor neurons and muscular atrophy (100). Pena-Shokeir syndrome type II manifests by arthrogryposis not associated with deficiency of motor neurons but is accompanied by microcephaly, ocular defects, and a variety of skeletal abnormalities (101). Several other malformation syndromes, some with chromosomal disorders, can be accompanied by arthrogryposis. These are listed in review articles by Hageman and coworkers (89), O'Flaherty (87), and Hall (102) and in the text by Jones (103).

Hall and coworkers (102,104) and Staheli and coworkers (105) distinguish several conditions termed *distal arthrogryposis*, which, in contrast to the proximal arthrogryposes, tend to be genetically transmitted and are marked by congenital contractures of hands and feet. The hand of such infants is characteristically tightly fisted with tight adduction of the thumb and medial overlapping of the fingers, similar to the position of the hand in the trisomy 18 syndrome (see Chapter 4). In some families, distal arthrogryposis is dominantly inherited and appears sporadically in others. A condition termed *distal arthrogryposis type II* also can have involvement of the proximal limb joints and associated congenital anomalies. In a significant proportion of families, arthrogryposis type II is dominantly inherited. One of the more common dominantly inherited conditions is the Freeman-Sheldon ("whistling facies") syndrome, in which arthrogryposis and a characteristic "whistling facies" is accompanied by microcephaly, mental retardation, and seizures (105,106). Generally, patients with distal arthrogryposis have a better prognosis in terms of limb function than those with mainly proximal joint involvement.

The reduced fetal movements of arthrogryposis permit an *in utero* diagnosis by ultrasonography and, if necessary, by fetoscopy (107).

Treatment of arthrogryposis should commence immediately after birth, with passive motion exercises, braces, and casts (87). Subsequently, surgery is usually necessary, particularly for contractions of the lower extremities and hips. These procedures are contraindicated in the presence of considerable weakness and amyoplasia. Generally, functional improvement of extension contractures is better than that of flexion contractures, and arthrogryposis secondary to maternal factors has a better outlook than that owing to neuromuscular disorders (102,108). In selected cases, a muscle biopsy may be indicated to rule out myopathies, such as congenital muscular dystrophy, often associated with multiple congenital contractures.

DISEASES OF THE AXON

Disorders of the axon result from genetic, infectious, postinfectious, traumatic, or toxic processes, and are, therefore, best discussed under their respective headings (see Chapters 3, 7, 8, 9, and 10, respectively).

In the differential diagnosis of muscular weakness, a polyneuritic process should always be considered. Although, supposedly, the presence of sensory loss in the affected area would easily distinguish polyneuritis from other disorders of the motor unit, an isolated motor neuropathy is far from rare. Commonly, motor weakness can overshadow sensory disturbances, the latter being particularly difficult to demonstrate in infants.

In general, the polyneuritides have a rapid onset, a feature they share only with the inflammatory muscular disorders: polymyositis and dermatomyositis. The site of muscular involvement is often a clue to the cause of the weakness; whereas the SMAs and the muscular dystrophies involve the proximal musculature preferentially, the polyneuritides usually affect the distal musculature. Ascending paralysis such as was originally described by Landry, Guillain, and Barré (see Chapter 8) is uncommon in infants. As a result of the predilection of the polyneuritides for the distal musculature, ankle reflexes are lost early in the illness; in the muscular dystrophies, they are retained.

The distinction between infectious polyneuritis and the hereditary motor and sensory neuropathies rests on the slower evolution of the neuropathies, their frequent association with skeletal deformities or cerebellar involvement, and the presence of a similar neuropathic condition in other members of the immediate family. In approximately two-thirds of children with infectious polyneuritis, the spinal fluid is abnormal. A classic picture of albuminocytologic dissociation, namely an elevated protein level in the absence of a cellular response, is common during the first 2 to 8 weeks of the illness. Motor nerve conduction times are usually slowed, although they can be normal during the initial phases of infectious polyneuritis. Although slowed motor conduction time, when present, is characteristic of infectious polyneuritis, it also can be seen with severe atrophy in anterior horn cell disease (poliomyelitis, West Nile encephalitis, and SMA type 1). In approximately one-half of the patients, the sensory nerve conduction times also are delayed. The histologic changes in affected muscle are rarely significant during the acute phase of infectious polyneuritis, whereas in chronic polyneuritis, the main abnormality is a widespread muscular atrophy.

DISEASES OF THE NEUROMUSCULAR JUNCTION

Myasthenia Gravis

Myasthenia gravis, a chronic disease characterized by unusual fatigability of voluntary muscles, was first described by Willis in 1672 (109). Three forms of myasthenia gravis are seen in childhood: juvenile myasthenia gravis, congenital myasthenia gravis, and transient neonatal myasthenia gravis. Aside from age of onset, there is no difference in terms of pathology and pathogenesis between juvenile myasthenia gravis and adult-onset myasthenia gravis.

Pathologic Anatomy

Microscopic changes in myasthenia gravis can be minute, even in severely affected muscles. On electron microscopy, the nerve terminals are small, and the cleft between the nerve and the subneural apparatus is widened. Additionally, the area reactive for acetylcholinesterase is reduced, but with no abnormality in the number or size of synaptic vesicles. In 70% to 80% of patients, there are pathologic changes in the thymus. Usually, these consist of lymphoid hyperplasia. Although thymomas occur in approximately 10% of all patients with myasthenia, they are rare in childhood. Myocardial abnormalities have been found in approximately half of autopsied patients.

Pathogenesis

The functional lesion in juvenile myasthenia gravis is located at the neuromuscular junction and is the consequence of an antibody-mediated autoimmune reaction against the postsynaptic acetylcholine receptors (AChR) in skeletal muscle (110). By contrast, the autoimmune response in Eaton-Lambert syndrome, a myasthenic syndrome seen almost exclusively in adults harboring a malignancy (most commonly a small cell carcinoma of the bronchus), is directed against the voltage-sensitive calcium channels on the presynaptic membrane.

Antibodies to the AChR protein have been demonstrated in the serum of a large proportion of patients with generalized juvenile myasthenia gravis (111), and the electrophysiologic features of the disease can be reproduced in animals by repeated injections of IgG derived from myasthenic subjects or by antibodies against the AChR (112). Several lines of evidence indicate that antibody production against AChR is T-cell dependent. Serum antibodies against AChR are usually absent in congenital myasthenia gravis (but not in the maternally transmitted neonatal form) and in many cases of myasthenia, that is limited to extraocular muscle involvement. A significant proportion of the small number of juvenile myasthenics who are AChR antibody negative have antibodies against a receptor tyrosine kinase (MuSK). MuSK has been localized to the neuromuscular junction and appears to be vital to its *in utero* development (112,113). Children and adults with anti-MuSK antibodies exhibit weakness of extraocular, pharyngeal and respiratory muscles and later should have shoulder girdle weakness. Plasma exchange and prednisone often are effective treatments, but cholinesterase inhibitors and thymectomy appear ineffective (113a). Some patients with congenital myasthenia gravis have been demonstrated to have anti-MuSK antibodies (113b). Still other congenital myasthenic infants with episodic apnea show mutations in the cholin acetyltransferase (*CHAT*) gene (113c).

By means of snake venom (bungarotoxin, which binds specifically to the AChR), AChRs have been localized to the postsynaptic folds. Myasthenic subjects show a 70% to 90% reduction in the number of functional AChR (114). The gross destruction of the AChR area, seen in subjects with long-standing myasthenia gravis, is probably the consequence of a cellular immune reaction. Three possible processes have been postulated to be operative: a complement-mediated lysis of the postsynaptic membrane, an IgG-induced accelerated rate of degradation by endocytosis of cross-linked acetylcholine receptors, or an antibody-mediated blockage of the active site of the receptors (112,114).

The factors that induce and sustain an autoimmune reaction against the AChR are still unknown, although there are some hints about the nature of the process. Administration of penicillamine to patients with rheumatoid arthritis can induce myasthenia that is reversible within a few months after withdrawal of the medication. Whereas this observation suggests an alteration of the AChR because of exogenous factors, Lindstrom and coworkers believe that patients with myasthenia gravis respond to some endogenous source of native AChR, rather than to a bacterial or viral coat protein that would not have the identical autoantibody specifications (110).

The initial anti-AChR sensitization probably occurs in the thymus. Extracts of thymic tissue have been found to contain acetylcholine receptors that are localized to myoid cells present in that tissue (115), and thymocytes of myasthenic patients produce AChR antibodies (116). In most instances, these antibodies are specific for the embryonic AChR (117). Whereas an environmental factor might initiate an immune response against the AChR in the thymus of genetically predisposed subjects, examination by immunofluorescence of thymus derived from patients with myasthenia gravis does not show these cells to be the foci of immunologic stimulation (118). Alternatively, a possibly viral-induced derangement of function or communication between the various types of cells that regulate the intensity and duration of an immune reaction (immune regulation) might be responsible for the breakdown in tolerance to AChR protein.

What appears most likely at present is that autoimmune myasthenia gravis is a heterogeneous group of diseases distinguishable by their clinical features, notably the age at onset of the illness and by their human leukocyte antigen types, with each entity having a different pathogenetic mechanism. Thus, in some 10% to 15% of adult myasthenic patients, antibodies against AChR cannot be detected, and evidence suggests that in these subjects, antibodies are directed to other parts of the end-plate, such as MuSK, rather than to the AChR (119). The immunopathology has been reviewed by Hughes and colleagues (120).

Whereas juvenile myasthenia gravis, like adult myasthenia gravis, appears to result from T-cell initiated antibodies directed against end-plate AChR protein, neonatal myasthenia is associated with the transfer of maternal AChR antibodies across the placenta. However, the story is not as simple as this. Maternal AChR antibodies are found in all infants of myasthenic mothers, whether infants are symptomatic or not, and myasthenic symptoms in an infant are not proportional to the amount of antibodies transferred to it from the mother (121,122). Rather, neonatal myasthenia appears to correlate with persistence of antibodies, possibly as a consequence of antibody synthesis by the myasthenic infant.

TABLE 16.5 Myasthenic Conditions of Infancy and Childhood

Condition	Clinical Features or Reference
Juvenile myasthenia	Girls more commonly affected, most have AChR antibodies
Neonatal myasthenia	Transient, affects 20% of infants of myasthenic mothers
Congenital myasthenia (CM)	
Presynaptic defects	
Choline acetyltransferase deficiency	Episodes of bulbar weakness triggered by stress or infections (128)
Paucity of synaptic vesicles	Only one known case (129)
Lambert-Eaton syndrome–like CM	Severe hypotonia; EMG reveals blocking that improves with increased rate of stimulation (130)
Synaptic defects	
Endplate ACh esterase deficiency	AR mutations of *ColQ*, the gene coding for tail of ACh esterase molecule; weakness, slowed papillary response to light, no response or worsens with ChE inhibitors; mutations in each of the domains described (131)
Postsynaptic defects	
Primary AChR deficiency with or without kinetic abnormality	
Reduced AChR expression due to AChR mutations	Severity varies and may improve with time (132)
Reduced AChR expression due to rapsyn mutations	Ptosis; weak facial, bulbar, limb muscles; good response to AChE treatment (133)
Reduced AChR expression with plectin deficiency	Epidermolysis bullosa; progressive ocular, facial, trunk weakness (134)
Primary AChR kinetic abnormality with or without AChR deficiency	
Slow-channel CM	Most common CM syndrome; neck muscles and distal regions of upper limbs more affected; worsens with ChE inhibitors; most are AD (135)
Fast-channel CM	Ptosis, ophthalmoplegia, dysphagia (136)
Sodium-channel CM	Single case: ptosis, bulbar and generalized weakness (137)

Ach, acetyl choline; ChE, choline esterase; AChR, acetylcholine receptor; rapsyn, receptor-associated protein at synapse; AD, autosomal dominant.
From Harper CM. Congenital myasthenic syndromes. *Semin Neurol* 2004;24:111–123.

Clinical Manifestations

> Before noon, the stores of the spirit which influenced the muscle being almost spent, they are scarcely able to move hand and foot. . . . [T]his person for some time speaks freely and readily enough, but after long, hasty or laborious speaking, presently she becomes mute as a fish and cannot bring forth a word.
>
> —*T. Willis (109)*

In the child, myasthenia gravis can take one of several forms (123,124).

Neonatal myasthenia is a transient disease seen in approximately one in five infants born to mothers who generally are suffering from active acquired myasthenia gravis (125). Symptoms usually appear during the first 24 hours or, at the latest, by the third day of life. All affected infants have a paresis of the lower bulbar muscles, causing a weak cry and difficulty in sucking or swallowing. Generalized hypotonia is found in approximately one-half of the infants. Antibody titers against the AChR are elevated in the mother and in most but not all infants. Symptoms respond promptly to anticholinesterase medication, and even if untreated, the illness usually lasts less than 5 weeks.

Congenital myasthenia gravis designates children with myasthenia born to mothers without the disease (126,127). Generally, antibodies against the AChR protein are undetectable. Several conditions have been recognized. These are outlined in Table 16.5 (126–137). Harper and Engel and coworkers have divided these into presynaptic, synaptic, and postsynaptic defects; primary AChR kinetic abnormalities; and the slow-channel congenital myasthenic syndrome (126,127).

Presynaptic defects include at least two autosomal recessive conditions caused by defects in acetylcholine resynthesis and mobilization (127,138,139). Postsynaptic defects include several forms associated with defects in the gene that codes for the collagenlike tail of acetylcholine esterase (131,140), and more than 60 mutations in one of the five genes coding for the adult or fetal subunits of the acetylcholine receptor (127). These entities are depicted in Table 16.5.

The most common congenital myasthenic syndrome is caused by a kinetic abnormality of AChR, the *slow-channel syndrome*. This is an autosomal dominant condition and is the consequence of an abnormally prolonged open-time of the acetylcholine-ion channels (127,135,141). Less common are the various mutations that cause the *fast-channel syndrome*. In these mutations, the postsynaptic

TABLE 16.6 Symptoms and Signs in 35 Patients with Juvenile Myasthenia Gravis

Symptom or Sign	*Number of Patients*
Ptosis	32
Diplopia	30
Facial weakness	29
Dysphonia	29
Weakness of arms	29
Weakness of legs	29
Chewing weakness	22
External ophthalmoplegia	18
Respiratory difficulties	12

Adapted from Millichap JG, Dodge PR. Diagnosis and treatment of myasthenia gravis in infancy, childhood and adolescence. *Neurology* 1960;10:1007.

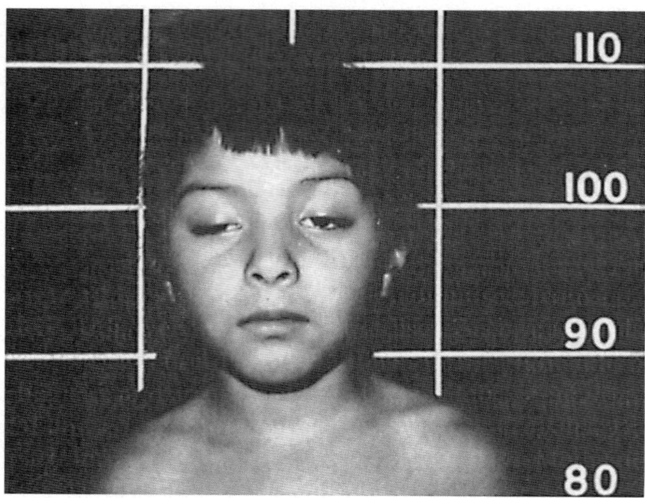

FIGURE 16.3. Girl with myasthenia gravis. She has bilateral ptosis, more marked on the right, and the typical myasthenic facies. (Courtesy of Dr. Christian Herrmann, Jr., Department of Neurology, University of California, Los Angeles, UCLA School of Medicine.)

response to acetylcholine is markedly diminished, although the number of acetylcholine receptors per endplate is normal (136,142). The numerous genetic defects that have been demonstrated in congenital myasthenic syndromes were recently summarized in tabular form, with references provided (143).

The clinical picture of congenital myasthenia also is heterogeneous. In approximately one-half of children, symptoms commence before 2 years of age, and more than one sibling can be affected (124,139). In many instances, fetal movements are reduced, and neonates can have feeding difficulties, ptosis, limitation of eye movements, and a weak cry. The initial symptoms in congenital myasthenia gravis are not as severe as in the neonatal variety, and the diagnosis is, therefore, more difficult. A few patients with congenital myasthenia have spontaneous remissions, but the course of the disease is usually protracted, with mild symptoms that often are refractory to both medical and surgical therapy (thymectomy).

Myasthenia can begin during childhood (juvenile myasthenia). In this form, girls are affected two to six times as frequently as boys. The onset of juvenile myasthenia can be insidious, although at times, it is rapid and often a sequel to an acute febrile illness. Generally, muscles innervated by the cranial nerves are affected first, with bilateral ptosis the most common presenting sign (Table 16.6 and Fig. 16.3). It was seen in 81% of children in the series of Afifi and Bell and was unilateral in 33% (111). Generalized weakness and dysphagia are less common presenting symptoms. The clinical course is highly variable. Approximately one-half of the patients experience one or more remissions, usually during the early years of the illness. In others, symptoms progress to a certain point and then become stationary. In 26% of cases in the series of Afifi and Bell, myasthenia was restricted to the extraocular musculature (111).

The characteristic feature of all forms of juvenile myasthenia gravis is the variability in muscular strength, with increasing weakness of the affected muscles with repeated contractions (Fig. 16.4). The child is usually at his or her best in the morning and becomes progressively weaker during the day, although partial or complete recovery may follow a nap. In approximately 10% to 20% of untreated cases, weakness becomes irreversible, and muscle wasting, particularly of the shoulder girdle and the extraocular muscles, becomes apparent. Despite hypotonia, tendon jerks are normal or even exaggerated, but they may disappear after repeated elicitation.

Other autoimmune diseases are sometimes associated with juvenile myasthenia gravis. The most common of these are rheumatoid arthritis, juvenile diabetes mellitus, and thyroid disease, usually thyrotoxicosis (144). For reasons as yet unexplained, seizures are seen in as many as 12.5% of patients (145,146). Malignancies were seen in 5%

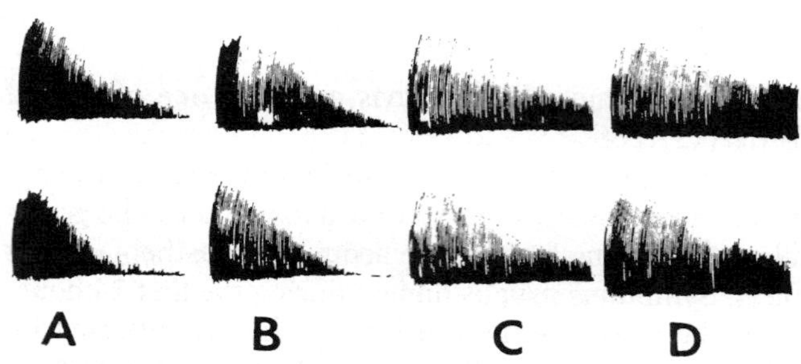

FIGURE 16.4. Muscle ergograph in a patient with myasthenia gravis. **A:** Resting state. **B:** After intravenous atropine (0.4 mg). **C:** After intravenous Tensilon (2.0 mg). **D:** After intravenous edrophonium chloride (8.0 mg). Note the progressive decrease in amplitude in A and B, partly or completely corrected by edrophonium chloride. (Courtesy of Dr. C. Herrmann, Jr., Department of Neurology, University of California, Los Angeles, UCLA School of Medicine.)

of the Mayo Clinic pediatric series (147). Postinfectious myasthenia gravis in children is transitory and usually follows a varicella-zoster infection in 2 to 5 weeks as an immune response (147a).

Myasthenia also can be seen in association with collagen vascular disease, notably systemic lupus erythematosus. Dobkin and Verity and Rodolico and others have described a familial limb girdle myasthenic syndrome transmitted through an autosomal recessive gene and characterized by cardiomyopathy, excessive muscle fatigability with a predilection for the proximal musculature, and improvement with anticholinesterase drugs (148,149). Muscle biopsy revealed hypoplasia of type 1 muscle fibers and tubular aggregates of types 1 and 2 fibers.

The Eaton-Lambert myasthenic syndrome is rarely encountered in children. It has been observed after the administration of antibiotics (most frequently neomycin), in conjunction with surgery (150,151), as a complication of allogeneic bone marrow transplantation (152), and in acute leukemia (153).

Diagnosis

The diagnosis of myasthenia gravis is based on a history of abnormal fatigability of voluntary muscles and evidence of a prompt improvement of muscle weakness with anticholinesterase drugs. It is supported by a history of remissions and exacerbations and by the absence of any concurrent illness that might contribute to the muscular weakness.

For diagnostic purposes, the most widely used drug is edrophonium chloride (Tensilon). Approximately 5 mg is given intravenously to a 3- to 5-year-old child. Within 1 minute after the injection, a transient improvement in muscle strength is observed, usually lasting 4 to 5 minutes. Positive responses are diagnostically reliable. In some infants, a positive response can be obscured by the response to the injection, in which case a longer-acting anticholinesterase drug such as neostigmine should be used. After intramuscular injection of 0.5 to 1.5 mg of neostigmine, muscle strength begins to improve in 10 to 15 minutes and reaches its peak by 30 minutes. Both tests are nearly 100% reliable in generalized myasthenia as well as in ocular myasthenia, which progresses to generalized myasthenia. Neostigmine should never be administered intravenously because it may induce fatal cardiac arrythmias. Edrophonium should be avoided in infancy for the same reason. In the series of Afifi and Bell, edrophonium gave positive test results in all cases of ocular myasthenia; neostigmine was positive only in 67% of cases (111). A number of conditions can give a false-positive result. These include drug-induced myasthenia gravis, botulism, brainstem gliomas, and Guillain-Barré syndrome (154). A confirmatory test, therefore, is required.

The presence of AChR antibodies in serum is the simplest diagnostic test in juvenile myasthenia, although false-negative results are not unusual, particularly in children whose symptoms are limited to the extraocular muscles. In the series of Afifi and Bell, AChR antibodies were found in 63% of cases (111). A similar incidence of positive serology has been reported in other series. When AChR antibodies are absent, it is necessary to consider one of the congenital myasthenic syndromes. This is not an academic exercise because in juvenile myasthenia gravis, therapy is not only supportive but also is directed against the immune-mediated response. Andrews and coworkers suggest that the rapid response to plasmapheresis frequently seen in children with juvenile myasthenia gravis can be used to distinguish this condition from congenital myasthenia gravis (155). It should be noted that antibody levels do not parallel disease severity.

Rapid stimulation of the distal (ulnar) or proximal (spinal, axillary, or facial) motor nerves produces a characteristic decrement in the amplitude of successive action potentials recorded from surface muscle electrodes and in the amplitudes of the mechanical excursions (see Fig. 16.4). This test is positive in some 80% of pediatric cases, but is usually negative in ocular myasthenia (156). Patients suspected of having myasthenia gravis on the basis of their clinical picture but who have a normal EMG study should undergo single-fiber EMG (157,158). The results of this study generally complement the results of the assay for AChR antibodies. Exceptions are seen in the various syndromes of congenital myasthenia gravis, in which single-fiber EMG is frequently positive; another exception is in children with the mild, predominantly ocular form of the disease (158).

In addition to penicillamine, a number of other drugs can induce or unmask myasthenia. These include β-adrenergic blockers, carnitine, aminoglycoside antibiotics, lithium carbonate, magnesium salts, trimethadione, and phenytoin (159).

Treatment

Treatment of the patient with juvenile myasthenia is generally lifelong, extending into all areas of activity. The three approaches to therapy are symptomatic, immunologic, and surgical. Treatment of the congenital myasthenias is solely symptomatic (160). As a rule, the first step is remission induction. This is usually accomplished through the use of high-dose corticosteroids, frequently in conjunction with intravenous immunoglobulin or plasmapheresis. Maintenance of the remission is then usually accomplished by slow tapering of the corticosteroids along with the use of "steroid-sparing" agents, which include thymectomy and immunosuppressants.

When juvenile myasthenia is mild or is restricted to the ocular musculature, treatment is generally symptomatic (i.e., using anticholinesterase drugs). At the University of California, Los Angeles, UCLA School of Medicine, pyridostigmine bromide (Mestinon) is the preferred drug. It is administered at a starting dosage of 15 mg two to three times a day (in tablet or syrup form) for a child 3 to 8 years old, or 0.5 to 1.0 mg/kg.

In the remaining patients, treatment should be as outlined above. Mann and coworkers and Vajsar suggest a course of oral prednisone, starting out at high dosages (1 mg/kg per day) and tapering when improvement is sustained or when side effects require reduction of the dosages (161,162). Sarnat and associates have advocated a starting dosage of 2 mg/kg given every other day (163). Cholinesterase inhibitors are used as needed while the patient is receiving corticosteroids. Exacerbation of myasthenia gravis can be seen during the early days of corticosteroid therapy, usually toward the end of the first week, and can last approximately 1 week. Improvement is noted within approximately 2 weeks and becomes maximal in approximately 3 months. Plasmapheresis lowers the level of antibodies against the acetylcholine receptor protein. Dau recommends this procedure to stabilize patients whose course worsens markedly during initiation of prednisone therapy and as primary therapy in combination with immunosuppressive drugs such as azathioprine (164). Plasmapheresis also has been used to treat patients who remain unresponsive to other forms of therapy, to improve respiratory function before thymectomy, and to hasten remission after thymectomy. Improvement, often dramatic, is seen within 1 to 3 days after the start of the course. Immunosuppression of refractory patients with azathioprine (2 to 3 mg/kg), cyclosporine, and cyclophosphamide (50 mg/kg per day) has been disappointing because of side effects such as bone marrow suppression and hepatotoxicity (162,165) and is not used at our institutions. Intravenous immune globulin has been used in conjunction with other modes of therapy, particularly corticosteroids and plasmapheresis, in rapidly deteriorating patients with bulbar symptoms (166). There is little difference between the efficacy of three plasma exchanges and intravenous immune globulin (0.4 mg/kg per day for 3 to 5 consecutive days), although as a rule, intravenous gammaglobulin is better tolerated (167). Intravenous immune globulin is ineffective in neonatal myasthenia gravis (168).

After establishment of maximal improvement, children should be considered for thymectomy (166,169,170), although the effectiveness of the procedure in the pediatric population has not been validated by controlled trials. In the German series of Lindner and coworkers, 82% of children were thymectomized (146). In general, the procedure is now indicated if symptoms recur after withdrawal of corticosteroids after 1 year of therapy or if corticosteroids fail to benefit the patient significantly. The best results from thymectomy may be predicted in children who have high titers of circulating antiacetylcholine receptor antibodies and who are symptomatic for less than 2 years. However, a long history of juvenile myasthenia gravis is not a contraindication to thymectomy; for both girls and boys, good operative results are possible. In the UCLA experience, the procedure is of considerable benefit when performed as early as the third year of life. The maximum benefit of thymectomy may be delayed for weeks or even several months, so absence of an immediate and dramatic postoperative improvement should not be discouraging.

Proceeding according to this treatment schedule, Mann and associates found that up to 90% of patients have significant improvement or complete remission of their myasthenic symptoms and that in some, corticosteroids and anticholinesterase drugs can even be tapered and discontinued (161). In the series of Lindner and colleagues, 60% of patients who underwent thymectomy went into remission, as compared with 29% of those who were not thymectomized (146). In the series of Rodriguez and coworkers, the remission rate was higher in children who underwent thymectomy within 12 months of the onset of symptoms. It also was higher in patients who had experienced bulbar symptoms before surgery, in those having involvement of extremities but neither ocular nor generalized weakness, and in those whose myasthenic symptoms presented between ages 12 and 16 years (147).

Patients with congenital forms of myasthenia may respond to anticholinesterases. When such treatment is unsatisfactory, Palace and colleagues have suggested 3,4-diaminopyridine. This substance blocks potassium conductance and increases the release of acetylcholine from the nerve terminal (171).

Toxic Disorders

The toxins of *Clostridium tetani* and *C. botulinum* and the venom of cobras and of arachnoideae such as the black widow spider affect the neuromuscular junction. These toxins are more extensively considered under their respective headings in Chapter 10.

DISEASES OF MUSCLE

Muscular Dystrophies

The muscular dystrophies are a group of diseases that are distinguished from other neuromuscular disorders by four obligatory criteria: (a) primary myopathies, not neurogenic; (b) genetically determined; (c) progressive diseases, some slowly progressive and compatible with normal longevity and others more rapidly progressive and leading to early death; and (d) myofiber degeneration at some stage in the disease (5).

An excellent review on the history of the terminology in muscular dystrophy was provided by Dubowitz (172). The name *muscular dystrophy*, meaning a growth disorder of muscle, was entrenched by Gowers in his "Clinical lecture on pseudohypertrophic muscular paralysis," a series of essays in *The Lancet* in 1879 (173).

From a clinical point of view, there are at least eight major forms of muscular dystrophy: Duchenne

(Aran-Duchenne) muscular dystrophy, Becker muscular dystrophy (now known to be merely a mild form of Duchenne dystrophy with the same genetic defect), Emery-Dreifuss (humeroperoneal) muscular dystrophy, facioscapulohumeral (Landouzy-Déjèrine) muscular dystrophy, the limb girdle dystrophies, oculopharyngeal muscular dystrophy, distal muscular dystrophy, and the congenital muscular dystrophies. The characteristic genetic and clinical features of each entity are presented in Table 16.7 (174;175–200).

Pathologic Anatomy

Despite differences in the clinical picture, the same pathologic findings are shared by all muscular dystrophies. The earliest stages of the disease show a dilated sarcoplasmic reticulum, with an irregular orientation of the triads (201). As the illness progresses, there are repeated episodes of necrosis and regeneration of muscle cells. This process is probably initiated by a breakdown of the muscle cell membrane, and electron microscopy may reveal the absence of the plasma membrane around all or part of the circumference of the muscle fibers (202). Small losses of membrane can be repaired, but generally, regeneration is inadequate. As a consequence of the membrane defect, an influx of calcium ions can occur, activating the endogenous proteases and inducing lysis of the Z-disc of the myofibril, which is probably the initial step in muscle breakdown. Subsequently, the number of muscle cells is reduced, and variability in fiber size is increased. Sarcolemmal nuclei are swollen and increased in number, a regenerative reaction to the injury of muscle fibers. Over the years, this reaction becomes more extreme, and muscle fibers appear enlarged, forked, hyalinized, or atrophied. With further progression of the disease, large accumulations of collagen and fat cells are seen between muscle fibers, and these cells are partly responsible for the muscular hypertrophy (Fig. 16.5) (45).

Neither heart nor smooth muscle is spared, and there is myocardial degeneration with fatty infiltration and fibrosis of the myocardial fibers.

When muscular dystrophy is associated with mental retardation, brain sections can be normal or can disclose various developmental anomalies of the cortex, such as pachygyria, heterotopia, and disorders of cortical architecture (203).

Pathogenesis

The elucidation of the gene defect in Duchenne and Becker muscular dystrophy represents one of the most important triumphs of molecular biology in the area of neurology, and was the first human disease whose nature was clarified by positional cloning (173). The gene for Duchenne and Becker muscular dystrophy is localized on Xq21.2. It is 10 times larger than any other gene characterized to date and consists of approximately 2 million base pairs; its product has been named *dystrophin*, a protein with a molecular weight of 427,000. The most common gene mutation in both Duchenne and Becker muscular dystrophies is a deletion. The phenotype of Duchenne and Becker muscular dystrophies does not always correlate with the size of the deletion in the dystrophin gene; some cases of undetectable dystrophin are paradoxically associated with only mild clinical manifestations (204). Rather, the effect of the deletion on dystrophin synthesis is important. If the deletion breaks up the codon triplet and thereby shifts the reading frame, a premature stop codon is quickly generated, and dystrophin synthesis comes to a halt, leaving a small, truncated protein molecule without its carboxy terminal, which is rapidly degraded. If the deletion removes a triplet codon in its entirety, the reading frame is maintained, resulting in the synthesis of a dystrophin molecule with a shortened rod domain but intact carboxy and amino domains. This is what occurs in Becker dystrophy (205).

Dystrophin is a low-abundance protein and constitutes but 0.002% of total muscle protein. It is a cytoskeletal protein with a globular amino domain, a central rodlike domain, and a globular carboxy domain. It is localized to the inner surface of the sarcolemma, aggregating as a homotetramer that is associated with actin at its amino terminus and with a glycoprotein complex at its carboxy terminus. The dystrophin-glycoprotein complex, by which the membrane cytoskeleton is linked to extracellular glycoproteins, consists of several dystrophin-associated glycoproteins and dystrophin-associated proteins (Fig. 16.6). The membrane complex is markedly reduced in Duchenne muscular dystrophy. Its synthesis is normal, but in the absence of dystrophin, the glycoproteins become unstable and are degraded (206). These associated glycoproteins include not only the dystroglycans and sarcoglycans, but also the syntrophin-dystrobrevin complex that is highly localized at the neuromuscular synaptic membrane and is later to appear in normal fetal development (206a).

Dystrophin is present not only in muscle, but in a variety of other cell types, including brain and retina (207–209). Although *in situ* hybridization demonstrates some expression of the gene in affected muscle (210), the complete dystrophin molecule is absent or is present in less than 3% of normal levels in more than 90% of patients with classic Duchenne muscular dystrophy. It is present in reduced amounts or in normal amounts but with an abnormal molecular configuration in boys with Becker muscular dystrophy (211).

The level of dystrophin expression in brain is lower than in muscle, and the structure of brain messenger RNA for dystrophin differs from that of muscle (212,213). This difference is because cortical dystrophin is transcribed from a promoter that is at least 90 kb upstream from the muscle promoter. Other, markedly truncated dystrophins can be found in normal brain and peripheral nerve. In particular, a 140-kD protein (Dp140) is found throughout the CNS (214,215).

TABLE 16.7 Clinical and Genetic Features of the Muscular Dystrophies

Disorder	Gene Locus	Protein Defect	Clinical Features	Reference
Duchenne	Xp21	Dystrophin	XR, onset 2 to 5 years, pelvic girdle, PH >80%, contractures, rapid progression, cardiac involvement	175
Becker	Xp21	Dystrophin	XR, childhood onset, pelvic girdle, PH 90%; slow progression, cardiac involvement in 15%	176
Emery-Dreifuss (XR)	Xq28	Emerin	Early contractures, slowly progressive weakness, proximal in UE, distal in LE, cardiomyopathy common, severe	177
Emery-Dreifuss (AD)	1q11–q23	Lamins A and C	Similar to X-linked form, but weakness presents before contractures	178
Emery-Dreifuss (AR)	1q11–q23	Lamins A and C	Severe muscle weakness	179
Fascioscapulohumeral	4q35 deletions	?	AD, variable age of onset, usually no cardiac involvement or contractures, retinal vascular disease and hearing loss can occur	180
LGD AD, 1A	5q31	Myotilin	Adult-onset, proximal muscle weakness	181
LGD AD 1B	1q21.2	Lamin A and C	Allelic with Emery-Dreifuss dystrophy, cardiac involvement common	182
LGD AD 1C	3p25	Caveolin-3	Onset in first decade, proximal muscle weakness, calf hypertrophy	183
LGD AD 1D	7q	?	Adult onset	184
LGD AD 1E	6q23	?	Adolescent-onset cardiomyopathy, adult-onset limb girdle weakness	185
LDG AD 1F	7q32.1–q32.2	?	Juvenile onset, no cardiac involvement, contractures, or pseudohypertrophy	186
LDG AR 2A	15q 15.1	Calpain-3	Mild form starting in first decade, unaccompanied by mental retardation or cardiomyopathy	187,188
LDG AR 2B	2p 13.3–p13.1	Dysferlin	Considerable variability—one type is Miyoshi myopathy, inflammatory changes in muscle	189
LDG AR 2C	13q12	γ-sarcoglycan	Early onset, Duchenne-like progression but longer survival	190
LDG AR 2D	17q12–q21.33	α-sarcoglycan (adhalin)	Considerable phenotypic variation, generally least severe of the sarcoglycanopathies	191,192
LDG AR 2E	4q12	β-sarcoglycan	Significant cardiac involvement	192,193
LDG AR 2F	5q33	δ-sarcoglycan	Significant cardiac involvement	194
LDG AR 2G	17q12	Telethonin	Not fully defined	195
LDG AR 2H	9q31–q34.1	TRIM 32, an E3-ubiquitin-ligase	Mild myopathy, first described in Manitoba Hutterites	196
LDG AR 2I	19q13.3	Fukutin-related protein (FKRP)	Variable age of onset—as early as first year, calf hypertrophy, elevated CK	197
LDGAR 2J	2q24.3	Titin	Severe myopathy starting in first to third decade is homozygous manifestation, heterozygotes show distal tibial myopathy	198
Oculopharyngeal muscular dystrophy	14q11.2–q13	Poly(A)-binding protein-2 (PAB 2)	Adult onset, extraocular muscles, face, dysphagia	199
Distal muscular dystrophy	14q,2,2,2p	?	AR and AD transmission, variable clinical picture	200

PH, pseudohypertrophy; XR, X-linked recessive; AD, autosomal dominant; AR, autosomal recessive; UE, upper extremities; LE, lower extremities; LGD, limb-girdle dystrophy.

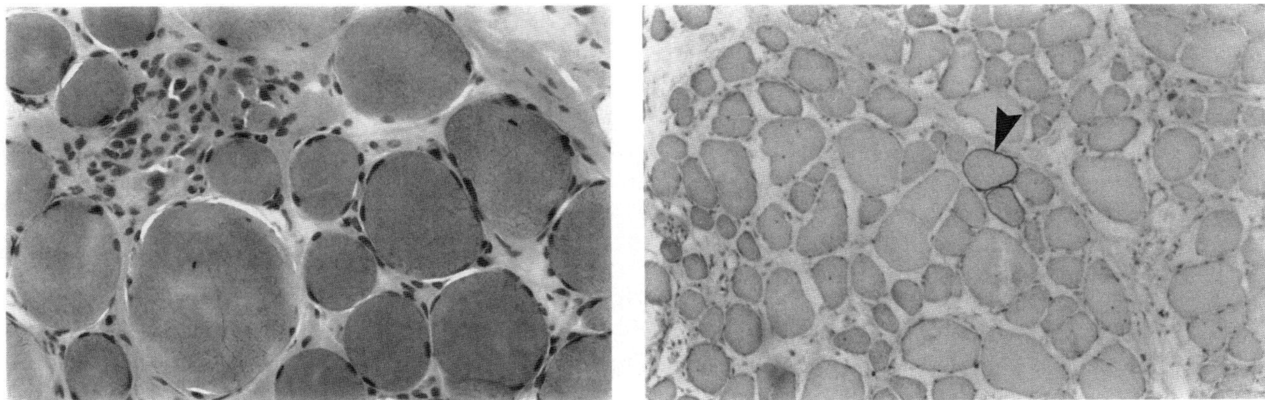

FIGURE 16.5. Muscle biopsy of a 5-year-old boy with Duchenne muscular dystrophy. **A:** Myofibers are extremely variable in size with both hypertrophic and atrophic forms. They have an abnormally rounded contour rather than the normal polygonal contour in the transverse section because of the proliferation of endomysial collagen that forms rigid sleeves around each fiber. A few fibers have internal nuclei. A zone of degenerating myofibers infiltrated by phagocytic cells is seen in the upper left of the figure. **B:** Immunocytochemistry shows absence of dystrophin at the sarcolemma of all myofibers, large and small, except for one (*arrowhead*) called a *revertant fiber* that expresses this protein as in normal fibers (**A,** hematoxylin and eosin, × 400; **B,** dystrophin, rod domain, × 250).

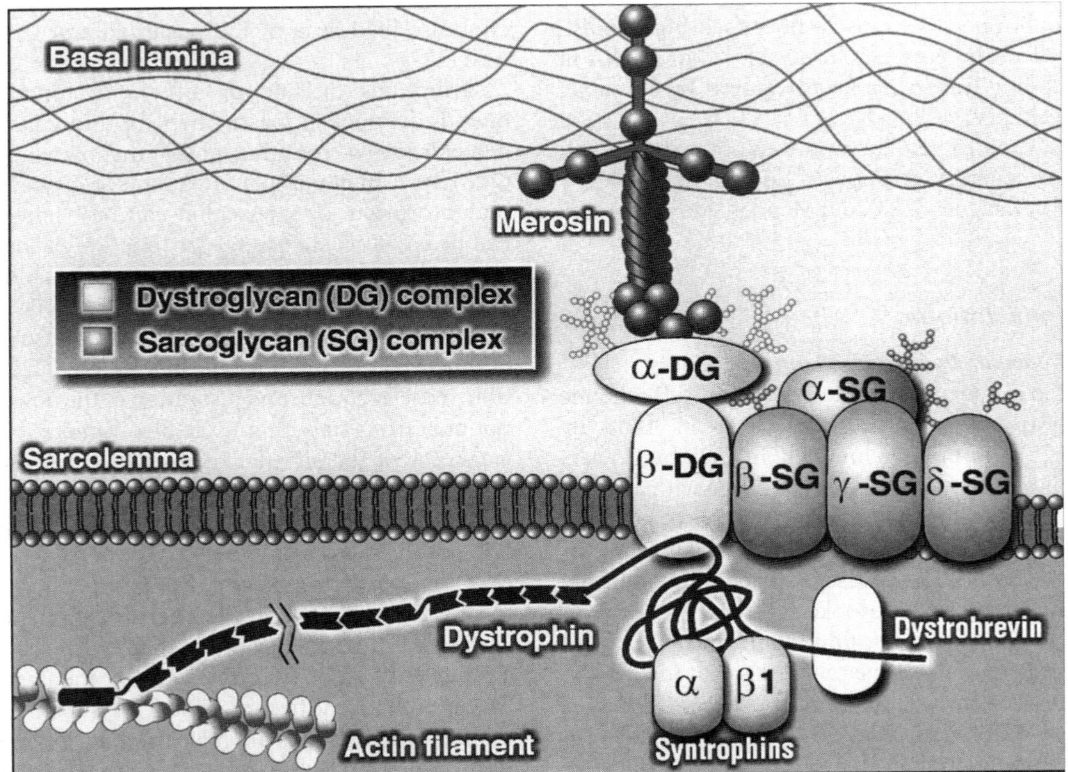

FIGURE 16.6. The dystrophin-glycoprotein complex. Dystrophin contacts F-actin in the cytoplasm of the cell, and the dystrophin-glycoprotein complex forms a bridge across the membrane to the merosin subunit of laminin in the extracellular matrix. (Courtesy of R. G. Worton, The Ottawa Hospital, Research Institute, Ottawa.)

Dystrophin is associated with other proteins at the sarcolemmal region, which also may be defective; these include α- and β-dystroglycans (216–219) and utrophin. Utrophin is an autosomal homologue of dystrophin, being encoded by a gene that has been mapped to the long arm of chromosome 6 (6q24). Like dystrophin, it is a large protein that is found at the neuromuscular synapse and the myotendinous junction and also is expressed in several other tissues, notably the lungs and intestines (220).

How the membrane defect results in the dystrophic process is not completely clear. It is likely that dystrophin stabilizes the muscle membrane during repeated cycles of muscle contraction. Lacking dystrophin, the normal interaction between sarcolemma and extracellular matrix is lost and as a consequence, osmotic fragility of muscle fibers increases (204). Possibly significant in the pathogenesis of the dystrophic process are the low potassium and high intrafiber sodium and calcium concentrations seen in dystrophic muscle (221). These electrolyte changes can reflect ionic leakage through the abnormal membrane of dystrophic fibers. Whether membrane leakage also is responsible for the elevation in serum CK activity is open to speculation. An incompletely explained finding is the presence in Duchenne muscular dystrophy of an occasional dystrophin-positive muscle fiber (see Fig. 16.5B). This could reflect the presence in muscle of an mRNA in which the reading frame has been restored by an as yet unknown mechanism (222).

Good reviews of the genetic variations of the dystrophin gene and its protein transcription products are provided by Muntoni and colleagues (223) and Mendell and colleagues (224).

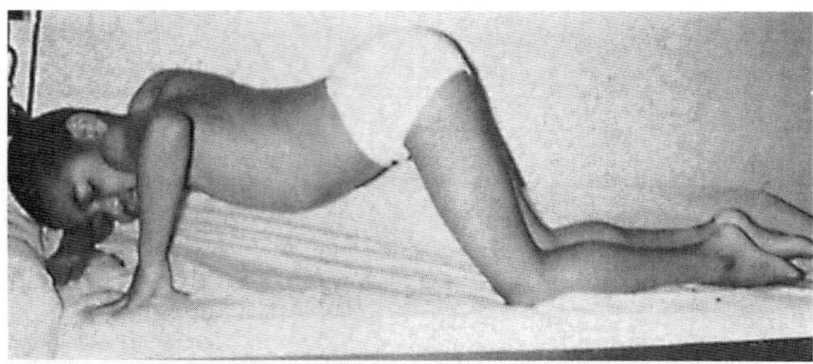

FIGURE 16.7. Boy with Duchenne muscular dystrophy. The atrophy of the proximal musculature and the pseudohypertrophy of the gastrocnemius become particularly evident when the patient attempts to rise from the prone position.

Clinical Manifestations

Duchenne Muscular Dystrophy (Aran-Duchenne)

Transmitted in a sex-linked recessive manner, Duchenne muscular dystrophy was first described in 1868 by Duchenne (225) and more definitively in 1879 by Gowers (171,226). It is a relatively common condition with a prevalence of 1 in 25,000. Clinically, it is the most clearly defined of the muscular dystrophies. The disease becomes apparent in early childhood. The course is so gradual that initial symptoms are commonly overlooked. At first, these are often confined to difficulty in climbing stairs, in arising from the floor, or in performing other activities that involve the pelvic muscles. An early indication of pelvic weakness is the manner by which patients arise from the floor, by progressively "climbing up their thighs" (Gowers' sign) (226). Lordosis commonly appears with progression of the disease, and the child "straddles as he stands and waddles as he walks." Muscular wasting and a progressive and early enfeeblement of deep tendon reflexes accompany the advance of the disease. Subsequent to the initial stages, muscular involvement is invariably symmetric. In contrast to the generalized atrophy, there is striking pseudohypertrophy of the calves and, less commonly, of the deltoids and infraspinati (Fig. 16.7). Contractures are common and occur chiefly at the hamstrings.

Enlargement of the heart, persistent tachycardia, and myocardial failure are seen in 50% to 80% of patients at some time during the disease and are reflected in significant electrocardiographic abnormalities. These result from metabolic abnormalities within a relatively circumscribed area of the posterolateral left ventricular wall (227).

Symptoms of smooth muscle dysfunction are frequently overlooked. Gastric hypomotility can result in sudden episodes of vomiting, abdominal pain, and distention (228). In a small number of patients, a history of diarrhea, malabsorption, or megacolon can be elicited, and there can be a disturbance in motor function of the esophagus. These clinical findings correspond to pathologic changes in smooth muscle, most characteristically a fatty infiltration of the myofibers, necrosis of the muscle fibers, and degenerative changes in the nuclei (228,229). Constipation, fecal retention, and distention of the bowel may result not only from smooth muscle involvement, but also from weakness of the striated rectus abdominus muscles that do not provide for a sufficient increase in intra-abdominal pressure during defecation to assist in the peristaltic emptying of the rectum.

A significant proportion of children with muscular dystrophy have defective intellectual development that affects verbal skills to a greater extent than nonverbal skills (230). This deficit can be accounted for by the presence of significant abnormalities in cortical architecture and abnormalities of dendrites in neurons that normally express dystrophin (201,206). Loss of the shorter isoforms, in particular Dp71 and Dp140, appears to be associated with severe intellectual impairment (223,231,232). The mean IQ of children with Duchenne muscular dystrophy is approximately 85, and its range appears to follow a normal (Gaussian) distribution curve (45). Retardation is nonprogressive, and its severity is unrelated to the severity of muscular weakness. It is accompanied by cerebral atrophy as

TABLE 16.8 Muscle Diseases with Central Nervous System Involvement

Condition	Central Nervous System Signs and Symptoms	Reference
Duchenne muscular dystrophy	Mental retardation	Dubowitz (45)
Myotonic dystrophy	Mental retardation	Harper (235)
Fascioscapulohumoral muscular dystrophy	Sensorineural hearing loss	Taylor et al. (178)
Centronuclear myopathy	Seizures, occasional mental retardation	Serratrice et al. (236)
Mitochondrial cytopathies	Protean CNS involvement	Ricci (237); Chapter 2
Glycerol kinase deficiency	Spasticity, mental retardation	Guggenheim et al. (238)
Systemic carnitine deficiency	Recurrent acute encephalopathy	Chapter 2
Glycogenosis type II (Pompe disease)	Dementia, seizures	Chapter 1
Debre-Sémélaigné syndrome	Cretinism	Spiro et al. (239); Chapter 17
De Lange syndrome	Mental retardation, extrapyramidal signs	De Lange (240)
Congenital muscular dystrophies		Van der Knaap et al. (241)
Walker-Warburg syndrome	Severe mental retardation, macrocephaly, various eye abnormalities, diffuse agyric cortex, hypoplasia cerebellar vermis, abnormal white matter	Dobyns et al. (242); Beltran-Valerode Bernabe (243)
Muscle-eye-brain disease	Mental retardation, microcephaly, eye abnormalities; cortical dysplasia less severe than in Walker-Warburg syndrome	Laverda et al. (244)
Fukuyama disease	Severe mental retardation, seizures, no eye abnormalities	Fukuyama et al. (245)

demonstrated by neuroimaging studies (233). It is of note that in mentally retarded patients with Becker dystrophy, the deletion also affects the Dp140 regulatory region (234).

Duchenne muscular dystrophy is but one of several muscle diseases in which the CNS also is involved, usually in the form of mental retardation. These various conditions are listed in Table 16.8 (235–245).

The course of the illness is steadily downhill. Death usually occurs in adolescence and results from secondary infections or intractable congestive heart failure.

The female carrier for muscular dystrophy is usually asymptomatic, but occasionally demonstrates pseudohypertrophy and mild weakness of the pelvic musculature. All gradations from apparent complete normality to a marked but focal dystrophy can be seen on biopsy (246). Both dystrophin-positive and dystrophin-negative fibers can be seen, a finding that supports the view, postulated by the Lyon hypothesis, that in the dystrophin-negative cells, the paternal X chromosome, on which the muscular dystrophy gene is located, is active. Cardiomyopathy can develop even in the absence of muscular weakness (172).

Becker Muscular Dystrophy

The incidence of Becker muscular dystrophy in the United Kingdom is 1 in 18,450 births, as compared with an incidence of 1 in 5,618 births for Duchenne muscular dystrophy. Because of the earlier demise of patients with Duchenne muscular dystrophy, the prevalence of the two diseases is about the same (247).

Symptoms begin somewhat later than in Duchenne muscular dystrophy, often after 8 years of age, and the ability to walk is retained beyond age 16 years (see Table 16.7). Pseudohypertrophy is less likely to be present, and the ankle reflexes are often lost. A diagnostic feature of this form of muscular dystrophy is the presence of pes cavus in 60% of subjects (176). The incidence of mental retardation and cardiac involvement is probably less than in Duchenne muscular dystrophy. Serum CK levels are markedly elevated. As has already been indicated, Becker muscular dystrophy results from a defect in the amount and structure of dystrophin.

A syndrome of X-linked myalgia and cramps with onset in early childhood and elevated serum CK levels is accompanied by normal amounts of muscle dystrophin that is truncated at the amino end of the molecule. The relatively mild symptoms in this condition contrast with the severe symptoms that result from deletions at the carboxy end of the dystrophin protein (248,249).

Emery-Dreifuss Muscular Dystrophy

Emery-Dreifuss muscular dystrophy, a rare myopathy, appears between ages 5 and 15 years. Inheritance is usually X-linked, but autosomal dominant and autosomal recessive pedigrees also have been encountered. The gene responsible for the X-linked form has been localized to the distal portion of the long arm (Xq28) (250). It encodes a single membrane spanning protein named *emerin*, which has been localized to the inner nuclear membrane. This protein is believed to stabilize the nuclear membrane against the mechanical stresses that develop during muscle contraction (251). The gene defective in the autosomal dominant form (*LMNA*) encodes lamins A and C, proteins that constitute part of the nuclear lamina, a fibrous layer on the nucleoplasmic side of the inner nuclear membrane.

Clinically, the X-linked and the dominant forms are similar. Weakness is diffuse or is maximal in the proximal muscles of the upper extremities: biceps, triceps, and the distal muscles of the lower extremities such as the peroneal muscles (177). Flexion contractures of the elbows, posterior cervical muscles, and Achilles tendons are prominent early in the course of the X-linked disease, but tend to occur somewhat later in the dominant form (178). The weakness progresses slowly, but all patients have severe and potentially fatal cardiac arrhythmias that can precede any apparent skeletal muscle weakness (see Table 16.7) (172,177). CK levels are only moderately elevated. Arrhythmias also can be seen in otherwise asymptomatic female carriers (252).

Facioscapulohumeral Muscular Dystrophy

As implied by its name, facioscapulohumeral muscular dystrophy (FSHD) comprises a group of diseases that affect the muscles of the face, shoulder, and upper arm. The classic form of the condition, described in 1885 by Landouzy and Déjèrine, is transmitted as an autosomal dominant trait with a frequency of 1 in 20,000 (252,253). Initial symptoms tend to appear at a somewhat later age than in the Duchenne form, with penetrance being approximately 50% by age 14 years (254). The gene for this condition has been localized to the subtelomeric portion of the long arm of chromosome 4 (4q35), and deletions of integral copies of 3.3.kb units from a tandem repeat located near the gene have been associated with the clinical expression of the disease. Genes located upstream from this deleted area are inappropriately overexpressed, suggesting that deletion of these units that are not transcribed induces an inappropriate derepression of one or more genes on 4p35 (253–255). In the experience of Wijmenga and coworkers, there was little genetic heterogeneity (256). This is somewhat surprising in view of the marked heterogeneity of clinical manifestations. The genetic phenomenon of *anticipation* often is demonstrated in families with this disease, a grandparent being only mildly involved from early adult life, a parent being more severely involved since late childhood or adolescence, and the infant or young child showing severe involvement since birth.

Pathologically, FSHD is a heterogeneous group, with a similar clinical picture being caused not only by muscular dystrophy, but also by neurogenic muscular atrophy, polymyositis, myasthenia gravis, myotubular myopathy, nemaline myopathy, and Möbius syndrome (infantile FSHD) (257). A lymphocytic inflammatory myopathy is not unusual, particularly in children with a rapidly progressive course (257), but subjects with this pathologic picture do not have an autoimmune disorder and do not respond to treatment with corticosteroids.

Initial symptoms usually include wasting of the shoulder girdle, prominent winging of the scapulae, and in many but not all families, development of myopathic facies. The lips cannot be pursed, and they protrude in what has been termed a *tapir's mouth*. The relative weakness of the zygomatic muscles results in an equally characteristic transverse smile. Muscular hypertrophy, contractures, and skeletal deformities are rare. Involvement tends to be symmetric, but asymmetric weakness is more common in this form than in any of the other dystrophies.

Although cardiac involvement has been encountered, it occurs rarely. Progression of FSHD is sufficiently slow and interrupted by periods of seeming remission, to allow a normal life span for a fairly large proportion of patients. When sought using fluorescence angiography, retinal vascular anomalies are not unusual and in one study were encountered in 75% of subjects, including some who lacked muscular symptoms (258). FSHD also may be accompanied by Coats disease (congenital retinal dysgenesis with telangiectasia and retinal detachment) (259) or sensorineural hearing loss (180).

Several other variants have been recognized. These include Erb muscular dystrophy (scapulohumeral muscular dystrophy) and scapuloperoneal dystrophy. In some subjects with the latter condition, sometimes known as Davidenkow syndrome, autopsy studies have disclosed evidence for both progressive neurogenic and myopathic forms. The condition is linked to chromosome 12, and onset of symptoms is usually during the third decade of life (260). In many instances, electrophysiologic and nerve biopsy document a motor neuropathy (261).

Limb-Girdle Muscular Dystrophies

Limb-girdle muscular dystrophies (LGMD) comprise a number of distinct clinical conditions, which are summarized in Table 16.7. An autosomal recessive transmission is much more common (*LGMD2*), but families in whom the condition is transmitted in a dominant manner (*LGMD1*) have been well documented (262,263). To date, at least six different gene loci for the autosomal dominant form and ten recessive forms have been described (172). They are well summarized in a recent review by Zatz and colleagues (264). Symptoms appear during the second or third decade, with muscles of either the shoulder or the pelvic girdle being affected initially. The rate of progression is highly variable, but generally, the course is far more benign than that of Duchenne muscular dystrophy. Approximately 30% of patients develop pseudohypertrophy, usually of the gastrocnemius, less commonly of the lateral vasti and deltoids. However, when examined with cDNA probes for the dystrophin gene, at least some of these patients have been found to have Becker muscular dystrophy (260). Cardiac involvement is rare except in type 1B of the autosomal dominant form, and intelligence is unaffected.

One of the more commonly encountered autosomal dominant LGMDs is 1C, which is associated with a mutation in *caveolin-3*. The caveolin-3 protein is expressed exclusively in muscle cells. The protein monomers oligomerize to form a high molecular weight scaffolding network that transforms certain regions of the sarcolemmal membranes into invaginated structures termed *caveolae*. Caveolae are enriched in several important muscle molecules, notably the dystrophin-glycoprotein complex, dysferlin, and neuronal nitric oxide synthase. Loss of caveolin-3 expression alters the proper function of these proteins and clinically is associated with four autosomal dominant conditions. In addition to limb-girdle dystrophy (1C), *caveolin-3* mutations are also seen in rippling muscle disease (265), distal muscular dystrophy, and hyperCKemia (266). Rippling muscle disease is usually encountered in adults; in children, the condition manifests itself with frequent falls, impaired gait, and percussion-induced painful muscle mounding and rippling (265).

The most frequently encountered autosomal recessive limb-girdle dystrophies are 2A and 2B (see Table 16.7). Type 2A is caused by a defect in the gene that encodes calpain-3 (198). Calpain-3 is a muscle-specific calcium-activated neutral protease whose deficiency is associated with a mild form of LGMD with onset of symptoms at approximately 10 years of age and unaccompanied by cardiomyopathy or mental retardation (198). This disorder is related to dysferlin deficiency and to defects in caleolin-3 and is associated with very high CK levels in blood that are disproportionate to the mild weakness seen clinically. Four autosomal dominant myopathies are documented as mutations in caveolin-3. Caveolin-3 is important in the Golgi apparatus of myocytes and the scaffolding of the cytoplasmic (inner) surface of the sarcolemma. These limb-girdle dystrophies are sometimes not expressed until adult life, but many cases are reported in prepubertal children as well (266).

LGMD 2B results from a defect in the gene that codes for dysferlin, a muscle-specific protein localized to the plasma membrane of muscle fibers. It interacts with calcium- and lipid-binding proteins and is believed to play a major role in calcium-dependent repair of sarcolemmal injury (267). The clinical picture is varied, but most often it tends to take the form of a distal myopathy. The condition is allelic with Miyoshi myopathy, in which weakness of the calf muscles becomes apparent during adolescence or early adult life (268).

In many cases of recessively transmitted limb-girdle syndrome, a deficiency of one of four sarcoglycans occurs (269,270). The first entity to be described was called *adhalen* as an anglicized version of the Arabic word for *muscle* because it was first reported in Tunisian families with consanguinity. Adhalen is now termed *α-sarcoglycan* (271). Other limb-girdle dystrophies are caused by defects in β-, γ-, or δ-sarcoglycan (190,197,272). In the series of Duggan and colleagues, mutations in the α-sarcoglycan gene (LGMD 2D) were the most common, with mutations in the β-sarcoglycan gene (LGMD 2E) the next most frequent (197). Immunocytochemical antibodies are now commercially available to demonstrate each of these sarcoglycans in frozen sections of muscle biopsy. Adhalen, or α-sarcoglycan, generally is secondarily deficient when any of the other sarcoglycans are not normally expressed, so deficiency of α-sarcoglycan alone does not prove that this defect is primary, but does provide a convenient screen for deficiency of any of the other sarcoglycans. Secondary deficiency of α-sarcoglycan also accompanies dystrophin deficiency in some cases of Duchenne muscular dystrophy. The genotype-phenotype correlation of the sarcoglycanopathies demonstrates that the pure α-form is the least severe with the slowest rate of progression. The condition is sometimes not expressed until adolescence or adult life. The other sarcoglycanopathies (LGMD 2C and LGMD 2F) are associated with a more severe clinical course that begins in the prepubertal years (190,272).

Oculopharyngeal Muscular Dystrophy

Oculopharyngeal muscular dystrophy has an adult onset. It affects the extraocular muscles and upper facial muscles as well as and induces dysphagia (199).

Distal Muscular Dystrophies

Distal muscular dystrophies present as a dominant, adult-onset form and an early onset autosomal recessive, slowly progressive form (200,273). Another form is characterized by the presence of rimmed vacuoles within muscle. This last disorder is allelic with hereditary inclusion body myopathy and, therefore, is not truly a muscular dystrophy (273,274). A hereditary infantile form of distal myopathy is discribed clinically (274), but its molecular basis is unknown. All these entities are rare, and Brooke has pointed out that myotonic dystrophy is the most common myopathy to affect the distal musculature in early life (2).

Congenital Muscular Dystrophies

Congenital muscular dystrophies (CMD), a heterogenous group of autosomally recessively transmitted disorders, are characterized by the presence at birth of a proximal muscular weakness, which progresses slowly and is accompanied by pathologic muscular changes that are consistent with muscular dystrophy (275) (Table 16.9; 243,276–285). Structural brain defects with or without mental retardation are seen in several of the disorders. The CMDs represent one of the less common causes of the floppy infant syndrome. Some authors classify CMDs with the "congenital myopathies," but this assertion is not consistent with a definition of congenital myopathies as nonprogressive diseases showing alterations in the muscle biopsy that exclude myofiber necrosis. CMD was first described in 1903 by Batten (286). The current classification and a recent update on the known genetic and histopathologic features were reviewed in 2004 by Muntoni and Voit (287).

Though the clinical presentation may be that of a pure myopathy, most CMDs are associated with brain malformations involving the cerebral cortex, cerebellum, and brainstem. The best-defined CMDs are Fukuyama muscular dystrophy, Walker-Warburg disease, muscle-eye-brain disease of Santavuori, Ullrich disease, and merosin-deficient CMD.

Approximately 40% of infants with CMD have a primary deficiency of the laminin α2 chain of merosin due to mutations in the *LAMA2* gene (CMD 1A) (172). In addition,

TABLE 16.9 Clinical and Genetic Features of the Congenital Muscular Dystrophies

Name	Gene Locus	Protein Defect	Clinical Features	Reference
1A	6q22–q23	Laminin α-2 (merosin)	40% of CMD	276
1B	1q42	?	Muscle hypertrophy, rigidity of spine, contractures of Achilles tendons	277
1C	19q13.3	Fukutin-related protein (FKRP)	Multiple small cysts throughout brain, also causes AR limb-girdle dystrophy	278
	12q13	Laminin receptor (α 7 integrin)	CMDS, cognitive impairment in some	279
Fukuyama muscular dystrophy	9q31–q33	Fukutin	Muscle weakness at birth, early contractures, massive decrease in WM density, also can cause the more severe Walker-Warburg syndrome	280
Rigid spine muscular dystrophy	1p35–p36	Selenoprotein N1 (SEPN1)	AR, limitation of flexion of dorsolumbar and cervical spine, nonprogressive	281
Muscle-eye-brain disease	1p32–p34	Glycosyltransferase	Congenital hypotonia, myopia, mental retardation	282,283
Ullrich variant	21q22.3	α2 chain of collagen VI	AR, slowly progressive muscle weakness, contractures of proximal joints	284,285
Walker-Warburg syndrome	9q31	protein *O*-mannosyl-transferase (POMT1) in about 20%	Lissencephaly, retinal abnormalities, CMD	243

CMDS, congenital muscular dystrophy; WM, white matter; AR, autosomal recessive.

a secondary laminin α2 deficiency is seen in several other CMD syndromes.

In one variant, first described by Fukuyama, severe mental retardation and seizures accompany muscular weakness (245). Although rare outside of Japan, this condition is second in frequency only to Duchenne muscular dystrophy in that country. It is transmitted as an autosomal recessive disorder with the gene localized to the long arm of chromosome 9 (9q31–q33). The gene codes for fukutin, one of the dystrophin-associated glycoproteins, which normally is expressed in both muscle and brain (275,288,289). The function of fukutin is not clear, but from its structure, it is believed to be involved in polysaccharide/phosphorylcholine modification and mannosyl phosphorylation (282).

In Fukuyama CMD, muscle weakness is present from birth, with contractures appearing early. In addition to generalized limb and trunk weakness, facial muscles are involved. CK levels are generally elevated and can reach 10 to 50 times normal after 6 months of age. Neuroimaging is often spectacular, with a massive decrease in the density of white matter in approximately one-third of infants (280). The electroencephalogram can show paroxysmal discharges, and the visual-evoked potentials also can be abnormal. Pathologic changes within the brain include pachygyria, micropolygyria, abnormal cortical lamination consistent with type II lissencephaly, and hypomyelination. The condition is progressive and is generally fatal by the end of the first decade.

The other CMDs may be divided into two groups, one with deficiency of merosin in muscle and another in which merosin is normally expressed. Merosin, the α_2 chain or M-chain of laminin, is an extracellular matrix protein that attaches the sarcolemma (i.e., the plasma membrane of the muscle fiber) to the basal lamina or basement membrane (see Fig. 16.6). Whereas primary merosin deficiency is associated with the *LAMA2* locus on 6q22, conditions with secondary merosin deficiency are genetically heterogenous, with some being linked to chromosome 1q42 (CMD 1B) (277). Reduced merosin also is seen in muscle-eye-brain disease and Fukuyama muscular dystrophy (290,291). In the absence of merosin, the basal lamina cannot form or disappear (Figs. 16.8 and 16.9), and the sarcolemma then degenerates secondarily, resulting in the eventual necrosis of the myofiber (292–294). Merosin can be demonstrated by immunocytochemistry in frozen sections of the muscle biopsy but also is present in skin and can be detected by skin biopsy. However, correlative studies of muscle and cutaneous merosin expression have not been documented sufficiently for the diagnosis to depend solely on skin biopsy. Merosin also is strongly expressed in Schwann cells, so peripheral nerve is immunoreactive for merosin both in muscle and skin biopsies. This is in contrast to dystrophin, sarcoglycans, and other sarcolemmal region proteins. When merosin is absent from myofibers, it also is not expressed in Schwann cells. Merosin also is expressed in brain and may contribute to pachygyria and other cerebral malformations in CMDs, but its role in neuroblast migration remains uncertain.

One of the prominent histopathologic features of the CMDs, with or without merosin deficiency, is a striking proliferation of endomysial collagen, evident even at birth,

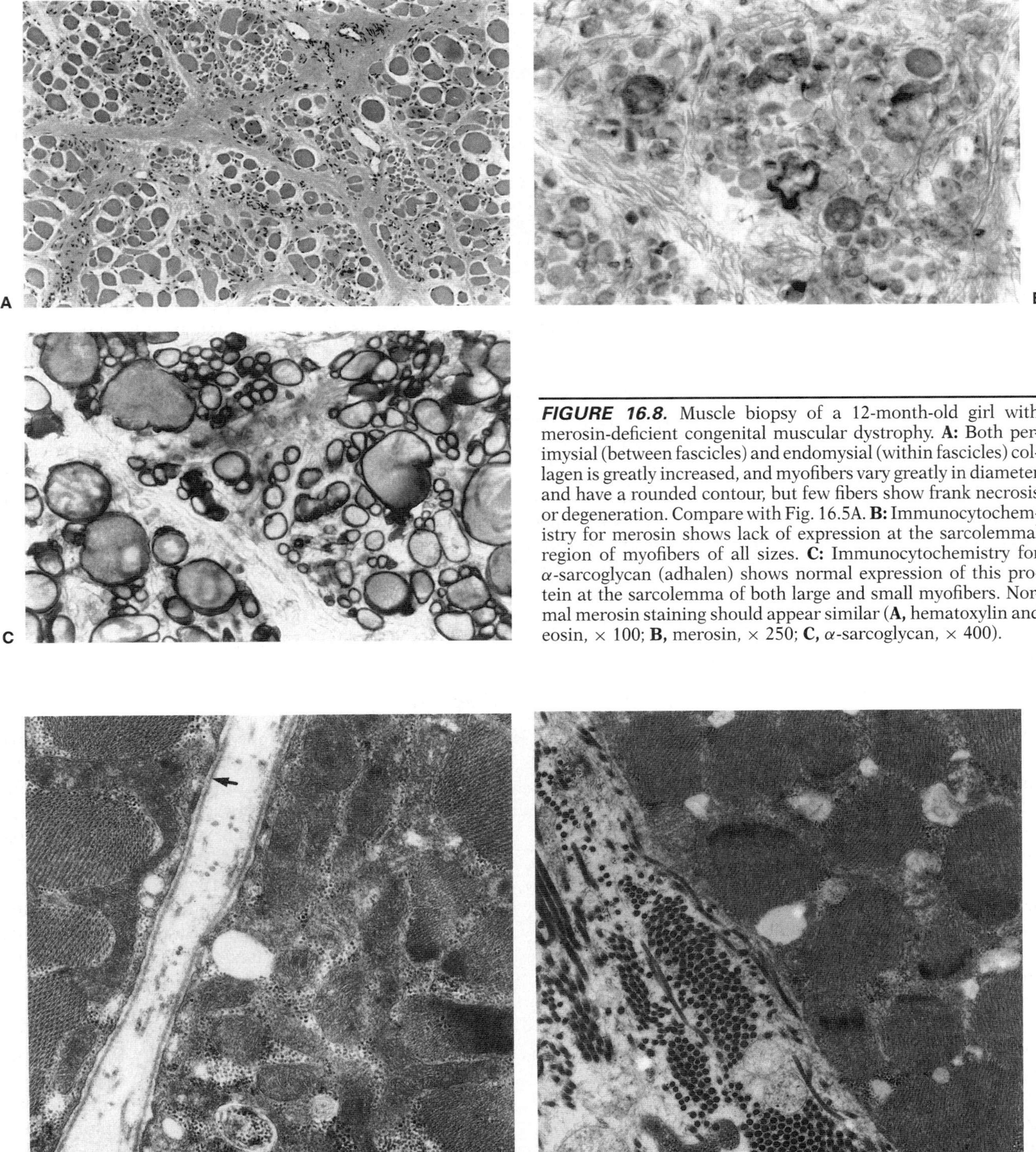

FIGURE 16.8. Muscle biopsy of a 12-month-old girl with merosin-deficient congenital muscular dystrophy. **A:** Both perimysial (between fascicles) and endomysial (within fascicles) collagen is greatly increased, and myofibers vary greatly in diameter and have a rounded contour, but few fibers show frank necrosis or degeneration. Compare with Fig. 16.5A. **B:** Immunocytochemistry for merosin shows lack of expression at the sarcolemmal region of myofibers of all sizes. **C:** Immunocytochemistry for α-sarcoglycan (adhalen) shows normal expression of this protein at the sarcolemma of both large and small myofibers. Normal merosin staining should appear similar (**A,** hematoxylin and eosin, $\times$ 100; **B,** merosin, $\times$ 250; **C,** α-sarcoglycan, $\times$ 400).

FIGURE 16.9. Electron micrographs of sarcolemmal region of **(A)** normal myofibers and **(B)** myofibers in merosin-deficient congenital muscular dystrophy, the biopsy shown in Figure 16.8. **A:** The sarcolemma is normally a well-defined plasma membrane of the myofiber; external to it is a thin gray line corresponding to the basal lamina or basement membrane (*arrow*). **B:** In merosin deficiency, the basal lamina is absent or discontinuous and the sarcolemma is less distinct than normal. Collagen is seen between myofibers (**A** and **B,** Uranyl acetate and lead citrate, $\times$ 16,000).

although the clinical progression of the disease may be slower than the neonatal muscle biopsy might have predicted. The number of frankly necrotic myofibers at any stage in the disease is never as great as in Duchenne dystrophy.

Infants with merosin deficiency (CMD 1A) manifest with a generalized weakness and dysphagia and often require a gastrostomy to prevent recurrent aspiration. Some infants also have apneic spells or respiratory insufficiency. CNS involvement, expressed as mental retardation, motor deficits, and cerebral cortical dysplasia, does not correlate well with the presence or absence of merosin or with the severity of the myopathy (295). Patients with merosin deficiency also show clinical and electrophysiologic evidence of peripheral neuropathy (296).

At least two of the other CMDs are the result of mutations in genes involved in *O*-mannosylation of α-dystroglycan (α-DG), *POMT1* and *POMGnT1*, respectively. α-DG is a major component of the sarcolemmal muscle membrane (see Fig. 16.6) (282). A defect in *POMT1* has been associated with Walker-Warburg syndrome. In this condition, a merosin-positive CMD transmitted as an autosomal recessive trait (242,297), the muscle disease is accompanied by type II lissencephaly (see Chapter 5), Dandy-Walker cyst, and cerebellar and retinal malformations. Muscle-eye-brain of Santavuori, a CMD found mainly in Finland, is due to mutations in the *POMGnT1* gene (283). This gene catalyzes the transfer of *N*-acetylglucosamine to *O*-mannose of glycoproteins, including dystroglycan that is linked to the dystrophin molecule at the sarcolemma and also is essential for neuroblast migration in the brain (298). Therefore, these CMDs are disorders of glycosylation. Muscle-eye-brain disease presents with congenital hypotonia, myopia, and mental retardation.

A defect in Fukutin-related protein (FKRP), another glycosylation enzyme, has been associated with a clinical picture of CMD, accompanied by microcephaly, cerebellar cysts, and vermian hypoplasia (299). So far, this condition has only been encountered in Tunisian children (300).

Another variant of CMD, Ullrich disease, is an autosomal recessive condition first recognized by Ullrich in 1930 (301). It is associated with recessive mutations in any one of the three collagen VI genes, *COL6A1*, *COL6A2* and *COL6A3* (284). Collagen VI is an ubiquitously expressed extracellular matrix protein composed of three chains: $\alpha 1$, $\alpha 2$ and $\alpha 3$, encoded by genes *COL6A1* and *COL6A2* on chromosome 21q22.3 and *COL6A3* with a locus at 2q37. The Ullrich phenotype is characterized by a nonprogressive or slowly advancing congenital muscle weakness, striking congenital contractures of the proximal joints, hyperextensibility of the distal joints, and normal intelligence (301–303). Hyperhidrosis and posterior protrusion of the calcaneus can be characteristic for this entity (303). One of the most constant and useful signs that provide a clinical clue and is not shared by most other neuromuscular diseases are congenital contractures, particularly of the elbows so that the forearm cannot be extended beyond about 160°. Torticollis also is frequently present at birth, and joint contractures may be multiple and involve both proximal and distal joints. These contractures are associated with hypotonia within the limited range of motion. A characteristic facial appearance of a round face with drooping of the lower eyelid and prominent ears is another clinical clue. The skin typically shows follicular hyperkeratosis, a sign already noted by Ullrich (301). Magnetic resonance imaging of thigh muscles in Ullrich disease shows a characteristic pattern of sparing of density changes in some muscles, such as the sartorius and gracilis, and may be a useful though not definitive clinical supplement in diagnosis (304). Merosin is always normal in Ullrich disease, but since the basis is a defect in collagen VI, there is a useful immunocytochemical antibody that can be used to demonstrate collagen VI in the muscle biopsy. There is no present means of detecting this defect in blood. Dominant mutations in the three collagen VI genes are associated with Bethlem myopathy, an early onset benign myopathy characterized by proximal muscular weakness and multiple flexion contractures (305).

The relationships between genotype and phenotype in the various CMDs is far from clear. They have been reviewed by Muntoni and Voit (287).

Diagnosis

Even though a fully developed case of muscular dystrophy can be readily diagnosed on clinical grounds (namely, by the proximal distribution of the involved muscles, the presence of pseudohypertrophy, and the absence of deep tendon reflexes at the proximal musculature), a complete investigation, including serum CK levels and a muscle biopsy, is the first step toward arriving at a diagnosis.

A qualitatively altered dystrophin is consistent with the diagnosis of Becker muscular dystrophy; absent dystrophin indicates the diagnosis of Duchenne muscular dystrophy (Fig. 16.10). Abnormal immunohistochemistry for dystrophin in a girl indicates a carrier state. Normal dystrophin points to another form of muscular dystrophy, such as the limb-girdle or Emery-Dreifuss types (306).

Muscle tissue (100 mg maintained at −70°C) suffices for quantitation of dystrophin and determination of molecular weight by Western blotting. For ELISA analysis, much smaller amounts (5 mg of tissue) suffice. Neither the site of the muscle biopsy nor the age of the patient is important in the evaluation of dystrophin (211). The anatomic appearance of the muscle biopsy and the elevation of muscle enzymes are less specific diagnostic parameters.

Because the early stages of the dystrophic process are accompanied by a marked outflow of muscle enzymes into the circulation, the serum level of many soluble enzymes normally present in muscle tissue is increased. These include aspartate aminotransferase, alanine

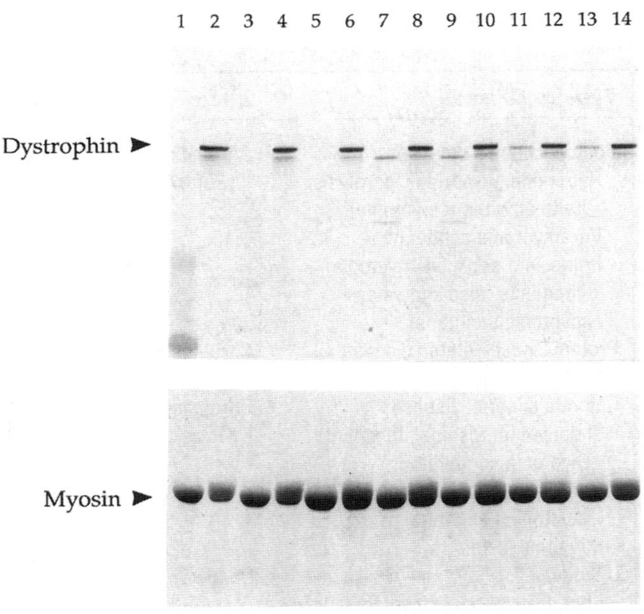

FIGURE 16.10. Western blot on muscle biopsies from patients with muscular dystrophies. The dystrophin assay is run with two different antibodies: antibody corresponding to amino acids 1991–3112 and a carboxyl terminus antibody corresponding to amino acids 3669–3685. Lanes 3, 5: Patient with Duchenne muscular dystrophy; dystrophin levels are virtually absent. Lanes 7, 9: Patient with mild to moderate Becker muscular dystrophy. Dystrophin is present in reduced amounts at an abnormal location. Lanes 11, 13: Patient with severe Becker muscular dystrophy. Marked reduction of dystrophin, which is in its normal location. Lane 1 shows molecular weight markers; even numbered lanes are control biopsies. (Courtesy of Genica Pharmaceuticals Corporation, Worcester, MA.)

aminotransferase, lactic dehydrogenase, aldolase, and CK. Of these enzymes, an elevation of CK MM isozyme is the most sensitive and specific for the presence of a dystrophic process (307).

In the early stages of Duchenne muscular dystrophy, and even before clinical signs appear, serum CK levels are strikingly increased. Neither liver disease nor hemolysis of blood samples changes the serum activity of this enzyme; this abnormality is fairly specific for a dystrophic process. With progression of the disease, enzyme levels decrease. Dystrophies other than the Duchenne form, with the exception of the Fukuyama type of congenital muscular dystrophy, show less striking enzyme abnormalities, and clinically typical cases of LGMD with normal serum enzymes are not rare.

DNA markers derived from within the dystrophin gene locus have been used in the prenatal diagnosis of Duchenne muscular dystrophy using amniocytes or chorionic villus cells. Despite the large number of intragenic DNA polymorphisms available, the diagnosis is still fraught with errors. For one, the large size of the gene permits crossovers within it (308). Furthermore, in the two-thirds of cases in which no previous family history of the disease is seen, linkage analysis is inadequate (309). Finally, deletion mutants are detectable only in some 65% of cases. For these reasons, other diagnostic means must be used (310). These include sonographically guided fetal muscle biopsy for dystrophin analysis by immunofluorescence, or measuring dystrophin by immunocytochemical analysis on amniocytes in which myogenesis was induced by infecting them with a retrovirus containing a gene that induces myogenesis (311).

In carriers of Duchenne or Becker muscular dystrophy, serum CK levels are elevated. This elevation is most striking in children younger than 16 years of age, and at that age, carrier detection, using the mean value of three or more separate CK estimations, is close to 100%. When mothers who are obligate carriers for Duchenne muscular dystrophy are screened by means of CK levels, the detection rate is approximately 70%. This discrepancy appears to be a function of the decrease in CK levels with age (312). The information obtained from the DNA probes can be correlated with the CK test data or immunohistochemistry for dystrophin on muscle biopsy to provide genetic information with 98% to 99% reliability (306).

Treatment

At present, no treatment is effective for any of the muscular dystrophies. The anecdotal effectiveness of courses of vitamin E and combinations of amino acids has not withstood controlled trial. A variety of corticosteroids slow the progression of the disease, in particular deflacort, a prednisolone derivative that appears to have the least side effects and has shown some benefit in well-controlled studies (314). Long-term treatment with corticosteroids, however, may actually make the patient weaker by the added weight of additional subcutaneous adipose tissue that the weakened muscles must overcome and because of other complications of chronic corticosteroid therapy in any patient. Varieties of the basic hydrocortisone molecule have been tried in an effort to reduce the undesirable side effects on a chronic basis, such as the substitution of deflazacort for prednisone in the treatment of Duchenne muscular dystrophy, with modest success (315), but the overall results were not as good as had been anticipated. Nevertheless, some children do seem to benefit long-term from the judicious use of low dose steroids, and this treatment should be considered early in the course of the disease. Even after a child is no longer ambulatory, deflazacort may stabilize the spine and delay scoliosis (315a).

The interesting observation that boys with growth hormone deficiency have a milder form of Duchenne muscular dystrophy has led to a randomized, double-blind controlled trial using mazindol, a growth hormone inhibitor. This did not show any slowing of the progression of muscular weakness (316). A significant proportion of patients with FSHD, when treated with corticosteroids, experience dramatic but often transient clinical improvement that is coupled with a striking decrease in previously elevated serum CK levels (317). Other potential therapeutic approaches include gene replacement, myoblast transplantation, or replacement of dystrophin by other, dystrophin-related proteins. The promises and problems inherent in these various approaches have been reviewed (175,318–320). Although there have been few adverse effects, less than 1% of the donor cells survived to express dystrophin (269). The reason for poor survival is unclear; it does not appear to be caused by immune rejection (320–322).

As stated by Brooke (2), "incurable and untreatable are not synonymous." A treatment program for the child with muscular dystrophy not only offers a positive attitude and hope to family and child, but also keeps the child as active as possible until such time, not too distant from now, when molecular biology will offer a more definitive approach. In the early stages of the illness, passive stretching of affected muscles and the application of night splints can delay contractures. Children are encouraged to take as much exercise as they desire. Physiotherapy can be helpful in preventing contractures of the ankles and hips in particular, but once the contractures appear, therapy alone cannot reverse them. Because of progressive fibrosis of muscle, contractures often appear despite conscientious physiotherapy. If physiotherapy is too rigorous, it may actually accelerate the rate of degeneration of the fragile myofibers with abnormal sarcolemmal membranes, reflected as a further increase in serum CK, so this therapy must be titrated to be forceful enough to prevent contractures without being excessive, causing further damage to the muscle.

While the child is still walking, major surgery is inadvisable. In the more advanced case, bracing is preferable to use of a wheelchair because the latter promotes curvature of the spine. Body jackets tend to delay these deformities. Orthopedic measures, particularly those followed by prolonged bed rest, seem to hasten the downhill process and should be resorted to only when absolutely necessary.

A small proportion of children with mild or clinically inapparent muscle disease develop anesthesia-induced malignant hyperpyrexia, also known as malignant hyperthermia (323,324). To prevent this complication, local or spinal anesthesia should be used for all procedures, or dantrolene sodium may be administered for several hours before the anesthetic, which effectively blocks this complication. If general anesthesia is unavoidable, thiopental sodium is the preferred agent, and body temperature should be monitored throughout surgery.

Myotonic Disorders

A number of genetically distinct conditions share the clinical feature of myotonia of the voluntary muscles. In some, the myotonic phenomenon is the most evident aspect of the disease; in others, it is overshadowed by other symptoms. Although in the past the myotonias were believed to represent various expressions of the same genetic disorder, it is now apparent that they have different underlying biochemical defects and can be classified as *channelopathies* of the sarcolemma, related to either sodium or chloride channels.

TABLE 16.10 Genetic Classification of the Myotonias

Type of Disease	*Locus*
Sodium channel diseases	Chromosome 17q23.1-q25.3 (*SCN4A* gene)
Hyperkalemic periodic paralysis (with or without myotonia)	
Paramyotonia congenita	
Potassium-sensitive myotonia congenita (also known as myotonia fluctuans)	
Protein kinase-related disease	Chromosome 19q13.3
Myotonic dystrophy	
Chloride channel diseases	Chromosome 7q32 (*CLCN1*)
Thomsen (autosomal dominant) myotonia congenita	
Becker (autosomal recessive) myotonia congenita	
Myotonia lesion	
Unknown	Unknown
Chondrodystrophic myotonia (autosomal dominant; also known as Schwartz-Jampel syndrome)	
Hyperkalemic periodic paralysis with dysrhythmias (Andersen syndrome)	

From Ptacek LJ, Johnson KJ, Griggs RC. Genetics and physiology of the myotonic muscle disorders. *N Engl J Med* 1993;328:482. With permission.

From a clinical point of view, the myotonias can be divided into nondystrophic and dystrophic types. The nondystrophic myotonias are further divided into myotonia congenita, paramyotonia congenita, hyperkalemic periodic paralysis, and the various syndromes of continuous motor discharges (Table 16.10).

Myotonia is characterized by a failure of voluntary muscle to relax after contraction ceases and by a slow, tonic response to mechanical and electric stimulation. This phenomenon is most readily observed in the muscles of the hand, face, and tongue. Patients are unable to relax their grasp, and percussion of the thenar eminence can produce a dimple lasting several seconds. Repetitive movements lessen myotonia; exposure to cold aggravates it. It is useful to ask the patient if the condition is aggravated or improved on entering a warm bath or shower or a cold swimming pool.

The defects of sodium and chloride channels may be distinguished by a careful history and physical examination. In sodium-channel disorders, the patient finds it increasingly difficult to relax muscle contractions with continued exercise; in chloride-channel disorders, by contrast, exercise improves the myotonia or abolishes it temporarily, so it is beneficial that patients learn to do warm-up exercises before undertaking physical tasks. Moxley and Meola have written an excellent review of the myotonic disorders that includes clinical, physiologic, and molecular genetic aspects (325).

Myotonic Dystrophies

Not a rare group of diseases (incidence at birth is 13.5 in 100,000), the myotonic dystrophies are transmitted as an autosomal dominant trait and are marked by the association of myotonia with a dystrophic process of muscle and multisystem involvement (235). Classic myotonic dystrophy (DM1) is caused by a cytosinethymineguanine (CTG) trinucleotide expansion on chromosome 19q13.3 in the 3' untranslated region of *DMPK*, the gene that encodes a serine-threonine protein kinase. DM2 is associated with unstable CTG repeat expansion on chromosome 3q21 of an intron of the zinc finger 9 protein gene. DM3 is not linked to either 19q13.3 or 3q21, but probably to chromosome 15q21–24. Neither DM2 or DM3 has been associated with congenital myotonic dystrophy (325).

Although DM1 myotonia usually appears in late adolescence or early adult life, it can manifest at birth (congenital myotonic dystrophy) or during the first decade (juvenile myotonic dystrophy). These congenital and juvenile forms of myotonic dystrophy constitute approximately 20% of all myotonic cases. As a rule, the disease shows an earlier onset and increasing severity of clinical manifestations in successive generations, a phenomenon termed *anticipation* (326).

In some patients, myotonia is severe and generalized, and dystrophic features are absent or develop late in life. In others, muscular atrophy and weakness are the prominent abnormalities, with myotonia difficult to elicit or completely absent on physical examination and recognized only on EMG studies. Sometimes, both clinical variants occur in the same family (327,328).

The distribution of muscular atrophy is characteristic for the disease. The face, sternocleidomastoids, and girdle musculature are the initial sites of atrophy. The wasted, weakened sternocleidomastoids and the facial atrophy marked by shrinkage of the masseter and temporal muscles produce a *hatchet face* appearance, which is distinctive even in a small child (Fig. 16.11). An inability to relax a smile, the *Cheshire cat smile*, also is characteristic (329). Myotonic dystrophy differs from most primary myopathies in that distal rather than proximal involvement predominates. This pattern is not caused by an accompanying neuropathy.

Smooth muscles, particularly those of the pharynx, esophagus, and gastrointestinal tract, are involved as well,

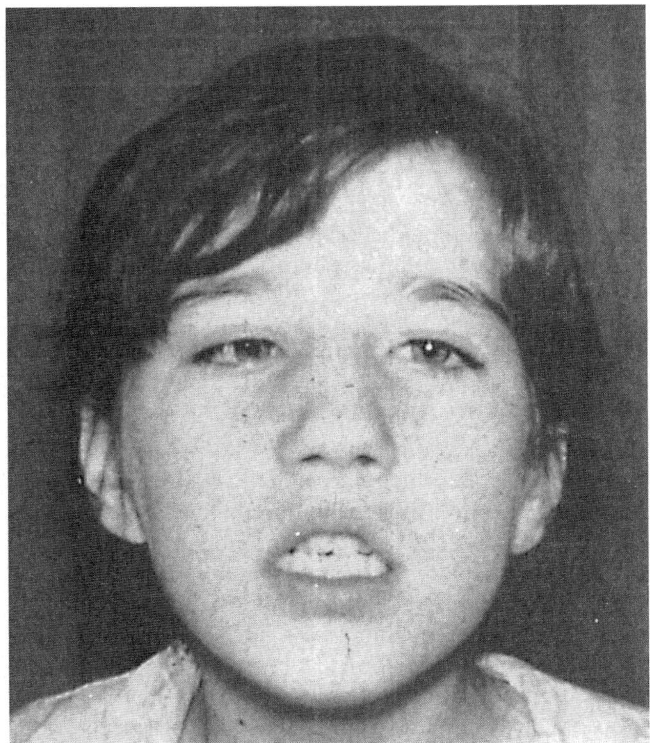

FIGURE 16.11. An 11-year-old girl with myotonic dystrophy. Note the distinctive snarling appearance of the face. Her presenting symptoms were impaired speech and mild mental dullness. Because of the atrophy of the neck muscles, the profile can have a "hatchet face" appearance.

and myotonia of the anal sphincter has been described (330). The involved neonate and young infant may have loss of peristalsis because of the smooth muscle involvement, leading to chronic obstipation, fecal retention, and distention of the bowel (331). Conduction velocities are slowed in several motor nerves, and biopsy reveals a preferential loss of the larger myelinated fibers. The cause of the polyneuropathy is still unknown; it is not the result of entrapment or secondary to muscle disease (235). Electrocardiographic abnormalities were seen in 86% of Harper's patients. These include cardiac conduction defects, mainly a prolonged PR interval (70%), and arrhythmias, mainly atrial flutter seen in 15% (235). Myotonic dystrophy is accompanied by excessive daytime sleepiness and is a common cause of this symptom in childhood.

Posterior cortical cataracts can regularly be demonstrated in the adult with myotonic dystrophy and can even occur in the absence of either myotonia or dystrophy in the guise of senile or presenile cataracts. In juvenile myotonic dystrophy, cataracts usually are not seen until after 10 years of age, but occasionally, neonates with symptomatic disease at birth have congenital cataracts in one or both eyes. The incidence in children with myotonic dystrophy is less than 30%, even when a careful slit-lamp examination is performed. Pigmentary retinal degeneration is relatively common; an abnormal electroretinogram (ERG) can predate muscular symptoms. Mental retardation is seen in 80% of patients with myotonic dystrophy and occurs almost invariably in congenital myotonic dystrophy. Cognitive impairment and learning disabilities in school-age childern are well documented (331a). In some instances, developmental delay is apparent before the onset of muscular symptoms. Mental retardation may be due to accumulations of mutant *DMPK* mRNA and aberrant alternative splicing in cerebral cortical neurons (331b).

Endocrine abnormalities such as frontal baldness, loss of body hair, and testicular atrophy are not seen in the affected child (332). Between 6.5% and 20.0% of patients ultimately develop an unusual insulin-resistant form of diabetes mellitus, which occasionally occurs before adolescence (333,334). Various immunologic abnormalities have been documented. Most consistent is an increased catabolism of IgG, which results in low serum concentrations of the immunoglobulin in approximately one-third of subjects, including some who have not yet developed muscle weakness (335,336).

The congenital form of myotonic dystrophy is almost invariably transmitted by an affected mother. In the DNA of infants, the number of CTG repeats ranges from 500 to 2,700, and the intergenerational expansion of the repeat depends on the sex of the transmitting parent (337). With maternal transmission of the myotonic dystrophy gene, there is marked expansion of the repeat, whereas with paternal transmission, there is reduced amplification or even contraction (338,339).

In congenital myotonic dystrophy, the disease expresses itself by a weak suck, delayed speech, retarded motor development, and generalized hypotonia especially involving the neck muscles. Infants are prone to perinatal asphyxia. Facial diplegia is evident in 87% of infants, delayed motor development in 87%, and mental retardation in 68% (234). Approximately one-half of mothers who carry an offspring with congenital myotonic dystrophy have polyhydramnios, sometimes sufficiently severe to require amniocentesis (331). Arthrogryposis can be noted at birth (95). Clinical myotonia is invariably absent before 1 year of age and is present in only 12% of 1- to 5-year-old children (235). MRI studies show white matter lesions and brain atrophy are often a reflection of perinatal asphyxial insults sustained by the infants (340).

The clinical course in the fully developed case of congenital myotonic dystrophy is one of gradual debilitation. Respiratory insufficiency, dysphagia and aspiration, and poor gastrointestinal motility may present life-threatening presentations in the neonatal period (331). Infants who survive the first year of life appear to improve over the course of the subsequent few years, only to deteriorate gradually with increasing muscular weakness, the appearance of myotonia, and the various other features of the adult form of the disease. Most significantly, these features include diabetes mellitus (334); cardiac involvement that usually takes the form of conduction defects; and ultimately, congestive heart failure (235) or sudden death as a consequence of tachyarrhythmias or bradyarrhythmias (341).

DM2 is prevalent in families of northern European ancestry, and in Germany, it is as common as DM1 (342). The clinical picture resembles adult-onset DM1, with electrographic myotonia, muscular dystrophy, cataracts, diabetes, and cardiac conduction defects. Initial symptoms in DM2 often involve proximal lower extremity musculature, whereas DM1 is more apt to be associated with severe muscle atrophy and symptomatic finger flexor weakness. DM2 is not associated with severely atrophic facial and forearm muscles. Clinical myotonia is rare, and to date, a congenital form of DM2 has not been recorded. Muscle biopsy findings are similar to those of DM1 in that there are increased central nuclei, ringed fibers, and subsarcolemmal masses. However, there is a preferential type 2 fiber atrophy in contrast to the type 1 atrophy seen in DM1 subjects (343).

The clinical picture of DM3 also resembles adult onset DM1 (325,344). It has an adult onset and in some families is accompanied by frontotemporal dementia (344).

Diagnosis

In a typical case of myotonic dystrophy affecting an older child, the facial appearance is striking, myotonic phenomena can be elicited, and the family history is often helpful. In the small child or infant, the diagnosis is less obvious, and myotonic phenomena are detected neither clinically nor, in most instances, by electromyogram (EMG) (345). Myotonia is never manifest in infancy and usually does not become evident, either clinically or by EMG, until 4 to 5 years of age. Rather, the characteristic aspects of the disease are facial diplegia and generalized hypotonia. Clinical and EMG examinations of the mother invariably show subclinical or overt signs of myotonic dystrophy (346).

Serum enzymes are usually normal. On EMG, prolonged trains of high-frequency discharges arising from single fibers or groups of muscle fibers occur in response to electrode insertion or movement. Amplified, their sound is highly characteristic, like that of a dive-bomber. Neuroimaging studies show ventricular enlargement, and in some instances hypoplasia of the corpus callosum, and abnormal myelination (347).

Myotonia occasionally is observed in hyperkalemic periodic paralysis, polyneuritis, and polymyositis. A slowing in muscular contraction and relaxation, resembling myotonia, also can be seen in hypothyroidism.

A DNA probe that is specific for more than 96% of patients is available for the diagnosis of myotonic dystrophy and obviates the need for linkage analyses (348). Muscle biopsy is generally not required because it is not definitively diagnostic, though characteristic changes such as large numbers of centronuclear fibers and selective type I fiber atrophy in children and many stages of arrested maturation in neonates are strongly suggestive of the diagnosis (349).

Treatment

When myotonic dystrophy occurs in childhood, myotonia is rarely severe enough to warrant intensive treatment, and there is no evidence that improvement of the myotonia affects the dystrophic process. Procaine amine, quinine, corticosteroids, antihistamines, and calcium-channel blockers such as nifedipine can be of benefit in children with myotonia caused by myotonic dystrophy or myotonia congenita (350,351). The side effects of these drugs at times are more disturbing than the myotonia. Medications that work at the sodium channel, such as carbamazepine, phenytoin, and especially mexiletine are often helpful in minimizing myotonia, but if the patient has predominantly weakness rather than myotonia, they are ineffective.

Pathologic Anatomy

Microscopic examination of muscle obtained from subjects with the adult form of myotonic dystrophy reveals nonspecific alterations in the appearance of the muscle fibers resembling that seen in other muscular dystrophies as a necrotizing myopathy, but usually with little or no connective tissue proliferation. The number of centronuclear fibers often is excessive. A characteristic finding shared only by a few other myopathies is selective type 1 myofibers atrophy, a feature shared with Emery-Dreifuss dystrophy but not seen in Duchenne, limb-girdle, or facioscapulohumeral dystrophy. Another of the histologic characteristics of the disease is a reorientation of peripheral myofibrils from a longitudinal disposition to one ringing the muscle fiber. The significance of this abnormality is uncertain; it is usually seen in long-standing myotonic dystrophy and never in the congenital or early forms of the disorder. It also occurs in hypothyroidism, limb-girdle, and FSHD, and can be the result of trauma to muscle. None of the ultrastructural features of myotonic muscle is specific (349). The sarcolemmal membrane and basal lamina (basement membrane) are well preserved. Immunocytochemical expression of sarcolemma-associated proteins such as dystrophin, merosin, and the sarcoglycans is normal.

In neonatal myotonic dystrophy, the muscle fibers present an apparent maturational arrest. They are arrested in maturation in various stages of development within the same fascicles: myoblasts, myotubes, incomplete histochemical differentiation into type 1 and type 2 fibers, and persistent expression of excessive fetal intermediate filament proteins such as desmin and vimentin (352,353). The ultrastructure in the congenital disease shows additional features not seen at the light microscopic level: persistent fetal orientation of triads parallel to the long axis of the myofibril and lack of registry of Z-bands of adjacent myofibrils, features that normally mature at approximately 30-weeks' gestation. In some cases of congenital myotonic dystrophy, congenital muscle fiber-type disproportion (see Congenital Myopathies, later in this chapter) is the dominant pattern of the muscle biopsy.

Pathogenesis

DMPK, the gene for myotonic dystrophy, is located on the long arm of chromosome 19 (19q13.3) and codes for serine-threonine protein kinase, a cyclic AMP-dependent protein kinase. Protein kinases modulate the activities of a variety of target proteins by phosphorylating some of their serine residues. In 1992, several groups who independently studied patients with myotonic dystrophy demonstrated an expansion on the 3' untranslated region of *DMPK* of a cytosinethymineguanine trinucleotide repeat (354,355). The CTG sequence is repeated between 5 and 35 times in DNA derived from healthy subjects, but between 40 and 1,500 times in DNA derived from patients with myotonic dystrophy (337), and 1,500 to 2,500 times in DNA derived from subjects with congenital myotonic dystrophy (338,339). Rare families with the characteristic picture of myotonic dystrophy but no triplet expansion have been encountered (356). With transmission of the gene to subsequent generations, the length of the CTG repeat tends to increase. This is especially the case when the gene is transmitted by an affected mother. Concomitant with this increase is a worsening of clinical symptoms in subsequent generations. When an affected father transmits the gene, on rare occasions, a contraction of the expanded repeat occurs into the normal range (357).

The mechanism by which the CTG expansion produces the multisystemic symptoms in DM1 has undergone considerable scrutiny. It is clear that the trinucleotide repeat does not affect the coding portion of the gene and that the mutation is transcribed into RNA but not translated into protein. Furthermore, the fact that no reported cases of DM1 have been caused by point mutations in the DMPK gene further suggests that the multisystemic features of DM1 are not caused simply by DMPK haploinsufficiency. Fluorescence *in situ* hybridization (FISH) experiments have demonstrated that CUG-containing nuclear RNA foci accumulate as foci in the nuclei of muscle and brain from DM1 subjects (358,359). These RNA-containing foci are believed exert a transdominant effect that disrupts splicing and possibly other cellular functions by binding to CUG-BP and ETR-3 like factor (CELF) and muscleblind proteins, cell-specific RNA-binding proteins involved in alternative splicing of messenger RNA (mRNA) (360). (The term *muscleblind* refers to the fact that this protein family is homologous to Drosophila, where these proteins are involved in myoblast and photoreceptor differentiation). CUG RNA expansions bind and sequester these transcription factors and in this manner disrupt regulation of a variety of genes including cardiac troponin T, the insulin receptor, and the chloride channel ClC-1, the main chloride channel in muscle (361,362).

DM2 also is caused by a transcribed but untranslated repeat expansion—but this time, a CCTG repeat expansion located in intron 1 of the zinc finger protein 9 (*ZNF9*) gene. Although DM2 is generally a milder disease than DM1, the DM2 CCTG expansions can be much larger than DM1 CTG expansions, with alleles ranging in size from ~75 to 11,000 CCTG repeats. As is the case in DM1, CCUG-containing RNA foci are found in DM2 muscle, and the RNA-binding proteins muscleblind colocalize to the repeat-containing foci (363).

Because DM1 patients have reduced reproductive ability, the gene pool needs to be replenished. This appears to happen by preferential transmission to offspring of alleles with greater than 19 CTG repeats (364).

Other Myotonic Disorders

Molecular biology has started to unravel the physiologic defects that underlie the various myotonic disorders (see Table 16.10). Mytonic disorders result from an abnormality of muscle membrane excitability. Two major subgroups have been recognized. In one, the mutations involve the skeletal muscle chloride channel (*CLCN1*), and in the other, they affect the gene that codes for the α-subunit of the skeletal muscle voltage-gated sodium channel (*SCN4A*) (365).

Two clinical entities are caused by a disorder of *CLCN1*. These are autosomal dominant myotonia congenita (Thompsen disease) and autosomal recessive Becker generalized myotonia (365,366). In both dominant and recessive forms of myotonia congenita, muscle membrane chloride conductance is abnormal in that the rate of repolarization after an action potential is excessively slow (367,368).

Numerous mutations in the gene coding for *SCN4A* have been recognized (365,369). They result in a number of phenotypes, of which hyperkalemic periodic paralysis and paramyotonia congenita are the most common (370–372). The presence of genetic defects altering sodium-channel function is consistent with the long-standing clinical observation that in both these diseases, inactivation of sodium channels in muscle is abnormal (373).

Myotonia Congenita (Thomsen Disease and Becker Disease)

Myotonia congenita (Thomsen disease and Becker disease) was first described in 1876 by Thomsen, an English physician, in himself and his own son (374). It is a rare condition, with the highest prevalence being in northern Finland, where it occurs in 7.3 per 100,000 (375). In myotonia congenita, myotonia and muscle stiffness are first observed in infancy. Occasional choking episodes are not uncommon, as is prolonged closure of eyes after sneezing. Myotonia improves with exercise and, in most instances, becomes less evident with increasing age. Muscular hypertrophy of the upper and lower extremities is commonly seen in later years (375). Thomsen disease is transmitted as a dominant disorder; a recessive form of myotonia congenita also is recognized and is known as Becker disease (not to be confused with the Becker form of dystrophinopathy related to Duchenne muscular dystrophy) (376). These two patterns of inheritance are different diseases, not only in the mendelian pattern of inheritance, but because of different mutations within the same voltage-gated chloride-channel gene (*CLCN1*) at the 7q32 locus (377). The recessive form is more common and is more severe (372). In some families, myotonia congenita is accompanied by hyperkalemic periodic paralysis, but this is yet another disease caused by a defect in the sodium rather than the chloride channels; this disorder is best classified as a form of paramyotonia congenita (see following discussion) (see Table 16.10).

The serum CK is normal or mildly elevated in the various forms of myotonia congenita. The muscle biopsy is normal or shows minimal, nonspecific alterations, such as excessive variation in myofiber diameter and poor differentiation of type II fiber subtypes with ATPase stains, but there is no myofiber degeneration; hence, unlike myotonic dystrophy, Thomsen and Becker diseases are not muscular dystrophies. The EMG discloses myotonic discharges.

Paramyotonia Congenita (Eulenburg Disease)

In paramyotonia congenita, a dominantly inherited disorder, myotonia is usually recognized during infancy. It is brought on or aggravated by exposure to cold and worsens with continued exercise (378). Many individuals also experience prolonged periods of weakness and develop muscular wasting (379). In some, weakness accompanies an increase in serum potassium, a feature that overlaps with hyperkalemic periodic paralysis (380). The condition is caused by a mutation in the α-subunit of the skeletal muscle voltage-gated sodium channel (*SCN4A*) (365,372).

Rippling muscle disease is a clinically unique condition that appears usually during adult life but may be encountered during the first or second decade. It is characterized by muscular stiffness and myalgia apparent after a period of rest. Symptoms abate with exercise. Generalized muscle hypertrophy occurs, especially in the calves, as well as grip myotonia. Tapping a muscle causes a peculiar rolling contraction across the muscle group that is unaccompanied by myotonic EMG discharges. One gene for this entity has been mapped to chromosome 1q41, but the condition also has been seen with *caveolin-3* mutations, and considerable genetic heterogeneity exists (381). A mutant of caveolin-3 is responsible for at least some cases of rippling muscle disease (382); this glycoprotein of the Golgi apparatus also is implicated in limb-girdle muscular dystrophy type 1C, distal myopathy, and in familial and sporadic hyperCKemia—each disease a different phenotype.

Hyperkalemic Periodic Paralysis

Atypical cases of hyperkalemic periodic paralysis (hyperPP) had been recognized for several years before Gamstorp's classic description of this condition (383). In her subjects, attacks started in early childhood, did not respond to potassium, and were unaccompanied by an electrolyte imbalance.

Attacks often begin in infancy, and in 90% of cases, the disease becomes established by 10 years of age. The condition affects both sexes equally and is transmitted by an autosomal dominant gene with a strong penetrance. The gene has been mapped to the long arm of chromosome 17 (17q23.1–q25.3) and codes for a subunit of the sodium channel (*SCN4A*). Attacks occur approximately once per week and are precipitated by rest after physical exertion or the administration of potassium. Weakness first affects the pelvic musculature but at times can become generalized. Average attacks last approximately 1 hour. During this time, the plasma potassium levels are usually higher than normal. Additionally, plasma phosphate levels tend to decrease, and patients respond to exercise with decreases in blood glucose and associated ketosis (384). Between attacks, muscle strength returns to normal, although a slowly progressive myopathy can develop in some families (385).

Hyperkalemic attacks can occur with myotonia or paramyotonia (cold-induced myotonia and weakness). The course of the paralytic attacks is similar in these conditions, and the disease also is transmitted in an autosomal dominant manner (386,387). When myotonia is present, it commonly affects the eyelids and produces a staring appearance. Percussion myotonia is noted occasionally, and in some families, potassium-induced paralysis and myotonia are jointly transmitted as a dominant disorder. Families in which hyperPP coexists with paramyotonia have been reported (388). These represent yet another mutation of the gene that codes for *SCN4A*.

Because hyperkalemia is not invariable, the diagnosis of hyperPP is best established by inducing an attack through the careful oral administration of potassium (25 mg/kg), with concomitant monitoring by electrocardiography.

Treatment

Most attacks of hyperkalemic periodic paralysis are mild and brief and do not require treatment. The administration of acetazolamide (125 mg per day for an 8-year-old child) has been successful in preventing attacks or reducing their severity (389). The drug has been postulated to achieve its benefits by activation of the calcium-activated potassium channel (390). Dichlorphenamide, another carbonic anhydrase inhibitor, also has been found to be effective (391). As well, inhalations of albuterol, a β-adrenergic stimulant, have been found to be effective in the treatment of paralytic episodes (392,393).

Hypokalemic Periodic Paralysis

The clinical picture of hypokalemic period paralysis (hypoPP), the acute transient paralysis of the musculature of the trunk and extremities with complete freedom from symptoms between attacks, was noted first by Shakhnovitch in 1882 (394) and by Westphal in 1885 (395). It is the most common of the inherited periodic paralyses (372).

Pathogenesis

In most instances, hypokalemic period paralysis is the consequence of mutations in the gene that encodes the dihydropyridine-sensitive L-type skeletal muscle calcium-channel α_1-subunit (*CACNA1S*). The gene has been mapped to chromosome 1q32. It encodes a dihydropyridine receptor that functions as a voltage-gated calcium channel (396). In about 10% of subjects, hypoPP is associated with mutations of *SCN4A* (372,397).

The importance of potassium and sodium metabolism in the clinical manifestations of the disease is well documented. Severe attacks are usually preceded by sodium retention in the body. During an attack, the plasma potassium decreases as weakness develops. Symptoms usually become evident at a serum potassium concentration of 3 mEq/L and are marked at between 2.5 and 2.0 mEq/L. Because healthy subjects do not develop significant muscle weakness when, as a result of electrolyte imbalance, their serum potassium drops to 2.5 mEq/L, it is unlikely that weakness results directly from a potassium deficiency. More likely, the converse actually takes place, for weakened muscle has a higher potassium concentration than the same muscle sampled between attacks.

It appears likely that muscle weakness results from an abnormal ratio between sodium and potassium conductances. Muscle sodium content is considerably elevated between attacks and remains unchanged or only slightly reduced with the development of paralysis. These findings suggest that potassium shifts into the muscle before or along with the onset of paralysis (398).

A muscle biopsy performed during a paralytic attack reveals marked vacuolization of the sarcoplasm (399). This abnormality is caused by an enormous dilatation of the endoplasmic reticulum and disappears once normal muscle function is regained.

Clinical Manifestations

Hypokalemic periodic paralysis is rare. In Finland, its current prevalence is 0.4 in 100,000 (400). It is transmitted as an autosomal dominant trait with 100% penetrance in male subjects and markedly reduced penetrance in female subjects. In 88% of cases, attacks first occur between the ages of 7 and 21 years. They can vary from slight transient weakness to almost complete paralysis (401). Most attacks last 6 to 24 hours and affect primarily the lower limbs. Bulbar and respiratory muscles are the last to become paralyzed, and death during an attack can occur in as many as 10% of patients. The most consistent factors predisposing to an attack are prolonged rest after vigorous exercise, a heavy carbohydrate meal, the administration of insulin, and exposure to cold. Administration of adrenocorticotropic hormone and a number of mineralocorticoid compounds, notably 2-methyl-9-α-fluorohydrocortisone, also induce paralysis.

During an attack, the subject has a flaccid paralysis that is most complete in the proximal musculature, a loss of deep tendon reflexes, and absent electric and mechanical excitability. Between attacks, patients are free of symptoms. However, permanent wasting and proximal and distal muscle weakness can develop even in patients who experience only rare attacks (402).

Treatment

Paralytic attacks are best treated by the oral administration of potassium. Prophylactically, a low carbohydrate diet and administration of supplemental potassium at bedtime is advisable. A low sodium intake and administration of diuretics, notably acetazolamide, also have been effective in preventing attacks or at least in reducing their frequency. Spironolactone, an aldosterone antagonist given in dosages of 100 to 200 mg per day, appears to be of benefit as well. None of these drugs, however, prevents the development of progressive muscular atrophy.

Normokalemic Periodic Paralysis

Periodic attacks of severe weakness, commencing in early childhood and lasting up to several weeks, are the characteristic features of a third, extremely rare type of periodic paralysis, normokalemic paralysis, transmitted as an autosomal dominant. Large amounts of sodium (460 mEq/24 hours for the average adult) can relieve the weakness in this condition, and attacks can occasionally be prevented by the prolonged administration of acetazolamide (403). The condition results from a mutation in *SCN4A*, and genetically, it represents a variant of hyperPP (404).

Differential Diagnosis

When a child experiences recurrent attacks of muscular weakness, a number of conditions should be considered. Hypokalemic periodic paralysis is diagnosed by the family history, a clinical response to potassium, and concurrent hypokalemia. In the absence of a family history, recurrent paralytic attacks can be caused by a sporadic form of the disease. In some sporadic cases of hypokalemic periodic paralysis, observed mainly in young male adults of Asian background, thyrotoxicosis appears to be a major predisposing factor (405). Renal tubular acidosis, ingestion of licorice extract (406), or barium poisoning incurred by ingestion of table salt contaminated with barium chloride or flour contaminated with barium carbonate also must be considered when muscle weakness is accompanied by hypokalemia (407,408). In barium poisoning, muscle weakness results from an interruption of the passive efflux of intracellular potassium, with a consequent net increase in muscle cell potassium (408). Periodic attacks of muscle weakness are seen also in primary hyperaldosteronism. The striking alkalosis, hypernatremia, and hypokalemia that accompany the attacks aid diagnosis.

Hyperkalemic periodic paralysis is distinguished by the early onset of brief but frequent attacks and their induction through the administration of potassium. In myasthenia gravis, weakness almost always affects the bulbar as well as the skeletal musculature, and deep tendon reflexes can be preserved during an attack. A clear-cut improvement in muscle strength after the administration of anticholinesterases confirms the diagnosis. Recurrent muscle weakness is seen also in myopathies associated with abnormal mitochondria and in polyneuropathies, particularly those accompanying intermittent acute porphyria. It is a prominent feature of paroxysmal myoglobinuria and muscle phosphorylase deficiency. Accidental or intentional ipecac ingestion can induce a reversible proximal myopathy (409,410).

Anderson syndrome is an autosomal dominant condition that is distinct from hypokalemic periodic paralysis. It is marked by periodic weakness, ventricular arrhythmias, short stature, and distinctive facial features, notably low-set ears, hypertelorism, and mandibular hypoplasia. A prolonged QT interval is seen in approximately 80% of subjects. Attacks of paralysis can be initiated by an oral potassium challenge, but the shifts in serum potassium are inconsistent, and hyperkalemia, normokalemia, or hypokalemia have been documented (411).

Syndromes of Continuous Motor Neuron Discharges

Several rarely encountered conditions are characterized by continuous motor neuron discharges.

Schwartz-Jampel Syndrome (Chondrodystrophic Myotonia)

Schwartz-Jampel syndrome (412) is an autosomal recessive disorder marked by clinical and EMG myotonia and muscular atrophy. The condition has been mapped to the short arm of chromosome 1 (1p34–p36). It codes for perlecan, a large heparan sulfate proteoglycan, which is a component of the basement membrane and other extracellular matrices (413).

There is considerable clinical and genetic heterogeneity. Giedion and coworkers have recognized three subtypes: 1A, apparent in childhood and marked by moderate bony dysplasia; 1B, which is apparent at birth with more striking bony changes; and type 2, which is manifest at birth and has increased mortality (414). Type 1A corresponds to the original patients of Schwartz and Jampel (415). In all forms, continuous motor neuron discharges involving the facial musculature produce blepharophimosis, a puckered mouth, and a characteristic pinched facies. Growth is retarded, and there is progressive limitation of joint movements in hips, wrists, fingers, and toes. Vertebral anomalies and deformities of chest and hips are almost always present. Mental development is generally normal (416). Myotonic EMG abnormalities have been observed in both parents (417). Procainamide hydrochloride produces considerable relief from the myotonia and the painful muscle spasms.

This condition should be distinguished from the Van Dyke–Hansen syndrome, in which continuous motor neuron discharges are accompanied by episodic ataxia (418).

Isaacs Syndrome (Acquired Neuromyotonia)

Isaacs syndrome (acquired neuromyotonia) is characterized by the appearance at any time of life of muscle stiffness and cramps, impaired muscular relaxation, and widespread myokymia or fasciculations (419). The condition can be acquired or can be inherited in an autosomal dominant manner, and in some families, it is associated with episodic ataxia type 1 (420). The acquired form is believed to result from antibodies mediated against the voltage-gated potassium channel (KCNA1) of the peripheral nerve (421,422). The motor neuron discharge is believed to arise from the peripheral motor axon because it is unaffected by peripheral nerve block and persists during sleep. Curare abolishes the abnormal discharges. EMG of the fully relaxed muscle discloses continuous discharges of normal motor unit potentials. Motor and sensory nerve conduction times are usually normal. The condition is nonprogressive and occasionally can improve. Relatively small amounts of phenytoin or carbamazepine decrease the abnormal muscle activity (423,424).

Isaacs syndrome is distinct from the stiff-man syndromes, one form of which is dominantly inherited and characterized by muscular symptoms at birth (stiff-baby syndrome or hyperekplexia) (see Chapter 3). The other form is sporadic and usually appears in adult life or, rarely, in adolescence (425). In both forms, the motor unit discharges disappear with sleep and are relieved with diazepam, a drug that is ineffective in Isaacs syndrome. Because a peripheral nerve block abolishes the rigidity, Layzer suggested that the abnormal motor unit discharges arise as a result of a defect in a descending spinal pathway that originates within the brainstem and inhibits muscle tone and exteroceptive spinal reflexes (426). This inhibition is enhanced by γ-aminobutyric acid and diminished by noradrenergic input, pointing to dysfunction of the inhibitory GABAergic or glycinergic interneurons (427,428). Autoantibodies against glutamic acid decarboxylase (GAD), the enzyme responsible for γ-aminobutyric acid synthesis within neurons, have been found in up to 80% of subjects (429). The duration of the illness is between 5 and 30 years, and there is no correlation between GAD antibody levels in blood or CSF and the severity of the illness (429).

Another condition to be considered in a child demonstrating continuous motor unit activity is malignant hyperthermia. Usually, this condition follows the administration of halothane or succinylcholine. It, too, is marked by generalized hypertonia, rigidity, and muscle fasciculation. Hyperthermia may not always be present, particularly in infants. The CK levels are markedly elevated, and a metabolic acidosis is usually demonstrable. Muscle biopsy in the acute stage or shortly thereafter shows a severe necrotizing myopathy. Malignant hyperthermia is, therefore, really acute rhabdomyolysis. Children with Duchenne muscular dystrophy, myotonic dystrophy, and especially central core disease are particularly prone to this condition, and mutations in the ryanodine receptor gene, the gene that is associated with central core disease, can be demonstrated in about 30% of subjects who experience malignant hyperthermia (430). Treatment is with dantrolene (7 mg/kg), more effective if given before the anesthetic is administered (431).

Dermatomyositis

The idiopathic inflammatory myopathies can be classified into three groups: dermatomyositis, polymyositis, and inclusion body myositis (432). In children, dermatomyositis is by far the most common of these conditions; inclusion body myositis is seen almost exclusively in late adult life (433,434). The existence of polymyositis as a distinct entity has been questioned, and many cases diagnosed as such may well represent inclusion body myositis (435).

Dermatomyositis is a systemic disease that involves many organs and is primarily characterized by low-grade fever, fatigue, anorexia, a typical skin rash, muscular weakness, and pain.

Pathologic Anatomy

The primary site of involvement in childhood dermatomyositis is the intramuscular microvasculature. As a consequence, the most striking anatomic abnormalities are found in the blood vessels of the muscles, fat, nerves, connective tissue, and gastrointestinal tract. Here, the endothelial cells undergo degeneration and regeneration, with inclusionlike reticulotubular aggregates within their cytoplasm; these structures probably are clusters of duplicated sarcoplasmic reticulum. Other changes include a markedly decreased number of pinocytotic vesicles in the endothelial cytoplasm, hyperplasia of the intima, and multiple vascular occlusions. These alterations produce areas of muscle infarction, which are often accompanied by denervation atrophy secondary to occlusion of the nutrient vessels to the peripheral nerves.

A characteristic feature of dermatomyositis is the presence of several layers of atrophic fibers at the periphery of fascicles, with relative preservation of myofibers in the centers of fascicles. This condition is known as *perifascicular atrophy*. Most of the atrophic fibers at the periphery of fascicles are regenerating, and only a few scattered degenerating fibers are demonstrated. This abnormality is seen in some 90% of children with dermatomyositis, but not in polymyositis. Degeneration of muscle fibers is disproportionately sparse in childhood dermatomyositis in contrast to polymyositis of adults and children (433,436). Another distinguishing feature in the muscle biopsy is the absence of lymphocytes infiltrating and phagocytosing myofibers in dermatomyositis, whereas this is a typical histopathologic feature in polymyositis. Immunocytochemical lymphocyte markers may be applied to sections of muscle biopsy tissue to demonstrate the specificity of B- and T-cells (see Pathogenesis, below). Perifascicular atrophy is characteristic but not necessarily diagnostic of dermatomyositis because it also occurs in other chronic small vessel ischemic diseases, such as in adults with diabetes mellitus and claudication of the legs.

Pathogenesis

The basic process that leads to dermatomyositis is an antibody or immune complex–mediated immune response against a vascular-endothelial component (432). The inflammatory cell in dermatomyositis is predominantly the B lymphocyte, and the immune reaction is mediated by circulating antibodies against endothelial cells, by contrast with the aggressive T cells of polymyositis that cause a cell-mediated immune reaction. Kissel and coworkers believe that the first pathologic event is complement activation in the microvasculature and have demonstrated a membrane attack complex in the walls of recently damaged muscle (437). A variety of cytokines and chemokines, notably interleukin-1α and 1β, and tumor growth factor-β are important in the mediation of the inflammatory response (432,438). This process is followed by ischemic muscle fiber damage and by a cellular inflammatory response. We do not know what process or processes activate the complement cascade. The importance of genetic factors in the evolution of dermatomyositis is underlined by the association with HLA-DQA1 0501 in children with dermatomyositis (439). The role of infectious agents such as enteroviruses, coxsackievirus, or toxoplasmosis in the evolution of the disease is less certain (432). Because of its resemblance to graft versus host disease, Reed and colleagues have suggested that nonself cells play a major role in the evolution of juvenile dermatomyositis (440,441). They identified maternally derived chimeric cells in blood lymphocytes, muscle biopsies, and skin biopsies more often in children with dermatomyositis than in their healthy siblings or unaffected controls, an indication that the maternal HLA genotype facilitates transfer and persistence of maternal cells in the fetal circulation (441).

TABLE 16.11 Clinical Data on 34 Children with Dermatomyositis

Symptom	*Number of Patients*
Weakness	32
Facial skin lesions	31
Fever	29
Contractures	29
Weakness of bulbar musculature	17
Death	10
Subcutaneous calcifications	8

After Wedgewood RJ, Cook C, Cohen J. Dermatomyositis: report of 26 cases in children with a discussion of endocrine therapy in 13. *Pediatrics* 1953;12:447; and Banker BQ. Dermatomyositis of childhood. *J Neuropathol Exp Neurol* 1975;34:46.

Clinical Manifestations

The onset of the disease can be insidious or acute and preceded by an infection. The most common early symptoms are weakness and easy fatigability (Table 16.11) (442). Typical skin changes, often at onset, include an erythematous, scaly, and occasionally violaceous discoloration of the upper eyelids. Subsequently, the skin of the periorbital region, malar areas, and extensor surfaces of the joints, particularly the knuckles (Gottron rash), elbows, and knees, also can become affected. The rash tends to spare the phalanges, in contrast to that seen in systemic lupus erythematosus, in which the phalanges are involved and the knuckles are spared. Less commonly, the rash involves the neck and the upper chest. It is exacerbated by sunlight. At times, the skin becomes edematous.

Muscle weakness usually is generalized but always is most marked proximally. Weakness of the flexor muscles of the neck is observed in approximately one-half of children. Involvement of the bulbar musculature is an unfavorable prognostic sign; in the series of Wedgewood and coworkers, reported in 1953, 75% of children with this sign died from the disease (442). Early flexion contractures at the ankles produce a tiptoe gait. The deep tendon reflexes are diminished or abolished.

When untreated, the course of the disease is extremely variable. In some children, particularly in those whose illness has an acute onset, the weakness advances rapidly

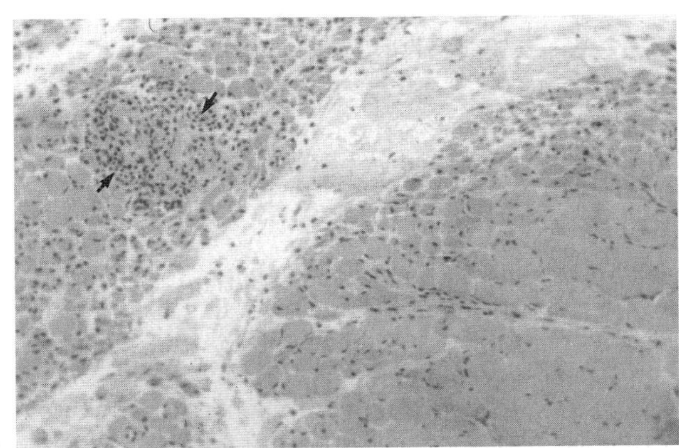

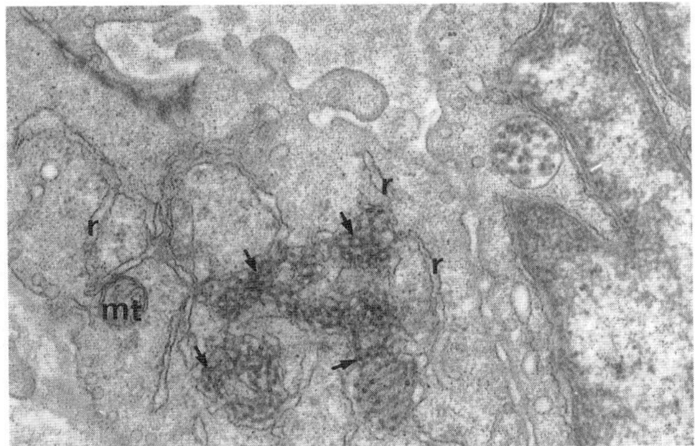

FIGURE 16.12. Muscle biopsy of a 9-year old girl with dermatomyositis, symptomatic with rash and proximal weakness for 3 months. **(A):** The characteristic *perifascicular atrophy* (*arrows*), a distribution of atrophic degenerating and regenerating myofibers at the edges, and more normal fibers at the centers of fascicles is due to small vessel ischemic myopathy and is not seen in polymyositis. Inflammatory cells, mainly B-lymphocytes, are seen in the endomysial connective tissue and around blood vessels. Hematoxylin-eosin, ×250. **(B):** Electron microscopy reveals *tubuloreticular aggregates* (*arrows*) within the cytoplasm of endothelial cells of intramuscular capillaries. These ultrastructural features are not viral inclusions, but rather proliferations of smooth endoplasmic reticulum, and occur only in dermatomyositis and lupus myositis, ×8000 (mt, mitochondrion; r, endoplasmic reticulum).

over a period of several months and, with involvement of the bulbar musculature, terminates fatally. Perforation of the gastrointestinal tract is a frequent cause of death. In other children, the disease does not progress but leaves the patient crippled by irreversible weakness, contractures, and subcutaneous calcium deposits.

Diagnosis

The diagnosis of dermatomyositis rests on (a) symmetric limb-girdle weakness, (b) muscle biopsy evidence of myositis and muscle necrosis, (c) increased levels of muscle enzymes in serum, (d) EMG changes of myositis, and (e) the presence of skin lesions (443,444). The appearance of cutaneous lesions may precede or follow the onset of myopathic weakness.

Routine laboratory studies are of little diagnostic help. In the active stage, the erythrocyte sedimentation rate is elevated, and the peripheral white cell count may be abnormal. Systemic lupus erythematosus cells are not demonstrated in peripheral blood, and the antistreptolysin titer is normal. The antinuclear antibody titer is occasionally positive, and the serum gamma globulins are increased in approximately one-half of patients. Serum enzymes can be normal or slightly elevated. EMG examination can reveal myopathic action potentials exclusively, a combination of fibrillation potentials within resting muscles and myopathic action potentials, or repetitive high-frequency discharges evoked by mechanical stimulation of muscle (445). MRI of muscle can be used to follow disease involvement. Involved muscles have increased signal on T2-weighted images and normal T1-weighted images. Perimuscular edema and inflammatory changes of subcutaneous fat are seen also (446). The muscle biopsy is usually diagnostic. In children who exhibit the typical dermatomyositis rash but who do not have apparent muscle weakness, the clinical diagnosis is amyopathic dermatomyositis (432).

Differential Diagnosis

The muscle weakness seen in dermatomyositis must be distinguished from that associated with muscular dystrophy and polymyositis. In muscular dystrophy, as in dermatomyositis, muscle weakness involves the proximal muscles of the shoulder and pelvic girdle. However, bulbar signs, in particular swallowing difficulties, are extremely rare in muscular dystrophy. The onset of weakness is far more gradual in muscular dystrophy, and contractures develop in its later stages. Finally, in childhood dermatomyositis, it is rare to see as striking an elevation in serum CK levels as occurs in the early phases of muscular dystrophy. Polymyositis is rare in childhood, and in pediatric subjects who have the characteristic weakness but no rash, the diagnosis of a slowly progressive myopathy, endocrine myopathies, and dermatomyositis sine dermatitis should be considered (432). Inclusion body myositis is a disease of adult life. A somewhat similar pathologic picture featuring inflammatory cell infiltrates but lacking the extensive vasculitis of dermatomyositis is seen in a number of collagen vascular diseases, including rheumatic fever, rheumatoid arthritis, systemic lupus erythematosus, and mixed connective tissue disease (see Chapter 8). An inflammatory, corticosteroid-responsive myopathy distinguished from dermatomyositis by the absence of vascular changes on muscle biopsy and unrelated to congenital muscular dystrophy is seen in infancy (447,448). In some instances, the condition is secondary to the injection of aluminium-containing vaccines (449). The eosinophilic myositis that resulted from toxic products in a tryptophan preparation is discussed in Chapter 9.

Treatment

Untreated, dermatomyositis has a poor prognosis. In the majority of affected children, however, the disease probably becomes quiescent after approximately 2 years, and treatment, therefore, is intended to carry the child through this period. The effectiveness of corticosteroid therapy in altering the course of dermatomyositis is still under dispute. However, most clinical centers, including our own, advocate instituting a regimen of prednisone (1.5 to 2.5 mg/kg per day for severe cases and 1.0 to 1.5 mg/kg per day for relatively mild cases). Dubowitz and his group, however, favor a starting dosage of 1 mg/kg per day for all patients. In their experience, and the experience of others, there are fewer relapses as well as less morbidity (45,444,445,450). This dosage is continued until remission has begun, as evidenced by a decrease in serum enzyme levels and by improvement in strength. It is then tapered and changed to alternate-day therapy at a level just sufficient to suppress symptoms. In many instances, corticosteroid therapy can be discontinued in 3 to 6 months by tapering the medication over the course of some 10 weeks. High dosed "pulsed" steroids are sometimes given to initiate treatment.

When the disease is life-threatening, when a high steroid dose cannot be tapered without a relapse, or when symptoms are not controlled with prednisone alone, immunosuppressive therapy is indicated (451,452). This can take the form of biweekly injections of methotrexate (2 to 3 mg/kg per dose), daily azathioprine (50 to 125 mg per day), or cyclosporine (2.5 to 7.5 mg/kg per day) (453). Later infertility is a risk with these drugs, in girls more than in boys. High-dose intravenous immune globulins have been used successfully. This management is indicated when there has been a relapse on previously effective therapy, when weakness persists despite high corticosteroid doses, or when corticosteroids cannot be reduced without precipitating a relapse. A dosage of 1 to 2 g/kg gamma globulins, given in divided amounts over the course of 3 to 5 days, is generally recommended for initial therapy (454). Side reactions include headache, fever, and gastrointestinal upset. Plasmapheresis has not been found to be helpful in a double-blind, placebo-controlled study (432).

In the experience of Spencer and coworkers, the course of the disease, when treated as indicated in this discussion, was chronic and continuous in 44% of children, chronic and polycyclic in 31%, and monocyclic in 25% (444). Although other series have not been as optimistic, these workers found that 78% of their patients were ultimately well and no longer taking medications.

Polymyositis

Polymyositis is uncommon in children. It is a chronic inflammatory process of muscles leading to the insidious onset of weakness, without the constitutional symptoms and skin changes that accompany dermatomyositis. In contrast to dermatomyositis, polymyositis is a cell-mediated disease associated with abnormal T-lymphocyte rather than B-lymphocyte infiltrates in muscle. Polymyositis can begin as early as the second year of life and usually first affects the pelvic musculature. Muscles are abnormally firm and occasionally painful. As the disease progresses, the weakness spreads to the upper limbs and the face. The clinical picture resembles that of muscular dystrophy and, from a clinical viewpoint, it is only the somewhat more rapid onset of muscle weakness and the arrest or retrogression of symptoms that suggest the diagnosis.

On microscopic examination, the affected muscles exhibit primary degeneration of muscle fibers, a considerable amount of regenerative activity, and round lymphocyte and macrophage infiltration, especially around blood vessels. In addition to perivascular cuffing by lymphocytes, there is often a true intramuscular vasculitis, with lymphocytes infiltrating the muscular wall of arterioles and small arteries, endothelial swelling and proliferation leading to occlusion of the lumen, and subintimal and muscularis (media) degeneration. The cause of the condition is obscure, but the presence of antibodies to myosin in some 90% of polymyositis patients suggests a virus-induced autoimmune process, but this theory of infectious induction remains unproved.

The course of the disease is generally downhill, and treatment of children with corticosteroids does not seem to alter the outlook (455).

Other Inflammatory Diseases of Muscle

Rheumatic fever, rheumatoid arthritis, and the collagen vascular diseases can all be associated with an interstitial polymyositis, which is characterized by focal round cell infiltrates but lacks the vasculitis seen in dermatomyositis. Eosinophilic fasciitis may involve perivascular infiltrates within muscle of both lymphocytes and eosinophils.

A number of chronic infections, notably tuberculosis and sarcoidosis, can produce myositis. Among the types of myositis caused by parasitic infections, trichinosis is the most common entity (see Chapter 7). Also, the presenting symptom of toxoplasmosis can be polymyositis.

A relatively common entity that is best grouped with the inflammatory myopathies is myalgia cruris epidemica (456,457). This condition is characterized by transient severe pain and weakness affecting mainly the gastrocnemius and beginning 1 to 2 days after an upper respiratory infection. As indicated by its name, the condition occurs epidemically, most commonly in association with influenza. Muscle biopsy reveals a polymorphonuclear and mononuclear infiltrate and muscle cell necrosis. EMG studies indicate that the myositis extends beyond the clinically affected calf muscles.

Myositis also can accompany various viral infections, with symptoms usually limited to muscular aches and pains (458). In epidemic pleurodynia, however, muscles of the chest, back, and shoulders are notably painful. The myositis that accompanies human immunodeficiency virus infection is considered in Chapter 7. In some instances, accompanying cerebrospinal fluid pleocytosis indicates meningeal involvement. Pleurodynia is usually caused by a variety of coxsackievirus B. Myositis also is a feature of various parasitic diseases and of tropical polymyositis. As well, a myopathy is seen subsequent to treatment with penicillamine, zidovudine, and various lipid-lowering drugs (459). Endomysial inflammation is seen in some of the muscular dystrophies, notably in FSHD; glycogen storage disease type II; and for approximately 1 month after the insertion of needle electrodes for EMG.

Congenital Myopathies

The term *congenital myopathy* encompasses a group of muscle diseases that present at birth and possess charateristic histopathologic findings on muscle biopsy that are distinct from necrotizing myopathies or muscular dystrophies. Nearly all the congenital myopathies are genetically determined, but some, such as congenital muscle fiber-type disproportion, are syndromes that may be associated with systemic metabolic disease or may represent aberrant developmental defects of muscle maturation. In the development of human striated muscle, more than 146 different genes are expressed at different times, but only 86 of these genes are involved in myogenesis in the mouse; hence, human muscle cell cultures are needed to study these genes in relation to their possible role in the pathogenesis of congenital myopathies (460).

The ambiguous term *benign congenital hypotonia* previously denoted an infant with hypotonia and mild, nonprogressive weakness who either improved with maturation or at least held his own. Oppenheim's poorly described patients with *amyotonia congenita*, a now obsolete term, would probably belong to this group (58), along with a number of new and pathologically well-defined muscular disorders (see Table 16.4). *Benign congenital hypotonia* now is used only as a convenient wastebasket term to describe an infant or child with generalized hypotonia without major weakness and in whom the muscle biopsy, EMG, and all other laboratory study results are normal. It is not a diagnosis of a disease.

Congenital Muscle Fiber-Type Disproportion

Congenital muscle fiber-type disproportion (CMFTD) is defined only by muscle biopsy and requires three principal obligatory criteria: (a) disproportion in the ratio of types I and II myofibers, with 80% or more predominance of type I fibers (type II predominance is not CMFTD); (b) type I fibers that are uniformly smaller than normal from birth, whereas type II fibers are of normal diameter or mildly hypertrophic to compensate; and (c) no myofiber degeneration or regeneration (461). Other minor criteria include that the hypoplastic type I fibers retain their normal polygonal contour in transverse section and are not angular as are atrophic fibers. In some cases, an excessive number of central nuclei are found in myofibers.

In cases not associated with other congenital myopathies or with systemic or neuromuscular metabolic diseases, the serum CK in CMFTD is invariably normal, and the EMG also is normal or shows minimal nonspecific myopathic features. In three unrelated families with this disorder, Laing and coworkers have found heterozygous missense mutations of the skeletal muscle α-actin gene (*ACTA1*)(462). It is not yet clear whether these patients do not represent cases of nemaline myopathy in which fiber size disproportion is particularly conspicuous (see discussion on Nemaline Myopathy).

The diagnosis can be suspected from clinical features, but confirmation requires muscle biopsy with histochemistry. The incidence is unknown, but it may be the most common of the congenital myopathies.

Pure CMFTD occurs in some families and appears to follow an autosomal recessive inheritance. An autosomal dominant trait is suspected in other rare families but is less certain. The clinical features are similar to those of nemaline rod myopathy and include dolichocephaly; high palate; a generalized small mass of axial, appendicular, and facial muscles; and occasionally, scoliosis. Failure to thrive is common (463). Pharyngeal, respiratory, and extraocular muscles are not generally involved to the extent of causing clinically detectable deficits. In the series of Clarke and North, congenital contractures were seen in 25% of patients (463). These respond well to gentle physiotherapy. Congenital subluxation of the hips is a rare complication, as is cardiac involvement. A quarter of patients with CMFTD follow a severe course, with death usually due to respiratory failure in childhood. If central nuclei occur in myofibers as well as the CMFTD pattern, the clinical myopathic features—particularly generalized weakness—are more severe, and ptosis and incomplete external ophthalmoplegia are often associated.

CMFTD also is seen as a syndrome or component of other diseases. Among neuromuscular and metabolic diseases, it is a regular part of globoid cell (Krabbe) leukodystrophy early in the course before the neuropathy produces changes of denervation-reinnervation (70,464). It is a reliable feature in the muscle biopsy of patients with nemaline rod disease (see following discussion) and is one of the patterns seen in the congenital form of myotonic dystrophy. CMFTD also is reported in some cases of glycogenoses II and III, multiple sulfatase deficiency, congenital hypothyroidism, fetal alcohol syndrome, rigid spine syndrome, minicore myopathy, and oculocerebrorenal disease of Lowe (213).

One of the most common nongenetic and nonneuromuscular etiologies of CMFTD is cerebellar hypoplasia and brainstem dysgeneses (71,465). Abnormal bulbospinal impulses that descend to influence the motor neuron during the histochemical stage of muscle maturation (20- to 28-weeks' gestation) apparently cause distortions in the suprasegmental innervation of the fetal motor unit that alters the ratio of fiber types and the differential growth of each type of fiber (461). Generalized muscular hypotonia is a constant clinical feature of cerebellar hypoplasia as well (see Chapter 5). Should CMFTD be reported in the muscle biopsy during the course of investigation for hypotonia and mild weakness and is unexplained, particularly if the child does not have the typical facies and body habitus of the pure myopathic CMFTD, an MRI of the brain is indicated with special attention to structures in the posterior fossa.

Nemaline Myopathy

First described in 1963 independently by Shy and coworkers (63) and Conen and coworkers (466), nemaline myopathy is another common congenital myopathy. To date, five genes have been associated with this condition (467). Three of these are transmitted as autosomal recessive conditions with variable penetrance, whereas two are transmitted as both autosomal dominant and autosomal recessive traits (467). One gene for the autosomal dominant condition has been localized to the long arm of chromosome 1 at the 1q21–q23 locus; it is called *NEM1* and is due to a defect in α-tropomyosin (468). Another gene for the autosomal recessive form is on the long arm of chromosome 2 at 2q21.2–q22; this form has been termed *NEM2* and involves a defective large protein, nebulin (469). It is most commmonly associated with the classic autosomal recessive form of the disease (469). *NEM3* is due to an α–actin defect in striated muscle, and both autosomal dominant and recessive varieties occur at the same 1q42.1 locus (470). *NEM4* is an autosomal dominantly inherited defect in β-tropomyosin at 9q13 (471). Mutations in the tropomyosin genes (α-tropomyosin and β-tropomyosin) are rare causes for nemaline myopathy and probably only account for 3% of patients (467,472). *NEM5* is an autosomal recessive troponin-T defect at 19q13 demonstrated in the Amish population (473). The genetic entities are indistinguishable by clinical history or muscle biopsy, so phenotype-genotype correlation is poor (474).

All these genes code for thin filament associated proteins, an indication that assembly of these structures is an essential factor in the development of nemaline rods.

Three clinical pictures have been recognized: a severe and almost always fatal neonatal form, which presents with hypotonia, weakness, and respiratory impairment; a milder form that also presents in the neonatal period, infancy, or early childhood and is either stationary or slowly progressive; and an adult-onset form (475). The last form can have a benign course or at times progress rapidly. Children have a dysmorphic appearance, and deformities of the palate, spine, and feet have been observed. A cardiomyopathy also has been noted.

Aggregates of threadlike, intracytoplasmic rods are present in most muscle fibers (476). In frozen sections, they may be demonstrated by the modified Gomori trichrome stain, in which they appear red against the green of the myofibrillar proteins, and in paraffin sections, they may be stained with phosphotungstic acid–hematoxylin or with the Luna-Parker acid fuscin stain. In electron microscopy, these rods are found to represent an excessive accumulation of Z-band material with the same geometric periodicity as the Z-band and often seen arising from Z-bands between sarcomeres (Fig. 16.13). In rare cases, intranuclear rods also are demonstrated, but how they form and become localized to sarcolemmal nuclei is unclear (477).

Chemical studies on the rod material suggest that it consists of several protein components, of which sarcomeric α-actinin is the most clearly defined, being present in increased amounts (478,479). Both tropomyosin-3 and nebulin are incorporated into the Z-band of the sarcomeres (480). Increased amounts of other normal components of the Z-band, such as actin and α-actinin, are probably secondary reactive changes.

An additional constant feature in the muscle biopsy is the presence of congenital muscle fiber–type disproportion (see previous discussion), particularly in infants. As the child grows older, and particularly in late childhood, adolescence, and early adult life, a slow but gradual conversion of more of the remaining type II myofibers to type I occurs, until the muscle may contain a uniform population of small type I myofibers. This histochemical conversion is not necessarily associated with clinical progression of the disease, but some cases do appear to show increased weakness (481).

The presence of nemaline bodies is not diagnostic of nemaline myopathy because it also may occur as a nonspecific finding. Nemaline bodies have been seen in skeletal muscle after experimental tenotomy and in a variety of human disease entities, including polymyositis, other autoimmune vascular disease, and in human immunodeficiency virus infection (482). An adult-onset nemaline rod

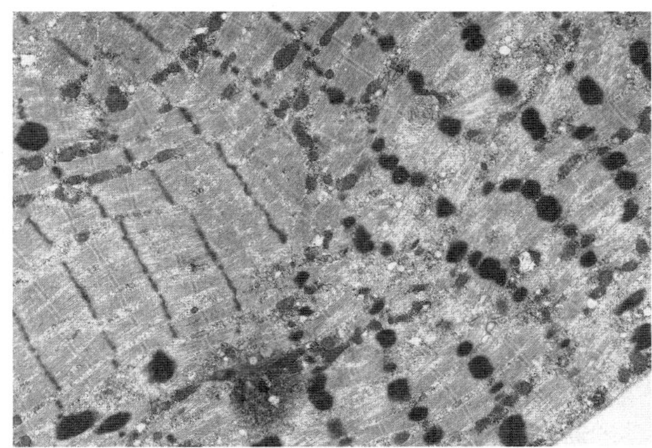

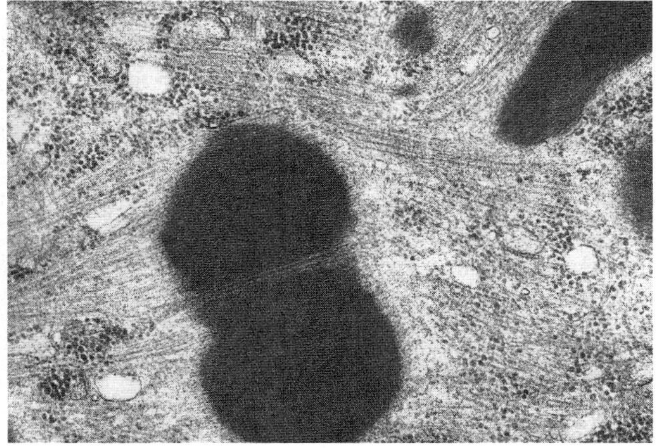

FIGURE 16.13. Vastus lateralis muscle biopsy of an 11-month-old girl with nemaline myopathy. Transmission electron microscopy shows (**A**) aggregates of electron-dense material appear to be arising from the Z-bands, but other Z-bands remain intact; (**B**) at higher magnification, the aggregates have an internal geometrical structure and periodicity identical to Z-bands. Uranyl acetate and lead citrate. (**A**) X3500; (**B**) X40,000.

myopathy is sporadic and not related to either of the two genetic forms found in children.

Central Core Disease

Central core disease, transmitted as both an autosomal dominant and an autosomal recessive trait, is characterized by mild and nonprogressive muscle weakness that is either proximal or generalized and is of early onset. The basic defect in this condition is located in the gene for the ryanodine receptor (*RYR1*). This gene codes for a tetramer receptor to a calcium channel found in the membrane of muscle sarcoplasmic reticulum. This nonvoltage-gated channel, which is characterized by its ability to bind ryanodine, a plant alkaloid, plays an important role in excitation-contraction coupling and calcium transport (483,484).

Central core disease is often associated with muscle contractures around the knees and hips and with various skeletal defects, including congenital dislocation of the hips and patella, kyphoscoliosis, and pes cavus. There is high incidence of cardiac abnormalities, and virtually all subjects are susceptible to malignant hypothermia (64). This observation has been explained by the finding that malignant hyperthermia, like central core disease, results from a mutation in the same ryanodine receptor gene (430,485). The serum CK is generally normal when the patient is not experiencing malignant hyperthermic rhabdomyolysis.

When muscle is stained with trichrome, the central areas of affected muscle fibers stain blue, whereas peripheral myofibrils appear red. With histochemical stains specific for the mitochondrial oxidative enzymes, the central area stains less intensively than the periphery of the fiber, and there is a type I fiber predominance, often so extensive that only a few scattered type II fibers remain or no fibers are found in the biopsy (486). Brooke has observed that the severity of the changes in muscle is unrelated to the clinical weakness (2). The central cores also exhibit prominent immunoreactivity for myotilin, a Z-disk protein that binds α-actinin and also is prominent in nemaline rods (487). The amino (N-) terminus of the dystrophin molecule, the end that attaches to actin (thin myofilaments and Z-disk), plays no known role in the pathogenesis of nemaline myopathy.

Because of the close clinical and genetic association with malignant hyperthermia, patients with central core disease who require a general anesthetic should be pretreated with dantrolene sodium before surgery as a precaution. A recent trial of salbutamol (Albuterol) therapy in 8 children with central core disease provided objective evidence of improved strength and forced vital capacity over a 6-month period (487a).

Minicore (Multicore) Myopathy

Minicore (multicore) myopathy is distinct from central core disease (488). The condition is mainly inherited as an autosomal recessive disorder, with mutations in the *RYR1* gene, and the selenoprotein-N *SEPN1* gene at locus lp 35–p36 having been documented (488a). This same gene and its transcription product are implicated in desmin-accumulating myofibrillar myopathy. The *SEPN1* gene also is implicated in rigid spine muscular dystrophy (281).

Minicore myopathy manifests shortly after birth with a rather benign nonprogressive generalized hypotonia. In about 30% of subjects, hypotonia appears to have a prenatal onset (489). Varying degrees of scoliosis are almost invariable, and in the sereis of Ferreiro and coworkers, 58% of subjects had an early onset of scoliosis (490). This was progressive even when the muscle disease was stable or improved. A large proportion of patients develop a rigid spine (489). Respiratory involvement was seen in 47% of patients (488a, 489). It was mainly due to involvement of the accessary respiratory muscles. Despite these involvements, almost all affected children walked by 2 years of age (490). The Swash-Schwartz variant of familial multicore disease is marked by a severe myopathy that also includes external ophthalmoplegia (491). Hypertrophic cardiomyopathy is reported rarely. Other inconstant complications include endocrinopathies, small stature, and severe mental retardation, but most patients are intellectually normal.

The diagnosis is supported by distinctive MRI findings in muscle (491a), and is confirmed by muscle biopsy, which shows multiple cores within myofibers with defects in histochemical enzymatic activities in the cores. CMFTD is reported in a few infants. Poor registry of Z-bands, disarray of myofilaments, and cores of amorphous granular material are seen ultrastructurally.

Myotubular (Centronuclear) Myopathy

A group of disorders characterized by rows of central nuclei in most myofibers have been termed *myotubular myopathies* because of their similarity to the architecture of the normal human fetal myotube at 8- to 15-weeks' gestation. However, few other features support the hypothesis of true maturational arrest (492). X-linked, autosomal dominant, and autosomal recessive forms of this condition have been described (467). Mutations in the myotubularin (*MTM1*) gene, mapped to chromosome Xq28, have been identified in up to 90% of subjects with the X-linked form (493,493a). Myotubularin belongs the phosphoinositide 3-phosphatase family, and it may be involved cell signalling and endocytic traffic (494).

The most common form of myotubular myopathy is transmitted as an autosomal dominant condition with variable penetrance. Children affected with this disorder show a slowly progressive weakness of the limb girdles and neck muscles, with acute fluctuations coinciding with respiratory illnesses (66). Although there is considerable clinical heterogeneity, ptosis and weakness of the extraocular muscles appear to be characteristic for most cases (495).

In the more severe, X-linked recessive form of hypotonia, diffuse weakness, inability to swallow, and respiratory failure appear during the neonatal period (496). The muscle biopsy is diagnostic and shows many abnormal features, but usually good histochemical differentiation is seen, although sometimes there is a predominance of type I fibers and registry of Z-bands, features that develop much later than the myotubular stage (488). The central nuclei in rows within the myofibers are always spaced with two to four nuclear diameters between them, unlike fetal myotubes, and the condensation of chromatin is that of the term neonate, not the fetus. Mothers, who are obligate carriers, can show mild muscle weakness and have minor changes in their muscle biopsy. Various X-inactivation patterns are shown in carriers of X-linked myotubular myopathy (497).

Myofibrillar Myopathies

The term *myofibrillary myopathy* subsumes a number of conditions that share pathologic changes of the Z-disks of the myofibril. A number of terms have been used to designate these conditions, including *desmin myopathy*, *spheroid body myopathy*, and *congenital myopathy with Mallory bodylike inclusions*. The disorder affects the intermediate filaments of muscle. These are protein fibers that are termed *intermediate* because their diameter is intermediate between the thin actin filaments and the thick myosin filaments of muscle cells. Desmin is a major polypeptide component of intermediate filaments. Some thirty diseases have been linked to disorders of the intermediate filaments (498,499). They include several disorders of keratin and the various disorders of lamins A and C, such as Emery Dreifuss muscular dystrophy and limb-girdle muscular dystrophy type 1B (see Table 16.7).

The muscle biopsy is diagnostic for this condition. It shows regions of abnormal fibers of varying size and shapes containing amorphous granular or hyaline structures. There is an accumulation of myofibrillar degradation products and an ectopic expression of multiple proteins including desmin, αB-crystallin, dystrophin, and congophilic amyloid material. On electron microscopy, abnormalities involve the myofibrils and characteristically the Z-disk. Alterations in cristae can be demonstrated in some mitochondria (500). In the series of patients reported by Olive and colleagues, an autosomal dominant transmission was more common (501). Molecular genetic studies have demonstrated mutations in the gene for desmin and less often in the gene for αB-crystallin and myotilin (502–504). In some families, mitochondrial defects in complex III, associated with 7.5-kb deletions of mtDNA are demonstrated (Sarnat HB and Marín-García J, unpublished), and mitochondrial dysfunctions of other types are demonstrated in other patients (505), but other families do not show mitochondrial defects.

The clinical picture is variable. The age of onset in most subjects is after the second decade of life, and symptoms are highlighted by progressive weakness involving both proximal and distal muscles. Cardiomyopathy and lens opacities also have been described (501). One of us (H.S.) has encountered an infantile form. It is primarily characterized clinically by dysphagia in early infancy that is disproportionately severe in relation to the mild generalized weakness, although respiratory muscle insufficiency sometimes occurs. Gastrostomy often is required, but patients gradually improve, and the gastrostomy can be removed by 3 to 4 years of age, when the child is able to swallow adequately. Mild axial weakness may persist, with a mild Gowers' sign and a hip-waddle gait. Intelligence and neurologic development proceed normally. Patients show a wide spectrum of clinical and laboratory findings, consistent with a multifactorial etiology (498,506). Cardiomyopathy is present in about 16% of patients (498), and in some, the cardiomyopathy is linked to chromosome 10q (507).

Mitochondrial Diseases (Mitochondrial Cytopathies)

Although muscle dysfunction is a prime feature in the majority of mitochondrial disorders, their discussion is found in a chapter devoted exclusively to mitochondrial encephalomyopathies (see Chapter 2).

Other Congenital Myopathies

A number of other rare congenital myopathies have now been recognized on the basis of their distinctive intramuscular structures. Their clinical and pathologic features are summarized in Table 16.4. Although these diseases were formerly termed *benign congenital hypotonias*, it is becoming clear that some are hardly benign and that respiratory or bulbar musculature weakness can prove fatal at an early age.

Congenital Absence of Specific Muscles and Segmental and Generalized Amyoplasia

Unilateral or bilateral congenital absence of muscle is more frequently observed in the pectoral group than elsewhere. Absence of the abdominal musculature is commonly associated with defects of the urinary tract and hydronephrosis (508). The palmaris longus muscle of the volar forearm is congenitally absent in approximately 30% of normal individuals and is asymptomatic, compensated in function by the flexor carpi ulnaris and flexor carpi radialis.

Segmental amyoplasia is absence of muscles derived from defective somites in a segmental distribution. The most common segmental amyoplasia is associated with sacral agenesis. In this condition, absent or defective myotomes belong to the same embryonic somites that fail to give rise to the sclerotomes that form the vertebral bodies at those same levels; dysplasia of the spinal cord occurs because of lack of induction by the notochord. Because all other components of muscle such as the connective tissue, blood vessels, nerves, and tendons are derived from the lateral mesoderm or from the neural crest, and the myotomes form only the myofibers themselves, the other components are present, but the myofibers are replaced by fat. Sacral agenesis is most commonly associated with maternal diabetes mellitus, and *rumpless chicks* are experimentally produced by injecting insulin into incubating eggs. In the autosomal dominant form of sacral agenesis, the defective *Sonic hedgehog* is the same gene that has a mutation in a common form of holoprosencephaly, at the other end of the neural tube (see Chapter 5).

Generalized amyoplasia is not compatible with life and is probably caused by defective myogenic gene expression, as occurs in a mouse model. There are four genes using basic helix-loop-helix transcription factors recognized as critical in myogenesis; these proto-oncogenes are known as myogenic factor 5 (*myf5*), *myogenin* (which promotes the fusion of myoblasts to form myotubes), *herculin* (also known as *mrf4* or *myf6*), and *MyoD1*. *MyoD1* and *myf5* may compensate for each other if either is defective, but loss of both gene expressions cannot be compensated, nor can loss of *myogenin* or *herculin* alone (5,509). The paired homeobox genes *Pax3* and *Pax7* also are essential in muscle progenitor cells (509a), and their defective expression may contribute to amyoplasia. The somitic origin of embryonic myoblasts and of satellite cells in adult muscle for regeneration is the same (509b).

Muscular Hypertrophy and Pseudohypertrophy

Hypertrophy of muscle is a physiologic process, such as work hypertrophy, the muscular enlargement induced by exercise. Pseudohypertrophy differs from hypertrophy because the enlargement of muscles is caused by a pathologic process.

Congenital muscular hypertrophy can be associated with several different conditions. Generalized pseudohypertrophy occurs in myotonia congenita (see previous discussion), and restricted pseudohypertrophy of the calves, tongue, and forearms occurs in Duchenne and Becker muscular dystrophies (see previous discussion). Pseudohypertrophy of muscle also may occur paradoxically in denervation, although neurogenic atrophy is the usual response. It sometimes occurs in hereditary sensory motor neuropathies.

In 1934, de Lange reported three children with generalized muscular enlargement, severe mental retardation, and widespread porencephaly (240). In some instances, the hypertrophy diminished as the children matured, but all patients remained severely mentally defective.

Hypothyroidism (Debre-Sémélaigne syndrome) (510, 511) and myotonic dystrophy are other rare causes of congenital muscular pseudohypertrophy. In muscular pseudohypertrophy associated with hypothyroidism, type I muscle fibers are atrophied and oxidative enzyme activity is abnormal, with a collection of glycogen in the subsarcolemmal areas (239). Finally, in Beckwith-Wiedemann syndrome, generalized or unilateral muscle hypertrophy is associated with generalized or unilateral macroglossia. Additional features include omphalocele, facial nevus flammeus, neonatal hypoglycemia with pancreatic hyperplasia, gigantism with increased bone age, and mild microcephaly. This condition is covered in Chapter 4.

DISORDERS OF MUSCLE METABOLISM

Muscle Phosphorylase Deficiency (Glycogenosis Type V, McArdle Disease)

Muscle phosphorylase deficiency, described by McArdle in 1951 (512), was the first inheritable myopathy for which the enzymatic abnormality, an absence of muscle phosphorylase activity, was recognized. Clinical onset is in childhood, with painful muscle cramps and weakness after exertion and episodes of myoglobulinuria. In a typical case, when the forearm muscle is exercised with its arterial circulation occluded, the flexor muscles go into contracture within a minute and remain in this state for an hour or longer after circulation is restored (513). In contrast to normal muscle, there is no increase in venous lactate.

A severe neonatal form of myophosphorylase usually results in neonatal death from respiratory muscle failure and severe generalized weakness. Muscle biopsy shows an excess of glycogen and only scattered myofibers that express phosphorylase.

The disease is transmitted as an autosomal recessive disorder with a predilection for male subjects. The gene has been localized to chromosome 11q13 (514). There is considerable genetic heterogeneity, and a high incidence of compound heterozygotes has been described (515). Several clinical variants have been reported including an infantile form, presenting with progressive muscular weakness (516).

Muscle biopsy shows an increased concentration of glycogen, and enzymatic studies reveal the specific defect in muscle phosphorylase activity. In some 85% of cases, immunologically reactive enzyme protein is undetectable. Some of the patients with biochemically inactive enzyme protein appear to have a defect in the enzyme-activating system, specifically in the cyclic AMP-dependent muscle phosphorylase b kinase. This autosomal recessive condition has been designated as glycogenosis type VIII (517,518).

Muscle phosphorylase deficiency was the first neuromuscular disorder diagnosed by nuclear MR spectroscopy. By means of this technique, it can be shown that intramuscular pH does not decrease with exercise, but the concentration of phosphocreatine decreases excessively. There is no depletion of adenosine triphosphate (519). Erythrocyte and liver phosphorylase, enzymes that are chemically different, are present in normal amounts.

The sequence of biochemical events leading to contractures and myoglobinuria is still unclear. There is some evidence that premature fatigue results from impaired excitation-contraction coupling caused by an accumulation of adenosine diphosphate (520). Because glycogenolysis is interrupted, energy for ordinary muscular effort must be derived from the oxidation of glucose or fatty acids.

Congenital Defect of Phosphofructokinase (Glycogenosis Type VII)

Congenital defect of phosphofructokinase is transmitted as an autosomal recessive trait with an increased incidence in male subjects. Subjects with a congenital defect of muscle phosphofructokinase tend to have a long history of easy fatigability and of weakness or stiffness induced by exertion (521). In addition, decreased insulin secretion occurs in response to glucose (522). An infantile form, presenting with congenital weakness and respiratory insufficiency, has been recognized also (523). CK levels are usually elevated and, as occurs in muscle phosphorylase deficiency, there is no increase in venous lactate with ischemic exercise. A mild hemolytic anemia is often present. In erythrocytes, enzyme activity is reduced by some 50%, but it is normal in leukocytes. Two subunits of phosphofructokinase M (muscle type) and L (liver type) have been recognized, with the muscle type subunit being inactive in this disease. The gene for phosphofructokinase has been mapped to chromosome 12q13.3, and numerous mutations have been described, with the disease being most frequent in the Ashkenazi Jewish population. Because the enzyme defect precludes glucose utilization in these individuals, energy for muscle contraction must be derived from fatty acid oxidation or, conceivably, from enhancement of the usually unimportant hexose monophosphate shunt.

Although many other defects of muscle carbohydrate metabolism are theoretically possible, the only well-documented ones at this time are caused by defects in phosphoglycerate mutase deficiency and aldolase A. Patients with phosphoglyceromutase deficiency have a lifelong history of muscle pains, cramps, and weakness after exercise (524). The enzyme defect also can result in hemolytic anemia, seizures, and mental retardation (520). Cramps respond to dantrolene, suggesting that they are caused by a high calcium release from the sarcoplasmic reticulum relative to calcium reuptake capacity (525). Subjects with aldolase A deficiency present with unexplained episodes of jaundice and anemia, accompanied by a marked elevation in CK and microcephaly. Muscle biopsy discloses lipid accumulation and distorted and vacuolated mitochondrial cristae (526).

Myoadenylate deaminase deficiency appears to be a relatively common autosomal recessive entity that can be asymptomatic or can present with exertional myalgia during the first or second decade of life (527).

Defects of Mitochondrial Transport (Lipid Storage Myopathies)

The lipid storage myopathies are mainly disorders of transport across the mitochondrial membrane and include disorders of carnitine and related enzymes, such as carnitine palmityltranferase. These diseases are discussed in Chapter 2, in relation to mitochondrial cytopathies.

Myoglobinuria

Myoglobinuria is a rare syndrome with a variety of causes, both hereditary and sporadic (45, 528,529).

Its causes include disorders resulting from defective energy production (e.g., exertional myoglobinuria), myoglobinuria accompanying convulsions, and the various hereditary enzymatic defects already discussed, notably muscle phosphorylase deficiency, phosphofructokinase deficiency, or deficient carnitine palmitoyl transferase activity (529). These conditions are reviewed by Tein and coworkers (530) and by Warren and coworkers (531). Exercise-induced myoglobinuria and progressive muscular weakness also can be caused by a mutation in the mitochondrial DNA coding for cytochrome b, and myoglobinuria precipitated by febrile illness can be transmitted as a dominant trait (532,533).

Sporadic myoglobinuria also can be caused by hypoxia, as occurs in carbon monoxide poisoning; by a primary muscle injury, such as accompanies trauma or burns; or after an infectious illness, notably viral illnesses with myalgic prodromes. Additionally, myoglobinuria can be encountered subsequent to exposure to a variety of toxins and medications (e.g., alcohol, barbiturates, amphotericin B, clozapine, colchicine, cyclohexanone, and licorice) (534). It also can follow insect bites and envenomation (535) (see Chapter10).

Patients characteristically have severe muscle pain and weakness accompanied by the passage of brown urine. Serum enzymes are strikingly elevated, and blood creatine kinase values of 50,000 units or higher have been reported. Occasionally, acute renal tubular necrosis accompanies the attack.

The presence of myoglobin is suggested by a positive benzidine test in an erythrocyte-free urine. The pigment is identified by acrylamide gel electrophoresis or immunodiffusion techniques or, more simply, albeit less specifically, by dipsticks such as Hemoccult (535).

In evaluating a child, often an adolescent, with muscle pain and easy fatigability, a creatine kinase determination and an erythrocyte sedimentation test are the two most helpful screening tests (536). In the experience of Mills and Edwards, a specific diagnosis could be made in almost every patient with an elevated creatine kinase or erythrocyte sedimentation rate (536). An enzymatic defect, the most common cause, was seen in 15% of patients. In half of these, a mitochondrial myopathy was diagnosed by muscle biopsy. The remaining patients had muscle phosphorylase deficiency or, less often, muscle phosphofructokinase deficiency. Of the nonmetabolic cases with muscle pain, inflammatory and endocrine myopathies and a neurogenic disorder were the major diagnostic categories. Most of the undiagnosed patients were found to be depressed.

REFERENCES

1. Engel AG, Franzini-Armstrong C. *Myology: basic and clinical*, 3rd ed. New York: McGraw–Hill, 2004.
2. Brooke MH. *A clinician's view of neuromuscular diseases*, 2nd ed. Baltimore: Williams & Wilkins, 1986.
3. Dubowitz V. *Muscle biopsy. A practical approach*, 2nd ed. London: Baillière Tindall, 1985.
4. Swash M. *Neuromuscular diseases. A practical approach to diagnosis and management*, 3rd ed. Berlin: Springer-Verlag, 1997.
5. Sarnat HB. Neuromuscular disorders. In: Behrman RE, Kliegman RM, Arvin AM, eds. *Nelson textbook of pediatrics*, 16th ed. Philadelphia: WB Saunders, 1999:1867–1893.
6. Ouvrier RA, McLeod JG, Pollard JD. *Peripheral neuropathy in childhood*, 2nd ed. London, UK: MacKeith Press, 1999.
7. Zuberi SM, Matta N, Nawaz S, et al. Muscle ultrasound in the assessment of suspected neuromuscular disease in childhood. *Neuromuscul Disord* 1999;9:203–207.
8. Pillen S, Scholten RR, Zwarts MJ, et al. Quantitataive skeletal muscle ultrasonography in children with suspected neuromuscular disease. *Muscle Nerve* 2003;27:699–705.
9. Byers TJ, Neumann PE, Beggs AH, Kunkel LM. ELISA quantitation of dystrophin for the diagnosis of Duchenne and Becker muscular dystrophies. *Neurology* 1992;42:570–576.
10. Fukuyama Y, Suzuki Y, Hirayama Y, et al. Percutaneous needle muscle biopsy in the diagnosis of neuromuscular disorders in children. Histological, histochemical and electron microscopic studies. *Brain Dev* 1981;3:277–287.
11. Voit T, Sewry CA, Meyer K, et al. Preserved merosin M-chain (or laminin-α2) expression in skeletal muscle distinguishes Walker-Warburg syndrome from Fukuyama muscular dystrophy and merosin-deficient congenital muscular dystrophy. *Neuropediatrics* 1995;26:148–155.
12. Al-Shekhlee A, Katirji B. Electrodiagnostic features of acute paralytic poliomyelitis associated with West Nile virus infection. *Muscle Nerve* 2004;29:376–380.
13. Wang CH. The molecular genetic basis of spinal musclar atrophies. In: Rosenberg RN, Prusiner SB, DiMauro S, et al., eds. *The molecular basis of neurologic and psychiatric disease*, 3rd ed. Philadelphia: Butterworth Heinemann, 2003:455–466.

13a. Kizilates SU, Talim B, Sel K, et al. Severe lethal spinal muscular atrophy variant with arthrogryposis. *Pediatr Neurol* 2005;32:201–204.

13b. Nadeau A, Anjou GD, Debray FG, et al. A newborn with spinal muscular atrophy type 0 presenting with a clinicopathological picture of centronuclear myopathy. *Can J Neurol Sci* 2005;32:S45 (*abstract*).

14. Lefebvre S, Burglen L, Reboullet S, et al. Identification and characterization of a spinal muscular atrophy-determining gene. *Cell* 1995;80:155–165.
15. Monani UR, Lorson CL, Parsons DW, et al. A single nucleotide difference that alters splicing patterns distinguishes the SMA gene SMN1 from the copy gene SMN2. *Hum Mol Genet* 1999;8:1177–1183.

16. Werdnig G. Zwei frühinfantile hereditäre Fälle von progressiver Muskelatrophie unter dem Bilde der Dystrophie, aber auf neurotischer Grundlage. *Arch Psychiat Nervenkr* 1891;22:437–481.
17. Hoffmann J. Über chronische spinale Muskelatrophie im Kindesalter auf familiärer Basis. *Dtsch Z Nervenheilk* 1893;3:427–470.
18. Biros I, Forrest S. Spinal muscular atrophy: untangling the knot? *J Med Genet* 1999;36:1–8.
19. Ogino S, Gao S, Leonard DG, et al. Inverse correlation between SMN1 and SMN2 copy numbers: evidence for gene conversion from SMN2 to SMN1. *Eur J Hum Genet* 2003;11:275–277.
20. Burghes AHM. When is a deletion not a deletion? When it is converted. *Am J Hum Genet* 1997;61:9–15.
21. Roy N, McLean MD, Besner-Johnston A, et al. Refined physical map of the spinal muscular atrophy gene (SMA) region at 5 q13 based on YAC and cosmid contiguous arrays. *Genomics* 1995;26:451–460.
22. Lorson CL, Hahnen E, Androphy EJ, et al. A single nucleotide in the SMN gene regulates splicing and is responsible for spinal muscular atrophy. *Proc Natl Acad Sci USA* 1999;96:6307–6311.
23. Scharf JM, Endrizzi MG, Wetter A, et al. Identification of a candidate modifying gene for spinal muscular atrophy by comparative genomics. *Nat Genet* 1998;20:83–86.
24. McAndrew PE, Parsons DW, Simard LR, et al. Identification of proximal spinal muscular atrophy carriers and patients by analysis of SMNT and SMNC gene copy number. *Am J Hum Genet* 1997;60:1411–1422.
25. Yamashita M, Nishio H, Harada Y, et al. Significant increase in the number of the SMN2 gene copies in an adult-onset type1 III spinal muscular atrophy patient with homozygous deletion of the NAIP gene. *Eur Neurol* 2004;52:101–106.
26. Battaglia G, Princivalle A, Forti F, et al. Expression of the SMN gene, the spinal muscular atrophy determining gene, in the mammalian central nervous system. *Hum Mol Genet* 1997;6:1961–1971.
27. Gubitz AK, Feng W, Dreyfuss G. The SMN complex. *Exp Cell Res* 2004;296:51–56.
28. Iwahashi H, Eguchi Y, Yasuhara N, et al. Synergistic anti-apoptotic activity between Bcl-2 and SMN implicated in spinal muscular atrophy. *Nature* 1997;390:413–417.
29. Sarnat HB. Research strategies in spinal muscular atrophy. In: Gamstorp I, Sarnat HB, eds. *Progressive spinal muscular atrophies*. New York: Raven Press, 1984:225–233.
30. Soler-Botija C, Ferrer I, Alvarez JL, et al. Down regulation of Bcl-2 proteins in type I spinal muscular atrophy motor neurons during fetal development. *J Neuropathol Exp Neurol* 2003;62:420–426.
31. Chou SM, Nonaka I. Werdnig-Hoffmann disease: proposal of a pathogenetic mechanism. *Acta Neuropathol* 1978;41:45–54.
32. Probst A, Ulrich J, Bischoff A, et al. Sensory ganglion neuropathy in infantile spinal muscular atrophy. Light and electron microscopic findings in two cases. *Neuropediatrics* 1981;12:215–231.
33. Kumagai T, Hashizume Y. Morphological and morphometric studies on the spinal cord lesion in Werdnig-Hoffmann disease. *Brain Dev* 1982;4:87–96.
34. Lowrie MB, Vrbovà G. Dependence of postnatal motoneurones on their targets: review and hypothesis. *Trends Neurosci* 1992;15:80–84.
35. Fidzianska A, Goebel HH, Warlo I. Acute infantile spinal muscular atrophy. Muscle apoptosis as a proposed pathogenetic mechanism. *Brain* 1990;113:433–445.
36. Altman J. Programmed cell death: the paths to suicide. *Trends Neurosci* 1992;15:278–280.
37. Kuzuhara S, Chou SM. Preservation of the phrenic motoneurons in Werdnig-Hoffmann disease. *Ann Neurol* 1981;9:506–510.
38. Brandt S. *Werdnig-Hoffmann's progressive muscular atrophy*. Copenhagen: Ejnar Munksgaard, 1950.
39. Mellins RB, Hays AP, Gold AP, et al. Respiratory distress as the initial manifestation of Werdnig-Hoffmann disease. *Pediatrics* 1974;53:33–40.
40. Rudnik-Schoneborn S, Goebel HH, Schlote W, et al. Classical infantile spinal muscular atrophy with SMN deficiency causes sensory neuronopathy. *Neurology* 2003;60:483–487.
41. Carpenter S, Karpati G, Rothman S, et al. Pathological involvement of primary sensory neurons in Werdnig-Hoffmann disease. *Acta Neuropathol (Berl)* 1978;42:91–97.
42. Pearce J, Harriman DG. Chronic spinal muscular atrophy. *J Neurol Neurosurg Psychiatry* 1966;29:509–520.
43. Dubowitz V. Infantile muscular atrophy: a prospective study with particular reference to a slowly progressive variety. *Brain* 1964;87:707–718.
44. Moosa A, Dubowitz V. Spinal muscular atrophy in childhood. Two clues to clinical diagnosis. *Arch Dis Child* 1973;48:386–388.
45. Dubowitz V. *Muscle disorders in childhood*, 2nd ed. Philadelphia: WB Saunders, 1995.
46. Van Wijngaarden GK, Bethlem J. Benign infantile spinal muscular atrophy. A prospective study. *Brain* 1973;96:163–170.
47. Wohlfart G, Fex J, Eliasson S. Hereditary proximal spinal muscular atrophy—a clinical entity simulating progressive muscular dystrophy. *Acta Psychiatr Neurol Scand* 1955;30:395–406.
48. Kugelberg E, Welander L. Heredofamilial juvenile muscular atrophy simulating muscular dystrophy. *Arch Neurol Psychiatry* 1956;75:500–509.
49. Müller B, Melki J, Burlet P, et al. Proximal spinal muscular atrophy (SMA) types II and III in the same sibship are not caused by different alleles at the SMA locus. *Am J Hum Genet* 1992;50:892–895.
50. Tsukagoshi H, Sugita H, Furukawa T, et al. Kugelberg-Welander syndrome with dominant inheritance. *Arch Neurol* 1966;14:378–381.
51. Dale AJ, Engel AG, Rudd NL. Familial hexosaminidase A deficiency with Kugelberg-Welander phenotype and mental changes. *Ann Neurol* 1983;14:109.
52. Grohmann K, Varon R, Stolz P, et al. Infantile spinal muscular atrophy with respiratory distress type 1 (SMARD1). *Ann Neurol* 2003;54:719–724.
53. van der Steege G, Grootscholten PM, van der Vlies P, et al. PCR-based DNA test to confirm clinical diagnosis of autosomal recessive spinal muscular atrophy. *Lancet* 1995;345:985–986.
53a. Tachi N, Kikuchi S, Nozuka N, et al. A new mutation of IGHmBP2 gene in spinal muscular atrophy with respiratory distress type 1. *Pediatr Neurol* 2005;32:288–290.
54. Denny-Brown D, Pennybacker JB. Fibrillation and fasciculation in voluntary muscle. *Brain* 1938;61:311–338.
54a. Hausmanowa-Petrusewicz I. Spinal Muscular Atrophy. Infantile and Juvenile Type. Warsaw: U.S. Dept. of Commerce, Translation and Publication, Springfield, VA. 1978, pp 52–64.
55. Buchthal F, Olsen PZ. Electromyography and muscle biopsy in infantile spinal muscular atrophy. *Brain* 1970;93:15–30.
56. Moosa A, Dubowitz V. Motor nerve conduction velocity in spinal muscular atrophy of childhood. *Arch Dis Child* 1976;51:974–977.
57. Walton JH. The limp child. *J Neurol Neurosurg Psychiatry* 1957;20:144–154.
58. Oppenheim H. Über allgemeine und localisierte Atonie der Muskulatur (Myatonia) im frühen Kindesalter. *Monatsschr Psychiatr Neurol* 1900;8:232–233.
59. Ford FR. Congenital laxity of ligaments. In: *Diseases of the nervous system in infancy, childhood and adolescence*, 5th ed. Springfield, IL: Charles C Thomas, 1966:1219–1221.
60. Lundberg A. Dissociated motor development—developmental patterns, clinical characteristics, causal factors and outcome, with special reference to later walking children. *Neuropaediatrie* 1979;10:161–182.
61. Iannaccone ST, Bove KE, Vogler CA, et al. Type 1 fiber size disproportion: morphometric data from 37 children with myopathic, neuropathic, or idiopathic hypotonia. *Pediatr Pathol* 1987;7:395–419.
62. Rapin I. Hypoactive labyrinths and motor development. *Clin Pediatr* 1974;13:922–923, 926–929, 934–937.
63. Shy GM, Engel WK, Somers JE, et al. Nemaline myopathy: a new congenital myopathy. *Brain* 1963;86:793–810.
64. Shuaib A, Paasuke RT, Brownell KW. Central core disease: clinical features in 13 patients. *Medicine* 1987;66:389–396.
65. Lynch PJ, Tong J, Lehane M, et al. A mutation in the transmembrane/luminal domain of the ryanodine receptor is associated with abnormal $Ca2^{+}$ release channel function and severe central core disease. *Proc Natl Acad Sci USA* 1999;96:4164–4169.
66. Spiro AJ, Shy GM, Gonatas NK. Myotubular myopathy. *Arch Neurol* 1966;14:1–14.

67. Kioschis P, Wiemann S, Heiss NS, et al. Genomic organization of a 225-kb region in Xq28 containing the gene for X-linked myotubular myopathy (MTM1) and a related gene (MTMR1). *Genomics* 1998;54:256–266.
68. Heffner R, Cohen M, Duffner P, et al. Multicore disease in twins. *J Neurol Neurosurg Psychiatry* 1976;39:602–606.
69. Cavanagh NPC, Lake BD, McMeniman P. Congenital fiber type disproportion myopathy: a histologic diagnosis with an uncertain clinical outlook. *Arch Dis Child* 1979;54:735–743.
70. Dehkharghani F, Sarnat HB, Brewster MA, et al. Congenital muscle fiber-type disproportion in Krabbe's leukodystrophy. *Arch Neurol* 1981;38:585–587.
71. Sarnat HB. Cerebral dysgeneses and their influence on fetal muscle development. *Brain Dev* 1986;8:495–499.
72. Engel AG, Angelini C, Gomez MR. Fingerprint body myopathy. *Mayo Clin Proc* 1972;47:377–388.
73. Jerusalem F, Engel AG, Gomez MR. Sarcotubular myopathy. *Neurology* 1973;23:897–906.
74. Lake BD, Wilson J. Zebra body myopathy: clinical, histochemical and ultrastructural studies. *J Neurol Sci* 1975;24:437–446.
75. Brooke MH, Neville HE. Reducing body myopathy. *Neurology* 1972;22:829–840.
76. Ringel S, Neville HE, Duster MC, et al. A new congenital neuromuscular disease with trilaminar muscle fibers. *Neurology* 1978;28: 282–289.
77. Rohkamm R, Boxler K, Ricker K, et al. A dominantly inherited myopathy with excessive tubular aggregates. *Neurology* 1983;33: 331–336.
78. Goebel HH, Schloon H, Lenard HG. Congenital myopathy with cytoplasmic bodies. *Neuropediatrics* 1981;12:166–180.
79. Mitrani-Rosenbaum S, Argov Z, Blumenfeld A, et al. Hereditary inclusion body myopathy maps to chromosome 9p1-q1. *Hum Mol Genet* 1996;5:159–163.
80. Bove KE, Iannaccone ST, Hilton PK, et al. Cylindrical spirals in a familial neuromuscular disorder. *Ann Neurol* 1980;7:550–556.
81. Kalimo H, Savontaus ML, Lang H, et al. X-linked myopathy with excessive autophagy: a new hereditary muscle disease. *Ann Neurol* 1988;23:258–265.
82. Thompson AJ, Swash M, Cox EL, et al. Polysaccharide storage myopathy. *Muscle Nerve* 1988;11:349–355.
83. Horowitz SH, Schmalbruch H. Autosomal dominant distal myopathy with desmin storage: a clinicopathologic and electrophysiologic study of a large kinship. *Muscle Nerve* 1994;17:151–160.
84. Goldfarb LG, Park KY, Cervenakova L, et al. Missense mutations in desmin associated with familial cardiac and skeletal myopathy. *Nat Genet* 1998;19:402–403.
85. Verity MA, Gao YH. Dysmaturation myopathy: correlation with minimal neuropathy in sural nerve biopsies. *J Child Neurol* 1988;3:276–291.
86. Andreassi C, Anbelozzi C, Tiziano FD, et al. Phenylbutyrate increases SMN expression in vitro: relevance for treatment of spinal muscular atrophy. *Eur J Hum Genet* 2004;12:59–65.
87. O'Flaherty P. Arthrogryposis multiplex congenita. *Neonatal Netw* 2001;20:13–20.
88. Hall JG. Arthrogryposis multiplex congenita: etiology, genetics, classification, diagnostic approach and general aspects. *J Pediatr Orthop B* 1997;6:159–166.
89. Hageman G, Willemse J, van Ketel BA, et al. The pathogenesis of fetal hypokinesia. A neurological study of 75 cases of congenital contractures with emphasis on cerebral lesions. *Neuropediatrics* 1987;18:22–33.
90. Wynne-Davies R, Williams PF, O'Connor JCB. The 1960 epidemic of arthrogryposis multiplex congenita. *J Bone Joint Surg* 1981;63B:76–82.
91. Strehl E, Vanasse M, Brochu P. EMG and needle muscle biopsy in arthrogryposis multiplex congenita. *Neuropediatrics* 1985;16: 225–227.
92. Clarren SK, Hall JG. Neuropathologic findings in the spinal cords of 10 infants with arthrogryposis. *J Neurol Sci* 1983;58:89–102.
93. Quinn CM, Wigglesworth JS, Heckmatt J. Lethal arthrogryposis multiplex congenita: a pathological study of 21 cases. *Histopathology* 1991;19:155–162.
93a. Castro-Gago M, Iglesias-Meliero JM, Blanco-Barca MO. Neurogenic arthrogryposis multiplex congenital and volopharyngeal incompetence associated with chromosome 22q11.2 deletion. *J Child Neurol* 2005;20:76–78.
94. Pearson CM, Fowler WG Jr. Hereditary nonprogressive muscular dystrophy inducing arthrogryposis syndrome. *Brain* 1963;86:75–88.
95. Dyken PR, Harper PS. Congenital dystrophica myotonica. *Neurology* 1973;24:465–473.
96. Muller JS, Abicht A, Christen JH, et al. A newly identified chromosomal microdeletion of the rapsyn gene causes congenital myasthenic syndrome. *Neuromuscul Disord* 2004;14:744–749.
97. Silberstein EP, Kakulas BA. Arthrogryposis multiplex congenita in Western Australia. *J Paediatr Child Health* 1998;34:518–523.
98. Jacobson L, Polizzi A, Morriss-Kay G, et al. Plasma from human mothers of fetuses with severe arthrogryposis multiplex congenita causes deformities in mice. *J Clin Invest* 1999;103:1031–1038.
99. Hageman G, Willemse J. Arthrogryposis multiplex congenita. Review with comment. *Neuropediatrics* 1983;14:6–11.
100. Hageman G, Willemse J, van Ketel BA, et al. The heterogeneity of the Pena-Shokeir syndrome. *Neuropediatrics* 1987;18:45–50.
101. Pena SDJ, Shokeir MHK. Autosomal recessive cerebro-oculo-facio-skeletal (COFS) syndrome. *Clin Genet* 1974;5:285–293.
102. Hall JG. Arthrogryposis and the other neuromuscular and motor neuron disorders. In: Hoffman HJ, Epstein F, eds. *Disorders of the developing nervous system*. Boston: Blackwell Scientific Publications, 1986:289–300.
103. Jones KL. *Smith's recognizable patterns of human malformation*, 5th ed. Philadelphia: W.B. Saunders Co., 1997.
104. Hall JG, Reed SD, Greene G. The distal arthrogryposes: delineation of new entities—review and nosologic discussion. *Am J Med Genet* 1982;11:185–239.
105. Staheli LT, Hall JG, Jaffe K, et al. *Arthrogryposis: a text atlas*. Cambridge, UK: Cambridge University Press, 1998.
106. Zampino G, Conti G, Balducci F, et al. Severe form of Freeman-Sheldon syndrome associated with brain anomalies and hearing loss. *Am J Med Genet* 1996;62:293–296.
107. Miskin M, Rothberg R, Rudd NL, et al. Arthrogryposis multiplex congenita: prenatal assessment with diagnostic ultrasound and fetoscopy. *J Pediatr* 1979;95:463–464.
108. Williams P. The management of arthrogryposis. *Orthop Clin North Am* 1978;9:67–88.
109. Willis T. De Anima Brutorum Quae Hominis Vitalis ac Sensitiva Est, Exercitationes Duae. Altera pathologica morbos qui ipsam, & sedem eius primariam, nempe cerebrum & nervosum genus afficiunt, explicat, eorumque therapeias instituit. Oxford: E theatro Sheldoniano. Impensis Ric. Davis, 1672; 565.
110. Lindstrom J, Shelton D, Fujii Y. Myasthenia gravis. *Adv Immunol* 1988;42:233–284.
111. Afifi AK, Bell WE. Tests for juvenile myasthenia gravis: comparative diagnostic yield and prediction of outcome. *J Child Neurol* 1993;8:403–411.
112. Vincent A, Palace J, Hilton-Jones D. Myasthenia gravis. *Lancet* 2001;357:2122–2128.
113. Vincent A, McConville J, Farrugia ME, et al. Seronegative myasthenia gravis. *Semin Neurol* 2004;24:125–133.
113a. Scheufele ML, Moore A, Iannaccone ST, et al. A series of myasthenia gravis patients with anti-MuSK antibodies. *J Child Neurol* 2005;20:264 [*abstract*].
113b. Moore AJ, Iannaccone ST. A closer look at congenital myasthenic syndromes. *J Child Neurol* 2005;20:271 [*abstract*].
113c. Barisic N, Müller JS, Paucic-Kirincic E, et al. Clinical variability of CMS-EA (congenital myasthenic syndrome with episodic apnea) due to identical *CHAT* mutations in two infants. *Eur J Paediatr Neurol* 2005;9:7–12.
114. Engel AG, Arahata K. The membrane attack complex of complement at the endplate in myasthenia gravis. *Ann NY Acad Sci* 1987;505:326–332.
115. Drachman DB, Adams RN, Josifek LF, et al. Functional activities of autoantibodies to acetylcholine receptors and the clinical severity of myasthenia gravis. *N Engl J Med* 1982;307:769–775.
116. Fujii Y, Monden Y, Nakahara K, et al. Antibody to acetylcholine receptor in myasthenia gravis: production by lymphocytes from thymus or thymoma. *Neurology* 1984;34:1182–1186.

117. Manfredi AA, Protti MP, Dalton MW, et al. T helper cell recognition of muscle acetylcholine receptor in myasthenia gravis. Epitopes on the gamma and delta subunits. *J Clin Invest* 1993;92:1055–1067.
118. Schluep M, Willcox N, Vincent A, et al. Acetylcholine receptors in human thymic myoid cells in situ: an immunohistological study. *Ann Neurol* 1987;22:212–222.
119. Andrews PL. Autoimmune myasthenia gravis in childhood. *Semin Neurol* 2004;24:101–110.
120. Hughes BW, De Casillas M, Kaminski JH. Pathophysiology of myasthenia gravis. *Semin Neurol* 2004;24:21–30.
121. Keesey J, Lindstrom J, Cokely H. Anti-acetylcholine receptor antibody in neonatal myasthenia gravis [Letter]. *N Engl J Med* 1977;296:55.
122. Lefvert AK, Osterman PO. Newborn infants to myasthenic mothers: a clinical study and an investigation of acetylcholine receptor antibodies in 17 children. *Neurology* 1983;13:133–138.
123. Millichap JG, Dodge PR. Diagnosis and treatment of myasthenia gravis in infancy, childhood and adolescence. *Neurology* 1960;10:1007–1014.
124. Fenichel GM. Clinical syndromes of myasthenia in infancy and childhood. A review. *Arch Neurol* 1978;35:97–103.
125. Papazian O. Transient neonatal myasthenia gravis. *J Child Neurol* 1992;7:135–141.
126. Harper CM. Congenital myasthenic syndromes. *Semin Neurol* 2004;24:111–123.
127. Engel AG, Ohno K, Sine SM. Congenital myasthenic syndromes: recent advances. *Arch Neurol* 1999;56:163–167.
128. Schmidt C, Abicht A, Krampfl K, et al. Congenital myasthenic syndrome due to a novel missense mutation in the gene encoding choline acetyltransferase. *Neuromuscul Disord* 2003;13:245–251.
129. Walls TJ, Engel AG, Nagel AS, et al. Congenital myasthenic syndrome associated with paucity of synaptic vesicles and reduced quantal release. *Ann NY Acad Sci* 1993;681:461–468.
130. Maselli RA, Kong DZ, Bowe CM, et al. Presysynaptic congenital myasthenic syndrome due to quantal release deficiency. *Neurology* 2001;57:279–289.
131. Ohno K, Engel AG, Brengman JM, et al. The spectrum of mutations causing end-plate acetylcholinesterase deficiency. *Ann Neurol* 2000;47:162–170.
132. Engel AG, Ohno K, Shen XM, et al. Congenital myasthenic syndromes: multiple molecular targets at the neuromuscular junction. *Ann NY Acad Sci* 2003;998:138–160.
133. Müller JS, Mildner G, Müller-Felber W, et al. Rapsyn N88K is a frequent cause of congenital myasthenic syndromes in European patients. *Neurology* 2003;60:1805–1810.
134. Banwell Bl, Russel J, Fukudome T, et al. Myopathy, myasthenic syndrome, and epidermolysis bullosa simplex due to plectin deficiency. *J Neuropathol Exp Neurol* 1999;58:832–846.
135. Harper CM, Engel AG. Quinidine sulfate therapy for the slow-channel congenital myasthenic syndrome. *Ann Neurol* 1998;43:480–484.
136. Brownlow S, Webster R, Croxen R, et al. Acetylcholine receptor delta subunit mutations underlie a fast-channel myasthenic syndrome and arthrogryposis multiplex congenita. *J Clin Invest* 2001;108:125–130.
137. Tsujino A, Maertense C, Ohno K, et al. Myasthenic syndrome caused by mutation of the SCN4A sodium channel. *Proc Natl Acad Sci USA* 2001;100:7377–7382.
138. Mora M, Lambert EH, Engel AG. Synaptic vesicle abnormality in familial infantile myasthenia. *Neurology* 1987;37:206–214.
139. Albers JW, Faulkner JA, Dorovini-Zis K, et al. Abnormal neuromuscular transmission in an infantile myasthenic syndrome. *Ann Neurol* 1984;16:28–34.
140. Ohno K, Brengman J, Tsujino A, et al. Human endplate acetylcholinesterase deficiency caused by mutations in the collagen-like tail subunit (ColQ) of the asymmetric enzyme. *Proc Natl Acad Sci USA* 1998;95:9654–9659.
141. Gomez CM, Maselli R, Gammack J, et al. A beta-subunit mutation in the acetylcholine receptor gate causes severe slow-channel syndrome. *Ann Neurol* 1996;39:712–723.
142. Ohno K, Wang HL, Milone M, et al. Congenital myasthenic syndrome caused by decreased agonist binding affinity due to a mutation in the acetylcholine receptor epsilon subunit. *Neuron* 1996;17:157–170.
143. Ohno K, Engel AG. Congenital myasthenic syndromes: gene mutations. *Neuromuscul Disord* 2003;13:8554–857.
144. Schlezinger NS, Corin MS. Myasthenia gravis associated with hyperthyroidism in childhood. *Neurology* 1968;18:1217–1222.
145. Snead OC, Benton JW, Dwyer D, et al. Juvenile myasthenia gravis. *Neurology* 1980;30:732–739.
146. Lindner A, Schalke B, Toyka KV. Outcome in juvenile-onset myasthenia gravis: a retrospective study with long-term follow-up of 79 patients *J Neurol* 1997;244:515–529.
147. Rodriguez M, Gomez MR, Howard FM Jr, et al. Myasthenia gravis in children. Long-term follow-up. *Ann Neurol* 1983;13:504–510.
147a. Felice KJ, DiMario F, Conway SR. Postinfectious myasthenia gnavis: report of 2 cases. *J Child Neurol* 2005;20:441–444.
148. Dobkin BH, Verity MA. Familial neuromuscular disease with type I fiber hypoplasia, tubular aggregates, cardiomyopathy, and myasthenic features. *Neurology* 1978;28:1135–1140.
149. Rodolico C, Toscano A, Autunno M, et al. Limb-girdle myasthenia: clinical, electrophysiological and morphological features in familial and autoimmune cases. *Neuromuscul Disord* 2002;12:964–969.
150. McQuillen MP, Cantor HE, O'Rourke JR. Myasthenic syndrome associated with antibiotics. *Arch Neurol* 1968;18:402–415.
151. Pittinger C, Adamson R. Antibiotic blockade of neuromuscular function. *Ann Rev Pharmacol* 1972;12:169–184.
152. Mackey JR, Desai S, Larratt L, et al. Myasthenia gravis in association with allogeneic bone marrow transplantation: clinical observations, therapeutic implications and review of the literature. *Bone Marrow Transplant* 1997;19:939–942.
153. Shapira Y, Cividalli G, Szabo G, et al. A myasthenic syndrome in childhood leukemia. *Dev Med Child Neurol* 1974;16:668–671.
154. Oh SJ, Cho HK. Edrophonium responsiveness not necessarily diagnostic of myasthenia gravis. *Muscle Nerve* 1990;13:187–191.
155. Andrews PI, Massey JM, Sanders DB. Acetylcholine receptor antibodies in juvenile myasthenia gravis. *Neurology* 1993;43:977–998.
156. Vial C, Charles N, Chauplannaz G, et al. Myasthenia gravis in childhood and infancy. Usefulness of electrophysiologic studies. *Arch Neurol* 1991;48:847–849.
157. Keesey JC. AAEE minimonograph 33: electrodiagnostic approach to defects of neuromuscular transmission. *Muscle Nerve* 1989;12:613–626.
158. Kelly JJ, Daube JR, Lennon VA, et al. The laboratory diagnosis of mild myasthenia gravis. *Ann Neurol* 1982;12:238–242.
159. Kaeser HE. Drug-induced myasthenic syndromes. *Acta Neurol Scand Suppl* 1984;100:39–47.
160. Keesey J. Myasthenia gravis. In: Raker RE, ed. *Conn's current therapy*. Philadelphia: WB Saunders, 1992:902–908.
161. Mann JD, Johns TR, Campa JF. Long-term administration of corticosteroids in myasthenia gravis. *Neurology* 1976;26:729–740.
162. Vajsar J. Neuromuscular junction disorders. In: Maria BL, *Current management in child neurology*, 2nd ed. Hamilton, London: BC Decker Inc, 2002; 368–373.
163. Sarnat HB, McGarry JD, Lewis JE. Effective treatment of infantile myasthenia gravis by combined prednisone and thymectomy. *Neurology* 1977;27:550–553.
164. Dau PC. Plasmapheresis therapy in myasthenia gravis. *Muscle Nerve* 1980;3:468–482.
165. Drachman DB, Jones RJ, Brodsky RA. Treatment of refractory myasthenia: "rebooting" with high-dose cyclophosphamide. *Ann Neurol* 2003;53:29–34.
166. Herrmann DN, Carney PR, Wald JJ. Juvenile myasthenia gravis: treatment with immune globulin and thymectomy. *Pediatr Neurol* 1998;18:63–66.
167. Gajdos P, Chevret S, Clair B, et al. Clinical trial of plasma exchange and high-dose intravenous immunoglobulin in myasthenia gravis. *Ann Neurol* 1997;41:789–796.
168. Tagher RJ, Baumann R, Desai N. Failure of intravenously administered immunoglobulin in the treatment of neonatal myasthenia gravis. *J Pediatr* 1999;134:233–235.
169. Youssef S. Thymectomy for myasthenia gravis in children. *J Pediatr Surg* 1983;18:537–541.
170. Fonkelsrud EW, Herrmann C, Mulder DG. Thymectomy for myasthenia gravis in children. *J Pediatr Surg* 1970;5:157–165.

171. Palace J, Wiles CM, Newsom-Davis J. 3,4-diaminopyridine in the treatment of congenital (hereditary) myasthenia. *J Neurol Neurosurg Psychiatr* 1991;54:1069–1072.
172. Dubowitz V. What's in a name? Muscular dystrophy revisited. *Eur J Paediatr Neurol* 1998;2:273–284.
173. Gowers WR. Clinical lecture on pseudohypertrophic muscular paralysis. *Lancet* 1879;2:1,37,73,113.
174. Emery AEF. The muscular dystrophies. *Lancet* 2002;359:687–695.
175. Hoffman EP. Dystrophinopathies. In: Rosenberg RN, Prusiner SB, DiMauro S, et al., eds. *The molecular basis of neurologic and psychiatric disease*, 3rd ed. Philadelphia: Butterworth Heinemann, 2003:467–478.
176. Ringel SP, Carroll JE, Schold SC. The spectrum of mild X-linked recessive muscular dystrophy. *Arch Neurol* 1977;34:408–416.
177. Emery AEH, Dreifuss FE. Unusual type of benign X-linked muscular dystrophy. *J Neurol Neurosurg Psychiatry* 1966;29:338–342.
178. Bonne G, Mercuri E, Muchir A, et al. Clinical and molecular genetic spectrum of autosomal dominant Emery-Dreifuss muscular dystrophy due to mutation of the lamin A/C gene. *Ann Neurol* 2000;48:170–180.
179. DiBarletta R, Ricci E, Galluzzi G, et al. Different mutations in the LMNA gene cause autosomal dominant and autosomal recessive Emery-Dreifuss muscular dystrophy. *Am J Hum Genet* 2000;66:1407–1412.
180. Taylor DA, Carroll JE, Smith ME, et al. Facioscapulohumeral dystrophy associated with hearing loss and Coats syndrome. *Ann Neurol* 1982;12:395–398.
181. Hauser MA, Horrigan SK, Salmikangas P, et al. Myotilin is mutated in limb girdle muscular dystrophy 1A. *Hum Mol Genet* 2000;9:2141–2147.
182. van der Kooi AJ, van Meegen M, Ledderhof TM, et al. Genetic localization of a newly recognized autosomal dominant limb-girdle muscular dystrophy with cardiac involvement (LGND1B) to chromosome 1q11-21. *Am J Hum Genet* 1997;60:891–895.
183. Minetti C, Sotgia F, Bruno C, et al. Mutations in the caveolin-3 gene cause autosomal dominant limb-girdle dystrophy. *Nat Genet* 1998;18:365–368.
184. Speer MC, Vance JM, Grubber JM, et al. Identification of a new autosomal dominant limb-girdle muscular dystrophy locus on chromosome 7. *Am J Hum Genet* 1999;64:556–562.
185. Messina DN, Speer MC, Pericak-Vance MA, et al. Linkage of familial dilated cardiomyopathy with conduction defect and muscular dystrophy to chromosome 6q23. *Am J Hum Genet* 1997;61:909–917.
186. Bushby KM. The limb-girdle muscular dystrophies—multiple genes, multiple mechanisms. *Hum Mol Genet* 1999;8:1875–1882.
187. Richard I, Roudaut C, Saenz A, et al. Calpainopathy—a survey of mutations and polymorphisms. *Am J Hum Genet* 1999;64:1524–1540.
188. Topaloglu H, Dincer P, Richard I, et al. Calpain-3 deficiency causes a mild muscular dystrophy in childhood. *Neuropediatrics* 1997;28:213–216.
189. McNally EM, Ly CT, Rosenmann H, et al. Splicing mutation in dysferlin produces limb-girdle muscular dystrophy inflammation. *Am J Med Genet* 2000;91:305–312.
190. Merlini L, Kaplan JC, Navarro C, et al. Homogenous phenotype of the gypsy limb-girdle MD with the gamma sarcoglycan C283Y mutation. *Neurology* 2000;54:1075–1079.
191. Angelini C, Fanin M, Freda MP, et al. The clinical spectrum of sarcoglycanopathies. *Neurology* 1999;52:176–179.
192. Duggan DJ, Gorospe JR, Fanin M, et al. Mutations in the sarcoglycan genes in patients with myopathy. *New Engl J Med* 1997;336:618–624.
193. Passos-Bueno MR, Vainzof M, Moreira ES, et al. Seven autosomal recessive limb-girdle dystrophies in the Brazilian population. *Am J Med Genet* 1999;82:392–398.
194. Moreira ES, Vainzof M, Marie SK, et al. A first missense mutation in the delta sarcoglycan gene associated with a severe phenotype and frequency of limb-girdle muscular dystrophy type 2F (LGND2F) in Brazilian sarcoglycanopathies. *J Med Genet* 1998;35:951–953.
195. Moreira ES, Wiltshire TJ, Faulkner G, et al. Limb-girdle muscular dystrophy type 2G is caused by mutations in the gene encoding the sarcomeric protein telethonin. *Nat Genet* 2000;24:163–166.
196. Frosk P, Weiler T, Nylen E, et al. Limb-girdle muscular dystrophy type 2H associated with mutations in TRIM32, a putative E3-ubiquitin-ligase gene. *Am J Hum Genet* 2002;70:663–672.
197. Mercuri E, Brockington M, Straub V, et al. Phenotypic spectrum associated with mutations in the fukutin-related protein gene. *Ann Neurol* 2003;53:537–542.
198. Bushby KM, Beckmann JS. The 105th ENMC-sponsored workshop: pathogenesis in the non-sarcoglycan limb-girdle muscular dystrophies. *Neuromuscul Disord* 2003;13:80–90.
199. Uyama E, Nohira O, Chateau D, et al. Oculopharyngeal muscular dystrophy in two unrelated Japanese families. *Neurology* 1996;46:773–778.
200. Barohn RJ, Miller RG, Griggs RC. Autosomal recessive distal dystrophy. *Neurology* 1991; 1365–1370.
201. Watkins SC, Cullen MJ. A qualitative and quantitative study of the ultrastructure of regenerating muscle fiber in Duchenne muscular dystrophy and polymyositis. *J Neurol Sci* 1987;82:181–192.
202. Carpenter S, Karpati G. Duchenne muscular dystrophy. Plasma membrane loss initiates muscle cell necrosis unless it is repaired. *Brain* 1979;102:147–161.
203. Rosman NP. The cerebral defect and myopathy in Duchenne muscular dystrophy. A comparative clinicopathologic study. *Neurology* 1970;20:329–335.
204. Blake DJ, Tinsley JM, Davies KE. Utrophin: a structural and functional comparison to dystrophin. *Brain Pathol* 1996;6:37–47.
205. England SB, Nicholson LV, Johnson MA, et al. Very mild muscular dystrophy associated with the deletion of 40% of dystrophin. *Nature* 1990;343:180–182.
206. Ibraghimov-Beskrovnaya O, Ervasti JM, Leveille CJ, et al. Primary structure of dystrophin-associated glycoproteins linking dystrophin to the extracellular matrix. *Nature* 1992;355:696–702.
206a. Compton AG, Cooper ST, Hill PM, et al. The syntrophin-dystrobrevin subcomplex in human neuromuscular disorders. *J Neuropathol Exp Neurol* 2005;64:350–361.
207. Zubrzykcka-Gaarn EE, Bulman DE, Karpati G, et al. The Duchenne muscular dystrophy gene product is localized in sarcolemma of human skeletal muscle. *Nature* 1988;333:466–469.
208. Anderson JL, Head SI, Rae C, et al. Brain function in Duchenne muscular dystrophy. *Brain* 2002;125:4–13.
209. Ueda H, Baba T, Ohno S. Current knowledge of dystrophin and dystrophin-associated proteins in retina. *Histol Histopathol* 2000;15:753–760.
210. Scott MO, Sylvester JE, Heiman-Patterson T, et al. Duchenne muscular dystrophy gene expression in normal and diseased human muscle. *Science* 1988;239:1418–1420.
211. Hoffman EP, Fischbeck KH, Brown RH, et al. Characterization of dystrophin in muscle-biopsy specimens from patients with Duchenne's or Becker's muscular dystrophy. *N Engl J Med* 1988;318:1363–1368.
212. Nudel U, Zuk D, Einat P, et al. Duchenne muscular dystrophy gene product is not identical in muscle and brain. *Nature* 1989;337:76–78.
213. Lidov HGW. Dystrophin in the nervous system. *Brain Pathol* 1996;6:63–77.
214. Ahn AH, Kunkel LM. The structural and functional diversity of dystrophin. *Nat Genet* 1993;3:283–291.
215. Lidov HGW, Selig S, Kunkel LM. Dp140: a novel 140 kDa CNS transcript from the dystrophin locus. *Hum Mol Genet* 1995;4:329–335.
216. Nigro V, Piluso G, Belsito A, et al. Gene redundancies in the dystrophin-associated protein complex. *Acta Myologica (Napoli)* 1998;2:29–31.
217. Hattori N, Kaido M, Nishigaki T, et al. Undetectable dystrophin can still result in a relatively benign phenotype of dystrophinopathy. *Neuromuscul Disord* 1999;9:220–226.
218. Salih MAM, Sunada Y, Al-Nasser M, et al. Muscular dystrophy associated with beta-dystroglycan deficiency. *Ann Neurol* 1996;40:925–928.
219. Brown RH Jr. Dystrophin-associated proteins and the muscular dystrophies: a glossary. *Brain Pathol* 1996;6:19–24.

220. Wilson J, Putt W, Jimenez C, Edwards YH. Up71 and Up140, two novel transcripts of utrophin that are homologues of short forms of dystrophin. *Hum Mol Genet* 1999;8:1271–1278.
221. Bodensteiner JB, Engel AG. Intracellular calcium accumulation in Duchenne dystrophy and other myopathies: a study of 567,000 muscle fibers in 114 biopsies. *Neurology* 1978;28:438–446.
222. Nicholson LVB, Johnson MA, Bushby KM, et al. Functional significance of dystrophin positive fibres in Duchenne muscular dystrophy. *Arch Dis Child* 1993;68:632–636.
223. Muntoni F, Torelli S, Ferlini A. Dystrophin and mutations: one gene, several proteins, multiple phenotypes. *Lancet Neurol* 2003;2:731–740.
224. Mendell JR, Sahenk Z, Prior TW. The childhood muscular dystrophies: diseases sharing a common pathogenesis of membrane instability. *J Child Neurol* 1995;10:150–159.
225. Duchenne G. *De la paralysis musculaire pseudohypertrophique ou paralysis myo-sclerotique*. Paris: P. Asselin, 1868.
226. Gowers WR. *Pseudo-hypertrophic muscular paralysis*. London: J & A Churchill, 1879.
227. Perloff JK. Cardiac rhythm and conduction in Duchenne's muscular dystrophy: a prospective study of 20 patients. *J Am Coll Cardiol* 1984;3:1263–1268.
228. Barohn RJ, Levine EJ, Olson JO, et al. Gastric hypomotility in Duchenne's muscular dystrophy. *N Engl J Med* 1988;319:15–18.
229. Huvos AG, Prudzanski W. Smooth muscle involvement in primary muscle disease. II. Progressive muscular dystrophy. *Arch Pathol* 1967;83:234–240.
230. Rosman NP, Kakulas BA. Mental deficiency associated with muscular dystrophy: a neuropathological study. *Brain* 1966;89:769–788.
231. Felisari G, Martinelli Boneschi F, Bardoni A, et al. Loss of Dp140 dystrophin isoform and intellectual impairment in Duchenne dystrophy. *Neurology* 2000;55:559–564.
232. Lidov HGW, Selig S, Kunkel LM. Dp140: a novel 140 kDa CNS transcript from the dystrophin locus. *Hum Mol Genet* 1995;4: 329–335.
233. Yoshioka M, Okuno T, Honda Y, et al. Central nervous system involvement in progressive muscular dystrophy. *Arch Dis Child* 1980;55:589–594.
234. Bardoni A, Sironi M, Felisari G, et al. Absence of brain Dp140 isoform and cognitive impairment in Becker muscular dystrophy. *Lancet* 1999;353:897–898.
235. Harper PS. *Myotonic dystrophy*. Philadelphia: WB Saunders, 2001.
236. Serratrice G, Pellissier JF, Faugere MC, et al. Centronuclear myopathy. Possible central nervous system origin. *Muscle Nerve* 1978;1:62–69.
237. Ricci E, Moraes CT, Servidei S, et al. Disorders associated with depletion of mitochondrial DNA. *Brain Pathol* 1992;2:141–147.
238. Guggenheim MA, McCabe ER, Roig M, et al. Glycerol kinase deficiency with neuromuscular, skeletal and adrenal abnormalities. *Ann Neurol* 1980;7:441–449.
239. Spiro AJ, Hirano A, Beilin RL, et al. Cretinism with muscular hypertrophy (Kocher-Debré-Sémélaigne syndrome). Histochemical and ultrastructural study of skeletal muscle. *Arch Neurol* 1970;23:340–349.
240. De Lange C. Congenital hypertrophy of the muscles, extrapyramidal motor disturbances and mental deficiency. *Am J Dis Child* 1934;48:243–268.
241. Van der Knaap MS, Smit LM, Barth PG, et al. Magnetic resonance imaging in classification of congenital muscular dystrophies with brain abnormalities. *Ann Neurol* 1997;42:50–59.
242. Dobyns WB, Pagon RA, Armstrong D, et al. Diagnostic criteria for Walker-Warburg syndrome. *Am J Med Genet* 1989;32:195–210.
243. Beltran-Valero de Bernabe D, Currier S, Steinbrecher A, et al. Mutations in the O-mannosyltransferase gene POMT1 give rise to the severe neuronal migration disorder Walker-Warburg syndrome. *Am J Hum Genet* 2002;71:1033–1043.
244. Laverda AM, Battaglia MA, Drigo P, et al. Congenital muscular dystrophy, brain and eye abnormalities: one or more clinical entities? *Child Nerv Syst* 1993;9:84–87.
245. Fukuyama Y, Osawa M, Suzuki H. Congenital progressive muscular dystrophy of the Fukuyama type—clinical, genetic and pathological considerations. *Brain Dev* 1981;3:1–29.
246. Pearce GW, Pearce JM, Walton JN. The Duchenne type muscular dystrophy: histopathologic studies of the carrier state. *Brain* 1966;89:109–120.
247. Bushby KMD, Thambyayah M, Gardner-Medwin D. Prevalence and incidence of Becker muscular dystrophy. *Lancet* 1991;337: 1022–1024.
248. Gospe SM, Lazaro RP, Lava NS, et al. Familial X-linked myalgia and cramps: a non-progressive myopathy associated with a deletion in the dystrophin gene. *Neurology* 1989;39:1277–1280.
249. Doriguzzi C, Palmucci L, Mongini T, et al. Exercise intolerance and recurrent myoglobinuria as the only expression of Xp21 Becker type muscular dystrophy. *J Neurol* 1993;240:269–271.
250. Yates JR, Warner JP, Smith JA, et al. Emery-Dreifuss muscular dystrophy: linkage to markers in distal Xq28. *J Med Genet* 1993;30:108–111.
251. Farley EA, Kendrick-Jones J, Ellis JA. The Emery-Dreifuss muscular dystrophy phenotype arises from aberrant targeting and binding of emerin at the inner nuclear membrane. *J Cell Sci* 1999;112:2571–2582.
252. Landouzy L, Dejerine J. De la myopathie atrophique progressive. *Rev Med Franc* 1885;5:811–817, 253–366;6:977–1027.
253. Tupler R, Perini G, Pellegrino MA, et al. Profound misregulation of muscle-specific gene expression in fascioscapulohumeral muscular dystrophy. *Proc Natl Acad Sci USA* 1999;96:12650–12654.
254. Lunt PW, Harper PS. Genetic counselling in facioscapulohumeral muscular dystrophy. *J Med Genet* 1991;28:655–664.
255. Gabellini D, Green MR, Tupler R. Inappropriate gene activation in FSHD: a repressor complex binds a chromosomal repeat deleted in dystrophic muscle. *Cell* 2002;110:339–348.
256. Wijmenga C, Padberg GW, Moerer P, et al. Mapping of facioscapulohumeral muscular dystrophy gene to chromosome 4q35-qter by multipoint linkage analysis and in situ hybridization. *Genomics* 1991;9:570–575.
257. Rothstein TL, Carlson CB, Sumi SM. Polymyositis with facioscapulohumeral distribution. *Arch Neurol* 1971;25:313–319.
258. Fitzsimons RB, Gurwin EB, Bird AC. Retinal vascular abnormalities in facioscapulohumeral muscular dystrophy. *Brain* 1987;110:631–648.
259. Wulff JD, Lin JT, Kepes JJ. Inflammatory facioscapulohumeral muscular dystrophy and Coats syndrome. *Ann Neurol* 1982;12:398–401.
260. Wilhelmsen KC, Blake DM, Lynch T, et al. Chromosome 12-linked autosomal dominant scapuloperoneal muscular dystrophy. *Ann Neurol* 1996;39:507–520.
261. Ronen GM, Lowry N, Wedge JH, et al. Hereditary motor sensory neuropathy type I presenting as scapuloperoneal atrophy (Davidenkow syndrome). Electrophysiological and pathological studies. *Can J Neurol Sci* 1986;13:264–266.
262. Mohire MD, Tandan R, Fries TJ, et al. Early-onset benign autosomal dominant limb-girdle myopathy with contractures (Bethlem myopathy). *Neurology* 1988;38:573–580.
263. Laval SH, Bushby KM. Limb-girdle muscular dystrophies—from genetics to molecular pathology. *Neuropathol Appl Neurobiol* 2004;30:91–105.
264. Zatz M, de Paula F, Starling A, et al. The 10 autosomal recessive limb-girdle muscular dystrophies. *Neuromuscul Disord* 2003;13:532–544.
265. Schara U, Vorgerd M, Popovic N, et al. Rippling muscle disease in childhood. *J Child Neurol* 2002;17:483–490.
266. Woodman SE, Sotgia F, Galbiati F, et al. Caveolinopathies: mutations in caveolin-3 cause four distinct autosomal dominant diseases. *Neurology* 2004;62:538–543.
267. Lennon NJ, Kho A, Bacsai BJ, et al. Dysferlin interacts with annexins A1 and A2 and mediates sarcolemmal wound healing. *J Biol Chem* 2003;278:50466–50473.
268. Ro LS, Lee-Chen GJ, Lin TC, et al. Phenotypic features and genetic findings in 2 Chinese families with Miyoshi distal myopathy. *Arch Neurol* 2004;61:1594–1599.
269. Worton R. Muscular dystrophies: diseases of the dystrophin-glycoprotein complex. *Science* 1995;270:755–756.
270. Bushby K. Muscular dystrophy and allied disorders: research strategies. *Trans Biochem Soc* 1996;24:489–496.
271. Ljunggren A, Duggan D, McNally E, et al. Primary adhalin

deficiency as a cause of muscular dystrophy in patients with normal dystrophin. *Ann Neurol* 1995;38:367–372.
272. Politano L, Nigro V, Passamano L, et al. Clinical and genetic findings in sarcoglycanopathies. *Acta Myologica (Napoli)* 1998;2:33–40.
273. Magee KR, DeJong RN. Hereditary distal myopathy with onset in infancy. *Arch Neurol* 1965;13:387–390.
274. Nishino I, Noguchi S, Murayama K, et al. Distal myopathy with rimmed vacuoles is allelic to hereditary inclusion body myopathy. *Neurology* 2002;59:1689–1693.
275. Matsumura K, Nonaka I, Campbell KP. Abnormal expression of dystrophin-associated proteins in Fukuyama-type congenital muscular dystrophy. *Lancet* 1993;341:521–523.
276. Coral-Vascquez RM, Rosas-Vargas H, Mexa-Espinosa P, et al. Severe congenital muscular dystrophy in a Mexican family with a new nonsense mutation (R2578X) in the laminin alpha-2 gene. *J Hum Genet* 2003;48:91–95.
277. Brockington M, Sewry CA, Herrmann R, et al. Assignment of a form of congenital muscular dystrophy with secondary merosin deficiency to chromosome 1q42. *Am J Hum Genet* 2000;66:428–435.
278. Brockington M, Blake DJ, Prandini P, et al. Mutations in the fukutin-related protein gene (FKRP) cause a form of congenital muscular dystrophy with secondary laminin (2 deficiency and abnormal glycosylation of α-dystroglycan. *Am J Hum Genet* 2001;69:1198–1209.
279. Hayashi YK, Chou FL, Engvall E. Mutations in the integrin alpha 7 gene cause congenital myopathy. *Nat Genet* 1998;19:94–97.
280. Barkovich AJ. Neuroimaging manifestations and classification of congenital muscular dystrophies. *Am J Neuroradiol* 1998;19:1389–1396.
281. Moghadaszadeh B, Petit N, Jaillard C, et al. Mutations in SEPN1 cause congenital muscular dystrophy with spinal rigidity and restrictive respiratory syndrome. *Nat Genet* 2001;29:17–18.
282. Grewal PK, Hewitt JE. Glycosylation defects: a new mechanism for muscular dystrophy? *Hum Mol Genet* 2003;12[Spec No 2]:R259–R264.
283. Yashida A, Kobayashi K, Manya H, et al. Muscular dystrophy and neuronal migration disorder caused by mutation in glycosyltransferase, POMGnT1. *Dev Cell* 2001;1:717–724.
284. Pan TC, Zhang RZ, Sudano DG, et al. New molecular mechanism for Ullrich congenital muscular dystrophy: a heterozygous in-frame deletion in the COL6A1 gene causes a severe phenotype. *Am J Hum Genet* 2003;73:355–369.
285. Higuchi I, Shiraishi T, Hashiguchi T, et al. Frameshift mutation in the collagen VI gene causes Ullrich's disease. *Ann Neurol* 2001;50:261–265.
286. Batten F. Three cases of myopathy, infantile type. *Brain* 1903;26:147–148.
287. Muntoni F, Voit T. The congenital muscular dystrophies in 2004: a century of exciting progress. *Neuromuscul Disord* 2004;14:635–649.
288. Saito Y, Mizuguchi M, Oka A, et al. Fukutin protein is expressed in neurons of the normal developing human brain but is reduced in Fukuyama-type congenital muscular dystrophy brain. *Ann Neurol* 2000;47:756–764.
289. Toda T, Segawa M, Nomura Y, et al. Localization of a gene for Fukuyama type congenital muscular dystrophy to chromosome 9q-31-33. *Nat Genet* 1993;5:283–286.
290. Yamamoto T, Shibata N, Kanazawa M, et al. Localization of laminin subunits in the central nervous system in Fukuyama congenital muscular dystrophy: an immunohistochemical investigation. *Acta Neuropathol* 1997;94:173–179.
291. Haltia M, Leivo I, Somer H, et al. Muscle-eye-brain disease: a neuropathological study. *Ann Neurol* 1997;41:173–180.
292. Osari S, Kobayashi O, Yamashita Y, et al. Basement membrane abnormality in merosin-negative congenital muscular dystrophy. *Acta Neuropathol* 1996;91:332–336.
293. North KN, Specht LA, Sethi RK, et al. Congenital muscular dystrophy associated with merosin deficiency. *J Child Neurol* 1996;11:291–295.
294. Tsao CY, Mendell JR, Rusin J, et al. Congenital muscular dystrophy with complete laminin-alpha2-deficiency, cortical dysplasia, and cerebral white-matter changes in children. *J Child Neurol* 1998;13:253–256.
295. Brett FM, Costigan D, Farrell MA, et al. Merosin-deficient congenital muscular dystrophy and cortical dysplasia. *Eur J Paediatr Neurol* 1998;2:77–82.
296. Di Muzio A, De Angelis MV, Di Fulvio P, et al. Dysmyelinating sensory-motor neuropathy in merosin-deficient congenital muscular dystrophy. *Muscle Nerve* 2003;27:500–506.
297. Voit T, Sewry CA, Meyer K, et al. Preserved merosin M-chain (or laminin-alpha2) expression in skeletal muscle distinguishes Walker-Warburg syndrome from Fukuyama muscular dystrophy and merosin-deficient congenital muscular dystrophy. *Neuropediatrics* 1995;26:148–155.
298. Yoshida A, Kobayashi K, Manya H, et al. Muscular dystrophy and neuronal migration disorder caused by mutations in a glycosyltransferase, *POMGnT1*. *Devel Cell* 2001;1:717–724.
299. Louhichi N, Triki C, Quijano-Roy S, et al. New FKRP mutations causing congenital muscular dystrophy associated with mental retardation and central nervous system abnormalities. Identification of a founder mutation in Tunisian families. *Neurogenetics* 2004;5:27–34.
300. Triki C, Louhichi N, Méziou M, et al. Merosin-deficient congenital muscular dystrophy with mental retardation and cerebellar cysts, unlinked to the LAMA2, FCMD, MEB and CMD1B loci, in three Tunisian patients. *Neuromuscul Disord* 2003;13:4–12.
301. Ullrich O. Kongenitale, atonisch-sklerotische Muskeldystrophie; ein weiterer Typus der heredodegenerativen Erkrankungen des neuromuskulären Systems. *Z Ges Neurol Psychiatrie* 1930;126:171–201.
302. Nonaka I, Une Y, Ishihara T, et al. A clinical and histological study of Ullrich's disease (congenital atonic-sclerotic muscular dystrophy). *Neuropediatrics* 1981;12:197–208.
303. Furukawa T, Toyokura Y. Congenital, hypotonic-sclerotic muscular dystrophy. *J Med Genet* 1977;14:426–429.
304. Mercuri E, Cini C, Pichiecchio A, et al. Muscle magnetic resonance imaging in patients with congenital muscular dystrophy and Ullrich phenotype. *Neuromuscul Disord* 2003;13:554–558.
305. Bertini E, Pepe G. Collagen type VI and related disorders: Bethlem myopathy and Ullrich scleroatonic muscular dystrophy. *Eur J Paediatr Neurol* 2002;6:193–198.
306. Beggs AH, Kunkel LM. Improved diagnosis of Duchenne/Becker muscular dystrophy. *J Clin Invest* 1990;85:613–619.
307. Nanji AA. Serum creatine kinase isoenzymes: a review. *Muscle Nerve* 1983;6:83–90.
308. Darras BT, Harper JF, Francke U. Prenatal diagnosis and detection of carriers with DNA probes in Duchenne's muscular dystrophy. *N Engl J Med* 1987;316:985–992.
309. Cole CG, Walker A, Coyne A, et al. Prenatal testing for Duchenne and Becker muscular dystrophy. *Lancet* 1988;1:262–266.
310. Kuller JA, Hoffman EP, Fries MH, et al. Prenatal diagnosis of Duchenne muscular dystrophy by fetal muscle biopsy. *Hum Genet* 1992;90:34–40.
311. Sancho S, Mongini T, Tanji K, et al. Analysis of dystrophin expression after activation of myogenesis in amniocytes, chorionic-villus cells, and fibroblasts. A new method for diagnosing Duchenne's muscular dystrophy. *N Engl J Med* 1993;329:915–920.
312. Nicholson GA, Gardner-Medwin D, Walton JN. Carrier detection in Duchenne muscular dystrophy: assessment of the effect of age on detection-rate with serum-creatine-kinase activity. *Lancet* 1979;1:692–694.
313. Flanigan KM, Kerr L, Bromberg MR, et al. Congenital muscular dystrophy with rigid spine syndrome: a clinical, pathological, radiological, and genetic study. *Ann Neurol* 2000;47:152–161.
314. Biggar WD, Gingras M, Fehlinger DL, et al. Deflacort treatment of Duchenne muscular dystrophy. *J Pediatr* 2001;138:45–50.
315. Biggar WD, Politano L, Harris VA, et al. Deflazacort in Duchenne muscular dystrophy: a comparison of two different protocols. *Neuromuscul Disord* 2004;14:476–482.
315a. Mah J, Lombardo K. Defalzacort stabilizes the spine in nonambulatory Duchenne muscular dystrophy patients. *Can J Neurol Sci* 2005;32:544 [*abstract*].

316. Griggs RC, Moxley RT 3rd, Mendell JR, et al. Randomized, double-blind trial of mazindol in Duchenne dystrophy. *Muscle Nerve* 1990;13:1169–1173.
317. Munsat TL. Inflammatory myopathy with facioscapulohumeral distribution. *Neurology* 1972;22:335–347.
318. Howell JM. Is there a future for gene therapy? *Neuromuscul Disord* 1999;9:102–107.
319. Fassati A, Murphy S, Dickson G. Gene therapy of Duchenne muscular dystrophy. *Adv Genet* 1997;35:117–153.
320. Qu Z, Balkir L, van Deutekom JC, et al. Development of approaches to improve cell survival in myoblast transfer therapy. *J Cell Biol* 1998;142:1257–1267.
321. Gussoni E, Blau HM, Kunkel LM. The fate of individual myoblasts after transplantation into muscles of DMD patients. *Nat Med* 1997;3:970–977.
322. Sammels LM, Bosio E, Fragall CT, et al. Innate inflammatory cells are not responsible for early death of donor myoblasts after myoblast transfer therapy. *Transplantation* 2004;77:1790–1797.
323. King JO, Denborough MA. Anesthetic-induced malignant hyperpyrexia in children. *J Pediatr* 1973;83:37–40.
324. Kleopa KA, Rosenberg H, Heiman-Patterson T. Malignant hyperthermia-like episode in Becker muscular dystrophy. *Anesthesiology* 2000;93:1535–1537.
325. Moxley RT, Meola G. The myotonic dystrophies. In: Rosenberg RN, Prusiner SB, DiMauro S, et al., eds. *The molecular basis of neurologic and psychiatric disease*, 3rd ed. Philadelphia: Butterworth Heinemann, 2003:511–518.
326. Harper PS, Harley HG, Reardon W, et al. Anticipation in myotonic dystrophy: new light on an old problem. *Am J Hum Genet* 1992;51:10–16.
327. Calderon R. Myotonic dystrophy: a neglected cause for mental retardation. *J Pediatr* 1966;68:423–431.
328. Pruzanski W. Variants of myotonic dystrophy in preadolescent life. *Brain* 1966;89:563–568.
329. Edwards JH. Sign of the Cheshire cat. *Lancet* 1987;2:581.
330. Camilleri M. Disorders of gastrointestinal motility in neurologic diseases. *Mayo Clin Proc* 1990;65:825–846.
331. Sarnat HB, O'Connor T, Byrne PA. Clinical effects of myotonic dystrophy on pregnancy and the neonate. *Arch Neurol* 1976;33: 459–465.
331a. Modoni A, Silvestri G, Pomponi MG, et al. Characterization of the pattern of cognitive impairment in myotonic dystrophy type 1. *Arch Neurol* 2004;61:1943–1947.
331b. Jiang H, Mankodi A, Swanson MS, et al. Myotonic dystrophy type 1 is associated with nuclear foci of mutant RNA, sequestration of muscleblind proteins and deregulated alternative splicing in neurons. *Hum Mol Genet* 2004;14:3079–3088.
332. Dodge PR, Gamstorp I, Byers RK, et al. Myotonic dystrophy in infancy and childhood. *Pediatrics* 1965;35:3–19.
333. Stuart CA, Armstrong RM, Provow SA, et al. Insulin resistance in patients with myotonic dystrophy. *Neurology* 1983;33:679–685.
334. Walsh JC, Turtle JR, Miller S, et al. Abnormalities of insulin secretion in dystrophia myotonica. *Brain* 1970;93:731–742.
335. Wochner RD, Drews G, Strober W, et al. Accelerated breakdown of immunoglobulin G (IgG) in myotonic dystrophy: a hereditary error of immunoglobulin catabolism. *J Clin Invest* 1966;45:321–329.
336. Bundey S. Clinical evidence for heterogeneity in myotonic dystrophy. *J Med Genet* 1982;19:341–348.
337. Lavedan C, Hofmann-Radvanyi H, Shelbourne P, et al. Myotonic dystrophy: size- and sex-dependent dynamics of CTG meiotic instability, and somatic mosaicism. *Am J Hum Genet* 1993;52:875–883.
338. Mulley JC, Staples A, Donnelly A, et al. Explanation for exclusive maternal origin for congenital form of myotonic dystrophy. *Lancet* 1993;341:236–237.
339. Hofmann-Radvanyi H, Lavedan C, Rabes JP, et al. Myotonic dystrophy: absence of CTG enlarged transcript in congenital forms, and low expression of the normal allele. *Hum Mol Genet* 1993;2:1263–1266.
340. Kornblum C, Reul J, Kress W, et al. Cranial magnetic resonance imaging in genetically proven myotonic dystrophy type 1 and 2. *J Neurol* 2004;251:710–714.
341. Moorman JR, Coleman RE, Packer DL, et al. Cardiac involvement in myotonic muscular dystrophy. *Medicine* 1985;64:371–378.
342. Day JW, Richater K, Jacobsen JF, et al. Myotonic dystrophy type 2: molecular, diagnostic and clinical spectrum. *Neurology* 2003;60:657–664.
343. Vihola A, Bassez G, Meola G, et al. Histopathological differences of myotonic dystrophy type 1 (DM1) and PROMM/DM2. *Neurology* 2003;60:1854–1857.
344. Le Ber I, Martinez M, Campion D, et al. A non-DM1, non-DM2 multisystem myotonic disorder with frontotemporal dementia: phenotype and suggestive mapping of the DM3 locus to chromosome 15q21-24. *Brain* 2004;127:1979–1992.
345. Dubowitz V. *The floppy infant*. London: William Heinemann Medical Books, 1980.
346. Koh TH. Do you shake hands with mothers of floppy babies? *BMJ* 1984;289:485.
347. Martinello F, Piazza A, Pastorello E, et al. Clinical and neuroimaging study of central nervous system in congenital myotonic dystrophy. *J Neurol* 1999;246:186–192.
348. Shelbourne P, Davies J, Buxton J, et al. Direct diagnosis of myotonic dystrophy with a disease-specific DNA marker. *N Engl J Med* 1993;328:471–475.
349. Schotland DL. An electron microscopic investigation of myotonic dystrophy. *J Neuropathol Exp Neurol* 1970;29:241–253.
350. Grant R, Sutton DL, Behan PO, et al. Nifedipine in the treatment of myotonia in myotonic dystrophy. *J Neurol Neurosurg Psychiatry* 1987;50:199–206.
351. Hughes EF, Wilson J. Response to treatment with antihistamines in a family with myotonia congenita. *Lancet* 1991;337:25–27.
352. Sarnat HB, Silbert SW. Maturational arrest of fetal muscle in neonatal myotonic dystrophy. *Arch Neurol* 1976;33:466–474.
353. Sarnat HB. Vimentin and desmin in maturing skeletal muscle and developmental myopathies. *Neurology* 1992;42:1616–1624.
354. Aslanidis C, Jansen G, Amemiya C, et al. Cloning of the essential myotonic dystrophy region and mapping of the putative defect. *Nature* 1992;355:548–551.
355. Brook JD, McCurrach ME, Harley HG, et al. Molecular basis of myotonic dystrophy: expansion of a trinucleotide (CTG) repeat at the 3′ end of a transcript encoding a protein kinase family member. *Cell* 1992;68:799–808.
356. Thornton CA, Griggs RC, Moxley RT. Myotonic dystrophy without trinucleotide repeat expansion. *Ann Neurol* 1994;35:269–272.
357. Brunner HG, Jansen G, Nillesen W, et al. Brief report: reverse mutation in myotonic dystrophy. *N Engl J Med* 1993;328:476–480.
358. Taneja KL, McCurrach M, Schalling M, et al. Foci of trinucleotide repeat transcripts in nuclei of myotonic dystrophy cells and tissues. *J Cell Biol* 1995;128:995–1002.
359. Jiang H, Mankodi A, Swandson MS, et al. Myotonic dystrophy type 1 is associated with nuclear foci of mutant RNA, sequestration of muscleblind proteins and deregulated alternative splicing in neurons. *Hum Mol Genet* 2004;13:3079–3088.
360. Ho TH, Charlet-B N, Poulos MG, et al. Muscleblind proteins regulate alternative splicing. *EMBO J* 2004;23:3103–3112.
361. Ebralidze A, Wang Y, Petkova V, et al. RNA leaching of transcription factors disrupts transcription in myotonic dystrophy. *Science* 2004;303:383–387.
362. Mankodi A, Takahashi MP, Jiang H, et al. Expanded CUG repeats trigger aberrant splicing of CIC-1 chloride channel pre-mRNA and hyperexcitability of skeletal muscle in myotonic dystrophy. *Mol Cell* 2002;10:35–44.
363. Ranum LPW, Day JW. Myotonic dystrophy: RNA pathogenesis comes into focus. *Am J Hum Genet* 2004;74:793–804.
364. Carey N, Johnson K, Nokelainen P, et al. Meiotic drive at the myotonic dystrophy locus? *Nat Genet* 1994;6:117–118.
365. Ackerman MJ, Clapham DJ. Ion channels—basic science and clinical disease. *N Engl J Med* 1997;336:1575–1586.
366. Lehmann-Horn F, Mailander V, Heine R, et al. Myotonia levior is a chloride channel disorder. *Hum Mol Genet* 1995;4:1397–1402.
367. Koch MC, Steinmeyer K, Lorenz C, et al. The skeletal muscle chloride channel in dominant and recessive human myotonia. *Science* 1992;257:797–800.
368. Grunnet M, Jespersen T, Colding-Jorgensen E, et al. Characterization of two new dominant CIC-1 channel mutations associated with myotonia. *Muscle Nerve* 2001;28:722–732.
369. Rosenfeld J, Sloan-Brown K, George AL. A novel muscle sodium

channel mutation causes painful congenital myotonia. *Ann Neurol* 1997;42:811–814.
370. Ptacek LJ, Johnson KJ, Griggs RC. Genetics and physiology of the myotonic muscle disorders. *N Engl J Med* 1993;328:482–489.
371. Wang J, Zhou J, Todorovic SM, et al. Molecular genetic and genetic correlations in sodium channelopathies: lack of founder effect and evidence for a second gene. *Am J Hum Genet* 1993;52:1074–1084.
372. Kleopa KA, Barchi RL. Ion channel disorders. In: Rosenberg RN, Prusiner SB, DiMauro S, et al., eds. *The molecular basis of neurologic and psychiatric disease*. 3rd ed. Philadelphia: Butterworth Heinemann, 2003:527–544.
373. Cannon SC, Brown RH, Corey DP. A sodium channel defect in hyperkalemic periodic paralysis: potassium-induced failure of inactivation. *Neuron* 1991;6:619–626.
374. Thomsen J. Tonische Krämpfe in willkürlich beweglichen Muskeln in Folge von ererbter psychischer Disposition: Ataxia muscularis? *Arch Psychiat Nervenkr* 1876;6:702–718.
375. Papponen H, Toppinen T, Baumann P, et al. Founder mutations and the high prevalence of myotonia congenita in northern Finland. *Neurology* 1999;53:297–302.
376. Becker PE. Neues zur Genetik und Klassifikation der Muskeldystrophien. *Humangenetik* 1972;17:1–22.
377. Moxley RT III. Myotonic disorders in childhood: diagnosis and treatment. *J Child Neurol* 1997;12:116–129.
378. Johnson T, Friis ML. Paramyotonia congenita (von Eulenberg) in Denmark. *Acta Neurol Scand* 1980;61:78–87.
379. Lundberg PO, Stalberg E, Thule B. Paralysis periodica paramyotonica: a clinical and neurophysiological study. *J Neurol Sci* 1974;21:309–321.
380. Auger RG, Daube JR, Gomez MR, et al. Hereditary form of sustained muscle activity of peripheral nerve origin causing generalized myokymia and muscle stiffness. *Ann Neurol* 1984;15:13–21.
381. Stephan DA, Buist NR, Chittenden AB, et al. A rippling muscle disease gene is localized to 1 q41: evidence for multiple genes. *Neurology* 1994;44:1915–1920.
382. Sotgia F, Woodman SE, Bonuccelli G, et al. Phenotypic behavior of caveolin-3 R26Q, a mutant associated with hyperCKemia, distal myopathy and rippling muscle disease. *Am J Physiol–Cell Physiol* 2003;285:C1150–C1160.
383. Gamstorp I. Adynamia episodica hereditaria. *Acta Paediatr Scand* 1956;[Suppl]108:11–26.
384. Hoskins B, Vroom FQ, Jarrell MA. Hyperkalemic periodic paralysis. Effects of potassium, exercise, glucose and acetazolamide on blood chemistry. *Arch Neurol* 1975;32:519–523.
385. Bradley WG, Taylor R, Rice DR, et al. Progressive myopathy in hyperkalemic periodic paralysis. *Arch Neurol* 1990;47:1013–1017.
386. Gamstorp I. Adynamia episodica hereditaria, and myotonia. *Acta Neurol Scand* 1963;39:41–58.
387. Ricker K, Rohkamm R, Bohlen R. Adynamia episodica and paralysis periodica paramyotonia. *Neurology* 1986;36:682–686.
388. Layzer RB, Lovelace RE, Rowland LP. Hyperkalemic periodic paralysis. *Arch Neurol* 1967;16:455–472.
389. McArdle B. Adynamia episodica hereditaria and its treatment. *Brain* 1962;85:121–148.
390. Tricarico D, Barbieri M, Camarino DC. Acetazolamide opens the muscular $KCa2^{+}$ channel: a novel mechanism of action that may explain the therapeutic effect of the drug in hypokalemic periodic paralysis. *Ann Neurol* 2000;48:304–312.
391. Tawil R, McDermott MP, Brown R, et al. Randomized trials of dichlorphenamide in the periodic paralyses. Work Group on Periodic Paralysis. *Ann Neurol* 2000;47:46–53.
392. Wang P, Clausen T. Treatment of attacks in hyperkalemic familial periodic paralysis by inhalation of salbutamol. *Lancet* 1976;1:221–223.
393. Meola G, Sansone V. Therapy in myotonic disorders and in muscle channelopathies. *Neurol Sci* 2000;21[5 Suppl]:S953–S961.
394. Shakhnovitch. On a case of intermittent paraplegia [Abstract]. *London Med Rec* 1884;12:130.
395. Westphal C. Über einen merkwürdigen Fall von periodischer Lähmung aller vier Extremitäten, mit gleichzeitigen Erlöschen der electrischen Erregbarkeit während der Lähmung. *Berl Klin Wochenschr* 1885;31:489–511.
396. Greenberg DA. Calcium channels in neurological disease. *Ann Neurol* 1997;42:275–282.
397. Sugiura Y, Makita N, Li L, et al. Cold induces shifts of voltage dependence in mutant SCN4A causing hypokalemic periodic paralysis. *Neurology* 2003;61:914–918.
398. Layzer RB. Periodic paralysis and the sodium-potassium pump. *Ann Neurol* 1982;11:547–552.
399. Ionasescu V, Schochet SS Jr, Powers JM, et al. Hypokalemic periodic paralysis. Low activity of sarcoplasmic reticulum and muscle ribosomes during an induced attack. *J Neurol Sci* 1974;21:419–429.
400. Kantola IM, Tarssanen LT. Familial hypokalaemic periodic paralysis in Finland. *J Neurol Neurosurg Psychiatry* 1992;55:322–324.
401. Dyken M, Zeman W, Rusche T. Hypokalemic periodic paralysis: children with permanent myopathic weakness. *Neurology* 1969;19:691–699.
402. Links TP, Zwarts MJ, Wilmink JT, et al. Permanent muscle weakness in familial hypokalaemic periodic paralysis. Clinical, radiological and pathological aspects. *Brain* 1990;113:1873–1889.
403. Poskanzer DC, Kerr DNS. A third type of periodic paralysis, with normokalemia and favourable response to sodium chloride. *Am J Med* 1961;31:328–342.
404. Chinnery PF, Walls TJ, Hanna MG, et al. Normokalemic periodic paralysis revisited: does it exist? *Ann Neurol* 2002;52:251–252.
405. Kelly DE, Gharib H, Kennedy FP, et al. Thyrotoxic periodic paralysis. Report of 10 cases and review of electromyographic findings. *Arch Intern Med* 1989;149:2597–2600.
406. Conn JW, Rovner DR, Cohen EL. Licorice-induced pseudoaldosteronism. Hypertension, hypokalemia, aldosteronopenia, and suppressed plasma renin activity. *JAMA* 1968;205:492–496.
407. Johnson CH, VanTassell VJ. Acute barium poisoning with respiratory failure and rhabdomyolysis. *Ann Emerg Med* 1991;20:1138–1142.
408. Stedwell RE, Allen KM, Binder LS. Hypokalemic paralyses: a review of the etiologies, pathophysiology, presentation, and therapy. *Am J Emerg Med* 1992;10:143–148.
409. Carraccio C, Blotny K, Ringer R. Sudden onset of profound weakness in a toddler. *J Pediatr* 1993;122:663–667.
410. Mateer JE, Farrell BJ, Chou SS, et al. Reversible ipecac myopathy. *Arch Neurol* 1985;42:188–190.
411. Sansone V, Griggs RC, Meola G, et al. Anderson's syndrome: a distinct periodic paralysis. *Ann Neurol* 1997;42:305–312.
412. Huttenlocher PR, Landwirth J, Hanson V, et al. Osteo-chondro-muscular dystrophy. *Pediatrics* 1969;44:945–958.
413. Arikawa-Hirasawa E, Le AH, Nishino I, et al. Structural and functional mutations of the perlecan gene cause Schwartz-Jampel syndrome, with myotonic myopathy and chondrodysplasia. *Am J Hum Genet* 2002;70:368–375.
414. Giedion A, Boltshauser E, Briner J, et al. Heterogeneity in Schwartz-Jampel chondrodystrophic myotonia. *Eur J Pediatr* 1997;156:214–223.
415. Schwartz O, Jampel RS. Congenital blepharophimosis associated with a unique generalized myopathy. *Arch Ophthalmol* 1962;68:52–57.
416. Aberfeld DC, Hinterbuchner LP, Schneider M. Myotonia, dwarfism, diffuse bone disease and unusual ocular and facial abnormalities (a new syndrome). *Brain* 1965;88:313–322.
417. Ferrannini E, Perniola T, Krajewska G, et al. Schwartz-Jampel syndrome with autosomal-dominant inheritance. *Europ Neurol* 1982;21:137–146.
418. Hansen PA, Martinez LB, Cassidy R. Contractures, continuous muscle discharges, and titubation. *Ann Neurol* 1977;1:120–124.
419. Isaacs H. Continuous muscle fibre activity in an Indian male with additional evidence of terminal motor fibre abnormality. *J Neurol Neurosurg Psychiatry* 1967;30:126–133.
420. Eunson LH, Rea R, Zuberi SM, et al. Clinical, genetic, and expression studies of mutations in the potassium channel gene KCNA1 reveal new phenotype variability. *Ann Neurol* 2000;48:647–656.
421. Arimura K, Sonoda Y, Watanabe O, et al. Isaacs' syndrome as a potassium channelopathy of the nerve. *Muscle Nerve* 2002;[Suppl 11]:S55–S58.
422. Benatar M. Neurological potassium channelopathies. *QJM* 2000;93:787–797.

423. Lutschg I, Jerusalem F, Ludin HP, et al. The syndrome of "continuous muscle fiber activity." *Arch Neurol* 1978;35:198–205.
424. Ashizawa T, Butler IJ, Harati Y, et al. A dominantly inherited syndrome with continuous motor neuron discharges. *Ann Neurol* 1983;13:285–290.
425. Daras M, Spiro AJ. "Stiff-man syndrome" in an adolescent. *Pediatrics* 1981;67:725–726.
426. Layzer RB. Stiff-man syndrome—an autoimmune disease? *N Engl J Med* 1988;318:1060–1062.
427. Solimena M, Folli F, Aparisi R, et al. Autoantibodies to GABA-ergic neurons and pancreatic β cells in stiff-man syndrome. *N Engl J Med* 1990;322:1555–1560.
428. Khasani S, Becker K, Meinck HM. Hyperekplexia and stiff-man syndrome: abnormal brainstem reflexes suggest a physiological relationship. *Neurol Neurosurg Psychiatry* 2004;73:1265–1269.
429. Rakocevic G, Raju R, Dalakas MC. Anti-glutamic acid decarboxylase antibodies in the serum and cerebrospinal fluid of patients with stiff-person syndrome: correlation with clinical severity. *Arch Neurol* 2004;61:902–904.
430. Robinson RL, Anetseder MJ, Brancadoro V, et al. Recent advances in the diagnosis of malignant hyperthermia susceptibility: how confident can we be of genetic testing? *Eur J Hum Genet* 2003;11:342–348.
431. Nelson TE, Flewellen EH. The malignant hyperthermia syndrome. *N Engl J Med* 1983;309:416–418.
432. Dalakas MC, Hohlfeld R. Polymyositis and dermatomyositis *Lancet* 2003;362:971–982.
433. Banker BQ. Dermatomyositis of childhood. *J Neuropathol Exp Neurol* 1975;34:46–75.
434. Riggs JE, Schochet SS Jr, Gutmann L, et al. Childhood onset inclusion body myositis mimicking limb-girdle muscular dystrophy. *J Child Neurol* 1989;4:283–285.
435. Amato AA, Griggs RC. Unicorns, dragons, polymyositis, and other mythological beasts. *Neurology* 2003;61:288–290.
436. Carpenter S, Karpati G, Rothman S, et al. The childhood type of dermatomyositis. *Neurology* 1976;26:952–962.
437. Kissel JT, Halterman RK, Rammohan KW, et al. The relationship of complement-mediated microvasculopathy to the histologic features and clinical duration of disease in dermatomyositis. *Arch Neurol* 1991;48:26–30.
438. Lundberg IE, Nyberg P. New developments in the role of cytokines and chemokines in inflammatory myopathies. *Curr Opin Rheumatol* 1998;10:521–529.
439. Reed AM, Ytterberg SR. Genetic and environmental risk factors for idiopathic inflammatory myopathies. *Rheum Dis Clin North Am* 2002;28:891–916.
440. Reed AM, Picornell YJ, Harwood A, Kredich DW. Chimerism in children with juvenile dermatomyositis. *Lancet* 2000;356:2156–2157.
441. Reed AM, McNallan K, Wettstein P, et al. Does HLA-dependent chimerism underlie the pathogenesis of juvenile dermatomyositis? *J Immunol* 2004;172:5041–5046.
442. Wedgewood RJ, Cook C, Cohen J. Dermatomyositis: report of 26 cases in children with a discussion of endocrine therapy in 13. *Pediatrics* 1953;12:447–466.
443. Malleson P. Juvenile dermatomyositis: a review. *J Roy Soc Med* 1982;75:33–37.
444. Spencer CH, Hanson V, Singsen BH, et al. Course of treated juvenile dermatomyositis. *J Pediatr* 1984;105:399–408.
445. Bohan A, Peter JB, Bowman RL, Pearson CM. A computer-assisted analysis of 153 patients with polymyositis and dermatomyositis. *Medicine* 1977;56:255–286.
446. Hernandez RJ, Sullivan DB, Chenevert TL, et al. MR findings in children with dermatomyositis: musculoskeletal findings and correlation with clinical and laboratory findings. *Am J Roentgenol* 1993;161:359–366.
447. Thompson CE. Infantile myositis. *Dev Med Child Neurol* 1982;24:307–313.
448. McNeil SM, Woulfe J, Ross C, et al. Congenital inflammatory myopathy: a demonstrative case and proposed diagnostic classification. *Muscle Nerve* 2002;25:259–264.
449. Di Muzio A, Capasso M, Verrotti A, et al. Macrophagic myofasciitis: an infantile Italian case. *Neuromuscul Disord* 2004;14:175–177.
450. Miller G, Heckmatt JZ, Dubowitz V. Drug treatment of juvenile dermatomyositis. *Arch Dis Child* 1983;58:445–450.
451. Jacobs JC. Methotrexate and azathioprine treatment of childhood dermatomyositis. *Pediatrics* 1977;59:212–218.
452. Wallace DJ, Metzger AL, White KK. Combination immunosuppressive treatment of steroid-resistant dermatomyositis/polymyositis. *Arthritis Rheum* 1985;28:590–592.
453. Heckmatt J, Hasson N, Saunders C, et al. Cyclosporin in juvenile dermatomyositis. *Lancet* 1989;1:1063–1066.
454. Sussman GL, Pruzanski W. Treatment of inflammatory myopathy with intravenous gamma globulin. *Curr Opin Rheumatol* 1995;7:510–515.
455. Bohan A, Peter JB. Polymyositis and dermatomyositis. *N Engl J Med* 1975;292:344–347,403–407.
456. Lundberg A. Myalgia cruris epidemica. *Acta Paediatr Scand* 1957;46:18–31.
457. Belardi C, Roberge R, Kelly M, et al. Myalgia cruris epidemica (benign acute childhood myositis) associated with Mycoplasma pneumonia infection. *Ann Emerg Med* 1987;16:579–581.
458. Ruff RL, Secrist D. Viral studies in benign acute childhood myositis. *Arch Neurol* 1982;39:261–263.
459. Bannwarth B. Drug-induced myopathies. *Expert Opin Drug Saf* 2002;1:65–70.
460. Sterrenburg E, Turk R, Hoen PAC, et al. Large-scale gene expression analysis of human skeletal myoblast differentiation. *Neuromuscul Disord* 2004;14:507–518.
461. Sarnat HB. *Congenital muscle fiber-type disproportion*. Neurobase (computer textbook), 1999.
462. Laing NC, Clarke NF, Dye DE, et al. Actin mutations are one cause of congenital fibre type disproportion. *Ann Neurol* 2004;56: 589–594.
463. Clarke NF, North KN. Congenital fiber type disproportion—30 years on. *J Neuropathol Exp Neurol* 2003;62:977–989.
464. Marjanovic B, Cvetkovic D, Dozic S, et al. Association of Krabbe leukodystrophy and congenital muscle fiber type disproportion. *Pediatr Neurol* 1996;15:79–82.
465. Sarnat HB. Le cerveau influence-t-il le développement musculaire du foetus humain? Mise en évidence de 21 cas. *Can J Neurol Sci* 1985;12:111–120.
466. Conen PE, Murphy EG, Donohue WL. Light and electron microscopic studies of "myogranules" in a child with hypotonia and muscle weakness. *Can Med Assoc J* 1963;9:618–625.
467. Jungbluth H, Sewry CA, Muntoni F. What's new in neuromuscular disorders? The congenital myopathies. *Eur J Paediatr Neurol* 2003;7:23–30.
468. Laing NG, Wilton SD, Akkari PA, et al. A mutation in the alpha tropomyosin gene TPM3 associated with autosomal dominant nemaline myopathy NEM1. *Nat Genet* 1995;9:75–79.
469. Wallgren-Pettersson C, Avela K, Marchand S, et al. A gene for autosomal recessive nemaline myopathy assigned to chromosome 2q by linkage analysis. *Neuromuscul Disord* 1995;5: 441–443.
470. Nowak KJ, Wattanasirichaigoon D, Goebel HH, et al. Mutations in the skeletal muscle alpha-actin gene in patients with actin myopathy and nemaline myopathy. *Nat Genet* 1999;23:208–212.
471. Donner K, Ollikainen M, Ridanpaa M, et al. Mutations in the beta-tropomyosin (TPM2) gene: a rare cause of nemaline myopathy. *Neuromuscul Disord* 2002;12:151–158.
472. Wattanasirichaigoon D, Swoboda KJ, Takada F, et al. Mutations of the slow muscle α-tropomyosin gene, TPM3, are a rare cause of nemaline myopathy. *Neurology* 2002;59:613–617.
473. Johnston JJ, Kelley RI, Crawford TO, et al. A novel nemaline myopathy in the Amish caused by a mutation in troponin T1. *Am J Hum Genet* 2000;67:814–821.
474. Wallgren-Pettersson C, Pelin K, Nowak KJ, et al. Genotype-phenotype correlations in nemaline myopathy caused by mutations in the genes for nebulin and skeletal muscle α-actin. *Neuromuscul Disord* 2004;14:461–470.
475. Wallgren-Pettersson C, Laing NG. Report of the 70th ENMC International Workshop: nemaline myopathy. *Neuromuscul Disord* 2000;10:299–306.
476. Rifai Z, Kazee AM, Kamp C, et al. Intranuclear rods in severe congenital nemaline myopathy. *Neurology* 1993;43:2372–2377.

477. Goebel HH, Warlo I. Nemaline myopathy with intranuclear rods: intranuclear rod myopathy. *J Child Neurol* 1997;7:13–19.
478. Jennekens FGI, Roord JJ, Veldman H, et al. Congenital nemaline myopathy. I. Defective organization of alpha-actinin is restricted to muscle. *Muscle Nerve* 1983;6:61–68.
479. Stuhlfauth I, Jennekens FG, Willemse J, et al. Congenital nemaline myopathy: II. Quantitative changes in alpha-actinin and myosin in skeletal muscle. *Muscle Nerve* 1983;6:69–74.
480. Pelin K, Hilpela P, Donner K, et al. Mutations in the nebulin gene associated with autosomal recessive nemaline myopathy. *Proc Natl Acad Sci USA* 1999;96:2305–2310.
481. Wallgren-Pettersson C, Rapola J, Donner M. Pathology of congenital nemaline myopathy. A follow-up study. *J Neurol Sci* 1988;83:243–257.
482. Feinberg DM, Spiro AJ, Weidenheim KM. Distinct light microscopic changes in human immunodeficiency virus–associated nemaline myopathy. *Neurology* 1998;50:529–531.
483. Zhang Y, Chen HS, Khanna VK, et al. A mutation in the human ryanodine receptor gene associated with central core disease. *Nat Genet* 1993;5:46–50.
484. Berridge MJ. Inositol trisphosphate and calcium signalling. *Nature* 1993;361:315–325.
485. Quane KA, Healy JM, Keating KE, et al. Mutations in the ryanodine receptor gene in central core disease and malignant hyperthermia. *Nat Genet* 1993;5:51–55.
486. Shy GM, Magee KR. A new congenital non-progressive myopathy. *Brain* 1956;79:610–621.
487. Schröder R, Reimann J, Salmikangas P, et al. Beyond LGMD1A: myotilin is a component of central core lesions and nemaline rods. *Neuromuscul Disord* 2003;13:451–455.
487a. Messina S, Hartley L, Main M, et al. Pilot trial of salbutamol in central core and multicore diseases. *Neuropediatrics* 2004;35: 262–266.
488. Panegyres PK, Kakulas BA. The natural history of minicore-multicore myopathy. *Muscle Nerve* 1991;14:411–415.
488a. Tajsharghi H, Darin N, Tulinius M, et al. Early onset myopathy with a novel mutation in the selenoprotein N gene (*SEPN1*). *Neuromuscul Disord* 2005;15:299–302.
489. Jungbluth H, Sewry C, Brown SC, et al. Minicore myopathy in children—a clinical and histopathological study of 19 cases. *Neuromuscul Disord* 2000;10:264–273.
490. Ferreiro A, Estournet B, Chateau D, et al. Multi-minicore disease—searching for boundaries: phenotype analysis of 38 cases. *Ann Neurol* 2000;48:745–748.
491. Swash M, Schwartz MS. Familial multicore disease with focal loss of cross-striations and ophthalmoplegia. *J Neurol Sci* 1981;52: 1–10.
491a. Jungbluth H, Davis MR, Müller C, et al. Magnetic resonance imaging of muscle in congenital myopathies associated with *RYR1* mutations. *Neuromuscul Disord* 2004;14:785–790.
492. Sarnat HB. Myotubular myopathy: arrest of morphogenesis of myofibres associated with persistence of fetal vimentin and desmin. Four cases compared with fetal and neonatal muscle. *Can J Neurol Sci* 1990;17:109–123.
493. Laporte J, Kress W, Mandel JL. Diagnosis of X-linked myotubular myopathy by detection of myotubularin. *Ann Neurol* 2001;50: 42–46.
493a. Tsai T-C, Horinouchi H, Noguchi S, et al. Characterization of MTMI mutations in 31 japanese families with myotubular myopathy, including a patient carrying a 240 kb deletion in Xq28 without male hypogenitalism. *Neuromuscul Disord* 2005;15:245–252.
494. Tsujita K, Itoh T, Ijuin T, et al. Myotubularin regulates the function of the late endosome through the gram domain-phosphatidylinositol 3,5-bisphosphate interaction. *J Biol Chem* 2004;279:13817–13824.
495. Campbell MJ, Rebeiz JJ, Walton JN. Myotubular, centronuclear or peri-centronuclear myopathy? *J Neurol Sci* 1969;8:425–443.
496. Barth PG, van Wijngaarden GK, Bethlen J. X-linked myotubular myopathy with fatal neonatal asphyxia. *Neurology* 1975;25: 531–536.
497. Kristiansen M, Knudsen GP, Tanner SM, et al. X-inactivation patterns in carriers of X-linked myotubular myopathy. *Neuromuscul Disord* 2003;13:468–471.
498. Selcen D, Ohno K, Engel AG. Myofibrillar myopathy: clinical, morphological and genetic studies in 63 patients. *Brain* 2004;127:439–451.
499. Goldfarb LG, Vicart P, Gobel HH, et al. Desmin myopathy. *Brain* 2004;127:723–734.
500. Omary MB, Coulombe PA, McLean WHI. Intermediate filament proteins and their associated diseases. *N Engl J Med* 2004;351:2087–2100.
501. Olive M, Goldfarb L, Moreno D. Desmine-related myopathy: clinical, electrophysiological, radiological, neuopathological and genetic studies. *J Neurol Sci* 2004;219:125–137.
502. Li M, Dalakas MC. Abnormal desmin protein in myofibrillar myopathies caused by desmin gene mutations. *Ann Neurol* 2001;49:532–536.
503. Selcen D, Engel AG. Myofibrillar myopathy caused by novel dominant negative alpha B-crystallin mutations. *Ann Neurol* 2003; 54:804–810.
504. Selcen D, Engel AG. Mutations in myotilin cause myofibrillar myopathy. *Neurology* 2004;62:1363–1371.
505. Reimann J, Kunz WS, Vielhaber S, et al. Mitochondrial dysfunction in myofibrillar myopathies. *Neuropathol Appl Neurobiol* 2003;29:45–51.
506. Amato AA, Kagan-Hallet K, Jackson CE, et al. The wide spectrum of myofibrillar myopathy suggests a multifactorial etiology and pathogenesis. *Neurology* 1998;51:1646–1655.
507. Melberg A, Oldfors A, Blomström-Lundqvist C. Autosomal dominant myofibrillar myopathy with arrhythmogenic right ventricular cardiomyopathy linked to chromosome 10q. *Ann Neurol* 1999; 46:684–692.
508. Dodge PR. Congenital neuromuscular disorders. *Res Publ Assoc Res Nerv Ment Dis* 1958;38:479–533.
509. Iannaccone ST. Myogenes and myotubes. *J Child Neurol* 1992;7: 180–187.
509a. Relaix F, Rocancourt D, Mansouri A, et al. A Pax3/Pax7-dependent population of skeletal muscle progenitor cells. *Nature* 2005;435:948–953.
509b. Gros J, Manceau M, Thomé V, et al. A common somitic origin for embryonic muscle progenitors and satellite cells. *Nature* 2005;435:954–958.
510. Wilson J, Walton JN. Some muscular manifestations of hypothyroidism. *J Neurol Neurosurg Psychiatry* 1959;22:320–324.
511. Debré R, Sémélaigne G. Syndrome of diffuse muscular hypertrophy in infants causing athletic appearance. *Am J Dis Child* 1935;50:1351–1361.
512. McArdle B. Myopathy due to a defect in muscle glycogen breakdown. *Clin Sci* 1951;10:13–33.
513. Rowland LP, Lovelace RE, Schotland DL, et al. The clinical diagnosis of McArdle's disease. Identification of another family with deficiency of muscle phosphorylase. *Neurology* 1966;16:93–100.
514. Lebo RV, Gorin F, Fletterick RJ, et al. High-resolution chromosome sorting and DNA spot-blot analysis assign McArdle's syndrome to chromosome 11. *Science* 1984;225:57–59.
515. Tsujino S, Shanske S, Nonaka I, et al. Three new mutations in patients with myophosphorylase deficiency (McArdle disease). *Am J Hum Genet* 1994;54:44–52.
516. DiMauro S, Hartlage PL. Fatal myopathic form of muscle phosphorylase deficiency. *Neurology* 1978;28:1124–1129.
517. Ohtani Y, Matsuda I, Iwamasa T, et al. Infantile glycogen storage myopathy in a girl with phosphorylase kinase deficiency. *Neurology* 1982;32:833–838.
518. van der Berg IET, Berger R. Phosphorylase b kinase deficiency in man: a review. *J Inherit Metab Dis* 1990;13:442–451.
519. Argov Z, Bank WJ. Phosphorus magnetic resonance spectroscopy (^{31}P MRS) in neuromuscular disorders. *Ann Neurol* 1991;30: 90–97.
520. DiMauro S, Servidei S, Tsujino S. Glycogen storage diseases. In: Rosenberg RN, Prusiner SB, DiMauro S, et al., eds. *The molecular and genetic basis of neurological and psychiatric disease*, 3rd ed. Philadelphia: Butterworth–Heinemann, 2003:583–589.
521. Layzer RB, Rowland LP, Ranney HM. Muscle phosphofructokinase deficiency. *Arch Neurol* 1967;17:512–523.
522. Ristow M, Vorgerd M, Mohlig M, et al. Deficiency of phosphofructo–1-kinase/muscle subtype in humans impairs

insulin secretion and causes insulin resistance. *J Clin Invest* 1997; 100:2833–2841.
523. Servidei S, Bonilla E, Diedrich RG, et al. Fatal infantile form of muscle phosphofructokinase deficiency. *Neurology* 1986;36:1465–1470.
524. DiMauro S, Miranda AF, Olarte M, et al. Muscle phosphoglycerate mutase deficiency. *Neurology* 1982;32:584–591.
525. Vissing J, Schmalbruch H, Haller RG, et al. Muscle phosphoglycerate mutase deficiency with tubular aggregates: treatment with dantrolene. *Ann Neurol* 1999;46:274–277.
526. Kreuder J, Borkhardt A, Repp R, et al. Brief report: inherited metabolic myopathy and hemolysis due to a mutation in aldolase A. *N Engl J Med* 1996;334:1100–1104.
527. Verzijl HT, van Engelen BG, Luyten JA, et al. Genetic characteristics of myoadenylate deaminase deficiency. *Ann Neurol* 1998;44:140–143.
528. Tonin P, Lewis P, Servidei S, et al. Metabolic causes of myoglobinuria. *Ann Neurol* 1990;27:181–185.
529. Herman J, Nadler HL. Recurrent myoglobinuria and muscle carnitine palmitoyl transferase deficiency. *J Pediatr* 1977;91:247–250.
530. Tein I, DiMauro S, DeVivo DC. Recurrent childhood myoglobinuria. *Adv Pediatr* 1990;37:77–156.
531. Warren JD, Blumbergs PC, Thompson PD. Rhabdomyolysis: a review. *Muscle Nerve* 2002;25:332–337.
532. Martin-Du Pan RC, Morris MA, Favre H, et al. Mitochondrial anomalies in a Swiss family with autosomal dominant myoglobinuria. *Am J Med Genet* 1997;69:365–369.
533. Andreu AL, Bruno C, Dunne TC, et al. A nonsense mutation (G15059A) in the cytochrome b gene in a patient with exercise intolerance and myoglobinuria. *Ann Neurol* 1999;45:127–130.
534. Coco TJ, Klasner AE. Drug-induced rhabdomyolysis. *Curr Opin Pediatr* 2004;16:206–210.
535. Knochel JP. Rhabdomyolysis and myoglobinuria. *Annu Rev Med* 1982;33:435–443.
536. Mills KR, Edwards RHT. Investigative strategies for muscle pain. *J Neurol Sci* 1983;58:73–78.

Chapter 17

Neurologic Manifestations of Systemic Illness

S. Robert Snodgrass

METABOLIC ENCEPHALOPATHIES

Extracerebral diseases and disturbances may interfere with neurologic function by impairing oxygen and glucose supply or by disturbing the ionic and humoral environment of neurons, glia, and synaptic processes. Neurons and supporting cells require specific chemical environments. Their ability to adapt to such mild deviations from the normal environment as life at high altitudes, elevated body temperature, or decreased serum sodium could hold the key to more effective future treatment for anoxic and metabolic encephalopathies.

Oxygen: Hypoxia and Hyperoxia

Pathophysiology

Hypoxia-ischemia, hypoglycemia, and status epilepticus induce energy failure with consequent brain damage (1–3). The significant differences in the time course and distribution of brain damage that result from these three insults are depicted in Table 17.1 and are reviewed by Auer and Sutherland (4). Brain consumes disproportionate amounts of oxygen, has scant glycogen stores, and tolerates hypoxia and hypoglycemia less well than most organs (5). Neurons need constant oxygen and glucose supply to maintain ion and neurotransmitter gradients.

Oxygen pressure is not uniform throughout the brain. It is higher in gray matter than in white matter, as is blood flow and glucose utilization. Brain glucose and oxygen consumption per gram of tissue are higher in neonatal than adult brain (4). The first effect of experimental cerebral hypoxia is an increase of intracellular pH. Subsequently, intracellular calcium content rises as consequence of calcium release from the endoplasmic reticulum. ATP concentration begins to fall, and when 50% to 70% of neuronal ATP is lost, the sodium pump fails and voltage-controlled ion channels open, permitting Na^+, K^+, Ca^{++} and Cl^- to flow down their concentration gradients and release stored neurotransmitters (6). Water follows because of increased osmolality, and cells swell. Neuronal intracellular calcium concentration can then increase by up to four orders of magnitude. These huge increases in cytosolic [Ca^{++}] activate lipases, proteases, and other catabolic enzymes.

Changes in oxygen pressure have rapid, direct effects on membrane ion channels, mostly phosphorylation-related (7). Some ion channels are down-regulated, reducing ion flux and cellular energy demands (8). Other ion channels are up-regulated, promoting depolarization and cell death (9). Hypoxia also induces a variety of molecules called hypoxia-inducible factors (HIF). HIFs are induced more slowly than the effects on ion channels. They are expressed in all tissues and activate transcription of genes that increase systemic O_2 delivery or provide cellular metabolic adaptation under conditions of hypoxia. Thus, they activate the transcription of the gene for erythropoietin, the genes for glycolytic enzymes, and genes involved in angiogenesis. Juul has reviewed the use of erythropoietin to protect against neonatal ischemic brain injury (10); a recent study reported that it decreased brain injury when given to very young rats before hypoxic-ischemic encaphalopathy (HIE) (11). Further investigation is warranted, but the dismal results of human neuroprotective drug trials to date imply that clinical use of these drugs may be far in the future (12). The factors that mediate the induction of HIFs are under intense investigation (13). They are related to the phenomenon of *ischemic tolerance*, or *preconditioning*. This term refers to the observation that a brief period of cerebral ischemia confers transient tolerance to a subsequent ischemic insult to the brain (14). The mechanisms underlying ischemic tolerance are not fully understood. Kirino has suggested two possibilities: (a) A cellular defense function against ischemia may be enhanced by the mechanisms inherent to neurons. They may arise by posttranslational modification of proteins or by expression of new proteins via a signal transduction system to the nucleus. These cascades of events could strengthen the influence of survival factors or could inhibit apoptosis; (b) a

TABLE 17.1 Neurobiological Differences Among Ischemia, Hypoglycemia, and Epilepsy

	Ischemia	*Hypoglycemia*[a]	*Epilepsy*
Energy level (% normal)	0–5	25	99
Predominant excitotoxin	Glutamate	Aspartate	Unknown
Lactic acidosis	Variable (depending on blood glucose)	Absent	Mildly elevated unless cerebral O_2 supply reduced
Duration of insult required to produce neuronal necrosis	2–10 min	10–20 min	45–120 min
Timing of neuronal death	2–4 d	1–8 hr postinsult	1–2 hr postinsult
Distribution of neuronal necrosis	Pan-necrosis	Selective neuronal necrosis	Selective neuronal necrosis and pan-necrosis
Location of brain damage			
Cerebral cortex	Middle laminae	Superficial laminae	Laminae 3 and 4
Hippocampus	CA 4, CA 1 pyramidal cells	Medial CA 1 cells dentate crest	CA 4 and CA 1
Basal ganglia, thalamus, midbrain	Thalamic reticular nucleus, caudate	Caudate	Caudate spared; globus pailidus, pars reticulata of substantia nigra

[a]We should emphasize that the studies on hypoglycemia were performed on adult animals and that the times noted to neuronal necrosis and neuronal death refer to times after an isoelectric electroencephalogram. The relevance of these studies to newborn animals or the neonate is unknown.

Adapted from Auer RN, Siesjö BK. Biological differences between ischemia, hypoglycemia, and epilepsy. *Ann Neurol* 1988;24:699.

cellular stress response and synthesis of stress proteins can lead to an increased capacity for health maintenance inside the cell (14). The mechanisms of ischemic tolerance or preconditioning may ultimately become relevant for therapy of HIE (15).

The mature brain requires both oxygen and glucose but can adapt to reduced serum glucose levels (16). The fetal and neonatal brain also uses ketone bodies as an energy source (17); these metabolic pathways can be increased by diet and fasting (18). *In vitro* studies show that low glucose media increase hypoxic injury and that this effect correlates well with tissue ATP content (19).

Hypoxic-Ischemic Encephalopathy

HIE as it pertains to neonates is covered in Chapter 6, while localized arterial and venous disease are discussed in Chapter 13.

Hypoxia means reduced blood oxygen content, and ischemia means reduced tissue perfusion. They often go hand in hand because sustained changes in tissue oxygenation have secondary circulatory effects. Asphyxia means impaired gas exchange, as carbon dioxide accumulates as oxygen falls. Mild experimental hypoxemia increases electroencephalogram (EEG) delta activity, prolongs reaction times, and impairs psychological test performance (20).

Acute severe hypoxia impairs consciousness. The duration and severity of hypoxia determines the magnitude of injury and residual impairment, but other factors influence the extent of neural injury. Transient hypoxic episodes may be seen in heart disease, with cardiac arrhythmias, and respiratory problems. Experimentally induced transient hypoxia impairs oculomotor and visual function and can be accompanied by brief nonfocal seizures. These result in no detectable sequelae (21). Stephenson reports "anoxic motor convulsions" with asystole induced by ocular compression (22).

Mild to moderate oxygen desaturation (oxygen saturation in the 80% to 90% range) need not be harmful, especially if brief in duration. The Collaborative Home Infant Monitoring Evaluation (CHIME) study found that 43% of 306 healthy term babies had at least one 20-second episode of apnea or bradycardia without evidence of neurological abnormality (23).

Longer periods of hypoxia produce cellular injury. Neurons are more vulnerable than glial cells to hypoxia and hypoglycemia, and oligodendrocytes are generally more vulnerable than astrocytes (24). Neurons in certain areas of the brain such as the basal ganglia and the hippocampal CA1 pyramidal neurons are particularly vulnerable to asphyxial injury. By contrast, spinal cord neurons tolerate longer periods of occlusion than do cerebral neurons (25). The factors that determine the selective vulnerability of certain neuronal populations are still incompletely understood. They are reviewed in Chapter 6.

How Cells Die

Two types of cell death have been recognized: apoptosis and necrosis. Biologists reported extensive cell death in developing organisms in the 19th century but did not consider cell death to be a central part of normal development

(26). Lockshin's 1965 PhD thesis on silkworm metamorphosis introduced the phrase "programmed cell death" (PCD) (27). The Australian pathologist John Kerr studied human liver disease and noted an orderly form of cell death characterized by cell shrinkage with nuclear compaction and no inflammation. He first called this *shrinkage necrosis* (28). Peripheral areas where shrinkage necrosis predominated sometimes surrounded a central zone of coagulation necrosis. Kerr and colleagues later replaced "shrinkage necrosis" with the Greek word *apoptosis* (29). They saw mitosis and apoptosis as opposing forces, postulating that apoptosis inhibited tumor growth and development. Wyllie reported DNA fragmentation in cells undergoing apoptosis (30). Gel electrophoresis revealed "DNA ladders." Apoptosis or PCD became a focus of attention, and studies of its cellular control mechanisms in the nematode *C. elegans* led to a Nobel Prize (31). Vertebrates produce too many neurons; programmed cell death prunes the numbers of neurons and glia. Mice with caspase gene knock-outs (caspases are proteases that trigger some forms of PCD) have gross central nervous system (CNS) malformations (32). Pathologists accepted the idea of qualitatively different forms of cell death, but they initially limited this to two types.

Lucas and Newhouse and Olney defined neuronal cell death caused by excessive glutamate receptor stimulation or "excitotoxicity" (33,34). It was characterized by swelling and bursting of cells, release of lysosomal enzymes, and subsequent inflammation. They called this phenomenon *necrosis*; any cell may suffer necrosis in the older sense of cell death followed by inflammation; excitotoxic cell death is a special form of necrosis limited to neural tissue with glutamate receptors. Standard teaching about HIE came to include the idea that glutamate leakage from presynaptic stores increased calcium and sodium influx and aggravated the brain injury (35). The characteristics of necrosis and apoptosis are summarized in Table 17.2. *Coagulation necrosis* refers to the death and disruption of a group of cells and is usually due to ischemia. It can often be detected by magnetic resonance imaging (MRI) in that inflammation and increased water content become visible in the T2 and spin-echo sequences, and contrast enhancement is common, due to breakdown of the blood brain barrier. Apoptosis is not associated with inflammatory changes and is generally invisible to MRI. Its demonstration in the postmortem brain can be difficult because of technical problems and because apoptotic cells are often cleared in minutes or hours, and can disappear within a few days (36). Karyorrhexis can indicate apoptosis but is not specific. The DNA digestion pattern recognized in apoptotic thymocytes by Wyllie gave rise to the TUNEL (terminal deoxynucleotidyl transferase dUTP nick end-labeling) method for identification of apoptosis (37). However, the specificity and sensitivity of the TUNEL method has been increasingly doubted (38), especially in postmortem brain tissue. Kerr defined apoptosis by electron microscopy; this technique is presently the best way to distinguish types of cell death (28). The various forms of PCD have been characterized by Clarke (39) (Table 17.3).

TABLE 17.2 Simple Dichotomy of Necrosis Versus Apoptosis

	Necrosis	*Apoptosis*
Cell swells	Yes	No
Plasma membrane disrupted	Yes	No
Nuclear compaction	No	Yes
Disrupts surrounding tissue	Yes	No
Inflammatory response	Yes	No
Blocked by caspase inhibition	No	Often
ATP dependent	No	Yes

Cell death morphology depends upon tissue, cell type, and age of the animal; severity and duration of asphyxia; and the density and characteristics of cellular receptors. These factors are reviewed in Chapter 6. Mixtures of necrosis and PCD may be found in the same section or same cell, with intermediate forms of cell death that include attributes of both PCD and necrosis (40,41). Inhibition of one form of cell death may appear to stimulate another form (42).

Pathologic Anatomy of Cerebral Anoxic-Ischemic Injury

Bakay and Lee (43) and Auer and Siesjö (1) have described the basic pathologic alterations in the hypoxic brain. Structural damage can be limited to neurons or, if the hypoxia is more severe, it also can involve glia and nerve fibers. The microscopic changes in neurons subjected to energy failure have been delineated by Auer and Beneviste (44). As a rule, associated glial cell damage is proportional to neuronal damage. In gray matter, astrocytes swell as a result of cellular overhydration, whereas in white matter, the intercellular space enlarges because of extracellular edema and alterations in the walls of the cerebral capillaries. These pathological alterations are summarized in Table 17.4.

Areas most sensitive to hypoxia, as occurs after sudden cardiac arrest, are the middle cortical layers of the occipital and parietal lobes, the hippocampus, amygdala, caudate nucleus, putamen, anterior and dorsomedial nuclei of the thalamus, and cerebellar Purkinje cells (45). Brainstem nuclei are more likely to be involved in infants than in older children.

Brierley and coworkers have studied the time course of these pathologic changes in adult and juvenile monkeys. The earliest changes seen at the light microscopic level included loss of Nissl substance (ribosomes), eosinophilia, and nuclear changes—the "red dead neurons" (46,47). The nuclear changes may be pyknosis or karyorhexis (fragmentation). Necrosis is accidental and

TABLE 17.3 Main Types of Cell Death

Names Used	Nuclear Change	Cell Membrane	Cytoplasm	Cellular Corpses Consumed by Phagocytes	Characteristic Signs
Preprogrammed Cell Death					
Type 1. Apoptosis or shrinkage necrosis	Nuclear condensation, chromatin clumping	Persists, but prominent bleb formation	Reduced volume, becomes electron dense	Prominent	Nuclear
Type 2. Autophagic cell death	Sometimes pyknosis, may separate, blebs may form	Sometimes blebs, endocytosis	Abundant autophagic vacuoles; dilated ER, Golgi, and mitochondria	Late	Cytoplasmic
Type 3. Nonlysosomal cell death	Various changes	Often breaks	Disintegration, empty spaces, dilated organelles	Sometimes	Cytoplasmic
Accidental or Unprogrammed Cell Death					
Necrosis or oncosis	Dark, may shrink	Bursts	Lysosomal rupture	Swelling, membrane rupture, late phagocytosis	

Modified from Clarke PGH. Developmental cell death: morphological diversity and multiple mechanisms. *Anat Embryol* 1990;181:195–213. With permission.

requires no energy, whereas programmed cell death requires energy-dependent sequential activation of highly conserved proteins. Coagulation necrosis and disruption of tissue architecture—for example, infarction—is expected in the most hypoxic area, with PCD in peripheral areas, where energy supply permits the execution of preprogrammed cell death routines. Experimental stroke studies report caspase-mediated delayed cell death in the region outside maximal injury, with apoptotic features (48). Benjelloun and colleagues found prominent caspase expression in experimental neonatal stroke; it was rare in adults (49). Caspase expression was prominent in neurons and astrocytes in ischemic regions of the neonatal sheep brain (50).

TABLE 17.4 Composite Brain Injury Resulting From Neonatal Asphyxia, Sepsis, Cardiac Surgery, and Other Forms of Hypoxia in Small Infants

Immediate
Cell death neurons, oligodendrocytes "necrotic type"
Later
Programmed cell death, variable involvement of neurons, astrocytes and oligodendrocytes
Gray matter growth is less because of isolation from corticopetal axons and loss of trophic chemical stimuli from injured white matter
Years later
Reduced volume of white matter, lesser reduction in volume of gray matter; distribution of shrinkage depends in part on vascular factors

Cardiac arrest or vascular obstruction of 15 minutes or more in duration is often followed by initially normal or supernormal cerebral blood flow that declines to subnormal values with regions devoid of perfusion. The causes of these progressive changes are unclear; they are common in children resuscitated from drowning or cardiac arrest with initial systemic pH values below 6.9 (51). In part, these changes can be due to increased cerebral vascular resistance with prolonged ischemia. Many other factors can contribute to this increased resistance, including release of intracellular potassium (52), increased blood viscosity, leukocyte margination, and mediators such as bradykinin and nitric oxide. Endothelial changes are often seen with prolonged ischemia and reperfusion (53,54). These processes can contribute to delayed encephalopathy and postanoxic deterioration. They could be part of the cerebral circulatory arrest seen in brain death, and they could be preventable.

Delayed Encephalopathy

The histologic manifestations of anoxic-ischemic brain injury take time to become evident (4,46). Sometimes, there is partial clinical recovery after anoxic events, followed by dramatic clinical deterioration. This syndrome occurs with strangulation (55) and with many forms of anoxia, including near drowning (56,57). It is most dramatic after carbon monoxide poisoning; this phenomenon is considered in Chapter 10. Most patients with delayed deterioration, whether their initial injury was due to anoxia or carbon monoxide poisoning, develop extensive deep white matter injury—"Grinker's myelinopathy"(58). However, some patients, such as Dooling and Richardson's 11-year-old patient (55) and other pediatric cases (59,60) have only gray matter lesions.

Clinical Manifestations

Hypoxia

A number of clinical features are shared by all metabolic encephalopathies (61). The earliest symptom is a gradual impairment of consciousness. In infants, this can take the form of irritability, loss of appetite, and diminished alertness. Periods of hyperpnea can progress to Cheyne-Stokes respiration, a pattern of periodic breathing in which hyperpnea regularly alternates with apnea. The eyes move randomly, but ultimately, as the coma deepens, they come to rest in the forward position.

When anoxia occurs acutely, consciousness is lost within seconds. In cyanotic congenital heart disease, anoxia can take the form of brief syncopal attacks, often after crying, exertion, or eating; most frequently, these occur during the second year of life. Usually, the child cries at the onset of the attack, then becomes deeply cyanotic and gasps for breath. Generalized seizures can terminate the more severe cyanotic episodes.

Should oxygen supply be restored immediately, recovery is quick, but when anoxia lasts longer than 1 to 2 minutes, neurologic signs persist transiently or permanently. These include impaired consciousness and decerebrate or decorticate rigidity. The prognosis for survival is relatively good for patients who after their anoxic episode exhibit intact brainstem function as manifested by normal vestibular responses, normal respiration, intact doll's eye movements, and pupillary light reactions (61).

The longer the duration of coma, the less likely the outlook for full recovery. In the series of Bell and Hodgson, which included all age groups, 17.5% of patients comatose for longer than 24 hours could be discharged from the hospital, but 70% of these subjects experienced significant and permanent neurologic impairment (62). There is fairly good evidence that some children who survive a major hypoxic episode without apparent gross neurologic residua are left with permanent visuoperceptual deficits (63).

The EEG is of assistance in predicting the outcome of coma after cardiorespiratory arrest. A phasic tracing early in the recovery period indicates a good prognosis, whereas a flat EEG is never associated with full recovery other than in cases of drug ingestion (64). Bilateral loss of cortical responses after median nerve stimulation on the somatosensory-evoked potential (SSEP) test is one of the best prognosticators for a poor outcome. Initial preservation of the cortical potentials does, however, not necessarily imply a good recovery (65,66). This is particularly true for small infants, and serial SSEPs are indicated to ascertain whether they continue to remain intact (67). In term neonates, the positive predictive value of an abnormal SSEP also is excellent, but in premature infants, a normal response after stimulation of the median nerve had a poor predictive value with respect to normal outcome (67,68). As a rule, evoked potentials, specifically somatosensory-evoked potentials, are much more useful indicators of prognosis in postanoxic coma than is the EEG (69). The outcome of pediatric patients resuscitated from cardiac arrest is reviewed in Table 17.5 (70,71).

TABLE 17.5 Combined Results of Two Controlled Trials of Hypothermia as Treatment for Adults Who Had Out-of-Hospital Cardiac Arrest

Outcome	*Control*	*Hypothermia*
Parra's Study (70)		
Good	54/137	75/136
Dead	76/138	56/137
Barnett's Study (71)		
Good	9/34	21/43
Dead	23/34	22/143
Combining both studies (not exactly the same: one used 12 hrs hypothermia, one used 24 hrs)	Overall $X^2 = 14.08$, $p < .01$	

Each study showed a statistically significant difference—more good outcomes and fewer deaths—in the hypothermia-treated patients. When the studies are combined with the null hypothesis that outcomes are equal between control and hypothermic groups, $X^2 = 14.08$, indicating that the null hypothesis can be rejected at the $p < .01$ level. Data reproduced with permission of the New England Journal of Medicine.

Near Drowning

In near drowning, the length of coma has even more significant prognostic implications than after cardiorespiratory arrest, and, as a rule, there is an all-or-nothing outcome, with few children experiencing mild degrees of neurologic damage. None of the patients still comatose in 15 to 30 minutes after their rescue survived without major neurologic residua, and 60% of subjects in this group died. In a Hawaiian series, all children who ultimately survived intact made spontaneous respiratory efforts within 5 minutes of rescue, and the majority of those did so within 2 minutes (72). The experiences from several other centers are similar in that all children who still required cardiopulmonary resuscitation on arrival at the hospital experienced permanent severe anoxic encephalopathy. Interestingly, the presence of convulsions does not indicate a bad prognosis, although their persistence beyond 12 hours does. However, the appearance of myoclonic status epilepticus after cardiac arrest is a poor prognostic sign (73). Fields lists the following factors that predict poor outcome: (a) submersion for more than 5 minutes; (b) serum pH below 7.0 at time of admission to the emergency room; (c) the need for cardiopulmonary resuscitation in the emergency room; (d) a delay before the first postresuscitation gasp; and (e) poor initial neurologic evaluation on resuscitation (74). Immersion in cold or icy water appears to give a better chance for survival (75).

SSEPs and an EEG obtained during the second 24 hours after the accident have been used as additional prognostic indicators (76).

A postanoxic dystonic syndrome has been recognized in children. It appears 1 week to 36 months after the anoxic insult and tends to worsen for several years. Dysarthria and dysphagia are common. Neuroimaging studies reveal putaminal lesions in the majority of such cases. Treatment is generally ineffectual. The pathophysiologic mechanism underlying this condition and the reason for its progression are totally unknown (77).

The *persistent vegetative state* (PVS) after near drowning is being seen with increasing frequency owing to the resuscitative facilities of most emergency rooms. According to data compiled in California and reported in 1994, survival of children in PVS is dependent on their age. Median survival of infants younger than 1 year of age was 2.6 years; of infants between 1 and 2 years, 4.2 years; and children between 2 and 6 years, 5.2 years (78). In 1999, it was found that in the mid-1990s, the mortality rate for infants in PVS was only one-third of that in the early 1980s. A smaller decrease in mortality rates was recorded for children ages 2 to 10 years (79). In the experience of Heindl and Laub, 55% of children who were in PVS as a result of an anoxic event became conscious within 19 months of the injury. The quality of life was fairly good for those who recovered from PVS; 9% recovered completely, and another 52% became independent in everyday life (80). After 9 months, less than 5% of children were able to recover from PVS (80). In the study of Ashwal and coworkers (78), children in PVS survive somewhat longer in institutions than at home; other studies have shown converse results (81). A consideration of PVS following head trauma can be found in Chapter 9.

Many factors are reported to influence the outcome of HIE. Anesthesia during HIE generally decreases the injury produced. Hypothermia has a consistent, albeit modest, beneficial effect (82,83), while even moderate hyperthermia increases the damage in human and animal ischemia (84).

Treatment

The goals of treatment for cardiac arrest and postanoxic coma whatever its cause are to stabilize cardiac function, prevent further brain injury including delayed encephalopathy, and to maximize recovery of function. Cardiac arrest typically occurs at unexpected and inopportune times. Therefore, advance protocols or treatment outlines are desirable. Numerous treatment regimens have been used for cerebral salvage. These include induced hypothermia, barbiturate coma, and intracranial pressure monitoring to control cytotoxic cerebral edema. None of these has been effective in improving the ultimate outcome (75,85). The neurologist attending a near-drowning victim should keep in mind that hypoglycemia and hyperglycemia can cause further neurologic damage. Hyperthermia should be avoided and seizures controlled, with phenytoin being the preferred anticonvulsant. Animal studies suggest that vasopressin may be superior to epinephrine for resuscitation after cardiac arrest, and some suggest using both drugs (86). However, a human study failed to show a clear difference in outcome when either vasopressin or epinephrine was used (87). A study of 68 pediatric patients found that high-dose epinephrine was no better than and possibly inferior to standard-dose epinephrine given after an initial unsuccessful standard epinephrine dose (88). Neither magnesium sulfate nor diazepam given after out-of-hospital resuscitation improved outcome (89). Moderate hypothermia (12 to 24 hr at 32° to 34°C) improved outcome of comatose survivors of out-of-hospital cardiac arrest in two small European studies (90,91). The details associated with hypothermia are important—such as use of paralysis and sedation and possible interaction between hypothermia and various other drugs. Volume restriction is generally unwise; Ginsberg (92) advises the use of albumin infusions not only to increase plasma volume and decrease blood viscosity (93), but also to bind fatty acids and other toxins. Glucocorticoids worsen the effects of HIE *in vivo* and oxygen-glucose deprivation *in vitro* in that they induce hyperinsulinemia and hyperglycemia and have complex effects on glucose transport and energy metabolism (94,95). They also impair neuronal and astrocytic glucose uptake and inhibit astrocytic uptake of excitatory amino acids promiscuously released during anoxic insults (96).

Although there are no current standards of practice or uniformly accepted regimens at this time, I recommend the following:

a. Hypothermia to 32.5° to 33°C for 24 to 36 hours starting soon after arrival in the pediatric intensive care unit (PICU).
b. Full fluid maintenance, unless there is renal, hepatic, or cardiac failure. In prior years, clinicians restricted the use of intravenous (IV) fluids, hoping to avoid cerebral edema. This encouraged sludging in cerebral microvessels and had little effect on the occurrence or severity of cerebral edema. Hypotonic fluid should be avoided. I use albumin if there is any reason to suspect that the patient has been volume depleted. Sometimes, I use full maintenance fluids with colloid and a loop diuretic.

c. Unless there is GI bleeding, I give rectal aspirin once daily, 5 to 7 mg/kg for the first three days plus an H_2 blocker to reduce gastric acid secretion until feeding begins. Celecoxib has been beneficial in experimental studies (97), but the selective COX-2 inhibitors appear to be more thrombogenic than aspirin, and I believe that aspirin antiplatelet actions are beneficial.
d. I resume ventilation with room air as soon as feasible—but if there is lung disease or arterial hypoxemia, I continue high oxygen ventilation because of the oxidative stress that it imposes. I urge avoidance of sustained hyperventilation, which may increase cerebral ischemia (98).
e. Use anticonvulsants or glucocorticoids only if there is a specific indication other than anoxic brain injury. Most and possibly all antiepileptic drugs cause apoptosis and death of neurons in very young rats (99). This risk in humans is probably greatest for infants less than 2 years old. I use antiepileptic drugs if there are clinical seizures. It is debatable as to whether treatment of electrographic seizures without clinical manifestations is helpful in hypoxic coma.
f. It is important to avoid hyperglycemia, which makes cerebral ischemia worse and increases edema in experimental brain hemorrhage (100).

Brain Death

The concept of brain death developed once it became possible to maintain vital functions in patients with massive brain injury. Studies during the 1960s suggested that patients without evidence of brain electrical activity did not recover unless their condition was due to drug overdose. However, those studies included few children and no neonates.

In 1987, the Ad Hoc Committee on Brain Death from the Children's Hospital, Boston, defined brain death as follows:

> Brain death has occurred when cerebral and brainstem functions are irreversibly absent. Absent cerebral function is recognized clinically as the lack of receptivity and responsivity, that is, no autonomic or somatic response to any sort of external stimulation, mediated through the brainstem. Absent brainstem function is recognized clinically when pupillary and respiratory reflexes are irreversibly absent.... Particularly in children, peripheral nervous activity, including spinal cord reflexes, may persist after brain death; however, decorticate or decerebrate posturing is inconsistent with brain death (101).

Recommendations made in 1987 by a special task force appointed to set guidelines for determining brain death in children have been published (102). Although it is generally recognized that particular caution should be exerted when diagnosing brain death in small children, the task force further emphasized this age distinction by recommending different brain death criteria for infants between 7 days and 2 months of age, between 2 months and 1 year, and those older than 1 year. The period of observation before declaration of brain death in the youngest group should be such that two examinations and EEGs to document electrocerebral silence are performed, separated by at least 48 hours. In the group from 2 months to 1 year of age, the interval between the two examinations and EEGs can be reduced to 24 hours. The clinical examination of the pediatric patient suspected of being brain dead is summarized in Table 17.6 (103–105). A repeat examination and EEG are not necessary in this group if radionuclide angiography demonstrates absent cerebral blood flow (106). In children older than 1 year, the task force recommended the period of observation be a minimum of 12 hours, unless corroborating tests added further support to the diagnosis of brain death. When the extent and reversibility of brain damage are difficult to assess because of the type of insult (e.g., hypoxic-ischemic encephalopathy), the observation period should be extended to at least 24 hours. The confounding problem today is that most children die in PICUs and receive many medications in the last days of life. It is likely that "therapeutic and falling" levels of barbiturates and other anticonvulsants do not invalidate ordinary clinical and EEG criteria for brain death (107), but drug metabolism can be very slow in the brain dead patient, and high levels of other drugs such as opioids are often present. EEG and evoked potentials may occasionally become unobtainable, only to return hours or days later (108).

TABLE 17.6 Clinical Evaluation of the Possibly Brain Dead Patient

Should not have:
Corneal reflexes
Eye movements with head turning or caloric irrigation of the ears
Should not breathe if disconnected from ventilator for 10 minutes
Should not have more than 10% change in heart rate when pinched
Should not close eyes on command
May have:
Deep tendon reflexes
Flexion response of UEs or LEs (103)
Undulating toe sign (104)
Lazarus movement of trunk with head turning, oculocephalic movements or disconnection from ventilator (105)

Dosemeci et al. reported spinal reflex movements in 18 of 134 brain dead patients (103). This is in agreement with the authors' experience. UEs, upper extremities; LEs, lower extremities.

An important aspect in diagnosing brain death is the documentation of apnea. During this procedure, it is vital to prevent hypoxemia. Administration of 100% oxygen for 10 minutes is recommended before withdrawal of respiratory support. A catheter should be inserted into the endotracheal or tracheostomy tube, and oxygen be continued at 6 L per minute during the test. The arterial pCO_2 level should be allowed to increase to 60 mm Hg. Patients who are hypothermic or receiving medications that suppress respiration cannot be reliably tested using this procedure (70).

Some authorities have therefore challenged these recommendations, and a survey of PICUs shows substantial variability, even within the same unit, with respect to criteria used by clinicians for the diagnosis of brain death (109). In a clinical and neuropathologic study of brain death, Fackler and coworkers found no support for employing distinct brain death criteria for infants between 2 months and 1 year of age (110). Other investigators question the validity of relying on the EEG to confirm brain death because EEG activity is occasionally seen after brain death (111). Conversely, phenobarbital levels above 25 to 35 μL can suppress EEG activity in neonates (112). The brainstem auditory-evoked response cannot be used as a confirmatory laboratory criterion of brain death. Its absence is not predictive of brain death, and persistence of peak I has occasionally been seen in brain dead infants (113).

Demonstration of cerebral circulatory arrest is the most convincing proof of brain death and is not influenced by drugs or hypothermia. In principle, this can be done by transcranial Doppler ultrasonography in the hands of an experienced technician (114), by radionuclide angiography (115), or by spiral CT (116). However, these methods are less precise than angiography or MRI. Ruiz-Garcia and colleagues compared EEG, radionuclide angiography, and evoked potentials in 125 brain dead Mexican children. There was considerable concordance, but only 61 of 76 children who were subjected to all three studies had positive results on all three (115). Although complete absence of cerebral blood flow is considered irrefutable evidence of brain death, it is necessary to consider that cerebral blood flow is extremely low in normal term or preterm newborns (117).

Although CT angiography (118) and MRI and MR angiography (119) offer even more precise demonstration of cerebral circulatory arrest, they require moving the patient to the radiology suite. High-resolution brain CT scans with contrast are quite satisfactory for this purpose. If there are no flow voids in a technically satisfactory MRI of the brain, the patient is brain dead.

I believe that as these more sophisticated imaging techniques are applied to the clinical evaluation of brain death in children, the criteria for making this diagnosis will become refined and perhaps simplified.

Hyperoxia

Hyperoxia is iatrogenic, the result of increased oxygen content of inspired air or hyperbaric oxygen therapy. The question is when and how hyperoxia under normal atmospheric pressure causes neuronal or glial cell death. Hyperoxia is well known to cause cell death in the eye and lung. Hu and coworkers found that both hypoxia and hyperoxia caused cell death with apoptotic features in 7-day-old rat cerebral cortex; hyperoxia after hypoxia did not prevent cell death (120). Several animal studies show mild deleterious effects of normobaric hyperoxia used for resuscitation, and hyperbaric oxygen treatment can cause seizures and permanent brain injury in adults (121,122). Children breathing 100% oxygen develop hyperintense cerebrospinal (CSF) signs on FLAIR (FLuid Attenuated Inversion Recovery) sequences. These partially or completely disappeared when FiO_2 was reduced to 30% (123). The controversies with respect to the value of oxygen in resuscitation have been reviewed by Saugstad (124).

Disorders of Glucose Homeostasis

Glucose is necessary for neuronal function. Lactate, pyruvate, and ketone bodies can partially support brain energy needs, but there is always a requirement for some glucose supply. Brain glucose content is less than blood glucose content and increases only slightly with hyperglycemia (125). This is because the delivery of glucose, lactate, and ketone bodies to the brain requires specific transporters, glucose and monocarboxylic acid transporter proteins (GLUTs and MCTs), respectively, and the number of transporter molecules available limits glucose penetration into cells. Neonates have less than half as many transporters per gram of brain tissue as adults (126). GLUT1 is located at the blood–brain barrier and GLUT3 at neuronal membranes (127). GLUT1 is the most widely distributed glucose transporter, with some expression being found in almost every organ. Mutations of GLUT1 produce a progressive encephalopathy with seizures appearing early in life, a condition covered in Chapter 1.

Hypoglycemia

Pathology

Many authorities state that hypoglycemia produces a different topography of cerebral lesions than HIE, in that gray matter is predominantly affected (4,128). There are many exceptions to this dictum, and brain imaging studies often show white matter and thalamic lesions associated with neonatal hypoglycemia (129–131). These lesions tend to resolve with prompt therapy (131).

Anatomical studies disclose a selective neuronal necrosis of the superficial cortical layers, the hippocampus, and dentate gyrus. The cerebral cortical lesions are most conspicuous in the insular and the parieto-occipital cortices (132). The thalamus and non-neuronal elements are spared unless hypoglycemia is severe and prolonged (133–135). Damage to Purkinje cells is less than occurs after hypoxia (4,136). Infarction or hemorrhage are usually absent, even after a severe hypoglycemic insult (137). As occurs in hypoxia, the accumulation of excitatory neurotransmitters plays an important pathogenetic role in neuronal damage and death (137). The predominant release of aspartate into extracellular fluid in response to hypoglycemia contrasts with the release of glutamate in hypoxia and may account for the differences in the distribution of neuronal damage. The presence of acidosis, as occurs in hypercapnia, aggravates hypoglycemic neuronal damage, as does concurrent hypoxia (136,138).

Clinical Manifestations

The clinical manifestations of neonatal hypoglycemia are distinct from those developing at a later stage in life. In a landmark paper published in 1937, Hartmann and Jaudon identified symptomatic hypoglycemia in a group of babies from St. Louis Children's Hospital (139). They pointed to symptoms of tetany, twitching, convulsion, sweating, and irregular respiration as signs of hypoglycemia. They noted that normal newborns had lower glucose values than adults and older children during the first days of life and reported 12 infants with "cryptogenic hypoglycemia" values below 50 mg/dL without symptoms. Infants of diabetic mothers were recognized as being especially prone to hypoglycemia (140).

The incidence of neonatal hypoglycemia is uncertain because the lower limit of normal for asymptomatic babies is open to dispute (141). Furthermore, we are still unsure whether asymptomatic hypoglycemia is harmful to newborns (142,143).

Symptoms of hypoglycemia in the neonate are nonspecific. Table 17.7 outlines the clinical picture of symptomatic hypoglycemia in term neonates, as recorded from a Finnish nursery (144).

Transient hypoglycemia has been observed in a relatively significant proportion of infants with intrauterine growth retardation, perinatal asphyxia, or other forms of perinatal stress (145,146) and in neonates born to mothers with diabetes or toxemia (147). The incidence of neonatal hypoglycemia is difficult to ascertain because of the different criteria used to define hypoglycemia as well as because of the varieties of feeding routines used in nurseries. Normal plasma glucose values during the first week of life have been published (148). With hypoglycemia defined as glucose levels of 20 mg/dL or less, the condition was identified in 5.7% of cases at the University of Illinois Hospital nursery (149). The incidence is higher in low-birth-weight infants than in term infants.

TABLE 17.7 Symptoms of Neonatal Hypoglycemia in 44 Newborn Patients[a]

Principal Symptoms	*Number of Infants*
Tremors	33
Apnea, cyanosis, tachypnea	22
Convulsions	13
Lethargy	9
No symptoms or symptoms masked by another condition	7

[a]Hypoglycemia was considered to be significant if the blood sugar was 20 mg/dL or less on at least two separate occasions.
From Raivio KO, Neonatal hypoglycemia. *Acta Pediatr Scand* 1968;57:540. With permission.

Symptoms of hypoglycemia may appear as early as 1 hour after birth, particularly in infants who are small for gestational age, but generally they are delayed until 3 to 24 hours. In approximately 25%, hypoglycemia does not become symptomatic until after 24 hours (144). An inconstant relationship exists between blood glucose levels and hypoglycemic symptoms. Some infants with blood sugar levels between 20 and 30 mg/dL develop hypoglycemic symptoms, whereas others whose levels fall below 20 mg/dL can remain asymptomatic (150). Hypothermia can be a useful sign of hypoglycemia. Tonic postures, chorea, and other movement disorders are occasionally seen during hypoglycemia. In rare cases, they become permanent after multiple hypoglycemic episodes (151). Recurrent hypoglycemia is more dangerous than is a single episode (152).

Evoked potentials have provided some evidence to suggest the critical value at which hypoglycemia affects the brain. Somatosensory-evoked potentials (SSEP) and brainstem auditory-evoked potentials (BAER) become abnormal in term infants when their blood sugar falls below 41.5 and 45.0 mg/dL, respectively (153). Visual-evoked responses remain normal at these levels. Koh and coworkers studied BAERs and SSEPs in 17 children during normal and subnormal glucose values (153). Only five of these children were less than 1 week old, two were teenagers, and 13 were hospitalized for investigation of possible endocrine or metabolic disorders. Many showed prolonged brain stem conduction (increased interval between waves I–V in the BAER) when blood sugar fell below 2.6 mmol/L (46 mg/dL). Data from this small and selected group without analogous studies on asymptomatic neonates cannot firmly establish normal or safe blood glucose values (154). From the point of view of a neurologist, it therefore seems prudent that any blood glucose value of 45 mg/dL or less should be emergently corrected and followed closely to ensure sustained normoglycemia.

A rapid compensatory increase in cerebral blood flow resulting from recruitment of previously unperfused capillaries mediated by an increase in plasma epinephrine levels occurs at or below blood glucose values of 30 mg/dL (155–157).

The clinical management of hypoglycemia in neonates is beyond the scope of this text. The reader is referred to a flow diagram by Cornblath and Schwartz (158).

It is difficult to know what the outlook is in terms of neurologic and cognitive deficits for neonates who develop symptomatic hypoglycemia. This is because of limitations of current definitions for neonatal hypoglycemia, our inability to determine at what glucose level hypoglycemia becomes symptomatic, and various other risk factors, which complicate the clinical course of hypoglycemic infants and confound every study on neurodevelopmental outcome (159). From a multitude of data derived from neonates without other major risk factors, who had severe hypoglycemia as a consequence of nesidioblastosis, it is clear that a significantly low plasma glucose level that persists over a prolonged period of time can indeed result in major brain damage. The risks of asymptomatic neonatal hypoglycemia are even more undefined because low-birth-weight and stressed infants, the group with the highest incidence of hypoglycemia, also are subject to a variety of other prenatal and perinatal risks, notably hypoxic ischemic encephalopathy (160). It is prudent to assume that blood sugars below 30 mg/dL can be harmful and should be treated in neonates. A higher critical value of 45 mg/dL or below is often cited for older children but is probably too high, since children placed on the ketogenic diet often have values much less than this without symptoms (161).

When older infants and children develop symptomatic hypoglycemia, the condition presents with autonomic symptoms, which accompany a progressive impairment of neurologic function. The serum glucose level at which symptoms appear varies, but any child with a blood glucose level of 46 mg/dL or less is suspect for symptomatic hypoglycemia (162). Autonomic symptoms are mainly caused by increased adrenaline secretion. They include anxiety, palpitations, pallor, sweating, irritability, and tremors (162). During the initial stages, impaired neurologic function is manifested by dizziness, headache, blurred vision, somnolence, and slowed intellectual activity. Transient cortical blindness is seen only rarely (163). In fact, if permanent blindness accompanies hypoglycemia, one must consider the diagnosis of congenital optic nerve hypoplasia associated with hypopituitarism (164). If hypoglycemia is prolonged, subcortical and diencephalic centers become inoperative. The brainstem, the area most resistant to hypoglycemia, is the last to be affected.

Almost all children develop generalized or focal seizures during a severe hypoglycemic episode. With even more prolonged involvement, tonic extensor spasms and shallow respirations develop. The response to intravenous glucose is immediate in patients who have not progressed to brain stem involvement. In children who have experienced prolonged unconsciousness or repeated hypoglycemic attacks, the prognosis for complete recovery is poor, and approximately one-half of patients remain mentally retarded (165).

Not uncommonly, the clinician encounters a child whose first seizure occurred in the setting of suspected hypoglycemia, but who continues to experience seizures in the absence of hypoglycemia. Although prolonged hypoglycemia can indeed induce hippocampal damage and thus set up a seizure focus, I believe that isolated hippocampal damage is quite rare and that, in the majority of such cases, both initial and subsequent seizures are unrelated to hypoglycemia. Transient hemiparesis or aphasia has been seen in diabetic children, often in association with documented hypoglycemia. The cause of these focal deficits is unclear, but they could reflect focal seizures followed by Todd's paralysis (166).

Hyperglycemia

Hyperglycemia aggravates ischemic brain injury. Rats made hyperglycemic before cerebral ischemia have greater brain damage and mortality (167). This is understandable from Myers's studies showing that feeding prior to cardiac arrest resulted in postischemic lactic acidosis (168). Even if hyperglycemia is induced after the ischemic period, recovery of function is impaired compared with normoglycemic controls (169). Therefore, normoglycemia is aimed for in acutely ill patients and patients undergoing cardiac surgery. In adult patients, hemiparesis, confusion, and movement disorders may be seen with either hypoglycemia or hyperglycemia (170).

Thermal Stress: Hyperthermia and Hypothermia

Increased body temperature is common in children, usually caused by infections. Children occasionally develop hyperthermia because of anesthesia-related malignant hyperthermia, drug effects, when sweating is impaired by extensive body casts and braces, or when children are left inside vehicles or covered in bed during hot weather (171). Children are more susceptible to heat illness than adults for many reasons, including a greater surface area to body mass ratio, a lower rate of sweating, and a slower rate of acclimatization. The drugs most often contributing to hyperthermia are cocaine and anticholinergic drugs. Life-threatening hyperthermia is less common; it can be seen with neuroleptic malignant syndrome (172), malignant hyperthermia (173), cocaine ingestion (174), and baclofen withdrawal (175). Baclofen withdrawal presents special problems because most such patients have intrathecal baclofen pumps that fail (176). The first sign of pump failure may be severe fever, tachycardia, and hypertension. There is no IV form of baclofen, but I have given such patients fluids, benzodiazepines, rectal baclofen, and cyproheptadine (177). Cocaine-induced hyperthermia is generally associated with exercise and/or warm ambient temperatures. Cocaine impairs sweating and cutaneous vasodilatation. It shares with Ecstasy and several other drugs the property of impairing subjective perception of overheating and need for fluids (174,178,179). Other drugs that can induce hyperthermia include zonisamide (180), topiramate (181), and less commonly, acetazolamide. Serotonin selective reuptake inhibitors (SSRIs) cause the serotonin syndrome, which can be associated with fever and sweating (182) but rarely induce renal failure and collapse.

The prevention of heat illness is based on recognizing and modifying risk factors, which include environmental conditions, clothing, hydration, and acclimatization.

Encephalopathy is prominent early in the course of heat injury and is required for the diagnosis of heat stroke. It may progress to renal failure and multiple organ dysfunction with disseminated intravascular coagulation unless vigorously treated (183). Bytomski and Squire (179) cover special issues related to children.

Hypothermia and Cold Injury

Infants are more susceptible to hypothermia than older children. As body temperature falls progressively, many complications ensue (184,185). Electrolyte abnormalities and disseminated intravascular coagulation are common in both sustained hyper- and hypothermia (186). Hypokalemia is the most common electrolyte abnormality seen with hypothermia and represents a shift of potassium into cells. If extra potassium is given, severe complications may arise when the patient is rewarmed (187). Hypothermia accompanied by vomiting and coma are common manifestations of alcohol intoxication in prepubertal children in cold climates (188). Several rare syndromes of periodic hypothermia exist (189,190), including periodic hypothermia and hyperhidrosis, sometimes associated with callosal abnormalities and called *Shapiro's syndrome* (191). These periodic diencephalic disorders may respond to clonidine or cyproheptadine and may be related to migraine (192).

Disorders of Acid–Base Metabolism

Brain function and excitability are pH sensitive. The pH of body fluids is tightly regulated, and permeability barriers separate the central nervous system from body fluids. Those barriers are more permeable to carbon dioxide than to protons. Brain extracellular fluid contains more protons and free or total Mg^{++} ions and less potassium than plasma; the intracellular compartments of neurons and astrocytes are quite different. The brain extracellular environment is regulated or programmed to contain more H^+ than plasma or most bodily fluids. This relative acidity of the CSF and brain interstitial fluid is due to metabolic acid production (193).

Many voltage-gated ion channels in the nervous system are pH sensitive. Falling pH (acidosis) inhibits voltage-gated ion channels and glutamate-activated ion channels such as NMDA receptors (194,195). Since voltage-regulated calcium and sodium channels are more sensitive to pH than are potassium channels, increasing pH (alkalosis) increases calcium and sodium entry into neurons, making them more excitable. Acute metabolic disturbances, whether primarily pH changes or changes in electrolyte content of body fluids, often cause seizures and disturbances of consciousness. Respiratory alkalosis may have various causes, including liver disease and acute respiratory distress syndrome (ARDS), and may aggravate seizures from any cause. Respiratory alkalosis is more likely to increase glutamate release than metabolic alkalosis. In general, CSF pH fluctuates less than arterial pH and is well maintained unless changes are acute and severe. The neurological component of acid–base disturbances is nonspecific and poorly correlated with blood or spinal fluid pH.

Electrolyte Disorders

Sodium

Hyponatremia

Sodium chloride (NaCl) is responsible for the largest fraction of osmoles in body fluids, except for cochlear endolymph, a most unusual fluid whose sodium–potassium ratio is about 0.01. Changes in plasma sodium concentration are the first and most obvious sign of water intoxication or water deficiency. Brain extracellular fluid is normally isotonic with plasma. If plasma osmolarity changes rapidly, the brain behaves like an osmometer—it swells when plasma osmolarity decreases and shrinks when plasma osmolarity rises due to water loss. Both hyponatremia and hypernatremia disturb CNS function by changing the osmolality of brain cells. The difference between osmolarity and osmolality is that the former refers to concentration per liter of solution (plasma or CSF), while the latter refers to concentrations per liter of solvent (in this case, water). Osmolarity neglects the effects of protein and lipid dissolved in plasma; this may be a problem if protein and lipid concentration exceeds 5–6% of plasma. The reader is referred to a review by Katzman and Pappius (196) for a full discussion of the pathogenesis of cerebral symptoms in electrolyte disorders and to a review by Strange on disorders of osmotic balance (197).

Hyponatremia

Low-sodium syndromes can result from an increase in body water with retention of a normal sodium store or can occur after reduction of sodium stores. It is the most common electrolyte disturbance, occurring in about 2.5% of hospitalized patients, and is even more frequent in neurological and neurosurgical inpatients (198). Hyponatremia is frequently associated with cerebral edema as well as with an increased mortality rate (199).

In the experience of Arieff and colleagues, the most common cause for symptomatic hyponatremia in the pediatric population was administration of hypotonic fluids combined with extensive extrarenal loss of electrolyte-containing fluids (199). Oral water intoxication from increased intake of tap water during the summer months also induces symptomatic hyponatremia (200). Table 17.8

TABLE 17.8 Clinical Conditions Producing Abnormalities of Sodium Concentration

Hyponatremia
- Administration of salt-poor solutions in the presence of impaired function, acute overload of solute-free water in infants
- Water retention (congestive heart failure, hepatic cirrhosis)
- Depletion of intracellular solutes (diuretics, protein energy malnutrition, cystic fibrosis, adrenogenital syndrome)
- Postoperative hyponatremia, associated with nonosmotic release of antidiuretic hormone
- Inappropriate secretion of antidiuretic hormone in diseases involving the central and peripheral nervous systems (anatomic isolation of supraoptic nucleus of hypothalamus resulting in released firing of osmoreceptors)
- Encephalitis, meningitis, polyneuritis, diffuse cerebral damage in infancy, cerebral infarction, supratentorial and infratentorial brain tumors, subarachnoid hemorrhage

Hypernatremia
- Limited water intake
- Excessive evaporative losses (hyperpnea, increased environmental temperature)
- Excessive excretory losses (diarrhea, diabetes insipidus)
- Salt loading (often accompanied by excessive water loss)
- Sodium retention (hyperaldosteronism and Cushing syndrome)

lists the major causes of salt loss in children, and Table 17.9 lists the clinical presentation of hyponatremia in children with CNS disease in the experience of Bussmann and colleagues (201).

Neurologic symptoms of hyponatremia include headache, nausea, incoordination, delirium, and, ultimately, generalized or focal seizures with apnea and opisthotonus (202,203). On autopsy, cerebral edema and transtentorial herniation are seen (199,200).

Generally, severe neurologic symptoms with permanent residua do not develop at sodium levels above 130 mEq/L, unless plasma sodium has decreased rapidly. Some have advocated rapid correction of hyponatremia in a patient with neurologic symptoms using urea in conjunction with salt supplements and water restriction (204).

TABLE 17.9 Hyponatremia in Children with Central Nervous System Disease

Total patients	195
Patients with hyponatremia (serum Na^+ <130)	20
Hyponatremia due to SIADH	7
Onset, median days after cerebral event	1
Hyponatremia due to CSW	9
Onset, median days after cerebral event	2
Mechanism undefined	4

See Bussman et al. (200) for details. Four patients with CSW were incorrectly treated with fluid restriction. Severity of hyponatremia did not differ between SIADH and CSW. SIADH, syndrome of inappropriate antidiuretic hormone secretion; CSW, cerebral salt wasting.

Central pontine myelinolysis was first reported in alcoholics in 1959. It is a frequently fatal disorder that typically appears after major encephalopathy has begun to improve. Clinically, it is characterized by confusion, cranial nerve dysfunction, and in larger lesions, a "locked in" syndrome and quadriparesis. Pathologically, central pontine myelinolysis is marked by symmetric destruction of myelin at the center of the pons. The pontile demyelination can be visualized by MRI (205). It has been associated with rapid correction of hyponatremia, although the exact rate of correction that is safe or dangerous is debated (206). According to Brunner and colleagues, central pontine myelinolysis is more likely to develop when the initial sodium level is less than 105 mEq/L, when hyponatremia has developed acutely, and when sodium levels are corrected too rapidly (207). Myelinolysis is not specific for hyponatremia. It may involve other structures in addition to the pons (207) and may be seen with correction rates of less than 12 meq/L per day (208).

Salt retention rather than salt loss occurs in the syndrome of inappropriate antidiuretic hormone (SIADH) secretion (209). Hyponatremia in the presence of neurologic disorder should not automatically be ascribed to the SIADH (201). It is often due to the syndrome of cerebral salt wasting (CSW). Both of these syndromes tend to begin within 1 or 2 days of the neurologic insult. Table 17.10 reviews the distinction between hyponatremia due to SIADH and that due to CSW.

Setting aside these two syndromes common in patients with neurologic disorders, hyponatremia is generally caused by water retention, as in congestive heart failure, excessive water intake, or loss of electrolytes in excess of water due to gastrointestinal (GI) or renal disease. Many psychotic patients drink excessive amounts of water, sometimes to the point of causing death (210). Hyponatremia also may be caused by excessive water intake in hot weather or after exercise (200). It is occasionally seen in children taking carbamazepine or oxcarbazepine, but few of those children have serum Na^+ values below 132 mEQ/L. In general, hyponatremia is not clinically significant until sodium falls below this level, with some exceptions if it develops rapidly (211).

Hypernatremia

Increased concentration of sodium in body fluids elevates fluid osmolality and induces severe cerebral manifestations. Major causes for hypernatremia are outlined in Table 17.8.

Luttrell and Finberg have delineated the factors responsible for neurologic symptoms. These are subdural hematomas, venous and capillary congestion, and hemorrhages, the last produced by shrinkage of the brain during dehydration (212).

Neurologic symptoms also can occur in the absence of any alterations in brain structure and are probably the direct result of hyperosmolality. Symptoms are caused by

TABLE 17.10 Differences Between the Syndrome of Inappropriate Antidiuretic Hormone Secretion and Cerebral Salt Wasting Syndrome

Factor	*Cerebral Salt Wasting*	*Inappropriate ADH Secretion*
Plasma volume	Decreased	Increased
Water balance	Negative	Positive or no change
Signs of dehydration	+	Absent
Central venous pressure	Decreased	Increased or normal
Osmolality	Increased or normal	Decreased
Serum potassium	Increased or no change	Decreased or no change

Adapted from Harrigan MR. Cerebral salt wasting syndrome. *Crit Care Clin* 2001;17:125–138.

cerebral edema, which is particularly likely to occur with rapid rehydration and is caused by an elevated content of chloride and potassium in the brain (213,214).

Hypernatremia is generally seen in infants younger than 6 months of age. Dunn and Butt compared 57 Australian pediatric inpatients with marked hypernatremia ($Na^+ > 165$) to children with hyponatremia ($Na^+ < 115$). The sodium disturbance developed after hospitalization in more than half, indicating management failures (215). Hypernatremic patients were more likely to have neurologic symptoms (79%) and death (37%) than hyponatremic children, of whom 58% had neurologic symptoms and 19% died. Gastroenteritis was the most frequent cause of hypernatremia. All had clear evidence of dehydration. Patients have varying degrees of impaired consciousness and hyperpyrexia. Approximately one-third experience generalized convulsions and spasticity. Focal neurologic abnormalities, notably hemiparesis, are seen in approximately 10% of patients. Finberg found subdural hematomas in many of his hypernatremic infants (216). In some, neurologic symptoms, notably seizures, do not appear until 24 to 48 hours after the start of fluid therapy. These symptoms have been ascribed to cerebral edema and a lowered convulsive threshold developing with rehydration of the brain (213).

Hypernatremia may develop in diabetes insipidus if patients are unconscious or do not have access to water. It is seen in patients with defective thirst mechanism, which is usually associated with other signs of hypothalamic dysfunction. This may be a complication of surgery for suprasellar tumors such as craniopharyngioma (217). Hypernatremic patients are often severely ill and may have intracranial hemorrhage (218), leading to suspicion of child abuse (219). Rhabdomyolysis and pontine and extrapontine myelinolysis can complicated severe hypernatremia (220,221).

Management of hypernatremia can be difficult because patients are often severely ill, and fluid replacement must be slow and careful (222,222). Kang and colleagues present formulas for calculating the volume of replacement solutions in these patients (223).

Potassium

Hypokalemia

Brain extracellular potassium concentration has major effects on cerebral excitability, but cerebral disturbances are extremely rare in patients with hypo- or hyperkalemia. Hypokalemia is a common metabolic disturbance but rarely causes or contributes to confusion and coma (224). Potassium depletion from any cause may produce muscle weakness. In severe cases, this progresses to quadriplegia and respiratory failure resembling Guillain-Barré syndrome (225). The effects of hypo- and hyperkalemia on muscle function and the periodic paralyses are covered in Chapter 16.

Hyperkalemia

Hyperkalemia is an often seen laboratory artifact due to hemolysis of red blood cells. True hyperkalemia is common in patients with renal or adrenal failure. Marked hyperkalemia can cause severe cardiac manifestations and weakness similar to that associated with hypokalemia. The latter can involve facial and pharyngeal muscles.

Chloride

Hypochloremia

A syndrome marked by anorexia, lethargy, failure to thrive, muscular weakness, and hypokalemic metabolic alkalosis was seen in infants who ingested a chloride-deficient formula for the preceding 1 or more months (226,227). Serum chloride as low as 61 mEq/L and arterial pH values as high as 7.74 were recorded (226). Usually, urinary chlorides were completely absent. Impaired growth of head circumference was documented in the majority of cases. Rehydration and chloride supplementation reversed all symptoms and resulted in a marked acceleration of motor milestones and in complete or partial recovery of the decelerated skull growth. Developmental testing in some of these children at 9 to 10 years of age indicated that children who had received this formula had significantly lower scores on the Wechsler Intelligence Scale for

Children (WISC) and significantly higher risks for receptive and expressive language disorders (228).

Kaleita and coworkers have recognized a clinical picture of an expressive language delay, coupled with visuomotor deficits and an attention deficit disorder that often assumes the overfocused pattern (see Chapter 18). When the defect is more severe, the language and visuomotor problems can expand to assume a picture of generalized mental retardation, and the attention disorder can exhibit autistic features (229). A similar condition has been seen in nursing infants whose mothers' milk was for unknown reasons deficient in chloride (230).

Familial chloride diarrhea, a rare hereditary disorder described in 1945, requires lifetime intake of huge amounts of chloride and responds to treatment with proton pump inhibitors (231).

Calcium

Calcium is the major extracellular divalent cation. Both high and low serum calcium levels are associated with neurologic symptoms. Total calcium in serum is found in three forms: protein bound (therefore nondiffusible, 30% to 55% of total); chelated (i.e., diffusible but nonionized, 15% of total); and ionized (remaining percentage). Generally, the appearance of neurologic symptoms correlates well with levels of ionized calcium of 2.5 mg/dL or less. The concentration of CSF calcium is normally approximately one-half that of serum calcium and represents the result of a secretory process, rather than the movement of diffusible and ionized calcium from the serum. Changes in the CSF concentration are relatively small, although large alterations in serum calcium values overcome homeostatic mechanisms.

Hypocalcemia

The clinical picture of hypocalcemia and its causes varies with the age of the affected child. Some of the syndromes that produce hypocalcemia are outlined in Table 17.11 (232–240).

In the last century, hypocalcemia was one of the more common causes of seizures during the neonatal period, and it is still encountered in premature infants or stressed term infants, typically in the first days of postnatal life (232,241). The condition can be defined by a level of serum calcium below 7 mg/dL or of ionized calcium below 3.5 mg/dL. Two forms of neonatal hypocalcemia are encountered. One occurs during the first 2 days of life in premature and critically ill term infants. It also is seen in infants who have suffered perinatal asphyxia and in infants of mothers with insulin-dependent diabetes. As many as 50% of very-low-birth-weight infants have serum calcium levels below 7 mg/dL (242). The exact mechanism of this form of hypocalcemia is still obscure. Impaired vitamin D

TABLE 17.11 Conditions Producing Hypocalcemia, Hypomagnesemia, and Neurologic Symptoms

Condition	*Symptoms*	*Reference*
Premature and critically ill term infants	Onset in first 48 hours of life, generalized neuromuscular hyperexcitability, convulsions, spontaneous attacks of apnea and cyanosis, hollow or squeaky cry, hyperactivity alternating with immobility	Hsu and Levine (232)
Transient neonatal hypoparathyroidism, decreased urinary excretion of phosphate (neonatal tetany)	Seen mainly in bottle-fed infants; appears at 5–8 days of age; convulsions and generalized neuromuscular hyperexcitability	Cockburn et al. (233)
Maternal hyperparathyroidism	Major motor convulsions, refractory to anticonvulsants; appears in second week of life	Hartenstein and Gardner (234)
Vitamin D deficiency	Convulsions, laryngospasm, carpopedal spasm, muscular hypotonia; appears at 3–12 months of age	Gessner et al. (235)
Hypoparathyroidism	Cataracts, photophobia, increased density of bones, ridging of teeth and nails, tetany and convulsions, increased intracranial pressure, mental deterioration, extrapyramidal disorder, calcification of basal ganglia	Simpson (236)
Pseudohypoparathyroidism	Obesity, dysmorphic appearance, round facies, stubby short hands and fingers, tetany and convulsions (88%), mental retardation (60%), syndrome unaltered by parathormone	Mallette (237) Cohen and Donnell (238)
Renal disease	Tetany, muscle cramps, fasciculations associated with moderate to severe acidosis, elevated serum potassium to calcium ratio, often unresponsive to calcium or magnesium administration	Tyler (239)
Hypomagnesemic tetany of infancy	Recurrent convulsions, appears first month of life, impaired magnesium absorption across gastrointestinal tract, transient hypoparathyroidism	Tsang (240)
DiGeorge syndrome	Cardiovascular defects, hypoplasia of parathyroids and thymus, seizures	Chapter 4

metabolism has been excluded as a pathogenetic factor. Increased levels of calcitonin have been suggested as an etiologic factor in the hypocalcemia of prematurity, but not for that seen in infants of diabetic mothers (232,243). Less often, maternal hyperparathyroidism, congenital absence of the parathyroid glands, or disturbed renal function induce neonatal hypocalcemia (see Table 17.11).

The second form of neonatal hypocalcemia is the classic neonatal tetany (late hypocalcemia), whose mechanism was first elucidated by Bakwin in 1937 (244). It occurs between the fifth and tenth days of life and results in part from intake of cow's milk, which induces an increased phosphate load. In this form of hypocalcemia, hyperphosphatemia and hypomagnesemia are commonly present. Additionally, low circulating parathyroid hormone levels are seen. With the widespread use of low-phosphate milk formulas, this condition has virtually disappeared. In the series of Lynch and Rust, congenital heart disease was seen in 47% of infants with hypocalcemic seizures and prematurity in 13%. Maternal hyperparathyroidism, idiopathic hypoparathyroidism, and DiGeorge syndrome were other causes. In 20% of infants, there was no obvious cause for the hypocalcemic seizures (245). In my experience, when hypocalcemia is found in a neonate with seizures, it is far more likely an association rather than its cause.

Neonatal hypomagnesemia has been recorded in connection with hypocalcemia resulting from maternal hyperparathyroidism (246). It also can be the result of a selective malabsorption of magnesium (243) (see Table 17.11).

Hypocalcemic seizures can be focal, multifocal, or generalized. In the series of Lynch and Rust, multifocal clonic seizures were the most common. True tonic seizures or tonic-clonic (grand mal) attacks are unusual, and the latter seizure type was not encountered by those researchers (245). In the interictal period, infants generally are alert, and seizures without apparent loss of consciousness are not uncommon (233). An increased extensor tone is relatively common, as are increased deep tendon reflexes and ankle clonus. Jitters were encountered in 35% of hypocalcemic infants in the 1971 series of Cockburn and coworkers (233) and in 27% of neonates in the series of Lynch and Rust (245). Patients looked relatively well between seizures, and most had good outcomes. In contrast to neonates suffering from seizures owing to nonmetabolic causes, persistent focal neurologic deficits are not observed. The classic signs of tetany seen in the older child are usually absent. Thus, carpopedal spasm was rare, and stridor owing to laryngospasm and Chvostek's sign (a brief contraction of the facial muscles elicited by tapping the face over the seventh nerve) were not noted in any of the hypocalcemic infants reported by Keen (247).

The EEG is frequently abnormal and can demonstrate electroencephalographic seizures (245).

The treatment of seizures caused by neonatal tetany consists primarily in the administration of calcium salts (see the section on neonatal seizures in Chapter 15). The long-term outlook for infants who have experienced seizures owing to late hypocalcemia is generally good, and in the absence of subsequent neurologic insults, the majority develop normally (233,245,247). Calcium deposition in necrotic areas of brains in stressed neonates has been related to the transient elevations of ionic calcium after parenteral administration of calcium gluconate (248).

In older infants and in children, neurologic symptoms of hypocalcemia include tetany and seizures. Tetany is characterized by episodes of muscular spasms and paresthesias mainly involving the distal portion of the peripheral nerves. Episodes appear abruptly and are precipitated by hyperventilation or ischemia. No alteration of consciousness occurs. Carpopedal spasm and laryngospasm are the two most frequent examples of tonic muscular spasms. Chvostek's sign is not diagnostic of tetany because it is seen in healthy infants and children. Seizures can occur in the absence of tetany and are occasionally focal. Headaches and extrapyramidal signs are less common and are confined to older children or adults with hypoparathyroidism (249). In this condition, CT scans can show symmetric bilateral punctate calcifications of the basal ganglia, although only 50% show an association between this finding and the occurrence of extrapyramidal signs (249). Other manifestations of hypocalcemia include laryngeal stridor (237) as well as a psychosis that responds poorly to antipsychotic drugs until calcium and magnesium have been normalized (250).

Pseudohypoparathyroidism is characterized by obesity, moon-shaped facies, mental retardation, cataracts, short and stumpy digits, enamel defects, and impaired taste and olfaction. Calcifications of the basal ganglia are seen in approximately one-third of instances. The condition is seen more commonly in females and is caused by an inability of renal tubules to respond to parathormone (251).

In neonates undergoing gastrostomy for various reasons, vitamin D malabsorption can lead to hypocalcemic seizures. This condition is treated by parenteral administration of vitamin D (252). Tetanic seizures also can result from sodium phosphate enemas (253). I have seen nonfocal seizures in the first year of life in exclusively breastfed infants whose mothers took no milk or dairy products (254). Nutritional rickets is an occasional cause of fractures and seizures in an infant, which at times leads to an incorrect diagnosis of child abuse (255).

Hypercalcemia

Hypercalcemia may be a result of hyperparathyroidism, which is rare in children, from idiopathic hypercalcemia of infancy, Williams syndrome (256), or several rare inborn errors of metabolism (257,258). As in adults, hypercalcemia may accompany malignant disease, including leukemia (259), and immobilization in patients with end-stage renal disease (260). Hypercalcemia may be the

TABLE 17.12 Hereditary Hypomagnesemic Syndromes

Syndrome	Chromosome	Gene
Primary hypomagnesemia with renal tubular defect	3q27	Claudin 16 gene
Renal magnesium wasting syndrome	11q23	HOMG2, subunit of Na, K ATPase
Familial intestinal hypomagnesemia*	9q22	TRPM6 gene
Bartter syndrome, type 1	15q15	SLC12A1, Na-K-Cl cotransporter-2 gene
Bartter syndrome, type 2	11q24	ROMK1, K channel gene
Bartter syndrome, type 3	1p36	CLCNKB, Cl channel gene
Gitelman variant of Bartter syndrome	16q13	SLC12A3
Albright hereditary osteodystrophy	20q13.2	GNAS1

*This is the disorder formerly called congenital hypomagnesemia. Although due to defective intestinal absorption of magnesium, serum magnesium can be normalized with supernormal magnesium intake (263).

first sign of childhood leukemia (261). Confusion, movement disorders, and coma are seen with hypercalcemia, as with many other electrolyte disturbances. Seizures are less frequent than in hypocalcemia; they have been associated with a reversible syndrome of confusion, blindness, and seizures (262).

Magnesium

Hypomagnesemia

Hypomagnesemia may be seen alone or together with hypocalcemia. Congenital hypomagnesemia is a classical cause of recurrent tetany and seizures beginning in the first weeks of life. Serum calcium and magnesium are both low, but only magnesium treatment is effective (240,263,264). The various rare hereditary syndromes associated with hypomagnesemia are listed in Table 17.12. Seizures due to renal magnesium wasting can present any time during the first year of life, although they are most common in the first week of life.

Magnesium depletion is common during cisplatin treatment and often is accompanied by significant potassium depletion (265). Cisplatin treatment may be followed by a permanent renal tubular defect with magnesium wasting, which becomes evident by convulsions or episodic encephalopathy (266). Various GI and hepatic diseases, severe malnutrition, and almost any primary disorder of calcium metabolism can cause hypomagnesemia.

Hypermagnesemia

Magnesium was once used as an anesthetic agent (267). Marked hypermagnesemia reduces transmitter release and causes muscle weakness, but not loss of consciousness (268). Magnesium is well established in the treatment of eclampsia of pregnancy (269) and also can be given intravenously for treatment of bronchospasm (270) and refractory convulsions (271). Hypermagnesemia is generally due to excessive magnesium intake that is often combined with renal failure. It has been seen in rhabdomyolysis and acute diabetic ketoacidosis. Hypermagnesemia aggravates myasthenia gravis and potentiates the effects of neuromuscular blocking agents. Calcium gluconate should be given intravenously for cardiac or respiratory manifestations of hypermagnesemia. Neonates are more sensitive to the neuromuscular blocking effects of magnesium than older children.

Phosphate

Phosphate depletion and hypophosphatemia has been associated with a rare and poorly defined encephalopathy (272–274). This is usually a complication of total parenteral nutrition (273,274). Patients may show tremor, confusion, agitation, ophthalmoplegia, and coma, and some are areflexic. Hypophosphatemia appears to contribute to central pontine myelinolysis in a few patients with Wernicke's encephalopathy, including patients with hyperemesis gravidarum as the primary problem (275). Hypophosphatemia and encephalopathy have been seen in anorexic patients receiving hyperalimentation.

Iron

The various disorders of iron and other metals are covered in Chapter 1.

NEUROLOGICAL COMPLICATIONS OF GASTROINTESTINAL DISORDERS

Gastroenteritis

Gastroenteritis is associated with clusters of seizures, even in the absence of fever. The first reports of this association came from Asia (276), but I have seen cases every year since 1998 that were not limited to children of Asian background (277). Typically, a previously normal child less than five years old begins to have GI symptoms, has a cluster of seizures with lethargy and perhaps ataxia, and recovers completely in 48 hours or so. EEG during the seizure cluster is normal or a bit slow. Encephalopathy often accompanies the seizures (278). Rotavirus is the cause in some cases (279). Rotavirus also may produce an encephalopathy with or without CSF pleocytosis. In the experience of Goldwater and coworkers, the presence of CSF pleocytosis is associated with a better outcome (280). Rotavirus also has been associated with the syndrome of hemorrhagic shock and encephalopathy (281).

Celiac Disease

Wheat, rye, and barley proteins induce celiac disease, an autoimmune type of gastrointestinal disorder, in genetically susceptible persons. Subjects with celiac disease can present with cerebellar ataxia, less often with progressive myoclonic ataxia, myelopathy, or cerebral, brainstem and peripheral nerve involvement (282,283). In many cases, there is no overt malabsorption or growth problem. Epilepsy, which is frequently associated with occipital lobe calcifications, also is encountered—even in patients who are not malnourished (284)—as is an inflammatory white matter disease resembling multiple sclerosis (285). Although neurologic complications of celiac disease are generally restricted to adult subjects, children with celiac disease are at greater risk for developing learning disorders, ADHD, and headaches than control subjects (286). Patients develop various antibodies, including antigliadin, antiendomysial, and antitissue transglutaminase antibodies (anti-tTG), of which anti-tTG may be the most specific for the condition (287).

Vitamin E Deficiency States

The recognition that vitamin E deficiency is associated with a number of neurologic manifestations points to the important role played by vitamin E in normal neurologic function. Generally, vitamin E deficiency induces a spinocerebellar degeneration, resembling that seen in spinocerebellar (Friedreich) ataxia. This picture is seen in a variety of conditions marked by chronic malabsorption such as occurs in chronic cholestatic liver disease (288), cystic fibrosis, short gut, blind loop, and other intestinal syndromes (289).

Children with chronic cholestatic liver disease can develop a syndrome characterized by areflexia, gait disturbance, decreased proprioception and vibratory sensation, and gaze paresis (290). Dystonia is seen less commonly (291). Nerve conduction velocities and nerve action potential amplitudes are decreased (292). In most instances, serum vitamin E levels have been low (293). In one series, 80% of children older than 5 years of age with chronic cholestasis and vitamin E deficiency developed clinically significant neurologic abnormalities, with areflexia being the earliest sign (294). A similar clinical picture is encountered in abetalipoproteinemia (295). Here, too, vitamin E levels can be strikingly reduced (see Chapter 1). However, a normal serum vitamin E level does not exclude a deficiency in the vitamin because hyperlipidemia can produce a false elevation in serum vitamin E levels. The ratio of vitamin E to total serum lipids (cholesterol, triglycerides, and phospholipids) is considered a better indicator of vitamin E deficiency. Oral vitamin E in large doses is usually satisfactory treatment, but some patients with severe problems require injectable forms of the vitamin (292,296).

A rare autosomal recessive disorder is caused by mutations in the gene for the alpha-tocopherol transfer protein. This protein incorporates alpha-tocopherol into lipoprotein particles during their assembly in liver cells. The defect results in a decrease in serum vitamin E levels (297,298). Several allelic variants have been recognized. In some, the clinical picture resembles that of spinocerebellar ataxia with peripheral neuropathy; in others, ataxia is accompanied by retinitis pigmentosa. The age of onset can be as early as the first decade, and the disease is relentlessly progressive. Vitamin E in large doses (400 to 1,200 IU) can stabilize or improve neurologic symptoms (299). However, a few patients have developed new neurologic symptoms while receiving vitamin E and maintaining satisfactory serum vitamin E levels (300). As a rule, the earlier treatment is begun the better the outcome.

The neuropathologic picture of vitamin E deficiency regardless of cause resembles that described for vitamin E deficiency in rats and monkeys. It includes a loss of large diameter myelinated sensory axons in the spinal cord and peripheral nerves, with spheroid formation. These findings are most pronounced in the posterior columns (301). The tocopherol content of biopsied peripheral nerve is reduced in vitamin E–deficient patients with peripheral neuropathy. In some cases, chemical changes precede anatomic evidence for peripheral nerve degeneration (302). Ultrastructural evidence of electron-dense accumulations in muscle fibers also has been reported (303,304).

Inflammatory Bowel Disease

Inflammatory bowel disease (Crohn disease and ulcerative colitis) is associated with an increased risk of cerebral venous thromboses, especially during times of crisis (295,296). Kao and colleagues describe four children who developed sinovenous thrombosis coinciding with flare-ups of their ulcerative colitis (305). Markers of coagulation and fibrinolysis are often abnormal in patients with inflammatory bowel disease (306). Cerebral vasculitis is associated with Crohn disease (307), and inflammatory bowel disease is associated with higher incidence of neuropathy, myelopathy, and myopathy more so than with other illnesses (308). Not all cases can be explained by intestinal malabsorption and an associated vitamin E deficiency. Prolonged use of metronizadole (Flagyl) for the treatment of the condition can result in a clinical or subclinical sensory polyneuropathy or a combined sensorimotor polyneuropathy.

White matter lesions similar to those of multiple sclerosis have been seen in Crohn disease patients who were treated with the tumor necrosis factor antagonists etanercept and infliximab (309).

The association of ileal lymphoid nodular hyperplasia (ILNH) with regressive autism is covered in Chapter 18.

Whipple Disease

Whipple disease is an unusual systemic illness caused by the culture-resistant organism *Tropheryma whipplei*. Although usually a disease of middle-aged men, the condition has been encountered in children; it causes CNS symptoms with or without obvious gastrointestinal disease (310,311). These include cognitive changes, supranuclear gaze palsy, altered consciousness, oculomasticatory and oculofacial skeletal myorhythmia, myoclonus, ataxia, and cranial nerve abnormalities (311). Some patients have CSF pleocytosis. Diagnosis usually requires brain or intestinal biopsy (312). The treatment of Whipple disease is beyond the scope of this text.

Abdominal Compartment Syndromes

Changes in intra-abdominal pressure can influence intracranial pressure, primarily through effects on cerebral venous pressure. Citerio and coworkers showed that placing weights on the abdomen of patients with head trauma produced measurable increases in intracranial pressure (313). Intra-abdominal pressure can be significant with ascites and other abdominal fluid collections (314) and may contribute to the evolution of pseudotumor cerebri in very obese patients (315).

Pancreatic Encephalopathy

Generalized encephalopathy complicates acute pancreatitis in up to one-third of cases (316,317). Features include confusion, depression of consciousness, and occasionally asymmetrical weakness. There can be slowing of the EEG. White matter lesions are sometimes evident on MRI studies (316). If the pancreatitis subsides, neurologic recovery is likely.

Intussusception

Intussusception is relatively common in early childhood, but its diagnosis can be difficult. The classical triad of abdominal pain, currant jelly stools, and palpable abdominal mass is seen in less than one-half of patients. Whereas lethargy in gastrointestinal disorders is unexpected, approximately one-half of patients present with the symptom. Lethargy is common in volvulus as well and is seen occasionally in bowel obstruction (318,319). Many have speculated that intestinal bacteria enter the circulation when the bowel is ischemic; however, blood cultures are usually negative, and the mechanism of brain dysfunction in this condition is unknown. In a few cases, lethargy can be so profound as to prompt lumbar puncture, neurologic consultation, and brain imaging studies (320,321).

Hepatic Failure and Hepatic Encephalopathy

Liver damage by acute or chronic disease initiates a characteristic set of neuropsychiatric symptoms termed *hepatic encephalopathy* (HE), a condition that was first delineated in 1952 by Adams and Foley (322). It is variable in severity and multifactorial in etiology (323,324).

Pathology and Pathogenesis

In acute liver failure, the morphologic changes in the brain are dominated by astrocytic alterations, notably astrocytic swelling and cytotoxic brain edema (325). With progression of brain edema, intracranial pressure increases and ultimately results in cerebral herniation. In chronic liver failure, the principal microscopic abnormalities include enlargement and an increased number of protoplasmic astrocytes. These cells (Alzheimer II cells) are astrocytes with an enlarged, pale nucleus and a marked diminution in glial fibrillary acidic protein. They are found throughout the cerebral cortex, basal ganglia, brainstem nuclei, and the Purkinje layer of the cerebellum (322,324). They also are seen in human immunodeficiency virus (HIV) encephalopathy (see Chapter 7). Neuronal changes are generally not seen. Less often, central pontine myelinolysis has been noted in children with hepatic failure (326).

According to current consensus, HE is multifactorial and in part represents a failure of glioneural communication and cooperation (327–329). The two most important factors in its pathogenesis are increased plasma and brain concentrations of ammonia. The brain:blood ratio of ammonia concentrations is markedly elevated, probably a consequence of a disrupted blood–brain barrier (324). In the brain, ammonia is converted to glutamine, which cycles from astrocytes to neurons, where it is further converted to glutamate. After release of glutamate into the synaptic cleft, its reuptake occurs in astrocytes. It has been postulated that the increased synthesis of glutamine depletes available amounts of α-ketoglutarate and reduces the concentration of high-energy phosphates, thus slowing the reactions in the Krebs tricarboxylic acid cycle. Decreased oxygen consumption and glucose metabolism, however, are secondary to HE rather than causative (328).

TABLE 17.13 Stages, Signs, and Symptoms of Hepatic Encephalopathy

Stage	Mental Status/Behavior	Motor/Reflexes
I	Confusion and irritability May be agitated, altered sleep pattern, disinterested in environment, inattentive	Fine tremor, slowed movements with poor coordination
II	Lethargy and drowsiness Personality changes, inappropriate behavior, time disorientation	Asterixis, hyperventilation, paratonia, ataxia, and other gait abnormalities
III	Gross delirium, somnolent if not stimulated, paranoia, severe disorientation, incoherent with dysarthric speech	Increased reflexes and tone Myoclonus, seizures, incontinence, hyperventilation
IV	Coma	Decerebrate postures, preserved eye movements on oculocephalic testing

Although in the past enhanced GABAergic neurotransmission was cited as a cause for hepatic encephalopathy, the evidence for this effect is far from convincing. In a vast majority of HE models, there are no alterations of GABA content in the brain tissue and/or extracellular space, and most of the substances in brain and other tissue with GABAergic properties can be traced to the ingestion of benzodiazepines (324).

HE is associated with multiple secondary biochemical abnormalities. MRI studies have shown increased signal in the globus pallidus in T1-weighted images, and an increased concentration of brain manganese is believed responsible for these findings. Brain copper concentrations also are increased, and as is the case in Wilson disease, the accumulation of the toxic metals can alter astrocyte function and morphology (324).

Evidence for the synergistic role of other neurotoxins such as mercaptans, short-chain fatty acids, and phenols as well as the generation of false neurotransmitters such as octopamine is currently less strong (328). Additionally, liver failure induces profound multisystem disturbances, which, in turn, can further impair neurologic function (330). Of significance are gut-derived bacteria and their toxic products, which are known to injure the liver and cause systemic illness (331–333). Serum levels of proinflammatory cytokines are increased in hepatic encephalopathy, and the severity of encephalopathy has been correlated with serum levels of tumor necrosis factor α (334).

Clinical Manifestations

HE can occur in two forms: acutely, as in fulminant hepatic failure, and as a chronic, progressive encephalopathy. In children, acute hepatic failure is primarily responsible for clinically important HE (335). The most common predisposing causes are acute infectious hepatitis; Wilson disease (336); the ingestion of various drugs such as valproic acid, acetaminophen, isoniazid, or halothane; and toxins, notably mushroom poisoning (337). In infancy, galactosemia, fructosemia, or tyrosinemia can present as fulminant hepatic failure (see Chapter 1). In the past, Reye syndrome and hemorrhagic shock syndrome presented with fulminant liver failure (see Chapter 7).

The onset of the encephalopathy usually coincides with a deterioration of the general clinical condition. The principal signs and symptoms of hepatic coma are related to disorders of consciousness. Neurologic symptoms in hepatic failure generally can be divided into six groups: those due to hypoglycemia; sepsis; intracranial bleeding resulting from coagulopathies; renal failure; electrolyte disturbances, notably hyponatremia, hypokalemia, and hypocalcemia; and cerebral edema. The various stages of HE are outlined in Table 17.13.

It is of utmost importance that the first signs of encephalopathy are recognized, as the progression from stages I to IV can be exceedingly rapid. Because the first evidence of encephalopathy may be outbursts of violent agitation or uncharacteristic behavior, the early stage of HE is frequently misdiagnosed. Hyperventilation can develop during stages II and III and can lead to alkalosis, low serum pCO_2, and a further deterioration of mental status. A fine tremor, and more characteristically coarse flapping movements, termed *asterixis*, can be present in stages I and II, respectively, whereas decorticate and decerebrate postural responses accompany stage IV of HE. Choreiform movements, a fluctuating rigidity of the limbs, parkinism, dystonia, and periods of noisy delirium are particularly frequent asian indian (338,339).

Poddar and colleagues reported 67 Asian-Indian children with fulminant hepatic failure treated without transplantation, 63 of whom were thought to have viral hepatitis (340). All children with stage I or II encephalopathy survived. Seventeen of 36 children with stage III or IV encephalopathy died. Ascites, peritonitis, and chemical evidence of severe hepatocellular dysfunction all increased the risk of death. Cerebral edema is a prominent part of the clinical picture of acute HE and is the principal cause of death, with brainstem herniation found in up to 80% of patients dying in fulminant hepatic failure (341).

Although severe liver disease is a prerequisite for the appearance of HE, ascites, jaundice, edema, or hepatomegaly do not invariably accompany the neurologic involvement. In fact, frequently, as irreversible liver failure supervenes, previously elevated serum transaminase levels decrease rapidly, the coagulopathy worsens, the initially enlarged liver shrinks, and the total bilirubin climbs while the conjugated portion decreases.

In a majority of patients, the EEG shows paroxysmal and diffuse bursts of high-voltage slow-wave activity, a pattern that is not specific for HE but is highly indicative of one of the metabolic encephalopathies. Triphasic waves, characteristic for HE, are common in adults but rare in children. Clinical or EEG evidence of seizures is associated with a poor outcome (342).

Treatment and Prognosis

The advent of successful liver transplantation, which offers a success rate of between 55% and 89%, has revolutionized the management, treatment, and prognosis of children with liver failure and HE (343,344). Liver transplantation is the definitive treatment in patients with acute or chronic hepatic failure, and in several major centers, including our own, results have been encouraging both in terms of survival rate and post-transplant complications. The decision of which patients to transplant and when surgery is to be done is beyond the scope of this text. Suffice it to say that the mortality of patients in stage IV HE is 63% to 80%. In particular, patients who have developed cerebral edema fare badly and are not suitable candidates for liver transplant (344). In the experience of the Children's Hospital of Pittsburgh, 70% of children who developed cerebral edema as demonstrated by computed tomography (CT) scan died, and 15% were left with severe to profound neurologic deficits. The remainder were left with moderate deficits that prevented them from an independent lifestyle (344).

The child with HE requires meticulous medical management until either the liver resumes adequate function or a replacement organ is found. Management of the precipitating event, dietary protein restriction, avoidance of constipation, and alteration of the intestinal flora are the major aspects of the therapeutic regimen (345). The therapeutic value of flumazenil, a benzodiazepine antagonist, appears to be minimal in the pediatric population (346). Response to flumazenil is transient, and the medication may precipitate an anaphylactic reaction.

Most commonly, the neurologist becomes involved in the treatment of a child with HE who has developed cerebral edema. Because cerebral edema mainly occurs on a cytotoxic basis, corticosteroids are not recommended for its treatment and were found to be ineffective in controlled trials. The best course of management is by fluid restriction and assisted hyperventilation. Hyperventilation is widely used and seems helpful early in the course of the illness. Cerebral blood flow tends to increase as encephalopathy develops if ventilation is not controlled, and this relative hyperemia contributes to intracranial hypertension (347). Late in the course of hepatic failure, cerebral blood flow tends to decrease, and hyperventilation at this stage can be harmful (348). Mannitol and related osmotic diuretics are helpful, but prolonged use of mannitol can cause hyperosmolality and aggravate renal problems (349,350). Minimizing stimulation (lights, sound, endotracheal suctioning) avoids sharp increases in intracranial pressure that are liable to become sustained and recalcitrant to therapeutic measures. Short-acting narcotics (fentanyl) can be administered to further blunt intracranial pressure increase from stimulation. Hypothermia and barbiturate coma have been advocated but should only be used if intracranial pressure is monitored.

Extradural or subdural monitoring devices are increasingly used for children in stage III or IV (350). These allow management of intracranial pressure and permit documentation of cerebral hypoperfusion and the rapid fluctuations of intracranial pressure encountered during the transplant procedure (351). Placement requires an experienced neurosurgeon and often necessitates simultaneous administration of fresh frozen plasma. In the experience of Blei and coworkers, a potentially fatal hemorrhage was the most common complication of cerebral pressure monitoring in fulminant hepatic failure (352).

This is not the place to discuss the complexities of artificial liver support (353) and the details of managing severe hepatic failure. For a comprehensive discussion of the therapy of hepatic failure, the interested reader is referred to reviews by Jalan (354), Sherlock (349), and DeVictor and coworkers (350).

Suffice it to say that hepatic transplantation is no solution unless intracranial pressure is controlled. Sustained increases in intracranial pressure resulting in diminished cerebral perfusion pressure (less than 40 torr for more than 2 hours) are generally accepted as a contraindication to liver transplantation (355). In addition, the cause of hepatic failure and a variety of other prognostic indicators must be considered (356). In particular, the longer the interval between the onset of jaundice and the development of HE, the worse the outcome (357). As a rule, somatosensory-evoked potentials are superior to EEG in terms of prognosis, and a lack of a thalamocortical potential presages a poor outcome (358).

NEUROLOGIC COMPLICATIONS OF LIVER TRANSPLANTATION

Transplantation has revolutionized the management of severe hepatic failure; however, neurologic complications of liver transplantation occur in 30% to 60% of patients

(359). As a rule, neurologic complications occur in the first months following transplantation (360). They can be categorized into problems related to the underlying disease, problems related to the transplant procedure, side effects of immunosuppressive drugs, and neurologic complications arising from immunosuppression (361).

The complications arising from the transplant procedure are related to the major fluid and electrolyte shifts that can occur during surgery when the diseased liver is removed and reperfusion of the new liver may produce a return of intracranial hypertension (362). Intracranial hemorrhage secondary to coagulopathy and severe ischemic injury secondary to hypoperfusion are uncommon but devastating consequences. Patients with fulminant hepatic failure can continue to experience encephalopathy and life-threatening cerebral edema for several days after the transplant. Intraoperative intracranial pressure can increase secondary to the stress of surgery, supine operating position, or fluid shifts.

Initial encephalopathy can occur in up to 60% of transplants (363). Seizures are less common (363); in a few instances, rapid shifts of sodium or other electrolytes during the perioperative period are associated with central pontine myelinolysis (364,365). Intracranial hemorrhage and ischemic strokes are most often encountered in patients with major infection (366,367).

In the pediatric age group, infectious complications resulting from immunosuppression are the most common, with the risk for CNS infections being the greatest between 1 and 6 months following transplantation (368,369). These may take the form of acute meningitis, subacute chronic meningitis, a meningoencephalitis, or a brain abscess. Conti and Rubin provide a timetable for the occurrence of infections in the transplant patient (368). Opportunistic infections of the CNS are rare during the first month after transplantation. The organisms responsible are different from those found in immunocompetent children. Four organisms—*Listeria monocytogenes*, *Aspergillus fumigatus*, herpesviruses, and *Cryptococcus neoformans*—account for most cases, although there is geographic variation (370). At 6 months post-transplant, patients are at risk for cryptococcal meningitis and cytomegalovirus. The most common organism to cause acute meningitis in the immunocompromised child is *Listeria monocytogenes*. *Cryptococcus*, *Listeria*, and *Mycobacterium tuberculosis* can be responsible for subacute infections. Brain abscesses are much more often due to fungal than bacterial infection in this special population (369).

Neurologic symptoms also can result from the use of immunosuppressive agents. Cyclosporine induces neurologic symptoms in some 10% to 25% of patients (370). The most common neurologic symptom is tremor. This can be caused by sympathetic activation, a leukoencephalopathy, or can be a part of generalized cerebellar dysfunction (371). Less often, one can observe seizures. In some patients, these appear to be related to metabolic derangements, notably hypomagnesemia. Seizures are more likely to occur with the intravenous form of cyclosporine (Sandimmune) than with the oral form of the drug. In such cases, the neurologic consultant is often asked whether to start anticonvulsant therapy as well as which anticonvulsant is most appropriate. By inducing the hepatic P450 system, most anticonvulsants interfere with the metabolism of immunosuppressive agents, thus increasing their required dosage. Benzodiazepines, gabapentin, and valproate are the drugs of choice in that they tend to have a lesser effect on cyclosporine metabolism (360).

A relatively frequent condition termed *reversible posterior encephalopathy* (RPE) has been seen in children receiving immunosuppressants such as cyclosporine or tacrolimus (372). This complication is more common when high doses are used, but there is no specific blood level that separates affected and unaffected patients receiving these drugs. Hypertension is almost invariably present, but it may be surprisingly mild. Its pathophysiology is similar to that of hypertensive encephalopathy in that the condition results when systemic blood pressure exceeds the autoregulatory capacity of the cerebral vasculature, with consequent breakdown of the blood–brain barrier and transudation of fluid into the brain. It is believed that the relative lack of sympathetic innervation of the posterior circulation may predispose the parietal occipital region to vasodilatation and breakdown of the blood–brain barrier. The condition is reversible upon lowering the blood pressure or discontinuation of immune suppressants. This entity presents with severe headache, depression of consciousness, seizures, confusion, or cortical visual deficits (373). It is rarely associated with papilledema or retinal hemorrhages. Many patients have seizures during the acute phase, but few have epileptiform discharges in their EEGs, and the majority can be withdrawn from anticonvulsant medication after 4 to 6 months. The CSF is generally normal (374). The neuroimaging picture is characteristic in that it demonstrates a symmetric bilateral subcortical/cortical hyperintensity in T2-weighted images typical of vasogenic edema (375) (Fig. 17.1). RPE is seen not only in patients on immunosuppressants, but also in a wide variety of other disorders that include acute glomerulonephritis with relatively normal creatinine, eclampsia of pregnancy, and uncontrolled hypertension. It also is encountered in patients receiving cancer chemotherapy (376–378). RPE is generally reversed after discontinuation or reduction of the immune suppressant. It has been linked to low serum cholesterol levels in that hypocholesterolemia upregulates the low-density lipoprotein receptor, which increases intracellular transport of cyclosporine (379). Although most patients do well, some are left with permanent neurologic deficits (380,381).

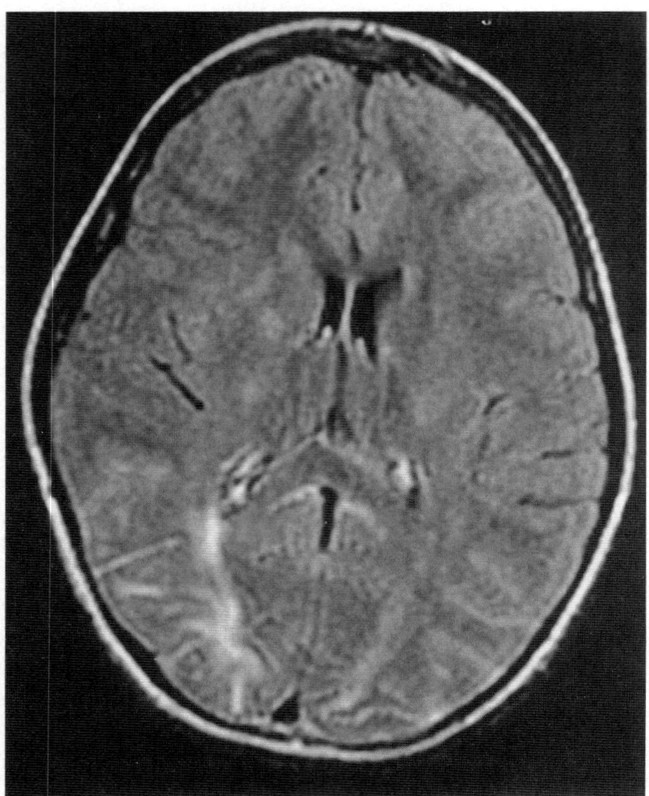

FIGURE 17.1. Reversible posterior encephalopathy. This T1-weighted axial magnetic resonance image demonstrates increased signal in the right occipital parietal region. The patient was a 9-year-old girl with chronic renal disease on home peritoneal dialysis. She developed status epilepticus after apparent fluid overload. On admission, her blood pressure was 195/140. She had hypotonia in the right upper extremity and hypertonia in the other extremities. There was no papilledema. (Courtesy of Dr. Franklin G. Moser, Department of Radiology, Cedars-Sinai Medical Center, Los Angeles.)

Patients taking immunosuppressant drugs should generally not receive enzyme-inducing antiepileptic drugs because they decrease the efficacy of the immunosuppressant agents. Benzodiazepines, valproate, gabapentin, and levetiracetam have been used successfully in transplant patients (382,383), but only the first two drugs are currently available in injectable form.

Other serious complications of immunosuppressant therapy include cerebellar symptoms, mental confusion, polyneuropathy, a motor spinal cord syndrome, and thromboembolic phenomena. A dose-dependent myopathy has been encountered some 5 to 25 months after initiation of cyclosporine therapy (384). In a small proportion of patients, cyclosporine induces a hemolytic uremic syndrome or thrombotic thrombocytopenic purpura with ensuing neurologic symptoms (385).

Tacrolimus is a newer immunosuppressant that is used increasingly in children. The spectrum and incidence of neurotoxicity is similar to that of cyclosporine. A severe postural tremor and, less frequently, mutism and speech apraxia as well as seizures are the most common manifestations (386,387). Headaches also are commonly seen, especially early after transplantation, a time when immunosuppression is highest. OKT3 is a monoclonal murine IgG immunoglobulin used for short courses in severe acute organ rejection. This agent can induce a sterile CSF pleocytosis. Symptoms include fever, headache, photophobia, meningism, cerebral edema, and transient hemiparesis. They are reversed by cessation of OKT3 treatment (388,389).

At dosages required for immune suppression, corticosteroids have the potential to induce mental status changes, a steroid myopathy, cerebrovascular changes owing to hypertension, and pseudotumor cerebri, which can develop after corticosteroid withdrawal. A primary CNS lymphoma is seen in some 2% of organ transplant patients.

Parkinsonian symptoms of bradykinesia and hypokinesia, cogwheel rigidity, and resting tremor have been noted after bone marrow transplantation (390). In the series of Martinez and colleagues, the most common pathologic findings in children dying after having undergone a liver transplantation were cerebral edema; a variety of ischemic and hemorrhagic vascular lesions; and infections, mainly caused by cytomegalovirus, aspergillosis, and candidiasis (391). A liver transplant series reported from the University of California, Los Angeles, UCLA School of Medicine shows similar neuropathologic sequelae (392).

Children who are long-term survivors of liver transplantation after chronic hepatic failure are at greater risk for intellectual and neuropsychologic deficits than are children with other chronic illnesses. Whether this is an effect on cognitive functioning of the pretransplant hepatic disease or the post-transplant immune suppressant therapy remains to be established (393,394). Cognitive outcome is influenced by many factors, including the severity of liver disease before transplantation, medication effects, and various socioenvironmental factors.

NEUROLOGIC COMPLICATIONS OF RENAL DISEASE

Uremia

Pathology

The molecular basis for uremic encephalopathy remains complex and poorly understood; it is generally accepted that several toxins are responsible. Urea is the most studied of these. However, it has been known for some time that the severity of cerebral symptoms correlates poorly with levels of serum urea, and hemodialysis sometimes reverses symptoms without lowering blood urea (395). Creatinine, p-cresol, the guanidines, organic acids, phosphates, and secondary hyperparathyroidism also are believed to contribute to the encephalopathy. Parathormone is believed to be responsible for some aspect of the various neurologic symptoms encountered in uremia, notably the peripheral neuropathy and the myopathy (396). Cerebral blood flow studies have shown a defect in oxygen use. In part, this defect might be caused by nonspecific increases in brain permeability and disordered membrane function, which could allow toxic products, possibly a variety of organic acids, to enter the brain. These acids could alter the function of the sodium-potassium ion pump. Disorders in blood and CSF electrolytes can aggravate the clinical picture, as can bouts of acute hypertensive encephalopathy (397).

Clinical Manifestations

The principal neurologic symptoms of uremia are abnormalities in mental status, tremor, myoclonus, asterixis, convulsions, and muscle cramps (239,398). As a rule, the more rapidly renal failure develops, the more prominent the motor symptoms, which may include unclassifiable twitches that are bilateral but asynchronous, and seizures. The motor disorder is usually relatively symmetrical. Peripheral nerve involvement is common in patients with uremia. Most frequently, it takes the form of a polyneuropathy. This can be a symptomatic mixed motor and sensory neuropathy, or it can be subclinical, detected only by nerve conduction studies. In one report, 76% of uremic children had a significantly reduced peroneal motor nerve conduction velocity without any clinical evidence of neuropathy (399). When symptoms develop, they begin with sensory abnormalities in the lower extremities. The condition can progress slowly to total flaccid quadriplegia. Nerve biopsy can reveal primarily an axonal neuropathy, progressive axonal neuropathy with secondary demyelination, or predominantly demyelinating neuropathy (400). Less commonly, patients develop a mononeuropathy, cranial nerve palsies, and choreoathetosis. Restless legs syndrome is seen in a large proportion of uremic patients (401). Signs of hypocalcemia and hypomagnesemia are often present. On rare occasions, one can encounter a primary myopathy (402).

EEGs are generally slowed and sometimes include spike-wave discharges in patients without clinical seizures (403). Rhythmical EEG discharges without clinical seizures are more common in renal failure than in children without renal disease; many of these patients do not demonstrate paroxysmal discharges when monitored (404).

In hypertensive encephalopathy, such as occurs with acute glomerulonephritis, patients develop symptoms and signs of increased intracranial pressure, with headache, vomiting, disturbance of vision, and papilledema. Seizures and transient focal cerebral syndromes, including hemiparesis and cortical blindness, also are common.

As a rule, developmental quotients of children who develop chronic renal failure before 1 year of age are more affected than those of children who go into uremia after 3 years of age (405). In the experience of McGraw and Haka-Ikse, more than 50% of patients with chronic renal failure present since infancy had significant developmental delay (406). This is accompanied by a significant reduction in the head circumference.

Neuroimaging studies of the brain of patients with end-stage uremia reveal a high incidence of cerebral atrophy, suggesting an adverse effect of uremia on brain development (407). MRI of patients with cortical blindness demonstrates increased signals in occipital white matter and cortex on T2-weighted images. With treatment, these tend to resolve over the ensuing weeks (408). The neurologic symptoms in uremia have been reviewed by Fraser and Arieff (409) and Smogorzewski (410).

Treatment and Prognosis

Treatment of uremia involves correction of electrolyte disturbance and maintenance of normal plasma composition. These have been greatly assisted by the use of dialysis. In some instances, neurologic symptoms can become aggravated after peritoneal dialysis or hemodialysis. Some workers have suggested that urea in the brain does not equilibrate freely with urea in blood, and therefore water enters the brain along an osmotic gradient. This is generally referred to as the *dialysis-dysequilibrium syndrome*. Gradual changes in blood electrolytes and earlier dialysis prevent some neurologic complications. In general, motor symptoms tend to improve once blood urea levels are lowered, whereas sensory symptoms tend to remain fixed. The sensory neuropathy does, however, respond dramatically to renal transplant (411). The correction of anemia by means of recombinant erythropoietin improves intellectual function (412).

Successful renal transplantation is associated with acceleration in head growth and improved intellectual functioning. Improvement can continue for more than 1 year after the transplant (413,414). Nevertheless, prospective studies of children with moderate to severe congenital renal disease indicate that both cognitive and motor developmental delay is common. Children who develop uremia in the first year of life often have microcephaly and significant cognitive impairment even if dialyzed and later transplanted (406,415). The younger the child, the greater the risk of this complication (416). This delay in brain growth reflects, in part, a toxic effect of uremia on brain growth and maturation, and, in part, chronic malnutrition, the various metabolic disturbances, and also any antecedent brain malformation. In the series of Bock and coworkers, approximately one-half of infants with congenital renal disease maintained normal development. In the remainder, development was delayed or deteriorated. Neither the cause for the renal disease nor its severity influenced the neurologic or cognitive status (417). Successful renal transplantation is associated with head growth and intellectual improvement (418,419). However, not all studies find better cognitive outcome following transplantation than that following dialysis (420).

Treatment of convulsions in uremic patients depends on the cause of the seizures. Seizures accompanying the dysequilibrium states are usually self-limiting and often can be prevented by close supervision of dialysis. Chronic seizures can be treated with phenobarbital or phenytoin, with recognition that serum protein binding, particularly for phenytoin, is reduced in uremia. As a result, therapeutic as well as toxic effects of the drug are encountered at lower serum levels than in patients who have normal renal function. Nevertheless, anticonvulsant activity can usually be achieved with the usual doses because the free fraction of phenytoin remains unchanged (421). No modification of carbamazepine clearance or bioavailability has been observed. In renal failure, the free fraction of valproate increases two- to threefold. However, the intrinsic metabolism of the drug is reduced so that the actual clearance remains normal. The metabolism of the various benzodiazepines is unaffected. Renal clearance of levetiracetam is up to 70% reduced in severe renal impairment; clearance of the drug generally correlates with creatinine clearance. Both phenytoin and phenobarbital are known to hasten the metabolism of corticosteroids and the immunosuppressant drugs cyclosporine and FK506. This causes ineffective immunosuppression in renal transplant recipients and reduced cadaver allograft survival (422). Hence, Wassner and coworkers have suggested that anticonvulsants not be administered to patients right after transplant unless absolutely essential, and if they are given, corticosteroid dosage should be increased accordingly (422). Alternatively, a benzodiazepine can be used. The various drug interactions are considered by Cutler (423). (See Chapter 14 for a discussion of anticonvulsant therapy of patients with renal failure.)

Complications of Treatment of Chronic Uremia

As a consequence of the various methods of therapy currently available for what at one time was considered an irreversible renal disease, various neurologic complications have been encountered.

Generally, neurologic complications are seen more frequently after hemodialysis than after peritoneal dialysis (424). Restlessness, headache, nausea, and vomiting are relatively common after more extreme adjustments of urea levels or acidosis. Seizures followed by impaired consciousness were seen in some 8% of patients subjected to dialysis before 1965, but they are now less common (424). These symptoms have been attributed to the osmotic gradient established when, as a consequence of the blood–brain barrier, urea is removed more rapidly from the blood than from the brain. Headaches also can be caused by impaired vascular regulation by damaged kidneys because bilateral nephrectomy resulted in complete relief of headaches in 70% of subjects despite continued dialysis (425).

Cerebral hemorrhages and central retinal vein occlusion are less common complications of hemodialysis (426).

With repeated dialyses, a variety of syndromes are encountered. Dialysis generally has little effect on brain water or on EEG (427). However, hemodialysis produces cytokine release (428), and patients may have headaches (429) or severe fatigue at the end of a session. As well, they may develop areas of osmotic demyelination or myelinolysis, notably central pontine myelinolysis (430). With time, these lesions generally disappear (431). Nutrition is a concern, and a few chronic dialysis patients have developed Wernicke's encephalopathy (432) that has been attributed to a deficiency of vitamins or other nutritional factors. Other nutritional deficiency syndromes include a peripheral sensorimotor neuropathy (burning feet or restless legs syndrome) (424) and leg cramps. Restless legs syndrome and leg cramps respond to vitamin supplementation; in particular, leg cramps respond to vitamin E, quinine, or to treatment with L-DOPA or dopamine agonists (433,434).

Eventually, almost all patients on chronic dialysis develop some electrophysiologic abnormalities, but these may be asymptomatic (435). Less often, patients develop mononeuropathy, cranial nerve palsies including optic neuropathy (436), and choreoathetosis. Patients may develop mononeuropathies resulting from placement of arteriovenous fistulas, including a rare but catastrophic ischemic monomelic neuropathy (437). Dialysis dementia is characterized by rapidly progressive speech disturbance, myoclonus, asterixis, seizures, and personality changes. Impaired bulbar function, weakness, and diffuse EEG abnormalities also can be seen (438). Untreated, the condition usually terminates in death within a few years (439). The role of aluminum in causing dialysis dementia is well established, and with modern techniques of water purification, this syndrome can be avoided (440).

A progressive encephalopathy with a clinical picture similar to dialysis dementia has been recognized in children who developed chronic renal insufficiency before 1 year of age and who have not been dialyzed. It is characterized by developmental delay, the evolution of microcephaly, seizures, hypotonia, and involuntary movements, including chorea and tremor (441,442). Various causes have been suggested for this clinical picture, including the oral ingestion of aluminum in the form of aluminum hydroxide, chronic malnutrition, and the neurotoxic effects of chronic renal failure during a vulnerable period of brain growth.

Another syndrome that is clinically indistinguishable from dialysis dementia is occasionally seen in uremic patients who develop acute hypercalcemia. It is easily reversed by normalizing calcium levels (443). The reversible posterior encephalopathy syndrome, mentioned in the preceding section, is common in children with glomerulonephritis and other rapidly evolving nephropathies. Seizures, cortical blindness, and unilateral motor deficits may accompany this. The patient may have normal or increased CSF pressure, normal fundi, or papilledema (444). Most children make a full neurologic recovery. The treatment of seizures associated with reversible posterial encephalopathy is usually not difficult; most patients respond to moderate doses of standard anticonvulsants.

The neurologic complications attending renal homotransplants are mainly the result of immunosuppressive therapy. Like the complications after hepatic transplants, considered earlier in this chapter, they include a variety of infections, notably fungal infections resulting from *Aspergillus* or *Candida* (445) and viral infections with cytomegalovirus and herpes simplex (446). The infectious and other complications of renal transplants are similar to those seen with liver transplants. Infection is the most frequent cause of late death in transplant patients.

In autopsy studies on renal transplant patients collected between 1968 and 1991, 58% of subjects who succumbed to infection died of bacterial infection, 27% of fungal infection, and 6% of viral infection (447). The clinical picture of these secondary infections is highlighted by disturbances of behavior and seizures. Fungal infections, in particular, are seen in children who have been on prolonged immunosuppressive therapy, and their appearance is unrelated to preexisting treatment with antibiotics. It is often difficult to establish an antemortem diagnosis. Imaging studies should be performed before lumbar puncture, which can be dangerous in the presence of a large brain abscess.

The neurologic complications of cyclosporine therapy for renal transplants are similar to those encountered after hepatic transplants but appear to be less frequent (448). Side effects of other immunosuppressants are covered in the section on liver transplantation.

Symptomatic hypoglycemia can develop in infants or children a few months to several years after transplantation. The etiology is probably multifactorial, but in the series of Wells and coworkers, almost all affected patients were receiving propranolol when they developed hypoglycemia. In such cases, propranolol should be discontinued and frequent feedings initiated (449).

Approximately 6% of renal homograft recipients, followed for up to 8 years, have developed neoplasms. The majority of these neoplasms has involved the CNS and includes reticulum cell sarcomas, lymphomas, and less commonly, Hodgkin disease (450,451).

Patients with chronic renal failure can develop nonconvulsive status epilepticus if they receive large doses of cephalosporins (452). The incidence of nonconvulsive seizures is increased in patients on chronic dialysis (453).

Hemolytic Uremic Syndrome

Hemolytic uremic syndrome, a heterogeneous group of disorders, is marked by microangiopathy, hemolytic anemia, and thrombocytopenia (454). Up to one-half of patients have neurologic symptoms, and some are left with permanent sequelae due to strokes and hemorrhages. A focally abnormal EEG may be prognostically useful (455). The classic or primary hemolytic uremic syndrome seen in infants or young children is in part the consequence of endothelial damage resulting from an infection, principally with the verotoxin-producing *Escherichia coli*, 0157:H7. Secondary hemolytic uremic syndrome, resulting from a variety of drugs, notably cyclosporine, is seen mainly in adults.

NEUROLOGIC COMPLICATIONS OF ENDOCRINE DISORDERS

Thyroid Gland

Pathology

The brain and thyroid act on each other reciprocally. The anterior hypothalamus controls the thyrotropic function of the pituitary by regulating thyroid-stimulating hormone secretion, which in turn is under feedback control by blood thyroxine or T_3 concentrations. Thyroid hormone is a major regulator of the various processes, such as dendritic arborization, axonal growth, synaptogenesis, neuronal migration, and myelination that are part of the final stage of brain differentiation. Thus, thyroid deficiency has an important effect on learning and behavior. A review of the role of thyroid hormone in brain development and of the molecular basis of the various actions of thyroid hormone in the developing brain is far beyond the scope of this book. The interested reader is referred to reviews by Dussault and Ruel (456), Bernal and coworkers (457), Oppenheimer and Schwartz (458), and Burrow and colleagues (459).

Thyroid Disease

Murray first reported the use of thyroid extracts for treatment of cretinism in 1891 (460). In 1972, Klein and coworkers reported that the timing of treatment for congenital hypothyroidism (CH) was crucial (461). In their experience, 78% of infants treated before 3 months of age had an IQ of 85 or better, whereas none of those treated after six months reached this level. Since clinical recognition of CH is difficult in the first days of life, it was not until the development of filter paper assays for thyroxine (T_4) and thyroid-stimulating hormone (TSH) that neonatal screening for CH became practical (462). Currently, all U.S. states and Canadian provinces screen for CH. Some regions use T_4 as their index, whereas others use TSH. Each approach has its limitations, but their discussion is beyond the scope of this text.

In essence, thyroid hormones act almost ubiquitously, but the brain's responsiveness to them is maximal during the last stages of development and maturation. During this period, thyroid hormones interact with specific receptors to alter genomic activity and affect synthesis of a variety of brain-specific proteins. In the human fetus, thyroxine is synthesized after 10 to 14 weeks' gestation. Because maternal thyroxine is unable to cross the placenta to any significant degree, an inability of the fetus to initiate or maintain thyroid synthesis can affect brain development during the latter part of gestation (463). Therefore, the degree of thyroid deficiency suffered by the athyrotic fetus influences the extent of intellectual retardation.

Structural abnormalities in the brain of hypothyroid individuals often incorporate characteristics of the immature organ. Both cerebrum and cerebellum partake of the developmental delay. As a consequence of increased neuronal cell death and defective oligodendrocyte differentiation, cortical neurons are smaller and fewer, axons and dendrites are hypoplastic, and myelination is retarded.

Hypothyroidism

Clinical Manifestations

The clinical picture of hypothyroidism depends on the degree of thyroid insufficiency and the time of its onset. With respect to neurologic symptoms, five clinical forms can be distinguished: (a) neonatal nongoitrous hypothyroidism, (b) congenital goitrous hypothyroidism, (c) goitrous hypothyroidism with deafness (Pendred syndrome), (d) endemic cretinism, and (e) congenital thyroid deficiency with muscular hypertrophy (Kocher-Debré-Sémélaigne syndrome). Central hypothyroidism due to brain abnormalities is unusual.

About 1 in 3500 newborns suffer from congenital hypothyroidism. In nongoitrous regions, approximately 80% to 85% of cases appear sporadically, while the remainder are hereditary (464). The most common sporadic etiology is thyroid dysgenesis (465). In this entity, the thyroid gland can be absent (agenesis), ectopically located, or hypoplastic. Most often, the thyroid gland is ectopic or hypoplastic rather than being totally aplastic. While in the majority of instances the pathogenesis of dysgenesis is unknown, some cases are the result of mutations in Dual oxidase (DUOX1) and the transcription factors PAX-8, TITF-1, and TTF-2. Loss of function mutations in the thyrotropin (TSH) receptor has been demonstrated in some familial forms of athyreosis. The various inborn errors of thyroxine T_4 biosynthesis are the most common hereditary causes for CH.

Almost all newborns with CH are asymptomatic. In neonatal nongoitrous hypothyroidism, the thyroid gland is absent or too small to keep the patient euthyroid. Only those with hereditary defects in thyroid hormone synthesis, maternal exposure to goitrogens, or iodine deficiency have large glands. At birth, symptoms of hypothyroidism are difficult to detect. A lingual thyroid may be visible at the base of the tongue, or a mass may be palpable in the neck. Affected infants tend to have a prolonged gestation and a birth weight greater than 4 kg. They also tend to have prolonged neonatal jaundice, abdominal distention, mottling of the skin, and decreased motor activity. The anterior and posterior fontanelles are typically large and are slow to close until thyroid replacement is started. Other causes for an unduly large anterior fontanel for age are cleidocranial dysostosis, achondroplasia, rickets, Down syndrome, and increased intracranial pressure. Osseous development is often retarded, and an umbilical hernia is present in approximately one-half of affected infants (466). Sensorineural hearing loss is present in at least 10% of these infants (467). Auditory brainstem-evoked responses can indicate a delayed wave I (468). The cause of the hearing loss is believed to result from developmental abnormalities of the cochlea.

Symptoms become more clear-cut by the second month of life. By then, infants are more obviously placid, with diminished spontaneous movements, generalized hypotonia, and a husky, grunting cry. The head appears large with coarse, lusterless hair and widely open sutures and fontanelle (Fig. 17.2). Motor and intellectual development is delayed. One-third of patients are spastic, uncoordinated, and experience cerebellar ataxia (469). The EEG also reflects delayed development of the brain (470).

A small proportion of CH patients have mutations of the TITF-1 (NKX2-1) gene and can have both CH and neonatal apnea and other respiratory problems, with subsequent development of choreoathetosis despite thyroid replacement (471,472).

When hypothyroidism develops after 3 years of age, intelligence is not irreversibly damaged. Impaired memory, poor school performance, and generalized slowing of movement and speech are prominent. The muscles are weak and pseudohypertrophic. A significant reduction in the speed of muscular contraction and relaxation can be demonstrated by electromyography (EMG) and can be visible on neurologic examination.

Several defects in the biosynthesis, storage, secretion, delivery, and use of thyroid hormone have been delineated. These entities are transmitted as autosomal recessive traits and are responsible for congenital goitrous hypothyroidism. De Felice and Di Lauro provide a detailed review of these conditions and their genetics (473).

The association of sensorineural deafness with goitrous hypothyroidism, Pendred syndrome, is transmitted as an autosomal recessive disorder (474–476). The condition is associated with mental retardation, developmental abnormalities of the cochlea, sensorineural hearing loss, and frequently, a diffuse thyroid enlargement or goiter. Most

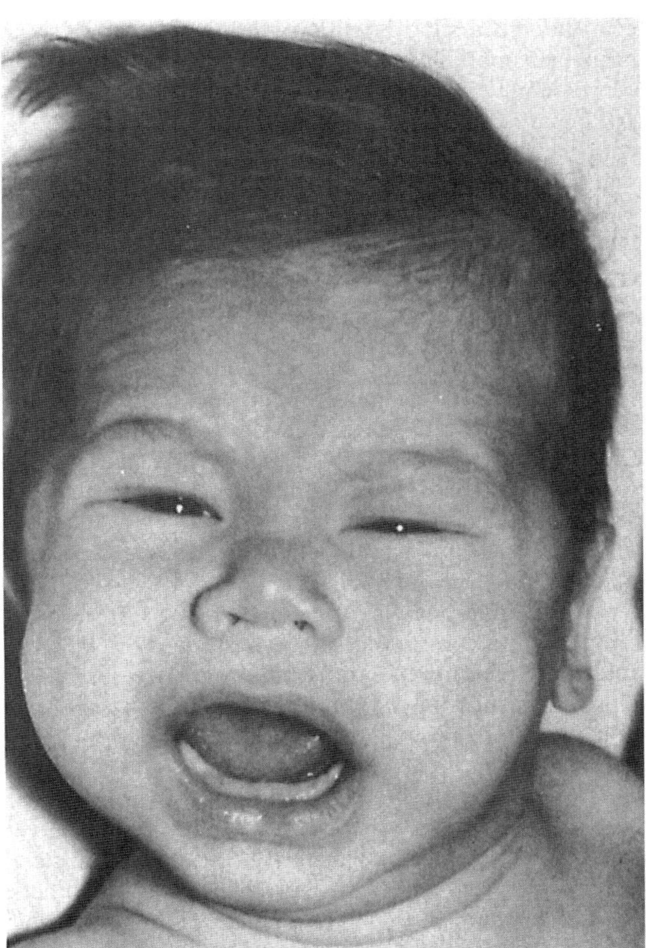

FIGURE 17.2. Congenital hypothyroidism. Five-month-old child presenting with developmental delay and hypotonia. Note the immature facies and coarse hair. Additionally, the anterior fontanelle was enlarged, the posterior fontanelle was still patent, and there was a hoarse cry and an umbilical hernia. A history of diminished motor activity was elicited as well.

subjects have enlargement of the vestibular aqueduct in their temporal bone (477). The condition, the most common syndromal form of deafness, accounts for an estimated 7.5% of childhood deafness. It is the consequence of a mutation in a gene coding for pendrin, an iodide transporter expressed in the apical membrane of thyroid follicular cells (478).

Endemic cretinism is by far the most prevalent form of hypothyroidism, affecting some 800 million people, mainly in Third World countries (479). It results from dietary iodine deficiency, which induces maternal hypothyroidism and deficient transfer of thyroid hormone across the placenta with ensuing fetal hypothyroidism. The neurologic picture includes a small head circumference; mental retardation; pyramidal tract signs; extrapyramidal deficits, notably focal or generalized dystonia; and a characteristic gait. The gait, which resembles that of parkinsonian patients, is marked by slow turning and reduced arm swing. Stance is broad based with flexion of hips and knees and knock-knees. Deafness, resulting from cochlear damage, is seen in as many as 90% of children with endemic cretinism and in some areas of the world can be the sole neurologic abnormality (480).

The CT scan discloses calcifications of the basal ganglia in 30% of subjects, principally those with severe and longstanding hypothyroidism. MRI demonstrates widening of the Sylvian fissures, a nonspecific developmental abnormality, and hyperintensity of the globus pallidus and substantia nigra on T1-weighted images (481). The selective vulnerability of these areas to thyroid deficiency has been postulated to reflect the density of T_3 receptors (482).

Supplementation of the maternal diet with iodine before the third trimester of pregnancy prevents the development of neurologic symptoms and improves psychologic development in offspring. Treatment during the third trimester is ineffective. These observations confirm experimental work showing the importance of thyroid hormone in neural differentiation and synaptogenesis (483).

Kocher, in 1892 (484), and Debré and Sémélaigne, in 1935 (485), described infants with an unusual combination of diffuse muscular hypertrophy and familial congenital thyroid deficiency. Cases continue to turn up (486), but they have never been seen in patients receiving adequate thyroid replacement. The condition is associated with a Herculean physique, but the child is not strong; rather, the muscles are stiff, and many children have cramps and mildly elevated serum creatine phosphokinase (CPK) values. The syndrome can be regarded as a special form of hypothyroid myopathy that improves greatly with thyroid replacement. The muscular hypertrophy is unexplained, for neither fiber enlargement nor an infiltrative process has been found with light or electron microscopy (487). Hoffman's syndrome of hypothyroidism, muscular pseudohypertrophy, and muscle stiffness (488) is a related adult disorder.

Transient hypothyroxinemia is common in premature infants and is believed to reflect hypothalamic-pituitary immaturity. In the study of Reuss and colleagues, preterm infants whose blood thyroxine concentrations were more than 2.6 standard deviations below the mean were at increased risk for cerebral palsy and developmental delay (489). The administration of thyroid hormone does not, however, improve neurodevelopmental outcome of these infants (490).

Untreated maternal hypothyroidism is known to adversely affect the child's intellectual development (491), and there is an inverse correlation between severity of maternal hypothyroidism and the child's IQ (492). In some cases, maternal antithyroid antibodies are responsible for CH (493). This antibody-mediated hypothyroidism can be transient (494).

Diagnosis

The diagnosis of congenital hypothyroidism should be considered in a child with developmental retardation. The infantile facies, protuberant abdomen, and dry hair and skin should evoke suspicion of the condition (495). The diagnosis can be confirmed by documenting retarded osseous development, delayed growth, and infantile bodily proportions. More specific are the determination of serum T_4 and T_3 concentrations and an elevated thyroid-stimulating hormone level.

In term babies, the suspicion of CH is aroused by the presence of at least two of its cardinal features: large size at birth, large posterior fontanel, respiratory distress, hypothermia, peripheral cyanosis, hypoactivity, poor feeding, delayed stooling, abdominal distension with vomiting, protracted icterus, and/or edema (466).

Treatment and Prognosis

Synthetic levothyroxine (Synthroid) is the accepted treatment of hypothyroidism. When treatment is started within the first weeks of life, somatic growth and head circumference is normal (496), but the prognosis for mental function is less clear-cut.

A meta-analysis of published data has concluded that in all studies, there was a trend toward lower IQ and poorer motor skills in infants with CH as compared with controls (497). The most important independent risk factor for eventual outcome was the severity of congenital hypothyroidism at the time of diagnosis as defined by the initial T_4 level and skeletal maturation. Age at start of treatment, dose of T_4, and plasma T_4 during treatment were less important in determining eventual cognitive development. It should be noted, however, that in the studies included for analysis, the mean age specified for the start of treatment ranged from 16 to 32 days (497). Children with CH who remain hypothyroid for the first 3 months of life frequently suffer residual cerebellar deficits and speech defects (498,499). One curious complication of excessive thyroid therapy for cretinism is the development of craniosynostosis (500).

Hyperthyroidism

Clinical Manifestations

Hyperthyroidism is frequently associated with neuromuscular disorders, but this is mostly a phenomenon of adult life. The condition is more common in girls than in boys; a quoted gender ratio is 6:1. Neuromuscular disorders seen in the course of hyperthyroidism include exophthalmic ophthalmoplegia, thyrotoxic myopathy, myasthenia gravis, and periodic paralysis (501–503). Some patients with hyperthyroidism can have ophthalmoplegia in the face of normal thyroid function (504).

Cerebral symptoms begin insidiously and at first are nonspecific. The child is irritable, nervous, unable to concentrate, has a short attention span, and does poorly in school. Exophthalmos is the most characteristic sign. It can be unilateral early in the disease and when severe is accompanied by papilledema and central scotomata. The chorea of hyperthyroidism can be continuous or paroxysmal (505); it is believed to be related to hypersensitivity of brain dopamine receptors in this condition (506). Tremors and increased deep tendon reflexes are seen in the more toxic children, and seizures, usually generalized, are encountered in a small proportion of children (507). Presentation in status epilepticus and coma also has been encountered (508). In some instances, previously diagnosed epilepsy can become more difficult to control. Cranial nerve palsies are rarely seen in childhood hyperthyroidism. Children with hyperthyroidism usually have enlarged thyroid glands, increased radioiodine uptake, and increased serum T_3 and T_4.

Thyrotoxicosis is occasionally associated with myasthenia gravis or with familial periodic paralysis (see Chapter 16). Antiadrenergic measures, such as β-blockers, are needed to control severe manifestations of hyperthyroidism in addition to antithyroid drugs. Details of treatment are beyond the scope of this text. Once thyroid function returns to normal, neuromuscular and most other neurologic symptoms remit.

Hyperthyroidism may cause premature closure of the sutures (craniosynostosis) (500).

Congenital hyperthyroidism is rare and often transient. The majority of such infants have hyperthyroid mothers. Others have gain of function mutations of the thyrotropin receptor gene (509,510). Long-term follow-up shows that a high proportion of infants with long-standing neonatal Graves disease have residual hyperactivity and major visuomotor deficits (511).

Thyroiditis may be associated with hyperthyroidism, or patients may be euthyroid or hypothyroid. Hashimoto's thyroiditis is an autoimmune thyroid disease associated with autoantibodies, such as antibodies to thyroid microsomal protein or thyroglobulin. The condition is at times accompanied by severe encephalopathy, confusion, seizures, abnormal CSF protein, and even increased intrathecal IgG synthesis (512–514). The encephalopathy is steroid responsive; seizures in these patients may respond to steroids and not to anticonvulsants (515). Thyroiditis is suggested by the presence of a symptomatic goiter in a euthyroid child. The clinical manifestations of thyroiditis can vary from symptoms suggesting hyperthyroidism to symptoms of hypothyroidism. The condition is uncommon in children, but the diagnosis should be kept in mind.

Parathyroid Gland

The neurologic symptoms of hypoparathyroidism and hyperparathyroidism are the direct or indirect result of disordered calcium metabolism and are, therefore, considered in the section dealing with the disturbances of electrolyte metabolism.

Adrenal Gland

Neurologic symptoms accompanying disorders of the adrenal gland are usually the result of disturbed serum electrolytes and osmolarity. They are referred to in another portion of this chapter. Adrenoleukodystrophy is discussed in Chapter 3. Addison's disease or adrenal insufficiency may be a feature of adrenoleukodystrophy or may have other etiologies. It has been associated with catatonia, vertigo, chorea, and papilledema (516). Some patients have encephalopathy, autoimmune thyroiditis, and adrenal insufficiency (517).

Allgrove syndrome is a rare, progressive autosomal recessive disorder that usually becomes symptomatic by age 10. Patients have adrenocorticotropic hormone (ACTH)–resistant adrenal insufficiency, achalasia, alacrima, hyperpigmentation, and hypoglycemia. Most subjects have mental retardation, pyramidal signs, ataxia, and other neurologic impairment (518). This disorder is due to mutations of the aladin or *AAAS* gene, whose function is unknown (519,520,520a).

Pituitary Gland

Neurologic symptoms associated with disorders of pituitary function can result from direct involvement of the perisellar and hypothalamic regions by a mass originating from the pituitary gland or neighboring structures (see Chapter 11). Less commonly, the neurologic picture evolves in conjunction with direct trauma or a destructive lesion affecting this area, such as occurs with histiocytosis X, sarcoidosis, or other granulomatous diseases.

MRI is superior to CT scans for detecting small masses in these regions. Cacciari and coworkers found that girls with precocious puberty who had its onset before age 2 are more likely to have lesions suggestive of hypothalamic hamartoma than those with precocious puberty of later onset, whose MRIs are generally normal (521). Reporting on a larger patient series, Ng and colleagues found that the age of onset of precocious puberty did not predict MRI results (522).

MRI is also useful in the evaluation of growth hormone deficiency (523–525). In a series of Agyropoulou and colleagues, approximately one-half of growth hormone–deficient children showed an interruption of the pituitary stalk with a gland of normal size (526). The significance of this finding is not clear, but interruption of the pituitary stalk can result from head injury, a prenatal developmental defect, or a perinatal insult (526,527). The likelihood of pituitary stalk interruption is greater when multiple hormones are deficient. In those cases, the adenohypophysis also is often absent or reduced in size (525). Other pituitary disorders are rarely associated with neurologic dysfunction. However, acromegaly is frequently accompanied by hypertrophic neuropathy (528) and lymphocytic or granulomatous hypophysitis (529). The latter condition can cause headache and visual field defects (530).

The Laurence-Moon-Bardet-Biedl syndrome is a clinically and genetically heterogeneous autosomal recessive disorder. As first described by Laurence and Moon, the condition is characterized by mental retardation, spinocerebellar ataxia, retinitis pigmentosa, progressive spastic paraparesis, and hypogonadism (531). Patients subsequently described by Bardet and Biedl suffered from mental retardation, retinitis pigmentosa, hypogonadism, obesity, and polydactyly (532). This group of disorders is clinically and genetically heterogeneous and has now been linked to at least eight different gene loci (533); most genes are associated with cilia, flagella, or centrioles. Inheritance is generally autosomal recessive. The Bardet-Biedl and Usher syndromes are the most prevalent syndromic forms of retinitis pigmentosa (RP) in North America; together, they make up almost a one-fourth of all RP patients (534).

Green and colleagues reviewed the syndrome in 28 Newfoundland patients (535); all had severe retinal dystrophy, but only 2 had typical RP. Obesity was seen in 96%, 58% had polydactyly, and 41% were mentally retarded. Many affected males had hypogonadism. Beales and coworkers studied 109 English patients and their families (536). In addition to the previously known signs and symptoms, they also identified neurologic, speech, and language deficits and behavioral traits, facial dysmorphism, and dental anomalies. Unaffected relatives had a significant incidence of renal anomalies and renal cell carcinoma. Beales and coworkers revised the diagnostic categorization to emphasize the phenotypical overlap with the disorder originally described by Laurence and Moon and proposed a unifying label: polydactyly-obesity-kidney-eye syndrome (536). Similar disorders are common in Arabs; many patients also have aminoaciduria and progressive renal failure as well as progressive visual failure (537). Most patients with the Bardet-Biedl and related syndromes have normal pituitary function; some, especially males, have hypothalamo-pituitary dysfunction, which is most marked in the realm of gonadotropins and gonadal function (538).

The Bardet-Biedl syndrome must be distinguished from the Alström syndrome, a condition in which RP, hypogonadism, obesity, and sensorineural hearing loss also are inherited in an autosomal recessive manner (539,540). The Biemond type II syndrome of iris coloboma, mental retardation, obesity, hypogenitalism, and postaxial polydactyly also is similar (541), as is the McKusick-Kaufman syndrome of hydrometrocolpos, hydronephrosis, postaxial polydactyly, and sometimes, Hirschsprung disease (542). The Online Mendelian Inheritance in Man (OMIM) Web site provides a good summary of these disorders and is regularly updated.

Polydactyly also is encountered as part of the various orofaciodigital syndromes (543,544). These disorders are often accompanied by cerebral defects, including callosal dysgenesis, heterotopic gray matter, hydrocephalus, and various posterior fossa anomalies, including agenesis or hypoplasia of the cerebellar vermis, or Dandy-Walker syndrome (545,546).

A syndrome of cerebral gigantism (Sotos syndrome), first described by Sotos in 1964 (547), is not rare. Sotos syndrome is associated with mental retardation and relatively distinctive facies with frontal bossing, hypertelorism, macrocrania, and prognathism. Birth weights usually exceed the 90th percentile, and growth is excessive in the first 4 to 5 years of life. Epilepsy and sexual precocity may be present (548). Cortical malformations can be demonstrated by MRI (549). School and learning difficulties are common, even if IQs fall in the normal range (550). These patients tend to improve as they become older.

The neuroimaging findings of Sotos syndrome often permit differentiation from other mental retardation syndromes with macrocephaly (549). In Sotos syndrome, the ventricles are almost always abnormal: Most common is a prominence of the trigone (90%), followed by prominence of the occipital horns (75%) and ventriculomegaly (63%). Various midline abnormalities also are noted; in particular, anomalies of the corpus callosum are quite common.

Most reported cases of Sotos syndrome have been sporadic and probably represent new mutations. Mutations, deletions and rearrangements of the NSD1 gene are found in almost all Sotos syndrome patients. This complex gene has many domains, one of which regulates the transcription of many other genes by histone acetylation. Sotos syndrome therefore is likely to be a genomic disorder, analogous to Rett syndrome (see Chapter 3) in which alterations of one gene derange the expression of other genes. One syndrome produces small heads and bodies; the other, large heads and bodies. De Boer and coworkers (551) found that facial appearance correlated with *NSD1* gene status patients with Sotos phenotypes. The best predictors for a *NSD1* alteration were frontal bossing, down-slanted palpebral fissures, pointed chin, and overgrowth. Patients with *NSD1* defects were more likely to have cardiac and feeding problems. No abnormality of pituitary hormone secretion has been found in Sotos syndrome.

The phenotypically overlapping but less common Weaver syndrome is marked by accelerated growth and osseous maturation, unusual craniofacial appearance, hoarse and low-pitched cry, and hypertonia with camptodactyly (552,553). Opitz and colleagues (553) reviewed the Sotos and Weaver syndromes and discussed the possibility that they represent a single genetic entity. From a phenotypic point of view, Weaver syndrome has more conspicuous contractures and a facial appearance that generally differs from that in Sotos syndrome. *NSD1* mutations are found in some patients with Weaver syndrome (554) as well as in a small minority of patients with the Beckwith-Wiedemann syndrome (BWS), another overgrowth syndrome (555). The cardinal features of the latter disorder are exomphalos, macroglossia, and neonatal gigantism. BWS patients are at increased risk of developing specific tumors, such as Wilms tumor, hepatoblastoma, and neuroblastoma (556). BWS also is covered in Chapter 4.

Septo-optic dysplasia (SOD) is a common congenital anomaly syndrome often associated with hypopituitarism and poor adrenal response to stress (557). It a heterogeneous disorder that varies greatly in severity and is loosely defined by any combination of optic nerve hypoplasia, pituitary gland hypoplasia, and midline abnormalities of the brain, including absence of the corpus callosum and septum pellucidum (558,559). As it frequently includes large defects of the cerebral mantle (schizencephaly), callosal defects, seizures, visual handicap, and variable degrees of mental retardation, the condition is covered in Chapter 5.

Growth failure is commonly seen in children who are severely retarded or who have other forms of serious and long-standing brain dysfunction. In the series of Castells and associates (560), the IQs of all children so affected were below 60, and the majority had severe microcephaly and a retarded bone age. In view of an impaired growth hormone response to a variety of stimuli, hypothalamic function appears to be faulty in at least some of these patients.

Several conditions in which delayed growth accompanies mental retardation have been described. Many of these also are associated with other neurologic features and with chromosomal disorders (see Chapter 4 for a more extensive discussion).

Diabetes

Of the neurologic complications of diabetes in children, the most common is an asymptomatic peripheral neuropathy. Its mechanism is discussed by Winegrad (561). Careful neurologic examination of juvenile diabetic patients can reveal slight distal weakness in the lower extremities, wasting of the interossei muscles, and diminished deep tendon reflexes. Conduction velocity in the peroneal nerve is abnormally slow in 11% of diabetic children between 8 and 15 years of age, even in the absence of clinical signs for peripheral neuropathy (562). Sensory changes are the most common electrophysiological findings. Somatosensory-evoked potentials from peroneal nerve stimulation are abnormal in some asymptomatic juvenile diabetics, suggesting additional abnormalities in spinal afferent transmission (563). The risk of diabetic neuropathy increases with patient age, duration of diabetes, and amount of hyperglycemia (564,565). In a study published in 1987, Kruger and colleagues found that proximal diabetic neuropathy was much better correlated with poor diabetic control than was peroneal or more distal neuropathy (566). This study confirmed the work of Hoffman and colleagues, which indicates that duration of diabetes, patient age, and diabetic control each significantly and independently influence the prevalence of delayed motor conduction in diabetic patients aged 6 to 23 years (565). Moreover, the presence of retinopathy in these patients correlates closely with the conduction velocity. Symptomatic diabetic polyradiculopathy is rare in juvenile diabetes (566,568). Nocturnal abdominal, leg, or foot pain may be troublesome. It can develop after rapid achievement of glycemic control. This is called *insulin neuritis*, and it occurs in type II diabetes as well (569). Diabetic cranial nerve palsies have not been seen in children.

Cognitive impairment may be seen in children whose diabetes begins before age 5 and who have frequent hypoglycemic episodes (570). Hypoglycemic episodes after age 5 are less clearly linked to cognitive impairment. A group of 90 Australian children with type I diabetes scored lower than control children on measures of intelligence, attention, processing speed, long-term memory, and executive skills. These effects were greatest in children whose diabetes began before age 4 (571).

Neurologic symptoms also are seen in diabetic coma, in the course of treatment of diabetic ketoacidosis, and in hyperosmolar nonketotic diabetic coma. The cause of neurologic impairment in diabetic ketoacidosis (DKA) is not well understood. Kety reported in 1948 that cerebral oxygen uptake was significantly reduced during DKA in adults despite increased cerebral blood flow and normal arterial oxygen saturation (572). The extent of decrease in cerebral oxygen uptake correlated with the degree of obtundation. The correlation between state of consciousness and pH was much weaker, and patients can remain alert even though there is marked acidosis during DKA (573). The concentration of ketone bodies, spinal fluid pH, and the degree of hyperosmolality also correlate poorly with mental status (574). It appears, therefore, that a multitude of factors, including brain intracellular pH, impaired oxygen use, hyperosmolality, and disseminated intravascular coagulation inducing localized areas of cerebral hyperperfusion act jointly to cause the depression of sensorium.

A number of deaths from irreversible cerebral edema have occurred in the course of apparently adequate treatment of DKA (575). About 1% of pediatric cases of DKA are associated with clinically obvious cerebral edema with compression of cerebral cisterns (576,577). These patients have significant mortality and risk of residual impairment (577) and often respond poorly to treatment (578). Neither the use of bicarbonate, nor the rate of decline of glucose, or excessive secretion of antidiuretic hormone, or the rate of fluid administration is responsible for the development of cerebral edema (579).

Duck and colleagues have proposed that a rapid reduction of blood hyperosmolality with treatment and a slower change in the cerebral hyperosmolality owing to the presence of substances termed *idiogenic osmoles* can result in the entrance of water into the brain and consequent cerebral edema (576). Van der Meulen and coworkers hypothesized that cell swelling during treatment of diabetic ketoacidosis results from conditions favoring the activation of the sodium-potassium exchanger, a plasma-membrane transport system that regulates cytoplasmic pH. Apparently, weak organic acids, such as ketoacids and free fatty acids, present in cytoplasm, are known to activate the exchanger, which, in the presence of extracellular sodium, leads to cell swelling (580). These theories all assume that cerebral edema is primarily intracellular. However, recent diffusion-perfusion MRI studies cast serious doubt on this concept (581). Glaser and colleagues studied 14 children during treatment for DKA and after recovery, using apparent diffusion coefficients (ADCs) and measures of cerebral perfusion. They found significantly elevated ADCs in all regions except the occipital gray matter, where it was decreased. Mean transit times were decreased, and the perfusion data suggested increased cerebral blood flow during DKA with normalization in the follow-up study. However, none of their patients had compression of cisterns or clinical evidence of cerebral edema, suggesting that symptomatic cerebral edema develops when a "second hit" is added to the initial clinically silent changes documented by Glaser and colleagues (581). The increased ADCs found in all patients during the acute stage suggest increased extracellular or interstitial fluid (vasogenic edema). The difference between increased extracellular fluid and blood flow in most brain regions and simultaneous decreases in ADC and perfusion in the occipital gray matter brings us back to reversible posterior encephalopathy, so common in renal disease and in patients on immunosuppressant treatment. The posterior cerebral circulation could be ischemic at the same time that excessive perfusion and extracellular fluid accumulation occurs in the carotid territory. This disparity can be explained by the different sympathetic innervations of the vertebro-basilar and carotid circulations (582). Our understanding of regional differences in cerebral autoregulation and autonomic control remains very limited, but if cerebral edema indeed results from hypoxic injury and cytotoxic mediators, additional treatment in addition to insulin and fluids could be of help (579).

Prediction and diagnosis of cerebral edema is difficult because characteristic clinical or biochemical features are lacking, and neuroimaging studies indicate that subclinical cerebral edema is fairly common during therapy of diabetic ketoacidosis in the pediatric age group but uncommon in patients over age 20 years (578). Rather, a patient's failure to recover consciousness, despite adequate treatment with insulin and fluids, will suggest the presence of cerebral edema.

Dexamethasone has been used in treatment of cerebral edema, but in my experience, it is usually given too late to be effective. Mannitol, administered as soon as cerebral edema is diagnosed, might be more beneficial (583). In any case, the incidence of death or neurologic handicap is quite high even with the most expert care.

Nonketotic hyperosmolal diabetic coma is rare in children. Neurologic symptoms are believed to result from brain swelling, but this is surely an oversimplification (584). In addition to impaired consciousness, patients can develop hemiparesis and generalized or focal seizures. Movement disorders, including eye movement disorders such as opsoclonus-myoclonus, may accompany nonketotic hyperglycemic coma or stupor more often in adults than in children (585).

Nonketotic hyperglycemic coma has been treated successfully with low-dose insulin infusion while intracranial pressure is monitored (586).

The neurologic complications of hypoglycemia are discussed at another point in this chapter.

The Wolfram syndrome is an autosomal recessive syndrome of early onset diabetes, progressive optic atrophy, sensorineural hearing loss, anosmia, ataxia, and peripheral neuropathy (587,588). Insulin-dependent diabetes mellitus and bilateral progressive optic atrophy are necessary to make this diagnosis. Both may present in childhood, adolescence, or early adult life; diabetes mellitus usually comes first. Other neurologic symptoms in Wolfram homozygotes include hearing loss, urinary retention, ataxia, peripheral neuropathy, mental retardation, dementia, and psychiatric illnesses (588).

Lipoatrophic diabetes or congenital generalized lipodystrophy, the Berardinelli-Seip syndrome, is a rare autosomal recessive disease characterized by a near total absence of adipose tissue from birth or early infancy and severe insulin resistance. Other features include acanthosis nigricans, accelerated linear growth, muscular hypertrophy, hepatomegaly, and mild mental retardation (589). This syndrome is usually due to mutations in *BSCL2*, the gene encoding seipin, an integral membrane protein of the endoplasmic reticulum (590). Mutations in this gene also are associated with a form of hereditary spastic paraparesis accompanied by amyotrophy of the hand muscles (Silver syndrome).

NEUROLOGIC COMPLICATIONS OF HEMATOLOGIC DISEASES

Anemia

Neurologic symptoms accompanying anemia usually result from cerebral hypoxia. They include irritability, listlessness, and impaired intellectual function. The relationship between the various hemoglobinopathies, coagulopathies, and stroke is reviewed by Grotta and coworkers (591) and by Chan and deVeber (592).

The effects on neurodevelopmental outcome of chronic iron deficiency anemia experienced during the first two years of life have been a matter of some debate. In the Chilean experience of Walter and colleagues, developmental test performance, particularly on language items, was impaired in children whose hemoglobin values had been below 10.5 g for more than three months. Correction of the iron deficiency failed to improve the performance scores (593). Similar results have been obtained from other parts of the world. Costa Rican children treated for iron deficiency anemia as infants still showed significant cognitive differences from controls at age 5, when all had normal hematological indices (594). Iron supplementation of relatively healthy elementary school children with iron deficiency anemia improved their cognitive function; this improvement correlated poorly with changes in hemoglobin (595). Supplementation of Third World infants with iron and zinc improves behavior and increases exploratory activity without measurable effects on hemoglobin (596). It is likely that iron has some effects on the brain independent of its red cell function and that chronic anemia of any cause has mild negative effects on development. Like the effects of lead, these results are confounded by a variety of environmental and particularly socioeconomic factors (597). Some of these aspects are covered in Chapter 18.

Congenital Aplastic Anemia (Fanconi's Anemia)

Congenital aplastic anemia is an autosomal recessive disorder is a heterogenous syndrome, with at least nine complementation groups having been delineated (598). It is characterized by the inadequate proliferation or differentiation of hematopoietic stem cells. Clinically, it is marked by association of pancytopenia and bone marrow hypoplasia with a variety of congenital anomalies (599). These include skeletal defects, growth retardation, microcephaly, microphthalmus, ptosis, facial weakness, strabismus, deafness, and malformations of ears, kidneys, and heart (600). Generalized hyperpigmentation and café-au-lait spots are seen in 51% and 23% of children, respectively. Both types of skin lesions can be present as well. Approximately 20% of children with Fanconi's anemia develop malignancies, including leukemia and brain tumors (601). Most patients are neurologically normal, but there is increased incidence of aqueductal stenosis, agenesis of the corpus callosum and septum pellucidum, and holoprosencephaly (602). A few children present with medulloblastoma as the first sign of Fanconi's anemia (603).

Hereditary Hemoglobinopathies

Sickle Cell Disease

Sickle cell (SC) disease results from a genetic, structural abnormality of hemoglobin that is found predominantly in individuals of African ancestry but also may be found in individuals of Mediterranean, Indian, and midwestern descent. In the United States, it occurs mainly in blacks (approximately 1 in 600) and in Hispanics of Caribbean or South American origins. Sickle cell in the homozygous state (SS) or in combination with another hemoglobin disorder may result in significant morbidity and mortality.

TABLE 17.14 First Adverse Events in 392 SS or Sickle-$\beta^{\circ}0$ Thalassemia Children Followed from Age 3 Months between 1988 and 1998

Incidence of First Adverse Events		
Adverse Event	*Number of Patients (%)*	*Mean Age Event First Occurred (yrs)*
More than 2 painful crises/yr	17 (24)	7.9 ± 3.7
More than 1 episode acute chest syndrome/yr	10 (14)	3.5 ± 1.0
Stroke	25 (36)	6.1 ± 3.4
Death	18 (26)	5.1 ± 3.7
Total having any events	70	5.9 ± 3.6

From Miller et al. (617).

SC disease has two harmful effects: Chronic hemolysis produces tissue hypoxia and cytokine activation, and a vaso-occlusive process produces focal ischemia in the brain and in many other organs. Serious neurologic problems occur primarily in patients with SS or S Beta$^+$ thalassemia (at least 29%) and less frequently in those with SC disease (approximately 5%) or S Beta$^+$ thalassemia (604–606). At least 25% of children with sickle cell have evidence of sickle-related neurovascular disease during the first decade of life, and some are younger than 2 years of age at diagnosis (607–609). Other problems, often associated with cerebral vascular disease, include an increased incidence of epilepsy and cognitive impairment, frequent headaches, myelopathy, and neuropathy (607).

The extent of the vascular occlusive problem can be delineated by neuroimaging studies. Wang and colleagues studied 39 SS children, 7 to 48 months old with MRI and magnetic resonance angiography (MRA) (610). None had a history of clinical stroke, although three had a history of seizures. The overall prevalence of CNS abnormalities in asymptomatic children was 11%. One patient had a silent infarct and a stenotic lesion on MRA; three others had arterial stenoses. The three seizure patients had infarcts. The results of this study illustrate the underlying problem, namely that although most SS patients do not have cerebral vascular disease, those who do often begin with silent infarcts (611) and have their first infarct before age 10 (612).

Kirkham and colleagues have attempted to predict strokes in SC disease by monitoring patients for nocturnal hypoxemia (613). In their experience, both mean overnight oxygen saturation and high flow velocity in the internal carotid or middle cerebral artery independently predicted CNS events. Sleep-disordered breathing is a known risk factor for stroke in the general population (614) and causes platelet activation and elevated serum C-reactive protein (615). Nocturnal oxygen desaturation also predicts a high incidence of pain crises in SC disease (616).

Sickle cell cerebral vascular disease (SCCVD) involves both large and small vessels and begins early in life. Miller and coworkers have documented the age at which the first adverse events make their appearance (Table 17.14) (617). In his series, 6.4% of children suffered a stroke by age 11 years. This was the most common major event, although a much larger number of children had at least one pain crisis.

The rate of clinical strokes is greatest in SS homozygotes and next highest in SC patients. The chances of a first clinically apparent stroke by age 20, 30, and 45 years of age is 11%, 15%, and 24% for SS and 2%, 4%, and 10% for SC patients. It is even lower for the S-^{2}-thalassemia patients (612). No protective effect of Hb F was found in this series, although it has been found in other studies.

Sickle hemoglobin causes neurovasculopathy by changing the shape and rheology of the red cell (618). Sickle red cells are more adherent to the endothelium than normal red cells, even when the hemoglobin is oxygenated. When it is deoxygenated, the process is markedly enhanced and the red cells become rigid and sickle in shape. There is evidence that under intra-arterial pressure the jet stream of blood containing sickle cells is sufficient to cause endothelial damage and start thrombosis (619). Intimal proliferation occurs, narrowing the vascular lumen. Blood flow, which is more rapid than normal because of the anemia, is even more rapid through the narrower lumen, bombarding the distal endothelium with sickle cells at an increasingly higher rate (619). The reason the young child is especially susceptible to CNS damage from sickling may be that the higher oxygen requirement of the child's brain necessitates a much higher blood flow than is required by the older child or adult (620).

Neuropathologic findings include widespread narrowing of the major cerebral arteries, smaller vessels, and distal microvasculature as a result of endothelial proliferation. This is sometimes accompanied by focal dilatation, thrombosis, neovascularization, and hemorrhage (609,619,620). Most infarcts are located in the major arterial border zones, confirming that the primary pathogenic mechanism is large vessel disease with distal hypoperfusion, and that distal small vessel disease accounts for only

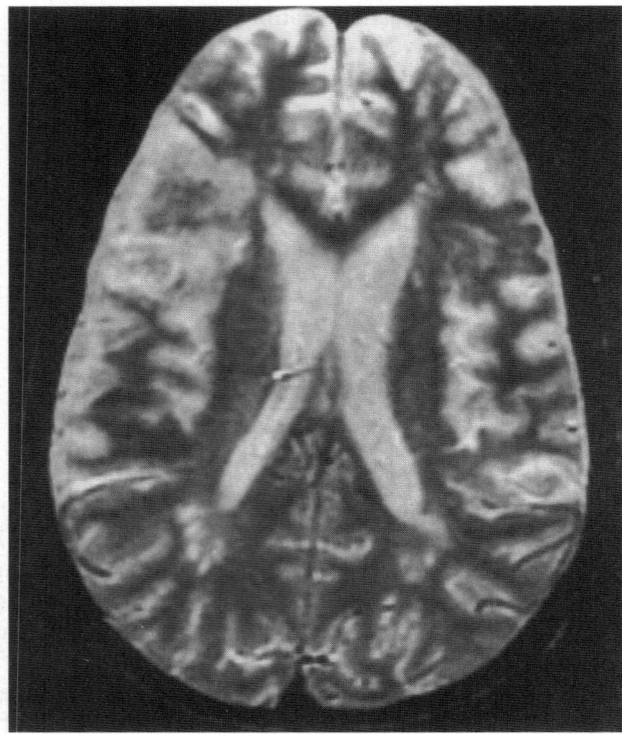

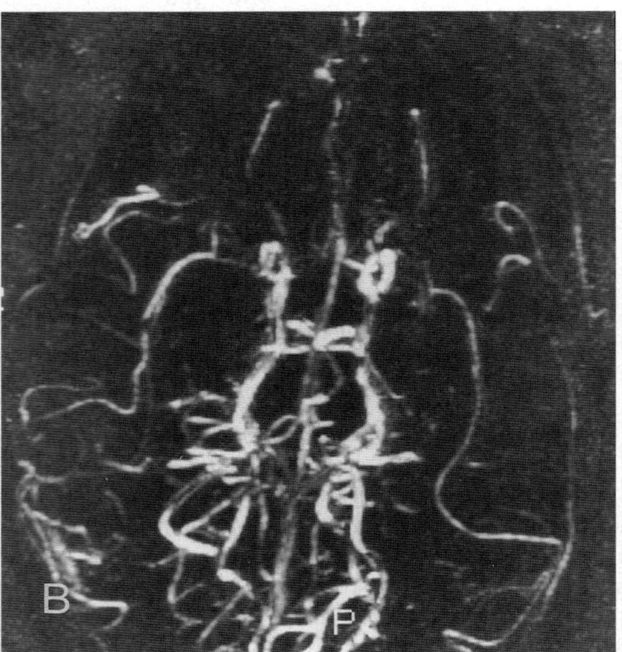

FIGURE 17.3. **A:** Sickle cell disease. This T2-weighted axial magnetic resonance image (2,000/80/1) demonstrates extensive patchy hyperintensity bilaterally in the distribution of the middle cerebral artery. The lesions are consistent with the clinical history of repeated episodes of stroke in this 9-year-old girl. (Courtesy of Dr. John Curran, Department of Radiology, UCLA Center for the Health Sciences, Los Angeles.) **B:** Magnetic resonance angiography in the same child demonstrates a severe loss of arterial supply in the middle cerebral artery distribution bilaterally. (Courtesy of Dr. John Curran, Department of Radiology, UCLA Center for the Health Sciences, Los Angeles.)

a minority of symptoms of cerebral ischemia (Fig. 17.3A) (621,622). In another neuropathologic study, infarcts were found in 50% of autopsied brains and were most extensive in the distal perfusion areas of the internal carotid arteries, particularly in the boundary zone between the anterior and middle cerebral artery boundary zone (623). For patients with a history of overt stroke, lesions were typically in the cortex and deep white matter, whereas in patients with silent stroke, they were confined to the deep white matter (624). The most common areas of infarction and ischemia were frontal lobe (78%), parietal lobe (51%), and temporal lobe (15%). Lesions in the occipital lobe, cerebellum, and brainstem were uncommon. However, posterior circulation infarcts and reversible posterior encephalopathy are seen in the special setting of acute chest syndrome (625). Serum levels of endothelin-1 are much increased in that setting (626). Among patients with lesions of infarction and ischemia, both hemispheres were affected in 60%, and 20% each had an affected right or left hemisphere. Generalized, focal, or both kinds of atrophy were present in 30 (14%) of the SS patients and 5 (5%) of the SC patients. Twenty of these also had lesions of infarction and ischemia (624).

Genetic factors influence the risk of SCCVD in patients with HbS; the stroke status of siblings is usually similar (627). Studies show an association between polymorphisms in TNF and IL4R (interleukin 4 receptor) genes and large vessel disease in SS, and between VCAM1, a cell adhesion molecule, and small vessel disease in SS patients (628). These data need confirmation from larger studies. These same genes could contribute to risk of stroke in neonatal and other hypoxic brain injuries. Alpha thalassemia is known to reduce the risk and severity of stroke in SC disease (629).

Occlusion or segmental narrowing of the larger arteries or veins can be demonstrated by MRI and MR angiography (Fig. 17.3B) (630). Both large and small vessel disease usually occur in combination (619). At times, neovascularization presents a moyamoya pattern (620,631). This picture of exuberant collaterals is associated with distal stenosis and occlusion of the internal carotid artery, and with risk for late hemorrhages (605,632). Transfusion therapy, if started early, reduces the risk of developing the moyamoya pattern, although once present, the risk of more strokes is high, even with transfusion therapy (632). Some SCCVD patients with moyamoya pattern have improved with encephaloduroarteriosynangiosis (EDAS) (633), but no controlled trials have been conducted.

Cerebral infarction is the most frequent complication in SC disease and occurs most often in children (634,635), whereas intracranial hemorrhage affects more adults than children. Both processes can occur simultaneously (605,619). Intracranial hemorrhage in children is usually subarachnoid and has a higher mortality than infarction (634). Hemorrhage may result from an aneurysm in the circle of Willis and be amenable to surgery (635).

Neurologic problems can be acute or chronic. The acute problems are emergencies and require immediate diagnosis and treatment. They include bacterial meningitis, the consequences of increased susceptibility to infection, overt stroke, or transient focal signs or symptoms of neurologic deficit. Stroke occurs most frequently and can be an isolated event or in combination with a sickle cell crisis, especially after a transient ischemic attack or acute chest syndrome, infection, transfusion, or other systemic illness. Findings include changes in sensorium, focal seizures, aphasia, transient weakness or inability to move an extremity, paresthesia of an extremity, ataxia, and homonymous hemianopia. These findings can be irreversible or transient, but those that are transient may be caused by vasospasm and in most instances precede an overt clinical stroke (605). As patients grow older, strokes in SS patients change from mostly ischemic to mostly hemorrhagic (612). Some of these hemorrhages are from aneurysms, which are more frequent in SC disease (636,637); others are late hemorrhages from moyamoya collaterals (605). Spinal cord infarction, mononeuropathies, and multiple cranial neuropathies also have been reported (638). Some patients have intracranial bruits because of hyperplastic marrow in the skull. Skull infarction and epidural hematomas may complicate SC disease (639). Proptosis and periorbital swelling may be manifestations of vaso-occlusive disease (640).

Chronic neurologic symptoms include headaches and the residua of prior infarcts or brain hypoperfusion such as seizures, and a variety of cognitive deficits including short attention span, delayed speech development, and behavior and school learning problems. Cognitive deficits occur more frequently in children with SC disease than in their siblings or in other healthy children (606). Imaging studies have confirmed that many of the children with cognitive deficits had experienced silent strokes (606,624,635). Seizures can result from an acute infarction or be part of a chronic process often in association with other neurologic abnormalities. Severe headaches can occur with intracranial hemorrhage, be related to increased cerebral blood flow, or be unrelated to SC disease (604,641).

In the acute stroke setting, SS patients should be transfused to reduce the percentage of HbS-containing cells. Exchange transfusion is best if feasible (610). However, no controlled trials comparing acute stroke treatments have been conducted. Because neurologic problems are among the most frequent and devastating complications and in many instances can be prevented, present-day management of SS patients is directed toward their prevention (604).

Transfusions are the mainstay of long-term therapy. Some patients revert to normal flow rates and vascular anatomy after years on transfusion therapy (642). Others continue to have abnormal transcranial Doppler (TCD) and MRA findings and are at risk for stroke if transfusions are stopped (643). Adams and others showed that SS children had flow abnormalities detectable by TCD before the appearance of infarcts and that transfusion therapy could prevent the development of infarcts and progressive cerebrovascular disease (644,645). This important finding means that the incidence of SCCVD can be reduced significantly with treatment. Hydroxyurea treatment was shown in 1995 to reduce the frequency of pain crises and acute chest syndrome, both more related to vaso-occlusive phenomena than to hemoglobin level (646). Hydroxyurea is believed to act by increasing fetal hemoglobin production, making the red cells less prone to sickling. Whether it can prevent or arrest the evolution of SCCVD is unknown (647). Chronic transfusion therapy has significant risks, including infection and iron overload (648). In addition, strokes and seizures can occur when patients are transfused for vaso-occlusive events such as priapism (649). Despite these adverse reactions, it has become evident that there is a return to high risk of stroke in children who stopped receiving the transfusions, and the National Heart Lung and Blood Institute has advised physicians that stopping transfusions cannot be recommended.

Bone marrow transplantation and stem cell transplants offer cures for SC disease, but at a price. Strokes and seizures occur during the peritransplant period (650). Allogeneic stem cell transplants come from another person and therefore require immunosuppression. If transplants are preceded by myeloablative chemotherapy to wipe out the host marrow, long-term adverse consequences are common because drugs that kill host marrow generally cause some CNS cell death. Adverse effects are most obvious in the growth and endocrine areas, but when children receive drugs like busulfan, brain ventricles enlarge, and delayed development is common. Nonmyeloablative protocols should have less negative effects on development. Anti-inflammatory drugs and endothelin antagonists are symptomatic treatments that have never been adequately evaluated in patients with SC disease.

We cannot expect transfusions to reduce late hemorrhages for many years because it takes years for the moyamoya pattern to evolve. Cerebral aneurysms in SC disease are unusual because they are often multiple and disproportionately involve the posterior circulation (637). Angiographic and imaging details of SCCVD are discussed by Moritani and coworkers (651). MRA shows smaller cerebral vessels less well than does CT angiography, which requires a contrast infusion (633).

SC disease patients often have pain crises and receive opioids for pain control. Use of meperidine in patients with a history of stroke, severe headache, or seizures is associated with greater risk of seizure than use of other opioids, such as morphine (652). This is because normeperidine, a major meperidine metabolite, is epileptogenic (653).

Fat embolism is another neurologic disorder associated with SC disease. Bone marrow necrosis may complicate leukemia and occurs in SC disease during acute chest wall syndrome and other vaso-occlusive crises (654). Fat from the marrow may embolize to the lungs, brain, and other organs with dire consequences (655,656). Cerebral fat embolism is most commonly seen in long bone fractures.

Recurrent headaches are common in SC disease and all severe anemias (608). Many patients describe pounding headaches consistent with migraine without aura. These respond well to nonsteroidal anti-inflammatory drugs (NSAID) and other remedies for migraine. The use of ergots and triptans is probably more risky in this patient group than in ordinary migraine patients. Headache in SC disease may be due to sinovenous thrombosis and occasionally to pseudotumor cerebri (657).

SC disease may be complicated by myelopathy and peripheral neuropathy. Spinal cord compression by bony disease, epidural abscess, or extramedullary hematopoiesis occurs in SC disease and thalassemia (658). Ischemic mononeuropathy is well known (659) and can involve the mental nerve, producing a non-neoplastic numb chin syndrome (660).

Sickle cell trait is generally not associated with shortening of the life span (661), but tolerance to high altitude, strenuous exercise, and severe hypoxia is reduced (662). Such patients have somewhat increased incidence of splenic infarcts (663) and possibly of strokes (664). They tolerate hyperventilation for EEG studies well, but SC disease patients should not be hyperventilated because this procedure occasionally precipitates a stroke (655).

Thalassemias

The thalassemias are a heterogeneous group of hemoglobin synthesis defects, mostly due to globin gene mutations. They vary greatly in severity and are less likely to be accompanied by neurologic problems than is SC disease. Readers may consult a comprehensive review by Orkin and Nathan for details (666). One-third of patients homozygous for β-thalassemia have myalgia, a myopathy with weakness and wasting of the proximal muscles in the lower extremities, hyporeflexia, and a myopathic EMG pattern (667). On muscle biopsy, a moderate variation in fiber size is seen, with fiber atrophy and preponderance of type 1 fibers (668). Because serum vitamin E levels are low in many such children, treatment with the vitamin should be considered. The incidence of strokes and venous thromboembolic events is somewhat higher in patients with moderate to severe thalassemia than in control subjects (669). High-dose deferoxamine, used for iron chelation in patients with thalassemia and congenital hypoplastic anemia, can lead to visual and auditory neurotoxicity characterized by decreased visual acuity, loss of color vision, deafness, and abnormal visual- and auditory-evoked potentials. Partial or complete recovery can be seen after discontinuation of the drug (670). A symmetrical motor sensory neuropathy is reported in some thalassemic patients (671). Spinal cord compression by extramedullary hematopoiesis has been reported (672). Neuroimaging studies demonstrate an extradural block. Surgical decompression and localized irradiation are recommended for this complication (672,672a). Some patients with thalassemia and this form of spinal cord compression respond well to transfusions or to hydroxyurea (672b).

The association of mental retardation and α-thalassemia was first reported by Weatherall and coworkers. The subjects were of northern European extraction, regions where thalassemia is rare (673). Two distinct syndromes have been recognized. In one group, extensive deletions of chromosome 16p could be detected. These subjects exhibit mild to moderate mental retardation accompanied by a variety of dysmorphic features. The other group is an X-linked condition in which mental retardation is more severe. In these children, the clinical features have been striking. They include microcephaly, hypertelorism, midface hypoplasia with a pouting lower lip, and hypotonia (Fig. 17.4A). Anemia is usually not severe, and this syndrome can best be diagnosed by demonstrating the presence of hemoglobin H in red cells. All affected cases have been male, and the condition is transmitted as an X-linked trait (674). It is caused by mutations of the ATRX gene at Xq13 (675). The protein is a helicase and functions as a global transcriptional regulator (676). It is associated with many mental retardation syndromes, including Carpenter syndrome (acrocephalopolysyndactyly type II) and Smith-Fineman-Myers syndrome. I suspect that the ATRX syndrome is not at all rare, but the anemia is frequently not marked, and hemoglobin H is not invariably detected by electrophoresis and requires special staining techniques. For this purpose, fresh venous blood is incubated for at least 4 hours or preferably overnight at room temperature, with an equal volume of 1% brilliant cresyl blue in 0.9% saline. Inclusions are seen in 0.8% to 40.0% of cells (Fig. 17.4B) (677). Hemoglobin H disease has a relatively high prevalence in Asians; it is seen sporadically in Mediterranean populations. Optimally, severely retarded male subjects in these ethnic groups should be screened for the presence of hemoglobin H.

Congenital Hemolytic Anemia

Several forms of congenital hemolytic anemia have been associated with neurologic deficits, most commonly

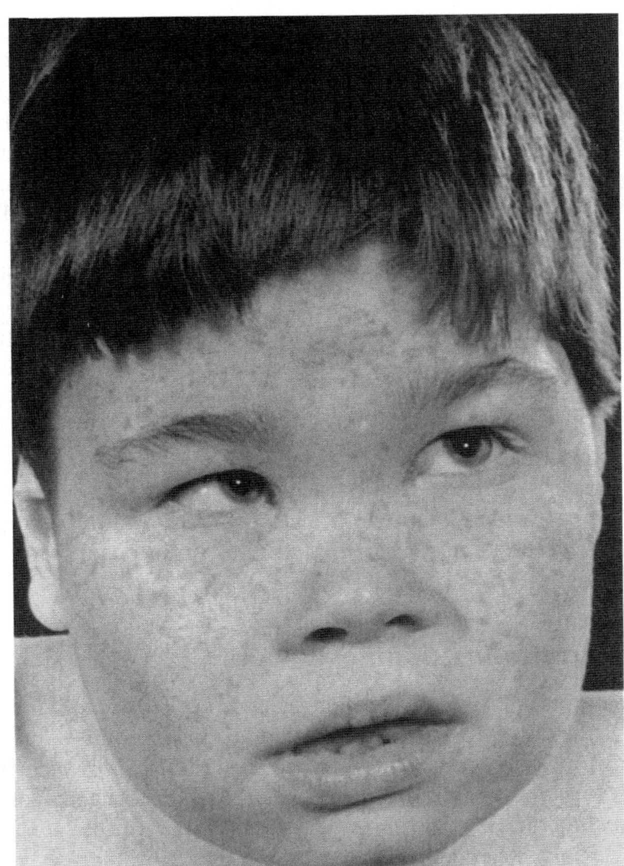

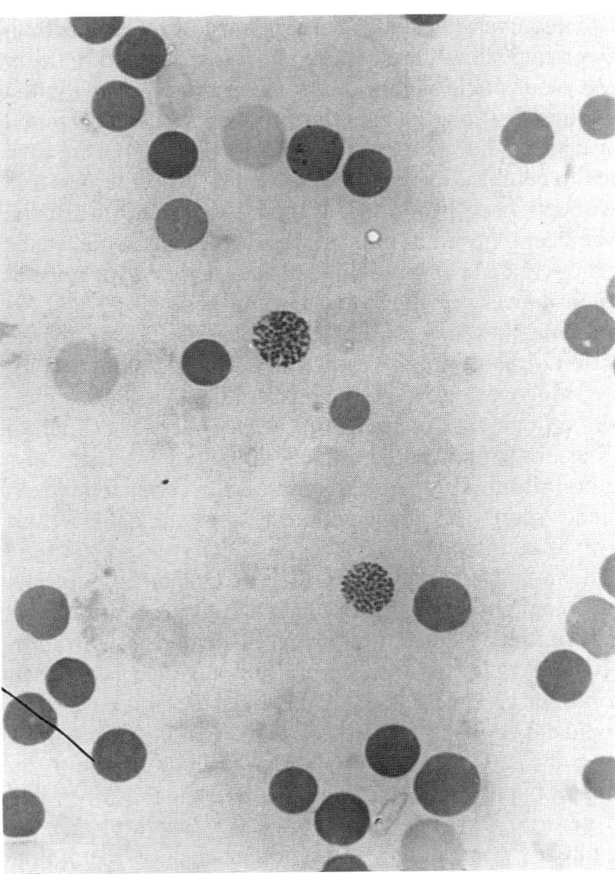

FIGURE 17.4. **A:** Eight-year-old boy with hemoglobin H disease. He has hypotonia, seizures, and severe mental retardation. Appearance is marked by microcephaly, relative hypertelorism, depressed nasal bridge, a pouting lower lip, and a small, triangular nose with anteverted nares. **B:** Blood smear stained with 1% brilliant cresyl blue, showing hemoglobin H inclusions. (Courtesy of Drs. Richard Gibbons and Douglas R. Higgs, MRC Molecular Haematology Unit, John Radcliffe Hospital, Oxford, England.)

developmental retardation. In all of these forms, the enzymatic defect affects red cell glycolysis. Muscle glycolysis also can be defective. In the most common of these disorders (pyruvate kinase deficiency), neurologic symptoms result from kernicterus as a consequence of severe neonatal jaundice. Deficiency of erythrocyte phosphoglycerate kinase, an X-linked disorder, causes hemolytic anemia of variable severity and is accompanied by a slowly progressive extrapyramidal disease characterized by a resting tremor, dystonic posturing of the extremities, and hyperlordosis (678). When the enzyme defect affects both red cells and muscle, patients also can present with recurrent myoglobinuria, mental retardation, and a seizure disorder. In some, no apparent hemolytic anemia is seen (679).

Triosephosphate isomerase deficiency also is accompanied by a progressive neurologic disorder with onset in infancy (680). Symptoms and signs are variable. They include dystonia, tremor, and involvement of the spinal motor neurons and pyramidal tract. Intellectual development is usually normal (681). A peripheral neuropathy has been encountered in this condition as well (682). In other families, the clinical picture is one of chronic hemolytic anemia, myopathy, and mental retardation (683). Muscle biopsy can show abnormalities in mitochondrial structure (684). Mutations of the TPI gene appear to induce protein misfolding and accumulation of toxic protein aggregates (685). This pathogenesis is analogous to that suspected to occur in disorders such as Alzheimer's disease and the trinucleotide repeat syndromes.

Acanthocytosis

At least six different mutations are associated with acanthocytosis or burr shaped red cells. These conditions are covered in Chapter 3.

Polycythemia

Neonatal polycythemia, defined by a hematocrit higher than 65% during the first week of life and hyperviscosity, is a common and heterogeneous syndrome. It occurs in up to

3% of neonates, caused by various intrauterine abnormalities or hypoxic complications during labor and delivery (686). Neurologic symptoms from neonatal polycythemia are generally thought to result from reduced cerebral blood flow caused by increased blood viscosity. This in turn leads to cerebral hypoxia and ischemia. Rosenkrantz and coworkers have postulated that the elevation of arterial oxygen content in infants with polycythemia compensates for the reduced cerebral blood flow and allows for normal oxygen delivery to the brain. On the basis of animal experiments, they suggest that the decreased plasma glucose fraction of blood in polycythemic animals results in a reduced glucose delivery to the brain and consequently a reduction in glucose metabolism (687). These experimental studies are supported by clinical data showing that polycythemic infants with concurrent hypoglycemia tend to experience more neurologic and developmental deficits than normoglycemic infants (688).

The most frequently encountered signs and symptoms of neonatal polycythemia are headache, paresthesias, vertigo, tinnitus, seizures, and visual disturbances. Intracranial hemorrhage is seen rarely (689). I also have seen thrombotic cerebrovascular accidents in neonates with unrecognized or poorly treated polycythemia. In one prospective study, 38% of newborns with polycythemia and the neonatal hyperviscosity syndrome had evidence of motor and neurologic abnormalities at 1 to 3 years of age. As has already been noted, in the experience of Black and coworkers, the presence of hypoglycemia posed an additional risk and raised this figure to 55% (688). Peripheral neuropathy has been noted as well. It probably is not an unusual complication, it but can only be detected by electrodiagnostic studies (690). Controlled studies show that partial exchange transfusions reverse many of the physiologic abnormalities and improve most symptoms, but do not improve the long-term neurologic and developmental outcome (691). The relatively poorer outcome of polycythemic infants could in part reflect the high incidence of antecedent fetal disorders in this group.

Coagulopathies

The Hemophilias

Hemophilia due to factor VIII deficiency usually presents after the newborn period. The risk and severity of bleeding depends upon the factor VIII level. The most common neurologic complication of hemophilia is compression of the lumbosacral plexus and peripheral nerves by hemorrhage into adjacent muscles. Intracranial hemorrhage is the leading cause of death (692). Difficult vaginal deliveries can produce subgalaeal and intracranial hemorrhage (683). Idiopathic intracranial hypertension or pseudotumor cerebri also has been reported (684). Newborns with hemophilia who are lethargic or unable to feed should have imaging studies to detect any intracranial bleeding. The prognosis of factor VIII deficiency has improved greatly with early use of factor VIII concentrates. The prognosis of subdural and subarachnoid bleeding is better than that of intracerebral bleeding. Neurosurgical intervention for large clots is feasible if adequate factor levels are maintained (695). Hemophilia has been associated with HIV infection.

Hemophilia B or Factor IX (plasma thromboplastin antecedent) deficiency is a sex-linked disorder that is less common than classical hemophilia. The clinical picture is identical, and bleeding is treated with factor IX concentrates. Intracranial hemorrhage is occasionally seen with factor VII deficiency and the von Willebrand diseases (696). Acquired hemophilia A due to factor VIII inhibitors may be seen as a postpartum complication, in hematologic malignancies, and some autoimmune states (697,698). It has been treated with immunosuppressant drugs (699).

Thrombocytopenic Purpuras

Idiopathic thrombocytopenic purpura (ITP) of childhood is usually an acute self-limited disorder. It may evolve into a chronic condition with remissions and exacerbations and a significant risk of CNS hemorrhage, greatest at the time of febrile illnesses (700). Chronic ITP, especially when complicated by multiple intracranial hemorrhages, can be associated with mental handicap (701), and patients also may have ischemic strokes. Mononeuritis multiplex due to nerve hemorrhages has been encountered (702). In patients with the chronic form of ITP, learning disorders and behavioral problems are common, and significant EEG abnormalities are seen in approximately 50% of cases. Minute, multiple capillary bleeding is believed to account for these findings (701). The treatment of thrombocytopenia is reviewed by Kaplan and Bussel (700).

The thrombocytopenia-absent radius or tetraphocomelia syndrome (703) is usually associated with normal intelligence, but patients may have abnormalities of the cerebellar vermis or corpus callosum (704). CNS hemorrhage from thrombocytopenia is more often subdural or subarachnoid than within the brain substance, but may occur in any location.

Neonatal Alloimmune Thrombocytopenia

Neonatal alloimmune thrombocytopenia is caused by infants having platelet antigen that differs from that of their mothers. Alloimmunization occurs during pregnancy, thereby inducing a transient severe thrombocytopenia. CNS hemorrhages develop in 10% to 15% of infants (705). The thrombocytopenia is transient, and maternal platelet transfusion or intravenous IgG improves the platelet count. A mother who has had one infant with this condition is at high risk for thrombocytopenia in subsequent pregnancies, and the likelihood of intracranial bleeding increases in later pregnancies as well.

Thrombotic Thrombocytopenic Purpura

In thrombotic thrombocytopenic purpura (TTP), a rare and occasionally familial condition usually confined to adult life, platelet aggregation in the microvasculature results in intracapillary and intra-arteriolar thrombi that are widespread throughout the brain. Rarely, thrombosis can involve the middle cerebral artery or other large arteries (706). The thromboses result in cerebral ischemia and a variety of neurologic symptoms. These have been reviewed by Lawlor and coworkers (707). The condition responds promptly to plasma exchange (708). TTP is related to the HELLP (hemolytic anemia, elevated liver enzymes, and low platelet count) syndrome of pregnancy, in which liver dysfunction is usually more prominent than neurologic symptoms (709), and to hemolytic uremic syndrome, an entity in which platelet aggregation occurs in the microvasculature.

Deficiency of the Von Willebrand factor cleaving metalloprotease, ADAMTS-13, is often associated with TTP (710), and familial TTP is due to mutations of the ADAMTS13 gene mapped to chromosome 9 and coding for a metalloproteinase (711,712). The condition can present in the newborn period (707).

Hemorrhagic Disease of the Newborn

Hemorrhagic disease of the newborn is associated with a deficiency in vitamin K. It is most common in fully breastfed infants who received no vitamin K after birth and in infants of mothers taking various anticonvulsants (713). Early and late forms of the condition have been described. In the early form of the disease, onset of bleeding occurs during the first day of life. Infants usually present with gastrointestinal bleeding. The peak age for the late form is 4 weeks. In the German series of Sutor and colleagues, 58% of infants had intracranial hemorrhage (714). Vitamin K–related prothrombin complex deficiency may develop after the newborn period, in which case CNS hemorrhages are frequent and devastating (715).

Henoch-Schoenlein Purpura

Neurologic complications occur in as many as 10% of children with Henoch-Schoenlein purpura, a self-limited disorder with hypertension, renal disease and vasculitis (716,716a). The disease also occurs in young adults. Immune complexes, mainly of IgA and C3, are deposited in various organ systems. Patients have nonthrombocytopenic purpura, arthritis or arthralgia, abdominal pain that may be complicated by intussusception, and glomerulonephritis. The disease usually lasts a few weeks. Recurrences are uncommon, but may occur, even years later. Most patients recover completely; prognosis depends primarily on the severity of renal involvement. The most frequently seen neurologic manifestations are headaches and mental status changes. Cerebral vasculitis can lead to ischemic strokes and intracerebral hemorrhage. A reversible encephalopathy typical of RPE (717), ataxia, and peripheral neuropathy also have been described (718). Other complications include seizures and focal neurologic deficits, notably hemiparesis, aphasia, chorea, ataxia, and cortical blindness. Peripheral nervous system involvement, manifested by a mononeuropathy (719), and polyradiculoneuropathy can be encountered as well (720).

Pernicious Anemia

Pernicious anemia is a classical hematologic syndrome that may present with neurologic symptoms. Childhood pernicious anemia is a rare but treatable cause of sensory ataxia (721). The various cobalamin-deficient and cobalamin-responsive states are covered in Chapter 1. Nutritional deficiencies of vitamin B_{12} are important; macrobiotic diets and maternal B_{12} deficiency may cause hematologic and neurologic problems in infants (722). Nitrous oxide, used for anesthesia or as a recreational drug, may cause dramatic neurologic symptoms in patients with unsuspected B12 deficiencies (723,724) because nitrous oxide oxidizes the cobalt prosthetic group, irreversibly inactivating the vitamin.

Paroxysmal Nocturnal Hemoglobinuria

Paroxysmal nocturnal hemoglobinuria (PNH) is an acquired genetic disorder with complement-mediated hemolysis and clonal expansion of affected cells of various hematopoietic lineages probably derived from an abnormal multipotential hematopoietic stem cell (725). Nocturnal hemolysis causes the classical dark urine on arising. Some patients have cerebral venous or arterial occlusions (726). PNH is one of the causes for moyamoya syndrome (727).

Sideroblastic Anemias

The sideroblastic anemias are a heterogeneous group of disorders with two common features: ring sideroblasts in the bone marrow (abnormal normoblasts with excessive mitochondrial iron) and impaired heme biosynthesis. Mitochondrial dysfunction underlies all of these anemias. Some are hereditary; others are due to toxins, such as lead. Several of the hereditary forms are associated with neurologic disease. Mitochondrial myopathy with lactic acidosis and sideroblastic anemia (MLSA) typically begins with progressive exercise intolerance during childhood, with lactic academia and onset of sideroblastic anemia around adolescence (728,729). An unusual X-linked non-progressive spinocerebellar ataxia of early onset is associated with mild anemia in the anemia, sideroblastic, and spinocerebellar ataxia (ASAT) syndrome, due to mutation of the *ABCB7* gene at Xq13.1 (730). Sideroblastic anemia associated metabolic myopathy and an axonal neuropathy that sometimes causes fatal respiratory failure also have been reported (731).

NEUROLOGIC COMPLICATIONS OF SYSTEMIC NEOPLASTIC DISEASE

This section deals only with neoplastic disease that arises outside the nervous system. Primary tumors of the nervous system are discussed in Chapter 11.

Leukemia

With the advent of effective antileukemic chemotherapy and, hence, longer patient survival, neurologic complications in acute leukemia have become more common, and their diagnosis and treatment have become major medical problems (732). Neurologic complications are of two kinds: those attending the disease and those resulting from the therapy used to control the disease.

Central Nervous System Leukemia

Some controversy exists as to what constitutes central nervous system (CNS) leukemia. The Children's Cancer Group (CCG) considers the diagnosis of CNS leukemia to be established when the cerebrospinal fluid cell count is greater than 5 and lymphoblast cells are found on microscopic examination or on cytospin counts (733).

Pathology

Neurologic complications result from leukemic infiltrations of the meninges, brain, and cranial or peripheral nerves or from intracranial hemorrhage and infections. In one neuropathologic study, published in 1978, CNS lesions were found in 93% of children who died from leukemia (734). The present incidence of CNS lesions is undoubtedly much lower. The most common lesion in the 1978 study was cerebral atrophy, seen in 65%, followed in frequency by leptomeningeal infiltrations and various forms of hemorrhage.

Meningeal leukemia (CNS leukemia) is seen in all types of acute leukemia and can occur at any stage of the disease. It is generally thought that CNS leukemia results from the entrance into the CNS of leukemic cells from the blood as a consequence of petechial hemorrhages and a failure of systemically administered chemotherapeutics to cross the blood–brain barrier. Leukemic cells are first seen in the walls of the superficial arachnoid veins. Cells then extend into the deeper arachnoid vessels, from there into the CSF, and finally they penetrate the vessel walls and invade brain parenchyma. The pathology of CNS leukemia and the neurologic complications of therapy have been reviewed by Price (732).

TABLE 17.15 Presenting Symptoms and Signs in 50 Episodes of Central Nervous System Leukemia Occurring in 29 Patients

Neurologic Symptoms or Signs	*Episodes (%)*
Vomiting	80
Headache	70
Papilledema	70
Increased appetite and weight gain	26
Cranial nerve palsies	16
Seizures	8
Visual disturbance	4
Ataxia	4

From Hardisty RM, Norman PM. Meningeal leukemia. *Arch Dis Child* 1967;42:441. With permission.

Clinical Manifestations

At the time when leukemia is first diagnosed, approximately 4% to 5% of children have CNS involvement (735). More often, CNS involvement occurs in the late stages of the disease and is frequently present at relapse. Leukemic deposits can be found in any region of the CNS and cause almost any neurologic symptom, ranging from hemiparesis to seizures to cortical blindness. Presenting symptoms and signs of CNS leukemia are shown in Table 17.15. The primary symptoms are headaches, nausea, and vomiting, often associated with lethargy, irritability, and cognitive impairment. Hydrocephalus and cranial nerve infiltration or compression may develop. Seizures are less frequent. Although nuchal rigidity was not noted by Hardisty and Norman (736), I have found it on numerous occasions. Cranial nerve palsies are relatively common and result from leukemic infiltration of the basilar meninges. Nerves most commonly affected are the second, third, sixth, seventh, and eighth cranial nerves. Pupil-sparing third nerve palsies have been seen (737), and patients can present with visual loss due to optic nerve infiltration (738) or facial palsy as the first sign of leukemia (739). In the series of Ingram and coworkers, facial nerve palsy was seen in over 90% of children who developed cranial nerve palsies as a part of the first CNS relapse (740). A numb chin can be the result of leukemic infiltration of the mental nerve (741). The numb chin sign is moderately common in Burkitt lymphoma and is often a sign of malignant disease in adults (742). Increased appetite and sudden weight gain, an indication of hypothalamic infiltration, also have been noted (736). Rarely, epidural spinal cord compression is seen at the time of diagnosis (743). This complication can be treated effectively with systemic chemotherapy and local radiation. Leukemic involvement of the spinal cord is much less common than that of the brain, and peripheral nerve infiltration is much less common than cranial nerve infiltration. However, occasional patients present with severe weakness due to leukemic nerve infiltration at the time of relapse (744).

Intracranial hemorrhage is common in leukemia, most often at times of relapse. It is usually multifocal, affecting meninges and brain or spinal cord, and almost invariably associated with thrombocytopenia, sometimes with additional features of disseminated intravascular coagulation (DIC) (745,746). Patients with both thrombocytopenia and markedly increased white cell counts (hyperleukocytosis) are at greatest risk. These patients are at major risk of spinal cord or cauda equina compression by bleeding if lumbar puncture (LP) is done (747). Brain herniation also can occur, even in the absence of an antecedent lumbar puncture (748). Wirtz and colleagues discuss platelet evaluation and therapy for thrombocytopenia before LP (747).

The hyperleukocytosis that occurs in chronic myelogenous leukemia and is occasionally encountered in acute lymphoblastic leukemia can induce a leukostatic syndrome. Neurologic signs include papilledema, hearing loss, impaired vestibular function, and a variety of focal neurologic deficits. Symptoms respond promptly when the leukocyte level is lowered (749).

Diagnosis

The diagnosis of meningeal leukemia can be difficult. The CSF pressure is often elevated, and the cell count is generally increased. The sugar content is reduced in approximately 60% of cases, and the protein content is increased in approximately 50% of children who present with CNS symptoms (750). With cytocentrifugation or "Cytospin," this diagnosis can be made even when the CSF cell count is less than 10 cells per mm^3 (751). Culture for opportunistic pathogens is very important. CT scans of the skull often show splitting of the sutures. MRI studies can demonstrate meningeal enhancement, particularly after the infusion of gadolinium (752). Imaging techniques often identify small CNS deposits (752) and are indispensable in the long-term management of leukemia and other malignant diseases (753,754). It should be noted that a traumatic lumbar puncture at the time of initial diagnostic workup adversely affects the treatment outcome, an indication that contamination of CSF with circulating leukemic blast cells must be avoided (755).

Prophylaxis and Treatment

Because leukemic cells are sequestered in the CNS even in the absence of overt clinical or CSF manifestations of CNS leukemia, CNS treatment is delivered as an early part of intervention (756). Treatment results of CNS leukemia continue to improve, and now, apparent cure rates approach 75% to 80 % (757). CNS leukemia is usually sensitive to chemotherapy, and there has been a trend to use intensive intrathecal chemotherapy and individualized systemic therapy with blood level monitoring of chemotherapeutic agents. Such a regimen prevents overt CNS leukemic manifestations in some 90% of cases and in part has contributed to the dramatic increase in long-term survival (758).

The presence of CNS leukemia at the time of diagnosis, however, is an ominous prognostic sign, even though with intensive therapy most of these children go into temporary remission. The ultimate outlook for children who experience an isolated CNS relapse after their initial remission has improved considerably, and the five-year survival rate now approaches 85% (759). Treatment requires intensive reinduction systemic chemotherapy using multiple agents, intrathecal therapy, and craniospinal irradiation.

Both acute and long-term complications of CNS prophylaxis are encountered when a combination of intrathecal therapy and cranial irradiation is used.

Neurologic complications seen in the course of intracranial irradiation include headache and, on rare occasion, seizures. These side effects have become uncommon with the lower radiation doses currently in use. On MRI, a transient, diffusely increased signal is seen on T2-weighted images. This finding probably reflects a reversible posterior encephalopathy (760). A transient episode of somnolence of fever has been seen 6 to 8 days after cranial irradiation. This condition clears spontaneously. It may be a predictor of later neuropsychologic deficits (761).

A subacute leukoencephalopathy is seen as a late effect of therapy. It frequently is the result of progressive multifocal leukoencephalopathy (PML). This is a progressive demyelinating disorder due to JC virus (JCV) reactivation in immunocompromised patients. The clinical picture is one of a rapid evolution of dementia, spasticity, and ataxia developing in the course of several days to weeks. Focal neurologic signs, including hemiparesis and blindness, also can be noted. Seizures and changes in consciousness are not uncommon (762–764). The diagnosis requires viral recovery or detection of viral DNA, usually from the CSF by polymerase chain reaction (PCR), but sometimes when the CSF is negative, a tissue biopsy is necessary. PML is usually rapidly fatal, but 7% to 9% of patients have survived longer than 12 months without specific therapy (764), and some patients have recovered after treatment with cytarabine and interferon-alpha (765). Elimination of immunosuppressant treatments, if possible, is helpful. Specific treatment for PML remains experimental.

It is important not to confuse PML with other atypical viral infections, which may have similar imaging profiles and to which children with leukemia are particularly prone. Thus, varicella-zoster virus may produce a clinical and imaging picture similar to PML and responds to acyclovir treatment (766). Cytomegalovirus (CMV) encephalitis and echoviral infections generally do not resemble PML.

Delayed effects appear several months to years after CNS prophylaxis and are marked focal neurologic signs, notably seizures or hemiparesis. Although clinical and neuroimaging correlates are poor, MRI shows progressive focal, multifocal, or diffusely increased signal in white matter (767). Additionally, CT scans reveal a calcifying microangiopathy (768). Changes are frequently bilateral and are most pronounced in the putamen and internal capsule, but also can affect the cerebral and cerebellar cortex (769). The cortical calcifications can resemble the "railroad tracks" of Sturge-Weber syndrome. They are most likely to be seen in children who received prophylactic irradiation before 5 years of age.

On rare occasions, one encounters isolated optic atrophy as a consequence of the combined use of cranial irradiation and chemotherapy (770). In addition, a large proportion of children develop secondary malignancies with a sevenfold increase in all second malignancies, and a 22-fold increase in the incidence of brain tumors over the general population (771).

Long-term follow-up of leukemic children has uncovered deficits in such areas as overall intellectual functioning, academic achievement, attention, concentration, and short-term memory (772). These deficits are more severe after cranial irradiation than after intrathecal or systemic chemotherapy and are particularly evident in children treated before 3 to 5 years of age. Children whose treatment regimen was restricted to systemic and intrathecal chemotherapy fared much better on follow-up studies; their deficits were generally limited to information processing, and they were equal to control children with respect to global IQ, sustained attention, and baseline speed (773,774).

In apparently asymptomatic children who have undergone cranial irradiation as treatment for leukemia, the incidence of neuroimaging abnormalities can be as high as 75%. Most commonly, there is cerebral atrophy. MRI studies can show increased white matter signal on T2-weighted images (775). On positron emission tomography, cerebral white matter glucose metabolism is reduced in subjects who had been treated with a combination of cranial irradiation and intrathecal chemotherapy but was normal in those who had received intrathecal therapy alone. Metabolic rates in cortical and subcortical gray matter were reduced, regardless of the mode of therapy (776). Radiation injury to the brain is more extensively covered in Chapter 11.

The use of immunosuppressants in the treatment of leukemia predisposes the child to a variety of infectious agents that can invade the CNS. Of the various viral encephalitides, herpes zoster, cytomegalovirus, and herpes simplex are the most common (750). Atypical subacute sclerosing panencephalitis also has been encountered with or without antecedent measles (777). Other infections of the CNS can be caused by a variety of organisms: *Staphylococcus aureus*, *Pseudomonas*, *Escherichia coli*, and a variety of fungi, most commonly *Candida* and *Cryptococcus*.

CNS involvement also occurs in acute nonlymphoblastic leukemia, a heterogeneous group of malignancies that accounts for some 20% of childhood leukemia and that is commonly accompanied by chromosome abnormalities (778). CNS involvement at diagnosis is more common in acute nonlymphoblastic leukemia than in acute lymphoblastic leukemia. At the time of diagnosis, some 5% to 15% have abnormal CSF. Neurologic symptoms at time of diagnosis are rare and are mainly limited to infants. The presence of CNS involvement at the time of diagnosis does not appear to have an adverse impact on the outcome in children with acute myelogenous leukemia (779).

Neurologic Complications from Antineoplastic Agents

A number of neurologic disorders result from the agents used in the treatment of leukemia. These are reviewed by Plotkin and Wen (780) and Armstrong and Gilbert (781). Acute encephalopathy with convulsions and coma may complicate induction chemotherapy for childhood leukemia (782). Disseminated leukoencephalopathy develops in some children treated with methotrexate (MTX) and cranial irradiation (783). This condition is most common with high doses of MTX or with intrathecal MTX. Patients may have mental status changes, obtundation, hemiplegia, ataxia, and evidence of cortical involvement such as seizures, aphasia, and hemianopia. On imaging studies, the lesions are usually subcortical and most prominent in the periventricular regions, but neither the imaging, the clinical, nor the CSF picture is entirely specific (784,785) (Fig. 17.5A,B). In the series of Rollins and coworkers, the abnormalities observed on diffusion-weighted imaging appeared to correlate best with the clinical deficits (786). Some patients with this entity die, others recover completely, and others yet are left with residual injury but may tolerate subsequent courses of MTX without additional problems. The variability in patient course and inability to validate this diagnosis makes the reports of "reversal of MTX neurotoxicity" with aminophylline and/or high-dose folinic acid difficult to evaluate (787). Even though there

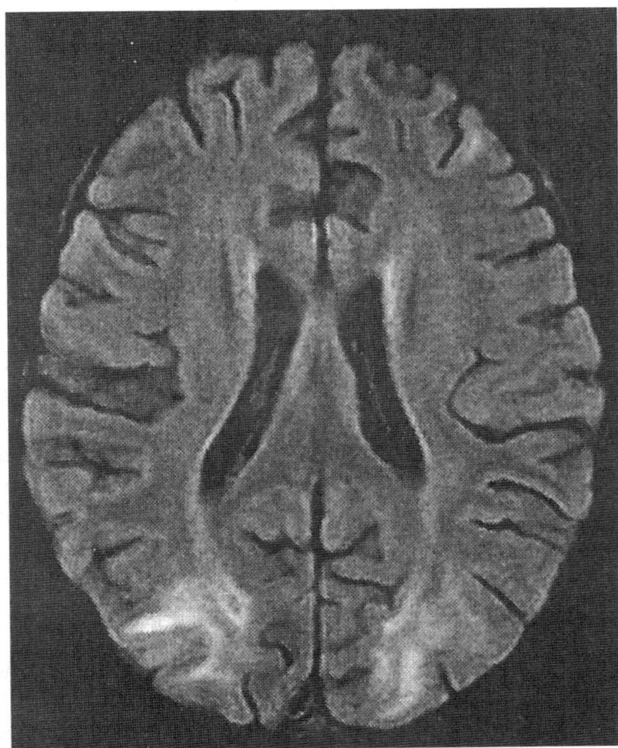

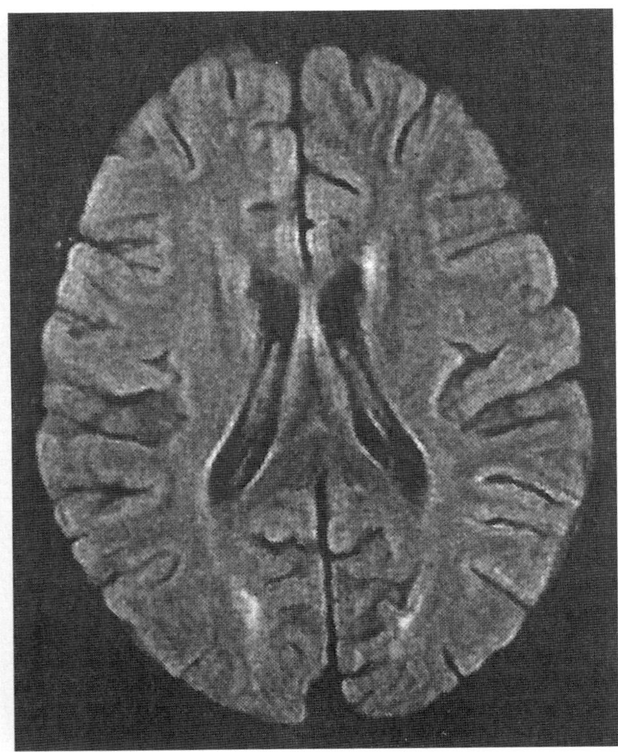

FIGURE 17.5. Methotrexate encephalopathy. **A:** Axial fluid inversion recovery MR sequence of brain demonstrates bilateral posterior parieto-occipital white matter abnormalities in addition to left frontal T2-weighted bright signal abnormality. **B:** A follow-up examination one month later shows almost complete resolution of the abnormalities. (Reproduced with permission from Shin RK, Stern JW, Janss AJ, et al. Reversible posterior leukoencephalopathy during the treatment of acute lymphoblastic leukemia. *Neurology* 2001;56:388–391.)

are theoretical reasons that folinic acid (leucovorin) might be helpful (788), I have used it in two cases, without definite benefit.

White matter disease is not the only neurologic syndrome associated with MTX treatment. Lumbar radiculopathy and paraplegia (789,790), ataxia, and confusion without imaging changes have been seen. Leukemic children have an increased risk of both reversible posterior encephalopathy (RPE) (372) and acute disseminated encephalomyelitis (ADEM), a highly variable entity further discussed in Chapter 8 (791,792).

Vincristine

Vincristine is used widely to induce the initial remission. Its neurologic side effects mainly are a dose-dependent peripheral neuropathy, with the drug's initial effect being on the muscle spindle (793). The Achilles tendon reflexes are depressed or lost in almost all patients. Less often, paroxysmal abdominal pain, weakness of the distal musculature of the lower extremities, and paresthesias in a stocking-glove distribution occur. Cranial nerve involvement, usually optic neuritis, ptosis, ophthalmoplegia, and facial palsy, has been noted less often and almost always in association with peripheral muscle weakness and atrophy. Autonomic disturbances, including constipation, paralytic ileus, bladder atony, and orthostatic hypotension, also have been encountered. The isolated appearance of cranial nerve signs in a leukemic child who has been treated with vincristine should suggest meningeal infiltration rather than a side effect of vincristine therapy.

The inadvertent intrathecal administration of vincristine results in an ascending and generally fatal myeloencephalopathy (794). Early irrigation of CSF and treatment with glutamic acid occasionally arrests the process (794,795). Vincristine produces a severe, even fatal, neuropathy in patients with hereditary neuropathies in the Charcot-Marie-Tooth family (CMT) (796,797) and in patients receiving vincristine together with itraconazole (798). Itraconazole is useful for fungal infection but is a potent inhibitor of CYP3A4, one of the families of cytochrome P450 mono-oxygenases. Several reports indicate that glutamic acid decreases vincristine neuropathy in patients (799). Painful neuropathies due to vincristine or paclitaxel also may be treated with gabapentin (800) or ethosuximide (801).

Cisplatin

Cisplatin induces a peripheral neuropathy in addition to many other toxic symptoms. Cisplatin neuropathy is dose-dependent and at times does not appear until after treatment has ended (802). Muscle cramps and Lhermitte's sign, a sudden electric-like sensation spreading down the body or into the limbs on flexion of the neck, can appear after cisplatin treatment (803). The drug usually affects large sensory fibers and can cause sensory ataxia. Strength is usually spared. Nerve conduction studies show evidence of a sensory axonopathy. Hearing loss is common. Cisplatin may contribute to vascular syndromes, including stroke.

Cytarabine or Cytosine Arabinoside (Ara-C)

Intrathecal Ara-C is sometimes followed by aseptic meningitis and/or myelopathy (804). It also can be associated with encephalopathy, seizures, and cranial nerve deficits; it can induce a significant neuropathy as well, although it does so less commonly than does vincristine (805,806). The drug is best known for its cerebellar toxicity, which can be permanent, and is seen more frequently in adults than in children (807).

L-Asparaginase

L-Asparaginase, an enzyme used in induction therapy for acute leukemia, has been associated with a variety of adverse reactions affecting the nervous system (808). The most serious of these complications, seen in 1% to 2% of children, are intracranial thromboses and hemorrhagic infarcts, which result in headache, obtundation, focal seizures, and hemiparesis (809). Symptoms occur a few weeks after L-asparaginase initiation and are believed to result from the enzyme-inducing deficiencies of antithrombin, plasminogen, and fibrinogen, with a subsequent disruption of plasma hemostasis. Because thrombosis of the cerebral veins or dural sinuses is common under these circumstances, MRI or angiography is required to establish the diagnosis. Administration of fibrinogen or fresh frozen plasma is the usual treatment. For unclear reasons, the risk of recurrence with further L-asparaginase therapy is low (810). The drug is yet another cause for the reversible posterior encephalopathy syndrome (811).

The immediate and long-term effects of radiation therapy are covered in Chapter 11.

Paraneoplastic Syndromes

Oppenheim proposed in 1883 that some neurologic disorders were due to release of toxic substances from distant cancers (811a). Some paraneoplastic syndromes, such as the Lambert-Eaton myasthenic syndrome, are so stereotyped that physicians may identify them from clinical observation. This syndrome, mostly seen in adults with small cell lung cancer, produces abnormal fatigability and proximal weakness in the absence of the bulbar involvement characteristic of myasthenia (812). Unlike myasthenia, tendon reflexes are often absent and may return with exercise. This autoimmune disorder can be treated by treating the tumor, if present, or by immunosuppressant measures. It is seen in children with leukemia and lymphoproliferative disorders (813) and in some children with autoimmune disease and no tumor (814).

Opsoclonus is a disorder of saccadic stability, often associated with myoclonus and cerebellar dysfunction, a clinical picture that is collectively termed the *opsoclonus-myoclonus* (OM) *syndrome*. The condition is a frequent accompaniment to neuroblastomas and other tumors of neural crest origin, such as ganglioneuroma and ganglioneuroblastoma. It is covered in Chapter 8.

Lymphoma and Hodgkin Disease

Primary CNS lymphoma is rare in children, and the neurologic complications of lymphomas generally result from an infiltration of the CNS and meninges. Symptoms and signs of increased intracranial pressure are present. A peripheral neuropathy also has been encountered (815). CNS involvement often presages a fatal outcome (816), and at diagnosis, it is encountered in approximately 20% of children with Burkitt lymphoma and develops despite prophylactic therapy (817). Paraplegia resulting from spinal cord compression, cranial neuropathies, and meningeal infiltration are the most common abnormalities. With intensive multidrug chemotherapy, the prognosis for 5-year survival has improved considerably (818).

Neurologic complications of Hodgkin disease are relatively unusual in childhood. They can take the form of infiltrations along the floor of the cranial cavity and the overlying meninges with an extension to the cranial nerves. Intracranial granulomas are rare (819). Progressive multifocal encephalopathy, an acute disseminated demyelination, also can be encountered in Hodgkin disease and lymphosarcoma.

NEUROLOGIC COMPLICATIONS OF CARDIAC DISEASE

In addition to the neurologic effects of hypoxia, cerebral complications can be encountered in a significant proportion of children with congenital or acquired heart disease. Such complications can be classified into those that occur as a consequence of the anatomic abnormality, and those that are at risk to develop after the treatment of such congenital or acquired abnormalities.

TABLE 17.16 Incidence of Neurologic Abnormalities in Various Types of Congenital Heart Disease[a]

Congenital Heart Disease	Incidence of Neurologic Abnormalities (%)
Transposition of the great arteries	2.3
Patent ductus arteriosus	11.0
Ventricular septal defects	8.6
Atrial septal defects	11.0
Tetralogy of Fallot	8.7
Coarctation of aorta	5.4
Aortic stenosis	0–5.0
Truncus arteriosus	5.4
Hypoplastic left-sided heart syndrome	29.0

[a]The high incidence of neurologic abnormalities in atrial septal defects and patent ductus arteriosus could reflect the fact that it was the central nervous system anomalies (e.g., postrubella syndrome) rather than the congenital heart disease that brought the child to the physician's attention.

Adapted from Greenwood RD, et al. Extracardiac abnormalities in infants with congenital heart disease. *Pediatrics* 1975;55:485; and Glauser TA, et al. Congenital brain anomalies associated with the hypoplastic left heart syndrome. *Pediatrics* 1990;85:984.

Congenital Heart Disease

A variety of developmental CNS anomalies can accompany many types of congenital heart disease. Malformations of the CNS are seen in approximately 7% of children with congenital heart disease (820). In a survey of children scheduled to undergo open-heart surgery, preoperative evaluation found neurologic and neurobehavioral abnormalities in more than one-half of the group. One-third of subjects were microcephalic, and 44% were hypotonic (821). The incidence of the neurologic abnormalities in the various major types of congenital heart disease is outlined in Table 17.16. A high incidence of CNS anomalies also is seen in patients with the hypoplastic left-sided heart syndrome (822). Trisomies 11, 18, and 21 are accompanied by both neurologic and cardiac dysfunction. About 40% of children with Down syndrome have congenital heart disease, most often endocardial cushion defects. Several of the contiguous gene syndromes such as the velocardiofacial syndrome, the DiGeorge syndrome, Rubinstein-Taybi syndrome, and the Williams syndrome have a high incidence of congenital heart disease. These conditions are covered in Chapter 4.

Left-to-Right Shunts

Patients with uncomplicated atrial septal defects, ventricular septal defects, or patent ductus arteriosus are, in the main, not at risk for neurologic complications. This is based on the basic physiology of a left-to-right shunt in which the pulmonary circuit serves as a buffer against insult to the brain. However, should patients with such lesions not be operated on and develop pulmonary vascular disease, the Eisenmenger's complex, a shunt reversal can develop, with consequent direct communication between the right side of the heart and the systemic circulation. This flow reversal puts the patient at risk for a cerebral embolus.

Cerebral embolization also can occur as a consequence of bacterial endocarditis. Currently, most cases of bacterial endocarditis are caused by congenital heart disease, notably ventricular septal defect and patent ductus arteriosus. Bacterial endocarditis has not been reported in a secundum atrial septal defect. Because the vegetations in a ventricular septal defect tend to occur on the right ventricular side, neurologic accidents secondary to this form of a congenital heart disease are rare. In the patient with a patent ductus arteriosus, vegetations also can occur on the pulmonary artery side but with a potential extension into the aorta. Children with unrepaired atrial septal defects are at risk for paradoxical emboli. In this defect, the right and left atrial pressures are generally equal. However, when intrathoracic pressures increase, the usual left-to-right shunt can then be reversed into a shunt from the right atrium to the left atrium. This exposes the patient to the possibility of an embolus, septic or otherwise, being routed to the brain with potential neurologic sequelae (823,824).

On the whole, with the widespread prophylactic use of antibiotics for dental surgery and for the treatment of bacterial infections, and with progressively earlier surgical correction of most cardiac malformations, bacterial endocarditis is seen rarely (824).

The clinical picture of cerebral embolization can be a sudden disturbance of consciousness, hemiparesis, seizures, or aphasia. Most patients show hematuria, the result of embolization to the kidneys. Rarely, cerebral embolization is the first sign of bacterial endocarditis or is secondary to the presence of immune complex.

The diagnosis of the cerebral embolization rests on the demonstration of sepsis by means of repeated blood cultures. Large intracardiac vegetations can be detected by echocardiography. Diffusion-weighted MRI and conventional MRI can demonstrate increased signal consistent with cerebral ischemia resulting from embolization. Treatment consists of parenteral antibacterial therapy against the invading organism, most commonly α- or γ-streptococcus or staphylococcus (824).

OBSTRUCTIVE LESIONS

In the obstructive lesions category, we consider the neurologic complications of aortic stenosis, pulmonary stenosis, and coarctation of the aorta. Each of these three lesions can be responsible for bacterial endocarditis and

Unique to aortic stenosis is the potential for an acutely decreasing cardiac output with reduced coronary artery flow leading to an arrhythmia such as ventricular tachycardia or fibrillation. Such an event in turn leads to diminished cerebral blood flow and the risk for seizures resulting from cerebral hypoxia.

Coarctation of the Aorta

The association of coarctation of the aorta with intracranial arterial aneurysms is well documented. Although intracranial arterial aneurysms are seen in only a small percentage of children with coarctation, they account for approximately one-fourth of aneurysms in childhood (825). Like arterial aneurysms in general, these are located around the circle of Willis and its major branches, particularly the anterior communicating artery. Arterial aneurysms are more fully discussed in Chapter 13.

A rare complication of surgery for repair of the coarctation is spinal cord damage. The nature of the repair requires occlusion proximally and distally to the site of the coarctation. Generally, children with fewer collateral vessels and the longest period of aortic occlusion are more disposed to this complication. Other factors, including the degree of compromise to the circulation of the spinal cord and variations in the anatomy of the blood supply to the spinal cord, play important roles (826,827).

The residua from spinal cord damage range from mild weakness and a picture resembling anterior spinal artery syndrome to complete paraplegia, with transection usually at the midthoracic level. Somatosensory-evoked potentials after posterior tibial nerve stimulation can be monitored during surgery to detect spinal cord ischemia (828). MRI studies can demonstrate a midthoracic hydromyelia.

Cyanotic Congenital Heart Disease

Cyanotic congenital heart disease includes the traditional *five T's*, namely, transposition of the great arteries, tetralogy of Fallot, truncus arteriosus, tricuspid atresia, and total anomalous pulmonary venous connection. Generally speaking, each of these lesions allows a connection between systemic venous blood passing into the heart and the cerebral circulation without the lungs acting as an intervening filter. As such, any peripheral infection could cause a neurologic event such as a brain abscess or a cerebral vascular accident.

Unique to the patient with tetralogy of Fallot is the additional risk of an acute hypoxic episode, known as "TET" spells. These result from a sudden increase in the infundibular stenosis, which then increases the flow of hypo-oxygenated blood from the right ventricle through the ventricular septal defect to the aorta and into the cerebral circulation. Attacks occur most frequently between 6 months and 3 years of age and are precipitated by crying, dehydration, and fever. Many attacks occur shortly after the child wakes up. In approximately one-half of the children, severe cyanotic attacks are followed by a generalized convulsion (829). The EEG during such an attack shows high-voltage slow-wave activity, but no spike discharges (830). These spells may be transient and short-lived. However, frequent spells lead to repeated cerebral insults and have the potential for permanent diminished cerebral function.

Brain abscesses are usually seen in children older than 2 years of age. Most often they occur as a complication of cyanotic congenital heart disease, sinus infections, or central lines. Early repair of most types of cyanotic cardiac lesions has reduced the incidence of brain abscess. Those with a residual right-to-left shunt remain at risk for this complication, however, and the risk of brain abscess is proportional to the degree of cyanosis (831). Anaerobic mouth organisms are the most common flora in immunocompetent patients without central lines. In the preimaging era, the distinction between ischemic stroke and abscess was often difficult. Patients with cyanotic heart disease have an increased risk of both complications. This distinction between the two diagnoses can generally be made with MR scanning (832). The mortality rate of brain abscess has improved greatly with the introduction of CT scanning (833). Prior to then, the diagnosis was frequently difficult. Fever generally is absent; only 20% of children with brain abscess seen at Boston Children's Hospital between 1981 and 2000 were febrile. Seizures were present in 27%, and 49% reported headaches. Thirteen patients (24%) in this series died, and of the survivors who returned for follow-up, more than one-half had epilepsy, cognitive, or motor handicaps. Almost all abscesses were in the cerebral hemispheres; 67% had single abscesses. Nearly all patients received both antibiotics and some type of surgical procedure. Eleven patients, seven of whom died, had fungal abscesses. Seven of the fungal abscess patients were immunosuppressed. No fungal abscesses had been seen at that institution before 1980 (833). Abscesses smaller than 2 cm in diameter in immunocompetent patients in good condition can often be successfully treated without surgery, as long as the elimination of the abscess is confirmed radiologically (834).

The diagnosis and treatment of brain abscesses in children with cyanotic heart disease are discussed more extensively in Chapter 7.

Any patient with inoperable cyanotic heart disease is at risk for progressive hemoconcentration with a potential increase in hematocrit to the high 60s or low 70s. This results in a small but recognizable risk of a cerebral vascular accident secondary to either embolic phenomenon or intrinsic vascular occlusion. The majority of cerebral infarcts in such children are caused by vascular occlusions, most often in the distribution of the middle cerebral artery. Venous thrombi are more common than arterial occlusions (835,836). Dehydration, fever, and iron deficiency anemia also play a role in the evolution of cerebrovascular accidents in nonsurgical patients (837).

A cerebrovascular accident is marked by a sudden onset of hemiplegia or aphasia. Seizures can accompany the acute episode; in some 10% of children, they can follow the cerebrovascular accident after a latent period of 6 months to 5 years. Approximately 20% of children, particularly those who incur a cerebrovascular accident during the early years of life, are left mentally retarded (838).

The differential diagnosis of hemiplegia and seizures in a child with cyanotic congenital heart disease is discussed in the section on brain abscess (see Chapter 7). We should point out that in cyanotic children, funduscopy is of little help in ascertaining the presence of increased intracranial pressure. Retinal changes consisting of dilated and tortuous veins and blurring of the disc margins can be observed in the majority of these children. This retinopathy is related to decreased oxygen tension and secondary polycythemia, rather than to retention of carbon dioxide or increased venous pressure (839).

Prolonged hypoxemia with pO_2 levels less than 25 torr in a patient with as yet unoperated cyanotic heart disease can lead to acidosis and potential cerebral vascular deficiencies. The symptoms may be seizures and, on a long-term basis, diminution in intellectual capability.

Acquired Heart Disease

Cardiomyopathy

This diagnosis applies to patients whose hearts are uncommonly dilated (dilated cardiomyopathy) or who demonstrate an abnormal hypertrophy, generally of the ventricular septum itself. The latter condition has been termed *asymmetric septal hypertrophy*, *hypertrophic cardiomyopathy*, or *idiopathic hypertrophic subaortic stenosis*. Dilated cardiomyopathy can be the aftermath of acute myocarditis or can be idiopathic. The presence of a chronically dilated heart can lead to stasis and clot formation, and the potential for emboli to enter the systemic circuit with a subsequent risk of a cerebral vascular accident. Hypertrophic cardiomyopathy can cause subtle or acute decrease in left ventricular output, decreased coronary blood flow, ventricular arrhythmia, syncope, and the potential of hypoxic brain damage.

Rheumatic Fever

Once a relatively common condition, rheumatic fever has gone through a phase of near nonrecognition, followed by a resurgence in the 1980s and. more recently, a quiescence. The principal neurologic complications of acute rheumatic fever and rheumatic heart disease are Sydenham chorea (see Chapter 8) and cerebral embolization secondary to bacterial endocarditis or cardiac arrhythmias.

Endocarditis

The bacteriology and diagnostic evaluation of endocarditis have changed greatly over the last few decades. Fifty years ago, most cases of endocarditis in the United States were due to rheumatic heart disease, which is now a minor contributor (840). Ventricular septal defect, patent ductus arteriosus, aortic valve disease, and tetralogy of Fallot are more likely predisposing conditions. Children with vascular patches, grafts, or prosthetic valves from previous surgery are at particularly high risk (840). Indwelling central lines in children without heart disease are responsible for about 10% of pediatric endocarditis today. Presentation of bacterial endocarditis is often indolent. Neurologists are involved when patients have seizures, or when there is a sudden onset of a focal neurologic deficit. The diagnostic evaluation of a youngster suspected of endocarditis is beyond the scope of this text. Suffice it to say that echocardiography is central to modern diagnostic evaluation.

Bacterial endocarditis can induce strokes, cerebral hemorrhage, and less commonly, mycotic aneurysms. Mycotic aneurysms can be identified by modern imaging techniques. Some are controlled with antibiotic therapy (841), or they can be surgically resected or treated by endovascular techniques (842).

Arrhythmias

It is well known that ventricular arrhythmias can develop during the postoperative period in patients who have undergone open-heart surgery in which the ventricle has been involved in the repair, such as tetralogy of Fallot, truncus arteriosus, or ventricular septal defect. The neurologist must remember that ventricular tachycardia can progress to fibrillation and to cardiac arrest with cerebral hypoxia.

The same sequence of events can occur in the patient with ventricular ectopy unrelated to surgery. Clinically, the presenting symptom is one of syncope. The differential diagnosis between cardiac and primary neurologic causes for syncope is considered in Chapter 15. Amiodarone and other drugs commonly used in the treatment of arrhythmias can induce a polyneuropathy (843).

Neurologic complications caused by hypertension, whether due to renal disease or to essential hypertension, are discussed more fully in a text on adult neurology. The interested reader is referred to a review by Wright and Mathews on hypertensive encephalopathy in a pediatric population (844). The condition is rare and generally develops in association with renal disease. As a rule, the percentage increase over base blood pressure rather than the actual magnitude of the level determines the development of neurologic symptoms. The most common presenting symptoms are focal or generalized seizures, headaches, and impaired vision. In the series of Wright and Mathews, papilledema was seen in approximately one-third of children whose discs were examined (844). Imaging studies are nonspecific or can demonstrate white matter hypodensity on CT, whereas MRI can show focal cortical and white matter increased signal on T2-weighted images. A reduction of the hypertension by 20% to 25% is usually adequate to improve or reverse neurologic symptoms within 24 to 48 hours.

The association of hypertension with lower motor neuron facial nerve palsy has been noted by several clinicians (845). The association of hypertension with pheochromocytoma and neurofibromatosis or pheochromocytoma with von Hippel–Lindau disease also is well recognized (see Chapter 12). Other neurologic conditions in which hypertension is not uncommon include familial dysautonomia, Guillain-Barré syndrome, increased intracranial pressure, and various viral diseases that can affect the brainstem, classically poliomyelitis.

The reversible posterior encephalopathy (RPE) syndrome, discussed in another part of this chapter, has been associated with hypertension, particularly with a rapid increase in blood pressure (376,846). MRI demonstrates hypointense T1 and hyperintense T2 signal involving gray and white matter mainly in the posterior regions (Fig. 17.1) (847). Systemic hypertension is moderately common in the NICU. It is most often associated with renovascular issues or parenchymal renal disease, and is surprisingly common in bronchopulmonary dysplasia (848,848a). It may be associated with ischemic stroke or cerebral hemorrhage. Marked reduction in blood pressure due to antihypertensive treatment may be less well tolerated by neonates than older children. Perlman and Volpe reported nine children with severe neonatal hypertension. Seven of them developed reversible renal (oliguria) and cerebral (seizures) symptoms associated with rapid treatment induced blood pressure reduction, even though the levels attained would generally be considered to be in the "normal rage" (849). The production of cerebral ischemia is a known risk of antihypertensive treatment, greatest in sick inpatients at the extremes of life, the very young and very old (849a).

Congestive heart failure in neonates has been observed secondary to large cerebral arteriovenous malformations (see Chapter 13). Although arteriovenous malformations are readily delineated by neuroimaging studies, their clinical recognition is often difficult. Audible bruits over the cranium can be heard in many of these patients but also are heard in approximately 15% of healthy infants younger than 1 year of age. Cutaneous abnormalities around the head and neck and dilated neck veins are perhaps more reliable indications of the diagnosis.

NEUROLOGIC SEQUELAE AFTER INTERVENTION TECHNIQUES

Cardiac Catheterization

Cardiac catheterization, originally primarily a diagnostic tool, now serves as both an avenue for diagnosis and treatment. Common to both purposes is the introduction of sheaths, catheters, balloons, and devices into arteries and veins. As a result, a significant risk exists of vessel compromise or occlusion and clot formation with emboli and air emboli. Further, the implanting of devices into the patent ductus arteriosus, atrial septum, and other vessels presents a nidus for thrombus, clots, and emboli. Neurologic complications rarely attend cardiac catheterization. When complications do develop in children, thromboembolic events predominate and appear most commonly when the procedure is performed in the first few months of life. Seizures and brachial plexus injuries also have been reported (850).

Neurologic Complications of Cardiac Surgery

Since the 1960s, we have witnessed improved diagnostic techniques and an increased aggressiveness in the surgical approach to the management of the child with heart disease. As a result, the incidence of neurologic complications attending cardiac surgery has become better defined. Also, improved survival of more serious types of heart disease has been accompanied by a more noticeable number of children with neurologic defects (851).

The basic technique of open-heart surgery initially isolated the heart for surgical repair and, at the same time, protected the other organs. Research demonstrated that lowering body temperatures permitted a longer time of perfusion with continued protection of the organs. Shortly thereafter, the technique of profound hypothermia with circulatory arrest was developed. With this technique, the patient's body temperature is decreased to 15° to 17°C. The blood volume is stored in the oxygenator compartment of the heart-lung system. Experimental work suggests that a window of safety for this technique is 1 hour (852–854).

After repair, the blood is returned to the patient, the patient is gradually rewarmed, and the surgical procedure completed. The parameters of this technique, in addition to standard open-heart surgical techniques, expose the patient to hypoxic-ischemic encephalopathy (HIE). Vanucci and colleagues have pointed out that HIE can be a sequel to inadequate blood flow to vital regions of the brain. The various causes include prolonged cardiac arrest beyond the perceived safety margin, intraoperative or postoperative systemic hypoxia and hypotension, and cerebral vascular occlusive insults secondary to thrombi or embolization (855). Several factors are responsible for impaired cerebral blood flow. Considerable evidence suggests that hypothermia, when used with cardiopulmonary bypass, produces a marked reduction in cerebral blood flow (856). Additionally, during deep hypothermia, there is a loss of cerebrovascular autoregulation. The reduction in cerebral blood flow is not immediately reversible postoperatively, and brain oxygenation remains impaired for some time after rewarming (857).

Clinically, one may see seizures in the immediate postoperative period. In a group of patients with transposition of the great arteries, Rappaport and coworkers spoke to the recognition of seizures and the potential risk of long-term neurologic and developmental sequelae (858). Although studying a different subset of patients, Uzark and colleagues reported a group of patients with single ventricle undergoing the Fontan procedure with no resultant deficiency in intellectual development, except for some deficits in visual motor integration (859). These patients, however, did not require circulatory arrest and were cyanotic before the onset of surgical intervention.

Actual figures on the incidence of neurologic complication after cardiac surgery vary, depending on the care and detail of the neurologic evaluation and on the period during which the series was collected. Currently, it is less than 5%. Menache and coworkers, reporting in 2002 of their experience from Boston Children's Hospital on 706 patients who underwent open-heart surgery, found a 2.3% incidence of early postoperative cerebral disorders, with clinical seizures being the most common complication (1.3%) (860). The effects of open heart surgery on ultimate developmental outcome are not as clear, and many factors—such as cross clamp time, complete or partial circulatory arrest, blood gas manipulation, and brain hypothermia—affect the supply and demand of oxygen in cerebral tissue and, as a consequence, developmental outcome (861–863). Thus, conclusions as to the incidence of cognitive complications must be drawn carefully and related specifically to the techniques used at a specific institution at a specific time. Furthermore, as was already noted, a significant proportion of infants who undergo open-heart surgery have preoperative neurologic and developmental deficits (863). Studies from Children's Hospital of Philadelphia show that white matter injury precedes surgery in some children; many more have white matter injury postoperatively. Postoperative white matter injury is much less frequent if surgery is done later than 12 weeks of age (864,865).

In the Boston Circulatory Arrest Study, patients at Boston Children's Hospital were randomized between deep hypothermic circulatory arrest (DHCA) and low-flow continuous cardiopulmonary bypass. Follow-up over an 8-year period showed no major difference between the two operative groups (866). Both techniques had some bad outcomes. If the patients whose DHCA time (period of circulatory arrest) exceeded 41 minutes would be removed from the series, most children would have had acceptable outcomes. The maximal tolerable duration of circulatory arrest depends on temperature, pH, and hematocrit (867). Perfusion with higher hematocrits improves brain outcomes. Adjustment to the needs of individual patients is facilitated by continuous EEG and near-infrared spectrometry (NIRS) monitoring during and after bypass. These techniques yield complex data; only the largest medical centers can make good use of them at present. Near-infrared spectroscopy can be used to monitor cerebral oxygenation in neonates and older children with closed fontanels. Oxygenated and deoxygenated hemoglobin are measured; it also is possible to measure the redox status of cytochrome oxidase. Wardle and coworkers provide details of this technique (868). NIRS or some measure of cerebral oxygenation is particularly useful in the immediate postbypass period, when electrical seizures or events that appear to be seizures are common. Most electrical events are not associated with clinical events; the availability of information about cerebral oxygenation can help in making a decision regarding anticonvulsant treatment (869). Patients with clinical or electrographic seizures in the perioperative period have statistically worse outcomes (858). It remains to be seen whether vigorous antiepileptic treatment improves those outcomes. Unfortunately, most common intravenous antiepileptic drugs decrease cardiac output and have other unwanted effects. Intravenous valproate has very little effect on cardiovascular or respiratory function and is good for older children after cardiac surgery but is hazardous in infants because of its metabolic effects.

Neuropathologic changes have been attributed to impaired cerebral blood flow; hypoxia or hypotension; reduced microvascular perfusion consequent to gas, microparticulate, or platelet embolization; a nonpulsatile blood flow; and the altered rheologic states of cardiopulmonary bypass and hypothermia (870).

The basic mechanisms of brain injury during cardiopulmonary bypass are reviewed by du Plessis (871).

During the immediate postoperative period, major neurologic deficits include alterations of consciousness, behavioral changes, and defects in intellectual function, particularly in recent memory and in those modalities that pertain to perception and synthesis of visual patterns. Additionally, several groups have observed a curious dyskinesia, which is frequently localized to the orofacial region and can be accompanied by developmental delay (872,873). In the large series of Medlock and coworkers, involuntary movements were seen in 1.2%; in other series, their incidence ranged from 1.1% to 18.0% (873). Although originally thought to be specific for children operated on with deep hypothermia and circulatory arrest, the choreoathetoid syndrome has been seen when this technique was not used.

After a latent period of several days, this syndrome generally begins with delirium; it varies in severity but can be devastating and irreversible. The movements vary and may include choreoathetosis, ballism, postural instability, and sometimes myoclonus. Imaging studies are uninformative, and neuroleptics, sedatives, and baclofen have been effective in only some patients (873). The cause for the dyskinesia is unknown. On neuropathologic examination, there is marked neuronal loss and gliosis in the globus pallidus, chiefly in the lateral segment (874). In the majority of children, the involuntary movements improve in the course of several days to three weeks and ultimately clear completely. However, du Plessis and colleagues reporting from Boston Children's Hospital found that 7 of 15 survivors had persistent dyskinesias, and many had IQs in the mentally retarded range (875).

When intraoperative hypoxic or hypotensive brain damage has been extensive, patients do not recover consciousness postoperatively. They often experience focal or generalized seizures. On examination, they are in extensor rigidity with papilledema and fixed, dilated pupils. Focal signs can be evident, even though autopsy reveals widespread anoxic changes throughout both hemispheres. Symptoms of cerebral emboli include hemiplegia, visual field defects, and seizures. These deficits are not likely to resolve spontaneously, and permanent residua are not unusual (876). As many patients undergo surgical repair in the early neonatal period or in infancy, signs of cerebral compromise are even more difficult to detect.

Other factors influence the ultimate outcome of infants and children subjected to open-heart surgery. The apolipoprotein e2 allele has been suggested as increasing the risk of neurologic injury in infants undergoing cardiopulmonary bypass (877). Cardiac surgery and bypass evoke strong inflammatory responses, which probably have undesirable CNS effects and could affect the ultimate outcome (878).

As is the case after renal or hepatic transplantation, neurologic sequelae of heart transplantation can be divided into perioperative and late complications.

The perioperative complications are those encountered with cardiopulmonary bypass surgery and hypothermia and have already been cited. Late complications are related to chronic immunosuppressants and include opportunistic intracranial infection and, less commonly, lymphoproliferative disorders as well as the complications that attend the use of cyclosporine and other immunosuppressive agents (879,880).

Chronic Complications

Evidence exists that prolonged hypoxia adversely affects the developing nervous system. Chronic hypoxia in children with cyanotic congenital heart disease is associated with motor dysfunction, poor attention span, and low academic achievement (881). In the experience of Bellinger and colleagues, the incidence of developmental sequelae is greater the longer the duration of circulatory arrest (882). Limperopoulos and his associates have come to the same conclusions (863). Neurocognitive abnormalities occur less frequently in children operated on before 14 months of age as compared with those who undergo surgery later. Newburger and associates also found that the age at which major cardiac surgery is performed correlates inversely with cognitive function (883). These data suggest that postponement of repair in a child with cyanotic congenital heart disease is associated with progressive impairment of postoperative cognitive abilities. It remains to be seen whether the best results come from using palliative procedures in neonates or the more aggressive approach currently in favor in North America with major operations using bypass or deep hypothermic circulatory arrest (DHCA) early in life.

Attacks of syncope occasionally occur in unrepaired patients with tetralogy of Fallot or after placement of a Blalock-Taussig shunt. This condition, called the *subclavian steal syndrome*, is caused by obstruction in the proximal portion of the vertebral artery and consequent siphoning off of blood from the vertebral-basilar system into the subclavian and, subsequently, the pulmonary artery. This shunt can be demonstrated by arteriography (884). Injuries to the brachial plexus can result from traction in the course of surgery. A postoperative polyneuropathy has been rarely encountered but is mainly seen in adults. This complication may be related to the duration of induced hypothermia. Unilateral or, more rarely, bilateral phrenic nerve injury with ensuing diaphragmatic paralysis and respiratory insufficiency is a moderately common complication of cardiac surgery, especially in smaller infants (885). It results from either packing the heart in ice or from nerve transection (886). Approximately one-half of the children require diaphragmatic plication or permanent diaphragmatic pacing (886,887).

Cardiac Tumors

The most common cardiac tumor is a rhabdomyoma, the majority of which are associated with tuberous sclerosis (888). Some are discovered prenatally because of fetal tachycardia or are seen on ultrasounds *in utero*. Rhabdomyomas generally involute with age and have relatively good prognoses—long-term outcome depends upon the associated abnormalities. Embolization from atrial myxomas may cause stroke in childhood (889).

NEUROLOGIC COMPLICATIONS OF PULMONARY DISEASE

Extracorporeal Membrane Oxygenation

Extracorporeal membrane oxygenation (ECMO) is being used in most medical centers to treat neonates with uncontrollable respiratory failure. This invasive, technically complicated procedure is designed to functionally bypass the lungs. It requires systemic anticoagulation and generally necessitates ligation of the right common carotid artery, the right internal jugular vein, or both. The carotid artery can be reconstructed after ECMO, but the efficacy of this procedure is unproven (890). Venovenous ECMO involves cannulation of only the jugular vein, sparing the carotid artery and maintaining pulsatile flow, which is lacking in venoarterial ECMO. Venovenous ECMO provides less cardiovascular support.

ECMO survival rates depend greatly on diagnosis; infants with persistent pulmonary hypertension (PPHN) and meconium aspiration syndrome do best, while those with cardiac conditions and congenital diaphragmatic hernia generally require more time on ECMO and have the highest mortalities (891). Even though there is a compensatory response that is anatomically mediated through the circle of Willis, approximately one-fourth of infants demonstrate focal parenchymal lesions on post-ECMO MRI (892). As a rule, these are right-sided ischemic lesions and contralateral hemorrhagic lesions consistent with hyperperfusion of the left cerebral hemisphere. In the experience of Mendoza and her group, 83% of ischemic lesions involved the right side, and 70% of the hemorrhagic lesions occurred solely or predominantly on the side opposite the carotid ligation (893). These abnormalities are demonstrable on head ultrasound studies performed during the course of ECMO (894). Additionally, there is a significant incidence of left hemiparesis and left focal seizures, and occasionally, a subclavian steal has been documented (895). Children must be anticoagulated during ECMO, which increases the risk of intraventricular hemorrhage (IVH). These deficits, seen during the neonatal period, however, do not always translate into focal functional disabilities in later life.

Follow up of ECMO patients has been relatively encouraging: Nield and colleagues studied cognitive function in 108 ECMO survivors at age 43 months (896). Sixty percent functioned in the normal range, including three children with obvious neurologic deficits. Eighty percent of those patients had relatively favorable conditions (meconium aspiration syndrome, sepsis, and PPHN). Hamrick and coworkers studied a less favorable group: 53 infants who required ECMO after cardiac surgery (897), most often because they could not be weaned from bypass. Eleven of 12 who had cardiac arrest before ECMO did not survive. Only 14 children survived; 10 of these functioned at their age levels. Three of the four with overt neurologic handicaps had hemorrhage and periventricular white matter abnormalities documented during the acute illness. On the other hand, five of the ten good outcome children also had abnormal imaging studies during the acute phase. Severe CNS hemorrhage led to withdrawal of support in one-fourth of nonsurvivors. Davis and colleagues reviewed outcomes in 73 neonates who received ECMO for congenital diaphragmatic hernia in the United Kingdom between 1991 and 2000 (898). Twenty-seven, or 37%, survived to age 1, and only six survivors were found to be neurodevelopmentally normal.

Asthma and Sleep-Disordered Breathing

Asthma and epilepsy are common episodic disorders; hypoxic seizures may occur during asthma attacks (899), or patients may lose consciousness from cough syncope (900). If these episodes occur only with asthma attacks, they are rarely epileptic in nature. Children with mild to moderate asthma are usually similar to controls on neuropsychologic testing (901), although those with many school absences often do poorly academically. Children with sleep apnea and sleep-disordered breathing seem to have more cognitive and behavior problems than those with asthma (902,903). Even if sleep apnea cannot be documented, children with disrupted sleep score below controls on neurocognitive tests (904). Adult criteria for sleep apnea apply poorly to children, many of whom have frequent arousals and oxygen desaturation with very rare apneas (905). The association of sleep-disordered breathing with chronic headache, stroke, inflammation, and elevated C-reactive protein (CRP) has been mentioned (615,905a).

Theophylline is commonly used for the treatment of asthma and other pulmonary conditions. The major neurologic complication of theophylline therapy is the appearance of seizures, which are seen in all age groups and are generally accompanied by elevated theophylline levels, although seizures have been observed at therapeutic or low toxic levels (906). Seizures can be focal or generalized. When they are focal, one should suspect an underlying focal cerebral lesion. Theophylline-induced seizures are often difficult to control with anticonvulsants, and in some instances, a toxic encephalopathy and permanent brain damage can ensue (907). Seizures are best avoided by careful monitoring of serum theophylline levels, and it would appear wise not to use the medication for the treatment of reactive airway disease in children who have an abnormally low seizure threshold.

In some children recovering from an acute episode of asthma, a flaccid paralysis resembling poliomyelitis has been encountered. This condition, first reported from Australia in 1974 (908), has been termed *Hopkins syndrome*. No consistent virus has been cultured from such patients, who generally have been successfully vaccinated against poliomyelitis. The disorder primarily involves the anterior horn cells. A rapid progression of paralysis usually affects one limb, leaving the child with a severe and permanent weakness. Sensation is preserved; the CSF usually shows moderate mononuclear pleocytosis, and the protein content can be slightly elevated (909). MR changes in the anterior horn have been documented (910). Some of the children have evidence for an underlying immune deficiency (911).

Another cause of amyotrophy associated with asthma is Hirayama disease (912), which is characterized by dilated posterior cervical venous plexuses, eosinophilia, and high serum IgE titers and high titer to mite antigens. A related and more symmetrical myelopathy associated with atopic dermatitis and allergy to mites (*mite myelopathy*) and observed in both children and adults has been reported only from Japan (913,914).

Pulmonary AV Fistula

Pulmonary arteriovenous fistulas may be part of the Osler-Weber-Rendu syndrome (915) or may be sporadic congenital anomalies (916). In either case, they may permit emboli from the body to enter the cerebral circulation, and they pose a risk for brain abscess (917). The Osler-Weber-Rendu syndrome or hereditary hemorrhagic telangiectasia is a dominantly inherited and highly variable syndrome with telangiectases and arteriovenous malformations of skin, mucosa, and viscera. This condition is considered in Chapter 13.

Other Pulmonary Conditions

Chronic lung disease, such as cystic fibrosis, may be complicated by pseudotumor cerebri (918). In some instances, pseudotumor cerebri can be explained by hypovitaminosis A, which commonly accompanies cystic fibrosis. However, a bulging fontanel in infants with cystic fibrosis is rarely due to vitamin A deficiency (919), and papilledema, confusion, and asterixis are common in older children with respiratory failure and carbon dioxide retention from any cause (920). Rapid correction of hypercapnia may cause seizures in patients (921). Hypophosphatemia may be a factor in this complication of mechanical ventilation (921).

CRITICAL ILLNESS POLYNEUROPATHY AND RELATED DISORDERS

Critical Illness Polyneuropathy

Bolton first described polyneuropathy associated with sepsis and ICU care in 1984 (922). Sepsis and multiorgan failure trigger a symmetrical polyneuropathy that often produces ventilatory muscle weakness but generally spares eye, face, and head movements (923). Patients may have received steroids, but they are not central to this complication of the sepsis syndrome. Electrodiagnostic studies show normal conduction velocities, reduced compound muscle action potential amplitude, and eventual muscle denervation changes. If sepsis and organ failure are controlled, prognosis for recovery is good. Van Mook and Hulsewe-Evers provide a good review of this common syndrome (924).

Major Weakness in the ICU Patient

Major weakness in ICU patients is easily overlooked. Severe weakness after asthma attacks that had been treated with large doses of intravenous corticosteroids was first reported in 1977 (925). The weakness is severe, proximal, and at times is accompanied by ophthalmoplegia. It has been termed *acute quadriplegic myopathy*. Most patients have received both high dose corticosteroids and neuromuscular blocking agents (926). Electrical studies show normal motor and sensory conduction velocity with low amplitude compound action potentials. Rhabdomyolysis and myoglobinuria are seen in the most severe cases, and serum CPK is often much increased (927). Muscle biopsy shows characteristic ultrastructural changes, including absence of myosin thick filaments (928), and denervation changes resembling those seen in steroid-associated ICU myopathies. Banwell and coworkers examined 830 PICU patients and found that fourteen had major weakness, including eight in whom acute quadriplegic myopathy followed organ transplant. Four of these patients failed repeated attempts at extubation; most had received corticosteroids, aminoglycosides, and neuromuscular blocking agents. Three patients died, and in the survivors, weakness persisted for at least 3 months (929). Not all patients with this syndrome have received steroids or neuromuscular blockers (930).

Hund has distinguished three kinds of ICU myopathies: a non-necrotizing "cachectic" myopathy (critical illness myopathy or atrophy), a myopathy with selective loss of myosin filaments (thick filament myopathy), and an acute necrotizing myopathy of intensive care (931). The first entity is a more benign muscle atrophy, whereas the latter two syndromes are usually associated with the use of steroids.

Muscle from patients with acute quadriplegic myopathy shows strong induction of transforming growth factor (TGF)-beta/MAPK (mitogen-activated protein kinase) pathways producing apoptosis. Acute stimulation of the TGF-beta/MAPK pathway, coupled with the inactivity-induced atrogin/proteosome pathway (932), may explain the acute muscle loss seen in these patients (933). There is no specific treatment, but patients generally improve.

Whether critical illness polyneuropathy or acute quadriplegic myopathy is more common in an ICU depends upon the mix of patients and the amount of high-dose steroids being used in the ICU. Table 17.17 provides a summary of the differences between acute quadriplegic myopathy, critical illness polyneuropathy, and Guillain-Barré syndrome.

Septic Encephalopathy

Encephalopathy and polyneuropathy develop in at least two-thirds of patients with sepsis leading to multiple organ failure. The syndrome of septic encephalopathy has been relatively well defined in adults (934,935). Clearly, this syndrome also occurs in children, and mental status changes can be the first sign of systemic infection. However, the condition is rarely mentioned, and it has not been well separated from parainfectious encephalopathies such as acute necrotizing encephalopathy. Its appearance coincides with fever and multiple organ failure, rather than coming after infection like a postinfectious disorder. The

TABLE 17.17 Clinical Features of Guillain Barré Syndrome (GBS), Acute Quadriplegic Myopathy (AQM), and Critical Illness Polyneuropathy (CIP)

Condition	Ophthalmoparesis	Serum CPK	Facial Weakness	Electrophysiological Features
GBS	No*	Normal or slightly increased	Usual if GBS is severe	Conduction block, reduced motor NCV**, abnormal F waves
AQM	Often	Marked increase	Often	Reduced CMAP amplitude, no response to direct muscle stimulation
CIP	No	Normal or slightly increased	Usually not	Reduced CMAP amplitude, fibrillation potentials and + sharp waves

* Except in Fisher syndrome; ** axonal forms of GBS exist. NCV = nerve conduction velocity; CMAP = compound muscle action potential.

EEG is slow and may progress to triphasic waves and a burst suppression pattern (936). Symmetrical deep abnormalities may be seen in MR scans (937). Patients with sepsis and major encephalopathy have higher mortality rates than those without encephalopathy. Cecal peritonitis in rats produces experimental septic encephalopathy. The rats develop encephalopathy, abnormal CNS amino acid patterns, and blood–brain barrier changes, which can be inhibited with adrenergic drugs, such as the β_2 agonist dopexamine (938,939).

REFERENCES

1. Auer RN, Siesjö BK. Biological differences between ischemia, hypoglycemia, and epilepsy. *Ann Neurol* 1988;24:699–707.
2. Siesjo BK. Mechanisms of ischemic brain damage. *Crit Care Med* 1988;16:954–963.
3. Santos MS, Moreno AJ, Carvalho AP. Relationships between ATP depletion, membrane potential, and the release of neurotransmitters in rat nerve terminals. An in vitro study under conditions that mimic anoxia, hypoglycemia, and ischemia. *Stroke* 1996;27:941–950.
4. Auer RN, Sutherland GR. Hypoxic brain damage. In: Graham DI, Lantos PL, eds. *Greenfield's Neuropathology,* 7th ed. London: Arnold, 2002:33–280.
5. Erecinska M, Silver IA. Tissue oxygen tension and brain sensitivity to hypoxia. *Respiration Physiol* 2001;128:263–276.
6. Seidl R, Stockler-Ipsiroglu S, Rolinski B. Energy metabolism in graded perinatal asphyxia of the rat. *Life Sci* 2000;67:421–435.
7. Fritz KI, Ashraf QM, Zubrow AB, et al. Expression of phosphorylation of N-methyl-D-aspartate receptor subunits during graded hypoxia in the cerebral cortex of newborn piglets. *Biol Neonate* 2004;85:128–137.
8. Kemp PJ, Peers C, Lewis A, et al. Regulation of recombinant human brain tandem P domain K^+ channels by hypoxia: a role for O2 in the control of neuronal excitability? *J Cell Mol Med* 2004;8:38–44.
9. Nieber K. Hypoxia and neuronal function under in vitro conditions. *Pharmacol Ther* 1999;82:71–86.
10. Juul S. Recombinant erythropoietin as a neuroprotective treatment: in vitro and in vivo models. *Clin Perinatol* 2004;31:129–142.
11. Sun Y, Zhou C, Polk P, et al. Mechanisms of erythropoietin-induced brain protection in neonatal hypoxia-ischemia rat model. *J Cerebr Blood Flow Metab* 2004;24:259–270.
12. DeGraba TJ, Pettigrew LC. Why do neuroprotective drugs work in animals but not humans? *Neurol Clin* 2000;18:475–493.
13. Lee HT, Chang YC, Wang LY, et al. cAmp response element-binding protein activation in ligation preconditioning in neonatal brain. *Ann Neurol* 2004;56:611–623.
14. Kirino T. Ischemic tolerance. *J Cereb Blood Flow Metab* 2002;22:1283–1296.
15. Dirnagl U, Simon RP, Hallenbeck JM. Ischemic tolerance and endogenous neuroprotection. *Trends Neurosci* 2003;26:248–254.
16. Owen OE, Morgan AP, Kemp HG, et al. Brain metabolism during fasting. *J Clin Invest* 1967;46:1589–1595.
17. Kraus H, Schlenker S, Schwedesky D. Developmental changes of cerebral ketone body utilization in human infants. *Hoppe Seylers Z Physiol Chem* 1974;355:164–170.
18. Aoki TT. Metabolic adaptations to starvation, semistarvation, and carbohydrate restriction. *Prog Clin Biol Res* 1981;67:161–177.
19. Wang J, Chambers G, Cottrell JE, Kass IS. Differential fall in ATP accounts for effects of temperature on hypoxic damage in rat hippocampal slices. *J Neurophysiol* 2000;83:3462–3472.
20. Van der Post J, Noordzji LAW, de Kam ML, et al. Evaluation of tests of central nervous system performance after hypoxemia for a model of cognitive impairment. *J Psychopharmacol* 2002;16:337–343.
21. Rossen R, Kabat H, Anderson JP. Acute arrest of cerebral circulation in man. *Arch Neurol Psychiat* 1943;50:510–528.
22. Stephenson JBP. *Fits and Faints*. London: Mac Keith Press; Philadelphia: Blackwell Scientific Publications; J. B. Lippincott Co., 1990.
23. Ramanathan R, Corwin MJ, Hunt CE, et al. Cardiorespiratory events recorded on home monitors. Comparison of healthy infants with those at increased risk of SIDS. *JAMA* 2001;285:2199–2207.
24. Petito CK, Olarte JP, Roberts B, et al. Selective glial vulnerability following transient global ischemia in rat brain. *J Neuropathol Exp Neurol* 1998;57:231–238.
25. Tureen LL. Effect of experimental temporary vascular occlusion of the spinal cord. I. Correlation between structural and functional changes. *Arch Neurol Psychiat* 1936;35:789–807.
26. Glucksman A. Cell deaths in normal vertebrate ontogeny. *Biol Rev* 1951;26:59–86.
27. Lockshin RA, Williams CM. Programmed cell death. I. Cytology of the degeneration of the intersegmental muscles of the Pernyl silkmoth. *J Insect Physiol* 1965;11:123–133.
28. Kerr JFR. Shrinkage necrosis: a distinct mode of cellular death. *J Pathol* 1971;101:13–20.
29. Kerr JFR, Wyllie AH, Currie AR. Apoptosis: a basic biological phenomenon with wide-ranging implications in tissue kinetics. *Br J Cancer* 1971;26:239–257.
30. Wyllie AH. Glucocorticoid-induced thymocyte apoptosis is associated with endogenous endonuclease activation. *Nature* 1980;284:555–556.
31. Horvitz HR. Worms, life, and death (Nobel lecture). *Chembiochem* 2003;4:697–711.
32. Leonard JR, Klocke BJ, D'Sa C. Strain-dependent neurodevelopmental abnormalities in caspase-3-deficient mice. *J Neuropathol Exp Neurol* 2002;61:673–677.
33. Lucas DR, Newhouse JP. The toxic effect of sodium L-glutamate on the inner layers of the retina. *Arch Opthalmol* 1957;58:193–201.

34. Olney JW. Glutamate-induced retinal degeneration in neonatal mice. Electron microscopy of the acutely evolving lesion. *J Neuropathol Exp Neurol* 1969;28:455–474.
35. Choi DW. Excitotoxic cell death. *J Neurobiol* 1992;23:1261–1276.
36. Parnaik R, Raff MC, Scholes J. Differences between the clearance of apoptotic cells by professional and non-professional phagocytes. *Curr Biol* 2000;10:857–860.
37. Gavrieli Y, Sherman Y, Ben-Sasson SA. Identification of programmed cell death in situ via specific labeling of nuclear DNA fragmentation. *J Cell Biol* 1992;119:493–501.
38. Labat-Moleur F, Guillermet C, Lorimie P. TUNEL apoptotic cell detection in tissue sections: critical evaluation and improvement. *J Histochem Cytochem* 1998;46:327–334.
39. Clarke PGH. Developmental cell death: morphological diversity and multiple mechanisms. *Anat Embryol* 1990;181:195–213.
40. Yakovlev AG, Faden AI. Mechanisms of neural cell death: implications for development of neuroprotective treatment strategies. *Neuro Rx* 2004;1:5–16.
41. Formigli L, Papucci L, Tani A, et al. Aponecrosis: morphological and biochemical exploration of a syncretic process of cell death sharing apoptosis and necrosis. *J Cell Physiol* 2000;182:41–49.
42. Pohl D, Bittigau P, Ishimaru MJ. N-Methyl-D-aspartate antagonists and apoptotic cell death triggered by head trauma in developing rat brain. *Proc Natl Acad Sci USA* 1999;96:2508–2513.
43. Bakay L, Lee JC. The effect of acute hypoxia and hypercapnia on the ultrastructure of the central nervous system. *Brain* 1968;91: 697–706.
44. Auer RN, Beneviste H. Hypoxia and related conditions. In: Graham DI, Lantos PL, eds. *Greenfield's neuropathology,* Vol. 1, 6th ed. New York: Oxford University Press, 1997:263–314.
45. Brierly JB, Graham DI, Adams JH, et al. Neocortical death after cardiac arrest. *Lancet* 1971;2:650–655.
46. Brierley JB, Meldrum BS, Brown AW. The threshold and neuropathology of cerebral "anoxic-ischemic" cell change. *Arch Neurol* 1973;29:367–374.
47. Brown AW, Brierley JB. The earliest alterations in rat neurones and astrocytes after anoxia-ischaemia. *Acta Neuropathol (Berl)* 1973;23:9–22.
48. Velier JJ, Ellison JA, Kikly KK. Caspase-8 and caspase-3 are expressed by different populations of cortical neurons undergoing delayed cell death after focal stroke in the rat. *J Neurosci* 1999;19:5932–5941.
49. Benjelloun N, Joly LM, Palmier B, et al. Apoptotic mitochondrial pathway in neurones and astrocytes after neonatal hypoxia-ischaemia in the rat brain. *Neuropathol Appl Neurobiol* 2003;29:350–360.
50. Duncan JR, Cock ML, Scheerlinck JP, et al. Extracellular glutamate levels and neuropathology in cerebral white matter following repeated umbilical cord occlusion in the near term fetal sheep. *Neuroscience* 2003;116:705–714.
51. Spack L, Gedeit R, Splaingard M, et al. Failure of aggressive therapy to alter outcome in pediatric near-drowning. *Pediatr Emerg Care* 1997;13:98–102.
52. Wade JG, Amtorp O, Sorensen SC. No-flow state following cerebral ischemia. Role of increase in potassium concentration in brain interstitial fluid. *Arch Neurol* 1975;32:381–384.
53. Okumura Y, Sakaki T, Hiramatsu K, et al. Microvascular changes associated with postischaemic hypoperfusion in rats. *Acta Neurochir (Wien)* 1997;139:670–676.
54. del Zoppo GJ, Mabuchi T. Cerebral microvessel responses to focal ischemia. *J Cereb Blood Flow Metab* 2003;23:879–894.
55. Dooling EC, Richardson EP. Delayed encephalopathy after strangling. *Arch Neurol* 1976;33:196–199.
56. Ginsberg MD, Hedley-Whyte T, Richardson EP. Hypoxic-ischemic leukoencephalopathy in man. *Arch Neurol* 1976;33:5–16.
57. Plum F, Posner JB, Hain RF. Delayed neurological deterioration after anoxia. *Arch Int Med* 1962;110:18–25.
58. Kim HY, Kim BJ, Moon SY, et al. Serial diffusion-weighted MR imaging in delayed postanoxic encephalopathy. A case study. *J Neuroradiol* 2002;29:211–215.
59. Gamper E, Stiefler G. Klinisches Bild und anatomischer Befund nach Drosselung. *Arch Psychiat Nervenkr* 1937;106:774–778.
60. Gascón Jiménez FJ, Navarro Gochicoa B, Velasco Jabalquinto MJ, et al. Encefalopatía postanóxica diferida. *An Esp Pediatr* 2000; 53:151–155.
61. Plum F, Posner JB. *Diagnosis of stupor and coma,* 3rd ed. Philadelphia: F. A. Davis Co., 1980.
62. Bell JA, Hodgson HJ. Coma after cardiac arrest. *Brain* 1974;97: 361–372.
63. Bell TS, Ellenberg L, McComb JC. Neuropsychological outcome after severe pediatric near-drowning. *Neurosurgery* 1985;17:604–608.
64. Pampiglione G, Chaloner J, Harden A, et al. Transitory ischemia/anoxia in young children and the prediction of quality of survival. *Ann NY Acad Sci* 1978;315:281–292.
65. Frank LM, Furgiuele TL, Etheridge JE. Prediction of chronic vegetative state in children using evoked potentials. *Neurology* 1985; 35:931–934.
66. Pohlmann-Eden B, Dingethal K, Bender HJ, et al. How reliable is the predictive value of SEP (somatosensory evoked potentials) patterns in severe brain damage with special regard to the bilateral loss of cortical responses? *Intensive Care Med* 1997;23:301–308.
67. Majnemer A, Rosenblatt B. Evoked potentials as predictors of outcome in neonatal intensive care unit survivors: review of the literature. *Pediatr Neurol* 1996;14:189–195.
68. Pierrat V, Eken P, de Vries LS. The predictive value of cranial ultrasound and of somatosensory evoked potentials after nerve stimulation for adverse neurological outcome in preterm infants. *Dev Med Child Neurol* 1997;39:398–403.
69. Chen R, Bolton CF, Young B. Prediction of outcome in patients with anoxic coma: a clinical and electrophysiologic study. *Crit Care Med* 1996;24:672–678.
70. Parra DA, Totapally BR, Zahn E, et al. Outcome of cardiopulmonary resuscitation in a pediatric cardiac intensive care unit. *Crit Care Med* 2000;28:296–300.
71. Horisberger T, Fischer E, Fanconi S. One-year survival and neurological outcome after pediatric cardiopulmonary resuscitation. *Intensive Care Med* 2002;28:365–368.
72. Fandel I, Bancalari E. Near-drowning in children: clinical aspects. *Pediatrics* 1976;58:573–579.
73. Wijdicks EF, Parisi JE, Sharbrough FW. Prognostic value of myoclonus status in comatose survivors of cardiac arrest. *Ann Neurol* 1994;35:239–243.
74. Fields AI. Near-drowning in the pediatric population. *Crit Care Clin* 1992;8:113–129.
75. DeNicola LK, Falk JL, Swanson ME, et al. Submersion injuries in children and adults. *Crit Care Clin* 1997;13:477–502.
76. Kruus S, Bergstrom L, Suutarinen T, et al. The prognosis of near-drowned children. *Acta Paediatr Scand* 1979;68:315–322.
77. Bhatt MH, Obeso JA, Marsden CD. Time course of postanoxic akinetic-rigid and dystonic syndromes. *Neurology* 1993;43:314–317.
78. Ashwal S, Eyman RK, Call TL. Life expectancy of children in a persistent vegetative state. *Pediatr Neurol* 1994;10:27–33.
79. Strauss DJ, Shavelle RM, Ashwal S. Life expectancy and median survival time in the permanent vegatative state. *Pediatr Neurol* 1999;21:626–631.
80. Heindl UT, Laub MC. Outcome of persistent vegetative state following hypoxia or traumatic brain injury in children and adolescents. *Neuropediatrics* 1996;27:94–100.
81. Wintermute GJ. Childhood drowning and near-drowning in the United States. *Am J Dis Child* 1990;144:663–669.
82. Holzer M, Sterz F. Hypothermia after Cardiac Arrest Study Group. Therapeutic hypothermia after cardiopulmonary resuscitation. *Expert Rev Cardiovasc Ther* 2003;1:317–325.
83. Agnew DM, Koehler RC, Guerguerian AM, et al. Hypothermia for 24 hours after asphyxic cardiac arrest in piglets provides striatal neuroprotection that is sustained 10 days after rewarming. *Pediatr Res* 2003;54:253–262.
84. Mishima K, Ikeda T, Yoshikawa T, et al. Effects of hypothermia and hyperthermia on attentional and spatial learning deficits following neonatal hypoxia-ischemic insult in rats. *Behav Brain Res* 2004;151:209–217.
85. Biggart MJ, Bohn DJ. Effect of hypothermia and cardiac arrest on outcome of near-drowning accidents in children. *J Pediatr* 1990;117:179–183.

86. Wenzel V, Lindner KH, Krismer AC, et al. Survival with full neurologic recovery and no cerebral pathology after prolonged cardiopulmonary resuscitation with vasopressin in pigs. *J Am Coll Cardiol* 2000;35:527–533.
87. Wenzel V, Krismer AC, Arntz HR, et al. A comparison of vasopressin and epinephrine for out-of-hospital cardiopulmonary resuscitation. *N Engl J Med* 2004;350:105–113.
88. Perondi MB, Reis AG, Paiva EF, et al. A comparison of high-dose and standard-dose epinephrine in children with cardiac arrest. *N Engl J Med* 2004;350:1722–1730.
89. Longstreth WT Jr, Fahrenbruch CE, Olsufka M, et al. Randomized clinical trial of magnesium, diazepam, or both after out-of-hospital cardiac arrest. *Neurology* 2002;27;59:506–514.
90. Bernard SA, Gray TW, Buist MD, et al. Treatment of comatose survivors of out-of-hospital cardiac arrest with induced hypothermia. *N Engl J Med* 2002;346:557–563.
91. Hypothermia after Cardiac Arrest Study Group. Mild therapeutic hypothermia to improve the neurologic outcome after cardiac arrest. *N Engl J Med* 2002;346:549–556.
92. Ginsberg MD. Adventures in the pathophysiology of brain ischemia: penumbra, gene expression, neuroprotection: the 2002 Thomas Willis Lecture. *Stroke* 2003;34:214–223.
93. Fischer M, Hossmann KA. Volume expansion during cardiopulmonary resuscitation reduces cerebral no-reflow. *Resuscitation* 1996;32:227–240.
94. Tombaugh GC, Yang SH, Swanson RA, et al. Glucocorticoids exacerbate hypoxic and hypoglycemic hippocampal injury in vitro: biochemical correlates and a role for astrocytes. *J Neurochem* 1992;59:137–146.
95. Chou YC. Corticosterone exacerbates cyanide-induced cell death in hippocampal cultures: role of astrocytes. *Neurochem Int* 1998;32:219–226.
96. Virgin CE Jr, Ha TP, Packan DR, et al. Glucocorticoids inhibit glucose transport and glutamate uptake in hippocampal astrocytes: implications for glucocorticoid neurotoxicity. *J Neurochem* 1991;57:1422–1428.
97. Chu K, Jeong SW, Jung KH, et al. Celecoxib induces functional recovery after intracerebral hemorrhage with reduction of brain edema and perihematomal cell death. *J Cereb Blood Flow Metab* 2004;24:926–933.
98. Ausina A, Baguena M, Nadal M, et al. Cerebral hemodynamic changes during sustained hypocapnia in severe head injury: can hyperventilation cause cerebral ischemia? *Acta Neurochir Suppl (Wien)* 1998;71:1–4.
99. Bittigau P, Sifringer M, Ikonomidou C. Antiepileptic drugs and apoptosis in the developing brain. *Ann NY Acad Sci* 2003;993:103–114.
100. Song EC, Chu K, Jeong SW, et al. Hyperglycemia exacerbates brain edema and perihematomal cell death after intracerebral hemorrhage. *Stroke* 2003;34:2215–2220.
101. Ad Hoc Committee on Brain Death, the Children's Hospital, Boston. Determination of brain death. *J Pediatr* 1987;110:15–19.
102. Task Force for the Determination of Brain Death in Children. Guidelines for the determination of brain death in children. *Neurology* 1987;37:1077–1078.
103. Dosemeci L, Cengiz M, Yilmaz M, et al. Frequency of spinal reflex movements in brain-dead patients. *Transplant Proc* 2004;36:17–19.
104. Saposnik G, Maurino J, Saizar R, et al. Undulating toe movements in brain death. *Eur J Neurol* 2004;11:723–727.
105. Bueri JA, Saposnik G, Maurino J, et al. Lazarus' sign in brain death. *Mov Disord* 2000;15:583–586.
106. Schwartz JA, Baxter J, Brill DR. Diagnosis of brain death in children by radionuclide cerebral imaging. *Pediatrics* 1984;73: 14–18.
107. LaMancusa J, Cooper R, Vieth R, et al. The effects of the falling therapeutic and subtherapeutic barbiturate blood levels on electrocerebral silence in clinically brain-dead children. *Clin Electroencephalogr* 1991;22:112–117.
108. Schmitt B, Simma B, Burger R, et al. Resuscitation after severe hypoxia in a young child: temporary isoelectric EEG and loss of BAEP components. *Intensive Care Med* 1993;19:420–422.
109. Mejia RA, Pollack MM. Variability in brain death determination practices in children. *JAMA* 1995;274:550–553.
110. Fackler JC, Troncoso JC, Gioia FR. Age-specific characteristics of brain death in children. *Am J Dis Child* 1988;142:999–1003.
111. Grigg MM, Kelly MA, Celesia GG, et al. Electroencephalographic activity after brain death. *Arch Neurol* 1987;44:948–954.
112. Ashwal S, Schneider S. Brain death in the newborn. *Pediatrics* 1989;84:429–437.
113. Ashwal S. Brain death in early infancy. *J Heart Lung Transplant* 1993;12:S176–S178.
114. Dosemeci L, Dora B, Yilmaz M, et al. Utility of transcranial doppler ultrasonography for confirmatory diagnosis of brain death: two sides of the coin. *Transplantation* 2004;77:71–75.
115. Ruiz-Garcia M, Gonzalez-Astiazaran A, Collado-Corona MA, et al. Brain death in children: clinical, neurophysiological and radioisotopic angiography findings in 125 patients. *Childs Nerv Syst* 2000;16:40–45.
116. Dupas B, Gayet-Delacroix M, Villers D, et al. Diagnosis of brain death using two-phase spiral CT. *AJNR Am J Neuroradiol* 1998;19:641–647.
117. Altman DI, Perlman JM, Volpe JJ, et al. Cerebral oxygen metabolism in newborns. *Pediatrics* 1993;92:99–104.
118. Qureshi AI, Kirmani JF, Xavier AR, et al. Computed tomographic angiography for diagnosis of brain death. *Neurology* 2004;62:652–653.
119. Karantanas AH, Hadjigeorgiou GM, Paterakis K, et al. Contribution of MRI and MR angiography in early diagnosis of brain death. *Eur Radiol* 2002;12:2710–2716.
120. Hu X, Qiu J, Grafe MR, et al. Bcl-2 family members make different contributions to cell death in hypoxia and/or hyperoxia in rat cerebral cortex. *Int J Dev Neurosci* 2003;21:371–377.
121. Bean JW, Siegfried EC. Transient and permanent after effects of exposure to oxygen at high pressure. *Am J Physiol* 1945;143:656–665.
122. Hampson N, Atik D. Central nervous system oxygen toxicity during routine hyperbaric oxygen therapy. *Undersea Hyperb Med* 2003;30:147–53.
123. Frigon C, Shaw DW, Heckbert SR, et al. Supplemental oxygen causes increased signal intensity in subarachnoid cerebrospinal fluid on brain FLAIR MR images obtained in children during general anesthesia. *Radiology* 2004;233:51–55.
124. Saugstad OD. The role of oxygen in neonatal resuscitation. *Clin Perinatol* 2004;31:431–443.
125. Hasselbalch SG, Knudsen GM, Capaldo B, et al. Blood–brain barrier transport and brain metabolism of glucose during acute hyperglycemia in humans. *J Clin Endocrinol Metab* 2001;86:1986–1990.
126. Powers WJ, Rosenbaum JL, Dence CS, et al. Cerebral glucose transport and metabolism in preterm human infants. *J Cereb Blood Flow Metab* 1998;18:632–638.
127. Nehlig A. Cerebral energy metabolism, glucose transport and blood flow: changes with maturation and adaptation to hypoglycaemia. *Diabetes Metab* 1997;23:18–29.
128. Banker BQ. The neuropathological effects of anoxia and hypoglycemia in the newborn. *Dev Med Child Neurol* 1967;9:544–550.
129. Barkovich AJ, Ali FA, Rowley HA, et al. Imaging patterns of neonatal hypoglycemia. *AJNR Am J Neuroradiol* 1998;19:523–528.
130. Efron D, South M, Volpe JJ, et al. Cerebral injury in association with profound iatrogenic hyperglycemia in a neonate. *Eur J Paediatr Neurol* 2003;7:167–171.
131. Kinnala A, Rikalainen H, Lapinleimu H, et al. Cerebral magnetic resonance imaging and ultrasonography findings after neonatal hypoglycemia. *Pediatrics* 1999;103:724–729.
132. Fujioka M, Okuchi K, Hiramatsu KI, et al. Specific changes in human brain after hypoglycemic injury. *Stroke* 1997;28:584–587.
133. Banker BQ. The neuropathological effects of anoxia and hypoglycemia in the newborn. *Dev Med Child Neurol* 1967;9:544–550.
134. Auer RN, Hugh J, Cosgrove E, et al. Neuropathologic findings in three cases of profound hypoglycemia. *Clin Neuropathol* 1989;8:63–68.
135. Auer RN, Siesjö BK. Hypoglycemia: brain neurochemistry and neuropathology. *Baillière Clin Endocrinol Metab* 1993;7:611–625.
136. Kristián T, Gidö G, Siesjö BK. The influence of acidosis on hypoglycemic brain damage. *J Cereb Blood Flow Metab* 1995;15:78–87.
137. Auer RN. Progress review: hypoglycemic brain damage. *Stroke* 1986;17:699–708.
138. Bachelard H, Badar-Goffer R, Ben-Yoseph O, et al. Studies on

metabolic regulation using NMR spectroscopy. *Dev Neurosci* 1993; 15:207–215.
139. Hartmann AF, Jaudon JC. Hypoglycemia. *J Pediatr* 1937;11:1–36.
140. Miller HC, Ross RA. Relation of hypoglycemia to the symptoms observed in infants of diabetic mothers. *J Pediatr* 1940;16:473–481.
141. Cornblath M, Hawdon JM, Williams AF, et al. Controversies regarding definition of neonatal hypoglycemia: suggested operational thresholds. *Pediatrics* 2000;105:1141–1145.
142. Cornblath M, Ichord R. Hypoglycemia in the neonate. *Semin Perinatol* 2000;24:136–149.
143. Kalhan S, Peter-Wohl S. Hypoglycemia: what is it for the neonate? *Am J Perinatol* 2000;17:11–18.
144. Raivio KO. Neonatal hypoglycemia. *Acta Paediatr Scand* 1968;57:540–546.
145. Lubchenco LO, Bard H. Incidence of hypoglycemia in newborn infants classified by birth weight and gestational age. *Pediatrics* 1971;47:831–838.
146. Gutberlet RL, Cornblath M. Neonatal hypoglycemia revisited, 1975. *Pediatrics* 1976;58:10–17.
147. Lubchenco LO. *The high risk infant*. Philadelphia: WB Saunders, 1976.
148. Srinivasan G, Pildes RS, Cattamanchi G, et al. Plasma glucose values in normal neonates: a new look. *J Pediatr* 1986;109:114–117.
149. Pildes R, Forbes AE, O'Connor SM, et al. The incidence of neonatal hypoglycemia: a completed survey. *J Pediatr* 1967;70:76–80.
150. Guthrie R, van Leeuwen GV. The frequency of asymptomatic hypoglycemia in high risk newborn infants. *Pediatrics* 1970;46:933–936.
151. Hefter H, Mayer P, Benecke R. Persistent chorea after recurrent hypoglycemia. A case report. *Eur Neurol* 1993;33:244–247.
152. Menni F, de Lonlay P, Sevin C, et al. Neurologic outcomes of 90 neonates and infants with persistent hyperinsulinemic hypoglycemia. *Pediatrics* 2001;107:476–479.
153. Koh THHG, Aynsley-Green A, Tarbit M, et al. Neural dysfunction during hypoglycaemia. *Arch Dis Child* 1988;63:1353–1358.
154. Cowett RM, Howard GM, Johnson J, et al. Brain stem auditory evoked response in relation to neonatal glucose metabolism. *Biol Neonate* 1997;71:31–36.
155. Skov L, Pryds O. Capillary recruitment for preservation of cerebral glucose influx in hypoglycemic, preterm newborns: evidence for a glucose sensor? *Pediatrics* 1992;90:193–195.
156. Pryds O, Greisen G, Friis-Hansen B. Compensatory increase of CBF in preterm infants during hypoglycemia. *Acta Paediatr Scand* 1988;77:632–637.
157. Pryds O, Christensen NJ, Friis-Hansen B. Increased cerebral blood flow and plasma epinephrine in hypoglycemic, preterm neonates. *Pediatrics* 1990;85:172–176.
158. Cornblath M, Schwartz R. Hypoglycemia in the neonate. *J Pediatr Endocrinol* 1993;6:113–129.
159. Cornblath M, Schwartz R, Aynsley-Green A, et al. Hypoglycemia in infancy: the need for a rational definition. *Pediatrics* 1990;85:834–837.
160. Haworth JC. Neonatal hypoglycemia: how much does it damage the brain? *Pediatrics* 1974;54:3–4.
161. Kang HC, Chung da E, Kim DW, et al. Early- and late-onset complications of the ketogenic diet for intractable epilepsy. *Epilepsia* 2004;45:1116–1123.
162. Gregory JW, Aynsley-Green A. Hypoglycemia in the infant and child. *Ba llière Clin Endocrinol Metab* 1993;7:683–704.
163. Garty BZ, Dinari G, Nitzan M. Transient acute cortical blindness associated with hypoglycemia. *Pediatr Neurol* 1987;3:169–170.
164. Costello JM, Gluckman PD. Neonatal hypopituitarism: a neurological perspective. *Dev Med Child Neurol* 1988;30:190–199.
165. Haworth JC, Coodin FJ. Idiopathic spontaneous hypoglycemia in children: report of seven cases and review of the literature. *Pediatrics* 1960;25:748–765.
166. Wayne EA, Dean HJ, Booth F, et al. Focal neurologic deficits associated with hypoglycemia in children with diabetes. *J Pediatr* 1990;117:575–577.
167. Siemkowicz E, Gjedde A. Post-ischemic coma in rat: effect of different pre-ischemic blood glucose levels on cerebral metabolic recovery after ischemia. *Acta Physiol Scand* 1980;110:225–232.
168. Myers RE, Yamaguchi S. Nervous system effects of cardiac arrest in monkeys, preservation of vision. *Arch Neurol* 1977;34:65–74.
169. Park WS, Chang YS, Lee M. Effects of hyperglycemia or hypoglycemia on brain cell membrane function and energy metabolism during the immediate reoxygenation-reperfusion period after acute transient global hypoxia-ischemia in the newborn piglet. *Brain Res* 2001;901:102–108.
170. Sorimachi T, Fujii Y, Tsuchiya N, et al. Striatal hyperintensity on T1-weighted magnetic resonance images and high-density signal on CT scans obtained in patients with hyperglycemia and no involuntary movement. Report of two cases. *J Neurosurg* 2004;101:343–346.
171. Krous HF, Nadeau JM, Fukumoto RI, et al. Environmental hyperthermic infant and early childhood death: circumstances, pathologic changes, and manner of death. *Am J Forensic Med Pathol* 2001;22:374–382.
172. Bhanushali MJ, Tuite PJ. The evaluation and management of patients with neuroleptic malignant syndrome. *Neurol Clin* 2004; 22:389–411.
173. Nelson TE. Malignant hyperthermia: a pharmacogenetic disease of Ca^{++} regulating proteins. *Curr Mol Med* 2002;2:347–369.
174. Crandall CG, Vongpatanasin W, Victor RG. Mechanism of cocaine-induced hyperthermia in humans. *Ann Intern Med* 2002;136:785–791.
175. Turner MR, Gainsborough N. Neuroleptic malignant-like syndrome after abrupt withdrawal of baclofen. *J Psychopharmacol* 2001;15:61–63.
176. Halloran LL, Bernard DW. Management of drug-induced hyperthermia. *Curr Opin Pediatr* 2004;16:211–215.
177. Meythaler JM, Roper JF, Brunner RC. Cyproheptadine for intrathecal baclofen withdrawal. *Arch Phys Med Rehabil* 2003;84: 638–642.
178. Lugo-Amador NM, Rothenhaus T, Moyer P. Heat-related illness. *Emerg Med Clin North Am* 2004;22:315–327.
179. Bytomski JR, Squire DL. Heat illness in children. *Curr Sports Med Rep* 2003;2:320–324.
180. Shimizu T, Yamashita Y, Satoi M, et al. Heat stroke-like episode in a child caused by zonisamide. *Brain Dev* 1997;19:366–368.
181. Ben-Zeev B, Watemberg N, Augarten A, et al. Oligohydrosis and hyperthermia: pilot study of a novel topiramate adverse effect. *J Child Neurol* 2003;18:254–257.
182. Skop BP, Finkelstein JA, Mareth TR, et al. The serotonin syndrome associated with paroxetine, an over-the-counter cold remedy, and vascular disease. *Am J Emerg Med* 1994;12:642–644.
183. Lugo-Amador NM, Rothenhaus T, Moyer P. Heat-related illness. *Emerg Med Clin North Am* 2004;22:315–327.
184. Ulrich AS, Rathlev NK. Hypothermia and localized cold injuries. *Emerg Med Clin North Am* 2004;22:281–298.
185. Cohen IJ. Cold injury in early infancy. *Isr J Med Sci* 1977;13:405–409.
186. Wetterberg T, Sjoberg T, Steen S. Effects of hypothermia with and without buffering in hypercapnia and hypercapnic hypoxemia. *Acta Anaesthesiol Scand* 1994;38:293–299.
187. Zydlewski AW, Hasbargen JA. Hypothermia-induced hypokalemia. *Mil Med* 1998;163:719–721.
188. Lamminpaa A. Acute alcohol intoxication among children and adolescents. *Eur J Pediatr* 1994;153:868–872.
189. Kloos RT. Spontaneous periodic hypothermia. *Medicine (Balt)* 1995;74:268–280.
190. Ruiz C, Gener B, Garaizar C, et al. Episodic spontaneous hypothermia: a periodic childhood syndrome. *Pediatr Neurol* 2003;28:304–306.
191. LeWitt PA, Newman RP, Greenberg HS, et al. Episodic hyperhidrosis, hypothermia, and agenesis of corpus callosum. *Neurology* 1983;33:1122–1129.
192. Arroyo HA, Di Blasi AM, Grinszpan GJ. A syndrome of hyperhidrosis, hypothermia, and bradycardia possibly due to central monoaminergic dysfunction. *Neurology* 1990;40:556–557.
193. Plum F, Siesjo BK. Recent advances in CSF physiology. *Anesthesiology* 1975;42:708–730.
194. Somjen GG. *Ions in the brain. Normal function, seizures and stroke*. New York: Oxford University Press, 2004.
195. Chesler M. Regulation and modulation of pH in the brain. *Physiol Rev* 2003;83:1183–1221.

196. Katzman R, Pappius H. *Brain electrolytes and fluid metabolism*. Baltimore: Williams & Wilkins, 1975.
197. Strange K. Regulation of solute and water balance and cell volume in the central nervous system. *J Am Soc Nephrol* 1992;3:12–27.
198. Anderson RJ, Chung HM, Kluge R, et al. Hyponatremia: a prospective analysis of its epidemiology and the pathogenetic role of vasopressin. *Ann Intern Med* 1985;102:164–168.
199. Arieff AI, Ayus JC, Fraser CL. Hyponatremia and death or permanent brain damage in healthy children. *BMJ* 1992;304:1218–1222.
200. Keating JP, Schears GJ, Dodge PR. Oral water intoxication in infants. An American epidemic. *Am J Dis Child* 1991;145:985–990.
201. Bussmann C, Bast T, Rating D. Hyponatraemia in children with acute CNS disease: SIADH or cerebral salt wasting? *Childs Nerv Syst* 2001;17:58–62.
202. Mangos JA, Lobeck CC. Studies of sustained hyponatremia due to central nervous system infection. *Pediatrics* 1964;34:503–510.
203. Editorial. Excess water administration and hyponatremic convulsions in infancy. *Lancet* 1992;339:153–155.
204. Decaux G, Unger J, Brimioulle S, et al. Hyponatremia in the syndrome of inappropriate secretion of antidiuretic hormone: rapid correction with urea, sodium chloride, and water restriction therapy. *JAMA* 1982;247:471–474.
205. Brunner JE, Redmond JM, Haggar AM, et al. Central pontine myelinolysis after rapid correction of hyponatremia: a magnetic resonance imaging study. *Ann Neurol* 1988;23:389–391.
206. Pirzada NA, Ali II. Central pontine myelinolysis. *Mayo Clin Proc* 2001;76:559–562.
207. Brunner JE, Redmond JM, Haggar AM, et al. Central pontine myelinolysis and pontine lesions after rapid correction of hyponatremia: a prospective magnetic resonance study. *Ann Neurol* 1990;27:61–66.
208. Karp BI, Laureno R. Pontine and extrapontine myelinolysis: a neurologic disorder following rapid correction of hyponatremia. *Medicine (Balt)* 1993;72:359–373.
209. Hoorn EJ, Geary D, Robb M, et al. Acute hyponatremia related to intravenous fluid administration in hospitalized children: an observational study. *Pediatrics* 2004;113:1279–1284.
210. Loas G, Mercier-Guidez E. Fatal self-induced water intoxication among schizophrenic inpatients. *Eur Psychiatry* 2002;17:307–310.
211. Arieff AI, Guisado R. Effects on the central nervous system of hypernatremic and hyponatremic states. *Kidney Int* 1976;10:104–116.
212. Luttrell CN, Finberg L. Hemorrhagic encephalopathy induced by hypernatremia. *Arch Neurol Psychiatr* 1959;81:424–432.
213. Hogan GR, Dodge PR, Gill SR, et al. Pathogenesis of seizures occurring during restoration of plasma tonicity to normal in animals previously chronically hypernatremic. *Pediatrics* 1969;43:54–64.
214. Swanson PD. Neurological manifestations of hypernatremia. In: Vinken PJ, Bruyn GW, eds. *Handbook of clinical neurology*, Vol. 28. New York: Elsevier Science, 1977:443–461.
215. Dunn K, Butt W. Extreme sodium derangement in a paediatric inpatient population. *J Paediatr Child Health* 1997;33:26–30.
216. Finberg L. Pathogenesis of lesions in the nervous system in hypernatremic states. I. Clinical observation of infants. *Pediatrics* 1959;23:40–45.
217. Smith D, Finucane F, Phillips J, et al. Abnormal regulation of thirst and vasopressin secretion following surgery for craniopharyngioma. *Clin Endocrinol (Oxf)* 2004;61:273–279.
218. Adrogue HJ, Madias NE. Hypernatremia. *N Engl J Med* 2000; 342:1493–1499.
219. Morris MW, Smith S, Cressman J, et al. Evaluation of infants with subdural hematoma who lack external evidence of abuse. *Pediatrics* 2000;105:549–553.
220. Brown WD, Caruso JM. Extrapontine myelinolysis with involvement of the hippocampus in three children with severe hypernatremia. *J Child Neurol* 1999;14:428–433.
221. Acquarone N, Garibotto G, Pontremoli R, et al. Hypernatremia associated with severe rhabdomyolysis. *Nephron* 1989;51:441–442.
222. Conley SB. Hypernatremia. *Pediatr Clin North Am* 1990;37:365–372.
223. Kang SK, Kim W, Oh MS. Pathogenesis and treatment of hypernatremia. *Nephron* 2002;92[Suppl 1]:14–17.
224. Phelan DM, Worthley LI. Hypokalaemic coma. *Intensive Care Med* 1985;11:257–258.
225. Haddad S, Arabi Y, Shimemeri AA. Hypokalemic paralysis mimicking Guillain-Barre syndrome and causing acute respiratory failure. *Middle East J Anesthesiol* 2004;17:891–897.
226. Grossman H, Duggan E, McCamman S, et al. The dietary chloride deficiency syndrome. *Pediatrics* 1980;66:366–374.
227. Rodriguez-Soriano J, Vallo A, Castillo G, et al. Biochemical features of dietary chloride deficiency syndrome: a comparative study of 30 cases. *J Pediatr* 1983;103:209–214.
228. Malloy MH. The follow-up of infants exposed to chloride-deficient formulas. *Adv Pediatr* 1993;40:141–158.
229. Kaleita TA, Kinsbourne M, Menkes JH. A neurobehavioral syndrome after failure to thrive on chloride-deficient formula. *Dev Med Child Neurol* 1991;33:626–635.
230. Hill ID, Bowie MD. Chloride deficiency syndrome due to chloride-deficient breast milk. *Arch Dis Child* 1983;58:224–226.
231. Aichbichler BW, Zerr CH, Santa Ana CA, et al. Proton-pump inhibition of gastric chloride secretion in congenital chloridorrhea. *N Engl J Med* 1997;336:106–109.
232. Hsu SC, Levine MA. Perinatal calcium metabolism: physiology and pathophysiology. *Semin Neonatol* 2004;9:23–36.
233. Cockburn F, Brown JK, Belton NR, et al. Neonatal convulsions associated with primary disturbance of calcium, phosphorus and magnesium metabolism. *Arch Dis Child* 1973;48:99–108.
234. Hartenstein H, Gardner LI. Tetany of the newborn associated with maternal parathyroid adenoma. *N Engl J Med* 1966;274:266–268.
235. Gessner BD, deSchweinitz E, Petersen KM, et al. Nutritional rickets among breast-fed black and Alaska native children. *Alaska Med* 1997;39:72–74.
236. Simpson JA. Neurologic manifestation of idiopathic hypoparathyroidism. *Brain* 1952;75:76–90.
237. Mallette LE. Pseudohypoparathyroidism. *Curr Ther Endocrinol Metab* 1997;6:577–581.
238. Cohen ML, Donnell GN. Pseudohypoparathyroidism and hypothyroidism: case report and review of the literature. *J Pediatr* 1960; 56:369–382.
239. Tyler RH. Neurologic disorders in renal failure. *Am J Med* 1968; 44:734–748.
240. Tsang RC. Neonatal magnesium disturbances. *Am J Dis Child* 1972;124:282–293.
241. Tsang RC, Steichen JJ, Chan GM. Neonatal hypocalcemia mechanism of occurrence and management. *Crit Care Med* 1977;5:56–61.
242. Koo WWK, Tsang RC. Calcium and magnesium homeostasis. In: Avery GB, Fletcher MA, MacDonald MG, eds. *Neonatology: pathophysiology and management of the newborn*, 4th ed. Philadelphia: JB Lippincott Co, 1994:585–604.
243. Venkataraman PS, Tsang RC, Chen IW, et al. Pathogenesis of early neonatal hypercalcemia: studies of serum calcitonin, gastrin, and plasma glucagon. *J Pediatr* 1987;110:599–603.
244. Bakwin H. Pathogenesis of tetany of the newborn. *Am J Dis Child* 1937;54:1211–1226.
245. Lynch BJ, Rust RS. Natural history and outcome of neonatal hypocalcemic and hypomagnesemic seizures. *Pediatr Neurol* 1994;11:23–27.
246. Mizrahi A, London RD, Gribetz D. Neonatal hypocalcemia: its causes and treatment. *N Engl J Med* 1968;278:1163–1165.
247. Keen JH. Significance of hypocalcemia in neonatal convulsions. *Arch Dis Child* 1969;44:356–361.
248. Changaris DG, Purohit DM, Balentine JD, et al. Brain calcification in severely stressed neonates receiving parenteral calcium. *J Pediatr* 1984;104:941–946.
249. Muenter MD, Whisnant JP. Basal ganglia calcification, hypoparathyroidism, and extrapyramidal motor manifestations. *Neurology* 1968;18:1075–1083.
250. Halterman JS, Smith SA. Hypocalcemia and stridor: an unusual presentation of vitamin D-deficient rickets. *J Emerg Med* 1998;16:41–43.
251. Ang AW, Ko SM, Tan CH. Calcium, magnesium, and psychotic symptoms in a girl with idiopathic hypoparathyroidism. *Psychosom Med* 1995;57:299–302.
251a. Levine MA, Germain-Lee E, Jan de Beur S. Genetic basis for resistance to parathyroid hormone. *Horm Res* 2003;60 Suppl 3:87–95.
251b. Bastepe M, Juppner H. GNAS locus and pseudohypoparathyroidism. *Horm Res* 2005;63:65–74.

252. Taitz LS, Wales JKH, Spitz L. Hypocalcaemic seizures following gastrectomy. *Eur J Pediatr* 1983;141:36–38.
253. Edmondson S, Almquist TD. Iatrogenic hypocalcemic tetany. *Ann Emerg Med* 1990;19:938–940.
254. Peng LF, Serwint JR. A comparison of breastfed children with nutritional rickets who present during and after the first year of life. *Clin Pediatr (Phila)* 2003;42:711–717.
255. Bloom E, Klein EJ, Shushan D, et al. Variable presentations of rickets in children in the emergency department. *Pediatr Emerg Care* 2004;20:126–130.
256. Wang MS, Schinzel A, Kotzot D, et al. Molecular and clinical correlation study of Williams-Beuren syndrome: no evidence of molecular factors in the deletion region or imprinting affecting clinical outcome. *Am J Med Genet* 1999;86:34–43.
257. Davies M, Adams PH, Lumb GA, et al. Familial hypocalciuric hypercalcaemia: evidence for continued enhanced renal tubular reabsorption of calcium following total parathyroidectomy. *Acta Endocr* 1984;106:499–504.
258. Drummond KN, Michael AF, Ulstrom RA, et al. The blue diaper syndrome: familial hypercalcemia with nephrocalcinosis and indicanuria. A new familial disease, with definition of the metabolic abnormality. *Am J Med* 1964;37:928–948.
259. Lankisch P, Kramm CM, Hermsen D, et al. Hypercalcemia with nephrocalcinosis and impaired renal function due to increased parathyroid hormone secretion at onset of childhood acute lymphoblastic leukemia. *Leuk Lymphoma* 2004;45:1695–1697.
260. Gopal H, Sklar AH, Sherrard DJ. Symptomatic hypercalcemia of immobilization in a patient with end-stage renal disease. *Am J Kidney Dis* 2000;35:969–972.
261. Turker M, Oren H, Yilmaz S, et al. Unusual presentation of childhood acute lymphoblastic leukemia: a case presenting with hypercalcemia symptoms only. *J Pediatr Hematol Oncol* 2004;26:116–117.
262. Kaplan PW. Reversible hypercalcemic cerebral vasoconstriction with seizures and blindness: a paradigm for eclampsia? *Clin Electroencephalogr* 1998;29:120–123.
263. Cole DE, Quamme GA. Inherited disorders of renal magnesium handling. *J Am Soc Nephrol* 2000;11:1937–1947.
264. Walder RY, Landau D, Meyer P, et al. Mutation of TRPM6 causes familial hypomagnesemia with secondary hypocalcemia. *Nat Genet* 2002;31:171–174.
265. Lajer H, Bundgaard H, Secher NH, et al. Severe intracellular magnesium and potassium depletion in patients after treatment with cisplatin. *Br J Cancer* 2003;89:1633–1637.
266. Goren MP. Cisplatin nephrotoxicity affects magnesium and calcium metabolism. *Med Pediatr Oncol* 2003;41:186–189.
267. Goodman LS, Gilman A. *The pharmacological basis of therapeutics*, 3rd ed. New York: MacMillan, 1965:803.
268. Somjen G, Hilmy M, Stephen CR. Failure to anesthetize human subjects by intravenous administration of magnesium sulfate. *J Pharmacol Exp Ther* 1966;154:652–659.
269. Lucas MJ, Leveno KJ, Cunningham FG. A comparison of magnesium sulfate with phenytoin for the prevention of eclampsia. *N Engl J Med* 1995;333:201–205.
270. Glover ML, Machado C, Totapally BR. Magnesium sulfate administered via continuous intravenous infusion in pediatric patients with refractory wheezing. *J Crit Care* 2002;17:255–258.
271. Wheless JW. Special treatments in epilepsy. In: Rho JM, Sankar R, Cavazos JE, eds. *Epilepsy: scientific foundations of clinical practice*. New York: Marcel Dekker, 2004.
272. Furlan AJ, Hanson M, Cooperman A, et al. Acute areflexic paralysis. Association with hyperalimentation and hypophosphatemia. *Arch Neurol* 1975;32:706–707.
273. Chudley AE, Ninan A, Young GB. Neurologic signs and hypophosphatemia with total parenteral nutrition. *Can Med Assoc J* 1981;125:604–607.
274. Subramanian R, Khardori R. Severe hypophosphatemia. Pathophysiologic implications, clinical presentations, and treatment. *Medicine (Balt)* 2000;79:1–8.
275. Falcone N, Compagnoni A, Meschini C, et al. Central pontine myelinolysis induced by hypophosphatemia following Wernicke's encephalopathy. *Neurol Sci* 2004;24:407–410.
276. Komori H, Wada M, Eto M, et al. Benign convulsions with mild gastroenteritis: a report of 10 recent cases detailing clinical varieties. *Brain Dev* 1995;17:334–337.
277. Narchi H. Benign afebrile cluster convulsions with gastroenteritis: an observational study. *BMC Pediatr* 2004;4:2–6.
278. Wong V. Acute gastroenteritis-related encephalopathy. *J Child Neurol* 2001;16:906–910.
279. Hung JJ, Wen HY, Yen MH, et al. Rotavirus gastroenteritis associated with afebrile convulsion in children: clinical analysis of 40 cases. *Chang Gung Med J* 2003;26:654–659.
280. Goldwater PN, Rowland K, Thesinger M, et al. Rotavirus encephalopathy: pathogenesis reviewed. *J Paediatr Child Health* 2001; 37:206–209.
281. Makino M, Tanabe Y, Shinozaki K, et al. Haemorrhagic shock and encephalopathy associated with rotavirus infection. *Acta Paediatr* 1996;85:632–634.
282. Hadjivassiliou M, Grunewald R, Sharrack B, et al. Gluten ataxia in perspective: epidemiology, genetic susceptibility and clinical characteristics. *Brain* 2003;126:685–691.
283. Hadjivassiliou M, Chattopadhyay AK, Davies-Jones GA, et al. Neuromuscular disorder as a presenting feature of coeliac disease. *J Neurol Neurosurg Psychiatry* 1997;63:770–775.
284. Arroyo HA, De Rosa S, Ruggieri V, et al. Epilepsy, occipital calcifications, and oligosymptomatic celiac disease in childhood. *J Child Neurol* 2002;17:800–806.
285. Kieslich M, Errazuriz G, Posselt HG, et al. Brain white-matter lesions in celiac disease: a prospective study of 75 diet-treated patients. *Pediatrics* 2001;108:E21.
286. Zelnik N, Pacht A, Obeid R, et al. Range of neurologic disorders in patients with celiac disease. *Pediatrics* 2004;113:1672–1676.
287. Baudon JJ, Johanet C, Absalon YB, et al. Diagnosing celiac disease: a comparison of human tissue transglutaminase antibodies with antigliadin and antiendomysium antibodies. *Arch Pediatr Adolesc Med* 2004;158:584–588.
288. Francavilla R, Miniello VL, Brunetti L, et al. Hepatitis and cholestasis in infancy: clinical and nutritional aspects. *Acta Paediatr Suppl* 2003;91(441):101–104.
289. Brin MF, Fetell MR, Green PH, et al. Blind loop syndrome, vitamin E malabsorption, and spinocerebellar degeneration. *Neurology* 1985;35:338–342.
290. Harding AE, Muller DP, Thomas PK, et al. Spinocerebellar degeneration secondary to chronic intestinal malabsorption: a vitamin E deficiency syndrome. *Ann Neurol* 1982;12:419–424.
291. Danks DM. Copper-induced dystonia secondary to cholestatic liver disease. *Lancet* 1990;335:410.
292. Sokol RJ, Butler-Simon N, Conner C, et al. Multicenter trial of d-alpha-tocopheryl polyethylene glycol 1000 succinate for treatment of vitamin E deficiency in children with chronic cholestasis. *Gastroenterology* 1993;104:1727–1735.
293. Gabsi S, Gouider-Khouja N, Belal S, et al. Effect of vitamin E supplementation in patients with ataxia with vitamin E deficiency. *Eur J Neurol* 2001;8:477–481.
294. Mariotti C, Gellera C, Rimoldi M, et al. Ataxia with isolated vitamin E deficiency: neurological phenotype, clinical follow-up and novel mutations in TTPA gene in Italian families. *Neurol Sci* 2004;25:130–137.
295. Harding AE, Muller DP, Thomas PK, et al. Spinocerebellar degeneration secondary to chronic intestinal malabsorption: a vitamin E deficiency syndrome. *Ann Neurol* 1982;12:419–424.
296. Sokol RJ, Butler-Simon NA, Bettis D, et al. Tocopheryl polyethylene glycol 1000 succinate therapy for vitamin E deficiency during chronic childhood cholestasis: neurologic outcome. *J Pediatr* 1987;111:830–836.
297. Gabsi S, Gouider-Khouja N, Belal S, et al. Effect of vitamin E supplementation in patients with ataxia with vitamin E deficiency. *Eur J Neurol* 2001;8:477–481.
298. Cavalier L, Ouahchi K, Kayden HJ, et al. Ataxia with isolated vitamin E deficiency: heterogeneity of mutations and phenotypic variability in a large number of families. *Am J Hum Genet* 1998;62:301–310.
299. Hentati A, Deng HX, Hung WY, et al. Human α-tocopherol transfer protein: gene structure and mutations in familial vitamin E deficiency. *Ann Neurol* 1996;39:295–300.
300. Mariotti C, Gellera C, Rimoldi M, et al. Ataxia with isolated vitamin

E deficiency: neurological phenotype, clinical follow-up and novel mutations in TTPA gene in Italian families. *Neurol Sci* 2004;25:130–137.
301. Larnaout A, Belal S, Zouari M, et al. Friedrich's ataxia with isolated vitamin E deficiency: a neuropathological study of a Tunisian patient. *Acta Neuropathol* 1997;93:633–637.
302. Traber MG, Sokol RJ, Ringel SP, et al. Lack of tocopherol in peripheral nerves of vitamin E-deficient patients with peripheral neuropathy. *N Engl J Med* 1987;317:262–265.
303. Werlin SL, Harb JM, Swick H, et al. Neuromuscular dysfunction and ultrastructural pathology in children with chronic cholestasis and vitamin E deficiency. *Ann Neurol* 1983;13:291–296.
304. Neville HE, Ringel SP, Guggenheim MA, et al. Ultrastructural and histochemical abnormalities of skeletal muscle in patients with chronic vitamin E deficiency. *Neurology* 1983;33:483–488.
305. Kao A, Dlugos D, Hunter JV, et al. Anticoagulation therapy in cerebral sinovenous thrombosis and ulcerative colitis in children. *J Child Neurol* 2002;17:479–482.
306. Vrij AA, Rijken J, van Wersch JW, et al. Coagulation and fibrinolysis in inflammatory bowel disease and in giant cell arteritis. *Pathophysiol Haemost Thromb* 2003;33:75–83.
307. Schluter A, Krasnianski M, Krivokuca M, et al. Magnetic resonance angiography in a patient with Crohn's disease associated cerebral vasculitis. *Clin Neurol Neurosurg* 2004;106:110–113.
308. Lossos A, River Y, Eliakim A, et al. Neurologic aspects of inflammatory bowel disease. *Neurology* 1995;45:416–421.
309. Thomas CW Jr, Weinshenker BG, Sandborn WJ. Demyelination during anti-tumor necrosis factor alpha therapy with infliximab for Crohn's disease. *Inflamm Bowel Dis* 2004;10:28–31.
310. Anderson M. Neurology of Whipple's disease. *J Neurol Neurosurg Psychiatry* 2000;68:2–5.
311. Brown AP, Lane JC, Murayama S, et al. Whipple's disease presenting with isolated neurological symptoms. Case report. *J Neurosurg* 1990;73:623–627.
312. Maiwald M, Relman D. Whipple's disease and Tropheryma whippelii: secrets slowly revealed. *Clin Infect Dis* 2001;32:457–463.
313. Citerio G, Vascotto E, Villa F, et al. Induced abdominal compartment syndrome increases intracranial pressure in neurotrauma patients: a prospective study. *Crit Care Med* 2001;29:1466–1471.
314. Bloomfield GL, Ridings PC, Blocher CR, et al. A proposed relationship between increased intra-abdominal, intrathoracic, and intracranial pressure. *Crit Care Med* 1997;25:496–503.
315. Sugerman HJ, DeMaria EJ, Felton WL 3rd, et al. Increased intra-abdominal pressure and cardiac filling pressures in obesity-associated pseudotumor cerebri. *Neurology* 1997;49:507–511.
316. Estrada RV, Moreno J, Martinez E, et al. Pancreatic encephalopathy. *Acta Neurol Scand* 1979;59:135–139.
317. Boon P, de Reuck J, Achten E, et al. Pancreatic encephalopathy. A case report and review of the literature. *Clin Neurol Neurosurg* 1991;93:137–141.
318. Godbole A, Concannon P, Glasson M. Intussusception presenting as profound lethargy. *J Paediatr Child Health* 2000;36:392–394.
319. Pumberger W, Dinhobl I, Dremsek P. Altered consciousness and lethargy from compromised intestinal blood flow in children. *Am J Emerg Med* 2004;22:307–309.
320. Goetting MG, Tiznado-Garcia E, Bakdash TF. Intussusception encephalopathy: an underrecognized cause of coma in children. *Pediatr Neurol* 1990;6:419–421.
321. Tenenbein M, Wiseman NE. Early coma in intussusception: endogenous opioid induced? *Pediatr Emerg Care* 1987;3:22–23.
322. Adams RD, Foley JM. The neurological disorder associated with liver disease. *Assoc Res Nerv Ment Dis* 1953;32:198–237.
323. Fraser CL, Arieff AI. Hepatic encephalopathy. *N Engl J Med* 1985; 313:865–873.
324. Butterworth RF. Role of circulating neurotoxins in the pathogenesis of hepatic encephalopathy: potential for improvement following their removal by liver assist devices. *Liver Internat* 2003;23[Suppl 3]:5–9.
325. Kato MD, Hughes RD, Keays RT, et al. Electron microscopic study of brain capillaries in cerebral edema from fulminant hepatic failure. *Hepatology* 1992;15:1060–1066.
326. Valsamis MP, Peress NS, Wright LD. Central pontine myelinolysis in childhood. *Arch Neurol* 1971;25:307–312.
327. Albrecht J, Faff L. Astrocyte-neuron interactions in hyperammonemia and hepatic encephalopathy. *Adv Exp Med Biol* 1994;368: 45–54.
328. Jones EA, Weissenborn K. Neurology and the liver. *J Neurol Neurosurg Psychiatry* 1997;63:279–293.
329. Blei AT, Butterworth RF. Hepatic encephalopathy. *Semin Liver Dis* 1996;16:233–239.
330. Butterworth RF, Pomier Layrargues G. Benzodiazepine receptors and hepatic encephalopathy. *Hepatology* 1990;11:499–501.
331. Kircheis G, Haussinger D. Management of hepatic encephalopathy. *J Gastroenterol Hepatol* 2002;17[Suppl 3]:S260–S267.
332. Solga SM, Diehl AM. Non-alcoholic fatty liver disease: lumen-liver interactions and possible role for probiotics. *J Hepatol* 2003;38:681–687.
333. Albillos A, de la Hera A. Multifactorial gut barrier failure in cirrhosis and bacterial translocation: working out the role of probiotics and antioxidants. *J Hepatol* 2002;37:523–526.
334. Odeh M, Sabo E, Srugo I, et al. Serum levels of tumor necrosis factor-alpha correlate with severity of hepatic encephalopathy due to chronic liver failure. *Liver Int* 2004;24:110–116.
335. McGuire BM. The critically ill liver patient: fulminant hepatic failure. *Semin Gastrointest Dis* 2003;14:39–42.
336. Klein AS, Hart J, Brems JJ, et al. Amanita poisoning: treatment and the role of liver transplantation. *Am J Med* 1989;86:187–193.
337. Riegler JL, Lake JR. Fulminant hepatic failure. *Med Clin North Am* 1993;77:1057–1083.
338. Burkhard PR, Delavelle J, Du Pasquier R, Spahr L. Chronic parkinsonism associated with cirrhosis: a distinct subset of acquired hepatocerebral degeneration. *Arch Neurol* 2003;60:521–528.
339. Danks DM. Copper-induced dystonia secondary to cholestatic liver disease. *Lancet* 1990;335:410.
340. Poddar U, Thapa BR, Prasad A, et al. Natural history and risk factors in fulminant hepatic failure. *Arch Dis Child* 2002;87:54–56.
341. Blei AT. Cerebral edema and intracranial hypertension in acute liver failure: distinct aspects of the same problem. *Hepatology* 1991;13:376–379.
342. Navelet Y, Girier B, Clouzeau J, et al. Insuffisance hepato-cellulaire aigue grave de l'enfant: aspects EEG prognostiques. *Neurophysiol Clin* 1990;20:237–245.
343. Schafer DF, Shaw BMJ. Fulminant hepatic failure and orthotopic liver transplantation. *Semin Liver Dis* 1989;9:189–194.
344. Alper G, Jarjour IT, Reyes JD, et al. Outcome of children with cerebral edema caused by fulminant hepatic failure. *Pediatr Neurol* 1998;18:299–304.
345. Lidofsky SD. Liver transplantation for fulminant hepatic failure. *Gastroenterol Clin North Am* 1993;22:257–269.
346. Devictor D, Tahiri C, Lanchier C, et al. Flumazenil in the treatment of hepatic encephalopathy in children with fulminant liver failure. *Intensive Care Med* 1995;21:253–256.
347. Strauss GI, Moller K, Larsen FS, et al. Cerebral glucose and oxygen metabolism in patients with fulminant hepatic failure. *Liver Transpl* 2003;9:1244–1252.
348. Ede RJ, Gimson AE, Bihari D, et al. Controlled hyperventilation in the prevention of cerebral oedema in fulminant hepatic failure. *J Hepatol* 1986;2:43–51.
349. Sherlock S. Fulminant hepatic failure. *Adv Intern Med* 1993;38: 245–267.
350. Devictor D, Tahiri C, Rousset A. Management of fulminant hepatic failure in children—an analysis of 56 cases. *Crit Care Med* 1993; 21:S348–S349.
351. Munoz SJ, Moritz MJ, Bell R, et al. Factors associated with severe intracranial hypertension in candidates for emergency liver transplantation. *Transplantation* 1993;55:1071–1074.
352. Blei AT, Olafsson S, Webster S, et al. Complications of intrapressure monitoring in fulminant hepatic failure. *Lancet* 1993;341:157–158.
353. Ichai P, Samuel D. Treatment of patients with hepatic failure: the difficult place of liver support systems. *J Hepatol* 2004;41:694–695.
354. Jalan R. Intracranial hypertension in acute liver failure: pathophysiological basis of rational management. *Semin Liver Dis* 2003; 23:271–282.
355. Hoofnagle JH, Carithers RL Jr, Shapiro C, et al. Fulminant hepatic failure: summary of a workshop. *Hepatology* 1995;21:240–252.

356. O'Grady JG, Alexander GJ, Hayllar KM, et al. Early indicators of prognosis in fulminant hepatic failure. *Gastroenterology* 1989; 97:439–445.
357. Rivera-Penera T, Moreno J, Skaff C, et al. Delayed encephalopathy in fulminant hepatic failure in the pediatric population and the role of liver transplantation. *J Pediatr Gastroenterol Nutr* 1997;24:128–134.
358. Kullmann F, Hollerbach S, Holstege A, et al. Subclinical hepatic encephalopathy: the diagnostic value of evoked potentials. *J Hepatol* 1995;22:101–110.
359. Gill RQ, Sterling RK. Acute liver failure. *J Clin Gastroenterol* 2001; 33:191–198.
360. Detry O, Arkadopoulos N, Ting P, et al. Intracranial pressure during liver transplantation for fulminant hepatic failure. *Transplantation* 1999;67:767–770.
361. Patchell R. Neurological complications of organ transplantation. *Ann Neurol* 1994;36:688–703.
362. Bronster DJ, Emre S, Boccagni P, et al. Central nervous system complications in liver transplant recipients—incidence, timing, and long-term follow-up. *Clin Transplant* 2000;14:1–7.
363. Ghaus N, Bohlega S, Rezeig M. Neurological complications in liver transplantation. *J Neurol* 2001;248:1042–1048.
364. Martinez AJ, Estol C, Faris AA. Neurologic complications of liver transplantation. *Neurol Clin* 1988;6:327–348.
365. Estol CJ, Faris AA, Martinez AJ, et al. Central pontine myelinolysis after liver transplantation. *Neurology* 1989;39:493–498.
366. Estol CJ, Pessin MS, Martinez AJ. Cerebrovascular complications after orthotopic liver transplantation: a clinicopathologic study. *Neurology* 1991;41:815–819.
367. McCarron KF, Prayson RA. The neuropathology of orthotopic liver transplantation: an autopsy series of 16 patients. *Arch Pathol Lab Med* 1998;122:726–731.
368. Conti DJ, Rubin RH. Infection of the central nervous system in organ transplant recipients. *Neurol Clin* 1988;6:241–260.
369. Singh N, Husain S. Infections of the central nervous system in transplant recipients. *Transpl Infect Dis* 2000;2:101–111.
370. Walker RW, Brochstein JA. Neurologic complications of immunosuppressive agents. *Neurol Clin* 1988;6:261–278.
371. Scherrer U, Vissing SF, Morgan BJ, et al. Cyclosporine-induced sympathetic activation and hypertension after heart transplantation. *N Engl J Med* 1990;323:693–699.
372. Cosottini M, Lazzarotti G, Ceravolo R, et al. Cyclosporine-related posterior reversible encephalopathy syndrome (PRES) in non-transplant patient: a case report and literature review. *Eur J Neurol* 2003;10:461–462.
373. Kiemeneij IM, de Leeuw FE, Ramos LM, et al. Acute headache as a presenting symptom of tacrolimus encephalopathy. *J Neurol Neurosurg Psychiatry* 2003;74:1126–1127.
374. Stein DP, Lederman RJ, Vogt DP, et al. Neurological complications following liver transplantation. *Ann Neurol* 1992;31:644–649.
375. Lamy C, Oppenheim C, Meder JF, et al. Neuroimaging in posterior reversible encephalopathy syndrome. *J Neuroimaging* 2004;14: 89–96.
376. Pavlakis SG, Frank Y, Chusid R. Hypertensive encephalopathy, reversible occipitoparietal encephalopathy, or reversible posterior leukoencephalopathy: three names for an old syndrome. *J Child Neurol* 1999;14:277–281.
377. Suminoe A, Matsuzaki A, Kira R, et al. Reversible posterior leukoencephalopathy syndrome in children with cancers. *J Pediatr Hematol Oncol* 2003;25:236–239.
378. Ito Y, Arahata Y, Goto Y, et al. Cisplatin neurotoxicity presenting as reversible posterior leukoencephalopathy syndrome. *AJNR Am J Neuroradiol* 1998;19:415–417.
379. Wijdicks EFM, Wiesner RH, Krom RAF. Neurotoxicity in liver transplant recipients with cyclosporine immunosuppression. *Neurology* 1995;45:1962–1964.
380. Antunes NL, Small TN, George D, et al. Posterior leukoencephalopathy syndrome may not be reversible. *Pediatr Neurol* 1999;20:241–243.
381. Prasad N, Gulati S, Gupta RK, et al. Is reversible posterior leukoencephalopathy with severe hypertension completely reversible in all patients? *Pediatr Nephrol* 2003;18:1161–1166.
382. Khan RB, Hunt DL, Thompson SJ. Gabapentin to control seizures in children undergoing cancer treatment. *J Child Neurol* 2004;19: 97–101.
383. Chabolla DR, Harnois DM, Meschia JF. Levetiracetam monotherapy for liver transplant patients with seizures. *Transplant Proc* 2003;35:1480–1481.
384. Arrelano F, Krupp P. Muscular disorder associated with cyclosporin. *Lancet* 1991;337:915.
385. Oursler DP, Holley KE, Wagoner RD. Hemolytic uremic syndrome after bone marrow transplantation without total body irradiation. *Am J Nephrol* 1993;13:167–170.
386. Eidelman BH, Abu-Elmagd K, Wilson J, et al. Neurologic complications of FK 506. *Transplant Proc* 1991;23:3175–3178.
387. Wijdicks EFM, Wiesner RH, Dahlke LJ, et al. FK506-induced neurotoxicity in liver transplantation. *Ann Neurol* 1994;35:498–501.
388. Osterman JD, Trauner DA, Reznik VM, et al. Transient hemiparesis associated with monoclonal CD3 antibody (OKT3) therapy. *Pediatr Neurol* 1993;9:482–484.
389. Strominger MB, Liu GT, Schatz NJ. Optic disk swelling and abducens palsies associated with OKT3. *Am J Ophthalmol* 1995;119: 664–665.
390. Mott SH, Packer RJ, Vezina LG, et al. Encephalopathy with parkinsonian features in children following bone marrow transplantations and high-dose amphotericin B. *Ann Neurol* 1995;37:810–814.
391. Martinez AJ, Estol C, Faris AA. Neurologic complications of liver transplantation. *Neurol Clin* 1988;6:327–348.
392. Ferreiro GA, Robert MA, Townsend J, et al. Neuropathologic findings after liver transplantation. *Acta Neuropathol* 1992;84: 1–14.
393. Krull K, Fuchs C, Yurk H, et al. Neurocognitive outcome in pediatric liver transplant recipients. *Pediatr Transplant* 2003;7:111–118.
394. Kennard BD, Stewart SM, Phelan-McAuliffe D, et al. Academic outcome in long-term survivors of pediatric liver transplantation. *J Dev Behav Pediatr* 1999;20:17–23.
395. Ringoir S. An update on uremic toxins. *Kidney Int* 1997;52[Suppl 62]:S2–S4.
396. Lazaro RP, Kirshner HS. Proximal muscle weakness in uremia: case reports and review of the literature. *Arch Neurol* 1980;37:555–558.
397. Raskin NH, Fishman RA. Neurologic disorders in renal failure. *N Engl J Med* 1976;294:143–148, 204–210.
398. Lockwood AH. Neurologic complications of renal disease. *Neurol Clin* 1989;7:617–627.
399. Mentser MI, Clay S, Malekzadeh MH, et al. Peripheral motor nerve conduction velocities in children undergoing chronic hemodialysis. *Nephron* 1978;22:337–341.
400. Said G, Boudier L, Selva J, et al. Different patterns of uremic polyneuropathy: clinicopathologic study. *Neurology* 1983;33:67–574.
401. Pirzada NA, Morgenlander JC. Peripheral neuropathy in patients with chronic renal failure. A treatable source of discomfort and disability. *Postgrad Med* 1997;249–261.
402. Berretta JS, Holbrook CT, Haller JS. Chronic renal failure presenting as proximal muscle weakness in a child. *J Child Neurol* 1986;1:50–52.
403. Hughes JR. Correlations between EEG and chemical changes in uremia. *Electroencephalogr Clin Neurophysiol* 1980;48:583–594.
404. Fusco L, Picca S, Rizzoni G, et al. Long-term EEG monitoring in uremic children on chronic dialysis treatment. *Eur Neurol* 1991;31:193–198.
405. Crittenden M, Holliday MA, Piel CF, et al. Intellectual development of children with renal insufficiency and end stage renal disease. *Int J Pediatr Nephrol* 1985;6:265–280.
406. McGraw ME, Haka-Ikse K. Neurologic-developmental sequelae of chronic renal failure in infancy. *J Pediatr* 1985;106:579–583.
407. Passer JA. Cerebral atrophy in end-stage uremia. *Proc Dialysis Transplant Forum* 1977;7:91–94.
408. Hauser RA, Lacey DM, Knight MR. Hypertensive encephalopathy. Magnetic resonance imaging demonstration of reversible cortical and white matter lesions. *Arch Neurol* 1988;45:1078–1083.
409. Fraser CL, Arieff AI. Nervous system complications in uremia. *Ann Intern Med* 1988;109:143–153.
410. Smogorzewski MJ. Central nervous dysfunction in uremia. *Am J Kidney Dis* 2001;38:S122–128.

411. Ibrahim MM, Barnes AD, Crosland JM, et al. Effect of renal transplantation on uraemic neuropathy. *Lancet* 1974;2:739–742.
412. Temple RM, Deary IJ, Winney RJ. Recombinant erythropoietin improves cognitive function in patients maintained on chronic ambulatory peritoneal dialysis. *Nephrol Dial Transplant* 1995;10: 1733–1738.
413. Davis ID, Chang PN, Nevins TE. Successful renal transplantation accelerates development in young uremic children. *Pediatrics* 1990;86:594–600.
414. So SKS, Chang PN, Najarian JS, et al. Growth and development of infants after renal transplantation. *J Pediatr* 1987;110:343–350.
415. Hulstijn-Dirkmaat GM, Damhuis IH, Jetten ML, et al. The cognitive development of pre-school children treated for chronic renal failure. *Pediatr Nephrol* 1995;9:464–469.
416. Madden SJ, Ledermann SE, Guerrero-Blanco M, et al. Cognitive and psychosocial outcome of infants dialysed in infancy. *Child Care Health Dev* 2003;29:55–61.
417. Bock GH, Conners CK, Ruley J, et al. Disturbances of brain maturation and neurodevelopment during chronic renal failure in infancy. *J Pediatr* 1989;114:231–238.
418. Davis ID, Chang PN, Nevins TE. Successful renal transplantation accelerates development in young uremic children. *Pediatrics* 1990;86:594–600.
419. Mendley SR, Zelko FA. Improvement in specific aspects of neurocognitive performance in children after renal transplantation. *Kidney Int* 1999;56:318–323.
420. Brouhard BH, Donaldson LA, Lawry KW, et al. Cognitive functioning in children on dialysis and post-transplantation. *Pediatr Transplant* 2000;4:261–267.
421. Dodson WE, Prensky AL, DeVivo DC, et al. Management of seizure disorders: selected aspects. *J Pediatr* 1974;89:527–540.
422. Wassner SJ, Malekzadeh MH, Pennisi AJ, et al. Allograft survival in patients receiving anticonvulsant medications. *Clin Nephrol* 1977;8:293–297.
423. Cutler RE. Cyclosporine drug interactions. *Dial Transplant* 1988;17:139–151.
424. Tyler HR. Neurological complications of dialysis, transplantation and other forms of treatment in chronic uremia. *Neurology* 1965;15:1081–1088.
425. Graham JR, Bana D, Yap A. Headache, hypertension and renal disease. *Res Clin Stud Headache* 1978;6:147–154.
426. Barton CH, Vaziri ND. Central retinal vein occlusion associated with hemodialysis. *Am J Med Sci* 1979;277:39–47.
427. Basile C, Miller JD, Koles ZJ, et al. The effects of dialysis on brain water and EEG in stable chronic uremia. *Am J Kidney Dis* 1987;9:462–469.
428. Tzanatos HA, Agroyannis B, Chondros C, et al. Cytokine release and serum lipoprotein (a) alterations during hemodialysis. *Artif Organs* 2000;24:329–333.
429. Goksan B, Karaali-Savrun F, Ertan S, et al. Haemodialysis-related headache. *Cephalalgia* 2004;24:284–287.
430. Aydin OF, Uner C, Senbil N, et al. Central pontine and extrapontine myelinolysis owing to disequilibrium syndrome. *J Child Neurol* 2003;18:292–296.
431. Tarhan NC, Agildere AM, Benli US, et al. Osmotic demyelination syndrome in end-stage renal disease after recent hemodialysis: MRI of the brain. *AJR Am J Roentgenol* 2004;182:809–816.
432. Ihara M, Ito T, Yanagihara C, et al. Wernicke's encephalopathy associated with hemodialysis: report of two cases and review of the literature. *Clin Neurol Neurosurg* 1999;101:118–121.
433. Pieta J, Millar T, Zacharias J, et al. Effect of pergolide on restless legs and leg movements in sleep in uremic patients. *Sleep* 1998;21:617–622.
434. Takaki J, Nishi T, Nangaku M, et al. Clinical and psychological aspects of restless legs syndrome in uremic patients on hemodialysis. *Am J Kidney Dis* 2003;41:833–839.
435. Van den Neucker K, Vanderstraeten G, Vanholder R. Peripheral motor and sensory nerve conduction studies in haemodialysis patients. A study of 54 patients. *Electromyogr Clin Neurophysiol* 1998;38:467–474.
436. Korzets Z, Zeltzer E, Rathaus M, et al. Uremic optic neuropathy. A uremic manifestation mandating dialysis. *Am J Nephrol* 1998; 18:240–242.
437. Pirzada NA, Morgenlander JC. Peripheral neuropathy in patients with chronic renal failure. A treatable source of discomfort and disability. *Postgrad Med* 1997;102:249–250, 255–257.
438. Hughes JR, Schreeder MT. EEG in dialysis encephalopathy. *Neurology* 1980;30:1148–1154.
439. Alfrey AC, Mishell JM, Burks J, et al. Syndrome of dyspraxia and multifocal seizures associated with chronic hemodialysis. *Trans Am Soc Artif Int Organs* 1972;18:257–261, 266–267.
440. Rob PM, Niederstadt C, Reusche E. Dementia in patients undergoing long-term dialysis: aetiology, differential diagnoses, epidemiology and management. *CNS Drugs* 2001;15:691–699.
441. Rotundo A, Nevins TE, Lipton M, et al. Progressive encephalopathy in children with chronic renal insufficiency in infancy. *Kidney Int* 1982;21:486–491.
442. Trompeter RS, Polinsky MS, Andreoli SA, et al. Neurologic complications of renal failure. *Am J Kidney Dis* 1986;7:318–328.
443. Rivera-Vazquez AB, Noriega-Sanchez A, Ramirez-Gonzalez R, et al. Acute hypercalcemia in hemodialysis patients: distinction from dialysis dementia. *Nephron* 1980;25:243–246.
444. Jellinek, EH, Painter M, Prineas J, et al. Hypertensive encephalopathy with cortical disorders of vision. *Quart J Med* 1964;33:239–256.
445. Rifkind D, Marchioro TL, Schneck SA, et al. Systemic fungal infections complicating renal transplantations and immunosuppressive therapy. *Am J Med* 1967;43:28–38.
446. Schneck SA. Neuropathological features of human organ transplantation. I. Probable cytomegalovirus infection. *J Neuropathol Exp Neurol* 1965;24:415–429.
447. Reis MA, Costa RS, Ferraz AS. Causes of death in renal transplant recipients: a study of 102 autopsies from 1968 to 1991. *J R Soc Med* 1995;88:24–27.
448. Grimm PC, Ettenger R. Pediatric renal transplantation. *Adv Pediatr* 1992;39:441–493.
449. Wells TG, Ulstrom RA, Nevins TE. Hypoglycemia in pediatric renal allograft recipients. *J Pediatr* 1988;113:1002–1007.
450. Gayal RK, McEvoy L, Wilson DB. Hodgkin disease after renal transplantation in childhood. *J Pediatr Hematol Oncol* 1996;18: 392–395.
451. Hoshida Y, Aozasa K. Malignancies in organ transplant recipients. *Pathol Int* 2004;54:649–658.
452. Chedrawi AK, Gharaybeh SI, Al-Ghwery SA, et al. Cephalosporin-induced nonconvulsive status epilepticus in a uremic child. *Pediatr Neurol* 2004;30:135–139.
453. Tanimu DZ, Obeid T, Awada A, et al. Absence status: an overlooked cause of acute confusion in hemodialysis patients. *J Nephrol* 1998;11:146–147.
454. Thorpe CM. Shiga toxin-producing Escherichia coli infection. *Clin Infect Dis* 2004;38:1298–1303.
455. Eriksson KJ, Boyd SG, Tasker RC. Acute neurology and neurophysiology of haemolytic-uraemic syndrome. *Arch Dis Child* 2001;84:434–435.
456. Dussault J, Ruel J. Thyroid hormones and brain development. *Annu Rev Physiol* 1987;49:321–334.
457. Bernal J, Guadano-Ferraz A, Morte B. Perspectives in the study of thyroid hormone action on brain development and function. *Thyroid* 2003;13:1005–1012.
458. Oppenheimer JH, Schwartz HL. Molecular basis of thyroid hormone-dependent brain development. *Endocr Rev* 1997;18:462–475.
459. Burrow GN, Fisher DA, Larsen PR. Maternal and fetal thyroid function. *N Engl J Med* 1994;331:1072–1078.
460. Murray GR. Note on the treatment of myxoedema by hypodermic injection of an extract of the thyroid gland of a sheep. *BMJ* 1891;2: 796.
461. Klein AH, Meltzer S, Kenny FM. Improved prognosis in congenital hypothyroidism treated before age three months. *J Pediatr* 1972;81:912–915.
462. Smith DW, Klein AM, Henderson JR, et al. Congenital hypothyroidism–signs and symptoms in the newborn period. *J Pediatr* 1975;87:958–962.
463. Fisher DA. Thyroid function in the fetus. In: Fisher DA, Burrow GN, eds. *Perinatal thyroid physiology and disease*. New York: Raven Press, 1975:21.

464. Kopp P. Perspective: genetic defects in the etiology of congenital hypothyroidism. *Endocrinology* 2002;143:2019–2024.
465. Macchia PE, Lapi P, Krude H, et al. PAX8 mutations associated with congenital hypothyroidism caused by thyroid dysgenesis. *Nat Genet* 1998;19:83–86.
466. Smith DW, Klein AM, Henderson JR, et al. Congenital hypothyroidism: signs and symptoms in newborn period. *J Pediatr* 1975;87:958–962.
467. Vanderschueren-Lodeweyckx M, Debruyne F, Dooms L, et al. Sensorineural hearing loss in sporadic congenital hypothyroidism. *Arch Dis Child* 1983;58:419–422.
468. Laureau E, Hebert R, Vanasse M, et al. Somatosensory evoked potentials and auditory brain-stem responses in congenital hypothyroidism. II. A cross-sectional study in childhood. Correlations with hormonal levels and developmental quotients. *Electroenceph Clin Neurophysiol* 1987;67:521–530.
469. Wilkins L. The effects of thyroid deficiency upon the development of the brain. *Assoc Res Nerv Ment Dis Proc* 1962;39:150–155.
470. Schultz MA, Schulte FJ, Akiyama Y, et al. Development of electroencephalographic sleep phenomena in hypothyroid infants. *Electroencephalogr Clin Neurophysiol* 1968;25:351–358.
471. Krude H, Schutz B, Biebermann H, et al. Choreoathetosis, hypothyroidism, and pulmonary alterations due to human NKX2-1 haploinsufficiency. *J Clin Invest* 2002;109:475–480.
472. Doyle DA, Gonzalez I, Thomas B, Scavina M. Autosomal dominant transmission of congenital hypothyroidism, neonatal respiratory distress, and ataxia caused by a mutation of NKX2–1. *J Pediatr* 2004;145:190–193.
473. De Felice M, Di Lauro R. Thyroid development and its disorders: genetics and molecular mechanisms. *Endocr Rev* 2004;25:722–746.
474. Batsakis JG, Nishiyama RH. Deafness with sporadic goiter. Pendred's syndrome. *Arch Otolaryngol* 1962;76:401–406.
475. Reardon W, Trembath RC. Pendred syndrome. *J Med Genet* 1996;33:1037–1040.
476. Reardon W, Coffey R, Chowdhury T, et al. Prevalence, age of onset, and natural history of thyroid disease in Pendred syndrome. *J Med Genet* 1999;36:595–598.
477. Reardon W, OMahoney CF, Trembath R, et al. Enlarged vestibular aqueduct: a radiological marker of Pendred syndrome, and mutation of the PDS gene. *QJM* 2000;93:99–104.
478. Yoshida A, Taniguchi S, Hisatome I, et al. Pendrin is an iodide-specific apical porter responsible for iodide efflux from thyroid cells. *J Clin Endocrinol Metab* 2002;87:3356–3361.
479. Halpern JP, Boyages SC, Maberly GF, et al. The neurology of endemic cretinism. A study of two endemias. *Brain* 1991;114:825–841.
480. Wang YY, Yang SH. Improvement in hearing among otherwise normal school children in iodine-deficient areas of Guizhou, China, following use of iodized salt. *Lancet* 1985;2:518–520.
481. Ma T, Lian ZC, Qi SP, et al. Magnetic resonance imaging of brain and the neuromotor disorder in endemic cretinism. *Ann Neurol* 1993;34:91–94.
482. Spano D, Branchi I, Rosica A, et al. Rhes is involved in striatal function. *Mol Cell Biol* 2004;24:5788–5796.
483. Morreale de Escobar G. The role of thyroid hormone in fetal neurodevelopment. *J Pediatr Endocrinol Metab* 2001;14[Suppl 6]:1453–1462.
484. Kocher T. Zur Verhütung des Cretinismus und cretinoider Zustände nach neuen Forschungen. *Dtsch Z Chir* 1892;34:556–626.
485. Debré R, Sémélaigne G. Syndrome of diffuse muscular hypertrophy in infants causing an athletic appearance. Its connection with congenital myxedema. *Am J Dis Child* 1935;50:1351–1361.
486. Tullu MS, Udgirkar VS, Muranjan MN. Kocher-Debre-Semelaigne syndrome: hypothyroidism with muscle pseudohypertrophy. *Indian J Pediatr* 2003;70:671–673.
487. Spiro AJ, Hirano A, Beilin RL, et al. Cretinism with muscular hypertrophy (Kocher-Debré-Sémélaigne syndrome): histochemical and ultrastructural study of skeletal muscle. *Arch Neurol* 1970;23:340–349.
488. Mastropasqua M, Spagna G, Baldini V, et al. Hoffman's syndrome: muscle stiffness, pseudohypertrophy and hypothyroidism. *Horm Res* 2003;59:105–108.
489. Reuss ML, Paneth N, Pinto-Martin JA, et al. The relation of transient hypothyroxinemia in preterm infants to neurologic development at two years of age. *N Engl J Med* 1996;334:821–827.
490. Osborn DA. Thyroid hormone for preventing of neurodevelopmental impairment in preterm infants. *Cochrone Database Syst Rev* 2000;2:CD001070.
491. Haddow JE, Palomaki GE, Allan WC, et al. Maternal thyroid deficiency during pregnancy and subsequent neuropsychological development of the child. *N Engl J Med* 1999;341:549–555.
492. Klein RZ, Sargent JD, Larsen PR. Relation of severity of maternal hypothyroidism to cognitive development of offspring. *J Med Screen* 2001;8:18–20.
493. Kung AW, Low LC. Thyrotrophin-blocking antibodies in congenital hypothyroidism. *J Paediatr Child Health* 1992;28:50–53.
494. Evans C, Jordan NJ, Owens G, et al. Potent thyrotrophin receptor-blocking antibodies: a cause of transient congenital hypothyroidism and delayed thyroid development. *Eur J Endocrinol* 2004;150:265–268.
495. Andersen HS. Studies in hypothyroidism in children. *Acta Paediatr* 1961;[Suppl]:125.
496. Aronson R, Ehrlich RM, Bailey JD, et al. Growth in children with congenital hypothyroidism detected by neonatal screening. *J Pediatr* 1990;116:33–37.
497. Derksen-Lubsen G, Verkerk PH. Neuropsychologic development in early treated congenital hypothyroidism: analysis of literature data. *Pediatr Res* 1996;39:561–566.
498. Wiebel J. Cerebellar-ataxic syndrome in children and adolescents with hypothyroidism under treatment. *Acta Paediatr Scand* 1976; 65:201–205.
499. MacFaul R, Dorner S, Brett EM, et al. Neurological abnormalities in patients treated for hypothyroidism from early life. *Arch Dis Child* 1978;53:611–619.
500. Penfold JL, Simpson DA. Premature craniosynostosis: a complication of thyroid replacement therapy. *J Pediatr* 1975;86:360–363.
501. Duyff RF, Van den Bosch J, Laman DM. Neuromuscular findings in thyroid dysfunction: a prospective clinical and electrodiagnostic study. *J Neurol Neurosurg Psychiatry* 2000;68:750–755.
502. Tanwani LK, Lohano V, Ewart R, et al. Myasthenia gravis in conjunction with Graves' disease: a diagnostic challenge. *Endocr Pract* 2001;7:275–278.
503. Swanson JW, Kelly JJ Jr, McConahey WM. Neurologic aspects of thyroid dysfunction. *Mayo Clin Proc* 1981;56:504–512.
504. Bartalena L, Wiersinga WM, Pinchera A, et al. Graves' ophthalmopathy: state of the art and perspectives. *J Endocrinol Invest* 2004;27:295–301.
505. Fishbeck KH, Layzer RB. Paroxysmal choreoathetosis associated with thyrotoxicosis. *Ann Neurol* 1979;6:453–454.
506. Klawans HL Jr, Shenker DM. Observations on the dopaminergic nature of hyperthyroid chorea. *J Neurol Transm* 1972;33:73–81.
507. Jabbari B, Huott AD. Seizures in thyrotoxicosis. *Epilepsia* 1980;21: 91–96.
508. Radetti G, Dordi B, Mengarda G, et al. Thyrotoxicosis presenting with seizures and coma in two children. *Am J Dis Child* 1993;147: 925–927.
509. Kopp P, van Sande J, Parma J, et al. Congenital hyperthyroidism caused by a mutation in the thyrotropin-receptor gene. *N Engl J Med* 1995;332:150–154.
510. Vaidya B, Campbell V, Tripp JH, et al. Premature birth and low birth weight associated with nonautoimmune hyperthyroidism due to an activating thyrotropin receptor gene mutation. *Clin Endocrinol (Oxf)* 2004;60:711–718.
511. Hollingsworth DR, Mabry CC. Congenital Graves' disease: four familial cases with long-term follow-up and perspective. *Am J Dis Child* 1976;130:148–155.
512. Byrne OC, Zuberi SM, Madigan CA, King MD. Hashimoto's thyroiditis—a rare but treatable cause of encephalopathy in children. *Eur J Paediatr Neurol* 2000;4:279–282.
513. Avila A, Serrado A, Reig L, et al. Early presentation of gait disturbance in a steroid-responsive encephalopathy associated with autoimmune thyroiditis. *Eur J Neurol* 2003;10:601.
514. Maydell B, Kopp M, Komorowski G, et al. Hashimoto's thyroiditis—a rare but treatable cause of encephalopathy in children. *Eur J Paediatr Neurol* 2000;4:279–282.
515. Gucuyener K, Serdaroglu A, Bideci A, et al. Tremor and myoclonus

heralding Hashimoto's encephalopathy. *J Pediatr Endocrinol Metab* 2000;13:1137–1141.
516. Jefferson A. A clinical correlation between encephalopathy and papilloedema in Addison's disease. *J Neurol Neurosurg Psychiatry* 1956;19:21–27.
517. Russell GA, Coulter JB, Isherwood DM, et al. Autoimmune Addison's disease and thyrotoxic thyroiditis presenting as encephalopathy in twins. *Arch Dis Child* 1991;66:350–352.
518. Kimber J, McLean BN, Prevett M, et al. Allgrove or 4 "A" syndrome: an autosomal recessive syndrome causing multisystem neurological disease. *J Neurol Neurosurg Psychiatry* 2003;74:654–657.
519. Huebner A, Kaindl AM, Braun R, et al. New insights into the molecular basis of the triple A syndrome. *Endocr Res* 2002;28:733–739.
520. Kinjo S, Takemoto M, Miyako K, et al. Two cases of Allgrove syndrome with mutations in the AAAS gene. *Endocr J* 2004;51:474–477.
520a. Salehi M, Houlden H, Sheikh A, Poretsky L. The diagnosis of adrenal insufficiency in a patient with Allgrove syndrome and a novel mutation in the ALADIN gene. *Metabolism* 2005;54:200–205.
521. Cacciari E, Zucchini S, Carla G, et al. Endocrine function and morphological findings in patients with disorders of the hypothalamo-pituitary area: a study with magnetic resonance. *Arch Dis Child* 1990;65:1199–1202.
522. Ng SM, Kumar Y, Cody D, et al. Cranial MRI scans are indicated in all girls with central precocious puberty. *Arch Dis Child* 2003;88:414–418.
523. Bozzola M, Adamsbaum C, Biscaldi I, et al. Role of magnetic resonance imaging in the diagnosis and prognosis of growth hormone deficiency. *Clin Endocrinol (Oxf)* 1996;45:21–26.
524. Arslanoglu I, Kutlu H, Isguven P, et al. Diagnostic value of pituitary MRI in differentiation of children with normal growth hormone secretion, isolated growth hormone deficiency and multiple pituitary hormone deficiency. *J Pediatr Endocrinol Metab* 2001;14:517–523.
525. Kornreich L, Horev G, Lazar L, et al. MR findings in growth hormone deficiency: correlation with severity of hypopituitarism. *AJNR Am J Neuroradiol* 1998;19:1495–1499.
526. Argyropoulou M, Perignon F, Brauner R, et al. Magnetic resonance imaging in the diagnosis of growth hormone deficiency. *J Pediatr* 1992;120:886–891.
527. Rappaport R. Magnetic resonance imaging in pituitary disease. *Growth Genet Hor* 1995;11:1–5.
528. Low PA, McLeod JG, Turtle JR, et al. Peripheral neuropathy in acromegaly. *Brain* 1974;97:139–152.
529. Vasile M, Marsot-Dupuch K, Kujas M, et al. Idiopathic granulomatous hypophysitis: clinical and imaging features. *Neuroradiology* 1997;39:7–11.
530. Leung GK, Lopes MB, Thorner MO, et al. Primary hypophysitis: a single-center experience in 16 cases. *J Neurosurg* 2004;101:262–271.
531. Laurence JZ, Moon RC. Four cases of retinitis pigmentosa occurring in the same family and accompanied by general imperfection of development. *Ophthal Rev* 1866;2:32–41.
532. Farag TI, Teebi AS. Bardet-Biedl and Laurence-Moon syndromes in a mixed Arab population. *Clin Genet* 1988;33:78–82.
533. Fan Y, Esmail MA, Ansley SJ, et al. Mutations in a member of the Ras superfamily of small GTP-binding proteins causes Bardet-Biedl syndrome. *Nat Genet* 2004;36:989–993.
534. Koenig R. Bardet-Biedl syndrome and Usher syndrome. *Dev Ophthalmol* 2003;37:126–140.
535. Green JS, Parfrey PS, Harnett JD, et al. The cardinal manifestations of Bardet-Biedl syndrome, a form of Laurence-Moon-Biedl syndrome. *N Engl J Med* 1989;321:1002–1009.
536. Beales PL, Elcioglu N, Woolf AS, et al. New criteria for improved diagnosis of Bardet-Biedl syndrome: results of a population survey. *J Med Genet* 1999;36:437–446.
537. Jacobson SG, Borruat FX, Apathy PP. Patterns of rod and cone dysfunction in Bardet-Biedl syndrome. *Am J Ophthalmol* 1990;109:676–688.
538. Soliman AT, Rajab A, AlSalmi I, et al. Empty sellae, impaired testosterone secretion, and defective hypothalamic-pituitary growth and gonadal axes in children with Bardet-Biedl syndrome. *Metabolism* 1996;45:1230–1234.
539. Goldstein JL, Fialkow PJ. The Alstrom syndrome. Report of three cases with further delineation of the clinical, pathophysiological, and genetic aspects of the disorder. *Medicine (Balt)* 1973;52:53–71.
540. Van den Abeele K, Craen M, Schuil J, et al. Ophthalmologic and systemic features of the Alstrom syndrome: report of 9 cases. *Bull Soc Belge Ophtalmol* 2001;281:67–72.
541. Verloes A, Temple IK, Bonnet S, et al. Coloboma, mental retardation, hypogonadism, and obesity: critical review of the so-called Biemond syndrome type 2, updated nosology, and delineation of three 'new' syndromes. *Am J Med Genet* 1997;69:370–379.
542. Slavotinek AM, Biesecker LG. Phenotypic overlap of McKusick-Kaufman syndrome with Bardet-Biedl syndrome: a literature review. *Am J Med Genet* 2000;95:208–215.
543. Gorlin RJ, Anderson VE, Scott CR. Hypertrophied frenuli, oligophrenia, familial trembling and anomalies of the hand. Report of four cases in one family and a forme fruste in another. *N Engl J Med* 1961;264:486–489.
544. Toriello HV. Heterogeneity and variability in the oral-facial-digital syndromes. *Am J Med Genet Suppl* 1988;4:149–159.
545. Leao MJ, Ribeiro-Silva ML. Orofaciodigital syndrome type I in a patient with severe CNS defects. *Pediatr Neurol* 1995;13:247–251.
546. Odent S, Le Marec B, Toutain A, et al. Central nervous system malformations and early end-stage renal disease in oro-facio-digital syndrome type I: a review. *Am J Med Genet* 1998;75:389–394.
547. Sotos JF, Dodge PR, Muirhead D, et al. Cerebral gigantism in childhood: a syndrome of excessively rapid growth with acromegalic features and a nonprogressive neurologic disorder. *N Engl J Med* 1964;271:109–116.
548. Ray M, Malhi P, Bhalla AK, Singhi PD. Cerebral gigantism with West syndrome. *Indian Pediatr* 2003;40:673–675.
549. Schaefer GB, Bodensteiner JB, Buehler BA, et al. The neuroimaging findings in Sotos syndrome. *Am J Med Genet* 1997;68:462–465.
550. Mouridsen SE, Hansen MB. Neuropsychiatric aspects of Sotos syndrome. A review and two case illustrations. *Eur Child Adolesc Psychiatry* 2002;11:43–48.
551. de Boer L, Kant SG, Karperien M, et al. Genotype-phenotype correlation in patients suspected of having Sotos syndrome. *Horm Res* 2004;62:197–207.
552. Cole TR, Dennis NR, Hughes HE. Weaver syndrome. *J Med Genet* 1992;29:332–337.
553. Opitz JM, Weaver DW, Reynolds JF Jr. The syndromes of Sotos and Weaver: reports and review. *Am J Med Genet* 1998;79:294–304.
554. Rio M, Clech L, Amiel J, et al. Spectrum of NSD1 mutations in Sotos and Weaver syndromes. *J Med Genet* 2003;40:436–440.
555. Baujat G, Rio M, Rossignol S, et al. Paradoxical NSD1 mutations in Beckwith-Wiedemann syndrome and 11p15 anomalies in Sotos syndrome. *Am J Hum Genet* 2004;74:715–720.
556. Elliott M, Bayly R, Cole T, et al. Clinical features and natural history of Beckwith-Wiedemann syndrome: presentation of 74 new cases. *Clin Genet* 1994;46:168–174.
557. Patel H, Tze WJ, Crichton JU, et al. Optic nerve hypoplasia with hypopituitarism: septo-optic dysplasia with hypopituitarism. *Am J Dis Child* 1975;129:175–180.
558. Kuban KC, Teele RL, Wallman J. Septo-optic-dysplasia-schizencephaly. Radiographic and clinical features. *Pediatr Radiol* 1989;19:145–150.
559. Sener RN. Septo-optic dysplasia associated with cerebral cortical dysplasia (cortico-septo-optic dysplasia). *J Neuroradiol* 1996;23:245–247.
560. Castells S, Reddy CM, Hashemi SE. Metabolic responses to human growth hormone in children with cerebral dwarfism. *J Pediatr* 1976;89:958–960.
561. Winegrad AL. Banting lecture 1986. Does a common mechanism induce the diverse complications of diabetes? *Diabetes* 1987;36:396–406.
562. Eeg-Olofsson O, Petersen I. Childhood diabetic neuropathy. *Acta Paediat Scand* 1966;53:163–176.
563. Cracco J, Castells S, Mark E. Spinal somatosensory evoked potentials in juvenile diabetes. *Ann Neurol* 1984;15:55–58.
564. el Bahri-Ben Mrad F, Gouider R, Fredj M. Childhood diabetic neuropathy: a clinical and electrophysiological study. *Funct Neurol* 2000;15:35–40.

565. Hoffman WH, Hart ZH, Frank RN. Correlates of delayed motor nerve conduction and retinopathy in juvenile-onset diabetes mellitus. *J Pediatr* 1983;102:351–356.
566. Kruger M, Brunko E, Dorchy H, et al. Femoral versus peroneal neuropathy in diabetic children and adolescents—relationships to clinical status, metabolic control and retinopathy. *Diabetes Metab* 1987;13:110–115.
567. Bastron JA, Thomas JE. Diabetic polyradiculopathy: clinical and electromyographic findings in 105 patients. *Mayo Clin Proc* 1981; 56:725–732.
568. Wilson JL, Sokol DK, Smith LH, et al. Acute painful neuropathy (insulin neuritis) in a boy following rapid glycemic control for type 1 diabetes mellitus. *J Child Neurol* 2003;18:365–367.
569. Takayama S, Takahashi Y, Osawa M, et al. Acute painful neuropathy restricted to the abdomen following rapid glycaemic control in type 2 diabetes. *J Int Med Res* 2004;32:558–562.
570. Rovet JF, Ehrlich RM. The effect of hypoglycemic seizures on cognitive function in children with diabetes: a 7-year prospective study. *J Pediatr* 1999;134:503–506.
571. Northam EA, Anderson PJ, Jacobs R, et al. Neuropsychological profiles of children with type 1 diabetes 6 years after disease onset. *Diabetes Care* 2001;24:1541–1546.
572. Kety SS, Polis BD, Nadler CS, et al. Blood flow and oxygen consumption of the human brain in diabetic acidosis and coma. *J Clin Invest* 1948;27:500–510.
573. Rosival V. The influence of blood hydrogen ion concentration on the level of consciousness in diabetic ketoacidosis. *Ann Clin Res* 1987;19:23–25.
574. Ohman JL Jr, Marliss EB, Aoki TT, et al. The cerebrospinal fluid in diabetic ketoacidosis. *N Engl J Med* 1971;284:283–290.
575. Rosenbloom AL. Intracerebral crises during treatment of diabetic ketoacidosis. *Diabetes Care* 1990;13:22–33.
576. Duck SC, Weldon VV, Pagliara AS, et al. Cerebral edema complicating therapy for diabetic ketoacidosis. *Diabetes* 1976;25:111–115.
577. Edge JA, Hawkins MM, Winter DL, et al. The risk and outcome of cerebral oedema developing during diabetic ketoacidosis. *Arch Dis Child* 2001;85:16–22.
578. Muir AB, Quisling RG, Yang MC, et al. Cerebral edema in childhood diabetic ketoacidosis: natural history, radiographic findings, and early identification. *Diabetes Care* 2004;27:1541–1546.
579. Levitsky LL. Symptomatic cerebral edema in diabetic ketoacidosis: the mechanism is clarified but still far from clear. *J Pediatr* 2004; 145:149–150.
580. Van der Meulen JA, Klip A, Grinstein S. Possible mechanism for cerebral oedema in diabetic ketoacidosis. *Lancet* 1987;2:306–308.
581. Glaser NS, Wootton-Gorges SL, Marcin JP. Mechanism of cerebral edema in children with diabetic ketoacidosis. *J Pediatr* 2004; 145:164–171.
582. Edvinsson L, Owman C, Sjoberg NO. Autonomic nerves, mast cells, and amine receptors in human brain vessels. A histochemical and pharmacological study. *Brain Res* 1976;115:377–393.
583. Franklin B, Liu J, Ginsberg-Fellner F. Cerebral edema and ophthalmoplegia reversed by mannitol in a new case of insulin-dependent diabetes mellitus. *Pediatrics* 1982;69:87–90.
584. Joosten R, Frank M, Hornchen H, et al. Hyperosmolar nonketotic diabetic coma. *Eur J Pediatr* 1981;137:233–236.
585. Morres CA, Dire DJ. Movement disorders as a manifestation of nonketotic hyperglycemia. *J Emerg Med* 1989;7:359–364.
586. Vernon DD, Postellon DC. Nonketotic hyperosmolal diabetic coma in a child: management with low-dose insulin infusion and intracranial pressure monitoring. *Pediatrics* 1986;77:770–772.
587. Hardy C, Khanim F, Torres R, et al. Clinical and molecular genetic analysis of 19 Wolfram syndrome kindreds demonstrating a wide spectrum of mutations in WFS1. *Am J Hum Genet* 1999;65:1279–1290.
588. Grosse Aldenhovel HB, Gallenkamp U, Sulemana CA. Juvenile onset diabetes mellitus, central diabetes insipidus and optic atrophy (Wolfram-syndrome)—neurological findings and prognostic implications. *Neuropediatrics* 1991;22:103–106.
588a. Osman AA, Saito M, Makepeace C, et al. Wolframin expression induces novel ion channel activity in endoplasmic reticulum membranes and increases intracellular calcium. *J Biol Chem* 2003;278:52755–52762.
589. Garg A. Acquired and inherited lipodystrophies. *N Engl J Med* 2004; 350:1220–1234.
590. Windpassinger C, Auer-Grumbach M, Irobi J, et al. Heterozygous missense mutations in BSCL2 arte associated with distal hereditary motor neuropathy and Silver syndrome. *Nat Genet* 2004;36:271–276.
591. Grotta JC, Manner C, Pettigrew LC, et al. Red blood cell disorders and stroke. *Stroke* 1986;17:811–817.
592. Chan AK, deVeber G. Prothrombotic disorders and ischemic stroke in children. *Semin Pediatr Neurol* 2000;7:301–308.
593. Walter T, Andraca I, Chadud P, et al. Iron deficiency anemia: adverse effects on infant psychomotor development. *Pediatrics* 1989; 84:7–17.
594. Lozoff B, Jimenez E, Wolf AW. Long-term developmental outcome of infants with iron deficiency. *N Engl J Med* 1991;325:687–694.
595. Metallinos-Katsaras E, Valassi-Adam E, Dewey KG, et al. Effect of iron supplementation on cognition in Greek preschoolers. *Eur J Clin Nutr* 2004;58:1532–1542.
596. Black MM, Baqui AH, Zaman K, et al. Iron and zinc supplementation promote motor development and exploratory behavior among Bangladeshi infants. *Am J Clin Nutr* 2004;80:903–910.
597. Wasserman G, Graziano JH, Factor-Litvak P, et al. Independent effects of lead exposure and iron deficiency anemia on developmental outcome at age 2 years. *J Pediatr* 1992;121:695–703.
598. Tischkowitz M, Dokal I. Fanconi anaemia and leukaemia—clinical and molecular aspects. *Br J Haematol* 2004;126:176–191.
599. Alter BP. Fanconi's anaemia and its variability. *Br J Haematol* 1993;85:9–14.
600. Minagi H, Steinbach HL. Roentgen appearance of anomalies associated with hypoplastic anemias of childhood: Fanconi's anemia and congenital hypoplastic anemia (erythrogenesis imperfecta). *AJR Am J Roentgenol* 1966;97:100–109.
601. Alter BP, Young NS. The bone marrow failure syndromes. In: Nathan DG, Orkin SH, eds. *Hematology of infancy and childhood*. Philadelphia: WB Saunders, 1998:259–273.
602. Pavlakis SG, Frissora CL, Giampietro PF, et al. Fanconi anemia: a model for genetic causes of abnormal brain development. *Dev Med Child Neurol* 1992;34:1081–1084.
603. Tischkowitz MD, Chisholm J, Gaze M, et al. Medulloblastoma as a first presentation of Fanconi anemia. *J Pediatr Hematol Oncol* 2004;26:52–55.
604. Adams JJ. Neurologic complications. In: Embury SH, Hebbel RP, Mohandas N, eds. *Sickle cell disease*. New York: Raven Press, 1994: 599–621.
605. Powars D, Wilson B, Imbus C. The natural history of stroke in sickle cell disease. *Am J Med* 1978;65:461–471.
606. Armstrong FD, Thompson RJ, Wang W. Cognitive functioning and brain magnetic resonance imaging in children with sickle cell disease. *Pediatrics* 1996;97:864–870.
607. Prengler M, Pavlakis SG, Prohovnik I, et al. Sickle cell disease: the neurological complications. *Ann Neurol* 2002;51:543–552.
608. Adams RJ, Ohene-Frempong K, Wang W. Sickle cell and the brain. *Hematology (Am Soc Hematol Educ Program)* 2001:31–46.
609. Powars D. Natural history of disease: the first two decades. In: Embury SH, Hebbel RP, Mohandas N, eds. *Sickle cell disease*. New York: Raven Press, 1994:395–412.
610. Wang WC, Langston JW, Steen RG, et al. Abnormalities of the central nervous system in very young children with sickle cell anemia. *J Pediatr* 1998;132:994–998.
611. Glauser TA, Siegel MJ, Lee BC, et al. Accuracy of neurologic examination and history in detecting evidence of MRI-diagnosed cerebral infarctions in children with sickle cell hemoglobinopathy. *J Child Neurol* 1995;10:88–92.
612. Ohene-Frempong K, Weiner SJ, Sleeper LA, et al. Cerebrovascular accidents in sickle cell disease: rates and risk factors. *Blood* 1998;91:288–294.
613. Kirkham FJ, Hewes DK, Prengler M, et al. Nocturnal hypoxaemia and central-nervous-system events in sickle-cell disease. *Lancet* 2001;357:1656–1659.
614. Yaggi H, Mohsenin V. Obstructive sleep apnoea and stroke. *Lancet Neurol* 2004;3:333–342.
615. Arter JL, Chi DS, Fitzgerald SM, et al. Obstructive sleep apnea, inflammation, and cardiopulmonary disease. *Front Biosci* 2004; 9:2892–2900.

616. Hargrave DR, Wade A, Evans JP, et al. Nocturnal oxygen saturation and painful sickle cell crises in children. *Blood* 2003;101:846–848.
617. Miller ST, Sleeper LA, Pegelow CH, et al. Prediction of adverse outcomes in children with sickle cell disease. *N Engl J Med* 2000;342: 83–89.
618. Huttenlocher PR, Moohr JW, Johns L. Cerebral blood flow in sickle cell cerebrovascular disease. *Pediatrics* 1984;73:615–621.
619. Koshy M, Thomas C, Goodwin J. Vascular lesions in the central nervous system in sickle cell disease [neuropathology]. *J Am Acad Min Phys* 1990;1:71–78.
620. Powars D, Adams RJ, Nichols FT. Delayed intracranial hemorrhage following cerebral infarction in sickle cell anemia. *J Assoc Acad Minor Phys* 1990;1:79–82.
621. Adams RJ, Nichols FT, McKie V, et al. Cerebral infarction in sickle cell anemia: mechanics based on CT and MRI. *Neurology* 1988;38:1012–1017.
622. Greer M, Schotland D. Abnormal hemoglobin as a cause of neurologic disease. *Neurology* 1962;12:114–123.
623. Rothman SM, Fulling KH, Nelson JS. Sickle cell anemia and cerebrovascular occlusion. *J Pediatr* 1978;93:808–810.
624. Moser FG, Miller ST, Bello JA. The spectrum of brain MR abnormalities in sickle-cell disease: a report from the cooperative study of sickle cell disease. *Am J Neuroradiol* 1996;17:965–972.
625. Henderson JN, Noetzel MJ, McKinstry RC, et al. Reversible posterior leukoencephalopathy syndrome and silent cerebral infarcts are associated with severe acute chest syndrome in children with sickle cell disease. *Blood* 2003;101:415–419.
626. Graido-Gonzalez E, Doherty JC, Bergreen EW, et al. Plasma endothelin-1, cytokine, and prostaglandin E2 levels in sickle cell disease and acute vaso-occlusive sickle crisis. *Blood* 1998;92:2551–2555.
627. Kwiatkowski JL, Hunter JV, Smith-Whitley K, et al. Transcranial Doppler ultrasonography in siblings with sickle cell disease. *Br J Haematol* 2003;121:932–937.
628. Hoppe C, Klitz W, Cheng S, et al. Gene interactions and stroke risk in children with sickle cell anemia. *Blood* 2004;103:2391–2396.
629. Hsu LL, Miller ST, Wright E, et al. Alpha thalassemia is associated with decreased risk of abnormal transcranial Doppler ultrasonography in children with sickle cell anemia. *J Pediatr Hematol Oncol* 2003;25:622–628.
630. Wiznitzer M, Ruggieri PM, Masaryk TJ, et al. Diagnosis of cerebrovascular disease in sickle cell anemia by magnetic resonance angiography. *J Pediatr* 1990;117:551–555.
631. Van Hoff J, Ritchey AK, Shaywitz BA. Intracranial hemorrhage in children with sickle cell disease. *Am J Dis Child* 1985;139:1120–1123.
632. Dobson SR, Holden KR, Nietert PJ, et al. Moyamoya syndrome in childhood sickle cell disease: a predictive factor for recurrent cerebrovascular events. *Blood* 2002;99:3144–3150.
633. Fryer RH, Anderson RC, Chiriboga CA, et al. Sickle cell anemia with Moyamoya disease: outcomes after EDAS procedure. *Pediatr Neurol* 2003;29:124–130.
634. Sarnaik SA, Lusher JM. Neurologic complications of sickle cell anemia. *Am J Pediatr Hematol Oncol* 1982;4:386–394.
635. Powars D. Sickle cell anemia and major organ failure. *Hemoglobin* 1990;14:573–598.
636. McQuaker IG, Jaspan T, McConachie NS, et al. Coil embolization of cerebral aneurysms in patients with sickling disorders. *Br J Haematol* 1999;106:388–390.
637. Preul MC, Cendes F, Just N, et al. Intracranial aneurysms and sickle cell anemia: multiplicity and propensity for the vertebrobasilar territory. *Neurosurgery* 1998;42:971–977.
638. Asher SW. Multiple cranial neuropathies, trigeminal neuralgia, and vascular headache in sickle cell disease, a possible common mechanism. *Neurology* 1980;30:210–211.
639. Resar LM, Oliva MM, Casella JF. Skull infarction and epidural hematomas in a patient with sickle cell anemia. *J Pediatr Hematol Oncol* 1996;18:413–415.
640. Ganesh A, William RR, Mitra S, et al. Orbital involvement in sickle cell disease: a report of five cases and review of the literature. *Eye* 2001;15:774–780.
641. Pavlakis SG, Prohovnik I, Piomelli S, et al. Neurologic complications of sickle cell disease. *Adv Pediatr* 1989;36:247–276.
642. Minniti CP, Gidvani VK, Bulas D, et al. Transcranial Doppler changes in children with sickle cell disease on transfusion therapy. *J Pediatr Hematol Oncol* 2004;26:626–630.
643. Wang WC, Kovnar EH, Tonkin IL, et al. High risk of recurrent stroke after discontinuance of five to twelve years of transfusion therapy in patients with sickle cell disease. *J Pediatr* 1991;118:377–382.
644. Adams RJ, McKie VC, Hsu L, et al. Prevention of a first stroke by transfusions in children with sickle cell anemia and abnormal results on transcranial Doppler ultrasonography. *N Engl J Med* 1998;339:5–11.
645. Seibert JJ, Glasier CM, Kirby RS, et al. Transcranial Doppler, MRA, and MRI as a screening examination for cerebrovascular disease in patients with sickle cell anemia: an 8-year study. *Pediatr Radiol* 1998;28:138–142.
646. Charache S, Terrin ML, Moore RD, et al. Effect of hydroxyurea on the frequency of painful crises in sickle cell anemia. Investigators of the Multicenter Study of Hydroxyurea in Sickle Cell Anemia. *N Engl J Med* 1995;332:1317–1322.
647. Kattamis A, Lagona E, Orfanou I, et al. Clinical response and adverse events in young patients with sickle cell disease treated with hydroxyurea. *Pediatr Hematol Oncol* 2004;21:335–342.
648. Harmatz P, Butensky E, Quirolo K, et al. Severity of iron overload in patients with sickle cell disease receiving chronic red blood cell transfusion therapy. *Blood* 2000;96:76–79.
649. Siegel JF, Rich MA, Brock WA. Association of sickle cell disease, priapism, exchange transfusion and neurological events: ASPEN syndrome. *J Urol* 1993;150:1480–1482.
650. Abboud MR, Jackson SM, Barredo J, et al. Neurologic complications following bone marrow transplantation for sickle cell disease. *Bone Marrow Transplant* 1996;17:405–407.
651. Moritani T, Numaguchi Y, Lemer NB, et al. Sickle cell cerebrovascular disease: usual and unusual findings on MR imaging and MR angiography. *Clin Imaging* 2004;28:173–186.
652. Pryle BJ, Grech H, Stoddart PA, et al. Toxicity of norpethidine in sickle cell crisis. *BMJ* 1992;304:1478–1479.
653. McHugh GH. Norpethidine accumulation and generalized seizure during pethidine patient-controlled analgesia. *Anaesth Intensive Care* 1999;27:289–291.
654. Ataga KI, Orringer EP. Bone marrow necrosis in sickle cell disease: a description of three cases and a review of the literature. *Am J Med Sci* 2000;320:342–347.
655. Horton DP, Ferriero DM, Mentzer WC. Nontraumatic fat embolism syndrome in sickle cell anemia. *Pediatr Neurol* 1995;12:77–80.
656. Parizel PM, Demey HE, Veeckmans G. Early diagnosis of cerebral fat embolism syndrome by diffusion-weighted MRI (starfield pattern). *Stroke* 2001;32:2942–2944.
657. Henry M, Driscoll MC, Miller M, et al. Pseudotumor cerebri in children with sickle cell disease: a case series. *Pediatrics* 2004;113:e265–269.
658. Lewkow LM, Shah I. Sickle cell anemia and epidural extramedullary hematopoiesis. *Am J Med* 1984;76:748–751.
659. Shields RW, Harris JW, Clark M. Mononeuropathy in sickle cell anemia: anatomical and pathophysiological basis for its rarity. *Muscle Nerve* 1991;14:370–374.
660. Friedlander AH, Genser L, Swerdloff M. Mental nerve neuropathy: a complication of sickle-cell crisis. *Oral Surg Oral Med Oral Pathol* 1980;49:15–17.
661. Castro O, Rana SR, Bang KM, et al. Age and prevalence of sickle-cell trait in a large ambulatory population. *Genet Epidemiol* 1987;4:307–311.
662. Kark JA, Posey DM, Schumacher HR, et al. Sickle-cell trait as a risk factor for sudden death in physical training. *N Engl J Med* 1987; 317:781–787.
663. Goldberg NM, Dorman JP, Riley CA, et al. Altitude-related specific infarction in sickle cell trait—case reports of a father and son. *West J Med* 1985;143:670–672.
664. Partington MD, Aronyk KE, Byrd SE. Sickle cell trait and stroke in children. *Pediatr Neurosurg* 1994;20:148–151.
665. Fatunde OJ, Sodeinde O, Familusi JB. Hyperventilation-precipitated cerebrovascular accident in a patient with sickle cell anaemia. *Afr J Med Sci* 2000;29:227–228.
666. Orkin SH, Nathan DG. The thalassemias. In: Nathan DG, Ginsburg

D, Orkin SH, Look AT, eds. *Nathan and Oski's hematology of infancy and childhood,* 6th ed. Philadelphia: Saunders, 2003:842–919.

667. Logothetis J, Constantoulakis M, Economidou J, et al. Thalassemia major (homozygous ?-thalassemia). A survey of 138 cases with emphasis on neurologic and muscular aspects. *Neurology* 1972;22:294–304.
668. Shapira Y, Glick B, Finsterbush A, et al. Myopathological findings in thalassemia major. *Eur Neurol* 1990;30:324–327.
669. Borgna Pignatti C, Carnelli V, Caruso V, et al. Thromboembolic events in beta thalassemia major: an Italian multicenter study. *Acta Haematol* 1998;99:76–79.
670. Olivieri NF, Buncic JR, Chew E, et al. Visual and auditory neurotoxicity in patients receiving subcutaneous deferoxamine infusions. *N Engl J Med* 1986;314:869–873.
671. Papanastasiou DA, Papanicolaou D, Magiakou AM. Peripheral neuropathy in patients with beta-thalassaemia. *J Neurol Neurosurg Psychiatry* 1991;54:997–1000.
672. Issaragrisil S, Piankijagum A, Wasi P. Spinal cord compression in thalassemia: report of 12 cases and recommendations for treatment. *Arch Intern Med* 1981;141:1033–1036.
672a. Niggemann P, Krings T, Hans F, Thron A. Fifteen-year follow-up of a patient with beta thalassaemia and extramedullary haematopoietic tissue compressing the spinal cord. *Neuroradiology* 2005;47:263–266.
672b. Rey J, Gagliano R, Christides C, et al. Spinal cord compression caused by extramedullary hematopoiesis foci in the course of thalassemia. *Presse Med* 2001;30:1351–1353.
673. Weatherall DJ, Higgs DR, Bunch C, et al. Hemoglobin H disease and mental retardation: a new syndrome or a remarkable coincidence? *N Engl J Med* 1981;305:607–612.
674. Gibbons RJ, Toutain A, Ronce N, et al. Clinical and hematological aspects of the X-linked alpha-thalassemia/mental retardation syndrome (ATR-X). *Am J Med Genet* 1995;55:288–299.
675. Gibbons RJ, Higgs DR. Molecular-clinical spectrum of the ATR-X syndrome. *Am J Med Genet* 2000;97:204–212.
676. Park DJ, Park AJ, Huynh K, et al. Comparative analysis of ATRX, a chromatin remodeling protein. *Gene* 2004;15:39–48.
677. Gibbons RJ, Wilkie AO, Weatherall DJ, et al. A newly defined X-linked mental retardation syndrome associated with a-thalassemia. *J Med Genet* 1991;28:729–733.
678. Konrad PN, McCarthy DJ, Mauer AM, et al. Erythrocyte and leukocyte phosphoglycerate kinase deficiency with neurologic disease. *J Pediatr* 1973;82:456–460.
679. Sugie H, Sugie Y, Nishida M, et al. Recurrent myoglobinuria in a child with mental retardation: phosphoglycerate kinase deficiency. *J Child Neurol* 1989;4:95–99.
680. Valentine WN, Hsieh HS, Paglia DE, et al. Hereditary hemolytic anemia associated with triosephosphate isomerase deficiency in erythrocytes and leukocytes. A probable X-chromosome-linked syndrome. *N Engl J Med* 1969;280:528–534.
681. Poll-The BT, Aicardi J, Girot R, et al. Neurological findings in triosephosphate isomerase deficiency. *Ann Neurol* 1985;17:439–443.
682. Wilmshurst JM, Wise GA, Pollard JD, et al. Chronic axonal neuropathy with triosephosphate isomerase deficiency. *Pediatr Neurol* 2004;30:146–148.
683. Eber SW, Pekrun A, Bardosi A, et al. Triosephosphate isomerase deficiency: haemolytic anaemia, myopathy with altered mitochondria and mental retardation due to a new variant with accelerated enzyme catabolism and diminished specific activity. *Eur J Pediatr* 1991;150:761–766.
684. Bardosi A, Eber SW, Hendrys M, et al. Myopathy with altered mitochondria due to a triosephosphate isomerase (TPI) deficiency. *Acta Neuropathol* 1990;79:387–394.
685. Olah J, Orosz F, Keseru GM, et al. Triosephosphate isomerase deficiency: a neurodegenerative misfolding disease. *Biochem Soc Trans* 2002;30:30–38.
686. Rosenkrantz TS. Polycythemia and hyperviscosity in the newborn. *Semin Thromb Hemost* 2003;29:515–527.
687. Rosenkrantz TS, Philipps AF, Skrzypczak PS, et al. Cerebral metabolism in the newborn lamb with polycythemia. *Pediatr Res* 1988;23:329–333.
688. Black VD, Lubchenco LO, Luckey DW, et al. Developmental and neurologic sequelae of neonatal hyperviscosity syndrome. *Pediatrics* 1982;69:426–431.
689. Wiswell TE, Cornish JD, Northam RS. Neonatal polycythemia: frequency of clinical manifestations and other associated findings. *Pediatrics* 1986;78:26–30.
690. Yiannikas C, McLeod JG, Walsh JC. Peripheral neuropathy associated with polycythemia vera. *Neurology* 1983;33:139–143.
691. Werner EJ. Neonatal polycythemia and hyperviscosity. *Clin Perinatol* 1995;22:693–710.
692. Lutschg J, Vassella F. Neurological complications in hemophilia. *Acta Paediatr Scand* 1981;70:235–241.
693. Chalmers EA. Haemophilia and the newborn. *Blood Rev* 2004;18:85–92.
694. Jacome DE. Idiopathic intracranial hypertension and hemophilia A. *Headache* 2001;41:595–598.
695. Hay CR, Doughty HI, Savidge GF. Continuous infusion of factor VIII for surgery and major bleeding. *Blood Coagul Fibrinolysis* 1996;7[Suppl 1]:S15–19.
696. Bhanchet P, Tuchinda S, Hathirat P, et al. A bleeding syndrome in infants due to acquired prothrombin complex deficiency: a survey of 93 affected infants. *Clin Pediatr (Phila)* 1977;16:992–998.
697. Sallah S, Nguyen NP, Abdallah JM, et al. Acquired hemophilia in patients with hematologic malignancies. *Arch Pathol Lab Med* 2000;124:730–734.
698. Tokarz VA, McGrory JE, Stewart JD, et al. Femoral neuropathy and iliopsoas hematoma as a result of postpartum factor-VIII inhibitor syndrome. A case report. *J Bone Joint Surg Am* 2003;85-A:1812–1815.
699. Collins PW. Management of acquired haemophilia A—more questions than answers. *Blood Coagul Fibrinolysis* 2003;14[Suppl 1]:S23–S27.
700. Kaplan RN, Bussel JB. Differential diagnosis and management of thrombocytopenia in childhood. *Pediatr Clin North Am* 2004;51:1109–1140.
701. Matoth Y, Zaizov R, Frankel JJ. Minimal cerebral dysfunction in children with chronic thrombocytopenia. *Pediatrics* 1971;47:698–706.
702. Ijichi T, Muranishi M, Shimura K, et al. Idiopathic thrombocytopenic purpura and mononeuropathy multiplex. *Acta Haemtol* 2003;110:33–35.
703. Greenhalgh KL, Howell RT, Bottani A, et al. Thrombocytopenia-absent radius syndrome: a clinical genetic study. *J Med Genet* 2002;39:876–881.
704. MacDonald MR, Schaefer GB, Olney AH, et al. Hypoplasia of the cerebellar vermis and corpus callosum in thrombocytopenia with absent radius syndrome on MRI studies. *Am J Med Genet* 1994;50:46–50.
705. Uhrynowska M, Maslanka K, Zupanska B. Neonatal thrombocytopenia: incidence, serological and clinical observations. *Am J Perinatol* 1997;14:415–418.
706. Kelly PJ, McDonald CT, Neill GO, et al. Middle cerebral artery main stem thrombosis in two siblings with familial thrombotic thrombocytopenic purpura. *Neurology* 1998;80:1157–1160.
707. Lawlor ER, Webb DW, Hill A, et al. Thrombotic thrombocytopenic purpura: a treatable cause of childhood encephalopathy. *J Pediatr* 1997;130:313–316.
708. Allford SL, Hunt BJ, Rose P, et al. Guidelines on the diagnosis and management of the thrombotic microangiopathic haemolytic anaemias. *Br J Haematol* 2003;120:556–573.
709. Knopp U, Kehler U, Rickmann H, et al. Cerebral haemodynamic pathologies in HELLP syndrome. *Clin Neurol Neurosurg* 2003;105:256–261.
710. Moake JL. von Willebrand factor, ADAMTS-13, and thrombotic thrombocytopenic purpura. *Semin Hematol* 2004;41:4–14.
711. Levy GG, Motto DG, Ginsburg D. ADAMTS13 turns 3. *Blood* 2005;106:11–17.
712. Veyradier A, Lavergne JM, Ribba AS, et al. Ten candidate ADAMTS13 mutations in six French families with congenital thrombotic thrombocytopenic purpura (Upshaw-Schulman syndrome). *J Thromb Haemost* 2004;2:424–429.
713. Cornelissen M, Steegers-Theunissen R, Kollee L, et al. Supplementation of vitamin K in pregnant women receiving anticonvulsant

therapy prevents neonatal vitamin K deficiency. *Am J Obstet Gynecol* 1993;168:884–888.
714. Sutor AH, Dagres N, Niederhoff H. Late form of vitamin K deficiency bleeding in Germany. *Klin Pädiatr* 1995;207:89–97.
715. Bor O, Akgun N, Yakut A, et al. Late hemorrhagic disease of the newborn. *Pediatr Int* 2000;42:64–66.
716. Gedalia A. Henloch-Schonlein purpura Curr. *Rheumatol Rep* 2004;6:195–202.
716a. Patrignelli R, Sheikh SH, Shaw-Stiffel TA. Henoch-Schonlein purpura. A multisystem disease also seen in adults. *Postgrad Med* 1995;97:123–124,127,131–134.
717. Woolfenden AR, Hukin J, Poskitt KJ, et al. Encephalopathy complicating Henoch-Schonlein purpura: reversible MRI changes. *Pediatr Neurol* 1998;19:74–77.
718. Bulun A, Topaloglu R, Duzova A, et al. Ataxia and peripheral neuropathy: rare manifestations in Henoch-Schonlein purpura. *Pediatr Nephrol* 2001;16:1139–1141.
719. Ritter FJ, Seay AR, Lahey ME. Peripheral mononeuropathy complicating anaphylactoid purpura. *J Pediatr* 1983;103:77–78.
720. Uhrynowska M, Maslanka K, Zupanska B. Neonatal thrombocytopenia: incidence, serological and clinical observations. *Am J Perinatol* 1997;14:415–418.
721. Facchini SA, Jami MM, Neuberg RW, et al. A treatable cause of ataxia in children. *Pediatr Neurol* 2001;24:135–138.
722. Weiss R, Fogelman Y, Bennett M. Severe vitamin B12 deficiency in an infant associated with maternal deficiency and a strict vegetarian diet. *J Pediatr Hematol Oncol* 2004;26:270–271.
723. Holloway KL, Alberico AM. Postoperative myeloneuropathy: a preventable complication in patients with B12 deficiency. *J Neurosurg* 1990;72:732–736.
724. Marie RM, Le Biez E, Busson P, et al. Nitrous oxide anesthesia-associated myelopathy. *Arch Neurol* 2000;57:380–382.
725. Nishimura J, Murakami Y, Kinoshita T. Paroxysmal nocturnal hemoglobinuria: An acquired genetic disease. *Am J Hematol* 1999; 62:175–182.
726. Hauser D, Barzilai N, Zalish M, et al. Bilateral papilledema with retinal hemorrhages in association with cerebral venous sinus thrombosis and paroxysmal nocturnal hemoglobinuria. *Am J Ophthalmol* 1996;122:592–593.
727. Lin HC, Chen RL, Wang PJ. Paroxysmal nocturnal hemoglobinuria presenting as moyamoya syndrome. *Brain Dev* 1996;18:157–159.
728. Casas KA, Fischel-Ghodsian N. Mitochondrial myopathy and sideroblastic anemia. *Am J Med Genet* 2004;125A:201–204.
729. Drugge U, Holmberg M, Holmgren G, et al. Hereditary myopathy with lactic acidosis, succinate dehydrogenase and aconitase deficiency in northern Sweden: a genealogical study. *J Med Genet* 1995;32:344–347.
730. Maguire A, Hellier K, Hammans S, et al. X-linked cerebellar ataxia and sideroblastic anaemia associated with a missense mutation in the ABC7 gene predicting V411L. *Br J Haematol* 2001;115:910–917.
731. Eckhardt SM, Hicks EM, Herron B. New form of autosomal-recessive axonal hereditary sensory motor neuropathy. *Pediatr Neurol* 1998;19:234–235.
732. Price RA. Histopathology of CNS leukemia and complications of therapy. *Am J Pediatr Hematol Oncol* 1979;1:21–30.
733. Smith M, Bleyer A, Crist W, et al. Uniform approach to risk classification and treatment assignment for children with acute lymphoblastic leukemia. *J Clin Oncol* 1996;14:4–6.
734. Crosley CJ, Rorke LB, Evans A, et al. Central nervous system lesions in childhood leukemia. *Neurology* 1978;28:678–685.
735. Gelber RD, Sallan SE, Cohen HJ, et al. Central nervous system treatment in childhood acute lymphoblastic leukemia. Long-term follow-up of patients diagnosed between 1973 and 1985. *Cancer* 1993;72:261–270.
736. Hardisty RM, Norman PM. Meningeal leukaemia. *Arch Dis Child* 1967;42:441–447.
737. Smith HP, Biller J, Kelly DL Jr. Oculomotor palsy with pupillary sparing, coincidental aneurysm, and chronic lymphocytic leukemic meningeal infiltration. *Surg Neurol* 1981;16:26–29.
738. Mayo GL, Carter JE, McKinnon SJ. Bilateral optic disk edema and blindness as initial presentation of acute lymphocytic leukemia. *Am J Ophthalmol* 2002;134:141–142.
739. Krishnamurthy S, Weinstock AL, Smith SH, et al. Facial palsy, an unusual presenting feature of childhood leukemia. *Pediatr Neurol* 2002;27:68–70.
740. Ingram LC. Cranial nerve palsy in childhood acute lymphoblastic leukemia. *Cancer* 1991;67:2262–2268.
741. Kuklok KB, Burton RG, Wilhelm ML. Numb chin syndrome leading to a diagnosis of acute lymphoblastic leukemia: report of a case. *J Oral Maxillofac Surg* 1997;55:1483–1485.
742. Laurencet FM, Anchisi S, Tullen E, et al. Mental neuropathy: report of five cases and review of the literature. *Crit Rev Oncol Hematol* 2000;34:71–79.
743. Kataoka A, Shimizu K, Matsumoto T, et al. Epidural spinal cord compression as an initial symptom in childhood acute lymphoblastic leukemia: rapid decompression by local irradiation and systemic chemotherapy. *Pediatr Hematol Oncol* 1995;12:179–184.
744. Boiron JM, Ellie E, Vital A, et al. Isolated peripheral nerve relapse masquerading as Guillain-Barre syndrome in a patient with acute lymphoblastic leukemia. *Leuk Lymphoma* 1993;10:489–491.
745. Creutzig U, Ritter J, Budde M, et al. Early deaths due to hemorrhage and leukostasis in childhood acute myelogenous leukemia. Associations with hyperleukocytosis and acute monocytic leukemia. *Cancer* 1987;60:3071–3079.
746. Barbui T, Falanga A. Disseminated intravascular coagulation in acute leukemia. *Semin Thromb Hemost* 2001;27:593–604.
747. Wirtz PW, Bloem BR, van der Meer FJ, et al. Paraparesis after lumbar puncture in a male with leukemia. *Pediatr Neurol* 2000;23:67–68.
748. Sinniah D, Looi LM, Ortega JA, et al. Cerebellar coning and uncal herniation in childhood acute leukaemia. *Lancet* 1982;2:702–704.
749. Maurer HS, Steinherz PG, Gaynon PS, et al. The effect of initial management of hyperleukocytosis on early complications and outcome of children with acute lymphoblastic leukemia. *J Clin Oncol* 1988;6:1425–1432.
750. Pierce MI. Neurologic complications in acute leukemia in children. *Pediatr Clin North Am* 1962;9:425–442.
751. Ricevuti G, Savoldi F, Piccolo G, et al. Meningeal leukemia diagnosed by cytocentrifuge study of cerebrospinal fluid. A study of 631 cerebrospinal fluid samples from 87 patients. *Arch Neurol* 1986;43:466–470.
752. Schumacher M, Orszagh M. Imaging techniques in neoplastic meningiosis. *J Neurooncol* 1998;38:111–120.
753. Chen CY, Zimmerman RA, Faro S, et al. Childhood leukemia: central nervous system abnormalities during and after treatment. *AJNR Am J Neuroradiol* 1996;17:295–310.
754. Vazquez E, Lucaya J, Castellote A, et al. Neuroimaging in pediatric leukemia and lymphoma: differential diagnosis. *Radiographics* 2002;22:1411–1428.
755. Gajjar A, Harrison PL, Sandlund JT, et al. Traumatic lumbar puncture at diagnosis adversely affects outcome in childhood actue lymphoblastic leukemia. *Blood* 2000;96:3381–3384.
756. Pinkel D, Woo S. Prevention and treatment of meningeal leukemia in children. *Blood* 1994;84:355–366.
757. Ravindranath Y. Recent advances in pediatric acute lymphoblastic and myeloid leukemia. *Curr Opin Oncol* 2003;15:23–35.
758. Steinherz PG. Radiotherapy vs. intrathecal chemotherapy for CNS prophylaxis in childhood ALL. *Oncology* 1989;3:47–53.
759. Unal Y, Yetgin S, Cetin M, et al. The prognosis and survival of childhood acute lymphoblastic leukemia with central nervous system relapse. *Pediatr Hematol Oncol* 2004;21:279–289.
760. Wilson DA, Nitschke R, Bowman ME, et al. Transient white matter changes on MR images in children undergoing chemotherapy for acute lymphocytic leukemia: correlation with neuropsychologic deficiencies. *Radiology* 1991;180:205–209.
761. Ch'ien LT, Aur RJ, Stagner S, et al. Long-term neurological implications of somnolence syndrome in children with acute lymphocytic leukemia. *Ann Neurol* 1980;8:273–277.
762. Safak M, Khalili K. An overview: human polyomavirus JC virus and its associated disorders. *J Neurovirol* 2003;9[Suppl 1]: 3–9.
763. Garcia De Viedma D, Diaz Infantes M, Miralles P, et al. JC virus load in progressive multifocal leukoencephalopathy: analysis of the correlation between the viral burden in cerebrospinal fluid, patient survival, and the volume of neurological lesions. *Clin Infect Dis* 2002;34:1568–1575.

764. Berger JR. Progressive multifocal leukoencephalopathy. *Curr Treat Options Neurol* 2000;2:361–368.
765. Aksamit AJ. Treatment of non-AIDS progressive multifocal leukoencephalopathy with cytosine arabinoside. *J Neurovirol* 2001;7:386–390.
766. Carmack MA, Twiss J, Enzmann DR, et al. Multifocal leukoencephalitis caused by varicella-zoster virus in a child with leukemia: successful treatment with acyclovir. *Pediatr Infect Dis J* 1993;12:402–406.
767. Curran WJ, Hecht-Leavitt C, Schut L, et al. Magnetic resonance imaging of cranial radiation lesions. *Int J Radiat Oncol Biol Phys* 1987;13:1093–1098.
768. Chen CY, Zimmerman RA, Faro S, et al. Childhood leukemia: central nervous system abnormalities during and after treatment. *Am J Neuroradiol* 1996;17:295–310.
769. Price RA, Birdwell DA. The central nervous system in childhood leukemia. III. Mineralizing microangiopathy and dystrophic calcification. *Cancer* 1978;42:717–728.
770. Fishman ML, Bean SC, Cogan DG. Optic atrophy following prophylactic chemotherapy and cranial radiation for acute lymphocytic leukemia. *Am J Ophthalmol* 1976;82:571–576.
771. Neglia JP, Meadows AT, Robison LL, et al. Second neoplasms after acute lymphoblastic leukemia in childhood. *N Engl J Med* 1991;325:1330–1336.
772. Stehbens JA, Kaleita TA, Noll RB, et al. CNS prophylaxis of childhood leukemia: what are the long-term neurological, neuropsychological, and behavioral effects? *Neuropsychol Rev* 1991;2:147–177.
773. von der Weid N, Mosimann I, Hirt A, et al. Intellectual outcome in children and adolescents with acute lymphoblast leukemia treated with chemotherapy alone: age- and sex-related differences. *Eur J Cancer* 2003;29:359–365.
774. Mennes M, Stiers R, Vandenbussche E, et al. Attention and information processing in survivors of childhood acute lymphoblastic leukemia treated with chemotherapy only. *Pediatr Blood Cancer* 2004;43:780–787.
775. Kramer JH, Norman D, Brant-Zawadzki M, et al. Absence of white matter changes on magnetic resonance imaging in children treated with CNS prophylaxis therapy for leukemia. *Cancer* 1988;61:928–930.
776. Phillips PC, Moeller JR, Sidtis JJ, et al. Abnormal cerebral glucose metabolism in long-term survivors of childhood acute lymphocytic leukemia. *Ann Neurol* 1991;29:263–271.
777. Sluga E, Budka H, Pichler E. Slow virus "Enzephalitis" nach Masern bei zytostatisch behandelter Leukämie im Kindesalter. *Wien Klin Wochenschr* 1975;87:248–251.
778. Mrózek K, Heinonen K, de la Chapelle A, et al. Clinical significance of cytogenetics in acute myeloid leukemia. *Semin Oncol* 1997; 17–34.
779. Abbott BL, Rubnitz JE, Tong X, et al. Clinical significance of central nervous system involvement at diagnosis of pediatric acute myeloid leukemia: a single institution's experience. *Leukemia* 2003;17:2090–2096.
780. Plotkin SR, Won PY. Neurologic complications of cancer therapy. *Neurol Clin* 2003;21:279–318.
781. Armstrong T, Gilbert MR. Central nervous system toxicity from cancer treatment. *Curr Oncol Rep* 2004;6:11–19.
782. Gerrard MP, Eden OB, Lilleyman JS. Acute encephalopathy during induction therapy for acute lymphoblastic leukemia. *Pediatr Hematol Oncol* 1986;3:49–58.
783. Sandoval C, Kutscher M, Jayabose S, et al. Neurotoxicity of intrathecal methotrexate: MR imaging findings. *AJNR Am J Neuroradiol* 2003;24:1887–1890.
784. Shuper A, Stark B, Kornreich L, et al. Methotrexate treatment protocols and the central nervous system: significant cure with significant neurotoxicity. *J Child Neurol* 2000;15:573–580.
785. Lovblad K, Kelkar P, Ozdoba C, et al. Pure methotrexate encephalopathy presenting with seizures: CT and MRI features. *Pediatr Radiol* 1998;28:86–91.
786. Rollins N, Winick N, Bash R, et al. Acute methotrexate neurotoxicity: findings on diffusion-weighted imaging and correlation with clinical outcome. *AJNR Am J Neuroradiol* 2004;25:1688–1695.
787. Jaksic W, Veljkovic D, Pozza C, et al. Methotrexate-induced leukoencephalopathy reversed by aminophylline and high-dose folinic acid. *Acta Haematol* 2004;111:230–232.
788. Cohen IJ. Defining the appropriate dosage of folinic acid after high-dose methotrexate for childhood acute lymphatic leukemia that will prevent neurotoxicity without rescuing malignant cells in the central nervous system. *J Pediatr Hematol Oncol* 2004;26:156–163.
789. Koh S, Nelson MD Jr, Kovanlikaya A, et al. Anterior lumbosacral radiculopathy after intrathecal methotrexate treatment. *Pediatr Neurol* 1999;21:576–578.
790. Watterson J, Toogood I, Nieder M, et al. Excessive spinal cord toxicity from intensive central nervous system-directed therapies. *Cancer* 1994;74:3034–3041.
791. Tardieu M, Mikaeloff Y. What is acute disseminated encephalomyelitis (ADEM)? *Eur J Paediatr Neurol* 2004;8:239–242.
792. Dale RC, de Sousa C, Chong WK, et al. Acute disseminated encephalomyelitis, multiphasic disseminated encephalomyelitis and multiple sclerosis in children. *Brain* 2000;123:2407–2422.
793. Quasthoff S, Hartung HP. Chemotherapy-induced peripheral neuropathy. *J Neurol* 2002;249:9–17.
794. Dyke RW. Treatment of inadvertent intrathecal injection of vincristine. *N Engl J Med* 1989;321:1270–1271.
795. Alcaraz A, Rey C, Concha A, et al. Intrathecal vincristine: fatal myeloencephalopathy despite cerebrospinal fluid perfusion. *J Toxicol Clin Toxicol* 2002;40:557–561.
796. Moudgil SS, Riggs JE. Fulminant peripheral neuropathy with severe quadriparesis associated with vincristine therapy. *Ann Pharmacother* 2000;34:1136–1138.
797. Chauvenet AR, Shashi V, Selsky C, et al. Vincristine-induced neuropathy as the initial presentation of Charcot-Marie-Tooth disease in acute lymphoblastic leukemia: a Pediatric Oncology Group study. *J Pediatr Hematol Oncol* 2003;25:316–320.
798. Jeng MR, Feusner J. Itraconazole-enhanced vincristine neurotoxicity in a child with acute lymphoblastic leukemia. *Pediatr Hematol Oncol* 2001;18:137–142.
799. Jackson DV, Wells HB, Atkins JN, et al. Amelioration of vincristine neurotoxicity by glutamic acid. *Am J Med* 1988;84:1016–1022.
800. La Spina I, Porazzi D, Maggiolo F, et al. Gabapentin in painful HIV-related neuropathy: a report of 19 patients, preliminary observations. *Eur J Neurol* 2001;8:71–75.
801. Flatters SJ, Bennett GJ. Ethosuximide reverses paclitaxel- and vincristine-induced painful peripheral neuropathy. *Pain* 2004; 109:150–161.
802. Boogerd W, ten Bokkel Huinink WW, Dalesio O, et al. Cisplatin-induced neuropathy: central, peripheral and autonomic nerve involvement. *J Neurooncol* 1990;9:255–263.
803. Roelofs RI, Hrushesky W, Rogin J, et al. Peripheral sensory neuropathy and cisplatin chemotherapy. *Neurology* 1984;34:934–938.
804. Thordarson H, Talstad I. Acute meningitis and cerebellar dysfunction complicating high-dose cytosine arabinoside therapy. *Acta Med Scand* 1986;220:493–495.
805. Hoffman DL, Howard JR, Sarma R, et al. Encephalopathy, myelopathy, optic neuropathy, and anosmia associated with intravenous cytosine arabinoside. *Clin Neuropharmacol* 1993;16:258–262.
806. Openshaw H, Slatkin NE, Stein AS, et al. Acute polyneuropathy after high dose cytosine arabinoside in patients with leukemia. *Cancer* 1996;78:1899–1905.
807. Herzig RH, Hines JD, Herzig GP, et al. Cerebellar toxicity with high-dose cytosine arabinoside. *J Clin Oncol* 1987;5:927–932.
808. Cairo MS. Adverse reactions of L-asparaginase. *Am J Pediatr Hematol Oncol* 1982;4:335–339.
809. Kieslich M, Porto L, Lanfermann H, et al. Cerebrovascular complications of L-asparaginase in the therapy of acute lymphoblastic leukemia. *J Pediatr Hematol Oncol* 2003;25:484–487.
810. Feinberg WM, Swenson MR. Cerebrovascular complications of L-asparaginase therapy. *Neurology* 1988;38:127–133.
811. Rathi B, Azad RK, Vasudha N, et al. L-asparaginase-induced reversible posterior leukoencephalopathy syndrome in a child with acute lymphoblastic leukemia. *Pediatr Neurosurg* 2002;37:203–205.
811a. Oppenheim H. Über Hirnsymptome bei Carcinomatose ohne nachweisbare Veränderungen im Gehirn. *Charité Annalen (Berlin)* 1888;13:335–344.
812. Wirtz PW, Sotodeh M, Nijnuis M, et al. Difference in distribution of muscle weakness between myasthenia gravis and the

Lambert-Eaton myasthenic syndrome. *J Neurol Neurosurg Psychiatry* 2002;73:766–768.
813. Argov Z, Shapira Y, Averbuch-Heller L, et al. Lambert-Eaton myasthenic syndrome (LEMS) in association with lymphoproliferative disorders. *Muscle Nerve* 1995;18:715–719.
814. Tsao CY, Mendell JR, Friemer ML, et al. Lambert-Eaton myasthenic syndrome in children. *J Child Neurol* 2002;17:74–76.
815. Woodman R, Shin K, Pineo G. Primary non-Hodgkins lymphoma of the brain. *Medicine* 1985;64:425–430.
816. Murphy SB. Childhood non-Hodgkin's lymphoma. *N Engl J Med* 1979;299:1446–1448.
817. Ziegler JL, Bluming AZ, Morrow RH, et al. Central nervous system involvement in Burkitt's lymphoma. *Blood* 1970;36:718–728.
818. Mazza JJ, Hines JD, Andersen JW, et al. Aggressive chemotherapy in the treatment of Burkitt's and non-Burkitt's undifferentiated lymphoma. *Leuk Lymphoma* 1995;18:289–296.
819. Sohn D, Valensi Q, Miller SP. Neurologic manifestations of Hodgkin's disease. *Arch Neurol* 1967;17:429–436.
820. Greenwood RD, Rosenthal A, Parisi L, et al. Extracardiac abnormalities in infants with congenital heart disease. *Pediatrics* 1975;55:485–492.
821. Limperopoulos C, Majnemer A, Shevell MI, et al. Neurologic status of newborns with congenital heart defects before open heart surgery. *Pediatrics* 1999;103:402–408.
822. Glauser TA, Rorke LB, Weinberg PM, et al. Congenital brain anomalies associated with the hypoplastic left heart syndrome. *Pediatrics* 1990;85:984–990.
823. Johnson DH, Rosenthal A, Nadas AS. A 40-year review of bacterial endocarditis in infancy and childhood. *Circulation* 1975;51:581–588.
824. Lerner PI. Neurologic complications of infective endocarditis. *Med Clin N Am* 1985;69:385–398.
825. Matson DD. Intracranial arterial aneurysms in childhood. *J Neurosurg* 1965;23:578–583.
826. Albert ML, Greer WE, Kantrowitz W. Paraplegia secondary to hypotension and cardiac arrest in a patient who has had previous thoracic surgery. *Neurology* 1969;19:915–918.
827. Ussia GP, Marasini M, Pongiglione G. Paraplegia following percutaneous balloon angioplasty of aortic coarctation: a case report. *Catheter Cardiovasc Interv* 2001;54:510–513.
828. Guerit JM, Witdoeckt C, Rubay J, et al. The usefulness of the spinal and subcortical components of the posterior tibial nerve SEP's for spinal cord monitoring during aortic coarctation repair. *Electroencephalogr Clin Neurophysiol* 1997;104:115–121.
829. Tyler HR, Clark DB. Incidence of neurological complications in congenital heart disease. *Arch Neurol Psychiatry* 1957;77:17–22.
830. Kalyanaraman K, Niedermeyer E, Rowe R, et al. The electroencephalogram in congenital heart disease. *Arch Neurol* 1968;18:98–106.
831. Fischbein CA, Rosenthal A, Fischer EG, et al. Risk factors for brain abscess in patients with congenital heart disease. *Am J Cardiol* 1974;34:97–102.
832. Nguyen JB, Black BR, Leimkuehler MM, et al. Intracranial pyogenic abscess: imaging diagnosis utilizing recent advances in computed tomography and magnetic resonance imaging. *Crit Rev Comput Tomogr* 2004;45:181–224.
833. Goodkin HP, Harper MB, Pomeroy SL. Intracerebral abscess in children: historical trends at Children's Hospital Boston. *Pediatrics* 2004;113:1765–1770.
834. Leys D, Christiaens JL, Derambure P, et al. Management of focal intracranial infections: is medical treatment better than surgery? *J Neurol Neurosurg Psychiatry* 1990;53:472–475.
835. Tyler HR, Clark DB. Cerebrovascular accidents in patients with congenital heart disease. *Arch Neurol Psychiatr* 1957;77:483–489.
836. Berthrong M, Sabiston DC Jr. Cerebral lesions in congenital heart disease. *Bull Hopkins Hosp* 1951;89:384–406.
837. Martelle RR, Linde LM. Cerebrovascular accidents with tetralogy of Fallot. *Am J Dis Child* 1961;101:206–209.
838. Cotrill CM, Kaplan S. Cerebral vascular accidents in cyanotic congenital heart disease. *Am J Dis Child* 1973;125:484–487.
839. Peterson RA, Rosenthal A. Retinopathy and papilledema in cyanotic congenital heart disease. *Pediatrics* 1972;49:243–249.
840. Ferrieri P, Gewitz MH, Gerber MA, et al. Unique features of infective endocarditis in childhood. *Circulation* 2002;105:2115–2126.
841. Diab KA, Richani R, Al Kutoubi A, et al. Cerebral mycotic aneurysm in a child with Down's syndrome: a unique association. *J Child Neurol* 2001;16:868–870.
842. Asai T, Usui A, Miyachi S, et al. Endovascular treatment for intracranial mycotic aneurysms prior to cardiac surgery. *Eur J Cardiothorac Surg* 2002;21:948–950.
843. The Collaborative Group for the Study of Polyneuropathy. Antiarrhythmic drugs and polyneuropathy. *J Neurol Neurosurg Psychiatry* 1994;57:340–343.
844. Wright RR, Mathews KD. Hypertensive encephalopathy in childhood. *J Child Neurol* 1996;11:193–196.
845. Lloyd AV, Jewitt DE, Still JD. Facial paralysis in children with hypertension. *Arch Dis Child* 1966;41:292–294.
846. Hinchey J, Chaves C, Appignani B, et al. A reversible posterior leukoencephalopathy syndrome. *N Engl J Med* 1996;334:494–500.
847. Jones BV, Egelhoff JC, Patterson RJ. Hypertensive encephalopathy in children. *Am J Neuroradiol* 1997;18:101–106.
848. Abman SH, Warady BA, Lum GM, et al. Systemic hypertension in infants with bronchopulmonary dysplasia. *J Pediatr* 1984;104:928–931.
848a. Flynn JT. Neonatal hypertension: diagnosis and management. *Pediatr Nephrol* 2000;14:332–41.
849. Perlman JM, Volpe JJ. Neurologic complications of captopril treatment of neonatal hypertension. *Pediatrics* 1989;83:47–52.
849a. Strandgaard S. Cerebral ischaemia caused by overzealous blood pressure lowering. *Dan Med Bull* 1987;34[Suppl 1]:5–7.
850. Liu XY, Wong V, Leung M. Neurologic complications due to catheterization. *Pediatr Neurol* 2001;24:270–275.
851. Bellinger D, Wernovsky G, Rappaport LA, et al. Cognitive development of children following early repair of transposition of the great arteries using deep hypothermic circulatory arrest. *Pediatrics* 1991;87:701–707.
852. Treasure T, Naftel DC, Conger KA, et al. The effect of hypothermic circulatory arrest time on cerebral function, morphology and biochemistry. An experimental study. *J Thorac Cardiovasc Surg* 1983;86:761–770.
853. Wells FC, Coghill S, Caplan HL, Lincoln C. Duration of circulatory arrest does influence the psychological development of children after cardiac operation in early life. *J Thorac Cardiovasc Surg* 1983;86:823–831.
854. Blackwood M, Haka-Ikse K, Steward DJ. Developmental outcome in children undergoing surgery with profound hypothermia. *Anesthesiology* 1986;85:437–440.
855. Vanucci R, Wasiewsk WW, Yager JY. Diagnosis and management of neurologic complications in infants and children. In: Waldhausen JA, Oringer MB (eds). *Complications in cardiothoracic surgery*. St. Louis: Mosby Year Book, 1991:68–74.
856. Greeley WJ, Ungerleider RM, Kern FH, et al. Effects of cardiopulmonary bypass on cerebral blood flow in neonates, infants and children. *Circulation* 1989;80:1209–1215.
857. Greeley WJ, Kern FH, Meliones JN, et al. The effect of deep hypothermia and circulatory arrest on cerebral blood flow and metabolism. *Ann Thorac Surg* 1993;56:1464–1466.
858. Rappaport L, Wypij D, Bellinger DC, et al. Relation of seizures after cardiac surgery in early infancy to neurodevelopmental outcome. Boston Circulatory Arrest Study Group. *Circulation* 1998;97:773–779.
859. Uzark K, Lincoln A, Lamberti JJ, et al. Neurodevelopmental outcomes in children with Fontan repair of functional single ventricle. *Pediatrics* 1998;101:630–633.
860. Menache CC, du Plessis AJ, Wessel DL, et al. Curent incidence of acute neurologic complications after open-heart operations in children. *Ann Thorac Surg* 2002;73:1752–1758.
861. Bellinger DC, Wypij D, Kuban KC, et al. Developmental and neurologic status of children at 4 years of age after heart surgery with hypothermic circulatory arrest or low-flow cardiopulmonary bypass. *Circulation* 1999;100:526–532.
862. Cottrell SM, Morris KP, Davies P, et al. Early postoperative body temperature and developmental outcome after open heart surgery in infants. *Ann Thorac Surg* 2004;77:66–71.
863. Limperopoulos C, Majnemer A, Shevell MI, et al. Predictors of developmental disabilities after open heart surgery in young children with congenital heart defects. *J Pediatr* 2002;141:51–58.

864. Gaynor JW. Periventricular leukomalacia following neonatal and infant cardiac surgery. *Semin Thorac Cardiovasc Surg Pediatr Card Surg Annu* 2004;7:133–140.
865. Galli KK, Zimmerman RA, Jarvik GP, et al. Periventricular leukomalacia is common after neonatal cardiac surgery. *J Thorac Cardiovasc Surg* 2004;127:692–704.
866. Ungerleider RM, Gaynor JW. The Boston Circulatory Arrest Study: an analysis. *J Thorac Cardiovasc Surg* 2004;127:1256–1261.
867. Sakamoto T, Zurakowski D, Duebener LF, et al. Interaction of temperature with hematocrit level and pH determines safe duration of hypothermic circulatory arrest. *J Thorac Cardiovasc Surg* 2004;128:220–232.
868. Wardle SP, Yoxall CW, Weindling AM. Cerebral oxygenation during cardiopulmonary bypass. *Arch Dis Child* 1998;78:26–32.
869. Clancy RR, Sharif U, Ichord R, et al. Electrographic neonatal seizures after infant heart surgery. *Epilepsia* 2005;46:84–90.
870. Moody DM, Brown WR, Challa VR, et al. Brain microemboli during cardiac surgery or aortography. *Ann Neurol* 1990;28:477–486.
871. du Plessis AJ. Mechanisms of brain injury during infant cardiac surgery. *Semin Pediatr Neurol* 1999;6:32–47.
872. Huntley DT, Al-Mateen M, Menkes JH. Unusual dyskinesia complicating cardiopulmonary bypass surgery. *Dev Med Child Neurol* 1993;35:631–641.
873. Medlock MD, Cruse RS, Winek SJ, et al. A 10-year experience with post-pump chorea. *Ann Neurol* 1993;34:820–826.
874. Kupsky WJ, Drozd MA, Barlow CF. Selective injury of the globus pallidus in children with post-cardiac surgery choreic syndrome. *Dev Med Child Neurol* 1995;37:135–144.
875. du Plessis AJ, Bellinger DC, Gauvreau K, et al. Neurologic outcome of choreoathetoid encephalopathy after cardiac surgery. *Pediatr Neurol* 2002;27:9–17.
876. Puntis JW, Green SH. Ischaemic spinal cord injury after cardiac surgery. *Arch Dis Child* 1985;60:517–520.
877. Gaynor JW, Gerdes M, Zackai EH, et al. Apolipoprotein E genotype and neurodevelopmental sequelae of infant cardiac surgery. *J Thorac Cardiovasc Surg* 2003;126:1736–1745.
878. Bjork V, Hultquist G. Contraindications to profound hypothermia in open heart surgery. *J Thorac Cardiovasc Surg* 1962;44:1–6.
879. Montero CG, Martinez AJ. Neuropathology of heart transplantation: 23 cases. *Neurology* 1986;36:1149–1154.
880. Hall WA, Martinez AJ, Dummer JS, et al. Central nervous system infections in heart and heart-lung transplant recipients. *Arch Neurol* 1989;46:173–177.
881. O'Dougherty M, Wright FS, Loewenson RB, et al. Cerebral dysfunction after chronic hypoxia in children. *Neurology* 1985;35:42–46.
882. Bellinger DC, Jonas RA, Rappaport LA, et al. Developmental and neurologic status of children after heart surgery with hypothermic circulatory arrest or low-flow cardiopulmonary bypass. *N Engl J Med* 1995;332:549–555.
883. Newburger JW, Silbert AR, Buckley LP, et al. Cognitive function and age at repair of transposition of the great arteries in children. *N Engl J Med* 1984;310:1495–1499.
884. Kurlan R, Krall RL, Deweese JA. Vertebrobasilar ischemia after total repair of tetralogy of Fallot. Significance of subclavian steal created by Blalock-Taussig anastomosis. *Stroke* 1984;15:359–362.
885. Tonz M, von Segesser LK, Mihaljevic T, et al. Clinical implications of phrenic nerve injury after pediatric cardiac surgery. *J Pediatr Surg* 1996;31:1265–1267.
886. Imai T, Shizukawa H, Imaizumi H, et al. Transient phrenic nerve palsy after cardiac operation in infants. *Clin Neurophysiol* 2004;115:1469–1472.
887. de Leeuw M, Williams JM, Freedom RM, et al. Impact of diaphragmatic paralysis after cardiothoracic surgery in children. *J Thorac Cardiovasc Surg* 1999;118:510–517.
888. Pipitone S, Mongiovi M, Grillo R, et al. Cardiac rhabdomyoma in intrauterine life: clinical features and natural history. A case series and review of published reports. *Ital Heart J* 2002;3:48–52.
889. Al-Mateen M, Hood M, Trippel D, et al. Cerebral embolism from atrial myxoma in pediatric patients. *Pediatrics* 2003;112:e162–167.
890. Desai SA, Stanley C, Gringlas M, et al. Five-year follow-up of neonates with reconstructed right common carotid arteries after extracorporeal membrane oxygenation. *J Pediatr* 1999;134:428–433.
891. Hansell DR. Extracorporeal membrane oxygenation for perinatal and pediatric patients. *Respir Care* 2003;48:352–362.
892. Lago P, Rebsamen S, Clancy RR, et al. MRI, MRA, and neurodevelopmental outcome following neonatal ECMO. *Pediatr Neurol* 1995;12:294–304.
893. Mendoza JC, Shearer LL, Cook LN. Lateralization of brain lesions following extracorporeal membrane oxygenation. *Pediatrics* 1991;88:1004–1009.
894. Lazar EL, Abramson SJ, Weinstein S, et al. Neuroimaging of brain injury in neonates treated with extracorporeal membrane oxygenation: lessons learned from serial examinations. *J Pediatr Surg* 1994;29:186–190.
895. Graziani LJ, Streletz LJ, Mitchell DG, et al. Electroencephalographic, neuroradiologic, and neurodevelopmental studies in infants with subclavian steal during ECMO. *Pediatr Neurol* 1994;10:97–103.
896. Nield TA, Langenbacher D, Poulsen MK, et al. Neurodevelopmental outcome at 3.5 years of age in children treated with extracorporeal life support: relationship to primary diagnosis. *J Pediatr* 2000;136:338–344.
897. Hamrick SE, Gremmels DB, Keet CA, et al. Neurodevelopmental outcome of infants supported with extracorporeal membrane oxygenation after cardiac surgery. *Pediatrics* 2003;111:e671–675.
898. Davis PJ, Firmin RK, Manktelow B, et al. Long-term outcome following extracorporeal membrane oxygenation for congenital diaphragmatic hernia: the UK experience. *J Pediatr* 2004;144:309–315.
899. Nellhaus G, Neuman I, Ellis E, et al. Asthma and seizures in children. *Pediatr Clin North Am* 1975;22:89–100.
900. Haslam RH, Freigang B. Cough syncope mimicking epilepsy in asthmatic children. *Can J Neurol Sci* 1985;12:45–47.
901. Annett RD, Aylward EH, Lapidus J, et al. Neurocognitive functioning in children with mild and moderate asthma in the childhood asthma management program. The Childhood Asthma Management Program (CAMP) Research Group. *J Allergy Clin Immunol* 2000;105:717–724.
902. Gottlieb DJ, Chase C, Vezina RM, et al. Sleep-disordered breathing symptoms are associated with poorer cognitive function in 5-year-old children. *J Pediatr* 2004;145:458–464.
903. Bass JL, Corwin M, Gozal D, et al. The effect of chronic or intermittent hypoxia on cognition in childhood: a review of the evidence. *Pediatrics* 2004;114:805–816.
904. O'Brien LM, Mervis CB, Holbrook CR, et al. Neurobehavioral correlates of sleep-disordered breathing in children. *J Sleep Res* 2004;13:165–172.
905. Rosen CL, D'Andrea L, Haddad GG. Adult criteria for obstructive sleep apnea do not identify children with serious obstruction. *Am Rev Respir Dis* 1992;146:1231–1234.
905a. Guilleminault C, Kirisoglu C, Ohayon MM. C-reactive protein and sleep-disordered breathing. *Sleep* 2004;27:1507–1511.
906. Bahls FH, Ma KK, Bird TD. Theophylline-associated seizures with "therapeutic" or low toxic serum concentrations: risk factors for serious outcome in adults. *Neurology* 1991;41:1309–1312.
907. Bigler ED. Theophylline neurotoxicity resulting in diffuse brain damage. *Dev Med Child Neurol* 1991;33:179–181.
908. Hopkins IJ. A new syndrome: Poliomyelitis-like illness associated with acute asthma in childhood. *Austral Paediatr J* 1974;10:273–276.
909. Beede HE, Newcomb RW. Lower motor neuron paralysis in association with asthma. *Johns Hopkins Med J* 1980;147:186–187.
910. Arita J, Nakae Y, Matsushima H, et al. Hopkins syndrome: T2-weighted high intensity of anterior horn on spinal MR imaging. *Pediatr Neurol* 1995;13:263–265.
911. Manson JI, Thong YH. Immunological abnormalities in the syndrome of poliomyelitis-like illness associated with acute bronchial asthma (Hopkin's syndrome). *Arch Dis Child* 1980;55:26–32.
912. Kira J, Ochi H. Juvenile muscular atrophy of the distal upper limb (Hirayama disease) associated with atopy. *J Neurol Neurosurg Psychiatry* 2001;70:798–801.

913. Horiuchi I, Yamasaki K, Osoegawa M, et al. Acute myelitis after asthma attacks with onset after puberty. *J Neurol Neurosurg Psychiatry* 2000;68:665–668.
914. Kira J, Kawano Y, Horiuchi I, et al. Clinical, immunological and MRI features of myelitis with atopic dermatitis (atopic myelitis). *J Neurol Sci* 1999;162:56–61.
915. Begbie ME, Wallace GM, Shovlin CL. Hereditary haemorrhagic telangiectasia (Osler-Weber-Rendu syndrome): a view from the 21st century. *Postgrad Med J* 2003;79:18–24.
916. Batinica S, Gagro A, Bradic I, et al. Congenital pulmonary arteriovenous fistula: a rare cause of cyanosis in childhood. *Thorac Cardiovasc Surg* 1991;39:105–106.
917. Moussouttas M, Fayad P, Rosenblatt M, et al. Pulmonary arteriovenous malformations: cerebral ischemia and neurologic manifestations. *Neurology* 2000;55:959–964.
918. Lucidi V, Di Capua M, Rosati P. Benign intracranial hypertension in an older child with cystic fibrosis. *Pediatr Neurol* 1993;9:494–495.
919. Roach ES, Sinal SH. Initial treatment of cystic fibrosis. Frequency of transient bulging fontanel. *Clin Pediatr (Phila)* 1989;28:371–373.
920. Jozefowicz RF. Neurologic manifestations of pulmonary disease. *Neurol Clin* 1989;7:605–616.
921. Laaban JP, Marsal L, Waked M. Seizures related to severe hypophosphatemia induced by mechanical ventilation. *Intensive Care Med* 1990;16:135–136.
922. Bolton CF, Gilbert JJ, Hahn AF, et al. Polyneuropathy in critically ill patients. *J Neurol Neurosurg Psychiatry* 1984;47:1223–1231.
923. Wijdicks EF, Litchy WJ, Harrison BA, et al. The clinical spectrum of critical illness polyneuropathy. *Mayo Clin Proc* 1994;69:955–959.
924. van Mook WN, Hulsewe-Evers RP. Critical illness polyneuropathy. *Curr Opin Crit Care* 2002;8:302–310.
925. MacFarlane IA, Rosenthal FD. Severe myopathy after status asthmaticus. *Lancet* 1977;2:615.
926. Barohn RJ, Jackson CE, Rogers SJ, et al. Prolonged paralysis due to nondepolarizing neuromuscular blocking agents and corticosteroids. *Muscle Nerve* 1994;17:647–654.
927. Williams TJ, O'Hehir RE, Czarny D, et al. Acute myopathy in severe acute asthma treated with intravenously administered corticosteroids. *Am Rev Respir Dis* 1988;137:460–463.
928. Sander HW, Golden M, Danon MJ. Quadriplegic areflexic ICU illness: selective thick filament loss and normal nerve histology. *Muscle Nerve* 2002;26:499–505.
929. Banwell BL, Mildner RJ, Hassall AC, et al. Muscle weakness in critically ill children. *Neurology* 2003;61:1779–1782.
930. Deconinck N, Van Parijs V, Beckers-Bleukx G, Van den Bergh P. Critical illness myopathy unrelated to corticosteroids or neuromuscular blocking agents. *Neuromuscul Disord* 1998;8:186–192.
931. Hund E. Neurological complications of sepsis: critical illness polyneuropathy and myopathy. *J Neurol* 2001;248:929–934.
932. Lecker SH, Jagoe RT, Gilbert A, et al. Multiple types of skeletal muscle atrophy involve a common program of changes in gene expression. *FASEB J* 2004;18:39–51.
933. Di Giovanni S, Molon A, Broccolini A, et al. Constitutive activation of MAPK cascade in acute quadriplegic myopathy. *Ann Neurol* 2004;55:195–206.
934. Young GB, Bolton CF, Austin TW, et al. The encephalopathy associated with septic illness. *Clin Invest Med* 1990;13:297–304.
935. Wilson JX, Young GB. Progress in clinical neurosciences: sepsis-associated encephalopathy: evolving concepts. *Can J Neurol Sci* 2003;30:98–105.
936. Young GB, Bolton CF, Archibald YM, et al. The electroencephalogram in sepsis-associated encephalopathy. *J Clin Neurophysiol* 1992;9:145–152.
937. Finelli PF, Uphoff DF. Magnetic resonance imaging abnormalities with septic encephalopathy. *J Neurol Neurosurg Psychiatry* 2004;75:1189–1191.
938. Davies DC. Blood–brain barrier breakdown in septic encephalopathy and brain tumours. *J Anat* 2002;200:639–646.
939. Moss RF, Parmar NK, Tighe D, et al. Adrenergic agents modify cerebral edema and microvessel ultrastructure in porcine sepsis. *Crit Care Med* 2004;32:1916–1921.

Disorders of Mental Development

Marcel Kinsbourne and Frank B. Wood

A host of neurologic disorders with onset early in life compromise mental development. The cognitive impairment may be one among many neurologic abnormalities, or it may be the dominant feature. Even in the latter case, less prominent neurologic signs and symptoms are usually also to be found, and no clear neurobiologic distinction can be made between syndromes of mental dysfunctions and other brain disorders. This chapter treats in detail those disorders in which the mental development component is key. Where disordered mental development is one of many abnormalities, the mental component is briefly summarized, and the reader is referred to other chapters for more comprehensive discussion of the entity in question.

A developmental disability is an impairment in behavioral development due to abnormality of the central nervous system. Developmental disabilities manifest during the developmental period and result in lifelong impairment in any combination of physical, cognitive, sensory, speech and language, and neuropsychologic functions. Beginning with the formation of the neuroectoderm, the developmental period is in principle not complete until the end of myelinization during the decade of the twenties. In practical terms, however, the general category of developmental disorders reflects alterations in neural maturation that manifest most often and most prominently in the preschool and early grade school years. This chapter considers the nature, diagnosis, and management of those developmental disorders and disabilities that implicate higher cortical function—that is, cognition and attention.

NATURE OF DEVELOPMENTAL DISORDERS

Postnatal neurologic maturation underwrites the gradual acquisition of an extensive repertoire of cognitive skills. The newborn is devoid of cerebrally controlled behavioral patterns, so that in the first 6 weeks of life it is hard to distinguish the normal newborn's behavior from that of an anencephalic infant. Different brain regions progressively assume control over specific functions in predictable sequence and timing—brainstem before cerebrum, sensorimotor projections before integrative cortex. Late-developing skills, typically subserved by late-maturing prefrontal cortex (1), develop over many years, at least until late adolescence, before the skill in question asymptotes to its ultimate adult level (2).

A developmental disorder typically becomes apparent when a specific ability fails to present within the normatively expected time frame. It induces an unexpected low point in the child's cognitive profile, a selective deficit. In the general childhood population, there is a high correlation between an individual's performance on a wide range of mental tests, a phenomenon that has given rise to the construct of *g*, or general intelligence. Some two-thirds of the interindividual variance in the overall intelligence quotient (IQ) of the general population reflects genetic diversity (3,4). Variations in the prenatal and postnatal environment account for the remainder. Even in the general population, aspects of brain structure correlate with IQ: Intracranial, cerebral, temporal lobe, hippocampal and cerebellar volume as well as gray matter volume account for between 12% and 31% of the variance in IQ (5). However, many adverse biologic, genetic, environmental, and gene-environment interactions can reduce the rate of intellectual development, either globally, causing mental retardation, or selectively, compromising some components of intelligence only. IQ tends to be higher in those who were heavier at birth or who grew taller in childhood and adolescence. In a study of normal nine-year-old children, IQ at age 9 rose by about two points for every standard deviation increase of head circumference at 9 months and by nearly three points for every standard deviation increase at 9 years. It appears that postnatal head growth, at asymptote between age 14 and 16, is more important than prenatal head growth in determining cognitive function. Postnatal head growth correlates positively with mothers' height and weight, socioeconomic status (SES), and educational level (6).

Selective cognitive deficit results in "intertest scatter," such that the child scores within the normal range on some tests, but disproportionately poorly on those that tap developmentally compromised cognitive processes. Such scatter between normally and slowly developing skills is typical of learning disabilities. Any cognitive skill may be selectively impaired, but it is the impairments that have social consequences that attract attention. Those selective cognitive deficits that result in delayed language development, abnormal play, and defective social skills commonly become apparent during the second and third years of life. Selective deficits in attention, concentration, and learning that leave a child lacking readiness for instruction in academic areas may not be recognized until the preschool or grade school period. Such disorders are usually diagnosed on functional and behavioral criteria, whether or not biologic validation of the diagnosis is feasible.

In some cognitive domains, normal development continues until late in adolescence. Examples of this include executive functions, such as the capacity of working memory and cognitive flexibility (7). A recent imaging finding that dorsolateral frontal activation continues to develop in adolescence (8) is provocative but may only show that adolescents tend to underutilize that cortex, rather than that they are as yet incapable of using it. Developmental delays usually reach an end-point of persisting cognitive deficits by late adolescence, within the same time frame as that in which normal development asymptotes. In general, gradual improvement is common, though some is due to statistical regression artifact. But some improvement reflects genuine progress as the child sorts out the most relevant and controlling stimuli of life, school, and work, thereby reserving the most effort at improvement for the areas that promise the most gain. A child's brain may compensate, reorganize, and mature, and special education may offer systematic practice of impaired skills, combined with alternative training that circumvents the cognitive limitation ("bypass"). In other instances, cognitive abilities gradually deteriorate, as in increasingly intractable seizure disorder and secondary behavioral disorder. Or development may be predestined genetically to decelerate gradually, as in Down syndrome. However, usually the child makes gains over time but with a ranking relative to his typically functioning peers that does not appreciably change. Notwithstanding that, the gap in adolescence is usually rather more obvious than it is around school entry. Such a child's level of functioning is quantitatively insufficient for his chronologic age and instead is as would have been expected in a younger child.

NEURODEVELOPMENTAL LAG

Normative cognitive and language developmental milestones are presented in Table 18.1. In neurodevelopmental lag, the effects of an early brain lesion or maldevelopment become increasingly apparent many months or years later as cognitive milestones are slow to be reached and immature patterns of sensorimotor control persist. The newborn has a limited repertoire of innate movement patterns. These synergisms subserve activities such as rooting, sucking, startle, and lateral orienting, which occur spontaneously or as reflexive responses to stimulation. Synergisms gradually disappear according to a well-delineated schedule in the course of infancy or childhood. The overall trend of motor development is toward increasingly precise control over an ever widening repertoire of discrete movement combinations (9); sensory development tends toward a finer, more exact differentiation between various stimuli (10).

TABLE 18.1 Typical Cognitive and Language Developmental Milestones of Infancy and Childhood

Age	*Early Cognitive Milestones*	*Early Language Milestones*
From birth	Interest in faces; begins to make eye contact	Phonologic discrimination
Few mo	A social smile should develop before 6 weeks of age Laughing out loud is a reliable milestone that should occur around 4 months of age	Responsive vocalization, turn-taking, cooing (vowels)
6–8 mo	Grabbing for objects, exploring surroundings	Babbling consonants/vowels, syllables, dada, baba
10–12 mo	Pointing to indicate wanted object; comprehension of words	2–3 words with meaning; imitation of animals
18–22 mo	Should follow simple commands, indicate body parts, ask for objects by pointing, and imitate actions	Vocabulary spurt; jargonizing develops interspersed with intelligent words; receptive language and understanding are more developed than speech
	Onlooker behavior, nonsocial activity, and solitary independent play	By 2 years: word combinations/many single words; expansion of comprehension
Around 2 yr	Limited social participation; parallel play	2-word utterances; mostly intelligible to family; comprehend many sentences
By 3 yr	Beginning social play (the child talks about play, borrows/lends toys, controls who may play in the group)	Speaks in grammatical sentences (with some errors); mostly intelligible to strangers (still makes phonologic errors)
Thereafter	Cooperative play; acts out make-believe themes	Phonology by school age; vocabulary increases lifelong

In neurodevelopmental lag, synergisms may persist, presenting as "soft signs" on the neurologic examination. Soft signs are signs that would have been normal had the child been younger. Motor soft signs are of two kinds: (a) unwanted movements (e.g., persistent asymmetrical tonic neck response, unwanted associated and mirror movements); and (b) imperfect execution, such as slowness in speeded sequential activities such as finger tapping or finger-thumb sequencing, or in alternating movements, such as pronation-supination of the forearm or flexion-extension at the ankle (dysdiadochokinesis). In the absence of long tract signs, dyspraxia, or clumsiness, is diagnostically nonspecific (see discussion of developmental coordination disorder below).

Delayed development proceeds through the same stages as normal development, although at a slower rate. Thus, with increasing age and neurologic maturation, scores on quantitative scales for soft signs decline, regardless of diagnosis (11). Considerable consistency in neuromotor developmental status has been demonstrated over periods as long as 10 years (12). Signs of sensorimotor immaturity are often lower-level analogues to later emerging cognitive immaturity, behavioral problems, and attention deficits. Early signs of developmental delay indicate a high risk of long-term functional developmental disabilities, depending on the distribution and severity of the underlying cause, but these associations do not provide an adequate basis for prognosis. For instance, an association exists between persisting mirror movements and aggressive psychopathology, perhaps because both are manifestations of disinhibition (13). Excessive, uncontrollable crying that persists beyond 3 months of age has been associated with a shortfall of some nine IQ points relative to controls with colic only in a prospective study (14).

Neurodevelopmental lags that involve both cognitive and sensorimotor control have been bracketed together as "minimal brain dysfunction" (MBD) (15). This construct was intended to indicate organicity, so as to counteract the now virtually extinct tendency to ascribe developmental delays to intrapsychic problems. A similar construct, intended to be descriptive rather than making hard-to-prove claims about the brain, has gained acceptance in Scandinavia. This is the collective labeling of children with childhood onset of deficits in attention, motor control, and perception with the acronym DAMP (16). These disparate neurocognitive immaturities may or may not affect specific academic skills. A clinical level of deficit is reached by 1.5% of the childhood population. The syndrome does not indicate any particular etiology (17), and its antecedents do not differ qualitatively from those of major brain dysfunctions such as cerebral palsy or mental retardation, which also are end results of a host of different neuropathologies. The extent to which development is impaired depends on the anatomical distribution and the severity of the insult, rather than its cause. Despite their substantial comorbidity (18), neuropsychologic testing does not reveal any functional overlap between the motor and the attentional components. The practical usefulness of the MBD/DAMP construct is limited by the fact that each component of the syndrome is managed in the same way when it coexists with the other ones, as when it is present in isolation.

CLASSIFICATION OF DEVELOPMENTAL DISORDERS AND DISABILITIES

Ideally, disorders of cognitive development are classified on both an etiologic and a descriptive and functional basis. However, many patients have developmental disorders "of uncertain etiology." In the absence of a precise medical diagnosis, it is preferable to record the chief characteristics of the abnormal developmental process rather than to make inferences such as "cerebral dysfunction," "organicity," or "static encephalopathy." The characteristics include qualitative and quantitative descriptions of the mental status, including use of language, play skills, visual and auditory recognition, reasoning, orientation to spatial relationships, impulse control, and the ability to sustain attention.

Most neurodevelopmental disorders that result in mild disability affect quality of life but do not curtail longevity. The children require no more than the customary standard of medical care throughout their lives. Any need for additional specific medical interventions for certain neurologic disorders (e.g., diets for metabolic disorders or epilepsy, pharmacologic treatment for severe behavioral problems), or for nonmedical therapy programs, should be re-evaluated periodically for evidence of cost-effectiveness on long-term outcome.

PRACTICAL APPROACHES TO NEURODEVELOPMENTAL DISORDERS

The medical model and the habilitation model (Fig. 18.1) are complementary, and both are fundamental to clinical practice. The habilitation model is particularly relevant when, as in disorders of mental development, there generally are few means of offering complete symptomatic relief and fewer still of outright cure. By federal law, the Individuals with Disabilities in Education Act (IDEA)—the habilitation/rehabilitation model for developmentally disabled children—is the programmatic and financial responsibility of local education authorities, assisted to a varying extent by federal funding.

Medical Diagnosis and Treatment

Developmental disorders have a wide variety of causes, and few have a specific, identifiable genetic or neurobiologic etiology. Different etiologies converge on identical

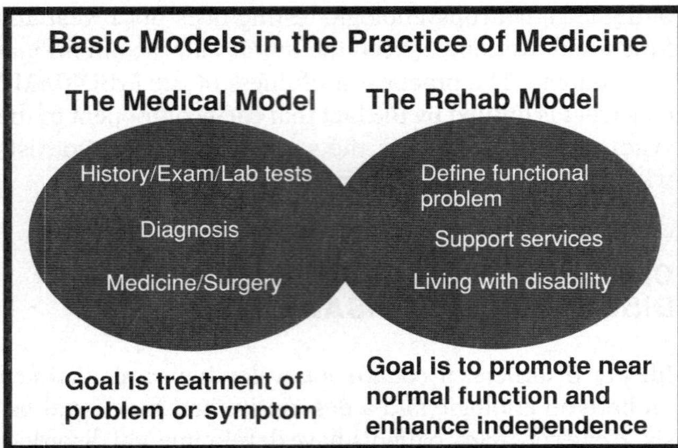

FIGURE 18.1. The practice of the medical model and the rehabilitation model should coincide.

behavioral phenotypes. The diagnostic yield is much greater if there is associated microcephaly, antenatal toxin exposure, or focal findings (19). In their absence, a thorough search for diagnostic clues includes family history with a three-generation pedigree and information from the prenatal, perinatal, and early postnatal periods. The development of motor skills; comprehension of speech; emergence of words and formed, intelligible sentences; and quality of social play skills are often relevant. The physical examination includes measuring head circumference as well as body size and growth; assessment of vision, hearing, and ocular funduscopy; searching for facial, skeletal, somatic, and dermatoglyphic anomalies and asymmetries; visceromegaly; neurocutaneous lesions and depigmentations; and other signs of chronic illness. Hand preference and pencil grip are noted as well as any abnormal postures and involuntary movements. Clinical clues in the evaluation of developmental disorders are presented in Table 18.2.

The mental status examination assesses the child's orientation, relatedness to, and interest in the examiner, caregiver, siblings, peers, and other people in the child's environment; the quality of reciprocal social exchange in verbal and nonverbal communication (e.g., eye contact, gestures, facial expression), ability to engage in reciprocal imaginative play with representational toys; presence of perseverative, stereotypic, and ritualistic behavior; and presence of problematic behaviors such as attention difficulties, overactivity, aggression, and self-injury.

The laboratory evaluation of choice for developmental disorders continues to evolve as increasingly detailed understanding of the human genome leads to improved delineation of syndromes and advances in cytogenetic,

TABLE 18.2 Clinical Clues in the Determination of Developmental Disorders and their Etiology

Clinical Clue	*Etiologic Category*	*Examples*
Family member with known condition, mental retardation, other developmental disabilities, multiple miscarriages	Genetic	Mendelian dominant, recessive, X-linked; some mitochondrial disorders; cytogenetic/chromosomal anomalies
Facial dysmorphism, severe central nervous system malformation	Genetic or acquired during embryogenesis	CHARGE syndrome, anencephaly, holoprosencephaly, septo-optic dysplasia
Evidence of neuroblast migrational disorder, hydrocephalus, congenital microcephaly	Genetic or acquired during the fetal period	Lissencephaly (Miller-Dieker syndrome), X-linked hydrocephalus
Born too soon, too small	Prematurity	Periventricular leukomalacia
Low Apgar scores, low cord pH, neonatal seizures	Perinatal	Hypoxic-ischemic encephalopathy
Acquired microcephaly, stagnation in developmental gain	Postnatal	Rett syndrome
Postnatal vomiting, failure to thrive, hypoglycemia	Metabolic	Phenylketonuria, urea cycle disorders, organic acidurias, other specific enzyme defects
Cerebral calcifications, congenital or acquired microcephaly	Infectious	Cytomegalovirus encephalopathy, toxoplasmosis, herpes simplex viruses, human immunodeficiency virus, bacterial meningitis
Hemorrhage, infarction, venous thrombosis	Cerebrovascular	Factor V Leiden deficiency, sickle cell disease
Failure to thrive	Nutritional	Prenatal and postnatal protein malnutrition, vitamin and essential element deficiency
Parental drug abuse, neonatal jaundice, acute encephalopathy	Prenatal, perinatal, postnatal toxic exposure	Fetal alcohol syndrome, neonatal hyperbilirubinemia, lead poisoning
Dry skin, hypotonia, hyporeflexia	Endocrine	Hypothyroidism
Extreme poverty, parental drug abuse, low parental educational level, severe plagiocephaly	Sociocultural/environmental	Nonaccidental head trauma, emotional deprivation, lack of infant stimulation
Nonspecific findings	Unknown	Up to one-half of all developmental disabilities

molecular, and neuroimaging techniques. Routine test batteries are not effective. The incidence of identifiable metabolic disorders in children with developmental delay is low, ranging from 0% to 5% (20,21). In addition, nonspecific, nondiagnostic, or false-positive "abnormalities" are common in routine nondirected laboratory testing. This can lead to further futile laboratory pursuits. Most infants and children with inborn errors of metabolism show signs or symptoms of their metabolic disorder such as hepatosplenomegaly, failure to thrive, intolerance of certain food groups, intermittent emesis, recurrent unexplained illnesses, seizures, intermittent somnolence, or fluctuating hypotonia. The relevant metabolic tests are reviewed in Chapter 1. In patients with developmental disorders who lack signs or symptoms of a metabolic disorder, metabolic screening should be deferred (22–24).

Many individuals with mental retardation have associated behavioral, emotional, and psychiatric disorders and nonneurologic congenital anomalies. A composite pattern recognition or cytogenetic testing may lead to a specific diagnosis (25). In these circumstances, the diagnostic label refers to the most salient aspect of the condition or is noted by an acronym, such as CHARGE association (of congenital anomalies) or eponym (e.g., Angelman syndrome), or by the underlying chromosomal abnormality, such as at chromosome 22q11.2. A specific molecular cytogenetic analysis, such as fluorescence *in situ* hybridization (FISH), may be indicated if the child has features of a known mental retardation syndrome (e.g., Williams or fragile X syndrome) or autism (e.g., chromosome 15q11 duplication) (see Chapter 4).

In most individuals with mild mental retardation, there are no specific neuropathologic correlates. Neuroimaging has a low diagnostic yield unless there are suspicious physical findings or localized neurologic deficits (26). Delayed myelination visualized on magnetic resonance imaging (MRI) is nonspecific in infants and children with neurodevelopmental delays (27). The diagnostic yield of neuroimaging increases considerably if the mental retardation is severe or complicated by microcephaly or macrocephaly, major motor abnormalities, features of a genetic syndrome, or seizures. MRI may reveal migrational disorders (e.g., lissencephaly), midline defects (e.g., holoprosencephaly or septo-optic dysplasia), or other brain malformations and disruptions (e.g., schizencephaly) (see Chapter 5). When the history suggests metabolic insult, vascular compromise, infection, or trauma, neuroimaging may reveal evidence of destructive central nervous system (CNS) changes.

There is no consensus on which children with developmental delay should be studied by imaging, and there are considerable variations in technique, methodology, demographics, and interpretation between the few available studies of computed tomography (CT) and MRI in children with mental retardation. Correspondingly, the reported frequency of abnormal neuroimaging findings in persons with mental retardation ranges from 9% to 80% (28–31). Positron emission tomography (PET), single photon emission CT (SPECT), functional MRI (fMRI) (32), and volumetric and morphometric MRI (33) provide insights into specific conditions but have limited overall application in the infant or child with a nonspecific developmental disorder. Formal audiologic testing is required to rule out hearing loss in all children who have language delay and may have isolated high-frequency hearing losses. Children with hearing impairment should be followed longitudinally for speech therapy and possible speech amplification.

Electroencephalography (EEG) is indicated if the history suggests seizures or regression or plateau in language acquisition (see Chapter 14). EEG can assist in the diagnosis of certain children with developmental disorders (34). Seizure disorders are often in their own right associated with diminishing IQ, as is their treatment with antiepileptic drugs (see Chapter 14). Memory may be deficient when the seizures are generalized. In complex partial seizure disorder, verbal and nonverbal memory may be impaired when there are left and right foci, respectively (35). Epileptic children as a group have inferior attention and general slowing of mental processes (36) as well as a varying degree of lag in language and reading ability (37). Children with frontal epileptic foci exhibited a relatively greater degree of impulsivity and disordered planning, verbal fluency, and motor coordination than generalized and temporal comparison groups (37). A comprehensive treatment of the neuropsychology of childhood epilepsy is available (38).

Habilitation and Rehabilitation

In habilitation, rehabilitation techniques are applied to individuals who, rather than having lost previously mastered skills, failed to master new skills at the expected age. This applies to children with developmental delay. For purposes of habilitation, the physician is less concerned about the level of function, and more with the implementation of evidence-based effective and enabling therapies, regardless of etiology. Schools are the primary venues of such therapies, and the consensus is swinging toward ever stricter demand for evidence-based justifications for such educational practices. For example, the Federal Department of Education maintains a "What Works Clearinghouse" that periodically reviews and reports educational efficacy evidence that meets high standards (39).

Children who are considered to have cognitive deficiency may come to attention because of poor academic achievement, abnormal behavior, or both. Is the lack of academic achievement due to limited cognitive ability, or does it represent underachievement relative to the child's potential for other (e.g., psychosocial or emotional) reasons? If the child appears to be achieving at his or her maximum level, consistent with that child's specific profile of cognitive or attentional strengths or weaknessess, then special needs are identified, and an individualized educational plan (IEP) is implemented. If the child is underachieving, the causes are sometimes found in the child's school and social setting or emotional well-being. In only a few developmental syndromes, notably attention-deficit hyperactivity disorder (ADHD), can cognitive potential be enhanced by medical means. In particular, there is as yet no evidence that learning disabilities, distinct from any comorbid attentional disorder, are pharmacologically treatable.

Most disorders of mental development are long lasting, if not permanent. Whether the child's condition declares itself at or before birth or during early childhood, the parents have to adjust their previous expectations of a perfectly healthy child to the current reality. This adjustment is traumatic, and not all parents navigate its difficulties with success. The problem is amplified if, as is commonly the case, a specific diagnosis as well as a specific prognosis cannot be formulated. Such opinions as "developmental disability" convey confusion and are no substitute for the clarity and credibility of a specific diagnosis. When the disability is chronic and not fully explained—for instance, as in mental retardation and in autism—the quality of the parent–child relationship may suffer for lack of clarity about what to expect in the future. The clinician cannot always persuade the parents of what appears to be the reality of the situation, or even of the diagnosis, when that can be ascertained. Continued uncertainty is detrimental to parent–child attachment as well as to the functioning of the family unit. Under such circumstances, encouragement to seek a second opinion can with advantage be accompanied by referral for psychological counseling.

Inclusion in Public Education

The Education for All Handicapped Children Act (EHA) was renamed the Individuals with Disabilities Education Act (IDEA) in 1990. This legislation requires schools to provide an appropriate individualized educational plan to students with disabilities, to be implemented in the "least restrictive environment." The IDEA mandates a nondiscriminatory assessment, active involvement of parents in the educational process with due-process rights and hearing, and access to indicated ancillary services such as physical therapy, counseling, and transportation. The reauthorization of IDEA requires that students with disabilities be educated with their nondisabled peers to the extent possible, and that schools actively plan for student transitions (and that traumatic brain injury and autism be considered separate categories). The word *handicapped* in the original version of the law was replaced with the word *disabled*. *Inclusion* refers to the effort to include students with disabilities in general classrooms while providing special services outside the general classroom as needed. Currently, approximately 70% of all students with disabilities attend mainstream classes during part of the school day.

Quantitative Measurement of Cognition (Standardized Scales)

In infancy and early childhood, receptive and expressive language and play skills are the best indices of cognitive level. The prognostic reliability of cognitive testing improves when children reach an age at which some language competence is expected and a wider range of testing modalities becomes available. Language development up to age 3 years can initially be documented in the clinical setting with the Early Language Milestone Scale (40). Early cognitive and language developmental milestones in infancy and childhood are summarized in Table 18.1.

The diagnosis of a cognitive deficiency requires that a clinical impression be validated by standard psychometric assessment or referral report. The assessment that is appropriate for infants and children with developmental delays or disabilities depends on the child's age, level of impairment, and the presence of additional sensory deficits. For clinical screening up to age 6 years, the Denver-II, formerly the Denver Developmental Screening Test–Revised (41), has been commonly used. The Denver-II draws on parent history, testing, and observation and takes approximately one-half hour to administer. However, for predictive value, the Battelle Developmental Inventory Screening Test (BDIST), which screens children up to age 8 years, is preferred (42) though it is not designed to identify specific learning disabilities. A trained infant psychometrist is likely to adminster the Bayley Scales of Infant Development II, which estimate the level of cognitive and motor deficits in infants (43). However, because infant cognition is limited, only sensorimotor functions can be evaluated accurately for normative purposes. These functions are nonspecifically correlated to an infant's later emerging cognitive skills, the lack of which may result in a developmental disability in later years. More specific information about selective deficits in cognitive operations can be gleaned from the results of neuropsychologic testing. A cognitive profile is established for diagnoses and functional evaluation, the monitoring of further development, and rehabilitation planning. Some commonly used measures of cognitive and adaptive behavioral development are summarized in Table 18.3.

Administered with proper reservation, an IQ test is by far the most valid means toward establishing a child's level of functioning—knowledge that has wide clinical application. Regardless of disagreements as to whether IQ is a valid measure of intellectual or educational potential (58), the IQ test result is unequivocably the best guide in estimating overall current levels of functioning. IQ within the normal range by definition eliminates mental retardation

TABLE 18.3 Common Measures of Cognitive and Adaptive Behavioral Development in Infancy and Childhood

Category of Test	*Test Name/Reference*	*Ages*	*Description*
Screening	Bayley Infant Neurodevelopment Screen (43)	3–24 mo	Assesses neurodevelopmental skills such as object permanence, imitation, and language
	Denver-II (41)	0–72 mo	Screens for language, fine motor, adaptive personal/social, and gross motor skills
Intelligence measures	Wechsler Preschool and Primary Scale of Intelligence, Revised (44)	Preschoolers	Measures verbal comprehension, perceptual organization, attention/concentration, and visual processing speed
	Wechsler Intelligence Scale for Children-III (45)	School-aged children	Both the Wechsler Preschool and the Wechsler Intelligence Scale give a verbal, performance, and full-scale IQ
	Stanford-Binet Intelligence Scale: Fourth Edition (46)	Variable for each subtest	Measures general intelligence, verbal reasoning, quantitative reasoning, abstract/visual reasoning, and short-term memory
Alternative cognitive measures	Goodenough-Harris Drawing Test (Draw-A-Man) (47)	3–16 yr	Easy to use as a screen of nonverbal intellectual abilities, especially useful for culturally diverse, low-functioning children
	Kaufman Assessment Battery for Children (48)	2.5–12.5 yr	Used to complement Stanford-Binet or Wechsler nonverbal estimates
	McCarthy Scales of Children's Abilities (McCarthy) (49)	2.5–8.5 yr	Provides information on young children with suspected learning disabilities
	Leiter International Performance Scale (50)	2 yr to adult	Often used with autistic children as a measure of nonverbal intelligence
Behavior rating scales	Achenbach Child Behavior Checklist (51)	2–3 yr	Allows parents or caregivers to rate a young child's social/emotional development
	Conners' Parent/Teacher Rating Scales (CPRS-48 and CPRS-28) (52)	3–17 yr	The CPRS-48 has 48 items and CPRS-28 items that assess conduct problems, learning problems, impulsivity/hyperactivity, and attention
Adaptive behavioral scales	Battelle Developmental Inventory (42)	Newborn to 8 yr	Assesses personal/social, adaptive, motor, communication, and cognition
	Vineland Adaptive Behavioral Scales (53)	Newborn to 18 yr	Parent questionnaire that assesses communication, daily living skills, socialization, motor skills, adaptive behavior, and maldevelopment; useful in children with cognitive disabilities
Achievement	Wide Range Achievement Test 3 (54)	5 yr to adult	Screening test of basic academic skills, including reading, spelling, and arithmetic
	Woodcock Johnson Psychoeducational Battery–Revised, Part II (55)	3 yr to adult	Psychometric test of academic abilities with subtests in reading, mathematics, and written language
Language	Early Language Milestone Scale (40)	Newborn to 3 yr	Examines listening, speaking, audition, and visual perception
	Peabody Picture Vocabulary Test–Revised (56)	2–6 yr	Vocabulary screening test for children with expressive language difficulties
Nonverbal	Developmental Test of Visual-Motor Integration (57)	4–18 yr	Tests child's abilities to integrate visual perception and motor output by requiring the child to copy increasingly complex geometric forms

as the reason for preschool or school achievement below the expected level. It does not exclude the possibility that specific learning disabilities are compromising the acquisition of some academic skills. Therefore, IQ has been withdrawn from the necessary definition of learning disability in the 2004 IDEA. Furthermore, no single IQ test measures all cognitive operations, and various subtests involve multiple cognitive processes. Therefore, a low score on a subtest would be unlikely to isolate the basic cognitive deficit that prevents the child from learning to read, write, or calculate.

Some "scatter" between the levels of subscale or subtest scores on an intelligence scale is normal. Only when it is statistically excessive might it reflect a disparity in the level of development of different intellectual skills. Verbal-performance discrepancy scores are often reported. Children with mild mental retardation tend to score somewhat lower on the Wechsler verbal subscale than on the performance subscale. A much lower verbal than performance IQ accompanies selective language delay; the converse discrepancy is often found in association with developmental difficulties in spatial orientation and visuomotor control, and to some extent in Asperger disorder.

The Stanford-Binet scale (46) and the Wechsler Preschool and Primary Scale of Intelligence (WPPSI) (44) are most commonly used for preschoolers. The Wechsler Intelligence Scale for Children (WISC-III) is available for school-aged children (45). These are well-standardized test batteries that call for the use of a range of different cognitive skills. For deaf children, the WISC-III performance scale and the Hiskey-Nebraska Test of Learning Aptitude have been specifically standardized (59). On such tests, deaf children without additional disabilities score close to the population average. The Perkins-Binet (60) and the Blind Learning Aptitude Test (61) are suitable for blind children. However, the most widely used psychometric instruments lack sensitivity in the mental retardation range. Even simple tests that use single words, such as the Peabody Picture Vocabulary Test (56), cannot be used if the patient is nonverbal. The Leiter International Performance Scale is useful for evaluating low functioning individuals (50). The interpretation of psychometric findings in mentally retarded subjects is complicated by uncertainties about the child's test orientation and motivation. Because IQ levels in children younger than 3 years are unstable, the low-scoring child should receive a more definitive evaluation at a later date.

Considerations in the Assessment of Learning, Emotion, and Behavior

The developmental history and physical findings in early infancy are unreliable bases for prognosis as to developmental outcome. For example, Apgar scores of 0 to 3 at 15 and 20 minutes are predictive of high mortality and high probability of disability; however, many of these infants score normally in later developmental assessment (see Chapter 6). Intelligence tests in infancy yield a developmental quotient (DQ) that is necessarily heavily loaded with factors that relate to motor development. Within a normal population, the DQ is a poor predictor of individual differences in cognitive development. It has some success, however, in distinguishing a normally functioning from a mentally retarded population. Infant testing is highly specialized and also calls for the child's cooperation. If this cannot be enlisted, the mother can be asked standard questions about her child's social development (53).

Taken literally, the IQ scores can underestimate the child's cognitive potential. Specific adaptive limitations often coexist with strengths in other adaptive skills or other personal capabilities. Limitations in adaptive skills may reflect the context of the child's community. Motivation to perform during testing cannot be taken for granted, particularly when the child's cultural or ethnic background has little understanding of and interest in cognitive testing and its uses. Anxiety can block the child's reasoning processes, alienation and withdrawal can render the child unavailable for the task, thought disorders can intrude, and impulsive behavior can disrupt test performance. Lapses of attention owing to subclinical absence seizures can interrupt concentration, and psychotropic and antiepileptic medication may impair some cognitive processes. The limited attention span of patients with ADHD can degrade performance on tasks that demand sustained attention and cognitive effort. In young children, even gross impairment of vision, hearing, or touch can go unrecognized, and the child's imperfect response to instruction or questions can be misattributed to defiance or cognitive deficiency. Other factors that complicate the interpretation of mental test performance are extremely low or high parental educational level, poor motivation with failure to expend mental effort on the test, depression, fatigue, and fear of failure with low self-esteem. Such potential sources of misinterpretation, which almost always lead to underestimation rather than overestimation, can never be fully ruled out, but conventional best practices expect the psychologist's report, usually in writing, to provide an estimate of the reliability of the reported score, taking such factors into consideration.

MENTAL RETARDATION

Terminology and Definitions

The terminology that is used to characterize persons with cognitive and adaptive behavioral disabilities has evolved, in repeated efforts to minimize social stigma. Terms such as *cognitive deficiency*, *intellectual disability*, and *learning disability* have been suggested to replace *mental retardation*, a term that misleadingly implies delay and therefore the possibility that the child will catch up. A similar term is *developmental delay*, which is nonspecific and is more of a chief complaint or a symptom complex than a diagnosis (62). Whereas children with mental retardation may learn new skills as they mature and are taught, most functional neurologic impairments are associated with intractable deficits of intellectual capacity. *Mental retardation* is a compendium term that does not refer to particular groups of diseases, syndromes, or medical disorders. It is not applied to cognitive deficiency that is a result of neurodegenerative and progressive neurometabolic diseases, or is secondary to psychiatric disorders.

The World Health Organization (ICD-10) characterizes developmental disabilities as due to *impairment* of the central nervous system, causing a functional *disability*, which consequently *handicaps* the individual in activities of daily living (63). It characterizes mental retardation as "incomplete or insufficient general development of mental capacities." Formal definitions of mental retardation that are currently recognized emphasize a descriptive diagnosis of persons with significant disability because of "subaverage intellectual functioning" and "concurrent deficits or impairments in present adaptive functioning [i.e., how effective persons are in meeting the standards expected for their age by their cultural group]" (64,65). In addition, the manifestation of brain dysfunction must originate during the developmental period of life. The three formal definitions differ slightly in their approach to the diagnosis because of differences in emphasis on adaptive skill symptom menus or underlying etiologic factors.

Because mental abilities are on a continuum, the quantitative definitions of mental retardation and its subdivisions based on the IQ are necessarily arbitrary cut-off points. The mental age (the age equivalent at which the child functions on the test) divided by the chronologic age is the IQ. The mean I.Q. for the general population is set at 100. Higher IQ predicts more academic success in such terms as higher grades, more years completed, and higher standardized test scores. It also predicts positive life outcomes, such as better mental health, lower divorce rate, lower level of criminality, and greater occupational success (66,67).

The standard deviation (SD) of a test refers to the distribution of scores around the mean. Mild, moderate, severe, and profound mental retardation have been traditionally associated with cutoff points in standard deviations below the mean of –2, –3, –4, and –5, respectively (68) (roughly corresponding to IQs of 70, 55, 40, and 25). IQ scores between 70 and 85 are sometimes referred to as borderline. But measured intelligence does not offer specific information about the individual's adaptive skills (Table 18.4). There is ongoing controversy on whether to emphasize IQ level or adaptive behavioral deficits as the central defining characteristic of mental retardation (69). The extent to which persons with mental retardation succeed in life is determined by their level of adaptive skills rather than by their IQ. However, there is no single measure of

TABLE 18.4 Classification of Mental Retardation by Measure of IQ and Level of Adaptive Behavior

Severity (Older Terminology)	Estimated IQ	Category of Support Required	Estimate of Cognitive/ Academic Level	Estimate of Adaptive Behavior as a Function of ADL
Borderline	70–85	Intermittent	Adequate language ability, but often develops late Variable learning disability	Independent in ADL Employable
Mild	50/55–70	Intermittent	Adequate language ability, but often develops late Severe learning disability May develop minimal reading ability	Most are independent in ADL Employable at simple jobs
Moderate	35/40–50/55	Limited	Simple language, develops late Most lack even minimal reading ability	Most are trainable in ADL (often need help) May be employable in a sheltered environment
Severe	20/25–35/40	Extensive	May speak some words or be nonverbal	May be trainable in some basic ADL
Profound	<20/25	Complete	May speak a few words; most are nonverbal	Dependent in all ADL

ADL, activities of daily living.

adaptive behavior. Newer efforts to define mental retardation have emphasized the amount of support needed for an individual to succeed or maintain basic activities of daily living, instead of focusing on global degrees of impairment (70). Support intensities are subdivided into four levels: intermittent, limited, extensive, and pervasive. Support functions are classified into eight categories: teaching, befriending, financial planning, behavioral support, in-home living assistance, community and school access and use, and health assistance. This categorization acknowledges that the diagnosis of mental retardation is useful only as a pointer toward providing the individual with additional supports for activities of everyday living beyond those that are considered to be customary for the child's age.

Further insight into the child' strengths and weaknesses is afforded by neuropsychological testing, which attempts to tease out of the cognitive spectrum different domains of functioning that can be differentially affected by brain damage, depending on which areas have borne the brunt of the insult. These techniques are most frequently used with normal functioning children who have school problems but also can be applied to mildly mentally retarded children. The resulting information may be helpful with respect to diagnosis, prognosis, and educational and vocational planning (e.g., 71). IQ labeling should not replace repeated educational and achievement assessments. Not only is the IQ score unreliable below age 3 years, but also deficits in visual, spatial, and motor function, as well as expressive language, may influence early testing. Underprivileged and understimulated children may perform poorly on language-based tests for reasons that are sociocultural rather than neurobiological. Such a child's level of functioning is better reflected in the results of nonverbal testing, as on the Culture-Fair Intelligence Test, Scale 2 (72), Raven's Progressive Matrices (73), and the Universal Nonverbal Intelligence Test (74). The interpretation of IQ test results should take into account cultural and linguistic diversity, differences in communication ability, and attentional and behavioral factors.

Behavioral Phenotypes of Mental Retardation Syndromes

A *syndrome* is a recognizable and consistent pattern of multiple manifestations that are known to have a specific etiology (75). More than 1,000 defined syndromes involve multiple congenital abnormalities (76). Most feature some pattern of impaired mental development. The degree of mental retardation is quite variable in most of these syndromes and is not indicated by the severity of neurobiologic concomitants, such as degree of abnormality of brain structure as visualized on MRI. Also, the deficit is often compounded by social factors. Dysmorphic facial features may give a misleading impression of low intelligence, and severe neurologic handicap may limit the children's ability to express their intellect. Striking instances are athetosis and *Lesch-Nyhan* syndrome. Teachers may underestimate the child's learning potential and offer a restricted number of learning opportunities. Nonetheless, some syndromes are characterized by specific behavioral phenotypes—of cognition, personality, and psychopathology—over and above the generally diminished level of functioning and any negative effects of the child's environment.

Behavioral phenotypes have been characterized as follows, "a number of conditions, recognizable by a common physical phenotype, single gene defect or chromosomal abnormality, seem also to have a constellation of behaviors or cognitive anomalies which are characteristic" (77). Although mentally retarded children are by definition impaired in all or most cognitive domains, certain mental retardation syndromes present striking cognitive and behavioral dissociations. Selective neuropsychological deficits can occur against a background of generally deficient intellect as well as in otherwise normally functioning children. The adverse influence, whether genetic or due to intercurrent insults, is widespread, but lowering the level of intelligence below normative expectations, is not homogeneous, perhaps reflecting unequal impact on areas of the brain that differ in functional specialization. Examples of dissociations follow.

Mentally retarded children with *autism* are disproportionately handicapped in the language and social domains, domains that are relatively spared in children with *Williams* syndrome (78 and see Chapter 4). Children with Williams syndrome speak with appropriate phonology and syntax, although their comprehension and pragmatics are weak (see Chapter 4). However, they are especially deficient in visual-spatial construction and number sense. Conversely, visuospatial skills are a strong point for children with *Prader-Willi* syndrome, who display a specific flair for jigsaw puzzles (79). *Down* syndrome children are particularly impaired in receptive and still more in expressive language, long-term memory (80,81), and gross and especially fine motor skills (82). Particularly with respect to language, these impairments become more obvious after the initial relatively rapid development of the first three years has decelerated. Some Down children become autistic, especially if there is an autistic spectrum disorder family history (83). Girls with Down syndrome as a group consistently perform better than boys (84). Children with *hydrocephalus* tend to be disproportionately strong in speech production, producing rapid uninformative "cocktail chatter," though not in speech comprehension and pragmatics. They are weak in face recognition and social cognition (85). Among X-linked chromosomal aberrations, *fragile X* syndrome (85a) is particularly handicapping in language development and social skills (86). Speech development is delayed, perseverative, and echolalic, and the children are shy, anxious, and show many autistic features. There is fine and gross motor delay. The language and social domains also are problematic for children with XXX (87), whereas *Turner* syndrome (XO) is associated with visuospatial, arithmetic, and memory deficits (88) as well as deficient recognition of faces and facial expressions (89), while language is intact. *XYY* syndrome is characterized behaviorally by language disability, lack of sociability and aggressiveness, and *Klinefelter* syndrome (XXY) boys tend to exhibit low verbal abilities, clumsiness, and introversion (90). In *Cornelia de Lange* syndrome, nonverbal abilities may be selectively impaired (91). Untreated, *phenylketonuria* results in severe mental retardation. Even when effectively treated, children with phenylketonuria exhibit impaired performance on executive function tests (92), apparently implicating dopaminergic projections to dorsolateral prefrontal cortex (93). The characterization of the selective deficit as involving executive functions is disputed, however (94). Untreated children with *congenital hypothyroidism* are severely mentally retarded. After early treatment, deficits are confined to the domains of visuospatial skills, attention, and fine motor control (95). In *galactosemia,* language and executive impairments as well as fine motor deficits have been reported. Some of the children are mentally retarded (96).

It is apparent from the highly diverse listing presented above that deficits in cases of atypical development are not interpretable in terms of selective loss with respect to a single behavioral module or a single functional domain. Rather, there is a suite of more impaired domains, and a suite of better functioning domains, in every type of affected child. The cognitive phenotypes associated with a specific genetic abnormality also can be quite diverse, as for instance in Williams syndrome (97). Therefore, the phenotypes even of genetically determined syndromes appear to be multiply determined, with some effect of environment, in the broad sense that encompasses both prenatal and postnatal factors, interacting with the genetically determined susceptibility. Notably, language ability does not fall out or remain intact in one piece (98). The classical dispute about whether language skill is modular and unique among cognitive skills (99) is not resolved by the study of atypical development.

Comorbid Psychiatric Disorders in Persons with Mental Retardation (Dual Diagnosis)

Persons with mental retardation are at increased risk for psychiatric disorders. Whereas the incidence of psychiatric disorders in the general childhood population is 7% to 10% (100), approximately one-third of all children with developmental disorders also have psychiatric disorders (100–103). In the severely retarded subpopulation, the frequency of psychiatric disorders is much higher and approaches two-thirds by adolescence (104). The broad spectrum of psychopathology includes affective disorders (105), anxiety disorders, autisticlike behaviors (106), conduct disorders (107), maladaptive behaviors (repetitive self-stimulation, self-injurious behavior, pica) (108,109), and psychosis. These emotional and behavioral disturbances are caused by multiple factors, both primary psychopathologies and neuropsychologic disorders and the secondary effects of illness, dependency, environmental deprivation, frustration, and low self-esteem (110).

The behavioral phenotypes of certain genetic syndromes are associated with typical personality characteristics and reproducible behavioral mannerisms (Table 18.5). Though otherwise often of even temperament, Down syndrome children may be irritable and inattentive because they are prone to obstructive sleep apnea (120), which in turn is a separate risk factor for neurocognitive (especially right hemisphere) deficits (121) and for depression (122). Specific personality differences also may occur in mental retardation syndromes, such as unusual sociability and distractibility in Williams syndrome and compulsivity, excessive talkativeness, impulsivity, and low activity level as well as compulsive eating and foraging for food in Prader-Willi syndrome (79).

Children with *velocardiofacial* syndrome have on average a borderline IQ, concrete thinking, bland affect, and little social interaction. They are highly susceptible to

TABLE 18.5 Examples of Genetic Syndromes with Characteristic Behavioral Phenotypes

Syndrome	*Behavioral Phenotype*	*References*
Fragile X	Poor eye contact, shy, withdrawn, hyperactive, self-injurious	See Chapter 4,85a, 86,150
Lesch-Nyhan syndrome	Self-injurious, especially compulsive lip and finger biting	111,112,126
Prader-Willi syndrome	Food seeking, hyperphagic, implusive, obstinate	79,113,114
Rett syndrome	Features of autism, stereotypical hand-wringing and hand-flapping, hyperventilation	115
Velocardiofacial syndrome	Ultrarapid cycling bipolar disorder, schizophrenialike condition	116,117,123,124
Williams syndrome	Superficial sociability, musically talented, shy, obsessive	78,118,119

psychiatric disorders, particularly schizophrenia, with which they may have a frequently occurring deletion on chromosome 22 in common (123). Twenty-five percent of children with velocardiofacial syndrome present with schizophrenia by early adulthood. A higher proportion still presents with ADHD in childhood and responds favorably to stimulant therapy (124). Girls with Turner syndrome tend to be unassertive and compliant and maintain poor and sparse social relationships (125). Children with Lesch-Nyhan syndrome have a unique form of compulsive behavior, which is expressed by an apparently involuntary drive toward self-injury and aggression. The children apologize and ask to be restrained in the act of attacking others or themselves (126). Abnormal dopamine functioning during early development may be implicated (126).

Epidemiology and Prevalence

Since the frequency with which a disorder arises in a population during a stated period of time is its incidence, and since its prevalence describes the amount within a population at a given time, the prevalence of the condition is the product of its incidence and its duration. The prevalence of a developmental disorder, therefore, may change over the years because of prenatal diagnosis and more frequent termination of pregnancy, changes in the maternal population, and changes in health care. For example, the prevalence of Down syndrome increased from the 1920s through the 1960s, as persons with this condition began to live much longer because of improvements in medical care. However, since 1980, further increases have been slight (127,128).

The prevalence of mental retardation is 6 to 20 per 1,000 (129–132). The published estimates vary on account of regional differences, ascertainment biases, and variations in diagnostic criteria and study methodology. Mild mental retardation is 10 to 12 times more common than severe retardation. Mental retardation is more common among males because of X-linked syndromes involving mental retardation, especially fragile X syndrome. The male to female ratio ranges from 1.3:1 to 1.9:1 (133). Morbidity and mortality are greater in persons with severe mental retardation, not due to the mental retardation itself, but because of the severe cerebral palsy that is often associated with it. Total immobility and feeding by nasogastric tube are the features that are most predictive of curtailed life span (134,135).

Causes of Mental Retardation

Timing

Mental retardation can be caused by genetic, environmental, and ecogenetic factors. A specific diagnosis can be determined in most children with global developmental delay [see (136) for recommendations as to which tests should routinely be used]. The diagnostic process is aided considerably if one can determine when the developmental insult occurred. Prenatal causes of mental retardation, with genetic etiologies as the major subset, account for approximately 60% to 80% of all developmental disorders. Perinatal causes include asphyxia and birth trauma. Mental retardation secondary to perinatal causes is almost invariably accompanied by cerebral palsy and/or epilepsy and probably accounts for at least 8% to 12% of all cases (137). Postnatal causes, including meningitis, encephalitis, trauma, and malnutrition, may account for up to 10% of cases. Some individuals may have more than one etiologic cause of their developmental disability, and the interacting causes may have occurred at different periods of development. For example, a fetus with hypotonia secondary to genetic causes is predisposed to perinatal injury (138–140). When individuals thought to have perinatal causes of their disabilities are later found to have a genetic etiology, the latter causation is likely to have been interactive with the perinatal stressors (141).

Severity

The more severe the mental retardation, the more likely it is that a specific etiologic diagnosis can be made [and the more likely the child is to be nonrighthanded (142)]. An identifiable cause is found in 70% to 80% of severe cases but in less than 50% of individuals with mild mental retardation. By neuroimaging or at autopsy, the brains of most severely mentally retarded individuals are found to be grossly abnormal. Mild mental retardation for which no specific cause can be uncovered is usually ascribed to polygenic inheritance. Subnormal head circumference may be the only abnormal physical sign in mentally retarded children. In a review of referrals to a child development center, some 15% of children were microcephalic. One-half of these children were mentally retarded. Prematurity, perinatal asphyxia, intrauterine growth retardation, respiratory distress syndrome, and intracerebral hemorrhage were associates of microcephaly (143) (see Chapter 5).

Diagnostic Categories

Chromosomal and Genetic

Chromosomal aberrations have been reported in 4% to 28% of persons with moderate to severe mental retardation, craniofacial differences, and other congenital anomalies (Table 18.6;143–148). The percentage of clinically relevant chromosomal abnormalities varies between studies because of differences in definitions, methodology, ascertainment (population-based versus institutional), and type of cytogenetic study. Down syndrome is by far the most common chromosomal disorder and accounts

TABLE 18.6 Cause of Mental Retardation by Diagnostic Category

	Percent
Chromosome abnormalities	4–28
Recognizable syndromes	3–9
Structural central nervous system malformations	3–17
Complications of prematurity	2–10
Perinatal conditions	8–13
Environmental/teratogenic causes	5–13
Cultural-familial mental retardation	3–12
Metabolic/endocrine causes	1–5
Unknown	30–50

Compiled references 22, 25, and 143–148.

for 4% to 7% of all cases of mental retardation (148,149). The fragile X syndrome (FXS) is considered in Chapter 4. In FXS, developmental testing reveals delays by 9 to 12 months of age (150). Cognitive deficits are milder in females than in males and often implicate math learning disability and frontal lobe–related deficits. Chromosomal disorders, including the contiguous gene syndromes, are considered in Chapter 4.

Primary malformations of the CNS result from multiple genetic and ecogenetic causes (see Chapter 5). Numerous major and minor developmental malformations result from disturbances in neuronal proliferation, migration, differentiation, axonal outgrowth, synapse formation, dendritic arborization, and process elimination, depending on the genetic condition or severity and timing of an environmental insult. In the prenatal period, it is often impossible to distinguish the extent to which an environmental insult causes vascular or parenchymal injury or disrupts gene and signaling molecule expression.

Prematurity and Cerebral Palsy

Technologic advances in neonatology have transformed survival rates and morbidity patterns. Outcomes differ notably between very-low-birth-weight infants (less than 1,500 g) and extremely low-birth-weight infants (less than 1,000 g). Outcomes in premature infants range from normal functioning to severe disability (151), lasting at least into the teenage years in the form of academic deficits (152). Cognitive deficits occur even if the neonatal course was uncomplicated. Difficulties in spatial memory, sustained attention, and visuospatial function were documented at 4 years of age in otherwise normal preterm children (153). A wide range of cognitive deficits as well as elevated scores on an ADHD rating scale were found in children aged 7 years who were born before 32 weeks of gestation and were being educated in mainstream schools (154). Very-low-birth-weight children do even worse if they also had bronchopulmonary dysplasia (BPD). At age 8 years, the presence of BPD and/or relatively long duration on oxygen were found to have predicted lower performance IQ, impaired perceptual organization, and motor and attentional skills as well as lower educational achievement, with more frequent special education placement (155). Twenty percent of BPD children had IQs below 70, in the mental retardation range, as compared with 11% of very-low-birth-weight children without BPD and 3% of term controls. However, even mild indications of risk for birth anoxia had significantly adverse effects on cognitive outcome (156). This result supports the view that the deficits following asphyxia at birth are a matter of degree, in proportion to the severity of the injury—"there is a continuum of brain injury in asphyxia" (157)—rather than supporting an all-or-none "threshold" model (158). Correspondingly, selective neuronal necrosis in asphyxiated sheep brain was directly proportional in its severity and extent to the duration/ischemic of the inflicted insult (159). Another recent study also found a continuum, such that the neuropsychologic outcome was inversely related to the birth weight among children born weighing less than 1,500 g (160). Verbal functions were relatively spared, whereas spatial recognition, working memory and attention shifting were most affected.

Bradycardia and apnea are postnatal causes of hypoxia. In one study, 256 preterm and term infants were monitored at home and then tested on an index of mental development 96 weeks after conception. Infants who had five or more episodes of apnea and/or bradycardia performed significantly worse than infants who did not meet that criterion (161). Furthermore, 5-year-old children with sleep-disordered breathing scored less well than controls on tests of overall intellectual ability as well as on attention, memory, and planning (162).

Nearly one-half of a group of premature children had ocular pathology associated with impaired acuity, stereopsis, contrast sensitivity, and color vision (163). Cognitive deficits may be associated with regional brain volume reductions revealed by neuroimaging. Episodic memory deficits were associated with diminution in hippocampal volume in otherwise normal very-low-birth-weight children (164). MRI studies of adolescents who were born after a gestation of 33 weeks or less reveal decreased brain volume and enlarged lateral ventricles (165). In premature infants scanned near term, regional volume reductions were documented. White matter volumes in the sensorimotor and midtemporal regions correlated strongly with neurodevelopmental outcome (166). Neurological complications of prematurity are reviewed in Chapter 6.

Those premature and term children who sustain damage that results in cerebral palsy frequently bear the additional burden of associated deficits in vision, hearing and the ability to learn. Independent of the frequently present mental retardation, children with bilateral spastic cerebral palsy were found to have selective difficulty on tasks that call for inhibitory control, and presumably rely on intact prefrontal function (167). More generally, cerebral palsied children have up to a 40% chance of learning disability or mental retardation. Most of this is accounted for by children with spastic quadriplegia. In hemiplegic cerebral palsy, early damage to either side has relatively more detrimental cognitive effects if it is complicated by seizure activity. The more severe deficits that accompany the seizure disorder group do not bear the usual qualitative relationship to the side of the lesion (168). Stroke before age 1 year has similar but greater effects on cognition than in adults (), calling into question the notion that children escape from the consequences of brain injury if it occurs very early (169). Both cerebral palsy (170) and childhood stroke (171) feature ADHD phenotypes among their sequelae. Methylphenidate is effective in treating the ADHD phenotype associated with cerebral palsy (172).

Toxins and Radiation

The long-term effects of exposure to alcohol, marijuana, cigarettes, cocaine, and other street drugs on cognition and behavior are difficult to determine separately because polydrug use is the rule. Also, the frequency, quantity, type of substance, and timing of exposure during pregnancy vary greatly. Moreover, drug habits are frequently associated with poor nutrition and lack of prenatal care. However, there are clear associations between maternal alcohol abuse and adverse effects on early brain development. Fetal alcohol syndrome (FAS) may be the most common among the identified causes of mental retardation in North America and Europe. Children with facial features of FAS and a history of maternal alcoholism during pregnancy have been described as inattentive and hyperactive, with disordered conduct and defective memory (173). Whether prenatal cocaine exposure has any adverse effect on long-term cognitive outcome is questionable (174). Any low functioning is more likely to be due to adverse conditions in the postnatal caretaking environment (175). Some children with fetal valproic acid syndrome have been reported to be autistic (176). Fetal alcohol syndrome and the effects of cocaine and opiates are discussed in Chapter 10.

Acute severe lead poisoning may cause mental retardation as a sequelae of an acute encephalopathy. Chronic subclinical lead poisoning is associated with an increased risk of antisocial and delinquent behavior as well as disorders of cognition and learning (177), but these outcomes are confounded by the effects of low socioeconomic status and stimulation level in the home environment (178) (see Chapter 10). The HOME questionnaire measures the stimulation a child receives at home. This type of variable is a crucial covariate in any population study on cognitive effects of potential toxins. When relevant covariates were held constant in a meta-analysis, the apparent detrimental effects of subclinical lead dwindled into insignificance (179). Maximum controversy centers on the clinical significance of the 10 to 19 ug/dL blood lead dose level, the Centers for Disease Control's (CDC) lowest "level of concern" (180,181). An attempt to show that lead levels below 10 ug/dL cause deficits in cognitive and academic skills (182,183) is controversial (184) and suffers from methodological shortcomings (185). The neurobiology of lead poisoning is discussed in Chapter 10.

Mercury nitrate is the toxin that caused "Mad Hatter's" disease (186). Children who were given a "teething" powder that contained mercury fell victim to acrodynia (pink disease), which in addition to physical signs caused severe irritability, anorexia, photophobia, and sleeplessness (187). A comprehensive resource for information about the toxic effects of methylmercury is available (188). Widely differing sensitivities to comparable levels of exposure draw attention to host factors in clinical susceptibility to mercury poisoning. Mercury is found in dangerous amounts in fish in certain geographic locations. When consumed in large amounts by pregnant women, it has led to cerebral palsy and mental retardation in their children (189). Symptoms of less severe exposure included muscle stiffness, dysesthesia, hand tremor, dizziness, loss of pain sensation, muscle cramps, arthralgia, chest pain, palpitations, fatigue, visual dimness, and staggering (190). Muscular atrophy was observed. Methylmercury is taken up by multiple organs. In the brain, it is gradually broken down to metallic mercury, which cannot be cleared. Over time, cerebral atrophy results. Other sources of intense mercury poisoning include skin whiteners and processing of mined gold. The recently withdrawn ethylmercury-containing vaccine preservative thimerosal was administered by routine vaccination (DPT, Hepatitis B, HiB) to infants in cumulative amounts well above the Environmental Protection Agency's (EPA) maximum sanctioned (benchmark) dose. Low-level prenatal exposure to methylmercury from maternal consumption of seafood poses a less severe but still increased neurodevelopmental risk (191–193). Neuropsychologic testing has implicated language, reading, attention, memory, and visuomotor function (194). The younger the child, the greater the risk. Susceptibility to low-grade poisoning also varies tremendously between individuals due to as yet unidentified host factors. Signs of mercury poisoning may present, weeks, months, or even years after exposure (195).

Prenatal polychlorinated biphenyls (PCB) and dioxin exposure have an apparent detrimental effect on children's mental development, which for reasons that are not clear spared children who were raised in optimal environments or breast-fed (196,197). Organophosphate pesticides also are under suspicion (198).

Pelvic nuclear (199) and x-irradiation (200) can lead to mental retardation of offspring, especially if applied between the seventh and fifteenth weeks of gestation. The degree of mental retardation is proportional to the amount of irradiation. The incidence of Down syndrome and other chromosomal abnormalities is greater among offspring of those women in their late reproductive years who were irradiated during pregnancy (201).

Poverty and Other Familial Factors

There is a complex relationship between genetics, nutrition, social environment, and learning (202). The adverse effects of psychosocial deprivation on socialization and motivation may impair performance even if the child has normal cognitive abilities. One American child in five lives in a family with income below the poverty threshold (203). The risk of mental retardation and inferior academic performance increases with decreasing socioeconomic status (204–206). However, on a population basis, the factors that mediate the effects of poverty on child health and development are uncertain (207). Parental nurturing, sociocultural influences, and educational environments are determinants of developmental outcome and ultimate adaptation to society (208). Less positive parenting contributes to adverse outcomes (208a). Some children are resilient and function better than one would expect based on their socioeconomic status. Resilience is partly heritable and partly mediated by maternal warmth and stimulating activities (209). In contrast, infants and children who are deprived of maternal attention and are institutionalized in a hospital or an orphanage often become depressed, and their cognitive skills decline or fail to advance (210–212). Children adopted from Romanian orphanages exhibited anomalies of attachment and personality (213). A positron emission tomography study of such adoptees revealed reduced brain activation in orbitofrontal, inferolimbic, and medial temporal cortex, including amygdala, structures involved both in cognition and emotion regulation (214). EEGs of Romanian adoptees showed diminished power in high frequency bands at frontal and temporal electrode sites and increased power in low-frequency bands posteriorly (215). These EEG abnormalities indicate cortical hypoarousal and/or delayed cerebral maturation. Adverse cognitive and academic consequences are to be expected in such children, but the outcome is never certain, let alone irremediable, in the individual case.

Hormones and Infections

Maternal hypothyroidism results in lowered IQ of the offspring (216). Congenital hypothyroidism causes mental retardation only in children who are left untreated after birth. Insulin-dependent diabetes mellitus is associated with declining verbal test scores (217). The neurologic complications of thyroid deficiency and diabetes are presented in Chapter 17. Nutritional disorders are discussed in Chapter 10.

CNS infection early in life is a major cause of mental retardation, especially in developing countries. Prenatal infections such as toxoplasmosis, syphilis, rubella, cytomegalovirus, herpes, and varicella are associated with microcephaly, intracranial calcifications, cataracts, growth retardation, sensorineural hearing loss, and seizures. Such infections may cause mild, moderate, or severe mental retardation. Bacterial, viral, and fungal meningitis and encephalitis—in particular, neonatal and childhood herpes simplex encephalitis—are perinatal and postnatal causes of mental retardation (see Chapter 7). Hookworm infection can contribute to iron deficiency, which is associated with decreased cognitive abilities (218) whether anemia is present or not (219).

Management

Medical

Stimulant medications, such as methylphenidate, may be beneficial for some mildly mentally retarded children who are hyperactive (220). Numerous other older and newer medications have been used with variable success to ameliorate adverse behaviors such as aggression, self-injury, and severe hyperactivity in persons with mental retardation. Neuroleptics, such as thioridazine in low doses, may have a calming effect in some children and when given at bedtime may assist sleep. Carbamazepine and propranolol can be beneficial for rage and episodic loss of control. Antidepressants, such as clomipramine and fluvoxamine, are often helpful in decreasing compulsive behaviors and stereotypies. Opioid antagonists, such as naltrexone, are occasionally successful in decreasing self-injurious behaviors (221,222). On withdrawal, some medications can give rise to tardive dyskinesias because of dopamine hypersensitivity (223). This tendency can be counteracted by GABAergic antiepileptic agents (224). Pharmacologic treatment of behavioral disorders in children with mental retardation should be coordinated with behavioral modification programs.

Nonmedical

Management includes family support and education, and the provision of early intervention and special education programs. There are no specific methods for improving the overall intelligence of most mentally retarded people, although improvement in some skill deficiencies is a feasible educational goal. There is disagreement about how the largest group, the mildly mentally retarded, should be taught, and even about whether that should be any different from how learning disabled children are taught. The efficacy of early intervention programs in enhancing mental development has not been validated (225). The primary goals are to provide a "least restricted environment," a placement that safeguards the child and at the same time permits the child to function at maximum potential. The child's temperament and level of socialization are important modifying factors that can differ widely among individuals at a given IQ level. A regular preschool with language therapy may be appropriate for mildly disabled preschool children with adequate comprehension and without behavioral problems. For children whose attention and concentration are limited, special education teachers use attention-focusing techniques to optimize learning. Best results are obtained in structured rather than flexible settings because individuals with mental retardation are usually deficient in judgment and problem-solving strategies. A child with mild mental retardation who is taught at an appropriate rate in suitably structured settings can become self-reliant in a considerable variety of work competencies, not strictly limited to manual and domestic occupations or routine industrial tasks such as assembly and production-line operations.

Children with mental retardation who in addition have significant language and social dysfunction often do not succeed in the typical classroom settings that are appropriate for students with specific learning disabilities. Self-contained classrooms usually provide a better environment for children with severe mental retardation and severe communication disorders or autistic behaviors. These classrooms ideally have a low teacher to student ratio with special education teachers who are familiar with interventions for students with nonverbal learning disabilities and social communication deficits. Some children with severe mental retardation require placements that offer behavioral modification programs and school time geared toward life skills such as basic hygiene and self-care. Public laws mandate that individual educational programs (IEP) be regularly reassessed.

Management involves many nonmedical disciplines. Caregivers may need to be trained in how to handle, feed, and toilet their child. Effective case management comprises health care planning that includes comprehensive diagnostic evaluation, an assessment of disabilities, and individualized treatment plans for educational, behavioral, pharmacologic, and medical interventions.

Declining Intellectual Function in Adolescence or Preadolescence

Infrequently, children are referred by psychologists, social workers, educators, or rarely, parents, based on the impression—with or without psychometric documentation—of declining intellect or IQ. Test-retest reliabilities on IQ tests are well established, and the findings must be taken seriously, especially when the psychologist's report rules out the usual motivational or sociocultural reasons for an occasional aberrantly low score. A progressive neurological disorder also must be ruled out. More commonly, drug abuse is responsible and should be investigated by serum drug screening, cocaine being the substance of greatest interest. Alternatively, prodromal changes heralding schizophrenia should be considered. By standard definition, schizophrenia involves declining function over a 6-month period, and declining IQ may be a warning sign. Particularly for a child with a history of schizophrenia spectrum disorder in the extended family, the appropriate syndromally based diagnostic interview is called for (over and beyond any global impression or score on a single scale). An outcome that falls short of being diagnostic of schizophrenia may still offer warning signs of an impending diagnosis if the decline persists. Prompt treatment may then forestall the more serious outcome.

Epilepsy

The mental functioning of children with epilepsy is at risk of impairment by the underlying brain malfunctions, the seizures themselves and the side effects of antiepileptic agents. Most children with epilepsy score within normal limits on IQ tests such as the WISC-R, but the distribution of IQs is skewed toward the lower end of the range. Lower IQ scores reflect the detrimental effects of the total number of seizures, which is compounded of age of onset and frequency of the seizures (226). Among seizure subtypes, minor motor and atypical seizure states are associated with lower mean IQs than other seizure types. Even in children with an IQ in the normal range, neuropsychological testing can pinpoint cognitive domains that present individual difficulty. Examples are the verbal learning and memory difficulty associated with complex partial seizures that arise from left-sided foci and the visuospatial learning and memory deficits that accompany right focal discharges. Left focal temporal discharges also may underlie dysnomia and circumlocution in speaking (227). A study of children with complex partial seizures found cognitive and linguistic deficits that were predicted by the duration and frequency of seizures and by the number of antiepileptic drugs that were used (228). Petit mal implicates sustained attention only. The more severe manifestations of epilepsy are often also associated with dysarthria, general inattentiveness, and slowing of responding. Seizures and antiepileptic drug treatments are discussed in Chapter 14.

AUTISTIC SPECTRUM DISORDERS

Autistic spectrum disorders (ASD) are a behaviorally defined set of developmental disorders that result from diverse biologic, genetic, and ecogenetic factors (229). Although the broad spectrum of cognitive and behavioral impairments defies a concise definition, clinicians tend to agree on its predominant features (230,231). Research into the neurobiology of ASDs is complicated by their broad heterogeneity in clinical and biological characteristics (see examples in Table 18.7; 232–304).

TABLE 18.7 Some Neurobiologic Clues to the Etiology of Idiopathic Autism

Etiologic Clue	Description of Findings in Studies of Autism	References
Environmental	Increased complications of pregnancy, labor, and delivery; perinatal problems/illness in some studies but not others	232–236
Genetic	Higher concordance for autism in monozygotic twin pairs Marked increase in prevalence of autism in siblings of children with autism Increased frequency of cognitive and learning disabilities in siblings of children with autism Increased frequency of mental health disorders in siblings and parents of children with autism Studies of potential susceptibility genes, such as genes within the 15q11–13 region, are ongoing	232,237,238,239–245
Chromosomal/ monogenetic	Numerous case reports and small series of patients with certain single-gene disorders and chromosomal anomalies are reported; these may account for 5% to 14% of all children with features of autism	246,247
Contiguous genes	Features of autism in some children with recognizable conditions such as Williams syndrome or Angelman syndrome; the most common cytogenetic finding in autism to date is the duplication of maternally derived chromosome 15q11–13	248–252
Mitochondrial	Possible effects of abnormal energy metabolism on central nervous system	253–255
DNA expansion	Features of autism in some children with fragile-X syndrome	256
Immunology	Abnormal immune function or presence or autoimmune antibodies in some studies of children with autism Reported improvement in some persons following nonspecific immunosuppressive or immunomodulating therapies	257–259
Infection	Features of autism in some children with congenital rubella and cytomegalovirus infections, among others; inflammatory bowel disease with intracellular measles virus genomic material in some autistic children	260–262,400
Metabolism	Features of autism in some children with phenylketonuria and other metabolic disorders Abnormal intestinal permeability	263–267 268
Neuroanatomy		
Cerebellum	Selective hypoplasia of the neocerebellar vermis (especially lobules VI and VII) in some autopsy and magnetic resonance imaging studies Developmental cellular abnormalities in the posterior inferior cerebellar hemispheres	269–275
Cerebrum	Associated abnormal neuronal migration, cortical cytoarchitecture in septum, hippocampi, amygdala, entorhinal cortex, and mamillary bodies Nonspecific differences in positron emission tomography and P nuclear magnetic resonance spectroscopic studies Variable morphologic differences in some magnetic resonance imaging studies Suppressed voluntary oculomotor responses attributed to prefrontal dysfunction	276–284
Electroenceph-alographic findings	Depending on associated brain dysfunction, seizures occur in 6% to 35%, and electroencephalographic abnormalities are reported in 35% to 65% of children with autism	285,286
Brainstem	Associated smaller pons in some studies	287–289
Neurochemistry		
Serotonin	Increased blood concentrations of serotonin in some children with autism Asymmetric serotonin metabolism by positron emission tomographic studies	290–293
Dopamine	Dopamine agonists worsen behavior, and dopamine antagonists improve behavior in some children with autism Increased CSF homovanillic in some studies	294–296
Norepinephrine	Increased plasma norepinephrine in some studies, but in others, normal plasma, urine, and CSF catecholamine metabolites are reported	296–299
Endorphin neuropeptides	Analogy to "insensitivity to pain" in those children with autism who show self-injurious behavior Increased CSF endorphin concentrations in some studies	300–304

When Kanner described and named autism in 1943 (305), he noted the following five characteristics in the 11 children he described: inability to relate to people, absent or abnormal and noncommunicative speech, obsessive desire to maintain sameness, but good cognitive potential and normal physical status. Autism was initially ascribed to dynamic causes, in line with the theoretical orientation of the times (cf. DSM I, DSM II). Reflecting the rise of biologic psychiatry, in 1980, the *Diagnostic and Statistical Manual of Mental Disorders*, Third Edition (DSM-III), abandoned the psychodynamic approach for the medical model and adopted an atheoretical nomenclature. The current criteria for autistic disorder in the DSM-IV include qualitative impairment in social interaction; qualitative impairment in communication; and restricted, repetitive, and stereotyped patterns of behavior, interest, and activities (48). By definition, onset is before 3 years of age. The World Health Organization's International Classification Diseases (ICD-10) invokes similar criteria (63). Rett syndrome, discussed in Chapter 3, and childhood disintegrative disorder (CDD) are separately classified. Autistic disorder, Asperger syndrome, Rett syndrome, and childhood disintegrative disorder are subsumed under the category of pervasive developmental disorders (PDD) in the DSM-IV (65).

The distinctions between the diagnostic categories are arbitrary and probably reflect differences in degree rather than kind (306). In family studies, different PDD subtypes cluster within the same pedigree, indicating that they share common causes. In the family of a proband with PDD, there is a 3% chance that another offspring has autistic disorder and a further 3% chance of an offspring with PDD or Asperger's disorder (307). Concordance between monozygotic twins is about 70% as opposed to 5% for dizygotic twins (308).

Approximately one-third of children appear to develop normally until the second year of life, at which time they gradually regress into autism (309,310), often in the context of seizures (312). Subtly abnormal signs may precede the overt regression (313). Some of these children may have become autistic after sustaining brain damage postnatally (314).

Clinical Characteristics

As a psychopathology, autism is profoundly internalizing. The children are deeply preoccupied with their internal states of mind and feeling and only minimally engage the outside world for purposes of activities of daily living. The majority of children with autism are to a varying degree atypical even at an early age, moving and crying little, averse to being held, and content to be alone. Scales that assist earlier diagnosis are available, and home videos reviewed retrospectively can reveal a previously unsuspected onset during infancy (315,316). The children may reject solid foods, and toys elicit little interest or are held onto with unusual obstinacy. Their motor development is usually normal, but minor physical anomalies are more frequently found in autistic children than in controls (317). During the second year of life, children with autism are typically unusually sensitive to auditory, visual, tactile, and movement stimulation, and repetitive mannerisms or gestures begin to appear. The older child with autism has restricted and stereotyped behaviors and activities and markedly impaired creativity, social relations, language, and perception. Disturbances in social relations are manifested by poor or absent eye contact and a lack of interest in people, whom the child uses instrumentally rather than interactively. Toys are handled bizarrely or are dropped when handed to the child. Mannerisms include repetitive, stereotyped movements, such as hand flapping, ear flicking, or head banging (318). Toe walking, whirling, and rocking also are common. These movements, often complex, increase when the child is anxious or is confronted with a novel situation (319).

Language disturbances can consist of complete lack of speech, failure to communicate by pointing, failure to imitate (320), perseveration, echolalia (repeating words or phrases out of communicative context), and lack of reciprocity in dialogue (321). If speech does develop, its prosody is often monotonal, pronouns are used poorly, and humor is not understood. Speech in children with autism differs qualitatively from the speech of children with mild mental retardation. Within the limits of a restricted vocabulary, children with mild mental retardation typically speak normally, whereas children with autism use abnormal prosody, syntax, semantics, and pragmatics (322). In some children, termed *hyperlexic*, mechanical reading skills develop out of proportion to spontaneous verbal expression or reading comprehension (323,324).

Children with autism may be oversensitive to stimuli, notably self-created sounds or spinning objects (325). This oversensitivity can alternate with periods of nonresponsiveness to speech, objects, or pain. Affected children frequently ignore sounds and are "aloof," provoking testing for possible hearing loss. Some have prolonged attention spans during self-initiated activity (326). Observational studies demonstrate hyperselectivity of attention in children with autism (319). They focus exclusively on a single distinctive aspect of a display, while ignoring its other features. They are impaired in broadening the spatial spread of visual attention (326a). Conversely, they excel as compared to their typical peers on tests that call for local perceptual processing, in which context has got to be discounted. An example is the Embedded Figures Task (326b). The propensity of some people with autism to achieve savant status on very narrowly defined skills (326c) also reflects their narrow focus. Children with autism also have been shown to be impaired in perceiving faces, but not objects (327). People's clothing was more salient to autistic children then their emotional expressions (328). They fail as compared to age-matched peers in inferring other people's perspectives and mental states, focusing narrowly on their own (326d).

Some children exhibit transitional or milder degrees of autistic behavior, within the PDD spectrum. After age 5 to 6 years, such behaviors may merge with those observed in mental retardation. Others deviate into childhood disintegrative disorder (329) or Asperger disorder (330). The natural history and outcome of autism is variable. Some 80% manifest a pronounced impairment in intelligence. Approximately one-third of children with autism do not develop communicative speech. Others develop rudimentary language, although their communication remains literal and concrete and their affect flat. In yet other affected children, characteristics of organic brain disease become apparent over subsequent years, including auditory or visuoperceptual impairment. A small subset of children with autism develops bizarre thoughts and even delusions. About 75% of children who fail to show language skills by age 5 years fail to adjust personally or socially. Other children with autism make a fairly adequate social adjustment but retain certain peculiarities of personality, lack of humor, and unawareness of social nuances (331). Neuropsychologic testing reveals deficits on problem-solving tasks (332). Standard diagnostic instruments include the ADI (332a) and the ADOS (332b). Early diagnosis is facilitated by the use of standard instruments such as the Checklist for Autism in Toddlers (CHAT) (333). It consists of nine questions asked of the parents, and five items that call for observation by the clinician. The latter include pointing and looking to where a parent is pointing and pretend play, activities that are available to a normal 18 month old. Approximately one-half of the population with autism have an IQ above 50, and one-fourth to one-third have an IQ above 70. Children who regressed into autism after initially developing normally generally are ultimately more impaired cognitively (312,334). Even when they are enrolled in treatment programs, only some children with ASD improve significantly. If children improve, they usually do so during the second half of their first decade.

Prevalence

Based on twin studies, autism is thought to have the heaviest genetic loading of the chief developmental disorders, with more than 50% hereditability for the narrowly defined autistic disorder (335), and as much as 90% for the wider range of ASD (336). Moreover, autistic individuals rarely reproduce (337). Autism would therefore be expected to have a stable incidence. On the contrary, its prevalence across the ASD spectrum has risen from 2 to 4 in 10,000 children in the 1970s to 60 in 10,000 children in recent years, that is, 0.6% of the population (338–345). The rate of increase in autism is highest in developed countries, in the United States among children of American rather than immigrant mothers, and for autistic children who are high-functioning (346). It has been argued that the rise in prevalence is due to relaxation in diagnostic criteria, diagnostic substitution [e.g., ASD diagnosis substituted for Developmental Language Disorder (DLD) diagnosis—(346)], changes in and increasing availability of special education services, mandatory notification of ASD diagnoses, and increasing awareness and earlier recognition of ASD. However, the rise in incidence is so worldwide that it cannot be attributed to regulatory changes in just one country. Potential alternative causes and a true rise in incidence are not mutually exclusive, and the explanatory power of the alternative factors is open to challenge (347,348). No published research has managed to determine how much of the variance in the spectacular increase in ASD diagnoses is attributable to each of the various factors that have been suggested. Pending such information, it is unwarranted to assume that the true incidence of ASD is not increasing.

Causes of Autism and Its Neurobiologic Basis

Pathogenesis

Autism clearly has genetic factors in its origins. Previous theories that certain family dynamics promote autism (349) have been refuted (238). However, autistic offspring are more frequent among mothers of relatively high intelligence (346) and perhaps social class (350). The importance of genetics in autism is illustrated by the four to one higher incidence of autism in males (336), a recurrence risk of up to 9% in families with one affected child (351), a high concordance of autism among monozygotic twins (336,352), an increased incidence of developmental and affective disorder in first-degree relatives (350), and the association of some disorders of known genetic etiology with autism. Susceptibility loci have been identified on distal 7q and 15q11–13 (353).

Increased head and brain size in autism contrasts with the frequent microcephaly of mentally retarded children (354). However, there is also an excess of microcephaly among autistic children who are mentally retarded and have diagnosable medical diseases. Autistic macrocephaly indicates an enlarged brain, according to measures of brain volume by MRI. The bulk of the increase is in cerebral and cerebellar white matter. It is not evident at birth, but develops throughout the first year of life (354a), and mostly consists of increased volume of the peripheral (radiate) cerebral white matter (355). It is perhaps the most consistently replicated neurobiologic feature of ASD (356). There is no consensus on the neural pathophysiology of autism (357). Structural abnormalities in various brain regions of autistic children may reflect etiologic heterogeneity. They include widespread abnormalities in the frontal and temporal cortices, cerebellar hemispheres, and vermis (358–362). An overview of neuropathologic findings (363) highlights the limbic system (increased cell packing density and smaller neurons in 9 of 14 cases), the cerebellum (21 of 29 had a decreased number of Purkinje cells), and cerebral cortex (more than half had dysgenesis). Purkinje cell loss in the cerebellum is the most consistent microscopic neurological abnormality found in autism. The high energy demands of these large neurons makes them vulnerable to damage following a variety of insults (364), and the associated presence of gliosis (362) opens up the possibility of damage rather than dysgenesis. The neural substrate of autistic disorders has typically been thought to be the medial temporal lobe and limbic structures (365,366). Bilateral excisions of amygdala and hippocampus of monkeys resulted in impairment of social interaction (367). The hypothesis that autistic behaviors are attempts to compensate for frequent phasic overarousal (368) has found support in recent neuroanatomic (369) and physiologic (370) findings that suggest that the cortical network is underconnected and therefore insufficiently inhibited (371).

Etiology

Many genetic syndromes feature autistic behavior, notably Rett syndrome (372), fragile X syndrome (373), and occasionally Down syndrome (see Chapters 3 and 4). An intriguing instance is Timothy syndrome, a rare multisystem disorder that features cardiac arrhythmias and both cognitive and physical deficits. It is caused by a mutation in the CaV1.2 calcium channel (374) that incurs the risk of excessive entry of calcium into the cell. That some children become autistic, and that others with the same mutation do not, suggests that the autistic phenotype requires some additional epigenetic or environmental factor. The raised incidence of autism in thalidomide (375) and valproic acid (176,398) embryopathies indicates that an abnormal event such as a poisoning can trigger autism as early as 20 to 24 days after conception (376). Children with autism often have recurrent seizures (377) and EEG abnormalities usually with onset in the first year of life (378). The neurological symptoms of tuberous sclerosis become apparent only after the onset of seizures. Seizures that interact with preexisting temporal lobe abnormalities may result in manifestations of autism. Tuberous sclerosis is discussed in Chapter 12. Perinatal injuries (232–236,379) and prematurity (380) are associated with autism with greater than chance frequency. However, the evidence more usually indicates prenatal maldevelopment even early in the first trimester (376). Rarely, an autistic syndrome arises during encephalitis (381), even at as late an age as 31 years (382). Therefore, autism is not always a developmental disorder.

Neurotransmitter levels have been extensively studied, with serotonin at the center of interest (290–293). Whole blood serotonin is elevated in more than 30% of patients with autism as well as in their first-degree relatives. Low binding site affinity of the 5-HT transporter may be related to distractibility (383). Serotonin synthesis also has been found to be abnormal in its distribution in the thalamus, cerebellum, and frontal cortex. Other research has implicated increased levels of norepinephrine, increases in opioid peptides, and decreased levels of oxytocin (383a), a substance shown to influence social behavior in animal studies. Neurotransmitter findings in autism were recently reviewed (384).

Abnormalities of immune response appear to be disproportionately frequent both in children with autism (259,384–388) and in their first-order relatives (385,389). In one study, 46% of families with autistic children had two or more family members with autoimmune disorders. The children of mothers with autoimmune disorders had the highest risk for developing autism. Autoantibodies to various components of the nervous system have been repeatedly demonstrated in a subset of autistic children participating in controlled studies (384,390). Recently, a sample of autistic children showed related elevations in the levels of antibodies against gliadin and cerebellar peptides, raising the possibility of immune-mediated attack against the brain and lending biologic plausibility to the anecdotal success of gluten-free dieting in minimizing symptoms of autism (391). A recent study of autopsied brains of autistic individuals revealed active inflammation in the cerebrum and cerebellum, with microglial and neuroglial activation but no adaptive immune response (392). In the same study, cerebrospinal fluid acquired from living autistic children contained markers of a neuroimmune reaction. This suggests that autism can be an active disorder over many years, rather than the static aftermath of prenatal dysgenesis, as is usually assumed. Table 18.7 presents genetic, immunologic, metabolic, neuroanatomic, and neurochemical findings associated with autism. Across varying diagnostic criteria and varying extent of medical evaluation, the specific etiology remains unknown in 70% to 90% of cases of autism (393). The etiology of autism in the diagnosable minority has recently been reviewed (394). Table 18.8 presents syndromes and other disorders that may be associated with autism.

External causes of autism subdivide into *toxic* [e.g., alcohol (395), cocaine (396), thalidomide (397)]; *in utero* exposure to valproate (398); *stress-related* (399); and *infectious* [e.g., cytomegalovirus (400), herpes simplex (401–403), rubella embryopathy (404)]. Viral infections are thought to contribute to the pathogenesis of neurodevelopmental disorders, including autism (405), and maternal viral infection has been cited as the "principal nongenetic cause of autism" (406). A mouse model of maternal influenza infection gives rise to macrocephalic offspring with abnormal cerebrum and hippocampus and atrophy of pyramidal cells (407) that are deficient in exploration and social interaction—perhaps a model for human autism (408).

There are many examples of gastrointestinal involvement in neurologic diseases (409). Many autistic children have gastrointestinal symptoms (410), and colitis and lymphoid nodular hyperplasia in the ileal region (ILNH) have been reported (260,411). Immunohistochemical

TABLE 18.8 Conditions Associated with Autism

Genetic
Fragile X
Rett syndrome
Tuberous sclerosis
Neurofibromatosis
Hypomelanosis of Ito
Phenylketonuria
Joubert syndrome
Prader-Willi syndrome
Angelman syndrome
Goldenhaar syndrome
Moebius syndrome
Cornelia de Lange syndrome
Lujan-Fryns syndrome
Sotos syndrome
Marker chromosome syndrome
Timothy syndrome
Metabolic and other
Landau-Kleffner
Tourette syndrome
Williams syndrome
Duchenne myopathy
Hypoythyroidism
Lactic acidosis
Mucopolysaccharidoses
Free fatty acid abnormalities
Autoimmune lymphoproliferative syndrome
Viral
Rubella embryopathy
Herpes simplex encephalitis
Cytomegalovirus
Toxic
Thalidomide
Valproic acid
Alcohol
Cocaine

studies of biopsy material from children with ILNH have revealed the hallmarks of dysregulated mucosal immunity (412). The enterocolitis has been attributed to infections with measles, mumps, or other paramyxoviruses (413). Despite apparent links between measles, mumps, and rubella (MMR) immunizations and autism (260), which have been vehemently disputed (414–416), the definitive epidemiologic study that would distinguish causation from chance association has not been performed. Measles vaccine virus genomic material has been reported in the gut mucosa of children with ILNH (417), as well as in blood and cerebrospinal fluid (418), consistent with a possible causal relationship of the MMR vaccine and late-presenting ("regressive") autism.

Differential Diagnosis

Classical autistic disorder is one of the five subtypes of pervasive developmental disorders listed in the DSM-IV. The four other subtypes are Rett syndrome (see Chapter 3), Asperger syndrome, childhood disintegrative disorder, and pervasive developmental disorder not otherwise specified (PDD-NOS). However, these subgroups may be better conceived as arranged along a spectrum of severity of autistic disorders (419).

Asperger Disorder

Possibly distinct from relatively high functioning autism but nonetheless highly similar to and possibly on a continuum with autism are individuals first described by Asperger (330) with flat affect, insensitivity to social cues, and obsessively indulged special interests. Their language skills develop normally, but their use of language and other means to communicate is aberrant. Their speech is formal, pedantic, and is uttered in a peculiar voice and with deviant prosody. Their gestures also are deviant, stiff, limited, inexpressive, and stilted. Their visuomotor development may be delayed, and they are clumsy and walk with a stiff gait. They are severely impaired in reciprocal social interaction, for which they have little enthusiasm. Their interests are quite circumscribed, and they impose many routines and rituals on themselves. Like autistic children, children with Asperger disorder seek sameness. They exhibit mannerisms such as hand or finger flapping or twisting. Children with this syndrome are of normal or near normal intelligence, and their self-help and adaptive behavioral skills are age appropriate. The prevalence of Asperger disorder in boys has recently risen to about one in five hundred. The male to female ratio is 4:1.

Childhood Disintegrative Disorder

First described by Heller (420) and alternatively known as Heller's disease, CDD appears after a child has developed normally for at least 2 to 3 years. The child regresses profoundly over weeks or months in at least two of the following domains: language, motor skills, play, and social or adaptive skills, including bowel and bladder control, to an autistic endpoint (330). CDD is rare. Averaged across four surveys, the prevalence of CDD was 1.7 per 100,000 (421).

Pervasive Developmental Disorder Not Otherwise Specified

PDD-NOS differs from autism in its later age of onset and in the subthreshold or atypical severity of communication, behavioral, and social impairment. Like Asperger syndrome, it may be on a continuum of social and cognitive impairment with autism (419).

Other Conditions with Autistic Features

Other conditions presenting with behavioral phenotypes that overlap those of autism include childhood schizophrenia, elective mutism, developmental language disorders, severe mental retardation, complex motor tics, and obsessive-compulsive disorder. Originally classified together with autism under the heading of childhood psychoses, *childhood schizophrenia* is now recognized to be quite distinct from the autistic spectrum disorders. Unlike autism, it is rare in the first decade (422). It is characterized by thought disorder, delusions, or hallucinations. The onset is gradual, initially presenting as shy, odd, and awkward behavior and social isolation (423). Once the psychotic symptoms emerge, the condition can be diagnosed by the same criteria as schizophrenia in adults (424). Children of schizophrenic mothers, who are at high risk to develop schizophrenia, tend to exhibit slow motor development and achieve poorly in school. They are described as being anxious in social situations and preferring solitary play (425). In early life, preschizophrenic children could be reliably retrospectively differentiated from healthy siblings based on home video recordings, mostly by their abnormal movements and reduced facial expressions (426). Prospective studies of "high risk" children (with a schizophrenic parent) consistently reveal deficits in attention, memory, and social skills (426a). Before schizophrenia becomes clinically obvious, the children increasingly manifest social withdrawal, anxiety, academic difficulties, and thought problems each year between the ages of 12 and 18 (427). Children with *elective mutism*, though generally mute, do by definition speak normally in some situations or to some people, typically a parent, and engage normally in play and nonverbal social interactions (428). *Developmental language disorder* is not associated with impaired social interaction and behavior. A few children with severe language disorders exhibit some aspects of autistic behavior but relate well, using gestures to communicate (429). Children with congenital ocular or cerebral *visual impairment*, such as retrolental fibroplasia and septo-optic dysplasia, respectively, may show stereotypic or self-injurious behavior. Autistic behavior is commonly seen in children with *congenital deafness* and with *mental retardation*. Milder cases described only as having some "autistic-like" features but exhibiting relatively normal intellectual functioning overlap the broad category of attention disorders (326 and see below).

Diagnostic Evaluation

High-resolution chromosome analysis leads to a diagnosis in approximately 5% of children with autistic traits. Brain imaging studies are indicated only if there are indications of progressive loss of function, localized neurologic deficits, or persistent focal seizures. An EEG is indicated if there is a suggestion of seizures. A spinal tap can assist in the differential diagnosis of new onset seizures or autistic regression. Approximately one-third of patients with autism experience one or more epileptic attacks during the first two decades of life. Various seizure types have been described. Of these, the most common are complex partial seizures (312). The question of subclinical seizures is frequently raised in the autistic subtype in which an acquired loss of receptive and communicative abilities occurs, as in Landau-Kleffner syndrome (see below and Chapter 14). For this reason, sleep electroencephalography has been advocated for children whose autistic symptoms develop after 2 to 3 years of age, in the hopes that antiepileptic drug therapy might improve their language and social skills (430,431). Magnetoencephalography appears to be more successful than electroencephalography in revealing the subclinical epileptiform discharges (432).

Metabolic studies, including serum copper and ceruloplasmin levels, are indicated if autistic symptoms develop in late childhood or are progressive. Cognitive, language, educational, and behavioral assessments establish the level of severity of the child's impairments and serve as a baseline for IEPs and additional therapies.

Prognosis

Outcomes are most favorable in the least severely affected children, who have normal or near normal intelligence and speak before they are 5 years old (433). There is a strong impression among clinicians that applied behavior analyses (ABA), has improved the chances of children with autistic spectrum disorder to function independently in the mainstream school and society. Whether such outcomes draw upon brain plasticity, or are strictly due to improved behavioral strategies, is unknown. In their adult years, high functioning autistic or Asperger patients usually achieve normal understanding of speech. However, their semantic and pragmatic deficits are lifelong and make it hard for them to converse normally while letting the listener take his turn or introduce a new topic (434).

Autistic Language Compared with Developmental Language Disorder

Autistic spectrum disorder and developmental language disorder are classified as distinct and separate entities. However, deficient or absent language skills are a major characteristic of ASD. Is autistic language similar to or distinct from language in DLD?

Until recently, autistic language has been assumed to be different from language in DLD. Whereas DLD is characterized by impairment in understanding and producing phonology (speech sounds) and syntax (grammar), the language deficit in autism was thought to be at the "pragmatic" level, at which one understands what is said and uses language communicatively (e.g., DSM-IV). However, a majority of ASD and DLD children exhibit both receptive and expressive language difficulties. Some children with ASD even exhibit these difficulties in their extreme form, verbal auditory agnosia (VAA) (433–435). Those whose language problems are limited to pragmatics are actually in the minority. DLD children do not have pragmatic disorder, whereas ASD children do not have expressive speech problems in isolation. Thus, most ASD children have a language impairment that is comparable to the receptive/expressive language impairment that stands alone in DLD.

The similarity in pattern of language deficit is accompanied by a similarity in the size and shape of the various parts of the cerebral hemisphere. Previously only seen at autopsy, these parameters can now be measured by structural MRI. On average, both ASD and DLD children have larger than expected brains in childhood, excess of cerebral white matter, and anomalous asymmetries between the right and left hemispheres. The volumetrics of ASD and DLD resemble each other more than either resembles the normal control state (436,437). So, the macroscopic structure of the brain in ASD and in DLD is quite similar.

The close relationship between DLD and ASD originates from closely associated abnormalities in the genome. Susceptibility loci on distal chromosome 7q are associated both with ASD and specific language impairment (SLI). When there are abnormalities in this chromosomal region, individuals with ASD, SLI, or both are characteristically found in the same extended family tree (438–442). Therefore, individuals with an abnormality on distal 7q have a genetic predisposition to both ASD and SLI and may express either one. The as yet unknown intervening variables that transform a risk into the reality of a language disorder might also be able to transform an ASD risk into overt ASD.

Management Strategies

Medical

Autism may be the most difficult developmental disability to manage. Impairments in cognition, communication, socialization, and behavior often result in lifelong disability and frustration. Fifty years of behavioral and pharmacologic treatment efforts for autism (433) have shown that none is potentially curative or even treats the core features of autism. Agents that modulate monoamine systems have had some success in ameliorating associated symptoms such as impulsivity, poor concentration, obsessive and compulsive actions, rituals and stereotypies, anxiety, depression, aggression, disordered sleep, and self-injury. These agents include serotonin reuptake inhibitors such as fluoxetine (443), dopamine and serotonin receptor antagonists such as risperidone (444,445), atypical antipsychotics (445a) tricyclic drugs such as clomipramine, antihypertensives such as propranolol and clonidine (446), and antiepileptic agents such as valproic acid (430). Dopamine antagonists such as haloperidol are used to reduce stereotypic behavior (447), whereas dopamine agonists such as stimulant drugs may reduce hyperactive behavior, though they increase stereotypies and mannerisms (448). The short- and long-term risks and benefits of corticosteroid regimens (431) await further investigation.

Little evidence exists that children with autism have nutritional deficiencies (449), but various dietary supplements, such as magnesium and pyridoxine, are commonly used (450). Gluten-free/casein-free diets (451,452) have gained wide public acceptance when, as is very common, autistic children have associated gastrointestinal symptoms, notably constipation with overflow, although evidence from controlled studies is still awaited. Those who believe that ethylmercury, which constitutes 49% of thimerosal, a now discontinued vaccine preservative, caused their child's autism, have used chelation in an attempt to reduce the body's mercury burden. The therapeutic use of secretin has been assessed in an open-label study, with negative outcome (453). On the theory that intestinal flora, notably Clostridia, can exacerbate autistic symptoms, oral vancomycin has been given to children whose late-onset autism was preceded by diarrhea, with apparent short-term success (454).

Nonmedical

Social skill training encounters unusual difficulty with autistic children, in that one cannot assume the usual infrastructure of social experiences and spontaneous learning (455). Autistic people create their own environment, comprised more of things than of people. Even if they master the principles of socialization in the abstract, they still may lack social pragmatics—the ability to recognize the situations in which the principles should be applied (456). The major intervention programs offer intensive training and often involve parents to the point of making them cotherapists. Five prominent programs are representative of the ongoing effort to ameliorate this allegedly untreatable condition with comprehensive behavior and educational treatment programs, ideally initiated in the preschool years. They are the UCLA Young Autism Project (YAP) (457), the Program for the Treatment and Education of Autistic and Related Communication Handicapped Children (TEACCH) (458–460), Learning Experiences . . . an Alternative Program (LEAP) (461), Applied Behavior Analysis (ABA) (462), and the Denver Health Sciences Program (DHSP) (463). YAP operates most intensively, on a 40-hour-per-week basis, and follows the lines of operant conditioning (454). TEACCH offers parents the opportunity of acting as cotherapists. All five programs report significant gains in measured IQ and in social skills, but none of these claims has been evaluated by rigorously designed research designs and methodologies. In particular, random assignment of subjects, verification of training at home, and long-term outcome assessment by independent observers are lacking. It is not clear whether less intensive programs are less effective. Demonstrations are lacking both of internal validity, that the methodology exerts its effects by actually ameliorating the autistic disorder rather than through other means, and external validity, that the gains achieved in the training program generalize to diverse real-world settings (464). Subject to this caution, clinicians and teachers increasingly prefer applied behavioral analysis. Education within the mainstream, so often encouraged for

TABLE 18.9 Conventional Strategies for Children with Autism

Therapy/Intervention	*Method*	*Rationale/Benefits*	*References*
Alleviate family distress	Provide diagnostic information Counseling (e.g., social worker)	Helps families deal with guilt and frustration Increases understanding of the cause and possible prognosis	465
Behavioral modification	Modify environmental factors Redirect maladaptive behaviors Engage children with solitary play Deter tantrums, aggression Restrain injurious behavior	Stereotypies, maladaptive and injurious behaviors occur less frequently in structured and stimulating environments	319,466
Communication therapy	Direct speech training Sign language Augmented communication	Increase all forms of communication, not just speech	467, 468
Individual education program	Structured teaching to promote communication, cognitive and social learning Limits overstimulation Direct social skills training Self-help, life skills training	Promotes directed cognitive, language, and social learning To help adaptation to new situations	319, 458–460
Pharmacologic trials	Individual medication trials should be symptom oriented, time-limited, beginning with low doses and gradual increases until the true benefits of the therapy are determined	May improve attention, impulsivity May decrease agitation, aggression, anxiety May enhance sleep Stops seizures	469

TABLE 18.10 Unproved Intervention Programs for Children with Autistic Spectrum Disorder

Therapy/Intervention	*Method*	*Rationale/Benefits/Outcomes*	*References*
Auditory integration training	Use filters to remove frequencies to which the individual is sensitive	Decrease sound sensitivity and hence behavioral disturbances Studies have not shown effectiveness of training	470,471
Cranial osteopathy	Gentle manipulation of cranial bones	No adequate outcome studies exist	
Facilitated communication	An augmented communication technique that requires a facilitator to provide physical assistance for writing or keyboarding	Leads to independent communication in few persons, communication is influenced by the facilitator	472,473
Nutritional restrictions or supplements	Includes numerous restriction diets (e.g., gluten casein) or supplements (e.g., vitamin B_6, magnesium, secretin)	Benefits remain unproven, side effects include sensory neuropathy and photosensitivity	450,451,474
Patterning exercises	Daily, extensive controlled stimulation of muscle activity	Claims to repair nonfunctional neural networks Little or no benefit from the treatment has been shown, places enormous demands on families	475
Sensory integration therapy	Attempts to improve sensory processing through exposure to auditory, olfactory, visual, and tactile stimuli	Unproven and probably ineffective treatment, but its current use is widespread	476,477

children with disabilities on account of their social deficits, offers little obvious benefit to most children with autism. It is not clear that they would learn by example in the mainstream classroom.

Spurious impressions of improvement abound with respect to all types of children with chronic developmental handicap, regardless of the specific therapy that has been applied. However, they seem to be particularly widespread in the case of the autistic spectrum disorders. This may be because of autistic children's perplexing variability in performance, which can give the impression that hidden skills are waiting to be released into activities of daily living. Be that as it may, efforts to identify the optimal education and behavior programs must rely on controlled long-term outcome studies.

Publicly funded special education programs and financial aid programs such as social security income (SSI) offer support, and developmental disability services provide funding for respite care. Family support groups, such as the National Society of Autism, offer additional information and family self-help services. The typical community-based support services, including education and communication (e.g., sign language, augmented communication) therapies, and behavioral modification programs are summarized alphabetically in Table 18.9 (319). Some unconventional and unproved interventions are summarized alphabetically in Table 18.10 (450,451,457).

SPEECH AND LANGUAGE DISORDERS

Prevalence

At least 5% to 7% of the school-aged children in the United States (aged 5 to 21 years) have serious deficits of speech or deficits of hearing, with which a speech disorder is associated. An additional 5% have relatively minor speech impairments (478,479). Approximately twice as many boys as girls are affected. Speech and language disorders overlap with academic underachievement and behavior problems in school-aged children (480,481).

Language Development

Precursors

Neonates can discriminate virtually all the speech contrasts that are used in natural languages. By the end of the first year, they begin to understand meaningful speech and then to produce it. At about the same time, they lose the ability to discriminate contrasts that do not occur in their own language (482).

Even in the first 6 weeks of life, infants vocalize when they orient by turning their head and gaze to a target and by hand pointing (asymmetrical tonic neck reflex), in response to a novel stimulus. Babbling begins between 2 and 6 months of age and soon includes all the phonemes in human languages. Babbling is both spontaneous and imitative of the speech of others. Although some severely mentally retarded children are late to begin babbling, the characteristics of babbling, when it occurs, cannot be used to predict the quality of the language that will follow. The act of babbling is not causally involved in the child's use of language. For instance, when babbling is prevented by long-term tracheotomy, this does not retard the development of speech once the aperture is closed. Babbling does not initially depend on auditory feedback; even profoundly deaf children babble (483). Toward the end of the first year, however, the deaf child babbles less and then falls silent.

Early Language

At around 11 to 13 months of age, children begin to utter single words, of which *mama* and *dada* are often, but unreliably, reported first by parents. They look and point with the right hand at the objects they are naming, and about two months later, they also monitor the listener's reaction (484). According to parental report, children produce approximately 4 words at 10 months, 12 words at 1 year, and 80 words at 16 months (485). When children acquire a vocabulary between 50 and 100 words, they begin to utter words in combination. There is a burst of vocabulary development toward the end of the second year (approximately 150 to 300 words by age 2 years) and of syntactic development in the third year (486). Girls show the language spurt earlier than boys. Simple sentences emerge at around 3 years and agreement between subject and verb toward the end of the fourth year. At all stages, children can understand more words and phrases than they can utter, and even children who cannot vocalize develop substantial comprehension of spoken speech. However, there is great variability; first words are aquired anywhere between 6 to 30 months and phrases between 10 to 44 months. Late talkers have a good prognosis as long as their receptive vocabularies are in the normal range (487).

Ontogenesis of Cerebral Dominance for Language

Lesion, stimulation, and metabolic activation effects show that in almost all right-handed individuals, the left hemisphere is primarily concerned with the neural process underlying language as well as the decoding of symbols and the programming of motor sequences. Some deficits in tasks that are not overtly verbal have been reported in children with language delay, notably discriminating the order of presentation of rapidly successive stimuli in various modalities (488). With respect to other nonverbal functions, such as spatial orientation and spatial organization of nonverbal patterns, there is a less striking but definite asymmetry in favor of the right hemisphere. As the child matures and new skills emerge, the laterality conforms to that of the child's precursor skills.

Left-handers are either genetic or pathologic (488a) in origin. The latter are thought to have incurred mild prenatal left hemisphere injury, not sufficient to result in an overt neurologic injury, but enough to impair right-hand dexterity sufficiently for preference to shift to the left hand. Conversely, those who incurred early right brain damage became unusually right-handed. Regardless of whether they are genetic or pathologic left-handers, about one-half are left lateralized for language, a third bilateralized, and a sixth right lateralized. A person's hand preference, right, left, or mixed, has little or no predictive value for cognitive development.

Although a newborn's cerebrum is barely functional, most newborns more often spontaneously turn their heads and eyes to the right rather than to the left, a tendency that subsequently comes under control of the left hemisphere. Congenital left hemispheric maldevelopment and injury in the first year do not invariably lead to the expected gross language disorder or delay (489a); the right hemisphere assumes language representation (489b). Preschoolers show transitory language deficits after left hemisphere injury, but usually only after the first decade does the language disorder assume the characteristic severity and persistence of adult aphasia (490). In very early lateralized lesions of either hemisphere, there is often contralateral compensation, but age, lesion site, lesion size, presence of seizures, and use of antiepileptic drugs or hemispherectomy contribute to variable outcomes (491,492).

Language lateralization was believed to be progressive, from bihemispheric origins toward the end-point of fully established left hemispheric dominance for language, only near the end of childhood. The weight of evidence is against this theory, however. Instead, it now appears that language processes and their antecedents are lateralized from the beginning, in conformity with how they will be lateralized in their mature adult state (491,493). This inference was directly validated when the location and extent of the language areas in young children were probed by intracranial electrical stimulation and found to be much like those of adults (494). Children are credited with more plasticity of the nervous systems than adults, in which their higher levels of brain glucose metabolism (495) and ongoing synaptic pruning (496) may be involved. Specifically with respect to language (497–499), young children show more recovery than older children and adults after unilateral brain damage. At any age, recovery after unilateral hemisphere injury can rely on adjoining ipsilateral areas (500), or homologous contralateral areas (501), to take over the compromised function (see also section on Acquired Childhood Aphasia, below).

The nonexistence of progressive lateralization invalidates a host of theories offered over the years that attribute a variety of language disabilities to delay in the "lateralization process." Because no such process exists, therapy programs that purport to jump-start or accelerate it by manipulating the side of entry of stimulation, the child's positioning, and which hand and eye the child is permitted to use (e.g., 475), are irrational.

Left hemispheric control of language involves inhibition of the potential language capability of the right hemisphere. Massive left hemispheric lesions release this inhibition. Disconnection of the hemispheres by section of the corpus callosum reveals that the right hemisphere can decode at least simple speech messages. The right hemisphere's ability to comprehend speech also emerges when the left hemisphere is temporarily anesthetized by intracarotid injection of amobarbital (502). The patient remains responsive to verbal commands, as indicated by left facial and left hand movements. This residual ability to comprehend and respond perhaps explains why permanent total receptive aphasia is so rare and hardly ever seen in children. Right hemisphere compensation for language disorder is more complete for language decoding than encoding (503). When the right hemisphere is involved in language from the start, rather than because the left hemisphere was malfunctioning, as happens in pathologic non–right-handers, language nonetheless develops in the normal manner. There is no basis for attributing language deficits, as in Down syndrome, to right-sided language lateralization per se. Agenesis of the corpus callosum yields few of the signs of hemispheric disconnection exhibited by patients who have undergone callosal section. Whether compensation for a prenatal injury involves brainstem commissures, redundant functional specialization in each cerebral hemisphere, or both, is not clear (504). Early right hemisphere damage, like later damage, results in sensory inattentiveness and motor impersistence, as well as negative affect, consonant with the early right-sided specialization for negative emotion (505).

Recent evidence also has implicated the cerebellum, and specifically its posterior lateral area, in developing language. A cerebellar cognitive affective syndrome has been proposed (506) and related to early language development by studies of the aftermath of cerebellar excisions during childhood (507). Transitory mutism is replaced by dysarthria and impaired spontaneity of speech. Neuropsychological deficits, including impaired executive functioning, are more severe with right-sided cerebellar involvement, perhaps reflecting the crossed organization of cerebral-cerebellar connections (508). In contrast, damage to the vermis is credited with causing disordered behaviors ranging from irritability to withdrawal (509). Congenital cerebellar hypoplasia may result in a similar profile of deficits, but obscured by the profound mental retardation that typically characterizes these children (510). The pattern of cognitive and emotional impairment described in children was previously established in adult postoperative cerebellar patients.

Disorders of Pronunciation and Stuttering

The prevalence of speech disorders is closely related to age. Speech disorders occur most commonly in young children and reach an incidence of 15% in kindergartners (511). Approximately 90% of children younger than 8 years of age outgrow their speech disorders, but those who still have a speech impairment by 14 years of age can expect improvement only with speech therapy.

The frequency of production of sounds normally increases up to 2.5 years of age, at which time the speech sound pattern closely resembles that of the adult. Children's phrases average 1.5 words at 18 months, 1.8 words at 2 years, 3.1 words at 2.5 years, and 4.1 words at 3 years. Ninety percent of children can correctly articulate all vowel sounds by 3 years of age. For boys, a 90% success rate for consonant sounds comes later; by age 3 years, they can pronounce *p*, *b*, *m*, *h*, *w*, *d*, *n*, *t*, and *k*; by age 4 years, *ng*; by age 5 years, *y*; by age 5 to 6 years, *j*; by age 6 years, *zh* and *wh*; and by age 7 years, *f*, *l*, *r*, *sh*, *ch*, *s*, *z*, *th*, and *v*. Girls achieve some of these sounds slightly sooner. Speech sounds are more accurately spoken when they are in the initial rather than a middle position. They are least well articulated at the end of the word. Impaired intelligibility is prognostically less ominous than depressed level of language use, and referral to speech therapy on its account can be delayed until 4 years of age. If speech also is sparse, however, as in the 2 year old who does not yet utter two-word phrases, earlier referral is justified. Even so, progress is slow, and a special effort by the parents is needed to offer the child experience by talking to him or her more than is usual.

Whereas immature central control of articulation is by far the most common cause of speech disorders in children, definable neurologic deficits contribute in some cases. Quadriplegia or double hemiplegia associated with suprabulbar palsy causes speech to be slurred, and athetosis renders it jerky, explosive, and indistinct. Congenital suprabulbar palsy is a major impediment of speech. A hyperactive jaw reflex distinguishes congenital suprabulbar palsy from acquired nuclear and infranuclear paralysis of muscles of articulation. Buccolingual apraxia affects voluntary tongue, lip, and palate movements but spares automatic movements (512).

Stuttering presents between the ages of 2 and 4 years, with maximal incidence at age 3 years. Many children stutter only transiently, but in some, the stutter persists. The underlying cause of stuttering in childhood is unknown. Rarely, it appears secondary to organic brain disease, such as focal dystonia. When stuttering is a symptom of an extrapyramidal disease, the patient is more likely to repeat an entire word, rather than a single sound (palilalia). Relatively more boys and left-handed persons stutter. The notion that stuttering is the result of left hemispheric dysfunction is supported by positron emission tomographic studies (513,514). Language representation may be bilateral in children who stutter, with rivalry between the hemispheres for control over speech (515). Stuttering cannot be a disorder of auditory feedback because speech, like any highly practiced and automatized process, is not under continual feedback control. However, stutterers do find it difficult to disengage their attention from their own speech, which then cannot be automatic. Stuttering is relieved by noise that is sufficiently loud to mask speech sounds, and it is rare among deaf persons.

The child who stutters has difficulty in passing smoothly from phoneme to phoneme, especially at the beginning of sentences, and with words of more than five letters. The child who stutters explosively reiterates a single sound or blocks speech completely. Moments of self-consciousness and embarrassment yield maximal dysfluency, whereas distraction can result in temporarily normal speech. Singing is spared. Speech therapies include awareness training, regulated breathing, and social support. Treatment outcomes are variable (516).

Distinct from stuttering is cluttering, in which speech is fast, slurred, and dysrhythmic, with omission, reduplication, and transposition of speech sounds and words. Like stuttering, it can rarely result from brain lesions (517).

Secondary Language Disorders

The DSM-IV differentiates developmental language disorders from those secondary etiologies such as epilepsy, mental retardation, autism, and severe brain injury that have other prognosis and treatment implications (48). Secondary language disorders may be associated with risk factors such as low socioeconomic status and other family and environmental adversities or with learning disabilities (518).

Twins who share a secret language, that sounds coherent though incomprehensible, rapidly transfer to normal language when they are separated. Blind children of normal intelligence tend to be slow to begin to learn to speak and often pass through an echolalic phase. Subsequently, their vocabulary grows at a normal rate, but they lack imitative gestures. Some "electively mute" children withhold speech, either totally or only outside the home (428), but comprehend well and otherwise act normally. Although some of them may be emotionally disturbed, the problem may be quite superficial, and the seriousness of the prognosis should not be overestimated. In autism, speech is not only limited but is pervaded by echolalia, stereotypic utterances, and avoidance of the personal pronoun *I*. Children with autism have less difficulty with articulation and more with comprehension than do children with DLD who are matched for nonverbal intelligence. Bilingual children, who have difficulty in acquiring the second language, are ones whose ability with the first language also is limited. A bilingual environment may explain some idiosyncratic uses modeled on the first language, but it does not explain delayed language development (519).

The language of culturally deprived children reflects local speaking patterns that are better described as different than impaired. On formal tests, such children score poorly relative to mainstream norms. The normally functioning child who has been totally deprived of language experience does not speak but rapidly learns once the opportunity is offered (unless the child is secondarily emotionally disturbed). Extreme instances of children isolated from language, such as "wolf children" (520), have been reported, but even 6 years of total deprivation can supposedly be overcome (521), although a striking counterexample exists (522). Evidence for a critical period for first language development is fragmentary. It is argued that second language learning results in lower ultimate competence the later it is begun, up to age 16 years. Beyond this age, there is no further relationship between age and ultimate level of proficiency in the second language (523). It also has been argued that children generally recover faster than adults from brain injury, including injury that causes aphasia, presumably because the brain is more "plastic" and better able to reorganize before maturity (524, but see 169).

Language in the Deaf

Three million American children have hearing deficits; 0.1% of the school population is deaf and 1.5% hard of hearing. Of cases of hearing deficits, the majority are congenital sensorineural, and related to genetic susceptibility factors. Children who are born with hearing loss in excess of 70 dB (severe) or even 90 dB (profound) cannot hear conversational speech and therefore do not learn to talk unassisted. Ostensibly, conflicting approaches to early intervention are the auditory-verbal and the bilingual-bicultural philosophies. When young deaf children are taught by the oral method, acquisition proceeds through the expected stages but falls far short of the expected eventual level of proficiency (525). In contrast, young children learn American Sign Language (ASL) spontaneously when exposed to it by their deaf parents. Their ultimate proficiency is an inverse function of the age at which learning began (526). Thus, it is essential to begin early. Consistent with the status of ASL as a natural language, its use depends on left hemisphere function, even though in execution it is visuospatial (527). However, ASL may not be particularly well suited to learning to read, since its gestures largely represent whole words, with less emphasis on individual phonemes. So-called "cued speech," wherein the individual gestures often represent individual parts of words, seems to provide more support for learning the underlying structure of the language, thereby facilitating learning to read. "Total communication" aims use both oral and sign approaches flexibly, depending on the needs of the child (528). It has become the most commonly used teaching method for deaf children (529).

Deafness often goes unnoticed, even by observant parents, particularly when a bright child uses contextual cues to compensate for not hearing words. It can be suspected, however, as early as 4.5 to 6 months of age, if a child fails to look toward a sound source beyond his or her visual field. In young children, free-field audiometry is used for definitive diagnosis. This study should take place as early as possible so that the child does not go without appropriate language training (after the fitting of a hearing aid, if it is shown to help) and does not acquire the habit of ignoring auditory stimuli. Rarely, the auditory processing disorder is central, calling for tests of auditory attention and discrimination of speech modified in various ways. Performance on central auditory processing tests also is impaired in children with ADHD and improves after stimulant therapy (530). Children with recurrent otitis media can be at risk for language delays (531).

Congenitally deaf children with the usual high-frequency deafness adopt a harsh "deaf tone." When children become deaf abruptly (usually owing to meningitis), the effect depends on the stage of their language development. Children who become deaf when younger than 5 years gradually lose their ability to control articulation and voice production, sounding increasingly like congenitally deaf persons. Children with as little as 1 year of language experience are substantially easier to train in language skills than the congenitally deaf, whereas children who become deaf before age 2 years become indistinguishable from the congenitally deaf. The early provision of hearing aids and training for all deaf children improves their language progress. The language skills and educational achievements of prelingually profoundly deaf children approximated the hearing population norms after cochlear implants (532).

Developmental Language Disorder

In the 3–10% (532a) of children who have *developmental language disorder* (DLD), alternatively named *specific language impairment* (SLI) (533), language develops abnormally slowly. The selective language delay results in speech that notably develops late, but also is semantically and syntactically impoverished. The diagnosis of developmental language disorder excludes secondary causes, unless the coexisting condition is unable to account for the severity of the language problem. Thus, an individual with mild mental retardation who is disproportionately impaired in verbal abilities can be considered to have developmental language disorder as well. However, the language impairment must not be explicable by other deficits, physical abnormalities, or disease processes, or by social or emotional deprivation. It is therefore a diagnosis of exclusion. Nonetheless, children with DLD exhibit subtle associated deficits in cognition, emotion, and motor performance (534).

The language of 2% to 3% of 3-year-old children is deficient in expression, reception, or both. Unlike speech in mental retardation, speech in DLD also is characterized by several articulatory disorders. These conditions differ from speech or articulation disorders such as stuttering, cluttering, lisping, and cleft palate nasality in that they are more severe, affect a wider range of phonemes, and involve a far greater difficulty in making the transition from phoneme to phoneme than in pronouncing the phonemes individually. This difficulty results in grossly curtailed word formation. Short binding words ("function" rather than "content" words) are frequently omitted.

In contrast to the relatively fixed deficits of speech disorder, delayed language is sensitive to context, and sound combinations that can be uttered at one time are unavailable at another. Greater mental effort often results in worse rather than better performance. The disorder is not limited to the spoken language; it affects writing, and even lip reading, manual alphabet, sign language, and Braille. Language delay invariably involves expressive speech. Verbal memory is impaired as well. In one subtype, speech comprehension can be relatively spared, although affected children have difficulty in discriminating speech sounds. In a less common subtype, semantic as well as syntactic comprehension is severely deficient. Rapin (535) distinguishes five subtypes:

1. Phonologic production and speech planning disorder: These are largely speech problems with other associated motor deficits. Utterances are sparse or fluent but contaminated by sequencing errors.
2. Lexical-syntactic deficit: Speech is sparse, though intelligible; word finding and paraphasic errors abound; and syntax is immature.
3. Phonologic-syntactic syndrome: Both speech sound formation and syntax are compromised and repetition is difficult. Speech is "telegraphic."
4. Verbal-auditory agnosia: Language expression and reception are generally disordered. The child cannot derive meaning from spoken language.
5. Semantic-pragmatic disorder: The child is fluent and talkative, and syntax is preserved, but comprehension and verbal reasoning are deficient. Language onset is delayed, and utterances are stereotyped and tangential. Speech is accompanied by echolalia, jargon, and auditory inattention.

When comprehension is severely affected, the problem is often initially mistaken for peripheral deafness. The impression that auditory acuity fluctuates, which leads parents to doubt that the learning disorder is genuine, is borne out by audiometry. Stable hearing thresholds are hard to obtain, and repeated testing is apt to lead to radically different audiometric profiles. Recording psychogalvanic skin responses to sound is informative. These instabilities are caused by inconstant focusing of attention on sound, a function that normally depends on the integrity of auditory cortex.

The claim has been made that a defect in auditory perception exists in some developmental language disorders, specifically, a difficulty in discriminating the patterns of transition from speech sound to speech sound (536). This problem is most common in verbal auditory agnosia as well as when phonology is permanently impaired. Affected persons may have variable degrees of difficulty in auditory, visual, and linguistic processing. Alternative mechanisms for the underlying nature of DLD remain controversial, however (537).

The neuropathology of developmental language disorder is poorly understood but it has been associated with a mild neuronal migrational disorder in left inferior frontal cortex (538). Children with semantic-pragmatic disorder sometimes exhibit autistic features that meet PDD criteria (429) and, like autistic children, perform poorly on tests of social cognition (539). Semantic-pragmatic disorder and autistic disorder also share neuropsychological features of right hemisphere dysfunction (540). The language characteristics of children with hydrocephalus and of children with Williams syndrome often fall into the semantic-pragmatic category.

A genetic susceptibility to language disorders is indicated by the aggregation of cases within extended families (541) and their co-occurrence in monozygotic twins (542). A common genetic basis for motor immaturity and DLD has been suggested (543). An abnormal gene, FOXP2 on chromosome 7q31, is associated with dyspraxic speech and FOXP2 may be fundamental to human expressive language ability (543a).

Developmental language disorder is associated with a substantially increased incidence of behavioral disorders (544,545). The psychiatric symptoms may occur secondary to social isolation. This isolation may be compounded by relative lack of early experience of language, when parents become discouraged and relinquish their attempts to converse with the child. In other cases, the language and behavioral disorders may arise in parallel from the same neurodevelopmental deficiency.

Acquired Childhood Aphasia

Aphasia is considered to be "acquired" when it results from a condition that occurs after language development has begun, generally after age 2 years (546). Whereas bacterial infections causing encephalopathy used to be the most common causes of acquired aphasia in children, traumatic lesions currently predominate (490). Stroke in childhood is another cause of acquired aphasia, when the dominant hemisphere is affected (547).

Acquired aphasia is almost always nonfluent, especially in the youngest children, and loss of spontaneous speech or even mutism occurs more commonly than in adults. Other syndromes analogous to those in adults also have been described in children, and with analogous lesion location. Right hemisphere lesions cause aphasia in children no more frequently than they do in adults (1% to 4%). When they precede the onset of language, lesions of either hemisphere can temporarily retard both language and spatial development (548). Of 10 children with extensive early left hemisphere insults, five showed bilateral or right language reorganization, whereas the other five compensated within the damaged hemisphere. All but two of the children were left-handed, indicating more frequent transfer of hand preference to the lift than of language to the right brain (549).

Unless the lesion is bilateral, recovery of fluent speech is more likely in children with acquired aphasia than in adults, and disorders of comprehension occur less commonly. Residual minor language deficits and consequent school problems are common, however (550,551).

A rare type of acquired aphasia in children, acquired epileptic aphasia (AEA), otherwise known as Landau-Kleffner syndrome (LKS) (552) in addition to the seizure, is discussed in Chapter 14, under the heading of nonconvulsive status epilepticus. There is a severe comprehension deficit as well as an agnosia for environmental sounds. Oral expression is poorer than written, although both are impaired. Nonverbal intelligence is normal. Children with AEA typically develop normally until they are about 4 to 8 years old, when they fairly rapidly and quite unexpectedly cease to understand what is said to them and soon also lose the ability to express themselves in words. At its onset, the language regression is associated with some seizures and temporal lobe spiking on the EEG, but epilepsy rarely becomes severe in AEA. The language deterioration is often accompanied by the development of an autistic syndrome, perhaps in relation to abnormal temporal lobe metabolism (553). Perhaps temporal lobe dysfunction is why DLD and ASD are frequently associated in AEA.

Seventy percent of children with AEA have an associated severe behavioral disorder, featuring hyperactivity, impulsivity, and oppositional behavior. The severity of disturbed behavior follows fluctuations in the severity of the language disorder (554). Long-term outcome is poor despite attempts at cure by antiepileptic therapy and intravenous immunoglobulin (IVIG).

Diagnosis of Speech and Language Disorders

Normal intellect in domains separate from language is assumed in speech and language disorders. However, it is sometimes difficult to demonstrate, on account of the great contribution of language to overall intellectual performance. Tests that are verbally based, such as the WISC verbal subscale and the Stanford-Binet, cannot be used to estimate the intellect of children with speech and language disorders. Nonverbal alternatives include Ravens Colored Progressive Matrices for Children (73), the Leiter International Performance Scale (34), the Test of Nonverbal-Intelligence (TONI), and the Hiskey-Nebraska Test of Learning Aptitude (46). While discrepancy between a child's language and nonverbal developmental levels is integral to the developmental language disorder diagnosis, there is no consensus on how great a differential is critical and how it might vary with age (555). Audiometry excludes cases secondary to high-frequency deafness, and it can reveal the fluctuating impairments of pure tone sensory threshold that are typical of cortical deafness. The language behavior itself is evaluated by one of the standard language test batteries, such as the Clinical Evaluation of Language Fundamentals (CELF). Physical examination reveals any mechanical or motor deficits of the vocal apparatus. In the rare instances in which receptive aphasia and deafness resist clinical differentiation, the ability to elicit auditory-evoked potentials confirms that the auditory projections to the auditory cortex are intact.

Electroencephalography and neuroimaging are often used to seek structural intracranial abnormalities but as a rule yield little information of practical use. Rarely, subclinical seizures thought to disrupt cognitive processes can be detected by EEG (556). In such cases, effective anticonvulsant management, and less often excision of circumscribed foci defined by electrocorticography, can improve cognition. Brain imaging techniques such as PET and functional MRI that index regional metabolic activity yield insights in language dysfunction (557,558), but their routine clinical value is still to be clarified. Molecular cytogenetic analysis can explain the susceptibility to developmental language disorders in a small minority of affected children (559–560).

Treatment of Speech and Language Disorders

Language delay with an organic basis resists remediation. Treating the commonly associated impairments of dexterity, attention, and impulse control has little effect on the language problems (561,562). Speech therapy is at its most effective in improving a child's articulatory skills, although such skills also are apt to improve spontaneously in most children with increasing age. However, the central problem of impoverished vocabulary and syntax and the resulting difficulty in thinking in words is harder to address, and the so-called enrichment techniques are at best marginal or inconsistent in the improvement they can provide. Syndrome-specific remediation may be more effective (563,564). A meta-analysis revealed that speech and language therapy is effective for children with phonologic and expressive language difficulties, mixed in outcome when there are expressive syntactic problems and ineffective for receptive language disorders (564). The parents' expectations need to be reconciled with the realities of what is often an enduring problem, and the children's education should be organized to enable them to learn optimally at their admittedly limited rate. Individual instruction is usually required as well as family therapy and behavioral modification on account of secondary emotional disorder, which involves the whole family.

When language skills remain inadequate, augmentation and alternative communication methods (AAC) may succeed (565). Beyond manual signing as used by the deaf, these methods are applied to children with disordered oral and verbal development caused by cerebral palsy, bulbar palsy, and dysarthria; developmental language disorder; autism; and mental retardation. The need first to verify that intensive speech training does not succeed is balanced against the advantage of starting AAC training early (566), keeping in mind that AAC training may even facilitate verbal production rather than merely replace it. AAC subdivides into unaided (manual signing, finger spelling) and aided (communication board displaying pictures, symbols, or words). Depending on the child's motor capabilities, the child responds with finger, head, or eye indicating; yes and no indicating; or through electronic devices. A frequently used symbol system is Blissymbolics (567). The additional placement of another's hand on the child's hand or arm, combined with an expectation of sophisticated latent communication skills, characterizes the method of facilitated communication (568). This treatment lacks both scientific basis and empirical validity (467,569).

LEARNING DISABILITIES

Definitions

Parents often seek clinical assessment when their child's performance in school is unexpectedly poor, based on the prevalent but inaccurate assumption that a child who deals intelligently with some topics also should be able to do so with others. Some children do not benefit as much as expected from conventional methods of education in specific subject areas. This failure of response to instruction (RTI) has now itself become one of the allowable defining criteria of learning disability in the 2004 IDEA.

The term *learning disability* conventionally refers to a developmentally determined impairment in acquisition of certain mental skills that are necessary for academic learning in the early grades. Historically, it was assumed that such skill deficits should be defined by reference to a significant discrepancy between observed low performance on an academic achievement test and significantly higher intellectual level, as estimated by the child's age or IQ (570,570a). An increasingly influential alternative formulation invokes depressed reading level alone, regardless of IQ (571–574). The educational prognosis and response to instruction is poorly, if at all, predicted from IQ. Therefore, the requirement for IQ to be significantly higher than achievement has not been empirically supported. In the 2004 reauthorization of IDEA, the federal policy has responded by permitting schools to disregard discrepancy from IQ in their definition of learning disability. Descriptors variously imply a neurologic basis (minimal cerebral dysfunction), a perceptual deficit (word blindness), or the isolated character of the disorder (selective reading disability or dyslexia). However, while a central nervous system role in the expression of the symptoms of dyslexia is certain, a preoccupation with the brain as the basis of the difficulty can lead to investigations that do not help in planning for the child's future. The isolated character of the deficit implied by the terms *selective*, *specific*, or *pure* also can be misleading, if it precludes a rational search for exactly what each affected child finds particularly difficult. Most dyslexic children have a scattering of other, nonreading disorders—often including ADHD—that are part of the overall constellation of academic difficulties. In particular, ADHD occurs along with dyslexia far more often than expected by chance alone (561,576), and it can have a significant independent role in diminishing long-term school achievement. Selective arithmetic disability, absent a coexisting reading (577) or attentional problem, is uncommon. Selective drawing disabilities, sometimes overinterpreted as "constructional apraxia," are more common but are much less frequently brought to clinical attention, unless the drawing disability includes poor handwriting and misshaping of letters.

Because social pressure is concentrated on reading, and schools use printed texts as vehicles for all forms of learning, especially as the child grows older, an early reading disability that is left uncorrected can broaden out into a general school and vocational failure. This is further aggravated by coexisting socioeconomic disadvantage. Such generalized failure retains its more specific etiology (see the genetic review below) and must therefore be distinguished from the consequences of global mental retardation, attentional problems, and severe hearing impairment causing severe delays in both reading and math achievement even for those who are skilled users of American Sign Language (578,579).

In addition to ADHD, other psychopathologies, including internalizing ones, are prominent and sometimes serious comorbid accompaniments of dyslexia and related learning disabilities (575). Anxiety is common (580–583), including phobic reactions. Depression, including suicidality, is the more serious and equally common comorbidity (584–590), and it is poorly recognized by parents and by teachers (585,591). For that reason, it behooves clinicians to monitor their dyslexic patients, from as early as age 8 or 9, for hitherto unexpressed or unrecognized symptoms of emerging depression. Children are often surprisingly frank to acknowledge depressive feelings to outsiders. Such feelings, coinciding with progressive withdrawal from school or life activities, as well as classic vegetative symptoms such as altered sleep and appetite, warn of potentially significant but treatable depression.

Prevalence

Approximately 11% of school-aged children (aged 6 to 21 years) in the United States are classified as disabled, and

52% (2.4 million) of these students have learning disabilities (592). Another 10% to 20% of all students have learning or behavioral problems that are not severe enough to be classified as disabilities. Other studies estimate that 7% to 8% of early grade-school students have reading disabilities (593).

Selective Reading Disability (Developmental Dyslexia)

Models of reading have progressed from the theoretical to the empirical, which has produced a recent consensus account—the National Reading Panel (594). Word decoding ability accounts for much variance in reading skills at all levels (596,597). Reading difficulties are not confined to any particular orthographic system; they are approximately equally prevalent among readers on all continents (598). Although selective reading disability was originally thought to be more frequent in males (599), current evidence favors little or no gender difference in prevalence. However, it remains controversial whether to regard children with reading disability as simply on the low end of a normally distributed function (593) rather than a distinctive group within the childhood population.

More advanced reading also requires fluent successive visual fixation and appropriate direction of eye movement as well as knowledge, explicit or implicit, of the phonologic structure of the language and the ability to construct meaning from the words in their context. Thus, a deficit that limits beginning readers, once overcome, does not prevent further acquisition of reading skill in a normal manner, whereas a deficit that limits advanced reading might not be foreshadowed in the early stages. Failing readers in early and later stages can show different patterns of cognitive deficit. Phonologic and fluency tests particularly describe the earliest stage (kindergarten through second grade); vocabulary increases in importance until the third grade, when it assumes a major role. In some cases, difficulty is limited to spelling (600).

Numerous cognitive components, acting together, represent the larger domain of reading and writing. Each component process is potentially subject to developmental immaturity. Thus, while phonologic, fluency, and vocabulary deficits remain central to dyslexia, slow readers are routinely reported to have numerous limitations. None is necessary or sufficient for dyslexia itself, but rather the overall academic difficulties are compounded. These implicate visual and auditory memory, the ability to store memories in terms of speech sounds and their linkage to visual information, left and right discrimination, auditory synthesis, analysis of words into speech sounds, rhyming judgments, temporal order judgment, fast sequential processing, and nonword reading (601–605). In the long-term, most individuals with reading disabilities face persistent global deficits in academics, underemployment, and problems with behavior, social skills, and emotional adjustment (606).

Many minor neurologic abnormalities have been uncovered in children with learning disabilities, but these seem haphazard in their occurrence. Soft signs of neuromotor immaturity are frequent in these children but do not predict problems in any particular cognitive or academic domain (607). Soft signs are less prevalent after puberty but remain in excess of those found in normally developed adults. MRI indicates a tendency toward decreased volume of the left posterior perisylvian region in children with learning disabilities. Topographic mapping of EEG activity has demonstrated differences between dyslexic and normal boys. These differences are localized not only to the cortical speech areas, but also in both supplementary motor areas (608). Regional cerebral blood flow is reportedly decreased in both parietal lobes (609). Additionally, multiple foci of microdysgenesis of cortical and thalamic architecture have been documented in the brains of dyslexic individuals (610). Widespread in the left hemisphere, they also extend into the right frontal territory. In contrast, CT scans are rarely revealing, even if there are abnormalities on neurologic examination (611). Structural imaging reveals a scattering of abnormalities, consistent for inferior parietal lobule, inferior frontal gyrus and cerebellum, but varying in degree (611a). In short, at none of the three levels of analysis (behavioral, physiologic, and anatomical) is the notion of "pure" dyslexia validated. Rather, a more widespread abnormality is indicated, particularly in dyslexic adults (612) and can be demonstrated by neuropsychologic studies of adult dyslexics (613) as well as by studies that document the various comorbid deficits that rather randomly accompany dyslexia (614). Still, even when adults are defined as selectively reading disabled by their childhood psychometric records, a notable degree of residual specific reading-related deficit is still observable.

Functional neuroimaging has proven unenlightening about the etiology of dyslexia and has yet to be related to the genetic evidence. Nonetheless, the studies are revealing with respect to how the disorder works: for example, by underactivity of the visual-verbal crossmodal association areas, particularly Brodmann's Area 37 in the vicinity of the left occipitotemporo incisura, and neighboring regions including anterior Area 19 on the ventral cerebrum near the fusiform gyrus (615). More superiorly on the lateral cortex, the angular gyrus has been implicated, sometimes as an abnormality of excess (616), sometimes as one of deficiency (617; see also 618–622). The abnormality of excess may reflect higher level cognitively or semantically based crossmodal associative processes that are being deployed to compensate for lower level perceptual deficits. Conversely, when the function being imaged calls for a higher level of semantic crossmodal processing, the angular gyrus may be underactive. Since the extant functional imaging studies describe a neurological accompaniment to the behavioral deficit, functional imaging studies also might reflect the improved functioning that results from successful remediation. In a study on adults with psychometrically documented childhood dyslexia, remediation as well as deficit was imaged.

Investigation of Failure in School

Ultimately dyslexia is an educational, not a medical, problem. Because the diagnosis of a learning disability is predicated on some specificity of deficit (thereby differing from global mild mental retardation), an array of psychometric tests is given to document the preserved and impaired functions. When these tests establish disproportionate difficulty in real word reading (both by phonologic decoding (sounding out) or sight word recognition, reading disability is appropriately diagnosed, either by the psychologist reporting the testing or by the responsible school committee. Since the highest correlations between IQ and reading achievement tests tend to range between 0.5 and 0.75, whereas the correlations between specific reading risk batteries and achievement can range above 0.8, specific skill-related testing is the sine qua non of reading disability diagnosis. Estimates of reading skill so derived are conventionally reported in standardized scores and in percentile ranks. It is when the percentile ranks range downward from about the 15th percentile, and especially when they descend below the tenth, that true disability is commonly diagnosed. However, many authorities recommend a threshold of educational concern at the 30th percentile, reflecting the fact that even children in this range have skill inefficiencies that, unless remediated, could substantially impair their future academic progress (624). If the child's motivation is inadequate, the reason may be a behavior deviancy that often involves the whole family, an impulsive or hurried approach to the task (as in ADHD), or a cultural alienation from middle-class educational aspirations. The lack of motivation also can derive from poor self-image and a sense of hopelessness secondary to cumulative failure. Psychologic or neuropsychologic assessment is expected to differentiate the motivational or attentional factors from those involving cognitive skill deficit, even when both are present, but the distinction can never be completely assured. Caution in the diagnosis of reading disability is always appropriate, particularly since the vast majority of children with reading disability, especially in the earliest grades, improve with proper remediation (624,625).

Genetics of Reading Disability

For over a century (626), reading disability has been known to be familial, at the least; and explicit models of genetic transmission extend back a full half-century (627). A large number of genetic studies have since confirmed a genetic transmission of risk, and clinicians can be entirely confident that a child has substantially heightened risk for dyslexia if a parent is affected (629,630)—especially so if both parents are affected. Mostly within the last decade and a half, a considerable range of specific genetic linkage and association studies have been done, suggesting multiple genes conferring risk for dyslexia. The best current evidence implicates loci on chromosomes 1, 2, 3, 6, 15, 18, and 21 (631–635). There is no consistent evidence for sex-linked transmission, and correspondingly, population-based studies (636) tend not to show a disproportionate gender prevalence in reading disability. In the genetic as well as the epidemiologic studies, phonologic decoding and its underlying skill of phonemic awareness are routinely implicated. However, the loci on chromosome 6 and 15 may implicate a risk profile that extends to include or even to emphasize fluency or single word reading, respectively (637). Fluency deficit alone is not usually considered an identifiable subtype of reading disability, but when reading problems coexist with fluency deficit, the prognosis is particularly guarded. Fluency is the single best predictor of later outcome for poor readers (615). Single word reading by definition includes some nonphonologic (sight word) skills, so it is possible that there are phenotypic differences across the various genetic loci that have been implicated. The distinctiveness of the phenotype is most prominent in the chromosome 2 studies, which appear to implicate a relatively uncommon but quite significant language disorder syndrome that includes reading disability in its phenotypic presentation (638).

Selective verbal or performance impairments on the Wechsler scales, for example, are neither necessary nor sufficient conditions for reading problems. In children with DLD, the impact on reading—once general language skill is accounted for—is somewhat unpredictable (638a). Children with nonverbal Wechsler deficit are especially unpredictable as to their reading skills. It has been proposed that a nonverbal learning disability explains a variety of symptoms ranging from arithmetic problems to social skills deficit (639). Arithmetic problems commonly occur with reading problems, and clinical experience suggests that their occurrence in isolation is often due only to attention problems. But specific arithmetic disability, apart from ADHD, is well known, with its own subtypes (640; see below). The assumed visuospatial component of some arithmetic disability may be plausibly related to social skills deficit, since social information processing particularly requires global integrative perception, often considered a particularly right hemisphere–related function.

Historically, visuospatial subtypes of reading disability were recognized (641), but these are confounded with comorbid ADHD and are not generally diagnosed in current practice. However, a specific version of this proposal is the subject of intense current research (642,643). Surprisingly, the dorsal stream of visual information, which is usually associated with visuospatial rather than with linguistic functioning, may be implicated in some aspects of reading disorder. This is perhaps because of the disproportionate involvement of the magnocellular visual system (644,645), or because this pathway specializes in visual "look ahead" anticipatory processing, hence fluency. The evidence does not implicate deficits in this pathway as sufficient to explain the reading disorder however, and is controversial (645a,645b).

The decoding needs not only to be accurate, it needs to be fluent. The ability to automatize retrieval of names is quantitated by the Rapid Naming test (RAN). There is a correlation of about 0.6 between RAN performance and reading rate (646,647). Scores in this test have substantial predictive value for poor readers (648).

Rare in the United States, a presumably left hemisphere–related disorder that implicates arithmetic is the developmental version of the Gerstmann syndrome, in which children make errors in manipulations (such as subtraction) that involve the relative position of digits, and in spelling that involve mistakes of letter sequence rather than letter choice (649). Failure on tests of "finger order sense" is similarly accounted for by difficulty in making use of information about relative position (650). Right-left discrimination difficulties may occur in severe cases, since typically developing children can distinguish between their right and left sides by about 7 years of age.

Another pattern is that of the child, often left-handed, who has a normal psychometric profile, but who occasionally reads or writes from right to left. Although these directional mistakes attract much attention, they are transient and of little consequence. Mirror-image reversals of letters are made by typical children who are not yet ready to learn to read.

As a group, slow readers have frequently been reported to show an excess of left-handedness, mixed-handedness, and inconsistency of side of preference for hand, foot, and eye. Some large series have shown no such relationship, however. In general, samples that yield a high proportion of left-handed subjects come from clinical sources, whereas samples that do not are drawn from the general school population (651). Samples from clinical sources are more likely to include children who have suffered early brain damage, which leads to pathologic left-handedness (489). The association between left-handedness and dyslexia also can encompass a vulnerability to autoimmune disease (652), and poor readers are more likely to have mothers with immune dysfunction (653), but current evidence distinguishes separable genetic bases for dyslexia and immune dysfunction (654). Eye preference, usually inferred from sighting dominance (655), bears no close relationship to hemisphere dominance. It is influenced by minor disparities of visual acuity between the eyes that are not neurologically significant. Anomalous lateral preference is too inconstant to be useful in diagnosis, and there is certainly no rationale for trying to correct a learning disability by interfering with a child's established limb preference or by guiding a younger child toward right-handedness. The evidence for the relationship between laterality and learning disability is tenuous (656).

Investigating reading disability with structural imaging such as MRI rarely yields useful information. The EEG is helpful only when absence seizures momentarily interrupt the child's attention often enough to interfere with the child's ability to follow trains of thought in class. On average, trains of generalized 3 per second spike-wave discharges that last 5.5 seconds or more can interfere with mental activity (see Chapter 14). Brain electrical activity mapping (608), using average evoked potentials, or mapping of brain activity using MEG (magnetoencephalography) reveal interesting group differences but are not suitable for individual diagnosis. This is partly because of the heightened sensitivity of these techniques to a wide variety of other variables that affect the evoked response but are less clearly related to the clinical syndromes themselves. Structural imaging reveals reversed hemisphere asymmetry no more frequently than in controls (657; but see reference 658).

Certain obvious genetic disorders impact reading other than by causing dyslexia. For example, children with Klinefelter syndrome have a language-based learning disability as well as executive dysfunction (659). Children with Duchenne muscular dystrophy have impaired verbal memory spans, which are detrimental to classroom learning (660). More broadly, gross deficits of hearing and vision must be ruled out as contributing to the problem; however, reading is only impaired when visual acuity is substantially reduced. Orthoptic investigation may reveal poor vergence control and stereoacuity, especially in children who report that the text is subjectively unstable (661). Six months of monocular occlusion reportedly results in better reading (662). Vestibular dysfunction is no more common among children with learning disabilities than in a control population (663).

Treatment

Treatment is at present altogether nonmedical. In order, it focuses first on phonemic awareness, then on matching phonemes to visual letters for decoding of words, then on sight words, and then on semantic aspects of the reading process. For early reading, the combination of phonemic awareness training (664) and direct instruction in alphabetic coding is the most effective and well-documented. Fluency training (665) is gaining a research base as well; vocabulary and comprehension training are earlier in development.

Ineffectual treatments for reading disability include optometric exercises (666), improvement of neuromuscular control (e.g., sensory integration therapy) (667,668), labyrinthine stimulation, attempts to change peripheral or central laterality (669), psychoactive drug treatment (670), and anti–motion sickness medication (671,672).

Physical training with a view to improving spatial orientation and body image has been claimed to improve mental performance. However, these techniques involve teaching the child accomplishments far removed from the area of the child's difficulty and giving him or her unaccustomed attention. This encouraging experience could improve self-concept and motivation, without specifically improving reading (673,674). Efforts to change hand preference do not address the basic deficits in learning disability and are ineffective. Eye-movement training ignores the fact that, except in rare cases of conjugate gaze palsies, rate of eye movement shift from fixation to fixation is not a limiting factor in reading skill. Visuomotor training is based on the view that early motor ability influences and predicts later intelligence. No evidence supports the claim that either visual training or perceptual training can improve the academic outcome of children with reading disabilities (675). A motor program based on "patterning" of locomotion (676) is not only ineffective but may be harmful and cause unnecessary expenses, delay in appropriate educational intervention, and engender a false sense of security. In general, the notion that cognitive deficits can be remediated by training ontogenetically earlier perceptuomotor skills has been abandoned.

Noneducational remedial methods have not been shown to have specific benefits for reading readiness. A systematic, analytic approach to reading itself is preferable, in which the information is presented stepwise, while distractions are minimized. Usually, this can only be achieved by individual instruction, to conform to the individual learning requirements of the child. "Language experience" approaches are generally unsuccessful.

To meet these requirements, some educators "teach to weakness" in the hopes of improving the efficiency of the process responsible for reading deficiency; others regard it as more realistic to circumvent ("bypass") the deficiency by teaching to residual strengths. In fact, neither position is supportable in isolation. Initial attempts must be to teach to weakness, since all but a very few children can and do learn the skills of reading if given the appropriate additional instruction and practice in the very things (phoneme-grapheme correspondence, for example) they initially find difficult. In this regard, the formal randomized prospective trials (677–679) are unambiguous, and there is therefore no rationale for withholding such instruction and practice from children who need it. Such instruction can, however, take time that in severe cases is measured in years, and the goal of education during this period must also be to develop the child's strengths. It is only rarely necessary or even helpful to remove the child totally from the regular classroom, though in severe cases such placements in "self-contained classrooms" of children with similar levels of need do maximize the instructional opportunity and can promote peer relationships with other similarly struggling students. There is the countervailing risk of negative self attributions by the child, who may complain that he or she has been put in the "dummy class." When otherwise indicated by the educators on the scene (who routinely avoid these placements when they can for cost reasons), children can usually be counseled and helped to focus on the prospect of improved reading and learning skills—which they will often value above the discomfort of the placement. Such counsel, of course, implies that the clinician also will follow the child's progress and expect evidence of improved learning from the schools, thereby to encourage the child and facilitate re-placement in a regular classroom when appropriate. In this context, the rare child who needs continued placement in a special class will become obvious to all parties. The more common case is that of a child needing individual or small-group services from specialist staff at the school, outside the main classroom. Sometimes termed *pull out* services, these occasions usually total at most a few hours a week. At times, children object to the adverse inference that they believe is implied by such services, but the prospect of improving their reading skills will override their social reservations.

Beyond identifying the child who needs individualized reading instruction, some educators attempt to subtype the reading disability and deploy special treatments for special needs ranging from visual recognition problems to auditory discrimination problems. If the diagnoses are about different degrees of phonologic, fluency, vocabulary, and sight word and text comprehension skills, then they can be useful in guiding efficiently individualized instruction in small groups and sometimes individually. However, suitably controlled randomized prospective efficacy evidence is not available to support allegedly specific but theoretically imprecise forms of sensory training for conditions such as "visual learner," "left hemisphere learner," or even "auditory discrimination deficit" (unless it involves actual deafness that prevents hearing of normal spoken discourse). The teaching of reading, like that of any other skill, has no shortcuts: The relevant underlying processes (phonemic awareness, phonologic letter-sound coding including spelling, fluent letter-sound-word associations, vocabulary, and text comprehension strategies) cannot be avoided and must not be replaced by expensive and unproven quick remedies. The state of the art in education now mirrors that in medicine: proper prospective randomized controlled studies of efficacy are required before new treatments can be endorsed. A recent review of the extant evidence is provided by the National Reading Panel Report (594).

Finally, lexical knowledge does not guarantee fluency. The child who has mastered phonics may nonetheless emerge as a halting, dysfunctional reader. Fluency training is a necessary sequel. Different children are led through these stages at different rates, encountering different problems on the way. This exacting, long-term effort is not substantially facilitated by any form of diagnostic testing at the time of the original assessment.

Prediction

Socioeconomic circumstances ultimately exert the most influence on success in learning to read (595). Holding these constant, preschool prediction of reading failure remains difficult, though less so by the second half of kindergarten (596). The predictive success of reading readiness tests naturally increases as early reading achievement itself—for example, knowledge of the alphabet—develops. Predictions from first grade forward therefore tend to be stronger than those predicted from kindergarten. Readiness testing is best performed by entry to first grade, soon enough to enable any necessary modifications in the classroom. Longitudinal studies indicate that learning disability persists into adulthood and even broadens into vocational and personal problems, and occasionally delinquency and depression, more often than generally realized.

NONVERBAL LEARNING DISABILITIES

Some children have selective difficulties that impede school performance in spite of satisfactory spoken and written language skills. In the long run, such nonverbal learning disabilities, NVLD (639) can be more handicapping for employment prospects than selective reading disability. They include children with developmental dyscalculia whose difficulty in mathematics is not explained by concurrent verbal difficulties, but instead is associated with visuospatial impairment (680–682). Some children with attention disorders have difficulty in achieving fluency in knowledge of arithmetic facts, such as tables (683). Children with dyscalculia also are described as experiencing difficulty in tactile discrimination, concept formation, fine motor coordination, and dysgraphia (684). Dyscalculia is as prevalent as dyslexia (685) but attracts little attention, perhaps because a fourth-grade arithmetic achievement level suffices for everyday activities (686). Four subtypes of mathematical disability have been suggested, corresponding to weakness in semantic memory, knowledge of mathematical procedures, visual and spatial processing, and working memory (687).

One formulation relates NVLD to hypothesized inadequacy of the right hemisphere (688) and invokes impaired social skills as yet another component. Shyness and social isolation are accompanied by lack of eye contact and impaired use of gestures with speech in flat intonation. Of the main groups of learning-disabled children, those with nonverbal learning disabilities experienced depression twice as often as children with reading disabilities (689). When soft neurological signs are present, they tend to be left-sided. An electrophysiological study reports diminished activity in the 36- to 44-Hz band over the right hemisphere during a face recognition task in dyscalculics (690). A group of children being treated for phenylketonuria conformed to such a neuropsychological pattern (691). Children with Turner's syndrome have impaired visuospatial, memory, and attentional skills (692). The behavioral phenotype of children with *velocardio* facial syndrome also suggests NVLD syndrome. Nonverbal learning disability is common in female carriers of fragile X (694). It is the most common type of learning disability in epilepsy (695). Some 50% of children with neurofibromatosis type 1 (NF1) have learning disabilities (696) that are described as being specifically visuospatial and visuomotor deficits and reading disabilities (697). However, a recent study has found the cognitive deficits in NF1 to be less specific and associated with low IQ and behavioral disorders (698). MRI studies that show basal ganglia and cerebellar lesions implicate subcortical structures in the etiology of NF1 (699–701).

Children with learning disabilities have low social status among their peers (702). This low status could result both from their associated social obliviousness, and from the school failure that children with learning disabilities experience, resulting in low self-concept and negative perception by others.

Social learning disability (703) comprises skill deficits, both in perception (of others' nonverbal communications) and performance (in the manner of outward behavior toward others). "Deficit" applies when the socially relevant skills or behaviors are not in the child's repertoire. Motivational failure is applicable when the skills are in the repertoire but not used (704). They might not be used because the child avoids interactions for reasons of fear or hostility or lacks adequate impulse control. In the rare cases, where the social deficit turns to aggressive expressions, the implication of dangerousness to others must be cautiously, but carefully, considered.

Developmental Coordination Disorder

Children who are so clumsy that they have difficulty coping with the demands of everyday tasks (such as dressing, feeding, writing, gym and playground activities) have been variously characterized as being physically awkward, developmentally dyspraxic, or subject to sensory integrative or perceptual motor dysfunction—the clumsy child syndrome (705). Named developmental coordination disorder (DCD) both in the DSM-IV and ICD-10, it was defined as existing when the child lacks the motor coordination necessary to perform age appropriate tasks, although intellectually normal and otherwise neurologically intact.

Previously believed to represent a temporary immaturity or lag that resolves with increasing age, it is now thought to persist at least into adulthood and probably to be lifelong, bringing in its wake health and fitness problems, disordered behavior, low self-esteem, and deficient social interactions (706). DCD is thought to be present in 5% to 6% of schoolchildren (707).

Movements are generally slow; DCD may involve timing difficulties related to dysfunction of the cerebellum. The child finds it particularly hard to inhibit moving toward salient external stimuli (708). Visuospatial deficits have been documented even in the absence of movement. When it is found in combination with ADHD, DCD persists into the adult years (709). The coordination deficits in ADHD children could not be attributed only to inattention (710). The poorly legible writing and copying of text found in writing disorder that is due to DCD differs from that in dysgraphia based on linguistic problems, in which spelling is poor but copying is preserved (711). When diverse physical interventions to remediate DCD are critically evaluated, it appears that any gains are slight and more probably accounted for by increased self-confidence than improvement in motor control (712).

ATTENTION-DEFICIT HYPERACTIVITY DISORDER

Characteristics

Attention-deficit hyperactivity disorder (ADHD) refers to the covariation of inattention, hyperactivity, and impulsivity. The DSM-IV describes three ADHD subtypes: (a) inattention alone, (b) hyperactivity-impulsivity alone, and (c) a combined type with significant inattention, hyperactivity, and impulsivity. Some 80% have the combined type, 15% the inattentive, and 5% hyperactivity and impulsivity only. Children may be restless during one stage of development but not subsequently. This two-factor model is a departure from the previous unidimensional model, and though it is far from validated, it does have some empirical basis (713). Correspondingly, hyperactivity/impulsivity is associated with externalizing psychopathology (e.g., conduct disorder, oppositional defiant disorder) and the inattentive subtype with internalizing psychopathology (e.g., anxiety, depression) (714). The DSM-IV does not include developmental qualifiers among its criteria for ADHD, but the listed behaviors, and particularly hyperactivity, typically decrease as the child grows older. This does not imply that the disorder grows milder with increasing age, but that its form of presentation changes during development. A synopsis of the current state of ADHD diagnosis and treatment is available (715).

According to the DSM-IV-TR (text revision), the major clinical manifestations of ADHD—namely developmentally maladaptive attention, activity, and impulse control—must be sufficient to cause impairment in social, academic, or occupational functioning (48). Signs of ADHD generally begin before age 7 years and should persist for at least 6 months in two or more settings (e.g., home, school, or play) before the diagnosis is made. However, some children may have a later onset of the signs of ADHD (716).

There is consensus on the behavioral characteristics of ADHD that are listed in DSM-IV criteria. The most frequently reported primary manifestations of ADHD include cognitive disorganization, distractibility, inattention, impulsivity, and hyperactivity. The most commonly reported secondary manifestations include disruptive behaviors, poor social skills, emotional immaturity, fidgeting, poor academic performance, and excessive talking.

The relationship between the level of motor activity in infants and subsequent hyperactivity is unknown. Mothers often observe in retrospect that their child with hyperactivity was unusually active from birth. Feeding difficulty and sleep disturbances in infancy and the preschool period are commonly reported precursors (717,718). A prospective study found the second year of life to be the earliest in which ADHD symptoms could be detected and age 3 to 5 years to be the peak time of onset (719). Young children with hyperactivity explore their environment with unusual persistence, which accounts for the increased frequency of accidental poisonings (720) and traumatic brain injury (721) in ADHD. In older children, gross motor exuberance can give way to a less flagrant but continual wriggling restlessness. More troublesome is the child's impulsive, distractible, and often antisocial behavior. The hyperactivity becomes less a source of adults' irritation at home and more an occasion for disapproval from teachers at times when schoolchildren are expected to sit still and pay attention. This disapproval may be partly responsible for the high stealing and truancy rates among hyperactive children. Girls and boys with ADHD are similar in their impulsivity, academic performance, social functioning, fine motor skills, parental education, and parental depression (722). Girls tend to be less hyperactive and externalizing, but more inattentive and cognitively impaired and more subject to rejection by peers (722,723).

Gross body movements are not uniformly more frequent in children with hyperactivity. In unstructured situations, many typical children are just as active, and children with hyperactivity do not stand out. In structured situations, differences appear both in the amount and the relevance of the activity. In a 24-hour study, an ADHD group did exhibit more overall activity than controls during the night and throughout the day (724). Recorded over as long as 1 week, boys with ADHD were significantly more restless than controls at ages 6 to 11 years, but rarely so at older ages. Some children manage to continue to be attentive (e.g., to a television program) while moving around a room. Mostly, however, each movement signals a more comprehensive reorientation of mental set. In infancy, and until the child walks, this continual reorientation appears not to cause concern. Subsequently, complaints gather as the child disrupts the orderly home or classroom while failing to pay the expected degree of attention to the teacher, the instructional materials, and homework assignments.

Young children with ADHD initially show no signs of distress, but negative reactions from adults and peers gradually engender feelings of inadequacy, and this can lead to withdrawal or aggression. Hyperactive children are seen as quarrelsome, irritable, defiant, untruthful, and destructive by their classmates as well as by adults (725). The discipline imposed by the school and the need to repeat grades further contribute to learning failure and social maladjustment. Nonhyperactive children with attention deficit are misperceived as undermotivated or lazy, and the diagnosis is often missed.

Schoolwork demands increasing effort and organization as of fourth grade (726), and the intermittency of attention interferes more with learning and becomes more troublesome to teachers. Some 10% to 50% of children with ADHD underachieve in reading (727,728). Whether this is due to the attention deficit, which can impair word attack (729), or to comorbid dyslexia is hard to determine in the individual case (730). Children with ADHD are not lower in IQ than attentionally normal children.

Neither restlessness nor inattention is the core of the ADHD syndrome. That ADHD is primarily a disinhibitory disorder (731) is questionable (732). A recent study failed to confirm a selective executive /inhibitory deficit in ADHD boys (733). There is experimental evidence that ADHD behavior is more variable than that of normal children and of children under stimulant control (734,735). Hyperactive children attend as efficiently as normal children to tasks that they find intrinsically interesting or rewarding. It is when the task is tedious and the incentive for doing it is remote in the future that their inattention is maximal. The hyperactive child understands consequences and professes the usual concern about them. However, the consequences make little impression on the child's behavior. But if the task is attractive or of interest to the child (i.e., intrinsically motivating), then the ADHD child performs as well as a child who is attentionally normal (736).

Diagnosis of Attention-Deficit Hyperactivity Disorder

There are no definitive diagnostic tests for ADHD. Rather, the diagnosis depends on determining (a) that the child is inattentive and/or impulsive and hyperactive to a degree that is excessive for the child's age and expected level of developmental maturity, and (b) that there is consequent impairment in social and school functioning. Corroborating information can be obtained through child, parental, and teacher interviews; standardized rating scales (737); direct observation; behavioral laboratory tests; and formal psychologic and educational evaluations. The child's history, physical, and neurologic examination should be complete enough to rule out any identifiable genetic or medical conditions that might simulate ADHD. Absent such conditions, and although it may uncover nonspecific soft signs, the neurological examination rarely contributes to the diagnosis. Neither physiological nor biochemical measures reliably identify ADHD children (738). Psychiatric consultation is indicated in children with more complex behavioral problems or who have comorbid depression or thought disorders. It is not known whether the three phenotypes presented in the DSM-IV-TR have different neurobiologic bases or are variants of the same underlying pathophysiology.

Prevalence

ADHD is the most common chronic behavioral disorder in children, with a prevalence that ranges between 3% and 5% of school-aged children worldwide (739). It is reported to be highest in inner city populations (740,741). It occurs far more frequently in boys than girls in clinic samples (742) as well as in approximately 3 to 1 ratio in population studies (722). Through the evolution of the diagnostic criteria and changes in the public's attitude toward the disorder, the prevalence of ADHD has gradually increased, particularly in girls, as has the use of stimulant therapy (743). In a more recent study, primary care providers identified behavioral problems in approximately one in five children, and attentional/hyperactivity problems in 9.2% of the entire study sample, but the diagnosis was commonly made solely by parental interview and without the benefit of standardized questionnaires (742).

Although it is most frequently diagnosed in North America, crosscultural studies have shown comparable levels of prevalence in all countries studied, even in the Third World (739), not only of ADHD, but also of internalizing and externalizing psychopathology in general (744). In Britain, the diagnostic label *hyperkinetic disorder* (745) is reserved for the most severe cases. Other children who would have been considered to have ADHD in the United States are termed *conduct disordered* in the United Kingdom (746). This difference is not only semantic. It reflects a difference in management, being that stimulant therapy is used sparingly in the United Kingdom. Whether ADHD and conduct disorder are truly separable is questionable (747). Those who use *aggressive conduct disorder* as a primary diagnosis find a majority of their patients to be hyperactive as well (747). Comorbidities affect both prognosis and treatment (748,749). In particular, aggressiveness in early childhood is a negative prognostic sign. The home environment plays a role. Aggressive children as a group tend to be ones reared by depressed mothers who offer less positive caregiving. Family income is lower than for unaggressive children continue to have more academic and social difficulty, and are seen as being angry, hostile, antisocial, and oppositional (750).

Neurobiologic Basis and Genetics

There is no single underlying cause of ADHD. It occurs both in the absence of any identifiable risk factors, and in association with numerous other childhood conditions such as motor dyspraxia, tics, learning problems, speech and language disorders, sleep disorders, oppositional behavior, enuresis, and encopresis. In addition, overactive and socially disruptive behavior is common in children who have evidence of injury from infections, head trauma (751), toxic exposures (752), and extreme prematurity (753,754). Minor physical anomalies are frequent (755).

In most cases, hyperactivity is already evident in infancy, although it is not necessarily recognized as such, and it frequently persists into adult life in the form of attentional and social problems (756). Thus, it has the characteristics of a stable personality trait or temperament, and for which there is a genetic link in most cases. Families of ADHD/conduct-disordered children are notable for the high incidence of sociopathy and alcoholism (757,758). ADHD is highly heritable, probably based on multiple genes, each with small effect size. Parents of children with ADHD have elevated ratings of ADHD symptoms (759). Compared with the general population, first-degree relatives are at a 4.6- to 7.6-fold risk of developing the disorder (760). Second-degree relatives also are at increased risk (761). Several linkage studies implicate a 7-repeat polymorphism of the dopamine receptor D4 (DRD4) gene, mapped to chromosome 11p 15.5 (762), and also a polymorphism of a dopamine transporter (DAT1) (763). The transporter is a target of many of the drugs used to treat ADHD (764). The density of dopamine transporters in the striatum is markedly increased, as measured by single photon emission computed tomography (SPECT) using labeled altropane, a specific ligand for dopamine transporter (765). This disorder in dopaminergic function results in a disinhibited sensation-seeking behavioral style (766).

Right frontostriatal circuitry has been invoked with respect to defective response inhibition. The right frontal lobe is reportedly smaller than normal in ADHD structural imaging (767), and the striatum has abnormal morphology (768–770). The cerebellar, temporal gray matter and total cerebral volume are smaller in ADHD individuals than attentionally normal controls, and these size variables correlate significantly with ratings of severity of ADHD behaviors (771). Corpus callosum size is reduced (772,773) as is the inferior cerebellar vermis, posterior lobe (773a). Regional cerebral blood flow is diminished in striatum and frontal lobes in ADHD, a deficiency that is partly reversible by methylphenidate (774, but see 775). Power spectrum analysis indicates prefrontal underactivation (776) and cerebral glucose metabolism is diminished generally, but most notably, in the prefrontal cortex (777). Some neuropsychologic deficits are consistent with prefrontal underactivity. The quantified EEG in ADHD has abnormal features (778). Event-related potential (ERP) studies suggest the presence of abnormalities in the right frontal (779) and parietal (780) regions. Some neurobiological clues to the etiology of ADHD are summarized in Table 18.11.

Differential Diagnosis

Restlessness and short attention span can be features of mental retardation and may conform to the child's developmental quotient. The presence of mental retardation can itself be hard to verify. If the validity of the intelligence testing is uncertain, the educational psychologist may qualify the IQ score with a warning that it could under-represent the child's cognitive potential, particularly for measures that require sustained attention rather than merely a quick response. Retesting after initiation of stimulant therapy can yield a more realistic estimate. Improvement can be conveniently documented by teachers and parents by means of the Conners rating scales (781). However, even correcting the attentional problem can leave the educational difficulty unresolved, given the 30% to 40% overlap between ADHD and learning disabilities (782).

When cognitive deficits do not explain the attentional problem, an alternative possibility is overanxious disorder. The anxious child is most restless under emotional stress, as in the classroom and consulting room, and least restless when unstressed, as on weekends or on vacation. The child is visibly unhappy, either characterologically or because of some maladjustment within the family. The hyperactive child, on the other hand, is typically in good spirits until he or she comes up against frustration and adverse attitudes from others. Whereas the time of onset of anxiety can usually be specified, hyperactivity often dates from early infancy. A favorable response to a stimulant supports the diagnosis of ADHD as opposed to anxiety. Anxiety is comorbid with ADHD in about one-third of cases. Its presence did not impair stimulant response in a large-scale study (783). Favorable response can be documented in the laboratory on a time-response and dose-response basis by use of a paired-associated learning task (784). The findings contribute to the design of an appropriate drug regimen for the child who responds favorably. Other tasks that can be used in a similar way are the Continuous Performance Test (CPT) (785) and the Test of Variables of Attention (TOVA) (786). CPT performance variables are significantly related to ADHD symptoms (787).

Overfocusing (326) is sometimes comorbid with ADHD and sometimes distinct. Children with overfocusing have difficulty in shifting mental set associated with perseveration and isolating tendencies. In addition to the social

TABLE 18.11 Neurobiologic Clues to the Etiology of Attention-Deficit-Hyperactivity Disorder (ADHD)

Etiologic Clue	Description of Findings in Studies of ADHD	References
Environmental	Increased incidence of behavioral disorders, sociopathy, and alcoholism in families of children with ADHD	757
Endocrine	Increased frequency of ADHD in patients with resistance to thyroid hormone in some studies	
Genetic	Increased concordance for hyperactivity/inattentiveness in monozygotic twins (59% to 81%) compared with dizygotic twins (approximately one-third). Increased incidence of ADHD in first-degree (up to 25%) and second-degree relatives of children with ADHD	758,759,761
Neuroanatomy		
Cerebrum	Some limited magnetic resonance imaging brain morphology and neuropsychologic studies suggest that children with ADHD have a smaller or functionally abnormal right frontal lobe; other studies show variable asymmetries and volumetric differences in the basal ganglia, corpus callosum, ventricular systems, and subcortical white matter	33,772,773
Electroencephalographic findings	Increased anterior absolute theta and decreased posterior relative beta activity in quantified electroencephalographic analysis suggests reduced cortical arousal in adolescents with ADHD	778
Brainstem	Prolonged latencies of waves III and V, and longer brainstem transmission of waves I–III and I–V in brainstem auditory-evoked potentials of children with ADHD suggest brainstem dysfunction in these children Activation of reticular midbrain formation and thalamic intralaminar nuclei increases on attention-demanding tasks in a positron emission tomographic study; executive functioning associated with greater subcortical activation in ADHD subjects	
Neurochemistry		
Dopaminergic and noradrenergic systems	Pharmacologic agents that are effective in ADHD (e.g., stimulants and tricyclic antidepressants) increase central nervous system dopamine and norepinephrine transmission Dopamine deficiency is postulated to account for lack of impulse control in ADHD; studies that measure catecholamines and their metabolites in blood, urine, and CSF in individuals with ADHD are inconclusive; regional dopamine inhibitory autoreceptors may play a role in central nervous system catecholamine metabolism Functional neuroimaging studies support the hypothesis that attention is regulated at multiple levels, especially frontal, parietal, or temporal cortex as well as subcortical structures within the basal ganglia and thalamus	762–765

withdrawal that is often manifest, overfocusing classically includes aversion to novelty, complexity, and time pressure. It bears some resemblance to high-level autistic behavior, though it is milder (325). A contrasting temperament of uncertain relation to overfocusing is exhibited by the behaviorally inhibited child (788). Irritable in infancy; shy and fearful as a toddler; and cautious, quiet, and introverted in grade school, these children are thought to have increased limbic-sympathetic tone and to be anxiety prone. Disordered sleep, especially caused by obstructive sleep apnea, can render a child inattentive and restless. Attention deficits are often found among children of schizophrenic parents, who are themselves at high risk for developing schizophrenia. They perform poorly on vigilance tasks but are not impulsive (789). Another potentially overlooked differential diagnosis of ADHD is occult mood disorder, notably bipolar disorder, particularly when it presents in adolescents with chronic rather than episodic symptomatology. The combination of dysphoric and irritable mood with aggressive conduct that is resistant to stimulant therapy as well as subjective report of elation, grandiosity, racing thoughts, flight of ideas, and decreased need for sleep (790) should prompt an examination of the family for bipolar disorder (791). However, a broad phenotype also is recognized: Children exhibit chronic nonepisodic disregulation, with severe irritability, hyperarousal, and increased reactivity to negative emotional stimuli (792). In one study of juvenile bipolar disorder, comorbidity with ADHD was 87% (793). Episodic loss of control is attributed to dysfunction in the limbic cortex (794). Whereas impulsive acts of aggression are common in ADHD, episodic explosive behavior is not. The restless movements of Sydenhams chorea are associated with ADHD in one-third of cases and are often accompanied by emotional lability and

TABLE 18.12 Pharmacologic Treatment of Attention Deficit-Hyperactivity Disorder

Medication	*Dose Ranges (mg/kg per day)*	*Maximum Dose (mg per day)*	*Formulations*	*Common Adverse Effects*
Stimulants				
D-amphetamine (Dexedrine)	0.1–0.5	40	5-mg tablets; 5-10-, 15-mg spansules	Insomnia, poor appetite, stomachache, tics
D-amphetamine/ L-amphetamine mixture (Adderall)	0.1–0.5	40	5-, 10-, 20-mg tablets	Insomnia, poor appetite, stomachache, tics
Methylphenidate (Ritalin)	0.5–1.0	60	5-, 10-, 20-mg tablets; 20-mg sustained release	Insomnia, poor appetite, stomachache, tics
Methylphenidate extended release (Concerta)	18 to 54 mg per day, given once a day in a.m.	54	18, 27, 36, 54 mg tablets	Headaches, abdominal pain, decreased appetite, sleeplessness
Pemoline (Cylert)	0.5–3.0	112.5	18.75-, 37.5-, 75-mg tablets	Insomnia, tics, stomachache, movement disorder; rarely: hypersensitivity and hepatic dysfunction
Others				
Clonidine (Catapres)	0.001–0.005	0.3–0.4	0.1-, 0.2-, 0.3-mg tablets 0.1-, 0.2-, 0.3-mg transdermal patch	Somnolence, fatigue, hypotension, bradycardia, headache, dry mouth, constipation
Desipramine (Norpramin)	1–3	100	10-, 75-, 100-mg tablets	Tachycardia, hypertension, arrhythmias; monitor electrocardiogram Rare, unexplained sudden death
Guanfacine (Tenex)	0.5–2 mg/d; 12 yr and older	2	1-, 2-mg tablets	Sedation, fatigue, headaches, insomnia, stomachache, decreased appetite
Imipramine (Tofranil)	0.5–3	100	10-, 25-, 50-mg tablets	Fatigue, dry mouth, blurred vision Rare, cardiac conduction block
Atomoxetine (Strattera) a selective norepinephrine reuptake inhibitor	0.5 to 12 mg as single dose in a.m. or divided doses in a.m. and after school	1.4 mg/kg or 100 mg per day, whichever is less	10, 18, 25, 40, and 60 mg capsules	Upset stomach, nausea, vomiting, dizziness, mood swings, rare liver failure

obsessive-compulsive symptoms (795). In addition to multiple motor and vocal tics, children with Tourette syndrome (TS) often exhibit symptoms that are diagnostic of ADHD. However, these symptoms represent comorbidity and are not inherent in TS. Learning disabilities and neuropsychologic deficits (796) have been reported in children with TS. With respect to executive functions, children with TS but without comorbid ADHD were impaired only in tests that call for response inhibition (797). The neurology of TS is considered in Chapter 3.

Management Strategies

Medical

Although behavioral modification may be a sufficient first-line therapy in mild cases of ADHD, it is advisable to consider a pharmacologic intervention trial before instituting extensive behavioral management therapies, home interventions, or changes in the educational program or curriculum (798). In fact, a large-scale cooperative study found that stimulant therapy was as effective alone as when combined with behavior modification (799). Doses and common adverse effects of medications used in the treatment of ADHD are listed in Table 18.12.

The most effective pharmaceutical agents for symptomatic control of hyperactivity are the stimulant medications. Therapy with stimulants leads to significant improvement in at least 70% to 80% of children with ADHD (800). At the effective dose, stimulants modify the child's activity, improve behavioral control, and permit a more adaptive disposition of attention in relation to the demands of the moment (801,802). A meta-analysis of effect size finds twice as much improvement of behavior as of classroom achievement (803). Stimulants also enhance performance in otherwise normal, healthy individuals when performance is impaired by disinterest, fatigue, or sleep deprivation. Methylphenidate may increase task salience, rendering it more motivating (804).

There is no empirical justification for the practice of prescribing stimulants according to the child's weight—for instance, at a dose of 0.3 mg/kg. Stimulant drugs have a strong affinity for the brain, which approximates its ultimate adult size by age 6 years, and the optimal dosage does not increase with increasing age or severity and is not a function of body weight (805).

Stimulant therapy usually remains useful for many years, if not indefinitely. Even after long periods of administration, discontinuing the drug leads to notable relapse within a day or less. Because most stimulants are short-acting, their effectiveness can be evaluated on a daily basis by comparing behavior on and off medication, without need for drug holidays.

Approximately 20% of children diagnosed with ADHD fail to respond to stimulants or respond adversely (806). In acute overdose, stimulants cause tics, which cease when the medication is stopped. The possibility that stimulant therapy can on rare occasions precipitate Tourette syndrome has been debated (807). If tics appear when stimulant therapy is begun, or if an existing tic disorder is aggravated by it, the medication should be discontinued. Approximately 50% of children with Tourette syndrome meet ADHD criteria, and one-third feel compulsions to perform risky acts (808,809). In up to one-half of these children, stimulant therapy exacerbates the tics (810). Desipramine or Risperidone are effective alternative treatments of symptoms in children with both ADHD and Tourette syndrome (811).

Dexedrine is preferred to the equally effective racemic amphetamine because it produces fewer side effects. The standard tablet is effective for 4 hours, but therapeutic effects can be distributed more evenly over time by using the longer-acting dextroamphetamine (Dexedrine Spansules). Any adverse effects are apparent within 3 days, and if these are worrisome, the dosage should be decreased or discontinued. If no change occurs at the initial dosage, an increase of 2.5 mg is introduced every 3 days until a favorable result occurs or until adverse effects supervene. Adverse effects are usually transient. Insomnia can be due to recurrence of hyperactivity after the stimulant has worn off or an effect of the stimulant itself. It can be controlled by adjusting dosage and timing. No long-term adverse effects have been substantiated. Stimulants may interfere with cartilage metabolism by inhibiting somatomedin-stimulated sulfate uptake by tissues (812). Nonetheless, the possibility that high dosages of stimulants retard growth (813) has not been confirmed (814,815, but see 816). The risk for substance abuse diminishes by as much as 50% in ADHD children who are receiving methylphenidate or amphetamine (817).

Methylphenidate probably inhibits receptor uptake of dopamine by blocking the dopamine transporter (DAT1) (818). A consensus group recommended that it be the first medication to use when treating ADHD (819). Optimal doses range between 10 and 50 mg per day (820). Methylphenidate is far more commonly used than dextroamphetamine. Both are effective, but are not necessarily effective in the same patients. The regimen is similar, but 5-mg doses are given in increments. Ideally, the drug is administered 30 minutes before meals because intestinal alkalinity is thought to degrade the product. The side effects are similar to, but less frequent than, those with dextroamphetamine. The long-acting methylphenidate preparation (Ritalin sustained release) is effective for approximately 6 hours. Other recently introduced long-acting methylphenidate preparations are trademarked as Concerta, Ritalin-LA, and Metadate CD. Their duration of action is in the 8 to 12 hour range, thereby reducing the variability of the stimulant effect and minimizing noncompliance. Scores on standardized IQ performance subscales may improve in some children who respond to methylphenidate, but stimulants do not treat comorbid learning disabilities. The drug assists performance by helping sustained attention, diminishing impulsiveness, and improving inhibition of hasty incorrect responses. Facility in creative thinking is unaffected (821). In some children, the medication improves motor control and handwriting. Methylphenidate can be used in ADHD children with seizure disorders. Double-blind medication and placebo crossover found that children whose seizure disorders had been well controlled on monotherapy did not relapse on methylphenidate, and their EEG tracings remained unchanged (822,823). The same applies for children with seizures and more severe underlying encephalopathy (824). A long-acting mixture of four amphetamine-based salts also is effective (825). Methylphenidate is also effective in adult ADHD, although brain activity remains abnormal (866).

The stimulant pemoline has a similar duration of action, similar beneficial effects on classroom behavior (826), and the additional advantage of lacking abuse potential. (Children with ADHD have not been reported to abuse their own prescribed stimulant medication.) Serum liver enzyme (aspartate aminotransferase/alanine aminotransferase) concentrations can be elevated during pemoline therapy (827). A few cases of liver failure attributed to pemoline have been reported (827,828).

Clonidine and guanfacine, α_2-adrenergic receptor agonists and antihypertensives, are alternative medications that ameliorate ADHD symptoms—in particular, the frequently associated aggression (829,830). Clonidine can cause cardiovascular complications, especially when combined with methylphenidate (831). Guanfacine appears to be less sedating and less apt to cause hypotension than clonidine, and it has a longer half-life (832). More recently, a norepinephrine reuptake inhibitor, atomoxetine, with a usual half-life of 5 hours, was found to ameliorate ADHD behavior (833,834). In preliminary studies, the benefits of atomoxetine and methylphenidate have been comparable (835), but a definitive comparative study has yet to appear. Theoretically, atomoxetine incurs less risk of leading to drug abuse, but this has not been demonstrated empirically. Atomoxetine may be beneficial in the treatment of nonresponders with the use of stimulants. Side effects such as anorexia and weight loss occur at frequencies comparable to methylphenidate. Acute liver failure is a rare complication.

Tricyclic antidepressants (836) or selective serotonin reuptake inhibitors (such as fluoxetine, sertraline, and paroxetine) (837) may assist in hyperactivity management, particularly in the presence of depressed affect (838). Barbiturates, used for antiepileptic therapy, have a sedative effect and aggravate hyperactivity (839). When this occurs, nonbarbiturate antiepileptic drugs should gradually be substituted. Methylxanthines such as caffeine and theophylline do not appear to have adverse behavioral effects in children. They may even have a mild positive effect on some externalizing behaviors (840).

Nonmedical Biological

Suggestions abound as to factors that might precipitate hyperactive behavior. These include fluorescent lighting; heavy metals; certain natural foods, notably sugar; and certain food additives, especially dyes. The most recent inconclusive claim is for attention problems due to prolonged television viewing (841). Food additives have been the most vigorously propagandized and therefore have been the most systematically studied (842).

Additive-free diets show little benefit in open clinical trials and even less in controlled studies. Although there is reliable evidence that an additive challenge in high dosage can impair learning in hyperactive children (843), an overview of available information suggests that restriction of additives is far less effective and less widely applicable than stimulant therapy. Nevertheless, it is occasionally worth trying. The most vigorous elimination diets appear to be the most successful (844,845), and desensitization to specific food substances also has been reported to be effective (846). An effect of sugar in rendering children irritable and restless has been reported anecdotally and in open trials but resists validation in controlled studies (847). A meta-analysis of 16 studies did not reveal any effect of sugar on children's behavior or cognition (848). The effects of sugar on brain function are complex and interact with whether a protein or carbohydrate meal preceded the challenge (849). A balance between factors promoting and opposing the availability of tryptophan as a serotonin substrate, carbohydrates versus amino acids, should be maintained. In contrast, megavitamin treatment and trace element replacement therapy are not supported by any acceptable evidence. There is no evidence that artificial sweeteners, such as aspartame, aggravate ADHD (850).

Nonmedical Behavioral

Short courses of supportive psychotherapy are often necessary for both the child and the child's family and can help to reduce intrafamily tensions that aggravate, or sometimes even precipitate, restless and impulsive behavior. A multimodality regime including intensive psychotherapy reduced the incidence of antisocial behavior in an ADHD cohort (851). However, in ADHD children without conduct disorder, adding multimodal psychosocial intervention did not further enhance the benefits of methylphenidate therapy (852). A recent study that compared ADHD children on stimulant therapy alone with children also afforded help through academic assistance, parent training, counseling, social skills training, and psychotherapy showed that a comprehensive outpatient treatment program for ADHD children is feasible and beneficial (853). For a detailed review of behavioral interventions, see Barkley (854).

Whereas underfocused, classically ADHD children benefit from the stimulative properties of many behavioral management techniques; the overfocused children do not. While the same structure and predictability that benefits ADHD children also benefits them, overfocused children do need less intrusive and confrontational approaches, the better to minimize their already excessive limbic arousal.

Rational management of children who are not relieved of their disability by medication rests on individual attention, frequent and consistent reward of socially acceptable behavior, consistent limit setting, and the gradual phasing in of material to be learned. Although it is possible to extinguish hyperactive behavior by operant conditioning, there is no evidence that this effect is lasting, that it generalizes, or that it is practicable to offer this labor-intensive individual management option to all but a few of the large number of ADHD children. In general, behavioral therapy should be an adjunct to effective stimulant therapy rather than the only treatment (855). Cognitive-behavioral therapy of ADHD is controversial (856,857), but parent training and school-based interventions may be effective (858,859). Children whose attentional, behavioral, or comorbid needs are not fully met by existing therapies are eligible for benefits under the Americans with Disabilities Act (860).

Prognosis

Whereas the overt restlessness of hyperactive children diminishes in adolescence, their impulsiveness and emotional lability usually persist, with a correspondingly mixed prognosis for long-term adaptive outcome. Long-term follow-up of children with ADHD shows an unfavorable outcome in many but not all. Adults who had ADHD in childhood often continue to show functional impairment (861). When aggressiveness is a feature, it particularly tends to persist (862) and appears to bear some association with early onset alcoholism (863). Impulsive aggressiveness is associated with low concentration of the serotonin metabolite 5-HIAA in cerebrospinal fluid (864). Thus, the ADHD prognosis is intermediate between that of control patients and the graver outlook for children with frank psychiatric disorder in childhood. Schizophrenia is not a major ADHD outcome. However, children of schizophrenic mothers, at high risk for adult schizophrenia, have been found to be prone to attentional dysfunction and poor social competence (789,865).

Attempts to relate the long-term prognosis of ADHD to psychoactive drug therapy have been so poorly controlled as to be uninterpretable. In the medium term, stimulant therapy is clearly beneficial for educational progress.

We gratefully acknowledge the contributions of Dr. William Graf, carried forward from the 2000 edition of this chapter.

REFERENCES

1. Giedd JN, Blumenthal J, Jeffries NO, et al. Brain development during childhood and adolescence: a longitudinal MRI study. *Nat Neurosci* 1999;2:861–863.
2. Luna B, Garver KE, Urban TA, et al. Maturation of cognitive processes from late childhood to adulthood. *Child Dev* 2004;75:1357–1372.
3. Bouchard TJ, Lykken DT, McGue M, et al. Sources of human psychological differences: the Minnesota study of twins reared apart. *Science* 1990;250:223–228.
4. Dickens WT, Flynn JR. Heritability estimates versus large environmental effects: the IQ paradox resolved. *Psychol Rev* 2001;108:346–369.
5. Andreasen NC, Flaum M, Swayze V 2nd, et al. Intelligence and brain structure in normal individuals. *Am J Psychiatry* 1993;150:130–134.
6. Gale CR, O'Callaghan FJ, Godfrey KM, et al. Critical periods of brain growth and cognitive function in children. *Brain* 2004;127:321–329.
7. Welsh MC, Pennington BF, Groisser DB. A normative-developmental study of executive function: a window on prefrontal function in children. *Dev Neuropsychology* 1991;7:131–149.
8. Bjork JM, Knutson B, Fong GW, et al. Incentive-elicited brain activation in adolescents: similarities and differences from young adults. *J Neurosci* 2004;24:1793–1802.
9. Denckla MB. Development of motor coordination in normal children. *Dev Med Child Neurol* 1974;16:729–741.
10. Kinsbourne M. Development of attention and metacognition. In: Rapin I, Segalowitz S, eds. *Handbook of Neuropsychology*. Amsterdam: Elsevier Science, 1993:261–278.
11. Mikkelsen EJ, Brown GL, Minichiello MD, et al. Neurological status in hyperactive, enuretic, encopretic, and normal boys. *J Am Acad Child Psychiatry* 1982;21:75–81.
12. Shaffer SQ, Stockman CJ, Shaffer D. Ten-year consistency in neurological test performance of children without focal neurological deficits. *Dev Med Child Neurol* 1986;28:417–427.
13. Woods BT, Eby MD. Excessive mirror movements and aggression. *Biol Psychiatry* 1982;17:23–32.
14. Rao MR, Brenner RA, Schisterman EF, et al. Long-term cognitive development in children with prolonged crying. *Arch Dis Childhood* 2004;89:989–992.
15. Rutter M. Syndromes attributed to "minimal brain dysfunction" in childhood. *Am J Psychiatry* 1982;139:21–33.
16. Gillberg C. Deficits in attention, motor control and perception: a brief review. *Arch Dis Child* 2003;88:904–910.
17. Gillberg C, Rasmussen P. Perceptual, motor and attentional deficits in seven-year-old children. Background factors. *Dev Med Child Neurol* 1982;24:752–770.
18. Piek JP, Dyek MJ, Nieman A, et al. The relationship between motor coordination, executive functioning and attention in school-aged children. *Arch Clin Neuropsychol* 2004;19:1063–1076.
19. Shevell MI, Majnemer A, Rosenbaum P, et al. Etiological determination of childhood developmental delay. *Brain Dev* 2001;23:228–235.
20. Wuu KD, Chin PC, Li SY. Chromosomal and biochemical screening of mentally retarded school children in Taiwan. *Japan J Hum Genet* 1991;36:267–274.
21. Allen WP, Taylor H. Mental retardation in South Carolina. VII. Inborn errors of metabolism. *Proc Greenwood Genet Ctr* 1996;15:76–79.
22. Schaefer GB, Bodensteiner JB. Evaluation of the child with idiopathic mental retardation. *Pediatr Clin North Am* 1992;39:929–943.
23. Levy SE, Hyman SL. Pediatric assessment of the child with developmental delay. *Pediatr Clin North Am* 1993;40:465–477.
24. First LR, Palfrey JS. The infant or young child with developmental delay. *N Engl J Med* 1994;330:478–483.
25. Curry CJ, Sandhu A, Fritos L, et al. Diagnostic yield of genetic evaluations in developmental delay/mental retardation. *Clin Res* 1996;44:130A.
26. Martin E, Boesch C, Zuerrer M, et al. MR imaging of brain maturation in normal and developmentally handicapped children. *J Comput Assist Tomogr* 1990;14:685–692.
27. Squires L, Krishnamoorthy KS, Natowitz MR. Delayed myelination in infants and young children: radiographic and clinical correlates. *J Child Neurology* 1995;10:100–104.
28. Moeschler J. The use of the CT scan in the medical evaluation of the mentally retarded child. *J Pediatr* 1981;98:63–65.
29. Lingham S, Kendall BE. Computed tomography in non-specific mental retardation and idiopathic epilepsy. *Arch Dis Child* 1983;58:628–643.
30. Root S, Carey JC. *Brain dysmorphology and developmental disabilities*. Proceedings of the Annual DW Smith Workshop on Malformation and Morphogenesis, 1996.
31. Kjos BO, Umansky R, Barkovich AJ. Brain MR imaging in children with developmental retardation of unknown cause: results in 76 cases. *Am J Neuroradiol* 1990;11:1035–1040.
32. O'Tuama LA, Dickstein DP, Neeper R, et al. Functional brain imaging in neuropsychiatric disorders of childhood. *J Child Neurol* 1999;14:207–221.
33. Filipek PA, Semrud-Clikeman M, Steingard RJ, et al. Volumetric MRI analysis comparing subjects having attention-deficit hyperactivity disorder with normal controls. *Neurology* 1997;48:589–601.
34. Prensky AL. An approach to the child with paroxysmal phenomena with emphasis on nonepileptic disorders. In: Dodson WE, Pellock JM, eds. *Pediatric epilepsy: diagnosis and therapy*. New York: Demos Publications, 1993.
35. Fedio P, Mirsky AF. Selective intellectual deficits in children with temporal lobe or centrencephalic epilepsy. *Neuropsychologia* 1969;7:287–300.
36. Stores G, Hart J, Piran N. Inattentiveness in school children with epilepsy. *Epilepsia* 1978;19:169–175.
37. Hernandez MT, Sauerwein HC, Jambaque I, et al. Deficits in executive functions and motor coordination in children with frontal lobe epilepsy. *Neuropsychologia* 2002;40:384–400.
38. Jambaque I, Lassonde M, Dulac O. *The neuropsychology of childhood epilepsy*. New York: Plenum, 1999.
39. www.whatworks.ed.gov
40. Coplan J, Gleason JR. Quantifying language development from birth to 3 years using the Early Language Milestone scale. *Pediatrics* 1990;86:963–971.
41. Frankenburg WK, Dodds J, Archer P, et al. The Denver II: a major revision and restandardization of the Denver Developmental Screening test. *Pediatrics* 1992;89:91–97.
42. Newborg J, Stock JR, Wnek L. *Batelle developmental inventory*. Allen, TX: DLM Teaching Resources, 1984.
43. Bayley N. *Bayley Scales of Infant Development II*. New York: The Psychological Corporation, 1993.
44. Wechsler D. *Wechsler preschool and primary scale of intelligence—revised*. New York: Psychological Corporation, 1989.
45. Wechsler D. *Wechsler intelligence scale for children*—III. New York: Psychological Corporation, 1991.
46. Thorndike RL, Hagen EP, Samer JM. *Guide for administering and scoring the Stanford-Binet Intelligence Scale*, 4th ed. Chicago: Riverside Publishing, 1986.
47. Goodenough FL, Harris DB. *Manual of the Goodenough-Harris drawing test*. San Antonio: Psychological Corporation, 1963.
48. Kaufman AS, Kaufman NL. Kaufman assessment battery for children. Circle Paines, NM: American Guidance Services, 1983.
49. McCarthy D. *Manual of the McCarthy scales of children's disabilities*. San Antonio: Psychological Corporation, 1972.

50. Leiter RG. *The Leiter International Performance scale*. California: Western Psychological Services, 1969.
51. Achenbach TM. *Manual for the Child Behavior Checklist/2–3 and 1992 profile*. Burlington, VT: University of Vermont Department of Psychiatry, 1992.
52. Conners CK. *Manual for Conners rating scales*. North Tonawanda, NY: Multi-Health Systems, 1989.
53. Sparrow SS, Balla DA, Ciccheui DV. *Vineland adaptive behavior scales*. Circle Pines, MN: American Guidance Services, 1985.
54. Wilkinson GS. *The wide range achievement test—revision 3, administration manual*. Wilmington, DE: Wide Range, 1993.
55. Woodcock RW, Mather N. *Woodcock-Johnson tests of achievement*. Allen, TX: DLM Teaching Resources, 1989.
56. Dunn LM, Dunn LM. *Peabody picture vocabulary test—revised*. Circle Pines, MN: American Guidance Services, 1981.
57. Beery KE. *The developmental test of visual-motor integration*, 3rd rev. Cleveland: Modern Curriculum Press, 1989.
58. Lyon GR, Fletcher JM, Shaywitz SE. Rethinking learning disabilities. In: Finn CE Jr, Rotherham AJ, Hokanson CR Jr, eds. *Rethinking special education for a new century*. Washington, DC: Thomas B. Fordham Foundation and the Progressive Policy Institute, 2001:259–287.
59. McQuaid F, Alovisetti M. School psychological services for hearing-impaired children in New York and the New England area. *Am Ann Deaf* 1981;126:37–43.
60. Davis CJ. *Perkins-Binet test of intelligence for the blind*. Watertown, MA: Perkins School for the Blind, 1980.
61. Newland TE. The blind learning aptitude test. *J Vis Impair Blind* 1979;73:134–139.
62. Petersen MC, Kube DA, Palmer FB. Classification of developmental delays. *Semin Pediatr Neurol* 1998;5:2–14.
63. World Health Organization. *The ICD-10: classification of mental and behavioural disorders: clinical descriptions and diagnostic guidelines*. Geneva: World Health Organization, 1992.
64. American Association on Mental Retardation. *Mental retardation: definition, classification, and systems of support*, 9th ed. Washington, DC: American Association on Mental Retardation, 1992.
65. American Psychiatric Association. *Diagnostic criteria from DSM-IV: diagnostic and statistical manual of mental disorders*. Washington, DC: American Psychiatric Association, 1994:63–66.
66. Hunt E. Will we be smart enough: cognitive changes in the coming workforce. New York: Russell Sage Foundation, 1995.
67. Hunter JE. Cognitive ability, cognitive aptitudes, job knowledge and job performance. *J Vocatl Behav* 1986;29:340–362.
68. Grossman H. *Manual on terminology and classification in mental retardation*. Washington, DC: American Association of Mental Retardation, 1973.
69. Reschly JD. Mental retardation: conceptual foundations, definitional criteria, and diagnostic operations. In: Hooper SR, Hynd GH, Mattison RE, eds. *Developmental disorders: diagnostic criteria and clinical assessment*. Hillsdale, NJ: Lawrence Erlbaum Associates, 1992:23–67.
70. Luckasson R, Borthwick-Duffy S. *Mental retardation: definition, classification, and systems of support*. Washington, DC: American Association on Mental Retardation, 1992.
71. Mattis S. Neuropsychological assessment of school-aged children. In: Rapin I, Segalowitz SJ, eds. *Handbook of neuropsychology*, Vol. 6. *Child neuropsychology*. Amsterdam: Elsevier, 1992:395–415.
72. Cattell RB, Cattell AKS. *Handbook for the Culture-Fair Intelligence Test, Scale 2*. Champaign, IL: Institute for Personality and Ability Testing, 1973.
73. Raven JC, Court JH, Raven J. *Manual for Raven's Progressive Matrices and Vocabulary Scales*. Oxford, UK: Oxford Psychologists' Press, 1996.
74. Bracken BA, McCallum RS. *The Universal Nonverbal Intelligence Test*. Chicago, IL, Riverside, 1997.
75. Carey JC, McMahon WM. Neurobehavioral disorders and medical genetics: an overview. In: Goldstein S, Reynolds CR, eds. *Handbook of neurodevelopmental and genetic disorders in children*. New York: Guilford, 1999:38–60.
76. Jones KL. *Smith's recognizable patterns of human malformation*, 5th ed. Philadelphia: Saunders, 1997.
77. Turk J, Hill P. Behavioral phenotypes in dysmorphic syndromes. *Clin Dysmorphol* 1995;4:105–115.
78. Udwin O. A survey of adults with Williams syndrome and idiopathic infantile hypercalcemia. *Dev Med Child Neurol* 1990;32:129–136.
79. Gabel S, Tarter RE, Gavaler J, et al. Neuropsychological capacity of Prader-Willi children: general and specific aspects of impairment. *Appl Res Ment Retard* 1996;7:459–466.
80. Dykens EM, Hodapp RM, Evans DW. Profiles and development of adaptive behavior in children with Down syndrome. *Am J Ment Retard* 1994;98:580–587.
81. Carlesimo GB, Marotta L, Vicari S. Long-term memory in mental retardation: evidence for a specific impairment in subjects with Down syndrome. *Neuropsychologia* 1997;35:71–79.
82. Spano M, Mercuri E, Rando T, et al. Motor and perceptual-motor competence in children with Down syndrome: variation in performance with age. *Eur J Paediatr Neurol* 1999;3:7–13.
83. Rasmussen P, Borjesson O, Wentz E, et al. Autistic disorders in Down syndrome: background factors and clinical correlates. *Dev Med Child Neurol* 2001;43:750–754.
84. Carr J. *Down's syndrome: children growing up*. Cambridge: Cambridge University Press, 1995.
85. Dennis M, Jacennik B, Barnes MA. The content of narrative discourse in children and adolescents after early-onset hydrocephalus and in normally developing age peers. *Brain Lang* 1994;46:129–165.
85a. Hessl Y, Rivera S, Reiss AL. The neuroanatomy and neuroendocrinology of Fragile X Syndrome. *Mental Retardation and Develop Disabilities Research Reviews* 2004;10:17–24.
86. Wisniewski KE, French JH, Fernando S, et al. Fragile-X syndrome: associated neurological abnormality and developmental disabilities. *Ann Neurol* 1985;18:665–669.
87. Pennington B, Puck M, Robinson A. Language and cognitive development in 47 XXX females followed since birth. *Behav Genet* 1980;10:31–41.
88. Rovet JF. The psychoeducational characteristics of children with Turner's syndrome. *J Learn Disabil* 1993;26:333–341.
89. Lawrence K, Kuntsi J, Coleman M, et al. Face and emotion recognition deficits in Turner syndrome: a possible role for X-linked genes in amygdala development. *Neuropsychology* 2003;17:39–49.
90. Rovet J, Netley C, Keenan M, et al. The psychoeducational profile of boys with Klinefelter Syndrome. *J Learn Disabil* 1996;29:180–196.
91. Stefanatos GA, Musikoff H. Specific neurocognitive deficits in Cornelia de Lange syndrome. *J Dev Behav Pediatr* 1994;15:39–43.
92. Antshel KM, Waisbren SE. Timing is everything: executive functions in children exposed to elevated levels of phenylalanine. *Neuropsychology* 2003;17:458–468.
93. Diamond A, Prevor M, Callender G, et al. Prefrontal cortex cognitive deficits in children treated early and continuously for PKU. *Monogr Soc Res Child Dev* 1997;62:i–v, 1–208.
94. Channon S, German E, Cassina C, et al. Executive functioning, memory and learning in phenylketonuria. *Neuropsychology* 2004;18:613–620.
95. Rovet JF. Long-term neuropsychological sequelae of early-treated congenital hypothyroidism. Effects in adolescence. *Acta Pediatrica* 1999;88:88–95.
96. Antshel KM, Epstein IO, Waisbren SE. Cognitive strengths and weaknesses in children and adolescents homozygous for the galactosemia Q188R mutation: a descriptive study. *Neuropsychology* 2004;18:658–664.
97. Dykens EM, Rosner BA. Refining behavioral phenotypes: personality-motivation in Williams and Prader-Willi syndromes. *Am J Ment Retard* 1999;104:158–169.
98. Stojanovik V, Perkins M, Howard S. Williams syndrome and specific language impairment do not support claims for developmental double dissociations and innate modularity. *J Neuroling* 2004;17:403–424.
99. Pinker S. *Words and rules*. London: Weidenfeld and Nicolson, 1999.
100. Rutter M, Graham P, Yule W. A neuropsychiatric study in childhood. *Clin Dev Med* 1970;35/36:1–272.
101. Borthwick-Duffy SA. Epidemiology and prevalence of psychopathology in people with mental retardation. *J Consult Clin Psychol* 1994;62:17–27.
102. Bregman JD. Current developments in the understanding of mental retardation: Part II. Psychopathology. *J Am Acad Child Adolesc Psychiatry* 1991;30:861–872.

103. Crews WDJ, Bonaventura S, Rowe F. Dual diagnosis: prevalence of psychiatric disorders in a large state residential facility for individuals with mental retardation. *Am J Ment Retard* 1994;98:724–731.
104. Gillberg C, Persson E, Grufman M, et al. Psychiatric disorders in mildly and severely mentally retarded urban children and adolescents: epidemiological aspects. *Br J Psychiatry* 1986;149:68–74.
105. Matson JL, Barrett RP, Helsel WJ. Depression in mentally retarded children. *Res Dev Disabil* 1988;9:39–46.
106. Dawson JE, Matson JL, Cherry KE. An analysis of maladaptive behaviors in persons with autism, PDD-NOS, and mental retardation. *Res Dev Disabil* 1998;19:439–448.
107. Gath H, Gumley D. Behavior problems in retarded children with special reference to Down syndrome. *Br J Psychiatry* 1986;149:156–161.
108. Matson JL, Hamilton M, Duncan D, et al. Characteristics of stereotypic movement disorder and self-injurious behavior assessed with the Diagnostic Assessment for the Severely Handicapped (DASH-II). *Res Dev Disabil* 1997;18:457–469.
109. Buitelaar JK. Self-injurious behavior in retarded children: clinical phenomena and biological mechanisms. *Acta Paedopsychiatrica* 1993;56:105–111.
110. Carr KG, Smith CE. Biological setting events for self-injury. *MRDD Research Reviews* 1995;1.
111. Anderson LT, Ernst M. Self-injury in Lesch-Nyhan disease. *J Autism Dev Disord* 1994;24:67–81.
112. Matthews WS, Solan A, Barabas G. Cognitive functioning in Lesch-Nyhan syndrome. *Dev Med Child Neurol* 1995;37:715–722.
113. Whitman BY, Accardo P. Emotional symptoms in Prader-Willi syndrome adolescents. *Am J Med Genet* 1987;28:897–905.
114. Curfs LM, Fryos JP. Prader-Willi syndrome: a review with special attention to the cognitive and behavioral profile. *Birth Defects: Original Article Series* 1992;28:99–104.
115. Hagberg B. Rett syndrome: clinical peculiarities and biological mysteries. *Acta Paediatrica* 1995;84:971–976.
116. Papolos DF, Faedda GL, Veit S, et al. Bipolar spectrum disorders in patients diagnosed with velo-cardiofacial syndrome: does a hemizygous deletion of chromosome 22q11 result in bipolar affective disorder? *Am J Psychiatry* 1996;153:1541–1547.
117. Motzkin B, Marion R, Goldberg R, et al. Variable phenotypes in velocardiofacial syndrome with chromosomal deletion. *J Pediatr* 1993;123:406–410.
118. Udwin O, Yule W. Expressive language of children with Williams syndrome. *Am J Med Genet* 1990;6:108–114.
119. Rossen ML, Samat HB. Why should neurologists be interested in Williams syndrome? [Editorial] *Neurology* 1998;5:8–9.
120. Marcus LC, Keens GT, Bautista BD, et al. Obstructive sleep apnea in children with Down Syndrome. *Pediatrics* 1991;88:132–139.
121. Andreou G, Galanopoulou C, Gourgoulianis K, et al. Cognitive status in Down syndrome individuals with sleep disordered breathing deficits (SDB). *Brain Cogn* 2002;50:145–149.
122. Ohayon MM. The effects of breathing-related sleep disorders on mood disturbances in the general population. *J Clin Psychiatry* 2003;64:1195–1200.
123. Bassett AS, Hodgkinson K, Chow EWC, et al. 22q11 deletion syndrome in adults with schizophrenia. *Am J Med Genet* 1998;81:328–337.
124. Gothelf D, Gruber R, Pesburger G, et al. Methylphenidate treatment for attention-deficit/hyperactivity disorder of children and adults with velocardiofacial syndrome: an open label study. *J Clin Psychiatry* 2003;64:1163–1169.
125. McAuley E, Ross R, Kushner H, et al. Self-esteem and behavior in girls with Turner syndrome. *J Dev Behav Ped* 1995;16:82–88.
126. Ernst M, Zametkin AJ, Matochik JA, et al. Presynaptic dopaminergic deficits in Lesch-Nyhan disease. *N Engl J Med* 1996;334:1568–1572.
127. Down syndrome prevalence at birth: United States 1983–1990. *MMWR Morb Mortal Wkly Rep* 1994;43:617–622.
128. Steele J, Stratford B. The United Kingdom population with Down syndrome: present and future projections. *Am J Ment Retard* 1995;99:664–682.
129. Strømme P, Valvatne K. Mental retardation in Norway: prevalence and sub-classification in a cohort of 30,037 children born between 1980 and 1985. *Acta Paediatr* 1998;87:291–296.
130. Hagberg B, Hagberg G, Lewerth A, et al. Mild mental retardation in Swedish school children. II. Etiologic and pathogenetic aspects. *Acta Paediatr Scand* 1981;70:445–452.
131. Murphy CC, Yeargin-Allsopp M, Decoufle P, et al. The administrative prevalence of mental retardation in 10-year-old children in Atlanta, 1985 through 1987. *Am J Public Health* 1995;85:319–323.
132. Brett EM, Goodman R. Mental retardation, infantile autism, and related disorders. In: Brett EM, ed. *Paediatric neurology*. London: Churchill Livingstone, 1997:406–423.
133. McLaren J, Bryson SE. Review of recent epidemiological studies of mental retardation: prevalence, associated disorders, and etiology. *Am J Ment Retard* 1987;92:243–254.
134. Eyman RK, Grossman HJ, Chaney RH, et al. Survival of profoundly disabled people with severe mental retardation. *Am J Dis Child* 1993;147:329–336.
135. Plioplys AV, Kasnocka I, Lewis S, et al. Survival rates among children with severe neurological disabilities. *South Med J* 1998;19:161–172.
136. Shevell M, Ashwal S, Donley D, et al. Practice parameter: evaluation of the child with global developmental delay. *Neurology* 2003;11:367–380.
137. Gustavson KH, Hagberg B, Hagberg G, et al. Severe mental retardation in a Swedish county. II. Etiologic and pathogenetic aspects of children born 1959–1970. *Neuropaediatrie* 1977;8:293–304.
138. Nelson KB. What proportion of cerebral palsy is related to birth asphyxia? *J Pediatr* 1988;112:572–573.
139. Gaffney G, Sellers S, Flavell V, et al. Case-control study of intrapartum care, cerebral palsy, and perinatal death. *BMJ* 1994;308:743–750.
140. Torfs CP, van den Berg B, Oechsli FW, et al. Prenatal and perinatal factors in the etiology of cerebral palsy. *J Pediatr* 1990;116:615–619.
141. Watemberg N, Silver S, Harel S, et al. Significance of microcephaly among children with developmental disabilities. *J Child Neurol* 2002;17:117–122.
142. McAnulty GB, Hicks RE, Kinsbourne M. Personal and familial sinistrality in relation to degree of mental retardation. *Brain Cogn* 1984;3:349–356.
143. Laxova R, Ridler MAC. An etiologic survey of the severely retarded Hertfordshire children who were born between January 1, 1965 and December 31, 1967. *Am J Med Genet* 1977;1:75–86.
144. Opitz JM, Kaveggia EG, Laxova R, et al. *The diagnosis and prevention of severe mental retardation*. Proceedings, lnternational Conference on Preventable Aspects of Genetic Morbidity, 1982, Cairo, ll.
145. Fryns JP, Kleczkowska A, Dereymaeker A, et al. A genetic diagnostic survey in an institutionalized population of 173 severely mentally retarded patients. *Clin Genet* 1986;30:315–323.
146. McQueen PC, Spence MW, Winsor EJ, et al. Causal origins of major mental handicap in the Canadian mountain provinces. *Dev Med Child Neurol* 1986;28:697–707.
147. Wellesley D, Hockey A, Stenely F. The aetiology of intellectual disability in westem Australia: a community-based study. *Dev Med Child Neurol* 1991;33:963–973.
148. Yeargin-Allsopp M, Murphy CC, Cordero JF, et al. Reported biomedical causes and associated medical conditions for mental retardation among 10-year-old children, metropolitan Atlanta, 1985 to 1987. *Dev Med Child Neurol* 1997;39:142–149.
149. Flint J, Wilkie AO. The genetics of mental retardation. *Br Med Bull* 1996;52:453–464.
150. Mirrett PL, Bailey DB, Roberts JE, et al. Developmental screening and detection of developmental delays in infants and toddlers with fragile X syndrome. *J Dev Behav Ped* 2004;25:21–27.
151. Mutch L, Leyland A, McGee A. Patterns of neuropsychological function in a low birth weight population. *Dev Med Child Neurol* 1993;35:943–956.
152. Breslau N, Paneth NS, Lucia VC. The lingering academic deficits of low birth weight children. *Pediatrics* 2004;114:1035–1040.
153. Vicari S, Caravale B, Carlesimo GA, et al. Spatial working memory in children at ages 3–4 who were low birth weight preterm infants. *Neuropsychology* 2004;18:673–678.
154. Hopkins-Golightly T, Raz S, Sander CJ. Influence of slight to moderate risk for birth anoxia on acquisition of cognitive and language function in the pretern infant: a cross-sectional comparison with preterm-birth controls. *Neuropsychology* 2003;17:3–13.
155. Short EJ, Klein NK, Lewis BA, et al. Cognitive and academic

consequences of bronchopulmonary dysplasia and very low birth weight: 8-year-old outcomes. *Pediatrics* 2003;112:e359.

156. Casaer P, de Vries L, Marlow N. Prenatal and perinatal risk factors for psychological development. In: M Rutter, P Casaer, eds. *Biological risk factors for psychosocial disorders*. Cambridge: Cambridge University Press, 1991:139–174.
157. Johnston MV, Trescher WH, Taylor GA. Hypoxic and ischemic nervous system disorders in infants and children. *Adv Pediatr* 1995;42:1–45.
158. Foulder-Hughes LA, Cooke RW. Motor, cognitive and behavioural disorders in children born very preterm. *Dev Med Child Neurol* 2003;45:97–103.
159. Williams CE, Gunn AJ, Mallard C, et al. Outcome after ischemia in the developing sheep brain: an electroencephalographic and histological study. *Ann Neurol* 1992;31:14–21.
160. Taylor HG, Minich N, Bangert B, et al. Long-term neuropsychological outcomes of very low birth weight: associations with early risks for periventricular brain insults. *J Int Neuropsychol Soc* 2004;10:987–1004.
161. Hunt CE, Corwin MJ, Baird T, et al. Cardiorespiratory events detected by home monitoring and one year neurodevelopmental outcome. *J Pediatr* 2004;145:465–471.
162. Gottlieb DL, Chase C, Vezina RM, et al. Sleep-disordered breathing symptoms are associated with poorer cognitive function in 5-year-old children. *J Pediatr* 2004;145:458–464.
163. Dowdeswell HJ, Slater AM, Broomhall J, et al. Visual deficits in children born at less than 32 weeks' gestation with and without major ocular pathology and cerebral damage. *Br J Ophthalmol* 1995;79:447–452.
164. Isaacs EB, Lucas A, Chong WK, et al. Hippocampal volume and everyday memory in children of very low birth weight. *Pediatr Res* 2000;47:713–720.
165. Nosarti C, Al-Asady MH, Frangou S, et al. Adolescents who were born very preterm have decreased brain volumes. *Brain* 2002; 125:1616–1623.
166. Peterson BS, Anderson AW, Ehrenkrantz R, et al. Regional brain volumes and their later neurodevelopmental correlates in term and preterm infants. *Pediatrics* 2003;111:939–948.
167. Christ SE, White DA, Brunstrom JE, et al. Inhibitory control following perinatal brain injury. *Neuropsychology* 2003;17: 171–178.
168. Vargha-Khadem F, Isaacs E, van der Werf S, et al. Development of intelligence and memory in children with hemiplegic cerebral palsy. The deleterious consequences of early seizures. *Brain* 1992;115:315–329.
169. Stiles J. Neural plasticity and cognitive development. *Dev Neuropsychol* 2000;18:237–272.
170. Breslau N, Chilcoat HD. Psychiatric sequelae of low birth weight at 11 years of age. *Biol Psychiatry* 2000;47:1005–1011.
171. Max JE, Mathews K, Manes FF, et al. Attention deficit hyperactivity disorder and neurocognitive correlates after childhood stroke. *J Int Neuropsychol Soc* 2003;9:815–829.
172. Gross-Tsur V, Shalev RS, Badihi N, et al. Efficacy of methylphenidate in patients with cerebral palsy and attention-deficit hyperactivity disorder (ADHD). *J Child Neurol* 2002;17:863–866.
173. Stratton K, Howe C, Bataglia F. *Fetal alcohol syndrome: diagnosis, epidemiology and treatment*. Washington, DC: National Academy Press, 1996.
174. Frank DA, Augustyn M, Knight WG, et al. Growth, development and behavior in early childhood following prenatal cocaine exposure: a systematic review. *JAMA* 2001;285:1613–1625.
175. Brown JV, Bakeman R, Coles CD, et al. Prenatal cocaine exposure: a comparison of 2-year-old children in parental and non-parental care. *Child Dev* 2004;1282–1295.
176. Christianson AL, Chesler N, Kromberg JGR. Fetal valproate syndrome: clinical and neuro-developmental features in two sibling pairs. *Devel Med Child Neurol* 1994;36:361–369.
177. Bellinger DC. Lead. *Pediatrics* 2004;113:1016–1022.
178. Schroeder SR, Hawk B, Otto DA, et al. Separating the effects of lead and social factors on IQ. *Environ Res* 1985;38:144–154.
179. Pocock SJ, Smith M, Baghurst P. Environmental lead and children's intelligence: a systematic review of the epidemiological literature. *BMJ* 1994;309:1189.
180. Kaufman AS. Do low levels of lead produce IQ loss in children? A careful examination of the literature. *Arch Clin Neuropsychology* 2001;6:403–431.
181. Needleman HL, Bellinger D. Studies of lead exposure and the developing central nervous system. A reply to Kaufman. *Arch Clin Neuropsychology* 2001;6:359–374.
182. Lanphear BP, Dietrich K, Auinger P, et al. Cognitive deficits associated with blood lead concentrations <10 ug/dl in US children and adolescents. *Public Health Report* 2000;115:521–529.
183. Canfield RL, Henderson CR, Cory-Slechta DA, et al. Intellectual impairment in children with blood lead concentrations below 10 ug per deciliter. *N Engl J Med* 2003;348:1517–1526.
184. Minder B, Das-Smaal EA, Orlebeke JF. Cognition in children does not suffer from very low lead exposure. *J Learn Disabil* 1998;31: 494–502.
185. Stone BM, Reynolds CR. Can the National Health and Nutrition Examination Survey III (NHANES III) data help resolve the controversy over low lead levels and neuropsychological development in children? *Arch Clinical Neuropsychology* 2003;18:219–244.
186. O'Carroll RE, Masterton G, Dougall N, et al. The neuropsychiatric sequelae of mercury poisoning. The mad hatter's disease revisited. *Brit J Psychiatry* 1995;167:95–98.
187. Warkany J, Hubbard DM. Acrodynia and mercury. *J Pediatrics* 1953;42:365–386.
188. National Research Council. *Toxicological effects of methylmercury*. Washington, DC: National Academy Press, 2000.
189. Takeuchi T, Eto K. *The pathology of Minimata disease*. Japan: Fukuoka Kyushi University Press, 1999.
190. Fukuda Y, Ushijima K, Kitano T, et al. An analysis of subjective complaints in a population living in a methylmercury-polluted area. *Environ Res* 1999;81:100–107.
191. Bakir F, Rustam H, Tikriti S, et al. Clinical and epidemiological aspects of methylmercury poisoning. *Postgrad Med J* 1980;56:1–10.
192. Davis LE, Kornfeld M, Mooney HS, et al. Methylmercury poisoning: long-term clinical, radiological, toxicological, and pathological studies of an affected family. *Ann Neurol* 1994;35:680–688.
193. Myers GJ, Davidson PW. Prenatal methylmercury exposure and children: neurologic, developmental, and behavioral research. *Environ Health Perspect* 1998;3:841–847.
194. Grandjean P, Weihe P, White RF, et al. Cognitive performance of children prenatally exposed to "safe" levels of methylmercury. *Environ Res A* 1998;77:165–172.
195. Weiss B, Clarkson TW, Simon W. Silent latency periods in methylmercury poisoning and in neurodegenerative disease. *Environ Health Perspect* 2002;5:851–854.
196. Jacobson JL, Jacobson SW. Prenatal exposure to polychlorinated biphenyls and attention at school age. *J Pediatr* 2003;143(6):780–788.
197. Vreugdenhil HJ, Lanting CI, Mulder PG, et al. Effects of prenatal PCB and dioxin background exposure on cognitive and motor abilities in Dutch children at school age. *J Pediatr* 2002;140: 48–56.
198. Eskenazi B, Bradman A, Castorina R. Exposures of children to organophosphate pesticides and their potential adverse health effects. *Environ Health Perspect* 1999;107:409–419.
199. Miller RW. Delayed radiation effects in atomic bomb survivors. *Science* 1969;166:569–574.
200. Dekaban AS. Abnormalities in children exposed to x-radiation and during various stages of gestation: tentative timetable of radiation injury to the human fetus, Part I. *J Nucl Med* 1968;9:471–477.
201. Uchida IA, Holunga R, Lawler C. Maternal radiation and chromosomal aberrations. *Lancet* 1968;2:1045–1049.
202. Lozoff B. Nutrition and behavior. *Am Psychol* 1989;44:231–236.
203. Bronfenbrenner U, McClelland PD, Ceci S, et al. *The state of Americans*. New York: The Free Press, 1996.
204. Kiely M. The prevalence of mental retardation. *Epidemiol Rev* 1987;9:194–228.
205. Roeleveld N, Zielhuis GA, Gabreels F. The prevalence of mental retardation: a critical review of recent literature. *Dev Med Child Neurol* 1997;39:125–132.
206. Patterson CJ, Kupersmidt JB, Vaden NA. Income level, gender, ethnicity, and household composition as predictors of children's school-based competence. *Child Dev* 1990;61:485–494.
207. Aber JL, Bennett NG, Conley DC, et al. The effects of poverty

on child health and development. *Annu Rev Public Health* 1997;18: 463–483.
208. Ramer JC, Miller G. Overview of mental retardation. In: Miller G, Ramer JC, eds. *Static encephalopathies of infancy and childhood.* New York: Raven Press, 1992:1–10.
208a. National Institute of Child Health and Human Development Early Child Care Research Network. Duration and developmental timing of children's cognitive and social development from birth through third grade. *Child Develop* 2005;76:795–810.
209. Kim-Cohen J, Moffitt TE, Caspi A, et al. Genetic and environmental processes in young children's resilience and vulnerability to socioeconomic deprivation. *Child Dev* 2004;75:651–668.
210. Spitz RA. Hospitalism. *Psychoanal Stud Child* 1945;1:53–74.
211. Gunnar MR. Effects of early deprivation: findings from orphanage-reared infants and children. In: Nelson CA, Luciani M, eds. *Handbook of developmental cognitive neuroscience*. Cambridge, MA: MIT Press, 2001:617–630.
212. Zeanah CH, Nelson CA, Fox NA, et al. Designing research to study the effects of institutionalization on brain and behavior development: the Bucharest Early Intervention Program. *Dev Psychopathol* 2003;15:885–907.
213. Chisholm K. A three-year follow-up of attachment and indiscriminate friendliness in children adopted from Romanian orphanages. *Child Dev* 1998;69:1092–1106.
214. Chugani HT, Behen ME, Muzik O, et al. Local brain functional activity following early deprivation: a study of postinstitutionalized Romanian orphans. *Neuroimage* 2001;14:290–301.
215. Marshall PJ, Fox NA, BEIP Core Group. A comparison of the electroencephalogram between institutionalized and community children in Romania. *J Cogn Neurosci* 2004;16:1327–1338.
216. Haddow JE, Palomaki GE, Allan WC, et al. Maternal thyroid deficiency during pregnancy and subsequent neuropsychological development of the child. *N Engl J Med* 1999;341:549–555.
217. Kovacs M, Goldstone D, Iyengar S. Intellectual development and academic performance of children with insulin-dependent diabetes mellitus: a longitudinal study. *Dev Psychol* 1992;28:676–684.
218. Grantham-McGregor SM, Ani C. A review of studies on the effect of iron deficiency on cognitive development in children. *J Nutr* 2001;131:649S–668S.
219. Halterman JS, Kaczorowsky JM, Aligne CA, et al. Iron deficiency and cognitive achievement among school-aged children and adolescents in the United States. *Pediatrics*107:1381–1386.
220. Aman MG, Kern RA, McGhee DE, et al. Fenfluramine and methylphenidate in children with mental retardation and ADHD: clinical and side effects. *J Am Acad Child Adolesc Psychiatry* 1993;32:851–859.
221. Campbell M, Cueva JE. Psychopharmacology in child and adolescent psychiatry: a review of the past seven years, Part I. *J Am Acad Child Adolesc Psychiatry* 1995;34:1124–1132.
222. Herman BH, Hammock MK, Arthur-Smith A, et al. Naltrexone decreases self-injurious behavior. *Ann Neurol* 1987;22:550–552.
223. Barnes TR. Tardive dyskinesia. *BMJ* 1988;296:150–151.
224. Swanson JM, Christian DL, Wigal T, et al. Tardive dyskinesia in a developmentally disabled population: manifestation during the initial stage of a minimal effective-dose program. *Exp Clin Psychopharmacol* 1996;4:1–6.
225. Ottenbacher K, Petersen P. The efficacy of early intervention programs for children with organic handicaps. *Eval Prog Plan* 1985;8:135.
226. Dodrill CB. Neuropsychology. In: Laidlaw J, Richens A, Chadwick D, eds. *A textbook of epilepsy,* 4th ed. New York: Churchill Livingstone, 1993:459–473.
227. Mayeux R, Brandt J, Rosen J, et al. Interictal and language impairment in temporal lobe epilepsy. *Neurology* 1980;30:120–125.
228. Caplan R, Siddarth P, Gurbani S, et al. Psychopathology and pediatric complex partial seizures: seizure-related, cognitive and linguistic variables. *Epilepsia* 2004;45:1273–1281.
229. Rapin I, Katzman R. Neurobiology of autism. *Ann Neurol* 1998;43:7–14.
230. Wing L. The autistic spectrum. *Lancet* 1997;350:1761–1766.
231. Pervasive developmental disorders. In: *Diagnostic and statistical manual of mental disorders,* 4th ed. Washington, DC: American Psychiatric Association, 1994:65–78.
232. Folstein SE, Rutter ML. Infantile autism: a genetic study of 21 twin pairs. *J Child Psychol Psychiatry* 1977;18:297–321.
232a. Bolton PF, Murphy M, Macdonald H, et al. Obstetric complications in autism. Consequences or causes of the condition. *J Aner Head Child Adoles Psychiat* 1997;36:272–281.
233. Gillberg C, Gillberg IC. Infantile autism: a total population study of reduced optimality in the pre-, peri-, and neonatal period. *J Autism Dev Disord* 1983;13:153–166.
234. Tsai LY, Stewart MA. Etiological implication of maternal age and birth order in infantile autism. *J Autism Dev Disord* 1983;13:57–65.
235. Bryson SE, Smith IM, Eastwood D. Obstetrical suboptimality in autistic children. *J Am Acad Child Adolesc Psychiatry* 1988;27:418–422.
236. Mason-Brothers A, Ritvo ER, Pingree C, et al. The UCLA–University of Utah epidemiologic survey of autism: prenatal, perinatal, and postnatal factors. *Pediatrics* 1990;86:514–519.
237. Ritvo ER, Jorde LB, Mason-Brothers A, et al. The UCLA–University of Utah epidemiologic survey of autism: recurrence risk estimates and genetic counseling. *Am J Psychiatry* 1989;146:1032–1036.
238. Wolff S, Narayan S, Moyes B. Personality characteristics of parents of autistic children: a controlled study. *J Child Psychol Psychiatry* 1988;29:143–153.
239. Steffenberg S, Gillberg C. Autism and autistic-like conditions in Swedish rural and urban areas: a population study. *Br J Psychiatry* 1986;149:81–87.
240. Bolton P, Macdonald H, Pickles A, et al. A case-control family history study of autism. *J Child Psychol Psychiatry* 1994;35:877–900.
241. Ritvo ER, Freeman BJ, Mason-Brothers A, et al. Concordance for the syndrome of autism in 40 pairs of afflicted twins. *Am J Psychiatry* 1985;142:74–77.
242. Steffenberg S, Gillberg C, Holmgren L. A twin study of autism in Denmark, Finland, Iceland, Norway, and Sweden. *J Child Psychol Psychiatry* 1989;30:405–416.
243. Piven J, Gayle J, Chase GA, et al. A family history study of neuropsychiatric disorders in the adult siblings of autistic individuals. *J Am Acad Child Adolesc Psychiatry* 1990;29:177–183.
244. Gillberg C, Gillberg IC, Steffenburg S. Siblings and parents of children with autism: a controlled population-based study. *Dev Med Child Neurol* 1992;34:389–398.
245. Philippe A, Martinez M, Guilloud-Bataille M, et al. Genome-wide scan for autism susceptibility genes. Paris Autism Research International Sibpair Study. *Hum Mol Genet* 1999;8:805–812.
246. Gillberg C, Coleman M. Autism and medical disorders: a review of the literature. *Dev Med Child Neurol* 1996;38:191–202.
247. Ritvo ER, Mason-Brothers A, Freeman BJ, et al. The UCLA–University of Utah epidemiologic survey of autism: the etiologic role of rare diseases. *Am J Psychiatry* 1990;147:1614–1621.
248. Schroer RJ, Phelan MC, Michaelis RC, et al. Autism and maternally derived aberrations of chromosome 15q. *Am J Med Genet* 1998;76:327–333.
249. Reiss AL, Feinstein C, Rosenbaum KN, et al. Autism associated with Williams syndrome. *J Pediatrics* 1985;106:247–249.
250. Gillberg C, Rasmussen P. Brief report: four case histories and a literature review of Williams syndrome and autistic behavior. *J Autism Dev Disord* 1994;24:381–393.
251. Bundey S, Hardy C, Vickers S, et al. Duplication of the 15q11-13 region in a patient with autism, epilepsy, and ataxia. *Dev Med Child Neurol* 1994;36:736–742.
252. Gurrieri F, Battaglia A, Torrisi L, et al. Pervasive developmental disorder and epilepsy due to maternally derived duplication of 15q11-q13. *Neurology* 1999;52:1694–1697.
253. Graf WD, Marin-Garcia J, Gao HG, et al. Autistic regression associated with a mutation in the mitochondrial tRNAlys gene (G8363A). *Ann Neurol* 1998;44:578.
254. Rogers SJ, Newhart-Larson S. Characteristics of infantile autism in five children with Leber's congenital amaurosis. *Dev Med Child Neurol* 1989;31:598–608.
255. McKusick VA. *Mendelian inheritance in man: catalogs of autosomal dominant, autosomal recessive, and X-linked phenotypes*. Baltimore: The Johns Hopkins University Press, 1992:1893–1894.
256. Reiss AL, Freund L. The behavioral phenotype of fragile X syndrome: DSM-111-R autistic behavior in males. *Am J Med Genet* 1992;43:35–46.

257. Ashwood P, Wills S, Van der Water J. The immune response in autism: A new frontier for autism research. *J Leukocyte Biology* 2006;80:1–15.
258. Zimmerman A, Frye V, Potter N. Immunological aspects of autism. *Int Pediatr* 1993;8:199–204.
259. Todd RD, Hickok JM, Anderson GM, et al. Antibrain antibodies in infantile autism. *Biol Psychiatry* 1988;23:644–647.
260. Wakefield AJ, Murch SH, Anthony A, et al. Ileal-lymphoid-nodular hyperplasia, non-specific colitis, and pervasive developmental disorder in children. *Lancet* 1998;351:637–641.
261. Chess S. Autism in children with congenital rubella. *J Autism Child Schizophr* 1971;1:33–47.
262. Ivarsson SA, Bjerre I, Vegfors P, et al. Autism as one of several disabilities in two children with congenital cytomegalovirus infection. *Neuropediatrics* 1990;21:102–103.
263. Lowe TL, Tanaka K, Seashore MR, et al. Detection of phenylketonuria in autistic and psychotic children. *JAMA* 1980;243:126–128.
264. Rutter M, Bartak L. Causes of infantile autism: some considerations from recent research. *J Autism Child Schizophr* 1971;1:20–32.
265. Kotsopoulos S, Kutty KM. Histidinemia and infantile autism. *J Autism Dev Disord* 1979;9:55–60.
266. Gillberg I, Gillberg C, Kopp S. Hypothyroidism and autism spectrum disorders. *J Child Psychol Psychiatry* 1992;33:531–542.
267. D'Eufemia P, Celli M, Finocchiaro R, et al. Abnormal intestinal permeability in children with autism. *Acta Pediatr* 1996;85:1076–1079.
268. Rapin I. Autism in search of a home in the brain. *Neurology* 1999;52:902–904.
269. Courchesne E, Yeung-Courchesne R, Press GA, et al. Hypoplasia of cerebellar lobules Vl and Vll in infantile autism. *N Engl J Med* 1988;318:1349–1354.
270. Murakami JW, Courchesne E, Press GA, et al. Reduced cerebellar hemisphere size and its relationship to vermal hypoplasia in autism. *Arch Neurol* 1989;46:689–694.
271. Holttum JR, Minshew NJ, Sanders RS, et al. Magnetic resonance imaging of the posterior fossa in autism. *Biol Psychiatry* 1992;32:1091–1101.
272. Kleiman MD, Neff S, Rosman NP. The brain in infantile autism: are posterior fossa structures abnormal? *Neurology* 1992;42:753–760.
273. Garber HJ, Ritvo ER. Magnetic resonance imaging of the posterior fossa in autistic adults. *Am J Psychiatry* 1992;149:245–247.
274. Piven J, Saliba K, Bailey J, et al. An MRI study of autism: the cerebellum revisited. *Neurology* 1997;49:546–551.
275. Kemper TL, Bauman M. Neuropathology of infantile autism. *J Neuropathol Exp Neurol* 1998;57:645–652.
276. Minshew NJ, Luna B, Sweeney JA. Oculomotor evidence for neocortical systems but not cerebellar dysfunction in autism. *Neurology* 1999;52:917–922.
277. Bailey A, Luthert P, Dean A. A clinicopathological study of autism. *Brain* 1998;121:889–905.
278. Piven J, Berthier ML, Starkstein SE, et al. Magnetic resonance imaging evidence for a defect of cerebral cortical development in autism. *Am J Psychiatry* 1990;147:734–739.
279. Bauman M, Kemper T. Neuroanatomic observations of the brain in autism. In: Bauman M, Kemper T, eds. *The neurobiology of autism*. Baltimore: The Johns Hopkins University Press, 1994:119–145.
280. Horwitz B, Rumsey JM, Grady CL, et al. The cerebral metabolic landscape in autism. Intercorrelations of regional glucose utilization. *Arch Neurol* 1988;45:749–755.
281. Jacobson R, Le Couteur A, Howlin P, et al. Selective subcortical abnormalities in autism. *Psychol Med* 1988;18:39–48.
282. Prior MR, Tress B, Hoffman WL, et al. Computed tomographic study of children with classic autism. *Arch Neurol* 1984;41.
283. Creasey H, Rumsey JM, Schwartz M, et al. Brain morphometry in autistic men as measured by volumetric computed tomography. *Arch Neurol* 1986;43:669–672.
284. Fombonne E, Roge B, Claverie J, et al. Microcephaly and macrocephaly in autism. *J Autism Dev Disord* 1999;29:113–119.
285. Minshew NJ. Indices of neural function in autism: clinical and biologic implications. *Pediatrics* 1991;87:774–780.
286. Tuchman RF, Rapin I, Shinnar S. Autistic and dysphasic children. II. Epilepsy. *Pediatrics* 1991;88:1219–1225.
287. Bauman ML, Kemper TL. Abnormal cerebellar circuitry in autism? *Neurology* 1989;39:186.
288. Gaffney GR, Kuperman S, Tsai LY, et al. Morphological evidence of brain stem involvement in infantile autism. *Biol Psychiatry* 1988;24:578–586.
289. Hsu M, Yeung-Courchesne R, Courchesne E, et al. Absence of magnetic resonance imaging evidence of pontine abnormalities in infantile autism. *Arch Neurol* 1991;48:1160–1163.
290. Anderson GM, Freedman DX, Cohen DJ, et al. Whole blood serotonin in autistic and normal subjects. *J Child Psychol Psychiatry* 1987;28:885–900.
291. McDougle CJ, Naylor ST, Goodman WK, et al. Acute tryptophan depletion in autistic disorder: a controlled case study. *Biol Psychiatry* 1993;33:547–550.
292. Cook EH, Leventhal BL. The serotonin system in autism. *Curr Opin Pediatr* 1996;8:348–354.
293. Chugani DC, Muzik O, Rothermel R, et al. Altered serotonin synthesis in the dentatothalamocortical pathway in autistic boys. *Ann Neurol* 1997;42:666–669.
294. Gillberg C, Svennerholm L. CSF monoamines in autistic syndromes and other pervasive developmental disorders of early childhood. *Br J Psychiatry* 1987;151:89–94.
295. Ross DL, Klykylo WM, Anderson GM. Cerebrospinal fluid indoleamine and monoamine effects in fenfluramine treatment of autism. *Ann Neurol* 1985;18:394.
296. Narayan M, Srinath S, Anderson GM, et al. Cerebrospinal fluid levels of homovanillic acid and 5-hydroxyindoleacetic acid in autism. *Biol Psychiatry* 1993;33:630–635.
297. Lake CR, Ziegler MG, Murphy DL. Increased norepinephrine levels and decreased dopamine-beta-hydroxylase activity in primary autism. *Arch Gen Psychiatry* 1977;34:553–556.
298. Leventhal BL, Cook EH Jr, Morford M, et al. Relationships of whole blood serotonin and plasma norepinephrine within families of autistic children. *J Autism Dev Disord* 1990;20:499–511.
299. Minderaa RB, Anderson GM, Volkmar FR, et al. Noradrenergic and adrenergic functioning in autism. *Biol Psychiatry* 1994;36:237–241.
300. Kalat JW. Speculation on similarities between autism and opiate addiction. *J Autism Child Schizophr* 1978;8:477–479.
301. Ross DL, Klykylo WM, Hitzemann R. Reduction of elevated CSF beta-endorphin by fenfluramine in infantile autism. *Pediatr Neurol* 1987;3:83–86.
302. Coid J, Allolio B, Rees LH. Raised plasma metenkephalin in patients who habitually mutilate themselves. *Lancet* 1983;2:545–546.
303. Herman B. A possible role of proopiomelanocortin peptides in self-injurious behavior. *Prog Neuropsychopharmacol Biol Psychiatry* 1990;14[Suppl]:S109–139.
304. Gillberg C. Endogenous opioids and opiate antagonists in autism: brief review of empirical findings and implications for clinicians. *Dev Med Child Neurol* 1995;37:239–245.
305. Kanner L. Autistic disturbances of affective contact. *Nervous Child* 1943;2:217–250.
306. Bishop DMV. Autism, Asperger's syndrome and semantic-pragmatic disorder: where are the boundaries? *Br J Disord Commun* 1989;24:107–121.
307. Bolton P, Macdonald H, Pickels A, et al. A case-control family history study of autism. *J Child Psychol Psychiatry* 1994;35:877–900.
308. Bailey A, LeCouteur A, Gottesman I, et al. Autism as a strongly genetic disorder: evidence from a British twin study. *Psychol Med* 1995;25:63–77.
309. Kurita H. Infantile autism with speech loss before the age of 30 months. *J Amer Acad Child Psychiatry* 1985;24:191–196.
310. Lord C, Shulman C, DiLavore P. Regression and word loss in autistic spectrum disorders. *J Child Psychol Psychiatry* 2004;45:936–955.
311. Richler J, Luyster R, Risi S, et al. Is there a "regressive phenotype" of autism spectrum disorder associated with the measles-mumps-rubella vaccine? A CPEA study. *J Autism Devel Disorders* 1006;36:299–316.
312. Tuchman RF, Rapin I. Regression in pervasive developmental disorders: seizures and epileptiform encephalogram correlates. *Pediatrics* 1997;99:560–566.
313. Rogers SJ. Developmental regression in autism spectrum disorders. *Ment Retard Dev Disabil Res Rev* 2004;10:139–143.

314. Rice D, Barone S. Critical periods of vulnerability for the developing nervous system: evidence from humans and animal models. *Environ Health Perspect* 2000;108[Suppl 3]:511–533.
315. Baron-Cohen S, Cox A, Baird G, et al. Psychological markers in the detection of autism in infancy in a large population. *Br J Psychiatry* 1996;168:158–163.
316. Osterling J, Dawson G. Early recognition of children with autism: a study of first birthday home video tapes. *J Autism Dev Disord* 1994;24:247–257.
317. Miles JH, Hillman RE. Value of a clinical morphology examination in autism. *Am J Med Genet* 2000;91:245–253.
318. Bauman ML. Motor dysfunction in autism. In: Joseph AB, Young RR, eds. *Movement disorders in neurology and neuropsychiatry*. Boston: Blackwell Science, 1992:658–661.
319. Lovaas O, Koegel R, Schreibman L. Stimulus overselectivity in autism: a review of research. *Psychol Bull* 1979;86:1236–1254.
320. Smith IM, Bryson SE. Imitation in autism. *Cogn Neuropsychol* 1998;15:747–771.
321. Tuchman RF, Rapin I, Shinnar S. Autistic and dysphasic children: clinical characteristics. *Pediatrics* 1991;88:1211–1218.
322. Rapin I, Dunn M. Language disorders in children with autism. *Semin Pediatr Neurol* 1997;4:86–92.
323. Tirosh E, Canby J. Autism with hyperlexia: a distinct syndrome? *Am J Ment Retard* 1993;98:84–92.
324. Grigorenko EL, Klin A, Pauls DL, et al. A descriptive study of hyperlexia in a clinically referred sample of children with developmental delays. *J Autism Dev Disord* 2003;32:3–12.
325. Liss C, Saulnier C, Fine D, et al. Sensory and attention abnormalities in autistic spectrum disorders. *Autism* 10:155–172.
326. Kinsbourne M. Overfocusing: an apparent subtype of attention-deficit hyperactivity disorder. In: Amir N, Rapin I, Branski D, eds. *Pediatric neurology: behavior and cognition of the child with brain dysfunction*. Basel: Karger, 1991:18–35.
326a. Mann TA, Walker P. Autism and a deficit in broadening the spread of visual attention. *J Child Psychol Psychiatry* 2003;44:274–284.
326b. Frith U. Autism explaing the enigma. Oxford, Blackwell, 1989.
326c. Hermelin B, O'Connor N. Idiot savant calendrical calculators: rules and regularities. *Psychol Med* 1986;16:885–893.
326d. Happe FGE. Central coherence and theory of mind in autism: reading homographs in context. *Brit J Develop Psychol* 1997;15:1–12.
327. Boucher J, Lewis V. Unfamiliar face recognition in relatively able autistic children. *J Child Psychol Psychiatry* 1992;33:843–859.
328. Dawson G, Meltzoff AN, Osterling J, et al. Children with autism fail to orient to naturally occurring social stimuli. *J Autism Dev Disord* 1998;28:479–485.
329. Volkmar FR. The disintegrative disorders: childhood disintegrative disorder and Rett's disorder. In: Volkmar FR, ed. *Psychoses and pervasive developmental disorders in childhood and adolescence*. Washington, DC: American Psychiatric Press, 1996:223–248.
330. Wing L. Asperger's syndrome: a clinical account. *Psych Rev* 1981; 11:115–129.
331. Baltaxe CAM, Simmons JQI. A comparison of language issues in high-functioning autism and related disorders with onset in childhood and adolescence. In: Schopler E, Mesibov GB, eds. *High-functioning individuals with autism*. New York: Plenum Publishing, 1991:201–225.
332. Rumsey JM, Hamburger SD. Neuropsychological findings in high-functioning men with infantile autism, residual state. *J Clin Exp Neuropsychol* 1988;10:201–222.
332a. Lord C, Rutter M, LeCouteur A. Interviw—Revised: a revised version of a diagnostic interview for caregivers of individuals with possible pervasive developmental disorders. *J Autism Dev Disord* 1994;24:659–685.
332b. Lord C, Risi S, Lambrecht L, et al. The Autism Diagnostic observation schedule—generic: A standard measure of social and communication deficits associated with the spectrum of autism. *J Autism Dev Disord* 2000;30:205–223.
333. Charman T, Baron-Cohen I, Baird G, et al. Commentary: the modified checklist for autism in toddlers. *J Autism Dev Disord* 2001;31:145–148.
334. Rogers SJ, DiLalla DL. Age of symptom onset in young children with pervasive developmental disorders. *J Am Acad Child Adolesc Psychiatry* 1990;29:863–872.
335. Bailey A, Le Couteur A, Gottesman I, et al. Autism as a strongly genetic disorder: evidence from a British twin study. *Psychol Med* 1995;25:63–77.
336. Wing L. The definition and prevalence of autism: a review. *Eur Child Adol Psychiatry* 1993;2:61–74.
337. Shapiro T, Hertzig ME. Social deviance in autism: a central integrative failure as a model for social nonengagement. *Psychiatr Clin North Am* 1991;14:19–32.
338. Ehlers S, Gillberg C. The epidemiology of Asperger's syndrome: a total population study. *J Child Psychol Psychiatry* 1993;34:1327–1350.
339. Honda H, Shimizu Y, Misumi K, et al. Cumulative incidence and prevalence of childhood autism in children in Japan. *Br J Psychiatry* 1996;169:228–235.
340. Webb EVJ, Lobo S, Hervas A, et al. The changing prevalence of autistic disorder in a Welsh health district. *Dev Med Child Neurol* 1997;39:150–152.
341. Bertrand J, Mars A, Boyle C, et al. Prevalence of autism in a United States population: the Brick township, New Jersey, investigation. *Pediatrics* 2001;108:1155–1161.
342. Chakrabarti S, Fombonne E. Pervasive developmental disorders in preschool children. *JAMA* 2001;285:3093–3099.
343. Wing L, Potter D. The epidemiology of autistic spectrum disorders: is the prevalence rising? *Ment Retard Dev Disabil Res Rev* 2002;8:151–161.
344. Fombonne E. Epidemiological surveys of autism and other pervasive developmental disorders: an update. *J Autism Dev Disord* 2003;33:365–382.
345. Yeargin-Allsopp M, Rice C, Karapurkar T, et al. Prevalence of autism in a US metropolitan area. *JAMA* 2003;289:49–55.
346. Croen LA, Grether JK, Selvin S. Descriptive epidemiology of autism in a California population: who is at risk? *J Autism Dev Disord* 2002;32:217–224.
347. Blaxill MF. What's going on? The question of time trends in autism. *Public Health Rep* 2004;119:536–551.
348. Mandell DS, Thompson WW, Weintraub ES, et al. Trends in diagnosis rates for autism and ADHD at hospital discharge in the context of other psychiatric diagnoses. *Psychiatr Serv* 2005;56:56–62.
349. Bettelheim B. *The empty fortress: infantile autism and the birth of the self*. New York: Free Press, 1967.
350. Baird TD, Augus TGJ. Familial heterogeneity in infantile autism. *J Autism Dev Disord* 1985;15:315–321.
351. Ritvo ER, Jorde LB, Mason-Brothers A, et al. The UCLA–University of Utah epidemiologic survey of autism: recurrence risk estimates and genetic counseling. *Am J Psychiatry* 1989;146:1032–1036.
352. Bailey A, Le Couteur A, Gottesman I, et al. Autism as a strongly genetic disorder: evidence from a British twin study. *Psychol Med* 1995;25:63–77.
353. Wassink TH, Piven J. The molecular genetics of autism. *Curr Psychiatry Rep* 2000;2:170–175.
354. Carper RA, Moses P, Tigue ZD, et al. Cerebral lobes in autism: early hyperplasia and abnormal age effects. *NeuroImage* 2002;1038–1051.
354a. Aylward EH, Minshew NJ, Field K, et al. Effects of age on brain volume and head circumference in autism. *Neurol* 2002;59:175–183.
355. Herbert MR, Ziegler DA, Makris N, et al. Localization of white matter volume increase in autism and developmental language disorder. *Annals Neurol* 2004;55:530–540.
356. Lainhart JE. Increased rate of head growth during infancy in autism. *JAMA* 2003;290:393–394.
357. Rapin I. Autism in search of a home in the brain. *Neurology* 1999;52:902–904.
358.
359. DeLong GR. Autism: new data suggest a new hypothesis. *Neurology* 1999;52:911–916.
360. Minshew NJ, Luna B, Sweeney JA. Oculomotor evidence for neocortical systems but not cerebellar dysfunction in autism. *Neurology* 1999;52:917–922.
361. Courchesne E, Townsend J, Saitoh O. The brain in infantile autism: posterior fossa structures are abnormal. *Neurology* 1994;44:214–223.
362. Bailey A, Luthert P, Dean A. A clinicopathological study of autism. *Brain* 1998;121:889–905.

363. Palmen SJMC, Engeland H van, Hop PR, et al. Neuropathological findings in autism. *Brain* 2004;127:2572–2583.
364. Kern JK. Purkinje cell vulnerability and autism: a possible etiological connection. *Brain Dev* 2003;25:377–382.
365. Damasio AR, Maurer RG. A neurological model for childhood autism. *Arch Neurol* 1978;35:777–786.
366. Bishop DVM. Autism, executive functions and theory of mind: a neurological perspective. *J Child Psychol Psychiatry* 1993;34:279–293.
367. Bachevalier J. An animal model for childhood autism: memory loss and socioemotional disturbances following damage to the limbic system in monkeys. In: Tammiga CA, Schultz SC, eds. *Advances in neuropsychiatry and psychopharmacology, Vol. 1. Schizophrenia Research.* New York: Raven Press, 1991:129–140.
368. Kinsbourne M. Cerebral-brain stem relations in infantile autism. In: Schopler E, Mesibov GB, eds. *Neurobiological issues in autism*. New York: Plenum, 1987:107–125.
369. Casanova MF, Buxhoeveden DP, Switala AE, et al. Minicolumnar pathology in autism. *Neurology* 2002;58:428–432.
370. Belmonte MK, Yurgelun-Todd DA. Functional anatomy of impaired selective attention and compensatory processing in autism. *Brain Res Cogn Brain Res* 2003;17:651–664.
371. Just MA, Cherkassky VL, Keller TA, et al. Cortical activation and synchronization during sentence completion in high-functioning autism: evidence of underconnectivity. *Brain* 2004;127:1811–1821.
372. Hagberg B, Aicardi J, Dias K, et al. A progressive syndrome of autism, dementia, ataxia, and loss of purposeful hand use in girls: Rett syndrome. Report of 35 cases. *Ann Neurol* 1983;14:471–479.
373. Bailey DB, Mesibov GB, Hatton DD, et al. Autistic behavior in young boys with fragile X syndrome. *J Autism Dev Disord* 1998;28:499–508.
374. Splawski, I, Timothy KW, Sharpe LM, et al. CaV1.2 calcium channel dysfunction causes a multisystem disorder including arrhythmia and autism. *Cell* 2004;119:19–31.
375. Stromland K, Nordin V, Miller M, et al. Autism in thalidomide embryopathy: a population study. *Devel Med Child Neurol* 1994;36:351–356.
376. Rodier SJ. The early origins of autism. *Sci Amer* 2000;282:56–63.
377. Volkmar FR, Douglas NS. Seizure disorders in autism. *J Am Acad Child Adolesc Psychiatry* 1990;29:127–129.
378. Wong V. Epilepsy in children with autistic spectrum disorder. *J Child Neurol* 1993;8:316–322.
379. Lord C, Mulloy C, Wendelboe M, et al. Pre- and perinatal factors in high-functioning females and males with autism. *J Autism Dev Disord* 1991;21:197–209.
380. Dunn HG, ed. Sequelae of low-birth-weight: the Vancouver Study. *Clin Dev Med* 1986;95/96:68–96.
381. DeLong GR, Bean SC, Brown FR. Acquired reversible autistic syndrome in acute encephalopathic illness in children. *Arch Neurol* 1981;38:191–194.
382. Gillberg IC. Autistic syndrome with onset at age 31 years: herpes encephalitis as a possible model for childhood autism. *Dev Med Child Neurol* 1991;920–924.
383. Oades RD, Slusarek M, Velling S, et al. Serotonin platelet-transporter measures in childhood attention-deficit/hyperactivity disorder (ADHD): clinical versus experimental measures of impulsivity. *World J Biol Psychiatry* 2002;3:96–100.
384. Korvatska E, Van der Water J, Anders TF, et al. Genetic and immunological considerations in autism. *Neurobiol Dis* 2002;9:107–125.
385. Jyonouchi H, Sun SN, Le H. Proinflammatory and regulatory cytokine production associated with innate and adaptive immune responses in children with autism spectrum disorder and developmental regression. *J Neuroimmunol* 2001;120:170–179.
386. Warren RP, Margaretten NC, Pace NC, et al. Immune abnormalities in patients with autism. *J Autism Dev Disorders* 1986;16:189–197.
387. Zimmerman A, Frye V, Potter N. Immunological aspects of autism. *Int Pediatr* 1993;8:199–204.
388. Todd RD, Hickok JM, Anderson GM, et al. Antibrain antibodies in infantile autism. *Biol Psychiatry* 1988;23:644–647.
389. Sweeten TL, Bowyer SL, Posey DJ, et al. Increased prevalence of familial autoimmunity in probands with pervasive developmental disorders. *Pediatrics* 2003;112:e420.
390. Silva SC, Correia C, Fesel C, et al. Autoantibody repertoires to brain tissue in autism nuclear families. *J Neuroimmunology* 2004;152:176–182.
391. Vojdani A, O'Bryan T, Green JA, et al. Immune response to dietary proteins, gliadin, and cerebellar peptides in children with autism. *Nutr Neurosci* 2004;7:151–161.
392. Vargas DL, Nascimbene C, Krishnan C, et al. Neuroglial activation and neuroinflammation in the brain of patients with autism. *Ann Neurol* 2005;57:67–81.
393. Gillberg C, Coleman M. Autism and medical disorders: a review of the literature. *Dev Med Child Neurol* 1996;38:191–202.
394. Trottier G, Srivastava L, Walker CD. Etiology of infantile autism: a review of recent advances in neurobiological esearch. *J Psychiatry Neurosci* 1999;24:103–115.
395. Nanson JL. Autism in fetal alcohol syndrome: a report of six cases. *Alcohol Clin Exp Res* 1992;16:558–565.
396. Davis E, Fennoy I, Laraque D, et al. Autism and developmental disabilities in children with perinatal cocaine exposure. *J Natl Med Assoc* 1992;84:315–319.
397. Stromland K, Nordin V, Miller M, et al. Autism in thalidomide embryopathy: a population study. *Dev Med Child Neurol* 1994;36:351–356.
398. Christianson AL, Chesler N, Kromberg JGR. Fetal valproate syndrome: clinical and neurodevelopmental features in two sibling pairs. *Dev Med Child Neurol* 1994;36:357–369.
399. Ward AJ. A comparison and analysis of the presence of family problems during pregnancy of mothers of "autistic" children and mothers of normal children. *Child Psychiatry Hum Dev* 1990;20:279–288.
400. Sweeten TL, Posey DJ, McDougle CJ. Brief report: autistic disorder in three children with cytomegalovirus infection. *J Autism Dev Disord* 2004;34:583–586.
401. Libbey JE, Sweeten TL, McMahon WM, and Fujinami RS. Autistic disorder and viral infections. *J Neuro Virology* 2005;11:1–10.
402. Gillberg IC. Autistic syndrome with onset at age 31 years: herpes encephalitis as a possible model for chidhood autism. *Dev Med Child Neurol* 1991;33:912–929.
403. Ghaziuddin M, Al-Khouri I, Ghaziuddin N. Autistic syndrome following herpes encephalitis. *Eur J Child Adolesc Psychiatry* 2002;11:142–146.
404. Desmond MM, Wilson GS, Melnick JL, et al. Congenital rubella encephalitis. Course and early sequelae. *J Pediatr* 1967;71:311–331.
405. Hornig M, Lipkin WI. Infectious and immune factors in the pathogenesis of neurodevelopmental disorders: epidemiology, hypotheses and animal models. *Ment Retard Devel Disabil Res Rev* 2001;7:200–210.
406. Ciaranello AL, Ciaranello RD. The neurobiology of infantile autism. *Ann Rev Neurosci* 1995;18:101–128.
407. Fatemi Sh, Earle J, Kamodia R, et al. Prenatal viral infection leads to pyramidal cell atrophy and macrocephaly in adulthood: implications for genesis of autism and schizophrenia. *Cell Mol Neurobiol* 2002;22:25–33.
408. Shi L, Fatemi SH, Sidwell RW, et al. Maternal influenza infection causes marked behavioral and pharmacological changes in the offspring. *J Neurosci* 2003;23:297–302.
409. Pfeiffer ZRF, Quigley EMM. Neurogastroenterology. *Semin Neurol* 1996;16.
410. Horvath K, Papadimitriou JC, Rabsztyn A. Gastrointestinal abnormalities in children with autistic disorder. *J Pediatr* 1999;135:559–563.
411. Torrente F, Ashwood P, Day R, et al. Small intestine enteropathy with epithelial IgG and complement deposition in children with regressive autism. *Mol Psychiatry* 2002;7:375–382,334.
412. Ashwood P, Anthony A, Torrente F, et al. Spontaneous mucosal lymphocyte cytokine profiles in children with autism and gastrointestinal symptoms: mucosal immune activation and reduced counter regulatory interleukin-10. *J Clin Immunol* 2004;24:664–673.
413. Montgomery SM, Morris DL, Pounder RE, et al. Paramyxovirus infections in childhood and subsequent inflammatory bowel disease. *Gastroenterology* 1999;116:796–803.
414. Chen RT, DeStefano F. Vaccine adverse events: causal or coincidental? *Lancet* 1998;351:611–612.
415. Lee JW, Melgaard B, Clements CJ, et al. Autism, inflammatory bowel disease, and MMR vaccine. *Lancet* 1998;351:905.

416. Taylor B, Miller E, Farrington CP, et al. Autism and measles, mumps, and rubella vaccine: no epidemiological evidence for a causal association. *Lancet* 1999;353:2026–2029.
417. Uhlmann V, Martin CM, Shiels O, et al. Potential viral; pathogenic mechanism for new variant inflammatory bowel disease. *Mol Pathol* 2002;55:84–90.
418. Bradstreet JJ, El Dahr J, Anthony A, et al. Detection of measles virus genomic RNA in cerebrospinal fluid of children with regressive autism: a report of three cases. *J Am Phys Surg* 2004;9: 38–45.
419. Prior M, Eisenmajer R, Leekam S, et al. Are there subgroups within the autistic spectrum? A cluster analysis of a group of children with autistic spectrum disorders. *J Child Psychol Psychiatry* 1998;39:893–902.
420. Heller T. Dementia infantilis. Zeitschrift für die Erforschung und Behandlung des Jugendlichen Schwachsinns 1908;2:141–165.
421. Fombonne E. Prevalence of childhood disintegrative disorder. *Autism* 2002;6:149–157.
422. Eggers C, Bunk D, Krause D. Schizophrenia with onset before age of eleven: clinical characteristics of onset and course. *J Autism Dev Disord* 2000;30:29–40.
423. Russell AT. The clinical presentation of childhood-onset schizophrenia. *Schizophr Bull* 1994;20:631–646.
424. McLellan JM, Werry J. Practice parameters for the assessment and treatment of children and adolescents with schizophrenia. *J Am Acad Child Adolesc Psychiatry* 1994;33:616–635.
425. Jones P, Rodgers B, Murray R, et al. Child developmental risk factors for adult schizophrenia in the British 1946 birth cohort. *Lancet* 1994;344:1398–1402.
426. Walker E, Lewine RJ. Prediction of adult-onset schizophrenia from childhood home movies of the patients. *Am J Psychiatry* 1990;147:1052–1056.
426a. Niemi L, Surisuari J, Tuulio-Henrikson A, et al. Childhood developmental abnormalities in schizophrenia: evidence from high-risk studies. *Schizophrenia Res* 2003;60:239–258.
427. Walker E, Baum K, Diforio D. Developmental changes in the behavioral expression of vulnerability for schizophrenia. In: Lenzenweger M, Dworkin R, eds. *Origins and development of schizophrenia*. Washington, DC: American Psychological Association Press, 1998:469–492.
428. Kolvin I, Fundudis T. Elective mute children: psychological development and background factors. *J Child Psychol Psychiatry* 1981;22:219–232.
429. Bartak L, Rutter M, Cox A. A comparative study of infantile autism and specific developmental receptive language disorder. I. The children. *Br J Psychiatry* 1975;126:127–145.
430. Plioplys AV. Autism: electroencephalogram abnormalities and clinical improvement with valproic acid. *Arch Pediatr Adolesc Med* 1994;148:220–222.
431. Stefanatos GA, Grover W, Geller E. Case study: corticosteroid treatment of language regession in pervasive developmental disorder. *J Am Acad Child Adolesc Psychiatry* 1995;34:1107–1111.
432. Lewine JD, Andrews R, Chez M, et al. Magnetoencephalographic patterns of epileptic form activity in children with regressive autism spectrum disorders. *Pediatrics* 1999;104:405–418.
433. Howlin P. Practitioner review: psychological and educational treatments for autism. *J Child Psychol Psychiatry* 1998;39:307–322.
434. Kjelgaard MM, Tager-Flusberg H. An investigation of language impairment in autism: implications for genetic subgroups. *Lang Cogn Proc* 2001;16:287–308.
435. Rapin I, Dunn M. Update on the language disorders of individuals on the autistic spectrum. *Brain Dev* 2003;25:166–172.
436. Herbert M, et al. MRI structural imaging of autism and developmental language disorder: a review and commentary. In: Sinha K, Chandra P, eds. *Advances in clinical neuroscience,* 2003.
437. Herbert MR, Ziegler DA, Deutsch C, et al. Brain asymmetries in autism and developmental language disorder: a nested whole-brain analysis. *Brain* 2005;128:213–226.
438. Folstein SE, Mankoski RE. Chromosome 7q: where autism meets language disorder? *Am J Hum Genet* 2000;67:278–281.
439. Warburton P, Baird G, Chen W, et al. Support for linkage of autism and specific language impairment to 7q3 from two chromosome rearrangements involving band 7q31. *Am J Med Genet* 2000;396:228–234.
440. Wassink TH, Piven J. The molecular genetics of autism. *Curr Psychiatry Rep* 2000;2:170–175.
441. Bradford Y, Haines J, Hutcheson H, et al. Incorporating language phenotypes strengthens evidence of linkage to autism. *Am J Med Genet* 2001;105:539–547.
442. Alarcon M, Cantor RM, Liu J, et al. Evidence for a language quantitative trait locus on chromosome 7q in multiplex autism families. *Am J Hum Genet* 2002;70:60–71.
443. DeLong GR, Teague LA, McSwain-Kamran M. Effects of fluoxetine treatment in young children with idiopathic autism: a case series. *Dev Med Child Neurol* 1998;40:551-562.
444. Nicholson R, Awad G, Sloman L. An open trial of risperidone in young autistic children. *J Am Acad Child Adolesc Psychiatry* 1998;37:372–376.
445. Shea S, Turgay A, Carroll A, et al. Risperidone in the treatment of disruptive behavioral symptoms in children with autistic and other pervasive developmental disorders. *Pediatrics* 2004;114:e634–e641.
455a. Barnard L, Young AH, Pearson J, et al. A systematic review of the use of atypical antipsychotics in autism. *J Psychopharm* 2002;16:93–101.
446. Fankhauser MP, Karumanchi VC, German ML, et al. A double-blind, placebo-controlled study of the efficacy of transdermal clonidine in autism. *J Clin Psychiatry* 1992;53:77–82.
447. Volkmar FR. Pharmacological interventions in autism: theoretical and practical issues. *J Clin Child Psychol* 2001;30:80–7.
448. Birmaher B, Quintana H, Greenhill L. Methylphenidate for the treatment of hyperactive autistic children. *J Am Acad Child Adolesc Psychiatry* 1988;27:248–251.
449. Raiten DJ, Massaro T. Perspectives on the nutritional ecology of autistic children. *J Autism Dev Disord* 1986;16:133–144.
450. Pfeiffer SI, Norton J, Nelson L, et al. Efficacy of vitamin B6 and magnesium in the treatment of autism: a methodology review and summary of outcomes. *J Autism Dev Disord* 1995;25:481–494.
451. Reichelt PM, Scott H, Ekrem J. Gluten, milk proteins and autism: the result of dietary intervention on behaviour and peptide secretion. *J Appl Nutr* 1990;42:1–11.
452. Knivsberg AM, Reichelt KL, Nodland M. Reports on dietary intervention in autistic disorders. *Nutr Neurosci* 2001;4:25–37.
453. Lightdale JR, Hayer C, Duer A, et al. Effects of intravenous secretin on language and behavior of children with autism and gastrointestinal symptoms: a single-blinded open label study. *Pediatrics* 2001;108:E90.
454. Sandler RH, Finegold SM, Bolte ER, et al. Short-term benefit from oral vancomycin treatment of regressive-onset autism. *J Child Neurol* 2000;15:429–435.
455. Klin A, Jones W, Schultz R, et al. The enactive mind, or from actions to cognition: lessons from autism. *Philos Trans R Soc Lond B Biol Sci* 2003;358:345–360.
456. Ozonoff S, Miller NJ. Teaching theory of mind: a new approach to social skills training for individuals with autism. *J Autism Dev Disord* 1995;25:415–433.
457. McEachin J, Smith T, Lovaas O. Long-term outcome for children with autism who received early intensive behavioral treatment. *Am J Ment Retard* 1993;4:359–372.
458. Schopler EA. Statewide program for the treatment and education of autistic and related communication handicapped children (TEACCH). In: Volkmar F, ed. *Child and adolescent psychiatric clinics of North America: psychoses and pervasive developmental disorders*. Philadelphia: WB Saunders, 1994:91–103.
459. Lord C. Facilitating social inclusion. In: Schopler E, Mesibov GB, eds. *Learning and cognition in autism*. New York: Plenum, 1995:221–239.
460. Mesibov GB. A comprehensive program for serving people with autism and their families: the TEACCH model. In: Matson JL, ed. *Autism in children and adults: etiology, assessment and intervention*. Belmont, CA: Brooks-Cole, 1995:85–97.
461. Strain PS, Cordisco L. LEAP preschool. In: Harris S, Handelman J, eds. *Preschool education programs for children with autism*. Austin, TX: PRO-ED, 1994:225–252.
462. Harris SL. Educational strategies in autism. In: Schopler E, Mesibov GB, eds. *Learning and cognition in autism*. New York: Plenum, 1995:293–309.
463. Rogers S, Lewis H. An effective day treatment model for young

children with pervasive developmental disorders. *J Am Acad Child Adolesc Psychiatry* 1989;28:207–214.
464. Gresham FM, Beebe-Frankenberger ME, MacMillan DL. A selective review of treatments for children with autism: description and methodological considerations. *School Psycholog Rev* 1999;28:559–575.
465. Howlin P. *Children with autism and Asperger syndrome: a guide for practitioners and carers*. Chichester: John Wiley & Sons, 1998.
466. Matson JL, Benavidez DA, Compton LS, et al. Behavioral treatment of autistic persons: a review of research from 1980 to the present. *Res Dev Disabil* 1996;17:433–465.
467. Quill K. *Enhancing children's social-communicative interactions. Teaching children with autism: strategies to enhance communication and socialization*. New York: Delmar, 1995:163–192.
468. Rutter M. Infantile autism. In: Shaffer D, Ehrhardt AA, Greenhill LL, eds. *The clinical guide to child psychiatry*. New York: Free Press, 1985:48–78.
469. Cohen DJ, Volkmar FR. *Autism and pervasive developmental disorders: a handbook*. New York: John Wiley, 1997.
470. Gillberg C, Johansson M, Steffenberg S, et al. Auditory integration training in children with autism: brief report of an open pilot study. *Autism* 1997;1:97–100.
471. Bettison S. The long-term effects of auditory training in children with autism. *J Autism Dev Disord* 1996;26:361–374.
472. Bebko JM, Perry A, Bryson S. Multiple method validation study of facilitated communication. II. Individual differences and subgroup results. *J Autism Dev Disord* 1996;26:19–42.
473. Howlin P. Prognosis in autism: do specialist treatments affect outcome? *Eur Child Adolesc Psychiatry* 1997;6:55–72.
474. Horvath K, Stefanatos G, Sokolski KN, et al. Improved social skills after secretin administration in patients with autistic spectrum disorders. *J Assoc Acad Minor Phys* 1998;9–15.
475. American Academy of Pediatrics. The Doman-Delacato treatment of neurologically handicapped children. *Pediatrics* 1982;70:810–812.
476. Mason SM, Iwata BA. Artifactual effects of sensory integrative therapy on self-injurious behaviour. *J Appl Behav Anal* 1990;26:361–370.
477. Hoehn TP, Baumeister M. A critique of the application of sensory integration therapy to children with learning disabilities. *J Learn Disabil* 1994;27:338–350.
478. Burden V, Stott CM, Forge J, et al. The Cambridge Language and Speech Project (CLASP). I. Detection of language difficulties at 36 to 39 months. *Dev Med Child Neurol* 1996;38:613–631.
479. Tomblin JB, Records NL, Buckwalter P, et al. Prevalence of specific language impairment in kindergarten children. *J Speech Lang Hear Res* 1997;40:1245–1260.
480. Stem LM, Connell TM, Lee M, et al. Adelaide preschool language unit: results of follow-up. *J Paediatr Child Health* 1995;31:207–212.
481. Silva PA, Williams S, McGee R. A longitudinal study of children with developmental language delay at age three: later intelligence, reading, and behaviour problems. *Dev Med Child Neurol* 1987;29:630–640.
482. Werker JF. The effects of multilingualism on phonetic perceptual flexibility. *Appl Psycholinguis* 1986;7:141–156.
483. Lenneberg EH, Rebelsky FG, Nichols IA. The vocalization of infants born to deaf and to hearing parents. *Vita Humana* 1965;8:23–37.
484. Franco F, Butterworth G. Pointing and social awareness: declaring and requesting in the second year. *J Child Lang* 1996;307–336.
485. Bates E, Thal D, Janowsky JS. Early language development and its neural correlates. In: Segalowitz SJ, Rapin I, eds. *Handbook of neuropsychology,* Vol. 7. New York: Elsevier Science, 1992:69–110.
486. Capute AJ, Accardo PJ. Linguistic and auditory milestones during the first two years of life: a language inventory for the practitioner. *Clin Pediatr* 1978;17:847–853.
487. Thal D, Tobias S, Morrison D. Language and gestures in late talkers: a one-year follow-up. *J Speech Hear Disord* 1991;34:604–612.
488. Tallal P, Stark RE, Mellits ED. Identification of language-impaired children on the basis of rapid perception and production skills. *Brain Lang* 1985;25:314–322.
488a. Silva DA, Satz P. Pathological left-handedness: evaluation of a model. *Brain & Lang* 1979;7:8–16.
489. Nass R. Language development in children with congenital strokes. *Semin Pediatr Neurol* 1997;4:109–116.
489a. Vicari S, Chilosi AM, et al. Plasticity and reorganization during language development in children with early brain injury. *Cortex* 2000;36:31–46.
489b. Jonas R, Nguyen S, Hu B, et al. Cerebral hemispherectomy: hospital course, seizure, developmental language and motor outcome. *Neurol* 2004;62:1712–1721.
490. Woods BT, Teuber HL. Changing patterns of childhood aphasia. *Ann Neurol* 1978;3:273–280.
491. Vargha-Khadem F, Isaacs EB, Papleloudi H. Development of language in six hemispherectomized patients. *Brain* 1991;114:473–495.
492. Dall'Oglio AM, Bates E, Volterra V, et al. Early cognition, communication, and language in children with focal brain injury. *Dev Med Child Neurol* 1994;36:1076–1098.
493. Hiscock M, Kinsbourne M. Phylogeny and ontogeny of cerebral lateralization. In: Davidson R, Hugdahl K, eds. *Brain asymmetry*. Cambridge, MA: MIT Press, 535–578.
494. Duchowny M, Jayakar P, Harvey AS, et al. Language cortex representation: effects of developmental versus acquired pathology. *Ann Neurol* 1996;40:37–38.
495. Chugani HT, Phelps ME, Mazziotta JC. Positron emission tomography of human brain functional development. *Ann Neurol* 1987;22:487–497.
496. Huttenlocher PR. Morphometric study of human cerebral cortex development. *Neuropsychologia* 1990;28:517–527.
497. Aram DM, Eisele JA. Intellectual stability in children with unilateral brain lesions. *Neuropsychologia* 1994;32:85–95.
498. Bates E, Thal D, Trauner D, et al. From first words to grammar in children with focal brain injury. *Dev Neuropsych* 1997;13:275–343.
499. Muter V, Taylor S, Vargha-Khadem F. A longitudinal study of early intellectual development in hemiplegic children. *Neuropsychologia* 1997;35:289–299.
500. Ramachandran VS. Behavioral and magnetoencephalographic correlates of plasticity in the adult human brain. *Proc Nat Acad Sciences* 1993;90:10413–10420.
501. Weiller C, Isenee C, Rijntjesz M, et al. Recovery from Wernicke's aphasia: a positron emission tomography study. *Ann Neurol* 1995;37:723–732.
502. Wada J, Rasmussen T. Intracarotid injections of sodium amytal for clinical observations. *J Neurosurg* 1960;17:266–282.
503. Kinsbourne M. The minor cerebral hemisphere as a source of aphasic speech. *Arch Neurol* 1971;25:302–306.
504. Chiarello C. A house divided? Cognitive functioning with callosal agenesis. *Brain Lang* 1980;11:128–158.
505. Nass R, Koch D. Differential effects of early unilateral brain damage on temperament. *Dev Neuropsychol* 1987;3:93–99.
506. Schmahmann JD, Sherman JC. The cerebellar cognitive-emotional syndrome. *Brain* 1998;121:561–579.
507. Riva D, Giorgi C. The cerebellum contributes to higher functions during development. *Brain* 2000;123:1051–1061.
508. Gottwald B, Wilde B, Mihajlovic Z, et al. Evidence for distinct cognitive deficits after focal cerebellar lesions. *J Neurol Neurosurg Psychiatry* 2004;75:1524–1531.
509. Levisohn L, Cronin-Golomb A, Schmahmann JD. Neuropsychological consequences of cerebellar tumour resection in children. *Brain* 2000;123:1041–1050.
510. Guzzetta F, Mercuri E, Bonanno S, et al. Autosomal recessive congential cerebellar atrophy: a clinical and neuropsychological study. *Brain Dev* 1993;15:439–445.
511. Travis LS. *Handbook of speech pathology and audiology*. New York: Appleton-Century-Crofts, 1971.
512. Kools JA, Williams AF, Vickers MJ, et al. Oral and limb apraxia in mentally retarded children with deviant articulation. *Cortex* 1971;7:387–400.
513. Braun AR, Varga M, Stager S, et al. Altered patterns of cerebral activity during speech and language production in developmental stuttering. An H2(15)O positron emission tomography study. *Brain* 1997;120:761–784.
514. Fox PT, Ingham RJ, Ingham JC, et al. A PET study of the neural systems of stuttering. *Nature* 1996;382:158–161.
515. Bishop DVM. *Handedness and developmental disorder: clinics in developmental medicine*. Oxford: Blackwell Science, 1990:110.
516. Hancock K, Craig A, McCready C, et al. Two- to six-year

controlled-trial stuttering outcomes for children and adolescents. *J Speech Lang Hear Res* 1998;41:1242–1252.
517. DeFusio EN, Menken M. Symptomatic cluttering in adults. *Brain Lang* 1979;8:25–33.
518. Mathinos DA. Communication competence of children with learning disabilities. *J Learn Disabil* 1988;21:437–443.
519. Kinsbourne M. The neuropsychology of bilingualism. *Ann NY Acad Sci* 1981;379:50–58.
520. Singh JA, Zingg RM. *Wolf children and feral man*. New York: Harper & Row, 1942.
521. Davis K. Final note on a case of extreme isolation. *Am J Sociol* 1947;52:432.
522. Curtis S. *Genie: a psycholinguistic study of a modern day "Wild Child."* New York: Academic Press, 1977.
523. Johnson J, Newport E. Critical period effects in second language learning: the influence of maturational state on the acquisition of English as a second language. *Cogn Psychol* 1989;21:60–99.
524. Stein DG, Brailovsky S, Will B. *Brain repair*. New York: Oxford University Press, 1995.
525. Mogford K. Oral language acquisition in the prelinguistically deaf. In: Bishop D, Mogford K, eds. *Language development in exceptional circumstances*. Edinburgh: Churchill Livingstone, 1988:110–131.
526. Mayberry RI, Eichen EB. The long-lasting advantage of learning sign language in childhood: another look at the critical period for language acquisition. *J Mem Lang* 1991;30:486–512.
527. Poizner J, Klima ES, Bellugi U. *What the hands reveal about the brain*. Cambridge, MA: MIT Press, 1987.
528. Mayer P, Lowenbraun S. Total communication use among elementary teachers of hearing-impaired children. *Am Ann Deaf* 1990;135:257–263.
529. Kaplan P. *Pathways for exceptional children*. Minneapolis, MN: West, 1996.
530. Gascon GG, Johnson R, Burd L. Central auditory processing and attention deficit disorders. *J Child Neurol* 1986;1:27–33.
531. Klein SK, Rapin I. Intermittent conductive hearing loss and language development. In: Bishop D, Mogford K, eds. *Language development in exceptional circumstances*. London: Churchill Livingstone, 1988:96–109.
532. Spencer LJ, Gantz BJ, Knutson JF. Outcomes and achievements of students who grew up with access to cochlear implants. *Laryngoscope* 2004;114:1576–1581.
532a. Tomblin JB, Records N, Buck water P, et al. Prevalence of specific language impairment in children. *J Speech and Hearing Research* 1997;39:1284–1294.
533. Leonard LB. Children with specific language impairment. Cambridge, MA: MIT Press, 1998.
534. Silva PA, McGee R, Williams S. Developmental language delay from three to seven years and its signficance for low intelligence and reading difficulties at age seven. *Dev Med Child Neurol* 1983;25:783–793.
535. Rapin I, Allen DA. Developmental language disorders: nosological considerations. In: Kirk U, ed. *Neuropsychology of language, reading, and spelling*. New York: Academic Press, 1983:155–184.
536. Tallal P, Stark RE, Mellits D. The relationship between auditory temporal analysis and receptive language development: evidence from studies of developmental language disorder. *Neuropsychologia* 1985;23:527–534.
537. Bishop DMV. The underlying nature of specific language impairment. *J Child Psychol Psychiat* 1992;23:3–66.
538. Cohen M, Campbell R, Yaghmai F. Neuropathological abnormalities in developmental dysphasia. *Ann Neurol* 1989;25:567–570.
539. Shields J, Varley R. Broks P, et al. Social cognition in developmental language disorders and high-level autism. *Dev Med Child Neurol* 1996;38:487–495.
540. Shields J, Varley R, Broks P, et al. Hemispheric function in developmental language disorders and autism. *Dev Med Child Neurol* 1996;38:473–486.
541. Hurst JA, Baraitser M, Auger E, et al. An extended family with an inherited speech disorder. *Dev Med Child Neurol* 1990;32:347–355.
542. Stromswold K. The heritability of language: a review and meta-analysis of twin, adoption and linkage studies. *Language* 2001;77:647–723.
543. Bishop DV. Motor immaturity and specific speech and language impairment: evidence for a common genetic basis. *Am J Med Genet* 2002;8:56–63.
543a. Marcus GF, Fisher SE. FOXP2 in focus: what can genes tell us about speech and language? *Trends in Cognitive Sciences* 2003;7:257–262.
544. Beichtman JH, Nair R, Clegg M, et al. Prevalence of psychiatric disorders in children with speech and language disorders. *J Am Acad Child Adolesc Psychiatry* 1993;32:595:603.
545. Willinger U, Brunner E, Diendorfer-Radner G, et al. Behaviour in children with language developmental disorders. *Can J Psychiatry* 2003;48:607–614.
546. Van Hout A. Acquired aphasia in children. *Semin Pediatr Neurol* 1997;4:102–108.
547. Cranberg LD, Filley CM, Hart EJ, et al. Acquired aphasia in childhood: clinical and CT investigations. *Neurology* 1987;37:1165–1172.
548. Stiles J. The effect of early brain injury on lateralization of cognitive function. *Curr Direct Psychol Science* 1998;7:21–26.
549. Liegeois F, Connelly A, Cross JH, et al. Language reorganization in children with early-onset lesions of the left hemisphere: an fMRI study. *Brain* 2004;127:1229–1236.
550. Van Dongen HR, Loonen MCB. Factors related to prognosis of acquired aphasia in children. *Cortex* 1977;13:131–136.
551. Cooper JA, Flowers CR. Children with a history of acquired aphasia: residual language and academic impairment. *J Speech Hear Disord* 1987;52:251–262.
552. Stefanatos GA, Kinsbourne M, Wasserstein J. Acquired epileptiform aphasia: a dimensional view of Landau-Kleffner syndrome and the relation to regressive autistic spectrum disorder. *Child Neuropsychology* 2002;8:195–228.
553. da Silva EA, Chugani DC, Muzik O, et al. Landau-Kleffner syndrome: metabolic abnormalities in temporal lobe are a common feature. *J Child Neurol* 1997;12:489–495.
554. Appleton RE. The Landau-Kleffner syndrome. *Arch Dis Child* 1995;72:386–387.
555. Lahey M. Who shall be called language disordered? Some reflections and one perspective. *J Speech Hear Disord* 1990;55:612–620.
556. Binnie CD, Kasteleijn-Nolst Trenite DG, Smit AM, et al. Interactions of epileptiform EEG discharges and cognition. *Epilepsy Res* 1987;1:239–245.
557. Kim KHS, Relkin NR, Lee KM, et al. Distinct cortical areas associated with native and second languages. *Nature* 1997;388:171–174.
558. Friedrich U, Dalby M, Staehelin-Jensen T, et al. Chromosomal studies of children and developmental language retardation. *Dev Med Child Neurol* 1982;24:645–652.
559. Ratcliffe SG. Speech and learning disorders in children with sex chromosome abnormalities. *Dev Med Child Neurol* 1982;24: 80–84.
560. Mazzocco MM, Myers GF, Hamner JL, et al. The prevalence of the FMR1 and FMR2 mutations among preschool children with language delay. *J Pediatr* 1998;132:795–801.
561. Cantwell DP, Baker C. Association between attention-deficit hyperactivity disorder and learning disorders. *J Learn Disabil* 1991;24:88–95.
562. Allen DA, Mendelson L, Rapin I. Syndrome-specific remediation in preschool developmental dysphasia. In: French JH, Havel S, Casser P, eds. *Child neurology and developmental disabilities*. Baltimore: Brooks, 1989:233–243.
563. Tallal P. Developmental language disorders. In: Kavanagh JF, Truss TJ, eds. *Learning disorders*. Parkton, MD: York Press, 1988:181–272.
564. Law J, Garrett Z, Nye C. The efficacy of treatment for children with developmental speech and language delay/disorder: a meta-analysis. *J Speech Lang Hear Res* 2004;47:924–943.
565. Owens RE, House LI. Decision-making process in augmentative communication. *J Speech Hearing Disord* 1984;47:18–25.
566. Amir N, Seligman-Wine J, Gross-Tsur V. The role of augmentative communication in impaired language acquisition. In: Amir N, Rapin I, Bianski D, eds. *Pediatric neurology: behavior and cognition of the child with brain dysfunction,* Vol 1. Basel: Karger, 1991:129–145.
567. Bilken D. Communication unbound. *Harv Educ Rev* 1990;60:291–314.
568. Cummus RA, Prior MP. Autism and assisted communication: a response to Bilken. *Harv Educ Rev* 1992;62:228–241.

569. Kavanagh JF, Truss TJ. *Learning disabilities*. Parkton, MD: York Press, 1988.
570. Lyon GR. Toward a definition of dyslexia. *Ann Dyslexia* 1995;45: 3–27.
570a. World Health Organization. The ICD-10 classification of mental and behavioural disorders. Geneva, World Health Organization.
571. Siegel L. IQ is irrelevant to the definition of learning disabilities. *J Learn Disabil* 1989;22:469–478.
572. Meyer MS. The ability-achievement discrepancy: does it contribute to an understanding of learning disabilities? *Edu Psychol Rev* 2000;12:315–337.
573. Flowers L, Meyer M, Lovato J, et al. Does third grade discrepancy status predict the course of reading development? *AnnDyslexia* 2001;50:1–23.
574. Lyon GR, Fletcher JM, Shaywitz SE, et al. Rethinking learning disabilities. In: Finn CE Jr, Rotherham AJ, Hokanson CR Jr, eds. *Rethinking special education for a new century*. Washington, DC: Thomas B. Fordham Foundation and the Progressive Policy Institute, 2001:259–287.
575. Willcutt EG, Pennington BF. Psychiatric comorbidity in children and adolescents with reading disability. *J Child Psychol Psychiatry,* 2000;41:1039–1048.
576. Wood FB, Felton RF. Separate linguistic and attentional factors in the development of reading. *Top Lang Disord* 1994;14(4):42–57.
577. Knopik VS, De Fries JC. Etiology of covariation between reading and mathematics performance: a twin study. *Twin Res (Engl),* 1999;2:226–34.
578. Moores DF. *Educating the deaf: psychology, principles, and practices,* 3rd ed. Boston: Houghton-Mifflin, 1987.
579. Ross M. *Hard-of-hearing children in regular schools*. Englewood Cliffs, NJ: Prentice-Hall, 1982.
580. Stein PA, Hoover JH. Manifest anxiety in children with learning disabilities. *J Learn Disabil* 1989;22:66–71.
581. Smith SL. *Succeeding against the odds: how the learning disabled can realize their promise*. New York, NY: G. P. Putnum's Sons, 1991.
582. Casey R, Levy SE, Brown K, et al. Impaired emotional health in children with mild reading disability. *J Dev Behav Pediatr* 1992;13:256–260.
583. Prior M, Smart D, Sanson A, et al. Relationships between learning difficulties and psychological problems in preadolescent children from a longitudinal sample. *J Am Acad Child Adolesc Psychiatry* 1999;38:429–436.
584. Maughan B, Rowe R, Loeber, R, et al. Reading problems and depressed mood. *J Abnorm Child Psychol* 2003;31:219–229.
585. Fristad MA, Topolosky S, Weller EB, et al. Depression and learning disabilities in children. *J Affect Disord* 1992;26:53–58.
586. Handwerk ML, Marshall RM. Behavioral and emotional problems of students with learning disabilities, serious emotional disturbance, or both conditions. *J Learn Disabil* 1998;31:327–338.
587. Maag JW, Behrens JT. Depression and cognitive self statements of learning disabled and seriously emotionally disturbed adolescents. *J Spec Ed* 1989;23:17–27.
588. Svetaz MV, Ireland M, Blum R. Adolescents with learning disabilities: risk and protective factors associated with emotional well being: findings from the National Longitudinal Study of Adolescent Health. *J Adolesc Health* 2000;27:340–348.
589. Wood F, Goldston D. Learning disabilities: a hidden source of suicidal thought and behaviour. In: Schlebusch L, Bosch BA, eds. Suicidal behavior 4. Proceedings of the Southern African conference on suicidology, Durban, South Africa.
590. Willcutt EG, Pennington BF. Psychiatric comorbidity in children and adolescents with reading disability. *J Child Psychol Psychiat* 2000;41:1039–1048.
591. Wright-Strawderman C, Watson BL. The prevalence of depressive symptoms in children with learning disabilities. *J Learn Disabil* 1992;25:258–264.
592. U. S. Department of Education. 17th annual report to Congress on the implementation of IDEA.
593. Shaywitz SE, Shaywitz BA, Fletcher JM, et al. Prevalence of reading disability in boys and girls. Results of the Connecticut Longitudinal Study. *JAMA* 1990;264:998–1002.
594. www.nationalreadingpanel.org
595. Nichols PL, Chen TC. *Minimal brain dysfunction: a prospective study*. Hillsdale, NJ: Erlbaum, 1981.
596. Liberman IY, Shankweiler D, Liberman AM. The alphabetic principle and learning to read. In: Shankweiler D, Liberman IY, eds. *Phonology and reading disability: solving the reading puzzle*. Ann Arbor, MI: University of MI Press, 1989:1–33.
597. Stanovitch K. Explaining the variance in reading ability in terms of psychological processes: what have we learned? *Ann Dyslexia* 1986;35:67–96.
598. Stevenson H. Orthography and reading disabilities. *J Learn Disabil* 1984;18:132–135.
599. Rutter M, Yule W. The concept of specific reading retardation. *J Child Psychol Psychiatry* 1975;16:181–197.
600. Nelson HE, Warrington EK. Developmental spelling retardation. In: Knights RM, Bakker DJ, eds. *The neuropsychology of learning disorders: theoretical approaches*. Baltimore: University Park Press, 1976:325–332.
601. Lyon GR. Research initiatives in learning disabilities: contributions from scientists supported by the National Institute of Child Health and Human Development. *J Child Neurol* 1995;10:120–S126.
602. Gleitman LR, Rozin P. The structure and acquisition of reading. I. Relations between orthographies and the structure of language. In: Reber AJ, Scarborough DL, eds. *Toward a psychology of reading*. Hillsdale, NJ: Erlbaum, 1977.
603. Bradley L, Bryant P. Categorizing sounds and learning to read—a causal connection. *Nature* 1983;301:419–421.
604. Tallal P. Auditory temporal perception, phonics, and reading disabilities in children. *Brain Lang* 1980;9:182–198.
605. Eden GF, Stein JF, Wood HM, et al. Temporal and spatial processing in reading disabled and normal children. *Cortex* 1995;31:451–468.
606. Reynolds AM, Elkonin N, Brown FRI. Specific reading disabilities: early identification and long-term outcome. *MRDD Res Rev* 1996;2:21–27.
607. Denckla M. Motor coordination in dyslexic children. In: Duffy F, Geschwind N, eds. *Dyslexia*. Boston: Little, Brown and Company, 1987.
608. Duffy FH, Denckla MB, Bartels PH, et al. Dyslexia: automated diagnosis by computerized classification of brain electrical activity. *Ann Neurol* 1980;7:421–428.
609. Lou HC, Hendrikson L, Bruhn P. Focal cerebral hypoperfusion in children with dysphasia and/or attention deficit disorder. *Arch Neurol* 1984;41:825–829.
610. Galaburda AM, Sherman GF, Rosen GD, et al. Developmental dyslexia: four consecutive patients with cortical anomalies. *Ann Neurol* 1985;18:222–233.
611. Denckla MB, LeMay M, Chapman CT. No CT scan abnormalities found even in neurologically impaired learning disabled children. *J Learn Disabil* 1985;18:132–135.
611a. EcKert M. Neuroanatomical markers for dyslexia: A review of dyslexia structural imaging studies. *The Neuroscientist* 2004;10: 362–371.
612. Johnson D, Balock J. *Adults with learning disabilities*. Orlando: Grune & Stratton, 1987.
613. Kinsbourne M, Rufo DT, Gamzu E, et al. Neuropsychological deficits in adults with dyslexia. *Dev Med Child Neurol* 1991;33:763–775.
614. Felton R, Naylor C, Wood F. Neuropsychological profile of adult dyslexics. *Brain Lang* 1990;39:485–497.
615. Wood FB, Flowers Dl, Grigorenko E. The functional neuroanatomy of fluency or why walking is just as important to reading as talking is. In: Wolf M, ed. *Dyslexia, fluency, and the brain*. Baltimore, MD: York Press, 2001:235–244.
616. Pugh KR, Mencl WE, Jenner AR, et al. Neurobiological studies of reading and reading disability. *J Commun Disord (USA),* Nov–Dec 2001;34:479–492).
617. Shaywitz SE, Shaywitz BA, Pugh KR, et al. Functional disruption in the organization of the brain for reading in dyslexia. *Proc Nat Acad Sci USA* 1998;95:2636–2641.
618. Flowers DL, Wood FB, Naylor CE. Regional cerebral blood flow correlates of language processes in reading disability. *Arch Neurol* 1991;48:637–643.
619. Gross-Glenn K, Duara R, Barker WW, et al. Positron emission tomographic studies during serial word-reading by normal and dyslexic adults. *J Clin Exp Neuropsychol* 1991;13:531–544.

620. Rumsey JM, Andreason P, Zametkin AJ, et al. Right frontotemporal activation by tonal memory in dyslexia, an O15 PET study. *Biol Psychiatry* 1994;36:171–180.
621. Rumsey JM, Zametkin AJ, Andreason P, et al. Normal activation of frontotemporal language cortex in dyslexia as measured with oxygen 15 positron emission tomography. *Arch Neurol* 1994;51: 27–38.
622. Rumsey JM, Nace K, Donohue B, et al. A positron emission tomographic study of impaired word recognition and phonological processing in dyslexic men. *Arch Neurol* 1997;54:562–573.
623. Eden GF, Jones KM, Cappell K, et al. Neural changes following remediation in adult developmental dyslexia [in process citation] *Neuron (USA)*, 2004;44:411–422.
624. Torgeson J. *Catch them before they fall. The American educator*. Spring/Summer, 1998.
625. Maughan B. Annotation: long-term outcomes of developmental reading problems. *J Psychol Psychiatry* 1995;36:357–371.
626. Thomas CJ. Congenital "word blindness" and its treatment. *Ophthalmoscope* 1905;3:380–385.
627. Hallgren B. Specific dyslexia (congenital word-blindness); a clinical and genetic study. *Acta Neurol Scand Suppl* 1950;65:1–287.
628. Yule W, Rutter M. Reading and intelligence. In: Knights R, Bakker J, eds. *Neuropsychology of language disorders: theoretical approaches*. Baltimore: University Park Press, 1976.
629. Finucci JM, Whitehouse CC, Isaacs SD, et al. Derivation and validation of a quantitative definition of specific reading disability for adults. *Dev Med Child Neurol* 1984;26:143–153.
630. Pennington BF. Using genetics to understand dyslexia. *Ann Dyslexia* 1989;39:81–93.
631. Tzenova J, Kaplan BJ, Petryshen TL, et al. Confirmation of a dyslexia susceptibility locus on chromosome 1p34-p36 in a set of 100 Canadian families. *Am J Med Genet* 2004;127B:117–124.
632. Fagerheim T, Raeymaekers P, Tonnessen FE, et al. A new gene (DYX3) for dyslexia is located on chromosome 2. *J Med Genet* 1999;36:664–669.
633. Fisher SE, Francks C, Marlow AJ, et al. Independent genome-wide scans identify a chromosome 18 quantitative-trait locus influencing dyslexia. *Nat Genet* 2002;30:86–91.
634. Deffenbacher KE, Kenyon JB, Hoover DM, et al. Refinement of the 6p21.3 quantitative trait locus influencing dyslexia: linkage and association analyses. *Hum Genet* 2004;115:128–138.
635. Morris DW, Robinson L, Turic D, et al. Family-based association mapping provides evidence for a gene for reading disability on chromosome 15q. *Hum Mol Genet* 2000;9:843–848.
636. Finucci J, Childs B. Are there really more dyslexic boys than girls? In: Ansarer A, Geschwind N, Galaburda A, eds. *Sex differences in dyslexia*. Baltimore, MD: The Orton Society, 1981.
637. Grigorenko EL, Wood FB, Meyer MS, et al. Susceptibility loci for distinct components of developmental dyslexia on chromosomes 6 and 15. *Am J Hum Genet* 1997;60:27–39.
638. Fagerheim T, Raeymaekers P, Tonnessen FE, et al. A new gene (DYX3) for dyslexia is located on chromosome 2. *J Med Genet* 1999;36:664–669.
638a. Bishop DVM, Snowling MJ. Developmental dyslexia and specific language impairment: Same or different? *Psychol Bull* 2004;130:858–886.
639. Harnadek MC, Rourke BP. Principal identifying features of the syndrome of nonverbal learning disabilities in children. *J Learn Disabil* 1994;27:144–154.
640. Geary DC. Mathematics and learning disabilities. *J Learn Disabil* 2004;37:4–15.
641. Satz P, Morris R. Learning disability subtypes: a review. In: Pirozzolo FJ, Wittrock MC, eds. *Neuropsychologic and cognitive processes in reading*. New York: Academic Press, 1981.
642. Geiger G, Lettvin JY. Peripheral vision in persons with dyslexia. *N Engl J Med* 1987;316:1238–1243.
643. Slaghuis WL, Lovegrove WJ. Spatial-frequency-dependent visible persistence and specific reading disability. *Brain Cogn* 1985;4:219–240.
644. Livingstone MS, Rosen GD, Drislane FW, et al. Physiological and anatomical evidence for a magnocellular defect in developmental dyslexia. *Proc Nat Acad Sci USA* 1991;88:7943–7947.
645. Lehmkuhle S, Garzia RP, Turner L, et al. A defective visual pathway in children with reading disability. *N Engl J Med* 1993;328:989–996.
645a. Greatrex JC, Drasdo N. The magnocellular deficit hypothesis in dyslexia: A review of reported evidence. *Opthal and Physiol Optics* 1995;15:501–506.
645b. Skottum BC. The magnocellular deficit theory of dyslexia: The evidence from contrast sensitivity. *Vision Res* 40:111–127.
646. Wolf M, Bowers PG. Naming-speed processes and developmental reading disabilities: an introduction to the special issue on the double-deficit hypothesis. *J Learn Disabil* 2000;33:322–324.
647. Huff E, Sorenson J, Dancer J. Relation of reading rate and rapid automatic naming in third graders. *Percept Mot Skills* 2002;95:925–926.
648. Meyer MS, Wood FB, Hart LA, et al. Selective predictive value of rapid automatized naming in poor readers. *J Learn Disabil* 1998;31:106–117.
649. Kinsbourne M, Warrington EK. Developmental factors in reading and writing backwardness. *Br J Psychol* 1963;54:145–156.
650. Kinsbourne M, Warrington EK. The development of finger differentiation. *Quarterly J Exper Psychol* 1964;15:132–137.
651. Hicks RE, Kinsbourne M. On the genesis of human handedness: a review. *J Mot Behav* 1976;8:257–266.
652. Geschwind N, Behan P. Left-handedness: association with immune disease, migraine, and developmental learning disorder. *Proc Natl Acad Sci USA* 1982;79:5097–5100.
653. Crawford SG, Kaplan BJ, Kinsbourne M. The effects of parental immunoreactivity on pregnancy, birth, and cognitive development: maternal immune attack on the fetus? *Cortex* 1992;28:483–491.
654. Gilger JW, Pennington BF, Harbeck RJ, et al. A twin and family study of the association between immune system dysfunction and dyslexia using blood serum immunoassay and survey data. *Brain Cogn* 1998;36:310–333.
655. Porac C, Cohen S. *Lateral preferences and human behavior*. New York: Springer-Verlag, 1981.
656. Hiscock M, Kinsbourne M. Progress in the measurement of laterality and implications for dyslexia research. *Ann Dyslexia* 1995;45:249–268.
657. Schultz RT, Cho NK, Staib LH, et al. Brain morphology in normal and dyslexic children: the influences of sex and age. *Ann Neurol* 1994;35:732–742.
658. Leonard CM, Voeller KK, Lombardino LJ, et al. Anomalous cerebral structure in dyslexia revealed with magnetic resonance imaging. *Arch Neurol* 1993;50:461–469.
659. Geschwind DH, Dykens E. Neurobehavioral and psychosocial issues in Klinefelter syndrome. *Learn Disabil Res Prac* 2004;19:166–173.
660. Hinton VJ, DeVivo DC, Fee R, et al. Investigation of poor academic achievement in children with Duchenne muscular dystrophy. *Learn Disabil Res Prac* 2004;19:146–154.
661. Stein JF, Riddell PM, Fowler S. Disordered vergence control in dyslexic children. *Br J Ophthalmol* 1988;72:162–166.
662. Comelissen P, Bradley L, Fowler S, et al. Covering one eye affects how some children read. *Dev Med Child Neurol* 1992;34:296–304.
663. Polatajko HJ. A critical look at vestibular dysfunction in learning disabled children. *Dev Med Child Neurol* 1985;27:283–292.
664. Ball EW, Blachman BA. Does phoneme awareness training in kindergarten make a difference in early word recognition and development of spelling? *Read Res Quart* 1991;26:49–66.
665. Meyer MS, Felton RH. Repeated reading to enhance fluency: old approaches and new directions. *Ann Dyslexia* 1999;49:284–306.
666. The 1986/87 Future of Visual Development/Performance Task Force Special Report. The efficacy of optometric vision therapy. *J Am Optom Assoc* 1988;59:95–105.
667. Carte E, Morrison D, Sublett J, et al. Sensory integration therapy: a trial of a specific neurodevelopmental therapy for the remediation of learning disabilities. *J Dev Behav Pediatr* 1984;5:189–194.
668. Cummins RA. Sensory integration and learning disabilities: Ayers' factor analyses reappraised. *J Learn Disabil* 1991;24:160–168.
669. Tomatis A. *Education and dyslexia*. France, Quebec: Les Editions, 1978.
670. Aman MG, Werry JS. Methylphenidate and diazepam in severe mental retardation. *J Am Acad Child Adolesc Psychiatry* 1982;21:31–37.
671. Levinson HN. *A solution to the riddle dyslexia*. New York: Springer-Verlag, 1980.
672. Fagan JE, Kaplan BJ, Raymond JE, et al. The failure of antimotion

sickness medication to improve reading in developmental dyslexia: results of a randomized trial. *J Dev Behav Pediatr* 1988;9:359–366.
673. McMahon JR, Gross RT. Physical and psychological effects of aerobic exercise in boys with learning disabilities. *J Dev Behav Pediatr* 1987;8:274–277.
674. Kohen-Raz RL. Learning disabilities and postural control. London: Freund, 1986.
675. American Academy of Ophthalmology. *Learning disabilities and children: what parents need to know*. San Francisco: American Academy of Ophthalmology, 1984.
676. Delacato CH. *The diagnosis and treatment of speech and reading problems*. Springfield, IL: Charles C Thomas, 1963.
677. Felton RH. Effects of instruction on the decoding skills of children with phonological-processing problems. *J Learn Disabil (USA)* 1993;26:583–589.
678. Foorman BR, Francis DJ, Fletcher JM, et al. The role of instruction in learning to read: preventing reading failure in at-risk children. *J Edu Psychol* 1998;90:37–55.
679. Juel C. What makes literacy tutoring effective? *Read Res Quart* 1996;31:268–289.
680. Fayol M, Barrouillet P, Mrinthe C. Predicting arithmetical achievement from neuropsychological performance: a longitudinal study. *Cognition* 1998;68:63–70.
681. Rourke B, Finlayson M. Neuropsychological significance of variations in patterns of academic performance: verbal and visuospatial abilities. *J Abnorm Child Psychol* 1978;6:121–133.
682. Shalev RS, Wurtmann R, Amir N. Developmental dyscalculia. *Cortex* 1988;24:555–561.
683. Ackerman P, Anhalt J, Dykman R. Arithmetic automatization failure in children with attention and reading disorders: associations and sequela. *J Learn Disabil* 1986;19:222–232.
684. Shalev RS, Manor O, Auerbach J, et al. Persistence of developmental dyscalculia: what counts? Results from a 3-year prospective follow-up study. *J Pediatr* 1998;133:320–321.
685. Shalev RS. Developmental dyscalculia. *J Child Neurol* 2004;19:756–771.
686. Chandler HN. Confusion confounded: a teacher tries to use research results to teach maths. *J Learn Disabil* 1987;11:361–369.
687. Semrud-Clikeman M, Hynd GW. Right hemisphere dysfunction in nonverbal learning disabilities: social, academic, and adaptive functioning in adults and children. *Psychol Bull* 1990;107:196–209.
688. Levin HS, Scheller J, Rickard T, et al. Dyscalculia and dyslexia after right hemisphere injury in infants. *Arch Neurol* 1996;53:88–96.
689. Cleaver RL, Whitman RD. Right hemisphere, white matter learning disabilities associated with depression in an adolescent amd young adult psychiatric population. *J Nerv Ment Dis* 1998;186:561–565.
690. Mattson AJ, Sheer DE, Fletcher JM. Electrophysiological evidence of lateralized disturbances in children with learning disabilities. *J Clin Exp Neuropsychol* 1992;14:707–716.
691. Pennington BF, van Doorninck WJ. Neuropsychological deficits in early treated phenylketonuric children. *Am J Ment Def* 1985;89:467–474.
692. Rovet J. Turner syndrome: genetic and hormonal factors contributing to a specific learning disability profile. *Learn Disabil Res Prac* 2004;19:133–145.
693. Swillen A, Devriendt K, Legius E, et al. The behavioural phenotype in velo-cardio-facial syndrome in adolescence. *Genet Couns* 1999;10:79–88.
694. Pennington BF. Genetics of learning disabilities. *Semin Neurol* 1991;11:28–34.
695. Aldenkamp HP, Alpherts WC, Dekker MJ, et al. Neuropsychological aspects of learning disabilities in epilepsy. *Epilepsia* 1990;31 [Suppl 4]:9–20.
696. Eliason MJ. Neuropsychological patterns: neurofibromatosis compared to developmental learning disorders. *Neurofibromatosis* 1987;6:17–25.
697. Cutting LE, Clements AM, Lightman AD, et al. Cognitive profile of neurofibromatosis type 1: rethinking nonverbal learning disabilities. *Learn Disabil Res Prac* 2004;19:155–165.
698. Ozonoff S. Cognitive impairment in neurofibromatosis type 1. *Am J Med Genet* 1999;89:45–52.
699. North K, Joy P, Yuille D, et al. Specific learning disability in children with neurofibromatosis type 1: significance of MRI abnormalities. *Neurology* 1994;44:878–883.
700. Sevick RJ, Barkovich AJ, Edwards MS, et al. Evolution of white-matter lesions in neurofibromatosis type 1: MR findings. *Am J Roentgenol* 1992;159:171–175.
701. Denckla MB. Neurofibromatosis type 1: a model for the pathogenesis of reading disability. *MRDD Res Rev* 1996;2:48–53.
702. Gresham FM, Reschly DJ. Social skills, deficits and low peer acceptance of mainstreamed learning disabled children. *Learn Disabil Quart* 1986;9:23–32.
703. Dudley-Marling C, Edmiaster R. Social status of learning disabled children and adolescents: a review. *Learn Disabil Quart* 1985;8:189.
704. Hazel JS, Schumaker JB. Social skills and learning disabilities: current issues and recommendations for future research. In: Kavanagh F, Truss TJ, eds. *Learning disabilities: proceedings of the national conference*. Parkton, MD: York Press, 1988:293–344.
705. Cratty BJ. Clumsy child syndromes: descriptions, evaluation and remediation. USA: Harwood Academic Publishers, 1994.
706. Smyth TR. Clumsiness: kinaesthetic perception and translation. *Child Care Health Dev* 1996;22:1–9.
707. Wilson PH, MacKenzie BE. Information processing deficits associated with developmental coordination disorder: a meta-analysis of research findings. *J Child Psychol Psychiatry* 1998;39:829–240.
708. Mandich A, Buckolz E, Polatajko H. On the ability of children with developmental coordination disorder (DCD) to inhibit response initiation: the Simon effect. *Brain Cogn* 2002;50:1501–1512.
709. Rasmussen P, Gilberg C. Natural outcomes of ADHD with developmental coordination disorder at age 22 years. A controlled longitudinal community-based study. *J Acad Child Adolesc Psychiatry* 2000;39:1424–1431.
710. Pitcher TM, Piek JP, Hay DA. Fine and gross motor ability in males with ADHD. *Dev Med Child Neurol* 2003;45:525–535.
711. Deuel RK. Developmental dysgraphia and motor skill disorder. *J Child Neurol* 1994;10:6–8.
712. Schoemaker MM, Hijlkema MGJ, Kalverboer AF. Physiotherapy for clumsy children: an evaluation study. *Dev Med Child Neurol* 1994;36:143–155.
713. Willcutt EG, Pennington BF, DeFries JC. Etiology of inattention and hyperactivity/impulsivity in a community sample of twins with learning disabilities. *J Abnorm Child Psychol* 2000;28:149–159.
714. DeQuiros GB, Kinsbourne M, Palmer RL, et al. Attention deficit disorder in children: three clinical variants. *J Devel Behav Pediatrics* 1994;15:311–319.
715. Rappley MD. Attention deficit-hyperactivity disorder. *N Engl J Med* 2005;352:165–173.
716. Applegate B, Lahey BB, Hart EL, et al. Validity of the age-of-onset criterion for ADHD: a report from the DSM-IV field trials. *J Am Acad Child Adolesc Psychiatry* 1997;36:1211–1221.
717. Kaplan BJ, McNicol J, Conte RA, et al. Sleep disturbances in preschool-aged hyperactive and nonhyperactive children. *Pediatrics* 1987;80:839–844.
718. Chervin RD, Dillon JE, Bassetti C, et al. Symptoms of sleep disorders, inattention, and hyperactivity in children. *Sleep* 1997;20:1185–1192.
719. Palfrey JS, Levine MD, Walker DK, et al. The emergence of attention deficits in early childhood: a prospective study. *J Dev Behav Pediatr* 1985;6:339–348.
720. Stewart MA, Thach BT, Freidin MR. Accidental poisoning and the hyperactive child. *Dis Nerv Syst* 1970;31:403–407.
721. Gerring JP, Brady KD, Chen A, et al. Premorbid prevalence of ADHD and development of secondary ADHD after closed head injury. *J Am Acad Child Adolesc Psychiatry* 1998;37:647–654.
722. Gaub M, Carlson CL. Gender differences in ADHD: a meta-analysis and critical review. *J Am Acad Child Adolesc Psychiatry* 1997;36:1036–1045.
723. Biederman J, Mick E, Faraone SV, et al. Influence of gender on attention deficit hyperactivity disorder in children referred to a psychiatric clinic. *Am J Psychiatry* 2002;159:36–42.
724. Porrino LJ, Rapoport JL, Behar D, et al. A naturalistic assessment of the motor activity of hyperactive boys. I. Comparison with normal controls. *Arch Gen Psychiatry* 1983;40:681–687.
725. Pelham W, Bender NE. Peer relationships in hyperactive children: description and treatment. *Adv Behav Disabil* 1982;1:365–435.

726. Levine MD, Oberklaid F, Meltzer L. Development output failure: a study of low productivity in school-age children. *Pediatrics* 1981;67:18–25.
727. Cantwell DP, Satterfield JH. The prevalence of academic underachievement in hyperactive children. *J Pediatr Psychol* 1978;3:168–197.
728. Lambert NM, Sandoval J. The prevalence of learning disabilities in a sample of children considered hyperactive. *J Abnorm Child Psychol* 1980;8:33–50.
729. Ackerman PT, Dykman RA, Gardner MY. ADD students with and without dyslexia differ in sensitivity to rhyme and alliteration. *J Learn Disabil* 1990;23:279–283.
730. Nigg JT, Hinshaw SP, Carte ET, et al. Neuropsychological correlates of childhood attention-deficit/hyperactivity disorder: explainable by comorbid disruptive behavior or reading problems? *J Abnorm Psychol* 1998;107:468–480.
731. Barkley RA. Behavioral inhibition, sustained attention and executive function: constructing a unified theory of ADHD. *Psychol Bull* 1997;121:65–94.
732. Nigg JT. Is ADHD a disinhibitory disorder? *Psychol Bull* 2001;127:571–598.
733. Scheres A, Oosterlaan J, Geurts H, et al. Executive functioning in boys with ADHD: primarily an inhibition deficit? *Arch Clin Neuropsychology* 2004;19:569–594.
734. Kinsbourne M. Testing models for attention deficit hyperactivity disorder in the behavioral laboratory. In: Conners C, Kinsbourne M, eds. *ADHD: attention deficit-hyperactivity disorder*. Munich: MMV Medizin Verlag, 1990:51–70.
735. Teicher MH, Ito Y, Glod CA, et al. Objective measurement of hyperactivity and attentional problems in ADHD. *J Am Acad Child Adolesc Psychiatry* 1996;35:334–342.
736. Kinsbourne M. Toward a model for the attention deficit disorder. In: Perlmutter M, ed. *Minnesota symposia in child development*. Hillsdale, NJ: Erlbaum, 1983:137–166.
737. Conners CK. Clinical use of rating scales in diagnosis and treatment of attention-deficit/hyperactivity disorder. *Pediatr Clin North Amer* 1999;46:857–870.
738. Zametkin A, Rapoport JL. The neurobiology of attention deficit disorder with hyperactivity: where have we come in 50 years? *J Am Acad Child Adolesc Psychiatry* 1987;26:676–686.
739. Bhatia MS, Nigam VR, Bohra N, et al. Attention deficit disorder with hyperactivity among paediatric outpatients. *J Child Psychol Psychiatry* 1991;32:297–306.
740. Wolraich ML, Hannah JN, Pinnock TY, et al. Comparison of diagnostic criteria for attention-deficit hyperactivity disorder in a county-wide sample. *J Am Acad Child Adolesc Psychiatry* 1996;35:319–324.
741. Szatmari P. The epidemiology of attention-deficit hyperactivity disorders. *Child Adolesc Psychiatry Clin North Am* 1992;1:361–371.
742. Wasserman RC, Kelleher KJ, Bocian A, et al. Identification of attentional and hyperactivity problems in primary care: a report from pediatric research in office settings and the ambulatory sentinel practice network. *Pediatrics* 1999;103:E38.
743. Robinson LM, Skaer JL, Sclar DA, et al. Is attention deficit hyperactivity disorder increasing among girls in the U.S? Trends in diagnosis and the prescribing of stimulants. *CNS Drugs* 2000;16:129–137.
744. Lambert MC, Knight F, Taylor R, et al. Epidemiology of behavioral and emotional problems among children of Jamaica and the United States: parent reports for ages 6 to 11. *J Abnorm Child Psychol* 1994;22:113–128.
745. The ICD-10 classification of mental and behavioral disorders: clinical descriptions and diagnostic guidelines. World Health Organization, 1992.
746. Prendergast M, Taylor E, Rapoport JL, et al. The diagnosis of childhood hyperactivity: a US-UK cross-national study of DSM-III and ICD-9. *J Child Psychol Psychiatry* 1988;29:289–300.
747. Hinshaw SP. On the distinction between attentional deficits/hyperactivity and conduct problems/aggression in childhood psychopathology. *Psychol Bull* 1987;101:443–463.
748. Stewart MA, Cummings C, Singer S, et al. The overlap between hyperactive and unsocialized aggressive children. *J Child Psychol Psychiatry* 1981;22:35–45.
749. Biederman J, Fararone SV, Laysey K. Comorbidity of diagnosis in attention-deficit hyperactivity disorder. *Child Adolesc Psychiatry Clin North Am* 1992;1:335–358.
750. NICHD early child care research network. Trajectories of physical aggression from toddlerhood to middle childhood. *Monographs Soc Res Child Dev* 2004;69:1–129.
751. Dennis M, Wilkinson M, Koski L, et al. Attention deficits in the long term after childhood head injury. In: Broman S, Michel ME, eds. *Traumatic brain injury in children*. New York: Oxford University Press, 1994.
752. Olson HC, Streissguth AP, Sampson PD, et al. Association of prenatal alcohol exposure with behavioral and learning problems in early adolescence. *J Am Acad Child Adolesc Psychiatry* 1997;36:1187–1194.
753. Astbury J, Orgill A, Bajuk B. Relationship between two-year behavior and neurodevelopmental outcome at five years of very low-birth-weight survivors. *Dev Med Child Neurol* 1987;29:370–379.
754. Klebanov PK, Brooks-Gunn J, McCormick MD. Classroom behavior of very-low-birth-weight elementary school children. *Pediatrics* 1994;94:700–708.
755. Krouse JP, Kaufman JM. Morphological anomalies in exceptional children: a review and critique of research. *J Abnorm Child Psychol* 1972;10:247–264.
756. Wasserman J, Wolf LE, LeFever F, eds. Adult Attention Deficit Disorder, Brain Mechanisms and Life Outcomes. *Ann NY Acad Sci* 2001.
757. Lahey BB, Piacentini JC, McBurnett K, et al. Psychopathology in the parents of children with conduct disorder and hyperactivity. *J Am Acad Child Adolesc Psychiatry* 1988;27:163–170.
758. Hechtman L. Families of children with attention deficit hyperactivity disorder: a review. *Can J Psychiatry* 1996;41:350–360.
759. Biederman J, Faraone SJV, Keenan K, et al. Family-genetic and psychosocial risk factors in DSM-III attention deficit disorder. *J Amer Acad Child Adolesc Psychiatry* 1990;29:526–533.
760. Epstein JN, Conners CK, Erhardt D, et al. Familial aggregation of ADHD characteristics. *J Abnorm Child Psychol* 2000;28:595–599.
761. Faraone SV, Biederman J, Milberger S. An exploratory study of ADHD among second-degree relatives of ADHD children. *Biol Psychiatry* 1994;35:398–402.
762. LaHoste GJ, Swanson JM, Wigal SB, et al. Dopamine D4 receptor gene polymorphism is associated with attention deficit hyperactivity disorder. *Mol Psychiatry* 1996;1:121–124.
763. Cook EHJ, Stein MA, Krasowski MD, et al. Association of attention-deficit disorder and the dopamine transporter gene. *Am J Hum Genet* 1995;56:993–998.
764. Gill M, Daly G, Heron S, et al. Confirmation of association between attention-deficit hyperactivity disorder and a dopamine transporter polymorphism. *Mol Psychiatry* 1997;2:311–313.
765. Doughety DD, Bonab AA, Spencer TJ, et al. Dopamine transporter density in patients with attention deficit hyperactivity disorder. *Lancet* 1999;354:2132–2133.
766. Zentall SS, Meyer MJ. Self-regulation of stimulation for ADD-H children during reading and vigilance task performance. *J Abnorm Child Psychol* 1987;15:519–536.
767. Filipek PA, Semrud-Clikeman M, Steingard RJ, et al. Volumetric MRI analysis comparing subjects having attention-deficit hyperactivity disorder with normal controls. *Neurology* 1997;48:589–601.
768. Castellanos FX, Giedd JN, Eckburg P, et al. Quantitative morphology of the caudate nucleus in attention-deficit hyperactivity disorder. *Am J Psychiatry* 1994;151:1791–1796.
769. Hynd GW, Hern KL, Novey ES, et al. Attention-deficit hyperactivity disorder and asymmetry of the caudate nucleus. *J Child Neurol* 1993;8:339–347.
770. Aylward EH, Reiss AL, Reader MJ, et al. Basal ganglia volumes in children with attention-deficit hyperactivity disorder. *J Child Neurol* 1996;11:112–115.
771. Castellanos FX, Lee PP, Sharp W, et al. Developmental trajectories of brain volume abnormalities in children and adolescents with attention-deficit/hyperactivity disorder. *JAMA* 2002;288: 1740–1748.
772. Baumgardner TL, Singer HS, Denckla MB, et al. Corpus callosum morphology in children with Tourette's syndrome and attention-deficit hyperactivity disorder. *Neurology* 1996;47:1–5.

773. Semrud-Clikeman M, Filipek PA, Biederman J, et al. Attention-deficit hyperactivity disorder: magnetic resonance imaging morphometric analysis of the corpus callosum. *J Am Acad Child Adolesc Psychiatry* 1994;33:875–881.

773a. Mostofsky SH, Reiss AL, Lockhart P, et al. Evaluation of cerebellar size in attention-deficit hyperactivity disorder. *J Child Neurol* 1998;13:434–439.

774. Lou HC, Henriksen L, Bruhn P, et al. Striatal dysfunction in attention deficit and hyperkinetic disorder. *Arch Neurol* 1990;46:48–52.

775. Matochik JA, Liebenauer LL, King AC, et al. Cerebral glucose metabolism in adults with attention-deficit hyperactivity disorder after chronic stimulant treatment. *Am J Psychiatry* 1994;151: 658–664.

776. Satterfield JH, Schell AM, Nicholas T, et al. Topographic study of auditory-event related potentials in normal boys and boys with attention deficit disorder with hyperactivity. *Psychophysiology* 1988;25:591–606.

777. Zametkin AJ, Liebenauer LL, Fitzgerald GA, et al. Brain metabolism in teenagers with attention-deficit hyperactivity disorder. *Arch Gen Psychiatry* 1993;50:333–340.

778. Lazzaro I, Gordon E, Whitmont S, et al. Quantified EEG activity in adolescent attention deficit hyperactivity disorder. *Clin Electroencephalogr* 1998;29:37–42.

779. Harter MR, Annelo-Vento L, Wood FB, et al. Separate brain potential characteristics in children with reading disability and attention deficit disorder. *Brain Cogn* 1988;7:115–140.

780. Robaey P, Breton F, Dugas M, et al. An event-related potential study of controlled and automatic processes in 6- to 8-year-old boys with ADHD. *Electroencephalogr Clin Neurophysiol* 1992;6:330–340.

781. Conners CK, March JS, Erhardt D, et al. Assessment of attention deficit disorders (ADHD): conceptual issues and future trends. *J Psychoeduc Assess* 1995;14:186–205.

782. Aylward EH, Whitehouse D. Learning disability with and without attention deficit disorders. In: Ceci SJ, ed. *Handbook of cognitive, social, and neuropsychological aspects of learning disabilities*. Hillsdale, NJ: Erlbaum Associates, 1986–1987:321–342.

783. March JS, Swanson JM, Arnold LE, et al. Anxiety as a predictor and outcome variable in the multimodel treatment study of children with ADHD (MTA). *J Abnorm Child Psychol* 2000;28:527–541.

784. Swanson J, Kinsbourne M, Roberts W, et al. A time-response analysis of the effect of stimulant medication on the learning ability of children referred for hyperactivity. *Pediatrics* 1978;61:21–29.

785. Epstein JN, Erkanli A, Conners CK, et al. Relations between continuous performance test performance measures and ADHD behaviors. *J Abnorm Child Psychol* 2003;31:543–554.

786. Greenberg LM, Waldman I. Developmental normative data on the test of variables of attention. *J Child Psychol Psychiatry* 1993;6: 1019–1030.

787. Epstein JN, Erkanli A, Conners CK, et al. Relations between continuous performance test measures and ADHD behaviors. *J Abnorm Child Psychol* 2003;31:543–554.

788. Kagan J, Reznick JS, Snidman N. Biological bases of childhood shyness. *Science* 1988;40:167–171.

789. Nuechterlein KM. Signal detection in vigilance tasks and behavioral attributes among offspring of schizophrenic mothers and hyperactive children. *J Abnorm Psychol* 1983;92:4–28.

790. Tillman R, Geller B, Craney JL, et al. Relationship of parent and child informants to prevalent mania symptoms in children with a prepubertal and early adolescent bipolar disorder phenotype. *Am J Psychiatry* 2004;161:1278–1284.

791. Akiskal HS, Downs J, Jordan P, et al. Affective disorders in referred children and younger siblings of manic depressives. *Arch Gen Psychiatry* 1985;42:996–1003.

792. Leibenluft E, Charney DS, Towbin KE, et al. Defining clinical phenotypes of juvenile mania. *Amer J Psychiatry* 2003;160:430–437.

793. Geller B, Zimerman B, Williams M, et al. *J Child Adolesc Psychopharmacology* 2002;12:11–25.

794. Rickler KC. Episodic dyscontrol. In: Benson F, Blumer A, eds. *Psychiatric aspects of neurologic disease*, Vol II. New York: Grune & Stratton, 1982.

795. Swedo SE, Leonard HL, Kiessling L. Speculations on antineuronal antibody-mediated neuropsychiatric disorders of childhood. *Pediatrics* 1994;93:323–326.

796. Yeates KO, Bornstein RA. Attention deficit disorder and neuropsychological functioning in children with Tourette's disorder. *Neuropsychology* 1994;8:65–74.

797. Channon S, Pratt P, Robertson MM. Executive function, memory and learning in Tourette's syndrome. *Neuropsychology* 2003;17:247–254.

798. American Academy of Pediatrics Committee on Children with Disabilities and Committee on Drugs. Medication for children with attentional disorders. *Pediatrics* 1996;98:301–304.

799. MTA Cooperative Group. National Institute of Mental Health multimodal treatment study of ADHD follow-up: 24 months outcomes of treatment strategies for attention-deficit hyperactivity disorder. *Pediatrics* 2004;113:754–761.

800. McDaniel KD. Pharmacologic treatment of psychiatric and neurodevelopmental disorders in children and adolescents, Part 1. *Clin Pediatr (Phila)* 1986;25:65–71.

801. Barkley RA. Hyperactive boys and girls: stimulant drug effects on mother-child interactions. *J Child Psychol Psychiatry* 1989;30:379–390.

802. Schachar R, Taylor E, Wieselberg M, et al. Changes in family function and relationships in children who respond to methylphenidate. *J Am Acad Child Adolesc Psychiatry* 1987;26:728–732.

803. Swanson JM, McBurnett K, Wigal T, et al. Effect of stimulant medication on children with attention deficit disorder: a "review of reviews."*Except Child* 1993;60:154–162.

804. Volkow ND, Wang GJ, Fowler JS, et al. Evidence that methylphenidate enhances the saliency of a mathematical task by increasing dopamine in the human brain. *Am J Psychiatry* 2004;161:1173–1180.

805. Lipkin PH, Goldstein IJ, Adesman AR. Tics and dyskinesias associated with stimulant treatment in attention-deficit/hyperactivity disorder. *Arch Pediatr Adolesc Med* 1994;148:859–861.

806. Rapport MD, duPaul GJ, Kelly KL. Attention-deficit hyperactivity disorder and methylphenidate: the relationship between gross body weight and drug response in children. *Psychopharm Bull* 1989;25:285–290.

807. Greenhill LL, Abikoff HB, Arnold LE, et al. Medication treatment strategies in the MTA study: relevance to clinicians and researchers. *J Am Acad Child Adolesc Psychiatry* 1996;35:1–10.

808. Comings DE, Comings BG. Tourette's syndrome and attention deficit disorder with hyperactivity. *Arch Gen Psychiatry* 1987;44:1023–1026.

809. Price RA, Leckman JF, Pauls DL, et al. Gilles de la Tourette's syndrome. Tics and central nervous system stimulants in twins and non-twins. *Neurology* 1986;36:232–237.

810. Cohen AJ, Leckman JF. Sensory phenomena associated with Gilles de la Tourette Syndrome. *J Clin Psychiatry* 1992;53:519–523.

811. Singer HS, Brown J, Quaskey S, et al. The treatment of attention-deficit hyperactivity disorder in Tourette's syndrome: a double-blind placebo-controlled study with clonidine and desipramine. *Pediatrics* 1995;95:74–81.

812. Kilgore BS, Dickinson LC, Burnett CR, et al. Alterations in cartilage metabolism by neurostimulant drugs. *J Pediatr* 1979;94:542–545.

813. Croche AF, Lipman RS, Overall JE, et al. The effects of stimulant medication on the growth of hyperkinetic children. *Pediatrics* 1979;63:847–850.

814. Gittelman-Klein R, Mannuzza S. Hyperactive boys almost grown up. III. Methylphenidate effects on ultimate height. *Arch Gen Psychiatry* 1988;45:1131–1134.

815. Kalachnik JE, Sprague RL, Sleator EK. Effect of methylphenidate hydrochloride on stature of hyperactive children. *Dev Med Child Neurol* 1982;24:586–595.

816. MTA Cooperative Group. National Institute of Mental Health multimodal treatment study of ADHD follow-up. Changes in effectiveness and growth after the end of treatment. *Pediatrics* 2004;113:762–769.

817. Faraone SV, Wilens T. Does stimulant treatment lead to substance abuse disorder? *J Clin Psychiatry* 2003;64[Suppl]11:9–13.

818. Volkow ND, Wang GJ, Fowler JS, et al. Dopamine transporter occupanciees in the human brain induced by therapeutic doses of oral methylphenidate. *Amer J Psychiatry* 1999;155:1325–1331.

819. Greenhill L, Beyer DH, Finkelstein J, et al. Guidelines and algorithms for the use of methylphenidate in children with

attention deficit/hyperactivity disorder. *J Attention Disord* 2000;6:S89–S100.
820. Greenhill LL, Swanson JM, Vitiello B, et al. Impairment and deportment responses to different methylphenidate doses in children with ADHD: the MTA titration trial. *J Amer Acad Child Adolesc Psychiatry* 2001;40:180–187.
821. Funk JB, Chessare JB, Weaver MT, et al. Attention deficit hyperactivity disorder, creativity, and the effects of methylphenidate. *Pediatrics* 1993;91:816–819.
822. Feldman H, Crumrine P, Handen BL, et al. Methylphenidate in children with seizures and attention-deficit disorder. *Am J Dis Child* 1989;143:1081–1086.
823. Gross-Tsur V, Manor O, vander Meere J, et al. Epilepsy and attention deficit disorder: is methylphenidate safe and effective? *J Pediatr* 1997;130:40–44.
824. Wroblewski BA, Leary JM, Phelan AM, et al. Methylphenidate and seizure frequency in brain injured patients with seizure disorders. *J Clin Psychiatry* 1992;53:86–89.
825. Spencer T, Biedermark J, Wilens T, et al. Efficacy of a mixed amphetamine salts compound in adults with attention deficit hyperactivity disorder. *Arch Gen Psychiatry* 2001;58:775–782.
826. Pelham WE, Swanson JM, Furman MB, et al. Pemoline effects on children with ADHD: a time-response by dose-response analysis on classroom measures. *J Am Acad Child Adolesc Psychiatry* 1995;34:1504–1513.
827. Shevell M, Schreiber R. Pemoline-associated hepatic failure: a critical analysis of the literature. *Pediatr Neurol* 1997;16:141–146.
828. Marotta PJ, Roberts EA. Pemoline hepatotoxicity in children. *J Pediatr* 1998;132:894–897.
829. Greenhill LL. Pharmacotherapy: stimulants. *Child Adolesc Psychiatry Clin North Am* 1992;1:411–447.
830. Chappell PB, Riddle MA, Scahill L, et al. Guanfacine treatment of comorbid attention-deficit hyperactivity disorder and Tourette's syndrome: preliminary clinical experience. *J Am Acad Child Adolesc Psychiatry* 1995;34:1140–1146.
831. Swanson JM, Flockhart D, Udrea D, et al. Clonidine in the treatment of ADHD: questions about safety and efficacy. *J Child Adolesc Psychopharmacol* 1995;5:301–304.
832. Balldin J, Berggren U, Erikson E, et al. Guanfacine as an alpha-2-agonist inducer of growth hormone secretion: a comparison with clonidine. *Psychoneuroendocrinology* 1993;18:45–55.
833. Michelson D, Farris D, Wernicke J, et al. Atomoxetine in the treatment of children and adolescents with attention-deficit/hyperactivity disorder a randomized, placebo-controlled dose-response study. *Pediatrics* 2001;108:E83.
834. Kelsey DK, Sumner CR, Casat CD, et al. Once-daily atomoxetine treatment for children with attention-deficit/hyperactivity disorder including an assessment of evening and morning behavior: a double-blind placebo-controlled trial. *Pediatrics* 2004;63:114. e1-e8.
835. Kratochvil CJ, Heiligenstein JH, Dittmann R, et al. Atomoxetine and methylphenidate treatment in children with ADHD: a prospective, randomized, open-label trial. *J Am Acad Child Adolescent Psychiatry* 2002;41:776–784.
836. Biederman J, Gastfriend DR, Jellinek MS. Desipramine in the treatment of children with attention deficit disorder. *J Clin Psychopharmacol* 1986;6:359–363.
837. Gammon GD, Brown TE. Fluoxetine and methylphenidate in combination for treatment of attention deficit disorder and comorbid depressive disorder. *J Child Adolesc Psychopharmacol* 1993;3: 1–10.
838. Popper CW. Antidepressants in the treatment of attention-deficit hyperactivity disorder. *J Clin Psychiatry* 1997;58:14–29.
839. Wolf SM, Forsythe A. Behavior disturbance, phenobarbital, and febrile seizures. *Pediatrics* 1978;61:728–731.
840. Stein MA, Krasowski M, Leventhal BL, et al. Behavioral and cognitive effects of methylxanthines. A meta-analysis of theophylline and caffeine. *Arch Pediatr Adolesc Med* 1996;150:284–288.
841. Christakis DA, Zimmerman FJ, DiGiuseppe DL, et al. Early television exposure and subsequent attentional problems in children. *Pediatrics* 2004;113:708–713.
842. Feingold BF. *Why your child is hyperactive*. New York: Random House, 1975.
843. Swanson JM, Kinsbourne M. Food dyes impair performance of hyperactive children on a laboratory learning test. *Science* 1980;207:1485–1487.
844. Egger J, Carter CM, Graham PJ, et al. Controlled trial of oligoantigenic treatment in the hyperkinetic syndrome. *Lancet* 1985;1:540–545.
845. Kaplan BJ, McNicol J, Conte RA, et al. Dietary replacement in preschool-aged hyperactive boys. *Pediatrics* 1989;83:7–17.
846. Egger J, Stolla A, McEwen LM. Controlled trial of hyposensitization in children with foot induced hyperkinetic syndrome. *Lancet* 1993;341:114–115.
847. Kinsbourne M. Sugar and the hyperactive child. *N Engl J Med* 1994;330:355–356.
848. Wolraich ML, Wilson DB, White JW. The effect of sugar on behavior or cognition in children. A meta-analysis. *JAMA* 1995;274:1617–1621.
849. Conners CK, Blouin AG. Nutritional effects on behavior of children. *J Psychiatr Res* 1982;17:193–201.
850. Shaywitz BA, Sullivan CM, Anderson GM, et al. Aspartame, behavior, and cognitive function in children with attention deficit disorder. *Pediatrics* 1994;93:70–75.
851. Satterfield JM, Satterfield BT, Schell AM. Therapeutic interventions to prevent delinquency in hyperactive boys. *J Am Acad Child Adolesc Psychiatry* 1987;26:56–64.
852. Abikoff H, Hechtman L, Klein RG, et al. Social functioning in children with ADHD treated with long-term methylphenidate and multimodal psychosocial treatment. *J Am Acad Child Adolesc Psychiatry* 2004;43:820–829.
853. Klein RG, Abikoff H, Hechtman L, et al. Design and rationale of controlled study of long-term methylphenidate and multimodal psychosocial treatment in children with ADHD. *J Am Acad Child Adolesc Psychiatry* 2004;43:792–801.
854. Barkley RA. *Attention deficit hyperactivity disorder: a handbook for diagnosis and treatmen*, 2nd ed. New York: Guilford Press, 1996.
855. Pelham WEJ, Carlson C, Sams SE, et al. Separate and combined effects of methylphenidate and behavior modification on boys with attention-deficit hyperactivity disorder in the classroom. *J Consult Clin Psychol* 1993;61:506–515.
856. Abikoff H. Cognitive training in ADHD children: less to it than meets the eye. *J Learn Disabil* 1991;24:204–209.
857. Wilens TE, McDermott SP, Biederman J, et al. Cognitive therapy in the treatment of adults with ADHD: a systematic chart review of 26 cases. *J Cogn Psychotherapy* 1999;13:215–226.
858. Braswell L, Bloomquist ML. *Cognitive-behavioral therapy with ADHD children: child, family and school interventions*. New York: Guilford, 1991.
859. Swanson JM. *School-based assessments and interventions for ADD students*. Irvine, CA: KC Publications, 1992.
860. Latham P, Latham P. Who has a disability under the ADA? *Attention* 1999;6:40–42.
861. Roy-Byrne P, Scheele L, Brinkley J, et al. Adult attention-deficit hyperactivity disorder: assessment guidelines based on clinical presentation to a specialty clinic. *Compr Psychiatry* 1997;38:133–140.
862. Loney J, Kramer J, Milich R. The hyperactive child grows up: predictors of symptoms, delinquency, and achievement at follow-up. In: Gadow J, Loney J, eds. *Psychosocial aspects of drug treatment for hyperactivity*. Boulder, CO: Westview, 1981:381–415.
863. Tarter RE, Alterman Al, Edwards KL. Vulnerability to alcoholism in men: a behavior-genetic perspective. *J Stud Alcohol* 1985;46:329–356.
864. Linnoila VI, Virkkunen M. Aggression, suicidality, and serotonin. *J Clin Psychiatry* 1992;53[Suppl]:46–51.
865. Marcus J, Hans SL, Nagler S, et al. Review of the NIMH Israeli Kibbutz-City Study and the Jerusalem Infant Development Study. *Schizophr Bull* 1987;13:425–438.
866. Schweitzer JB, Lee DO, Handford RB, et al. Effect of methylphenidate on executive functioning in adults with attention-deficit/hyperactivity disorder: normalization of behavior but not related brain activity. *Biol Psychiatr* 2004;56:597–606.

INDEX

Page numbers followed by t and f indicate tables and figures, respectively.

A

C

D

E

F

G

H

J

K

L

M

N

O

P

Q

R

S

T